Manson's
TROPICAL
DISEASES

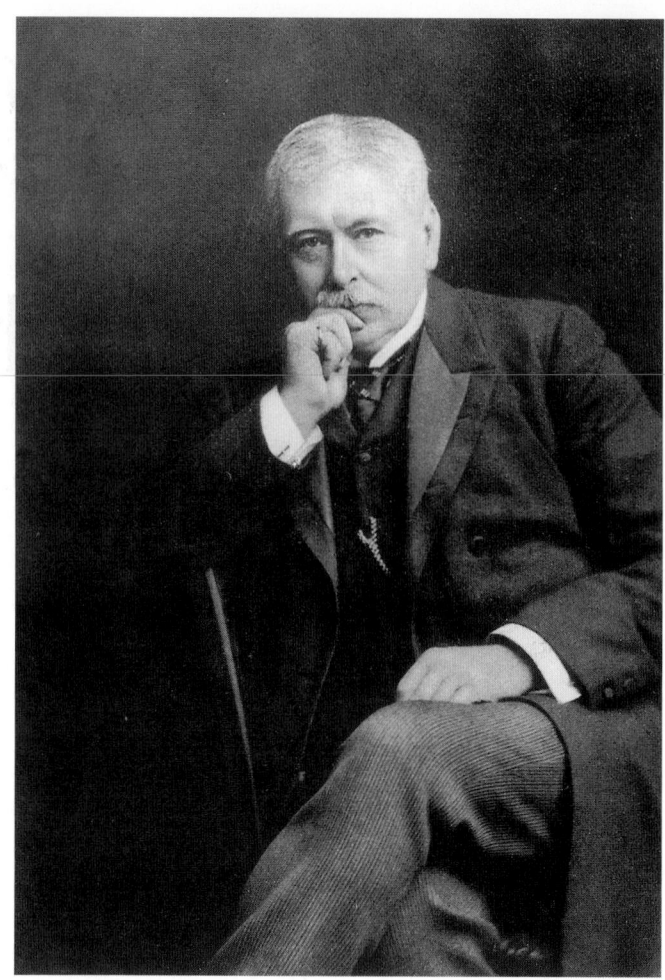

Sir Patrick Manson, (1844–1922), GCMG FRS

Manson's
TROPICAL
DISEASES

Twenty-first edition

Gordon C. Cook
MD DSc FRCP(Lond) FRCP(Edin) FRACP FLS

Visiting Professor, Department of Medical Microbiology and Centre for Infectious Diseases, Royal Free and University College London Medical School, London, UK

President, The Fellowship of Postgraduate Medicine, London, UK

President Elect, History of Medicine Section, Royal Society of Medicine, UK

President, The Royal Society of Tropical Medicine and Hygiene (1993–1995)

Formerly: Professor of Medicine, the Universities of Zambia, Riyadh (Saudi Arabia) and Papua New Guinea; Consultant Physician at University College Hospitals Trust, Hospital for Topical Diseases, London; St.Luke's Hospital for the Clergy and Senior Lecturer at the London School of Hygiene and Tropical Medicine, London, UK

Alimuddin I. Zumla
BSc MBChB MSc PhD FRCP(Lond) FRCP(Edin)

Professor of Infectious Diseases and International Health, University College London, Royal Free and University College London Medical School, and Director, Centre for Infectious Diseases and International Health, Windeyer Institute of Medical Sciences, University College London, London, UK

Honorary Consultant in Infectious Diseases, University College London Hospitals NHS Trust, London, UK

Honorary Professor, Liverpool School of Tropical Medicine, University of Liverpool, UK

Honorary Professor, Centre for International Child Health, Institute of Child Health, London, UK

Visiting Professor, University of Zambia School of Medicine, Lusaka, Zambia

Formerly, Associate Professor, Center for Infectious Diseases, University of Texas Health Science Center at Houston, School of Medicine and Public Health, Houston, Texas, USA

SAUNDERS

First published in 1898
Eighteenth edition 1982
Nineteenth edition 1987
Twentieth edition 1996
Twenty-first edition 2003

ISBN 0 70202 6409

British Library Cataloguing in Publication Data
A catalogue record for this book is available from the British Library

Library of Congress Cataloging in Publication Data
A catalog record for this book is available from the Library of Congress

Note
Medical knowledge is constantly changing. As new information becomes available, changes in treatment, procedures, equipment and the use of drugs become necessary. The contributors and the publishers have taken care to ensure that the information given in this text is accurate and up to date. However, readers are strongly advised to confirm that the information, especially with regard to drug usage, complies with the latest legislation and standards of practice.

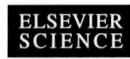

ELSEVIER SCIENCE your source for books, journals and multimedia in the health sciences
www.elsevierhealth.com

The publisher's policy is to use paper manufactured from sustainable forests

Printed in China by RDC Group Limited

Acquisitions Editor: Quincy McDonald
Associate Editor: Paul Fam
Project Development Manager: Firiel Benson
Project Manager: Cheryl Brant
Designer: Andy Chapman
Illustrations Manager: Mick Ruddy
Illustrator: Robin Dean

Contents

Contributors

Adewale O. Adebajo MB BS MSc FWACP FACP FRCP
Honorary Clinical Lecturer, Academic, Rheumatology
Group, Division of Molecular and Genetic Medicine,
University of Sheffield Medical School, Sheffield, UK

Dwomoa Adu MD FRCP
Consultant Physician and Nephrologist, Queen
Elizabeth Medical Centre, Birmingham, UK

Yusuf Ahmed BSc BM MRCOG
Senior Lecturer, Department of Obstetrics and
Gynaecology, School Of Medicine, Lusaka, Zambia

K. George M.M. Alberti MA DPhil BMBCh PRCP FRCP(Ed)
FRCP(G) FRCPath DMed (Hon Caus. Aarhus)
Professor of Medicine, Department of Diabetes and
Metabolism, School of Clinical Medical Sciences,
Newcastle Upon Tyne, UK

Sandra Amor PhD
Senior Scientist, Department of Neuroinflammation,
Division of Neuroscience, Imperial College School of
Medicine, London, UK

Felix Idowu Anjorin MB BS FMCP FWACP
Consultant Physician and Cardiologist, Medical
Department(East), Shell Petroleum Development
Company Ltd, Port Harcourt, Nigeria

Jeffrey K. Aronson MA Dphil MB ChB FRCP
Clinical Reader in Clinical Pharmacology, University
Department of Clinical Pharmacology, Radcliffe
Infirmary, Oxford, UK

Masharip Atadzhanov MD PhD DSc
Professor of Neurology, Department of Internal
Medicine, University of Zambia School of Medicine,
Lusaka, Zambia

Guy Baily MD FRCP
Consultant Physician, Department of Infection and
Immunity, Barts and The London NHS Trust, London,
UK

John R. Baker BSc PhD DSc MA FIBiol
Professor, c/o Royal Society of Tropical Medicine and
Hygiene, Manson House, London, UK

Anthony H. Barnett BSc (Hons) MD FRCP
Professor of Medicine and Honorary Consultant
Physician, Birmingham Heartlands Hospital,
Birmingham, UK

Imelda Bates BSc MB BS MRCP DTM&H MRCPath
Senior Lecturer in Tropical Haematology, Liverpool
School of Tropical Medicine, Liverpool, UK

Raman Bedi BDS MSc DDS FDSRCS DipHE
Professor and Head, National Centre for Transcultural
Oral Health, Eastman Dental Institute and Hospital for
Oral, Health Sciences, University College London,
London, UK

D. Gareth Beevers MB ChB FRCP
Professor of Medicine and Honorary Consultant
Physician, Department of Medicine, City Hospital,
Birmingham, UK

Ron Behrens BSc MRCS MB ChB MD FRCP
Consultant Physician in Tropical and Travel Medicine,
Hospital for Tropical Diseases; Senior Lecturer, Infectious
and Tropical Disease, Department of Hygiene and
Tropical Medicine, London, UK

Soloman R. Benatar MB ChB FFA (SA) FRCP FACP (Hon) FRS SAfr
Professor of Medicine, University of Cape Town, Cape
Town, South Africa

Gerard Bodeker BPsych MPsych EdM EdD
Senior Lecturer in Public Health, Green College,
University of Oxford, Oxford, UK

Bernard J. Brabin MB ChB MSc PhD FRCPC FRCPCH
Senior Lecturer in Tropical Paediatrics, Tropical Child
Health Group, Liverpool School of Tropical Medicine,
Liverpool, UK

Rodney A. Bray BA PhD C Biol MI Biol FLS
Researcher, Department of Zoology, The Natural History
Museum, London, UK

Joseph S. Bresee MD
Medical Epidemiologist Respiratory and Enteric Virus
Branch, National Center for Infectious Diseases, Centers
for Disease Control and Prevention, Atlanta, Georgia, USA

Annette K. Broom BSc PhD
Senior Research Officer, Department of Microbiology, The
University of Western Australia, Nedlands, Perth, Australia

Reto Brun PhD
Research Group Leader, Protozoology Laboratory Swiss Tropical Institute, Basel, Switzerland

James E.G. Bunn MD ChB MRCP
Lecturer in Tropical Paediatrics, Liverpool School of Tropical Medicine, Liverpool, UK

Christian Burri MSc PhD
Deputy Head of Department, Operations, Swiss Tropical Institute, Basel, Switzerland

David A. Cavan DM FRCP
Consultant Physician, Honorary Senior Lecturer, Royal Bournemouth Hospital, Bournemouth, UK

Ana-Maria Cevallos PhD
St Bartholomew's Hospital, London, UK

Peter L. Chiodini BSc MB BS PhD FRCP
Consultant Parasitologist, Department of Clinical Parasitology, The Hospital for Tropical Diseases, London, UK

Sunil Chopra BSc MRCP
Consultant Dermatologist, Barking, Havering and Redbridge Hospital NHS Trust; Honorary Consultant Dermatologist, Bart's and Royal London Hospitals, London, UK

Timothy J. Coleman MB BS PhD
Head, Public Health Laboratory Service Leptospira Reference Unit, Public Health Laboratory County Hospital, Hereford, UK

Ken J. Collins MB BS DPhil (Oxon) FRCP
Consultant (Retired), Guildford, UK

Gordon C. Cook MD DSc FRCP(Lond) FRACP FRCP(Edin) FLS
Visiting Professor, Department of Medical Microbiology and Centre for Infectious Diseases, Royal Free and University College London Medical School, London, UK; President, The Fellowship of Postgraduate Medicine, London, UK; President elect, History of Medicine Section, Royal Society of Medicine, UK; President, The Royal Society of Tropical Medicine and Hygiene (1993–1995); Formerly: Professor of Medicine at the Universities of Zambia, Riyadh (Saudi Arabia) and Papua New Guinea; Consultant Physician at University College Hospitals Trust, Hospital for Topical Diseases, London; St.Luke's Hospital for the Clergy and Senior Lecturer at the London School of Hygiene and Tropical Medicine

John B.S. Coulter MD FRCPI FRCPCH
Senior Lecturer in Tropical Paediatrics, Liverpool School of Tropical Medicine, Liverpool, Merseyside, UK

George O. Cowan OBE FRCP
Linacre Fellow, Royal College of Physicians of London. Formerly Dean of Postgraduate Medicine, North Thames Department of Postgraduate Medical and Dental Education, University of London, London, UK.

Dorothy H. Crawford PhD MD DSc FRCPath
Professor of Medical Microbiology, Division of Biomedical and Clinical Lab Sciences, University of Edinburgh, Edinburgh, UK

J. Kennedy Cruickshank BSc MB ChB MSc MD FRCP
Senior Lecturer in Clinical Epidemiology, Manchester University Medical School, Manchester, UK

Luis E. Cuevas MD MTrop Med
Senior Lecturer in International Child Health, Liverpool School of Tropical Medicine, Pembroke Place, Liverpool

Nigel A. Cunliffe BSc(Hons) MB ChB PhD MRCP DTM&H
Clinical Lecturer in Microbiology, Department of Medical Microbiology and Genito-Urinary, Medicine, The University of Liverpool, Liverpool

David A. Dance MB ChB MSc FRCPath DLSHTM
Director Consultant Microbiologist, Public Health Laboratory, Derriford Hospital, Plymouth, UK

Denis Daumerie MD PhD
Group Leader (Leprosy), WHO/CDS/CPE/CEE/LEP, World Health Organization, Geneva, Switzerland

Andrew Davis MD FRCP FFPHM DTM&H
Former Director, Parasitic Diseases Programme, World Health Organization, Geneva, Switzerland

P. Shanthamali de Silva MB BS DCH MRCP(Paed) FRCP FSLCP
Consultant Paediatrician, Nugegoda, Sri Lanka

Jean-Pierre Dedet MD MSc
Professor of Parasitology, Laboratoire de Parasitologie and Centre National de Référence des Leishmanioses, Montpellier, France

John E. Eyers BA MLS MIInfSc
Deputy Librarian, London School of Hygiene and Tropical Medicine, London, UK

Michael J.G. Farthing MD FRCP
Executive Dean, Faculty of Medicine, University of Glasgow, Glasgow, Scotland

Alan F. Fleming MA MD FRCPath
Consultant Haematologist, Kilmersdon Common Farmhouse, Radstock, Somerset, UK

Susan Foster PhD
Professor and Acting Chair, Boston University School of Public Health, Boston, USA

Neil French MB ChB MRCP
Wellcome Fellow and Honorary Consultant in Infectious

Diseases, Liverpool School of Tropical Medicine/Aintree, University Hospital, Liverpool, UK

Charles Gilks DPhil FRCP DTM&H
Professor, Department of HIV/AIDS, World Health Organization, Geneva, Switzerland

Herbert M. Gilles MD MSc FRCP FFPHM DSc DmedSc
Emeritus Professor of Tropical Medicine, University of Liverpool, Liverpool, Merseyside, UK

Stephen H. Gillespie MD FRCP(Edin) FRCPath
Professor of Medical Microbiology, Department of Microbiology, Royal Free Campus, Royal Free & University College Medical School, London

Bruno Gottstein PhD
Professor and Director, Institute of Parasitology, Faculty of Veterinary Medicine and Faculty of Medicine, University of Berne, Laenggass-Strasse 122, CH-3001 Bern, Switzerland

Stephen M. Graham MB BS FRACP DTCH
Clinical Research Fellow, Wellcome Trust Research Laboratories, Blantyre, Malawi

John M. Grange MB MD MSc
Visiting Professor, Department of Medical Microbiology and Centre for Infectious Disease , Royal Free and University College Medical School, Windeyer Institute of Medical Science, London, UK

Roy A. Hall PhD
Department of Microbiology and Parasitology, School of Molecular and Microbial Sciences, University of Queensland, St Lucia, Queensland, Australia

Tony Hart MB BS BSc PhD FRCPCH FRCPath
Professor of Medical Microbiology, Department of Medical Microbiology, University of Liverpool Medical School, Liverpool , UK

Melissa R. Haswell-Elkins BA MSc PhD
North Queensland Coordinator, Indigenous Health Division, School of Population Health, The University of Queensland, Cairns, Queensland, Australia

Alan Haworth OBE, FRCPsych, DPM
Professor, National Mental Health Resource Centre, Lusaka, Zambia

Roderick J. Hay DM FRCP FRCPath
Professor of Cutaneous Medicine, Guy's King's and St Thomas School of Medicine, St John's Institute of Dermatology, London, UK

Tran Tinh Hien MD
University of Oxford Research Unit, Centre for Tropical Diseases, Cho Quan Hospital, Ho Chi Minh City, Viet Nam

Richard E. Holliman BSc MB BS MSc MD FRCPath DSc
Consultant Medical Microbiologist, Reader in Clinical Microbiology, Department of Medical Microbiology, °University of London, London, UK

Cheryl A. Johansen BSc MSc
Research Officer, Arbovirus Research and Surveillance Laboratory, Department of Microbiology, The University of Western Australia, Nedlands, Perth, Western Australia, Australia

John J.E. Jellis MB BS LRCP FRCS
Honorary Professor in Orthopaedic Surgery, University of Zambia School of Medicine, Lusaka, Zambia

Moses Kapembwa PhD BSc FRCP(Lond) FRCP(Edin)
Consultant Physician and Senior Lecturer (Hon), Department of Genitourinary and HIV Medicine, Northwick Park and St Marks Hospitals, Harrow, UK

Paul Kelly MA MD FRCP
Senior Lecturer in Gastroenterology, Department of Adult and Paediatric Gastroenterology, Barts and the London School of Medicine, London, UK

Dominic Kwiatkowski FRCP FRCPCH F Med Sci
Professor, University Department of Paediatrics, John Radcliffe Hospital, Oxford, UK

Edward P. Levri PhD
Assistant Professor of Biology, Division of Mathematics and Natural Science, Penn State Altoona, Altoona, Pennsylvania, USA

Chewe Luo MB ChB MMed(Paed) MTropPaed PhD
HIV/AIDS (PMTCT) Officer, UNICEF, Gaborone, Botswana

Gary Maartens FCP(SA) MMed DTM&H
Head, Infectious Diseases Unit, Department of Medicine, University of Cape Town, Cape Town, South Africa

David C.W. Mabey DM FRCP
Professor, Department of Infectious and Tropical Diseases, London School of Hygiene & Tropical Medicine, London, UK

John S. Mackenzie BSc PhD FASM FACTM
Professor, Department of Microbiology and Parasitology, School of Molecular and Microbial Sciences, The University of Queensland, Brisbane, Queensland, Australia

Charles R. Madeley MD FRCPath
Professor Emeritus of Clinical Virology, University of Newcastle upon Tyne, Northumberland, UK

Jean Claude Mbanya MD PhD MRCP (UK)
Department of Internal Medicine and Specialities, Faculty of Medicine and Biomedical Sciences, University of Yaounde, Yaounde, Cameroon

D. Murray McGavin MD FRCS (Ed) FRCOphth DCH
Editor, Journal of Community Eye Health , Medical
Director, International Resource Centre, International
Centre for Eye Health, Institute of Opthalmology,
London, UK

Michael A. Miles MSc PhD DSc FRCPath
Professor of Medical Protozoology, Department of
Infectious & Tropical Diseases, London School of
Hygiene and Tropical Medicine, London, UK

James S. Milledge MD FRCP
Physician Emeritus (Retired), Northwick Park Hospital,
Harrow, UK

Robert F. Miller MB BS MIBiol FRCP
Reader in Clinical Infection, Royal Free and University
College Medical School, University College London,
London, UK

Anthony Moody M Phil MIBiol FIBMS DLSHTM
Head BMS and Laboratory Manager, Department of
Clinical Parasitology, Hospital for Tropical Diseases,
London, UK

Peter Mwaba MMed PhD (Lond)
Head of Department of Medicine, University of Zambia
School of Medicine, Lusaka, Zambia

Nguyen T.N.Nga MB BS
Vice-Director, Tetanus Unit, Centre for Tropical Diseases,
Ho Chi Minh City, Viet Nam

Suchitra Nimmannitya MD MPH
Senior Consultant, Pediatric Infectious Diseases, Queen
Sirikit National Institute of Child Health, (Children's
Hospital), Bangkok, Thailand

Charles L.M. Olweny MB ChB MMed FRACP
Professor of Medicine Manitoba University and, Site Co-
ordinator, Section of Hematology Oncology, Manitoba
Cancer Treatment and Research, Foundation, Winnipeg,
Canada

John H. Orley DM FRCPsych
Senior Medical Officer, WHO, Geneva, Switzerland,
Les Olivets, St Martins, Guernsey, Channel Islands

Eldryd H.O. Parry OBE FRCP
Professor, The Tropical Health and Education Trust,
London, UK

Joseph S.M. Peiris MB BS FRCPath Dphil
Associate Professor, Department of Microbiology, The
University of Hong Kong, Hong Kong

Francine Pratlong PhD
Maître de Conférence, Laboratoire de Parasitologie and
Centre National de Référence des Leishmanioses,
Montpellier, France

Jurg Reichen MD PhD
Professor of Clinical Pharmacology, Department of
Clinical Pharmacology, University of Berne, Berne,
Switzerland

Tristan I.L. Richardson MB BS BSc MRCP
Specialist Registrar, Bournemouth Diabetes and Endocrine
Centre, Royal Bournemouth Hospital, Bournemouth, UK

Jonathan L. Richenberg MA MRCP FRCR
Consultant in Radiology, Royal Sussex County Hospital,
Brighton, UK

John Richens MA MB BS MSc FRCPE
Clinical Lecturer, Department of Sexually Transmitted
Diseases, Royal Free and University College Medical,
Schools, London, UK

Ivan M. Roitt DSc HonFRCP FRCPath FRS
Emeritus Professor of Immunology, Royal Free &
University College Medical School, London, UK

Alfa Sa'adu MSc PhD FRCP DTM&H
Honorary Senior Lecturer, Centre for Infectious Diseases,
Royal Free and University College London, Medical
School, London, UK

Geoff Scott MD FRCP FRCPath DTM&H
Consultant Microbiologist, University College London
Hospitals NHS Trust, London, UK

Crispian Scully MD PhD MDS FDSRCS FFDRCSI FRCPath FMedSci
Dean, Director of Studies and Research, International
Centres for Excellence in Dentistry and Eastman Dental
Institute for Oral Health Care Sciences, London, UK

Paul Shears MD FRCPath
Senior Lecturer, Tropical Microbiologist , University of
Liverpool, Liverpool, UK

Nandini P. Shetty MD MRCPath Dip HIC
Consultant Microbiologist, Department of Clinical
Microbiology, University College London Hospital,
London, UK

Prakash Shetty MD PhD
Professor of Human Nutrition, Department of
Epidemiology and Population, Health, London School
of Hygiene & Tropical Medicine, London, UK

P.E. Simonsen PhD
Danish Bilharziasis Laboratory, Charlottenlund, Denmark

David W. Smith BMedSc MB BS FRCPA
Clinical Director, Division of Microbiology & Infectious
Diseases, The Western Australian Centre for Pathology
and Medical Research, Nederlands, Western Australia,
Australia

Michael David Smith BM MRCP FRCPath
Consultant Microbiologist, Public Health Laboratory,
Taunton and Somerset Hospital, Taunton, UK

Tom Solomon MRCP PhD
Wellcome Trust Career Development Fellow, WHO
Collaborating Center for Tropical Diseases, University of
Texas Medical Branch, Galveston, Texas, USA

Vaughan R. Southgate BSc PhD CBiol FIBiol FLS
Head Biomedical Parasitology Divison, Merit Researcher,
Wolfson Wellcome Biomedical Laboratories, Department
of Zoology, The Natural History Museum, London, UK

Robert Steffen MD
Head, Division of Communicable Diseases; Director,
World Health Organization for Travellers' Health,
University of Zurich/ISPM, Zurich, Switzerland

Eric J. Threlfall BSc PhD
Head of Antibiotic Resistance/Epidemiology Laboratory,
Central Public Health Laboratory, Laboratory of Enteric
Pathogens, London, UK

Raj C. Thuraisingham MB BS MRCP
Consultant Nephrologist, Renal Unit, Royal London
Hospital, London, UK

Catherine Thwaites MB BS
Research Registrar, Wellcome Trust Clinical Research
Unit, Centre for Tropical Diseases, Cho Quan Hospital,
Ho Chi Minh City, Viet Nam

Eli Tumba Tshibwabwa, MD PhD
RSNA International Visiting Professor and Consultant
Radiologist, Department of Radiology, McMaster
University Medical Sciences, Hamilton, Ontario, Canada

Nigel Unwin BA MSc BM BCh FRCP MFPHM
Senior Lecturer, School of Clinical Medical Sciences and
the School of Population Health Sciences, University of
Newcastle upon Tyne, Newcastle upon Tyne, UK

Francisco Vega-López MD MSc PhD
Consultant Dermatologist and Honorary Senior
Lecturer, University College London Hospitals NHS
Trust, London School of Hygiene and Tropical Medicine,
London, UK

David C. Warhurst BSc PhD DSc FRCPath
Professor of Protozoan Chemotherapy, Department of
Infections and Tropical Diseases, London School of
Hygiene & Tropical Medicine, London, UK

David A. Warrell MA DM DSc FRCP FRCPE FMedSci
Professor of Tropical Medicine and Infectious Diseases;
Director Centre for Tropical Medicine, Centre for
Tropical Medicine, Headington, Oxford, UK

Mary J. Warrell MB BS MRCP FRCPath
Clinical Virologist, The Centre for Tropical Medicine,
John Radcliffe Hospital, Headington, Oxford, UK

Graham B. White MB ChB
AFYA Health Partners, Richmond, Surrey, United Kingdom

Nicholas J. White OBE FRCP
Professor and Wellcome Trust Principal Fellow,
Wellcome Trust Research Laboratories, Faculty of
Tropical Medicine, Bangkok, Thailand

Hilary Williams MB ChB BMedSci MRCP
Department of Medical Microbiology, The Royal Dick
Veterinary School, University of Edinburgh, UK

Stephen G. Wright MB FRCP
Consultant Physician, Hospital for Tropical Diseases,
London; Honorary Senior Lecturer, Department of
Infectious and Tropical Diseases, London School of
Hygiene & Tropical Medicine, London, UK

Sarah Wyllie PhD
Microbiologist, Department of Clinical
Microbiology, University College London Hospitals,
London, UK

Arie J. Zuckerman MD DSc FRCP FRCPath
Professor of Medical Microbiology, Academic Centre for
Travel Medicine and Vaccines, London; Former Dean,
Royal Free Hospital Medical School, London, UK

Jane Zuckerman MB BS MD
Senior Lecturer and Honorary Consultant, Academic
Centre for Travel Medicine and, Vaccines, Royal Free
Hospital Medical School, London, UK

Alimuddin Zumla BSc MB ChB (Zambia) MSc(Lond) PhD(Lond)
FRCP(Lond) FRCP(Edin)
Professor of Infectious Diseases and International
Health, University College London, Royal Free and
University College London Medical School, and
Director, Centre for Infectious Diseases and
International Health, Windeyer Institute of Medical
Sciences, University College London, London, UK;
Honorary Consultant Infectious Diseases Physician,
University College London Hospitals NHS Trust,
London, UK; Honorary Professor, Liverpool School of
Tropical Medicine, University of Liverpool, UK;
Honorary Professor, Centre for International Child
Health, Institute of Child Health, London, UK; Visiting
Professor, University of Zambia School of Medicine,
Lusaka, Zambia; Formerly, Associate Professor, Center for
Infectious Diseases, University of Texas Health Science
Center at Houston, School of Medicine and Public
Health, Houston, Texas, USA

Preface to the First Edition (1898)

A manual on the diseases of warm climates, of handy size, and yet giving adequate information, has long been a want; for the exigencies of travel and tropical life are, as a rule, incompatible with big volumes and large libraries. This is the reason for the present work.

While it is hoped that the book may prove of practical service, it makes no pretension to being anything more than an introduction to the important department of medicine of which it treats; in no sense is it put forward as a complete treatise, or as being in this respect comparable to the more elaborate works by Davidson, Scheube, Rho, Laveran, Corre, Roux , and other systematic writers in the same field. The author avails himself of this opportunity to acknowledge the valuable assistance he has received, in revising the text, from Dr. L. Westenra Sambon and Mr. David Rees, M.R.C.P, L.R.C.P., lately Senior House Surgeon, Seamen's Hospital, Albert Docks, London. He would also acknowledge his great obligation to Mr. Richard Muir, Pathological Laboratory, Edinburgh University, for his care and skill in preparing the illustrations.

Patrick Manson
April 1898

Preface to the Twenty-first Edition

Sir Patrick Manson GCMG, FRS (1844–1922) produced the first edition of this text, *Tropical Diseases: A Manual of the Diseases of Warm Climates* in 1898. Many books had previously been written on disease(s) in various tropical locations, but Manson had by then amassed a wealth of factual material from all parts of the tropics. He subsequently wrote a further five editions of this book between 1898 and 1921, distilling into it his immense experience and wisdom. Manson's son-in-law Sir Philip Manson-Bahr CMG, DSO (1881–1966) then became editor until the 16th edition. His son, (Manson's grandson), Dr P.E.C.Manson-Bahr was the joint editor for the 17th-19th editions. For the 104 years since its origin, 'Manson's' has become the classic text covering tropical medicine.

Manson's original work was a monograph focussed mainly on helminthic and protozoan infections. Since then the book has grown with each subsequent edition. The first editor of the present edition undertook a radical overhaul for the 20th edition incorporating chapters on the related medical specialities and on non-infectious diseases. This signified a change in direction for 'Manson's'. In this 21st edition we consolidate the direction pursued in the 20th edition, and have made the overhaul complete. All previous chapters have been revised and updated; several have been re-written, and very importantly, we have included ten new chapters to keep pace with the rapid advancement in knowledge and the changing practice of medicine in the tropics; these include: Primary Care; Epidemiology; Traditional Medicine; Genetics; Economics; Ethics; Blood Transfusion; Tropical Oral Health; Pneumococcal Disease; and Sources of Information on Tropical Medicine. Many new authors from all continents have contributed to this 21st edition, imparting a truly international flavour to this very well established 'British' text.

'Manson's' will inevitably remain 'the bible' of Tropical Medicine, and provide a reference guide for physicians worldwide. Although 'Manson's' is of necessity orientated towards infective conditions, the contributions on surgery, obstetrics, paediatrics, radiology, oral health, blood transfusion, ethics, economics, traditional medicine, as well as system-based coverage of disease, make it a major text covering 'medicine in the tropics'. We express our gratitude to the 119 international authors who contributed to this present edition; the many patients who consented to having their photographs included in this book; and the publishers Saunders/Elsevier Science Ltd for their co-operation, in particular Ms Deborah Russell, Mr Paul Fam and Ms Cheryl Brant. Finally, we are indebted to our wives (Farzana and Jane) for their patience whilst we were working on this project.

The 21st edition completes a change in direction for *Manson's Tropical Diseases* and we believe it will be of immense value to physicians, scientists, nurses and paramedical personnel worldwide.

Gordon C. Cook
Alimuddin I. Zumla
October 2002

Section 1

Underlying Factors in Tropical Medicine

Seven new chapters have been included in this section: 'Primary Care' focuses on the provision of promotive, preventive, curative and rehabilitation services in the tropics. Disease control programmes, including the management of the sick child; maternal health and safe motherhood initiative; nutritional supplementation and provision of clean and safe water supply, are all addressed.

'Epidemiology of Disease' discusses the distribution and determinants of disease in the tropics; the main causes of mortality are detailed with a focus on six deadly diseases —pneumonia, tuberculosis, diarrhoeal illnesses, malaria, measles and HIV/AIDS. Seventeen 'new' infectious diseases have emerged since 1973. Some of these have caused media hysteria due to their high fatality rates; examples are Ebola, Legionnaire's disease; toxic shock syndrome; HIV/AIDS; *E.coli* O157:H7 infection; Hantavirus and Nipah virus.

Traditional medicine healers are frequently the first point of contact for patients in the tropics. They play a significant role in access to health care, although the health sectors of most countries have not fully appreciated their input. Recently, the emergence of a global political consensus that traditional medicine in developing countries must take a role in health sector development is a major step forward in recognition of the role played by traditional healers (and their medicines). This chapter illustrates the importance of traditional medicine, and lays down the framework for what traditional medicine is, who uses it and why, as well as its use in the treatment of common tropical illnesses.

'Genetics' covers several aspects of patterns of autosomal and sex-linked inheritance, the diversity of the human genome, selective pressures on the human genome such as haemoglobinopathies, and genetic contribution(s) to common diseases, including single gene defects, DNA polymorphisms and HLA types that confer resistance or susceptibility.

'Immunological Aspects of Tropical Diseases' gives an overview of the constant battle between the human host and the multitude of organisms in his/her own immediate environment. It illustrates the delicate balance involving the host and invading pathogens. Mechanisms involved in host susceptibility and parasite evasion of the human immune system are also described.

The chapter covering 'the economics and financing of tropical and infectious disease programmes' focuses on the effects of poverty and inadequate resources, particularly on the inability of many developing countries to reduce the burden of disease due to economic reasons. Poverty is the most important factor underlying poor health in the tropics; poor people are more vulnerable to disease, and institutional poverty leads, in turn, to poor health services. Also covered in this chapter are: concepts of efficiency; types of economic evaluations (a cost-effective, benefit and utility analysis); and the financing of infectious disease control activities. The chapter concludes with a discussion of how to develop a strategy for funding tropical disease control.

'Ethics and Tropical Diseases' discusses some global considerations on the issue of equity, fairness, the 'North-South' divide and morality of the current world order.

Chapter 1
History of Tropical Medicine, and 'Medicine in the Tropics'

G. C. Cook

Numerous European doctors (British included) practised in tropical countries as early as the seventeenth and eighteenth centuries: in the English West Indies (the 'Sugar Islands'), India, the East Indies and later Africa, the western coast of which was widely termed the 'white man's grave'.[1,2] Many also produced monographs describing their experiences, with an outline of the disease pattern at these various locations. Many infections which now fall under the 'tropical' umbrella were widely distributed in northern Europe and northern America during the seventeenth to nineteenth centuries. For example, Shakespeare was well aware of malaria in England: 'he is so shak'd by the burning quotidian tertian that it is most lamentable to behold' (*Henry V*, II. i. 123). Thomas Sydenham (1624–1689) successfully used fever-tree bark (quinine) in the management of the 'intermittent fevers' during the seventeenth century.[3] Indigenous *Plasmodium vivax* infection remained a clinical problem in south-east England well into the twentieth century. Plague, typhoid, cholera, typhus and smallpox were major health hazards in Britain, London included, during the Victorian era.[4] John Bunyon (1628–1688) was well aware of the consumption (tuberculosis)—now such a dominant disease in 'tropical' countries—which so often 'took him down to the grave' (*The Life and Death of Mr Badman*).

What then is tropical medicine? Balfour[2] summarized the position as he saw it, in his Presidential Address to the Royal Society of Tropical Medicine and Hygiene in 1925: 'there is in one sense no such thing as tropical medicine, and in any case many of the most erudite writings of Hippocrates are concerned with maladies which nowadays are chiefly encountered under tropical or subtropical conditions'. Some, including many historians, consider that 'tropical medicine' originated as a by-product of the British Empire and Raj.[5] The truth of the matter is that the discipline was exploited by the Colonialists in order that the health of British personnel, both overseas and following return to the UK, could be improved (see below).[1] The specialty, in fact, had its origin(s) in a multidisciplinary background: major areas of progress during the nineteenth century were public health (and hygiene), travel and exploration, natural history, evolutionary theory, and a precise knowledge of the causation of disease (the 'germ theory').[6,7] The miasmatists and contagionists were previously at logger heads. The development of clinical parasitology following the work of Manson, Ross and others (see below), and superimposed on this complex backcloth, led to the inevitable genesis of 'tropical medicine'.[6,8,9]

Development of tropical medicine in London
The Seamen's Hospital Society

In London, the Seamen's Hospital Society (SHS) (the 'foster mother of clinical tropical medicine') was formed in 1821, its predecessor being the Committee for Distressed (or destitute) Seaman which was set up in the winter of 1817–1818; the *raison d'être* was to provide temporary relief to sick members of the mercantile marine then roaming in large number on London's streets.[1,10] The major objective was thus largely targeted at the management of illnesses (especially fevers and sexually transmitted diseases), many of which had been introduced into London from tropical and subtropical countries.[4] At a meeting held at the City of London Tavern on 8 March 1821 (William Wilberforce M.P. was amongst those present), the committee resolved to establish a permanent floating hospital on the Thames for the exclusive use of sick and distressed seamen; the venture was to be supported by voluntary contributions. A series of hulks, HMS *Grampus* (commissioned in 1821) (Figure 1.1), HMS *Dreadnought* (1831–1857) and HMS *Caledonia* (renamed *Dreadnought*, also) (1857–1870) were anchored in Greenwich Reach and used successively; they had been 48, 98, and 120-gun vessels, respectively.[1,10] Although they served a valuable function, major practical problems arose: ventilation was poor, and nosocomial spread of disease occurred; lack of light was a major drawback during the winter months; and other problems (not least noise) associated with being situated in the midst of an extremely busy part of the River Thames proved tiresome.[11] In 1870, after protracted negotiations, the Commissioners of the Admiralty granted the SHS a 99-year lease of the Infirmary (and adjoining Somerset Ward) of the Royal Hospital, Greenwich, in lieu of the loan of the ship(s).[1,10] This move was made possible by a sharp decline in the number of pensioners residing in the Hospital during the the peaceful years following the battle of Waterloo (in 1815); the Infirmary was therefore no longer required. (In 1873 the Hospital ceased being a permanent home for Naval

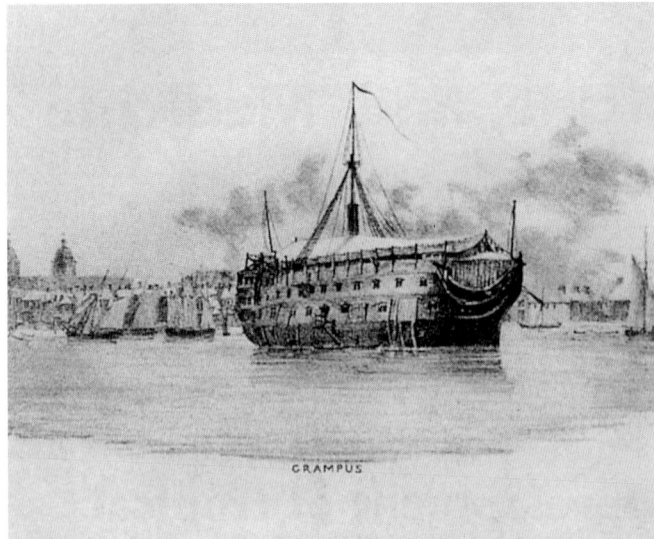

Figure 1.1: HMS *Grampus*. The first of three hospital ships sponsored by the Seamen's Hospital Society, anchored on Greenwich Reach. This disused 48-gun warship served in this capacity from October 1821 to October 1831.

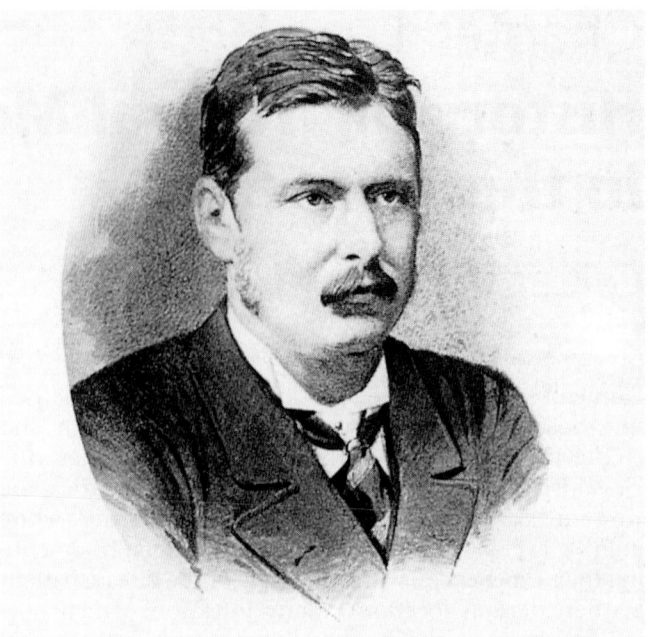

Figure 1.2: Dr (later Sir) Patrick Manson (1844–1922) aged 31 years. This photograph was probably taken whilst he was on leave in Britain from Amoy in 1875.

pensioners and became the Royal Naval College (previously based at Portsmouth). The Royal Hospital[12] had been founded in 1694 by William and Mary as the Naval equivalent of the Royal Hospital, Chelsea (founded by King Charles II), which remains in use for Army pensioners today.

Emergence of the specialty in London

Following his return to London from Formosa, Amoy (where he had made his seminal discovery of the man-mosquito cycle of the nematode *Filaria sanguinis hominis* (*Wuchereria bancrofti*), the causative agent of lymphatic filariasis) and Hong Kong, Patrick Manson (1844–1922)[7,13] (Figure 1.2) embarked on a series of lectures devoted to 'tropical medicine' at several London medical schools.[7,14] The Rt Hon Joseph Chamberlain, Secretary of State for the Colonies, was immediately impressed at the possibility of sending the Colonial medical staff on leave in Britain to these lectures, to give an update in the prevention and management of those diseases which seriously affected the servants of Empire.[1] Regular trade, efficient administration and agricultural production were all seriously hampered by disease; furthermore, Chamberlain's concept of 'constructive imperialism' could not be adequately developed in the presence of such a great deal of morbidity and mortality. Despite a great deal of opposition,[15] *clinical tropical medicine* emerged as both an important medical specialty and scientific discipline (the importance of parasites and their vector transmission in disease had recently become clear—see above), Chamberlain considered that 'tropical medicine' was an essential component in the future development of British economic and social

imperialism. It was, in fact, to become a 'colonial science'.[1,11] At the 1898 meeting of the British Medical Association held in Edinburgh, at which Ronald Ross' work on the rôle of the mosquito in avian malaria was announced (his initial demonstration of *Plasmodium* spp. development in the mosquito had been published in the *British Medical Journal* the previous year), a new section devoted to Tropical Medicine was inaugurated.[9] There were several reasons why the discipline had *not* previously emerged. Many 'tropical diseases' had formerly existed in northern Europe (including England) and northern America (see above). There was also a widespread feeling that the high mortality rate affecting the white man in the tropics was inevitable, and that he would never be able to live and work there successfully. The 'miasmatic theory' held sway. Furthermore, there was an understandable pessimism regarding the possibility of significant environmental improvement in the foreseeable future, most British colonies being situated on unhealthy coastlines. Also, research had until then taken a very low priority for medical staff working in the tropics; their perceived task was solely to provide medical advice and clinical care to the local British community.

The Manson–Chamberlain collaboration

In order to implement effective development of the 'new' discipline, Manson was appointed Medical Officer to the Colonial Office in 1897. Here, with Chamberlain's whole-hearted support, he set about establishing a School of Tropical Medicine in London (LSTM).[1,15] A major problem related to the venue of the proposed institution. Manson favoured the Branch (Seamen's) Hospital of the Greenwich Hospital, situated near the Royal Albert Dock.[16] However, hostility to this suggestion arose from several quarters. The War Office favoured the Royal Victoria Hospital, Netley, which, situated on Southampton Water, had been founded in 1863;[1,17] it had been established primarily for soldiers invalided from the Crimea and was then staffed by officers of the Royal Army Medical Corps. Manson considered this option unacceptable: the atmosphere and remote situation from London were, in his opinion, incompatible with the teaching of clinical tropical medicine. The Royal College of Physicians was of the opinion that a new school was uncalled for! The senior medical staff of the Greenwich Hospital felt that removal of the 'tropical' cases to the Albert Dock Hospital was a slight on their professional ability and was in any case undesirable because medical students from London's teaching hospitals were accustomed to visiting Greenwich for tuition in the diagnosis and management of these illnesses.[15] The end result was an outburst of acrimonious correspondence in the columns of the *Lancet*, the *British Medical Journal* and *The Times*, which later involved, amongst others, Sir William Broadbent, Sir William Church, Sir Jonathan Hutchinson and Sir Joseph Fayrer, the doyen of the Indian Medical Service. However, staunch determination from Manson and Herbert Read (Assistant Private Secretary to Chamberlain) to proceed with the project, of course strongly supported by Chamberlain himself, led to the rapid establishment of the proposed school at the Albert Dock Hospital;[1,18] financial assistance to the tune of £3550 came from the Colonial Office. A subcommittee was set up to 'formulate a scheme for organisation and management of the LSTM in connection with the SHS'; the committee of management was composed of equal numbers of personnel from the SHS, the medical and surgical staff of the Branch Hospital, and teachers from the LSTM.

School and Hospital in Close Proximity

The LSTM was officially opened on 2 October 1899.[1] The hospital (under SHS supervision) and teaching and research facilities (LSTM) were on the same site (Figure 1.3). With Sir Perceval Nairne (Chairman of the SHS) presiding, the inaugural address—written by Manson—was read in his absence. He later declared: 'the school strikes, and strikes effectively, at the root of the principal difficulty of most of our Colonies—disease. It will cheapen government and make it more efficient. It will encourage and cheapen commercial enterprise. It will conciliate and foster the native.'[19] Meanwhile continuous funding was necessary, and several sources of income were exploited; two charity dinners, at which Chamberlain presided, were held at the Hotel Cecil in 1899 and 1905; they raised £12 000 and £11 000 respectively. At the former, Chamberlain declared:[1] 'The man who shall successfully

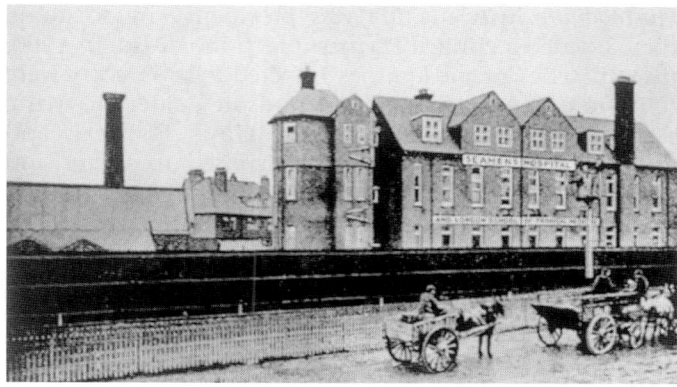

Figure 1.3: Newly opened London School of Tropical Medicine—situated on an adjoining site to the Seamen's Hospital Society's Branch (Albert Dock) Hospital—in October 1899.

grapple with this foe of humanity and find the cure for malaria, for the fever desolating our colonies. . . and shall make the tropics livable for white men. . . will do more for the world, more for the British Empire, than the man who adds a new province to the wide Dominions of the Queen.' A 'Tropical Diseases Research Fund' was set up, and the Dean—Sir Francis Lovell—raised funds on several overseas trips. In 1912 the school was enlarged and a new wing opened by Their Majesties King George V and Queen Mary. 'Tropical' cases were relatively few in the early days of the LSTM;[20] in fact, the Albert Dock Hospital had been founded to care for seafarers and others in the London Docks—most of whom suffered from injuries.

In 1919 a decision was taken to relocate the school and hospital in central London; Endsleigh Palace Hotel, 25 Gordon Street, WC1, was purchased (by the SHS) for £70 000 and on 11 Novembr 1920 the Duke of York (later King George VI) opened the joint LSTM and Hospital for Tropical Diseases in this building.[1,11] The structure, which remains extant, provided five floors (at the top) for clinical tropical medicine, and four for the basic sciences; a radiology department was situated in the basement. Sir Philip Manson-Bahr (1881–1966)[11] considered the building 'dark, awkward and inconvenient, with multitudes of doors and narrow passages', but never before had there been 'more unanimity or good fellowship amongst the staff of the school and the hospital'. The Wellcome Tropical Museum was nearby and provided invaluable teaching resources.

Between 1899 and 1929 the clinical specialty and the basic sciences were thus on the same site—first at the Albert Dock Hospital[16] and later London, WC1;[18] the close proximity was both valuable and productive, and a great deal of teaching and clinical research was accomplished. For example, two research projects carried out by the clinical staff clinched the mosquito transmission of malaria saga in *Homo sapiens*. Dr G. C. Low (1872–1952) (later largely responsible for establishing the Royal Society of Tropical Medicine and Hygiene)[21,22] and three other investigators slept between dusk and dawn, for 3 months, in a mosquito-proof hut about 7 km from Rome, Italy (where

Plasmodium vivax malaria was prevalent); by so doing they avoided a clinical *P. vivax* infection.[1,7] Also, in 1900, three batches of mosquitoes infected with *P. vivax* were sent from Rome to London; Manson's elder surviving son—then a medical student at Guy's Hospital, and captain of rugby football—was exposed to them, and duly acquired a clinical attack of *P. vivax* infection, which responded to quinine.[1,7]

Foundation of the London School of Hygiene and Tropical Medicine: the close relationship between tropical physicians and basic scientific staff ends

In 1921 the Postgraduate Medical Committee recommended that an Institute of State Medicine be created in the University of London; the Rockefeller Foundation was persuaded by Professor R. T. Leiper (1881–1969) to donate \$2 million to the Ministry of Health for the development of this project.[1,11,18] In 1929, the London School of Hygiene and Tropical Medicine (LSHTM) was officially opened at Keppel Street (Gower Street) by the Prince of Wales (later King Edward VIII). Some years after this the SHS ceased managing the School, and *clinical* tropical medicine became detached from the basic sciences.

Clinical tropical medicine in London suffered a further temporary setback when the Ross Institute and Hospital for Tropical Diseases (Director: Sir Ronald Ross (1857–1932)—see below) was opened at Putney in 1926.[1,11,23,24] It was, however, clear from the outset that there was insufficient clinical material in London to justify two separate hospitals devoted to the management of tropical disease; the project therefore had no chance of becoming viable from a clinical viewpoint! The institution ultimately became incorporated into the LSHTM, as the Ross Institute for Tropical Hygiene, in 1934; the Director had died two years before.[24]

The itinerant saga of *clinical* tropical medicine in London continued unabated and the survival of Manson's original concept seemed at times in serious jeopardy— not least during World War II (1939–45) when the specialty had to make do with a mere ten beds—with no teaching facilities, at the Dreadnought (the SHS's flagship) Hospital, Greenwich. For a brief period after the war a nursing home in Devonshire Street, W1, housed the discipline. In 1951 a Hospital for Tropical Diseases was opened at St Pancras, NW1 on 24 May (Empire Day) by the Duchess of Kent.[1,18] In late 1999, the latest (and possibly the final) move of the clinical discipline, to University College Hospital, took place;[18] regrettably, the facilities in that overcrowded vicinity are extremely limited.

Regarding the *clinical* discipline in London, Manson-Bahr[11] later concluded: 'In recounting the chequered history of this institution, the Hospital for Tropical Diseases, a venture one would have thought essential to the greatest of all Empires, there runs the thread of insecurity . . . the hospital became the whipping boy of medical politics . . . The Board of the SHS was always a representative body of admirals whose interest lay in the sailor, but *not* in (clinical) tropical medicine.' The future of the *clinical* discipline in London remains anyone's guess![1,25]

Development of tropical medicine in Liverpool

The Liverpool School of Tropical Medicine had opened about six months before that in London.[1,26,27] Although the concept of a School of Tropical Medicine in Liverpool developed after that in London, the plan of action proceeded more rapidly, and the School was opened to students on 21 April 1899. The initial momentum had originated in a circular from Chamberlain to the General Medical Council and leading British medical schools (11 March 1898), and a letter to the Governors of the Colonies (14 June 1898). The timescale of the first appointments was impressive:[26,28] 20 January 1899—Dean appointed; 7 February—Demonstrator in tropical pathology (Dr H. E. Annett); 10 April—Lecturer in tropical medicine (Major Ronald Ross, IMS); 22 April—School officially opened by Lord Lister (1827–1912); May 1899—teaching started. The Liverpool School was not a 'brainchild' of Manson/ Chamberlain (unlike the LSTM), and it did not therefore receive Government support—a source of irritation (and perhaps even anger) at the time. It owed its inception to the initiative(s) of Mr (later Sir) Alfred Jones KCMG (1845–1909), a prominent Liverpool (like London, an important seaport) figure, and an energetic leader in the development of Liverpool's overseas trade with the West African Colonies; he controlled the Elder Dempster shipping line, which traded with the Canary Islands and West Africa (and had a thriving business in bananas, groundnuts and oil nuts); local commerce had previously involved the *'triangular trade'*. Together with several extremely wealthy and generous Liverpool merchants he also provided the finance for the School's foundation. The other major personality in the project was Dr (later Sir) Rubert Boyce, FRS (1863–1911).

The project was supported by the Royal Society, whose Secretary wrote to the Principal of University College, Liverpool (18 November 1898):[26,27] 'I think the idea of starting something at Liverpool about Tropical Diseases in connection with the College, most admirable. The opportunities of studying Tropical Diseases are greater at Liverpool than anywhere else in England, excepting perhaps London. You have to arrange: 1. For teaching. 2. For investigation. No. 2 wants, I think, more support than No. 1. If you had a ward, say at the Southern Hospital, one of the physicians might take charge of it, and give lectures, clinical at the Hospital, and general say at the College—I suppose you might give him a title. For investigation you do not, I think, need a separate Laboratory at College, but a small Clinical Laboratory and the

Hospital itself . . . The next point, I am in doubt about. I am inclined to think that the Pathology of Tropical Diseases should belong to the *Professor of Pathology*, who should, by virtue of this have some connection with the Tropical Diseases Ward in the Hospital, have access to the cases,. . . This system of a Pathologist working with the Physician or Surgeon in Clinical charge of the sick is being very largely worked with great success in America, and in this Tropical Disease seems to offer an opportunity for it. I have talked with Lord Lister [President of the Royal Society], and he generally approves of what I have proposed, at least, thinks it most desirable that the Hospital and College should lay hold of Tropical Diseases. I myself feel very strong that it is an opportunity of *study* of these diseases. When the experts on Malaria sent out to Africa get to work on the West Coast, as they will in time do, it will be a great advantage to have an Institution for Tropical Diseases already in work at Liverpool. The experts abroad can work with the men at home.'

At a meeting convened at the offices of Messrs Elder, Dempster & Co on 23 November 1898, the following were present:[26,27] Alfred L. Jones; William Adamson, President of the Royal Southern Hospital; R. T. Glazebrook, Principal of University College; William Alexander, Senior Surgeon of the Royal Southern Hospital; William Carter, Physician to the Royal Southern Hospital, Professor of Therapeutics, University College; and Boyce. 'The following resolutions were unanimously passed: 1. That the gentlemen present form themselves into a Committee, with the approval of their various boards, for promoting the study of Tropical Diseases and to consider the best means of carrying out . . . Jones' intentions in the munificent offer he has made to further the above object. 2. That Mr Charles W. Jones (of Messrs Lamport and Holt) be asked to serve on this Committee. It was decided that the above resolutions should be printed, and that Jones would hand a copy to . . . Chamberlain . . . The Committee recommended that before the next meeting, the Professional Members should meet together to consider and suggest the best means for . . . carrying out these objects.' At a second meeting (12 December 1898) a letter from Lord Ampthill (Colonial Office) to the Chairman (1 December) was read:[26] 'I have shown your letter of the 28th ult. with regard to the School of Tropical Medicine [to] Chamberlain. He was much interested and very glad to hear of the important work you have thus commenced. You are no doubt aware of what . . . Chamberlain has been doing himself with regard to the establishment of a School of Tropical Medicine [in London] and he considers it a great advantage that Liverpool should be co-operating on similar lines. If it would interest you, I should be very glad to send you particulars of the Colonial Office scheme and information as to what has been done already, but I dare say you have learnt all that is essential from the newspapers.'

In December 1898 the *Lancet*[28] reported: '. . . Chamberlain's scheme for the teaching of tropical diseases to colonial surgeons . . . has already born practical fruit. Mr Alfred Jones of Liverpool has offered £350 annually to establish and maintain a laboratory in Liverpool for the study of tropical diseases and the scheme will be carried out by a joint committee of the Royal Southern Hospital and of University College. A laboratory for immediate investigation will be built opposite the hospital, whilst prolonged research will be carried out in the pathological laboratory of University College, under the direction of Professor Boyce. A large number of cases from the West Coast of Africa are taken into the wards of the Royal Southern Hospital, as Liverpool, being the centre of the African trade, is in constant communication with West Africa. We again have to congratulate Liverpool on the munificence of her citizens and would direct the attention of medical men about to practice in any capacity on the West Coast of Africa to the opportunity that is being afforded them for obtaining invaluable information.'

In a letter (1 February 1899) from the Colonial Office,[26] read to a Committee meeting, it was stated that 'Chamberlain was very glad to learn that it had been decided to establish this School, but regretting that the Government could not grant any financial aid; however, in the selection of candidates for medical appointments in the Colonies, preference would be given to those who had receive instruction in tropical medicine, such as that provided in the Liverpool School'. A further letter from Chamberlain (23 February) stated, however, that 'all doctors appointed to the Colonial Service must be attached to the Albert Docks' Hospital[16] for at least 2 months'. The Committee resolved to: (1) write to the Colonial Office and express regret that Chamberlain did not see his way to dispense with the latter condition in the case of students from the Liverpool School; and (2) approach the Colonial Office on the subject. On 20 March, Professor Boyce announced that Lord Lister had written stating that he intended to approach Chamberlain on behalf of the School, and it was therefore resolved to postpone further action in the matter pending receipt of information concerning the result of this interview. However, Government funding was never forthcoming and there can be no doubt that this led to a significant souring of relationships (some rivalry still exists) between Liverpool and London.

Foundation of the Liverpool school

In 1899, The *Lancet*[29] summarized the opening of the Liverpool School (Figure 1.4): 'This School was inaugurated under fortunate auspices on April 22nd of this year by Lord Lister. "At the annual dinner of the Royal Southern Hospital on Nov. 12th, 1898, Mr. Alfred L. Jones, a prominent Liverpool citizen and West Africa merchant, made an offer of £350 a year to start a school in Liverpool for the study of tropical diseases. The offer was made in the presence of Professor Rubert Boyce of University College, Liverpool, and Dr. William Alexander of the Royal Southern Hospital". . . "The great interest subsequently taken in the project by Mr. Alfred L. Jones,

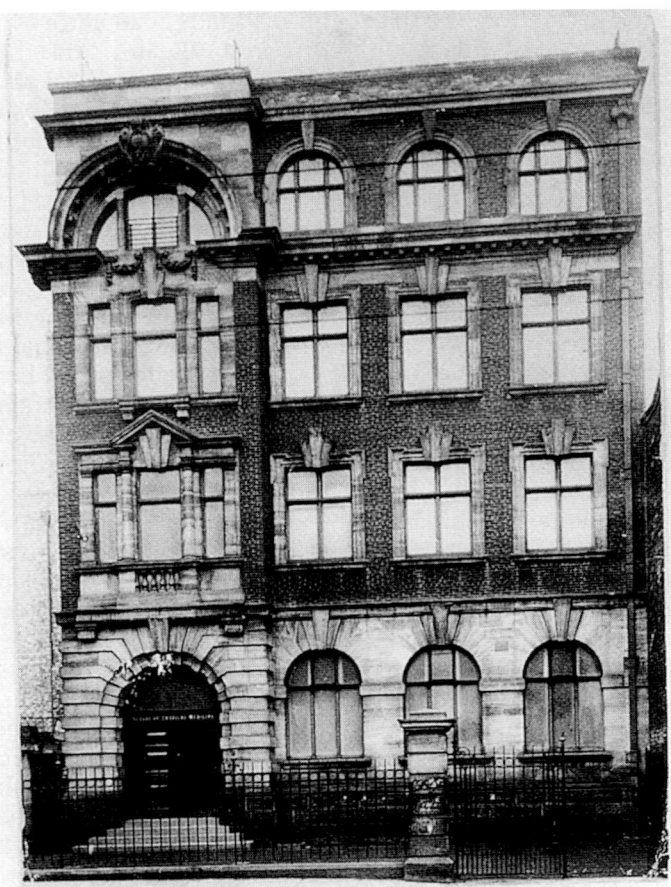

Figure 1.4: Liverpool School of Tropical Medicine; this building opened in 1920.

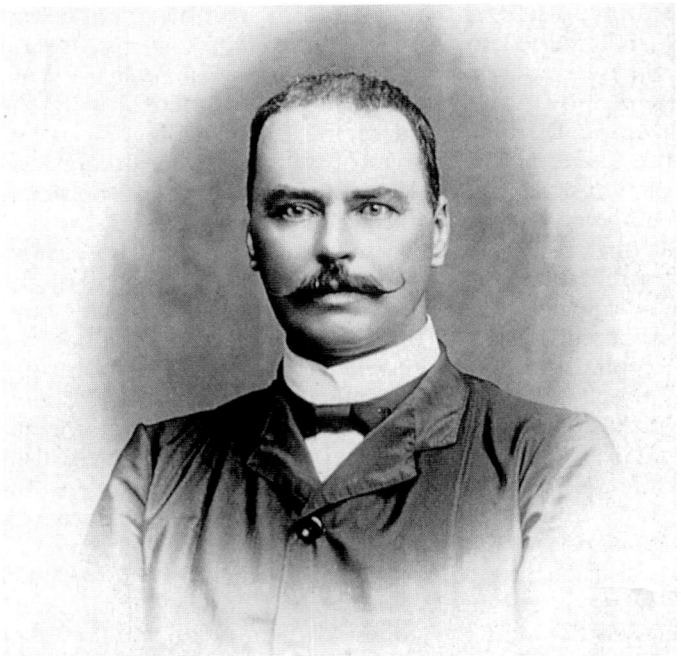

Figure 1.5: Major (later Sir) Ronald Ross (1857–1932).[35] The photograph was probably taken around 1900.

aided by the indomitable energy of Professor Boyce, resulted in subscription and donations coming in from all quarters towards the expenses of the proposed school. To those two gentlemen, warmly supported by the committee and medical staff of the Royal Southern Hospital, is due the establishment of the Liverpool School of Tropical Diseases. The management of the school is in the hands of a strong committee, of which Mr. Alfred L. Jones is the chairman and Mr. William Adamson . . . the vice-chairman. The committee also consists of duly appointed representative of University College, Liverpool, the Royal Southern Hospital, the Liverpool Chamber of Commerce, the Steamship Owners' Association, and the Shipowners' Association. A sum of over £1700 has already been promised, partly in annual subscriptions and partly in donations, in support of the school", but more pecuniary support is urgently needed if the practical work already begun is to be maintained at its excellent level. "A large floor in the Royal Southern Hospital has been set apart for tropical cases. This floor includes a cheerful ward containing 12 beds, now fully occupied, also an extensive laboratory for the examination of blood, urine, faeces, &c., and furnished with the apparatus applicable to modern research". Professor Boyce superintends "the pathological department of the school, with Dr. Annett as

pathological demonstrator. The committee have been fortunate in securing the services of Major Ronald Ross, IMS, as special lecturer on tropical diseases. . . The number of malarial cases treated in Liverpool in 1898 amounted to 294. In the previous year . . . there were 242 cases of malaria, 14 of beri-beri, 30 of dysentery, and 39 of tropical anaemia. With the means of instruction in the varied forms of tropical diseases thus afforded there will be no need for Liverpool students to proceed to London [where there were fewer cases[20]] to obtain that which is ready to hand at their own doors". The authorities of the Liverpool School of Tropical Medicine have lost no time in getting to real work.'

In June 1899, Ross (Figure 1.5) gave an inaugural lecture: he committed himself to the *practical* application of his malaria researches; extirpation of the mosquito, he envisaged, was the answer to the 'great malaria problem'. Ross had thus embarked on the 'sanitation' (or hygiene) tack which was to dominate much of the Liverpool School's work for the forthcoming century.[27]

Subsequent developments in Liverpool

Shortly after its opening (in April 1899), the Liverpool School set up a series of 'expeditions': the first embarked for Sierra Leone in July, and 11 more had been carried out by the end of 1903. Between its foundation and 1914, a total of 32 scientific expeditions to the tropics had taken place.[26,30] The *Annals of Tropical Medicine and Parasitology* was founded by the School's staff in 1907. The School was compelled, however, to survive by subscription; there was therefore no year-to-year stability.

At the outbreak of the Great War in 1914, teaching had been in full swing for 15 years;[31] two full courses were being given annually. An advanced practical course (one month duration) was designed to meet the convenience of practitioners when at home on leave; those who attended this were excused the first month of the other course. Special courses on entomology designed for officers in the West African Medical Service and others were also given three times annually. Special research work was carried out at the School and the Runcorn Research Laboratories (about 16 miles from Liverpool).

Historical accounts of the Liverpool School of Tropical Medicine are due to Miller[27] and Maegraith.[32] The School (unlike that in London) has established close collaborative links with some of the recently created Universities and Medical Schools of Africa, and other newly 'emergent' developing countries.

Medicine in the tropics and tropical medicine

The practice of medicine in a tropical country differs in many ways from that in a temperate one—where the classical specialty (exemplified by the London and Liverpool Schools) has dominated the scenario. A major problem arises in the *definition* of 'tropical medicine'; this was addressed by Manson[8] in the preface to the first edition of this textbook in 1898: 'The title I have elected to give to this work, TROPICAL DISEASES, is more convenient than accurate. If by 'tropical diseases' be meant diseases peculiar to, and confined to, the tropics, then half a dozen pages might have sufficed for their description . . . If . . . the expression 'tropical diseases' be held to include all diseases occurring in the tropics, then the work would require to cover almost the entire range of medicine.' The tropical practitioner (he continued): 'enjoys opportunities for original research and discovery far superior in novelty and interest to those at the command of his fellow inquirer in the well-worked field of European and American research.' Figures 1.6 and 1.7 summarize some of the highlights in the development of these separate disciplines.[6]

In Britain (and other European countries) and northern America, infectious diseases dominated the medical scene until well into the last century (see Figure 1.6); however, following the introduction of improved sanitation/hygiene in Victorian England, their prevalence slowly declined,[1,33] the downward trend continuing with the introduction of antibiotics in the 1940s and 1950s. Only recently has prevalence tended to increase—largely as a result of the HIV/AIDS pandemic. *Tropical medicine*, as an organized discipline, took off in the 1890s (see above) and reached a peak during the first half of the last century. Following World War II (1939–1945) a downward trend set in; as a result, this specialty continues to decline

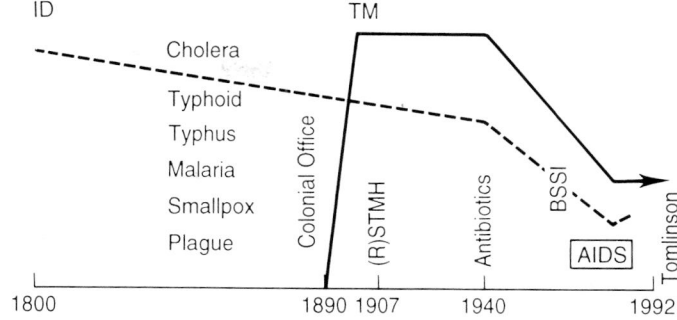

Figure 1.6: Approximate sequence of events in the foundation and development of the classical discipline. Tropical medicine (TM). ID, infectious diseases; (R)STMH, (Royal) Society of Tropical Medicine and Hygiene; BSSI, British Society for the Study of Infection; AIDS, acquired immune deficiency syndrome; Tomlinson Report, published in 1992, which gave rise to sweeping changes in the British National Health Service.

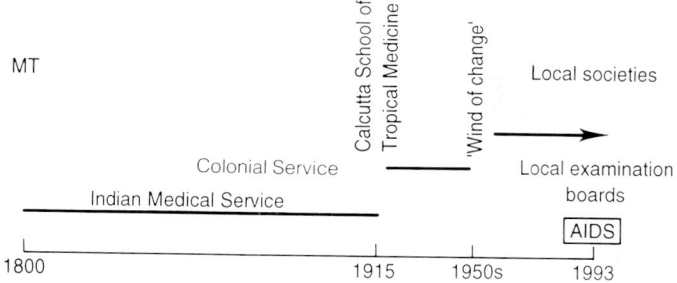

Figure 1.7: Approximate sequence of events in the progress of teaching/research in tropical (developing) countries. Medicine in the tropics (MT). AIDS, acquired immune deficiency syndrome.

as a *specific* entity. Introduction of National Health Service 'reforms', following the Tomlinson report (published in 1992), rendered the future of the relatively small discipline extremely vulnerable. The major priority at present is to maintain a cadre of physicians well versed in the more 'exotic' infections encountered in the UK (e.g. trypanosomiasis, leishmaniasis and schistosomiasis), a requirement which also applies to other 'temperate' countries.

In *tropical* countries (Figure 1.7), the scenario is entirely different.[6] Organized medical services began with the Indian Medical Service; this was followed by the Colonial Medical Service—with a far wider influence. Although Manson had started a Medical School in Hong Kong in 1887, the first School of Tropical Medicine in a tropical country was established by Sir Leonard Rogers (1868–1962) at Calcutta in 1920; this was a pioneering achievement. When the former British Colonies acquired 'independence' in the 1950s and later, the 'wind of change' brought in its wake many newly created (indigenous) universities and medical schools, e.g. Makerere University College, Kampala; Ibadan University, Nigeria; and the University (and University Teaching Hospital), Lusaka. This led to much local teaching and research, and also simultaneously the introduction of local medical societies and examining boards. These are changing times, and the future of the specialty *Tropical Medicine* is at present uncertain! But that must on no account be confused with 'medicine in the tropics'.[34]

REFERENCES

1 Cook G C. *From the Greenwich Hulks to Old St Pancras: A History of Tropical Disease in London.* London: Athlone Press, 1992: 338.

2 Balfour A. Some British and American pioneers in tropical medicine and hygiene. *Trans R Soc Trop Med Hyg* 1925; 19:189–231.

3 Dewhurst K. *Dr Thomas Sydenham (1624–1689): His Life and Original Writings.* London: Wellcome Historical Medical Library, 1966: 131–139.

4 Singer C & Underwood E A. *A Short History of Medicine,* 2nd edn. Oxford: Oxford University Press, 1962: 221–223.

5 Arnold D. Introduction: diseases, medicine and empire. In Arnold D (ed.) *Imperial Medicine and Indigenous Societies.* Manchester: Manchester University Press, 1988: 1–26.

6 Cook G C. Presidential Address. Evolution: the art of survival. *Trans R Soc Trop Med Hyg* 1994; 89:4–18.

7 Cook G C. Some early British contributions to tropical disease. *J Infect* 1993; 27:325–333.

8 Manson P. *Tropical Diseases: A Manual of the Diseases of Warm Climates.* London: Cassell, 1898: 624.

9 Ross R. *Memoirs: With a Full Account of the Great Malaria Problem and its Solution.* London: John Murray, 1923: 547.

10 Cook G C. The Seamen's Hospital Society: a progenitor of the tropical institutions. *Postgrad Med J* 1999; 75:715–717.

11 Manson-Bahr P. *History of the School of Tropical Medicine in London: 1899–1949.* London: H K Lewis, 1956: 328.

12 Cook G C. Changing rôle(s) for the Royal Hospital, Greenwich. *Hist Hosp* 2001; 22:35–46.

13 Manson-Bahr P H & Alcock A. *The Life and Work of Sir Patrick Manson.* London: Cassell, 1927: 273.

14 Manson P. The necessity for special education in tropical medicine. *Lancet* 1897; ii:842–845.

15 Cook G C. Doctor Patrick Manson's leading opposition in the establishment of the London School of Tropical Medicine: Curnow, Anderson, and Turner. *J Med Biog* 1995; 3:170–177.

16 Cook G C & Webb A J. The Albert Dock Hospital, London: the original site (in 1899) of Tropical Medicine as a new discipline. *Acta Tropica* 2001; 79:249–255.

17 Hoare P. *Spike Island: The Memory of a Military Hospital.* London: Fourth Estate, 2001: 417.

18 May A. *London School of Hygiene & Tropical Medicine 1899–1999.* London: LSHTM, 1999: 40.

19 Manson P. London School of Tropical Medicine: the need for special training in tropical disease. *J Trop Med* 1899; 2:57–62.

20 Cook G C. 'Tropical' cases admitted to the Albert Dock Hospital in the early years of the London School of Tropical Medicine. *Trans R Soc Trop Med Hyg* 1999; 93:675–677.

21 Low G C. The history of the foundation of the Society of Tropical Medicine and Hygiene. *Trans R Soc Trop Med Hyg* 1928; 22:197–202.

22 Cook G C. George Carmichael Low FRCP: twelfth President of the Society and underrated pioneer of tropical medicine. *Trans R Soc Trop Med Hyg* 1993; 87: 355–360.

23 Cook G C. Aldo Castellani FRCP (1877–1971) and the founding of the Ross Institute & Hospital for Tropical Diseases at Putney. *J Med Biog* 2000; 8:198–205.

24 Cook G C. A difficult metamorphosis: the incorporation of the Ross Institute & Hospital for Tropical Diseases into the London School of Hygiene and Tropical Medicine. *Med Hist* 2001; 45:483–506.

25 Cook G C. Future structure of clinical tropical medicine in the United Kingdom. *Br Med J* 1982; 284:1460–1461.

26 *Liverpool School of Tropical Medicine: Historical Record 1898–1920.* Liverpool: University Press, 1920: 103.

27 Miller P J. *'Malaria, Liverpool': An Illustrated History of the Liverpool School of Tropical Medicine 1898–1998.* Liverpool: Liverpool School of Tropical Medicine 1898: 78.

28 The study of tropical diseases in Liverpool. *Lancet* 1898; ii: 1495.

29 The Liverpool School of Tropical Medicine. *Lancet* 1899; i: 1174–1176.

30 Worboys M. Manson, Ross and colonial medical policy: tropical medicine in London and Liverpool, 1899–1914. In Macleod R & Lewis M (eds) *Disease, Medicine and Empire: Perspectives on Western Medicine and the Experience of European Expansion.* London: Routledge, 1988: 21–37.

31 Liverpool School of Tropical Medicine. *Br Med J* 1914; i: 324.

32 Maegraith B G. History of the Liverpool School of Tropical Medicine. *Med Hist* 1972; 16:354–368.

33 Cook G C. Joseph William Bazalgette (1819–1891): a major figure in the health improvements of Victorian London. *J Med Biog* 1999; 7:17–24.

34 Cook G C. Tropical Medicine. *Lancet* 1997; 350:813.

35 Cook G C. Ronald Ross (1857–1932): 100 years since the demonstration of mosquito transmission of *Plasmodium spp.* – on 20 August 1897. *Trans R Soc Trop Med Hyg* 1997; 91: 487–488.

Chapter 2
Primary Care and Disease Prevention and Control

N. Shetty and P. S. Shetty

Introduction

In 1978, the International Conference on Primary Health Care was held in Alma-Ata, USSR, and endorsed by the World Health Organization (WHO). This conference called for urgent and effective national and international action to develop and implement primary health care throughout the world, particularly in developing countries, in a spirit of technical cooperation and in keeping with a new international economic order. The Alma-Ata Declaration of 1978 states that the main social target should be the attainment by all peoples of the world, by the year 2000, of a level of health that will permit them to lead a socially and economically productive life.[1] However, the world more than 20 years on from the Alma-Ata Declaration is vastly different from that which saw the signing of the Declaration. Significant global changes—new epidemics, economic instability, continuing civil unrest and conflict, and triumph of the free market enterprise that has meant more pressure to produce profits—have all resulted in health care delivery systems across the world that are vastly different and hugely inequitable.[2]

Definition of primary health care

The Alma-Ata Declaration describes primary health care (PHC) as essential health care based on practical, scientific and socially acceptable methods and technology. It is made universally accessible to individuals and families in the community through their full participation and at a cost that the community and country can afford to maintain at every stage of their development in the spirit of self-reliance and self-determination. It is the first level of contact of individuals, the family and community with the national health system, bringing health care as close as possible to where people live and work, and constitutes the first element of a continuing health care process.[1]

The key elements of primary health care

PHC addresses the main health problems in the community, providing promotive, preventive, curative and rehabilitative services accordingly. Key elements of the programme are:[1]

- Education concerning prevailing health problems and the methods of preventing and controlling them.
- Promotion of food supply and proper nutrition.
- An adequate supply of safe water and basic sanitation.
- Maternal and child health care, including family planning.
- Immunization against the major infectious diseases.
- Prevention and control of locally endemic diseases.
- Appropriate treatment of common diseases and injuries.
- Provision of essential drugs.

Basic concepts drawn from the programme are summarized as follows:

- Primary health care should be shaped around the life patterns of the population.
- It should both meet the needs of the local community and be an integral part of the national health care system.
- Preventive, promotional and rehabilitative services for the individual, family and community need to be integrated.
- The majority of health interventions should be undertaken as close to the community as possible by suitably trained workers.
- The balance among these services should vary according to the community needs and may well change over time.
- The local population should be involved in the formulation and implementation of health care activities.
- Decisions about the community's needs and solutions to its problems should be based on a continuing dialogue between the people and the health professionals who serve them.

Primary health care workers

Based on experience of the success in Thailand, it was recognized that potential human resources exist in the community and are waiting to be mobilized. Two types of primary health care workers have thus been developed: village health communicators (VHCs) and village health volunteers (VHVs), who promote rural health and other development efforts through an organized community. The VHCs are responsible for a cluster of 8–15 households, the VHVs for the whole village. The functions of VHCs are to impart health education (prevention and promotion), and to disseminate and obtain health information from the villagers. The VHVs perform the same functions as VHCs, but also have the duty of caring for people who have had simple accidents or injuries and those with common diseases. Both VHCs and VHVs work on a voluntary basis. However, the government provides them with free medical services and a certificate when their training is completed. Other intangible incentives such as recognition from their peer group are also present. An informal 5-day training course for VHCs, covering the use of self-instruction modules, health problem identification, team working, etc., is organized by subdistrict health personnel. The 35 self-instruction modules for VHCs cover curative, preventive and promotive measures. The VHCs are expected to be able to disseminate such knowledge and gather information from villagers. VHVs obtain 17 additional modules on simple curative care and are trained for an additional 2 weeks.[3]

In India, multi-purpose health workers (MPWs) perform the role of village health workers. An evaluation of their role in a PHC in Kerala, India, revealed that MPWs apportion time to some national health programmes such as the malaria eradication programme and family welfare and immunization programmes to the detriment of others such as tuberculosis and acute respiratory infection. This demonstrated the need for continued training and evaluation of grass-root level workers to fulfil their multi-purpose role.[4]

The PHC programme in Thailand is often hailed as a success since it was responsible for solving many of the health problems of underserved people in rural areas. The concept of community participation—consisting of the contribution of ideas, manpower, money and materials by the community—was fundamental and provided the key to success of the PHC programme. To educate the community to be self-reliant or self-supportive is another basic concept that the Thai PHC programme fostered. Their Ministry of Public Health was also a key player in that it recognized that strengthening of a health service delivery system and the development of a referral system were essential to support PHC activities.[5]

Integrated management of the sick child

While a great deal has been learned from disease-specific control programmes during the past 15 years, the challenge remained of how to combine the lessons learned into a single method for more efficient and effective management of childhood illness. WHO and UNICEF responded by jointly developing an approach referred to as integrated management of childhood illnesses (IMCI).[6]

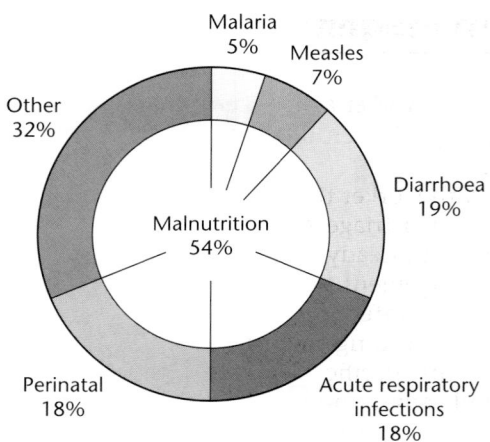

Figure 2.1: Distribution of 11.6 million deaths among children less than 5 years old in all developing countries, 1995. (Source: World Health Organization.)

According to the World Bank's *World Development Report 1993*, integrated management of the sick child is seen as the intervention likely to have the greatest impact in reducing the global burden of disease. It is also among the most cost-effective health interventions in low- and middle-income countries. Indeed, adoption and implementation of this approach were deemed essential to reaching the goal set in the 1990 World Summit for Children of reducing childhood mortality by 50% by the year 2000.[5] Every year some 12 million children die before reaching their fifth birthday, many of them during their first year of life. Of these, 70% are killed by one of five causes—diarrhoea, pneumonia, measles, malaria or malnutrition—and often in combination (Figure 2.1). Because their signs and symptoms may overlap, recognizing which of these conditions is present in a sick child can be difficult and a single diagnosis is often inappropriate. Treatment of the sick child may also be complicated by the need to combine therapies for several conditions. The situation argues for child health programmes which address the sick child as a whole, not just single diseases.

Integrated management presents several key advantages. It leads to more accurate diagnoses in outpatient settings; ensures more appropriate and, where possible, combined treatment of major illnesses; and speeds referral of severely ill children. The approach gives due attention both to prevention of childhood disease as well as to treatment, emphasizing immunization, vitamin A supplementation if needed, and improved infant feeding, including exclusive breast-feeding. The role of the voluntary health worker or multi-purpose health worker is immediately evident in the IMCI programme.

Newly developed treatment guidelines for the sick child cover the most common potentially fatal conditions. The health worker is trained to assess every child for non-specific danger signs; for the four main symptoms of cough or difficult breathing, diarrhoea, fever and ear problems; for nutritional status; and for immunization status.

Case management process

1. The health worker assesses the child—asking questions, examining the child and checking immunization status.
2. The health worker then classifies the illness based on a colour-coded triage system, with which many health workers are already familiar through use of the WHO case management guidelines for diarrhoea and acute respiratory infections (ARI). The system classifies illnesses according to whether they require (a) urgent referral, (b) specific medical treatment and advice, or (c) simple advice on home management.
3. After classifying the illness, the health worker identifies specific treatments. If the child is being urgently referred, the health worker gives only urgent treatments beforehand.
4. The health worker then provides practical instructions, such as how to administer oral drugs, increase fluids during diarrhoea and treat local infections at home. Mothers are advised on the signs which indicate the child should immediately be brought back to the clinic and when to return for follow-up.
5. For children under 2 years of age and those who are malnourished, the health worker assesses feeding, notes any feeding problems and provides counselling on feeding problems.

Training

Training health workers is a key activity in the long-term undertaking to improve the system for providing care to sick children. The WHO/UNICEF course *Management of Childhood Illness* trains health workers in first-level facilities (outpatient clinics and health centres), enabling them to effectively manage illnesses in an integrated fashion in sick children between the ages of 1 week and 5 years. The course also teaches them to communicate key health messages to mothers, helping them to understand how best to ensure the health of their children. The training course is based on the treatment guidelines and emphasizes hands-on practice. But course materials must be adapted to local situations so that, for example, local foods and drinks can be mentioned or locally appropriate drugs recommended.

Research

Research is an essential component of all programmes to reduce mortality and morbidity in children. WHO has drawn up a list of future research priorities related to integrated management of the sick child in order to improve the detection and treatment of the five major illnesses. Examples of areas where more information is needed are:

- Detection and management of anaemia and meningitis.
- Management of malnutrition and feeding problems.

- Management of severe disease in very young infants.
- Identification of high-risk children.
- Adequacy of clinical management in first-level health facilities.
- Reasons why families do not seek health care for sick children.

While much research is concerned with biomedical questions, there is also a need for further behavioural research on issues such as communicating with mothers and adaptation of advice on feeding to local conditions. Training of health care workers in Gondar, Ethiopia, and their performance in the delivery of IMCI was evaluated by Simoes et al.[7] The training course, just 9 days in duration, and with a few modifications of the IMCI guidelines to local conditions resulted in significant improvement in treatment outcomes of sick children in the area. IMCI treatment algorithms were evaluated in Kenya,[8] where malaria transmission is high, and in the Gambia,[9] where malaria is seasonal. The study in Kenya provided important technical validation of the IMCI guidelines with changes to incorporate local health problems, and continuous monitoring of health care workers was underscored. In the Gambia, the IMCI algorithm was found to be useful for the diagnosis of pneumonia, gastroenteritis, measles and malnutrition but not malaria. Microscopy was deemed to be essential to prevent over-diagnosis of malaria, especially during periods of low transmission. The impact of PHC services on infant mortality was assessed in the Gambia[10] and in rural Niger.[11] In both studies PHC programmes had a significant impact on infant mortality particularly when they were well supported and effectively mounted over a short time period. Significant impact of PHC on maternal and child mortality and morbidity could also be demonstrated in the Gomoa experience in rural Ghana.[12]

Shearley,[13] while commenting on the societal value of vaccination in developing countries, made the observation that vaccination forms the basis of village operated PHC activity. Vaccination programmes provide an opportunity for the provision of other primary care services, as it can be the only recurring activity in primary care that brings mother and child into contact with health services on a predictable and frequent basis. Vaccination leads to a direct and measurable reduction of child mortality rates. This encourages smaller families and contributes to success of family planning programmes. Protecting the lives of children directly through vaccination and other PHC activities is a major strategy towards improving the lives of women as it liberates their time, energy and resources. It empowers women to protect their own health and that of their children through their own actions. Therefore vaccination services are best delivered along with other services needed by children in the first year of their life and by pregnant women—the persons who constitute the priority groups for PHC services in the developing world.

Maternal health

The global Safe Motherhood Initiative was launched in 1987 to improve maternal health and cut the number of maternal deaths in half by the year 2000.[14] Services for safe motherhood should be readily available through a network of linked community health care providers, clinics and hospitals. The integrated services that policy-makers from around the world have pledged to provide include:

- Community education on safe motherhood.
- Prenatal care and counselling, including the promotion of maternal nutrition.
- Skilled assistance during childbirth.
- Care for obstetric complications, including emergencies.
- Postpartum care.
- Management of abortion complications, postabortion care and, where abortion is not against the law, safe services for the termination of pregnancy.
- Family planning counselling, information and services.
- Reproductive health education and services for adolescents.

Important lessons learned from the collaborative effort of several agencies highlight the following:

1. *Empower women, ensure their choices.* Gender inequalities and discrimination, especially in the developing world, limit women's choices and contribute directly to their ill-health and death (Figure 2.2). Legal reform and community mobilization can help women safeguard their reproductive health by enabling them to understand and articulate their health needs, and to seek services with confidence and without delay.
2. *Every pregnancy faces risks* (Figure 2.3). Every pregnant woman—even if she is well nourished and well educated—can develop sudden, life-threatening complications that require high-quality obstetric care. Attempts to predict these problems before they occur have not been successful, since most complications are unexpected and the majority of women with poor pregnancy outcomes do not fall into any high-risk categories. Therefore, maternal health programmes

must aim to ensure that *all* women have access to essential services.
3. *Ensure skilled attendance during childbirth.* The single most effective way to reduce maternal death is to ensure that a health professional with the skills to conduct a safe, normal delivery and manage complications is present during childbirth. Unfortunately, there is a chronic shortage of these professionals in poor and rural communities in the developing world. Research has shown that even trained traditional birth attendants (TBAs) have not significantly reduced a woman's risk of dying in childbirth, largely because they are unable to treat pregnancy complications. As an interim strategy for settings where TBAs attend a significant proportion of deliveries, programme planners may want to provide TBAs with adequate training and support to help them refer complicated cases effectively. In all settings, however, skilled attendance at delivery should continue to be the long-term goal.
4. *Improve access to high-quality maternal health services.* A large number of women in developing countries do not have access to maternal health services (Figure 2.4). Many of them cannot get to, or afford, high-quality care. Cultural customs and beliefs can also prevent women from understanding the importance of health services, and from seeking them. In addition to legal reform and efforts to build support within communities, health systems must work to address a range of clinical, interpersonal and logistical problems that affect the quality, sensitivity and accessibility of the services they provide.
5. *Address unwanted pregnancy and unsafe abortion.* Unsafe abortion is the most neglected—and most easily preventable—cause of maternal death. These deaths can be significantly reduced by ensuring that safe motherhood programmes include client-centred family planning services to prevent unwanted pregnancy, contraceptive counselling for women who have had an induced abortion, the use of appropriate technologies for women who experience abortion complications and, where not against the law, safe services for pregnancy termination.

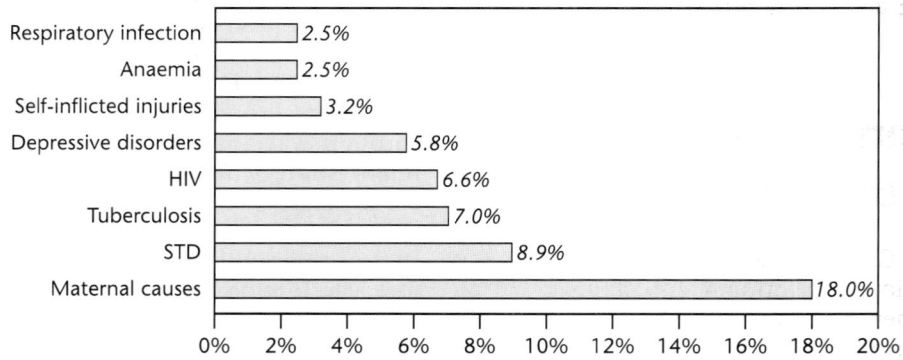

Figure 2.2: Leading causes of the burden of disease in women aged 15–44 in the developing world, 1990. (Source: World Development Report, 1993: *Investing in health.* World Bank, Washington, 1993.)

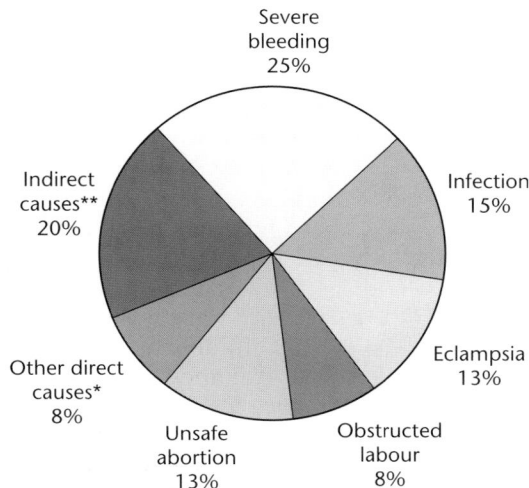

Figure 2.3: Causes of maternal deaths. (Source: *Maternal Health Around the World* poster; World Health Organization and the World Bank, 1997.) *Other direct causes including, for example, ectopic pregnancy, embolism, anaesthesia related; **indirect causes including, for example, anaemia, malaria, heart disease.

6. *Measure progress.* Governments around the world have pledged to reduce maternal mortality by 50% by the year 2000. However, maternal mortality is difficult to measure, due to problems with identification, classification and reporting. Therefore, safe motherhood partners have developed alternative means for measuring the impact and effectiveness of programmes; for example, by recording the proportion of births attended by a skilled health provider. These indicators can identify weaknesses and suggest programmatic priorities so that maternal deaths can be better prevented in the future.

Female health workers in Pakistan, given appropriate training, have been shown to substantially reduce infant, child and maternal mortality and to generate positive perceptions of family planning in the community.[15] Non-governmental organizations in some urban areas have incorporated the management of sexually transmitted diseases (STD) into primary health care provision for women.[16] This is particularly relevant for commercial sex workers and other vulnerable groups; it also provides a platform for training and awareness of STD as a health risk for women.

Management of specific infectious diseases

Since 1990 the WHO Global Tuberculosis Programme has promoted the revision of national tuberculosis programmes to strengthen the focus on directly observed treatment, short course (DOTS). With direct observation of treatment, the patient does not bear the sole responsibility of adhering to treatment. Health care workers, public health officials, governments and communities must all share the responsibility and provide a range of support services patients need to continue and finish treatment. One of the aims of effective TB control is to organize TB services which are an integral part of PHC systems so that the patient has flexibility in where he or she receives treatment, for example in the home or at the workplace. Treatment observers can be anyone who is willing, trained, responsible, acceptable to the patient and accountable to the TB control services. The recording and reporting system is used to systematically evaluate patient progress and treatment outcome. The system consists of: a laboratory register that contains a log of all patients who have had a smear test done; patient treatment cards that detail the regular intake of medication and follow-up sputum examinations; the TB register, which lists patients starting treatment and monitors their individual and collective progress towards cure; and reporting from districts to the national level, which allows assessment of control efforts. Yet, DOTS is still not used widely. Although some progress has been made, only about 24% of all TB patients were treated through the DOTS strategy in 1999. The consequences of not using DOTS more widely are alarming. TB cases and deaths will certainly continue, the global epidemic will remain uncontrolled, and harder-to-manage multidrug-resistant TB (MDR-TB) will be created. To address the problem of MDR-TB in areas where it has emerged, WHO is piloting a research initiative known as DOTS-Plus.[17]

The DOTS strategy has been successful in several centres in Asia and Africa. In Bangladesh[18] success was attributed to decentralizing sputum smear microscopy and treatment delivery services to peripheral health facilities utilizing the existing PHC network. Maintaining the quality of implementation, keeping it convenient and safeguarding confidentiality were important factors for its success in key centres in India.[19,20] In Thailand DOTS was performed by supervised family members and contributed to effective and widespread implementation of the programme.[21] Community-based delivery systems for DOTS have been found to be successful in Ethiopia and other parts of sub-Saharan Africa. The community-based delivery systems used patients themselves in the form of 'TB Clubs'[22] or 'guardians' in the community,[23,24] thus effectively decentralizing the programme and empowering the community itself.

Utilizing PHC workers has been a successful strategy for case detection and control of leprosy[25] and visceral leishmaniasis[26] in remote districts in Bihar, India.

Water sanitation and health

Deficiencies in water and sanitation contribute to the heavy disease burden imposed by diarrhoea, poliomyelitis, hepatitis, intestinal nematodes like hookworm and tropical diseases such as leishmaniasis. Food safety and hygiene are important factors in the prevalence of these illnesses.

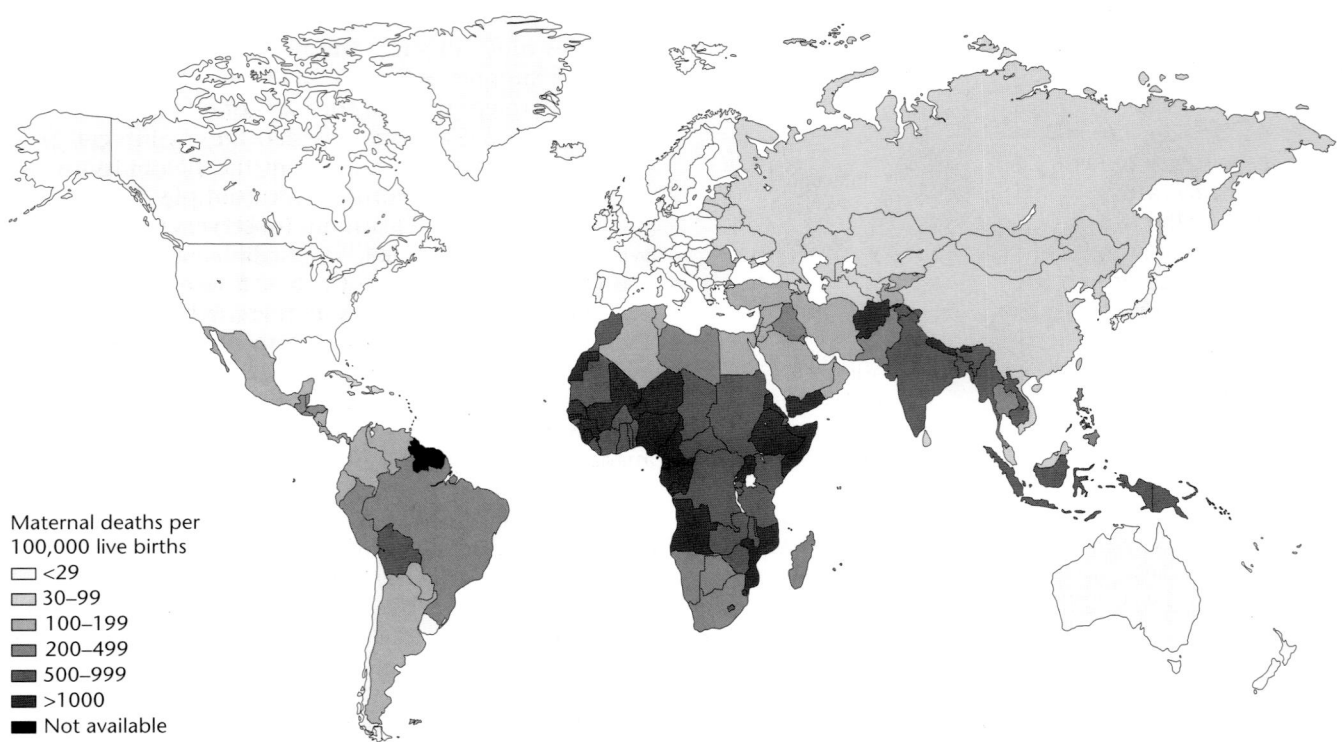

Maternal deaths per
100,000 live births
- [ ] <29
- 30–99
- 100–199
- 200–499
- 500–999
- >1000
- Not available

Figure 2.4: Maternal mortality ratios, 1990. (Source: *Maternal Health Around the World* poster; World Health Organization and the World Bank, 1997.)

Few persons would dispute, however, that water and sanitation are also important contributing factors. Furthermore, chemical contamination of drinking water is the main cause of important illnesses such as arsenicosis and fluorosis. It has been suggested that local communities should be trained as guardians of sound water management practices—such as monitoring quality, protecting water sources from pollutants, and identifying and penalizing polluters. Consumers could even take the initiative, such as in many local communities, of mobilizing demand for proper sanitation and sewerage systems and implementing schemes.[27]

Nutrition in primary health care

Nutrition is an important element of PHC, and is a major determinant of the health of the community and optimum growth of children. Nutrition and health are not synonymous, but without good nutrition health cannot be optimal. An essential prerequisite to prevent malnutrition or more appropriately undernutrition (since overnutrition and an unbalanced diet can also lead to poor health and disease) in a household or a community is to assure availability and access to adequate quantity, good quality and safe food to meet the nutrient needs of all people. However, the recognition that malnutrition is not just a food problem has been realized more recently, with due importance now being given to considerations of health, education and care. UNICEF in 1997 developed a conceptual framework on the causes of malnutrition as part of their nutrition strategy.[28] The framework shows that causes of malnutrition are multisectoral, embracing food, health and caring practices. They are also classified as immediate, underlying and basic, whereby factors at one level influence other levels. While inadequate dietary intake may be an immediate cause of childhood malnutrition, the underlying causes at the household or family level may be insufficient access to food, inadequate maternal and childcare, poor water or sanitation and inadequate access to health care and health services. The basic causes are much broader and include political, social, cultural, religious and economic systems in which the community or household exists. Malnutrition may manifest as a health problem and health professionals can provide some answers, although health professionals alone cannot solve the problem. Agricultural professionals are needed to ensure enough production of the right kinds of foods, while educators, both formal and non-formal, are required to assist people, particularly women, in achieving and ensuring good nutrition.

Breast-feeding

Promotion of exclusive breast-feeding at the primary health care level is crucial. This may include preparing the pregnant mother and helping her to decide to breast-feed the child. It also includes support in the postpartum period, through formal and informal activities, which may help women to have confidence in their ability to breast-feed and relieve doubts and anxieties they may have about it. Protection of breast-feeding should be aimed at guarding women who normally would successfully breast-feed against forces and situations that might cause them to alter this practice. Promotion of breast-feeding which must be part of primary health care includes motivating or re-educating mothers who might not be inclined to breast-feeding, although promotion is difficult given changing work patterns of women in developing societies and changing demands on their time. The Baby Friendly Hospital Initiative (BFHI) launched in 1992 by UNICEF and WHO[28] to help protect, support and promote breast-feeding by addressing problems in hospitals may be less relevant for countries and communities where most babies are born outside hospital settings. However, there are lessons to be learned for application in PHC settings.

Complementary feeding

With a healthy mother providing adequate breast milk, breast-feeding alone should ensure good growth, nutrition and health of an infant up to 6 months of life. Continued breast-feeding with the addition of safe high-quality complementary foods into the second year of life provides the best nourishment and protects children from infections.[28] Thus at 6 months of age, complementary feeding should be introduced gradually while the infant continues to be breast-fed. The introduction of complementary feeds is a critical stage in a child's life. A child must have additional complementary feeds at 6 months of age since breast milk is no longer able to provide all the nutrients the child needs. Hence delaying the introduction of complementary feeds can cause a child's growth to falter. However, too early introduction can also increase the risk of malnutrition and infection in a child, particularly if the preparation and storage of food are not hygienic. From 6 to 18 months of age the child needs frequent feeding and will need meals that are dense in energy and nutrients and are also easily digestible. Foods the rest of the family normally eat will have to be adapted to suit the need of a growing child. Emphasis on hygiene in preparation and storage of complementary feeds can never be adequate. The health worker at the PHC level can be an important player in educating the mother not only of the importance of good and nutritious complementary feeds, but also in promoting hygienic practices in the preparation, storage and handling of complementary feeds based on local foods for the child and in the imparting of knowledge of transmission of infectious agents.

Care

Of the three underlying causes of malnutrition, namely food, health and care, care is the one least investigated,

least understood and least emphasized.[29] Adequate care is not only important for the child's survival but also for optimal physical and mental development. Care also contributes to the child's general well-being and happiness. Child care may be influenced by external factors such as war, conflict and civil unrest, by local factors such as equity and access to health services at the PHC level and availability of educational facilities, as well as factors within a family or household such as adequate housing, safe water, household hygiene and mother's knowledge and educational achievement. Care is manifested in the ways a child is fed, nurtured, taught and guided. It is the expression by individuals and families of the domestic and cultural values that guide them.[28] Nutritionally, care encompasses all measures and behaviours that transmit available food and health resources into good child growth and development. In most developing countries the mother is the care-giver for the infant and the very young child although in extended families older relatives often play an important role. Care-giving behaviour is often mistakenly assumed to be the exclusive domain of mothers; it should in fact be the responsibility of the entire family.

Care-giving behaviour that contributes to good nutrition and health varies enormously between societies and cultures. While the assumption that all societies value children and wish to see them grow in a healthy manner to become valuable assets of their society is very largely true, the assumption that societies have evolved with traditional or culturally determined caring practices which are mostly good is often questioned. Identification of child-caring practices that are desirable should be the first step in any health promotion strategy that involves care. Protection of good practices that promote childcare from erosion or loss due to the developmental process is essential. Support is essential when good traditional practices of mothers or families is threatened or eroded by changes in society. A good example is the decline in breast-feeding that is seen in developing societies with urbanization. The PHC setting is obviously the focal point for integrating activities related to childcare in the community.

Promotion of growth monitoring

Growth monitoring was the first of UNICEF's GOBI (growth monitoring, oral rehydration, breast-feeding and immunization) strategy to improve child health and nutrition. Growth monitoring itself does not improve health or promote adequate and appropriate growth in children. It ensures that children are growing well and in a healthy manner. It helps the early detection of the onset of malnutrition either because of inadequate and poor-quality food or because proper growth is affected adversely by other factors such as episodes of infections. Hence the promotion of growth monitoring should form an important part of the PHC system. It should be closely integrated into primary health care activities and should not, as far as possible, be a separate programme. It should focus on maintaining and monitoring good and appropriate growth in infants and children in the community and help detect the early signs of growth faltering. It should not merely be used for following up and rehabilitating children who are recovering from malnutrition and whose growth is poor. Hence it is important that growth-monitoring promotion when integrated into PHC activities should be aimed at all children in the community. In order to do that, it is essential that all children are entered into the growth-monitoring programme soon after birth, since all infants up to about 6 months who are exclusively breast-fed show satisfactory growth. Growth monitoring also derives other indirect benefits, since good physical growth is often related to other aspects of good child development and environments that promote good child development usually help promote optimum physical growth. The proper promotion of growth monitoring requires not only that the health worker at the PHC level is trained adequately in techniques used to measure and monitor growth in infants and children, but also has access to good, simple equipment for measuring length or height and weight, appropriate growth charts and record-keeping facilities. Above all, the health worker should have a good understanding of existing child-rearing practices and the cultural, social and dietary environment of the community. Growth-monitoring promotion is viewed as a strategy to empower mothers to maintain good nutritional status in their children and to prevent growth faltering or growth retardation. It is a preventive strategy designed to promote optimum growth and good health and not merely to help diagnose malnutrition and ill-health.

The promotion of good nutrition for health at the primary care level is an important role that can be played by the PHC-level health worker. Nutrition information and education are essential to improve nutrition knowledge for application during pregnancy to ensure the best possible birth outcome along with other aspects of antenatal care. This process of empowering communities with the requisite knowledge to promote the health and nutrition of their families should continue with the birth of the infant and the growth and development of the child. Special emphasis needs to be placed on promoting breast-feeding, the timely introduction of complementary feeding and the crucial role that growth monitoring plays in ensuring the optimum health of children. Increasing the awareness of food and nutrition and their important role in the good health of the entire household, good food hygiene practices and correction of false food beliefs and taboos is a role health workers at the PHC level can readily play. Providing adequate training in nutrition and the necessary resources along with support is crucial for the important role these workers at the community level can fulfil. Thailand has been a beacon to most countries in integrating nutritional activities into primary care and in empowering and involving the community in promoting the nutrition and health of its population.

Conclusion

It has been argued that broad PHC cannot be afforded by developing countries in the present constrained economic circumstances. The counter-argument is that the PHC approach is viable even with slow economic growth if there is the political will to effect resource allocations according to PHC priorities.

In an unprecedented 'Declaration of Commitment' against HIV/AIDS the United Nations in June 2001 pledged an annual target expenditure of $7–10 billion on access to medicines as a fundamental element in tackling infection in middle- and low-income countries. In many low-income countries over 70% of the population live in rural areas that do not have access to the most basic facilities. The devastation caused by HIV/AIDS and other infections is as a result of complex health issues. Far more crucial than the delivery of antiretroviral and antituberculosis drugs is a sustainable infrastructure of PHC dealing with comprehensive basic health issues. Without this most basic requirement, the delivery of drugs would fail to contain the spread of human misery as a result of HIV/AIDS, TB and malaria, to name just the top three.

REFERENCES

1 World Health Organization. Declaration of Alma-Ata. International Conference on Primary Health Care, Alma-Ata, 1978.

2 World Health Organization. Primary Health Care in the 21st century is everybody's business. Press release WHO/89, November 1998. Available: http://www.who.int/inf-pr-1998/en/pr98-89.html [27 November 1998].

3 Nondasuta A, Ningsanon P, Chandavimol P & Tantlwongse P. Nutrition in primary health care. In Andersen J & Valyasevi A (eds) *Effective Communications for Nutrition in Primary Health Care*. Washington, DC: United Nations University Press, 1988: 6.

4 Nair V, Thankappan K, Sarma P & Vasan R. Changing roles of grass-root level health workers in Kerala, India. Health Policy Plan 2001; 16:171–179.

5 Nondasuta A. Primary health care and nutrition. In Winichagoon P, Kachondham Y, Attig G A & Tontisirin K (eds) *Integrating Food and Nutrition into development*. Bangkok: UNICEF and Mahidol University, 1992: 56–62.

6 World Health Organization–UNICEF. Integrated management of the sick child. Division of Child Health and Development (CHD), 2001. Available: http://www.who.int/chd/publications/sickchi/sickchi3.htm [24 April 2001].

7 Simoes E, Desta T, Tessema T et al. Performance of health workers after training in integrated management of childhood illness in Gondar, Ethiopia. *Bull World Health Organ* 1997; 75(suppl. 1):43–53.

8 Perkins B, Zucker J, Otieno J et al. Evaluation of an algorithm for integrated management of childhood illness in an area of Kenya with high malaria transmission. *Bull World Health Organ* 1997; 75(suppl. 1):33–42.

9 Weber M, Mulholland E, Jakar S et al. Evaluation of an algorithm for the integrated management of childhood illness in an area with seasonal malaria in the Gambia. *Bull World Health Organ* 1997; 75(suppl. 1):25–32.

10 Hill A, MacLeod W, Joof D et al. Decline of mortality in children in rural Gambia: the influence of village-level primary health care. *Trop Med Int Health* 2000; 5:107–118.

11 Magnani R, Rice J, Mock N et al. The impact of primary health care services on under-five mortality in rural Niger. *Int J Epidemiol* 1996; 25:568–577.

12 Afari E, Nkrumah F, Nakana T et al. Impact of primary health care on child morbidity and mortality in rural Ghana: the Gomoa experience. *Cent Afr J Med* 1995; 41:148–153.

13 Shearley A. The societal value of vaccination in developing countries. *Vaccine* 1999; 17(suppl. 3):S109–112.

14 Safe Motherhood Inter Agency Group. What is safe motherhood, 2001. Available: http://www.safemotherhood.org/init_what_is.htm [22 June 2001].

15 Barzgar M, Sheikh M & Bile M. Female health workers boost primary care. *World Health Forum* 1997; 18:202–210.

16 Baksi C, Harper I & Raj M. A 'Well Woman Clinic' in Bangalore: one strategy to attempt to decrease the transmission of HIV infection. *Int J STD AIDS* 1998; 9:418–423.

17 World Health Organization. Tuberculosis strategy and operations: DOTS. 2000. Available: http://www.who.int/gtb/dots/index.htm [March 2000].

18 Kumaresan J, Ahsan Ali A & Parkkali L. Tuberculosis control in Bangladesh: success of the DOTS strategy. *Int J Tuberc Lung Dis* 1998; 2:992–998.

19 Khatri G R & Frieden T R. The status and prospects of tuberculosis control in India. *Int J Tuberc Lung Dis* 2000; 4:193–200.

20 Balasubramanian V N, Oommen K & Samuel R. DOT or not? Direct observation of anti-tuberculosis treatment and patient outcomes, Kerala State, India. *Int J Tuberc Lung Dis* 2000; 4:409–413.

21 Akkslip S, Rasmithat S, Maher D & Sawert H. Direct observation of tuberculosis treatment by supervised family members in Yasothorn Province, Thailand. *Int J Tuberc Lung Dis* 1999; 3:1061–1065.

22 Getahun H & Maher D. Contribution of 'TB clubs' to tuberculosis control in a rural district in Ethiopia. *Int J Tuberc Lung Dis* 2000; 4:174–178.

23 Maher D, Hausler H P, Raviglione M C et al. Tuberculosis care in community care organizations in sub-Saharan Africa: practice and potential. *Int J Tuberc Lung Dis* 1997; 1:276–283.

24 Banerjee A, Harries A D, Mphasa N et al. Evaluation of a unified treatment regimen for all new cases of tuberculosis using guardian-based supervision. *Int J Tuberc Lung Dis* 2000; 4:333–339.

25 Vijayakumaran P, Reddy N B, Krishnamurthy P et al. Utilizing primary health are workers for case detection. *Indian J Lepr* 1998; 2:203–210.

26 Saxena N B, Aggarwal V, Dhillon G P et al. Visceral leishmaniasis control in India through primary health care system: a successful experiment of district level planning. *J Commun Dis* 1996; 28:122–128.

27 World Health Organization. Global Water Supply and Sanitation Assessment 2000 Report. Available: http://www.who.int/water_sanitation_health/Globassessment/GlasspdfTOC.htm [24April 2001].

28 UNICEF. *State of the World's Children 1998*. New York: UNICEF, 1998.

29 Latham M C. *Human Nutrition in the Developing World*. FAO Food & Nutrition Series 29. Rome: Food and Agriculture Organisation, 1997.

Chapter 3
Epidemiology of Disease in the Tropics

N. Shetty and P. S. Shetty

'Ingenuity, knowledge, and organization alter but cannot cancel humanity's vulnerability to invasion by parasitic forms of life. Infectious disease which antedated the emergence of humankind will last as long as humanity itself, and will surely remain, as it has been hitherto, one of the fundamental parameters and determinants of human history.' William H. McNeill in *Plagues and Peoples*, 1976

Introduction

The study of epidemiology in the tropics has undergone major changes since its infancy when it was largely a documentation of epidemics. It has now evolved into a dynamic phenomenon involving the ecology of the infectious agent, the host, reservoirs and vectors as well as the complex mechanisms concerned in the spread of infection and the extent to which this spread occurs.[1] Similar concepts in the study of epidemiology apply to communicable as well as non-communicable diseases. The understanding of epidemiological principles has its origins in the study of the great epidemics. Arguably the most powerful example of this is the study of that ancient scourge of mankind, the so-called black death or plague. A study of any of the plague epidemics throughout history has all the factors that govern current epidemiological analysis: infectious agent, host, vector, reservoir, complex population dynamics including migration, famine, fire

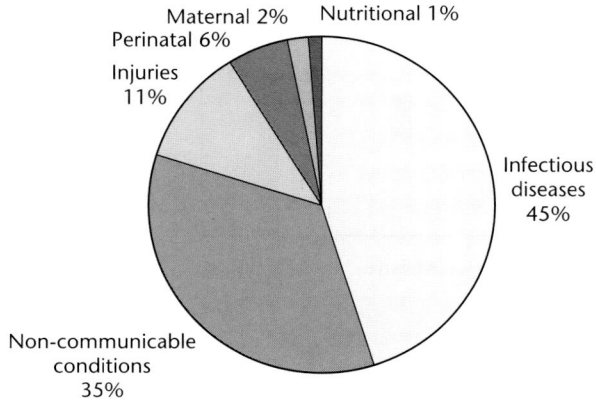

Figure 3.1: Main causes of death in low-income countries in South-East Asia and Africa. Estimates for 1998. (Source: WHO, 1999.)

Table 3.1 Examples of pathogenic microbes and the diseases they cause, identified since 1973.

Year	Microbe	Type	Disease
1973	Rotavirus	Virus	Infantile diarrhoea
1977	Ebola virus	Virus	Acute haemorrhagic fever
1977	*Legionella pneumophila*	Bacterium	Legionnaires' disease
1980	Human T-lymphotrophic virus I (HTLV 1)	Virus	T cell lymphoma/leukaemia
1981	Toxin-producing *Staphylococcus aureus*	Bacterium	Toxic shock syndrome
1982	*Escherichia coli* O157:H7	Bacterium	Haemorrhagic colitis; haemolytic uraemic syndrome
1982	*Borrelia burgdorferi*	Bacterium	Lyme disease
1983	Human immuno-deficiency virus (HIV)	Virus	Acquired immuno-deficiency syndrome (AIDS)
1983	*Helicobacter pylori*	Bacterium	Peptic ulcer disease
1989	Hepatitis C	Virus	Parentally transmitted non-A, non-B liver infection
1992	*Vibrio cholerae* O139	Bacterium	New strain associated with epidemic cholera
1993	Hantavirus	Virus	Adult respiratory distress syndrome
1994	*Cryptosporidium parvum*	Protozoa	Enteric disease
1995	Ehrlichiosis	Bacterium	Severe arthritis?
1996	nvCJD	Prion	New variant Creutzfeldt–Jakob disease
1997	HVN1	Virus	Influenza
1999	Nipah	Virus	Severe encephalitis

Source: WHO. (1999)[3]

and war; resulting in spread followed by quarantine and control.

The World Health Report 1996—'Fighting disease, fostering development'—states that infectious diseases are the world's leading cause of premature death.[2] Infectious diseases account for 45% of deaths in low-income countries (Figure 3.1) and up to 63% of deaths in children under 4 years of age worldwide. In addition, new and emerging infections pose a rising global threat (Table 3.1).[3]

The six deadly killers

No more than six deadly infectious diseases—pneumonia, tuberculosis, diarrhoeal diseases, malaria, measles and more recently HIV/AIDS—account for half of all premature deaths, killing mostly children and young adults (Figure 3.2).

Acute respiratory infections

Acute respiratory infections (ARIs) constitute the leading cause of death of infectious aetiology, killing more than 4 million people a year.[4] This range of infections, which includes pneumonia in its most serious form, accounts for more than 8% of the global burden of disease. Most of these deaths (99%) occur in developing countries. Pneumonia often affects children with low birth weight or those whose immune systems are weakened by malnutrition or other diseases. Caused by different

viruses or bacteria, ARI is closely associated with poverty, overcrowding and unsanitary household conditions. Several other factors seem to exacerbate the disease. Exposure to tobacco smoke increases the risk of contracting these infections, and many studies implicate both indoor and outdoor air pollution. Indoor air pollution has been the focus of particular concern: specifically, the soot and smoke associated with the burning of biomass fuels such as wood, coal, or dung. Many people in the developing world, mostly in rural areas, rely on biomass fuels for heating or cooking. A cause-and-effect relationship between indoor air pollution and ARI has been difficult to prove. Even so, the World Bank estimated in 1992 that switching to better fuels could halve the number of pneumonia deaths.[5] Approaches to management of childhood pneumonia in the tropics are hampered by the lack of diagnostic facilities to identify the aetiological agent. The WHO has devised a simple algorithm for use in field situations, by primary health care workers, using clinical criteria such as respiratory rate and in-drawing of ribs to decide whether a child needs hospitalization. Proper implementation of this strategy has been shown to reduce the mortality from childhood pneumonias by 25–50%.[6]

HIV/AIDS

The AIDS pandemic has emerged as the single most defining occurrence in the history of infectious diseases of the late twentieth and early twenty-first centuries.

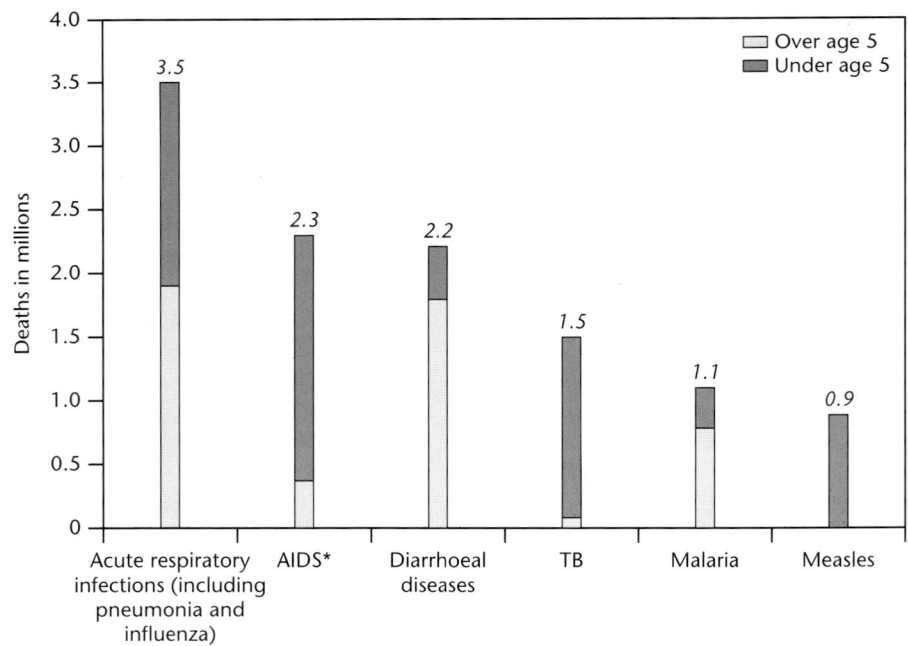

* HIV-positive people who died with TB have been included among AIDS deaths

Figure 3.2: Leading infectious killers (millions of deaths, worldwide, all ages, 1998). HIV positive people who died with TB have been included in AIDS deaths.

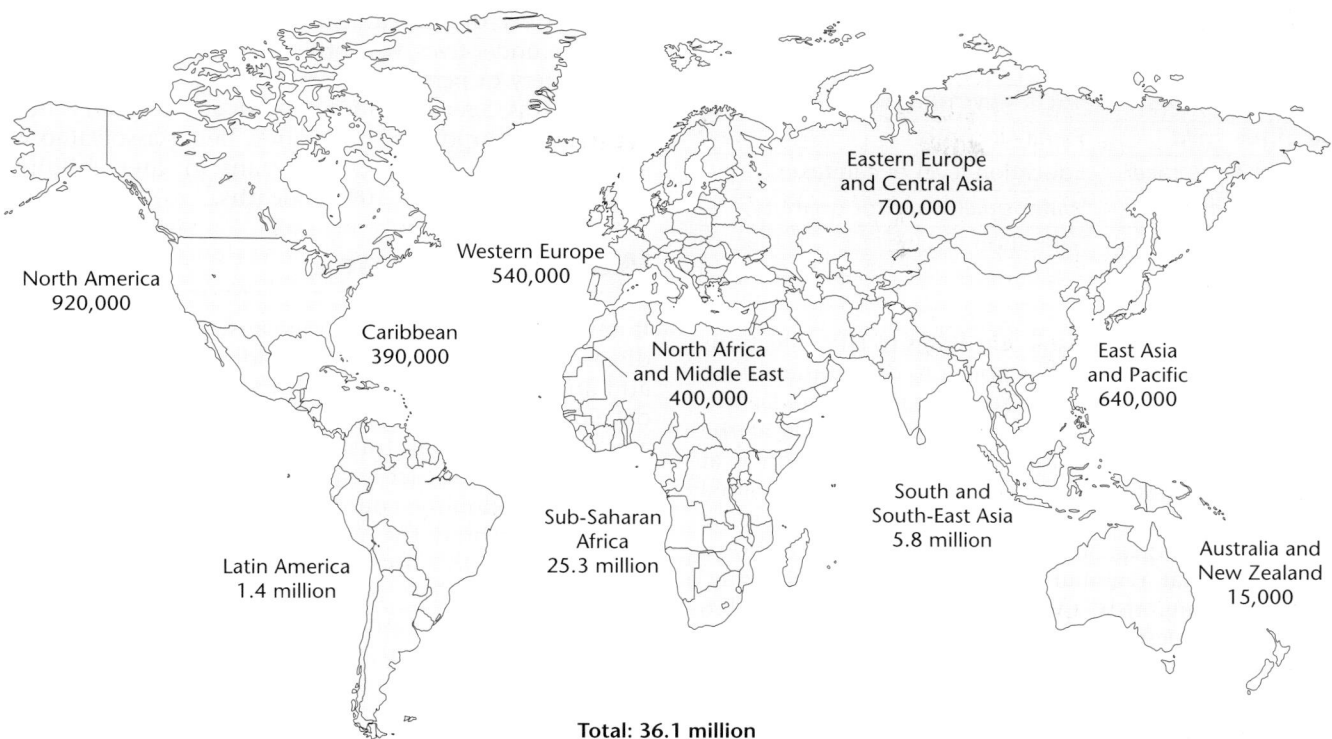

North America
920,000

Western Europe
540,000

Eastern Europe
and Central Asia
700,000

Caribbean
390,000

North Africa
and Middle East
400,000

East Asia
and Pacific
640,000

Latin America
1.4 million

Sub-Saharan
Africa
25.3 million

South and
South-East Asia
5.8 million

Australia and
New Zealand
15,000

Total: 36.1 million

Figure 3.3: Adults and children estimated to be living with HIV/AIDS as of end 2000. (Source: WHO/UNAIDS, December 2000.)

According to the AIDS epidemic update of December 2000 (UNAIDS and WHO),[7] the epidemiology of HIV in the tropics varies enormously from place to place (Figure 3.3).

Asia

An estimated 700 000 adults, 450 000 of them men, have become infected in South and South-East Asia in the course of the year 2000. These estimates are in line with known risk behaviour in this region, where men account for the majority of injecting drug users, and are responsible for sexual transmission of HIV, largely through commercial sex. Overall, as of the end of 2000, the region is estimated to have 5.8 million adults and children living with HIV or AIDS.

The region of East Asia and the Pacific is still keeping HIV at bay in most of its huge population. The number of people living with HIV or AIDS at the end of 2000 is estimated to be 640 000, representing just 0.07% of the region's adult population, as compared with the prevalence rate of 0.56% in South and South-East Asia. Having practically eradicated sexually transmitted infections by the 1960s, China is now seeing a steep rise in these rates, which could lead to higher HIV spread as a consequence.

North Africa and the Middle East

Because of insufficient data, few new country estimates of HIV infection were produced for this region between

1994 and 1999. Recent evidence, however, suggests that new infections are on the rise. For example, localized studies in southern Algeria show rates of around 1% in pregnant women attending antenatal clinics, and surveillance sites in both northern and southern Sudan indicate that HIV is spreading among the general population. With an estimated 80 000 new infections in the region during 2000, the number of adults and children living with HIV or AIDS had reached 400 000 by the end of 2000.

Latin America and the Caribbean

The epidemic in Latin America is a complex mosaic of transmission patterns in which HIV continues to spread through male-to-male sex, sex between men and women, and injecting drug use. By the end of year 2000 some 1.4 million adults and children in the region were estimated to be living with HIV or AIDS, as compared with 1.3 million at the end of 1999. In places where HIV is transmitted through sex between men and women, a far larger proportion of the whole population is immediately at risk. This is the transmission pattern in the Caribbean, where HIV rates are the highest in the world outside Africa.

Sub-Saharan Africa

In all parts of the world except sub-Saharan Africa, there are more men infected with HIV and dying of AIDS than

Table 3.2 Factors contributing to diarrhoea morbidity and mortality.[8]

Biological factors	Socio-environmental factors
Age of the child	Family income
Age of the caretaker	Education level of caretaker
Birth order of child	Water quality and/or quantity
Feeding mode	Sanitation facilities

women. Male behaviour also contributes to HIV infections in women, who often have less power to determine where, when and how sex takes place. South of the Sahara Desert, the total number of people living with HIV/AIDS at the end of 2000 rose to 25.3 million, and 2.4 million people at a more advanced stage of infection died of HIV-related illness. Though sub-Saharan Africa heads the list as the region with the largest annual number of new infections, it is thought that regional HIV incidence is stabilizing. Overall, therefore, new infections in 2000 totalled 3.8 million, slightly less than the 1999 regional total of 4.0 million. However, AIDS deaths in 2000 totalled 2.4 million, as compared with 2.2 million in 1999.

Diarrhoeal disease

Diarrhoea remains one of the most common diseases afflicting children under 5 years of age and accounts for 15–30% of under-five deaths in childhood. The number of episodes per year among these children varies according to the area and country, and is reported to be between two and four. The lowest reports come from East Asia and the highest from South Asia (Bangladesh). Diarrhoea remains a disease of poverty afflicting malnourished children in crowded and contaminated environments. Efforts to immunize children against measles, provide safe water and adequate sanitation facilities, and to encourage mothers to exclusively breast-feed infants through 6 months of age can blunt an increase in diarrhoea morbidity and mortality. Preventive strategies to limit the transmission of diarrhoeal disease need to go hand in hand with national diarrhoea disease control programmes that concentrate on effective diarrhoea case management and the prevention of dehydration.[8] The factors contributing to childhood mortality and morbidity due to diarrhoea are described in Table 3.2.[8]

Studies in Asia and Africa have clearly shown that establishment of an oral rehydration therapy (ORT) unit with training of hospital staff can significantly reduce diarrhoea case fatality rates. For instance, at Mama Yemo Hospital in Kinshasa, Zaire, there was a 69% decline in diarrhoea deaths after creation of an ORT unit.[9] On a community level, studies in Teknaf, Bangladesh, have demonstrated that intensive campaigns to increase effective use of oral rehydration therapy can reduce mortality.[10]

Changing patterns in the epidemiology of diarrhoea have been noted in many studies. In Matlab, Bangladesh, acute watery diarrhoea accounted for 34% of diarrhoea deaths in under-fives, while the remaining 66% were related to dysentery or persistent diarrhoea and malnutrition. This pattern was age dependent, with acute watery deaths being more important in infancy, being associated with 40% of deaths, and less important in later childhood, being associated with 10% of deaths.[11]

Watery diarrhoea

Rotavirus is the most common cause of severe diarrhoeal disease in infants and young children all over the world, and an important public health problem, particularly in developing countries where 600 000 deaths each year are associated with this infection. More than 125 million cases of diarrhoea each year are attributed to rotavirus. In tropical developing countries, rotavirus disease occurs either throughout the year or in the cold dry season. Almost all children are already infected by the age of 3–5 years. Although the infection is usually mild, severe disease may rapidly result in life-threatening dehydration if not appropriately treated. The only control measure likely to have a significant impact on the incidence of severe disease is vaccination. Natural infection protects children against subsequent severe disease. Globally, four serotypes are responsible for the majority of rotaviral disease, but additional serotypes are prevalent in some countries. Only one rotavirus vaccine candidate, namely the RRV-TV vaccine, is currently licensed. Encouraging results of vaccine efficacy have been obtained from Venezuela and from many industrialized countries. The RRV-TV vaccine was, however, withdrawn from routine use in the United States because of the perceived risk of intussusception. Before rotavirus vaccines may be recommended for large-scale immunization in developing countries, it is essential that protective efficacy be documented in the concerned areas. If affordable prices for the vaccines can be achieved, rotavirus immunization is likely to be given high priority in all areas where rotavirus infection is recognized as a public health problem.[12]

Dysentery

Man is both the reservoir and natural host of *Shigella*, the commonest cause of dysentery in the tropics. The most severe infections are caused by the *S. dysenteriae* type 1 (also known as Shiga's bacillus); it is also the only serotype implicated in epidemics. Infection is by the faecal–oral route and is usually spread by person-to-person transmission. It takes only 10–100 shigella organisms to produce dysentery, a low infectious dose, whereas 1 million to 10 million organisms may need to be swallowed to cause cholera. During the late 1960s, Shiga's bacillus was responsible for a series of devastating epidemics of dysentery in Latin America, Asia and Africa. In 1967 it was detected in the Mexican–Guatemalan border area and spread into much of Central America. An estimated half a million cases, with 20 000 deaths, were reported in the region between 1967 and 1971. In some villages the case fatality rate was as high as 15%; delayed diagnosis and incorrect treatment may have been responsible for this high death rate. One particularly disturbing feature was the resistance of the bacteria to the most commonly used antibacterial drugs: sulfonamides, tetracycline and chloramphenicol.

Serious epidemics due to the multiple-drug resistant *S. dysenteriae* type 1 have occurred recently in Bangladesh, Somalia, South India, Burma, Sri Lanka, Nepal, Bhutan, Rwanda and Zaire. West Bengal in India has always been an endemic area for bacillary dysentery. Preventive measures include boiling or chlorination of drinking water, covering faeces with soil, protecting food from flies, avoiding eating exposed raw vegetables and cut fruits, and washing hands with soap and water before eating and after using the latrine. However, such measures are not easy to implement in most areas. Consequently epidemics take their own course and subside only gradually.[13]

Tuberculosis

Tuberculosis (TB) is the leading cause of death associated with infectious diseases globally. The incidence of TB is expected to increase substantially worldwide during the next 10 years because of the interaction between the TB and HIV epidemics. There were an estimated 8.4 million new TB cases in 1999, up from 8.0 million in 1997; the rise is due largely to a 20% increase in incidence in African countries most affected by the epidemic of HIV/ AIDS. If present trends continue, 10.2 million new cases are expected in 2005, and Africa will have more cases than any other WHO region. At the end of 2000, it was estimated that 3.5 million TB deaths would occur (39% more than in 1990), approximately 0.5 million would be associated with HIV infection and almost half of these HIV-associated deaths would occur in sub-Saharan Africa.[14]

In many developing countries, TB is mainly a disease of young adults affecting carers and wage-earners in a household, thus placing a huge economic burden on society as a whole. Chemotherapy, if properly used, can reduce the burden of TB in the community, but because of the fragile structure of treatment programmes in many countries TB cases are not completely cured and patients remain infectious for a much longer time. Another important consequence of poor treatment compliance is development of drug resistance in many developing countries. Resistance to tuberculosis drugs is probably present everywhere in the world. Multidrug-resistant TB (MDR-TB) is now present in five continents; a third of the countries surveyed had levels above 2% among new patients. In Latvia 30% of all patients presenting for treatment had MDR-TB. Russia reported 5% of TB patients with MDR-TB. In the Dominican Republic, 10% of TB patients had MDR-TB. In Africa, Ivory Coast

has also witnessed the emergence of MDR-TB. Preliminary reports from Asia (India and China) show high levels of drug resistance. In the state of Delhi, India, 13% of all TB patients had MDR-TB.[15]

Directly observed treatment, short course (DOTS), is the most effective strategy available for controlling the TB epidemic today. DOTS uses sound technology and packages it with good management practices for widespread use through the existing primary health care network. It has proven to be a successful, innovative approach to TB control in countries such as China, Bangladesh, Vietnam, Peru and countries of West Africa. However, new challenges to the implementation of DOTS include health sector reforms, the worsening HIV epidemic, and the emergence of drug-resistant strains of TB. The technical, logistical, operational and political aspects of DOTS work together to ensure its success and applicability in a wide variety of contexts.[14]

The current TB situation with regard to DOTS (from WHO Report 2001, Global Tuberculosis Control)[14] is as follows:

- If current trends are maintained, the target of 70% case detection under DOTS will not be reached until 2013; to get to the target by 2005, DOTS programmes must collectively recruit at least 300 000 additional smear-positive cases each year.
- Almost all (92%) of the progress in DOTS expansion, as judged by smear-positive case notifications, was made in just five countries; 65% of these additional cases were found in two countries: India and South Africa.
- In 1999, Peru and Vietnam were still the only high-burden countries to have exceeded both WHO targets of 70% case detection and 85% treatment success.

A number of smaller countries appear to have declining TB incidence rates that are linked to high rates of case detection and cure; these include Cuba, Lebanon, the Maldives, Nicaragua, Oman and Uruguay.

Malaria

Close to 100 countries or territories in the world are considered malarious, almost half of which are in Africa, south of the Sahara (Figure 3.4).

The incidence of malaria worldwide is estimated to be 300–500 million clinical cases each year, with about 90% of these occurring in sub-Saharan Africa, where *Plasmodium falciparum* predominates. Malaria is thought to kill between 1.1 and 2.7 million people worldwide each year, of whom about 1 million are children under the age of 5 years in Africa. These childhood deaths, resulting mainly from cerebral malaria and anaemia, constitute nearly 25% of child mortality in Africa. One of the greatest challenges facing malaria control worldwide is the spread and intensification of parasite resistance to antimalarial drugs. The limited number of such drugs has led to increasing difficulties in the development of antimalarial drug policies and adequate disease management.[16]

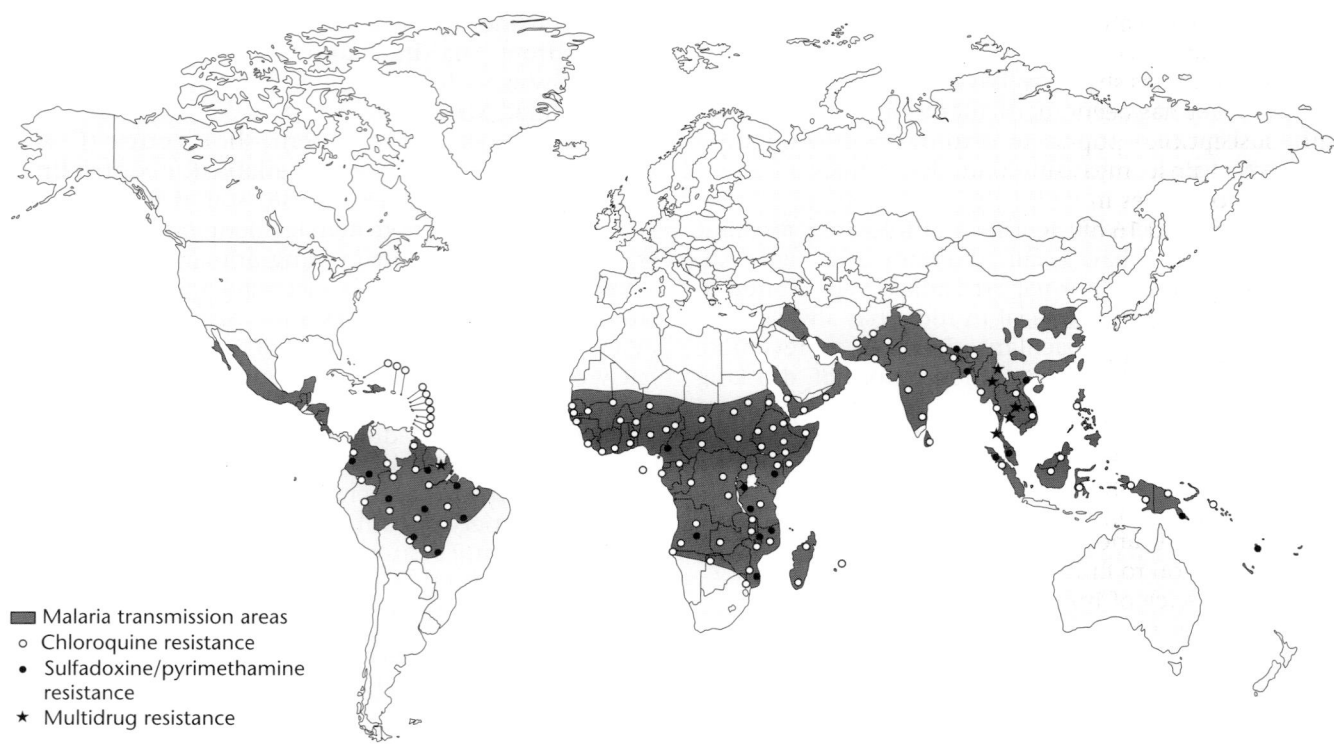

Figure 3.4: Reported *P.falciparum* drug resistance 1998. (Source: WHO, 1998.)
Main causes of death in low-income countries in South-East Asia and Africa. Estimates for 1998. (Source: WHO, 1999.)

Resistance of *P. falciparum* to chloroquine is now common in practically all malaria-endemic countries of Africa (Figure 3.4), especially in East Africa. Resistance to sulfadoxine/pyrimethamine, the main alternative to chloroquine, is widespread in South-East Asia and South America. Mefloquine resistance is now common in the border areas of Thailand with Cambodia and Myanmar. Parasite sensitivity to quinine is declining in several other countries of South-East Asia and in the Amazon region, where it has been used in combination with tetracycline for the treatment of uncomplicated malaria. Consequently, artemisinin and its derivatives are now increasingly being used as first-line treatment in some of these areas. Resistance of *P. vivax* to chloroquine has now been reported from Indonesia (Irian Jaya), Myanmar, Papua New Guinea and Vanuatu.[17]

Urban and periurban malaria are on the increase in South Asia and in many areas of Africa. Military conflicts and civil unrest, along with unfavourable ecological changes, have greatly contributed to malaria epidemics, as large numbers of unprotected, non-immune and physically weakened refugees move into malarious areas. Such population movements contribute to new malaria outbreaks and make epidemic-prone situations more explosive.[16] Another disquieting factor is the re-emergence of malaria in areas where it had been eradicated (e.g., Democratic People's Republic of Korea, Republic of Korea and Tadjikistan), or its increase in countries where it was nearly eradicated (e.g., Azerbaijan, northern Iraq and Turkey). Current malaria epidemics in a majority of these countries are the result of a rapid deterioration of malaria prevention and control operations. Climatic changes have also been implicated in the re-emergence of malaria. In the past 5 years, the worldwide incidence of malaria has quadrupled, influenced by changes in both land development and regional climate. In Brazil, satellite images depict a 'fish bone' pattern where roads have opened the tropical forest to localized development. In these 'edge' areas malaria has resurged. Temperature changes have encouraged a redistribution of the disease; malaria is now found at higher elevations in central Africa and could threaten cities such as Nairobi, Kenya. This threat has been hypothesized to extend to temperate regions of the world that are now experiencing hotter summers year on year.[18]

Vaccine-preventable infectious diseases
Measles

Despite the widespread availability of safe and effective measles vaccines since 1963, measles still accounts for approximately one million deaths annually. Measles was the sixth leading cause of death worldwide in 1998. Measles remains highly endemic in several countries in Europe, Asia and Africa, irrespective of the level of economic development. However, measles-related deaths occur almost exclusively in developing countries. Routine measles vaccination coverage at the global level reached 80% in 1990, and has shown minimal progress from 1990 through 1997. It has been estimated that more than 90% of the susceptible population must be adequately immunized against measles to interrupt transmission. There are 19 countries in which measles vaccine coverage is less than 50% and 16 of these countries are in Africa.[19,20]

Hepatitis B

In much of the world, particularly sub-Saharan Africa, South-East Asia, China and the Pacific Basin, infection with hepatitis B virus (HBV) is very widespread. The carrier rate in some of these populations may be as high as 10–20%. In developing countries most hepatitis B transmission occurs during the perinatal period. Infection between children is another common route of infection; it is not uncommon to find up to 90% of 15-year-olds have serological evidence of infection with HBV. Intermediate levels of infection (2–7%) are seen in parts of the former Soviet Union, South Asia, Central America and the northern zones of South America. These high rates of infection lead to a high burden of disease, mainly from the clinical consequences of long-term carriage of the virus, which may include chronic hepatitis, cirrhosis and liver cancer. It has been estimated that HBV infection is the second most common cause of cancer deaths in the world (after tobacco consumption). In India hepatitis B is linked to 60% of cases of hepatocellular carcinoma and 80% of cases of cirrhosis of the liver.[21]

Although there is no cheap and effective cure for HBV infection, there is a safe and effective vaccine. In 1992 the World Health Assembly endorsed the value of universal hepatitis B immunization for infants. Infant immunization has been shown to reduce the prevalence of chronic infection by 80–90% and to reduce the frequency of hepatocellular carcinoma in Taiwanese children by 50%. Unfortunately, the vaccine requires three doses, and is still expensive compared to other vaccines commonly given in childhood. Nevertheless a large number of countries have begun mass HBV immunization, and WHO recommended all countries begin mass infant immunization by the year 1997.[22]

Neonatal tetanus

Tetanus occurs worldwide and is endemic in 90 developing countries, but its incidence varies considerably. The most common form, neonatal (umbilical) tetanus, kills approximately 500 000 infants each year because the mother was not immunized; about 80% of these deaths occur in just 12 tropical Asian and African countries. In addition, an estimated 15 000–30 000 non-immunized women worldwide die each year from maternal tetanus that results from postpartum, postabortal or postsurgical wound infection with *Clostridium tetani*. Immunization of women with tetanus toxoid prevents neonatal tetanus, and the World Health Organization is currently engaged in a global programme for the elimination of neonatal tetanus through maternal immunization with at least two doses of antenatal tetanus toxoid.[23]

Vaccination against a range of bacterial and viral diseases is an integral part of communicable disease control worldwide. Vaccination against a specific disease not only reduces the incidence of that disease, but it also reduces the social and economic burden of the disease on communities. Very high immunization coverage can lead

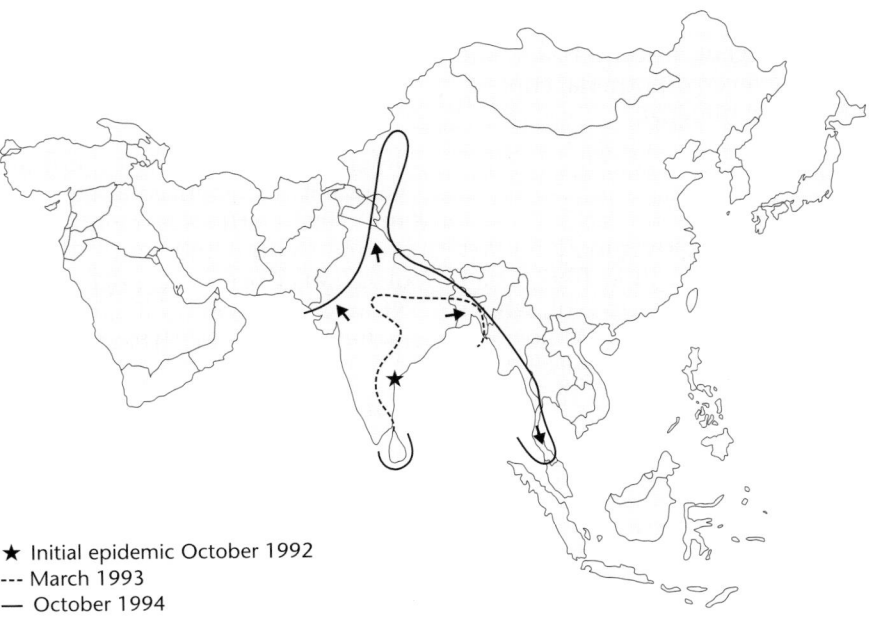

★ Initial epidemic October 1992
--- March 1993
— October 1994

Figure 3.5: Spread of *Vibrio cholerae* O139–Asia, 1992–1994. (Source: CDC MMWR Weekly, March 1995.)

to complete blocking of transmission for many vaccine-preventable diseases. The worldwide eradication of smallpox and the near-eradication of polio from many countries provide excellent examples of the role of immunization in disease control. Despite these advances many of the world's poorest countries do not have access to vaccines and these infections remain among the leading global causes of death.

Emerging and resurgent infectious diseases

Since 1991 resurgent and emerging infectious disease outbreaks have occurred worldwide. In addition many diseases widely believed to be under control, such as cholera, dengue and diphtheria, have re-emerged in many areas or spread to new regions or populations throughout the world (Figure 3.5).[24] A growing population and increasing urbanization contribute to emerging infectious disease problems. In many parts of the world, urban population growth has been accompanied by overcrowding, poor hygiene, inadequate sanitation and unclean drinking water. Urban development has also caused ecological damage. In these circumstances, certain disease-causing organisms and some of the vectors that transmit them have thrived, making it more likely that people will be infected with new or re-emerging pathogens. The existing public health infrastructure is already overtaxed and ill prepared to deal with new health threats. Breakdown of public health measures due to civil unrest, war and the movement of refugees has also contributed to the re-emergence of infectious diseases (Table 3.3).[24] International travel and commerce have made it possible for pathogens to be quickly transported from one side of the globe to the other (Figure 3.6).[24]

Examples of new and resurgent infections include Ebola, dengue fever, Rift Valley fever, diphtheria, cholera, Nipah virus infection and avian influenza.

Ebola

In 1976 Ebola (named after the Ebola River in Zaire) first emerged in Sudan and Zaire. Through June 1997, 1054 cases had been reported to the WHO, 754 of which proved fatal mainly from Côte d'Ivoire, Democratic Republic of Congo, Gabon and Sudan. In October 2000 the first ever cases of Ebola were reported to the WHO from Uganda. By January 2001 there were 426 cases and 224 deaths in Uganda.[25]

Dengue fever

Dengue fever and dengue haemorrhagic fever (DHF), widespread in many parts of South-East Asia since the 1950s, re-emerged in the Americas in the 1990s following

Table 3.3 Factors in emergence and re-emergence of infectious diseases.[24]

Categories	Specific examples
Societal events	Economic impoverishment; war or civil conflict; population growth and migration; urban decay
Health care	New medical devices; organ or tissue transplantation; drugs causing immunosuppression; widespread use of antibiotics
Food production	Globalization of food supplies; changes in food processing and packaging
Human behaviour	Sexual behaviour; drug use; travel; diet; outdoor recreation; use of childcare facilities
Environmental changes	Deforestation/reforestation; changes in water ecosystems; flood/drought; famine; global warming
Public health	Curtailment or reduction in prevention programmes; infrastructure and communicable disease surveillance inadequate; lack of trained personnel (epidemiologists, laboratory scientists, vector and rodent control specialists)
Microbial adaptation	Changes in virulence and toxin production; development and change of drug resistance; microbes as cofactors in chronic diseases

deterioration in active mosquito control. In 1990 Venezuela experienced a major epidemic. Between 1995 and 1997, DHF was reported in 24 countries in and around Central and South America. During the summer of 2000 Costa Rica, El Salvador Guatemala, and Nicaragua experienced outbreaks of dengue fever that included cases of DHF and deaths.[26]

Rift Valley fever

Rift Valley fever (RVF) is a zoonotic disease typically affecting sheep and cattle in Africa. Mosquitoes are the principal means by which RVF virus is transmitted among animals and to humans. Following abnormally heavy rainfall in Kenya and Somalia in late 1997 and early 1998, RVF occurred over vast areas, producing disease in livestock and causing haemorrhagic fever and

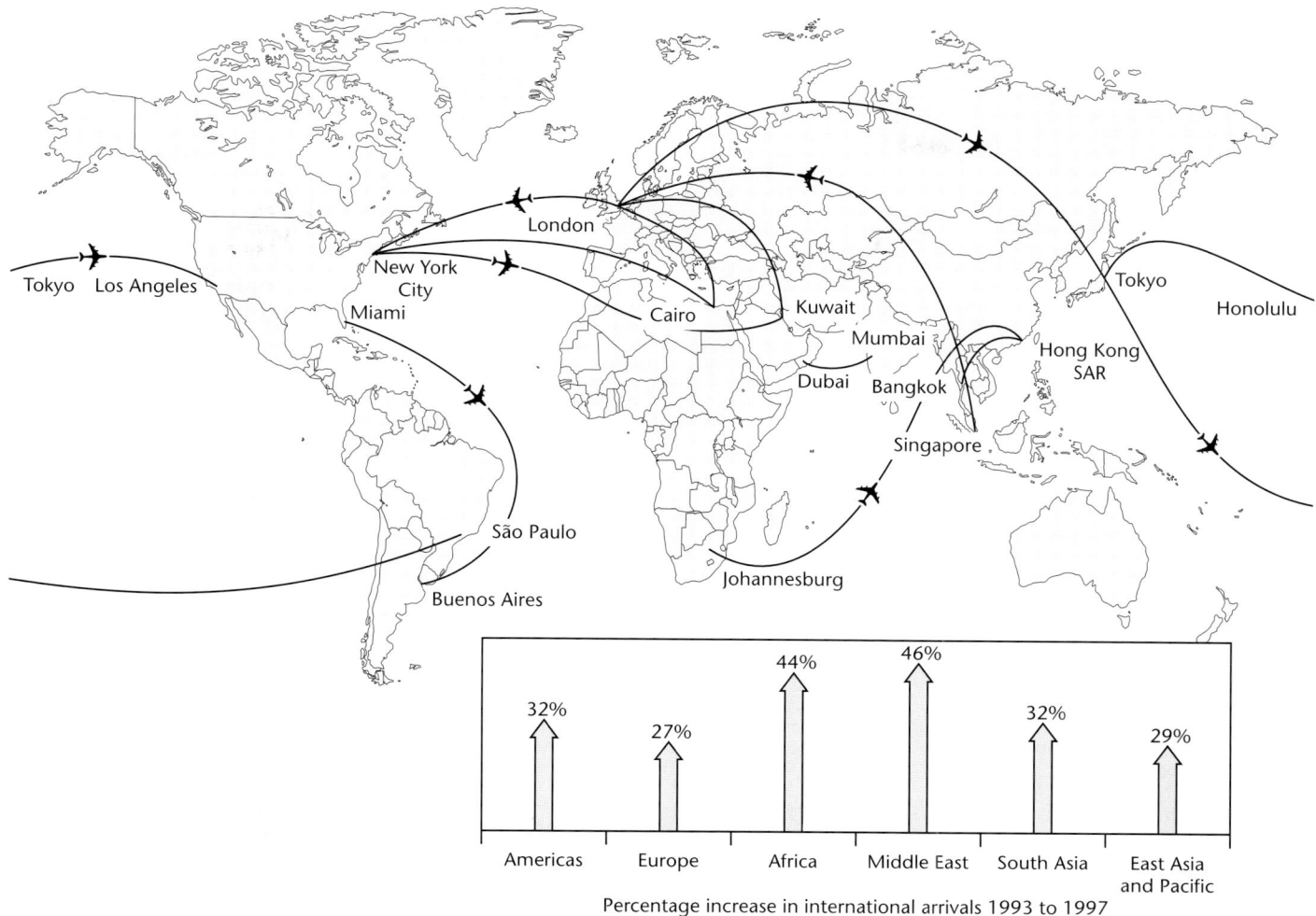

Figure 3.6: Most popular air routes between continents, 1997. (Source: WHO, 1999.)

death among the human population. In September 2000 WHO documented the first ever RVF outbreak outside Africa, in Yemen and the Kingdom of Saudi Arabia (KSA). RNA sequencing of the virus from KSA indicated that it was similar to the RVF viruses isolated from East Africa in 1998. 1087 suspected cases were identified, of which 121 (11%) persons died. Of the 1087, 815 (75%) cases reported exposure to sick animals, handling an abortus or slaughtering animals in the week before onset of illness.[27]

Diphtheria

Diphtheria re-emerged in the Russian Federation and some other republics of the former Soviet Union in 1994 and culminated in 1995, with over 50 000 cases reported. The re-emergence was linked to a dramatic decline in immunization programmes following the disruption of health services during the unsettled times immediately after the break-up of the Soviet Union. Since then immunization services have been re-established, reversing the upward trend: in 1996, 13 687 cases were reported in the Russian Federation.[28]

Cholera

Cholera (biotype El Tor) broke out explosively in Peru in 1991, after an absence of 100 years, and spread rapidly in Central and South America, with recurrent epidemics in 1992 and 1993. From the onset of the epidemic in January 1991 through 1 September 1994, a total of 1 041 422 cases and 9642 deaths (overall case fatality rate 0.9%) were reported from countries in the Western Hemisphere to the Pan American Health Organization. In December 1992 a large epidemic of a new strain of cholera *V. cholerae* 0139 began in South India, and spread rapidly through the subcontinent. (Figure 3.5). This strain has changed its antigenic structure such that there is no existing immunity and all ages, even in endemic areas, are susceptible. The epidemic has continued to spread and *V. cholerae* O139 has been reported from 11 countries in South Asia. Because humans are the only reservoirs, survival of the cholera vibrios during inter-epidemic periods probably depends on low-level undiagnosed cases and transiently infected, asymptomatic individuals. Recent studies have suggested that cholera vibrios can

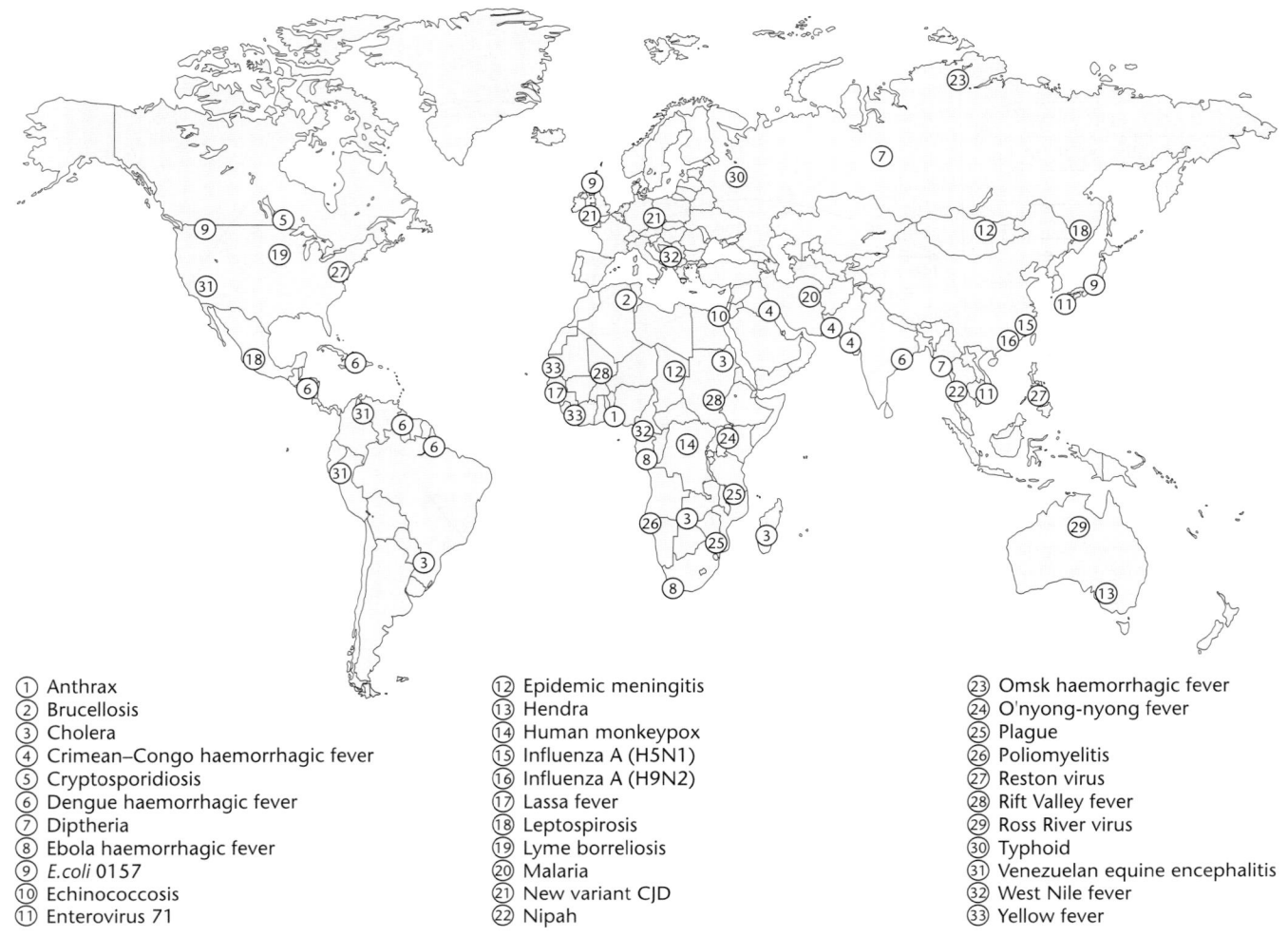

Figure 3.7: Examples of emerging and re-emerging infectious diseases 1994–1999. (Source: WHO, 1999.)

① Anthrax
② Brucellosis
③ Cholera
④ Crimean–Congo haemorrhagic fever
⑤ Cryptosporidiosis
⑥ Dengue haemorrhagic fever
⑦ Diptheria
⑧ Ebola haemorrhagic fever
⑨ E.coli 0157
⑩ Echinococcosis
⑪ Enterovirus 71

⑫ Epidemic meningitis
⑬ Hendra
⑭ Human monkeypox
⑮ Influenza A (H5N1)
⑯ Influenza A (H9N2)
⑰ Lassa fever
⑱ Leptospirosis
⑲ Lyme borreliosis
⑳ Malaria
㉑ New variant CJD
㉒ Nipah

㉓ Omsk haemorrhagic fever
㉔ O'nyong-nyong fever
㉕ Plague
㉖ Poliomyelitis
㉗ Reston virus
㉘ Rift Valley fever
㉙ Ross River virus
㉚ Typhoid
㉛ Venezuelan equine encephalitis
㉜ West Nile fever
㉝ Yellow fever

persist for some time in shellfish, algae or plankton in coastal regions of infected areas and it has been claimed that they can exist in a viable but non-culturable state.[29]

Nipah virus

In early 1999 health officials in Malaysia and Singapore investigated reports of febrile encephalitis and respiratory illnesses among workers who had been exposed to pigs. A previously unrecognized paramyxovirus (formerly known as Hendra-like virus), now called Nipah virus, was implicated by laboratory testing in many of these cases.

As of April 1999, 257 cases of febrile encephalitis were reported to the Malaysian Ministry of Health, including 100 deaths. Laboratory results from 65 patients who died suggested recent Nipah virus infection. The apparent source of infection among most human cases continues to be exposure to pigs. Human-to-human transmission of Nipah virus has not been documented. Outbreak control in Malaysia has focused on culling pigs; approximately 890 000 pigs have been killed. Other measures include a ban on transporting pigs within the country, education

about contact with pigs, use of personal protective equipment among persons exposed to pigs, and a national surveillance and control system to detect and cull additional infected herds.[30]

Avian influenza virus in humans in Hong Kong

In May 1997 a 3-year-old boy in Hong Kong contracted an influenza-like illness, was treated with salicylates, and died 12 days later with complications consistent with Reye's syndrome. Laboratory diagnosis included the isolation in cell culture of a virus that was identified locally as influenza type A but could not be further characterized with reagents distributed for diagnosis of human influenza viruses. By August, further investigation with serological and molecular techniques in the Netherlands and in the United States had confirmed that the isolate was A/Hong Kong/156/97 (H5N1), which was very closely related to isolate A/Chicken/Hong Kong/258/97 (H5N1). The latter virus was considered representative of those responsible

Table 3.4 Distribution of deaths from three groups of causes by region.

Region	Number of deaths, attributed (per cent)		
	Infectious causes	Non-communicable causes	Injuries
Established market economies	6.2	87.6	6.2
Former socialist economies	3.6	86.8	9.6
China	15.1	73.4	11.5
Latin America	32.3	57.9	9.8
Middle Eastern crescent	46.2	44.8	8.9
India	43.3	50.2	6.5
Sub-Saharan Africa	68.2	23.9	7.9
Other Asia and islands	41.8	49.6	8.6
World	33.4	58.1	8.5

Adapted from Murray and Lopez.[33]

for severe outbreaks of disease on three rural chicken farms in Hong Kong during March 1997, during which several thousand chickens had died. Molecular analysis of the viral haemagglutinins showed a proteolytic cleavage site of the type found in highly pathogenic avian influenza viruses.

By late December, the total number of confirmed new human cases had climbed to 17, of which five were fatal; the case fatality rates were 18% in children and 57% in adults older than 17 years. Almost all laboratory evidence of infection was in patients who had been near live chickens (e.g., in market-places) in the days before onset of illness, which suggested direct transmission of virus from chicken to human rather than person-to-person spread. In December 1997 veterinary authorities began to slaughter all (1.6 million) chickens present in wholesale facilities or with vendors within Hong Kong, and importation of chickens from neighbouring areas was stopped. Subsequently, no more human cases caused by avian influenza virus were detected. Because these cases occurred at the beginning of the usual influenza season in Hong Kong, public health officials were concerned that human strains might co-circulate with the avian influenza to generate human and avian reassortant viruses with capacity for efficient person-to-person spread. This has so far not been documented.[31]

Emerging non-infectious killers in the tropics

Non-infectious diseases take an enormous toll on lives and health worldwide. Non-communicable diseases (NCDs) account for nearly 60% of deaths globally, mostly due to heart disease, stroke, cancer, diabetes and lung diseases. The rapid rise of NCDs represents one of the major health challenges to global development in the twenty-first century and threatens economic and social development of nations as well as the lives and health of millions of their subjects. In 1998 alone, NCDs were estimated to have contributed to 31.7 million deaths globally and 43% of the global burden of disease.[32] Based on current trends, it is expected that by the year 2020 NCDs will account for 73% of deaths and 60% of the disease burden.

Until recently it was believed that NCDs were a minor or even non-existent problem in developing countries in the tropics. A recent analysis of mortality trends from NCDs suggests that large increases in NCDs have occurred in developing countries,[33] particularly those in rapid transition like China and India (Table 3.4). According to these estimates at least 40% of all deaths in the tropical developing countries are attributable to NCDs, while in industrialized countries NCDs account for 75% of all deaths. Low- and middle-income countries suffer the greatest impact of NCDs. The rapid increase in these diseases is seen disproportionately in poor and disadvantaged populations and is contributing to widening health gaps between and within countries. In 1998, of the total number of deaths attributable to NCDs 77% occurred in developing countries, and of the disease burden they represent 85% was borne by low- and middle-income countries.[32]

It is important to recognize that these trends, indicative of an increase in NCDs, may be partly confounded by factors such as an increase in life expectancy, a progressive reduction in deaths due to communicable diseases in adulthood, and improvements in case detection and reporting in the tropics. However, increase in the incidence of these chronic degenerative diseases is real. The complex range of determinants (below) that interact to determine the nature and course of this epidemic[34] needs to be understood in order to adopt preventive strategies to help developing societies in the tropics to deal with this burgeoning problem.

The determinants of non-communicable diseases in developing societies are as follows:[1]

• Demographic changes in population.
• Epidemiological transition.
• Urbanization and internal migration.

- Changes in dietary and food consumption patterns.
- Lifestyle changes (changes in physical activity patterns, socio-cultural milieu and stress as well as increased tobacco consumption).
- Adult-onset effects of low birth weight and the effects of early life programming.
- Infections and their associations with chronic disease risk.
- Effect of malnutrition and nutrient deficiencies.
- Poverty, inequalities and social exclusion.
- Deleterious effects of environmental degradation.
- Impacts of globalization.

Four of the most prominent NCDs—cardiovascular disease, cancer, chronic obstructive pulmonary disease and diabetes—are linked to common preventable risk factors related to diet and lifestyle. These factors are tobacco use, unhealthy diet and lack of physical activity. Interventions to prevent these diseases should focus on controlling these risk factors in an integrated manner and at the family and community level since the causal risk factors are deeply entrenched in the social and cultural framework of society. Developing countries in the tropics have to recognize that the emerging accelerated epidemic of NCDs is a cause for concern and that it needs to be dealt with as a national priority. They have to learn from the experience of industrialized and affluent countries to tackle the emerging crisis of chronic diseases that they are likely to face in the near future. The emerging health burden of chronic disease affecting mainly the economically productive adult population will consume scarce resources. It is important, however, to realize that the poorer countries will be burdened even more in the long run, if attempts are not made to evolve and implement interventions to address these emerging health issues on an urgent basis.

Conclusion

The world we live in is constantly changing. In the past 25 years, we have witnessed significant progress in sustainable and technological development. However, increases in mass population movements, continuing civil unrest and deforestation have helped carry diseases into areas where they have never been seen before. This has been aided by the massive growth in international travel. Effective medicines and control strategies are available to dramatically reduce the deaths and suffering caused by communicable and non-communicable diseases. Despite reduced global military spending many governments are failing to ensure that these strategies receive enough funding to succeed. WHO priorities for the control of infectious diseases in developing countries include childhood immunization, integrated management of childhood illnesses, use of the DOTS strategy to control TB, a package of interventions to control malaria, a package of interventions to prevent HIV/AIDS, access to essential drugs, and the overall strengthening of surveillance and health service delivery systems. Over 10% of all preventable ill-health today is due to poor environmental quality—conditions such as bad housing, overcrowding, indoor air pollution, poor sanitation and unsafe water. The challenge of disease in the tropics has continued into the new millennium—never before have we been so well equipped to deal with disease threats. It remains for humankind to summon the collective will to pursue these challenges and break the chain of infection and disease.

REFERENCES

1 Raska K. National and international surveillance of communicable diseases. *World Health Organ Chron* 1966; 20:315–321.

2 World Health Organization. *World Health Report: Fighting Disease Fostering Development.* Geneva: WHO, 1996.

3 World Health Organization. *Report on Infectious Diseases: Removing Obstacles to Healthy Development.* Geneva: WHO, 1999.

4 World Health Organization. *Acute Respiratory Infections.* Geneva: WHO, 1990.

5 World Bank Group. *Indoor Air Pollution Energy and Health for the Poor.* Washington, DC, 2000.

6 Reyes H, Perez-Cuevas R, Salmeron R et al. Infant mortality due to acute respiratory infections: the influence of primary care processes. *Health Policy Plan* 1997; 12(3):214–223.

7 WHO–UNAIDS. *AIDS Epidemic Update.* Geneva: UNAIDS, 2000.

8 UNICEF Staff Working Papers. Evaluation, Policy and Planning Series. Number EVL-97-002. A Global Review of Diarrhoeal Disease Control. New York: UNICEF, 1997.

9 Moore M, Davachi F, Bongo L et al. New parameters for evaluating oral rehydration therapy: one year's experience in a major urban hospital in Zaire. *J Trop Pediatr* 1989; 35(4):179–184.

10 Rahaman M M, Aziz K M, Patwari Y et al. Diarrhoeal mortality in two Bangladeshi villages with and without community ORT. *Lancet* 1979; ii:809–812.

11 Fauveau V, Yunus M, Zaman K et al. Diarrhoea mortality in rural Bangladeshi children. *J Trop Pediatr* 1991; 37:31–36.

12 Rotavirus vaccines: WHO Position Paper. *Wkly Epidemiol Rec* 1999; 74:33–40.

13 World Health Organization. Guidelines for the control of epidemics due to *Shigella dysenteriae* 1. Publication no. WHO/CDR/95.4. *Epidemiology of Dysentery Caused by Shigella.* Geneva: WHO, 1995.

14 World Health Organization. Global tuberculosis control. WHO Report WHO/CDS/TB/2000.287. Geneva: WHO, 2001.

15 Raviglione M. *Anti-Tuberculosis Drug Resistance in the World.* WHO/IUATLD Global Project on Anti-tuberculosis Drug Resistance Surveillance 1994–1997. Available: http://www.who.int/gtb/publications/dritw/index.htm [5 March 2001].

16 WHO Expert Committee on Malaria. 20th report. Geneva: WHO, 1998.

17 WHO Expert Committee on Malaria. *World Health Organ Tech Rep Ser* 2000; 892:i–v, 1–74.

18 Epstein P R. Climate, ecology and human health. *Consequences* 1997; 3:3–12. Available: http://www.gcrio.org/CONSEQUENCES/vol3no2/climhealth.html [2 November 1997].

19 Christopher J L & Lopez A D (eds). The global burden of disease: a comprehensive assessment of mortality and disability from diseases, injuries, and risk factors in 1990 and projected to 2020—summary. Geneva, WHO, 1996: 17–26.

20 Morbidity and Mortality Weekly Report. Progress toward global measles control and regional elimination, 1990–1997. *MMWR* 1998; 47(48):1049–1054.

21 World Health Organization. Towards the elimination of hepatitis B: a guide to the implementation of National Immunization Programs in the Developing World. The International Task Force on hepatitis B Immunization. Geneva: WHO, 1991.

22 Maynard J E. Hepatitis B: global importance and need for control. *Vaccine* 1990; 8(suppl.):S18.

23 Morbidity and Mortality Weekly Report. Expanded program on immunization: progress toward the global elimination of neonatal tetanus, 1989–1993. *MMWR* 1994; 43:885–887, 893–894.

24 Centers for Disease Control and Prevention. Addressing emerging infectious disease threats: a prevention strategy for the United States. Atlanta, Georgia: US Department of Health and Human Services, Public Health Service, 1994.

25 World Health Organization. WHO Fact Sheet: Ebola haemorrhagic fever. Fact sheet no. 103. Geneva: WHO, 2000.

26 Gubler D J & Clark G G. Dengue/dengue hemorrhagic fever: the emergence of a global health problem. *Emerg Infect Dis* 1995; 1(2):55–57.

27 World Health Organization. WHO Fact Sheet: Rift Valley fever. Fact sheet no. 207. Geneva: WHO, 2000.

28 Expanded programme on Immunization. Update: diphtheria epidemic in the newly independent states of the former USSR, January 1995–March 1996. *Wkly Epidemiol Rec* 1996; 71:245–250.

29 Morbidity and Mortality Weekly Report. Update: *Vibrio cholerae* O1—Western Hemisphere, 1991–1994, and *V. cholerae* O139—Asia, 1994. *MMWR* 1995; 44(11):215–219.

30 Morbidity and Mortality Weekly Report. Update: outbreak of Nipah virus: Malaysia and Singapore, 1999. *MMWR* 1999; 48(16):335–337.

31 Snacken R, Kendal A P, Haaheim L R & Wood J M. The next influenza pandemic: lessons from Hong Kong, 1997. *Emerg Infect Dis* 1999; 5(2):195–203.

32 World Health Organization. *Global Strategy for the Prevention and Control of Non-communicable Diseases*. Geneva: WHO, 2000.

33 Murray C J L & Lopez A D. *Global Comparative Assessments in the Health Sector*. Geneva: WHO, 1994.

34 Shetty P S. Diet and life-style and chronic non-communicable diseases: what determines the epidemic in developing societies? In Krishnaswami K (ed.) *Nutrition Research: Current Scenario and Future Trends*. New Delhi: Oxford & IBH Publishing, 2000: 153–167.

Chapter 4
Traditional Medicine

G. Bodeker

Why should tropical medicine practitioners be informed about traditional medicine?

In Britain the General Medical Council has requested all medical schools to establish introductory courses on complementary medicine for medical students, in order to bridge the gap between patients and doctors in this field. In tropical countries, where a greater percentage of the population use traditional medicine than use conventional medicine, or than use complementary medicine in Britain, the need is even greater.

There has been a historic mistrust between traditional health practitioners (THPs) and modern medical doctors. This has come in part from colonial policies which have attempted to suppress and replace traditional medicine. It also comes from the modern medical view that traditional medicine is at best of low therapeutic value and at worst dangerous. In reality, what appears to happen is that each side sees the other's worst cases and builds their impressions based on this sample. With the emergence of a global political consensus that traditional medicine in developing countries—and complementary medicine in industrialized countries—must take a role in comprehensive health sector development, an understanding of traditional medicine is necessary on the part of mainstream health personnel.

At the local level, there will be questions of whether particular traditional medicines are responsible for presenting renal or liver pathology. There will also be questions about interactive effects of traditional and conventional drugs. There may also be consideration of whether traditional means can be used in the management of common conditions such as wounds and tropical ulcers when conventional means are not available or have not worked.

This chapter attempts to provide an introduction to some of the above issues, but within the available space clearly they will not be able to be addressed in their entirety or in any real depth. This will be up to the clinician, by a combination of open enquiry with local THPs, via searches of relevant databases such as CABI, Medline, the British Library's AMED database, SOCIOFILE and EMBASE.

Chapter overview

The field of traditional medicine is as diverse as the societies in which it is found. *Materia medica* differ, and diagnosis, treatments and theories of disease also vary. In view of this immense diversity of traditional practice, it is clearly unrealistic to attempt to provide a comprehensive review of the various systems of traditional medicine found in tropical countries or to review their various clinical applications. What this chapter aims to do is to provide a framework for understanding what traditional medicine is, who uses it and why, and how it is moving towards being given a place in the formal health care systems of many countries. There is also a review of the use of traditional medicine in the management of common conditions: malaria, HIV/AIDS, wounds and eye disease. These have been selected for consideration as they are among the commonest reasons for people seeking treatment—from both modern and traditional health professionals. Other areas which have not been able to be included in this chapter, but which are of importance, include traditional birth practices, the use of traditional anthelmintics and traditional orthopaedics. Each is a subject in itself and each has been subject of review and policy consideration. Searches of the relevant databases will yield literature for those interested in further exploring these and related fields.

What is missing in the international literature is a body of sound clinical research. This is due to the low value ascribed to this sector by funders and health authorities, despite the fact that the majority of the public continue to use medical approaches about which little is known with respect to safety, efficacy, dosage or mechanisms of action. Clearly, the call for evidence must be matched by a commitment of resources to enable high-quality, sound research to be conducted. This is necessary to determine what constitutes best practice and safe practice as well as to open up the possibility of new discoveries for health care generally. These may be discoveries such as has been found for the evaluation of the traditional Chinese febrifuge, *Artemisia annua*, which has given rise to artemisinin and the class of antimalarial drugs derived from this compound. Or they may be discoveries such as the clinical study by Homsy et al.[1] cited in the section on HIV/AIDS, where a Ugandan herbal preparation has been found to be more effective and considerably cheaper than the conventional treatment for herpes zoster.

For information on safety/toxicity issues, the reader is referred to Chapter 26.

While many of the studies presented in this chapter may need further replication, better trial design etc., they do point to general trends in efficacy and safety as well as highlight the importance of further research and investment in the traditional health care sector.

Traditional health systems

The World Health Organization estimates that the majority of the population of most non-industrial countries still relies on traditional forms of medicine for their everyday health care. In many countries up to 80–90% of the population are in this category.

Traditions vary from region to region and even within a single country. Attempts to classify these traditions into meaningful systems and sets of practices have generally adopted a twofold classification.

In Asia, traditional medical knowledge has often been classified into two broad groupings: codified and folk traditions.[2] The codified traditions of Asia typically have a written *materia medica* and clinical texts, a systematic theory of pathogenesis and treatments based on a formal diagnostic system, and a pharmacological tradition with precise standards of dosage and an awareness of toxicity and its management. These traditions include the Ayurvedic medical system of India and South Asia, traditional Chinese medicine and its related systems in Vietnam and Korea, Unani medicine, and the Graeco-Arabic tradition found in Pakistan, India and many other countries with Islamic traditions.

Folk traditions are generally seen as the collection of community knowledge about the use of plants in the management of common illness, non-pharmacological interventions such as massage, meditation, the use of steam and other physical means of effecting cure.

In studying Mayan medicine of Mexico, Berlin and Berlin have adopted Foster's[3] dual division of medical systems into *naturalistic* and *personalistic* frameworks. In the *naturalistic* system, a health condition is empirically determined. Diagnosis is based primarily on immediately apparent *signs* and *symptoms*. For a condition such as bloody diarrhoea, it is the norm for people to treat themselves with medicinal plants or to seek local expert advice in the use of plants as treatment. However, diagnosis of a *personalistic* condition is based on a retrospective analysis of possible causative factors, such as an encounter with ancestral spirits.

Berlin and Berlin[4] have noted in their study of Mayan traditional medicine that 'such cases are first treated with plant medicinals, and later classed as personalistic in cases that are unresponsive to herbal remedies or that are either prolonged or progressively worsen. These patterns of diagnosis have been extensively described by virtually everyone who has studied the subject. Diagnosis and treatment frequently involve the intervention of healers with special powers, such as a pulser or diviner. While personalistic conditions may at times also be treated with herbal medications, Maya curers normally employ remedies that require ceremonial healing rituals and special prayers.'

In the context of tropical medicine, it is sufficient to note that what may appear to the clinician as the practice of herbal medicine, with varying degrees of competence, is often grounded in theoretical assumptions, beliefs about disease and its origins, and what constitutes a real cure as opposed to simply the management of symptoms. An understanding of these perspectives is necessary to understand the beliefs and health practices of patients, many of whom will use both conventional and traditional medicine in the management of a condition. Accordingly, this chapter will give an introduction to the prevailing views of what traditional medicine is, how widely it is used, by whom and for what, some examples of the use of traditional medicine for commonly occurring conditions in the tropics, and how the clinician may gain more information about traditional medicine.

Definitions and conceptualizations of traditional medicine

The following is a selection of definitions and characterizations of traditional medicine.

On the basis of a community's or a country's culture, history and beliefs, traditional medicine came into being long before the development and spread of Western medicine that originated in Europe after the development of modern science and technology. The knowledge of traditional medicine is often passed on verbally from generation to generation. Nevertheless, in some cases a sophisticated theory and system is involved.[5]

Traditional medicine is widespread throughout the world. As its name implies, it is part of the tradition of each country and employs practices that are handed down from generation to generation of healer. Its acceptance by people receiving care is also inherited from generation to generation. Traditional medicine originated aeons before the modern medical era.[6]

WHO definition of herbal medicines: Finished, labelled medicinal products that contain as active ingredients aerial or underground parts of plants, or other plant material, or combinations thereof, whether in the crude state or as plant preparations.

Plant material includes juices, gums, fatty oils, essential oils, and any other substances of this nature. Herbal medicines may contain excipients in addition to the active ingredients. Medicines containing plant material combined with chemically defined active substances, including chemically defined, isolated constituents of plants, are not considered to be herbal medicines.[7]

Traditional medicine is the totality of all knowledge and practices, whether explicable or not, used in diagnosing, preventing or eliminating a physical, mental or social disequilibrium and which rely exclusively on past experience and observation handed down verbally from generation to generation (Good *et al.*, cited in Troskie[8]).

African Traditional Medicine: The sum total of all knowledge and practices, whether explicable or not, used in diagnosis, prevention and elimination of physical, mental, or societal imbalance, and relying exclusively on practical experience and observation handed down from generation to generation, whether verbally or in writing. Traditional medicine might also be considered to be the sum total of all practices, measures, ingredients and procedures of all kinds, whether material or not, which from time immemorial had enabled the African to guard against disease, to alleviate his suffering and to cure himself.[9]

The above definitions characterize traditional medicine as a collection of knowledge and skills. While these are aspects of the traditional systems that can be the subject of training, regulation and formalization, other aspects such as the traditional theory of physiological function and disease, and the role of spiritual practice and belief, are more elusive yet perhaps more fundamental to most traditional health care systems.

Theoretical framework

An essential feature of traditional health systems is that they are based in theories or cosmologies that take into account mental, social, spiritual, physical and ecological dimensions of health and well-being. A fundamental concept found in many systems is that of balance—the balance between mind and body, between different dimensions of individual bodily functioning and need, between individual and community, individual/community and environment, and individual and the universe. The breaking of this interconnectedness of life is a fundamental source of *dis-ease*, which can progress to stages of illness and epidemic. Treatments, therefore, are designed not only to address the locus of the disease but also to restore a state of systemic balance to the individual and his or her inner and outer environment.

The World Health Organization has referred to the world's traditional health systems as *holistic*, i.e., 'that of viewing man in his totality within a wide ecological spectrum, and of emphasizing the view that ill health or disease is brought about by an imbalance, or disequilibrium, of man in his total ecological system and not only by the causative agent and pathogenic evolution'.[10]

Arthur Kleinman, of Harvard University's Center for Culture and Medicine, has noted that 'for members of non-Western societies, the body is an open system linking social relations, the self, a vital balance between interrelated elements in a holistic cosmos. Emotion and cognition are integrated into bodily processes. The body-self is not a secularized private domain of the individual person, but an organic part of a sacred, sociocentric world, a communication system involving exchanges with others (including the divine).'[11]

The natural world is thus not only imbued with non-material attributes but also, in many traditions, is an expression of a more fundamental level of spiritual reality with which the individual is linked. Vitalistic traditions were present in the early days of Western medicine in ancient Greece. Aesculapian traditions drew on spiritual healing as a basis for complete recovery. Subsequently, the systematic, natural science approach of Hippocrates, while emphasizing the observable, acknowledged the value of the sacred in the healing process.

In Ayurvedic medicine, the classical health care system of India, consciousness is of primary significance and matter is deemed secondary. Accordingly, Ayurvedic medical treatment, when practised according to the high traditions of Ayurveda, will first address the spiritual and mental state of the individual—through meditation,[12] intellectual understanding of the problem, behavioural and lifestyle advice, etc.—and then address the physical problem by means of diet, medicine and other therapeutic modalities.[13]

In the shamanic traditions of the Americas, spiritual healing is fundamental to the recovery process. 'Traditional health practices are part of a cultural identity that goes from the particular to the collective and vice versa. The forces which allow traditional health practices to function are based on spirituality, the wholeness of the person, the maintenance of balance and harmony with habitat and Nature. The practice strengthens and reinforces family and community connections. Therefore the traditional doctor re-establishes the patient's lost harmony.'[14]

Utilization

The widespread demand for traditional medical services has been recognized as an enduring phenomenon. Earlier calls for traditional medicine to be replaced by modern medical services have now given way to recognition that some degree of formalization of these health services might offer the public increased standards of quality and safety.

In many countries, life begins with the support of traditional medicine. An estimated 60–70% of births in developing countries still take place with the sole help of traditional birth attendants (Mangay-Maglacas and Simons; cited in Stephens[15]).

Africa

There have been many general estimates of the extent of use of traditional medicine in Africa. Bannerman[16] estimated that traditional medicine caters for the health needs of 80% of the African population. This figure echoes an earlier estimate of 80% made by Koumare (cited in Shai-Mahoko[17]).

However, some estimates of use are strikingly low. Shiferaw,[18] for example, reports on an interview survey of perceived morbidity in a rural community in south-western Ethiopia, where 55.4% of those reporting illness took no action at all; 30.3% applied to health institutions, 9.2% reported self-care and only 5.2% visited a traditional healer. By contrast, research done at Mogopane Hospital in north-eastern Transvaal, South Africa, showed that nine out of ten patients who come to the outpatients department first consult traditional healers.[19]

Clearly, studies of community groups and of hospital populations address the needs and choices of different populations with different health profiles. In planning services such differences need to be accounted for.

Age and gender are factors in utilization of traditional health care services. A study of visitors to traditional healers in central Sudan indicated that children under 10 years did not take part in visits. Most visitors were between 21 and 40 years (61%) and were women (62%). They were less educated compared to the general population in the area. The main reasons given for attending traditional healers were treatment (60%) and blessing (26%).[20]

In Mali, men are more likely to prefer traditional treatments for malaria than women,[21] and more boys than girls believed in herbal medicine in a survey in the Sudan.[22] It has been suggested that women are less likely to be treated at modern facilities, and are more likely to resort to traditional medicines.[23] Travel time can be a factor in the choice of traditional over modern medical services.

People with a serious health condition may seek traditional health care before accepting modern medical services. In Malawi, 37% of tuberculosis patients reported attending a traditional healer prior to attending the health service. By the time a final diagnosis of tuberculosis had been made, most patients had visited several different care providers: private practitioner (69 visits), village clinic (64) and traditional healer (40), and 32 patients reported taking some form of traditional remedy at home (Brouwer et al.; cited in Wilkinson et al.[24]) (see Table 4.1).

Among comments made by traditional midwives in South Africa, in a study by Troskie,[8] was that 'the nearest hospital is 20 kilometres far'. Similar responses were recorded from clients. In Kwale district, Kenya, which has one health service facility for 12 000 people, it has been estimated that 24% of the population has a health facility

Table 4.1 Adult conditions taken to the indigenous healers.

Condition	No. of respondents (healers)	%
Infertility	32	91
Septic sores	31	89
Impotence	30	86
STDs	28	80
Deliveries	28	80
Asthma	23	66
Mental illness	21	60
High blood pressure	20	57
Palpitations	15	43
TB	14	40
Alcoholism	12	34
Diabetes	9	26
Cancer	9	26

From Shai-Mahoko.[17]

within 2 km distance, 58% within 5 km and 83% within 10 km (Ministry of Health, Kenya; cited in Boerma & Baya[25]). By contrast, traditional health care services are readily available. Every village has a number of traditional healers and birth attendants, each with their own specializations.[25]

Similarly, in India, rural women in Gujarat were more likely to use services which were closer to home, other things being equal. The 'travel' variable (including time and travel costs) is a more important factor determining use of modern and traditional services among women in the study area than the actual direct costs of the service.[26]

In the case of malaria, selection of first-line treatment varies from area to area. Sometimes, herbal remedies are given at home as the first-line treatment,[27,28] especially in mild cases of malaria.[29,30] Sometimes, herbs are the second-line treatment when chemotherapy has failed.[31–33] Munguti[34] found that in a rural area of Kenya 7% used herbs as first choice of treatment, 17% as second choice and 14% as third choice.

There can be contrasting patterns of use across countries and regions. Whereas young children in the Sudan were found not to attend traditional healers, in Kenya 40% of sick children were taken to the *mganga* (traditional healer) and 55% to the clinic; 26% of the mothers said that both sources of treatment were consulted.[25]

There are usually differences between urban and rural populations in their use of traditional and modern medicine. While 95% of urban women who attended modern medical clinics in South Africa strongly advocated mixing traditional and Western antenatal care, only 63% of rural clinic attenders found this practice acceptable. All groups favoured Western over traditional care in cases of serious pregnancy complications.[35]

Asia

In India, it has been found that the influence of family structure is significant. The presence of the mother-in-law is associated with a greater use of traditional healers.[26]

Inadequacies in and scarcity of modern medical services can contribute to the use of traditional health services. Less than half (44%) of Chinese immigrants studied in the United States had used Western health services in the United States within the previous 12 months; 20% reported that they had never used them. Chinese physicians stated that many Chinese patients are not satisfied with American doctors because of the inflexibility of appointments, short visit, long waiting, distrust and miscommunication.[36]

In a study of health service utilization in four villages in India, the most common complaint by a majority of those surveyed was that 'medicines are never available' at the Primary Health Centre, followed by discourteous behaviour of the staff and health personnel, 'doctors never available', 'doctors demand money for better treatment', and so on. Almost a quarter of the women initially tried homeopathic treatment, followed by 9% who administered Western medicine at home, while 2% opted for traditional home remedies for cure and treatment, before visiting and consulting a trained medical practitioner. Medical pluralism was found to be flourishing as people switched from one medical system to another depending on affordability and time.[37]

In Sri Lanka, two patterns of health care seeking which cut across modern and traditional medical systems have been identified. The first involved patients who searched for a medicine which could cure. The second pattern involved the search for a practitioner who had the power of the hand to cure one's illness.[38]

Medical pluralism is common worldwide and consumers practise integrated health care irrespective of whether or not it is present at the formal level. In Taiwan, 60% of the public have been found to be users of multiple healing systems, including modern Western medicine, Chinese medicine and religious healing.[39]

Indigenous communities

Native American communities incorporate traditional forms of treatment into the US Indian Health Service (IHS) alcohol rehabilitation programmes. In a study of 190 IHS contract programmes, it was found that 50% of these offered a traditional sweat lodge or encouraged its use. Treatment outcomes were found to be better for alcoholic patients when a sweat lodge was available. In addition, the presence of medicine men or healers, when used in combination with the sweat lodge, greatly improved the outcome.[40]

In the tropical regions of Australia, traditional Aboriginal medicine is widely practised (Taylor et al.; cited in Maher[41]). In most regions of the Northern Territory, more than 22% of indigenous people had used bush medicine in the last 6 months when surveyed (McLennan; cited in Maher[41]). A decrease in use of traditional medicine seems to be because Western medicine is easier to access, not because of a lack of faith in its efficacy (Scarlett et al.; cited in Maher[41]). Indigenous Australian medicine includes herbal preparations, diet, rest, massage, restricted diet and external remedies such as ochre, smoke, steam and heat (Peile; cited in Maher[41]).

Traditional medicine and the formal health sector in Africa

Healers have for long been treated like trees on savanna farms—not formally cultivated, yet valued and used, particularly by women and children.[42]

There has been a long-reported willingness on the part of traditional healers in Africa to collaborate with the formal sector and to establish joint training. Burnett et al.[43] note that 37 of the 39 traditional healers (94%) and 14 of the 27 formal health workers (52%) interviewed in a Zambian study were keen to collaborate in training and patient care relating to HIV/AIDS.

However, this is not generally a reciprocal view. Although 1% of nurses in South Africa are reported to be traditional healers, rural nurses in Swaziland perceived themselves as being teachers to healers, but not learning from healers. They saw themselves as a source of referral for healers, but not the reverse.[44]

One view is that it may be more appropriate to work towards a system of cooperation between two independent systems, with each recognizing and respecting the character of the other (Staugard; cited in Last & Chavanduka[42]). This has been the policy in Botswana, where parallel development has been encouraged, since it is felt that one or other of the two systems might suffer in the process of integration (WHO; cited in Burnett et al.[43]).

WHO policies of the late 1970s and 1980s have promoted the establishment of associations of traditional healers in Africa. During the 1990s, NGOs of traditional health practitioners—associations, small groups, clinics, etc.—have grown exponentially in Africa, playing a partnership role in HIV/AIDS education and care,[45] in delivering child survival messages and in managing endemic disease in partnership with modern health care workers.

A Parliamentary Committee on Social Services in South Africa proposed that the profession of traditional healing should be divided into four categories: the *inyanga* (traditional doctors or herbalists); the *sangoma* (diviner); birth attendants or midwives; and traditional surgeons who mainly do circumcision. Spiritual healers were not included because their training and accreditation were considered 'unclear' and 'ill defined'.[46]

In South Africa, many traditional healers are members of well-organized national organizations that are seeking formal recognition from the government. In one instance of WHO-sponsored collaboration, it has been recognized that the rapid increase in TB caseload, especially in African countries heavily affected by the HIV epidemic, requires a search for effective ways to treat patients outside hospital. As a component of the WHO's Community Care for Tuberculosis in Africa Project, Wilkinson et al.[24] studied the potential role for collaboration between the health service and traditional healers, especially as tuberculosis treatment supervisors, and examined what precedent and potential exist for traditional healers to act in this role.

Before commencing collaborative effort in health care between modern and traditional sectors, a careful assessment of potential benefits and obstacles should be made. The medical services utilization patterns of the communities need to be ascertained and the specific role of traditional health practitioners considered. In such efforts the ideas of healers themselves about possible collaboration are crucial.[25]

Ghana has recently passed the Traditional Medicine Practice Act 2000, Act 595, to establish a Council to regulate and control the practice of traditional medicine. The primary draft of this Act originated from the traditional healers themselves. The Act defines traditional medicine as 'practice based on beliefs and ideas recognized by the community to provide health care by using herbs and other naturally occurring substances', and herbal medicine as 'any finished labelled medicinal products that contain as active ingredients aerial or underground parts of plants or other plant materials or the combination of them whether in crude state or plant preparation'. It is arranged into four sections, namely the establishment and functions of the Traditional Medicine Practice Council; registration of practitioners; licensing of practices; and miscellaneous provisions.

Ghana's Ministry of Health has incorporated a Traditional Medicine Unit since 1991, and in 1999 this was upgraded to the status of a Directorate. The Ministry, in collaboration with the Ghana Federation of Traditional Medicine Practitioners Associations and other stakeholders, has now developed a 5-year strategic plan for traditional medicine. This plan outlines activities to be carried out from 2000 to 2004, and will be reviewed every 2 years. It proposes, among other aspects, the need to develop comprehensive training in traditional medicine from basic and secondary to tertiary levels.

A 'Ghana Herbal Pharmacopoeia', containing scientific information on 50 medicinal plants, has been published. A second volume is currently in preparation. Efforts are being made to integrate traditional medicine into the official public health system and it is expected that by the year 2004 certified and efficacious herbal medicines will be prescribed and dispensed in hospitals and pharmacies. The Ghanaian government has set aside the third week of March every year as a Traditional Medicine Week, starting from the year 2000.

In Nigeria, the National Agency for Food and Drug Administration and Control (NAFDAC) has taken steps to regulate and control traditional medicine products with a view to ensuring their safety, efficacy and quality. In consultation with traditional healers and researchers NAFDAC has developed guidelines on regulating herbal medicines. Recently, the government of Nigeria approved

a national policy on a Traditional Medicine Code of Ethics. Draft legislation has been prepared to establish national and state Traditional Medicine Boards to enhance the regulation of traditional medicine practice and promote cooperation and research in traditional medicine.[47]

As a further reflection of the trend towards greater recognition of traditional medicine, in July 2001 the Organization of African Unity's Heads of Government meeting in Lusaka, Zambia, declared a Decade for the Development of Traditional African Medicine. The African heads of government recognized the cultural significance of traditional medicine and its ongoing role as part of health care in Africa. The Decade will focus on the development of standards of practice, training, research and the protection of indigenous intellectual property rights over traditional medicinal knowledge.

Priority disease areas: HIV/AIDS and malaria

Traditional medicine has a central role to play in combating new and re-emerging diseases. Global priority is currently placed on combating malaria and HIV/AIDS and new partnerships between the communities of traditional medicine, public health and health research are being formed. Two diseases are addressed below, but partnerships are being developed with other diseases such as tuberculosis and control of vector-borne diseases such as trypanosomiasis.

Partnership with the traditional sector in HIV/AIDS prevention and management

As the AIDS crisis leads an increasing number of countries to question their priorities in health expenditures, there is an emerging awareness that traditional health practitioners (THPs) can play an important role in delivering an AIDS prevention message. There is growing recognition that some THPs may be able to offer treatment for opportunistic infections. At the same time, there are concerns about unsafe practices and a growth in claims of traditional cures for AIDS. Partnerships between the modern and traditional health sectors are a cornerstone for building a comprehensive strategy to manage the AIDS crisis.

Africa

In Uganda, where there is only one doctor for every 20 000 people, there is one traditional health practitioner per 200–400 people.[48] In such settings, partnerships may be the only way that effective health care coverage can be achieved in managing the twin epidemics of AIDS and malaria. Clearly, such partnerships not only make good public health sense but, based on a growing body of pharmacological evidence, may also yield important preventive and treatment modalities.

In light of the widespread availability of traditional health care services and the reliance of the population on these services, it is inevitable that people suffering from AIDS will turn to THPs for treatment. Collaborative AIDS programmes have been established in many African countries, including Malawi, Mozambique, Uganda, Senegal, South Africa, Swaziland, Zambia and Zimbabwe.

Information sharing and educational programmes in South Africa have resulted in THPs providing correct HIV/AIDS advice as well as demonstrations of condom use. One such programme trained 1510 THPs and it was calculated that during the first 10 months of the programme some 845 600 of their clients may have been reached with AIDS/STD prevention messages. In similar programmes in Mozambique, traditional healers learned that AIDS is transmitted by sexual contact, by blood and non-sterile razor blades used in traditional practice. In a follow-up evaluation, 81% of those trained reported that they had promoted condom use with at least their STD patients.[49]

One of the challenges in such workshop situations is to move beyond 'training' to genuine information sharing. It has been noted that it is difficult to modify the manner in which health professionals teach about AIDS—a style that tends towards the didactic and use of scientific jargon. Removing communication barriers such as these is a necessary first step in ensuring that training is an effective tool in mobilizing traditional health practitioners as partners in AIDS control.

An important example of how this may be done was conducted in Brazil, where a face-to-face educational intervention by healers blended traditional healing— with its language, codes, symbols and images—with scientific medicine, and simultaneously addressed social injustices and discrimination. New information about HIV/AIDS transmission was conveyed using languages and concepts intimately familiar to traditional health practitioners. A controlled evaluation found significant increases in AIDS awareness, knowledge about risky HIV behaviour, information about correct condom use, and acceptance of lower-risk, alternative ritual blood practices among the 126 members of the trainee group compared to 100 untrained controls. There were significant decreases in prejudicial attitudes related to HIV transmission among the trainee group compared to controls.[50]

The Ugandan NGO, Traditional and Modern Health Practitioners Together Against AIDS (THETA), was established in 1992 to conduct research on potentially useful traditional medicines with HIV-related illness and to promote a mutually respectful collaboration between traditional and modern health workers in the fight against AIDS. THETA has conducted workshops to share knowledge on AIDS prevention and also treatment of opportunistic infections using local herbal remedies.

Traditional healers participating in clinical observational studies of their herbal medicines have subsequently sought training in prevention, education and counselling issues, as well as in basic clinical diagnostic skills. A 1998 UNAIDS-sponsored evaluation of THETA found that it had reached 125 THPs (44 women and 81 men) in five districts of Uganda. Fifty thousand people were found to have benefited from the improved services offered by traditional health practitioners over a period of 2 years.[45]

THETA director Dr Donna Kabatesi[45] has outlined the challenges entailed in such partnership-building programmes:

- Many health workers expressed scepticism about this kind of collaboration, while healers feared losing their treatment secrets to scientists and researchers.
- Major questions remain to be researched on the identity and processing of useful herbs.
- Healers feared that doctors would not respect their rights and knowledge because of previous experience with other researchers.
- Medical doctors continued to misunderstand traditional medical practice by attempting to apply the scientific model of biomedicine to traditional medicine.
- Traditional healers feared talking about AIDS and discussing death with their patients because this would indicate failure and possibly also because they were not sure how to deal with the situation after that. Training them in counselling has since improved their skills in talking about AIDS.
- For those healers whose herbal treatments had no efficacy, THETA clinical study results were not so easily accepted.
- Traditional healer associations that initially agreed to work together have continued to have internal power wrangles, which have sometimes interfered with project activities.
- The projects raised many unmet expectations, such as immediate official recognition by the Ministry of Health.
- Methodological issues, including the consistency of herbal preparations used during the study, availability of sufficient herbs for study subjects, and noncompliance by patients of each study arm, were major concerns.

In South Africa, a follow-up of educational workshops found that some THPs reported that local medical staff had begun referring HIV-positive and STD patients to them for condom demonstrations and HIV counselling. All THPs reported having given condom demonstrations not only to clients but also to any member of their communities with potential interest.

Giving a perspective on the benefits from investment in this involvement of local traditional health practitioners in AIDS prevention exercises, Edward C. Green, an organizer of the workshops, reported that: '630 second generation healers had been trained in 12 workshops held in diverse parts of South Africa. The total direct cost of training these 630 was about $23.30 per healer, or $5.90 per day per healer. In addition to these 630 direct beneficiaries of training, up to 229 320 patients or clients of these healers may have benefited from AIDS education within 7 months of the first generation training (calculated as 26 weeks times an average of 14 patients a week per healer [see below] times 630 healers trained). Not all these healers specialize in STDs or AIDS, but most of them see a great number of at least STD patients. Finally, an inestimable number of friends, family members, and others in the local community (local associations, sports teams, youth groups, etc.) benefited from informal AIDS education.'[48]

Research

Health care consumers and THPs want information on the safety and efficacy of local treatments, their effect on opportunistic infections, and how to test claims of cure in an efficient and cost-effective manner.

There has been little official response from governments on this front. However, in one of the more forward-looking national programmes, the Uganda AIDS Commission and the Joint Clinical Research Centre in Kampala have worked with traditional healers in evaluating several traditional treatments used locally for OIs. The research has found traditional medicine to be 'better suited to the treatment of some AIDS symptoms such as herpes zoster (HZ), chronic diarrhoea, shingles and weight loss.' THETA has conducted controlled clinical trials on a Ugandan herbal treatment for HZ. Comparing subjects with herbal treatments with controls using acyclovir, the conventional treatment for HZ, both groups were found to experience similar rates of resolution of HZ attacks. The traditional medicine group had less super-infection and showed less keloid formation than did subjects on acyclovir. HZ pain resolved significantly faster in the herbal group. The investigators concluded that herbal treatment is an important local and affordable alternative in managing HZ in HIV-infected patients in Uganda.[1]

A study conducted by the Blair Research Institute Clinic in Harare, Zimbabwe, evaluated the impact of traditional medicine in persons with HIV infection and assessed their quality of life with respect to HIV disease progression. There were 105 HIV-infected persons in the study, at various stages of HIV infection, of whom 79% were on traditional herbal medicine and 21% were on conventional medical care (CMC). Using the WHO Quality of Life Scale, it was found that the proportions of scores on five domains measuring different aspects of quality of life for patients on traditional medicine were much lower than those on conventional therapy ($p < 0.0001$, for all variables). The research team concluded that the data supported the role of traditional medicine in improving the quality of life of HIV-1 infected patients, although its pharmacological basis is unknown.[51]

While clinical research has been slow to begin in the evaluation of traditional herbal treatments for HIV-related illness, there has been screening for antiviral effects of locally used plants since the early 1990s. A recent study reported promising antiviral effects from selected Ethiopian medicinal plants. Asres et al.[52] found that the highest selective inhibition of HIV-1 replication was found with the acetone fraction of *Combretum paniculatum* Vent., and the methanol fraction of *Dodonaea angustifolia* L.f.[52] These showed selectivity indices (ratio of 50% cytotoxic concentration to 50% effective antiviral concentration) of 6.4 and 4.9, and afforded cell protection of viral-induced cytopathic effect of 100% and 99%, respectively, when compared with control samples. Asres et al. found that the greatest degree of antiviral activity against HIV-2 was achieved with the acetone extract of *C. paniculatum* (EC(50): 3 µg/ml), which also showed the highest selectivity index (32). The 50% cytotoxic concentration ranged from 0.5 µg/ml for the hexane extract of *D. angustifolia* L.f., the most cytotoxic of the extracts tested, to > 250 µg/ml for some extracts such as the methanol fraction of *Alcea rosea* L., the least toxic tested. While there is the obvious potential for commercial development of fractions of these plants as pharmaceutical leads, there is growing recognition of the need to evaluate such plants clinically in order to determined the viability of affordable, locally available medicines for managing HIV-related illness.

A new Traditional Medicine and AIDS in East and Southern Task Force, established in Kampala in early 2000, aims to build a research programme which will identify, assess and develop safe and effective local treatments for HIV-related illnesses. The programme will use simplified but controlled clinical protocols to conduct rapid evaluations of promising treatments.[53]

In a parallel development, Nigeria has taken an important step towards addressing the research needs in this field. The Nigerian health minister, Hon. Tim Menakaya, announced on 30 March 2000 that 'the government has significantly increased its budget for verifying HIV/AIDS cure claims, after a recommendation by the World Bank and UNAIDS'.

Asia

While much of the international focus on AIDS in the developing world has been on Africa, there has been growing awareness of the rapid spread of the disease in Asia. Reflecting the concerns now beginning to be addressed in many African countries, India's national AIDS policy states:

In a scenario where anti-retroviral drugs are extremely expensive, there is a great need to look into the indigenous systems of medicine (ISM), like Ayurveda, Unani and Siddha. Some of the medicines in these systems have the potential of reducing the viral load in the body of the patient thus ensuring a healthier and longer life with the infection. The Government has sponsored research projects in ISM and is receiving encouraging response. It will pursue a policy of sponsoring research in ISM for development of drugs which can serve the purpose of anti-retrovirals.

The policy statement cautions about false claims of cures among unscrupulous practitioners and makes the point that 'Any medicine or system of treatment which cannot stand the test of scrutiny by the professional organizations like the Ayurveda Council cannot be accepted as a drug or a system of treatment in the country.' Clearly, drugs which are shown by rigorous research methods to have an effect can become part of a system of treatment in India.[54]

Traditional Chinese medicine is also being used in HIV management, not only in China but also in Africa and in other parts of Asia, where traditional Chinese medicines are exported. In one study, qian-kun-nin, a Chinese herbal formulation considered to have anti-infection, anti-tumour, antiretroviral and immunomodulatory properties, was evaluated for its anti-HIV effects.

Eight HIV-positive subjects were given oral qian-kun-nin capsules for 24 consecutive weeks in a single-blind design. Compared to baseline level, the plasma virus load decreased significantly at the end of week 12 ($p < 0.01$) and week 24 ($p < 0.01$), respectively. Four weeks after cessation of qian-kun-nin treatment, plasma virus load was still significantly lower compared to baseline ($p < 0.01$). Blood CD4 cell counts were increased significantly at the end of the 12th week compared to the baseline level ($p < 0.01$). No adverse effects were observed, and no significant side effects were recorded in any subjects.[55]

This is one of many emerging studies that require adequate funding to ensure that the research methodology is sound. While these data appear to suggest that qian-kun-nin has therapeutic potential in the treatment of HIV-positive patients clearly, the trial design and the sample size make it difficult to draw solid conclusions from the study. What this study does highlight is the potential for anti-HIV effects in traditional medicines and the need for standard operating procedures for the clinical evaluation of these medicines.

In Africa, Asia and elsewhere in the world, partnerships between modern and traditional health systems are being seen to be the clear way forward to build on existing community resources and to harness the potential therapeutic benefit of local and affordable treatments for HIV-related illness, as well as to screen out false claims and unsafe medicines and practices.

A meeting on Indian Systems of Medicine and the response to HIV/AIDS held in Delhi in November 2000 addressed research needs in this field and a clinical protocol has subsequently been published for use in the clinical evaluation of herbal medicines with HIV-related illness.[56]

Malaria

The emergence of multidrug-resistant strains of malaria which has accompanied each new class of antimalarial drugs may be viewed as one of most significant threats to the health of people in tropical countries. While there is widespread agreement that a fresh approach to the prevention and treatment of malaria is urgently needed, solutions have tended to focus on the development of new classes of drugs. More recently, there has been an emphasis on promoting combination therapy of existing drugs as a means of preventing resistance.

Historically, however, local communities in tropical regions have used local flora as a means of preventing and treating malaria.[57] It can be argued that these traditional medicines, based on the use of whole plants with multiple ingredients or of complex mixtures of plant materials, constitute combination therapies that may well combat the development of resistance to antimalarial therapy.

Resistance, synergism and traditional medicines

While combination therapy in malaria, cancer and AIDS is based on the principle of synergistic action among multiple drugs, little significance has as yet being given to the obvious point that all of the major antimalarials have been derived from plants and that combination existed in the traditional formulations before the process of extraction took place. For example, flavinoids in *Artemisia annua*, which are structurally unrelated to the antimalarial drug *artemisinin*, enhance the in vitro antiplasmodial activity of artemisinin (Phillipson et al.; cited in Kirby[57]).

Elsewhere, synergism has been observed between the alkaloids of the antimalarial plant *Ancistrocladus peltatum*. A total alkaloid extract of this plant had far greater antiparasitic activity than any of the six alkaloids isolated subsequently. In studies on antimalarial plants from Madagascar, the alkaloids bisbenzylisoquinoline, novel pavine and benzyl tetrahydroisoquinolines, all were found to potentiate the antiparasitic activity of chloroquine in vitro and, in some cases, in vivo. Preparations of these plants are currently being tested as adjuvants to chloroquine therapy in Madagascar.[57] In Uganda, there are data from clinical case reports and a cohort study that a traditional Ugandan herbal remedy is effective against malaria.[33,58]

As with other conditions, people with malaria will often combine conventional drugs and traditional medicines, sometimes simultaneously or as first- or second-line treatments,[27,59-64] with herbalists reporting their view that this combination gives an additional therapeutic effect.[65] Perceived efficacy is an important reason for people using traditional antimalarial medicines. Affordability is another. However, when patients themselves were asked why they choose traditional medicine over conventional drugs, a study in Burkina Faso found that the cost of medicines accounted for only 50% of respondents. Lack of faith in doctors was the reason for the other 50% resorting to traditional medicine.[66] Elsewhere it has been reported that medical staff at Burkina Faso hospitals are less trusted as they are frequently young, do not speak the local languages, and are not courteous or welcoming to patients.[59]

Several cohort studies have been conducted to evaluate the outcomes of traditional herbal treatments used by herbalists in managing malaria. A few of these have shown complete parasite clearance by day 7 (Phetsouvanh; Makinde et al; Mueller et al.; all cited in Willcox & Bodeker[67]). Phetsouvanh's study of the antimalarial effects of *Alocaci macrorhiza* root decoction showed 100% parasite clearance by day 7, without any recrudescence for the duration of follow-up (21 days), although this study has not been published or replicated. Makinde et al. showed 100% parasite clearance in adults by a leaf extract of *Morinda lucida*. However, there was not full parasite clearance from infected children. Further clinical studies on the antimalarial effects of plants have been reviewed by Willcox & Bodeker.[67]

The research initiative for traditional antimalarial methods (RITAM)

To redress this situation, a partnership was established in December 1999 between the Global Initiative for Traditional Systems (GIFTS) of Health, the Tropical Disease Research Programme of WHO.[68] Through the Research Initiative for Traditional Antimalarial Methods (RITAM) <http://mim.nih.gov/english/partnerships/ritam_repotr.pdf>, individual scientists, traditional health practitioners and others have formed a partnership to investigate, evaluate and, where appropriate, develop traditional herbal medicines to combat malaria. Standard operating procedures have been developed for experimental, toxicological and clinical research on traditional antimalarials. A research network to evaluate the potential of classically prepared *Artemisia annua* has also been established by RITAM.[69]

Wounds

Dermatological problems are the third most common reason for people seeking medical care in developing countries.[70] Among the most common dermatological problems of non-industrialized countries are non-healing tropical ulcers, particularly among young men of working age.[71] Tropical or seasonal environments with occupational exposure to the damp are typical for tropical ulcer,[72] where malnutrition may also be a factor.

Many wounds are inadequately treated in these countries because of issues of treatment cost, storage, manufacture and supply.[73,74] Bacterial and viral contamination of wounds is usual and some form of antisepsis is helpful. Reliance on imported agents in health centres and from pharmacies is expensive and unsustainable and the widespread casual use of antibiotics should be discouraged. The use of hypochlorite, iodine or gentian violet in the tropics follows now-questionable conventional Western therapies.

This has led to calls for research and rationalization of wound treatment in this setting.[75] In non-industrial countries the majority of the population uses traditional health care, and commonly uses herbal treatment for wounds.[76–78] These treatments warrant investigation for this reason and because they may be more readily available and efficacious than the alternatives.[79]

There is growing evidence that a number of plant treatments are useful in a variety of dermatological conditions, including wounds.[70,80,81] *Centella asiatica* extract is one of the most widely studied plant-based wound treatments. It is used in Madagascar and several other tropical countries. In vivo laboratory studies have shown its topical application to significantly accelerate wound healing, and in vitro studies of treated granulating tissues have demonstrated a significant increase in fibroblast activity, total DNA and collagen content.[82,83]

Recent research on *Aloe barbadensis* has shown it to be a powerful wound-healing agent.[84] Extracts from *Aloe barbadensis*, or *aloe vera* as it is commonly known, have been found to penetrate tissue, have anaesthetic properties, have antibacterial, antifungal and antiviral properties, serve as an anti-inflammatory agent, and dilate capillaries and increase blood flow.[85,86]

Research at the National Institute for Traditional Medicine in Hanoi has examined the mechanism by which *Cudrania cochinchinensis* (Moraceae), commonly used in Vietnam as a traditional wound-healing agent, produces a wound-healing effect. Tran et al.[87] examined its effect on fibroblast proliferation and the protection of both fibroblast and endothelial cells against oxidative damage. An ethyl acetate extract of the plant was found to protect fibroblasts and endothelial cells against hydrogen peroxide-induced damage. The research team have suggested that stimulation of fibroblast proliferation and protection of cells against destruction by mediators of inflammatory processes may be ways in which the polyphenolic substances from this plant contribute to wound healing.

Phan et al.[88] studied the wound-healing properties of Eupolin, a topical agent produced from the leaves of *Chromolaena odorata*, and which is used widely for the treatment of burns and soft tissue wounds in Vietnam. Eupolin was found to enhance haemostasis, stimulate granulation tissue and re-epithelialization, and inhibit collagen contraction. These results suggest a mechanism for clinical reports on the effectiveness of Eupolin in reducing wound contraction and scarring, which are critical complications in post-burn trauma. Other studies have found Eupolin to have antibacterial properties.[89]

Chen et al.[90] studied the effects of 'dragon's blood', sap from the bark of *Croton lechleri* used as a wound-healing agent in South America. The researchers found that *Croton lechleri* has no isolable 'wound-healing principle', but acts as a natural dressing which forms an occlusive layer with an antimicrobial environment and cell proliferative effects. This is due to the combined effects of several compounds. This synergistic effect was further investigated by Pieters et al.,[91] who compared the in vivo effects of dragon's blood on wound repair with a polyphenolic fraction of dragon's blood and with a solution of artificial polyphenols. Wound repair was defined as the percentage of the wound volume filled with new tissue. Pieters et al. found:

- 90% wound repair with traditionally prepared dragon's blood.
- 50% with a polyphenolic fraction of dragon's blood.
- 40% when a solution of artificial polyphenols was used.

This finding lends support to the traditional practice of the complex mixture of compounds found in the bark rather than an isolated 'active ingredient' approach to the development of an effective wound treatment typical of conventional natural products research.

Ophthalmic conditions

Traditional eye treatment (TET) in Africa has been the cause of much concern due to serious eye infections and injury associated with many traditional treatments.

Public health programmes have focused on training traditional practitioners to refer patients for eye treatment.

Research in Tanzania found that of 26 corneal ulcers present in a sample of TET users, 58% (*n* = 15) had no other identified cause of ulceration apart from TET use. There was a trend to more central and dense corneal scarring in the TET users group (42% vs. 23%, *p* = 0.06).[92]

A subsequent clinical study at Muhimbili Medical Centre in Tanzania looked over a period of 1 year at the visual impact of using traditional medicine in a sample of 257 patients with eye injury.[93] The study examined the causes, presenting visual acuity and associated ocular complications, use of traditional eye medicine on the injured eye and the visual outcome of these effects. It was reported that stones, sticks and metallic objects were the major causes of ocular trauma. The study found that traditional medicine was used by half of the patients (49%) and that the principal types of traditional medicines were plant juices, milk mixed with black powder and pounded roots. These were mainly applied via instillation into the conjunctival sac. Keratitis, endophthalmitis and panophthalmitis were the main ocular complications presented and were seen more in patients with a positive history of using traditional eye medicines than in patients with a negative history. The study found poor visual outcome more in patients who used traditional eye medicines than in those who did not use them. These results led to the recommendation for intensive community health education to create awareness of the dangers of using traditional medicine on injured eyes.

Courtright and co-workers[94] have assessed the rates of corneal disease in a district in Malawi following an interactive training programme with traditional healers, based on a collaborative approach to eye care. In addition to directly contributing to corneal disease, use of traditional medicine has been found often to delay the use of modern medical treatment for eye disease. Courtright et al. found that among the 175 pre-intervention

and 97 post-intervention patients, delay in presentation improved only slightly. However, blindness among patients using TEM decreased from 44% to 21% and bilateral corneal disease in patients using TEM decreased from 31% to 10%. Despite this success, the research team note that distance to a hospital continues to be a barrier to the use of modern medical approaches to eye care.

Safety

A primary concern regarding traditional and complementary therapies is 'Are they safe?' As noted above, traditional eye medicine in Africa has been found to have serious effects on eye health.

Recent studies in the UK have found that there has been adulteration with steroids of some traditional Chinese dermatological preparations. In an analysis of Chinese herbal creams prescribed for dermatological conditions, Keane et al.[95] found that eight of eleven creams analysed contained steroids.

In Japan, contrary to popular belief, traditional Kampo medicines can create adverse effects. In 1992, adverse effects were associated with 48 Kampo prescriptions by doctors and with 47 drugs purchased from pharmacies in Japan. Syo-saiko-to has been reported to cause interstitial pneumonia, alone and in combination with interferon-α.[96]

One prominent example of dangerous plant-based medicines is plant species which contain pyrrolizidine alkaloids, widely known to produce adverse effects. In a number of countries, plants containing alkaloids are prohibited from use in herbal medicines intended for internal use. This is due to the hepatotoxic effect of these alkaloids. Following absorption from the gut, pyrrolizidine alkaloids are carried to the liver, where they are converted by microsomal mixed function oxygenation to highly reactive pyrrole esters, which are the primarily toxic metabolites. At high doses these compounds bind to liver cell proteins and other macromolecules and cause extensive periacinar hepatocellular necrosis and hepatic failure. With lower, repeated doses, the progressive damage to liver cells results in a gradual increase in connective tissue in the liver and cirrhosis develops (Seawright; cited in Noller et al.[97]).

Chapter 33 further elaborates the risks associated with ingestion of or contact with poisonous plants.

Safety must be the starting point for national drug development strategies for herbal medicines. While most of the published research on herbal medicine is pharmacological, the WHO's *1993 Guidelines on the Evaluation of Herbal Medicines* consider that clinical evaluation is ethical where drugs have long been in traditional use. Roy Chaudhury has offered a model for the clinical evaluation of herbal medicines:

1. Toxicity testing of the plant in two species of animal for acute and subacute toxicity.
2. A modified, shorter toxicity testing if the plant has already been used in man or is in such use now.

3. Administration of the total extract or combination of plants, if used, in exactly the same way as it is prepared and used by the population.

The differences between this approach and that of conventional drug evaluation methodology are that:

- Efficacy testing is carried out on humans rather than on animals; human studies are undertaken subsequent to modified, shortened toxicology studies having shown that the substance is not toxic in animals.
- The duration of the toxicity studies is reduced to 6 weeks for plants that are already in common use.
- The plant or mixture of plants is administered to subjects in the same manner in which it is used in traditional medicine.[98]

Research should consider best evidence for safety, including evidence for adverse effects from treatments (including magnitude, percentage of people so affected, etc.), as well as from inappropriate applications of traditional therapies. Postmarket surveillance studies can provide information on adverse effects of botanical herbal preparations. Pharmacognostic and pharmacological research can provide information on the quality, efficacy, safety or toxicity of botanical/herbal medicinal preparations.

It is also important to keep a balanced perspective on the issue of safety of herbal medicines, while recognizing the very real risks associated with a number of these and with the untrained use of plants as medicines. A basic question often asked in addressing safety in herbal medicines is 'Safe with respect to what?' Research has found that in the United States 51% of FDA-approved drugs have serious adverse effects not detected prior to their approval. One and a half million people are sufficiently injured by prescription drugs annually that they require hospitalization.[99] Once in hospital, the problem may be compounded. The incidence of serious and fatal adverse drug reactions (ADRs) in US hospitals is now ranked as between the fourth and the sixth leading cause of death in the United States, after heart disease, cancer, pulmonary disease and accidents.[100]

Clearly, the safety of and risks associated with medical interventions is an issue across all categories of health care. A regulatory response is necessary on the part of governments.

In developing health systems for traditional medicine, safety and quality control of herbal medicines go hand in hand. A case in point is the development of new standards of safety and quality for herbal medicines produced in India. New regulations were introduced in India in July 2000 to improve the standard and quality of Indian herbal medicines. Regulations will establish standard manufacturing practices and quality control. The new regulations outline requirements for infrastructure, manpower, quality control and raw material authenticity and absence of contamination. Of the 9000 licensed manufacturers of traditional medicines, those who qualify can immediately seek GMP certification. The remainder have

2 years to come into compliance with the regulations and to obtain certification. The government has also set up 10 new drug-testing laboratories for ISM and upgraded existing ones to provide high-quality evidence to licencing authorities of the safety and quality of herbal medicines. This replaces an ad hoc system of testing that was considered by the Department of ISM to be unreliable. Randomized controlled clinical trials of selected ISM prescriptions have been initiated to document their safety and efficacy and to provide the basis for their international licensure as medicines rather than simply as food supplements (Sanjay Kumar, *Reuters*, 13 July 2000).

Research and policy priorities

In July 2001, a Global Forum on the Safety of Herbal and Traditional Medicine was established in association with the Commonwealth Working Group on Traditional and Complementary Health Systems.[97] The recommendations of the Global Forum are to:

1. Establish as a high priority a global database to consolidate and develop further the international literature on traditional and complementary medicine, including the translation of non-English sources into English to provide a one-stop resource centre for information on the safety of those medicines.
2. Carry out critical evaluation of available knowledge where possible by a systematic review of this information, aimed at a summary of the current knowledge on specific plants or plant combinations.
3. With full respect for customary resource and intellectual property rights, document the knowledge of traditional healers who work within oral traditions and hold valuable information on the benefits of the world's biodiversity.
4. Establish a system for the evaluation of the toxicity and safety that should be different from, but run in parallel, to the system required for pharmaceutical drugs.
5. Provide protocols, advice and training in methods to evaluate safety of herbal and traditional medicines.
6. Offer toxicological services to countries, companies and communities via the Global Forum's hub, which will be based at the Australian National Institute of Environmental Toxicology in Brisbane, and through a number of linked regional centres.
7. Generate publications—hard copy and electronic in this field—possibly a journal, a news bulletin, and regular symposia at international toxicology conferences.

The Global Forum also recommended that an international centre be urgently established to implement the needs and knowledge gaps in the good manufacture and safe use of herbal and traditional medicine.

These recommendations are being developed by a partnership between the Commonwealth, the Global Forum on the Safety of Herbal and Traditional Medicine and the member institutes of the Forum in both developing and industrialized countries.[97] As the databases develop, they will be accessible via the Commonwealth Working Group on Traditional and Complementary Health Systems[101] and the Australian National Institute for Environmental Toxicology.

Food and medicine

A final consideration in the understanding of traditional health systems is the relationship between food and medicine that exists in these traditions.

In many traditional societies, and also in urban communities where traditional medicine is used and traditional medical theory influences household cooking and self-medication practices, food is considered central to health and the management of disease. Typically, there is not a clear distinction made between food and medicine, as food is often viewed medicinally and many plants used for medicine may also be included in the diet according to seasonal changes and family requirements.

The Hausa of Nigeria use certain plants as both food and medicine, including plants identified as having antimalarial effects. Nina Etkin of the University of Hawaii has reported that the use of plants with anti-malarial effects 'as both food and medicine exposes individuals to more pharmacologically remarkable constituents than does either category of use alone. Thus of the 54 most commonly used Hausa antimalarials, 82% also appeared in diet, and among those there was 89% concordance that the same plant structure (root, leaves, etc.) served as both antimalarial and food. Further, among those 39 plants, 67% were maximally available during the period of highest risk of malaria infection.'[102]

In Cameroon and the Central African Republic, the Aka and Baka Pygmies have a view of illness that includes both physical causes and a more fundamental view of equilibrium having been disturbed. Disequilibrium may pertain to the relationships between an individual and the worlds of which he or she is a part, including nature, society, the cosmos and the invisible. The Aka search for balance extends to food, where moderation in taste and quantity is preferred. Excess intake of food is considered to be life-threatening. The feeling of well-being associated with balance can only, in the Aka view, be obtained through a diet based around meat and honey. Meat is a sign of the hunter's prowess and is considered essential for health. Meat is obtained through hunting and skill in hunting requires clarity or peace of mind. Vital energy, intuition and keenness of eye are all attributes of the skilled hunter.[103]

The Masai of East Africa cook the bark of *Acacia goetzei* (Mimosaceae) and *Albizia anthelmintica* (Mimosaceae) with their traditional diet of boiled meat, milk and blood—sometimes described as 'the world's worst diet'. Research by Timothy Johns of McGill University has shown that combining the bark with the other foods results in cholesterol levels one-third that of the average American. Unique saponins in these plants are considered to be implicated in producing the cholesterol-lowering effects.[104]

The impact of traditional diet on health has been studied in Japan, where a high variety of foods, especially plant foods, is characteristic of a traditional Japanese diet. A Japanese survey of the diets of 200 elderly women revealed that they consumed a variety of over 100 biologically different foods per week. By contrast, in most Western countries the recommended minimum is only 30. The higher the variety, the less risk of many diseases, including cardiovascular disease, diabetes and many cancers. A high intake of soy products is also found in Japan: approximately 40 times more than the Western intake. Green tea, common in traditional Japanese diet, is rich in antioxidants (http://members.tripod.com).

Japanese who move overseas and adopt a Western-style diet have an increased risk of breast cancer, coronary heart disease and diabetes. Breast cancer is rare in Japan due to a low dietary fat intake, and a high intake of soy (with protective phyto-oestrogens), antioxidants and fibre. In addition, high food variety may be involved, as well as a possible genetic element. A low intake of meat is a major factor in the low bowel cancer rate in Japan. The traditional diet is based on the healthy combination of a high food variety, with minimal saturated fat, more fish, less meat, and especially more fruit, vegetables and grains.

In the context of tropical medicine, an understanding of traditional dietary practices can be helpful in the management and possibly the prevention of certain common conditions. It is an area worth enquiring into when taking a patient's history, as diet may include herbal ingredients that may influence the course of conventional treatment. More generally, the role of diet in the management of illness in the tropics is worthy of evaluation. While it will be complex to design dietary studies due to the multiple components in traditional diet, clinical and epidemiological research into the preventive and nutritional effects of traditional diet could examine their impact on the diseases which they have been used to combat in the tropics as well as on the emerging diseases of urban communities related to Western-style diet and lifestyle—particularly, diabetes, hypertension, stroke, heart disease and cancer.

Conclusion

Traditional medicine continues to exist in the tropics as a major source of health care for the majority of the population. National and international policies are calling for partnerships between conventional and traditional health practitioners in order to provide adequate health care coverage in the face of limited resources.

The tropical medicine practitioner may be faced with the negative effects of traditional medicine practice, such as renal and liver failure associated with improper use of traditional medicine; or, faced with unavailability of conventional medicines for common conditions, the tropical medicine practitioner might consider that partnerships with traditional practitioners in research-based practice are called for to evaluate possible traditional treatments for common conditions. In all cases, research ethics and medical ethics clearly take priority in evaluating and applying traditional treatments.

The move towards partnerships is clearly justified in the face of beneficial outcomes of such programmes in the fields of AIDS prevention and care and in reducing eye disease associated with traditional practices. Other research suggests that important discoveries may also result from such collaborative partnerships, expanding the range of treatment options available for the management of disease in the tropics.

REFERENCES

1   Homsy J, Katabira E, Kabatesi D, Mubiru F, Kwamya L, Tusaba C, Kasolo S, Mwebe D, Ssentamu L, Okello M & King R. Evaluating herbal medicine for the management of Herpes zoster in human immunodeficiency virus-infected patients in Kampala, Uganda. *J Altern Complement Med* 2000; 6(1):1–2.

2   Shankar D. The spiritual dimensions of medicinal plants in the Vedic tradition of India. In Posey D (ed.) *Cultural and Spiritual Values in Biodiversity*. Nairobi: UN Environment Programme, 2000.

3   Foster G Disease etiologies in non-western medical systems. *Am Anthropol* 1976; 78:773–782.

4   Berlin E & Berlin B. General overview Of Maya ethnomedicine. In Posey D (ed.) *Cultural and Spiritual Values in Biodiversity*. Nairobi: UN Environment Programme, 2000.

5   Zhang X. Integration of traditional and complementary medicine into national health care systems. *J Manipulative Physiol Ther* 2000; 23(2):139–140.

6   WHO SEARO (2000).

7   WHO. Guidelines for training traditional health practitioners in primary health care. Geneva: WHO Division of Strengthening of Health Services and Traditional Medicine, 1995 (unpublished).

8   Troskie T R. The importance of traditional midwives in the delivery of health care in the Republic of South Africa. *Curationis* 1997; 20(1):15–20.

9   WHO Regional Office for Africa. Report of a consultation on the coordination of activities relating to traditional medicine in the African region, Brazzaville, 2–6 July 1984. Brazzaville: WHO-AFRO (unpublished, ref. AFR/TRM/3).

10 WHO/UNICEF. *Primary Health Care: A Joint Report*. Geneva: WHO, 1978.

11 Kleinman A. *The Illness Narratives*. New York: Basic Books, 1988: 12.

12 Herron R E & Hillis S L. The impact of the Transcendental Meditation program on government payments to physicians in Quebec: an update. *Am J Health Promotion* 2000; 14(5):284–291.

13 Sharma H & Clarke C. Contemporary Ayurveda. London: Churchill-Livingstone, 1998.

14 Alderete W & Guevara G. South and Central America regional workshop on traditional health systems: GIFTS of health. Conclusions and recommendations, *J Altern Complement Med* 1996; 2(3):398–401.

15 Stephens C. Training urban traditional birth attendants: balancing international policy and local reality. Preliminary evidence from the slums of India on the attitudes and practice of clients and practitioners. *Soc Sci Med* 1992; 35(6):811–817.

16 Bannerman R H. *Traditional Medicine and Healthcare Coverage*. Geneva: WHO, 1983.

17 Shai-Mahoko S N. Indigenous healers in the North West Province: a survey of their clinical activities in health care in the rural areas. *Curationis* 1996; 19(4):31–34.

18 Shiferaw T (1993). Illness burden and use of health services in a rural community, southwestern Ethiopia. *East Afr Med J* 1993; 70(11):717–720.

19 Oskowitz B. Bridging the communication gap between traditional healers and nurses. *Nursing RSA* 1991; 6(7):20–22.

20 Ahmed I M, Bremer J J, Magzoub M M & Nouri A M. Characteristics of visitors to traditional healers in central Sudan. *Eastern Mediterranean Health J* 1999; 5(1):79–85.

21 Traore S, Coulibaly S O & Sidibe M. Comportements et coûts liés au Paludisme chez les femmes des campements de pêcheurs dans la zone de Sélingué au Mali. Institut National de Recherche en Santé Publique, Bamako, Mali. TDR/SER/PRS/12, 1993.

22 Elzubier AG, Ansari EHH, El Nour MH, Bella H. Knowledge and misconceptions about malaria among secondary school students and teachers in Kassala, Eastern Sudan. *J R Soc Health* 1997; 117(6):381–385.

23 Tanner M & Vlassoff C. Treatment-seeking behaviour for malaria: a typology based on endemicity and gender. *Soc Sci Med* 1998; 46(4–5):523–532.

24 Wilkinson D, Gcabashe L & Lurie M. Traditional healers as tuberculosis treatment supervisors: precedent and potential. *Int J Tuberc Lung Dis* 1999; 3(9):838–842.

25 Boerma J T & Baya M S. Maternal and child health in an ethnomedical perspective: traditional and modern medicine in coastal Kenya. *Health Policy Plann* 1990; 5(4):347–357.

26 Vissandjee B, Barlow R & Fraser D W. Utilization of health services among rural women in Gujarat, India. *Public Health* 1997; 111(3):135–148.

27 Agyepong I A & Manderson L. The diagnosis and management of fever at household level in the Greater Accra Region, Ghana. *Acta Tropica* 1994; 58:317–330.

28 Ruebush T K, Kern M K, Campbell C C & Oloo A J. Self-treatment of malaria in a rural of western Kenya. *Bull World Health Organ* 1995; 73:229–236.

29 Miguel C A, Manderson L & Lansang M A. Patterns of treatment for malaria in Tayabas, the Philippines: implications for control. *Trop Med Int Health* 1998; 3(5):413–421.

30 Miguel C A, Tallo V L, Manderson L & Lansang M A. Local knowledge and treatment of malaria in Agusan del Sur, the Philippines. *Soc Sci Med* 1999; 48:607–618.

31 Théra M A, Sissoko M S, Heuschkel C et al. Village level treatment of presumptive malaria: experiences with the training of mothers and traditional healers as resource persons in the Region of Mopti, Mali. In *Clone, Cure and Control: Tropical Health for the 21st Century: Second European Congress on Tropical Medicine*, Liverpool. Poster P72, 1999: 139.

32 Hausmann Muela S, Muela Ribera J, Tanner M. Fake malaria and hidden parasites – the ambiguity of malaria. *Anthropol Med* 1998; 5:43–61.

33 Bitahwa N, Tumwesigye O, Kabariime P, Tayebwa A K M, Tumwesigye S & Ogwal-Okeng J W. Herbal treatment of malaria: four case reports from the Rukararwe Partnership Workshop for Rural Development (Uganda). *Trop Doct* 1997; (suppl. 1):17–19.

34 Munguti K J. Community perceptions and treatment seeking for malaria in Baringo District, Kenya: implications for disease control. *East African Med J* 1998; 75(12):687–691.

35 Varga C A & Veale D J H. *Isihlambezo*: utilization patterns and potential health effects of pregnancy-related traditional herbal medicine. *Soc Sci Med* 1997; 44(7):911–924.

36 Ma G X. Between two worlds: the use of traditional and Western health services by Chinese immigrants. *J Commun Health* 1999; 24(6):421–437.

37 Bandyopadhyay M & MacPherson S. *Women and Health: Tradition and Culture in Rural India.* 1998.

38 Nichter M. Ethnomedicine: diverse trends, common linkages. Commentary. *Med Anthropol* 1991; 13:137–171.

39 Chi C. Integrating traditional medicine into modern health care systems: examining the role of Chinese medicine in Taiwan. *Soc Sci Med* 1994; 39(3):307–321.

40 Hall R L. Alcohol treatment in American Indian populations: an indigenous treatment modality compared with traditional approaches. *Ann NY Acad Sci* 1986; 472:168–178.

41 Maher P. A review of 'traditional' aboriginal health beliefs. *Aust J Rural Health* 1999; 7(4):229–236.

42 Last M & Chavanduka G L. *The Professionalisation of African Medicine.* Manchester: Manchester University Press, 1986.

43 Burnett A, Baggaley R, Ndovi-MacMillan M, Sulwe J, Hang'omba B & Bennett J. Caring for people with HIV in Zambia: are traditional healers and formal health workers willing to work together? *AIDS Care* 1999; 11(4):481–491.

44 Upvall M J. Nursing perceptions of collaboration with indigenous healers in Swaziland. *Int J Nurs Stud* 1992; 29(1):27–36.

45 Kabatesi D. Use of traditional treatments for AIDS-associated diseases in resource-constrained settings. In Robertson L, Bell K, Laypang L & Blake B (eds) *Health in the Commonwealth: Challenges and Solutions 1998/99.* London: Kensington Publications, 1998.

46 Baleta A. South Africa to bring traditional healers into mainstream medicine (news). *Lancet* 1998; 352:554.

47 Osuide G E. Regulation of herbal medicines in Nigeria: the role of the National Agency for Food and Drug Administration and Control (NAFDAC). Paper presented at the International Conference on Ethnomedicine and Drug Discovery, Silver Spring, MD, 3–5 November 1999.

48 Green E C. *AIDS and STDs in Africa: Bridging the Gap Between Traditional Healers and Modern Medicine.* Boulder, CO: Westview Press, 1994. (South African edition published by University of Natal Press, 1994).

49 Green E C. The participation of African traditional healers in AIDS/STD prevention programmes. *Trop Doct* 1997; 27(suppl. 1):56–59.

50 Nations M K, & de Souza M A. *Umbanda* healers as effective AIDS educators: case–control study in Brazilian urban slums (*favelas*). *Trop Doct* 1997; 27(suppl. 1):60–66.

51 Sebit M B, Chandiwana S K, Latif A S, Gomo E, Acuda S W, Makoni F & Vushe J. Quality of life evaluation in patients with HIV-1 infection: the impact of traditional medicine in Zimbabwe. *Cent Afr J Med* 2000; 46(8):208–213.

52 Asres K, Bucar F, Kartnig T, Witvrouw M, Pannecouque C & De Clercq E. Antiviral activity against human immunodeficiency virus type 1 (HIV-1) and type 2 (HIV-2) of ethnobotanically selected Ethiopian medicinal plants. *Phytother Res* 2001; 15(1):62–69.

53 Bodeker G, Kabatesi D, Homsy J & King R. A regional task force on traditional medicine and AIDS in East and Southern Africa. *Lancet* 2000; 355:1284.

54 Government of India. Indian Health Policy, 1999.

55 Zhan L, Yue S T, Xue Y X, Attele A S & Yuan C S. Effects of qian-kun-nin, a Chinese herbal medicine formulation, on HIV positive subjects: a pilot study. *Am J Chin Med* 2000; 28(3–4):305–312.

56 Chaudhury RR. A clinical protocol for the study of traditional medicine and human immunodeficiency virus-related illness.

Altern Complement Ther 2001; 7(5):553–566.

57 Kirby G C. Malaria and vector control. *Trop Doct* 1997; 27(suppl. 1):5–25.

58 Willcox M L. A clinical trial of 'AM', a Ugandan herbal remedy for malaria. *J Public Health Med* 1999; 21(3):318–324.

59 Bugmann N. Le concept du paludisme, l'usage et l'efficacité in vivo de trois traitements traditionnels antipalustres dans la région de Dori, Burkina Faso. Inaugural doctoral dissertation, Faculty of Medicine, University of Basel, 2000.

60 Gessler M C, Msuya D E, Nkunya M H, Schar A, Heinrich M & Tanner M. Traditional healers in Tanzania: sociocultural profile and three short portraits. *J Ethnopharmacol* 1995; 48(3):145–160.

61 Jayawardene R. Illness perception: social cost and coping strategies of malaria cases. *Soc Sci Med* 1993; 37:1169–1176.

62 Lipowsky R, Kroeger A & Vazquez M L. Sociomedical aspects of malaria control in Colombia. *Soc Sci Med* 1992; 34:625–637.

63 McCombie S C. Treatment seeking for malaria: a review of recent research. *Soc Sci Med* 1996; 43:933–945.

64 Pagnoni F, Convelbo N, Tiendrebeogo J, Cousens S & Esposito F. A community-based programme to provide prompt and adequate treatment of presumptive malaria in children. *Trans R Soc Trop Med Hyg* 1997; 91:512–517.

65 Rasoanaivo P, Ratsimamanga-Urverg S & Milijaona R. *In vitro* and *in vivo* chloroquine-potentiating action of *Strychnos myrtoides* alkaloids against chloroquine-resistant strains of Plasmodium malaria. *Planta Medica* 1994; 60:13–16.

66 Abyan I M & Osman A A. Social and behavioural factors affecting malaria in Somalia. TDR/SER/PRS/11, 1993.

67 Willcox & Bodeker. Herbal remedies for malaria: an overview of clinical studies. In Willcox M, Rasoanaivo P, Bodeker G (eds) *Traditional Medicine, Medicinal Plants and Malaria.* London: Harwood Press, 2002.

68 Bodeker G & Willcox M. New research initiative on plant-based antimalarials. *Lancet* 2000; 355:761.

69 Willcox M L, Cosentino M J, Pink R, Bodeker G & Wayling S. Natural products for the treatment of tropical diseases. *Trends Parasitol* 2001; 17(2):58–60.

70 Ryan T J. Global curriculum for wound management. *Trop Doct* 1997; 27(suppl. 1):31–35.

71 Ryan T J. The epidemiology of leg ulcers. In Westerhof W (ed.) *Leg Ulcers: Diagnosis and Treatment.* Amsterdam: Elsevier Science, 1993.

72 Robinson D C, Adriaans B, Hay R J & Yesudian P. The clinical and epidemiological features of the tropical ulcer (tropical phagedenic ulcer). *Int J Dermatol* 1988; 27:49–53.

73 Ryan T J. Wound healing in the developing world. *Dermatol Clin* 1993; 11:791–799.

74 Zeina B, Zohra B I, al-Assad S. The effects of honey on *Leishmania* parasites: an *in vitro* study. *Trop Doct* 1997; 27(suppl 1):36–38.

75 Ryan T J. International Foundation for Dermatology: solving the problems of skin disease in the developing world. *Trop Doct* 1992; 22(suppl. 1):42–43.

76 Hamman (1991).

77 Bodeker G & Hughes M A. Wound healing, traditional treatments and research policy. In Etkin N, Prendergast H & Houghton P (eds). *Modern Medicine and Traditional Remedies.* London: Kew Press, 1998.

78 Bodeker G. Lessons on integration from the developing world's experience. *BMJ* 2001; 322:164–167.

79 Bodeker G, Ryan T J & Ong C-K. Traditional approaches to wound healing. *Clin Dermatol* 1999; 17(1):93–98.

80 Bakhiet A & Adam S. Therapeutic utility, constituents and toxicity of some medicinal plants: a review. *Vet Hum Toxicol* 1995; 37(3):255–258.

81 Brantner A & Grein E. The antibacterial activity of plant

extracts used externally in traditional medicine. *J Ethnopharmacol* 1994; 44(1):35–40.

82 Sasaki S, Shinkai H, Akashi Y & Kishihara Y. Studies on the mechanism of action of asiaticoside (Madecassol) on experimental granulation tissue and cultured fibroblasts and its clinical application in systemic scleroderma. *Acta Dermato-Venerol* 1972; 52(2):141–150.

83 Suguna L, Sivakumar P & Chandrakasan G. Effects of *Centella asiatica* on dermal wound healing in rats. Indian *J Exp Biol* 1996; 34(12):1208–1211.

84 Heggers J P, Pelley R P & Robson M C. Beneficial effects of *Aloe* in wound healing. *Phytother Res* 1993; 7:S48–52.

85 Grindlay D, Reynolds T. The *Aloe Vera* phenomenon: a review of the properties and modern uses. *J Ethnopharmacol* 1986; 16:117–151.

86 Robson M C, Heggers J P & Hagstrom W J. Myth, magic, witchcraft or fact? *Aloe vera* revisited. *JBCR* 1982; 3:157–163.

87 Tran V H, Hughes M A & Cherry G W. *In vitro* studies on the antioxidant and growth stimulatory activities of a polyphenolic extract from *Cudrania cochinchinensis* used in the treatment of wounds in Vietnam. *Wound Repair Regen* 1997; 5:159–167.

88 Phan T T, Hughes M A, Cherry G W, Le T T & Pham H M. An aqueous extract of the leaves of *Chromolaena odorata* (Eupolin) inhibits hydrated collagen lattice contraction by normal human dermal fibroblasts. *J Altern Complement Med* 1996; 2:349–358.

89 Irobi O N. Activities of *Chromolaena odorata* (Compositae) cus faecallis. *J Ethnopharmacol* 1992; 37:81–83.

90 Chen Z P, Cai Y & Phillipson J D (1994). Studies on the antitumour, antibacterial and wound healing properties of dragon's blood. *Planta Med* 1994; 60:541–545.

91 Pieters L, de Bruyne T, van Poel B et al. *In vivo* wound healing of Dragon's blood (*Croton* spp.), a traditional South American drug, and its constituents. *Phytomedicine* 1995; 2:17–22.

92 Yorston D & Foster A. Traditional eye medicines and corneal ulceration in Tanzania. *J Trop Med Hyg* 1994; 97(4):211–214.

93 Mselle J. Visual impact of using traditional medicine on the injured eye in Africa. *Acta Trop* 1998; 70(2):185–192.

94 Courtright P, Lewallen S & Kanjaloti S. Changing patterns of corneal disease and associated vision loss at a rural African hospital following a training programme for traditional healers. *Br J Ophthalmol* 1996; 80(8):694–697.

95 Keane F M, Munn S E, du Vivier A W P, Taylor N F & Higgins E M. Analysis of Chinese herbal creams prescribed for dermatological conditions. *BMJ* 1999; 318:563–564.

96 Okada F. Kampo medicine, a source of drugs waiting to be exploited. *Lancet* 1996; 6 July.

97 Noller B N, Myers S, Abegaz B, Mohinder Singh M, Kronenberg F & Bodeker G. Report on the Global Forum on Safety of Herbal & Traditional Medicine. *J. Altern Complement Med* 2001; 7(5):583–601.

98 Roy Chaudhury R. *Herbal Medicine for Human Health*. New Delhi: WHO Regional Office for SE Asia, 1992.

99 Moore T J, Psaty B M & Furberg C D. Time to act on drug safety. *JAMA* 1998; 279(19):1571–1573.

100 Lazarou J, Pomeranz B H & Corey P N. Incidence of adverse drug reactions in hospitalized patients: a meta-analysis of prospective studies. *JAMA* 1998; 279(15):1200–1205.

101 Bodeker G. Traditional (i.e. indigenous) and complementary medicine in the Commonwealth: new partnerships planned with the formal health sector. *J Altern Complement Med* 1999; 5(1):97–101.

102 Etkin N. Antimalarial plants used by Hausa in northern Nigeria. *Trop Doct* 1997; 27(suppl.1):12–16.

103 Motte-Florac, Bahuchet S and Thomas J M C. The role of food in the therapeutics of the Central African Republic. In Hladik C M, Hladik A, Linars O F, Pagezy H, Semple A & Hadley M (eds). *Tropical Forests, People and Food: Biocultural Interactions and Applications to Development*. Man and the Biosphere Series, vol. 13. Paris: UNESCO and Parthenon Press, 1993.

104 Johns T, Mahunnah R L, Sanaya P et al. Saponins and phenolic content in plant dietary additives of a traditional subsistence community, the Batemi of Ngorongoro District, Tanzania. *J Ethnopharmacol* 1999; 66(1):1–10.

Chapter 5
Genetics

D. Kwiatkowski

Individual variation

Apart from identical twins, no two human beings are exactly alike. A range of variation is found in almost every characteristic that it is possible to quantify, whether it is a simple physical attribute such as height or something that is more complicated to measure, such as a hormone level. Sometimes there are striking differences between populations, for example in skin colour. But the phenomenon of human individuality goes much deeper than ethnic differences, and the vast majority of characteristics show significant variation within a single village or even within a single family. In this chapter, the characteristics that interest us are those that determine susceptibility to disease.

Since ancient times it has been debated whether nature or nurture is primarily responsible for individual variation—i.e., how much is due to genetics as opposed to environment. A substantial proportion of disease in the tropics is caused by environmental factors such as infectious agents or inadequate diet, so it might be thought that genetics would play a very small role, at least for the common ailments. Two lines of epidemiological evidence indicate that this view is incorrect. If a parent dies prematurely of infection then the children are more likely to die of infection, even if they are adopted in childhood and thus live in a different environment from the parent.[1] And the risk of developing tuberculosis,[2] leprosy[3] or malaria[4] has been demonstrated to have a significant heritable component by comparing monozygous twins (who are genetically identical) with dizygous twins (who are genetically related but not identical). Such observations, together with a growing body of molecular data, have led to the view that genetic factors play a role in almost all human disease, even if the primary cause is environmental. For example, genetic variation may partly explain why one child develops fatal cerebral malaria, or kwashiorkor, while other children living in the same compound are equally exposed to malaria parasites and to poor diet but do not develop these severe clinical syndromes. A huge amount of scientific effort is now being put into investigating the many different genetic factors that influence susceptibility to common diseases, in the hope that this will provide fundamental insights into molecular pathogenesis and ultimately lead to better methods of disease prevention.

Human disease genetics in the twentieth century was dominated by a set of rules deduced by Gregor Mendel in 1865. The observable characteristics that Mendel measured in his flowering peas, and that epidemiologists measure in human subjects, comprise the 'phenotype' of the individual. Mendelian rules apply when a specific genetic variant, for example a deletion or change in part of a DNA sequence, causes a predictable phenotypic change.[5] Humans normally have two copies of each gene: one from the mother and one from the father. A genetic effect is termed dominant if the phenotypic effect is observed in the heterozygote, i.e., when one copy of the gene is affected and the other copy is not. In this case, affected individuals typically receive the genetic variant from only one parent who is themselves affected. In contrast, a recessive effect is one where the affected phenotype is observed only in the homozygous state, i.e., when both copies of the gene are of the variant type. Here the affected individual must receive the genetic variant from both parents, who may or may not be affected themselves. Genes on the X and Y chromosomes are a special case, as females carry two copies of the X chromosome while males carry one X plus one Y chromosome: thus only one copy of a recessive X-linked genetic character is sufficient to cause the affected phenotype in a male. Based on these principles, clinical investigators have identified many major genetic diseases simply by analysing how the phenotype segregates in affected families. A classical example of a recessive effect is sickle cell disease, caused by a mutation that substitutes valine for glutamic acid in the sixth position of the β-globin chain. In homozygotes this causes anaemia and severe clinical complications resulting from major erythrocyte deformities at low oxygen saturations. Heterozygotes have a much milder phenotype and are normally asymptomatic. Thus the typical patient with sickle cell disease is born to heterozygous parents, who each carry one copy of the affected gene but have no overt manifestations of the disease. Molecular geneticists have now identified over 7000 forms of DNA variation that act in a Mendelian fashion to alter human phenotype.[6] Mendelian genetic diseases are mostly at low prevalence in the general population, with the notable exception of erythrocyte defects such as sickle cell disease and thalassaemia.

The challenge for the twenty-first century is to unravel the genetic basis of common human diseases which do not show a Mendelian pattern of inheritance. These include major infectious diseases such as malaria, HIV/AIDS and tuberculosis, as well as non-infectious conditions such as hypertension, diabetes, dementia and the different cancers. The lack of Mendelian inheritance simply indicates that these conditions are not determined by a single major gene. Probably hundreds of different genes are involved, interacting with each other as well as with multiple environmental risk factors. Up until now such complexity has been impossible to dissect, but this field has recently been revolutionized by the sequencing of the human genome, and by novel technologies that will permit analysis of many thousands of genetic variants at the epidemiological level.

Diversity of the human genome

A draft sequence of the human genome was published in early 2001 and should be completed by 2003.[7,8] The sequence is publicly available on Internet sites, which contain utilities for querying the database as well as much useful information about genetic aspects of common human diseases.[9,10] The total size of our genome is approximately 3000 million base pairs but genes that encode protein account for only a small proportion of this, and most of our DNA has no obvious useful function. Surprisingly we are estimated to have only about 30 000 genes, which seems a small number given that the fly has 13 000 and the worm has 18 000. This highlights the potential importance of gene regulation in determining uniquely human attributes. By the same token, a large part of human phenotypic diversity may stem from DNA polymorphisms that alter gene regulation rather than protein structure.

The term polymorphism is used to describe genetic variants that are found in a significant proportion (e.g. >1%) of the general population. The most common form of DNA variation, where one nucleotide is substituted for another, is called a single nucleotide polymorphism or SNP (pronounced 'snip'). Variation also commonly occurs in the number of repeat elements within highly repetitive areas of DNA sequence. This is known as a microsatellite polymorphism if the length of the repeated element is very small, while for larger elements it is known as a minisatellite or variable number tandem repeat (VNTR) polymorphism. Another type of variation is deletion or insertion of a segment of DNA which may range from one or two nucleotides to several kilobases.

Despite the recent explosion in the number of known polymorphisms[11] it will be many years before we have a comprehensive catalogue of common genetic variants. Extrapolating from existing data, it seems likely that the whole genome contains in the order of 10 million polymorphisms. A useful statistical measure is nucleotide diversity, which gives an estimate of how many differ-

ences are likely to be observed if the DNA sequences of two randomly selected chromosomes are compared. Typical values are around 1 difference per 2000 nucleotides, meaning that if the maternal and paternal chromosomes were compared within a single individual then over a million differences would probably be observed. Remarkably, the level of nucleotide diversity within an single African village is not much less that the values observed when chromosomes are randomly sampled from around the world. This reinforces a point which population geneticists have known for some time, namely that the level of genetic differentiation between human populations is low, relative to the amount of genetic diversity that is typically present within a single population. Overall, nucleotide diversity within Africa tends to be greater than in other populations, consistent with the view that modern humans migrated out of Africa relatively recently in our evolutionary history.

Selective pressure of infectious disease on the human genome

By far the most common group of genetic disorders worldwide are those that involve the red blood cell. They include disorders of haemoglobin regulation (α- and β-thalassaemia due to mutations that suppress production of α- and β-globin respectively); haemoglobin structure (sickle cell disease due to haemoglobin S, and other structural mutations of β-globin such as haemoglobin C and haemoglobin E), red cell enzymes (glucose-6-phosphate dehydrogenase deficiency due to *G6PD* mutations) and red cell ultrastructure (ovalocytosis due to mutations of the gene encoding band III protein). Although these genetic variants have different geographic distributions they share one remarkable feature, namely that all are commonest in populations whose ancestors were highly exposed to malaria. Over 50 years ago Haldane proposed an explanation, namely that these polymorphisms confer protection against malaria.[12]

There is now substantial evidence that Haldane's hypothesis is correct. The *HbS* allele, which encodes haemoglobin S, is a classical example of the evolutionary scenario known as balanced polymorphism, whereby heterozygotes are protected against malaria while the harmful genetic effects are restricted to homozygotes. African children who are heterozygous for *HbS* are 10 times less likely to develop life-threatening complications of *Plasmodium falciparum* infection than those who lack this allele, but they suffer none of the severe clinical problems seen in *HbS* homozygotes.[13] Different degrees of protection against severe malaria have been documented for the *HbC* allele and for *G6PD* variants in African populations, and for band III polymorphisms in Papua

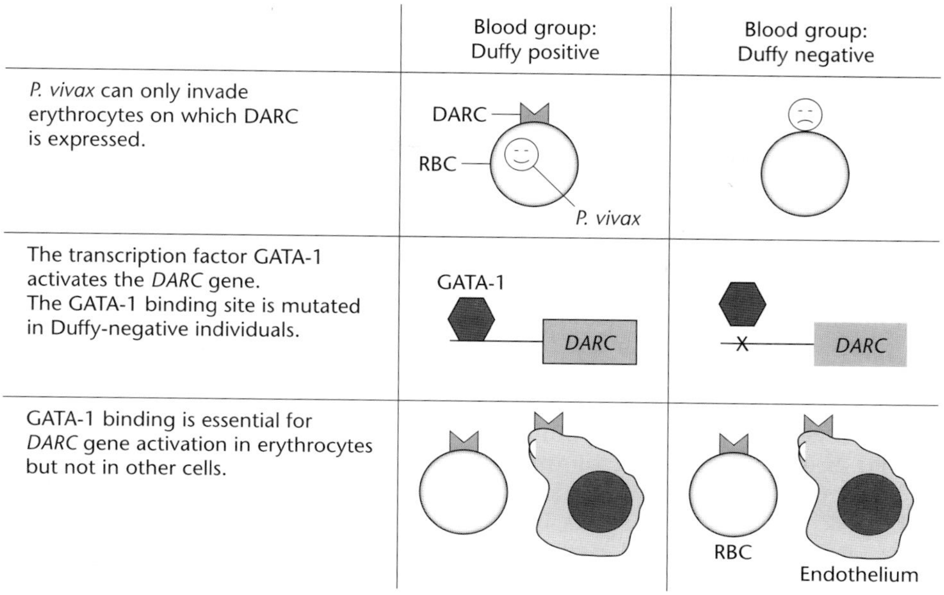

	Blood group: Duffy positive	Blood group: Duffy negative
P. vivax can only invade erythrocytes on which DARC is expressed.		
The transcription factor GATA-1 activates the *DARC* gene. The GATA-1 binding site is mutated in Duffy-negative individuals.		
GATA-1 binding is essential for *DARC* gene activation in erythrocytes but not in other cells.		

Figure 5.1: The malaria parasite *Plasmodium vivax* invades human erythrocytes by binding to Duffy antigen/chemokine receptor (DARC) expressed on the erythrocyte surface. Other parasite species such as *Plasmodium falciparum* invade erythrocytes through different receptors. Many West Africans have a single nucleotide polymorphism in the *DARC* promoter region that prevents binding of the erythroid transcription factor GATA-1, thus suppressing *DARC* expression in erythrocytes and leucocytes but not other cell types. This confers complete protection against infection with *P. vivax* but not against any other species of malaria parasite.[20,21]

New Guinea.[14–16] For α-thalassaemia there is a remarkably close epidemiological relationship between gene frequency and malarial endemicity,[17] but the precise protective role of this common genetic variant remains open to debate.[18,19]

The potential value of population genetics in elucidating fundamental aspects of infectious disease is beautifully illustrated by the story of Duffy blood group antigen. West Africans lack Duffy antigen on their erythrocytes because of a SNP in the corresponding gene, and this makes them highly resistant to infection with *P. vivax*.[20,21] (Figure 5.1). This discovery has yielded fundamental insights into the molecular mechanism by which malaria parasites invade human erythrocytes,[22] the type of information which could be invaluable in the development of an effective vaccine.

How has the selective pressure of infectious disease affected genetic diversity of the immune system? Certain HLA types appear to have risen to a high frequency in West Africa because of their protective effect against malaria,[13] but this is just the tip of the iceberg, and many similar examples for other infectious agents and for other immune genes undoubtedly remain to be discovered. It is also possible that non-infectious diseases are exacerbated by genetic factors that have been selected by infections suffered by previous generations. For example, the observation that *CD36* determines insulin resistance in hypertensive rats as well as being a host receptor for *P. falciparum*-infected erythrocytes has fuelled speculation about possible evolutionary relationships between malaria and susceptibility to diabetes or hypertensive disease.[23]

Genetic contribution to common diseases

There is now much information about those human diseases that are primarily caused by a major defect in a single gene.[6] They include a large number of fatal or highly debilitating diseases, such as muscular dystrophy, cystic fibrosis and Tay–Sachs disease, which are of huge consequence for the affected family, but fortunately they are relatively uncommon. From the perspective of the developing world, sickle cell disease and thalassaemia are of great importance but most other single-gene disorders are not major public health priorities. The commonest infectious and non-infectious diseases of the developing world are influenced by many different environmental factors plus a genetic component which is largely unknown but undoubtedly complex. Here we will consider two different ways in which genetic factors may contribute to common disease of complex aetiology.

At one end of the spectrum, even if many environmental and genetic variables influence the disease process, there may exist certain families where the predominant factor is a single gene. For example, in a population with an extremely high prevalence of *P. vivax* infection, where a small minority of individuals are Duffy negative, complete resistance to *P. vivax* is a rare phenomenon which segregates in certain families according to classical Mendelian rules. Another example is the group of genetic defects that result in severe immunodeficiency. In parts of the world with a high burden of infectious disease, it is extremely difficult for doctors and nurses to distinguish the child with congenital severe immunodeficiency from all the other infants and children who die of infectious causes. Thus a clinical syndrome such as 'infant death due to disseminated staphylococcal infection' is a highly complex phenotype, of which a small subgroup may come from families afflicted with a major genetic defect. Table 5.1 gives some examples of the 100 or so major genetic defects of the immune system that have been identified, mostly due to a rare mutation of a single gene. Apart from the importance of this information for affected families, it has provided valuable insights into the molecular and cellular basis of host immunity against different microbial species.

At the other end of the spectrum are genetic variants with a much more modest effect on disease susceptibility. In recent years there has been an explosion of information about DNA polymorphisms that appear to increase or decrease the risk of common diseases by a factor of 2 or even less. Being only a small part of a complex picture, such genetic effects do not show Mendelian segregation within families, but they can be detected by large-scale epidemiological studies such as case–control analysis. Why are scientists concerned about such weak genetic effects? Even a modest genetic effect may be of considerable public health importance if it acts on an extremely common disease, and if many different genes each make a modest contribution then the overall genetic effect may be huge. And even modest association with specific genetic variants may be sufficient to gain novel insights into the molecular pathogenesis of common diseases—by providing categorical evidence about the host factors that are involved—that may point to new strategies for treating or preventing the disease. Table 5.2 lists some genetic polymorphisms that have

been associated with susceptibility to common infectious diseases, and here we will discuss the possible significance of a few of these associations.

Table 5.1 Severe immunodeficiency disorders.

System involved	Typical clinical syndrome	Example of genetic defect
B lymphocyte	Recurrent bacterial infection due to defective antibody production	B cell cytoplasmic tyrosine kinase CD40 ligand
T lymphocyte	Severe bacterial, viral and fungal infection due to defective humoral and cellular immunity	Interleukin-2 receptor γ chain Adenosine deaminase
Neutrophil	Severe bacterial infection due to defective phagocytosis	Cytochrome b558 Integrin β chain
Macrophage	Extreme susceptibility to infection with environmental mycobacteria	Interferon-γ receptor
Complement	Recurrent *Neisseria* infection	Terminal complement

Almost 100 severe deficiency disorders have been identified. Each is caused by a rare mutation of a single gene. Different mutations in the same gene may cause subtle variations in clinical phenotype. Mutations of different genes may lead to similar clinical syndromes if they disrupt a common immune pathway.

Table 5.2 Examples of candidate gene associations with common infectious diseases.

Infection	Candidate gene region		Selected references
HIV/AIDS	CCR5/CCR2	chemokine receptor	25, 33
	HLA class I	antigen presentation	
Hepatitis B	HLA class II	antigen presentation	28
Meningococcal disease	C5 to C9	terminal complement pathway	49
	MBL	opsonization	
Tuberculosis	HLA-DR	antigen presentation	26, 44
	NRAMP1	divalent cation transporter	
	VDR	vitamin D receptor	
Leprosy	HLA class II	antigen presentation	27, 36
	TNF	pro-inflammatory cytokine	
Malaria	DARC	chemokine receptor	13, 15, 17, 20, 21, 35
	α- and β-globin	haemoglobin subunits	
	G6PD	carbohydrate metabolism	
	HLA class I and II	antigen presentation	
	TNF	pro-inflammatory cytokine	
Leishmaniasis	TNF	pro-inflammatory cytokine	38

Gene regions in which allelic variants have been associated with increased or decreased susceptibility to infectious disease. Often the variant allele is common in the population (e.g., above 10%) but the alteration in disease risk is relatively modest (e.g., two- to fourfold). These examples probably represent a small minority of the total number of genetic factors involved. By dissecting the functional basis of such genetic associations, through detailed epidemiological and experimental analyses of the candidate gene regions in question, it may be possible to gain important insights into the molecular basis of immunity and pathogenesis.

The great diversity of human leucocyte antigens (HLA), which act to present antigens for recognition by T lymphocytes, is postulated to have arisen as a host strategy to counter antigenic diversity in infectious organisms. The theory that heterozygosity of HLA alleles is an advantage, as it allows the immune system to 'see' a wider range of antigens, is supported by recent investigations of persistent hepatitis B infection[24] and HIV-1[25] although it was not evident in a large study of susceptibility to severe malaria.[13] Attempts to identify HLA types that confer resistance or susceptibility to specific pathogens have for the most part been inconclusive, possibly reflecting geographical and temporal fluctuation in critical microbial antigens, but a few general themes have emerged. Several studies in Asian populations and elsewhere have identified HLA-DR2 as a risk factor for susceptibility to tuberculosis and leprosy.[26,27] HLA-DRB1*1302 has been associated with resistance to chronic hepatitis B infection in both African and European populations.[28,29] HLA-B*35 is associated with rapid progression of HIV-1 infection in Caucasian populations[25,30,31] and other associations have also been reported. HLA-B*5301 and HLA-DRB1*1302 show independent and highly significant associations with protection from severe malaria in West Africa[13] but these associations do not appear to hold in East Africa.

The human chemokine receptors CCR5 and CCR2 serve as co-receptors with CD4 for entry as a virus into macrophages. Several studies have found that common variants in these genes confer resistance to AIDS progression after infection.[32] Current evidence suggests that this is a complex effect arising from at least three independent loci within the CCR5 and CCR2 gene regions, including a possibly functional variant of the CCR5 promoter region which (unlike the other variant alleles) appears to increase the rate of AIDS progression.[33]

Pro-inflammatory cytokines such as tumour necrosis factor (TNF) which act as powerful agents of innate immunity against infection, but which are also responsible for severe pathological complications of infectious disease if secreted in excess, have attracted considerable interest as potential susceptibility genes in a range of infectious diseases. Three different SNPs located within a short stretch of the TNF promoter region appear to be independently associated with susceptibility to severe malaria in African children.[34,35] Since the TNF gene is located within the major histocompatibility complex (MHC) it is important to note that these associations appear to be independent of HLA class 1 and class 2 types which, as noted above, are associated with protection from severe malaria. TNF promoter polymorphisms have also been associated with susceptibility to lepromatous leprosy,[36] scaring trachoma,[37] mucocutaneous leishmaniasis[38] and susceptibility to fatal outcome in patients with meningococcal septicaemia.[39] However the precise functional significance of these polymorphisms remains uncertain; some experimental studies indicate that they alter levels of TNF production but the evidence is not conclusive at present.

One approach to discovering human disease genes for complex diseases is to identify mouse strains that differ in disease susceptibility and then, by a process of cross-breeding and genetic mapping, to track down some of the genes responsible. A classical example is a gene identified through a laborious and systematic effort to identify genetic locus for resistance to infection with mycobacteria, *Salmonella* and *Leishmania* in certain inbred strains of mice[40] (*Salmonella typhimurium*)[41] (*Leishmania*).[42,43] The gene responsible was located by positional cloning: it is known as natural resistance-associated macrophage protein 1 (*NRAMP1*), and it seems to be divalent cation transporter. What do these elegant and comprehensive studies tell us about human susceptibility to mycobacterial, salmonella and leishmanial infections? From available data it would seem that humans do not commonly possess major disruptive muations of *NRAMP1* as seen in susceptible mouse strains, but more subtle mutations in areas of DNA that may be involved in *NRAMP1* regulation have been associated with susceptibility to pulmonary tuberculosis in West Africans.[44] This provides yet another example of the novel information about host defence mechanisms that can be gained through the genetic approach.

The future of genetic epidemiology

The classical genetic approach used to study Mendelian disease, i.e., single gene defects with major clinical consequences, is known as linkage analysis. This has two essential components. Firstly, it requires families with more than one case of the disease, ideally extensive pedigrees with several affected individuals. Secondly, it requires highly polymorphic genetic markers distributed throughout the genome, which are used to localize chromosomal regions that segregate with disease susceptibility within families. Of the thousands of major single gene defects that are now known, most have been discovered through this approach. These include severe defects of the immune system, some of which are given in Table 5.1, and important diseases such as cystic fibrosis and muscular dystrophy.

Over the past decade much effort has gone into applying the genetic linkage approach to common diseases which lack Mendelian inheritance patterns but which are known from epidemiological evidence, e.g., twin studies, to have a significant heritable component. Since it can be difficult to ascertain pedigrees with large numbers of affected individuals, one popular strategy has been to recruit a large number of families with just two or more affected siblings, and to apply a statistical technique known as affected sib-pair analysis. This approach has recently scored some major successes, including the identification of *calpain* as a susceptibility gene for maturity-onset diabetes, and *NOD2* as a susceptibility gene for Crohn's disease. However, this approach is not without difficulties, as it may miss genes with complex or modest effects on the disease phenotype, and it is a huge amount of work to progress from the initial observation of a susceptibility locus (typically a chromosomal region of around 10 million bases, which may harbour over a hundred genes) to the formal identification of the mutation or mutations responsible, within a specific gene. Genetic linkage studies of affected families in the tropics have revealed susceptibility loci for schistosomiasis (in the chromosomal region 5q31–33), malaria (also on chromosome 5), leprosy and tuberculosis (on the X chromosome). These are important findings and major efforts are now being made to find the genes responsible. However, it is becoming increasingly clear that common diseases could be determined by a large number of different genetic factors, most of which would not be apparent using the genetic linkage approach unless the sample size was vast.

A more statistically powerful method of detecting a genetic effect is to test for disease association. The simplest approach is a case–control study, where the frequency of a particular genetic variant is measured in diseased individuals, and compared with controls recruited from exactly the same ethnic group. To understand why ethnic matching is so important, consider a mixed population within which a certain ethnic group is liable to develop a specific disease for entirely sociocultural reasons. In this case, a random sample of disease cases will contain a higher proportion of this ethnic group than is found in the general population, and there is a danger that apparent 'genetic associations' may simply reflect ethnic differences rather than true disease susceptibility genes. In most of the disease association studies described in Table 5.2, some attempt has been made to ensure ethnic matching of cases and controls, but this can be difficult to achieve with certainty. This has led to growing interest in intrafamilial association studies, where the distribution of genotypes amongst index cases is compared with that predicted from their parental genotypes using statistical techniques such as the transmission disequilibrium test.[45] This method, although somewhat less statistically powerful than a well-conducted case–control study, excludes the possibility of ethnic artifact.[46] As the number of polymorphisms under investigation grows dramatically, there is increasing requirement for a large sample size to permit multiple comparisons: clearly a P value of 0.05 may be of little significance if this is only one of 100 polymorphisms that are being assessed in the same study. With a realistic prospect that, within the next decade, it will become feasible to screen for association with polymorphic markers in every known human gene, sample sizes in the order of 2000 are likely to be required to validate genetic associations that give a doubling or a halving of relative risk.[47,48]

Discovering a genetic association is not the end of the story. Every polymorphism shows a greater or lesser degree of association with neighbouring polymorphisms (a phenomenon known as linkage disequilibrium). So when we find a disease association with a polymorphism in gene X, the next step is to search for other polymorphisms in the region of X, and then to compare the strength of disease association with different combinations of linked polymorphisms (known as haplotypes), in order to dissect the causative polymorphism from linked markers that are functionally irrelevant. If gene X is just one of a large number of environmental and genetic factors that determine disease susceptibility, then the process of fine-mapping may be extremely complex (e.g., it is much more difficult for diabetes than for cystic fibrosis) and this is the area where the most questions remain about the feasibility of the new genetic approach to the analysis of common human diseases.

How is genetics going to shape medical practice?

What is the practical purpose of understanding the molecular genetic basis of susceptibility to infection? Efforts to develop vaccines and improved treatments for major diseases such as tuberculosis, HIV/AIDS and malaria are hindered by our poor understanding of the molecular and cellular mechanisms that determine clinical outcome. Genetic epidemiology may identify novel molecular mechanisms and improve understanding of critical events in the evolution of disease. For example, if an infectious disease is associated with high levels of factor X in the blood, it is often difficult to know whether this is of pathogenic importance or simply an epiphenomenon of the disease process. But if the production of factor X is known to be determined by a genetic polymorphism, and if this polymorphism is shown to predispose to the disease in question, then there is a much stronger case for factor X playing a causal role.

The human genome project has generated huge expectations but it will take decades for the full clinical implications to be revealed. For severe genetic disorders, detailed understanding of the molecular causes will improve diagnostic screening and genetic counselling, and will spawn novel therapeutic strategies including gene therapy. But for common human diseases, the long-term impact of genetic research will be at the level of the population rather than the individual patient. Genetic epidemiology provides a potentially powerful way of identifying the critical molecular events required for an infectious agent to invade the human host, and for the host to eradicate or succumb to the infection. This information is likely to revolutionize the process of drug discovery and vaccine development, a point that has already been taken on board by many of the major pharmaceutical agencies.

Humankind has evolved in a hostile microbial environment, and natural selection by infectious disease may be one of the major causes of human genetic diversity, particularly in the immune system. The high frequency of the sickle haemoglobin gene in West Africa, which has arisen because of its protective effect against malaria and despite the lethal nature of the homozygous state, gives some idea of the strength of genetic selection that may be involved. It is possible that some Western ailments such as atopy and autoimmune disease are a legacy of the evolutionary impact of infectious disease, where immune gene variants selected for protection against parasites and other infectious pathogens may have deleterious effects in an increasingly hygienic environment. A deeper understanding of the genetic factors that determine susceptibility to major infectious diseases in the tropics may eventually provide clues to the prevention of wide range of non-infectious diseases in populations around the world.

REFERENCES

1 Sorensen T I, Nielsen G G, Andersen P K & Teasdale T W. Genetic and environmental influences on premature death in adult adoptees. *N Engl J Med* 1988; 318(12):727–732.

2 Comstock G W. Tuberculosis in twins: a re-analysis of the Prophit survey. *Am Rev Respir Dis* 1978; 117(4):621–624.

3 Fine P E. Immunogenetics of susceptibility to leprosy, tuberculosis, and leishmaniasis: an epidemiological perspective. *Int J Lepr Other Mycobact Dis* 1981; 49(4):437–454.

4 Jepson A P, Banya W A, Sisay-Joof F, Hassan-King M, Bennett S & Whittle H C. Genetic regulation of fever in Plasmodium falciparum malaria in Gambian twin children. *J Infect Dis* 1995; 172(1):316–319.

5 Strachan T & Read A P. *Human Molecular Genetics*, 2nd edn. Oxford, UK: BIOS Scientific Publishers, 1999.

6 http://www.ncbi.nlm.nih.gov/Omim/. Online Mendelian inheritance in man.

7 Lander E S, Linton L M, Birren B et al. Initial sequencing and analysis of the human genome. *Nature* 2001; 409(6822):860–921.

8 Venter J C, Adams M D, Myers E W et al. The sequence of the human genome. *Science* 2001; 291(5507):1304–1351.

9 http://www.ncbi.nlm.nih.gov/genome/guide/. Human Genome Resources.

10 http://www.wellcome.ac.uk/en/genome/.

11 http://snp.cshl.org/. The SNP Consortium.

12 Haldane J B S. Disease and evolution. *Ricerca Sci* 1949; 19 (suppl. 1):3–10.

13 Hill A V, Allsopp C E, Kwiatkowski D et al. Common west African HLA antigens are associated with protection from severe malaria. *Nature* 1991; 352(6336):595–600.

14 Agarwal A, Guindo A, Cissoko Y et al. Hemoglobin C associated with protection from severe malaria in the Dogon of Mali, a west African population with a low prevalence of hemoglobin S. *Blood* 2000; 96(7):2358–2363.

15 Ruwende C, Khoo S C, Snow R W et al. Natural selection of hemi- and heterozygotes for G6PD deficiency in Africa by resistance to severe malaria. *Nature* 1995; 376(6537):246–249.

16 Genton B, al-Yaman F, Mgone C S et al. Ovalocytosis and cerebral malaria (letter). *Nature* 1995; 378(6557):564–565.

17 Flint J, Hill A V, Bowden D K et al. High frequencies of alpha-thalassaemia are the result of natural selection by malaria. *Nature* 1986; 321(6072):744–750.

18 Williams T N, Maitland K, Bennett S et al. High incidence of malaria in alpha-thalassaemic children. *Nature* 1996; 383(6600):522–525.

19 Allen S J, O'Donnell A, Alexander N D et al. alpha+-Thalassemia protects children against disease caused by other infections as well as malaria. *Proc Natl Acad Sci USA* 1997; 94(26):14736–14741.

20 Miller L H, Mason S J, Clyde D F & McGinniss M H. The resistance factor to Plasmodium vivax in blacks: the Duffy-blood-group genotype, FyFy. *N Engl J Med* 1976; 295(6):302–304.

21 Tournamille C, Colin Y, Cartron J P & Le Van Kim C. Disruption of a GATA motif in the Duffy gene promoter abolishes erythroid gene expression in Duffy-negative individuals. *Nat Genet* 1995; 10(2):224–228.

22 Chitnis C E & Miller L H. Identification of the erythrocyte binding domains of Plasmodium vivax and Plasmodium knowlesi proteins involved in erythrocyte invasion. *J Exp Med* 1994; 180(2):497–506.

23 Aitman T J, Cooper L D, Norsworthy P J et al. Malaria susceptibility and CD36 mutation. *Nature* 2000; 405(6790):1015–1016.

24 Thursz M R, Thomas H C, Greenwood B M & Hill A V. Heterozygote advantage for HLA class-II type in hepatitis B virus infection (letter; published erratum appears in *Nat Genet* 1998; 18(1):88). *Nat Genet* 1997; 17(1):11–12.

25 Carrington M, Nelson G W, Martin M P et al. HLA and HIV-1: heterozygote advantage and B*35-Cw*04 disadvantage. *Science* 1999; 283(5408):1748–1752.

26 Singh S P, Mehra N K, Dingley H B, Pande J N & Vaidya M C. Human leukocyte antigen (HLA)-linked control of susceptibility to pulmonary tuberculosis and association with HLA-DR types. *J Infect Dis* 1983; 148(4):676–681.

27 Todd J R, West B C & McDonald J C. Human leukocyte antigen and leprosy: study in northern Louisiana and review. *Rev Infect Dis* 1990; 12(1):63–74.

28 Thursz M R, Kwiatkowski D, Allsopp C E, Greenwood B M, Thomas H C & Hill A V. Association between an MHC class II allele and clearance of hepatitis B virus in the Gambia. *N Engl J Med* 1995; 332(16):1065–1069.

29 Hohler T, Gerken G, Notghi A et al. HLA-DRB1*1301 and *1302 protect against chronic hepatitis B. *J Hepatol* 1997; 26(3):503–507.

30 Itescu S, Mathur-Wagh U, Skovron M L et al. HLA-B35 is associated with accelerated progression to AIDS. *J Acquir Immune Defic Syndr* 1992; 5(1):37–45.

31 Sahmoud T, Laurian Y, Gazengel C, Sultan Y, Gautreau C & Costagliola D. Progression to AIDS in French haemophiliacs: association with HLA-B35. *Aids* 1993; 7(4):497–500.

32 Dean M, Carrington M, Winkler C et al. Genetic restriction of HIV-1 infection and progression to AIDS by a deletion allele of the CKR5 structural gene. Hemophilia Growth and Development Study, Multicenter AIDS Cohort Study, Multicenter Hemophilia Cohort Study, San Francisco City Cohort, ALIVE Study (published erratum appears in *Science* 1996; 274(5290):1069). *Science* 1996; 273(5283):1856–1862.

33 Martin M P, Dean M, Smith M W et al. Genetic acceleration of AIDS progression by a promoter variant of CCR5. *Science* 1998; 282(5395):1907–1911.

34 McGuire W, Hill A V, Allsopp C E, Greenwood B M & Kwiatkowski D. Variation in the TNF-alpha promoter region associated with susceptibility to cerebral malaria. *Nature* 1994; 371(6497):508–510.

35 Knight J C, Udalova I, Hill A V et al. A polymorphism that affects OCT-1 binding to the TNF promoter region is associated with severe malaria. *Nat Genet* 1999; 22(2):145–150.

36 Roy S, McGuire W, Mascie-Taylor C G et al. Tumor necrosis factor promoter polymorphism and susceptibility to lepromatous leprosy. *J Infect Dis* 1997; 176(2):530–532.

37 Conway D J, Holland M J, Bailey R L et al. Scarring trachoma is associated with polymorphism in the tumor necrosis factor

alpha (TNF-alpha) gene promoter and with elevated TNF-alpha levels in tear fluid. *Infect Immun* 1997; 65(3):1003–1006.

38 Cabrera M, Shaw M A, Sharples C et al. Polymorphism in tumor necrosis factor genes associated with mucocutaneous leishmaniasis. *J Exp Med* 1995; 182(5):1259–1264.

39 Nadel S, Newport M J, Booy R & Levin M. Variation in the tumor necrosis factor-alpha gene promoter region may be associated with death from meningococcal disease. *J Infect Dis* 1996; 174(4):878–880.

40 Plant J & Glynn A A. Genetics of resistance to infection with Salmonella typhimurium in mice. *J Infect Dis* 1976; 133(1):72–78.

41 Bradley D J. Regulation of Leishmania populations within the host. II. Genetic control of acute susceptibility of mice to Leishmania donovani infection. *Clin Exp Immunol* 1977; 30(1):130–140.

42 Vidal S M, Malo D, Vogan K, Skamene E & Gros P. Natural resistance to infection with intracellular parasites: isolation of a candidate for Bcg. *Cell* 1993; 73(3):469–485.

43 Blackwell J M, Barton C H, White J K et al. Genomic organization and sequence of the human NRAMP gene: identification and mapping of a promoter region polymorphism. *Mol Med* 1995; 1(2):194–205.

44 Bellamy R, Ruwende C, Corrah T, McAdam K P, Whittle H C & Hill A V. Variations in the NRAMP1 gene and susceptibility to tuberculosis in West Africans. *N Engl J Med* 1998; 338(10):640–644.

45 Spielman R S, McGinnis R E & Ewens W J. Transmission test for linkage disequilibrium: the insulin gene region and insulin-dependent diabetes mellitus (IDDM). *Am J Hum Genet* 1993; 52(3):506–516.

46 Lander E S & Schork N J. Genetic dissection of complex traits (published erratum appears in *Science* 1994; 266(5184):353). *Science* 1994; 265(5181):2037–2048.

47 Risch N & Merikangas K. The future of genetic studies of complex human diseases. *Science* 1996; 273(5281):1516–1517.

48 Risch N J. Searching for genetic determinants in the new millennium. *Nature* 2000; 405(6788):847–856.

49 Hibberd M L, Sumiya M, Summerfield J A, Booy R & Levin M. Association of variants of the gene for mannose-binding lectin with susceptibility to meningococcal disease. Meningococcal Research Group. *Lancet* 1999; 353(9158):1049–1053.

Chapter 6
Immunological Aspects of Tropical Diseases

A. Zumla, A. Sa'adu and I. Roitt

Introduction

The host is a continuous battleground between the immune system of the body[1] and invading antigens, whether they are micro-organisms,[2] chemicals or cancer cells. At-risk patients are commonplace in the tropics because of malnutrition, HIV/AIDS, high parasite load, cancers, alcoholism, chronic renal and hepatic diseases, famine and poverty. While a vast amount of literature is accumulating on the subject of immune responses to pathogens,[3] the mechanisms underlying specific immunity to many micro-organisms remain unknown.[4] Paradoxically, while the immune response has evolved to confer protection against invading antigens, much human pathology arises when the immune responses are evoked[5–8] (Tables 6.1 and 6.2).

Immunology impinges on the practice of tropical medicine[4] in four main ways:

1. Firstly, protective immunity to particular tropical parasitic infections is frequently inadequate and sometimes non-existent; this affects both the normal course of the disease and the prospects for vaccination.
2. Secondly, the prolonged ineffective immune responses can give rise to serious immunopathological consequences.
3. Thirdly, people afflicted with tropical infections often suffer a general immunodeficiency that weakens their response to normally mild infections.
4. Fourthly, the monitoring of immune responses, even when they are not protective, can often be of help in diagnosis and management.

Components of the immune system

The human immune system, which has evolved to resist infection by micro-organisms, has traditionally been classified into two parts:

Table 6.1 Immunopathological consequences of tropical infections.

Hypersensitivity type*	Mechanism involved	Examples
Type I (allergic) (anaphylactic)	IgE Mast cells, basophils IgE, mast cells	*Ascaris* larvae (lung) Schistosomiasis (swimmers' itch) Hydatid cyst leak/rupture
Type II (antibody-mediated)	IgG Complement Autoantibody	Malaria anaemia? Goodpasture's syndrome Chagas' disease (*T. cruzi*) Streptococci (rheumatic heart disease, glomerulonephritis)
Type III (immune complex)	Immune complexes Complement Neutrophils	Malaria (kidney) Trypanosomiasis Schistosomiasis (Katayama fever) Streptococci Serum sickness Pulmonary eosinophilia
Type IV (cell-mediated)	T cells Cytokines Macrophages	Schistosomiasis (egg granuloma) Tuberculosis Tuberculoid leprosy Lymphatic filariasis Lung flukes (paragonimiasis)

*Gell and Coombs' classification.

Table 6.2 Immunopathology associated with acute bacterial infections.

Bacteria	Toxins	Disease
Staphylococci	Enterotoxin A Enterotoxin B Enterotoxin C1–3 Enterotoxin D Enterotoxin E	Food poisoning

	Toxin shock
	  syndrome toxins
		Toxic shock
		  syndrome

	Exfoliating toxin A	Scaled-skin syndrome
	Exfoliating toxin B	

Group A
streptococci
	Pyrogenic
	  exotoxin A
		Streptococcal sore
		  throat

	Pyrogenic exotoxin B	
	Pyrogenic exotoxin C	
	Pyrogenic exotoxin D	
	Erythrogenic exotoxin	Scarlet fever
	Haemolysis exotoxin	Erysipelas
Clostridium perfringens	enterotoxin	Gas gangrene
Yersinia enterocolitica	enterotoxin	Terminal ileitis
Mycoplasma arthritidis	exotoxin	Arthritis
Gram-negative bacteria	(Endotoxin, LPS)	Gram-negative shock

1. The *non-specific immune system* consisting of:
   (a) External barriers.
   (b) Innate immune system.
2. The *specific immune system*, or the acquired immune response.

Non-specific immunity: external barriers

External barriers (Figure 6.1) are normal mechanical and physiological properties of the host, which include:

(a) Skin (e.g., keratin, sebum, normal flora).
(b) Mucosal surfaces (e.g., intestinal, vaginal, cornea).
(c) Flushing mechanisms (e.g., urinating, ciliary movement).
(d) Enzymes (e.g., gut, tears).
(e) Normal microbial flora (e.g., commensals in skin, gut, vagina).

Skin

The skin is probably the most important physical barrier to invading micro-organisms. The skin secretes sebum which inhibits growth of mico-organisms. The skin's normal microflora compete with pathogenic organisms.

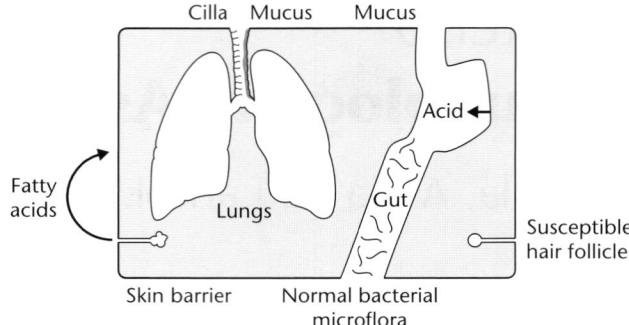

Figure 6.1: The first lines of defence against infection: protection at the external body surfaces. (Redrawn with permission from Roitt, I. & Delves, P., *Roitt's Essential Immunology*, 10th edn, © 2001 Blackwell Science Inc., Oxford.)

This effect, called 'colonization inhibition', is also seen in the gut and pharynx. The physical barrier of the skin is usually only overcome when it is breached by scratches, wounds, bites, burns, trauma or injections.

Abrasions, ulcers, trauma
Breach in the continuity of the skin permits entry of skin pathogens such as staphylococci, streptococci or leptospira.

Insect bites
A number of infectious agents have used the vehicle of blood-sucking insects to get through the skin. Transmission by blood-sucking insects is a good example of how a resourceful parasite overcomes the external skin barrier and simultaneously solves the problem of spreading in a thinly populated country, but of course it also restricts the parasite to areas where the vector flourishes. They are further restricted to flourish in warmer parts of the world because they are not able to complete their life cycles in colder climates when their insect hosts assume the temperature of the environment. Nevertheless, only a tiny minority of potential parasites actually succeed in gaining a foothold in man. When they do, the responsibility for dislodging them passes to the adaptive immune system.

Active penetration by parasite larvae
Helminth parasites such as hookworm larvae and schistosome cercariae invade the human skin by use of proteolytic enzymes before gaining entry into the bloodstream.

Injections and razors
The use of contaminated needles and razors (traditional medicine cuts) breaches the skin and may enable bacteria and fungi to cause septicaemia. They may also transmit hepatitis viruses, HIV, malaria and trypanosomes.

Mucosal surfaces
Mucosal surfaces are not keratinized and thus are prone to invasion by bacteria and viruses. However, natural defences occur at mucosal surfaces[9] and these include:

(a) Ciliary movement to expel the debris.
(b) Surface phagocytes.
(c) Enzymes and surface antibody (secretory IgA).
(d) Mechanical washing by tears or urine.
(e) Bacteriocins from normal flora.

There are a number of physico-chemical barriers which provide important mechanisms for limiting infectious agents. These include the tears from the eyes, lysozyme in saliva, ear wax and vaginal acidity. The mechanical barrier produced by the cilia and mucus of the respiratory tract traps 95% of inhaled organisms. The constant flow of bile in the biliary system as well as continuous production and flow of urine are other important mechanisms by which invading micro-organisms may be kept at bay.

Commensal microbial flora

The role of the normal flora of the mouth, the vagina and the alimentary and urinary tracts deserves special mention. The human host provides a safe haven for these less harmful bacteria, which are then able to antagonize and prevent the flourishing of pathogenic bacteria. The facultative and obligate aerobes produce potent inhibitors of bacterial growth called bacteriocins, which act to inhibit the growth of competing organisms. In addition, many obligate anaerobes produce free fatty acids and alter the local redox potential, making the environment less supportive to other micro-organisms. This delicate balance can be upset by disease or by the use of antibiotics. There is an increasing scientific and commercial interest in the use of beneficial micro-organisms, or 'probiotics', for the prevention and treatment of disease. The micro-organisms more frequently used as probiotic agents are lactic acid bacteria such as *Lactobacillus rhamnosus* GG

(LGG), which has been extensively studied in recent literature. Multiple mechanisms of action have been postulated, including lactose digestion, productive anti-microbial agents, competition for space or nutrients and immunomodulation. Studies of paediatric diarrhoea show substantial evidence of clinical benefits from probiotic therapy in patients with viral gastroenteritis, and data on LGG treatment for *Clostridium difficile* diarrhoea appear promising. However, data to support use of probiotics for prevention of traveller's diarrhoea are more limited.[10]

Parasite evasion mechanisms for avoiding innate immunity

Complex multicellular micro-organisms such as helminths have developed extensive strategies, not only for gaining access through direct intact skin, but also for migrating through subcutaneous tissues of the body until they reach their favourite habitats where they can thrive and multiply. In the tropics most infectious agents (apart from a few helminths such as cercariae of schistosomes and larvae of hookworm) use the faecal—oral route to overcome the external barriers. This route is more effective in tropical areas where clean water supplies are not highly organized and where sanitary facilities are often rudimentary. Clearly external barriers, while highly effective in preventing infections with harmless agents, are relatively ineffective against highly virulent organisms.

Non-specific immune system: innate immune responses

These can be divided into those that are mediated by:

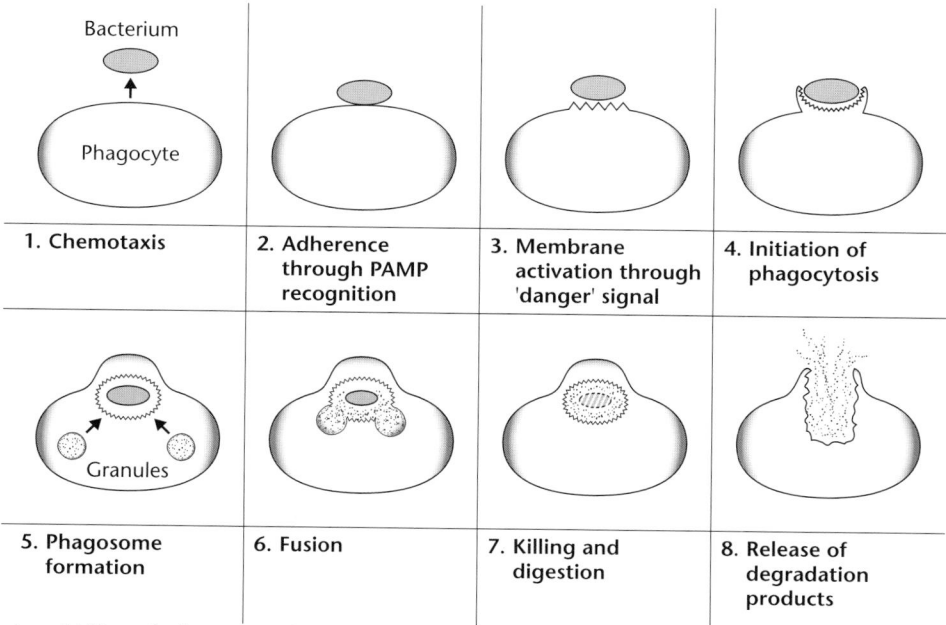

Figure 6.2: Phagocytosis and killing of a bacterium. Stage 3/4, respiratory burst and activation of NADPH oxidase; stage 5, damage by reactive oxygen intermediates; stage 6/7, damage by peroxidase, cationic proteins, antibiotic peptide defensins, lysozyme and lactoferrin. (Redrawn with permission from Roitt, I. & Delves, P., *Roitt's Essential Immunology*, 10th edn, © 2001 Blackwell Science Inc., Oxford.)

(a) Phagocytic cells.
(b) Natural killer (NK) cells.
(c) Soluble factors.
(d) Complement system.

Phagocytic cells

The cells of the innate immune system are collectively termed phagocytic cells because they are able to ingest simple unicellular organisms such as viruses, bacteria and rickettsiae and kill them by a variety of different mechanisms. These cells include (a) neutrophil leucocytes[11] and (b) monocytes/macrophages.[11,12] Phagocytosis of invading organisms occurs when phagocytic cells are attracted to sites of invasion/inflammation by soluble mediators. The efficiency of phagocytosis is enhanced when organisms are covered or 'opsonized' by complement or antibody which provide receptors for the attachment for antibody. Organisms are phagocytosed and taken up into phagosomes which fuse with the lysosomes containing free radicals and lytic enzymes, resulting in killing (Figure 6.2).

The *neutrophils* are produced in large numbers (10^{11} per day) but circulate for only a few hours before passing through capillary walls into the extravascular space. Peripheral blood neutrophils are appropriately placed to prevent infections with circulating micro-organisms, especially bacteria. Patients with deficiencies in neutrophil phagocyte function are prone to repeated pyogenic infections or develop chronic pyogenic granuloma.

Monocytes are larger phagocytic cells produced in the bone marrow. They circulate for hours to days in the peripheral blood, before differentiating into tissue macrophages.[12,13] They acquire specific characters depending on the tissue in which they reside, e.g., liver Kupffer cells, lung alveolar macrophages, synovial membrane A cells. Macrophages secrete lysozyme, neutral proteases, interleukin 1 (IL-1), tumour necrosis factor (TNF), superoxidases, leukotrienes and complement components. They can ingest bacteria via the macrophage mannose receptor or the macrophage scavenger receptor. They are also capable of ingesting other micro-organisms, opsonized by IgG and/or complement. They kill the ingested organisms by using oxygen-dependent mechanisms. Macrophages are also capable of processing antigens and presenting them to T cells as peptides bound to major histocompatibility complex (MHC) molecules. All three functions of macrophages, i.e., secretion, phagocytosis and antigen presentation, are enhanced when macrophages become 'activated' by exogenous stimuli, particularly the lipopolysaccharide (LPS) of invading micro-organisms and interferon-α (IFNα) derived from virally infected cells.

Natural killer cells are large granular lymphocytes derived from the bone marrow that circulate in the blood.[14,15] They recognise and kill targets in the absence of antigenic stimulation and antibody. This killing is not MHC restricted. Many NK cells have surface Fc receptors through which they are able to mediate antibody-dependent cellular cytotoxicity (ADCC). NK cells seem to recognize virus-infected and tumour-derived cells, through

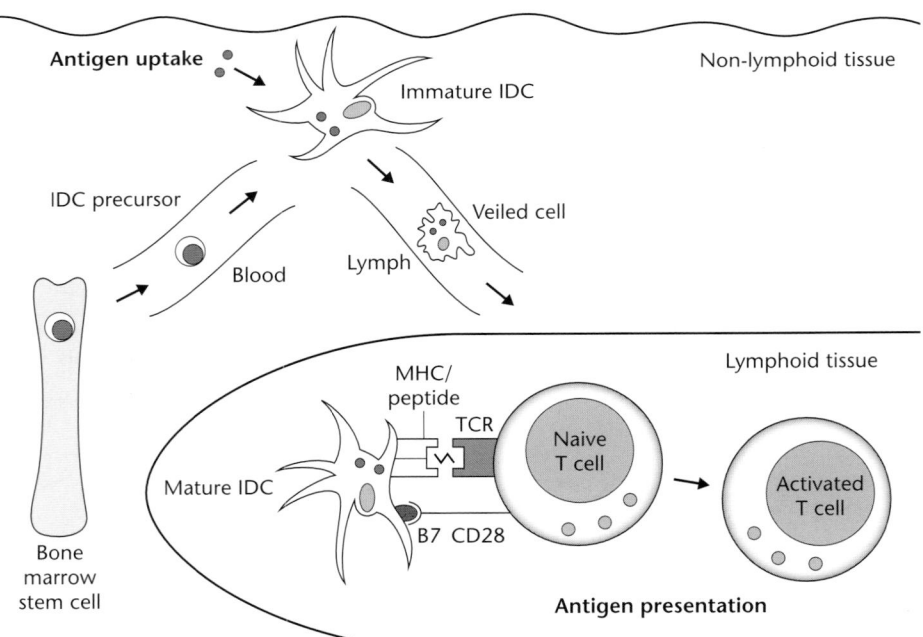

Figure 6.3: Migration and maturation of interdigitating dendritic cells (IDC). The precursors of these cells are derived from bone marrow stem cells. They travel via the blood to non-lymphoid tissues. These immature dendritic cells, e.g., Langerhans' cells in skin, are specialized for antigen uptake. Subsequently they travel via the afferent lymphatics as veiled cells to take up residence within secondary lymphoid tissues, where they express high levels of MHC class II and co-stimulatory molecules such as B7. These cells are highly specialized for the activation of naive T cells. (Redrawn with permission from Roitt, I. & Delves, P., *Roitt's Essential Immunology*, 10th edn, © 2001 Blackwell Science Inc., Oxford.)

targets that are carbohydrate, glycolipid or glycoprotein. The cytotoxicity of NK cells is also enhanced by IFN and IL-2. NK cells are not a homogeneous population, each one containing a combination of different inhibitory and activating receptors which promote killing.

Dendritic cells are specialized antigen-presenting cells (APCs) derived from the bone marrow.[16,17] They are distributed throughout the tissues and when activated by inflammatory stimuli take up and process antigen and migrate to the local lymph nodes where they present the antigen to naive T cells (Figure 6.3). Dendritic cells express high levels of MHC class 1 and class 2 molecules and are highly susceptible to infection by human immunodeficiency virus (HIV) because they express CD4.

Evasion of killing by phagocytic cells by micro-organisms

A number of both unicellular and multicellular micro-organisms have developed evasion mechanisms to enable them to survive inside the normally destructive phagocytic cells (Table 6.3). For instance, *Haemophilus* bacteria are able to do so by developing an outer capsular coat. The special cell wall of *Mycobacteria* also renders them difficult

Table 6.3 Some important persistent intracellular infections.

Parasite	Site of persistence	Clinical manifestation
Herpes simplex virus	Dorsal root ganglia	Recurrent herpes simplex
Varicella zoster virus	Dorsal root ganglia	Recurrent shingles
Hepatitis B	Liver	Chronic hepatitis Carrier state Hepatoma
Epstein–Barr virus	B cells Nasal epithelium	Burkitt's lymphoma Nasopharyngeal cancer
Human immuno-deficiency virus (HIV)	T cells Macrophages	AIDS
Mycobacterium tuberculosis	Macrophages	Reactivation
Salmonella typhi	Macrophages	Systemic spread Carrier state
Brucella	Macrophages	Chronic infection
Toxoplasma	Macrophages	Chronic infection or reactivation
Trypanosoma cruzi	Macrophages	Chronic infection
Leishmania spp.	Macrophages	Chronic infection
Plasmodium vivax	Hepatocytes	Recurrence

to kill by phagocytic cells. The bacteria *Staphylococcus* are able to destroy phagocytes by producing toxins which reduce their number. The protozoan *Leishmania* and the bacteria *Listeria* and *Rickettsia* are able to prevent phagocytosis by escaping from the phagosome into the cytoplasm of the phagocytic cell. The protozoan *Toxoplasma* is able to prevent intracellular killing by preventing phagolysosome fusion. The bacteria *Legionella* demonstrates a similar ability. Some bacteria, namely *Legionella*, *Salmonella* and *Mycobacterium* spp, can survive and replicate within the phagolysosome in a location specifically designed to kill them by somehow remodelling the phagosome.

The ability of a wide variety of infectious micro-organisms to survive and sometimes thrive in the intracellular environment in which they are meant to be killed is the mechanism by which many of them become chronic infections (Table 6.3). In this intracellular 'haven' they are able to escape other immune mechanisms which would lead to their destruction. Herpes simplex virus and the varicella zoster virus cause recurrent infections by persisting in the intracellular environment of the dorsal root ganglia. Persisting viruses may act as co-factors in the development of certain malignancies (Table 6.4). The Hepatitis B virus (HBV) is able to cause chronic hepatitis and hepatoma, not only by persisting in hepatocytes but also by integrating its genome within the host cells. The Epstein–Barr virus (EBV) is able to persist in B lymphocytes and in malarial areas gives rise to Burkitt's lymphoma. The persistence of the same virus in nasal epithelium is associated with the development of nasopharyngeal carcinoma. It is the ability of HIV to persist intracellularly in T cells 'amongst other cells' that leads to the development of the acquired immunodeficiency syndrome (AIDS).

Viruses are not alone in their ability to cause chronic infection by persisting in intracellular sites. Chronic infection with *Brucella* is possible because of the ability of this bacterium to survive in macrophages. Similarly, the reactivation of previously healed *Mycobacterium tuberculosis* infections is due to the ability of this organism to lie dormant within macrophages.[18] The ability of *Salmonella typhi* to persist in macrophages is partially responsible for the carrier state although the importance of the

Table 6.4 Viruses, cancer and immunity.

Virus implicated	Tumour	Immune or other component
EB virus	Burkitt's lymphoma Nasopharyngeal carcinoma	Immunosuppression by malaria? High EB virus antibody Dietary carcinogens?
Hepatitis B	Hepatic carcinoma	Neonatal tolerance to virus? Aflatoxins
Papilloma	Cervical carcinoma	
KSAHV (HHV8)	Kaposi's sarcoma	Immunosuppression by HIV

enterohepatic cycle via the biliary system should not be underestimated.

The protozoa *Leishmania* species[8] and *Trypanosoma cruzi* cause chronic infection by persisting within macrophages although this is a pretty precarious strategy. Under certain conditions, the infected macrophages become activated and become capable of killing these intracellular parasites. Not only have IFNα and IL-4 been demonstrated to be important for this activation process, but the macrophage divalent cation transporter, natural resistance-associated macrophage protein (NRAMP-1), has been demonstrated in mice to play an important role.[1] The ability of certain strains of the protozoan *Plasmodium* species, especially *Plasmodium vivax*, to remain dormant within infected hepatocytes, has been responsible for the recurrence of attacks of malaria in individuals many years after leaving malaria endemic areas.[19]

Soluble factors

Just as there are many different types of phagocytic cells making up the innate immune defences, numerous families of soluble factors (Table 6.5) are also involved in antimicrobial activity.[20,21]

Interferons

The interferons[22–24] (IFNα, β and γ), originally described through their antiviral effect, are now recognized to have antiproliferative and immunomodulatory roles. In response to viral infections IFNα and IFNβ are released from a wide variety of virus-infected cells. They react with specific receptors on neighbouring uninfected cells, rendering them immune to virus infection. This binding induces the production of protein kinase and double-stranded RNA (dsRNA)-activated inhibitor of translation (DAI). In the presence of viral dsRNA, DAI inactivates the cellular protein (eIF-2α) required for translation of messenger RNA (mRNA) which inhibits protein synthesis and therefore viral replication.

IFNγ is a cytokine produced by T cells that activates both macrophages and natural killer cells. Although the IFNs are used in cancer therapy and in multiple sclerosis, it is their use as antiviral agents against chronic hepatitis B and chronic hepatitis C infections that is most relevant to tropical diseases.

Defensins and *cathelicidins* are two major families of antimicrobial peptides.[25] They are positively charged polar molecules which have a high affinity for negatively charged phospholipids in microbial cell membranes. They insert and disrupt the cell membrane, causing lysis of the micro-organism. In response to microbial invasion, exposure to bacterial LPS and TNF, α-defensins are produced by neutrophils and intestinal Paneth cells. Under similar provocation β-defensins are produced by epithelial cells of the skin, pancreas, kidney and respiratory tract. In addition to their anti-membrane effects, both α- and β-defensins chemo-attract memory T cells to sites of infection. β-Defensins also chemo-attract immature dendritic cells which then develop and take up antigens and present them to T cell-dependent regions of local lymph nodes, initiating acquired immune responses.

Acute-phase proteins are an assorted group of plasma proteins which are synthesized by the liver in response to infection.[26] They are normally present at undetectable levels but rapidly increase, some by over a thousand times, during the process of acute inflammatory responses.[27] C-reactive protein (CRP), α-1 acid glycoprotein (AGP) and fibrinogen are amongst this group of proteins. Albumin is unusual in being a negative acute-phase protein; i.e., it is present in detectable amounts but the levels fall precipitously during infection with invading micro-organisms. CRP is probably the most widely studied. It is so called because it binds to the C polysaccharide of *Streptococcus*, rendering the bacterium opsonized for phagocytosis and intracellular killing. AGP increases fourfold in malaria and has been demonstrated to inhibit invasion of red blood cells by *Plasmodium* species by up to 80%, probably by blocking the merozoite binding site.

The complement system is a complex system of serum proteins and serum enzymes working as an amplification cascade system which has important inflammatory and antimicrobial function.[28–30] There are two pathways of complement activation: the antibody-dependent *classical* pathway and the phylogenetically older antibody-independent *alternative* pathway, both of which generate enzymes (C3 convertases) capable of splitting the most abundant complement component, C3, into C3a and C3b fragments.

The net result of both mechanisms of activation is the deposition of C3b on micro-organisms, opsonizing them for phagocytosis by neutrophils which are attracted to the site by chemotactic factors associated with C3a and the later fragment C5a, together with mast cells. Figure 6.4 shows the basis of these mechanisms which underline the defensive acute inflammatory response. Deposition of the C3b cleavage product C3d greatly enhances the uptake and presentation of microbial antigen by antigen-specific B cells and so potentiates the development of strong antibody responses. Finally, activation of the terminal components C5–9 is associated with the lysis of the cell walls of micro-organisms.

Table 6.5 Some activities of T lymphocytes that are mediated by cytokines.

Cytokine	Target cell	Result
IFNγ, IL-4	Macrophage	Activation Parasite killing MHC class II increased
IFNγ, IL-2	NK cell	Activation Virus killing
IL-1 to-6	B cell	Antibody formation
IL-5	Eosinophil	Activation Worm killing
IL-2	CD4 T cell CD8 T cell	Clonal T cell growth Clonal T cell activation

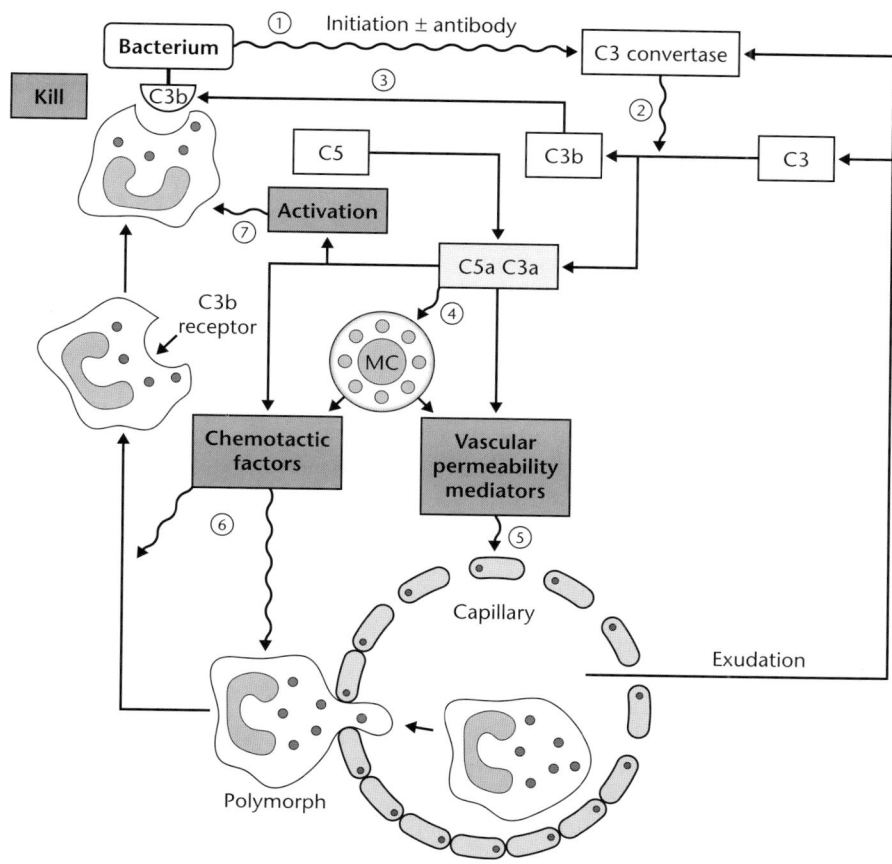

Figure 6.4: The defensive strategy of the acute inflammatory reaction initiated by bacterial activation of the complement system. Directions: (1) start with the activation of the *alternative pathway* C3 convertase through stabilization of the C3b Factor Bb complex by microbial polysaccharides or of the *classical pathway* C3 convertase through formation of the C142 complex by IgG or IgM opsonized microbes, (2) notice the generation of C3b, (3) which binds to the bacterium, C3a and C5a, (4) which recruit mast cell mediators, (5) follow their effect on capillary dilatation and exudation of plasma proteins and (6) their chemotactic attraction of neutrophils to the C3b-coated bacterium and triumph in (7) the adherence and final activation of neutrophils for the kill. (Redrawn with permission from Roitt, I. & Delves, P., *Roitt's Essential Immunology*, 10th edn, © 2001 Blackwell Science Inc., Oxford.)

Complement activation by the classical pathway is more highly effective than by the alternative pathway and genetic deficiencies of C3 are associated with severe bacterial infections. Deficiencies of the terminal components C5–9 are specifically associated with meningococcal septicaemia.

Specific acquired immune responses

The specific immune responses are mediated by T and B lymphocytes. These responses are generally more effective than innate immune responses and are much more antigen specific. Acquired immune responses also generate a large population of antigen-specific memory cells that mediate stronger and more rapid responses on re-exposure to the same infectious agent. These more rapid and exaggerated responses are always referred to as secondary immune responses, even after repeated exposure to the same antigen (i.e., not the primary immune response).

T lymphocytes are derived from the bone marrow but undergo maturation in the thymus gland. They bear a T cell receptor which can recognize a peptide bound to an MHC molecule on the surface of other cells (c.f. Figure 6.3).[20] Generally peptides derived from protein synthesized in the cytoplasm bind to MHC class I molecules (HLA A, B and C) and are usually recognized by CD8+ cytotoxic T lymphocytes (CTL). Peptides derived from extracellular proteins that are taken into APCs by endocytosis bind to MHC class II molecules (HLA DP, DQ and DR) and are usually recognized by CD4+ helper T lymphocytes (Th). The MHC molecules that an individual possesses, therefore, determine which peptides are efficiently presented to T cells and hence determine the strength of the acquired immune responses against a given infection. The MHC class I molecule (HLA-B53), which is common in West Africa, is associated with increased resistance to the malaria parasite, *Plamodium*. HLA-B53 binds to specific peptides derived from malaria sporozoites and generates CTLs which destroy the infected hepatocytes and inhibit malaria infection within the liver. Individuals with the MHC class II molecule DR7 mount weak immune responses against HBV and are more likely to become chronic carriers, whereas those with the DR13 allele are more likely to eradicate HBV infection permanently.

Cell-mediated immune responses

Cell-mediated immunity describes immune responses that involve T lymphocytes without the need for antibody.[31] They are dependent on the recognition of antigens from intracellular parasites which are otherwise hidden from view. CTLs reduce the severity of infections by killing cells infected with intracellular micro-organisms. The abundant 'atypical lymphocytes' seen in the peripheral blood of patients with infectious mononucleosis represent EBV-specific CTLs responsible for killing the EBV-infected B cells and terminating the disease. If this protective cytotoxicity does not materialize then malignant transformation of the chronically infected B cells may occur, giving rise to Burkitt's lymphoma. The malaria parasite is postulated to inhibit the development of this protective cytotoxicity. In persistent viral infections with EBV, cytomegalovirus (CMV) and HIV, large numbers of memory CTLs continue to circulate in the blood and participate in the control of virus reactivation from latent infections.

CTLs have been implicated in leprosy, where they have been demonstrated in vitro to kill neuronal Schwann cells and liberate intracellular *Myobacterium leprae*, which can then be taken up by macrophages and killed. Similarly CTLs have been implicated in the killing of lymphocytes harbouring the protozoa *Theileria* (East Coast fever) in cattle. While the importance of CTLs in limiting episodes of infection is not in doubt, there is no established example of CTLs directly killing an infectious agent.

CD4+ helper T cells (Th) are classified as either Th0, Th1 or Th2, according to the pattern of soluble factors or cytokines they secrete. Most human Th cells are Th0, producing a broad range of cytokines, including IL-2, IFNγ, IL-4, IL-5, IL-6 and IL-10. Highly differentiated Th1 and Th2 cells secrete a narrow, non-overlapping range of cytokines which tend to have mutually antagonistic biological actions. For optimum control on intracellular infections the Th1 subset is required. They are generated during strong cell-mediated immune responses in response to IL-12 secreted by macrophages. Th1 cells secrete IL-2 and IFNγ and induce delayed hypersensitivity skin reactions to antigens from the organism in question. In certain situations it is the Th2 subset which is preferentially stimulated, resulting in the secretion of IL-4 (induces IgE synthesis in B cells), IL-5 (activates eosinophils), IL-6 and IL-10 (inhibits Th1 cells). Th2 cell stimulation results in copious antibody production (which is usually of no benefit against intracellular parasites), while macrophage activation and intracellular parasite killing are reduced or absent (Figure 6.5).

Impaired T cell immunity is associated with susceptibility to severe infections with intracellular organisms including viruses, bacteria (*Mycobacteria*, *Brucella* and *Salmonella typhi*), protozoa (*Toxoplasma*, *Leishmania* and *Plasmodium vivax*) and fungi such as *Pneumocystis* and *Cryptosporidium*.

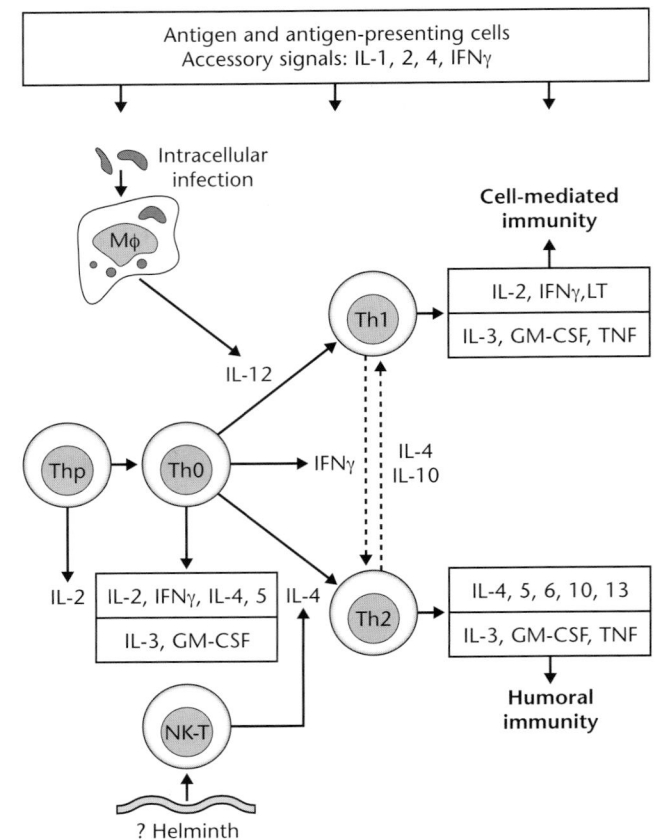

Figure 6.5: The generation of Th1 and Th2 CD4 subsets. It is envisaged that, following the initial stimulation of T cells, a range of cells producing a spectrum of cytokine patterns emerges. Under different conditions, the resulting population can be biased towards two extremes. IL-12, possibly produced through an 'innate'-type effect of an intracellular infection on macrophages, encourages the development of Th1 cells which produce the cytokines characteristic of *cell-mediated immunity*. IL-4 possible produced by interaction of micro-organisms with the lectin-like NK1.1⁺ receptor on NK-T cells skews the development to the production of Th2 cells, whose cytokines assist the progression of B cells to antibody secretion and the provision of *humoral immunity*. Cytokines produced by polarized Th1 and Th2 subpopulations are mutually inhibitory. LT, lymphotoxin (TNFβ); THp, T helper precursor; Th0, early helper cell producing a spectrum of cytokines; GM-CSF, granulocyte–macrophage colony-stimulating factor. (Redrawn with permission from Roitt, I. & Delves, P., *Roitt's Essential Immunology*, 10th edn, © 2001 Blackwell Science Inc., Oxford.)

A study of the immune response in leprosy provides an example of the distinction between Th1 and Th2 immune responses. Tuberculoid leprosy represents a Th1 pattern of response where the micro-organisms are kept to small numbers at the expense of serious tissue damage to the host, while lepromatous leprosy represents a Th2 pattern of response where the host tissues are teeming with mycobacteria but there is little host tissue destruction. The study of leishmaniasis provides another example of these two extremes of response. The study of healthy contacts of people with leprosy and leishmaniasis would appear to indicate sufficient immune response to keep the organism in check without causing severe tissue damage.

The concept of antagonism between the Th1 and Th2 cell cytokines is gaining broad acceptance and may account for many instances of immune suppression. The possibility that we may be able to switch an immune response from one spectrum to another is something that makes this hypothesis an attractive one. A number of academic units as well as pharmaceutical companies are trying to produce monoclonal antibodies and other immunological tools that will enable us to be able to modulate immune responses in whichever direction we choose.

Humoral (antibody) responses

The bone marrow and spleen produce in the region of 10^9 new B lymphocytes daily. These cells recognize antigens through their specific surface immunoglobulin (Ig or antibody) receptor, which is a product of the single light and heavy chain Ig genes which each B lymphocyte has been programmed to express. Sometimes when this surface immunoglobulin binds to the antigens (usually with repeating motifs such as polysaccharides) of invading micro-organisms, the B cell is induced to proliferate and change to plasma cells, producing specific antibody[21] to the antigen in question. The antigens that are capable of doing this directly are referred to as T cell-independent antigens and tend to give rise to the production of low-affinity IgM antibodies which, however, have high 'functional affinity' (avidity) for the repeating groups on these polymeric antigens.

More commonly when antigens bind to the surface antibody of B cells, the complex becomes internalized inside the cell and antigenic peptides are presented to Th cells. This induces B cell proliferation and somatic mutation, resulting in the production of high-affinity IgG antibodies. This so-called 'isotype' class switching can also result in the production of other classes of immunoglobulin with different effector functions (i.e., IgA and IgE). Th cells also induce the differentiation of antigen-specific B cells into plasma cells and the production of memory B cells.

The different classes of immunoglobulin serve different functions. IgM circulates in the bloodstream and is responsible for immune surveillance in the vascular compartment. IgG provides defence against extracellular micro-organisms in both intravascular and extravascular body fluids. IgA is usually secreted on to the mucosal surfaces of the respiratory, alimentary and genital tracts, where it is responsible for mucosal immunity. IgE is usually to be found in the tissues bound to mast cells, where it mediates immune responses against invading helminths, but is also intimately involved in allergic reactions.

The antiviral effect of antibody is easy to understand. In *neutralization*, the antibody binds to specific regions of the virion of the virus that is responsible for binding and penetration into cells. The virus is said to be neutralized as it can no longer gain entry into the cell and cause infection. Similarly, envelope viruses that have an LPS coat can be neutralized when antibody binds to their coat and induces antibody-dependent lysis of the viral envelope involving complement activation by the classic pathway. Also, viruses with attached antibody can be more readily destroyed by phagocytosis through binding the Fc receptor region of the antibody molecule. A word of caution here: one rather undesirable effect of antibody is, via binding to Fc receptors, the enhanced uptake into macrophages of organisms that thrive there, the most striking example of this being dengue virus.

The antibacterial affect of antibody includes the mechanism of opsonization and phagocytosis just described for viruses as well as the complement-dependent lysis of bacterial cell walls. Antibody can also have an antibacterial affect by neutralizing their extracellular toxins. Obviously, this mechanism is particularly important in limiting the clinical effects of the infections with bacteria whose clinical symptoms are caused mainly through the production of toxins, e.g., scarlet fever, diphtheria, tetanus and cholera.

In the past we have made use of the production of these antitoxin antibodies in animals to ameliorate clinical disease. Antitoxin antibodies have also been used to alleviate the symptoms of snake bites. Unfortunately antibodies produced in other animals are in themselves immunogenic to humans. Therapy with these agents is therefore limited as repeated exposure will either give rise to anaphylactic reactions in humans or to such rapid immune elimination of the antibodies as to render them non-effective. So far, attempts to generate human monoclonal antibodies that will have such an effect has met with very limited success. Attempts have therefore been made to 'humanize' monoclonal antibodies generated in laboratory animals by genetically engineering the antigen binding sites of murine monoclonal antibodies into human monoclonal immunoglobulin molecules. Interestingly, it is not in the field of tropical or infectious disease that these humanized antibodies are being commonly used, as these diseases caused by bacterial toxins have been very effectively controlled by vaccination programmes.

It is very rare for a parasite not to induce an antibody response. Even the higher eukaryotic organisms such as protozoa and helminths display large numbers of antigens foreign to humans, who as a general rule make antibody to most of them. Indeed, serum antibody is a most useful guide to infection, the general principle being that a predominance of IgM is a sign of recent infection. As mentioned earlier, antibody is only likely to provide effective defence when the parasite (or a parasite product such as a toxin) is in the extracellular compartment—blood, tissue spaces, secretions, etc. Even then, however, the existence of an antibody response does not ensure parasite disposal. The antibody may be of the wrong class or subclass (isotype) or of inadequate amount or affinity. Many of the effects of antibody rely on attachment of the antibody molecule not only to the antigen but also to phagocytes and/or complement, and here IgG is the most desirable isotype. Isotype switching and affinity maturation are both dependent on help from T cells, as is the development of memory. The involvement of T as well as B cells in antibody responses is therefore crucial, and protein antigen sequences from parasites are increasingly being analysed for antigenic portions, or 'epitopes', with the characteristic B cell or T cell recognition patterns; this is felt to be particularly important when identifying antigens for incorporation into vaccines (see below). Circulating antibody leads to the destruction of blood forms of *Trypanosoma brucei*, blocks invasion of erythrocytes by *Plasmodium* merozoites which it opsonizes for phagocytosis, and helps to limit the spread of *Trypanosoma cruzi* and *Leishmania* infections.

There tend to be vigorous Th2 responses to helminths generating copious IgE synthesis and chemoattraction of eosinophils through IL-5 production. Thus eosinophils binding to the larvae of *Schistosoma mansoni* or *Trichinella*

spiralis coated with specific IgE or IgG bring about their killing through release of the crystalloid major basic protein and activation of oxygen-dependent microbicidal mechanisms. Th2 responses also facilitate the expulsion of intestinal nematodes by the mechanisms set out in Figure 6.6.

Granuloma formation

Granulomas form as a consequence of the body's defence mechanism for walling off pathogens.[32] A granuloma can be defined as a 'focal, compact collection of inflammatory cells in which mononuclears predominate and are usually formed as a result of undegradable or persisting micro-organisms, or due to hypersensitivity responses to the

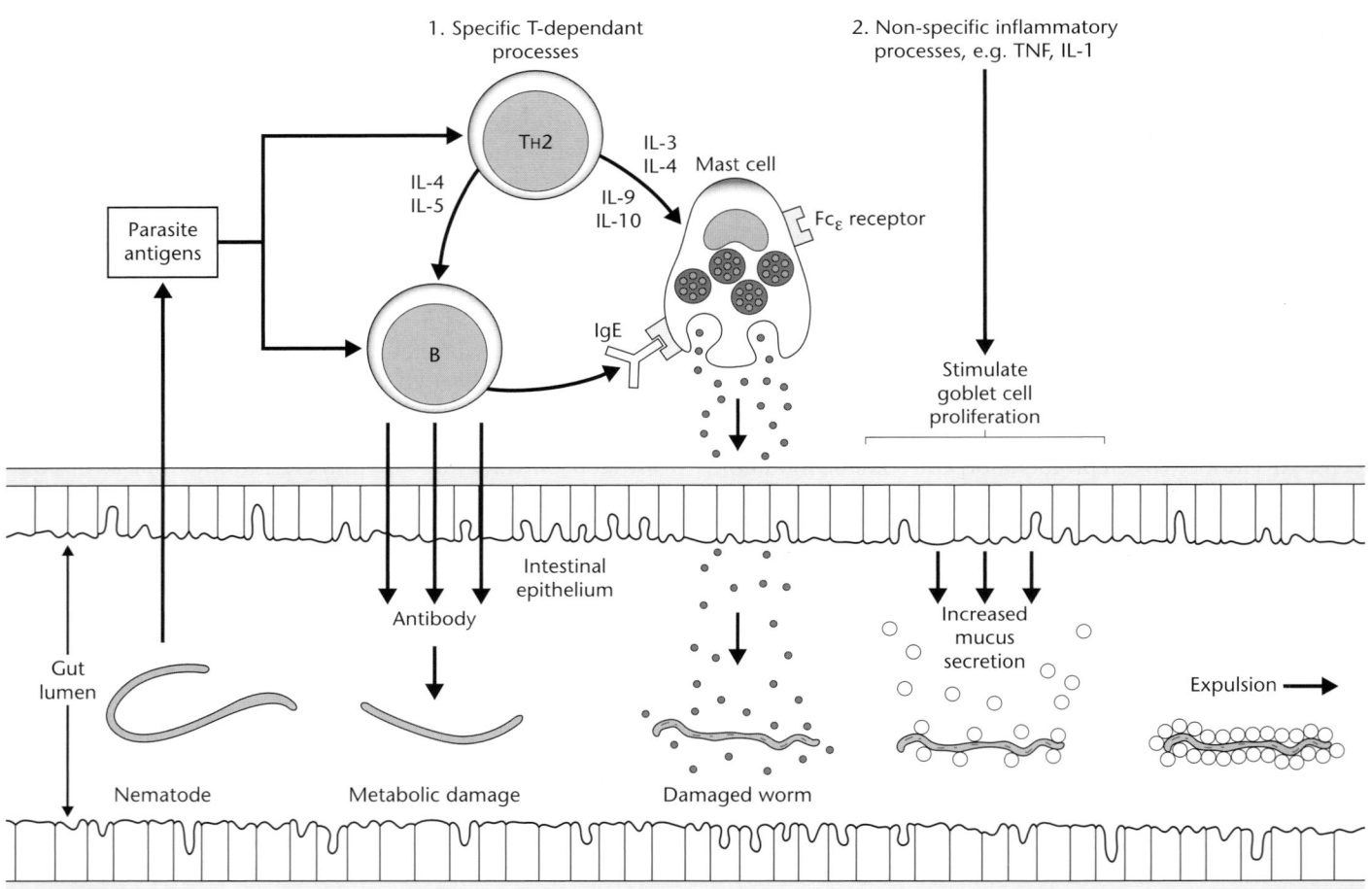

Figure 6.6: The expulsion of some intestinal nematodes occurs spontaneously a few weeks after primary infection. There seem to be two stages in the expulsion, which is achieved by a combination of T-dependent and T-independent mechanisms. (1) T cells (predominantly Th2 cells) respond to parasite antigens and induce (a) the production of antibody by B cells that have proliferated in response to IL-4 and IL-5, (b) the proliferation of mucosal mast cells, in response to IL-3, IL-4, IL-9 and IL-10, and (c) hyperplasia of mucus-secreting goblet cells in the intestinal epithelium. The worms are damaged by antibody together with products of IgE-sensitized mast cells which degranulate following contact with antigen, and so release histamine which increases the permeability of the intestinal epithelium. These processes are not sufficient to eliminate the worms. (2) Non-specific inflammatory molecules secreted by macrophages, including TNF and IL-1, contribute to goblet cell proliferation and cause increased secretion of mucus. The mucus coats the worms and leads to their expulsion. The numbers of goblet cells in the jejunal epithelium and the secretion of mucus increase in proportion to the worm burden. The antigen-specific effector T cells are generated early in infection and the rate-limiting step is the onset of antibody damage. The relative importance of these various processes varies with the infecting nematode. (From Roitt, I., Brostoff, J. & Male, D., *Immunology*, 6th edn, © 2001 Mosby International Publishers, London.

organism antigens. Table 6.6 groups the infectious aetiologies of granulomatous disorders. The granuloma form by a stepwise series of events and is the end result of a complex interplay between invading organism, prolonged antigenaemia, macrophage activity, T cell responses, B cell overactivity, circulating immune complexes and a vast array of biological mediators. Areas of inflamation of immunological reactivity attract monocyte–macrophages which may fuse to form multinucleated giant cells. Further cellular transformation of macrophages to epithelioid cells may occur. The granuloma is an active site of numerous enzymes and cytokines and, with ageing, fibronectin and progression factors such as platelet-derived growth factor (PDGF), transforming growth factor β (TGFβ), insulin-like growth factor (IGF-1) and tumour necrosis factor alpha (TNFα). There is a close relationship between activated macrophages bearing increased expression of major histocompatibility (MHC) Class II molecules and CD4+ T lymphocytes. These T helper cells recognize protein peptides

presented to it by APCs bearing MHC class II molecules. The T cell induces IL-1 on the macrophage and thereafter a cavalcade of chemotactic factors promotes granulo-magenesis. IFNγ) increases the expression of MHC Class II molecules on macrophages, and activated macrophage receptors carry an Fc fraction of IgG to potentiate their ability to phagocytose. The end result is the epithelioid granuloma, which progresses under the impact of transforming and platelet-derived growth factor towards fibrosis.

Granulomas of various infections may have different immunoregulatory mechanisms governing their formation and resolution. Granulomas which synthesize predominantly Th2-type cytokines, such as those that form in response to parasite ova, make only small quantities of Th1-type cytokines chronically, whereas granulomas such as those of tuberculoid leprosy make large quantities of Th1-type cytokines and less of the Th2-type cytokines.

Table 6.6 Infectious causes of granulomatous disorders.

Group 1 Granulomatous disorders with well-recognized causal agents	
Mycobacteria	(tuberculosis, leprosy, BCGiosis, Buruli ulcer, fish tank granuloma)
Bacteria	(brucellosis, melioidosis, actinomycosis, nocardiosis, granuloma inguinale, tularaemia, listeriosis)
Viruses	(infectious mononucleosis, CMV, measles, mumps)
Chlamydia	(lymphogranuloma venereum, trachoma)
Fungi	(cryptococcosis, candidiasis, aspergillosis, chromoblastomycosis, mycetoma, histoplasmosis, coccidiodomycosis, sporotrichosis)
Protozoa	(leishmaniasis, toxoplasmosis, amoeboma)
Rickettsia	(Q fever)
Spirochaetes	(syphilis, yaws, pinta)
Nematodes	(ascariasis, toxocariasis)
Trematodes	(schistosomiasis, paragonomiasis, fascioliasis, opisthorciasis, clonorchiasis)
Cestodes	(echinococcosis, cryptococcosis, sparganosis)
Group 2 Granulomatous disorders with recently identified causal agents	
Bacteria	(cat scratch disease: *Bartonella henselae*)
Actinomyces	(Whipple's disease: *Tropheryma whippelli*)

Parasite evasion of host defense mechanisms

Infectious agents have developed a number of mechanisms for evading the body's immune system (Table 6.7). Many infectious microbes avoid antibody responses by adapting to an intracellular environment where it is impossible for them to come into contact with antibody. The helminth, *Schistosoma* species and the protozoan, *Trypanosoma cruzi*, have been demonstrated to cleave the Fc portion of antibody and evade antibody responses by this mechanism.

In malaria, where the *Plasmodium* undergoes a complicated life cycle within the infected host, different antigens are being produced at different stages and antibody responses are constantly having to adapt. *Schistosoma* represent another example of this 'stage-specific' immune response, because the adult worms seem to provoke very little immune response, while their eggs are highly immunological and induce immunopathology.[33]

It has often been proposed that parasites adapt to their host by mimicking their antigens. The acquisition of the ABO blood group antigen on the surface of mature *Schistosoma* may be one mechanism where the mature worms evade antibody reactions. However if this 'antigenic mimicry' is not fully effective, then the development of antibodies to the infection may cross-react with auto-antigens in the host and give rise to immunopathology. Such mechanisms may be responsible for the rheumatic carditis seen in Group A β-haemolytic streptococcal infections and the carditis and neuritis of Chagas' disease seen in *Trypanosoma cruzi* infections.

Infectious agents also evade antibody responses through the mechanism of 'antigenic drift' and 'antigenic shift'. Thus the influenza virus can escape neutralizing antibody by subtly changing its antigens, not only in going from patient to patient but also within the individual. 'Antigenic shift' is said to occur when a completely new haemagglutinin gene is incorporated into a new influenza

Table 6.7 Some parasite evasion mechanisms.

Immune mechanism	Evasion strategy	Examples
Complement	Cell wall protected	*Salmonella* spp.
	Lytic complex expelled	*Leishmania* spp.
Phagocytosis	Capsule formation	*Haemophilus* spp.
	Phagolysosome blocked	Toxoplasmosis
	Oxygen radicals neutralized	Malaria
	Escape into cytoplasm	*Leishmania* spp.
	Difficult to kill	Mycobacteria
	Phagocytes destroyed	*Staphylococcus* spp. (toxins)
Antibody	Intracellular habitat	Mycobacteria
		Viruses
	Cyst formation	*Echinococcus granulosus*
		Paragonimus westermanii
	Antigenic variation	
	by mutation	Influenza, poliovirus, HIV
	by recombination	Influenza
	by gene switching	Trypanosomes
		Borrelia spp.
		Brucella spp.
	Antibody binding factors	Staphylococcus protein A
	Antibody destroyed	Bacterial proteases
T cells	Inhibition of MHC expression	Herpesvirus
		Adenovirus
	Th2 stimulation	Leprosy
	Polyclonal activation	*Staphylococcus* spp. (enterotoxins)
T and B cells	Host antigen uptake	Schistosomiasis
	Tolerance	Congenital cytomegalovirus?
	Immunosuppression	Measles, HIV
		EB virus
		Trypanosomes
		Malaria
		Toxoplasmosis

strain and gives rise to the pandemic that occurs from time to time. Similar antigenic shift is seen in the envelope proteins of HIV and makes the epidemiological tracing of infections that much more difficult. The variation in the pilin genes of gonococci is a good example of antigenic variation in bacteria. In relapsing fever, the spirochaete *Borrelia hermsi* changes its surface major protein with each episode of fever. Similarly in African sleeping sickness, the protozoa *Trypanosoma brucei* constantly changes its variant antigenic type (VAT) and its variant specific glycoprotein (VSG) during the infection.[34] In this way the antibody response tends to be primarily of the IgM class, which has low affinity for the organism. The protozoa *Entamoeba histolytica*, which causes amoebiasis, constantly sheds its surface antigen thereby evading antibody responses.

Exposure to infective larvae of the filarial nematode *Onchocerca volvulus* (Ov) either results in patent infection (microfilaridermia) or it leads to a status called putative immunity, characterized by resistance to infection. Similar to other chronic helminth infections, there are T cell proliferative hyporesponsiveness to Ov antigen (OvAg) by peripheral blood mononuclear cells (PBMC) from individuals with patent infections, i.e., generalized onchocerciasis, compared to PBMC from putatively immune individuals. Recent studies argue against a general shift towards a Th2 response being the cause of hyporesponsiveness.[35]

Concomitant infections

Concomitant infections (existence of two or more parasites in one host) occur in nature and a number of interactions between protozoa and viruses; protozoa and bacteria; protozoa and other protozoa, protozoa and helminths; helminths and viruses; helminths and bacteria and helminths and other helminths have been described.[36] The interactions vary and the burden of one or both of the infectious agents may be increased; one or both may be suppressed, or one may be increased and the other suppressed. These interactions may be explained by the effects of parasites on the immune system, particularly parasite-induced immunosupression, parasite-induced cytokine production and effects of cytokines controlling polarization to the Th1 or Th2 type T cell responses.

Immunopathology

Immune responses that do not achieve their purpose within a few weeks very often cause tissue damage to the host, and nowhere is this more true than with chronic tropical infections. All four types of hypersensitivity reaction are seen in chronic tropical infections (Table 6.1) and sometimes they are responsible for almost all the symptoms of infection. Schistosomiasis is an example where, judging by single-sex experiments in animals, the worms themselves are perfectly well tolerated but their eggs, deposited in the liver or bladder wall, induce T cell-mediated granulomas that can ultimately kill the patient. Hydatid disease is an infection in which the symptoms are due mainly to the large space-occupying cysts (essentially a host fibrotic response to the worms), with the added possibility, upon cyst rupture, of life-threatening anaphylaxis due to the encounter of massive amounts of worm antigen and IgE-loaded mast cells. In *Plasmodium falciparum* malaria there has always been debate as to the cause of the very diverse symptoms, and interest is currently being focused on the possibility that many of them may be secondary to the overproduction of cytokines, notably tumour necrosis factor (TNF). TNF has been found in the blood of severely ill malaria patients, and the levels correlate with the incidence of cerebral malaria and of hypoglycaemia. In animal models, evidence has also been obtained for a role of TNF in pulmonary oedema and anaemia. The roles of other cytokines such as IL-1, which resembles TNF in many of its actions, and of IFNγ, also deserve investigation.

Bacterial toxins and the immune system

Acute bacterial infections can also cause immunopathology through the actions of their exo- and endotoxins.[5,37] It is thought that the activation of large numbers of T cells with a subsequent release of cytokines, especially TNF and IL-1, are responsible (Table 6.2). Bacterial endotoxin or LPS, a component of the cell wall of Gram-negative bacteria, comprises an outer polysaccharide and an inner lipid A moiety, and is responsible for the features of Gram-negative shock. When LPS is bound by the acute-phase protein, LPS-binding protein, it activates macrophages through a series of complex surface proteins comprising CD14, toll-like receptor and MD-2 to release TNF and IL-1. LPS can activate complement by the alternative pathway and is a powerful polyclonal B cell activator. The Jarisch–Herxheimer reaction is seen when human spirochaete infections are treated with antibiotics. The sudden killing of large numbers of spirochaetes produces severe hypotension as a result of the release of LPS from dead bacteria. The fact that this reaction can be attenuated by treatment with neutralizing antibody against TNF implicates this as the main cytokine involved in this reaction.

Malnutrition, immune responses and infection

A complex two-way interaction exists between infection and malnutrition[38] (Figure 6.7). There are two aspects:

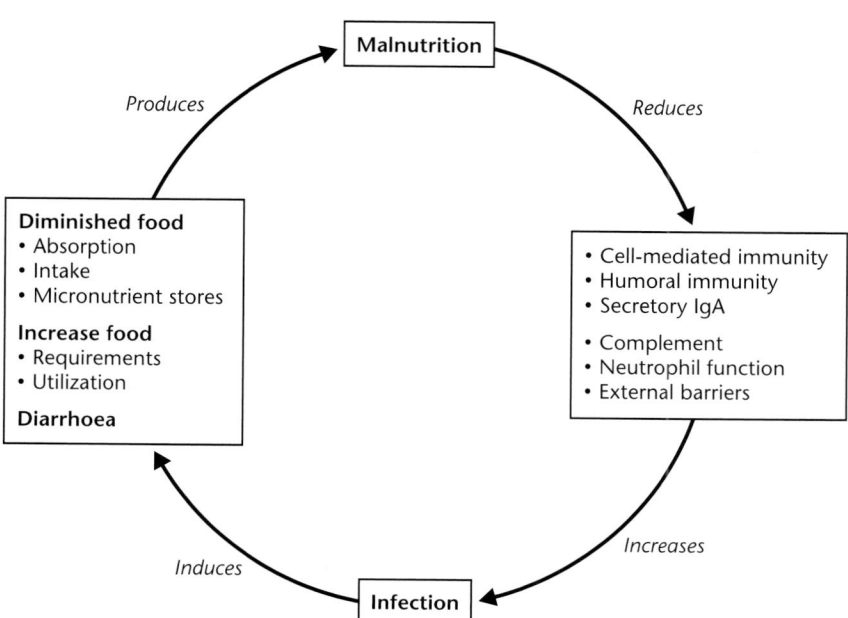

Figure 6.7: The malnutrition–infection cycle.

Table 6.8 Some immunodeficiency syndromes secondary to malnutrition.

Deficiency	Immune components affected	Effect on disease
Calorie (marasmus)	Neutrophils Complement T cells	Susceptibility to bacterial and viral infections Tuberculosis
Protein–calorie (kwashiorkor)	T cells Antibody Macrophages	Susceptibility to all infections
Iron	Neutrophils	Bacterial infections Malaria reduced?
Zinc, copper	T cells	Susceptibility to most infections
Selenium	T cells	Susceptibility to bacterial and viral infections
Vitamin A	T cells	Susceptibility to most infections

Table 6.9 Some infections that cause immunodeficiency.

Infection	Immune components affected	Effect on disease
HIV	CD4 T cells, macrophages	Opportunistic infections, e.g., *Pneumocystis carinii Toxoplasma gondii Mycobacterium tuberculosis*
Measles	T cells, neutrophils	Pneumonia, otitis media
Malaria	Antibody T cells	? increased infections ? Burkitt's lymphoma
Trypanosomiasis (African)	Antibody	Bacterial infection

the effect of infection on metabolism and the nutritional state and the effect of malnutrition on the susceptibility and severity of infections. Malnutrition causes depression of cell-mediated and humoral immune responses. The term 'malnutrition' usually refers to deficiency of macronutrients such as carbohydrate, protein and lipid, but may also be used for deficiencies of micronutrients such as vitamins, minerals and trace elements. Immunodeficiency syndromes secondary to malnutrition are shown in Table 6.8. Classically patients, who are calorie deficient (marasmus), are prone to viral, bacterial and tuberculosis infections; whereas those who suffer the more severe protein–calorie deficiency (kwashiorkor) are prone to all infections and have an impaired response to vaccination. Deficiency of zinc, copper and vitamin A also makes the host susceptible to infections, especially tuberculosis and fungal infection. While iron deficiency may seem to render people susceptible to bacterial infections,[39] it has been suggested that it can keep malarial infection at bay. It is not unusual for people who are having their nutrition restored or who are receiving iron therapy for anaemia to experience a flare-up of malarial infection.

Infections causing immunodeficiency

Infections which cause immunodeficiency are listed in Table 6.9. The much more serious course run by certain worldwide diseases in tropical countries, for example measles, meningococcal infection and gastroenteritis, is mainly due to the lowered immune status of the patients. Often it is not possible to pinpoint the reason for this, since inhabitants of the tropics are exposed to such a large number of different causes of immunodeficiency. The links between nutrition and immunity are much more complex than might be supposed. Many diseases are undoubtedly more severe in patients who are malnourished or underweight, measles being among the most striking examples. Occasionally the opposite is true, as in the case of malaria, where iron deficiency inhibits the growth of the parasite and restoration of nutrition may induce a flare-up of the infection. A distinction is usually made between calorie deprivation and protein deprivation, the latter being generally more serious because both cell-mediated and antibody responses are impaired. There are also specific effects of deficiencies of iron, zinc, copper and vitamins on immune performance (Table 6.8).

Immunosuppression as a result of infection is extremely common, though it has usually proved very difficult to analyse the precise mechanisms involved, some of which have only been properly demonstrated in vitro. Thanks to the existence of animal models, malaria and African trypanosomiasis have been studied in particular detail, and the reality of the problem is well illustrated by the finding that treatment of even quite mild malaria improves the ability of patients to respond to unrelated vaccines (pneumococcal and meningococcal). Measles has long been known to suppress T cell responses and predispose to secondary infection, but all previous examples have been put in the shade by HIV, the most immunosuppressive and the most intensively studied parasite ever. Measles infection is undoubtedly more severe in the underweight or malnourished children in the tropics. Once they have caught the infection they are much more likely to develop pneumonia and otitis media.

AIDS and tropical infections

The impact of AIDS in the tropics has, of course, been catastrophic (see Chapter 20). The original assumption that all the complications were due to a simple infection and destruction of CD4 T cells has turned out to be greatly oversimplified, and current research is also focused on the effects of HIV on macrophages, antigen-presenting cells, B cells and the cytokine network. It was a protozoan (or perhaps, according to recent data, fungal) infection, *Pneumocystis carinii*, that first drew attention, at the beginning of the 1980s, to the impending AIDS epidemic, and this strange parasite remains a major cause of death in AIDS patients in the developed world, along with *Toxoplasma*, *Cryptococcus*, *Cryptosporidium* and other previously rare organisms. However, in tropical countries it is mycobacterial infections which have been most dramatically enhanced by AIDS, not only *Mycobacterium tuberculosis* but also the normally well-controlled *M. avium*, while some other parasites have been surprisingly unaffected. Malaria, for instance, shows virtually no change in either the density or the severity of infection, and nor, so far, do intestinal parasites such as *Entamoeba* or *Giardia*, or the major helminths.[8] Parasite immunologists are still digesting the implications of these unexpected findings, which seem to point to a particularly suppressive effect of HIV on those T cells that are concerned with parasites inhabiting macrophages, though *Pneumocystis* remains a puzzle because the parasite lives extracellularly in the lung alveoli. A sinister aspect of the relationship between HIV and *M. avium* is that each infection appears to enhance both the growth of the other within macrophages and the clinical progress of the disease, and it has been proposed that these effects are mediated by cytokines such as IL-1 and TNF. Infection with HIV makes people in tropical areas susceptible to a whole range of bacterial, viral and fungal infections. Mycobacterial infections, acute bacterial sepsis, cryptococcal meningitis, *Pneumocystis carinii* and *Cryptosporidium* diarrhoea are important opportunistic infections in AIDS patients worldwide.

Immunodeficiency and cancer

Some of the best evidence for a role of the immune system in preventing malignancy comes from tropical conditions. In four tropical tumours a virus has been implicated, and in two, Burkitt's lymphoma and Kaposi's sarcoma, immunodeficiency appears to be a contributory factor (Table 6.4). Burkitt's lymphoma was recognized by Burkitt himself to have a very similar distribution to malaria in Africa and Papua New Guinea, and although the full aetiology is still not established, one plausible theory is that malaria suppresses the normal cytotoxic T cell response against the EB virus-infected B cells. The precise stage at which the well-known translocation of the c-*myc* proto-oncogene to one or other of the immunoglobulin gene loci occurs is not clear. Kaposi's sarcoma is found mainly in patients with T cell deficiencies, including AIDS. However Kaposi's sarcoma is not particularly associated with malaria, nor is Burkitt's lymphoma with AIDS, which again emphasizes the range of different defects to which T cells are susceptible. Chronic infection with the human papilloma virus (HPV) can lead to cervical carcinoma, not only in the tropics but throughout the world.

Immunodiagnosis

While the diagnosis of tropical infections is undoubtedly heavily reliant on clinical skills of history taking and physical examination, a number of laboratory tests are extremely helpful in confirming the diagnosis. However, as microbiological and pathological procedures are tedious, time consuming and relatively inefficient, several immunodiagnostic procedures[40] have found their way into general use. The five main immunodiagnostic tests for detection of antigen or antibody are:

1. ELISA test (enzyme-linked immunosorbant assay).
2. Fluorescent antibody test.
3. Radioimmunoassay.
4. Complement fixation test.
5. Agglutination test.

Unfortunately, many of the early serological tests, although sensitive, lacked specificity and have been replaced by the detection of parasite antigens using monoclonal antibodies. The advent of the molecular biological tool of polymerase chain reaction, which allows the detection of small amounts of microbial DNA and RNA, has increased the sensitivity of immunodiagnosis. This tool has moved from the experimental to clinical laboratory, but is hampered by the problems of cross-contamination and false positive results, in addition to the enormous cost of performing the tests.

Is immunity ever protective?

The combination of inappropriate immune responses with sophisticated parasite evasion ensures that virtually all protozoa and helminths can avoid elimination; the only case of 'proper' self-cure with resulting immunity, in the sense that we expect it with, for example, the childhood viruses (e.g., chickenpox, measles, mumps), is seen with Old World cutaneous leishmaniasis (oriental sore). However, it is nowadays accepted that the reduced parasite load with age in malaria and schistosomiasis is genuinely due to the development of a partial state of immunity, though the exact mechanisms in both cases are controversial. It should be remembered that there are

Table 6.10 WHO recommended vaccines.

Vaccines against viruses	Vaccines against bacteria
Polio	Tetanus
Measles	Diphtheria
Hepatitis A—not for <12 year	Typhoid
Mumps	Meningococcal meningitis
Rubella	Tuberculosis (BCG)
Hepatitis B	Cholera
Rabies	
Japanese B encephalitis	
Influenza	

also bacterial infections where immunity is precarious (e.g., tuberculosis) or non-existent (e.g., syphilis), and viral infections where it is ineffective in practice because of extensive antigenic variation (e.g., influenza, HIV).

Immunization

A number of infectious diseases can now be controlled by immunization.[41] Generally speaking, immunization is likely to succeed in diseases in which good protective immunity follows natural infection. Sometimes immunization may result in better immunity than that seen after natural infection. In tetanus, the patient is only immune for about 3 or 4 months after recovery from infection. However, vaccination with three doses of tetanus toxoid induces a state of immunity that lasts between 5 and 10 years.

Table 6.10 shows the list of infections that are currently controlled by immunization programmes and is dominated by viruses and other simple organisms. Eradication of certain viral infections through vaccines (e.g., smallpox) have been a great success. Immunization may not always evoke a protective immune response. In dengue fever, an arthropod-borne virus infection, immunization can give rise to more serious infection. Similarly in natural infections, previous infection to one strain of Dengue seems to give rise to a more exaggerated clinical course when one is exposed to another strain of Dengue, possibly due to Fc-mediated uptake of antibody-coated virus into productive macrophages, as mentioned

earlier. Generally speaking, the longer the infection the more common is the likelihood of immunopathology.

The question is whether vaccines will ever succeed against infections that do not induce good immune responses. Opinion fluctuates on this point, but is at present guardedly optimistic. Great efforts are going into the production and testing of vaccines[42–47] against HIV/AIDS, malaria, schistosomiasis, leishmaniasis, tuberculosis and leprosy and at the research level filariasis and trypanosomiasis are targeted, though with less certain prospects. Unfortunately vaccine development programmes have only had limited success against more complicated multicellular organisms such as protozoa and helminths and against the more elusive HIV.

The advent of molecular and genetic techniques and availability of sophisticated methods for identifying and modifying genes which produce immunogenic proteins have revolutionalized vaccine development. As more infectious agents become targets for immunization programmes, the spectrum of adverse events linked to vaccines has been widening.[43] Although some of these are tenuous, relatively little is known about the immuno-pathogenesis of even the best characterized vaccine-associated adverse events (VAAEs). The range of possible use of active immunization is rapidly expanding to include vaccines against infectious diseases that require cellular responses to provide protection (e.g., HIV infection, viral hepatitis B and C), and vaccines against non-infectious conditions (e.g., cancer, autoimmune disease). Less virulent pathogens (e.g., varicella, rotavirus in the developed world) are also beginning to be targeted, and vaccine use is being justified in terms of societal and parental 'costs' rather than in straightforward morbidity and morality costs. In the developed world, the paediatric immunization schedule is becoming crowded, with pressure to administer increased numbers of antigens simultaneously in ever simpler forms (e.g., subcomponent, peptide and DNA vaccines). This trend, while attractive in many ways, brings hypothetical risks (e.g., genetic restriction, narrowed shield of protection and loss of randomness), which will need to be evaluated and monitored. The available epidemiological and laboratory tools to address issues outlined above are somewhat limited. As immunological and genetic tools improve, VAAEs will decrease and perhaps even avoid some of them.[43]

REFERENCES

1 Reynolds H Y. Defense mechanisms against infections. *Current Opin Pulmon Med* 1999; 5:136–142.

2 Mimms C, Playfair J H L, Roitt, IM et al. *Medical Microbiology*, 2nd edn. London: Mosby, 1998.

3 Kotwal G J. Microorganisms and their interaction with the immune system. *J Leucocyte Biology* 1997; 62:415–429.

4 Zumla A & James D G. Lung immunology in the tropics. In Sharma O P (ed.) *Lung Disease in the Tropics*. New York: Marcel Dekker, 1991: 1–64.

5 Zumla A. T cells, superantigens and microbes. *Clin Infect Dis* 1992; 15(2):313–320.

6 Penninger J M & Bachmaier K. Review of microbial infections

and the immune response to cardiac antigens. *J Infect Dis* 2000; 181:S498–S504.

7 Ong R K & Doyle R L. Tropical pulmonary eosinophilia. *Chest* 1998; 113:1673–1679.

8 Mosser D M & Brittingham A. Leishmania, macrophages and complement: a tale of subversion and exploitation. *Parasitology* 1997; 115:S9–S23.

9 Freihorst J & Ogra P L. Mucosal immunity to viral infections. *Ann Med* 2001; 33:172–177.

10 Alvarez-Olmos M I & Oberhelman R A. Probiotic agents and infectious diseases: a modern perspective on a traditional therapy. *Clin Infect Dis* 2001; 32:1567–1576.

11 Burg N D & Pillinger M H. The neutrophil: function and regaulation in innate and humoral immunity. *Clin Immunol* 2001; 99:7–17.

12 Paulnock D M & Collier S P. Analysis of macrophage activation in African Trypanosomiasis. *J Leuco Biol* 2001; 69(5):685–690.

13 Pieters J. Entry and survival of pathogenic mycobacteria in macrophages. *Microbes Infect* 2001; 3:249–255.

14 Brooks A G, Boyington J C & Sun P D. Natural killer cell recognition of HLA class I molecules. *Rev Immunogenet* 2000; 2:433–448.

15 Tefferi A, Morice W G & Leibson P J. Natural killer cells and the syndrome of chronic natural killer cell lymphocytosis. *Leuk Lymphoma* 2001; 41:277–284.

16 Steinman R M. Dendritic cells and the control of immunity. *Mount Sinai J Med* 2001; 68(3): 160–166.

17 Sousa C R. Dendritic cells as sensors of infection. *Immunity* 2001; 14:495–498.

18 Collins H L & Kaufmann S H. The many faces of host responses to tuberculosis. *Immunology* 2001; 103:1–9.

19 Plebanski M & Hill A V. The immunology of malarial infection. *Curr Opin Immunol* 2000; 12:437–441.

20 Matsukawa A, Hogaboam C M, Lukacs N W & Kunkel S L. Chemokines and innate immunity. *Rev Immunogenet* 2000; 2:339–358.

21 Banyer J L, Hamilton N H, Ramshaw I A & Ramsay A J. Cytokines in innate and adaptive immunity. *Rev Immunogenet* 2000; 2:359–373.

22 Le Page C, Genin P, Baines M G & Hiscott J. Interferon activation and innate immunity. *Rev Immunogenet* 2000; 2:374–386.

23 Levy D E & Garcia-Sastre A. The virus battles: IFN induction of the antiviral state and mechanisms of viral evasion. *Cytokine Growth Factor Rev* 2001;12: 143–156.

24 Shtrichman R & Samuel C E. The role of gamma interferon in antimicrobial immunity. *Curr Opin Microbiol* 2001; 4:251–259.

25 Yang D, Chertov & Oppenheim J J. Participation of mammalian defensins and cathelicidins in antimicrobial immunity: receptors and activities of human defensins and cathelicidin (LL-37). *J Leukoc Biol* 2001; 69:691–697.

26 Dhainaut J F, Marin N, Mignon A & Vinsonneau C. Hepatic response to sepsis: interaction between coagulation and inflammatory processes. *Crit Care Med* 2001; 29:S42–S47.

27 Thorn J. The inflammatory response in humans after inhalation of bacterial endotoxin: a review. *Inflamm Res* 2001; 50:254–261.

28 Walport M J. Complement: Part I *N Engl J Med* 2001; 344:1058–1066.

29 Walport M J. Complement: Part II *N Engl J Med* 2001: 344:1140–1144.

30 Jokiranta T S, Jokipii and Meri S. Complement resistance to parasites. *Scand J Immunol* 1995; 42:9–20.

31 Johnson R M & Brown E J. Cell-mediated immunity in host defense against infectious diseases. In Mandell G L, Bennett J E & Dolin R (eds) *Principles and Practice of Infectious Diseases*, 5th edn. Edinburgh: Churchill Livingstone, 2000: 31–155.

32 Zumla A & James G. Granulomatous infections: an overview. In James D G & Zumla A (eds) *Granulomatous Disorders*. Cambridge, UK: Cambridge University Press, 2000: 103–122.

33 Boros D L. The role of cytokines in the formation of the schistosome egg granuloma. *Immunobiology* 1994; 191:441–450.

34 Donelson J E, Hill K L & El-Sayed N M. Multiple mechanisms of immune evasion by African trypanosomiases. *Mol Biochem Parasitol* 1998; 91:51–66.

35 Doetze A, Satoguina J, Burchard G, Rau T, Loliger C, Fleischer B & Hoerauf A. Antigen-specific cellular hyporesponsiveness in a chronic human helminth infection is mediated by T(h)3/T(r)1-type cytokines IL-10 and transforming growth factor-beta but not by T(h)1 to T(h)2 shift. *Int Immunol* 2000; 12:623–630.

36 Cox F E. Concomittant infections, parasites and immune responses. *Parasitology* 2001; 122:S23–S38.

37 Lencer W I. Microbes and microbial toxins: paradigms for microbial–mucosal interactions. *Am J Physiol Gastrointest Liver Physiol* 2001; 280(5):G781–786.

38 Watzl B. Review of nutrition and immunity in man. *Am J Clin Nutr* 2001; 73:11–14.

39 Oppenheimer S J. Iron and infection in the tropics: paediatric clinical correlates. *Ann Trop Paediatr* 1998; 18:S81–S87.

40 Harnett W, Bradley J E & Garate T. Molecular and immunodiagnosis of human filarial nematode infections. *Parasitology* 1998; 117:S59–S71.

41 Wenger J. Vaccines for the developing world: current status and future directions. *Vaccine* 2001; 19:1588–1591.

42 Minoprio P. Parasite polyclonal activators: new targets for vaccination approaches? *Int J Parasitol* 2001; 31:587–590.

43 Ward B J. Vaccine adverse events in the new millenium: is there reason for concern? *Bull World Health Organ* 2000; 78:205–215.

44 Rowland-Jones S. Vaccines out of Africa. *Biologist* 2001; 48:64–66.

45 Tsuji M, Rodrigues E G & Nussenweig S. Progress towards a malaria vaccine: efficient induction of protective anti-malaria immunity. *Biol Chem* 2001; 382: 553–570.

46 Moore J P, Parren P W & Burton D R. Genetic subtypes, humoral immunity and human immunodeficiency virus type 1 vaccine development. *J Virol* 2001; 75:5721–5729.

47 Cohen J. 'Breeding' antigens for new vaccines. *Science* 2001; 293:236–239.

Chapter 7

The Economics and Financing of Tropical and Infectious Disease Programmes

S. D. Foster

Introduction

Infectious diseases including malaria, tuberculosis and HIV/AIDS are leading causes of mortality of both children and adults worldwide, and are the most important causes of the global burden of disease. Yet in many countries the resources available to prevent, diagnose and treat infectious disease have not been sufficient to reduce this burden. Projections show that the burden of TB is expected to continue to increase in the next decade despite the availability of effective treatment. Malaria continues to cause over 1 million deaths per year; over 36 million people are infected with HIV and will progress to AIDS eventually. It is not coincidental that the highest disease burdens occur in the poorest countries—poverty plays a major role in ill health. But ill health can also be a direct cause of poverty—families can face financial catastrophe as a result of illness and slip into poverty as a result. When this happens on a national scale, economic growth can be slowed, and as this often coincides with rapid population growth, over time the result is a decline in the welfare and income for everyone.

The growth in the infectious disease burden in terms of new cases is much greater in some countries than the growth in the resources available for treatment and control. These resources will always be scarce—there will never be enough to produce all the goods and services that people need to cope with all possible sources of ill health. This is not just a problem of infectious disease control programmes or the health sector or the public sector alone but is common to all types of activities regardless of whether they are public or private.

Managers of infectious disease control programmes, and health care providers, face a number of key questions where economic thinking and methodology can provide useful insights. For example:

- The President, or Minister of Health or Minister of Finance might ask, how much does it cost the country's economy to have a high rate of a particular disease among the population? Should more money go to the transport sector, to agriculture, to education or to health? Within the health budget, how much should be allocated to treatment or prevention of the different prevalent diseases?
- A disease control programme manager might ask, how much does it cost to treat the cases of this particular disease in the people? How much of this burden is borne by the health services, and how much by patients?
- What is the role of various diagnostic techniques—for example, in TB diagnosis, what is the role of sputum smears, of radiography, of culture, and of new methods such as polymerase chain reaction (PCR)? Which is the best way to diagnose TB given the resources available?
- Which is the best way to treat a particular disease? Is prevention more effective than cure? Are various types of treatment programme—DOTS for TB for example—more cost-effective than standard treatment programmes?
- In case of resistance to drugs or pesticides, when it is appropriate to switch to a newer and more effective, but more expensive alternative? Where resistance to chloroquine is high, should the malaria control programme switch to sulfadoxine–pyrimethamine (SP), which is relatively cheap but where resistance has also developed, or should it switch to a higher-cost alternative for which resistance is lower?
- What is the appropriate role of other non-medical interventions, e.g., vector control, environmental interventions and nutrition interventions?

I have written this chapter to help those responsible for disease control and prevention to better understand the language and the thinking of economics, to make them more effective advocates for the resources they need, and to help with problem solving at national and local level.

Concepts of efficiency

Every TB control manager and health professional treating TB patients will have to compete for scarce health resources with other programmes and activities. That TB control manager will need to justify the use of resources for TB, and the person responsible for deciding on final resource allocations will need to choose between a wide range of other possible uses—would it be better to subsidize the treatment of tuberculosis, to increase the distribution of impregnated mosquito nets, to construct a primary care facility in an isolated community, or a tertiary referral hospital in the capital, for example? Accountability in the public sector demands that in distributing or allocating the scarce resources we must ensure the provision of the mix of goods and services which society values most highly—we seek to achieve *allocative efficiency*.

Once a programme has been chosen, for example to reduce the burden associated with TB, we refer to a narrower, but complementary version of 'best' use of resources: the concept of *technical efficiency*. There are always alternative ways of meeting a specific goal (e.g., reducing the burden imposed by tuberculosis) and this provides a way to determine which of the alternative strategies would achieve this goal more effectively for a given expenditure of resources. Another way of saying the same thing is that this approach identifies the strategy which uses the fewest resources (the least cost method) to produce a benefit of a given size (e.g., reduce the number of deaths due to tuberculosis by 10%).

Depending on how severe the resource constraints are, a manager or clinician may have had to choose between alternative effective interventions, leaving some not implemented. And as we will show later, 'cost-effective' unfortunately is not synonymous with 'affordable'. When resources are scarce, many potentially beneficial interventions cannot be afforded. The overall goal of economics is to choose the best possible use of available resources. And each choice we make means that other worthwhile programmes and activities cannot be implemented. Economists are concerned with the 'lost opportunity' that each choice represents and use the specific term *'opportunity cost'*: the cost of the choice you made measured in terms of what you have given up. So how can a manager or clinician make the best decision regarding the use of limited resources for, say, TB control? What options or activities are given up if a particular decision is made—what is the opportunity cost of that decision? If money and human resources are spent on active case finding, will anything have to be given up in terms of supporting patients already on treatment? A laboratory technician can only work well for so many hours a day. If a technician is asked to carry out three sputum smears on each patient when most cases are detected by the first smear, what are the alternative uses of that technician's time? Would this time be better used on more careful examination of two smears or on examining blood slides for malaria?

Economic evaluation (sometimes also called efficiency analysis) aims to provide a transparent and methodical way to compare different alternatives and to help guide the decision-making process. This is where the disciplines of economics and financing come into the picture. *Economics* is the study of how scarce resources are used to produce goods and services, and how those goods and services are distributed and used by members of society. *Financing* looks primarily at how resources are generated—through taxation of various types, user fees and other methods. This chapter presents a brief introduction to the methods of these disciplines as they apply to some of the important questions about infectious and tropical disease in the world today.

Economic analysis
Types of economic evaluations

All forms of economic evaluation require calculating the resources used by an intervention (*inputs*) and the benefits (*outputs and outcomes*) that are produced. Many assumptions must be made in carrying out an economic analysis, and it is important for the analyst to be clear about what assumptions have been made and what alternative assumptions were rejected. Economic evaluations can be classified according to how they express the outputs and outcomes.

Cost-benefit analysis (CBA) focuses on allocative efficiency. It examines whether the proposed use of resources is better than all possible alternatives. It does this by valuing the outputs and inputs in money terms. The costs, at least in theory, are the benefits which would have been earned, and which now must be foregone, if the inputs had been used in the best alternative way. If the benefits of the proposed alternative exceed the costs, the proposed alternative is allocatively efficient and the investment should be made. There are major problems in applying CBA to health, one of them being measuring health improvements—the benefit of an intervention—in money terms. If an intervention saves a life of a patient, how does one attach a monetary value to this benefit? The two most common ways of doing this are the human capital approach and the use of 'willingness to pay' estimates. The former approach values the benefit of saving a life as the value of the goods and services the person would have produced had they lived (or sometimes the production minus the consumption). The latter values benefits in terms of the amounts that people are willing to pay to avoid the risk of death or ill health, often derived from asking respondents hypothetical questions (called contingent valuation).

Both have methodological problems, and both also raise ethical issues. For example, the former would value the lives of employed people more highly than the unemployed, while the latter would value the lives of richer people more highly than the poor. That is because ability to pay, and therefore willingness to pay, is higher in the rich. The ethical implications of either method of valuing benefits in money terms are a major reason why cost-effectivensess analysis has been used more commonly than CBA in the health sector. CBA can, however, be used in a more limited fashion to examine savings to the health services, for example; screening blood donations for HIV in a high-prevalence area saves not only lives but also future health service costs, which may on their own justify the intervention.[1]

In *cost-effectiveness analysis* (CEA), costs are measured in the same way as in CBA but benefits are measured in physical units chosen to capture the improvement in health status. Different types of outcome indicators are used to reflect the health improvement. *Final outcome indicators* represent the actual improvement in health—

e.g., the number of lives or years of life saved. They can explore both allocative and technical efficiency. *Intermediate outcome indicators*, or *output indicators*, reflect a stage in the process of improvement which is believed to be directly proportional to the final outcome—e.g., the number of TB patients with negative smears on completing treatment reflects the success of the TB programme on the grounds that the resultant improvement in population health is directly proportional to the number of patients completing treatment with negative smears. These outcome indicators explore technical efficiency. They are often problematic, but in some cases they are the only option for measurement; consider the case of condom distribution. It is possible to measure the number of condoms distributed for HIV prevention, but it is not possible to directly observe that they have been correctly used and that they have thus had the predicted impact on health.

A limitation of CEA as defined above is that it is difficult to consider allocative efficiency, or the appropriate mix of interventions. For example, whether it is better to use additional resources to distribute condoms or to increase the coverage of childhood vaccinations cannot be done using intermediate outcome indicators—it makes little sense to compare the cost per condom distributed with the cost per additional child fully immunized. To do this requires an outcome indicator which takes into account the impact of interventions on quality of life as well as, or instead of, duration and it has traditionally been difficult to incorporate the improvements in both quantity and quality into one outcome indicator. Recently, Quality Adjusted Life Years (QALYs), Disability Adjusted Life Years (DALYs) and a number of variations of the theme (e.g., Healthy Year Equivalents) have been developed to do this. The outcome indicator combines morbidity and mortality by putting death at one end of a scale (e.g., on a 0–1 scale) and perfect health in the other end. Morbid states are weighted somewhere in between these two anchoring states. CEA based on QALYs has often been referred to as a *cost-utility analysis* (CUA) although it is simply a special case of CEA.

Steps in CEA analysis

CEA can be used at the national, sub-national and facility levels. At the national level, some governments, with assistance from external agencies such as the World Bank, have defined a basic package of services which should be available to all people. WHO is in the process of defining a menu of cost-effective interventions from which countries could choose according to their resources and other social goals. CEA in both cases is used to decide which interventions to include in the menu or basic package—and which to exclude—on the grounds that those which improve public health standards more efficiently should be given preference.

While CEA of this nature can require technical skills, financial resources and possibly clinical or field studies to collect data, there are ways of learning from the experience of others. The results of studies undertaken in other settings can sometimes be adapted. Often effectiveness (or efficacy) data will be available from field or clinical trials. Adjustments might need to be made for local variations in compliance and coverage, or for a different group of patients likely to avail themselves of the intervention. Costs will generally differ across sites, but estimates of local costs can often be made from studies published in other areas if those studies provide details of the physical use of resources as well as their money values or prices.

A CEA can be divided into five main steps.

Step 1: Define alternatives

All CEA requires a comparison of alternatives, so it is important to specify clearly those under consideration. Most commonly this involves a straight comparison of alternatives (e.g., directly observed treatment, short course versus conventionally delivered short-course chemotherapy), but it is also possible to compare a proposed or existing intervention with the option of doing nothing. The former type of analysis is more common, called incremental analysis. It asks how much additional benefit (in physical units) a proposed variant on an intervention will produce compared to current practice, and at what additional cost. The latter has been called generalized CEA and allows current interventions to be evaluated at the same time as proposed new or modified interventions.[2] The analyst should clarify the nature of the interventions and the types of people who are expected to benefit from them, the current status quo for approaching the disease/condition, and the exact manner in which the intervention will be, or is, organized.

Step 2: Identify and measure outcomes

What is the intervention hoping to achieve? In CEA, effectiveness is measured in terms of natural effects or physical units, such as 'years of life gained' or 'cases correctly diagnosed or treated'. Defining the most appropriate measure is a critical step, and as noted above, although it is not ideal, the analyst might be limited to measurable output indicators, rather than final outcome indicators. The final choice depends on the purpose of the analysis. If it is to improve allocative efficiency, an indicator like the DALY is required.

Step 3: Identify and measure costs
Perspective of the analysis
CEA is often used for decisions about how best to use public resources.[3] The viewpoint guiding the overall decision about cost-effectiveness therefore should be that of society as a whole—and all costs, regardless of who pays them, should be included. For budgeting purposes, however, governments might wish to know how much

an intervention will cost them over time and they would also estimate costs from the more limited perspective of the government. And in some cases it might even be appropriate to estimate costs from the perspective of only one part of government—e.g., in countries where drugs are funded by a separate part of government from those which fund the rest of the health sector. In any case, the important contribution made by patients in terms of time, transport costs, expenditures on medicines and other inputs should not be omitted from the analysis.

Cost concepts
Intervention costs
Costs estimated in the numerator of a cost-effectiveness study generally are the costs of undertaking the intervention. These are sometimes called direct costs, although the term is confusing because accountants use the term in a different way. Tropical disease interventions typically require drugs, diagnostic equipment and supplies, pesticides, staff, vehicles and running costs, buildings, training, supervision, and health education and promotion. From the viewpoint of the patient, costs of transport, seeking care, and possibly accommodation, special food etc. should be included. Care should be taken not to double count costs—for example, patients might pay for part of the cost of drugs. Sometimes analysts add the cost paid by the patient to the full cost of the drugs estimated as part of provider costs. This is clearly incorrect and overestimates the costs of the drugs.

Capital and recurrent costs
The costs of the intervention are the resources used to produce it. They are usually divided into *capital* and *recurrent* costs. Capital items are those which have a comparatively long useful life, usually defined as a year. An example of this is a microscope or a vehicle. The economic costs of such items include not only the rate at which the equipment deteriorates but also the potential benefits forgone by investing resources in the capital goods rather than elsewhere. Recurrent costs are those elements which are consumed and for which payments recur on a periodic, regular basis—usually items which must be purchased or paid weekly, monthly or frequently: staff salaries, drugs, vehicle running costs. There are several methods of measuring and valuing capital costs; the method we mostly use is to annualize the initial capital outlay over the expected useful life of the asset, which gives the equivalent annual cost. There are well-established formulae for deriving the annual equivalent value of a capital item based on the replacement cost, the expected lifetime of the good and the discount rate.[4,5] Recurrent costs are typically underestimated; a typical health facility will require an annual recurrent expenditure of about 25–33% of the initial capital cost.

Fixed and variable costs
Some costs such as buildings, salaried staff and electricity generally do not vary over the short term with the number of people served by an intervention; these are termed fixed costs. Others, however, such as drugs, vaccines, laboratory supplies and reagents, vehicle fuel, food for patients and stationery clearly do vary according to the number of people using the service; these are termed variable costs.

Shared costs
Some costs, both capital and recurrent, are not unique to one intervention. These are *shared or overhead costs*. For example, a malaria control programme might share offices and administrative staff, or laboratory space and staff with the schistosomiasis programme. In undertaking a CEA of malaria control strategies, some of the time of the administrative staff and some of the office space should be charged to the schistosomiasis interventions, using an appropriate unit of allocation.

Average and marginal costs
Related to the concept of shared costs is the fact that the unit costs of expanding or contracting a service—known as *marginal costs*—are not the same as the *average costs* of the current intervention. Average costs are the total costs of the intervention divided by the number of units produced—bed days, smears examined, patients treated. The average cost of a day in hospital includes a component of shared costs, such as the costs of buildings, equipment and administrative staff. These costs contain a large element of fixed costs, which are incurred regardless of the level of output.

The marginal cost is a very useful tool to measure the impact of making a change to the status quo. It is defined as the cost of producing one additional unit. Marginal costs change depending on the situation. Consider the situation of a hospital which has only 50% of its beds full. Adding one more patient entails very little additional, *marginal* cost—the nurses, doctors, and other staff are already there, the lights are on, the kitchen and laundry are functioning. However, if the hospital was already operating at full capacity, expansion to serve even one more patient might require the construction of a new facility, hiring of new staff, etc. The costs of that additional patient would be considerably higher than the currently observed average cost—and higher than the marginal cost of the other 50% situation.

Discounting
Many types of health intervention do not produce immediate results—costs are incurred in advance of the benefits. Consider an immunization programme against hepatitis B. Children are immunized around the age of 2 years in order to protect them from a disease which would probably occur at age 30 or above. How do we take account of this in CEA? We have to take account of *time preference*. In general, if offered a choice, people will prefer to receive $1000 today rather than in 1 year; and they would rather put off paying $1000 for a year instead of paying it today—in part because of the potential earnings available if the money was invested for the intervening year. The further into the future the $1000

cost must be paid, the better it is from the perspective of the payer.

In order to compare costs and benefits or effects which occur at different times in the future, economists use a method called discounting, to translate future costs and benefits into a common time frame which reflects time preference, which is called their 'present values'. For example, if a discount rate of 3% is chosen, then for each successive year in the future the analyst will reduce the costs and the benefits by 3% annually. A cost (or benefit) of $100 in our base year will be $97 in year 1, and so on. In year 10, the same cost which would have been $100 in year 1 is only $74 for purposes of our analysis; and in year 28, when our child vaccinated against hepatitis B might be expected to develop liver disease, the benefit is worth only $41. Formulae and tables for discounting at different times in the future can be found in many texts (e.g. Drummond et al.[5]). Discounting on costs is routinely undertaken and is not controversial, although the *rate* at which future costs should be discounted is controversial, with the general consensus being that somewhere between 2.5% and 5% is appropriate when real (inflation free) rather than nominal (allowing for inflation) costs are used.[6] Gold et al. recommend using both 3% and 5%. The discounting of benefits is more controversial, although common practice is to use the same rate as for costs.[6]

The choice of discount rate can have an impact on the overall result: returning to the hepatitis B immunization example above, if the costs are incurred in the present, but the benefits in terms of prevention of liver disease occur far in the future and are discounted (even at a modest rate), we would probably choose not to vaccinate—despite the considerable benefits to be obtained by doing so.

Cost controversies

Analysts do not all agree on the appropriate way to measure costs in a cost-effectiveness analysis. The two major sources of controversy involve the question of cost offsets, and whether or not to include the costs of lost production. Cost offsets usually involve preventive interventions. Analysts argue that BCG vaccination will prevent some TB cases in the future, for example, and that there will be savings in health care costs as a result of not having to treat so many patients in the future. In this case, they usually deduct the present value of future savings from the cost of the intervention.

Losses, or gains, in productivity as a result of our intervention are sometimes called indirect costs or benefits to distinguish them from direct costs. The time involved in seeking and obtaining care has an opportunity cost in the sense that people (including their carers and accompanying family members) could have been doing something else. In addition, the extra time available because people are cured could be used to benefit the patient. There is controversy about whether to include either production losses in seeking care or production gains from cure in the numerator, and different text books recommend different solutions.

Step 4: Interpreting results

The results of CEA are presented in the form of a cost-effectiveness ratio showing the costs incurred per unit of 'success' or benefit. In principle, the lower the (discounted) cost per unit of (discounted) benefit, the more efficient is the programme. This is, however, only strictly true where one intervention is both less costly and more effective than the alternatives. In many cases, an intervention will be more costly but will produce more benefits than the alternative. If the interventions are mutually exclusive—only one can be done but not both—an incremental analysis must be performed. An incremental cost-effectiveness ratio compares the extra benefit with the extra cost that would be involved by switching from the intervention with the lowest cost-effectiveness ratio to the intervention with the next lowest ratio.

Step 5: Account for uncertainties

As we noted above, the analyst must make many assumptions and predictions about such things as effectiveness of certain drugs, patient compliance, prices, etc. And because many of the critical parameters in CEA are not known with certainty, or may take a range of values, *sensitivity analysis* can be used to find out whether the results would be different if there were changes in critical assumptions. Although traditionally studies have considered changes in each critical parameter separately, computer programs increasingly allow analysts to undertake multivariable sensitivity analysis showing the range of values of a cost-effectiveness ratio when many parameters vary at the same time. This is sometimes also referred to as *scenario analysis*. At the end of the chapter, some references are given as additional readings for those who are interested in knowing more about cost-effectiveness analysis.

The policy use of CEA

CEA shows the mix of interventions which would maximize population health for the available resources. However, most governments and societies have additional goals to which they expect their health system to contribute, such as reducing health inequalities or ensuring financial fairness in contributions.[7] Accordingly, CEA should be used as a guide to decision making rather than a substitute for it. Policy-makers certainly require information on the mix of interventions that will improve population health most efficiently, but they will then choose the final mix based on their contribution to the other social goals as well.

The financing of infectious disease control activities

The context of health care financing

Interest in health care financing in developing countries

increased dramatically in the late 1970s when it became clearer that existing financing mechanisms were inadequate to meet demand. Several factors contributed to this: among them the 1970s recession, demographic changes, rising expectations and changes in disease patterns, equity concerns and cost escalation. These factors were present to differing degrees in different countries—in Europe and the USA cost escalation has been a driving force, and in many developing countries recession made it impossible for ministries of health to continue the level of service they had previously provided—but the reader will probably recognize several of them as contributing to a drive towards a reform of health care financing in his or her own country. The upheaval of health care financing in 'transitional economies'—moving from a 'command economy' under Communism towards a more market-oriented economy—raises many of the same issues.

Financing issues

Andrew Green (1992) mentions three options for improving health care financing. These include improving efficiency, reallocation of resources within the health sector and reallocation of resources to the health sector from other sectors. The likely obstacles to improving efficiency would include that it takes time and training and better management, which may be scarce in many settings. There may also be opposition from groups who benefit from the inefficiency—for example, pharmaceutical companies may benefit from the fact that the national pharmacy stores do not know their annual needs for certain drugs, and they may therefore purchase more than is needed. Lax controls on the food allocations or drugs and supplies for patients in hospitals may mean that the health staff are able to use some of it themselves.

The reallocation *within* the health sector may involve opposition from the medical profession and urban consumers, especially if the reallocation is from urban hospitals to rural primary health care clinics, as is the likely direction. Reallocation from outside the health sector will be opposed by the other ministries and typically the ministry of health is relatively weak in comparison with other ministries (although that is changing) and unable to make a good case for its needs in hard economic terms (although this too is changing!). The military typically has its own health services and thus is unaffected by weakness in the public health system—and is quite competent at making claims on resources.

The weakness of support for health care financing has had an impact on infectious disease, including TB. During the 1970s the main infectious diseases appeared to be under control in the USA and in the UK. The Republicans in the USA and the Conservatives in the UK both had a strong private sector orientation, and it was comparatively easy for them to justify cuts in funding of public health interventions. Accordingly public health funds were cut; this coincided with a resurgence in tuberculosis and other

diseases which had been thought to be under control. This decline in interest, and funding, had an impact on the international and bilateral funding agencies. Legislatures which were reluctant to allocate funds for infectious disease in their own countries, and which had little interest in foreign assistance, were not enthusiastic about spending money in other countries.

Thus countries which lacked sufficient resources on their own, and which relied at least partially on external funding, found this lack of resources meant that their own efforts had to be curtailed. The enthusiasm shown by major donors for family planning was not matched by enthusiasm for health promotion and disease control. To some extent developing country politicians took their cue from their northern counterparts, and complacency became a global phenomenon. The world was woken from its complacency by the arrival of HIV/AIDS, which has spread so rapidly throughout the world, and which has had major consequences for worldwide efforts to control TB, sexually transmitted diseases, leishmaniasis and other infectious diseases.

So it should be clear that the availability of resources for health is very relevant to the control of infectious disease. The financing of health interventions is *key* not only to the way services are delivered, but also to the overall level of activity that is possible. The major issue, then, is who will pay for public health interventions?

Who will pay for public health interventions?

Public health professionals usually have no problem seeing the benefit of public health interventions and the rationale for devoting financial resources to these interventions. But this logic is not always apparent to people outside the field of public health, and one of the key skills of the public health professional is to be able to form a more coherent argument for making additional resources available. A few concepts will be useful in that regard, and their application to infectious diseases drawn out.

The notion of a 'public good'

Many public health measures—health education over the radio, or environmental control of mosquitoes—are interventions which benefit everyone, whether or not they agree to pay. Even if they refuse to pay, they will receive the benefits. It is difficult therefore to charge people for such 'public goods' since the number of 'free riders'—people who benefit without paying—may be considerable. Other examples of public goods are the national defence, bridges or a weather forecasting centre.

Another key concept is that of 'externality'. Treatment of communicable disease—tuberculosis and sexually transmitted diseases are excellent examples—are things which benefit both the individual who receives the treatment and the population as a whole. To deprive any one individual from getting treatment for TB or STDs would have negative implications which could go beyond that individual—the disease would continue to spread. In some cases the benefit of prevention or treatment to the society would exceed the benefit to the individual patient. In such cases, it may benefit society to provide incentives for people to consume enough of these services—immunizations, for example—to ensure that society as a whole is protected.

The relevance for public health

The relevance of the public/private good distinction for public health is that many public health interventions, especially those involving primary prevention through health promotion, have many 'public good' characteristics and positive externalities for society as a whole. Individual health care of a curative nature usually has no public good characteristics and no externalities. Yet people are generally more willing to pay for services which are not public goods and have no externalities, and for which there are no 'free riders'. Which is easier to get people to pay for: a health promotion campaign about a healthy diet to avoid heart attacks, or a coronary artery bypass graft (CABG) for people with heart disease? Of course it is easier to get people to pay for things which will benefit them specifically—and which they would not obtain without paying.

Since many of the most effective public health interventions are essentially public goods or have significant externalities, it becomes clearer why funding of public health can pose problems. Everyone wants these services, but people, and their political representatives, are not always willing to pay for them, particularly since someone who does not pay will usually not be excluded from benefiting from the services. (Some would argue, however, that political representatives often underestimate the willingness to pay for the health of their constituents.) And the more 'free riders' are visible in the system, the less incentive individuals have to pay themselves. In some cases, where the positive externalities are significant, we may even *pay* people to consume public health services—for example, an incentive to TB patients to complete their TB treatment, or transportation to and from the STD clinic, or to complete immunizations. People are willing to pay for the private benefit, but not for the public benefit, so the consumption of that service may be less than the optimal level. Asking poor people to pay for such services may preclude them from using them, and the public health suffers as a result. So when, if ever, is it appropriate to ask infectious disease patients to pay substantially for their treatment? First, let us consider where funds for health come from. An estimated $4.8 billion were disbursed internationally for health assistance in 1990. At international level the sources of health finance are numerous: major sources include the bilateral aid agencies such as the UK's Department for International Development (DFID), the United States Agency for International Development (USAID), and the international and multilateral agencies such as WHO, UNICEF and UNFPA. The biggest single source of external funding now is the World Bank, whose lending for health has now reached US $1–2 billion each year. Non-governmental agencies (NGOs) also provide a substantial amount of funding, and some of their funding comes from the bilateral and multilateral agencies.

Internal sources of health care financing

What are the major options available for the domestic or internal financing of health services? There are four main methods: fees for service and health insurance; tax revenue and national insurance; community financing; and loans and grants.[8] Many European countries and Canada use a predominantly tax revenue-based health care financing system, some with public provision of services and others with privately provided services. In the USA the system is primarily based on fees for service and insurance. Most developing country systems, depending on the level of income, rely primarily on fees for service, with varying degrees of insurance cover, although a large part of the population in many Latin American countries is covered by social security and receives care in that sector. Transitional economies are often attempting to move from a tax-based centrally funded system towards a privately funded system, but are encountering difficulties in getting people to pay significant charges for services which used to be at least nominally free.

The range of financing mechanisms

When considering the range of available financing mechanisms, it may be useful to distinguish between public mechanisms and private mechanisms.

Public mechanisms include:

- *Tax revenues*: income tax, local taxes, property tax, sales tax, value-added tax, taxes on business, and export and import duties.
- *Social insurance*: compulsory insurance, usually paid by deduction 'at source' from people's pay cheques.
- *Lotteries and betting proceeds*: in a few countries lottery and betting proceeds are spent on health, such as in the State of New Jersey, where a portion of revenues from the Atlantic City gambling casinos was devoted to a fund for paying prescription fees for the elderly residents of the State.
- *Earmarked or hypothecated taxes*: proceeds of a tax on alcohol or tobacco may be 'earmarked' for spending on health care to offset the costs they impose on society.
- *Deficit financing*: a country may borrow to cover some of its health care financing needs, either for capital expenditure such as a new hospital or for recurrent financing of everyday costs.

Private mechanisms include:

- *Direct household expenditures*: this is the largest single source of private funding in many countries, and includes patient and household expenditures on seeking and obtaining care, including user fees, hospital charges, drugs, supplies and lab tests. Household expenditures also include transportation to and from the health provider, and other costs of accessing care.

- *Private health insurance*: expenditures made by private people for health insurance cover health maintenance or 'managed care' organizations. People who have joined an HMO will be paying a monthly or yearly fee (possibly co-financed by their employer). In the HMO model, the health provider also takes on the role of insurer.
- *Employer-financed schemes or care*: in some settings the employer provides health care, such as in mines, large farms or plantations and factories.
- *Charity and voluntary contributions*: these may constitute a large fraction of the revenues available to NGOs and even to multilateral agencies such as UNICEF, which relies on contributions and sales of items such as Christmas cards for a part of its funding.
- *Community financing and self-help schemes*: this category would include community efforts to raise funds for a clinic, a piece of equipment or even on behalf of an individual patient.

Within these broad categories there are many possibilities, and most health systems use a combination of several mechanisms.

Which are the best options for paying the cost of infectious disease treatment and control? One of the most important elements to keep in mind is that infectious and tropical diseases are often most prevalent among the poorest groups of society. Tropical and infectious diseases occur more frequently in low-income and marginalized groups owing to environmental, nutritional, social and economic factors. The causation can go in the other direction as well: becoming ill can force a family or individual into poverty through loss of labour and wages, expenditure on medicines and treatment, and diversion of labour to the care of the sick person. Thus relying on patients and their families to fund the treatment of these diseases is likely to prove infeasible.

A World Bank study found that choice of payment methods can have a direct and negative effect on efforts to control a disease. In China, when a policy of requiring TB patients to pay for the treatment was instituted, many low-income TB patients did not come for treatment, or stopped treatment early. Higher income patients were prescribed many more examinations and tests than previously, and more expensive antibiotics which could have been kept for resistant cases. The overall result was an estimated additional 1–1.5 million infectious TB cases during the 1980s, and many additional infections which will require treatment later. The World Bank has claimed that an estimated 3 million people who died from TB during the 1980s would have been treated and saved if the policy had been different.[9]

Developing a strategy for funding of tropical disease control

From the brief review above, it is clear that there is no obvious answer to the problem of how to fund infectious disease control and treatment. In many cases the only suitable source of funding will be the government—and any given public health intervention, including infectious and tropical disease treatment and control, will have to compete not only with other public health interventions, but possibly with other needs such as supplies for the military, food imports, spare parts for agricultural machinery, and debt service. Within the health sector the pressure from both doctors and patients for more money for curative care will be quite intense, and it will be hard to make the case for funds for public health.

Within this constrained framework, there are three approaches to take. The first is to be able to demonstrate that the existing control and treatment programme is functioning as efficiently as possible, and is using available resources very effectively. This includes paying the lowest possible price for drugs consistent with acceptable quality. The second is to take advantage of existing sources of funding for public health such as grants from bilateral agencies, and from international agencies such as WHO and UNICEF. It is worth remembering that the generous assistance available through the World Bank comes in the form of loans, not grants, and thus adds to the national debt. Such international assistance often tends to be geared more towards public health than private care—it will pay for things people are unwilling to pay for collectively and which they otherwise might under-consume, while making room for the natural tendency for people to pay for curative care. International cooperation can reduce the duplication of efforts on surveillance and monitoring and make better use of existing resources for such activities—and thus possibly free up additional resources for other uses. Sectoral assessment and evaluation work provided by external funders can be very useful in maximizing effectiveness of existing programmes.

The third approach is for public health professionals to become more skilled at making the case for tropical and infectious disease control and other public health interventions. Much is to be gained by more effective advocacy to increase the public's understanding of and support for public health. Two particularly useful skills are an understanding of economic evaluation, such as cost-effectiveness analysis, and effective communications, including use of the media and negotiations. Skill in these areas will help to make sure that existing funds are being used as efficiently as possible, and to make the case for public health more clearly and convincingly.

Conclusion

In this chapter we have explained some of the key methods and ways of thinking of economics, to enable the interested tropical medicine specialist to understand economics and to put it to use in managing and funding a tropical disease programme. Concepts such as opportunity cost, marginal cost and public good should prove invaluable in thinking through the best strategy to obtain and manage effectively the funds required to reduce the suffering from tropical diseases and their consequences.

Acknowledgements

I am indebted to David Evans for his input to this chapter.

REFERENCES

1   Foster S & Buvé A. Benefits of HIV screening of blood transfusions in Zambia. *Lancet* 1995; 346(8969):225–227.

2   Murray C J L, Evans D B, Acharya A & Baltussen R M P M. Development of WHO guidelines on generalized cost-effectiveness analysis. *Health Econ* 2000; 9(3):235–251.

3   Evans D B & Hurley S F. The application of economic evaluation techniques in the health sector: the state of the art. *J Int Dev* 1995; 7(3):503–524.

4   Phillips M, Mills A & Dye C. *Guidelines for Cost-Effectiveness Analysis of Vector Control*. Geneva: World Health Organization, 1993.

5   Drummond M F, O'Brien B J, Stoddart G L & Torrance G. 1997. *Methods for the Economic Evaluation of Health Care Programmes*, 2nd edn. New York: Oxford University Press, 1997.

6   Gold R M, Siegel J E, Russell L B & Weinstein M C. *Cost Effectiveness in Health and Medicine*. New York: Oxford University Press, 1996.

7   World Health Organization. *The World Health Report 2000. Health Systems: Improving Performance*. Geneva: World Health Organization, 2000.

8   Green A T. *An Introduction to Health Planning in Developing Countries*. Oxford: Oxford University Press, 1992.

9   World Bank. *World Development Report: Investing in Health*. Oxford: Oxford University Press, 1993.

Chapter 8
Ethics and Tropical Diseases
Some global considerations

S. R. Benatar

Introduction

A proper understanding of the distribution and impact of infectious diseases on humankind in the broadest temporal and spatial context requires some knowledge of the trajectory of history over thousands of years.[1] A less ambitious perspective on the forces promoting and sustaining tropical diseases would acknowledge the influence of imperialistic and colonial forces over the past 500 years.[2–4] However, such historical considerations tend to be eclipsed by spectacular advances in science and technology during the twentieth century. The extent to which infectious diseases have been controlled in industrialized countries favours a selective and somewhat narrower focus on the prospects offered by modern vaccines and drugs to rid the world of infectious diseases.[5] Indeed a few decades ago the World Health Organization's success in eradicating smallpox provided hope that many other major infectious diseases that plagued humankind could be largely eliminated.

The persistence of many diseases, for example malaria and tuberculosis, the emergence of multi-drug resistance to both of these and the appearance of HIV (and other new infections) illustrate the limitations of a strictly scientific approach to public health.[4,6–8] Infections have no respect for geographic boundaries, particularly in a globalizing world in which new ecological niches are being created and where speed of travel and transport allow enhanced transmission. Control of infectious diseases thus poses not merely a scientific challenge for individual nations but rather global political and economic challenges that carry moral implications. Developing solutions to tropical diseases requires transdisciplinary attention to the social conditions that determine the burden of tropical diseases that science and medicine alone cannot address.

The aim in this chapter are modest: to provide a synoptic overview of powerful global forces that play a dominant role in perpetuating inequities that impair human flourishing and frustrate the control of infectious diseases, to identify some challenging ethical imperatives and to offer some potential solutions. The chapter shares that gross inequalities in wealth, and how these have arisen and are perpetuated, lie at the heart of inequality and inequity in health between nations; and that the major ethical imperatives of our time are to narrow these gaps by striving towards structuring more just societies in which premature death and unnecessary suffering from tropical diseases could be diminished.

A starting point: the facts
Widening economic disparities, hunger and extreme poverty

The gap between the richest 20% and the poorest 20% of the world's population has widened from 9 × at the beginning of the century to over 80 × by 1997. The scale of absolute poverty has also increased.[9] The number of extremely poor people in the world has more than doubled between 1975 and 1990. Over 50% of the world's population live on less than $300 a year, and more than a quarter of the world's population live under conditions of 'absolute poverty' defined as 'a condition of life so limited by malnutrition, illiteracy, disease, squalid surroundings, high infant mortality, and low life expectancy as to be beneath any reasonable definition of human decency'.[10]

The burden of disease and widening disparities in health

Growing inequalities and inequities in the burden of disease and premature death are associated with the growing economic disparities described. The inappropriateness of health care delivery is revealed by the fact that 89% of annual global expenditure on health care is spent on 16% of the world's population who account for 7% of global disability adjusted life years (DALYs),[11] and 90% of expenditure on health research is on those diseases accounting for 10% of the global burden of disease.[12] As a result millions of people in the world lack access to even basic essential drugs—a tragedy that has long been ignored but is now achieving a well-deserved profile as multi-drug resistant tuberculosis becomes a growing threat and millions of patients cannot benefit from advances in the treatment of AIDS.[13]

The social construction of human rights abuses

The persistence and even growth of human rights abuses

(even in countries with a long history of commitment to human rights), and the failure of human rights advocacy to sustain human dignity and decent living conditions, should encourage critical perspectives on the powerful economic and military forces that frustrate sincere human rights endeavours.[10,14–16]

Ecological degradation

Population growth and excessive consumption of the earth's limited resources are having adverse ecological effects that are among our major causes of concern at the beginning of the twenty-first century. During the past 100 years the world's population has increased from 1.6 billion to almost 6 billion, and the annual consumption of energy (natural resources) has increased 30-fold. While population growth in poor countries has been the main focus of concern for industrialized countries, consumption patterns in rich countries now pose risks of equal or greater magnitude. 'Environmental capital' is being consumed more rapidly than it can be regenerated by nature and new ecological niches are favouring the emergence of new infectious diseases. Future generations will pay the price in terms of disease, impaired quality of life and reduced longevity.[17,18]

Moral justification for change

These facts arouse moral indignation and must be addressed for several reasons. First, and foremost is the ethical imperative to respect equally the dignity of all people. Having recently celebrated the 50th anniversary of the Universal Declaration of Human Rights it is necessary to reflect on its content (and that of subsequent supportive covenants and declarations) and on the extent to which these aspirations have not been achieved. Moreover, concerns about human rights become magnified in an era in which there will be the potential to modify nature by applying genetic engineering techniques to all forms of life.[19–21]

Second is the need to promote the social stability necessary for human flourishing in a complex world. While the twentieth century was characterized by spectacular scientific and technological progress from which many have benefited greatly, it was also characterized by ongoing wars since 1945, especially in the developing world. While wars have complex causes, they were certainly fuelled by the economic and ideological interests of the great powers during the Cold War, and continue under the influence of powerful global economic forces driving the extraction of human and material resources from poor regions to promote economic growth of the rich. Consequent hunger, miserable living conditions, lack of education, illiteracy and lack of control over personal destiny have bred anger, violence, crime, drug dealing

and abuse of vulnerable humans—all of which reflect injustice and erode the fabric of society.[8,22–27]

Third is the need to be aware of the adverse ecological effects of modern life and to develop processes necessary to protect the environment for the well-being of future generations.[17,18]

Causes of widening disparities

Disparities in wealth and health are symptoms of an unjust world—a well-known fact that is widely stated, but about which most privileged people have become complacent in pursuit of their own economic goals,[28] and in the deluded belief that we live in a just world.[29] Some believe that poverty is not the fault of wealthy countries, but rather the result of bad government elsewhere, and can be alleviated by market forces. Others believe either that the problems are of such great magnitude that there is little that can be done to ameliorate them, or that there is too much disagreement about values to focus on solutions. These views are all contestable. The extent of injustice, the underlying causes of such injustice (described synoptically below) and potential solutions suggested in this chapter should be constructively addressed by scholars, politicians and policy-makers. Progress towards reducing inequalities and the burden of preventable diseases will be limited if these causes of injustice are ignored and a merely biological approach adopted to addressing inequalities in health. The World Health Organization's renewal strategy[30] indirectly acknowledges these issues but its approach is inadequate and a bolder thrust is required.

Economic exploitation and the debt problem

During the second half of the twentieth century, the evolution towards a globalized economy has perpetuated and aggravated centuries of exploitative processes that facilitate the enrichment of some people at the expense of others—within and between nations. Such exploitation (made possible by the processes that devalue and dehumanize the 'other', relegating them to lower standards of life) overtly underpinned slavery, racism and industrial labour abuse. Over the past 50 years, covert erosion of the economies of many poor countries, under the impact of the neo-liberal economic policies driving globalization, has obstructed real development and prevented the introduction of effective forms of modern medicine into many poor countries and the achievement of widespread access to even basic health care for billions of people. Average national per capita GNP has risen to above US $25 000 in some countries and remained static or dropped to less than US $200 in others—and similar gaps can be observed within many societies.[22,27,30–33] The debt owed to rich countries by the poor amounted to $2.2 trillion in 1997—a debt developed and perpetuated through arms trading and ill-conceived 'development projects' that did more harm than good and usually benefited developed nations more than those they were allegedly 'developing'. Such debt can never be repaid and perpetuates economic slavery and human misery in more covert guises.[24,25]

The adverse effects of globalization on health and health policy are evident in the policies of the World Bank and IMF—institutions that have held the balance of power for over 20 years in formulating global health policy. Liberalization of economies, reduced subsidies from basic foods and shifts in agricultural policy that promote growing export crops to the detriment of home-grown food production have resulted in devastating malnutrition and starvation that have caused billions to suffer, especially in Africa. It is an indictment of the IMF's and World Bank's structural adjustment programmes that they impose reduced government expenditure on health care, education and other social services and encourage privatization, even within health care. Availability of condoms, STD treatments, antituberculosis therapy and treatments for co-infections of HIV are subject to user charges introduced and still encouraged by the World Bank in many African countries. The whole Public Health Agenda (information surveillance, epidemiology, research and behavioural surveillance) has been reduced to a skeleton by the privatization of health care. Structural adjustment programmes, debt repayments, cuts in aid budgets (especially by the USA), discrimination against African trade, increasing malnutrition and the Cold War activities of the great powers have all played a significant part in sustaining high rates of infectious disease and in fanning the AIDS pandemic.[34,35]

Further privatization of public health services through the recently described endeavours by the World Trade Organization to 'outlaw the use of cross subsidization, universal risk pooling, solidarity, and public accountability in the design, funding, and delivery of public services' will adversely affect health care in many countries.[36,37]

Military expenditure

A concept of security that relies on force has resulted in industrialized countries spending vast sums of money on the military. In the 1990s such expenditure averaged 5.3% of GNP (as contrasted with 0.3% on aid for developing countries). By deflecting resources away from true human development over many decades such militarization and the associated militarism have compromised the health of individuals and nations directly and indirectly—killing, maiming, torture, refugeeism, destruction of livelihoods, starvation, rape, impoverishment of physical, social and mental health, environmental damage and social destabilization, most especially within developing countries where children too have become hardened warriors. Even though military expenditure has been falling since 1990 it remains exorbitant.[10,38]

Social justice

Assuming that economic disparities and the causal processes behind these are a major global problem, the dilemma becomes one of addressing the question of economic or distributive justice. This involves consideration of such overlapping notions as: rights, fairness (equity), equality and desert. Each of these are complex notions and they may be in conflict with each other. No attempt will be made here to review the many theories of justice that have been formulated as potentially coherent, comprehensive and plausible unifying solutions to such complex issues,[39–41] except to say that none have provided workable solutions.

While it is unrealistic to imagine that economic equality can be achieved globally, it is increasingly agreed that extreme poverty should be alleviated and prevented, and that it is necessary to address social injustice within societies and across national boundaries. Some have suggested that the only way to achieve social justice is to abandon the capitalist system.[37] Others have argued that this is both implausible and impossible, yet agree that major changes are required in the way in which economic systems operate.[26,27]

The absence of definitive answers to such complex questions should not engender paralysis. Moral solutions can be identified at the level of institutions and nations. For example, in the context of the American health care system, which is manifestly unjust, inefficient and extraordinarily expensive, a philosophically coherent and practically applicable proposal has been made for progress towards greater justice in health care.[42] If a powerful and wealthy country were to set such an example the global impact could be profound. It is also necessary to move beyond considerations of justice within nations and attempt to reduce injustice at a global level by reconsidering the ethics of international relations.

Ethics at the level of international relations

Searching for solutions to the problems of poverty, inequality and inequity requires some understanding of how relationships between nations have fostered global disparities and of how such relationships could be further changed—hopefully for the better.[22,43–46]

Over many centuries there have been three basic forms of world politics: imperialism, feudal systems and anarchic state systems.[43] Each has taken several forms over the centuries. Prior to the Peace of Westphalia in 1648 (following the Thirty Years War in Germany) there was no respect for the sovereignty of states. After the treaty it gradually became accepted in Europe that states should be recognized as sovereign, territorial, political units. Interference by one state in the affairs of another was a violation of state sovereignty. With no overarching governing system above states, the system was essentially 'an-archic' (without a ruler) and states could treat their citizens as they wished. While Hobbes viewed this as a non-benign 'state of nature', John Locke, writing half a century later, saw the possibility of the development of ties and contracts that would make anarchy less threatening to individuals and to other states. These two views of the state of nature are the philosophical precursors of two current views of international politics—one more pessimistic (realism) and the other more optimistic (liberalism).[43] It is important to note that the idea of sovereignty of states only applied to so-called civilized countries and that the European powers at the time felt totally justified in structuring such relationships for themselves while scrambling for colonial territories in Africa.[47]

Realism, as the dominant tradition, views war and the use of force as the central problems of international politics. Liberalism conceives of the possibility of a global society in which states can function alongside each other—with economic and intellectual interdependence reducing the likelihood of war. The catastrophe of the Great War in 1914–18, following 40 years of relative peace in Europe, vindicated the realists. Interest in international politics was reactivated and led to new ideas about war and international relations. International Relations Theory, as a relatively new discipline, emerged in its modern form following the Versailles conference (1919) and the formation of the League of Nations at the end of the First World War.[46]

Liberal Internationalism, the first orthodoxy of this new discipline, was based on advocacy of national self-determination and the need to develop mechanisms and institutions to prevent war. Despite the many widely shared values it represented, liberal internationalism was an incoherent and flawed doctrine, and a Second World War could not be averted. Its failure gave rise to further conflict between realists who believed in the sovereignty of states with diplomatic strategic relations (predominantly concerned with military security) at the core of international relations. Realists viewed liberal internationalism as 'utopianism' and expressed concern about the capacities of collectivities, such as states, to behave in moral ways. At the same time the universal human rights doctrine being promulgated allowed criticism of the behaviour of states towards their citizens and even interference across state borders if necessary.[14]

By the 1960s, circumstances in the world led to the major European powers recognizing the damage they had done to their colonies and the need to give them independence. In the 1960s and 1970s changes in great power diplomacy and in global socio-economics were also leading to new theories of international relations that have become more dominant during the past 20 years. Not only were human rights being promoted more vigorously but other challenges to the state-centric system (which characterized both neo-liberal internationalism and neo-realism) were arising as a result of many globalizing forces that progressively reduced the influence of states on issues of national and international importance. Multinational corporations and non-governmental organizations emerged as powerful global actors, the Bretton Woods System weakened and transformed, and a global financial network created the potential for manipulating markets. Western states became increasingly pluralistic, and the possibility of the Cold War turning into a Hot War diminished and faded.[46] It should be noted that for developing countries the 'Cold War' was actually a 'Hot War' with loss of 23 million lives due to small-scale wars fuelled by the competing interests of the East and West in the Third World.[31]

In the 1990s following the end of the Cold War, as military security became a less dominant issue and new interactions developed between state and non-state actors, it became increasingly important to set agendas that go beyond military security. New agendas, of common interest to those who have been marginalized to the 'periphery' (a concept that also includes the marginalized and minorities within wealthy societies) focus on multiculturalism, gender issues, mass unemployment, the resurgence of infectious diseases, refugeeism, large-scale drug trafficking, widespread human rights abuses and ecological threats.

With these changes it is becoming clear that the anarchic state system that has prevailed since the peace of Westphalia cannot be sustained deep into the future. The gradual emergence of (albeit weak) aspects of global governance reflects this process of transition towards a state of complex interdependence between states. An emancipatory transdisciplinary discourse emphasizing complex interdependence of nations is emerging. Despite all the adverse effects of globalization hope is being generated that this discourse will offer new insights and methods of dealing with modern challenges.[46,48] Now, perhaps more than ever before, opportunities can be seen for developing inclusive cooperative alliances across the globe that could improve the ability of states to meet the human rights and needs of their citizens.[49] The mindset shift that allowed South Africa to move peacefully from pariah status to fledgling democracy is an example of what can be achieved if imaginative solutions are sought to intractable problems.[8]

International law and human rights

Cutting across these complex political, social and economic developments there has been growing support for the concept of universal human rights. Donnelly has suggested that Universal Human Rights is now becoming a new standard of civilization, superseding those standards of civilization that dominated over many centuries. These range from common culture and language in Ancient Greece, through religion in the medieval era to the concept of the 'white man's civilization' during the age of empire, and the sovereignty of states. Since 1945 an extensive body of international human rights law has been developed.[14]

This new inclusive standard, adherence to which is required for full membership of international society, is now advocated to prevent the violation of human rights within states, and to allow intervention where required to protect the rights of the vulnerable and abused. The UDHR and international human rights law are considered to be capable of playing this role. Human rights considerations have indeed become an everyday (allegedly) non-partisan part of foreign policy and are of greatest concern in cases of shocking barbarism—for example, in Rwanda and in Bosnia, but regrettably also in prisons in the highly industrialized and privileged world.[50,51]

Whether states can respond to moral issues remains contentious. Sceptics doubt that moral behaviour can be expected of states. Moralists insist on the highest standard of morality from states. Both extremes seem untenable and yet it seems reasonable to expect at least some degree of moral behaviour from states. Such expectations lie behind the UDHR, international law and the rules of war. NATO attacks on Serbia (without United Nations approval), in response to the crisis in Kosovo, illustrate the potential for the use and abuse of power and the implications of actions seemingly based on 'humanitarian concerns'.[46]

The impact of globalization on human rights

Globalization describes the development of a complex web of material, institutional and ideological forces that influence the balance of power, and effectively blur the boundaries between states. Globalization has been ostensibly spearheaded by a few hundred corporate giants, the development of earth-spanning technologies and products that can be produced anywhere and sold everywhere, and the spreading of credit through pervasively penetrating global channels of communication. However, globalization is both a more complex and an ambiguous concept than this, going beyond economics to include social, cultural and ecological dimensions. Nor is it, indeed, a new phenomenon, but rather the outcome of a long and interwoven economic and political history, involving a wide range of actors. Its effects are both beneficial and damaging—although it is arguable that, like population growth, adverse manifestations are now becoming starkly apparent.

Positive manifestations of progress associated with globalization include advances in science and technology; increased longevity; enhanced economic growth; greater freedom and prosperity for many; improvements in the speed and cost of communications and transport; and popularization of the concept of human rights.

Negative effects of globalization include widening economic disparities between rich and poor (within and between nations), and increases in both absolute and relative poverty. The power of massive multinational corporations in a globalizing world has profound impli-

cations for the accumulation of capital and for the way in which resources are controlled. In 1970, 70% of all money that changed hands on a daily basis was payment for work, while speculative financial transactions accounted for 30%. By 1997 these proportions had changed to 5% and 95% respectively. Such a striking shift in the distribution of money arguably reflects devaluation of the lives and work of most people in the world. The influence of the shift in the locus of economic power from the nation-state to global corporations thus alters the balance of power in the world, effectively blurring boundaries between states, and between foreign and domestic policies—in the process undermining small states' control over their own economies, and threatening their ability to provide for their citizens. Economic disparities have become so marked and their adverse effects so apparent that a very significant degree of incompatibility has arisen between neo-liberal economic policies and the goals of democracy.[16,52,53]

Because the concept of rights was developed in an era in which national sovereignty was respected it becomes clear that another level of complexity is introduced when there is a need to implement human rights under conditions in which the power of states to deliver the rights expected by its citizens is being diluted by the adverse effect of globalizing forces on national economies. Even the extent to which states can control warfare is being diminished and independent warlords and militant groups are capable of waging uncontrollable conflict.[54] As all gradually become citizens of the world, as well as of states, so the ability to deliver on human rights requires both capacity and responsibility that extend beyond the state.[55,56]

World views: understanding other cultures

Optimism for the role of a universal concept of human rights within a state-centric system is not only reduced by globalizing forces. Donnelly, a champion of the human rights approach, has suggested that it can also reasonably be doubted whether universal human rights can constitute an effective international morality, given the degrees of ideological and political diversity that remain in the world. He expresses concern that even if the UDHR appears to be widely accepted it is not clear that its values have genuine significance for all.[14] It is thus necessary to acknowledge that there are many world views and that the West has not worked hard enough to understand the implications of these for making real progress towards a more peaceful world. Attempts by theologians to find the common ground on which all world religions can meet,[57] approaches to understanding how world views are constructed[58] and attention to human needs[59] offer at least some hope that there may be some potential for facilitating processes of peaceful interaction between diverse peoples.

Reflections on some ethical imperatives in our modern world

The major ethical imperatives of our time—and we should have no difficulty recognizing these unless we are morally blind—are to relieve hunger, alleviate profound poverty, sustainably improve the lives of those living under abominable conditions and to foster global peace and ecological security. Several United Nations conferences—Rio 1992, Cairo 1994, Copenhagen and Beijing 1995—and others testify to the growing acknowledgement of these ethical imperatives and the need to enable the processes by educating and empowering women and children. However, insufficient attention has been devoted to the ways in which resources can be generated to achieve these ambitious goals. Scholarly attention and political action directed at ethical and effective use of resources are central to the imperatives to be faced. Some suggestions follow.

Demilitarization

Given the amount of money spent globally on military activities (US $750 billion per year in the 1990s) saving even a modest proportion could generate considerable resources for diversion to development. Associated reduction in conflict and the promotion of peace could further contribute to sustainable progress towards better lives for many, and encourage new visions of global security. Demilitarization and progressive diversion of resources from activities of war to making peace is one of the ethical imperatives that must be faced.[10,38]

Debt restructuring

Debts that can never be repaid must surely be abolished.[24,25] Maintenance of Third World debt in the knowledge that this was to a large extent created through inappropriate arms trading and defective development projects undermines both the humanity of the those who demand repayment, and the lives and dignity of the those who are effectively enslaved by debt. Expenditure of up to $15 per citizen each year in some developing countries on debt repayment, while spending only $2.5 per person per year on health care[60] is an indictment of the integrity of wealthy nations that claim to be concerned about universal human rights and the equality of all people. Debt relief will not remove the need for loans and financial assistance but will require that these be restructured on more accountable grounds to ensure their legitimacy in the future. Deposits of large sums of

money by despots in Swiss banks, and other forms of fraud with the full knowledge and collusion of arms dealers and other powerful traders should also no longer be possible. The transparency and accountability that the rich require of the poor through structural adjustment programmes should also apply to their own financial transactions that have such profound effects on the lives of billions.

Implementation of appropriate international taxation

Given that less than 10% of the $1 trillion daily global financial transactions are for services rendered and that the remainder represents repackaging and reselling of money within what has been called a 'casino economy',[52,61] it is difficult to contest the legitimacy of taxing electronic monetary transactions for a global development fund. Similarly it is being acknowledged that there is a need to modify current concepts of free trade to include environmental costs in business activities—indicating acceptance that we cannot have free access to the 'natural commons' in our respective countries to the disadvantage of distant others or future generations.[18,27,62]

Developing imaginative new sustainable development programmes

The achievement of real development within poor countries is also an ethical imperative.[63,64] The risks for all are becoming apparent if this is not achieved—extreme poverty giving rise to 'violence from below', new and old infectious diseases spreading rapidly across the world, and the environment becoming irrevocably compromised. With 50% of the world's population lacking access to even the most basic essential drugs, millions of impoverished people are becoming desperate because of lack of concern for their lives and basic human dignity. In the face of this and increasingly evident ecological threats, rational self-interest alone provides sufficient reason for promoting sustainable development programmes, even if the need for altruism and reparations is denied.[65,66] Ordinary citizens, health care professionals and informal organizations, such as NGOs, can build a process of 'globalization from below' that could contribute to sustainable development.[27,49]

Restructuring international relations

The inability and failure of the great powers to shape successfully a fair, just and peaceful world is evident from the scale and magnitude of war, ethnic conflict, and the disparities and associated human misery that have characterized the twentieth century.[33] Lives of comfort and luxury seem to have dulled the moral sensitivity of many to the needs of fellow humans. In a world of rapid and comprehensive information transfer it is neither possible to plead ignorance of the plight of billions, nor to ignore the implications of this for all in the long term— even the most privileged. Highly egoistic notions of humanity, reflected in selfish individualism and long-standing concepts of state-centricity with considerations of security limited to military issues, have run their course.

New ways of looking at the world and at how states should interact are gradually being shaped. A deeper understanding of what it means to be a citizen in an increasingly interdependent world will need to embrace renewed concepts of civic citizenship, solidarity and concern for others, even those very distant from our own daily lives. New ways of thinking about ourselves, and our relationship to others are also necessary in order to link concepts of human rights to human needs and to the ethics of social justice within and between nations. New paradigms of thinking would embrace concern for population well-being as well as individual well-being; deeper insights into how complex systems function; and development of an ethic for institutions and international relations that recognizes the responsibility to balance individual goods and social goods, and not to harm weak and poor nations or groups of people through economic and other forms of exploitation that frustrate the achievement of human rights and well-being.[46,67–69]

An ecological approach to justice

In recent years it has been cogently argued that neither well-respected theories of justice nor the individualistic human rights approach have taken into consideration the adverse effects of population growth and of ecological degradation. As a result the environment has become a commons that has been abused and severely compromised. Loss of biodiversity, global warming, damage to the ozone layer, soil erosion, pollution of the air and the sea have all been allowed to escalate without sufficient attention to their implications for the future of life on our planet.[17,18] The persistence of tropical diseases must be seen against this background.

It is not only redistribution of resources that must be faced but also overpopulation and overconsumption. An ecological approach to justice requires a shift from a predominantly anthropocentric view of the world to an ecocentric world view that includes concern for nature and for all forms of life. A long-term perspective on life and a concern for rights that extends to include the well-being of future generations are essential to this viewpoint. The age-old concept of stewardship of nature here replaces the idea of the subjugation of nature. Consideration of all costs associated with consumerism—rigorous economics—is required to operationalize these concerns.

Setting a moral example

As powerful as human rights and other moral languages

may be, the power of wealthy countries setting a moral example is potentially more influential. Amnesty International's report on the extent of human rights violations in the USA[50] and Cassese's description of such violations in the prisons of Europe[51] provide insight both into how such abuses can continue even in wealthy democratic countries, and into the great need for setting moral examples. Neglect of the poor within rich societies, perpetuation of unsustainable consumerist lifestyles, lack of universal access to health care within the USA and the continuing production of weapons of mass destruction are also poor examples for other nations. A shift from the idea that 'might is right' to the idea that 'right is might' is needed. South Africa's peaceful political transition illustrates the possibility of such change. The Jubilee 2000 programme to relieve poor nations of crippling debts exemplifies the need for moral leadership at a global level. Widespread support for this endeavour could provide evidence of the power of rational persuasion and illustrate sincere belief in the role of human rights in dealing with poverty and associated intense human misery.[14–16]

Conclusions

Reducing the burden of tropical diseases and fostering greater human well-being on a global scale will require acknowledgement that unbridled materialism and wasteful consumerism are associated with impoverishment of the human spirit and threaten the lives of billions. Perpetual economic growth for some cannot continue at the expense of others without sacrificing our humanity. The root causes of poverty should be studied more seriously and constructively addressed. The poor are not poor because they are lazy, incompetent or corrupt. While poor countries must also accept some blame for their condition, the causes of poverty are much more complex. Wealthy industrialized nations are deeply implicated in creating and sustaining poverty.*

Powerful nations need to resolve to deal with the root causes of intolerable economic disparities through such processes as described above. Their wealth, their sense of entitlement and their moral insensitivity are as problematic as the existence of poverty.

Crucial to a new approach will be the recognition that it is not merely altruism that is called for but more importantly a long-term perspective on rational

---

*The facts and interpretations offered above are not intended to imply that the wealthy, productive and fortunate in the world should bear the whole burden of the blame for the complex series of historical developments that polarize the world. Political realities within developing countries, including corruption, ruthless dictatorships, ostentatious expenditure by elites and underinvestment in education and health, have contributed greatly to the suffering of billions. However, it is vital for privileged people to have insight into the extent to which these deficiencies in many developing countries have been facilitated by the policies of wealthy nations in pursuit of their own interests. Insight into how favoured lives are sustained by overt and covert exploitation of unseen others could allow those of us who live comfortable lives anywhere in the world to appreciate that we do not have a monopoly of entitlement to the benefits of progress.[70]

self-interest in an increasingly interdependent world. To achieve this will require a broader approach to morality that firmly embraces but also goes beyond the concept of human rights, and includes concern for human needs worldwide and for the environment on which all life is crucially dependent. Sustainable development and respect for human rights and human dignity are in the interest of all worldwide. These can only be achieved through a combination of analytically incisive and honest thinking about global problems; and the active promotion of solidarity devoid of economic, cultural and ethical imperialism. Is should also be acknowledged that all people and cultures have something to contribute to the development of a more just world and a true form of universalism. The goal of achieving a global mindset to which all can contribute is the challenge for the twenty-first century.[71] If this can be achieved the prospects of reducing suffering from tropical diseases will be greatly enhanced.

Acknowledgements

I am grateful to Allen Buchanan for constructive comments.

REFERENCES

1 McMichael T. *Human Frontiers, Environments and Disease: Past Patterns, Uncertain Futures.* Cambridge: Cambridge University Press, 2001.

2 McNeill W H. *Plagues and Peoples.* New York: Anchor, 1976.

3 Karlen A. *Plagues Progress: A Social History of Man and Disease.* London: Victor Gollancz, 1995.

4 Garrett L. *Betrayal of Trust: The Collapse of Public Health.* New York: Hyperion, 2000.

5 Fauci A. AIDS in the 21st century. *N Engl J Med* 1999; 341: 1046–1050.

6 Benatar S R. Prospects for global health: lessons from tuberculosis. *Thorax* 1995; 50:487–489.

7 Lee K & Zwi A B. A global political economy approach to AIDS: ideology, interest and implications. *New Political Economy* 1996; 1:355–373.

8 Benatar S R. South Africa's transition in a globalising world: HIV/AIDS as a window and a mirror. *Int Affairs* 2001; 77:347–375.

9 United Nations Development Program. *Human Development Report.* 1998, New York: Oxford University Press.

10 Sivard R L. *World Military and Social Expenditure,* 16th edn. Washington, DC: World Priorities Press, 1996.

11 Iglehart J K. The American health care system: expenditures. *N Engl J Med* 1999; 340:70–76.

12 World Health Organization. *Investing in Health, Research and Development. Report of the ad-hoc Committee on Health's Research Relating to Future Intervention Options.* Geneva: WHO, 1996.

13 Gellman B. The belated global response to AIDS in Africa. *The Washington Post* 5 July 2000, PA01. An unequal calculus of life and death. *The Washington Post* 27 December 2000, PA01.

14 Donnelly J. Human rights: a new standard of civilisation? *Int Relations* 1998; 74:1–24.

15 Aiken W & La Follette H (eds). *World Hunger and Morality.* London: Prentice-Hall, 1996.

16 Falk R. *Human Rights Horizons: The Pursuit of Global Justice.* New York: Routledge, 2000.

17 McMichael A J. *Planetary Overload: Global Environmental Change and the Health of the Human Species.* Cambridge, UK: Cambridge University Press, 1993.

18 Lou N & Gleeson B. *Justice, Society and Nature.* London: Routledge, 1998.

19 Burley J (ed.). *The Genetic Revolution and Human Rights.* Oxford: Oxford University Press, 1999.

20 Benatar S R. A perspective from Africa on human rights and genetic engineering. In Burley J (ed.) *The Genetic Revolution and Human Rights.* Oxford: Oxford University Press, 1999: 159–208.

21 Benatar S R. Human rights in the biotechnology era: a story of two lives and two worlds. In Bhatia G S, O'Neil J S, Gall G L & Bendin P O (eds) *Peace, Justice and Freedom.* Edmonton: University of Alberta Press, 1998: 245–257.

22 Alexander T. *Unravelling Global Apartheid: An Overview of World Politics.* Cambridge, UK: Polity Press, 1996.

23 Richmond A H. *Global Apartheid: Refugees, Racism and the New World Order.* Toronto: Oxford University Press, 1996.

24 George S. *A Fate Worse than Debt.* London: Pelican, 1988.

25 Pettifor A. *Debt, the Most Potent Form of Slavery: A Discussion of the Role of Western Lending Policies in Supporting the Economies of Poor Countries.* London: Debt Crisis Network, 1996.

26 Heilbroner R. *Twenty-first Century Capitalism.* London: W W Norton, 1993.

27 Falk R. *Predatory Globalisation: A Critique.* Cambridge, UK: Polity Press, 1999.

28 Galbraith J K. *The Culture of Contentment.* Boston, MA: Houghton Mifflin, 1992.

29 Lerner M. *The Belief in a Just World: A Fundamental Delusion.* New York, Plenun Press, 1980.

30 World Health Organization. *Renewing Health for all Strategy: Elaboration of a Policy for Equity, Solidarity and Health.* Geneva: WHO, 1995.

31 Comaroff J & Comaroff J L. Millennial capitalism: first thoughts on a second coming. *Public Culture* 2000; 12:291–343.

32 Teeple G. *Globalisation and the Decline of Social Reform: Into the 21st Century,* 2nd edn. Aurora, Ontario: Garamond, 2000.

33 Hobsbawm E. *The Age of Extremes: A History of the World 1914–1991.* New York: Patheon Books, 1994.

34 Abbasi K. The World Bank and health. *BMJ* 1999; 318:1132–1135.

35 Nandy S, Scott R, Logie T E & Benatar S R. Realistic priorities for AIDS control. *Lancet* 2000; 356:1525–1526.

36 Price D, Pollock A & Shaoul J. How the world trade organisation is shaping domestic policies in health care. *Lancet* 1999; 354:1889–1892.

37 Pollock A M & Price D. Revising the regulations: how the World Trade Organisation could accelerate privatisation of healthcare systems. Lancet 2000; 356:1995.

38 Kiefer C. Militarism and world health. *Social Sci Med* 1992; 34:719–784.

39 Graham G. *Contemporary Social Philosophy.* Oxford: Blackwell, 1988.

40 Arthur J, Shaw W H. *Justice and Economic Distribution,* 2nd edn. Englewood Cliffs, NJ: Prentice-Hall, 1991.

41 Nielsen K. Global justice, capitalism and the third world. *J Appl Philos* 1984;175–186.

42 Buchanan A E. Privatisation and just health care. *Bioethics* 1995; 9:220–239.

43 Nye J. *Understanding International Conflicts.* New York: Harper Collins, 1993.

44 Mansbach R W. *The Global Puzzle: Issues and Actors in World Politics.* Boston, MA: Houghton Mifflin, 1994.

45 Ray J L. *Global Politics,* 6th edn. Boston, MA: Houghton Mifflin, 1996.

46 Brown C. *Understanding International Relations*. London: Macmillan, 1997.

47 Pakenham T. *The Scramble for Africa*. Johannesburg: J Ball, 1991.

48 Somerville MA & Rapport DJ (eds). *Transdisciplinarity: Recreating Integrated Knowledge*. Oxford: EOLSS, 2000.

49 Brecher J, Costello T & Smith B. *Globalisation from Below: The Power of Solidarity*. Cambridge, MA: South End Press, 2000.

50 Amnesty International. *The United States of America: Rights for All*. London: Amnesty International, 1998.

51 Cassese A. *Inhuman States: Imprisonment, Torture and Detention in Europe Today*. Cambridge, UK: Polity Press, 1996.

52 Barnet R J & Cavanagh J. *Global Dreams: Imperial Corporations and the New World Order*. New York: Simon & Schuster, 1994.

53 Ralph J. American democracy and democracy promotion. Review article. *Int Affairs* 2001; 77:129–140.

54 Friman H R & Andreas P (eds). *The Illicit Global Economy and State Power*. Oxford: Rowman & Littlefield, 1999.

55 Rotblat J (ed.). *World Citizenship: Allegiance to Humanity*. London: Macmillan, 1997.

56 Felice W. *Taking Suffering Seriously: The Importance of Collective Human Rights*. New York: State University of New York Press, 1996.

57 Kung H. *Global Responsibility: In Search of a New World Ethic*. New York: Continuum Press, 1993.

58 Smart N. *World Views Cross-Cultural Explorations of Human Beliefs*, 2nd edn. Englewood Cliffs, NJ: Prentice-Hall, 1995.

59 Doyal L & Gough I. *A Theory of Human Need*. London: Macmillan, 1991.

60 *The Oxfam Poverty Report*. Oxford: Oxfam, 1996.

61 Strange S. *Casino Capitalism*. Oxford: Blackwell, 1986.

62 *Health and Sustainable Development: 5 Years after the Earth Summit*. Geneva: WHO, 1997.

63 Shue H. *Basic Rights: Subsistence, Affluence and US Foreign Policy*. Princeton, NJ: Princeton University Press, 1980.

64 Rist G. *The History of Development: From Western Origins to Global Faith*. London: Zed Books, 1997.

65 Raspail F. *The Camp of the Saints*. Petoskey, MI: Social Contract Press, 1982.

66 Hosle V. The third world as a philosophical problem. *Social Res* 1992; 59:227–262.

67 Elfstrom G. *Ethics for a Shrinking World*. London: Macmillan, 1990.

68 Benatar S R. Towards social justice in a new South Africa. *Med Conflict Survival* 1997; 13:229–239.s

69 Benatar S R. Streams of global change. In Bankowski Z, Bryant J H & Gallagher J G (eds) *Ethics, Equity and Health for All*. Geneva: Council for the International Organization of Medical Sciences, 1997, 75–85.

70 Benatar S R. Respiratory health in a globalizing world. *Am J Resp Crit Care Med* 2001; 163:1064–1067.

71 Benatar S R, Daar A & Singer P A. Global health ethics: a rationale for mutual caring (in preparation).

Section 2

Symptoms and Signs

The fundamental practice of clinical medicine in the tropics remains more of an 'art' than science. Despite technological advances of the past two decades, history taking and physical examination remain the mainstay of clinical practice. Clinical acumen is of paramount importance when arriving at a correct diagnosis where there is poor laboratory back-up. Even where technological facilities are available, the health practitioner can enhance patient management by meticulous evaluation, and by the recognition of multiple (often asymptomatic) pathologies. Furthermore, the increasing frequency of diseases associated with urbanization and globalization (such as diabetes, hypertension, obesity and ischaemic heart disease) is acknowledged. HIV/AIDS can present with protean clinical manifestations and should be in the mind of every practitioner. The chapter on general approach to the patient discusses several important aspects of the history and physical examination of the tropical patient. Logical evaluation of patients with fever are described, and causes of splenomegaly and lymphadenopathy in the tropics are detailed. This chapter emphasises that multiple pathology is common, and the clinician should not be surprised to find abnormalities which are additional to those anticipated from the primary complaint.

Chapter 9
General Approach to the Patient

G. Maartens, P. Mwaba and A. Zumla

Introduction

The knowledge base of medicine in the tropics has grown rapidly[1,2] yet the fundamental practice of clinical medicine in the tropics remains more of an 'art' than a 'science'. The ability to establish a sympathetic rapport with the patient, understand the social, cultural and economic reasons underlying the patient's ill health, elicit the important parts of the history, identify the important physical signs and make sound judgements in the absence of sophisticated technological help, and maintain the highest ethical standards when dealing with patients from different ethnic and cultural backgrounds constitutes the 'art' of the practice of medicine in the tropics.

Despite the technological advances of the past two decades,[3] history taking and physical examination remain the mainstay of the practice of medicine.[4–6] Clinical acumen is of paramount importance in arriving at a correct diagnosis when medicine is practised in rural areas of the tropics or where laboratory backup is scarce or unavailable. Even when modern technology is available, the medical practitioner can greatly enhance patient management by meticulous evaluation and by recognizing the multiple, often asymptomatic, pathologies that are a frequent feature of disease in the tropical context. Furthermore, non-infectious medical conditions are also common and may easily be overlooked (for examples, see Figures 9.9–9.19).

The spectrum of diseases in tropical areas has changed considerably in the last two decades.[1] Rapid urbanization in the tropics has led to a rise in diseases associated with obesity, smoking and reduced physical activity. There has been increased detection of non-infectious diseases such as diabetes, hypertension and cardiovascular diseases (see Chapters 37, 38 and 12).[7] The rapid and devastating spread of the human immunodeficiency virus (HIV) epidemic has substantially changed the practice of medicine in the tropics and has added another complex dimension to the interpretation of symptoms and signs.[8,9] HIV/AIDS should be at the back of every clinician's mind and must now enter the differential diagnosis of any problematic clinical condition. At the same time there have been successful campaigns that have reduced the incidence of many diseases—examples include polio, onchocerciasis and leprosy.

Medical practitioners, particularly those in temperate countries, need to recognize travel to endemic areas by their patient early in their consultation. Those practising in the tropics must be meticulous in their history taking and general examination and must be aware of the rare complications of common diseases and common manifestations of rare diseases. This chapter attempts to cover 'a general approach' to the patient who lives in the tropics or acquired the disease whilst visiting the tropics.

Clinical history

There are several important aspects of the history to which particular attention should be given irrespective of whether the patient lives in the tropics or is a returning traveller. A check-list for important components of the history is presented in Table 9.1.

Travel

A precise list of places visited in chronological order, together with the extent of rural travel and exposure to water (rivers, streams, lakes) and animals, must be obtained, as many diseases show a marked geographical variation in endemicity and prevalence. For instance, in the differential diagnosis of a feverish illness, bartonellosis would only be considered in visitors to, or residents of, Andean valleys in Peru, Ecuador or Colombia, whereas malaria and typhoid are so widespread as to necessitate consideration after any tropical or subtropical exposure. Some infections are common and widespread but are only acquired in certain well-defined circumstances or exposures. For example: (a) mosquitoes are widespread in the tropics and a range of infections can be transmitted by them including malaria (Chapter 71), arboviruses (Chapter 41) and filariasis (Chapter 82); (b) tick bites can transmit typhus, Colorado tick fever, Lyme disease and relapsing fever (see Chapter 50); (c) dog bites may be responsible for rabies (Chapter 45) or bacterial sepsis, sometimes with esoteric bacteria such as *Capnocytophaga canimorsus*; (d) schistosomiasis after contact with fresh water (see Chapter 80), (e) rickettsial diseases following the bite of specific arthropod vectors in restricted ecological niches, (f) variant Creutzfeldt–Jakob disease after contact with bovine spongiform encephalopathy-infected cattle products (although not yet a problem in tropical

Table 9.1 Check-list in history taking.

Ethnic origin	
Occupation	e.g., farmer, fisherman, abattoir worker, cave explorer
Travel history	e.g., countries and places visited, contact with rivers, lakes, animals
Prophylaxis	e.g., immunizations, malaria prophylaxis, insect repellants, sunscreens, PCP prophylaxis
Treatment	e.g., antimalarials, antibiotics, antihypertensives, analgesics hypoglycaemics; blood transfusions, injections; traditional medicine, scarification, tattoos; splenectomy, gastrectomy
Drugs	e.g., intravenous drug abuse, other addictive drugs; traditional medicines, over-the-counter medications; smoking
Diet	e.g., vegans, food fads, seafood; undercooked meat/fish/snails; traditional brews; water source
Sex	e.g., sexual orientation, unprotected sex, multiple sexual partners, commercial sex
Allergies	e.g., seasonal, antibiotic, food, insect bite, plant
Bites	insect (e.g., mosquito, fleas, lice, tick, mite, tsetse-fly, blackfly, horsefly); snake (see Chapter 32); carnivore (e.g., dog, cat, mongoose, jackal, leopard); arachnid (e.g., spider, scorpion, tarantula); monkey; human
Pets	birds (e.g., parakeets, budgies); dogs; cats
Family history	e.g., diabetes, sickle cell, tuberculosis, asthma, hypertension, epilepsy, partner with HIV/AIDS
Detailed systems review of symptoms	

countries, a tropical student studying in Britain may have contracted it). It follows that the physician should be aware of the epidemiology of the disease(s) under consideration.

Ethnic origin, gender issues and cultural factors

There are marked ethnic differences in disease incidence. Some of these differences are due to genetic disorders. Familial Mediterranean fever may present with acute fever and pain in certain Middle Eastern races, whereas a similar presentation in a West African would bring sickle

cell disease to mind. Other ethnic differences in incidence are related more to exposure to pathogens than to genetic predisposition—for instance, tuberculosis in the United Kingdom is more common in patients originating from the Indian subcontinent.

The presentation of disease is greatly influenced by cultural factors and gender issues.[10] Sensitivity to different cultures and the role of gender is of paramount importance for all clinicians in tropical areas, especially when the clinician is from a different cultural background. In many cultures diseases are believed to result from bewitchment or disturbed ancestors. Although these beliefs contradict scientific understanding, they must be respected. It can be very difficult to distinguish appropriate but exaggerated religious experiences from psychiatric disease in certain ethnic groups and a great deal of reliance must be placed on the opinions of others from the same culture. Many patients will first consult a traditional healer. This, together with the fact that access to health care facilities is often poor, frequently results in late presentation of disease. It is clearly desirable to speak and understand a patient's language when taking a history, but this is not always possible. Interpreters who have not undergone medical training may unintentionally change the patient's or clinician's intended meaning.

Diet

Malnutrition is common in tropical areas, particularly in children who may present with marasmus or kwashiorkor (see Chapter 23). 'Road to health' height and weight charts are essential tools in tropical paediatrics. Malnutrition becomes almost universal in extended droughts or when large groups of people are displaced by war or persecution. Vitamin deficiencies are frequently seen in areas where people depend on limited staple foods—beriberi is common in areas where rice is a staple food and pellagra where maize is a staple. Nutritional megaloblastic anaemia is common in pregnancy or lactation due to folate deficiency or in vegans due to vitamin B_{12} deficiency. Iron deficiency anaemia is very common in children and menstruating women due to a combination of poor diet and hookworm infestation. Abdominal pain in a Muslim patient during Ramadan may be caused by renal colic due to ureteric stones after self-imposed water deprivation during daylight hours in a hot environment. Diseases due to dietary excess are becoming increasingly common in the tropics. Obesity occurs frequently with urbanization, resulting in increased frequency and severity of diabetes and hypertension. Dietary iron overload is common in central and southern Africa due to cooking and beer brewing in iron pots.

Ingestion of contaminated water or unwashed fruit and vegetables can lead to several infections such as amoebiasis, hepatitis A and E, leptospirosis, typhoid, cholera, salmonellosis and shigellosis. Unpasteurized milk and dairy products are responsible for the transmission of brucellosis, listeriosis, Q fever and tuberculosis. Undercooked meat may transmit a range of infections, including tapeworm, trichinosis, salmonellosis and toxoplasmosis. Fish or shellfish, particularly if uncooked, can transmit infections such as cholera, gastroenteritis (e.g. *Vibrio parahaemolyticus*), hepatitis A or parasites (e.g., anisakiasis, gnathostomiasis, diphyllobothriasis or paragonimiasis). Ciguatera poisoning is caused by the consumption of fish that have accumulated toxic dinoflagellates in certain tropical areas.

Sexual contacts

Sexually transmitted diseases (STDs) are rampant world-wide (see Chapter 21). Several STDs occur much more frequently in the tropics—e.g., chancroid. Care and sensitivity are required in approaching a patient with sexually transmitted disease and patients must be encouraged to bring their partners for treatment. STDs frequently present with extragenital manifestations; hence, poly-arthropathy, papular skin rash and fever may be the presenting features of gonococcaemia; likewise, an illness that includes a generalized rash and lymphadenopathy could be caused by secondary syphilis. HIV is endemic throughout the tropics, where it is mainly transmitted by heterosexual coitus, and should be suspected as a cause or co-factor in virtually any febrile illness.

Vaccines, drugs and traditional medicines

A history of relevant vaccination should not be used as a reason to exclude any infection from the differential diagnosis, since vaccination is never 100% effective and errors within the vaccine chain do occur. In the same way, the appropriate use of antimalarial prophylactic drugs does not eliminate all risk for this infection but may decrease blood parasite counts to undetectable levels, thereby delaying diagnosis. Broad-spectrum antibiotics are freely available to the general public without prescription in many parts of the world and their prior use may prevent microbiological diagnosis in bacterial disease, as well as actually causing ill-health through side effects, such as diarrhoea. Patients often consult traditional medicine healers (see Chapter 4) and use herbal remedies but they may be reluctant to admit this. There are undoubtedly many effective traditional therapies. The highly efficacious Chinese antimalarial qinghaosu is an example. However, some herbal preparations can also cause ill-health, especially when impurities such as heavy metals are present, and severe symptoms may ensue. Acute toxicities which have been described in patients after consuming substances from traditional healers include confusion, coma, renal failure, haemorrhagic gastro-enteritis and fulminant hepatic failure. Chronic toxicities include hepatic fibrosis and hepatic veno-occlusion.

Weight loss, anorexia and malaise

These are relatively common presenting complaints and, for the most part, are readily attributable to associated disease; however, they may dominate the clinical presen-

Table 9.2 Cryptic causes of weight loss.

Weight loss and malaise with anorexia
Acquired immune deficiency syndrome
Tuberculosis
Malignancy (hepatoma, lymphoma, cervical carcinoma, colon and others)
Extrapulmonary tuberculosis
Visceral leishmaniasis
Brucellosis
Giardiasis
Hydatid disease
Schistosomiasis
Anaemia
Weight loss and malaise without anorexia
Gut helminths
Diabetes mellitus
Thyrotoxicosis
Malabsorption
Drugs

tation in situations where the aetiology is not obvious. Diseases to be considered in this circumstance are listed in Table 9.2.

Diarrhoea and vomiting

Most symptoms in tropical practice are system specific. The physician's knowledge of clinical syndromes, disease epidemiology and geographical medicine will often lead to a specific diagnosis. Diarrhoea is a frequent presenting complaint and in most patients will be caused by an acute primary gut infection (Table 9.3). Gasterointestinal symptoms are frequent in patients infected with HIV or who have full-blown AIDS. Unfortunately, some extra-intestinal diseases, such as legionnaires' disease, pneumo-coccal pneumonia or streptococcal septicaemia, measles, Addison's disease or diabetic ketoacidosis, can occasionally masquerade as gastroenteritis. Vomiting commonly accompanies diarrhoea in many gut infections but toxin-associated food poisoning (*Staphylococcus aureus*, *Bacillus cereus*, ciguatera poisoning), plant or marine food toxin ingestion, drugs, malaria, meningitis, renal failure, acute hypotension (septicaemia, haemorrhage), peptic ulceration and other severe systemic illnesses should also be considered.

General examination

(See Figures 9.1–9.19)

Multiple pathology is common within the context of tropical disease[11] and the clinician should not be surprised to find physical abnormalities additional to those expected from the primary complaint. The general examination

Table 9.3 Common aetiologies of diarrhoea (and vomiting).

Acute watery diarrhoea (duration < 2 weeks)	
Bacterial infections	*Vibrio cholerae* *Salmonella* spp. *Campylobacter jejuni* *Escherichia coli* (enterotoxigenic, enteropathogenic and enteroadherant) *Shigella sonnei* *Yersinia enterocolitica* *Legionella pneumopilia*
Viral infections	HIV enteropathy Rotavirus and other enteric viruses
Protozoal infections	Malaria (*Plasmodium* spp.) *Giardia lamblia* *Cryptosporidium parvum* *Microsporidia* spp. *Isospora belli* *Sarcocystis* spp.
Toxin diarrhoea	
	Clostridium perfringens (toxin) *Staphylococcus aureus* (toxin) *Bacillus cereus* (stable toxin) Ciguatera fish poisoning
Bloody diarrhoea	
	Shigella spp. *Campylobacter jejuni* *Salmonella* spp. Enteroinvasive and enterohaemorrhagic *E. coli* *Clostridium perfringens* (necrotizing enterocolitis, pigbel) *Yersinia* spp. *Clostridium difficile* (pseudomembranous colitis) *Schistosoma* spp. (intestinal schistosomiasis) *Entamoeba histolytica* (amoebiasis) *Balantidium coli* Inflammatory bowel disease (Crohn's disease or ulcerative colitis)
Chronic diarrhoea (duration > 3 weeks)	
	Giardia lamblia *Entamoeba histolytica* Tropical enteropathy and tropical 'sprue' HIV enteropathy Ileocaecal tuberculosis *Shigella* spp. Enteroadherent *E. coli* *Strongyloides stercoralis* *Trichuris trichiura* *Capillaria philippinensis* Chronic pancreatitis Schistosomiasis Disaccharide intolerance Lactose intolerance Postinfective irritable bowel syndrome (IBS) Inflammatory bowel disease (IBD) Coeliac disease

should include an assessment of nutritional status. Wasting or failure to thrive due to HIV/AIDS, the cachexia of chronic disease (especially tuberculosis), malnutrition or malabsorption is a common finding. Anaemia, often on a nutritional basis, is common. Several vitamin deficiencies (pellagra, rickets and scurvy) produce characteristic

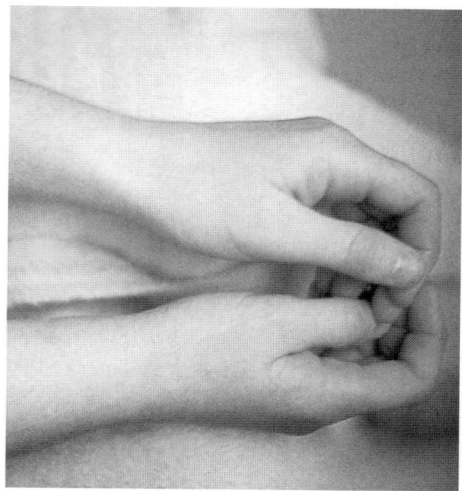

Figure 9.1: Transient swelling over the wrist in *Loa loa* infection.

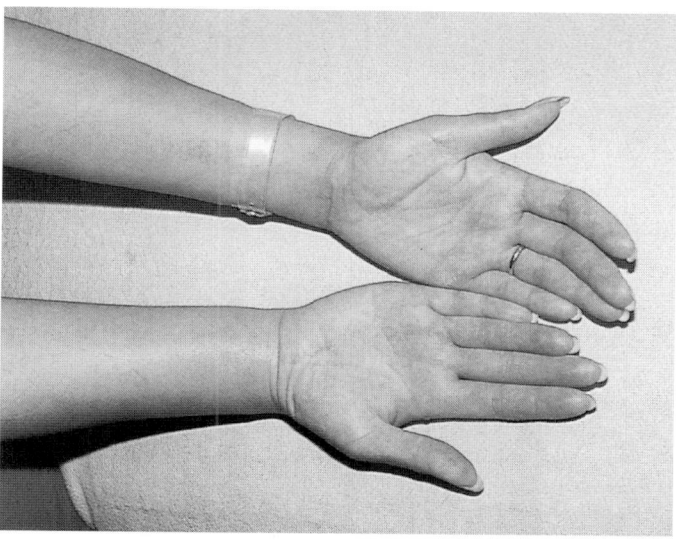

Figure 9.2: Transient swelling over the wrist in gnathostomiasis.

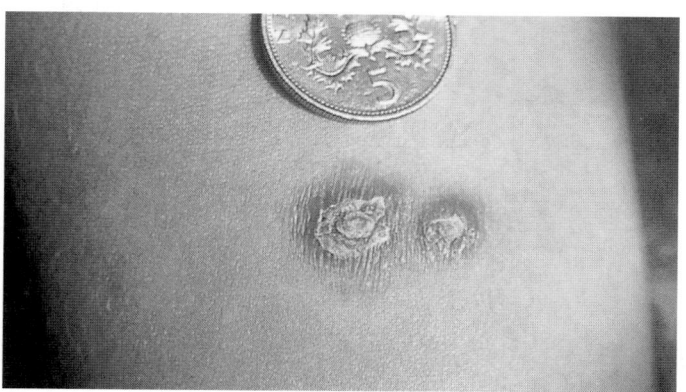

Figure 9.3: Crusted ulcers in cutaneous leishmaniasis.

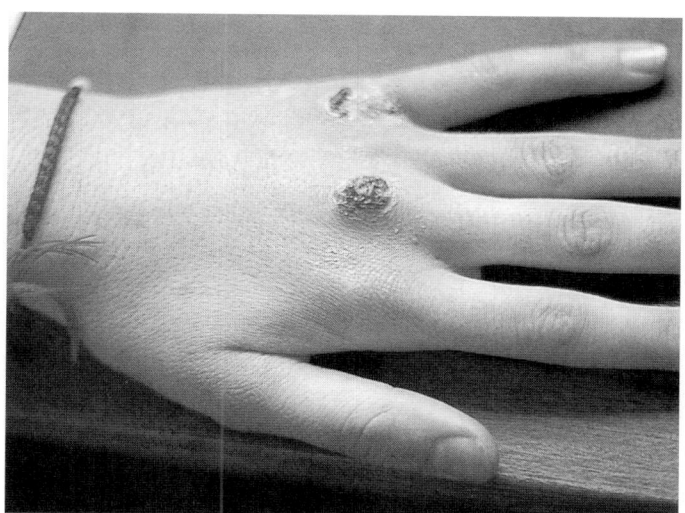

Figure 9.4: Crusted ulcers in *Staphylococcus* species: infected insect bites.

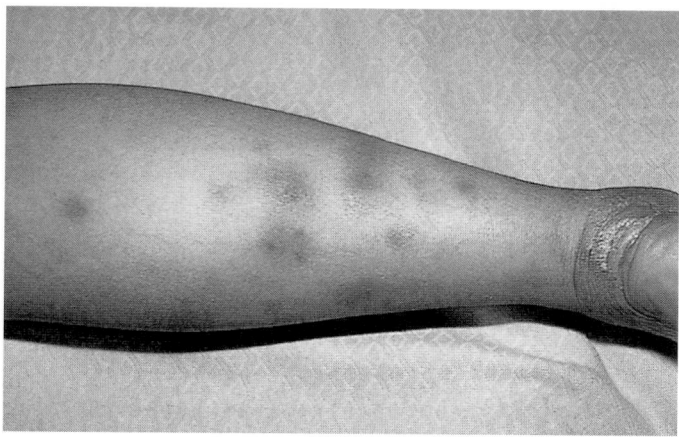

Figure 9.5: Painful nodules on the legs in erythema induratum (Bazin's disease)—related to tuberculosis.

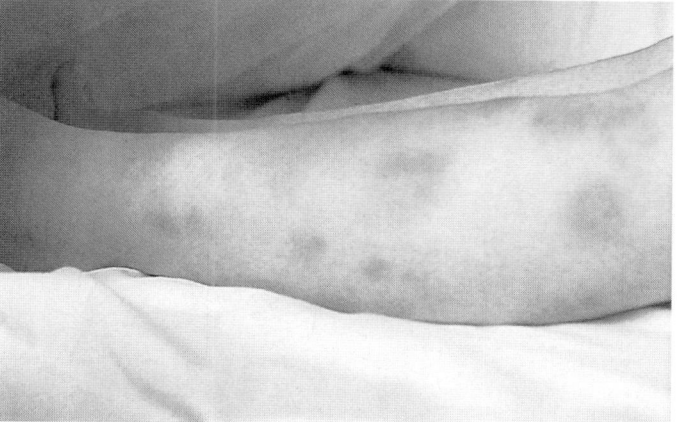

Figure 9.6: Painful nodules on the legs in erythema nodosum—related to tuberculosis.

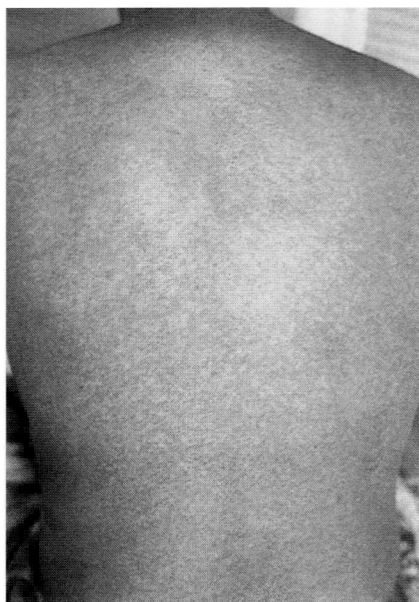

Figure 9.7: Non-confluent maculopapular rash due to dengue fever.

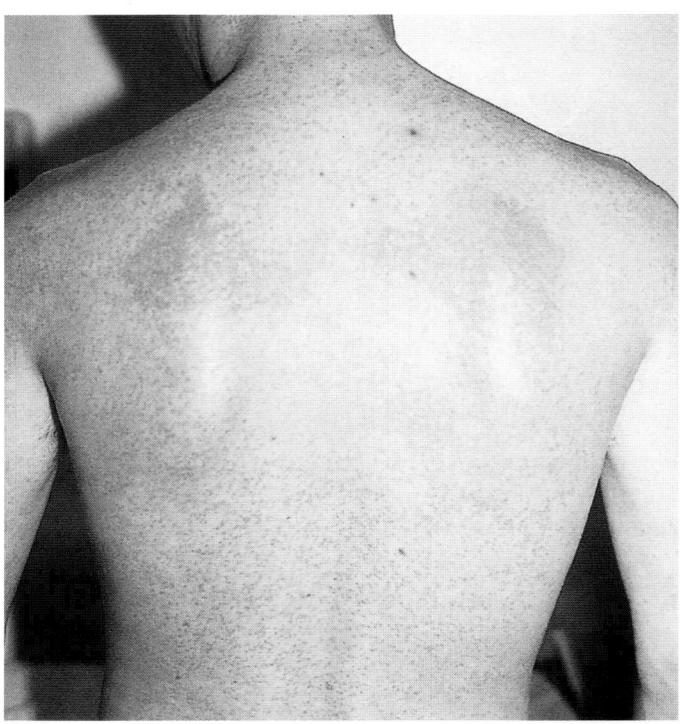

Figure 9.8: Non-confluent maculopapular rash due to rubella infection.

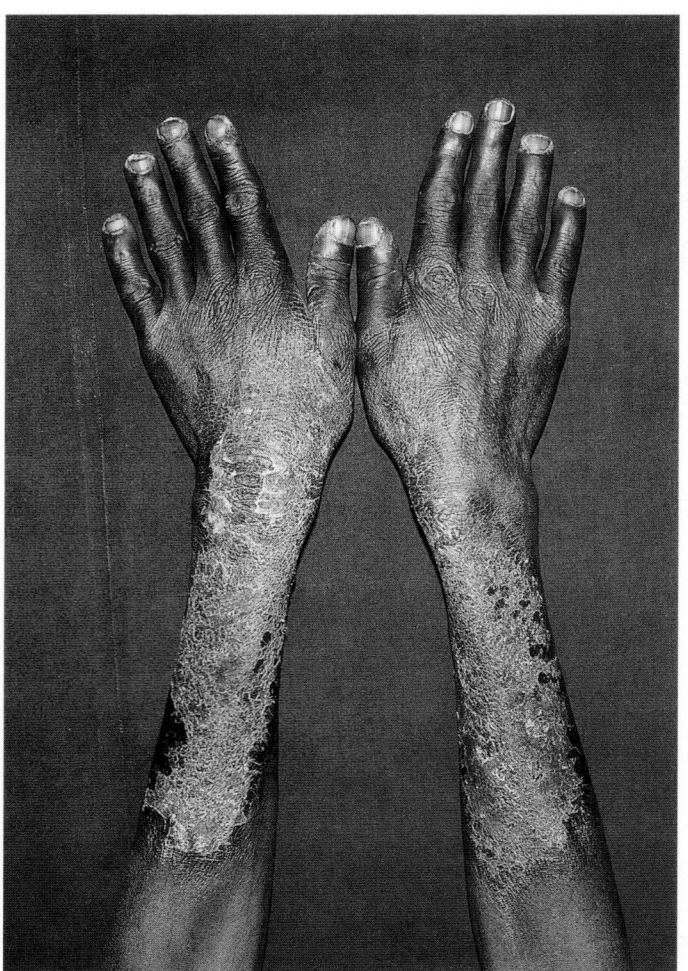

Figure 9.9: Skin rash (dermatitis) in pellagra.

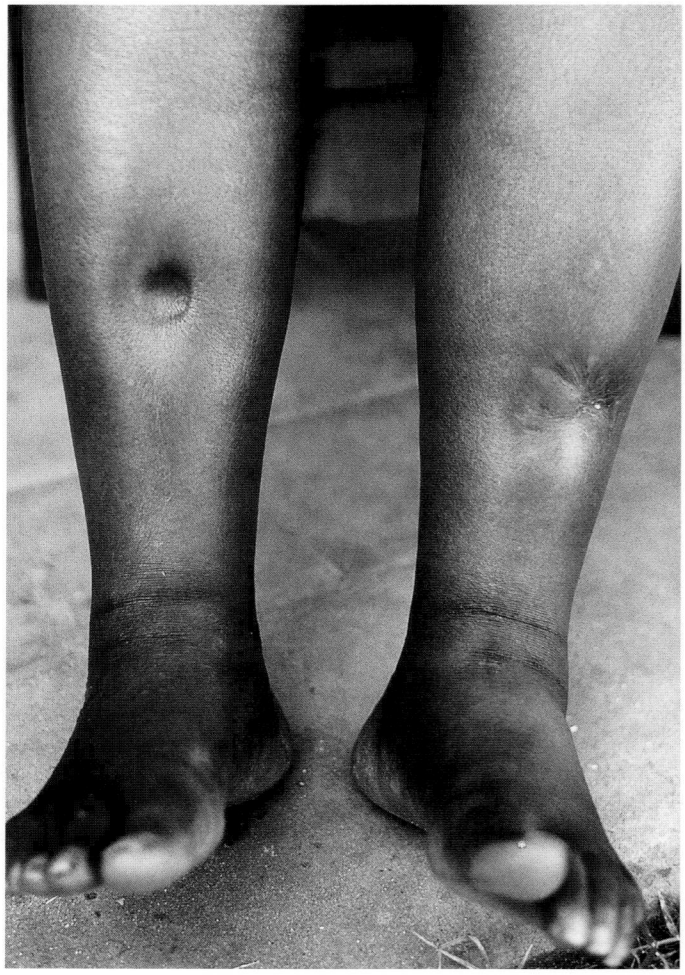

Figure 9.10: Pitting leg oedema in a patient with nephrotic syndrome.

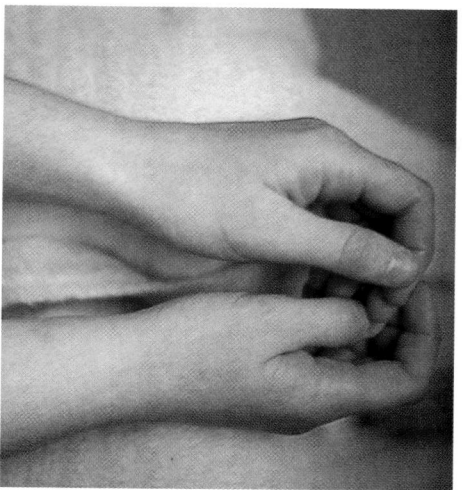

Plate 9.1: Transient swelling over the wrist in *Loa loa* infection.

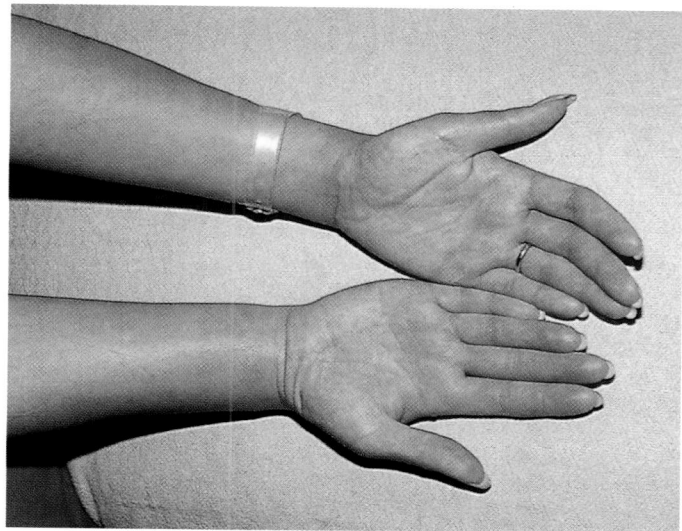

Plate 9.2: Transient swelling over the wrist in gnathostomiasis.

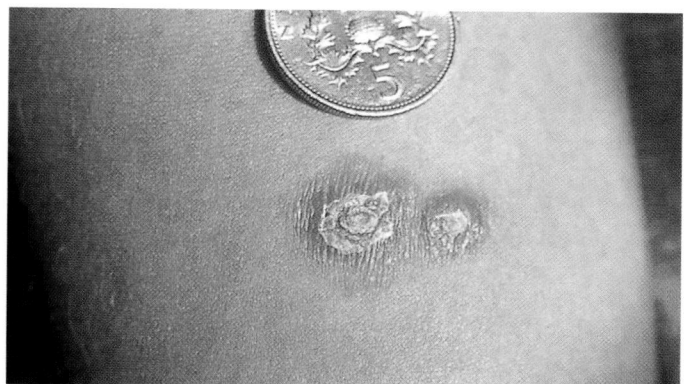

Plate 9.3: Crusted ulcers in cutaneous leishmaniasis.

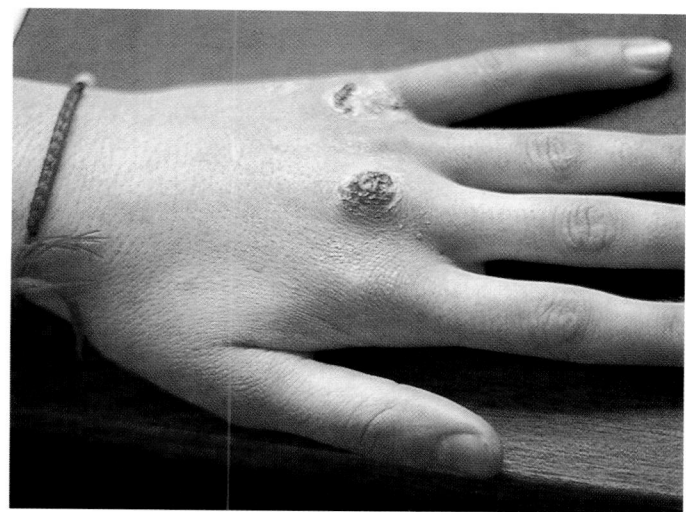

Plate 9.4: Crusted ulcers in *Staphylococcus* species: infected insect bites.

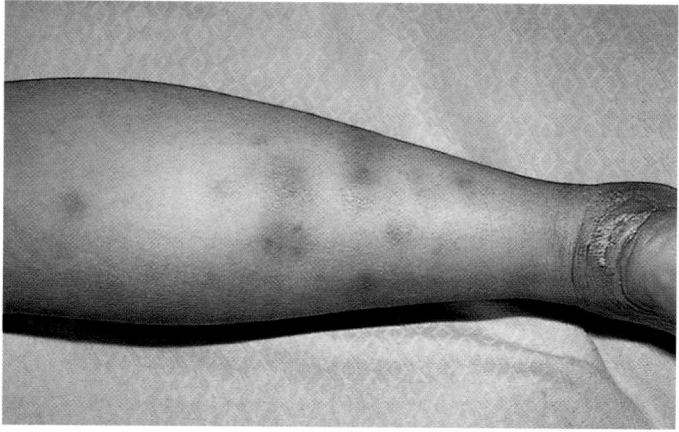

Plate 9.5: Painful nodules on the legs in erythema induratum (Bazin's disease)—related to tuberculosis.

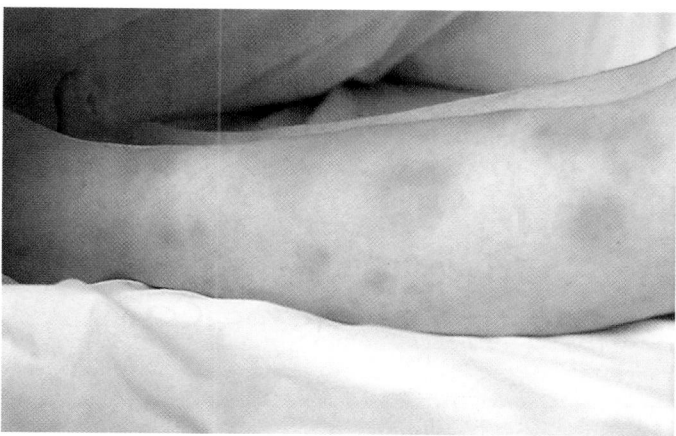

Plate 9.6: Painful nodules on the legs in erythema nodosum—related to tuberculosis.

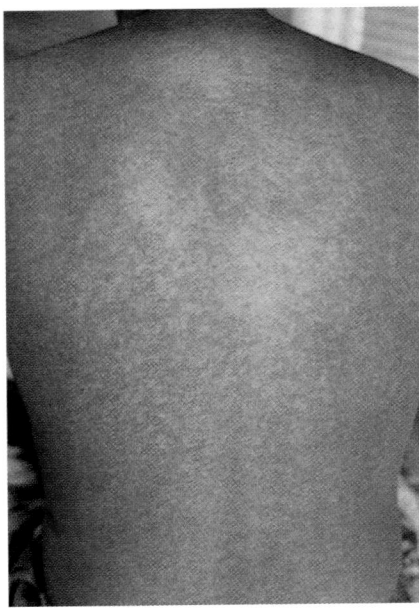

Plate 9.7: Non-confluent maculopapular rash due to dengue fever.

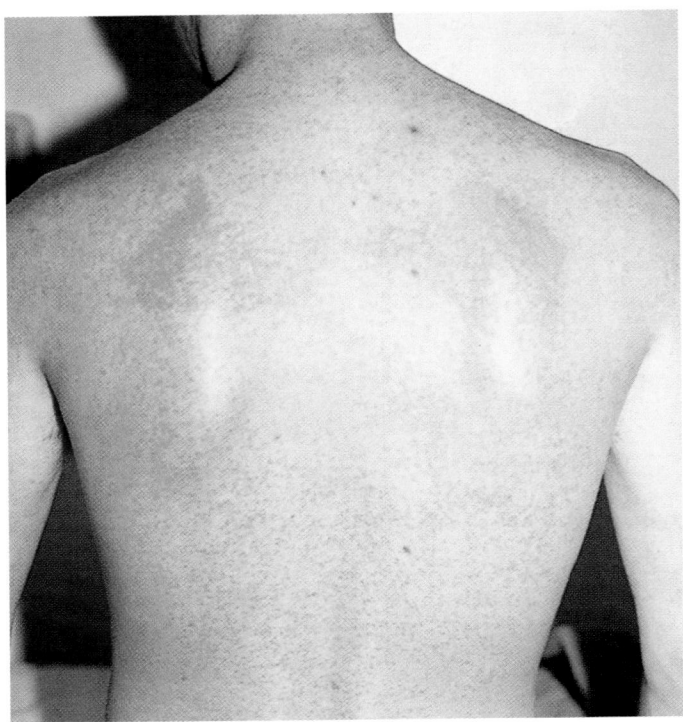

Plate 9.8: Non-confluent maculopapular rash due to rubella infection.

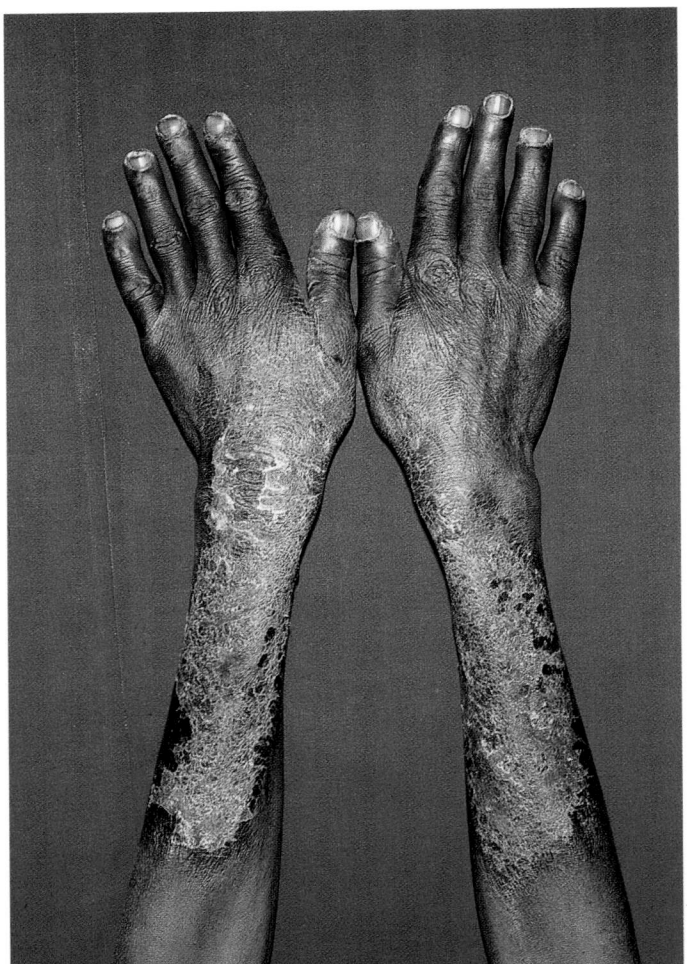

Plate 9.9: Skin rash (dermatitis) in pellagra.

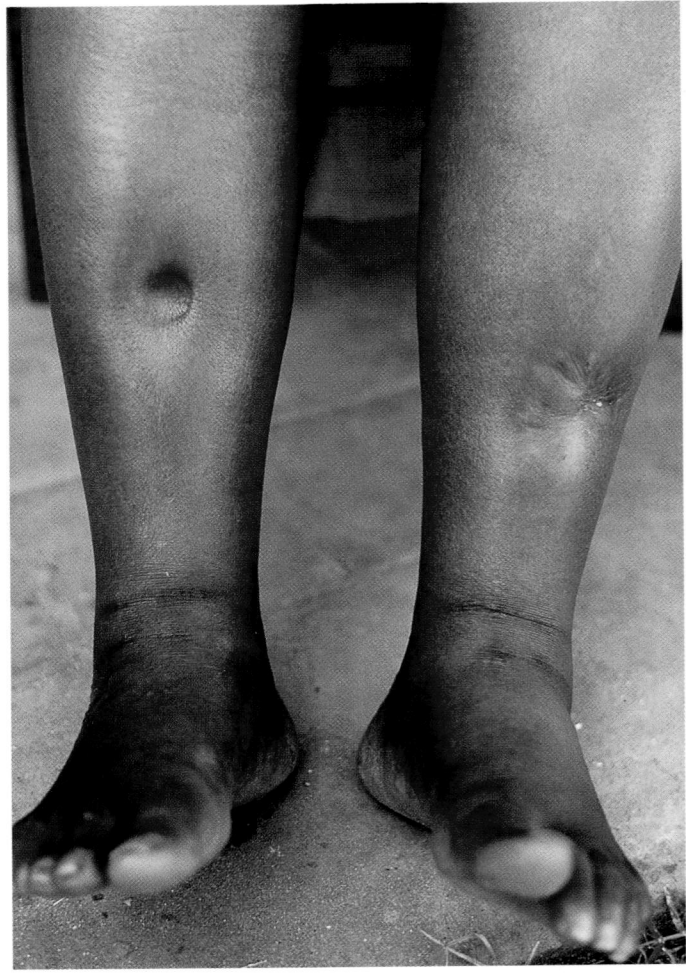

Plate 9.10: Pitting leg oedema in a patient with nephrotic syndrome.

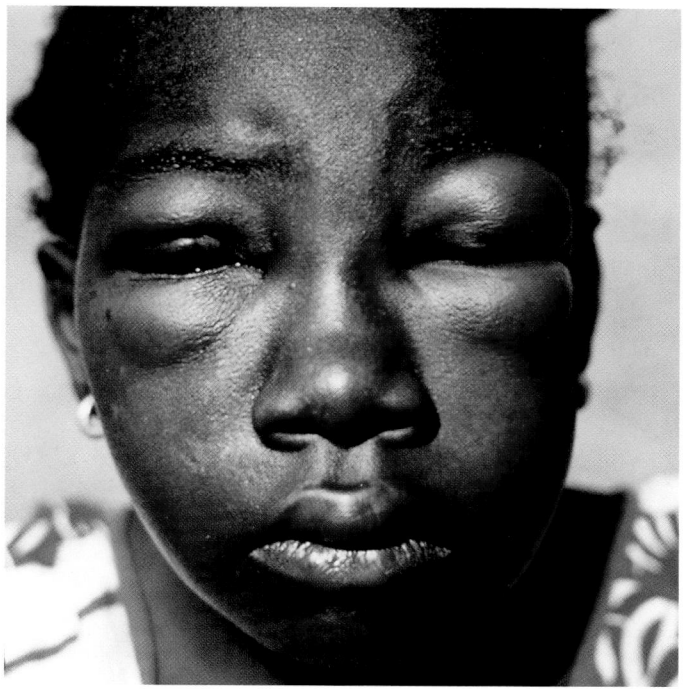

Plate 9.11: Bilateral facial oedema in nephrotic syndrome.

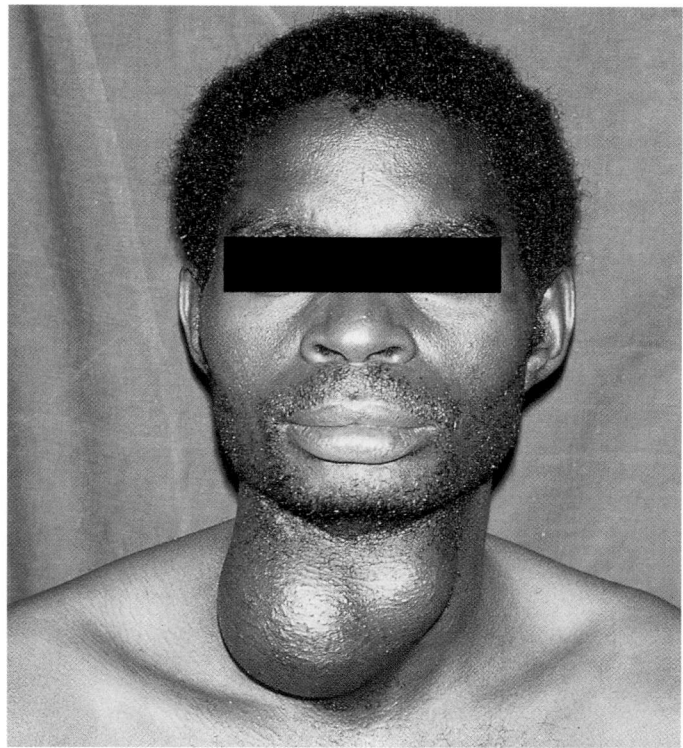

Plate 9.12: Endemic goitre.

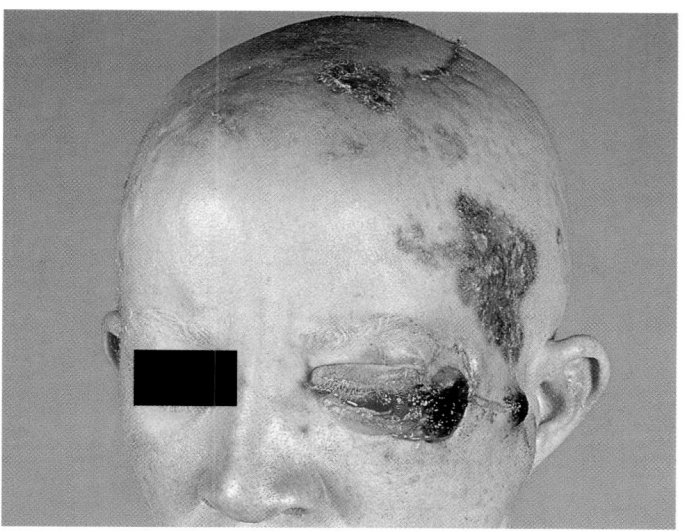

Plate 9.13: Squamous cell carcinoma in an African patient with albinism.

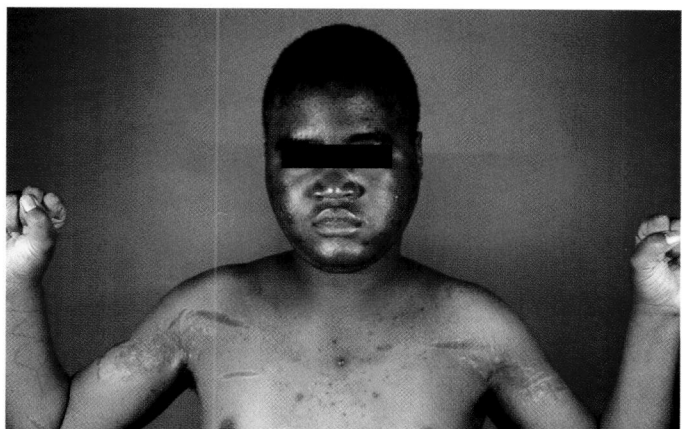

Plate 9.14: Cushingoid facies with cutaneous striae.

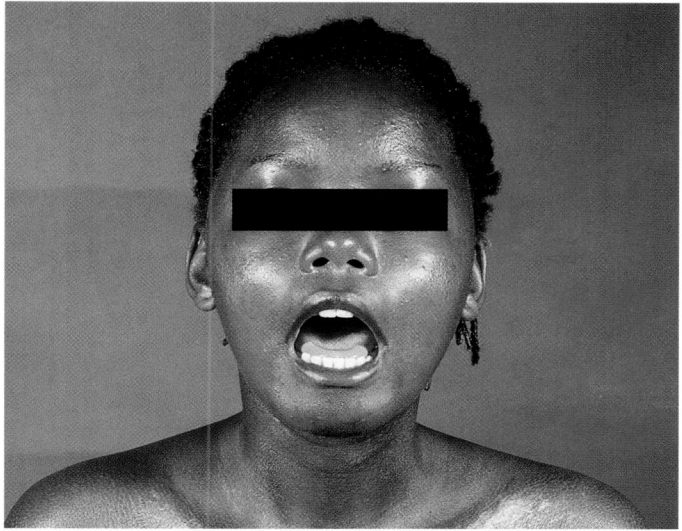

Plate 9.15: Systemic sclerosis restricting mouth opening.

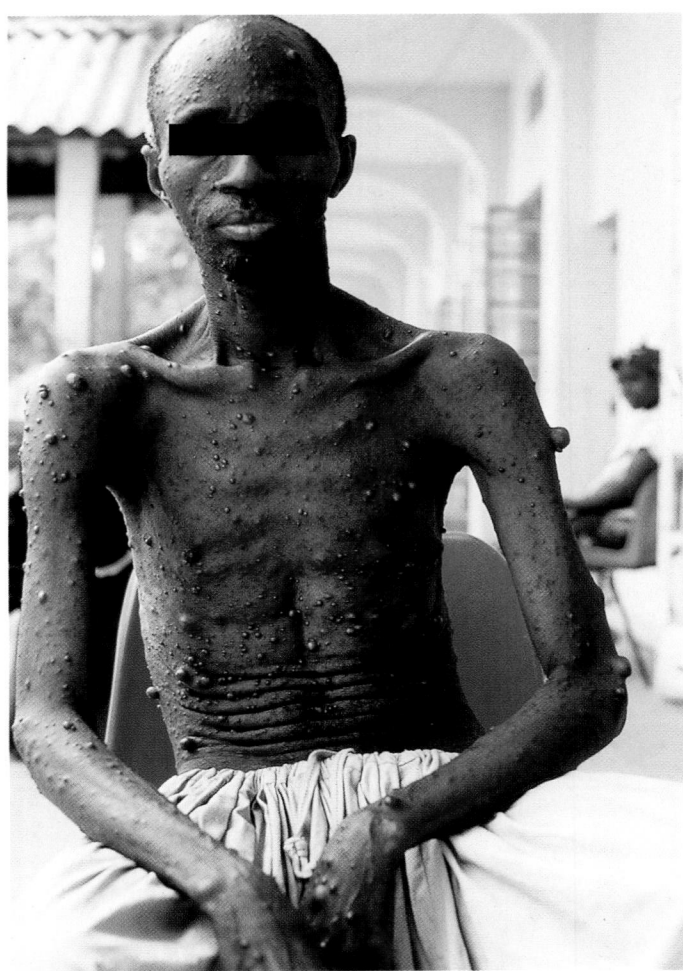

Plate 9.16: Multiple nodules of neurofibromatosis.

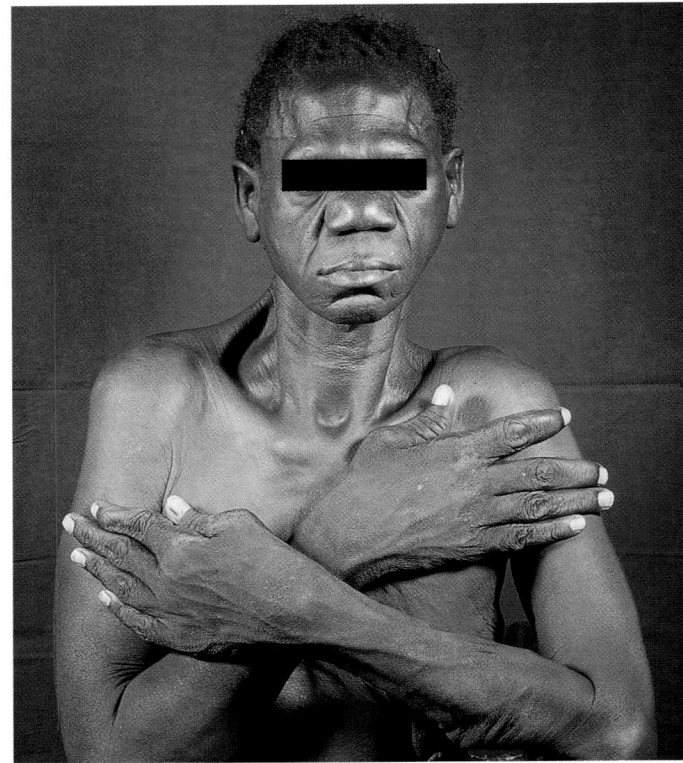

Plate 9.17: Acromegaly (large hands and prominent facial features).

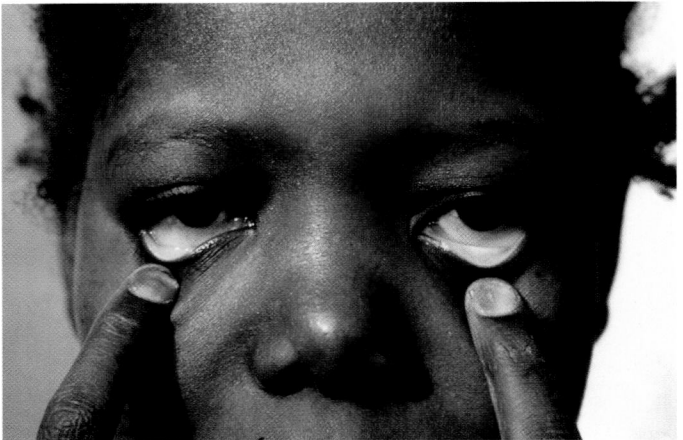

Plate 9.18: Pallor (anaemia) and koilonychia due to iron deficiency anaemia resulting from hookworm infestation.

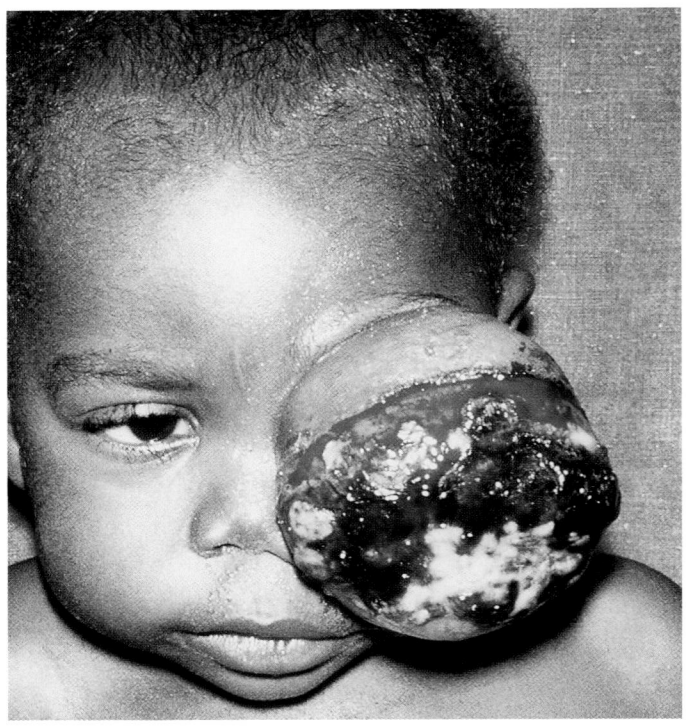

Plate 9.19: Retinoblastoma in a Zambian child.

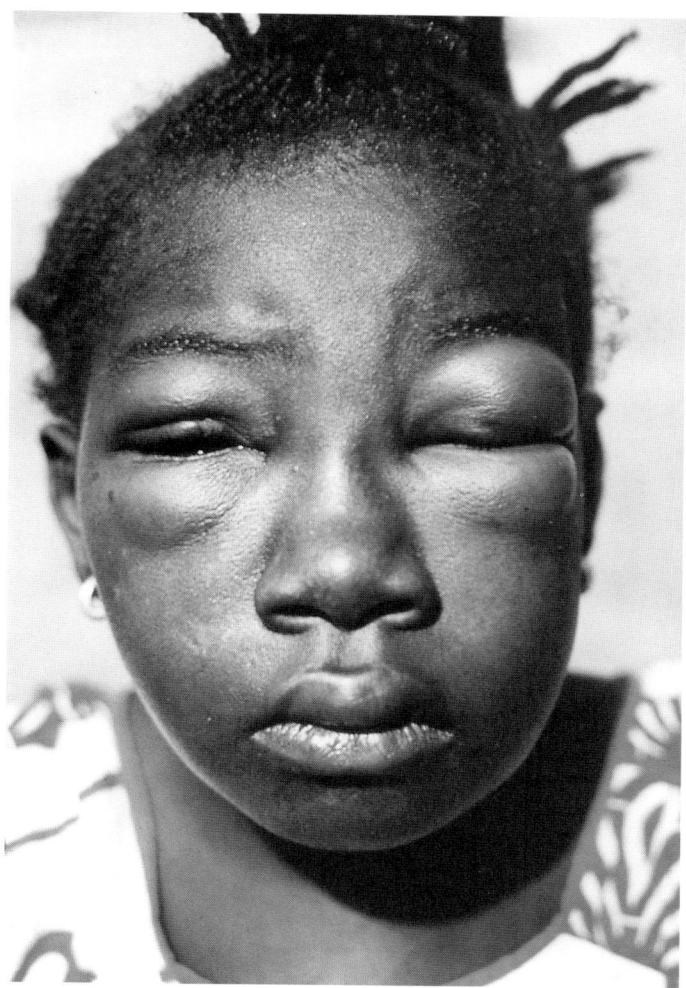

Figure 9.11: Bilateral facial oedema in nephrotic syndrome.

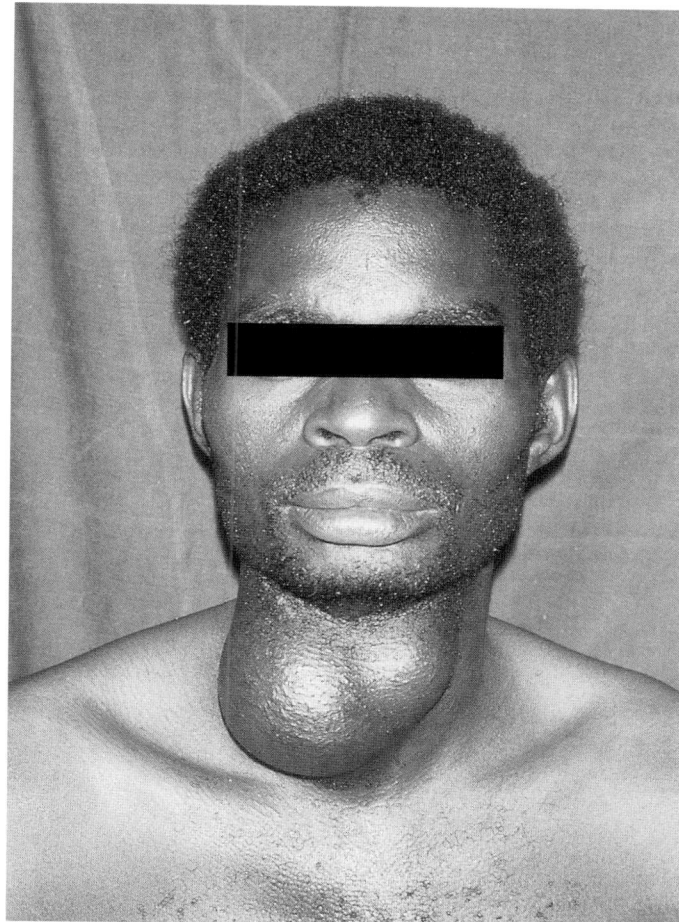

Figure 9.12: Endemic goitre.

features on general examination (described in Chapter 31). Angular stomatitis and glossitis may suggest associated vitamin B deficiencies. Clinical features of kwashiorkor include oedema, thin hypopigmented hair and dermatological lesions (described in Chapter 31).

Other common causes of generalized oedema are the same clinical syndromes as those in industrialized countries (cardiac failure, glomerulonephritis, nephrotic syndrome and cirrhosis) but with a different aetiological spectrum (see Chapters 12, 15 and 10). Lymphoedema in the tropics may be due to filariasis (see Chapter 82) or Kaposi's sarcoma. Focal migratory oedema, typically on the limbs, occurs in loiasis (Calabar swellings) and gnathostomiasis. Unilateral orbital oedema (Romaña's sign) suggests acute Chagas' disease in endemic areas. Bilateral periorbital oedema is a feature of trichinosis but more commonly found in renal disease and malnutrition.

Classic facies of selected diseases in the tropics include frontal bossing (associated with sickle cell anaemia or β-thalassaemia major), risus sardonicus (tetanus), leonine facies (lepromatous leprosy), lupus vulgaris (tuberculosis) and saddle nose (congenital syphilis).

Erythema nodosum has a wide differential diagnosis—in the tropics streptococcal infection, primary tuberculosis, leprosy, yersiniosis, lymphogranuloma venereum and the endemic mycoses should be considered.

Several features on general examination are highly suggestive of HIV/AIDS (see Chapter 20): generalized lymphadenopathy (see below), bilateral cystic parotidomegaly, oral hairy leucoplakia, oral candidiasis, zoster in patients younger than 50 years, papular pruritic eruption (associated marked postinflammatory hyperpigmentation is particularly common in Africa), extensive seborrhoeic dermatitis, giant mucocutaneous herpes simplex virus ulcers and Kaposi's sarcoma.

Skin

The skin is frequently involved in systemic disease: e.g., petechiae in meningococcal sespsis, the hypopigmentation and flaking appearance of kwashiorkor, and the photosensitive dermatitis of pellagra. Many problems in tropical disease practice may manifest themselves dermatologically

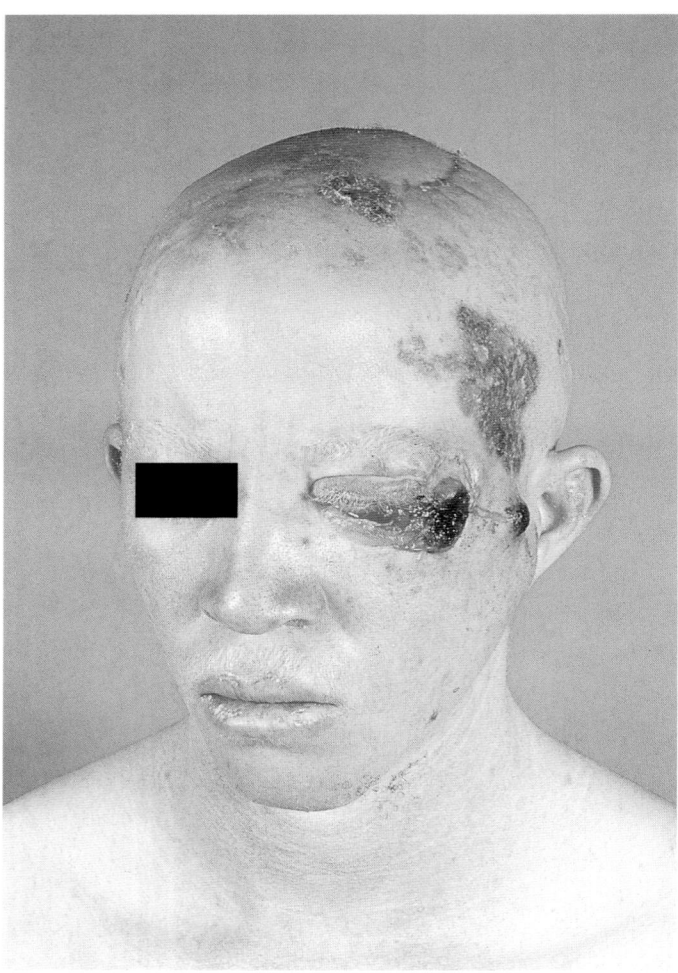

Figure 9.13: Squamous cell carcinoma in an African patient with albinism.

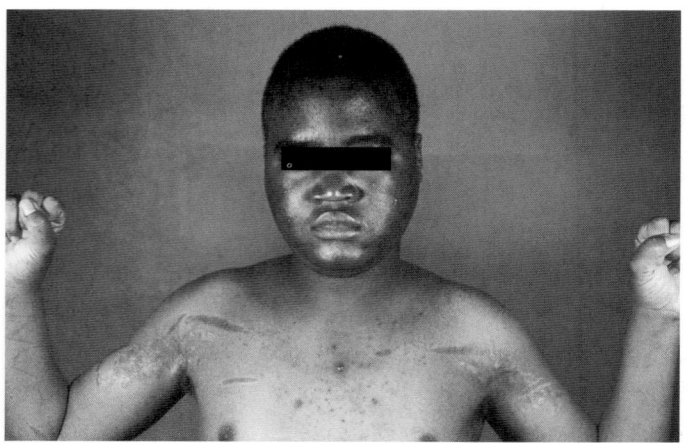

Figure 9.14: Cushingoid facies with cutaneous striae.

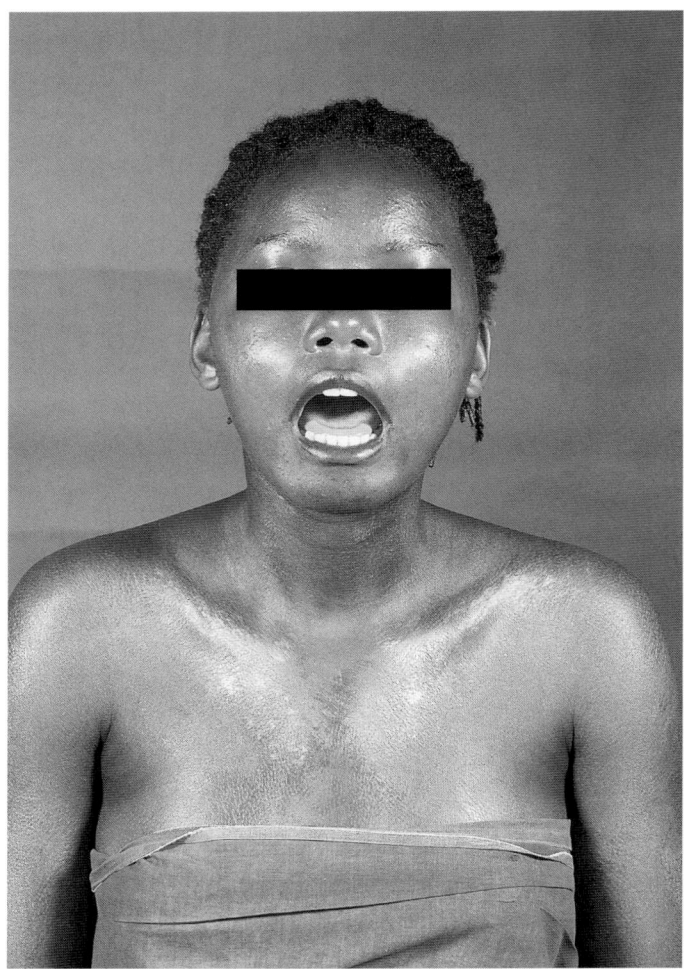

Figure 9.15: Systemic sclerosis restricting mouth opening.

and infections of the skin are especially common. It is often difficult to recognize many of the exanthemas on a dark-coloured skin. This subject is extensively dealt with in Chapter 19.

Fever

The symptom of fever should always be confirmed by measuring the temperature. Normal temperature is < 37.2°C, but fever is generally diagnosed when it is 38°C or more. Most patients with significant fever will have an infection, but non-infectious diseases may also cause fever; this is particularly true of patients presenting with chronic fever (> 2 weeks duration). Absence of fever does not exclude severe infection, particularly in the elderly. Hypothermia may occur in severe sepsis. Many patients present with fever with no obvious focus of infection.

Fever patterns

The pattern of fever may be helpful in determining the underlying cause but 'classical' patterns are not seen

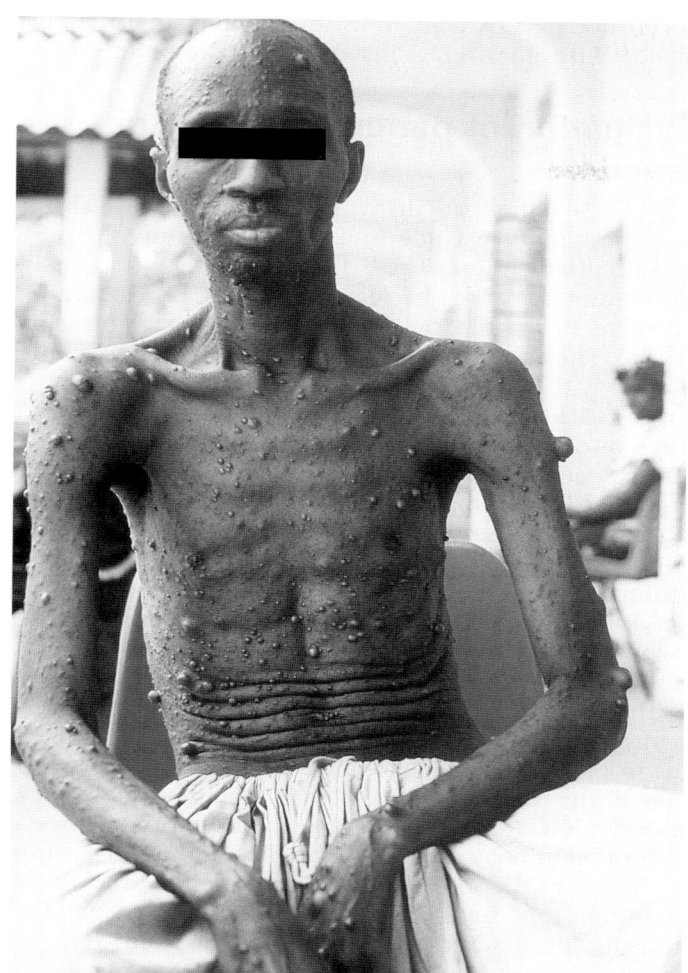

Figure 9.16: Multiple nodules of neurofibromatosis.

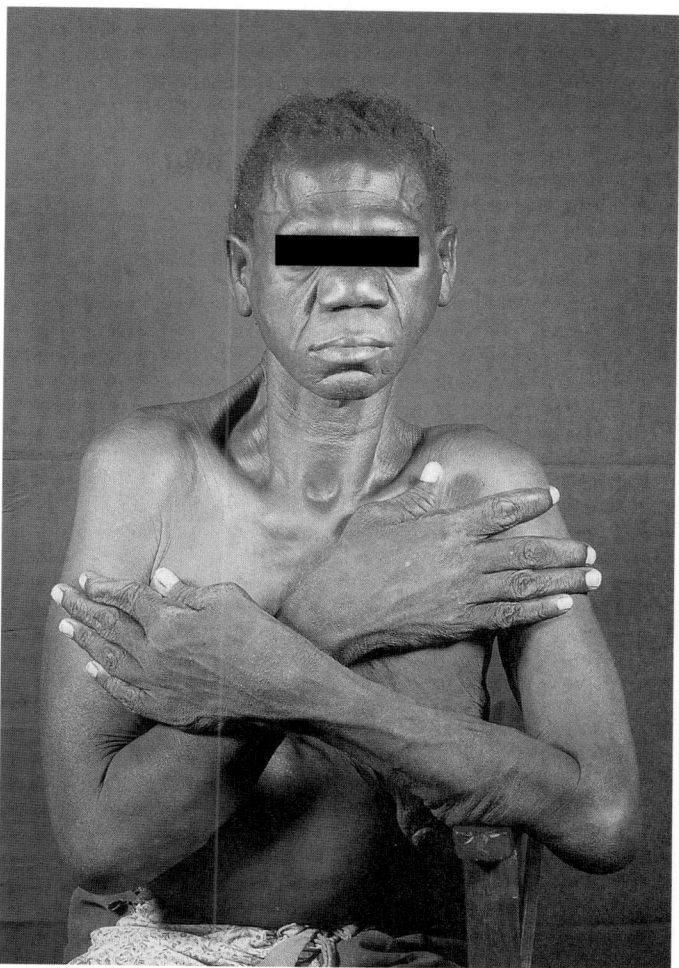

Figure 9.17: Acromegaly (large hands and prominent facial features).

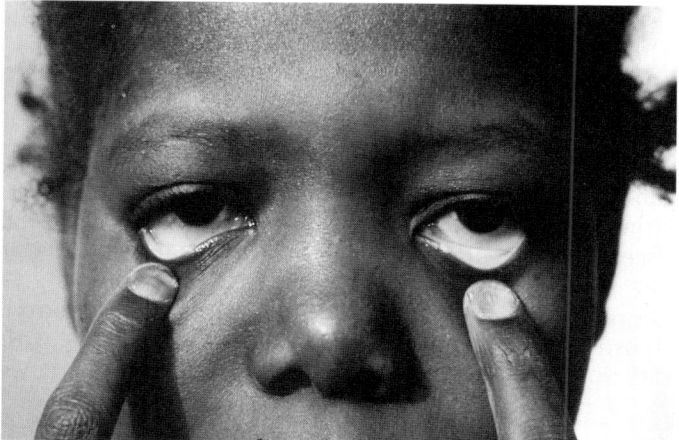

Figure 9.18: Pallor (anaemia) and koilonychia due to iron deficiency anaemia resulting from hookworm infestation.

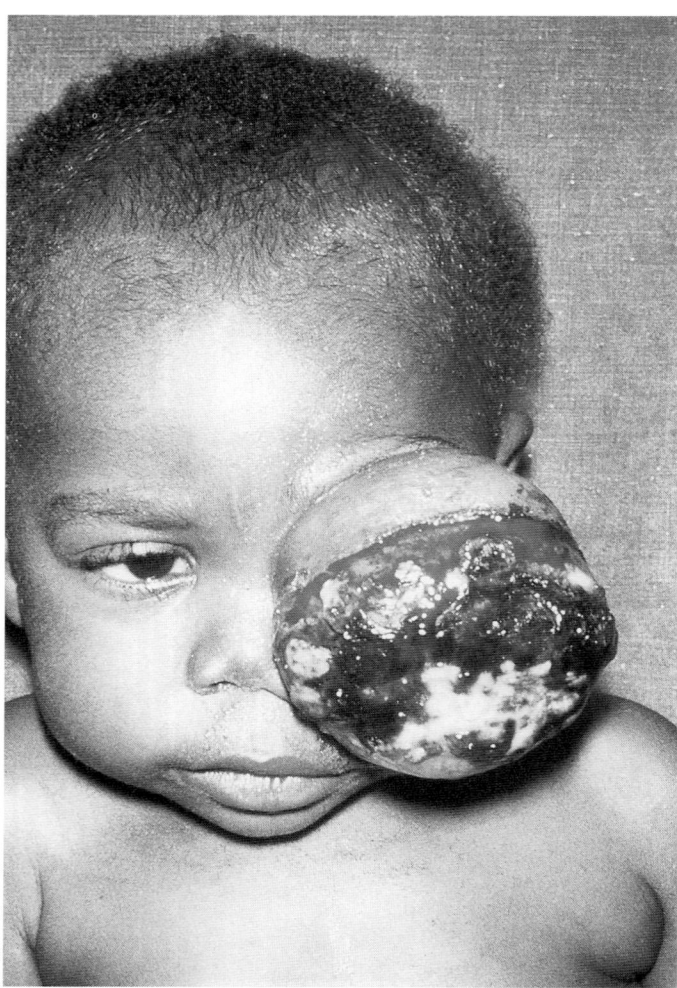

Figure 9.19: Retinoblastoma in a Zambian child.

frequently in clinical practice. The most characteristic pattern is periodic fever every second or third day in tertian or quartan malaria respectively (see Figure 9.20). In malaria the tertian or quartan fever patterns are not present at the onset and the tertian pattern is generally not present in non-immune patients with *Plasmodium falciparum* malaria. A biphasic or 'saddle-back' fever pattern with a short afebrile interval occurs in dengue and leptospirosis. Undulant fever that waxes and wanes over days may occur in brucellosis, visceral leishmaniasis and lymphoma (Pel–Ebstein fever). Fever that settles spontaneously with recurrences after intervals of a few days or weeks is characteristic of relapsing fever. Relative bradycardia (pulse rate increase less than the expected 15 beats per minute for each 1°C rise in temperature) is associated with several infections, particularly typhoid, yellow fever and legionnaires' disease.

Incubation periods

Knowledge of the incubation period of infections can be very helpful in differential diagnosis if the exposure period is known. This applies particularly to travellers.

Incubation periods are most useful in ruling out infections. Table 9.4 lists the average incubation periods of infections.

Evaluation of patients with acute fever

When evaluating patients with acute fever (< 2 weeks) it is important to exclude infections which may require urgent intervention. These include malaria (especially falciparum malaria), bacteraemia (especially meningococcaemia), typhoid, rickettsioses and viral haemorrhagic fevers. The latter must be considered in any febrile patient with a bleeding tendency. The presence of rigors suggests bacteraemia, severe viral infections or malaria. The skin should be carefully examined for early petechial lesions suggesting meningococcaemia, rose spots of typhoid (difficult to see on dark skin), eschars suggesting rickettsiosis (these are usually found on the legs or the perineum), sparse papular or pustular lesions of disseminated gonococcal infection and stigmata of infective endocarditis. Features indicating severe sepsis include tachycardia with low volume pulse, tachypnoea, confusion, hypotension and organ failure.

The extent of laboratory work-up of patients with acute fever in the tropics or the returning traveller from the tropics[12–14] will depend on the available facilities and how ill the patient is. Microscopic examination of thick and thin blood smears is the most important initial investigation and may identify malaria, *Borrelia* (relapsing fever) and African trypanosomiasis. However, it is important to recognize that the identification of malarial parasites in the indigenous population from a holo-endemic area does not necessarily mean that malaria is the cause of fever as asymptomatic parasitaemia is common in this context. A complete blood count is often helpful. Significant anaemia suggests malaria, bartonellosis or acute haemolytic anaemia complicating sickle cell disease or glucose-6-phosphate dehydrogenase deficiency. Neutrophilia is present in many infections and is not of diagnostic value. However, neutropenia suggests viral infections, typhoid or fulminant sepsis. Eosinophilia suggests acute parasite invasion or drug hypersensitivity reaction (see below). Thrombocytopenia is common in severe sepsis, viral infections and malaria. Urinalysis and chest radiography may indicate the source of infection. A blood culture should be done if there is no clear diagnosis. Liver function tests may suggest viral hepatitis, which typically presents with fever in the pre-icteric phase. Arterial blood gas analysis and renal function should be done in patients with features of severe sepsis.

Fever and generalized rash

Many infections present as an acute febrile illness with a generalized rash. The pattern of the rash is important in the differential diagnosis. The least specific pattern is maculopapular. Other patterns are diffuse erythroderma, vesicular and haemorrhagic lesions (petechiae, purpura or ecchymoses). Table 9.5 lists infections that typically

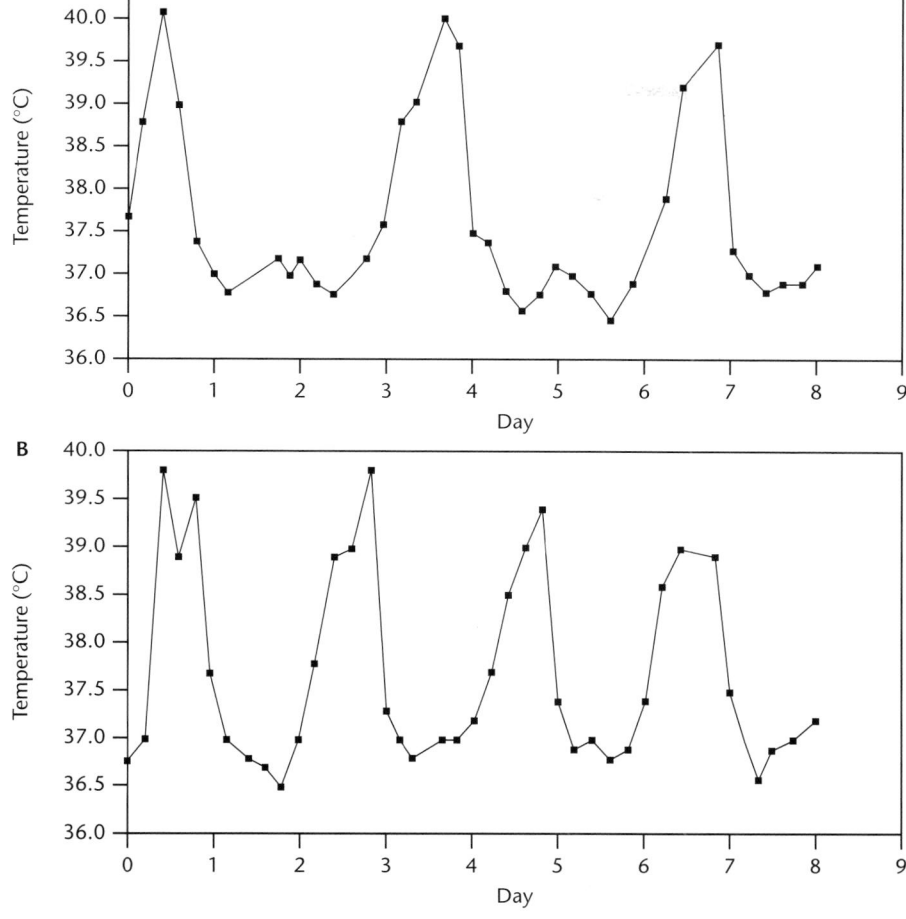

Figure 9.20: On rare occasions a fever pattern can be so characteristic as to be virtually diagnostic as in (**A**) the quartan (2-day gap) fever of *Plasmodium malariae* infection, or (**B**) the tertian (1-day gap) fever of *Plasmodium vivax* infection.

Table 9.4 Average incubation periods of selected infections.

Short (< 10 days)	Arboviruses
	Bacillary dysentery
	Rickettsial spotted fever
	Rickettsialpox
	Scrub typhus
	Relapsing fever
	Plague
Intermediate (10–21 days)	Typhoid
	Falciparum malaria
	Leptospirosis
	HIV
	Brucellosis
	Typhus (louse-borne)
	Q fever
	African trypanosomiasis
	Acute Chagas' disease
Long (> 21 days)	Viral hepatitis
	Malaria (including
	P. falciparum)
	Amoebic liver abscess
	Visceral leishmaniasis

present with these patterns. Drug hypersensitivity reactions and connective tissue diseases should also be considered.

Fever and jaundice

There are several pitfalls in managing the patient with jaundice.[6] The primary viral hepatitides (A–E) are febrile illnesses primarily in the prodromal, non-icteric phase. Fever normally subsides with the onset of jaundice but may persist for a few days after the development of jaundice. A patient who is febrile and jaundiced concurrently is more likely to be afflicted with another, usually more severe condition, such as *P. falciparum* malaria, typhoid or leptospirosis (Table 9.6). In view of the appreciable mortality of the latter conditions, their diagnosis should always be carefully considered.

Fever and eosinophilia

This is usually due to immature parasites that migrate through tissue. This clinical syndrome is generally called visceral larva migrans. Pulmonary symptoms or infiltrates commonly also occur, as many parasites which present

Table 9.5 Infections typically presenting with acute fever and generalized rash.

Maculopapular	Measles Rubella Dengue Rickettsial spotted fevers Primary HIV Louse-borne typhus Scrub typhus Chikungunya O'nyong-nyong
Vesicular	Chickenpox Disseminated zoster Disseminated herpes simplex Monkeypox
Erythroderma	Scarlet fever Kawasaki's disease Toxic shock syndrome
Haemorrhagic	Meningococcaemia Viral haemorrhagic fevers Disseminated intravascular coagulation Louse-borne typhus (severe) Rickettsial spotted fevers (severe) Chickenpox (haemorrhagic)

Table 9.6 Jaundice with concurrent fever.

Hepatic	Severe *P. falciparum* malaria Typhoid Leptospirosis (Weil's disease) Viral hepatitis A–E (fever usually settles before jaundice) Septicaemia Pneumococcal pneumonia Relapsing fever Yellow fever (and other viral haemorrhagic fevers) Typhus Alcoholic hepatitis
Posthepatic	Ascending cholangitis (may complicate liver flukes or ascariasis) Cholecystitis (bacterial, *Cryptosporidium parvum*), cytomegalovirus
Haemolytic	Malaria Haemoglobinopathies (especially sickle cell disease) Glucose-6-phosphate dehydrogenase deficiency (favism, drug-induced crisis) *Bartonella bacilliformis* Haemolytic–uraemic syndrome (*Shigella dysenteriae, E. coli*)

with fever and eosinophilia migrate through the lungs. Diagnosis of the specific parasite involved is difficult as the parasites have not yet arrived at their final destination and laid eggs—serological tests are available for some parasites. The commonest diseases presenting with fever and eosinophilia in the tropics are acute schistosomiasis (Katayama fever) and ascariasis. Other diseases include toxocariasis, hookworm, trichinosis, fascioliasis, gnathostomiasis and paragonimiasis. Hypersensitivity reactions to drugs should always be considered.

HIV-associated fever of unknown origin (FUO)

This has been defined as FUO in an HIV-infected person with no diagnosis after 3 days of inpatient investigation. HIV itself can cause a fever, but this is a diagnosis by exclusion as the vast majority of patients will have another treatable cause. Mycobacterial infections account for almost half of these. Table 9.7 lists the likely causes of FUO in the HIV-infected patient in the tropics. Bacteraemias are listed in the table as blood culture results in resource-poor settings often take longer than 3 days.

Classical FUO

Classical FUO is chronic fever (> 2 weeks) with no cause identified after initial investigations on two outpatient visits or three inpatient days.[13] In industrialized countries malignancies (particularly lymphoproliferative disorders), infections and connective tissue disorders are collectively the cause in about three-quarters of cases of classical FUO, with malignancies being the commonest. In the tropics infectious causes are far more important and connective tissue diseases are relatively uncommon. Extrapulmonary tuberculosis is the commonest cause. Table 9.8 lists some important infections presenting as classical FUO in the tropics.

Table 9.7 Common causes of HIV-associated FUO in the tropics.

Tuberculosis
Bacteraemia (*Salmonella* spp. and *S. pneumoniae*)
Pneumocystis carinii pneumonia
Community-acquired pneumonia
Cryptococcosis
Toxoplasmosis
Visceral leishmaniasis
Disseminated atypical mycobacteriosis
Disseminated endemic mycoses
Non-Hodgkin's lymphoma
Cytomegalovirus

Table 9.8 Important infectious causes of classical FUO in the tropics.

Extrapulmonary tuberculosis
Typhoid fever
Amoebic liver abscess
Infective endocarditis
Pyogenic intra-abdominal abscesses
Brucellosis
Relapsing fever
Visceral leishmaniasis
Cryptococcosis
Strongyloides hyperinfection syndrome
Katayama fever
Visceral larva migrans
Q fever
Trypanosomiasis
Toxoplasmosis
Histoplasmosis
Coccidioidomycosis

Lymphadenopathy

Residents of the tropics are frequently exposed to infectious disease and palpable shotty lymph nodes are a common finding that does not necessarily indicate active pathology. Larger palpable inguinal nodes of no clinical significance are particularly common in people who walk barefoot. However, inguinal nodes should always be examined as several important diseases typically cause inguinal lymphadenitis (many STDs, bubonic plague and lymphatic filariasis). Lymphadenopathy may be generalized or regional, acute or chronic, and accompanied by suppuration (with bubo formation) or caseation. Table 9.9 lists diseases in the tropics that may present with lymphadenopathy. The majority of diseases causing generalized lymphadenopathy also cause splenomegaly.

HIV-associated persistent generalized lymphadenopathy is very common in early disease, but in advanced disease the nodes regress. Lymphadenopathy at this stage of the illness is usually due to opportunistic infections (overwhelmingly tuberculosis) or malignancies (Kaposi's sarcoma or lymphoma). Tuberculosis may present with generalized adenopathy, nodes matted together or with large asymmetrical nodes, which may be fluctuant if there is extensive caseation necrosis. Sinus formation is

Table 9.9 Diseases associated with lymphadenopathy.

	Acute	Chronic
Generalized	Measles Dengue Primary HIV Cytomegalovirus Epstein–Barr virus Rubella Scrub typhus Leptospirosis Leukaemia	HIV Disseminated tuberculosis Secondary syphilis Brucellosis Toxoplasmosis African trypanosomiasis Chagas' disease Kala azar Leprosy Disseminated endemic mycoses Sarcoidois Connective tissue diseases

Regional	Pyogenic adenitis*
	Adenovirus
	STD:
	    Chancroid*
	    Primary genital herpes
	    Primary syphilis
	    Lymphogranuloma venereum*
	Rickettsia:
	    R. conorii
	    R. africae
	    R. akari
	Recurrent lymphatic filariasis
	Diphtheria
	Bubonic plague*
	Tularaemia*
	Anthrax
		Tuberculosis*
		Lymphoma
		Metastatic carcinoma/sarcoma
		Non-tuberculous mycobacteria*
		Endemic mycoses
		Chronic lymphatic filariasis
		Onchocerciasis
		Loiasis
		Cat scratch disease*
		Meliodosis*
		Kawasaki's disease
		Kikuchi's disease*

*Denotes that suppuration or caseation may occur

common; in the neck this may present with 'collar stud' abscesses.

Ulceroglandular syndromes present with a lesion at the site of inoculation (occasionally this may be the eye, producing the oculoglandular syndrome) associated with regional lymphadenitis. The classic example is tularaemia, but this pattern is also seen with anthrax, cat scratch disease (the site of inoculation is usually a papule rather than an ulcer) and rickettsiae that are associated with an eschar.

Lymphangitis is inflamed subcutaneous lymphatic vessels. Acutely these are commonly associated with subcutaneous pyogenic infections or with recurrent attacks of lymphatic filariasis. Chronic nodular lymphangitis presents with granulomatous nodules along thickened lymphatic vessels. Sporotrichosis is the classic cause, but non-tuberculous mycobacteria (especially *Mycobacterium marinum*) and *Nocardia* species can also present in this way.

Glandular fever in the tropics is not common as Epstein–Barr virus and cytomegalovirus are typically subclinical diseases of early childhood. Primary HIV infections should be considered in sexually active patients with a glandular fever-type illness. Features that strongly suggest this diagnosis are a maculopapular rash (without a history of prior aminopenicillin use) and small orogenital ulcers.

Splenomegaly

Splenomegaly and hepatomegaly or hepatosplenomegaly are common findings in patients living in the tropics.[15] A wide range of tropical infections and other systemic diseases can cause these signs (Table 9.10). The common causes of a very large spleen reaching the right iliac fossa are (a) tropical splenomegaly syndrome due to malaria, (b) visceral leishmaniasis, (c) portal hypertension (schistosomal), (d) myelofibrosis and (e) lymphoma/chronic myeloid leukaemia.

Conclusion

History taking and physical examination remain the

Table 9.10 Common causes of splenomegaly, hepatomegaly or hepatosplenomegaly.

Malaria*
Typhoid
Brucellosis
Relapsing fever (louse and tick borne)
Typhus
Visceral leishmaniasis*
Trypanosomiasis
Schistosomiasis (portal hypertension)
Haemoglobinopathies
HIV infection
Hepatitis B infection
Hydatid disease
Lymphoma*
Chronic myeloid leukaemia*
Myelofibrosis*
Leptospirosis
Bartonellosis

*May cause massive splenomegaly.

mainstay of the practice of medicine. Clinical acumen is of paramount importance in arriving at a correct diagnosis when medicine is practised in rural areas of the tropics or where laboratory backup is scarce or unavailable. Medical practitioners in the tropics must take a practical and common-sense approach to the diagnosis and management of patients who present with infectious and non-infectious conditions. Where the diagnosis is uncertain the answer often lies in retaking a history and redoing the physical examination. In problematic cases, they should know where to seek assistance to obtain information on diseases specific to certain geographical areas (see Appendix V). Subsequent chapters in this book highlight the main symptoms and signs of infectious and non-infectious diseases relating to each system of the body.

REFERENCES

1   Gilles H M & Lucas A O. Tropical medicine: 100 years of progress. *Br Med Bull* 1998; 54:269–280.

2   Murray H, Pépin J, Nutman T, Hoffman S & Mahmoud A. Tropical medicine. *BMJ* 2000; 320:490–494.

3   Weatherall D. The future role of molecular and cell biology in medical practice in the tropical countries. *Br Med Bull* 1998; 54:489–501.

4   Cook G C. Dealing with disease related to tropical exposure. In Toghill P J (ed.) *Examining Patients: An Introduction to Clinical Medicine*, 2nd edn. London: Edward Arnold, 1995: 245–258.

5   Hoffman S H. Tropical medicine and the acute abdomen. *Emerg Med Clin North Am* 1989; 7:591–609.

6   Maher D & Harries A. Pitfalls in the diagnosis and management of the jaundiced patient in the tropics. *Trop Doctor* 1994; 24:128–130.

7   Holocombe C, Weedon R & Llwin M. The differential diagnosis and management of breast lumps in the tropics. *Trop Doctor* 1999; 29:42–46.

8   Karp C L & Neva F A. Tropical infectious diseases in human immunodeficiency virus-infected patients. *Clin Infect Dis* 1999; 28:947–965.

9   Polsky B, Kotler D & Steinhart C. HIV-associated wasting in the HAART era:guidelines for assessment, diagnosis, and treatment. *AIDS Patient Care STDS* 2001; 15:411–423.

10 Dias J C. Tropical diseases and the gender approach. *Bull Pan*

Am Health Organ 1996; 30:242–260.

11 Peters W & Gilles H M. *Tropical Medicine and Parasitology*, 5th edn. Philadelphia: Mosby-Wolfe, 2000.

12 Suh K N, Kozarsky P E & Keystone J S. Evaluation of fever in the returned traveler. *Med Clin North Am* 1999; 83: 997–1017.

13 Durack D & Street A C. Fever of unknown origin re-examined and redefined. *Curr Clin Top Infect Dis* 1991; 11:35–51.

14 Norman G, Joseph A, Theodore A & Maruthamuthu M. Community-based teaching of tropical diseases: an experience with filariasis. *Trop Doctor* 1999; 29:86–89.

15 Onuigbo M A & Mbah A U. Tropical splenomegaly syndrome in Nigerian adults. *West Afr J Med* 1992; 11:72–78.

16 Scheidler M D & Giannella R A. Practical management of acute diarrhea. *Hosp Pract* 2001; 36:49–56.

Section 3

System-oriented Diseases

The discipline of 'tropical medicine' was traditionally dominated by infectious diseases. With modernization and globalization, the practice of medicine in the tropics has incorporated the non-infectious diseases. This section covers system-orientated diseases involving all the main body systems—STIs and HIV/AIDS are included in this section since they can affect every system in the body and can present to any specialty within medicine. A new chapter dealing with blood transfusion is included in this section to compliment that on haematology in the tropics; blood transfusions are vital components of every country's health service. Transfusion or injection of unsafe blood is responsible for betwen 8 and 16 million cases of hepatitis B virus infections, as well as 80–160,000 HIV infections each year! Twenty-five per cent of maternal deaths are linked to blood loss.

Chapter 10
Tropical Gastroenterological Problems

G. C. Cook

The portals of entry for organisms responsible for most infections which dominate medicine in tropical countries (as elsewhere) are the skin, and respiratory and intestinal tracts. In fact a very high proportion of infections of warm climes originate from ingestion of contaminated water and foodstuffs; many resultant diseases therefore fall into the subspecialty *tropical gastroenterology.*[1–3]

Most gastroenterological emergencies which occur in a temperate climate can also occur in tropical and subtropical countries. However, there are notable differences in prevalence.[4] Some problems are probably ethnically related (although elimination of environmental factors is often difficult), but the majority are superimposed upon an underlying communicable (infective) disease; important examples are ileal perforation or haemorrhage resulting from typhoid (enteric) fever, colonic perforation—and less often haemorrhage—in amoebic colitis and shigellosis, and hepatic 'abscess' in *invasive* amoebiasis.[4]

Mouth and pharynx

The mouth and rectum are the most accessible parts of the gastrointestinal tract from a clinical viewpoint;[5] therefore, where endoscopic procedures are impossible (that applies to many tropical and subtropical countries), as much information as possible should be derived from careful examination of these organs.

Viral, bacterial, mycotic and parasitic infections all give rise to oropharyngeal pathology, which is often most pronounced in the presence of associate malnutrition (especially in infants and children). Herpes simplex virus, Epstein–Barr virus (EBV) (see Chapter 44) and many enteroviruses can produce a stomatitis; oral ulceration is also a frequent manifestation of Behçet's syndrome—common in the Middle East and Japan. Lassa fever (see Chapter 41) and diphtheria (see Chapter 65) are frequently characterized by severe pharyngeal involvement, and in rabies (see Chapter 45) dysphagia caused by spasm of the pharyngeal muscles is an important feature of the disease. In addition to acute bacterial infections, tuberculosis, leprosy, syphilis and yaws all exert oral manifestations. Candidiasis (exceedingly common in the acquired immune deficiency syndrome (AIDS)) (Chapter 20), histoplasmosis, South American blastomycosis and coccidioidomycosis can also produce buccal lesions. Acute pharyngitis caused by infection with young adult *Fasciola hepatica* (ingested in raw sheep or goat liver—reported from the Middle East and India—and known locally as 'halzoun' (Chapter 81)) is caused by pentastomids.[1] Therapeutic agents such as sulfinamides (included in some antimalarial prophylactics, e.g., pyrimethamine + sulfamethoxazole ('Fansidar')) can give rise to the Stevens–Johnson sydrome, in which oral ulceration is common. Manifestations of specific malnutrition states (vitamin B and C deficits, and iron deficiency anaemia) are usually obvious, whereas in kwashiorkor these are frequently combined with infective complications. Cancrum oris is a gangrenous condition involving the gums and cheeks and is associated with *Borrelia vincenti* and *Fusiformis fusiformis* infection; it is especially common in malnourished children,[1] especially in West Africa. Descriptions of the mouth, especially the tongue, in postinfective malabsorption (tropical sprue) (see below) were dominant in *clinical* accounts of this disease in the nineteenth century (i.e., before the advent of laboratory investigation).

Periodontal disease and dental caries are also a major problem in tropical countries.[1] Oral submucous fibrosis—a chronic disease of unknown aetiology—may affect any part of the oral cavity;[1] most reports are from the Indian subcontinent and South-East Asia. Fibroelastosis of the submucous tissues, accompanied by epithelial atrophy, are important sequelae and are probably premalignant.

Of malignant disease(s), buccal carcinoma is pre-eminent;[5] Burkitt's lymphoma (Chapter 44), ameloblastoma and nasopharyngeal carcinoma (Chapter 36) are other malignancies which have important geographical distributions in tropical countries.

Hypertrophy of the salivary glands is common in malnourished children; it can also be associated with *Ascaris lumbricoides* infection and chronic calcific pancreatitis (see below).[1] Tumours of the salivary glands are probably no more common than in temperate regions.

Oesophagus

The most important disease to involve this organ is oesophageal carcinoma[6] (Figure 10.1) (Chapter 36); this malignancy possesses an enigmatic geographical distribution. It has a high prevalence in some geographical locations:[1,6] Central and East Africa (western Kenya, Malawi and eastern Zambia have the highest rates), the

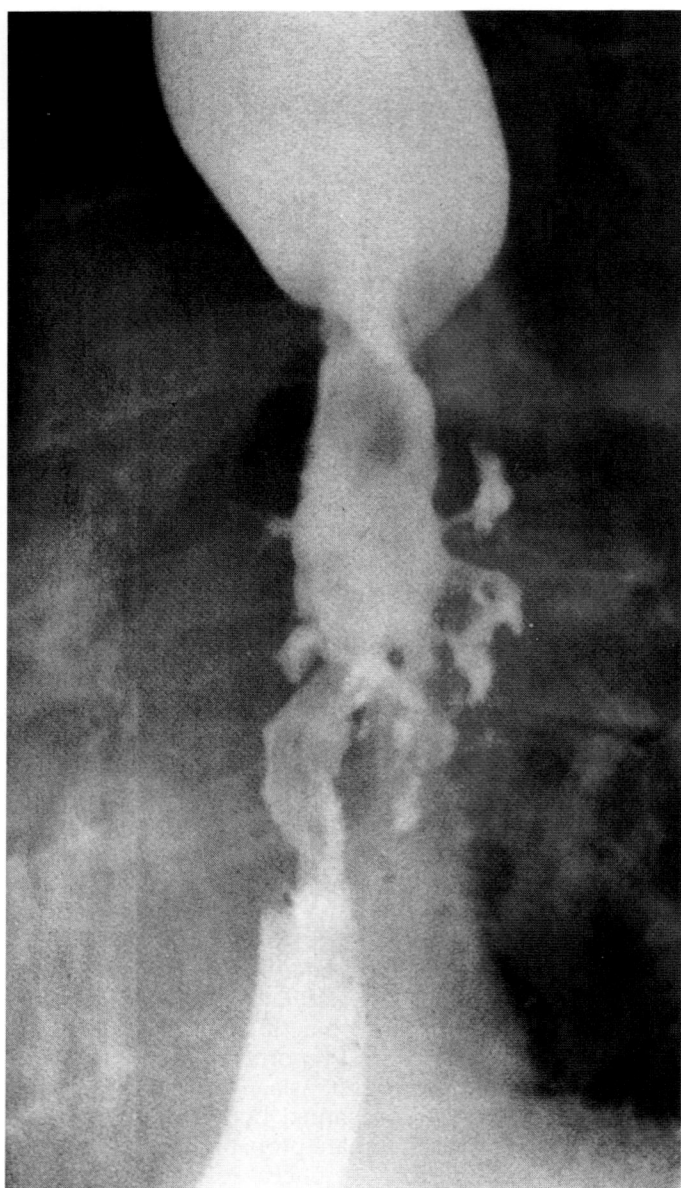

Figure 10.1: Barium swallow showing oesophageal carcinoma with gross mediastinal invasion.

Table 10.1 Some causes of dysphagia in tropical countries.

Trauma	Gastritis Foreign bodies Corrosive agents
Infection	South American trypanosomiasis (Chagas' disease) Candidiasis (usually associated with AIDS) *Rhizopus, Absidia* (mucormycosis)
Neoplasia	Oesophageal carcinoma
Oesophageal	Macronodular cirrhosis (usually varices postviral) Schistosomiasis Portal vein thrombosis Hyperreactive malarious splenomegaly
Others	Achalasia Peptic oesophagitis Hiatus hernia
Extrinsic pressure	Endemic goitre

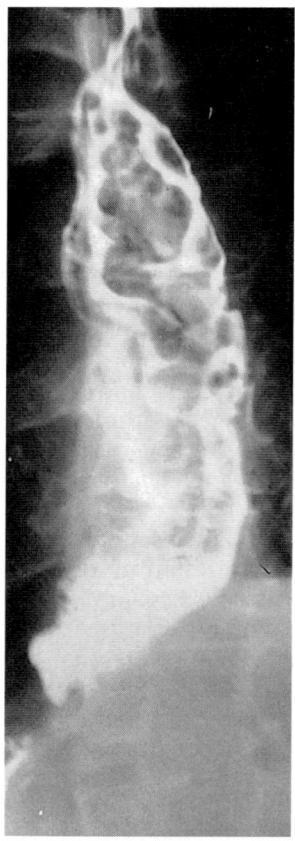

Figure 10.2: Advanced oesophageal varices in a Zambian woman with severe macronodular cirrhosis associated with HBV infection; barium swallow examination.

southern Caspian littoral (especially north-eastern Iran) and northern China (in and around the Taihand mountains). Various hypotheses have been advanced to explain the high incidence of this tumour in these areas (Chapter 36).[1,6]

Megaoesophagus, a feature of chronic *Trypanosoma cruzi* infection (Chagas' disease), is described in Chapter 74. Table 10.1 lists some major causes of dysphagia in a tropical environment.

Oesophageal varices (Figure 10.2) usually result from advanced macronodular cirrhosis (see below); however, hepatic schistosomiasis (caused by *Schistosoma mansoni, Schist. japonicum, Schist. intercalatum, Schist. matthei* and *Schist. mekongi*) are also important (Chapter 80). Portal vein obstruction (see below) is also common in some parts of Africa and Asia; this probably results in most cases from umbilical sepsis in the neonatal period;[1] it is occasionally a sequel to hepatocellular carcinoma. A very high splenic blood flow associated with hyperreactive malarious splenomegaly (HMS; tropical splenomegaly syndrome) can also give rise to oesophageal varices (see below).[1] Where and when available, upper gastro-intestinal endoscopic sclerotherapy is of enormous value in the management of oesophageal varices, but an ideal method of dealing with bleeding varices has yet to appear; in most tropical countries, older methods (see below) remain extant.

Oesophageal trauma is a major problem in several African countries; foreign bodies (e.g., kola nuts and fish bones) and corrosive agents—which give rise to strictures— are also relatively common.[1] Achalasia, peptic oesophagitis and hiatus hernia are all encountered, but are not unduly common.

In HIV/AIDS infection, oesophageal candidiasis is a common manifestation; other systemic mycoses (Chapter 69) can also produce an oesophagitis.

Emergencies

The most common oesophageal lesions in tropical countries are varices (Table 10.1 summarizes the major causes) and carcinoma (see above);[4] resultant *acute* complications are upper gastrointestinal haemorrhage and obstruction, respectively. Hookworm and *Ascaris lumbricoides* infections (Chapter 83) should not be neglected in this context.[7] Of lesser importance, foreign bodies in the oesophagus (e.g., kola nuts) cause dysphagia; corrosive lesions can result in stricture formation.[1]

Oesophageal varices

Reported prevalences for bleeding oesophageal varices in tropical countries are unreliable.[4] Transport facilities are usually exceedingly unsatisfactory; therefore, the majority of those afflicted die before reaching medical care. Also, high technology (e.g., endoscopic sclerotherapy) and blood transfusion are less often available; outcome following medical intervention is therefore frequently less satisfactory than in a Western country.[8] The cause of upper gastrointestinal bleeding in 131 successive patients admitted with haematemesis or melaena to a hospital at Harare, Zimbabwe, has been analysed;[9] in 36 (27%) admissions (mean age 42 years) oesophageal varices were responsible. In 21, conservative management was followed by cessation of bleeding; however, nine suffered continuous bleeding, and six rebleeding; five patients died (four within 24 hours of admission) from haemorrhagic shock. Vasopressin infusions were used in four with the addition of oesophageal tamponade in two.

The pathophysiological mechanisms underlying oesophageal bleeding have been addressed on numerous occasions.[10] Both erosive and eruptive bases seem the most likely explanations; in addition, pressure and variceal size are probably important. In Egypt, endoscopic biopsies obtained from intervariceal mucosa (within 5 cm of the cardia) in 20 individuals with, and 30 without, a history of variceal bleeding (most suffered from schistosomal liver disease) were examined histologically;[11] they showed dilated intraepithelial blood-filled channels within the squamous epithelium and lamina propria in all of the 'bleeders' and in 15 (50%) of the 'non-bleeders'. Furthermore, oesophagitis was more pronounced in the bleeders compared with the non-bleeders: 11 (55%) and 7 (23%), respectively.

The role of upper gastrointestinal endoscopy in a developing country has been studied in Kuwait;[12] 345 (4%) of 8680 patients examined successively using this technique had evidence of oesophageal varices, the usual cause being chronic schistosomal liver disease (usually in Egyptian labourers). By examining 718 successive patients who presented with upper gastrointestinal bleeding within 24 hours of admission, the exact site of the haemorrhage was delineated in 651 (91%), and the responsible lesion detected in 685 (97%). At Ibadan, Nigeria, a recent study has indicated that endoscopy gives a superior result to radiology in the diagnosis of variceal disease resulting in upper gastrointestinal haemorrhage;[13] endoscopy was successful in 64 (85%), but a barium meal correctly located the source of bleeding in only 38 (51%) of 75 patients.

Three reports from New Delhi, India, have focused on the role of endoscopic sclerotherapy in the management of bleeding oesophageal varices.[14–16] Seventy-nine patients underwent treatment (with either absolute or 50% alcohol) every 3 weeks, for oesophageal varices; active bleeding was controlled in 14 of 15 (93%) and 5 of 13 (54%) using the two fluids, respectively ($P < 0.05$); the sole disadvantage of absolute alcohol was that it produced a higher incidence of retrosternal pain. In another study, using a similar regimen, 5% ethanolamine oleate was compared with absolute alcohol in 47 randomly allocated patients; the latter solution eradicated oeso-phageal varices earlier (12.9 versus 8.2 weeks, respectively) ($p < 0.001$); the mean number of injection courses and necessary amount of sclerosant were also lower in the alcohol-treated group ($p < 0.001$), but the frequency of rebleeding did not differ significantly ($p > 0.05$). Thirty-one children with variceal bleeding caused by extrahepatic portal vein obstruction (19), non-cirrhotic portal fibrosis (5) or cirrhosis (7) were treated by sclerotherapy using absolute alcohol; arrest of acute bleeding was achieved in 10 by emergency sclerotherapy, and a 3-week schedule was able to achieve variceal obliteration in all of them; during a 23-month follow-up period, recurrent varices occurred in three (two with cirrhosis and one with non-cirrhotic portal fibrosis) patients; a rebleed was successfully controlled with emergency sclerotherapy in five, and an oesophageal stricture in four of them (which was easily dilated) were the only significant complications.

Although now rarely used in the Western world, oeso-phageal compression using a Sengstaken tube is often the only technique available. Intravenous pitressin is of limited value in acute bleeding. In long-term management, propranolol undoubtedly has a place in a developing country context.

In an attempt to provide clinical guidelines for the prediction of outcome of upper gastrointestinal bleeding in a developing country, Clamp et al.[8] carried out a multicentre study based on two centres, in Sikkim and China; in the former country, 60 (69%) of the patients put into the 'high-risk' group (by applying Bayes' theorem using a computer system) for rebleeding experienced this event (27 (54%) died), whereas this complication occurred in only six (2%) in the 'low-risk' group; furthermore, a simplified scoring system (little computer technology was available at Sikkim) gave almost exactly the same predictive accuracy. The authors suggest that, by using one of these systems, patients in remote areas can be categorized in order that scarce resources (which are available there) can be put to the best use.

The optimal means of managing haemorrhage resulting from extrahepatic portal venous obstruction is summarized in the section on liver disease (see below).

Oesophageal carcinoma

Presence of histologically diagnosed chronic oesophagitis (using upper gastrointestinal endoscopy) has been shown to be common in a high-risk population (15–26 years) in China.[17] This lesion was significantly associated with: (1) consumption of 'burning hot' beverages; (2) a family history of oesophageal carcinoma (including second-degree relatives); (3) infrequent consumption of fresh fruit; and (4) infrequent consumption of dietary staples, other than maize. Associated factors which have been recorded in that population include: (1) positive cytological smears (568 individuals > 30 years of 42 190 had a positive result); and (2) a high prevalence of pharyngeal carcinoma in free-range chickens which lived off domestic scraps[18] in the local environment.

This tumour often presents late in its clinical course in the heavily affected areas; in fact, complete luminal obstruction (accompanied by inability to swallow saliva) is not uncommon at presentation. Passage of a Celestin latex rubber tube (a palliative technique) is often the only available procedure;[6] however, blockage is a frequent problem resulting largely from the bulky African (or other) diet. Chemotherapy and radiotherapy (when available) are of very limited value.

Stomach and duodenum

Peptic ulceration was at one time considered an unusual cause of abdominal pain in tropical countries; it was felt by many physicians to be a rare disease.[1] It is now clear, however, that this is not the case; many difficulties facing the clinical epidemiologist in a developing country are highlighted by studies of the geographical distribution of this disease. Because sophisticated methods of diagnosis,

including barium meal and upper gastrointestinal endoscopy, have not until recently been widely used in developing countries, diagnosis and attempts at establishing accurate prevalence rates have depended upon recording incidence rates of complications, especially pyloric stenosis; upper gastrointestinal haemorrhage seems an unusual presentation overall, but this probably results from the fact that such patients do not reach hospital before exsanguinations occurs. Therefore, serious deficiencies exist in knowledge regarding the true prevalence of peptic ulceration, and it is currently impossible to draw accurate conclusions on regional and rural/urban patterns, and also on variations with time, i.e., during the course of 'westernization'.

As recently as the 1950s, duodenal ulcer (DU) was considered a rare disease in Africa;[1] this is not so, because satisfactory radiological, and more recently endoscopic, investigations have yielded accurate facts on true prevalence rate(s). Prevalence of DU in Africa has been reviewed using the available literature;[1,19] high-prevalence areas seem to exist in parts of West Africa, Rwanda, Burundi, eastern Zaire, western Tanzania, south-western Uganda and the Ethiopian highlands. In southern India[19] (and Fijians descended from this population[20]) and Papua New Guinea the disease also seems relatively common. It has a marked male predominance; it is frequently postbulbar, and presentation with pyloric obstruction is relatively usual. Genetic factors might be important;[19] the role of diet remains difficult to assess. Whether low rates of presentation resulting from haemorrhage and/or perforation accurately reflect incidence, or are biased by the inability to transport a sick patient to hospital, is also impossible to evaluate. Evidence for a causative role for *Helicobacter pylori* in chronic active gastritis, peptic ulceration and possibly gastric malignancy has escalated during the last decade;[19] however, Koch's postulates have not all been satisfied, and infection rate with this organism frequently approaches 100% at an early age in an affected population.

Overall, gastric ulcer (GU) is uncommon in developing countries.[1] When it occurs it usually has a male predominance, is most common in the fifth and sixth decades, and afflicts predominantly the lower social strata. Pyloric obstruction is a common presentation, due frequently to late-stage disease at presentation.

Management of a bleeding peptic ulcer has been reviewed.[1,4]

Gastritis, often resulting from alcohol and spicy foods, is a major cause of abdominal pain/discomfort[21] (Table 10.2). Infective causes (including tuberculosis) are rare overall, although are occasionally encountered; infections which involve predominantly lower sections of the gastrointestinal tract (e.g., *Salmonella typhi* and *Shigella* species) occasionally produce significant gastric pathology. A heavy infection with hookworm and/or *Ascaris lumbricoides* can also account for epigastric discomfort (see below) and must be differentiated from peptic ulceration.

When H_2-receptor antagonists (e.g., cimetidine and ranitidine) are used in developing countries, a possibility

Table 10.2 Some causes of severe abdominal pain (without features of intestinal obstruction) in relation to tropical exposure.

Site of pain	Cause
Epigastrium	Heavy nematode infection (e.g., *Ascaris lumbricoides*, hookworm) Mesenteric adenitis (helminthic eggs or tuberculosis) Acute pancreatitis (helminth related)
Generalized	Peritonitis Typhoid perforation Amoebic colitis perforation (appendix, perforated peptic ulcer or diverticulitis) Abdominal tuberculosis Ruptured hydatid cyst Sickle cell crisis Recurrent familial polyserositis (familial Mediterranean fever) Hyperinfective syndrome caused by *Strongyloides stercoralis* *Angiostrongylus costaricensis*
Right upper quadrant	Helminthic infection involving biliary system
Left upper quadrant	Splenomegaly (e.g., hyperreactive malarious splenomegaly) Splenic rupture Solitary splenic abscess
Right iliac fossa	Appendicitis *Anisakis* spp. infection

exists that they will encourage proliferation of intestinal pathogen(s)—bacterial and parasitic—for the gastric acid defence mechanism is largely removed;[22] available data are, however, presently inadequate for assessing the practical importance of this. Several studies of gastric acid production indicate that mean acid production probably varies little in different ethnic groups. Hypochlorhydria is relatively common in the tropics;[1] whether it is the cause or consequence of intestinal infection (of bacterial, including *S. typhi*, and/or parasitic origin) remains far from clear.

Gastric carcinoma is overall an uncommon malignancy in tropical countries (Chapter 36). At Sura, Fiji, gastric ulcer and carcinoma have been shown to be more common in Fijians than Indians.

Emergencies

Many facts remain unclear regarding upper gastrointestinal haemorrhage in tropical countries. For example, DU is apparently common in descendants of southern Indians in Fiji (see above); however, haematemesis from a chronic DU is more common in Fijians.

Many data suggest that pyloric obstruction is the most common complication of DU in developing countries. A report from Zaire, northern Nigeria, indicates that at that location perforation is by no means uncommon;[24] between 1971 and 1983, 74 (24%) of 302 patients operated for DU, and 29 (58%) of 50 for GU, presented with perforation; furthermore, there was a progressive increase in the years 1971–1974 to 1979–1983 of from 16% to 45%, respectively. A rare case report from India has recorded massive haematemesis and melaena from a cholecystoduodenal fistula secondary to DU in a 24-year-old man;[25] he was successfully managed surgically.

Ideally, management of the complications of gastritis and peptic ulceration is exactly the same as in a Western country.

Although usually associated with oesophageal varices, gastric varices also occur alone. In New Delhi, India, 48 (16%) out of 309 patients with portal hypertension were shown to have gastric varices;[26] in six (12%) there was no evidence of associated oesophageal varices. In 11 (28%) of 40 patients who completed endoscopic sclerotherapy for oesophageal varices, gastric varices disappeared concurrently with the former, or during the following 6 months. In the light of their experience, these authors considered that 'if they persist for 6 months after eradication of oesophageal varices, a combination of paravariceal and intravariceal sclerotherapy should be attempted for their obliteration'.

Abdominal pain

Epigastric pain/discomfort is a common presenting symptom in medical practice in tropical countries (see above);[1,27] this frequently results from heavy small-intestinal helminthic infections, especially with *A. lumbricoides* and hookworm. Mesenteric adenitis as a sequel to the presence of helminthic ova, and tuberculosis, are further causes. Helminth-related acute pancreatitis is another possibility.

Table 10.2 summarizes some causes of *severe* generalized abdominal pain. This most commonly results from peritonitis, which has numerous aetiologies. Right upper quadrant pain is less likely to result from biliary tract disease than in a 'temperate' area of the world (see below); nevertheless, helminthic infections of the biliary system are occasionally encountered. Left upper quadrant pain can result from splenomegaly (following numerous 'tropical' infections; see below); an extreme example (HMS) occurs in most areas which are endemic for human *Plasmodium* species. Ruptured spleen is a further cause of left hypochondrial pain; this event usually presents acutely. Solitary splenic abscess is by no means an uncommon event in West and Central Africa; the aetiology remains unclear.

Right iliac fossa pain is less likely to be caused by appendicitis (see below) than in most Western countries. However, an appendix-like syndrome has been recorded in *Yersinia* species, and *Anisakis* species infections and ileocaecal tuberculosis (see below). *Enterobius vermicularis* is not infrequently detected in an appendicectomy specimen; whether there is a cause–effect relationship to acute appendicitis is frequently unclear. Less common parasites involving the appendix include *Taenia* species, *Trichuris trichiura* and *Angiostrongylus costaricensis* (see below). A peripheral blood eosinophilia is often (but by no means always) present when a helminthiasis is causatively related to appendicitis. Ileocaecal tuberculosis can account for chronic right iliac fossa pain; an ileocaecal mass is often palpable clinically (this can be confirmed by ultrasonography when this technique is available). A colonic amoeboma represents a possible source of diagnostic confusion.

Small intestine

Tropical enteropathy and subclinical malabsorption

The small-intestinal mucosa of an individual living in a developing country possesses minor structural differences compared with that in one always resident in a temperate zone.[1,28,29] Changes are not related to the clinical syndrome postinfective malabsorption (tropical sprue; see below). Although the cause of these changes is not entirely clear, they seem to result from repeated low-grade viral and bacterial infection(s). Similarly, marginal xylose and glucose malabsorption has been demonstrated in large numbers of people indigenous to tropical countries; these abnormalities are certainly greater in lower socioeconomic groups. Subclinical malabsorption exists in many people in developing countries;[1] xylose and B_{12} malabsorption have been demonstrated in 39% and 52%, respectively, of Peace Corps workers living under rural conditions in Pakistan. Apart from repeated small-intestinal infections, other factors are probably also important.[30] Xylose, glucose and folic acid absorption have been shown to be impaired in individuals with systemic bacterial infections, e.g., pulmonary tuberculosis and pneumococcal pneumonia. Dietary folate depletion also results in xylose malabsorption. Marginal malnutrition and pellagra have both been suggested as causing subclinical malabsorption, but evidence is contradictory.

The practical importance of subclinical malabsorption is unclear.[1,28,29] It seems likely that it significantly contributes to malnutrition in people in developing countries who subsist on a marginally adequate dietary intake consisting largely of carbohydrate. Before any rigid conclusions are drawn, however, it should be appreciated that the small intestine has a very substantial functional reserve, and that the role of the colon in absorption of carbohydrate (and other substances) (see above) remains unclear.

Diarrhoea resulting from small-intestinal disease consists of two main types;[1,29] (1) profuse watery (e.g., cholera), and (2) steatorrhoeic (exemplified by post-infective tropical malabsorption (tropical sprue)). Table 10.3 summarizes the most important causes; several of

Table 10.3 Small-intestine diarrhoea.

Watery diarrhoea (large volume, fluid stool(s))
Travellers' diarrhoea (TD) (turista)
Vibrio cholerae (and other vibrios)
Escherichia coli (enterotoxigenic)
Salmonella spp.
Campylobacter jejuni
Rotavirus (and other enteric viruses)
Cryptosporidium spp.
(Food poisoning—*Staphylococcus*, *Clostridium perfringens*)
Hypolactasia: (1) primary—genetically determined
(2) secondary—resulting from enterocyte damage

Steatorrhoeic diarrhoea (malabsorption)
(characteristically large pale, fatty, offensive stools; microscopy often shows fat globules in faecal smear)
Postinfective tropical malabsorption ('tropical sprue')
Intestinal parasites
 Giardia lamblia
 Strongyloides stercoralis
 Capillaria philippinensis
 Coccidia: *Cryptosporidium parvum*
  Isospora belli
  Sarcocystis hominis
  Microsporidium spp.
  Cyclospora cayetanensis
HIV enteropathy
Trauma—short bowel syndrome (e.g., recovered pigbel disease)
Lymphoma—Burkitt's, Mediterranean lymphomas
Ileocaecal tuberculosis
Chronic calcific pancreatitis
Acute and chronic liver disease

(Gluten-induced enteropathy (coeliac disease) seems to be uncommon or even rare in most tropical populations. Occasionally it can become clinically obvious in visitors from Western countries to the tropics)

those responsible for the former type are infective, and then exert their pathogenic effect via an enterotoxin (either heat stable or heat labile); invasive disease involving the enterocyte is less important. The role of intestinal hormones—especially vasoactive intestinal peptide—in the production of watery diarrhoea has become clearer.[29] The pathogenesis of diarrhoea in AIDS has a multifactorial basis, and is often by no means clear;[31] some but not all cases are associated with an opportunistic infection(s), especially *Cryptosporidium parvum* (Chapter 77).[29] The bacteria *Escherichia coli*, fungi *Candida albicans* and *Histoplasma capsulatum*, and the astroviruses and caliciviruses are also relevant. Other opportunistic infections in this syndrome include cytomegalovirus, *Mycobacterium avium intracellulare*, *Salmonella* species, and the protozoa *Isospora belli*, *Cyclospora cayatenensis*, *Sarcocystis hominis* and *Microsporidium* species infections; in addition, Kaposi's sarcoma (Chapter 36) causes severe small-intestinal disease.

Many of the problems encountered in management, including chemoprophylaxis and chemotherapy, are exemplified by travellers' diarrhoea (see below).

Travellers' diarrhoea

The clinical syndrome traveller's diarrhoea (TD)[1,32–36] is arguably the world's most common disease entity; only rarely is it associated with mortality (usually in the presence of debility, or at the extremes of life), but the significant morbidity with which it is associated not infrequently interferes with a crowded schedule or a leisure or sporting activity. Numerous titles have been applied, including 'turista', 'Montezuma's revenge', 'Hong Kong dog' and 'Delhi belly'. One estimate is that 12 million individuals travel annually from an industrialized (Western) country to one in the tropics or subtropics;[37] in this group incidence of TD varies from around 20% to 50%. There is a highly significant geographical variation in prevalence; high-risk areas include North Africa, sub-Saharan Africa, the Indian sub-continent, South-East Asia, South America, Mexico and the Middle East; intermediate ones include the north Mediterranean, Canary Islands and the Caribbean islands; low-risk ones include North America, Western Europe and Australia. In a retrospective study carried out in Switzerland, a large group of travellers were asked to complete a questionnaire after travelling abroad; incidence of the disease varied greatly, the highest figure (50%) being associated with travel to Tunisia. (No detailed study exists of TD acquired in a European country.[38])

The disease tends to become less common with advancing years; it is unclear whether this is due to the fact that older travellers (≥60 years) have a more discerning lifestyle, or whether relative immunity increases with advancing age.[32] Individuals resident for substantial periods in areas where TD is common seem to experience it less frequently than those not previously exposed.[32,33]

Clinical features

TD is contracted by ingestion of contaminated water/food; it is characterized by acute-onset watery diarrhoea (usually of small-intestinal origin);[32–36] when colorectal involvement exists, diarrhoea is often bloody (see below). Abdominal colic, nausea and vomiting may be present; fever is unusual, being recorded in 1–10% of infected individuals. Prostration and resultant dehydration (with electrolyte imbalance) cause major problems in a *severe* case. Rarely, symptoms become chronic, and it seems likely that a small proportion of cases of TD proceed to postinfective malabsorption (see below).[28] Unfortunately for the investigator, by the time disease has become clinically overt, the initiating infection(s) has invariably been cleared. Chronic diarrhoea of lesser severity is a relatively common problem following recovery from

acute disease; this can usually be attributed to (1) *tropical enteropathy* (in which there is major derangement of enterocyte structure and function) (see above) or (2) the *irritable bowel syndrome* (see below).

On clinical grounds, an important differential diagnosis is inflammatory bowel disease—presenting for the first time during, or immediately after, tropical exposure.[39,40] In a retrospective review of UK residents presenting at the Hospital for Tropical Diseases, London, with acute onset/bloody diarrhoea, the majority had inflammatory bowel disease (usually ulcerative colitis); it was numerically more important than shigellosis and amoebic colitis.[39]

Acute disease pursues an especially virulent course in certain high-risk groups,[32,33] e.g., those suffering from achlorhydria (*Salmonella* species and *Vibrio* species infections are known to be significantly more common in this group), known inflammatory bowel disease (see below), previous gastrointestinal tract surgery, a malignancy involving the gastrointestinal tract, and acquired or congenital immunodeficiency (including immunosuppressive therapy and HIV/AIDS). In addition, individuals on diuretic therapy (in whom maintenance of electrolyte balance is precarious) and others at the extremes of life also fall within the high-risk group. It is important to recognize these factors when advising chemoprophylaxis (see below).

Aetiology

In 1970, Rowe et al.[41] recorded results of a study involving British soldiers newly arrived in Aden; in 19 (54.3%) of 33 cases in which a recognized pathogen was not apparent, a 'new' serotype of *Escherichia coli* was isolated in the acute phase of TD; in a further 14 (40%), several different *E. coli* serotypes were also isolated. (B. H. Keane had suggested in the 1950s (on circumstantial evidence) that bacterial pathogens were implicated.[32,33]) Sack[42] recorded the identity of *E. coli* serotypes isolated from US Peace Corps volunteers serving in various countries: Kenya 06:H16, 06H⁻, 027:H7, 0159:H4 and 0159:H34; Morocco 06:H16, 0128:H12, 027:H20 and 0169:H⁻; Honduras 08:H9, 015:H49, 015:H⁻ and 027:H20. Therefore, many common strains of enterotoxigenic *E. coli* (ETEC) are relevant. Many other micro-organisms are also involved. *Salmonella* species, *Shigella* species, *Campylobacter jejuni*, enteroadherent *E. coli* (EAEC) (Chapter 52) and *Vibrio* species (see Chapter 52); rotavirus and Norwalk virus (Chapter 46), and *Giardia lamblia*, *Coccidia* species (including *Cryptosporidium* species, *I. belli* and *Blastocystis hominis*) and *Entamoeba histolytica* (Chapter 77). Other bacteria which have been implicated include *Aeromonas hydrophila*, *Plesiomonas shigelloides* and *Yersinia enterocolitica*. The causative agent(s) vary significantly in different locations, e.g., in an affected individual in Asia, Central America or Africa the likely organism is different on statistical grounds, although not relevant to a specific case. Furthermore, more than one organism is frequently present; in a study involving US Peace Corps workers in Thailand, 33% were infected by two to four different pathogens.[32] Although protozoan parasites are usually incorporated in the list of aetiological agents, the incubation period is usually somewhat longer than is usual in TD; this applies especially to *G. lamblia*. When the colorectum is predominantly involved, *Shigella* species, enteroinvasive *E. coli* (EIEC), enterohaemorrhagic *E. coli* (EHEC) and *Ent. histolytica* may be responsible. Rarely, herpes simplex virus and *Chlamydia trachomatis* have been implicated. New pathogens will doubtless emerge in future years.

Pathophysiology

The pathophysiology varies and depends on the site within the gastrointestinal tract to be involved.[1,32–35] Whereas in the small intestine toxigenic diarrhoeas predominate (see above), in the colorectum (see below) invasive disease is more common.

ETEC are characterized by both toxin production and mucosal adherence (via specific fimbriae); the latter property is required for disease production, for toxin-producing non-adherent mutants do not cause disease. Enteropathogenic *E. coli* (EPEC) (probably not a major cause of TD) adhere to intestinal mucosal cells and although they do not invade, destroy microvilli. EAEC (detected in up to 15% of patients suffering from TD) do not belong to classical serotypes of EPEC, but adhere to Hep-2 cells in culture; they neither produce a toxin nor invade.[43] EIEC behave similarly to *Shigella* species and account for up to 5% of cases; the main site of action is the colorectum, and the major clinical manifestation is therefore dysentery resulting from epithelial cell invasion and intracellular multiplication; there is resultant mucosal inflammation and ulceration.[43] EHEC (an uncommon cause of TD) produces disease via verotoxin production.

Prophylaxis

Travellers should take maximal care to avoid water/food likely to be contaminated; common sense is of paramount importance! Use of prophylactic agents is controversial. Many chemoprophylactics have been used: doxycycline, co-trimoxazole, trimethoprim, mecillinam, bicozamycin and the fluroquinolone compounds (norfloxacin and ciprofloxacin). High protection rates (≥90%) have been claimed for co-trimoxazole and the fluroquinolones; for trimethoprim a rate of around 50% has been recorded. Most cases of TD therefore possess a bacterial aetiology. The major problem with antibiotic chemoprophylaxis, however, is the risk of significant side effects, dominated by dermatological reactions (including Stevens–Johnson syndrome) and pseudomembranous colitis (see below); using co-trimoxazole, a rate of up to 20% of significant skin reactions, necessitating discontinuation of prophylaxis, has been recorded. Also, the acquisition of resistant faecal *E. coli* during chemoprophylaxis has been recorded in several studies; an increase from 21% to 100% has been recorded using doxycycline in Kenya, and one of 3% to 100% with co-trimoxazole in Mexico. When chemoprophylaxis is used, either norfloxacin or ciprofloxacin seems to be the most appropriate, although strains of *Campylobacter jejuni* rapidly acquire resistance.[38] In a recent study in Egypt, two of 105 individuals on norfloxacin developed TD, compared with 30 (26%) of 117 given a placebo.[43] (Ciprofloxacin should be avoided in children because of experimental evidence indicating cartilaginous damage in young experimental animals; there is no evidence in *Homo sapiens*.)

Should chemoprophylaxis be recommended widely in this essentially *benign* clinical syndrome? In addition to the objections so far outlined (see above), there is a possibility of inducing a false sense of security, resulting in increased exposure to other infections, e.g., viral hepatitis.[43] The following groups should be seriously considered for chemoprophylaxis (for < 3 weeks):

- Travellers with a bad 'history' of TD.[32–35]
- Those in whom hypochlorhydria is proven (or a possibility).
- Individuals suffering from inflammatory bowel disease.
- HIV-infected patients.
- Those in whom electrolyte balance is precarious (e.g., those receiving diuretic therapy), and others with chronic renal failure.
- The 'elderly' (not easily defined!).
- A nebulous group in whom TD is professionally embarrassing (e.g., members of the armed services, airline pilots, athletes, politicians, businessmen and other professionals on tight schedules, etc.).

The role of prophylactic antiperistaltic agents is likewise controversial: action is unphysiological. It has been suggested that they can mask a more serious infection, e.g., *S. typhi*, although in this disease diarrhoea is an unusual presenting symptom (Chapter 53). By delaying excretion of pathogen(s) it is also possible that clinical disease is prolonged. In children, paralytic ileus is a major complication and has occasionally precipitated mortality.[44]

Bismuth subsalicylate has a role in prophylaxis; the bismuth moiety possesses antimicrobial activity and salicylate antisecretory properties.[33] Early studies in Mexico by DuPont et al.[45] showed that, given as a suspension (the sheer bulk required precluded its use by travellers), this agent significantly reduced TD; the same group, also working in Mexico, has demonstrated that, when given in tablet form (two tablets four times daily for ≤ 3 weeks, i.e., 2.1 g daily), a 65% protection rate can be achieved;[45] at half that dose, efficacy was greatly reduced. Number(s) of pathogen-positive TD cases in a group of treated patients was seven of 29, compared with 35 of 59, in a placebo group; ETEC was present in three and 22 respectively, and *Shigella* species in two and eight, respectively.[45]

A B-subunit/whole-cell (BS-WC) cholera vaccine has been shown to produce relative protection.[46] In a study involving Finnish tourists to Morocco, BS-WC induced

52% protection against diarrhoea caused by ETEC, 65% with mixed infection, 71% when ETEC was present with another pathogen, and 82% when ETEC and *S. enterica* were present concurrently. (Sack[42] has concluded that 'any advances in prevention and treatment of diarrhoea in travellers will be directly applicable to the worldwide problem of diarrhoea in children, which is far more important on a global scale'. This statement does not apply to this BS-WC vaccine, because protection only lasts for about 3 months.) A further approach under consideration consists of oral administration of colostrum-derived antibodies against ETEC.[33]

A recent experimental investigation indicates that lactobacilli, which have the ability to adhere to the intestinal mucosa, can prevent *E. coli* colonization. In a limited clinical study, *Lactobacillus* GG reduced prevalence of TD by up to 40%.[33]

Management

Treatment (as in cholera, see below) devolves around oral rehydration (see below); all travellers should carry suitable preparations.[1,35,47] When properly constituted, Dioralyte (Rhône-Poulenc Rorer) solution contains glucose 90, Na$^+$ 60, K$^+$ 25, Cl$^-$ 45 and citrate 20 mmol/litre. Corresponding concentrations for another proprietary preparation, Rapolyte (Janssen), are 111, 60, 20, 50 and 10 mmol/litre. WHO/UNICEF rehydration fluid contains glucose 111, Na$^+$ 90, K$^+$ 20, Cl$^-$ 80 and citrate 10 mmol/litre. In a mild case adequate rehydration can usually be achieved using ordinary mineral water.

The role of chemotherapy in established TD remains controversial. Early work carried out by DuPont et al.[45] in Mexico showed that both co-trimoxazole and trimethoprim reduced the length of symptoms. Recent trials, using antibiotics which have been given for chemoprophylaxis (see above), have also indicated that the length of symptoms can be shortened; in Mexico, ofloxacin (600 mg daily for 3 days) produced cure in 77 (95%) of 81, compared with 56 (71%) patients who received placebo ($p = 0.0001$).[48] Short-course chemotherapy can only be justified in a *severe* case; this applies at the extremes of life and in high-risk groups (see above), especially HIV-infected individuals.[34]

Cholera (See also Chapter 52)

This represents the archetypal disease in the context of small-intestinal secretory (watery) diarrhoea.[29,49,50]

The causative organism, *Vibrio cholerae*, is not invasive and exerts its effect by means of an enterotoxin.[49] If untreated, the disease has a 20–80% mortality; with modern oral rehydration regimens that figure should be less than 1%. Death results from dehydration, vascular collapse and renal failure.

Historically, cholera was not confined to tropical countries and involved many temperate areas, including much of northern Europe. An epidemic in 1854 in London was traced to contaminated water supplied from the Broad Street pump in Soho. According to legend, when the handle of the pump was tied down by Dr John Snow, the London anaesthetist, a rapid decline in the incidence of new cases was recorded.[51]

Epidemiology

Cholera is endemic in India, Pakistan, Bangladesh, Afghanistan and many other countries of South-East Asia. Nosocomial transmission is reported. In recent years, epidemics have occurred in the Middle East, South America and Africa;[49] most have been localized. Cholera is endemic along the Gulf Coast of the USA. The disease is closely associated with poverty, overcrowding and low socio-economic status.

In former times cholera was spread by population movements such as the annual hadj to Mecca; outbreaks involving air travellers have been recorded. Overall, however, the disease is rare in British travellers.[52] It tends to affect young people more often than the elderly.

Aetiology and pathogenesis

There is probably a genetic predisposition: blood group O is associated with a higher infection rate than group A.[29]

Classical cholera is caused by *V. cholerae*, which is now localized to the Indian subcontinent, particularly the deltas of the Ganges and Brahmaputra rivers. Elsewhere, the El Tor biotype, which originated in Indonesia around 1960, and the 0139 strain have been responsible for most epidemics. *Vibrio* species are curved, Gram-negative, flagellated rods approximately 2 µm in length. Each biotype of cholera contains three serotypes: Inaba, Ogawa and Hikojima.

For details of the organism and its pathophysiological effects see Chapter 52.

Pathology

Histologically, the small-intestinal mucosa is intact. Light and electron microscopical appearances are normal. Following circulatory collapse following gross dehydration, renal tubular necrosis can be demonstrated.

Clinical features

There are no prodromal symptoms. The incubation period varies from a few hours to 5 days. The disease is similar whichever biotype is involved, but there is a wide spectrum of severity. When the El To biotype is responsible, a higher proportion of patients are asymptomatic. Onset is sudden, and mild diarrhoea rapidly gives way to the passage of a large volume of opalescent fluid—the classic 'rice-water' stools. Up to 30 litres of fluid, containing a high concentration of *Vibrio* species organisms, may be passed in 24 hours.[50] Vomiting of fluid of a similar composition is a later feature. Thirst, muscle cramps, hoarseness and anuria follow.

Clinical signs of severe dehydration may be present by 24 hours after onset in an untreated case. The body temperature is normal or mildly elevated. Circulatory failure and acute renal failure follow. Confusion, disorientation and hypoglycaemic convulsions may occur. Mortality rate is directly related to the degree of dehydration. Relative immunity is short lived. A carrier state, which lasts a few weeks, may occur, and gallbladder foci have been identified.

Investigations

Vibrio species organisms are easily identified in a faecal specimen; material should be transported to the laboratory in alkaline peptone water (pH 9.0). A rapid diagnostic technique for field use has been described. For accurate serological identification of *V. cholerae*, rigid criteria are necessary. With classic cholera, organisms are present during the incubation period and up to 5 days after an attack; in the El Tor variety, *Vibrio* species can persist for weeks or months.

Faecal samples are isotonic, with a protein concentration of approximately 10 g/litre; pH is about 7.5; typical electrolyte concentrations are sodium 139 mmol/litre, potassium 23 mmol/litre, chloride 106 mmol/litre and bicarbonate 48 mmol/litre. Specimens contain a high concentration of IgA. Serum IgA and IgM are elevated, the former most markedly in patients with an El Tor infection. In in vitro animal studies, cholera toxin enhances IgA secretion from crypt epithelium to ileal lumen.[53]

Serum electrolyte, urea and creatinine concentrations vary with the stage and severity of the disease. Excessive potassium loss exacerbates metabolic acidosis. Urine is concentrated; its composition depends on the severity of the disease.

Differential diagnosis

Diagnosis is usually straightforward; however, all other causes of small-intestinal diarrhoea (with and without vomiting) of acute onset (see below) should be considered. These include travellers' diarrhoea, *E. coli*, *Staphylococcus* species, *Clostridium perfringens*, *Cl. botulinum*, *Campylobacter jejuni* and viral causes (e.g., rotavirus, Norwalk agent). *Salmonella* and *Shigella* species should also be considered. *Vibrio parahaemolyticus* (conveyed by infected raw seafood) and other non-cholera *Vibrio* species can produce a similar disease. Very occasionally, *Plasmodium falciparum* malaria presents with severe watery diarrhoea, especially in infants and children. Food poisoning, caused by toxic agents, should be added to the list of differential diagnoses.

Prevention

Basic sanitation and public health procedures should be improved.[54] Sterility of water supplies is of paramount importance. Contacts of proven cases should be vaccinated; all faeces and bed linen should be destroyed. Vaccination with inactivated (dead) *Vibrio* species organisms gives only limited protection;[55] 0.5 ml and 1.0 ml vaccine should be given at an interval of 1 week, and a 0.5 ml booster every 6 months.

The 26th Assembly of the WHO recommended, in 1973, that cholera vaccination should *not* be compulsory, due to its limited public health value. Despite this, a few countries continue to demand vaccination before entry. Important progress is being made towards an effective oral bivalent cholera–typhoid vaccine.[56]

Management
Rehydration regimens

Treatment was revolutionized by the introduction of oral rehydration regimens.[47,57–59] The enterocyte sodium–glucose carrier system is not affected by cyclic AMP, and thus glucose (and glycine)-stimulated membrane transport takes place normally.

It is impossible to overload the circulation by the oral route in a previously fit person. Quantity of ingested fluid should be regulated by faecal loss, best measured 2-hourly. Rehydration should be accomplished within 48 hours. In an unsophisticated situation, sucrose is often more easily obtainable than glucose; results are usually good, although if severe mucosal damage pre-exists, sucrase concentration is lowered and satisfactory rehydration is less readily achieved. Cereal-based electrolyte solutions have also given satisfactory results.[58]

In a severe case, intravenous fluids may be necessary for initial rehydration.[58] A widely used formula consists of sodium chloride 5.0 g, sodium bicarbonate 4.0 g, potassium chloride 1.0 g, made up to 1 litre. Severity of dehydration should be assessed on clinical grounds; in a case of average severity, 5 litres should be given (the first litre within 10 minutes) to a 50 kg subject.

Drug treatment

Analgesics may be necessary for severe muscle cramps. Intravenous calcium gluconate is of value for tetany.

Tetracycline hydrochloride, 1 g/day for 5 days, shortens duration of diarrhoea and clears the luminal content of *Vibrio* species organisms in the case of the El Tor biotype.[59] A single dose (1 g or 2 g) has also been shown to be effective in *V. cholerae* infection, but is associated with asymptomatic bacteriological relapse.[60,61] Tetracycline should be started several hours after rehydration therapy has begun. Single-dose doxycycline (300 mg) is probably as effective as tetracycline. There is clear evidence that in epidemics the El Tor biotype rapidly develops resistance not only to tetracycline, but also to several other antibiotics (including trimethoprim plus sulfamethoxazole), and is therefore of very limited value. Recently, *Vibrio cholera* 01 biotype El Tor strains have proved resistant to furazolidone and co-trimoxazole.[63]

Prognosis

If cholera is adequately treated, there should be zero mortality, and complete recovery. A suggestion has been made that individuals who have suffered from cholera might be predisposed to α-chain disease (see below).

Malabsorption in the tropics

Apart from infective causes, *primary* hypolactasia (lactase deficiency)[1,64] accounts for watery small-intestinal diarrhoea in some people indigenous to tropical countries. A low concentration of this enzyme in the enterocyte brush border is normal for adult *Homo sapiens* (as for other species within the mammalian kingdom); the enzyme is under genetic control. In a minority of the world's population, i.e., northern Europeans, Africans with an Hamitic ancestry, certain Middle Eastern populations (e.g., Saudi Arabians) and others in northern parts of the Indian subcontinent, a high concentration continues into adult life. *Secondary* hypolactasia results from brush border damage;[1,64] concentration of all disaccharidases (and other digestive enzymes) is reduced, and slow recovery occurs after the initiating insult has disappeared. Thus, whenever there is enterocyte destruction (this includes postinfective malabsorption, see below) hypolactasia develops.

Following ingestion of milk or another milk produce, in which lactose is incompletely hydrolysed, osmotic diarrhoea results; this is accompanied by abdominal colic, distension and flatulence ('lactose intolerance'). Yoghurt contains adequate bacterial lactase to hydrolyse the lactose component and is usually well tolerated. Lactic acid production (derived from hydrolysis of lactose by colonic bacteria) produces irritative diarrhoea—which contributes to the symptoms. The precise role of the colon in adaptation remains unclear; carbohydrate, in the form of free fatty acid(s) (and also nitrogen and electrolytes), can be absorbed from this organ. Investigation of hypolactasia most often utilizes the breath hydrogen test; lactose 'tolerance' test and lactase assay in a jejunal biopsy specimen are alternatives. In management, milk and all lactose-containing dairy products should be eliminated from the diet;[1,64] individuals in countries with a high prevalence of *primary* hypolactasia can regulate bowel function by varying lactose ingestion.

Postinfective malabsorption (PIM) (tropical sprue)

Relatively little is known about the prevalence and severity of malabsorption in acute infective conditions of the small intestine (viral, bacterial and parasitic) and the duration for which it can continue *after* the specific organism(s) has been eliminated.

In some cases, malabsorption persists in the presence of *mixed* luminal flora, and a single infective agent cannot be detected. In others the recognizable initiating infective cause (or causes) may continue, culminating in a *chronic* form; a more precise term is therefore 'post*acute* infective' malabsorption. As with all infective diseases, the clinical spectrum of disease varies from subclinical to gross pathology (malabsorption). PIM is of particular clinical significance in tropical countries, where small (and large) intestinal infections are exceedingly common.

PIM related to tropical exposure has been reviewed by Cook,[1,28,24,65] Tomkins,[66] Baker[67] and Mathan.[68]

History and definition

Confusion has existed between PIM and tropical sprue; however, in tropical and subtropical countries these entities are synonymous, and the difficulty is primarily one of semantics.[1,28] Patrick Manson first coined the term tropical sprue (derived from a word used by Dutch workers in the East Indies) in 1880.[69] The term was rapidly applied to all cases of malabsorption in tropical countries—undoubtedly including some resulting from tuberculosis and various parasitoses (both protozoan and helminthic). Historically, chronic diarrhoea accompanied by wasting was recognized in India before 600 BC; although the Englishman William Hillary is often credited with the first precise description of tropical sprue at Barbados,[70] it now seems likely that he described either epidemic *G. lamblia* infection, or possibly strongyloidiasis. The *clinical* syndrome was well known to British physicians in India during the eighteenth and nineteenth centuries; most descriptions were made in British expatriate populations. It was in the early 1960s that reports of a high prevalence of epidemic PIM in indigenous Indians became available.[1,67,68] Despite early suggestions that chronic tropical diarrhoea had an *insidious* onset, it is clear (after careful assessment) that the vast majority of cases always presented *acutely*. Confusion has been compounded further when acute epidemic cases of small-intestinal infection, associated with gross dehydration (in addition to xylose and fat malabsorption) and acute mortality, have been designated tropical sprue, as in numerous reports from southen India.[68] It is essential to include a *time factor* in the definition of this clinical *syndrome*, e.g., chronic diarrhoea and malabsorption, with weight loss, of at least 3–4 months duration. The term *tropical sprue* (if used at all) would be better reserved for a condition where malabsorption of nutrients is quantitatively more important than that of water and electrolytes. Although the aetiology of PIM is not yet completely clear (see below), in most cases it undoubtedly follows an *acute* small-intestinal insult by either a bacterial, viral or parasitic (or mixed) pathogen.

Overall, evidence for PIM following a small-intestinal insult is most complete for bacterial and parasitic infections; those of viral origin might, however, be more important numerically. Lack of precise data can be largely attributed to the fact that virology remains a relatively neglected discipline in most developing countries, where infections of all types are far more common than in the Western world.

The effect of malabsorption on overall nutritional status is largely unknown (see above); children are especially at risk. The magnitude of energy loss is unclear; a deficit of 10% of dietary energy (one estimate) is substantial in tropical populations subsisting on a 'marginal' diet. The importance of anorexia in exacerbating associated malnutrition is also underexplored.

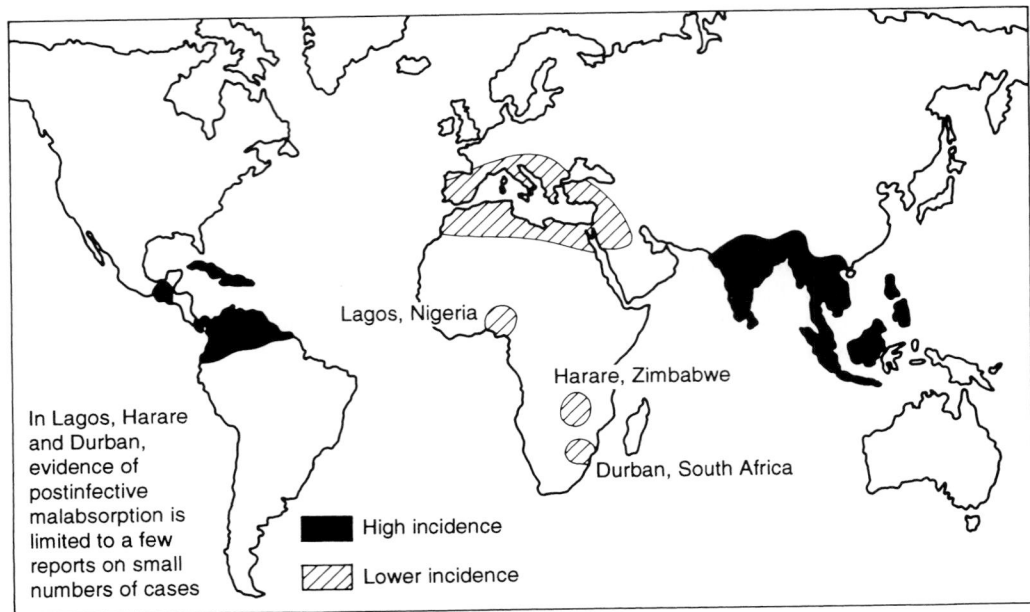

Figure 10.3: World map showing areas where postinfective tropical malabsorption is a significant problem.

Geographical distribution

Figure 10.3 summarizes the geographical localities where PIM has been reported either commonly or less frequently;[28,29] the map does *not* include areas where sporadic cases have been rarely recorded. Although the disease is common (and endemic) in Asia and the northern part of South America, it is a very unusual condition in tropical Africa. It remains a problem in travellers to many tropical locations.[71–73] Until recently it was a common entity in overland travellers from the UK to Asia; the fact that it is now rarely seen is probably associated with early antibiotic administration. In the Middle East and Mediterranean littoral PIM is unusual, but undoubtedly occurs.[65]

Aetiology

There can now be no reasonable doubt that PIM has an *infective* basis (see above): it is (1) more common in geographical areas where enteric infection abounds; (2) epidemic in certain areas, including southern India; (3) the small-intestinal lumen is colonized by aerobic enterobacteria; and (4) recovery usually occurs rapidly (and dramatically) following initiation of broad-spectrum antibiotic treatment. Despite this, however, Mathan[68] is of the opinion that in southern India the primary lesion is enterocyte damage resulting from a 'persistent' lesion of the stem cell compartment on a 'background of tropical enteropathy'. He further considers that 'an immunity-conferring agent may be responsible for the initiating damage'. The widely used definition for this *clinical syndrome* in southern India, 'intestinal malabsorption of at lease two nutrients and the exclusion of diseases that give rise to secondary malabsorption in a tropical environment', is inadequate; it does not exclude *tropical enteropathy* (see above), nor does it introduce a time (chronicity) factor.

Genetic predisposition

All infective diseases, without exception, have a genetic background. In a limited study at Puerto Rico, 25 of 27 patients with PIM (not well defined) had at least one antigen of the HLA-Aw19 series;[74] the strongest associated link was with Aw31. In India, a high frequency of HLA-B8 was documented;[75] HLA-A1, A28 and Bw35 were significantly decreased in the affected group. More data are undoubtedly required on genetic markers in PIM.

Infection

In severe PIM (in the absence of parasites) bacterial colonization has been demonstrated both within the jejunal lumen and in biopsy specimens. The importance of adhesive properties of bacteria in pathogenesis is unclear; many bacteria, including *E. coli*, *S. typhimurium* and *V. cholerae*, possess such properties, mediated by a transmissible plasmid. In tropical PIM, several groups have demonstrated a higher concentration of aerobic enterobacteria in relation to the enterocyte compared with luminal fluid. (In the normal individual, anaerobes outnumber aerobes by about 1000-fold.) It seems likely that a variety of toxins released by these enterobacteria induce net water secretion and malabsorption. In the blind-loop syndrome, enterobacteria (which are invariably obligate anaerobes) do *not produce toxins*. Several months after tropical exposure the upper small-intestinal intraluminal bacterial flora (mucosal biopsy or luminal fluid) remains abnormal;[77] seven of 11 patients studied had enterobacteria in numbers ranging from 10^3 to 10^8/g or ml. The most common organisms were *Klebsiella pneumoniae*, *Enterobacter cloacae* and *E. coli*;

Citrobacter feundii, Serratia marcescens and *Psuedomonas* species have also been detected. It seems highly likely, therefore, that these organisms were present since the onset of disease. In southern India, a viral aetiology has been sought, but there is little evidence for this. The origin of continuing overgrowth has not been adequately studied in tropical PIM; in patients in England with small-intestinal bacterial overgrowth, faecal flora account for most of the organisms, but salivary flora are probably important in some cases.

Jejunal morphology

Morphological changes are non-specific and range in severity.[65] Blunting of villi ('partial villous atrophy') with increased lymphocyte and plasma cell infiltration (not a feature of *tropical enteropathy*) are present to a variable degree; a 'flat' mucosa is exceedingly unusual. Although the number of plasma cells is increased, distribution of IgA-, IgM- and IgG-containing cells is normal.[78] In untreated gluten-induced enteropathy, T cells expressing T cell receptor γ/δ heterodimers are disproportionately raised; this is not so in PIM.[98] The significance of elevated jejunal surface pH (demonstrated in southern India) is unclear, but is probably merely an indicator of enterocyte damage. Crypt *hyperplasia* has been demonstrated.

Although a predisposing immunological deficit has been postulated in tropical PIM, there is no good evidence for this; immunological changes (increased IgG, IgE, C4 and orosomucoid, gastric parietal cell antibodies, and lymphopenia with a low peripheral blood T-cell count) seem to be *sequelae* of mucosal damage, and are not causally related.

Small-intestine stasis

In southern India whole-gut transit time (using a radio-opaque marker technique) has been shown to be unaltered in tropical PIM, despite a striking increase in faecal weight. Small-intestinal stasis has, however, been well documented in tropical PIM and might result from excessive enteroglucagon production in response to ileal (and colonic) mucosal injury (see below).[79] However, many patients with PIM have received diphenoxylate or loperamide for acute diarrhoea; both agents produce relative small-intestinal stasis. Both of these agents interfere with iperistalsis and prevent prostaglandin-induced diarrhoea; inhibition of small-intestinal secretion also occurs. Such stasis is of particular interest because peristalsis is usually *increased* in the presence of intraluminal bacteria.

Gut hormones

Gut hormones have been studied in tropical PIM in the fasting state and following a standard meal.[79] Fasting and postprandial plasma enteroglucagon concentrations (produced by cells in the distal ileum and colon) and motilin were markedly elevated; furthermore, the elevated enteroglucagon concentration is significantly correlated with a reduction in small-intestinal transit (using the H_2 breath test). Both enteroglucagon and motilin concen-

trations fall after treatment. Concentration of another gut hormone, plasma peptide YY (also produced by endocrine cells in the ileum and colon and known to delay gastric emptying and small-intestinal transit, and to reduce gastric and pancreatic secretion) has been shown to be grossly elevated in PIM;[80] it seems possible that this results from a change in peptide YY secretion, resulting from malabsorption, and is a compensatory mechanism in diarrhoea. Patients with PIM also have a reduced postprandial rise in gastric inhibiting polypeptide; gastrin and pancreatic polypeptide are normal.

Role of the colon

The colonic mucosa, in addition to that of the small intestine, is abnormal in tropical PIM ('tropical colonopathy').[81] Few causes of diarrhoea are strictly confined to one or other of these organs; for example, shigellosis frequently involves the small intestine, and salmonellosis and *Campylobacter jejuni* infection of the colon.

The normal colon is able to absorb 4–7 litres of water per 24 hours,[82] together with 100–160 mmol carbohydrate (as volatile fatty acid(s)). Failure of the diseased colon to 'salvage' the increased ileal effluent must increase the intensity of diarrhoea.

Colonic abnormalities have been reported in tropical sprue; using a colonic perfusion system, impaired water and sodium absorption was demonstrated.[83]

Colonic function has *not* been investigated in tropical PIM investigated and treated in London.

Animal model

A clinical syndrome which exhibits very close similarities to PIM has been described in the German shepherd dog.[84] Jejunal biopsy specimens show villous atrophy with a variable infiltration of lymphocytes and plasma cells in the lamina propria. Aerobic bacteria are involved; both clinical and laboratory recovery take place after broad-spectrum antibiotic therapy.

Clinical aspects

This is dominated by *chronic* diarrhoea with large, pale, fatty stools, and sometime excessive flatulence, usually following an *acute* intestinal infection.[1,28,29,65] Weight loss is sometimes gross and is probably related to anorexia as much as to intestinal disease. Figure 10.4 shows an affected patient before and after chemotherapy. A wide range of clinical presentation exists, however, varying from the *acute* onset type (not strictly postinfective), described by Baker and Mathan as occurring in epidemics (with vomiting and pyrexia in up to 50%) at Vellore, India, to a far more *chronic* entity. Other clinical features, such as glossitis (aphthous ulceration was common in nineteenth-century reports), megaloblastic anaemia, fluid retention, depression, apathy, amenorrhoea and infertility, occur only after several months duration.

Table 10.3 summarizes the more important differential diagnoses of chronic malabsorption in relation to

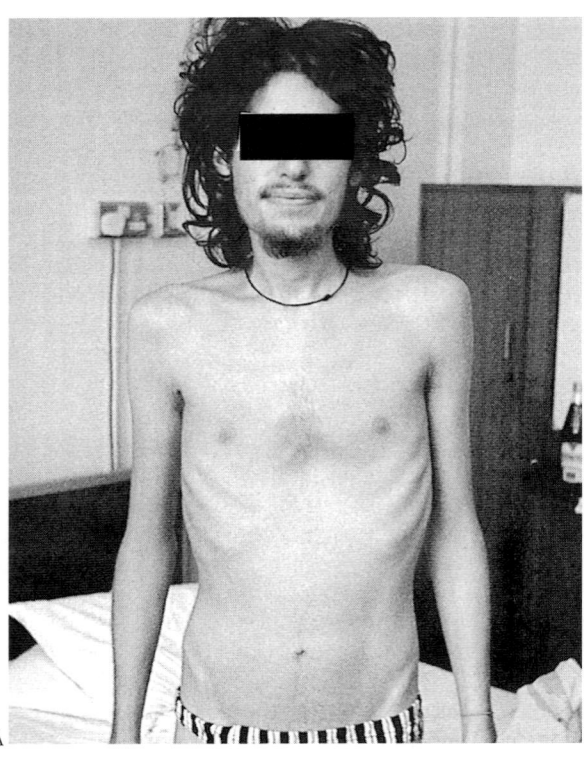
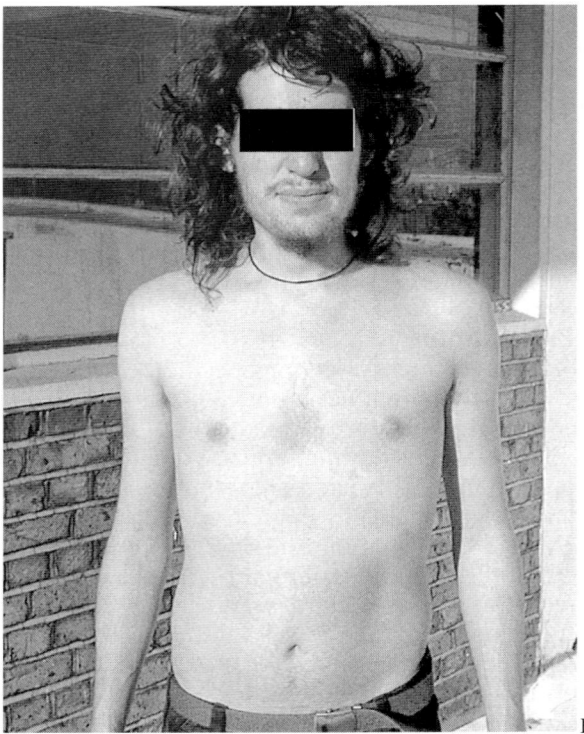
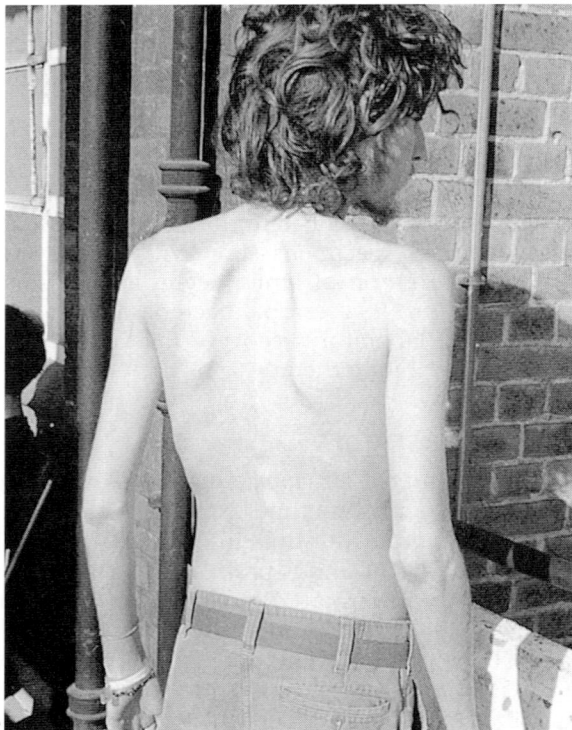
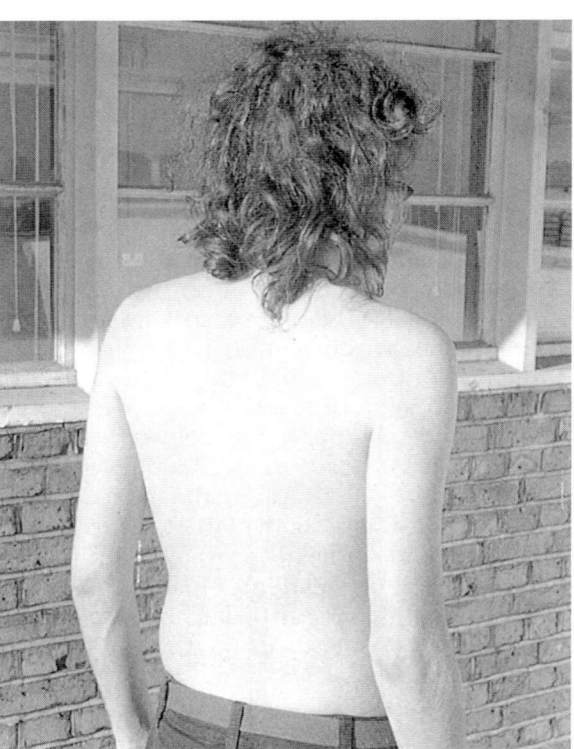

Figure 10.4: (**A** and **C**) A 19-year-old Englishman presented in London with postinfective tropical malabsorption (tropical sprue). Acute diarrhoea started soon after his arrival in Nepal and he lost approximately 12 kg in weight during the subsequent 2 months. The total urinary xylose excretion after a 25 g oral load was 2.5 mmol/5 hours (normal range 8.0–16.0 mmol/5 hours); the 24-hour faecal fat was 83 mmol (normal range 11–18 mmol); the Schilling test result was 0.16% urinary excretion at 24 hours (normal >10%) and the 8-hour serum concentration was 0% (normal >0.6%) of the loading dose. Jejunal biopsy histology showed marked villous blunting with increased lymphocytes in the lamina propria. Parasites were not found in several faecal samples. Serum albumin 36 g/litre; haemoglobin 13.2 g/dl; mean corpuscular volume 102.9; red blood cell folate 113 ng/litre (normal >150 ng/litre); serum vitamin B$_{12}$ 322 pg/litre (normal >150 pg/litre). The patient responded rapidly to treatment with oral tetracycline and folic acid. (**B** and **D**) The same man 4 weeks after initiation of treatment.

tropical exposure (see below).[71] There are also many non-infective causes of malabsorption in the tropics and subtropics; these should be excluded systematically.[85]

During, and immediately after, an acute small-intestinal infection, xylose, glucose, fat, B_{12} and filate malabsorption frequently is usual (see above). After 4 months or so, moderate/severe morphological change occurs in the jejunal mucosa; serum filate and later B_{12} concentrations decline—often to very low concentrations. Hypoalbuminaemia and oedema are late signs.

Gastric acid secretion is often depressed, but whether this precedes, or is a sequel to, the initiating infection is unknown. The role of hypochlorhydria in the production of small-intestinal infection remains unclear. In a small proportion of cases in southern India, B_{12} absorption either improved or became normal with addition of intrinsic factor.[81] Secondary hypolactasia may be present (see above).[64]

There is no good evidence that PIM predisposes to any gastrointestinal malignancy.

Investigations

Investigations should include urinary D-xylose excretion, 72-hour faecal fat estimation, a Schilling test and jejunal biopsy; faecal parasites should be excluded (1-hour blood xylose concentration is in practice probably superior to a 5-hour urinary collection in a tropical environment[86]): serum B_{12} and red blood cell folate concentrations should be estimated; after 4 months of illness most patients have a low folate concentration. Serum albumin and globulin concentrations are often depressed. Monosaccharide absorption is impaired to a greater extent than that of amino acids.[78] Barium meal and follow-through examination show dilated loops of jejunum with clumping of barium, in addition to reduced transit rate.

Jejunal mucosal changes are variable, depending on the duration of the disease. By 3 or 4 months most biopsies are ridged and/or convoluted; a flat mucosa is extremely unusual and, if present, gluten-induced enteropathy[85] should be suspected. Submucosal invasion with lymphocytes (predominantly T cells) and plasma cells is usual.

Ultrastructural changes in jejunal biopsy specimens have been studied;[87] although lysosomes, peroxisomes and mitochondrial enzymes are not depressed, the organelles are more fragile. Endoplasmic reticulum is unchanged. A significant reduction in 5-nucleotidase in the basolateral (plasma) membrane persists after recovery. The latter finding might reflect an underlying abnormality in the enterocyte of individuals susceptible to PIM.

Intestinal permeability has also been investigated;[30,88] abnormalities in urinary excretion of lactulose and rhamnose following an oral load are similar to results obtained in gluten-induced enteropathy.

Aetiology and treatment

A hypothesis to account for the aetiology of tropical PIM is summarized in Figure 10.5.[89] The 'vicious cycle' can be

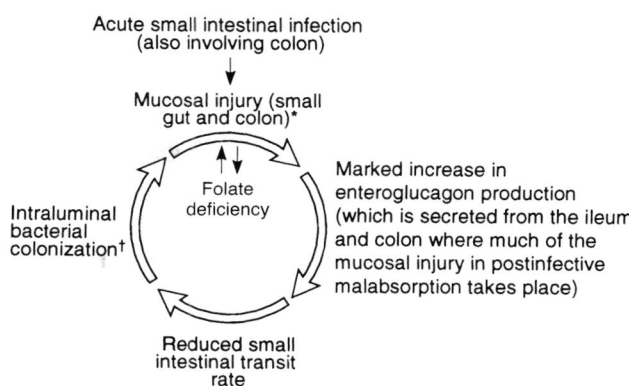

Figure 10.5: Hypothetical scheme to illustrate the pathogenesis of postinfective malabsorption. The open arrows indicate the vicious cycle which, once set in motion, is only broken by elimination of the abnormal luminal flora, and hastening of enterocyte recovery.

broken by (1) eliminating bacterial overgrowth, and (2) aiding mucosal recovery (with folic acid supplements). While this hypothesis has been challenged,[90] a satisfactory alternative has not been produced. An adequate diet should be combined with tetracycline (250 mg three times a day for at least 2 weeks) and folic acid (5 mg three times a day for 1 month). Evidence of susceptibility of the responsible flora to antibiotics other than tetracycline is limited. Symptomatic treatment may be necessary in the *acute* stage of the disease; codeine phosphate (30 mg three times a day), diphenoxylate (2.5–5 mg four times daily), or loperamide (5–10 mg four times daily) are of value if stool frequency is excessive. Mild cases respond without treatment, but this may take several months. Recovery is usually rapid and straightforward;[1,65,89] in the pre-antibiotic era a mortality rate of 10–20% was usual.

Evidence from south India suggests that response to antibiotics is less satisfactory;[67,68] this has been used as evidence to support a *viral* rather than a *bacterial* aetiology is causative in that locality.

Conclusion

The aetiology of PIM—especially that presenting in association with tropical exposure—is becoming clearer. It is probable that several primary insults to the enterocyte (of an infective nature) are involved. Whereas PIM resulting from most viral, bacterial and parasitic causes is usually self-limiting, this does not apply to the 'tropical sprue' syndrome, when well established. The reason why only a minority of affected individuals who suffer an acute small-intestinal infection are susceptible to PIM is unknown; a genetic (or ethnic) basis for susceptibility seems likely.

Other causes of malabsorption in the tropics

Table 10.3 summarizes some of these. The role of parasitic infection has been highlighted by AIDS, in which prolonged diarrhoea accompanied by malabsorption and weight loss can be very troublesome.[31] Incontrovertible evidence exists that HIV itself causes chronic enteropathy with villous blunting; crypt hypoplasia results from a direct effect of the viruses on cell replication, or by an unknown immunological reaction. This is a very common cause of persisting malabsorption in Africa. In this context, *Cryptosporidium parvum* and *Isospora belli* have recently come to the fore and it is now also clear that these organisms can produce a self-limiting illness stimulating TD in immunocompetent adults and children (see below). *G. lamblia* (see below) is undoubtedly the most common cause of parasitic malabsorption.[65,91,92] *Strongyloides stercoralis* (see below), which is widespread in tropical countries, was until very recently still present in approximately 15–30% of former prisoners of war in South-East Asia during the Second World War; it is an underdiagnosed cause.[1]

Of all causes of malabsorption related to tropical exposure, *intestinal tuberculosis*—usually involving the ileocaecal region—is probably that with the lowest index of suspicion amongst medical personnel.[65,94] Abdominal tuberculosis can assume several clinical forms: apart from the hypertrophic ileocaecal form, glandular (involving the mesenteric glands), peritoneal (sometimes with ascites) and hepatic involvement (with granulomatous disease) are relatively common. With the first of these presentations, weight loss and diarrhoea are often accompanied by a low-grade febrile illness; in severe cases stools are large, pale and bulky. Examination reveals an ileocaecal mass in 35–50% of cases,[94] and occasionally enlargement of one or more lymph glands; however, there is often no clinical abnormality. Late presentation can be as adult kwashiorkor. Anaemia and hypo-albuminaemia are common.[94] Chest radiography is usually normal. Absorption tests are frequently abnormal; fat and B_{12} absorption are affected most severely. A protein-losing enteropathy may be present. Pathologically, the disease results either from miliary dissemination, or follows ileal ulceration. Malabsorption is caused by chronic bile salt loss; unabsorbed bile salts (normally reabsorbed in the terminal ileum) in turn interfere with colonic absorption. Barium meal and follow-through examination shows ileal strictures,[94] frequently multiple, in a high percentage of cases; the ascending colon may also be shortened. The major differential is Crohn's disease, which is statistically much less common in people indigenous to the tropics. *Yersinia* infection should also be considered. Chest radiography is usually normal. The tuberculin test is positive in 70–90% of cases.[94] A needle liver biopsy specimen occasionally shows hepatic granulomas with caseation. Diagnostic laparotomy or peritoneoscopy (and peritoneal biopsy) is sometimes necessary in order to obtain a tissue diagnosis.[94] Treatment is with an antituberculosis regimen (Chapter 57). Resection of stricture(s) and occasionally hemicolectomy are sometimes necessary; chemotherapy should be initiated before surgical intervention.

A further cause of malabsorption in a tropical environment consists of the Mediterranean (α-chain) lymphoma,[95,96] which occurs sporadically in many parts of the tropics. If started early, tetracycline usually produces a good result, but not always so.

Other small-intestinal infections

Viral infections

Significant intestinal protein loss (mean 1.7 g daily) and xylose malabsorption have been demonstrated in northern Nigerian children with measles (see Chapter 23); approximately 25% also had lactose malabsorption.[97] Other infections in children caused by enteroviruses and herpes simplex viruses are also associated with diarrhoea and weight loss; malnutrition may result; the mechanism(s) (involving enterocyte damage) is probably similar to that in measles.

Volunteers infected with enteric viruses develop small-intestinal morphological lesions which are not always associated with symptoms.

Jejunal mucosal changes giving rise to severe malabsorption have been well documented in viral hepatitis;[98] these may persist for a considerable time after resolution of the hepatic abnormalities. The Norwalk agent (a 27 nm piconavirus) can also produce mucosal damage and malabsorption.[99] Rotavirus infections give rise to morphological abnormalities and (especially in children) malabsorption.[100]

These viral infections are invasive, and the resulting diarrhoea and malabsorption are caused by enterocyte destruction. Malabsorption usually occurs after the virus has been shed into the intestinal lumen; the villi contain immature crypt-type enterocytes. In coronavirus infection(s) in piglets, which resemble human rotavirus infections, glucose absorption is significantly impaired.[101] This has practical importance in management because sodium and water secretion cannot be reversed by glucose; oral rehydration fluids, commonly used in small-intestinal (including travellers') diarrhoea (see above), contain a high glucose concentration which overwhelms the limited absorptive capacity.

Baker et al. have suggested that coronavirus infections are responsible for at least some cases of 'tropical sprue' in southern India (see above); this might be the case, but asymptomatic individuals often excrete these viruses and this does therefore indicate a cause–effect relationship. Also at Vellore, a search for evidence of Berne virus infection in 'epidemic tropical sprue' proved negative.[102]

Bacterial infections

Moderate to severe malabsorption is commonplace during acute intestinal infections of bacterial origins; subnormal absorptive capacity persists for variable periods after termination of the diarrhoea and apparent clinical recovery. In a study in Bangladesh, approximately 70% of patients had evidence of xylose malabsorption

1 week after the diarrhoea had ceased; this was less common after cholera than *Shigella* species, *Salmonella* species and/or *Staphlococcus* species infections; xylose and B$_{12}$ malabsorption persisted for up to 378 and 196 days, respectively, after the diarrhoea had cleared.

Although many different infective insults to the enterocyte are probably important in PIM (see above), evidence for bacteria being responsible currently has more solid support than that involving other agents.

Escherichia coli

These organisms (with varying modes of pathogenicity) produce a spectrum of disease from TD to malabsorption by enterotoxin production and mucosal invasion— similar to that caused by *Shigella* species (Chapter 52). They are frequently food or water borne, and may cause outbreaks of gastroenteritis. Heat-labile enterotoxins exert an effect by activating adenylcyclase by a mechanism(s) similar to *V. cholerae*. Both heat-labile and heat-stable enterotoxins are probably important in TD (see above). A large pool of resistant *E. coli* (often showing resistance to multiple antimicrobials) now exists in the community. Enterotoxin production by *E. coli* may be transferred simultaneously with antibiotic resistance (Chapter 54); in a study, 72% and 44% of ETEC isolated in South-East Asia were resistant to one or more, and four or more antibiotics, respectively.[141] Enterocyte adhesiveness of *E. coli* is also a property of some strains and that might be important in continuing colonization and subsequent malabsorption. The relationship between adherence and verotoxin production remains unclear.[104] Attachment of micro-organisms to the enterocyte prevents clearance by peristaltic activity; such mucosal receptors may be determined genetically.[145] Ultrastructural studies have shown *E. coli* adherent to mucosal cells, with flattering of the microvilli, loss of the cellular terminal web and cupping of the plasma membrane around individual bacteria; intracellular damage was marked in the most heavily colonized cells. Histological improvement was demonstrated following clearing of *E. coli* with neomycin

and nutritional support. This mechanism can lead to protracted diarrhoea in infants. In most cases, resultant malabsorption is short lived.

Salmonellosis

Malabsorption occasionally follows infection with *Salmonella* species (Chapter 53),[105] but the frequency is unknown.

Campylobacter jejuni

Although unusual, dysenteric disease (bloody diarrhoea) has for long been known to predispose to tropical PIM;[65] in addition to shigellosis it is clear that some cases are caused by *E. coli* (see above) and others by *Campylobacter jejuni* (Chapter 52).

Although most cases of *Campylobacter jejuni* infection are acute, present with gastroenteritis and are self-limiting, initial symptoms can be prolonged.[106] The disease is a zoonosis; poultry are frequently contaminated. Many outbreaks have been traced to infected cow's milk. Dogs also constitute a reservoir of infection. Although the infection is self-limiting, erythromycin probably hastens recovery when given early in a severe case. The carrier state is common.

Enteritis necroticans (pigbel disease)

Although described in Germany at the end of the Second World War (1939–1945), and named Darmbrand,[4,29] this acute infection (Figure 10.6), which is more common in children than adults, occus in several tropical countries, notably the highlands of Papua New Guinea (where it is endemic),[107] Thailand and Uganda. Recently, enteritis necroticans has been recorded in Khmer children at an evacuation site on the Thai–Kampuchean border of Thailand; in the former report 36 (58%) out of 62 affected children (10 months to 10 (mean 4) years) died.[4] It seems likely that a disease termed 'necrotizing jejunitis' in rural areas of Bihar, India—which also affects children— represents the same entity; this condition ('segmental necrotizing enteritis') has also been recorded in Jaipur,

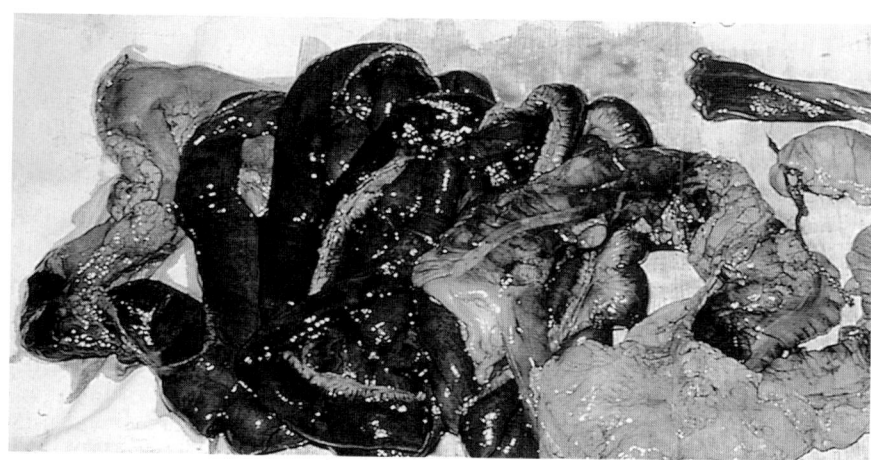

Figure 10.6: Gangrenous small intestine at post-mortem in a Papua New Guinean child who had died from necrotizing enteritis (pigbel disease).

India, and in Sri Lanka.[4] Scanty reports of a similar condition have also been made from northern Europe, which suggests that the disease exists worldwide, but only reaches epidemic proportions when suitable conditions exist, most importantly for the β-toxin of *Clostridium perfringens* type C (ingested in contaminated foodstuffs) to take its toll. Murrell[108] has suggested (in the light of historical evidence) that the disease was widespread in medieval Europe when 'human habitats, food hygiene, protein deficiency and periodic meat feasting formed the basics of village life as they do in many Third World cultures today'. Enteritis necroticans is now known to be caused by the ingestion (often at pig feasts or 'mumus') of food contaminated by *Cl. perfringens* type C.[107] The pathophysiology of the disease is complex, but the presenece of a low concentration of trypsin (resulting from trypsin inhibitors in foodstuffs and chronic protein–energy malnutrition) allows the β-toxin of *Cl. perfringens* to survive and produce mucosal injury.[29] It is sometimes associated with persisting structural changes in the small intestine; malabsorption may be a sequel.

Fluid and electrolyte replacement are essential (see below). Tetracycline or chloramphenicol, and type C gas gangrene antisera are of value; laparotomy is often indicated. In Papua New Guinea, immunization against *Cl. perfringens* type C has given good results;[29] in a controlled trial, marked reduction in incidence and mortality was demonstrated in the treatment group. A management strategy has been outlined.[109]

Parasitic infections
Giardiasis
The spectrum of disease caused by this flagellated protozoan is broad.[1,65,91,92] Symptoms vary from subclinical cases to those with severe malabsorption and malnutrition. The reason why some individuals are prone to symptomatic giardiasis is not clear; size of infecting dose, strain variability, genetic predisposition, acquired immunity factors, achlorhydria, a local secretory IgA deficiency and the presence of blood group A phenotype have all been considered. An increase in IgE and IgD cell numbers has been reported in the jejunal mucosa of 20 affected patients;[109] the former reversed after treatment, when an increase in IgA cell numbers was also recorded. The actual mechanism by which the trophozoites cause an absorptive defect is also unclear. Mucosal injury, with or without invasion, bacterial overgrowth in association with parasitization, and bile salt deconjugation by bacteria and/or parasites have all been considered. The extent of jejunal morphological abnormality varies widely.

Clinical presentation is usually between 1 and 3 weeks after infection; contaminated water and, less commonly, food are the usual sources of infection. Infection occurs both endemically and epidemically. The disease can probably be contracted from domestic animals.[110] It is more common in male homosexuals, but is *not* an opportunistic infection in AIDS sufferers. Diarrhoea of acute onset, flatus and weight loss may all be present; the stools have the characteristics of *malabsorption*. The disease is clinically indistinguishable from PIM; investigations also give similar results. A full-blown case has all of the clinical and laboratory features of the classical (historical) reports of 'tropical sprue' (see above). Cysts may be found in a faecal specimen; trophozoites can be detected in either a jejunal biopsy or jejunal fluid, or with the string test ('Enterotest'). If mucosal changes and malabsorption exist, circulating antibodies to *G. lamblia* cysts can often be detected.

Treatment is with metronizadole (2 g on three consecutive days); alcohol should be avoided during the treatment period. A single dose of tinidazole (2 g orally) has been used with success. Two 5-nitroimidazoles—ornidazole and tinidazole (as a single 1.5 g dose)—have been compared;[111] recurrence of infection during the subsequent 2 months was similar in each case (about 10%). Nimorazole has also been used. An alternative is mepacrine (100 mg three times daily for 10 days), which is less often used.

Cryptosporidium parvum
Like *G. lamblia*, this organism produces a broad spectrum of disease; prolonged infection usually, but not always, occurs in the immunosuppressed (including AIDS) sufferer where the organism is opportunistic. Diagnosis is similar to that for *G. lamblia* infection; oocysts are usually detectable in a faecal sample. Treatment (rarely indicated in the immunointact) is with spiramycin, but is usually ineffective in the immunosuppressed; although at least 70 other compounds have been tested, none, including spiramycin, has proven efficiency in vitro.

Other parasites
The vast majority of small-intestinal parasitic infections do not result in signs/symptoms unless present at a high concentration.[27] In a heavy infection, hookworm is responsible for hypochromic anaemia; *A. lumbricoides* rarely accounts for obstruction in the small intestine and biliary and pancreatic ducts (Chapter 83). The major clinical sequel of tapeworm infection is neurocysticercosis (*Taenia solium*) (Chapter 85)—a complication unrelated to the intestinal tract.

Although *A. lumbricoides*, *Ancylostoma duodenale* and *Necator americanus* have at various times been implicated in malabsorption, there is no clear evidence except in rare or anecdotal case reports.[112] *Diphyllobothrium latum* infections are occasionally associated with a low serum B_{12} concentration; however, this is caused by B_{12} uptake within the small-intestinal lumen, and is not an example of true malabsorption.

Clear evidence exists that *Strongyloides stercoralis* is causally related to malabsorption.[1,29,65,93] This helminth can survive in the human host for several decades; some 10–20% of ex-prisoners of war in South-East Asia during the Second World War (1939–1945) remained infected until recently. Onset of diarrhoea is less acute than with *G. lamblia*. Larvae can be demonstrated by the 'Enterotest', and less often by jejunal biopsy. Ova and larvae can occasionally be detected in faecal specimens. Eosinophilia may be gross; however, it is often absent. The immuno-fluorescent antibody test (IFAT) is positive in approximately 70% of cases; however, cross-reaction with filaria is common. The enzyme-linked immunosorbent assay (ELISA) test, when available, is more specific. A negative serological result is common in the immunosuppressed patient. Treatment is with thiabendazole (1.5 g twice daily on three successive days); repeated courses may be required. Albendazole (400 mg daily for 3 days) seems less effective. In animal experiments, cambendazole has given encouraging results; this has also been the case in limited clinical studies, but the compound has not been officially released for human use. Other *Strongyloides* species are important, especially in children. *Stongyloides fülleborni* has been implicated in the pathogenesis of severe PIM (see above) in Zambia and Papua New Guinea, where a significant mortality rate has been recorded.[65]

In the northern Philippines and Thailand, *Capillaria philippinensis* has been causally associated with PIM.[1,79] It can occur in epidemics. Diarrhoea of acute onset is followed by malabsorption and, if untreated, infection carries a substantial mortality rate. Protein-losing entero-pathy may also be present. Treatment with one of the benzimidazole compounds has given good results.

The protozoa *Isospora belli* and *Sarcocystis hominis* (usually conveyed by undercooked pork and beef)[113] also cause malabsorption. These organisms replicate within the enterocyte. *I. belli*, like *Crytosporidium parvum*, causes a spectrum of disease, from TD to PIM, and is more common in the immunosuppressed individual. Pyrimethamine + sulfadiazine, and co-trimoxazole + nitrofurantoin, have been used with some success. Other protozoan parasites, such as *P. falciparum* (in an acute infection) and visceral leishmaniasis (kala azar), can also produce significant malabsorption. Other protozoa which have assumed practical importance in the wake of the HIV/AIDS pandemic are *Cyclospora cayetanensis*,[114–116] micro-sporidiosis,[117,118] and *Blastocystis hominis*.[119] All can be implicated in a wide range of small-intestinal problems ranging from travellers' diarrhoea to malabsorption.

Emergencies

Severe dehydration consequent upon secretory watery diarrhoea accounts for enormous amounts of acute morbidity throughout the tropics; this applies especially to infants and children. Intravenous replacement therapy has been in use for more than 150 years; Dr Robert Lewins MD FRCP, of Leith, recorded that he had witnessed Dr Thomas Latta inject saline intravenously into a patient suffering from cholera (see above) in 1832,[58] and George Leith Roupell,[120] a physician at St Bartholomew's Hospital, London, seems to have been an early user of this technique. It is unlikely, however, that these were the first attempts at intravenous rehydration (in fact, Sir Christopher Wren, better known for his

architectural achievements, had used the technique experimentally in 1657). Nearly three-quarters of a century passed before Sir Leonard Rogers, working at Calcutta, demonstrated a reduction in the mortality rate in cholera patients from 70% to 20% by use of this technique. Introduction of *oral* rehydration regimens had to wait much longer, in fact until the latter half of the twentieth century. Introduction of this form of management, which followed upon important basic applied physiological observations, was, in a world context, one of the most important medical advances during the twentieth century.[1] In many acute medical conditions, gastric emptying is delayed; however, this is not the case in cholera (and presumably other acute small-intestinal infections) and does not constitute a barrier to oral rehydration, even when fluid and electrolyte loss (in the stool) is severe.[121] Oral rehydration therapy remains grossly underused,[122] however, and infants and children in developing countries with acute gastroenteritis continue to die unnecessarily because this simple technique is not readily applied. The authors of this latter article have concluded: 'the impediment to its wide acceptance may be that it is counterintuitive for a simpler and much less expensive treatment to be an improvement over an effective but more complicated technology'!

Enteritis necroticans (pigbel disease)

This acute small-intestinal emergency (see above), which usually affects infants and children (see above) is characterized by gangrenous changes in the small-intestinal wall (in patchy distribution); the jejunum is most markedly affected, but the ileum is also involved. Presentation is usually as an acute abdominal (surgical) emergency, with abdominal pain, fever and bloody diarrhoea (see above). A chronic stage of the disease may ensue in which there is narrowing of the small-intestinal lumen (in one or more places) by a fibrotic stenosis or adhesion; clinical presentation is with subacute obstruction, often accompanied by malabsorption and malnutrition. Fluid and electrolyte replacement are vitally important in management; gastric suction is also required. Penicillin or another antibiotic should be given (see above). Laparotomy is frequently indicated to confirm the diagnosis and to resect the necrotized, haemorrhagic segment(s) of small intestine. Fortunately, active immunization against the β-toxin has proved effective prophylaxis in Papua New Guinea; hospital admissions for pigbel in one area of the country fell to less than one-fifth of the previous figure ($p < 0.001$) when a vaccination programme was introduced.[123] Morbidity due to this acute abdominal emergency (with a very high mortality rate) should eventually fall in the seriously affected countries.

Paralytic ileus and acute obstruction

In Pakistan, paralytic ileus has recently been recorded as a late complication of acute diarrhoeal disease in infants;[124]

despite rehydration and total parenteral nutrition, the mortality rate was 25%. When compared with others who did not develop ileus (following acute diarrhoeal disease), these infants were shown to have had significantly more antimotility agents preceding the ileus; furthermore, more had a depressed serum potassium concentration. The potential dangers associated with antiperistaltic agents, especially in infancy and childhood, are thus re-emphasized.

Acute intestinal obstruction constitutes a common surgical emergency in both children and adults in many parts of the tropics, including Africa. Strangulated hernia (usually of inguinal origin) is usually the most common cause; volvulus and intussusception are relatively common in tropical Africa; tuberculosis is a further cause—due either to stenosis or to pressure on the third part of the duodenum or jejunum. A heavy *A. lumbricoides* infection (especially in children) can also produce small-intestinal obstruction;[125] when diagnosed clinically, laparotomy can usually be avoided. Management consists of intravenous hydration, nasogastric suction and appropriate anthelmintic chemotherapy. Strangulated hernia, volvulus and intussusception nearly always require laparotomy.[125] In a report from southern India, 904 children presented with intestinal obstruction;[126] the most common causes in order of frequency were necrotizing enteritis (see above), acute intussusception, band obstruction, subacute obstruction, and remnants of the vitello-intestinal duct. Rare causes of small-intestinal obstruction include: Burkitt's lymphoma, Mediterranean lymphoma (α-chain disease) (see above) and intestinal schistosomiasis. Small-intestinal trauma—caused by a road accident or knife, arrow or gunshot wound—is also important in a tropical context.

Typhoid (enteric) fever (See also Chapters 53 and 54)

In most areas within the developing world, typhoid (and to a lesser extent tuberculosis) accounts for much small-intestinal disease encountered in surgical practice;[127] perforation, obstruction and less often haemorrhage constitute acute surgical emergencies. This seems especially important in West Africa. *S. typhi* infection is also an increasing problem in travellers from industrialized countries to the tropics; in the USA, 2666 cases (fatality rate 1–3%) of acute enteric fever were officially notified between 1975 and 1984; 62% of them were imported, the majority of infections having originated in either Mexico or India.[128] Statistically, surgical complications are unusual; thus in a series of 82 culture-positive cases in The Gambia there were no surgical complications;[129] this was also the case in a series of 192 cases of enteric fever— most caused by *S. typhi*—in Thailand.[130] Despite its relative rarity, however, (perhaps 2–4% of cases worldwide), typhoid perforation is an extremely serious event, accounting for 20–60% of deaths in this disease (a statistic which is increased by late presentation, female sex, age ≥ 40 years and the presence of multiple

perforations). Late perforation is often indistinguishable from a perforated appendix, amoebic liver abscess, tuberculous peritonitis, an infected ruptured ectopic pregnancy or intestinal strangulation. The optimal form of management seems to be surgical, provided the patient is not too shocked to endure such a procedure (a prolonged period of preoperative resuscitation is often required). There is as yet no general agreement, however, regarding the ideal type of operative intervention;[131] simple closure, ulcer excision and closure, wedge excision and closure, ileal resection and anastomosis, resection and transverse ileotransverse colostomy, and right hemicolectomy have all found favour. When the perforation is single, simple closure (with or without excision) is the procedure of choice; an area(s) of impending perforation should not be overseen; closure should always be in two layers: an inner one of chromic catgut and an outer of silk. When there are three or more perforations, bowel resection is probably advisable. Peritoneal lavage with a copious amount of washing with normal saline should be carried out. The incidence of postoperative complications is high, and includes peripheral vascular failure, respiratory infections, anaemia, sepsis, abscess formation, burst abdomen and intestinal obstruction.[131] Re-perforation or a new perforation is possible. In a series of 108 consecutive cases of perforated typhoid enteritis managed in western Nigeria, 100 (93%) underwent 'debridement of the perforation and two-layer bowel closure';[132] 35 patients died, usually from overwhelming sepsis. In addition to specific chemotherapy— although chloramphenicol (1 g four times daily in an average adult, reduced to 1 g twice daily when body temperature is normal) remains the agent of choice, increasing numbers of reports of multiple-antibiotic-resistant strains of *S. typhi* are being reported (especially from India)—metronidazole, and possibly corticosteroids, seem to improve the prognosis.[175] Alternative chemotherapeutic agents include amoxycillin, co-trimoxazole, trimethoprim and ciprofloxacin; the last agent is indicated when there are serious doubts about sensitivity to the other compounds, as is frequently the case when infection has resulted in Asia. Despite these advances therefore, ileal perforation in enteric fever remains a potentially lethal complication—especially in children.[133]

Haemorrhage is rarely life threatening, although recorded;[134] whereas the majority of cases can be treated conservatively (blood transfusion is indicated), when selective angiography, fibreoptic endoscopy and high-resolution radionuclide imaging are available, localization of the bleeding site can be delineated and appropriate surgery instituted.

Emergencies associated with helminthiases

Abdominal discomfort (and pain) are common sequelae to heavy small-intestinal nematode infections (see above), especially ancylostomiasis and *A. lumbricoides* (see above), but serious acute complications (see above) are fortunately rare.[135] Anisakiasis, for example—usually acquired from ingestion of undercooked or raw infected fish (sushi and sashimi)—can present with an acute appendicitis-like illness.[136] Invasive disease caused by this organism is usually localized to the ileocaecal region; there is no satisfactory parasitological or serological test, and chemotherapy is not effective. A diagnostic laparotomy is often necessary.

Eosinophilic enteritis is an entity of multiple aetiology.[137] A recent report from Townsville, Australia, suggested that *Ancylostoma caninum* (the dog hookworm) was responsible for an epidemic (93 cases) encountered there;[138] nine were subjected to diagnostic laparotomy: eosinophilic infiltration involving a segment of ileum with indurated thickening of the distal small intestine and proximal dilatation was the usual underlying pathology. A rare case of acute mesenteric ischaemia (accompanied by segmental small-intestinal infarction and gangrene) caused by *Schist. mansoni* has been reported from Baghdad, Iraq.[139] The small intestine can also be involved in *Schist. japonicum* infection; intestinal obstruction resulting from mesenteric ischaemia, an intussuscepting polypoid mass or fibrotic stenosis are possible sequelae. Intestinal perforation resulting from infection with the acanthocephalan worm *Macracanthorhynchus hirudinaceus*, a natural intestinal parasite of the pig, has been described in Bangkok, Thailand[140] (eight other cases are on record); this infection has also been reported from several other parts of the world, including China and southern Europe. Fatal gastrointestinal haemorrhage (associated with fluctuating jaundice, a tender liver, palpable gallbladder and an eosinophilia) has been attributed to *Fasciola hepatica* (liver fluke) infection in Harare, Zimbabwe;[141] the site of bleeding was probably the biliary tree.

Colorectum

Most cases of colorectal disease occurring in a tropical environment have an infective basis (Table 10.4); they are dominated by bacterial (*Shigella* species (Chapter 52) (Figure 10.7), *Campylobacter jejuni* and invasive *E. coli*) and protozoan (*Ent. histolytica* (Chapter 77) and *Balantidium coli*) infections. Amoebic colitis and shigellosis present classically with bloody diarrhoea; this should be differentiated from carcinoma, necrotizing colitis, antibiotic-associated colitis and inflammatory bowel disease (which is overall not very common in tropical countries). Whether or not amoebic colitis can proceed to inflammatory bowel disease is debatable; however, misdiagnosis of amoebic colitis as inflammatory bowel disease (with subsequent corticosteroid therapy) can result in fatality. In AIDS, cytomegalovirus colitis is common; *Cryptosporidium* is usually a small-intestinal parasite, but colonic involvement can also occur. In addition, megacolon resulting from South American trypanosomiasis (Chagas' disease) (Chapter 74) is another cause of colonic pathology. Of diseases localized to the

Table 10.4 Colorectal diarrhoea.*

Bacterial infection
    Shigellosis
    Campylobacter jejuni
    Escherichia coli (enteroinvasive)

Protozoan infection
    Entamoeba histolytica
    Balantidium coli

Schistosomiasis (usually *Schistosoma mansoni* and *Schist. japonicum*)

Unusual causes
    Non-specific ulcerative colitis—inflammatory bowel disease[†]
    Crohn's disease[†]
    Appendicitis
    Diverticulitis
    Haemorrhoids
    Colonic carcinoma
    Irritable bowel syndrome

*Characteristically, numerous small stools containing mucus, pus and blood; microscopy shows pus cells and/or red blood cells in a faecal smear.
[†]Although these diseases are uncommon, or even rare, in most tropical populations, they can become clinically overt for the first time in visitors from Western countries to the tropics.

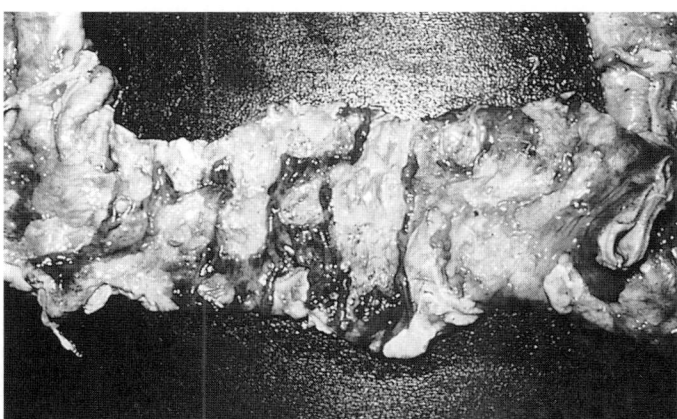

Figure 10.7: Severe amoebic colitis: operative specimen obtained from an Australian nurse misdiagnosed as having non-specific ulcerative colitis (inflammatory bowel disease) while working in Papua New Guinea.

anal region, lymphogranuloma is perhaps the most important although bacterial (including donovanosis, syphilis and gonorrhoea (Chapter 21)) and parasitic (including *Ent. histolytica*, *Schistosoma* species and *Enterobius vermicularis*) infections constitute differential diagnoses.

Overall, diseases of the colorectum are far less common in indigenous people in developing countries compared with individuals in industrialized ones;[1,144] colonic carcinoma seems, for example, to be an unusual lesion in rural communities. Good evidence now exists that frequency of these diseases is increasing as urbanization advances—in Africa especially. Hypotheses to account for these differences include high dietary fibre consumption in most tropical countries; however, such associations rarely have a proven cause–effect relationship.

Many data have been collected on colonic function in indigenous inhabitants of developing countries;[1] it seems likely that mean 24-hour faecal weight and volume is higher in Africa, and constipation unusual. Overall, intestinal transit rate also seems more rapid. Limited evidence indicates that colorectal histology is mildly different in indigenous people in developing countries, and is comparable to *tropical enteropathy* (see above). In PIM in India (see above) in vivo colonic functional abnormalities have been demonstrated. Whether colonic pathology is important in a nutritional context remains difficult to evaluate (see above): evidence now exists that this organ is important in the absorption of nitrogen and free (volatile) fatty acids.

Inflammatory bowel disease (non-specific ulcerative colitis and Crohn's disease)[145] is less common overall in indigenous people in developing countries compared with the UK and other Western countries. The aetiology of this disease is unknown, although an infective basis has frequently been suggested; satisfactory evidence for a viral or bacterial (possibly mycobacterial) origin is at present lacking. A handful of reports of ulcerative colitis have been made from African countries, and a few more from Asia.[145] In individuals in the UK with an ancestry in the Caribbean or Indian subcontinent this disease clearly exists but is unusual. Such differences also apply to Crohn's disease, although this disease also is well recognized in Caribbean people in the UK. Although Crohn's disease behaves very much like intestinal tuberculosis in clinical practice, response to antituberculous therapy is disappointing. When inflammatory bowel disease occurs, it seems to behave similarly to that in the indigenous population of the UK. It is a common cause of bloody diarrhoea in travellers who have returned to temperate from tropical countries (Figure 10.8).[38-40] Similarly, appendicitis, diverticular disease and haemorrhoids are overall less common in a developing country population, where a high-fibre intake has been implicated in their prevention; a causative association has not, however, been proved.

Although irritable bowel (IBD) syndrome (spastic colon)[146] is extremely common in UK residents (and others) following an intestinal infection acquired in a tropical country, it seems to be far less significant in indigenous peoples in Africa and Asia. Whether this constitutes a genuine difference is unclear because so many of the latter have more severe symptoms of different origin(s) which might mask symptoms resulting from IBD. This syndrome does not constitute a single entity; although some cases respond to mebeverine or peppermint oil, many do not.

Enterobius vermicularis infection (Chapter 83) is arguably the most common gastrointestinal infection in the world;[147] it exists in both tropical and temperate areas.

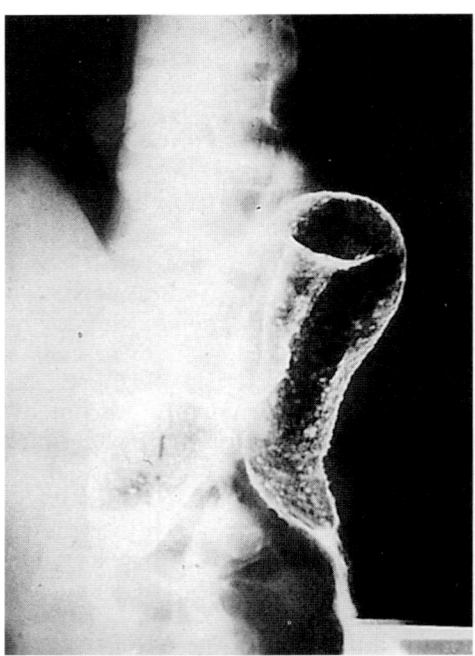

Figure 10.8: Barium enema in a 35-year-old woman who experienced bloody diarrhoea during a visit to Africa; she had not previously had significant gastrointestinal problems. Colonic biopsy specimen obtained at colonoscopy confirmed the diagnosis.

Colonoscopy is an endoscopic technique which is now available in some, but by no means all, developing countries; frequently, it is available only at the teaching hospital and/or other (tertiary referral) centre(s).

Emergencies

Invasive amoebic colitis

Perforation—although a rare event—can complicate this disease, with the production of amoebic peritonitis;[1] there may be diffusion of *Ent. histolytica* from a 'blotting-paper'-like colon, and perforation (especially in the rectosigmoid or caecal regions or to the retroperitoneal tissues) or leakage into a confined space (resulting in a pericolic abscess or internal intestinal fistula). Management consists of gastric suction and intravenous fluid replacement; metronizadole, 500 mg 8-hourly (preferably by the intravenous route), and a broad-spectrum antibiotic should immediately be given. The colon is extremely fragile; laparotomy is usually best avoided;[148] overall, mortality is of the order of 50% and after surgery close on 100%. Two reports have recorded results of surgical intervention in 15 patients with fulminant amoebic colitis.[149,150] In the first, five out of six patients (four had a subtotal colectomy with ileostomy, and two a right hemicolectomy and ileostomy) subsequently died (none was diagnosed either preoperatively or during surgery); in the second, three out of nine died, all of whom had exteriorization of the cut ends of the bowel following resection of the necrotic segment (four of those who died had end-to-end anastomoses, and two peritoneal drainage).

Shigellosis

Although perforation is less common in shigellosis compared with amoebic colitis, haemorrhage is well documented. The most recent pandemic of this disease in the Western Hemisphere began in Guatemala in 1969 and ended in 1973. It spread rapidly to Nicaragua, Belize, Honduras, Costa Rica, Panama and Mexico; with an estimated 500 000 affected, of whom 20 000 died.[151]

Appendicitis

Overall, this entity is less common in developing compared with 'westernised' countries. Nevertheless it certainly exists, and a predominance of appendicectomies in women has recently been recorded.[152] Confusion with an acute gynaecological condition is a real problem and more widespread use of ultrasound and laparoscopy might be the solution.[153] In Calabar, Nigeria, 603 consecutive cases were investigated prospectively during a 5-year period;[154] there were no major differences from this disease in industrialized countries, and it constituted the second most common abdominal emergency during the study period, being less common than acute intestinal obstruction. Many causative agents have been implicated; in a retrospective review of 2921 appendicectomies carried out at Allahabad, India, during a 25-year period, 153 produced histological evidence of a specific infection:[155] tuberculosis (70), *Ent. histolytica* (17), *A. lumbricoides* (13), *A. lumbricoides* and *Trichuris trichiura* (2), *Enterobius vermicularis* (41), and *Taenia* species (2). This acute disease should be differentiated from pelvic inflammatory disease, typhoid enteritis, ruptured ectopic pregnancy, psoas abscess, acute amoebic colitis, and *Schist. mansoni* colitis. Although the vast majority of cases of appendicitis in developing countries result from a bacterial cause, helminths, including *Schist. mansoni*, *Strongloides stercoralis* and *Trichuris trichiura*, have also been implicated.[1]

Volvulus of the colon

This is a disease with clear geographical differences; it is common in much of Central and East Africa, India and South America;[1] numerous reports have been made from Uganda and Zimbabwe. Although genetic factors have been suggested for these high rates, a high-fibre diet, common in most of Africa, has also been implicated. The major complication is strangulation, and gangrene of a colonic segment; this should be differentiated from primary volvulus of the small intestine, compound volvulus (usually ileosigmoid) and internal herniae. Distention can be relieved with a flatus tube; at laparotomy the nature of the operation, and extent of resection, depends on the length of gangrenous colon. With simple volvulus, mortality rate should be low. Zimmerman et al.[156] have emphasized the value of emergency colonoscopy in the diagnosis of colonic volvulus; when the mucosa is ischaemic or necrotic, emergency laparotomy is indicated, but when appearances are normal relief of flatus (with a flatus tube passed per rectum) together with medical management followed by elective surgery (resection and anastomosis) 10 days later is recommended.

Colonic intussusception

The common variety, especially in West Africa, is the caecocolic one; although children may be afflicted, the vast majority are in adults.[1] Aetiology—as with that of volvulus—is conjectural; while an intestinal polyp or amoeboma accounts for some, there is no obvious clue in most cases. Gangrene is about three times more common with the ileoileal and ileocaecal varieties compared with the caecocolic type.

Acute colonic dilatation

Several gastrointestinal infections can cause toxic megacolon. These include: *Salmonella* species, *Campylobacter* species and *Y. enterocolitica* infection; recently, however, there has been a growing recognition of *Shigella* species in this potentially lethal condition.[157] Correct diagnosis is essential; an unnecessary laparotomy can thus usually be avoided. If the condition is misdiagnosed as ulcerative colitis, and corticosteroids administered, potentially fatal consequences can ensue. Diagnostically, the causative organism can usually be identified in a faecal sample. Choice of an appropriate antibiotic is often difficult; in *Shigella* species infection, a fluoroquinolone, e.g., ciprofloxacin (200 mg intravenously 12-hourly for 10 days), seems most appropriate. Toxic dilatation of the colon has also been reported, albeit rarely, in *Ent. histolytica* infection;[158] these authors recorded a single case (in which total colectomy, and administration of metronidazole and emetine, was followed by recovery); they were able to detect seven cases in the world literature.

Other colorectal lesions

Anorectal infections in relation to tropical exposure have been reviewed.[159] Trauma to the colon, often resulting from road accidence, constitutes a medical emergency in most tropical countries.[1] Necrotizing colitis (the pathology is similar to that of enteritis necroticans; see above) is rarely encountered. Colonic obstruction is rarely caused by carcinoma (a rare tumour in the rural tropics[160]) but is recorded following introduction of a foreign body per rectum. Colorectal tuberculosis is an unusual cause of stricture formation, which occasionally requires surgical intervention.[161]

Liver and biliary system

Liver histology in an individual indigenous to a tropical country differs from that in one who has spent his/her life in a temperate region of the world.[1] This organ is subjected to numerous systemic infections—viral, bacterial and parasitic—and it lies at the distal end of the portal circulation; it is therefore bathed with portal blood containing viruses, bacteria, parasites, ova, products of digestion and other antigens. Thus, Kupffer cell hyperplasia and periportal infiltration (with lymphocytes, plasma cells and eosinophils) are more common, and stellate fibrosis occurs more frequently. Also, nuclear pleomorphism in hepatocytes and sinusoidal lymphocytes are frequently prominent; these appearances are unusual in biopsies obtained in a temperate country. Malaria and schistosomal pigment are often also present. Granulomas are common (Figure 10.9) and a large number of differential diagnoses exist; Table 10.5 lists some of them.

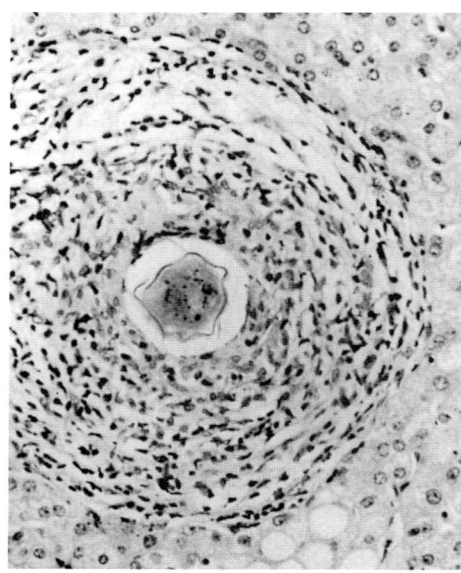

Figure 10.9: Liver biopsy specimen from a 30-year-old Zambian woman. A degenerating *Schistosoma mansoni* egg is surrounded by a well-formed granuloma.

Table 10.5 Some causes of hepatic granulomas in tropical countries.

Infection	Viral cytomegalovirus, Epstein–Barr virus
Bacterial	Tuberculosis and atypical mycobacteria, leprosy, syphilis, Q fever, brucellosis
Parasitic	Schistosomiasis, ascariasis, strongyloidiasis, toxocariasis, filariasis, enterobiasis, visceral leishmaniasis
Fungi	Histoplasmosis, cocidioidomycosis, aspergillosis, actinomycosis, candidiasis
Neoplasms	Lymphomas—especially intra-abdominal Hodgkin's disease
Others	(sarcoidosis) therapeutic agents—especially sulfonamides

Acute liver infections

Jaundice in a tropical context (Table 10.6) is most commonly a result of viral hepatitis (types A,[162,163] B (sometimes a combined infection with D), C,[164] E[165–168] and F) (Chapter 40), but other causes should also be considered; Table 10.6 summarizes some of them. An important cause is the jaundice of *acute bacterial infection*—most commonly caused by pneumococcal lobar pneumonia or pyomyositis.[1] The mechanism of this form of jaundice is complex and consists of hepatocellular, cholestatic and haemolytic elements; the importance of the latter depends on the underlying prevalence of glucose-6-phosphate dehydrogenase (G6PD) deficiency in the population under consideration (Chapter 13). It is important to differentiate this form of jaundice from viral hepatitis, otherwise the appropriate antibiotic will not be administered for an underlying bacterial infection. In addition to yellow fever, several other viruses are implicated;[164] dengue fever, Kyasanur Forest disease, herpes simplex and Coxsackie virus should also be considered.

In AIDS, the liver is affected by many opportunistic organisms. These include viruses; hepatitis B (HBV) and C (HCV) infections can be especially virulent. A liver biopsy specimen may also yield evidence of cytomegalovirus,

Table 10.6 Some causes of jaundice in the tropics.

Jaundice of acute bacterial infection: pneumococcal lobar pneumonia, pyomyositis	
Viruses	Hepatitis (A–F) Yellow fever Epstein–Barr virus Cytomegalovirus Marburg and Ebola diseases Lassa fever
Bacteria	Leptospirosis Typhoid fever Syphilis Gonococcal disease Bartonellosis
Parasites	Malaria (acute *Plasmodium falciparum* and *P. vivax*) Schistosomiasis Amoebiasis (rarely) Toxoplasmosis Trichinellosis Fascioliasis ⎫ Clonorchiasis ⎬ predominantly large-duct obstructive jaundice Opisthorchiasis ⎭ Ascariasis Hydatidosis (rarely)
Genetic	Sickle cell disease Glucose-6-phosphate dehydrogenase deficiency Dubin–Johnson syndrome

Mycobacterium tuberculosis, M. avium intracellulare, atypical mycobacteria, *Cryptosporidium parvum, Pneumocystis carinii, Cryptococcus* species and/or Kaposi's sarcoma. Cholestatic features are common.

In addition to septicaemia, several bacterial infections can produce jaundice;[1,169] leptospirosis is frequently accompanied by renal involvement, while overt jaundice in typhoid fever 'hepatitis' is unusual.[171,172] Melioidosis, plague, tularaemia and relapsing fever can also produce hepatitis. Of parasitic causes, acute *P. falciparum* infection is probably the most important. In acute (Katayama syndrome) and *severe* chronic schistosomiasis jaundice may be present, but is rare in invasive hepatic amoebiasis. Most parasitic infections, including African trypanosomiasis (Chapter 73) and visceral leishmaniasis (Chapter 75), can produce significant hepatitis and deranged hepatocellular function—often in the absence of *clinical* jaundice.

Several parasites produce large duct biliary obstruction; for practical purposes, *A. lumbricoides* is the most important to recognize and treat urgently.

Sickle cell disease and haemoglobinopathies (Chapter 13) are important causes of haemolytic jaundice; they possess a genetic basis. Jaundice in the presence of G6PD deficiency is frequently precipitated (or worsened) by therapeutic agents and/or toxins. In some parts of the tropics, especially Indonesia and Papua New Guinea, the Dubin–Johnson syndrome seems unusually common.

Chronic liver disease

Most cases of *chronic active hepatitis* in tropical countries result from HBV and HCV infections;[174] corticosteroids should *not* be administered for they exacerbate hepatocyte viral infection; interferon γ and adenine arabinoside have given encouraging results, but ethnic factors are probably important. There is no reliable evidence that either malnutrition (including kwashiorkor) or *Plasmodium* species infection are aetiologically important, although such beliefs linger.[1]

In tropical countries most cases of macronodular cirrhosis result from viral hepatitis—most commonly HBV, and to a lesser extent HCV hepatitis.[170] The sequence of events is: acute hepatitis → chronic active hepatitis → macronodular cirrhosis → and, ultimately, hepatocellular carcinoma[175–178] (hepatoma) (acute viral hepatitis is covered in Chapter 40 and hepatoma in Chapter 36). HBV and HCV are undoubtedly the most important aetiological factors in hepatoma, but the role of aflatoxin[1] should not be totally disregarded.

An important and probably underrated cause of chronic liver disease in a tropical context is schistosomiasis (Chapter 80).[179,180] Although hepatocellular function is preserved until late in the disease, portal hypertension and its various complications (see below) are as important as in the various forms of cirrhosis.

Clinically, cutaneous stigmata of chronic hepatocellular disease are difficult to detect in brown or black skins;[1] similarly, other cutaneous stigmata of chronic liver disease may be absent. Diagnosis is often first suspected by abnormal liver function tests; a needle liver biopsy specimen is usually diagnostic. Peritoneoscopy is relatively simple and underused in developing countries; refined diagnostic techniques are rarely available. No treatment is of any avail in established cirrhosis, but some of the chormalitics in chronic schistosomal disease of the liver are reversible after treatment (Chapter 80). Major complications (see below) resulting from portal hypertension are: (1) haemorrhage, from oesophageal varices (see below); (2) fluid retention, including ascites; and (3) hepatic encephalopathy. Fluid retention is a major long-term problem, largely the result of a very low serum albumin concentration. This complication is often difficult to manage, largely because salt restriction is virtually impossible to impose in a tropical setting; diuretics, e.g., frusemide (Lasix) (40–120 mg daily) and spironolactone (Aldactone) (100 mg daily), usually achieve success. Paracentesis abdominis should rarely be undertaken; this procedure depletes albumin stores further and electrolyte balance can be seriously disturbed; tapping ascitic fluid should be reserved for: (1) diagnostic purposes—to understand whether a bacterial infection, tuberculous peritonitis or hepatocellular carcinoma is present concurrently; and (2) management of *tense* ascites, accompanied by respiratory embarrassment. Hepatic encephalopathy is managed by accepted methods: oral neomycin (6 g daily) and/or lactulose (20–35 g three times daily); in the presence of hypolactasia lactose can be substituted for lactulose.

Other forms of chronic liver disease (with subsequent decompensation) (see below) include those resulting from excessive alcohol ingestion, Indian childhood cirrhosis, haemosiderosis and veno-occlusive disease. Wilson's disease (hepatolenticular degeneration) and other genetically determined forms of cirrhosis are of limited importance numerically in the tropics, although they too should enter the list of differential diagnoses.

Alcoholic liver disease

Alcohol-related disease (including cirrhosis) is common in both indigenous and expatriate populations in tropical countries.[1,181] Genetic factors are undoubtedly involved; HBsAg carriers are especially vulnerable. The liver in chronic alcoholic disease is classically micronodular, but not always so; liver biopsy histology sometimes shows characteristic Mallory's hyaline deposits, and haemosiderin may be present in excess. There are no major differences from the disease in temperate climates. The quantity of daily alcohol required to produce this disease is not known with accuracy, and estimates differ widely; an individual variation exists, and women seem to tolerate chronic alcohol ingestion less well than men. Acute alcoholic hepatitis is underdiagnosed and possesses a high mortality rate; the role of corticosteroids continues to be disputed;[1,181] any beneficial effect is at best marginal and administration should probably be confined to severe and advanced cases.

Indian childhood cirrhosis

Indian childhood cirrhosis[182] is largely confined to India (especially south India, Calcutta and the Punjab) and surrounding countries; it is frequently familial. Diagnosis is usually made between 1.5 and 3 years of age; members of the upper strata of Hindu society are often affected. The disease may pursue fulminant, acute or subacute courses, and carries a high mortality rate. The clinical course therefore varies widely and is comparable to viral hepatitis (see above), with acute fulminant viral hepatitis at one extreme of the spectrum and cirrhosis (with one or all of its classic complications) (Figure 10.10) at the other. Histologically, there is usually progressive fibrosis, with absence of regeneration; macronodular and micro-nodular cirrhosis result. Hepatocellular carcinoma is an uncommon complication. The disease is associated with a high copper intake; epidemiological evidence suggests that early weaning followed by milk-feeding from copper vessels imparts an excessive copper intake.[183] However, the possibility of an inherited defect resulting in excess copper absorption and/or metabolism has not been eliminated. There is no adequate treatment; in prevention, non-human milk for infant and childhood consumption should *not* be stored in copper-containing vessels.

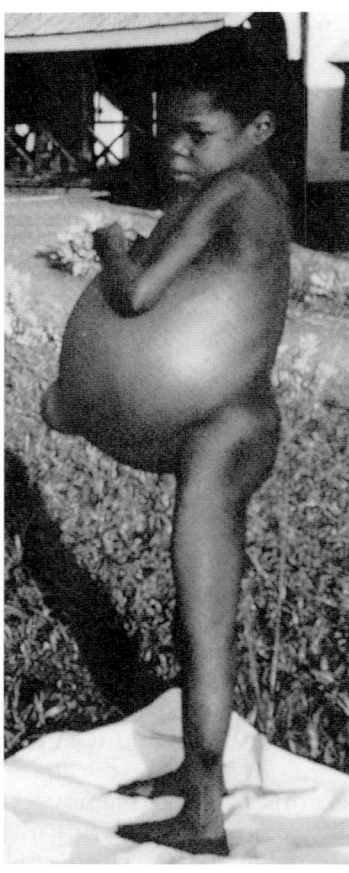

Figure 10.10: Indian child suffering from decompensated chronic liver disease—Indian childhood cirrhosis.

Haemosiderosis

Haemosiderosis (African or Bantu siderosis) is a disease of southern, and to a lesser extent other (tropical) parts of East and West Africa.[184] Whether it can proceed to clear-cut cirrhosis is arguable; heavy alcohol intake is commonplace in many geographical areas where the disease is common; it is frequently impossible to exclude this as an aetiological factor (as with haemochromatosis). Iron-containing pots for cooking are commonly used in most areas, such as Zimbabwe, where haemosiderosis is common, but other factors also seem relevant.[185] Also, chronic pancreatitis is relatively common in these areas; evidence exists that an excess of hepatocyte iron (and fat) is common.

Veno-occlusive disease

Although first described in Jamaica, distribution of veno-occlusive disease is now known to be much wider.[186] Bush-teas, which contain pyrrolizidine alkaloids (*Heliotropium*, *Crotalaria* and *Senecio*) are important aetiologically. Veno-occlusive disease occurs in many localized areas of the tropics, and is certainly not confined to the Caribbean.

Other chronic liver diseases

The liver is involved in most chronic infective diseases; tuberculosis, leprosy, syphilis, actinomycosis, visceral leishmaniasis and African histoplasmosis are examples. It is, however, unusual for decompensation (and liver failure) to result. Major space-occupying lesions involving the liver are amoebic abscess (see below), pyogenic abscess and hydatid disease; tuberculomas, cysticercosis and melioidosis are of lesser importance. Of non-infective diseases, sickle cell disease, β-thalassaemia, haemoglobin-H disease, porphyria and α_1-antitrypsin deficiency produce significant hepatic pathology.

Portal hypertension

Portal hypertension[1,187] is a sequel to any form of chronic liver disease; Table 10.7 summarizes some causes in a tropical country. Cirrhosis and schistosomal liver disease (Chapter 80) are numerically very important; however, in the latter entity hepatocellular function is preserved to a greater extent, and for longer in the course of disease than in cirrhosis; therefore, fluid retention and more importantly encephalopathy are less common. A form of non-cirrhotic chronic liver disease—sometimes associated with portal hypertension—exists in India; despite various suggestions (including arsenic poisoning), the aetiology remains unclear. Of prehepatic causes, HMS is the most common; portal hypertension results from an increased splenic blood flow. Portal/splenic vein obstructions, probably resulting from neonatal umbilical sepsis, are important causes throughout tropical countries, and are undoubtedly underdiagnosed;[187] hepatocellular function is usually intact. Posthepatic causes of portal

Table 10.7 Causes of portal hypertension and oesophageal (and gastric) varices, showing those which are more common in developing countries.

Level of obstruction	Cause
Prehepatic	Hyperreactive malarious splenomegaly (HMS) (increased portal blood flow)* Portal vein occlusion* Splenic vein occlusion
Hepatic macronodular cirrhosis*	Hepatosplenic schistosomiasis* Veno-occlusive disease* Congenital hepatic fibrosis
Posthepatic	Cardiac failure (secondary to chronic rheumatic disease)* Endomyocardial fibrosis* Constructive pericarditis* Inferior vena caval obstruction Hepatic vein thrombosis (Budd–Chiari syndrome)

*More common in a developing country.

hypertension include (Table 10.7) cardiac failure (usually resulting from chronic rheumatic cardiac disease), right-sided endomyocardial fibrosis (Chapter 12) and constrictive pericarditis, usually but not always resulting from tuberculosis. Other causes of portal hypertension are hepatocellular carcinoma (see above) and various dehydrating diseases, including dysentery and cholera. Splenomegaly is present whatever the cause of portal hypertension (which should be distinguished from other causes of enlargement of this organ in a tropical country). Barium swallow or upper gastrointestinal endoscopy usually confirms the presence of oesophageal varices. When available, ultrasonography is valuable in assessing portal vein patency.

Biliary tract disease

In tropical countries biliary pathology is largely attributable to parasites[1,173,188]—ascariasis (Chapter 83), clonorchiasis and opisthorchiasis (Chapter 81); pigment stones (often intrahepatic) occasionally complicate sickle cell disease. A. lumbricoides infection (Chapter 83) is an under-diagnosed cause of large-duct obstruction. It should always be considered in this clinical situation, for it may be confused with pancreatic carcinoma. Endoscopy, if available, is of value; medical treatment is usually successful. Clonorchiasis and opisthorchiasis (Chapter 81), acquired from ingestion of raw fresh-water fish, may result in cholangiohepatitis and biliary obstruction; cholangiocarcinoma is a late complication of both infections. F. hepatica infection (Chapter 81) can give rise to tender hepatomegaly accompanied by jaundice; difficulty in diagnosis from viral hepatitis may be a problem; an eosinophilia is, however, common with this and all biliary trematode infections. Praziquantel is of no

value in treatment; triclabendazole has now replaced it.[189-191] Overall, cholesterol stones (and associated secondary infection) are uncommon in rural populations, especially in Africa. Gallbladder infection by *S. typhi* can result in the typhoid carrier state (Chapter 53); the focus of infection is usually intrahepatic. Gallbladder carcinoma is unusual.

Emergencies

Acute hepatocellular failure

Acute liver failure (acute hepatic necrosis) is a major clinical problem in all developing countries (see above);[4] various hepatitis viruses (most commonly B, C, D and E, and to lesser extent A) are involved (see above), but some cases are caused by other viruses, bacteria or toxins. Although acute hepatocellular failure has been recorded in severe acute *P. falciparum* infection, this is of very limited clinical importance; it occurs as a terminal event but is of far less importance than other major organ failure.[192]

The role of several viruses involved in the production of acute liver injury has been summarized.[170] Reports highlight the aetiological basis of hepatitis in tropical countries; in Egypt, HBV and hepatitis A virus (HAV) accounted for 47% and 0.7% of cases of acute hepatitis (there was serological evidence of both viral infections in a further 1.4%), whereas 14.2% of cases were HBsAg carriers, 31% 'non-A, non-B' hepatitis and 6% were drug-induced.[193] In other locations, however, hepatitis D virus (HDV) is important—especially southern America, South-East Asia (and probably India) and northern Africa. Thus in Thailand, HDV is frequently present in drug abusers; it is also endemic in Chandigarh, India,[194] and has been described in an epidemic of acute hepatitis in the Himalayan foothills in south Kashmir.[195] In India and South-East Asia, hepatitis E virus (HEV) (see above) is responsible for most cases of the entity previously termed 'non-A, non-B' hepatitis; a similar situation probably pertains in Africa and South America. This virus is transmitted by the faecal–oral route and is transmitted in contaminated drinking water; the major importance of this infection is that it produces a high incidence of hepatocellular failure in pregnant women. HCV also causes severe disease—including acute hepatic failure—similar to that produced by HBV (Chapter 40).

Differential diagnosis

Many other viruses present in tropical and subtropical regions may also produce acute hepatic necrosis; these include herpes simplex type 1, herpes virus 6,[196] Epstein–Barr virus, cytomegalovirus, yellow fever[197] and the haemorrhagic fever viruses, which include the Lassa fever virus, the Marburg agent, Ebola virus and Rift Valley fever virus (see above).[198,199] Of bacterial causes of hepatitis, enteric fever is common, but rarely (if ever) proceeds to hepatocellular necrosis (see above). The jaundice of systemic bacterial infection[1] often follows pyomyositis, especially in Africa. *P. falciparum* malaria causes deranged liver function tests resulting from centrilobular necrosis (see above). Hepatotoxicity resulting from herbal remedies is not confined to tropical countries.[200] Alcoholic hepatitis is a significant clinical problem in both indigenous and expatriate populations.

Management

Tandon et al.[201] have outlined their experience of acute hepatic failure (resulting from viral hepatitis) in 145 (> 12 years old) patients managed by them using a 'simple supportive therapeutic regimen' during a 5.5-year period at New Delhi, India. Criteria for inclusion were:

- Development of hepatic encephalopathy within 4 weeks of onset of symptoms and signs of acute hepatitis; and
- Absence of evidence of pre-existent liver disease.

There were 65 men and 80 women; 46 of them were pregnant and presumably infected by HEV infections.

They used a simple intensive support mechanism; this consisted of:

1. Isolation in an intensive care room.
2. Attention to general hygiene and care of a comatose patient.
3. Intravenous fluid to provide 1000–1500 calories daily using 10% dextrose, supplemented, if necessary, by 20% dextrose.
4. Nasogastric tube for aspiration of gastric contents and instillation of drugs.
5. Gut sterilization by ampicillin (1.5 g 6-hourly via nasogastric tube); bowel washes twice daily.
6. Liquid antacids (30 ml 2-hourly).
7. 'Lactisyn' (1 ampoule = *Lactobacillus lactus* 490 million, *L. acidophilus* 490 million, *Streptococcus lactus* 10 million) three times daily.
8. Condom or catheter drainage of the urinary bladder.
9. Maintenance of electrolyte and fluid balance by intravenous supplementation.

Complications were managed as follows:

- Infection (diagnosis was based on clinical findings, leucocyte count > 15 10^9/1itre, and/or chest radiograph abnormality): gentamicin 3.5 mg/kg body weight (as three divided doses), and/or cephalexin (2 g daily as four divided doses).
- Cerebral oedema (criteria for diagnosis were: focal or generalized seizures, abnormal reactive or unequal pupils, decerebrate posture of the body after minor stimuli, and/or sudden deterioration of vital signs): intravenous mannitol (200 ml administered during 30 minutes and repeated three or four times per 24 hours).
- Gastrointestinal bleeding (diagnosed by aspiration of fresh or altered blood via nasogastric tube): liquid antacid (30–45 ml every 2 hours), gastric lavage (with 100 ml cold saline containing 8 mg noradrenaline every 30 minutes) and occasionally cimetidine. (When the prothrombin time was > 7 s compared with a control, fresh frozen plasma was administered.)

- Renal failure (the criterion used was: oliguria (urine output < 400 mg/24 h, and rising blood urea) despite adequate hydration): diuretics (judiciously used!).

Overall 42 (28.9%) survived; of those ≤ 40 years old 41 (33%) recovered, compared with only one (4.8%) of those ≥ 40 years; survival was not affected by pregnancy. Indicators of poor prognosis were: grade IV coma, presence of HBsAg, serum bilirubin concentration > 20 mg/100 ml and sodium < 119 mmol/litre. In fatal cases the immediate complications resulting in death were cerebral oedema (65), bleeding (31), renal failure (11) and infection (8). The authors concluded that these results were comparable with results from centres using a variety of complex therapeutic regimens (e.g., exchange blood transfusion, charcoal perfusion and haemodialysis).

Chronic hepatocellular failure

Cirrhosis, generally resulting from one of the hepatitis viruses (see above), is a very common problem throughout tropical and subtropical countries. A study carried out at New Delhi, India, has addressed the problem of survival in young (< 35 years old) and older patients with cirrhosis;[202] numbers in the two groups were 63 and 106, respectively. Aetiology of cirrhosis in the young and adult groups was: HBV-related (32 and 51), alcohol-related (10 and 28), while 19 and 21, respectively, were labelled 'cryptogenic'; in the former group, one had Wilson's disease and another α_1-antitrypsin deficiency. During the surveillance period 27 and 47 deaths occurred: 40% and 64% from hepatic failure, and 52% and 26% from variceal bleeding. The 5-year survival (62% and 56%) and probability of survival within a similar grade of liver disease (Child's classification) were comparable. As anticipated, probability of survival was significantly higher in grade A and lowest in C. Aetiology of cirrhosis did not significantly influence prognosis in this study.

Hepatocellular carcinoma usually presents as a rapidly progressive malignancy; however, an acute or chronic presentation can occur due to internal necrosis and haemorrhage.[125] Such a lesion can in fact rupture into the peritoneal cavity, posing problems in differential diagnosis.

In a patient with actively bleeding oesophageal varices, differentiation of the aetiology of underlying liver disease (from postviral (or another aetiology) cirrhosis and chronic schistomsomal disease) is usually impossible on clinical grounds alone. In a study carried out at Cairo, Egypt, liver ultrasonography was undertaken in 50 patients who were undergoing an operation for bleeding oesophageal varices;[203] ultrasonographic diagnosis was compared with a surgically obtained wedge biopsy specimen. The authors concluded that ultrasonography gave the more accurate diagnosis; the findings in schistosomal periportal (pipe-stem) fibrosis were characteristic and were not mimicked by other liver diseases (including cirrhosis); ultrasonography agreed with the histological diagnosis in 44 cases.

Role of ultrasonography in management

The overall value of ultrasonographic scanning and scintigraphy in the diagnosis of *chronic* liver disease in developing countries has been addressed.[204] Needle biopsy is frequently necessary to diagnose diffuse disease, but a high degree of specificity can be anticipated with a space-occupying lesion.[136] A further problem surrounding ultrasonography has been highlighted:[204] in Africa and other developing countries, focal lesions 'often present so late that lesions revealed by ultrasound are huge and bizarre', and the inexperienced radiologist may therefore be baffled.

Portal hypertension and its complications

The major causes of portal hytertension (and oesophageal varices) are summarized in Table 10.7. Some geographical variations have been reviewed.[1,9] While in many parts of the world cirrhosis is the most common cause, in India non-cirrhotic portal fibrosis is relatively common.[9] Indian childhood cirrhosis (see above) also accounts for cases in the younger age group(s). Extrahepatic portal vein obstruction is common in some countries (including India);[187,205] however, in Egypt, Africa, the Middle East, South America and China, *Schist. mansoni* and *Schist. japonicum*, respectively, are frequently responsible. In Jamaica, South Africa, central Asia and the south-western USA, epidemic veno-occlusive disease (see above) (caused by *Heliotropium*, *Crotalaria*, *Senecio* and other alkaloids; see above) is important.

Pitressin (vasopressin) forms the basis of management of variceal haemorrhage; if and where available, upper gastrointestinal endoscopic sclerotherapy is of value, but this technique usually has to be repeated at 6-month intervals. The Sengstaken tube (for variceal compression) still has a place in developing countries. Haemorrhage is not a major presenting feature at most tropical hospitals (see above).

Bleeding varices resulting from extrahepatic portal obstruction

The cause of portal vein thrombosis in developing countries remains unclear; it is, however, a relatively common condition, and neonatal umbilical sepsis is usually cited as the likely aetiological factor.[1] During an 8.5-year period, 136 patients with extrahepatic portal hypertension were treated surgically at New Delhi, India;[205] in 22 it was carried out as an emergency (for variceal bleeding), and in 114 as an elective procedure (in 104 for a past haematemesis and in 10 for massive splenomegaly). The emergency strategy consisted of: splenectomy and splenorenal shunt (14), transoesophageal variceal ligation (4), splenectomy and gastro-oesophageal devascularization (3) and mesocaval shunt (1). Elective procedures were: splenectomy and splenorenal shunt (94), mesocaval shunt (8) and splenectomy and gastro-oesophageal devascularization (12). Operative mortality was 2 (9%) and 1 (1%), respectively; none of the survivors developed encephalopathy or postsplenectomy sepsis. One hundred and seventeen (86%) were followed up for 2–10 years; 17 had a further haematemesis, but 90% and 75% were alive at 5 and 10 years, respectively. Patients experiencing haematemesis are often far from medical facilities in a developing country; the authors therefore considered that in this setting operative intervention was more satisfactory than endoscopic sclerotherapy or management with propranolol (variceal compression was not considered).

Space-occupying hepatic lesions
Invasive hepatic amoebiasis

Amoebic liver abscess is a cause of right upper quadrant pain (and hepatomegaly); this is usually accompanied by fever, and not infrequently right shoulder-tip pain. Travellers to infected areas as well as the indigenous population(s) of the tropics may be affected.[1,206] Pathogenesis is dependent on an oral infection with a potentially invasive strain (zymodeme) of *Ent. histolytica*.[207] The mode of evolution remains unclear.[208] Diagnosis is based on an appropriate serological technique (IFAT, cellulose acetate or countercurrent immunoelectrophoresis) and hepatic ultrasonography or computed tomography.

Clinical characteristics in a group of 52 patients suffering from amoebic liver abscesses have been recorded at Cairo, Egypt;[209] while 22 (42%) presented with an acute illness (see above), 30 (58%) had a more chronic illness with dull aching in the right hypochondria, weight loss, fatigue, moderate to low-grade pyrexia and anaemia. A right-sided pleural effusion, emphysema, ascites and jaundice were present in three (6%), four (8%), seven (13%) and seven (13%), respectively. Forty-two (81%) abscesses were solitary and in the right lobe; 29 (43%) were initially solid or heterogeneous. Response to metronidazole (750 mg three times daily for 10 days) was described as good in 50; in four aspiration was carried out on account of the large abscess size.

Whether needle aspiration of an amoebic abscess (in addition to satisfactory chemotherapy) is indicated remains controversial. A prospective, randomized controlled study carried out at New Delhi, India, has addressed this issue;[210] in 17 of 37 patients (all received appropriate chemotherapy, 2–4 g metronizadole for 10 days) who completed the study, aspiration was carried out on the day of hospital admission; clinical improvement (and cure) was similar to that in 20 controls. 'Abscess' diameter was slightly lower in those who underwent aspiration (54 versus 72 mm). However, at Benin, Nigeria, needle aspiration was considered to 'enhance clinical recovery';[211] in a non-randomized trial, 19 patients were managed by needle aspiration in addition to chemotherapy, and 17 were given chemotherapy (metronidazole, diloxanide and chloroquine) alone; 18 and 10, respectively, experienced complete resolution (as shown by ultrasonography) after 21 days ($p < 0.021$), and clinical response was also considered more rapid ($p < 0.01$), especially when the abscess was >6 cm in diameter. Delay in ultrasonographic 'recovery' is not important, there being good evidence that a residual abnormality after a year or more is compatible with complete, uncomplicated resolution.

Although no in vitro evidence of *Ent. histolytica* resistance to the 5-nitroimidazole compounds exists, reports continue to be made from India of drug-resistant cases. The main problem with such reports is that, in few (if any) has diloxanide furoate (500 mg three times daily for 10 days) been administered; this is essential for a definitive cure because it is a far superior luminal amoebicide compared with the 5-nitroimidazole compounds—and therefore kills the cysts (which could belong to invasive zymodemes). In a prospective randomized study of 50 such 'resistant' cases at New Delhi, four management regimens were used:[212] (1) a repeat course of conservative therapy (with 1.25 mg/kg dehydroemetine given intramuscularly daily for 10 days); (2) needle aspiration (under ultrasonographic guidance); (3) percutaneous catheter drainage (under ultrasonographic guidance); and (4) open surgical drainage with catheter insertion. The authors concluded that 'the most impressive results' were obtained with regimen 3.

To summarize, in the uncomplicated case needle aspiration (under cover of a 5-nitroimidazole compound) is indicated when: (1) the abscess(es) cavity is large and the patient seriously ill; and (2) the site of the lesion is such that perforation into a nearby viscus (most importantly the pericardium) seems probable. All cases of invasive amoebiasis should receive a course of the luminal amoebicide diloxanide furoate (500 mg three times daily for 10 days) *after* metronidazole (800 mg three times daily for 10 days) or tinidazole (2 g daily for 3 days). If this regimen is omitted, *Ent. histolytica* cysts remain in the colonic lumen and, in the event of their being of a pathogenic zymodeme, further tissue invasion (including liver abscess) might occur.

Spontaneous perforation of an amoebic liver abscess is a serious complication which is associated with high morbidity and mortality rates;[206] this applies especially when perforation takes place into the pericardial cavity. Successful percutaneous drainage (for 7–34 days) of a perforated abscess in five 'severely ill' patients (with a total of 11 lesions) under metronidazole cover has been recorded;[213] there were resultant abscesses in the subhepatic space, pelvis, chest, right and left paracolic gutters, lesser sac, retroperitoneum and flank, and associated fistulas were demonstrated with the bile duct, duodenum and the colon; all healed completely. No patient required a laparotomy. These authors recommend wider use of catheter drainage for this serious complication of hepatic amoebiasis.

Pyogenic liver abscess
Although in a tropical context it is far less common than invasive amoebiasis (see above), pyogenic abscess is a serious disease with high morbidity and mortality—even when managed in experienced hands.[1] In most cases, a primary intra-abdominal focus of infection can be detected. Differentiation from invasive hepatic amoebiasis

is usually straightforward, the patient being more severely and acutely ill; jaundice, septicaemia and renal impairment are common accompaniments. Ultrasonography is usually diagnostic. In Kuala Lumpur, 25 pyogenic abscesses were encountered between 1970 and 1985;[214] during the same period, there were 90 amoebic and one tuberculous abscesses, while in 89 others the cause of the abscess was not determined. At Kingston, Jamaica, fever and abdominal pain were present in 21 (80%) out of 24 cases of pyogenic abscess encountered between 1977 and 1986;[215] the most common signs were right upper quadrant tenderness and hepatomegaly; leucocytosis, elevated alkaline phosphatase and hypoalbuminaemia were common. Reports from London[216] and California[217] have given encouraging reports of management by needle aspiration under antibiotic (usually gentamicin and metranidazole or clindamycin) cover. Another study has also recorded satisfactory results in 18 of 21 patients using this form of percutaneous drainage. Other authors have intimated, however, that this form of management should be reserved for selected patients.[218] A report from Riyadh, Saudi Arabia, has provided results which were less encouraging. In Jamaica surgical drainage using a guided percutaneous technique gave comparable results.[219] Taking all reports into account, it seems wise to perform a laparotomy and to institute surgical drainage as soon as possible after diagnosis. Using ultrasonographic control, a pyogenic abscess can be seen to 'resolve' significantly more rapidly than an amoebic abscess. It should be appreciated, however, that this disease carries a significant mortality rate; between 1975 and 1986, these authors treated 109 children with pyogenic liver abscess; the mortality rate was 15%.[220] There is limited (suggestive) evidence that the overall prognosis is improving.

Hydatid disease and schistosomiasis involving the liver
Only rarely, usually following trauma, does hydatidosis[173,221] present as an abdominal emergency. Perforation into the peritoneal cavity may produce an anaphylactoid reaction with hypotension, and/or seeding of daughter hydatid cysts within the peritoneal cavity. Secondary bacterial infection is an unusually event. Chemotherapy is with albendazole and/or praziquantel (Chapter 84).

Hepatic schistosomiasis[14,222] is complicated by portal hypertension and oesophageal varices in an advanced case; however, hepatocellular function is maintained late into the course of disease and hepatic encephalopathy and ascites occur as advanced (usually terminal) signs. Praziquantel is the chemotherapeutic agent of choice; evidence of reversal of fibrotic changes is now available.

Pancreas

The two major diseases involving this organ encountered in tropical countries, and which differ from those in temperate ones, are (1) 'J-type' diabetes, first reported in Jamaica (Chapter 37) and (2) chronic calcific pancreatitis.

Diabetes, which is *not* associated with pancreatic calcification in young people, is encountered throughout tropical countries; those affected are usually thin, and require high doses of insulin; however, they do not rapidly develop ketosis when insulin is discontinued. J-type diabetes might have a viral aetiology, a Coxsackie virus being involved; a raised incidence of antibody to Coxsackie B₄ has been demonstrated in affected patients in India. A suggestion has been made that these patients, especially those in Africa, are less susceptible to chronic diabetic complications than Europeans; this now seems unlikely.

A popular Indian and Chinese vegetable, karela (*Momordica charantia*) possesses hypoglycaemic properties; these are enhanced by chlorpropamide, a fact that should be taken into account in the management of diabetes in a number of Asian countries.

A syndrome consisting of pancreatic calcification associated with both exocrine and endocrine impairment is common in many tropical countries (Figure 10.11);[1,223,224] most observations have been made in Africa (East and West), southern India and Indonesia. The aetiology of *chronic calcific pancreatitis* remains unknown. Pancreatic disruption in childhood kwashiorkor can be severe and might be relevant. Cassava (*Manihot esculenta*) has also been implicated. Long-standing pancreatic damage can also follow viral hepatitis. A further hypothesis is that pancreatic ducts blocked by secretions and inspissated mucous plugs later calcify; this might be more common after starvation, gastroenteritis and dehydration. Presentation is with weight loss and malabsorption (in some parts of Africa, this is the most common cause of overt malabsorption); diabetes mellitus and pancreatic pain are important features. Management consists of providing pancreatic supplements (e.g., pancreatin BP, 6 g orally with meals) together with diabetic control.[1] Pain is often difficult to manage and may be so severe that suicide is a sequel.

The pancreas can also be involved in many infections including *Schist. mansoni* and *Schist. japonicum*, trichinellosis, cysticercosis and hydatid disease.

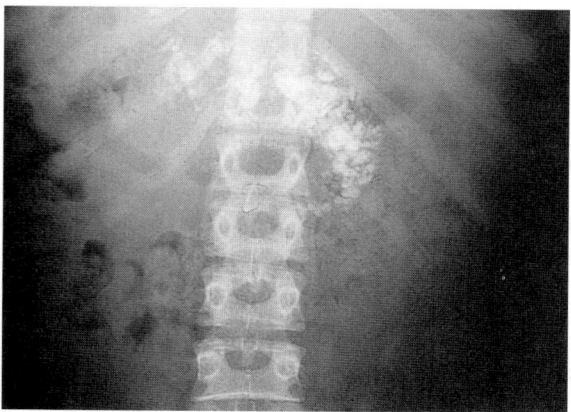

Figure 10.11: Abdominal radiograph showing calcified pancreas in the chronic calcific pancreatitis syndrome. There was no history of alcohol excess or infant malnutrition; aetiology was therefore undetermined.

Pancreatic duct obstruction, complicated by acute pancreatitis, is most commonly a sequel to *A. lumbricoides* infection (see below); tapeworms are rarely implicated. Clonorchiasis and opisthorchiasis may involve the pancreatic duct system.

Emergencies: pancreas, and biliary system

One of the most widely distributed nematodes in tropical and subtropical countries is *A. lumbricoides*. By entering the biliary system (from the duodenum) this parasite can cause several acute medical and surgical conditions. Reporting from Kashmir, India, Khuroo et al.[225] collected 500 cases in which *A. lumbricoides* involved the liver, biliary tract and pancreas; biliary ascariasis was present in 171 cases, and in 140 there was hepatic, in eight gall-bladder and in seven pancreatic involvement. These authors recognized five clinical presentations: acute cholecystitis (64), acute cholangitis (121), biliary colic (280), acute pancreatitis (31) and hepatic abscess (4). Twenty-seven had a pyogenic cholangitis which was treated by decompression and drainage—surgically in two and endoscopically in 25; removal of adult worms from the ampullary orifice (with extraction per os) led to rapid relief of biliary colic in 214, and acute pancreatitis in 16; four patients died, from acute pancreatitis (2), pyogenic cholangitis (1) and hepatic abscess (1). Worms persisted at 3 weeks in the biliary tree in 12 patients; dead worms were removed either by surgery (5) or by using an endoscopic basket (7). *A. lumbricoides* moved out of the ductal system in 211 cases. The patients were followed up for a mean of 48 months; 76 became reinfected and had reinvasion of the biliary tree; in seven cases intrahepatic duct and bile duct calculi (superimposed on dead worms) were present.

In South-East Asia, the two most common biliary parasites are *Clonorchis sinensis* and *Opisthorchis* species. Although these cause chronic problems, notably secondary bacterial cholangitis[125] and adenocarcinoma of the biliary system, an acute presentation[1] is unusual.

In most indigenous people of developing countries, gallstones are unusual; when they occur they are usually of the pigment variety, and often associated with haemolysis. A report from Saudi Arabia, where the average lifestyle has rapidly become westernized (with striking changes in diet) over the last two to three decades, indicates that cholecystectomy for cholelithiasis is now one of the most common major abdominal operations to be carried out;[226] between 1977 and 1986, 2854 individuals (most of them young Saudis) underwent this operation at 14 hospitals in the Eastern Province of the country.

Acute pancreatitis is uncommon overall in developing countries, although severe abdominal pain caused by chronic calcific pancreatitis[1] can give rise to problems in differential diagnosis. The pain may be so severe that suicide is attempted. Biliary involvement by *A. lumbricoides* can result in acute pancreatitis.[1,125] Other helminths, including *Clonorchis sinensis*, *Opisthorchis* and *Anisakis* species have also been associated with this condition.

Spleen

Table 10.8 summarizes some causes of splenomegaly in the tropics.[1] Most of these receive attention in other chapters. The most extreme form of splenomegaly (HMS) (Figure 10.12) is covered in Chapters 13 and 70; those caused by various viral, bacterial and parasitic infections are dealt with under these respective headings.

Table 10.8 Some causes of splenomegaly in the tropics.

Infections
Viral Epstein–Barr virus, cytomegalovirus, viral hepatitis and other virus diseases
Bacterial   typhoid fever, brucellosis, tuberculosis
Parasitic   malaria (especially hyperreactive malarious splenomegaly (HMS)), schistosomiasis, visceral leishmaniasis, trypanosomiasis
Portal hypertension
Haemopoietic diseases
Sickle cell disease, thalassaemia
Reticuloendothelial diseases
Burkitt's lymphoma, leukaemia, reticuloses
Cystic lesions
Hydatid disease
Abscess
Amoebic; unknown aetiology
Spontaneous haemorrhage and rupture
Metabolic
Amyloidosis

The spleen is an extremely important line of defence against many infections, especially pneumococcal and *Plasmodium* species infections. Splenectomized individuals in tropical countries should receive pneumococcal vaccine; prudent advice regarding malaria prophylaxis is mandatory.

Splenic abscess is a well-documented tropical disease.[1] Aetiology is unknown; underlying viral and parasitic diseases have been suggested, but not proved. A connection with carriage of the sickle cell gene has also been suggested, but this has also not been proved. Most reports have been made in West Africa and Zimbabwe. In most, the aetiology is unknown, but some undoubtedly result

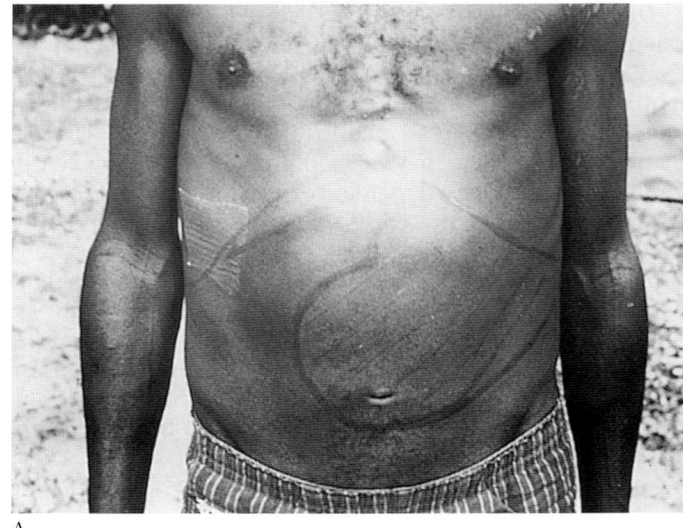

A

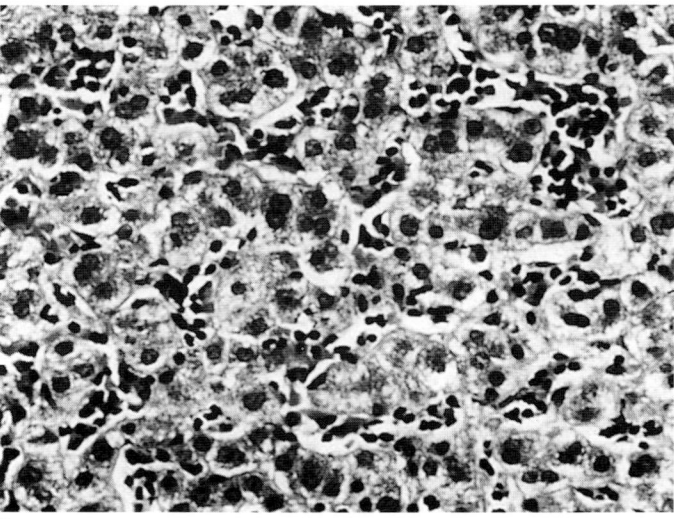

B

Figure 10.12: (**A**) Papua New Guinea man suffering from hyperreactive malarious splenomegaly (HMS); all of the features of this syndrome were present. (**B**) Liver biopsy specimen showing severe sinusoidal lymphocytosis, a component of the HMS syndrome.

from *S. typhi* infection. The clinical history is usually one of 2–3 weeks duration, and consists of pain/swelling in the left hypochondrium, associated with pyrexia. The splenic swelling is tender, often exquisitely so, and fluctuant. A radiograph may show gas within the abscess. Untreated, the abscess can rupture into the peritoneal cavity; splenectomy therefore has an important role in management. Should the condition become chronic—an unusual sequel—splenectomy is also the correct course of management.

REFERENCES

1   Cook G C. *Tropical Gastroenterology*. Oxford: Oxford University Press, 1980: 484.

2   Cook G C (ed.). *Gastroenterological Problems from the Tropics*. London: BMJ Publishing Group, 1995: 146.

3   Cook G C (ed.). *Travel-Associated Disease*. London: Royal College of Physicians 1995: 179.

4   Cook G C. Gastroenterological emergencies in the tropics. *Bailliere's Clin Gastroenterol* 1991; 5:861–886.

5   Ferguson R. Diseases of the mouth. In Misiewicz J J, Pounder R E & Venables C W (eds) *Diseases of the Gut and Pancreas*, 2nd edn. Oxford: Blackwell, 1994: 93–101.

6   Watson A. Carcinoma of the oesophagus. In Misiewicz J J, Pounder R E & Venables C W (eds) *Diseases of the Gut and Pancreas*, 2nd edn. Oxford: Blackwell, 1994: 159–172.

7   Sharma B C, Bhasin D K, Bhatti H S, Das G & Singh K. Gastrointestinal bleeding due to worm infestation, with negative upper gastrointestinal endoscopy findings: impact of enteroscopy. *Endoscopy* 2000; 32:314–316.

8   Clamp S E, Morgan A G, Kotwal M R et al. Use of a multinational survey to provide clinical guidelines for upper gastrointestinal bleeding in developing countries. *Scand J Gastroenterol* 1988; 23(suppl. 144):63–66.

9   Kiire C F, Kitai I, Sigola L & Ternouth I. Upper gastrointestinal bleeding in an African setting. *J R Coll Physicians Lond* 1987; 21:107–110.

10 Okumura H, Aramaki T & Katsuta Y. Pathophysiology and epidemiology of portal hypertension. *Drugs* 1989; 37(suppl. 2):2–12.

11 El-Zayadi A, Montasser M F, Girgis F, El-Okby S, Botros B & Mohran Z. Histological changes of the esophageal mucus in bleeding versus non-bleeding varices. *Endoscopy* 1989; 21:205–207.

12 Nakib B A I, Radhakrishnan S, Liddawi H A I, Jacob G S & Ruwaih A A I. The role of gastrointestinal endoscopy in a developing country. *Endoscopy* 1986; 18:37–39.

13 Atoba M A, Ayoola E A & Olubuyide I O. Radiological and endoscopic correlation in upper gastrointestinal haemorrhage and malignancy. *Scand J Gastroenterol* 1986; 21(suppl. 124): 149–151.

14 Sarin S K, Nanda R & Sachdev G. Relative efficacy and safety of absolute alcohol and 50% alcohol as variceal sclerosants. *Gastrointest Endosc* 1987; 33:362–365.

15 Sarin S K, Mishra S P, Sachdev G K, Thorat V, Dalal L & Broor S L. Ethanolamine oleate *versus* absolute alcohol as a variceal sclerosant: a prospective, randomised, controlled trial. *Am J Gastroenterol* 1988; 83:526–530.

16 Sarin S K, Misra S P, Singal A K, Thorat V & Broor S L. Endoscopic sclerotherapy for varices in children. *J Pediatr Gastroenterol Nutr* 1988; 7:662–666.

17 Wahrendorf J, Chang-Claude J, Liang Q S et al. Precursor lesions of oesophageal cancer in young people in a high-risk population in China. *Lancet* 1989; ii:1239–1241.

18 Clarke C A & Bodmer W F. Oesophageal cancer in China. *Lancet* 1989; ii:1525.

19 Langman M J S. Aetiologies of peptic ulcer. In Misiewicz J J, Pounder R E & Venables C W (eds) *Diseases of the Gut and Pancreas*, 2nd edn. Oxford: Blackwell, 1994: 249–259.

20 Scobie B A, Beg F & Oldmeadows M. Peptic diseases compared endoscopically in indigenous Fijians and Indians. *N Z Med J* 1987; 100:683–684.

21 Tytgat G N J. Gastritis. In Misiewicz J J, Pounder R E & Venables C W (eds) *Diseases of the Gut and Pancreas*, 2nd edn. Oxford: Blackwell, 1994: 221–235.

22 Cook G C. Hypochlorhydria and vulnerability to intestinal infection. *Eur J Gastroenterol Hepatol* 1994; 6:693–695.

23 Craven J L. Carcinoma of the stomach. In Misiewicz J J, Pounder R E & Venables C W (eds) *Diseases of the Gut and Pancreas*, 2nd edn. Oxford: Blackwell, 1994: 335–352.

24 Mabogunje C A. Perorated duodenal and gastric ulcers in the Nigeria savannah. *Int Surg* 1985; 70:327–330.

25 Kochhar R, Krishna P R, Gupta N M & Mehta S K. Massive gastrointestinal bleeding due to cholecystoduodenal fistula. *Acta Chir Scand* 1988; 154:471–472.

26 Sarin S K, Sachdev G, Nanda R, Misra S P & Broor S L. Endoscopic sclerotherapy in the treatment of gastric varices. *Br J Surg* 1988; 75:747–750.

27 Jernigan J, Guerrant R L & Pearson R D. Parasitic infections of the small intestine. *Gut* 1994; 35:289–293.

28 Cook G C. The small intestine and its role in chronic diarrheal disease in the tropics. In Gracey M (ed.) *Diarrhea*. Boca Raton, FL: CRC Press, 1991: 127–162.

29 Cook G C. Tropical disease and the small intestine. In Misiewicz J J, Pounder R E & Venables C W (eds) *Diseases of the Gut and Pancreas*, 2nd edn. Oxford: Blackwell, 1994: 597–615.

30 Menzies I S, Zuckerman M J, Nukajam W S et al. Geography of intestinal permeability and absorption. *Gut* 1999; 44:483–489.

31 Ramakrishna B S. Prevalence of intestinal pathogens in HIV patients with diarrhea: implications for treatment. *Indian J Pediatr* 1999; 66:85–91.

32 DuPont H L. Travelers' diarrhea. In Gracey M (ed.) *Diarrhea*. Boca Raton, FL: CRC Press, 1991: 115–126.

33 Gorbach S L. Travelers' diarrhea. In Gorbach S L, Barlett J G & Blacklow N R (eds) *Infectious Diseases*. Philadelphia: W B Saunders, 1992: 622–628.

34 Okhuysen P C & Ericsson C D. Travelers' diarrhea. *Curr Opin Gastroenterol* 1992; 8:110–114.

35 Farthing M J G. Travellers' diarrhoea. *Gut* 1994; 35:1–4.

36 Ansdell V E & Ericson C D. Prevention and empiric treatment of traveler's diarrhea. *Med Clin North Am* 1999; vi: 83:945–973.

37 Black R E. Epidemiology of travelers' diarrhea and relative importance of various pathogens. *Rev Infect Dis* 1990; 12(suppl. 1):S73–S79.

38 Ljungh A H. Travellers' diarrhoea and the European tourist. *Eur J Gastroenterol Hepatol* 1992; 4:764–770.

39 Harries A D, Myers B & Cook G C. Inflammatory bowel disease: a common cause of bloody diarrhoea in visitors to the tropics. *BMJ* 1985; 291:1686–1687.

40 Schumacher G, Kollberg B & Ljungh A. Inflammatory bowel disease presenting as travellers' diarrhoea. *Lancet* 1993; 341:241–242.

41 Rowe B, Taylor J & Bettelheim K A. An investigation of travellers' diarrhoea. *Lancet* 1970; i:1–4.

42 Sack R B. Travelers' diarrhea: microbiologic bases for prevention and treatment. *Rev Infect Dis* 1990; 12(suppl. 1):S59–S63.

43 Tellier R & Keystone J S. Prevention of travelers' diarrhoea. *Infect Dis Clin North Am* 1992; 6(2):333–354.

44 Bhutta T I & Tahir K I. Loperamide poisoning in children. *Lancet* 1990; 353:363.

45 DuPont H L, Ericsson C D, Johnson P C & de la Cabada F J. Use of bismuth subsalicylate for the prevention of travelers' diarrhea. *Rev Infect Dis* 1990; 12(suppl. 1):S65–S67.

46 Peltola H, Siitonen A, Kyronseppa H et al. Prevention of travellers' diarrhoea by oral B-subunit/whole cell cholera vaccine. *Lancet* 1991; 338:1285–1289.

47 CHOICE Study Group. Multicenter, randomised, double-blind clinical trial to evaluate the efficacy and safety of a reduced osmolarity oral rehydration salts solution in children with acute watery diarrhea. *Pediatrics* 2001; 107:613–618.

48   DuPont H L, Ericsson C D, Matthewson J J & DuPont M W. Five versus three days of ofloxacin therapy for travelers' diarrhea: a placebo-controlled study. *Antimicrob Agents Chemother* 1992; 36:87–91.

49   Nalin D R. Cholera and severe toxigenic diarrhoeas. *Gut* 1994; 35:145–149.

50   Phillips S F. Asiatic cholera: nature's experiment? *Gastroenterology* 1986; 91:1304–1307.

51   Cook G C. The Asiatic cholera: an historical determinant of human genomic and social structure. In Drasar B S (ed.) *Cholera*. London: Chapman & Hall, 1995 (in press).

52   Steffen R. Epidemiologic studies of travelers' diarrhea, severe gastrointestinal infections, and cholera. *Rev Infect Dis* 1986; 8:S122–S130.

53   Hamilton S K, Keren D F, Boitnott J K, Robertson S M & Yardley J H. Enhancement of cholera toxin of IgA secretion from intestinal crypt epithelium. *Gut* 1980; 21:365–369.

54   Cook G C. Preventive strategies for the avoidance of infectious diarrhoea. In Gracey M & Bouchier I A D (eds) *Infectious Diarrhoea*, vol. 7(2). London: Baillière Tindall, 1993: 519–545.

55   Levine M M. Modern vaccines: enteric infections. *Lancet* 1990; 335:958–961.

56   Kaper J B. *Vibrio cholerae* vaccines. *Rev Infect Dis* 1989; 11:S568–S573.

57   Avery M E & Snyder J C. Oral therapy for acute diarrhea: the underused single solution. *N Engl J Med* 1990; 323:891–894.

58   Cosnett J E. The origins of intravenous fluid therapy. *Lancet* 1989; ii:768–771.

59   Cook G C. Management of cholera: the vital role of rehydration. In Drasar B S (ed.) *Cholera*. London: Chapman & Hall, 1995 (in press).

60   Islam M R. Single-dose tetracycline in cholera. *Gut* 1987; 28:1029–1032.

61   Rabbani G H, Islam M R, Butler T, Shahrier M & Alam K. Single-dose treatment of cholera and furazolidone or tetracycline in a double-blind randomised trial. *Antimicrob Agents Chemother* 1989; 33:1447–1450.

62   Alam A N, Alam N H, Ahmed T & Sack D A. Randomized double blind trial of single dose doxycycline for treating cholera in adults. *BMJ* 1990; 300:1619–1621.

63   Sengupta P G, Niyogi S K & Bhattacharya S K. An outbreak of Eltor cholera in Aizwal town of Mizoram, India. *J Commun Dis* 2000; 32:207–211.

64   Cook G C. Hypolactasia: geographical distribution, diagnosis, and practical significance. In Chandra R K (ed.) *Critical Reviews in Tropical Medicine*, vol. 2. New York: Plenum Press, 1984: 117–139.

65   Cook G C. Persisting diarrhoea and malabsorption. *Gut* 1994; 35:582–586.

66   Tomkins A. Tropical malabsorption: recent concepts in pathogenesis and nutritional significance. *Clin Sci* 1981; 60:131–137.

67   Baker S J. Idiopathic small intestinal disease in the tropics. In Chandra R K (ed.) *Critical Reviews in Tropical Medicine*, vol. 1. New York: Plenum Press, 1982:197–245.

68   Mathan V I. Tropical sprue in southern India. *Trans R Soc Trop Med Hyg* 1988; 82:10–14.

69   Manson P. Notes on sprue. *Medical Reports for the half year ended 31 March 1880*, 19th issue. Imperial Maritime Customs 11, spec. ser. 2. Shanghai: Statistical Department of the Inspectorate General, 1880: 33–37.

70   Hillary W. Of chronical diseases. In *Observations on the Changes of the Air and the Concomitant Epidemical Diseases, in the Island of Barbados*, 2nd edn. Hawes, Clarke & Collins, 1799: 276–297.

71   Taylor D N, Connor B A & Shlim D R. Chronic diarrhea in the returned traveler. *Med Clin North Am* 1999; vii:83:1033–1052.

72   Gerson C D. The small intestine. *Mt Sinai J Med* 2000; 67:241–244.

73   Peetermans W E & Vonck A. Tropical sprue after travel to Tanzania. *J Travel Med* 2000; 7:33–34.

74   Menendez-Corrada R, Netthleship E & Santiago-Delpin E A. HLA and tropical sprue. *Lancet* 1986; ii:1183–1185.

75   Naik S. HLA and gastrointestinal disorders. *Indian J Gastroenterol* 1986; 5:121–124.

76   Klipstein F A, Engert R F & B Short H B. Enterotoxigenicity of colonising coliform bacteria in tropical sprue and blind-loop syndrome. *Lancet* 1978; ii:342–344.

77   Tomkins A M, Wright S G & Drasar B S. Bacterial colonization of the upper intestine in mild tropical malabsorption. *Trans R Soc Trop Med Hyg* 1980; 74:752–755.

78   Spencer J, Isaacson P G, Diss T C & MacDonald T T. Expression of disulfide-linked and non-disulfide-linked forms of the T cell receptor γ/δ heterodimer in human intestinal intraepithelial lymphocytes. *Eur J Immunol* 1989; 14:1335–1338.

79   Besterman H S, Cook G C, Sarson D L et al. Gut hormones in tropical malabsorption. *BMJ* 1979; ii:1252–1255.

80   Adrian T E, Savage A P, Bacarese-Hamilton A J, Wolfe K, Besterman H S & Bloom S R. Peptide YY abnormalities in gastrointestinal disease. *Gastroenterology* 1986; 90:379–384.

81   Mathan V I. Tropical sprue in southern India. *Trans R Soc Trop Med Hyg* 1988; 82:10–14.

82   Read N W. Diarrhoea: the failure of colonic salvage. *Lancet* 1982; 11:481–483.

83   Ramakrishna B S & Mathan V I. Role of bacterial toxins, bile acids, and free fatty acids in colonic water malabsorption in tropical sprue. *Dig Dis Sci* 1987; 32:500–505.

84   Batt R M & McLean L. Comparison of the biochemical changes in the jejunal mucosa of dogs with aerobic and anaerobic bacterial overgrowth. *Gastroenterology* 1987; 93:986–993.

85   Catassi C, Ratsch I M, Gandolfi L et al. Why is coeliac disease endemic in the people of the Sahara? *Lancet* 1999; 354:647–648.

86   Gupta B, Narru N & Dhar K L. Evaluation of surface area corrected peak blood xylose as a screening test of intestinal malabsorption in the tropics. *Indian J Gastroenterol* 1987; 6:89–91.

87   Peters T J, Jones P E, Wells G & Cook G C. Sequential enzyme and subcellular fractionation studies on jejunal biopsy specimens from patients with post-infective tropical malabsorption. *Clin Sci Mol Med* 1979; 56:479–486.

88   Cook G C & Menzies I S. Intestinal absorption and unmediated permeation of sugars in post-infective tropical malabsorption (tropical sprue). *Digestion* 1986; 33:109–116.

89   Cook G C. Aetiology and pathogenesis of post-infective tropical malabsorption (tropical sprue). *Lancet* 1984; i:721–723.

90   Glynn J. Tropical sprue: its aetiology and pathogenesis. *J R Soc Med* 1988; 79:599–606.

91   Jelinek T & Loscher T. Epidemiology of giardiasis in German travellers. *J Travel Med* 2000; 7:70–73.

92   Yong T S, Park S J, Hwang U W et al. Genotyping of Giardia lamblia isolates from humans in China and Korea using ribosomal DNA sequences. *J Parasitol* 2000; 86:887–891.

93   Grove D I. Strongyloidiasis: a conundrum for gastroenterologists. *Gut* 1994; 35:437–440.

94   Tandon R K. Abdominal tuberculosis. In Bouchier I A D, Allan R N, Hodgson H J F & Keighley M R B (eds) *Gastroenterology: Clinical Science and Practice*, 2nd edn. London: W B Saunders, 1993: 1459–1468.

95   Rambaud J-C & Ruskoné-Fourmestraux A. Small intestinal lymphomas: immunoproliferative small intestinal disease, α-chain disease and Mediterranean lymphomas. In Bouchier I A D, Allan R N, Hodgson H J F & Keighley M R B (eds)

Gastroenterology: Clinical Science and Practice, 2nd end. London: W B Saunders, 1993: 636–643.

96 Ghoshal U C, Chetri K, Banerjee P K et al. Is immunoproliferative small intestinal disease uncommon in India? *Trop Gastroenterol* 2001; 22:14–17.

97 Dossetor J F B & White H C. Protein-losing enteropathy and malabsorption in acute measles enteritis. *BMJ* 1975; 2:592–593.

98 Conrad M E, Schwartz F D & Young A A. Infectious hepatitis: a generalised disease. *Am J Med* 1964; 37:789–801.

99 Schreiber D S, Blacklow N R & Trier J S. The intestinal lesion of the proximal small intestine in acute infectious nonbacterial gastroenteritis. *N Engl J Med* 1973; 288:1318–1323.

100 McCormack J G. Clinical features of rotavirus gastroenteritis. *J Infect* 1982; 4:167–174.

101 Telch J, Shephard R W, Butler D G et al. Intestinal glucose transport in acute viral enteritis in piglets. *Clin Sci* 1981; 61:29–34.

102 Brown D W G, Selvakumar R, Daniel D J & Mathan V I. Prevalence of neutralising antibodies to Berne virus in animals and humans in Vellore, South India. *Arch Virol* 1988; 98:267–269.

103 Lindenbaum J. Malabsorption during and after recovery from acute intestinal infection. *BMJ* 1965; ii:326–329.

104 Editorial. Mechanisms in enteropathogenic *Escherichia coli* diarrhoea. *Lancet* 1983; i:1254–1256.

105 Mandal B K. *Salmonella typhi* and other salmonellas. *Gut* 1994; 35:726–728.

106 Editorial. Campylobacter enteritis. *Lancet* 1982; ii:1437–1438.

107 Murrell T G C & Walker P D. The pigbel story of Papua New Guinea. *Trans R Soc Trop Med Hyg* 1991; 85:119–122.

108 Murrell T G C. Pigbel disease in Papua New Guinea: an ancient disease rediscovered. *Int J Epidemiol* 1983; 12:211–214.

109 Gillon J, Andre C, Descos L et al. Changes in mucosal immunoglobulin-containing cells in patients with giardiasis before and after treatment. *J Infect* 1982; 5:67–72.

110 Farthing M J G. *Giardia lamblia*. In Farthing M J G & Keusch G T (eds) *Enteric Infection: Mechanisms, Manifestations and Management*. London: Chapman & Hall, 1988: 397–413.

111 Jokipii L & Jokipii A M M. Treatment of giardiasis: comparative evaluation of ornidazole and tinidazole as a single oral dose. *Gastroenterology* 1982; 83:399–404.

112 Crosby W H. The deadly hookworm: why did the Puerto-Ricans die? *Arch Intern Med* 1987; 147:577–578.

113 Bunyaratvej S, Bunyawongwiroj P & Nitiyanant P. Human intestinal sarcosporidiosis: report of six cases. *Am J Trop Med Hyg* 1982; 31:36–41.

114 Eberhard M L, Nace E K, Freeman A R, Streit T G, da Silva A J & Lammie P J. Cyclospora cayetanensis infections in Haiti: a common occurrence in the absence of watery diarrhea. *Am J Trop Med Hyg* 1999; 60:584–586.

115 Green S T, McKendrick M W, Mohsen A H, Schmid M L & Prakasam S F. Two simultaneous cases of Cyclospora cayatensis enteritis returning from the Dominican Republic. *J Travel Med* 2000; 7:41–42.

116 Verdier R I, Fitzgerald D W, Johnson W D & Pape J W. Trimethoprim–sulfamethoxazole compared with ciprofloxacin for treatment and prophylaxis of Isospora belli and Cyclospora cayetanensis infection in HIV-infected patients: a randomised, controlled trial. *Ann Intern Med* 2000; 132:885–888.

117 Lopez-Velez R, Turrientes M C, Garron C, Montilla P, Navajas R, Fenoy S & del Aguila C. Microsporidiosis in travellers with diarrhea from the tropics. *J Travel Med* 1999; 6:223–227.

118 Bicart-See A, Massip P, Linas M D & Datry A. Successful treatment with nitazoxanide of Enterocytozoon bieneusi microsporidiosis in a patient with AIDS. *Antimicrob Agents Chemother* 2000; 44:167–168.

119 Vdovenko A A. Blastocystis hominis: origin and significance of vacuolar and granular forms. *Parasitol Res* 2000; 86:8–10.

120 George Leith Roupell FRS (1797–1854): significant contributions to the early nineteenth-century understanding of cholera and typhus. *J Med Biog* 2000; 8:1–7.

121 Collins B J, van Loon F P L, Molla A et al. Gastric emptying or oral rehydration solutions in acute cholera. *J Trop Med Hyg* 1989; 92:290–294.

122 Avery M E & Snyder J D. Oral therapy for acute diarrhea: the underused simple solution. *N Engl J Med* 1990; 323:891–894.

123 Lawrence G W, Lehmann D, Anian G et al. Impact of active immunisation against enteritis necroticans in Papua New Guinea. *Lancet* 1990; 336:1165–1167.

124 Murtaza A, Khan S R, Butt K S, Finkel Y & Aperia A. Paralytic ileus, a serious complication in acute diarrhoeal disease among infants in developing countries. *Acta Paediatr Scand* 1989; 78:701–705.

125 Hoffman S H. Tropical medicine and the acute abdomen. *Emerg Med Clin North Am* 1989; 7:591–609.

126 Gopi V K, Joseph T P & Varma K K. Acute intestinal obstruction. *Indian Pediatr* 1989; 26:525–530.

127 Archampong E Q. Tropical diseases of the small bowel. *World J Surg* 1985; 9:887–896.

128 Ryan C A, Hargrett-Bean N T & Blake P A. *Salmonella typhi* infections in the United States, 1975–1984: increasing role of foreign travel. *Rev Infect Dis* 1989; 11:1–8.

129 Weeramanthri T S, Corrah P T, Mabey D C W & Greenwood B M. Clinical experience with enteric fever in The Gambia, West Africa 1981–1986. *J Trop Med Hyg* 1989; 92:272–275.

130 Thisyakorn U, Mansuwan P & Taylor D N. Typhoid and paratyphoid fever in 192 hospitalized children in Thailand. *Am J Dis Child* 1987; 141:862–865.

131 Gibney E J. Typhoid perforation. *Br J Surg* 1989; 76:887–889.

132 Meier D E, Imediegwu O O & Tarpley J L. Perforated typhoid enteritis: operative experience with 108 cases. *Am J Surg* 1989; 157:423–427.

133 Ameh E A. Typhoid ileal perforation in children: a scourge in developing countries. *Ann Trop Paediatr* 1999; 19:267–272.

134 Rubin C M E & Fairhurst J J. Life-threatening haemorrhage from typhoid fever. *Br J Radiol* 1988; 61:415–416.

135 Raj S M, Sivakumaran S & Vijayakumari S. Morbidity due to intestinal helminthiasis. *Lancet* 1990; 336:811–812.

136 Cook G C. *Parasitic Disease in Clinical Practice*. London: Springer, 1990: 272.

137 Hepburn N C. Aetiology of eosinophilic enteritis. *Lancet* 1990; 336:571.

138 Prociv P & Croese J. Human eosinophilic enteritis caused by dog hookworm *Ancylostoma caninum*. Lancet 1990; 335:1299–1302.

139 Anayi S & Al-Nasiri N. Acute mesenteric ischaemia caused by *Schistosoma mansoni* infection. BMJ 1987; 294:1197.

140 Radomyos P, Chobchuanchom A & Tungtrongchitr A. Intestinal perforation due to *Macracanthorhynchus hirudinaceus* infection in Thailand. *Trop Med Parasitol* 1989; 40:476–477.

141 Bannerman C & Manzur A Y. Fluctuating jaundice and intestinal bleeding in a 6-year-old girl with fascioliasis. *Trop Geogr Med* 1986; 38:429–431.

142 Acheson D W K & Keusch G T. The shigella paradigm and colitis due to enterohaemorrhagic *Escherichia coli*. *Gut* 1994; 35:872–874.

143 Ravdin J I. Diagnosis of invasive amoebiasis: time to end the morphology era. *Gut* 1994; 35:1018–1021.

144 Fielding L & Padmanabhan A. Clinical features of colorectal cancer. In Misiewicz J J, Pounder R E & Venables C W (eds) *Diseases of the Gut and Pancreas*, 2nd edn. Oxford: Blackwell, 1994: 877–892.

145 Misiewicz J J, Pounder R E & Venables C W (eds). *Diseases of the Gut and Pancreas*, 2nd edn. Oxford: Blackwell, 1994: 675–804.

146 Holdsworth C D. Irritable bowel syndrome. In Misiewicz J J, Pounder R E & Venables C W (eds) *Diseases of the Gut and Pancreas*, 2nd edn. Oxford: Blackwell, 1994: 921–930.

147 Cook G C. *Enterobius vermicularis* infection. *Gut* 1994; 35:1159–1162.

148 Ravdin J I. Intentional disease caused by *Entamoeba histolytica*. In Ravdin J I (ed.) *Amebiasis: Human Infection by Entamoeba histolytica*. New York: Churchill Livingstone, 1988: 495–510.

149 Ellyson J H, Bezmalinovic Z, Parks S N & Lewis F R. Necrotizing amebic colitis: a frequently fatal complication. *Am J Surg* 1986; 152:21–26.

150 Shukla V K, Roy S K, Vaidya M P & Mehrotra M L. Fulminant amebic colitis. *Dis Colon Rectum* 1986; 29:398–401.

151 Parsonnet J, Greene K D, Gerber A R, Tauxe R V, Aguilar O J V & Blake P A. *Shigella dysenteriae* type 1 infections in US travellers to Mexico. *Lancet* 1989; ii:543–545.

152 Lanenscheidt P, Lang C, Puschel W & Feifel G. High rates of appendicectomy in a developing country: an attempt to contribute to a more rational use of surgical resources. *Eur J Surg* 1999; 165:248–252.

153 Ameh E A. Appendicitis versus genital disease in young women in tropical Africa. *Trop Doct* 2000; 30:103–104.

154 Out A A. Tropical surgical emergencies: acute appendicitis. *Trop Geogr Med* 1989; 41:118–122.

155 Gupta S C, Gupta A K, Keswani N K, Singh P A, Tripathy A K & Krishna V. Pathology of tropical appendicitis. *J Clin Pathol* 1989; 42:1169–1172.

156 Zimmerman J-M, de Graeve B, Coblence J-F & Colonna M-A. Attitude thèrapeutique actuelle devant le volvulus du colon pelvien en milieu tropical. *Méd Trop* 1989; 49:371–374.

157 Wilson A P R, Ridgway G L, Sarner M, Boulos P B, Brook B C & Cook G C. Toxic dilatation of the colon in shigellosis. *BMJ* 1990; 301:1325–1326.

158 Gradon J D & Lutwick L I. Toxic dilation and amebiasis. *Am J Gastroenterol* 1988; 83:206–207.

159 Cook G C. Anorectal infections in relation to tropical exposure. In Demling L & Frühmorgan P (eds) *Non-Neoplastic Diseases of the Anorecturm*. Dordrecht: Kluwer, 1992:187–226.

160 Segal I, Edwards C A & Walker A R. Continuing low colon cancer incidence in African populations. *Am J Gastroenterol* 2000; 95:859–860.

161 Misra S P, Misra V, Dwivedi M & Gupta S C. Colonic tuberculosis: clinical features, endoscopic appearance and management. *J Gastroenterol Hepatol* 1999; 14:723–729.

162 Kunasol P, Cooksley G, Chan V F et al. Hepatitis A virus: declining seroprevalence in children and adolescents in Southeast Asia. *Southeast Asian J Trop Med Public Health* 1998; 29:255–262.

163 Shah U, Habib Z & Kleinman R E. Liver failure attributable to hepatitis A virus infection in a developing country. *Pediatrics* 2000; 105:436–438.

164 Anonymous. Hepatitis C: global prevalence (update). *Wkly Epidemiol Rec* 1999 74(10 December):425–427.

165 Coursaget P, Buisson Y, N'Gawara M N, Van Cuyck Gandre H & Roue R. Role of hepatitis E virus in sporadic cases of acute and fulminant hepatitis in an endemic area. *Am J Trop Med Hyg* 1998; 58:330–334.

166 Labrique A B, Thomas D L, Stoszek S K & Nelson K E. Hepatitis E: an emerging infectious disease. *Epidemiol Rev* 1999; 21:162–179.

167 Potasman I, Koren L, Peterman M & Srugo I. Lack of hepatitis E infection among backpackers to tropical countries. *J Travel Med* 2000; 7:208–210.

168 Tarrago D, Lopez-Velez R, Turrientes C, Baquero F & Mateos M L. Prevalence of hepatitis E antibodies in immigrants from developing countries. *Eur J Clin Microbiol Infect Dis* 2000; 19:309–311.

169 Bircher J, Benhamou J-P, McIntyre N, Rizzetto M & Rodes J (eds) Viral infections of the liver. In *Oxford Textbook of Clinical Hepatology*, 2nd edn, vol. 2. Oxford: Oxford University Press, 1999: 825–985.

170 Summerfield J A. Virus hepatitis update. *J R Coll Physicians Lond* 2000; 34:381–385.

171 Pramoolsinsap C & Viranuvatti V. Salmonella hepatitis. *J Gastroenterol Hepatol* 1998; 13:745–750.

172 Shetty A K, Mital S R, Bahrainwala A H, Khubchandani R P & Kumta N B. Typhoid hepatitis in children. *J Trop Pediatr* 1999; 45:287–290.

173 Da Dilva L C, Chieffi P P & Carrilho F J. Protozoal and helminthic diseases of the liver. In Prieto J, Rodes J & Shafritz D A (eds) *Hepatobiliary Disease*. Berlin: Springer, 1992:631–664.

174 Bircher J, Benhamou J-P, McIntyre N, Rizzetto M & Rodes J (eds) Cirrhosis. In *Oxford Textbook of Clinical Hepatology*, 2nd edn, vol. 1. Oxford: Oxford University Press, 1999: 605–641.

175 Okuda K & Okuda H. Primary liver cell carcinoma. In Bircher J, Benhamou J-P, McIntyre N, Rizzetto M & Rodes J (eds) *Oxford Textbook of Clinical Hepatology*, 2nd edn, vol. 2. Oxford: Oxford University Press, 1999: 1491–1530.

176 Bosch F X, Ribes J & Borras J. Epidemiology of primary liver cancer. *Semin Liver Dis* 1999; 19:271–285.

177 Haworth E A, Soni-Raleigh V & Balarajan R. Cirrhosis and primary liver cancer amongst first generation migrants in England and Wales. *Ethn Health* 1999; 4:93–99.

178 Wild C P & Hall A J. Primary prevention of hepatocellular carcinoma in developing countries. *Mutat Res* 2000; 462:381–393.

179 Pan K T, Hung C F, Tseng J H, Lui K W & Wan Y L. Hepatic calcification by sequelae of chronic schistosomiasis japonica: report of four cases. *Changgeng Yi Xue Za Zhi* 1999; 22:265–270.

180 El-Hawey A M, Amr M M, Abdel-Rahman A H et al. The epidemiology of schistosomiasis in Egypt: Gharbia Governorate. *Am J Trop Med Hyg* 2000; 62(suppl. 2):42–48.

181 Bircher J, Benhamou J-P, McIntyre N, Rizzetto M & Rodes J (eds) Alcoholic liver disease. In *Oxford Textbook of Clinical Hepatology*, 2nd edn, vol. 2. Oxford: Oxford University Press, 1999: 1155–1247.

182 Mowat A P. Paediatric liver disease. In Bircher J, Benhamou J-P, McIntyre N, Rizzetto M & Rodes J (eds) *Oxford Textbook of Clinical Hepatology*, 2nd edn, vol. 2. Oxford: Oxford University Press, 1999: 1875–1889.

183 Scheinberg I H & Sternlieb I. Is non-Indian childhood cirrhosis caused by excess dietary copper? *Lancet* 1994; 344:1002–1004.

184 Brissot P & Deugnier Y. Genetic haemochromatosis. In McIntyre N, Benhamou J-P, Bircher J, Rizzetto M & Rodes J (eds) *Oxford Textbook of Hepatology*. Oxford: Oxford University Press, 1991: 948–958.

185 Gordeuk V R. Bantu siderosis. *Lancet* 1986; i:1310.

186 Valla D & Benhamou J-P. Vascular abnormalities. In Bircher J, Benhamou J-P, McIntyre N, Rizzetto M & Rodes J (eds) *Oxford Textbook of Clinical Hepatology*, 2nd edn, vol. 2. Oxford: Oxford University Press, 1999: 1457–1479.

187 Arora N K, Lodha R, Gulati S et al. Portal hypertension in north Indian children. *Indian J Pediatr* 1998; 65:585–591.

188 Osman M, Lausten S B, El-Sefi T, Boghdadi I, Rashed M Y & Jensen S L. Biliary parasites. *Dig Surg* 1998; 15:287–296.

189 Richter J, Freise S, Mull R & Millan J C. Fascioliasis: sonographic abnormalities of the biliary tract and evolution after treatment with triclabendazole. *Trop Med Int Health* 1999; 4:774–781.

190 El-Morshedy H, Farghaly A, Sharaf S, Abou-Basha L & Barakat R. Triclabendazole in the treatment of human fascioliasis: a community-based study. *East Mediterr Health J* 2000; 5:888–894.

191 Millan J C, Mull R, Freise S & Richter J. The efficacy and tolerability of triclabendazole in Cuban patients with latent and chronic Fasciola hepatica infection. *Am J Trop Med Hyg* 2000; 63:264–269.

192 Cook G C. Hepatic structure and function in experimental and human malaria. In Bianchi L, Gerok W, Maier K-P & Dienhardt F (eds) *Infectious Diseases of the Liver (Falk Symposium 54)*. Dordrecht: Kluwer, 1990: 191–213.

193 Zakaria S, Goldsmith R S, Kamel M A & El-Raziky E H. The etiology of acute hepatitis in adults in Egypt. *Trop Geogr Med* 1988; 40:285-292.

194 Pal S R & Prasad S R. Delta virus infections in and around Chandigarh, Northern India: evidence for endemicity. *Trop Geogr Med* 1987; 39:123–125.

195 Khuroo M S, Zargar S A, Mahajan R, Javid G & Lai R. An epidemic of hepatitis D in the foothills of the Himalayas in South Kashmir. *J Hepatol* 1988; 7:151–156.

196 Asano Y, Yoshikawa T, Suga S et al. Fatal fulminant hepatitis in an infant with human herpesvirus-6 infection. *Lancet* 1990; 335:862–863.

197 Boulos M, Segurado A A C & Shiroma M. Severe yellow fever with a 23-day survival. *Trop Geogr Med* 1988; 40:356–358.

198 Holmes G P, McCormick J B, Trock S C et al. Lassa fever in the United States: investigation of a case and new guidelines for management. *N Engl J Med* 1990; 323:1120–1123.

199 Lucia H L, Coppenhaver D H, Harrison R L & Baron S. The effect of an arenavirus infection on liver morphology and function. *Am J Trop Med Hyg* 1990; 43:93–98.

200 MacGregor F B, Abernethy V E, Dahabra S, Cobden I & Hayes P C. Hepatoxicity of herbal remedies. *BMJ* 1989; 299:1156–1157.

201 Tandon B N, Joshi Y K & Tandon M. Acute liver failure: experience with 145 patients. *J Clin Gastroenterol* 1986; 8:664–668.

202 Sarin S K, Chari S, Sundaram K R, Ahuja R K, Anand B S & Broor S L. Young *v* adult cirrhotics: a prospective, comparative analysis of the clinical profile, natural course and survival. *Gut* 1988; 29:101–107.

203 Abdel-Wahab M F, Esmat G, Milad M, Abdel-Razek S & Strickland G T. Characteristic sonographic pattern of schistosomal hepatic fibrosis. *Am J Trop Med Hyg* 1989; 40:72–76.

204 Editorial. Clinical ultrasound in developing countries. *Lancet* 1990; 336:1225–1226.

205 Pande G K, Reddy V M, Kar P et al. Operations for portal hypertension due to extrahepatic obstruction: results and 10 year follow-up. *BMJ* 1987; 295:1115–1117.

206 Reed S L & Braude A I. Extraintestinal disease: clinical syndromes, diagnostic profile, and therapy. In Ravdin J I (ed.) *Amebiasis: Human Infection by Entamoeba histolytica*. New York: Churchill Livingstone, 1988: 511–532.

207 Sargeaunt P G. Zymodemes of *Entamoeba histolytica*. In Ravdin J I (ed.) *Amebiasis: Human Infection by Entamoeba histolytica*. New York: Churchill Livingstone, 1988: 370–387.

208 Robinson S P, Remedios D & Davidson R N. Do amoebic liver abscesses start as large lesions? Case report of an evolving amoebic liver abscess. *J Infect* 1998; 36:338–340.

209 Ahmed L, Rooby A E I, Kassem M I, Salama Z A & Strickland G T. Ultrasonography in the diagnosis and management of 52 patients with amebic liver abscess in Cairo. *Rev Infect Dis* 1990; 12:330–337.

210 Sharma M P, Rai R R, Acharya S K, Ray J C S & Tandom B N. Needle aspiration of amoebic liver abscess. *BMJ* 1989; 299:1308–1309.

211 Freeman O, Akamaguna A & Jarikre L N. Amoebic liver abscess: the effect of aspiration on the resolution or healing time. *Ann Trop Med Parasitol* 1990; 84:281–287.

212 Singh J P & Kashyap A. A comparative evaluation of percutaneous catheter drainage for resistant amebic liver abscesses. *Am J Surg* 1989; 158:58–62.

213 Ken J G, van Sonnenberg E, Casola G, Christensen R & Polanski A M. Perforated amebic liver abscesses: successful percutaneous treatment. *Radiology* 1989; 170:195–197.

214 Goh K L, Wong N W, Paramsothy M, Nojeg M & Somasundaram K. Liver abscess in the tropics: experience in the University Hospital, Kuala Lumpur. *Postgrad Med J* 1987; 63:551–554.

215 Bansal A S & Prabhakar P. Clinical aspects of pyogenic liver abscess: the University Hospital of the West Indies experience. *J Trop Med Hyg* 1988; 91:87–93.

216 Berger L A & Osborne D R. Treatment of pyogenic liver abscesses by percutaneous needle aspiration. *Lancet* 1982; i:132–134.

217 Herbert D A, Fogel D A, Rothman J, Wilson S, Simmons F & Ruskin J. Pyogenic liver abscesses: successful non-surgical therapy. *Lancet* 1982; i:134–136.

218 Bowers E D, Robison D J & Doberneck R C. Pyogenic liver abscess. *World J Surg* 1990; 14:128–132.

219 McCorkell S J & Niles N L. Pyogenic liver abscesses: another look at medical management. *Lancet* 1985; i:803–806.

220 Pineiro-Carrero V M & Andres J M. Morbidity and mortality in children with pyogenic liver abscess. *Am J Dis Child* 1989; 143:1424–1427.

221 Franchi C, Di Vico B & Teggi A. Long-term evaluation of patients with hydatidosis treated with benzimidazole carbamates. *Clin Infect Dis* 1999; 29:304–309.

222 Strickland G T. Gastrointestinal manifestations of schistosomiasis. *Gut* 1994; 35:1334–1337.

223 Castillo C F del, Richter J M & Warshaw A L. Chronic pancreatitis. In Bouchier I A D, Allan R N, Hodgson H J F & Keighley M R B (eds) *Gastroenterology: Clinical Science and Practice*, 2nd edn. London: W B Saunders, 1993:1615–1634.

224 Chattopadhyay P S, Chattopadhyay R, Goswami R & Gupta S K. Observations on hepatic structure and function in fibro-calculous pancreatic diabetes (FCPD) vis-à-vis other diabetic subtypes. *Indian J Pathol Microbiol* 1998; 41:141–146.

225 Khuroo M S, Zarger S A & Mahajan R. Hepatobiliary and pancreatic ascariasis in India. *Lancet* 1990; 335:1503–1506.

226 Tamimi T M, Wosornu L, Al-Khozaim A & Abdul-Ghani A. Increased cholecystectomy rates in Saudi Arabia. *Lancet* 1990; 336:1235–1237.

Chapter 11
Respiratory Problems in the Tropics

S. M. Graham

Respiratory diseases are major causes of illness and death throughout the world. Clinicians in the tropics have to deal with a large number of patients with respiratory disease, and often do so without the diagnostic devices available to those working in richer nations. Fortunately a great deal can be achieved through careful history-taking and physical examination, judicious choice of which tests to do and which not to do, and a thorough knowledge of which diseases are important in the patient's environment.

The age of the patient and duration of symptoms will be important in determining clinical approach, likely aetiology and appropriate diagnostic options. Within the tropics, the pattern of respiratory disease differs greatly from one region to another. Patients may be suffering from diseases that are common in low- and middle-income tropical countries such as bacterial pneumonia or pulmonary tuberculosis (PTB), or are peculiar to a region, e.g. melioidosis, paracoccidioidomycosis or pulmonary schistosomiasis. Others have conditions such as chronic obstructive airways disease (COAD), asthma or viral bronchiolitis that are usually more frequent outside the tropics. The human immunodeficiency virus (HIV) epidemic has had a major impact, particularly on the incidence and manifestations of tuberculosis in African adults.[1]

In an average outpatient department, 20–50% of patients have come with respiratory complaints, and 20–30% of hospital medical admissions are for disorders predominantly affecting the lungs. The incidence is highest in infants and young children, especially for those living in urban areas. It is estimated that acute respiratory infection (ARI) is responsible for one-third of deaths of children under 5 years of age globally and the majority of these deaths occur in children from tropical countries. The clinical challenge is to identify and effectively treat the patient who requires specific therapy or hospitalized management from among the far greater number that present with mild acute disease. Frequently, this must be done in an extremely congested outpatient setting with limited time and no investigations.

In those who are very sick or who have recurrent, chronic or unresponsive symptoms a full clinical assessment is essential. A consequence of the resurgence of tuberculosis (TB), especially among HIV-infected individuals, is that many people with other causes of chronic cough suffer unwarranted lengthy therapeutic trials of anti-TB drugs. The therapeutic trial for 'possible tuberculosis' is sometimes sensible, but must only be embarked upon after all available attempts have been made to diagnose PTB, such as by sputum smear, and other diagnoses have been carefully considered.

Clinical assessment in adults

The history may give useful clues. In a patient with cough, associated symptoms may help with diagnosis or management: fever, haemoptysis, wheeze, breathlessness, night sweats, weight loss, chest pain. Ask about previous anti-TB therapy and the adequacy thereof: this may not be mentioned by the patient and is easily neglected by the doctor. It would help to know whether PTB was proven or merely suspected. Look for previous events or current symptoms that might suggest immunosuppression, especially HIV infection. Look for any history of an episode of unconsciousness preceding the symptoms, e.g. general anaesthesia, epilepsy, alcoholic coma or trauma; inhalation at such a time is a common cause of localized pulmonary infection or lung abscess. Remember that bronchial asthma and left ventricular failure may each give rise to cough as the major symptom, or the only one the patient mentions; other clues if sought will usually point to the diagnosis. Mitral valve disease is much more common in developing than in industrial countries and cardiomyopathy is not uncommon.

The environmental or family context may suggest important possibilities. Ask about contacts known to have TB, but also about any close contact known to have died recently of undiagnosed respiratory disease—TB is a strong possibility. Frequent and severe disease of spouse or children may be strongly suggestive of HIV infection. Certain occupations indicate a high risk of HIV infection. In the traveller who has recently returned from tropical countries where HIV is endemic, consider the possibility of HIV seroconversion illness, which may present with respiratory disease. Pneumonic plague is contracted by inhalation from a close contact dying of septicaemic plague.

There may have been frequent exposure to smoke from indoor hut fires and cigarette smoking is now increasing in many tropical countries. Smoke increases susceptibility to acute or chronic pulmonary infection and causes COAD and lung cancer. Enquire about place and conditions of work, with particular emphasis on dusts (e.g. silicosis, asbestosis or berylliosis) and the relation of symptoms to the time of work. Work in mines, even in the distant past, may have been responsible for fibrotic lung disease. Exposure to asbestos or other industrial air pollutants is associated with an increased risk of lung cancer. Most cases of melioidosis in South-East Asia occur in rice farmers. A patient who works with animals or birds may be exposed to zoonotic diseases that sometimes have a pulmonary component: histoplasmosis, brucellosis, tularaemia, Q fever, leptospirosis or psittacosis. In areas where paragonimiasis and gnathostomiasis occur, enquire about eating raw or undercooked fish; where schistosomiasis is prevalent consider the likelihood of environmental contact.

In the physical examination note the general condition and severity of respiratory distress. Because so many patients have advanced disease by the time they reach medical attention, a variety of physical signs are encountered that are seldom seen in industrialized countries. Abnormalities of chest movement or shape and mediastinal (tracheal) shift may indicate contraction from chronic fibrosis within the chest. A hydro-pneumothorax or pyopneumothorax can be identified clinically by the succussion splash and shifting dullness (percussion over the fifth intercostal space anteriorly is dull with the patient erect, and hollow when supine). Amphoric breathing and post-tussive crackles may be heard over a large cavity. Amoebic liver abscess may present as cough and haemoptysis—which may be acute or chronic. This possibility should be deliberately looked for by palpating for intercostal tenderness over the right lower chest (the liver below the costal margin may be non-tender and is sometimes not palpable, especially when an abscess has discharged some of its contents upwards). A diagnosis of lung abscess can often be made from the characteristic pungent fetor that may fill a ward. COAD is common everywhere; the characteristic physical signs should indicate the diagnosis, but remember that other pulmonary disease such as PTB may be difficult to detect in the presence of COAD.

Look for features suggestive of chronic lung disease such as a barrel-shaped chest or finger clubbing. Marked wasting, generalized lymphadenopathy and enlarged non-tender parotid glands are consistent with HIV infection but may also occur with disseminated TB, sarcoidosis or malignancy. Severe fungal infections such as histoplasmosis, cryptococcosis or paracoccidioidomycosis can also present as pneumonia in an emaciated patient and occur more commonly, but not exclusively, in HIV-infected individuals. Palpable lymph nodes may provide a source of diagnostic material and should be sought routinely.

Carefully examine the skin, mouth and eyes. HIV infection is suggested by current or recent herpes zoster infection, by oral candidiasis or an extensive fungal skin rash. Typical reddish-purple nodules of Kaposi's sarcoma are commonly found on the skin or palate, and in children may present with conjunctival lesions and peri-orbital ecchymoses. Infectious and auto-immune disorders that cause granulomatous lesions in the lungs often present with ocular or skin lesions, e.g. erythema nodosum might suggest sarcoidosis or histoplasmosis. Other conditions with cutaneous manifestations include TB, melioidosis or systemic mycoses.

Finally, look carefully for evidence of cardiac or abdominal abnormalities. Pericardial constriction or effusion may mimic or complicate pulmonary disease such as TB. Right ventricular hypertrophy with cor pulmonale may develop secondary to chronic pulmonary disease, e.g. pulmonary schistosomiasis or chronic pulmonary histoplasmosis. Liver abscesses may present with respiratory symptoms and right-sided chest signs.

Clinical assessment in children

Most of the morbidity and mortality due to ARI in children occurs in infants and children of less than 4 years of age. This influences clinical approach as there is less detail of symptoms than for older children and adults, and abnormalities of auscultation or percussion may be absent or hard to define in small chests. The child usually presents with cough and/or difficulty breathing. The presence of stridor suggests large airway obstruction (e.g. croup), while wheeze indicates small airway obstruction (e.g. asthma).

A raised respiratory rate is consistently the most reliable clinical sign for lower respiratory tract infection. There is some clinical overlap with the presentation of other common childhood illnesses such as malaria or septicaemia. More severe pneumonia is indicated by chest indrawing, difficulty with feeding in infants or cyanosis. School-aged children often present with acute lobar pneumonia and initially cough may not be a prominent symptom. They may complain of pleuritic chest pain and sometimes present with acute abdominal pain or with headache and neck pain, depending on the site of lobar involvement.

Factors that increase the incidence and severity of childhood pneumonia include young age, low birth weight, malnutrition, exposure to indoor smoke and underlying disease such as HIV infection, cardiac abnormalities or cerebral palsy. Poor immunization coverage for measles and whooping cough may be a factor in some regions.

In children with persistent cough or wheeze not responding to standard treatment consider tuberculosis, foreign body, HIV-related lung disease or cardiac failure. A history of TB contact (or of household contacts with chronic cough) is important. A history of a choking episode in a child with persistent wheeze suggests foreign body aspiration. In HIV endemic regions, consider *Pneumocystis carinii* pneumonia (PCP) in an infant with severe pneumonia not responding to standard antibiotic treatment. PCP is usually the first presentation of HIV-related disease. Lymphoid interstitial pneumonitis (LIP) is an HIV-related lung disease that usually presents in older children and is often misdiagnosed as TB. Children with congenital or acquired heart disease often present with recurrent or persistent respiratory symptoms.

Investigations

The diagnosis of bacterial pneumonia is clinical. Blood culture is often not available, has a low sensitivity (less than 30%) and a decision to treat with antibiotics must be made before the result is available. Transthoracic needle aspiration of consolidated lung has a higher yield and has been an important research technique for studies of aetiology that guide standard management policy, but usually is not practical for routine clinical management.

Sputum smear microscopy for acid-fast bacilli is the initial investigation of choice for PTB diagnosis. Appropriate patient selection, proper sputum collection and optimal specimen processing are important; indeed, they are all critical components of a successful TB control programme.[2] In HIV-infected patients, pulmonary tuberculosis is more likely to be sputum-negative than in other people. The likelihood of getting useful information from the sputum is proportional to the quality of sputum sampling. Children of less than 6–8 years of age are unable to expectorate sputum and so the diagnosis of PTB can be particularly difficult. Improved samples can be obtained in adults by initiating a deep cough using nebulized hypertonic saline (i.e. induced sputum technique). Induced sputum is also showing promise as a diagnostic technique for infants and young children.[3]

Good sputum samples may yield other information, depending on available microbiology services. Note the quantity and appearance, e.g. mucoid, purulent or blood-stained. Bacterial culture is of limited value because of the plentiful commensal flora in the pharynx. Culture for tubercle bacilli yields a delayed diagnosis in a small proportion of smear-negative subjects. Nocardiosis is difficult to distinguish clinically and radiologically from PTB but *Nocardia asteroides* is identifiable by Gram stain or culture of the sputum. Other organisms that are identifiable from sputum include *Burkholderia pseudomallei* (causing melioidosis), *Pneumocystis carinii*, *Histoplasma capsulatum*, *Cryptococcus neoformans* and *Paracoccidioides brasiliensis*. Sputum microscopy may occasionally reveal larval helminths, *Strongyloides*, *Paragonimus* ova, hydatid scolices or fungal hyphae (aspergilloma).

Lymph node aspiration and biopsy can provide useful diagnostic information. HIV serology helps to clarify a suspected diagnosis of AIDS; but remember that not every clinical problem is attributable to HIV infection in seropositive individuals. A peak flow-meter provides an index of airways obstruction, both for diagnosis and for observing changes and response to treatment. Pulse oximetry is a useful method for determining severity of hypoxia and response to oxygen therapy.

Chest radiographs are important but expensive: use with discretion and with a clear idea of what they can and cannot do. Never use a radiograph as a short cut to the correct diagnosis. It is often rendered unnecessary by proper clinical evaluation of the patient and is highly susceptible to misinterpretation. There is no point in taking a chest radiograph to demonstrate what is clearly deducible from clinical features, as in lobar pneumonia, massive pleural effusion or sputum-positive tuberculosis. It is better to reserve radiography for circumstances such as the management of pneumothorax or the investigation of unresolving pneumonia. HIV infection has affected the specificity and sensitivity of chest X-ray abnormalities for patients with PTB. The appearance may be atypical, e.g. lower zone infiltrates, or even normal, especially in the severely immunocompromised patient.

A positive tuberculin test strongly supports a diagnosis of PTB in children but a negative test does not exclude the diagnosis. The presence of severe disseminated disease, malnutrition or HIV infection further reduces sensitivity. TB is the predominant cause of pleural effusion in African adults. If a large effusion is present, a pleural tap is often helpful to differentiate causes such as tuberculosis (straw-coloured fluid), empyema (thick purulent fluid) or pulmonary Kaposi's sarcoma (bloody tap). The protein content of the fluid will determine whether it is an exudate or transudate. Pleural biopsy, using an Abrams' needle and taking two or three specimens in different directions at the same site, assists with histological diagnosis.

If available, fibreoptic bronchoscopy may provide useful additional diagnostic information: by identifying causes of local bronchial obstruction (e.g. foreign bodies, tumours) or obtaining secretions and specimens by bronchoalveolar lavage and transbronchial biopsy. As for sputum sampling, the value of fibreoptic bronchoscopy is limited by the quality of laboratory facilities that can be applied to fluid or tissues obtained. It is rarely indicated in young children except for foreign body removal.

Acute respiratory infection in children

The urban child suffers an average of five to eight episodes of ARI per year and the rural child three to four episodes per year, whether in the tropics or non-tropics. The majority are mild upper respiratory tract infections due to viruses. The important difference in epidemiology between the regions is that acute lower respiratory tract infection (pneumonia) is more common, more frequently due to bacteria, more severe and much more likely to be lethal in the tropics. Although respiratory diseases are seasonal, especially in temperate regions, the contrast in severity is a reflection of socio-economic differences rather than differences in climate.

Simple clinical criteria such as breathing rate and the presence of subcostal indrawing are very useful in determining severity of ARI. Bacteria are responsible for up to 60% of severe pneumonia cases and for the majority of pneumonia-related deaths. The most common bacteria in children older than 2 months of age are *Streptococcus pneumoniae* and *Haemophilus influenzae*. These facts provided the foundation for the case management approach that aimed to reduce pneumonia deaths by identification and appropriate antibiotic (and supportive, i.e. oxygen/feeding) management of children with severe pneumonia and to reduce unnecessary use of antibiotics in children with mild ARI.[4]

There is increasing resistance of pneumococcus and *Haemophilus* to co-trimoxazole, penicillin and chloramphenicol, common first-line antibiotics for children with suspected acute bacterial pneumonia in low-income countries. As the bacteria are rarely isolated in cases of pneumonia, useful information of the pattern of resistance in the community can be obtained from nasopharyngeal sampling of healthy young children or by reviewing the pattern of resistance among isolates from children with bacterial meningitis. However, unlike for meningitis, in vitro resistance may not necessarily affect treatment response for bacterial pneumonia.

Pneumonia is due to a wider range of bacteria in neonates, malnourished children and HIV-infected children, and they are at greater risk of death. *Staphylococcus aureus* and Gram negatives such as *Klebsiella, Escherichia coli* or *Salmonella* are also important in these children. Staphylococcal pneumonia with pneumatoceles seems to be less common than it was and this may in part be due to less frequent and less severe measles in many countries.

Of the responsible viruses causing pneumonia, respiratory syncytial virus (RSV), the influenza and parainfluenza viruses and measles are numerically most important. Bronchiolitis and croup occur but are less seasonal and less common than in cooler climates. Again, nutritional state affects presentation and outcome. RSV is the commonest viral cause of childhood pneumonia in tropical countries. The typical clinical picture of RSV bronchiolitis in infants is recognized but in malnourished and HIV-infected children wheeze is unusual and secondary bacterial infection more common. Common and often fatal complications of measles were severe laryngotracheitis and/or pneumonia. However, measles is now less common owing to effective immunization and vitamin A supplementation and treatment has further reduced the frequency of such complications in children with measles.

Mycoplasma pneumoniae and *Chlamydia pneumoniae* cause atypical pneumonia, particularly in school-aged children, usually not severe, and characterized by a protracted course over a few weeks and fine crackles on auscultation. Their relative importance in the tropics is not clear. Treatment of choice is erythromycin. *Chlamydia trachomatis* causes pneumonia in up to 20% of infants born to infected women and presents between 1 and 3 months of age. There is often a history of neonatal conjunctivitis. Finally, remember that tuberculosis does present as acute pneumonia, particularly in infants. The contact will usually be the mother.

Immunization against measles and pertussis, breast-feeding and improved socio-economic circumstances can reduce the incidence and mortality of childhood ARI. The successful development of effective conjugate vaccines against invasive pneumococcus and haemophilus strains means that there is great potential for prevention of severe bacterial pneumonia.[5] These vaccines are not likely to be available in most tropical countries in the near future.

Acute pneumonia in adults

Acute pneumonia is common in adults in tropical countries and *Streptococcus pneumoniae* is the usual cause. Bacterial pneumonia is often preceded by a viral infection such as influenza that presumably alters the susceptibility of the host or damages local defence mechanisms. Lobar pneumonia occurs in previously healthy adults or may present as a complication of another disorder (e.g. structural defect) or circumstance (e.g. period of unconsciousness with aspiration or atelectasis). Note the immune status of the host: the HIV-infected individual, the auto-splenectomized sickler, the postsplenectomy patient, the pregnant woman, the alcoholic, the diabetic and the malnourished all have an increased susceptibility to bacterial infection. Other causes of acute bacterial pneumonia are similar to those mentioned above for children and may be difficult to distinguish from pneumococcal disease on the basis of the clinical features.

The symptoms and signs of lobar pneumonia are well known but sometimes confusing. In early pneumonia, the diagnosis may have to be deduced from the symptoms and the presence of fever and shallow tachypnoea in the absence of any auscultatory signs. The site of consolidation may be more reliably predicted by the 'pointing sign' than by auscultation; the patient is asked to cough and point to the place where this causes pain. When pleurisy is diaphragmatic, the patient may present with suspected abdominal disease. In some populations a considerable proportion of patients with lobar pneumonia develop jaundice. This may be deep, is of mixed type and usually fades rapidly with treatment of the pneumonia.

Mycoplasma pneumoniae, Chlamydia pneumoniae and *Legionella pneumophila* are recognized causes of atypical pneumonia in adults. In *Legionella* pneumonia, there may be mental confusion, diarrhoea or hypotension; hyponatraemia and haematuria are common. These features, together with failure to respond to initial antibiotic treatment, should indicate the possibility of this diagnosis, for which erythromycin is the drug of choice. The incidence of *Legionella* pneumonia in the tropics is not well known. The propensity of the organism to multiply in warm water and the fact that about a third of

UK patients have acquired the infection after travel in southern Europe suggest that *Legionella* may be responsible for more of the pneumonia occurring in the tropics than is generally recognized. *Mycoplasma* may be complicated by erythema multiforme, haemolytic anaemia or arthritis.

In some areas, particularly South-East Asia and northern Australia, melioidosis should be considered as a possible cause of both acute and of unresolving pneumonia, especially in the debilitated or immunocompromised. Appropriate media are needed to culture the organism, *Burkholderia pseudomallei*. Paracoccidioidomycosis is common in Latin America and may present with pulmonary disease. Histoplasmosis and blastomycosis are also endemic in the Americas.

It is important to remember that PTB may present with a clinical syndrome indistinguishable from acute bacterial pneumonia. William Osler recognized this when working in Boston in 1900, where tuberculosis was as common as it is in many tropical areas today. He taught that every patient with lobar pneumonia should be considered to have tuberculosis until clinical progress proved otherwise. This advice is much more important today when specific therapy is available.

Pulmonary tuberculosis

Mycobacterium tuberculosis is the leading cause of death due to infectious disease in the world. PTB is very common in tropical countries because it is closely related to poverty, and there has been a dramatic resurgence in some regions in the wake of the HIV pandemic.[1,2] It is frequently a disease of young adults and children. Epidemiology and clinical management are covered in detail in Chapter 57.

PTB often presents with a history of chronic respiratory symptoms that have not resolved with usual antibiotic treatment. However, as mentioned, the presentation is sometimes acute. This is often the case in infants who are particularly susceptible to severe, disseminated disease. The clinical findings are typically few, although wasting is common. On the other hand, when the auscultatory or radiographic abnormalities are surprisingly marked in comparison to a lack of respiratory distress, think of PTB.

Diagnosis is confirmed by sputum examination. When sputum is not readily available, as in young children, or is smear-negative as is more likely with HIV-infected patients with PTB, clinical score charts or algorithms may be helpful in deciding which patient should receive TB treatment. Chest radiograph may be helpful if the patient does not respond to TB treatment. Differential diagnoses include a range of fungal diseases, parasitic diseases and non-infectious granulomatous disorders (Table 11.1).

The HIV pandemic has had a profound effect on epidemiology, clinical presentation, diagnosis, drug treatment and treatment response. Most cases of tuberculosis in HIV-infected individuals are pulmonary with a positive

Table 11.1 Differential diagnoses of pulmonary tuberculosis

Fungal Disease	PCP
	Cryptococcosis
	Aspergillosis
	Histoplasmosis
	Candidiasis
	Paracoccidioidomycocsis[a]
	Coccidioidomycosis[a]
	Penicilliosis[b]
Bacterial Disease	Nocardiosis
	Melioidosis[b]
	Lung Abscess
	Brucellosis
	Actinomycosis
Parasitic Disease	Paragonimiasis
	Amoebiasis
	Echinococcosis
	Strongyloidiasis
Non-Infectious	Sarcoidosis
	Emphysema
	Cardiac Disease
	Neoplasm

a: in Central or South America
b: in South-East Asia

sputum smear and typical radiological features. However, the presentation of PTB in HIV-infected adults is more commonly atypical (e.g. diffuse, miliary or basal in its distribution) than in HIV-uninfected adults, and there is considerable overlap of clinical and epidemiological features of PTB with other HIV-related lung disease. This makes the confirmation of the diagnosis difficult in many patients, and presumptive treatment is commonly necessary. Drug reactions are more common among patients with HIV-related disease and thiacetazone is associated with severe and often fatal Stevens–Johnson syndrome. The case fatality of PTB is consistently higher in HIV-infected patients than in individuals without HIV. The immunosuppressed patient with PTB is more liable to develop additional pulmonary infections.

The impact of HIV infection

HIV infection is common in many regions of the tropics, particularly in sub-Saharan Africa. This subject is dealt with in detail in Chapter 20. Peak prevalence is among young adults and mother-to-child transmission is common. Respiratory disease, acute or chronic, is the commonest cause of morbidity and mortality in HIV-infected adults and children. Pulmonary symptoms are often the first clinical manifestation of the disease, but clinical evidence of underlying immunosuppression should be sought.

There are important differences in the pattern of HIV-related pneumonia between adults and children within

Table 11.2 Causes of HIV-related lung disease in low-income tropical regions

Age group	Most common	Less common
INFANTS	Bacteria pneumonia PCP	Viral pneumonia (e.g. CMV) Tuberculosis
CHILDREN	Bacterial pneumonia LIP Tuberculosis	Viral pneumonia (e.g. measles) Pulmonary Kaposi's sarcoma Nocardiosis Candidiasis
ADULTS	Bacterial pneumonia Tuberculosis	PCP Cryptococcosis Nocardiosis Pulmonary Kaposi's sarcoma Penicilliosis[a] Melioidosis[a] Paracoccidioidomycocsis[b] Histoplasmosis[b]

a: in Sout-East Asia
b: in Central and South America

the tropics, and in comparison to non-tropical regions (Table 11.2).[6,7] PTB and bacterial pneumonia are the major causes of respiratory morbidity in HIV-infected adults living in the poorer regions of the tropics. The clinical features of bacterial pneumonia are similar to those in HIV-seronegative patients, although bacteraemia is more common.[8] Less common diseases in HIV-infected adults living in tropical Africa include cryptococcosis, PCP, nocardiosis and pulmonary Kaposi's sarcoma.[6] The clinical presentation of PCP is described in Chapter 70. HIV-related infections in other tropical regions include paracoccidioidomycosis in tropical America and *Penicillium marneffei* in South-East Asia.[9,10]

In contrast, PCP is a common cause of severe pneumonia in HIV-infected African infants but is rare beyond 6 months of age.[7] In comparison to bacterial pneumonia, PCP is characterized by a low-grade or absent fever, a clear chest with good air entry or diffuse rather than focal abnormalities, severe and persistent hypoxia, and a poor clinical response to usual broad-spectrum antibiotics (e.g. chloramphenicol) and to oxygen.[11] Hyperinflation and diffuse interstitial infiltration are the usual radiographic abnormalities. PCP is usually fatal even when treated with high-dose co-trimoxazole, prednisolone and oxygen. Co-trimoxazole prophylaxis is effective in preventing PCP in HIV-infected infants.

The incidence of bacterial pneumonia is also greatly increased in HIV-infected children.[12] The range of causative organisms is similar to that which occurs in HIV-uninfected children of similar nutritional status. Although HIV-infected children are more susceptible to PTB, the actual incidence of PTB is low. A common cause of chronic lung disease in HIV-infected children, which is often misdiagnosed as PTB or miliary TB, is LIP.[7] LIP is an HIV-related disease that usually occurs in children, and health workers in regions where childhood HIV infection is endemic need to be familiar with the typical clinical presentation of LIP. Common clinical markers include marked generalized lymphadenopathy, finger clubbing, enlarged parotid glands and massive hepatomegaly. The typical radiographic abnormalities are diffuse reticulo-nodular infiltration with bilateral hilar lymphadenopathy, which contrasts with the focal and often unilateral abnormalities of PTB. Bronchiectasis presents with a chronic cough productive of copious purulent and sometimes blood-stained sputum, finger clubbing and halitosis. Bronchiectasis may complicate LIP or PTB.

Although a variety of parasites causes lung problems in the tropics (see below), these infections do not appear to be increased in frequency or altered in their clinical manifestations by concomitant HIV infection or AIDS.

Mixed infection

It is not unusual that acute bacterial pneumonia complicating underlying chronic lung disease such as PTB or LIP is the illness which has persuaded the patient to seek medical care. Persistence of symptoms following an adequate course of antibiotics or the finding of clinical signs suggestive of chronic lung disease is an indicator for further investigation such as sputum collection. Mixed infections requiring different therapies, such as PCP, bacterial pneumonia and PTB, are described in HIV-infected adults and children.[6,7] Organisms of normally low pathogenicity such as *Aspergillus fumigatus* are able to colonize already damaged airways and can form abscesses, such as in old tuberculous cavities.[13] A chest radiograph can be useful in assessing the patient with proven or presumed PTB who is not responding to antituberculous therapy.

Asthma

Asthma is not as common in the tropics as it is in some temperate regions and there are differences in the pattern of presentation.[14] However, the prevalence in tropical countries is increasing, particularly in urban communities. Many asthmatics first develop symptoms in adult life and there is less likely to be a history of other atopic conditions. The low but increasing incidence of atopic disease and asthma in tropical countries is an area of current research interest with the hope that it may provide important information as to why such diseases have become so common in more affluent countries. Nutrition is likely to be one factor: asthma is extremely rare in malnourished children. Relationship to infections more prevalent in the tropics such as the higher burden of parasitic disease may also be important.

Each patient should be assessed for and advised of possible precipitating factors or circumstances: season, time of day, exercise, dust, drugs (e.g. salicylates—present in innumerable mixtures and tablets available from grocery stores), animals, bedding. Progress can be monitored by symptom indices and measurements of peak flow rate.

Treatment should be appropriate to the frequency and severity of attacks but often the range of therapeutic options available is limited. Oral salbutamol or aminophylline are perhaps the most widely available but have limited efficacy. Inhaled β_2-agonists such as salbutamol or terbutaline are very useful but patients should be taught to use the inhaler effectively either by direct delivery or via a spacer. This can be difficult in practice. Cromoglycate may be assessed for prophylactic efficacy over a period of weeks for those suffering frequent attacks or exercise-induced asthma. Severe episodes can be treated with nebulized β_2-agonists and short courses of oral corticosteroids. Subcutaneous adrenaline can be very useful for the life-threatening episode especially as it is usually available.

Tropical pulmonary eosinophilia

In areas where *Wuchereria bancrofti* and *Brugia malayi* are common, patients with cough or wheeze may have tropical pulmonary eosinophilia, in which marked eosinophilia (eosinophil count often greater than 3000 per mm^3) and lung shadows on radiography are supported by a positive filarial antibody test. The condition improves rapidly with antifilarial treatment (see Chapter 81).[15,16] Filariasis is most common in Southern and Eastern Asia, the Pacific and Brazil. The condition is uncommon in Africa, but a similar combination of cough, wheeze and eosinophilia may occur due to the migrating larval stages of *Ascaris*, hookworm, schistosomiasis or *Strongyloides* infection (see Chapter 82).[17]

Sarcoidosis

In many tropical countries, sarcoidosis has never been identified. However, in temperate countries, Africans,

West Indians and Asians have a much higher incidence of sarcoidosis than do Caucasians living in the same vicinity. Caucasians are also found to have less severe disease, with fewer systemic manifestations, than the other ethnic groups. There is now evidence that sarcoidosis has been under-reported from tropical countries and is often misdiagnosed as tuberculosis.[18] The possibility of sarcoidosis should be considered in patients with unresolving lung disease, especially if there are accompanying extrathoracic features such as iridocyclitis, lymphadenopathy, central nervous system complications or hypercalcaemia.

Pulmonary problems in common parasitic diseases

Those working in a tropical area, or having to deal with travellers, must be aware of pulmonary aspects of most of the common parasitic diseases; lung involvement may complicate other more usual features of those infections, or may sometimes be the major mode of presentation. In some parasitic diseases the lung is the predominant organ involved. Paragonimiasis (see Chapter 81) may present with cough, haemoptysis and cavitating lung disease. It is often mistaken for PTB and must be considered in areas where raw fish is eaten. Hydatid cysts (see Chapter 84) may produce a variety of lung problems as a result of mechanical compression of intrathoracic structures. In a number of helminth infections (hookworm, *Ascaris*, *Strongyloides*, schistosomiasis) a larval stage of the parasite migrates through the lungs, when it may cause cough, fever, dyspnoea and sometimes wheeze or haemoptysis (see Chapter 83).

The severity of the illness probably depends on how many larvae are migrating at one time; the classical self-experiment of Koino illustrated this. He swallowed 2000 viable *Ascaris* eggs, and within a week suffered a severe illness with high fever, dyspnoea, cyanosis, severe cough and frothy, blood-stained sputum lasting for 7 days. There was eosinophilia, and many *Ascaris* larvae were recovered from his sputum. It would be unusual for such a large number of eggs to be ingested simultaneously in natural circumstances. In schistosomiasis, especially where portal hypertension has led to venous shunts bypassing the liver, eggs may be deposited in pulmonary capillaries and arterioles, eliciting a granulomatous reaction resulting either in pulmonary hypertension or the accumulation of large masses of granulation tissue (see Chapter 80).

Malaria may be complicated by pulmonary problems; cough is not uncommonly a symptom, even in moderately severe malaria, and in severe *Plasmodium falciparum* malaria pulmonary problems have been reported in 5–15% of cases. Although pulmonary oedema due to therapeutic fluid overload, or bronchopneumonia complicating deep coma, may occur, a more specific malarial lesion indistinguishable from adult respiratory distress syndrome has been recognized in which there is septal oedema, endothelial cell swelling and hyaline membrane formation within the alveoli (see Chapter 71). In children in endemic areas, anaemia and acidosis with resultant tachypnoea are common in severe malaria, but respiratory distress syndrome is rare.

Smoking in the tropics

The impact of indoor smoke on the incidence of respiratory disease in developing countries is enormous but, until recently, cigarette smoking was not common.[19] Many developing countries have a tobacco industry that contributes to revenue, employment and trade. The end-product is increasingly finding its way back to the countries of origin. Tobacco companies are now bound by strict advertising regulations and have suffered from costly litigation in rich countries, and are now targeting middle- and low-income countries. Particularly alarming are figures from secondary schools: 30–40% of pupils in some areas have been found to be regular smokers.[20]

Smoking-related diseases have increased in tandem. Emphysema and lung cancers are becoming more common in China, Nigeria, India and Malaysia. Because of the delayed effects of smoking, a great increase of these and other smoking-related diseases can be expected within the coming decade in tropical countries.

REFERENCES

1   Johnson J L & Ellner J J. Adult tuberculosis overview: African versus Western perspectives. *Curr Opin Pulm Med* 2000; 6:180–186.

2   Harries A D, Graham S M & Maher D. *TB/HIV: A Clinical Manual*, 2nd edn. Geneva: WHO, 2001.

3   Zar H J, Tannebaum E, Apolles P, Roux P, Hanslo D & Hussey G. Sputum induction for the diagnosis of pulmonary tuberculosis in infants and young children in an urban setting in South Africa. *Arch Dis Child* 2000; 82:305–308.

4   Rasmussen Z, Pio A & Enarson P. Case management of childhood pneumonia in developing countries: recent relevant research and current initiatives. *Int J Tuberc Lung Dis* 2000; 4:807–826.

5   Mulholland K, Levine O, Nohynek H & Greenwood B M. Evaluation of vaccines for the prevention of pneumonia in children in developing countries. *Epidemiol Rev* 1999; 21:43–55.

6   Daley C L. Pulmonary infections in the tropics: impact of HIV infection. *Thorax* 1994; 49:370–378.

7   Graham S M, Coulter J B S & Gilks C F. Pulmonary disease in HIV-infected African children. *Int J Tuberc Lung Dis* 2001; 5:1–12.

8   Scott J A, Hall A J, Muyodi C et al. Aetiology, outcome and risk factors for mortality among adults with acute pneumonia in Kenya. *Lancet* 2000: 355:1225–1230.

9   Levi G C. Management of opportunistic infections in HIV (+) patients: contrasts between Europe and South America. *Braz J Infect Dis* 1998; 2:118–127.

10 Sirisanthana T & Supparatpinyo K. Epidemiology and management of penicilliosis in human immunodeficiency virus-infected patients. *Int J Infect Dis* 1998; 3:48–53.

11 Graham S M, Mtitimila E I, Kamanga H S, Walsh A L, Hart C A & Molyneux M E. The clinical presentation and outcome of *Pneumocystis carinii* pneumonia in Malawian children. *Lancet* 2000; 355:369–373.

12 Madhi S A, Petersen K, Madhi A, Khoosal M & Klugman K P. Increased disease burden and antibiotic resistance of bacteria causing severe community-acquired lower respiratory tract infections in human immunodeficiency type 1-infected children. *Clin Infect Dis* 2000; 31:170–176.

13 Saubolle M A. Fungal pneumonias. *Semin Respir Infect* 2000; 15:162–177.

14 Beasley R, Crane J, Lai C K & Pearce N. Prevalence and etiology of asthma. *J Allergy Clin Immunol* 2000; 105:S466–472.

15 Ong RK, Doyle R L. Tropical pulmonary eosinophilia. *Chest* 1998; 113:1673–1679.

16 Cooray J H & Ismail M M. Re-examination of the diagnostic criteria of tropical pulmonary eosinophilia. *Respir Med* 1999; 93:655–659.

17 Sarinas P S & Chitkara R K. Ascariasis and hookworm. *Semin Respir Infect* 1997; 12:130–137.

18 Jindal S K, Gupta D & Aggarwal A N. Sarcoidosis in developing countries. *Curr Opin Pulm Med* 2000; 6:448–454.

19 Bruce N, Perez-Padilla R & Albalak R. Indoor air pollution in developing countries: a major environmental and public health challenge. *Bull World Health Org* 2000; 78:1078–1092.

20 Warren C W, Riley L, Asma S et al. Tobacco use by youth: a surveillance report from the Global Youth Tobacco Survey project. *Bull World Health Org* 2000; 78:868–876.

Chapter 12
Cardiovascular Disease in the Tropics

E. H. O. Parry and F. I. Anjorin

Cardiovascular disease is changing continuously in the tropics,[1-4] and so the pattern of disease described in any country describes point prevalence and no more. In Abidjan and Accra[5] coronary arterial disease now accounts for about 10% of cardiovascular cases, but this is not seen in rural people,[6] and the predictions of the World Health Report of 1993 were made without reliable data. HIV infection now dominates clinical practice in many countries[7] and is responsible for the rise of cases of tuberculous pericarditis.

Some cardiac diseases depend on the local environment and/or its microbes:[8] Chagas' disease in Latin America, schistosomal cor pulmonale in Egypt, Sudan and Brazil,[9] and cor pulmonale in parts of India and Papua New Guinea, sometimes associated with smoke pollution inside small huts and repeated bronchitis. The chief diseases are still rheumatic heart disease, dilated cardiomyopathy, hypertension, pericardial tuberculosis associated with HIV and, with urbanization, coronary arterial disease.

Rheumatic heart disease

This important disease accounts for from 12% to about 30% of cardiovascular admissions. It prevails among the poorly housed and is an indicator of their plight.[10-13] Rheumatic fever in poor communities in the tropics differs from the formerly familiar pattern in the industrialized countries:[14] it affects young children;[15] it has different clinical features;[16,17] it affects the heart more commonly both in the first attack and in recurrences; and, on account of weak health services, its secondary prevention is very difficult indeed,[18] and comprehensive programmes are needed to control it.[19]

Epidemiology

Risk factors are poverty and overcrowded housing in the drier areas of the tropics. This is presumably due to easier transmission and/or acquisition of *Streptococcus pyogenes* in a hot dry climate. WHO has used, as a baseline for further studies,[20] a mean prevalence of 10/1000 for established rheumatic heart disease and an incidence of rheumatic fever of 100/100 000, but methods of study vary greatly.

Criteria for diagnosis

The Duckett Jones criteria have been successively modified because chorea, subcutaneous nodules and erythema marginatum are rare in the tropics: carditis is allowed as the only major manifestation,[21] and arthralgia instead of arthritis. Rheumatic fever[20] follows infection with *Strep. pyogenes*. For every 100 cases of sore throat, 20 are caused by *Strep. pyogenes*. For every 100 of those caused by *Strep. pyogenes*, 20 are symptomatic with fever and cervical lymph nodes. Out of the 20 symptomatic cases, two of rheumatic fever may develop, whereas only one case may develop in the 80 without symptoms, except during an epidemic, when the numbers are increased five times.

Clinical features

Echocardiography is important for confirming a diagnosis and for following the evolution of the disease.[22]

Rheumatic fever
Carditis in a child may present as a low-grade fever and a tachycardia and nothing else. Dissociation between the height of the temperature and the tachycardia, and a cardiac murmur—systolic or diastolic, at the apex of the heart may help in diagnosis.

Rheumatic heart disease
Established disease affects (1) the mitral valve alone, which leads to mitral incompetence, the most common lesion; next, mitral stenosis or mixed stenosis and incompetence; (2) both mitral and aortic valves; and (3) least commonly, the aortic valve alone (Figure 12.1)

Streptococcal sore throat
A clinical episode may precede some cases of acute rheumatic fever, and it must be recognized in the community if primary prevention is to have any hope of success. The distinction between a streptococcal and a viral infection may be difficult (Table 12.1).

Prevention

The fundamental aims are as follows:

1. *Environment:* to improve homes and housing, food and health care.

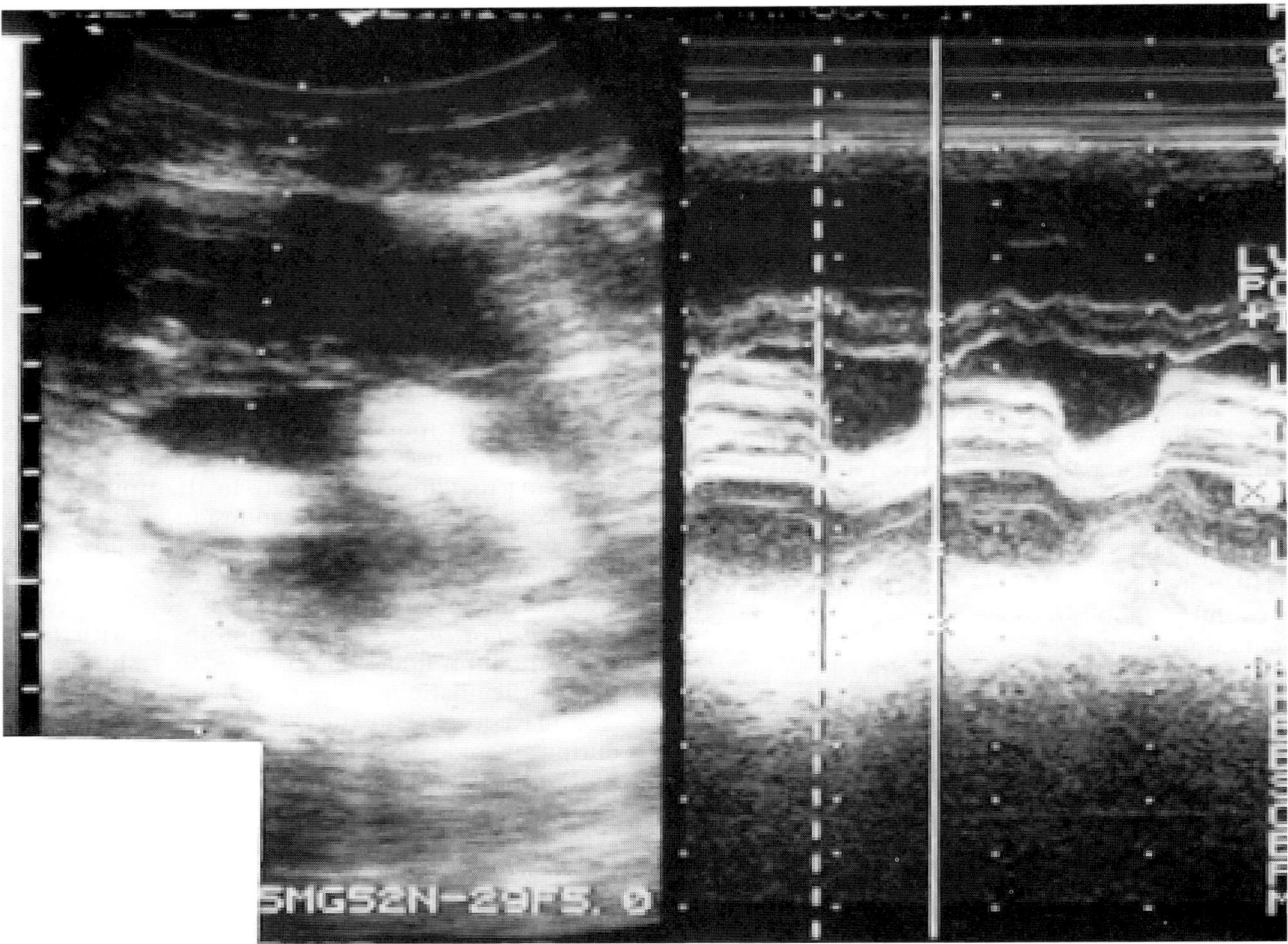

Figure 12.1: Echocardiogram of a 39-year-old Nigerian male showing mitral valve (MV) stenosis with dense calcification. He subsequently underwent a successful mitral valve replacement.

Table 12.1 Comparison of streptococcal and viral sore throat.

Feature	Streptococcal	Viral
Onset	Abrupt	Gradual
Throat	Painful	Uncomfortable
Cervical nodes	Enlarged, tender	Not enlarged
Eyes and nose	Not affected	Watery eyes, runny nose
Throat/tonsils	Red, swollen, exudate	Red, vesicles, ulcers

2. *Primary prevention:* to detect and treat symptomatic *Strep. pyogenes* sore throat—with either benzathine penicillin 1.2 megaunits, penicillin V for 10 days, or benzyl penicillin.
3. *Secondary prophylaxis:* to prevent streptococcal infection, with benzathine penicillin every 3 weeks, in those with known rheumatic heart disease through dedicated community nurses.

Management
Acute rheumatic fever
Eradicate *Strep. pyogenes* with benzyl penicillin and establish maintenance prophylaxis with benzathine penicillin. Manage cardiac failure with bed-rest for acute carditis and give aspirin or corticosteroids, for as long as there is evidence of carditis, provided there is no evidence of cardiac failure.

Chronic rheumatic heart disease
Maintain penicillin prophylaxis to prevent recurrences (and infective endocarditis), and give standard treatment for valvular disease, disorders of rhythm or cardiac failure.

Dilated cardiomyopathy

In some tropical countries, patients who have a dilated heart, without any identifiable cause, account for about 20% of cardiovascular cases.

Pathogenesis

There are many possible factors and this is, at best, a syndrome.[23] Men are affected more than women, predominantly in the age group 40–49 years.

Poverty and social class

The condition is much more common in patients of low social class in West Africa than is found with other types of heart disease.[23]

Anaemia

While severe anaemia may be associated with cardiac failure it does not appear to be a causal factor in dilated cardiomyopathy in the tropics.

Toxins

These are often suggested but rarely incriminated.

Alcohol

Alcohol, often a strong traditional brew, is an important cause of dilated cardiomyopathy in many areas of the tropics.

Nutrition and micronutrients

There is no evidence for a direct nutritional cause of dilated cardiomyopathy in the tropics, except the rare cases of beriberi, and micronutrient deficiency (for example, selenium) has not yet been proved. The wasting associated with HIV infection is associated with a loss of left ventricular mass and of diastolic function.[24]

Myocarditis

A previous viral myocarditis may prove to be more significant than is currently appreciated.

Hypertension

There is evidence that some patients may be former hypertensives: the age groups of those with hypertensive cardiac failure and dilated cardiomyopathy are similar; the aortic arch diameter in all cases of dilated cardiomyopathy is intermediate between that of hypertensive and normal individuals; in some cases the blood pressure rises to abnormal levels as cardiac failure responds to treatment; and in East Africa formerly proved hypertensives presented years later with dilated cardiomyopathy but with normal blood pressures.

Clinical features

Most patients have symptoms of pulmonary and/or systemic oedema for up to 2 years and thus often present with pulmonary oedema or dependent oedema, ascites and a large liver, a large left ventricle and signs of atrioventricular valvular incompetence. Some patients present with systemic embolization, for example a 'cerebrovascular accident', from an intracavitary left ventricular thrombus.

Diagnosis

In a man with normal arterial pressure and no evidence of valvular disease the diagnosis is not difficult, but if there is raised arterial pressure, retinal arterial changes and a left ventricle which is thickened but dilated, the distinction from hypertensive cardiac failure may be difficult. Similarly, mitral incompetence in a younger patient may indicate rheumatic heart disease or even endomyocardial fibrosis, but the mitral valvular incompetence in cardiomyopathy may be reversed by treatment of the cardiac failure.

Management and prognosis

Management depends on the resources and drugs available. In district hospitals, diuretics, with digoxin when there is an atrial arrhythmia, are essential. Other forms of treatment are available at specialist hospitals. The prognosis depends on the function of the left ventricle: those who do worst have a high left ventricular end-diastolic pressure, end-systolic volume and end-diastolic volume with a reduced ejection fraction. If alcohol is incriminated as a causative factor then somehow the patient has to stop drinking it.

Peripartum cardiac failure (PPCF)

The definition of PPCF varies but only in the time interval related to delivery. In Nigeria the following definition has been used: 'cardiac failure, with symptoms beginning in pregnancy or up to 6 months post partum—of up to 6 months duration, with no history of cardiac failure other than PPCF itself, and with no discernible cause for cardiac failure other than anaemia or hypertension, presumed to be acute'.[25]

Distribution

The syndrome has been reported from tropical Latin America,[26] the Caribbean, East, West[27] and South Africa,[28] India, China and Korea. Occasional cases are also seen in temperate countries and some important series of cases have been reported in the USA,[29] almost exclusively among black women.

Factors in the pathogenesis

This syndrome may conceal a number of conditions: some cases resemble dilated cardiomyopathy and therefore its possible causes have to be considered in PPCF.

Race

The largest reported series have been in West Africans and black Americans. The syndrome is apparently also common in Korea, and cases are reported in all races.

Parity

PPCF is more common in multiparous women, and this appears to be independent of age, although increasing age is itself a risk factor.

Twin births

Data are few but the risk has been reported to be twofold in a twin pregnancy.

Blood pressure

The question therefore arises as to whether PPCF patients are a potentially hypertensive cohort and whether PPCF is a form of hypertensive heart failure, as suggested in southern Nigeria, or can the hypertension is some cases be explained by some other mechanism? There is persuasive evidence from northern Nigeria that this is indeed the case in some patients. Some women develop hypertension soon after treatment for their cardiac failure and, although the numbers were small, more Nigrian PPCF women had hypertensive immediate family members than controls. Similarly a highly significant number took extra salt compared with controls and so there may be a genetically determined disorder of salt taste resulting in excess salt intake. The group probably represents a salt-sensitive subset with resultant actual or potential hypertension, masquerading as PPCF but revealed as hypertension later in life.

Infection

There is a rapidly advancing myocarditis, possibly viral, in some non-tropical cases, confirmed by endomyocardial biopsy in over 50% of such cases, but its mechanism is not known.[30,31]

The northern Nigerian PPCF syndrome

Cultural practices

After delivery, the Hausa women around Zaria traditionally take *kanwa*, a rock salt rich in sodium and potassium, in order to promote the flow of breast milk. They also lie on a heated bed for at least 40 days post partum and take hot 'baths' twice daily to prevent themselves from becoming diseased from cold.

Seasonal variation

The peak of admissions follows about 2 months after the hottest humid season.

The Nigerian syndrome: a possible mechanism

The factors are postpartum state, hot season and hot beds and baths, and ingestion of a sodium-rich rock salt. The heat causes vasodilatation so that the cardiac output rises in order to maintain flow and arterial pressure, but the excessive sodium load demands a high renal arterial pressure for its excretion. This can only be at best partially achieved by a further rise of cardiac output and blood pressure.[32] Oedema therefore develops and the cycle is set for it to increase daily. The syndrome is thus established with a high output state and vasodilatation, oedema, and systemic and pulmonary venous congestion. Physiologically it is not true cardiac failure because the stroke volume can rise in response to a rise in filling pressure. This group responds rapidly with a massive diuresis, but it does not include a smaller number whose heart is dilated and who do not respond with a diuresis.

Clinical picture

Symptoms of pulmonary and/or systemic venous congestion develop, often with massive swelling of body and face. The blood pressure is often raised when the patient is first seen, but falls within a few days during diuretic treatment. Systemic and pulmonary emboli are seen when the heart is very large. Imaging shows a dilated heart, pulmonary venous congestion and oedema.

Disordered physiology

There is no homogeneous pattern of cardiac function. Most Brazilian patients showed a raised ventricular filling pressure with low cardiac output but a subset, similar to the Nigerian group, had high output 'failure'.[26] Volume overload was thought to be responsible: this hypervolaemia, when cured by diuretics, can leave a normal heart.[33] Some cases, however, have irreversible cardiac damage.

Evolution and treatment

The prognosis of this syndrome varies with its pathogenesis, from the rapidly progressive myocarditis for which cardiac transplantation may be needed, to a syndrome of oedema and uncomplicated cardiomegaly, which resolves very quickly with treatment by diuretics. Bad signs are an arrhythmia, persistent hypertension, cardiomegaly, or systemic or pulmonary emboli.[34] There is no reason to take the baby off the breast, and as soon as the mother has had a major diuresis she can be treated at home.

Subsequent pregnancies

The syndrome may recur,[8,34] but if the heart returns to normal after the first episode[35] there is no reason to advise against subsequent pregnancy.

Hypertension and hypertensive heart disease

Most people in the tropics with high blood pressure (defined by the WHO criteria) do not know that they are hypertensive, and even if they were aware and sought treatment, in many countries the public budget cannot possibly stretch to supply the ideal combination of anti-hypertension drugs.

Blood pressure in rural and urban societies (See also Chapter 38)

In isolated people the prevalence of hypertension is very low and blood pressure levels remain within a remarkably narrow range throughout adult life, whereas they may rise modestly with age in rural people and rise even more in those who live in cities[36,37] among whom the prevalence of hypertension is high. Migration apparently affects the blood pressure in women less than men.

Body weight is an important determinant of blood pressure, as are indices relating weight to height and sodium (from common salt) intake.[38] There is an associated lower intake of potassium. There are now very many such studies: some examples are given in the reference list.[39–42] Indeed, in Tanzania, blood pressure in normotensive urban men, who normally take a relatively low amount of salt, was found to be peculiarly sensitive to a high salt intake.[43] Salt sensitivity has also been related to the survival of those who were transported from Africa: they survived because they could conserve sodium.

Race

Different origins apparently govern both the prevalence and pattern of hypertension. In any society those of black African origin are most susceptible and, as discussed below, they are vulnerable to stroke; low renin hypertension is also more common.

Sequelae of hypertension

Stroke is a common problem in hospital practice in the tropics and it is closely correlated with hypertension:[44] in one study, over 27 years, stroke mortality was 11.4% in hypertensives but only 1.8% in normotensives. It is often the presenting feature of hypertension, particularly if this has not been detected previously, and so, if much hypertension goes undetected, numerous strokes can be expected.

Hypertensive cardiac disease and failure[45] have already been discussed in relation to dilated cardiomyopathy; in some cases of hypertensive heart disease left ventricular hypertrophy is asymmetrical. It accounts for 20–35% of cases of cardiovascular admissions in many tropical countries.

Malignant hypertension is well recognized and renal failure with severe hypertension is also often seen,[46] but without a definite diagnosis of the underlying renal disease the cause for this remains conjectural. Retinopathy occurs in hypertension, as it does in northern countries.

Coronary arterial events are much more common in Asian hypertensives than among those of black African origin.

The problem of management

As life expectancy increases, there are inevitably more untreated and later disabled victims of hypertension. Severe hypertension may be detected if there is an efficient primary health care service, but few tropical countries can afford to treat hypertension in all those who need drugs. This problem is compounded because

angiotensin-converting enzyme (ACE) inhibitors are less efficacious in black people than they are in white people.

For the individual who needs drugs it is essential both to establish that drug supply can be sustained indefinitely, and to ensure that treatment will be followed.[47] The drug regimen will depend on national drug policy, the essential drug list, and thus what drugs are available at each level of health care. Follow-up with good records can be handled by a well-trained medical assistant or nurse, who has defined criteria for referral if there is an unexpected change.

Endomyocardial fibrosis

Endomyocardial fibrosis (EMF) has distinctive clinical and pathological features[48,49] and a novel pathogenesis,[50] but even in specialist centres in endemic areas it comprises only about 1–5% of cases. Nevertheless, in some parts of the hot and humid tropics—Kerala, Malaysia, West and Central Africa and Brazil[51]—EMF is seen much more commonly than in other areas.

What is EMF?

Endocardial thickening of the ventricle leads to cardiac constriction or restriction and atrioventricular valvular incompetence, leading to regurgitation. In the left ventricle dense fibrous tissue at the apex spreads around the cavity of the ventricle or may first appear around the papillary muscle of the posterior cusp of the mitral valve. This muscle is anchored so that the valve becomes incompetent. The right ventricular cavity is obliterated from below by the advancing fibrosis of layered mural thrombi. In late cases the papillary muscles are lost in a bed of fibrous tissue, the tricuspid valve becomes functionless and the right atrium becomes aneurysmal. The left, right or both ventricles can be affected. Chronic pericardial effusion can complicate right ventricular EMF; a pleural effusion is more common with left or biventricular disease.

The anatomical changes explain physiological dysfunction and the physical signs in established disease. Dense avascular fibrous tissue, often sharply defined from or 'dipping into' the myocardium, is characteristic of established disease. In acute disease, however, the pericardium, myocardium and endocardium show active inflammation with lymphocytes, eosinophils which may be degranulated,[50] and many small blood vessels packed with cells. In addition, irregularly scattered throughout the myocardium, and often unrelated to overlying endocardial change, there are foci where myocardial fibres are disappearing and fibroblasts are evident.

Pathogenesis

The term eosinophilic endomyocardial disease has been suggested to replace endomyocardial fibrosis because the cardiac changes are explained in terms of the eosinophil and its constituents.[4,52] Thus EMF has changes similar to those found in the heart in patients with hypereosinophilic syndromes.[53] The critical questions are: what is the trigger for an eosinophilia in EMF,[17] and is it found consistently? Eosinophilia is not consistent, but that could be because the disease is often not present until its pathogenetic process is burnt out. Early reports from West Africa linked filariasis with EMF, and particularly *Loa loa*, or any other helminth which provokes an eosinophilia.[53] A clear initial illness[54,55] has been described, when there may be a significant eosinophilia.

The suggested sequence is as follows: a trigger to eosinophilia (helminthic or other infection) leads to hypereosinophilia and liberation of eosinophilic major basic proteins and cationic protein which are toxic to a wide range of cells, including endocardial and myocardial cells. The damaged endocardium serves as a focus for mural thrombi which are themselves promoted by the release of platelet activation factor(s) from the eosinophils. Further mural thrombi are then laid down at the original and adjacent sites, and a fibrotic mass, sometimes calcified,[56] results. This is a logical and clear sequence following hypereosinophilia but the difficulty lies in reconciling it with all the data, particularly from Uganda, where for example the prevalence of EMF differed between immigrant Rwanda and native Baganda, in a ratio of about 4–5 to 1, whereas rheumatic heart disease was just the reverse.[57] Similarly, in a kindred with the tropical splenomegaly syndrome, EMF was apparently more prevalent.[58] Causes of eosinophilia are abundant in the tropics but EMF is not. Additionally, it appears to be much less prevalent in dry grassland areas—but why? On the whole, available evidence suggests that hypereosinophilia in a hot and humid environment promotes features leading to the development of endomyocardial fibrosis. The role of trace elements is not yet established.[59]

Clinical features
These depend on the stage of the disease and the anatomical distortion of the affected ventricle(s), together with the resultant effects on cardiac function.

Initial illness
Some patients have a febrile illness with facial swelling, and symptoms of pulmonary venous congestion. This can be fatal within months, but little is known about this phase of the disease.[54]

Left ventricular disease
The ventricle is not enlarged and there are inevitably, in almost every case, signs of mitral valvular incompetence with a loud pulmonary closure sound, and progressive pulmonary hypertension. A third heart sound is usual—early and crisp, and is dominant when the physiological pattern is a restricted ventricle.

Right ventricular disease
The classical picture, described from Ibadan, is of a young patient, often with delayed puberty, slight exophthalmos, central cyanosis, no peripheral oedema and massive ascites. Many cases of established right ventricular EMF are at first missed because the ascites is so dominant and the jugular pressure so high that it is missed clinically. The jugular systolic wave, secondary to tricuspid regurgitation, may even move the ear lobe. The arterial pulse has a small pulse pressure and atrial fibrillation is common. The heart may be impalpable either because there is a large pericardial effusion or because it is rotated by the massive right atrium, which lies under the sternum, so that the left ventricle lies more posteriorly. There may be no murmur at the defunct tricuspid valve but only an abrupt third heart sound.

Investigations
The stage and site of disease determine findings on the chest radiograph; these vary from a massive cardiac shadow (aneurysmal right atrium or pericardial effusion) (Figure 12.2) to an almost normal heart with perhaps a prominent pulmonary artery. Echocardiography[60] is valuable as it shows distinctive patterns.

Management
Established disease
Cardiac surgery[61] is economically adventurous, but it is clinically logical in deforming inactive disease.

The acute illness
Treatment aims to maintain cardiac function and possibly suppress the eosinophilia with corticosteroids.

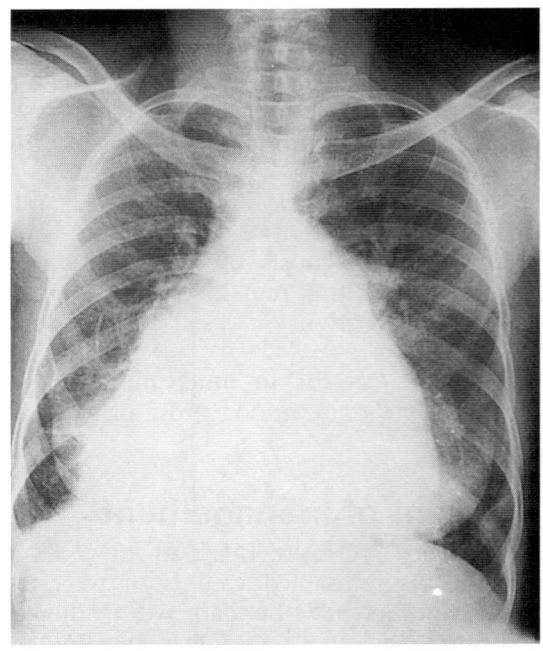

Figure 12.2: Biventricular endomyocardial fibrosis: the cardiac shadow is totally distorted with the enlarged right atrium prominent.

Pericardial disease

In the tropics the two important forms of pericarditis are both secondary to a major infection: (1) acute pyogenic pericarditis; and (2) tuberculous pericarditis, which has been catapulted into prominence by HIV. Rarely, pericarditis complicates amoebic liver abscess.

Pyogenic pericarditis

The pericardium is affected in a bacteraemia associated with a pyogenic infection, for example pyomyositis, lobar pneumonia or pelvic infection, when local and systemic signs are dominant and pericarditis may not be recognized until it causes circulatory effects.

Clinical features

These depend on whether or not there is a pericardial effusion and the speed at which this has formed. If the fluid forms quickly, the parietal pericardium cannot stretch adequately to accommodate it and symptoms and signs of cardiac tamponade develop. The heart is compressed and the signs therefore depend on obstruction to venous inflow and a subsequent fall in stroke output, cardiac tamponade. There may be evidence of pericarditis—a pericardial rub, or signs of fluid, dullness to percussion at the right border of the sternum, an impalpable cardiac impulse and very quiet heart sounds.

Management

In an uncomplicated effusion, in a district hospital without echocardiography, a chest radiograph may reveal a large cardiac shadow but this may be difficult to interpret if there is lobar pneumonia or a pleural effusion (Figure 12.3). Pericardial purulent fluid confirms the diagnosis; it should be aspirated totally by the epigastric approach, with the patient sitting up in bed. Use a 50 ml or 20 ml syringe with a long needle fitted with a two-way tap so that fluid can easily be expelled. Aspirate daily, but be prepared to transfer the patient to a cardiac surgical unit if there are persistent signs of fluid or cardiac compression. Early diagnosis with aspiration and instillation of the appropriate antibiotic into the pericardial sac may prevent this.

In pericardial effusion with cardiac tamponade the fluid must be aspirated immediately and completely.

Tuberculous pericarditis

This is now a major problem in patients with HIV infection. Before the HIV epidemic an unusually high prevalence was described in Transkei.[21] *Mycobacterium tuberculosis* reaches the pericardium from adjacent lymph nodes or possibly pleura.

Clinical picture

This depends on the stage of the disease. Many patients

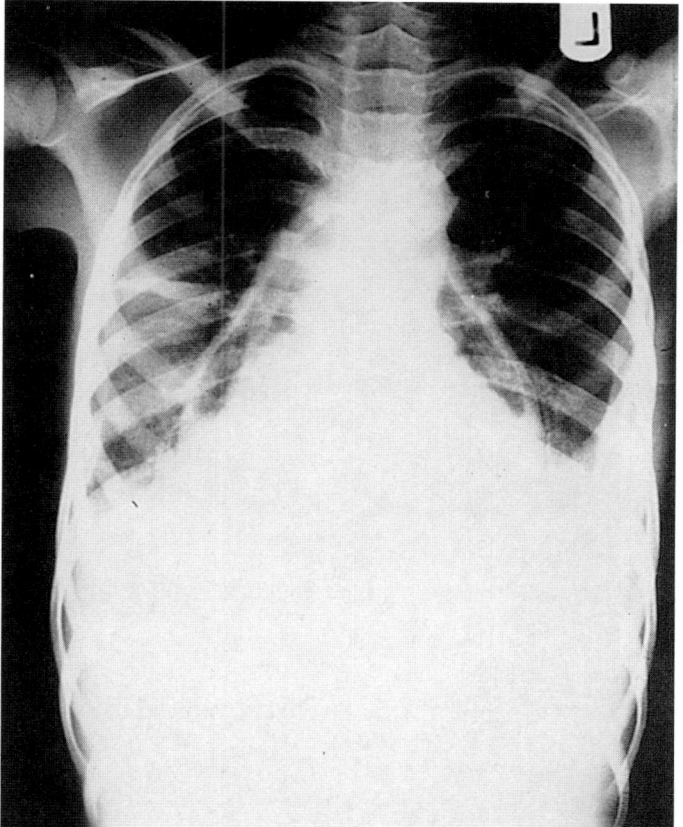

Figure 12.3: Pyogenic pericarditis. Note thickness of pericardium and the associated pleural effusion and pulmonary changes.

present late and are thought to have liver disease because they are wasted and have tense ascites, or because the jugular venous pressure is not examined, or is very high. Those who have HIV/AIDS often show evidence of early pericardial infection, with a pericardial rub and some precordial pain. Most patients have a pericardial effusion which may be large or small, with underlying pericardial fibrosis. This is constrictive pericarditis with its distinctive signs: a small arterial pulse pressure, sometimes with pulsus paradoxus, and a venous pulse which has a high pressure and can be seen to fall sharply immediately after carotid pulsation (*y* descent): the heart may be impalpable and, when constriction is established, a third heart sound is audible.

Diagnosis

In patients with HIV/AIDS, signs of pericarditis must be assumed to be caused by tuberculosis. Aspiration of pericardial fluid is helpful: the fluid has a high protein content around 40 g/litre and in about 80% of cases it is bloodstained; the cells are lymphocytes. There is no characteristic chest radiograph: this depends on the volume of pericardial fluid, the presence of a pleural effusion, and whether the pericardium has calcified or not (Figure 12.4).

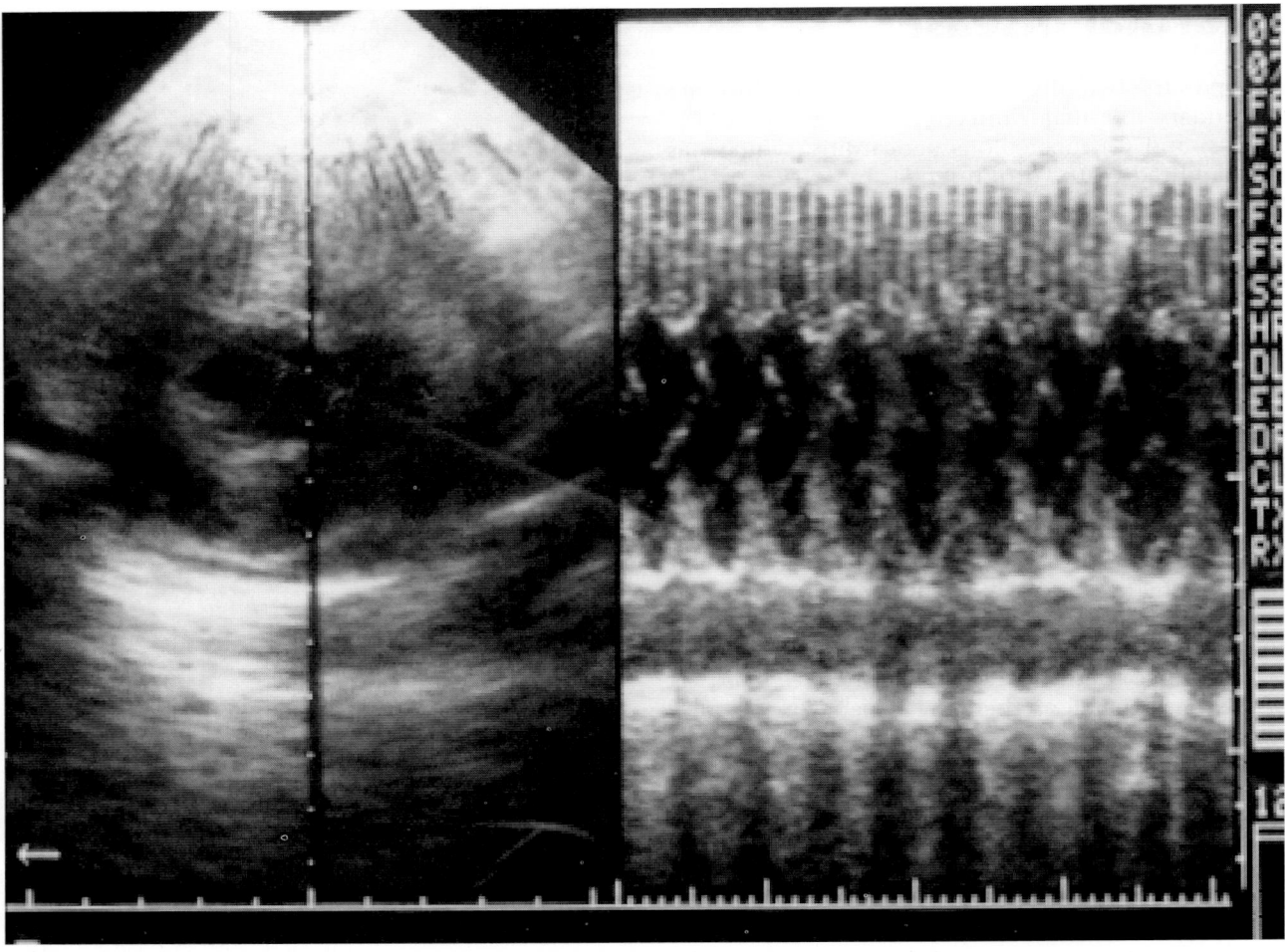

Figure 12.4: Echocardiogram of a 37-year-old Nigerian woman showing a large pericardial effusion (PE) due to tuberculous pericarditis. She had an effusive, constrictive pericarditis; there was a good response to antituberculosis therapy and pericardiectomy.

Management

Give antituberculosis drugs with corticosteroids—Strang showed that steroids prevent constriction.[62,63] The currently recommended initial dose is prednisolone 2 mg/kg. The course of steroids is 11 weeks. This makes patients rapidly better, constriction is prevented, and pericardial fluid disappears.

Other Infections

Viruses

There is nothing distinctive about viral pericarditis in the tropics.

Meningococcus

Signs of pericarditis may be detected in patients with meningococcal disease who have bacteraemia and antigenaemia. Immune complexes are formed and are deposited on the pericardium. The pericarditis is transient and the prognosis is dominated by the severity of infection.

Parasites

Rarely trophozoites of *Entamoeba histolytica* reach the pericardium from an adjacent liver abscess. The prognosis is bad. Pericardial tamponade demands urgent aspiration. Metronidazole and chloroquine orally, and metronidazole injected into the pericardial sac, have been advocated for treatment.

Arterial disease
Aorta and large arteries

Idiopathic 'tropical' aortitis is more common in the tropics, particularly in Asian countries: Malaysia,[64] Thailand, Singapore, Korea, China and India,[65] where some cases are named Takayasu's disease. It has been described in many African countries, with notable studies in South Africa.[66,67] Whether the disease in Asia is the same as that seen in African countries is not known. The question is: what are the triggers for the disease?

The clinical features are determined by the pathological/ anatomical damage to the aorta and its large branches, so that regional ischaemia in a tissue or organ is the most common clinical presentation. Imaging shows aneurysmally dilated or stenosed segments of aorta with an irregular lumen so that the orifices of any of its branches may be occluded.

The disease affects the abdominal aorta in over 90% of cases, the subclavian arteries in over 60%, and renal arteries in over 80%.

Pathogenesis

The cause of the arteritis is not known. There is a systemic inflammatory phase in some patients, and the morphological changes are those of a giant-cell arteritis. Therefore, while an immune mechanism has been suggested (an associated glomerulonephritis in some patients may be suggestive evidence), there are no consistent markers of an immune reaction. HLA-B5 has been linked to both Takayasu's disease and HLA-DRB1 in Buerger's disease.

Clinical features

The symptoms depend on the artery affected. Most patients are young adults; in some series women predominate. About one-third have hypertension,[65] and another third have visual symptoms. Physical signs depend on the vessel affected, for example, a renal arterial bruit.

Management

The arteritis is widespread and treatment is unlikely to help, but in advanced hospitals angioplasty or an arterial bypass can be advised for limited disease, for example renal arterial disease with severe hypertension.

Coronary arterial disease

The remarkable differences in the prevalence of coronary artery diseases between different countries in the tropics have led to many comparative studies. Similarly, the pattern of disease is changing as countries become industrialized and where habits and diet are changing.

Clinically, coronary arterial disease causes the same symptoms, whether in tropical or temperate countries. Cardiac pain on effort, however, in a patient who is at low risk—a young adult from a rural African community—may cause a problem with diagnosis. Severe anaemia from untreated heavy hookworm infection can lead to a qualitative defect in coronary arterial flow in spite of a greatly increased cardiac output. In a patient who is not anaemic the orifices of the coronary arteries or their lumina may be occluded or stenosed. Tropical or syphilitic aortitis may involve the orifice(s); the lumen may be occluded by emboli in rheumatic cardiac disease or dilated cardiomyopathy with a left ventricular mural or cavitary thrombus. A rare curiosity which may distort a coronary artery is annular subvalvular aneurysm of the left ventricle.[68] This has been seen in a number of tropical countries; a pouch forms and enlarges so that it may stretch the circumflex branch of the left coronary artery, appear as a rounded shadow on the left ventricle—in a chest radiograph—or grow into the septum. Mural thrombi form and may partially fill the aneurysm and lead to systemic emboli.

Left ventricular cavitary thrombus

Originally described at autopsy in Senegal in patients with dilated cardiomyopathy, these thrombi are now being detected by echocardiography in similar cases in West Africa and in patients with peripartum cardiac failure. In some, streptokinase has been remarkably effective.

REFERENCES

1 Astagneau P, Lang T, Delarocque E et al. Arterial hypertension in urban Africa: an epidemiological study on a representative sample of Dakar inhabitants in Senegal. *J Hypertens* 1992; 10:1095–1101.

2 Hakim J G & Manyemba J. Cardiac disease distribution among patients referred for echocardiography in Harare, Zimbabwe. *Cent Afr J Med* 1998; 44:140–144.

3 Lodenyo H A, McLigeyo S O & Ogola E N. Cardiovascular disease in elderly in-patients at the Kenyatta National Hospital, Nairobi, Kenya. *E Afr Med J* 1997; 647–651.

4 Stephen S J. Changing patterns of mitral stenosis in childhood and pregnancy in Sri Lanka. *J Am Coll Cardiol* 1992; 19:1276–1284.

5 Amoah G B & Kallen C. Aetiology of heart failure as seen from a national cardiac referral centre in Africa. *Cardiology* 2000; 93:11–18.

6 Swai A B, McLarty D G, Kitange H M et al. Low prevalence of risk factors for coronary heart disease in rural Tanzania. *Int J Epidemiol* 1993; 22: 651–659.

7 Silva-Cardoso J, Moura B, Martins L et al. Pericardial involvement in human immunodeficiency virus infection *Chest* 1999; 18: 415–422.

8 Adoh A, Kouassi-Yapo F, N'Dori R et al. Etiologie des artériopathies des membres inférieurs chez les Noirs Africains à Abidjan. *Cardiol Trop* 1991; 17:59–65.

9 Barbosa M M, Lamounier J A, Oliveira E C et al. Pulmonary hypertension in schistosomiasis mansoni. *Trans R Soc Trop Med Hyg* 1996; 90:663–665.

10 Carapetris J R, Wolf D R & Currie B J. Acute rheumatic fever and rheumatic heart disease in Top End of Australia's Northern Territory. *Med J Aust* 1996; 164:146–149.

11 Ibrahim Khalil S, Elhaq M, Ali E et al. An epidemiological survey of rheumatic fever and rheumatic heart disease in Sahafa Town, Sudan. *J Epidemiol Community Health* 1992; 46:477–479.

12 Ilyas M, Peracha M A, Ahmed R et al. Prevalence and pattern of rheumatic heart disease in the frontier province of Pakistan. *JPMA* 1979; 29:165–198.

13 Quinn R W. Comprehensive review of morbidity and mortality trends for rheumatic fever, streptococcal disease, and scarlet fever: the decline of rheumatic fever. *Rev Infect Dis* 1989; 11:928–953.

14 Majeed H A, Batnager S, Yousof A M et al. Acute rheumatic fever and the evolution of rheumatic heart disease: a prospective 12 year follow-up report. *J Clin Epidemiol* 1992; 45:871–875.

15 Chauvet J, Kakou Guikahue M, Aka F et al. La gravité des cardites rheumatismales à Abidjan. A propos de 52 cas à Abidjan chez les enfants de moins de 15 ans. *Cardiol Trop* 1989; 15:77–81.

16 Serme D. Etude épidémiologique, clinique et évolutive de valvulopathies rheumatismales observées à Ouagadougou. *Cardiol Trop* 1992; 18:93–99.

17 Rutakingirwa M, Ziegler J L, Newton R et al. Poverty and eosinophilia are risk factors for endomyocardial fibrosis in Uganda. *Trop Med Int Health* 1999; 4:229–235.

18 Edington M E & Gear J S S. Rheumatic heart disease in Soweto: a programme for secondary prevention. *S Afr Med J* 1982; 62:523–525.

19 Bach J F, Chalons S, Forier E et al. 10-year educational programme aimed at rheumatic fever in two French Caribbean islands. *Lancet* 1996; 347:644–648.

20 Stollerman G H. Rheumatic fever. *Lancet* 1997;349: 935–942.

21 Strang J I G. Tuberculous pericarditis in Transkei. *Clin Cardiol* 1984; 7:667–670.

22 Sagie A, Frietas N, Padial L R et al. Doppler echocardiographic assessment of long term progression of mitral stenosis in 103 patients: valve area and right heart disease. *J Am Coll Cardiol* 1996; 28:472–479.

23 Malu K, Ticolat R, Renambot I et al. Enquête épidémiologique sur les myocardopathies chroniques dilatées primitives: 69 cas. *Cardiol Trop* 1991; 17:127–132.

24 Martinez-Garcia T, Sobrino JM, Pujol E et al. Ventricular mass and diastolic function in patients infected by the human immunodeficiency virus. *Heart* 2000; 84:620–624.

25 Davidson N McD & Parry E H O. Peripartum cardiac failure. *Q J Med* 1979; 47:431–461.

26 Marin-Neto J A, Maciel B C, Teran Urbanetz L L et al. High output failure in patients with peripartum cardiomyopathy: a comparative study with dilated cardiomyopathy. *Am Heart J* 1991; 121:134–140.

27 Cenac A & Djibo A. Postpartum cardiac failure in Sudanese–Sahelian Africa: clinical prevalence in western Niger. *Am J Trop Med Hyg* 1998; 58:319–323.

28 Desai D, Moodley J, Naidoo D. Peripartum cardiomyopathy: experiences at King Edward VIII Hospital, Durban, South Africa and a review of the literature. *Trop Doct* 1995; 25:118–123.

29 Homans D C. Current concepts: peripartum cardiomyopathy. *N Engl J Med* 1985; 312:1432–1437.

30 Midei M G, De Ment S H, Feldman A M et al. Peripartum myocarditis and cardiomyopathy. *Circulation* 1990; 81:922–926.

31 Sanderson J E, Olsen E G J & Gatei D. Peripartum heart disease: an endomyocardial biopsy study. *Br Heart J* 1986; 56:285–291.

32 Sanderson J E, Adesanya C O, Anjorin F I et al. Postpartum cardiac failure—heart failure due to volume overload? *Am Heart J* 1979; 97:613–621.

33 Albanesi Filho F M & da Silva T T. Natural course of subsequent pregnancy after peripartum cardiomyopathy. *Arq Bras Cardiol* 1999; 73:47–57.

34 Ford L, Abdullahi A, Anjorin F I et al. The outcome of peripartum cardiac failure in Zaria, Nigeria. *Q J Med* 1998; 91:93–103.

35 Sutton M St J, Cole P & Plappert M. Effects of subsequent pregnancy on left ventricular function in peripartum cardiomyopathy. *Am Heart J* 1991; 121:1776–1778.

36 Edwards R, Unwin N, Mugusi F et al. Hypertension prevalence and care in an urban and rural area of Tanzania. *J Hypertens* 2000; 18:145–152.

37 Poulter N R, Khaw K T, Hopwood B E C et al. The Kenya Luo migration study: observations of the initiation of a rise in blood pressure. *BMJ* 1990; 309:967–972.

38 Olubodun J O, Akingbade O A & Abiola O O. Salt intake and blood pressure in Nigerian hypertensive patients. *Int J Cardiol* 1997; 59:185–188.

39 Cooper R S, Rotimi C N, Ataman S L et al. The prevalence of hypertension in seven populations of West African origin. *Am J Public Health* 1997; 87:160–168.

40 Cooper R S, Rotimi C N, Kaufman J S et al. Hypertension treatment and control in sub-Saharan Africa: the epidemiological basis for policy. *BMJ* 1998; 316:614–617.

41 James S A, de Almeida-Filho N & Kaufman J S. Hypertension in Brazil: a review of the epidemiological evidence. *Ethn Dis* 1991; 1:91–98.

42 Kaufman J S, Rotimi C N, Brieger W R, Oladokum M A, Kadiri S, Osotimehin B O & Cooper R S. The mortality risk associated with hypertension: preliminary results of a prospective study in rural Nigeria. *J Hum Hypertens* 1996; 10:461–464.

43 Mtabaji J P, Nara Y & Yamori Y. The cardiac study in Tanzania: salt intake in the causation and treatment of hypertension. *J Hum Hypertens* 1990; 4:80–81.

44 Walker R W, McLarty D G, Kitange H M et al. Stroke mortality in urban and rural Tanzania *Lancet* 2000; 355:1684–1687.

45 Falase A O, Ayeni O, Sekoni G A et al. Heart failure in Nigerian hypertensives. *Afr J Med Sci* 1983; 12:7–15.

46 Plange-Rhule J, Phillips R, Achaempong J et al. Hypertension and renal failure in Kumasi, Ghana. *J Hum Hypertens* 1999; 13:37–40.

47 Maro E E & Lwakatare J. Medication compliance among Tanzanian hypertensives. *E Afr Med J* 1997; 539–542.

48 Connor D H, Somers K, Hutt M S R et al. Endomyocardial fibrosis in Uganda (Davises' disease). *Am Heart J* 1968; 75:107–124.

49 Connor D H, Somers K, Hutt M S R et al. Endomyocardial fibrosis in Uganda (Davises' disease). *Am Heart J* 1967; 74:687–700.

50 Po-chun Tai, Spry C J F, Olsen E G J et al. Deposits of eosinophil granule proteins in cardiac tissues of patients with endomyocardial fibrosis. *Lancet* 1987; i:643–647.

51 Guimaraes A C, Esteves J P, Filho A S et al. Clinical aspects of endomyocardial fibrosis in Bahia, Brazil. *Am Heart J* 1971; 81:7–19.

52 Spry C J F. Eosinophils in eosinophilic endomyocardial disease. *Postgrad Med J* 1987; 62:609–613.

53 Andy J J, Ogunowo P O, Akpan N A et al. Helminth associated hypereosinophilia and tropical endomyocardial fibrosis (EMF) in Nigeria. *Acta Trop* 1998; 69:127–140.

54 Andy J J, Bishara F F. Observations on clinical features of early disease of African endomyocardial fibrosis. *Cardiol Trop* 1982; 8:23–33.

55 Parry E H O & Abrahams D G. The natural history of endomyocardial fibrosis. *Q J Med* 1965; 34:383–408.

56 Canesin M F, Gama R F, Smith D L et al. Endomyocardial fibrosis associated with massive calcification of the left ventricle. *Arq Bras Cardiol* 1999; 73:499–506.

57 Shaper A G & Coles R M. The tribal distribution of endomyocardial fibrosis in Uganda. *Br Heart J* 1965; 27:121–127.

58 Patel A K, Ziegler J L, D'Arbela P G et al. Familial cases of endomyocardial fibrosis in Uganda. *BMJ* 1971; 4:331–334.

59 Kartha C C, Eapen J T, Radhakumary C et al. Pattern of cardiac fibrosis in rabbits periodically fed a magnesium-restricted diet and administered rare earth chloride through drinking water. *Biol Trace Elem Res* 1998; 63:19–30.

60 Berenzstein C, Pineiro D, Marcotegui M et al. Usefulness of echocardiography and Doppler echocardiography in endomyocardial fibrosis. *J Am Soc Echocardiogr* 2000; 13:385–392.

61 Moraes F, Lapa C, Hazin S et al. Surgery for endomyocardial fibrosis revisited. *Eur J Cardiothorac Surg* 1999; 15:309–312.

62 Strang J I G, Gibson D G, Nunn A J et al. Controlled trial of prednisolone as adjuvant in treatment of tuberculous constrictive pericarditis in Transkei. *Lancet* 1987; i:1418–1422.

63 Strang J I G, Gibson D G, Mitchison D A et al. Controlled clinical trial of complete open surgical drainage and of prednisolone in treatment of tuberculous pericardial effusion in Transkei. *Lancet* 1988; ii:759–764.

64 Danaraj T J, Wong H O & Thomas M A. Primary arteritis of aorta causing renal artery stenosis and hypertension. *Br Heart J* 1963; 25:153–165.

65 Chugh K S, Jain S, Sakhuja V et al. Renovascular hypertension due to Takayasu's arteritis among Indian patients. *Q J Med* 1992; 85:833–843.

66 Isaacson C A. An idiopathic aortitis in young Africans. *J Pathol Bacteriol* 1961; 81:69–79.

67 Schrire V & Asherson R A. Arteritis of the aorta and its major branches. *Q J Med* 1964; 33:439–463.

68 Abrahams D G, Barton J, Cockshott W P et al. Annular subvalvular left ventricular aneurysms. *Q J Med* 1962; 31:345–360.

Chapter 13
Haematological Diseases in the Tropics

A. F. Fleming and P. S. de Silva

Reference ranges

The normal values of red cell counts and indices, white cell counts, platelet counts and activities of haemostatic mechanisms vary with age, sex and pregnancy state.[1,2] There are also genetic and common environmental factors which can affect the reference ranges in certain populations.[3] It is especially important that the difference in reference ranges in all stages of life be appreciated by health workers in tropical countries, where up to half the population are aged under 15 years and women experience numerous and often complicated pregnancies.

Red cell values

Age
Full-term infants
Red cell values of the fetus are almost unchanged during the last trimester of pregnancy. The full-term infant is born with a high haemoglobin (Hb) concentration, red blood cell (RBC) count and mean cell volume (MCV) (Table 13.1). A rapid rate of red cell production and low splenic function are shown by the presence of nucleated RBCs, occasional Howell–Jolly bodies (red cell nuclear fragments), polychromasia, a high reticulocyte count (mean 150×10^9/litre) and target cells in the peripheral blood. In the first few hours of life, the Hb concentration of capillary blood is on average 35 g/litre higher than in venous blood, due to haemoconcentration. If the blood from the placenta is allowed to transfuse into the infant, the Hb rises about 10–20 g/litre.

The blood volume ranges from 50 to 100 ml (mean 85 ml) per kilogram body weight.

During the first few weeks of life, the ability of the blood to deliver oxygen is in excess of what is required, so that erythropoietin secretion is low and the bone marrow is relatively hypoplastic. Red cell survival is short: 80–100 days compared with 90–150 (mean 120) days in adults. Plasma volume increases as the infant grows. As a consequence, the Hb, packed cell volume (PCV) and RBC count decline to reach a nadir between 8 and 12 weeks of life. The large fetal red cells are replaced, and the MCV declines (Table 13.1). Fetal haemoglobin (HbF) is replaced by adult haemoglobin (HbA) (Table 13.2).[4]

Premature infants
Infants born prematurely during the third trimester have red cell values initially the same as those of full-term infants. However, their basal metabolic rates, oxygen consumption, erythropoietin secretion, red cell production and red cell survival (60–80 days) are all lower. After birth, red cell values fall faster and to lower levels than in mature infants: at around 8 weeks of life the most premature but otherwise normal and well-nourished infant can have an Hb as low as 70 g/litre (Table 13.3).[2]

Table 13.1 Red blood cell values at various ages.

	Hb (g/l)	PCV (l/l)	RBC (× 10¹²/l)	MCV (fl)	MCH (pg)	MCHC (g/l)
Birth (cord blood)	165 ± 30	0.54 ± 0.10	6.0 ± 1.0	120 (mean)	–	300 ± 27
3 months	115 ± 20	0.38 ± 0.04	4.0 ± 0.8	95 (mean)	29 ± 5	325 ± 25
1 year	120 ± 15	–	4.4 ± 0.08	78 ± 8	27 ± 4	325 ± 25
3–6 years	130 ± 10	0.40 ± 0.04	4.8 ± 0.7	84 ± 8	27 ± 3	325 ± 25
10–12 years	130 ± 15	0.41 ± 0.04	4.7 ± 0.7	84 ± 7	27 ± 3	325 ± 25
Men	155 ± 25	0.47 ± 0.07	5.5 ± 1.0	86 ± 10	29.5 ± 2.5	325 ± 25
Women	140 ± 25	0.42 ± 0.05	4.8 ± 1.0	86 ± 10	29.5 ± 2.5	325 ± 25

Values are mean ± 2 SD (95% range).
Hb, haemoglobin; MCH, mean cell haemoglobin; MCHC, mean cell haemoglobin concentration; MCV, mean cell volume; PCV, packed cell volume (haematocrit); RBC, red blood cell count.
Reproduced with permission of the authors and publishers from Lewis et al. (eds) Dacie & Lewis's Practical Haematology 9th edn, London: Churchill Livingstone, 2001.[1]

Table 13.2 Proportion of haemoglobin F found at various ages.

Age	HbF (%)
Birth	70–90
1 month	50–75
2 months	25–60
3 months	10–35
4 months	5–20
6 months	<8
9 months	<5
1 year	<2
Adults	<0.4

Reproduced with permission of the author and publishers from Huehns.[4]

Table 13.3 Haemoglobin (g/litre) observed in iron-sufficient preterm infants.

Age	Birthweight (g) 1000–1500	1501–2000
2 weeks	163 (117–184)	148 (188–196)
1 month	109 (87–152)	115 (82–150)
2 months	88 (71–115)	94 (80–114)
3 months	98 (89–112)	102 (93–118)
4 months	113 (91–131)	113 (91–131)
5 months	116 (102–143)	118 (104–130)
6 months	120 (94–138)	118 (107–126)

Values are mean (range).
Reproduced with permission of the authors and publishers from Lundström U, Siimes M A & Dallman P R. *J. Pediatr* 1977; 91:878–883.

Childhood

After the third month of life, oxygen needs exceed oxygen delivery and provide the necessary stimulus to erythropoietin secretion and red cell production: the Hb, PCV and RBC count rise steadily until puberty (Table 13.1).

Sex

The Hb continues to rise in boys but levels off in girls at puberty, so that men have on average Hb 15 g/litre higher than non-pregnant women (Table 13.1). Red cell volumes are 30 ± 5 ml/kg in men and 25 ± 5 ml/kg in women; plasma volume (45 ± 5 ml/kg) and total blood volume (70 ± 10 ml/kg) are the same in both sexes. Testosterone is the stimulus to additional erythropoiesis in men, whereas oestrogen depresses erythropoiesis.

Pregnancy

From the 12th week of gestation there is an increase of erythropoietin secretion, erythroid hyperplasia, reticulocytosis (2–6%) and an increase of the total red cell volume by 400–450 ml in normal and iron-sufficient pregnant women. The plasma volume increases also, by

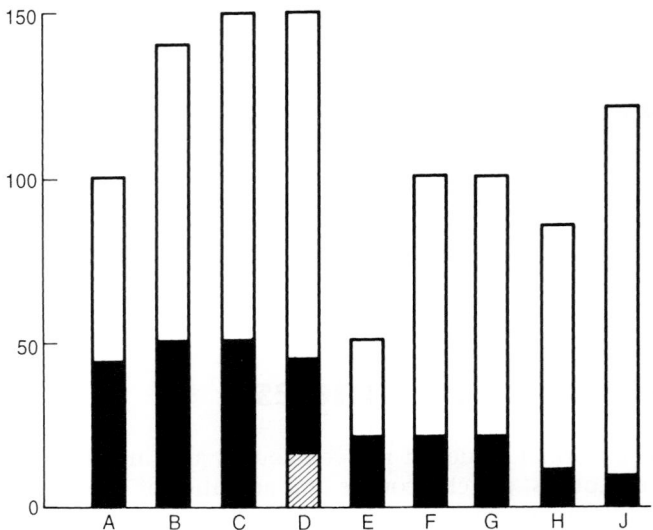

Figure 13.1: Blood volume changes in health and disease. (**A**) Normal (non-pregnant) adult. (**B**) Normal single pregnancy. (**C**) Normal twin pregnancy. (**D**) Hypersplenism, not anaemic. (**E**) Acute haemorrhage. (**F**) Acute haemorrhage, 48 hours later. (**G**) Moderate anaemia. (**H**) Severe anaemia. (**J**) Severe anaemia with circulatory congestion. Note that two or more of these conditions may be present in the same patient; in particular E–J are variations on A (non-pregnant), but could be shown again as variants on B (pregnant), C (multiple pregnancy) or D (hypersplenism). Solid bars, red cells; hatched bar, red cells sequestered in the spleen; white bars, plasma. (Reproduced with permission of the publisher from Fleming A F. In Parry E H O (ed.) *Principles of Medicine of Africa,* 2nd edn. Oxford: Oxford University Press, 1984: 706).

about 1250 ml in primigravidae and 1500 ml in multigravidae. As the increase in plasma volume is greater than that of the red cell volume, there is haemodilution (Figure 13.1 B, C): Hb 110 g/litre and PCV 0.31 are the accepted lower limits of normal. There is a mild macrocytosis (increase of MCV) during pregnancy.[5]

Genetic and environmental differences

When large series of persons of European descent (whites) and of sub-Saharan African descent (blacks) have been matched for age, sex, pregnant state and socio-economic status, it has been found that at all ages and in both sexes blacks have on average Hb 5–10 g/litre lower than whites, and that this difference is independent of environment. A high frequency of α^+ thalassaemia, up to 50% of some black populations, explains this small genetically determined difference.

Of much greater importance are environmental factors, including malaria, other intercurrent infections and malnutrition, especially deficiencies of iron and folic acid. Apparently healthy members of communities living in the tropics frequently show an average Hb 20 g/litre lower at all ages and in both sexes than the internationally accepted reference means. The control of malaria, improvements in hygiene and nutrition, and rises in social class are all associated with the range of Hb concentrations increasing towards the standard ranges.[3]

Altitude
For every 1000 m above sea level, the Hb increases on average by 2.5 g/litre, due to low oxygen tension stimulating erythropoietin production.

Miscellaneous factors
The Hb rises slightly with muscular exercise and in assuming the upright posture. It is somewhat higher in the morning than the evening. It is lower in athletes in training, and is raised in tobacco-smokers.

White cell count

Neutrophils

Age
There is a transiently high total white blood cell (WBC) count and a neutrophil leucocytosis at and following birth, peaking at about 12 hours of life (Table 13.4), with a high number of non-segmented neutrophils (up to 1.8×10^9/litre). The number of neutrophils declines and is exceeded by the lymphocyte count after 2 weeks. From 2 years, the number of circulating neutrophils increases with age until adult life, when they contribute 40–75% of the total count of $4.0–11.0 \times 10^9$/litre in Caucasian adults.[2]

Sex
Women during their reproductive period of life have slightly higher WBC and neutrophil counts (average difference 0.66×10^9/litre) than men, and oral contraceptives increase counts further: there are two peaks of neutrophil leucocytosis coinciding with peaks of oestrogen secretion and a fall following menstruation. Postmenopausal women have counts slightly lower than men.

Pregnancy
The WBC and neutrophil counts rise to a plateau by the second trimester (WBC mean 9.0×10^9/litre, range $5.0–16.0 \times 10^9$/litre; neutrophils mean 7.0×10^9/litre, range $2.5–14.0 \times 10^9$/litre) (Figure 13.2).[5] There is a sharp peak of neutrophil leucocytosis during obstetric delivery, when the total WBC count may reach 40×10^9/litre in an uninfected patient. Neutrophil and total WBC counts fall to non-pregnant levels by the sixth day post partum. The circulating neutrophils in pregnant women are relatively young, with a shift to the left (< 3% metamyelocytes and myelocytes), raised activity of neutrophil alkaline phosphatase and other enzymes and enhanced bactericidal function.

Genetic and environmental factors
A relative and absolute neutropenia has been described in children over 6 months and adults who are black Africans or of black African descent in the Americas and Europe (Table 13.5),[3] and in Palestinians, Yemeni Jews and Saudi Arabians. The total body neutrophils have been found to be the same in adults of West Indian origin living in the UK as in the white Britons, but the West Indians have a greater number of neutrophils in the bone marrow storage pool, while Europeans have more in circulation; provocation of a neutrophil response, either experimentally or by natural infection, leads to rises to the

Table 13.4 Normal leucocyte counts.

Age	Total leucocytes Mean	(range)	Neutrophils Mean	(range)	%	Lymphocytes Mean	range	%	Monocytes Mean	%	Eosinophils Mean	%
Birth	18.1	(9.0–30.0)	11.0	(6.0–26.0)	61	5.5	(2.0–11.0)	31	1.1	6	0.4	2
12 hours	22.8	(13.0–38.0)	15.5	(6.0–28.0)	68	5.5	(2.0–11.0)	24	1.2	5	0.5	2
24 hours	18.9	(9.4–34.0)	11.5	(5.0–21.0)	61	5.8	(2.0–11.5)	31	1.1	6	0.5	2
1 week	12.2	(5.0–21.0)	5.5	(1.5–10.0)	45	5.0	(2.0–17.0)	41	1.1	9	0.5	4
2 weeks	11.4	(5.0–20.0)	4.5	(1.0–9.5)	40	5.5	(2.0–17.0)	48	1.0	9	0.4	3
1 month	10.8	(5.0–19.5)	3.8	(1.0–9.0)	35	6.0	(2.0–16.5)	56	0.7	7	0.3	3
6 months	11.9	(6.0–17.5)	3.8	(1.0–8.5)	32	7.3	(4.0–13.5)	61	0.6	5	0.3	3
1 year	11.4	(6.0–17.5)	3.5	(1.5–8.5)	31	7.0	(4.0–10.5)	61	0.6	5	0.3	3
2 years	10.6	(6.0–17.0)	3.5	(1.5–8.5)	33	6.3	(3.0–9.5)	59	0.5	5	0.3	3
4 years	9.1	(5.5–15.5)	3.8	(1.5–8.5)	42	4.5	(2.0–8.0)	50	0.5	5	0.3	3
6 years	8.5	(5.0–14.5)	4.3	(1.5–8.0)	51	3.5	(1.5–7.0)	42	0.4	5	0.2	3
8 years	8.3	(4.5–13.5)	4.4	(1.5–8.0)	53	3.3	(1.5–6.8)	39	0.4	4	0.2	2
10 years	8.1	(4.5–13.5)	4.4	(1.8–8.0)	54	3.1	(1.5–6.5)	38	0.4	4	0.2	2
16 years	7.8	(4.5–13.0)	4.4	(1.8–8.0)	57	2.8	(1.2–5.2)	35	0.4	5	0.2	3
21 years	7.4	(4.5–11.0)	4.4	(1.8–7.7)	59	2.5	(1.0–4.8)	34	0.3	4	0.2	3

Values are mean (95% confidence limits) $\times 10^9$/litre and mean percentage of differential counts.
Reproduced with permission of the author, the publisher and W B Saunders. From Dallman P R. In Rudolph A M (ed.) *Pediatrics*, 16th edn. New York: Appleton-Century-Crofts, 1977:1178.

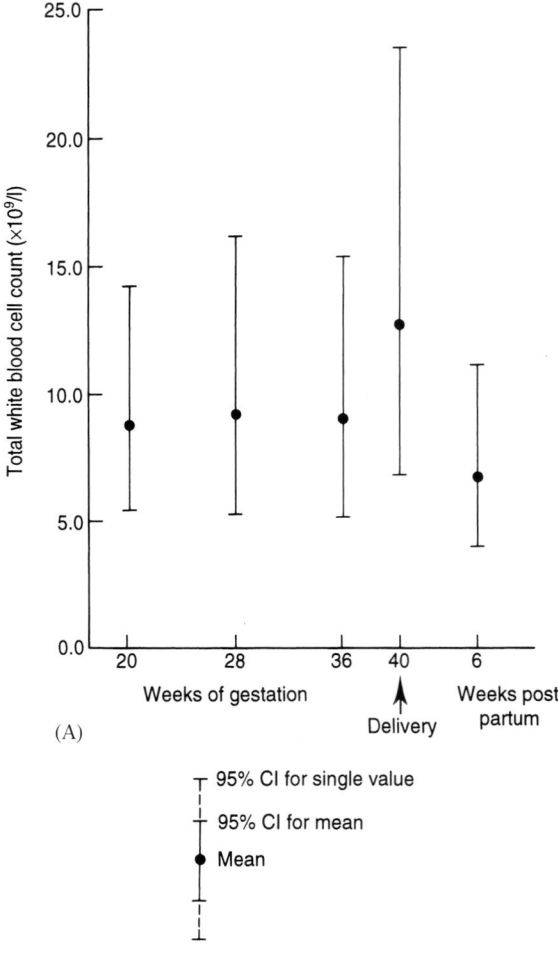

(A)

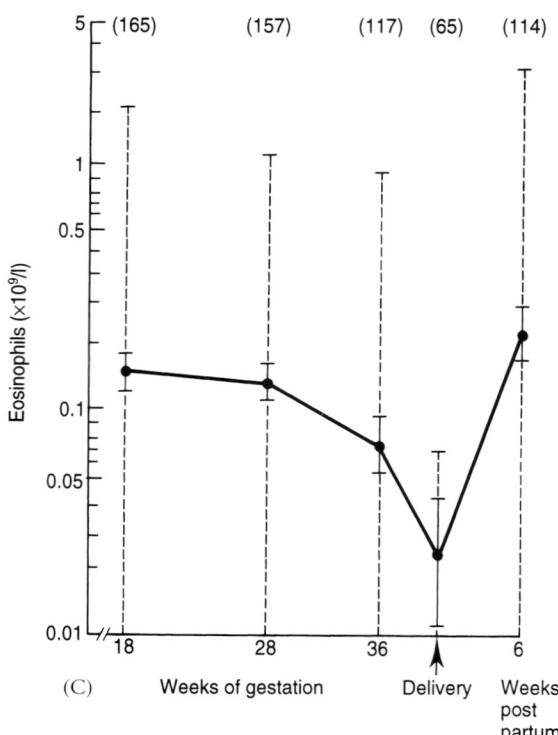

(C)

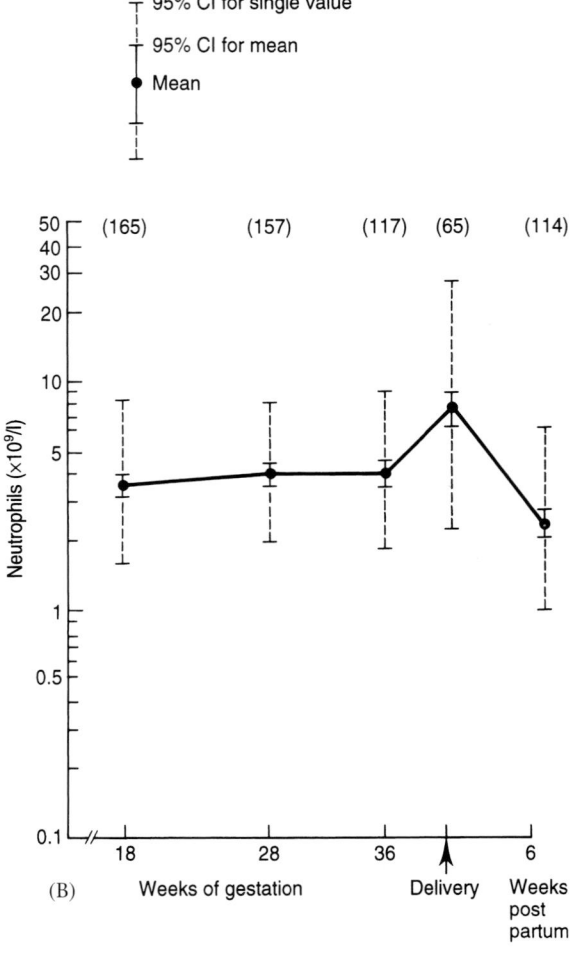

(B)

Figure 13.2: (**A**) Total white blood cell count (mean and 95% confidence limits for a single value) in 67 white Australian women during pregnancy. From Fleming.[5] (**B**) Absolute neutrophil counts and (**C**) absolute eosinophil counts in Nigerian primigravidae during pregnancy and the puerperium: numbers of observations are in parentheses. (Reproduced with permission from Fleming A F, Akintunde E A, Harrision K A & Dunn D. *E Afr Med J* 1985; 62:175–184.)

Table 13.5 Leucocyte counts in 123 non-elite male Nigerian blood donors in Zaria.

	Mean	(Range)	%
Total white cells	5.1	(2.6–10.2)	–
Neutrophils	2.8	(1.1–7.1)	30–85
Eosinophils	0.11	(0–2.0)	1–30
Basophils	0.002	(0–0.02)	0–1
Lymphocytes	2.1	(0.7–3.1)	15–60
Monocytes	0.13	(0–1.3)	0–8

Values are mean (95% confidence limits) $\times 10^9$/litre and range of percentage of differential counts.

same level in both races. There is probably a genetic factor underlying this ethnic neutropenia, but environmental factors may also play a role, for example those causing splenomegaly and hypersplenism. The neutrophil count rises with higher socioeconomic status in Africans, and declines in Europeans living in West Africa.

The WBC and neutrophil counts rise during pregnancy in African women, but remain about 3.0×10^9/litre lower than in pregnant Caucasians (Figure 13.2).

Miscellaneous factors

Counts are higher in the afternoon than in the morning, by about 0.5×10^9/litre. Exercise mobilizes the cells marginated on the endothelium, and so raises the number of circulating cells, even up to a WBC count of 30×10^9/litre with the most strenuous exertion. Emotional stress can raise counts transiently. Tobacco-smokers have persistently higher neutrophil counts.

Acute reactive neutrophil leucocytosis is seen most commonly in response to pyogenic infections (Table 13.6): immature neutrophils (metamyelocytes) are released from the bone marrow; there is an excess of deeply purple-staining primary cytoplasmic granules ('toxic granulation'); occasionally oval blue-staining Döhle bodies, which are RNA, are present in the cytoplasm. Neutrophil damage shows as ragged and vacuolated cytoplasm and pyknotic nuclei. With severe infections there can be a leukaemoid reaction, when the total count is above 80×10^9/litre with a shift to the left as far as promyelocytes and blast cells.

Eosinophils and basophils

The eosinophil count is high at birth and declines slowly throughout childhood to less than 0.4×10^9/litre in adult life (see Table 13.4).[2] There is a diurnal variation, more considerable than that of neutrophils. The eosinophil count is lower during pregnancy; the stress of obstetric delivery causes the eosinophils to vanish from the peripheral blood almost entirely, even if there was an initially high count (Figure 13.2). Symptom-free individuals living in the tropics often have high eosinophil counts due to subclinical infections by helminths (see Table 13.5); counts are higher in rural and non-elite groups than in urban and elite groups. In the tropics eosinophilia is more likely to be a response to

Table 13.6 Some causes of reactive leucocytosis.

Leucocytosis	Causes
Neutrophilia	Acute viral infections (e.g. poliomyelitis) Acute bacterial infections (e.g. staphylococcal) Tissue damage Haemorrhage Malignancies Stress states Diabetic ketoacidosis Miscellaneous (drugs, corticosteroids, chemicals, renal failure, collagen diseases) Pregnancy and delivery
Eosinophilia	Helminthic infections of tissues Löffler's syndrome (larval migration of nematodes) Convalescence from viral or other infections Malignancies Cytotoxic therapy Allergic disorders Miscellaneous (post splenectomy, familial, lead ingestion, polyarteritis nodosa, pulmonary aspergillosis, rheumatoid arthritis)
Basophilia	Miscellaneous (hypersensitivity, myxoedema, iron deficiency, chronic haemolysis)
Lymphocytosis	Childhood infections generally Protozoan infections (malaria, toxoplasmosis) Viral infections
Monocytosis	Protozoan infections (malaria) Rickettsial infections Subacute/chronic bacterial infections (tuberculosis, brucellosis, subacute bacterial endocarditis)

helminthic infection than to be an indication of allergy (Table 13.6).

The basophil count is normally low (see Table 13.4); accurate electronic counting demonstrates diminished counts during stress, pregnancy, acute infections and the administration of corticosteroids. A raised count is always suggestive of leukaemia or a myeloproliferative disorder, but may be seen in some allergic conditions (Table 13.6).

Lymphocytes

The lymphocyte count is normally high in the first year of life and then declines to adult levels (see Table 13.4). There are no reported differences between adult males and non-pregnant females, but the total lymphocyte count declines slightly during pregnancy; of more importance is a functional reduction of T cell-mediated immunity during pregnancy.

A proliferation of B cell lymphocytes is commonly seen in the tropics in response to malaria and other intercurrent infections, especially in childhood in rural and non-elite groups (Table 13.6). An absolute lympho-cytosis with numerous activated lymphocytes (plasmacytoid cells) is frequently seen in children in the tropics. Atypical lymphocytes with slate-grey or blue cytoplasm are suggestive of viral infections. African adults have a relative lymphocytosis, due to neutropenia, and often an absolute lymphocytosis (see Table 13.5). Of peripheral blood lymphocytes of adults in the industrialized countries, approximately 80% are T cells, 10–15% B cells and 5–10% null cells; rural Nigerians have been reported to have higher proportions of B cells (about 30%), whereas elite Nigerians and Europeans had similar distribution of lymphocyte subsets.

Monocytes

The monocyte count is highest during the first 2 weeks of life (see Table 13.4); there is no other significant physiological change, except a fall during obstetric delivery. In the tropics counts may be raised in association with subclinical protozoan or other infections or lowered in subjects with splenomegaly (see Tables 13.5 and 13.6).

Haemostasis

Age

Platelet counts (normal $150–400 \times 10^9$/litre) and function do not vary with age to any clinically significant degree.

Vitamin K is a fat-soluble vitamin, widely distributed in both vegetable and animal foods as well as being absorbed from that produced by the microbiological flora of the normal gut. Vitamin K levels of infants, especially premature infants, are critically low in the first 3 days of life because of a slow rate of transport across the placenta, low hepatic stores, the absence of an intestinal bacterial flora, and low concentrations in colostrum and breast

Table 13.7 Haemostatic measurements in the newborn and adults.

	Preterm infants	Full-term infants	Children over 2 months and adults
Platelets $\times 10^9$/litre	150–400	150–400	150–400
Prothrombin time (s)	13–18	12–16	11–14
Partial thromboplastin time (s)	35–50	30–45	23–35
Fibrinogen (g/litre)	2–4	2–4	2–4
FDP (mg/litre)	< 10	< 10	< 10

Reproduced with permission of the author and publishers from Buchanan G R. *Clin Haematol* 1978; 7:85–109.

milk. In addition, the immature liver has limited capacity for the synthesis of clotting factors. Vitamin K is essential for the synthesis by the liver of clotting factors (II, VII, IX and X) and protein C and protein S; these have low activity in umbilical cord blood, especially in preterm infants, so that the prothrombin time (PT) and partial thromboplastin time (PTT) are prolonged (Table 13.7).[2] Vitamin K-producing bacteria colonize the bowel and the deficiency is rectified usually by 72–120 hours. However, a few infants, especially the preterm, progress to haemor-rhagic disease of the newborn. Fibrinolytic activity is essentially functional in infants.

Sex

Platelet counts are higher in women than men by about 20%, and fall following menstruation.[1]

Pregnancy

Plasma volume expansion causes the platelet count to fall about 20% during pregnancy, but function remains unchanged. The activity of the extrinsic pathway is enhanced during pregnancy, with high levels of factors VII, X and fibrinogen. On the intrinsic pathway, activity of factors XII, IX and VIII are also moderately raised, but factor XI decreases. A decline of antithrombin III (AT III) adds to hypercoagulability in pregnancy, so that the thromboplastin generation time and PT are accelerated. This potential hypercoagulability is balanced by lower levels of factor XIII. Plasminogen levels are increased parallel to the rise of fibrinogen, while antiplasmin activity is unchanged. This potential for fibrinolysis is suppressed normally by the placenta producing inhibitors to plasminogen activator synthesis and release by endo-thelium. Fibrin/fibrinogen degradation products (FDPs) are present in plasma in low concentrations in the third trimester only.

During obstetric delivery and following separation of the placenta there is activation and consumption of platelets and coagulation factors; the fibrinolytic pathway is activated, with a transient appearance of FDPs reaching a maximum in the first 4 hours post partum. There is a return of all haemostatic factors to non-pregnant levels by the end of the second week of the puerperium.

Genetic and environmental differences

The platelet counts in the African newborns up to around 6 months of age do not differ significantly from those of European newborns and adults. Older children and adults throughout tropical Africa have a moderate thrombocytopenia, for example $70–370 \times 10^9$/litre in symptom-free adult male Nigerians. This is probably the result of increased pooling of platelets in subclinically enlarged spleens.[1,3]

Platelets from non-elite Nigerians have been shown to be relatively resistant to aggregation by ADP, thrombin and ristocetin: aggregation can be induced either by increasing concentrations of the agonists or by resuspending the platelets in European plasma, suggesting that there are inhibitory plasma factors; these could be merely high levels of macroglobulins in response to intercurrent infections. The bleeding time and clot retraction are within standard reference ranges and there is no tendency to purpura, but the inhibition of platelet adhesion and aggregation could contribute to the low incidence of atheroma and thrombosis.[6]

Factor VIII coagulant activity of Africans is commonly greater than 150% of the activity of pooled European plasma. Levels in plasma of fibrinogen, plasminogen activators and spontaneous fibrinolysis are high in Africans and Papua New Guineans who perform heavy manual work, but levels fall with rising economic status and a more sedentary life. In Kenya and Papua New Guinea the frequency distribution of PT was shown to be skewed to the right; that is, there was a subpopulation with prolonged times; subclinical hepatic disease is a probable cause, and this is likely to apply to other tropical populations.

Anaemia
Definition

Anaemia is defined as a condition in which the Hb concentration in peripheral blood is lower than normal for age, sex and pregnancy state of the subject (Table 13.8).[7] The Hb is usually directly related to the total red cell volume, but there are exceptional circumstances: (1) during the first hours of life, when there is haemo-concentration in the capillaries, capillary blood samples will underestimate anaemia, especially in premature, acidotic, hypotensive or hypovolaemic infants; (2) immediately following acute haemorrhage, the Hb remains unchanged until there has been compensatory expansion of the plasma volume over the following 48 hours (see Figure 13.1 E, F); (3) with splenomegaly there is both an expansion of plasma volume and sequestration of red cells, so that patients with massive splenomegaly may have a Hb 80 g/litre, for example, while the total red cell mass is normal (see Figure 13.1 D).

Table 13.8 Haemoglobin concentrations below which anaemia is likely to be present in populations living at sea level.

	Hb (g/litre)
Newborn infants	140
6 months–6 years	110
6–14 years	120
Adult males	130
Adult females (non-pregnant)	120
Adult females (pregnant)	110

For each increment of 1000 m above sea level, add 2.5 g/litre (2 g/litre per 2500 feet). Reproduced from various sources, including the World Health Organization.[7]

Aetiology

Anaemia results from three basic mechanisms: (1) blood loss (haemorrhage); (2) decreased production of red cells; and (3) increased destruction of red cells (haemolysis) (Table 13.9). Only those causes which are of major public health importance in the tropics will be discussed. These include: (1) infections such as malaria, the human immunodeficiency viruses (HIV-1 and HIV-2), tuberculosis, hookworm and schistosomiasis; (2) nutritional deficiencies of iron and folate; and (3) inherited disorders of red cells, including the thalassaemias, sickle cell disease, glucose-6-phosphate dehydrogenase (G6PD) deficiency and ovalocytosis.

Table 13.9 Aetiology of anaemia.

1 Blood loss	
(a) *Acute*	(b) *Chronic* (e.g. hookworm) leading to iron deficiency
2 Decreased red cell production	
(a) *Nutritional deficiencies*	(b) *Depressed bone marrow function*
Iron	Secondary anaemias
Folate	HIV/AIDS
Vitamin B$_{12}$	tuberculosis
Various	other chronic infections
protein–energy,	chronic hepatic disease
vitamin A,	chronic renal disease
vitamin C,	carcinomatosis
vitamin E, riboflavin,	Aplastic anaemia
pyridoxine, Cu	drugs and chemicals
	infiltration
	idiopathic
	irradiation
	congenital
	Thalassaemias
	α thalassaemias
	β thalassaemias
3 Increased red cell destruction	
(a) *Abnormalities of red cells*	(b) *Abnormal haemolysis*
Haemoglobin	Immune haemolysis
sickle-cell disease	autoimmune
Enzymes	fetomaternal
G6PD deficiency	incompatibility
Membrane	incompatible blood
elliptocytosis	transfusion
ovalocytosis	Non-immune haemolysis
spherocytosis	infections (e.g. malaria)
	hypersplenism
	drugs and chemicals
	venoms
	burns
	mechanical

Table 13.10 Estimated prevalence of anaemia by geographic region and age/sex category, around 1980 (population data in millions).

	Children						Men			Women					
	0–4 years			5–12 years			15–59 years			15–49 years					
										Pregnant			All		
	No.	Anaemic		No.	Anaemic		No.	Anaemic		No.	Anaemic		No.	Anaemic	
Region		%	No.		%	No.		%	No.		%	No.		%	No.
Africa	85.7	56	48.0	96.6	49	47.3	116.8	20	23.4	17.9	63	11.3	106.4	44	46.8
Northern America	19.6	8	1.6	27.5	13	3.6	76.3	4	3.1	3.4	–	–	64.2	8	5.1
Latin America	52.9	26	13.7	69.8	26	18.1	98.1	13	12.8	9.9	30	3.0	86.5	17	14.7
East Africa	16.1	20	3.2	25.4	22	5.6	55.8	11	6.1	2.7	20	0.5	46.9	18	8.4
South Asia	212.0	56	118.7	278.4	50	139.2	386.3	32	123.6	41.7	65	27.1	329.4	58	191.0
Europe	33.4	14	4.7	55.0	5	3.0	147.2	2	3.0	5.7	14	0.8	117.5	12	14.1
Oceania	2.3	18	0.4	3.6	15	0.5	6.9	7	0.5	0.4	25	0.1	5.5	19	0.1
Former Soviet Union	23.1	–	–	31.1	–	–	80.3	–	–	4.0	–	–	68.7	–	–
World*	445.1	43	193.5	587.6	37	217.4	967.7	18	174.2	85.8	51	43.9	825.0	35	288.4
Developed regions	86.1	12	10.3	130.7	7	9.1	346.5	3	12.0	14.8	14	2.0	285.5	11	32.7
Developing regions*	395.0	51	183.2	456.8	46	208.3	621.2	26	162.2	71.0	59	41.9	539.5	47	255.7

*Excluding China.
Reproduced by permission of the World Health Organization from DeMaeyer and Adiels-Tegman.[8]

Epidemiology

Anaemia is the most common manifestation of disease observed in the tropics (Table 13.10).[8] Prevalence and morbidity are greatest in preschool children and pregnant women, in whom it is usual to find about half to be anaemic in rural and impoverished communities. The most common causes in preschool children are iron deficiency, malaria, thalassaemias (in Asia) and sickle cell disease (in Africa). The conditions leading most frequently to an anaemia in pregnancy are iron and folate deficiencies, malaria, thalassaemia minor (in Asia) and milder forms of sickle cell disease (in Africa). Although anaemia is less common and usually less severe in school children, men and non-pregnant women, it is still a major health problem in these groups: in them, anaemia is often secondary to tuberculosis or other chronic infections. HIV infection is now an extremely common cause of anaemia in men and women in the sexually active age range, but also in children: it is now the commonest cause of anaemia in adults requiring admission to hospital in sub-Saharan Africa.

Pathophysiology

Anaemia reduces the oxygen-carrying capacity of the blood. The body compensates for this by: (1) increasing the release of oxygen from Hb to the tissues; (2) increasing cardiac output; (3) enhancing blood flow to vital tissues with high oxygen requirements, while reducing flow to other organs; and (4) increasing respiration. The severity of anaemia is best considered as passing through three stages: (1) compensated, (2) decompensated and (3) life-threatening anaemia. The severity of anaemia does not depend on the Hb concentration alone, so that cut-off points of Hb 70 g/litre and 30 g/litre for when decompensation and cardiac failure respectively are likely must be taken as very approximate. Older patients are more likely to progress to decompensation or heart failure than the young; infants and young children are able to tolerate extremely low Hb concentrations with few complaints. Patients who develop an anaemia acutely have less time to compensate than patients with chronic anaemias such as sickle cell disease or aplastic anaemia. Patients who are hypervolaemic as a result of pregnancy (see Figure 13.1 B), especially multiple pregnancy (see 13.1 C), or of splenomegaly (see Figure 13.1 D) are more liable to progress as far as congestive cardiac failure, as are patients with underlying cardiac, vascular or respiratory diseases. In contrast, patients with low levels of activity, including the bedridden, are less likely to become decompensated.

Compensated anaemia

The major compensatory mechanism in mild to moderate anaemia is the increase of 2,3-diphosphoglycerate (2,3-DPG) concentration in red cells: this binds to deoxyhaemoglobin, shifts the oxygen dissociation curve of Hb to the right (decreased oxygen affinity) and increases oxygen release to tissue by up to 40%.[9] Cardiac output is raised by an increase in stroke volume at rest: on exertion there is both an exaggerated tachycardia and further rise in stroke volume. Vasodilatation enhances the blood flow to the myocardium, skeletal muscle and brain, while there is vasoconstriction in the skin and kidneys. The plasma volume expands, but the total blood volume remains normal (see Figure 13.1 G).

Patients complain of breathlessness on exertion only, and there are no physical signs except pallor, unless there are symptoms and signs from the underlying cause of the anaemia.

Work capacity

Maximal work capacity, as measured by the Harvard Step Test (HST), correlates directly with Hb at all levels, and is reduced by even mild anaemia: the average HST of Guatemalan labourers was 65 at Hb 130–150 g/litre and 30 at Hb 70–90 g/litre.[10]

Productivity and earnings of anaemic male manual workers are seriously reduced.[11,12] The earnings of anaemic women performing less strenuous factory work are also reduced.[13] Anaemia in either parent has an adverse effect on the family through low food production, low income and poor care for children; village life suffers from there being less ground under cultivation, and the national economy declines from overall low productivity.

The incidence of low birthweight and perinatal mortality rise rapidly when the maternal haematocrit (Hct) falls below 0.30.[14]

In childhood, anaemia is associated with slow growth, delayed development and poor cognitive abilities.

Decompensated anaemia

When the Hb falls below about 70 g/litre, the major mechanism for improving oxygen delivery is an increase in cardiac output.[9] Both stroke volume and the heart rate are raised at rest. The work of the ventricles is reduced by the low viscosity of anaemic blood and by peripheral vasodilatation; the circulation time is short. The blood volume is reduced in about 25% of patients (see Figure 13.1 H).

Patients are breathless even at rest. There is tachycardia, arterial and capillary pulsation, a wide pulse pressure and haemic ejection systolic murmurs. It is common experience that patients who are subsistence farmers, or others wholly dependent on their own manual labour, do not seek treatment until they have reached this stage of anaemia.

Life-threatening anaemia
Hypoxia and acidosis
If anaemia progresses in children with malaria until Hb falls to < 50 g/litre, respiratory distress develops, showing as tachypnea and at least one of the signs of nasal flaring, indrawing of the chest wall or diaphragm, grunting or deep breathing. The children are hypovolaemic (Fig. 13.1 H) and acidotic with lactic acidaemia.[15] Without appropriate treatment, mortality is high.

Anaemic heart failure
If anaemia progresses (Hb < 30 g/litre approximately), the oxygen supply to the myocardium is insufficient, no further increase of cardiac output is possible, and high-output cardiac failure develops. The plasma volume expands (see Figure 13.1 J): patients who are already hypervolaemic from pregnancy or splenomegaly are most liable to develop anaemic heart failure.

Patients are severely breathless and may complain of angina, night cramps or claudication. There is cardiomegaly, engorgement of jugular veins, pulmonary oedema, hepatomegaly, peripheral oedema and sometimes ascites. Without appropriate treatment there is a high morbidity rate. Maternal deaths rise sharply when the Hct is below 0.20 at the time of delivery: up to 20% of maternal deaths in Africa and India used to be due to anaemic heart failure, and this may still be true where obstetric and blood transfusion services have not developed.[16]

Management

The first principle of management is the diagnosis and treatment of the cause of the anaemia. The transfusion of concentrated red cells is required by anaemic patients in three circumstances only: (1) a patient is in danger of dying of anaemic heart failure or hypoxia before specific medication can raise the Hb; (2) a patient is about to experience stress, such as emergency major surgery, obstetric delivery or cytotoxic therapy; and (3) the anaemia is incurable, for example thalassaemia or aplastic anaemia, as will be discussed under these conditions. Children with severe malarial anaemia are *hypovolaemic*, not *hypervolaemic*, and should be transfused whole blood, *not* concentrated red cells, when the Hb is less than 50 g/litre and there is respiratory distress or when the Hb is less than 40 g/litre with or without respiratory distress. (Management of severe malaria is discussed in Chapter 71.) The inappropriate use of blood transfusion is not to be condoned, especially since the advent of HIV and the acquired immunodeficiency syndrome (AIDS).[17]

Haemolytic anaemias

This is a group of anaemias in which there is an increase of red cell turnover due to a shortening of the red cell lifespan from the normal range of 90–150 (mean 120) days. Haemolysis may be the consequence of an abnormal haemolytic process, or of abnormalities (usually congenital) of the red cells (see Table 13.9). Clinical and laboratory features common to all haemolytic anaemias are due to the increased breakdown of haemoglobin and the compensatory mechanisms of increased red cell production (Table 13.11). Haemolysis may be extravascular, that is, within the reticuloendothelial system (RES), when the breakdown products of haemoglobin follow the

Table 13.11 Features of the haemolytic anaemias.

Features of extravascular and intravascular haemolysis
Jaundice
Hyperbilirubinaemia (unconjugated)
Increased urinary urobilinogen
Increased faecal urobilinogen (stercobilinogen)
Features of intravascular haemolysis
Reduced/absent haptoglobins
Reduced haemopexin
Haem/methaemoglobinaemia
Methaemalbumin (positive Schumm's test)
Haem/methaemoglobinuria
Haemosiderinuria
Features of increased RBC production
Polychromasia
Reticulocytosis
Bone marrow erythroid hyperplasia

normal metabolic pathways of bilirubin. Lysis of red cells within the circulation results in the release of haemoglobin into plasma, the saturation and removal of haemoglobin- and haem-binding proteins (haptoglobins and haemopexin), and the presence of haemoglobin and its degradation products in the plasma and urine. Chronic haemolysis can lead to the formation of pigment stones in the gallbladder.

The bone marrow is capable of increasing red cell production around eight times the normal rate. Compensatory erythroid hyperplasia may be sufficient to maintain a normal or near-normal Hb, but is insufficient when rates of haemolysis are most rapid. Often the haemolytic process is accompanied not by erythroid hyperplasia, but by depression of marrow activity, either as part of the pathology of the disease (e.g., malaria) or due to complicating infections, such as parvovirus B19, which precipitates the so-called aplastic crises of sickle cell disease. A rapid rate of red cell production leads to high demands for folic acid, and long-standing haemolytic anaemias are frequently complicated by folate deficiency and megaloblastic erythropoiesis, followed by more profound anaemia. Chronic erythroid hyperplasia, as in sickle cell disease and the thalassaemias, results in expansion of the bone marrow cavity, seen clinically as bossing of the vault of the skull and projection of the maxilla (gnathopathy), and on radiography of the skull—as the hair-on-end appearance (see Figure 13.10).

Splenomegaly and hypersplenism

Palpable enlargement of the spleen is a common clinical finding in the tropics, especially where malaria is endemic (Table 13.12). In many instances splenomegaly is accompanied by the syndrome of hypersplenism, when there is pancytopenia, the severity of which is usually related to the size of the spleen. The anaemia is due to: (1) increased red cell pooling in the spleen, (2) shortened red cell lifespan with increased destruction of the spleen, and (3) haemodilution from an increased plasma volume (see Figure 13.1 D). The mechanisms of granulocytopenia and thrombocytopenia are similar: an eosinophilic response to helminthic infection may not be apparent in

Table 13.12 Some causes of splenomegaly (See also Chapter 10).

Generally slight (< 5 cm below the costal margin)	
Acute infections	• malaria, septicaemias, viraemias, hepatitis, trypanosomiasis, brucellosis, toxoplasmosis, typhus
Subacute, chronic infections	• tuberculosis, **brucellosis**, syphilis, hydatid, meningococcal septicaemia, histoplasmosis, bacterial endocarditis
Miscellaneous	• megaloblastic anaemia, iron deficiency anaemia, immune thrombocytopenia, **rheumatoid arthritis**, hyperthyroidism, myeloma, disseminated lupus erythematosus, **sarcoidosis**, amyloidosis
Generally moderate (5–10 cm below the costal margin)	
Chronic haemolysis	• **recurrent malaria**, haemoglobinopathies, spherocytosis
Portal hypertension	• hepatic cirrhosis
Haematological malignancies	• **chronic lymphocytic leukaemia, lymphomas**, acute leukaemias, polycythaemia vera
Usually gross (> 10 cm below the costal margin)	
Hyperreactive malarial splenomegaly (HMS)	
Schistosomiasis	
Kala-azar	
Thalassaemia major	
Haematological malignancies	• chronic granulocytic leukaemia, **myelofibrosis**
Miscellaneous	• splenic cysts and tumours, lipid storage diseases

Conditions in bold print are commonly associated with hypersplenism.

the peripheral blood because the eosinophils are held in the spleen, but it will be obvious in the bone marrow. The anaemia is usually normocytic and normochromic, there is a reticulocytosis and the bone marrow shows hyperplasia.

Malaria (See also Chapter 71)

The features of malaria are described in detail in Chapter 71; here are discussed only the haematological consequences, which include anaemia, changes in the white cells and disorders of haemostasis.[18,19] Of the different species of parasite, *Plasmodium falciparum* is the most common and has the most profound haematological consequences; this species of malaria is implied except where stated otherwise.

Malarial anaemia

Where malaria is endemic, for example in tropical Africa, the severity and pathology (including anaemia) progress through three phases as individuals acquire partial immune protection: (1) acute malaria in non-immune children after about 6 months of age when maternally derived immunity is lost; (2) recurrent malaria in children less than about 5 years of age; and (3) recurrent mild parasitaemia in partially immune older children and adults. Malaria in non-immune adults, such as expatriate visitors to endemic areas or inhabitants of countries where malaria is unstable, have haematological complications of acute or recurrent malaria essentially similar to those of children in the endemic areas.

Acute malaria

In non-immune individuals there is usually no anaemia within 24–48 hours of the onset of fever, but there is then a rapid fall of the Hb and Hct over 4–5 days, with the degree of anaemia corresponding approximately to the intensity of parasitaemia. The anaemia is normochromic and normocytic. The reticulocyte count is low at this stage, although the bone marrow shows erythroid hyperplasia with minimal dyserythropoietic changes. The total plasma bilirubin and unconjugated fraction are raised: increased conjugated bilirubin indicates complicating hepatic dysfunction. Haptoglobins are reduced or absent (see Table 13.11).

A major mechanism of haemolysis is rupture of red cells at the time of release of merozoites, but anaemia is often more severe and more persistent than can be accounted for directly by parasitaemia. The Hb may continue to fall for between 7 and 21 days following clearing of the parasites, due apparently to both continued haemolysis and delayed release of red cells from the marrow. Survival of both autologous non-parasitized red cells and donated red cells is shortened. There is phagocytosis of the parasitized and unparasitized red cells, seen easily in the bone marrow. The direct Coombs' test (DCT) is frequently positive, associated with adsorption by red cells of immunoglobulin (Ig) G and the C3 component of complement; however, auto-immune haemolysis is not an important mechanism, although

IgG-coated red cells are more rapidly removed by the RES than uncoated cells. Haemolysis of unparasitized red cells appears, therefore, to be due to a non-specific activation of the RES, hypersplenism and Fc receptor-mediated uptake.

Malaria is immunosuppressive and is frequently complicated by secondary infections, such as broncho-pneumonia, urinary tract infections and Gram-negative septicaemias; anaemia is generally more profound when there is secondary infection, especially with non-typhoid *Salmonella* septicaemia. It has been suggested that profound anaemia in some children may be the result of concurrent infection by parvovirus B19, which infects early red cell precursors preferentially and causes a transient red cell hypoplasia.

During acute malaria there is immobilization of iron in the macrophages, and low serum iron concentrations: serum ferritin is massively increased, being an acute reactive protein. Red cell folate levels are raised above normal through mechanisms which are uncertain, but possibly due to synthesis of folate by the parasites themselves.

Following clearance of the parasitaemia and during recovery, the peripheral blood shows a reticulocytosis, anisocytosis, macrocytosis and polychromasia (see Table 13.11).

Recurrent malaria

Children living where malaria is endemic suffer from recurrent attacks: they complain of intermittent fever and general ill health, and on examination often have moderate splenomegaly. They have a chronic normocytic, normochromic anaemia with a low reticulocyte count; anaemia may be profound during acute exacerbations but there is only a scanty parasitaemia, although gameto-cytes and malarial pigment may be seen in the mono-cytes. The anaemia is a result of both hypersplenism and severe dyserythropoietic disturbance of the bone marrow (Figure 13.3). The mechanism of dyserythropoiesis is uncertain, but it could be secondary to hypoxia from the packing of bone marrow sinusoids with parasitized red cells, or be mediated by an imbalance of cytokines.

Serum tumour necrosis factor (TNF) and interferon γ (IFNγ) are raised in acute malaria: they play an essential role in the control of parasitaemia and in inflammatory reactions. Interleukin 10 (IL-10) is also raised, and modulates the inflammatory responses. Low IL-10 concentrations have been found in African children with severe malaria, and it has been suggested that a failure of IL-10 may allow the uncontrolled actions of TNF in promoting dyserythropoiesis and erythrophagocytosis.

Disturbed marrow function is reversed by successful antimalarial treatment, which is followed by a brisk reticulocytosis and rise in Hb.

Haemoglobinuria and blackwater fever

The majority of patients presenting with haemo-globinuria seen today are G6PD deficient and have been treated with oxidant drugs (see below). However, some

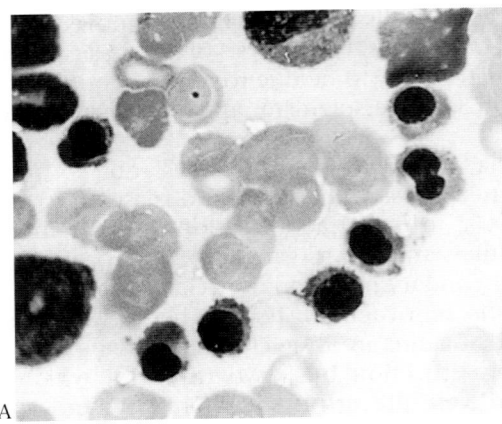

A

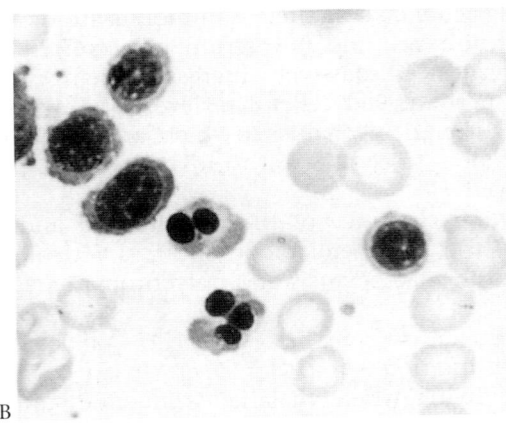

B

Figure 13.3: (**A**) and (**B**) Dyserythropoiesis: a term used to describe specific morphological changes in bone marrow which usually denotes ineffective erythropoiesis. These changes include cytoplasmic vacuolation, basophilic stippling, intracytoplasmic bridges, nuclear fragmentation (karyorrhexis), incomplete and unequal nuclear division and multinuclearity.

are G6PD normal and the trigger to severe intravascular haemolysis cannot be found. In the past patients were not infrequently seen with blackwater fever. Typically such a patient was a non-immune adult expatriate who had been taking quinine irregularly as prophylaxis. The patient complained of loin pain, vomiting and diarrhoea; initially there was polyuria, but later oliguria with dark-brown or black urine. There was tender hepato-splenomegaly, jaundice and profound anaemia; malarial parasites were scanty or even absent. There was massive haemoglobinuria and all other features of intravascular haemolysis (see Table 13.11). The mechanism was probably quinine-induced immune haemolysis. Blackwater fever is increasing in incidence as quinine comes back into use, and may be triggered also by mefloquine, artemisinin and halofantrine.

Malaria in the partially immune
Where malaria is endemic, older children and adults experience recurrent malarial parasitaemia contained by acquired immunity, with moderate haemolysis and compensatory erythroid hyperplasia. This contributes

largely to the mean Hb being about 20 g/litre lower than accepted reference figures in both sexes in many communities.[3] There is moderate anisocytosis, macro-cytosis and polychromasia. The balance between haemolysis and erythroid hyperplasia is disturbed during pregnancy (see below), after splenectomy and immune anergy, for example from malignant disease, and with hyperreactive malarial splenomegaly (HMS) (see below).

HIV infection is associated with increased parasite densities and incidence of clinical malaria, which has significance particularly during pregnancy (see below).[20]

Leucocytes in malaria
Lymphocytes
From about the third day of fever onwards there are, in the peripheral blood, numerous transformed lympho-cytes or plasmacytoid cells with dark blue cytoplasm and large nuclei with nucleoli. These are activated B cells. Sometimes in African children a leukaemoid reaction is seen, difficult to distinguish on simple blood film exam-ination from acute lymphoblastic leukaemia.[21]

Neutrophils
Many patients with acute malaria show a neutropenia due to margination to the endothelial surface of neutrophils in the circulation. During recovery from uncomplicated malaria there is often a leucocytosis with a shift to the left, toxic granulation, vacuolation and ragged cytoplasm. A neutrophil leucocytosis is seen often in reaction to secondary infections, and carries a poor prognosis.[18] Rarely there is a myeloid leukaemoid reaction, with an extremely high neutrophil count and shift to the left as far as myelocytes or promyelocytes and blast cells.[21]

Eosinophils
The eosinophil count is low during acute malaria, even if the initial count is high in response to helminthic infections. During recovery, there may be an eosinophilia.[21]

Monocytes
The monocyte count is raised; the cells are frequently vacuolated, and erythrophagocytosis and malarial pig-ment may be seen. The examination of monocytes in a thin blood film is most valuable in diagnosis as malarial pigment persists for several days after the clearance of parasitaemia; pigment remains in bone marrow macro-phages for up to 20 weeks after infection.

Disorders of haemostasis in malaria
Platelets
The platelet count is reduced regularly in acute malaria; for example, in 105 Nigerian children with malaria, the mean platelet count was 132×10^9/litre, as compared to 234×10^9/litre in the same subjects 12 days later after receiving treatment with chloroquine. However, severe thrombocytopenia ($< 50 \times 10^9$/litre) was observed in only 5%. Platelet survival is reduced to 2–4 days; probable mechanisms include reduced membrane sialic acid leading

to rapid clearance, an immune mechanism involving anti-platelet IgG and hypersplenism. There may be some megakaryocyte dysfunction with the release of giant platelets, but usually megakaryocytes are numerous, normal in appearance and actively budding in the bone marrow. Platelet function is enhanced generally, including aggregation induced by ADP, adrenaline, thrombin and thromboxane A_2 (TXA_2).[18,22]

Coagulation

AT III levels are reduced in proportion to the severity of the parasitaemia. PT may be prolonged as a consequence of hepatic dysfunction.

In a small proportion, for example less than 10% of Thai adults, acute malaria may be complicated by disseminated intravascular coagulation (DIC). The process is triggered by the release of thromboplastin during massive haemolysis, toxic destruction of endothelium and the activation of complement. DIC is reversed usually following active antimalarial therapy: patients may require transfusion with fresh whole blood, or even exchange transfusion; the use of heparin is controversial.[18,21]

Management of severe malarial anaemia

The management of acute malaria and its complications is discussed in Chapter 71. Malarial anaemia generally responds to antimalarial therapy, but is a major cause of morbidity and of mortality. In different series between 10% and 16% of all deaths in childhood in Africa have been attributed to malarial anaemia, but these are certain to be underestimates.

In the past there has been far too great a willingness to treat malarial anaemia by blood transfusion. With the advent of HIV in Africa many thousands of children have been treated successfully for anaemia, but at the cost of developing AIDS later. Even where blood donations are screened for anti-HIV, donors may be in the window between infection and seroconversion, so that more stringent criteria for transfusion must be applied, which will prevent mortality from anaemia but minimize the transmission of HIV.[15,19]

1. Hb > 50 g/litre *with* or *without* respiratory distress: intravenous normal saline in aliquots of 10 ml/kg.
2. Hb 40–50 g/litre *without* respiratory distress: intravenous saline as above, with careful monitoring and reviewing over 48 hours.
3. Hb < 50 g/litre *with* respiratory distress or impaired consciousness: transfusion of whole blood 20 ml/kg, without a diuretic; with mild distress (nasal flaring) transfuse over 4–6 hours; with severe distress, transfuse 10 ml/kg over 1 hour and the remaining 10 ml/kg over the next 2–4 hours.
4. Hb < 40 g/litre *with* or *without* respiratory distress: transfuse as in (3).

Malaria in pregnancy

There is a reduction in resistance to malaria during pregnancy.[23] The mechanisms of increased susceptibility may include (1) a physiological suppression of cell-mediated immunity, (2) high serum cortisol and oestrogen concentrations, (3) cytoadherence of parasites in the placenta,[24] leading to intense infection within the placenta and extensive placental damage, and (4) a higher risk of mosquito bites during pregnancy.[25] Humoral immunity to malaria is unaltered. The presentation of malaria during pregnancy varies enormously according to the woman's previous exposure and level of acquired immunity to malaria.[25,26]

Women with no or low levels of acquired immunity to malaria, if infected during pregnancy, suffer from severe malaria, frequently complicated by cerebral malaria, renal failure, blackwater fever, profound anaemia and DIC. Women of all ages and parities are affected equally. Maternal and fetal morbidity and mortality are heavy.

In women who live where malaria is stable (hyper- or holoendemic), and who have acquired high levels of immunity to *P. falciparum*, the frequency and density of parasitaemia rise to plateaux early in the second trimester, especially in primigravidae, or women in their second pregnancies to a less extent. The densities of parasitaemias do not reach levels seen in early childhood, and the women are generally asymptomatic or have mild symptoms only. However, there is haemolysis and anaemia, seen most commonly in the mid-second trimester and in primigravidae. Compensatory erythroid hyperplasia leads to high demands for folate, demands which are already increased because of pregnancy. The haemolytic process is often complicated by megaloblastic erythropoiesis, and profound anaemia follows.

The frequency of palpable splenomegaly increases during pregnancy in all gravida classes, and a peak spleen rate about double that of non-pregnant women can be reached at around 16 weeks of gestation. Even higher spleen rates (e.g., 70% in Nigeria) are seen in anaemic pregnant women; in Nigeria about 25% of severe anaemias in pregnancy were complicated by HMS (see below) and hypersplenism. About 5% of women in the same series had a severe haemolytic process which was not controlled by antimalarials but responded to prednisolone and was presumed to be due to an immune process triggered by malaria.[26,27]

The presentation of malaria in pregnancy is intermediate between the two patterns where malaria is unstable (mesoendemic), as for example in Thailand and Zambia.

Patterns of resistance to malaria during pregnancy are further complicated by co-infection with HIV; in Malawi, for example, women attending antenatal clinic for the first time during their present pregnancy were found to be around 30% HIV infected and more than 40% with malarial parasitaemia. HIV positivity in pregnancy was associated with increased prevalence and density of *P. falciparum* parasitaemia and placental infection, increased incidence of clinical malaria and decreased effectiveness of prophylactic antimalarials, in women of all parities.[28]

The peripheral blood picture of malarial plus folate deficiency anaemia in pregnancy is characterized by great anisocytosis, macrocytosis and polychromasia with or without nucleated red cells, but no poikilocytosis; there is a reticulocytosis; malarial parasites are usually absent or scanty. The white cell count is variable and there may be a myeloid leukaemoid reaction; the expected hypersegmentation of folate deficiency is often masked by a shift to the left. The bone marrow shows megaloblastic changes which may be gross; malarial pigment is present in the macrophages; iron stores tend to be increased unless there is concurrent iron deficiency.

Maternal and fetal morbidity and mortality are extremely high (see Anaemia: Pathophysiology).

Blood transfusion is indicated only if the patient is in incipient or established cardiac failure, or if the patient is approaching delivery with an Hb < 70 g/litre.[17] Anaemia responds rapidly in most patients following antimalarial therapy and folic acid; the haematocrit tends not to rise, but remains steady in patients with HMS;[26] in the few patients with immune haemolysis the haematocrit rises rapidly following treatment with prednisolone 60 mg/day for 1 week, 45 mg/day for 1 week and 30 mg/day maintenance in three divided doses, up to about 36 weeks of gestation.[27]

Malaria and anaemia can be effectively prevented by the administration of prophylactic antimalarials and folic acid supplements to pregnant women.[26] There are, however, great problems in the delivery of effective regimens to more than the few who attend antenatal clinics regularly: malaria chemoprophylaxis (Maloprim) has been given by traditional birth attendants in The Gambia, with beneficial effects on parasite rates, the haematocrit and birthweight, especially in primigravidae and also grandes multigravidae.[29]

Administration of sulfadoxin/pyrimethamine (Fansidar®) in two or more intermittent doses from first attendance to the third trimester has the advantages of practicality and cost-effectiveness, and results in higher maternal Hb, decreased placental malaria and decreased low birthweight. This strategy should be applicable in remote communities.[30]

The efficacy of insecticide-impregnated bed-nets (IIBN) (see Chapter 71) during pregnancy, alone or in combination with prophylactics, in the reduction of malaria and its consequences for mothers and infants, needs research in the field, as reports so far are contradictory.

The prevention of malaria in pregnancy in endemic areas has focused on first (or second) pregnancies as being the worst affected. With advent of HIV, however, more attention should be given to multigravidae as well, because HIV infection decreases the ability to control malaria in women of all parities, and it is possible that malaria infection may also increase vertical transmission of HIV.[31]

Hyperreactive malarious splenomegaly (See also Chapter 71)

In malarious areas a varying proportion of children (and non-immune adult visitors) have splenomegaly associated with intermittent parasitaemia, and regressing with the gradual acquisition of relative immunity. In some, however, the spleen does not regress but enlarges progressively with increasing age. This condition is known as hyperreactive malarious splenomegaly (HMS), and was previously called the tropical splenomegaly syndrome (TSS). Its defining features are: (1) residence in a malarious area; (2) chronic splenomegaly, often massive; (3) serum IgM elevated to more than 2 standard deviations above the local reference mean; (4) high malarial antibody titres; (5) hepatic sinusoidal lymphocytosis; and (6) clinical and immunological response to long-term antimalarial prophylaxis.[32,33]

Pathophysiology

Central to the pathophysiology of HMS is the overproduction of IgM in response to recurrent infection by *P. falciparum*, *P. malariae* or *P. vivax*. There is familial and ethnic clustering suggesting a genetic basis. It is seen most often in groups who have migrated relatively recently to endemic malarial areas, and so are likely to lack genetic polymorphisms which confer partial protection against malaria. Such polymorphisms could include HLA-linked genetically controlled processing of malarial antigens and antibody production.[34,35] During acute malaria, there is transient production of IgM lymphocytotoxic antibodies which are specific for activated suppressor T lymphocytes (CD8+), which normally downregulate synthesis of IgM by B cells. It has been shown in Indonesian patients with HMS that these lymphocytotoxic antibodies persist, with consequent imbalance between helper T cells (CD4+) which are normal, and suppressor T cells which are greatly reduced, so that there is a lack of inhibition of B cell activity.[36] Recurrent antigenic and mitogenic stimuli from malaria to the B cells result in gross overproduction of polyclonal IgM, of which only a small part has antimalarial specificity. The IgM forms aggregates (cryoglobulins) and immune complexes. These are phagocytosed by the RES, including the macrophages of the liver (Kupffer cells), spleen and bone marrow, stimulating macrophage hyperplasia and T cell proliferation, seen as hepatic sinusoidal infiltration and the lymphocytosis of spleen and bone marrow. Overproduction of IgM and its complexes precedes and is the stimulus to progressive and eventual massive splenomegaly and hepatomegaly. Pancytopenia of variable severity results from hypersplenism. The apparent anaemia is caused mainly by the expansion of plasma volume (up to 130 ml/kg) and sequestration of up to one-third of the total red cells in the spleen (see Figure 13.1D). There is haemolysis of cells pooled in the spleen, and erythrophagocytosis mediated by the adsorption of immune complexes; haemolytic crises are associated with pregnancy and infection. Patients are liable to frequent and prolonged infections related to neutropenia and disturbed immune function.[37,38]

Distribution and clinical presentation

HMS has been described in Africa (Nigeria, Uganda, Kenya and Zambia), western Asia (Aden), the Indian subcontinent (Bengal, Sri Lanka), South-East Asia (Vietnam, Thailand, Indonesia), Oceania (Papua New Guinea) and South America (Amazon basin). High incidences are reported in the Fulani in northern Nigeria, Rwandan immigrants in Uganda, the Angas of Upper Watut Valley and the related Menya of Tauri Valley (Papua New Guinea), and the Yanomani in Venezuela. Prevalence rates of over 50% have been reported only in the Papua New Guinea groups and the Indonesians of the island of Flores.[32–38]

Presentation is usually in young to middle-aged adults, but can occur as early as 8 years of age and in old age. In some series women have outnumbered men, but in others there is an equal sex incidence. Patients complain most commonly of abdominal swelling and a dragging feeling or pain from the enlarged spleen. The spleen may be huge, reaching to the left iliac fossa and across the midline. There is usually hepatomegaly. Lymphadenopathy is not a feature.[33,36]

Haematology

The anaemia is generally moderate, but may be severe during pregnancy or following acute infections; it is normocytic, but there may be macrocytosis and polychromasia with a reticulocytosis. The total WBC is generally low, with granulocytopenia. However, in West Africa in about 10% of patients there is a lymphocytosis which may mimic chronic lymphocytic leukaemia (CLL). There is a mild thrombocytopenia, but not usually sufficient to lead to haemorrhage. Malarial parasites are absent as a rule.

Sickle cell trait confers significant but partial protection against the development of HMS.

The bone marrow shows hyperactivity of erythroid, granulocyte and megakaryocyte lines. Megaloblastic changes are rare. An excess of normal lymphocytes is observed in West African patients. The frequency of depleted iron stores is not different from that of the population. Malaria pigment is not seen.[33,37]

Diagnosis

The defining feature is excessively high serum IgM. When there is a leukaemoid reaction, HMS may be distinguished from CLL by (1) the absence of lymphadenopathy, (2) the high serum IgM, whereas levels are lower than normal in CLL except when there is a monoclonal paraprotein, (3) normal lymphocyte transformation with phytohaemagglutinin (PHA), whereas transformation is reduced in CLL, (4) polyclonal lymphoproliferation and polycolonal Ig heavy chain gene rearrangement, as compared to monoclonal proliferation in CLL.[32,33,37,39]

Prognosis

The condition appears benign in most patients when seen first, but there is a high mortality without treatment; for example 46% over 15 years rising to nearly 90% in those with gross splenomegaly in the Upper Watut Valley. Death is usually from acute bacterial or other overwhelming infections.[38]

Some patients show a haematological and immune status suggestive of transition to a clonal lymphoproliferation, sometimes called 'African CLL' or 'tropical splenic lymphoma' (see 'Chronic lymphocytic leukaemia'). It is probable that the polyclonal expansion of B lymphocytes provides targets for somatic mutation, followed by selection of a single clone. A previous suggestion that 'African CLL' was splenic lymphoma with villous lymphocytes (SLVL) has not be supported as the cells have an origin from naive B cells:[40] surface markers of cells from a small series of Zambian patients are consistent with B cell prolymphocytic leukaemia.[41] Multicentre studies into the nature of HMS and its transition to malignancy are much needed.

Management

The treatment of choice is the administration of antimalarial chemoprophylaxis for life. The choice of prophylactic depends on the local pattern of sensitivity of the malarial parasites: proguanil has been the most effective agent in tropical Africa. After about 3 months of treatment there is a steady decrease in splenomegaly over many months and a return of all immunological and haematological parameters to normal. Failure of treatment suggests non-compliance, ineffectiveness of the prescribed antimalarial prophylactic, malignant transformation or incorrect diagnosis. Non-compliance leads to relapse, morbidity and increased mortality.

There is no place for splenectomy, despite the immediate improvement it causes, because of high operative and later mortality, the transfer of disease from splenomegaly to hepatomegaly, and the need in any case for lifelong antimalarial prophylaxis to prevent acute malaria.[33,37]

Other protozoa

Visceral leishmaniasis (See also Chapter 75)

Infection by *Leishmania donovani* is followed by hyperplasia of macrophages and lymphocytes, massive production of IgG and progressive hepatosplenomegaly (kala-azar). The size of the spleen is related directly to the duration of infection and to the severity of pancytopenia.[21,42] Anaemia is due primarily to hypersplenism (expansion of plasma volume, haemodilution, splenic sequestration and haemolysis) (see Figure 13.1 D). There are plasma cold anti-I agglutinins, the adsorption of IgG by red cells and the fixation of complement, but no convincing evidence that autoimmune haemolysis contributes to the severity of anaemia in kala-azar.[43] Dyserythropoiesis and ineffective erythropoiesis have a role in the causation of anaemia in at least some patients.[44] In India about half of patients are reported to have moderate to severe megaloblastosis, due to folate deficiency secondary to increased demands from haemolysis.[45] Pancytopenia is particularly severe in subjects who are also infected by HIV.

In the early stages there may be leucocytosis with a shift to the left, but neutropenia becomes increasingly severe with advancing disease. Neutrophil function has been reported to be normal by some, but Italian workers have reported reduced phagocytic and bactericidal activity.[46] Neutropenia may become profound: children in particular are liable to secondary bacterial infections, or the development of cancrum oris. The eosinophil count is reduced; lymphocyte and monocyte counts are raised and occasionally there may be leukaemoid reactions.[21]

Platelets are sequestered in the spleen and platelet survival is short: thrombocytopenia may be sufficiently severe to cause mucosal bleeding but cutaneous purpura is unusual. Hepatic dysfunction can lead to hypoprothrombinaemia with prolonged coagulation time and PT. There is increased fibrinolytic activity and reduced fibrinogen concentration in some patients with advanced disease.[21] Immune complex-mediated vasculitis and DIC have been reported from Sudan.[47]

The bone marrow is usually hyperplastic and often megaloblastic, with increased erythroid, granulocytic and megakaryocytic activity; lymphocytes and plasma cells are numerous, as are macrophages, many of which contain Leishman–Donovan bodies. In long-standing chronic kala-azar there may be bone marrow hypoplasia and fibrosis; gelatinous transformation of bone marrow has been described in one patient.[48] Pure red cell aplasia has been reported, which could have been due to coincidental infection by parvovirus B19.[49]

Successful treatment of leishmaniasis is followed by regression of the spleen and a return to haematological normality over 9 months following cure. The Hb response may be delayed due to the anaemia of chronic disorder (see below).[50,51]

Trypanosomiasis (See also Chapters 73 and 74)
African trypanosomiasis is accompanied by a haemolytic anaemia, which is usually moderate but may be severe.[21] Haemolysis has several mechanisms: (1) trypanosomes release haemolysins, which enables the parasites to utilize haem and other nutrients from the red cells; (2) there is adsorption of IgM immune complexes on to red cells with fixation of complement, and the sensitized red cells are phagocytosed throughout the RES; and (3) there is hypersplenism. There is a moderate leucocytosis, with raised lymphocyte and monocyte counts, but a neutropenia from hypersplenism. Thrombocytopenia is usual during acute infections, and may be profound due to hypersplenism. With *Trypsanosoma brucei rhodesiense* infections there is, in addition, platelet aggregation and destruction, and in some patients DIC.

In infections with *T. cruzi* (American trypanosomiasis, Chagas' disease) there may be a normocytic anaemia, leucocytosis, lymphocytosis and hypoprothrombinaemia.

Toxoplasmosis
There is a high rate of transmission of *Toxoplasma gondii* in childhood in the developing countries, causing only mild disease generally; some patients may have a persistent lymphocytosis with atypical mononuclear cells like glandular fever cells and a thrombocytopenia.[21] Congenital toxoplasmosis is rare as women are almost invariably immune. Severe and congenital toxoplasmosis may be seen more commonly as a result of the AIDS pandemic.

Amoebiasis
Patients with chronic disease have a hypochromic microcytic anaemia as a result of either chronic blood loss and iron deficiency, and/or the anaemia of chronic disorders. Neutrophil leucocytosis, sometimes amounting to a leukaemoid reaction, is associated with perforation of the bowel, peritonitis, secondary bacterial infections and amoebic liver abscesses. Hepatic disease results in prolonged PT and excessively high serum vitamin B_{12} levels.

Giardiasis
Acute diarrhoea due to *Giardia lamblia* causes a malabsorption of folate, whereas about half of the patients with chronic infections have impaired absorption of vitamin B_{12} which is multifactorial, including damage to ileal receptors, utilization of the vitamin by the parasite, and bacterial overgrowth of the bowel.[21]

Haemoglobinopathies
The inherited disorders of haemoglobin synthesis, the haemoglobinopathies, form by far the largest group of single-gene disorders in the world population, and also the largest group of genetically determined anaemias. There are hundreds of millions of carriers, and each year 200 000–300 000 severely affected homozygotes or compound heterozygotes are born.[52,53]

In many of the developing countries, where there is still a very high mortality from infection and malnutrition in the first years of life, these conditions are not yet recognized as important public health problems. However, once economic conditions improve and the infant death rates fall, the genetic disorders of haemoglobin will start to place a major burden on the health services. They occur most frequently in Asia, Africa and the Mediterranean region and in the immigrant population from these areas, but can be encountered in every ethnic group.

Normal human haemoglobins
The oxygen-carrying pigment in the RBC of vertebrates is haemoglobin, a globular protein molecule (molecular weight 64 450), made up of four subunits (Figure 13.4). Each subunit contains a haem moiety (iron-containing porphyrin) conjugated to a polypeptide (globin) chain. The four polypeptide chains consist of two identical pairs each of over 140 amino acids. One pair belong to the α family (α or ζ chains) and other to the β family (β, γ, δ or ε chains). The productions of the α and β families are controlled by gene clusters on chromosome 16 and chromosome 11 respectively (Fig. 13.5).

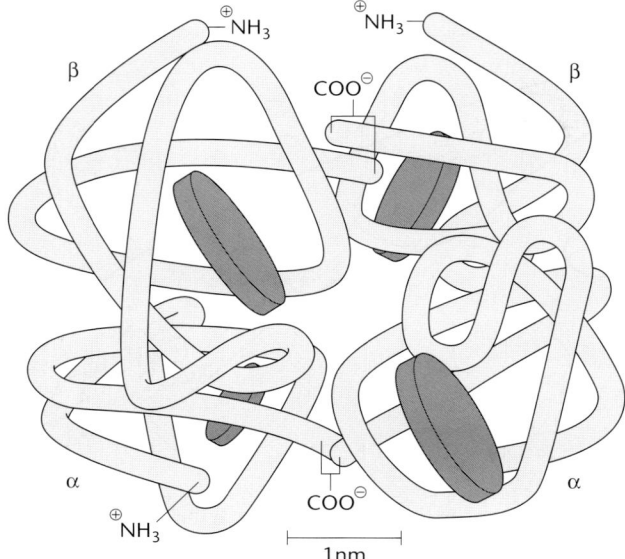

Figure 13.4: The structure of haemoglobin. Diagrammatic representation of adult haemoglobin (HbA) showing four subunits. There are two α and two β polypeptide chains, each containing a haem moiety, represented by disks.

The embryonic haemoglobins consist of Hb Gower 1 ($\zeta_2\varepsilon_2$), Hb Portland ($\zeta_2\gamma_2$) and Hb Gower 2 ($\alpha_2\varepsilon_2$). They are produced in the yolk sac before the tenth week of embryonic–fetal life. Fetal haemoglobin (HbF) is $\alpha_2\gamma_2$: it has a higher oxygen affinity than the adult haemoglobin and hence allows efficient extraction of oxygen from the maternal circulation. It is produced by the liver and

spleen from about the tenth week of fetal life and declines from about the thirtieth week to reach the adult level by 1–2 years of age (see Table 13.2). In certain pathological conditions, the embryonic and fetal globin chain synthesis persists to a later period.

In the adult, two types of haemoglobin are present— HbA and HbA$_2$—constituting 95% and 1–3% respectively. HbA is composed of two α and two β chains ($\alpha_2\beta_2$), and HbA$_2$ of two α and two δ chains ($\alpha_2\delta_2$). The α chain consists of 141 amino acid residues, and the β chain contains 146 amino acid residues. The δ chain also has 146 amino acids but 10 individual residues differ from those in the β chains. HbA is detectable at the eleventh week of fetal life. By the eighteenth week of gestation, it comprises approximately 8%. It replaces HbF during late gestation and infancy, reaching adult levels by 6 months of age. HbA$_2$ begins to appear at birth and increases over the 2 years of life. Because it is present in such low concentrations, it is of no practical use as an oxygen carrier. However, it is a useful diagnostic tool for evaluating patients with certain types of thalassaemia.

Inherited disorders of haemoglobin synthesis

The mutations leading to abnormalities of haemoglobin synthesis may result from either a deletion of a gene or part of the gene, as seen in most α thalassaemias, or may result in a single base change (point mutation), as seen in most β thalassaemias. In point mutations there is a deletion, substitution or insertion of one or two bases in the nucleotide strand of the gene. The haemoglobinopathies are inherited in a single Mendelian codominant fashion: the carriers are relatively symptom free and the homozygotes manifest the disease.

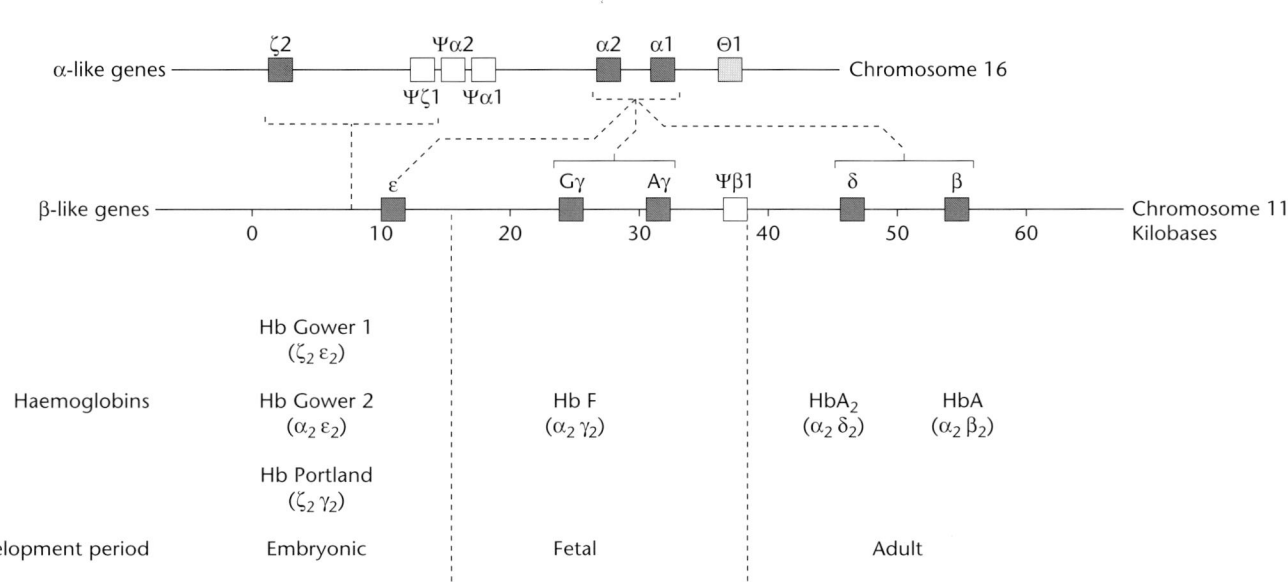

Figure 13.5: Chromosomal organization of the globin genes and their expression during development. The solid boxes indicate functional globin genes, whereas the open boxes indicate pseudo genes. The scale of the depicted chromosomal segment is in kilobases of DNA (Kb). The switch from the embryonic to fetal haemoglobin occurs between 6 and 10 weeks of gestation, and the switch from the fetal to adult haemoglobin occurs at about the time of birth. (Reproduced with the permission of the publishers from Nathan D G & Oski F A (editors). *Hematology of Infancy and Childhood*, 4th edn. Philadelphia: W B Saunders, 1993.)

The main genetic disorders of haemoglobin productions are due to (1) either a complete absence or reduced production of α or β polypeptides chains, the thalassaemias, or (2) a structural defect of the polypeptide chains, the haemoglobin variants, leading to instability of the molecule or abnormal oxygen transport. In addition, there is a harmless group of mutations which interfere with the normal switching of fetal to adult haemoglobin production, called hereditary persistence of fetal haemoglobin (HPFH).

The common thalassaemias are the β thalassaemias, when there is a defective rate of synthesis of β chains, and the α thalassaemias, when there is defective synthesis of α chains. Of the structural defects, variants of the β chain are the most common and clinically important: they include HbS, HbC, HbD, HbE and HbO, which occur in certain populations at polymorphic frequencies. These populations all live in regions where *P. falciparum* malaria is or was endemic or are migrant populations from these areas. On geographical evidence, and in some instances demographic and parasitological evidence as well, it is thought that heterozygous inheritance of these abnormalities of haemoglobin synthesis renders the red cell less favourable than normal for the development of malarial parasites. Carriers enjoy, therefore, some protection against severe malaria, and hence survival and genetic advantages, which balance in the population the genetic disadvantages arising from the ill health and early deaths in the homozygotes.[35,52,53]

Thalassaemia syndromes

The thalassaemias are a heterogeneous group of disorders of haemoglobin synthesis, all of which result from an absent or a reduced rate of production of one or more of the globin chains. They are divided in to α, β, δβ or γδβ thalassaemias according to which globin is deficient. When globin chains are not synthesized at all, they are designated as $α^0$ or $β^0$ thalassaemias, and when globin chains are produced at a reduced rate it is called $α^+$ or $β^+$ thalassaemias. δβ and γδβ thalassaemias are always characterized by absence of chain synthesis: thus they are $(δβ)^0$ and $(γδβ)^0$ thalassaemias.

Because thalassaemias occur in populations in which structural haemoglobin variants are also common, it is not unusual for an individual to receive a thalassaemia gene from one parent and a gene for a structural variant from the other. Furthermore, both α and β thalassaemia occur commonly in some countries, and hence individuals may receive genes for both types. These different interactions produce an extremely complex and clinically diverse series of genetic disorders, which range in severity from death in utero to extremely mild, symptomless hypochromic anaemia.

Clinically thalassaemias are classified according to their severity into major, intermedia and minor forms. Thalassaemia major is a severe transfusion-dependent disorder. Thalassaemias intermedia are characterized by anaemia and splenomegaly but not so severe to require regular blood transfusions. Thalassaemia minor is a symptomless carrier state.

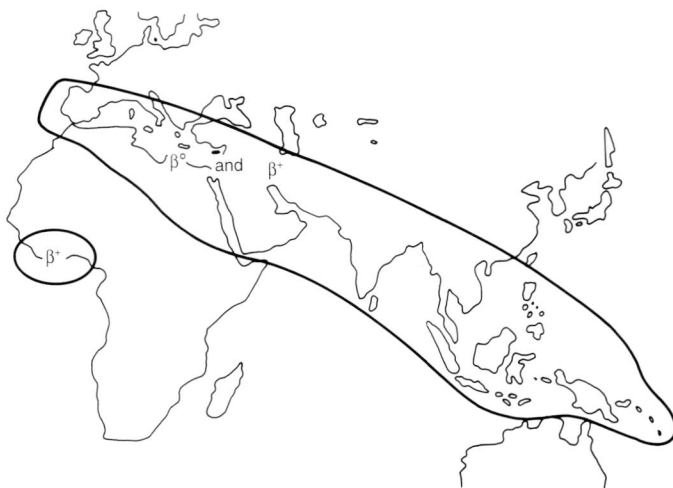

Figure 13.6: Areas of the Old World where β thalassaemias reach polymorphic frequencies. (Reproduced with permission of the publishers from Fleming A F. In Strickland G T (ed.) *Hunter's Tropical Medicine*, 7th edn. Philadelphia: W B Saunders, 1991: 36–64.)

The β thalassaemias

The β thalassaemias are the most important types of thalassaemia because they are so common and produce severe anaemia in their homozygous and compound heterozygous states. They occur commonly in a broad belt ranging from the Mediterranean and parts of North and West Africa through the Middle East and the Indian subcontinent to South-East Asia (Figure 13.6). The disease is particularly common in South-East Asia, where it occurs in a line starting in southern China and stretching down through Thailand, the Malay Peninsula and Indonesia to the Pacific islands.

The carrier frequency for various forms of the disease ranges between 2% and 30%. About 3% of the world's population, or over 150 million individuals, mostly in Asia, are carriers. Over 50 000 infants are born annually with β thalassaemias major. In many of these regions β thalassaemia is a major public health problem and a drain on medical resources.

Molecular pathology

The molecular lesions responsible for the defective synthesis of the β chains are extremely heterogeneous: nearly 200 different mutations, mostly point mutations, can produce the clinical phenotype of β thalassaemia but only about 20 alleles account for 90% of all β thalassaemia genes (Table 13.13).[35,52–54]

Pathophysiology

The basic molecular defect in β thalassaemia results in absent or reduced β chain production: α chain synthesis proceeds at the normal rate and hence there is an excess of α chains (Figure 13.7). In the absence of their partner β chains, α chains are unstable and precipitate in the red

Table 13.13 Some examples of point mutations in β thalassaemia.

Mutant class	Genotype	Origin
I Non-functional mRNA		
(a) Nonsense mutants		
Codon 17 (A–T)	β°	Chinese
Codon 15 (G–A)	β°	Indian
Codon 37 (G–A)	β°	Saudi Arabian
Codon 39 (C–T)	β°	Mediterranean
(b) Frameshift mutants		
Codon 41/42	β°	Indian, Chinese, Sri Lanka
Codon 8/9	β°	Indian, Sri Lanka
Codons 71/72	β°	Chinese
Codon 6	β°	Mediterranean
II RNA processing mutations		
(a) Splice junction alteration		
IVS1–1 (G–A)	β+	Mediterranean
IVS1–1 (G–T)	β°	Indian, Chinese
IVS1–5 (G–C)	β+	Indians, Sri Lanka, Chinese, Mediterranean
IVS2–1 (G–A)	β°	American black, Mediterranean
(b) Creation of new splice signals in IVS		
IVS1–110 (G–A)	β+	Mediterranean
IVS2–654 (C–T)	β°	Chinese
(c) Coding region substitution after the RNA processing		
Codon 26 (G–A)	HbE	SE Asian
Sri Lanka		
Codon 24 (T–A)	β+	American black
III Transcriptional mutations		
–88 C–T	β+	Indian
–31 A–G	β+	Japanese
–28 A–G	β+	Chinese
IV RNA cleavage = polyadenylation mutants		
AATAAA-AACAAA	β+	American black
V Cap site mutations		
+1 A–C	β+	Indian
VI Unstable globins due to missense mutations		
Codon 112	β+	European
Codon 10	β+	Japanese

cell precursors, giving rise to large intracellular inclusions, demonstrable on methyl violet staining of the peripheral blood of splenectomized patients. In non-splenectomized individuals, the inclusions are difficult to demonstrate as they are removed during passage of RBC through the splenic sinusoids, generating fragments and teardrops. The inclusions have several detrimental effects on red cells. They interfere with the division of RBC precursors causing ineffective erythropoiesis: they damage the cell membrane and contribute to the intramedullary death of red cells; and they disturb red cell deformability, interfering with the egress of cells from the bone marrow spaces. Red cells which do mature and enter the circulation contain α chain inclusions, which interfere with their passage through the microcirculation particularly in the spleen, leading to their premature destruction. Thus the anaemia of β thalassaemia results from both ineffective erythropoiesis and a shortened red cell survival.

The anaemia is a stimulus for erythropoietin production, which causes a massive expansion of the bone marrow and leads to serious deformities of the skull and long bones. Because the spleen is constantly bombarded with abnormal red cells, it hypertrophies and the resulting splenomegaly gives rise to a massive increase of the plasma volume, which exacerbates an already severe degree of anaemia.

Normally HbF production decreases to a low level over the first 6 months of postuterine life. However, some adult red cells precursors retain the ability to produce a small number of γ chains. Because the latter can combine with excess α chains to form HbF, cells which make relatively more γ chains in the bone marrow of β thalassaemia are partially protected against the

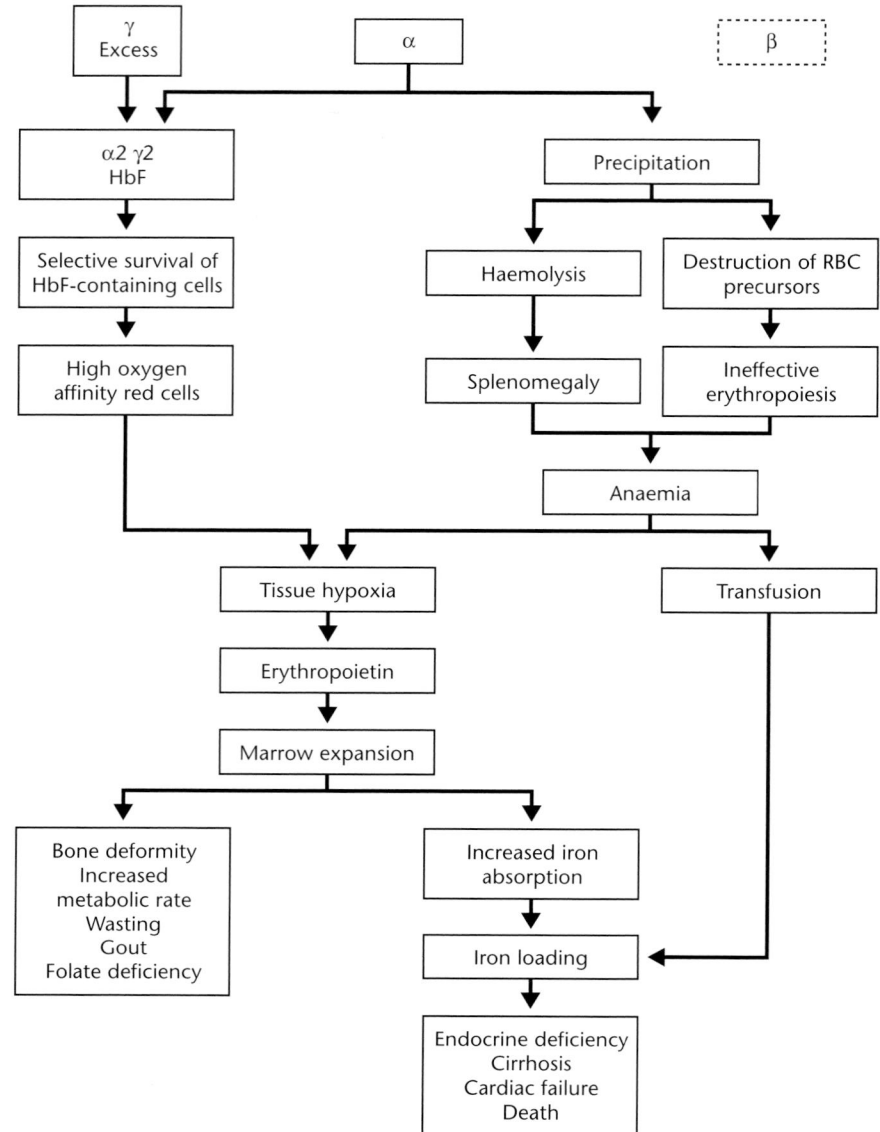

Figure 13.7: The pathophysiology of β thalassaemia.

deleterious effects of α chain precipitation. Hence the red cell precursors which produce HbF are selected in the marrow, and there are relatively large amounts of HbF in the peripheral blood RBC. Because δ chain synthesis is unaffected the disorder is characterized by increased HbA_2 production.

β Thalassaemia major

Clinical features

Patients with most severe forms of β thalassaemia present within the first year of life with a failure to thrive, poor feeding, intermittent fever and intercurrent infections. At this stage the affected infant is pale with splenomegaly. There are no other specific clinical signs and the diagnosis depends on the haematology.

If the anaemia is not corrected the child will die of complications due to anaemia by the age of 5 years (Figure 13.8). If the anaemia is corrected with blood transfusions the erythropoietic drive is shut off, growth and development are normal and bone deformities do not occur. However, each unit of blood contains 200 mg of iron; with regular transfusions there is a steady accumulation of iron in the liver, endocrine glands and myocardium. Thus, although well-transfused thalassaemic children grow and develop normally until puberty , they die of iron overload unless steps are taken to remove iron.

The clinical picture in children who are inadequately transfused is of growth retardation, progressive spleno-megaly and hypersplenism which causes a worsening of the anaemia, sometimes associated with thrombo-cytopenia and a bleeding tendency (Figures 13.7, 13.9). Because of the bone marrow expansion, there are deformities of the skull, marked bossing and overgrowth of the zygomata, giving rise to the classical facies of β thalassaemia (Figure 13.10). Expansion of medullary

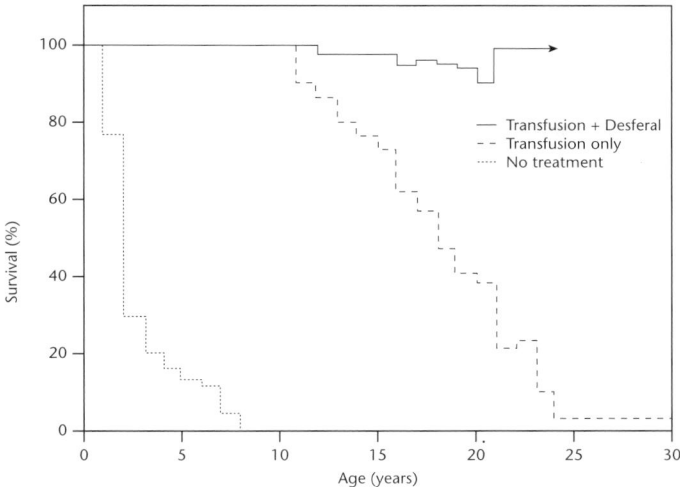

Figure 13.8: The prognosis of patients with β thalassaemia major.

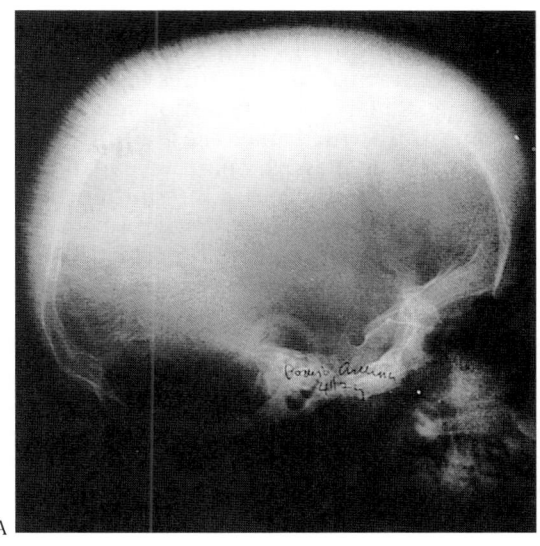

A

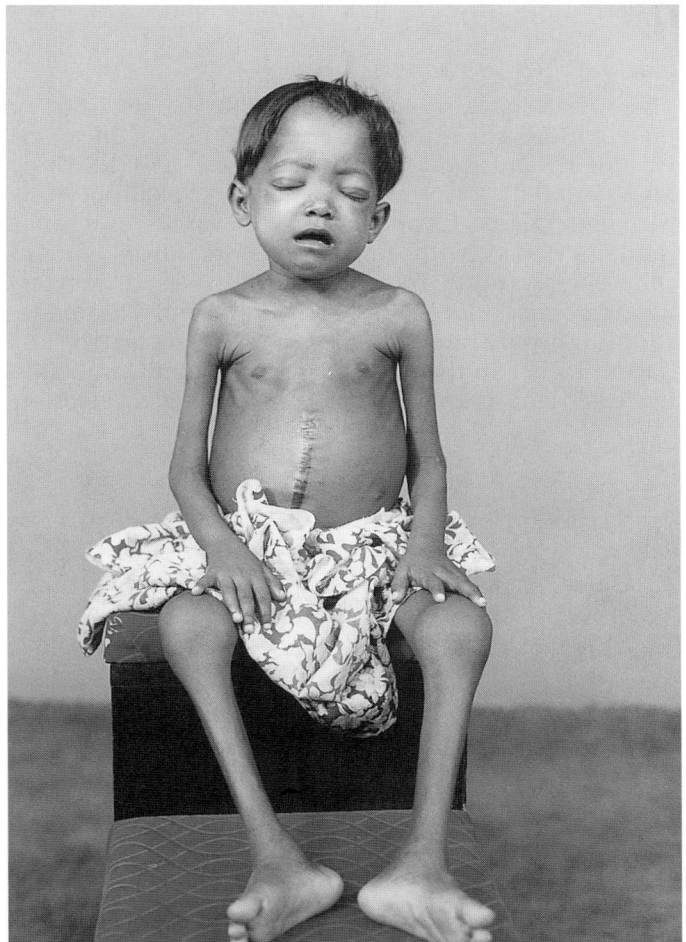

Figure 13.9: Typical features of a poorly transfused child with homozygous β thalassaemia, with severe wasting and an enlarged abdomen with a splenectomy scar. She is grossly iron loaded with a liver iron 30 mg/dry weight of liver, and has diabetes.

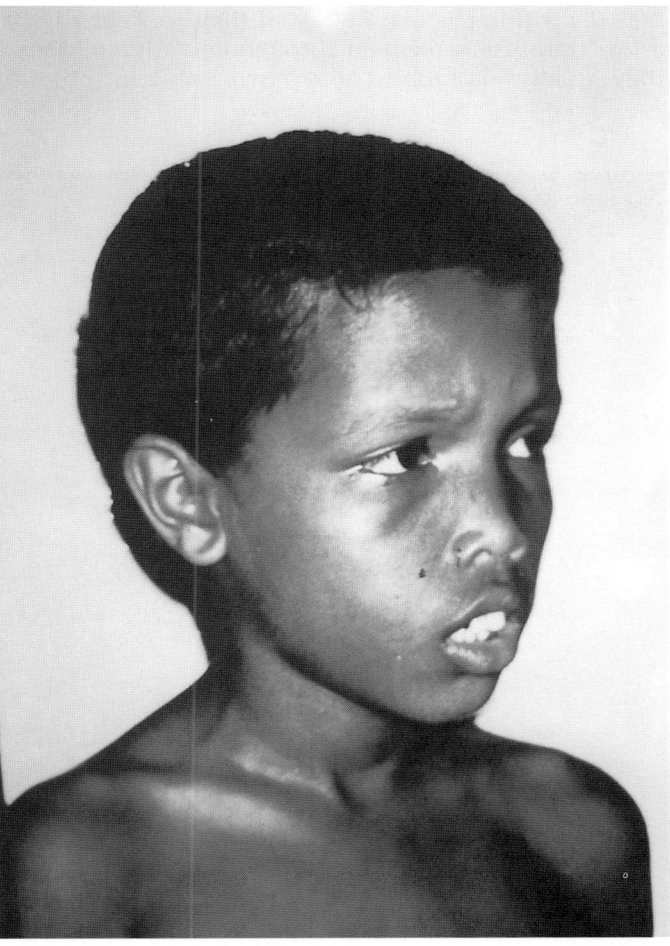

B

Figure 13.10: (**A**) Skull radiograph in β thalassaemia major, showing hair-on-end appearance which is the result of massive expansion of the bone marrow cavity. (**B**) Thalassaemia facies, with permission of the patient.

cavities by bone marrow and thinning of cortical bone in bones of arms, hands, legs and feet lead to structural weakness and recurrent fractures (Figure 13.11). Osteoporosis is a major cause of morbidity.[55] They are prone to infection, which may cause a further drop in Hb. Because of the massive marrow expansion these children are hypermetabolic, run intermittent fevers and lose weight. Folic acid deficiency develops because of low dietary intake, decreased absorption and the enormous demands for the vitamin by the expanded bone marrow: folate depletion leads to worsening of the anaemia. Because of the increased turnover of red cell precursors, hyperuricaemia and secondary gout occur occasionally. If these unfortunate children survive to puberty, they develop in addition the complications of iron loading: some of the iron accumulation results from increased rate of gastrointestinal iron absorption as well as from transfused blood.

The prognosis for the poorly transfused thalassaemic children is bad. If they receive no transfusions at all they may die within the first 2 years; if they are kept alive by a low transfusion regimen throughout early childhood, they usually succumb to an overwhelming infection by 10 years. If they reach puberty, they die of the effects of iron accumulation with acute or chronic cardiac failure or diabetes.

In the well-transfused thalassaemic child, early growth and development are normal and splenomegaly is minimal. There is, however, gradual accumulation of iron and the effects of tissue siderosis start to appear by the end of the first decade. The normal adolescent growth spurt fails to occur and hepatic, endocrine and cardiac complications of iron overloading produce a variety of problems including diabetes, hypoparathyroidism, adrenal insufficiency and progressive liver failure. Secondary sexual development is delayed, or does not occur at all. The short stature and lack of sexual development may lead to serious psychological problems. By far the commonest cause of death, which usually occurs towards the end of the second or early in the third decade, is progressive cardiac damage. Patients die ultimately either from protracted cardiac failure or suddenly from an acute arrhythmia. The use of intensive chelation may prevent or delay this distressing termination (Figure 13.8).

Haematological changes

There is always a severe anaemia and the Hb value on presentation ranges from 20 to 80 g/litre. The mean cell Hb (MCH) and the MCV are reduced (MCH 12–18 pg; MCV 50–60 fl). RBC show variation in size (anisocytosis) with both microcytes and macrocytes; variations in shape (poikilocytosis) with target cells, teardrops, microspherocytes and fragmented cells (schistocytes); hypochromia; blue-stained red cells (polychromasia), stippling (punctate basophilia) and nucleated RBC (Figure 13.12). In the post-splenectomy film many of the nucleated and mature red cells show ragged inclusions

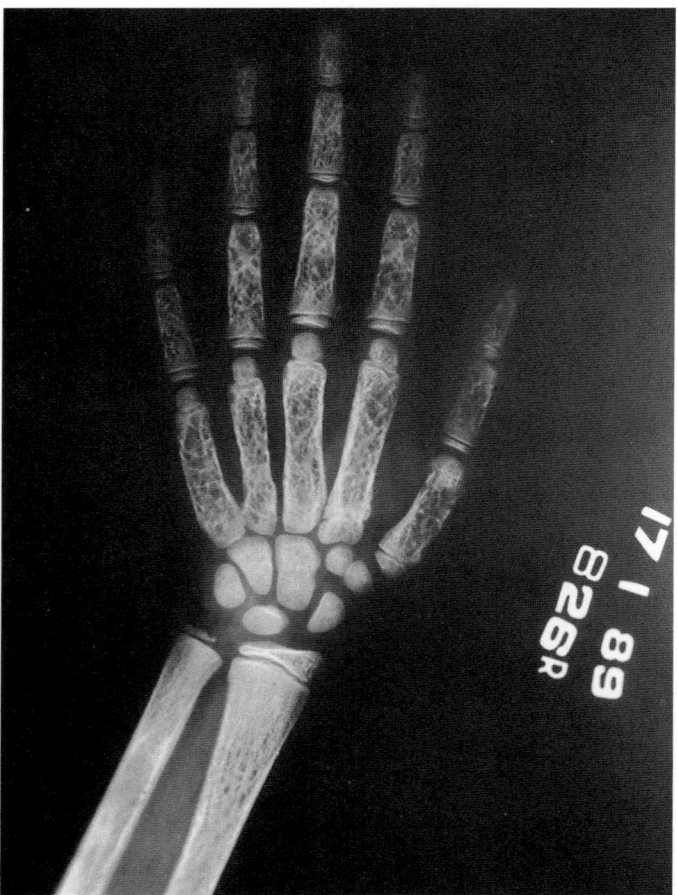

Figure 13.11: X-ray of the hand of a homozygous β thalassaemia patient showing the lace-like appearance, and the thinning of cortical bone.

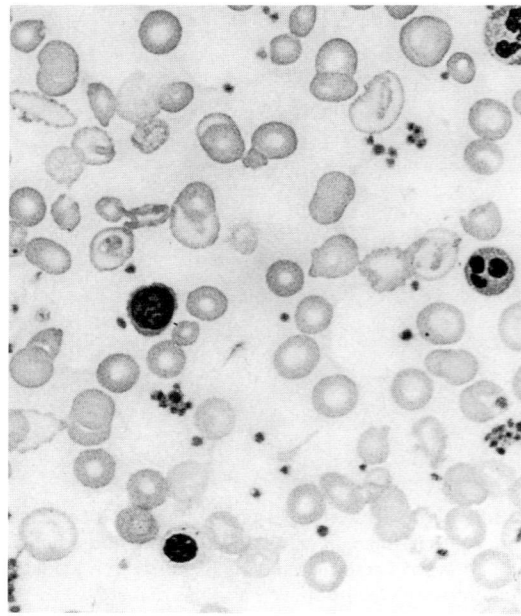

Figure 13.12: Peripheral blood film in β thalassaemia major, showing gross hypochromia, numerous target cells and nucleated red cells.

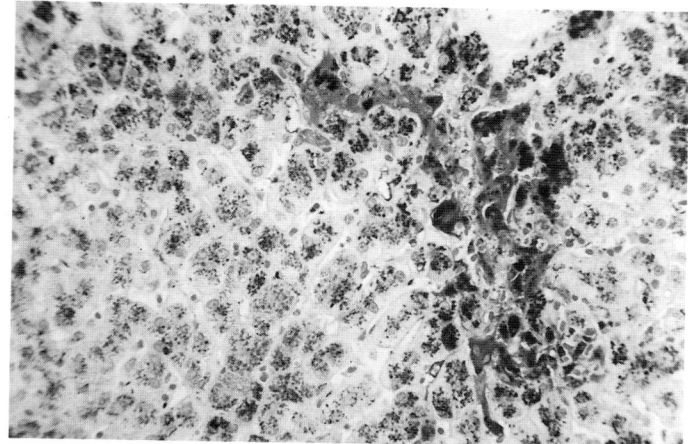

Figure 13.13: Histological appearance of the liver in homozygous β thalassaemia showing gross iron deposition.

after incubation of blood with methyl violet. The reticulocyte count is slightly elevated. The white cells and platelets are normal, unless there is hypersplenism when they are reduced, or the white cells are raised during infection. Bone marrow shows marked erythroid hyperplasia with a myeloid/erythroid (M/E) ratio of unity or less. Many red cell precursors show ragged inclusions after incubation of the marrow with methyl violet. Serum bilirubin is raised and haptoglobins are absent. Red cell survival is shortened. The serum iron rises progressively and the iron binding capacity is saturated. Plasma ferritin is high and the liver biopsy shows a marked increase in iron in both RES and parenchymal cells (Figure 13.13).

Haemoglobin changes

HbF level is always elevated. In β^0 thalassaemia there is no HbA and the haemoglobin consists of HbF and HbA_2 only. In β^+ thalassaemia some HbA is present, and the level of HbF ranges from 30% to 90% of the total; the HbA_2 level is usually normal.

Management

The management of β thalassaemia major needs a multidisciplinary team, which should include (1) dedicated physicians who give continuity of care, (2) dedicated nurses to allow the critically important relationship to develop with each patient, (3) other specialists such as cardiologists, endocrinologists, ophthalmologists, orthopaedic surgeons, general surgeons, hepatologists, neurologists, obstetricians and psychologists and (4) social workers.

The principles of management are (1) a regular blood transfusion regimen, (2) the administration of chelating agents to reduce iron overload, (3) splenectomy when hypersplenism develops, (4) folic acid supplementations, 1 mg per day, (5) psychological and financial support, (6) bone marrow transplantation and (7) genetic counselling.

Blood transfusion

The decision to initiate regular transfusions in patients with β thalassaemia may be difficult and should be based on the presence and severity of symptoms and signs of anaemia, including failure of growth and development. Even when the Hb is 70 g/litre, if the child has no symptoms of anaemia and is thriving the patient need not be transfused.

It is important to have an accurate diagnosis prior to starting treatment. The clinical and haematological diagnosis should be confirmed by DNA studies whenever possible. This is mainly to distinguish β thalassaemia major from thalassaemia intermedia and to permit prenatal diagnosis in subsequent pregnancies. Countries where facilities for DNA studies are not available embark on regular blood transfusion to all the phenotypical thalassaemics, thus giving unnecessary transfusions to thalassaemia intermedia patients and increasing the financial burden to the country unnecessarily.

The current recommendation for thalassaemia major is to maintain a pre-transfusion Hb concentration at 95–100 g/litre. This prevents chronic hypoxaemia, reduces compensatory marrow hyperplasia, promotes normal physical activity and growth, prevents bone changes, hypersplenism and hypervolaemia, and reduces gastrointestinal iron absorption. The post-transfusion Hb should not rise above 155 g/litre, as higher Hb levels raise blood viscosity, reduce tissue oxygenation and increase the risk of thrombosis, especially in the presence of other risk factors such as infections, metabolic acidosis, diabetes, or high platelet count following splenectomy. Higher Hb levels also increase blood consumption and accelerate iron overload. This regimen requires blood to be given at 4- to 6-weekly intervals throughout the patient's life.

Unless one gives good-quality and safe blood, patients are exposed to risks of (1) alloimunization against donor red cell, platelet and white cell antigens, (2) allergic reactions to plasma and (3) transmission of infections. The aim is to give red cells with the smallest possible amount of white blood cells or plasma. Antibody reactions manifest as fever during or 8 hours after transfusions without any other apparent cause. Allergic reactions to plasma show as urticaria during the transfusion. Leucocytes can also transmit leucocyte-borne viruses, including cytomegalovirus (CMV), Epstein–Barr virus (EBV), hepatitis B and C viruses (HBV, HCV) and human T-lymphotropic virus type 1 (HTLV-1). Leucocytes induce graft-versus-host disease and may be immunosuppressive. Therefore, it is best to give packed red cells via leucodepleting filters as this removes 99.9% of the white cells and platelets. An Italian and a Greek study showed that by using filters there was a 90% reduction of febrile illness in thalassaemias. Transmission of HBV, HCV, HIV, HTLV-1, syphilis and malaria are reduced to a minimum through donor selection, donor screening and immunization of the patient against HBV.

The volume of blood to transfuse is calculated according to the patient's weight, Hct of the available blood preparation and the patient's pre-transfusion Hb level. The rate at which blood can be transfused without overloading the circulation depends on the patient's Hb level and cardiovascular status. If there is no cardiac problem, it is acceptable to give 5–7 ml of packed red cells per kilogram body weight per hour. If cardiac failure is present it is advisable to give 2 ml/kg per hour. Hypertension, convulsions and cerebral haemorrhage have been observed in patients whose Hb is raised rapidly, especially when they were maintained at a very low Hb level.

It is important to evaluate the annual mean Hb level and the annual red cell consumption. The usual red cell consumption for splenectomized patients with a mean Hb of 120 g/litre ranges from 100 to 200 ml/kg per year. An unsplenectomized patient may consume 130–240 ml/kg per year. If the consumption of red cells is higher than this, the cause should be identified and corrected. The main causes of increased blood consumption are hypersplenism, red cell incompatibility and poor quality of transfused blood.

Chelation therapy

Regular chelation with desferrioxamine has proved remarkably effective in reducing the iron burden of transfused patients.[54] Cardiac disease is delayed or prevented and life expectancy is significantly extended, but endocrinopathy may develop and persist (Figure 13.8). Unfortunately, effective use of the drug requires devotion to a mechanical pump that slowly infuses the medication into a subcutaneous site. (Figure 13.14). Nearly normal concentration of hepatic iron can be maintained with modern regimens of desferrioxamine, and the progression of hepatic fibrosis to cirrhosis can be arrested. There are relatively low prevalences of thyroid, parathyroid and adrenal abnormalities. Early and intensive desferrioxamine therapy increases the incidence of normal sexual maturation, but it apparently does not reverse established abnormalities. Desferrioxamine prevents diabetes mellitus, but does not reverse this complication.

A balance between the effectiveness of desferrioxamine and its toxicity (the later observed primarily in the presence of relatively low body iron burden) can be maintained through regular determination of body iron burden. The serum ferritin concentration, measured 6-monthly, is commonly used to assess the effectiveness of treatment, but this test may lead to errors in the management; many factors influence ferritin levels such as presence of inflammatory disease, liver disease or vitamin C deficiency. By contrast, the annual or biannual measurement of hepatic stores, whose concentrations are highly correlated with total body iron stores, provides the best quantitative, specific and sensitive method of evaluating iron burden in patients with thalassaemia. Determination of hepatic iron concentration in liver biopsy specimens obtained with ultrasonographic guidance is safe and permits rational adjustments in iron chelating therapy (Figure 13.13).

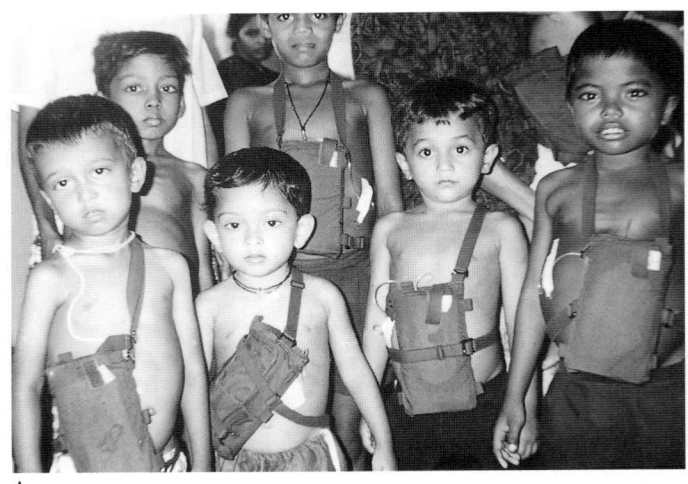

A

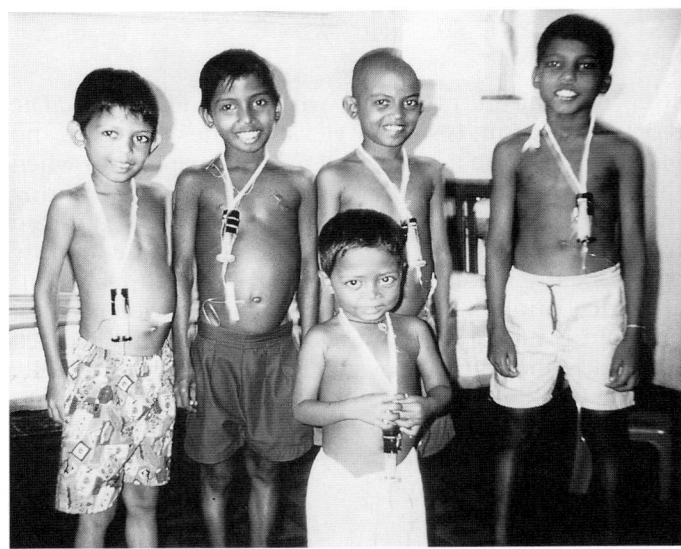

B

Figure 13.14: (**A**) A group of thalassaemic patients using infusion pumps (cost US $260 per pump). (**B**) Using hand-made pumps (cost quarter of a dollar).

Chelation therapy should be started as soon as transfusions have deposited enough iron to protect against desferrioxamine toxicity. The current recommendation is to start therapy when serum transferrin is completely saturated, which happens usually after 10–20 transfusions, or when the ferritin level rises above 1000 ng/ml, or at least by the age of 3 years. Administration recommended is by slow subcutaneous infusion via a thin needle inserted subcutaneously, over 8–12 hours using an infusion pump, given five to seven times per week at a mean daily dose of 20–50 mg/kg body weight. The dose is adjusted according to hepatic iron value or serum ferritin levels. If the patient's serum ferritin is < 2000 ng/ml about 25 mg/kg per day is required; if the ferritin level is 2000–3000 ng/ml about 35 mg/kg per day is required; patients with a higher serum level require up to 55 mg/kg per day.

Continuous infusion of desferrioxamine is more beneficial than periodic infusions, because of the constant removal of toxic free iron which returns to the pretreatment levels within minutes of stopping a continuous intravenous infusion. When intensive chelation is needed an implanted intravenous delivery system (portacath) can be used. Patients who have cardiac problems secondary to iron overload will benefit with continuous intravenous desferrioxamine as this removes large quantities of iron. It can reverse deteriorating cardiac function by removing the toxic non-transferrin bound iron. The recommended dose is 50–70 mg/kg per day for 5–6 days. Individuals with refractory congestive cardiac failure or hypotension due to cardiac disease are poor candidates for intravenous desferrioxamine.

It is best to avoid desferrioxamine during pregnancy. Treatment can be resumed at full dosage during lactation, as the drug is not absorbed orally.

Desferrioxamine treatment is burdensome and can be painful, and non-compliance is an important and common problem. Compliance requires a constant and secure relationship between doctor, patient and parents, and regular discussion of its importance.

Complications of desferrioxamine administration

Infection with *Yersinia enterocolitis* is the most important acute risk associated with desferrioxamine treatment. Treatment should be discontinued temporarily in any patient with an acute febrile illness, especially if any or all of the following symptoms are present: sore throat, high fever, acute abdominal pain or severe diarrhoea.

Rashes of more or less intense hyperaemia are common. They may be due to the injection of a concentrated solution of desferrioxamine (usually 500 mg in 5 ml of distilled water for injection). It is better to dilute the preparation further. If the rash persists, adding hydrocortisone to the infusion should be tried. Severe allergic reactions to desferrioxamine are rare.

Desferrioxamine overdose is seen if it is administered in high doses to patients who are not heavily iron loaded. The complications are toxic effects on the eye, including night blindness, reduction in visual fields and reduction of visual acuity. These usually regress when treatment is stopped. High tone deafness is seen particularly in the young; this is usually not reversible. Patients should be questioned frequently regarding the symptoms and formal audiometry and ophthalmological examination should be performed regularly. There may be retardation of growth, with skeletal changes such as short trunk, genu valgum and short stature, which can be reversible with dose reduction.

Other ways to reduce the iron overload

The oral iron chelating drug deferiprone is effective in removing iron, at least in the short term.[56] Long-term studies have suggested that hepatic iron may stabilize at or rise to concentrations associated with hepatic fibrosis, an increased risk of cardiac disease and early death in approximately half of patients. Previously recognized adverse effects of deferiprone include embryo toxicity, teratogenicity, neutropenia and agranulocytosis.

The results of long-term follow-up of the effectiveness of other modes of administration of desferrioxamine are awaited. These include desferrioxamine attached to high-molecular starch, or given in a lipid vehicle permitting slow release.

Role of vitamin C

Iron-loaded patients usually become vitamin C deficient, probably because iron oxidizes the vitamin. When this is the case, administration of vitamin C increases the availability of iron and so increases its toxicity if large doses are taken without simultaneous desferrioxamine infusion. Vitamin C supplements should be started only if the patient is receiving desferrioxamine regularly. The minimum effective dose is 5 mg/kg (50 mg for children under 10 years and 100 mg for children over 10 years) and should be given after starting the desferrioxamine.

Splenectomy

Massive splenomegaly with hypersplenism that causes leucopenia, thrombocytopenia and an increasing transfusion requirement is frequent at a relatively early age in patients on moderate transfusion regimens. Early splenectomy is required. The benefits of splenectomy on iron balance occur if the transfusion requirements exceed 200–250 ml/kg per year of packed red cells when the minimum Hb is maintained at 100 g/litre; a spleen which is very large, in the absence of overt hypersplenism, accounts for a relatively large portion of the total blood volume, and its removal often leads to a marked reduction in blood requirement. The surgical risks in experienced hands are minimal. Removal of the spleen may blunt the primary immune response to encapsulated organisms *Diplococcus pneumoniae*, *Haemophilus influenzae* or *Neisseria meningitidis*, and therefore delay of splenectomy until after 4 or 5 years of age is most desirable, so that the child has an opportunity to develop some resistance to these organisms. It advisable to immunize patients with the appropriate vaccines against these organisms about 2 weeks prior to surgery, and to prescribe long-term prophylactic oral penicillin to prevent colonization by strains of pneumococcus not covered by the vaccine, especially in young children. Any illness accompanied by high fever of uncertain aetiology should be treated aggressively with parenteral antibiotics, usually an ampicillin derivative such as amoxycillin, until culture results become known. Splenectomized patients are also more susceptible to malaria, and should receive lifelong prophylaxis when living in endemic regions.

Splenectomy usually results in a transitory or persistent thrombocytosis. As a rule this carries no risk for patients, possibly because it is balanced by a simultaneous reduction in platelet aggregation, but studies in Thailand claim that splenectomized patients have evidence of pulmonary vascular disease due to thrombocytosis.

Low-dose prophylactic aspirin may be considered for patients whose platelet count exceeds 800×10^9/litre.

Psychological support

The inherited nature of the disease, its appearance during the first year of life, the possibility of physical deformity and the need for continuous punishing treatment have important implications for the child's emotional development and relationships with the rest of the family. An appropriately constituted therapeutic team can help patients to cope successfully with the psychological consequences of their illness, to integrate themselves into society and to see themselves as essentially normal people.

All members of the management team, especially nursing staff, should remain the same for as long as possible and should have a thalassaemia-oriented training. The team should reserve time and space for meeting with both patients and parents before, during or after the visit to the treatment centre. Patients should be helped to understand and accept their illness, so that they can also accept the necessary treatment.

Integration into school constitutes a critical step in psychological development. The ultimate goal is the development into an adult who can actively participate in society. In general, school staff should be advised to avoid limiting the patient's activity or allowing special privileges (unless they are medically indicated) which could lead to continued dependency. Patients' overriding right not to inform teachers or peers that they have thalassaemia should always be respected.

Patients' and parents' associations help families to feel less isolated, and offer them the help and comfort of others in the same situation. Participation helps patients and families to comply with the treatment regimen.

Bone marrow transplant

Over 1000 patients have received bone marrow transplants in several highly experienced centres.[52-54] The donor should be an HLA-matched sibling, or occasionally a parent. When a patient has an HLA-compatible donor, if transplantation is chosen it should be done as soon as possible. Transplantation from an unrelated donor carries a substantially increased risk, and should be considered only in exceptional circumstances. Graft-versus-host disease (GVHD) is less common in children than in adults: in the largest series in Italy mild GVHD occurred in 10% of cases, moderate GVHD in 8% and serious GVHD in 2%. Graft rejection can occur up to 3–5 years after transplantation. The chance of success is highest when patients are well chelated, with normal liver size and histology, and free of cardiac complications. Hepatic fibrosis and the presence of iron overload are important risk factors. In countries where it is available, marrow transplantation should be considered for all patients with a suitable donor (30–40% of patients in most populations) and who have a low score of these risk factors.

Cord blood transplantation

Cord blood contains haemopoietic stem cells that can be used for transplantation. Preliminary experience is encouraging and all new siblings of thalassaemic patients should have cord blood preserved for possible future use.

Augmentation of fetal haemoglobin synthesis

Several trials have attempted to augment the synthesis of HbF in an effort to ameliorate the severity of thalassaemia.[52-54] Therapy with hydroxyurea, butyric acid compounds and these agents in combination has reduced or eliminated transfusion requirements in some patients. Other studies have reported only a small increase in HbF and total Hb concentrations during the administration of oral hydroxyurea and intravenous or oral butyrates. Erythropoietin has not been proved useful in thalassaemia, either alone or in combination with hydroxyurea. Therapies to increase the synthesis of HbF in β thalassaemia have, with few exceptions, proved disappointing to date.

Gene therapy

Permanent correction of genetic deficit of the haemopoietic system requires the transfer of genes into stem cells, with long-term, high-level and lineage-specific expression of these cells after autologous transplantation. Over the last decade, there has been progress in the development of transduction methods and vectors, but many problems remain.[54]

Thalassaemia Intermedia

The term thalassaemia intermedia is used to describe patients with clinical thalassaemia which, although not transfusion dependent, is associated with a much more severe degree of anaemia than that found in heterozygous carriers for α and β thalassaemia. This clinical course is seen in β+ thalassaemia homozygotes with mild decrease in the β globin expression (e.g., in West Africa and Afro-Americans), HbC β[0] thalassaemia and various δβ thalassaemias. It is also seen in homozygous thalassaemia patients who have inherited an α thalassaemia determinant, thereby reducing the overall degree of globin chain imbalance. Co-inheritance of a triplicated α globin locus with heterozygous β thalassaemia also causes thalassaemia intermedia phenotype (Table 13.14).

Table 13.14 Molecular basis of thalassaemia intermedia.

- **Homozygous β thalassaemia**
  Mild β+ point mutation
  Co-inheritance α+ thalassaemia
  Enhanced production of HbF
- **δβ thalassaemia**
  Homozygous δβ thalassaemia
- **Heterozygous β thalassaemia**
  Co-inheritance of triplicated α globin loci (ααα)

The clinical features of the intermedia forms are extremely variable. At one end of the spectrum are individuals who are virtually symptom free except for moderate anaemia. At the other end there are patients who have Hb in the range 50–70 g/litre, who develop marked splenomegaly, severe skeletal deformities due to expansion of bone marrow and, as they get older, become heavily iron loaded because of increased intestinal absorption of iron. Recurrent leg ulcers, folate deficiency, symptoms due to extramedullary haemopoietic tumour masses in the chest and skull, gallstones and a marked proneness to infection are particularly characteristic of this group of thalassaemics. Many of them are identified with anaemia later in life than is usual for homozygous β thalassaemia.

β Thalassaemia minor

Heterozygous inheritance of either $β^0$ or $β^+$ thalassaemia genes results in β thalassaemia minor; there are over 150 million such carriers alive today.

Clinical

The condition is asymptomatic. A small proportion of subjects have just palpable splenomegaly. The moderate but persistent anaemia during pregnancy causes fetal hypoxia, compensatory placental hypertrophy, mild intrauterine growth retardation, low urinary oestradiol excretion, an increased frequency of fetal distress during delivery and a high frequency, about 12%, of Apgar scores of 3 or less at 1 minute, but no significant increase of perinatal mortality.[57]

Haematology

The Hb is in the range 90–110 g/litre, and during pregnancy about 20 g/litre lower; the MCV and MCH are low, especially with $β^0$ thalassaemia (Table 13.15), and the blood film shows moderate anisocytosis, microcytosis and hypochromia with occasional target cells and a few cells with punctate basophilia; the red cell changes are greater than expected for the mild degree of anaemia. There is mild to moderate erythroid hyperplasia in the bone marrow; there is no tendency to iron overload unless the patient has received inappropriate parenteral iron therapy, and the prevalence of iron deficiency is the same as that of the general population.

The diagnosis is made by observing that the HbA_2 is raised to 4–6%; the HbF is also raised to about 3% in approximately half of the subjects. Osmotic fragility is reduced.

Management

It is important for the diagnosis to be made so as to avoid unnecessary treatment of the hypochromic anaemia with iron. Subjects should be reassured as to the benign nature of the condition and be offered genetic counselling (see below).

Malaria

J. B. S. Haldane was the first to hypothesize that the geographical coincidence of malaria and β thalassaemia could be due to the heterozygotes being at genetic advantage through a partial protection against *P. falciparum*. A relative resistance to malaria was confirmed in Liberian children with thalassaemia minor.[58] Suggested mechanisms of limiting parasitaemia have included: (1) a slower than normal decline of HbF in the first 2 years of life;[59] (2) a greater rigidity of red cell membranes resisting parasite invasion; (3) modified expression of parasite-induced neoantigens on red cell surfaces enhancing the development of protective cell mediated immunity;[60] and (4) high oxidant stress in thalassaemic cells inhibiting parasite growth.[61]

β Thalassaemia in association with Hb variants

In many populations, because there is a high incidence of both β thalassaemia and Hb variants, it is quite common for an individual to inherit a β thalassaemia gene from one parent and a gene for structural Hb variant from the other, e.g., HbS β thalassaemia (discussed under 'Sickle cell disease') HbC β thalassaemia, HbE β thalassaemia and HbD β thalassaemia.

Haemoglobin C thalassaemia

This disorder is restricted to West African, some North African, southern Mediterranean and American populations. HbC $β^+$ thalassaemia in West Africans is characterized by a mild haemolytic anaemia associated with splenomegaly: the peripheral blood film shows numerous target cells and thalassaemic red cell changes with a moderately elevated reticulocyte count. Hb electrophoresis shows a preponderance of HbC, some HbA and HbF. HbC $β^0$ thalassaemia, in Mediterranean people and Americans, is somewhat more severe clinically, resembling thalassaemia intermedia: there is only HbC and HbF. (HbA_2 cannot be separated from HbC.) Diagnosis is confirmed by checking the parents.

Table 13.15 Red cell indices in iron deficiency and in thalassaemia compared with normal individuals.

Red blood cell indices	Normal range	Iron deficiency	Typical α or β thalassaemia trait
Red blood cell count × 10^{12}/litre	4–5	< 4	6.32
Mean corpuscular volume (MCV) fl	75–99	< 76	63
Mean cellular haemoglobin (MCH) pg	27–31	27.5	20.3
Mean corpuscular haemoglobin concentration (MCHC) g/dl	32–36	30	32.2

Haemoglobin E thalassaemia

This is the commonest severe form of thalassaemia in South-East Asia and eastern India. HbE is inefficiently synthesized, and hence when a HbE gene is inherited together with a β^0 thalassaemia determinant, there is a marked deficiency of β chain production. The resulting clinical picture can closely resemble homozygous β^0 thalassaemia, and is seen commonly in South-East Asia.[62]

In contrast, in Sri Lanka, where HbE thalassaemia constitutes 40% of all thalassaemias, the clinical picture varies from an almost normal to a mild anaemia to a severe anaemia.[63] The majority in Sri Lanka have a mild anaemia with splenomegaly: they grow and develop normally with few complications, and there are many recorded cases of pregnancy in women with this disorder. They usually have an average Hb of 60–70 g/litre, are rarely symptomatic because the Hb O_2 dissociation curve is shifted to the right and more oxygen is released to tissues than from HbF in β thalassaemia major, and may not be transfusion dependent. They are liable to become more anaemic and may require transfusions during an infection, to which these patients are more prone. These patients continue to become iron overloaded in spite of not receiving blood transfusions, probably due to increased gastrointestinal absorption of iron.

The diagnosis of HbE β thalassaemia is confirmed by finding only HbE and HbF on electrophoresis, and by demonstrating the HbE trait in one parent and β thalassaemia trait in the other parent.

The $\delta\beta$ thalassaemias

The disorders due to reduced β and δ chain synthesis are much less common than those due to defective β chain production alone. They result from deletions of the β and δ globin genes or may be due to unequal crossing over between the δ and β globin gene loci with the production of $\delta\beta$ fusion genes. The latter produce $\delta\beta$ fusion chains which combine with α chains to form haemoglobin variants called Lepore haemoglobins.

Clinical features

The $\delta\beta$ thalassaemias have been reported in many populations although there are no high-frequency areas. In the homozygous state there is a mild degree of anaemia with Hb values of 80–100 g/litre. There is often a moderate degree of splenomegaly, but these patients are usually symptomless except during periods of stress, such as infections or pregnancy. Haemoglobin analysis shows 100% HbF in homozygotes; heterozygous carriers have a thalassaemic blood picture, elevated levels of HbF of 5–20% and normal levels of HbA_2.

The homozygous state for Hb Lepore is characterized by a clinical picture which is usually similar to that of homozygous β thalassaemia, although in some cases it might be milder and not transfusion dependent. The clinical and haematological findings are similar to those of β thalassaemia. The haemoglobin consists of HbF and Hb Lepore only.

Hereditary persistence of fetal haemoglobin (HPFH)

HPFH results from a combined deletion of the δ and β chains, but the deficit of β globin chains is compensated for by a high rate of synthesis of γ chains. Heterozygotes have no clinical or haematological abnormalities except that they have HbF 20–30%; acid elution and staining for HbF on a peripheral blood film shows that HbF is homogeneously distributed in all red cells, so distinguishing this from other conditions such as β^+ thalassaemia, where HbF is distributed unevenly in the erythrocytes. The homozygotes are entirely asymptomatic, but have a thalassaemic-like appearance in the red cells and 100% HbF.

$\gamma\delta\beta$ thalassaemia

This rare thalassaemia results from long deletion of β globin gene clusters which, as well as removing the entire β gene, removes the γ and δ genes. There is no output of globin from this gene cluster at all. The homozygous state leads to an absence of HbF and is not compatible with fetal survival; heterozygotes have severe haemolytic disease of the newborn with anaemia and jaundice. If they survive the neonatal period, they grow and develop normally; in adult life they have a haematological picture resembling heterozygous β thalassaemia.

The α thalassaemias

Although the α thalassaemias are commoner than the β thalassaemias they pose less of a public health problem, because the severe homozygous forms cause death in utero or in the neonatal period and the milder forms do not produce major disability.

The α thalassaemias occur widely throughout the Mediterranean region, Sub-Saharan Africa, the Middle East, isolated parts of the Indian subcontinent, and throughout South-East Asia in a line stretching from south China through Thailand, Malaysia and Indonesia (Figure 13.15).

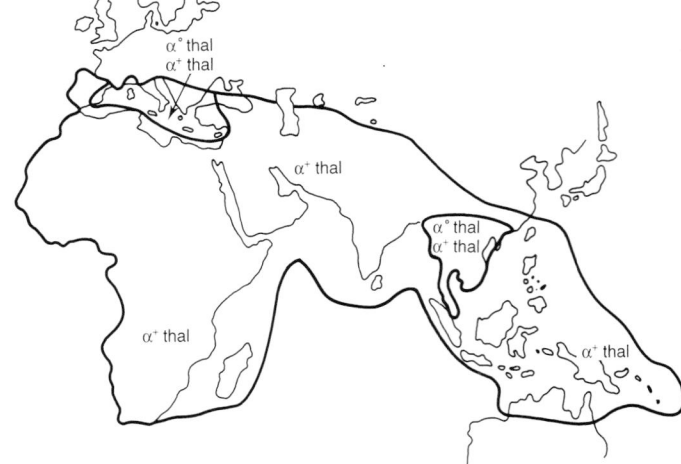

Figure 13.15: Areas of the Old World where α thalassaemias reach polymorphic frequency.

Definition and inheritance

Genetic disease of α chain synthesis results in defective HbF and HbA production, as both contain α chains. In the fetus the deficiency of α chains leads to the production of excess γ chains, which form γ_4 tetramers or Hb Bart's. In the adult a deficiency of α chains leads to an excess of β chains which forms β_4 tetramers or HbH. Hb Bart's and HbH are the hallmarks of α thalassaemia, but the carrier states of different forms of α thalassaemia are difficult to diagnose as only trace amounts of these haemoglobins are produced.

Genetically determined reductions of α globin synthesis are most often the outcomes of a variety of deletions from α globin clusters on chromosome 16 (Figure 13.5).[52,53,64] There are two α genes (α_2 and α_1) responsible for the production of α globin chain in the chromosome. Thus there are four genes in a human diploid cell, two coming from each parent, represented as $\alpha\alpha/\alpha\alpha$. Deletion of one of the two α globulin genes is denoted as ($-\alpha$) and this results in α^+ thalassaemia, with partial suppression of the α globin synthesis: this is caused by unequal crossover events, generating at the same time a triple α gene ($\alpha\alpha\alpha$), which can be observed in the normal population. Deletions of both genes, denoted as ($-$ $-$), results in α^0 thalassaemia with total absence of α globin synthesis. A further refinement of this nomenclature includes the designation of specific mutations; ($-$ $-^{SEA}$) signifies the α^0 deletion mutation that is confined to South-East Asia, while ($-\alpha^{3.7}$) symbolizes the α^+ rightward gene deletion common in Africa.

A few α^+ thalassaemias are due to point mutations, giving rise to more severe reduction of α globulin synthesis than due to the single gene deletions. These are designated by the superscript T ($\alpha\alpha^T$). The most important non-deletional α thalassaemia gene is a termination codon mutation on α_2 globin gene, designated as ($\alpha^{CS}\alpha$), leading to the production of an elongated α chain which combines with β chains to form Hb Constant Spring: the abnormal mRNA is unstable so that only low levels of Hb Constant Spring are synthesized and the phenotype is a moderately severe α thalassaemia.

Genetics of α thalassaemia

Three genotypes are associated with clinically asymptomatic states: (1) heterozygous α^+ thalassaemia ($-\alpha/\alpha\alpha$); (2) homozygous α^+ thalassaemia ($-\alpha/-\alpha$); and (3) heterozygous α^0 thalassaemia ($-$ $-/\alpha\alpha$) (Table 13.16).

Doubly heterozygous α^0 thalassaemia/α^+ thalassaemia ($-$ $-/-\alpha$) leaves only one active α globulin gene. Both Hb Bart's and HbH have high oxygen affinity, resulting in tissue hypoxia; in addition, HbH is unstable and is precipitated as intracellular inclusion bodies, causing haemolysis and the clinical condition of HbH disease.

Homozygous α^0 thalassaemia ($-$ $-/-$ $-$) allows for only Hb Bart's to be formed in fetal life; because of its high oxygen affinity, infants are hypoxic and hydropic, inevitably dying in utero or shortly after delivery.

Geographical distribution

The α^0 thalassaemia gene frequencies are highest in South-East Asia and China (Figure 13.15);[64] in Thailand, for example, gene frequency for α^0 thalassaemia is 0.025, for α^+ thalassaemia 0.10–0.15, and for Hb Constant Spring 0.05–0.15. In consequence, Hb Bart's hydrops fetalis affecting 25 000 infants each year, and HbH disease affecting about 68 000 infants each year, are major health problems.

Both α^+ thalassaemia and α^0 thalassaemia deletions are seen at low frequencies in the Mediterranean region, so that HbH disease and hydrops fetalis can occur: in addition, HbH disease arises rarely from non-deletional mutations. The α^+ thalassaemias are common in Saudi

Table 13.16 The α thalassaemia syndromes.

Genotype (Normal $\alpha\alpha/\alpha\alpha$, $\beta\beta$)	Globin genes affected by mutations	Syndrome	Clinical features	Haemoglobin pattern
$\alpha-/\alpha\alpha$. $\beta\beta$	1 (α_2)	Silent carrier	No anaemia Normal red cell	Hb Bart's 1–2% at birth HbCS 1–2% Remainder HbA
$-$ $-/\alpha\alpha$. $\beta\beta$ or $\alpha-/\alpha-$. $\beta\beta$	2 (α_2 α_1) or 2 (α_2)	Thalassaemia trait	Mild anaemia Hypochromic microcytic red cells	Hb Barts 5–10% HbCS 1–2% Remainder HbA
$-$ $-/-\alpha$. $\beta\beta$	3 (α genes)	HbH disease	Moderate anaemia Hypochromic microcytic, fragmented red cells. May demonstrate inclusion bodies	Hb Bart's 5–30% HbCS 1–2% Remainder HbA
$-$ $-/-$ $-$. $\beta\beta$	4 (α genes)	Hydrops fetalis	Severe anaemia Death in utero	Mainly Hb Bart's (γ_4)

HbCS: haemoglobin Constant Spring.

Arabia (frequency 0.37), as is a severe non-deletional form of α thalassaemia resulting in HbH disease.

On the Indian subcontinent α⁺ thalassaemia gene frequencies are extremely high (above 0.70) in tribal or scheduled groups and in the Tharu of Nepal. In Sri Lanka 15.5% of the population are heterozygous for α⁺ thalassaemia and about 3% of the population were heterozygous for the triplicated α-globin gene arrangement (ααα).[63] Similarly the α⁺ thalassaemia gene frequency reaches up to 0.70 on coastal areas of Papua New Guinea. α⁺ thalassaemia gene frequencies are in the range 0.10–0.27 throughout sub–Saharan Africa.[65] However, α⁰ thalassaemia is not present in these populations and there is no disease.

Pathophysiology

The pathophysiology of α thalassaemia is different from that of β thalassaemia. Hb Bart's and HbH respectively do not precipitate in the marrow and hence there is less intramedullary destruction of red cell precursors, and erythropoiesis is more effective than in β thalassaemia. However, HbH is unstable and precipitates in red cells as they age. The resulting inclusion bodies are trapped in the spleen and other parts of the microcirculation, leading to shortened red cell survival. Furthermore, both Hb Bart's and HbH have a very high oxygen affinity. Thus the pathology of severe forms of α thalassaemia is based on defective haemoglobin production, the synthesis of homotetramers which are physiologically useless, and the haemolytic component due to their precipitation in older red cells.

Haemoglobin Bart's hydrops syndrome

The homozygous state for α⁰ thalassaemia (– –/– –) is a common cause of fetal loss throughout South-East Asia, Greece and Cyprus. Affected infants do not produce HbF or HbA. The infants are usually stillborn between 28 and 40 weeks or die within a few hours after delivery.[52,53] They have the typical features of hydrops fetalis with gross pallor, generalized oedema and massive hepatosplenomegaly. There is a very large friable placenta. All these findings are due to severe intrauterine anaemia. The Hb values are in the 60–80 g/litre range, and there are gross thalassaemic changes of the peripheral blood film with many nucleated red cells. The haemoglobin consists of approximately 80% Hb Bart's and 20% of embryonic Hb Portland ($\zeta_2\gamma_2$). It is believed that these infants survive to term because they continue to produce embryonic haemoglobin which transports oxygen functionally.

The syndrome is characterized also by a high incidence of toxaemia of pregnancy and considerable obstetric difficulties due to the presence of the large, friable placenta. Both parents have minor thalassaemic red cell changes with normal HbA_2 values, which is a characteristic finding of the heterozygous state of α⁰ thalassaemia.

Haemoglobin H disease

HbH disease usually results from the inheritance of doubly heterozygous α⁰ thalassaemia/α⁺ thalassaemia

(– –/–α), or from the inheritance of α⁰ thalassaemia and Hb Constant Spring (– –/α^{cs}α), or from the homozygous state for severe non-deletion form of α thalassaemia particularly common in Saudi Arabia.[52,53]

There is a variable degree of anaemia and splenomegaly, but it is most unusual to see severe thalassaemic bone changes or growth retardation. Affected patients survive into adult life as they have sufficient HbA, but their course may be interspersed with severe episodes of haemolysis associated with infection, or worsening of the anaemia due to progressive hypersplenism. In addition, oxidant drugs such as sulfonamides, or pregnancy, may increase the rate of precipitation of HbH and exacerbate the anaemia. Iron overload is uncommon.

The Hb values range from 70 to 100 g/litre and the blood film shows typical thalassaemic changes. There is moderate reticulocytosis, and on incubating the red cell with brilliant cresyl blue numerous inclusion bodies are generated by precipitation of the HbH under the redox action of the dye. Haemoglobin analysis reveals from 5% to 40% HbH, together with HbA and normal or reduced level of HbA_2.

Consistent with the mild nature of the disease, treatment is primarily supportive.

Asymptomatic α thalassaemia

The silent carrier state (–α/αα) is due to the presence of a mutation affecting the deletion of a single α globin gene. α Thalassaemia trait is commonly associated with two genotypes: (– –/αα) and (–α/–α). Point mutation affecting the α_2 gene ($\alpha^T\alpha/\alpha\alpha$) may also lead to α thalassaemia trait. Subjects develop mild hypochromic, microcytic anaemia. At birth, Hb Bart's contributes about 2.5% of the total Hb in heterozygous α⁰ thalassaemia (– –/αα) and homozygous α⁺ thalassaemia (–α/–α), and may be seen in trace amounts in about 10% of heterozygous α⁺ thalassaemia (–α/αα). HbH is not detected.

α⁺ Thalassaemia is of some importance in Africa as, besides causing a slight anaemia, it ameliorates the severity of sickle cell disease as well as the anaemia of homozygous β⁺ thalassaemia, and is associated with lower proportion of HbS in sickle cell trait.

Malaria

The strongest evidence that α⁺ thalassaemia has been selected for by malaria is epidemiological: for example, gene frequency is closely and positively correlated with endemicity of malaria in Papua New Guinea and of island Melanesia.[66] As the disadvantage of α⁺ thalassaemia, or even α⁰ thalassaemia, is not great, only mild selective pressure would be required to achieve polymorphism. In fact, no increased fitness or control of parasitaemia has been demonstrated in heterozygotes. However, in α⁺ thalassaemia increased amounts of malaria-induced neoantigens are displayed on red cell surfaces, and rapid immune clearance of parasitized cells is one probable mechanism of advantage.[60] Also, an *increased* incidence of mild *P. falciparum* malaria has been described in children with α thalassaemia, stimulating high levels of immunity.[66]

Screening for thalassaemia syndromes Thalassaemia syndromes may be easily recognized from clinical presentation of anaemia, growth retardation, jaundice and splenomegaly, and changes in the red cell morphology. However, carrier detection including genotype determination requires certain laboratory investigations.[67]

Usually, Hb levels of 100 g/litre and below are considered as indications for the screening of thalassaemia for subjects without iron deficiency. However, the Hb level may be normal in the carrier or heterozygous states. In all cases, iron deficiency must be ruled out before the diagnosis is made since its interference can cause misdiagnosis (Table 13.15).

Routine haemoglobinopathy screening includes the measurement of red cell indices, electrophoresis and measurement of haemoglobins, and analysis of globin chains. An MCV < 80 fl, MCH < 27 pg and/or Hct < 36% suggest thalassaemia: the mean cell haemoglobin concentration (MCHC) generally remains within normal range. Although MCV, MCH and/or PCV are decreased in most cases of thalassaemia, the values are within the normal range for α thalassaemias, HbE and Hb Constant Spring.

Prevention Thalassaemias produce severe public health problems and are serious drains on medical resources in many populations. Since there is no definitive treatment and supportive treatment is extremely expensive, most countries in which the disease is common are putting a major effort into prevention.

There are two major approaches to the prevention of thalassaemia. Since the carrier states for β thalassaemia can be recognized easily, it is possible to screen populations and offer genetic counselling about the choice of marriage partners. If a β thalassaemic heterozygote marries another carrier, one in four (on average) of their children will have the severe transfusion-dependent homozygous disorder. It is well to remember that this risk applies to each pregnancy. Large-scale programmes of this type have had variable outcomes.

Most countries are developing screening programmes at antenatal clinics. When heterozygous carrier mothers are found their husbands are tested, and if they are also carriers the couple is offered the possibility of prenatal diagnosis and termination of pregnancies carrying fetuses with severe forms of thalassaemia.

In view of the considerable burden of the disease, most parents of children with thalassaemia major find the 25% risk of recurrence to be unacceptable. They prefer to have prenatal diagnosis of the disease in the next pregnancy. It has been observed that where the prenatal diagnosis is not available, most of the couples at risk restrict family size subsequent to the birth of an affected child.

Prenatal diagnosis Prenatal diagnosis is by DNA studies on chorionic villus sampling at 9–12 weeks of gestation or by testing the fetal blood obtained at 18–20 weeks of gestation. The preferred method is through DNA studies: the diagnosis is highly accurate, and in the event of an affected fetus preventive abortion can be undertaken early and easily.[68]

Chorionic villus sampling can be done as an outpatient investigation either transcervically or transabdominally with ultrasound guidance. There is a 2–4% risk of a miscarriage. There is always a 1–2% chance of error of DNA diagnosis because of mixing with some maternal cells; therefore collection, cleaning and selection of villi is critically important. Prenatal diagnosis of thalassaemia is now well established in many countries, and in Sardinia, Greece and Cyprus has already reduced by up to 97% the number of new cases of thalassaemia major in the community.[68]

The control of thalassaemia in the community In developing countries optimal management of all patients having β thalassaemia is extremely difficult, if not impossible, to provide. This is not to deny that there are many individual success stories where affected children have received the optimal management, have excellent growth, and can even go on to marry and have children. However, the availability of blood for transfusion is always limited, while desferrioxamine and pumps for infusing are expensive and unaffordable by the vast majority.

Strategy for control involves: (1) educating the community to the problem, and making people aware of the burden of the disease and the desirability of control; (2) screening the community to identify carriers of β thalassaemia genes, and to recognize couples at risk of having homozygous children. Carrier screening can be done at various times, such as at birth, in school, in college, before marriage, just after marriage or during pregnancy. Many scientists have suggested that carrier screening be done at high school or college, so that counselling may prevent marriage between carriers. In most Asian countries this strategy is not satisfactory and it would be better to permit free choice of partner, and then to screen the couple. If they are carriers, they can be counselled appropriately.

It is essential for success that all the components of the programme (health education, carrier screening and prenatal diagnosis) be in place for proper implementation. Such a community programme requires two other essential ingredients: a strong political will and active participation by the community and by parents and children with thalassaemia. People for their part must be motivated enough to accept a screening and control programme. Health education to all sections of the population—politicians, bureaucrats, professionals and the community as a whole—is the key to success.

Sickle cell disease

A point mutation replaces glutamic acid with valine at position 6 on the β globin. The combination of normal α chains with the abnormal $β^S$ chains forms sickle haemoglobin (HbS).[53,69–71] *Sickle cell disease* is defined as the condition resulting from the inheritance of two abnormal allelomorphic genes controlling β globin formation, of which at least one is the β^S gene. Sickle cell disease includes the most common type, homozygous HbSS (referred to as *sickle cell anaemia*), and the compound heterozygous conditions of HbS β thalassaemias, HbSC, HbSD, HbSO^{Arab} and others. *Sickle cell trait* (HbAS) is the condition arising from the inheritance of one normal β globin gene and one β^S gene.

There were about 78 million carriers of sickle cell trait in the world in 1992; of these, 65 million were in Africa south of the Sahara and north of the Zambesi River and Kalahari Desert. In tropical Africa β^S gene frequencies reach to over 0.15; that is, more than 30% of the adult population have HbAS (Figure 13.16).[72] The β^S gene is found at polymorphic frequencies also in the tribal (scheduled) groups of India, in the Arabian peninsula and the Mediterranean region. High gene frequencies are encountered also in populations derived from the slave trade or voluntary emigration from Africa and the Mediterranean, such as in the Americas, the UK, other northern European countries and Australia.

DNA analysis of the β globin gene cluster has shown that the β^S gene is linked to various β chain haplotypes, each with a distinct geographical distribution (Figure 13.16). This implies that the sickle mutation arose independently at different times, linked to the different haplotypes. The Arab–India haplotype is found throughout the Indian tribal groups and in eastern Saudi Arabia. The Senegal haplotype is confined to the western seaboard of West Africa. The Benin haplotype is common in central West Africa, and would seem to have spread through the trans-Saharan slave trade to North Africa, the Mediterranean region and western Arabia. The Bantu haplotype (previously called Central African Republic or CAR haplotype) is found uniformly throughout the Bantu speakers of central and southern Africa. The fourth African β^S mutation, linked to the Cameroon haplotype, is restricted to the Eton ethnic group of central Cameroon.[72] These distributions are of interest not only in our understanding of selective pressures and human evolution, but also because clinical expression is modified by haplotype linkages.

Each year about 156 000 infants are born with sickle cell disease, of whom 130 000 are in Africa and 33 000 in Nigeria alone. Most have sickle cell anaemia (HbSS); HbSC is also common in central West Africa (Burkina Faso, Ghana, Benin and south-western Nigeria); HbS β$^+$ thalassaemia is seen in West Africa, especially Liberia; HbS β^0 thalassaemia occurs in North African, the Mediterranean and mixed populations of the Americas; HbSD is seen most in the Punjab (see Figures 13.6, 13.16 and 13.18).

Pathophysiology

Valine is a hydrophobic amino acid, whereas glutamic acid is hydrophilic: as position 6 of the β globin is externally situated, the solubility of the HbS molecule is much reduced compared to HbA, especially in the deoxygenated state. Deoxy-HbS polymerizes the contact points between molecules involving the β6 valines. The polymers form long chains of haemoglobin molecules; in cross-section, each chain consists of 14 molecules. The polymers align in parallel, and this is the probable mechanism for the distortion of red cells into the characteristic sickle cell shape (Figure 13.17), as the polymers lie parallel to the long axis of the sickled cells. With alternating deoxygenation and oxygenation, the red cell sickles and unsickles, but eventually ill-defined losses and changes of membrane lipids and proteins lead to the membrane becoming rigid in the sickle form. The red cell is then an irreversible sickled cell, although within the

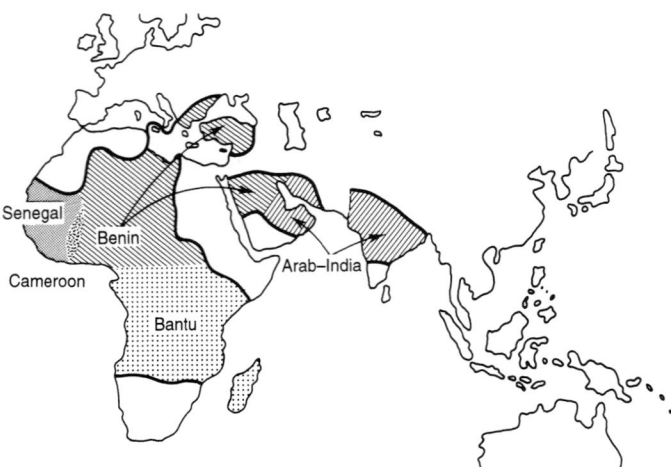

Figure 13.16: Areas of the Old World where haemoglobin S gene frequency is >0.02, and distribution of β^s haplotypes. Heavy arrows indicate probable spread of the Benin haplotype to the Mediterranean and western Asia.

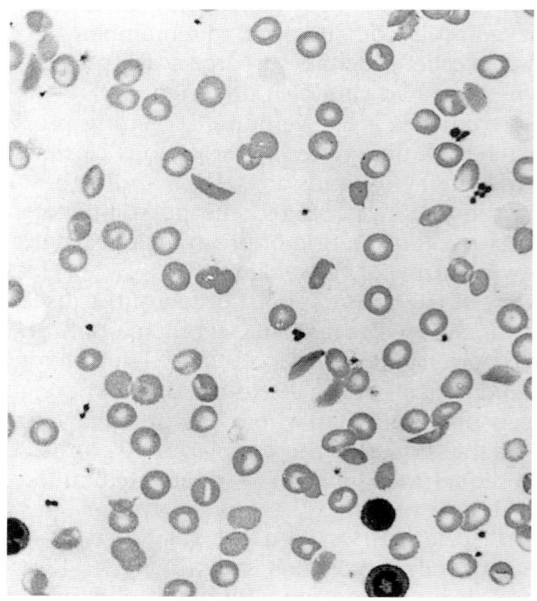

Figure 13.17: Peripheral blood film in sickle cell anaemia.

membrane the haemoglobin is still capable of degelling on oxygenation. Failure of transmembrane ion exchange mechanisms leads to the loss of K$^+$ and water from the cell, while intracellular concentrations of Na$^+$ and Ca^{2+} rise.

Sickled cells are fragile and are phagocytosed by cells of the RES, so that there is both intravascular and extravascular haemolysis. Sickled cells adhere to each other and to the endothelium, so causing blockage of small blood vessels, infarction and death of tissues. Important secondary effects include an increased susceptibility to infection, which has several mechanisms: (1) mucosal and skin integrity may be breached following infarction; (2) haemoglobinaemia activates and consumes complement, so that there is a chronic defect of the alternative pathway of activation and diminished opsonization and phagocytosis of, for example, pneumococci; (3) recurrent infarction in the spleen leads to destruction of the organ (autosplenectomy) and functional hyposplenism; and (4) postinfarctive tissue necrosis provides a microenvironment favouring bacterial growth, and precedes the development of osteomyelitis and pyelonephritis. Recurrent infections and chronic ill health are associated with retardation of growth and development: chronic haemolysis creates high demands for folate, and deficiency contributes to the impaired growth and development besides leading to anaemic crisis.

Disease is worst in HbSS and HbS β^0 thalassaemia, and is in diminishing order of severity in HbSC, HbSD, HbSO^{Arab} and HbS β$^+$ thalassaemia. Sickle cell trait (HbAS) and HbS/HPFH are essentially without clinical abnormality except when under extreme stress.

Clinical presentation

Infants with HbSS have complications only rarely in the early months of life, while HbF concentrations remain high. The disease is manifest clinically from the third month onwards: the earliest presentation is frequently the 'hand–foot' syndrome of painful swelling of the dorsum of the hands or feet, often symmetrical, resulting from infarctions into the small bones. Due to parents coming late for advice and limited diagnostic skills at the first levels of care, the diagnosis is commonly delayed in tropical Africa (where about five out of six patients are born with sickle cell anaemia) with consequent morbidity and mortality, which could have been prevented.[73] The diagnosis is made in the first year of life in only about 10% of Nigerian children with sickle cell anaemia receiving hospital care. The most common age is 1–3 years, but up to 20% of patients are over 10 years at the time of diagnosis.

Patients suffer from chronic ill health interspersed with acute anaemic, infarctive and infective crises.

The steady state

Height and weight are below average for age throughout childhood. There is little body fat. The limbs are long and thin, and much of the loss of height is in the spinal column; there is an exaggerated lumbar lordosis and the chest is often barrel shaped due to an increase in the anteroposterior distance. The bones of the vault of the skull and the face show bossing similar to that of β thalassaemia major (see Figure 13.10a): rounding of the forehead causes exaggeration of the supraorbital sulcus; the bridge of the nose appears sunken because of expansion of the bones around it; expansion of the maxilla causes the upper teeth to protrude. Bossing is much more pronounced in African than American patients; it is largely reversible with long-term antimalarial prophylactics, which suggests that malarial haemolysis is a contributory factor.

There is pallor and usually clinically obvious jaundice. The liver is invariably enlarged. Gallstones can be demonstrated in about 10% of African and 30% of American adult patients, but only rarely do they cause symptoms. The spleen is large in early childhood, but shrinks due to infarction, and is palpable in about 7% of patients only after puberty. In only the occasional patient is there hypersplenism. Moderate chronic cervical adenopathy is usual.

The heart is enlarged: the apex beat is displaced laterally and may be visible. The pulse rate is normal at rest but is rapid after minimal exertion or with apprehension and excitement. Mid-systolic murmurs are heard in most patients, and third heart sounds are common. Patients complain of polydipsia and polyuria, related to renal medullary infarction and loss of ability to concentrate urine; enuresis in childhood and nocturia are usual.

Most patients are remarkably well adapted psychologically, and perform their schooling well, although achievement may be poor from loss of time through ill health.

After the age of about 11 years skeletal maturation is delayed. Fusion of the epiphyses is late, and growth may continue for longer than normal, so that postpubertal HbSS subjects catch up on growth and a few even go on to reach well above average height (e.g., 190 cm). Puberty is delayed, and menarche occurs in girls on average 1 year later than in the normal population. Postadolescent patients, girls in particular, persist in a non-adult lifestyle, so that first sexual experience and marriage are often at a relatively late age; many men are impotent following priapism (see below). Rarely, growth and development are so retarded that the patient has the appearance of a pituitary dwarf.

Haematology in the steady state

The Hb is generally in the range 60–100 g/litre; patients are not in distress, even with levels constantly lower than this range, as they are compensated by high levels of erythrocyte 2,3-DPG and efficient oxygen delivery to the tissues. The red cells show great anisocytosis, macrocytosis with microcytosis, sickle cell forms, target cells, poikilocytes, polychromasia and a variable number of nucleated red cells (Figure 13.17); with hyposplenism the red cell appearance is more abnormal, and punctate basophilia and Howell–Jolly bodies may be seen. The reticulocyte count is raised up to 20%. The total white cell count is generally raised, showing a neutrophil leucocytosis with a shift to the left and toxic granulation, or a lymphocytosis with activated forms, even in the absence of obvious infection. The platelet count is high, especially when there has been autosplenectomy and foliowing an infarctive crisis.

Haemoglobin electrophoresis shows the major fraction in the position of HbS, with a variable proportion of HbF and normal HbA_2. That the major haemoglobin is HbS can be confirmed by the solubility test.[1,67]

The biochemical features of both intravascular and extravascular haemolysis are present (see Table 13.11); conjugated bilirubin is usually raised due to liver dysfunction.

Anaemic crises

Catastrophic declines of Hb are the result of (1) malaria, (2) acute splenic sequestration, (3) folate deficiency and (4) aplastic crises.[73]

Acute *P. falciparum* malaria in subjects with sickle cell disease causes a severe haemolytic crisis and profound anaemia, often leading to anaemic cardiac failure, which used to be the most common observed cause of death in Africa. The most severe anaemias in acute illness are still associated with malaria, even in patients who are supposedly receiving prophylactics.

A sequestration crisis is characterized by an acutely enlarging spleen and a precipitate fall of Hb by more than 20 g/litre, with a high reticulocyte count. It is most frequent in the second 6 months of life but can occur at older ages, even adulthood, in subjects who retain their spleens. Anaemic cardiac failure can develop, and it is the single most common cause of death in early life in non-malarial areas such as the West Indies.[69]

More than 10% of untreated African patients have megaloblastic erythropoiesis from folic acid deficiency when seen first. Megaloblastosis is almost inevitable during pregnancy unless prevented. Life-threatening anaemia develops rapidly.

During almost any acute infection erythropoiesis is depressed, and as patients with sickle cell anaemia are dependent on abnormally high rates of erythropoiesis the Hb drops rapidly. Of greater severity is infection by parvovirus B19 (see below). 'Aplastic' crises occur in clusters in patients with sickle cell anaemia, associated with epidemic transmission of parvovirus B19 and outbreaks of erythema infectiosum in the population of normal children.

Infarctive crises

Sickling can lead to infarction in almost any organ or tissue in the body. The common sites of infarction crises are the bones, chest and abdomen.[53,69,70,73]

Up to 90% of African children seen with sickle cell anaemia between 6 months and 2 years of age have the hand–foot syndrome. If the swelling is hot, red and fluctuant, a superimposed osteomyelitis must be suspected. After about 2 years of age the sites of bone pain crises shift to the long bones. Pain is frequently localized around the joints, may be in multiple sites, be symmetrical in its distribution, and move from site to site. Onset is sudden; severity is variable, but often intense; duration is also variable, but usually there is spontaneous resolution within 5 days. Often there are no physical signs except warmth and tenderness over the affected bone, and the unwary physician is liable to underestimate the severity of the pain and overestimate the patient's reaction. Malaria, other infections, cold or damp (in the rainy season) are recognized precipitating factors, but often crises start for no apparent reason. Necrosis can lead rarely to emboli of bone marrow fat or bone to the lungs, brain, kidneys or other tissues.

Acute severe pain in the chest can be due to (1) lower respiratory tract infection, (2) bone marrow fat embolism, (3) pulmonary infarction, (4) acute pulmonary sequestration and (5) bone pain crisis in the thoracic cage.[71,74] The first four conditions are serious and often difficult to distinguish clinically or radiologically; as one may precede and precipitate the others, the phrase 'acute chest syndrome' is used. Lobar pneumonia and infection by the pneumococcus are more likely in early childhood, and infarction to be the primary pathology in adults.

Patients commonly complain of recurrent mild abdominal pain, but this may be severe and require admission to hospital. Pain is usually localized centrally or in the epigastrium. The patient may be vomiting. There is a history of constipation; bowel sounds are reduced and fluid levels can be seen radiologically. Aetiology is obscure, but is thought to be due to mesenteric infarcts. The condition resolves spontaneously, usually within 5 days. Other abdominal painful crises related to sickle cell disease are splenic infarction, infarction in lumbar vertebrae, duodenal ulceration, acute cholecystitis, obstruction of cystic or bile ducts and pancreatitis. Patients may also present with abdominal crises unrelated to sickle cell disease, for example acute appendicitis.

Sickling in cerebral vessels can cause obstruction, infarction and haemorrhage. The immediate consequences of stroke include convulsions, coma, paralyses of varying extent and depth, or death. The late sequelae are contractions of limbs if no physiotherapy is available, faecal and urinary incontinence, speech defects and serious impairment of intellectual function. Two-thirds of untreated children have recurrent clinical strokes.[75]

Older patients can complain of blurred vision: examination reveals tortuous retinal vessels, proliferation of the retinal vessels, intraocular haemorrhages and sometimes retinal detachment. Pathology can develop until there is severe or total loss of vision.

Leg ulceration is a most common complication in the West Indies and North America, starting most often between 10 and 20 years of age. For reasons which remain obscure, ulcers are uncommon (less than 10%) in Africa even in those above 12 years of age; males are affected six times more often than females. The ulcers are usually on the lower third of the leg above the medial or lateral malleoli. They start as infarcts into the skin which show as small blisters; these develop into necrotic sloughs after

2 weeks and ulcers in about 3 weeks. Small ulcers may heal or may spread to up to 10 cm in diameter, causing serious incapacity.

Infarction in the renal pelvis leads to papillary necrosis, often complicated by haematuria and bacteriuria. Priapism is seen in adolescent or young adult males, but can occur in childhood; severity can vary from mild and transient, to moderate which resolves with 24 hours, to when the penis is hot and exquisitely tender, with pain referred to the perineum and lower abdomen. Untreated, severe priapism subsides over about 2 weeks but leads to fibrosis of the corpora cavernosa and permanent impotence.

Bacterial infections

The pneumococcus (*Streptococcus pneumoniae*) is the most common infectious cause of death in non-malarial areas; its frequency in Africa has been underestimated, and it is probably second only to malaria as a cause of morbidity and mortality.[73] Pneumococcal pneumonia, septicaemia and meningitis are seen in children between 5 months and 5 years old, and most frequently under the age of 2 years; the children have high fevers (> 39.5°C) and are liable to convulsions, coma, shock and the Waterhouse–Friderichsen syndrome. Without appropriate treatment mortality is greater than 50%.

Other organisms commonly associated with acute upper or lower respiratory tract infections and bacteraemia are *Haemophilus influenzae*, staphylococci, streptococci and various Gram-negative bacilli. Bone infarction is complicated by acute osteomyelitis in less than 10% of all patients; invading organisms in Africa are *Salmonella* (usually *S. typhi*) in about half, other coliforms in less than half and *Staph. pyogenes* in about one-fifth.

Chronic degenerative disease

As more patients live into adult life, chronic and irreversible degenerative changes after the age of 20 years are becoming increasingly important. Irreversible organ damage leading to death includes hepatic failure, renal failure, stroke and pulmonary fibrosis, pulmonary hypertension and respiratory failure.[69-71] Major debilitation is the result of (1) avascular necrosis of bones, which can lead to loss of mobility when affecting the head of the femur or vertebral bodies, (2) retinopathy with loss of vision and (3) leg ulcers. Men over 25 years commonly present with duodenal ulcers (over 30% in Jamaica), which have complicated clinical courses, including pyloric stenosis.[69] There can be a progressive bone marrow failure after the age of 40.[76]

Pregnancy

African women with sickle cell anaemia invariably become severely depleted of folic acid by mid-pregnancy if they are without medical supervision. About one-quarter may experience sequestration crises. Shortly before and shortly after delivery they are liable to severe bone pain crises, which may be complicated by marrow and bone embolus and systolic hypertension with albuminuria ('pseudotoxaemia'). They have high frequencies of urinary tract and other infections.

Obstetric delivery is often complicated by pelvic disproportion, the result of impaired growth during childhood. In Nigeria about half are delivered by caesarean section. During the puerperium they are liable to infection, especially wound sepsis.

Maternal mortality rates depend largely on the obstetric care available: in early series it was about 33%, but this has been reduced to nearly zero in the USA. In Nigeria mortality remains around 12%.

There is fetal growth retardation, and one-third of infants are of low birthweight. Perinatal mortality can be as high as 33% but can be reduced to around 10% with good antenatal care and careful supervision of delivery and the puerperium.[77]

Prognosis

The pattern and severity of disease are governed by both environmental and genetic factors.[73] In Africa the environmental factors are of far greater importance in determining prognosis; in the USA the impact of the environment is largely controlled and the severity of disease depends more on the inherited factors.

In Jamaica, where there has been a long-running intensive, nationwide and successful programme of sickle cell care, calculated mean survival for men is 53 years and for women 58.5 years.[78] In contrast in rural tropical Africa, when there was inadequate nutrition, poor hygiene, no avoidance of mosquitoes and no practice of modern medicine, less than 2% of infants born with sickle cell anaemia survived beyond 4 years.[79] The family are all-important: when they are caring, intelligent, educated and wealthy, children with HbSS do much better, even without regular medical care. The principal role of the medical profession is to support the family in the maintenance of the good health of family members with sickle cell disease (see below). Since the 1960s the provision of care has spread and improved throughout much of tropical Africa, so that it is now not unusual to see African patients with HbSS entering professional life (e.g., law, medicine, nursing) and achieving parenthood.

The expression of sickle cell disease is modified by a range of other mutations on the β globin gene cluster, the so-called β globin haplotypes (Figure 13.16).[72] The Arab–India and the Senegal haplotypes are linked to determinants of high levels of persisting HbF (means 20% and 12% respectively) in subjects with HbSS. The Benin and Bantu haplotypes are associated with lower levels of HbF (means 8%), but for reasons which are not yet understood disease is more severe with the Bantu than the Benin haplotype. Sickle cell anaemia with high levels of HbF, linked to Arab–India and Senegal haplotypes, is associated with a more normal body build, more subcutaneous fat, less dactylitis, less acute chest pain, less splenic atrophy and less major organ failure in adult life; Hb concentrations are higher, red cell survival is longer, there are fewer sickled cells, and reticulocyte and platelet counts are lower.

Coincidental inheritance of homozygous α^+ thalassaemia ($-\alpha/-\alpha$) with HbSS results in less anaemia, less haemolysis, lower MCH and MCV, fewer sickled cells and lower reticulocyte counts. Values with heterozygous α^+ thalassaemia are intermediate between those with $-\alpha/-\alpha$ and $\alpha\alpha/\alpha\alpha$. α Gene deletions do not seem to have much influence on the severity of acute complications of sickle cell disease but do decrease the risks of chronic organ damage in adults.

Maintenance of health

Wherever the β^S gene has high frequency, priority should be given to a system for maintaining patients in a steady state of good health through early diagnosis, supportive care at sickle cell clinics and obstetric units, easy access to appropriate care in crises, and education of the public, patients and health professionals (Table 13.17).[73]

To facilitate early diagnosis all pregnant women should be screened by Serjeants' HbS solubility test, with confirmation of positive results by haemoglobin electrophoresis; screening of fathers would identify couples at risk of having affected infants but it is more practical if a woman has HbS to test the newborn infant by electrophoresis (on citrate agar at pH 6–6.5). Other children at risk and to be screened are all with severe anaemia and the ill siblings of known patients with sickle cell disease. Serjeants' HbS solubility test is preferable by far to the sickling test as it distinguishes heterozygotes from homozygotes and is simpler to perform; it is the test of choice in the primary health care setting. Haemoglobin electrophoresis should be set up in all hospitals of around 100 beds or more in tropical Africa and should be available for all clinicians.

Once diagnosed, sickle cell disease should be explained in detail to parents, guardians and patients in a language and phraseology they can understand. Their knowledge and comprehension must be reinforced with the aid of pamphlets and further discussions. The first essential intervention is the prevention of malaria: patients should receive a curative course of antimalarials at first attendance or following any break in attendance at the sickle cell clinic; they must be kept free from malaria through regular antimalarial prophylaxis, the choice of prophylactic depending on the prevailing pattern of resistance in *P. falciparum* strains and national policies. A regimen of once-daily folic acid supplement and once-daily proguanil is easy to remember and comply with. Prophylactic oral penicillin V potassium 125 mg twice daily up to the age of 5 years (or to adolescence) has substantially reduced the morbidity and mortality associated with pneumococcal septicaemia in the USA and the UK.[80] Controlled trials are needed in Africa but present problems of cost and logistics. Widespread immunization against the pneumococcus is not an option for reasons of cost, difficulties of the cold chain and the inadequate response of children under 3 years. On the other hand it is import-

Table 13.17 Maintenance of health in sickle cell disease.

Early diagnosis	Laboratory techniques	• HbS solubility • Hb electrophoresis
	Screening	• pregnant women • newborn of mothers with S gene • anaemic children • siblings of patients
	Clinical awareness	
Education	Parents and patients Health professionals General public	
Sickle cell clinics	Prevent infection	• prophylactic antimalarials • immunization • prophylactic penicillin
	Nutrition	• folic acid supplements • general nutritional advice
	Advice	• avoid cold, fatigue, dehydration, excessive alcohol • no useless treatment • attend clinic regularly • report when ill • report when pregnant
Induction of fetal haemoglobin	Hydroxyurea	
Hospital	Prompt treatment of crises	
Obstetrics	Supervision of pregnancy, delivery, puerperium Family limitation to ≤ 3 viable children	

ant for children with sickle cell disease to receive the expanded programme of immunization against other common infections.[73]

The coincidence of the area of Africa where the β^S gene has high frequency and where HIV is now epidemic makes it more important than ever that the health of patients with sickle cell disease be maintained so as to avoid situations where it is necessary to transfuse blood. Where there are no programmes of health care for sickle cell disease sufferers, but merely treatment of crises, which often involves transfusions of blood (appropriate and inappropriate), 20% or more of patients with sickle cell disease have been infected with HIV. In Africa 130 000 infants are born each year with sickle cell disease, and only 400 with haemophilia, who are at risk of infection by HIV through blood and blood products.[73]

Induction of fetal haemoglobin

Various agents have been tried for their efficacy in raising the concentration of HbF in patients with sickle cell disease. The oral cytotoxic agent hydroxyurea is the only one to date which has an established place in the management of sickle cell disease. [80]

Treatment with hydroxyurea for 2 years: (1) increases the concentration of HbF up to 15–20% of the total haemoglobin; (2) decreases the number of granulocytes and monocytes, and hence the release of oxidative radicals; and (3) reduces the adherence of sickled cells to the endothelium. Clinically, hydroxyurea reduces the frequency of painful crises, of acute chest syndrome, of hospitalization and of the need for blood transfusion.

Treatment is started with hydroxyurea 500 mg per day (10–15 mg/kg body weight). If this is tolerated, the dosage is increased to 1000 mg per day after 6–8 weeks; the dose can be increased further to 2000 mg (20–30 mg/kg body weight). The full blood count HbF renal function and hepatic function need to be monitored.

Short-term toxicity is minimal, but the long-term effects of hydroxyurea are not known, and it may be mutagenic.

In Africa, hydroxyurea is available at present only to those who are able to purchase it: the current price (March 2002) in the UK is £2.39 sterling for 20 tablets of 500 mg.

Management of the patient in crisis

Prompt treatment is essential and arrangements should be made for patients in crisis to be able to report and receive attention without having to compete with the mass of sick people seen in the outpatient clinics of equatorial Africa. Regardless of the nature of the crisis it should be assumed that the patient has malaria, and treatment started without waiting for the results from a thick blood film. Antimalarial prophylaxis and supplementary folic acid should continue.

Anaemic crises

In the great majority of patients the haematocrit will cease to fall and will rise rapidly following treatment with antimalarials, folic acid and antibiotics if indicated. Blood transfusion is necessary only if (1) there is respiratory distress, or incipient or established heart failure, (2) there is a sequestration crisis, with Hb < 60 g/litre and falling rapidly, (3) obstetric delivery is imminent, with Hb < 80 g/litre, or (4) there are coincidental indications, such as haemorrhage or emergency surgery.[17,73]

Infarctive crises

Management is based on three principles: (1) the control of pain; (2) the restoration and maintenance of hydration and acid–base balance; and (3) the treatment of infection.[53,69,73,80]

The physician should assess the severity of pain and prescribe appropriate analgesics to be given at determined dosage and intervals; the physician must reassess pain at regular intervals and be prepared to increase or decrease the analgesics. Analgesic dosage should never be left to the judgement of different ward staff and the persuasive powers of the patients. Mild pain can be controlled with paracetamol, moderately severe pain with dihydrocodeine tartrate (DF118) and severe pain with opiates, such as diamorphine 10 mg at once, followed by an infusion, assessed by body size and the patient's response.[80]

Hydration is maintained by encouraging the mildly affected patient to drink; a more severely ill patient may be treated with nasogastric fluids if bowel sounds can be heard, or by intravenous fluids.

Acute infections

Antibiotics should be withheld unless there are clear indications for their use. If there are indications, antibiotics should be given promptly and in adequate dosage. Treatment must be started before results of bacteriological investigations are completed when there is (1) fever of > 39°C, unless due to malaria, (2) the acute pulmonary syndrome, or (3) suspected meningitis. Initial treatment could be with cefuroxime sodium 150 mg/kg per 24 hours, or alternatively ampicillin or penicillin plus chloramphenicol. Treatment of acute osteomyelitis can commence with chloramphenicol and cloxacillin.[73]

Cerebrovascular accidents

Patients should be rehydrated immediately. Some physicians advocate exchange blood transfusion but it is not possible to give general advice on this question.[75,80] Patients should be managed individually, taking into consideration the safety of blood transfusion in the locality. Repeated transfusions, aimed at reducing HbS concentrations to less than 30%, largely prevent recurrent strokes, but such a regimen can only be embarked upon if there is an assured supply of safe blood.

Priapism

Treatment is aimed at relieving pain and preventing fibrosis of the corpora cavernosa. Mild or 'stuttering' priapism can be relieved by micturition, walking around, avoiding sexual arousal and bathing in cold water.

Moderately severe priapism will respond, usually within 24 hours, to bed-rest, sedation, analgesics, intravenous hydration, and cyproterone or stilboestrol. Initial therapy of severe priapism should include opiate analgesics and rehydration; under general or spinal anaesthetic, a wide-bore needle is inserted into the lateral side of the base of the penis and the viscous blood aspirated; this is followed by repeated irrigation with adrenaline $1:10^6$ in saline and aspiration until fresh blood only is obtained.

Leg ulceration

Small and clean ulcers are treated successfully with daily antiseptic washing and dressing. Large ulcers will heal slowly with (1) prolonged bed-rest with the affected leg raised, (2) appropriate antibiotic therapy, (3) hydrogen peroxide lotion or surgical debridement to remove the slough, and (4) antitetanus prophylaxis. Larger ulcers or those which fail to heal require skin grafts. Once healed, the legs should be protected by crepe or elastic stockings.[70]

Management during pregnancy

Health must be maintained through careful antenatal supervision and the insistence on prophylactic anti-malarials and supplementary folic acid.[17] Prophylactic red cell transfusions has been advocated, but benefits are slight, if any, and are certainly outweighed by the risk of complications from transfusion in the tropics. Transfusion of red cells is indicated if a patient approaches obstetric delivery with Hb < 80 g/litre.[17] Patients should be assessed as to the danger of pelvic disproportion, and elective caesarean delivery planned if necessary.

Prevention of sickle cell disease

Strategies for prevention of sickle cell disease include (1) screening to recognize couples at risk, (2) genetic counselling, and (3) prenatal diagnosis followed by termination of homozygous or doubly heterozygous fetuses. Postmarital screening and counselling are widely available for African couples who have had affected children already: in Nigeria in particular, there have been attempts to educate the population and to make premarital counselling available.[81]

Prenatal diagnosis is technically possible and is becoming relatively inexpensive to apply in a few centres.[53] National programmes in Africa suffer restraints of low priority from government, lack of knowledge in the whole community, lack of trained staff, lack of facilities and the illegality or ethical non-acceptance of termination of pregnancy.

Haemoglobin SC disease

The compound heterozygous inheritance of HbS and HbC occurs often in West Africa and in populations derived from West Africa (see Figures 13.16 and 13.18). The pathophysiology and clinical features are similar to those of HbSS, but the severity is much less, and some patients are nearly asymptomatic.[69] Age at presentation is generally later. Because many girls survive childhood,

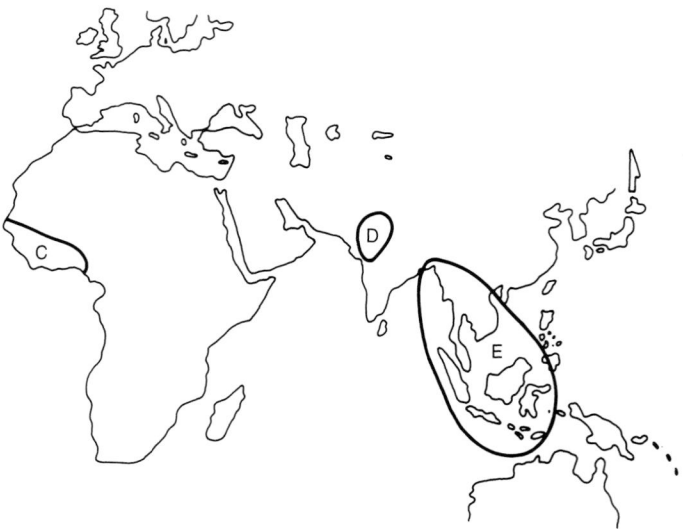

Figure 13.18: Areas of the Old World where haemoglobins C, D (Punjab or Los Angles) and E reach polymorphic frequencies. (Reproduced with permission of the publishers from Fleming A F. In Strickland G T (ed.) *Hunter's Tropical Medicine*, 7th edn. Philadelphia: W B Saunders, 1991: 36–64.)

HbSC is the most common form of sickle cell disease to present with complications during pregnancy in West Africa.[77] Eye disease is more frequent, related to the higher Hb concentration. Because the spleen is not destroyed, acute sequestration crises and splenic infarcts during flight, including in pressurized aircraft, occur during adult life.

The Hb concentration is intermediate between that of HbSS and normals. The MCV is lower than in HbSS; reticulocyte counts are moderately raised. The red cell appearance is of anisocytosis, some macrocytes, some microspherocytes, numerous target cells, occasional sickle cell forms but with rounded ends, and occasional intraerythrocytic crystals of precipitated HbC (Figure 13.19). Electrophoresis shows two major fractions in the position of HbS and HbC.

The condition of combined inheritance of HbSS plus the α globin variant HbG[Philadelphia] is commonly mistaken for HbSC in West Africa. On electrophoresis the subject with HbSS + G shows HbS and the hybrid HbS/G, which moves into the position of HbC; HbS solubility easily differentiates between the two, showing the heterozygous pattern (half precipitated) with HbSC and the homozygous pattern (all haemoglobin precipitated) with HbSS + G.

Haemoglobin S β⁰ thalassaemia

The inheritance of both HbS and β^0 thalassaemia occurs most often in North Africa, Sicily and in the mixed population of the Americas (see Figures 13.6 and 13.16).[69,70,72]

The clinical course is very similar to that of HbSS. Haematologically the two conditions are difficult to distinguish: the peripheral blood pictures are similar, the

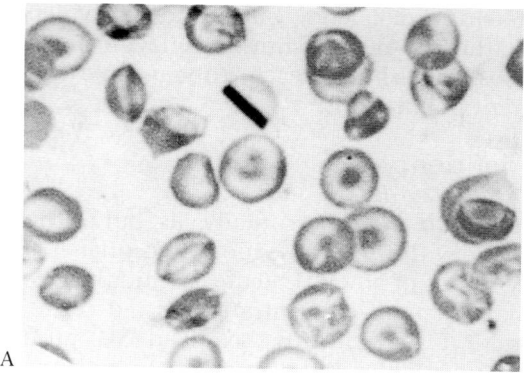

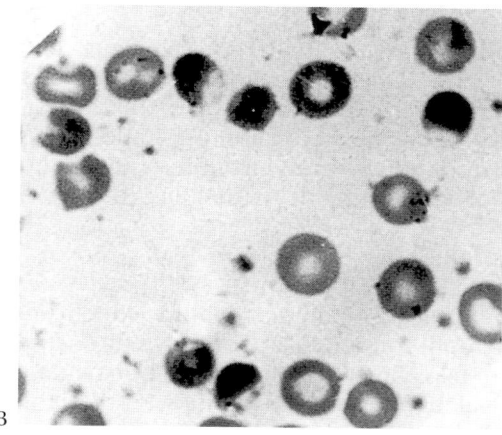

Figure 13.19: Peripheral blood films. (**A**) Haemoglobin C disease: there are numerous target cells and one red cell shows intracellular crystal formation. (**B**) G6PD deficiency: red cells showing oxidative damage. The haemoglobin seems to be separated from the membrane of the cells in certain areas ('blister' cells) and 'bite' cells where the Heinz bodies have been removed in the spleen; the rest of the cell looks dense. These changes occur only during a haemolytic episode.

MCV and MCH are lower in HbS β⁰ thalassaemia; HbS is the only major fraction and the HbF is raised in both conditions, but HbA₂ is raised only in HbS β⁰ thalassaemia. The diagnosis is made with certainty when one parent carries the βˢ gene and the other has β⁰ thalassaemia trait.

Haemoglobin S β⁺ thalassaemia

This doubly heterozygous condition is most common in Liberia and other parts of West Africa (see Figures 13.6 and 13.16). The clinical course is mild. Anaemia is often slight, and irreversibly sickled cells are seen rarely in the blood. Haemoglobin electrophoresis shows HbA 5–30%, and HbS greater than 50%. It is important not to mistake HbS β⁺ thalassaemia for HbAS, in which the HbS is always less than 50%.

Haemoglobin S D^Punjab

There are several HbDs, but only HbD^Punjab interacts with HbS, leading to a disease similar to HbSS, and is seen amongst Sikhs and mixed populations (see Figures 13.16 and 13.18).[69,70] There is moderately severe haemolytic anaemia; the peripheral blood picture resembles HbSS;

electrophoresis at alkaline pH shows a single band in the position of HbS, but the HbS solubility test yields the heterozygous pattern, and electrophoresis on agar gel separates HbS from HbD (in the position of HbA).

Sickle cell trait

The inheritance of HbAS results in what is essentially a benign condition, which is not associated with decreased life expectancy or with any haematological abnormalities except for the presence of HbS. There are, however, some complications resulting from microinfarcts in the renal medulla and spleen.[53,69,70]

There is a progressive decrease in the ability to concentrate urine, which could lead to an increased tendency to dehydration during extreme exertion. This is the probable explanation for the relative risk of sudden unexplained death in enlisted recruits during basic training in the US Armed Forces being 28–40 times higher among those with HbAS as compared with black recruits or recruits of all races; the relative risk increased with age.[82] These sudden deaths are rare, however, as there were only 12 deaths among 38 600 HbAS individuals in over 2 million recruits. Other renal complications include a doubling of the expected frequency of significant bacteriuria during pregnancy, and rarely painless haematuria following renal papillary necrosis.

Incidents are reported of splenic infarcts following exertion at high altitudes. Earlier reports of splenic infarcts while flying at high altitudes in unpressurized aircraft have been largely discounted as being before haemoglobin electrophoresis and differentiation from HbS β⁺ thalassaemia or even HbSC was possible.

In the absence of other causes of anaemia, the Hb, red cell indices and reticulocyte count are normal. Electrophoresis shows HbA and HbS: the proportion that is HbS has a trimodal distribution associated with the coincidental inheritance of α-thalassaemia genes; HbS is 34–38% with αα/αα, 28–34% with –α/αα and 20–28% with –α/–α. HbS above 45% is suggestive of HbS β⁺ thalassaemia.

A partial protection against *P. falciparum* malaria has been more clearly demonstrated to be associated with sickle cell trait than it has with any other inherited abnormality of the red cells.[35,72] In the non-immune, parasite densities, the frequency of severe malaria (e.g., cerebral malaria or malarial anaemia) and the frequency of death from severe malaria are all lower, and survival rates in childhood are higher. In areas of low endemicity female fertility is higher. In areas of stable malaria HbAS gives partial protection against HMS and severe anaemia associated with HMS during pregnancy.[26,33] There appear to be several mechanisms by which the density of parasitaemias is controlled:[35,72] (1) there is an increase of sickling of parasitized red cells, with subsequent removal of the parasitized and sickled cells by the spleen, so limiting the number of early parasite forms; (2) the intraerythrocyte growth during schizogony is inhibited by HbS gelling during the last 12 hours of the cycle spent in relatively hypoxic deep tissues; (3) enhancement of cell-mediated immune responses against *P. falciparum* antigens has been described, possibly related to a modified expression of parasite antigens.[83]

Other haemoglobinopathies associated with haemolytic anaemia

The other common haemolytic haemoglobin disorders are Hbs C, D and E diseases (see Figure 13.18).[53]

HbC disease occurs commonly in West Africa, the carrier rate being highest in northern Ghana, with an incidence of 16–28%. The homozygous disorder is characterized by a mild haemolytic anaemia and splenomegaly. It can be recognized by examination of a blood film which shows up to 100% target cell formation with intracellular crystals (Figure 13.19A). Mild microcytosis is a common but not universal feature of HbC trait and disease. Folic acid deficiency and megaloblastic erythropoiesis frequently complicate the course of pregnancy. The diagnosis can be confirmed by haemoglobin electrophoresis.

HbD disease has been found in several racial groups. The clinical picture is that of a moderately severe haemolytic anaemia with splenomegaly. The blood film usually shows moderate numbers of target cells. There are several different types of HbD, all of which have the same rate of electrophoretic migration as HbS but do not precipitate with the HbS solubility test or result in sickling. HbD^{Punjab} is the one which is associated with the most marked clinical symptoms.

HbE disease is extremely common in South-East Asia and also occurs in Burma, India, Sri Lanka and Pakistan.[62] It is occasionally associated with splenomegaly, and is characterized by a mild haemolytic anaemia with hypochromic red cells. HbE migrates in the same position as HbC and HbA$_2$.

Enzymopathies

Erythrocytes are non-nucleated but living cells dependent on several enzymatic pathways. They obtain energy from the breakdown of glucose, 95% of which is metabolized by anaerobic glycolysis to lactate and in the process adenosine triphosphate (ATP) is produced. Five per cent of glucose is metabolized via the hexose monophosphate (pentose phosphate) shunt, during which reduced nicotinamide adenine dinucleotide phosphate (NADPH) is produced. There are many enzymopathies or inherited defects of enzymes affecting the red cells, for example pyruvate kinase deficiency, but of these only deficiencies of G6PD, the first and rate-limiting enzyme of the hexose monophosphate shunt, reach polymorphic frequencies in different populations.[84,85]

G6PD deficiency
Role of the enzyme

G6PD is vital to and occurs in all cells, but in the red cell this enzyme with the hexose monophosphate pathway is the only source of NADPH. Reduced glutathione (GSH) is synthesized at high concentration in red cells, and has the function of restoring oxidized SH groups and reducing superoxides and peroxides (through the actions of superoxide dismutase and glutathione peroxidase), but is itself oxidized to GSSG. NADPH is essential for the regeneration of GSH (with the enzyme glutathione reductase). G6PD deficiency and a reduction of synthesis of NADPH expose the red cell to oxidation of haemoglobin with the intracellular precipitation of globin as Heinz bodies, of several enzymes and of lipids and proteins of the membrane, with consequent haemolysis.

G6PD variants

Over 400 allelic variants of G6PD have been differentiated by electrophoretic mobility, kinetic properties and spectrophotometric assay of enzymatic activity. They have been classified according to their enzymatic activity and clinical manifestations (Table 13.18). Variants of class I, causing chronic non-spherocytic haemolytic anaemias, occur sporadically in all populations. Variants of class II (e.g., Gd^{Mediterranean}) and of class III (e.g., GdA$^-$) are associated with intermittent haemolytic crises triggered by oxidant stresses: all variants of major public health importance are in these two groups. Class IV includes GdB, the most common enzyme and referred to as the normal: other variants with normal activity achieve polymorphic frequency, for example GdA in Africa.

The gene controlling G6PD structure is carried on the X chromosome. Males who inherit an abnormal gene (X̄Y) will have the variant enzyme in all their erythrocytes, as will homozygous females (X̄X̄). Heterozygous females (X̄X) will have on average half of their red cells containing normal enzyme and half containing variant enzyme, due to the random suppression of one X chromosome in all female somatic cells. Clinically significant enzyme deficiency will be seen most often in hemizygous males; homozygous females contribute about 10% of those genetically deficient, and about 10% of female

Table 13.18 Classification of variants of G6PD.

Class	G6PD activity	Haematological manifestations	Polymorphic variants
I	Nearly absent	Congenital non-spherocytic haemolytic anaemia	–
II	Severe < 10%	Intermittent haemolysis	Mediterranean, Mali, Union
III	Moderate 10–60%	Less severe intermittent haemolysis	A⁻, Canton, Mahidol
IV	Normal 60–100%	None	B, A, Gambia
V	Increased > 150%	None	

heterozygotes are also effectively deficient due to unequal inactivation of their X chromosomes. Frequency in populations is usually expressed as a percentage of males who are hemizygotes.

World distribution

About 400 million of the world's population carry one or two genes for G6PD deficiency: the highest frequencies are in sub-Saharan Africa (e.g., 32% of males among the Luo on the shores of Lake Victoria), Saudi Arabia and South-East Asia (Figure 13.20). There are populations, for example Sardinians and Kurdish Jews, in which the frequency of G6PD deficiency in males exceeds 50%. The Old World can be divided into three zones according to which G6PD variants achieve polymorphic frequency. In zone I, covering the Mediterranean, North Africa, western Asia and the Indian subcontinent, the severely deficient (class II) Gd^{Mediterranean} is prevalent. In zone II, covering South-East Asia, China, Korea and Oceania, two class II variants (Gd^{Mediterranean} and Gd^{Union}) and two moderately severely deficient (class III) variants (Gd^{Mahidol} and Gd^{Canton}) are common: Asia is remarkable for the number of variants, for example in the population of Taiwan there are at least nine different deficient enzymes, of which Gd$^{Taiwan-Hakka}$ is the most prevalent.[86] In the third zone, sub-Saharan Africa, the class III enzyme GdA$^-$ is frequent, the class II Gd^{Mali} achieves local polymorphic frequency, and up to 40% carry the GdA variant with normal activity. G6PD deficiency is not found in the indigenous populations of America or Australia, but deficient variants occur commonly in the descendants of African, Mediterranean and Asian immigrants.

About 4.5 million infants born each year are at risk for the complications of G6PD deficiency.

Clinical manifestations

Episodes of haemolysis and jaundice occur in four situations: (1) the neonatal period; (2) severe viral and bacterial infections; (3) following ingestion of certain foods; and (4) following exposure to various drugs and chemicals (Table 13.19). These intermittent episodes tend to be more severe with class II (e.g., Gd^{Mediterranean}) than class III (e.g., GdA$^-$) variants.

Neonatal jaundice

Newborn infants are frequently jaundiced (defined as serum bilirubin > 250 µmol/litre (15 mg/dl) on about the fourth day of life in all parts of the world where G6PD deficiency is common (see Figure 13.20), and neonatal jaundice is recognized as a major public health problem in Greece, Saudi Arabia, tropical Africa, the Caribbean, South-East Asia and China, although incidence figures are not often available; in Hong Kong 12% and Singapore 10% of newborns were jaundiced before the introduction

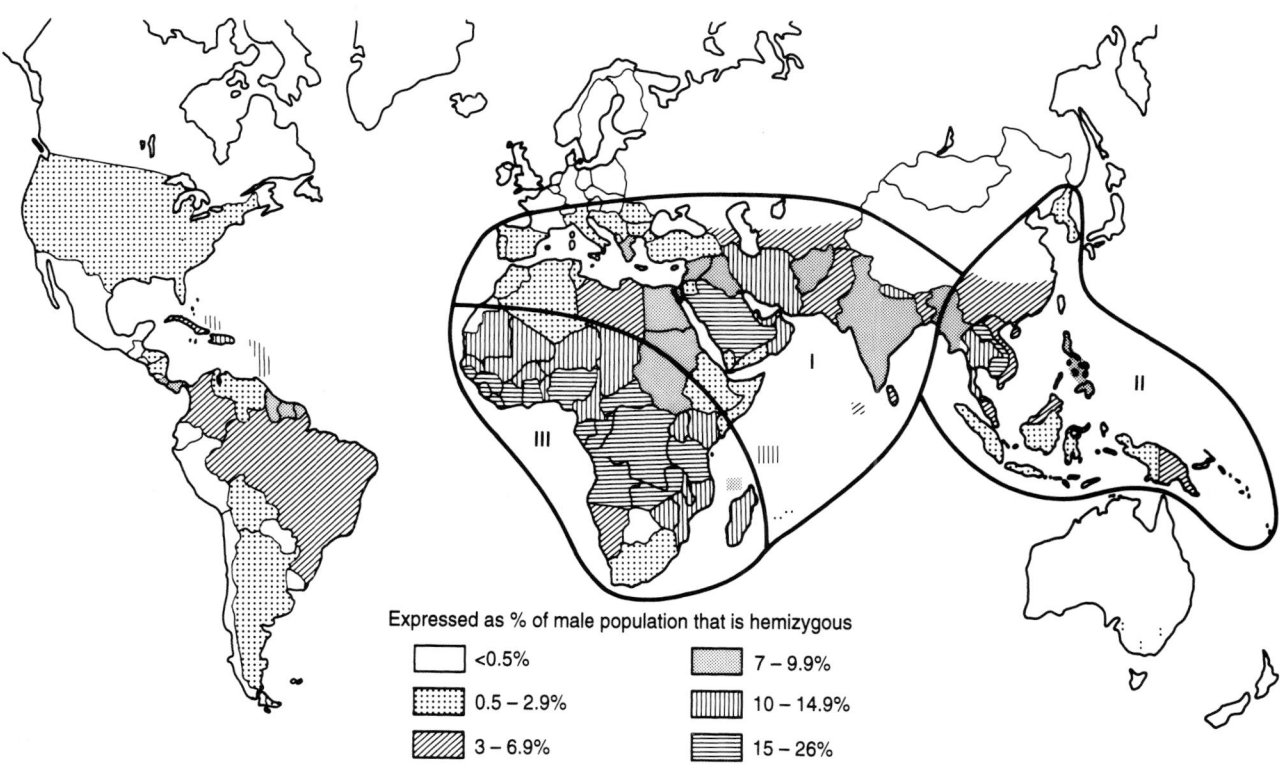

Expressed as % of male population that is hemizygous

<0.5%	7 – 9.9%
0.5 – 2.9%	10 – 14.9%
3 – 6.9%	15 – 26%

Figure 13.20: World distribution of G6PD deficiency. Superimposed are three zones where different G6PD variants reach polymorphic frequencies: Zone I, Gd^{Mediterranean}; zone II, Gd^{Mediterranean}, Gd^{Canton}, Gd^{Union}, Gd^{Mahidol}; Zone III, Gd A$^-$. (Reproduced with permission of the World Health Organization from WHO Working Group[84]).

of successful control programmes.[87] Jaundice is often multifactorial: common causes include sepsis, prematurity, G6PD deficiency, fetomaternal ABO incompatibility, and haematomas from birth trauma. G6PD deficiency contributes in 30–80% of patients. Globally, infant mortality due to jaundice associated with G6PD deficiency is 0.7–1.6 per 1000 births, with an equal number suffering lifelong morbidity.

Identified variables which potentiate jaundice due to G6PD deficiency are: (1) the severity of the enzyme deficiency (e.g., Mediterranean versus African variants) and lower levels of G6PD in the liver; (2) prematurity; (3) genetically determined slower maturity of the liver in Asians; (4) infections, such as umbilical sepsis, septicaemia and pneumonia; (5) exposure of either the mother or the infant to oxidant drugs (Table 13.19), e.g., mothballs (in the preservation of towelling saved from an older infant), herbal medicines (e.g., Chinese *hung lian*), 'mentholated' powders applied to the umbilical cord, vitamin K analogues, sulfonamides and nitrofurantoins; and (6) breast-feeding, which, however, should not be discouraged unless there are exceptional circumstances. Jaundice results from both haemolysis and poor hepatic function. Anaemia is generally moderate (e.g., Hb 130 g/litre), with red cell anisocytosis, spherocytosis, polychromasia and numerous nucleated cells. Total unconjugated bilirubin levels are raised, and when above 300 µmol/litre there is the danger of kernicterus and severe permanent brain damage.

While the serum bilirubin is in the range of 250–300 µmol/litre in mature and otherwise healthy infants, treatment should be with phototherapy. In the absence of designed equipment, sufficient irradiance can be obtained from a unit of at least seven 20-watt fluorescent tubes placed 40 cm above the naked infant, whose eyes are shielded.[85] Alternatively, exposure to the morning sunlight, with cooling of the body and shielding of the eyes, is effective. When the unconjugated bilirubin rises above 300 µmol/litre, treatment is by exchange blood transfusion with blood from G6PD normal donors compatible with both mother and infant, at a volume twice that of the infant's blood volume (i.e., 2×85 ml/kg body weight), in 20 ml aliquots over 2 hours. Phototherapy and exchange transfusion are indicated at lower bilirubin levels in low-weight and ill infants.[85-88]

Neonatal jaundice has been controlled and kernicterus virtually abolished in Singapore by a highly successful national campaign in which (1) G6PD activity is screened in cord blood of all infants; (2) all those deficient are observed in hospital for 2 weeks, and treated promptly if jaundice develops; (3) both the general public and health professionals are informed and educated; (4) letters are given to parents with G6PD deficiency addressed to the obstetrician who delivers the next baby; and (5) G6PD-deficient infants are issued with cards warning against potentially haemolysing drugs.[87] Other measures preventing neonatal jaundice include: (1) adequate prenatal care, so avoiding many premature deliveries; (2) non-traumatic

Table 13.19 Drugs and other agents commonly associated with oxidative damage to red cells.

Drugs and chemicals which cause oxidative damage to red cells in normal subjects and more severe haemolysis in G6PD-deficient subjects
Phenylhydrazine
Dapsone and other sulfones
Naphthalene (moth balls)
Phenacetin and acetanilide (in large doses only)
Sulfasalazine (Salazopyrin)
Drugs and chemicals which are shown to cause haemolysis in G6PD-deficient subjects
Acetanilide and phenacetin (therapeutic doses)
Henna dye
Methylene blue
Nalidixic acid
Niridazole (Ambilhar)
Nitrofurantoins
Orange RN (red suya food colouring)
Pamaquine
Primaquine
Pentaquine

Sulfonamides: sulfacetamide
                          sulfamethoxale/co-trimoxazole
                          sulfanilamide
                          sulfapyridine

Thiazosulfone
Toluidine blue
Trinitrotoluene (TNT)
Vicia faba (broad beans)
Drugs and chemicals that may cause haemolysis in some types of G6PD-deficent subject but not shown to be haemolytic in GdA⁻ type
Aspirin (in large doses)
Chloroquine
Quinine
Quinidine
Vitamin K analogues
Chloramphenicol
Dimercaprol (BAL)

This list is not comprehensive. In addition there are many isolated unconfirmed reports of other drugs causing haemolysis in G6PD deficiency.

delivery, so avoiding extensive haematomas; and (3) hygiene in the puerperium, so avoiding sepsis.

Infection-induced jaundice

Viral infections, including hepatitis, infections of the respiratory and gastrointestinal tracts, and bacterial infections, including lobar pneumonia, typhoid, paratyphoid and septicaemia, may cause severe jaundice in G6PD-deficient subjects.[85] Possible mechanisms are the generation of H_2O_2 by activated neutrophils and macrophages triggering haemolysis of G6PD-deficient cells, and liver dysfunction leading to hepatocellular jaundice. Anaemia will be more severe as a result of suppression of erythropoiesis by infection. The course may be complicated in adults, but only rarely in children, by renal failure, which can be the result of pre-existing renal disease, nephrotoxic drugs, urinary tract infection, hepatic virus infection, renal ischaemia and tubular obstruction by haemoglobin. The administration of oxidant drugs may lead to further intravascular haemolysis and life-threatening renal failure.

Management is supportive: the treatment of the primary infection, the avoidance of oxidative drugs (Table 13.19) and a regimen for renal failure.

Food-induced haemolysis

Favism is a condition of severe intravascular haemolysis precipitated by eating fava beans (*Vicia faba*) or inhalation of the pollen; it occurs commonly in G6PD-deficient inhabitants of the Mediterranean area, North Africa and western and eastern Asia. It had been thought to be associated only with class II variants (e.g., Gd^{Mediterranean}), but has been described with other variants including GdA$^-$.[89] Favism occurs with the ingestion of fresh, dried or frozen beans, but fresh young beans in the spring are the most potent. Haemolysis in breast-fed infants may follow when mothers eat fava beans. Which ingredients trigger haemolysis is not proven.

Favism affects children under 5 years most commonly. Its pathogenesis is uncertain, as some G6PD subjects are spared altogether, while others have attacks for the first time after eating beans for years without trouble. There is intravascular haemolysis of sudden onset 24–48 hours after ingestion of beans: patients show pallor and haemoglobinuria; jaundice is less pronounced than with the haemolysis triggered by infections or drugs. Anaemia may be profound and renal failure can develop.

There is no specific treatment: transfusion of G6PD normal blood may be required if there is incipient or established cardiac failure.

Haemolytic episodes are best prevented by screening of G6PD deficiency in populations with high frequency, education and avoiding eating beans.

Milder acute haemolytic episodes have followed eating red suya, a peppered kebab-like roasted meat, in Nigeria; the offending substance was Orange RN (monosodium salt of 1-phenylazo-2-naphthol-6-sulfonic acid) used as colouring. It can be predicted that other foods could have the same effect in developing countries where there is inadequate control of additives.[90]

Drug-induced haemolysis

Ingestion of a wide variety of drugs and chemicals induces haemolysis in G6PD-deficient subjects (Table 13.19). The range of precipitating substances and the severity of the crises are greater with class II (e.g., Gd^{Mediterranean}) than class III (e.g., GdA$^-$) variants. There is also considerable intrapatient variability of severity between subjects with the same G6PD variant and drug exposure.[84,85,88]

Starting from between a few hours and 3 days after exposure, there may be only transient mild anaemia, or in some there is a rapidly progressive severe anaemia reaching a nadir at 7–8 days. Patients can complain of loin and abdominal pain; there is jaundice, haemoglobinuria and transient splenomegaly. Recovery is marked by a reticulocytosis and a rise of haemoglobin after 8–9 days.

Continued exposure to the drug can lead to fatal anaemia or renal failure in the case of class II variants. However, in the milder haemolysis of GdA$^-$ it is sometimes possible to continue with essential therapy, for example dapsone in the treatment of leprosy; patients have a transient haemolytic anaemia, followed by a state of compensated haemolysis.

Treatment is supportive and by withdrawal of the offending agent. Further attacks can be prevented by giving the patient a list of drugs to be avoided. Community strategies include screening and education.

Diagnosis

Haematology

During the steady state, subjects with the common forms of G6PD deficiency have a very mild chronic haemolysis, with a red cell lifespan of around 100 days. With Gd^{Mediterranean} the mean Hb in males is slightly decreased (141 versus 157 g/litre in controls in one series). Red cell indices and appearance on blood film are normal, but there is a slight reticulocytosis (±1.5%).

During a haemolytic crisis there are all the features of intravascular haemolysis (see Table 13.11) and a characteristic peripheral blood film appearance (see Figure 13.19B): supravital staining shows the presence of Heinz bodies.

G6PD screening and identification

There are several screening tests available that depend on NADPH production and its detection by direct fluorescence or by reduction of a coloured dye (e.g., methylene blue) to its colourless form.[85] These are simple, inexpensive and sensitive for the detection of hemizygous males and homozygous females when in the steady state. However, immediately following haemolytic crises, when there is a high population of young red cells, G6PD activity of whole blood may be normal, especially with class III (e.g., GdA$^-$) variants; in this situation blood should be centrifuged and the older cells at the bottom of the column tested, or the test delayed for about 6 weeks.

G6PD activity can be measured quantitatively by the spectrophotometric assay of NADPH formation by red cells: this requires a basic biochemistry laboratory. Male hemizygotes, female homozygotes and more than 80% of female heterozygotes can be identified.

The different G6PD variants are identified by several techniques, including electrophoresis and enzyme kinetic studies: these investigations are performed in reference or research laboratories only.

G6PD and malaria

Evidence that G6PD deficiency may confer advantage is derived from geography, parasitology of patients and in vitro cultures of *P. falciparum*.[84,85] Globally, G6PD deficiency reaches polymorphic frequency only where *P. falciparum* is or was endemic (see Figure 13.20), suggesting that in these areas deficient subjects have a genetic advantage; this view is supported by micro-mapping, for example in Sardinia where deficient gene frequency declines with increasing altitude and decreasing transmission of malaria. In a clinical study, female Nigerian children with GdB/GdA⁻ had significantly lower *P. falciparum* densities than normal children with malaria; furthermore, GdB (normal) red cells were much more often parasitized than GdA⁻ (deficient) red cells in the same individual.[85] It had been thought that limitation of malaria was confined to female heterozygotes only and was not enjoyed by male hemizyotes, but large case–control studies of children in West and East Africa have shown that both female heterozygotes and male hemizygotes had significant protection against severe malaria (about 46% and 58% respectively), but protection against mild malaria was statistically significant only in female heterozygotes.[91] In vitro cultures of *P. falciparum* have demonstrated that parasite growth is impaired in G6PD-deficient compared with normal red cells, but in some studies additional oxidative stress was needed before the difference became apparent. Oxidant radicals in parasitized red cells could lead to both impaired parasite development and to damage to the red cell membrane with early phagocytosis.[92]

Membrane defects

The red cell membrane is supported by a protein skeleton consisting of a lattice of hexagons, the sides of which are spectrin tetramers: these are linked at the corners of the hexagons by actin, tropomyosin and protein 4.1, and attached to the lipid bilayer by ankyrin and protein band 3 (the major transmembrane protein and anion transporter), as well as by glycoproteins such as glycophorin C. Inherited variants of either the integral or skeletal proteins of the red cell membrane may be manifest as abnormalities of shape, such as hereditary spherocytosis, elliptocytosis and ovalocytosis.[93] Membrane defects occur sporadically in all populations, hereditary spherocytosis being the most studied; only ovalocytosis in South-East Asia and Oceania achieves polymorphic frequency, but elliptocytosis is approaching polymorphic frequency in West and North Africa (see Figure 13.21).

South-East Asian ovalocytosis

The molecular basis of South-East Asian ovalocytosis (SAO) is a deletion of 27 nucleotides, resulting in the deletion of nine amino acids from band 3: the abnormal SAO band 3 has a higher than normal affinity for ankyrin, resulting in increased membrane rigidity and the oval shape (Figure 13.22A).[93,94] Inheritance is autosomal and dominant. Homozygotes have not been observed and this condition is probably lethal.

Ovalocytosis is seen at high frequency in populations of Malaysia, Indonesia, the Philippines, Papua New Guinea and the Solomon Islands, and possibly in

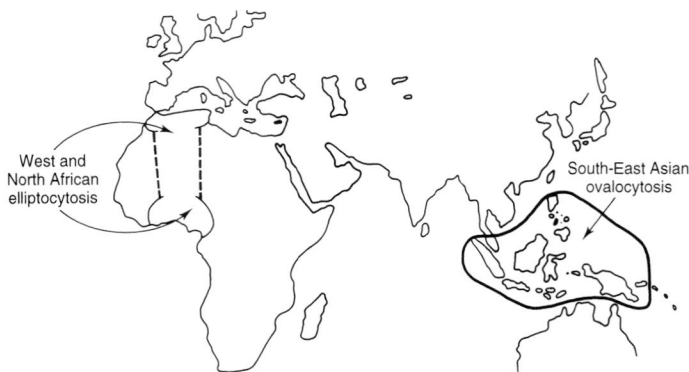

Figure 13.21: Areas of the Old World where ovalocytosis and elliptocytosis achieve (or approach) a polymorphic frequency.

Micronesian populations further out into the Pacific (see Figure 13.21). The distribution is extremely uneven within this area, but reaches up to 50% in Sulawesi (Celebes) and 27% in coastal Papua New Guinea.

A high proportion of red cells are ovalocytes (with a long axis less than twice the transverse axis), stomatocytes and knizocytes (with duplicated central pallor) (Figure 13.22A). Osmotic fragility is reduced. In otherwise healthy children, SAO is not associated with haemolysis or anaemia.

It had been reported earlier that in vivo both *P. falciparum* and *P. vivax* parasite rates were significantly lower in subjects with ovalocytes than in those with normal red cells, and that in vitro there was reduced parasite invasion of the rigid membranes of ovalocytes. More recently, however, when the diagnosis was made by detection of the SAO band 3 and not by subjective microscopy, similar rates of densities of both *P. falciparum* and *P. vivax* parasitaemias have been observed in community controls with and without SAO. Malarial anaemia was exacerbated by ovalocytosis, the median Hb being 12 g/litre lower during acute malaria in subjects with SAO than in controls. On the other hand, SAO prevented cerebral malaria, being observed in none of 68 children with cerebral malaria and in 6 (8.8%) of 68 matched controls in Papua New Guinea.[95] The mechanism of protection is likely to be related to differences of adherence of parasitized RBC to endothelium.

Elliptocytosis in West and North Africa

There are many mutations which result in elliptocytosis, and several have been described in West and North Africa.[94] Two variants of spectrin ($Sp\alpha^{I/65}$, $Sp\alpha^{I/46-50a}$) are at least approaching polymorphic frequency. Spectrin $\alpha I/65$ is the more common, but both are found throughout West Africa, the Maghreb (Tunisia, Algeria and Morocco), southern Italy and the Americas;[96] Tuaregs who inhabit the Sahara between West and North Africa have elliptocytosis, but this has not been characterized (see Figure 13.22). Up to 2–3% of both northern and southern Nigerians have an uncharacterized elliptocytosis. Inheritance is dominant. The condition is usually symptomless, but there may be mild haemolysis,

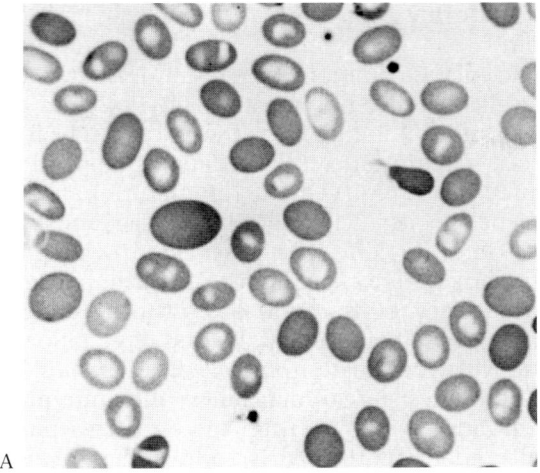

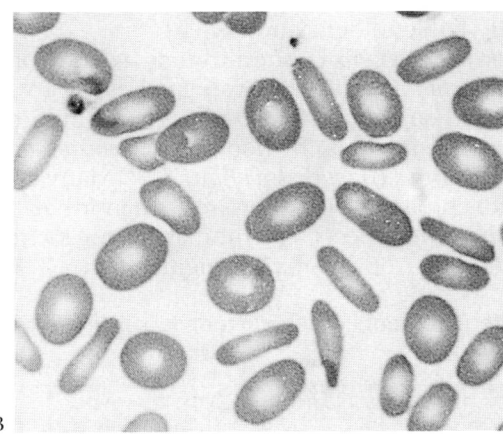

Figure 13.22: Peripheral blood films. (**A**) South-East Asian ovalocytosis. A high proportion of cells have a long axis which is less than twice the transverse axis (ovalocytosis). Some have two areas of central pallor (knizocytes), e.g., on the horizontal midline, towards the right edge. Some have mouth-like slits of pallor (stomatocytes), e.g., near the lower edge towards the left. (Reproduced with permission of the author and publisher from Dacie JV. *The Haemolytic Anaemias* 1, 3rd edn. Edinburgh: Churchill Livingstone, 1985.) (**B**) Elliptocytosis. The long axis is more than twice the transverse axis.

especially in homozygotes with the spectrin αI/65 variant. Red cells have a long axis more than twice the transverse axis (Figure 13.22B). There can be periodic episodes of slight jaundice and moderate splenomegaly following intercurrent infections; children with elliptocytosis and malaria sometimes develop profound anaemia (personal observations). Some elliptocyte variants in vitro are resistant to invasion by *P. falciparum*,[97] but there is no evidence at present as to whether there is selection for elliptocytosis in West Africa.

Nutritional anaemias

Iron

Iron is essential for the formation of haemoglobin, myoglobin and various enzymes. Its deficiency is the most common of all nutritional disorders: about 1000 million individuals suffer from anaemia due to iron deficiency (see Table 13.10), while an even larger number have iron depletion which has not reached the stage of anaemia.[98,99]

Dietary iron and absorption

In early postnatal life iron is derived normally from breast milk, which contains 0.3–0.5 mg/litre in a readily available form (50% absorbed). Iron in all other foods is in three forms: (1) haem iron, (2) non-haem iron and (3) contamination iron.

Haem iron is a constituent of haemoglobin and myoglobin in meat, poultry, fish and blood products; it is readily absorbed (20–30%) by the duodenal mucosal cells and utilized.

Non-haem iron is found in varying concentrations in all foods of plant origin, including cereals, tubers, vegetables and pulses. It is poorly absorbed (<5%) from common staples such as rice, maize, wheat, sorghum and millet when eaten alone. Absorption is inhibited by many vegetable ligands, including phytates in cereals, polyphenols in nuts and legumes, tannin in tea and soy protein, and by fibre; other inhibitors are egg phosphoproteins, and in those with pica, ash and clay. Absorption may be enhanced to up to 20% by consumption during the same meal of (1) fresh fruits and vegetables rich in ascorbic acid (e.g., guava, citrus, pineapple, mango, green or red peppers, cauliflower, some green leaves, potato, sweet potato, tomato and turnip), (2) amino acids from meat, poultry, fish and other seafoods, and (3) acids (e.g., lactic, citric).

Contamination iron is from two sources: dirt and iron cooking vessels. An adult male can take in 40–500 mg of contaminating iron on rice, sorghum or tef (*Eragrostis abyssinica*, a staple of the Ethiopian highlands) from the dirt picked up during threshing on earth floors and the dust of the marketplace; little of this is absorbable. Cooking food in iron pots may increase the iron content several fold, especially with soups containing acid-rich vegetables which are simmered for a long time. Beer brewed in iron pots is rich in available iron, and nutritional iron overload can follow after years of steady consumption (see below).

Absorption is by duodenal mucosal cells and is regulated by the iron status of the individual, being more efficient in the iron depleted than in the iron replete.

Iron balance

The iron in the body is in four compartments: (1) haemoglobin iron 1.5–3.0 g, (2) storage iron 1.0–1.5 g as ferritin and haemosiderin, (3) 'essential' iron 300 mg in myoglobin and numerous enzymes, and (4) transport iron 3–4 mg as transferrin, all quantities relating to adult males. The turnover of iron is rapid, about 23 mg entering and leaving the haemoglobin compartment of an adult each day, but iron is highly conserved and basal losses by desquamation in faeces, urine and skin for adult men and postmenopausal women are only about

1 mg/day (Table 13.20). Infants have low requirements while the red cell mass diminishes during the first 4–6 months, and these are met by breast-feeding. Iron needs are high relative to body size during growth in older infancy, childhood and the adolescent growth spurt. Menstruation approximately doubles the basal demand. Requirements are low during the first trimester of pregnancy but rise rapidly in the second trimester, to reach around 6–7 mg/day; approximately 1000 mg of iron is needed over the whole of one pregnancy. Lactating women secrete about 0.3 mg of iron per day in breast milk, but while they have amenorrhoea daily requirements are relatively low.

Diets with high contents of bioavailable iron are eaten by most populations in industrialized countries, and also, until recently, surviving communities of hunter–gatherers, pastoralists who eat meat and blood (e.g., Masai in Kenya) and some groups with high ascorbic acid intake (e.g., Yoruba in Nigeria); physiological demands for iron are usually met, except during pregnancy when negative balance and some depletion of stores is inevitable. The majority of the world's population eat food with intermediate, low or very low bioavailable iron, from which it is impossible to meet the basic physiological requirements for iron (Table 13.20).[99]

Iron deficiency
Aetiology
Iron deficiency is commonly the result of *inadequate intake* of bioavailable iron not meeting physiological requirements. Ligands inhibiting iron absorption can be increased in special circumstances: food taboos applied during pregnancy; the replacement of traditional diets by convenience foods including wheat-bread and eggs; the drinking of tea (or coffee to a lesser extent) with the meal. Premature infants are a special case of nutritional deficiency as the transplacental transport of iron to the infant takes place almost wholly in the last 4 weeks of gestation.

Those with the greatest *physiological demands* for iron are at the highest risk of deficiency; these are preschool children, adolescents during the growth spurt, and especially menstruating girls, and pregnant women. Women who have many pregnancies, closely spaced, are especially liable to deficiency.

As normal red cells contain iron as haemoglobin 1 mg per 1 ml, *chronic blood loss* can lead easily to negative balance and depletion of iron stores. Common causes in the tropics are infection by hookworm, *Schistosoma* species and whipworm (*Trichuris trichiura*).[98–100] Many conditions leading to chronic haemorrhage (e.g., menorrhagia, aspirin ingestion, peptic ulcers, carcinomas) occur in tropical as well as in non-tropical environments.

Table 13.20 FAO/WHO recommended iron intakes (mg/day) to cover requirements of 97.5% individuals in each age/sex group for diets with different bioavailabilities (after ref. 98).

| Age/sex group | Absorbed iron required | Bioavailability of dietary iron (% of iron absorbed) | | | |
		Very low[1] (< 5%)	Low[2] (5–10%)	Intermediate[3] (11–18%)	High[4] (> 19%)
Children, both sexes					
0–4 months	0.5	*	*	*	*
4–12 months	0.96	24	13	6	4
13–24 months	0.61	15	8	4	3
2–5 years	0.70	17	9	5	3
6–11 years	1.17	29	16	8	5
Adolescents					
12–16 years (girls)	2.02	50	27	13	9
12–16 years (boys)	1.82	45	24	12	8
Adults					
Men	1.14	28	15	8	5
Women					
Menstruating	2.38	59	32	16	11
Pregnant:					
1st trimester	0.8	–	–	–	–
3rd trimester	6.3	†	†	†	–
Lactating	1.31	33	17	9	6
Postmenopausal	0.96	24	13	6	4

*Iron from breast milk is sufficient for about the first 6 months.
†Supplementation essential.
[1]*Very low bioavailability*. Diet composed almost entirely of cereals (e.g., in India).
[2]*Low bioavailability*. Monotonous diet based on cereals, roots and tubers, with a preponderance of foods which inhibit iron absorption (maize, rice, beans, wheat, sorghum) and with negligible quantities of meat, fish or ascorbic acid.
[3]*Intermediate bioavailability diet*. Similar to above, but including some foods of animal origin and/or ascorbic acid.
[4]*High bioavailability*. A diversified diet containing generous quantities of meat, poultry, fish or foods rich in ascorbic acid: typical of most populations in industrialized countries. The regular consumption with meals of inhibitors of absorption (e.g., tea or coffee) can reduce bioavailability to the intermediate level.

Hookworm

Infections with *Ancylostoma duodenale* and *Necator americanus* are widespread, and approximately 1200 million individuals, almost a quarter of the world's population, are infected (see Chapter 83).[100] Prevalence of 80–90% in the population in the moist tropics is not unusual.

The adult worms ingest, detach and digest the host's intestinal mucosa, causing bleeding. The daily loss of iron has been calculated as 1.2 mg and 0.8 mg per 1000 ova per gram of faeces for *A. duodenale* and *N. americanus* respectively, but as both species are now found more or less worldwide and mixed infections are common, the daily loss of iron of 1 mg per 1000 ova per gram of faeces regardless of species is a good working figure.[99,100]

Depletion of iron stores depends on (1) the daily absorption of iron, (2) the size of the body's iron stores and (3) the intensity of the hookworm infection. Subjects with diets poor in bioavailable iron and with low or no stores need only light infections to deplete them of iron; in contrast, adults in West Africa on traditional diets had a threshold of at least 20 000 ova per gram of faeces, equivalent to an iron loss of 20 mg/day, above which they went into negative balance. Women have lower thresholds than men. Children expose their whole body surfaces to infection when playing on the ground, and have heavy hookworm loads in relation to their body weights; the resultant *subacute hookworm anaemia* has an element of acute haemorrhage in its aetiology.

Acute hookworm anaemia is rare but follows extremely heavy infections, usually in infants but sometimes in older children or even adults. *A. duodenale* is able to cross the placenta and infect the infant in utero. Anaemia is from acute blood loss, shows a normochromic picture and may be severe and life threatening.[21,100]

Schistosomiasis

About 200 million people are infected by *Schistosoma*, and transmission is increasing with the spread of irrigation (see Chapter 80).

The haematuria from *S. haematobium* is short lived but can give rise to a loss of 30–40 mg of iron per day and contribute significantly to iron deficiency, especially in adolescent boys, for example in Somalia and coastal East Africa.

The mechanisms of anaemia caused by *S. mansoni* and *S. japonicum* infections are complex. Ulcers and polyps in the colon bleed and can result in a chronic loss of iron of 7–8 mg/day. Infection of the liver is followed by hepatic fibrosis and the anaemia of chronic disorders; portal hypertension leads to splenomegaly and the pancytopenia of hypersplenism; oesophageal varices may bleed acutely or intermittently, leading to iron loss.[21,100]

Trichuriasis

T. trichiura is one of the most prevalent helminths in the world, infecting about 1000 million people (see Chapter 83).[100] Blood is lost from the inflamed colonic mucosa.

Heavy infections in excess of 800 worms (16 000 ova per gram of faeces) result in a blood loss of 4 ml, or iron loss of 1.5 mg, per day. Trichuriasis can contribute to iron deficiency, or be a major cause in children, as has been reported from Central America and Malaysia.[100]

Stages of iron deficiency

Iron deficiency passes through three stages. In the first stage, *iron depletion*, iron stores are reduced, but haemopoiesis remains unaffected: plasma ferritin is below normal and staining for iron in a bone marrow aspirate shows scanty (1+) or zero iron in the macrophages of a cellular fragment; plasma iron is low normal, plasma transferrin raised and its percentage saturation reduced within the normal range. In the second stage, *iron-deficient erythropoiesis*, iron stores have been exhausted: plasma ferritin is reduced further, iron is absent from the bone marrow and there are no sideroblasts; plasma iron and transferrin saturation are below normal and red cell protoporphyrin is raised; the Hb is likely to be within the normal range or there may be a slight normochromic anaemia. With further depletion, iron is not available for haemoglobin synthesis, and *iron deficiency anaemia* develops.

Iron deficiency anaemia
Clinical

Patients present with symptoms and signs of anaemia from any cause; in addition they may show angular stomatitis, koilonychia and loss of melanin skin pigmentation.

Iron is essential for many metabolic processes, and its deficiency even without anaemia has adverse effects on development during childhood, the outcome of pregnancy and work capacity. In practice it is not feasible to distinguish the results of iron deficiency per se from those of anaemia. The consequences of iron deficiency, and especially iron deficiency anaemia are: *in infants, children and adolescents*, impaired motor development, coordination, language development and scholastic achievement, psychological and behavioural effects (inattention, fatigue, insecurity, etc.) and decreased physical activity;[101] *in adults of both sexes*, decreased physical work, earning capacity and resistance to fatigue; *in pregnant women*, increased maternal and infant morbidity and mortality, placental hypertrophy premature delivery, and risk of low birthweight.[98,99,102,103] There is no convincing evidence that iron deficiency either enhances or significantly impairs resistance to infections, although there is some reduction of cellular immune responses.[99]

Haematology

Anaemia varies from mild to profound. The MCV, MCH and MCHC are all reduced; the peripheral blood film shows microcytic hypochromic red cells and sometimes numerous target cells (Figure 13.23). In the bone marrow aspirate there are micronormoblastic red cell precursors

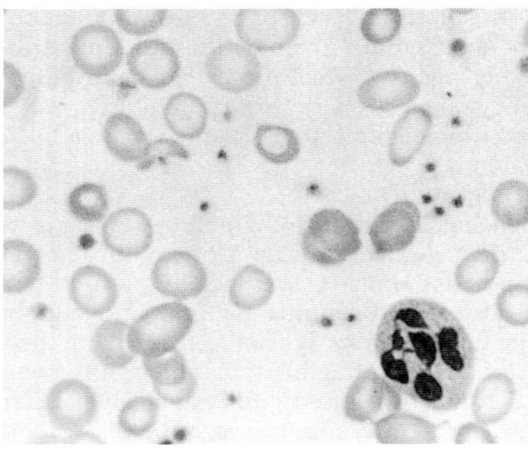

Figure 13.23: Peripheral blood film. Iron deficiency anaemia: there is variation in size of the red cells (anisocytosis) with many small cells (microcytosis), variation of shape (poikilocytosis) and hypersegmented neutrophil, suggestive but not diagnostic of folate or vitamin B_{12} deficiency; there are numerous platelets (thrombocytosis) which are likely to be a response to chronic haemorrhage.

and the total absence of storage iron. Plasma, for example in a microhaematocrit tube, is nearly colourless and water clear.

There are three considerations in confirming the diagnosis of iron deficiency anaemia: (1) limited laboratory facilities; (2) biochemical measurements of iron status giving misleading results in patients with multiple pathology; and (3) differentiation from the microcytic hypochromic anaemias of chronic disorders and β thalassaemia minor.

With a limited laboratory the diagnosis of iron deficiency anaemia can be usually made with certainty from the blood film appearance, colourless plasma and the absence of iron in the bone marrow. However, iron is immobilized in the RES in the anaemia of chronic disorders, megaloblastic anaemia and protein–energy malnutrition (PEM); although iron is seen in the bone marrow and iron deficiency is not limiting erythropoiesis at the time, treatment of the primary condition can lead to the mobilization of all iron and the uncovering of iron deficiency.

Ferritin is an acute reactive protein and plasma ferritin levels are generally raised in rural populations in the tropics, and although levels correlate with the body iron stores, higher cut-off points have to be applied. Malaria, other recurrent infection and chronic hepatic disease can be accompanied by abnormally high plasma ferritins even in the face of severe iron deficiency, making the measurement of plasma ferritin of limited diagnostic value, especially in children.

In iron deficiency, the plasma iron is low and the plasma transferrin is raised, so that transferrin saturation is < 16% in adults, < 14% in children and < 12% in infants. In contrast, in anaemia of chronic disorders and PEM, both plasma iron and plasma ferritin are reduced, and although the saturation of transferrin is decreased it remains > 15%.

In β thalassaemia minor the red cell count is higher ($> 5.0 \times 10^{12}$/litre), there is less anisocytosis (normal RBC distribution width (RDW)), greater microcytosis and less hypochromia than with iron deficiency (Table 13.15). From these characteristics are derived several formulae to differentiate the two conditions; for example, the ratio MCV:RBC is > 14 in iron deficiency and < 14 in thalassaemia.

Management

Oral treatment

Tablets of ferrous salts (for example, exsiccated ferrous sulfate 200 mg, containing 60 mg of elemental iron) taken orally are the cheapest effective treatment.[98,104] For adults and adolescents the recommended dosage is 60 mg of elemental iron per day for mild anaemia and 120 mg (plus folic acid 400 µg) per day for moderate or severe anaemia. Absorption is best if the tablets are taken on an empty stomach. Treatment should continue until the Hb has reached normal limits and ceased to rise, and then for at least another 4–6 weeks in order to build up body stores.

Pregnant women should receive a combination tablet containing 400 µg of folic acid and 60 mg of iron twice a day; suitable tablets are supplied by UNICEF for US $1 per 1000 tablets.

Infants and children may be treated with liquid preparations in divided doses to provide 5 mg of iron per kilogram body weight (plus folic acid 100–400 µg) per day.

Oral iron can cause upper gastrointestinal side effects (epigastric discomfort, nausea and vomiting), or lower gastrointestinal side effects (diarrhoea or constipation). The frequency of adverse reactions is related directly to the dosage of iron and not to the ferrous compound prescribed. Oral treatment must continue if possible: dosage should be reduced and then stepped up again slowly within the patient's tolerance, or the tablets taken with meals (although this reduces absorption), or the formulation changed to a better tolerated but much more expensive slow-release preparation.

Where folate intake is poor, deficiency may develop during the response to iron therapy: folic acid 5 mg/day for 3 weeks should be given.

Parenteral treatment

A parenteral route is justified when (1) oral treatment has not been tolerated, (2) there is persistent non-compliance, (3) it is nearly impossible for a patient to comply because of the severity of the iron deficiency and the length of time required for oral therapy, and (4) an advanced period of gestation does not allow for full oral treatment before obstetric delivery. The extra cost of parenteral preparations is offset by savings on hospital bed occupancy and staff time, and by the rapid return of the patient to productive life.[100]

Complementary parasite treatment

Where hookworm is endemic (prevalence greater than 20%), those above 2 years of age should receive albendazole 400 mg in a single dose as the simplest to administer effective anthelmintic; treatment should be withheld during the first trimester of pregnancy. Where urinary schistosomiasis is endemic, any person over 5 years of age who has visible haematuria should be treated with oral praziquantel 50 mg/kg body weight in a single dose. Recovery may be delayed by coincidental malaria: children under 5 years of age in malaria endemic areas should receive curative antimalarial therapy followed by prophylaxis for 3 weeks, appropriate to the area.[104]

Prevention

There are four strategies for the prevention of iron deficiency: (1) iron supplementation; (2) fortification of a staple food with iron; (3) measures to increase dietary intake of bioavailable iron; and (4) the control of hookworm and other helminthic infections.[98,100]

Supplementation

Supplementation with medicinal iron has the advantages of having immediate impact and of being targeted on specific groups which are known to be liable to deficiency, including pregnant women, premature infants, preschool children and adolescent girls.[104]

Iron supplementation for pregnant women should be given the highest priority in all national programmes of prenatal care delivery.[26,98,102] A successful programme must involve policy makers, planners, managers, educators, workers, midwives, obstetricians, the pregnant women themselves and their families, in order to ensure the utilization of antenatal services, the provision of medication and compliance by pregnant women; administration of iron supplements by traditional birth attendants reduced the prevalence of iron deficiency and anaemia and increased the mean birthweight, without enhancing peripheral blood or placental malaria, in The Gambia.[105] Pregnant women with sickle cell trait and their infants may not benefit from iron supplementation, through mechanisms which are not understood.[106] Recommended supplementation is the UNICEF combined tablet of elemental iron 60 mg (as ferrous sulfate) and folic acid 400 µg, taken twice daily without food throughout the second half of pregnancy; if compliance is poor or if there are unacceptable side effects, the two tablets can be taken together, or taken with meals or reduced to one per day. Where malaria is endemic, antimalarial prophylaxis should start from the time of first antenatal attendance. Where women are exposed to heavy hookworm infestations, albendazole 400 mg should be given orally on first attendance after the first trimester. Vitamin A (2.4 mg retinol/day) supplements dramatically enhanced the efficacy of iron in the prevention of anaemia in pregnancy in Indonesia.[100]

Breast-feeding for 6 months or more protects full-term infants; breast-fed preterm infants require iron supplements by not later than 2 months of age. Recommended dosage is 2 mg/kg body weight, up to a maximum of 15 mg/day until iron-fortified cereal foods can be introduced. Parents must be warned about the toxicity of iron overdosage. Bottle-fed infants should receive formulae containing iron 12 mg/litre and vitamin E 10 iu/litre;[2] unfortified brands are still being sold by the unscrupulous in developing countries. Children aged 6–24 months of age can be given supplements of 12.5 mg iron plus 50 µg folic acid daily.[104] It is the consensus that this does not increase significantly the risk of malaria.[107]

Food fortification

The fortification with iron of widely consumed and centrally processed staple foods is the main strategy for anaemia control in many countries.[11,99] Vehicles for fortification have included acidified milk formulae and biscuits (with added bovine haemoglobin) in Chile, sugar in Guatemala, salt in India and fish sauce in Thailand. Fortification has been followed by a slow but steady decrease of prevalence of anaemia at low cost. Fortification programmes require industrial infrastructure and organized marketing which do not exist in many countries, particularly in Africa.

Dietary modification

In the long term the ideal is for people to eat food from which they can absorb sufficient iron for normal physiological requirements.[98] Improved iron status can be achieved by increasing enhancers of iron absorption (e.g., ascorbic acid and animal protein), decreasing inhibitors (e.g., tannin and phytic acid), or by increasing total food intake so that energy needs are met fully and total iron intake improved by up to 30%. Ethiopian children fed on food cooked in iron pots had lower rates of anaemia and improved growth than children whose food was cooked in aluminium pots: provision of iron pots may be a cheap and effective way of preventing iron deficiency anaemia.[108]

Even when the value of ascorbic acid-rich foods is understood, there are restraints of cost if purchased, and of limited water supply and expense of fencing if grown in home gardens. As ascorbic acid is destroyed by heat, encouragement should be given to eating food raw or cooked only lightly and not reheated. Germination, malting and fermentation of grains both increase ascorbic acid and decrease tannin and phytates. Attempts to increase intake of animal protein are restrained by high costs and by religious objections, for example Hinduism.

Control of helminthic infections

It has been shown, for example in Korea, that transmission of hookworm can be reduced highly effectively and cheaply by simple sanitary measures, such as pit latrines, wearing plastic sandals and abandoning human faeces as fertilizer[99] (see also Chapter 83 and Appendix II).

Iron overload

There are many congenital and acquired conditions leading to systemic iron overload, including hereditary haemochromatosis and thalassaemia.[109] In sub-Saharan

Africa, dietary iron overload is associated with drinking regularly for many years beers brewed from sorghum, millet and maize (Chapter 10). The beers are fermented in iron pots or, in more recent times, steel (oil) barrels, and contain absorbable iron at a concentration of up to 80 mg/litre; as acid and alcohol stimulate gastric acid secretion, absorption is enhanced further.[110] Men especially commonly drink several litres at weekends.

Dietary iron overload, as defined as hepatic iron > 360 µmol/g dry weight (normal < 17 µmol/g), was present in 26% of male and 8% of female black South Africans over 40 years of age in necropsies at Baragwanath Hospital, Soweto, in 1959–1960. The 'liberalization' of the drinking laws, allowing black South Africans to drink bottled beer, was followed by a substantial decline in prevalence of the condition. However, dietary iron overload remains common in rural areas of much of southern Africa; for example, 21% of Zimbabwean men aged 45 years or more had high serum ferritins and transferrin saturation > 70% in 1986, and the condition is reported in several countries of East and West Africa. It seems probable that a high dietary intake is not the only factor but that it is interacting with an inborn error of metabolism in the causation of iron overload in Africa.[111]

Once the hepatic iron is above 360 µmol/g dry weight, portal fibrosis and cirrhosis develop. Other complications include pancreatic fibrosis and diabetes mellitus, cardiac fibrosis and heart failure, chronic scurvy and osteoporosis. Patients have a history of beer consumption over years, hepatomegaly with or without ascites and hyperpigmentation. The diagnosis is confirmed by finding excessively high serum iron, transferrin saturation and ferritin, and excessive iron in a liver biopsy. Benefit is described from repeated venesections; chelating agents have had no extensive trials.

Folic acid
Normal metabolism
The vitamin folic acid is not found naturally in the form of the core molecule pteroylglutamic acid (PGA), but as active folates, which are reduced, conjugated and condensed forms of PGA.[112] The enzyme dihydrofolate reductase, found in mammalian liver cells, reduces PGA to dihydro- and tetrahydrofolates. Folates are transported and absorbed as monoglutamates, but intracellularly are often conjugated to form polyglutamates. Folates are metabolically active when condensed with one-carbon radicals (e.g., methyl, methenyl, methylene, formyl); folates function as cofactors for the transfer of these one-carbon radicals in the synthesis of purines and pyrimidines (and hence nucleic acids) and in amino acid interconversions (e.g., histidine/glutamic acid, homocysteine/methionine and glycine/serine). Folate is essential for the conversion of uridine to thymidine required for DNA synthesis; therefore, folate is necessary for normal cell division, and tissues with rapid rates of cell division, for example bone marrow and gastrointestinal mucosa, have the highest requirements.

Folates are found in a wide variety of both animal and vegetable foods. Good sources include liver, green vegetables, tubers (e.g., yams, sweet potatoes), bananas and plantains, mangoes, fresh green and red peppers, locust beans, eggs, cheese and yeast products (e.g., bread and beer). Red meat and poultry are moderately good sources. Poor sources are grains (e.g., rice, maize, sorghum, millet), roots (e.g., cassava), non-green vegetables and distilled alcohols. Folates are heat labile and water soluble, so that prolonged cooking, reheating or boiling in large volumes of water greatly reduces the available folate.

Polyglutamates are deconjugated and folates are absorbed actively as monoglutamates in the upper jejunum. Serum transport is as N-5-methyltetra-hydrofolate. Storage is mainly in the liver, and is normally sufficient to meet requirements for about 3 months only. Folate is excreted in bile, but most of this is reabsorbed. There is a small loss in urine; faeces are rich in folate, but this is derived from bacterial synthesis in the colon and is extraneous to the body's metabolism. Folate is consumed in intermediary metabolism: requirements are highest during growth, pregnancy and lactation (Table 13.21).

Folate deficiency
Aetiology
Despite folates being found in a wide range of commonly eaten foods, dietary deficiency is common, often related to food shortages, destruction by cooking or eating of inappropriate foods (Table 13.22).[112,113] In some communities of subsistence farmers, folate deficiency is seen most frequently at the end of the dry season and in the early rainy season before the new harvest. Sometimes all the folate-rich foods are cooked in a soup or relish added to the bulky staple; this may be cooked for several hours and reheated many times before being finished, so destroying most of the folate. Individuals with highest requirements, especially pregnant women and premature infants, are the most likely to be severely deficient.[26]

Table 13.21 Daily dietary requirements for folates and vitamin B$_{12}$ (after ref. 7).

Nutrient	Group	Daily dietary requirement (µg)
Folate	0–6 months	40–50
	7–12 months	120
	1–12 years	200
	≥ 13 years	400
	Pregnant women	800
	Lactating women	600
Vitamin B$_{12}$	0–12 months	0.3
	1–3 years	0.9
	4–9 years	1.5
	≥ 10 years	2.0
	Pregnant women	3.0
	Lactating women	2.5

Table 13.22 Some causes of folate and vitamin B$_{12}$ deficiencies.

	Folate	Vitamin B$_{12}$
Inadequate intake	Boiling of bottle feeds Goats' milk feeding of infants Inappropriate weaning foods Anorexia (recurrent infection, old age) Seasonal shortage (end of dry season) Prolonged cooking/reheating Prolonged storage of food Famine Taboos and food fads Alcoholism	Breast-feeding by B$_{12}$-deficient women Veganism
Malabsorption	Diarrhoea in infancy Acute enteric infections *Giardia lamblia* Ileocaecal tuberculosis Systemic infections (pneumonia, tuberculosis) Coeliac disease Tropical sprue (acute) Crohn's disease	Pernicious anaemia Gastrectomy Chronic *Giardia lamblia* *Diphyllobothrium latum* Stagnant loop syndrome Tropical sprue (chronic) (Chapter 10) Crohn's disease
High physiological demands	Growth (permaturity, infancy, adolescence) Pregnancy Lactation	(Pregnancy)
Pathologically high demands	Haemolysis (sickle cell, thalassaemia, etc.; recurrent malaria) Malignant disease (Burkitt's, choriocarcinoma)	
Disturbed metabolism	Pyrexia Overdosage of antagonists (pyrimethamine, trimethoprim)	Nitrous oxide Chronic cyanide intoxication (cassava)

Malabsorption of folate results from tropical sprue and from acute or chronic intestinal infections (e.g., giardiasis), and may also complicate systemic infections, including acute pneumonias, tuberculosis and malaria.

Haemolysis leads to erythroid hyperplasia and high demands for folate: patients with severe chronic haemolytic anaemias (e.g., sickle cell disease, thalassaemia major, spherocytosis) are almost inevitably seriously deficient if untreated. Recurrent malaria in childhood leads to dyserythropoiesis but not folate deficiency; in contrast, the main pathology of malaria in partially immune pregnant women is haemolysis and an anaemia which is normocytic at first but can progress to a profound folate deficiency megaloblastic anaemia.[26]

Dihydrofolate reductase is inactive at 39°C: high or prolonged pyrexia can lead to acute megaloblastic arrest of erythropoiesis due to this block in folate metabolism. The 2,4-diaminopyrimidines (pyrimethamine and trimethoprim) are analogues of PGA and competitive inhibitors of dihydrofolate reductase. Their affinities for the enzymes of protozoa or bacteria are high and for the enzymes of mammals low, but overdosage can lead to severe disturbance of folate metabolism and megaloblastic anaemia. This has occurred in epidemics in China following the addition of pyrimethamine to table salt. Infants are liable to be overdosed, and individuals may overtreat themselves with antimalarial prophylactics (e.g., pyrimethamine daily instead of weekly), or with therapies containing pyrimethamine (e.g., Fansidar), or with simultaneous antimalarials and co-trimoxazole in high dose.

Aetiology is often multiple. In infancy and childhood, folate deficiency commonly complicates prematurity, feeding with boiled cows' milk or with goats' milk (which contains only folate unavailable for man), poor weaning foods, diarrhoea, repeated systemic infections, and haemoglobinopathies;[112] in West Africa, for example, about one-third of children with either PEM or moderate to severe anaemia are folate deficient. Factors leading to folate deficiency during pregnancy are commonly low intake, high demands from pregnancy, especially multiple pregnancy, malarial haemolysis, especially in primigravidae, pyrexia and haemoglobinopathies; folate deficiency is a major aetiological factor in severe anaemias in pregnancy in around three-quarters of West African patients and two-thirds of Indian patients.[11,26] In southern Africa women present commonly about 6 months post partum with megaloblastic anaemia due to a low intake of folate from a maize-based diet not meeting the high demands of repeated pregnancies and prolonged lactation.[113]

Clinical

Patients with folate deficiency present with the symptoms and signs of anaemia. They have an increased susceptibility to infection related to neutropenia and immune deficiency. Rarely, there is a history of purpura or menorrhagia associated with thrombocytopenia. Mild splenomegaly is not unusual. Patients may have depression of mood and mental alertness, but not the major neurological signs of vitamin B_{12} deficiency. Long-standing folate deficiency can cause hyperpigmentation of the skin, but this is not so obvious as with vitamin B_{12} deficiency. Changes in the intestinal tract are glossitis, angular cheilosis, mild malabsorption and delayed regeneration of liver cells. Chronic deficiency causes sterility in both sexes and retarded growth and development in childhood, for example in patients with sickle cell disease. Folate deficiency in early pregnancy has an association with neural tube defects in the infants, and in later pregnancy with fetal growth retardation, premature delivery and low birthweight.[114]

Haematology

Anaemia varies in severity but may be profound. The MCV and MCH are raised, but the MCHC is normal. Macrocytosis may be masked if there is a coincidental cause for microcytosis, such as iron deficiency or thalassaemia trait. The reticulocyte count is high if the underlying cause is haemolysis, but otherwise is normal or low. The red cells show anisocytosis and macrocytosis; there is a tendency to oval forms, but poikilocytosis is unusual unless the anaemia is long-standing; cells are normochromic; there is polychromasia, punctate basophilia occasionally, nucleated cells (which may be obvious megaloblasts) and Howell–Jolly bodies (Figure 13.24A). Macrocytosis and raised MCV may not be apparent in patients who have concomitant iron deficiency or α thalassaemia. The total WBC and neutrophil counts are usually low, with hypersegmented neutrophils in the peripheral blood (Figure 13.24B); however, with complicating infections, as are common in the tropics, there may be leukaemoid reactions, with excessively high total WBC and neutrophil counts, showing a shift to the left as far as the promyelocytes or even blasts, and numerous giant metamyelocytes. The platelet count is moderately reduced commonly, but sometimes severely. Bone marrow aspirates reveal megaloblastic haemopoiesis (Figure 13.25); iron stores tend to be raised due to immobilization, but in patients with dual deficiencies megaloblastic changes can be masked and iron absent from the marrow. Serum lactate dehydrogenase levels are extremely high; serum bilirubin is moderately raised.

With many patients, for example pregnant women or patients with sickle cell disease, it is obvious that megaloblastic erythropoiesis is the result of folate deficiency, but with others it is necessary to distinguish folate from vitamin B_{12} deficiency by assaying serum folate, red cell

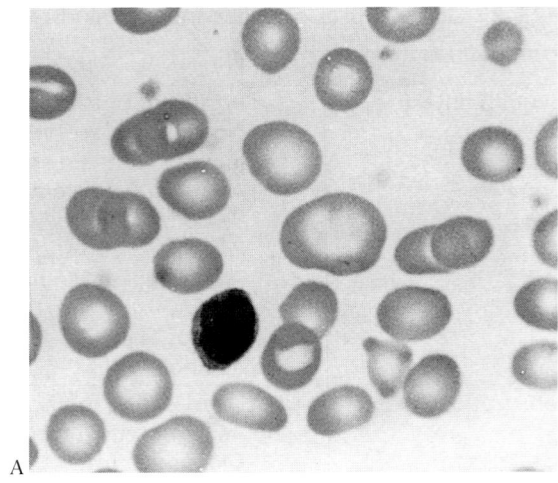

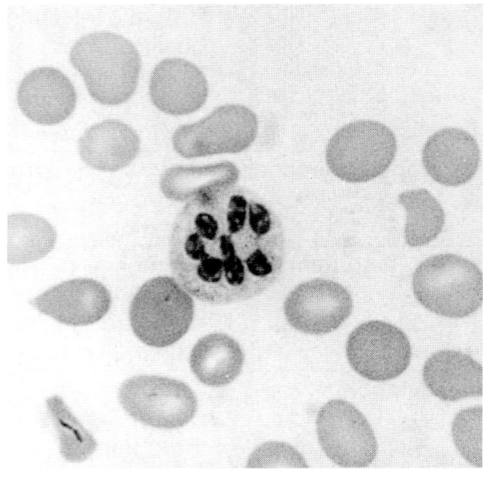

Figure 13.24: Peripheral blood films. (**A**) Macrocytic megaloblastic anaemia. Red cells show variation of size (anisocytosis) and large cells (macrocytes), some of which are oval. (**B**) Hypersegmented neutrophil of a patient with dietary vitamin B_{12} deficiency.

folate and serum vitamin B_{12} levels. If assays are not available, the two deficiencies can be distinguished by a therapeutic trial of physiological doses of folic acid 50 μg/day: if there is no reticulocyte or haemoglobin response within 1 week, vitamin B_{12} 1 μg/day intramuscularly is tried; coincidental infections suppress haematological responses, making results difficult to interpret.

Management

Folic acid 5 mg/day is followed by a reticulocyte response after about 5 days, and the slow restoration of normal haematology; treatment for 3 weeks is sufficient to replace the body stores but should be continued if there are ongoing high demands or malabsorption. This dosage is in excess of requirements and there is never any need to increase to 15 mg/day; parenteral treatment is indicated only rarely with severe malabsorption, and the reduced form folinic acid is needed only to counteract dihydrofolate reductase inhibitors.

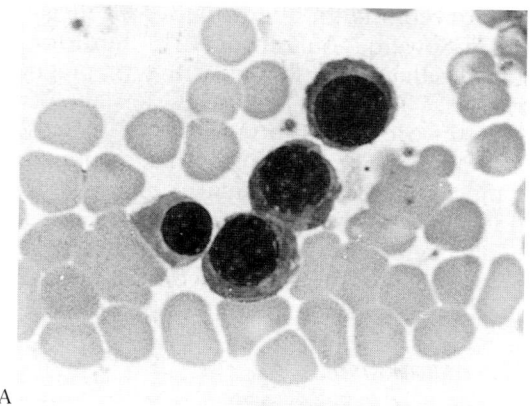

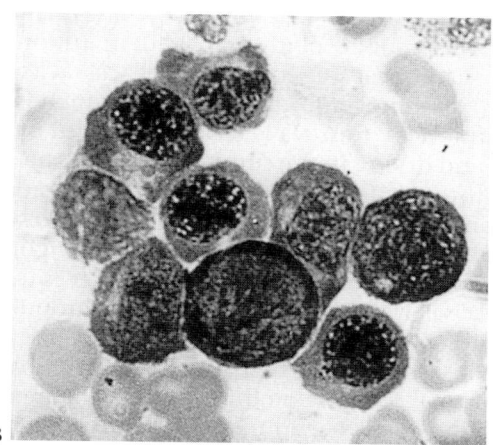

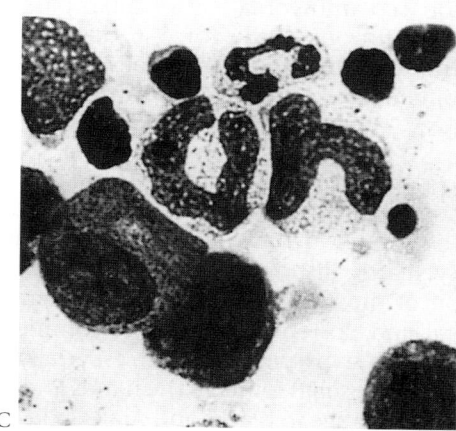

Figure 13.25: Bone marrow. (**A**) Normoblastic erythroid hyperplasia from a patient with haemolytic anaemia, to show the normal stages of maturation of erythroblasts. (*B*) Megaloblastic bone marrow: the erythroblasts are large; the nuclei are grainy (deficient in chromatin); the nuclei remain immature whereas the cytoplasm continues to develop (nuclear–cytoplasmic dissociation); there are bizarre-shaped nuclei and Howell–Jolly bodies; there is a high proportion of early forms which do not develop to late forms, but suffer intramedullary destruction. (**C**) Giant metamyelocytes: these are about twice the size of normal metamyelocytes and characteristic of megaloblastic bone marrows, but may be seen also following cytotoxic therapy.

Patients with a megaloblastic anaemia can be treated initially with both folic acid and vitamin B_{12} while awaiting the results of vitamin assays, provided all blood and marrow samples have been collected for necessary investigations.

Prevention

The same three strategies of supplementation, fortification of food and dietary modification apply as in the prevention of iron deficiency.

Premature infants should be given supplements of $50\,\mu g$/day. Infants with diarrhoea should receive $50\,\mu g$ in addition. Deficiency in pregnancy is prevented with the combined iron ($60\,mg$) and folic acid ($400\,\mu g$) tablets twice a day. Preconceptional supplements of folic acid are required to prevent recurrence of neural tube defects.[114] Patients with chronic haemolytic anaemias (e.g., thalassaemia, sickle cell disease, congenital spherocytosis) are generally given folic acid $5\,mg$/day, this large dose being the pharmaceutical preparation usually available.

For populations with high frequencies of nutritional deficiency there is a strong case for the fortification of the staple with folic acid, for example maize flour in southern Africa; however, this has not yet been enforced.[113]

The natural folate content of food can be enhanced by cultivating and eating folate-rich vegetables, which are generally those which are also rich in ascorbic acid (see 'Prevention of iron deficiency'). Encouragement should also be given to eating raw or only lightly cooked vegetables and fruit.

Vitamin B_{12}

The natural forms of vitamin B_{12} in mammals are: (1) deoxyadenosylcobalamin, which accounts for about 80% of intracellular vitamin B_{12}; (2) methylcobalamin, which is the main form in plasma; and (3) hydroxocobalamin, which occurs in small quantities both intracellularly and extracellularly.[112] Cyanocobalamin occurs naturally in trace amounts only, but is stable and so finds diagnostic and therapeutic applications. There are only three biochemical reactions known to involve vitamin B_{12} in man: (1) the isomerization of methylmalonyl CoA to succinyl CoA; (2) the isomerization of α-leucine to β-leucine; (3) the methylation of homocysteine to methionine, a reaction which results in conversion of methyltetrahydrofolate to tetrahydrofolate. Vitamin B_{12} is vital for normal folate metabolism and for the myelination of nerve fibres.

Vitamin B_{12} is synthesized by micro-organisms and is available to man in animal foods, especially liver, and animal products, including milk and its derivatives and eggs. Vitamin B_{12} is not found in vegetables: it is available, however, from faecally contaminated water, and this source is important in the poorest vegetarian societies.[115] Requirements are extremely low, and are met by very small intakes of animal food (Table 13.21).

Vitamin B_{12} is released from food in the stomach, and then bound to intrinsic factor (IF), a glycoprotein secreted by parietal cells. The IF–B_{12} complex is adsorbed by means of a specific receptor on to the mucosal cells of the terminal ileum; the vitamin B_{12} is absorbed and transported to the liver by the plasma protein transcobalamin II (TC-II). Storage, mainly in the liver, amounts to 3–5 mg and is sufficient to meet requirements for 3–4 years. There is an enterohepatic circulation: there is a minimal loss in urine; faeces are rich in vitamin B_{12}, but this is synthesized by colonic bacteria and not absorbed.

Serum vitamin B_{12} is bound about 80% to TC-I, derived from neutrophils; the function of this fraction is not understood. TC-II, derived from macrophages and hepatocytes, carries metabolically available vitamin B_{12} between tissues. The reference range of serum vitamin B_{12} is usually given as 150–900 ng/litre, but higher levels (160–2250 ng/litre) are normal in blacks, who have a genetically determined higher TC-II binding capacity.[116] High serum vitamin B_{12} is associated also with PEM, hepatic disease and granulocytic proliferations.

Vitamin B_{12} deficiency
Aetiology
Vitamin B_{12} deficiency can be the result of (1) inadequate intake, (2) malabsorption due to a failure of IF secretion by gastric parietal cells, (3) disease of the ileum, (4) competition by the fish tapeworm, *Diphyllobothrium latum*, and (5) disturbed metabolism (Table 13.22).[112,115] Demands are raised during pregnancy and lactation (Table 13.21), but this precipitates overt deficiency only in those whose status was marginal before pregnancy.

Dietary inadequacy
The requirements for vitamin B_{12} are so low that nutritional deficiency is rare. It is seen most commonly in infants born to and breast-fed by women who are vitamin B_{12} deficient; the disorder occurs predominantly in Indians whose mothers have tropical sprue and/or inadequate nutrition, but can result from maternal pernicious anaemia.[115]

Strictly vegan diets, which exclude all animal products such as milk and eggs, contain inadequate vitamin B_{12} and deficiency occurs in some impoverished Indian Hindu populations and other vegans such as Rastafarians. Indian immigrants in the UK seem to be at an increased risk of deficiency, possibly because there is less bacterial contamination of water and food. Severe vitamin B_{12} deficiency has been described in long-term prisoners of oppressive governments.

Malabsorption
Classical Addisonian pernicious anaemia (PA) is an autoimmune disease characterized by antiparietal cell and/or anti-IF antibodies, and a failure of IF secretion. It has the highest incidence in populations of northern European descent, but it is being diagnosed with increasing frequency in Arabs, Asians and blacks.[116,117] Undefined environmental factors appear to protect against the development of PA in tropical Africa, as it is rare in Zambia (personal observations) and Nigeria.[118] In contrast, PA accounts for about half of all megaloblastic anaemias in Soweto, South Africa,[113,116] and for 86% of megaloblastic anaemias not occurring in pregnancy in Zimbabwe.[119]

Sprue is the most common cause of malabsorption, probably as a result of interfering with adsorption of IF–B_{12} by ileal mucosal cells. Subnormal serum vitamin B_{12} is reported in up to 40% of people with AIDS; this may not be a true deficiency but the result of neutropenia and low synthesis of TC-I.[120] The fish tapeworm is a rare cause of deficiency, even where the infestation is common.

Disturbed metabolism
Cassava flour is an important staple in sub-Saharan Africa, especially in Mozambique, Tanzania and the Democratic Republic of Congo, and in Indonesia and Brazil.[121] The peel of the roots of cassava contains linamarin, a cyanogenic glycoside from which is released hydrocyanic acid. Cassava is usually prepared by peeling, washing and drying in the sun; this destroys the source of cyanide through fermentation. Chronic cyanide intoxication can follow drought, for example in Mozambique, when the linamarin content is excessively high, or from imperfect preparation, for example in refugees during the Nigerian civil war. Patients suffer from chronic cyanide intoxication, leading to tropical amblyopia. Urinary thiocyanate excretion is high, serum cyanocobalamin is raised but total serum vitamin B_{12} is low. The neurological complications have been linked to disturbed metabolism of vitamin B_{12}, but megaloblastic anaemia has not been reported. Tobacco amblyopia has a similar pathogenesis.

Exposure to nitrous oxide for 5–6 days or recurrent exposure induces megaloblastic anaemia through the oxidation of cobalamins to inactive forms.

Clinical
Vitamin B_{12} deficiency has the same haematological and systemic consequences as folate deficiency. In addition, the course can be complicated by peripheral neuropathy, optic atrophy, psychiatric disturbances and subacute combined degeneration of the cord, characterized by demyelination in the lateral and posterior columns. A common clinical finding is melanin hyperpigmentation, especially of palms, soles and across the small joints of the hands and feet.[115] PA is seen at a younger age in blacks and Arabs, and the rate of progression of the disease may be more rapid than in other ethnic groups.[116,117]

Neonatal deficiency, as seen in Indian infants, shows as a failure of normal development, involuntary movements, loss of muscle tone, pallor and hyperpigmentation of skin and mucous membranes; untreated the condition can progress to coma and death.[115]

Haematology
The peripheral blood and bone marrow findings are identical to those of folate deficiency, except that as vitamin B_{12} deficiency is likely to be more long standing, there tends to be more poikilocytosis and thrombocytopenia. Diagnosis is confirmed by the serum vitamin

B_{12} level being well below the reference range. Measurement of vitamin B_{12} absorption, without and with IF (the Schilling test), is cumbersome, expensive, involves radioactivity and is generally not available in developing countries. Both blacks and Arabs with PA have high frequencies of anti-IF antibodies.[116,117] A diagnosis of PA is established without resorting to the Schilling test, in a patient with megaloblastic anaemia, low serum vitamin B_{12} and anti-IF antibodies, a test shown to have high sensitivity in black South Africans.[122]

Management
Normal stores are restored with hydroxocobalamin 1000 μg intramuscularly, six times over 1–2 weeks; thereafter, 1000 μg is given every 3 months to all patients with permanent malabsorption. Vegans may be treated orally, or be encouraged to eat some vitamin B_{12}-containing food. Infants should receive 0.1 μg per day orally, and deficient mothers treated at the same time.

Cyanocobalamin is still used in some developing countries but is not as satisfactory because maintenance doses have to be given monthly, and it is useless in the treatment of cyanide intoxication.

Other deficiencies
Vitamin A deficiency
About 250 million children worldwide are at risk of vitamin A deficiency. Vitamin A deficiency has distinct haematological actions: (1) there is immobilization of iron in the reticuloendothelial system; (2) there is increased susceptibility to infection, and hence anaemia and further immobilization of iron. Vitamin A may also have a role in red cell differentiation. Simultaneous supplementation with iron and with vitamin A results in greater haemopoietic benefit than supplementation with iron alone to children, pregnant women and non-pregnant adults.

Vitamin A deficiency in children should be improved by (1) breast-feeding, (2) dietary improvements, (3) food fortification, (4) supplementation to the child, and (5) supplementation to the mother. It is recommended that children at risk of vitamin A deficiency should receive vitamin A 100 000 IU at 9 months at the time of measles vaccination, and 200 000 IU between 15 and 21 months. Women should receive 10 000 IU daily or 25 000 IU weekly while pregnant, and 200 000 IU once after delivery.[123]

Riboflavin deficiency
Low dietary intake and overcooking are the usual causes of deficiency of riboflavin: high prevalences of deficiency have been reported amongst children and pregnant or lactating women in West Africa. Riboflavin deficiency is associated with erythroid hypoplasia and immobilization of iron.[124] Supplementation with riboflavin has enhanced the response to supplementation with iron in children, women who are pregnant or lactating, and men with anaemia in West Africa.[125,126]

Protein–energy malnutrition
PEM is a serious cause of disease, but not of anaemia. Anaemia is usually moderate (Hb 80–90 g/litre), normocytic and normochromic, although the MCV may be slightly elevated.[124] The reticulocyte count is low and the marrow shows a normoblastic erythroid hypoplasia. Erythropoietin levels are increased appropriately for the degree of anaemia but there is an impaired response by erythroid precursors. Red cell survival may be moderately shortened, especially in kwashiorkor. Anaemia is more severe when there is concomitant infection related to impaired cell-mediated immunity, and deficiencies of iron and folate, as occur commonly.

Vitamin C deficiency
Severe scurvy is associated with normochromic normocytic anaemia.[124] Vitamin C-deficient diets are certainly deficient in folate and bioavailable iron as well, and anaemia of multiple deficiencies is usual.

Vitamin E deficiency
Premature infants bottle-fed with milk rich in poly-unsaturated fatty acids, deficient in vitamin E and supplemented with iron, develop a haemolytic anaemia due to oxidation of the red cell membrane.

Pyridoxine deficiency
Naturally occurring pyridoxine deficiency is rare, but administration of pyridoxine antagonists, such as cycloserine and pyrazinamide, causes a failure of incorporation of iron into haemoglobin and sideroblastic anaemia.[127]

Copper deficiency
Premature infants and infants or children with severe chronic diarrhoea and malnutrition may become deficient of copper.[124] There is anaemia and severe neutropenia. The marrow shows vacuolated erythroid cells, megaloblasts and ringed sideroblasts; myeloid cells are also vacuolated and have an arrest of maturation at the myelocyte stage.

Anaemia due to marrow depression
Acute infections
Any acute infection may result in a temporary depression of erythropoiesis, which generally goes unnoticed. Significant anaemia results if the patient is dependent on a rapid rate of erythropoiesis (e.g., sickle cell disease), or if the infection causes haemolysis as well; mechanisms of haemolysis may be: (1) specific to the infection (e.g., malaria, the lecithinases of *Clostridium*); (2) DIC and microangiopathic haemolysis following septicaemias or viraemias; (3) immune, for example complicating infection by *Mycoplasma pneumoniae*; or (4) idiosyncrasies of the patient, for example G6PD deficiency.

Anaemia of chronic disorders

With chronic infections, and also malignant disease and some collagen diseases (e.g., rheumatoid arthritis), anaemia can progress over weeks to reach a constant state known as the *anaemia of chronic disorders*. There are at least four mechanisms: (1) there are factors which depress erythropoiesis and reduce the sensitivity to erythropoietin; (2) there is a depression of production of erythropoietin; (3) there is moderate reduction of red cell lifespan; (4) iron is sequestered into the RES; possibly this is mediated at sites of inflammation through the release from granulocytes of lactoferrin, a protein with a high affinity for iron and for which there is a specific receptor on macrophages.

The anaemia is usually moderate (Hb > 80 g/litre, Hct > 0.30) and normocytic, but may progress to being hypochromic and rarely microcytic. The plasma iron is reduced (< 12 μmol/litre), plasma transferrin is low (unlike iron deficiency) and the saturation of transferrin is low (15–25%) but generally higher than in iron deficiency; serum ferritin is raised (> 200 μg/litre) (unlike iron deficiency). In the bone marrow, iron is seen in increased quantities in the macrophages (unlike iron deficiency), but the number of siderocytic granules in normoblasts (sideroblasts) is low; erythropoiesis is normoblastic with occasional mild dyserythropoietic changes; there tends to be granulocytic hyperplasia and often an obvious increase in the number of plasma cells.

The haematological complications of three infections—tuberculosis, HIV and parvovirus B19—need to be discussed in detail because they show certain features and because of their public health importance. The anaemias of protozoal and helminthic infections have already been discussed.

Tuberculosis (See also Chapter 57)

Approximately one-third of the world's population is infected by *Mycobacterium tuberculosis*. It is estimated that 8 million develop tuberculosis each year, of whom more than 4.5 million are in Asia, including China; 2.6–2.9 million die each year. The highest incidence (220/100 000 per year) was in sub-Saharan Africa, and this has now risen further to about 400/100 000 per year, due to the pandemic of HIV. It is predicted that during the next decade the incidence of tuberculosis will continue to rise in Africa, and as it seems inevitable that the incidence of HIV infections in Asia will overtake that of Africa, the impact of AIDS on tuberculosis in Asia will be catastrophic.

Tuberculosis is one of the most common causes of anaemia in adult males and non-pregnant females in the developing world, probably the most common cause amongst adults requiring hospital care, and in some communities, for example in southern Africa, the most common underlying disease leading to the need to administer blood transfusions in the management of anaemia.[127]

The major mechanism is the anaemia of chronic disorders: anaemia is more common and tends to be more severe in patients with extrapulmonary and disseminated disease. Patients, especially vegetarians, are frequently undernourished, with specific deficiencies of vitamin B_{12}, folate, iron and protein, both as predisposing factors through impairment of cell-mediated immunity and as complications of tuberculosis through anorexia and malabsorption, especially with abdominal tuberculosis. Metastatic fibrocaseous granulomas in the bone marrow give rise to a leucoerythroblastic picture and severe anaemia.

Abnormalities of the white cells are most pronounced with disseminated non-reactive miliary tuberculosis. These include: a neutrophil leucocytosis with a shift to the left and toxic granulation, and this may amount to a leukaemoid reaction; eosinophilic reactions, which are likely to reflect coincidental helminthic infections; increased basophils, which are suggestive of an underlying myeloproliferative disease; monocytosis and lymphocytosis. Many patients have reactive thrombocytosis, sometimes exceeding 1000×10^9/litre. Other patients have neutropenia, lymphopenia or thrombocytopenia due to inhibition of production related to tuberculosis, hypersplenism of tuberculous splenomegaly, or HIV infection.

The bone marrow is commonly normoblastic but may show micronormoblastic, dyserythropoietic or megaloblastic features; granulocytic and megakaryocytic hyperplasia and plasma cell excess are usual; there is an excess of iron in the macrophages unless the patient is iron deficient. Some patients may show hypoplasia of one or more cell lines, associated with severe anaemia, neutropenia and thrombocytopenia.

The various therapeutic agents used in the management of tuberculosis can lead to haematological complications. These include: (1) the sideroblastic anaemia of pyridoxine inhibitors (isoniazid, pyrazinamide, cycloserine); (2) hypoplasia or aplasia of one or more of the cell lines; (3) disturbances of folate or vitamin B_{12} metabolism; and (4) immune haemolysis.[127]

Immune deficiency states predispose to the reactivation of latent tuberculosis. For many years it has been known that tuberculosis is associated with lymphomas, leukaemias (especially chronic myeloid leukaemia), the myeloproliferative diseases and aplastic anaemia. Currently in Africa, one-third of patients presenting with AIDS have active tuberculosis; where the HIV epidemic is mature, up to 60% of all patients newly diagnosed as having pulmonary tuberculosis and a higher proportion with extrapulmonary tuberculosis are anti-HIV seropositive.

Human immunodeficiency virus

(See also Chapter 20)

The pattern of disorders of the blood, and the practice of haematology as with other disciplines in medicine, has been changed profoundly in sub-Saharan Africa by the epidemic of HIV. AIDS is now the commonest cause of anaemia, leucopenia and thrombocytopenia encountered both in patients and in the community.[128]

There is often an infectious mononucleosis-like illness 6–8 weeks following infection by HIV, at the time of acute viraemia and seroconversion: the peripheral blood shows initially lymphopenia, but after a few days there is a lymphocytosis with atypical mononuclear cells (virocytes); moderate neutropenia, thrombocytopenia or anaemia can occur, but resolve over 2 weeks.[129]

During the asymptomatic period of HIV infection, which lasts on average 8–10 years, the only haematological abnormality which are commonly detected are thrombocytopenia in up to 12% of subjects due to immune destruction and significant neutropenia in 5–10%.[129]

Patients who have progressed to AIDS commonly have an absolute lymphopenia; atypical lymphocytes and lymphocytes with lobulated nuclei are usual. Around half of patients have a neutropenia from marrow dysfunction. There are two patterns seen: some neutrophils show the hypogranularity and non-segmented forms typical of myelodysplasia; some neutrophils have toxic granulation, a shift to the left (sometimes with the presence of myelocytes, promyelocytes or blasts) and vacuolated and ragged cytoplasm in response to intercurrent infection.[129]

Anaemia becomes increasingly common (up to 95%) and more severe (Hb < 50 g/litre in terminal stages) with the progression of AIDS. Anaemia is not uncommonly the first presentation of AIDS in Africa. The anaemia is normochronic and normocytic, but anisocytosis and macrocytosis are not infrequent. The main mechanism of anaemia is probably infection by HIV of bone marrow stromal cells, disturbed production of haemopoietic growth factors and hence dyserythropoiesis. Other mechanisms include (1) the anaemia of chronic disorders secondary to opportunistic infections or activation of latent infection such as tuberculosis, (2) chronic parvovirus B19 infection (see below), (3) folate deficiency from inadequate intake, malabsorption and self-medication with overdosage of trimethoprim (in co-trimoxazole) or pyrimethamine (in Maloprim® and Fansidar®) (Table 13.22), (4) vitamin A deficiency, (5) microangiopathic haemolysis associated with DIC or a thrombotic thrombocytopenic purpura (TTP)-like syndrome, and (6) autoimmune haemolysis, which is rare although the DCT is commonly positive. Serum vitamin B$_{12}$ is low in up to 40% of people with AIDS, but this is thought not to reflect a true deficiency (see above).[120,129]

Up to 70% of people with AIDS develop thrombocytopenia as a consequence of immune destruction, low production and, in some, hypersplenism. Spontaneous haemorrhage or purpura is uncommon, but there can be excessive bleeding following trauma and surgery. Severe thrombocytopenia is seen when the rare TTP-like syndrome develops.[129]

In early stages of HIV/AIDS, the bone marrow is hypercellular but there is a decline of cellularity as disease progresses, and hypocellularity is usual in the late stages. Red cell and granulocyte precursors and megakaryocytes are increasingly dysplastic with severity of AIDS. Macrophage numbers are commonly raised; haemophagocytosis is often present. There is frequently a markedly increased number of plasma cells: this may lead to a mistaken diagnosis of myeloma, especially if there is also hyper-gammaglobulinaemia. There may be heavy deposits of iron in macrophages as a result of immobilization of iron with infections and of high intake, for example from traditional beers. Tuberculosis of the marrow was diagnosed in about a half of South Africans with AIDS, either by culture or the presence of granulomas.[130] The bone marrow may be infiltrated by AIDS-related Burkitt's lymphoma.[131]

Patients with AIDS and haematological cytopenias should receive supportive management with red cell and platelet transfusions when required, treatment of opportunistic infections, and antiretrovirals if these are available.

Treatment with nucleoside reverse transcriptase inhibitors, for example zidovudine or stavudine, causes dose-related macrocytosis, megaloblastosis and pancytopenia, limiting their usefulness in the already anaemic patient. Overdosage of trimethroprim-containing therapies can precipitate profound megaloblastosis and pancytopenia. Dapsone, in the management of pneumocystis, may precipitate haemolysis in G6PD-deficient or, more rarely, G6PD-normal subjects.[129]

AIDS-related lymphomas
The increased risk of developing lymphomas is well documented in the industrialized countries.[129,131] Non-Hodgkin's lymphomas (NHL) are 60–200 times more common in HIV-positive patients than in the general population. The incidence of Hodgkin's disease (HD) is increased by eight times.

AIDS-related NHL has been observed in Africans, but relatively infrequently. Possible reasons for the low frequency in sub-Saharan Africa are (1) lack of diagnostic facilities, (2) a high death rate from infection early in the course of AIDS, (3) the absence of antiretroviral therapy which prolongs life until lymphomas develop, and (4) genetic factors. The chemokine stromal cell-derived factor 1 (SDF-1) is polymorphic: 37% of Caucasians and only 11% of Afro-Americans carry the 3^{1}A variant; the risk of AIDS-related lymphoma is doubled in heterozygotes for SDF1-3^{1}A and quadrupled in homozygotes.[131]

Over 90% of AIDS-related lymphomas are high-grade B cell tumours. About two-thirds are diffuse large cell lymphomas, and about one-third are Burkitt's lymphomas. In these tumours there are two recognized factors associated with tumorigenesis: (1) reactivation of latent EBV, contributing to 70% of diffuse large lymphomas and 30% of Burkitt's lymphomas, and (2) HIV-induced production of cytokines that cause B cell stimulation, proliferation and activation. Causative factors in other rarer AIDS-related lymphomas are (1) the human herpes virus 8 (HHV8, also known as the Kaposi's sarcoma-associated virus) plus EBV in body cavity lymphoma (also called primary effusion lymphoma), (2) HHV8 and sometimes coinfection with EBV in multicentric Castleman's disease, (3) HIV acting as an oncogenic virus in peripheral T cell lymphoma, and (4) EBV in HD.

Prognosis remains poor for all persons with AIDS-related lymphomas, despite management which involves cytotoxic and antiretroviral therapy, and the treatment of opportunistic infections.[131]

Parvovirus B19

Parvovirus B19 is a single-stranded DNA virus which is common and distributed worldwide.[132] Transmission is by respiratory droplets, but also transplacentally and by exchange of blood. In tropical countries children are usually infected in the first 2 years of life, and protective antibodies are present in about 90% of adults. Between 7 and 10 days after infection there is a transient viraemia for not more than 2 weeks; this may be symptomless in up to 30%, or be accompanied by flu-like symptoms, or cause self-limiting erythema infectiosum (fifth disease) after 1 week, or in adults arthritis or arthralgia; vascular purpura is a rare complication.

The virus has a tropism for early erythroid cells: during viraemia there is an absence of reticulocytes, a great reduction of erythroid progenitors and the presence of giant pronormoblasts in the bone marrow. In subjects with previously normal erythropoiesis and normal immunocompetence there is only a transient depression of erythropoiesis coinciding with the viraemia, but this is tolerated and usually unnoticed. There are three situations in which parvovirus B19 has serious consequences: pregnancy, haemolytic anaemias and immune deficiency.

When parvovirus B19 infection is acquired for the first time during the first half of pregnancy, there is transplacental transmission which can cause spontaneous abortion or hydrops fetalis or congenital anaemia, increasing by 20 times the risk of fetal wastage.

Patients with a short red cell life are dependent on a compensatory rapid rate of erythropoiesis and suffer from 'aplastic crises' when infected by parvovirus B19; morbidity and mortality rates are high. This was described first with sickle cell disease but has been observed with thalassaemia, spherocytosis, enzymopathies and acquired haemolytic anaemias.[69] It has been suggested that concomitant infection with parvovirus B19 could be a cause of severe anaemia and death in children with malaria.[133]

Parvovirus B19 viraemia can persist in patients who are immunocompromised, including those with leukaemias, lymphomas and HIV disease. There is severe chronic anaemia due to erythroid hypoplasia; occasionally there is also neutropenia and thrombocytopenia. It is certain that parvovirus B19 infections are occurring frequently in infants and young children already infected transplacentally with HIV, and it is probable that this is a common cause of profound anaemia in Africa and elsewhere.

During epidemics of parvovirus B19, susceptible subjects, such as patients with sickle cell disease and non-immune pregnant women, can be protected with intravenous normal immunoglobulin. Immunoglobulin therapy is curative of persistent viraemia and chronic anaemia in immunocompromised patients, but failures have been reported with AIDS. Vaccines are being developed.

Aplastic anaemia

Aplastic anaemia is a rare condition. The annual incidence is $2-3/10^6$ in the Western world, with peaks at 10–24 years and in old age, and a male predominance. High annual incidence is observed in Thailand, up to 5.0 $\times 10^6$ in the north of the country; there is a male predominance, a peak incidence in young adults (15–24 years) and an association with low socioeconomic status.[134] This high incidence is probably to be found also in Japan and other Far Eastern countries, for unknown reasons. No cause is found in the majority of patients, but in some exposure to antibiotics (e.g., chloramphenicol), non-steroidal anti-inflammatory drugs (e.g., indomethacin, butazones), paint, benzene and irradiation have proven aetiological associations. The easy availability of potent pharmaceuticals without prescription, and the constant exposure to benzene of unofficial vendors of petrol and sweatshop factory workers are serious, if unmeasured, risk factors in developing countries.[135] The role of hepatitis and other viruses remains unclear.

Alcoholism

Excessive consumption of alcohol is a large and growing social and health problem in tropical communities whose traditional ways of life have been disrupted. The haematological consequences are anaemia, macrocytosis, vacuolation of the normoblasts and excess sideroblasts, as a direct result of the toxicity of alcohol on early red cell precursors (CFU-E and BFU-E). Thrombocytopenia is common, but leucopenia is unusual. Other results of alcoholism include malnutrition leading to folate deficiency and megaloblastic anaemia, and haemosiderosis (see 'Iron overload'). Hepatic failure can be complicated by hypoprothrombinaemia (see below).

Disorders of white cells

The peripheral blood white cell counts of healthy individuals (see Tables 13.4, 13.5 and Figure 13.2) and the causes of reactive leucocytosis (see Table 13.6) have been discussed under 'Reference ranges'.

Leucopenia

The number of circulating WBCs may be abnormally low as a result of failure of production, inhibition of release, increased margination in the circulation, pooling in an enlarged spleen or excessive consumption, and there is often a combination of these factors in one patient. Both neutropenia and lymphopenia are common in the tropics, usually as the direct or indirect result of infections (Table 13.23).

Lymphomas and paraproteinaemias

Only the epidemiological and possible aetiological factors in the tropics will be discussed; lymphomas are described in detail in Chapter 36 and in standard texts.

Table 13.23 Some causes of leucopenia in the tropics.

Neutropenia: $< 2.0 \times 10^9$/litre
  AIDS
  Viral infections in early stages
  Acute malaria
  Typhoid
  Brucellosis
  Overwhelming bacterial infections
  Megaloblastosis
  Hypersplenism
  Bone marrow infiltration (e.g., leukaemia)
  Exposure to chemicals (e.g., benzene)
  Idiosyncratic reactions to drugs and herbal remedies
  Acute leukaemias
  Aplastic anaemia
  Felty's syndrome
  Miscellaneous (racial, familial, cyclic, chronic, idiopathic)
Lymphopenia: $< 1.5 \times 10^9$/litre
  AIDS
  Viral infections in prodromal stages
  Corticosteroids
  Lymphoma
  Acute leukaemias

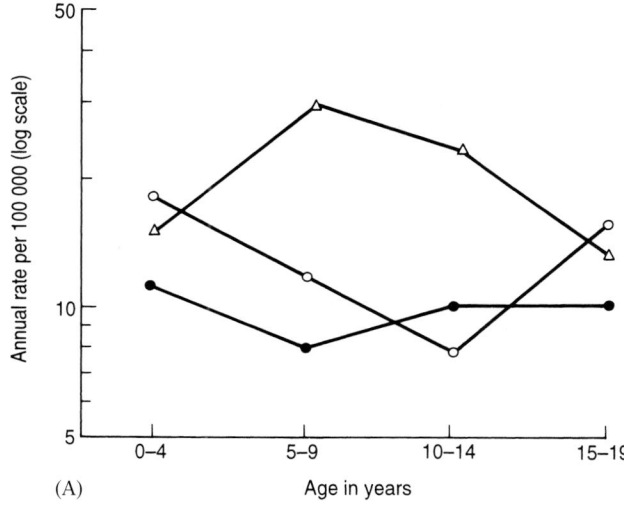

(A)

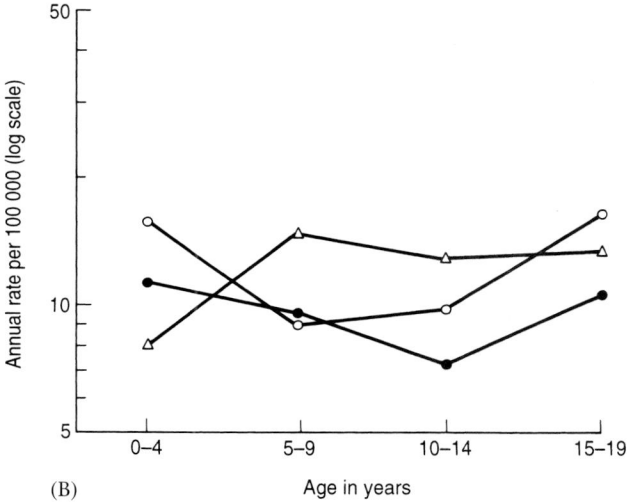

(B)

Figure 13.26: Age-specific incidence of childhood cancer (all types) in (**A**) males and (**B**) females in US whites (○) and blacks (●) (Michigan) and Nigerians (△) (Ibadan). (From data in ref. 136.)

Burkitt's lymphoma (See also Chapter 44)

The highest age-specific incidence of cancers (all types) in childhood has been reported from tropical Africa; there is a peak of incidence between the ages of 5 and 9 years, more marked in boys than girls and predominantly due to Burkitt's lymphoma (BL) (Figure 13.26).[136] There are three epidemiological patterns: (1) BL is *endemic* in tropical Africa and Papua New Guinea, where annual incidence is 8–12/100 000, with a peak at 4–9 years of age; (2) *intermediate* incidence of 1–2/100 000 per year is found in North Africa, western Asia and South America; (3) BL occurs *sporadically*, <0.1/100 000 per year, in the Western world.[137]

The causation of endemic BL may be summarized: the majority of children in developing countries are infected by the EBV before the age of 1 year; infection by EBV immortalizes B cells, resulting in their proliferation; where *P. falciparum* is endemic, recurrent infections suppress T cell regulation of B cell proliferation, and also stimulates antigenically and mitogenically further B cell proliferation; somatic mutations are more probable the larger is the polyclonal pool of proliferating B cells; one such mutation is a translocation involving chromosome 8 at the site of the c-*myc* proto-oncogene, with its juxtaposition to an immunoglobulin heavy chain gene sequence on chromosome 14; BL is the result of the monoclonal proliferation of cells with t8:14 in 85% of cases, or in the minority of cases the juxtaposition of the chromosome 8 c-*myc* to immunoglobulin κ or λ light chain sequences on chromosomes 2 and 22 respectively. In areas of intermediate endemicity there are high rates of EBV transmission in early childhood, but no or low malaria transmission. Less than 20% of sporadic cases of BL are associated with EBV. BL also results as a complication of AIDS (see above).

Hodgkin's disease

There are four histological types of Hodgkin's disease (HD): nodular sclerosing (NS), mixed cellularity (MC), lymphocyte depleted (LD) and lymphocyte predominant (LP). The last form, LP, may be a distinct and separate entity. HD is not common, having a crude annual incidence of 2.4–3.0/100 000 in North America and Western Europe; overall, the male to female ratio is 1:1.5. There are four epidemiological patterns. Pattern I: there are high incidences (or relative frequencies) of HD in childhood in Central and South America, North Africa, western Asia and sub-Saharan Africa; there is a predominance of MC and LD, which carry poor prognoses.[138]

Pattern III: in developed countries, there is a peak of incidence in young adults (20–34 years), in whom NS is the predominant type; a second peak of HD in middle age has been described in the past, but this may have been due to overdiagnosis. Pattern II: this is intermediate between patterns I and III, and is found in rural areas of developed countries, including Eastern Europe and southern USA. Pattern IV: HD has a low incidence in eastern Asia.[139]

EBV genomes are expressed by the malignant Reed–Sternberg cells from a high proportion (50–70%) of HD patients aged under 15 or over 50 years, and it is most probable that EBV plays an aetiological role in these patients. In contrast, EBV genome positivity is rare in patients aged 15–34 years and with NS, suggesting a different aetiology.[139] HIV-infected persons appear to be at greater risk of developing HD (see above).

Non-Hodgkin's, non-Burkitt's lymphomas

The remaining lymphomas, excluding BL and HD, are a heterogeneous group of tumours of B cell and T cell origin, the classification of which is complex and not wholly agreed. The combined incidence of all non-Hodgkin's lymphomas (NHLs) generally exceeds the incidence of HD, for example 4.9/100 000 per year for males and 4.1/100000 per year for females in England and Wales; incidence rises with age to peak at 55–74 years.

In developed countries, follicle centre cell lymphomas with follicular pattern are the most common NHL, with increasing incidence with age. About 75% have a translocation of chromosomes 14 and 18, juxtaposing the immunoglobulin heavy chain locus and the *bcl*-2 putative proto-oncogene. In contrast, these low or intermediate grade tumours are relatively rare in developing countries.[137] High-grade NHLs have higher frequencies in Asia and Africa: a strong association has been reported in Africa between frequency of high-grade NHLs and malarial endemicity, but as high incidence persists into the second generation of immigrants in Israel, there may be some inherited susceptibility.[140–142]

Immunoproliferative small intestinal disease

This is a condition which occurs at high incidence in children and young adults in North Africa, western Asia, eastern Asia and sub-Saharan Africa. Sporadic cases have been reported in South, Central and North America, and Europe.[137,143] It is associated with low socioeconomic status and recurrent or chronic enteric infections. Prolonged antigenic stimulation of intestinal lymphoid tissues and a genetic predisposition are proposed mechanisms. In its premalignant phase, there is steatorrhoea, malabsorption and weight loss; histologically there is a lymphoproliferation and plasma cell infiltration of the small bowel mucosa and mesenteric lymph glands. The proliferating cells are IgA-producing B cells, which synthesize defective immunoglobulin α heavy chains (α heavy chain disease). The condition responds at this stage to ampicillin, metronidazole and anthelmintic agents, followed by long-term tetracycline. Untreated, the condition may progress to a high-grade malignant lymphoma of large cell immunoblastic plasmacytoid type (sometimes called 'Mediterranean lymphoma'). The annual incidence of intestinal lymphoma used to be as high as $4.8/10^6$ in Israel, but this has now dropped; the male to female ratio is around 2:1. The anaemia of chronic disorders is usual and is complicated in about 40% of patients by malabsorption of iron, folate or vitamin B_{12}. The lymphoma responds to combination chemotherapy, e.g., cyclophosphamide, adriamycin, vincristine and prednisolone (CHOP).

Adult T cell leukaemia/lymphoma

Epidemiology

The human T cell lymphotropic virus type 1 (HTLV-1) is a type C retrovirus which is causative of adult T cell leukaemia/lymphoma (ATL) and tropical spastic paraparesis/HTLV-1-associated myelopathy (TSP/HAM) in a small number of infected individuals.[144,145] HTLV-1 is transmitted by sexual intercourse, through breast-feeding and by the exchange of blood. Male to female transmission is more efficient than female to male, and is enhanced by other concomitant sexually transmitted diseases: female prostitutes have higher seroprevalence than the general population. Unidentified receptors for HTLV-1 are on surfaces of CD4 +ve T cells, CD8 +ve T cells and monocyte-derived cells. After invasion of cells and transcription, proviral DNA is integrated into the DNA of host cells.

HTLV-1 is endemic in geographical clusters in Asia, Africa, the Americas, Australasia and Oceania. Seroprevalence is high (up to 30%) in south-west Japan, especially on Kyusha and Shikoku islands. HTLV-1-associated ATL is encountered sporadically in other parts of Japan and on Taiwan, and only occasionally in other Asian countries.[141] The largest pool of the virus is in sub-Saharan Africa, where there are probably about 10 million infected subjects. The highest rates of seropositivity are in the rainforests of west Central Africa: up to 15% has been reported in the Equateur region of the Democratic Republic of Congo, and 10% in Gabon and southern Cameroon; prevalence declines northwards into the savannah and sahel. In West Africa seroprevalence is 3–6% in the savannah of Nigeria and Benin; rates are lower (1–2%) in coastal areas and further west as far as Senegal. HTLV-1 has low endemicity (about 1%) in populations of East and Central Africa, except in the Seychelles, where overall frequency is 6.2%. There is a geographical cluster in northern Kwazulu (3.5%), northern Transkei and Free State of South Africa. The virus is also endemic in populations of African descent in the Caribbean, Central America, southern USA and Britain (e.g., 3–6% amongst Jamaican adults). Clusters have been reported amongst Iranian Jews, Iraqis, Georgians of the Caucasus, Australian Aborigines and the inhabitants of Papua New Guinea and the Solomon Islands. Seroprevalence rises slowly with age, compatible with the slow rate of transmission in endemic areas.[146]

HTLV-1 is spreading epidemically amongst intravenous drug users and male homosexuals in North and South America and Western Europe.

The structurally similar HTLV-2 is endemic amongst groups of the aboriginal population of Central America, and is being spread epidemically amongst blood transfusion recipients and intravenous drug users in the USA and Italy. Associations with disease, such as hairy cell leukaemia, cutaneous T cell lymphoma, chronic neurodegenerative disease or the chronic fatigue syndrome, remain indefinite.

Pathogenesis
HTLV-1 (and HTLV-2) induces a latent infection in a small subset of cells predominantly CD4 +ve T cells. HTLV-1 does not possess oncogenes, but the regulatory gene *tax* has oncogenic potentials through inducing expression of both IL2 and IL2 receptor. The lifetime risk of developing ATL is about 5% in subjects infected by HTLV-1 before 20 years of age. The incubation period is decades: the mean age of onset is 40–45 years, but it can be seen rarely in adolescence; women are affected more often than men in Africa and the Americas. In contrast, in Japan the mean age at diagnosis is nearly 60 years, and men are affected more often than women. It is possible that HIV accelerates progression to ATL.

T cell function is defective; *Strongyloides stercoralis* hyperinfection and other opportunistic infections are associated with HTLV-1 infection at any stage.

The pathogenesis of TSP/HAM is discussed in Chapter 16.

Clinical
Five clinical phases are recognized: (1) asymptomatic, (2) acute ATL, (3) chronic ATL, (4) smouldering ATL, and (5) lymphoma type. Some asymptomatic patients show a preleukaemic condition, diagnosed from the incidental observation of lymphocytosis, with abnormal cells characterized by pleomorphism, multilobed nuclei ('flower' or 'clover-leaf' cells), or cytoplasmic vacuoles; pre-ATL is transient in about half of patients, but may persist and progress to ATL.

About half of African and Caribbean patients have acute ATL. Predominant clinical findings are lymphadenopathy, hepatosplenomegaly and skin lesions, which include papules, nodules, plaques, tumours and ulcers.

Histology of the lymph nodes and of skin lesions is of a high-grade NHL. The cells originate usually from helper T cells (CD4 +ve, CD8 –ve) with functional suppressor activity. Radiology shows pulmonary infiltration and osteolytic lesions which are associated with hypercalcaemia. Anaemia and thrombocytopenia are rare. The WBC count is raised, $30–130 \times 10^9$/litre, with a predominance of the characteristic abnormal lymphocytes; the bone marrow shows infiltration, but less than would be expected from the leukaemic blood picture. The disease is generally resistant to aggressive cytotoxic therapy, and patients die within 12 months of diagnosis. The most effective treatment is IFNα in combination with zidovudine, but relapses are frequent.[144] Patients should receive anthelmintic, antifungal, antibacterial, antimalarial and antiviral treatment and prevention, as indicated clinically or by assessment of risk.

Chronic ATL, seen in about one-fifth of African and Caribbean patients, is associated with skin lesions, mild lymphocytosis only, and a prolonged course. Smouldering ATL, seen in about 5% of patients, shows as skin rashes and a low count of ATL cells, and remains stable for many years. The lymphoma type, seen in about one-fifth of patients, is clinically like NHL, without the leukaemic manifestations; prognosis is poor.

ATL (and TSP/HAM) develops amongst individuals wherever HTLV-1 is endemic: the low reported frequency, for example in tropical Africa, reflects a low rate of diagnosis.

Myeloma in black Africans
The age-adjusted incidence rates of myeloma have been reported to be 9.9/100 000 in blacks and 4.3/100 000 in whites in the USA. Similar high incidence is observed in black South Africans, and the diagnosis is made at high frequencies in the Caribbean and tropical Africa.[147,148] The high incidence in black Africans and those of black African descent may be genetically determined. The disease is seen in sub-Saharan Africa not infrequently in patients of 30–39 years of age, and around 65% of patients are 40–60 years old. Plasmacytomas are not uncommon.

Leukaemias
The crude incidence of all leukaemias is probably very much the same in tropical and non-tropical regions, but there are distinct differences in the age and gender distribution of the four main types: (1) acute lymphoblastic leukaemia (ALL), (2) acute myeloblastic leukaemia (AML), (3) chronic myeloid leukaemia (CML), and (4) chronic lymphocytic leukaemia (CLL). There are only a few clinical and haematological manifestations and diagnostic problems peculiar to the tropics, but there are severe limitations to their management, especially of the acute leukaemias, in the developing countries.

Acute lymphoblastic leukaemias
Immunophenotypic markers distinguish ALL according to the cells of origin of the blast cells, as precursor B-ALL (including null-ALL, common ALL (c-ALL) and pre-B-ALL), B-ALL and T-ALL. There are three epidemiological patterns of childhood ALL.[149] Pattern I: in countries with the poorest economic development, for example much of tropical Africa and Asia, the incidence of diagnosed ALL is low (< 0.1/100 000 per year). Pattern II: in countries of intermediate economic development and where there has been the establishment of some haematological services, for example North Africa, Nigeria, Kenya and southern Africa, ALL remains uncommon (< 1/100 000 per year), cALL is rare but there is a peak of T-ALL at 5–14 years of age. Pattern III: in the developed or Western

countries, the incidence of ALL is 2–3/100 000 per year, with a marked peak of cALL at 2–4 years of age. ALL of all types is seen at low incidence in adults at all ages. The male to female ratio is generally 2:1. Pattern I is largely the result of the lack of medical facilities and diagnostic abilities. The rarity of cALL in pattern II is true; T-ALL has only a relatively high incidence, due to the absence of cALL, not an absolutely high incidence. It is unlikely that the deficit of cALL in developing countries compared to industrialized countries is genetically determined, as the peak of cALL in childhood is now emerging in Arabia, South-East Asia, Afro-Americans, black South Africans and Zimbabweans.[150–152] It is postulated that cALL is the rare consequence of an unidentified virus, or other agent, of high infectivity but low pathogenicity. The risk of cALL is increased in the industrialized countries as a consequence of delayed exposure to the infection, associated with reduced infection rates in childhood, deficit of social contacts in infancy and possibly the absence of prolonged breast-feeding.[153,154] Small epidemics of cALL in childhood follow mixing of populations, which exposes a non-immune, often remote, population to infection introduced by another population, often urban, carrying the infection.[155] The factors increasing the risk of cALL in childhood may be becoming prevalent in South Africa and Zimbabwe, but not yet in Zambia, where cALL is still rare.[41] The children of immigrants (for example, Asians and West Indians in the UK) have patterns of incidence similar to the population of their country of residence, illustrating the importance of the environment.

Clinical

The symptoms and signs of ALL are those arising from malignant infiltration (lymphadenopathy, hepatosplenomegaly, bone pain), anaemia, haemorrhage or thrombosis, and infections from immune depression. Being uncommon in the developed countries, these symptoms and signs arouse the suspicion of leukaemia, but in the tropical world the diagnosis may be overlooked in the mass of children with anaemia, infection and hepatosplenomegaly.

Diagnosis

The total WBC count is raised in around two-thirds, but may be normal or low in one-third of patients. The leukaemic blast cells can be mistaken for activated or transformed lymphocytes in response to malaria, viral or other infections, and the diagnosis missed in the laboratory. The bone marrow is infiltrated with blasts. ALL is classified according to the French–American–British (FAB) criteria by the light microscopic appearance of the blasts: L1, the blasts are uniformly small and have little or no cytoplasm; L2, the blasts are pleomorphic with more abundant, agranular cytoplasm; L3, the blasts have dark-blue staining cytoplasm with vacuoles in both cytoplasm and nucleus. L3 often corresponds to B-ALL or the leukaemic presentation of BL.

Management and prognosis

Supportive treatment includes red cell transfusion for anaemia, platelet transfusion for haemorrhage from thrombocytopenia, antibiotics for infection, allopurinol for hyperuricacidaemia, and antimalarial therapy and prophylaxis. Specific treatment is with complex regimens of cytotoxic agents and radiotherapy of the central nervous system: it is highly effective, especially for cALL in childhood, but cannot be undertaken except in specialized units. Regrettably, patients in most of the developing world have not benefited from the strides made in leukaemia management during the last 30 years, because of both social and biological handicaps. Patients, or parents, are not able to comply with therapeutic regimens because of their complexity, cost, distances of travel, lack of comprehension or distrust of modern medicine. Supplies of cytotoxic drugs are uncertain and radiotherapy usually wholly unavailable. Patients often show indicators of poor prognosis, including late presentation, poor nutrition, high leucocyte counts, severe thrombocytopenia, L2 blasts, T cell markers and mediastinal masses.

Acute myeloblastic leukaemias

AML is classified by FAB criteria as: M0 and M1, with malignant blast cells that have few or no granules; M2, with blasts that have granules and Auer rods; M3, promyelocytic leukaemia, of hyper- or hypogranular variants; M4, myelomonocytic leukaemia; M5, monocytic leukaemia; M6, erythroleukaemia; and M7, megakaryocytic leukaemia, the last two being rarities.

AML is diagnosed at equal frequency as ALL in childhood in tropical Africa, whereas in the Western world there are four cases of ALL to one of AML; this is due in part to the low incidence of cALL in Africa, but there is also a high frequency of AML in boys (male to female ratio as high as 3.8:1), associated with low socioeconomic status.[41,149] AML in adults has about equal gender frequency and no association with economic status. Recognized risk factors in adults include cigarette smoking, which may account for up to 20% of AML in some communities;[156] a rising incidence of AML will be one part of the large increases of cancer, mostly tobacco related, predicted for developing countries during the next few decades. Exposure to chemicals and toxic or radioactive waste at work and in the environment is increasing and is uncontrolled in the Third World; factors related causatively to AML include benzene, to which are exposed informal petrol vendors and workers in the rubber, shoe, petroleum, leather, printing and chemical industries, asbestos, chemical fertilizers, pesticides and irradiation.[135,155] As alkylating agents (e.g., cyclophosphamide) are associated causatively with AML and as they are used in the treatment of BL, NHL, HD, myeloma and CLL, all of which occur in the young or relatively young in the tropics, it may be anticipated that AML will be observed at higher than expected incidence in patients who have received cytotoxic therapy.[149] The myelodysplastic syndromes are not diagnosed often in tropical countries, but are significant causes of anaemia, have the same environmental risk factors as AML (tobacco, benzene, myelotoxic agents) and are preleukaemic conditions.[135,153,156,157]

Clinical
AML is indistinguishable from ALL clinically, except that in tropical Africa between 10% and 25% of all patients and about one-third of boys may present with a chloroma.[149] Chloromas are solid tumours usually arising in the orbit but occurring at other sites: the freshly cut surface is characteristically green (hence the name); histologically the tumour is a myeloblastic deposit.[41]

Diagnosis
Monocytic and myelomonocytic leukaemoid reactions from tuberculosis may be mistaken sometimes for M4 and M5 AML.[127] L2 ALL and M1 AML are differentiated by the myeloperoxidase and Sudan black reactions, which are positive with AML. The non-specific esterase reaction is strongly positive with M5 and positive with M4 AML.

Management and prognosis
Supportive treatment should be given as with ALL (see above). Survival without specific treatment is about 2 months. Cytotoxic therapy should be undertaken in specialist centres only: conventional chemotherapy allows for a median survival of about 9 months. Marrow ablation followed by bone marrow transplant carries much better prognosis and the possibility of cure, but needs sophisticated and expensive facilities.

In promyelocytic leukaemia (M3) there is a specific translocation which fuses the retinoic acid receptor α gene on chromosome 17 to a locus, PML on chromosome 15. All-*trans*-retinoic therapy has been followed by differentiation of M3 blasts down the neutrophil pathway, a treatment which it is possible to administer and control with limited resources.

Chronic myeloid leukaemia
Over 90% of CMLs have cells with the Philadelphia (Ph[1]) chromosome, which is a chromosome 22 that has lost much of its long arm in reciprocal translocation with chromosome 9. The translocation juxtaposes the Abelson proto-oncogene (*Abl*) from the long arm of chromosome 9 with a breakpoint cluster region (*bcr*) on chromosome 22. *Bcr/Abl* may be detected by polymerase chain reaction in many patients in whom the Ph[1] chromosome cannot be demonstrated. The combination produces a chimeric mRNA, which translates a protein with tyrosine kinase activity able to confer independence from control by growth factors on several cell lines.

Annual incidence is about 1/100 000 throughout the world, with a slightly higher rate in male blacks; males are affected more often than females. Age-specific incidence rises progressively with age from childhood; frequency peaks in the industrialized countries in the fifth decade, but in the developing countries with younger populations more patients are seen under 40 years than over. CML is the third leukaemia of childhood, and in Africa between 10% and 20% of cases occur in patients below the age of 15 years.[41,149] Environmental factors associated with CML are excessive exposure to ionizing irradiation and benzene.[149]

Clinical
Patients complain most often of abdominal discomfort from gross hepatosplenomegaly. They may be emaciated, have generalized lymphadenopathy, and be anaemic. African patients have on average larger spleens and more severe anaemia than European patients.

Diagnosis
The WBC count is raised up to 500×10^9/litre; all stages of granulocyte development are present in increasing proportions from blasts to mature granulocytes, with neutrophils predominating usually, but eosinophils and basophils are also present. Tuberculosis, meningococcal meningitis, septicaemia, megaloblastosis in pregnancy, eclampsia, acute liver necrosis, amoebic liver abscess, burns, mercury poisoning from skin-lightening ointments, and severe haemorrhages may give leukaemoid reactions resembling CML. CML and leukaemoid reactions can be distinguished by: (1) a gap in the progression of granulocyte development in CML, e.g., relatively few metamyelocytes; (2) a high basophil count in CML; (3) toxic granulation and other reactive features in leukaemoid reactions; and (4) the neutrophil leucocyte alkaline phosphatase reaction, which is strongly positive with leukaemoid reactions and negative with CML.

Management and prognosis
Supportive therapy should include initial antimalarial treatment and prophylaxis for life in endemic regions, and allopurinol. There are five therapeutic options. (1) Oral busulfan reduces the WBC and splenomegaly, improves the quality of life, but does not prolong survival. Median survival is 40–47 months from diagnosis, with the most usual cause of death being transformation of CML to AML or ALL. Busulfan is wholly superseded in the developed countries, but it still has a place in the tropics as it is inexpensive and the control of WBC is easy, so allowing patients to travel long distances to their homes and to have long intervals between blood counts and reassessment. (2) Oral hydroxyurea reduces the WBC more rapidly and may prolong life slightly, but it is more difficult to control myelotoxicity; it is to be preferred to chlorambucil when the patient has easy access to the hospital and laboratory monitoring. (3) Subcutaneous IFNα, in combination with hydroxyurea or cytosine arabinoside, has resulted in definite prolongation of life, and rarely in the elimination of detectable *bcr/abl*. This represents an advance in the management of CML, but IFNα is too expensive for use in most developing countries. (4) Imatinib is a recently synthesized inhibitor of the *bcr/abl* tyrosine kinase.[158] Oral administration is impressively effective against CML, including blastic

crisis, and also *bcr/abl*-positive ALL. It is well tolerated. It promises to be an agent which could be administered with a minimum of laboratory monitoring, as in the developing world. The cost is very high. (5) Bone marrow transplant, which if successful is curative.

Chronic lymphocytic leukaemia

In 90–95% of CLLs the cells are of mature B cell origin; other variants are hairy cell leukaemias (5–10%) usually of B cell origin, T-CLL (about 1%) and B- or T-prolymphocytic leukaemias (<1%). Age-adjusted incidence rates differ more than 10-fold among populations, showing greater variation than any other major leukaemia type. There are three main epidemiological patterns.

Pattern I: the highest age-adjusted rates (> 3/100 000 per year for males) are in Canada and Scandinavia; the rest of the Western world has intermediate rates (> 2/100 000 per year for males); lower rates (about 1/100 000 per year for males) are found in Central and South America. CLL is rare under 40 years of age, and thereafter incidence rises rapidly with age. The male to female ratio is about 2:1.

Pattern II: in tropical Africa, CLL occurs from the age of about 17 years, with equal numbers of men and women affected.[149,159] There is a bimodal distribution. About half the patients are aged less than 45 years; in these younger adults CLL is associated with low socioeconomic status and rural habitation; females predominate by about 2:1 in most West African series, but not in some East and Central African series; frequency rises with age in females to peak at the end of reproductive life. Over the age of 45 years the male to female ratio is 2:1, as in pattern I.

It is hypothesized that the probability of somatic mutation in B cells is increased in an enlarged pool of proliferating B cells resulting from recurrent malaria and other infections; probability is greatest in individuals of low socioeconomic status and high rates of exposure to infection, and in women whose cell-mediated immunity has been depressed repeatedly during pregnancies; the probability is further enhanced in individuals with HMS (see above). A second genetic event could follow infection by a virus, whose transmission is more likely in poor communities and whose proliferation may be more rapid with depression of immunity by malaria and pregnancy; HTLV-1, EBV, HCV and HHV8 have been excluded as likely causative agents.[159,160] The condition is referred to variously as 'tropical splenic lymphoma' or 'African CLL'. Analysis of V_H genes showed that the cells have an origin from naive B cells which have not undergone somatic mutation in the germinal centres; this is not consistent with the lymphoma/leukaemia being splenic lymphoma with villous lymphocytes as had been suggested.[161] Immunophenotyping of cells in Zambian patients was consistent with B cell prolymphocytic leukaemia.[41]

Pattern III: CLL is rare throughout the Indian subcontinent, South-East Asia and the Far East. Genetic factors are important determinants, as Asian immigrants to Hawaii, North America and Europe have continued low incidence.

Clinical
Onset is insidious. Patients present with hepatosplenomegaly and lymphadenopathy. Spleens tend to be larger where malaria is endemic and may reach across to the right iliac fossa.

Diagnosis
The WBC count is commonly > 40×10^9/litre, with the majority of cells mature lymphocytes. Following acute malaria, cells are marginated and the count in the peripheral blood falls temporarily. It is common to see two populations of lymphocytes in the blood: one representing the malignant clone, the other reactive to recurrent malaria or other infections. The bone marrow is infiltrated with the malignant clone only.

The only condition which can give a CLL leukaemoid reaction is HMS (see above); the differentiation of the two conditions has been discussed.

Management and prognosis
Initial curative antimalarial therapy followed by long-term prophylaxis, for example with proguanil, is followed by a partial reduction of spleen size and peripheral lymphocyte count, supporting the view that patients with CLL have a loss of acquired immunity to malaria. In mild disease this may be the only necessary treatment. Most patients will require reduction of tumour mass by chlorambucil or chlorambucil plus prednisolone, following standard regimens. Response can be monitored and treatment controlled wherever there is a minimum of laboratory support. Median survival is about 8 years, but is dependent on the stage of disease, and is certainly shorter in tropical countries. Infections are often the terminal events.

Haemato-oncology services
Most patients with leukaemias in tropical countries have not benefited from the great advances in management which have occurred in the past 30 years. Diagnostic facilities are often not developed; supplies of cytotoxic agents are insufficient for the protocols which are now standard; radiotherapy units are few, and liable to break down; staff in all disciplines have not received appropriate training. Sustainable haemato-oncology services can be established through the twinning of centres in the developing world with centres in the industrialized countries, as shown by the successful Italian–Swiss cooperative with Nicaragua in the La Mascota Programme.[162] The developing country benefits from (1) rational treatment of patients, (2) training of different cadres in oncology practice, and (3) training in research methods. The centre in the developed country gains advantage from (1) the experience in the range of malignant disease seen in the tropics, (2) research opportunities, (3) the intellectual stimuli derived from living in a different community and environment and (4) a sense of fulfilment.[41]

Disorders of haemostasis

Abnormal bleeding can arise from disorders of: (1) the initiation of haemostasis, involving the vascular endothelium and platelets, and manifest as purpura and haemorrhage from or into superficial surfaces; and (2) the consolidation of haemostasis, involving the coagulation and fibrinolytic pathways, and showing clinically as uncontrolled haemorrhages from or into deeper tissues. The pathogenesis of haemorrhage is often multiple; for example, a viraemia can cause damage to both endothelium and platelets, and this can lead to the consumption of platelets and coagulation factors, and the activation of fibrinolysis.

Purpuras

Disorders of the initiation of haemostasis result from (1) abnormalities of the endothelium, (2) abnormalities of platelet function or (3) thrombocytopenia.

Vascular purpuras

Damage to endothelium is a common cause of purpura and haemorrhage in the tropics (Table 13.24). Infections are important, leading to haemorrhage through either direct toxicity to the endothelium (the haemorrhagic fevers), or to an immune damage during convalescence from several of the common childhood diseases, or to late immune damage as in Henoch–Schönlein purpura. The viral haemorrhagic fevers include dengue, yellow fever, Lassa fever, Rift Valley, Argentinian, Bolivian, Venezuelan, Crimea–Congo, Omsk, Kyasanur Forest, Korean, Marburg and Ebola haemorrhagic fevers. In immunocompromised individuals, herpes viruses (simplex and varicella) and arboviruses (O'nyong-nyong, African chikungunya) can cause haemorrhages which are sometimes fatal. Dengue is the most common of the haemorrhagic fevers, being hyperendemic in South-East Asia and spreading epidemically, especially to the Americas and China: the annual incidence in Thailand was 345/100 000 in 1987.

Defective platelet function

Purpura resulting from disordered platelet function (thrombopathy) can complicate the course of some of the haemorrhagic fevers (Lassa, dengue, Marburg, Ebola), alcoholism, hepatic cirrhosis, uraemia, paraproteinaemias, leukaemias and myeloproliferative disorders, or can result from ingestion of non-steroidal anti-inflammatory agents (aspirin, indomethacin) and other drugs. The bleeding tendency of patients with uraemia can be corrected temporarily by cryoprecipitate (see under 'Haemophilia').

Thrombocytopenia

An abnormally low platelet count may result from defective production, destruction or consumption in the peripheral blood, splenic pooling, or a combination of these mechanisms. Many of the common causes in the tropics have been discussed already (viral, bacterial and protozoal infections, AIDS, hypersplenism, megaloblastosis, alcoholism, overdosage with pyrimethamine and trimethoprim, benzene exposure) (Table 13.25). Other conditions, such as idiopathic thrombocytopenic purpura (ITP), have no epidemiological or clinical features peculiar to the tropics, except that patients tend to have splenomegaly and anaemia.[22]

Onyalai

The word *onyalai* means blood blister in the language of the Kimbundu in western Angola.[163] It is an acquired immune thrombocytopenia which differs epidemiologically, immunologically and clinically from ITP.

Epidemiology

Onyalai has been described only in Africa south of the equator. The geographical area of distribution has shrunk over the last 60 years, due partly to the discontinuation of the habit of calling any thrombocytopenia an African onyalai, and probably because changing lifestyles have removed unknown aetiological factors. Onyalai is encountered commonly in Kavango and Ovambo territories of northern Namibia and in neighbouring southern Angola. Onyalai accounts for over 1% of all hospital admissions in Kavango, where the minimum annual incidence has been calculated to be 151/100 000.

Table 13.24 Some causes of haemorrhage due to vascular endothelial disorders in the tropics.

Infections	—direct toxicity:	viraemias (dengue, yellow fever, Lassa fever, other haemorrhagic fevers)
		bacteria (typhoid, Gram-negative septicaemia, meningococcal septicaemia)
	—early immune damage:	measles, scarlet fever, chickenpox, rubella, tuberculosis
	—late immune damage:	Henoch–Schönlein purpura, purpura fulminans
Drugs	—idiosyncratic reactions:	streptomycin, isoniazid, penicillin, sulfonamides, aspirin, quinine, etc.
Uraemia		
Scurvy		
Dysproteinaemias (e.g., myeloma)		
Fat embolism (e.g., marrow embolism in sickle cell disease)		
Congenital (Ehlers–Danlos, Osler–Rendu–Weber, etc.)		
Miscellaneous (purpura simplex, senile purpura, factitious bleeding)		

Table 13.25 Some causes of thrombocytopenia in the tropics.

Primarily low production	
Infections (e.g., typhoid, brucellosis)	
Megaloblastic anaemia	
Alcoholism	
Marrow infiltration (e.g., leukaemia)	
Aplastic anaemia	
Drugs and chemicals	— cytoxic drugs
	— overdosage (e.g., pyrimethamine, trimethoprim)
	— idiosyncratic reactions
	— occupational exposure (e.g., benzene)
Miscellaneous (cyclic, congenital)	
Primary increased consumption or destruction	
Infections (e.g., acute malaria, trypanosomiasis, dengue)	
Hypersplenism (see Table 13.12)	
Chronic hepatic disease	
Disseminated intravascular coagulation (see Table 13.26)	
Immune	— idiopathic thrombocytopenia (ITP)
	— acute viral infections
	— drugs (e.g., quinine, penicillin)
	— AIDS
	— onyalai
	— other autoimmune diseases
	— lymphomas, CLL

There is no significant seasonal variation of frequency. Over half of all patients are aged under 20 years, which may not differ from the age structure of the whole population. The male to female ratio is 1:1.5.

Aetiology is linked clearly to some factor(s) in rural life in the Okavango valley, where millet is the main staple, and mycotoxins from fungal contamination of grain are suspected. Recently, autoantibodies to glycoprotein (GP) IIb/IIIa of platelets have been demonstrated in 12 out of 14 patients with onyalai; both IgG and IgM antibodies were present. In contrast, anti-GPIIb/IIIa is found in only about one-third of patients with ITP, and it is mainly IgG.[163]

Clinical

The clinical hallmark is the acute appearance of haemorrhagic bullae in the mucous membranes of the mouth, tongue and palate, and less frequently on the skin, including the soles of the feet. Epistaxis is often present and may be severe. Blood loss can lead to haemorrhagic shock. The median duration of haemorrhage is about 8 days, but the condition may persist for months and tends to recur.

Haematology

Patients have profound thrombocytopenia, and many are anaemic from blood loss. The bone marrow shows hyperplasia of the erythron and megakaryocytes. Platelets are morphologically normal.

Management and prognosis

Mortality in the acute phase used to be about 10%: patients dying of haemorrhagic shock or from cerebral haemorrhage. Treatment with transfusions of whole blood for haemorrhagic shock and of platelets, and supportive measures including oral hygiene, has reduced mortality to less than 3%. Prednisolone is not effective. Splenectomy is indicated for otherwise uncontrollable bleeding, and is followed by a return to normal platelet counts, but the condition has recurred fatally in some splenectomized patients. Intravenous immunoglobulin has been effective in four patients, but the cost is prohibitive. Vincristine may benefit some patients.

Coagulation disorders

The disorders of blood coagulation may be acquired or congenital. The acquired disorders occur more commonly in clinical practice, but have not attracted the intense medicoscientific interest given to the congenital diseases such as haemophilia.[164]

Acquired coagulopathies
Hypoprothrombinaemias
Vitamin K deficiency

Haemorrhagic disease of the newborn

The newborn, especially the premature, have normally low levels of vitamin K and somewhat prolonged PTs (see 'Reference ranges'; Table 13.7).[165] Classical haemorrhagic disease of the newborn (HDN) is the result of vitamin K deficiency: premature infants and infants of mothers receiving antituberculous therapy, anticonvulsants or warfarin are at increased risk; bleeding is usually into skin, mucosal surfaces, the gastrointestinal tract, or from the umbilical stump or from circumcision. Infants may present between 1 and 3 months with intracranial haemorrhage of late HDN due to vitamin K deficiency: they are exclusively breast-fed and may have received antibiotics.

The incidence of HDN is not known, but is obviously high where premature infants are breast-fed exclusively; late HDN has been estimated to occur in 3/1000 Thai infants. The diagnosis is confirmed by a prolonged PT. HDN is prevented by prophylactic vitamin K, 1 mg intramuscularly on the first day of life; in treatment, vitamin K should be given intravenously.

Malabsorption

Patients with biliary obstruction or small bowel disease become deficient of the fat-soluble vitamin. Gut sterilization by antibiotics can contribute to but does not cause deficiency alone. Diagnosis is based on a prolonged PT, which reverts rapidly to normal following vitamin K, 10 mg intravenously; the response will be partial only if there is liver disease.

Vitamin K antagonism

Warfarin is a competitive inhibitor of vitamin K. Haemorrhage follows inadvertent overdosage, self-administration by the psychiatrically disturbed, the simultaneous administration of medications which potentiate warfarin (e.g., co-trimoxazole, chloramphenicol), or the eating by children of warfarin laid out as rat poison. Patients remain anticoagulated for several days after warfarin has been stopped, so that severe over-dosage or poisoning has to be reversed by intravenous vitamin K.

Hepatic disease

Bleeding in liver disease is multifactorial. During acute infectious hepatitis, a mild disorder of haemostasis, consisting of reduced levels of V, VII and X and a prolonged PT, is not unusual. In association with liver failure, there is severe factor deficiency, afibrinogenaemia and DIC (see below). Patients with chronic hepatic disease or cirrhosis show impairment of synthesis of all vitamin K-dependent factors and fibrinogen and reduced platelet function; some patients show a reduced clearance of FDPs, which contributes to chronic DIC.

The PT is prolonged and vitamin K has little or no effect. If the PT is four times the normal or more, it is hazardous to perform a percutaneous liver biopsy. Bleeding with liver disease should be treated by transfusion of cryosupernate (residual plasma following removal of cryoprecipitate), or fresh frozen plasma or factor concentrates (if available).[17]

Disseminated intravascular coagulation

The widespread or uncontrolled deposition of fibrin in the circulation may be triggered by a large range of conditions (Table 13.26).[164,166] Pathogenesis starts with (1) damage to the endothelium, often from infectious causes in the tropics or (2) the release of tissue factor from traumatized tissues with the activation of platelets and coagulation or (3) the injection of procoagulants of various snake venoms (Table 13.27) or contact by South American rubber-tappers with caterpillars of the moths *Lonomia achelous* and *L. obliqua*, which feed on the leaves of rubber trees. During pregnancy there is normally a potential hypercoagulable and hyperfibrinolytic state (see 'Reference ranges') and a wide range of obstetric disorders can trigger severe DIC (see Table 13.26).

The dominant feature of acute DIC is haemorrhage, which is multifactorial (Figure 13.27): there is endothelial damage, and consumption of platelets, coagulation factors and fibrinogen, rendering the blood incoagulable; plasmin is activated, both fibrin and fibrinogen are degraded, and FDPs are released into the circulation; FDPs have antithrombin activity and are incorporated into clot

Table 13.26 Main causes of DIC encountered in clinical practice in the tropics.

Acute	Subacute	Chronic
Infections	*Obstetric*	*Metabolic*
Viraemias	Pre-eclampsia/eclampsia	Liver disease
Septicaemias (Gram-negative, typhoid, meningococcal)	Retention of dead fetus	Renal disease
Protozoan (African trypanosomiasis)	Hydatidiform mole	*Malignancy*
Obstetric disorders	*Malignancy*	Prostatic carcinoma
Septic abortions	Acute leukaemias (M3)	*Others*
Abruptio placentae	*Others*	Purpura fulminans
Ruptured uterus	Purpura fulminans	
Amniotic fluid embolus		
Shock		
Accidental trauma (birth trauma or anoxia, head injuries, thoracic, fractured femur)		
Surgical trauma (thoracic)		
Burns		
Heat stroke		
Envenomation		
Snake bites (see Table 13.27)		
Lonomia achelous caterpillars		
Others		
Acute hepatic necrosis		
Cytotoxic therapy		
Incompatible blood transfusion		

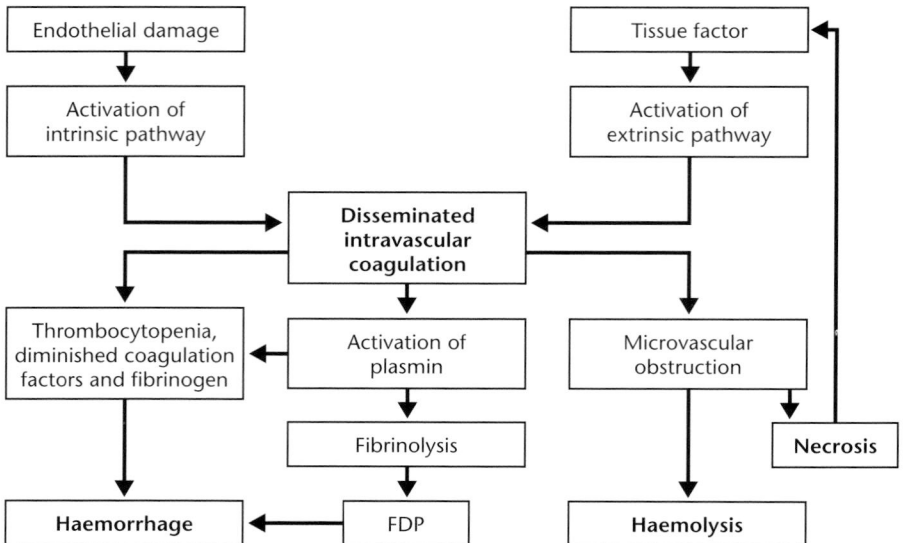

Figure 13.27: The pathogenesis of disseminated intravascular coagulation (DIC). (Reproduced with permission of the publishers from Fleming A F. In Parry E H O (ed.) *Principles of Medicine in Africa,* 2nd edn. Oxford University Press, 1984: 733.)

rendering it friable. In subacute and chronic DIC red cells are ruptured by being forced through fibrin networks in small blood vessels, resulting in microangiopathic haemolytic anaemia. The obstruction of small blood vessels can cause ischaemia, tissue necrosis and renal failure; pituitary and suprarenal failure are rarer complications.

Clinical

Patients have the clinical features of their primary condition. DIC can range from a minor derangement of coagulation without bleeding to a severe haemorrhagic state. It is a dynamic condition which can progress rapidly, so that attention must be paid to minor abnormalities of clotting tests. The most usual presentation is bleeding from mucous membranes, skin, venepuncture sites or from the uterus.

Diagnosis

The platelet count is reduced, kaolin–cephalin clotting time (KCCT), PT and thrombin times are prolonged, and the plasma FDPs are raised. In severe DIC the simple clotting time is prolonged or the blood may be incoagulable or nearly so, allowing for confirmation of the diagnosis in the absence of other laboratory tests. Microangiopathic haemolytic anaemia shows the features of intravascular haemolysis (see Table 13.11); in the peripheral blood there are many small fragmented red cells with bizarre shapes (schizocytes).

Subacute or chronic DIC is confirmed when there are thrombocytopenia, raised plasma FDPs, moderate decreases in coagulation factors and evidence of micro-angiopathic haemolysis.

Management

The first principle is to treat the primary cause. If the underlying disease responds rapidly (e.g., meningococcal septicaemia to antibiotics, snake envenomation to

specific antivenom, or abruptio placentae to the completion of obstetric delivery), DIC will correct spontaneously in most instances.

Secondly, the blood volume must be restored and maintained with the transfusion of whole blood (or if not available, concentrated red cells plus saline, or saline and colloids).

Thirdly, if haemorrhage cannot be controlled, platelets, fresh frozen plasma and cryoprecipitate may have to be transfused to restore the missing factors.[17]

Fourthly, in subacute or chronic conditions in which the primary cause cannot be cured, the patient may be heparinized, with the aim of keeping the clotting time just above 15 minutes, in order to break the chain of pathogenesis.

Snake envenomation (See also Chapter 32)

Snake bites are of major public health importance in many communities as causes of haemorrhage, other morbidity and mortality, but are largely neglected in health care planning (Table 13.27).[164] Those at highest risk of envenomation include: (1) farmers working in paddy fields, or at the beginning of the rains in dryer climates, when small rodents and reptiles attract the snakes to the fields at the same time as farmers are digging; (2) nomadic herdsmen; (3) hunter–gatherers; (4) workers on development sites. Epidemics of snake bites follow floods, when human and snake populations are concentrated together. Snake venoms contain up to about 20 components with a wide range of toxicity (see Chapter 32); only snake venoms causing haemorrhage through procoagulant activities are discussed here briefly (Figure 13.28).

Africa

Echis ocellatus

The carpet or saw-scale viper is probably the most

Table 13.27 Species of snake commonly responsible for morbidity or death from haemorrhage (See also Chapter 32).

Area		Latin name	Vernacular names
Africa		*Echis ocellatus*‡	Carpet or saw-scale viper
		Bitis arietans	Puff adder
		Naja nigricollis	Spitting cobra
		Dispholidus typus	Boomslang
Asia			
	Middle East	*E. ocellatus*‡	Carpet or saw-scale viper
	South-East	*Daboia russelii**	Russell's viper
		E. carinatus	Carpet or saw-scale viper
		Calloselasma rhodostoma†	Malayan pit viper
		Trimeresurus species	Green pit viper
Australia			
		Notechis scutatus	Tiger snake
		Oxyuranus scutellatus	Taipan
		Pseudonaja textilis	Eastern brown snake
America			
	North	*Crotalus adamanteus*	Eastern diamond-backed rattlesnake
		C. atrox	Western diamond-backed rattlesnake
	Central	*C. durissus durissus*	Central American rattlesnake
		Bothrops asper	Terciopelo, caissaca
	South	*B. atrox*	Fer-de-lance, barba amirilla
		B. jararaca	Jararaca
		C. durissus terrificus	South American rattlesnake

*Formerly *Vipera russellii*.
†Formerly *Agkistrodon rhodostoma*.
‡Formerly *Echis carinatus*

dangerous snake in the world, and is found throughout Africa north of the equator, as well as in the Middle East, the Indian subcontinent and South-East Asia. The snake is particularly prevalent in West Africa, where in rural areas during the early rains up to one-third of adult male hospital beds may be occupied by envenomed farmers. The annual incidence in the Bambur area of the Benue valley, Nigeria, has been estimated to be 600/100 000: mortality is 10–20% in those who attend hospital but do not receive appropriate attention; this has been projected to an estimated 23 000 deaths annually in West Africa.

The venom contains an activator of thrombin (Figure 13.28), causing consumption of coagulation factors, but not usually of platelets, and high levels of FDPs. The blood is incoagulable, which is diagnostic of severe *E. ocellatus* envenomation where this is common. Death follows intracranial haemorrhage after 1 or 2 days, or haemorrhagic shock and renal failure after 1 week.

Therapy is with an antivenom which must be known to be effective in the locality because antigenic specificity

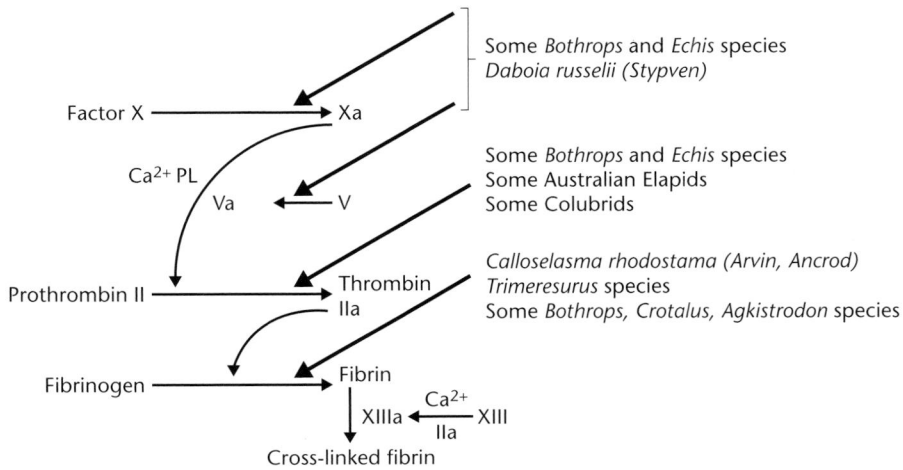

Figure 13.28: Sites of action of some snake procoagulants. (Reproduced with the kind permission of D A Warrell.)

of venoms varies, for example between East and West Africa. Both Pasteur Paris *Echis* and South African Institute for Medical Research (SAIMR) antivenoms are reliable in West Africa.

Naja nigricollis

The spitting cobra is common throughout sub-Saharan Africa, except in the central African forest and the temperate south. Besides spitting, the snakes bite, and about one-fifth of systematically envenomed victims have spontaneous haemorrhages, which may be fatal.

Procoagulant activity has been shown in vitro, but is probably not important. FDPs can be raised from about the fifth day, associated with tissue necrosis, but DIC is not a serious feature. One specific action is the destruction of platelet actin and a failure of clot retraction. In the clotting time test, clot forms normally (unlike with *E. carinatus*), but fails to retract on standing.

Polyvalent antivenoms are not effective.

Bitis arietans

The puff adder is found throughout sub-Saharan Africa except in dense forest, and occurs also up the west Atlantic seaboard to Morocco and in western Arabia. The main effects of envenomation are cytotoxic on the heart, the automatic nervous system and the kidney. Some patients have spontaneous haemorrhages, usually of gums and nose, as a result of endothelial damage, consumption of platelets and thrombocytopenia; DIC is not usual, but may occur and be complicated by microangiopathic haemolytic anaemia.

Bites by the Gaboon viper (*B. gabonica*) found throughout sub-Saharan Africa, and by the rhinoceros-horned viper (*B. nasicornis*) found in a belt between West Africa and western Kenya, have similar effects.

Treatment includes specific polyvalent antivenom.

Dispholidus typus

The green African tree-snake or boomslang is widespread in wooded areas of sub-Saharan Africa, except in the dense central African forest. It is not aggressive and is inefficient in envenomation as it is back-fanged. Only those who handle snakes are liable to be bitten. Envenomation is followed after 1–2 days by spontaneous haemorrhage, due to the activation of factors II, X and XIII leading to DIC. The course may be complicated by microangiopathic haemolysis and renal failure. Mortality without treatment is high, but antivenoms are effective.

Asia

Daboia russelii

Russell's viper is widely but discontinuously distributed in South-East Asia; it is a major health problem in the rice-growing areas of the Indian subcontinent, Myanmar (Burma) and Thailand. Annual incidence of fatal snake bites in Sri Lanka is 6/100 000 and in Myanmar

3.3/100 000, of which about three-quarters are due to *D. russelii*.

Venom is cytotoxic for endothelium, platelets, red cells, muscles, nerve cells and liver; there is vasodilatation and increased capillary permeability. Two major procoagulants activate factors X and V (Figure 13.28), causing consumption coagulopathy, DIC, deposition of fibrin in the kidneys and other organs, and fibrinolysis. With severe systemic envenomation there are widespread spontaneous haemorrhages. Causes of death include: (1) early shock from haemorrhage, vasodilatation and increased capillary permeability; (2) intracerebral and subarachnoid haemorrhages; (3) late shock from massive gastrointestinal bleeding; (4) late shock from pituitary–adrenal insufficiency following haemorrhage or infarction; and (5) acute renal failure.

Blood is usually incoagulable, FDPs are high and there is often thrombocytopenia.

Antivenom restores haemostasis but does not prevent the complications of renal failure.

Asian pit vipers

Calloselasma rhodostoma, the Malayan pit viper, is the second most important cause of envenomation in South-East Asia. There is more local swelling, pain, lymphadenopathy and tissue necrosis than with *D. russelii* bites. The proteolytic enzyme 'arvin' or 'ancrod' cleaves fibrinogen (Figure 13.28), defibrinating the victim in about half an hour: platelets are damaged, fibrinolysis is activated and the FDPs raised. Haemorrhage may be local, spread up the bitten limb or become generalized.

Many species of *Trimeresurus*, the green pit vipers, bite frequently but with less serious effects than with the Malayan pit viper.

Central and South America

About 200 deaths in Brazil and 100 in Venezuela each year are due to bites by *Crotalus* species (rattlesnakes) and *Bothrops* species (Table 13.27). Envenomation causes (1) extensive tissue necrosis, (2) defibrination from cleavage of fibrinopeptide A from fibrinogen (Figure 13.28), (3) intravascular haemolysis, (4) renal failure, and (5) neurotoxicity.

Antivenom should be administered in all cases of rattlesnake bite, even before there is evidence of systemic envenomation.

Congenital disorders

The prevalence of haemophilia A (congenital deficiency of factor VIII) is about 10/100 000, that of von Willebrand's disease (congenital deficiency or abnormality of factor VIII-related antigen) is greater than 10/100 000, and that of haemophilia B (congenital deficiency of factor IX) is about 0.1/100 000 population.[164] All other congenital disorders of coagulation are rarities. Except in consanguineous communities, there is probably little true variation of incidence between populations in the world, although the rate of diagnosis may be low in developing countries due to early death, low clinical suspicion and lack of laboratory facilities.[167]

The clinical presentation of these disorders is much the same in the tropics as in the temperate zones. Boys present not infrequently following circumcision, and cerebral haemorrhages can result from the raised intracranial pressure of persistent coughing.

The specific treatment of choice for haemophilia A is factor VIII concentrate, but this is costly and not available in many developing countries. Cryoprecipitate, which is rich in factor VIII, can be prepared simply with a minimum of equipment. Donor blood is collected into a multipack plastic blood collection set: the unit is centrifuged or allowed to sediment, and the plasma separated into the second pack, which is separated and frozen at − 20°C or colder for 24 hours; the plasma is thawed at 4°C and centrifuged; the cryoprecipitate is retained in the second bag and the cryosupernate separated into a third bag; both are stored at − 20°C until used. Because factor VIII coagulant activity is high in normal subjects in the tropics (e.g., Africans have > 150% activity of pooled European plasma), cryoprecipitate of high activity can be produced with no more than a domestic deep-freezer.

During the first half of the 1980s a large number of haemophiliacs treated with factor VIII concentrates were infected with HIV through this product. Patients escaped infection when they were treated only with locally produced cryoprecipitate from donors in communities which were not yet infected by HIV, for example in Nigeria. The present situation (2002) is that factor VIII concentrates are non-infective if the virus is correctly inactivated, whereas cryoprecipitate is potentially infective. In the future, many haemophiliacs in tropical Africa, America and Asia are liable to be infected through contaminated cryoprecipitate, unless virus-inactivated concentrates or the more expensive recombinant factors VIII and IX are made available.

Haemophilia B is best treated with virus-inactivated factor IX concentrate; cryosupernate and fresh frozen plasma can be given in the absence of the concentrate, but are potentially infectious for HIV.

Wherever possible, von Willebrand's disease should be managed with desmopressin, but cryoprecipitate may be necessary.

All blood products which are not heat inactivated are potentially infectious for HIV, HBV (if donors are not screened for HBsAg), HCV and other micro-organisms. Blood and blood products should be used appropriately: that is, only when there are definite indications for which the advantages are judged to outweigh the risks of infection.[17]

Haemophilia care in developing countries

Only about 25% of people with haemophilia in the world are receiving adequate comprehensive care. National programmes for haemophilia care can be launched and be successful, with the guidance and support of the World Federation of Hemophilia (Contact: Executive Director, WFH Secretariat, 1310 Greene Avenue, Suite 500, Montreal, Quebec, Canada H3Z 2BZ. Tel.: 1-514-933-7944; fax: 1-514-933-8916; email: wfh@wfh.org).[168]

Components of a national programme of comprehensive care include (1) the establishment of centres for care, (2) the training of care providers, (3) diagnosis and registration of people with haemophilia, (4) the education of patients and their families, (5) education of the whole community, (6) the provision of safe and effective therapeutic products, and (7) the prevention of haemophilia through counselling and antenatal diagnosis.

REFERENCES

1   Lewis S M, Bain B, Bates I. Dacie & Lewis's *Practical Haematology*, 9th edn. Edinburgh: Churchill Livingstone, 2001.

2   Lubin B H. Reference values in infancy and childhood. In Nathan D G & Oski F A (eds) *Hematology of Infancy and Childhood*, 4th edn. Philadelphia: W B Saunders, 1993: Appendix i–xx.

3   Gilles H M. Normal haematological values in tropical areas. *Clin Haematol* 1981; 10:697–706.

4   Huehns E R. The structure and function of haemoglobin: clinical disorders due to abnormal haemoglobin structure. In Hardisty R M & Weatherall D J (eds) *Blood and its Disorders*. Oxford: Blackwell, 1974: 526–629.

5   Fleming A F. Haematological changes in pregnancy. *Clin Obstet Gynecol* 1975; 2:269–283.

6   Dupuy E, Fleming A F & Caen J P. Platelet function, factor VIII, fibrinogen, and fibrinolysis in Nigerians and Europeans, in relation to atheroma and thrombosis. *J Clin Pathol* 1978; 31:1094–1101.

7   World Health Organization. Nutritional anaemias. *WHO Tech Rep Ser* 1972; 503.

8   DeMaeyer E & Adiels-Tegman M. The prevalence of anaemia in the world. *World Health Stat Q* 1985; 38:302–316.

9   Bellingham A J. The red cell in adaption to anaemic hypoxia.

Clin Haematol 1974; 3:577–594.

10 Viteri F E & Torún B. Anaemia and physical work capacity. *Clin Haematol* 1974; 3:609–626.

11 Baker S J & DeMaeyer E M. Nutritional anemia: its understanding and control with special reference to the work of the World Health Organization. *Am J Clin Nutr* 1979; 32:368–417.

12 Wolgemuth J C, Latham, M C, Hall A et al. Worker productivity and nutritional status of Kenyan road construction laborers. *Am J Clin Nutr* 1982; 36:68–78.

13 Florencio C A. Effects of iron and ascorbic acid supplementation on hemoglobin level and work efficiency of anemic women. *J Occup Med* 1981; 23:699–704.

14 Harrison K A, Lister U G, Rossiter D E & Chang H. Perinatal mortality. *Br J Obstet Gynaecol* 1985; 92(suppl. 5):86–99.

15 English M. Life-threatening severe malarial anaemia. *Trans R Soc Trop Med Hyg* 2000; 94:585–588.

16 Harrison K A & Rossiter C E. Maternal mortality. *Br J Obstet Gynaecol* 1985; 92(suppl. 5):100–115.

17 World Health Organization, Global Programme on AIDS, Global Blood Safety Initiative. *Guidelines for the Appropriate Use of Blood*. WHO/GPA/Inf/ 89; 18. Geneva: WHO, 1989.

18 World Health Organization. Severe falciparum malaria. *Trans R Soc Trop Med Hyg* 2000; 94(suppl. 1).

19 Mendendez C, Fleming A F & Alonso P. Malaria-related anaemia. *Parasitol Today* 2000; 16:469–476.

20 French N & Gilks C F. HIV and malaria, do they interact? *Trans R Soc Trop Med Hyg* 2000; 94:233–237.

21 Fleming A F. Haematological manifestations of malaria and other parasitic diseases. *Clin Haematol* 1981; 10:983–1011.

22 Essien E M. Platelets and platelet disorders in Africa. *Baillière's Clin Haematol* 1992; 5:441–456.

23 Menendez C. Malaria during pregnancy: a priority area of malaria research and control. *Parasitol Today* 1995; 11:178–183.

24 Wahlgren M & Spillman D. Sticky sugars attract malaria to the fetus. *Nature Med* 2000; 6:25–26.

25 Lindsay S, Ansell J, Selman C et al. Effect of pregnancy on exposure to malaria mosquitoes. *Lancet* 2000; 355:1972.

26 Fleming A F. Tropical obstetrics and gynaecology. 1. Anaemia in pregnancy in tropical Africa. *Trans R Soc Trop Med Hyg* 1989; 83:441–448.

27 Fleming A F & Allan N C. Severe haemolytic anaemia in pregnancy in Nigerians treated with prednisolone. *BMJ* 1969; iv:461–466.

28 Steketee R W, Wirima J J, Bloland P B et al. Impairment of a pregnant woman's acquired ability to limit *Plasmodium falciparum* by infection with human immunodeficiency virus type-1. *Am J Trop Med Parasitol* 1996: 55(suppl. 1):42–49.

29 Greenwood B M, Greenwood A M, Snow R W et al. The effects of malaria chemoprophylaxis given by traditional birth attendants on the course and outcome of pregnancy. *Trans R Soc Trop Med Hyg* 1989; 83:589–594.

30 Rogerson S J, Chaluluka E, Kanjala M et al. Intermittent sulfadoxine–pyrimethamine in pregnancy: effectiveness against malaria morbidity in Blantyre, Malawi, in 1977–99. *Trans R Soc Trop Med Hyg* 2000; 94:549–553.

31 Fleming A F, MacIntyre J A & Johnstone F D. HIV infection and AIDS in pregnancy. In Lawson J B, Harrison K A & Bergström S (eds) *Maternity Care in the Developing Countries*. London: Royal College of Obstetricians and Gynaecologists, 2001: 337–359.

32 Bryceson A, Fakunle Y M, Fleming A F et al. Malaria and splenomegaly. *Trans R Soc Trop Med Hyg* 1983; 77:879.

33 Bryceson A D M, Fleming A F & Edington G M. Splenomegaly in northern Nigeria. *Acta Trop* 1976; 33:185–214.

34 Crane G. The genetic basic of hyperreactive malarial splenomegaly. *Papua New Guinea Med J* 1989; 32:269–276.

35 Hill A V S. Malaria resistance genes: a natural selection. *Trans R Soc Trop Med Hyg* 1992; 86:225–226, 232.

36 Piessens W F, Hoffman S L, Wadee A A et al. Antibody-mediated killing of suppressor T lymphocytes as a possible cause of macroglobulinemia in the tropical splenomegaly syndrome. *J Clin Invest* 1985; 75:1821–1827.

37 Fakunle Y M. Tropical splenomegly. Part 1: tropical Africa. *Clin Haematol* 1981; 10:963–973.

38 Crane G G. Hyperreactive malarious splenomegaly (tropical splenomegaly syndrome). *Parasitol Today* 1986; 2:4–9.

39 Jimmy E O, Bedu-Addo G, Bates I et al. Immunoglobulin gene polymerase chain reaction to distinguish hyperreactive malarial splenomegaly from 'African' chronic lymphocytic leukaemia and splenic lymphoma. *Trans R Soc Trop Med Hyg* 1996; 90:37–39.

40 Zhu A, Thompsett A R, Bedu-Addo G et al. V_H genes sequences from a novel tropical splenic lymphoma reveal a naïve B cell as the cell of origin. *Br J Haematol* 1999; 107:114–120.

41 Fleming A F, Terunuma H, Tembo C & Mantini H. Leukaemias in Zambia. *Leukemia* 1999; 13:1292–1293.

42 Cartwright G E, Chung H-L & Chang A. Studies on the pancytopenia of kala-azar. *Blood* 1948; 3:249–275.

43 Kager P A, van der Plas-van Dalen C, Rees P H et al. Red cell, white cell and platelet autoantibodies in visceral leishmaniasis. *Trop Geogr Med* 1984; 36:143–150.

44 Wickramasinghe S N, Abdalla S H & Kasili E G. Ultrastructure of bone marrow in patients with visceral leishmaniasis. *J Clin Pathol* 1987; 40:267–275.

45 Marwaha N, Sarode R, Gupta R K et al. Clinico-hematological characteristics in patients with kala azar. *Trop Geogr Med* 1991; 43:357–362.

46 Lazzarin A, Esposito R & Almaviva M. Modifications of leucocyte function in visceral leishmaniasis. *Boll Ist Sieroter Milan* 1981; 60:222–224.

47 El-Hassan A M, Ahmed M A M, Rahim A A et al. Visceral leishmaniasis in the Sudan: clinical and hematological features. *Ann Saudi Med* 1990; 10:51–56.

48 Varma N, Bhoria U, Bambery P & Dash S. Gelatinous transformation of the bone marrow and *Leishmania donovani* infection. *J Trop Med Hyg* 1991; 94:310–312.

49 Solano C, Gomez-Reino F & Fernandez-Rañada J M. Pure red cell aplasia in kala azar. *Acta Haematol* 1984; 72:205–207.

50 Kager P A & Rees P H. Haematological investigations in visceral leishmaniasis. *Trop Geogr Med* 1986; 38:371–379.

51 Pippard M J, Moir D & Weatherall D J. Mechanism of anaemia in resistant visceral leishmaniasis. *Ann Trop Med Parasitol* 1986; 80:317–323.

52 Weatherall D J & Clegg J B. *The Thalassaemia Syndromes*, 4th edn. Oxford: Blackwell Science, 2000.

53 Steinberg M H, Forget B G, Higgs D R & Nagel R L. *Disorders of Hemoglobin*. Cambridge: Cambridge University Press, 2001.

54 Olivieri N F. The β-thalassaemias. *N Engl J Med* 1999; 341:99–109.

55 Wonke B. Bone disease in β-thalassaemia major. *Br J Haematol* 1998; 103:897–901.

56 Pippard M J & Weatherall D J. Oral iron chelation therapy for thalassaemia: an uncertain scene. *Br J Haematol* 2000; 111:2–5.

57 Fleming A F. Maternal anemia and fetal outcome in pregnancies complicated by thalassemia minor and 'stomatocytosis'. *Am J Obstet Gynecol* 1973; 116:309–319.

58 Willcox M, Björkman A & Brohult J. Falciparum malaria and β-thalassaemia trait in northern Liberia. *Ann Trop Med Parasitol* 1983; 77:335–347.

59 Metaxotou-Mavromati A D, Antonopoulou H K Laskari S S et al. Developmental changes in hemoglobin F levels during the first two years of life in normal and heterozygous β-thalassemia infants. *Pediatrics* 1982; 69:734–738.

60 Luzzi G A, Merry A H, Newbold C I et al. Surface antigen expression of *Plasmodium falciparum*-infected erythrocytes is modified in alpha- and beta-thalassemia. *J Exp Med* 1991; 173:785–791.

61 Senok A C, Nelson E A S, Li K & Oppenheimer S J. Thalassaemia trait, red blood cell age and oxidant stress: effects on *Plasmodium falciparum* growth and sensitivity to artemisinin. *Trans R Soc Trop Med Hyg* 1997; 91:585–589.

62 Fucharoen S & Winichagoon P. Clinical and hematologic aspects of hemoglobin E β-thalassemia. *Current Opinions Hematol* 2000; 7:106–112.

63 de Silva S, Fisher C A, Premawardhena A et al. Thalassaemia in Sri Lanka: implications for the future health burden of Asian populations. *Lancet* 2000; 355:786–791.

64 Chen F E, Ooi C, Ha S Y et al. Genetic and clinical features of hemoglobin H disease in Chinese patients.– *N Engl J Med* 2000; 343:544–550.

65 Muklwala E C, Banda J, Siziya S et al. Alpha thalassaemia in Zambian newborn. *Clin Lab Haematol* 1989; 11:1–6.

66 Williams T N, Maitland K, Bennett S et al. High incidence of malaria in α-thalassaemic children. *Nature* 1996; 383:522–525.

67 Bain B J. *Haemoglobinopathy Diagnosis*. Oxford: Blackwell Science, 2001.

68 Modell B & Bulyzhenkov V. Distribution and control of some genetic disorders. *World Health Stat Q* 1988; 41:209–218.

69 Serjeant G R & Serjeant B E. *Sickle Cell Disease*, 3rd edn. Oxford: Oxford University Press, 2001.

70 Platt O S & Dover G J. Sickle cell disease. In Nathan D G & Oski F A (eds) *Hematology of Infancy and Childhood*, 4th edn. Philadelphia: W B Saunders, 1993: 732–782.

71 Serjeant G R. The emerging understanding of sickle cell disease. *Br J Haematol* 2001; 112:3–18.

72 Nagel R L & Fleming A F. Genetic epidemiology of the β^s gene. *Baillière's Clin Haematol* 1992; 5:331–365.

73 Fleming A F. The presentation, management and prevention of crisis in sickle cell disease in Africa. *Blood Rev* 1989; 3:18–28.

74 Vichinsky E P, Neumayr L D, Earles A N et al. Causes and outcomes of the acute chest syndrome in sickle cell disease. *N Engl J Med* 2000; 342:1855–1865.

75 Powars D R. Management of cerebral vasculopathy in children with sickle cell disease. *Br J Haematol* 2000; 108:666–678.

76 Morris J, Dunn D, Beckford M et al. The haematology of homozygous sickle cell disease after the age of 40 years. *Br J Haematol* 1991; 77:382–385.

77 Harrison K A. Haemoglobinopathies in pregnancy. In Lawson J B, Harrison K A & Bergström S (eds) *Maternity Care in Developing Countries*. London: Royal College of Obstetricians and Gynaecology, 2001, pp. 129–145.

78 Wierenga K J J, Hambleton I R & Lewis N A. Survival estimates for patients with homozygous sickle-cell disease in Jamaica: a clinic-based population study. *Lancet* 2001; 357:680–683.

79 Molineaux L, Fleming A F, Cornille-Brøgger R et al. Abnormal haemoglobins in the sudan savanna of Nigeria. III. Malaria, immunoglobulins and antimalarial antibodies in sickle cell disease. *Ann Trop Med Parasitol* 1979; 73:301–310.

80 Steinberg M H. Management of sickle cell disease. *N Engl J Med* 1999; 340:1021–1030.

81 Akinyanju O O & Anionwu E N. Training of counsellors in sickle-cell disorders in Africa. *Lancet* 1989; i:653–654.

82 Kark J A, Posey D M, Schumacher H R & Ruehle C J. Sickle-cell trait as a risk factor for sudden death in physical training. *N Engl J Med* 1987; 317:781–787.

83 Abu-Zeid Y A, Abdulhadi N H, Theander T G et al. Seasonal changes in cell mediated immune responses to soluble *Plasmodium falciparum* antigens in children with haemoglobin AA and haemoglobin AS. *Trans R Soc Trop Med Hyg* 1992; 86:20–22.

84 WHO Working Group. Glucose-6-phosphate dehydrogenase deficiency. *Bull World Health Organ* 1989; 67:601–611.

85 Luzzatto L. G6PD deficiency and hemolytic anemia. In Nathan D G & Oski F A (eds) *Hematology of Infancy and Childhood*, 4th edn. Philadelphia: W B Saunders, 1993: 674–695.

86 Huang C-S, Hung K-L, Huang M-J et al. Neonatal jaundice and molecular mutations in glucose-6-phosphate dehydrogenase deficient newborn infants. *Am J Hematol* 1996; 51:19–25.

87 Ho N K. Neonatal jaundice in Asia. *Baillière's Clin Haematol* 1992; 5:131–142.

88 Chan M C K. Glucose-6-phosphate dehydrogenase (G6PD) deficiency. *Postgrad Doct Middle East* 1992; 15:10–15.

89 Galiano S, Gaetani G F, Barabino A et al. Favism in the African type of glucose-6-phosphate dehydrogenase deficiency (A⁻). *BMJ* 1990; 300:236.

90 Williams C K O, Osotimehim B O, Ogunmola G B & Awotedu A A. Haemolytic anaemia associated with Nigerian barbecued meat (red suya). *Afr J Med Med Sci* 1988; 17:71–75.

91 Ruwende C & Hill A. Glucose-6-phosphate dehydrogenase deficiency and malaria. *J Mol Med* 1998; 76:581–588.

92 Cappadora M, Giribaldi G, O'Brien E et al. Early phagocytosis of glucose-6-phosphate dehydrogense (G6PD)-deficient erythrocytes parasitized by *Plasmodium falciparum* may explain malaria protection in G6PD deficiency. *Blood* 1998; 92:2527–2534.

93 Tse W T & Lux S E. Red blood cell membrane disorders. *Br J Haematol* 1999; 104:2–13.

94 Nurse G T, Coetzer T L & Palek J. The elliptocytoses, ovalocytosis and related disorders. *Baillière's Clin Haematol* 1992; 5:187–207.

95 Allen S J, O'Donnell A, Alexander N D E et al. Prevention of cerebral malaria in children in Papua New Guinea by Southeast Asian ovalocytosis band 3. *Am J Trop Med Hyg* 1999; 60:1056–1060.

96 Glele-Kakai C, Garbarz M, Lecomte M-C et al. Epidemiological studies of spectrin mutations related to hereditary elliptocytosis and spectrin polymorphisms in Benin. *Br J Haematol* 1996; 95:57–66.

97 Chishti A H, Palek J, Fisher D et al. Reduced invasion and growth of *Plasmodium falciparum* into elliptocytic red blood cells with a combined deficiency of protein 4.1, glycophorin C, and p 55. *Blood* 1996; 87:3462–3469.

98 DeMaeyer E M, Dallman P, Gurney J M et al. *Preventing and Controlling Iron Deficiency Anaemia through Primary Health Care*. Geneva: WHO, 1989.

99 Fleming A F. Iron deficiency in the tropics. *Clin Haematol* 1982; 11:365–388.

100 *Report of the WHO Informal Consultation on Hookworm Infection and Anaemia in Girls and Women*. WHO/CTD/SIP/96.1. Geneva: World Health Organization, 1996.

101 Bruner A B, Joffe A, Duggan A K et al. Randomised study of cognitive effects of iron supplementation in non-anaemic iron-deficient adolescent girls. *Lancet* 1996; 348:992–996.

102 Allen L H. Anemia and iron deficiency: effects on pregnancy outcome. *Am J Clin Nutr* 2000; 71(suppl.):1280S–1284S.

103 Hindmarsh P C, Geary M P P, Rodeck C H et al. Effect of maternal iron stores on placental weight and structure. *Lancet* 2000; 356:719–723.

104 Stoltzfus R J & Dreyfuss M L. *Guidelines for the Use of Iron Supplements to Prevent and Treat Iron Deficiency Anemia*. INACG/WHO/UNICEF Washington: ILSA Press, 1998.

105 Menendez C, Todd J, Alonso P L et al. The effect of iron supplementation during pregnancy, given by traditional birth attendants, on the prevalence of anaemia and malaria. *Trans R Soc Trop Med Hyg* 1994; 88:590–593.

106 Menendez C, Todd J, Alonso P L et al. The response to iron supplementation of pregnant women with the haemoglobin genotype AA or AS. *Trans R Soc Trop Med Hyg* 1995; 89:289–292.

107 INACG. *Safety of Iron Supplementation Programs in Malaria-Endemic Regions*. Washington: INACG, 1999.

108 Adish A A, Esrey S A, Gyorkos T W et al. Effect of consumption of food cooked in iron pots on iron status and growth of children: a randomized trial. *Lancet* 1999; 353:712–716.

109 Gordeuk V. Hereditary and nutritional iron overload. *Baillière's Clin Haematol* 1992; 5:169–186.

110 Saungweme T, Khumalo H, Mvundura E et al. Iron and alcohol content of traditional beers in rural Zimbabwe. *Centr Afr J Med* 1999; 45:136–140.

111 Moyo V M, Mandishona E, Hasstedt S J et al. Evidence of genetic transmission in African iron overload. *Blood* 1998; 91:1076–1082.

112 Cooper B A, Rosenblatt D S & Whitehead V M. Megaloblastic anemia. In Nathan D G & Oski F A (eds) *Hematology of Infancy and Childhood*, 4th edn. Philadelphia: W B Saunders, 1993:354–390.

113 Ingram C F, Fleming A F, Patel M & Galpin J S. Pregnancy- and lactation-related folate deficiency in South Africa: a case for folate food fortfication. *S Afr Med J* 1999; 89:1279–1284.

114 Scholl T O & Johnson W G. Folic acid: influence on the outcome of pregnancy. *Am J Clin Nutr* 2000; 71(suppl.):1295S–1303S.

115 Baker S J. Nutritional anaemias. Part 2. Tropical Asia *Clin Haematol* 1981; 10:843–871.

116 Carmel R. Ethnic and racial factors in cobalamin metabolism and its disorders. *Semin Hematol* 1999; 36:88–100.

117 Harakati M S E. Pernicious anaemia in Arabs. *Blood Cells Mol Dis* 1996; 22:98–103.

118 Akinyanju O O & Okany C C. Pernicious anaemia in Africans. *Clin Lab Haematol* 1992; 14:33–40.

119 Savage D, Gangaidzo I, Lindenbaum J et al. Vitamin B_{12} deficiency is the primary cause of megaloblastic anaemia in Zimbabwe. *Br J Haematol* 1994; 86:844–850.

120 Remacha A F & Cadafalch J. Cobalamin deficiency in patients infected with the human immunodeficiency virus. *Semin Hematol* 1999; 36:75–87.

121 Cardosa A P, Ernesto M, Cliff J et al. Cyanogenic potential of cassava flour: field trial in Mozambique of a simple kit. *Int J Food Sci Nutr* 1998; 49:93–99.

122 Ingram C F, Fleming A F, Patel M & Galpin J S. The value of the intrinsic factor antibody test in diagnosing pernicious anaemia. *Cent Afr J Med* 1999; 44:178–181.

123 WHO/UNICEF/IVACG/HKI. *Vitamin A Supplements: A Guide to their Use in the Treatment and Prevention of Vitamin A Deficiency*, 3rd edn. Geneva: World Health Organization, 2001.

124 Wickramasinghe S N. Nutritional anaemias. *Clin Lab Haematol* 1988; 10:117–134.

125 Powers H J, Bates C J, Prentice A M et al. The relative effectiveness of iron with riboflavin in correcting a microcytic anaemia in men and children in rural Gambia. *Hum Nutr Clin Nutr* 1983; 37C:413–425.

126 Power H J, Bayes C J & Lamb W H. Haematological response to supplements of iron and riboflavin to pregnant and lactating women in rural Gambia. *Hum Nutr Clin Nutr* 1984; 39C:117–129.

127 Knox-Macaulay H H M. Tuberculosis and the haemopoietic system. *Baillière's Clin Haematol* 1992; 5:101–129.

128 Malyanga E, Abayomi E A, Adewuyi J & Coutts A M. AIDS is now the commonest clinical condition associated with multilineage blood cytopenia in a central referral hospital in Zimbabwe. *Cent Afr J Med* 2000; 46:59–61.

129 Bain B J. The haematological features of HIV infection. *Brit J Haematol* 1997; 99:1–8.

130 Karstaedt A D, Pantanowitz L, Gavalakis C & Stevens W. Bone marrow morphology in human immunodeficiency virus-infected South Africans with and without tuberculosis. *Br J Haematol* 2001; 112:824–827.

131 Bower M. Acquired immunodeficiency syndrome-related systemic non-Hodgkin's lymphoma. *Br J Haematol* 2001; 112:863–873.

132 Alter B P & Young N S. The bone marrow failure syndromes. In Nathan D G & Oski F A (eds) *Hematology of Infancy and Childhood*, 4th edn. Philadelphia: W B Saunders, 1993: 216–316.

133 Yeats J, Daley H & Hardie D. Parvovirus B19 infection does not contribute significantly to severe anaemia in children with malaria in Malawi. *Eur J Haematol*; 1999; 63:276–277.

134 Issaragrisil S, Leaverton P E, Chansung K et al. Regional patterns in the incidence of aplastic anemia in Thailand. *Am J Hematol* 1999; 61:164–168.

135 Niazi G A, Fleming A F & Siziya S. Blood dyscrasia in unofficial vendors of petrol and heavy oil and motor mechanics in Nigeria. *Trop Doct* 1989; 19:55–58.

136 Waterhouse J, Muir C, Correa P & Powell J. *Cancer Incidence in Five Continents*, 3. Lyon: International Agency for Research on Cancer, 1976.

137 Ramot B & Rechavi G. Non-Hodgkin's lymphomas and paraproteinaemias. *Baillière's Clin Haematol* 1992; 5:81–99.

138 Glaser S L. Hodgkin's disease in black populations: a review of the epidemiologic literature. *Semin Hematol* 1990; 17:643–659.

139 Jarrett R F. Hodgkins disease. *Baillière's Clin Haematol* 1992; 5:57–79.

140 Schmauz R, Mugerwa J W & Wright D H. The distribution of non-Burkitt, non-Hodgkin's lymphomas in Uganda in relation to malarial endemicity. *Int J Cancer* 1990; 45:650–653.

141 Shih L-Y & Liang D-C. Non-Hodgkins lymphomas in Asia. *Hematol Oncol Clin North Am* 1991; 5:983–1001.

142 Iscovich J & Parkin D M. Risk of cancer in migrants and their descendants in Israel: I. Leukaemias and lymphomas. *Int J Cancer* 1997; 70:649–653.

143 Foerster J. Heavy chain disease. In Nathan D G & Oski F A (eds). *Hematology in Infancy and Childhood*, 4th edn. Philadelphia: W B Saunders, 1993:2693–2704.

144 Pawson R, Mufti G J & Pagliuca A. Management of adult T-cell leukaemia/lymphoma. *Br J Haematol* 1998; 100:453–458.

145 Manns A, Hisada M & La Grenade L. Human T-lymphotropic virus type 1 infection. *Lancet* 1999; 353:1951–1958.

146 Weber T, Hunsmann G, Stevens W & Fleming A F. Human retroviruses. *Baillière's Clin Haematol* 1992; 5:273–314.

147 Blattner W A, Jacobson R J & Shulman G. Multiple myeloma in South African Blacks. *Lancet* 1979; i:928–929.

148 Mukiibi J M & Mkwananzi J B. Multiple myeloma in Zimbabweans. *East Afr Med J* 1987; 64:471–481.

149 Fleming A F. Leukaemias in Africa. *Leukemia* 1993; 7(suppl.):S138–S141.

150 Greaves M F, Colman S M, Beard M E J et al. Geographical distribution of acute lymphoblastic leukaemia subtypes: second report of the Collaborative Group study. *Leukemia* 1993; 7:27–34.

151 Fleming A F, Glencross D K, Adam F et al. Acute lymphoblastic leukaemia in Johannesburg: distribution of phenotypes by race, age and sex. *24th Congress of the International Society of Haematology, London*. 1992, Abstract 144:382.

152 Paul B, Mukiibi J M, Mandisodsa A, Levy L & Nkrumah F K. A three-year prospective study of 137 cases of acute leukaemia in Zimbabwe. *Cent Afr J Med* 1992; 38:95–99.

153 Greaves M F. Aetiology of acute leukaemia. *Lancet* 1997; 349:344–349.

154 Greaves M. Childhood leukaemia. *Br Med J* 2002; 324:283–287.

155 Kinlen L J & Balkwill A. Infective cause of childhood leukaemia and wartime population mixing in Orkney and Shetland, UK. *Lancet* 2001; 357:858.

156 Pasqualetti P, Festuccia V, Acitelli P et al. Tobacco smoking and risk of haematological malignancies in adults: a case–control study. *Br J Haematol* 1997; 97:659–662.

157 Mukiibi J M & Paul B. Myelodysplastic syndromes (MDS) in Central Africans. *Trop Geog Med* 1994; 46:17–19.

158 Goldman J M & Melo J V. Targeting the BCR-ABL tyrosine kinase in chronic myeloid leukemia. *N Engl J Med* 2001; 344:1084–1086.

159 Fleming A F. Chronic lymphocytic leukaemia in tropical Africa: a review. *Leuk Lymphoma* 1990; 1:169–173.

160 Bates I, Bedu-Addo G, Jarrett R F et al. B-lymphotropic viruses in a novel tropical splenic lymphoma. *Br J Haematol* 2001; 112:161–166.

161 Zhu D, Thompsett A R, Bedu-Addo G et al. V_H gene sequences from a novel tropical splenic lymphoma reveal a naïve B cell as the cell of origin. *Br J Haematol* 1999; 107:114–120.

162 Masera G, Baez F, Biondi A et al. North–South twinning in paediatric haemato-oncology. The La Mascota programme, Nicaragua. *Lancet* 1998; 352:1923–1926.

163 Hesseling P B. Onyalai. *Baillière's Clin Haematol* 1992; 5:457–473.

164 Nathwani A C & Tuddenham E G D. Epidemiology of coagulation disorders. *Baillière's Clin Haematol* 1992; 5:383–439.

165 Zipursky A. Prevention of vitamin K deficiency bleeding in newborns. *Br J Haematol* 1999; 104:430–437.

166 Levi M & ten Cate H. Disseminated intravascular coagulation. *N Engl J Med* 1999; 341:586–592.

167 Adewuyi J O, Coutts A M, Levy L & Lloyd S E. Haemophilia care in Zimbabwe. *Cent Afr J Med* 1996; 42:153–156.

168 Word Health Organization. *Control of Haemophilia:Haemophilia Care in Developing Countries. Report of a Joint WHO/World Federation of Haemophilia Meeting.* WHO/HGN/WFH/WG/98.3 Geneva: World Health Organization, 1998.

Chapter 14
Blood Transfusion

I. Bates

'17% of the global population has access to 60% of the global blood supply'[1]

Blood transfusion is a vital component of every country's health service (Table 14.1). It can be a life-saving intervention for severe, acute anaemia, but mistakes in the transfusion process can be life threatening, either immediately or years later through transmission of infectious agents. It is imperative that clinicians have a good understanding of how blood is acquired and prepared for transfusion, and when it should be used, and that governments put in place mechanisms to guarantee that blood for transfusion is safe.

The four key objectives of any strategy to ensure that blood is safe for transfusion are:[1]

- Establish a co-ordinated blood transfusion service that can provide adequate and timely supplies of safe blood for all patients in need.
- Collect blood only from voluntary non-remunerated blood donors from low-risk populations and use stringent donor selection procedures.
- Screen all blood for transfusion-transmissible infections and have standardized procedures in place for grouping and compatibility testing.
- Reduce unnecessary transfusions through the appropriate clinical use of blood, including the use of intravenous replacement fluids and other simple alternatives to transfusion, wherever possible.

Effective quality assurance should be in place for all aspects of the transfusion process.

Blood transfusion service at the national level

Transfusion medicine is a distinct and multi-disciplinary sector of the health service and should be incorporated into all national health plans. Less than 70 out of the 191 member states meet the World Health Organization's (WHO) recommendations for a national blood programme.[1] At the national level the transfusion service should have a director, an advisory committee and clear transfusion policies and strategies. Blood collection, testing and distribution need to be standardized. Although centralization of these services may offer the best guarantee of

Table 14.1 Global facts about blood transfusion

80% of the world's population has access to 20% of the world's safe blood supply
Transfusion or injection of unsafe blood accounts for 8–16 million hepatitis B virus infections, 2.3–4.7 million hepatitis C virus infections, and 80,000–160,000 HIV infections each year
25% of maternal deaths from pregnancy-related causes are linked with loss of blood

quality, it is often not practical in countries with poorly developed communications and transport infrastructure. In such countries each hospital organizes its own blood transfusion service and it is then difficult to ensure national standardization and quality.

When a transfusion service is provided by individual hospitals it places an enormous burden on laboratory resources. In a typical district hospital in Malawi in 1997, 39% of all tests performed by the laboratory were transfusion-related. The overall cost of the transfusion service, including consumables, proportional amounts for capital equipment, staff time and overheads, was 36% of total laboratory costs (Figure 14.1). Extrapolating from these figures, each unit of whole blood cost the laboratory approximately £10 to collect and process.[2]

In countries where the transfusion service is nationally or regionally centralized, blood donor recruitment, and screening and processing of donated blood, is physically separated from the hospitals where blood is transfused. It is carried out in purpose-built centres that operate to good manufacturing standards similar to those laid down for the pharmaceutical industry. After donation and exclusion of potentially infected units, the blood is generally separated into various components and filtered to remove white cells. In some centres the whole process is computerized and individual components are bar-coded so that they can be tracked back to the original donor. Hospitals are proficient at predicting how much blood they will require and they receive regular consignments though a well-established delivery network. The efficiency of the system means that one donor centre may provide blood to many hospitals and cover a population of several million. This process is expensive and one unit of blood currently costs almost £100.[3]

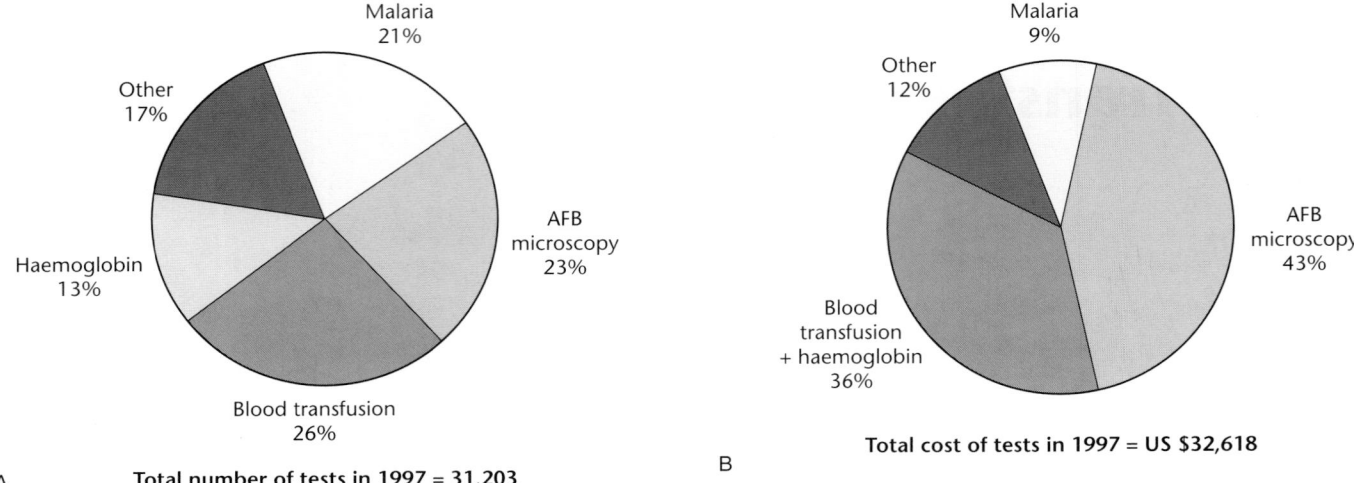

Figure 14.1: (**A**) Tests performed by a district hospital in Malawi. 'Other' includes urine and stool microscopy, syphilis serology and CSF examination. (**B**) Cost of tests performed by a district hospital in Malawi. 'Other' includes urine and stool microscopy, syphilis serology and CSF examination.

Separation of whole blood into components

In wealthy countries it is standard practice to optimize the use of each donation of blood by separating it into individual components. These components, which may include plasma, platelets and cryoprecipitate, are prepared by centrifugation using a closed, sterile system. Each component has different storage requirements. Plasma and cryoprecipitate are kept frozen, red cells are stored at 1–5°C, and platelets at 18–22°C with constant agitation.

Separation of blood, even into simple components such as cells and plasma, requires equipment and expertise that may not be available in the poorest countries. Furthermore, blood should not be separated if the residual risk of infection is high as this will increase the number of potentially infected recipients. Blood components are therefore usually not available in poorer countries, or are only accessible to those living close to a central hospital with blood separation facilities.

Ensuring safety of blood for transfusion

An unsafe blood supply is costly in both human and economic terms. Transfusion of infected blood causes morbidity and mortality in the recipients, and has an economic and emotional impact on their families and communities. Those who become infected through blood transfusion are infectious to others and contribute to the spread of disease throughout the wider population. This increases the burden on health services and reduces productive labour. Investment in safe supplies of blood is therefore a cost-effective investment for every country, even those with few resources.

Selecting low-risk blood donors

Strategies for recruiting blood donors have to balance supply with demand, and yet ensure that the blood is as safe as possible. The safest sources of blood, which comprise 98% of donors in the wealthiest countries, are altruistic voluntary unpaid donors who should be anonymous to the recipient. Only 16% of the global supply of blood is donated by such low-risk blood donors in developing countries.[1]

In countries without a national transfusion service each hospital is responsible for finding its own donors and processing blood for transfusion. Recruiting voluntary donors from the community is expensive and logistically complicated, requiring resources such as a local education programme, dedicated venesection team, vehicles and cold storage. Paid donors or 'loan' systems, where family members are responsible for providing blood for their relatives in the hospital, are therefore widespread in poorer countries. Cultural taboos and misinformation about donating blood (e.g., 'men will become impotent if they donate blood'; 'HIV can be caught from the blood bag needle') mean that relatives may be reluctant to donate. They are open to exploitation by 'professional donors' who charge relatives a fee to donate in their place. By the time a donor has been found, screened and venesected, and the blood is transfused into the patient, several hours or even days can elapse. Because patients in poorer countries often present late in the course of their disease, severely anaemic patients may die in hospital without ever receiving a blood transfusion. It is unfortunate that in many countries where the majority of transfusions are performed as an emergency and where it is imperative to have a good stock of blood in the blood bank, the 'loan' system, with its inherent delays, predominates. The feasibility of using placental blood as a novel source of blood for small children is currently being investigated.[4] The placenta containing this blood is normally discarded after delivery but the high haematocrit and easy availability may make it suitable for small volume emergency transfusions.

Potential donors should be rejected if they are considered to be at 'high risk' of HIV infection. This group includes commercial sex workers or those having frequent contact with these individuals, intravenous drug abusers, or persons with itinerant or fluctuating activities such as traders, drivers and military personnel.[5] Even in areas where HIV infection rates in the general population are high, donor deferral can be effective in excluding HIV-infected donors.[6]

The whole donation process, including the fact that they will be tested for HIV and other infections, should be explained to the donor before blood is collected. They should have the option of knowing the results and receiving counselling. It is imperative that complete confidentiality is maintained throughout all procedures.

Screening for transfusion-transmitted infections

Infections with HIV-1 and 2, hepatitis A, B, C and δ, cytomegalovirus, syphilis, lyme borreliosis, malaria, babesiosis, American trypanosomiasis (Chagas' disease) and toxoplasmosis can all be acquired through blood transfusions. At the present time there have been no cases of transmission of Creutzfeldt-Jakob disease by the intravenous route. WHO recommends that all donated blood should be screened for HIV, hepatitis B and syphilis and, where feasible and appropriate, for hepatitis C, malaria and Chagas' disease. Current routine screening processes in the USA have reduced the risk of transmission of HIV and hepatitis B virus through transfusion to 1:493,000 and 1:63,000, respectively.[7]

Between 5 and 10% of HIV infections worldwide are transmitted through the transfusion of infected blood and blood products.[1] HIV testing of blood donors needs to be highly sensitive, and blood which tests positive should be rejected. Before informing the donor of the outcome, all positive results should be confirmed using a test with a high degree of specificity. Where blood donation is organized locally, the confirmatory test is often performed at a central laboratory so there may be delay in informing the donor of the result.

Malaria can also be transmitted by transfusion and has an incubation period between 7 and 50 days depending on the species. In areas of low or no malaria transmission, screening for the parasite is important, as recipients are likely to have no immunity. It is unclear whether malaria screening is necessary in regions where the disease is common. In countries where malaria is highly endemic, a policy of excluding donors with low-grade parasitaemia would lead to a significant loss of donors. Furthermore, in this setting, most of the blood is given to hospitalized children with malaria who are likely to be receiving antimalarial drugs, or adults who are clinically immune.

Further research to assess the risks and benefits of screening blood for malaria is needed, particularly as the proportion of HIV-positive transfusion recipients is increasing.

Screening for hepatitis B surface antigen should be carried out on all donated blood, as hepatitis B-infected blood is almost 100% infectious. Although the risk of acquiring syphilis from infected blood is low, it is used as a marker of HIV risk. Fresh blood is potentially infectious for syphilis but storage at 4°C can inactivate the bacterium *Treponema pallidum*. Globally, the prevalence of hepatitis C, HTLV-1 and 2 and Chagas' disease, is variable and the decision to introduce donor screening for these infections will be based on local assessments of the risks, benefits, feasibility and costs.

It is common practice for blood to be taken from donors and stored in the blood bank until screening tests for infections have been completed. This system has several drawbacks: potentially infected blood may be mixed up with units that have already been screened; donors may donate blood unnecessarily, thereby increasing their risk of anaemia; and the whole process of venesection with wastage of blood collection bags is costly. Predonation screening, by which potential donors are tested for HIV, hepatitis B and possibly hepatitis C at the site of donation before being venesected, may be a more cost-effective way of ensuring safe blood and the results of ongoing studies are awaited.[8]

Clinical use of blood
Reasons for transfusion in poorer countries

In wealthy countries the majority of transfusions are planned and carried out electively. By contrast, in poorer countries, and particularly those where the malaria transmission rate is high, most transfusions are given for life-threatening emergencies. In these countries 50-80% of transfusions are administered to children predominantly for malaria-related anaemia. Transfusion can significantly reduce the mortality of children with severe anaemia but it may not have any benefit unless it is given within the first two days of hospital admission.[9] In areas of high HIV prevalence, young children have a relatively low risk of being infected with HIV and potentially have a long life expectancy. However, this is the age group which is predominantly affected by severe malaria-related anaemia and so they are particularly at risk of transfusion-acquired HIV infection.[10] Pregnant women are the second most common recipients of blood, particularly for haemorrhagic emergencies.[11,12] Other specialities which are significant users of blood are surgery, trauma and general medicine.

Avoiding unnecessary transfusions

Whether a patient needs a blood transfusion or not is ultimately a clinical decision. Emergency transfusions can be life saving for patients in whom the anaemia has developed too quickly to allow physiological compensation. Examples of such emergencies include severe malaria-related anaemia in children, and sudden, severe obstetric bleeding. In contrast, if the anaemia has developed slowly, such as that due to hookworm infestation or nutritional deficiency, patients can generally be managed conservatively by treating the cause of the anaemia and prescribing haematinic replacements. These should be continued for at least three months after the haemoglobin has returned to normal so that body stores can be replenished.

Guidelines for transfusion practice

It is possible to avoid unnecessary transfusions through the use of clinical transfusion guidelines and most institutions or organizations have developed guidelines to help clinicians make rational decisions about the use of blood transfusions (Table 14.2). Strict enforcement of a transfusion protocol in a Malawian hospital reduced the number of transfusions by 75% without any adverse effect on the mortality rate.[13] While the details may vary, the principles underlying most transfusion guidelines are similar and combine a clinical assessment of whether the patient is developing complications of inadequate oxygenation, with measurement of their haemoglobin. The haemoglobin level is used as a surrogate measure for

Table 14.2 Prescribing blood: a checklist for clinicians[1]

Always ask yourself the following questions before prescribing blood or blood products for a patient:
1. What improvement in the patient's clinical condition am I aiming to achieve?
2. Can I minimise blood loss to reduce this patient's need for transfusion?
3. Are there any other treatments I should give before making the decision to transfuse, such as intravenous replacement fluids or oxygen?
4. What are the specific clinical or laboratory indications for transfusion in this patient?
5. What are the risks of transmitting HIV, hepatitis, syphilis or other infectious agents through the blood products that are available for this patient?
6. Do the benefits of transfusion outweigh the risks for this particular patient?
7. What other options are there if no blood is available in time?
8. Will a trained person monitor this patient and respond immediately if any acute transfusion reactions occur?
9. Have I recorded my decision and reasons for transfusion on the patient's chart and the blood request form?
Finally, if in doubt ask yourself the following question: If this blood was for myself or my child, would I accept the transfusion under these circumstances?

intracellular oxygen concentration. Increasingly, transfusion guidelines are making use of evidence which shows that adequate oxygen delivery to the tissues can be achieved at haemoglobin levels that are significantly lower than the normal range.[14]

It is easier to develop guidelines than to ensure that they are used in routine practice. Implementation of transfusion guidelines is even more difficult if clinicians do not have confidence in the quality of haemoglobin measurements. It has been shown that when the quality of haemoglobin result is in doubt, clinicians will rely entirely on clinical judgement to guide transfusion practice. This may lead to significant numbers of inappropriate transfusions.[15] In a typical district hospital in Africa the cost of providing a unit of blood is approximately 40 times the cost of a quality-assured haemoglobin test. This demonstrates how a lack of investment in assuring the quality of a basic but critical test such as haemoglobin can result in a significant waste of resources downstream in the transfusion process, with the additional unnecessary exposure of recipients to the risk of transfusion-related infections.

Haemoglobin thresholds for transfusion

In resource-poor countries, the recommended haemoglobin threshold for transfusions is often well below that which would be accepted in more wealthy countries. For example, American anaesthetists suggest that transfusions are almost always indicated when the haemoglobin level is less than 6 g/dl,[16] whereas in Malawi transfusions are recommended for children with haemoglobin levels less than 4 g/dl providing there are no other clinical complications.[17] Complications such as cardiac failure or infection may necessitate transfusion at a higher haemoglobin level. Transfusion should be combined with adequate iron and folate replacements so that a normal haemoglobin count can be achieved during the weeks following transfusion.

Any transfusion service must be able to guarantee the quality of haemoglobin results. They are crucial in donor selection and are also used to guide the decision to transfuse patients. Although it is the most commonly performed test, accurate haemoglobin estimation is difficult to achieve in laboratories without automated blood analysers.[2,18] The reference technique for haemoglobin measurement is the haemiglobincyanide method.[19] Not only does this method need a constant electricity source for the spectrophotometer, but it also depends on the technicians having mathematical skills necessary to calculate dilutions and draw calibration curves, and on accuracy of dilutions that is difficult to achieve without automatic pipetting devices. In under-resourced countries district hospitals may use simpler, cheaper and less accurate methods of haemoglobin measurement, many of which are based on visual colour comparisons. While individual laboratories within poor countries may be registered with an external system to monitor the quality of laboratory tests, almost none has a nationwide programme. This means that for many laboratories and their users, the quality of tests, including haemoglobin and those used in the blood transfusion process, is unknown.

Complications of blood transfusion

Complications can occur immediately during transfusion, within a few hours of its completion, or be delayed for many years, as in the case of viral infections.

Acute and delayed haemolysis due to red cell incompatibility

Transfusion of blood into a recipient who possesses antibodies to the donor's red cells can cause an acute, and occasionally fatal, intravascular haemolysis. This could occur, for example, if group A cells are transfused into a group O recipient who has naturally occurring antibodies to group A cells. The profound haemolysis induces renal vasoconstriction and acute tubular necrosis. Treatment involves stopping the transfusion, cardiorespiratory support and inducing a brisk diuresis. In addition to abnormalities indicating renal failure, laboratory findings include haemoglobinuria and haemoglobinaemia. Proof of the diagnosis involves rechecking the whole transfusion process including all documentation stages, re-grouping the donor and the recipient, and screening for antibodies on red cells with a direct antiglobulin test. These tests are usually available in any hospital laboratory capable of providing a transfusion service. Delayed haemolysis has a similar physiological basis to acute intravascular haemolysis. The antibody–antigen reaction develops 7–10 days after the transfusion and it is less likely to present as a clinical emergency.

Bacterial contamination

Bacteria can enter the blood bag during venesection or if the bag is perforated at a later stage perhaps to reduce the volume for a paediatric recipient or during component preparation. Gram-negative bacteria, including *Pseudomonas* and *Yersinia,* grow optimally at refrigerator temperatures and infected blood may not necessarily appear abnormal. Reactions following infusion of infected blood are often due to endotoxins and may occur several hours after the transfusion has finished. Although these reactions are rare they can be severe and fatal. If bacterial contamination is suspected, the transfusion should be stopped and samples from the patient and the blood bag sent to the laboratory for culture. Cardiorespiratory support may be needed and broad-spectrum antibiotics should be started immediately and continued until culture results are available.

Non-haemolytic febrile reactions

These are episodes of fever (i.e., ≥1°C rise in temperature) and chills for which no other cause can be found. They are due to recipient's antibodies reacting against antigens present on the donor's white cells or platelets. These reactions are most common in patients who have received multiple transfusions in the past and have therefore been exposed to a broad range of antigens. Mild febrile reactions usually respond to simple anti-pyretics such as paracetamol. More severe reactions may be the first indication of a haemolytic transfusion reaction or bacterial contamination and should be investigated and managed accordingly.

Allergic reactions

These are due to infusion of plasma proteins and manifestations include erythema, rash, pruritus, bronchospasm and anaphylaxis. The transfusion should be stopped and the patient treated with antihistamines. If the reaction is mild and the symptoms and signs completely disappear, the transfusion can be re-started. If this type of mild reaction occurs repeatedly with more than one unit of blood, the red cells can be washed before transfusion. This should only be done if absolutely necessary as it carries the risk of introducing potentially fatal bacterial infection. Severe allergic reactions with evidence of systemic toxicity should be managed as acute anaphylaxis.

Circulatory overload

Blood should always be transfused slowly to avoid overloading the circulation unless the patient is actively and severely bleeding. Overload may be a particular problem when paediatric blood bags are not available as children may be over-transfused due to miscalculation of the required volume or inadvertent administration of an adult-sized unit of blood.

Transfusion-transmitted infections

In tropical practice, blood transmission of hepatitis B, HIV-1 and 2, and in some areas, American trypanosomiasis (Chagas' disease) is of particular concern. In general, transfusions are not the major route of transmission of these infections and they may not cause clinical problems until many months or years after the transfusion.

Haemosiderosis

Four units of blood contain the equivalent of the amount of iron stored in the bone marrow (approximately 1 g). Repeated transfusions for chronic haemolytic anaemia, as in thalassaemia major and sickle cell disease, lead to iron deposition in parenchymal cells. Eventually failure of the heart, liver and other organs supersede. Adequate doses of iron chelators, such as desferrioxamine or the newer oral chelator, deferiprone, are able to maintain acceptable iron balance in patients with chronic anaemia receiving regular transfusions.

Hypothermia

It is not usually necessary to warm blood unless rapid transfusion of large quantities is needed. This may lower the temperature of the sino-atrial node to below 30°C at which point ventricular fibrillation can occur. If blood needs to be warmed, an electric blood warmer specifically designed for the purpose should be used. This keeps the temperature below 38°C thereby avoiding the haemolysis associated with overheating blood.

Graft-versus-host disease

Graft-versus-host disease occurs when donor lymphocytes engraft in an immune suppressed recipient. The lymphocytes recognize the recipient's bone marrow as foreign and induce aplasia. Graft-versus-host disease is almost universally fatal and can be prevented by irradiating the donor blood, which inactivates the donor lymphocytes.

Reducing the use of transfusions
Minimizing surgical blood loss

Where blood is in short supply it is particularly important to ensure that the best anaesthetic and surgical techniques are used to minimize blood loss during surgery. Drugs which improve haemostasis or reduce fibrinolysis, such as aprotinin and Cyclokapron, and fibrin sealants, can be effective in reducing perioperative blood loss and hence the need for blood transfusion. Cost is a major limiting factor to the use of these therapies in poorer countries, and surgical blood loss is generally not a major contributor to the overall transfusion needs.

Autologous blood donation

Patients undergoing planned surgery who are likely to require a blood transfusion can have units of their own blood removed and stored prior to surgery for use by themselves only, if required.[20] Autologous donation requires careful organization: the surgeon needs to predict how much blood will be required, the patient has to be fit enough to withstand removal of one or more units of blood over the weeks preceding the surgery, and the surgery must take place within the shelf-life of the blood. As the blood has to be stored in the blood bank there is still a risk that they may receive blood which is not their own or that the blood may be bacterially infected.

Intra-operative blood salvage

This involves collecting surgical blood lost during the operation and re-infusing it into the patient either during or after surgery. Although this technique is practical and safe, and reduces the need for donor blood, it requires specialized equipment and training and is more expensive than routinely donated blood.[21]

Other methods

Normal saline or intravenous replacement fluids can be used judiciously in acute blood loss and in certain circumstances may be as effective as whole blood, red cells or plasma. Erythropoietin, which stimulates endogenous red cell production, has well-established uses in chronic anaemias such as those due to renal failure and cancer. Its delayed action makes it unsuitable for use in acute anaemias, the major reason for transfusions in poorer countries. The development of synthetic oxygen carriers, generally perfluorocarbons, has been fraught with problems and it is likely that they may only be useful for specific indications within intensive care units.[22]

In under-resourced countries, especially those with a heavy burden of malaria, the most effective way to avoid unnecessary transfusions is to reduce the prevalence of anaemia in the community. Studies on the ability and cost of combined interventions such as the provision of bed nets, nutritional supplements and antihelmintic drugs to children to prevent anaemia and reduce transfusion requirements, are yet to be done. When resources are very limited, governments may need to make some difficult decisions in order to achieve an equitable balance between investing in a transfusion service and improving public health.

REFERENCES

1   World Health Organisation. Blood Safety for too few. Press release WHO/25. 7 April 2000.
2   Mundy C, Bates I, Floyd K et al. District hospital laboratory services in an HIV endemic area in Malawi. Presented at International Society of Haematology, Durban 1999.
3   Provan D. Better blood transfusion. *Br Med J* 1999; 381: 1435–1436.

4   Hassall O, Bedu-Addo G, Adarkwa M et al. Feasibility of cord blood transfusions for severe paediatric anaemia in under-resourced countries. *Trans R Soc Trop Med Hyg* (abstract in press 2002).
5   European Commission. Safe blood in developing countries. European Commission. Edited by C Gerard, D Sondag-Thull, E J Watson-Williams & L Fransen. Published by European

Commissions, Brussels, 1995, 48.

6 Schutz R, Savarit D, Kadjo J-C et al. Excluding blood donors at high risk of HIV infection in a West African city. *Br Med J* 1993; 307: 1517–1519.

7 Schreiber G, Busch M, Kleinman S et al. The risk of transfusion-transmitted viral infections. *New Engl J Med* 1996; 334: 1685–1690.

8 Allain J-P, Adarkwa M, Sarkodie F et al. Pre-donation screening: improving cost-efficiency in resource poor, highly endemic areas. VIIth European Congress of the International Society of Blood Transfusion. Paris. In: *Transf Clin Biol* 2001; 8 suppl 1: S12.003.

9 Lackritz E, Campbell C, Ruebush T et al. Effect of blood transfusion on survival among children in a Kenyan hospital. *Lancet* 1992; 340: 524–528.

10 Shaffer N, Hedberg K, Davachi F et al. Trends and risk factors of HIV-1 seropositivity among outpatient children, Kinshasa, Zaire. *AIDS* 1990; 4: 1231-1236.

11 European Commission. Safe blood in developing countries. European Commission. Editied by C Gerard, D Sondag-Thull, E J Watson-Williams & L Fransen. Published by European Commissions, Brussels, 1995, 95.

12 Zucker J, Lackritz T, Ruebush T et al. Anaemia, blood transfusion practices, HIV and mortality among women of reproductive age in western Kenya. *Trans R Soc Trop Med Hyg* 1994; 88: 173–176.

13 Craighead J & Knowles J. Prevention of transfusion-associated HIV transmissions with the use of a transfusion for under 5s. *Trop Doc* 1993; 23: 59–61.

14 Weiskopf R, Viele M, Feiner J et al. Human cardiovascular and metabolic response to acute, severe isovolemic anemia. *J Am Med Assoc* 1998; 279: 217–221.

15 Bates I, Mundy C, Pendame R et al. Use of clinical judgement to guide administration of blood transfusions in Malawi. *Trans R Soc Trop Med Hyg* 2001; 95: 510–512.

16 American Society of Anesthesiologists Task Force. Practice guidelines for blood component therapy. *Anesthesiology* 1996; 84: 732–747.

17 Ministry of Health and Population, Malawi. AIDS control programme. Recommended guidelines for the practice of safe blood transfusion in Malawi, 1997.

18 Ministry of Health, Ghana. Regional Laboratory In-service Training. Programme. Workshop Report 4. June 2001

19 World Health Organisation. Methods recommended for essential clinical chemistry and haematological tests for intermediate hospital laboratories. *WHO/LAB/86.3*, 1986, 22–24.

20 Voak D, Finney R, Forman K et al. Guidelines for autologous transfusion. *Transf Med* 1997; 3:307–316.

21 Napier J, Bruce A, Chapman J et al. Guidelines for autologous transfusion. *Br J Anaesth* 1997; 78: 768–771.

22 Prowse C. Alternatives to standard blood transfusion: availability and promise. *Transfusion Medicine* 1999; 9: 287–299.

Chapter 15
Renal Disease in the Tropics

R. Thuraisingham and D. Adu

There are variations in the causes of renal diseases in different parts of the world and this is most marked between temperate and tropical regions. Even within tropical regions differences are seen in the pattern of renal diseases. The main factor that differentiates renal disease in the tropics from that in temperate regions of the world is the much higher frequency with an infectious aetiology. Much renal disease in the tropics is, however, idiopathic and similar to renal disease found elsewhere in the world. Whether caused by infections or not, the principles underlying the understanding of renal disease are the same in all parts of the world.

Glomerulonephritis

Glomerulonephritis is more common in the tropics than in temperate countries. It has been calculated that the incidence of nephrotic syndrome is 60–100 times higher in some tropical countries than in the USA and UK.[1] In tropical areas infections are a major cause of both acute and chronic glomerulonephritis. In most instances infection-induced acute glomerulonephritis resolves when the infection is cured, although glomerulonephritis resulting from chronic infection (e.g., malaria and schistosomiasis) is not reversed following measures that eradicate the infection.

Pathogenesis of infection-associated glomerulonephritis

The classical studies of Dixon et al.[2] established that glomerulonephritis could be induced in experimental animals following immunization with antigen. The development of glomerulonephritis coincided with the rise in specific antibody titres and the development of circulating immune complexes. Renal tissue studied by immunofluorescence showed glomerular mesangial or capillary wall deposits of immunoglobulin (Ig), complement and antigen. These studies provided the theoretical basis for the concept of immune complex-mediated glomerulonephritis. Subsequent studies, however, showed that it was difficult to induce a glomerulonephritis by the injection of preformed antigen–antibody complexes in 'naive' animals. It therefore seems unlikely that circulating immune complexes are important in the pathogenesis of glomerulonephritis. Other factors are likely to be responsible for the development of nephritis.[3] Cationic antigen or antibody is more likely to bind to the anionic surface of glomerular basement membrane and induce a glomerulonephritis. In situ antigen–antibody complexes formed following prior fixation of antigen or antibody to glomerular structures have been shown experimentally to lead to the development of a glomerulonephritis. Finally, some antibodies formed in response to non-renal antigens have been shown to bind to glomerular structures. Only a minority of individuals with a given infection develop a glomerulonephritis, demonstrating the importance of host factors in pathogenesis. Often with a single infecting organism a variety of glomerulonephritides is seen in different individuals (Table 15.1).

Classification

The most helpful classification is one based on aetiology

Table 15.1 Infection-associated glomerulonephritis.

Glomerulonephritis	Infection
Membranous nephropathy	Hepatitis B *Schistosoma mansoni* Leprosy *Loa loa* Syphilis
Mesangiocapillary glomerulonephritis	*Schistosoma mansoni* Leprosy *Loa loa* Onchocerciasis Tuberculosis Candidiasis
Focal segmental glomerulosclerosis	HIV *Schistosoma mansoni*
Proliferative glomerulonephritis	*Streptococcus* spp. *Staphylococcus* spp. *Schistosoma mansoni* Leprosy *Wuchereria bancrofti* Onchocerciasis Syphilis
Amyloid	Leprosy *Schistosoma mansoni*

Table 15.2 Clinical presentation of glomerulonephritis.

Persistent microscopic haematuria
Persistent proteinuria
Nephrotic syndrome
Acute nephritic syndrome
Acute renal failure
Chronic renal failure

and histology. The histological changes may be of unknown aetiology (idiopathic), or secondary to well-defined aetiological factors. The types and clinical features of idiopathic glomerulonephritis have been reviewed elsewhere.[4]

Clinical presentation

The ways in which glomerulonephritis may present are fairly limited and are summarized in Table 15.2. Patients with glomerulonephritis can present with asymptomatic proteinuria and/or haematuria, with proteinuria that is heavy enough to cause a nephrotic syndrome, with an acute nephritic syndrome which may be severe enough to cause acute renal failure, or with chronic renal failure.

Diagnosis

Definitive diagnosis of most forms of glomerulonephritis is dependent on a renal biopsy with careful interpretation of the renal histology in the light of clinical, biochemical and immunological features of the disorder.

Overview of management of glomerulonephritis

Conservative management of the nephrotic syndrome is with salt restriction, careful use of diuretics and of angiotensin converting enzyme inhibitors (ACEI). There is now good evidence that a reduction in blood pressure and in urine protein retards the rate at which renal function deteriorates. ACE inhibition is more effective than other hypotensive drugs in reducing proteinuria and the rate of decline in renal function in patients with a glomerulonephritis and proteinuria. There have been real improvements in the long-term prognosis of patients with a glomerulonephritis although the evidence base in terms of randomized controlled trials of therapy is small. The trials that have been done are few and often the numbers of patients in each trial are small. The treatment of glomerulonephritis is often with steroids and immuno-suppressants and these drugs have major toxicities which need to be offset against any benefit. The aims of treatment of glomerulonephritis are the induction of remission, the maintenance of remission and the prevention of progression of glomerular injury. Choice of treatment is based on the clinical syndrome as well as on the acuteness and hence potential reversibility of the glomerular lesion and the extent of scarring which is irreversible.

Pattern of glomerular disease in the tropics

This has been reviewed by Chugh and Sakhuja.[5] In most tropical countries primary glomerular diseases are more common than secondary glomerular disease. In Jamaica, however, 54% of patients with a nephrotic syndrome have secondary glomerular disease, usually lupus nephritis.[6] In Zimbabwe, 80% of children with a nephrotic syndrome have hepatitis B or streptococcal infection[7] although in a later study these aetiologies were uncommon.[8] This emphasizes the point that the aeti-pathogenesis of glomerulonephritis in tropical countries does seem to be changing. Over the last two decades there have been only infrequent reports of quartan malarial nephropathy, which had been a common cause of the nephrotic syndrome in children in Nigeria and Uganda.[9] In Ghana, Kenya, the Indian subcontinent and South-East Asia, however, 70–90% of adults with a nephrotic syndrome have a primary glomerular disease.[10–16] Indeed there is now increasing evidence that idiopathic glomerulonephritis is common in tropical countries, making the diagnosis and treatment of these disorders important.

Idiopathic glomerulonephritis

Minimal change nephropathy

This is uncommon in tropical Africa, where it is found in between 4% and 30% of cases.[7–9,13,15] Seventy-seven per cent of children in India with a nephrotic syndrome have minimal change nephropathy, an incidence comparable with that seen in Europe and North America.[14] The glomeruli are normal on light microscopy and there are no glomerular deposits of immunoglobulin and complement.

Management
Children
The standard treatment is with prednisolone $60 \, mg/m^2$ per day for 4 weeks and then $40 \, mg/m^2$ per day for 4 weeks. Of children treated in this way 94% go into remission within 8 weeks. The major problem is that approximately 40–50% of patients develop a frequently relapsing course requiring repeated courses of steroids. A longer initial course of steroids (12 weeks) leads to a lower relapse rate but is accompanied by greater toxicity. In frequent relapsers an 8-week course of cyclophosphamide (2 mg/kg) will lead to a sustained remission in 30–60% of patients for up to 5 years. Patients who run a frequently relapsing course after cyclophosphamide treatment often respond to cyclosporin A (to maintain blood levels of 100 ng/litre) but the remission induced is not long lasting and cyclosporin A is nephrotoxic.[4] In a controlled study levamisole provided marginal benefit but can cause leucopenia. The long-term prognosis for renal function in minimal change nephropathy is excellent.

Adults

Adults with minimal change nephropathy go into remission more slowly and less completely than children and at 6 months only 75% are in remission. Adults therefore require a longer period of treatment than children. Fewer adults than children run a frequently relapsing course, and when they do the response to cyclophosphamide is better.

Focal segmental glomerulosclerosis

This is particularly common in Ghana,[11] Senegal,[17] Zaire[18] and South Africa.[19] Renal biopsies from the patients described in Senegal had an unusual fibrillary splitting of glomerular capillary walls with interposition of basement membrane-like material. Immunohistochemistry reveals deposits of IgM and C3 in sclerosed areas.

Management

Focal segmental sclerosing glomerular lesions are seen in a wide range of disorders in which there is proteinuria and/or haematuria with or without renal impairment. Some patients with an idiopathic nephrotic syndrome have renal biopsies that show segmental areas of glomerular sclerosis with IgM and C3 deposits. There is now good, although uncontrolled evidence that the nephrotic syndrome in 30% of such patients will go into remission with steroids and, of importance, the long-term prognosis for renal function in such patients is good. By contrast, of the patients who do not respond to steroids, 50% develop end-stage renal failure over a period of 5–8 years. Several uncontrolled studies suggest that more intensive treatment with alkylating agents (chlorambucil and cyclophosphamide) as well as steroids increases the proportion of patients going into remission. In the absence of controlled trials and with the toxicity of alkylating agents this treatment cannot be recommended.

Membranous nephropathy

This is common in children in Zimbabwe,[7] Namibia[20] and South Africa,[21,22] and also in adults in Sudan[15] and Pakistan.[16] In both Africa and Asia it is frequently a complication of hepatitis B infection. The glomerular basement membranes are uniformly thickened in membranous nephropathy with regular spikes on the epithelial side when stained with periodic acid–methenamine silver. Immunohistology shows uniform granular deposition of IgG and complement on the epithelial side of glomerular basement membranes.

Management

About 70% of patients with membranous nephropathy and a nephrotic syndrome survive free of end-stage renal failure at 10 years. Therefore any therapy that benefits the 30% of patients who develop renal failure exposes the other 70% to unnecessary toxicity. The evidence from randomized controlled trials is that prednisolone on its own is not effective in inducing remission of the nephrotic syndrome or reducing the development of end-stage renal failure in membranous nephropathy. A regime of treatment at alternating months of prednisolone and chlorambucil or cyclophosphamide has been shown to be significantly more effective in inducing remission of the nephrotic syndrome, and probably improving renal survival, than prednisolone alone or no treatment. A small-scale study suggested that cyclosporin A might play a role in reducing the rate of decline of renal function in high-risk patients. It remains to be established whether any of these treatment options are of benefit in patients with membranous nephropathy whose renal function is deteriorating. Treatment of patients with membranous nephropathy and a nephrotic syndrome requires a careful trade-off between likely benefit and toxicity.

Mesangiocapillary glomerulonephritis

This has been described in Indonesia, India, Ghana and Nigeria, and may be idiopathic but is also commonly seen in postinfectious glomerulonephritis.[5] Most cases of mesangiocapillary glomerulonephritis (MCGN) in the tropics are of the Type I (subendothelial) variety. Here immunohistology reveals subendothelial deposits of IgG and less frequently of IgM and IgA and C3. In Type II MCGN (dense-deposit disease), basement membrane and mesangial deposits of C3 are found.

Management

Approximately 40% of patients with MCGN go into renal failure over a period of 10 years. In one study, children with MCGN who were treated with prednisone ($40\,\text{mg/m}^2$ on alternate days for a mean of 41 months) had less deterioration of renal function than those treated with placebo but the difference was not significant. In other studies adults with MCGN were treated with different combinations of cyclophosphamide, anticoagulants, dipyridamole or aspirin with no convincing evidence of benefit. At present no treatment can be recommended for the management of MCGN.

IgA nephropathy

This is common in Singapore, Malaysia, Hong Kong and Taiwan; in Singapore 75% of patients with more than 1 g of proteinuria per 24 hours have IgA nephropathy.[10,23] IgA nephropathy is, however, uncommon in blacks in Africa.[24] Renal histology is characterized by the presence of diffuse mesangial deposits of IgA and C3.

Management

Between 20% and 30% of patients with IgA nephropathy will develop end-stage renal failure by 20 years. Adverse prognostic features for renal function include proteinuria in excess of 1.0 g per 24 hours, renal impairment at the time of diagnosis and possibly hypertension. The options for treatment of patients with IgA nephropathy, and proteinuria > 1.0 g/24 hours and serum creatinine < 250 μmol/litre are (a) supportive treatment only with ACE inhibitors, (b) prednisolone (methylprednisolone 1 g intravenously daily for 3 days at 0, 2 and 4 months and oral prednisolone 0.5 mg/kg on alternate days for 6 months, or (c) fish-oil (MaxEPA) 6 g twice daily for 2 years. Further randomized clinical trials are necessary to establish the effectiveness of these treatments.

Mesangial IgM proliferative glomerulonephritis

Mesangial IgM proliferative glomerulonephritis is a major cause of the nephrotic syndrome in Thailand and other parts of South-East Asia[25] and in parts of Africa.[8] This type of glomerulonephritis can also present with asymptomatic proteinuria and haematuria.

Secondary glomerulonephritis

Systemic lupus erythematosus

Lupus nephritis is common in Malaysia and Singapore and other parts of South-East Asia, and in these areas is found mostly in people of Chinese origin.[26] Lupus nephritis is also common in Jamaica[6] and also in black Americans but is relatively uncommon in blacks in Africa.[11,27] Clinically apparent nephritis develops in about 40–75% of patients with systemic lupus erythematosus. The renal manifestations of lupus nephritis are heterogeneous both in clinical presentation and in histology. Patients with minimal changes or mesangial glomerulonephritis (WHO Class I and II lesions) usually have an inherently low rate of progressive renal failure. Patients with membranous nephropathy (WHO Class V) have an intermediate prognosis for renal function. In contrast, patients with focal or diffuse proliferative glomerulonephritis (WHO Classes III and IV) have a high risk of progressive renal failure.

Management
Lupus mesangial proliferative glomerulonephritis
In the absence of controlled trials to guide treatment, it is reasonable to treat such patients with corticosteroids in the hope that this will prevent progression to a more severe glomerulonephritis, although that is not certain.

Lupus membranous nephropathy
Here again there are no controlled trials of treatment and thus there is no consensus on treatment. Patients with pure lupus membranous nephropathy will respond to treatment with prednisolone only and azathioprine may be used as a steroid sparing agent in these patients. Patients with lupus membranous nephropathy and proliferative glomerulonephritis lesions are at high risk of developing progressive renal failure and should be treated as for patients with a proliferative lupus nephritis.

Focal and diffuse lupus proliferative glomerulonephritis
There is now good evidence from meta-analyses of randomized controlled trials that the addition of cyclophosphamide to prednisolone confers benefit when compared with patients treated with prednisolone alone. The evidence that azathioprine confers such benefit is less good although this agent may have a role in maintaining remission. A series of clinical trials from the National Institutes of Health (NIH) provided evidence of the effectiveness of intermittent intravenous cyclophosphamide together with oral prednisolone in preserving renal function in patients with severe lupus nephritis. This regime is preferable to continuous oral cyclophosphamide as it has less bladder toxicity, although the frequency of gonadal toxicity is unaffected. It is not yet known whether pulse cyclophosphamide is less carcinogenic than continuous oral therapy. From the NIH data, monthly pulse cyclophosphamide (0.5–0.75 g/m^2) adjusted for the glomerular filtration rate and leucocyte count at 10–14 days is given monthly for the first 6 months, then quarterly for 18–24 months. The longer course of cyclophosphamide was associated with fewer relapses than a shorter 6-month course but carries a higher rate of gonadal toxicity. The risk of bladder toxicity with intravenous cyclophosphamide is reduced by hydration and the administration of mesna. Prednisolone is given together with the cyclophosphamide at an initial dose of (0.5–1 mg/kg per day) for 6–8 weeks with gradual tapering, preferably to an alternate-day regime to minimize toxicity.

Controlled trials of plasmapheresis in patients with all types of proliferative lupus glomerulonephritis showed no benefit over treatment with prednisolone and immunosuppressants alone and this cannot be recommended.

Crescentic glomerulonephritis
Most renal biopsy series from the tropics report that between 4% and 7% of patients have a crescentic glomerulonephritis with extracapillary proliferation. This is seen in a wide variety of disorders, including poststreptococcal glomerulonephritis, hepatitis B and C-associated glomerulonephritis, microscopic polyarteritis (polyangiitis), Wegener's granulomatosis and lupus nephritis. The importance a crescentic glomerulonephritis is that it is usually associated with a rapid decline in renal function. Treatment is usually with prednisolone and cyclophosphamide.

Infection-associated glomerulonephritis

Acute endocapillary proliferative glomerulonephritis

The most common cause of acute proliferative glomerulonephritis (APGN) is an infection with group A streptococci. This is common in Africa,[7] the Caribbean countries[28] and in India.[29] A similar type of glomerulonephritis has been reported with other bacteria in patients with infective endocarditis, shunt nephritis and visceral abscesses. APGN commonly develops 1–2 weeks after a streptococcal pharyngitis and 3–6 weeks after a skin infection (impetigo). With both sites of infection the risk of an ensuing glomerulonephritis is higher in children aged between 2 and 12 years. APGN has become quite rare in Western countries but epidemic outbreaks following skin infections with streptococci still occur in tropical countries.[30]

Pathogenesis

Only certain M types (cell wall protein antigens) of Lancefield group A streptococcal infections are followed by the development of glomerulonephritis. This is an immune-mediated nephritis and would by convention be termed an immune complex nephritis. The frequent observation of hypocomplementaemia fits in with antigen–antibody-mediated nephritis. The candidate 'nephritogenic' antigen is as yet not known. Some studies have suggested that this is a soluble water-extractable antigen called endostreptosin. Other studies have suggested that M proteins or M-associated proteins may be pathogenic antigens, and in yet others a cationic streptococcal proteinase has been suggested. The sera of patients with poststreptococcal glomerulonephritis also contain rheumatoid factors and antinuclear antibodies and the role of these autoantibodies in the pathogenesis of the nephritis is unclear.

Pathology

This is the classical endocapillary proliferative glomerulonephritis. There is increased hypercellularity of glomeruli from mesangial proliferation and an influx of polymorphonuclear leucocytes, monocytes and T lymphocytes (Figure 15.1). Subepithelial humps on electron microscopy are characteristic of this disorder. Extracapillary proliferation (crescents) is infrequent. Renal biopsies show deposits of C3, IgG and sometimes IgM in the glomerular mesangium and also large sub-epithelial deposits (humps) on immunofluorescence and electron microscopy.

Serology

Antibodies to various streptococcal antigens form the basis of diagnosis in culture-negative cases: after pharyngitis 95% of children will have an antibody response to streptolysin O, deoxyribonuclease, deoxyribonuclease B,

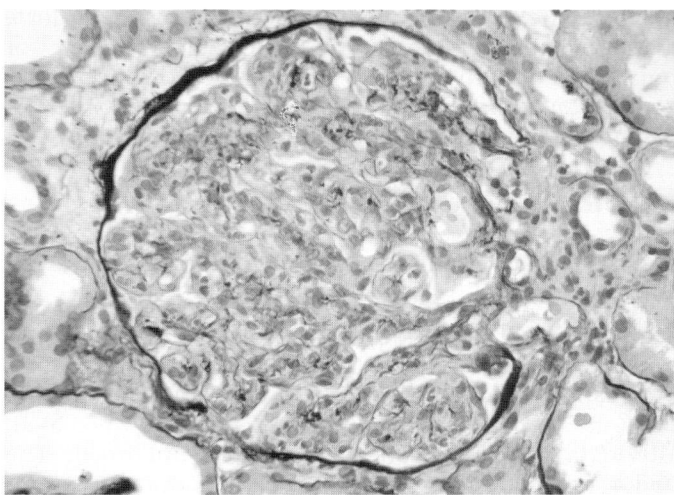

Figure 15.1: Acute postinfective glomerulonephritis. Acute nephritic syndrome: solid-looking tuft filled with neutrophil polymorphs. (Courtesy of A. J. Howie.)

hyaluronidase and streptokinase. After pyoderma antibody responses to deoxyribonuclease B are found, while responses to streptolysin O are infrequent.

Clinical

The clinical presentation ranges from asymptomatic haematuria and proteinuria, through an acute nephritic syndrome, at times accompanied by a nephrotic syndrome, and rarely a rapidly progressive glomerulonephritis. The patient with an acute nephritic syndrome presents with oliguria, reddish-brown urine due to haematuria, proteinuria, a puffy face and ankle oedema, and this is often accompanied by hypertension. Hypertension and cardiac failure are usually due to salt and water overload. Headache, vomiting and fits may complicate the rise in blood pressure. A full-blown nephrotic syndrome is infrequent and acute renal failure from extracapillary glomerulonephritis is rare, being found in less than 2% of affected children.

Management

All patients should be given a 10-day course of penicillin or erythromycin to eradicate the organism and prevent secondary spread, although this treatment has no effect on the outcome of the renal illness. The management of the acute nephritic illness is based on conventional treatment, with meticulous attention to fluid balance, together with diuretics and hypotensive drug therapy as necessary. Rarely there may be the development of a crescentic glomerulonephritis and if renal failure is severe then treatment with prednisolone and cyclophosphamide should be considered.

Outcome

The long-term prognosis of poststreptococcal glomerulo-nephritis is good and there are few reports of end-stage chronic renal failure as a long-term sequel. Long-term prospective studies of epidemic poststreptococcal glomerulonephritis following skin infection showed little evidence of progressive chronic renal failure or hypertension. Other studies of sporadic postpharyngitic glomerulonephritis, however, showed that up to 50% of patients have some evidence of chronic renal damage.[20]

Hepatitis B infection and renal disease[31,32]

The renal complications of hepatitis B infection are found mainly in individuals who are chronically infected. The observation by immunological techniques of hepatitis B antigen or its antibody in glomeruli strongly suggests that the renal injury is immune mediated, although the precise mechanisms are unknown. The major renal lesions of hepatitis B infection are membranous nephropathy, which is more common in children, and less commonly a mesangiocapillary glomerulonephritis, IgA nephropathy (more common in adults) and polyarteritis.

Hepatitis B-associated membranous nephropathy

This is seen particularly in children who are chronic carriers of hepatitis B virus. The frequency of hepatitis B as a cause of membranous nephropathy parallels the general carrier rate of this virus in the population. Between 60% and 100% of children with membranous nephropathy in Japan, Hong Kong, South Africa and Zimbabwe have HBsAg,[5,7,21,22,32] and by contrast this is infrequent in the USA and the UK. In children the age of onset is between 2 and 12 years, and over 80% of affected children are male. The clinical presentation is usually with a nephrotic syndrome. Most affected children have no clinical evidence of liver disease; this is more common in adults.

Serology

Sera from almost all patients with hepatitis B-associated membranous nephropathy show evidence of infection in the form of HB_sAg, HB_c antibodies, HB_eAg, and HB_e antibodies.

Pathology

The histological lesion of hepatitis B-associated membranous nephropathy differs from the idiopathic variety in that in addition to subepithelial immune deposits there are often subendothelial and mesangial deposits. Glomerular capillary deposits of the hepatitis B antigens HB_sAg, HB_cAg and HB_eAg have been demonstrated in renal biopsies.

Management and outcome

There is no treatment of proven benefit in hepatitis B-associated membranous nephropathy. There is no evidence that corticosteroids are beneficial and indeed their use and withdrawal may lead to rebound hepatitis. The antiviral agents interferon α and lamivudine may be of benefit in this disorder but there are no controlled trials of treatment. The prognosis in children is good, with reported spontaneous remissions of the nephrotic syndrome in up to two-thirds of cases. Approximately 5% of children progress to end-stage renal failure, while adults fare worse with 10% developing renal failure. Vaccination of all neonates has been shown to reduce the rate of hepatitis B carriage and hepatitis B-associated glomerulonephritis.

Hepatitis B-associated polyarteritis nodosa

HBsAg has been reported in 10–40% of patients in the USA, 18–50% of patients in France and 4–8% of patients in the UK who have classical polyarteritis. This association is uncommon in tropical countries.

Hepatitis C-associated nephropathy

Hepatitis C virus infection is found in less than 0.6% of the population of North America and Northern Europe but is more common in southern Europe and Africa and has a high prevalence in haemophiliacs and intravenous drug abusers. Hepatitis C infection may lead to chronic active hepatitis and cirrhosis. Hepatitis C infection is the main cause of mixed essential cryoglobulinaemia. The clinical presentation is with a fever, purpuric rash, arthralgia and peripheral neuropathy. The renal presentation is with proteinuria or a nephrotic syndrome often accompanied by mild to moderate renal impairment.[33]

Pathology

The renal lesion in cryoglobulinaemic glomerulonephritis is a type of membranoproliferative glomerulonephritis characterized by intraluminal and subendothelial deposits (Figure 15.2) but other types of glomerulonephritis, e.g., a mesangioproliferative glomerulonephritis, has been reported and rarely there is a renal arteritis. Immunofluorescent microscopy shows subendothelial as well as mesangial and capillary wall deposits of IgM, IgG and C3. On electron microscopy these deposits may show the characteristics of cryoglobulins.

Management

Treatment with interferon α improves proteinuria and possibly renal function in patients with hepatitis C-associated mesangiocapillary glomerulonephritis although renal disease and viraemia mostly relapse after cessation of therapy. Treatment of acute cryoglobulinaemic glomerulonephritis and vasculitis has usually been with prednisolone and cyclophosphamide. Interpretation of

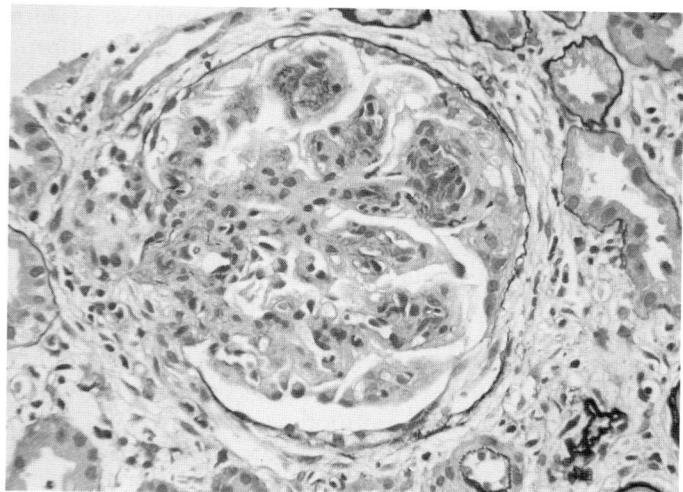

Figure 15.2: Glomerulus showing changes associated with hepatitis C infection and cryoglobulinaemia. There is the appearance of subendothelial membranoproliferative/mesangiocapillary glomerulonephritis with an acute segmental lesion of vasculitic type. (Courtesy of A. J. Howie.)

these studies of treatment is complicated by the lack of controlled studies and also by the fact that many of these studies were performed prior to the recognition of the role of HCV infection in the pathogenesis of mixed cryoglobulinaemia. Plasma exchange reduces cryoglobulin and immune complex levels and has been reported to lead to an improvement of renal function. However, the effects are usually temporary, since depletion of cryoglobulins leads to rapid rebound immunoglobulin synthesis.

Human immunodeficiency virus-associated glomerulonephritis[34]

A variety of renal disorders occur in patients with HIV infection. Acute deterioration of renal function may develop as a result of volume depletion from renal salt wasting or from diarrhoea and vomiting. In addition, some of the antiviral drugs used in therapy are potentially nephrotoxic, as are some of the drugs used to treat opportunistic infections. In addition there may be renal disease from coexistent hepatitis B or C infection, postinfectious glomerulonephritis or an IgA nephropathy. A major clinical problem in these patients is the development of proteinuria, a nephrotic syndrome and renal impairment.[35] This complication appears to be more common in the USA than in Europe and affects blacks predominantly. There is little data from Africa but HIV-associated nephropathy has been reported from South Africa and from the Ivory Coast.[36,37] HIV-associated nephropathy appears to be uncommon in Asia.[38]

Clinical presentation

The clinical presentation is with a nephrotic syndrome

and renal impairment. Hypertension is uncommon and ultrasound examination shows large echogenic kidneys. The clinical evolution in patients with HIV-associated collapsing glomerulopathy is with rapid evolution to end-stage renal failure within weeks to months.

Pathology

Collapsing glomerulopathy was initially described in patients with HIV-associated nephropathy, where it was associated with a severe nephrotic syndrome and rapid progression to end-stage renal failure. The characteristic histological lesion in HIV glomerulonephritis is a type of focal segmental sclerosing glomerulonephritis characterized by segmental or global collapse of glomerular capillaries with basement membrane wrinkling and crowding of glomerular epithelial cells (Figure 15.3). There is often a marked interstitial infiltrate of lymphocytes and plasma cells with microcysts. In addition there are endothelial tubuloreticular inclusions. On immunofluorescent microscopy mesangial and capillary wall deposits of IgM and C3 are seen. Collapsing glomerulopathy may also be seen in patients without HIV infection and here an association has been described with parvovirus B19 infection.

Management

There is as yet no proven evidence of benefit from treatment with combined highly active antiretroviral agents, although this has not been systematically studied. Some studies suggested benefits from the use of steroids but this cannot be recommended because of the risks of infection. As with other proteinuric renal diseases there is evidence that treatment with ACEI may be of long-term benefit. Patients with HIV infection and end-stage renal failure have been treated with chronic haemodialysis with benefit.

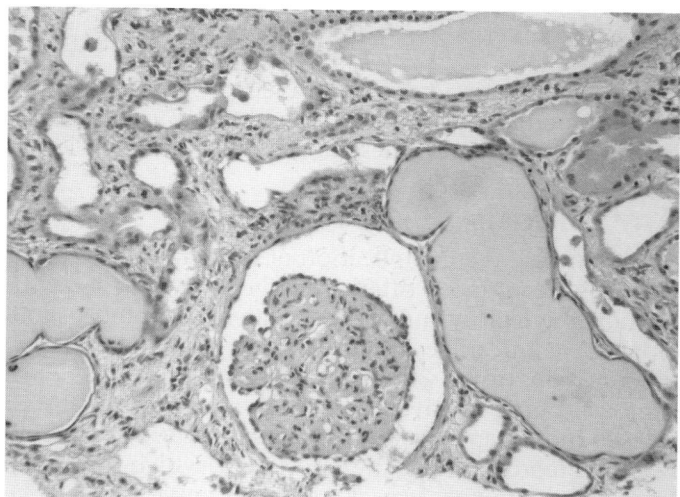

Figure 15.3: Renal cortex in HIV nephropathy. Tubules are dilated and contain casts. Glomeruli have changes of collapsing glomerulopathy. (Courtesy of A. J. Howie.)

Schistosomiasis (See also Chapter 80)

Schistosomiasis is widespread in the tropics. *Schistosoma haematobium* affects the urinary tract, and *S. mansoni* and *S. japonicum* the intestine(s) and liver. Significant glomerular disease has been reported only in patients with *S. mansoni* infection and hepatosplenic disease.[39,40] Overall just under 5% of patients with *S. mansoni* infection have hepatosplenic disease, and of these about 10–15% develop glomerular lesions over a period of up to 10 years. The clinical presentation is with proteinuria or nephrotic syndrome. In Egypt there is evidence that schistosomal glomerulonephritis is more common in individuals with concomitant chronic infections with *Salmonella* species.[41]

Pathology

A mesangial proliferative glomerulonephritis is seen in mild or early cases and the most common histological change in advanced cases is a mesangiocapillary glomerulonephritis, seen in about 50% of patients. The next most frequently seen histological lesion is a focal segmental glomerulosclerosis. There are also infrequent reports of a membranous nephropathy and a proliferative glomerulonephritis. Immunofluorescent microscopy of renal biopsies shows granular deposits, predominantly of IgM but also of IgG, IgA, IgE and C3 in the mesangium and the subepithelial and subendothelial sites. Renal amyloidosis has been described in patients with *S. mansoni* infection in Sudan and in Egypt.[42]

Management

Treatment of schistosomal glomerulonephritis with antischistosomal drugs, prednisolone and cyclophospamide has been of no benefit and progression to renal failure is usual.

Leprosy (See also Chapter 59)

The major renal lesions found in leprosy are amyloidosis and glomerulonephritis, although chronic interstitial nephritis has also been described.

Amyloidosis

Renal amyloid is a complication of long-standing leprosy and has been most often described in patients with lepromatous leprosy and rarely in patients with tuberculoid leprosy.[43,44] In earlier autopsy studies, renal amyloid was described in up to 30% of cases in North and South America, but is relatively uncommon (less than 10% of cases in India, Papua New Guinea and Africa). The amyloid fibrils in leprosy are of the AA variety, which is derived from the acute-phase reactant serum amyloid A (SAA). Serum levels of SAA rise in patients with erythema nodosum leprosum (ENL) reactions and there are suggestions that amyloidosis is more common in patients with recurrent ENL.[43] The clinical presentation is with proteinuria, microscopic haematuria and the nephrotic syndrome, and progression to renal failure is common.

Glomerulonephritis

Glomerulonephritis is found in up to 10% of patients with leprosy at autopsy. It tends to be more common in patients with lepromatous than with tuberculoid leprosy, and the onset of glomerulonephritis may coincide with an episode of ENL. The most common glomerular lesions are a mesangial proliferative glomerulonephritis and a focal or diffuse proliferative glomerulonephritis. Rarely a membranous nephropathy or mesangiocapillary glomerulonephritis is seen. Immunofluorescent microscopy shows granular glomerular deposits of IgG, IgM and C3 in the mesangium or on capillary walls.[44,45] The renal disease progresses to renal failure and it is unclear whether treatment for leprosy influences progression.

Filariasis

There are several reports of an association between filariasis and glomerulonephritis from India and Cameroon.[46,47] The clinical presentation is usually with nephrotic syndrome and rarely with an acute nephritic syndrome. Patients with *Wuchereria bancrofti* infection may develop a mesangial proliferative or a diffuse proliferative glomerulonephritis.[46] In patients with *Loa loa* infections a membranous and a mesangiocapillary glomerulonephritis have been reported. Onchocerciasis infections have been reported to be associated with a nephrotic syndrome due to minimal-change nephropathy, mesangial proliferative glomerulonephritis and a mesangiocapillary glomerulonephritis.[46]

Pathology

On immunofluorescent microscopy glomerular deposits of IgG, IgM and C3 are seen in the mesangium and capillary walls, and in one study onchocercal antigens were identified on glomerular capillaries.

Management

Treatment with diethylcarbamazine probably hastens recovery in those patients with an acute nephritic presentation but has no effect in patients presenting with nephrotic syndrome.

Malaria (See also Chapter 71)

Malaria is widespread in the tropics and is a major cause of death. In the 1930s in British Guyana Giglioli[48] established the long-suspected association between *Plasmodium malariae* infection and a nephrotic syndrome. Proteinuria, nephritis and deaths from nephritis were common in British Guyana. Patients with nephrotic syndrome in this area had a higher incidence of *P. malariae* parasitaemia than unaffected individuals, who more often had *P. vivax* and *P. falciparum* infection. In 1962 Giglioli[49] summarized his observations that following eradication of malaria from British Guiana there was a reduction in the incidence of proteinuria and nephritis and deaths from malaria.

Quartan malarial nephropathy

The association between *P. malariae* infection and glomerulonephritis was confirmed by clinicopathological studies from Nigeria and Uganda in children with nephrotic syndrome. These children mostly had an incidence of *P. malariae* parasitaemia (up to 88% of children) that was significantly higher than in healthy controls (20%).[1,50,51] There have, however, been few recent reports of quartan malarial nephropathy from tropical Africa.

Sickle cell disease[52,53]

Patients with sickle cell disease often have an impaired ability to concentrate and acidify urine and to excrete a potassium load but these changes are minor and usually of no clinical significance. Glomerular filtration rate (GFR) and effective renal plasma flow are increased in children with sickle disease and it is suggested that the increased GFR may lead to glomerular damage in later life.

Haematuria

Microscopic haematuria is common in patients with both sickle cell disease and trait, and less commonly macroscopic haematuria, that may be persistent, is seen. The management is with conservative measures only. It is worthwhile screening for other causes of haematuria in these patients, e.g., schistosomiasis.

Renal papillary necrosis

This is found in both sickle cell disease and sickle cell trait. The clinical presentation is with haematuria that on occasion may be complicated by clot colic. Diagnosis is confirmed by intravenous pyelography, showing changes ranging from clubbing of calyces to a ring sign in which an often calcified, partly attached papilla is surrounded by a ring of contrast.

Glomerulonephritis
Focal segmental glomerulosclerosis[54]
This is the most frequently described lesion. It is found in older patients, usually aged over 30 years. The incidence of this lesion is unclear. Histologically the glomeruli are larger than normal and show segmental areas of glomerular sclerosis. Because the GFR is raised in early life in patients with sickle cell disease, it has been suggested that the segmental sclerosis is a consequence of hyperfiltration and intraglomerular hypertension. The clinical presen-

tation is with proteinuria and the clinical course is with progressive renal impairment. The proteinuria reduces with treatment with angiotensin converting inhibitors and it is possible that these agents, by reducing intraglomerular pressures, might reduce the rate at which renal function declines.

Mesangiocapillary glomerulonephritis[55]
The second most commonly described lesion in patients with sickle cell anaemia and proteinuria is a mesangiocapillary glomerulonephritis. The pathogenesis of this is unclear and suggestions that it is caused by the glomerular deposition of renal tubular epithelial cell antibodies and antigen await confirmation.

Acute proliferative glomerulonephritis[52]
An increased predisposition to poststreptococcal glomerulonephritis from infected leg ulcers has also been reported in older patients with sickle cell anaemia.

End-stage renal failure in sickle cell anaemia
Both continuous ambulatory peritoneal dialysis and haemodialysis have been successfully used in these patients. Anaemia is a major problem and is not helped by erythropoietin which, by increasing the levels of sickle haemoglobin, may worsen the clinical condition. Patients with sickle cell anaemia have had successful renal transplants. It is necessary to perform exchange transfusion with AA blood prior to transplantation to prevent sickling of the renal graft.

Acute renal failure[56,57]

Acute renal failure complicates a wide variety of diseases. The abrupt cessation of renal function leads to uraemia, with abnormalities of fluid and electrolyte balance. The persistently high mortality in these patients leaves no room for complacency in management. Patients with acute renal failure do not necessarily present in neat diagnostic categories but more often as unexplained acute uraemic emergencies. Investigation, diagnosis and initial management must often be compressed into a few hours. The priorities in this early phase are to manage acute uraemia and electrolyte abnormalities, in particular hyperkalaemia, to establish the reversibility of the renal failure and to define its cause.

Causes of acute uraemia

The main cause of acute renal failure in the tropics is acute tubular necrosis, often as a result of infection, with glomerulonephritis presenting less commonly. Of all cases of acute renal failure in the tropics, 60% have a medical cause, 25% a surgical cause and 15% an obstetric cause.[58,59] In the more developed areas the pattern is akin to that found in the West,[60] where medical and surgical causes predominate and obstetric cases are rare.[61] The

Table 15.3 Causes of acute renal failure.

Prerenal
Renal hypoperfusion (leading to acute tubular necrosis)
Hypovolaemia
Septicaemia
Obstetric accidents
Massive intravascular necrosis
Rhabdomyolysis
Renal
Acute tubular necrosis
Acute interstitial nephritis
Diffuse extracapillary glomerulonephritis
Acute pyelonephritis
Nephrotoxins
Haemolytic–uraemic syndrome
Postrenal
Obstructive uropathy
Renal tubule blockage
Myeloma (light chains)
Uric acid, sulfadiazine
Bilateral urinary tract blockage
Calculi
Schistosoma haematobium
Urethral stricture
Prostatic hypertrophy
Pelvic malignancy
Posterior urethral valves

differences in aetiology are largely dependent on socio-economic factors and the availability of abortion services. The classification of the causes of acute renal failure into prerenal, intrinsic and postrenal categories remains clinically useful in that it allows a structured approach to diagnosis and management. In an Egyptian series 38% had prerenal, 24% postrenal and the rest intrinsic renal disease as a cause of their acute renal failure.[62] The major causes of acute renal failure are summarized in Table 15.3. This list is not exhaustive and is meant to emphasize the importance of seeking an aetiology in a patient with unexplained acute renal failure.

Clinical syndromes

Acute tubular necrosis

A variety of infections and hypovolaemia may lead to renal ischaemia with renal vasoconstriction and tubular cell damage with a reduction in GFR. In addition there may be tubular obstruction and back-leakage of filtrate. A similar outcome may be the result of nephrotoxic drugs, such as aminoglycosides, and also traditional herbal remedies. There has been considerable research into the mediators involved in this injurious process. Nitric oxide, oxygen radicals, endothelin and free iron have all been implicated. To date there has been little convincing data to suggest that manipulation of these systems improves

outcome, although some preliminary studies have shown N-acetylcysteine to be beneficial in a nephrotoxic model of acute tubular necrosis (radio contrast-induced acute renal failure).[63]

The clinical consequence of acute tubular necrosis is uraemia, which is usually associated with oliguria, although some patients may be non-oliguric, producing urine volumes of 1–2 litres or higher. In the vast majority of cases acute tubular necrosis is self-limiting and with spontaneous recovery occurring between 10 days and 6 weeks provided the initial insult is treated. When the initial insult is very severe, cortical necrosis may occur, leading to irreversible renal failure.

Renal parenchymal causes

Acute glomerulonephritis, especially when accompanied by extracapillary proliferation (crescent formation), may lead to acute renal failure. Acute interstitial nephritis is seen in leptospirosis and may also be a complication of drugs such as the penicillins, sulfonamides, thiazide diuretics and frusemide as well as non-steroidal anti-inflammatory drugs.

Obstructive uropathy

Obstruction to the urinary tract is important because it is a common and potentially reversible cause of acute renal failure. The most common site of obstruction is at the bladder outlet due to prostatic hypertrophy or cancer, and urethral stricture. Urethral stricture is particularly common in tropical Africa.[64] Pelvic tumours in women (cervical and disseminated ovarian tumours), and in both sexes bladder cancer and less commonly retroperitoneal fibrosis or malignancy, may also obstruct the urinary tract. Obstruction at the level of the ureters or higher must be bilateral, unless there is a solitary functioning kidney, to cause acute renal failure. This is usually due to renal calculi or schistosomal-induced ureteric stenosis. Renal tubules may become blocked by uric acid crystals, particularly in patients with hyperuricaemia following chemotherapy for lymphoma, leukaemia or myeloma. Prophylactic treatment with allopurinol, hydration and alkalinization of urine in these patients now make this an infrequent cause of acute renal failure. Other causes of renal tubular obstruction include sulfadiazine therapy and high-dose methotrexate treatment.

Causes of acute renal failure in the tropics

Acute renal failure in pregnancy

Acute renal failure from obstetric causes is common in the tropics. In the West, 3% of all causes of acute renal failure have an obstetric aetiology, whereas this figure is much higher in the tropics: 25% in Ghana[65] and 15% in India.[66] The actual cause varies according to the different stages of pregnancy. In the first trimester septic abortions account for the vast majority of cases. This is common because of the lack of legal abortion services in many tropical countries, resulting in a high prevalence of 'back street' abortions. In the third trimester the causes include pre-eclampsia and eclampsia, HELLP syndrome, puerperal sepsis, haemorrhage and abruptio placentae. The most common histological lesion found is acute tubular necrosis, although cortical necrosis is found more frequently in the tropics. The striking decline in the incidence of acute renal failure during pregnancy in some developing countries can be attributed to improved obstetric care and also to liberalization of abortion laws.[67]

Massive intravascular haemolysis

Glucose-6-phosphate dehydrogenase deficiency

Glucose-6-phosphate dehydrogenase (G6PD) deficiency is a red cell abnormality which is inherited as a sex-linked gene of partial dominance. The gene abnormality is widespread in tropical Africa, India and South-East Asia. The product of the G6PD reaction is NADPH, which is essential for the function of enzymes that protect against oxidants (catalase and glutathione peroxidase). Hence in G6PD deficiency, erythrocytes are susceptible to the effects of oxidant stress. The major clinical consequence of this is haemolysis due to infections and drugs. Acute renal failure has been reported in G6PD-deficient individuals following haemolysis due to drugs[68,69] and infections such as typhoid fever, malaria and hepatitis.[70,71]

Malaria

Acute renal failure is a well-recognized complication of malarial infection by *Plasmodium falciparum*.[72] The prevalence of acute renal failure is of the order of 1% but in cases of severe infection can be as high as 60%.[73] The major causes of acute renal failure are severe parasitaemia and blackwater fever from massive intravascular haemolysis.[74,75] The latter may be a consequence of severe infection alone although this is rare. More usually it is triggered by drugs such as quinine, or caused by G6PD deficiency. The acute renal failure seen in *P. falciparum* infection usually occurs 4–7 days after the onset of fever. It can be of the oliguric or non-oliguric type and most patients are hypercatabolic. Cholestatic jaundice is often seen and there have been reports of disseminated intravascular coagulation. Jaundice, oliguria, hypotension and multiple organ failure signify a poor prognosis.

The mechanism of acute renal failure has recently been reviewed.[76] Erythrocytes containing *P. falciparum* become adherent to capillaries and venules and hence are sequestered in organs such as the kidney, causing alterations in the microcirculation. The infected red cells also display reduced deformability, which results in predominantly extravascular haemolysis. The combination of these two phenomena causes renal vasoconstriction, renal tubular toxicity and activation of intravascular coagulation. Activation of cytokines also contributes to the increased adhesion and alteration of the renal microcirculation.

The histological changes are those of acute tubular necrosis, more marked in the distal tubule, and there may be casts of haemoglobin and malarial pigment. Quinine is the drug of choice in the treatment of severe *P. falciparum* malaria in most areas and the renal failure should be treated along standard lines. Exchange transfusions are effective when used with quinine in patients with sustained heavy parasitaemia and/or jaundice. Of the patients that develop acute renal failure, 60% will require dialysis but the overall mortality is less than 10%.

Diarrhoeal diseases

The acute renal failure that occurs with diarrhoeal disease is usually due to volume depletion. In one study in India 53% of cases of acute renal failure in infants and 22% in adults were due to a diarrhoeal illness.[77]

Typhoid fever

Renal complications occur in around 10% of cases of typhoid fever. Acute renal failure may be caused by massive intravascular haemolysis and this is particularly common in patients with G6PD deficiency.[78,79] There have been reports of haemolytic–uraemic syndrome in association with *Salmonella* species infections,[80] and also of a transient mesangial proliferative glomerulonephritis with glomerular deposits of IgM, C3 and Vi antigen.[81]

Shigella species

Shigella dysentry accounts for up to 65% of childhood acute renal failure in the tropics.[82] In severe *Shigella* species infection volume depletion and toxaemia can lead to acute renal failure from acute tubular necrosis. Acute renal failure may also occur from a haemolytic–uraemic syndrome during the diarrhoeal phase of the illness.[83] The mortality from this condition is high at 70%, with 14% of the survivors going on to develop chronic renal impairment as a result of chronic interstitial nephritis and cortical necrosis.[84]

Cholera[85]

The WHO received reports of over 250 000 cases of cholera worldwide in 1999, of which there were over 9000 deaths. The vast majority of these are due to renal failure secondary to volume depletion as a result of the profuse diarrhoea. This can usually be prevented by adequate fluid replacement. Given the degree of diarrhoea in cholera, hypokalaemia is frequently present, and in addition to acute tubular necrosis there may also be evidence of vacuolation of the proximal tubular epithelium.

Leptospirosis[86]

Leptospirosis is contracted following exposure to contaminated water, either in rivers or sewage. The clinical presentation is with myalgia, pyrexia, conjunctival congestion, headache and jaundice. There may be a bleeding diathesis with gastrointestinal and pulmonary haemorrhage. Acute renal failure occurs during the acute leptospiraemia stage and is usually accompanied by jaundice (Weil's syndrome). Aproximately 50% of patients develop acute renal failure and the major histological lesion is an acute interstitial nephritis with acute tubular necrosis. Minor glomerular mesangial proliferation may be seen. Characteristic features of the acute renal failure are that it is hypercatabolic and that hyperuricaemia, hyperkalaemia and the rise in blood urea are disproportionate to the serum creatinine. Dark-field microscopy of urine may reveal leptospires and they may also be grown from blood culture specimens. The diagnosis may also be established by serological tests. Treatment of leptospirosis when there is renal failure is with penicillin or erythromycin. The use of penicillin may be complicated by a Jarisch–Herxheimer reaction and in certain studies has been ineffective in preventing the need for dialysis.[87] Patients with severe renal failure require treatment with haemodialysis or peritoneal dialysis.

Poststreptococcal glomerulonephritis

β-Haemolytic streptococcal infections of the throat or skin can be complicated by an endocapillary proliferative glomerulonephritis. In Ethiopia 5% of children with these infections developed renal complications. There is evidence that the incidence is decreasing in some tropical countries; however, it still accounts for up to 13% of all paediatric acute renal failure cases.[88] This disease is discussed in more detail above.

Heatstroke[89]

Heatstroke occurs in hot climates, usually in association with exertion and poor fluid input, and can lead to acute renal failure. The mechanism of the renal failure is rhabdomyolysis and disseminated intravascular coagulation. Fulminant hepatic failure may also occur, contributing to the coagulopathy and renal failure. Investigations reveal evidence of haemoconcentration with a raised creatinine kinase, hyperuricaemia, myoglobinuria, hyperkalaemia, hypocalcaemia, proteinuria and often microscopic haematuria. Renal failure is treated along standard lines.

Melioidosis

This infection is caused by *Burkholeria pseudomallei*, an organism found in soil and water, and the infection is endemic in South-East Asia, Central and South America and the West Indies.[90] Patients with diabetes mellitus and tuberculosis have an increased susceptibility to this infection. There is a marked seasonal variation in this disease, with the majority of cases occurring in the rainy season. In northern Thailand it accounts for 20% of all community-acquired septicaemias. Patients can present with a localized form of the illness with discrete foci of infection or they can present with septicaemia without any obvious site of infection. Acute renal failure is more common in patients with septicaemia (60%) than in those with the localized form of the infection (35%). In the septicaemic form the presentation is usually one with a short history of a high temperature with diarrhoea,

shock and a metabolic acidosis. There is usually radiological evidence of pneumonia, although there may be no symptoms or signs to support this. Microabscesses are sometimes seen in the skin. Other features include hypoglycaemia, hyponatraemia and a low white cell count. In patients with acute renal failure the mortality is high. The renal lesion is most often acute tubular necrosis but an interstitial nephritis and renal microabscesses have been seen. Treatment is with ceftazidime or a combination of ceftazidime and trimethoprim–sulfamethoxazole. Imipenem can also be used but this is not as readily available. The organism is resistant to gentamicin and penicillin.

Snake bite (See also Chapter 32)

Acute renal failure is a well-recognized complication of snake bites. In a series from Chandrigah in India, out of 1862 patients with snake bites 3% developed acute renal failure.[91] Acute renal failure has been reported in patients bitten by snakes of the viper, colubrid and sea snake class. Following the bite of a Russell's viper between 3% and 30% of patients go on to develop renal failure; the figure following rattlesnake envenomation is around 15%. The risk of developing acute renal failure depends on the venom dose and the time between the bite and the administration of antivenom. Gastrointestinal bleeding and also bleeding into the muscle, viscera and subarachnoid space may develop. Acute renal failure develops within hours to 3 days after envenomation. The mechanism for the acute renal failure differs among the various snake families. Vipers cause intravascular haemolysis and disseminated intravascular coagulation but there is also evidence for direct nephrotoxicity. The mechanism whereby sea snake bites cause acute renal failure is rhabdomyolysis and myoglobinuria. The most common renal histological change seen is acute tubular necrosis, but cortical necrosis may be seen in up to 3% of cases. Other renal lesions reported include proliferative glomerulonephritis (occasionally with crescents), arteritis and renal infarcts. The main aim of treatment is adequate volume replacement and the administration of as specific an antivenom as is available as soon as possible. Treatment of renal failure is along standard lines.

Nephrotoxins[92] (See also Chapter 33)

A wide variety of plants used as herbal remedies in the tropics have been reported to be nephrotoxic. Renal failure has also been reported following multiple bee and wasp stings, spider bite and scorpion sting. In addition to direct nephrotoxicity the causes of acute renal failure include haemolysis and disseminated intravascular coagulation. Other causes of nephrotoxic acute renal failure include paraquat and copper sulphate poisoning.

Haemolytic–uraemic syndrome

This is a syndrome of thrombocytopenia, microangiopathic haemolytic anaemia with fragmented red blood cells and acute renal failure. The main cause of epidemic diarrhoea-associated haemolytic–uraemic syndrome (HUS) is vero-cytotoxin-producing *Escherichia coli* (VTEC) although HUS can occur as part of many other disease processes including HIV infection. Mortality from this condition can be as high as 40% in some countries. The clinical syndromes of VTEC infections include mild diarrhoea, haemorrhagic colitis and in 7–24% of patients HUS. Sporadic cases of HUS also occur and this is more common in adults. In the Indian subcontinent HUS may complicate *Shigella dysenteriae* type I infection.[93] Rare infective causes of HUS include neuraminidase-producing pneumococci and also *Salmonella typhi* infection.[94] Most cases of endemic HUS occur in infants and young children. There is usually a prodromal bloody diarrhoeal illness followed by renal failure and bleeding from the gut. Hypertension is common and focal neurological abnormalities such as fits and strokes may develop.

The pathological lesion is caused by the preferential binding of verotoxin to renal endothelial cells, increasing adhesion molecule expression and hence neutrophil and monocyte adhesion. It is thought that these activated neutrophils release free radicals that cause endothelial injury. This insult results in a variety of histological abnormalities including glomerular changes such as endothelial swelling, proliferation and capillary loop thrombosis. Afferent glomerular arterioles may show fibrin deposition and may be thrombosed. In some patients a deficiency of prostacyclin-stimulating factor has been found in the plasma. The consequent defect in endothelial prostacyclin synthesis would lead to platelet aggregation and intrarenal coagulation. This provides the basis for the use of fresh plasma infusions or prostacyclin in patients with HUS. Uncontrolled studies suggest that these measures may improve the outcome in these patients. The use of antibiotics in preventing patients with *E. coli* infection from developing HUS, however, is more controversial, with some studies showing benefit and others a detrimental effect.

Investigations in acute renal failure

These are aimed at establishing the presence and severity of acute renal failure and its aetiology, together with the history and physical examination; it is then possible to plan rational management for these patients.

Urine
Microscopic haematuria with red cell casts in the presence of proteinuria points strongly to a glomerulonephritis, while eosinophiluria suggests a drug-induced acute interstitial nephritis. The presence of urinary myoglobin is diagnostic of rhabdomyolysis.

Haematology
In acute renal failure an elevated neutrophil count usually suggests underlying sepsis. In either VTEC or *Shigella*-associated HUS the neutrophil count also correlates with disease severity. Anaemia with thrombocytopenia and fragmented red cells in the presence of normal clotting indices is also indicative of HUS, whereas the presence of a coagulopathy and raised serum levels of fibrinogen degradation products suggests disseminated intravascular coagulation. In severe drug-induced interstitial nephritis there may be an increase in the circulating peripheral blood eosinophil count. Blood should also be examined for the presence of malarial parasites.

Chemistry
An elevation of blood urea and creatinine will be found in acute renal failure. An inappropriately elevated urea compared to creatinine, however, may suggest volume depletion and a prerenal aeitology. Gastrointestinal haemorrhage in the presence of acute renal failure will also produce a similar picture. If rhabdomyolysis is suspected the blood creatinine phosphokinase concentrations should also be measured as these are grossly elevated in this condition.

Radiological investigations
A chest radiograph should be performed in all patients with acute renal failure and a plain abdominal radiograph may reveal renal or ureteric calculi. An ultrasound examination of the kidneys helps to exclude obstruction and determine renal size. In patients with an obstructive uropathy, percutaneous antegrade pyelography allows visualization of the pelvis and ureter, defines the site of obstruction and allows both drainage and decompression, allowing recovery of renal function. If access to the renal pelvis is not achieved the site of the obstruction may be determined using retrograde pyelography. Computed tomography is another useful tool for defining the nature and the level of obstruction in obstructive nephropathy. Radionuclide scanning with DTPA or DMSA demonstrates renal perfusion.

Renal biopsy
Renal histology is useful in all patients with unexplained acute renal failure and normal-sized unobstructed kidneys, especially if they have features suggestive of glomerulonephritis or other systemic diseases.

Management[95]

Prevention of acute tubular necrosis
Many patients develop acute tubular necrosis after a severe infection. It is likely that many of these cases can be prevented by paying careful attention to fluid balance and avoiding nephrotoxic drugs. In this early phase acute renal failure may be potentially reversible. Oliguria, with a low urinary Na^+ (< 10 mmol/l), a low fractional excretion of Na^+ and urine that is more concentrated than plasma, is indicative of incipient or prerenal acute renal failure. The ability of these urinary indices to differentiate reversible from established renal failure is imprecise and

is invalidated by loop diuretics. We and others find them of little value in practice. In patients with oliguria the first step is to correct hypovolaemia and a low cardiac output. The use of central venous or pulmonary capillary wedge pressure monitoring may be helpful in difficult cases. A potential pitfall is that if the patient remains oliguric pulmonary oedema may be precipitated. There is now accumulating evidence that low-dose dopamine does not improve the outcome of patients with acute renal failure even in the context of diseases such as malaria. Frusemide may make fluid overload easier to manage and avoid the need for dialysis but some studies suggest a poorer outcome for patients treated in this way.

Fluid balance

A daily weight chart is valuable in assessing the fluid balance of patients with acute renal failure. Volume depletion is usually present if the jugular venous pressure is not visible, there is a resting tachycardia and a postural drop in blood pressure. Skin turgor is more difficult to interpret as it depends on other factors such as age. The amount of fluids given to a patient in acute renal failure is based on: (1) measured fluid losses; (2) insensible losses minus metabolically produced water (about 600 ml/day in an adult); and (3) fluid removed by dialysis. Crystalloids such as either normal saline or isotonic sodium bicarbonate should be used unless there has been blood loss, in which case blood transfusions are required. Colloids should only be used to treat hypotension in the presence of severe volume depletion (hypovolaemic shock).

Hyperkalaemia and acidosis

Serum potassium can rise rapidly in patients who are hypercatabolic or acidotic or who have rhabdomyolysis. Hyperkalaemia is cardiotoxic and the electrocardiographic features include tall peaked T waves, prolongation of the PR interval, broadening of the QRS complex, which merges into the T wave, and ventricular arrhythmias with cardiac arrest. The serum potassium must be measured daily in patients with acute renal failure and more frequently in patients who are hypercatabolic. With milder degrees of hyperkalaemia (K^+ less than 6.0 mmol/l) cation exchange resins may be used to increase faecal potassium excretion, although these can lead to severe constipation and should be administered with laxatives. Serum potassium levels higher than 6.0 mmol/l are an indication for urgent dialysis. Intravenous glucose and soluble insulin are often helpful in reducing serum potassium pending dialysis. Most patients with acute renal failure have a metabolic acidosis and this can be severe in patients who are hypercatabolic. Intravenous isotonic sodium bicarbonate is useful in that it can be administered peripherally, corrects the acidosis and by doing so also lowers serum potassium. It should only be used in patients who are volume depleted and should not be used in the presence of hypocalcaemia as it will lower ionized calcium and provoke tetany and convulsions.

Dialysis

There are now a variety of techniques for treating uraemia and removing fluid from patients with acute renal failure. These include haemodialysis, peritoneal dialysis, haemofiltration, continuous arteriovenous haemofiltration, and continuous veno-venous haemodialysis (CVVHD).

Peritoneal dialysis

This has the advantage of being widely available, easy to set up and easy to run. The advent of percutaneous peritoneal dialysis catheter insertion techniques has made this procedure safer. It is effective in patients with milder degrees of renal failure who are not hypercatabolic. It has the advantage of not needing specialized equipment, avoids anticoagulation and is carried out at the bedside. Because it is a continuous process it is suitable for patients who are cardiovascularly unstable. The main complication of peritoneal dialysis is peritonitis.

Haemodialysis

Haemodialysis is now the mainstay of treatment for acute renal failure in the non-ITU setting. Access to the circulation is achieved by means of temporary or semi-permanent central venous catheters. Ideally these should be placed in the internal jugular vein. The femoral vein can be used if the patient is unable to lie flat but this route is prone to infective complications. Tunnelled semi-permanent venous catheters should be employed if prolonged dialysis is likely to be required.

Patients are usually dialysed for between 3 and 4 hours either daily or every other day. This is an extremely efficient form of treatment as it has the ability to clear large quantities of catabolic products and fluid over a relatively short period of time. Its intermittent nature also means that patients do not require the continuous anticoagulation needed for the other forms of haemodialysis (discussed below). The disadvantages of intermittent haemodialysis are that patients who are hypotensive or cardiovascularly unstable are often not able to tolerate the procedure.

In the unstable patient continuous forms of dialysis are better tolerated. Peritoneal dialysis has been discussed above. Continuous forms of haemodialysis are also available but usually require intensive care. Continuous arteriovenous haemofiltration utilizes the patient's own blood pressure to 'pump' blood through an artificial kidney. Access to the circulation is achieved usually by cannulating the femoral artery and vein. It does not require dialysis machinery. There is a risk of bleeding from the arterial site and in hypotensive subjects it is often inefficient. Rapid fluid removal is also difficult to achieve. The more popular mode of continuous haemodialysis is CVVHD. A dual-lumen venous catheter is required and blood is pumped through an artificial kidney. It requires continuous anticoagulation and hence cannot be used in the presence of a bleeding diathesis.

Fluid removal takes place constantly, making this suitable treatment for unstable patients.

Nutrition

Patients with acute renal failure should be given adequate nutrition in an attempt to minimize muscle catabolism and reduce malnutrition with the added risks of delayed wound healing and impaired resistance to infection.

Sepsis

Sepsis is important both as a cause and as a complication: most studies show that sepsis is still a major cause of death in patients with acute renal failure. The major sites of sepsis are intra-abdominal and pulmonary, and septicaemia is a frequent complication. Antibiotic doses may need to be adjusted as many are cleared by the kidney. More importantly, if drugs such as gentamycin and vancomycin are required strict monitoring of trough levels is required almost on a daily basis.

Drugs

Many drugs used in patients with acute renal failure are excreted by the kidneys and, unless their dose is modified, will accumulate with potentially toxic effects. It is therefore essential to know the precise pharmacokinetics of any drug before it is given to a patient with acute renal failure. Detailed guidelines of drug treatment in these patients are available.

Chronic renal failure

Chronic renal failure results from the progressive and irreversible loss of kidney function. The remarkable reserve in renal function means that the kidneys can support life with as little as 10% of the original functioning nephrons. Below this level of function patients develop uraemic symptoms and dialysis and/or transplantation is required for survival.

Chronic renal failure prevalence rates vary widely in the tropics. The vast majority of surveys, however, equate dialysis with chronic renal failure. As this data is garnered from dialysis units, the numbers of patients with chronic renal failure are generally underestimated as dialysis is not offered until end-stage renal failure is reached and even then, in many places, to a minority of patients only. The prevalence of end-stage renal failure in UK is 539 per million of the population, whereas in the USA it is over 1000 per million population. In these countries the incidence of end-stage renal failure in patients originating from the Indian subcontinent and Africa is three times that of the Caucasian population.[96,97] It can be argued that these population groups have higher rates of renal disease; however, socio-economic factors may also play a major role. In the tropics the prevalence of patients receiving dialysis is largely governed by socio-economic forces. In Singapore approximately 500 per million popu-

lation are on dialysis, whereas dialysis prevalence rates are lower in countries such as Eygpt (264 per million population), the Phillipines (40 per million population), and Pakistan (15 per million population).[98] In many tropical countries patients have to pay for their dialysis, which obviously limits numbers.

Aetiology

There are many causes of chronic renal failure in the tropics and these are summarized in Table 15.4. In tropical countries, glomerulonephritis, hypertension and diabetic nephropathy are major causes of chronic renal failure, as is an obstructive uropathy.[99–101] Disease patterns are changing and increasingly diabetic nephropathy is becoming the commonest causes of renal failure.

Pathophysiology

Hyperfiltration injury forms the basis of progressive renal damage in chronic renal failure once the initial insult has passed. In all renal diseases, when a critical portion of functioning renal tissue is lost progressive injury to the remaining kidney ensues. Studies in rats that had undergone a five-sixths nephrectomy suggested that the consequences of nephron loss, in particular glomerular hypertrophy, were responsible for progressive renal damage.[102] Glomerular hypertrophy resulting from nephron loss was accompanied by glomerular hyperperfusion, hyperfiltration and hypertension and these in turn led to progressive glomerular sclerosis, tubulointerstitial atrophy and scarring. In rats reduction of intraglomerular pressures, either by a low protein diet or by an angiotensin-converting enzyme inhibitor (ACEI) (which reduces intraglomerular pressures by afferent arteriolar vasodilatation), slowed down the rate at which renal failure progressed.

A common consequence of hyperfiltration injury is proteinuria. Proteinuria itself may be injurious to the nephron. Numerous studies have shown that patients

Table 15.4 Causes of chronic renal failure in the tropics.

Cause	Africa[72]	India[11,71]	Malaysia[73]
Hypertensive renal disease (nephrosclerosis)	32–49	5–23	?
Glomerulonephritis	25–62	35–65	30
Pyelonephritis	2–29	7–18	2
Diabetic nephropathy	3–9	7–23	9
Obstructive uropathy	?	3–14	6
Renal calculi	12	7	?
Tuberculosis	?	1–5	?
Polycystic kidney disease	?	1–6	0.5

Values are percentages.

with proteinuria are more likely to progress to end-stage renal failure independent of initial diagnosis.[103] There is also increasing laboratory evidence that proteins such as albumin lead to proximal tubular cell injury and dysfunction.[104]

Arguably the most important factor in progression is hypertension. Large clinical trials have shown that blood pressure control successfully reduces the rate of progression of chronic renal failure in both diabetic and non-diabetic renal disease.

Diabetic nephropathy

The numbers of patients with type 2 diabetes is growing rapidly. WHO estimates the numbers will increase from 140 million to 300 million in 25 years. The prevalence of diabetes in the general population of some tropical countries is staggering, with up to 23% of those between 30 and 64 years being affected. This appears to be, in part at least, a problem related to urbanization. In South India around 3% of men aged 30–64 years in rural areas have diabetes, whereas the figure is closer to 12% in the urban population.

The pathogenesis of diabetic nephropathy has and is being studied extensively and is too large a subject to be covered here in detail. Direct effects of glucose on mesangial and tubular cells have been identified. Reactive oxygen species and free radicals have been implicated, as has endothelial dysfunction. Abnormal glycation of proteins occurs in diabetes, resulting in the formation of advanced glycation end products (AGEs). AGEs have been shown to cause a wide range of changes in cellular function and may also prove to be of great importance. There are also genetic factors placing certain diabetic patients at increased risk of developing nephropathy.

Diabetic nephropathy has been reported in tropical Africa, the Caribbean, the Indian subcontinent and South-East Asia. In most areas the prevalence of diabetic nephropathy in patients with diabetes mellitus varies between 10% and 20%. The progressive nature of diabetic nephropathy makes this likely to be a major cause of end-stage renal failure in these areas. In the USA diabetes now accounts for 31% of all patients with end-stage renal disease receiving renal replacement therapy. In the tropics the prevalence of diabetics on dialysis varies from country to country. In Egypt and Brazil diabetes accounts for 9% and 18% of their dialysis populations, respectively, whereas in more affluent tropical countries such as Singapore this figure may be as high as 40%.

Biochemistry

Serum creatinine and urea do not rise above normal until the GFR falls below 50 ml/min, i.e., until renal function is halved. This makes them inaccurate markers of renal function in mild renal impairment. Below a GFR of 30 ml/min the serum creatinine rise is approximately linear to decline in GFR. Indeed, because of tubular

secretion of creatinine, serum creatinine levels become a better marker of renal function than the creatinine clearance at low levels of renal function.

Hyperkalaemia and acidosis

These are not marked until the GFR falls below 20 ml/min. Exceptions to this are patients with tubulointerstitial disorders.

Salt and water handling

In most patients, salt and water balance is maintained until the GFR falls below 15% of normal, although in diabetes this may occur earlier. Nevertheless some individuals with tubulointerstitial disease are salt and water losers and tend to dehydration at a higher GFR. Others with glomerular disease and hypertension, especially with hypertensive heart disease, may retain salt and water and develop heart failure.

Bone[105]

Increased blood levels of parathormone are found in very early renal failure when GFR falls below 50–60 ml/min. This is probably due to inappropriately low levels of 1,25-dihydroxycholecalciferol and not to hyperphosphataemia with consequent hypocalcaemia, as previously thought. With advanced renal failure there is impaired renal synthesis of 1,25-cholecalciferol from its precursor 25-cholecalciferol. A reduction in intestinal absorption of calcium and also hyperphosphataemia increase the tendency to hypocalcaemia. This stimulates the parathyroid glands to hyperplasia and in severe cases to adenoma formation. The consequences of this are renal osteodystrophy. Vitamin D deficiency leads to osteomalacia, and hyperparathyroidism to the development of bone erosions and osteitis fibrosa.

Aluminium intoxication

This arises from dialysis against fluid containing aluminium and to a lesser extent absorption of aluminium-containing phosphate binders. The bony consequences are osteomalacia. Aluminium intoxication can also cause an encephalopathy.

Anaemia[106]

Haemoglobin concentrations tend to be maintained until the GFR falls below 30 ml/min. At this time anaemia ensues. There are several reasons for the anaemia of chronic renal failure. Perhaps the most important is the failing kidney's inability to produce sufficient quantities of erythropoietin, the hormone that drives the bone marrow to produce red blood cells. Other factors such as reduced red cell survival are also important. In addition, the uraemic environment renders the bone marrow relatively resistant to the action of erythropoietin, especially if inflammation and infection are present. Recombinant human erythropoietin is now readily available but at considerable cost.

Management

The causes of chronic renal failure are varied and its clinical presentation differs between patients. Management must therefore be guided by the assessment of individual patients.

Conservative management

This is effective in individuals with a GFR of 10 ml/min or greater. The first objective is to identify and correct potentially reversible causes of progressive renal failure. Examples of this include obstructive uropathy and the use of potentially nephrotoxic drugs such as non-steroidal anti-inflammatory drugs.

There are certain basic principles that can be applied to all patients to retard the rate of progression of chronic renal failure. The most important of these is blood pressure control. There is now little doubt that good control of blood pressure will slow down the progression to end-stage renal failure of both diabetic and non-diabetic renal disease.[107] The MDRD study in the USA demonstrated that lower than normal blood pressure (mean arterial pressure < 97 mmHg) resulted in a slower rate of progression in patients with proteinuria and chronic renal failure.[108] The REIN study suggested that ACEIs may provide additional benefit over and above blood pressure reduction in both proteinuric and non-proteinuric non-diabetic renal diseases.[109] There does not seem to be a lower limit to blood pressure targets. These studies suggest that targets may be as low as 120/70. In diabetes large studies in both type 1 (DCCT)[110] and type 2 (UKPDS)[111] have clearly shown that good glycaemic controls will slow the rate of progression of chronic renal failure. The UKPDS further emphasizes the importance of blood pressure control in retarding progression of renal failure in type 2 diabetes.[112]

Most nephrologists now advocate the use of ACEIs in the treatment of hypertension in chronic renal failure. Caution, however, needs to be exercised in patients with both large and small vessel renal disease as in this setting these drugs may cause an acute but usually reversible deterioration in renal function. Because of this, high-risk patients require close monitoring of renal function after the initiation of therapy.

A low-protein diet reduces the progression of renal damage in rats and possibly in humans. We arbitrarily restrict protein intake to 0.6 g/kg with a serum creatinine over 400 μmol/litre and to 0.5 g/kg when the serum creatinine rises to over 600 μmol/litre.

The maintenance of GFR in advanced renal failure is critically dependent on salt and water balance. Salt and water overload leads to heart failure, a reduction in cardiac output and worsening of renal function. Salt and water depletion leads to volume depletion, a reduction in cardiac output and a reduction in GFR. Each patient must have careful regular assessments of their fluid status and salt and water intake and this is then optimized, if necessary, using diuretics. Once the GFR falls below 20 ml/min plasma potassium tends to rise, justifying a reduction in dietary potassium intake. Expert dietetic help adjusted to the local foods is invaluable in the management of these patients.

Renal osteodystrophy was relatively uncommon in most parts of the tropics but is becoming more of a problem as more patients are now receiving maintenance dialysis. Key principles in management include control of hyperphosphataemia with phosphate binders which binds ingested phosphate and the use of 1α-hydroxycholecalciferol or 1,25-dihydroxycholecalciferol in patients who are (1) hypocalcaemic, (2) have a raised alkaline phosphatase, and/or (3) have a raised parathormone. The dose of calcium carbonate must be adjusted to avoid hypercalcaemia.

Careful monitoring of anaemia is also required so that treatment can begin early. The use of subcutaneous recombinant human erythropoeitin on a regular basis can be initiated in order to achieve haemoglobin levels of between 11 and 13 g/dl. Adequate utilizable iron is required to minimize erythropoeitin dosage and many centres in the West now administer regular intravenous iron to dialysis patients.

Dialysis and transplantation

Once the GFR falls below 10 ml/min, renal replacement with either dialysis or a renal transplant is necessary if life is to be maintained. The costs of dialysis—both continuous ambulatory dialysis and haemodialysis—are substantial but increasingly tropical countries are providing chronic dialysis facilities. In the more developed tropical countries the level of dialysis provision approaches that of the West. Singapore, for instance, has 500 dialysis patients per million population and neighbouring Malaysia has 253 dialysis per million population; however, other countries lag far behind, with figures of between 15 and 40 per million population (Pakistan and Philippines). Renal transplantation once set up is less costly in the long term.

Haemodialysis

This is the most popular method for the delivering of long-term dialysis worldwide. In the USA, nearly 90% of all patients on dialysis receive haemodialysis. In the UK the proportion receiving haemodialysis is somewhat lower at 60%. In tropical countries the majority with chronic dialysis programmes have more patients on haemodialysis. This method of dialysis delivery has the advantage of being able to treat a large number of patients and is fast and efficient. Technique survival is only limited by vascular access. It is, however, limited by staff, space and availability of machines. Also patients have to travel to centres to have this treatment as very few tropical countries have home haemodialysis programmes.

Peritoneal dialysis

Several techniques are now on offer: continuous ambulatory peritoneal dialysis (CAPD), automated peritoneal dialysis

(APD) and intermittent peritoneal dialysis (IPD). Both CAPD and APD are domiciliary treatments and hence are less dependent on staff or space. Patients living far from dialysis centres may benefit from these modalities although provision and delivery of dialysate may prove difficult. Unfortunately most commercially produced dialysates are expensive and hence render this treatment no cheaper than haemodialysis. Because of membrane failure median technique survival for CAPD is 7–8 years.

Transplantation

This form of renal replacement therapy provides patients with the best long-term outlook, with living donation providing the best graft survival figures. Many tropical countries have established live donor programmes but cadaveric programmes are also being established in some. The previous practice of 'organ trade' is now illegal in countries such as India following the passage of Act 42: The Transplantation of Human Organs Act. Transplantation provides patients with a near-normal lifestyle, most of the complications occurring as a result of side effects of the immunosuppressive therapy. The mainstay of immuno-suppression is steroids, azathioprine and calcineurin inhibition with drugs such as cyclosporin and tacrolimus. The patent on cyclosporin has recently expired, resulting in numerous cheaper generic forms. This will hopefully afford greater access to this drug. This is especially important when graft failure secondary to poor compliance, for economic reasons, is common. Newer and more expensive drugs such as mycophenalate mofetil and rapamycin are now available but it is not yet clear whether they provide better results than those listed above.

Obstructive uropathy

Renal tuberculosis[113]

Tuberculosis can affect the urinary tract in three ways. Most commonly there is parenchymal renal involvement with ureteric and bladder involvement. Parenchymal renal involvement often leads to cavitation, seen on intravenous urography as papillary ulceration or cavities in the parenchyma, and these may communicate with the pelvicalyceal system. Advanced parenchymal lesions lead to a non-functioning kidney—so-called auto-nephrectomy. On plain abdominal radiographs renal calcification is often a clue to the diagnosis of tuber-culosis. Bladder involvement leads to ulceration and there may be inflammation of the ureters. In advanced disease the bladder becomes obstructed and fibrosed and this, together with ureteric stricture or incompetence of the vesico-ureteric junction, can lead to an obstructive uropathy. Extrarenal tuberculosis may lead to the late development of glomerular amyloid. The clinical presen-tation is that of renal amyloid from any other cause. Rarely tuberculosis has been associated with the develop-ment of a mesangiocapillary glomerulonephritis.

Renal calculi[114]

Renal and ureteric calculi tend to be uncommon in blacks in tropical Africa but is common in the Middle East, the Indian subcontinent and the rest of Asia. The overall probability of forming stones ranges from 1–5% in Asia to 20% in Saudi Arabia compared to 5–9% in Europe and 13% in North America. The Indian population of Fiji is noted for their high incidence of renal calculi, unlike their native Fijian counterparts.

In areas with a high incidence of schistosomiasis bladder stones may be common. It is suggested that a high temperature, inadequate fluid intake and low urine volume predispose to stone formation in some areas. Bladder stones are common in Central Africa and parts of South-East Asia.

Schistosoma haematobium[80,115]

S. haematobium infections are widespread in the tropics. *Schistosoma*-mediated inflammation of the bladder and ureters can lead to fibrosis and to obstructive uropathy. The bladder and the juxtavesical ureter are initially involved by granuloma formation. Ureteric involvement leads to ureteric dilatation, stricture and vesico-ureteric reflux. Functionally these abnormalities may lead to renal failure. Diagnosis is by examining the urine for *S. haematobium* ova. A calcified bladder or ureters may be seen on abdominal radiographs (Figure 15.4). Intravenous urography shows a variety of changes including segmental dilatation of the ureter, ureteric stenosis and dilatation of the upper tracts. More recently the ultrasonographic features have been described and this technique is gaining popularity. Treatment with praziquantel results in high cure rates and when used community wide in endemic areas has been shown to reduce the prevalence of urinary tract abnormalities. There is good evidence of an association between *S. haematobium* infection and the subsequent development of bladder cancer. The majority of these tumours are squamous cell carcinomas.

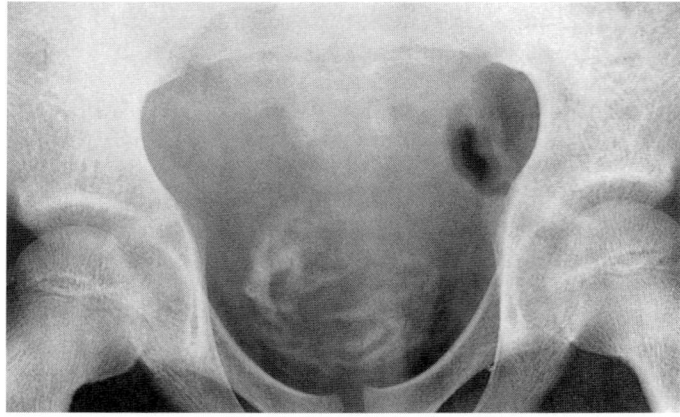

Figure 15.4: Bladder wall calcification in schistosomiasis. (Courtesy of Judy Webb, St Bartholomew's Hospital.)

REFERENCES

1   Kibukamusoke J W, Hutt M S R & Wilks N E. The nephrotic syndrome in Uganda and its association with quartan malaria. *Q J Med* 1967; 36:393–407.

2   Dixon F J, Vasquez J J, Weigle W O & Cochrane C G. Pathogenesis of serum sickness. *Arch Pathol* 1958: 65:18–28.

3   Glotz D & Druet P. Immune mechanisms of glomerular damage. In Davison A M, Cameron J S, , Grunfeld J-P, Kerr D N S, Ritz E & Winearls C G. (eds) *Oxford Textbook of Clinical Nephrology*, 2nd edn. Oxford: Oxford University Press, 1998: 375.

4   Adu D. Idiopathic glomerulonephritis. In Weatherall D J, Ledingham J G G , Warell D A (eds) *Oxford Textbook of Medicine*, 3rd edn. Oxford: Oxford University Press, 1996: 20.4.2.

5   Chugh K S & Sakhuja V. Glomerular disease in the tropics. In Davison A M, Cameron J S, , Grunfeld J-P, Kerr D N S, Ritz E, Winearls C G (eds) *Oxford Textbook of Clinical Nephrology*, 2nd edn. Oxford: Oxford University Press, 1998: 703.

6   Morgan A G, Shah D J, Williams W & Forrester T E. Proteinuria and glomerular disease in Jamaica. *Clin Nephrol* 1984; 21:205–209.

7   Seggie J, Davies P G, Ninin D & Henry J. Pattern of glomerulonephritis in Zimbabwe: survey of disease characterised by nephrotic proteinuria. *Q J Med* 1984; 53:109–118.

8   Borok M Z, Nathoo K J, Gabriel R & Porter K A. Clinicopathological features of Zimbabwean patients with sustained proteinuria. *Cent Afr J Med* 1997; 43:152–158.

9   Seggie J L & Adu D. Nephrotic syndrome in the tropics. In Cameron J S & Glassock R J (eds) *The Nephrotic Syndrome*. New York: Marcel Dekker, 1988: 653–695.

10 Sinniah R & Khoo O T. The pathology and immunopathology of glomerulonephritis in Singapore. In *Proceedings of the 1st Asian Pacific Congress of Nephrology*, Tokyo, 1979: 114.

11 Adu D, Anim-Addo Y, Foli A K et al. The nephrotic syndrome in Ghana: clinical and pathological aspects. *Q J Med* 1981; 50:297–306.

12 Chugh K S & Sakhuja V. Renal disease in northern India. In Kibukamusoke J W (ed.) *Tropical Nephrology*. Canberra: Citforge, 1984: 428–440.

13 McLigeyo, S O. Glomerular diseases in Kenya: another look at diseases characterised by nephrotic proteinuria. *Afr J Health Sci* 1994; 4:185–190.

14 Srivastava R N, Mayekar G, Anand R, Choudhury V, Ghai O P & Tandon H. Nephrotic syndrome in Indian children. *Arch Dis Child* 1975; 50:626–630.

15 Musa A R M, Veress B, Kordofani A M, Asha H A, Satir A & Hassan A M E. Pattern of the nephrotic syndrome in the Sudan. *Ann Trop Med Parasitol* 1980; 74:37–42.

16 Sadiq S, Jafrey N A & Naqvi S A J. An analysis of percutaneous renal biopsies in fifty cases of nephrotic syndrome. *J Pakistan Med Assoc* 1978; 28:121–124.

17 Morel-Maroger L, Saimot A G, Sloper J C et al. 'Tropical nephropathy' and 'tropical extramembranous glomerulonephritis ' of unknown aetiology in Senegal. *BMJ* 1975; 1:541–546.

18 Pakasa M, Mangani N & Dikassa L. Focal and segmental glomerulosclerosis in nephrotic syndrome: a new profile of adult nephrotic syndrome in Zaire. *Mod Pathol* 1993; 6125–6128.

19 Adhikari M, Bhimma R & Coovadia H M. Focal segmental glomerulosclerosis in children from KwaZulu/Natal, South Africa. *Clin Nephrol* 2001; 5516–5524.

20 van Buuren A J, Bates W D & Muller N. Nephrotic syndrome in Namibian children. *S Afr Med J* 1999; 89:1088–1091.

21 Bhimma R, Coovadia H M & Adhikari M. Hepatitis B virus-associated nephropathy in black South African children. *Pediatr Nephrol* 1998; 12:479–484.

22 Gilbert R D & Wiggelinkhuizen J. The clinical course of hepatitis B virus-associated nephropathy. *Pediatr Nephrol* 1994; 8:1–14.

23 Levy M & Berger J. Worldwide perspective of IgA nephropathy. *Am J Kidney Dis* 1988; 12:340–347.

24 Swanepoel C R, Madaus S, Cassidy M J, Temple-Camp C, Van Diggelen N T, Pascoe M D & van Zyl-Smit R. IgA nephropathy: Groote Schuur Hospital experience. *Nephron* 1989; 53:61–64.

25 Sitprija V. The kidney in acute tropical disease. In Kibukamusoke J W (ed.) *Tropical Nephrology*. Canberra: Citforge, 1984: 148–169.

26 Prathap K & Looi L M. Morphological patterns of glomerular disease in renal biopsies from 1000 Malaysian patients. *Ann Acad Med Singapore* 1982; 11:52–56.

27 Seedat Y K, Parag K B & Ramsaroop R. Systemic lupus erythematosus and renal involvement: a South African experience. *Nephron* 1994; 66:426–430.

28 Poon-King T, Potter E V, Svartman M et al. Epidemic acute nephritis with reappearance of M-type 55 streptococci in Trinidad. *Lancet* 1973; i:475–479.

29 Chugh K S, Malhotra H S & Sakhuja V. Progression to end-stage renal disease in poststreptococcal glomerulonephritis. *Int J Artif Organs* 1987; 10:189–194.

30 Rodriguez-Iturbe B. Acute endocapillary glomerulonephritis. In Davison A M, Cameron J S, , Grunfeld J-P, Kerr D N S, Ritz E & Winearls C G (eds) *Oxford Textbook of Clinical Nephrology*, 2nd edn. Oxford: Oxford University Press, 1998: 613.

31 Johnson R J & Couser W G. Hepatitis B infection and renal disease: clinical, immunopathogenetic and therapeutic considerations. *Kidney Int* 1990; 37:663–676.

32 Lai K N, Lai F M, Chan K W, Chow C B, Tong K L & Vallance-Owen J. The clinico-pathological features of hepatitis B virus-associated glomerulonephritis. *Q J Med* 1987; 240:323–333.

33 D'Amico G & Fornasieri A. Cryoglobulinemic glomerulonephritis: a membrano-proliferative glomerulonephritis induced by hepatitis C virus. *Am J Kidney Dis* 1995; 25:361–369.

34 Bourgoignie J J. Renal complications of human immunodeficiency virus type 1. *Kidney Int* 1990; 37:1571–1584.

35 Klotman P E. HIV-associated nephropathy. *Kidney Int* 1999; 56:1161.

36 Pantanowitz L, Goetsch B, Butker O & Katz J J. Renal biopsies of HIV positive patients at Baragwanath Hospital (1989–1997). Abstracts of Congress of the South African Association of Nephrology. *Kidney Int* 1999; 55:2130.

37 Diallo AD, Niamkey E & Yao Beda B. Etiologic aspects of nephrotic syndrome in Black African adults in a hospital setting in Abidjan. *Bull Soc Pathol Exot* 1997; 90:345.

38 Praditpornsilpa K, Napathorn S, Yenrudi S et al. Renal pathology and HIV infection in Thailand. *Am J Kidney Dis* 1999; 33:282.

39 Andrade Z A & Rocha H. Schistosomal glomerulopathy. *Kidney Int* 1979; 16:23–29.

40 Barsoum R S. Schistosomiasis. In Davison A M, Cameron J S, Grunfeld J-P, Kerr D N S, Ritz E & Winearls C G (eds) *Oxford Textbook of Clinical Nephrology*, 2nd edn. Oxford: Oxford University Press, 1998: 1287.

41 Barsoum R S, Bassily S, Baligh O K et al. Renal disease in hepatosplenic schistosomiasis: a clinicopathological study. *Trans R Soc Trop Med Hyg* 1977; 71:387–391.

42 Omer H O & Wahab S M A. Secondary amyloidosis due to *Schistosoma mansoni* infection. *BMJ* 1976; i:375–377.

43 McAdam K P W J, Anders R F, Smith S R, Russell D A & Price M A. Association of amyloidosis with erythema nodosum leprosum reactions and recurrent neutrophil leucocytosis in leprosy. *Lancet* 1975; ii:572–575.

44 Chugh K S, Damle P B, Kaur S et al. Renal lesions in leprosy amongst north Indian patients. *Postgrad Med J* 1983; 59:707–711.

45 Johny K V, Karat A B A, Rao P S S & Date A. Glomerulonephritis in leprosy: a percutaneous renal biopsy study. *Lepr Rev* 1975; 46:29–37.

46 Ngu J L, Chatelanat F, Leke R, Ndumbe P & Youmbissi J. Nephropathy in Cameroon: evidence for filarial derived immune complex pathogenesis in some cases. *Clin Nephrol* 1985; 24:128–134.

47 Chugh K S, Singhal P C & Tewari S C. Acute glomerulonephritis associated with filariasis. *Am J Trop Med Hyg* 1978; 27:630–631.

48 Giglioli G. Malarial nephritis: epidemiological and clinical notes on malaria. In *Blackwater Fever, Albuminuria and Nephritis in the Interior of British Guiana, Based on Seven Years' Continual Observation*. London: Churchill, 1930.

49 Giglioli G. Malaria and renal disease with special reference to British Guiana. II. The effect of malaria eradication on the incidence of renal disease in British Guiana. *Ann Trop Med Parasitol* 1962; 56:225–241.

50 Hendrickse R G, Adeniyi A, Edington G M, Glasgow E F, White R H R & Houba V. Quartan malarial nephrotic syndrome: collaborative clinicopathological study in Nigerian children. *Lancet* 1972; i:1143–1149.

51 Adeniyi A, Hendrickse R G & Houba V. Selectivity of proteinuria and response to prednisolone or immunosuppressive drugs in children with malarial nephrosis. *Lancet* 1970; i:644–648.

52 Nicholson G D. Kidney in sickle cell disease. In Kibukamusoke J W (ed.) *Tropical Nephrology*. Canberra: Citforge, 1984: 272–286.

53 Caruana R J. The patient with sickle cell disease. In Davison A M, Cameron J S, Grunfeld J-P, Kerr D N S, Ritz E & Winearls C G (eds) *Oxford Textbook of Clinical Nephrology*, 2nd edn. Oxford: Oxford University Press, 1998: 995.

54 Falk R J, Scheinman J, Phillips G, Orringer E, Johnson A & Jennette J C. Prevalence and pathologic features of sickle cell nephropathy and response to inhibition of angiotensin-converting enzyme. *N Engl J Med* 1992; 326:910–915.

55 McCoy R C. Ultrastructural alterations in the kidney of patients with sickle cell disease and the nephrotic syndrome. *Lab Invest* 1969; 21:85–95.

56 Adu D & Kibukamusoke J W. Acute renal failure in the tropics. In Kibukamusoke J W (ed.) *Tropical Nephrology*. Canberra: Citforge, 1984: 199–215.

57 Beaman M & Adu D. Acute renal failure. In Tinker J & Zapol W M (eds) *Care of the Critically Ill Patient*. Berlin: Springer, 1992: 515–532.

58 Chugh K S & Kjellstrand C M. The changing epidemiology of acute renal failure: patterns in economically advanced and developing countries. In Andreucci V E (ed.), Fine L G, Hatano M & Kjellstrand C M (co-eds) *International Yearbook of Nephrology*. Boston: Kluwer, 1989: 207–226.

59 Adu D, Anim-Addo Y, Foli A K, Yeboah E D, Quartey J K M & Riberio B F. Acute renal failure in tropical Africa. *BMJ* 1976; i:89–91.

60 Beaman M, Turney J H, Rodger R S C, McGonigle R S, Adu D & Michael J. Changing pattern of acute renal failure. *Q J Med* 1987; 237:15–23.

61 Sural S, Sharma R K, Singhal M K, Kher V, Gupta A, Arora P & Gulati S. Acute renal failure in an intensive care unit in India: prognostic factors and outcome. *J Nephrol* 1999; 12(6):390–394.

62 Essamie M A, Soliman A, Fayad T M, Barsoum S & Kjellstrand C M. Serious renal disease in Egypt. *Int J Artif Organs* 1995; 18:254–260.

63 Tepel M, van der Giet M, Schwarzfeld C, Laufer U, Liermann D & Zidek W. Prevention of radiographic-contrast-agent-induced reductions in renal function by acetylcysteine . *N Engl J Med* 2000; 343:180–184.

64 Yeboah E D. Acute retention of urine at Korle Bu Teaching Hospital. *Ghana Med J* 1980; 19:152–155.

65 Adu D, Anim-Addo Y, Foli A K, Yeboah E D, Quartey J K M & Riberio B F. Acute renal failure in tropical Africa. *BMJ* 1976; i:89–91.

66 Chugh K S, Singhal P C, Sharma B K et al. Acute renal failure of obstetric origin. *Obstet Gynecol* 1976; 48:642–646.

67 Utas C, Yalcindag C, Taskapan H, Guven M, Oymak O & Yucesoy M. Acute renal failure in Central Anatolia. *Nephrol Dial Transplant* 2000; 15:152–155.

68 Chugh K S, Singhal P C, Sharma B K et al. Acute renal failure due to intravascular hemolysis in the North Indian patients. *Am J Med Sci* 1977; 274:139–146.

69 Owosu S K, Addy J H, Foli A K et al. Acute reversible renal failure associated with glucose-6-phosphate dehydrogenase deficiency. *Lancet* 1972; i:1255–1257.

70 Lwanga D & Wing A J. Renal complications associated with typhoid fever. *East Afr Med J* 1970; 47:146–152.

71 Adu D, Anim-Addo Y, Foli A K, Yeboah E D, Quartey J K M & Ribeiro B F. Acute renal failure and typhoid fever. *Ghana Med J* 1975; 4:172.

72 Boonpucknavig V & Sitprija V. Renal disease in acute *Plasmodium falciparum* infection in man. *Kidney Int* 1979; 16:44–52.

73 Lim T O, Lim Y N. Seventh annual report of the Malaysian Dialysis and Transplant Registry, 1999.

74 Dukes D C, Sealey B J & Forbes J I. Oliguric renal failure in blackwater fever. *Am J Med* 1968; 45:899–903.

75 Canfield C J, Miller L H, Bastelloni P J, Eichler P & Barry K B. Acute renal failure in *Plasmodium falciparum* malaria. *Arch Intern Med* 1968; 122:199–203.

76 Eiam-Ong S, Sitprija V. Falciparum malaria and the kidney: a model of inflammation. *Am J Kidney Dis* 1998; 32:361–375.

77 Chugh K S. Etiopathogenesis of acute renal failure in the tropics. *Ann Natl Acad Med Sci (India)* 1987; 23:89–99.

78 Lwanga D & Wing A J. Renal complications associated with typhoid fever. *East Afr Med J* 1970; 47:146–152.

79 Adu D, Anim-Addo Y, Foli A K, Yeboah E D, Quartey J K M & Ribeiro B F. Acute renal failure and typhoid fever. *Ghana Med J* 1975; 4:172.

80 Baker N M, Mills A F, Rachman I & Thomas J E P. Haemolytic uraemic syndrome in typhoid fever. *BMJ* 1974; ii:84–87.

81 Musa A M, Salch S Y & Abu Asha H. Transient nephritis during typhoid fever in five Sudanese patients. *Ann Trop Med Parasitol* 1981; 75:181–188.

82 Raghupathy P, Date A, Shastry J C, Sudarsanam A & Jadhav M. Haemolytic–uraemic syndrome complicating shigella dystentery in south Indian children. *BMJ* 1978; i:1518–1521.

83 Bhuyan U N, Srivastava R N & Choudhry V P. Pathology of acute renal failure and haemolytic uraemic syndrome in acute dysentery in children. *Indian J Med Res* 1985; 81:402–408.

84 Srivastava R N, Moudgil A, Bagga A & Vasudev A S. Hemolytic uremic syndrome in children in northern India. *Pediatr Nephrol* 1991; 5(3):284–288.

85 Benyajati C, Keoplung M, Beisel W R, Gangarosa E J, Spring H & Sitprija V. Acute renal failure in Asiatic cholera: clinicopathological correlations with acute tubular necrosis and hypokalemic nephropathy. *Ann Intern Med* 1960; 52:960–975.

86 Sitprija V. Renal involvement in leptospirosis. In Robinson R

R (ed.) *Tropical Nephrology*. New York: Springer, 1984: 1041–1052.

87 Daher E D & Nogueira C B. Evaluation of penicillin therapy in patients with leptospirosis and acute renal failure. *Rev Inst Med Trop Sao Paulo* 2000; 42:327–332.

88 Srivastava R N, Bagga A & Moudgil A. Acute renal failure in north Indian children. *Indian J Med Res* 1990; 92:404–408.

89 Shibolet S, Coll R, Gilat T & Sohar E. Heatstroke: its clinical picture and mechanism in 36 cases. *Q J Med* 1967; 36:525–548.

90 Susaengrat W, Dhiensiri T, Sinavatana P & Sitprija V. Renal failure in melioidosis. *Nephron* 1987; 46:167–169.

91 Chugh K S, Aikat B K, Sharma B K, Dash K C, Mathew M T & Das K C. Acute renal failure following snakebite. *Am J Trop Med Hyg* 1975; 24:692–697.

92 Sitprija V. The kidney in acute tropical disease. In Kibukamusoke J W (ed.) *Tropical Nephrology*. Canberra: Citforge, 1984: 148–169.

93 Raghupathy P, Date A, Shastry J C, Sudarsanam A & Jadhav M. Haemolytic–uraemic syndrome complicating shigella dysentery in south Indian children. *BMJ* 1978; i:1518–1521.

94 Baker N M, Mills A F, Rachman I & Thomas J E P. Haemolytic uraemic syndrome in typhoid fever. *BMJ* 1974; ii:84–87.

95 Beaman M & Adu D. Acute renal failure. In Tinker J & Zapol W M (eds) *Care of the Critically Ill Patient*. Berlin: Springer, 1992: 515–532.

96 Roderick P J, Raleigh V S, Hallam L & Mallick N P. The need and demand for renal replacement therapy in ethnic minorities in England. *J Epidemiol Community Health* 1996; 50(3):334–339.

97 Easterling R E. Racial factors in the incidence and causation of end-stage renal disease (ESRD). *Trans Am Soc Artif Intern Organs* 1977; 23:28–33.

98 Naqvi S A J. Nephrology services in Pakistan. *Nephrol. Dial Transplant* 2000; 15:769–771.

99 Chugh K S & Sakhuja V. Renal disease in northern India. In Kibukamusoke J W (ed.) *Tropical Nephrology*. Canberra: Citforge, 1984: 428–440.

100 Kirubakaran M G. Renal disease in South India. In Kibukamusoke J W (ed.) *Tropical Nephrology*. Canberra: Citforge, 1984: 448–456.

101 Matekole M, Affram K, Lee S J, Howie A J, Michael J & Adu D. Hypertension and end-stage renal failure in tropical Africa. *J. Hum Hypertens* 1993; 7(5):443–446.

102 Brenner B M, Meyer T W & Hostetter T H. Dietary protein intake and the progressive nature of kidney disease: the role of haemodynamically mediated glomerular injury in the pathogenesis of progressive glomerular sclerosis in aging,

renal ablation and intrinsic renal disease. *N Engl J Med* 1982; 307:652–659.

103 Remuzzi G & Bertani T. Pathophysiology of progressive nephropathies. *N Engl J Med* 1998; 339:1448–1456.

104 Erkan E, De Leon M & Devarajan P. Albumin overload induces apoptosis in LLC-PK(1) cells. *Am J Physiol Renal Physiol* 2001; 280(6):F1107–1114.

105 Reichel H, Drüeke T & Ritz E. Skeletal disorders. In Davison A M, Cameron J S, Grunfeld J-P, Kerr D N S, Ritz E & Winearls C G (eds) *Oxford Textbook of Clinical Nephrology*. Oxford: Oxford University Press, 1998: 1954–1981.

106 MacDougall I C & Eckardt K-U. Haematological disorders. In Davison A M, Cameron J S, Grunfeld J-P, Kerr D N S, Ritz E & Winearls C G (eds) *Oxford Textbook of Clinical Nephrology*. Oxford: Oxford University Press, 1998: 1935–1953.

107 Ruggenenti P, Schieppati A & Remuzzi G. Progression, remission, regression of chronic renal diseases. *Lancet* 2001; 357(9268):1601–1608.

108 Klahr S, Levey A S, Beck G J, Caggiula A W, Hunsicker L, Kusek J W & Striker G. The effects of dietary protein restriction and blood-pressure control on the progression of chronic renal disease: Modification of diet in Renal Disease Study Group. *N Engl J Med* 1994; 330(13):877–884.

109 The GISEN Group. Randomized placebo-controlled trial of effect of ramipril on decline in glomerular filtration rate and risk of terminal renal failure in proteinuric, non-diabetic nephropathy. *Lancet* 1997; 349:1857–1863.

110 DCCT Research Group. The absence of a glycemic threshold for the development of long-term complications: the perspective of the diabetes control and complications trial. *Diabetes* 1996; 45:1289–1298.

111 Stratton I M, Adler A I, Neil H A W et al. Association of glycaemia with macrovascular and microvascular complications of type 2 diabetes (UKPDS 35): prospective observational study. *BMJ* 2000; 321:405–412.

112 Adler AI, Stratton I M, Neil H A W et al. Association of systolic blood pressure with macrovascular and microvascular complications of type 2 diabetes (UKPDS 36): prospective observational study. *BMJ* 2000; 321:412–419.

113 Eastwood J B, Corbishley C M & Grange J M. Tuberculosis and the kidney. *J Am Soc Nephrol* 2001; 12:1307–1314.

114 Robertson W G. Urolithiasis: epidemiology and pathogenesis. In Husain I (ed.) *Tropical Urology and Renal Disease*. Edinburgh: Churchill Livingstone, 1984: 143–164.

115 Barsoum R S. Schistosomaisis. In Davison A M, Cameron J S, Grunfeld J-P, Kerr D N S, Ritz E & Winearls C G (eds) *Oxford Textbook of Clinical Nephrology*. Oxford: Oxford University Press, 1998: 1287–1301.

Chapter 16
Tropical Neurology

M. Atadzhanov

Introduction

Applying equally to other chapters in this book is the problem of a comprehensive yet pragmatic definition of tropical medicine—for which there appears to be no simple resolution. Even the nineteenth-century rubric—those diseases which prevail between the tropics of Cancer and Capricorn—was unsatisfactory because illnesses such as cholera, typhoid, typhus and malaria occurred widely in Europe until the beginning of the twentieth century. Now, when speed and facility of travel can dramatically influence presentation of disease, definitions must be appropriately elastic. No doubt controversy will continue concerning a more suitable, precise and contemporary name for this specialty. Maurice King's term 'the medicine of poverty' is probably as succinct as can be presently contrived—to embrace afflictions arising from primitive social conditions, malnutrition, high population growth, ignorance of 'overly traditional societies', high infant mortality rates and low life expectation, all fundamentally determined by major factors beyond the powers of physicians; only the economist, engineer, agriculturalist and those who can alter the distribution of global wealth can make a significant impact.

Tropical neurology encompasses a wide range of infectious and non-infectious clinical presentations. It is not limited to bizarre manifestations of viral, bacterial and parasitic infections, but also reflects the expression of many non-infectious diseases in a particular environment where malnutrition, trauma, perinatal injury and cerebrovascular and degenerative diseases tend to show patterns of nineteenth-century Western proportions; 'younger' societies may show different disease distributions. These are among the many factors that must be taken into consideration when assessing and comparing epidemiological surveys. Consider, for example, epilepsy: this is a major neurological disorder in the tropics and has important medical and social implications (Table 16.1).[1] Attempts to determine accurately the magnitude of the problem have encountered considerable difficulties, including differences in definition and methods of case detection. It is therefore difficult to determine what significance should be attributed to the reported relatively low prevalence in India and the fact that certain regions of Africa and Latin America have a very high prevalence,

Table 16.1 Causes of fits/convulsions.

Infections
Meningitis
Encephalitis
HIV/AIDS
Cerebral malaria
Tuberculous meningitis/tuberculoma
Neurocysticerosis
Schistosomiasis
Cerebral hydatid diseases
Paragonimiasis
Cerebral toxoplasmosis
Cerebral amoebiasis
Tetanus (pseudoepilepsy)
Alcohol
Trauma (cerebral concussion, contusion, laceration, extradural or intracerebral haemorrhage)
Cerebrovascular accident (thrombosis, haemorrhage, embolism)
Aneurysm
Metabolic (hypoglycaemia, hyperglycaemia, insulinoma, uraemia)
Drugs (opiates, overdose)
Space-occupying lesions (primary and secondary tumours, cysts, abscesses, tuberculoma, hydatid)
Hydrocephalus

sometimes as much as ten times the average for industrialized countries. It would appear that rural prevalence is lower than in urban areas, partial seizures more common than primary generalized ones and mortality rates for epilepsy appear to be higher in tropical countries in comparison to those in industrialized areas. Known aetiological factors present a bewildering spectrum.[2] Cysticercosis accounts for about half the cases of epilepsy of late onset in several countries. Other parasitic infections known to cause epilepsy include schistosomiasis, paragonimiasis, sparganosis, hydatid disease, toxoplasmosis, trypanosomiasis, cerebral malaria, cerebral amoebiasis and *Gnathostoma spinigerum*. Tuberculous, pyogenic, viral and fungal infections can also cause epilepsy as a late sequel as well as being a feature of the acute illness. Poor antenatal and perinatal care resulting in perinatal brain damage probably contributes to a higher prevalence. Despite these problems there have been impressive attempts to sharpen the epidemiological profile of epilepsy. Thus a recent survey[3] of a rural Tanzanian population showed a prevalence of 11.4 per thousand in a population of 18 183. It was possible to study 203 of these in detail: 32.5% had partial seizures, 85.2% tonic–clonic ones and 8.4% had unclassifiable fits; 95% initially sought aid from outside the immediate family—a traditional healer, a priest—and 80% had consulted traditional healers. Fewer than 20% of the patients were receiving regular anti-convulsants. The authors stress the importance of improving patient attitudes and, in particular, acceptance of anticonvulsant therapy. The epidemic of human immunodeficiency virus (HIV) has had some effect on the epidemiology, clinical and pathological presentation of epilepsy. New-onset seizures are frequent manifestations of the central nervous system (CNS) disorders in patients infected with HIV.[4] In some patients the HIV infection itself may be the cause of the seizure.[5]

On 12 October 1999 the world's population reached an estimated 6 billion[6] and by the year 2050 is likely to be 9.3 billion. 'The growth of the earth's population has been like a long thin powder fuse that burns slowly and haltingly until it finally reaches the charge and explodes' (Kingsley Davis). To this potential explosion must be added the impact of global environmental change[7] on disease patterns.[8] Thus the effects of global warming on the distribution of parasitic and other infectious diseases—disequilibrium in physical and biological ecosystems—and the potential impact of climate changes on world food supply indicate that the developing countries are likely to bear the brunt of the problem. The disparity between developed and developing countries may become even more conspicuous. Famine is as old as humanity and 'tropical diseases' and their neurological complications are likely to increase. The past three decades have seen the rapid spread of the HIV epidemic throughout the tropics and neurological manifestations of infection with HIV are common.

Nutritional and toxic factors

The clinical features of the major classical nutritional disorders of the central and peripheral nervous systems are well known, as is the importance of the vitamin B complex for the development and functioning of the nervous system. Thus beriberi ('I can't, I can't', depicting profound weakness), usually due to the discarded germinal layer of polished rice, presents clinically in the wet or dry form: the salient neurological features are painful poly-neuropathy with tender calves and sensitive soles. Pellagra, due to a similar dietary deficiency mainly involving the nicotinic acid obtained in white maize, presents clinically—often in endemic spring attacks—with diarrhoea, a light-sensitive erythematous rash progressing to thickening

and atrophy with glossitis, diplopia, dysarthria, myelo-pathy and neuropathy with psychological and behavioural changes. Wernicke's encephalopathy may be acute or insidious, with vomiting, nystagmus, diplopia, confusion, ophthalmoplegia, retinal haemorrhages, polyneuropathy, and a dramatic Korsakoff's syndrome with amnesia and confabulation. Alcoholism is the most frequent pre-disposing factor for Wernicke's encephalopathy. High levels of alcohol consumption and abuse were found in some tropical countries.[9] The effects of excessive alcohol consumption, and its relationship to current neurological practice, are a potentially important area of future research in these countries. It will be appreciated that even in communities known to be thiamine deficient from the consumption of processed rice, or in maize-eating populations known to be vulnerable to pellagra from niacin deficiency, it is common to see the con-sequences of the lack of thiamine, pyridoxine and niacin and perhaps also pantothenic acid in combination, necessitating appropriate blunderbuss therapy. The manner in which thiamine depletion produces neurological dis-orders is unknown.

It will also be appreciated that there are numerous local and usually well-recognized (yet to appear in classical textbooks) nutritional syndromes. For example, among certain hill tribes in north-east Burma it is tra-ditional for women to consume only polished rice while pregnant; their infants may develop an unusual pattern of beriberi with congestive heart failure, hepato-splenomegaly and aphonia due to bilateral recurrent laryngeal nerve lesions which respond promptly to parenteral pyridoxine. Strachan's syndrome (visual failure, painful neuropathy and oral, perianal and scrotal dermatitis and ulceration) has been described in several parts of the world and is another probable consequence of multiple nutritional deficiencies including riboflavin, thiamine, niacin and pyridoxine. The painful burning feet described in prisoner-of-war camps was probably another example of multiple nutritional deficiency.

Clinically and epidemiologically it is often difficult to separate the consequences of nutritional deficiency from environmental toxins because they tend to occur in similar settings and the manifestations may be indistinguishable. The problem is further compounded by the increasing quantities of chemicals, often indiscriminately used in industry and agriculture as well as medicine. Toxic pesticides merit particular attention and many of the hazards arise from the lack of precautions and facilities for handling and storing these neurotoxic products safely.

The peripheral nervous system is commonly affected and has been frequently studied because it is easier to recognize clinically and to investigate electrodiagnostically and by nerve biopsy. While the pathophysiology may vary according to the putative toxin, distal axonal degeneration—so-called 'dying back' phenomenon[10]—is the most common mechanism; initially, longer or larger nerve fibres are involved, then degeneration begins in the distal regions of the nerve fibres, progressing proximally with time. However, mechanisms are probably more complex: experimental evidence suggests that many toxic agents act at the level of the axon rather than the cell body,[11] impairing axonal transport; others may disturb anabolic mechanisms in the region of the neuronal perikaryon. Whatever the precise mechanism, clinical features are similar. Early symptoms are usually sensory with paraesthesiae, suprasensitivity, hyperalgesia and pain, followed later by peripheral weakness and wasting. Impairment of tendon reflexes occurs early and all sensory modalities may be variably affected. Some have associated myelopathic disturbances with spasticity and extensor plantar responses. Involvement of the autonomic nervous system with defective sweating and vasomotor disturbances commonly occurs.

The list of known aetiological agents is legion (Table 16.2). Heavy metals such as arsenic, lead and thallium are

Table 16.2 Causes of neuropathy/weakness.

Infections
Leprosy
HIV
Spinal schistosomiasis
Spinal tuberculosis
Spinal brucellosis
Tropical spastic paraparesis (HTLV-1)
Postinfectious ascending neuropathy (Guillain–Barré syndrome)
Diphtheria
Botulism

Metabolic
Diabetes mellitus
Uraemia
Amyloidosis
Porphyria

Toxins/metals
Ciguatera fish
Snake (see Chapter 32)
Cassava (cyanide)
Lathyrism and cycad poisoning (plant toxins)
Heavy metals (lead, arsenic, thallium)

Nutritional deficiencies
Vitamin B complex
    Vitamin B_{12} deficiency (subacute combined degeneration of spinal cord)
    Thiamine (beriberi, alcoholism)
    Nicotinic acid (pellagra)
Pyridoxine deficiency

Drugs/chemicals
Isoniazid, nitrofurantoin, vincristine, chloroquine

Mechanical
Trauma, compression, stretching

Miscellaneous
Sarcoidosis
Rheumatoid arthritis
Malignancy
Hereditary neuropathies

often found in traditional folklore medications.[12] For example, arsenical polyneuropathy (acute, or more commonly chronic) occurs very widely. Acute symptoms may include vomiting, diarrhoea, burning discomfort in the eyes, excessive tears, photophobia, congestion and facial swelling, followed by a predominantly sensory neuropathy. Mees' lines (transverse white bands across the fingernails) frequently occur, as does increased pigmentation of the extremities with patches of depigmentation, hyperkeratosis and desquamation of palms and soles. Here the diagnosis may be confirmed, if facilities permit, by demonstrating high concentrations of arsenic in scalp hairs and nail clippings. Illicit liquor, crude arbortifacients and well water deliberately contaminated by an enemy have all been reported.[13] It will also be recalled that certain ocean fish and marine crustacea, such as the pomfret, plaice, halua and hilsa, may contain relatively high concentrations of arsenic. Another source of arsenical poisoning is said to be contaminated opium. The mechanism is thought to be direct reaction of arsenical compounds with the sulfhydryl group of proteins; electrophysiologically the signs of distal axonal degeneration and nerve biopsies show loss of myelinated fibres and degeneration of myelin into rows of myelin ovoids;[14] segmental demyelination and inflammatory changes do not occur. In the acute stages dimercaprol and/or penicillamine must be given early; when there is a delay, response may be poor.

Lead may cause a peripheral neuropathy in adults and an encephalopathy in children. Lead neuropathy tends to be predominantly motor, more evident in the upper limbs where the extensors of the wrists and fingers are affected early and asymmetrically, tending to affect the dominant hand.[15] Proximal involvement is slow and occurs later, and sensory disturbances are minimal or absent. Associated abdominal colic and the characteristic anaemia with punctate basophilia, when present, may suggest the diagnosis. Potential sources include reconditioning of car batteries and burning lead-containing batteries for cooking, illicit liquor distillation by means of lead pipes or radiators, and contaminated water.

Thallium may be a constituent of rodenticides. The acute painful neuropathy may be associated with gastrointestinal symptoms—non-specific signs—but the occurrence of alopecia within 3 weeks should suggest the diagnosis.[16] Potassium ferrocyanide, given orally, is the present treatment of choice.

Of the many conventional medications that may provoke peripheral neuropathy brief mention will be made of those drugs widely used in the treatment of tropical bacterial and parasitic infections. Peripheral neuropathy, particularly in those genetically disposed to slow acetylation of isoniazid for the treatment of tuberculosis, is well known, as is the similar hazard of ethionamide, from sulfonamides widely used in bacillary dysentery and urinary tract infections; similarly the optic neuritis related to ethambutol. Chloroquine, a standard antimalarial agent, may produce a neuromyopathy after prolonged use, with muscle fibres showing vacuolation and peripheral nerves showing involvement of terminal axons with Schwann cell defects.[17] Clioquinol—previously widely used in the symptomatic treatment of diarrhoea and intestinal amoebiasis—is now known to be the causative agent of subacute myelo-optic neuropathy;[18] unfortunately clioquinol continues to be prescribed in certain countries and the complication is still sporadically encountered. The aromatic diamidines used in the treatment of leishmaniasis and trypanosomiasis have been associated with an odd, uncommon focal disturbance of sensory function of the trigeminal nerve.

Industrial chemicals of known potential neurotoxicity rarely cause hazards in developed societies; it is where appropriate safety measures and conditions are not practised that outbreaks continue to occur. Well known is trio-ortho-creasyl phosphate; commonly used as an industrial solvent, it has been the culprit in many reported outbreaks.[19] Accidental contamination of food, particularly edible oils, may produce not only classical peripheral mixed neuropathy, but also signs of cord involvement. Unfortunately, the damage is permanent and there is no curative or generally available protective agent. In unprotected environments, carbon disulfide and acrylamide may produce similar hazards. Insecticides widely dispensed in tropical countries are a common cause. The most common culprit is the group of organophosphorous insecticides; the defect is believed to be mainly at the postsynaptic border of the neuromuscular junction. Clinically the onset may be acute or delayed.

Particularly well documented in recent years are the toxic effects of the root crop cassava, a major crop sustaining millions of people in Africa.[20] Flour made from cassava roots may contain a high concentration of linamarin, a cyanogenic glycoside, resulting in chronic cyanide intoxication and clinically 'tropical ataxic neuropathy'. The clinical features in addition to painful neuropathy and ataxia may include blurred vision and impaired hearing of cochlear type; occasionally upper motor neurone lesions are seen. This pattern of illness is usually slowly progressive.

Konzo is a clinically distinct pattern of tropical myelopathy because of its abrupt onset and dominant upper motor neurone pattern of involvement.[21] A recent study in rural Zaire[22] was able to determine the cyanergine content of the locally used cassava flour and blood cyanide concentrations in cases and controls. This detailed study indicated that not only was there a significant sustained high blood cyanide concentration, but also that the deficient sulfur intake impaired the conversion of cyanide to thiocyanate. Even though the immediate causes are poverty and shortage of food, a relatively minor change in traditional cooking habits could prevent much disability.

Lathyrism and *cycad* poisoning are two other well-known examples of neurotoxic plant poisons affecting the CNS. Lathyrism, endemic in parts of India, Bangladesh and Ethiopia, is caused by excessive consumption of peas of the lathyrus family (chickpeas). It presents as a slowly progressive spastic paraparesis: neuropathological studies have shown selective atrophy of the pyramidal, spinocerebellar and dorsal columns of the spinal cord. The neurotoxin is an amino acid β-*N*-oxalylamino-L-alanine, which is thought to act by excessive and prolonged exhaustion stimulation—a so-called excitatory amino acid. Once damage has occurred there is no effective treatment. In a similar manner excessive consumption of the seed of the false-sago palm—either as a foodstuff or as a medicinal component—may have an excitatory neurotoxic effect and may be one of the constellation of factors responsible for the occurrence of amyotrophic lateral sclerosis and Parkinsonism–dementia complex in the Pacific Mariana Islands.[23]

Rarer plant toxins include that of *Gloriosa superba* (glory lily):[24] accidental ingestion may cause alopecia, aplastic anaemia and polyneuropathy due to colchicine, which impairs exoplasmic transport in peripheral nerves and also damages skeletal muscle. Podophyllin (from the dried rhizome and root of the mandrake) also has neurotoxic properties. A recent report from Hong Kong[25] described encephalopathy and sensorimotor polyneuropathy and autonomic changes after ingestion of a broth containing herbal guyjiu. Another poisonous shrub of the buckthorn family (*Karwinskia humboldtiana*), which grows freely in Mexico and Texas, may cause a progressive polyneuropathy, terminating in respiratory and bulbar paralysis.[26]

All these essentially irreversible and disabling toxic disturbances of the central autonomic and peripheral nervous systems are preventable and presumably will continue to be observed and reported in the developing world until nutritional, economic and educational disparities are resolved.

CNS infections

The variety of infectious agents which can damage the nervous system is vast and their clinical manifestations are protean. Table 16.3 lists those which cause meningitis and encephalitis, and Table 16.4 lists infectious and non-infectious causes of decreased consciousness and confusion. Symptoms related to CNS infections are (a) headache, (b) fever, (c) irritability, (d) confusion, (e) photophobia, (f) vomiting, (g) deteriorating conscious levels and (h) fits; in addition, children may have listlessness and failure to feed.

In addition to the general predisposing factors mentioned above—poverty, ignorance, deprivation, inadequate education—is the prevalence and persistence of insect and other vectors which thrive in humid climates and which survive throughout the seasons. In a limited review it is possible to indicate only certain salient clinical features of some of these numerous disorders, which will be discussed under conventional categories.

Viruses (See also Chapters 20, 41, 45 and 49)

The acute exanthemas of childhood—measles, mumps

Table 16.3 Causes of meningitis and encephalitis.

Meningitis
Bacterial
Neisseria meningitidis
Streptococcus pneumoniae
Haemophilus influenzae
Mycobacterium tuberculosis
Listeria monocytogenes
Escherichia coli
Brucella spp.
Viral
Enterovirus (polio, echo, Coxsackie)
Mumps virus
HIV (also *Cryptococcus neoformans* in AIDS)
Protozoal
Amoebae (*Naegleria fowleri*, Acanthamoebae)
Helminths
Strongyloides stercoralis (hyperinfection syndrome)
Angiostrongylus cantonensis
Gnathostoma spp.
Encephalitis
Acute
Arboviruses
Herpes simplex
Measles
Chickenpox
Yellow fever
Rabies
Trichinella spiralis
Subacute/chronic
African trypanosomiasis
AIDS (cryptococcal, toxoplasmosis)
Rickettsia spp.
Kuru

Table 16.4 Confusion/decreased conscious level.

Infective	Non-infective
Meningitis	Drugs/alcohol/herbal medicines
Encephalitis	Dehydration
Cerebral malaria	Liver failure (acute fulminant hepatitis)
AIDS (e.g. HIV encephalopathy)	Hypoglycaemia (e.g. in malaria)
Viral haemorrhagic fever, e.g. dengue	Hypertensive stroke
Legionnaires' disease	Head injury
Leptospirosis	Renal failure
Typhus	Psychiatric illness (hysterical conversion)
Relapsing fever	
Septicaemia	
Viral haemorrhagic fevers	
Rabies	
Neurocysticercosis	

and chickenpox—are still major killers, especially when epidemics occur in the presence of severe malnutrition. The clinical scene and the therapeutic possibilities have changed considerably in recent years. Thus acute poliomyelitis (see below) is now rarely seen—an impressive example of the power of truly effective preventive medicine. Similarly subacute sclerosing panencephalitis (SSPE) is disappearing in many parts of the world where measles vaccination is available, but is still prevalent and fatal in many parts of the Middle East, Far East, India, Africa and South America; the eradication of measles should greatly diminish the incidence of SSPE. There are conflicting reports on its pathogenesis and management.[27,28] Several authors have reported the use of intraventricular interferon α or the combined use of interferon α plus isoprinosin.[29]

Acute viral encephalitis

Acute viral encephalitis—due to direct invasion of the brain parenchyma—is indistinguishable clinically from the postinfectious encephalitides where perivenous

demyelination is probably triggered by allergic or immune reactions caused by a latent viral infection. Globally, viruses are by far the most common cause of encephalitis. The arboviruses cause epidemic encephalitides in many parts of the world. The majority are perpetuated by zoonoses, often inconspicuous infections obtained from birds and smaller vertebrates; transmission is by an arthropod vector such as a mosquito or tick. After replication and viraemia, encephalitis of unpredictable gravity develops. Many patients recover spontaneously after a mild attack; others may deteriorate and die within days or weeks. The clinical features are common to all: prodromal myalgia, fever and malaise, then headache, mental changes, drowsiness, with or without signs of meningeal irritation; focal neurological abnormalities such as disturbances of behaviour, mood, disorientation, deterioration of speech, level of consciousness, fits (focal or generalized), raised intracranial pressure and a deepening coma. Even when sophisticated diagnostic neuroimaging techniques such as computed tomography (CT) or magnetic resonance imaging (MRI) are available, there may be no specific features and the EEG and cerebrospinal fluid (CSF) may not be diagnostically helpful. The demonstration of sequential changes in antibody titre in samples of serum or CSF may be the only means of establishing the true agent in sporadic cases and usually the illness has taken its course by the time the agent is confirmed.

Eastern equine encephalitis

Eastern equine encephalitis—mainly on the Atlantic and Gulf coasts of America—tends to occur in summer and autumn and the mortality may be as high as 70%;[30]

Western equine encephalitis, which despite its name occurs throughout the USA and eastern South America, tends to be less severe.

Japanese encephalitis is a mosquito-borne arboviral infection which still claims many lives in South-East Asia. The virus is antigenically related to the flaviviruses of St Louis encephalitis and Murray Valley encephalitis and to the West Nile virus. The illness is usually severe, and fatal in about 25% of cases, with neuropsychiatric sequelae in a further 30%. It mainly affects the young, but a shift now to the elderly may be due to early immunization. CT and MRI show thalamic involvement (Figure 16.1). An inactivated Japanese encephalitis virus vaccine is now available and its use should reduce the incidence in due course.[31] Sporadic and epidemic attacks of encephalitis continue to be reported from different parts of the world and often the reasons for these fluctuations remain obscure. For example,

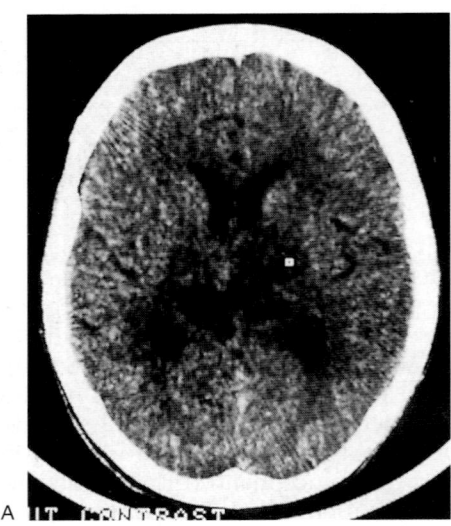

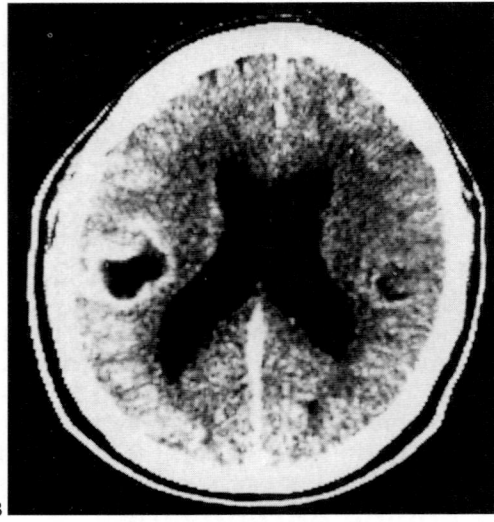

Figure 16.1: Japanese encephalitis. Brain scan (**A**) before and (**B**) after contrast showing thalamic lesions. (Courtesy of M. Gourie-Devi, National Institute of Mental Health and Neurosciences, Bangalore, India.)

Rift Valley fever has recently been recorded in Egypt after an absence of over 12 years. In 1993, patients began to complain of a febrile illness with headaches, retro-orbital pain, nausea, vomiting and loss of vision with or without features of a generalized encephalitis.[32] In this pattern of illness a reasonably firm clinical diagnosis can be made because of the frequent finding of macular and paramacular retinal lesions, often with haemorrhage and oedema, occurring at a time when there has been an abnormally high number of abortions in cattle and buffalo, but the true reason(s) for the recurrence remain cryptic.

Poliomyelitis

At the end of 2000, 20 countries remained endemic for polio and fewer than 2900 cases were reported. Wild polio-virus circulation is now concentrated in South Asia, the horn of Africa and West and Central Africa.[33] The America region was certified free of polio in 1994 and the western Pacific region in October 2000.[34]

Although the initial 2000 target for polio eradication was overly optimistic, progress has been steady. WHO and its partners have recently recommitted to achieving global eradication by the end of 2005.

Vaccine-associated paralytic poliomyelitis is the prominent form of the disease not only in Western countries, but also in the developing world. In those vaccine-related cases reported in the USA there were three high-risk groups: infants receiving the first oral polio vaccine dose, unvaccinated or inadequately vaccinated adults who are in contact with receipients of oral polio vaccine, and immunocompromised individuals. Wild poliovirus causing disease is still a problem in small pockets of individuals in Western Europe who for religious reasons refuse vaccination, as exemplified by the 1992 outbreak in Holland. While apparent outbreaks are still reported worldwide,[33,35,36] and persisting low-level transmission in Egypt threatens to undermine the idea of eradication.

Dengue

Dengue, especially the haemorrhagic variety, still causes considerable morbidity and fatality in South-East Asia, and yellow fever similarly in Africa and South America.

Lassa fever

Lassa fever, an acute haemorrhagic febrile illness occurring in West Africa, carries a fatality of up to 20%. It is caused by an arenavirus spread by a rodent (*Mastomys natalensis*) and causes a wide spectrum of clinical disease, from asymptomatic or trivial malaise to fatal illness, and is often associated with neurological manifestations during the acute disease or in early convalescence. Delirium, convulsions and coma occur in critically ill patients; deafness may occur towards the end of an acute illness and is believed to be the result of cochlear nerve damage. The importance of metabolic encephalopathy, severe tremor, self-limiting encephalitis, late ataxia and subacute or chronic neuropsychiatric sequelae has been emphasized.[37]

Rabies

Rabies remains endemic throughout the world[38] except for the UK, Australasia, the Caribbean and Scandinavia. In Indonesia about 700 000 people are treated for exposure to the virus each year and worldwide more than 1 million receive rabies vaccine annually. No patient has survived the established disease. Whereas vaccines derived from cell cultures are now much safer and more effective than animal-derived preparations,[39] sadly the vast majority of human exposure to rabies occurs in developing countries, most of whom cannot afford cell culture vaccines. The majority will have access only to vaccines derived from animal neural tissue, which unfortunately may result in a disabling immune response. Reports of such neurological complications range from 1:1200[40] to 1:120.[41] Consequently many people in developing countries who are bitten and potentially exposed to rabies will deliberately avoid vaccination, fully aware of the possible hazards. Attempts to control the animal reservoir of rabies have not been successful and even in developed countries wildlife reservoirs affecting racoons and foxes still persist. The need for low-cost safe rabies vaccines equally acceptable in the developed and developing world remains a technological challenge. The WHO recently recommended a rabies vaccine pre-exposure schedule using three intradermal injections of one-fifth the standard intermuscular dose of current cell culture vaccines as a cost-reducing alternative for developing countries.[42]

HIV

HIV infection is causing major morbidity and mortality in Africa and there is a similar trend in South-East Asia. The nervous system is among the most frequent and serious targets of HIV infection. Forty per cent to 70% of all persons infected with HIV develop symptomatic neurological disorders.[43] Despite more than 15 years of extensive investigative efforts, a complete understanding of the neurological consequences of HIV infection remains elusive. Illnesses affecting the nervous system because of HIV may be separated into primary illnesses, which may be the direct result of the virus, and secondary illnesses, which result from other identifiable causes. Primary HIV-asssociated disorders include encephalopathy (dementia), myelopathy, distal sensory polyneuropathy and myopathy. Secondary complications are chiefly as a consequence of the severe abnormalities of cellular immunity accompanying AIDS. The main infectious complications are cerebral toxoplasmosis, cryptoccocal meninigitis, cytomegalovirus infection and progressive mutifocal leucoencephalopathy.[44] All neurology complications of HIV infection cannot be adequately covered in a short review. One of the most frequent primary complications of HIV infection is HIV dementia (HIV encephalopathy). The symptoms of HIV dementia are characterized by deterioration of mental status, motor signs and behavioural abnormalities. Cerebral toxoplasmosis is the most common secondary complication

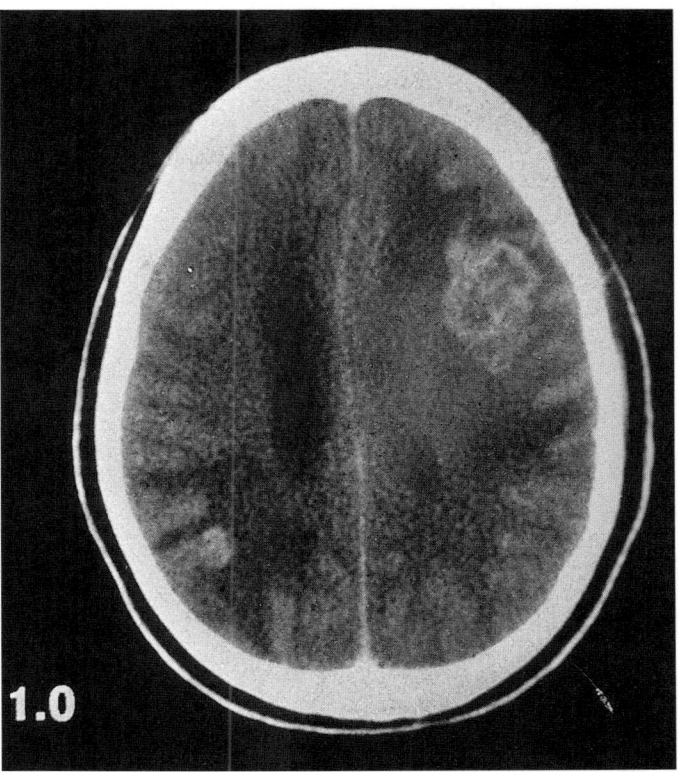

A

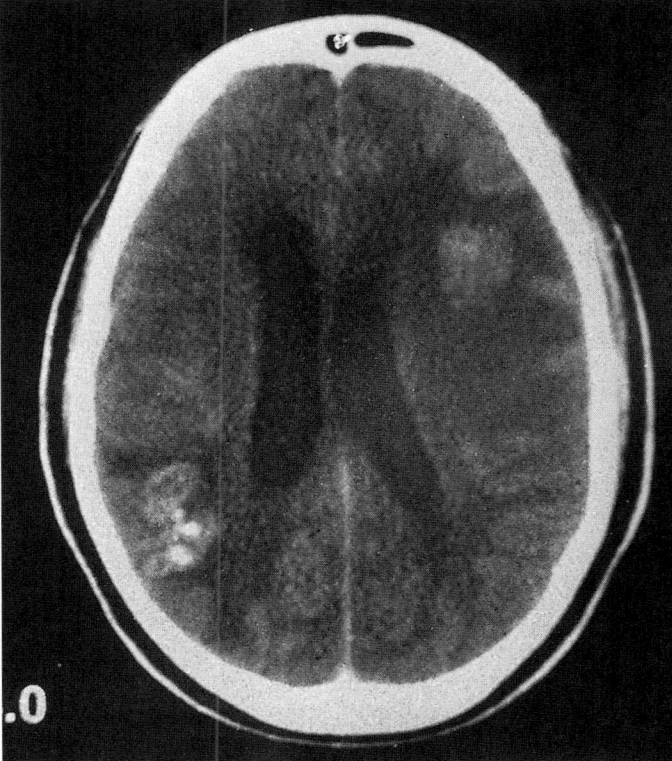

B

Figure 16.2: CT scan of the brain showing multifocal (left tempoparietal (**A**) and right posterior supratentorial (**B**) areas) ringenhancing lesions with surrounding oedema in a Zambian patient with cysticercosis.

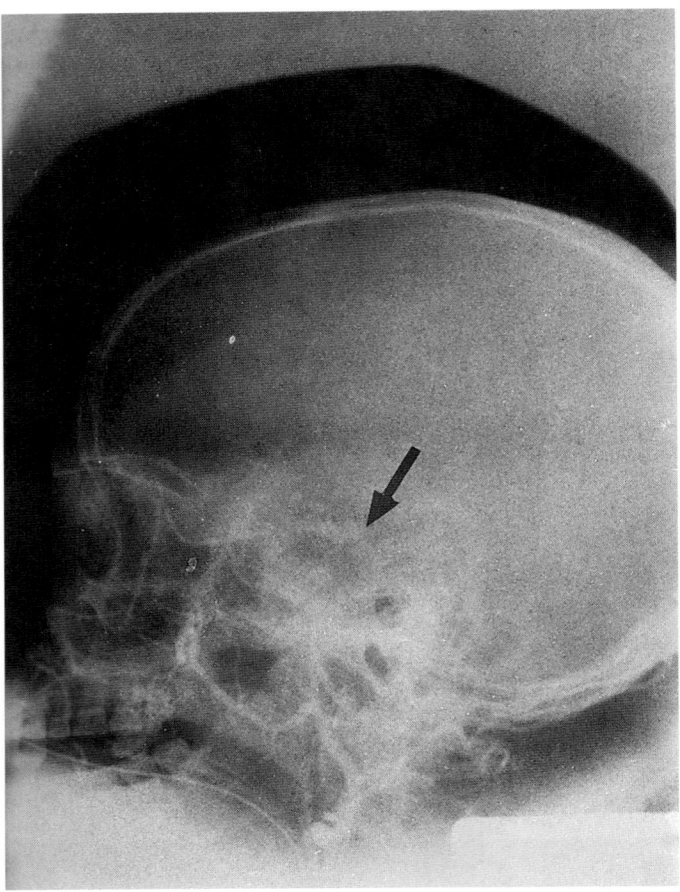

Figure 16.3: Carotid angiography showing the posterior communicating artery aneurism. (Courtesy of Dr T. K. Lambart, University Teaching Hospital, Lusaka, Zambia.)

of HIV infection. The most frequent clinical manifestations of toxoplasmic encephalitis may present as generalized symptoms (headache, disturbances of consciousness and seizures) and focal neurological signs (hemiparesis, ataxia, and cranial nerve palsies). Brain CT scan reveals single or multiple ring-enhancing lesions (Figure 16.2). Other neurological manifestations of HIV infection include aseptic meningitis, primary and secondary neoplasms, neurosyphilis and cerebrovascular complications (Figure 16.3).

Human T lymphotropic virus

A recent discovery concerns the related human T lymphotropic virus (HTLV)-I, which may be responsible for certain patterns of chronic myelopathy seen in the tropics, separating this group of illnesses from the tropical paraparesis and ataxic neuropathic group. HTLV-I-associated myelopathy was first described in the Caribbean[45] and Japan, and is also found in many parts of Africa.[46] Previously described under many guises, including tropical paraparesis and ataxic neuropathy,[47] its relation to adult T cell leukaemia and clinical progress is now well established.[48]

HTLV-I-associated myelopathy/tropical spastic paraplegia (HAM/TSP) is a condition which appears in the fifth decade as a slowly progressive spastic paraparesis. There is usually sphincter involvement with some sensory changes. HTLV-I-specific uveitis can present acutely or subacutely with vitreous opacities, mild iritis and retinal vasculitis.[49] There may be some mild pleocytosis with raised IgG and positive oligoclonal bands on a CSF study. HTLV-I-specific cytotoxic T lymphocytes were isolated in the CSF of HAM/TSP patients.[50] The transmission of HTLV-I virus is reported to be through infected T lymphocytes (this can occur sexually), through blood transfusions, or vertically from mother to infant through milk.[51]

HAM/TSP has been reported not only in the tropics but also in immigrants in Europe and the USA[52] and needs to be differentiated from multiple sclerosis,[53] subacute combined degeneration, syphilis and Behçet's disease. The neuroimaging of patients with HAM/TSP shows normal myelography and periventricular low density with ventricular enlargement on brain CT; MRI shows high-intensity signals in the periventricular and subcortical white matter. Features of spinal cord atrophy have been described.[54] HTLV-II is a close relative of HTLV-I—structurally similar but molecularly distinct—and has been associated with chronic spastic paraparesis and high titres of HTLV-II antibodies in the serum and CSF.

Clearly the full spectrum of human illnesses due to this family of retroviruses is yet to be determined. All human retroviruses studied to date have been lymphotropic; whether they will all prove to cause disease of the nervous system remains to be elucidated. From the clinical point of view, presentations may be multiple; toxoplasmosis, lymphoma, progressive leucoencephalopathy and HIV encephalopathy may all overlap in the same individual. Thus multiple focal brain lesions may be due to the simultaneous development of lymphoma, toxoplasma abscesses or tuberculosis. Opportunistic infections, including parasites, fungi, bacteria as well as viruses, may cause diagnostic difficulties of unparalleled complexity.

Rickettsia (See also Chapter 50)

This group of illnesses,[55] which usually present as an acute meningoencephalitis, are transmitted to man by the bites of ticks or mites and occur throughout the world except in Antarctica. Mediterranean spotted fever (*Rickettsia conorii*) in Africa, Asia and the Mediterranean basin,[56] scrub typhus (*R. tsutsugamushi*) in Asia and the Pacific, typhus (*R. prowazekii*) and Q fever (*Coxiella burnetii*) are ubiquitous. Whereas the incubation period and clinical features vary between organisms, all patients manifest high fever, rash and headache, with meningoencephalitis developing during the second week of the illness.[57] Nonfocal neurological features include headache, neck stiffness and photophobia, confusion, impairment of consciousness and fits. When present, the distinctive eschar at the site of the bite may suggest the diagnosis. CSF examination is rarely helpful and treatment should be started on clinical suspicion. The response to tetracycline or chloramphenicol is usually gratifying.

Bacterial infections (See also Chapters 56, 57, 59, 60 and 67)

The organisms that produce bacterial infections of the nervous system in tropical regions are similar to those existing in the rest of the world. Despite the diagnosis of acute bacterial meningitis, which is an important cause of morbidity and mortality both in children and adults, there remains difficulty in tropical countries due to inadequate laboratory facilities.[58] Timely detection of meningitis epidemics in the tropics is still a serious problem. It became obvious in 1996 when the worst recorded meningococcal epidemics in history occurred in Africa.[59] In view of field experience and new evidence in 2000 WHO revised its guidelines for detecting meningococcal meningitis epidemics in highly endemic countries of Africa.[60] *Haemophilus influenzae* and meningococcus cause more than four-fifths of the cases of childhood meningitis in Africa.[61] Neonatal meningitis may be caused by almost any organism and most frequently by *Escherichia coli* and other enteric bacilli.[62] In the elderly, Gram-negative bacilli and *Listeria* species should be considered. Confirmatory CSF examination should not delay treatment. In the search for an early appropriate antibiotic in a high-incidence part of Africa, long-acting chloramphenicol injections were found to be as effective as ampicillin four times a day for 8 days. Vaccination remains the only real hope for preventing epidemics of meningitis. Recently data of the effectiveness of conjugate vaccine for *Haemophilus influenzae* type b and meningococcus infection has been obtained for the first time.[63]

Tuberculosis

The HIV epidemic has had a major impact on the worldwide incidence of tuberculosis.[64] In some tropical countries where tuberculosis is endemic and HIV incidence has markedly increased, tuberculosis has become the major opportunistic infection among HIV-infected persons, contributing to high mortality rates.[65] Tuberculosis involvement of the nervous system remains common, and despite the now worldwide availability of effective antituberculous therapy the classical syndromes—spinal cord compression from tuberculous osteitis, tuberculous meningitis, and intracranial tuberculomas—continue to cause significant morbidity and mortality.[66] As far as tuberculous osteitis is concerned it is important to appreciate that this may occur at any spinal level and is not restricted to the dorsal vertebrae; whereas in the early stages of the granulomatous process involving adjacent vertebrae and the intervening disc the cord is usually compressed anteriorly, this is not invariably so. There

may be one or more posterior compressive lesions arising from tuberculous osteitis in the laminae and pedicles, and epidural tuberculomas can easily be confused with epidural tumours and other focal pathologies.

Intracranial tuberculoma—single or multiple—remains the most common cause of a space-occupying lesion in many parts of the world. CT facilities are now more widespread and the most common finding is a hypodense lesion on an unenhanced scan with a ring or disc-like enhancement with contrast and surrounding hypodensity. Where tuberculosis is common, physicians frequently promptly embark on a course of antituberculous therapy without histological verification. After 3 months of treatment a repeat brain scan will show clearing of the lesion. While there are regional differences in the optimal combination of antituberculous drugs, chemotherapy is usually given for 6–12 months, depending upon the severity of the disease and response to treatment; corticosteroids are not given routinely, but dexamethasone in high doses during the acute phase of raised pressure may be helpful in reducing cerebral oedema. Obstructive hydrocephalus may develop at any stage of the illness, sometimes acutely; it is the most likely explanation for sudden neurological deterioration and should be treated promptly by surgical drainage.

Leprosy

Leprosy remains by far the most common cause of chronic mononeuritis multiplex in the world.[67] The WHO currently estimates that there are 5.5 million patients with leprosy worldwide, a fall of about 50% since the 1980s. Nevertheless, despite much publicity and public health measures, the disease is frequently overlooked or misdiagnosed, often neglected and still generally feared. Thus the extent of the illness in a community may be difficult to estimate, but all reasonable attempts to do so indicate that, despite the availability of effective treatments, prevalence throughout the world is essentially unaltered. It remains true[68] that 'leprosy should be considered whenever confronted by a chronic and symptomless skin rash that does not correspond with a common dermatosis or which does not respond to standard treatment for similar lesions. Leprosy should be considered in all cases of transient, recurrent or persistent numbness of paraesthesiae especially when this is localized to a more or less well-defined area of skin.' Hypopigmentation, with impaired sensitivity to light touch and pinprick, and particularly focal impairment or absence of sweating, should strongly suggest the diagnosis and a careful search should be made for thickening of peripheral nerves. Most commonly palpable are the great auricular nerve in the neck, the ulnar nerve just above the medial epicondyle, the median nerve at the wrist, the lateral popliteal nerve below the head of the fibula and the sural nerve on the dorsum of the foot. Early thickening may be difficult to clinch. Trained paramedical staff often become expert in detecting and confirming the presence of leprosy in suspects. Even those with advanced disease, severe neuropathy, deformity and incapacity may be helped by skilled reconstructive surgery.

Brucellosis

Brucellosis occurs in many tropical and subtropical areas and the nervous system may be affected in up to 5% of patients in a variety of ways.[69] It can cause an acute meningoencephalitis with papilloedema, convulsions and coma. Spinal presentation is with spastic or flaccid paraparesis due to cord compression or myeloradiculo-pathy, and central involvement with hemiparesis and ataxia. Diagnosis depends on blood or CSF culture of brucella, or more commonly on enzyme-linked immuno-sorbent assay (ELISA) of the blood and CSF.[70] Treatment with rifampicin, tetracycline and streptomycin should be for 3 months in those presenting with the subacute or chronic forms.

Spirochaetes

Neurosyphilis is again on the march and is increasingly occurring in the wake of HIV infection. The old clinical adage remains true—'to know all the manifestations of syphilis is to know the whole of medicine'—but even here there are new twists to perplex even experienced physicians. When a young and apparently otherwise healthy male presents with acute onset of unilateral neural deafness, who would immediately suspect secondary syphilis? Other frequently occurring spirochaetal infections affecting the nervous system include borreliosis or relapsing fever (*Borrelia recurrentis*—louse-borne; *B. duttonii*—tick-borne), usually presenting as a febrile meningoencephalitis. Leptospirosis may affect any part of the nervous system, including an acute neuropathy.[71] Lyme disease (*B. burgdorferi*) is spread to man by infected ticks. While there is a very extensive literature[72] on its diverse neurological and systemic manifestations—now recognized as the leading vector-borne disease in the USA—this malady occurs mainly in temperate climates. The neural manifestations span from meningitis, encephalitis, focal cranial neuropathies, radiculitis neuropathy, encephalopathy and post-borreliosis syndromes.

Protozoa (See also Chapters 71, 73, 74, 77 and 78)

Plasmodium falciparum

The problems of malaria are considered in detail elsewhere in this book. From the neurological aspect cerebral malaria is a major life-threatening complication of *Plasmodium falciparum* in humans, responsible for up to 2 million deaths annually.[73] It is characterized by a marked elevation in body temperature, disturbances of consciousness and coma along with convulsions, acute delirium and symmetrical motor signs. Children, pregnant women and non-immune adults are more susceptible to have cerebral malaria.[74] Cerebral malaria-associated neurological sequelae and systemic complications

like hypoglycaemia, hypovolaemia, hyperpyrexia, renal failure, bleeding disorders, anaemia, lactic acidosis and respiratory distress may contribute to the pathogenisis of coma, and are responsible for high mortality.[75] The mechanisms underlying the fatal cerebral complications of *P. falciparum* are still not fully understood. Studies in murine cerebral malaria models and recent studies of human cerebral malaria indicate a role for the immune system in the neurological complications.[76] However, it is likely that multiple mechanisms are involved in the induction of cerebral complications and both the presence of parasitized erythrocytes in the CNS and immuno-pathological processes contribute to the pathogenesis of cerebral malaria. Despite introducing new antimalaria drugs to clinical practice an effective and practical vaccine is still urgently required.[77] A minor but poorly recognized clinical point: *P. falciparum* can cause polymyositis[78] with muscle pain and weakness. Thus to the list of manifestations of 'malaria the mimic' should be added myositis. The management of postcerebral malaria syndromes (mental and physical retardation in young children, seizures, cranial neuropathies, encephalopathy, tremor and cerebellar dysfunction, sensory and motor deficit, and cerebrovascular disorders) remains a challenge for neurologists in the tropics.

Trypanosomiasis

African trypanosomiasis produces progressive CNS damage which if untreated results in death. Involvement occurs within a few weeks in the case of *Trypanosoma rhodesiense*, but usually takes much longer in the case of *T. gambiense*—months or even years. Leptomeningitis with distended ventricles, demyelination and perivascular cuffing develops and trypanosomes aggregate in the choroid plexus with an eosinophilic CSF reaction. In experimental studies trypanosomes shelter in the ependymal cells. It is also suggested that after clearing the parasite from outside the CNS with chemotherapy there may be an immune-mediated reaction against the intracellular parasite from outside the CNS and this may explain the encephalopathy noted with melarsoprol use and its prevention with steroids. Early clinical symptoms are those of an encephalopathy—with lassitude, sleepiness, walking difficulty, ataxia, tremor, dysarthria and back and neck stiffness; headaches and papilloedema may also occur.[79] The CSF is usually under pressure, with high protein and pleocystosis and the appearance of a modified plasma cell containing a large eosinophilic inclusion of IgG (morular or Mott cells). Therapy for African trypanosomiasis has been transformed by the introduction of eflornithine,[80] which is best given intravenously and has been shown to be effective in late stages of the disease when the CNS is involved, which is not the case with pentamidine and suramin. The problems of early diagnosis and introduction of cheap, safe and effective therapy before irreversible cerebral damage occurs are immense; meanwhile the prognosis for established sleeping sickness must remain grim.

Chagas' disease (American trypanosomiasis) remains a major cause of morbidity and mortality in developing countries; the myocardium is usually heavily parasitized, frequently associated with complicated cardiac arrhythmias and presenting clinically with syncope. American trypanosomiasis caused by *T. cruzi* can involve the nervous system in the acute stage with trypanosomes in the CSF.[81] In its chronic stage enlargement of hollow organs is the diagnostic hallmark. Myositis and neuritis due to demyelination and axonal degeneration with remyelination and regeneration have been described.[82] Recent reports of the occurrence of acute Chagas' disease in patients with the acquired immune deficiency syndrome (AIDS) are usually due to reactivation of chronic or dormant infection. Fatal meningoencephalitis in patients with AIDS, as well as other causes of depressed immunity, are well recognized.[83]

Amoebiasis

Amoebic cerebral abscesses, although uncommon, have been recognized since 1849[84] and, provided the possibility of *Entamoeba histolytica* is considered early, the response to a 5-nitroimidazole compound can be impressive. *E. histolytica* can cause single or multiple cerebral abscesses which are noted on CT and may be clinically silent. Granulomatous amoebic meningoencephalitis commonly occurs in immunocompromised and debilitated individuals, including patients with AIDS. The disease has a subacute course and is generally fatal.[85] Amoebic serology is usually positive with immunofluoroescence, cellulose acetate precipitation and countercurrent immunoelectrophoresis. Brain biopsy occasionally shows *E. histolytica* trophozoites. Oral or intravenous metronidazole should be started and followed by diloxanide furoate to eliminate colonic cysts; the latter may not be successful. Surgical excision of cerebral granulomas has been reported, but the general condition of the patient should be taken into consideration carrying out invasive procedures. Most patients die despite treatment, but survival following early treatment with metronidazole supplemented with rifampicin and tetracycline has been described.

Naegleria fowleri can cause amoebic meningoencephalitis in both tropical and temperate climates. The organism prospers in moist soil and cases have been reported in children who have been swimming or playing in stagnant water. It is presumed that amoebae cross the nasal epithelium and extend to the brain through the olfactory nerves.[86] The neurological complications of meningoencephalitis may be subacute or acute. Amoebae can be isolated from the CSF, with neutrophilia and low glucose content. The changes may not be florid in patients with a subacute course due to acanthamoeba. The organisms can be identified if kept at room temperature. Treatment should start immediately with intravenous amphotericin B for 10 days; miconazole, rifampicin and tetracycline may enhance the effect of amphtericin B.

Helminths (See also Chapters 80–85)

The diversity and complexity of the life cycles of the numerous parasites that may affect the nervous system are considered elsewhere in this book. Here, brief consideration will be given only to the salient clinical features.

Cysticercosis

This is an infection caused by *Taenia solium* larvae (cysticerci), the most common parasite to invade the CNS. When the cysticercus is lodged in the CNS the disease is known as neurocysticercosis. Neurocysticercosis is the most frequent and most widely disseminated neuroparasitosis. It is endemic in many parts of the world, particularly in Latin America, Africa and Asia.[87] Presumably improvements in sanitation and meat inspection since the 1960s have been largely responsible. However, other cestodes such as the fish tapeworm (*Diphyllobothrium*) should not be completely forgotten because of increased consumption of sashimi and sushi from raw salmon.[88] It is believed that the fish tapeworm infects about 10% of people living in Scandanavia.[89] There, megaloblastic anaemia and its associated neurological complications may occur as a long-term consequence of infection because the adult tapeworm competes with the host for dietary vitamin B_{12}.

The larval form of *T. solium* is probably the most common cause of cystic lesions in the brain worldwide. The cysticercus, a fluid-filled bladder containing the invaginated head or scolex of the larval form, may infect all parts of the CNS, including the subarachnoid spaces and cisterns and, rarely, the sella turcica. Hydrocephalus is common and chronic meningitis with a lymphocytic or occasionally eosinophilic pleocytosis may be found when cysts are present in the subarachnoid space or ventricles in close proximity to the meninges.[90] CT and MRI have greatly facilitated diagnosis (Figure 16.4). The cystic lesions may be seen to contain more dense nodules, corresponding to the scolex; calcifications where cysts have died and cysts on nodules may enhance with contrast material as the cysticerci degenerate. However, there may be no radiological evidence of parasitic lesions and a negative scan does not eliminate the diagnosis if other clinical evidence is persuasive.

A less common pattern is the racemose (bunch of grapes) cluster of cysts within the cisterns.[91] The proliferating form consists of multiple interconnecting bladders of different sizes, but lacks scolices. These tend to occur in parts of the nervous system where the parasite is not closely confined by host tissue; the bladders may become large and extend into the spinal column. Careful examination may be required to reveal the degenerating scolex. It may be that recemose cysticerci are aberrant cysticerci of *T. solium* or other cestodes such as *T. multiceps* or *T. serialis* (the latter two are canine tapeworms of which the larval forms infect sheep and rabbits). Coenuri contain multiple scolices and may bud off daughter

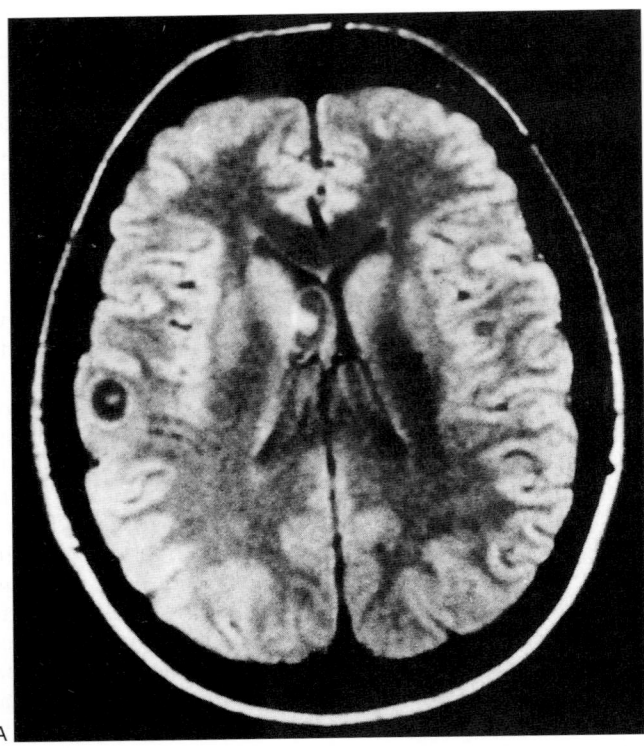
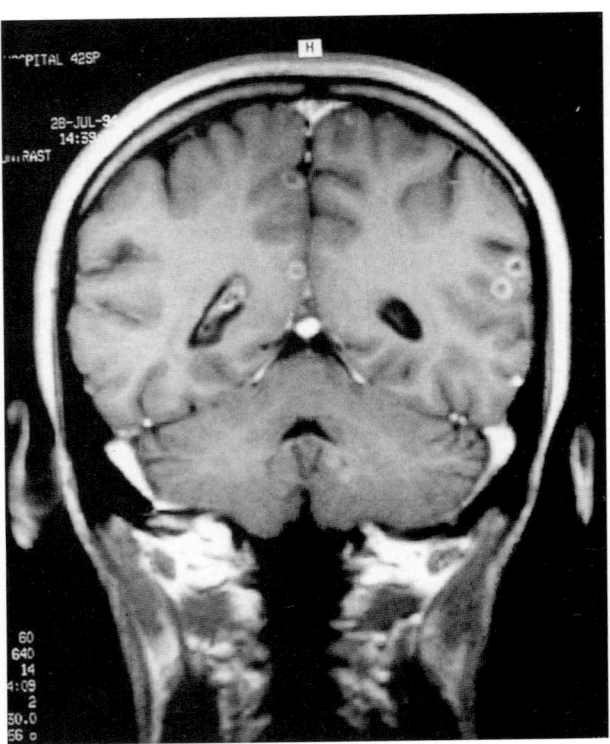

Figure 16.4: Neurocysticercosis. (**A**) Cysts in different stages of maturation. (**B**) Two cysts containing scolices.

bladders; this condition is rare. Confirmation of the diagnosis of racemose cysticercosis requires pathological examination of the cystic lesion. When plain radiographs of soft tissues fail to reveal calcified lesions a number of available serological tests have been described. A recently introduced enzyme-linked immunoelectrotransfer blot assay is sensitive and specific. Cisternal, parenchymal and intraventricular cysticerci may occur in the same patient, causing local disturbances, of which the most common is focal epilepsy. Larger cysts may produce mass effects: hydrocephalus commonly occurs and inflammation of blood vessels adjacent to cysts may cause brain thrombosis and infarction. Cysticercosis involving the basilar cisterns carries a poor prognosis.

Treatment of racemose and cisternal cysticercosis is difficult[92] and there are few satisfactory controlled trials to guide management. Anticysticercal drugs, corticosteroids, shunting procedures and surgical removal or decompression of cysts have been recommended. Praziquantel, an isoquinolone, and albendazole and imidazole have been used extensively in the treatment of parenchymal disease. Serial scans indicate that cysticerci are frequently eliminated or at least markedly reduced in numbers; the drugs are less effective for the cisternal and racemose manifestation. It is still not known whether albendazole is superior to praziquantel and in refractory cases both drugs are used. Praziquantel has been associated with a more adverse reaction that may be due to the host's inflammatory reaction to dying parasites, and headache, nausea and frequent seizures are common. Corticosteroids may ameliorate some of these effects and are usually prescribed, but there are few controlled trials to support this strategy.

Those with hydrocephalus due to cisternal disease and arachnoiditis will require shunting if there are symptoms and if serial scans indicate deterioration; some have recommended that a ventricular shunt should be considered in all patients with hydrocephalus before medical therapy is attempted.[93] If racemose and cisternal cysts are focally impairing the egress of CSF, surgical removal is sometimes recommended, but such procedures may be difficult and at times hazardous.

Ischaemic cerebrovascular disease is an under-recognized and relatively common complication.[94] Inflammatory occlusion of the arteries at the base of the brain is secondary to arachnoiditis. The involved vessels are usually of small diameter provoking lacunar infarcts. However, occlusion of larger vessels such as the middle cerebral artery or even the internal carotid artery has been reported as well as transient ischaemic attacks and 'brain stem syndromes'.

While neurocysticercosis commonly seen in Latin America, Asia and Africa and in Mexico is the main cause of late-onset epilepsy, it should be borne in mind even in those whose sojourn in endemic areas has been brief and even when there is no history of possible exposure. This was clearly illustrated in a description of an outbreak of neurocysticercosis in an orthodox Jewish community residing in New York City[95] traced to a domestic employee who was found to have active parasitic infection probably acquired in her native Mexico. As man can clearly be an intermediate host through the ingestion of eggs in human faeces, it follows that the relatives of any patient with established disease should be examined—no matter how improbable the diagnosis.

Filariasis

Human filariasis may be due to *Loa loa*, *Dracunculus medinensis* or *Onchocerca volvulus*. Loiasis can cause meningoencephalitis with microfilariae in the CSF. Encephalitis with retinal haemorrhages has been described, probably as a reaction to the dying filariae with diethylcarbamazine used for treatment.[96] *D. medinensis* has been isolated from thickened peripheral nerves and can also cause paraspinal abscess by penetrating the extradural space.[97]

Wuchereria bancrofti is the cause of lymphatic filariasis. Recurrent Guillain–Barré syndrome has been reported after flare-ups of acute filariasis over a period of several years.[98]

Onchocerciasis

River blindness, endemic in large areas of Africa and Central America and caused by the filarial worm *Onchocerca volvulus*, is transmitted by an insect vector. This breeds in fast-flowing rivers. Adult worms can survive in humans for many years, intermittently releasing microfilariae into the skin. More calamitous is migration into the anterior and posterior segments of the eye causing irreversible blindness, making onchocerciasis the most common cause of blindness in the world. The parasite occurs in both rainforests and savanna, where it is more likely to invade the eye. The anterior segment disease[99]—sclerosing keratitis and uveitis—is usually evident but the extent of posterior segment damage is more difficult to ascertain. In rainforest areas blindness is more likely to be due to posterior segment involvement with choreoretinitis and optic nerve lesions. The introduction of the antiparasitic agent ivermectin for the insect vector (*Simulium* species) was promising; spraying rivers with larvicide is very expensive and vector reinvasion after the discontinuation of spraying has occurred. Mass treatment with ivermectin (a semi-synthetic macrocyclic lactone) is most encouraging. The drug is safe, well tolerated and effective in reducing microfilarial counts. A recent study concluded that annual ivermectin treatment may reduce the incidence of blindness by up to 80% in a savanna region. While most of the studies of onchocerciasis relate to blindness, a possible relationship with seizures has been suspected. Recent evidence[100] from western Uganda describes an improvement in seizure activity after ivermectin treatment in a community with demonstrable microfilariasis (*O. volvulus*). It may be that further studies will indicate more widespread systemic and CNS involvement than is currently suspected.

Nematode infections

While the adult form of *Gnathostoma spinigerum* has been known since the nineteenth century, when it was discovered in the stomach of a tiger in the London Zoo, the neurological manifestations of the mature parasite in man have been recognized more recently.[101] Those who prefer uncooked fish, shrimps and frogs in the tropics may acquire the larval third stage and present with a curious and sometimes fatal multifocal neurological illness (Figure 16.5). During the acute stage there may be a febrile illness with headache, neck stiffness and a rash; on occasions the parasite can be extracted from a skin lesion. A painful radiculomyelopathy may then develop with intensive girdle pain, paraparesis and eosinophilia in blood and CSF.[102] This phase may subside, but if unrecognized or untreated the parasite may then migrate through the spinal cord into the brain. Death may occur because of brain stem involvement and at autopsy the live gnathostome may be seen emerging. A patient seen recently in London had spent only a few weeks in Hong Kong on business; he had developed a complete paraplegia with a wheelchair existence and a dense hemianopia as a consequence of his preference for fresh crustacea in exotic restaurants. *Angiostrongylus cantonensis* (rat lungworm) similarly affects those in South-East Asia who consume poorly cooked snails, prawns and crabs. Neurological complications include meningitis, papilloedema

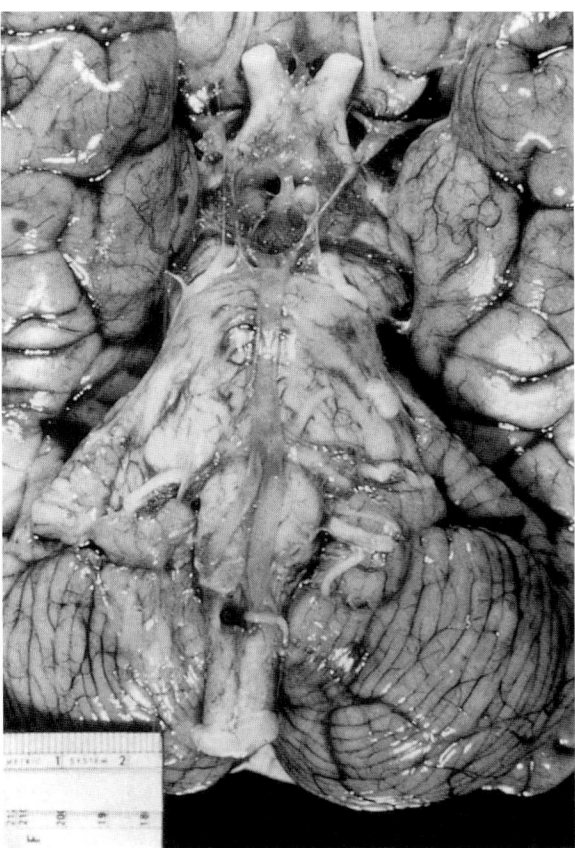

Figure 16.5: Gnathostomiasis. On the ventral surface of the lower medulla the nematodes can be seen emerging from a cavity (seen at autopsy). (Courtesy of Athasit Vejjajiva, Department of Neurology, Ramathibodi Hospital, Thailand.)

and extraocular palsies with an eosinophilic CSF pleocytosis. Brain abscesses may occur and CT shows well-circumscribed enhancing lesions. Both these nematodes are treated with albendazole with steroid cover.

Strongyloides stercoralis, another nematode affecting the nervous system with an eosinophilic meningitis, usually occurs as part of the 'hyperinfection syndrome' with multiple cerebral infarcts, vasculitis and larval depositions.[103]

Hydatid disease

This may present as intracranial cysts, occasionally spectacularly large with the features of space-occupying lesions and obstructive hydrocephalus, or with a basal arachnoiditis due to multiple smaller lesions.[104] CT and MRI (Figure 16.6) may reveal the diagnostic daughter cysts. Surgical excision and shunting are usually required. When hydatid disease affects the spine, paraplegia may result and it is usually impossible to excise all the diseased bone effectively. In consequence the prognosis is poor. Albendazole reduces cyst size and, at least in the gerbil,[105] is more effective than mebendazole and praziquantel.

Schistosomiasis

This long-known parasite of man—the earliest case known to have occurred was 5000 years ago in an Egyptian adolescent from the predynastic period[106]—

continues to afflict mankind and it is believed that at present more than 250 million people worldwide are affected. Of the schistosomia species, *S. mansoni*, *S. hematobium* and *S. japonicum* are the most important to man and the most widely distributed. The CNS involvement may be observed with any of the clinical forms of the infection. Acute schistosomiasis (Katayama fever) presents as fever, cough, arthralgia, abdominal pain and urticaria; the neurological manifestations may be conspicuous headache, neck stiffness, evidence of raised intracranial pressure and fits. Involvement of the lower spinal cord and conus medullaris and/or cauda equina due to *Schistosoma mansoni* or *S. haematobium* has been well described,[107] but the diagnosis may be elusive even when suspected. Ova may be absent from stool and urine; available serological tests may be negative and eosinophilia absent.[108] However, eosinophilia in the CSF is usually present and the CT and MRI findings (Figure 16.7) may clinch the diagnosis. Most of the cases of neuroschistosomiasis associated with the hepatosplenic and cardiopulmonary chronic forms, or with severe urinary schistosomiasis, though more frequent, are asymptomatic.[109] The interval of time between exposure and neurological presentation may be many years. It is recommended that all denizens where *S. mansoni* and *S. haematobium* prevail, and all travellers even with a remote history of recreational exposure to fresh water who present with a painful cauda equina or spinal syndrome, should commence praziquantel and corticosteroids without waiting for the results of laboratory or imaging tests.[110]

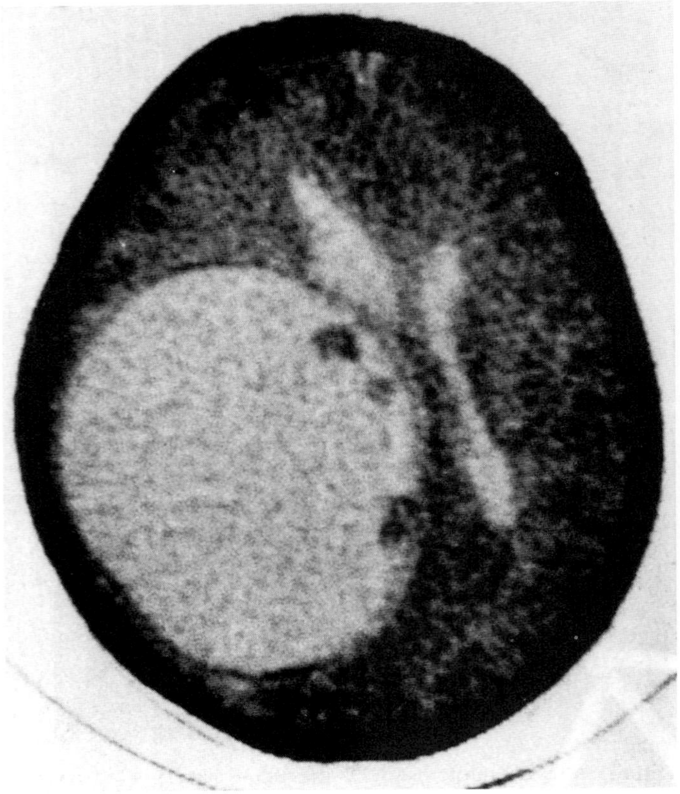

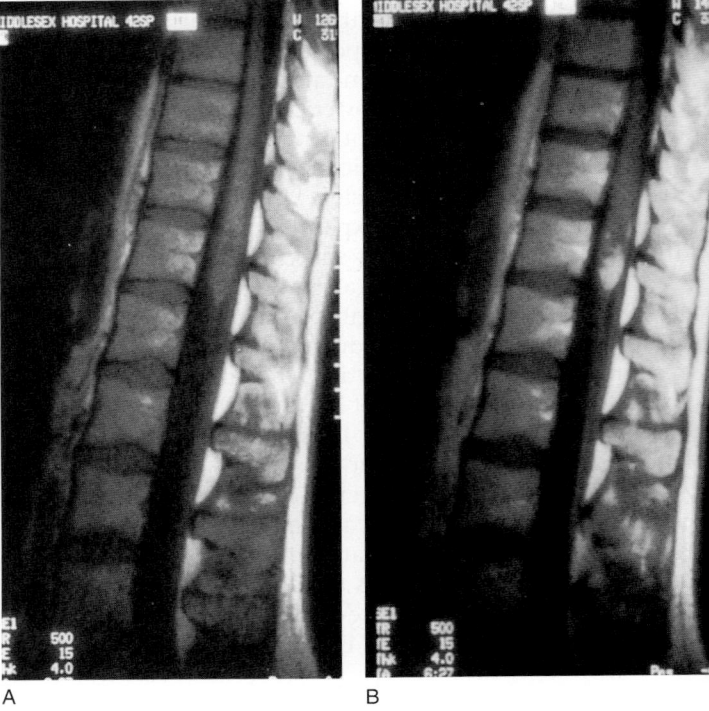

Figure 16.6: Brain scan showing large hydatid cyst with daughter cysts.

Figure 16.7: Schistosomiasis of the lower spinal cord and conus. (**A**) Before contrast. (**B**) After contrast with an irregular area of altered signal in surrounding oedema.

Toxocariasis

Toxocara canis transferred from dogs to humans through the eggs and the worm occasionally involves the CNS; unilateral retinal disease may occur in children; encephalitis and encephalomyelitis[111] have been reported in adults. Serious and persistent organic neurological and psychological deficits have been described and related to multiple brain infarcts from vasculitic lesions and eosinophilic granulomas. Myelitis with larvae in CSF and small arterial lesions may occur. Immune vasculitis should be prevented by early anthelmintic treatment, but there is a paucity of evidence of therapeutic efficacy.

Trichinosis

This parasitic disease, which develops after ingestion of undercooked meat contaminated with larvae of *Trichinella spiralis*, occurs both in tropical and temperate climates, and there have been large outbreaks in France related to the ingestion of horse meat.[112] The acute illness, with fever, headaches, myalgia, periorbital oedema, nausea and diarrhoea with a marked blood eosinophilia, increased serum muscle enzymes and specific antibodies, is well known. Less so are the neurological manifestations which are protean, making sporadic cases difficult to identify. Encephalopathy with a wide variety of focal deficits and numerous small hypodense CT changes in cortex and white matter has been clearly described.[113] The brain shows multiple small ischaemic cavities throughout the white matter and pons. Arteriolar microthrombi are present without an inflammatory infiltrate or remnants of *Trichinella* larvae. Toxaemic, allergic and larval pathogenic mechanisms have been proposed and a recent study suggests that hypereosinophilia may be implicated in the genesis of cerebral lesions. Early diagnosis and prompt treatment with anthelmintic therapy such as diffusible benzimidazole with corticosteroids is mandatory.

Paragonimiasis

This trematode causes major neurological problems in the Far East, especially Korea. It presents as an intracranial space-occupying lesion. *Paragonimus westermani* is transmitted to man through ingestion of crab and crayfish; the metacercariae travel to the lungs and mature. The adult can live in the lung for several years and is usually asymptomatic. It can produce pulmonary symptoms, the most characteristic of which is cough with rusty sputum.[114] Neurological presentation is due to cerebral involvement as a result of the development of cysts in ectopic sites; various intracranial sites can be affected.[115] The diagnosis is established by demonstrating *P. westermani* eggs in sputum, faeces and pleural fluid. A monoclonal antibody assay has recently been reported. Treatment with praziquantel may be successful.[116]

Conclusion

This short chapter has briefly described an exceedingly diverse and fascinating group of illnesses which affect the CNS in tropical patients. While this extent and somewhat idiosyncratic depth of coverage will not be beyond the criticism of the specialist, there is sufficient detail for clinical neurologists to be aware of CNS diseases that may affect many patients throughout the tropics and subtropics. Neurological manifestations are early and common in HIV-positive patients and early counselling and testing should be offered to the patient. For more specialist discussion of the subject the reader is referred to a recently published book *Tropical Neurology*.[117]

REFERENCES

1   Senanayake N & Roman G C. Epidemiology of epilepsy in the tropics. *J Trop Geogr Neurol* 1992; 2:10–19.

2   Senanayake N & Roman G C. Aetiological factors of epilepsy in the tropics. *J Trop Geogr Neurol* 1991; 1:69–80.

3   Rwiza H T, Matuja W B P & Mteza I. The past medical profile of epilepsy patients in an African rural community. *J Trop Geogr Neurol* 1992; 2:146–150.

4   Garg R K. HIV infection and seizures. *Postgrad Med J* 1999; 75:387–390.

5   Modi G, Modi M, Martinus I et al. New-onset seizures associated with HIV infection. *Neurology* 2000; 55:1558–1560.

6   World Population Prospects. The 2000 Revision. Available at www.un.org/esa/population/wpp2000.htm.

7   Rozenzweig C & Parry M L. Potential impact of climate change on world food supply. *Nature* 1994; 367:133–137.

8   Cook G C. Effect of global warming on the distribution of parasitic and other infectious diseases: a review. *J R Soc Med* 1992; 85:688–691.

9   London L. Alcohol consumption amongst South African farm workers: a challenge for post apartheid health sector transformation. *Drug Alcohol Depend* 2000; 59(2):199–206.

10 Cavanagh J B. The 'dying back' process: a common denominator in many naturally occurring and toxic neuropathies. *Arch Pathol Lab Med* 1979; 103:659–664.

11 Spencer P S, Sabri M I, Schaumburg H H & Moore C L. Does a defect of energy metabolism in the nerve fibre underlie axonal degeneration in polyneuropathies? *Ann Neurol* 1979; 5:501–507.

12 Senanayake N & Roman G C. Toxic neuropathies in the tropics. *J Trop Geogr Neurol* 1991; 1:3–15.

13 Senanayake N, de Silva W A S & Salgado M S L. Arsenical polyneuropathy: a clinical study. *Ceylon Med J* 1972; 17:195–203.

14 Le Quesne P M & McLeod J G. Peripheral neuropathy following a single exposure to arsenic. *J Neurol Sci* 1977; 32:437–451.

15 Windebank A J, McCall J T & Dyck P J. Metal neuropathy. In Dyck P J, Thomas P K, Lambert E H & Bunge R P (eds) *Peripheral Neuropathy*. Philadelphia: W B Saunders, 1984: 2133–2161.

16 Cavanagh J B, Fuller N H, Johnson H R M & Rudge P. The effect of thallium salts with particular reference to the nervous system. *Q J Med* 1974; 43:293–319.

17 Loftus L R. Peripheral neuropathy following chloroquine therapy. *Can Med Assoc J* 1963; 89:917–920.

18 Nakae K, Yamamoto S, Shigematsu I & Kono R. Relation

between subacute myelooptic neuropathy (SMON) and clioquinol: a nationwide survey. *Lancet* 1973; i:171–174.

19 Vora D D, Dastur D K, Braganca B M et al. Toxic polyneuritis in Bombay due to ortho-cresyl phosphate poisoning. *J Neurol Neurosurg Psychiatry* 1962; 25:234–242.

20 Roman G C, Spencer P S & Schoenberg B S. Tropical myeloneuropathies: the hidden endemias. *Neurology* 1985; 35:1158–1170.

21 Howlett W P, Brubaker G, Mlingi N & Rosling H. A geographical cluster of konzo in Tanzania. *J Trop Geogr Neurol* 1992; 2:102–108.

22 Tylleskar T, Banea M, Bikangi N, Cooke R D, Poulter N H & Rosling H. Cassava cyanogens and konzo, an upper motorneurone disease found in Africa. *Lancet* 1992; 339:208–211.

23 Spencer P S, Ohta M & Palmer V S. Cycad use and motor neurone disease in Kii peninsula of Japan. *Lancet* 1987; ii:1462–1463.

24 Angunawela R M & Fernando H A. Acute ascending polyneuropathy and dermatitis following poisoning by tubers of *Gloriosa superba. Ceylon Med J* 1971; 16:233–235.

25 Ng T H K, Chan Y W, Yu Y L et al. Encephalopathy and neuropathy following ingestion of a Chinese herbal broth containing podophyllin. *J Neurol Sci* 1991; 101:107–115.

26 Calderon-Gonzalez R & Rizzi-Hernandez H. Buckthorn polyneuropathy. *N Engl J Med* 1967; 277:69–71.

27 Gascon G G, Crowell J, Stigsby B et al. Subacute sclerosing panencephalitis. *Neurology* 1992; 43:454–455.

28 Schoub B D, Johnson S & McAnerney J M. Observations of subacute sclerosing panencephalitis in South Africa. *Trans R Soc Trop Med Hyg* 1992; 86:550–551.

29 Steiner I, Wirguin I, Morag A et al. Intraventricular interferon treatment for subacute sclerosing panencephalitis. *J Child Neurol* 1989; 4:20–24.

30 Freier J E. Eastern equine encephalomyelitis. *Lancet* 1993; 342:1281–1286.

31 Thongchareon P. Japanese encephalitic virus encephalitis: an overview. *Southeast Asian J Trop Med Public Health* 1989; 20:559–573.

32 Arthur R R, El-Sharkawy M S, Cope S E et al. Recurrence of Rift Valley fever in Egypt. *Lancet* 1993; 342:1149–1150.

33 Hull H F. The future of polio eradication. The Lancet. Infectious Diseases 2001; 1(5):299–303

34 Anon. Certification of poliomyelitis eradication – Western Pacific Region, October 2000. MMWR Morb Mortal Wkly Rep 2001; 50:1–3.

35 Sutter R W, Patriarca PA, Brogan S et al. Outbreak of paralytic poliomyelitis in Oman: evidence of widespread transmission among fully vaccinated children. *Lancet* 1991; 338:715–720.

36 Otten M W, Denning M S, Jaiteh K O et al. Epidemic poliomyelitis in the Gambia following the control of poliomyelitis as an endemic disease. 1. Descriptive findings. *Am J Epidemiol* 1992; 135:381–392.

37 Solbrig M V & McCormick J B. Lassa fever: central nervous system manifestations. *J Trop Geogr Neurol* 1991; 1:23–30.

38 Warrell D A & Warrell M J. Human rabies and its prevention: an overview. *Rev Infect Dis* 1988; 10(Suppl. 4):5726–5731.

39 Petricciani J C. Ongoing tragedy of rabies. *Lancet* 1993; 342:1067.

40 Nicholson K G. Rabies. *Lancet* 1990; 335:1201–1206.

41 Swaddiwuthipong W, Weniger B G, Wattanasi S & Warrell M J. A high rate of neurological complications following Semple anti-rabies vaccine. *Trans R Soc Trop Med Hyg* 1988; 82:472–475.

42 Lang J, Duong Q H, Nguyen V G et al Immunogenicity and safety of low-dose intradermal rabies vaccination given during an Expanded Programme on Immunisation session in Viet Nam. *Trans R Soc Trop Med Hyg* 1999; 93(2):208–213.

43 Krebs F C, Ross H, McAllister J & Wigdahl B. HIV-I-associated central nervous system dysfunction. *Adv Pharmacol* 2000; 49:315–385.

44 Simpson D M & Berger J R. Neurological manifestations of HIV infection. *Med Clin North Am* 1996; 80(6):1363–1394.

45 Gessain A, Barin F, Vernant J C et al. Antibodies to human T-lymphotrophic type 1 in patients with tropical spastic paraparesis. *Lancet* 1985; ii:407–409.

46 Roman G C. The neuroepidemiology of tropical spastic paraparesis. *Ann Neurol* 1988; 23(Suppl.):113–120.

47 Montgomery R D. The epidemiology of myelopathy associated with human T-lymphotrophic virus 1. *Trans R Soc Trop Med Hyg* 1993; 87:154–159.

48 Yamaguchi K. Human T-lymphotropic virus type 1 in Japan. *Lancet* 1994; 343:213–216.

49 Mochizuki M, Watanabe T, Yamaguchi H et al. Uveitis associated with human T-lymphotrophic virus type 1. *Am J Ophthalmol* 1992; 114:123–129.

50 Jacobson S, McFarlin D E, Robinson S et al. HTLV-1-specific cytotoxic T lymphocytes in the cerebrospinal fluid of patients with HTLV-1-associated neurological disease. *Ann Neurol* 1992; 32:651–657.

51 Hino S & Hiroshi D. Mechanisms of HTLV-1 transmission. In Roman G C, Vernant J C & Osame M (eds) *HTLV-1 and the Nervous System.* New York: Alan R Liss, 1989:495–501.

52 Cruickshank J K, Rudge P, Dalgleish A G et al. Tropical spastic paraparesis and human T cell lymphotrophic virus type 1 in the United Kingdom. *Brain* 1989; 112:1057–1090.

53 Poser C M, Roman G C & Vernant J C. Multiple sclerosis or HTLV-1 myelitis? *Neurology* 1990; 40:1020–1022.

54 Alcindor F, Valderrama R, Canaveggio M et al. Imaging of human T-lymphotrophic virus type 1-associated chronic progressive myeloneuropathies. *Neuroradiology* 1992; 35:69–74.

55 Shaked Y. Rickettsial infections of the central nervous system: the role of prompt antimicrobial therapy. *Q J Med* 1991; 79:301–306.

56 Raoult D, Zuchelli P, Weiller P J et al. Incidence, clinical observations and risk factors in the severe form of Mediterranean spotted fever among patients admitted to hospital in Marseilles 1983–1984. *J Infect* 1986; 12:111–116.

57 Kirk I J, Fine P D, Sexton J D & Muchmore G. Rocky Mountain spotted fever: a clinical review based on 48 confirmed cases 1943–1986. *Medicine* 1990; 69:35–45.

58 Berkley J A, Mwangi I, Ngetsa C J et al. Diagnosis of acute bacterial meningitis in children at a district hospital in sub-Saharan Africa. *Lancet* 2001; 357:1753–1757.

59 Lewis R, Nathan N, Diarra L et al. Timely detection of meningococcal meningitis epidemics in Africa. *Lancet* 2001; 358:287–293.

60 WHO. Detecting meningococcal meningitis epidemics in highly-endemic African countries. *Wkly Epidemiol Res* 2000; 75:306–309.

61 Peltola H. Burden of meningitis and other severe bacterial infections of children in Africa: implications for prevention. *Clin Infect Dis* 2001; 32:64–75.

62 Ross K L, Tunkel A R & Scheld W M. Acute bacterial meningitis in children and adults. In Scheld W M, Whitley R J & Durck D T (eds) *Infections in the Central Nervous System.* New York: Raven Press, 1991: 335–409.

63 Adeghola R A, Usen S O. Weber M et al. Haemophilus Influenzae type b meningitis in Gambia after intorudction of a conjucate vaccine. *Lancet* 1999; 354:1091–1092.

64 Zumla A, Mwaba P, Rook G & Lukas S. Tuberculosis. In James D G, Zumla A (eds) *The Granulomatous Disorders.* Cambridge, UK: Cambridge University Press, 1999: 132–160.

65 WHO. *Global Tuberculosis Control 1999.* Geneva: WHO, 1999.

66 Wood M & Anderson M. CNS tuberculosis. In Walton J (ed.) *Neurological Infections.* London: W B Saunders, 1988: 172–196.

67 Zhang G, Li W, Yan L et al. An epidemiological survey of deformities and disabilities among 14257 leprosy patients in 11 countries. *Chin Med J* 1992; 7:216–220.

68 Browne S G. Leprosy. *BMJ* 1968, 3:725–728.

69 Shakir R A, Al-Din A S N, Araj G F et al. Clinical categories of neurobrucellosis. *Brain* 1987; 110:213–223.

70 Araj G F, Lulu A R, Khateeb M I et al. ELISA versus routine tests in the diagnosis of patients with systemic and neurobrucellosis. *Acta Pathol Microbiol Immunol Scand* 1988; 96:171–176.

71 Turner L H. Leptospirosis. *BMJ* 1973; 1:537–540.

72 Finkel M J & Halperin J J. Nervous system borreliosis—revisited. *Arch Neurol* 1992; 49:102–107.

73 Medana I M, Chaudhri G, Chan-Ling T & Hunt N H. Central nervous system in cerebral malaria: 'innocent bystander' or active participation in the induction of immunopathology? *Immunol Cell Biol* 2001; 79(2):101–120.

74 Garg R K. Cerebral malaria. *J Assoc Phys India* 2000; 48:1004–1013.

75 Muphy S C, Breman J G. Gaps in the childhood malaria burden in Africa. *Am J Trop Med Hyg* 2001; 64(Suppl. 1–2):57–67.

76 Tuner G. Cerebral malaria. *Brain Pathol* 1997; 7(1):569–582.

77 Lockwood D N J & Pasvol G. Recent Advances in tropical Medicine. *BMJ* 1994;308:1559–1562.

78 De Silva H J, Goonetilleke A K E, Senaratna N et al. Skeletal muscle necrosis in severe falciparum malaria. *BMJ* 1988; 296:1039.

79 Chimelli L & Scaravilli F. Trypanosomiasis. *Brain Pathol* 1997; 7(1):599–611.

80 Milord F, Pepin J, Loko L, Ethier L & Mpia B. Efficacy and toxicity of eflornithine for treatment of *Trypanosoma brucei gambiense* sleeping sickness. *Lancet* 1992; 340:652–655.

81 Spina-Franca A & Mattosinho-Franca L S. American trypanosomiasis (Chagas' disease). In Vinken P J & Bruyn G W (eds) *Handbook of Clinical Neurology*, vol. 35, part III. Amsterdam: North-Holland, 1978: 85–114.

82 Woodhouse J I J. The prevalence of clinical peripheral neuropathies in human chronic Chagas disease. *J R Army Med Corps* 1993; 139:54–55.

83 Rosenberg S, Chaves C J, Higuchi N M L et al. Fatal meningoencephalitis caused by reactivation of *Trypanosoma cruzi* infection in patients with AIDS. *Neurology* 1992; 42:640–642.

84 Morehead C. Notes on the pathology and treatment of diseases of the brain, as observed in the European General Hospital at Bombay. *Trans Med Phys Soc Bombay* 1849; 9:112–115.

85 Gardner H A R, Martinez A J, Visvesvara G S et al. Granulomatous amoebic encephalitis in an AIDS patient. *Neurology* 1991; 41:1993–1995.

86 Peral I M, Visvesvara G S, Martinez A J et al. Naegleria and acanthomoeba infections: review. *Rev Infect Dis* 1990; 12:490–513.

87 Pittella J E H. Neurocysticercosis. *Brain Pathol* 1997; 7(1):681–693.

88 Schantz P M & McAley I. Current status of foodborne parasitic zoonoses in the United States. *Southeast Asian J Trop Med Public Health* 1991; 22(Suppl.):65–71.

89 Salokannel J. Intrinsic factor in tapeworm anaemia. *Acta Med Scand Suppl* 1987; 517:1–51.

90 Del Brutto O H & Sotelo J. Neurocysticercosis: an update. *Rev Infect Dis* 1988; 10:1075–1087.

91 Jung R C, Rodriguez M A, Beaver P C, Schenthal J E & Levy R W. Racemose cysticercus in human brain: a case report. *Am J Trop Med Hyg* 1981; 30:620–624.

92 Earnest M P, Reller L B, Filley C M & Grek A J. Neurocysticercosis in the United States: 35 cases and a review. *Rev Infect Dis* 1987; 9:961–979.

93 Lobato R D, Lamsa E M, Portillo J M et al. Hydrocephalus in cerebral cysticercosis: pathogenic and therapeutic considerations. *J Neurosurg* 1981; 55:786–79.

94 Del Brutto O H. Cysticercosis and cerebrovascular disease: a review. *J Neurol Neurosurg Psychiatry* 1992; 55:252–254.

95 Schantz P M, Moore A C, Munoz J L et al. Neurocysticercosis in an orthodox Jewish community in New York City. *N Engl J Med* 1992; 327:692–695.

96 Negess Y, Lanoie L O, Neafie R C et al. Loiasis: 'calabar' swellings and involvement of deep organs. *Am J Trop Med Hyg* 1985; 34:537–546.

97 Brown W J & Voge M. *Neuropathology of Parasitic Infections*. Oxford: Oxford University Press, 1982: 240.

98 Bhatia B & Misra S. Recurrent Guillain–Barré syndrome following acute filiariasis. *J Neurol Neurosurg Psychiatry* 1993; 56:1133–1134.

99 Mabey D. Onchocerciasis: ivermectin and onchocercal optic nerve lesions. *Lancet* 1993; 341:153–154.

100 Kipp W, Kasoro S & Burnham G. Onchocerciasis and epilepsy in Uganda. (Letter.) *Lancet* 1994; 343:182–184.

101 Schmutzhard E, Boongird P & Vejjajiva A. Eosinophilic meningitis and radiculomyelitis in Thailand caused by CNS invasion of *Gnasthostoma spinigerum* and *Angiostrongylus cantonensis*. *J Neurol Neurosurg Psychiatry* 1988; 51:80–87.

102 Punyagupta S, Juttijudata P & Bunnag T. Eosinophilic meningitis in Thailand. *Am J Trop Med Hyg* 1975; 24:921–931.

103 Belani A, Leptrone D & Shands J W. Strongyloides meningitis. *South Med J* 1987; 80:916–918.

104 Cataltepe O, Colak A, Ozcan O E et al. Intracranial hydatid cyst: experience with surgical treatment in 120 patients. *Neurochirurgia* 1992; 35:108–111.

105 Taylor D H, Morris D L, Reffin D et al. Comparison of albendazole, mebendazole and praziquantel chemotherapy of *Echinococcus multilocularis* in a gerbil model. *Gut* 1989; 30:1401–1405.

106 Miller R J, Armelagos G J, Ikram S, De Jonge N, Krijger F W & Deelder A M. Palaeoepidemiology of schistosomasa infection in mummies. *BMJ* 1992; 304:555–556.

107 Haribhai H C, Bhigee A I, Bill P L A et al. Spinal cord schistosomiasis: a clinical laboratory and radiological study with a note on therapeutic aspects. *Brain* 1991; 114:709–726.

108 Blunt S B, Boulton J & Wise R. MRI in schistosomiasis of conus medullaris and lumbar spinal cord. *Lancet* 1993; 341:557.

109 Pittella J E. Neuroschistomiasis. *Brain Pathol* 1997; 7(1):649–662.

110 Blanchard T J, Milne L M, Pollok R & Cook G C. Early chemotherapy of imported neuroschistosomiasis. (Letter.) *Lancet* 1993; 341:959.

111 Sommer C, Ringelstein E B, Biniek R & Glockner W M. Adult *Toxocara canis* encephalitis. *J Neurol Neurosurg Psychiatry* 1994; 57:229–231.

112 Ancelle T, Dupouy-Camet J, Bougnoux M E et al. Two outbreaks of trichinosis caused by horsemeat in France in 1985. *Am J Epidemiol* 1988; 127:1302–1311.

113 Fourestie V, Douceron H, Brugieres P, Ancelle T, Lejonc J L & Gherardi R K. Neurotrichinosis: a cerebrovascular disease associated with myocardial injury and hypereosinophilia. *Brain* 1993; 116:603–616.

114 Cook G C. Protozoan and helminthic infections. In Lambert H P (ed.) *Infections of the Central Nervous System*. New York: Marcel Decker, 1991: 264–282.

115 Toyonaga S, Kurisaka M, Mori K et al. Cerebral paragonimiasis: report of five cases. *Neurol Med Chir* 1992; 32:157–162.

116 Zhang Z, Zhang Y, Shi Z et al. Diagnosis of active *Paragonimus westermani* infections with a monoclonal antibody-based antigen detection assay. *Am J Trop Med Hyg* 1993; 49:329–334.

117 Misra U K, Kalita J & Shakir R A (eds). *Tropical Neurology*. Georgetown, TX: Landes Bioscience, 2001.

Chapter 17
Psychiatry

A. Haworth and J. H. Orley

Psychiatric disorders account for more morbidity than is often recognized. The World Health Organization's 1999 World Health Report states that neuropsychiatric conditions make up an estimated 11.5% of the global burden of disease and on average these conditions account for 28% of total years lived with disability. A large proportion of the burden is attributable to major depression. Five of the ten leading causes of disability worldwide are mental disorders and suicide is the tenth leading cause of death in the world.[1] Natural disasters with their psychosocial consequences tend to occur with more frequency in tropical countries. Malnutrition and its consequences affect both prenatal and postnatal growth in the child. Malnutrition and other physical stresses such as chronic anaemia, parasitic infections and the burden, for example, of trying to grow one's own food in drought conditions make their contribution to the occurrence of psychiatric morbidity generally. While psychiatric disorders such as schizophrenia and affective disorders are as common in tropical countries as elsewhere in the world, patients are more likely to have focal cerebral changes and cerebral atrophy has been noted at a much younger age. There are higher levels of head trauma and of intracranial infections such as neurosyphilis and human immunodeficiency virus and associated opportunistic infections. In the past a simple dichotomy between urban and rural was described but the situation is much more complex and there is, for example, no clear definition applicable worldwide of the term 'urban'. In some countries settlements with more than a population of 1000 are considered to be urban, while in many the lower limit is 20 000 and some tropical countries also have very large cities. Much emphasis was in the past put on the many stresses of living in an urban environment with somewhat simplistic conceptualizations of rural serenity but more recent studies show that the main social determinant of psychiatric disorder remains poverty and its concomitants. Many of the migrants to vibrant urban centres move there because of the poverty and other stresses of rural life.[2]

Systematic psychiatry is covered in the standard textbooks on the subject. The aim of this chapter is to consider those aspects which are particularly relevant to practitioners who have to deal with psychiatric problems in the tropics but who have not had special training in the subject. Although psychiatrists working in the tropics are scarce (about one per million population in most of sub-Saharan Africa, for example) some countries also employ professional psychiatric nurses or medical auxiliaries with experience in the field who can be called upon to assist and advise in the management of the mentally ill.[3] It should be stressed, however, that most

Table 17.1 Polar attributes of traditional and modern societies

Traditional society	Modern society
Group oriented	Individual oriented
Extended family	Nuclear family
Income-producing linked to kinship ties	Income-producing independent of kinship ties
Economic functions non-specialized	Economic functions specialized
High mortality, high fertility	Low mortality, low fertility
Status determined by age and position in family	Status achieved by own efforts
Relationships between kin obligatory	Relationships between kin permissive
Relationships determined by role and position in family	Relationships determined by individual choice
Arranged marriages	Choice of marital partner
Individuals can be replaced by others filling same roles	Individuals unique and irreplaceable
Extensive classification terminology for distant relatives	Restricted classification terminology for close relatives only
Behaviour to specific kin prescribed	Great variation in kin behaviour
Emotional relationships stereotyped	Emotional relationships differentiated

mentally disturbed patients can be managed by the general medical officer in the wards of a district hospital or in the community. Most medical schools now give more time to psychiatry than in the past and doctors are better equipped to recognize psychiatric disorders. But most courses and many major general textbooks of psychiatry do not give sufficient attention to the 'cultural' element, which is so important in psychiatric practice. We use the word 'culture' in a very broad sense as referring to any socially determined influence impinging upon a person's lifestyle, means of coping with problems and conceptualization of illnesses. Table 17.1 lists some polar attributes of traditional and modern societies. These attributes vary in the extent of their application to any particular society, and not all would apply in any particular location. The concept of cultural sensitivity concerns the differences, of which any doctor should be aware, between his own cultural background, including his values and attitudes, and those of any patient coming from a different background, even in his own country. While practitioners who are foreign to a particular culture should not be expected to 'master' the culture (one can speak of culture as well as language-learning), they should make themselves skilled in working with local staff who have the knowledge to make sense when all might seem confusion. Knowledge of a language must include an appreciation of idiom and of the emotional loading attached to particular words in different contexts. In multi-ethnic societies no single practitioner will be able to communicate directly with all patients in their own vernaculars. Hence the skilful use of interpreters becomes essential in practice. It is frequently found that, say, in a large cosmopolitan city local residents may claim to speak several languages; caution should be employed with such a claim since this knowledge may be very superficial.[4]

Alternative and complementary healing practices

Traditional healers are an important aspect of life in most tropical areas. The term 'traditional healer' is misleading, however, and it tends to lump all non-Western-trained healers together. Much depends on the part of the world—India has its great tradition of Ayurvedic practice, for example. A comprehensive classification is impossible in a chapter of this length. The term 'alternative medicine' has come into more general usage and its techniques, successes and failures are being scrutinized more closely; traditional healing should be looked upon as part of alternative medicine. If many patients consult local healers, it is wise to learn something of their techniques and ways of interpreting illness. Some healers use trance states (spirit possession, sometimes called shamanistic healing) or other means of divination. Spiritual healing also includes activities taking place within a formal religious context—for instance, casting out of demons. It should not be assumed that the traditional healer can

always communicate better with patients or their families than orthodox medical workers, especially in an urban setting where they might accept patients from any ethnic group. Because a healer may often look to interpersonal conflict and jealousy as the cause of illness, some individual may be blamed, resulting in family or other social disruption. While a patient's belief in having been bewitched or affected by a magical charm may be understandable in terms of 'culture', it may equally well be a symptom which needs assessment within the total clinical context. The type of healer available for consultation, be he 'Western' oriented, traditional or religious, is also part of the individual's culture. Some traditional healers are men and women of experience and wisdom and some know of herbs that seem to have potent neuroleptic or tranquillizing effects. It is wise to ask a patient if they have consulted a healer, or are currently receiving treatment or are intending to do so. Some of the constituents of herbs given by traditional healers may interact with prescribed medications or have other toxic effects[5] but it appears that the majority probably have only a placebo effect.[6] Should the doctor encourage or allow his patients to consult traditional healers? Clinical judgement must determine the response. One cannot prevent a patient seeking alternative help but should at least warn where this is seen as inappropriate or dangerous. Patients with organic disorders and those with psychotic symptoms and the severely depressed should be advised not to seek such help. Many healers tend to avoid looking after such patients.

Terminology and classification

There are currently two main systems of classification used in psychiatry. Although the 4th edition of the American Psychiatric Association's Diagnostic and Statistical Manual[7] (DSM-IV) is comprehensive and detailed in its definitions the International Classification of Diseases, 10th edition[8] (ICD-10), has the advantage of being truly international and of being concise in its definitions while being very largely consistent with the larger American volume. All references to diagnostic categories in this chapter will be to ICD-10. Modern classifications have all but abandoned certain well-known but ill-defined terms. There is no advantage in saying that someone is suffering from a psychosis when a definite diagnosis is available, although the word 'psychotic' is useful when drawing attention to symptoms such as delusions, hallucinations and loss of contact with reality. Likewise the term 'neurosis' is not used in ICD-10 and the word 'neurotic' is found only in the title of a chapter. As an adjective, the word tends sometimes to carry a pejorative connotation and implies some form of innate weakness of character or inability to cope. It should never be used in this sense. The word 'hysteria' has also been abandoned since it had become ambiguous in its meaning and 'puerperal psychosis' is also redundant since a diagnosis should almost always be possible under some other heading. There are in addition a number of culture-bound symptoms or symptom complexes which have been described in the past. Such terms should now be looked upon as essentially obsolete. Making a more specific diagnosis enables all factors to be taken into account (as with many psychiatric conditions, the aetiology may be multiple) and should lead to more focused management. The use of local terminology in describing an illness can be justified in its increasing understanding of underlying social processes.

Organic, including symptomatic, mental disorders

Acute organic states

Although brief episodes of apparent clouding of consciousness may occur in psychoses such as schizophrenia or during an acute polymorphic psychiatric disorder (sometimes called a brief psychotic episode), it is best to assume that all such states are caused by organic dysfunction. It is wise to avoid the term 'confusional state', often used for acute organic states, since the expression is generally used to refer to muddled thinking, which is found in other psychiatric disorders. Delirium may occur as a result of primary cerebral disorders or of systemic disease.

Common systemic conditions causing delirium in the tropics include:

- Heat: high fever, heat stroke, heat exhaustion
- Dehydration, electrolyte imbalance
- Infections, especially malaria, pneumonia, septicaemia, typhoid, typhus, urinary tract infection
- Poisons including carbon monoxide
- Vitamin deficiency, thiamine, niacine, B_{12}, folate
- Alcohol, drug intoxication or withdrawal
- Prescribed drugs, herbal remedies
- Endocrine and metabolic disorders, hypoglycaemia.

Disorders primarily affecting the central nervous system and causing delirium include:

- Infection: meningitis, encephalitis, brain abscess, tuberculoma, cerebral schistosomiasis, cysticercosis, hydatid disease, paragonimiasis
- Epilepsy and postepileptic states
- Head injury and its sequelae including cerebral haemorrhage, subdural haematoma
- Intracranial space-occupying lesions
- Raised intracranial pressure.

Since delirium refers to a constellation of psychiatric symptoms occurring in individuals suffering from some other underlying illness, the nature of this illness will also determine the presentation and may be a main feature; or the illness may present as a delirium and steps have to taken to determine its cause. The main feature—impairment of consciousness—may be very mild and may vary, both according to the time of day (usually worse at night) and from moment to moment. It is characterized by disorientation in time and place and by an inability to recognize familiar people. There are typically visual hallucinations and possibly illusions or other disturbances of perception; the mood is often anxious, irritable or simply one of perplexity but often very labile; thinking is slow and muddled and there may be some paranoid ideation and such a degree of suspiciousness that it is difficult to nurse the patient. The patient can give little information about himself and registration of new memories is impaired.

The treatment of any delirious episode needs to be both general and specific. The general treatment must include adequate nursing and this is best complemented by the presence of family members. Nursing should be done in an environment where the patient is neither under- nor over-stimulated and is rapidly able to recognize those who are caring for him. Drug treatment should not sedate during the day and should assist sleep at night. While chlordiazepoxide is often the drug of choice in delirium tremens it may sometimes prove to be too sedative with other types of delirium (for example, in an individual recovering from unconsciousness due to head injury) and in this case a neuroleptic such as haloperidol may be preferred during the day. Since alcohol withdrawal and vitamin deficiency states so often coexist and may also be factors in a person who has been concussed after a road traffic accident, it is wise to give the full spectrum of B vitamins to all delirious patients. Delirium tremens should be treated, if severe, as a medical emergency. There may be severe dehydration and disturbance of electrolyte balance, seizures may occur and there may be hepatic pathology and a cardiomyopathy. Infusing glucose without ensuring an adequate supply of thiamine can precipitate Wernicke's encephalopathy. Other specific treatments will depend on the cause of the delirium.

Chronic organic mental disorders and dementia (chronic brain syndrome)

Dementia is a syndrome due to disease of the brain, usually of a chronic or progressive nature, in which there is a disturbance of multiple functions including memory, thinking, orientation, comprehension, calculation, learning capacity, language and judgement. Consciousness is not clouded although episodes of clouding may occur during the course of a dementing process. Although there is no specific therapy for some forms of dementia it is important to be able to recognize those cases in which effective treatment can be given. Because some of the main causes of dementia arise from degenerative conditions (such as Alzheimer's disease, Huntington's chorea and cerebrovascular disease), they are more commonly seen in older patients and thus are less common in those countries with a lower life expectancy. As the population structure changes, so does the spectrum of diseases. It is likely that Alzheimer's dementia will become more common, although in some countries HIV infection has taken over as one of the commonest causes of a dementing process. Especially in younger persons, however, treatable forms of dementia may occur, such as that due to chronic subdural haematoma, syphilis or prolonged lack of vitamin B$_{12}$. The dementia of HIV infection tends to occur late in the disease when the patient is seriously ill from other manifestations of AIDS. Other opportunistic infections such as toxoplasmosis, tuberculous meningitis or cytomegalovirus may also lead to a dementing process and should also be kept in mind, especially with a view to possible treatment. In case one of these is found without any prior suspicion of HIV infection, the question of counselling and testing becomes part of the overall management. Depression may be mistaken for dementia, especially when older patients are admitted to the foreign environment of a hospital and their natural perplexity (perhaps confounded by inability to communicate well in the local lingua franca) gives a false impression of intellectual deterioration.

Mental and behavioural disorders due to psychoactive substance use

Alcohol remains the main substance of abuse in most countries. Since the consumption of alcohol is linked to so many forms of morbidity, it is advisable for practitioners in any tropical country to make themselves acquainted with locally consumed beverages and the consumption style of the population. Alcoholic beverages may be very cheap, especially grain-based opaque beers, whether commercial or home-brewed, which are drunk without previous filtration. While a country may have laws concerning the production and distribution of alcoholic beverages, these laws may often not be enforced and in remote rural areas their enforcement is in any case largely impractical. The definition of an illicit beverage is usually determined locally but the fact of being illicit unfortunately seldom deters either producers or drinkers. More importantly, there is no formal quality control over such products and potency-enhancing contaminants may be added. Illicitly distilled beverages often contain about 20–30% or more alcohol by volume. When a spirit has been made, the most common and dangerous contaminant is methyl alcohol, which can lead to sudden death or bilateral optic neuritis and blindness. The drinking style of the population may be very heterogeneous in that different age and income bands may have different patterns, while there may be a sharp differentiation between the sexes. Consumption patterns are often related to cost as well as to availability. Many drinkers do not realize how much harm alcohol can do to the body but its social disruptiveness can often be mitigated by established customs in drinking.[9]

The concept of the alcohol dependence syndrome is now well established, but the common style of drinking may not usually lead to this particular complication. For a person to become dependent, it is usually necessary for there to be a high intake of alcohol on a daily basis over a long period. The main features of alcohol dependence include a strong desire or compulsion to take alcohol, difficulties in controlling drinking behaviour in terms of its onset, termination or levels of use; a physiological withdrawal state; evidence of tolerance; neglect of alternative pleasures or interests; and persisting with drinking despite clear evidence of overtly harmful consequences. Disorders related to thiamine deficiency (Wernicke's encephalopathy and Korsakov psychosis) may occur less commonly than, for example, pellagra. In some countries pellagra is seen when a heavy-drinking man is deprived for a time of the food provided by his wife and he turns to a diet of bread and an illicit spirit. There is often a mixed vitamin deficiency state, with either niacin or thiamine deficiency the more prominent. Although the features of Wernicke's encephalopathy are well known, those of niacin deficiency are not. The medical student's triad of three Ds is incorrect. There is no dementia but an acute organic state. While the skin changes may be typical, there may be no history of gastrointestinal symptoms. The clouding of consciousness is usually very labile and within a matter of a minute or so a patient may be able to give some personal details and then become inaccessible. Neurological signs are commonly present, with a marked snout reflex and increased deep-tendon reflexes but with (usually) downgoing plantar reflexes. There may be features of a peripheral neuropathy from thiamine deficiency. It is common for health workers to successfully treat the pellagra while ignoring the underlying cause. Following up the patient and helping him with his drinking problem is an example of how prevention should be incorporated into all health programmes and practice.

Cannabis is often implicated as a cause of acute mental disorder in countries where it is grown and used. The plant *Cannabis sativa* (Indian hemp) is easily grown in the tropics and is widely available. Besides the well-known synonyms for cannabis products there is a constantly changing list of new names invented by current users in any locality. The main active ingredient is tetrahydrocannabinol; it enters the body usually by being smoked or sometimes by being eaten, and induces in most people a pleasant, dreamy state of altered perception. However, some people experience a panic attack or feel depressed. An acute psychotic state may be induced by heavy intoxication but it is generally agreed that there is no cannabis psychosis as such. It seems likely, however, that cannabis use may precipitate a schizophrenic episode in especially vulnerable persons. In countries where there is widespread use of cannabis, mental illness is often attributed to its use in a very uncritical way. Careful history taking will more often reveal that there is no association. Longer-term psychological effects include interference with memory and learning. Psychological dependence may occur in regular users. The concept of a cannabis amotivational syndrome has not been confirmed. Cannabis slows down reaction time and hence when combined with alcohol can be responsible for traffic or other accidents. Cannabis use is not especially associated with violence but this may occur when it is used at the same time as alcohol. There are no pharmacological effects producing fatal consequences.[10]

Alcohol and cannabis are widely available and relatively inexpensive. Many other drugs are much more expensive—but the scene is a constantly changing one. In countries swept by war, other drugs may be introduced (amphetamines for example) or tablets like diazepam looted from stores may be widely distributed. The taking of a drug like diazepam or an amphetamine may become fashionable in any country and particularly in schools and colleges. The drug 'ecstasy' is making its way round the world. Doctors should be aware of the effects of these drugs and be prepared to advise the authorities as well as treat individuals.

Psychotic states
Schizophrenia

The most characteristic symptoms of schizophrenia are remarkably consistent all over the world, whatever the culture. ICD-10 states that although there are no strictly pathognomonic symptoms of schizophrenia, the following often occur together: thought echo, thought insertion or withdrawal, and thought broadcasting; delusions of control, influence or passivity clearly referred to body movement, specific thoughts action or sensations; hallucinatory voices, commenting, discussing the patient among themselves, or other types of voice coming from some part of the body; persistent culturally inappropriate or impossible delusions; breaks or interpolations in the train of thought, resulting in incoherent or irrelevant speech or neologisms. Catatonic behaviour with excitement, posturing, waxy flexibility, negativism, mutism or stupor is uncommon.

Negative symptoms may also be present, including marked apathy, paucity of speech, blunting or incongruity of emotional responses. They usually result in withdrawal and lowering of social performance, with a significant change in the overall quality of personal behaviour, manifest in loss of interest, aimlessness, idleness and a self-absorbed attitude. Paranoid schizophrenia is the commonest type in most parts of the world but many patients present with an undifferentiated form. A dilemma presents itself with regard to diagnosis. On the one hand, making an early diagnosis and instituting treatment early improves the prognosis but, on the other hand, one should not be too hasty in attaching this diagnosis to an individual. However, if the symptoms are quite typical and there is no question of prior drug use or any other organic factor, a provisional diagnosis should be made and treatment instituted. Schizophrenia can run

a variety of different courses. The typical, but fortunately not the most frequent, is one in which the symptoms continue unremittingly, with a progressive decline in the patient's condition. In others the symptoms remit after an initial episode but, following this, the patients may relapse periodically and some, but not all, again run a downhill course. In an appreciable number of cases, however, the patients recover and remain well. Favourable prognostic factors include a negative family history, good premorbid personality, an acute onset and a good response to treatment. Prognosis in the tropics is said to be better, perhaps because those schizophrenics who are brought for treatment are the ones whose onset was acute, and also because of a tolerant and positive attitude by the patients' families.

While a biochemical basis for schizophrenia involving dopamine neurotransmission is postulated, it is evident that the neurological mechanisms involved are extremely complex and other neurotransmitters and neuropeptides will be found to have a role to play. Any drugs which are prescribed will inevitably have some unwanted effects and some may be dangerous. The patient's tolerance for these unwanted effects will be an important factor in compliance, as will the cost of treatment. Attending to psychosocial factors is important in helping the schizophrenic patient. Counselling for the family is especially important; for instance, many patients cannot tolerate highly emotional situations and are unwilling to be pushed into strong social interaction. The patient and his family must understand why the drugs are being given and know the difference between those given for the illness and those given to prevent unwanted effects. There is a new generation of neuroleptic drugs which are generally tolerated much better by patients, although there is as yet little evidence that they are more effective therapeutically.[11] Unfortunately drugs such as risperidone and olanzapine are very expensive compared with the older neuroleptics such as chlorpromazine, trifluoperazine and haloperidol. Chlorpromazine is still a drug of first choice in the treatment of an acute schizophrenic episode and it generally does not need to be given with an antiparkinsonian drug such as trihexyphenidyl (benzhexol). For many patients the drug of choice will be a depot preparation such as fluphenazine decanoate. An injection may need to be given only once per month and sometimes even less frequently. This drug requires an antiparkinsonian and, with prolonged therapy, a watch needs to be made for the symptoms of tardive dyskinesia.

Mania and bipolar manic–depressive affective disorders

Mania is one pole of the affective disorder spectrum and its main feature is elevation of mood, often amounting to elation, although irritability is often present when attempts at restraining an overactive patient are made. There is reduced sleep—which others complain about, not the patient, and there is increased appetite. Behaviour is often socially inappropriate. On examination there are expansive ideas or actual grandiose delusions, pressure of speech with flight of ideas are present and hallucinations may occur. Insight is impaired and may not be fully recovered, even by a compliant patient receiving a mood-stabilizing drug. There will often be a family history of similar episodes, or of depression and suicide, and the patient may have suffered from a previous episode or episodes, either of mania or depression. A first episode should be differentiated from schizophrenia or an acute transient psychotic episode, since long-term management differs in the three conditions. Even without treatment manic episodes are self-limiting after a few weeks or months, and the patients are able to live normal sociable lives between the episodes. Treatment of the acute episode is essentially the same as that for schizophrenia. Haloperidol is the drug of choice. There is usually no need to guard against a recurrence after a first episode of mania, but if two or more recur at relatively short intervals continuing medication will be advisable. While it may be possible to institute lithium treatment in larger centres with the necessary flame photometric facilities, it should not be used when relying only on clinical monitoring. The therapeutic window of acceptable blood concentration is far too narrow and the situation is made more hazardous in hot climates with a high turnover of body water. Positive reports have been made of the effectiveness of carbamazepine and possibly sodium valproate as mood stabilizers and although they are moderately expensive some families may be willing to take the burden rather than cope with further manic episodes.

Acute transient psychotic episodes

The concept of the parasuicidal 'cry for help' has proved to be very useful in some cultures but it needs some modification where a strong sense of group membership rather than self-identity is fostered (see Table 17.1.) Instead of violence directed against the self, it is directed towards the family and community. A common picture is of a young woman who, quite often in the evening, begins to sing and dance and may exhibit destructive or exhibitionistic behaviour such as running outside the house naked. This behaviour may continue for many hours and even for 2 or 3 days, while the patient is taken to a traditional healer or church leaders. Admission or detention of such patients is usually desirable, not only because their behaviour is unacceptable at home and they need care and treatment, but also because observation of their clinical course over the next few hours and days will provide essential information for future management. Such episodes are often incorrectly diagnosed as manic but the typical elevation of affect, pressure of speech and flight of ideas are not seen. The condition may settle very quickly, even without drug treatment, after admission to hospital, but if sedation is required either a neuroleptic or a benzodiazepine may be used.

The length of treatment is likely to be short. Once the patient is able to communicate, the psychological and social causes need to be explored. Not infrequently symptoms of depression will be found to be present or there may be some history of an acute traumatic episode or of conflict within the family. This is the point at which familiarity with the patient's culture is especially important.

Some patients are brought for medical attention because they are currently or have been violently aggressive. A common cause is the patient's fear of others and this may well have been realistic, since the family or members of the public and especially the police may have attempted forceful restraint. A struggling, seemingly violent patient can often be left in the capable hands of an experienced nurse who is ready to listen and reassure. Where a patient is manifestly violent and no communication can be established, sufficient staff members experienced in working together should hold the patient so that intramuscular chlorpromazine or haloperidol may be administered. It should be kept in mind that chlorpromazine tends to cause local tissue necrosis. This should be looked upon as an exceptional act, carried out only in the best interests of the patient as well as of his family or community.

Depression

There have been numerous attempts at the classification of depressive disorders. The niceties of classification in practice are less important than the ability to recognize depression in its milder as well as more extreme forms and the ability to offer appropriate therapy. While depression may form one pole of bipolar affective disorder, it may also be found as a component of many other disorders, including schizophrenia and dementia. Depression can have many causes and several may be operating at the same time—for example, in a woman who is at the menopause, is taking antihypertensive drugs, is just recovering from an attack of influenza and has a daughter with an unwanted pregnancy. The fact that both physical and psychological factors are involved, as well as genetic, supports an aetiology involving monoamine neurotransmitters but also admits of the influences of psychosocial factors.

Depression is characterized by depressed mood or sadness, loss of interest and enjoyment, reduced energy, increased fatiguability and diminished activity. Some of the following may also be present: reduced concentration and attention, reduced self-esteem and self-confidence, ideas of guilt and unworthiness, bleak and pessimistic views of the future, ideas or acts of self-harm or suicide, disturbed sleep, diminished appetite (including desire for sex). Some patients may feel worse at the end of the day and have difficulty getting off to sleep. Others feel worse on waking, sometimes linked with early-morning waking. Depression is often a hidden and unmentioned cause of distress and disability, particularly in housewives. Although depression in the tropics is similar to that seen elsewhere, it is thought to be harder to recognize because, it is claimed, the symptoms tend to be more somatic and less psychological than in the West. While there is a lack of typical presenting symptoms, there is a tendency of patients to make complaints only of somatic symptoms such as aches and pains, burning sensations on the top of the head and sometimes symptoms attributable to the working of magic or spirits. Once the condition is suspected the presence of both typical psychological and vegetative symptoms of depression will rapidly confirm the diagnosis. Often a single question about 'thinking too much' will give an initial clue.

Both drugs and psychosocial therapy may be beneficial. In an emergency, say when a patient is actively suicidal, electroconvulsive therapy (ECT) may be used. As with the older neuroleptics, the older tricylic antidepressants are much less well tolerated than newer products such as the selective serotonin reuptake inhibitors. The antimuscarinic side effects of the older tricyclics discourage many patients from continuing with an adequate dose—and too low a dose is one of the commoner causes for failure to respond to treatment. The newer drugs are better tolerated but more expensive. When only the older tricyclics, such as amitriptyline, are available, it is best to start with a relatively small dose and work up to the dose required while explaining and offering reassurance about the side effects. The drug can be given in a single dose before going to bed and there is the double advantage of better sleep and less experience of side effects. Patients should always be informed that there will be a delay of up to 2 weeks in feeling the full antidepressant effect.

Suicide

Recognizing suicidal intent can be life-saving, since suicide is mostly preventable when its possibility is kept in mind. It is not always possible after a 'failed attempt' to determine whether an individual really wished to die or not but there are many indications. It is particularly important to be able to assess risk before any act is carried out. In these days, with the wide availability of pharmaceutical and poisonous domestic products, carrying out a suicidal act is far easier than in the past, when resort might have been had to hanging, drowning or self-immolation. When an individual talks of or threatens suicide the risk must be assessed. The patient who is depressed should always be asked about suicidal ideation or plans. There is never any risk in doing so. Indicators of risk include: if an individual talks of committing suicide or killing themselves, has made definite plans including putting affairs in order; the presence of a psychiatric disorder such as schizophrenia but especially severe depression; alcohol or drug dependence; being older, especially if suffering from any chronic illness or disability; and being socially isolated. Those who are less suicidal are more likely to be young, female, less commonly suffer from a psychiatric disorder, have usually acted on impulse and used a less dangerous method.

Neurotic disorders

Anxiety disorders

The term *phobia* refers to anxiety occuring in relation to specific situations. Since phobic states appear to be uncommon in tropical countries, and their management (mainly psychological) requires specialist training, they are not dealt with further. Panic attacks are brief episodes of severe anxiety when the patient suddenly experiences autonomic symptoms accompanied by a fear of being about to die or lose control or become mad. Imipramine may be effective in suppressing attacks, with doses gradually increased up to 150 mg daily being taken for several months. Generalized anxiety disorder manifests with persistent autonomic symptoms as well as somatic complaints such as abdominal discomfort and constriction of the chest, and accompanied by vague fears, irritability and poor concentration. Sometimes there is a more specific complaint such as tension headache (which must be distinguished from migraine). Generalized anxiety may occur with depression and often in clinical practice it is unnecessary to distinguish between the two; the designation 'common mental disorders' has been found useful for this group of disorders[12] but this is not a 'diagnosis' in the ICD sense. In all patients with a provisional diagnosis of anxiety or depression, a thorough physical examination is an important procedure, which can be reassuringly therapeutic. Anxiolytic drugs such as the benzodiazepines are only suitable for the relief of acute anxiety in the short term. Since many patients also have depressive symptoms, an antidepressant may prove helpful. Symptomatic treatment will not remove the need for intervention at the social level and counselling but can be an important component of treatment.[13] Although it is often stated that the traditional healer can be especially helpful it will often be found that the patient has already visited several, with little practical help having been obtained.

Reference has been made to the strong pressure to conform in traditional society. In the modern world there is also strong pressure from parents for their children to fulfil frustrated parental ambitions and many children are ambitious to go far in their schooling. This led in Nigeria to the naming of a syndrome which still merits attention, if not the special name (brain fag syndrome).[14] The symptoms (complained of more often by boys) may be attributed diagnostically to a mild anxiety/depressive disorder with marked somatization and they include difficulty in concentrating or retaining what has been read and blurred vision. Relating mainly to problems of study, symptoms tend to increase as examination time approaches. Medical intervention is rarely necessary and much distress can be prevented if the school can appoint a trained counsellor, able to give guidance on good study habits and deal with the problems of adolescence and of boarding school life, as well as giving guidance to parents.

Dissociative (conversion) disorders

The word 'hysteria' has practically been dropped. This is because it has had many meanings attached to it, some implying a particular theory of aetiology (e.g. in Freudian psychoanalysis), referring to personality (the designation is now 'histrionic') or to a constellation of physical complaints while often having a pejorative meaning. The mechanism of dissociation implies a loss of conscious (and therefore voluntary) control over the integration of memories, current experiences and current behaviour, which results in psychological or apparent neurological dysfunction—the latter being designated 'conversion'. It is assumed that psychological discomfort has been converted to physical symptoms, thus allowing relief of distress and secondary gain.[15] Of psychological symptoms dissociative amnesia and fugue states are most often seen and of conversion disorders, aphonia and paralysis. More dramatic manifestations are rare. The mechanism of dissociation is sometimes encountered in states of possession, which often serve a useful function in allowing expression of psychosocial problems in socially acceptable ways.

Epidemic hysteria

One type of disorder which a doctor may be called upon to deal with can still conveniently be called 'epidemic hysteria'. Reports are regularly made of tens of even scores of school children being inflicted with a disease causing bizarre symptoms and defying immediate diagnosis in terms of any infectious agent, although the rapidity of spread of the symptoms suggests an 'epidemic'. Usually there is some cause of common distress or concern in the establishment, e.g. regarding the quality of food, or dislike for a particular staff member. A prominent figure (such as a head girl) may provide an example of easily imitated symptoms. Rapid isolation of the afflicted and an understanding that perpetuation of the symptoms will result in leaving school quickly cure the epidemic.

Post-traumatic stress disorder

Unfortunately natural and man-made disasters (including war and civil conflict) are common causes of stress to large numbers of people, including refugees, and many individuals are also subject to overwhelming stress in their personal lives, for example because of a serious traffic accident, involvement in a fire or being assaulted. Post-traumatic stress disorder is a reaction that can affect anyone, and not only the especially vulnerable. It often appears after a delay of some days or weeks and then persists with anxiety, insomnia and nightmares. Although there is difficulty in remembering details of the traumatic event, patients are troubled by intrusive and unwanted memories of what happened and try to avoid reminders of the event. There are also complaints of irritability, poor concentration and in some cases a feeling of detachment and of an inability to feel emotion. Early treatment is likely to be most effective and should be aimed first at reducing severe anxiety and restoring sleep by use of appropriate drugs over a short period while increasingly enabling individuals to recall their experiences and express their emotions in a supportive relationship.

REFERENCES

1 Mubbashar M H. Epidemiology of mental disorder in developing countries. In Tantam D, Appleby L & Duncan A (eds). *Psychiatry for the Developing World*. London: Gaskell, 1996: 3–9.

2 Satterthwaite D. Will most people live in cities? *BMJ* 2000; 321:1143–1145.

3 Murthy R S. Reaching the unreached. *The Lancet Perspectives* 2000; 356:s39.

4 Swartz L. *Culture and Mental health: A South African View*. Cape Town: Oxford University Press, 1998, Ch. 2.

5 Escher M, Desmeules J, Giatra E et al. Drug points: hepatitis associated with Kava herbal remedy for anxiety. *BMJ* 2001; 322:139.

6 Ernst E. The role of complementary and alternative medicine. *BMJ* 2000; 321:1133–1135.

7 American Psychiatric Association. *Diagnostic and Statistical Manual of Mental Disorder*, 4th edn. Washington, DC: American Psychiatric Association, 1994.

8 World Health Organization. *ICD-10 Classification of Mental and Behavioural Disorders*. Geneva: WHO, 1992.

9 Haworth A & Acuda S W. Sub-Saharan Africa. In Grant M (ed.). *Alcohol and Emerging Markets*. Philadelphia: Brunner/Mazel, 1998: 19–90.

10 World Health Organization. *Cannabis: A Health Perspective and Research Agenda*. Geneva: WHO, 1997.

11 Frangou S & Byrne P. How to manage the first episode of schizophrenia. *BMJ* 2000; 321:522–523.

12 Goldberg D & Huxley P. *Common Mental Disorders*. London: Routledge, 1992.

13 Patel V, Todd C, Winston M et al. Outcome of common mental disorders in Harare, Zimbabwe. *Br J Psychiatry* 1998; 172:53–57.

14 Prince R. Concept of culture bound syndromes: anorexia and brain fag. *Soc Sci Med* 1985; 21:197–203.

15 Kendell R E. Hysteria, somatisation and the sick role. *Med Int* 1991; 95:3944–3947.

Chapter 18
Ophthalmology in the Tropics and Subtropics

D. D. Murray McGavin

World blindness

The World Health Organization (WHO) Programme for the Prevention of Blindness and Deafness estimates that the number of people blind in the world is now around 50 million. The figure does not take into account the many millions who have only partial sight, an estimated further 145 million. Over 80% of blindness is in countries of the developing world and 80% of this blindness could be 'avoided', that is, either prevented or cured.

WHO categories of visual impairment

Approximately 25 years ago, it was realized that there were over 70 different definitions of blindness amongst United Nations member states. Five categories of visual impairment were later defined (Table 18.1).

By definition, 'blindness' is recognized in a person whose best-corrected binocular visual acuity is less than 3/60 (less than counting fingers at 3 metres) or where the central visual field is less than 10° around fixation in the better eye. Agreed definitions allow comparisons between countries and regions, and between the main causes of blindness affecting different populations. It then becomes possible to consider the ophthalmic personnel and equipment required to provide eye care services.

Patterns of blindness

The prevalence of blindness around the world is influenced by a number of factors, including age, sex, ethnic origin, environment and geographical location.

Age

Life expectancy is increasing in developing countries, and with the increase in numbers of old people there is a corresponding increase of those who are blind. In the countries of the so-called developed (industrialized) world, increased longevity has also resulted in more older people with chronic blinding diseases. There is, however, a contrast in the common causes of blindness between

Table 18.1 Categories of visual impairment (adapted from the International Classification of Diseases, ninth (1975) revision).

Categories*	Visual acuity† with best possible correction	
	Maximum less than:	Minimum equal to; or better than:
1 Visual impairment	6/18 20/70 3/10 (0.3)	6/60 20/200 1/10 (0.1)
2 Severe visual impairment	6/60 20/200 1/10 (0.1)	3/60 (finger counting at 3 metres) 20/400 1/20 (0.05)
3 Blindness	3/60 (finger counting at 3 metres) 20/400 1/20 (0.05)	1/60 (finger counting at 1 metre) 5/300 (20/1200) 1/50 (0.02)
4 Blindness	1/60 (finger counting at 1 metre) 5/300 (20/1200) 1/50 (0.02)	Light perception
5 Blindness	No light perception	

'*If the extent of the visual field is taken into account, patients with a visual field radius no greater than 10° but greater than 5° around central fixation should be placed in category 3. Patients with a field no greater than 5° around central fixation should be placed in category 4, even if the central acuity is not impaired.
†For the first four categories of visual impairment, the different figures in each box of the visual acuity columns represent the same level of acuity expressed according to different notations. The first line gives the notation used with the Snellen 6-metre scale (and, where applicable, the corresponding ability to count extended fingers at a set distance); the second line gives the equivalent notation used with the 20-foot scale; the third gives the decimal notation.

Table 18.2 Major causes of blindness (after ref. 1).

	United Kingdom	Tanzania
Children (0–15 years)	Genetic diseases Retrolental fibroplasia Congenital anomalies	Vitamin A deficiency (measles) Congenital cataract Ophthalmia neonatorum
Adults (45 years +)	Age-related macular degeneration Chronic glaucoma Diabetic retinopathy	Cataract Trachoma Chronic glaucoma

the developed and the developing world. Similarly, blinding eye disease amongst children (0–15 years) shows quite different causes of visual impairment (Table 18.2).[1]

Sex

Blinding eye disease throughout the world shows some differences between males and females (Table 18.3).[1] Trachoma is four to five times more common amongst women compared with men, primarily due to the recurrent cycle of reinfection affecting children and mothers (Figure 18.1). Onchocerciasis (river blindness), as a blinding disease, is more common in men who are more exposed to the bites of the black biting fly (genus *Simulium*). However, in Burkina Faso, amongst the Dagara tribe, where women have worked alongside men in the fields, the prevalence of blinding eye disease is the same between the sexes.

Angle closure glaucoma in Eskimo women is found three to four times more often when compared with

Table 18.3 Major causes of blindness (after ref. 1).

More common in women	More common in men
Trachoma	Onchocerciasis
Acute glaucoma	Chronic glaucoma
Cataract	Climatic keratopathy
Diabetic retinopathy	

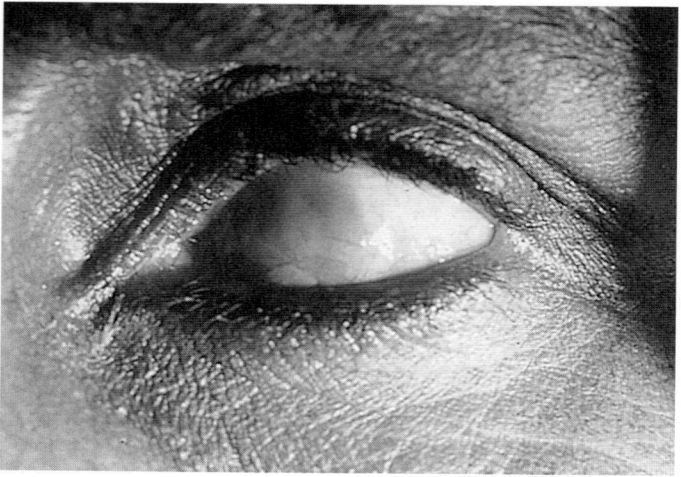

Figure 18.1: A blind eye due to trachoma in a 44-year-old woman. (Photo: John D. C. Anderson.)

Eskimo men. Conversely, open angle glaucoma amongst Africans seems to be more common in men than women.

Climatic keratopathy, due to exposure to direct or reflected ultraviolet light, is up to five times more common amongst men than women. This relates to the exposure to sunlight of men working out of doors, and is common in desert areas.

Hospital and clinic records consistently show that more men seek help for their eye problems. However, population-based surveys reveal a more even pattern of disease distribution between the sexes.

Ethnic origin

Glaucoma, in its two primary forms, shows considerable variation amongst broad ethnic regions around the world. Primary angle closure glaucoma is more common amongst Eskimos, Chinese and other races with mongoloid facial characteristics. In contrast, primary open angle glaucoma is recognized as common amongst Africans, often presenting in younger patients as compared with Caucasian races. This pattern of distribution of open angle glaucoma is also recognized amongst black Americans and in the Caribbean.

Environmental factors

Many environmental factors affect the prevalence of blindness in communities, and provide a huge variety of influences on eye disease. Of the common blinding diseases, both cataract and trachoma are found in populations where there are poor primary sources of water. Acute dehydration, which may have been due to acute diarrhoeal disease, is recognized as a risk factor for the later onset of cataract. The closer a community is to a good primary water source, the less likely it is that trachoma will be a major blinding scourge within that community.

A village situated close to a river with turbulent, frothy water is more likely to have blinding eye disease due to onchocerciasis. The *Simulium* fly, which carries the micro-filariae of the worm *Onchocerca volvulus*, breeds at the margins of these rivers—hence the name river blindness.

Poor environmental sources of fruits and vegetables, or lack of basic health education where these vitamin A-rich foods may be available, place children, particularly between the ages of 1 and 6 years, at risk of xerophthalmia.

Geographical location

Prevalence rates of blindness in the developing countries of the world are higher when compared with those in the developed world. Estimates of the number of blind people in different regions of the world (see below) reflect population densities as well as available eye care services.

In the developed countries, better perinatal care allows infants to survive, but with occasional eye abnormalities such as genetic defects and retinopathy of prematurity. In countries where obstetric and neonatal care is less advanced, many premature babies do not survive.

In adult and ageing populations in the developed world, diabetic retinopathy, age-related macular degeneration and glaucoma are major causes of blindness. In the developing world, besides glaucoma, the most common eye diseases are cataract and the gross scarring effects of trachoma.

Onchocerciasis (river blindness) is found in West and Central Africa, and there are pockets of infection in Sudan, Ethiopia, Tanzania and the Yemen. It is also found in isolated foci in Central America and the northern regions of South America.

Common causes of worldwide blindness (Table 18.4)

We have briefly discussed the definition of blindness and some significant factors which influence blindness in the world. Table 18.4 gives estimates of world blindness from different sources including the WHO World Health Report (1998) estimates for cataract, the glaucomas, trachoma, vitamin A deficiency (children under 5 years) and onchocerciasis.[2]

Eye care services

There is a huge imbalance in the provision of eye care services when comparing the developed and the developing countries of our world. In Europe and North America, there is one ophthalmologist for populations

Table 18.4 Major causes of blindness worldwide: estimates in millions.

Cataract	19.3
The glaucomas	6.4
Trachoma	5.6
Vitamin A deficiency (under 5 years)	2.7
Age-related macular disease	2.7
Diabetes	2.5
Injuries	1.5
Onchocerciasis	0.29
Leprosy	0.1
Others	3.5

ranging from 20 000 up to 100 000. In sub-Saharan Africa, on average, there is one ophthalmologist for one million people.

The countries of Asia reveal great variety in the provision of eye care services. India has over 100 medical schools and many trained ophthalmologists who carry out large cataract surgical lists. Eye camps may accommodate 50 or more cataract operations each day. One research paper indicated an incidence of blinding cataract in India in 1 year of 3.8 million.[3] This figure of 3.8 million may only reflect the picture in certain parts of India. Approaching 3 million cataract operations are carried out each year in India, and even allowing for the recognized increased mortality amongst patients with blinding cataract, compared with controls of the same age and sex, there is an increasing pool of unoperated blinding cataract. Other countries in Asia and around the world have the same traditional method of reaching the rural populations through eye camps. However, in some countries there is little recognition of the huge numbers of patients requiring eye care who may live and die in remote areas of a country without specialist help.

A universal feature of eye care services throughout the world is the 'urbanization' of ophthalmologists—drawn to the major cities by the attractions of lifestyle and financial reward. This gives a different picture when considering statistics for eye specialists in relation to populations, where the ratio in rural areas consistently reveals inadequate eye care facilities and expertise. Some of those who have specialized in ophthalmology do contribute generously, giving their time and resources in visiting distant and often impoverished communities, whether within their own countries or by arranged visits from the more advantaged countries of the world.

If we consider that 80% of the world's blindness is in developing countries and that 80% of this blindness could be either prevented or cured, then the message of need and responsibility is clear.

However, there are over 100 countries in the world that have a programme/committee/focal point for the prevention of blindness—a tribute to the considerable efforts of the team leading the WHO Programme for Prevention of Blindness and Deafness.

To meet the needs of the huge numbers of cataract blind patients in Africa, surgeons are being trained who may not be medically qualified. Ophthalmic medical assistants (ophthalmic clinical officers) who have an interest and aptitude, possessing the hand and coordination skills required for eye surgery, make excellent surgeons. Good hands and surgical skills are not confined only to those who are medically trained!

The best and most effective organization of eye care services, in most developing countries, has a structure of primary health care workers, trained in the recognition of eye disease, who can provide basic treatment and advice for patients and recognize those patients who should be referred to secondary eye care units. Secondary eye care facilities will provide routine eye surgery, but should have the option of referring patients to tertiary eye care

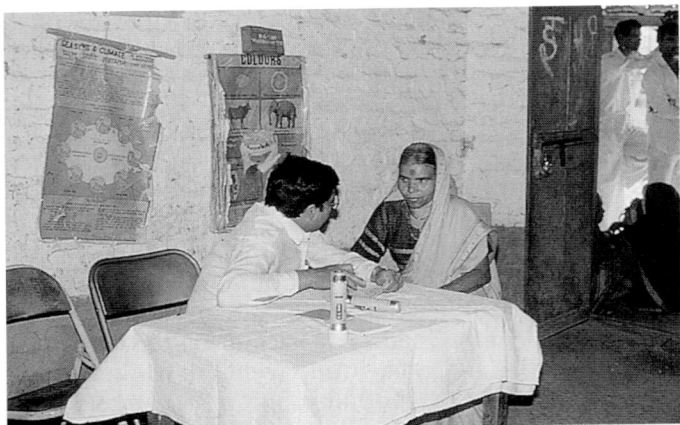

Figure 18.2: A screening/diagnostic eye camp in a school near Pune, India. (Photo: Murray McGavin.)

centres. These centres should be well staffed with trained ophthalmologists, ophthalmic medical assistants, optometrists, nurses and support staff, and also be equipped with necessary diagnostic and surgical instruments.

At all levels of expertise and experience, ongoing training should be given high priority. Training materials such as textbooks, manuals, videos, CD ROMs, teaching slide sets and posters should be made widely available. These eye health care workers can in turn develop their own programmes to provide health education for the general public.

Eye camps

Eye camps (Figure 18.2) may be planned and instituted in several forms. These ophthalmic outreach programmes may be described in three broad categories:

- Screening/diagnostic eye camps with referral to the base hospital.
- Permanent peripheral eye clinics.
- Traditional surgical/operational eye camps.

Examination of the eyes

One of the real advantages in ophthalmology is the opportunity to visualize eye abnormalities of both the anterior and posterior segments of the eye. Thus, with a focal light and magnification, the anterior eye can be examined, and, with an ophthalmoscope, the vitreous, optic nerve, retina and blood vessels can be seen.

Basic equipment and diagnostic materials

For effective examination of the eyes, only a few basic items are required.

- A test chart, e.g., Snellen's E chart.
- A pin-hole disc to screen for refractive errors.
- A hand torch (flashlight).
- A magnifying lens or loupe—uniocular or binocular.
- A direct ophthalmoscope.
- A lid speculum or retractor(s) (suitably shaped paper-clips may be used).
- A Schiotz tonometer.
- Eye drops: local anaesthetic drops, e.g., amethocaine 1%, benoxinate 0.4%; short-acting mydriatics (to dilate the pupil), e.g., tropicamide 1%, cyclopentolate 1%; fluorescein dye, e.g., minims (very small, disposable); paper strips. (Do not use fluorescein eye drops from bottles as pathogenic organisms may contaminate these bottles.)

Other equipment and medicines for treatment of eye patients

A few basic requirements for the removal of conjunctival or corneal foreign bodies, corneal abrasions, eyelid and periorbital lacerations, infection of the eyelids, conjunctiva and cornea are as follows:

- Sterile hypodermic needles.
- Fine suture material, needle-holding forceps, plain forceps.
- Cotton-wool 'buds'.
- Eye pads, adhesive tape, bandages.
- Scissors.
- Antibiotic eye drops and ointments, e.g., tetracycline 1% eye ointment, chloramphenicol 0.5% eye drops; systemic antibiotics, e.g., ampicillin 250 mg; vitamin A capsules (200 000 iu).

This chapter on eye diseases in the tropics and subtropics cannot describe the methods of examination in detail, which are always best taught by demonstration. However, a systematic approach to examination should always be followed.

1. History of the complaint
Symptoms and signs should be requested and described. What is the nature of the complaint? How long has the condition been present? Is vision affected? Is there pain, irritation, itching or discharge? What is the nature of the pain? Is the condition improving or worsening? Is there a family history of a similar complaint?

2. Measurement of visual acuity
Visual acuity should be assessed both for distance and near. Distance visual acuity should be recorded for each eye separately (Figure 18.3). If spectacles are worn for distance vision, visual acuity should be recorded with the spectacles on. If vision is reduced and there is no clear evidence of any eye disease, the pin-hole disc should be used. An improvement in vision in one or both eyes using the pin-hole indicates a likely refractive error—spectacles should improve vision.

3. Observe the general health of the patient
Does the patient, whether adult or child, appear healthy? Is the patient pale? Is the child distressed? A general

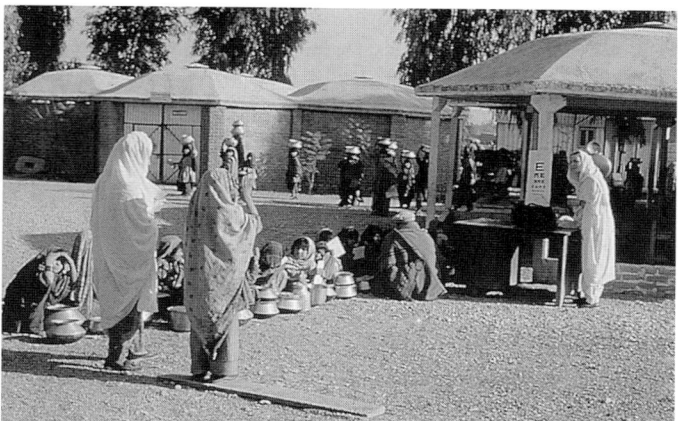

Figure 18.3: Testing the distance visual acuity of Afghan refugee children in Pakistan. (Photo: Murray McGavin.)

impression of health or systemic disease is most important.

4. Examine the periorbital region of each eye
Is there swelling or inflammation—for example in the region of the lacrimal sac? Are the eyelids in the normal position, or are they everted (ectropion) or inverted (entropion)?

5. Examine both eyes together
Is there any squint (strabismus)? Is there evidence of proptosis of either eye?

6. Examine the anterior eye with a focal light and magnification
Systematic examination of each eye—the conjunctiva (bulbar and tarsal), cornea, anterior chamber, iris and pupil—should be carried out using the hand-held torch. To observe the upper tarsal conjunctiva, the eyelid should be everted.

7. Examination of the posterior eye
Using the ophthalmoscope and rotating different lens powers into the eyepiece, examination from the anterior vitreous through the substance of the vitreous to the retina, optic nerve and retinal blood vessels can be carried out.

8. Examination of the intraocular pressure
A crude assessment of the intraocular pressure can be effected by gently palpating the upper eyeball through the eyelid, using the two index fingers, with alternating compression. This rough method will indicate only a very hard eye with increased intraocular pressure, or a very soft eye. Much more accurate readings may be obtained using a Schiotz tonometer or an applanation tonometer. Extreme care should be observed in manipulation should there be an eye injury, particularly if perforation is a possibility.

These simple procedures can be carried out very quickly by a primary health care worker trained to examine the eyes.

Vision 2020: The Right to Sight

The Global Initiative for the Prevention of Blindness—Vision 2020: The Right to Sight—was officially endorsed by Gro Harlem Brundtland MD MPH, Director-General, World Health Organization on 18 February 1999.

Recognizing that 100 million people will needlessly go blind by the year 2020 without joint global action, Vision 2020's mission is 'to eliminate the main causes of blindness in order to give all people of the world, particularly the millions of needlessly blind, the right to sight'.

This global partnership involves the World Health Organization and the Task Force of the International Agency for the Prevention of Blindness incorporating the leading international non-governmental development organizations.

Vision 2020 focuses on three areas requiring action:[4]

1. Disease control.
2. Human resource development.
3. Infrastructure development and appropriate technology.

Disease control
Cataract is the first priority amongst the major causes of blindness with an estimated backlog of around 20 million unoperated patients.

Trachoma is the most common infective cause of blindness with around 5.6 million blind or at risk of blindness, and active disease affecting 146 million. The 'SAFE' strategy (Surgery, Antibiotics, Facial cleanliness and Environmental factors) has provided impetus in the programme to eliminate this eye disease.

Onchocerciasis provides cause for some optimism that the disease can be eradicated by 2010 through community directed distribution of ivermectin (Mectizan).

The prevention of *childhood blindness* requires more initiatives for success although progress is being made with xerophthalmia and measles through 'child survival' programmes. Other causes of blindness include conjunctivitis of the newborn, congenital cataract and retinopathy of prematurity.

Refractive errors and low vision require new efforts to meet the huge needs worldwide. These will include services within primary health care, in schools and in the provision of spectacles and low-vision devices.

Human resource development
Recognizing a primary health care approach in blindness prevention, there is an emphasis on primary eye care training. Efforts will be made to train more ophthalmologists, to achieve, in Africa, one ophthalmologist for 250 000 people by the year 2020. In Asia the equivalent figures would be from the present one ophthalmologist for 200 000 today to one per 50 000 in the year 2020. Of equal importance is the training of ophthalmic medical assistants and ophthalmic nurses to reach a ratio of one in 100 000 in Africa and one in 50 000 in Asia by the year 2020. Further, basic eye care must be taught in all medical

schools worldwide by 2020. Other specialist personnel requiring training include refractionists, managers and equipment technicians.

Infrastructure and appropriate technology

Standards require to be set for availability, access and affordability in the provision of eye beds, refraction facilities and basic eye medicines.

Emphases will be placed on local production of instruments and consumables for cataract surgery, basic eye examination equipment and facilities, instrumentation for trichiasis surgery, spectacles and other optical devices, together with computers and communication systems for effective management and coordination.

Cataract

Cataract is found worldwide and is the most common cause of blindness (Figure 18.4). It is estimated that up to 20 million people in the world are blind due to cataract. By definition, this means that the vast majority of these patients have bilateral mature or maturing cataracts. Many millions more have early or immature cataract. Most of the backlog of blind people requiring surgery is in Asia (70%), followed by Africa (20%).

The number of bilaterally blind people in the world due to cataract is increasing dramatically due to two factors:

- Population growth.
- Increasing longevity.

The world population over 60 years old will double during the next 20 years to around 800 million by 2020, with a corresponding increase in patients who are bilaterally blind because of cataract. It is likely that the global incidence of cataract blindness is in the region of 5 million.

Cataract may be described as congenital/developmental, traumatic, secondary or age-related. Table 18.5 gives the causes of cataract within these categories.[5]

The only treatment for established cataract is the surgical removal of the lens of the eye, either as a whole (intracapsular cataract extraction) or in part (extracapsular cataract extraction) with the insertion of an intraocular lens implant. The second method is recognized as the

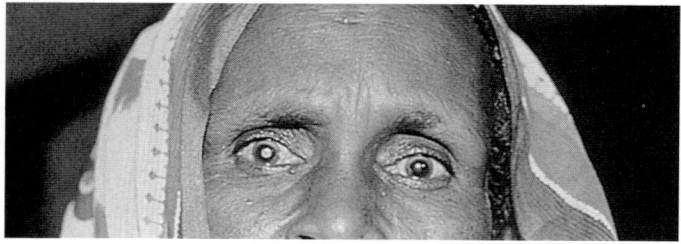

Figure 18.4: Bilateral cataract in a Somali woman. (Photo: Murray McGavin.)

Table 18.5 Common causes of cataract (after ref. 5).

Developmental:	due to genetic factors, or intrauterine infection (especially rubella)
Traumatic:	due to blunt or perforating injuries
Secondary:	due to intraocular inflammation, systemic diseases or drugs
Age-related:	due to largely unknown factors associated with ageing

best method, which should be made available worldwide, provided the surgeon has the skill and training required, together with the necessary surgical instruments and appropriate operating microscope.

Aetiology

Nutrition

A number of nutrients have been cited as playing a role in the development of cataract, based on animal and in vitro studies. These include: riboflavin, total protein, amino acids (especially tryptophan), vitamin C, vitamin E, selenium, calcium and zinc. The question of whether malnutrition predisposes to the development of cataract is difficult to elucidate. Chatterjee and his colleagues[6] in Punjab associated a higher prevalence of cataract with inadequate diet of proteins, including beans, lentils, milk, eggs and curd. In this study short height and low weight were also linked with the higher prevalence of cataract.

The converse of this and other studies is the question of whether the regular taking of multivitamins provides protection against the development of cataract. The Lens Opacities Case Control Study in the USA has indicated a decreased risk for all cataract types with regular use of multivitamins.[7]

Diarrhoea/dehydrational crises

Evidence has accumulated that episodes of acute dehydration, as with severe diarrhoea or heatstroke, is a risk factor for the later onset of cataract, at least in some localities. The author was advised by a former professor of ophthalmology in Calcutta, India, that he recalled the 'acute' onset of cataract during epidemics of cholera. A history of severe diarrhoeal disease, sufficient to confine a patient to bed or mattress for 3 days, greatly increases the risk of the onset of cataract. It should be said that not all studies implicate acute dehydration so dramatically. However, the value of providing vulnerable communities with good water supplies is obvious. The best ophthalmologist for a community may well be the engineer who digs a deep well!

Sunlight

There are differing views as to the significance of sunlight in the aetiology of cataract. In 1937, Wright[8] reported his study of 4000 labourers in two areas of India—one area typically with clear blue skies, and the other recognized as more cloudy. Cataract was more common in the cloudier area.

Epidemiological studies have been conducted in the USA. A cross-sectional survey of 838 watermen in Chesapeake Bay reported that lifetime sunlight exposure was associated with cortical but not nuclear cataracts. Only ultraviolet B light (295–320 nm) was associated with a weak increased risk of cortical cataract formation.[9]

A further 168 patients who required surgery for posterior subcapsular cataracts during 12 months in Maryland were compared with controls without posterior subcapsular cataracts selected from the same area and matched for age, sex and referral patterns. An association which was statistically significant was found between ultraviolet B and posterior subcapsular cataracts.[10]

Health authorities in Australia and Canada encourage health campaigns directed at reducing exposure to sunlight, to prevent both skin carcinoma and cataract. An environmental factor which demands our attention is the recognized thinning of the ozone layer which reduces the barrier protecting our planet from potentially harmful ultraviolet rays.

Smoking

A number of reports indicate an association between smoking and increased risk of nuclear cataracts and possibly posterior subcapsular cataracts. These studies suggest a two to three times increased risk of cataract with smoking. However, it is possible that smokers can reduce the risk by stopping the habit.[11]

Other risk factors for cataract

Diabetes and impaired glucose tolerance, glaucoma, hypertension, myopia and alcohol consumption are all described as increasing the risk of cataract in the developed world.

Surgery

Barriers to cataract surgery[12]

In a number of countries, including India, Brazil and Malawi, it has been shown that many patients remain cataract blind even if cataract surgery is available. There is increasing recognition that a number of factors provide barriers to effective cataract surgery. These include:

- Cost of surgery.
- Distance to the hospital.
- Cultural and social barriers.
- Knowledge of services.
- Trust in the outcome of surgery.
- Lack of eye surgeons, particularly in Africa.

These issues must be addressed to achieve effective cataract surgical services.

Cataract surgical rate

In order to reduce the backlog of cataract blindness it will be necessary to operate at least on the total number of new blind patients from cataract which present each year. The cataract surgical rate (CSR) is the number of cataract operations performed per year, per million population. In the industrialized countries of the world the CSR is usually between 4000 and 6000 cataract operations per million population per year. India has significantly increased its CSR in the last 10 years from less than 1500 to a figure of around 3000 today. However, this is still insufficient to keep pace with the incidence of cataract in India.

Cataract surgical coverage

Together with prevalence data, cataract surgical coverage (CSC) can provide important information on the impact of cataract intervention programmes. CSC may be measured for both 'persons' and/or 'eyes'. CSC indicates the extent to which services have covered the needs in communities/populations. It measures the effectiveness of the cataract intervention programme. Thus, it is an output indicator and does not measure the quality of cataract surgery.

For example, CSC (eyes) can be measured by the following equation:

$$\text{Cataract surgical coverage (eyes)} = \frac{a}{a+b} \times 100$$

where a = pseudophakic and aphakic eyes, and b = eyes with operable cataract.

The CSC (eyes) and the CSC (persons) are given as a percentage, where the percentage findings for eyes will be lower than that found for persons.

Surgical technique and postoperative care

During the last 10 years, the debate as to which surgical method should be used in countries of the developing world has continued, with the overwhelming preference now for extracapsular cataract extraction with an intraocular lens implant (ECCE + IOL).

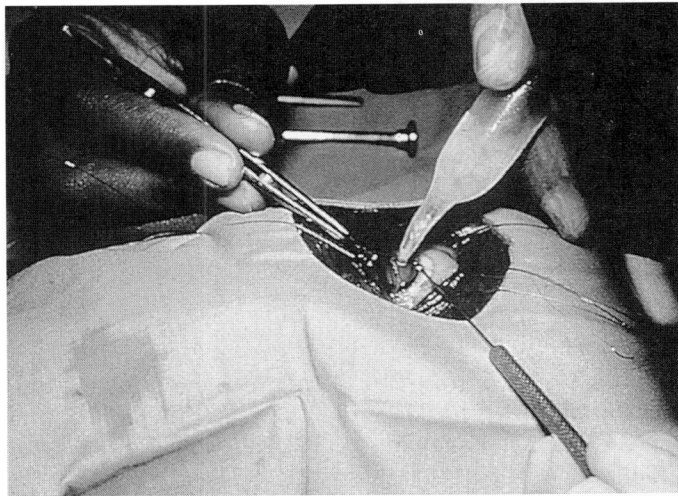

Figure 18.5: Intracapsular extraction using a cryoprobe. (Photo: John D. C. Anderson.)

The traditional method used for very many years to provide high-volume cataract surgery has been intra-capsular cataract extraction (ICCE), where the entire lens is removed within its capsule. This has been effected by a variety of methods, including the use of capsule forceps and the safer procedure using the cryoprobe (Figure 18.5). The particular disadvantage of this method is the need for spectacle aphakic correction. Aphakic spectacles give a magnified, distorted image; in addition, they are often broken, lost and sometimes expensive (see below).

The extracapsular cataract extraction (ECCE) leaves the posterior capsule of the lens in position, removing the nucleus and cortex of the lens. In the industrialized world and in much of the emerging surgical practice through-out the world, the posterior chamber intraocular lens (IOL) implant is placed within the capsular bag. Optically, this is by far the best method. In recent years, the cost of high-quality IOLs has reduced considerably—to less than US $10 for each IOL. There is no need postoperatively for relatively thick, convex magnifying aphakic spectacles. Further, this type of cataract operation (ECCE + IOL) may be used for a unilateral cataract which may occur, for example, after trauma. The disadvantages of ECCE + IOL are the extra time taken to carry out surgery, the need for sophisticated magnification with coaxial illumination of the surgical field, and more expensive instrumentation.

Surgeons in developing countries are rightly keen to develop more advanced and better techniques and thus, in most centres throughout the world, ECCE + IOL is being routinely performed. The problem of necessary surgical intervention still exists, however, where vast numbers in rural areas require routine cataract surgery, sometimes involving operating lists of up to 50 patients each day.

A suitable compromise solution which may be appropriate in certain circumstances is the combination of intracapsular cataract extraction (ICCE) with an anterior chamber IOL (ACIOL).

The glaucomas

Glaucoma is not a single disease entity and therefore, the group of conditions with different mechanisms involved is best described as 'the glaucomas'. The abnormal mechanisms involved may be the result of raised intraocular pressure (although not invariably), damage to the vascular supply of the optic nerve head which may result in cupping and corresponding visual field defects.

Glaucoma presents in two primary forms:

- Primary open angle glaucoma.
- Primary angle closure glaucoma.

A congenital form of glaucoma may also occur (buphthalmos).

There are a number of secondary forms of glaucoma. Examples are:

- Glaucoma due to iridocyclitis.
- Glaucoma after haemorrhage in the anterior chamber.

- Phacomorphic glaucoma.
- Phacolytic glaucoma.
- Pigmentary glaucoma.
- Pseudoexfoliative glaucoma.
- Neovascular glaucoma.
- Steroid-induced glaucoma.
- Epidemic dropsy.

Epidemiology of the primary glaucomas

Glaucoma is found throughout the world. It is a blinding disease with probably over 6 million blind worldwide. Estimated figures have suggested 13.5 million with open angle glaucoma, 6 million with angle closure glaucoma, 2.7 million with secondary glaucoma and 300 000 children with congenital glaucoma.[13]

Open angle glaucoma is especially prevalent amongst Africans, where the disease process occurs relatively early in life, even in teenagers, with a correspondingly serious prognosis if treatment is not sought or is unavailable. However, open angle glaucoma in Africa appears to occur in clusters, with some variety in prevalence rates in different countries and regions of the African continent. The significance of this disorder amongst ethnic black races 'carries over' to the countries of the Caribbean and also within the black populations of North America. The prevalence of open angle glaucoma amongst black Americans is 8–10 times higher than their white American compatriots. However, it is interesting that very high prevalences of open angle glaucoma have not been found in populations in West Africa. It should be noted that angle closure glaucoma does occur in some populations in Africa, including Nigeria, South Africa, Somalia and Uganda. Open angle glaucoma is more common amongst the Caucasian populations of the industrialized world when compared with angle closure glaucoma.

Very late diagnosis of open angle glaucoma in most of the developing countries of the world is borne out in the author's experience. In one country in Central Asia, of patients examined during one calendar year in whom the diagnosis proved to be glaucoma, nearly 50% were already completely blind or nearly blind in one eye, with vision at no light perception or only slightly better, and in the second eye the vision was commonly reduced to counting fingers.

Angle closure glaucoma presents particularly amongst Asian races of mongoloid origin, such as those in China, Myanmar and Singapore. The Inuits (Eskimos) have high prevalence rates of angle closure glaucoma.

It should be noted, however, that these separately described primary forms of glaucoma, in general, may occur amongst all races and there may be great variety in presentation. Thus, an intermittent angle closure form of glaucoma may occur. Clearly, the conditions described are not always absolute, falling into one category or another, and there may be some overlap in clinical presentation, still resulting, however, in damage to the eye.

Anatomy and physiology of aqueous fluid circulation

The production of aqueous fluid is through the ciliary processes of the ciliary body. The aqueous fluid circulates around the lens of the eye and passes through the pupil, with most of the drainage of fluid being filtered through the trabecular meshwork at the angle of the anterior chamber. Any form of blockage of drainage, whether due to the root of the iris, blood, inflammatory cells, pigment, etc., can disturb the free drainage of aqueous from the eye, with a consequent rise in intraocular pressure.

Open angle glaucoma

Ocular features which have long been recognized in relation to open angle glaucoma should help us in our understanding of some of the factors which contribute to this eye abnormality:

1. Intraocular pressure.
2. Optic nerve head damage.
3. Central visual fields defects.
4. Drainage angle of the anterior chamber.

The onset of open angle glaucoma is typically insidious and may be unassociated with pain or headache. However, if a patient does complain of some headache then glaucoma must be considered in the differential diagnosis. The anterior segments of each eye are usually entirely normal in appearance. The intraocular pressure is characteristically raised, usually above 21 mmHg, and this is measured by tonometry. However, it should be noted that raised intraocular pressure alone does not necessarily mean that the patient has glaucoma. Glaucoma may be present, with visual field loss, associated with normal pressure (normal tension glaucoma) and moderately raised pressures can occur in eyes that do not have classical open angle glaucoma (ocular hypertension).

Examination of the optic nerve head in each eye, using the ophthalmoscope, is of great importance in the diagnosis of glaucoma, particularly open angle glaucoma. An abnormally cupped optic nerve head can often be diagnostic of open angle glaucoma (Figure 18.6). A vertically cupped disc is more likely to be a glaucomatous cup. Borderline cupping of the optic disc, when the cup:disc ratio may be around 0.5, requires further investigation, with examination of central visual fields. The finding of typical 'glaucomatous' visual field defects will often confirm the diagnosis.

Gonioscopy is the technique used to examine the angle of the anterior chamber using a specially designed contact lens with a small mirror. Thus, the diagnosis of 'open angle', 'narrow angle', 'closed angle', 'secondary' glaucoma may be confirmed.

The central visual fields may be examined by a variety of methods from simple techniques to highly sophisticated computerized methods.

Primary open angle glaucoma (POAG) is typically a bilateral condition.

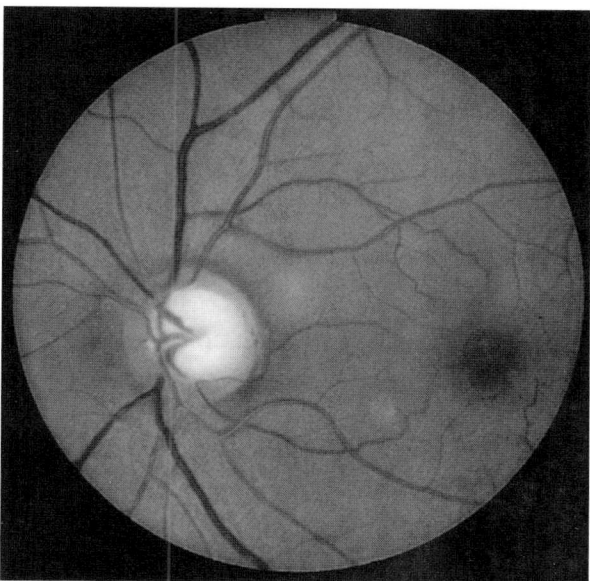

Figure 18.6: Cupping of the optic nerve head. (Photo: Gordon Johnson.)

Other risk factors for open angle glaucoma which are recognized include increasing age, ethnic groups (see before), myopia, family history, evidence of vascular spasm elsewhere (e.g., Raynaud's syndrome, migraine) and possibly diabetes and hypertension (in older age).

It is recognized that 50% or more of POAG cases in a population remain undiagnosed.

Management

The treatment of open angle glaucoma is to lower the intraocular pressure. There is a choice between surgical intervention and medical therapy. In developing countries, the approach should generally be surgical. This is for a number of reasons. Many patients, unfamiliar with the use of eye drops, may be confused by the instructions given, will also be very irregular in the instillation of the antiglaucoma eye drops and will not replace them when finished. This example of patient non-compliance is not confined only to developing countries. Eye drops, if used, will be instilled for many years, often for the lifetime of the patient, and these are costly. Also, experience in recent studies in industrialized countries has indicated that early surgery is beneficial in arresting the progress of glaucoma.

If medical therapy is given, even for a short period of time, the following eye drops may be used:

- Pilocarpine 1%, 2% or 4%, three to four times daily (alternative: carbachol 0.75 or 3%, three times daily).
- Timolol maleate (Timoptol) 0.25% or 0.5%, twice daily (alternatives: levobunolol 0.5%, twice daily; carteolol, 1% or 2%, twice daily; metipranolol 0.1% or 0.3% twice daily).
- Adrenaline 1%, twice daily (alternative: depivefrine, 0.1% twice daily).

Latanoprost (50 μg/ml drops) is a prostaglandin analogue which can be given as one drop daily (preferably evening) for open angle glaucoma or ocular hypertension where other treatments have failed.

Topical treatment with eye drops may be supplemented with oral acetazolamide tablets and these may be given in doses of 125 mg or 250 mg, ranging from one to four times daily. However, acetazolamide should only be used as a short-term measure; if required for a longer period of time, the patient should also be given a potassium supplement. Side effects of acetazolamide include paraesthesiae, gastrointestinal disturbance and kidney stones.

The surgical procedure that is commonly used for open angle glaucoma is trabeculectomy. This filtering procedure allows escape of the aqueous fluid into the subconjunctival space. African patients may have an inflammatory postoperative response with consequent scarring and blockage of the filtering site. This can be dealt with by using antimetabolites at the time of surgery.

Angle closure glaucoma

Although angle closure glaucoma may occur in an intermittent form with occasional blurring of vision, the characteristic presentation of this acute eye condition is with severe pain, headache and, in extreme forms, even vomiting and disorientation. The intraocular pressure may be considerably raised, sometimes to 60 or 70 mmHg, and this must be reduced as soon as possible.

Angle closure glaucoma can be an ophthalmic emergency—delay can result in permanent loss of vision. Furthermore, without any treatment, the second eye has a greater than 50% chance of developing angle closure glaucoma within 5 years.

Clinical presentation

An 'acute' presentation will find a patient who is distressed with severe pain and headache. The affected eye is red and congested. The cornea is often hazy due to corneal oedema and there may be awareness of coloured haloes around lights. Closer examination reveals a shallow or 'flat' anterior chamber, with the iris close against the corneal endothelium. The pupil may be dilated or semi-dilated and fixed, not responding to light. It may not be possible to view the posterior segment of the eye, in particular the optic nerve head, through the hazy cornea.

It should be noted that the 'angle closure' variety of glaucoma may also be 'intermittent' or even 'latent' in its presentation, always with the potential for an acute episode to occur.

The second eye, in comparison, is usually quiet and appears entirely normal. Close examination is likely to reveal a shallow anterior chamber. A shallow anterior chamber can be viewed by shining a light from the side of the eye across the anterior segment of the eye.

Visual acuity is usually considerably reduced in the glaucomatous eye, while often normal in the unaffected eye. Using the two index fingers, and gently palpating the upper surface of the affected eye 'through' the upper eyelid, with the patient looking down, may give a sense of a hard eye when compared with the other eye. Tonometry will confirm the likely diagnosis.

Predisposing factors for angle closure glaucoma include 'crowding' of the anterior segment of the eye—a smaller corneal diameter, an enlarged lens and a smaller axial length of the eye.

Risk factors for angle closure glaucoma are increasing age, gender (women are generally more often affected, e.g., amongst Eskimos, Europeans and South African blacks), race in general (see earlier), refractive error (hypermetropia), side effects of drugs (e.g., atropine, hyoscine) and possibly stress.

Management

Treatment must be immediate. Acetazolamide, taken orally if possible, should be given in high doses, 250 mg four times daily. If the patient is not able to take acetazolamide orally, the drug may be given by slow intravenous infusion or by injection intramuscularly. Alternatives to acetazolamide, providing systemic treatment for markedly raised intraocular pressure, are oral glycerol or intravenous mannitol. This systemic treatment is supplemented with Gutt. timolol maleate 0.5% twice daily. Pilocarpine should be given when the intraocular pressure has started to come down, and then three to four times daily while longer-term treatment is considered.

When the eye has quietened and the intraocular pressure has returned to normal, a surgical procedure is planned. In the eye which has had the acute attack, the likely procedure is a trabeculectomy. It is of particular importance that the second eye also has surgery as a prophylactic measure. Here the procedure is an iridectomy or an iridotomy. The iridotomy can be done using the laser. This procedure creates another opening through which aqueous fluid can pass (the other opening is the pupil) and deepens the anterior chamber of the eye, drawing the root of the iris away from the trabecular meshwork and thus allowing escape of aqueous fluid which previously had been blocked.

Normal tension glaucoma

It should be noted that typical glaucomatous field defects may occur in association with a glaucomatous cup of the optic nerve head but the intraocular pressure is consistently recorded within the normal range. This is normal tension (or 'low' tension) glaucoma and indicates poor blood circulation at the optic nerve head, resulting in progressive optic nerve atrophy. Treatment may be difficult, but lowering the intraocular pressure further is the only approach we have at present.

Central visual fields and medical treatment of glaucoma

If medical therapy with eye drops is used, it is most important that the central visual fields are carefully recorded at regular intervals, often every 3–4 months. This regular attendance at the glaucoma clinic will necessarily continue for the rest of the patient's lifetime. However, surgery is usually carried out in most developing countries of the world, and now more commonly in the industrialized world.

Secondary glaucomas

Glaucoma presents secondarily to a number of different predisposing conditions. These include the following.

Iridocyclitis

Iridocyclitis can be a complication of a number of systemic disorders, including leprosy, tuberculosis, syphilis, onchocerciasis and many others. Cells and proteins in the anterior chamber disturb the normal outflow of aqueous fluid through the trabecular meshwork. Using a focal light and magnification a 'flare' may be seen in the anterior chamber—like a shaft of sunlight streaming into a room full of dust. The presence of these cells and proteins in the anterior chamber may secondarily cause a rise of intraocular pressure. As a result of the inflammatory reaction within the eye there may be adhesions between the pupil margin and the anterior lens surface (posterior synechiae) and/or in the angle of the anterior chamber (peripheral anterior synechiae). The pupil will dilate irregularly if posterior synechiae are present. Occasionally the adhesions may be total, affecting the entire pupil margin, and this is described as seclusio pupillae. The iris bows forward as aqueous fluid cannot pass through the pupil and this further embarrasses the drainage angle of the anterior chamber—described as 'iris bombé'.

Haemorrhage into the anterior chamber (hyphaema)

Degenerate red blood cells may block the trabecular meshwork at the angle of the anterior chamber and there is a secondary rise in intraocular pressure. Further, if the haemorrhage has been a result of a severe blunt injury, for example, with damage to the trabecular meshwork and the angle of the anterior chamber, later healing with fibrosis may cause a severe type of secondary raised intraocular pressure (post-traumatic angle recession).

Phacomorphic glaucoma

The cataractous lens may become swollen (intumescent) which causes relative pupil block, the iris root is moved forward and this may result in blockage of outflow of aqueous fluid at the angle of the anterior chamber (Figure 18.7). This is a secondary form of angle closure glaucoma.

Phacolytic glaucoma

Lens material may cause blockage of outflow of the aqueous at the drainage angle and this may occur after injury (including cataract surgery) or when lens material leaks through the lens capsule of a mature/hypermature lens. Macrophages, attempting to remove this abnormal

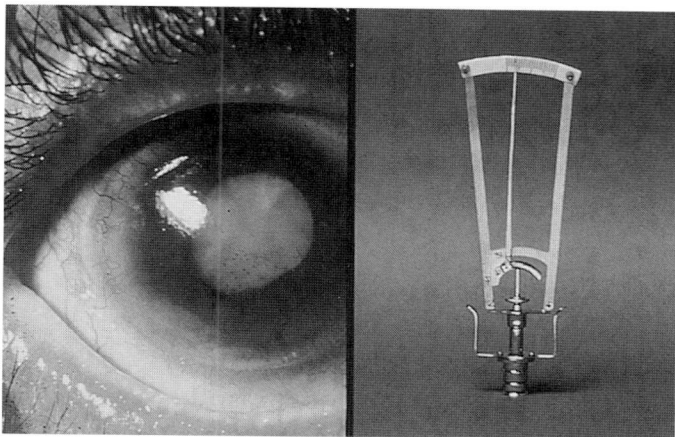

Figure 18.7: Secondary glaucoma caused by an intumescent cataract. A Schiotz tonometer is shown on the right. (Photos: John D. C. Anderson and David's Studio.)

material, together with the abnormal lens material itself may cause blockage at the angle of the anterior chamber.

Pigmentary glaucoma

In certain eyes, pigment particles may circulate abnormally in the aqueous fluid, and these in turn may cause blockage at the drainage angle.

Pseudoexfoliative glaucoma

Abnormal accumulation of white particles (not unlike dandruff in appearance) may accumulate in the anterior eye. This abnormal material can cause secondary blockage of the drainage angle. Pseudoexfoliative glaucoma is particularly found in Sudan, Somalia, Ethiopia and Tanzania. It is less common in West Africa.

Neovascular glaucoma (rubeotic glaucoma)

A thrombosis of the central retinal vein will result in disturbance of the circulation within the eye and this may result in new vessel formation within the anterior segment of the eye. These abnormal blood vessels may affect the angle of the anterior chamber, where the blood vessels can be visualized, and a form of secondary glaucoma can result. Also, neovascular glaucoma may occur in diabetics where abnormal new blood vessel formation has occurred, similarly causing disturbance to the outflow of aqueous at the angle of the anterior chamber.

Corticosteroid-induced glaucoma

The longer-term use of topical corticosteroids can result in a rise of intraocular pressure in patients in whom there is a genetically determined susceptibility to this complication of treatment. Usually the raised intraocular pressure is reduced on discontinuing the use of topical corticosteroids.

Epidemic dropsy

This acute toxic disease is caused by the unintentional ingestion of *Argemone mexicana* oil, an adulterant of cooking oils. It has been reported in India, Mauritius, Fiji,

Bangladesh and southern Africa. Rash, oedema of the lower limbs and gastrointestinal and cardiovascular disturbances may be accompanied by a secondary form of glaucoma and retinal vascular abnormalities.

Treatment of the secondary glaucomas

The intraocular pressure should be reduced with acetazolamide, 125 mg or 250 mg, two to four times each day.

The predisposing primary condition should be treated appropriately, for example the treatment of inflammation in iridocyclitis by mydriasis and cycloplegia with atropine sulfate 1% and an anti-inflammatory agent such as a topical corticosteroid.

Blood should be removed from the anterior chamber where there is total or almost total haemorrhage (hyphaema).

An eye which has a cataractous intumescent lens should have cataract extraction. The same procedure should be followed where the diagnosis is phacolytic glaucoma.

Neovascularization within the drainage angle can be improved with panretinal laser photocoagulation. This procedure will apply both to thrombotic glaucoma and proliferative diabetic retinopathy.

Congenital glaucoma (buphthalmos, 'ox eye')

Congenital glaucoma occurs throughout the world. There is failure of normal development within the angle of the anterior chamber resulting in some blockage of aqueous fluid outflow. This blockage will vary according to the cause and severity of the condition. The intraocular pressure rises as a result and in these small children the eyeball, which has less rigid 'walls', can enlarge. Cupping of the optic disc may be evident.

If the condition affects only one eye, the diagnosis is usually an easy one. A larger cornea and a bigger eye is quickly recognized. However, bilateral buphthalmos may not be so immediately obvious. Other clinical features include photosensitivity and corneal oedema.

Management

Pilocarpine eye drops and acetazolamide are often given before surgery. The traditional surgical procedure is a goniotomy, in which a goniotomy knife is introduced into and across the anterior chamber of the eye to effect sweeping incisions along the abnormal tissue within the angle of the anterior chamber. Other surgical procedures which may be used are trabeculotomy or trabeculectomy. These are necessary if the cornea is already too cloudy to see the anterior chamber angle for goniotomy.

It is important that children have surgery which is skilled—preferably by a surgeon who is a specialist in paediatric surgery.

Trachoma

Trachoma is one of the major blinding diseases of the world. It is the most common infectious cause of blindness. Active trachoma is believed to affect around 146 million people. About 5.6 million are blind or at risk of blindness as a consequence of trachoma. This eye disease is a serious public health problem in many parts of Africa, the Middle East, Central Asia, India and South-East Asia. It is also found in focal areas of Latin America and the Pacific region.

This eye disease is a recurrent, chronic eye infection. The infecting organism is *Chlamydia trachomatis*—one of a group of organisms which share characteristics of both viruses and bacteria. Of the different types of *C. trachomatis*, serotypes A, B, Ba and C cause the eye infection. Serotypes D–K mainly cause urogenital infection, where a secondary eye infection may occur, either due to infection transmitted to the newborn child during delivery (conjunctivitis of the newborn) or to a conjunctivitis occurring in association with urogenital infection in an adult. Unlike the eye-to-eye infection (serotypes A–C) which we are discussing here, chlamydial infection with serotypes D–K is a sexually transmitted disease.

Eye infection often begins in early childhood. Children a few months old may be infected with *C. trachomatis*. Recurrent episodes of reinfection, together with secondary bacterial infection, may, after 10 or 20 years, lead to scarring of the eyelids. Typically, the upper eyelid turns inwards (entropion), and distortion of the eyelashes occurs. These rub on the eyeball (trichiasis) with consequent disturbance of the corneal surface, inflammation (keratitis) and eventually corneal scarring and blindness.

Risk factors

Communities which typically have endemic trachoma are those where the environment is dry and dusty, personal hygiene is poor, and there is lack of adequate

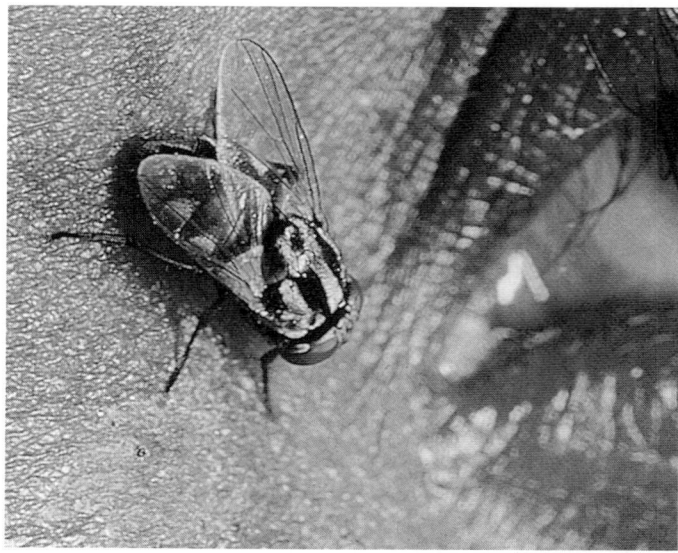

Figure 18.8: An eye-seeking fly which carries the organism *Chlamydia trachomatis*. (Photo: John D. C. Anderson.)

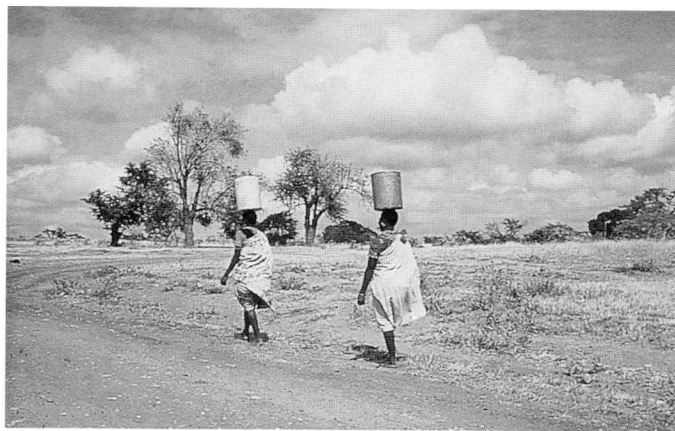

Figure 18.9: Collecting water—at a distance. (Photo: Erika Sutter.)

sanitation, overcrowding in the homes and especially a large fly population.

Flies carry the organism *C. trachomatis*. Transmission of infection from child to child by flies has been demonstrated. Eyes which have discharge attract flies (Figure 18.8). Nasal discharge attracts flies. Dirty, unwashed faces and fingers amongst children create an environment which predisposes to trachoma.

The presence of faeces lying exposed, whether human or animal, will also attract flies. Well-designed ventilated pit latrines within communities, which are properly used, will reduce the prevalence of trachoma within a community. Rubbish lying in open places is a further attraction for flies.

An inadequate or far-distant primary water source is a further risk factor for trachoma. There is a correlation between the distance travelled to collect water and the prevalence of trachoma within a community (Figure 18.9). It is evident that a good local water supply must improve the personal hygiene of individuals within communities.

Lack of education, especially of mothers, is recognized as a risk factor for trachoma. Health education for parents and children should include advice about contaminated materials, for example, a cloth or a part of clothing, which might be used to wipe away the discharge from a child's eyes. This can so easily be passed on to another child within the family.

One can summarize the mainly environmental risk factors for trachoma by listing the six Ds:

- Dry
- Dusty
- Dirty
- Dung
- Discharge
- Density (overcrowding in the home).

Another way of helping to remember agents of transmission of the eye disease is by listing the five Fs:

- Flies
- Faeces
- Faces
- Fingers
- Fomites (contaminated material or objects such as clothing or towels).

Clinical examination

Examination of each eye should be carried out with at least 2.5× magnification and with a good light.

1. After a brief examination of each eye for evidence of any discharge or inflammation of the conjunctiva, the eyelids should be carefully examined to see if any eyelashes are rubbing against the cornea.
2. It should be noted if any eyelashes have been removed (epilation).
3. The cornea is then examined for evidence of inflammation and/or corneal opacity.
4. The upper eyelid should now be turned over (everted). Ask the patient to look down, but keep the eyes open. The eyelashes are gently grasped between finger and thumb, while the other hand places a glass rod or similar object on the skin at the upper aspect of the tarsal plate of the upper eyelid, parallel to the lid margin. The upper eyelid is rotated against the slim rod and will evert. This provides a view of the upper tarsal conjunctiva.
5. The tarsal conjunctiva is examined for evidence of follicles, intense inflammation or conjunctival scarring.

Simple grading system (Figures 18.10–18.15)

A new simplified grading classification for trachoma looks for the presence or absence of five selected signs. The order of examination for these five signs is given above.

Trachomatous inflammation—follicular (TF)

The presence of five or more follicles in the upper tarsal conjunctiva. Follicles must be at least 0.5 mm in diameter and should be situated on the flat surface of the tarsal

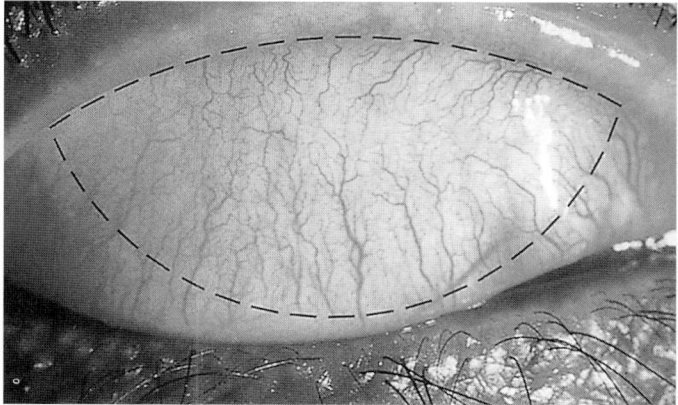

Figure 18.10: Normal upper eyelid. (The area to be examined for inflammatory changes is outlined.) (Courtesy of *Journal of Community Eye Health*, International Centre for Eye Health, Institute of Ophthalmology, London.)

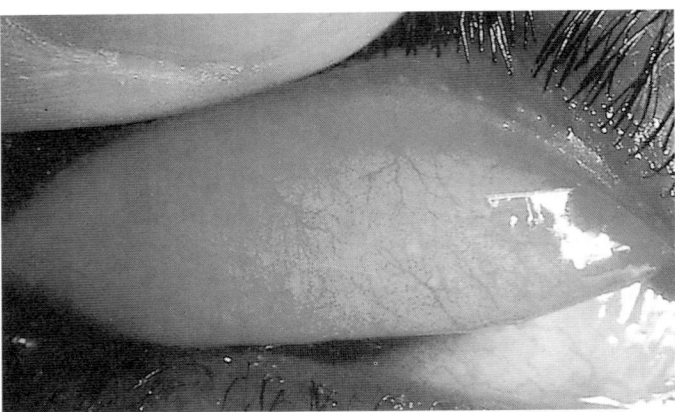

Figure 18.11: Trachomatous inflammation—follicular (TF): the presence of five or more follicles (each of which must be >0.5 mm diameter) on the flat surface of the upper tarsal conjunctiva. (Courtesy of John DC Anderson and the *Journal of Community Eye Health*, International Centre for Eye Health, Institute of Ophthalmology, London.)

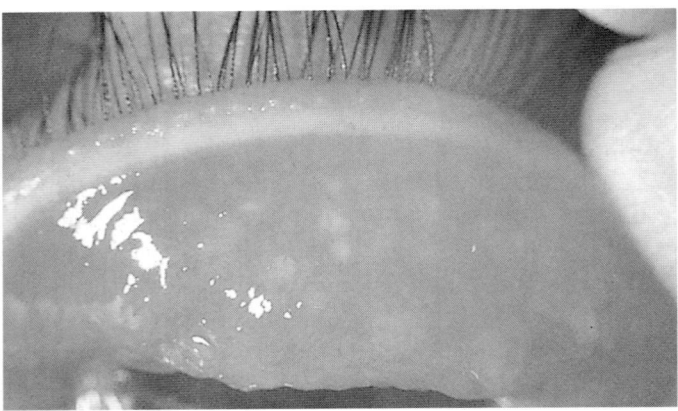

Figure 18.12: Trachomatous inflammation—intense (TI): marked inflammatory thickening of the upper tarsal conjunctiva; this obscures more than half he normal deep tarsal vessels. (Courtesy of Allen Foster and the *Journal of Community Eye Health*, International Centre for Eye Health, Institute of Ophthalmology, London.)

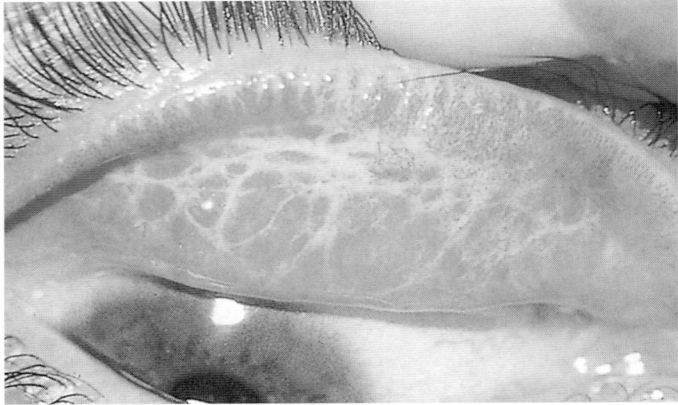

Figure 18.13: Trachomatous scarring (TS): involving the tarsal conjunctiva. (Courtesy of Hugh Taylor and the *Journal of Community Eye Health*, International Centre for Eye Health, Institute of Ophthalmology, London.)

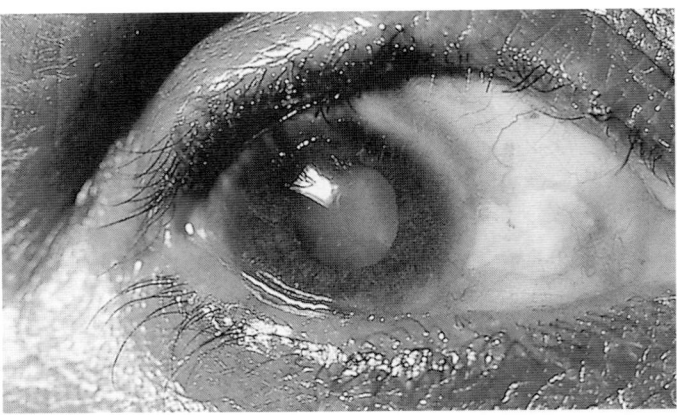

Figure 18.14: Trachomatous trichiasis (TT): evidence of one or more eyelashes rubbing on the eyeball. If one or a number of eyelashes have recently been removed, this should be graded trachomatous trichiasis. (Courtesy of John DC Anderson and the *Journal of Community Eye Health*, International Centre for Eye Health, Institute of Ophthalmology, London.)

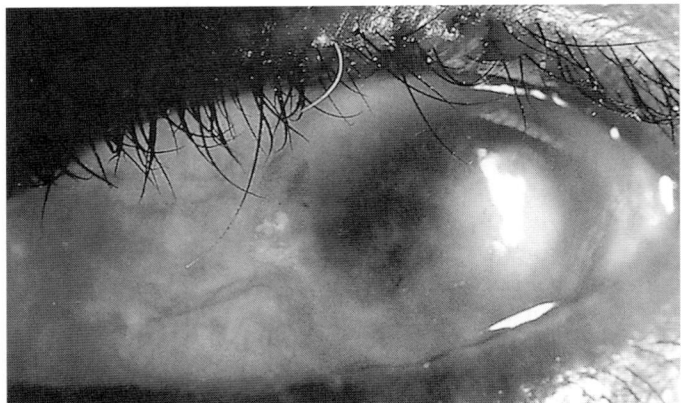

Figure 18.15: Corneal opacity (CO): corneal scarring due to trachoma where the scarring is central and sufficiently dense to obscure part of the pupil. (Courtesy of John DC Anderson and the *Journal of Community Eye Health*, International Centre for Eye Health, Institute of Ophthalmology, London.)

conjunctiva. Follicles are small spots or lumps, yellowish or white and paler than the rest of the conjunctiva, which are accumulations of lymphoid cells.

Trachomatous inflammation—intense (TI)

Pronounced inflammatory thickening of the upper tarsal conjunctiva that obscures more than half of the deep tarsal vessels. In severe inflammation, the tarsal conjunctiva will appear red, rough and thickened. There is diffuse inflammatory infiltration, oedema and vascular papillary hypertrophy. There may also be many follicles present. This is an extremely infective stage of trachoma.

Trachomatous scarring (TS)

The presence of scarring in the tarsal conjunctiva. White lines in the tarsal conjunctiva show early signs of the scarring stage of trachoma. The scarring may also appear as bands or sheets and may sometimes look like the edge of a feather.

Trachomatous trichiasis (TT)
At least one eyelash rubbing on the eyeball. Evidence of removal of an eyelash(es) (epilation) should also be included within this category in the grading system.

Corneal opacity (CO)
Easily visible corneal opacity over at least part of the pupil. The pupil margin should be blurred when examining an eye with this size of corneal opacity. Thus, there should be some degree of visual impairment.

Trachoma control and the SAFE strategy[14]

A new strategy with the acronym SAFE provides an appropriate and focused approach in control measures which involve tertiary prevention (surgery), secondary prevention (antibiotic treatment) and primary prevention (facial hygiene and environmental change). These three elements are contained within the SAFE strategy, but in reverse order:

- **S**urgery to prevent blindness in those who have trichiasis/entropion.
- **A**ntibiotics (tetracycline eye ointment/orally or doxycycline/orally or azythromycin/orally).
- **F**acial hygiene.
- **E**nvironmental change.

It has been suggested that the final 'E' should include not just environmental change but education and economic development—perhaps SAFE3![14]

Management
Medical treatment
Treatment of active trachoma requires the application of tetracycline 1% eye ointment to both eyes. There are different regimens of treatment but, in practice, the usual regimen is:

- Two times each day for 6 weeks.

Clearly, the ointment is only effective against active trachoma, particularly follicular trachoma and intense inflammatory trachoma. However, the upper eyelid which shows conjunctival scarring may also have active inflammation as well. Whenever there is any possibility of active trachoma, a full course of tetracycline 1% eye ointment should be given.

Where there is intense inflammatory activity, a systemic antibiotic may be used:

- Doxycycline 100 mg, once each day for 21 days, or
- Tetracycline 250 mg, four times each day for 21 days, or
- Azithromycin 20 mg/kg as a single dose.

Important: These systemic antibiotics should not be given to women during pregnancy. If treatment is necessary for a woman of childbearing age, erythromycin 500 mg twice a day is a safe alternative.

Doxycycline and tetracycline should not be given to children under the age of 7 years. A single dose of the new systemic antibiotic, azithromycin, has been shown in field trials to be as effective in treating trachoma as 6 weeks of topical tetracycline ointment.[15] The dose is 20 mg/kg to a maximum of 1 g. Although it should not be used in pregnancy, it may be given to children over 6 months of age. The drug is, however, expensive.

Trichiasis and epilation
When an occasional eyelash, or eyelashes rub against the cornea or conjunctiva causing extreme irritation, many patients remove the eyelash using forceps. They may carry a small mirror or other polished mirror-like surface to help them in this procedure. The disadvantage of this method is that the eyelashes will grow again in 4–6 weeks.

A more permanent and effective method for dealing with isolated ingrowing eyelashes is to apply cautery at the base of the eyelash with the intention that the hair follicle will be destroyed. This method requires local anaesthesia by injection at the base of the eyelash.

Surgery for trachomatous entropion
There are a number of surgical procedures which have been designed to effect rotation of the eyelashes away from the eyeball by surgery to the eyelid, including the tarsal plate. In skilled hands the procedure can be most effective, and in a study carried out in Oman the most effective surgical method was bilamellar tarsal rotation.[16] Sometimes visual acuity will improve slightly following surgery for entropion, where there is some clearing of the corneal haze.

Surgery after corneal opacity
The severity of corneal scarring, which is often bilateral, usually precludes a good surgical result by corneal grafting, although this surgical procedure should not be excluded as a possible intervention in a tertiary centre.

If an area of cornea does remain clear, despite bilateral corneal scarring, one possible surgical procedure is an optical iridectomy. The pupil is surgically enlarged behind clear cornea by removing a sector of the iris. Visual acuity can improve from hand movements to counting fingers at 3 or 4 metres following this surgical intervention.

Prevention
Recent studies have shown that regimens of topical treatment with tetracycline 1% eye ointment used within communities do not eradicate this eye disease. Within months the infection may return, with further inflammation and potential scarring.

Communities must be educated in the prevention of trachoma. The following advice should be given:

- Secure a suitable water supply.
- Regular daily face washing (and hand washing).

- Use of well-designed ventilated pit latrines.
- Rubbish lying in the open should be burned.
- Animals, especially cattle, should be housed some distance from the family home.
- Health education should be arranged for the community.

There is little anticipation at present of a vaccine that would prevent trachoma.

In many countries of the world, trachoma as an eye-to-eye condition has been eradicated due to improved social, environmental and economic conditions. Foci of severe trachoma, however, remain. The message in preventing trachoma becomes clear: raise the standard of living and life for so many impoverished and disadvantaged communities around the world.

Diabetes mellitus

Diabetes is increasing in countries of the developing world, and this is sufficiently widespread for King and Rewers to describe an 'apparent epidemic amongst adult populations of disadvantaged communities, both in developing countries and also in the industrialized world'. Certain ethnic groups have a very high prevalence of diabetes. The Pima Indians of Arizona, USA, have up to one-half of the population in the age range 30–64 years with diabetes. Impaired glucose tolerance is almost 30% in Arab Omanis and also among blacks in the USA.[17]

Earlier estimates by the WHO indicate that up to 2.5 million people worldwide are blind due to the complications of diabetes, in particular diabetic retinopathy, although the survey data is too limited to reach accurate figures. This estimate, however, would make blindness due to diabetes fourth in the 'league' of causes of worldwide blindness. At least 60 million have the disease, with 40 million in developing countries. For every person who is known to have the disease, another has diabetes but is unaware of their diabetic state.

Diabetic retinopathy

Twenty years after the onset of diabetes, nearly all patients with Type I diabetes (insulin-dependent) and more than 60% of those with Type II diabetes (non-insulin-dependent) will have retinopathy. Diabetic retinopathy is the leading cause of blindness amongst people of working age in industrialized countries (Figure 18.16).

A patient's diabetic condition must be well controlled, whether with or without insulin. It is a well-recognized fact that poor control is associated with retinopathy.

Retinal changes which cause visual loss are:

- Oedema of the macula.
- Proliferative diabetic retinopathy, with haemorrhage from new blood vessels, which may be retinal, preretinal or intravitreal.
- Proliferative diabetic retinopathy, with contraction of associated fibrous tissue leading to tractional retinal detachment.

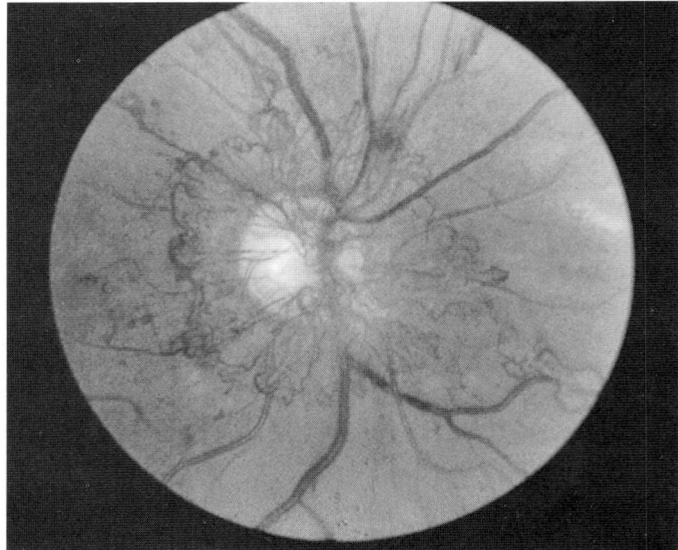

Figure 18.16: Proliferative diabetic retinopathy. (Photo: Gordon Johnson.)

Screening for diabetic retinopathy will become increasingly important in developing countries. Thus the technique of ophthalmoscopy should be taught widely and not only to those involved with eye care services. Relatively new descriptive terms for diabetic retinopathy have been used by the Early Treatment of Diabetic Retinopathy Study (ETDRS). This classification is set against standard photographs which are beyond our needs in this chapter. However, an attempt is made (following) to describe these categories and use these terms.

Background diabetic retinopathy: mild and moderate non-proliferative retinopathy

1. Mild non-proliferative retinopathy: the mildest form of non-proliferative diabetic retinopathy, characterized by the presence of at least one microaneurysm and also by dot, blot or flame-shaped haemorrhages in all four fundus quadrants.
2. Moderate non-proliferative retinopathy: characterized by intraretinal microaneurysms and dot and blot haemorrhages in one to three quadrants. Cotton wool spots, venous calibre changes, including venous beading and some intraretinal microvascular abnormalities (IRMA), occur.

Preproliferative diabetic retinopathy: severe non-proliferative retinopathy

At least one of the following should be present:

- Haemorrhages and microaneurysms in all four quadrants of the fundus.
- Venous beading in at least two quadrants.
- Intraretinal microvascular abnormalities in at least one quadrant.

Proliferative diabetic retinopathy

Within this category there are widespread areas of retinal

capillary closure and non-perfusion. New vessel formation from the venous end of capillaries, with endothelial budding, occur. Fragile new vessels bleed easily. Fibrovascular abnormalities develop. Vitreous haemorrhage or contraction bands may lead to retinal detachment. This is more common in insulin-dependent diabetes. High-risk proliferative retinopathy involves new vessels on the optic disc or elsewhere in the fundus and vitreous haemorrhage.

Diabetic maculopathy

The terms 'diffuse', 'exudative' and 'ischaemic diabetic maculopathy' were not used in the new terminology of diabetic retinopathy. Instead, patients were given macular focal laser therapy based on whether 'clinically significant macular oedema' was present or not.

This is the most common cause of visual loss in diabetes mellitus. It is more common in Type II disease. Exudates may be isolated or in groups or form a circinate pattern. Fluorescein angiography shows areas of capillary non-perfusion, indicating ischaemia.

Treatment of diabetic retinopathy

Control of diabetes:

- Good control of blood glucose levels.
- Reduce alcohol intake, smoking.
- Treat high blood pressure, renal disease, hyperlipidaemia.

Photocoagulation

Laser photocoagulation can be sight preserving in patients with severe diabetic retinopathy. With advanced new vessel formation, particularly new vessels at the optic nerve head or where neovascularization has taken place in the anterior segment of the eye, the patient is likely to require panretinal photocoagulation. With the laser, tiny focal burns may be distributed throughout the peripheral retina with 3000 or more applications. Focal laser applications in expert hands can be beneficial for clinically significant macular oedema. Also, focal laser to leaking spots associated with exudates threatening the macula may be applied. These applications should be made as far as possible before visual loss has been established.

The portable diode laser attached to a slit-lamp is now being widely used for diabetic retinopathy.

Pars plana vitrectomy

Vitrectomy is indicated for vitreous haemorrhage, which should be performed early for insulin-dependent diabetics. If the patient is non-insulin-dependent the procedure should be undertaken if the haemorrhage fails to clear after 6 months.

Vitreoretinal surgery is indicated if the macula is detached or threatens to detach and this should be performed early.

Screening for diabetic retinopathy

Insulin-dependent/juvenile-onset diabetes

- Dilated examination of the fundi every year beginning 5 years after diagnosis.

- Examinations more frequently once diabetic retinopathy is diagnosed.

Non-insulin-dependent/maturity-onset diabetes

- Dilated examination of the fundi every year once diabetes is diagnosed.
- Examination more often once diabetic retinopathy is diagnosed.

Vitamin A deficiency disorders (VADD) and the eye

Vitamin A deficiency, affecting young children throughout the developing world, is an example of a condition where the simple remedy is well known but many thousands of children still become blind.

Vitamin A deficiency disorders[18]

During the past 10 years or so, the huge relevance of subclinical vitamin A deficiency on the health of the young child has become evident. Morbidity and mortality, immune status, growth and haemopoiesis can be significantly affected. This evidence also relates to maternal health and survival in childbirth. Thus, the new term, vitamin A deficiency disorders, brings a wider perspective in recognition and treatment of this widespread nutritional deficiency.

Magnitude of VADD worldwide and blindness

Vitamin A deficiency affecting the eye, which has been described by the term xerophthalmia ('dry eye'), is the most common cause of blindness in children. Seventy per cent of blindness in children is due to corneal scarring, and the vast majority of these young patients have a history of vitamin A deficiency. In many of these cases, this acute nutritional deficiency earlier in their lives has been associated with measles.

Table 18.6 Magnitude of VADD worldwide (after ref. 19).

- Approximately 300 000 preschool-age children are blind from xerophthalmia and up to 60% of these die within 1 year
- About 3 million children are blind worldwide
- Approximately 3 million children have clinical xerophthalmia which includes night blindness and Bitot's spots
- In the region of 250 million preschool-age children are subclinically vitamin A deficient, with the corresponding consequences of morbidity and mortality
- Around 500 000 women die in childbirth annually and an unknown percentage of these die because of impaired vitamin A status

The magnitude of VADD worldwide is indicated in Table 18.6.[19]

Malnourished children are found in many countries of Asia and Africa, as well as in some areas of the Americas (Table 18.7).[18]

There have been some encouragements that countries with large numbers of children and a history of widespread VADD have shown distinct improvement in vitamin A status in recent years, particularly India, Indonesia and Bangladesh.

Table 18.7 Countries categorized by degree of public health importance of vitamin A deficiency, by WHO region (from information available to WHO as of February 1997) (after ref. 18).

WHO region	Clinical	Severe	Subclinical Moderate	Mild	No data available	VAD—under control/no problem likely
Africa	Angola Benin Burkina Faso Cameroon Chad Comoros Ethiopia Ghana Kenya Malawi Mali Mauritania Mozambique Niger Nigeria Rwanda United Republic of Tanzania Zambia Zimbabwe	Burundi Cape Verde Congo Côte d'Ivoire Gambia Lesotho Senegal	Botswana Namibia Sierra Leone Eritrea	Madagascar	Algeria Central African Republic Equatorial Guinea Gabon Guinea Guinea-Bissau Liberia Mauritius Sao Tome and Principe Seychelles Swaziland Zaire	
Americas	Dominican Republic Haiti	Brazil Colombia El Salvador Mexico Nicaragua Peru	Belize Bolivia Ecuador Guatemala Honduras	Guyana Panama	Argentina Cuba Dominica Paraguay Puerto Rico Suriname Uruguay Venezuela	Antigua and Barbuda Bahamas Barbados Canada Chile Costa Rica Grenada Jamaica St Kitts and Nevis St Lucia St Vincent and the Grenadines Trinidad and Tobago United States of America
South-East Asia	Bangladesh Bhutan India Nepal Sri Lanka	Indonesia Myanmar	Thailand		Maldives Mongolia	Democratic People's Rep. Of Korea

Vitamin A (retinol)

Vitamin A plays an important part in the body's defences against infection. Deficiency of the vitamin results in an impaired immune response with decreased resistance to infection. Squamous metaplasia of epithelial surfaces allows, for example, a greater susceptibility to lung infection.

The stores of vitamin A are mainly found in the liver, where 90% of the body's vitamin A is retained. Vitamin A undernutrition is typically associated with other nutritional deficits, which makes the young patient vulnerable to systemic disease.

Infection with the measles virus is particularly important in relation to vitamin A deficiency. The measles virus is found in the corneal epithelium and conjunctiva, respiratory tract and alimentary tract. When a child has an acute infection with measles, the depleted body stores of vitamin A are quickly used up and dramatic and distressing eye changes, with corneal damage (keratomalacia), may occur.

In older children and adults, where a more accurate history may be obtained, a description of night blindness is a common presenting symptom. Vitamin A is required for the production of rhodopsin (visual purple) of the rods of the retina.

The importance of early recognition of vitamin A deficiency, particularly in the young child, is therefore not only in the preservation of sight but in many instances the saving of a young life.

Eye changes in vitamin A deficiency

The following are the eye symptoms and signs (Figure 18.17) of xerophthalmia (Table 18.8).

1. *Night blindness (XN).* Rhodopsin (visual purple) is required by the retina of the eye to allow night vision.

Vitamin A is needed to replace and restore the rhodopsin of the retina. Although adults and older children may describe this symptom, it is necessary to ask the mother of a small child whether the infant bumps into objects in the evening or when it is dark.

2. *Conjunctival xerosis (X1A).* This typically dry appearance of the conjunctival (and corneal) surfaces indicates the importance of vitamin A in maintaining healthy epithelium with adequate secretions on the surface of the eye. This dry appearance provides the term xerophthalmia, which is commonly used to describe the condition of vitamin A deficiency affecting the eye.

3. *Bitot's spots (X1B).* Bitot's spots are found on the surface of the conjunctiva—most often on the temporal bulbar conjunctiva. The typical appearance is foamy and spots may present in triangular form with the base at the corneoscleral margin. Bitot's spots may be found in both eyes. They may occur in children under the age of 5 years, but can also persist in older children. Often the foamy spot may be removed quite easily. However, it should be noted that the appearance can remain in older children beyond the period during which the child was vitamin A deficient. Bitot's spots may take various shapes and sizes and are not always triangular in appearance. Some may contain pigment. Bitot's spots indicate changes in the squamous epithelium of the conjunctiva overlying areas of dryness (xerosis).

4. *Corneal xerosis (X2).* The cornea can become dry and appear lustreless indicating changes in the corneal epithelium consequent to vitamin A deficiency. It is the corneal changes which will begin to affect vision in the child.

5. *Corneal ulceration with xerosis (X3A).* The development of corneal xerosis and consequent damage to the

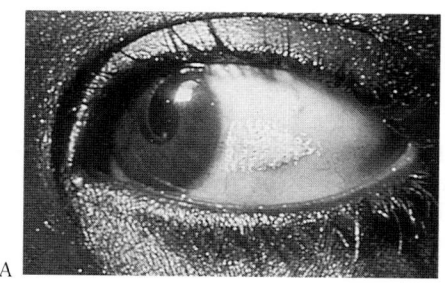
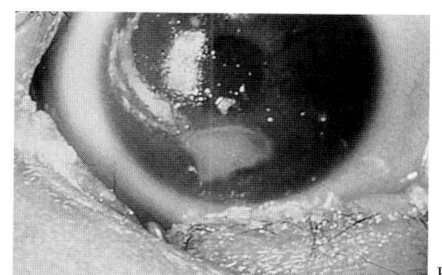
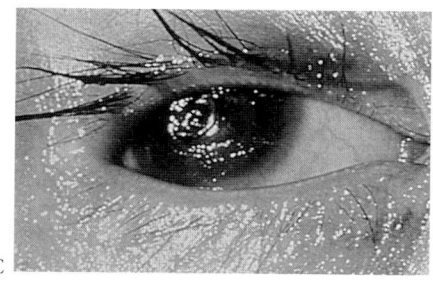
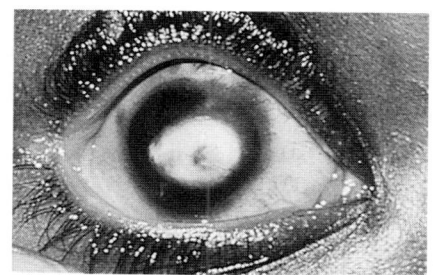

Figure 18.17: (**A**) Bitot's spots; (**B**) corneal xerosis with early ulceration; (**C**) corneal ulceration/keratomalacia; (**D**) corneal scarring. (Photos: (**A**) Simon Franken; (**B**) Allen Foster; (**C**) Donald McLaren; (**D**) Gordon Johnson.)

Table 18.8 Eye changes and vitamin A status.

Eye lesion	Vitamin A status*	Comments
Night blindness (XN)	Mild–moderate decrease (over 1 per 100)	Sensitive sign of low body vitamin A stores; still associated with increased illness and mortality Prevalence often increases into early school-age years Boys may be more affected than girls Cause is chemical deficiency in retina
Conjunctival xerosis (X1A)	Mild–moderate decrease (not used in WHO classification)	Dryness of conjunctiva due to decrease in goblet cells and epithelial change Difficult to diagnose reliably by clinincal examination
Bitot's spots (X1B)	Mild–moderate decrease (over 5 per 1000)	White 'foamy' or 'cheese-like' spots on the conjunctiva: usually bilateral and temporal Caused by change in squamous epithelium with underlying xerosis In older children may not disappear with vitamin A treatment
Active corneal changes (X2/X3)	Severe decrease (over 1 per 10 000)	Danger signs of permanent loss of sight Cornea may 'melt' (keratomalacia) in a few hours Most common at age 2–4 years No sex differences
Corneal scars (XS)	Depends on examination timing (over 5 per 10 000)	End-stage of malnutrition eye damage Scarring (leucoma) often allows some residual vision Blinded eyes may be protuberant (anterior staphyloma) or shrunken (phthisis)

*Public Health problem criteria as defined by the WHO in children aged between 6 months and 6 years.
Source: WHO Programme for Prevention of Blindness.

corneal epithelium may progress to involve the deeper layers of the cornea, resulting in corneal ulceration, which can be superficial or deep. A centrally situated corneal ulcer will profoundly affect vision.

6. *Corneal ulceration/keratomalacia (X3B).* The cornea may 'melt' dramatically (keratomalacia), with an acute onset, even over a few hours. Younger children are particularly susceptible to this development, which is most often found in infants aged 1–3 years. Treatment must be given as an emergency intervention, often to protect the other, less affected eye. Sadly, keratomalacia may present as a bilateral condition.

7. *Corneal scarring (XS).* The healed state following severe vitamin A deficiency with corneal ulceration and keratomalacia can result in marked corneal scarring which will often affect both eyes. Vision is greatly reduced. Many children who have this severe form of vitamin A deficiency will not survive beyond some months after the acute episode because they are particularly susceptible to intercurrent infections, such as respiratory infections and diarrhoea. For those who live through this acute phase, both their eyes, and inevitably their lives, may be scarred.

Severe damage to the anterior eye may result in unsightly, bulging eyes (anterior staphylomas) or the reverse occurs and the eye begins to shrink (phthisis bulbi).

The progression of eye signs that we have described may not occur in the sequence given.

Evidence of vitamin A deficiency affecting children who appear for examination indicates that others in the same family and community are likely to be vitamin A deficient.

The human immunodeficiency virus (HIV) is more readily transmitted to the fetus in mothers with low vitamin A status.

Treatment of xerophthalmia

The recommended treatment of recognized vitamin A deficiency affecting all age groups except women of reproductive age is given in Table 18.9.[19]

Table 18.9 Treatment schedule for xerophthalmia for all age groups except women of reproductive age[a] (after ref. 19).

Timing	Vitamin A dosage[b]
Immediately on diagnosis:	
• <6 months of age	50 000 iu
• 6–12 months of age	100 000 iu
• >12 months of age	200 000 iu
Next day	Same age-specific dose[c]
At least 2 weeks later	Same age-specific dose[d]

[a]Caution: women of reproductive age with night blindness or Bitot's spots should receive daily doses ≤25 000 iu. However, all women of childbearing age, whether or not pregnant, who exhibit severe signs of active xerophthalmia (i.e., acute corneal lesions) should be treated as above.
[b]For oral administration, preferably in an oil-based preparation.
[c]The mother or other responsible person can administer the next-day dose at home.
[d]To be administered at a subsequent health service contact with the individual.

If there is vomiting which would render the oral treatment useless, an intramuscular injection of 100 000 iu of water-soluble vitamin A (not an oil-based preparation) may be used instead of the first oral dose.

At the commencement of treatment with vitamin A, a topical antibiotic eye ointment, for example tetracycline 1% or chloramphenicol 1%, each given three times daily, is advised to prevent bacterial infection of the eye. Any affected eye(s) should be covered with an eye pad if the cornea is involved, making sure that the eyelid is gently closed before applying the eye pad.

The patient should be referred immediately to an eye specialist.

Prevention of xerophthalmia

A high-dose schedule for prevention of vitamin A deficiency is given in Table 18.10.[19]

Treatment of vitamin A-deficient women during the reproductive years, including pregnancy

High doses of vitamin A are contraindicated in pregnancy, as there have been concerns about the effects of vitamin A on the unborn child.

Vitamin A is contained within breast milk, and this will also provide a protective supply for the newborn child.

Communities which have a recognized problem of vitamin A deficiency should be given well-planned instructions outlining the consequences of vitamin A deficiency, especially for their children. The advantages of prevention, very often with remedies which are readily available, should be carefully explained (Figure 18.18).

Education about nutritional needs should be emphasized:

- Encourage breast-feeding.

Table 18.10 High-dose universal-distribution schedule for prevention of vitamin A deficiency (after ref. 19).

Age	Vitamin A dosage
Infants <6 months of age[a] • Non-breast-fed infants • Breast-fed infants whose mothers have not received supplemental vitamin A	50 000 iu orally 50 000 iu orally
Infants 6–12 months of age	100 000 iu orally, every 4–6 months[a]
Children > 12 months of age	200 000 iu orally, every 4–6 months[b]
Mothers	200 000 iu orally, within 8 weeks of delivery

[a]Programmes should ensure that infants < 6 months of age do not receive the larger dose intended for mothers. It may therefore be preferable to dose infants with a liquid dispenser to avoid possible confusion between capsules of different dosages.
[b]Evidence suggests vitamin A reserves in deficient individuals can fall below optimal levels 3–6 months following a high dose: however, dosing at 4–6-month intervals should be sufficient to prevent serious consequences of vitamin A deficiency.

- Mothers should supplement the feeding of infants by 6 months with fruits such as mango or papaya. Children aged 1 year or older can be given dark-green leafy vegetables, which are rich in vitamin A.
- Health workers, mothers and children, and the whole community, should receive instruction about foods that have a high content of vitamin A. Examples are spinach, carrots, sweet potatoes, certain fruits and green leafy vegetables. Dairy products and eggs contain vitamin A. Red palm oil, which is used especially by populations of West Africa, has a high content of

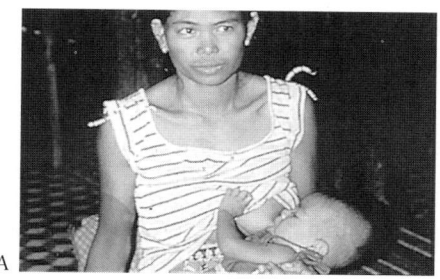
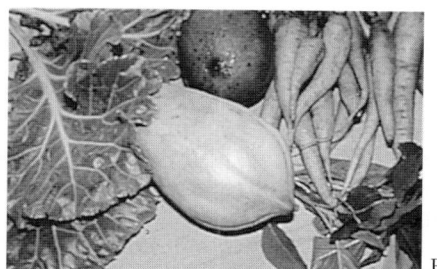
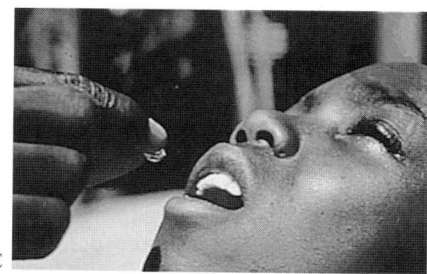
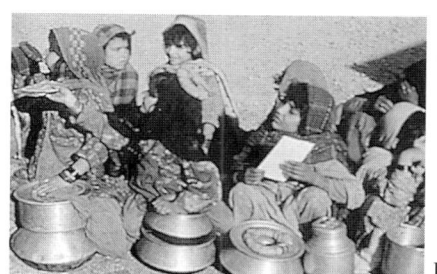

Figure 18.18: (**A**) Breast-feeding; (**B**) vitamin A-rich fruit and vegetables; (**C**) vitamin A capsule; (**D**) milk fortified with vitamin A. (Photos: (**A**, **B**, **D**) Murray McGavin; (**C**) Christoffel Blindenmission.)

vitamin A. Vitamin A, which is mainly stored in the liver, can be found in animal liver and fish liver oils.

- Encouragement should be given to farmers and all members of the community to plant appropriate foodstuffs, whether in small gardens or in larger plantations.

Interventions by the health authorities:

- Foods which are widely used may be fortified with vitamin A, for example sugar and milk.
- Public awareness of vitamin A deficiency and its consequences should be consistently emphasized by posters, by health education at mother and child health clinics and in schools. Radio can be used to pass on information and knowledge.

Measles and the eye

Measles is a serious infection, especially in the developing world. Estimates have suggested 1 million deaths due to measles annually. Most of these are children. A child is 400 times more likely to die as a consequence of measles if living in a developing country. Measles infection has often been associated with the acute onset of eye problems earlier in the life of a child or young person who presents with corneal scarring.

Clinical presentation

A child with measles will often have photosensitivity (sensitivity to light), watering and red eyes. There may be evidence of a punctate keratitis. Some children can develop corneal ulceration.

The measles virus is present in the superficial cornea and conjunctiva, but it is the secondary complications which can be disastrous for the eye or eyes.

- In a child with low reserves of vitamin A (mostly in the liver), where the clinical picture is characterized by poor appetite and gastroenteritis with inadequate intake of vitamin A and protein, acute vitamin A deficiency can result in corneal ulceration and keratomalacia (X3B).
- There may be depression of the immune system in association with measles infection. Secondary infection with herpes simplex virus may complicate the picture.
- A child who is ill with measles, vitamin deficient and dehydrated may be listless and fail to close the eyelids adequately. Corneal dryness due to exposure can result in corneal ulceration. A topical antibiotic eye ointment should be used at least four times daily during the illness.
- A previous visit to a traditional healer may confuse the clinical picture. Often the mother will be reluctant to admit that they have first attended the traditional healer.

Treatment of measles and its eye complications

1. Vitamin A 200 000 iu orally should be given at least once. If there is a known risk of vitamin A deficiency

in the community or if there are any symptoms or signs of vitamin A deficiency affecting the eyes of the child, the full regimen of three doses of vitamin A should be prescribed.
2. A topical antibiotic should be given to each eye at least four times each day. Avoid corneal exposure.
3. Systemic treatment should be given as appropriate, for example for gastroenteritis or respiratory infection.
4. Admission to hospital may be necessary.

Prevention

In Africa, it has been considered that about one half of childhood blindness has some relation to measles infection.

A programme of immunization should be instituted as soon as possible for the community or communities at risk. The WHO Expanded Programme on Immunization is promoting increased coverage of immunization around the world.

Onchocerciasis

Onchocerciasis is a parasitic disease caused by the filarial worm *Onchocerca volvulus*. The worm is transmitted by a vector, one of several species of the *Simulium* blackfly. The 'black biting fly' breeds in rivers, with a preference for turbulent and highly oxygenated waters. Thus, there is a high prevalence of disease near to rock-strewn rivers, with turbulent streams. Both the skin and the eyes are particularly affected by the disease, commonly known as 'river blindness'.

Epidemiology

The WHO Expert Committee has estimated that the number of people infected by *O. volvulus* is approximately 18 million. About 125 million people have been at risk. Around 270 000 are blind due to the disease.[20,21]

It is estimated that 40 000 new blind people are added each year. Once blind, affected individuals have a life expectancy of only one third of that of the sighted. Most die within 10 years. Of the 37 countries where the disease is endemic, 30 are in sub-Saharan Africa and 6 are in the Americas. Recent studies in Ethiopia, Nigeria and Sudan have shown that the disease is responsible for poor school performance and a higher drop-out rate among infected children.

Over 17 million of those infected with *O. volvulus* live in West and Central Africa. There are pockets of infection found in Yemen. Areas of infection are also found in Central America and northern countries of South America.

The social and economic consequences of this disease are huge, with considerable human suffering. The prevalence of blindness in villages near to fast-flowing rivers may reach 15%, often affecting men of working age. The impact of this disabling infection can be such that villages have been deserted when situated close to rivers.

The development of blindness will typically affect a relatively young man, perhaps 30–40 years old, who has lived and worked near to a fast-flowing, turbulent river in West or Central Africa. During the years of childhood and early adult life he will have been bitten many times by the *Simulium* fly and will have been infected and reinfected with the microfilariae of *O. volvulus*. He may be a farmer, a fisherman or a ferryman. Gradually, over the years, the distressing symptoms and signs of onchocerciasis develop. Scarring affects both the anterior and posterior segments of the eye. The eye condition is usually bilateral; visual field is gradually lost in each eye, and vision is severely reduced, leading to blindness.

The vector: the *Simulium* fly

The disease is spread from person to person by the blackfly of the genus *Simulium*. The female *Simulium* lays her eggs on rocks and vegetation where rivers are fast flowing and 'white' through turbulence because the eggs and larvae of the fly need oxygen for their development.

The female fly can travel up to 80 km in 1 day, although this is unusual and she is more likely to fly 5–10 km on either side of a river. During the rainy season the flies may travel to new breeding sites but when the season is dry they are more localized to permanent rivers and streams.

Around mating time, the female fly requires a blood meal to ensure development of her eggs, and as the disease is transmitted through the bite of the female fly, it is most dangerous to be living and working near to breeding sites. The female fly particularly feeds on human blood at dawn and dusk.

Life cycle of *O. volvulus*

When a person is already infected by the worm *O. volvulus* and is bitten by the *Simulium* fly, the small embryo worms (microfilariae) present in the skin of the infected person enter the body of the fly. There they pass through the gut wall and travel to the thoracic muscles. Further development takes place and after about 7 days the larvae move to the head of the fly, ready to be transmitted to the next human host when the fly requires another blood meal.

In this way the microfilariae of *O. volvulus* are transmitted to another person. They will take 1–3 years to develop into adult worms. One female worm can produce 0.5–1 million microfilariae in 1 year. The cycle of transmission from person to person continues.

Clinical presentation

The microfilariae of *O. volvulus* have a particular predilection for the skin and the eyes of the infected person but may also give rise to musculoskeletal pain interpreted as 'rheumatism'.

Skin complications

Itching is one of the first symptoms of onchocerciasis and this can be very severe, disturbing sleep. There is a rash which may occur on most parts of the body but often affects the buttocks. Very obvious scratch marks may indicate the severity of the itching.

A feature of onchocercal skin disease is depigmentation, described as 'leopard skin', which follows repeated episodes of skin inflammation associated with the death of microfilariae. There is subcutaneous fibrosis, skin atrophy and pigmentary changes. The skin may look and feel like the skin of a very old person. This clinical feature has been described as 'lizard skin'.

Lymphoedema of the skin can result in chronic thickened and often blackened skin, the result of severe, reactive onchodermatitis. Lymph node enlargement in the inguinal areas can disturb lymphatic drainage and the skin of the region is greatly enlarged. These folds of skin may not retract to the original, more normal situation and remain as the 'hanging groin' of onchocerciasis.

Subcutaneous nodules are found in different parts of the body, often around the hips or on the head. They are firm, discrete and painless. A nodule is formed by a fibrous reaction around coiled adult worms. Surgical removal of nodules (nodulectomy) may be considered, particularly where nodules are situated in the region of the head or shoulders.

Eye complications

Most of the symptoms and signs characteristic of onchocerciasis, including those affecting the eyes, are caused by the microfilariae of *O. volvulus*. Typically both eyes will be involved. As with the skin changes, it is the dead microfilariae which cause most inflammatory reaction within the eye. Microfilariae may be seen circulating in the aqueous fluid behind the cornea if sufficient magnification is available for close observation.

Eye inflammation can affect both the anterior and the posterior eye.

'Snowflake' and punctate keratitis

White-grey spots may be seen in the superficial cornea and these indicate a reaction to dead microfilariae within the cornea. Inflammatory cells accumulate around the dead microfilariae, resulting in opacities. There may be a red eye with photosensitivity and watering. Topical corticosteroids may be used, but these must only be given by the eye specialist as corticosteroids have their own complications for which follow-up is required.

Sclerosing keratitis

Sclerosing keratitis is one of the common inflammatory features of onchocerciasis which can cause blindness (Figure 18.19). Typically, sclerosing keratitis is seen at the nasal and temporal aspects of the cornea, and the opacity then extends throughout the lower part of the cornea. Advanced sclerosing keratitis can result in a total corneal scar. There is no specific treatment.

Iridocyclitis

Inflammation of the iris (iritis) and of the ciliary body (cyclitis) can contribute to reduced vision. The pupil may be drawn down in its lower aspect due to inflammatory

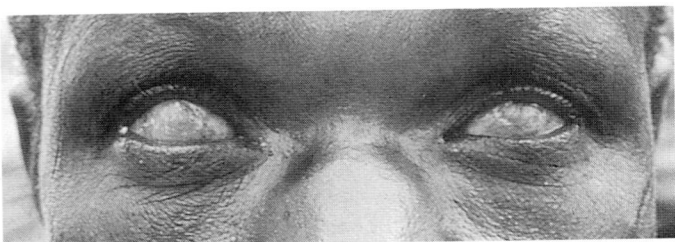

Figure 18.19: Sclerosing keratitis in onchocerciasis. (Photo: Pak Sang Lee.)

reaction where accumulated dead microfilariae may be found. In association with iridocyclitis, or incidental to it, a cataract can occur. These patients should be referred to the eye specialist. Iridocyclitis will be treated with a topical mydriatic and cycloplegic, often using atropine sulfate 1% eye drops and anti-inflammatory agents. A cataract will need to be removed, preferably in an eye which is quiet without active inflammation.

Optic neuritis and choroidoretinitis
Onchocerciasis affecting the posterior eye may show optic nerve atrophy and choroidoretinal atrophy. In severe optic atrophy, the optic nerve head is abnormally pale and white, whereas the normal optic disc is a faint pink colour, although slightly paler in its central part. Areas of the retina may be pale with scattered clumps of pigmentation (Figure 18.20). There is no treatment for optic atrophy and choroidoretinal atrophy.

Diagnosis
Clinical features
The symptoms and signs of onchocerciasis are often sufficient to make a certain diagnosis: onchodermatitis,

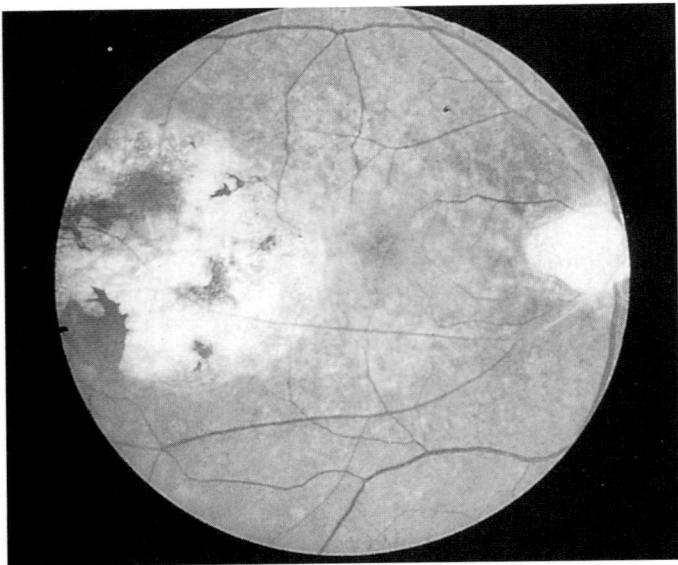

Figure 18.20: Choroidoretinal atrophy and optic nerve atrophy after onchocerciasis. (Photo: Ian Murdoch.)

signs of scratching, depigmentation of the skin, 'lizard' skin and subcutaneous nodules. Further, the eye changes and the presence of microfilariae in the anterior chamber may confirm the diagnosis.

The skin snip
A small piece of superficial skin may be removed, often from the region of the iliac crest or from the shoulder, using a sterile needle with a razor blade. Alternatively, a purpose-designed skin punch may remove the superficial skin. The tiny piece of skin is placed on a dry microscope slide and a drop of saline is added. After at least 30 minutes, and if possible sometime later, the skin and saline are visualized through the microscope. Mobile microfilariae can be seen moving in the fluid when using 40× magnification. However, the skin snip is used less often now because of the risk of spreading hepatitis B and HIV/AIDS.

Control
Onchocerciasis control can be effected in four ways:

1. By inhibiting the development of the *Simulium* flies:
    (a) Vector control to stop breeding.
    (b) Removal of obstacles which cause white, turbulent water. This may include removing rocks or even structures made by man.
2. By reducing the number of bites by the *Simulium* fly on man:
    (a) Wearing clothing which covers most of the skin surface.
    (b) Communities removing from sites near to the breeding areas of the *Simulium* fly.
3. By killing the microfilariae: chemotherapy with microfilaricides.
4. By killing the adult worms:
    (a) Removal of the subcutaneous nodules (nodulectomy).
    (b) Chemotherapy with macrofilaricides.

Vector control
Vector control involves spraying larvicides to kill the larvae of the *Simulium* fly and this has been most effectively carried out in West Africa by the huge Onchocerciasis Control Project (OCP). The OCP has organized this programme in 11 countries of West Africa, with vector control and more recently ivermectin distribution.

There has been a significant expansion of onchocerciasis control activities due to the combined efforts of WHO and other UN agencies, together with the World Bank and non-governmental development organizations. Three regional programmes have been established, one in Central and Latin America, the Onchocerciasis Control Programme of the Americas (OEPA), and two in Africa, the OCP as described above, and the African Programme for Onchocerciasis Control (APOC).[20,21]

Nodulectomy
Removal of the coiled mass of adult worms within the fibrous nodule which forms the subcutaneous lump, often

in the region of the head, is thought to be beneficial, particularly where nodules are situated near to the eyes. The rationale for this procedure is that it will reduce the number of microfilariae which are produced.

Macrofilaricides

In the past suramin has been used, given in weekly intravenous injections. However, suramin is toxic and can cause serious systemic and ocular reactions. It is not routinely recommended.

A new macrofilaricide is being field tested at the present time. Moxidectin is presently only available in veterinary preparations but plans are underway to start clinical trials in humans.

Microfilaricides

Formerly, the established treatment by the oral route used diethylcarbamizine which kills microfilariae. However, diethylcarbamazine can also produce a severe systemic and ocular reaction with intense itching, a rash with skin eruption, fever, headache and joint pains. This is described as the Mazzotti reaction. The effective killing of microfilariae within the eye, while ultimately producing systemic benefit, could result in further ocular damage and loss of sight. Diethylcarbamazine is no longer routinely used.

Ivermectin ('Mectizan')

Ivermectin kills the microfilariae of the worm O. volvulus but typically with only mild reactions, unlike diethylcarbamizine. Of particular significance is the knowledge that ocular damage does not routinely occur. Ivermectin has made an enormous impact in the treatment of onchocerciasis and brings hope for eradication of the disease by the year 2010.

Ivermectin has the following advantages:

- It kills microfilariae.
- It has been shown to prevent blindness due to optic nerve disease by 50%.
- The production of microfilariae by the adult female worm is inhibited for some months.
- The tablet or tablets need only to be taken every 6–12 months.
- There is usually no severe ocular reaction.
- The oral route provides easy delivery of the drug.
- Ivermectin has been donated free of any charge by Merck & Co.

The main logistical problem in treating populations with ivermectin is the provision of resource personnel and facilities to distribute the drug to communities in need.

The most recent strategy for the distribution of ivermectin is described as community-directed treatment with ivermectin (CDTI). This involves affected communities themselves in the planning, implementation and monitoring of treatment activities. CDTI is the recognized and official method used throughout Africa by both OCP and APOC.[21]

The drug is given every 6–12 months by mouth. The dose is 150 µg per kg by weight. It should not be given to the following groups of patients:

- Children under 5 years old or weighing less than 15 kg or less than 90 cm in height.
- Women who are pregnant.
- Women who are breast-feeding a child under 1 week old.
- Patients who are severely ill.

Ivermetin should be used with extreme caution in areas co-endemic with *Loa loa*.

Side effects of ivermectin include mild itching, fever, rash, headache, oedema, lymphadenopathy, myalgia and generalized body aches. More severe reactions, which are uncommon, include hypotension, asthma attacks in known asthmatics and bullous skin lesions after 1–2 weeks (Table 18.11). Most reactions occur within the first 2 or 3 days. Aspirin or an antihistamine may be given.

Age-related macular disease

Age-related macular disease (AMD) is a common cause of bilateral blindness in the industrialized world (Figure 18.21). As the name suggests the main risk factor is age—the condition becomes more common with advancing years. By definition, the patient with bilateral AMD may be registered as blind, but the great reassurance that may be given to the patient who has these changes affecting the central retina is that 'total' blindness will not occur. The patient will be able to see to move around, because peripheral vision is retained, although central vision can be severely affected.

Epidemiology

Age-related macular disease accounts for about 50% of registered blindness in England and Wales.

There is good evidence of a genetic predisposition to AMD from twin and sibling studies, presumably in the presence of appropriate environmental influences.

In non-Caucasians there is evidence that AMD has become more common, for example, in Japan, at least in urban communities. In other parts of eastern Asia and amongst the elderly Inuit in Greenland, AMD has become more in evidence.[22]

Table 18.11 Adverse reactions to ivermection ('Mectizan') therapy.

Mild	Severe
Pruritus	Hypotension
Fever	Asthma attacks (in known
Rash	patients)
Headache	Bullous skin lesions (afer 1–2
Oedema	weeks)
Lymphadenopathy	
Myalgia	
Generalized body aches	

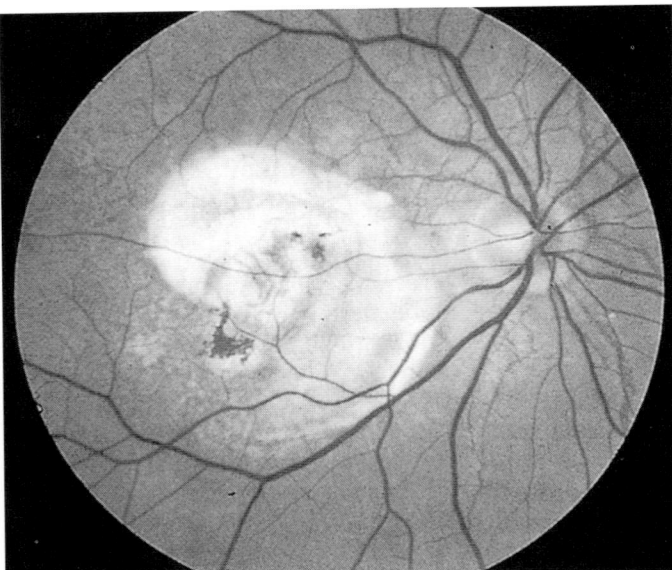

Figure 18.21: Age-related macular degeneration. (Photo: Gordon Johnson.)

AMD occurs more often in Caucasians, in females, where there is a family history of the eye disease, and is associated with cigarette smoking.

Clinical appearance and treatment

AMD is a degenerative disorder of the central retina. In the early stages there are drusen, pigmentary changes and degeneration of the retinal pigment epithelium. Later, there is atrophy of the photoreceptors and the retinal pigment epithelium (geographic atrophy or dry form) and/or choroidal neovascularization (CNV or wet form), which may result in a typical disciform scar. Choroidal neovascularization can be treated with focal laser photocoagulation. Present techniques and treatment with the laser may not have the major impact on blindness that was originally hoped. Less than 20% of the macular lesions present are suitable for laser treatment. The subretinal neovascular membrane which may form must be extrafoveal for the applications of laser burns to be possible.

Prevention

Dietary supplements with antioxidants have some promise of benefit in preventing the development of new vessels at the macula. These have been given with or without zinc supplementation. Further, low-intensity laser treatment to eyes with large diffuse drusen, in the prevention of choroidal neovascularization, have shown some delay in loss of vision in treated eyes. In general, however, age-related maculopathy is a bilateral and progressive eye disease. Low vision aids may benefit these patients.

Leprosy and the eye

Epidemiology

At the beginning of 2000, active disease in 640 000 leprosy patients was being treated with multidrug therapy (MDT) worldwide. Around 680 000 newly detected patients were registered in 1999. More than 10 million previous leprosy patients had been released from treatment (RFT). It is estimated that around 100 000 leprosy patients are blind due to the disease. It should be recognized that many thousands of leprosy patients, who may be receiving little medical advice and care, are blind due to non-leprosy-associated eye disease.[23]

Clinical presentation

Leprosy is a chronic bacterial disease caused by *Mycobacterium leprae*, which is an acid-fast bacillus of low-grade infectivity, and a preference for cooler temperatures. Thus, the slightly cooler anterior segment of the eye is particularly affected by the presence of the organism.

Subdivisions of clinical leprosy

The clinical picture of leprosy is determined by the immune response of the individual.

If the immune response is high, the corresponding bacterial count will be low, and so-called paucibacillary (PB) leprosy will develop. PB leprosy is divided into PB single-lesion leprosy (one skin lesion) and PB two to five lesions leprosy (two to five skin lesions).

If the cellular immune response is low, the corresponding bacterial count will be high, and so-called multibacillary (MB) leprosy will develop (more than five skin lesions).

Type of leprosy:

- PB leprosy: single skin lesion.
- PB leprosy: two to five skin lesions.
- MB leprosy: more than five skin lesions.

MB leprosy patients may spread the disease. PB leprosy patients do not spread the disease.

The type of leprosy is important for both the treatment regimens and the type and patterns of systemic complications which may occur.

Multidrug therapy for leprosy

Adults: PB leprosy (single skin lesion):

- Rifampicin 600 mg as a single dose.
- Ofloxacin 400 mg as a single dose.
- Minocycline 100 mg as a single dose.

PB leprosy (two to five skin lesions):

- DDS (dapsone) 100 mg unsupervised once daily.
- Rifampicin, 600 mg supervised, once per month, six doses to be completed in a maximum of 9 months.

MB leprosy:

- DDS (dapsone) 100 mg and clofazimine (lamprene) 50 mg, unsupervised once daily.

- Rifampicin 600 mg with clofazimine 300 mg, supervised, once per month, 12 doses to be completed in a maximum of 18 months.

  Children: Should receive adjusted doses.

  Two mechanisms are responsible for nerve damage and various disabilities in leprosy. These are described as Type I and Type II reactions.

Type I reaction (reversal reaction)

(Table 18.12)[24]

A Type I reaction occurs as a result of a sudden increase in cellular immunity (paucibacillary leprosy patients).

Acute redness and thickening in the skin and certain peripheral nerves can cause both motor and sensory nerve loss. Involvement of both the fifth and seventh cranial nerves can result in corneal hypoaesthesia (fifth nerve) and lagophthalmos (seventh nerve), where the patient is unable to close the eyelids. The facial skin patch which occurs may be red and raised (in reaction)— or be paler than the surrounding skin.

Eye complications associated with a Type I reaction

Lagophthalmos (seventh cranial nerve)
Lagophthalmos is the most common eye complication found in leprosy and may be associated with all forms of the disease (Figure 18.22). However, lagophthalmos and corneal hypoaesthesia are the expected complications found in association with a Type I reaction. Lagophthalmos is diagnosed when there is inability to close the eyelids, which can be found with both gentle and attempted forced closure of the eyelids.

Corneal hypoaesthesia (fifth cranial nerve)
Corneal hypoaesthesia may occur in association with lagophthalmos, and the combined effect of inadequate lid closure and corneal insensitivity provides considerable danger to the eye through exposure and the effects of minor (or more severe) trauma.

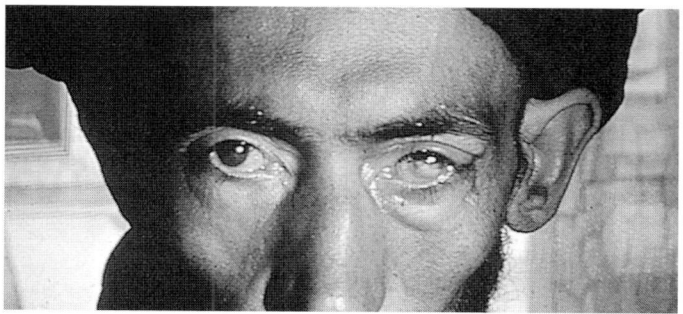

Figure 18.22: Bilateral facial paralysis due to leprosy. Temporal tarsorrhaphies have been carried out, but the left eye has severe corneal ulceration. (Photo: John D. C. Anderson.)

Treatment of eye complications associated with Type I reaction

1. Treatment of an acute Type I reaction requires systemic corticosteroids for 4–6 months (e.g., prednisolone 30 mg per day decreasing over 6 months).
2. Treatment of lagophthalmos and corneal hypoaesthesia is recorded in Table 18.13. The patient must be taught to 'think blink'—that is, the regular and deliberate blinking of both eyes many times each day.
3. Protective spectacles may be worn during the day.
4. Any possibility of exposure, particularly involving the cornea, requires an antibiotic eye ointment as a protective measure at night.
5. A tarsorrhaphy, often a lateral tarsorrhaphy, where the upper and lower eyelids are permanently sutured together, must be considered. Other surgical methods which are used include correction of ectropion (the lower eyelid turning out and drooping).

Type II reaction (erythema nodusum leprosum: ENL) (Table 18.12)[24]

ENL reactions occur only in multibacillary leprosy patients and are due to antigen–antibody reactions.

Table 18.12 Eye complications in leprosy, related to classification* (after ref. 24).

Cause of complications	Complications	Paucibacillary	Multibacillary
Type I reaction	Lagophthalmos	+	+
	Corneal hypoaesthesia	+	+
Type II reaction	Acute iritis	–	+
	Scleritis	–	+
	Chronic iritis	–	+
Bacilli in high numbers	Madarosis	–	+
	Blepharochalasis	–	+
	Blocked lacrimal sac	–	+
	Limbal leproma	–	+
	Leprous keratitis	–	+
	Iris pearls	–	+
	Neuroparalytic iritis	–	+
	Iris atrophy	–	+

*Exceptions may occur due to variations in the grading of patients.

Table 18.13 Treatment of lagophthalmos (after ref. 24).

Duration	Treatment
<6 months	Prednisolone (30 mg/day), decreasing over 6 months Blinking exercises Protective spectacles
>6 months No exposure keratitis Normal corneal sensation With exposure keratitis/ectropion and /or corneal sensation reduced	Eye health education Protective spectacles and other protective measures 'Think-blink habit' Permanent tarsorrhaphy Ectropion surgical correction

The clinical presentation of a Type II reaction typically has fever, subcutaneous nodules, swelling of nerves and inflammatory foci. A Type II reaction affecting the eye can cause acute iridocyclitis, episcleritis and scleritis. Massive infiltration with *M. leprae* can cause secondary atrophy of the involved tissues leading to madarosis, collapse of the nose and thin ear lobes.

Eye complications associated with a Type II reaction
Acute iridocyclitis
Treatment of acute iridocyclitis is similar to treatment of this inflammation due to many other causes. Atropine sulfate 1% eye drops together with corticosteroid eye drops should be given. Systemic corticosteroids should not be required.

Episcleritis and scleritis
An episcleritis will respond quickly to topical cortico-steroids. The deeper inflammation of scleritis, particularly severe bilateral scleritis, which is often associated with an anterior iridocyclitis (anterior uveitis), is a well-recognized complication of severe Type II reactions. Topical treatment should be given as described above, with atropine sulfate 1% and corticosteroids, but short courses of systemic corticosteroids—together with clofazimine—will be required. There is always the danger of scleral staphyloma formation (bulging of the inflamed sclera with adherent choroid and ciliary body behind), sometimes associated with scleral thinning.

Chronic iridocyclitis
This less acute form of iridocyclitis presents with some haziness of the aqueous fluid within the anterior chamber of the eye due to the presence of cells and protein (Figure 18.23). While posterior synechiae formation (adherence of the pupil margin to the anterior lens face) is not common, the pupils may become small (miosis) and resist dilatation with mydriatics. Keratic precipitates may be found on the corneal endothelium. These are foci of cells adherent to the back of the cornea. In treating chronic iridocyclitis, attempt to keep the pupil as dilated and active as possible using phenylephrine 2.5–5% eye drops.

Other eye signs
Thus far we have discussed the eye complications of

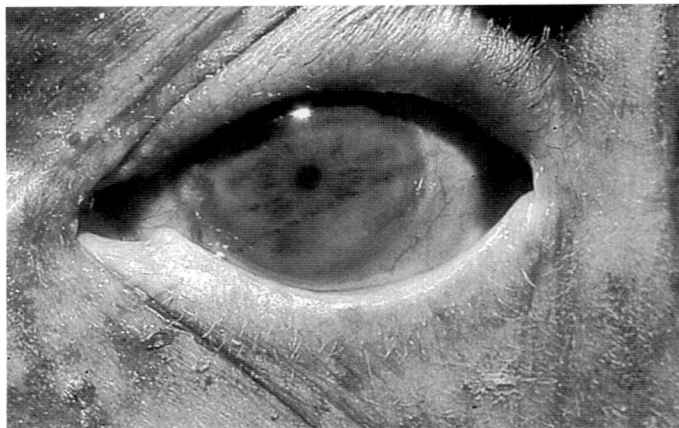

Figure 18.23: Chronic iridocyclitis in leprosy. (Photo: Hans Limburg.)

leprosy which can result in visual loss and blindness. We shall now look briefly at other features which present clinically and can confirm the diagnosis of systemic leprosy with eye complications.

Madarosis
There is loss of eyebrow hair which may be associated with loss of eyelashes. A hair-bearing skin graft may be used to provide a 'new' eyebrow. Alternatively a dark pencil may be used.

Blepharochalasis
Excessive folds of the skin of the upper eyelid can occur after inflammatory reactions deep to the eyelid skin have disappeared. The treatment is surgical.

Lacrimal duct obstruction
This usually results in excessive watering of the affected eye (epiphora) and may occur following inflammation of the nasal mucosa and sometimes collapse of the nasal cartilage. Removal of the tear sac (dacryocystectomy) may be required.

Limbal leproma
A painless pinkish or yellowish nodule may present at the corneoscleral margin (limbus). This should resolve slowly with supervised multiple systemic drug treatment.

Leprous keratitis

Corneal deposits which are chalk-like in appearance may occur, often in both eyes and at the upper aspect or outer quadrant of the cornea. These usually do not affect visual acuity and are evidence of corneal invasion by *M. leprae*.

Iris atrophy

In long-standing multibacillary leprosy the iris stroma may become thin and atrophic, with the dilator muscle of the iris affected. The result is that the pupils become miotic and 'pin-point' in appearance. Irregular atrophy of the iris may result in pupil distortion.

Iris pearls

Small white nodules may appear on the surface of the iris. These are pathognomonic for leprosy and are formed by calcified foci of dead leprosy bacillae.

Age-related cataract in leprosy patients

Age-related (senile) cataract is a most important cause of blindness amongst leprosy patients. Often these patients do not receive the attention given to others with age-related cataract who do not have leprosy. It is a sensible precaution to require that a patient has had 6 months of systemic antileprosy treatment, without any recognized reaction, prior to intraocular surgery. Where intraocular lens implant surgery is available this is to be recommended for the patient who has had treatment for leprosy.

Leprosy and the intraocular pressure

Raised intraocular pressure may occur in association with iridocyclitis. However, the intraocular pressure is often slightly lower than average (ocular hypotension) where atrophy of the ciliary body has occurred.

Summary: examination of the eyes in leprosy and eye health education

In examining the patient with leprosy take particular note of the following:[23,25]

- Visual acuity of each eye.
- Lagophthalmos.
- Red eye.
- Facial skin patch.
- Cataract.

1. Record the visual acuity in each eye. Where visual acuity is reduced below 6/12 in either eye, refer to the eye specialist.
2. Note if the patient blinks regularly. Ask the patient to gently close the eyes. If necessary, ask the patient to close the eyelids forcibly. Record any evidence of lagophthalmos. If there is evidence of a lid-gap > 5 mm the patient should certainly be referred for surgery.
3. The patient with lagophthalmos or corneal hypoaesthesia should be taught to think-blink—many times each day. This patient requires referral to the eye surgeon.
4. Note any redness of either eye. Any patient who has a red eye should be referred to the eye specialist.

5. Test the corneal sensation with a fine tip of 'rolled' cotton wool.
6. Examine, with magnification, the anterior chamber of the eye for evidence of any haziness suggesting circulating cells and proteins.
7. Note any evidence of a grey-white pupil which can suggest the presence of cataract.
8. Dilate the pupil with a short-acting mydriatic (e.g., cyclopentolate 1% eye drops). The pupil's response to the mydriatic, together with evidence of haziness of the aqueous fluid behind the cornea, may suggest acute or chronic iridocyclitis. Evidence of posterior synechiae or a miotic pupil which fails to dilate will indicate the presence of active or previous iridocyclitis.
9. It should be confirmed with each patient that they are on the correct systemic treatment for their leprosy.

Leprosy programmes are becoming integrated[23,25]

Because there has been success in reducing the prevalence of leprosy, this has resulted in specialized leprosy programmes being closed and some leprosy workers moving on to other employment. In India, Tamil Nadu is the first state where leprosy control has become fully integrated into the general health services and other states and countries are following this example. There is a danger in this in that new cases will be missed and disabilities in leprosy patients will not receive good and proper care. This, therefore, means that the guidelines and responsibilities of general health workers must be clarified and appropriate training instituted.

Close collaboration between former leprosy control and prevention of blindness programmes will be required, at national, regional and local levels.

Suppurative keratitis

Suppurative corneal ulceration, due to either bacteria or fungi, is a common and often difficult problem in many countries (Figure 18.24). The cornea has been described as the 'battleground for sight', and central ulceration, when healing does occur, will usually leave a central corneal scar with marked reduction of vision. The clinical treatment of this problem can often be made difficult by lack of antibiotics and particularly antifungal agents.

Damage to the corneal epithelium alone, without corneal stromal involvement, can result in healing without scarring. However, damaged epithelium may allow entry of a variety of organisms, with consequent deep ulceration and later scarring. Further, if the infection penetrates within the eye, pus cells may accumulate and settle at the lower aspect of the anterior chamber (hypopyon), and more severe involvement can result in endophthalmitis with irreversible damage and eventual shrinkage of the eyeball (phthisis).

Many organisms may cause suppurative keratitis. Bacterial keratitis can often be caused by *Streptococcus*

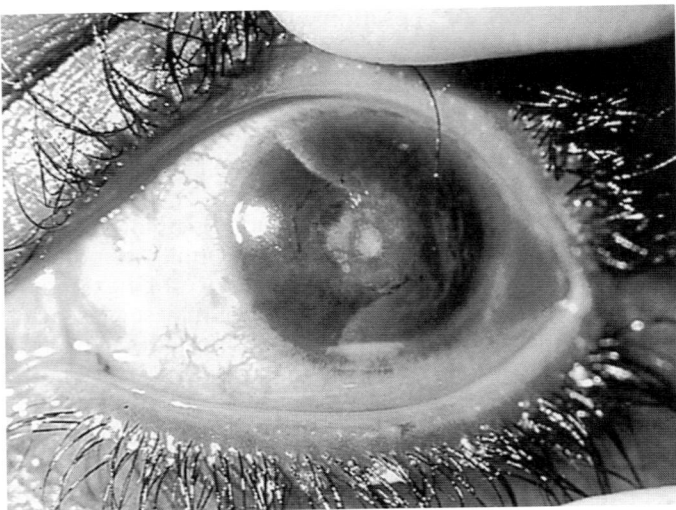

Figure 18.24: Corneal ulceration with hypopyon formation. (Photo: Allen Foster.)

pneumoniae, Pseudomonas species and *Staphylococcus aureus*. Fungi which may cause a suppurative keratitis most commonly are *Aspergillus, Fusarium* and *Candida albicans*. Fungi are often found in humid tropical areas such as coastal West Africa and South-East Asia. Agricultural accidents and injuries with vegetable matter predispose to fungal infection.

Clinical appearance

It is not possible, clinically, to be certain whether a corneal ulcer is due to bacterial or fungal infection. However, a demarcated or multifocal ulceration with central and satellite foci may suggest infection due to a fungus.

Laboratory diagnosis

Gram staining and microscope examination are possible within half an hour. The procedure for obtaining and examining material from a corneal scrape is shown in Table 18.14.[26] This procedure will demonstrate the presence of bacteria or fungi. Bacteria will be shown as Gram positive or Gram negative, as rods or cocci, under a 100× oil emersion objective. Fungal hyphae are seen under a 40× objective.

Management

The treatment of suppurative keratitis/corneal ulceration is urgent. Initial treatment may be given according to Gram stain results. Treatment can be changed if culture and sensitivity tests are available, although at least 24 hours will be required to obtain results.

Different regimens of treatment are given in Tables 18.15 and 18.16.[26]

Gentamicin should be used where the infection is recognized as due to *Pseudomonas* species. Many strains of *Neisseria gonorrhoea* and *Staph. aureus* are resistant to penicillin G.

Ciprofloxacin has very good activity against all Gram-negative organisms, including *Pseudomonas*. It also has good activity against many Gram-positive species and is an acceptable treatment to use initially.

Topical treatment may be supplemented with subconjunctival injections. Examples are gentamicin 40 mg or penicillin G 500 000 units.

Natamycin and econazole are the antifungals of choice. Natamycin, however, penetrates the cornea poorly, while econazole is more irritant to the corneal epithelium. Amphotericin B may be tried, but it is toxic to the cornea.

Table 18.14 Materials and procedure for a corneal scrape (after ref. 26).

Material
Topical anaesthetic (ideally preservative-free if culture is to be performed)
Scalpel blades, needles or platinum spatula
Alcohol or gas burner
Matches or lighter
Clean glass microscope slides (labelled)
Wax or diamond marker
Culture media (labelled)

Procedure
Put nothing in the eye except anaesthetic until the specimen is taken
Explain the procedure to the patient
Children require sedation
Apply topical anaesthetic if required
Use sterile, cooled blade or needle to sample representative areas of ulcer (a spirit lamp may be used for sterilization)
Avoid touching lids and lashes
Use each scrape to prepare one smear or culture
Spread material thinly on to microscope slides
Resterilize and cool instrument between scrapes
Fix slides for microscopy with gentle heat (or alcohol)
Label slides and cultures with name and date

Table 18.15 Topical treatment of suppurative keratitis according to results of Gram stain.

	Ideal circumstances	Practical alternatives
Gram-positive cocci	Cefuroxime 50 mg/ml *or* Ciprofloxacin 0.3%	Gentamicin 14 mg/ml *or* Chloramphenicol 0.5% *or* Enriched tetracycline 1% (with polymyxin)
Gram-negative rods	Ciprofloxacin 0.3% *or* Gentamicin 14 mg/ml	Gentamicin 14 mg/ml *or* Chloramphenicol 0.5% *or* Enriched tetracycline 1% (with polymyxin)
Gram-negative cocci	Ciprofloxacin 0.3% *or* Cefuroxime 50 mg/ml	Enriched tetracycline 1% (with polymyxin)
Fungal elements	Econazole 1% *or* Natamycin 5%	

Table 18.16 Treatment of suppurative keratitis of unknown aetiology.

Ciprofloxacin 0.3% drops
or
Gentamicin drops (14 mg/ml) + cefuroxime drops (50 mg/ml)
or
Gentamicin drops (14 mg/ml) + chloramphenicol drops 0.5%
or
Gentamicin drops (14 mg/ml) + enriched tetracycline 1%

If there is no response to therapy in 48 hours then an antifungal should be added:
Econazole 1% drops or natamycin 5%

Flucytosine is active against *Candida albicans* but should be used in conjunction with an imidazole to prevent acquired resistance.

Antifungal eye drops are preparations of ketaconozale 2%, natamycin 5%, fluconazole 3 mg/ml and clotrimazole 1% and these have become available in India and Bangladesh where they are under assessment.

Any eye with corneal ulceration should also be given a mydriatic/cycloplegic, such as atropine sulfate 1%, used at least once daily.

If the corneal ulceration heals with central scarring, a penetrating keratoplasty (corneal graft) may be considered.

Eye injuries

In many countries of the world, trauma results in a great deal of eye pathology and human distress. Mine blasts often cause damage to limbs and eyes, in many cases involving young people and children.

Injuries to the eye may be superficial or deep. They may be due to penetrating injury or blunt injury. Burns, which may be chemical or due to excessive heat, may affect one or both eyes.

Corneal abrasion

Superficial injury to the cornea can have many causes. It may be due to the scraping of the nail of a child against the mother's cornea, catching the eye on a twig, or injury with a contact lens. If the corneal epithelium only is involved, this can heal without any scarring.

Management

Instil antibiotic drops or ointment for at least 5 days. Give a mydriatic/cycloplegic drop, e.g., cyclopentolate 1% once. Pad and bandage the eye with the eyelid carefully closed, until the epithelium heals, but at least for 24 hours. If vegetable matter is involved in causing the injury, remember the possibility of fungal infection complicating the injury.

Superficial retained foreign body

A great variety of foreign bodies may cause superficial injury. These are often metallic but may also be stone, wood, an eyelash, etc. The foreign body may be situated on the tarsal conjunctiva and be revealed by everting the eyelid.

Management

Instil local anaesthetic drops, e.g., amethocaine 1% or benoxinate 0.4%. Remove the foreign body with a cotton-wool bud or a sterile hypodermic needle. If the foreign body is metallic, there may be some surrounding rust present. Do not be energetic in removing this as the central cornea is only about 0.5 mm in depth. Give antibiotic drops or ointment for at least 5 days. Give a mydriatic/cycloplegic drop, e.g., cyclopentolate 1% once. Pad and bandage for at least 24 hours.

Penetrating injuries

A penetrating injury may be due to a retained intraocular foreign body or any sharp object, such as a thorn, which penetrates the eye.

The evidence of injury may not, at first sight, be obvious. In some instances only careful examination will reveal the track of a retained intraocular foreign body. Very occasionally the patient may be quite unaware that a foreign body has entered the eye.

Clinical examination

There is no substitute for careful examination of the disturbed eye, using magnification. A retained foreign body which is radio-opaque should be shown on X-ray. However, the localization of a foreign body prior to surgery requires exact localizing methods.

Management

Where a penetrating injury is evident, or suspected, the patient should be given antibiotic cover, both topically and systemically, and referred to the eye specialist. The damaged eye should be protected with a shield, either a Cartella shield or an improvised shield using radiographic film.

Blunt injury

A blunt injury, or non-penetrating injury, can cause considerable damage to an eye. Injuries may be caused by objects such as a stone or a fist.

It is good clinical practice to examine the eye from the front through to the back of the eye, beginning, however, with the periorbital region and eyelids. Fractures may occur at the orbital margin and the bony floor of the orbit may fracture (a blow-out fracture), which may result in adherence of the inferior extraocular muscles. Bruising may occur affecting the eyelids and the conjunctiva and there may be bleeding into the anterior chamber of the eye (hyphaema). The cornea can be damaged, resulting in oedema. Intraocular tissues may be torn, such as a tear of the root of the iris (iridodialysis). A cataract may form. The lens itself may be dislocated. Bleeding in the posterior segment of the eye may result in vitreous haemorrhage and there can be isolated or associated retinal haemorrhages. Retinal oedema may be apparent on ophthalmoscopy.

Management

In most instances the correct treatment of a blunt injury is rest until the condition resolves. Should there be a total or near total hyphaema in the anterior chamber of the eye, the intraocular pressure must be carefully monitored. A pressure rise in the presence of a hyphaema may result in blood elements entering the corneal stroma, with consequent corneal blood staining. Any suggestion of a rise in intraocular pressure in the presence of a large hyphaema is a clear indication for a paracentesis, with release of the blood from the anterior chamber.

As rest is indicated in these patients, it will not be sensible to ask a patient to travel any distance, perhaps over uneven roads, for further assessment. It is advisable to provide topical antibiotic eye drops and possibly a systemic antibiotic. A mydriatic/cycloplegic such as cyclopentolate 1% may be given. In the presence of bleeding from the iris, movement of the iris should be avoided. Any moderate intraocular pressure rise can be controlled by oral acetazolamide.

Burns of the eye

Burns of the eye may be due to chemicals or fire. In the case of chemical injury, both acid or alkali may be involved, with alkali burns generally being more serious.

Management

Where a burn of the eye(s) has occurred, *immediately* begin thorough irrigation of the eye(s) with water. Keep washing, even for 15–20 minutes, until you feel all the substance which has caused the burn has been washed out. Remember to irrigate under the eyelids as well. Any fragments of chemical or ash, or other material, may be picked off with plain forceps. Antibiotic drops and ointment should be applied frequently, at least hourly, during the first day or two. Eyelids should be kept mobile with deliberate movement of the lids a number of times each day. If there is any question of possible permanent damage, such as corneal haze or adhesions between the eyelids and the eyeball, the patient should be urgently referred to the eye specialist.

Snake venom conjunctivitis

In regions of the world where the spitting cobra is found snake venom can cause a conjunctivitis.

Solar burn (eclipse retinopathy)

Our natural precaution is to avoid the direct glare of the sun's rays, but in certain situations this does not happen. An eclipse of the sun should only be viewed, if at all, with appropriate and adequate filters, otherwise a macular burn will follow because sunlight will focus on the retina.

In at least one central Asian country, children play a 'game', competing with each other to see who can gaze longest at the sun! A macular burn may occur resulting in a permanent central scotoma.

Caterpillar hair conjunctivitis (ophthalmia nodosum)

The conjunctival reaction to an unusual foreign body, a caterpillar hair, is recognized as an entity in ophthalmology, described as *ophthalmia nodosum*. A granuloma or granulomas may form around each caterpillar hair. Treatment requires removal of the hair, otherwise deeper invasion may occur.

Landmine injuries

Antipersonnel landmines (APLs) inflict horrendous injuries and so often kill or maim civilians who have no or very little part in any conflict. In the 10 years up until 1997, the hospitals of the International Committee of the Red Cross (ICRC) had treated about 15 000 mine-injured patients, many of them in Cambodia and Afghanistan. Afghanistan is said to have 8–10 million unmarked mines. The problem is repeated in Cambodia, Angola, Mozambique, Kurdistan and northern Somalia. It is also present in Rwanda, Bosnia, Laos and El Salvador and more than 50 other countries. One estimate gives a figure of more than 100 million mines laid worldwide.[27]

Writing in the *Journal of Community Eye Health*, Heather Jackson described 29 patients with ocular trauma due to APLs who presented to a hospital eye department in northwest Cambodia during 9 months of 1994.[28] Fourteen of these patients were bilaterally blind. Clare Gilbert described a blind school in Tirana, Albania, where nine of the children (24% of the pupils) had previously had injuries when playing with landmines.[29]

Each mine may cost around five dollars and, with current techniques of mine clearance, about US $1000 to remove.

Climatic droplet keratopathy

Climatic droplet keratopathy is a degenerative condition in which translucent droplets accumulate in the superficial stroma of the cornea (Figure 18.25). It has been described in many countries and regions[30] including Eritrea, southern Africa, India, New Guinea, Australia, Labrador, Greenland, Iceland, Somalia and Mongolia.

It is considered that high exposure to ultraviolet sunlight is the main aetiological factor in the pathogenesis of this corneal disease, which can cause significant visual impairment.

Treatment, where necessary, can involve sector iridectomy, debridement (scraping) of the central cornea, lamellar or penetrating keratoplasty and more recently ablation by excimer laser.

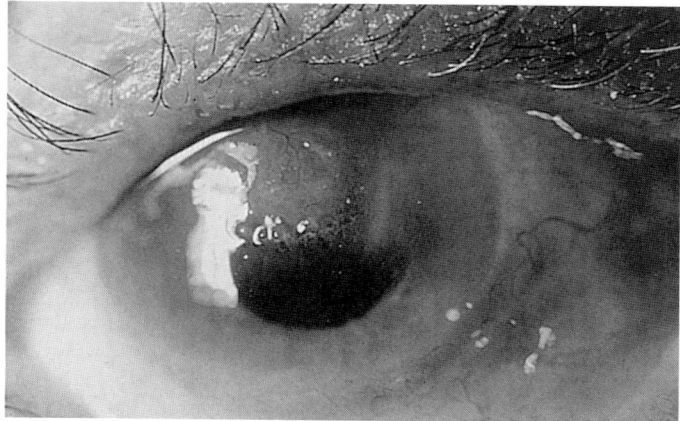

Figure 18.25: Climatic droplet keratopathy. (Photo: Gordon Johnson.)

Toxins and the optic nerve

In patients with nutritional deficiency, particularly of the vitamin B complex, the optic nerve is susceptible to toxic damage.

Tobacco smoking in excess, often with considerable *alcohol* consumption and relatively poor nutrition, can result in a toxic optic neuropathy. Pipe smokers have long been recognized to be at risk of this condition. Methyl alcohol is sometimes drunk with disastrous effects, including optic neuropathy and subsequent blindness. The author was called to examine a senior official in an Asian country because of the possibility of eye damage after drinking methyl alcohol. The patient did not survive the toxic effects of this bout of drinking.

Cassava is eaten in many tropical countries. Inadequately prepared cassava can cause optic neuropathy and peripheral nerve abnormalities due to cyanide toxicity. Cyanide is found particularly in the roots. Water used for soaking cassava must be discarded, together with any fermenting cassava; then the cassava must be dried before grinding into flour.

Drugs which may cause a toxic optic neuropathy include ethambutol, quinine and isoniazid.

An epidemic of bilateral optic neuropathy has been affecting large numbers of people between 10 and 40 years in Dar es Salaam, Tanzania. The condition has an acute onset with accompanying impairment of colour vision and temporal pallor of the optic discs. There may be associated peripheral neuropathy and sensorineural hearing loss.[31]

The pigment beneath the macula was dispersed and clumped, sometimes forming a small ring. Thus far this eye disease has been noted only in indigenous Africans, but of 35 different tribes. There is as yet no clear evidence as to the cause, although the history and clinical appearance suggest some unidentified toxic agent.

An epidemic of general neuropathy occurred in Cuba during 1992–1994. More than 50 000 cases were reported. Most patients were middle-aged and males were slightly more often affected (3:2). Painful paraesthesiae, mainly in the legs, with ataxia were reported. The number of patients with optic nerve involvement is uncertain, but some estimates suggested nearly 50% of cases. The aetiology is obscure but factors considered are poor nutrition, toxic influences such as tobacco or alcohol, or a virus. Patients did seem to benefit by receiving B complex vitamins and the number of new cases declined dramatically.[32]

Eye disease in children

Although the exact number of blind children in the world is not known, it is estimated that the figure is approximately 1.4 million, with up to 500 000 new cases every year. Approximately 75% of these children live in Africa and Asia.[33] Up to 60% die within 1–2 years after blindness occurs. In many developing countries 70% of blindness in childhood (0–15 years) is due to corneal scarring. Most of these patients with corneal scarring have had acute episodes of vitamin A deficiency, often associated with measles infection. Other causes of corneal scarring include newborn conjunctivitis (ophthalmia neonatorum), herpes simplex keratitis and the use of harmful traditional eye medicines.

In certain countries, rubella infection in mothers during pregnancy can result in the congenital rubella syndrome which, amongst other abnormalities, may result in blinding bilateral cataract. Inherited genetic factors may also result in congenital cataract and retinal dystrophies may cause visual loss. Premature babies are at risk of retinopathy of prematurity.

Major causes and strategies for prevention

The major causes of blindness vary from region to region, and accurate data are difficult to obtain. In industrialized countries blind registers are one source, although these records often lack detail and may not include all children who are blind. Indications of the common causes of blindness in children can be obtained from schools for the blind in developing countries, although this information is likely to be biased for a number of reasons.

Aetiological classification (Table 18.17)

A form developed by the International Centre for Eye Health, London, and accepted by the World Health Organization, is available providing classification of blindness in children, with coding instructions, definitions, description of methods and guidelines.

Table 18.17 Aetiological classification of childhood blindness (after ref. 33).

Factors operating at conception:	• Genetic and chromosomal abnormalities
Intrauterine factors:	• Infections (e.g., rubella), toxins (e.g., alcohol)
Perinatal factors:	• Infections (e.g., ophthalmia neonatorum)
	• Prematurity (e.g., retinopathy of prematurity)
Childhood factors:	• Measles, vitamin A deficiency, use of harmful traditonal eye medicines, trauma, meningitis
Unclassifiable:	• This includes conditions, often present since birth, where the underlying cause is not known and where the abnormality cannot be attributed to genetic disease or intrauterine events

Vitamin A deficiency disorders and the eye

See Chapter 31.

Newborn conjunctivitis (ophthalmia neonatorum)

Newborn conjunctivitis, where infection of the child's eyes occurs during the birth of the child, is a very serious problem in many parts of the developing world. Infection involving the conjunctiva is usually the first evidence, sometimes with purulent discharge, and danger to the cornea with subsequent perforation or scarring and blindness is our first concern.

By definition, newborn conjunctivitis occurs in a child within the first 30 days of life. Two organisms commonly cause newborn conjunctivitis: *Neisseria gonorrhoea* and *Chlamydia trachomatis* (Table 18.18).[34] Between 25% and 50% of infants exposed to *N. gonorrhoea* or *C. trachomatis* during birth develop the corresponding eye infection, if no eye prophylaxis is given.

The World Health Organization has estimated a yearly adult incidence of 62 million cases of gonorrhoea and 89 million of genital chlamydial infection.[2] The prevalence of gonorrhoea amongst antenatal attenders in African countries is disturbingly high, at between 4% and 15%. However, the global incidence of newborn conjunctivitis is not known.

Gonococcal newborn conjunctivitis due to *N. gonorrhoea* typically has a dramatic onset with bilateral purulent conjunctivitis and profuse discharge of pus, associated with tense and swollen eyelids (Figure 18.26). The condition usually presents within the first few days of birth. This is an eye emergency and treatment must be started immediately. For treatment of newborn conjunctivitis due to *N. gonorrhoea*, see Table 18.19.[34]

Newborn conjunctivitis due to *C. trachomatis* is less dramatic in onset, presenting as irritable, red eyes but without purulent discharge unless secondary bacterial

Table 18.18 Causes of newborn conjunctivitis (after ref. 34)

Microbial
Sexually transmitted diseases (STD)
Chlamydia trachomatis
Neisseria gonorrhoeae
Other micro-organisms, often mixed
Haemophilus spp.
Staphylococcus spp.
Streptococcus pneumoniae
Streptococcus group D
Escherichia coli
Pseudomonas spp.
Chemical
Silver nitrate

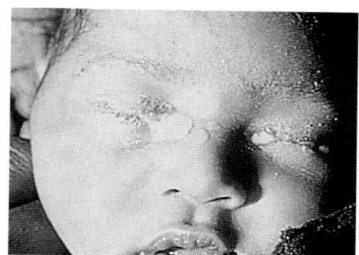

Figure 18.26: Newborn conjunctivitis due to *Neisseria gonorrhoeae*. (Photo: John D. C. Anderson.)

Table 18.19 Management of newborn conjunctivitis (after ref. 34).

Gonococcal
A. Admission to hospital
    Penicillin i.m. or i.v.
    Topical antimicrobial therapy, e.g., tetracycline 1% ointment, intensively at first (hourly) then reducing to three times a day for 14 days

B. *If PPNG* prevalence more than 1%*   Single i.m. injection of cefotaxime 100 mg/kg or kanamycin 25 mg/kg plus tetracycline 1% ointment or erythromycin 0.5% ointment as indicated in (A)
Chlamydial: systemic treatment Erythromycin estolate orally (syrup) 5 mg/kg per day for 14 days
Non-gonococcal, non-chlamydial Tetracycline 1% ointment or erythromycin 0.5% ointment four times a day for 14 days
Treatment of parents

*Penicillinase-producing N. gonorrhoeae.

Table 18.20 Prevention of newborn conjunctivitis (after ref. 34).

Detection and treatment of infected pregnant women Screening of all pregnant women is difficult in most countries and expensive May be possible to screen high-risk groups
Eye prophylaxis in the neonate at birth Mechanical cleaning of the eyelids immediately at birth, plus tetracycline 1% ointment or silver nitrate 1% drops
Treatment of the neonate as an index case Only applicable where: • prevalence of gonococcal infection low • main sexually transmitted disease causing newborn conjunctivitis is *Chlamydia trachomatis* • all infected infants can be detected and treated • facilities exist for diagnosis of *C. trachomatis*

infection occurs. Often the infection presents some days later than with the gonococcal infection. Treatment for newborn conjunctivitis due to *C. trachomatis* is given in Table 18.19.

Spectinomycin may prove equally effective, if available. A single dose of 75 mg kanamycin with topical gentamicin ointment for 7 days may also give good results.

It is important to remember that treatment for these infective conditions should include systemic therapy because the infection is not confined to the eyes alone. Systemic treatment must also be given to both parents. Also, it should be kept in mind that parents of babies with newborn conjunctivitis are at high risk of other sexually transmitted diseases.

Other bacteria which may cause newborn conjunctivitis include *Haemophilus*, *Str. pneumoniae*, *Staphylococcus* and *Pseudomonas*.

Prevention of newborn conjunctivitis requires prophylactic treatment of the newborn child (Table 18.20).[34] The eyelids of both eyes should be carefully swabbed with sterile saline *as soon as each child is born*. A single application of tetracycline 1% eye ointment is given to each eye. Alternatively, silver nitrate 1% eye drops may be used, but the silver nitrate must be well preserved, avoiding any exposure to light or evaporation. Silver nitrate may cause a chemical conjunctivitis.

Retinitis pigmentosa

The hereditary dystrophies of the retina can be sporadic, autosomal recessive, autosomal dominant or X-linked recessive in inheritance. These dystrophies are characterized by progressive loss of photoreceptor and retinal pigment epithelium function.

Symptoms include night blindness (nyctalopia) and gradual loss of vision due to field defects. Dark adaption is affected, a typical ring scotoma is the recognized visual field abnormality, and progressive disease causes characteristic 'bone corpuscle' pigmentary disturbance of the peripheral and equatorial retina. The blood vessels become attenuated and the optic nerve head has a pale appearance. The condition may be associated with a number of other disorders or syndromes. It may also present with atypical forms.

The visual prognosis is variable. Before the age of 20 years, few patients will have a visual acuity of 6/60 or worse. By the age of 50 years most will have poor vision.

There is no specific treatment. Close intermarriage (consanguinity) in many countries increases the risk of this disorder and genetic counselling should be offered to affected families.

Sickle cell disease

Hereditary abnormalities affecting haemoglobin are found almost exclusively in blacks, with red blood cells developing a sickle shape in conditions where low oxygen tension exists. Eye changes include conjunctival vascular abnormalities, focal iris ischaemia, peripheral retinal vascular disturbance with new blood vessel formation, haemorrhages, fibrosis and sometimes a detached retina.

Laser photocoagulation should be used to 'treat' any peripheral retinal neovascularization. Late-stage disease with vitreous haemorrhage may require surgical removal of the vitreous (vitrectomy). Retinal detachment surgery may also be necessary.

Thalassaemia

Also a hereditary disorder of haemoglobin, thalassaemia is found mainly in the Mediterranean region, Middle East, India and South-East Asia.

Congenital cataract

It is important to recognize congenital cataract (present at birth) as early as possible so that treatment can be given, thus avoiding the danger of amblyopia or 'lazy' eye. Many different types of congenital cataract may present, and the cataract can affect the whole lens or only part of the lens.

Congenital cataract may be the result of rubella during the early months of the mother's pregnancy (Figure 18.27). Chickenpox and toxoplasmosis affecting the mother may also cause cataract in the unborn child. Cytomegalovirus and herpes simplex infections may have the same effect. Congenital cataract may be the result of inherited genetic factors so that brothers and sisters may also be born with cataract. Down's syndrome (mongolism), and other recognized syndromes, may be associated with congenital cataract.

Other causes of cataract include metabolic disorders with abnormal biochemical functions, for example, galactosaemia, although this is strictly a newborn (neonatal) cataract which develops in the first few days or weeks of life.

Prevention of congenital cataract can especially be effected by immunization against rubella. Vaccination may be given to all babies in infancy, often together with immunization against mumps and measles. Alternatively, young girls can be vaccinated at puberty.

Treatment of congenital cataract requires surgery. A child with congenital cataract, whether unilateral or bilateral, should be referred to the eye surgeon as soon as the diagnosis is made. The eye surgeon should be an expert in paediatric eye surgery. If both eyes are involved, the surgeon will operate on each eye, as early as possible, with the second operation sometimes within a few days of the first.

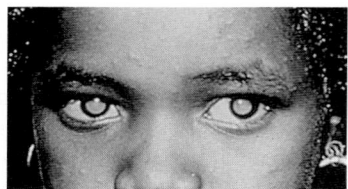

Figure 18.27: Bilateral congenital cataract after rubella infection during the mother's pregnancy. (Photo: John D. C. Anderson.)

In most developing countries the child who has had surgery for bilateral congenital cataract will be provided with aphakic spectacles. Refraction should be carried out every 6 months to maintain accuracy in the lenses provided. Methods which may also be considered are contact lenses (although compliance in the growing child usually proves a considerable problem) and intraocular lens implants (IOLs). IOLs are being used increasingly worldwide—but this surgery must be in specialist surgical hands. An IOL (or possibly contact lens) is necessary where the congenital cataract is unilateral as an aphakic spectacle correction for one eye will cause double vision.

Congenital glaucoma (buphthalmos)

Glaucoma in childhood may be present at birth or can develop during the first few years of life. Increased intraocular pressure in a young child causes the more elastic tissues of the eyeball to stretch and so the eye enlarges. For this reason the description of buphthalmos, or 'ox eye', is used. Congenital glaucoma may be unilateral or bilateral. The unilateral enlarged eye is usually more quickly recognized.

The condition may cause discomfort, with photosensitivity (avoidance of bright light), and reduced vision may also be evident. On examination it may be obvious that the cornea is larger than it should be and in some instances the cornea may be hazy. With examination under anaesthesia, a cupped optic nerve head may be seen.

Treatment requires surgery to allow the aqueous fluid to drain out of the eye. Often persistent congenital remnants in the drainage angle of the anterior chamber of the eye have caused some degree of obstruction to the outflow of aqueous.

Retinopathy of prematurity

There is evidence that retinopathy of prematurity is again becoming a cause of childhood blindness in the USA and Europe. Increasingly sophisticated neonatal care has resulted in the survival of tiny, premature babies who can develop the condition. In moderately developed countries, with improving neonatal care, babies who now survive premature birth are also at risk of retinopathy of prematurity.

Retinopathy of prematurity is a proliferative retinopathy in premature babies with immature retinal blood vessels. There is often a history of exposure to high oxygen concentration. Spasm of the retinal vessels is followed by dilated vessels, new vessel formation, vitreous haemorrhage, vitreous traction, retinal folds and retinal detachment.

Treatment in expert hands, using cryotherapy or laser, can prevent progression of the disease when applied in the early stages.

Clinical trials have shown that 'threshold' stage III 'plus' disease can be prevented from progressing to blinding disease (stages IV and V) in approximately 50% of cases, by prompt and appropriate cryotherapy. Recent results with laser treatment are even better, with advanced disease being prevented in over 90% of babies.[33]

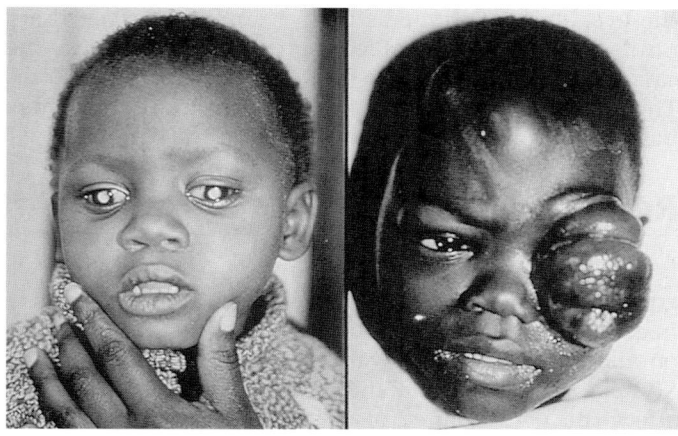

Figure 18.28: Bilateral retinoblastoma (left). Advanced retinoblastoma (right). (Photos: Volker Klauss.)

Retinoblastoma[35]

Retinoblastoma is the most common malignant eye tumour of childhood. The tumour arises in the retinal cells.

Most children in developing countries present for examination and treatment too late, with the tumour far advanced, commonly extraocular and often extraorbital (Figure 18.28). The tumour extends along the optic nerve to the brain. In the later stages, metastases occur to other parts of the body.

Retinoblastoma will usually first be noticed because of the presentation of a white pupil. Tumour tissue in this presentation is situated behind the lens in the eye. Other eye abnormalities which may lead to a discovery of retinoblastoma include a squint, glaucoma, visual loss, a painful red eye and orbital cellulitis. The tumour may present at any time during the first 5 years of life.

In the child a developing retinal cell can lose both of a pair of 'antioncogenes' or tumour-suppressing genes. These are situated on the long arm of chromosome 13. Two-thirds of children with retinoblastoma develop the tumour because of random somatic mutations. These children present with a single, unilateral tumour, typically at a relatively older age than other children with retino-blastoma. If they survive, these children do not pass on a genetic defect to their offspring.

The remaining one-third of children who develop retinoblastoma have lost one of each antioncogene pair in every cell in the body. Either the defect is inherited or this abnormality occurs at the time of conception. A random mutation will then occur affecting the second antioncogene, often in more than one retinal cell. Thus, foci of retinoblastoma are multiple, normally bilateral and occur at a relatively younger age.

Multiple or bilateral tumours can be considered to be genetically determined.

It is most important, following the discovery of a single tumour, that both eyes are examined very carefully. Examinations must continue regularly, every 3–6 months, until at least the age of 5 years.

Adults who have had multiple retinoblastoma, and survived, must be advised that there is a one in two chance of their children being affected.

Occasionally a tumour regresses spontaneously. The parents of a child with retinoblastoma should be examined, together with each of the siblings.

Differential diagnosis

The differential diagnosis of this whitish, raised tumour (when still intraocular) includes infestations such as toxocariasis, retinopathy of prematurity and other causes of a 'white' pupil. Investigations should involve ultra-sonography or computed tomography, if available.

Management

Effective treatment of retinoblastoma is largely dependent on early recognition of the tumour while it is still contained within the eye. The patient must be referred immediately to the specialist. In most eye centres in developing countries the correct treatment requires surgical excision of the eye (enucleation), removing as much of the attached optic nerve as possible. Some specialist centres will be able to provide chemotherapy and radiotherapy for these children. Chemotherapy uses vincristine, carboplatin and etoposide. These may be combined with cyclosporin. Cyclophosphamide and doxorubicin are alternatives in appropriate regimens in experienced hands.

For smaller intraocular tumours, where the tumour does not extend to the ora serrata, or where there is no vitreous seeding, lens-sparing radiotherapy may be used. Focal radiotherapy can use surgically inserted scleral plaques, such as cobalt-60 or iodine-125. Cryotherapy can also be applied directly to a small tumour, and indirect xenon photocoagulation can be placed *around* a tumour less than 5 mm in diameter and situated away from the optic disc. It should be noted that an eye which has the original tumour can often be retained and, after expert treatment for more than one focus of retinoblastoma, the first affected eye may have better vision than the other affected eye.

Harmful (traditional) eye medicines and practices

Many patients will attend the local traditional healer before considering a visit to the health worker trained in what we consider to be standard medical practice. It should be recognized that traditional healing can provide considerable benefit to patients and some centres, for example in India, have a traditional healer at the local health centres. However, some applications to the eyes used by these local healers can cause severe adverse reactions.

The clinical picture which does not provide a clear diagnosis when seen by the health worker may have been confused by the superimposed application of harmful eye medicines into an eye already suffering the original disease. In these situations the history of the eye problem will be important. It should be kept in mind that the patient, or the parent who has brought a child, may be very hesitant to admit that a traditional eye medicine has been used.

A variety of harmful medications may be used: the juice of squeezed plant leaves, lime juice, kerosene, toothpaste and urine (either animal or human). A chemical or caustic keratoconjunctivitis may occur, or infection, such as with *N. gonorrhoea* from human urine. In Zimbabwe, tomato juice may be given for mild conjunctivitis and lemon peel juice for discharging eyes. Powdered herbs can be blown into a diseased eye.[36]

Treatment is often difficult. Topical therapy with an antibiotic three to four times each day, and a mydriatic/cycloplegic such as atropine sulfate 0.5% or 1%, once daily, may be used. The original eye disease, if identified, should be treated accordingly.

The constructive approach of discussion with traditional healers and herbalists has been encouraged in a number of countries. Programmes to develop dialogue and cooperation with traditional healers have been developed in Zimbabwe, Malawi and Nepal where it has been demonstrated that traditional healers can be a positive force in the prevention of blindness. The purpose of these programmes has been to encourage the following:

- Encourage healers to change specific practices that may be harmful and encourage those that are not harmful.
- Improve the ability of healers to recognize and refer patients with cataract.
- Build upon existing respect given to healers by the community.
- Develop programmes in collaboration with healers, using their pre-existing knowledge and skills.
- Maintain interaction between healers and eye care providers, establishing collaborative activities.

Couching

Couching is a common procedure for the treatment of blinding cataract in many countries of the developing world. Indeed, John Sandford-Smith, writing in the *Journal of Community Eye Health*[37] following a visit in Northern Nigeria, said that the method of cataract surgery which had increased in recent years is couching!

Two methods of couching are reported;

1. 'Sharp' method: the eye is perforated and the lens is pushed backwards by a sharp instrument, for example a long thorn.
2. 'Blunt' method: the lens is pushed into the vitreous by massage or by, effectively, blunt injury. In this method the eye is not perforated and it is, therefore, assumed to be safer.

The author had a 'blunt' method described when visiting Sudan in recent years. The traditional healer would place the spent cartridge of a bullet filled with sand or gravel against the patient's closed eye. The end of the cartridge was struck sharply and the 'bolus' of sand or gravel hit the eye. This was done as many times as was necessary until the patient described better vision because the cataractous lens had been dislocated into the vitreous. There was no mention of the other injuries which may have occurred due to blunt injury!

Refractive errors

It is beyond the scope of this chapter to discuss refractive errors in any detail. However, the recognition of refractive needs and the provision of spectacles is vital to most populations during the various stages and ages of life. Myopia, hypermetropia and/or astigmatism can severely affect the performance of a child in school. Successful school screening programmes have been implemented, for example in India. For screening purposes a pin-hole disc can indicate if poor vision is due to a refractive error. Middle and old age brings the need for presbyopic correction—for reading, for sewing, or for picking stones out of rice! Aphakic spectacle corrections are required if intracapsular cataract surgery is carried out.

Further, it has been increasingly appreciated that the provision of low-vision optical aids must be energetically pursued so that patients who are visually impaired can have the opportunity of considerably improved visual capacity.[38]

It is estimated that 2.3 billion people worldwide have refractive errors. The vast majority of these could have their sight restored by spectacles, but only 1.8 billion people have access to eye examinations and affordable correction. Therefore, around 500 million people, mostly in developing countries, remain with uncorrected refractive errors.[39]

The author recalls watching an excellent refraction carried out by an ophthalmic 'tecnico' in Mozambique, admiring the steady hand of the woman who had been given presbyopic lenses, as she carefully threaded a needle. The disappointment was profound when I heard that was the end of the matter—no spectacles were available for her and she probably could not afford them anyway.

According to Brien Holden and colleagues, spectacles should be of good quality, be in ready supply, distributed effectively, have low or no cost and be acceptable to individuals.[39]

The Refractive Error Study in Children (RESC) was designed to assess the prevalence of refractive errors and vision impairment in children (5–15 years of age) of different ethnic origins and cultural settings.

These initiatives are part of the strategy of Vision 2020: The Right to Sight, which includes refractive errors and low vision. This strategy seeks to develop the following:

- Create awareness and demand for refractive services through community-based services/primary eye care and school screening.
- Develop accessible refractive services for individuals identified with significant refractive errors, which will require training and refraction and dispensing.
- Ensure that affordable spectacles are made available for individuals with significant refractive errors.

- Develop and make available low-vision services and optical devices for all those in need, including children in blind schools and integrated education.
- Include comprehensive low-vision care as an integral part of national programmes for the prevention of blindness and rehabilitation services for the visually disabled.

Differential diagnosis of the red eye

Inflammation of the eyelids
Blepharitis
Inflammation of the eyelids is a common complaint which is typically chronic in character. Chronic seborrhoeic blepharitis presents with redness of the lid margins with crusts on and at the base of eyelashes. *Staph. aureus* may be involved. Treatment of this chronic condition can be difficult and the inflammation will often recur. Crusts should be removed with moist cotton wool (warm water) or a 25% solution of baby shampoo. An antibiotic eye ointment should be applied to the lid margins. If there is a severe infective blepharitis a systemic antibiotic, such as tetracycline 250 mg orally, four times daily for 1 week and then twice daily, for 6–12 weeks, may be considered. As tetracycline stains teeth in children under 12 years of age, it should not be given in this age group. Alternatives are doxycycline 100 mg twice daily for 1 week and then once daily, or minocycline 100 mg once daily.

Inflammation of the eyelid skin or eyelid margins may also be due to a virus or be allergic in origin. Viruses associated with this type of inflammation include the common wart, herpes simplex, herpes zoster ophthalmicus and molluscum contagiosum.

Stye (hordeolum)
A localized staphylococcal abscess at or near the base of an eyelash follicle requires treatment with heat and antibiotic eye ointment. A wooden spoon wrapped in cotton wool and a bandage, dipped in boiling water, can then be held close to the eyelid (not against the eyelid), so that the steam can 'bathe' the lesion. Epilation of the eyelash may speed resolution of the infection.

Ectropion and Entropion
Abnormal positions of the eyelids, such as an eyelid which turns out (ectropion) or turns in (entropion), may result in considerable discomfort and inflammation.

Ectropion, which usually involves the lower eyelid, results in exposure of the tarsal conjunctiva. Epiphora (overflow of tears) usually occurs. Ectropion can follow weakness of the orbicularis oculi or facial nerve paralysis. Injury or infection with associated scarring can cause a cicatricial ectropion.

Entropion can commonly affect both upper and lower eyelids. The scarring of trachoma is often associated with upper eyelid entropion. Injuries may cause entropion. In older age, a spastic lower eyelid may turn in, causing considerable irritation due to eyelashes rubbing on the cornea.

Chalazion (meibomian cyst, tarsal cyst, lipogranuloma)
The meibomian glands, which are situated in the tarsal plates of each eyelid, open along the lid margins. Ducts may become blocked, resulting in a retention cyst with ensuing inflammatory reaction. Often a chalazion will require incision. Following local anaesthetic injection beside the cyst and eversion of the eyelid with a chalazion clamp, an incision is made into the cyst vertically, towards the lid margin. The contents of the cyst are curetted out. A topical antibiotic eye ointment is given for some days.

Eyelid tumours
Both basal cell carcinoma and squamous cell carcinoma may result in nodular or ulcerating lesions on the eyelids.

Other eyelid inflammations
Considerable inflammation and scarring of the eyelids may be caused by conditions such as anthrax, actinomycosis, leishmaniasis and yaws.

Orbital cellulitis
Inflammation within the bony orbit of the eye can result in swelling of the eyelids, with proptosis of the eye. Conjunctival chemosis (oedema of the conjunctiva) is usually present. The patient may have a fever and be very unwell.

Complications of acute orbital cellulitis include corneal ulceration, endophthalmitis, septicaemia and cavernous sinus thrombosis.

Treatment is with high doses of a systemic antibiotic. A topical antibiotic eye ointment may be given, mainly to protect the eye.

A characteristic presentation of orbital cellulitis is described with infection by *Loa loa*, also known as Calabar swelling.

Dacryocystitis
Inflammation of the tear sac can result in swelling at the side of the nose near to the inner canthus of the eye. This can progress to an acutely inflamed abscess or may become chronic in nature.

Blockage of the tear ducts, which often occurs in the nasolacrimal duct running from the tear sac to below the inferior turbinate of the nose, may be a precursor of this type of inflammation. Blockage may also occur in the superior or inferior canaliculi and also the common canaliculus, which runs from the inner canthus of the eye into the tear sac.

Treatment is with topical and systemic antibiotics and subsequent syringing of the tear ducts with normal saline. Failure to open the tear ducts by this method will subsequently require surgery. Blockage of the nasolacrimal duct will require a dacryocystorhinostomy.

Inflammation of the conjunctiva and cornea

A large variety of organisms may cause inflammation of the conjunctiva (conjunctivitis) and/or of the cornea (keratitis).

Bacterial or fungal infections typically present with a red eye and discharge. Both bacteria and fungi may cause suppurative conjunctivitis and keratitis. Infection with viruses more usually presents with a red eye and watering, although secondary infection with bacteria is not uncommon, causing subsequent discharge with pus.

Allergic conjunctivitis is characterized by a slightly red eye, extreme itching and watering. This may be associated with conditions such as hay fever.

Vernal keratoconjunctivitis (spring catarrh)

This common disorder, which often affects children and teenagers, has a typical presentation affecting both the tarsal conjunctivae and the limbal region (corneoscleral margin). The eyes are red, irritable and may show strands of mucus. Severe itching is typical. Papillae may be pronounced and often have an appearance like 'cobblestones'. The exact cause is unknown and it is difficult to treat. IgE and cell-mediated immune mechanisms play an important role.

Treatment of vernal keratoconjunctivitis is most effective using topical corticosteroids. If possible, a weaker steroid such as fluorometholone should be used instead of dexamethasone or prednisolone. This treatment must be continued under strict specialist ophthalmic supervision. Topical corticosteroids can have dangerous side effects. A *steroid-induced glaucoma* can result in damage to the optic nerve due to raised intraocular pressure. The author vividly recalls a young man of 18 years presenting at the eye hospital in Kabul, Afghanistan, blind due to bilaterally cupped optic nerve heads. This young man had been troubled with vernal keratoconjunctivitis and had been treated intermittently with topical corticosteroids. Further, it should be noted that topical corticosteroids can be a disaster where a red eye is caused by infective agents. Thus, a herpes simplex keratitis, treated with topical corticosteroids, can cause great harm to the eye, with corneal scarring and consequent severe visual loss.

Other forms of treatment for vernal conjunctivitis are topical antihistamines or sometimes a systemic antihistamine in the late evening. If available, topical sodium cromoglycate 2% (Opticrom, Aarane, Intal) may be used four times or more each day. Alternative treatment may be given with nedocromil 2% drops twice daily. Acetylcysteine 5% drops given four times daily have mucolytic properties. Symptomatic relief may be obtained to some extent with eye drops such as zinc sulfate. Cold compresses may be of some benefit.

If trachoma is present as well this should be treated before topical corticosteroids are given.

Pinguecula

The accumulation of yellow-white fatty deposits at the nasal or temporal conjunctival limbus is a common finding in middle or older age. Calcium deposits may sometimes occur. Occasionally the pinguecula may become inflamed, when a topical anti-inflammatory agent may be used. The best form of treatment is to leave them alone.

Pterygium

A pterygium is a 'wing' of conjunctival and subconjunctival fibrovascular tissue which grows across the cornea from either the temporal or the nasal side (Figure 18.29). Although poorly understood, its presence in the interpalpebral area suggests external influences such as ultraviolet light, irritation and chronic dryness, or different climates, especially hot, dry and dusty conditions. Some pterygia are pale and flat and cause few problems. Others are fleshy, more often inflamed and, if surgery is required, tend to recur. Anti-inflammatory agents may be used topically if required. Surgery should be avoided if at all possible but may become necessary if the pterygium begins to approach the visual axis.

Phlyctenulosis

A phlycten appears most commonly at or near to the limbus and is evidence of bacterial allergy, for many years associated with the tubercle bacillus. It may also be associated with hypersensitivity reactions to staphylococci or other bacterial allergens. A phlycten is a microabscess which appears as a raised, pinkish-yellow nodule. It responds quickly to topical corticosteroids. Again, the diagnosis should be certain and any use of topical corticosteroids should be carefully monitored. Any patient with a phlycten should be examined for possible systemic disease.

Keratoconjunctivitis sicca (dry eye, xerosis)

Keratoconjunctivitis sicca (KCS) is a common condition where dryness of the eyes causes symptoms of irritation,

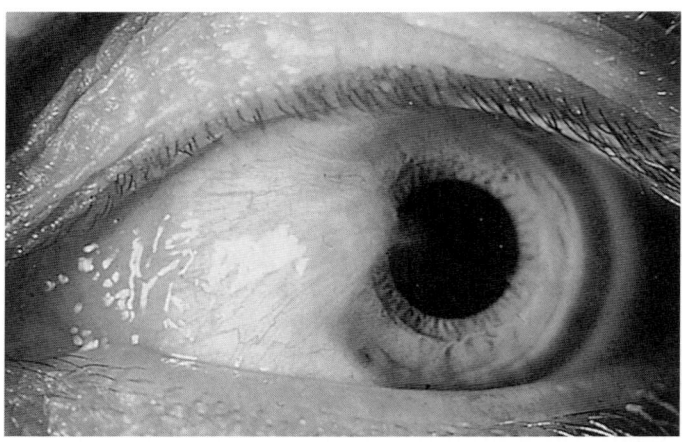

Figure 18.29: Nasal pterygium. (Photo: Murray McGavin.)

with grittiness (like sand in the eye) and redness. It is more common with advancing years. There is a recognized association with rheumatoid arthritis (Sjögren's syndrome: KCS, dry mouth and rheumatoid arthritis/other systemic disease). In tropical countries dry eyes can follow trachoma, in which conjunctival glands are damaged.

The diagnosis may be confirmed using a Schirmer's tear test in which strips of filter paper are hooked over the lower eyelid and the length of wetting of the strip is measured after 5 minutes. A drop of Rose Bengal 1% eye drops will reveal punctate staining of the cornea and conjunctiva and filaments of epithelium on the cornea (filamentary keratitis). In an eye with severe dryness, Rose Bengal will cause considerable discomfort.

Treatment is with artificial tear preparations such as hypromellose 0.3% eye drops.

In extreme cases of dry eyes, temporary occlusion of the lacrimal canaliculi (using plugs) or permanent occlusion (using cautery) can be very effective in preserving tears. However, permanent occlusion should only be done in patients who have extreme dryness.

Trachoma
See pp. 312–316.

Corneal ulcers and corneal scarring
See pp. 329–331.

Vitamin A deficiency (xerophthalmia, keratomalacia)
Although xerophthalmia is often apparent in a quiet eye, a devitalized anterior eye may be subject to other influences, such as infection, which will result in a red eye.

Inflammation of the episclera and sclera

Episcleritis
Episcleritis is essentially a self-limiting condition in which the aetiology is often uncertain. It has been associated with herpes zoster ophthalmicus, gout and rheumatoid arthritis and is a recognized complication of leprosy. Topical corticosteroids can be used when required.

Scleritis
Inflammation of the sclera is often associated with uveal tract inflammation, resulting in a sclero-uveitis. Scleritis is most commonly associated with rheumatoid arthritis and 30% of patients presenting with scleritis are found to have rheumatoid disease. Infective conditions associated with a scleritis are leprosy, tuberculosis and herpes zoster ophthalmicus.

Scleritis requires systemic treatment, either with non-steroidal anti-inflammatory agents or systemic corticosteroids. Other immunosuppressive agents may also be used. Subconjunctival injections of corticosteroids should *not* be used because focal necrosis can occur.

When the scleral inflammation has settled, the area of sclera may appear faintly translucent. This area of sclera may be thinned although not invariably so.

Inflammation of the anterior uvea (anterior uveitis, iridocyclitis)
Inflammation of the iris (iritis) and of the ciliary body (cyclitis) may be described as iridocyclitis or anterior uveitis.

Iridocyclitis presents typically with pain, redness, photophobia and blurred vision. The condition may be unilateral or bilateral. Examination with magnification will reveal a haziness of the aqueous fluid in the anterior chamber of the eye due to the presence of circulating proteins and inflammatory cells. Deposits of cells may be found on the endothelium of the cornea (keratic precipitates). Inflammation of the iris and its pupil margin may result in adherence of parts of the pupil to the anterior lens face. These are posterior synechiae. Synechiae may also occur at the base of the iris, across the angle of the anterior chamber to the base of the cornea, described as peripheral anterior synechiae.

This inflammation can result in a secondary glaucoma and, in some instances, secondary cataract formation.

The causes of iridocyclitis are many. Systemic diseases which present with a classical granulomatous type of iridocyclitis with large keratic precipitates include sarcoidosis and tuberculosis.

Injury to an eye can occasionally result in a 'sympathetic' inflammation of the second eye. It is said that this may occur days, months or even years after the original injury. Topical and systemic corticosteroid therapy is required.

There are a variety of factors influencing the onset of iridocyclitis which may relate to genetic characteristics, sex and race. For example, the presence of the HLA-B27 antigen is often associated with ankylosing spondylitis and uveitis. Males are more likely to develop ankylosing spondylitis or Reiter's syndrome. Reiter's syndrome is recognized by non-specific urethritis, polyarthritis, conjunctivitis or possibly iridocyclitis. Certain racial factors influence uveitis in conditions such as Behçet's syndrome, which is more common in eastern Mediterranean people and the Japanese. Behçet's syndrome typically presents with recurrent ulcers of the mouth and genitalia associated with a severe uveitis. The iridocyclitis of sarcoidosis is more common in the black population of North America.

Acute angle closure glaucoma
See pp. 309–310.

Eye injuries
See pp. 331–333.

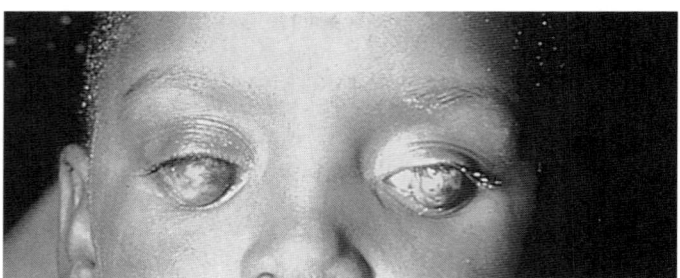

Figure 18.30: Gross staphylomata after measles and vitamin A deficiency. A blind unsightly eye will usually be enucleated. (Photo: Simon Franken.)

Inflammation of the eyeball
Endophthalmitis
Infection which develops in the interior of the eye, for example when a bacterial or fungal corneal ulcer perforates or when a penetrating foreign body enters the eye, often stone, wood or coal, may result in a severe intraocular inflammatory reaction. Often this is disastrous for the eye. Vigorous treatment is required with systemic and local antibiotics and often systemic corticosteroids. Subconjunctival and intravitreal antibiotic injections may be required.

Staphyloma
A staphyloma is a bulging of the eye where, by definition, uveal tissue is adherent behind the bulging wall of the eye; thus a staphyloma may be a corneal staphyloma or a scleral staphyloma. In its initial stages the eye is usually severely inflamed with a weakened cornea or sclera. This appearance may be associated with vitamin A deficiency (Figure 18.30), in which inflammation will be minimal, or possibly follow severe injury.

Phthisis bulbi
A shrunken eye may follow severe inflammation, such as endophthalmitis or panophthalmitis, and injury from a variety of causes. The intraocular pressure is low (hypotony). The resulting shrunken eye can be quiet but during the damaging process, of whatever origin, the eye is usually inflamed.

If the patient is not complaining, nothing needs to be done. However, an artificial eye may be inserted either on top of the phthisical eye or after the eye has been removed surgically. The appearance can be greatly improved.

Subconjunctival haemorrhage
Apart from this form of haemorrhage after injury, a *subconjunctival haemorrhage* may occur spontaneously and is evident as a dramatic red area over the white sclera. This will resolve in 2–3 weeks. Unless the patient has similar haemorrhages elsewhere, it is likely to be an isolated episode of no consequence. If in any doubt, however, the blood pressure and blood picture should be determined.

Systemic infections and the eye
Systemic bacterial infections and the eye

Brucellosis (undulant fever; Mediterranean fever)
Brucellosis is caused by infection with organisms which are Gram-negative bacilli: *Brucella abortus*, *B. melitensis* or *B. suis*. The disease is widespread throughout the world and can include eye changes.

Eye complications
A uveitis which is chronic and granulomatous in character is described. Keratitic precipitates with cells and circulating proteins in the anterior chamber indicate an iridocyclitis. A posterior uveitis may occur also.

Keratitis may occur with epithelial opacities. An optic neuritis is rare. Extraocular muscle abnormalities can appear, either due to local inflammation or sixth cranial nerve paralysis due to a basal meningoencephalitis.

The diagnosis of brucellosis is based on the isolation of the organism from blood, urine or pus, or serological tests.

Management
Treatment of the eye disease is that given for an anterior uveitis, with topical mydriasis/cycloplegia, using eye drops such as atropine sulfate 1%, and topical corticosteroids.

Treatment of the systemic disease is described in Chapter 60.

Tularaemia
Tularaemia is caused by a small Gram-negative bacillus, *Francisella tularensis (Pasteurella tularensis)*. The human infection is found in Europe, Japan and North America.

The systemic disease and its transmission from animals such as rabbits and other rodents are described in Chapter 62.

Eye complications
The eye changes associated with tularaemia occur when the organism penetrates the conjunctiva. After a period of up to 2 weeks, itching, photosensitivity and pain, together with redness and conjunctival oedema (chemosis), may present. Granulomas may appear and the regional lymph nodes become enlarged. This clinical picture is one description of Parinaud's oculoglandular syndrome.

Treatment
Details of systemic treatment are given in Chapter 62.

Tuberculosis
Tuberculosis is widespread and there is an increase in the infection worldwide. The WHO estimates over 7 million

new cases each year, with nearly 3 million deaths.[2] In countries where HIV/AIDS is endemic, tuberculosis is showing a disturbing increase. The causative organism is an acid-fast bacillus, *Mycobacterium tuberculosis*.

Eye complications

The disease may affect all systems of the body, including the eyes. Infection of the skin (lupus vulgaris) can result in eyelid scarring and secondary corneal involvement due to exposure. A papillary conjunctivitis can occur. Phlyctenular keratoconjunctivitis can be a hypersensitivity reaction to the tuberculoprotein, presenting as small yellow/pink nodules, often situated on the corneoscleral margin. This nodule is a microabscess and any patient, often a child, presenting with this allergic response should have a systemic examination for tuberculosis. An 'interstitial' keratitis is described. Scleritis, may be either anterior or posterior. The latter, posterior scleritis, may be associated with considerable thickening of the sclera due to granuloma formation.

An anterior uveitis (iridocyclitis) is typically granulomatous in type with large keratitic precipitates, described as 'mutton fat' keratic precipitates (KP). Examination with magnification may reveal small white nodules at the pupil margin or on the iris stroma (Koeppe nodules). Posterior uveitis (choroiditis) and a panuveitis can result in considerable disturbance to the eye. Miliary choroidal tubercles can be present as part of widespread disease. Both optic neuritis and consequent atrophy are described.

Management

The systemic treatment of tuberculosis with isoniazid, together with rifampicin or ethambutol and other medications, in a variety of regimens, is described in Chapter 57.

A phlycten responds quickly to topical corticosteroid therapy.

Periphlebitis retinae

In developing countries, it has been considered that periphlebitis retinae is often associated with systemic tuberculosis. However, association with other systemic diseases is well recognized (see below). The vascular disturbance may vary, from mild retinal vasculitis, evident on examination of the retinal periphery, to new vessel formation and gross bilateral vitreous haemorrhages. The condition is also described as Eales' disease, now recognized as a group of diseases with different aetiologies. The author has seen both forms of the disease and in one Central Asian country (Afghanistan), Eales' disease is found in the more florid form. Other causes of retinal neovascularization and vitreous haemorrhage must be excluded.

Retinal vasculitis may be associated with sarcoidosis, Behçet's disease, systemic lupus erythematosus and multiple sclerosis.

Meningococcal meningitis

Epidemics of meningococcal meningitis (cerebrospinal meningitis) occur in tropical countries, although the disease

is found worldwide. Each year 50 000 patients will die of meningococcal meningitis.[2] A 'meningitis belt' has been described across the savannah of sub-Saharan Africa, from Sudan to The Gambia. The organism is the Gram-negative *N. meningitidis*, which typically is shown on microscopy as pairs of cocci or as a single coccus.

Eye complications

Extraocular muscle imbalance can occur due to involvement of the cranial nerves, in particular the sixth nerve, although a partial third nerve paralysis is not uncommon. Encephalitis with optic neuritis may result in postneuritic atrophy. These features are associated with basal meningitis.

A conjunctivitis and also an anterior uveitis can occur associated with meningococcaemia.

The pupils react in a variety of ways according to the particular site of inflammation intracranially. In the early stages there may be miosis but mydriasis will occur with the onset of coma.

Involvement of the visual cortex can result in loss of vision with entirely normal ocular features and reactions. This visual disturbance or blindness ('cortical blindness') may have some recovery of sight in time, following treatment.

Management

The treatment of the systemic disease with penicillin or chloramphenicol is described in Chapter 56.

Local inflammation involving the eye or eyes should be treated appropriately.

Diphtheria

Diphtheria is caused by infection with a Gram-positive bacillus, *Corynebacterium diphtheriae*.

The disease is a public health problem in some developing countries, for example Sudan and India. Due to immunization, diphtheria has been reduced in distribution and effects worldwide.

Eye complications

A membranous conjunctivitis may present with eyelid oedema, discharge and local lymph node enlargement. Corneal ulceration can occur.

The classical sign of the infection with the bacillus is a 'dirty' grey membrane which forms where infection has occurred. The discharge can be bloodstained. On removal of the membrane the surface uncovered is raw and often has petechial haemorrhages.

The exotoxins formed by the organisms are particularly damaging to the heart, kidneys and central nervous system. Cranial nerve paralysis can occur, affecting the extraocular muscles, particularly the sixth cranial nerve, but with the fourth and third nerves sometimes also affected.

It should be noted that a membrane may form with other infections, such as *Streptococcus* or *Pneumococcus*.

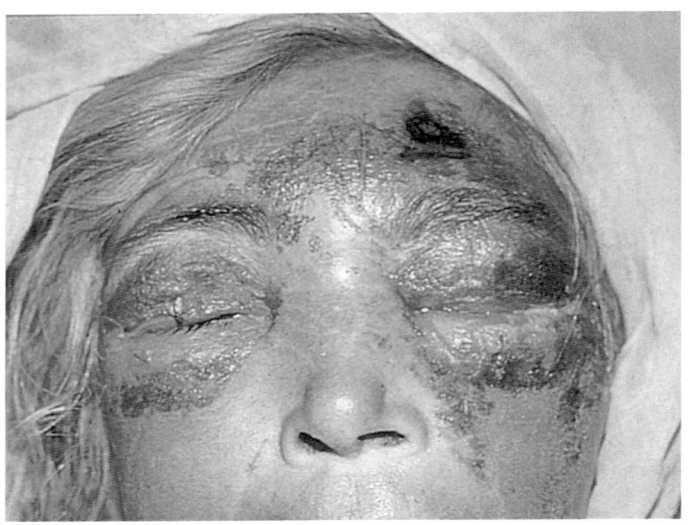

Figure 18.31: Anthrax in Central Asia. Notice the black eschar on the forehead. (Photo: Murray McGavin.)

Management
Diphtheria antitoxin should be used and then treatment with penicillin or erythromycin. Treatment of the disease is given in Chapter 65.

Anthrax
Cutaneous anthrax can involve the eyelids and periorbital regions. Infection is by direct contact with contaminated skins and other animal products, most often amongst those who work with live or dead animals. The organism can also be transmitted by insects. A red papule forms at the site of inoculation with the organism, *B. anthracis*. The area of inoculation becomes black (eschar) and gangrenous. The woman from Central Asia shown in Figure 18.31 said that an insect had bitten her forehead and a dark eschar can be seen at the site. Typically the patient is very ill.

Eye complications
Eschar formation affecting the eyelids can progress to considerable scarring, resulting in dramatic cicatricial ectropion—the eyelid can turn 'inside out'.

Management
Systemic treatment with the penicillins is described in Chapter 61.

Eyelid surgery requires horizontal division of the scar tissue externally—to allow the eyelid to resume its original position—with a full-thickness skin graft in the region of divided scar tissue.

Cholera
Cholera is a gastrointestinal disease caused by the bacillus *Vibrio cholerae*. The disease is widespread in tropical countries and has occurred in devastating epidemics. Profuse watery diarrhoea and vomiting results in acute dehydration.

A cholera pandemic, beginning in the East, gradually spread westwards over 30 years, reaching Latin America by 1991. The disease is described in Chapters 10 and 52.

Eye complications
The severely dehydrated patient will present with 'sunken' eyes. Conjunctivitis, corneal ulceration and corneal oedema have been reported. The great danger to the eyes is in the severely ill patient where the eyelids are left open, with consequent dehydration, exposure keratoconjunctivitis and corneal ulceration.

Of particular importance is the increased risk of cataract due to acute systemic dehydration. The author has discussed with Professor I. S. Roy, of Calcutta, the acute onset of cataract which he has described during cholera epidemics in India.

Management
Treatment details are given in Chapters 10 and 52.

Typhoid fever
Infection with the bacterial organism *Salmonella typhi* causes fever, abdominal pain and prostration. The bacilli may be harboured by a carrier of the infection and the organism is also found in water, milk, ice-cream and other foodstuffs.

Eye complications
Classically, rose spots may be described on the conjunctiva of patients with typhoid fever. They are found in association with similar rose spots on the trunk and limbs. During epidemics, cataract may form, possibly related, at least in part, to the associated dehydration. Involvement of the nervous system may result in a variety of complications, including extraocular muscle involvement and pupillary abnormalities.

Management
For a full description of treatment options in typhoid fever see Chapter 65.

Spirochaetal diseases and the eye

Syphilis
Syphilis is caused by the spirochaete *Treponema pallidum* which may be transmitted by venereal contact or, in the congenital form of the disease, from the mother to the unborn child. An annual incidence of 12 million with a worldwide prevalence of 28 million is reported by the WHO.[2]

Congenital syphilis
A great variety of symptoms and signs may occur in congenital syphilis and the disease may be sufficiently severe to cause abortion. The distinctly ocular changes of congenital syphilis can be relatively mild, although severe ocular defects are well recognized. These include

inflamed eyelids, dacryocystitis, conjunctivitis, extraocular muscle paresis, interstitial keratitis, iridocyclitis, pupil abnormalities (an Argyll Robertson pupil may be seen occasionally), choroidoretinitis with the classical appearance of pigment granules and yellow/red spots (the 'salt and pepper' fundus), and optic neuritis and optic atrophy. Typically, congenital syphilis becomes latent and then reactivates, often during the teenage years, and may 'reappear' as an interstitial keratitis. The patient then complains of severe discomfort or pain with photosensitivity and a red eye or eyes. The area of the cornea so affected may attract fine new blood vessels and the oedematous and inflamed area appears pink, which has been described as a 'salmon patch' appearance. Associated inflammation can include an iridocyclitis. Corneal scarring may also be a consequence. Later, tiny, empty blood vessels in the cornea are described as 'ghost vessels'.

Adult acquired syphilis

In acquired syphilis the primary stage of the disease is manifest as a painless, ulcerated 'chancre', where the spirochaete has gained entry, and this may be associated with local lymphadenopathy. The chancre will heal and some time later second-stage syphilis develops. Eye changes associated with this stage of syphilis can include iridocyclitis, retinal vasculitis and optic neuritis. Inflammation of the iris (iritis) may be obviously hyperaemic (roseolae). Tertiary-stage syphilis may ensue after a variable period of time and can have similar clinical features. Also, the classical Argyll Robertson pupil may occur. Bilateral involvement of the pupils usually causes irregular pupils, and the affected pupil does not react to either direct or consensual light stimulation but will constrict on accommodation. Optic atrophy may be found.

Management

Treatment of the inflammatory disease of the anterior eye will require mydriasis and cycloplegia using eye drops such as atropine sulfate 1%, together with topical corticosteroids.

A description of the general treatment of syphilis, using penicillin, is given in Chapter 21.

Leptospirosis

Leptospirosis is caused by spirochaetes of the genus *Leptospira*. The organisms are found worldwide. Man is infected by contact with a variety of domestic and wild animals, including rats, pigs, dogs and cattle, mostly due to contact with urine-contaminated water and soil. After an incubation period of 8–12 days, the patient develops fever and chills with general malaise and photosensitivity.

Eye complications

The conjunctival vessels may be dilated and there may be subconjunctival haemorrhages. An iridocyclitis can occur, although the onset of the intraocular inflammation may be weeks or some months after the initial infective phase

has passed. In its severe systemic form leptospirosis has been described as Weil's disease, with jaundice and an enlarged liver and severe kidney disease.

See Chapter 68 for details of appropriate treatment. Antibiotics in high doses are indicated.

Relapsing fever

Relapsing fever is caused by the spirochaetes *Borrelia recurrentis* and *Borrelia duttoni*, which may be louse borne or tick borne, respectively. The disease is widespread.

The patient has a recurring fever with severe headache, photosensitivity, muscle and joint pains, upper respiratory tract inflammation, nausea and vomiting. A rash is common.

Eye complications

Eye complications of relapsing fever include anterior uveitis, which may be acute or chronic in character. Haemorrhages and exudates of the retina have been described. A meningitis may result in ptosis and extraocular muscle abnormalities due to cranial nerve paralysis.

Management

A full description of the systemic disease, diagnostic tests and treatment is given in Chapter 67.

Yaws

Yaws is caused by the spirochaete *Treponema pertenue*, which is found in many geographical locations including Asia, Africa, South America and the Caribbean. An ulcerating papilloma forms the primary lesion.

As the disease progresses there may be the appearance of papules at a variety of sites. During the later stages the characteristic lesion is an ulcerating granuloma (gumma) which heals with scarring. This lesion, affecting the nose or orbit, can destroy bone and cartilage in the region (gangosa).

Eye complications

Eye changes particularly involving the eyelids are due to scarring. Consequent deformities may cause the lower eyelid to turn out due to scar tissue formation (cicatricial ectropion). However, there can be considerable destruction in the region of the eye and orbit.

Chlamydial infections and the eye

Trachoma

Infection with *Chlamydia trachomatis* is described on pp. 312–313.

Lymphogranuloma venereum

Lymphogranuloma venereum is caused by an organism of the *Chlamydia* (or *Bedsonia*) group of infective agents. It is a venereal disease, transmitted by sexual contact. The organism is widespread geographically.

The initial lesion, the primary sore, is usually in the genital region and within days there follows a regional lymphadenitis, with fever, headache, malaise, nausea and skin changes.

Eye complications

Eye changes include a follicular conjunctivitis with a lymphadenopathy, particularly of the preauricular lymph node. This is also the clinical picture of Parinaud's oculoglandular syndrome. A keratitis may be associated with corneal infiltration and new vessel formation. An iridocyclitis has been described. Posterior eye changes include dilatation of the retinal veins, some retinal haemorrhages and oedema at the optic nerve head.

Management

Tetracyclines are the drugs of choice. A description of the treatment of lymphogranuloma venereum is given in Chapter 21.

Rickettsial infections and the eye

Typhus

Typhus fever may be louse borne, where the infecting organism is *Rickettsia prowazeki*, or tick, mite or flea borne.

Eye complications

Eye complications associated with typhus fever can include conjunctivitis with photosensitivity. Subconjunctival haemorrhages may occur. Other complications include iridocyclitis, retinal changes with haemorrhages and optic nerve oedema. Optic atrophy may ensue.

Management

Chloramphenicol, doxycycline and tetracycline are the drugs of choice.

Rocky Mountain spotted fever

This rickettsial disease is caused by *R. rickettsii* and is found in the Western Hemisphere. The vector is the tick—carried by wild rodents and dogs.

A conjunctivitis with photosensitivity and petechial haemorrhages of the bulbar and tarsal conjunctivae is described.

Treatment is with chloramphenicol, doxycycline or tetracycline.

Viral infections and the eye

Measles

Measles and the eye and its association with vitamin A deficiency disorders are discussed on p. 322

Rubella

The disease is caused by an RNA virus of the arbovirus group. It is most often diagnosed when it appears in epidemics. The disease presents with a maculopapular rash, which is pink/red, on the face, trunk and extremities.

Rubella infection in susceptible mothers during the first 3 months of a pregnancy has an 80% chance of affecting the unborn child. The congenital rubella syndrome can have both minimal and severe effects. Apart from eye complications, the child may be deaf or mentally retarded and there may be cardiovascular abnormalities. Growth of the fetus may be inhibited, and in the most severe form the fetus may be aborted or the child stillborn.

Eye complications

Cataract may occur in around half of all children affected by rubella in utero. This form of congenital cataract may be unilateral or bilateral. The virus may remain in the lens for some years after birth and surgical removal of the cataract may result in a uveitis. Other eye defects include congenital glaucoma (buphthalmos), rubella retinopathy, which can have a 'salt and pepper' appearance, optic atrophy, squint, nystagmus and microphthalmos.

Management

The treatment of rubella is preventive. Young females should be immunized; immunization may be carried out at 1 year of age or before puberty. This provides lasting immunity.

Herpes simplex and the eye

The herpes simplex virus (HSV) is distributed worldwide and can have severe effects on the eye. The virus contains a DNA core and this insinuates itself into the cell and the cell nucleus, where it is able to reproduce itself. Most individuals will have experienced a 'cold sore' on the face, but the effect on the cornea is clearly much more significant. It may cause a keratitis and, with the inappropriate use of topical corticosteroids which are contraindicated in this infection unless used by the experienced eye specialist, the results can be disastrous for the eye. Most herpes simplex keratitis is caused by Type I infection, although occasionally Type II infections occur, particularly in the newborn—when infection occurs in the mother's birth canal.

It appears that the virus can remain latent for a long time within the nervous system, particularly the ganglion of the fifth cranial nerve (trigeminal). It should be noted that herpes simplex infection is more severe in immunocompromised individuals and may, for example, complicate the picture of measles keratitis and vitamin A deficiency.

In one study in Tanzania, HSV was responsible for 36% of corneal ulcers found in children (1981–1985).[40]

Although herpes simplex keratitis may be immediately obvious due to the presence of the classical dendritic figure, confusion may occur as the ulcer often presents in developing countries with an atypical appearance. The ulcer may be larger and geographic or amoeboid in appearance (Figure 18.32). These presentations may

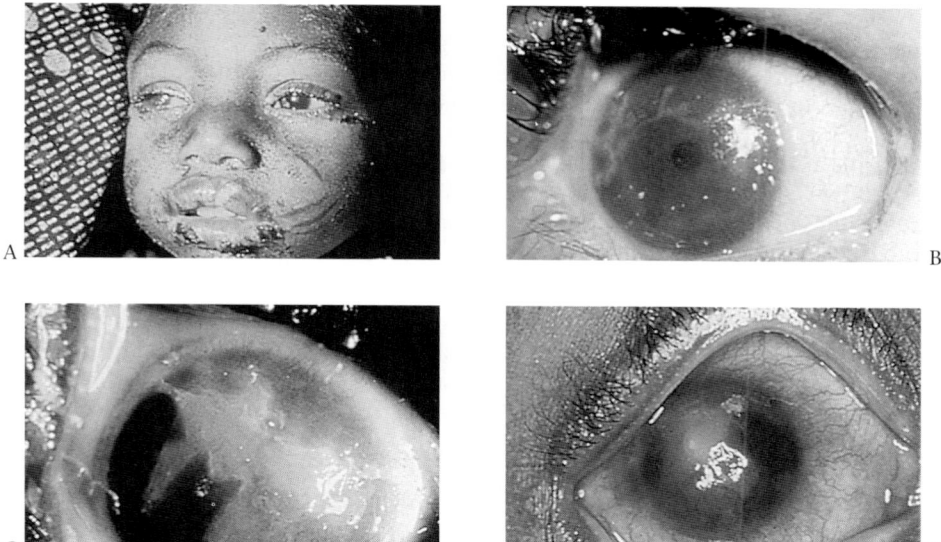

Figure 18.32: Herpes simplex keratitis. (Photos: (**A**, **C**) John Sandford-Smith; (**B**) Allen Foster; (**D**) David Yorston.)

relate to the length of time before treatment is sought, but may also be the result of wrong diagnosis and wrong treatment, particularly with corticosteroids, or the consequence of treatment with inappropriate traditional eye medicines.

Eye complications

Herpes simplex ulceration of the cornea has a tendency to recur and, should the infection and inflammation spread deeper than the corneal epithelium, corneal scarring is likely to result. Recurrence may be stimulated by a number of factors, including fever, exposure to ultraviolet light, minor trauma, measles and psychological factors. Herpes simplex keratitis is often found in association with malaria and other causes of high fever.

Symptoms of HSV keratitis include pain and photo-sensitivity. Signs (Table 18.21) include watering (lacrimation), a red eye with circumcorneal injection and, in the classic presentation, a branching dendritic figure. This appearance is well delineated by instilling fluorescein dye. The same dye will, of course, also outline

Table 18.21 Distinguishing signs of herpetic corneal ulcers.

Typical, narrow branching dendritic ulcer
Large, irregular geographic ulcer
Intense corneal vascularization
Dense stromal infiltrate
Stromal necrosis and/or facetting
Reduced corneal sensation
Scarring/facetting/vascularization from previous attacks
Central corneal oedema, with keratitic precipitates (disciform)

Reproduced from Yorston D. Measles and childhood blindness. *J Community Eye Health* 1991; 4: 2–4.

a larger ulcer, such as the geographic ulcer previously noted. A severe host immune reaction to the presence of the virus in the stroma of the cornea can result in considerable inflammation. Neovascularization is likely to develop, particularly with ulcers close to the limbus. When healing occurs a scar remains and can also result in an irregular corneal surface. Corneal hypoaesthesia may be a feature. Deep inflammation of the cornea due to HSV infection provides a complicated problem in treatment. A uveitis may develop and sometimes the evidence of previous corneal epithelial infection can only be found with careful examination under magnification.

Management

Previously, treatment of superficial HSV keratitis affecting only the corneal epithelium was mechanical removal of the infected cells of the epithelium.

Idoxuridine (IDU) was the first antiviral agent used, either as IDU 0.1% drops or 0.5% eye ointment. Unfortunately, long-term use can result in occlusion of the lacrimal puncta.

Other forms of treatment are now more commonly used. These include acyclovir 3% eye ointment, which should be given five times daily, or vidarabine eye ointment, five times daily, or trifluorothymidine 1% solution, five times daily. Acyclovir is also available for systemic treatment, either orally or intravenously. It is expensive. Cycloplegic eye drops should be given while the eye is painful.

In experienced hands only, it may be necessary to use topical corticosteroids in a patient in whom there has been an immune response resulting in a deep disciform keratitis. The weakest effective dose of steroid should be used and (only) after treatment with an antiviral agent has been started and probably continued.

The eye health worker should refer any patient with herpes simplex keratitis to an experienced colleague after beginning treatment with a topical antiviral agent only, if this is available.

In the longer term, an unhealed HSV ulcer may require a conjunctival flap or a tarsorrhaphy to effect healing. (A tarsorrhaphy is a surgical procedure, in this situation usually temporary, in which the eyelids are partially sutured together.)

Scarring may require a later corneal graft which can be highly successful, although recurrence of the HSV infection can occur within the graft itself.

Herpes zoster ophthalmicus

The virus of herpes zoster is a DNA virus which lies dormant in sensory nerve root ganglia after a previous infection with chickenpox (varicella). A variety of stimuli may cause the development of herpes zoster (shingles) but, most commonly, herpes zoster affects the older age group and the immunocompromised individual. The development of shingles may be the first evidence of infection with the HIV/AIDS virus. Most often shingles affects the trunk but herpes zoster ophthalmicus, affecting the periorbital region and eye, occurs in less than 10% of patients who develop shingles. In these patients the ophthalmic division of the fifth cranial nerve is affected.

The clinical features of herpes zoster ophthalmicus include the classical rash, which is red and vesicular, develops crusts and later resolves with multiple tiny scars. The rash is typically 'one sided' in the region of the eyelids, supraorbital region and to a variable extent backwards above the hairline. The patient is generally unwell with headache and often depression. A distressing characteristic of the infection is postherpetic neuralgia which can persist for a year or two or more.

Eye complications

Eye complications occur in around 50% of patients with herpes zoster ophthalmicus and these can be expected if the nasociliary branch of the ophthalmic division of the fifth nerve is affected, with vesicles on the side of the nose. There may be lid scarring, a conjunctivitis, episcleritis, scleritis, keratitis and loss of corneal sensation (neuroparalytic keratitis), anterior uveitis, secondary glaucoma, extraocular nerve and muscle involvement and optic neuritis. Herpes zoster keratitis may take a variety of forms, including punctate epithelial erosions, filamentary keratitis and disciform keratitis.

Management

The patient requires rest, adequate fluids and analgesia to allow relief of the often severe pain. Antiviral drugs should be applied topically, both to the skin and to the eye. Acyclovir is most commonly used as a cream to the skin and as an ointment for the eye. Acyclovir may also be given systemically, especially if a patient is immuno-compromised. Alternatives for systemic treatment, if available, are valacyclovir 1 g three times daily for 1 week or famcyclovir 250 mg three times daily for 1 week. A topical cycloplegic, such as atropine sulfate 1% eye drops,

should be given. A topical corticosteroid may also be given if there is deep inflammation of the cornea or an iridocyclitis, but this must be under supervision of an eye specialist.

Chickenpox (varicella)

This common virus infection of childhood is characterized by fever, malaise and rash, which appears 12–16 days after infection has occurred. The rash is erythematous with vesicles occurring in groups which are widespread over the body surface. It may, however, occur at any age and can be a complicated and serious disease. The virus is a DNA virus identical to the herpes virus group. The patient has immunity to varicella following infection.

Eye complications

Vesicles may occur on the eyelids, conjunctiva and at the corneoscleral margin(s). Superficial punctate keratitis, deeper inflammation of the corneal stroma (interstitial keratitis) and iridocyclitis have been described. Occasionally, extraocular muscle involvement, pupil abnormalities and optic neuritis have occurred. The retina can be involved in immunocompromised individuals.

Management

Antibiotic ointment can prevent secondary bacterial infection of skin lesions. Any systemic complication, such as a pneumonia, will require suitable antibiotic cover for secondary bacterial infection.

Mumps

An acute fever associated with a parotitis is the typical presentation, sometimes involving other organs, causing orchitis, oophoritis and pancreatitis. It is due to a virus which, following infection, provides long-term immunity.

Eye complications include dacryoadenitis, conjunctivitis, keratitis, iridocyclitis, scleritis, retinitis and optic neuritis. Treatment is supportive with analgesics and appropriate treatment of any eye complications.

Molluscum contagiosum

Molluscum contagiosum is caused by a DNA virus which usually infects children. Infection in adults, especially in Africa, may be a sentinel lesion for HIV infection. A small papule with a central umbilicus is the typical lesion. There may be an isolated lesion or groups of papules. When situated on the eyelid, or possibly the conjunctiva, a follicular conjunctivitis or sometimes a keratitis may occur. Curetting of the lesions, after local anaesthesia, with the application of chemical cautery using tincture of iodine or carbolic acid is usually successful.

Cytomegalovirus

Infection with this virus has been particularly associated in recent years with the HIV/AIDS epidemic. Thus, it is a relatively common infection in the immunocompromised host. 'HIV/AIDS and the eye' is discussed further below.

Eye complications

Eye changes associated with the infection include an anterior uveitis, retinal oedema and necrosis, retinitis with widespread haemorrhages and sometimes retinal detachment. The optic nerve may be involved, with progressive optic atrophy. Opacities may occur in the vitreous and a posterior uveitis may also occur.

Infection affecting a woman who is pregnant can result in general and ocular abnormalities in the fetus. General features include low birthweight, purpura, deafness, mental retardation, pneumonitis, and an enlarged liver and spleen. Eye changes include a cataract, uveitis, optic nerve atrophy, choriodoretinitis and microphthalmos.

Burkitt's lymphoma

The Epstein–Barr virus has been implicated in this form of lymphoma although no direct proof is available. The tumour is found especially in sub-Saharan, middle Africa, but also in South America, Papua New Guinea and sporadically elsewhere.

Most commonly found in children under 10 years old, the maxillary region and orbit are often involved. The abdomen is often affected and also the central nervous system. A cranial nerve palsy can occur. The considerable upper jaw swelling can involve the eyelids and the anterior eye surfaces.

Treatment is by surgery, radiotherapy and chemotherapy (see Chapters 36 and 44).

HIV/AIDS and the eye

HIV infection is most often a sexually transmitted disease caused by the human immunodeficiency virus. It can also be transmitted by transfusion of contaminated blood and by unsterile needles associated with drug abuse.

While HIV infection in industrialized countries occurs particularly in homosexual populations and amongst drug users, in Africa it is mainly transmitted by heterosexual activity. Seropositivity is significantly linked with a history of sexually transmitted disease, genital ulcer disease, contact with prostitutes and lack of male circumcision. Age-specific peaks of HIV infection are found amongst children under the age of 5 and amongst young adults.

Epidemiology of HIV/AIDS[41]

HIV/AIDS emerged in the late 1970s and spread in America, Europe and Australia, mainly among homosexual and bisexual man and intravenous drug users. At the same time an epidemic occurred in East and Central Africa and in the Caribbean, but in these regions the infections have been mainly among heterosexual men and women with multiple sexual partners. It is now estimated that there are more than 34 million people infected with HIV and AIDS cases have been reported from about 190 countries (WHO, 2000).

It does seem that the rate of progression from HIV seropositivity to clinical AIDS and death advances more quickly in Africans than in Americans.

Modes of transmission

HIV has been isolated from most body fluids, with semen, vaginal secretions and blood of most importance in transmission of the disease.

Thus, the different routes of transmission can be described as follows:

1. Sexual transmission (86%)
   (a) heterosexual (71%)
   (b) homosexual (15%)
2. Blood and blood products (12%)
   (a) transfusion (5%)
   (b) injections: drug abuse (7%)

HIV-infected women may transmit the disease to their babies. The risk that a baby born to a seropositive mother will be infected is probably between 25% and 40% in Africa and around 15–20% in the industrialized world.

HIV has been found in the tears, conjunctiva, the cornea, the aqueous humour and the vascular endothelium of the retinal vessels. These findings, in relation to potential transmission of the infection, are important, for example when examining patients with an applanation tonometer. However, there is no report of transmission occurring through tears. Isopropyl alcohol swabbing of the tonometer tip is an adequate means of sterilization. The possible transmission of HIV as a result of corneal transplant surgery is an obvious concern.

Clinical stages of the disease and ocular complications (Table 18.22)

Herpes zoster ophthalmicus

Herpes zoster ophthalmicus is a marker for HIV infection in Africa. The course of this disease is more severe in HIV-positive patients, with more subjective discomfort. It also occurs in a younger age group. Intravenous or oral

Table 18.22 Clinical stages of the disease and ocular complications.

Group 1	Asymptomatic or generalized lymphadenopathy
Group 2	Early-stage disease (minor opportunistic infections) HZO, molluscum contagiosum, papillomata
Group 3	Intermediate-stage disease HIV-related retinopathy
Group 4	AIDS (opportunistic infections) CMV retinitis, cryptococcal meningitis Kaposi's sarcoma

acyclovir is the preferred treatment, but the drug is expensive. Retinal necrosis may occur in association with herpes zoster and this can present in two clinical forms. The typical form has necrotic areas in the peripheral fundus, with vasculitis, haemorrhages and vitreous and anterior chamber involvement. The other presentation, more often found with HIV seropositivity, shows many yellowish lesions scattered throughout the fundus and less often vitreous and anterior chamber inflammation. Treatment is with high doses of acyclovir or foscarnet intravenously. Prognosis is very poor.

Molluscum contagiosum and papillomata

The eyelids may have multiple warts or the umbilicated papules of molluscum contagiosum, both suggestive of HIV/AIDS infection.

Other infective agents which may take advantage of the depressed immune state in AIDS include *Cryptococcus neoformans*, *Pneumocystis carinii*, *Mycobacterium avium-intracellulare*, *Toxoplasma gondii*, *Histoplasma capsulatum* and *Candida albicans*.

HIV-related retinopathy

The most common ocular manifestation of HIV-infected patients are abnormalities of the small vessels of the retina. These can be found in around one-third of AIDS patients. These lesions consist of small necrotic spots ('cotton-wool' spots), small haemorrhages and micro-aneurysms and telangiectasias. Generally, these lesions do not cause visual loss.

AIDS and cytomegalovirus (CMV) retinitis

CMV is one of the herpes viruses. In HIV patients with severe immunodepression, reactivation of earlier infection with CMV may cause gastrointestinal disease, pneumonitis, encephalitis and retinitis. CMV retinitis will affect up to 30% of AIDS patients in the industralized world, while in developing countries the prevalence seems to be lower, between 5% and 10%. CMV retinitis typically affects patients with profound immune depression (CD4 count less than 50/mm^3). AIDS patients in developing countries will often die from other diseases, such as malaria or cryptococcal meningitis, before they develop CMV retinitis.

The classical appearance of CMV retinitis is that of a haemorrhagic retinal necrosis—sometimes described as ketchup (tomato sauce) on cottage cheese, with extension of the lesions along the vascular arcades (Figure 18.33). The disease is bilateral in about 50% of patients. It is severely progressive and if no treatment is provided the whole retina may be destroyed within 6 months.

Two drugs which are available for treatment of CMV retinitis are ganciclovir and foscarnet. Ganciclovir suppresses the bone marrow, while foscarnet is nephrotoxic.

An alternative drug to ganciclovir and foscarnet is cidofavir, which does have the advantage of once-weekly treatment.

Treatment with ganciclovir and foscarnet is as follows:

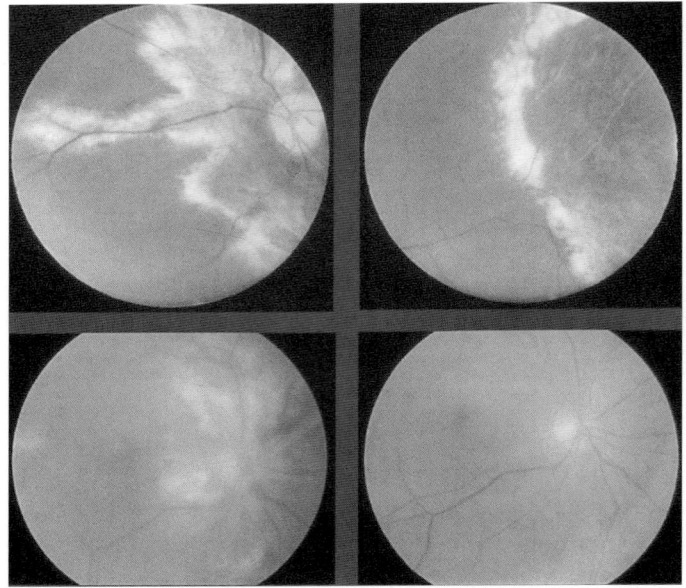

Figure 18.33: AIDS and cytomegalovirus (CMV) retinitis. (Photos: Philippe Kestelyn.)

	Ganciclovir	Foscarnet
Induction	5 mg/kg IV twice daily for 2 to 3 weeks	60 mg/kg IV three times daily for 2 to 3 weeks
Maintenance	5 mg/kg IV once every day or 6 mg/kg IV once daily for five days a week	90 to 120 mg/kg IV once daily

HIV/AIDS and syphilis

All patients with syphilis should be tested for HIV and vice versa. Ocular manifestations of syphilis and HIV-seropositive patients include uveitis, retinal vasculitis and optic nerve disease.

The recommended treatment for ocular syphilis in HIV-seropositive patients is 12–24 million units of aqueous crystalline penicillin G intravenously per day for 10–14 days.

HIV/AIDS and tuberculosis

Because of the profound depression of cell-mediated immunity in AIDS patients the organism cannot be held in check and rapid multiplication occurs with dissemination to multiple organs (miliary disease). The alarming rise in the prevalence of tuberculosis parallels the spread of the HIV epidemic. In developing countries, 30–50% of adults have latent tuberculosis that will be reactivated in the presence of HIV infection. In patients with profound immune depression, the presentation may be atypical, with extrapulmonary involvement and a negative tuberculin test. In patients with HIV/AIDS massive choroidal invasion may lead to secondary retinal necrosis and blindness. Most patients die within a few months.

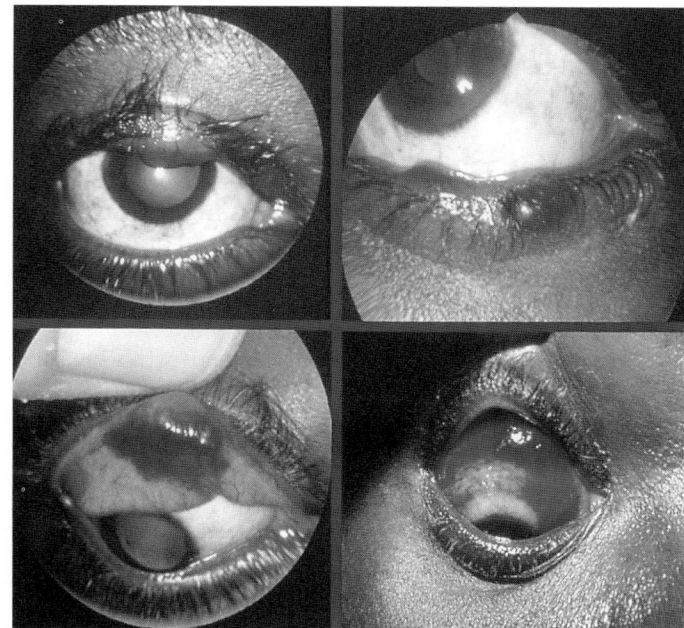

Figure 18.34: HIV/AIDS and tumours: Kaposi's sarcoma. (Photos: Philippe Kestelyn.)

The treatment of tuberculosis is the same as in patients who are not HIV infected, with isoniazid, rifampicin and pyrazinamide for at least 6 months.

HIV/AIDS and tumours

Kaposi's sarcoma and B cell lymphoma are the two most common malignancies reported in association with HIV infection and are considered diagnostic of AIDS.

Kaposi's sarcoma is a malignant vascular tumour which occurs in 15–24% of patients with AIDS, at least in the developing world. This tumour can present on any cutaneous surface and also on mucous membranes. It may develop on the eyelid skin, on the eyelid margins, on the conjunctiva and rarely within the orbit. The clinical presentation of the tumour appears as a deep purple-red nodule (Figure 18.34). Typically, multifocal skin lesions appear which later ulcerate. They are usually slow growing and rarely invasive. The tumours can be excised or given focal radiation therapy.

Squamous cell carcinomas have been reported with greater frequency in HIV-infected individuals. These tumours may be anal, oral, cervical and conjunctival. It may be that the oncogenic potential of the human papilloma virus acts as a co-factor. The presence of a greyish-white keratinized mass surrounded by a blood supply of engorged conjunctival vessels, sometimes with pigmentation, is typical of the tumour. The tumour is often aggressive. Prompt and complete surgical excision is required.

Fungal infections and the eye

Over 100 fungal species, whether filamentous fungi, yeasts or dimorphic organisms, have been associated with eye infections. Difficulties in management of the oculomycoses relate to problems in diagnosis and often an inadequate resource of antifungal agents. A suppurative keratitis, for example, may be due to either bacteria or fungi but this cannot be firmly decided on clinical grounds alone. A simple measure for determining the type of organism involved is to carry out a Gram stain.

Pathogenic fungi and eye infection (oculomycoses)

Fungi causing eye infections are most commonly filamentous fungi and yeasts.

- *Filamentous fungi.* These are multicellular organisms with projections known as hyphae. Hyphae may have divisions or be non-septate. Septate filamentous fungi include important organisms causing eye infections: *Fusarium*, *Aspergillus* and *Penicillium*. Non-septate filamentous fungi, for example *Rhizopus* and *Phycomycetes*, less commonly involve the eye.
- *Yeasts.* *Candida albicans* and *Cryptococcus neoformans* are species of yeasts that may be involved in eye infections. They are distinguished by the fact that they are unicellular organisms that reproduce by budding.
- *Dimorphic fungi.* These fungi, such as *Blastomyces dermatitidis*, may be responsible for ocular and orbital disease following blood and lymphatic spread.

Oculomycoses are found worldwide but particularly in countries with hot and humid climates. The geographical pattern of these infections is gradually emerging as the literature on mycotic infections of the eye increases. In some parts of the tropics, between a third and a half of adult corneal ulcers are caused by fungi. The filamentous fungi *Aspergillus* and *Fusarium* are most commonly found affecting the eye. *Candida albicans* is also found worldwide.

In terms of the treatment of fungal eye infections, the most significant anatomical site is the cornea, where suppurative keratitis, ulceration, hypopyon formation and possible corneal perforation mean that early recognition of the infection and prompt treatment are vital.

A fungal corneal ulcer is suggested by a dry, slowly worsening, necrotic ulcer with stromal infiltrate and multifocal lesions, particularly if the ulcer fails to respond to antibiotic treatment. However, these signs are not consistently present.

Fungi are associated with vegetable matter, so injuries, such as abrasions of the cornea with twigs, thorns and husks, must always be examined with an awareness of possible fungal infection.

Fungi may also involve the canaliculi of the lacrimal duct system.

Aspergillosis

The genus *Aspergillus* contains over 300 identified species and is common in warm and humid climates. The nose and paranasal sinuses are often infected, which can lead on to ocular involvement with extraocular muscle palsies. Intracerebral abscess formation can cause eye complications due to a space-occupying lesion.

Fusariosis

Fusarium species may cause a suppurative keratitis, with or without hypopyon formation. As with any suppurative keratitis, corneal scarring is likely when the area of infection and inflammation heals. At a later time corneal grafting may be indicated.

Candidiasis (moniliasis)

Candida albicans is an organism commonly found in the mouth, throat and vulva.

The fungus may affect the eyelids, lacrimal system, conjunctiva and cornea. Often infection will follow injury to the eye, whether accidental or (sometimes) surgical.

Cryptococcosis

Cryptococcosis neoformans is a yeast-like fungus which may have systemic effects involving the skin, lungs and meninges. It may cause a mycotic corneal ulceration and hypopyon may form. Endogenous spread through the bloodstream results in involvement of either the anterior or posterior uveal tract. Infection of the meninges may cause raised intracerebral pressure with the ocular sign of papilloedema and subsequent optic atrophy. Cranial nerve abnormalities also occur.

Blastomycosis

Blastomycosis dermatitidis is found in the Americas and Africa and affects the skin, lungs and various other organs. The infection is characterized by suppurative granulomas which may be found in the mouth, nose and also sometimes involving the eyelids. The orbit, lacrimal canaliculi, conjunctiva and cornea may be affected.

Coccidioidomycosis

Infection with *Coccidioides immitis* usually begins with inhalation of the organism causing a pneumonitis. The disease may also involve skin, subcutaneous tissues, bone and meninges. Eye involvement can include a hypersensitivity response manifest as a phlyctenular conjunctivitis. The eyelids may be affected, and intraocular involvement has been recorded, causing a posterior uveitis. As with many fungi an endophthalmitis can occur.

Histoplasmosis

Infection by the fungus *Histoplasma capsulatum* is widespread. The organism is found in the soil and is inhaled.

The eye changes associated with this infection are described as 'presumed ocular histoplasmosis syndrome' (POHS), and based on evidence of infection elsewhere, but no organism has been isolated from the eye. It is presumed that histoplasmosis has a predilection for the posterior uvea and the characteristic lesions are multifocal atrophic choroidal and disciform macular changes.

If subretinal neovascular membranes form, treatment is with argon laser photocoagulation.

Treatment of fungal infections

If possible, immediate empirical antifungal treatment should be avoided and a Gram stain of a corneal scrape carried out. If a mycotic corneal ulcer is suspected, when antibacterial therapy has been unresponsive after 48 hours, an antifungal agent should be used.

Natamycin 5% eye drops are most effective against filamentous fungi, including *Aspergillus* and *Fusarium*, but may not always achieve good results. Dosage is one drop half-hourly, then six to eight times per day after 3–4 days.

Amphotericin B is most effective against yeasts, particularly *Candida* and *Cryptococcus*. It may be given intravenously and topically.

Flucytosine 1% is effective against yeasts, including *Candida* and *Cryptococcus*, although some strains are resistant. It must therefore be given with an imidazole. It may be given in oral form and topically.

The imidazoles have a broad spectrum of antifungal activity. All are used topically. Clotrimazole 1%, miconazole 1%, ketoconazole 2% and econazole 1% are often used in treatment of the keratomycoses caused by filamentous fungi and yeasts. They do not invariably achieve a good result.

Recent studies from India and Bangladesh have reported beneficial results with 0.2% aqueous chlorhexidine.

Silver sulfadiazine 1% eye ointment has proved beneficial in treating *Aspergillus* and *Fusarium*.

Systemic antifungal treatment will be necessary in endogenous infections, such as with *Candida*, where flucytosine orally 200 mg/kg per day or ketoconazole orally 200 mg once per day or 2 weeks may be given. Alternatively, amphotericin B can be administered intravenously over several days.

Diseases caused by protozoa

Toxoplasmosis

Toxoplasmosis is caused by *Toxoplasma gondii*. The distribution of toxoplasmosis is worldwide, with as many as one-third of adults infected. There is some geographical variation which mainly relates to the dietary habits of populations, particularly consumption of uncooked or raw meat, and the presence of cats, often domestic pets, which are the recognized hosts of the organism.

Eye complications

Toxoplasmic retinochoroiditis is the common manifestation of the disease affecting the eyes. Typically the condition is seen in a quiescent form, with scarring affecting the posterior segment of the eye. By far the most common presentation is the result of congenital toxoplasmosis, with infection of the fetus during pregnancy. Descriptions

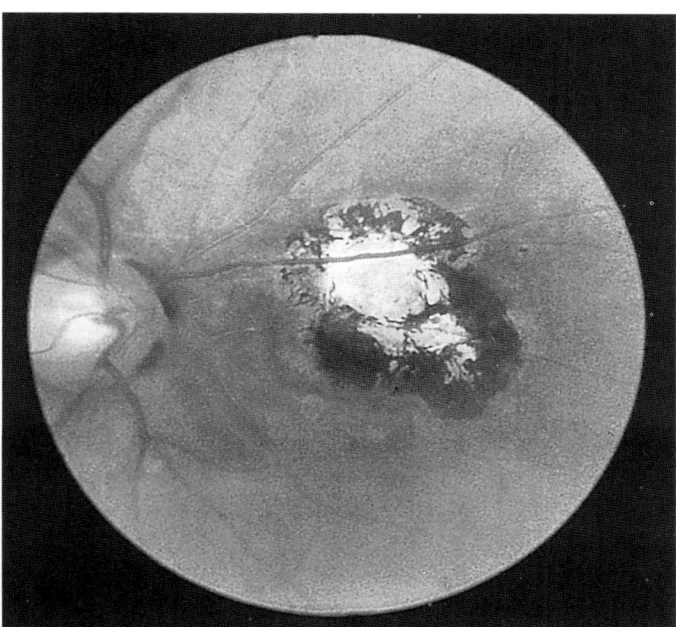

Figure 18.35: Old toxoplasmic retinochoroidal atrophy. (Photo: Gordon Johnson.)

of acquired toxoplasmic retinochoroiditis have been reported but these are uncommon. Eye disease due to toxoplasmosis is found more commonly in patients with AIDS.

Congenital toxoplasmosis which has caused a retinochoroiditis may present with a squint or nystagmus. Most eye changes affecting the retina and choroid are situated at the posterior pole of the eye, often in the region of the macula, and the patient may complain of poor vision (Figure 18.35). However, the typical scarring of old retinochoroidal atrophy is also found during routine eye examinations in teenage or adult life where vision has not been significantly affected.

The acute, 'acquired' infection is characterized by focal, necrotizing retinitis. The patient may complain of blurred vision, floaters and photosensitivity. The lesions may be multifocal, although the final 'punched-out' scar may be seen as an isolated lesion. In the acute phase the foci of inflammation are 'fluffy' white with hazy margins. Vitritis and iridocyclitis may be associated. Cystoid macular oedema can develop.

Treatment
A full description of systemic treatment is given in Chapter 66.

Leishmaniasis

Leishmaniasis is a protozoan disease caused by parasites of the genus *Leishmania*. The insect vector which transmits the parasite is the sandfly. It is found in many developing countries, with up to 2.5 million cases of 'visceral' disease and 9.5 million of the cutaneous form estimated.[2]

Eye complications (visceral leishmaniasis)
The visceral form of leishmaniasis is known as kala-azar and eye disease is uncommon with this condition. Retinal haemorrhages have been described, typically bilateral and multiple in distribution. Iridocyclitis has been reported, with occasional descriptions of keratitis.

Eye complications (cutaneous leishmaniasis)
Cutaneous leishmaniasis has been described as tropical sore (oriental sore), mucocutaneous leishmaniasis (espundia) and disseminated anergic cutaneous leishmaniasis.

Eye changes commonly affect the eyelids, with occasional involvement of the lacrimal ducts or conjunctiva. The cutaneous lesion has a variety of appearances, with ulcer formation after the initial appearance of nodules or papules, often situated on the face, sometimes affecting the eyelids. Skin involvement leaves a characteristic scar.

Treatment
Details of treatment regimens are given in Chapter 75.

Amoebiasis

Amoebiasis is an intestinal protozoal disease due to the organism *Entamoeba histolytica*.

The disease is found worldwide, with possibly 500 million infected and an incidence of 48 million new cases each year.[2] It is found in deprived communities, being associated with poverty and inadequate sanitation. It is a major health problem in parts of Africa, Asia and Latin America, where highly virulent strains may exist. Around 70 000 deaths probably occur each year.[2]

Eye complications
In many populations where infection with *Entamoeba histolytica* is endemic, or even epidemic, it is difficult to determine whether eye changes are specifically associated with the systemic infection. A relatively uncommon but well-recognized complication of amoebiasis is a cerebral focus of infection, and reports of improvement in eye lesions, for example keratitis, associated with systemic treatment of amoebiasis, do suggest an occasional association. Braley and Hamilton[42] described cysts in the region of the macula with associated small retinal haemorrhages and disturbance of the retinal pigment epithelium. King and his colleagues[43] described five patients with a similar appearance, three of whom also had opaque, yellow foci within the cysts described.

Management
A description of systemic treatment is given in Chapter 77.

Giardiasis

Giardiasis is an infective condition of the intestine caused by the protozoan organism, *Giardia lamblia*. Giardiasis is found in populations worldwide and typically results in gastroenteritis following ingestion of contaminated food or water, particularly water where contamination with faecal matter has occurred. It is believed that around 200 million people are infected, with a yearly incidence of 500 000.[2]

Eye complications

Presumed giardiasis affecting the eyes has most commonly involved anterior and posterior uveitis with iridocyclitis, choroiditis, retinal and subretinal haemorrhages and macular disturbance. However, it should be noted that these descriptions of giardiasis affecting the eyes have no definite evidence. Patients responded to systemic treatment for the disease with improvement in the eye abnormalities.

Management

Systemic treatment details are given in Chapter 77.

African trypanosomiasis

Trypanosomiasis in Africa is caused by two protozoa, *Trypanosoma brucei gambiense* and *T. b. rhodesiense*. The insect vector for the disease is the tsetse fly of the genus *Glossina*.

The distribution of the disease, commonly known as 'sleeping sickness', is in Africa, between latitudes 15°N and 15°S. As many as 50 million people are at risk and there is an estimated prevalence of active disease in 400 000 people.[2]

Eye complications

A variety of clinical eye abnormalities have been reported. Eyelid oedema with conjunctival redness and photosensitivity may occur. Interstitial keratitis and iridocyclitis are reported. In the severe form of the disease, with the onset of meningoencephalopathy, there may be widespread neurological changes, ptosis, extraocular muscle involvement, optic neuritis and papilloedema.[44]

Management

A description of the treatment of African trypanosomiasis is given in Chapter 73.

American trypanosomiasis

Also known as Chagas' disease, American trypanosomiasis is caused by a protozoan parasite, *T. cruzi*. The insect vectors transmitting the organism are the blood-sucking reduviid bugs of the genera *Triatoma*, *Rhodnius* and *Panstrongylus*.

Geographically the disease is found in Central and South America, extending from Mexico to Argentina. Up to 18 million people are estimated to be infected, with 45 000 deaths each year.

Eye complications

Characteristic evidence of Chagas' disease, where the inoculation site is in the region of the eye, is oedema of the eyelids, which is typically unilateral (Romana's sign). The lacrimal gland can be involved in the inflammation. A single report in 1981 described granulomatous uveitis in a premature child.

Management

Please see Chapter 74 for details.

Malaria

Malaria is caused by protozoan infection with organisms of the *Plasmodium* species, the cause of the severe form of the disease in the tropics, *P. falciparum*. Other species are: *P. vivax*, *P. ovale* and *P. malariae*. It remains a devastating disease in tropical countries and has an incidence of 300–500 million cases each year with 1.5–2.7 million deaths.[2]

Eye complications

Retinal haemorrhages are seen in association with malaria. In some patients the retinal haemorrhages may have associated retinal exudates.

In severe cerebral malaria there may be extraocular muscle pareses, optic neuritis and cortical blindness due to brain damage.

An important eye abnormality associated with the treatment of malaria is the rare complication of chloroquine retinopathy. Chloroquine is used routinely in the treatment of malaria, but in a number of countries individuals who are unwell for a variety of different reasons will regularly take chloroquine. Chloroquine can damage the central retina, disturbing the macula and producing a pathognomonic 'bull's eye' maculopathy. The disturbed retinal pigment epithelium forms a ring or oval which provides the reason for the descriptive term. Central vision is affected.

Management

The treatment of malaria is described in Chapter 71.

Pneumocystosis

Pneumocystosis is caused by the organism *Pneumocystis carinii*. There is some debate as to whether the organism should have a protozoan classification or be associated with fungi.

In recent years *Pn. carinii* has caused infection, particularly a pneumonia, in immunodeficient individuals. Those with AIDS are particularly susceptible.

Eye complications

It is accepted that at least some of the retinal changes found in patients with AIDS during recent years are associated with *Pn. carinii* infection. These appearances are described as cotton-wool spots, which appear as fluffy, whitish foci in the retina. A choroiditis due to *Pn. carinii* is recognized.

Management

A description of systemic treatment is given in Chapter 70.

Diseases caused by nematodes

Onchocerciasis

By far the most common cause of blindness within this group of infections, onchocerciasis and its effects on the eye are discussed in Chapter 82.

Toxocariasis

Toxocariasis is caused mainly by the organism *Toxocara canis*; it results from contact with the host, especially puppies. Occasionally toxocariasis is caused by *Toxocara cati*, where the host is the cat.

Toxocariasis is distributed worldwide, and is found in both developing and industrialized countries.

The systemic disease is described as *visceral larva migrans*, which is further discussed in Chapter 83.

Eye complications

Ocular larva migrans may present with an eye problem such as squint or a white pupil (leucocoria). The typical abnormality is a single isolated granuloma at the posterior pole of the eye, although the lesion may occur peripherally and more than one focus may be evident. Intraretinal tracks of 'wandering' larvae may be seen on ophthalmoscopic examination. The presence of granulomatous inflammation may result in a variety of other clinical features, including keratitis, iridocyclitis, chronic endophthalmitis, detached retina and optic neuritis. In the 'quiet state' the retina and choroid may show atrophic scarring.

It is important to differentiate ocular toxocariasis from the malignant intraocular tumour of childhood, retinoblastoma. Both of these eye abnormalities may present with leucocoria. It should be noted that ocular larva migrans may occur as a congenital infection.

Management

Most eye lesions are quiescent and no therapy is indicated. Eye inflammation should be treated appropriately. If severe intraocular inflammation is present, systemic or periocular corticosteroids may also be required. Intraocular inflammation can result in endophthalmitis, membrane formation or traction on the retina and retinal detachment. Expert surgical intervention can involve vitrectomy, division of membranes and retinal detachment surgery.

Treatment details are also described in Chapter 83.

Loiasis

Loiasis is found in West and Central Africa and is caused by the filarial helminth *Loa loa*. The insect vector of the worm is the fly of the genus *Chrysops*.

Eye complications

The most typical evidence of infection with *L. loa* is the presence of the worm under the conjunctiva of the eyeball. There may be conjunctival redness and some discomfort. The more dramatic presentation shows considerable swelling due to oedema of the eyelids (Calabar swelling), caused by the presence of the worm subcutaneously. Usually this swelling will settle in a few days.

Other eye features described include the presence of worms in the anterior chamber, a uveitis and a retinopathy.

Management

The regimen of treatment is described in Chapter 82.

The presence of a subconjunctival worm first requires topical anaesthesia. A suture is passed under the worm and tied tightly and the worm is dissected out. Alternatively a cryoprobe may immobilize the worm before surgical removal.

Thelaziasis

The oriental eye worm, *Thelazia callipaeda*, has principally been reported in patients from Japan and other countries in the Far East. Transmission is possibly by flies.

Eye complications

Typically the patient complains of irritation and watering with a congested eye, often associated with pain. The worm may be seen within the conjunctival sac. An intraocular infection was described in an 8-year-old Pakistani girl in whom the worm was found on the endothelial surface of the cornea.[45] Following instillation of cocaine drops the worm was removed surgically.

Management

Any worm present on the surface of the eye can be removed after the application of a local anaesthetic.

Bancroftian and Brugian filariasis

Filariasis caused by *Wuchereria bancrofti* has a widespread distribution in Africa, Asia and Latin America, with 119 million infected (WHO).[2] *Brugia malayi* occurs principally in South-East Asia, while *Brugia timori* is found in Indonesia. These lymphatic filariases have a wide variety of clinical presentations.

Transmission is by mosquitoes.

Eye complications

Adult worms have been isolated in the conjunctiva, with associated pain and redness. A subretinal adult worm has been found and larvae can infiltrate the anterior chamber, iris, lens capsule, retina and choroid. Worms have been found in the eyelid and also the lacrimal gland.

Management

An adult worm may be removed from beneath the conjunctiva after the application of topical anaesthetic to the bulbar conjunctiva.

The preferred treatment is described in Chapter 82.

Dracunculiasis

Dracontiasis (dracunculosis) due to the guinea worm, *Dracunculus medinensis*, is widely distributed, mainly in sub-Saharan Africa but also in southern Asia. It is estimated by the WHO that the number of people infected is now around 70 000.[2] Few die of the disease. Water which is contaminated with the small crustacean, *Cyclops*, is ingested and the patient becomes infected. After an incubation period of up to 1 year a worm will often emerge through the skin.

Eye complications

In one 12-year-old girl from India, who had an irritable, watering eye and swelling of the conjunctiva, an adult female guinea worm was removed surgically.[46] The older literature has reported involvement of the orbit in association with dracunculiasis.

Management

A description of treatment is given in Chapter 82.

Trichinosis

Trichinosis is caused by infection with the larvae of *Trichinella spiralis*.

Trichinosis is commonly the result of eating infected, uncooked meat, most often pork. A great variety of other animals are also infected, including dogs, rodents, bears and jackals. The disease is found worldwide, including both Europe and America, where raw meat may be eaten.

Eye complications

The most common sign which may present to an eye specialist is bilateral eyelid oedema. This may be a consequence of invasion of the extraocular muscles with the organism, and pain on eye movement can be a feature. There may be associated oedema of the conjunctiva (chemosis).

Photosensitivity and blurring of vision can occur. Small haemorrhages may occur. These may present subconjunctivally and also within the eye, for example as a retinal haemorrhage. There may be an optic neuritis and optic nerve oedema.

Management

Treatment of the eyes is with a cycloplegic, such as atropine sulfate 1%, and topical corticosteroids. Swelling may be reduced with the application of cold compresses.

The systemic treatment of trichinosis with thiabendazole is described in Chapter 83.

Gnathostomiasis

Most reports of gnathostomiasis have been from Thailand and Japan, although other reports have been recorded from a number of countries, principally in Asia.

Infection is caused by eating uncooked fish, chicken or pork.

The human disease has been mainly due to infection with *Gnathostoma spinigerum*, the inflammatory consequences being caused by the larvae, with hypersensitivity reactions within the tissues. Central nervous system involvement may present with pain in the limbs followed by permanent paraplegia.

Eye complications

A great variety of eye complications may occur in association with the systemic disease. The eyelids, the anterior surface of the eye and intraocular tissues may be involved, and there may be an orbital cellulitis. Corneal ulceration, uveitis, worms in the anterior or posterior chambers, cataract and secondary glaucoma are described. The worm may cause retinal disturbance and inflammatory changes can occur along the track made by the moving worm.

Management

The only well-recognized form of treatment is the removal of the worm after anaesthesia. It has been suggested that cryotherapy could be used to immobilize the worm before surgery.

Angiostrongyliasis

The form of angiostrongyliasis which causes eye disease is caused by the worm *Angiostrongylus cantonensis*. Also described as eosinophilic meningitis, the transmission of the disease to humans follows the ingestion of snails, prawns, crabs or vegetables which are uncooked. Areas for preparing food should be kept clean. Angiostrongyliasis is a disease of rodents and is found mainly in Asia and the Pacific region. The parasite has been identified in Egypt and Cuba.

Eye complications

The adult worm has been found in the anterior chamber of the eye and reports have identified a worm under the retina. The third-stage larva has been found in the vitreous in two patients.

Symptoms and signs have included visual loss, pain, blepharospasm and evidence of iridocyclitis. Posterior segment inflammatory consequences, including retinal pigment disturbance or retinal detachment, can occur.

Optic neuritis occurs in association with eosinophilic meningitis and the sixth cranial nerve can be affected.

Management

Surgical removal of the worm is indicated. One method of removing the worm from the posterior segment is to use a cryoprobe to immobilize the worm before incision and removal.

Anterior segment inflammation will require treatment with topical atropine sulfate 1% and topical corticosteroids.

Diseases caused by cestodes

Cysticercosis

Cysticercosis is associated with the encysted form of the larvae of the tapeworm *Taenia solium*, and occasionally *T. saginata*. Faecal contamination of food and water is the most common cause of the acquired form of the disease, although the consumption of raw pork or beef means that the infection is widespread throughout the world. Muslims and Jews do not eat pork and therefore the disease is less common in these communities.

T. solium cysticerci have been found in many tissues, including brain, spinal cord, muscles, lungs, subcutaneous tissues and eyes.

Eye complications

Cysticercosis affecting the eye is commonly intraocular and is particularly found in the posterior segment of the eye, either subretinally or within the vitreous. *T. solium* cysticerci may also occur in the anterior chamber and other eye tissues. The typical form of the intraocular cyst may show movement and the protoscolex may move 'in or out' of the cyst.

Symptoms and signs include pain, double vision, blurring of vision and sometimes flashes of light.

Management

The systemic treatment of cysticercosis with praziquantel is described in Chapter 85. Corticosteroids may be used in association with praziquantel.

It is necessary to attempt removal of the intraocular cyst surgically.

Echinococcosis

Also described as hydatid disease, this infection is most often due to the larvae of the tapeworm *Echinococcus granulosus*. The disease is widespread and other species are found in particular geographical locations. Most cysts are found in the liver and lungs.

Eye complications

Typically ocular echinococcosis is found within the bony orbit. The most common sign is proptosis. There may be associated conjunctival chemosis, congestion and exposure keratitis.

Management

Treatment of the orbital cyst is by surgical removal.

The treatment of the systemic disease is described in Chapter 84.

Sparganosis

Sparganosis, due to infection with larvae of the cestode of the genus *Spirometra*, is found worldwide, but particularly in the Far East.

Humans can develop sparganosis by drinking contaminated water or eating infected snakes, birds or mammals. The flesh of an infected frog may be placed on ulcers and eye problems are usually caused by direct contact. For example, in China raw flesh may be applied to the eyes of patients who have fever.

Eye complications

The application of the flesh of a frog to inflamed or painful eyes can result in infection with the parasite, and eyelid oedema, watering and extreme irritation may develop. A worm may be found subconjunctivally and retrobulbar invasion can occur. The larva has been identified in the anterior chamber of the eye.

Management

The worm or nodule should be removed surgically.

Diseases caused by trematodes

Paragonomiasis

A number of lung flukes of the genus *Paragonimus* have been implicated in this infection, which is particularly prevalent in the Far East but is also found in Africa and Latin America. The organism is carried by many animals and human infection may follow the consumption of uncooked meats, including crab and other crustaceans.

Eye complications

Typically the onset of eye inflammation is characterized by severe pain which is intermittent in nature. There is a uveitis leading to considerable intraocular inflammation. The immature worm may cause anterior segment inflammation with hypopyon formation. There may be vitreous and retinal haemorrhages.

Management

In ocular paragonomiasis the helminth should be removed surgically.

Treatment of the systemic disease is described in Chapter 81.

Schistosomiasis

Schistosomiasis (bilharziasis) probably affects around 200 million people, with as many as 600 million at risk and 20 000 deaths each year.[2] This helminthic infection is mainly caused by *Schistosoma japonicum*, *S. mansoni* and *S. haematobium*. Dams and irrigation canals have increased the spread of schistosomiasis because these waters contain the snail which is the intermediate host for the worm.

Eye complications

Egg granulomas are found on the conjunctiva but also in the choroid and in the lacrimal gland. The most frequent infecting agent is *S. haematobium*.

An *S. mansoni* adult has been found in the anterior chamber of an eye.

There are records of uveitis and retinal haemorrhages that have been observed in patients with schistosomiasis.

Management

Systemic treatment regimens are given in Chapter 80.

Disease caused by arthropods

Myiasis

The larvae (maggots) of certain flies may cause ocular myiasis. These infestations are found in the Mediterranean region, Central America and Africa but also in temperate regions. Orbital involvement has been reported in many countries around the world.

Eye complications

External ocular myiasis can affect the eyelids, nasolacrimal ducts, lacrimal sac and conjunctiva. There is acute redness with irritation and discharge. This extremely unpleasant infection requires surgical removal of the larvae.

Internal ocular myiasis may result in uveitis, which can be severe. Usually the inflammation is due to a single larva and the prognosis is relatively good.

Orbital myiasis is often found in patients with poor personal hygiene; maggots invade the periorbital regions.

Management

External ocular myiasis requires the careful removal of the larvae after applying local anaesthetic eye drops.

Internal ocular myiasis requires treatment of any inflammation with topical therapy, including cortico-steroids. Occasionally it may be necessary to remove the larvae surgically.

Orbital myiasis requires removal of the maggots with the application of antiseptic solutions and the likely need of systemic antibiotics to deal with secondary bacterial infection.

Essential eye drugs

Table 18.23 gives details of medications routinely used in ophthalmic practice. Many of these drugs can be locally manufactured from ready-prepared materials.[47]

Glossary

Abrasion: injury to the cells lining the surface of the anterior eye, often describing superficial injury of the corneal epithelium.
Amblyopia ex anopsia: also described as a 'lazy' eye; the result of inadequate stimulus to the retina in the child, often in an eye that squints.
Anterior uveitis: inflammation of the anterior uveal tract.
Aphakia: an eye in which the lens has been removed or has dislocated.
Band keratopathy: deposition of calcium between the epithelium and Bowman's membrane across the middle and lower part of the cornea.
Bitot's spot: an often triangular foam-like plaque on the bulbar conjunctiva associated with vitamin A deficiency.
Blepharitis: inflammation of the eyelids.
Blepharospasm: tonic contraction of the eyelids.
Bowman's membrane: the interface between the corneal epithelium and the corneal stroma.
Buphthalmos: congenital glaucoma ('ox eye').
Cataract: opacity in the lens of the eye.
Chalazion: a cyst in the region of the meibomian glands of the eyelid.
Chemosis: oedema of the conjunctiva.
Chlamydia: the genus of micro-organisms that includes those causing trachoma.

Table 18.23 Essential eye drugs* (after ref. 47).

Topical antimicrobial agents	Antibiotic† Antiherpetic† Pan antiinfective†	0.5% Chloramphenicol eye drops 0.1% Idoxuridine eye drops 5% Povidone-iodine 1% Tetracycline eye ointment (enriched with polymyxin B) This last, being an ointment, has to be purchased in bulk
Local anaesthetic	Topical†	0.5% Amethocaine hydrochloride eye drops
Mydriatic	Diagnostic† Therapeutic†	1% Cyclopentolate hydrochloride 1% Atropine sulphate
Topical steroids	Weak† Normal† Strong†	0.1% Prednisolone 0.5% Prednisolone 1.0% Prednisolone
Corneal stain		Fluorescein paper strips
Subconjunctival drugs	Antibiotic Steroid Mydriatics	Gentamicin 40 mg/ml Hydrocortisone succinate 100 mg ampoule Methyl prednisolone 40 mg/ml (Depo-prep) Atropine sulphate 1 mg/ml Adrenaline hydrochloride 1/1000
Oral agents		Tab. Acetazolamide 250 mg Tab. Predinisolone 5 mg Tab./Amp. Vitamin A 200 000 iu Tab. Ivermectin (in areas where onchocerciasis occurs)

*Many of these can be locally made and are already in use by some National Prevention of Blindness programmes.
†These drops can be locally prepared from raw materials.

Choroiditis: inflammation of the choroid.

Choroidoretinitis: inflammation of the choroid and retina.

Climatic keratopathy (solar keratopathy, Labrador keratopathy): corneal changes and opacities caused by excessive exposure to ultraviolet light.

Cobblestones: a descriptive term used for the papillae of the tarsal conjunctiva found in vernal (spring) catarrh.

Conjunctivitis: inflammation of the conjunctiva.

Corneal anaesthesia: loss of corneal sensitivity.

Corneal grafting: the surgical technique used to replace a centrally scarred cornea with a donor graft.

Corneal stroma: the main thickness of the cornea (9/10) between Bowman's and Descemet's membranes.

Cryotherapy: treatment by freezing.

Cycloplegia: paralysis of the ciliary muscle of the eye.

Dacryocystectomy: surgical removal of the lacrimal sac.

Dacryocystitis: inflammation of the lacrimal sac.

Dacryocystorhinostomy (DCR): surgery to create a new opening from the lacrimal sac into the nose to allow tears to drain into the nose.

Dendritic ulcer: the typical appearance of a primary corneal ulcer caused by the herpes simplex virus.

Descemet's membrane: the membrane in the cornea between the stroma and the corneal endothelium.

Ectasia: outward bulge of thinned tissue.

Ectropion: outward turning of the eyelid.

Endophthalmitis: extensive inflammation inside the eye.

Entropion: inward turning of the eyelid.

Enucleation: removal of the eyeball, most often as a surgical procedure.

Epilation: removal of an eyelash.

Epiphora: overflow of tears.

Episcleritis: inflammation of the episclera.

Evert: turning inside out; for example, turning the upper eyelid to examine the tarsal conjunctiva.

Evisceration: removal of the contents of the eye by curettage, leaving the sclera, optic nerve and extraocular muscles.

Extraocular: outside the eye.

Facial nerve palsy: paralysis of the facial (seventh cranial) nerve.

Filtration angle: the region between the base of the iris and the cornea where aqueous fluid drains through the trabecular meshwork.

Fluorescein: a dye used topically on the surface of the eye to stain an area of corneal ulceration. The dye is also used by injection to view vascular and other abnormalities of the retina and choroid (fluorescein angiography).

Follicles: small yellow/white lumps on the conjunctiva which vary from 0.2 to 2 mm in diameter. Histologically they consist of lymphoid tissue.

Foreign body: usually a tiny fragment causing eye injury; it may be metal, dust, wood, stone, etc.

Gonioscopy: examination of the filtration angle of the anterior chamber of the eye with a contact lens (gonioscope).

Goniotomy: a surgical procedure with a goniotomy knife used in congenital glaucoma.

Gram stain: a stain used to identify organisms, both bacteria and fungi, microscopically.

Halo: a diffuse circle of rainbow-like colours around a light when corneal oedema is present.

Hypermetropia: long sight.

Hyphaema: blood in the anterior chamber of the eye.

Hypopyon: pus in the anterior chamber of the eye.

Hypotony: low intraocular pressure.

Intumescent: swollen; often used to describe an enlarged hypermature cataractous lens.

Iridocyclitis: inflammation of the iris and the ciliary body.

Keratic precipitates (KP): clumps of cells and/or pigment on the corneal endothelium due to inflammation of the iris and possibly ciliary body.

Keratitis: inflammation of the cornea.

Keratoconjunctivitis: inflammation of the cornea and the conjunctiva.

Keratoconjunctivitis sicca: dry eyes due to a reduced and abnormal precorneal tear film.

Keratomalacia: destructive melting of the cornea associated with vitamin A deficiency.

Keratomycosis: fungal infection of the cornea.

Lacrimation: secretion and flow of tears.

Lagophthalmos: inability to close the eyelids; may be associated with facial nerve paralysis, e.g., in leprosy.

Laser iridotomy: the creation of a hole in the iris using the laser.

Lens-induced uveitis: inflammation of the uvea due to leakage of protein through the lens capsule.

Leucoma: a white scar of the cornea.

Madarosis: loss of eyebrow hair and/or eyelashes.

Mazzotti reaction: systemic reaction following the use of diethylcarbamazine and suramin for onchocerciasis.

Miosis: constriction of the pupil.

Molluscum contagiosum: a virus-induced small papilloma.

Mydriasis: dilatation of the pupil.

Myopia: short sight.

Night blindness: poor vision at night.

Nodulectomy: surgical removal of nodules (onchocercomas) in onchocerciasis.

Onchocercomas: nodules formed by the encapsulated mass of adult worms in onchocerciasis.

Ophthalmia neonatorum: infection of a newborn child's eyes within 30 days of birth.

Optical iridectomy: surgical enlargement of the pupil to improve vision.

Optic neuritis: inflammation of the optic nerve.

Orbit: the bony skeleton (part of the skull) which contains the eye and extraocular muscles, nerves, blood vessels and fat.

Pannus: a superficial fibrovascular membrane of the upper cornea, associated with trachoma.

Panretinal photocoagulation: multiple small burns of the retina with the laser photocoagulator; commonly used for proliferative diabetic retinopathy.

Papilloedema: oedema of the optic nerve head.

Peripheral anterior synechiae (PAS): inflammatory adhesions in the angle of the anterior chamber of the eye.

Peripheral iridectomy: the surgical removal of a small piece of peripheral iris.

Phacolytic glaucoma: raised intraocular pressure due to macrophages and lens protein blocking the filtration angle, often associated with hypermature cataract.

Phlycten: a microabscess, usually at the corneoscleral margin, often associated with an allergic reaction to the tubercle bacillus.

Photophobia: fear (dislike) of light.

Phthisis bulbi: shrunken eye.

Pinguecula: fatty deposit on the bulbar conjunctiva.

Pin-hole disc: a tiny aperture or multiple apertures in a card or plastic disc; used to assess visual acuity.

Posterior synechiae: inflammatory adhesions between the pupil margin and the anterior surface of the lens.

Proptosis: forward displacement of the eye.

Pseudoexfoliation: the accumulation of white particles within the anterior segment of the eye, collecting on the anterior lens capsule, pupillary margin, ciliary body and zonule.

Pterygium: fleshy growth which grows across the cornea from the conjunctiva and subconjunctiva.

Ptosis: drooping of the eyelid.

Refractive error: a variation from the accepted normal optics of an eye, usually corrected by suitable spectacles.

Retinoblastoma: a malignant tumour of the retina found in young children.

Rhodopsin (visual purple): a substance required by the rods of the retina to allow some vision at night.

Schiotz tonometer: an instrument designed to measure intraocular pressure.

Scleritis: inflammation of the sclera.

Sclerosing keratitis: scarring of the peripheral cornea in association with inflammation.

Snellen 'E' chart: a standard chart to measure visual acuity.

Staphyloma: outward bulge of the cornea or the sclera with the uvea adherent behind.

Stye: infection at or near an eyelash follicle.

Subconjunctival haemorrhage: bleeding under the conjunctiva.

Subluxated: partial dislocation, usually describing a lens which is out of position.

Tarsal conjunctiva: conjunctiva lining the inner surface of the eyelids.

Tarsorrhaphy: stitching together of the eyelids, usually partial and often a temporary measure.

Trabecular meshwork: a connective tissue network in the angle of the anterior chamber through which the aqueous fluid drains out of the eye.

Trabeculectomy: a surgical filtering procedure, usually for open angle glaucoma.

Trabeculotomy: a surgical procedure for congenital glaucoma.

Trachoma: eye infection caused by the micro-organism *Chlamydia trachomatis*.

Traditional eye medicines (TEM): medicines used by traditional healers in developing countries.

Trichiasis: eyelashes turning inwards and scratching the external surface of the eyeball.

Vernal catarrh (spring catarrh): a type of allergic conjunctivitis.

Visual acuity: the measurement of vision.

Xerophthalmia: 'dry eye'; used to describe the eye changes associated with vitamin A deficiency.

Xerosis: dryness of the surface of the eye, often associated with vitamin A deficiency.

Acknowledgements

The author is very grateful to Professor Gordon Johnson and Ms Sue Stevens, who reviewed the original manuscript for the 20th edition. Review articles from the *Journal of Community Eye Health*, for which publication the author is editor, have provided abundant material and resources—which have been very much appreciated (please see references). An authoritative source on parasites and the eye, *Ophthalmic Parasitology* by B. H. Kean, Tsieh Sun and Robert M. Ellsworth (Igaku-Shoin), is the standard text in the field to which the author constantly referred for that section of the chapter.

I am particularly thankful to Mrs Anita Shah, Mr Andrew McGavin and Ms Caroline McGavin who typed the script, made excellent suggestions and coped admirably with many rethinks and changes as the text was brought up to date.

The original references for the 20th edition were compiled by Ms Susan M. Stevens RGN RM OND FETC.

REFERENCES

1 Foster A. World distribution of blindness. *J Commun Eye Health* 1988; 1:2–3.

2 World Health Organization. *The World Health Report 1998. Life in the 21st century: A vision for All*. Geneva: WHO, 1998.

3 Minassian D C & Mehra V. 3.8 million blinded by cataract each year: projections from the first epidemiological study of incidence of cataract blindness in India. *Br J Ophthalmol* 1990; 74:341–343.

4 Thylefors B. A Global initiative for the elimination of avoidable blindness. *J Commun Eye Health* 1998; 11:1–3.

5 Foster A & Johnson G J. Treatable blindness. *Trop Doc* 1988; 18:112–115.

6 Chatterjee A, Milton R C & Thyle S. Prevalence and aetiology of cataract in Punjab. *Br J Ophthalmol* 1982; 66:35–42.

7 Leske M C, Chylack L T & Wu S Y. The Lens Opacities Case–Control Study Group. The lens opacities case–control study: risk factors for cataract. *Arch Ophthalmol* 1991; 109:244–251.

8 Wright R E. The possible influence of solar radiation on the production of cataract in certain districts of Southern India: a preliminary investigation. *Indian J Med Res* 1937; 24:917–920.

9 Taylor H R, West S K, Rosenthal F S et al. Effect of ultraviolet radiation on cataract formation. *N Engl J Med* 1988; 319:1429–1433.

10 Bochow T W, West S K, Azar A, Munoz B, Sommer A & Taylor H R. Ultraviolet light exposure and risk of posterior subcapsular cataracts. *Arch Ophthalmol* 1989; 107:369–372.

11 West S K. Cataract: a challenge for public health ophthalmology. *J Commun Eye Health* 1992; 5:1–2.

12 Lewallen S & Courtright P. Recognizing and reducing barriers to cataract surgery. *J Commun Eye Health* 2000; 13:20–21.

13 Thylefors B & Negrel A-D. The global impact of glaucoma. *Bull World Health Organ* 1994; 72:323–326.

14 Cook J A. Trachoma and the SAFE strategy. *J Commun Eye Health* 1999; 12:49–51.

15 West S K. Azithromycin for control of trachoma. *J Commun Eye Health* 1999; 12:55–56.

16 Reacher M H, Huber M J E, Camarearathnam R & Alehassany A. A trial of surgery for trichiasis of the upper lid from trachoma. *Br J Ophthalmol* 1990; 74:109–113.

17 King H & Rewers M. Diabetes in adults is not a third world problem. *Bull World Heath Organ* 1991; 69:643–648.

18 McLaren D S & Frigg M. *Sight and Life Manual on Vitamin A Deficiency Disorders (VADD)*, 2nd edn. Basel: Task Force Sight and Life, 2001.

19 McLaren D S. Vitamin A deficiency disorders (VADD): new name, challenge and opportunity. *Global Prevention of Blindness Rev* (in press).

20 Thylefors B. Onchocerciasis: impact of interventions. *J Commun Eye Health* 2001; 14:17–19.

21 Etya'ale D. Vision 2020: update on onchocerciasis. *J Commun Eye Health* 2001; 14:19–21.

22 Bird A C. Age-related macular disease: aetiology and clinical management. *J Commun Eye Health* 1999; 12:8–9.

23 Johnson G J. Update on ocular leprosy. *J Commun Eye Health* 2001; 14:25–26.

24 Hogeweg M. Leprosy and the eye. *J Commun Eye Health* 1989; 2:2–5.

25 Courtright P. Recommendations of a workshop on ocular leprosy. *J Commun Eye Health* 2001; 14:26.

26 Wright E & Foster A. Suppurative keratitis: a blinding corneal infection. *J Commun Eye Health* 1988; 2:5–7.

27 Coupland R. Antipersonnel mines: why a ban? *J Commun Eye Health* 1997; 10:33–35.

28 Jackson H. Severe ocular trauma due to landmines and other weapons in Cambodia. *J Commun Eye Health* 1997; 10:37–39.

29 Gilbert C. Childhood blindness due to landmines. *J Commun Eye Health* 1997; 10:40.

30 Gray R H, Johnson G J & Freedman A. Climatic droplet keratopathy. *Surv Ophthalmol* 1992; 36:241–253.

31 Bourne R R, Dolin P J, Mtanda A T, Plant G T & Mohamed A A. Epidemic optic neuropathy in primary school children in Dar es Salaam, Tanzania. *Br J Ophthalmol* 1998; 82:232–234.

32 Hedges T R, Hirano M, Tucker K & Caballero B. Epidemic optic and peripheral neuropathy in Cuba: a unique geopolitical public health problem. *Surv Ophthalmol* 1997; 41:341–353.

33 Gilbert C. Childhood blindness: major causes and strategies for prevention. *Global Prevention of Blindness Rev* (in press).

34 Klauss V. Newborn conjunctivitis (ophthalmia neonatorum). *J Commun Eye Health* 1988; 1:2–4.

35 Hungerford J. Retinoblastoma. *J Commun Eye Health* 1990; 3:2–6.

36 Chana H S. Traditional eye medicine in Zimbabwe. *J Commun Eye Health* 1989; 2:10.

37 Sandford-Smith J. Is there still a place for intracapsular cataract extraction or should it be relegated to the history books? *J Commun Eye Health* 2000; 13:62.

38 Ager L. Optical services for visually impaired children. *J Commun Eye Health* 1998; 11:38–40.

39 Holden B A, Sulaiman S & Knox K. The challenge of providing spectacles in the developing world. *J Commun Eye Health* 2000; 13:9–10.

40 Foster A & Sommer A. Corneal ulceration, measles, and childhood blindness in Tanzania. *Br J Ophthalmol* 1987; 71:331–343.

41 Kestelyn P. HIV/AIDS and the eye. Slides/Text Teaching Series. London: International Centre for Eye Health, 2001.

42 Braley A E & Hamilton H E. Central serous choroidosis associated with amebiasis: a record of 9 cases. *Arch Ophthalmol* 1957; 58:1–14.

43 King R E, Praeger D L & Hallett J W. Amebic choroidosis. *Arch Ophthalmol* 1964; 72:16–22.

44 Kean B H, Sun T & Ellsworth R M. *Ophthalmic Parasitology*. New York: Igaku-Shoin, 1991.

45 Choudry A R. Thelaziasis. *Am J Ophthalmol* 1969; 67:773–774.

46 Verma A K. Ocular dracontiasis. *Int Surg* 1968; 50:508–509.

47 Taylor J. Appropriate eye drugs for developing countries. *J Commun Eye Health* 1991; 4:2–6.

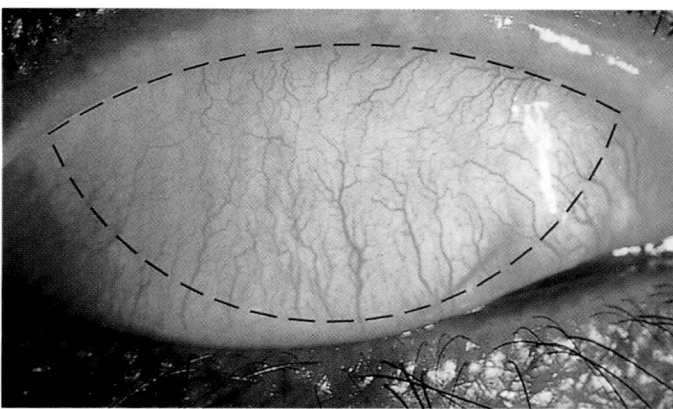

Plate 18.10: Normal upper eyelid. (The area to be examined for inflammatory changes is outlined.) (Courtesy of *Journal of Community Eye Health*, International Centre for Eye Health, Institute of Ophthalmology, London.)

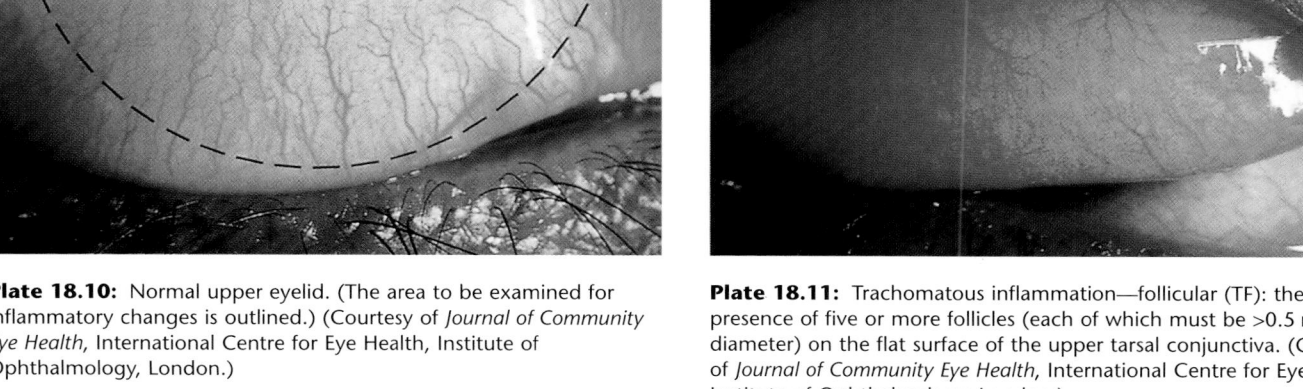

Plate 18.11: Trachomatous inflammation—follicular (TF): the presence of five or more follicles (each of which must be >0.5 mm diameter) on the flat surface of the upper tarsal conjunctiva. (Courtesy of *Journal of Community Eye Health*, International Centre for Eye Health, Institute of Ophthalmology, London.)

Plate 18.12: Trachomatous inflammation—intense (TI): marked inflammatory thickening of the upper tarsal conjunctiva; this obscures more than half the normal deep tarsal vessels. (Courtesy of *Journal of Community Eye Health*, International Centre for Eye Health, Institute of Ophthalmology, London.)

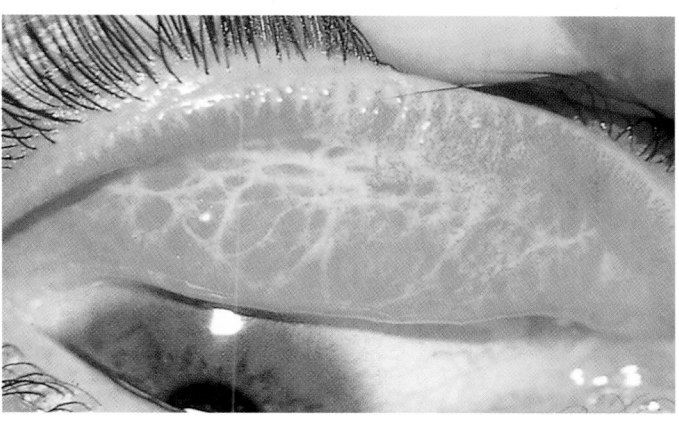

Plate 18.13: Trachomatous scarring (TS): involving the tarsal conjunctiva. (Courtesy of *Journal of Community Eye Health*, International Centre for Eye Health, Institute of Ophthalmology, London.)

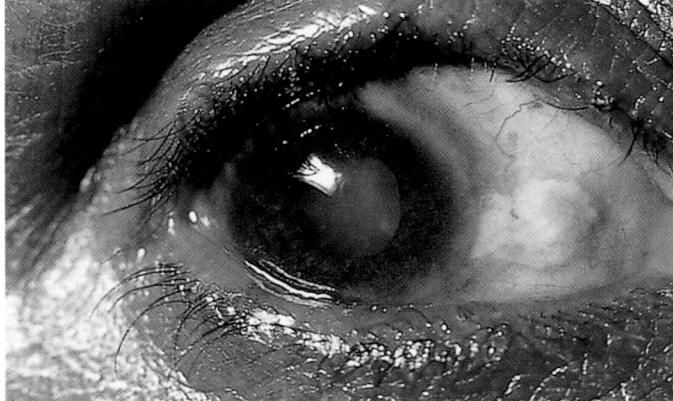

Plate 18.14: Trachomatous trichiasis (TT): evidence of one or more eyelashes rubbing on the eyeball. If one or a number of eyelashes have recently been removed, this should be graded trachomatous trichiasis. (Courtesy of *Journal of Community Eye Health*, International Centre for Eye Health, Institute of Ophthalmology, London.)

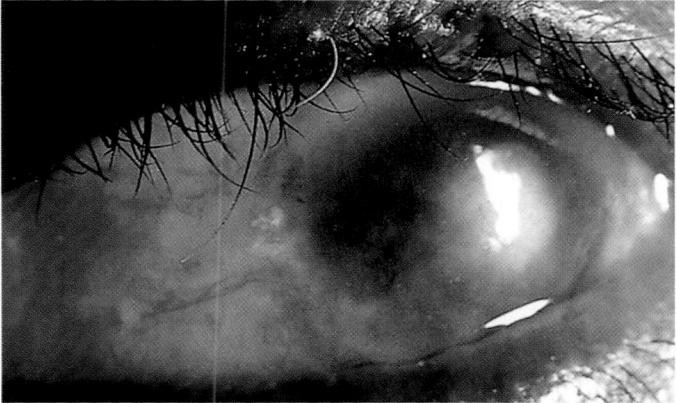

Plate 18.15: Corneal opacity (CO): corneal scarring due to trachoma where the scarring is central and sufficiently dense to obscure part of the pupil. (Courtesy of *Journal of Community Eye Health*, International Centre for Eye Health, Institute of Ophthalmology, London.)

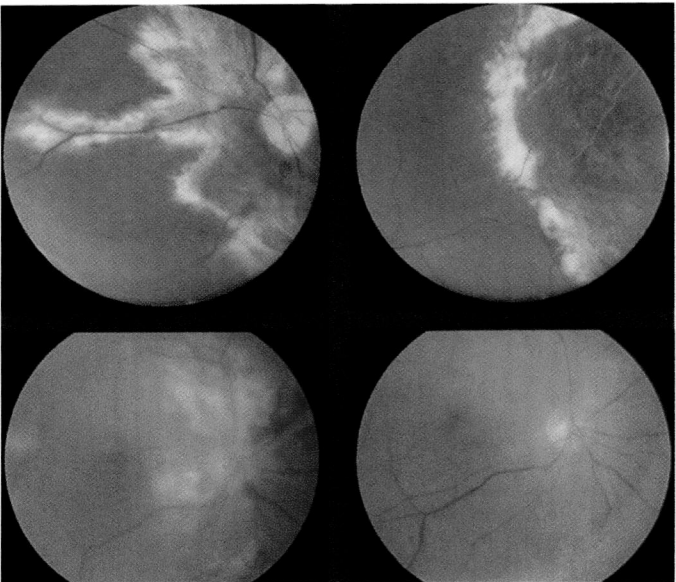

Plate 18.33: AIDS and cytomegalovirus (CMV) retinitis. Photos: Philippe Kestelyn.

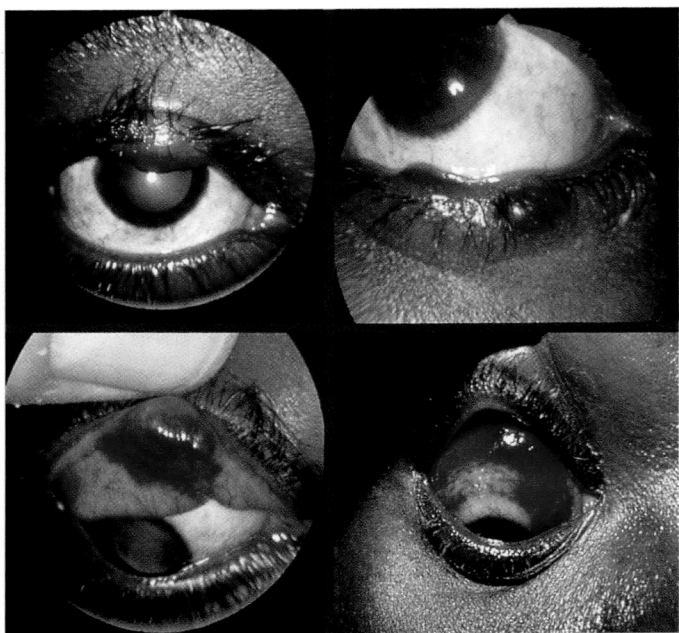

Plate 18.34: HIV/AIDS and tumours: Kaposi's sarcoma. Photos: Philippe Kestelyn.

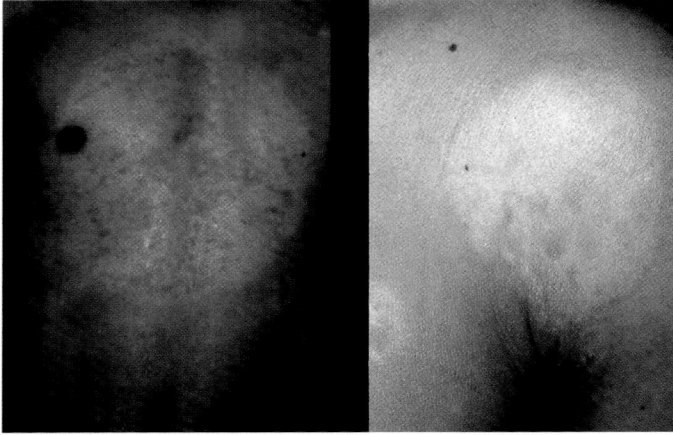

Plate 19.6: Circumscribed patches of hypopigmented truncal skin in 'mal del pinto'. (Courtesy of Professor Amado Saúl, Mexico.)

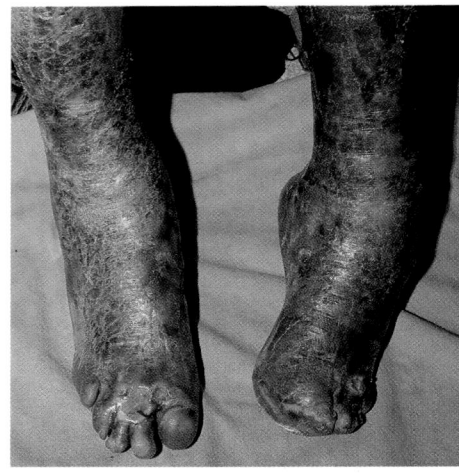

Plate 19.8: Pigmentary atrophic changes of the skin and mutilation in severe bilateral leprosy neuropathy.

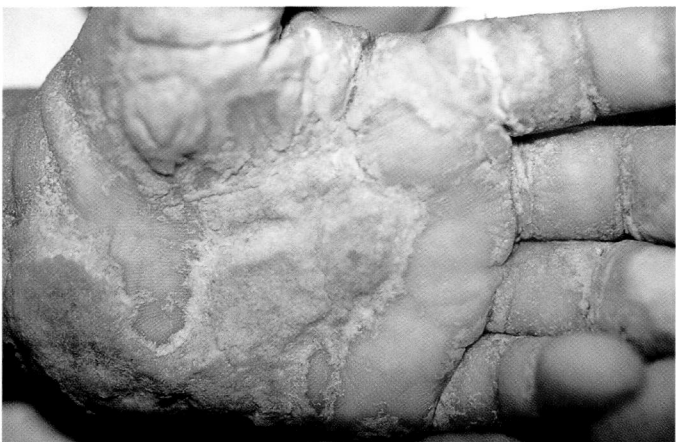

Plate 19.19: Disseminated crusted scabies in an immunodeficient child. (Courtesy of Dr Edmundo Velázquez, Mexico.)

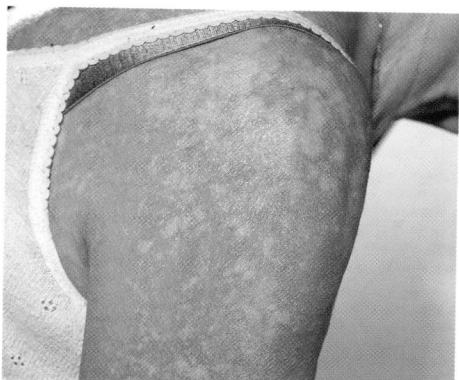

Plate 19.27: Hypo- and hyperpigmented small coalescing patches of pityriasis versicolor.

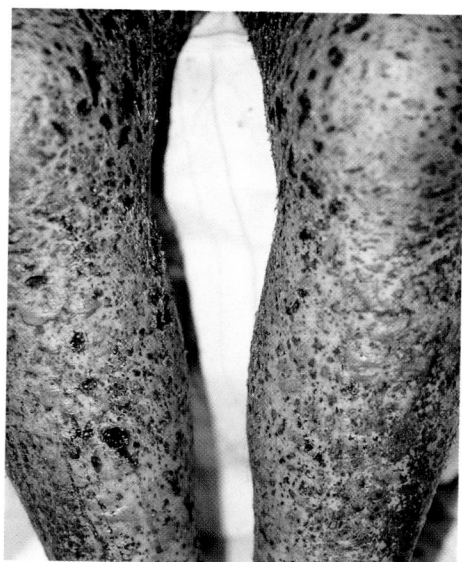

Plate 19.32: Disseminated blistering and crusting in a case of varicella infection.

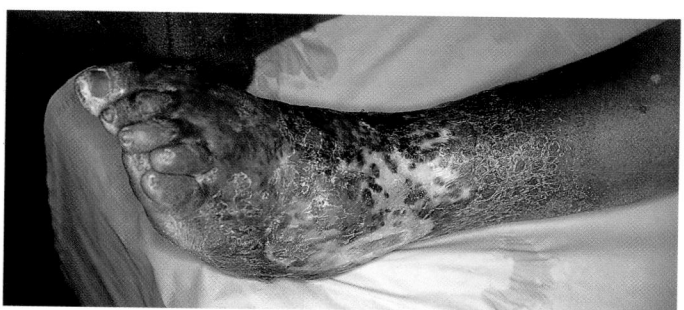

Plate 19.28: Deformity, atrophy, sinus tract formation, scarring and pigment disorder in fungal mycetoma.

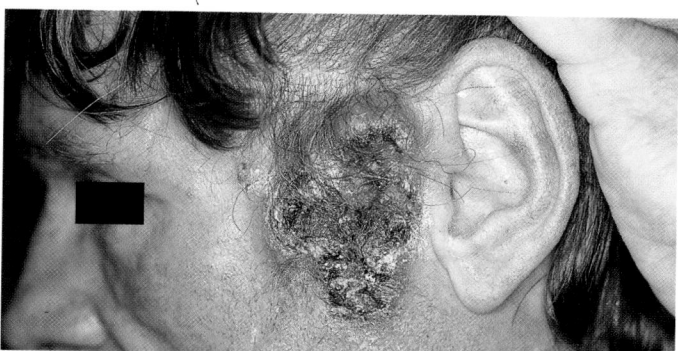

Plate 19.37: Ulcerated and exophytic large squamous cell carcinoma in a Caucasian patient with AIDS.

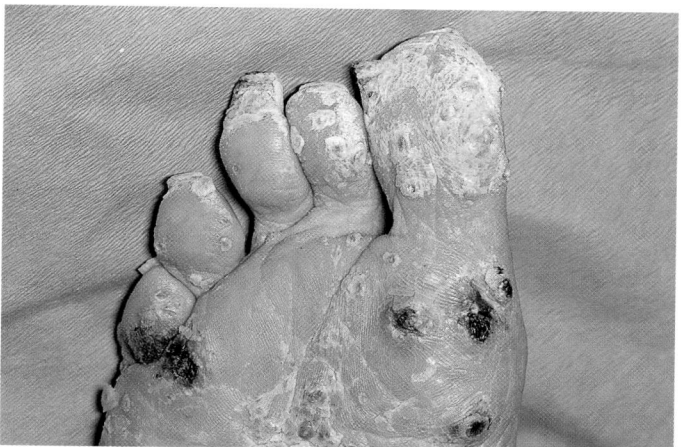

Plate 19.31: Hyperkeratotic, verrucous, ulcerated and crusted lesions on the feet in a patient with paracoccidioidomycosis.

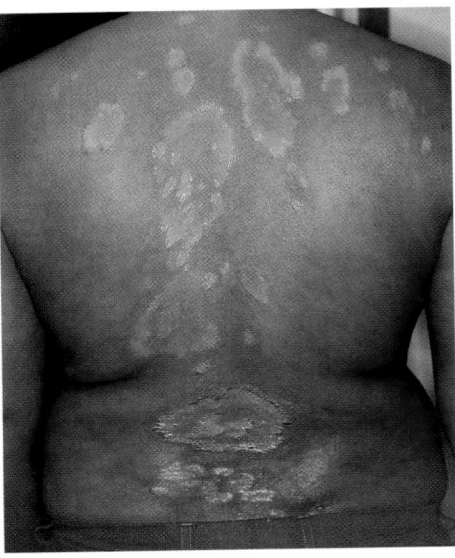

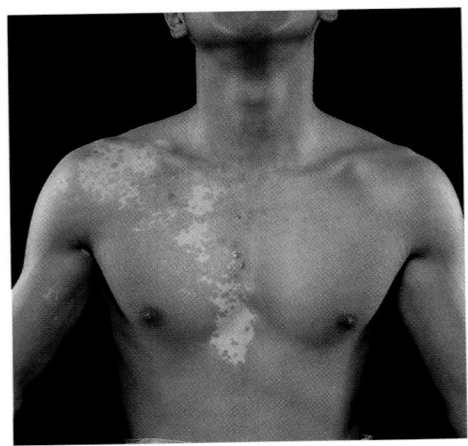

Plate 19.54: Segmental hypopigmentation of trunkal vitiligo.

Plate 19.41: Circumscribed plaques of erythema, thickening and scale in plaque psoriasis.

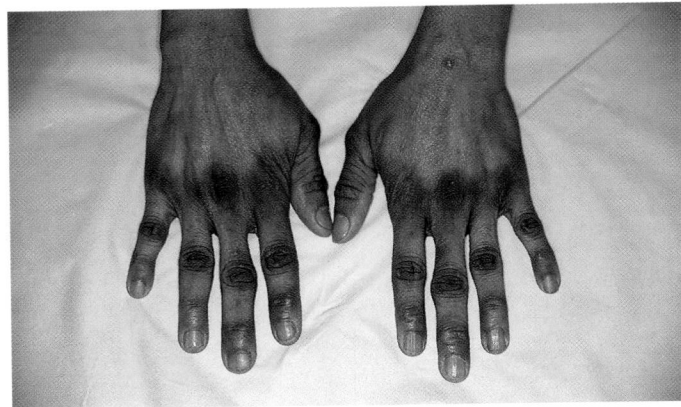

Plate 19.51: Pruritic plaque of lichen amyloid on the shin.

Plate 19.55: Postinflammatory hyperpigmentation of the hands in a patient with atopic eczema.

Chapter 19
Dermatological Problems

F. Vega-López and S. Chopra

Introduction

Skin diseases are highly prevalent in the general population and represent one of the main causes of consultation for the general practitioner and other members of the health team. In tropical regions of the world this high prevalence is in sharp contrast with the paucity or absence of specialist services. Moreover, the undergraduate medical curriculum is quite poor in both the quality and quantity of contents dedicated to dermatology in many universities around not only the tropical, but also the developed world. Patient care and education in dermatology should consequently become priorities for those involved in leadership and policy-making.

Poverty and disability are two main characteristics of the individual patient and the community affected by skin disease in the tropics. A number of quantitative and qualitative epidemiological studies as well as individual observations by clinicians support the aetiological role of

poverty in skin conditions such as fungal diseases, leprosy, scabies and impetigo. The vicious circle is closed as chronic or recurrent skin disease results in further disability and loss of economic activity. Clear examples of this complex problem are overtly manifest in those individuals suffering from superficial pyogenic infections, cutaneous leishmaniasis, leprosy, scabies and fungal diseases, amongst others.

Skin infectious and tropical diseases may present as a primary condition or as a secondary manifestation of illness elsewhere in the body. Madura foot, cutaneous larva migrans and localized cutaneous simple leishmaniasis are examples of the former, whereas the latter can be exemplified by systemic conditions such as leprosy, disseminated leishmaniasis secondary to kala azar, and coccidioidomycosis. The clinical approach to a patient with skin tropical disease involves a thorough exercise in history-taking that leads to establishing a morphological and topographical diagnosis. The identification of primary and secondary elementary skin lesions as well as

Table 19.1 Skin lesions and symptoms suggesting a variety of diagnoses.

Clinical features	Working diagnosis
Itchy papules in clusters	Arthropod bites
Asymptomatic palmoplantar papules	Syphilis
Single ulcerated nodule on exposed skin	Cutaneous leishmaniasis
Asymptomatic chronic verrucous plaque	Tuberculosis or chromoblastomycosis
Dysautonomic changes and ulceration	Leprosy
Hyper/hypopigmented patch/plaques with atrophy and ulceration	Leprosy
Erythematous or hypopigmented plaques or nodules with peripheral neuropathy	Leprosy
Excoriated papules and burrows	Scabies
Ulcerated nodule and lymphangitis	Sporotrichosis or cutaneous leishmaniasis
Chronic scarring and sinus tracts	Mycetoma
Itchy serpiginous track	Cutaneous larva migrans
Haemorrhagic eschar, rash and fever	Tick typhus, Lyme disease
Pruritic lichenification, nodules and dyschromic changes	Onchocerciasis
Recurrent swellings	Loa loa or gnathostomiasis
Patchy alopecia and boggy inflammation	Scalp ringworm
Acute urticaria, fever and abdominal pain	Acute schistosomiasis (Katayama fever)
Painful, pruritic, plantar blisters	Acute tinea pedis or acute eczema
Furunculoid painful lesions	Myasis
Erythema, or urticaria, or exfoliative skin lesions with/without mucosal involvement	Drug reactions

the anatomical region affected score high in terms of diagnostic sensitivity and specificity. Table 19.1 shows examples of lesions and symptoms that suggest or establish a particular diagnosis in clinical practice.

The dermatological history must include detailed information on previous skin disease, travel history, activities while travelling, occupation, drugs, duration of signs and symptoms, evolution of clinical signs, symptoms in relatives or household contacts, wild or domestic animal contacts, and a fast practical assessment of the patient's immune status. The identification of extracutaneous signs such as fever, enlarged lymph nodes, hepatosplenomegaly and general malaise indicates systemic illness and these findings should prompt immediate action for further investigations or an appropriate referral. Particular epidemiological settings in the tropics determine exposure and attack rates from specific diseases and, hence, an in-depth understanding of the global geographical pathology and living conditions of the overseas population is required in the practice of tropical dermatology.

Table 19.2 summarizes the main outpatient dermatological problems diagnosed in a Latin American hospital. The main differences found in tropical dermatology when compared to the practice of this speciality in northern European hospitals are a higher incidence of endemic infectious diseases, a lower frequency of skin malignancy, and the lack or decreased availability of dermatological services.

Our specialized clinic in 'Tropical Dermatology and Skin Infections' was established in 1997 at the Hospital for Tropical Diseases in London and provides a clinical service for travellers as well as for individuals with HIV/AIDS-related skin conditions. Our experience from this tertiary centre indicates that 75% of the total of referrals present with a skin condition related to a travelling event. Most patients are travellers returning from the Caribbean, Latin America, India, South-East Asia, northern, central and eastern Africa, but cases returning from other tropical regions are also well represented. A third of our cases travel to the tropics for professional or

Table 19.2 Common dermatological problems at the National Medical Center, IMSS, Mexico City, 1993–2001.

Eczema (acute, chronic, contact, atopic, others)
Psoriasis
Pyogenic infections
Pemphigus
Dermatophyte infections
Benign tumours
Lupus erythematosus
Viral infections
Drug reactions
Leprosy
Other fungal diseases
Leg ulcers
Malignant tumours
HIV-related skin conditions

Table 19.3 Frequency of tropical skin conditions in 1857 travellers referred to the Hospital for Tropical Diseases in London.

Pyogenic infections	24%
Eczema and eczematization	17%
Urticaria	11%
Arthropod bites and bite reactions	9%
Dermatophyte and other fungal infections	9%
Cutaneous larva migrans	7%
Leishmaniasis, schistosomiasis, onchocerciasis	6%
Pruritus, scabies, prurigo and other	17%

family reasons. The relative frequencies and most common diagnoses in a case series of travellers referred to our clinic are presented in Table 19.3.

This chapter presents a description of the most relevant conditions in tropical dermatology grouped by aetiological agents, with an emphasis on the clinical findings and diagnosis, to provide a practical guide for everyday work. Pathogenesis of disease and management of conditions have also been included, and the chapter concludes with a brief description of non-infectious skin conditions that are relevant in tropical medicine.

Skin diseases caused by bacteria
Pyogenic infections

Aetiology and pathogenesis

Common skin bacterial infections in the tropics are caused by *Staphylococcus* and *Streptococcus* species. These infectious agents are ubiquitous in both urban as well as rural environments and are capable of causing disease in all age groups. Healthy and immunocompromised hosts develop pyogenic infections of the skin following direct inoculation of bacteria. Less often haematogenous dissemination and even a septicaemic state may develop as a result of a minor skin injury. The port of entry for these pathogenic organisms is often unnoticed by both the patient and doctor, but minor injuries, insect bites, friction blisters or superficial fungal infection are the commonest found in clinical practice. Other clinical circumstances such as burns, use of indwelling catheters in children and minor surgical procedures also play a role as risk factors for these infections.

Pyogenic bacteria cause damage in the infected tissue by the pathogenic action of proteases, haemolysins, lipoteichoic acid and coagulases. Erythrogenic toxins are responsible for the erythema commonly observed in infections by *Streptococcus* species.[1]

Clinical findings and diagnosis

The clinical spectrum of skin pyogenic infections includes folliculitis, furuncle and carbuncle formation on areas with hair follicles. Plaques of impetigo (Figure 19.1) and infiltrated thickened dermis commonly affect the lower limbs (Figure 19.2) and are respectively caused by *Staphylococcus* and *Streptococcus* species. Abscess formation, cellulitis and necrotic ulceration represent the more severe end of the spectrum.

By far, the perimalleolar regions are more commonly affected than other areas of the lower limb as they are exposed to mechanical trauma; however, other common pyogenic infections may present on the upper limbs, face (Figure 19.3) and trunk. Common clinical signs of pyogenic infections include a variety of manifestations such as erythema, inflammation, pus discharge, abscess formation, ulceration, blistering, necrotizing lesions and gangrene. Severe scarring may result from pyogenic ulcers caused by friction injury or else in cases of ecthyma (Figure 19.4). Most pyogenic skin infections are painful and the diagnosis is based on the clinical history and findings. Bacteriological investigations and sensitivity profile to antibiotics must be carried out if available. Disseminated, chronic or severe infections require an immediate referral

to a dermatologist or to an infectious disease specialist. Uncommon cases of streptococcal infection of the throat may express clinically with a sudden eruption of guttate psoriasis as a result of bacterial superantigen stimulation.

Management

Mild infections are successfully treated with bathing or soaking of the affected skin in potassium permanganate solution (1:10 000 dilution in water) for 20 minutes daily. Other mild superficial infections like isolated plaques of impetigo or impetiginized eczema respond well to antiseptic or antimicrobial creams and ointments containing cetrimide, chlorhexidine, fucidic acid or mupirocin. Acute or chronic eczema requires treatment with potent topical steroids in order to eliminate risk factors for infection. Infections with multiple lesions or those involving larger areas of the skin require a complete course of systemic β-lactam or macrolide antibiotics in addition to the above topical treatments. Recurrent episodes of cellulitis require longer courses of these

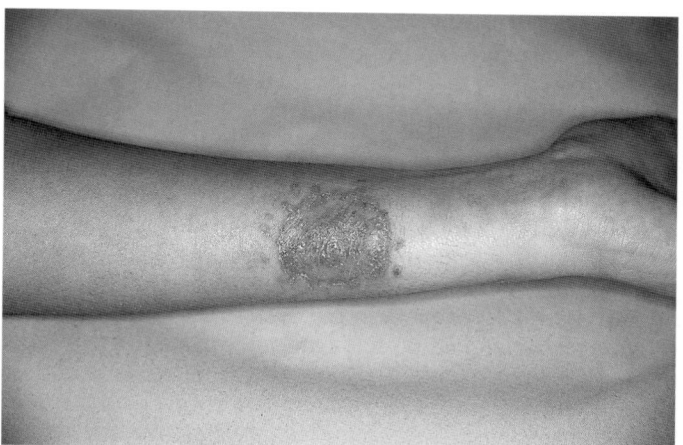

Figure 19.1: Erythematous plaque of superficial impetigo with satellite lesions.

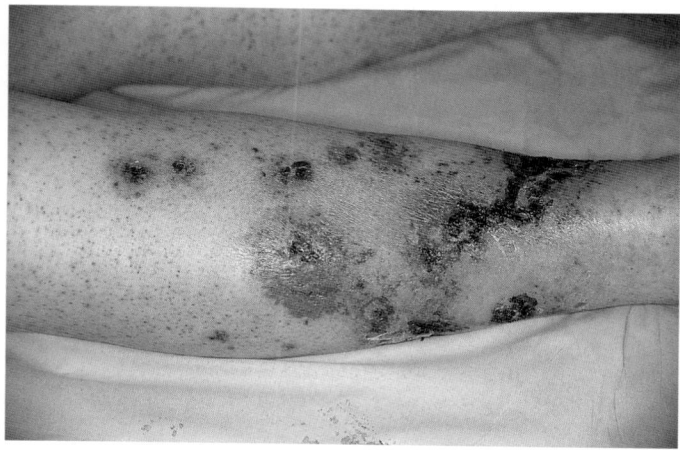

Figure 19.2: Pyogenic superficial lesions with purpuric plaques of cellulitis and proximal dissemination.

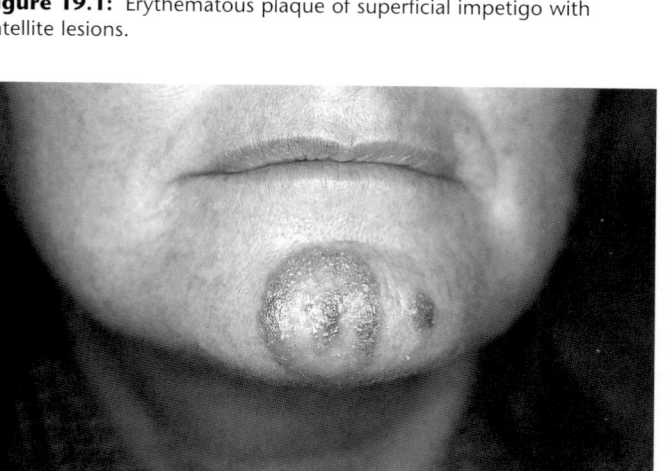

Figure 19.3: Circular plaque of staphylococcal pustular impetigo on the chin with satellite lesions.

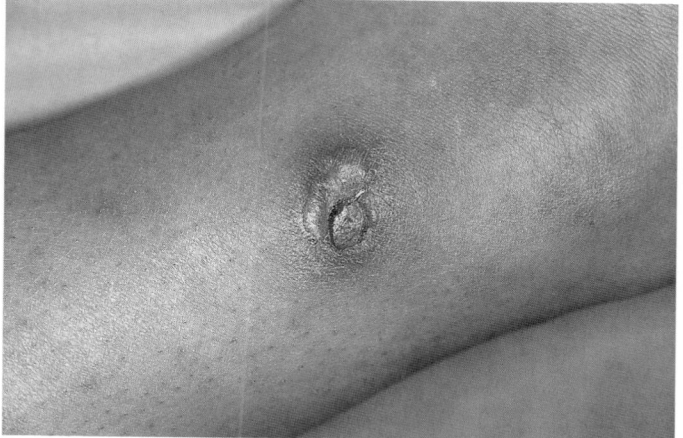

Figure 19.4: Localized ecthyma with surrounding cellulitis on the lower limb.

antibiotics, and hospitalization followed by surgical debridement is mandatory in necrotic lesions, gangrenous plaques and deeper infections with severe fasciitis. Superficial infections of the foot skin complicated by deeper involvement with necrosis of soft tissues carry a high mortality rate up to 25%.[2]

Treponemal infections

Cosmopolitan treponemal diseases such as secondary *syphilis* present with an asymptomatic, symmetrical papular eruption and scaling of palmoplantar regions. Other clinical features such as the history of a primary chancre, the characteristic truncal rash or the presence of gummata (Figure 19.5) confirm the clinical suspicion. A definitive diagnosis can be established by specific tests such as positive dark-field microscopy from early skin lesions, as well as from highly sensitive treponemal serology.[3] Despite the fact that syphilis is not strictly a tropical disease, it represents a significant problem for the returning traveller involved in high-risk sexual activities while in the tropics.[4] The treatment of choice is penicillin but allergic individuals respond to erythromycin or tetracyclines.

Yaws is a treponemal tropical disease manifesting on the feet and periorificial skin on the face. This condition affects mainly the male rural population in South America, sub-Saharan Africa and South-East Asia. This disease is associated with poverty in the humid tropics[5] and one of the characteristic clinical presentations is that of plantar hyperkeratosis. Late tertiary infection results in asymptomatic palmoplantar keratoderma that develops nodular

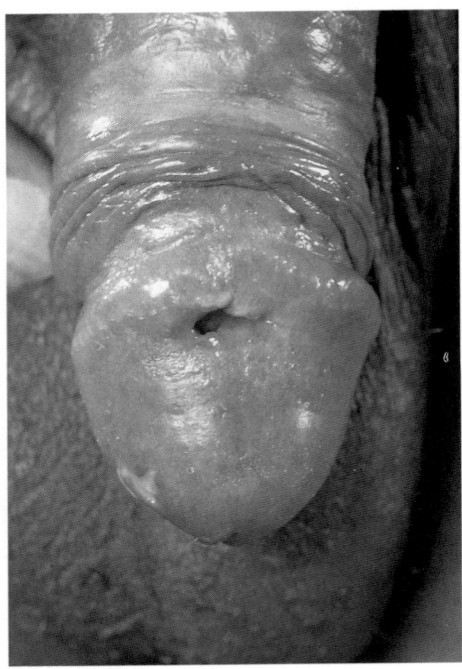

Figure 19.5: Asymptomatic exudative gummata of the penis in syphilis.

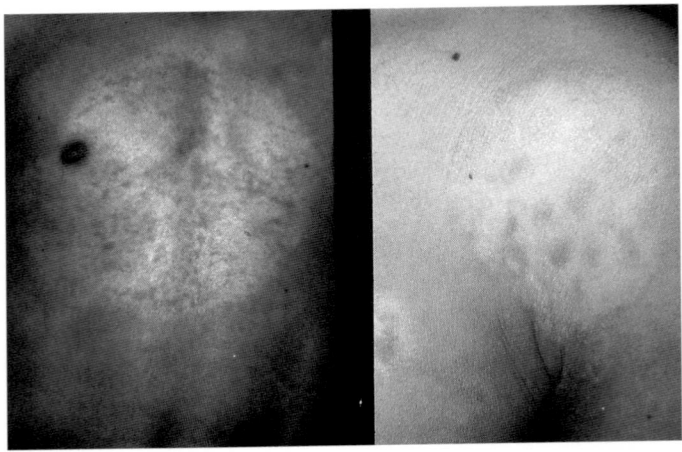

Figure 19.6: Circumscribed patches of hypopigmented truncal skin in 'mal del pinto'.

hyperkeratotic lesions leading to painful disability; hence the characteristic walk known as 'crab yaws'. The clinical picture can be difficult to differentiate from other types of infectious and non-infectious plantar keratodermas. Tests for diagnosis include dark-field microscopy of early lesions and treponemal serology. The treatment of choice is penicillin but *Treponema pallidum pertenue* also responds to tetracyclines and macrolides.

Pinta or *mal del pinto* is caused by *T. carateum* and cases have been mainly reported from Philippines, Mexico, and Colombia, where children and young adults are the main victims. Clinically it presents with a papular eruption or more commonly with progressive dyschromic patches and plantar keratoderma. Asymmetrical hypo- and hyperpigmented lesions affect the limbs, trunk (Figure 19.6), neck and face. Late hypopigmented lesions or frank leukoderma with geometrical patterns manifest on the elbows, wrists or other areas subject to trauma. Treponemal organisms can be found in the early dyschromic lesions and cross-reactive positive serology is very helpful in establishing the diagnosis. Benzyl-penicillin is the treatment of choice.

Mycobacterial infections

Aetiology and pathogenesis

A number of mycobacterial species can cause primary or secondary infection of the skin. The 'swimming' or 'fish tank granuloma' is an infection caused by *Mycobacterium marinum*. Other common chronic mycobacterial tropical infections include leprosy, tuberculosis and Buruli ulcer. These are respectively caused by *M. leprae*, *M. tuberculosis* and *M. ulcerans*. Other opportunistic mycobacteria can cause clinical disease in the immunocompromised host. Such is the case for infections by *M. avium-intracellulare*, *M. chelonae* and *M. kansasii*. Mycobacterial skin diseases can be acquired by direct skin contact with a patient, by direct accidental or occupational inoculation and by inhalation of the infective organisms. Particular clinical forms of cutaneous tuberculosis result following haematogenous dissemination from a primary infection elsewhere. The respiratory route is particularly important for leprosy and diverse forms of pulmonary tuberculosis. In the case of Buruli ulcer it has recently been suggested that contact with infected water in rural areas of Africa may represent the main source of infection. A toxin called mycolactone seems to be responsible for the severe tissue destruction and ulceration seen in patients with Buruli ulcer.[6] In general, however, it is accepted that agents causing mycobacterial skin diseases have a low pathogenic potential as most infected individuals in endemic regions do not suffer from overt clinical mycobacterial diseases.

Mycobacteria are very complex organisms, most of them ubiquitous in nature as saprophytes, but a number of species cause disease in other animals. A very thick wall surrounds the cytoplasmic membrane of mycobacteria and contains virulence factors such as proteins and glycolipids. Mycobacteria can inhibit an efficient phagocytosis and intracellular killing by macrophages and also interact with the host's immune cells. This interaction results in chronic inflammation, tissue damage and immunopathology, all of which account for the signs and symptoms observed in the wide range of mycobacterial diseases.

Clinical findings and diagnosis

The *fish tank granuloma* affects more commonly the fingers or hand dorsum but it has also been described on the foot and other anatomical sites. *M. marinum* frequently infects freshwater fish and, hence, individuals handling fish tanks represent the main population at risk.[7] The disease manifests as a localized progressing swelling with variable pain, and the appearance, within a few weeks, of nodular or verrucous skin lesions on the affected area (Figure 19.7). These lesions can show ulceration and bleeding from the disease process itself but also from mechanical trauma. The nodular lesions

measuring a few millimetres up to 2 or 3 cm may resolve spontaneously after a few months, but they can also disseminate proximally by haematogenous or lymphatic spread. The dorsal aspects of the hand, foot and the malleolar regions are exposed to trauma and therefore direct inoculation commonly takes place on these regions. Once the condition is suspected, microbiological and histopathological investigations represent the most sensitive tests to confirm the clinical diagnosis.

Leprosy is a chronic disease that affects not only the skin but particularly the peripheral nerves bilaterally. The hands and feet are the anatomical sites where inflammation and nerve damage occur in the course of leprosy. The commonest skin lesions are nodules, erythematous plaques or hypopigmented patches. Symptoms like hypo- or dysaesthesia, together with motor/sensitive nerve abnormalities and obvious thickening of peripheral nerve branches, suggest the characteristic demyelinating neuropathy of leprosy. Advanced disease manifests with skin atrophy, pigmentary changes, and in severe cases chronic ulceration leading to mutilation and disability (Figure 19.8). Mutilating lesions of the hands and feet result from bone resorption, mechanical trauma and secondary bacterial infection.

The clinical diagnosis of leprosy can be easily established in most cases that occur in endemic regions of the world.[8] Epidemiological, clinical, histopathological, bacteriological and immunological criteria have been used for many years to diagnose and classify the cases of leprosy within a disease spectrum. This spectrum considers two polar groups or forms, called tuberculoid and lepromatous, as well as intermediate forms of the disease defined as

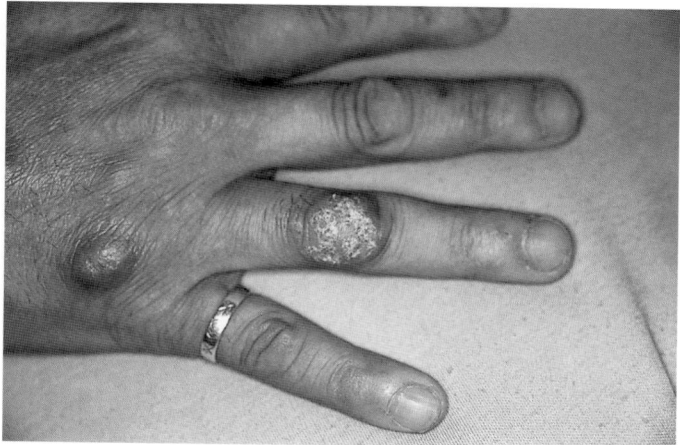

Figure 19.7: Nodular verrucous violaceous lesions with proximal dissemination caused by *Mycobacterium marinum*.

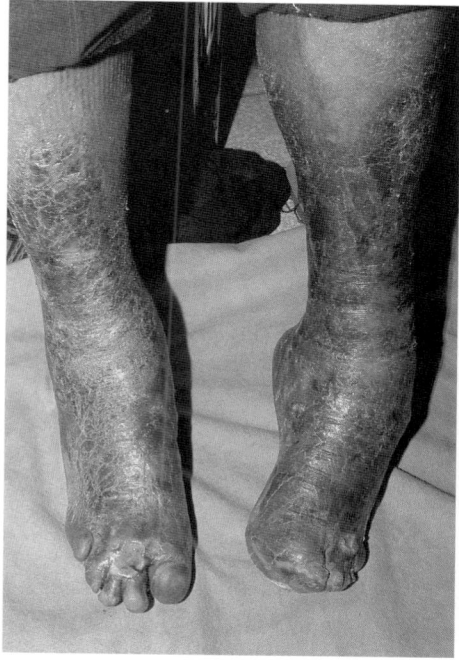

Figure 19.8: Pigmentary atrophic changes of the skin and mutilation in severe bilateral leprosy neuropathy.

borderline. Early disease may not present characteristics of any of the above groups and such cases are called indeterminate. The evolution of leprosy is a dynamic process and a significant number of cases cannot be easily classified at the time of diagnosis. All patients require long-term follow-up as their place within the spectrum involves not only therapeutic but, most importantly, prognostic implications. Patients with early disease and particularly those presenting to the travel specialist in non-endemic countries for leprosy often pose diagnostic difficulties. The delay in establishing an accurate diagnosis and treatment inevitably results in irreversible nerve damage and chronic complications with variable degrees of disability.

Skin tuberculosis affects individuals of all ages and both sexes presenting with a variety of clinical pictures that frequently affect the lower limbs and particularly one or both feet.[9] However, lupus vulgaris and papulo-necrotic tuberculide are more common in females, whereas tuberculosis verrucosa cutis is rare in children. By far the main clinical presentation of cutaneous tuberculosis affecting the adult foot is called tuberculosis verrucosa cutis, whereas cases of lupus vulgaris are commonly observed on the face. The tuberculous bacilli cause disease following direct inoculation into the skin but clinical disease can also result from haematogenous dissemination. Unilateral and asymmetrical involvement is the rule in almost the totality of cases with skin tuberculosis. Commonly observed asymptomatic lesions include dry patches of atrophic skin, pigmentary changes, nodules and plaques of verrucous lesions (Figure 19.9). The typical plaque of tuberculosis can measure between 2 and 12 cm in diameter, but chronic and larger lesions can involve most of the foot dorsum and lateral aspects. The course of cutaneous tuberculosis is indolent and chronic, but determines skin atrophy and scarring with a consequent degree of local skin insufficiency. The clinical diagnosis can be confirmed by histopathology,

bacteriology and polymerase chain reaction (PCR) investigations.

Buruli ulcer affects mainly young individuals in rural Africa and particularly in West Africa, where an increase in incidence has been reported.[6] More than two-thirds of the total of cases present in children below age 15. The initial lesions present as papules or small nodules that slowly increase in size to the point of causing an area of inflammation and subsequently ulceration of the skin. The ulcer characteristically presents with undermined edges and manifests as active indolent phagedenism often involving large areas of the affected limb. A single ulcer or else smaller coalescing ulcers present more frequently on the lower leg above the ankles but other regions of the foot can be involved as well. Oedematous forms may progress rapidly and cause a panniculitis with destruction of underlying tissues such as fascia and bone. In cases where a large ulceration is followed by healing, contractures of the affected limb result from scarring. Severe scarring and contractures have been identified as a high morbidity factor for disability and up to 10% of them require amputation of the deformed limb.[10]

Mycobacterial diseases in the immunocompromised host include infections by *M. avium-intracellulare*, *M. chelonae* and *M.kansasii* amongst others. Patients with AIDS, advanced diabetes mellitus, transplant recipients or cases with severe kidney failure are at particular risk for these infections. Clinically they manifest as symmetrical or asymmetrical asymptomatic papules, nodules (Figure 19.10), cold abscess, ulcerating or scarring lesions. The picture can be monomorphic; however, polymorphic chronic eruptions are not uncommon. Proximal

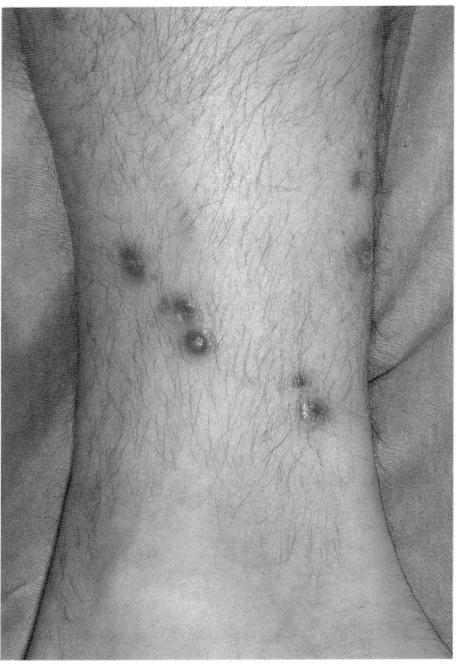

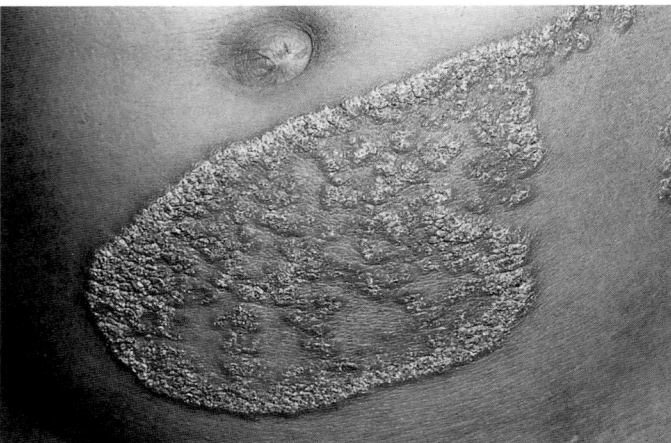

Figure 19.9: Circumscribed large verrucous plaque with erythematous islets in chronic tuberculosis verrucosa cutis. (Courtesy of Professor Amado Saúl, Mexico.)

Figure 19.10: Erythematous papules, nodules, and scarring caused by MAIS complex infection in a patient with AIDS.

dissemination on a limb is quite a characteristic feature and once the diagnosis is clinically suspected the histopathological investigation reveals abundant intracellular and extracellular acid-fast bacilli in the dermis of lesional skin with a poorly organized granulomatous inflammation and necrosis. A positive culture is more frequently successful than in the case of other mycobacterial infections such as tuberculosis or fish tank granuloma.

Management of mycobacterial infections

All mycobacterial diseases require highly specialized diagnostic investigations that in many cases can only be carried out in a tertiary hospital setting. Most mycobacterial diseases affecting the skin represent public health priorities not only for the endemic countries where they occur, but also at an international level as established by the WHO. Following the diagnosis of individual cases a long-term multi-drug therapeutic regimen can be prescribed only by specialized physicians. Mycobacteria are known to develop resistance to antibiotics and it is imperative that all cases are treated with combinations of at least two drugs. The main drugs with antimycobacterial activity are rifampin, ethambutol, pirazinamide, clofazimine, sulfone, isoniazide, macrolide antibiotics, tetracyclines and quinolones. Established combinations for particular infections are routinely administered according to international and local guidelines. The management of all mycobacterial diseases must consider not only the medical treatment but also a full range of educational initiatives aimed at the patient, the community and health personnel. Early lesions of fish tank granuloma, skin tuberculosis and particularly those caused by Buruli ulcer require surgical excision.

Bacterial mycetoma

Aetiology and pathogenesis

Nocardia, *Actinomadura* and *Streptomyces* species are the common aetiological agents of 'Madura foot' or actinomycetoma. This form of mycetoma occurs in tropical countries and the main case series have been reported from Sudan, Senegal, Nigeria, Saudi Arabia, India and Mexico. The infection is acquired by direct inoculation of bacteria into the skin and does not seem to represent a risk for travellers. Young male individuals living in endemic regions and dedicated to agricultural activities have been reported with the highest incidence of actinomycetoma.[11] Bacteria causing actinomycetoma have a thick wall surrounding the cytoplasmic membrane which is rich in lipid and carbohydrate compounds. Some of these compounds such as lipoarabinomannan and mycolic acids have been identified as virulence factors. These bacteria are capable of blocking the adequate killing mechanisms by the cells of the infected host; however, it is considered that they have a low pathogenic potential and most of them live as saprophytes in the soil.

Clinical findings and diagnosis

The clinical disease is characterized by a chronic course with inflammation, formation of sinus tracts discharging 'grains' and progressive deformity of the affected foot. Healing of discharging sinus tracts throughout years determines scarring with atrophic skin plaques and secondary pigmentary changes. Asymptomatic nodular or verrucous lesions can also be found and in a few cases a variable range of symptoms is present. These include pain that often results from superimposed pyogenic infection, acute inflammation and bone involvement. The chronic infection with deformity of the foot determines periosteal involvement and subsequently osteomyelitis. Variable but often severe degrees of disability complete the chronic course of actinomycetoma (Figure 19.11). The clinical picture manifested on one foot is highly suggestive of the diagnosis. The main differential diagnosis includes mycetoma caused by fungi (see 'Eumycetoma' below) but other forms of 'cold abscess' formation, histoplasmosis, chromoblastomycosis, cutaneous tuberculosis and sarcoidosis are the other main conditions to consider. Direct microscopy to disclose the 'grains' discharged from sinus tracts confirms the diagnosis and the culture of this material also provides a definite diagnosis of actinomycetoma.

Management

Effective drugs against the agents of bacterial mycetoma include streptomycin, dapsone and trimethoprim/sulfamethoxasol.[12] Recently, a report revealed efficacy with a combination of cefotaxime, amikacin and

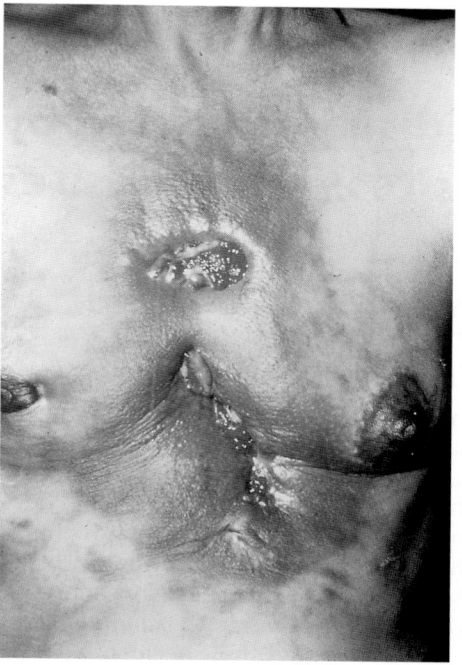

Figure 19.11: Sinus tract formation and severe scarring in chest actinomycetoma. (Courtesy of Dr Ruben López, Mexico.)

immunomodulators.[13] The treatment for mycetoma has to be administered for several months and the therapeutic response is variable. Early cases with small single lesions can be cured by surgical excision. In contrast, advanced cases with periosteal involvement and those with osteomyelitis do not respond to medical treatment and radical surgery of the foot represents the only therapeutic option.

Other bacterial infections

Tropical *seaborne infections* by halophilic *Vibrio vulnificus* can produce localized or systemic disease manifested by acute and painful erythema, purpura, oedema and necrosis, particularly affecting the lower limbs. Cases of returning travellers presenting in inland metropolitan areas can be very difficult to diagnose and these patients carry a high mortality risk. Fatal septicaemia manifests with coalescing purpuric patches on one or both lower limbs that subsequently spread to the periumbilical region. The infection is acquired by direct traumatic inoculation in estuaries and seawater, or by ingestion of raw seafood, particularly oysters. Male individuals with a history of liver disease and iron overload states are the group at highest risk for this infection.[14] Severe cases require immediate referral to a specialist hospital physician as intravenous antibiotics and early surgical debridement represent the treatment of choice.

Exfoliation of the face, truncal and palmoplantar skin is part of the complex and severe picture in cosmopolitan cases with *staphylococcal scalded skin syndrome* (SSSS),[15] whereas necrotic ulceration on a limb can result from tropical *cutaneous diphtheria* caused by *Corynebacterium diphtheriae*.[16] Cutaneous diphtheria commonly manifests as a non-healing single ulcerated lesion on the toe or toe cleft lasting between 4 and 12 weeks.

Skin diseases caused by parasites, ectoparasites and bites

Cutaneous larva migrans

Aetiology and pathogenesis

This dermatosis results from the accidental penetration of the human skin by parasitic larvae from domestic canine, bovine and feline hosts. Animals pass ova of these helminths with the stools and larval stages develop in the soil or beach sand. A close contact with human skin allows the infective larvae to burrow into the epidermis and cause clinical disease. The main aetiological agents are *Ancylostoma brasiliense*, *A. caninum*, *A. ceylanicum* and *A. stenocephalae* but other species affecting ruminants and pigs can also cause human disease. Following penetration into the skin, the larvae are incapable of

crossing the human epidermodermal barrier and stay in the epidermis creeping across spongiotic vesicles until they die a few days or weeks later. Multiple infections can, however, last for several months. Cases of systemic invasion with a Loeffler's syndrome have been exceptionally described.

Clinical findings and diagnosis

The plantar regions of one or both feet represent the main anatomical site affected by cutaneous larva migrans (Figure 19.12), but any part of the body in contact with infested soil or sand can be involved. Individuals of all age groups and both sexes can be affected and the disease is a common problem for tourists on beach holidays where they walk on bare feet or lay naked on the infested sand. A report of 44 cases presenting in returning travellers attending our specialized clinic in London revealed that 70% of the lesions were located on one foot, but the buttocks were also commonly affected.[17] The initial lesion is a pruriginous papule at the site of penetration that appears within a day following the infestation. An erythematous, raised larval track measuring 1–3 mm in width and height starts progressing in a curved or looped fashion. New segments of larval track reveal that the organism can advance at a speed of 2–5 cm daily. Commonly, the larval track measures between a few millimetres up to several centimetres in the region adjacent to the penetration site, but uncommon cases may present long larval tracks surrounding large areas of the foot with a well-defined perimalleolar distribution. Localized clinical pictures on the toes may present with only papular lesions but other presentations include eczematous plaques, blisters and urticarial wheals. Secondary complications to the presence of the parasite in the epidermis include an inflammatory reaction, eczematization, impetiginized tracks or papules and even deeper pyogenic infections. Variable in severity, but most commonly intense pruritus and burning sensation, are the main symptoms.

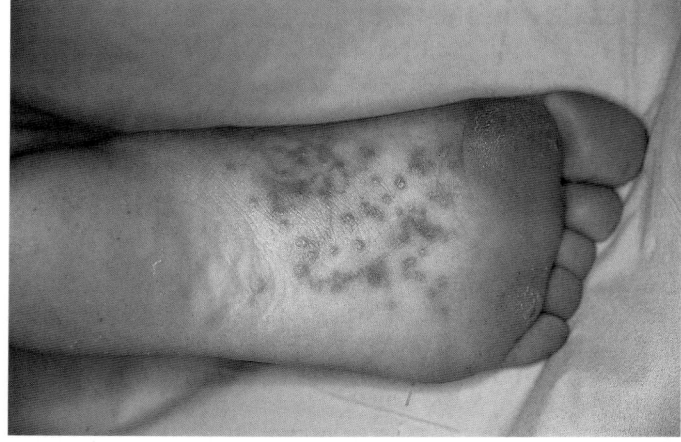

Figure 19.12: Erythematous larval track and papulovesicular eruption in unilateral cutaneous larva migrans of the plantar region.

The diagnosis is based on the clinical history and physical findings on the affected skin. The histopathological investigation has little if any value in the diagnosis of cutaneous larva migrans. The study of 332 cases in central Mexico throughout 10 years in the 1980s (Orozco, personal communication, 1993) revealed that HE preparations of affected skin show a spongiotic acute or subacute dermatitis with a variable presence of larval structures. A mild perivascular lymphocytic infiltrate was frequently observed in the dermis and a low proportion of cases may develop peripheral eosinophilia but this is not a constant finding.

Management

The treatment of choice is the oral administration of albendazol for 3 days. Topical options include a 10% thiabendazol cream applied several times daily for 10 days, and one or more sessions of cryotherapy with liquid nitrogen. Resistant cases may respond to a single oral dose of ivermectin.[18]

Leishmaniasis

Aetiology and pathogenesis

Leishmania species parasites are protozoan organisms transmitted to humans and other vertebrates by the bite of female sandflies of the genera *Phlebotomus* or *Lutzomya*. Most *Leishmania* species can cause skin or mucocutaneous disease, but a few of them affect internal organs as well. It is estimated that 15 million individuals are infected by *Leishmania* in 88 countries and 1.5 million new cases of cutaneous leishmaniasis occur every year. The main endemic foci are found in Asia, the Middle East, India, Northern Africa, Southern Europe, Mediterranean basin and Latin America. A hot and humid environment such as that found in rainforest jungles provides adequate habitat for the animal reservoirs and vectors in Latin America. In contrast, desert conditions favour breeding sites for the vectors in the Middle Eastern and north African endemic regions.[19]

Following the bite from a *Leishmania*-infected sandfly the human skin can heal spontaneously or else develop localized or disseminated disease. Sandfly and *Leishmania* species causing skin disease in humans have been classified in geographical terms as Old World and New World cutaneous leishmaniasis. Both can affect one area of exposed thin skin but multiple infective bites or disseminated forms may present with lesions on several anatomical regions. Common inoculation sites include facial bone prominent regions, external aspects of wrists and malleolar regions. The bite of the sandfly commonly targets exposed areas such as the external ankles during sleep or else medial regions of the foot when the host is at rest. *Leishmania* parasites can resist phagocytosis and damage by complement proteins from the host by the action of lipophosphoglycan and glycoprotein antigens. Following phagocytosis, the intracellular forms of leishmania parasites induce a delayed type hypersensitive granulomatous reaction which adds to the tissue damage.[20]

Clinical findings and diagnosis

The bite of a sandfly may induce an inflammatory papular or nodular lesion that slowly progresses for several weeks. The incubation period can be as short as 15 days but commonly it is estimated at around 4–6 weeks. Certain forms may take longer to develop clinically. A non-healing papule with surrounding erythema and pain may also indicate superimposed bacterial infection that subsequently develops ulceration. On average 6–8 weeks after the sandfly bite a violaceous nodule starts enlargement and ulceration. The ulcer is partially or completely covered by a thick crust that following curettage reveals a haemorrhagic and vegetating bed. Cutaneous leishmaniasis can be clinically manifest as nodules covered with crust, ulceration with a raised inflamed solid border, tissue necrosis and lymphangitic forms. Advanced late forms present with scarring, skin atrophy and pigmentary changes. A particular localized form caused by *L. mexicana* or *L. braziliensis* is called 'chiclero ulcer' (Figure 19.13) and affects the helix of one ear; however, *L. braziliensis* more commonly manifests as a single destructive violaceous ulceration of the skin (Figure 19.14).

Other regions of the body surface may be affected by pigmented and hyperkeratotic lesions in patches and plaques in the clinical form named post-kala-azar dermal leishmaniasis (PKDL). This clinical form presents after an episode of visceral leishmaniasis by *L. donovani* in cases originating from India and Africa. Other common and

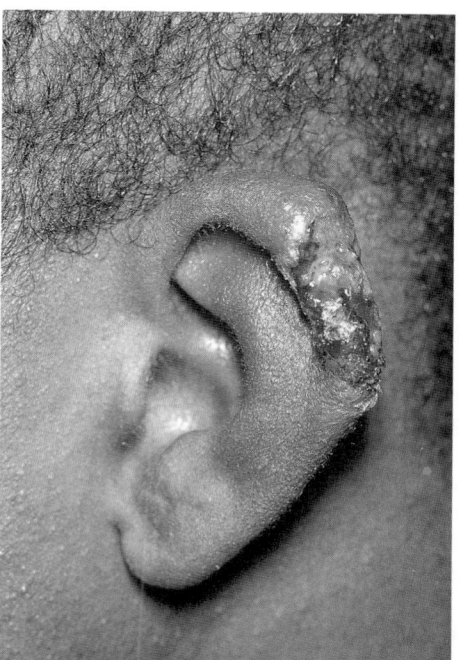

Figure 19.13: Chiclero ulcer in American cutaneous leishmaniasis by *Leishmania braziliensis*.

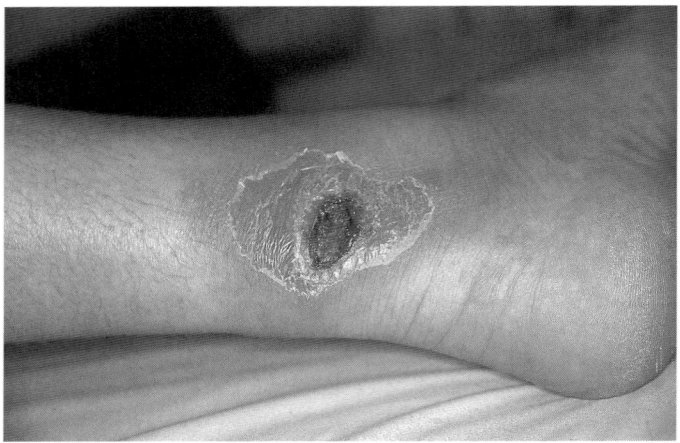

Figure 19.14: Erythemato-violaceous nodular ulceration with surrounding cellulitis by *Leishmania braziliensis*.

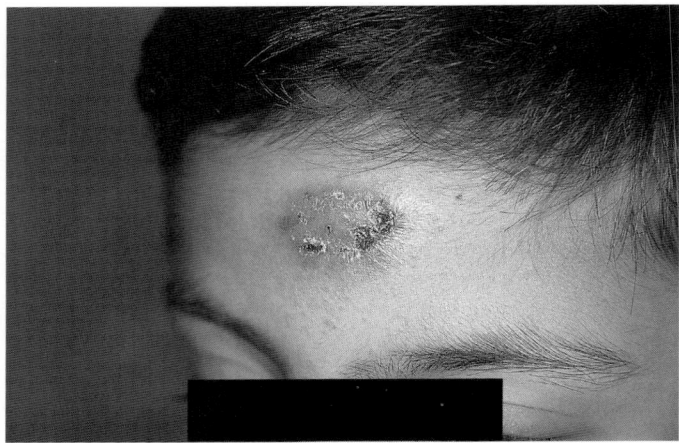

Figure 19.15: Single scarring erythematous sore with crusting in Old World leishmaniasis by *Leishmania tropica*.

characteristic clinical pictures include dry, single oriental sore by *L. tropica* (Figure 19.15), wet destructive single ulcer by *L. major*, diffuse anergic cases by *L. aethiopica* or *L. mexicana*, and cases of mucocutaneous leishmaniasis by *L. braziliensis* or *L. mexicana*.

The clinical picture of cutaneous leishmaniasis and the history of exposure in an endemic region of the world strongly suggest the diagnosis and the species involved. Complementary tests include histology of lesional skin, slit skin smears stained with Giemsa for direct microscopy, tissue samples for culture in NNN medium, and genetic analysis by PCR techniques. In our experience at the Hospital for Tropical Diseases we have found that in the context of a positive history of exposure and a typical clinical picture the sensitivity for the histopathological diagnosis with dermal granulomata is 100%.

Management

The general public and health personnel easily establish the diagnosis of cutaneous leishmaniasis in endemic areas of the world and, following referral to a physician, one or more treatment options are locally available. However, in non-endemic regions, and particularly in non-tropical countries, the returning traveller requires attention by an experienced doctor in tropical medicine, infectious diseases or dermatology. Several drugs are effective against leishmania parasites and these include pentavalent antimonials, amphotericin B, triazole and allylamine antifungal compounds. However, the only treatment of choice for a number of species is the intravenous administration of antimonials carefully monitored in hospital and administered only by experienced personnel. In our experience, a dose of 20 mg/kg body weight daily for 3 weeks has been effective to cure most of our cases with New World cutaneous leishmaniasis caused by *L. braziliensis*. Patients require long-term follow-up as leishmaniasis may relapse in some cases. Educational interventions targeting travellers planning to visit leishmania-endemic regions

must emphasize the use of protective clothing, bed nets at night and the frequent use of insect repellents, particularly between dusk and dawn. Other strategies for control and protection of the population at risk in endemic areas include reservoir surveillance, vector control and health checks of domestic animals—dogs in particular—that play a significant role as reservoirs of parasites.

Onchocerciasis

Aetiology and pathogenesis

This filarial disease is acquired through the inoculation into the skin of *Onchocerca volvulus* by black flies of the genus *Simulium*. This infection, also named 'river blindness' and 'Robles disease', is highly prevalent in Africa within latitudes 15°N and 15°S, and affects tropical countries in Central and South America. Fast-flowing brooks and small rivers provide breeding sites for the black fly vectors and only the female individuals are haematophagous. They can bite potential hosts throughout the day and principally those pursuing outdoor activities. Holiday-makers as well as those travelling for professional reasons have a risk of acquiring this parasitic disease, but it is the local population that suffers the highest toll from both clinical disease and subsequent disability.

Following an incubation period of approximately 1 year, the adult worms live freely in the skin or within fibrotic nodules or cysts named onchocercomata. The female adult worm releases microfilaria into the dermis and they are disseminated by the lymphatic system. Adult worms may live and reproduce for up to 15 years in the human host.

Clinical findings and diagnosis

The main clinical manifestations include pruritus and skin lesions with lichenified plaques, papular or prurigo

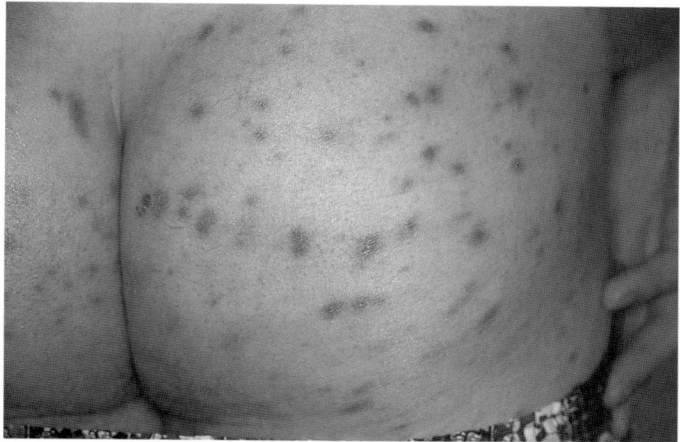
Figure 19.16: Pruritic papules and nodules on the buttocks in a patient with eosinophilia caused by onchocerciasis.

eruptions, nodules, atrophic changes and pigmentary abnormalities. Early symptoms include fever, arthralgia and transient urticaria affecting face and trunk. Pruritus and scratching lead to eczematization revealed as patches of lichenified and excoriated skin on the trunk and lower limbs. The buttocks are commonly involved (Figure 19.16) and oedematous plaques are characteristic in Latin American cases, locally named 'mal morado'. Late skin lesions show atrophy, hyper- and hypopigmented patches giving the appearance of 'leopard skin' described in African cases. The presence of filaria in the ocular anterior chamber causes acute symptoms and late ocular lesions lead to blindness.

The parasitological diagnosis includes the identification of microfilaria in samples taken from skin snips from the back, hips and thighs, specimens for histopathological investigation and serology. Most patients develop peripheral hypereosinophilia.

Management

The treatment of choice for onchocerciasis is a single dose of oral ivermectin every 6 months. The surgical excision of nodules is indicated and all patients require specialized attention in tertiary medical centres including a comprehensive ophthalmological assessment. An active programme of mass therapy for individuals living in endemic regions of the world has been in place for more than a decade and other control strategies include the rotational spraying of breeding sites with insecticides.

Gnathostomiasis

Aetiology and pathogenesis

Several *Gnathostoma* species live as adult worms in the intestine of domestic cats and humans can acquire the disease by eating contaminated fish that have ingested small crustaceans acting as intermediary hosts in this condition. The larval stages do not reach maturation in the human body; however, they are capable of causing disease in several internal organs as well as in the skin. The disease is prevalent in South-East Asia, China, Japan, Indonesia, Australia and Mexico.

Clinical findings and diagnosis

Episodes of migrating intermittent subcutaneous oedema with pruritus constitute the main clinical picture and cases can adopt a chronic protracted course for years. The trunk and proximal limbs are commonly affected. The episodes of oedema can be quite inflammatory and painful and the larvae can erupt out from the affected skin. Peripheral eosinophilia and positive serology support the clinical diagnosis.

Management

The surgical extraction of the larva from the skin results in cure.[21]

Tungiasis

Aetiology and pathogenesis

Tungiasis is a localized skin disease commonly affecting one foot and caused by the burrowing flea *Tunga penetrans*. This is also known as chigoe infestation, jigger, sandflea, chigoe and puce chique (Fr). It has been described that this flea originated in Central and South America[22] and was subsequently distributed in Africa, Madagascar, India and Pakistan. It is a very small organism as it measures ~1 mm in length and lives in the soil nearby pigsties and cattle sheds. Fecundated females require blood and their head and mouthparts penetrate the epidermis to reach the blood from the superficial dermis. After nourishment through several days eggs are laid to the exterior and the flea dies.

Clinical findings and diagnosis

These fleas commonly affect one foot, penetrating the soft skin on the toe web spaces, but other areas of toes and plantar aspects on the foot can be affected.[23] The initial burrow and the flea body can be evident in early lesions but within 3–4 weeks a crateriform single nodule develops with a central haemorrhagic punctum (Figure 19.17). Superimposed bacterial infections may be responsible for impetigo, ecthyma, cellulitis and gangrenous lesions.

The diagnosis is clinical but skin specimens for direct microscopy and histopathology with HE stain reveal structures of the flea and eggs.

Management

Curettage, cryotherapy, surgical excision, or else careful removal of the flea and eggs are the curative choices. Early treatment and avoidance of secondary infection are of the utmost importance in all infested hosts, and

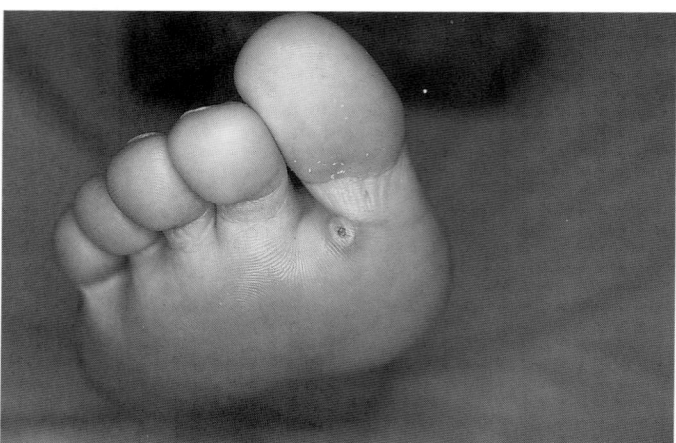

Figure 19.17: Single nodular lesion with central hemorrhage by *Tunga penetrans* acquired in Tanzania.

particularly in individuals with diabetes mellitus, leprosy or other debilitating conditions of the feet. A haemorrhagic nodule by *Tunga penetrans* may pose a diagnostic difficulty with an inflammed common wart or a malignant melanoma, but the short duration of the lesion and the history of exposure indicate the acute nature of this parasitic disease.

Myasis

Aetiology and pathogenesis

Several dipteran species in larval stages (maggots) are capable of colonizing the human skin. The infestation mechanism involves direct deposition of eggs, contamination by soil or dirty clothes, other insects acting as vectors, or else actual penetration of larvae into the skin. Drying clothes on a line can be a common target where eggs become attached and subsequently reach contact with human skin. Species of *Dermatobia* and *Cordylobia* are the commonest found in the tropics, respectively in the Americas and Africa, whereas European cases originate from *Hypoderma* species.[24] A local inflammatory reaction to the larvae with secondary infection is responsible for the signs and symptoms of disease.

Clinical findings and diagnosis

Elderly and debilitated individuals of both sexes with exposed chronic wounds or ulcers are at a higher risk of suffering from this infestation; however, most affected hosts are in good general health. Furunculoid and subcutaneous forms may affect any part of the body, but in children the scalp is a commonly affected site. Chronic ulcers of the lower legs and feet represent a predisposing factor and myasis can complicate severe infections by bacteria or fungi. Larvae feed on tissue debris and may not cause discomfort or symptoms at all; however, cases with secondary local or systemic pyogenic infections can result from myasis. Cases are observed throughout the year in tropical regions where the standards of hygiene, nutrition and general health are poor. The diagnosis is based on clinical suspicion and physical findings.

Management

The treatment of choice is the mechanical removal or surgical excision of the larvae.[24] Single furunculoid lesions can be covered by thick Vaseline or paste to suffocate the larvae, which, following death, can be subsequently extracted. Superficial infestations respond to repeated topical soaks or baths in potassium permanganate at a 1:10 000 dilution in water carried out for a few days. Cases with secondary pyogenic infection require a full course of β-lactam or macrolide antibiotics.

Scabies

Aetiology and pathogenesis

Scabies is a cosmopolitan problem but individuals in poor tropical countries with low standards of hygiene and particularly overcrowding suffer from cyclical outbreaks of severe and chronic forms. This infestation is acquired by personal direct skin contact. The human scabies mite *Sarcoptes scabiei* commonly affects the skin of both feet of infants and children. Adults rarely manifest scabies on the lower limbs below the knees (Hebra lines), but exceptional cases of crusted scabies may present with lesions on both feet. The scabies mite burrows a tunnel of up to 4 mm into the superficial layer of the epidermis, where eggs are laid. The eggs hatch and reach the stage of nymph and subsequently become an adult male or female mite. Female individuals live up to 6 weeks and lay up to 50 eggs. A new generation of fecundated females penetrates the skin in adjacent regions to the nesting burrow, but the mite infestation can also be perpetuated by clothes or by reinfestation from another host in the household.

Clinical findings and diagnosis

Papules, with or without excoriation, and S-shaped burrows are the elementary classical lesions of scabies. Infants and young children present with papular, vesicular and/or nodular lesions on both plantar regions but other parts of the feet can be affected. In contrast, adults present with bilateral lesions on fingers, finger web spaces, anterior wrists, upper limbs, anterior axillary lines, periumbilical region, external genitalia and buttocks. A high proportion of males suffer involvement on prepuce and scrotum (Figure 19.18). Patients of all age groups suffering from chronic crusted scabies may present with eczematization, impetiginized plaques and hyperkeratosis masking the typical clinical signs of this infestation. Large crusts (Figure 19.19) covering inflammatory papular lesions contain a high number of parasites and a careful examination is required to prevent health personnel from acquiring the infestation.

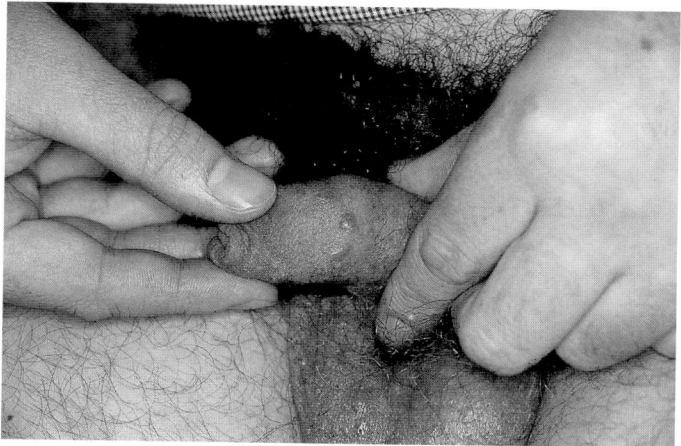

Figure 19.18: Pruritic erythematous papules of scabies on the prepuce and scrotum.

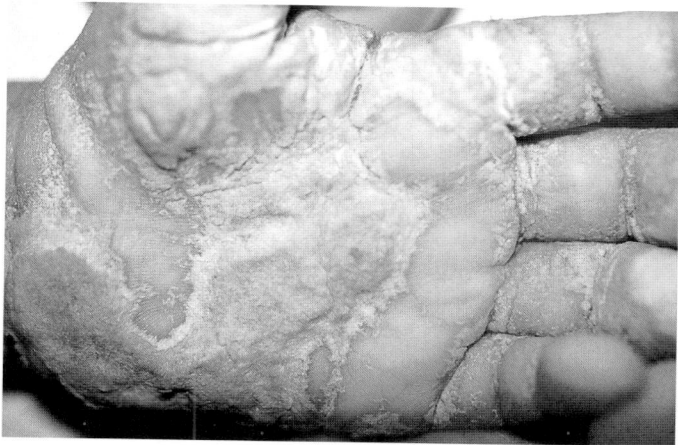

Figure 19.19: Disseminated crusted scabies in an immunodeficient child. (Courtesy of Dr Edmundo Velázquez, Mexico.)

The clinical findings and intense pruritus support the diagnosis. Confirmation is obtained by direct microscopy of skin scrapings from a burrow revealing the structures or faecal pellets of the mite. This test is carried out on a glass slide and 10–15% KOH solution under low power and has a low sensitivity if carried out by non-experienced hands.

Management

Topical treatment overnight with benzyl benzoate, malathion, lindane or permethrine, lotion or cream, is usually effective and trials have reported similar efficacy of between 65% and 80% for any of the above. A second application 10–14 days after the original treatment must be prescribed and all the affected members of a household or community require treatment at the same time to prevent cyclical reinfestations. Severe cases or individuals in particular communal settings such as homes for the elderly, orphans, prisons or psychiatric wards may require oral treatment with a single dose of ivermectin as originally described by Macotela in 1991 (personal communication). Severe outbreaks require a second dose of ivermectin at a 2-week interval (150–200 µg/kg body weight). Other therapeutic measures are directed to control the symptoms, inflammation and secondary bacterial infection. Clothes and bed-linen require washing at high temperature to kill all young fecundated females but a number of authors have demonstrated that this is not necessary, as the mites die from dehydration shortly after losing a niche on human skin. In the right epidemiological context scabies may represent a venereal disease. Pruritus may last for several weeks after cure.

Ticks

Aetiology and pathogenesis

Ticks are cosmopolitan ectoparasites capable of transmitting severe viral, rickettsial, bacterial and parasitic diseases. The transmission of infectious agents takes place at the time of taking a blood meal from a human host that becomes infested accidentaly. Soft ticks of the Argasidae family are more prevalent in the tropics and subtropical regions of the world and transmit agents of tick-borne relapsing fever. The main genera of hard ticks are *Ixodes*, *Dermacentor*, *Haemaphysalis* and *Amblyomma* and these can transmit arboviral, bacterial and rickettsial diseases.

Clinical findings and diagnosis

The bite of a tick is painful and the patient is aware of this episode. The bite produces a local inflammatory reaction suggesting initially an ordinary papular insect bite that subsequently causes localized superficial vascular damage with necrosis. The characteristic clinical picture manifested as an eschar can be easily recognized on careful physical examination (Figure 19.20). This area of circular scaling of the skin surrounding the original haemorrhagic bite can be seen after a week or 10 days. Residual chronic lesions may leave hyperpigmentated patches with a central induration.

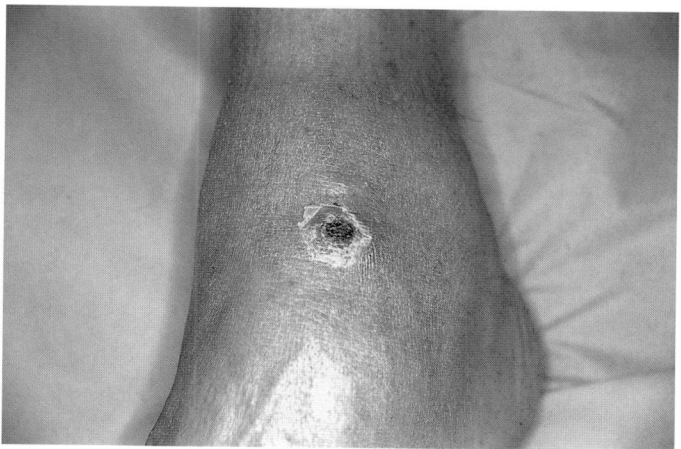

Figure 19.20: Small erythematous patch surrounding a haemorrhagic ulceration characteristic of an eschar produced by tick bite.

Management

Careful removal of the tick can be carried out by applying a tight dressing or cloth impregnated with chloroform, petrol or ether on the tick body. The organism is carefully removed a few minutes later, avoiding the rupture of head and mouth-parts, which can be left behind in the skin. A careful follow-up and self-surveillance are indicated as systemic illness may start a few days or weeks following the tick bite. Symptoms such as a fever, skin rash, lymph node enlargement, fatigue and night sweats indicate systemic disease and the patient requires referral to a hospital physician or to a specialist in tropical or travel medicine.

Fleas

Aetiology and pathogenesis

The common human flea *Pulex irritans* is cosmopolitan but a number of other species show preference for tropical climates. Such is the case of the tropical rat flea *Xenopsylla cheopis*. Fleas bite humans in order to obtain a blood meal and in doing so produce a localized inflammatory reaction. History of exposure can reveal an individual host or family members recently moving house or acquiring a second-hand piece of wooden furniture where fleas can live for months without taking blood meals.

Clinical findings and diagnosis

A clinical picture of prurigo with papules, vesicles or small nodules on both feet and lower legs is characteristic and the lesions are often found in clusters (Figure 19.21).

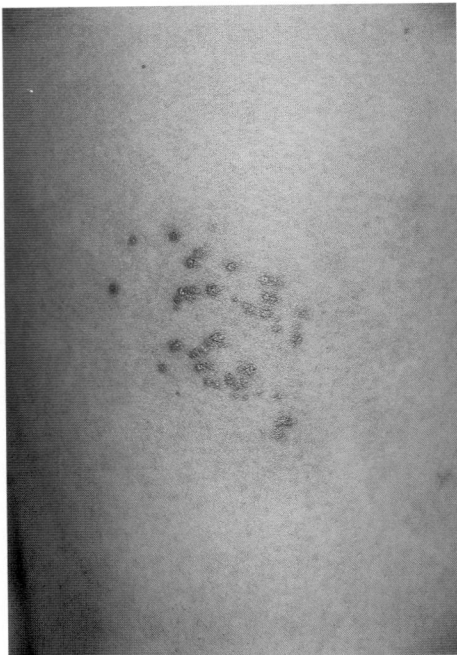

Figure 19.21: Cluster of pruritic erythematous papules on a thigh caused by *Pulex irritans*.

The papular discrete lesions may reveal a central haemorrhagic punctum and the lesions in clusters often show a remarkable asymmetry. Modification of the initial pruriginous lesions may result from intense scratching and superimposed secondary bacterial infection.

Management

Fumigation can be successfully achieved by using common insecticide products approved for domestic use. Severe reactions of prurigo require a topical steroid cream and impetiginized cases topical or systemic antibiotics. Antihistamine lotions or tablets may provide symptomatic relief. Severe cases are treated with a single dose or short course of systemic corticosteroids.

Skin diseases caused by fungi
Dermatophytes and malasseziosis

Aetiology and pathogenesis

Superficial fungal infections by dermatophytes are cosmopolitan and affect any anatomical site including scalp and nails; however, one of the commonest presentations occurs in one or both feet. These fungi are transmitted to humans by direct skin contact from their habitat in the soil, vegetation, animals or other individuals. Local conditions on the skin such as moist and hot environment are predisposing factors and therefore these infections are highly prevalent in tropical climates. The main genera involved in human infections are *Trychophyton*, *Epidermophyton* and *Microsporum*, and there are more than 25 pathogenic species. Common infections of the foot and toenails are particularly caused by *T. rubrum*, *T. mentagrophytes* and *E. floccosum*, whereas *Microsporum* and *Trychophyton* species are responsible for scalp infections. *E. floccosum* is the causative organism of tinea on the trunk, groin, hand and feet. Dermatophytes are keratinophylic organisms and exert their pathogenesis through attachment to the skin, nail or hair surfaces by the action of acid proteinases, keratinase, elastase and lipolytical enzymes.

Clinical findings and diagnosis

Individuals of both sexes and all age groups are affected by dermatophytes; however, children under the age of 10 rarely present with tinea pedis. The main clinical pictures are those of localized tinea pedis (Figure 19.22), intertriginous, plantar hyperkeratotic, and onychomycosis. Common names for these conditions include ringworm and athlete's foot. Dermatophyte infections can manifest as localized single (Figure 19.23) or multiple coalescing circinate plaques with erythema and variable degrees of scaling on the body in cases of tinea corporis (Figure 19.24). Athlete's foot can involve the dorsum or

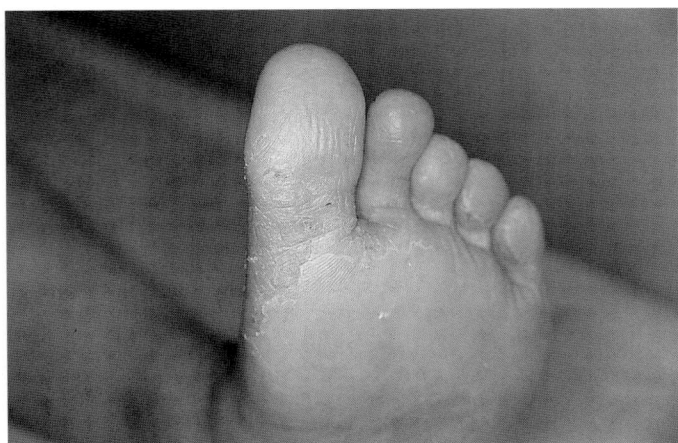

Figure 19.22: Scaling and diffuse erythema in tinea pedis.

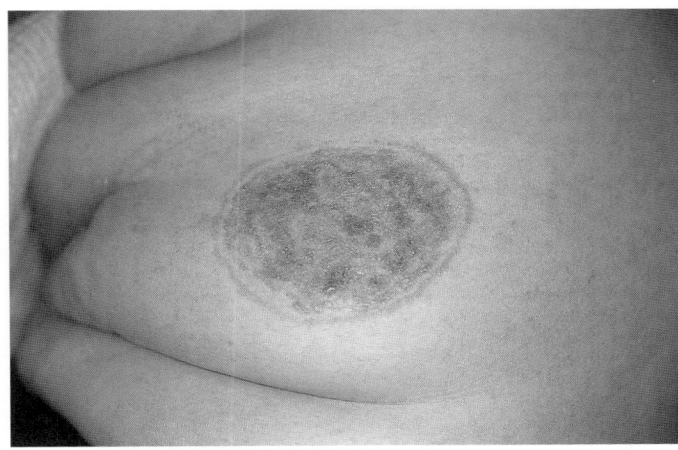

Figure 19.23: Pruritic erythematous and inflammatory localized plaque of tinea corporis.

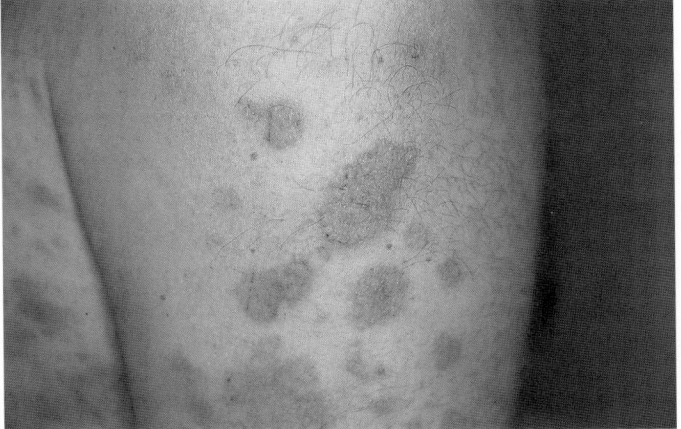

Figure 19.24: Coalescing small erythematous plaques with a microvesicular border in tinea corporis.

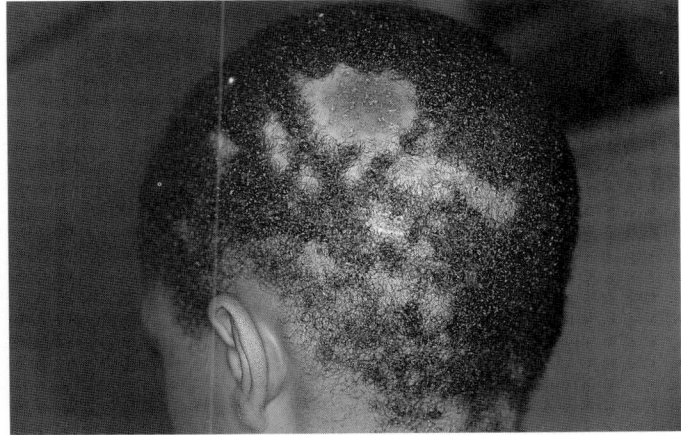

Figure 19.25: Non-scarring patchy alopecia and boggy inflammation in Celsus' kerion.

perimalleolar regions. Toe-web involvement is commonly bilateral, presenting with erythema, burning sensation, pruritus and scaling particularly of the fourth interdigital toe-web space. Severe acute forms present with painful erythema and blistering in a similar pattern to that found in cases of acute eczema or pompholyx. Patients with a history of atopy are predisposed to superficial infections by dermatophytes, and in these cases erythematous inflammatory fungal lesions coexist with patches of eczematous skin. Chronic plantar lesions develop asymptomatic large hyperkeratotic plaques and a particular form of toenail infection by *T. rubrum* manifests clinically as a subungual white onychomycosis. Varying degrees of temporary disability may result from severe infections. Children manifest scalp infections under the kerion clinical form with patches of non-scarring alopecia and boggy inflammation of the skin (Figure 19.25). Less commonly, adults manifest granulomatous inflammation with varying degrees of scarring in pustular infections caused by other species of *Trychophyton* (Figure 19.26).

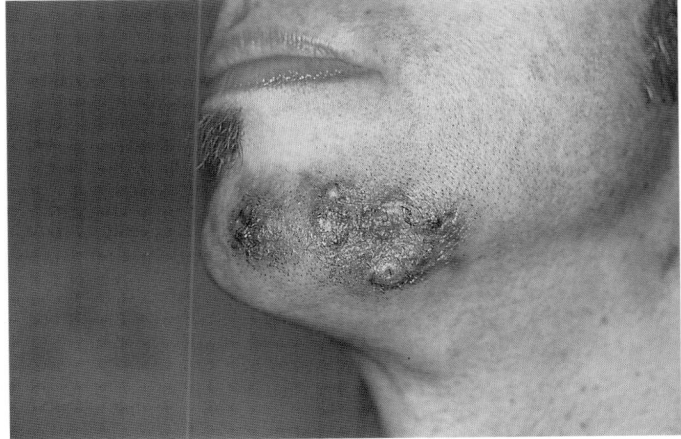

Figure 19.26: Erythematous plaque with nodules and pustules in tinea barbae by *Trichophyton mentagrophytes*.

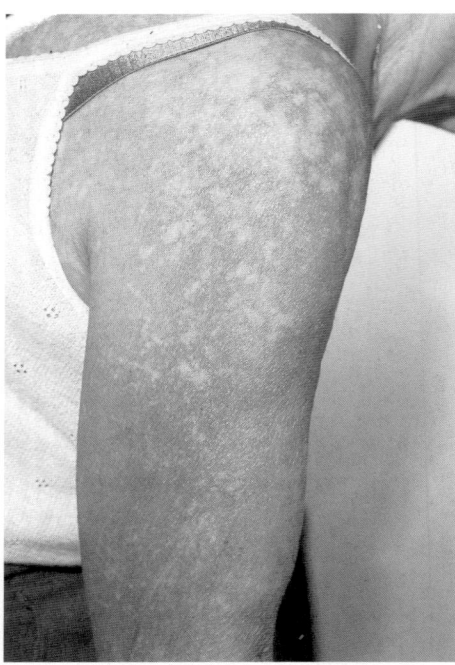

Figure 19.27: Hypo- and hyperpigmented small coalescing patches of pityriasis versicolor.

Discrete plaques of granuloma annulare have to be considered in the differential diagnosis of localized ringworm, whereas thickened plaques of plantar psoriasis may pose diagnostic difficulties with chronic hyper-keratotic infections by dermatophytes. Other superficial skin and nail infections of the foot such as those caused by *Candida* and *Scytalidium* species may also represent a diagnostic difficulty. The returning traveller from the tropics often is referred to our specialized clinic with severe or recurrent superficial yeast infections by *Malassezia furfur* called pityriasis versicolor (Figure 19.27). This is characterized by small coalescing patches or plaques on upper truncal skin and shoulders showing hyper- or hypopigmentation and furfuraceous scaling.

The diagnosis of dermatophyte infection on the skin is made on clinical grounds. Additional diagnostic measures include direct microscopy of skin scrapings in 10–12% KOH solution, and the identification by culture in Sabouraud's medium of the causative organism. A similar strategy is recommended for the laboratory diagnosis of pityriasis versicolor (malasseziosis) that requires special oily additives for a successful isolation in culture.

Management and treatment

The therapy of choice includes the use of topical and/or systemic azole or allylamine antifungal compounds. Localized infections require topical therapy for 3–4 weeks but cases with intertriginous athlethe's foot may require up to 6–8 weeks. Topical steroids are often required to control the inflammatory picture, but are administered only when effective antifungal treatment is already in place. Oral therapy with antifungals is indicated in severe

or disseminated skin infections, scalp ringworm and onychomycosis. Triazole and allylamine compounds have a similar efficacy in the treatment of tinea skin and nail infections; however, reports indicate that triazoles induce less adverse side effects and serious complications. Drug resistance rarely occurs with both groups of antifungals. *Malassezia furfur* infection responds to selenium sulfur topical preparations, ketoconazol shampoo, and other imidazolic or allylamine topical compounds applied for 6 weeks. Cases also respond to oral triazoles; however, recurrence is common. Other therapeutic measures should address the control of symptoms, secondary eczematization and superimposed bacterial infection. Measures of general hygiene and appropriate footwear can be useful to treat and prevent infections; however, the frequency of reinfections, particularly onychomycosis and athlete's foot, is a common problem in the tropics. Superficial lesions and broken skin on the lower limbs can be the port of entry for pyogenic or other bacteria and this is particularly dangerous in patients with diabetes and/or leprosy.

Sporotrichosis

Aetiology and pathogenesis

This infection is acquired by direct inoculation into the skin or subcutaneous tissue of mycelia or conidia from *Sporothrix schenckii*. Inhalation of infective organisms can also produce clinical disease and the accidental exposure takes place outdoors as a result of an accidental or professional contact involving splinters, thorns, straw, wood shavings or other sharp objects. This dimorphic fungus is ubiquitous in nature and lives in the soil, bark of trees, shrubs and plant detritus. This is a disease of temperate humid and tropical areas and represents a risk for travellers. *S. schenckii* has a low pathogenic potential and causes disease by virulence factors that include extracellular enzymes and polysaccharides as well as thermotolerance. The infective structures display a strong acid phosphatase activity and mannan compounds are capable of inhibiting phagocytosis by macrophages.

Clinical findings and diagnosis

Sporotrichosis may manifest as a systemic illness in pulmonary forms but in most cases the disease is limited to the skin, subcutaneous and lymphatic tissues. The upper and lower limbs are the usual sites of inoculation. Following the traumatic episode the disease manifests with a localized skin nodule involving only the affected limb. This inoculation chancre develops a suppurative and granulomatous infection that remains fixed, or else disseminates proximally via the lymphatic system. Super-imposed bacterial infection may occur and verrucous lesions show a tendency to ulceration. The gold standard of laboratory diagnosis is the identification of the fungus in culture, but direct microscopy and histopathological investigations also have some diagnostic value.

Outbreaks in parties of travellers require full epidemiological investigation.

Management

Potassium iodide in increasing daily oral doses from a saturated stock solution is the treatment of choice in the tropics; however, oral itraconazole or intravenous amphotericin B have also resulted in cure in a hospital context. In view of the fact that the disease is acquired by direct inoculation into the skin, preventive measures are of the utmost importance. Protective footwear, clothing and avoidance of skin contact with splinters, rough bark, plant detritus and soil are the most efficient methods to prevent the disease. Activities such as tree-planting, gardening, hay handling and soil removal carry a risk for the infection either by direct skin inoculation or by inhalation of the infective forms.

Eumycetoma

Aetiology and pathogenesis

Madurella mycetomatis, *Pseudallescheria boydii* and *Leptosphaeria senegalensis* are the main aetiological agents of true fungal mycetoma, also known as eumycetoma. A generic term, 'Madura foot', is currently used to describe all forms of bacterial and fungal mycetoma (see 'Bacterial mycetoma' above). Eumycetoma occurs in Sudan, Senegal and Saudi Arabia, particularly in arid or semi-arid regions.[25] Cases also occur in India and Central and South America. Infective organisms penetrate the skin of the foot or other exposed regions by direct traumatic inoculation and in the host's tissue the agents multiply and infect adjacent structures. Changes in the fungus cell wall and melanin production are the main virulent factors involved in local pathogenesis.

Clinical findings and diagnosis

Eumycetoma affects predominantly young male individuals between 20 and 50 years of age. It has been estimated that more than 70% of cases with eumycetoma manifest on one foot (Figure 19.28). Other anatomical regions for the accidental, professional or traumatic inoculation include the trunk, face and scalp. The perimalleolar region and the foot dorsum are the most commonly affected sites but any region of the foot can suffer the direct inoculation of infective organisms. The characteristic clinical signs include a nodule or irregular swelling followed by sinus tract formation and discharge of purulent material containing the characteristic grains. Pigmentary changes of the skin and scarring result from the persistent and chronic inflammatory process over months or years. Periosteal involvement is the starting point of bone resorption, osteolysis and irreversible osteomyelitis.

The epidemiological context and characteristic clinical picture are diagnostic. This is confirmed by direct microscopy revealing pale or black grains that measure

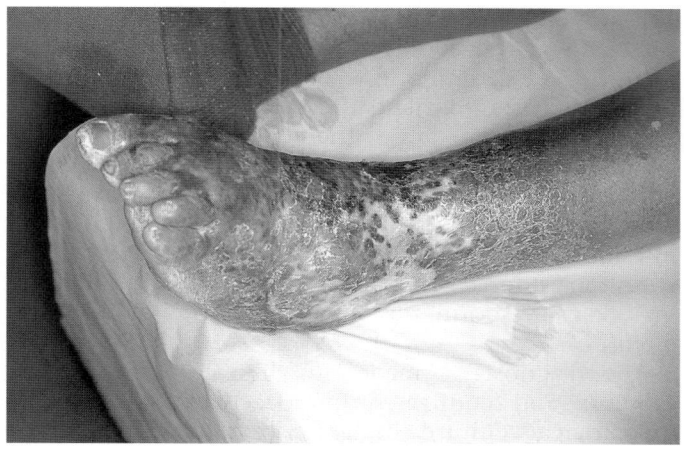

Figure 19.28: Deformity, atrophy, sinus tract formation, scarring and pigment disorder in fungal mycetoma.

between 0.5 and 1 mm containing fungal structures measuring 2–4 μm. This material grows in agar containing glucose and peptone, and the histological sections of deep skin specimens reveal the characteristic and in many cases pathognomonic grains of particular fungal species. Radiological investigation of the affected region discloses periosteal involvement, cortical resorption and osteolysis.

Management and treatment

Early nodular lesions or small papular forms called 'micromycetoma' can be treated by complete surgical excision. However, the delay in diagnosis results in advanced cases that respond poorly to medical treatment. Systemic antibiotics in combination such as streptomycin, cotrimoxazol, amikacin, dapsone and rifampin are the drugs of choice that require long-term administration. Nearly two-thirds of cases caused by *M. mycetomatis* respond to ketoconazole.[26] Severe cases with bone involvement can only be cured by radical surgery. Education and use of protective footwear are the main strategies for prevention.

Chromoblastomycosis

Aetiology and pathogenesis

This is a chronic infection caused by pigmented fungi of *Fonsecaea*, *Cladosporium* and *Phialophora* species. The disease is widely distributed in the tropics and affects predominantly agricultural workers who acquire the infection through direct inoculation into the skin. Numerous cases have been reported mainly from Costa Rica, Cuba, Brazil, Mexico, Indonesia and Madagascar.

Clinical findings and diagnosis

The initial lesion starts as a papular or nodular inflammatory reaction that subsequently develops a warty appearance. In time this lesion enlarges at a slow rate and becomes characteristically a large verrucous asymptomatic plaque. The commonest site affected in sporadic infections is the foot and the chronic verrucous plaque appears on the dorsum or the perimalleolar region. The plaque may become very thick in several years, and cause gross deformity of the affected foot. Varying degrees of disability and recurrent secondary infections and/or infestations are a common problem for the foot with chromoblastomycosis. Less characteristic clinical forms include psoriasiform, rupioid and sporotrichoid localized pictures.

The diagnosis is made on clinical–epidemiological grounds and confirmed by direct microscopy and mycological culture in glucose–peptone agar. The histopathology of skin specimens is characteristic, showing acanthosis with a granuloma formation and the presence of typical fungal structures known as fumagoid or muriform cells.

Management

Flucytosine and thiabendazol have been used in combination without consistent efficacy. Several months' treatment with oral triazole compounds such as itraconazol has resulted in cure but in general it is recognized that chromoblastomycosis is not easy to treat medically, and patients require long-term treatment. Localized and early cases respond successfully to complete surgical excision of the lesion, and thermosurgery has also been reported of benefit. A new antifungal compound, voriconazole, has shown efficacy in chromoblastomycosis. All patients affected by chromoblastomycosis require follow-up by specialists in mycology, infectious diseases and/or dermatology.

Systemic mycosis manifesting on the skin

Infections by *Coccidioides immitis*, *Histoplasma capsulatum* and *Paracoccidioides brasiliensis* commonly manifest with disease of the lungs but haematogenous dissemination results in the appearance of skin lesions.

Coccidioidomycosis is acquired through inhalation of infective spores in tropical but also subtropical desert regions of the world, particularly in the American continent. South and western states in the USA and north-western regions of Mexico represent well-recognized endemic regions, and the disease is acquired most commonly in urban areas. Travellers acquire the infection in urban areas where a high proportion of the resident population manifest a positive intradermal reaction on skin testing using coccidioidin. This systemic mycosis presents a risk particularly for the immuno-compromised traveller. The skin becomes involved in a small proportion of cases and lesions manifest as erythematous, verrucous, scarring or scaling nodules on the face, trunk (Figure 19.29), upper or lower limbs. A

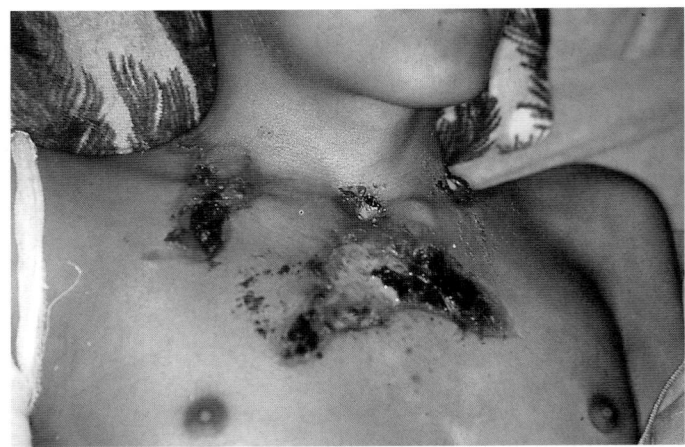

Figure 19.29: Ulcerated plaques and scarring of the trunk in coccidioidomycosis. (Courtesy of Dr Sergio González, Monterrey, Mexico.)

history of exposure in endemic regions followed by an episode of erythema nodosum supports the diagnostic possibility. Other investigations such as serology, chest X-rays and culture for the isolation of the organism confirm the diagnosis. Culture of agents causing systemic mycoses should only be carried out in specialized laboratories as they represent a serious biological hazard. Systemic therapeutic options for coccidioidomycosis include amphotericin B and triazole compounds.

Histoplasmosis is highly prevalent in the American continent but species occur as saprophytes in other parts of the world. This fungus is found in birds' and bats' excreta (guano) and is highly prevalent in caves and abandoned mines. This infection is caused by the dimorphic fungus *Histoplasma capsulatum* var. *capsulatum* (American) or var. *duboisii* (African), acquired by inhalation. Most cases have been reported from the USA, Mexico, Colombia, Venezuela, Argentina and the Caribbean; however, the disease also occurs in the Far East, South-East Asia, India, Middle East, central and southern Africa, Europe, Australia and the South Pacific. Acute or chronic pulmonary forms may be asymptomatic or severe, with high mortality rates. The main differential diagnosis is pulmonary tuberculosis. A low proportion of chronic forms may result in haematogenous dissemination to the skin and mucosal regions, presenting as ulcerations or erythematous exudative nodules (Figure 19.30). Diagnosis is made by history of exposure, clinical picture, chest X-rays, direct microscopy and culture in Sabouraud's medium. Successful treatment has been achieved with itraconazole, fluconazole or amphotericin B. Immuno-compromised individuals are at a higher risk for this infection.

Paracoccidioidomycosis occurs in Mexico, Central and South America, predominantly affecting male individuals who live and acquire the infection in rural areas. Actual evidence of the mode of transmission is incomplete but the respiratory route seems to be common in acquiring the infection. Following a chronic picture of lung involvement, weight loss and fatigue, the skin of the face, particularly periorificial, or else of other anatomical location on lower limbs, becomes affected. Painful nodular, haemorrhagic, ulcerated and verrucous lesions can be observed covered by a thick crust (Figure 19.31), and severe disability results in advanced forms of the disease. The diagnosis is based on the history of exposure in an endemic region and the clinical picture supported by investigations to reveal the presence of the typical large budding yeast cells. These can be observed in direct microscopy from skin lesions, bronchoalveolar lavage and HE preparations for histology, and are easily identified in culture. Effective systemic treatment has been reported with triazole compounds and amphotericin B.

Patients with foot involvement from systemic fungal disease require immediate referral to an experienced hospital physician or specialist in mycology, infectious diseases or dermatology.

Diseases caused by viruses

Most common viral skin diseases are cosmopolitan but the onset may coincide with a trip to the tropics and pose problems in the differential diagnosis of the returning traveller. Viral infections that are prevalent in the tropics include *molluscum contagiosum* in children, plantar warts in adults, *Kaposi's sarcoma* in patients with AIDS and severe blistering forms by *varicella* (Figure 19.32). Severe cases require a full diagnostic protocol with specimens for culture, electron microscopy, serology and histopathology, followed by specialized treatment in tertiary referral centres.

For the last decade we have observed that 100% of our patients with HIV infection suffer from one or more skin conditions at some stage of their evolution. Severe forms of eczema, seborrheic dermatitis, recalcitrant viral warts (Figure 19.33) or worsening of psoriasis are commonly found in clinical practice. The frequency and number of skin problems increase with progressing AIDS established illness. In the early to mid-1990s, prior to the introduction of new antiretroviral regimens, skin infections and vasculitis by cytomegalovirus were frequently observed. Severe dermatophyte infections, cutaneous

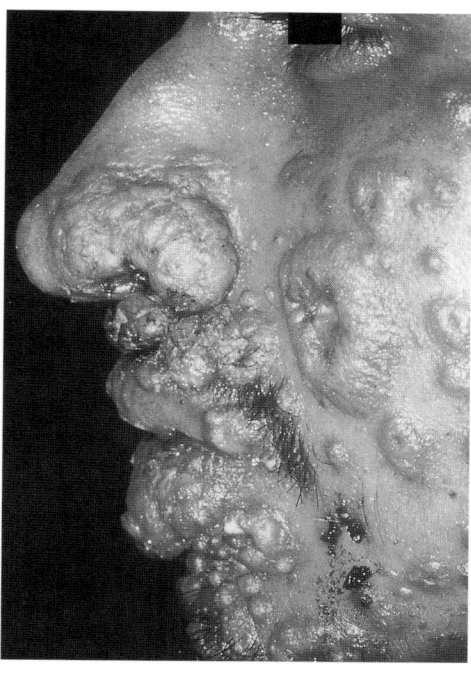

Figure 19.30: Nodular lesions and plaques with exudate on the face in a case with histoplasmosis. (Courtesy of Dr Alexandro Bonifaz, Mexico.)

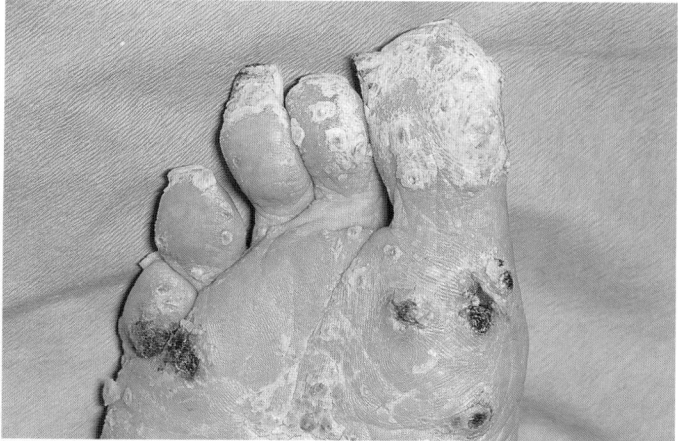

Figure 19.31: Hyperkeratotic, verrucous, ulcerated and crusted lesions on the feet in a patient with paracoccidioidomycosis.

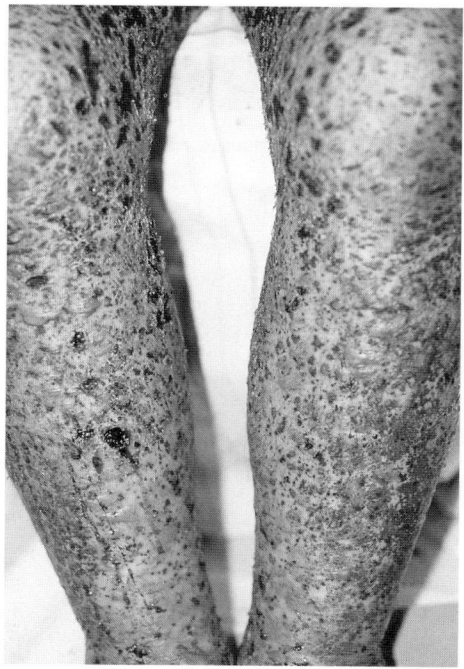

Figure 19.32: Disseminated blistering and crusting in a case of varicella infection.

cryptococcosis (Figure 19.34) and Kaposi's sarcoma (Figure 19.35) were more commonly diagnosed as well. However, in recent years where survival is approaching figures found in the general population without HIV infection, skin malignancy is expected to increase, particularly in Caucasian individuals of developed countries (Figures 19.36 and 19.37).

Non-infectious skin problems in the tropics

Cutaneous disorders that present to the tropical doctor may vary according to the ethnic background of the patient. It is well recognized that skin conditions that occur in people of different ethnic backgrounds are modified or influenced by the characteristic differences in pigment, follicular response, curved, flat hair and fibroblast reactivity. In addition the tropical environment may also lead to a different presentation of common skin

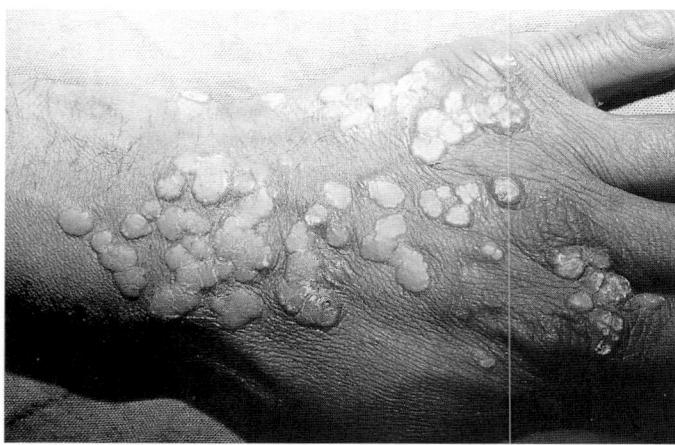

Figure 19.33: Chronic warty plaques on the hand's dorsa by HPV in a patient with AIDS.

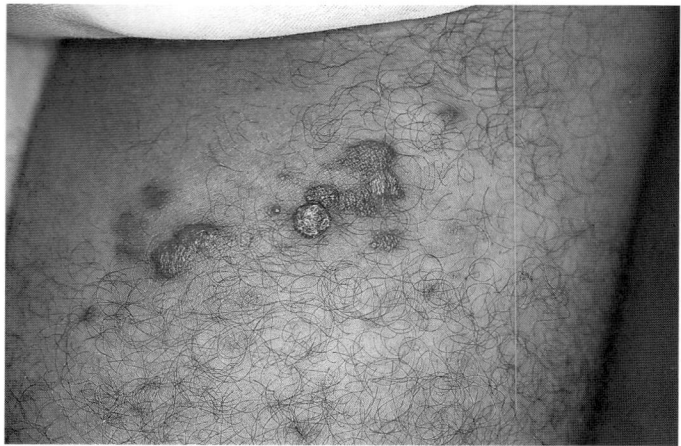

Figure 19.35: Violaceous plaques and nodules of Kaposi's sarcoma in a patient with AIDS.

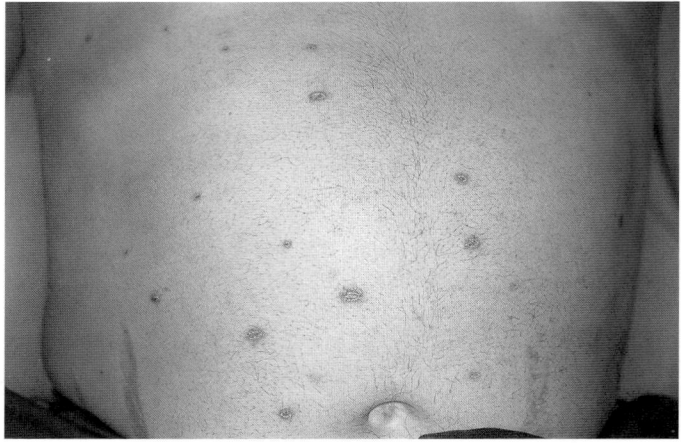

Figure 19.34: Erythematous lesions with central ulceration in cutaneous cryptococcosis.

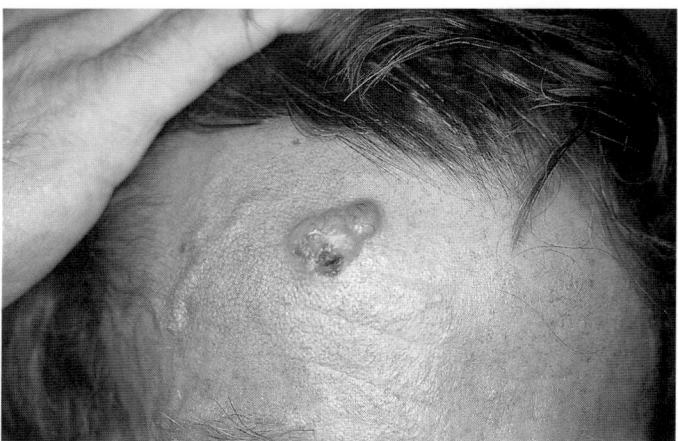

Figure 19.36: Large nodular basal cell carcinoma in a Caucasian patient with AIDS.

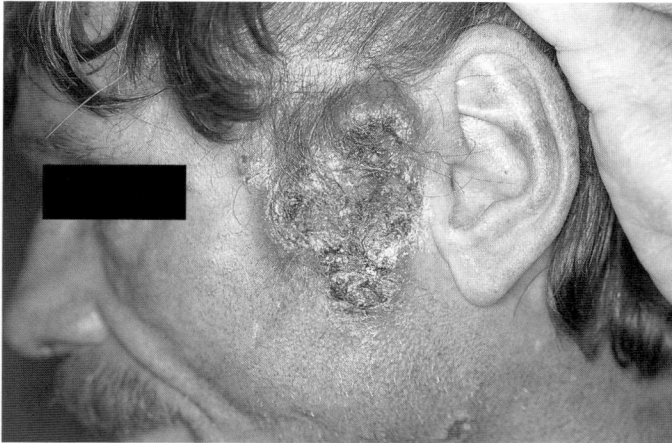

Figure 19.37: Ulcerated and exophytic large squamous cell carcinoma in a Caucasian patient with AIDS.

diseases and also may require a different approach to treatment.

Acne vulgaris

Acne vulgaris is the most common skin disease and affects 80% of all people at some time between age 11–30 years. It begins from age 10–13 at a time when a child is undergoing puberty. It therefore can have far-reaching psychosocial consequences as well as result in permanent disfigurement.

Aetiology and clinical manifestations

Acne is a disease of the pilosebaceous unit and four pathophysiological interrelated factors are involved: excess sebum production, blockage of the pilosebaceous duct, *Propionibacteriun acnes* and inflammation.

The adrenal glands mature in the prepubertal period and thereby produce increasing amounts of adrenal androgens. Gonadal development adds to this increased androgen production still further. The sebaceous gland contains the enzyme 5α-reductase, which converts testosterone to 5α-dihydroxytestosterone. There is good evidence to suggest that 5α-dihydroxytestosterone increases sebum production. Androgens may also have an important part in controlling ductal hyperproliferation, leading to blockage of the pilosebaceous duct. In addition, patients with acne seem to have decreased sebaceous linoleic acid; such a decrease is known to cause scaling of the skin in animal models and therefore it is thought that abnormal levels of linoleic acid in sebum may enhance accumulation of scale in the pilosebaceous duct and also lead to blockage. Clinically this excess sebum production and blockage results in the formation of a microcomedone that evolves either into a comedone or an inflammatory lesion. The excess sebum and blockage of drainage is an ideal environment for the proliferation of *Propionibacterium acnes*, which results in the release of pro-inflammatory mediators resulting in the clinical expression of an inflammatory lesion. Therefore one can explain the clinical appearance of acne vulgaris with the comedones presenting as blackheads and whiteheads, and the inflammatory lesions present-ing as inflamed papules, pustules and cystic nodules. A patient may have a mixture of all lesions or a predominance of either comedones or inflamed lesions. In the tropics the environment causes increased sebum production, and patients may find either an exacerbation or the first initial presentation of acne when they travel from a temperate zone to a tropical zone. There is a great deal of variation in the incidence of acne throughout the world, with South-Eastern Asians having less sebaceous gland activity and tending to show a decreased incidence of acne as well as it being less severe. Black-skinned patients are more likely to form comedones, and white-skinned patients more likely to have inflammatory acne. It is thought that the pilosebaceous duct is more likely to respond by epidermal cell proliferation within the duct in black patients, whereas in white patients the pilo-

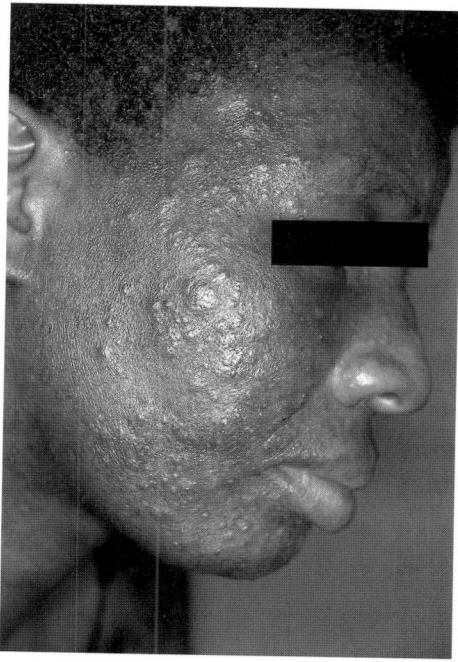

Figure 19.38: Papular, nodular, and cystic facial late-onset acne.

sebaceous duct is more likely to disintegrate and rupture into the surrounding tissue and thereby produce an inflammatory reaction. Patients with black skin may respond to inflammatory acne by forming keloid scars which can result in gross disfigurement. The distribution of acne occurs where the density of sebaceous glands is greatest, namely the forehead, cheeks, chin (Figure 19.38), upper chest and upper back.

Management of acne vulgaris in the tropics

Mainly comedonal acne

This form of acne is very common in pre-teenage or early teenage years. Treatment at this stage may prevent further development of the acne: topical tretinoin or adaptaline used once daily at night. We prefer to use retinoids at night as they can photosensitize the skin and therefore are best washed off in the morning before going into the tropical sunshine. Topical retinoids are effective against comedogenesis and may also benefit patients with hyperpigmentation. If such retinoids are not available, a solution of salicylate to wash the face twice a day may be used, although it is not as effective. Topical azelaic acid can also be effective. A specific form of comedomal acne that is very common in black patients is pomade acne, due to the application of waxes, greases and oils to the hair, resulting in pilosebaceous duct blockage and therefore comedogenesis. Ideally the patient should cease from using such materials on the hair.

Mainly inflammatory acne

Mild inflammatory acne may be treated by either 5–10% benzyl peroxide on its own, or benzyl peroxide combined with erythromycin. This treatment is ideal as it is the most effective topical antimicrobial therapy. Topical clindamycin and erythromycin are also effective and can be used twice daily. More severe inflammatory acne will require systemic antibiotics such as minocycline, doxycycline, tetracycline, erythromycin or a combination of trimethoprim plus sulfamethoxazole. Systemic retinoids in the form of isotretinoin is the treatment of choice for severe cases. A 4–6-month course of 0.5–1.0 mg/kg per day causes complete remission in most cases.

Eczema/dermatitis

It has to be appreciated that eczema is not a single disease, but rather a family of conditions. The hallmark of these conditions is epidermal oedema (spongiosis) and pruritus. This epidermal oedema may be caused by numerous factors, both endogenous and exogenous. Traditionally the eczemas have been classified into the exogenous and endogenous forms, although there is a great deal of interaction between the various factors. The main exogenous eczemas are contact dermatitis, either primary irritant or allergic contact dermatitis. Primary irritant dermatitis occurs due to the application of a normally irritant substance to the skin and is most often occupationally related. Individuals vary in their susceptibility to such irritation and the vast majority of cases of contact dermatitis/eczema are of the primary irritant type. About a quarter of all contact dermatitis is due to allergy to a specific substance. In this case epidermal spongiosis occurs due to the occurrence of a Type IV hypersensitivity reaction (DTH) to the allergen. In such cases patch testing has to be performed to identify the appropriate antigen. Endogenous causes of eczema include atopic dermatitis, seborrhoeic dermatitis, varicose eczema, xerotic eczema, discoid eczema and endogenous hand eczema.

Pruritus leads to chronic scratching and the epidermis becomes hyperkeratotic, thickened and more scaly. Acute eczema may have epidermal oedema which clinically manifests as vesicles; if these vesicles rupture onto the surface of the skin the extracellular fluid accumulates and evaporation of water leaves protein behind, leading to crusting on the surface of the skin.

Atopic dermatitis

A typical atopic individual suffers from some combination of asthma, hayfever, atopic dermatitis and elevated serum IgE. The British prevalence of atopic dermatitis has been estimated to be from 10% to 15% of the population. Interestingly migrant Asians or Africans tend to first express their atopic dermatitis when they arrive in Britain. Therefore it is thought that the incidence of atopic dermatitis is higher in Asians and Africans living in Britain than the incidence in their original countries of residence. In addition it seems to be a condition of more affluent groups and more common in urban environments than in rural environments.

Aetiology

Over 80% of patients with atopic dermatitis have a personal or family history of atopic disease. Twin and family studies have shown that the inheritance of atopic dermatitis is polygenic and that the clinical expression of atopy is dependent on the interaction of genetic and environmental factors. Currently there is evidence pointing to a genetic linkage between atopy and the IgE high-affinity receptor gene at chromosome 11q13. It is well recognized that there is an increase in both non-antigen-specific IgE levels and antigen-specific IgE levels in atopic dermatitis; therefore, it is postulated that genetic control is responsible for determining the overall risk for allergy and the total level of serum IgE whereas environmental factors may be more important in determining antigen specificity. However, the immunohistological features of atopic dermatitis are more inconsistent with a Type IV hypersensitivity reaction than a Type I reaction. Indeed, epidermal Langerhans cells in clinically involved skin of atopic dermatitis patients have been found to bind IgE. It is therefore hypothesized that cutaneous antigens may bind to allergen-specific IgE on the surface of these Langerhans cells and thereby present such antigens to T helper cells, leading to T lymphocyte activation and the eczematous reaction. The T cells that do proliferate have been found to have a Th2 predominance of clonal T cells, which produce cytokines such as IL-4, IL-5, IL-10 and IL-13. Such cytokines are meant to promote B cell proliferation and further IgE synthesis while at the same time suppressing the Th1 cell-mediated response. This diminished Th1-mediated response is expressed clinically by an increase in susceptibility of the atopic dermatitis patient to viral and bacterial infection. A particularly important bacterial colonization in exacerbations of atopic dermatitis is infection with *Staphylococcus aureus*. Staphylococcal superantigens have been implicated in stimulating a Th2 cell proliferation in the skin and also in inducing resistance to topical corticosteroid therapy. A small section of the atopic population may have reactions to *Malassezia furfur* as specific IgE antibodies to such an organism have been found. Indeed, in some atopic exacerbations may be controlled with oral ketoconazole or itraconazole. *Trichophyton rubrum* infection has also been similarly implicated. Since fungal infections are extremely common in the tropics, fungal infection is an important factor in the exacerbation of atopic dermatitis and should not be overlooked. Much has been written about the role of food allergy in atopic dermatitis. Most cases of food allergy occur in children under 1 year of age, and almost certainly most children with dermatitis significantly affected by food allergy have lost such an association by the age of 4. Indeed, data from dietary restriction trials have shown little benefit from such manoeuvres in atopic dermatitis. This is important as the nutritional levels of patients in the tropics may already be low and dietary restriction may not only not help the atopic dermatitis but also further diminish the nutritional status of the patient.

Clinical manifestations

Presentation can be very varied or may be classic. When the lesions are characteristic and there is a personal or family history of atopy, a diagnosis is easily made. Most clinical manifestations of atopic dermatitis are a result of the secondary skin lesion caused by the patient continually scratching. The earliest manifestations of atopic dermatitis are dryness and transient redness of the skin. Acutely there is then the eruption of vesicles on an erythematous basis. These burst leaving a honey-coloured crust on the surface. The accompanied scratching leads to thickness (lichenification) of the epidermis and results in accentuation of the normal skin lines as a result of this scratching. The distribution of atopic dermatitis is bilateral and symmetrical and varies with age at presentation. Infants have involvement of areas that are in contact with the floor by crawling and in areas where the infant can reach to scratch such as the extensor extremities, the scalp, neck and face. Once the child is over 4 years old facial involvement is uncommon and such children present with lesions in the antecubital and popliteal fossae, the neck, wrists and the ankles. Adult involvement tends to be flexural and less severe than in infants. In darker-skinned patients constant scratching may produce follicular papules instead of lichenification and it is important to note that in dark-skinned patients all the reaction may be follicular; such follicular papules are commonly found para-umbilically and on the extensor surface of the elbows. Darker-skinned patients may also undergo postinflammatory hyperpigmentation, which may take several years to resolve. The patient should be warned and educated about such pigmentation as it is often a cause of great concern.

Complications

These include eyelid dermatitis, atopic keratoconjunctivitis, anterior subcapsular cataracts, posterior cataracts (probably as a result of chronic corticosteroid usage) and retinal detachment. Abnormal cell-mediated immunity may lead to ocular herpes simplex virus infection and corneal damage. Generalized infection with herpes simplex virus can occur and can be rapidly fatal if not treated. Such an infection is called eczema herpeticum; the patient is unwell with a fever and has the appearance of numerous punched-out erosions on the skin. Atopics are also more susceptible to infection with molluscum contagiosum virus as well as the human papilloma virus. Acute exacerbations, as mentioned before, may be caused by infection with *S. aureus*, *M. furfur* and *T. rubrum*.

Management

Avoidance of precipitant factors for pruritus such as heat and perspiration is especially relevant in the tropical environment. Ninety per cent of patients are intolerant to wool and this should be avoided, with plain cotton being the cloth of choice. The most important foods which the patient may be intolerant to are eggs, cow's milk, soya beans, nuts and wheat, but this is more likely to be relevant in a child under the age of 4. There is some evidence to suggest that measures to decrease the amount of house dust mite may be of relevance but the measures required to decrease them are extreme and the benefits quite marginal.

Emollients should be used as a soap substitute and to moisturize the skin several times daily. Topical steroids are the mainstays of therapy for atopic dermatitis. They are classified into weak, moderate and potent strengths. The patient is instructed to apply the required strength of topical steroid twice a day until the symptoms have subsided. Topical steroids are then slowly tapered to aim for treatment twice a week. In general, weaker steroids should be used on the face and flexures, with stronger steroids being used on the more lichenified areas. In adults where flexures are more likely to be colonized by fungi it may be wise to use a preparation that contains an antifungal component, such as Trimovate or Daktacort.

Exacerbating factors such as secondary infections require therapy with antifungals and/or antibiotics. Antihistamines are commonly prescribed in atopic dermatitis; however, there is no role for non-sedating antihistamines in this condition.

Phototherapy with UVA combined with Psoralen is called PUVA. PUVA is very effective in atopic dermatitis but requires the use of specialized facilities often not available in the tropics. UVB both in a broad band and in a narrow band have been used and are also effective, but these too require specialized equipment. However, one of the advantages of the tropics is that such radiation is freely available and if cultural factors permit the patient should be instructed to expose the body to sunlight, beginning with small periods of time such as 10–15 minutes and building up over weeks to 1 or 2 hours.

Azathioprine is reasonably safe and easy to monitor and is commonly used in the treatment of atopic dermatitis, although there have been no controlled trials. Doses of 50–150 mg per day are used and may, in very selected cases, be combined with systemic steroids in short courses. Cyclosporin A has been shown to be highly effective in both childhood and adult atopic dermatitis in clinically controlled trials. It is started at a dose of 2.5–5 mg/kg, and the dose adjusted according to clinical efficacy and safety.

Chinese herbal medicine has been found to be highly effective in atopic dermatitis but it is expensive and is found to be highly unpalatable by many patients. In addition, liver toxicity has been reported.

Contact dermatitis

This is divided into irritant and allergic contact dermatitis. All irritants when applied in sufficient concentration in frequent enough applications should cause an irritant dermatitis. Therefore, those in professions which require immersion of hands in detergents, chemicals or dyes are more likely to get such a reaction. The commonest irritants are strong acids or alkalis and detergents. In such cases considered advice about careers has to be given and all measures taken to avoid further irritation. Treatment requires avoidance of irritant or allergen as well as using emollients instead of soap, and topical steroids. A DTH reaction may occur in response to metal such as nickel (Figure 19.39), and fragrances. In Europe there is a standard battery of the commonest allergens in the form of a patch test. Patch tests are applied on a suitable

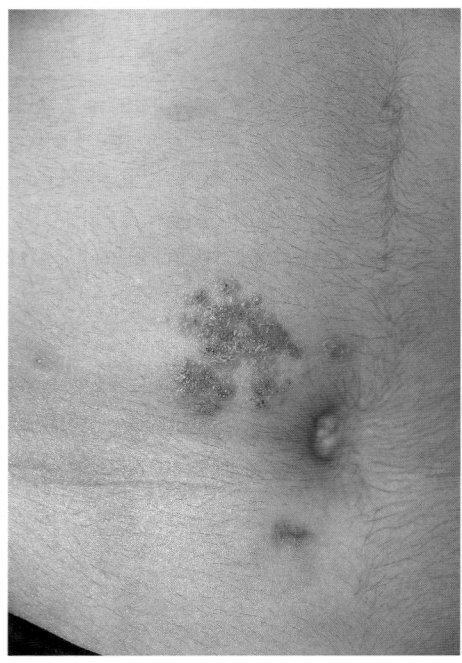

Figure 19.39: Acute allergic contact dermatitis to nickel from the metal button and buckle of blue jeans.

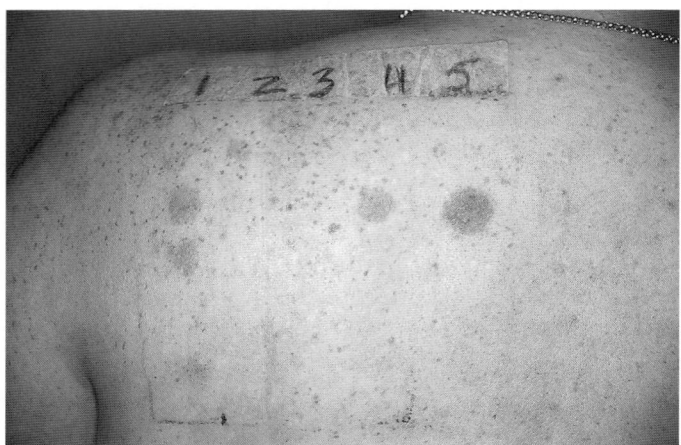

Figure 19.40: Erythema and induration of positive patch testing read at 96 hours.

anatomical location for a period of 48 hours and then removed. Any area of redness under each patch is graded as a positive result (Figure 19.40). Patches are then reviewed a further 48 hours later in order to identify a positive reaction. Latex products are commonly involved in contact dermatitis and a Type I hypersensitivity reaction with urticaria and angioedema.

Pompholyx

This is very common in the tropics, being associated with sweating of the hands and feet. The initial pathophysiological process of epidermal oedema causes superficial vesicles and since the keratin layer of the palmoplantar skin is especially thick they do not burst or form crusts. The condition is variably itchy and begins on the sides of the fingers and may be associated with atopy and other forms of endogenous eczema. Treatment is to avoid sweating of the hands, use of emollients instead of soap and potent topical corticosteroids. Secondary fungal infection can be a complication.

Discoid eczema

This consists of a bilateral symmetrical itchy eruption. The lesions themselves are rather atypical of most eczemas in that they are well defined and up to 2 cm in diameter. When they first present as solitary lesions they may be mistaken for cutaneous fungal infection. They are commonly found on the arms and legs and vary in the degree of pruritus. There have been no aetiological factors described in this condition and treatment consists of emollients and topical steroids; it tends to respond to the same treatments as atopic dermatitis.

Keloid

The aetiology of keloid formation is unknown although trauma may play a major part. Keloids are likely to occur after surgical procedures and are defined by their extension beyond the area first traumatized. Clinically keloids are dense and hard with a shiny erythematous or hyperpigmented surface. The borders are usually smooth and they have claw-like extensions. The commonest sites are the ear lobes, upper back, mid chest and shoulders. Symptomatically they can be painful and itchy.

Acne keloidalis nuchae is a chronic progressive keloidal scarring process on the nape of the neck that affects mainly black men. Patients present in their twenties and thirties and often after a short haircut. It is not associated with acne vulgaris. The initial patho-physiological process is follicular inflammation leading to a weak follicular wall and rupture of the hair follicle. This rupture elicits a foreign body inflammatory reaction in the dermis, where scarring leads to keloidal formation. The process may be exacerbated by superimposed infection. Clinically a follicular pustular eruption is found on the nape of the neck. Unlike acne, comedones and blackheads are not seen. Such a process may cause a scarring alopecia.

Treatment of keloids may be medical and/or surgical. Keloid scars may be excised as long as there is not too much tension on the postoperative wound; however, the patient should be warned that such a procedure has a 50% recurrence rate. They may be shaved down to follicular level and then injected with potent intralesional steroids postoperatively with a single dose, followed up by four weekly injections until control of the scar is attained. Intralesional steroids may be used on their own in order to induce atrophy of smaller scars. Lesions of acne keloidalis nuchae may be excised, injected with intralesional steroid, or shaved with the postoperative injection of intralesional steroid. Active inflammation may also be controlled by tetracyclines combined with a topical dose of a potent topical steroid twice daily.

Psoriasis

Psoriasis is a chronic hyperproliferative condition of the skin of unknown aetiology. It can present in numerous morphological forms and it can affect a few areas to total skin surface involvement.

Epidemiology and aetiology

Psoriasis is said to affect up to 1% of the whole world's population. Although it was thought to be less common in Africans and Afro-Caribbeans it is now known that this is not the case, but that psoriasis is often less severe due to the therapeutic effects of a tropical environment. One-third of patients have a positive family history of psoriasis and it is in association with HLAB 13 and HLAB 17. It tends to develop in two different age groups: between 20 and 30 years, and between the ages of 50 and 60 years. It is postulated that activated T cells may play a major role in the pathogenesis of psoriasis and this is evidenced by the efficacy of cyclosporin A therapy.

Clinical features

In making a diagnosis of psoriasis one has to consider the morphology of each lesion present as well as its distribution and extent of involvement. The condition tends to remit and exacerbate in a chronic manner throughout the patient's life. In some patients it may go into complete remission whereas in others it may continue in a chronic form. The classic psoriasis lesion is well defined and raised. It has a red colour with a thick white silvery scale on its surface. Clinically psoriasis may be divided into four general forms:

- *Plaque psoriasis (psoriasis vulgaris)*. This is the commonest form, with involvement of the scalp, trunk (Figure 19.41), elbows and knees, the sacrum and the nails.
- *Erythrodermic psoriasis*. The skin is red and has a fine scale over the entire surface. There may be small areas of uninvolved skin but the vast majority will be affected. This form commonly arises in a patient with

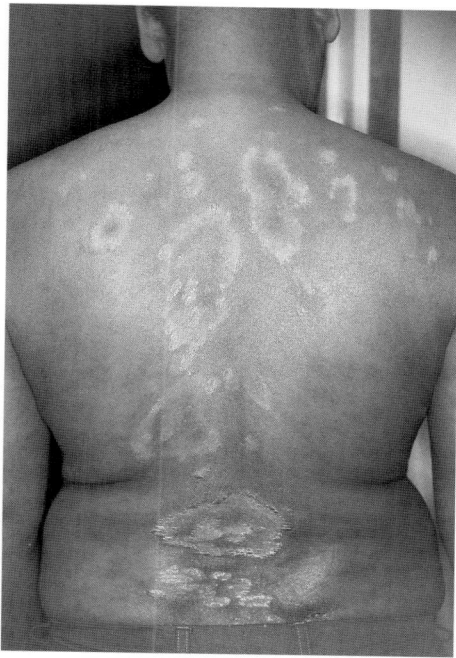

Figure 19.41: Circumscribed plaques of erythema, thickening and scale in plaque psoriasis.

pre-existent plaque psoriasis but may occur as a first presentation. It may also occur as a result of medication with corticosteroids, lithium, β-blockers, non-steroidal anti-inflammatory drugs and antimalarials. The condition can be fatal and the patient should be hospitalized and kept warm, with particular attention paid to fluid and electrolyte imbalance as well as the risk of infection and septicaemia.
- *Guttate psoriasis*. This is characterized by the sudden onset of pink droplets or flat papules, which appear in crops principally on the trunk (Figure 19.42) and proximal extremities. It is strongly associated with recent or active β-haemolytic streptococcal infection.
- *Pustular psoriasis*. This may be a localized form on the palms and soles or it may be generalized. The palmoplantar form is relatively common, with the appearance of sterile yellow pustules on an erythematous background on the palms and soles (Figure 19.43). The generalized form can be fatal and it may be precipitated by treatment with corticosteroids or potent topical steroids if they are withdrawn rapidly. In the generalized form there are extensive sheets of sterile yellow pustules, which become painful and sore. The patient may have constitutional symptoms such as a fever and tachycardia.

Psoriatic arthropathy

There are five clinical patterns of joint involvement:

1. An arthritis similar in distribution to osteoarthritis, with distal interphalangeal joint involvement and the clinical manifestations of Heberdens notes.

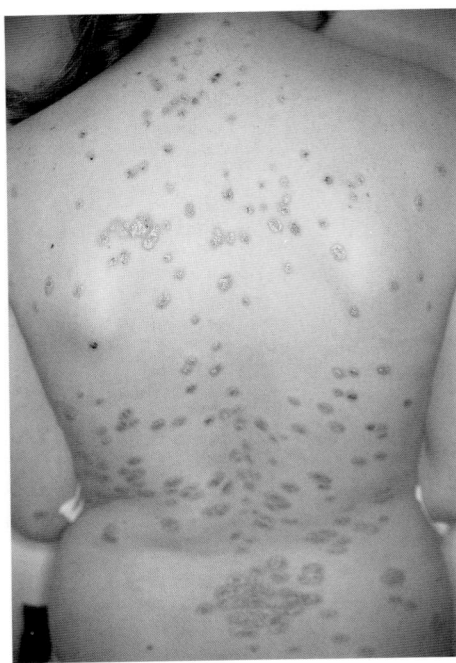

Figure 19.42: Guttate erythemato-scaling small plaques of guttate psoriasis.

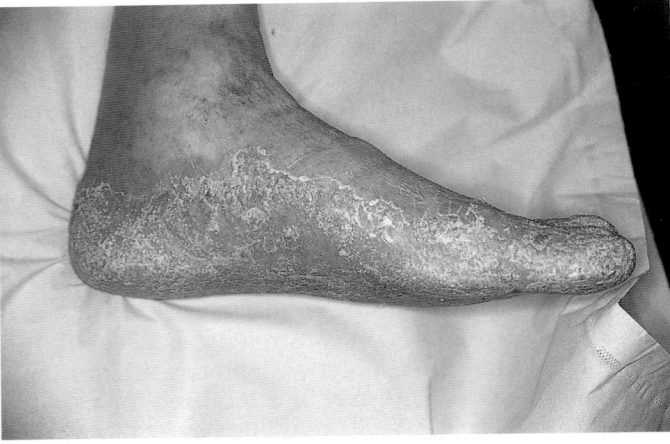

Figure 19.43: Erythema, scaling, hyperkeratosis and pustules in pustular plantar psoriasis.

2. Rheumatoid arthritis distribution with involvement of the metacarpal and metatarsal joints.
3. Mono- or oligo-arthropathy with one joint being involved, most commonly the knee or ankle.
4. Arthritis mutilans. This is a particularly severe form of psoriatic arthritis where the phalanges are eroded leading to telescoping of the skin of the fingers and a destructive arthropathy.
5. Sacroileitis.

Treatment

It has already been mentioned that the tropical environment may be beneficial to psoriasis and all that patients may really need is an extended period of sun exposure. However, there are numerous treatments for psoriasis reflecting the fact that none of them is a cure. Treatments are often used in combination and tailored to the anatomical distribution and extent of the disease and the availability of therapy. The patient should be instructed to stop using soap on their skin and to use an emollient instead. The patient is always instructed to moisturise the skin regularly with an emollient.

Tar has been used for several decades in a solution of 5%, 10% or 20% in some form of vehicle. A popular vehicle is Lassar's paste. This is applied once or twice daily but has the disadvantage of being extremely smelly and also tends to stain clothing. It can be especially effective in combination with ultraviolet therapy or simple sun exposure. It may be combined with a topical steroid for added potency.

Topical potent steroids should only be used for very small periods of time in psoriasis as rapid withdrawal can lead to a rebound effect with a more severe psoriasis. They are especially indicated for the face or the flexures, and scalp psoriasis.

Dithranol is derived from the bark of the aroroba tree. It has been used in psoriasis for several decades and is often made up in Lassar's paste in different concentrations varying from 0.1% to 1%, with higher concentrations being used for inpatients. The dithranol treatment may be applied for 24 hours and then washed off with arachis oil the next day. Other dithranol protocols require contact for 30 minutes and then the dithranol is washed off. This treatment has several disadvantages and causes erythema and burning, it stains clothing, and the patient's skin tends to have a characteristic staining which lasts for up to 2 weeks. It cannot be used in flexures or on pustular psoriasis.

Phototherapy with PUVA or UVB has been found to be effective in psoriasis. However, such treatment often is not available in the tropics and an alternative is graduated sun exposure if local traditions allow. If psoralens are available locally a methoxypsoralen may be taken and the patient instructed to expose their skin to sunlight for 30–60 minutes three times weekly.

Calcipotriol is a vitamin D analogue and has to be used thickly twice a day on the psoriatic plaques. It may be combined with a weak topical steroid in order to increase its potency.

Systemic therapy for psoriasis involves the use of agents such as cyclosporin A, methotrexate, hydroxyurea and micofenolate. Methotrexate has been highly effective in psoriasis for more than 25 years and is considered the gold standard of systemic therapy. Doses are given weekly, ranging from 2.5 mg to up to 25 mg per week. Baseline liver function tests and levels of procollagen peptide should be performed and monitored throughout therapy. A full blood count has to be performed regularly as methotrexate can cause bone marrow aplasia. Cyclosporin A has been shown in a clinical controlled trial to be highly effective in psoriasis but it is very expensive and often not available in the tropics. Systemic retinoids have been used successfully in the form of acitretin at a daily dose of 30–40 mg daily; however, these are expensive drugs that require close monitoring for renal and liver toxicity. Teratogenesis is a main concern.

Photosensitivity disorders

The photosensitivity diseases are a group of dermatoses characterized by the development of cutaneous eruption after exposure to UVB, UVA and/or visible light. In practice the results of sun exposure are one of the commonest cutaneous disorders that patients will complain of after having visited a tropical environment. Photodermatoses can be classified into four main groups: idiopathic; those due to exogenous agents, such as phototoxicity and photoallergy; those secondary to endogenous agents such as the porphyrias; and dermatoses that are made worse by sunlight. The classic photoreactive eruption occurs on exposed sides such as the forehead, nose, cheeks, the V of the neck (Figure 19.44), the forearms and the dorsa of the hands.

Clinical evaluation in photosensitivity

Ask if the condition is photoexacerbated and ascertain the distribution of the eruption, the duration, the age of onset and whether the eruption occurs seasonally. It is also important to assess how much sun exposure is required to produce the eruption, how long after exposure the eruption occurs and how long it lasts. Clues as to which wavelengths may be causing the photodermatosis may be sought as to whether the eruption occurs through window glass or in the presence of a UVB or broad-spectrum sunscreen. An occupational and social history should be taken to exclude any topical photosensitizers that have been applied. A family history is sought of autoimmune disorder, porphyrias or any genetic disorders. Physical examination has to obtain a description of the distribution of the rash. Morphology is a very good clue as to aetiology, with urticarial plaques

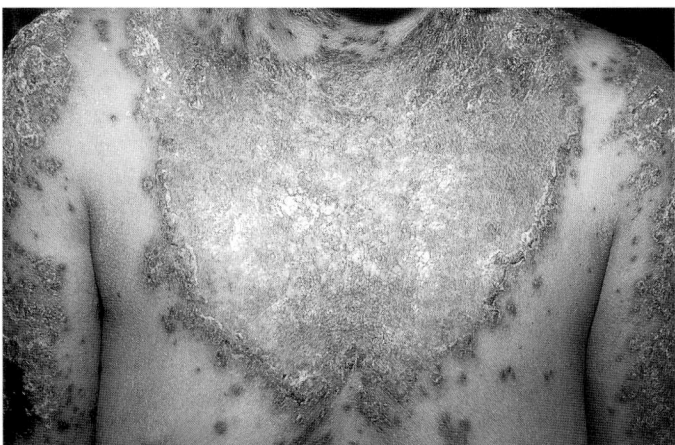

Figure 19.44: Severe erythema and inflammation on the neck V following sun exposure in a case of photosensitive dermatosis.

being common in erythropoetic porphyria, and solar urticaria with papules, vesicles and plaques common in polymorphic light eruption. Vesicles, scarring and pigment disorder are commonly found in porphyria cutanea tarda.

Polymorphic light eruption

This is the most common idiopathic photodermatosis and it commonly occurs when patients go from a temperate environment to a tropical environment; it can also be caused by change in season within a temperate environment. Its onset is commonly from childhood to late adult life and is more common in women than in men. It is common in all races and skin types. It presents clinically with polymorphic lesions including erythematous papules, vesicles, nodules, plaques, purpura and target-like lesions. Thankfully only one type of lesion tends to predominate in any one patient. Unfortunately it tends to recur indefinitely on sudden exposure to sunlight. It is crucial that serology be performed to exclude systemic lupus erythematosus. Treatment includes photoprotection by covering up and sunscreens; as topical corticosteroids are only partially effective, systemic corticosteroids may be used for severe flares. UVB phototherapy may be used prophylactically and is to be preferred to PUVA therapy as it has fewer side effects. Antimalarials are disappointing and azathioprine has been used for severe cases.

Erythropoetic porphyria

This is an autosomal dominant condition with variable penetrance and presents in childhood with a burning and stinging sensation on exposure to sunlight. The photosensitive eruption consists of erythema, oedema and urticated lesions, with blisters only occurring rarely. The skin has a pebble-like appearance on the interphalangeal joint and there may be scar formation. There may be an associated anaemia and hepatic decompensation. The defective enzyme is the ferokelotase gene on chromosome 18. Investigations reveal elevated photoporphyrin in erythrocytes with normal protoporphyrin in plasma, faeces and urine. The treatment is by photoprotection, β-carotenes and liver transplantation in those that develop hepatic failure.

Porphyria cutanea tarda

This is the most common type of porphyria and is due to defective hepatic uroporphyrinogen decarboxylase activity. Most cases are sporadic, with a small amount being autosomal dominantly inherited. Precipitating factors may include alcohol, exogenous oestrogens, iron and chlorinated hydrocarbons. It may also be associated with hepatitis C and HIV infection. Clinically it presents with skin fragility, vesicles, milia on sun exposed areas, periorbital hypertrichosis and mottled hyperpigmentation, and hypopigmentation with sclerodematous changes of the hands. Investigations reveal an elevated neuroporphyrin in the urine, and elevated isocoproporphyrin in the stool. Treatment is with phlebotomy, low-dose hydroxychloroquine, colestyramine and erythropoietin.

Drugs that cause photosensitivity

There is a large group of drugs that may cause photosensitivity; the commonest are the tetracyclines, thiazide diuretics and sulfamide compounds.

Skin malignancies

Cutaneous cancer is rare in dark-skinned patients. Historical migrations of lighter-skinned peoples to the more tropical parts of the world have led to a large increase in the amount of skin cancer being diagnosed. Indeed, one of the major hazards of light-skinned people travelling even for short periods to the tropics is in fact skin carcinogenesis. The various skin cancers are easy to diagnose often by morphology alone, with histology being the gold standard. Most commonly cutaneous cancers are not fatal; however, those that arise from melanocytes are highly invasive and aggressive and are called malignant melanoma. Therefore it is practical to divide skin cancer into non-melanoma skin cancer and malignant melanoma skin cancer.

Non-melanoma skin cancer

The main and commonest groups are actinic keratoses, basal cell carcinomas and squamous cell carcinomas.

Actinic keratoses

These are poorly circumscribed erythematous macules and flat plaques variable in diameter from several millimetres to a few centimetres (Figure 19.45). A scale on the surface is adherent and rough. Lesions arising from the ears, dorsum of hands and forearms tend to be thicker and more hyperkeratotic than those on the face. Some actinic keratoses can be tender or hyperpigmented. Actinic keratoses arising on the lip present as confluent scaliness with focal erosion and fissures and loss of definition of the vermilion border. The natural history of actinic keratosis is controversial and estimates of progression to squamous cell carcinoma range from 3% to 20%.

Isolated lesions may easily be treated using cryotherapy, with two freeze/thaw cycles required for curative therapy. However, if the lesions are widespread topical 5-fluorouracil (Efudix) may be used once or even twice daily to the rough areas for 3 weeks. The patient should be warned that there is intense inflammatory response as apoptosis of abnormal cells occurs and that this is a normal part of the treatment. The inflammation can be so intense as to extremely distress the patient. The patient should be reassured and if the areas are painful a moderate topical steroid may be used in the mornings, with the Efudix being used at night. A more recent therapy has been the introduction of topical glycosenac, which needs to be used for a minimum of 3 months. The advantage of this treatment is that there is no intense inflammatory reaction and efficacy can be as high as 50% in 3 months, rising to higher curative rates the longer the cream is used.

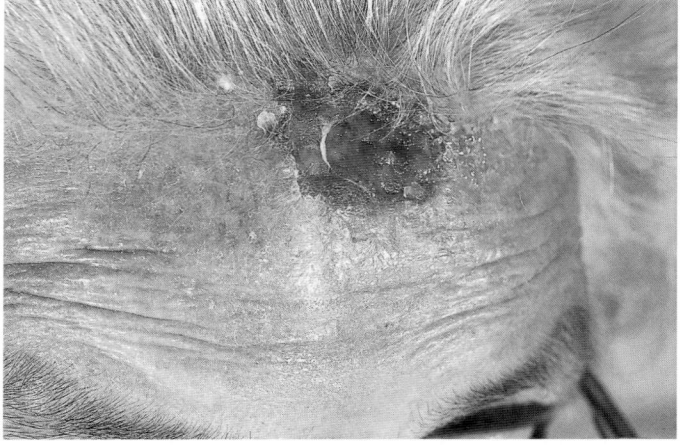

Figure 19.45: Erythema, superficial ulceration and scaling in actinic keratosis.

Squamous cell carcinoma (SCC)

This malignant tumour arises from epithelial keratinocytes whose cells usually show some degree of maturation toward keratin formation. The epidemiology of actinic keratoses mirrors that of SCC. The incidence of actinic keratoses and SCC is dependent on the combination of cumulative sun exposure and photosensitivity. Most actinic keratoses and SCCs occur in areas that receive the most solar radiation, with the vast majority occurring on the upper limbs, head and neck. Those with an outdoor job and those living closer to the equator are also more severely affected. The classic SCC is a hyperkeratotic, skin-coloured erythematous papule, nodule or plaque arising on sun-damaged skin. Invasive lesions may have a soft cutaneous extension.

Aetiology

Most actinic keratoses and SCCs will contain mutations of the p53 tumour suppressor gene. p53 is a negative cancer regulator and normally acts to prevent cells from proliferating uncontrollably. It is hypothesized that ultraviolet radiation causes mutations in the p53 gene, leading to clonal keratinocyte proliferation in an uncontrolled way. At the early stages of clonal expansion one would see the lesion clinically as an actinic keratosis. However, when the clonal proliferation advances, an SCC would develop.

Metastases and natural history

The actinic keratosis is the initial lesion in a disease continuum that progresses to invasive SCC. Eighty per cent of SCCs will have a concomitant AK giving rise to or in close proximity to the SCC. Such high prevalence of concomitant actinic keratosis and cutaneous SCC suggests a strong correlation between these two lesions. Invasive SCC may grow slowly or rapidly and may metastasize, usually to the regional lymph nodes with a metastatic rate of 5%, an overall mortality of 3% and a 70% mortality in the metastatic group. Local recurrence and regional metastasis are dependent on treatment modality, previous treatment, location, size, depth, histological differentiation, histological evidence of perineural involvement, precipitating factors other than ultraviolet light and host immunosuppression. Lesions found on the ears and lip are known to be at higher risk of local recurrence and metastasis. SCCs presenting on the lip have an especially high local and metastatic rate, with 8% of patients presenting with clinically positive lymph-node involvement with an overall 5-year mortality rate of 17%. Indeed combined with poor histology the metastatic rate at presentation can be as high as 23%.

The surgical treatment of SCC requires a 4 mm margin; however, certain tumor characteristics are associated with a greater risk of subclinical tumour extension and include size of 2 cm or larger, aggresive histology—especially invasion of the subcutaneous tissue and perineural spread—and location in high-risk areas, in which case at least a 6 mm margin is recommended. However, carcinomas with a diameter of more than 20 mm involve a much higher risk of recurrence of 9.8%, because of local micrometastases, which require more generous local excision with a safety margin of about 10 mm.

Basal cell carcinoma (BCC)

This tumour is also called rodent ulcer or basal cell epithelioma and is a malignancy derived from the keratinocytes and stroma of the pilosebaceous follicle. BCCs are the most common human cancer, affecting an estimated 750,000 US inhabitants per year. Estimates predict that 28% of Caucasians born after 1994 will develop a BCC in their lifetime.

Aetiology

Epidemiological data implicates UV radiation exposure in BCC tumorigenesis. Sixty-six per cent of BCCs occur on the head and neck. The incidence is much greater in those with fair skin and they only very rarely occur in Africans. Most BCCs present on the face and upper trunk. The inner canthus and eyelids, which are more shielded from sunlight than other parts of the face, are frequently involved. Rare cases of vulval BCC also occur. This occurrence of BCCs in relatively sun-protected sites suggests that other co-factors may be important (Figure 19.46). Arsenic salts are a factor and arsenic-induced tumours are usually multiple and occur mainly on the trunk (see 'Arsenism', below). Molecular studies of the basal cell naevus syndrome and sporadic BCCs have led to the identification of an important tumour suppressor gene—the Patched gene—which is thought to be crucial

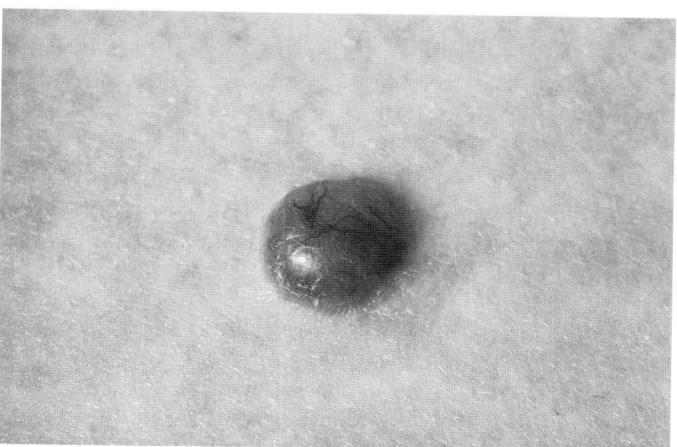

Figure 19.46: Nodular basal cell carcinoma on the chest.

in the pathogenesis of BCCs and that inactivation of patch is a necessary step in the evolution of BCCs.

Metastasis, progress and clinical features

The course of BCCs is slow but steady and progression results in local destruction of structures if left untreated. In immunosupprosed patients, tumours may be more aggressive. Metastases are extremely rare, with an estimated risk as low as 0.1%. There are six main clinical types of BCC.

1. *Rodent ulcer* commences as a small papule that subsequently becomes nodular and undergoes central ulceration. The margins of the tumour are well defined, slightly raised with a rolled border and with a pearly, shiny appearance. Blood vessels traversing over the margin give it a telangiectatic appearance.
2. *Pigmented BCC* is clinically similar to the rodent ulcer but the margins of the tumour are pigmented. Such pigmented BCCs may easily be mistaken clinically for malignant melanoma.
3. *Cystic BCC* is a well-defined papule which attains a pearly-coloured lobulated appearance with a telangiectatic surface earlier on, with the central part of the tumour ulcerating later on in its evolution.
4. *Morphoeic (sclerosing) BCC* may be difficult to eradicate, as clinically it is often impossible to determine the margins. Indeed, the tumour may have the clinical appearance of a scar; however, the pearly colour is maintained in certain areas of the tumour and telangiectasia is often present.
5. *Superficial BCC* often occurs on the trunk or limbs. It is a well-defined, slightly raised red plaque with an adherent scaly surface. Most lesions are solitary and may be pigmented. Over many years, the lesion may thicken and appear more like the rodent ulcer; however, early on, the margin of the tumour does have a lightly rolled, pearly-looking border with the characteristic telangiectasia present. Such tumours, when multiple, may suggest arsenic ingestion as an aetiological factor.

6. *Linear BCC* is an uncommon variant, first described in 1985. Clinically it is a linear, pearly and telengiectatic lesion and is located most often on the head and neck. On average this variant is thought to belong to a more aggresive subtype with subclinical dissemination.

Diagnosis and management of BCC

The diagnosis of BCC is based upon the clinical findings; however, if clinical doubt exists, a preoperative biopsy is advised. There are four generally accepted methods for obtaining tissue for diagnosis: shave biopsy, punch biopsy, cytology or definitive surgery. Almost all BCCs begin as small easily managed lesions that can be treated in several different ways, resulting in minimal morbidity and a highly favourable outcome. Treatment by curretage and cautery, surgical exicision, radiotherapy, cryotherapy and Moh's chemosurgery all have cure rates of well over 90%. Tumours in certain sites have a greater risk of recurrence, namely the nasae alae, nasolabilal fold, tragus and retro-auricular area.

Follow-up

The main aims of follow-up are detection of tumour recurrence, early detection and treatment of new lesions. Indeed 36% of patients who have a previous BCC will develop a further BCC. Those especially at risk of BCCs are those with very fair skin and excess sun exposure. These patients with multiple BCCs are found in as many as 20% of such high-risk patients .

Most BCCs that will recur will recur within 3 years. It is a matter of the resources available, whether in an outpatient dermatology department or in general practice, as to how frequent or for how long the follow-up surveillance should be. Obviously patients with multiple BCCs and at high risk of developing further BCCs should be followed up at least 6-monthly for the patient's remaining lifetime. However, it may not be economically justifiable to follow up every BCC, especially if it is a single isolated BCC in the older age group. One major advantage of regular follow-up is continued patient education regarding sun avoidance.

Malignant melanoma

The incidence of malignant melanoma is increasing in developed countries and also in those fair-skinned persons who live in the tropics. Epidemiological studies suggest that sunlight is a major cause of melanoma. Worldwide the incidence of melanoma correlates inversely with latitude, with high rates closest to the equator and lower rates closer to the poles. Although pale-skinned patients are most at risk, rare forms such as the acral lentiginous malignant melanoma are equally distributed throughout all skin types. Five per cent of patients with a melanoma have a family history of malignant melanoma. Other risk factors are the existence of numerous dysplastic naevi, higher than average number of benign naevi, the existence of a congenital naevus, previous cutaneous melanoma, immunosupression, excessive sun exposure and excessive sun sensitivity. Experimentally melanocytes demonstrate resistance to UVB-induced apoptosis and therefore are at a higher risk of incorporating UV-induced mutations. Mutations have been found in susceptibility genes such as the CDKN2A gene or in genes implicated in control of the cell cycle or maintenance of cell integrity. However, the molecular basis of malignant melanoma still remains to be elucidated.

Metastasis and natural history of malignant melanoma

There is an inverse relationship between tumour thickness and survival. Therefore the more superficial the lesion at presentation the more likely is a cure. The thickness of the tumour is defined by the Breslow scale, which is measured in millimetres from the granular cell layer of the epidermis to the deepest tumour cells. Those tumours that have a Breslow thickness of 1.5 mm or less have a 93% 5-year survival rate, whereas those with a Breslow thickness of more than 3.5 mm have a 5-year survival rate of 37%. Metastasis is first to regional lymph nodes and then to lung, liver, brain, bone and peritoneum.

Clinical presentation

Most malignant melanomas appear de novo as pigmented lesions. A fifth of malignant melanomas are thought to arise from pre-existent naevi. Any pigmented lesion that is asymmetric, has an irregular border, a variegated or dark colour, and a diameter of more than 0.6 cm and rapid elevation are all signs of malignant melanoma. Although most melanomas are typically asymptomatic, presentation may include itching and bleeding of existent naevi. There are four major types of malignant melanoma described clinically. These are superficial spreading malignant melanoma, lentigo maligna melanoma, acral lentiginous malignant melanoma and nodular melanoma. Lentigo maligna occurs in patients who are over 50 years old and is found mainly on sun-damaged skin of the head and neck. Clinically it appears as an irregularly bordered tan or brown macule which enlarges slowly over many years (Figure 19.47). It is commonly mistaken for another similar-looking lesion that occurs on the head and neck called a seborrhoeic keratosis and may even be mistaken for a solar lentigo. The prognosis of lentigo maligna is extremely good; however, if palpable areas develop within it this means that this relatively non-aggressive tumour may have developed into a nodular malignant melanoma, which has a far worse prognosis. The superficial spreading malignant melanoma occurs after the age of 40 and the diameters are often more than 1 cm and are palpable. There is a great variability in the colour of these lesions, from shades of pink, red, brown and black (Figure 19.48). Since the prognosis of malignant melanoma is dependent on tumour thickness, this tumour has a very good

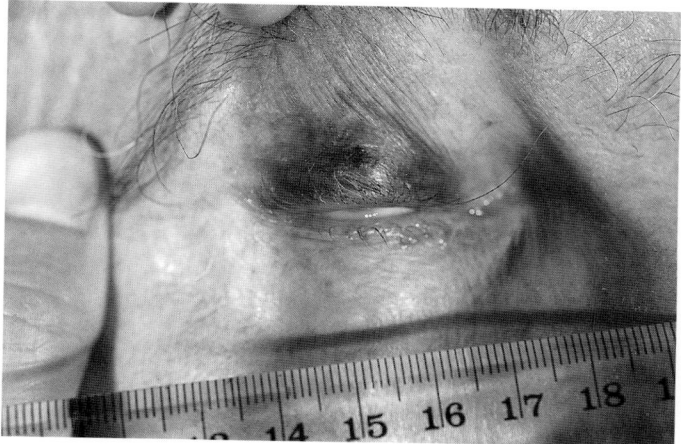

Figure 19.47: Chronic lentigo maligna melanoma on the upper eyelid of an elderly patient.

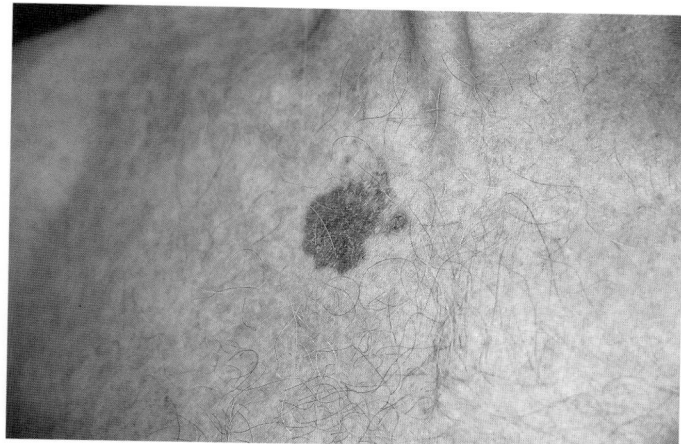

Figure 19.48: Superficially spreading malignant melanoma of the chest.

prognosis. However, the appearance of nodular areas signifies the development of a more aggressive tumour. Nodular malignant melanoma appears as a papule or a nodule and in men commonly occurs on the trunk and in women on the legs. It grows rapidly and is seen to elevate over a few months. Unfortunately this form of malignant melanoma has the worst prognosis. Acral lentiginous malignant melanoma is found on the palms, sole and nail-beds. Although this is a rare tumour it is of equal incidence in all races and therefore may be seen in the tropics. This form of malignant melanoma has the poorest prognosis and it is vital that it is recognized early.

Management

The definitive treatment for malignant melanoma is excision. This means that diagnosis has to be made early in order to ensure a cure. The margins for excision should be of at least 1 cm and should include subcutaneous fat for thin melanomas of less than 1.5 mm. However, for the lentigo maligna a 2–5 mm margin of clinically normal skin should be sufficient. In cases of thick melanoma of 1.5 mm or more it is suggested that a 2 cm margin of normal skin be used to ensure complete excision. Once the melanoma has metastasized there are no known therapies at present which affect long-term prognosis.

Urticaria

This is a family of conditions characterized by the appearance of itchy wheals. Internationally, prevalence is thought to be as high as 20%. Clinically it can be divided into acute and chronic urticaria. The lesions themselves are transient and in the Caucasian patient they may be pink or red skin swellings surrounded by erythema. Such erythema and skin redness may not be apparent in the darker-skinned patient. The shape and size of the lesions vary considerably and can occur anywhere on the body (Figure 19.49). By definition an urticarial attack will last

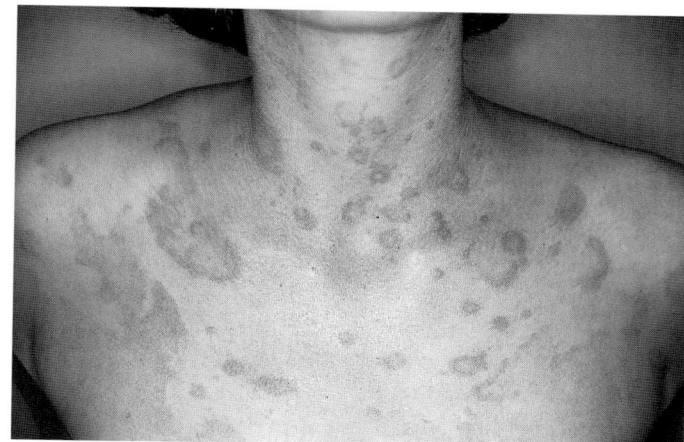

Figure 19.49: Pruritic urticarial wheals on the trunk.

less than 24 hours. Another associated condition called angio-oedema may coexist with urticaria and in this case the oedema is actually deeper in the dermis and subcutaneous tissues. The lesions last longer, resulting in swelling of the lips, eyelids, tongue and internal organs.

Acute urticaria

This is defined as urticaria occurring for less than 6 weeks. The commonest cause of acute urticaria is the ingestion or parenteral administration of drugs. The commonest involved drugs are antibiotics, sedatives, tranquillizers, analgesics, laxatives and diuretics. The pathogenesis of this process is thought to be IgE mediated, in which case they would need to be preformed IgE to the exposed allergen. However, drugs may cause acute urticaria in a non-immunological way, with opioid type drugs being thought to release mast cell histamine by a direct mechanism. Other drugs such as aspirin and non-steroidal anti-inflammatory drugs may also cause an acute angio-oedema. A minority of patients may have a food allergy and the commonest substances are nuts, fish, shellfish, eggs, milk, chocolate, tomatoes and certain food additives such as tartrazine and benzoic acid derivatives. When a patient's urticaria appears during spring and summer the role of inhaled allergens such as pollens and spores should be considered as a cause of acute urticaria. Certain infectious agents such as viral infections and streptococcal pharyngitis in children may also cause a transient urticaria over weeks. The commonest acute contact urticarial reaction is to latex. This is especially a problem in health care workers, in which case non-latex gloves should be used.

Any possible precipitants or exacerbation factors such as drug therapy should be removed. The patient should be started on a non-sedating antihistamine and this is usually sufficient to treat an acute urticaria. If the patient is non-responsive to treatment or the whealing attacks seem to last longer than 6 weeks, then the patient should be treated as if they have a chronic urticaria.

Chronic urticaria

This is said to occur when whealing attacks last more than 6 weeks. By far the largest group are of the chronic idiopathic form with no immediate cause found. However, a careful history and examination should be carried out and appropriate tests performed in order to elicit a possible cause. The chronic urticarias may be divided into the physical urticarias, chronic idiopathic urticaria, angio-oedema and urticarial vasculitis.

Physical urticaria

This may be caused by physical pressure (Figure 19.50), vibration during exercise, or periods in a hot environment, periods of cold and cooling of the skin, in response to sunlight, and aquagenic urticaria, where the wheals occur in response to contact with water. In most cases the type of physical urticaria can be elucidated by the detailed history, with pressure urticaria occurring under tight clothing and cholinergic urticaria occurring at times

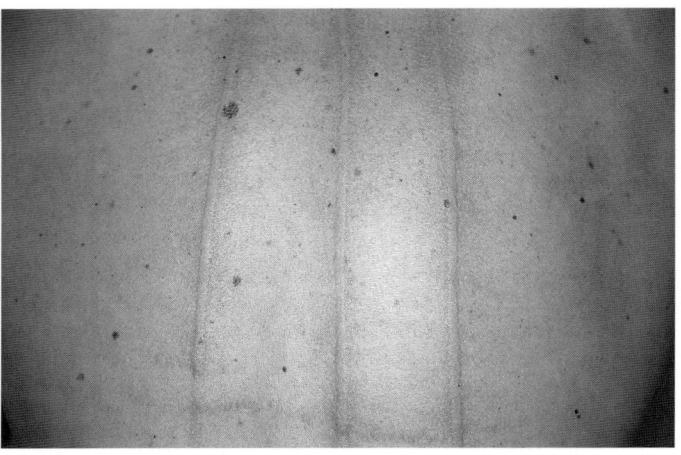

Figure 19.50: Pressure urticaria or dermographism.

of emotion and sweating. Patients with cold urticaria may complain of lesions as soon as they exit a hot bath. Solar urticaria is very rare and occurs in response to natural or artificial sunlight. Cold urticaria may be tested for by placing an ice cube on the skin for 10 minutes and then observing a wheal appearing 5–10 minutes later.

Chronic idiopathic urticaria

This is a diagnosis made once all the previous aetiological factors have been excluded. However, in the tropics common causes of long-standing urticaria may be hookworm, tapeworms and roundworms, and thus the stools should be examined in such patients. In addition the patient should be examined for evidence of trichinoses, dracunculosis, lymphatic filariasis and strongyloidiasis. A small minority of patients labelled as having chronic idiopathic urticaria may in fact have circulating histamine-releasing autoantibodies. In such patients autologous serum injected intradermally produces an intense whealing reaction.

Angio-oedema

This is a deeper form of urticaria and may be associated with urticarial wheals. It results in swollen lips, eyelids, tongue, hands and feet, with involvement of the upper airways causing respiratory arrest and fatal respiratory failure. Less than 1% of cases of angio-oedema may be hereditary in autosomal dominant fashion, in which case a plasma complement C4 should be measured and if this is low more detailed investigations of C1 esterase activity should be instituted.

Urticarial vasculitis

The lesions in this case may be painful and last for several days. Such an urticarial vasculitis should be investigated histologically and the biopsy should include both lesional and non-lesional skin. Biopsy will show a vasculitis or a leucocytoklastic vasculitis. A leucocytoklastic vasculitis is more likely to be associated with systemic diseases such as the autoimmune connective tissue diseases and the oral and parenteral administration of drugs.

Management of chronic idiopathic urticaria

Any identifiable causes should be removed and the patient should be educated to avoid drugs that may cause histamine release such as aspirin, non-steroidal anti-inflammatory drugs and the opioid drugs. The patient should be started on a non-sedating antihistamine and if there is a poor response a further sedating antihistamine should be added at night. If the patient still has not responded an H_2 antagonist such as cimetidine may be added. Resistant forms of urticaria may need short courses of systemic steroids and patients with hereditary angio-oedema or severe angio-oedema may need adrenaline pens for emergency situations. Refractory cases may require immunosupression with cyclosporin A, intravenous immunoglobulin and even in extreme cases plasmapheresis.

Other non-infective dermatoses mainly limited to the tropics

Arsenism

Although arsenic was commonly used in medications in the past this had stopped by the first half of the twentieth century. Today arsenic is widely used in its inorganic form in insecticides, fungicides, herbicides, and in the manufacture of glass and fireworks. Inorganic arsenic compounds exist in the form of arsenites and arsenates. Arsenites are thought to be the most toxic; such arsenites are normally detoxified in the liver and excreted in the urine. However, this detoxification process may be subject to genetic polymorphisms, resulting in the inability of a proportion of the population to detoxify arsenite, and thereby cause carcinogenicity and toxicity in humans. The commonest form of arsenism is now due to water contamination and cases have been reported in Chile, Taiwan, Mexico, Argentina, Thailand and the Ganges delta in India. Cutaneous changes begin with hyper-pigmentation in the groin and areolae. These hyper-pigmented areas may develop hypopigmented areas within them, giving rise to a characteristic raindrop appearance. As many as 30% of patients may have pigmentation in the oral cavity. Hyperkeratotic papules on the palms and soles occur in up to 70% of patients; patients may have an associated cutaneous malignancy such as Bowen's disease, BCC, SCC or keratoacanthomas. These tumours mainly occur on sun-exposed sites and suspicion of arsenism should be aroused as such tumours are rare in dark-skinned patients. The clinical management of these patients needs careful long-term monitoring for the development of cutaneous neoplasms and also associated internal malignancy. The hyperkeratotic areas on the palms and soles may be treated by a 10% salicylate ointment twice daily. In more affluent areas systemic retinoids may be given to prevent the onset of cutaneous malignancy.

Brazilian pemphigus foliaceus (fogo selvagem—wild fire)

This is an autoimmune bullous dermatosis. It is characterized by antibodies to the epidermal desmosomes, specifically desmoglein 1 (Dsg1). It is clinically identical to the non-endemic form of pemphigus foliaceus, which is found throughout the world. Pemphigus foliaceus itself is a variant of pemphigus vulgaris, which is one of the commonest forms of blistering disease causing intra-epidermal vesicles. Fogo selvagem, unlike the non-endemic form of pemphigus foliaceus, is endemic to certain regions of Brazil and some areas of Colombia, Bolivia, Paraguay and Argentina. It is associated with recent areas of colonization and cases tend to decrease with increasing urbanization. The sex and race incidence is the same within an endemic area. The vast majority of patients live near rivers and within flying range of black flies (*Simulium pruinosum*). Clinically the lesions of fogo selvagem are a superficial vesicle which can be mistaken for impetigo. The blisters rupture easily, leaving superficial erosions. The lesions begin on the face, scalp, upper chest and abdomen and then spread to the limbs. Unlike pemphigus vulgaris oral or mucosal lesions are extremely uncommon in pemphigus foliaceus and fogo selvagem. The dermatosis evolves gradually over a period of several weeks or months. Fogo selvagem may present as a localized form of disease in which the seborrhoeic areas of the face and trunk are involved and this may lead to diagnostic confusion with discoid lupus erythematosus, but patients with fogo selvagem have no positive lupus serology and can be distinguished by skin biopsy. The localized form may stay localized or eventually become generalized. Patients with generalized fogo selvagem may present in one of three ways: an acute aggressive form; those with exfoliative erythroderma; and a more slowly aggressive form. Patients with the acute aggressive form have a predominance of blisters and it may be associated with fever, arthralgias and malaise. It is thought that patients who have this form of disease are susceptible to life-threatening herpes simplex virus infections. In those patients who develop exfoliative erythroderma the main clinical lesions are superficial erosions and crusting. The third form includes those patients in whom localized fogo selvagem has become generalized and clinically consists of keratotic plaques and nodular lesions in the seborrhoeic and acral areas. There is a rarer, hyper-pigmented, form of fogo selvagem which often occurs when the patient is recovering from fogo selvagem after treatment.

It is especially important that this condition is diagnosed early in childhood as delay in diagnosis can lead to dwarfism and azoospermia as an adult. It is thought that fogo selvagem may also have psychiatric effects and may be associated with depression. This form may be differentiated from pemphigus foliaces by distinct epidemiological features. It may be distinguished from pemphigus vulgaris due to its lack of oral lesions. The gold test for diagnosis is indirect and direct immunofluorescence for Dsg1. However, if such investigations are not available a Tzank smear may show acantholytic cells suggestive of fogo selvagem. Skin biopsy may also suggest the diagnosis.

Management

Left untreated 40% of patients die within 2 years. High-dose systemic steroid is the treatment of choice and is slowly tapered in dosage according to response. Steroid-sparing agents such as azathioprine are useful and cyclophosphamide has been used with good results. Useful adjunctive therapies include antimalarials and dapsone. An important consideration before starting systemic corticosteroids is to rule out the possibility of concurrent tuberculosis. Fatal cases of disseminated strongyloidiasis have also been reported after steroid therapy for this condition.

Amyloid and amyloidosis

Amyloidosis is the abnormal extracellular deposition of a group of unrelated proteins that may show green birefringence on Congo Red staining when viewed under polarized light. Light microscopy shows amyloid to be an amorphous homogeneous eosinophilic material. Electron microscopy shows it to be made of linear non-branching paired fibrils of protein arranged in a loose meshwork. Cutaneous lesions are common in patients with primary amyloid and myeloma-associated systemic amyloidosis. They may occur in up to 40% of patients. Clinically, these consist of waxy purpuric lesions on the skin and mucosae and should result in an investigation for a plasma cell dyscrasia. Associated features include carpal tunnel syndrome, macroglossia and hepatomegaly.

Cutaneous involvement in secondary systemic amyloidosis is uncommon but when it does occur presents with petechiae, purpura and ecchymoses occurring spontaneously after minor trauma and is the result of amyloid infiltration of blood vessel walls. Purpuric lesions are likely to be found in the flexural region such as eyelids, nasolabial folds, neck, axillae, umbilicus, anogenital area as well as orally. A third form of amyloidosis is the group of localized cutaneous amyloidosis. This may present as a nodular localized cutaneous amyloidosis, lichen amyloidosus and a macular amyloidosis.

Nodular localized cutaneous amyloidosis

This is uncommon and presents with single or multiple lesions on the limbs, face, trunk or genitalia. Clinically, the lesions may be identical to those of plasma cell dyscrasia and systemic amyloidosis. The lesions may vary in size from a few millimetres to several centimetres. Some patients develop a paraproteinaemia and overt systemic amyloidosis.

Lichen amyloidosus

This presents with an itchy eruption of multiple discrete hyperkeratotic papules distributed on the shins that coalesce to form plaques (Figure 19.51). Rarely, lesions may be found on the calves, ankles, dorsa of the feet and the thighs. There has been a great deal of debate as to the aetiology of lichen amyloidosus, with some researchers finding Epstein–Barr virus using in situ hybridization within the keratinocytes. It is also thought that it may occur as a result of an abnormal reaction to scratching as most people with lichen amyloidosus have concomitant lichenified eczema around the plaques. Indeed treatment with steroids, which decreases the itch, tends to improve the condition although only minimally.

Macular amyloidosis

This is an itchy eruption of dusky brown-greyish macules, symmetrically distributed on the upper back

Figure 19.51: Pruritic plaque of lichen amyloid on the shin.

and limbs. After constant scratching the macules assume a rippled appearance. Macular amyloid and lichen amyloidosus may coexist, leading to the hypothesis that they are the result of a single pathological process. Lichen amyloidosus is commoner among Chinese whereas macular amyloidosis is commoner among Central and South Americans, Middle Easterners and South Asians. Familial cases have been described.

Treatment

Deposits of nodular primary localized cutaneous amyloidosis can be treated surgically but they may recur locally. Lichen and macular amyloid are treated with a topical steroid mainly under occlusion but results are disappointing. There has been some success using dermabrasion as well as topical dimethylsulfonamide and systemic retinoids.

Lichen planus and lichenoid eruptions

Lichen planus is a relatively common disease with a worldwide dermatology referral prevalence of 1–2%. The classic lesion presents on both skin and mucosae. Cutaneous lesions present with flat-topped polygonal, pruritic shiny papules with a violaceous hue. In darker skin purple, brown or black are more typical colours than violet (Figure 19.52). Postinflammatory hyperpigmentation is prominent and persistent in darker-skinned patients. It is thought that lichen planus itself is more common in darker-skinned patients. Variants of classical lichen planus include hypertrophic, atrophic and linear lichen planus. Classical lichen planus begins most frequently on the limbs, especially around the ankles and wrists, and a quarter have involvement of the oral cavity, which may present in the form of white Wickham's striae or as erosive painful lesions (Figure 19.53). A quarter of patients have truncal involvement and small number (5%) have face and neck involvement. The two types of lichen planus which are most relevant to the tropical physician are hypertrophic lichen planus and actinic lichen planus.

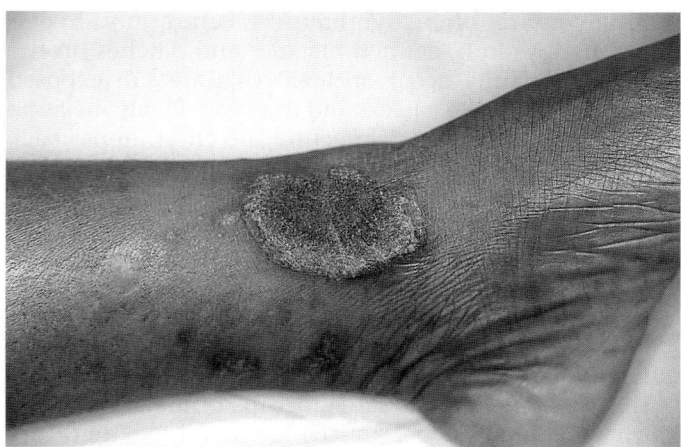

Figure 19.52: Isolated papules and large plaque of lichen planus with Wickham's striae.

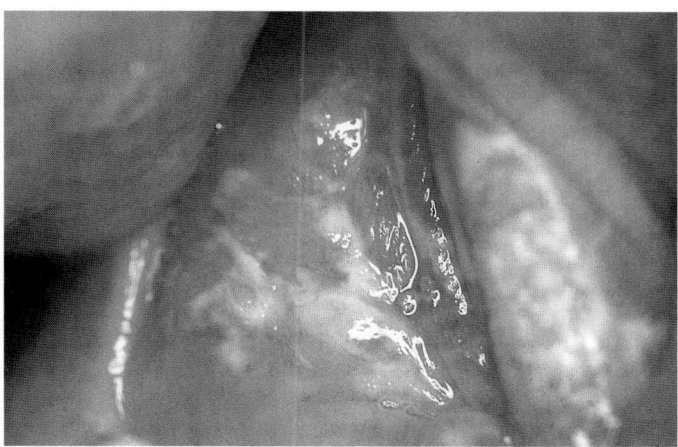

Figure 19.53: Erosive oral lichen planus.

Hypertrophic lichen planus

This presents with red, brown or violaceous lichenified verrucous plaques which are extremely itchy. The lesions primarily occur on the lower legs and ankles. It is especially common in inhabitants of southern India and Sri Lanka.

Actinic lichen planus

This occurs in a photodistribution (see section on 'Photosensitivity disorders', above) and is induced by sun exposure. In countries such as India actinic lichen planus forms as little as 5% of all cases of lichen planus, whereas in the Middle East it can be as high as 30–40% of cases. The main group of patients that are affected are children and young adults. There are three clinical presentations: annular, dyschromic and pigmented. The commonest form is the annular type, which presents as brownish plaques with an annular configuration most commonly affecting the lateral aspects of the forehead, dorsum of the hands, forearms, lower lip, cheeks and the V-shaped area of the neck. With time the annular lesion develops hypopigmentation centrally and some subtle atrophy. This form of lichen planus typically occurs in dark-skinned individuals, with women being affected more than men and occurring at a younger age of onset than classic lichen planus. It is not associated with positive autoimmune serology.

Treatment

Spontaneous remissions of cutaneous lichen planus occur in up to 70% of cases after 1 year. However, oral lesions tend not to resolve spontaneously, with the erosive form remission rate being as low as 3%. Other forms of oral involvement may last about 5 years and then resolve; however, such resolution only occurs in up to 40%.

Precipitant factors such as scratching or sun exposure should be avoided and patients advised to use a broad-spectrum, high-factor sunscreen. Topical steroids, topical steroids with occlusion and intralesional steroids are all used. Systemic steroids may be used when lichen planus is acute in onset and rapidly progressive. However, it is not recommended for long periods of treatment. Systemic retinoids have been used successfully in widespread lichen planus as well as cyclosporin A, dapsone and antimalarials. Actinic lichen planus has been reported to respond particularly well to systemic antimalarials. Hypertrophic lichen planus can be treated with intralesional steroids and topical steroids under occlusion. The authors find that a potent steroid combined with 5% or 10% salicylate is particularly effective applied twice a day for a period of at least 4–6 weeks. Oral lichen planus especially if it is erosive will particularly require systemic treatments. Phototherapy can be used to treat most cutaneous forms of lichen planus apart from actinic lichen planus.

Disorders of pigmentation

The majority of the world's population is brown skinned and therefore hyper- or hypopigmentation is of major concern to dermatologists worldwide and to tropical physicians. Inflammatory disease of the skin is extremely common and therefore postinflammatory hyper-pigmentation is also common. The unfortunate and widespread use of depigmenting creams in Africa and parts of Asia in order to lighten the complexion has led to significant morbidity and in some cases permanent disfigurement. Treatments for hyperpigmentation disorders is difficult and prolonged and requires a great deal of patience and patient education.

Vitiligo

This is a condition characterized by the complete loss of pigment within skin. Initially it was thought that vitiligo was more common in dark-skinned patients but it is much more likely that vitiligo is more clearly seen in such patients and therefore they are more likely to present. Males and females are equally affected and the condition most commonly occurs in the first to third decades, with congenital cases being described. It is thought that the aetiology of vitiligo is autoimmunity

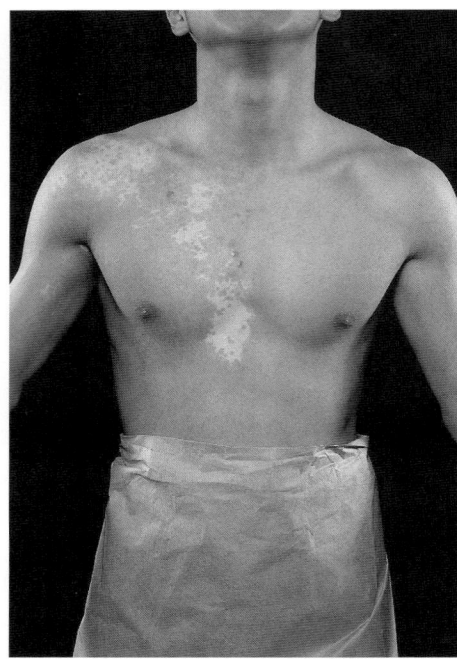

Figure 19.54: Segmental hypopigmentation of trunkal vitiligo.

because of its strong association with organ-specific auto-immune disease. Depigmentation starts suddenly, with the commonest sites being the hands, feet, genitalia, and periocular and perioral areas of the face. The pigmentation may form a generalized symmetrical pattern or a segmental pattern which follows a dermatome, and it ceases to progress after one year (Figure 19.54). The focal form may be an isolated lesion which progresses slowly. Vitiligo is usually symptomless but some patients may complain of pruritus. Diagnosis is clinical and confusion can sometimes be with pityriasis versicolor, post-inflammatory hypopigmentation, scleroderma and lichen sclerosus et atrophicus.

Management
Unfortunately, due to the slow mobility of melanocytes treatment of vitiligo can last more than a year. Melanocytes migrate from the margins and also from hair follicles. Therefore when repigmentation occurs it is around hair follicles and the periphery of the lesion. Unfortunately most of the therapies for vitiligo are largely unsuccessful. However, potent topical steroids may cause repigmentation in between 15% and 55% of patients. A commonly used treatment is an oral psoralen with exposure to UVA radiation; this is, however, a prolonged treatment and risks the development of skin cancers in the depigmented areas. A newly developed treatment called narrow band UVB has been found to be up to 60% successful in vitiligo. Surgical treatments include minigrafting with melanocytes.

Melasma
There are three patterns of melasma that are recognized clinically: centrofacial, malar and mandibular. The lesions

themselves are often symmetrical, uniformly hyper-pigmented, sharply defined macules and patches on the face. They mainly occur on areas that are sun exposed such as the upper lip, cheeks and forehead. Rarely melasma can be more widespread, affecting the chest, upper back and the sun-exposed side of the arms. The centrofacial variant consists of lesions on the cheeks, forehead, upper lip, nose and chin, whereas in the malar variant the lesions are found on the cheeks and nose. When lesions are found on the ramus of the mandible this is described as the mandibular distribution.

Melasma may be further subdivided into three different histological types. An increase predominantly in the basal and superbasal epidermis of melanin occurs in the epidermal type. In the dermal type there are melanin-laden macrophages in the superficial and deep dermis, with some of these melanin-laden macrophages being found in a perivascular distribution. The mixed type shows a histology that is a mixture of the previous two types. Clinically the epidermal type of melasma is accentuated by Wood's light examination of the skin. Wood's light accentuation only occurs on the epidermal components in the mixed type. This examination is highly relevant to therapy as the epidermal type is much more amenable to therapy than the dermal types. African women are more likely to have onset of melasma at an older age and to have the malar type distribution and this group of patients may also have higher incidence of the dermal type histology.

Epidemiology and aetiology
Ninety per cent of affected patients are women although when men are affected the characteristics are identical in both sexes. The disease is most common in Hispanic, South Asian and South-East Asian people, and those who live in areas of high-intensity UV radiation. Black-skinned patients may be affected but melasma may not be easily noticed. Interestingly, up to 70% of patients can have a family history suggesting a predisposition as well as UV exposure being of aetiological importance. The commonest causes, however, are oral contraceptives, hormone replacement therapy, pregnancy and rarely thyroid dysfunction. Some authorities have found elevated levels of luteinizing hormone in a small group of patients and have suggested that subclinical ovarian dysfunction may be of significance.

Treatment
The most useful treatment is hydroquinone, which is a hydroxyphenolic chemical that inhibits the conversion of dopa to melanin by inhibiting the tyrosinase enzyme. Thankfully this is widely available in the tropics and concentrations vary from 2% to 10%. It is suggested that the hydroquinone is used twice daily for 12 weeks. The authors cannot help but warn the reader that mono-benzyl ether of hydroquinone, which is a permanent depigmenting agent, should never be used to treat melasma, as it causes irreversible loss of pigment. It is important to be aware of the side effects of hydroquinone

as it may cause local skin irritation and thereby lead to postinflammatory hyperpigmentation, making the skin appear worse. However, this is uncommon. The patient should be warned that if the hydroquinone happens to go onto surrounding normal skin this may lighten as well, and may give the patient a sort of leopard skin appearance. Exogenous ochronosis is thought to be a rare side effect of hydroquinone therapy.

Hydroquinone may be combined with topical tretinoin and 1% dexamethasone in an ointment form and this is applied once a day at night for a minimum of 4–6 months. There may be an irritant dermatitis about which the patient should be warned. Azelaic acid may be used twice daily for 6 months and is tolerated very well, with very few side effects.

The most important treatment for melasma is to remove any exacerbating causes such as medication and contraceptives; patients should be advised to wear a broad-spectrum sun block when going out and to cover up thoroughly, wearing a hat in the sun. More recent therapy for melasma has included glycolic acid peels, tretinoin peels and laser treatment.

Postinflammatory hyperpigmentation

This is an acquired excess of pigment in skin that develops after an inflammatory dermatosis. The distribution of melanin synthesis is determined by the distribution of the preceding inflammation. Such inflammation may be caused by infections, allergic reactions, conditions such as eczema and psoriasis (Figure 19.55), reactions to medications, phototoxic eruptions and physical agents. The condition seems to be much worse in cases that disrupt the basement membrane layer such as in discoid lupus erythematosus and lichen planus. As in melasma, the melanin may be epidermal, dermal or mixed, in which case a Wood's light examination is helpful. Treatment of postinflammatory hyperpigmentation may take 6–12 months and involves the use of hydroquinone, tretinoin cream, glycolic acid and azelaic acid.

Phrynoderma

This is a distinctive form of follicular hyperkeratosis, which was initially described in association with vitamin A deficiency. The condition presents as small papules and nodules with central intrafollicular plugs to large papules. Some of the larger papules may have massive hyper-

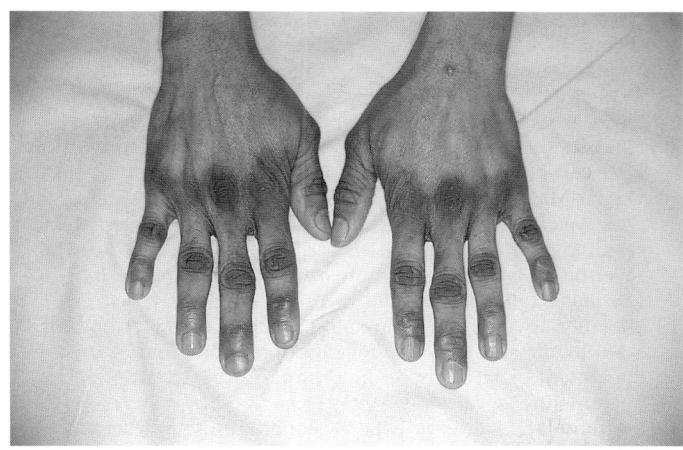

Figure 19.55: Postinflammatory hyperpigmentation of the hands in a patient with atopic eczema.

keratosis which when shed leaves large crateriform lesions. Clinically the lesions first appear on the extensor surfaces of the extremities, shoulders and buttocks, and sometimes may spread to most of the body. The lesions are flesh coloured but may be slightly hyperpigmented. Interestingly the most recent and comprehensive study has shown that only 5% of patients have lower than normal serum vitamin A levels and these patients present with lesions localized around the knees and elbows only. Those patients with normal vitamin A levels had more widespread lesions. Unfortunately there is no good evidence that adults with vitamin A deficiency respond to replacement therapy. However, children with phrynoderma seem to show signs of deficiency of both vitamin A and B; the B complex deficiency is more significant in Nigeria, whereas studies in India on affected children suggest an interaction of the vitamin B group and unsaturated fatty acids. Therefore it has been suggested that phrynoderma may be caused by a fat-soluble vitamin deficiency. A study from Thailand has shown that those children with vitamin deficiency respond well to vitamin A therapy. Those that do not have a vitamin A deficiency can be treated with a 5–10% salicylate ointment twice a day, a potent topical steroid on its own or in a combination with salicylate; 10–20% urea in a cream base has been used effectively. Most of the lesions tend to disappear before age 18 without treatment.

REFERENCES

1 Bisno A L & Stevens D L. Streptococcal infections of skin and soft tissues. *N Engl J Med* 1996; 334:240.
2 Elliot D C, Kufera J A & Myers R A. Necrotizing soft tissue infections: risk factors for mortality and strategies for management. *Ann Surg* 1996; 224:672–683.
3 Young H. Syphilis: new diagnostic directions. *Int J Sex Transm Dis AIDS* 1992; 3:391–413.
4 WHO. *Expert Committee on Venereal Diseases and Treponematoses*, 6th report. Technical Report Series, no. 736. Geneva: World Health Organization, 1986.
5 Sehgal V N, Jain S, Bhattacharya S N & Thappa D M. Yaws control and eradication. *Int J Dermatol* 1994; 33:16–20.
6 Thangaraj H S, Evans M R W & Wansbrough-Jones M H. *Mycobacterium ulcerans* disease; Buruli ulcer. *Trans R Soc Trop Med Hyg* 1999; 93:337–340.
7 Gray S F, Smith R S & Reynolds N J. Fish tank granuloma. *BMJ* 1990; 300:1069–1070.
8 Bryceson A & Pfaltzgraff R E. Symptoms and signs. In *Leprosy*, 3rd edn. Edinburgh: Churchill Livingstone, 1990: 25–55.
9 Chopra S & Vega-López F. Skin granulomas in clinical practice.

In James & Zumla (eds) *The Granulomatous Disorders*. Cambridge, UK: Cambridge University Press, 1999: ch. 33 (cutaneous tuberculosis: 507–510; cutaneous leishmaniasis: 513–517).

10   Josse R, Guedenon A, Aguiar J, Anagonou S & Zinsou C. Buruli's ulcer, a pathology little known in Benin: apropos of 227 cases. *Bull Soc Pathol Exot* 1994; 87:170–175.

11   López-Martínez R, Méndez-Tovar L J, Lavalle P, Welsh O, Saúl A & Macotela-Ruiz E. Epidemiología del micetoma en México: estudio de 2105 casos. *Gaceta Med Mex* 1992; 128:477–481.

12   Welsh O. Mycetoma: current concepts in treatment. *Int J Dermatol* 1991; 30:387–398.

13   Méndez-Tovar L J, Serrano-Jaen L, Ameida-Arvizu. Combined cefotaxime and amikacin for immunomodulation in the treatment of actinomycetoma-resistant to conventional treatment. *Gac Med Mex* 1999; 135:517–521.

14   Serrano-Jaén L & Vega-López F. Fulminating septicaemia caused by *Vibrio vulnificus*. *Br J Dermatol* 2000; 142:386–387.

15   Cribier B, Piemont Y & Grosshans E. Staphylococcal scalded skin syndrome in adults. *J Am Acad Dermatol* 1994; 30:319–324.

16   Belsey M A & LeBlanc D R. Skin infections and the epidemiology of diphtheria: acquisition and persistence of C. diphtheria infections. *Am J Epidemiol* 1975; 102:179–184.

17   Blackwell V & Vega-López F. Cutaneous larva migrans: clinical features and management of 44 cases presenting in the returning traveller. *Br J Dermatol* 2001; 145:434–437.

18   Caumes E, Datry A & Paris L. Efficacy of ivermectin in the therapy of cutaneous larva migrans. *Arch Dermatol* 1992; 128:995–996.

19   WHO. *Control of Leishmaniasis*. Report of a WHO Expert Committee. Technical Report Series, no. 793. Geneva: World Health Organization, 1990.

20   Tapia E J, Cáceres-Dittmar G & Sánchez M A. In *Molecular and Immune Mechanisms in the Pathogenesis of Cutaneous Leishmaniasis*. Heidelberg: Springer, 1996: pp 1–21, 25–47.

21   Taniguchi Y, Ando K & Isoda K. Human gnathostomiasis: successful removal of Gnathostoma hispidum. *Int J Dermatol* 1992; 31:175–177.

22   Ibanez-Bernal S & Velasco-Castrejón O. New records of human tungiasis in Mexico (Siphonaptera: Tungidae). *J Med Entomol* 1996; 33:988–999.

23   Douglas-Jones A G, Llewelyn M B & Mills C M. Cutaneous infection with *Tunga penetrans*. *Br J Dermatol* 1995; 133:125–127.

24   Lui H & Buck W. Cutaneous myasis: a simple and effective technique for extraction of Dermatobia hominis larvae. *Int J Dermatol* 1992; 31:657–659.

25   Abbott P H. Mycetoma in the Sudan. *Trans R Soc Trop M Hyg* 1956; 50:11–24.

26   Mahgoub E S & Gumaa S A. Ketoconazole in the treatment of eumycetoma due to Madurella mycetomi. *Trans R Soc Trop Med Hyg* 1984; 78:376–379.

Br J Dermatol 2000; 142 (in press).

Chapter 20
HIV/AIDS – with an emphasis on Africa

C. F. Gilks

Introduction

Human immunodeficiency virus (HIV) infection causes progressive destruction of part of the immune system. With time, a characteristic and relatively specific group of infections and malignancies develops; for surveillance purposes, these make up the acquired immunodeficiency syndrome (AIDS). These unusual problems were first recognized in 1981 in the USA to be clustering in individuals who had a damaged immune system for no obvious reason. By 1983–84, the virus had been identified and cultured. With this rapid advance came screening tests and the shocking realization that HIV was already widely spread, particularly in sub-Saharan Africa, and was epidemic. Following this a second variant, HIV type 2 was indentified and characterized. Now, 20 years later, it is (perhaps conservatively) estimated that about 60 million people have been infected with HIV and, of those, 25 million have already died. Today, about 16 000 new diagnoses of HIV infection are made daily; the vast majority (95%) are in people from resource-poor countries of the tropics.

No other disease has had such a profound impact on tropical medicine. Almost overnight, wards have become full of young men and women chronically sick and wasting away, with little prospect of adequate care and support. Suffering on this scale with the attendant clinical impotence has profoundly disillusioned many health professionals, a consequence rarely recognized but of increasing concern. AIDS burnout is contributing to difficulties in staff retention and increasingly also to recruitment. Furthermore, as the demand for care escalates sharply, clinical staff themselves are falling sick and dying from HIV/AIDS. Sadly, there are no data to suggest that health-care workers have used superior knowledge to reduce their own risk of infection.

HIV/AIDS has also shattered the comfortable dichotomy between temperate and tropical, rich and poor medicine. For the first time a serious and visible disease is a top public health problem in both the USA and Malawi. Very costly and highly effective antiretroviral therapy (ART) and high-technology therapeutic monitoring is standard of care in the West, but is not affordable or achievable at the moment in high-prevalence, low-income countries facing the brunt of the epidemic. The huge disparity in responses generated—dictated by resource availability rather than need—is clearly inequitable. The only similar health issue is multidrug-resistant tuberculosis, which is almost invisible in low-income countries because of laboratory constraints in identifying most cases.

Most knowledge about HIV/AIDS has come from the West, which has had the resources and capacity to research and react comprehensively to the clinical challenges posed by the disease. Unfortunately much of this information, and the innumerable textbooks and chapters, is of little relevance to clinicians facing HIV in a resource-poor environment. This chapter tries to redress the balance to some extent. It has an explicit focus on how poverty impacts on HIV-related immunosuppression, and how illness can be managed in a low-technology setting. The emphasis is on Africa because most published data come from that region. However, the clinical issues discussed are likely to be relevant in other poor regions of the developing world. Clearly not all people with HIV/AIDS in Africa are poor, and some physicians have the luxury of practising in well equipped and resourced (private) hospitals. For them, standard HIV/AIDS textbooks may be more relevant.

History and origins of the epidemic

The first definite serological evidence of human infection dates to a stored blood sample taken from an unidentified African man resident in Leopoldville (now Kinshasa) taken in 1959 and unequivocally positive for HIV-1.[1] Events around then in the Congo are unclear, and the serological record remains patchy until the late 1970s. The early history of the epidemic, and in particular the early African cases, are best described by Hooper.[2] The first reliable evidence of HIV-2 infection is of a person who was probably infected in Guinea Bissau in the early 1960s.[3]

There is no doubt that HIV types 1 and 2 were originally African primate viruses of the chimpanzee *Pan troglotydes* and sooty mangabey *Cercocebus atys*, respectively. It is also clear that these viruses have crossed the species barrier several times this century. What has in the past been controversial was when and how this occurred. Several theories have been advanced. They have included HIV contamination of oral polio vaccine stocks through use of

African monkey kidney cell lines,[2] and experiments involving human infection with various African primate malaria species.[4] Some theories, involving bizarre use of monkey blood in obscure rites and initiation ceremonies, have caused great offence.

There is now general consensus that the virus crossed over into humans as a result of people hunting and butchering monkeys in the bush meat trade. This must have happened many times over the centuries but previously resulted in an evolutionary dead-end, but was in the twentieth century able to spread as a result of the profound social changes accompanying colonization, urbanization and, more recently, easy international travel. Molecular typing seems, with reasonable accuracy, to have dated the time of the most important cross-species transmission (the ancestor of the HIV-1 M group) to the 1930s.[5]

In seeking the origins of the epidemic, it is important not to lay blame but to understand where the most important and prototypic 'emerging' infection to date actually came from, and to learn lessons for the future. It is also important to know where the ancestors of HIV naturally exist, particularly in the struggle to develop effective vaccines.

The virus

HIV is classified as a lentevirus in the Retroviridae. Decoded, this means that it is a virus with RNA as its genetic material, thus making it dependent on reverse transcriptase to infect mammalian cells, and that it produces pathological changes slowly. There are two variants of HIV, types 1 and 2, which have significant (approximately 30%) genetic differences. Each type is further subdivided into different groups, and subtypes or clades. These are assigned letters of the alphabet. Replication in retroviruses is error-prone and there is a rapid evolution of HIV subtypes with new mutations.

HIV-1 group M is the cause of the pandemic. It has several different clades, from type A to type K (type I does not exist). This probably represents rapid evolution (a starburst) from one founder M-group ancestor virus. To complicate matters, some wild viruses seem to be recombinations and subtype mosaics. Thus, subtype E (which is common in drug users in Thailand) is more correctly now referred to as circulating recombinant form CRF_01AE. In Africa, the complete alphabet of subtypes exists in west central Africa (Cameroon, Gabon, the Congo), whereas more restricted subtypes are epidemic outside the central focus. In South Africa subtype C predominates, whereas in Uganda types A and D are both epidemic. In West Africa, type A is most commonly identified. Subtype B, which predominates in the West, is uncommon in most regions of the tropics. Two rare HIV-1 groups, N and O, are recognized in west central Africa. These probably represent different cross-species transfer events, but appear not to have the epidemic potential of group M viruses and are very uncommon.[6]

HIV-2 is largely restricted to West Africa. It has several different subgroups (A–E) and this heterogeneity may represent more frequent monkey-to-human infections rather than a single starburst. For reasons that are unclear, HIV-2 is transmitted less efficiently from person to person than HIV-1 and has a longer natural history. However, it causes the same type of immunosuppression as HIV-1, and once disease develops the clinical manifestations are the same.[7] Across its range, HIV-2 is being outcompeted by HIV-1. The rest of this chapter refers to HIV-1 infection unless otherwise stated.

Pathogenesis and immune responses

A detailed description of pathogenesis is outside the scope of this chapter and can be found in standard US or European textbooks of virology or infectious diseases. Broadly speaking, the main damage caused by HIV is brought about by active viral replication, which causes cell death. The main target cells for infection by HIV are those that have on their surface a cell surface molecule called CD4, usually T lymphocytes. This receptor is recognized by the HIV envelope glycoprotein to which the virus binds before fusing and entering the susceptible host cell. Initially host immune responses manage to keep the virus in check and viral levels are low. Even so, there is a very high rate of cell infection and thus cell killing. Eventually viral replication takes over, depleting and eventually exhausting the infected individual's CD4 T-lymphocyte population.[8]

The rate of decline of CD4 cells varies considerably from person to person. With waning CD4 cell numbers, a specific immunodeficiency emerges, which permits infection with a relatively limited range of virulent diseases (to which immunocompetent individuals are also susceptible) and opportunistic infections (those capable of causing disease only in immunosuppressed individuals). Susceptibility to infection comes from defects in cell-mediated immune responses (e.g., tuberculosis may develop), and with loss of control over antibody production increasing susceptibility to pneumococcal infection, for instance, may develop. Viral loads also vary considerably person to person. They peak with initial infection, fall to a plateau for several years, and then rise as symptomatic disease develops (Figure 20.1). Viral loads rise with many acute intercurrent infections as well as some vaccinations, but usually fall back quickly to baseline levels. They are useful for monitoring the therapeutic response to ART.[9]

Both CD4 counts and viral load measurements are good markers of disease status and are useful prognostic indicators. However, they can be measured only by means of expensive high-technology equipment. A clinical staging classification has been developed by the World Health Organization (WHO) for use in clinics without access to CD4 counts or viral loads (Table 20.1).[10] Patients with asymptomatic disease or minor clinical problems are classified as having stage 1 and 2 disease, respectively. The importance of high-grade virulent pathogens early on in the disease process is encompassed; pulmonary tuberculosis (now classified as an AIDS-defining disease in the USA) and severe bacterial infections are stage 3 problems. Opportunistic infections characteristic of classical AIDS are classified as stage 4 events. The staging system has recently been validated against CD4 counts in Uganda and is useful for predicting survival.[11]

Total lymphocyte count may also be a useful prognostic indicator, particularly if combined with WHO clinical staging, and may therefore be useful as a guide to starting ART when CD4 counts are not readily available.[12]

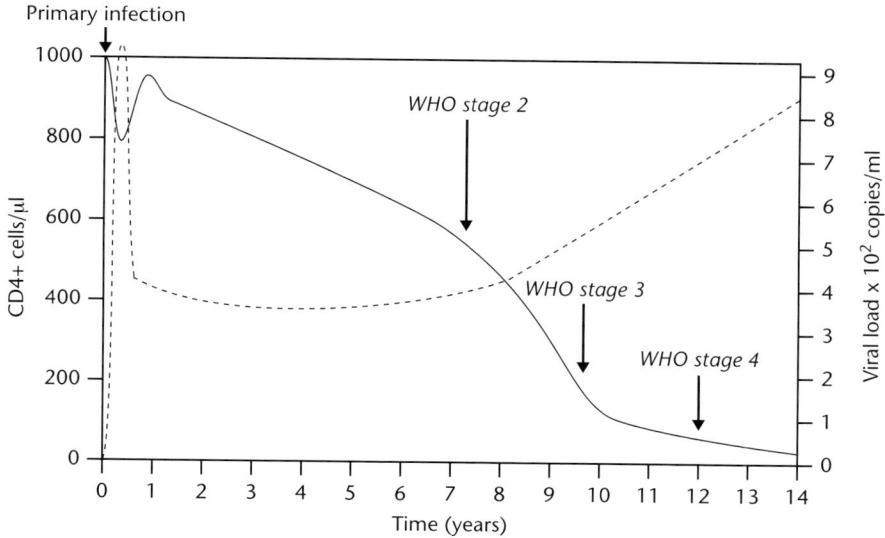

Figure 20.1: Natural history of untreated HIV-1 infection. WHO stage 2, minor symptoms and infections; stage 3, virulent and early opportunistic infections; stage 4, late opportunistic infections.

Table 20.1 WHO clinical staging for HIV/AIDS

	Clinical findings
Stage 1	1. Asymptomatic 2. Persistent generalized lymphadenopathy (PGL) Performance scale 1: asymptomatic, normal activity
Stage 2	3. Weight loss, < 10% of body weight 4. Minor mucocutaneous manifestations (seborrheic dermatitis, prurigo, fungal nail infections, recurrent oral ulcerations, angular cheilitis) 5. Herpes zoster within the last 5 years 6. Recurrent upper respiratory tract infections (e.g., bacterial sinusitis) and/or performance scale 2: symptomatic, normal activity
Stage 3	7. Weight loss, > 10% of body weight 8. Unexplained chronic diarrhoea, >1 month 9. Unexplained prolonged fever (intermittent or constant), > 1 month 10. Oral candidiasis (thrush) 11. Oral hairy leucoplakia 12. Pulmonary tuberculosis, within the past year 13. Severe bacterial infections (i.e., pneumonia, pyomyositis) and/or performance scale 3: bedridden, < 50% of the day during the last month

Table 20.1 (*Cont'd*)

	Clinical findings
Stage 4	14. HIV wasting syndrome, as defined by CDC[a]
	15. *Pneumocystis carinii* pneumonia
	16. Toxoplasmosis of the brain
	17. Cryptosporidiosis with diarrhoea, > 1 month
	18. Cryptococcosis, extrapulmonary
	19. Cytomegalovirus (CMV) disease of an organ other than liver, spleen or lymph nodes
	20. Herpes simplex virus (HSV) infection, mucocutaneous > 1 month, or visceral any duration
	21. Progressive multifocal leucoencephalopathy (PML)
	22. Any disseminated endemic mycosis (e.g., histoplasmosis, coccidioidomycosis)
	23. Candidiasis of the oesophagus, trachea, bronchi or lungs
	24. Atypical mycobacteriosis, disseminated
	25. Non-typhoid salmonella septicaemia
	26. Extrapulmonary tuberculosis
	27. Lymphoma
	28. Kaposi's sarcoma (KS)
	29. HIV encephalopathy, as defined by CDC[b] and/or performance scale 4: bedridden, > 50% of the day during the last month (Note: both definitive and presumptive diagnoses are acceptable)

[a]HIV wasting syndrome: weight loss > 10% of body weight, plus either unexplained chronic diarrhoea (> 1 month), or chronic weakness and unexplained prolonged fever (> 1 month).
[b]HIV encephalopathy: clinical finding of disabling cognitive and/or motor dysfunction interfering with activities of daily living, progressing over weeks to months, in the absence of a concurrent illness of condition other than HIV infection that could explain the findings.

Immunity is at least partly type specific, and important elements may also be subtype specific. This has great bearing on vaccine development because the full geographical distribution of subtypes must be included or covered by any putative vaccine construct. Multiple infections can occur, although their frequency is not well documented. They have, however, been sufficiently common to allow the emergence of at least four well-documented circulating recombinant forms. Dual infections with both HIV-1 and HIV-2 also occur, suggesting that there is little cross-type immunity. It appears that immunity is not sterilizing, because infection is never eliminated. The virus can hide in privileged sites or remain in latently infected cells. Even after several years of highly active ART, which fully controls viral replication and allows immune reconstitution to occur, productive infection still ensues when latently HIV-infected cells are activated. Also, critically, when therapy is stopped, virus re-emerges and viral loads rise.

Diagnosis of HIV

Most HIV diagnoses are made with serological tests. All commercially available HIV test kits can identify both HIV-1 and HIV-2 infection. There was concern that the rare HIV-1 groups N and O might be difficult to diagnose with standard kits, but this has been rectified and in reality was of little relevance. It is rarely necessary to differentiate between HIV-1 and HIV-2 infection, or to document dual infection, outside research settings. Viral load testing will also diagnose infection but such tests are more usually done to monitor drug therapy. Infection can also be diagnosed by viral culture, but this is extremely laborious, expensive and time consuming, and is not used outside research laboratories.

When serum samples can be batched up, the most cost-effective way to conduct HIV testing is by enzyme immunoassay (EIA). However, for economy of scale, the full plate has to be used and a properly equipped laboratory with trained personnel is required. Results are available only after a few hours with the full cycle of washing and rinsing and incubation of substrate. A whole new generation of rapid and simple-to-use, single-sample test kits is now available, which can be used on whole blood, serum, or even saliva or urine. Although more costly than a single EIA test, the so-called rapid tests are very easy to use and can be performed by a counsellor, for instance, with little training. They also, as the name suggests, produce a result within a few minutes and can be used for individual patients or, for instance, to screen single units of blood or blood donors. Nowadays, few laboratories other than in research settings bother with Western blotting. Once regarded as obligatory to confirm infection identified with first- and second-generation EIA kits, the newest generation of serological test kits, both rapid and EIA, is extremely sensitive and specific. Nowadays some countries accept a single test result, whereas others promote a dual-test algorithm using a second, different, serological test.

Epidemiology and current status of the epidemic

Surveillance for HIV infection (prevalence) is conducted by active serological surveys of core groups, such as sex workers and genitourinary clinic attenders, and representative samples of adults—usually pregnant women attending for antenatal care or military recruits. Figures on HIV incidence are notoriously difficult to collect and are highly context specific. Data on disease burden relates to documented AIDS cases and, in some areas, HIV prevalence rates in patients admitted to hospital or diagnosed with active tuberculosis; data are gathered passively, relying on physicians to identify and report cases. A clinical case definition for African AIDS has been developed. The impact on mortality could theoretically be collected from vital registration of deaths and causes of death. Epidemiological data are usually broken down by sex and are increasingly reported according to age bands. Data collection is the responsibility of individual ministries of health, and is often supported by external assistance. Global data are collated and updated annually by the WHO, and are often released on 1 December to coincide with World AIDS Day.

In the calendar year 2000, WHO/UNAIDS estimates based on national surveys were 5.3 million incident cases globally compared with 3 million deaths, and 36.1 million people living with HIV/AIDS infection (Figure 20.2).[13] The force of the pandemic is illustrated by the excess number of new cases over deaths. Most people infected with HIV (90%) live in tropical regions; Africa is disproportionately infected and affected. Making up about 12% of the world's population, the majority of deaths (80%) and people living with HIV (75%) are African. In Africa,

55% of prevalent HIV infection is in women, with 6% in children under 15 years. The burden in adolescents is less clear, but may be 15%. Women tend to become infected sexually several years earlier than men, and have a peak prevalence at 15–24 years of age, compared with the 25–34 years age band for men. This appears to be a consistent finding across the developing world.

HIV data for individual countries vary in quality and are patchy and incomplete in both time and populations surveyed; see the UNAIDS website (www.unaids.org) for the most detailed and up-to-date country-specific information. Prevalence figures across countries are usually given for adults rather than total populations; thus about 9% of South African adults are thought to be infected with HIV. There also may be wide variation within countries by region and between urban and rural populations—with towns and cities usually recording higher rates. These may not be captured or reflected well in national figures. Nevertheless, there are sufficient data for reasonably accurate estimates to be made about current HIV prevalence in the developing world and particularly in Africa, and for epidemic trends in some countries to be identified. Ominously, the virus is continuing to spread rapidly in highly populous regions of India and southern China, and in the Russian Federation. India has the largest pool of HIV infection, estimated to be well over 4 million people. In parts of east and central Africa, prevalence is stabilizing, sometimes at rates in excess of 30%, and the 'HIV endemic' is emerging. In Uganda and Thailand, recent

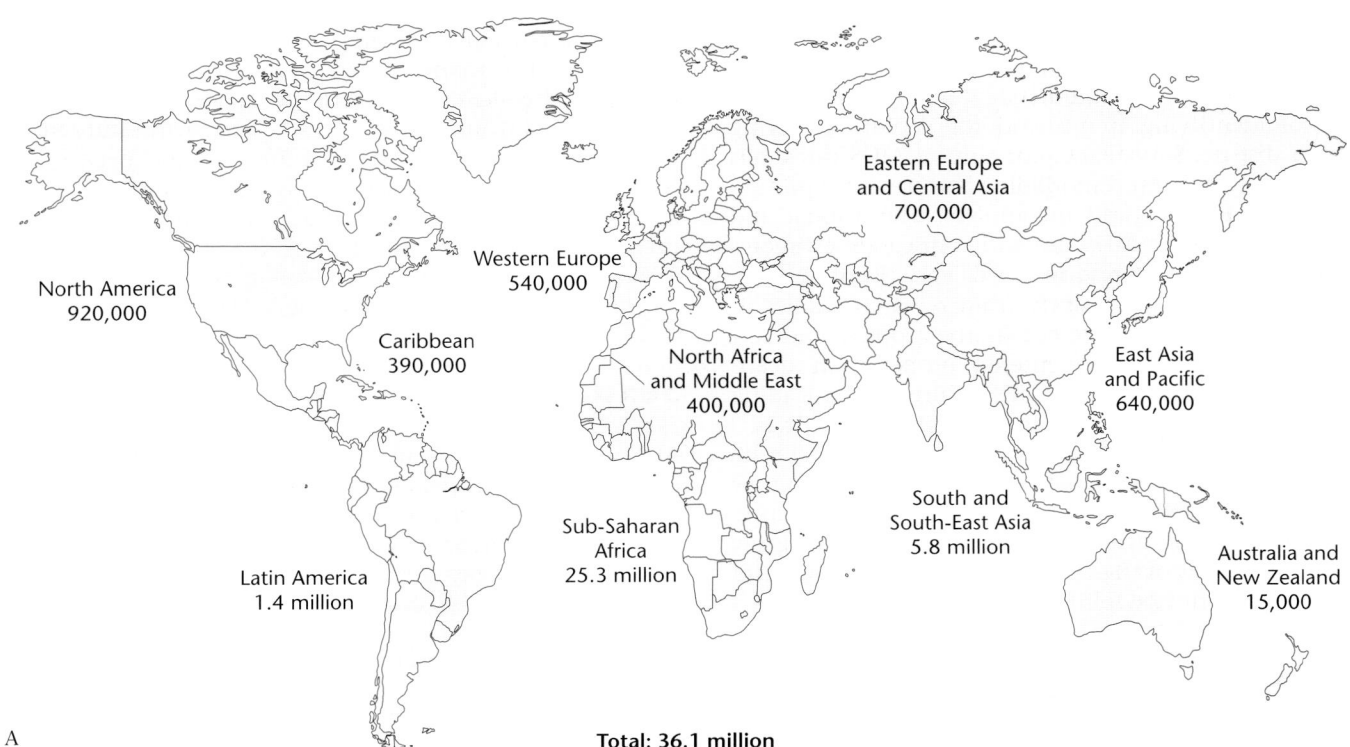

A   Total: 36.1 million

Figure 20.2: Two world maps from UNAIDS and WHO. (**A**) Adults and children estimated to be living with HIV/AIDS at the end of 2000 (total 36.1 million).

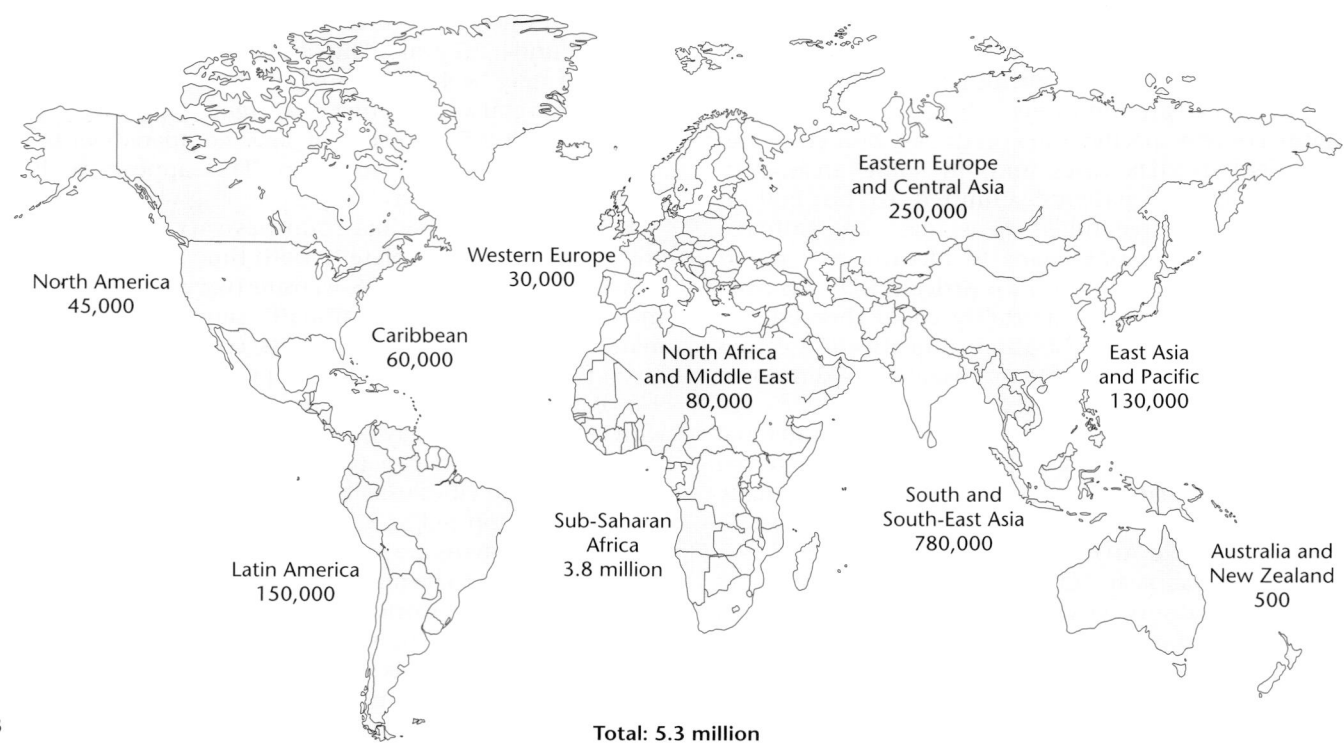

B

Total: 5.3 million

Figure 20.2: (*Cont'd*) (**B**) Estimated number of adults and children newly infected with HIV during 2000 (total 5.3 million).

declines in HIV prevalence have been ascribed to behavioural change and successful control programmes.[14]

Data on burden of disease are usually inadequate or absent (Figure 20.3). Information on HIV-tuberculosis co-infection is collected sporadically, usually in research projects rather than as routine practice. Most surveys of hospital patients are single studies; few are longitudinal and capable of identifying trends and the rapidly changing burden of disease. Surveillance for clinical AIDS cases fails to capture early non-AIDS morbidity, and passive reporting is woefully inaccurate and incomplete. The annual and cumulative figures for AIDS deaths in Africa are estimates based on several assumptions and very limited data. Mortality data come exclusively from research studies as vital registration is very limited in the tropics, and few deaths from HIV/AIDS are entered properly on death certificates. It is clear that HIV/AIDS is already the leading cause of death for adults in many African countries.[15] Despite this, there is no developing country yet where the epidemic is in a steady state (i.e., where the number of new cases equals the number of HIV-related deaths). The future burden of HIV/AIDS disease will thus continue to grow and the full impact of the epidemic on development and civil society will not be felt for many years.

Modes of transmission

HIV can be transmitted from person to person in three quite distinct ways: (1) through sexual intercourse, in all its permutations; (2) through blood or blood products, including contamination during intravenous drug use; and (3) vertically from mother to infant. Some groups may be particularly vulnerable, and sex inequality may often exacerbate the risk. The contribution made by each different route in a particular geographical region is variable and dependent on many different factors. In developing countries, heterosexual sex is the major route of transmission and from this follows a significant burden of paediatric infection. Substantial inroads have been made in almost all countries in reducing transfusion-associated cases. In some areas drug use is widespread, but this practice is at present unusual in Africa. An understanding of the different risk factors involved can be used to develop appropriate interventions to reduce HIV transmission.

Sexual transmission

Although almost all adults have sex, and often quite regularly, it is universally considered a private act. Taboos on open discussion are commonplace, and reliable information on sexual behaviour and practices is very difficult to obtain. These restraints have bedevilled understanding of the risk factors involved in sexual transmission and the implementation of interventions around safer sex. Nevertheless several facts are clear.

HIV-1 is more readily transmitted than HIV-2, but the biological basis for this is not understood.[7] It is unclear whether different HIV-1 clades differ in transmissibility. It has been estimated that the individual probability of transmission is about 0.1% with each act of heterosexual

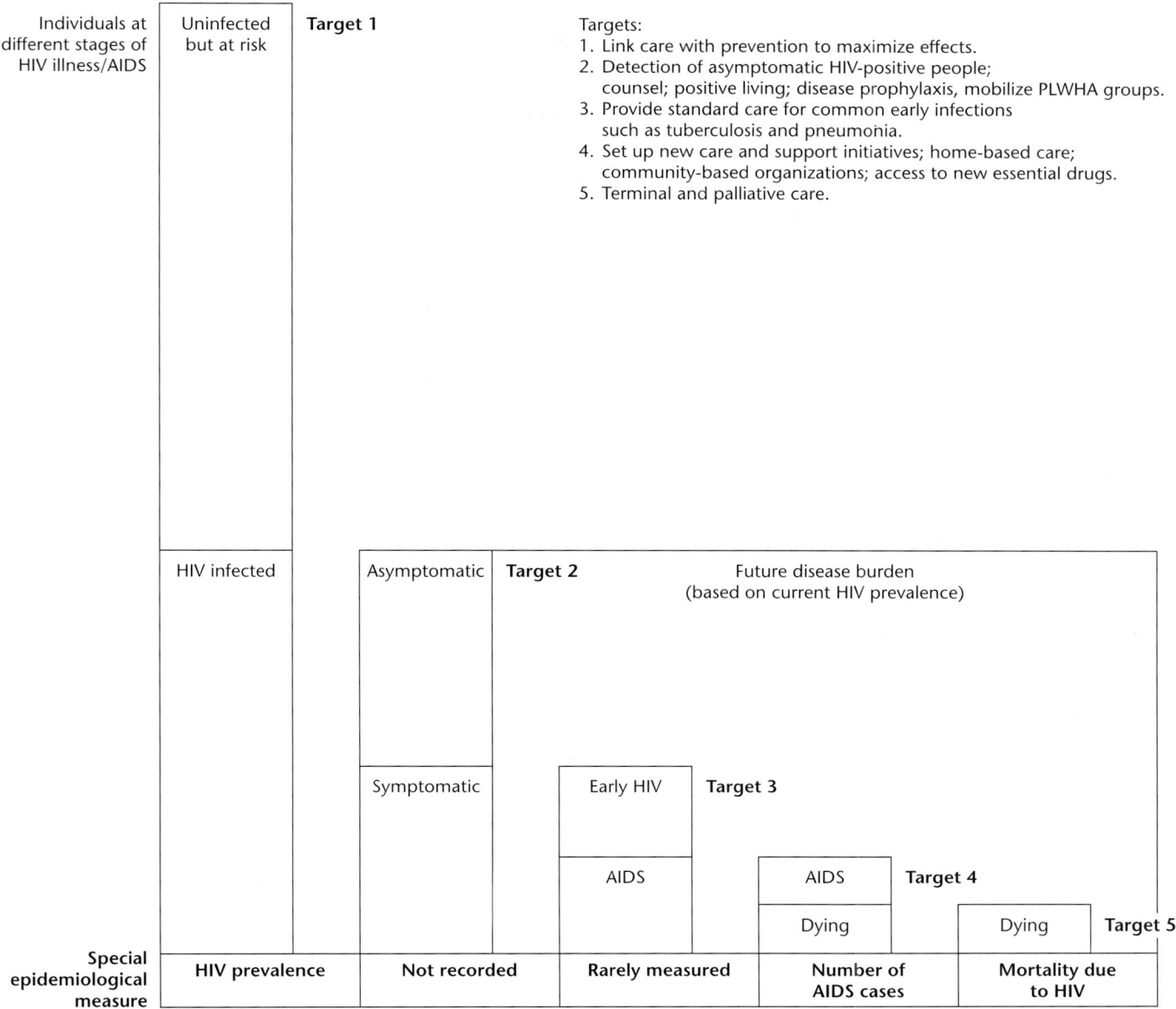

Figure 20.3: The HIV/AIDS care burden in a community. PLWHA, person living with HIV/AIDS.

intercourse. The overall risk, however, depends on the stage of infection and, critically, the viral load of the infected individual: around seroconversion and with advancing disease, the chances of transmission are greater.[16] In discordant couples, women (receptive partners) are slightly more susceptible to infection than men (penetrative partners). Adolescent women may be at higher risk of infection than older women because of the anatomy and physiology of the immature female genital tract; this is one reason why prevalence peaks at an earlier age in female than in male populations. In males, being uncircumcised seems to increase the risk of acquiring infection, although the precise impact of this is hard to measure.[17]

The presence of an active sexually transmitted disease (STD) substantially increases the risk of both transmission and acquisition of HIV. Ulcerative STDs such as chancroid

or genital herpes increase the risks of transmission by threefold or more, and inflammatory STDs such as gonorrhoea may at least double the risk.[18] Intact skin is an effective barrier to HIV, and any ulceration or breach is an easy portal of entry for the virus. HIV loads in genital secretions are higher in people with inflammation or in inflammatory exudates.[19] Asymptomatic sexually transmitted infections may also increase the risk of HIV transmission, but to a lesser extent.

Frequent partner change obviously increases the likelihood of being sexually exposed to HIV infection. Prostitutes are at most risk, and many studies have documented extremely high rates of infection.[20] Clients who purchase sex are also at significant risk of infection, especially if condoms are not used. Prostitutes are a very important 'core transmitter' group for HIV, and the reporting of commercial sex (i.e., purchasing sex with a sex worker) is a commonly identified risk factor in infected men. Serial monogamy, changing one regular sex partner at frequent intervals, may be equally risky because it is the overall frequency of sexual acts as well as the risk of encountering an infected partner that counts. Migrant workers and single men who travel widely (e.g., long-distance lorry drivers) are often at risk. Adolescents may under some circumstances be particularly vulnerable to HIV, especially as they start sexual relationships with little experience.[21]

Parenteral transmission

Direct inoculation of infected blood is the most effective way of transmitting infection. The parameters are the viral load, the route of inoculation and the volume of blood involved. Having a transfusion, or blood products of any kind, used to be a major risk factor for HIV transmission. With careful donor selection and universally practised, rigorous, quality-controlled blood screening, it is very unusual nowadays to document a case of transfusion-associated, or blood-product related, HIV infection in industrialized countries. In resource-poor regions, quality assurance is less easy to implement. Furthermore, in high-prevalence countries a small but significant (0.5–1%) proportion of donors who are sexually active may have just become infected. Such new cases may be impossible or impractical to identify by routine serology—the so-called window period. HIV transmission through blood transfusion is therefore still a problem in many parts of Africa.[22]

In some countries commercial blood banks have proved a major problem and risk for HIV transmission. Uncommon in Africa, their use is widespread in parts of Asia. In India it has been difficult to supervise commercial blood banks, and some unscrupulous blood bank owners have managed in the past fraudulently to pass off infected blood as safe. In China the risks have been to the paid donors, often impoverished villagers who sell their blood to commercial blood product companies, which in turn use poorly sterilized equipment or reuse single-use devices time and time again.

Injecting drug users who share injection paraphenalia run the risk of being infected with the whole range of bloodborne infections. Explosive outbreaks of HIV, hepatitis C, etc. may occur and sometimes involve large groups of users. At present there are few injecting drug users in Africa, but in parts of Asia and the Russian Federation this is a major route of infection.[23] Secondary sexual epidemics may frequently be seen in female users who resort to prostitution to pay for their drug habit.

The final issue is nosocomial transmission of HIV. This is usually from infected patient to the health-care worker through needlestick injuries or cuts during surgical procedures, but may occasionally be from patient to patient when inadequate care is taken and needles and syringes are reused without proper sterilization. The risks depend on the type of incident and the volume of blood involved. The overall risks of seroconversion are low (aggregate about 0.5% per incident where the skin is breached), but are still of huge concern to the exposed individual and often generate considerable psychological strain. The overall risks also increase with recurrent events experienced during a surgical or obstetrical career.[24] This may be starting to affect graduate choice of specialty training.

Mother-to-child transmission

An infected mother can transmit HIV to her offspring by three quite distinct biological processes: *in utero* across the placenta, during the birth process itself, and through breast milk. Stage of infection and viral load are the main parameters in mother-to-child transmission. For unknown reasons, HIV-2 is very rarely transmitted vertically.[7] Viral subtype may be a minor determinant. Initial data suggested that maternal vitamin A deficiency was an important (correctable) risk factor for perinatal transmission, but this has subsequently been shown not to be the case. Each process is additive and combines to give an overall rate of vertical transmission that may average out at about 20–30% overall.[25]

It is very important to note that the majority of infants escape infection. On average, about 10% of fetuses may become infected transplacentally. Given that the virus readily spreads to most organs in an infected individual, it is entirely unclear why the placenta presents such an efficient barrier to HIV. In the birth process, direct exposure to maternal blood and body fluids seems to be the key determinant. The duration of labour, either with prolonged rupture of membranes or a lengthy second stage, is important. Thus the second twin has a lower risk of being infected than the first-born because labour is usually more rapid. The aggregate risk may be about 5% for transmission during a normal delivery.[26]

Transmission through breast-feeding depends on how long this is carried out for: there is still an appreciable and measurable risk of infection if breast-feeding is carried on beyond 6 months.[27] Exclusive breast-feeding may result in significantly less transmission than supplementary feeding. However, the data from one research group in South Africa need to be confirmed and are not universally accepted.[28] The overall contribution of breast-feeding alone to vertical transmission may be about 10%.

Interventions to reduce HIV transmission

The absolute priority of HIV prevention cannot be over-emphasized, given the misery of disease, the costs of therapy, and the social and economic consequences of ill-health and premature death. Knowledge of the different biological risk factors for HIV transmission, and an adequate evidence base, is of fundamental importance in the design of specific interventions to reduce or prevent HIV infection. A wide range of interventions is now available, many field tried and tested. From this basket, each country can put together its own best control programme based on local need and circumstances. However, it is not just biomedical interventions that are important. The social and political context cannot be ignored if any sustainable gains are to be made in averting infection and controlling HIV effectively. Until society has a more normal and accepting attitude to HIV/AIDS, it is difficult to see how interventions can be fully effective. UNAIDS widely advocates that people living with HIV/AIDS are seen not as the problem but as part of the solution. Political commitment and leadership is vital.

The political environment

Uganda is the only country in Africa to date that has managed to reduce the incidence and reverse the epidemic.[14] Crucial in this has been the political leadership and commitment shown by President Museveni. In Asia, Thailand's similar achievements are a tribute to effective political leadership. Sadly, these are isolated examples. Elsewhere, leaders have ignored or denied that HIV is present in their own countries, or have only recognized— or been forced to acknowledge—the impact that HIV/AIDS is having very late on, until it is almost too late to make a difference. There is even confusion in some politicians' minds about the exact role that HIV, as opposed to poverty, actually plays in causing AIDS. Such lack of political leadership is unacceptable, but is not an issue easily addressable by public health practitioners. The lack of commitment severely hampers the workings and effectiveness of national HIV/AIDS control programmes.

Linking prevention with care

To date, many African countries, and many donors, have concentrated almost exclusively on prevention and have ignored the downstream consequences of infection. However, it is becoming increasingly evident that intervention strategies that define HIV simply in terms of how it is transmitted (as an STD or a blood contaminant) are unbalanced, and that this adversely affects uptake and efficacy of interventions across the board. As with most major disease control programmes in the tropics, prevention needs to be combined with care to be relevant to individuals and affected communities. Thus control of tuberculosis is based on case detection and treatment, and malaria control includes as a mainstay the diagnosis and treatment of the sick patient. HIV prevention needs to be promoted not by itself but as part of a comprehensive programme of HIV/AIDS care and control.[29]

Basic information and education

HIV is a new disease and one that has arrived with considerable misinformation, fear and stigmatization. One immediate priority is an appropriate public health and education campaign to inform and assist—in local languages and through appropriate media outlets. More people in Africa listen to the radio than watch television, for instance. The days are hopefully long gone when scare tactics were used to inform and terrorize communities, emphasizing what a terrible disease AIDS was to have, and thus reinforcing the fear of finding out one's status through voluntary counselling and testing (VCT), for instance. Messages need to be thought out very carefully if they are to be culturally sensitive and appropriate, but not so anodyne as to miss the point. HIV is also transmitted sexually, which means that many people are uncomfortable about talking openly about how it is spread or prevented. Such taboos and prejudices are hard to overcome, but without dealing with them effectively it is almost impossible to generate real and sustained sexual behaviour change sufficient to reduce HIV transmission. Any information and education programme needs constantly to be revised to keep up to date and to maintain relevance.

Reducing sexual transmission

Two interventions currently form the mainstay of efforts to reduce sexual transmission of HIV in the tropics: (1) control, and better treatment of sexually transmitted infections; and (2) the promotion of latex condoms. Both require an element of behaviour change in the individual, geared towards practising safer sex. It is important to note that it is safer rather than safe sex that is promoted. These days sex can never be considered entirely risk free.

The rationale for improving STD treatment to control HIV is based on the increased risks that any STD, inflammatory or ulcerative, generates for person-to-person transmission of HIV. Initial enthusiasm for this was based on a single randomized controlled trial in East Africa (Mwanza, Tanzania) which documented a 42% (95% confidence interval 21–58%) reduction in HIV transmission.[30] A larger study (Rakai, Uganda) subsequently showed no effects with mass community-wide STD treatment.[31] One further randomized controlled trial has recently ended (Masaka, Uganda), but initial results seem inconclusive (J. Whitworth, personal communication).[32] It may be that differences relate to the stage of the epidemic. Improved STD treatment may have most impact where the virus is still epidemic rather than endemic, and where sexual contact with high-risk core transmitter groups is more important than transmission from spouse or regular partner.[33]

Whatever the exact impact on HIV transmission, it is beyond doubt that reducing STD morbidity is an important public health goal in itself, and justifies financing. Most resource-poor countries are introducing syndromic management for STDs: patients are treated for logistical reasons according to presenting symptoms rather than aetiology. Such an approach means that effective STD management can be delivered at the health centre level, by nurses and clinical officers, provided the necessary drugs are made available.

The male latex condom is an effective barrier to all sexually transmitted pathogens. It is thought that condoms, when used properly, can reduce HIV transmission by as much as 70%;[34] if anyone produced a vaccine with such efficacy it would be hailed as a major breakthrough. Condoms can be distributed without cost, or sold by local traders who buy at discounted wholesale prices, a process known as social marketing. This encourages the condom market and accepts that clients are more likely to use condoms that have been bought rather than given away. In some countries social marketing has helped greatly to expand the uptake of condoms. In others, male reluctance still inhibits widespread usage. In Asia it has been easier to scale up condom usage because communities are far more familiar with them as they have been widely promoted for family planning. In African programmes, much less use was made of condoms for contraception.

One problem with the male latex condom is that use is at the say of the man. It can be very difficult, and often impossible, for women to make their male partner use a condom. A female condom is available which is also an effective barrier to HIV and other STDs. Although more cumbersome and more expensive, it has the advantage of being controlled by the woman. Use in Africa is relatively limited at present.

Novel approaches are being evaluated. Vaginal microbicides are agents that have the potential *in vitro* to interfere with viral attachment to mucous membranes and thus reduce transmission. Initial enthusiasm for one agent, nonoxynol 9 (also a spermicide), was shattered in a large trial which showed that it increased the risk of acquiring HIV infection, probably by irritating the vaginal wall.[35] Current efforts focus on much less irritant agents, such as dextrin sulfate and PRO 2000.[36] Field trials are under way in several sites in Africa. If effective, they offer a simple female-controlled method.

Reducing parenteral transmission

Great strides in blood safety have been made in many African countries. Widespread provision of EIA testing equipment and the advent of rapid single-use HIV test kits have meant that almost all blood transfused is (or should be) tested for HIV. Quality control remains the single most important issue in maintaining the integrity of the blood supply. The 'window period' means that appreciable risk may exist if unselected donors are used.[22] Many blood transfusion services now seek donors from schools or institutions where sexual activity is likely to be low, so minimizing the number of units possibly in the window period. Where the safety of a unit of blood cannot be guaranteed, another important strategy to reduce transfusion-acquired HIV is to develop stringent clinical protocols for triggering transfusion, and then regularly auditing or monitoring their use. This is particularly important in malaria-endemic regions where the majority of transfusions are given to children for malarial anaemia. Where this has been done, the use of transfusion may fall by 50%.[37]

The most effective intervention for reducing the risk of HIV spread in intravenous drug use communities is to make clean and sterile injection equipment widely available. Unfortunately, the decision to implement open-access needle exchange schemes is often taken (or avoided) on political rather than public health grounds. There are very few countries that implement these schemes in the general community, and almost none that has faced up to the problem in prisons, where many inmates may inject illicit drugs.

Reducing the risk of needlestick injury involves simple safety measures such as the provision of adequate numbers of sharps bins, safe disposal of sharps (by incineration or burial), care with sharps during every procedure, and having appropriate equipment such as needle holders for suturing. It is depressing to see the general lack of simple, locally made, sharps bins or the poor disposal procedures for sharps in many hospitals across the continent. Disposable single-use needles and syringes are not always affordable or available, and many hospitals still use reusable needles and glass syringes. As with more expensive (reused) surgical equipment, the critical issue is proper cleaning and autoclaving, which removes any risk of patient-to-patient spread.

Post-exposure prophylaxis (PEP) will markedly reduce the risk of seroconversion if started soon, within 24–48 hours. It is usually given for 4 weeks. Although most efficacy data come from AZT monotherapy, most PEP protocols specify dual or triple therapy as this is likely to be more effective.[38] Dual-combination preparations such as lamivudine–zidovudine (Combivir®) taken for 2–4 weeks have advantages with respect to adherence and low toxicity. Protocols for the use of PEP are now standard of care in industrialized countries where ART is affordable. Although many African countries also have PEP protocols, they are rarely implemented because antiretroviral drugs are not available and access to VCT cannot be assumed. Even in countries such as South Africa where drugs are readily accessible for PEP and VCT is widely available, uptake may be very low because staff are reluctant to undergo HIV testing. Many are fatalistic and seem to believe they are already infected.

Reducing mother-to-child transmission

In the West, mother-to-child transmission can be virtually eliminated with comprehensive antenatal counselling and HIV testing, antiretroviral therapy, caesarian section and avoidance of breast-feeding.[39] In high-prevalence developing countries, where need is greatest, the financial resources and capacity to implement such interventions are woefully lacking. The promise of simple, cheap therapy with nevirapine,[40] or simplified regimens with AZT,[41] reduces the cost barrier and has created a wide-ranging international debate with calls for charitable donations or concerted bilateral aid. There is considerable debate about whether also to provide formula feeding to mothers rather than to continue to promote breast-feeding as usual. There are clear risks of HIV transmission with breast-feeding; formula feeding also carries significant risks of disease and malnutrition when the mother cannot afford to buy enough tins to nourish the child.[27,42] In a fair world, the mother would not just be seen as a conduit for transmitting the virus, but as a person living with HIV and meriting treatment when clinically indicated (an obvious example of linking prevention with care). Averting infection in the baby will increase the numbers of AIDS orphans in the absence of maternal ART.

Some countries are trying to develop policy guidelines, and pilot sites are being planned. It is as yet unclear how such programmes will work from day to day, and how any workable models will actually be rolled out. The limiting factor is likely to be not drug costs but the capacity to implement any package broadly and equitably in urban and rural areas. The staff time required, particularly to provide counselling and testing, is significant.[43] In other countries, even though cost-effective,[44] reducing mother-to-child transmission is not considered to be a leading public health priority, particularly without robust policies to cope with AIDS orphans.

Natural history of HIV/AIDS

High morbidity, not rapid early disease progression

One feature distinguishes the natural history of HIV in developing countries from that described in rich industrialized societies: dealing with the consequences of progressive ill-health and immunosuppression on a background of poverty and lack of resources. The environment for most poor people is unhygienic and unhealthy, characterized by high exposure to ordinary as well as opportunistic pathogens. With such exposure, it is well recognized that infants in the tropics suffer far higher rates of acute respiratory infections, tuberculosis, skin infections and diarrhoeal disease than those in the West. Adults are similarly exposed, and it should come as no surprise that in the slums and shanties of the developing world tuberculosis, pneumococcal disease and non-typhi salmonellosis are all leading clinical problems.[45]

These virulent pathogens are quite capable of causing disease in the immunocompetent adult as well as in children, and may develop relatively soon after seroconversion. They cause significant morbidity in the early stages of disease progression, which according to the WHO clinical classification would be either stage 2 or stage 3 disease.[10] If time to the different stages is considered (e.g., from seroconversion to stage 2, median 29 months; and to stage 3, 46 months[46]), transition time can be interpreted as showing rapid disease progression. This happens particularly in cohorts where individuals are known to be HIV positive, and where staging data may be backed up by limited clinical investigation of morbid events, because clinical manifestations can be – and are – often overfitted into AIDS diagnoses.[47] Furthermore, several stage 2 (weight loss, minor mucocutaneous manifestations) and stage 3 events (marked weight loss, unexplained prolonged fever) are common in HIV-uninfected community controls when included, and these events occur at relatively high frequencies irrespective of HIV status.[46]

When staging is carefully conducted and matched with CD4 counts, it is clear that survival times for patients in the early stages of HIV do not indicate rapid progression.[11]

Survival following specific early disease events may also be relatively good. Thus one meticulous cohort study in Uganda noted a median survival in excess of 4.1 years following pulmonary tuberculosis, and 3.36 years following acute bacterial infection.[46] The median survival in this unique seroincident cohort (i.e., a cohort in which the time of acquisition of HIV infection is known) has recently been established, and is over 10 years.[48] None of these data are consistent with the notion of rapid disease progression in African patients with HIV disease, at least in the early stages of disease.

Several groups have proposed that the high background rates of endemic disease, in particular helminth infections, tuberculosis, sexually transmitted infections and, in many areas, malaria, generate 'immune activation' which drives rapid progression. While this may be demonstrated in vitro in both HIV-infected and uninfected Africans (in and out of Africa),[49] it is difficult to reconcile this with lack of evidence that it occurs in the early stages of HIV. Whilst viral loads may go up with acute malaria, this may be only transient and associated with acute febrile episodes; the impact this may have on progression is likely to be limited.[50] The most likely candidate disease significantly to disturb the immune system is tuberculosis. Even here, whilst particular individual studies may show worse survival with tuberculosis, the control groups may not be strictly comparable.[51] A recent comprehensive review found little evidence epidemiologically of a significant interaction.[52] In African patients in the UK there is no difference in survival with tuberculosis – indeed survival is better if tuberculosis is the first AIDS indicator disease.[53]

Poor survival with clinical AIDS

Poverty also influences disease presentation and quality of care. With few resources at hand, health-seeking behaviour may be significantly compromised, with delay resulting in late clinical presentation, and this is likely to increase mortality even in readily treatable conditions. It is extremely hard to quantify this in any fashion. Household studies would need to be very large, and identifying morbidity in any ethical study requires that the event is properly managed and treated. An indirect measure of this is the much higher mortality rate for community-acquired pneumonia in predominantly young adults in

Kenya of 10%;[54] in the UK, comparable age-adjusted rates would be only 1–2%.

Whatever impact late presentation may have, it is compounded by inadequate health-care services in which the facilities may be very basic and the quality of care provided highly compromised. The supply of essential drugs cannot always be maintained, and simple diagnostic tests and radiology may not be available because of lack of supplies or machine faults. Trained staff may not be on hand to deliver even a limited basic package of care, either because they are not paid a living wage and need second jobs, or because HIV/AIDS is itself taking a toll on clinical staff. There is little primary medical care, and continuity of care in the community on discharge can rarely be organized.[29]

These issues are likely to be critical with more severe ill health and immunosuppression. There are far more data from Africa on mortality with an AIDS-defining illness, or when a patient develops stage 4 illness. All studies suggest that survival is far shorter than in the West.[55] In a rural Ugandan cohort, median survival with stage 4 clinical AIDS was 9 months.[56] In an urban Ugandan cohort, median survival with a CD4 count less than 200 was 9 months, whereas that in an urban US cohort before the introduction of highly active ART was 19–20 months.[11] Whether this is all just inadequate health care, or whether inadequately treated virulent infections significantly upregulate viral replication, lower CD4 counts and hasten death is not clear.

Clearly, some patients do present with profound immunosuppression,[57] but it is unclear how long they have been in this state: whether it is recent and a consequence of viral activation, or long-standing. In some patients with virulent infections, low CD4 counts rise on therapy.[58] It must also be remembered that these data do not indicate rapid progression to the point of development of AIDS, but only impaired survival with AIDS. Unfortunately many authors look just at time to death and conclude that rapid disease progression throughout the course of HIV infection must be taking place,[59] assuming that all death occurs at a similar point in the disease process.[60]

Rarity of the classical Western opportunistic infections

With high early morbidity and mortality in developing countries, it is to be expected that fewer people will survive long enough to develop profound immunosuppression than in the West, or will survive long in such a state. Thus, even with the ubiquitous exposure to opportunistic infections in the environment, the rate of developing such conditions will be far lower in resource-poor countries for people who are poor and use government facilities. It is important to point out that the more affluent users of private hospitals are likely to experience a more typical Western pattern of opportunistic infection, but these groups are just a small minority in all developing countries.

Pneumocystis carinii pneumonia (PCP) occurs but is consistently identified only in small numbers of adult patients who are from highly selected populations and bronchoscoped,[61] or at autopsy.[62] In contrast, PCP is very common in HIV-infected infants in Africa in the first few months of life. Whilst *Mycobacterium avium* infection does occur in Kenya, it is estimated to occur in only about 1% of patients with HIV/AIDS admitted to hospital.[63] Autopsy data suggest, in some areas at least, that *Toxoplasma* lesions may be common,[62] but clinical studies indicate that far fewer patients actually present with encephalitis; it seems that many of these lesions may be clinically silent, contributing little to clinical outcome. Geography may play some role here with potentially different rates of *Toxoplasma* exposure, although in Kenya, where rates of clinical disease are very low, the majority of adults have *Toxoplasma* antibodies.[64] The most important true opportunists seem to be fungal, with *Cryptococcus neoformans* a problem across the tropics[65] and *Penicillium marnefii* restricted to South-East Asia.[66] Clinically cytomegalovirus disease is very rarely seen.

Individual clinical problems

Bacterial and mycobacterial infections

Tuberculosis

Tuberculosis is the most important HIV-associated disease in poor communities.[67] Because the majority of adults in developing countries are infected with *Mycobacterium tuberculosis* and HIV is an important trigger for the reactivation of latent tuberculous infection, it is widely assumed that most active disease develops from previous (childhood) exposure. HIV-infected adults are also highly susceptible to acute primary infection. Given the intense exposure to tuberculosis in most overcrowded populations, it seems likely that substantial numbers of cases also arise from acute infection, super- or reinfection. The underlying mechanisms of the interaction between HIV and tuberculosis are poorly understood.

The majority of patients present with pulmonary tuberculosis. Classical sputum smear-positive upper lobe cavitary disease is seen in the early stages of HIV. With more advanced immunosuppression, extensive, often bilateral, lower-lobe consolidation is found, and sputum microscopy is usually negative although culture is positive. Extrapulmonary disease is common, particularly in patients with advanced HIV infection. A broad range of presentations is seen: localized adenopathy with caseation, pleural effusion, meningitis, tuberculoma, visceral abscesses, pericardial effusions, peritoneal disease, miliary spread and disseminated anergic tuberculosis with mycobacteraemia.[68] The clinical features suggest that both acute primary disease and reactivation are occurring.[69]

Diagnosis can be difficult when only radiology and microscopy are available, particularly in paucibacillary pulmonary tuberculosis. Negative sputum smears take far longer to examine than positive specimens, and laboratory staff may be overwhelmed. Pleural tap is done to exclude haemorrhage (Kaposi's sarcoma) or pus (empyema). Gland aspiration and microscopy is useful in tuberculous adenitis. In chronic meningitis, microscopy of cerebrospinal fluid can confirm lymphocytes and exclude yeasts. Even if mycobacterial culture is available, several weeks are needed to make a positive diagnosis. Most patients will receive empirical therapy pending results or on clinical suspicion alone. Much treatable disease is undoubtedly being missed.

Patients with early HIV infection usually respond well to standard short- or long-course therapy. National treatment guidelines should be followed and all cases notified to the tuberculosis control services. Thiacetazone is associated with high rates of hypersensitivity and should be avoided if possible; if not, close monitoring for skin problems during the first 2 months of therapy will identify most cases early, preventing evolution into Stevens–Johnson syndrome.[70] Patients with disseminated or advanced disease often do poorly, especially if myco-bacteraemia is present. Rifampicin-containing regimens may improve the outcome with mycobacteraemia.[71]

Unfortunately, 25–30% of patients in Africa with HIV tuberculosis may die during or soon after completing appropriate therapy.[72] Most deaths are due to community-acquired bacterial infections rather than failure of anti-tuberculosis treatment.[73] Failure to respond or deterioration on standard first-line therapy should prompt the search for additional HIV-related co-morbidity rather than trigger a change to second-line drugs. Treatment failure because of drug resistance is not a major problem in Africa.[74] Tuberculosis frequently recurs following therapy; short-course therapy with rifampicin may result in fewer relapses.[75] It can be difficult to establish whether relapse or reinfection has occurred; both have been described.[69,76]

In a cross-sectional autopsy study in Abidjan, nearly 40% of HIV-seropositive adults had evidence of active tuberculosis at post-mortem examination, and tuberculosis was the leading attributable cause of death.[62] No clinical data were available on these patients and it is unclear why so many had failed to be diagnosed, or perhaps did not adhere to treatment. In contrast, in one large Ugandan cohort using standard guidelines and therapy, the case fatality rate for tuberculosis was 18%, and tuberculosis was considered to be the cause of death in just 5% of 481 deaths.[77] These contrasting results show the potential impact that standard tuberculosis control measures, if properly implemented, can have on HIV tuberculosis co-infection. Tuberculosis should not be seen as the biggest killer in HIV, but the most important disease to treat – the starting point for any care package.

Pneumococcal infection

Streptococcus pneumoniae infection is strongly associated with HIV; the risk of acquiring disease increases progressively following seroconversion. The relative risk of developing invasive disease with HIV in one cohort in Nairobi was 18.9.[58] Lobar pneumonia accounts for about two-thirds of cases; acute sinusitis, occult bacteraemia, meningitis, pericarditis, pyomyositis, skin sepsis and conjunctivitis are also seen. In immunocompetent adults almost all disease would be pneumonia, so HIV clearly widens the clinical spectrum of infection, making its presentation more like infection in children. The radiographic appearance of pneumonia is not changed significantly with HIV.[78] In patients with HIV, most community-acquired pneumonia is pneumococcal in aetiology, but co-infection with *M. tuberculosis*, *Haemophilus influenzae* or non-typhi salmonellae is increasingly being recognized. Recurrent disease, mainly reinfection, is extremely common and about 25% of patients in East Africa who survive will develop a second episode within a year.[58,79] In the USA, recurrent bacterial pneumonia within a year is an AIDS-defining event.[80]

The majority of patients with pneumonia are bacteraemic,[81] and Gram-positive diplococci are abundant in sputum. Percutaneous lung aspiration has been used safely in several studies.[54,58] Without a bacteriology laboratory all cases of lobar pneumonia can be considered pneumococcal and the patients should be given empirical penicillin therapy. Although patients with non-pulmonary presentations will respond well to penicillin, it may be difficult to establish a diagnosis of pneumococcal disease without culture facilities. Because other pathogens may be responsible, broad-spectrum therapy should be used for suspected septicaemia, sinusitis, meningitis and pericarditis in the absence of an aetiological diagnosis.

Patients respond well to standard penicillin therapy given for 7 days, although mortality rates are consistently higher in patients who are HIV positive than in those who are not HIV infected. In Abidjan, nearly 25% of HIV-seropositive adults had bacterial pneumonia at autopsy.[62] In Nairobi, penicillin resistance appears to be more frequent in pneumococcal isolates derived from HIV-infected patients.[82] As intermediate resistance is already widespread in several parts of sub-Saharan Africa, the worrying possibility exists that HIV will facilitate the evolution and spread of drug resistance. Once therapy is started, it is important to complete the full course. Ampicillin, chloramphenicol and erythromycin are also effective. Lack of response within 48–72 hours suggests a second problem or an alternative pathogen.

The salmonellae

Systemic salmonellosis and probably gastroenteritis are highly associated with HIV infection.[83] Both *Salmonella typhimurium* and *S. enteritidis* are frequently isolated; other non-typhi salmonellae are less important and HIV does not significantly predispose to or worsen *S. typhi* infection.[71,84] It seems that HIV infection increases the susceptibility to severe and invasive disease in those non-typhi salmonellae with limited invasive potential in immunocompetent adults, whereas *S. typhi* is invasive regardless of immunosuppression. The associated defects in cell-mediated immunity are poorly defined. There are probably many environmental sources and therefore no obvious ways to prevent exposure.

Most patients present with an enteric fever-like illness that is clinically indistinguishable from typhoid fever.[85] In the majority of cases salmonellae can be isolated from blood. Non-typhi salmonellae co-infection can also occur in patients with tuberculosis or pneumococcal pneumonia. It is unclear whether asymptomatic stool carriage and acute gastroenteritis or dysentery is more common in HIV infection. As with classical typhoid fever, relapse following appropriate therapy is common.[58,86] With HIV-related non-typhi salmonellosis, it may occur in 30% of those who survive the initial event. In Nairobi 10% of patients with chronic diarrhoea and wasting have salmonellae in their stool, and many have no features of systemic involvement.[87] These patients may improve with therapy, but this is often not sustained and the wasting is not reversed.

Diagnosis requires culture of blood or stool. Treatment can be severely compromised without knowledge of drug sensitivities. Many hospitals in developing countries do not have a microbiology laboratory; few cases are identified and there is generally poor recognition of the importance of non-typhi salmonellae in HIV disease. Antimicrobial resistance is common, especially to the affordable and widely used broad-spectrum antibiotics.[88] Chloramphenicol is widely used as first-line therapy, or ampicillin with gentamicin. If available or affordable, a quinolone or fourth-generation cephalosporin should be used for therapy. Unfortunately these agents are not on the essential drug lists for salmonellosis in many African countries (although they are available for syndromic management of STDs). Therapy is given for 2 weeks. Recommendations for treatment will vary according to local data on drug resistance and on what antimicrobials can be afforded. Quinolone maintenance therapy is effective in preventing relapse but is too costly for most developing countries. It is important, therefore, to advise the patient to re-present if symptoms recur.

Patients with bacteraemic disease may respond poorly, especially if therapy is delayed, the diagnosis is missed or the organism is resistant. In Nairobi, when salmonella bacteraemia was first noted in seropositive patients the mortality rate was 80%. With better recognition and therapy, the rate has been reduced to 30%.[71] Gross evidence of bacteraemia was seen in over 15% of HIV-infected adults autopsied in Abidjan; although not cultured, the majority were probably salmonellae.[62]

Other pathogenic bacteria

Although *Staphylococcus aureus* skin infections are common in HIV-positive patients, few studies have been published. Limited access to clean water for washing may be one risk factor. Extensive local necrosis may develop and infection can disseminate. Regular wound cleaning and dressing is important. If the lesion is not healing or is developing atypically, penicillinase-resistant penicillins are necessary. Several studies have linked pyomyositis

with HIV,[89] although endocarditis appears common only in intravenous drug users; it is uncommon in Africa.

Escherichia coli is the third leading cause of community-acquired bacteraemia in Africa.[57,71] It is assumed that most infections come from the bowel, although urinary tract infection is more common in both male and female HIV-positive patients. It usually presents as an enteric fever-like illness. Antimicrobial resistance is widespread; chloramphenicol is suitable first-line therapy. The role of the various pathogenic *E. coli* types in diarrhoea is unclear; when looked for, they can all be recovered from 'slim' patients with chronic diarrhoea,[87] and adherent strains are also found in HIV-positive patients with acute diarrhoea.[90]

Shigella species are widely distributed in the community, and exposure is presumably intense in areas with limited sanitation. They may frequently be isolated from the stool of HIV-positive patients with acute and chronic diarrhoea but, as with non-typhi salmonellae, it has not yet been established whether they cause the diarrhoea. HIV infection predisposes to bacteraemia but it is uncommonly identified.[91] Chloramphenicol is also suitable first-line therapy, modified by clinical response and drug sensitivities.

H. influenzae is occasionally isolated from the blood or lung aspirate of patients with acute pneumonia, either as the sole pathogen or with *Streptococcus pneumoniae*.[70] It is responsible for less than 5% of cases of HIV-related community-acquired pneumonia and can be treated effectively with ampicillin.[92]

Rhodococcus equi is occasionally identified in patients with either lymphadenopathy or chronic lung disease.[93] *Nocardia* also is occasionally seen in patients with chronic lung disease and HIV.[94] It is likely that both of these are underdiagnosed, being mistaken for smear-negative pulmonary tuberculosis.

There does not appear to be any important interaction between *Mycobacterium leprae* and HIV immunosuppression. Neither meningococcal disease[95] nor brucellosis[96] seems to be associated with or exacerbated by HIV infection. There are no data on an association between HIV and anaerobic infections, anthrax, bartonellosis, borreliosis, cholera, leptospirosis, listeriosis, melioidosis, mycoplasma diseases, pertussis, plague, group B streptococcal infections, tetanus or any of the rickettsial diseases from Africa.

Parasitic infections

Malaria

It has long been unclear whether there is any important interaction between malaria and HIV. Some people have begun to assume that the lack of any published data means that there really is no significant interaction, rather than this being a complex issue that is difficult to investigate properly. Recent studies have shattered any optimism that existed.

Studies in pregnant women living in malaria-endemic areas of Malawi[97] and Kenya[98,99] have consistently shown higher rates of parasitaemia and parasite density, and a possibly clinically important negative impact on perinatal outcome and response to sulfadoxine–pyrimethamine (Fansidar) therapy.[100] It also seems that placental parasitaemia is higher with HIV infection and that this may increase the risk of vertical transmission of HIV. More recently, two detailed studies of adults living in endemic malaria areas of Uganda have noted that rates of malaria fever increase with advancing immunosuppression, and that parasite densities also increase with falling CD4 counts.[101,102] Whatever protective antimalarial immune responses develop with repeated exposure, they clearly are reduced with HIV infection. Neither study had sufficient disease episodes to indicate whether underlying HIV infection in adults with pre-existing immunity to malaria affected the risks of developing severe complicated disease. Any association would be of great public health significance.

It also seems that HIV is an important risk factor for severe complicated disease in adults without acquired immunity to malaria who live in unstable malaria transmission areas. Unpublished data from a recent epidemic of *Plasmodium falciparum* malaria in KwaZulu Natal noted that HIV-infected adults were significantly more likely to be admitted to hospital with malaria, to develop severe complicated disease and to die (K. Grimwade, personal communication). The additional risks for death with HIV were substantial.

Clearly the data are inadequate and partial. It is unclear what happens to HIV-infected children as they are exposed to malaria in endemic areas.[103] It seems plausible that they may develop more serious disease and perhaps be more likely to die, if the adult data can be extrapolated. What impact HIV has on the generation of acquired immunity is quite unclear. Given that, in Africa, the main burden of malaria disease and death is in children, these questions need to be addressed urgently.

Cryptosporidium parvum

Acute self-limiting cryptosporidial infection is recognized in adults with HIV infection in Africa. Infection persists in patients with marked immunosuppression and is an AIDS-defining and a WHO stage 4 condition.[104] The chronic diarrhoea is usually watery but this is not a wholly reliable indication of cryptosporidiosis. Although *Cryptosporidium* is ubiquitous, there is marked seasonal and perhaps geographical variation. The prevalence of cyst excretion in cross-sectional studies of seropositive African patients with chronic diarrhoea ranges from 5% to 48%, and *Cryptosporidium* is usually the most commonly identified pathogen in patients with 'slim' disease.[105]

There is at present no effective treatment, although several agents have been tried. Imodium or codeine phosphate may initially reduce the frequency of diarrhoea; whether such benefit is maintained during chronic therapy is not known. Despite the importance of this, no trials have been conducted to evaluate the role of simple antidiarrhoeal agents in patients with 'slim' disease. It is

difficult to avoid exposure. *Cryptosporidium* is zoonotic in many large domestic animals and municipal water supplies may be contaminated even after filtration. It is not known whether human cyst excretors are an important reservoir, but isolation is not recommended. The cysts can withstand chemical treatment and it is necessary to boil water for several minutes to ensure killing.

Isospora belli

Isospora belli is widespread in the tropics and is an important cause of chronic diarrhoea. In most case series it is identified less frequently than *Cryptosporidium*[105] and appears to be absent in some areas of Africa.[87] It is common in the Caribbean, where the prevalence in chronic diarrhoea is 15%.[106] Isosporiasis is important to identify because it can be treated effectively with high-dose co-trimoxazole (800 mg sulfamethoxazole and 160 mg trimethoprim four times daily for 10 days). Recurrences are common and lifelong maintenance therapy is recommended.[106]

Toxoplasma gondii

Toxoplasma gondii occurs throughout the developing world and many adults have latent infection. With advanced immunosuppression (AIDS), latent foci in the brain can reactivate and cause encephalitis. In Nairobi 20% of HIV-positive hospital patients have serological evidence of reactivation, but clinically obvious encephalitis consistent with *Toxoplasma* is uncommon[64] and it has not been seen at autopsy.[107] Few groups across Africa have reported significant rates of encephalitis in comprehensive case series or in cohort studies, although in Abidjan nearly 20% of patients at autopsy had cerebral toxoplasmosis.[62] The autopsy data are difficult to reconcile with the clinical data. Perhaps the initial reactivation is clinically silent and the autopsy findings incidental; early disease with non-specific or diffuse signs may be missed; or there may be geographical variation.

Toxoplasma encephalitis is difficult to diagnose definitively, usually requiring a brain biopsy. There are characteristic findings with computed tomography, but this is not widely available in the developing world. Treatment is expensive; initial therapy is with pyrimethamine and sulfadiazine, supplemented with folinic acid, and should be followed by lifelong maintenance to prevent relapses. Fansidar is occasionally used when first-line therapy is not available, but is of unproven benefit. In many developing countries it may not be cost effective to attempt to diagnose and treat *Toxoplasma* encephalitis.

Microsporidium spp

In industrialized countries, microsporidial infections may be identified in 10–20% of patients with chronic diarrhoea. However, fairly special techniques are required: either a modified trichrome stain or Uvitex B, or a specific polymerase chain reaction (PCR) test. Only a few cross-sectional studies, and no cohort studies, from Africa have been technically able to look properly for microsporidial infection in patients with chronic diarrhoea. Those that have been reported suggest infection rates of the order of 10% or more.[108] It is not known whether there is marked variation in geographical distribution.

Microsporidia can be treated with albendazole, although patients tend to relapse even with maintenance therapy. One interesting recent trial compared initial albendazole treatment (800 mg twice daily for 2 weeks) with placebo in the treatment of persistent diarrhoea without any parasitological investigations. Significant symptomatic relief was noted in the albendazole arm over placebo, but with no impact on survival.[109] Albendazole is relatively expensive, and these results have not been pursued elsewhere or become standard management practice.

Endemic tropical parasitic diseases

Visceral leishmaniasis is well described in patients with AIDS from southern Europe, arising from both acute exposure and reactivation of latent infection. Some cases are clearly transmitted from intravenous drug user to intravenous drug user, complicating interpretation of the overall importance in an endemic temperate area. There have been few case reports from endemic tropical areas.[110] Seroprevalence is at present low (but rising) in many of the rural foci; the disease is difficult to diagnose and patients may die before becoming sufficiently immunosuppressed to develop visceral leishmaniasis. Any significant interaction would be of great importance, particularly in the kala-azar belt of India.

There is no recognized association between African trypanosomiasis and HIV. Odd case reports have described unusual manifestations of Chagas' disease in seropositive adults. Neither pathogenic amoebae nor giardia are thought to be important in 'slim' disease, or are exacerbated by HIV infection.

A few cases of hyperinfection and disseminated disease caused by *Strongyloides stercoralis* have been described.[111] Although AIDS defining, this appears to be a rare problem. Helminths have not been implicated in 'slim' disease. There are no data suggesting any important interaction between HIV and schistosomiasis (except perhaps to reduce inflammation and increase egg excretion),[112] other flukes, hookworm, ascaris, filariasis or any of the cestode (tapeworm) infections.

Viral infections

Herpes zoster

Reactivation of varicella-zoster virus is very common in adult HIV infection, and is often the first indication of underlying HIV infection in a young person. In several communities with a high burden of disease, zoster is well recognized as being HIV related, and vernacular words have developed for it, such as Chisipe in Bugandan, and Tetemaji in kiSwahili. It is important to remember this when managing a patient with zoster, as it is often

equivalent to being given a positive HIV test result out of the blue and without any pretest counselling.

The annual rate of developing zoster is about 5%, and perhaps one-third of patients overall can expect to have at least one episode of infection.[113] Recurrent disease, usually in a different dermatome, is also common. Although not life threatening, it can be extremely painful. No particular dermatomes are involved, but ophthalmic zoster may be seen more frequently in hospital. Extensive necrosis and secondary bacterial infections can develop, but generalized dissemination is unusual. Although lesions can be extensive within one dermatome, the area of single dermatomes is broad and it is incorrect to talk about multidermatomal disease. Keloid scars commonly develop in black patients.

High-dose acyclovir will reduce the duration and extent of the eruption but is costly and not widely available. Codeine phosphate, 30–60 mg 6-hourly, provides reasonable analgesia. Care is needed to avoid secondary bacterial infection.

Herpes simplex

Persistent or recurrent genital herpetic ulcers which are often extremely painful are seen. There is increasing evidence that HSV type 2 is important as a cofactor in HIV transmission. Analgesia can be provided and secondary bacterial infections treated promptly, even if acyclovir is not available. In contrast, nasolabial cold sores (often with HSV type 1), although common, appear to be no more frequent in HIV-positive adults with pneumonia or meningitis than in HIV-uninfected adults.

Enteric viruses

The role of enteric viruses in HIV-associated diarrhoea and enteropathy remains unclear. Limited studies from developing countries have not shown a major association between acute or chronic diarrhoea, HIV infection and stool carriage of rotavirus, small round structured viruses, coronavirus or adenovirus. There are no data on the novel enteric viruses such as astrovirus or picobirnavirus that may be of limited importance in North America. In children in Malawi, rotavirus infection was less common in children with HIV infection.[114]

Fungal infections

Candidiasis

Oral candida or thrush is a common and often painful problem in many patients with moderate or advanced HIV immunosuppression. It may present in several ways: as angular cheilitis, which is a stage 2 event, or as whitish plaques (pseudomembranous) or flat erythematous lesions (atrophic candidiasis), both of which are stage 3-defining events. Genital candidiasis is also common, especially in women. It is unclear how many patients develop oesophageal candida; the pain of extensive oral candidiasis may be difficult to differentiate from true oesphageal disease, which is a stage 4 event. Systemic spread with candidaemia is uncommon.

Infection is relatively easy, although expensive, to control with amphotericin lozenges, nystatin or clotrimazole pessaries, or daily ketoconazole. Gentian violet is cheap and also effective. However, many people now associate both thrush and its therapy with HIV infection, and purple lips can easily stigmatize the patient. Oral candida may become refractory to imidazole therapy, which indicates resistance or overgrowth with drug-resistant species.

Cryptococcus neoformans

Infection with cryptococcus is highly associated with HIV, and across the tropics it is the leading invasive fungal infection described. Even in South-East Asia where *Penicillium marneffei* is endemic, case series show more episodes of cryptococcal fungaemia.[115] Nearly all cases are of variety *neoformans*, although a handful of cases of variety *gattii* have been described. There may be wide regional variation in disease prevalence in cross-sectional studies: in Rwanda the cryptococcus accounts for over 20% of pathogens isolated by blood culture,[116] but in Nairobi it is less than 5% in acute medical admissions.[71] In Uganda most (95%) episodes of cryptococcal disease occurred in people with CD4 counts below 200 per ml, and rates of disease were 10% when CD4 counts fell below 100 per ml.[117]

Clinical presentation in some is with acute fungaemia, occasionally with an associated pulmonary focus. The great majority present with chronic meningitis and have often been unwell for weeks. Headache, often debilitating and intractible, and mood changes are very common.[65] Cutaneous nodules are occasionally seen,[117] but other manifestations are rare. Diagnosis can be made without culture by microscopy of an Indian ink preparation of cerebrospinal fluid or by a simple latex agglutination kit. Few centres routinely perform blood or sputum culture, so there is an inherent bias towards identifying meningitis rather than pulmonary or generalized disseminated disease.

Both amphotericin B and fluconazole are effective. Following initial treatment, lifelong maintenance therapy is recommended. Headaches can be intractible and very difficult to control; sedation and opiates may be required in the agitated and confused patient. Antifungal drugs are expensive and are not usually on essential drug lists or stocked in government pharmacies. In the absence of antifungal therapy, death is inevitable. In the autopsy series from Abidjan, evidence of infection was seen in only 2.5% of post-mortem examinations. One cohort study in Uganda noted that *Cryptococcus* was the leading identified cause of death, responsible for nearly 20% of over 400 deaths investigated.[117]

Currently it is very dispiriting to manage patients with cryptococcal disease in the absence of the effective drugs. However, Pfizer has donated large stocks to some African countries and generic preparations are available at a fraction of the cost of the proprietary drug. This, hopefully, will soon revolutionize outcome following disease, and even opens up the possibility of primary prophylaxis for patients with advanced HIV/AIDS disease.

Other fungi

P. marneffei infection is emerging as an important systemic mycosis in HIV-positive adults in South-East Asia.[66] *Histoplasma duboisii* has been reported in seropositive patients in central Africa,[118] and *Histoplasma capsulatum* in Central America and the Caribbean.[119] Coccidioidomycosis and paracoccidioidomycosis have been associated with HIV infection in South America.[119] It is likely that several other fungal diseases ecologically or geographically restricted to parts of the tropics will be recognized as HIV-associated pathogens. They may never be common as they are usually seen only in advanced immunosuppression.

Malignancies

Kaposi's sarcoma

Kaposi's sarcoma (KS) has always been endemic and relatively common in sub-Saharan Africa; it was the leading malignancy on tumour registers in many parts of Africa before HIV. With HIV infection, a different pattern of disease has emerged. Women are more likely to be affected, although there is still a male preponderance. Lesions are more extensive, frequently involve the mucosae, and often visceralize.[120] Disease is more aggressive and can progress rapidly, carrying a poor prognosis. However, despite being endemic, KS has been reported in less than 5% of African patients with AIDS[121] The reasons why, despite being epidemic, it has never been as prevalent in African adults as it was in North American homosexual men (up to 30% of AIDS-defining events in some cohorts) have not been established. It may relate to the epidemiology and age or route of acquisition of the KS virus, human herpesvirus 8.

Patients are usually diagnosed clinically. Biopsy confirmation is seldom required or performed, although the histological appearances are typical. Patients with just a few cutaneous lesions may develop few problems with KS. However, those with visceral disease (palatal lesions or organ involvement) may deteriorate rapidly, and would benefit from treatment. Unfortunately, many patients do not receive cytotoxic therapy as it is expensive and not widely available in district hospitals in Africa. Few regional cancer centres will accept patients with HIV-related KS. A relatively cheap and simple regimen using actinomycin D and vincristine has proved to have some efficacy in HIV-positive patients in Zambia[122] and is being evaluated at the district hospital level in South Africa.

Other malignancies

Lymphomas have been recorded in life and at autopsy in Africa, but are uncommon and occur much less frequently than in industrialized countries.[62,107] Few patients with AIDS live long enough to develop such late-stage complications. So far, little work has been done on cervical neoplasia and HIV infection; no cases were seen in the Abidjan autopsy series. A novel malignancy of the conjunctival sac has been reported from Uganda. It is rare.[123]

The evolving and growing HIV/AIDS disease burden

All HIV-related disease is 'new' in the sense that it would not have developed without the HIV epidemic. In high-prevalence countries, this additional, new burden of disease presenting for care may be very large and growing, and may have a significant impact on health-care services themselves. This is because the existing, pre-AIDS, disease burden has not diminished in any way as the epidemic of HIV/AIDS disease has taken off. It is complex to understand and to plan for, because disease burden and clinical needs change with the evolution of disease (Figure 20.4). Few high-prevalence countries have been able to increase health spend in anticipation of this additional burden of disease; indeed, some health budgets have actually diminished in real terms. Another problem with inadequate disease surveillance is that it is quite unclear how such unprecedented shifts in the burden of disease have been met by health services.[124]

The evolving and ever-growing disease burden

To date, there have been only two longitudinal studies in hospitals facing large HIV care burdens have been published; one served a rural district, Hlabisa in KwaZulu Natal,[125] and the other a government facility in an urban centre, Nairobi.[71,126] The earliest evidence of the impact of HIV is the rapid and sustained rise in the number of cases of tuberculosis. In Hlabisa, the tuberculosis workload had doubled within 3 years of HIV being identified in the district, in 1990, and by 1997 57% of all cases of tuberculosis were attributable to HIV, with an HIV prevalence in new patients of 67% (when a condition such as HIV is common in the background population, it must be assumed that some patients with tuberculosis are coincidentally HIV-positive).[125] In contrast, clinical AIDS cases were relatively rare in 1997, indicating the relatively long period the later-stage diseases take to develop, and perhaps that a significant proportion of people die before developing clinical AIDS.

In Nairobi, the trends with time are equally revealing. Over a decade (1988–1997) the number of HIV-infected patients admitted daily to one hospital increased steadily from 4.3 to 13.9.[126] There was a consistent pattern of disease over the study period, with bacteraemia and

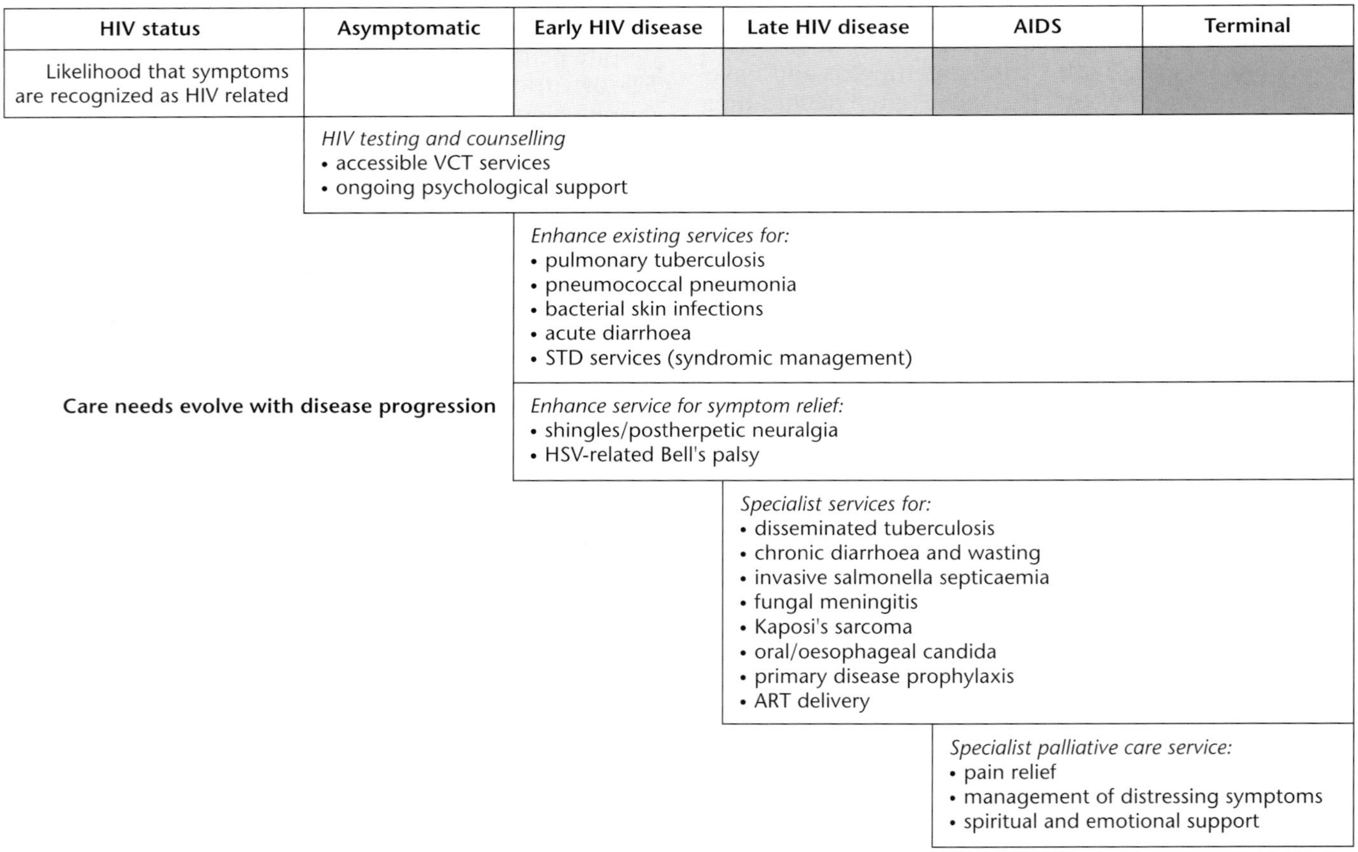

HIV status	Asymptomatic	Early HIV disease	Late HIV disease	AIDS	Terminal
Likelihood that symptoms are recognized as HIV related					

HIV testing and counselling
• accessible VCT services
• ongoing psychological support

Care needs evolve with disease progression

Enhance existing services for:
• pulmonary tuberculosis
• pneumococcal pneumonia
• bacterial skin infections
• acute diarrhoea
• STD services (syndromic management)

Enhance service for symptom relief:
• shingles/postherpetic neuralgia
• HSV-related Bell's palsy

Specialist services for:
• disseminated tuberculosis
• chronic diarrhoea and wasting
• invasive salmonella septicaemia
• fungal meningitis
• Kaposi's sarcoma
• oral/oesophageal candida
• primary disease prophylaxis
• ART delivery

Specialist palliative care service:
• pain relief
• management of distressing symptoms
• spiritual and emotional support

Figure 20.4: Evolving care needs with stage of HIV/AIDS disease. ART, antiretroviral therapy; HSV, herpes simplex virus; VCT, voluntary counselling and testing.

mycobacteraemia predominating, and there was no evidence of the classical Western opportunistic infections emerging as the AIDS epidemic matured.[71] HIV prevalence in patients hospitalized in Nairobi doubled from 19% in 1988–89 to 39% in 1992. Initial trends suggested that the sick patients with HIV/AIDS were crowding out the HIV-uninfected patients and that mortality rates were rising, effects that had been widely predicted.[127] However, in 1997 admissions increased irrespective of HIV status, so the HIV prevalence stabilized at 40% whilst hospital bed occupancy nearly doubled, from 105% to 190%. Far fewer patients with clinical AIDS were admitted over the decade (39% of HIV-positive patients initially, falling to 24% in 1997), probably because of changes in health-seeking behaviour. Carers seem less likely to bring in potential AIDS sufferers because of perceived stigmatization or lack of confidence that much can be achieved. With a changing spectrum of early versus late disease/AIDS over the time period, the inpatient mortality rate actually fell significantly, from 36% to 23%, despite the rise in bed occupancy.[126] These counterintuitive results may be unique to Nairobi, or a common feature in developing countries. It is frustrating to note that there are no other comparable longitudinal studies or databases to refer to. If these responses are common, they have important implications for care, particularly if patients with end-stage disease remain in the community.

Relevant HIV/AIDS care services in resource-poor settings

Spectrum of clinical needs

HIV is a complex disease process in which several different clinical stages can be seen. Care needs relate to the different stages and evolve with the stage of disease (Figure 20.4). A comprehensive response would ideally provide all these care services as and when they are needed. Some of the clinical services (e.g., treatment for tuberculosis, inpatient management for acute pneumonia or Gram-negative sepsis) are already provided in all health services, and the challenge is to provide more standard care to meet the extra demand generated by the HIV epidemic. Other services such as counselling, HIV testing, disease prophylaxis and ART are new, and were not needed or provided in the pre-HIV era. The challenge here is to set up these new services, which is often a difficult and costly exercise.

Prioritizing care needs

Developing countries are invariably short of financial resources and many cannot afford to implement all of these initiatives in a comprehensive and rational care package. There is a clear need to prioritize the more critical

from those less vital, which depends on what already is in place.[128] For instance, VCT is the entry point for care and is a critical link between effective care and prevention. With this in mind, it is possible to construct a hierarchy of care services (Table 20.2).

Such a practical approach may appear to be inimical, and indeed some AIDS activists dispute the validity and morality of such an approach: specialist services including ART must be made available now, as in the West. Others feel that this is grounded in reality and that, although it is important to press for more resources just for HIV/AIDS, in the real world there are competing needs in public health and disease care, and priorities have to be selected. It would seem sensible to advocate widespread specialist services only when other more basic services for patients with HIV/AIDS can be assured. The most relevant specialist interventions are primary disease prophylaxis and ART.

Voluntary testing and counselling

VCT for HIV is a new service being developed and introduced across the tropics.[129] It acts as the entry point both to effective prevention work and to any HIV/AIDS care package.[130] This individual one-to-one approach to the epidemic is now being adopted as government strategy in many countries, such as Kenya, that have seen little impact from traditional health education and prevention messages over the past two decades. It is also clear that any interventions to reduce mother-to-child transmission or to deliver ART will require people to know their HIV status.

Private testing facilites and 'stand-alone' sites (government or non-governmental organization facilities that provide only counselling and testing services) have developed in urban areas and appear to be cost-effective.[131] Such approaches are less cost-effective in rural areas where population density is far lower. Here, the integration of VCT into primary health-care facilities may constitute a less costly alternative which is easier to sustain.[132] The counsellors are trained extensively in confidentiality, professional before and after test counselling, and assisting clients to develop personal risk reduction plans. The key to sustainability in integrated settings has been the recognition of counsellor burn-out as a significant problem and the provision of ongoing support supervision from the outset. As the counsellors are seen regularly and are able to share their problems in a safe environment, they develop and grow as counsellors as well as a group. In all such services the quality of the counselling is critical: if a quality message is not delivered, the expected gains in behavioural change and reduced HIV transmission will not be generated.

Disease prophylaxis in Africa

In the West, primary and secondary disease prophylaxis was implemented early. Initially for pneumocystis

Table 20.2 Hierarchy of care for a resource-poor country

Care level	Services	Comments
The essential minimum *To deliver any form of HIV/AIDS care and support, a certain minimum level of specific services needs to be provided*	Universally accessible HIV testing Support and counselling for the person with HIV/AIDS Information and education which includes clear prognosis and advice on care and support issues Access to PWHIV/AIDS groups	Most countries in Africa have started implementing these basic minimum essential services Once implemented, the provision of basic HIV/AIDS education and information, and training staff in counselling and support skills, is relatively cheap and sustainable
Basic care delivery within the existing health-care services *Most HIV/AIDS clinical care in Africa is delivered by the existing health services, which are under increasing pressure as demand grows. Extra capacity must be developed; if not, services will deteriorate or collapse and the whole community will suffer*	Restructured tuberculosis control services with the capacity to cope with rising demand Restructured hospital services with the capacity to cope with rising and changing caseload in equitable fashion (HIV/AIDS and non-HIV considered equally) Improved primary health-care services (health centres, clinics and dispensaries) to include specific HIV/AIDS care packages More resources for terminal care	DOTs is being introduced and will improve the capacity for tuberculosis control to be delivered Where confidence exists in hospital care, crowding out of patients and reduced quality of services are becoming evident. No solutions are yet identified Often spare capacity in clinics and health centres; little yet done to develop existing potential or improve referral patterns
Introducing specific HIV/AIDS clinical services *It will usually be appropriate to set up specific (new) HIV/AIDS clinical services only if basic level services are in place, and the existing health services are delivering effective basic care*	The purchase and provision of drugs for opportunistic infections that are not on essential drugs list Establishment of technology to diagnose and manage common opportunistic infections Provision of clinics and centres from where primary/secondary prophylaxis can be delivered	To pay for such services, more money has to be voted to the health sector or redistributed within existing health budget For many African countries the initial stumbling block has been the treatment of fungal infection Equity and access issues are complex and largely unresolved
Providing disease-modifying antiretroviral therapy *At present this is very expensive to implement; it is likely to be more cost-effective to increase lifespan in Africa by reducing the incidence and improving outcome of specific HIV/AIDS infections, particularly tuberculosis*	The purchase and provision of antiretroviral drugs in keeping with current consensus guidelines Establishment of technology to manage HIV/AIDS patients on antiretroviral therapy Expansion of existing HIV/AIDS treatment clinics to accommodate antiretroviral therapy	Massive investment necessary to finance such a new initiative, and sustain it once implemented If poorly implemented, threat of drug resistance is a major concern Equity and access issues are complex and largely unexplored

PWHIV, person with HIV; DOTs, directly observed therapy—short-course.

infection, its use widened to cover all the important AIDS-defining opportunistic infections,[133] until the advent of highly active ART obviated its use in most patients. It is important to note that, even when widely used, there was no dramatic impact on survival, although clearly a significant impact on quality of life was achieved. The burden of HIV-related disease is very different in developing countries and the potential for prophylaxis is relatively limited. Three interventions are relevant and have been evaluated. Given the changes in global drug pricing, it will be important to trial new interventions. The most important is fluconazole for cryptococcal prophylaxis. A trial is currently planned for Uganda.

Several randomized placebo-controlled trials have shown that tuberculosis, at least in patients with positive Mantoux tests, can be prevented by chemoprophylaxis (isoniazid for 6 months). Despite this knowledge and consensus policy statements,[134] few people across Africa with HIV infection are receiving or have received prophylaxis. Logistically it is difficult to implement because of the need to exclude incipient active disease; giving isoniazid alone as monotherapy for such patients is likely to produce drug resistance.[135] Many tuberculosis control programmes prefer to continue to concentrate on case detection and follow-up.

Two recent placebo-controlled trials of co-trimoxazole in HIV-infected adults, conducted by independent groups but in the same city, have both shown important positive impacts. One study in which the co-trimoxazole or placebo was given to tuberculosis–HIV co-infected patients showed a significant reduction in mortality;[136] the second study with a similar protocol, in HIV-infected patients without major co-morbitity at trial entry, showed a significant reduction in morbidity but no effect on mortality.[137] These data have been interpreted by some as conclusive enough to recommend co-trimoxazole for all people with HIV/AIDS in Africa.[138] Others have been more cautious, noting that Abidjan has an atypically low rate of co-trimoxazole resistance among bacterial pathogens, and consider more data are needed before such a sweeping policy decision can be made.[139] Recent data from Senegal showed no benefit, but this trial, like several others, was terminated prematurely because the investigators considered it unethical to continue once the Abidjan results had been released.[140] Concern has also emerged that with the similarity of sulfamethoxazole–pyrimethamine (Fansidar) and co-trimoxazole, widescale use of the latter may help select for resistance to Fansidar.[141] The situation is somewhat confused and confusing, and policies differ across Africa. More data are required on efficacy and effectiveness, and the results of several ongoing trials and evaluations are awaited.

The pneumococcus is the only important HIV-associated pathogen for which a vaccine is available. It is recommended (without efficacy data) in the USA for all HIV-seropositive adults. A placebo-controlled trial of the 23-valent polysaccharide vaccine in Uganda has been undertaken. Not only did the vaccine fail to prevent invasive disease, significantly more vaccine recipients developed pneumonia than placebo recipients.[77] Use of the polysaccharide vaccine cannot therefore be recommended in Africa. Whether the new conjugate vaccines will protect remains to be seen. A clinical trial is under way in Malawi evaluating efficacy as secondary prophylaxis.

Access to antiretroviral therapy

To many in the West, the main issue about HIV/AIDS care is to address the huge inequity in access to ART in the developing world, which bears the main brunt of the HIV epidemic. Somehow, mechanisms must be found to purchase drugs so that the single global standard of care for HIV/AIDS (that practised in the West) can be adopted, because only triple drug therapy will significantly alter HIV disease progression.[142] Drug prices have fallen dramatically recently, and may fall even further over the next few years. Indeed, we are facing in some countries the bizarre scenario of the costs of laboratory monitoring for ART being more expensive that the drugs themselves. Together with the creation of the global fund for AIDS, tuberculosis and malaria drugs, pleas for action that once seemed so unrealistic and utopian are now on the verge of being implemented.[143]

However, price has been only one of several problems in broadening access to ART. More challenging issues remain: how to develop the human resources and health system capacity to use such drugs properly (training, laboratory monitoring, drug distribution); and how to reduce the price and technology of the laboratory monitoring needed to monitor ART for safety and maximal efficacy so that it can be used in laboratories with a limited infrastructure. Programmes are needed that focus on strengthening the health-care system itself, within which HIV/AIDS care, including ART, is provided. Only when AIDS care is integrated into mainstream clinical practice can any African government realistically hope to improve equitability in access to care. This is far more difficult than is realized and it will be many years before we have sufficient real data, knowledge and experience to be able clearly to lay down the simple rules for effective ART as part of general clinical practice in resource-constrained environments. Nevertheless, the lack of knowledge should not constrain the implementation of ART in carefully monitored situations, in order that that best practice can be developed—by identifying what works, and what does not work and why. Then at least some of the therapeutic advances made over the past decade in the West will have a significant impact in tropical countries.

Several issues will be of great importance in any country where ART is implemented. All must clearly realize and accept that ART does not cure infection: it just holds the virus in check for as long as the drugs are taken correctly. Poor adherence will result in drug resistance and, if not carefully controlled, this may threaten the effectiveness of those ARTs that are most suitable for resource-poor situations. Potentially the most worrying concern is the possible negative impact on HIV control and the promotion of safer sex—behavioural disinhibition with reduced concerns about HIV infection born out of false optimism of the benefits of care. Such a threat is well recognized in some communities in the USA and Europe, and may negate the potential benefits of reducing HIV transmission that ART may achieve through viral load suppression.

HIV vaccines

The development of an HIV vaccine that stimulated effective immunity would be of enormous importance to world health, and could be used in two different ways. The most important way—and the strategy that most groups are investigating—is as a protective vaccine.[144] Some, however, are exploring the use of candidate agents as therapeutic agents. To date, no vaccine has completed phase 3 efficacy trials and been shown to work. The best hope for an effective vaccine is to induce antibodies that can both neutralize most (if not all) subtypes of HIV-1 and induce T cells, with the ability to inhibit viral replication by secretion of effector molecules and by directly killing HIV-infected cells. Efforts to produce high-titre neutralizing antibodies across different clades have been disappointing in animal models. Nevertheless, some candidate envelope vaccine constructs are in trials in Thailand, and data are eagerly awaited. Data from animal studies are more encouraging for inducing both effector and killer T cells, either with DNA vaccines or with subunit vaccines expressed in viral vectors such as canarypox. Several phase 1 and 2 trials are underway with such constructs, but it will be a long time before any phase 3 trials are completed.[145]

International research efforts in the early stages of the epidemic were disappointing in the attention given to HIV vaccines. That has changed recently, with initiatives such as the International AIDS Vaccine Initiative (IAVI) coupled with large grants and donations from individual philanthropists and foundations. Whether such a cash influx alone will be sufficient to guarantee success in this critical venture remains to be seen. Some HIV vaccinologists are optimistic. Others are more pessimistic. Only time will tell.

REFERENCES

1   Nahmias AJ, Weiss J, Xao X et al. Evidence for human infection with an HTLV-III/LAV like virus in central Africa 1959. *Lancet* 1986; i:1279–1280.

2   Hooper E. *The Virus: A Journey Back to the Source of HIV and AIDS.* Boston MA: Little, Brown, 1999.

3   Bryceson A, Tomkins A, Ridley D et al. HIV-2-associated AIDS in the 1970s. *Lancet* 1988; ii:221.

4   Gilks CF. AIDS, monkeys and malaria. *Nature* 1991; 354:262.

5   Sharp P, Bailes E, Chaudhuri RR et al. The origins of acquired immune deficiency syndrome virus: where and when? *Phil Trans R Soc Lond B* 2001; 356:867–876.

6   McCutchan FE. Understanding the genetic diversity of HIV-1. *AIDS* 2000; 14 (Supplement 3):s31–44.

7   Marlink R. Lessons from the second AIDS virus, HIV-2. *AIDS* 1996; 10:689–699.

8   Weber J. The pathogenesis of HIV-1 infection. *Br Med Bull* 2001; 58:61–72.

9   Mellors J, Rinaldo C, Gupta P et al. Prognosis in HIV-1 infection predicted by the quantity of virus in plasma. *Science* 1996; 272:1167–1170.

10 World Health Organization. Interim proposal for a WHO staging system for HIV infection and disease. *Wkly Epidemiol Rec* 1990; 65:221–228.

11 French N, Mujugira A, Nakiyingi J, Mulder D, Janoff EN & Gilks CF. Imunological and clinical staging in HIV-1-infected Ugandan adults are comparable and provide no evidence of rapid progression but poor survival with advanced disease. *J Acquir Immune Defic Syndr* 1999; 22:509–516.

12 Post FA, Wood R & Maartens G. CD4 and total lymphocyte counts as predictors of HIV disease progression. *Q J Med* 1996; 89:505–508.

13 UNAIDS/WHO. *AIDS Epidemic Update.* Geneva: WHO, December 2000.

14 Asiimwe-Okiror G, Opio AA, Musinguzi J et al. Change in sexual behaviour and decline in HIV infection among young pregnant women in urban Uganda. *AIDS* 1997; 11:1757–1163.

15 Timaeus I M. Impact of the HIV epidemic on mortality in sub-Saharan Africa: evidence from national surveys and censuses. *AIDS* 1998; 12 (Supplement 1): s15–s27.

16 Quinn TC, Wawer MJ, Sewankambo N et al. Viral load and heterosexual transmission of human immunodeficiency virus type 1. *N Engl J Med* 2000; 342:921–929.

17 Van Howe RS. Circumcision and HIV infection: review of literature and meta-analysis. *Int J STD AIDS* 1999; 10:8–16.

18 Fleming DT & Wasserheit JN. From epidemiological synergy to public health policy and practice: the contribution of other sexually transmitted diseases to sexual transmission of HIV infection. *Sex Transm Inf* 1999; 75:3–17.

19 Cohen MS, Hoffman IF, Royce RA et al. Reduction of concentration of HIV-1 in semen after treatment of urethritis: implications for prevention of sexual transmission of HIV-1. *Lancet* 1997; 349:1868–1873.

20 Kreiss JK, Koech D, Plummer FA et al. AIDS virus infection in Nairobi prostitutes; spread of the epidemic to East Africa. *N Engl J Med* 1986; 314:414–418.

21 Rotheram-Borus M J. Expanding the range of interventions to reduce HIV among adolescents. *AIDS* 2000; 14 (Supplement 1):s33–s40.

22 Savarit D, De Cock KM, Schutz R, Konate S, Lackritz E & Bondurand A. Risk of HIV infection from transfusion with blood negative for HIV antibody in a West African city. *BMJ* 1992; 305:498–501.

23 Des Jarlais DC, Friedman SR, Choopanya K, Vanichseni S & Ward TP. International epidemiology of HIV and AIDS among injecting drug users. *AIDS* 1992; 6:1053–1068.

24 Consten ECJ, van Lanschot JB, Henny PC, Tinnemans JGM & van der Meer JTM. A prospective study on the risk of exposure to HIV during surgery in Zambia. *AIDS* 1995; 9:585–588.

25 Newell ML. Mechanisms and timing of mother-to-child transmission of HIV-1. *AIDS* 1998; 12:831–837.

26 The International Perinatal HIV Group. The mode of delivery and the risk of vertical transmission of HIV type 1. *N Engl J Med* 1999; 340:977–987.

27 Leroy V, Newell ML, Dabis F et al. International multicentre pooled analysis of late postnatal mother-to-child transmission of HIV-1 infection. *Lancet* 1998; 352:597–600.

28 Coutsoudis A, Pillay D, Spooner E et al. Influence of infant-feeding patterns on early mother-to-child transmission of HIV-1 in Durban, South Africa: a prospective cohort study. *Lancet* 1999; 354:471–476.

29 Gilks CF, Floyd K, Haran D, Kemp J, Squire B & Wilkinson D. *Care and Support for People with HIV/AIDS in Resource-poor Settings.* Health and Population Occasional Paper in Sexual and Reproductive Health. London: Department for International Development, June 1997.

30 Grosskurth H, Mosha F, Todd J et al. Impact of improved treatment of sexually transmitted diseases on HIV infection in rural Tanzania: randomised controlled clinical trial. *Lancet* 1995; 346:530–536.

31 Wawer MJ, Sewankambo NK, Serwadda D et al. Control of sexually transmitted diseases for AIDS prevention in Uganda: a randomised community trial. Rakai Project Study Group. *Lancet* 1999; 353:525–535.

32 Whitworth J (personal communication).

33 UNAIDS/WHO. *Consultation on STD Interventions for Preventing HIV: What is the Evidence?* WHO/HSI/2000.02. Geneva: UNAIDS/WHO, 2000.

34 Weller SC. A meta-analysis of condom effectiveness in reducing sexually transmitted HIV. *Soc Sci Med* 1993; 36:1635–1644.

35 Traore E, Gyhs PD, Diallo MO et al. Safe sex behaviour among female sex workers enrolled in a microbicide trial in Abidjan. *XII International AIDS Conference*, Durban, South Africa, 9–14 July 2000. Abstract TnOrC660.

36 Weber J & Lacey CJN. The development of novel vaginal microbicides: from bench to clinic. *J Acquir Immune Defic Syndr* 2001; 15(Suppl 1): S35–S37.

37 Lackritz EM, Ruebush TK, Zucker JR et al. Blood transfusion practices and blood banking services in a Kenyan hospital. *AIDS* 1993; 7:995–999.

38 Cardo DM, Culver DH, Ciesielski CA et al. Case–control study of HIV seroconversion in health care workers after percutaneous exposure. *N Engl J Med* 1997; 337:1485–1490.

39 Mofenson LM & McIntyre JA. Advances and research directions in the prevention of mother-to-child HIV-1 transmission. *Lancet* 2000; 355:2237–2244.

40 Guay LA, Musoke P, Fleming T et al. Intrapartum and neonatal single-dose nevirapine compared with zidovudine for prevention of mother-to-child transmission of HIV-1 in Kampala, Uganda: HIVNET 012 randomised trial. *Lancet* 1999; 354:795–802.

41 De Cock K, Fowler MG, Mercier E et al. Prevention of mother-to-child HIV transmission in resource-poor countries. *JAMA* 2000; 283:1175–1182.

42 Fowler MG, Bertolli J & Niebirg P. When is breastfeeding not best? The dilemma facing HIV-infected women in resource-poor settings. *JAMA* 1999; 282:781–783.

43 Wilkinson D, Floyd K & Gilks CF. Antiretroviral drugs as a public health intervention for pregnant HIV-infected women in rural South Africa: an issue of cost-effectiveness and capacity. *AIDS* 1998; 12:1675–1682.

44 Marseille E, Kahn JG, Mmiro F et al. Cost effectiveness of single dose nevirapine regimen for mothers and babies to reduce vertical HIV-1 transmission in sub-Saharan Africa. *Lancet* 1999; 354:1084–1089.

45 Gilks CF. Acute bacterial infections and HIV disease. *Br Med Bull* 1998; 54:383–393.

46 Morgan D, Ross A, Malamba S & Whitworth J. Early manifestations of HIV-1 infection in Uganda. *AIDS* 1998; 12:591–596.

47 Anzala OA, Nagelkerke NJD, Bwayo JJ et al. Rapid progression to disease in African sex workers with HIV-1 infection. *J Infect Dis* 1995; 171:686–689.

48 Morgan D, Mahe D, Mayanja B et al. HIV-1 infections in rural Africa: is there a difference in median time to AIDS and survival compared with that in industrialised countries? AIDS 2002; 16:597–603.

49 Rizzardini G, Trabattoni D, Saresella M et al. Immune activation in HIV-infected African individuals. *AIDS* 1998; 12:2387–2396.

50 Hoffman IF, Jere CS, Taylor TE et al. The effect of *Plasmodium falciparum* malaria on HIV-1 RNA blood plasma concentration. *AIDS* 1999; 13:487–494.

51 Whalen CC, Nsubuga P, Okwera A et al. Impact of pulmonary tuberculosis on survival of HIV-infected adults: a prospective epidemiologic study in Uganda. *AIDS* 2000; 14:1219–1228.

52 Del Amo J, Malin A, Pozniak A & de Cock KM. Does tuberculosis accelerate the progression of HIV disease? Evidence from basic science and epidemiology. *AIDS* 1999; 13:1151–1158.

53 Del Amo J, Petruckevitch A, Phillips A et al. Disease progression and survival in HIV-1-infected Africans in London. *AIDS* 1998; 12:1203–1209.

54 Scott JAG, Hall AJ, Muyodi C et al. Aetiology, outcome and risk factors for mortality among adults with acute pneumonia in Kenya. *Lancet* 2000; 355:1225–1230.

55 Grant AD, Djomand G & de Cock K. Natural history and spectrum of disease in adults with HIV/AIDS in Africa. *AIDS* 1997; 11 (Supplement B): s43–s54.

56 Morgan D, Maude GH, Malamba SS et al. HIV-1 disease progression and AIDS-defining disorders in rural Uganda. *Lancet* 1997; 350:245–250.

57 Grant D, Djomand G, Smets P et al. Profound immunosuppression across the spectrum of opportunistic disease amongst hospitalized HIV-infected adults in Abidjan, Cote d'Ivoire. *AIDS* 1997; 11:1357–1364.

58 Gilks CF, Ojoo SA, Ojoo JC et al. Invasive pneumococcal disease in a cohort of predominantly HIV-1 infected female sex workers in Nairobi, Kenya. *Lancet* 1996; 347:718–724.

59 Deschamps M, Fitzgerald DW, Pape JW & Johnson WD. HIV infection in Haiti: natural history and disease progression. *AIDS* 2000; 14:2515–2521.

60 Gilks CF. The clinical challenge of the HIV epidemic in the developing world. *Lancet* 1993; 342:1037–1039.

61 Kamanfu G, Mlika-Cabanne N, Girard P-G et al. Pulmonary complications of HIV infection in Bujumbura, Burundi. *Am Rev Respir Dis* 1993; 147:658–663.

62 Lucas SB, Hounnou A, Peacock C et al. The mortality and pathology of HIV infection in a West African city. *AIDS* 1993; **7**:1569–1579.

63 Gilks CF, Brindle RJ, Mwachari C et al. Disseminated *Mycobacterium avium* infection among HIV-infected patients in Kenya. *J Acquir Immune Defic Syndr* 1995; 8:195–198.

64 Brindle R, Holliman R, Gilks C & Waiyaki P. *Toxoplasma* antibodies in HIV-positive patients from Nairobi. *Trans R Soc Trop Med Hyg* 1991; 85:750–751.

65 Heyderman RS, Gangaidzo IT, Hakim JG et al. Cryptococcal meningitis in human immunodeficiency virus-infected patients in Harare, Zimbabwe. *Clin Infect Dis* 1998; 26:284–289.

66 Supparatpinyo K, Khamwan C, Baosoung V, Nelson KE & Sirisanthana T. Disseminated *Penicillium marneffei* infection in Southeast Asia. *Lancet* 1994; 344:110–113.

67 Raviglione MC, Harries AD, Msiska R, Wilkinson D & Nunn P. Tuberculosis and HIV: current status in Africa. *AIDS* 1997; 11 (Supplement B):s115–s123.

68 De Cock KM, Soro B, Coulibaly IM & Lucas SB. Tuberculosis and HIV infection in sub-Saharan Africa. *JAMA* 1992; 268:1581–1587.

69 Gilks C F, Godfrey-Faussett P, Batchelor B I F et al. Recent transmission of tuberculosis in a cohort of HIV-1 infected female prostitutes in Nairobi, Kenya. *AIDS* 1997; 11:911–918.

70 Nunn P, Kibuga D, Gathua S et al. Thiacetazone commonly causes cutaneous hypersensitivity reactions in HIV-1 seropositive patients treated for tuberculosis. *Lancet* 1991; 337:627–630.

71 Arthur G, Nduba VN, Kariyuki S, Kimari J, Bhatt S & Gilks CF. Trends in blood-stream infections among human immunodeficiency virus-infected adults admitted to a hospital in Nairobi, Kenya during the last decade. *Clin Infect Dis* 2001; 33:248–256.

72 Nunn P, Brindle R, Carpenter L et al. Cohort study of human immunodeficiency virus infection in patients with tuberculosis in Nairobi, Kenya. *Am Rev Respir Dis* 1992; 146:849–854.

73 Brindle RJ, Nunn PP, Batchelor BIF et al. Infection and morbidity in patients with tuberculosis in Nairobi, Kenya. *AIDS* 1993; 7:1469–1474.

74 Pablos-Mendez A, Raviglione MC, Laszlo A et al. Global surveillance for antituberculosis-drug resistance 1994–97. *N Engl J Med* 1998; 338:1641–1649.

75 Perriens JH, St Louis ME, Mukadi YB et al. Pulmonary tuberculosis in HIV-infected patients in Zaire; a controlled trial of treatment for either 6 or 12 months. *N Engl J Med* 1995; 332:779–784.

76 Sonnenberg P, Murray J, Glynn JR, Shearer S, Kambashi B & Godfrey-Faussett P. HIV-1 and recurrence, relapse and reinfection of tuberculosis after cure: a cohort study in South African mineworkers. *Lancet* 2001; 358:1687–1693.

77 French N, Nakiyingi J, Whitworth J & Gilks CF. A description of tuberculosis in HIV-infected African adults and its impact on survival. Third Annual Meeting of the British Infection Society, May 2000. Abstract 27.

78 French N, Williams G, Williamson V et al. The radiographic appearance of pneumococcal pneumonia is unaltered by HIV-1 infection in hospitalized Kenyans *AIDS* 2002; in press

79 French N, Nakiyingi J, Carpenter LM et al. 23-valent pneumococcal polysaccharide vaccine in HIV-1-infected Ugandan adults: double-blind, randomised and placebo controlled trial. *Lancet* 2000; 355: 2106–2111.

80 Centers for Disease Control and Prevention. 1993 Revised classification system for HIV infection and expanded surveillance case definition for AIDS among adolescents and adults. *MMWR Morb Mortal Wkly Rep* 1992; 41(RR-17): 1–19.

81 Feldman C, Glatthaar M, Morar R et al. Bacteraemic pneumococcal pneumonia in HIV-seropositive and HIV-seronegative adults. *Chest* 1999; 116:107–114.

82 Paul J, Kimari J & Gilks C F. *Streptococcus pneumoniae* resistant to penicillin and tetracycline associated with HIV seropositivity. *Lancet* 1995; 346:1034–1035.

83 Gilks CF, Brindle RJ, Otieno LS et al. Life-threatening bacteraemia in HIV-1 seropositive adults admitted to hospital in Nairobi, Kenya. *Lancet* 1990; 336:545–549.

84 Vugia DJ, Kiehlbauch JA, Yeboue K et al. Pathogens and predictors of fatal septicaemia associated with human immunodeficiency virus infection in Ivory Coast, West Africa. *J Infect Dis* 1993; 168:564–570.

85 Gilks CF, Brindle RJ, Otieno L et al. The presentation and outcome of HIV-related disease in Nairobi. *Q J Med* 1992; 82:25–32.

86 Gordon MA, Banda HT, Gondwe M et al. Non-typhoidal *Salmonella* bacteraemia among HIV-infected Malawian adults: high mortality and frequent recrudescence. *AIDS* 2002; in press.

87 Mwachari C, Batchelor B, Paul J, Waiyaki P & Gilks CF. Chronic diarrhoea among HIV-infected adult patients in Nairobi, Kenya. *J Infect* 1998; 37:48–53.

88 Kariuki S, Gilks CF, Corkhill J et al. Multidrug-resistant non-typhi salmonellae in Kenya. *J Antimicrob Chemother* 1996; 38:425–434.

89 Pallangyo K, Hakanson A, Lema L et al. High HIV seroprevalence and increased HIV-associated mortality among hospitalized patients with deep bacterial infections in Dar es Salaam, Tanzania. *AIDS* 1992; 6:971–976.

90 Mathewson JJ, Jiang ZD, Zumla A et al. HEp-2 cell-adherent *Escherichia coli* in patients with human immunodeficiency virus-associated diarrhoea. *J Infect Dis* 1995; 171:1636–1639.

91 Angulo FJ & Swerdlow DL. Bacterial enteric infections in persons infected with human immunodeficiency virus. *Clin Infect Dis* 1995; 21 (Supplement 1): s84–s93.

92 Koulla-Shiro S, Kuaban L & Belec L. Acute community-acquired bacterial pneumonia in human immunodeficiency virus (HIV) infected and non-HIV-infected adult patients in Cameroon: aetiology and outcome. *Tubercle Lung Dis* 1996; 77:47–51.

93 Gray KJ, French N, Lugada E, Watera C & Gilks CF. *Rhodococcus equi* and HIV-1 infection in Uganda. *J Infect* 2000; 41:227–231.

94 Jones N, Khoosal M, Louw M & Karstaedt A. Nocardial infection as a complication of HIV in South Africa. *J Infect* 2000; 41:232–239.

95 Brindle R, Simani P, Newnham R, Waiyaki P & Gilks C. No association between meningococcal disease and human immunodeficiency virus in adults in Nairobi, Kenya. *Trans R Soc Trop Med Hyg* 1991; 85:651.

96 Paul J, Gilks C, Batchelor B, Ojoo J, Amir M & Selkon JB. Serological responses to brucellosis in HIV-seropositive patients. *Trans R Soc Trop Med Hyg* 1995; 89:228–230.

97 Steketee RW, Wirima JJ, Slutsker L et al. Malaria parasite infection during pregnancy and at delivery in mother, placenta, and newborn: efficacy of chloroquine and mefloquine in rural Malawi. *Am J Trop Med Hyg* 1996; 55:24–32.

98 Steketee RW, Wirima JJ, Bloland PB et al. Impairment of a pregnant woman's acquired ability to limit *Plasmodium falciparum* by infection with human immunodeficiency virus type-1. *Am J Trop Med Hyg* 1996; 55:42–49.

99 Steketee RW, Nahlen BD, Ayisi J, Van Eijk A & Misore A. HIV and malaria overlap and do interact in sub-Saharan African pregnant women. Proceedings of the XIIth International conference on AIDS, Geneva, 1998: Abstract 145.

100 Verhoeff FH, Brabin BJ, Hart CA, Chimsuku L, Kazembe P & Broadhead RL. Increased prevalence of malaria in HIV-infected pregnant women and its implications for malaria control. *Trop Med Int Health* 1999; 4:5–12.

101 Whitworth JAG, Morgan D, Quigley M et al. Effect of HIV-1 and increasing immunosuppression on malaria parasitaemia and clinical episodes in adults in rural Uganda: a cohort study. *Lancet* 2000; 356:1051–1056.

102 French N, Nakiyingi J, Lugada E, Watera C, Whitworth JAG & Gilks CF. Increasing rates of malarial fever with deteriorating immune status in HIV-1-infected Ugandan adults. *AIDS* 2001; 15:899–906.

103 French N & Gilks CF. HIV and malaria, do they interact? *Trans R Soc Trop Med Hyg* 2000; 94:233–237.

104 Gowan IM, Hawkins AS & Weller IVD. The natural history of cryptosporidial diarrhoea in HIV-infected patients. *AIDS* 1993; 7:349–354.

105 Conlon CP, Pinching AJ, Perera CU, Moody A, Luo NP & Lucas SB. HIV-related enteropathy in Zambia: a clinical, microbiological and histological study. *Am J Trop Med Hyg* 1990; 42:83–88.

106 Pape JW, Verdier R & Johnson WD. Treatment and prophylaxis of *Isospora belli* infection in patients with the acquired immunodeficiency syndrome. *N Engl J Med* 1989; 320:1044–1447.

107 Rana FS, Hawken MP, Mwachari C et al. Autopsy study of HIV-1-positive and HIV-1-negative adult medical patients in Nairobi, Kenya. *J Acquir Immune Defic Syndr* 2000; 24:23–29.

108 van Gool T, Luderhoff E, Nathoo KJ, Kiire CF, Dankert J & Mason PR. High prevalence of *Enterocytozoon bieneusi* infections among HIV-positive individuals with persistent diarrhoea in Harare, Zimbabwe. *Trans R Soc Trop Med Hyg* 1995; 89:478–480.

109 Kelly P, Lungu F, Keane E et al. Albendazole chemotherapy for treatment of diarrhoea in patients with AIDS in Zambia: a randomised double blind controlled trial. *BMJ* 1996; 312:1187–1191.

110 World Health Organization. *Leishmania* and HIV in gridlock. WHO/CTD/Leish/98.9. Geneva: WHO, 1998.

111 Ferreira MS, NishiokaS de A, Borges AS et al. Strongyloidiasis and infection due to human immunodeficiency virus: 25 cases at a Brazilian teaching hospital including seven cases of hyperinfection syndrome. *Clin Infect Dis* 1999; 28:154–155.

112 Karanja DMS, Colley DG, Nahlen BL, Ouma JH & Secor WE. Studies on schistosomiasis in western Kenya: 1. Evidence for immune-facilitated excretion of schistosome eggs from patients with *Schistosoma mansoni* and human immunodeficiency virus coinfections. *Am J Trop Med Hyg* 1997; 56:515–521.

113 Morgan D, Mahe C, Malamba S, Okongo M, Mayanja B & Whitworth J. Herpes zoster and HIV-1 infection in a rural Ugandan cohort. *AIDS* 2001; 15:223–229.

114 Cunliffe NA, Gondwe JS, Kirkwood CD et al. Effect of concomitant HIV infection on presentation and outcome of rotavirus gastroenteritis in Malawian children. *Lancet* 2001; 358:550–555.

115 Archibald LK, Mcdonald LC, Rheanpumikankit S et al. Fever and HIV infection as sentinels for emerging mycobacterial and fungal bloodstream infections in hospitalized patients > 15 years old, Bangkok. *J Infect Dis* 1999; 180:87–92.

116 Taelman H, Bogaerts J, Batungwanayo J et al. Community-acquired bacteraemia, fungaemia and parasitaemia in febrile adults infected with HIV in central Africa. *Vth International Conference on AIDS in Africa*, Kinshasa, October 1990 (FOD1).

117 French N, Watera C, Lugada E et al. Cryptococcal disease in an urban Ugandan cohort. *AIDS* 2002; (in press).

118 Carme B, Ngaporo A I, Ngolet A et al. Disseminated African histoplasmosis in a Congolese patient with AIDS. *J Med Vet Mycol* 1992; 30:245–248.

119 Cunliffe NA & Denning DW. Uncommon invasive mycoses in AIDS. *AIDS* 1995; 9:411–420.

120 Bayley AC, Downing RG, Cheingsong-Popov R, Tedder R S, Dalgleish AG & Weiss RA. HTLV-III serology distinguishes atypical and endemic Kaposi's sarcoma in Africa. *Lancet* 1985; i:359–361.

121 Berkley S, Okware S & Naamara W. Surveillance for AIDS in Uganda. *AIDS* 1989; 3:79–85.

122 Bayley AC. Aggressive Kaposi's sarcoma in Zambia, 1983. *Lancet* 1984; i:1318–1320.

123 Ateenyi-Agaba C. Conjunctival squamous-cell carcinoma associated with HIV infection in Kampala, Uganda. *Lancet* 1995; 345:695–696.

124 Gilks CF. Improving HIV/AIDS disease surveillance in low-income countries. *AIDS* 1997; 11:1881–1882.

125 Floyd K, Reid A, Wilkinson D & Gilks CF. Admission trends in a rural South African hospital during the early years of the HIV epidemic. *JAMA* 1999; 282:1087–1091.

126 Arthur G, Bhatt SM, Muhindi D, Achia J, Kariuki S & Gilks CF. The changing impact of HIV/AIDS on Kenyatta National Hospital, Nairobi from 1988/9 through 1992 to 1997. *AIDS* 2000; 14:1625–1631.

127 Gilks CF, Floyd K, Otieno LS, Adam AM, Bhatt SM & Warrell DA. Some effects of a rising case-load of adult HIV-related disease on a hospital in Nairobi. *J Acquir Immune Defic Syndr* 1998; 18:234–240.

128 Gilks CF, Katabira E & de Cock KM. The challenge of providing effective care for HIV/AIDS in Africa. *AIDS* 1997; 11 (Supplement B):s99–s106.

129 World Health Organization. *Global Programme on AIDS. Counselling for HIV/AIDS: A Key to Caring.* WHO/GPA/TCO/HCS/95.15. Geneva: WHO, 1995.

130 Voluntary HIV-1 Counselling and Testing Efficacy Study Group. Efficacy of voluntary HIV-1 counselling and testing in individuals and couples in Kenya, Tanzania and Trinidad: a randomised trial. *Lancet* 2000; 356:103–112.

131 Sweat M, Gregorich S, Sangiwa G et al. Cost-effectiveness of voluntary HIV-1 counselling and testing in reducing sexual transmission of HIV-1 in Kenya and Tanzania. *Lancet* 2000; 356:11–21.

132 Forsythe S, Arthur G, Ngatia G, Mutemi R, Odhiambo J &

Gilks CF. Assessing the cost of VCT in Kenya. *Health Policy Planning* 2001 (in press).

133 US Public Health Service and Infectious Diseases Society of America. 1999 USPHS/IDSA guidelines for the prevention of opportunistic infections in persons infected with human immunodeficiency virus. *MMWR Morb Mortal Wkly Rep* 1999; 48(RR-10):1–66.

134 Wilkinson D, Squire SB & Garner P. Effect of preventive treatment for tuberculosis in adults infected with HIV: systematic review of randomised placebo controlled trials. *BMJ* 1998; 317:625–629.

135 World Health Organization. Preventive therapy against tuberculosis in people living with HIV. *Wkly Epidemiol Rec* 1999; 74:385–398.

136 Wiktor SZ, Sassan-Morokro M, Grand AD et al. Efficacy of trimethoprim–sulphamethoxazole prophylaxis to decrease morbidity and mortality in HIV-1-infected patients with tuberculosis in Abidjan, Cote d'Ivoire: a randomised controlled trial. *Lancet* 1999; 353:1469–1475.

137 Anglaret X, Chene G, Attia A et al. Early chemoprophylaxis with trimethoprim–sulphamethoxazole for HIV-1-infected adults in Abidjan, Cote d'Ivoire: a randomised trial. Lancet 1999; 353:1463–1468.

138 WHO/UNAIDS. *Provisional WHO/UNAIDS Secretariat Recommendations on the Use of Cotrimoxazole Prophylaxis in Adults and Children Living with HIV/AIDS in Africa.* Geneva: UNAIDS, 2000.

139 Grimwade K & Gilks CF. Cotrimoxazole prophylaxis in adults infected with HIV in low-income countries. *Curr Opin Infect Dis* 2001; 14:507–512.

140 Maynart M, Lièvre L, Salif PS et al. Primary prevention with cotrimoxazole for HIV-1 infected adults: results of the pilot study in Dakar, Senegal. *J Acquir Immune Defic Syndr* 2001; 26:130–136.

141 Iyer JK, Milhous WK, Cortese JF, Kiblin JG & Plowe CV. *Plasmodium falciparum* cross-resistance between trimethoprim and pyrimethamine. *Lancet* 2001; 358:1066–1067.

142 Carpenter CCJ, Cooper DJ, Fischl M A et al. Antiretroviral therapy in adults: updated recommendations of the International AIDS Society – USA panel. *JAMA* 2000; 283:381–390.

143 World Health Organization. Scaling up antiretroviral therapy in resource-limited settings: guidelines or a public health approach. 2002; http://www.who.int/HIVAIDS/HIVAIDScare/ARVDraftApril2000.pdf

144 Hanke T. Prospect of a prophylactic vaccine for HIV. *Br Med Bull* 2001; 58:205–218.

145 Heeney JL & Hahn B. Vaccines and immunology: elucidating immunity to HIV-1 and current prospects for AIDS vaccine development. *AIDS* 2000; 14 (Supplement 3):s125–s128.

Chapter 21
Sexually Transmitted Infections (Excluding HIV)

D. Mabey and J. Richens

Sexually transmitted infections (STIs) are among the most common reasons for seeking medical care in developing countries, accounting for 10% or more of medical consultations in some parts of Africa.[1] Nevertheless, and in spite of their serious consequences (particularly for women and children), and increasing evidence that they facilitate the transmission of human immunodeficiency virus (HIV) through sexual contact, they have often been accorded low priority by medical professionals and health planners. The consequent lack of good facilities for their management has led many patients with these conditions to seek treatment outside the formal health sector, with inadequate treatment regimens leading to increasing antimicrobial resistance among sexually transmitted pathogens. Because no statistics are available for patients treated outside the formal health sector, the extent of the problem continues to be underestimated.

Epidemiology of sexually transmitted diseases

Certain broad generalizations can be made about the epidemiology of sexually transmitted diseases (STIs). Clearly they are diseases of the sexually active, although mother-to-child transmission also occurs. None of the sexually transmitted agents described in this chapter has an epidemiologically significant non-human reservoir. They are more common among young adults, among single people of both sexes, and among those who travel. Although no sexually active individual is immune, certain groups can be identified whose behaviour places them at higher risk than others. Such groups include sex workers and their clients, bar workers, adolescents, the military, truck drivers and sailors.

Accurate STI prevalence figures are not available for any developing country, but studies in Swaziland and Uganda have estimated the incidence of gonorrhoea to be 3000 and 15 000, respectively, per 100 000 total population per annum.[2] For comparison, the annual incidence of gonorrhoea in England and Wales is less than 50 per 100 000.

The prevalence of certain STIs among antenatal clinic attenders in a variety of developing countries is shown in Table 21.1.[3-7] In rural Uganda, a community-based survey of adults aged 15–59 years found the prevalence of syphilis to be 10%, of gonorrhoea 1.6% and of chlamydial infection 3%; 24% of women had *Trichomonas vaginalis* infection and 51% had bacterial vaginosis.[8] Table 21.2 shows a number of factors which may explain the higher incidence and prevalence of STIs in developing compared with industrialized countries. Lack of access to effective treatment probably explains much of the difference in the case of the curable STIs.

The relative importance of certain STIs is much greater in developing countries. For example, chancroid remains a common cause of genital ulceration in many African countries but has almost disappeared from Europe. Sporadic outbreaks among impoverished communities in North America in the 1980s suggest that this has more to do with socio-economic factors than with climate. Donovanosis (granuloma inguinale) is highly prevalent in certain parts of Papua New Guinea, India and South Africa but appears to be rare outside these areas. The lack of reliable and cheap diagnostic tests for the three classical 'tropical STIs'—chancroid, donovanosis and lymphogranuloma venereum (LGV)—has hindered attempts to study their epidemiology.

Table 21.1 Prevalence of STIs among antenatal clinic attenders in developing countries.

Country	Neisseria gonorrhoeae (%)	Chlamydia trachomatis (%)	Treponema pallidum (%)	Trichomonas vaginalis (%)
Gambia[3]	6.7	6.9	1	32
Kenya[4]	6.6	10.0	–	–
Swaziland[5]	3.9	–	14	23
Zambia[6]	11.2	–	12.5	38
Ghana[7]	3.4	7.7	–	–

Table 21.2 Factors contributing to the high incidence of STIs in developing countries.

1. Demographic factors (high proportion of population are young adults)
2. Rural–urban migration with breakdown of traditional customs
3. Prostitution
4. Lack of adequate medical services
5. High prevalence of antibiotic-resistant strains of *Neisseria gonorrhoeae, Haemophilus ducreyi*
6. Polygamy

Because of the lack of adequate diagnostic and treatment facilities for STIs in many developing countries, complications are commonly seen, particularly among women and children. Pelvic inflammatory disease (PID), due in the majority of cases to gonorrhoea or chlamydial infection, is the most common cause of admission to gynaecology wards in Africa.[9] Ectopic pregnancy as a sequela of PID is up to three times as common in Africa as in Europe, and tubal infertility, another common sequela, is widespread, with up to 20% of women affected in some regions of Africa.[10] The incidence of carcinoma of the cervix is extremely high in many developing countries. Of infants born in many African cities, 2–3% develop gonococcal ophthalmia neonatorum, and congenital syphilis has been an important cause of hospital admission among infants aged less than 3 months in Lusaka, Zambia.[11,12]

Table 21.3 lists organisms transmissible by sexual contact and the diseases they cause. In this chapter only those responsible for major morbidity in developing countries will be considered further.

Control of STIs

Strategies for the the control of STIs include primary and secondary prevention, and, in the case of bacterial and protozoal infections, improving access to curative treatment. Primary prevention is health education given to young people before they are exposed to the risk of STIs, emphasizing the importance of delaying the onset of sexual activity, limiting the number of their sexual partners, and using condoms to reduce risk. Secondary prevention refers to health education given to individuals with STIs, aimed at reducing the risk to their sexual partners, and the likelihood of their becoming reinfected. Improved case management, in which accessible, affordable and effective treatment is made available to patients with symptomatic STIs, is a cornerstone of STI control. Effective treatment should be given at the first visit, to reduce onward transmission and the likelihood of complications. The treatment of sexual partners of STI patients is also of critical importance for STI control. Since many STIs are asymptomatic, especially in women, screening programmes can play an important role in STI control;

for example, screening of pregnant women is an important strategy for the prevention of congenital syphilis. Effective control of STIs cannot be achieved by health ministries in isolation. Coordinated multisectoral interventions which attempt to address broader societal issues that allow STIs to thrive (e.g., migrant labour and prostitution) also need to be tackled vigorously.

STIs and HIV infection

There is no doubt that other STIs, by causing inflammation and ulceration of the genital tract, facilitate the transmission of HIV infection through sexual contact.[13] Ulcerative STIs, in particular, increase both the infectivity of HIV-positive individuals, and the susceptibility of HIV negatives, by a factor of 10–100 per sexual exposure.[14] Gonococcal and chlamydial infection have been shown to increase the shedding of HIV at the cervix, and gonorrhoea to increase the shedding of HIV in seminal fluid.[15] An intervention trial in Tanzania showed that the incidence of HIV infection was reduced by 40% following the introduction of improved case management of STIs, using the syndromic approach, in rural health centres.[16] These studies have given renewed impetus to STI control programmes.

History-taking and examination in the STI clinic

It is not possible to provide a good clinical service for STIs unless one gains the confidence of the patient(s). This requires *privacy* and the *avoidance of a moralistic attitude*.

It is usually possible to take a history and examine a patient with an STI in 10 minutes. When taking a *history*, the following information should be collected:

1. The nature and duration of the symptoms.
2. The nature of any treatment already taken for this condition.
3. A sexual history, which should indicate when and with whom the patient has had sexual intercourse. This information is essential in order to attempt contact tracing and/or partner notification. Information about the type of sexual activity and condom use will assist in examination, collection of specimens and preventive counselling.
4. Past medical history and history of previous STIs and HIV testing.
5. History of drug allergy.
6. In female patients a menstrual and obstetric history should be taken.

STI patients should always be counselled concerning risk reduction, including the promotion of condom use; the importance of compliance with the full course of

Table 21.3 Sexually transmitted infections in humans.

	Agent	Disease
STDs producing genital lesions		
Viruses	Herpes simplex virus	Genital herpes, disseminated and neonatal herpes infection
	Human papilloma virus	Genital warts, juvenile laryngeal papillomatosis, squamous carcinoma in anogenital area
	Molluscum contagiosum virus	Molluscum contagiosum
Bacteria	*Neisseria gonorrhoeae*	Gonococcal infections of urethra, epididymis, pharynx, rectum, conjunctiva, upper genital tract of women, disseminated gonorrhoeal infection
	Chlamydia trachomatis, serotypes D–K	As for gonorrhoea, except for disseminated infection; also infantile pneumonia and reactive arthritis
	Chlamydia trachomatis, L1,2,3 serotypes	Lymphogranuloma venereum
	Ureaplasma urealyticum	Non-gonococcal urethritis
	Mycoplasma hominis	Salpingitis, postpartum fever
	Haemophilus ducreyi	Chancroid
	Treponema pallidum	Syphilis
	Gardnerella vaginalis and anaerobes	Bacterial vaginosis
	Klebsiella (formerly Calymmatobacterium) granulomatis	Donovanosis (granuloma inguinale)
Fungi	*Candida albicans*	Genital candidiasis
Protozoa	*Trichomonas vaginalis*	Trichomoniasis
Arthropods	*Phthirus pubis*	Pediculosis
	Sarcoptes scabiei	Scabies
Infections which can be sexually transmitted but which do not generally produce genital lesions		
Viruses	Hepatitis viruses	Hepatitis A–D
	Cytomegalovirus (CMV)	CMV infections of newborn and immunosuppressed
	HIV	Acquired immune deficiency syndrome
	HTLV-1	Tropical spastic paraparesis, T cell leukaemia/lymphoma
Bacteria	*Shigella* spp.	Shigellosis
	Campylobacter spp.	Campylobacter enteritis
	Salmonella spp.	Salmonellosis
	Group B streptococcus	Neonatal sepsis
Protozoa	*Giardia lamblia*	Giardiasis
	Cryptosporidium spp.	Cryptosporidosis
	Entamoeba histolytica	Amoebiasis*
Helminths	*Enterobius vermicularis*	Enterobiasis
	Strongyloides stercoralis	Strongyloidiasis
	Trichuris trichiura	Trichuriasis

*Occasionally produces anogenital ulceration in tropical countries.
Source: World Health Organization.

treatment if directly observed single-dose treatment is not given; and the importance of referring sexual contacts for treatment.

The *examination* should be carried out in private in a good light. After examination of the mouth and palms, patients should be exposed from the umbilicus to the knees. The skin of the abdomen, groins and perineum should be examined in particular for evidence of scabies and pediculosis, and the inguinal glands palpated. In males the penis should be inspected, after retraction of the foreskin in uncircumcised patients. If a urethral discharge is not apparent, evidence of urethritis can be sought by milking the urethra forward and examining the meatus for discharge. The scrotum should be palpated for evidence of epididymitis. Female patients should be examined in the lithotomy position. The lower abdomen should be palpated for evidence of PID (masses and/or tenderness) and, after inspection of the vulva, a vaginal speculum should be passed. The cervix should be examined and the speculum then slowly withdrawn while the walls of the vagina are examined. Bimanual examination should then be performed to identify pelvic masses and/or tenderness.

The presence of pain on moving the cervix (cervical excitation tenderness) suggests the presence of PID. In both sexes the perianal skin should also be inspected, and proctoscopy may be performed to check for rectal infections.

The *laboratory investigations* requested will depend on the facilities available. In general they should be selected on the principle that a patient with one STI is also at increased risk of other STIs; that is, they should not be limited to tests designed to identify the cause of the present symptoms. All patients with an STI should be screened for syphilis. Whether they should also be screened for HIV depends on the availability of counselling and of treatment for those found to be positive.

In settings where laboratory diagnosis is not feasible, the World Health Organization (WHO) recommends *syndromic management*, in which patients with a syndrome such as urethral discharge or genital ulcer are treated for all the likely causes of that syndrome.[17] Even when laboratory diagnosis is available, syndromic management has the advantage that treatment is given at the first visit, rather than relying on the patient to return for his/her results. Effective syndromic treatment depends on knowledge of local disease patterns and antimicrobial susceptibilities; a laboratory is required to monitor these, preferably in each country or province.[18] WHO syndromic treatment flow charts for eight common STI syndromes are shown in Figure 21.1. The advantages and disadvantages of syndromic management are shown in Table 21.4. The flow chart for vaginal discharge is the least satisfactory, as many women with this complaint are not suffering from an STI. This not only leads to over-treatment, but can also jeopardize relationships if such women are asked to refer their partners for STI treatment.

Table 21.4 Advantages and disadvantages of syndromic management of STIs.

Advantages
Simple
Rapid
No laboratory required
Treatment given a first visit, preventing complications and further transmission
Simplifies reporting and supervision

Disadvantages
Leads to over-treatment, especially in women
May lead to problems with partner notification, especially in women who are told they have an STI when they do not
Only symptomatic STIs treated

Diseases causing a genital discharge

Urethral discharge in males

Urethritis in males is either gonococcal, non-gonococcal or of mixed aetiology; the presence of gonococci is easily demonstrated by Gram stain. When the Gram stain is negative the presence of > 5 polymorphs per high-power field is accepted as evidence of non-gonococcal urethritis. In most developing countries the majority of cases presenting to hospital are gonococcal. Up to 50% of cases of non-gonococcal urethritis are due to *Chlamydia trachomatis*; a proportion of the remaining cases are associated with *Ureaplasma* or *Mycoplasma* species, and a

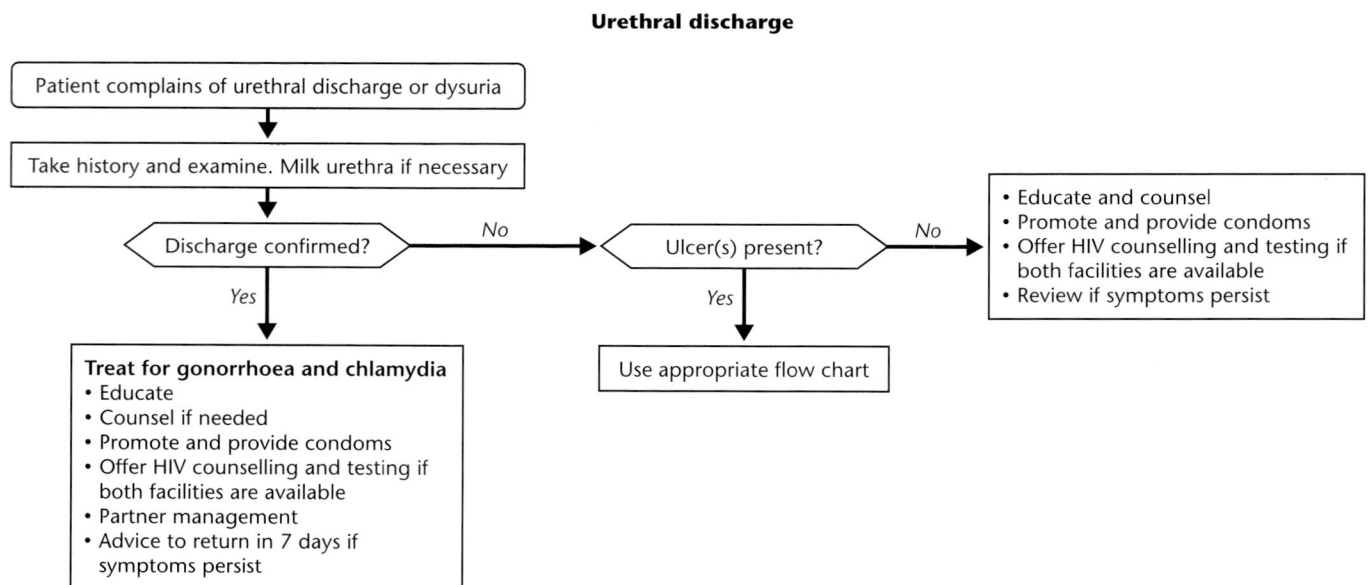

Figure 21.1: WHO flow charts for the management of common STI-associated syndromes. (© 2001 World Health Organization.)

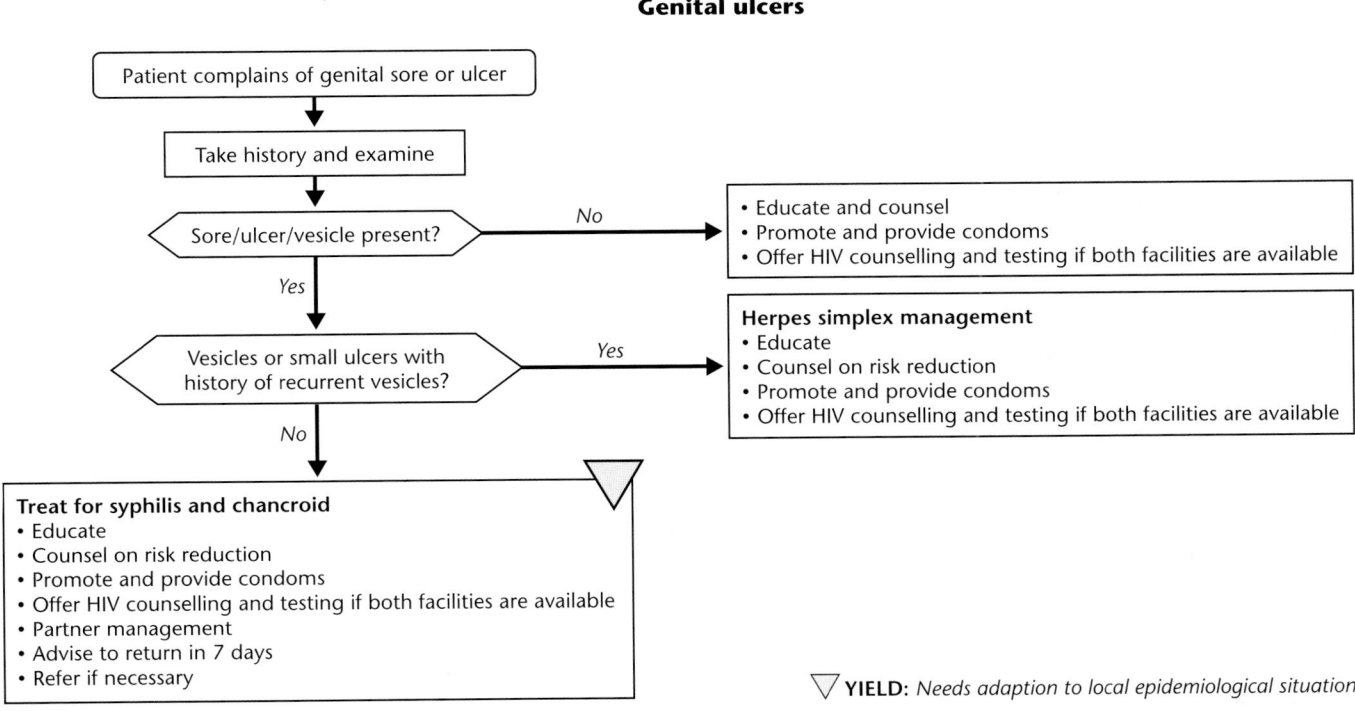

Persistent/recurrent urethral discharge in men

NB: This flow chart assumes effective therapy for gonorrhoea and chlamydia to have been received and taken by the patient prior to this consultation

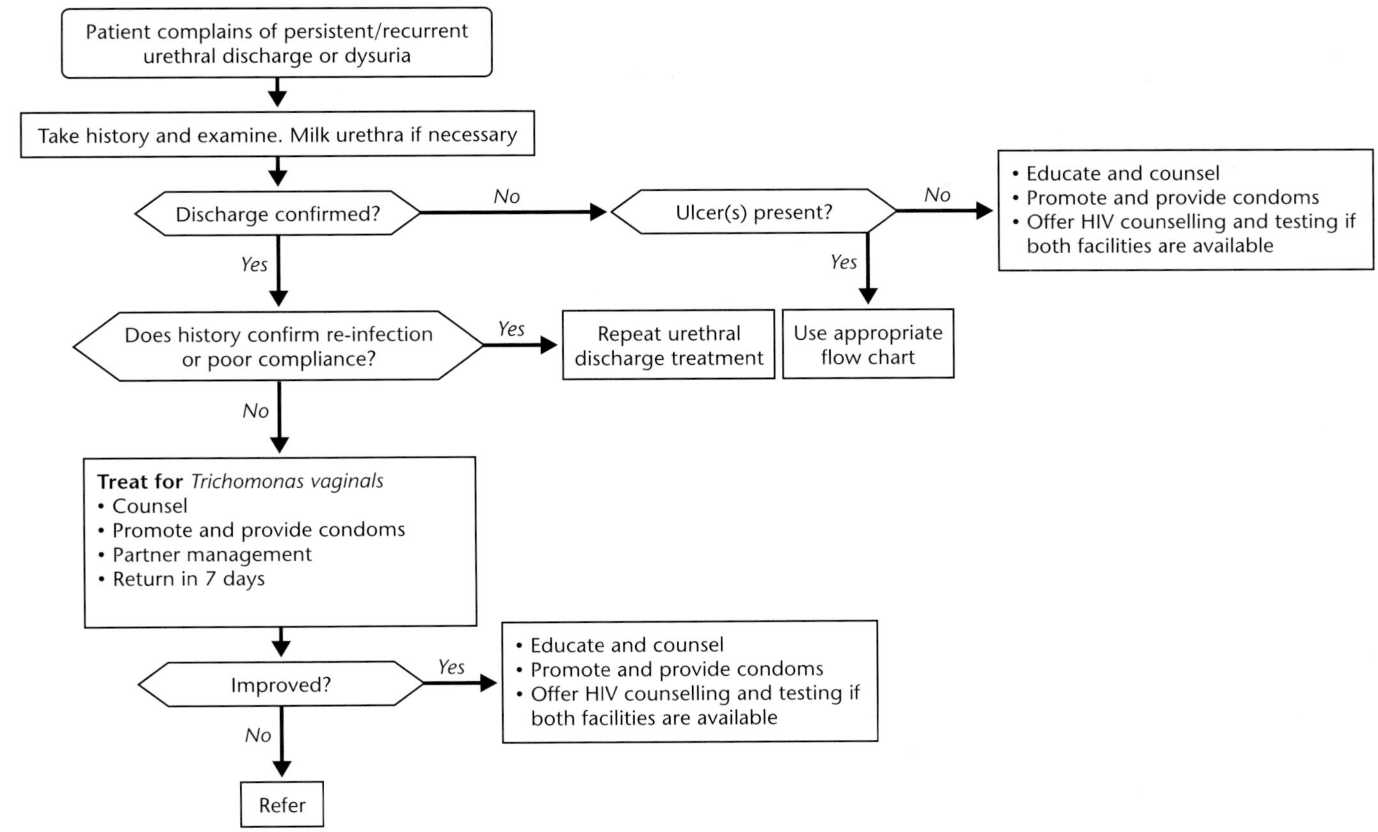

Patient complains of persistent/recurrent urethral discharge or dysuria

Take history and examine. Milk urethra if necessary

Discharge confirmed?

No → Ulcer(s) present? → No →
- Educate and counsel
- Promote and provide condoms
- Offer HIV counselling and testing if both facilities are available

Yes ↓

Yes ↓

Does history confirm re-infection or poor compliance? → Yes → Repeat urethral discharge treatment   Use appropriate flow chart

No ↓

Treat for *Trichomonas vaginals*
- Counsel
- Promote and provide condoms
- Partner management
- Return in 7 days

Improved? → Yes →
- Educate and counsel
- Promote and provide condoms
- Offer HIV counselling and testing if both facilities are available

No ↓

Refer

Figure 21.1: Part 2

Genital ulcers

Patient complains of genital sore or ulcer

Take history and examine

Sore/ulcer/vesicle present? → No →
- Educate and counsel
- Promote and provide condoms
- Offer HIV counselling and testing if both facilities are available

Yes ↓

Vesicles or small ulcers with history of recurrent vesicles? → Yes →
Herpes simplex management
- Educate
- Counsel on risk reduction
- Promote and provide condoms
- Offer HIV counselling and testing if both facilities are available

No ↓

Treat for syphilis and chancroid
- Educate
- Counsel on risk reduction
- Promote and provide condoms
- Offer HIV counselling and testing if both facilities are available
- Partner management
- Advise to return in 7 days
- Refer if necessary

▽ **YIELD:** *Needs adaption to local epidemiological situation*

Figure 21.1: Part 3

Inguinal bubo

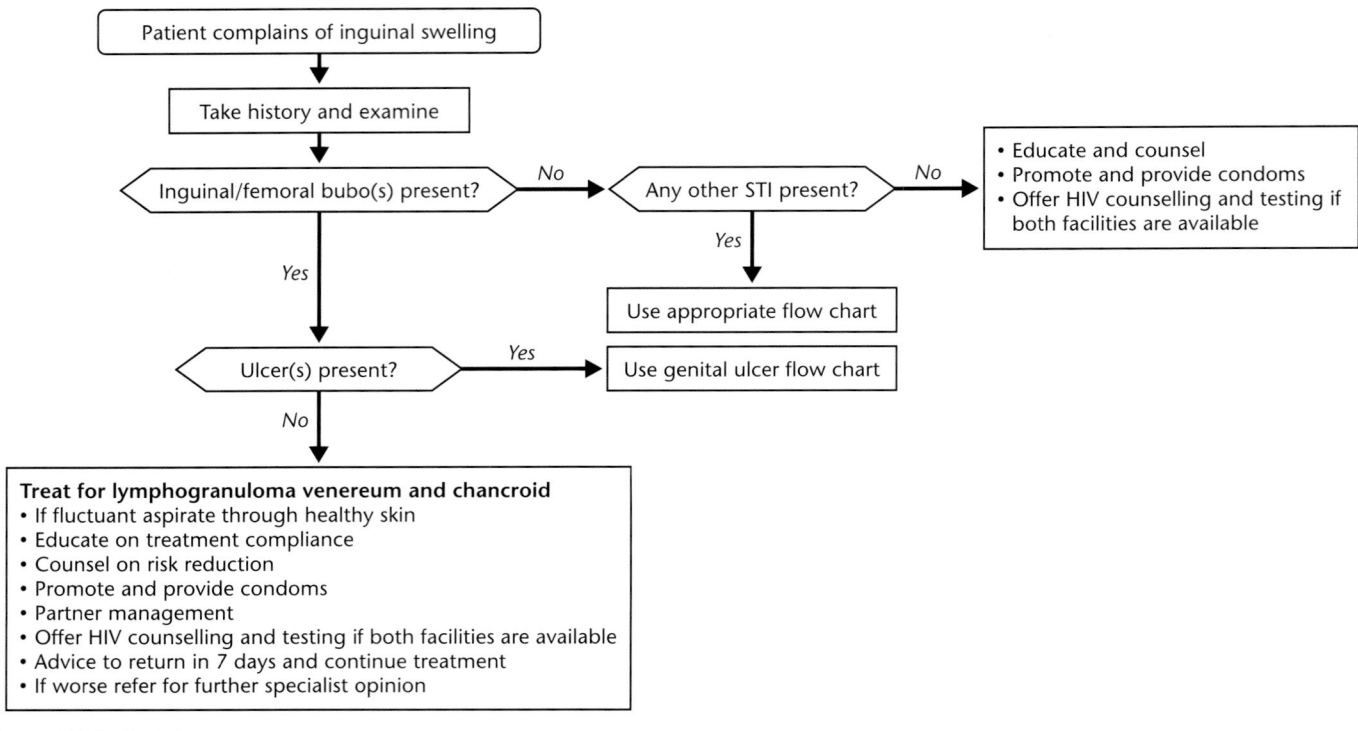

Figure 21.1: Part 4

Scrotal swelling

Patient complains of scrotal swelling/pain

↓

Take history and examine

↓

Swelling/pain confirmed? —No→
- Reassure patient and educate
- Provide analgesics if necessary
- Promote and provide condoms
- Offer HIV counselling and testing if both facilities are available

↓ Yes

Testis rotated or elevated, or history of trauma? —No→
Treat for gonorrhoea and chlamydia
- Educate
- Counsel if needed
- Promote and provide condoms
- Partner management
- Offer HIV counselling and testing if both facilities are available
- Review in 7 days or earlier if necessary; if worse then refer

↓ No

Refer immediately for a surgical opinion

Figure 21.1: Part 5

Vaginal discharge

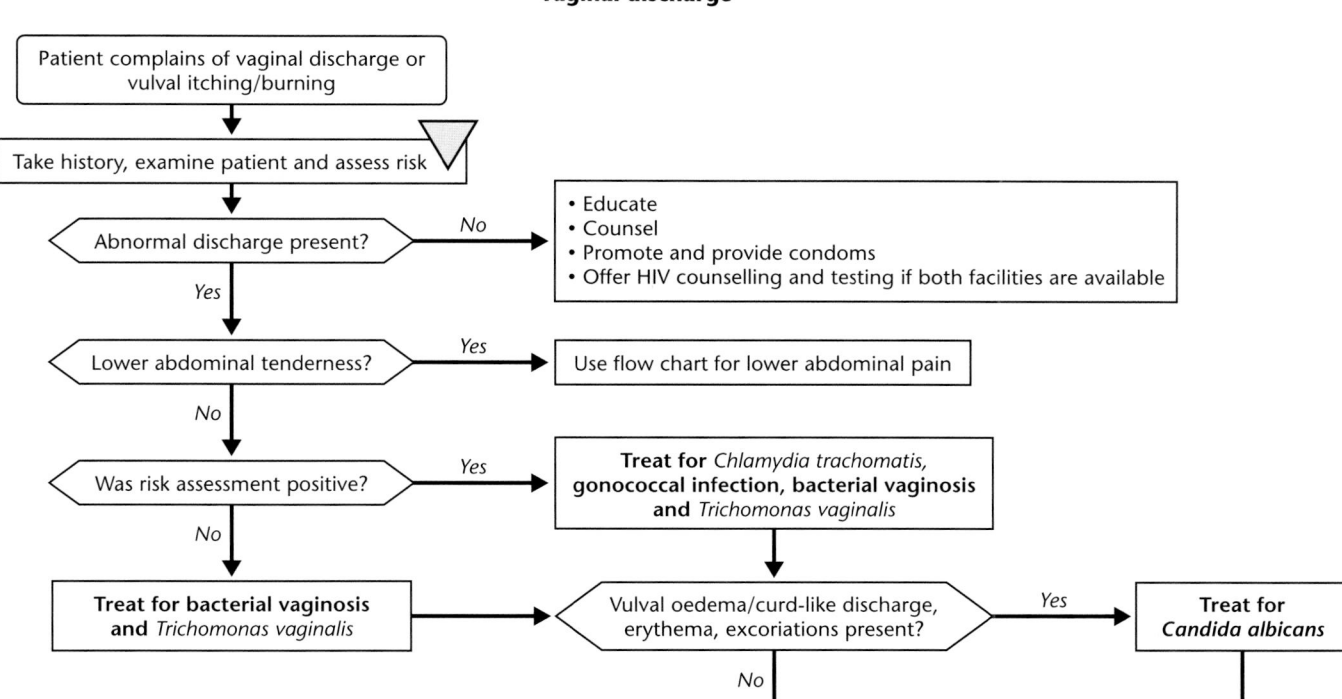

YIELD: *Needs adaption to local social and behavioural epidemiological situation*

Figure 21.1: Part 6

small percentage may harbour *Trichomonas vaginalis*. According to the WHO syndromic management guidelines, men with urethral discharge should be treated for both gonorrhoea and chlamydial infection (this will also cover most cases of *Ureaplasma* and *Mycoplasma* infection). Cases in which it is possible to exclude gonorrhoea by microscopy of a Gram stain can be treated for chlamydial infection alone.

Gonorrhoea

Gonorrhoea is the most prevalent bacterial STI in the tropics. The causative organism, *Neisseria gonorrhoea*, a Gram-negative oval diplococcus found only in man, is especially adept at colonizing the epithelial surfaces of the male and female urogenital tract, conjunctiva, pharynx, rectum and synovium.

Pathogenesis

Virulence is conferred by the presence of pili which mediate adherence, sufficient to withstand hydrodynamic forces within the urethra, and which also inhibit uptake by phagocytes. Invasion and multiplication have been demonstrated in mucus-secreting non-ciliated cells of the Fallopian tubes. No specific toxins produced by *N. gonorrhoea* have been identified but the lipo-oligosaccharide and peptidoglycan components have

been implicated in inhibition of ciliary function and the genesis of synovitis respectively. *N. gonorrhoea* is highly adept at avoiding the host immune response. The pilus antigens, the protein designated P.II and the lipo-oligosaccharide are all capable of antigenic variation sufficient to permit repeated reinfection of the same host within a short period. Antibodies to the P.III protein do not fix complement and can block bactericidal, complement-fixing antibodies to the lipo-oligosaccharide. The bacteria produce an IgA_1 protease which may impair the host mucosal immune response. The mucosal immune response to infection is characterized by the production of IgA, IgM and IgE, which can inhibit adherence and facilitates opsonization. These responses have been demonstrated in both infected and non-infected, exposed contacts of infected individuals. Strains responsible for disseminated gonococcal infection have been shown to be less susceptible to killing by human serum, are less chemotactic to neutrophils and elicit greater amounts of blocking antibody.

Clinical features

The risk of contracting gonorrhoea after a single exposure is about 20% for males and probably higher for females. Typically men develop symptoms after a 2–5-day incubation period, with 90% of symptomatic infections manifesting within 14 days. Asymptomatic infections are

Vaginal discharge (speculum and bimanual)

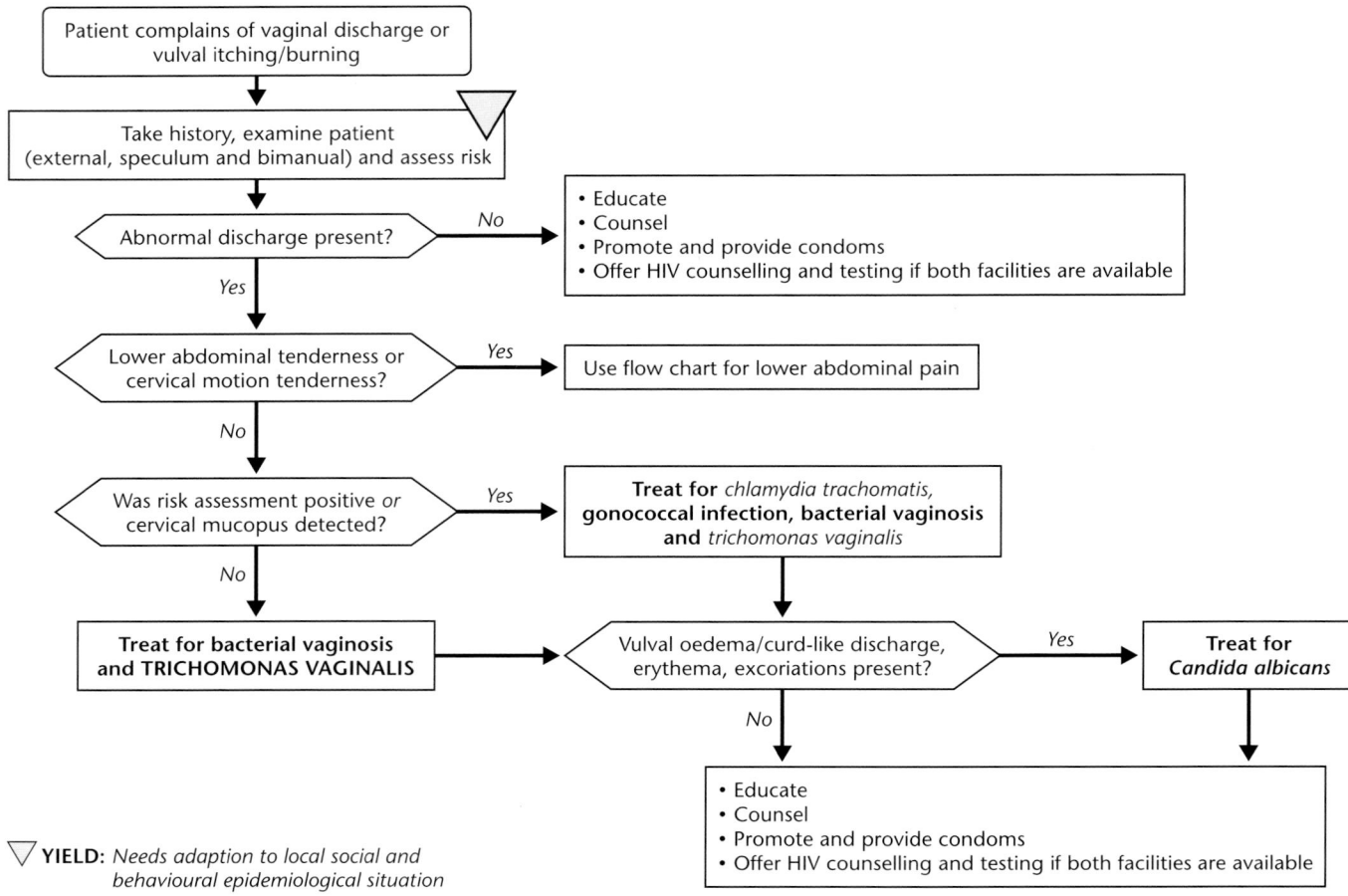

Figure 21.1: Part 7

frequent in women—up to 80% of infections detected in contacts of symptomatic partners. Recent community-based studies from Tanzania have indicated much higher levels of asymptomatic gonorrhoea in males than previously recorded (about 85%).[19]

Symptomatic uncomplicated infections in males manifest typically a thick, yellow urethral discharge. In females vaginal discharge or dysuria are the major symptoms. Accompanying symptoms include a variable degree of meatal itching, burning, dysuria, frequency and oedema. Infections of the pharynx and rectum (mostly asymptomatic) can result from orogenital and genitoanal sexual contact in males, but in females the rectum is easily infected by contamination from an infected vaginal discharge. Gonococcal infection may present as vulvovaginitis in children infected by sexual abuse or by infected fomites.

Complications in men
In males, spread of the infection to the epididymis, usually unilaterally, is the most common complication (20% of patients not receiving antibiotics). Acute epididymitis has initially to be distinguished from acute torsion. Because it is often difficult to establish an aetio-

logical diagnosis, sexually active males should be given treatment that is effective for gonorrhoea and chlamydia. Some cases will be due to mumps virus infection, and in older men Gram-negative bacilli from the urinary tract may be responsible.

The older literature on gonorrhoea describes a number of complications seldom encountered in industrialized countries but which may still be seen in the tropics.[20] These include abscess and fistula formation resulting from spread of infection to various glands associated with the genitourinary tract (prostate, glands of Tyson, Littré, Cowper). Ultimately these may lead to urethral stricture, a difficult complication to manage, which appears to show marked geographical variation in the tropics.[21,22]

Complications in women
In women, common local complications are infections of the paraurethral (Skene's) glands and Bartholin's glands (Figure 21.2). Much more serious complications may ensue when infection spreads into the uterus and Fallopian tubes. Abortion, delivery and insertion of intrauterine devices are risk factors for ascending infection. Unusual uterine bleeding in sexually active women should prompt consideration of a possible gonococcal endometritis.

Vaginal discharge (speculum and microscope)

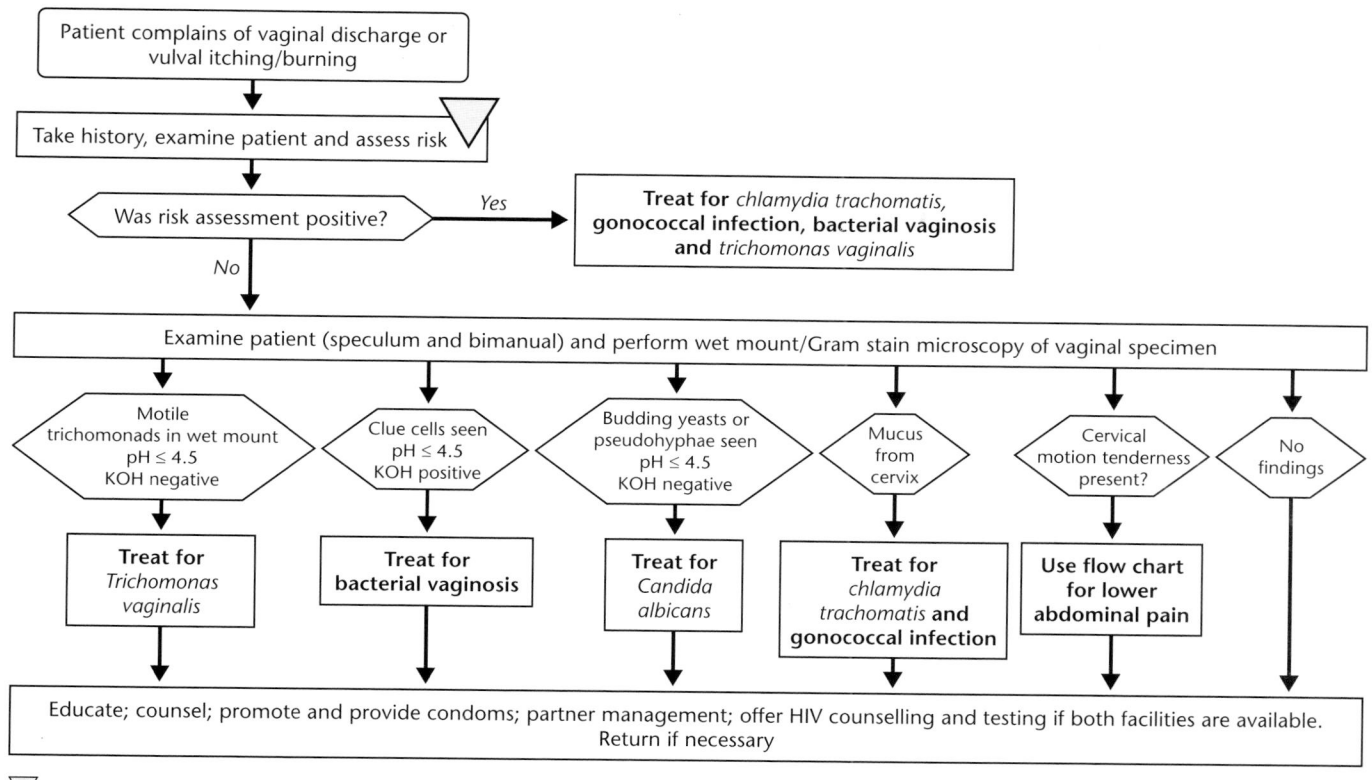

Figure 21.1: Part 8

Lower abdominal pain

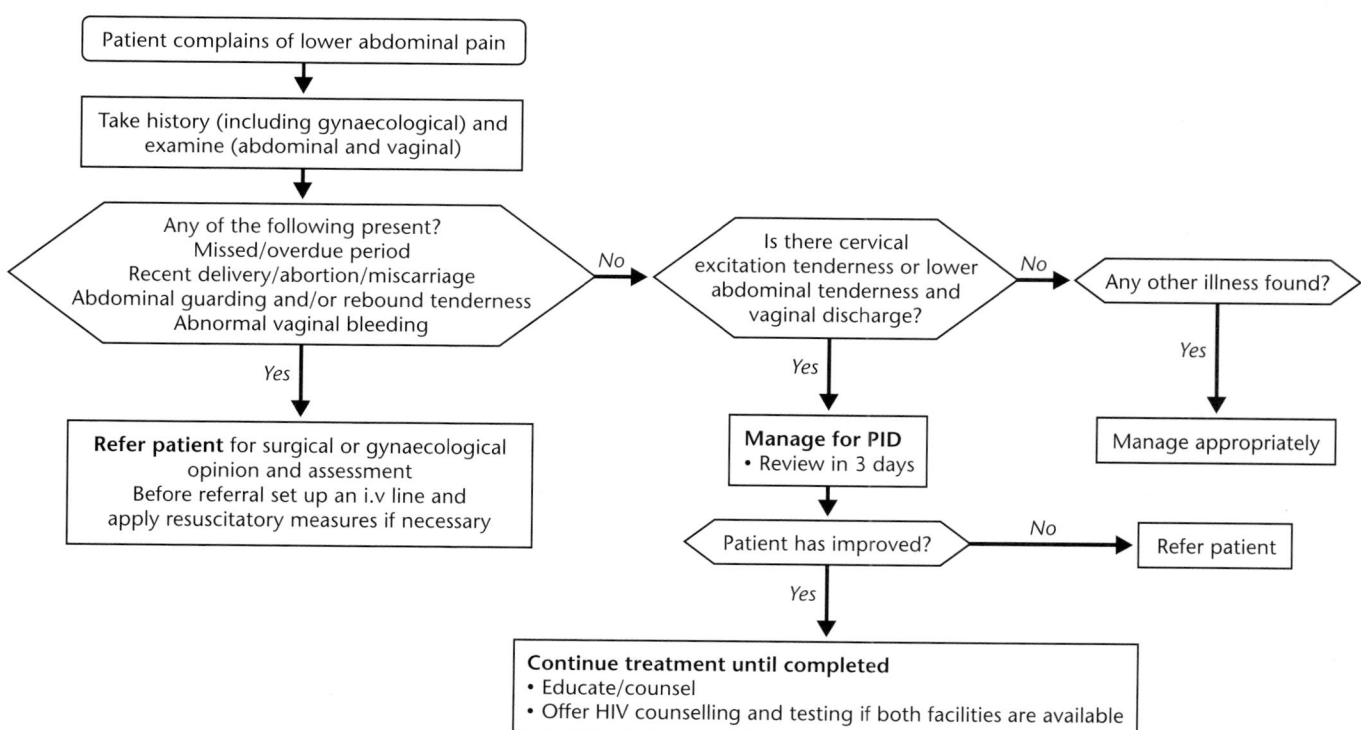

Figure 21.1: Part 9

Neonatal conjunctivitis

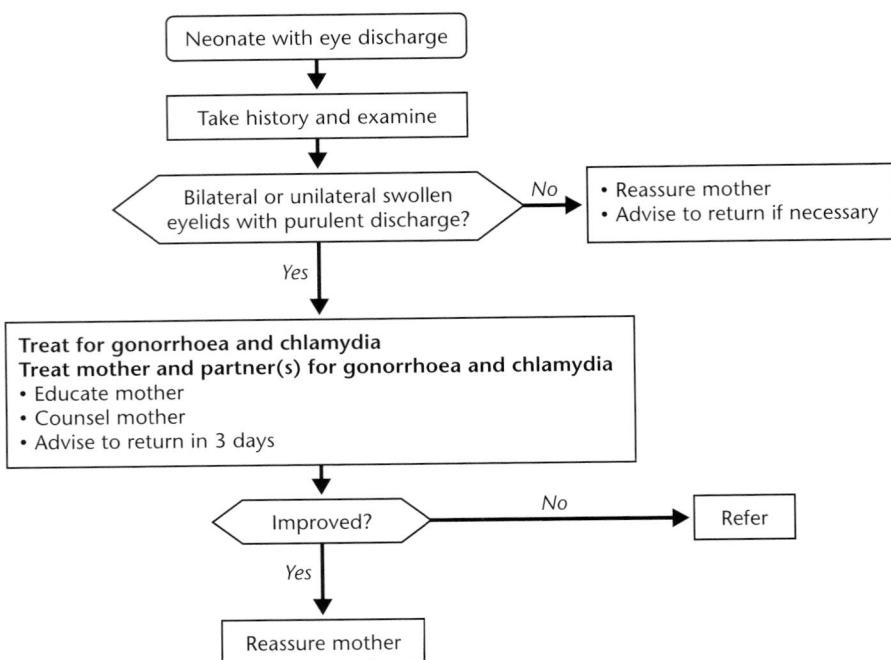

Figure 21.1: Part 10

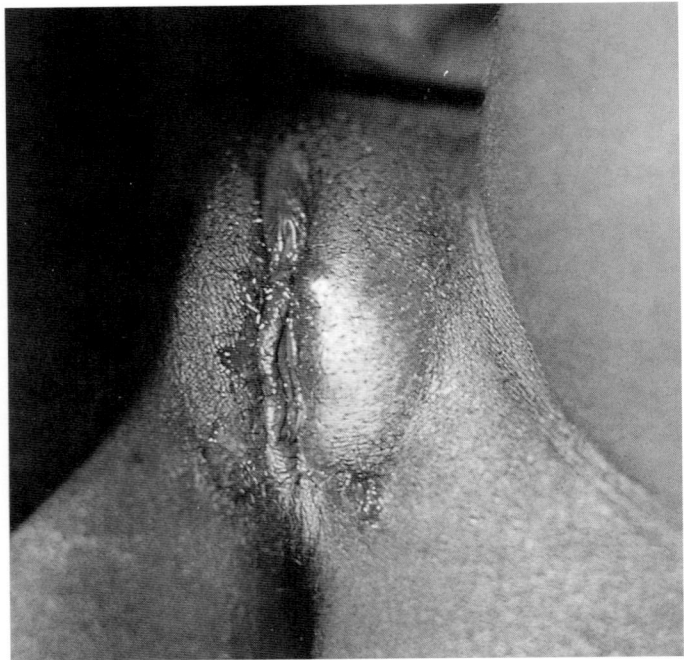

Figure 21.2: Acute bartholinitis due to gonorrhoea. (© 2001 World Health Organization.)

Further spread may lead to acute complications such as acute salpingitis and abscess formation or long-term problems of chronic PID, and increased risk of ectopic pregnancy (increased 10-fold after one episode of salpingitis). Acute salpingitis has to be differentiated clinically from ectopic pregnancy (pregnancy test, ultrasonography) and acute appendicitis (laparoscopy).

Sterility may complicate both overt and silent infection in either sex. In a study from central Africa Fallopian tube occlusion was present in 83% of infertile women.[23] Acute salpingitis has been estimated to produce sterility in 17% of patients, the risk rising with multiple episodes of infection, in older patients and with more severe inflammation. Gonorrhoea in pregnancy has been associated with low birth weight,[24] premature rupture of membranes, chorioamnionitis and postpartum upper genital tract infection.[25] There is also a higher risk of disseminated gonococcal infection.

Disseminated infection

Disseminated gonococcal infection may arise in about 2% of patients with gonorrhoea overall. The local infection from which it originates is often asymptomatic. It manifests most often as an asymmetric oligoarthritis with a predilection for knees, ankles, and large and small joints of the upper limb. Tenosynovitis occurs frequently. The skin lesions (classically the tender necrotic pustule, but many other forms also occur) often noted in white skins are rare in dark-skinned patients. Gonococcal arthritis accounts for as much as 20% of acute arthritis in young adults in the tropics.[26] It has to be differentiated from other septic arthritides, and in particular from reactive arthritis, which is also often sexually acquired. Rarer manifestations of disseminated gonococcal infection include endocarditis and meningitis. Disseminated infections can no longer be expected to respond to penicillin as in the past. Treatment effective against penicillinase-producing strains is required. Seven days therapy is recommended.

Ocular gonococcal infections

Ocular gonococcal infection in adults, which is presumed to follow autoinoculation with a contaminated finger in most cases, is a common and potentially blinding complication in developing countries.[27] It presents as an acute purulent conjunctivitis which may progress rapidly to corneal perforation in the absence of adequate systemic and topical antimicrobial treatment.

Ophthalmia neonatorum

Ophthalmia neonatorum is defined as an acute conjunctivitis occurring in the first month of life. The high prevalence of infection with *N. gonorrhoea* and *C. trachomatis* among pregnant women in many tropical countries is reflected in a correspondingly high incidence of ophthalmia neonatorum, which occurs in 30–50% of children born to infected mothers if prophylaxis is not administered.

Ophthalmia neonatorum usually presents as an acute bilateral purulent conjunctivitis (Figure 21.3). Gonococcal infections frequently present in the first week and can lead to blindness. The diagnosis can often be made by microscopy (Gram stain for gonorrhoea, Giemsa stain for chlamydial inclusions). Cultures should be made when possible. Systemic and topical treatment (Tables 21.5 and 21.6) should be administered to the neonate, and the mother and her sexual partner(s) should also be treated.

The use of ocular prophylaxis in countries where the prevalence of gonorrhoea in antenatal women exceeds 1% is highly cost-effective. A trial in Kenya showed that the instillation of 1% silver nitrate or 1% tetracycline ointment into the eyes of infants at delivery was equally effective in preventing gonococcal ophthalmia neonatorum,[28] but since it was conducted the prevalence of tetracycline-resistant strains of *N. gonorrhoea* has increased greatly in developing coutries; in some studies 90% or more of strains were found to be resistant.[29] A later trial suggested that 2.5% povidone–iodine was as effective as 1% silver nitrate in preventing chlamydial and gonococcal ophthalmia.[30]

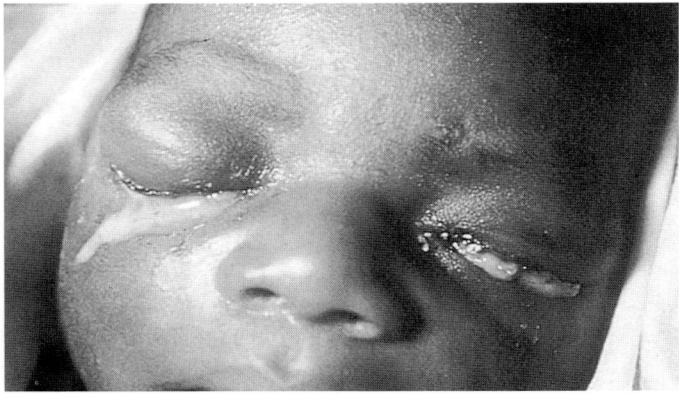

Figure 21.3: Gonococcal ophthalmia in a 7-day-old neonate. (© 2001 World Health Organization.)

Laboratory diagnosis

The definitive diagnosis of gonorrhoea rests on the isolation of *N. gonorrhoea*. In many parts of the tropics this is not feasible. The demonstration of Gram-negative diplococci in urethral smears (Figure 21.4) has a sensitivity and specificity of >95% for the diagnosis of gonorrhoea in males, but both sensitivity and specificity are considerably lower in females, where culture is the method of choice. In disseminated infection specimens from joints, blood or skin lesions give a rather poor yield and the organism may be isolated more readily from the genital tract.

When cultures are to be made, the sites for swabbing should be determined by the history and examination findings. In males it is best to obtain a urethral specimen by insertion and rotation of a swab in the urethra for 5 seconds. For women the ectocervix should be wiped clean and a swab should be inserted into the cervical os and rotated for 10 seconds. Rectal swabs are best obtained through a proctoscope. *N. gonorrhoea* is a delicate organism, highly susceptible to drying, and prompt inoculation of media and careful adherence to recommended laboratory technique is important to maximize isolation rates. Of newer reported methods for the diagnosis of gonorrhoea (e.g., antigen detection by immunofluorescence or enzyme immunassay, serology, detection of gonococcal DNA), none has so far been shown to be superior to traditional methods.[31]

Treatment (Tables 21.5 and 21.6)

Gonorrhoea is treated ideally with a single dose of supervised oral treatment. The dose administered should give a serum level of at least three times the minimum inhibitory concentration for 8 or more hours. Throughout the tropics an increasing proportion of isolates of *N. gonorrhoea* show both plasmid- and chromosomally mediated resistance to penicillin and other cheap antibiotics such as tetracycline and co-trimoxazole.[29] Penicillinase-producing *N. gonorrhoea* (PPNG) accounts for more than 50% of isolates in many tropical countries. WHO recommendations for the treatment of uncomplicated gonorrhoea are shown in Table 21.5.[17] Test of cure 3–5 days after treatment is undertaken where resources permit.

Treatment of contacts should extend to all individuals exposed within 2 weeks of the onset of symptoms in the index case and within 4 weeks of diagnosis of asymptomatic infected individuals. The issue of whether to give blind treatment for chlamydial infection to all patients with gonorrhoea is controversial but certainly worth serious consideration. This practice has been officially recommended in some developed countries.

Prevention

The major obstacle to the control of gonorrhoea is the large reservoir of asymptomatic or clinically non-specific infections in women and the difficulty of establishing the diagnosis in women. The greatly increased cost of effective treatment for PPNG is an added burden for tropical

Table 21.5 Recommended treatment for STIs.

Disease	Recommended treatment	Schedule*	Alternatives	Schedule	Notes
Gonorrhoea	Ciprofloxacin Azithromycin Ceftriaxone Cefixime Spectinomycin	1 1 1 1 1	Kanamycin Co-trimoxazole	1 1	Treatment for chlamydia is also recommended Azithromycin should be used in 2 g rather than 1 g dose to protect against the emergence of resistance
Ophthalmia neonatorum (gonococcal)	Ceftriaxone	2	Kanamycin i.m. Spectinomycin	2 2	Special precautions need to be taken to avoid nosocomial spread of the infecton
Chlamydial infection	Doxycycline Azithromycin	1 1	Amoxycillin Erythromycin Ofloxacin Tetracycline	1 1 1	
Chlamydial ophthalmia	Erythromycin syrup	–	Co-trimoxazole	2	
Early syphilis (i.e. primary, secondary or latent < 2 years duration)	Benzathine benzylpenicillin		Doxycycline[1] Procaine benzylpenicillin Tetracycline hydrochloride[1] Erythromycin[2]	3 1 1 3 3	[1]Suitable for non-pregnant penicillin-allergic individuals. [2]Efficacy questionable. Late syphilis requires longer therapy
Congenital syphilis up to age 2 years	Aqueous benzylpenicillin Procaine benzylpenicillin	– 2	Erythromycin syrup –	2 –	
Chancroid	Ciprofloxacin Erythromycin Azithromycin	2 1 2	Ceftriaxone	3	
Lymphogranuloma venereum	Doxycycline Erythromycin	2 2	Tetracycline	2	Repeated courses of antibiotics may help in difficult cases
Donovanosis	Azithromycin Doxycycline	3 4	Erythromycin Tetracycline Co-trimoxazole	4 4 3	The addition of a parenteral aminoglycoside such as gentamicin should be strongly considered for HIV-infected patients.
Trichomoniasis	Metronidazole Tinidazole	1 1	Tinidazole Metronidazole	2 3 or 4	
Bacterial vaginosis	Metronidazole	2	Metronidazole Clindamycin	1 or 4 1 or 2	Only symptomatic women require treatment
Candidiasis	Miconazole Clotrimazole Fluconazole	 1 or 2	Nystatin		Other imidazoles may be used Only topical azoles should be used to treat pregnant women
Primary genital herpes	Acyclovir Famciclovir Valaciclovir	1 or 2 1 1	–	–	There is no known cure. Topical therapy with acyclovir produces only minimal shortening of the duration of symptomatic episodes and is not recommended

Table 21.5 (Cont'd)

Disease	Recommended treatment	Schedule*	Alternatives	Schedule	Notes
Complicated herpes	Acyclovir	3	–	–	–
Recurrent herpes	Acyclovir Famciclovir Valaciclovir	4, 5 or 6 2 2	–	–	
Pelvic inflammatory disease	1. Treatment for gonorrhoea + 2. tetracycline or Doxycycline + 3. Metronidazole	2 2 2	1. Treatment for gonorrhoea + 2. Erythromycin + 3. Metronidazole	2 3	
Epididymitis	1. Treatment for gonorrhoea + 2. Treatment for chlamydia				

Details of dosage schedules are given in Table 21.6
Source: World Health Organization[17]

countries. Given these constraints it is more appropriate to direct resources to condom promotion and other safe sex messages rather than costly strategies to increase case-finding and treatment. The development of vaccines for gonorrhoea has been hindered by the antigenic variation manifest by the organism.

Chlamydial infections

The demonstration in 1909 of chlamydial inclusions in cervical scrapings from the mother of an infant with inclusion conjunctivitis and in urethral scrapings from her male partner laid the basis for our understanding of genital chlamydial infections, but it was not until it became possible to isolate *C. trachomatis* in tissue culture in 1965 that the extent of the morbidity due to this organism became clear.

Epidemiology

C. trachomatis is the most prevalent sexually transmitted bacterial pathogen in industrialized countries,[32] and appears to be at least equally prevalent in developing countries (see Table 21.1). Studies in industrialized countries have shown that genital chlamydial infection is more prevalent in younger age groups, even after taking account of differences in sexual activity, implying that some degree of protective immunity may develop after natural infection.

Aetiology

C. trachomatis is a Gram-negative bacterium which is an obligate parasite of eukaryotic cells. The genus *Chlamydia* has a unique life cycle. The metabolically inert infectious elementary body has a rigid cell wall and is adapted for extracellular survival. It appears to infect preferentially columnar epithelial cells, by which it is actively taken up.

After entering the host cell it differentiates over a number of hours to the metabolically active reticulate body, which divides by binary fission until an intracellular inclusion is formed, which may contain several thousand organisms. The life cycle is completed when reticulate bodies condense to form elementary bodies, which are released from the inclusion after lysis of the host cell.

A number of serotypes of *C. trachomatis* have been identified by the microimmunofluorescence test of Wang and Grayston. Serotypes A–C cause ocular infection in trachoma endemic areas, whereas serotypes D–K cause genital tract infections worldwide. Serotypes L1, L2 and L3 are more invasive both in vitro and in vivo, and cause lymphogranuloma venereum (LGV).

Pathology

The pathological hallmarks of infection with *C. trachomatis* are: (1) the subepithelial lymphoid follicle; and (2) fibrosis and scarring. The latter may progress for months and years even in the absence of chlamydial organisms demonstrable by conventional means. The host immune system is believed to play an important part in the pathogenesis of chlamydial infections, and a chlamydial heat shock protein of 57 kDa which has been shown to elicit a delayed hypersensitivity reaction in previously infected animals may also be a determinant of immuno-pathology in humans.[33]

Clinical features

The clinical spectrum of disease due to chlamydial infection is similar to that seen in gonococcal infection. Although in general chlamydial infections are less likely than gonococcal to cause severe symptoms, they are more likely to cause serious sequelae, particularly in women.[34]

In males, chlamydial infection causes urethritis and, in a proportion of cases, epididymo-orchitis. It is possible

Table 21.6 Dosage schedules for drug treatment of STIs.

Drug	Route	Schedule	Dose	Duration	Notes
Aciclovir	Oral	1	200 mg 5 times daily	7 days	
	Oral	2	400 mg 3 times daily	7 days	
	i.v.	3	5–10 mg/kg 8-hourly	5–7 days	
	Oral	4	200 mg 5 times daily	5 days	
	Oral	5	800 mg twice daily	5 days	
	Oral	6	400 mg 3 times daily	5 days	
Amoxycillin	Oral	1	500 mg 3 times daily	7 days	
Aqueous benzylpenicillin	i.m.		50 000 iu/kg in 2 divided doses	10 days	Infants with CSF abnormalities should receive 50 000 iu/kg i.v for 7 days then 8 hourly for a further 3 days
Azithromycin	Oral	1	2 grams in a single dose		
	Oral	2	1 gram in a single dose		
	Oral	3	1 gram on the first day, then 500 mg once a day	Till cured	
Benzathine penicillin	i.m.		2.4 million iu, split between two injection sites	1 dose	HIV +ve patients may require ↑ doses
Cefixime	Oral	1	400 mg as a single dose		
Ceftriaxone	i.m.	1	125 mg	1 dose	
		2	50 mg/kg	1 dose	
		3	(max. 125 mg) 250 mg	1 dose	
Ciprofloxacin	Oral	1	500 mg	1 dose	Contraindicated in pregnancy Ciprofloxacin is superior to other quinolones for gonorrhoea
		2	500 mg twice daily	3 days	
Clindamycin	Oral	1	300 mg twice daily	7 days	
	Intra-vaginal	2	5 g of 2% cream at night	7 days	
Clotrimazole	Intra-vaginal	1	200 mg once daily	3 days	
		2	500 mg	1 dose	
Co-trimoxazole (tablets of trimethoprim 80 mg, sulphamethoxazole 400 mg) or syrup	Oral	1	10 tablets daily	3 days	
		2	240 mg twice daily	7 days	
		3	2 tablets twice daily	till healed	
Doxycycline	Oral	1	100 mg twice daily	7 days	Contraindicated in pregnancy and lactation.
		2		14 days	
		3		15 days	
		4		Till cured	
Erythromycin	Oral	1	500 mg 4 times daily	7 days	Use only erythromycin or ethylsuccinate in pregnancy Should not be taken on empty stomach
		2	500 mg 4 times daily	14 days	
		3	500 mg 4 times daily	15 days	
		4	500 mg 4 times daily	till healed	
Erythromycin syrup	Oral	1	500 mg/kg per day in 4 divided doses	2 weeks	
		2	7.5–12 mg/kg 4 times daily	30 days	
Famciclovir	Oral	1	250 mg 3 times daily	7 days	
		2	125 mg twice daily	5 days	
Fluconazole	Oral		150 mg as a single dose		

Table 21.6 (*Cont'd*)

Drug	Route	Schedule	Dose	Duration	Notes
Kanamycin	i.m.	1	2 g	1 dose	
		2	25 mg/kg (max. 75 g)	1 dose	
Metronidazole	Oral	1	2 g	1 dose	Avoid alcohol while taking the drug and for 24 hours after the last dose
		2	400–500 mg twice daily	7 days	
		3	400–500 mg twice daily	14 days	Not recommended in the first trimester.
	Intra-vaginal	4	5 g of 0.75% gel twice daily	5 days	Use minimum effective dose in second and third trimesters.
Miconazole	Intra-vaginal	1	200 mg daily	3 days	
Nystatin	Intra-vaginal		100 000 iu daily	14 days	
Ofloxacin	Oral		300 mg twice daily	7 days	Contraindicated in pregnancy
Procaine penicillin	i.m.	1	1.2 million iu daily	10 days	
		2	50 000 iu/kg daily	10 days	
Spectinomycin	i.m.	1	2 g	1 dose	
		2	25 mg/kg (max. 75 mg)	1 dose	
Tetracycline hydrochloride	Oral	1	500 mg 4 times daily	7 days	Contraindicated in pregnancy and lactation
		2		14 days	
		3		15 days	
		4		till healed	
Tinidazole	Oral	1	2 g	1 dose	See metronidazole
		2	500 mg twice daily	5 days	
Valaciclovir	Oral	1	1 g twice daily	7 days	
		2	500 mg twice daily	5 days	
		3	1000 mg once daily	5 days	

Source: World Health Organization.[17]

that urethral stricture is a late sequela of chlamydial urethritis.

In females, chlamydial cervicitis is often asymptomatic. Sometimes patients will complain of vaginal discharge, and the finding of a mucopurulent discharge at the cervical os is suggestive of chlamydial or gonococcal cervicitis. Ascending infection of the female genital tract may lead to endometritis, salpingitis or PID and this is facilitated by trauma to the cervix, for example during childbirth, insertion of an intrauterine device or termination of pregnancy. Because the symptoms of chlamydial PID are often mild, patients may present only when the sequelae of irreversible damage to the Fallopian tubes (infertility, ectopic pregnancy) become apparent. Infection may track to the right upper quadrant, giving rise to a peri-hepatitis with characteristic adhesions between the liver capsule and peritoneum (Curtis–FitzHugh syndrome).

Some 30% of infants born to infected mothers become infected. In the majority of cases the only consequence of this is a self-limiting conjunctivitis presenting within the first 2 weeks of life, but occasionally chlamydial ophthalmia is more severe and if it persists it may give rise to conjunctival scarring. A small proportion of infected infants develop chlamydial pneumonitis, presenting usually between the ages of 6 weeks and 3 months with a paroxysmal cough and tachypnoea in the absence of fever. Rales may be heard on clinical examination, and a chest radiograph often reveals extensive bilateral pulmonary infiltrates with hyperinflation. There is characteristically a raised serum total IgG and IgM, and a mild eosinophilia.[35]

Diagnosis

DNA amplification tests (e.g., polymerase chain reaction (PCR) or ligase chain reaction (LCR)) are now the gold standard for the diagnosis of genital chlamydial infection. Several are on the market, but they are expensive, and require expensive equipment as well as careful laboratory practice. DNA amplification techniques are more sensitive than antigen detection test or isolation, the sensitivity of which is only approximately 70%.[36] This means that the type of specimen taken is less critical. Whereas for culture and antigen detection it was essential to collect intra-urethral or endocervical samples, PCR and LCR give good results in first-catch urine samples or self-administered vaginal swabs.

Serology has no place in the diagnosis of uncomplicated chlamydial infections with the exception of the more

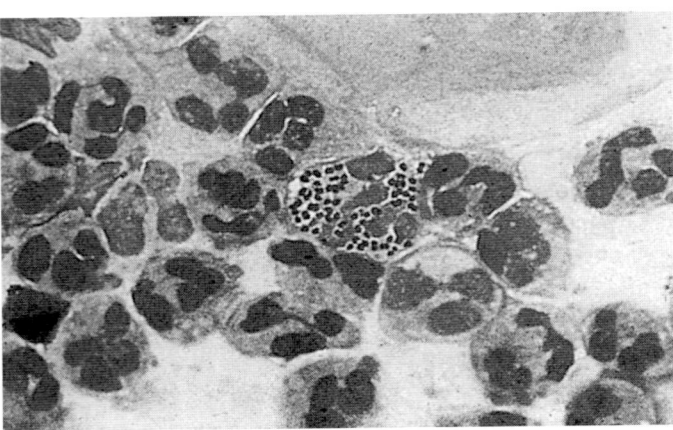

Figure 21.4: Appearance of *Neisseria gonorrhoeae* in a Gram-stained smear of urethral discharge. (© 2001 World Health Organization.)

invasive LGV, but may be helpful in the diagnosis of suspected PID and is the method of choice for the diagnosis of neonatal chlamydial pneumonia. It is only possible to distinguish between antibodies to the various species of *Chlamydia* by the micro-immunofluorescence test, which is subjective and labour intensive. Other serological tests may give positive results due to infection with the highly prevalent respiratory tract pathogen, *Chlamydia pneumoniae*.

Management

C. trachomatis remains sensitive to tetracyclines and erythromycin, and single-dose treatment with azithromycin is effective in uncomplicated chlamydial infection (see Tables 21.5 and 21.6).[37]

Vaginal discharge in women

The three most prevalent causes of vaginal discharge are *Candida albicans*, *Trichomonas vaginalis* and bacterial vaginosis. *Neisseria gonorrhoea* and *Chlamydia trachomatis*, which infect the endocervix rather than the vagina, are less commonly associated with symptomatic discharge. Unfortunately it is not possible to distinguish reliably between these infections on clinical grounds, although the presence of mucopurulent discharge at the cervical os has been proposed as a marker of gonococcal or chlamydial infection. A wet preparation made from a swab collected from the posterior fornix, examined with a phase-contrast microscope, can usually distinguish between candidiasis, trichomoniasis and bacterial vaginosis. Sexual transmission is not considered important in vulvovaginal candidiasis and bacterial vaginosis, and treatment of sexual partners of affected women has not been shown help women who develop repeated episodes of these infections.

Vulvovaginal candidiasis

Candida albicans can be isolated from the vagina of up to 50% of sexually active women, the majority of whom are asymptomatic. Although sexual transmission may occur, the gastrointestinal tract has also been implicated as a source of infection. Symptomatic disease is associated with an increase in the number of yeasts present in the vagina; factors which predispose to this are pregnancy, antimicrobial therapy, oral contraceptive use, immunosuppression (e.g., HIV related) and glycosuria. It has also been suggested that tight, poorly ventilated nylon underclothing, by increasing perineal moisture, may predispose to symptomatic disease in warm climates.

The cardinal clinical features of vulvovaginal candidiasis are pruritus vulvae and vaginal discharge. The discharge is typically whitish, with curd-like plaques adhering to the vaginal wall, and does not smell. There may be erythema and/or oedema of the vulva and vaginal walls.

The diagnosis can be made on a wet preparation made from the vaginal discharge, the sensitivity of which can be increased by adding 10% potassium hydroxide. Typical mycelia and yeast cells are seen. For the treatment of vulvovaginal candidiasis, see Table 21.5.

Trichomoniasis (Chapter 79)

Trichomonas vaginalis has been found in the vagina of up to 30% of antenatal clinic attenders in certain African centres (see Table 21.1). Studies in the USA have shown that its prevalence is higher among women with many partners, and that it can be isolated from a high proportion of male contacts of infected women, suggesting that transmission is primarily through sexual contact. In males most infections are believed to be asymptomatic and self-limiting, although occasionally it may give rise to urethritis. Recent studies using more sensitive diagnostic techniques have shown substantially higher rates of infection in males in developing countries.[38]

Up to 75% of women attending STI clinics with *T. vaginalis* infection complain of vaginal discharge. Pruritus vulvae, dyspareunia and dysuria are also common symptoms. On examination a profuse yellow-green frothy discharge, which is not malodorous, is typically noted. The vulva and vaginal walls may be excoriated and erythematous in severe cases, and punctate haemorrhages may be seen on the cervix.[39]

The diagnosis can be made on a wet preparation collected from the posterior fornix. Under phase contrast, increased numbers of polymorphonuclear leucocytes are usually seen, and motile flagellated parasites, slightly larger than polymorphonuclear leucocytes, are present. Compared with culture, direct microscopy is less than 80% sensitive, so that culture should also be performed when available. Culture using the In-pouch kit and diagnosis by PCR show considerably higher sensitivity than older methods. For the treatment of trichomoniasis, see Table 21.5.

Bacterial vaginosis

Bacterial vaginosis is a syndrome in which a malodorous vaginal discharge is associated with characteristic changes in the vaginal bacterial flora. There is an increase in numbers of anaerobes, *Gardnerella vaginalis* and *Mycoplasma hominis*, such that lactobacilli are no longer predominant. Bacterial vaginosis appears to be more prevalent among women with many sexual partners, but since it has been found in sexually inexperienced women it is not clear that it is a sexually transmitted condition.

The discharge of bacterial vaginosis is typically homogeneous and white, and associated with increased vaginal pH (> 4.5). The characteristic fishy smell is more easily detectable after the addition of a drop of 10% potassium hydroxide to a drop of discharge on a slide. Bacterial vaginosis has been shown to be associated with adverse pregnancy outcome (premature labour, chorioamnionitis, postpartum endometritis).[40]

The diagnosis of bacterial vaginosis can be made on Gram stain of a vaginal swab, according to Nugent's criteria, in which a score is given depending on the relative proportion of lactobacilli and Gram-negaitve rods and coccobacilli,[41] or on a combination of clinical signs and microscopy (Amsel's criteria).[42] To diagnose bacterial vaginosis according to Amsel's criteria, three of the following four signs must be present: increased homogeneous vaginal discharge; amine odour on adding a drop of 10% KOH to a drop of the discharge; vaginal pH > 4.5; and the presence of 'clue cells' (epithelial cells to which many bacteria are attached) in a wet preparation. For the treatment of bacterial vaginosis, see Table 21.5.

Diseases causing genital ulceration

Chancroid

Chancroid, or soft sore, was first distinguished from the hard chancre of syphilis by Ricord in 1838. In 1889 Ducrey, in Naples, showed that the inoculation of material from chancroidal ulcers into the skin of the forearm caused ulceration which could be serially passaged, and identified the causative organism which now bears his name. The development of defined solid media for the isolation of *Haemophilus ducreyi* in the 1970s enabled detailed epidemiological studies of chancroid to be carried out for the first time.[43,44]

Epidemiology

Chancroid is an important cause of genital ulceration in Africa. Before the HIV epidemic it accounted for more than 60% of genital ulcers seen in hospital, but in the 1990s hospital-based studies in several countries found that the proportion of ulcers due to *Herpes simplex* had increased, and that the proportion due to chancroid had decreased correspondingly.[45] Although generally rare in industrialized countries, there have been several well-documented outbreaks in North America since the 1970s. Characteristic features of these outbreaks have been a high male-to-female case ratio, the involvement of

prostitutes and the low socio-economic status of the populations affected. A study in Nairobi investigated the role of asymptomatic females in the transmission of the disease and concluded that they were of little importance.[46] Studies among Australian solders during the Vietnam war suggest that chancroid is more common among uncircumcised than circumcised males.[47]

The prevalence of chancroid is high among commercial sex workers in the cities of Africa (Figure 21.5), as is the prevalence of HIV infection. Prospective studies among both males and females at high risk of HIV infection in Nairobi have suggested that chancroid significantly increases the risk of transmission of HIV via heterosexual contact, either by increasing infectivity, susceptibility or both.[48,49]

Aetiology

Chancroid is caused by *Haemophilus ducreyi*, a small facultatively anaerobic Gram-negative bacillus which requires haemin (X factor), reduces nitrate to nitrite and forms typical streptobacillary chains on Gram stain. It is a fastidious organism which will only grow on enriched media and grows best at 30–33°C in an atmosphere of 5% carbon dioxide.

Pathogenesis

Histopathologically, chancroidal ulcers contain three distinct zones: a superficial zone consisting of necrotic tissue, fibrin and numerous bacteria; an intermediate zone showing oedema and new vessel formation; and a deep zone containing a dense infiltrate of neutrophils and plasma cells with fibroblastic proliferation.

Studies involving the inoculation of human volunteers have improved our understanding of the pathogenesis of

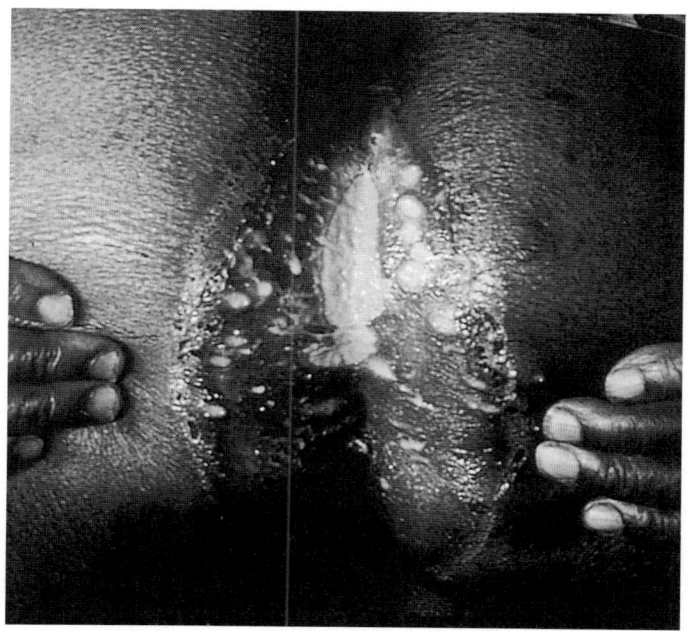

Figure 21.5: Extensive perianal ulceration resulting from an *Haemophilus ducreyi* infection in a sex worker. (© 2001 World Health Organization.)

chancroid.[50] The application of *H. ducreyi* to the human forearm does not produce a lesion unless the skin is traumatized. There is some evidence that virulent strains are relatively resistant to phagocytosis by human polymorphonuclear leucocytes and to complement-mediated killing by normal human and rabbit serum. An isogenic mutant lacking a receptor for haemoglobin showed reduced virulence in humans.[51] Two toxins have been characterized: one is a cell-associated haemolysin, similar to those produced by *Proteus mirabilis*, toxic to human foreskin fibroblasts but not to HeLa cells in tissue culture. The other is a soluble toxin, homologous to the cytolethal distending toxin produced by a number of enteric organisms, which is toxic to a variety of cell lines.[52] The suppurating lymphadenopathy of chancroid is notable for the large number of neutrophils and small number of bacilli present.

Clinical features

After an incubation period of 3–7 days, a papule appears at the site of inoculation which soon ulcerates. The typical ulcer of chancroid (Figure 21.6) is painful and soft, has a purulent base with an undermined edge, and bleeds on contact. Multiple ulcers are commonly present, and there is painful inguinal lymphadenopathy (Figure 21.7) in some 50% of cases, often unilateral. Atypical presentations are, however, common, and even in experienced hands chancroid cannot reliably be distinguished from primary syphilis on clinical grounds.[53] *Herpes simplex*, LGV and donovanosis must also be considered in the differential diagnosis of chancroid.

Chancroid may cause extensive local destruction (Figure 21.8), particularly in HIV-infected individuals who may fail to respond to antimicrobial treatment, but the infection does not disseminate.

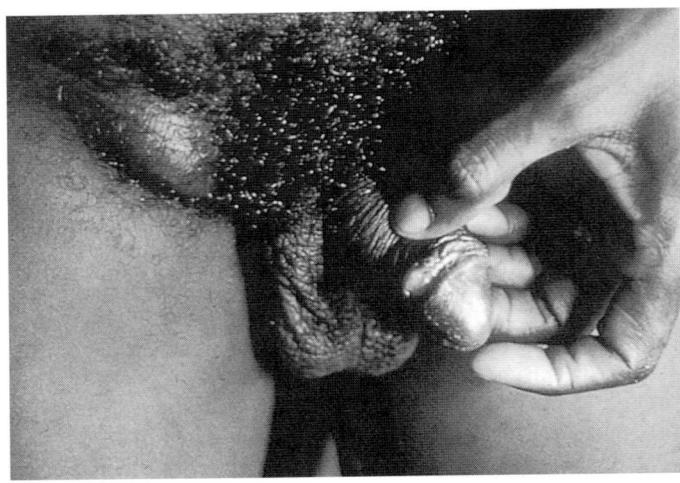

Figure 21.7: Chancroid: ulcer of corona accompanied by a painful bubo. (© 2001 World Health Organization.)

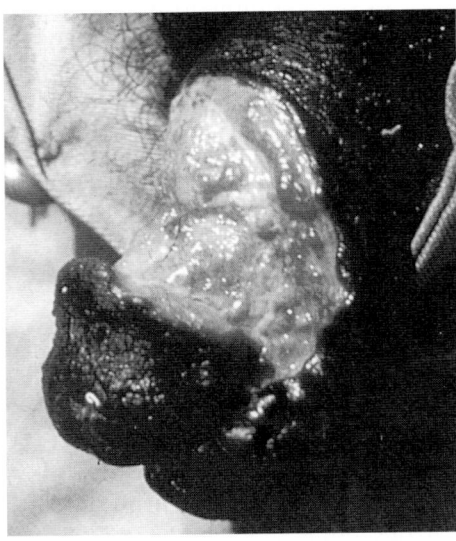

Figure 21.8: Phagaedenic chancroid: destructive ulcer of penile shaft. (© 2001 World Health Organization.)

Diagnosis

Gram stain of smears obtained from ulcers has been advocated in the past for the diagnosis of chancroid, but this lacks both sensitivity and specificity. The laboratory diagnosis of chancroid depends on the isolation of *Haemophilus ducreyi* from the ulcer. Swabs should be taken from the ulcer base or its undermined edge and plated directly on appropriate blood-containing media enriched with fetal calf serum and Vitox and made selective with vancomycin. For optimal rates of isolation media made up from both GC agar and Mueller–Hinton agar base should be inoculated. Plates should be incubated for at least 72 hours in an atmosphere of 5% carbon dioxide at 33°C. *H. ducreyi* is identified by its typical colonial morphology (colonies are difficult to break up and can be moved intact across the surface of the agar), Gram stain and inability to ferment sugars.

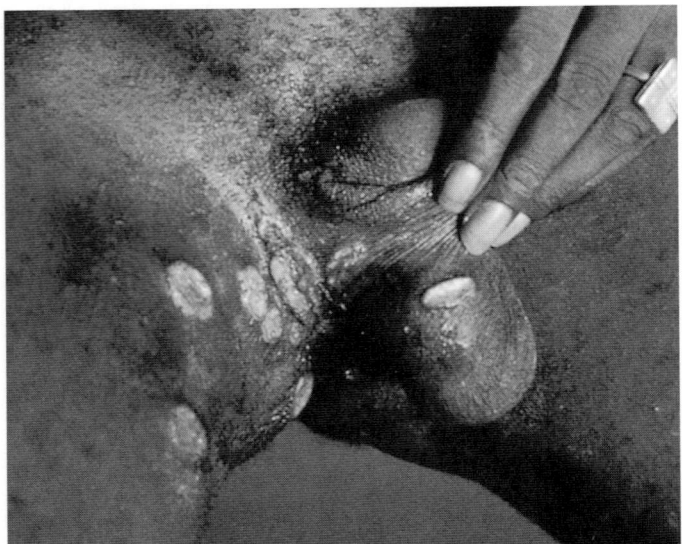

Figure 21.6: Chancroid: multiple soft painful ulcers. (© 2001 World Health Organization.)

Management (Tables 21.5 and 21.6)

Chancroidal ulcers should be kept clean and dry, with regular washing in soapy water. The mainstay of anti-microbial treatment has for a number of years been co-trimoxazole or erythromycin in standard dosage given by mouth for 7 days. However, an increasing proportion of strains worldwide are now resistant to sulfonamides, and many trimethoprim-resistant strains have been isolated in Thailand and Kenya. Ciprofloxacin 500 mg daily for 3 days by mouth and ceftriaxone 500 mg as a single intramuscular dose and azithromycin as a single 1 g oral dose appear to be effective alternatives, although in HIV-infected patients longer courses of treatment may be required.

Syphilis

History

Syphilis, a young shepherd boy, was the eponymous hero of a Latin poem written in 1530 by the Italian G. Fracastorio. He succumbed to an apparently new disease which had swept across Europe a few years earlier in the wake of the French army's retreat from Naples. The timing of this epidemic led to the suggestion that syphilis had been brought back from the New World by Columbus and his men in 1493. An alternative hypothesis put forward by E. H. Hudson, a physician working in the 1930s in Mesopotamia (now Iraq), was that syphilis originated as an endemic infection of childhood (yaws) in the hot humid tropics, and that venereal transmission only became important when living standards improved sufficiently to prevent transmission in childhood giving rise to long-lasting immunity. This so-called unitarian hypothesis is supported by recent evidence of very close DNA homology between *Treponema pallidum* and *T. pertenue* (recently reclassified as *T. pallidum* subsp. *pertenue*).[54]

Although syphilis in all its clinical aspects had been described in detail by nineteenth-century physicians, notably Hutchinson in Britain and Fournier in France, it was not until 1905 that the causative organism, *T. pallidum*, was first identified by Schaudin and Hoffman; in 1906 Wasserman described the first serological test for the diagnosis of syphilis. Complete sequencing of the *T. pallidum* genome was completed recently.

Epidemiology

The incidence of syphilis has declined steadily for most of the twentieth century in Western Europe and North America, with the exception of a brief rise during and immediately after each world war.

There are no reliable incidence figures for developing countries. Seroprevalence surveys have shown high rates of positivity among antenatal clinic attenders and in the general population in many African countries (see Table 21.1).[2,54–56] The relative rarity of late syphilis in parts of Africa where early syphilis is common has led to speculation that the disease has become more common in recent years, perhaps reflecting loss of herd immunity following the mass treatment campaigns against endemic treponemal disease in the 1950s and 1960s.

Transmission by sexual contact requires exposure to moist mucosal or cutaneous lesions; experiments in the rabbit suggest that an inoculum of some 50 organisms is sufficient to initiate infection. The rate of transmission from an infected partner is approximately 30%.

Aetiology

Syphilis is caused by *T. pallidum*, one of a small group of treponemas (of the order Spirochaetales) pathogenic to man. It cannot be distinguished in the laboratory from the agents responsible for yaws and pinta (*T. pallidum* subsp. *pertenue* and *T. carateum* respectively). It is a spiral organism 6–15 µm in length and 0.15 µm in width, visible by light microscopy only under conditions of dark-field illumination, and cannot be grown on artificial media. In tissue culture and in animal models it divides slowly, with a replication time of approximately 30 hours. The cell wall of *T. pallidum* is remarkable for a very low density of outer membrane proteins, which probably contributes to the organism's ability to persist in its host for lengthy periods. It is highly susceptible to drying.

Pathogenesis

T. pallidum has not been shown to produce either exotoxins or endotoxins. Following experimental infection in the rabbit, *T. pallidum* begins to replicate once it has passed through the epithelium. An initial polymorphonuclear leucocyte response at the lesion is soon replaced by an infiltrate of T and B lymphocytes. The primary chancre also contains mucoid material, mainly hyaluronic acid and chondroitin sulfate, which may modulate the host immune response. Both circulating *T. pallidum* specific T cells and specific antibody can be found in the majority of cases of primary syphilis. At the same time as these are first noted, the number of organisms in the lesion decreases and the ulcer begins to heal, suggesting that the immune system is controlling the infection.

The appearance of secondary lesions some weeks later, due to the dissemination of organisms and circulating immune complexes, indicates that this is not the case, although the mechanism by which such a slow-growing organism evades the host immune response is not clear. Much of the pathology of secondary syphilis may be immune complex mediated. High levels of antitreponemal antibody are present in the circulation, but cell-mediated immune responses are depressed.

Eventually cell-mediated immune responses to *T. pallidum* are restored as the lesions are brought under control, leading to the latent stage. Follow-up studies in the pre-penicillin era showed that relapse of infectious secondary lesions occurred in up to 25% of cases. The organism can survive in the body for many years thereafter, causing tertiary lesions characterized by the presence of a small number of organisms and a lymphocytic host response giving rise to an endarteritis.

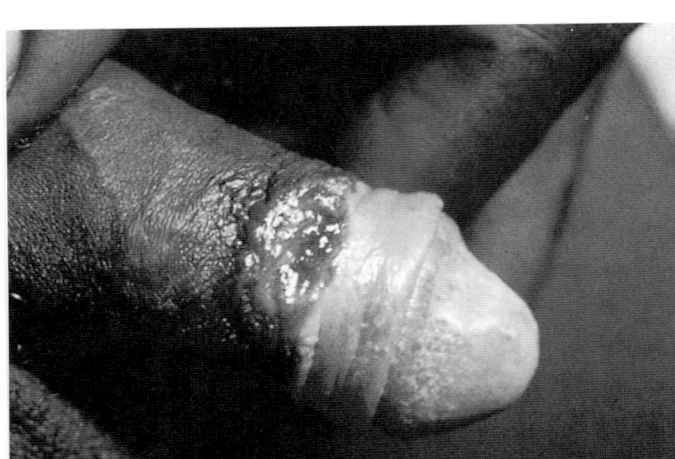

Figure 21.9: Syphilis: primary chancre. (© 2001 World Health Organization.)

Clinical features

After an incubation period of 10–70 days (median 21 days), a *primary chancre* (Figure 21.9) develops at the site of inoculation. The chancre is typically painless, indurated, with a clean base and a raised edge, and does not bleed on contact. There is usually only a single lesion; in the male it is most commonly on the glans, the foreskin, the coronal sulcus or the shaft of the penis, and in the female on the cervix or vulva. The primary chancre is often accompanied by inguinal lymphadenopathy; the glands are characteristically hard (the 'bullet bubo' of Hutchinson) and painless.

The primary chancre generally resolves spontaneously over several weeks. Between 3 and 6 weeks after its first appearance the features of *secondary syphilis* appear. The rash of secondary syphilis may take many forms: papular, macular or pustular; annular lesions are not uncommon. It often desquamates, but in moist areas of the body (e.g., perineum, axilla) soft raised condylomata lata may be seen (Figures 21.10 and 21.11). It generally affects the palms (Figure 21.12) and soles, and does not itch. The mucous membranes may be involved, with mucous patches or oral ulceration sometimes in the form of the characteristic 'snail track' ulcer. In addition to its cutaneous manifestations secondary syphilis may cause systemic illness (fever, malaise), generalized lymphadenopathy, nephritis, hepatitis, meningitis or uveitis.

The lesions of secondary syphilis generally resolve after several weeks, although relapses commonly occurred in the pre-antibiotic era. In the absence of adequate treatment the patient then enters the latent stage of the disease, and is liable to develop *tertiary syphilis* at some time in the future.

The lesions of tertiary syphilis fall into three categories: the gumma, cardiovascular disease and central nervous system disease. The classic Oslo study of untreated syphilis,

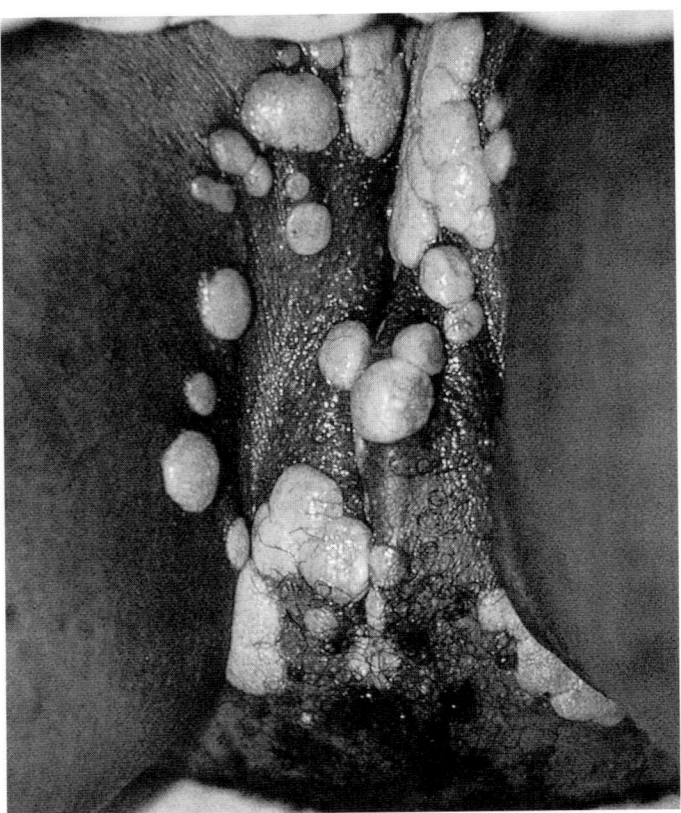

Figure 21.10: Secondary syphilis: condylomata lata.

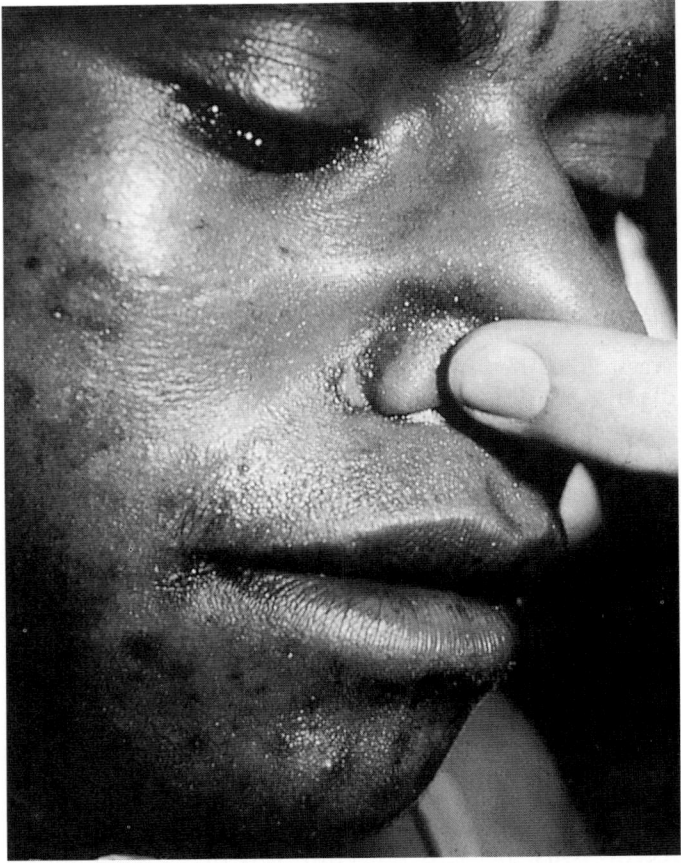

Figure 21.11: Secondary syphilis: condyloma abutting on ala nasi.

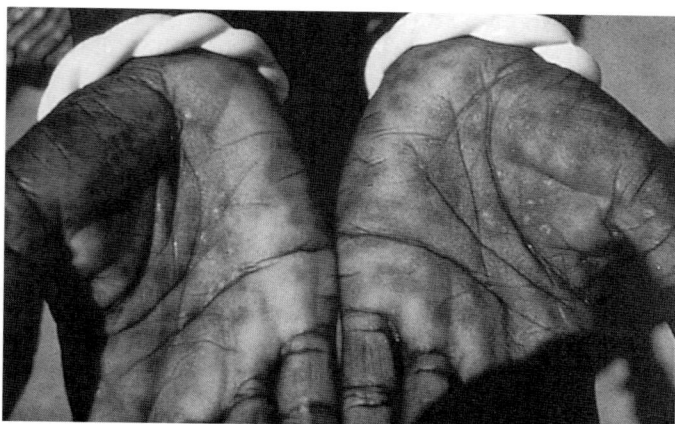

Figure 21.12: Secondary syphilis: typical palmar rash.

in which some 1400 patients were followed for up to 50 years, found that the most common manifestation was the gumma, a painless 'punched out' ulcer with little or no inflammatory reaction, which developed in 15%: 70% were cutaneous, 10% involved bone and rarely the viscera were involved. Most cases occurred in the first 15 years following infection. Cardiovascular lesions (aortitis, aortic valve disease or coronary ostial occlusion) were seen in 15% of males and 8% of females, with onset typically 30–40 years after infection. Neurological manifestations were seen in 9% of males and 5% of females, with meningovascular disease typically occurring after 15–20 years and tabes dorsalis or general paresis after 20–30 years.[57] The Tuskegee study of untreated black Americans showed similar results. It is therefore surprising that tertiary syphilis, and in particular neurosyphilis, appears rather uncommon in Africa in spite of the high incidence of early syphilis.

Congenital syphilis

Early congenital syphilis
Pregnant women with untreated early or latent syphilis are liable to give birth to congenitally infected infants. The risk is highest among those with primary or secondary syphilis during pregnancy, and diminishes as the duration of latent syphilis increases. Studies conducted in the pre-antibiotic era found that untreated early syphilis in the mother led to stillbirth in 25% of cases, neonatal death in some 15% of cases and a syphilitic infant in about 40% of cases. Corresponding figures for untreated late syphilis were 12%, 9% and 2%.[58]

Signs of congenital syphilis in the neonate include a bullous rash (Figure 21.13), anaemia, jaundice and hepatosplenomegaly. The infant is often small for dates and may have feeding difficulties. The prognosis is poor in infants with signs of congenital syphilis at birth. More commonly, the syphilitic infant appears normal at birth, and presents in the first 3 months of life with: failure to thrive; a rash which resembles that of secondary syphilis, with desquamation usually involving the palms (Figure 21.14) and soles; persistent nasal discharge (sometimes blood-stained); and anaemia or hepatosplenomegaly (Figure 21.15). Periostitis of the long bones, with or without metaphyseal abnormalities, is radiologically evident in more than 90% of cases, and may present clinically as pseudoparalysis of one or more limbs. The prognosis is very much better in those presenting in the postnatal period.[59]

Late congenital syphilis
Late congenital syphilis in the child or adolescent corresponds to tertiary syphilis in the adult, although the cardiovascular system is seldom involved. Manifestations include bony and dental abnormalities (skull bossing, Hutchinson's teeth) and inflammatory lesions of the cornea (interstitial keratitis) and joints (Clutton's joints). Eighth nerve deafness is commonly seen, and symptomatic neurosyphilis may occur, corresponding to tabes dorsalis or general paresis in the adult. In view of the high incidence of early congenital syphilis in many African cities, late manifestations of the disease are surprisingly rare in Africa.

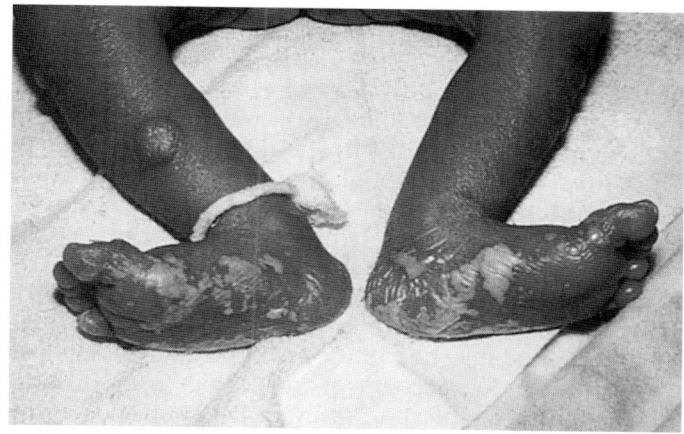

Figure 21.13: Congenital syphilis in a neonate: bullous lesions of feet.

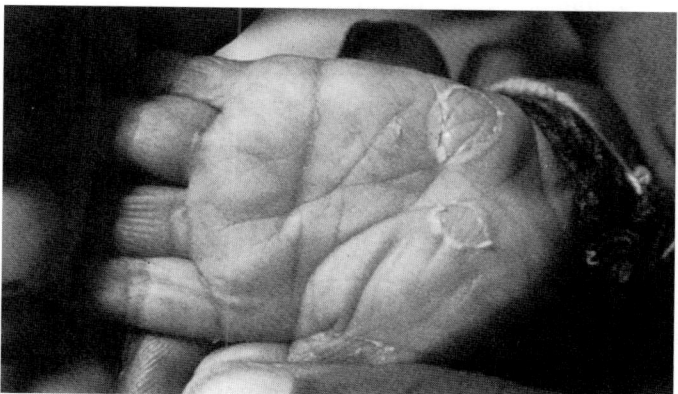

Figure 21.14: Congenital syphilis in a 3-month-old infant: desquamating lesion of palm.

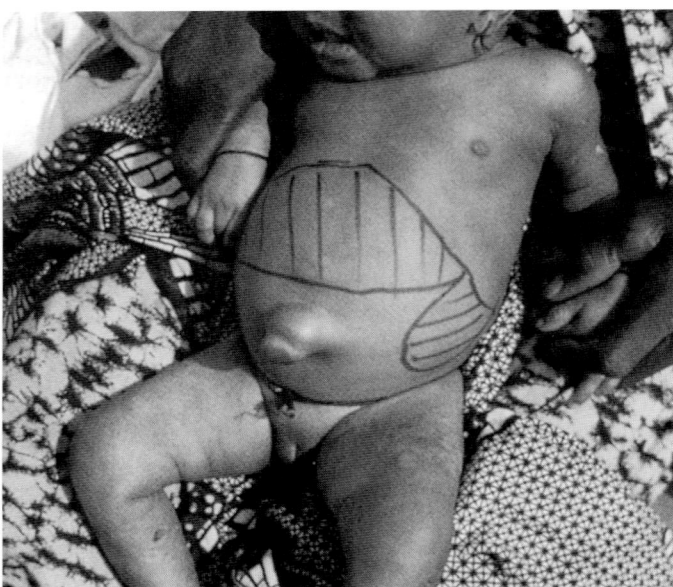

Figure 21.15: Congenital syphilis in a 3-month-old infant: hepatosplenomegaly.

Diagnosis

Clinically it may not be possible to distinguish a syphilitic primary chancre from other causes of genital ulceration. In most parts of Africa chancroid is the most important differential diagnosis, but in areas where donovanosis is prevalent this should also be considered. The primary chancre should also be distinguished from LGV, herpes and non-venereal causes of genital ulceration. Secondary syphilis may resemble a variety of other skin conditions, but rashes which do not itch and affect the palms and soles should be considered syphilitic until proved otherwise. Early congenital syphilis in the neonatal period may be confused with perinatally acquired herpes simplex on account of the bullous rash, or with other intrauterine infections causing hepatosplenomegaly, anaemia and jaundice (e.g., cytomegalovirus, toxoplasmosis, rubella).

Dark-field microscopy

T. pallidum may be demonstrated by dark-field microscopy in fluid from ulcerated or moist lesions of early syphilis, or in bulla fluid from lesions of early congenital syphilis. It can be distinguished from other spirochaetes which may be present under the foreskin by its characteristic shape and motility. Dark-field microscopy is likely to be negative in patients who have applied antiseptics to the lesion or taken antibiotics.

Serological diagnosis

Two categories of test are available for the serological diagnosis of syphilis: non-specific or reagin tests (e.g., Venereal Disease Research Laboratory (VDRL), rapid plasma reagin (RPR)) and treponemal tests (*T. pallidum* haemagglutination (TPHA), fluorescent treponemal antibody (FTA)). The reagin tests are useful for monitor-ing the response to treatment because they exhibit a falling titre after successful therapy, but they may give false positive reactions in subjects with other chronic infections. The treponemal tests generally remain positive for life, and cannot therefore distinguish between a current and a past infection. They are more specific than the reagin tests but cannot distinguish between sexually acquired and endemic treponemal infections. The RPR and TPHA tests are simple to perform and do not require sophisticated laboratory equipment. In the neonate it is necessary to demonstrate IgM antibodies by the FTA test in order to distinguish between true infection and passively acquired maternal antibody; however, in an infant with signs of congenital syphilis, a positive maternal reagin test is sufficient grounds for treatment. A new generation of specific IgM EIA tests shows promise as a new tool for recognizing recently acquired active infection.[60,61]

Management (Tables 21.5 and 21.6)

T. pallidum remains fully sensitive to penicillin. Because it is a slowly dividing organism it is necessary to ensure adequate circulating penicillin levels for at least 10 days. Recommended treatment regimens are shown in Table 21.5. It has been suggested that single-dose benzathine penicillin does not ensure adequate levels in the cerebrospinal fluid, and recent anecdotal evidence suggests that it may be ineffective in some HIV-infected patients and pregnant women. If it is possible to ensure compliance, 10 daily doses of aqueous procaine penicillin 1.2 million units may be preferable although a recent randomized trial showed no differences in outcomes between patients treated with single-dose and extended high-dose penicillin, regardless of HIV status.[62] Epidemiological treatment is recommended for sexual contacts.

Early congenital syphilis should be treated with procaine penicillin 50 000 units/kg i.m. daily for 10 days. If compliance is considered unlikely, benzathine penicillin 50 000 units/kg i.m. as a single dose may be given, although this does not give therapeutic levels in the cerebrospinal fluid. The mother and her sexual partner(s) should be investigated and treated appropriately. If possible, infants should be followed up after 6 months to ensure that the RPR or VDRL test has reverted to negative.

Prevention

Congenital syphilis can be prevented by serological screening of pregnant women at antenatal clinics. Experience in Lusaka, Zambia, has shown that in a developing country setting this is only successful if serological tests are performed in the clinic and treatment given immediately.

Lymphogranuloma venereum

Lymphogranuloma venereum (LGV) is also known as lymphogranuloma inguinale, lymphopathia venereum, tropical or climatic bubo and Durand–Nicolas–Favre disease.

Epidemiology

The epidemiology of LGV is not well defined owing to the lack of a sensitive and specific diagnostic test. It is an STI largely confined to the tropics. In most places it accounts for only a small proportion of patients with STIs. The disease is seen more often in men than women, although the late anorectal complications are more prevalent in women.

Aetiology

LGV is caused by the invasive L1, L2 and L3 strains of *Chlamydia trachomatis.*

Pathology

The characteristic pathological features are a thrombo-lymphangitis and perilymphangitis with proliferation of the endothelial cells of the lymphatics. In the lymph nodes prominent migration of neutrophils leads to characteristic stellate abscess formation.

Clinical features

The disease is important chiefly as a cause of bubo. When a sexually active adult presents with an inguinal bubo not associated with genital ulcer, LGV is an important diagnosis to consider. The initial event in infection, occurring 3–30 days after exposure, is typically a small, painless, usually herpetiform ulcer of the genitalia which may pass unrecognized and resolves spontaneously. It is thought likely that some patients develop asymptomatic infections of the urethra and cervix. The second phase of the illness is the development of increasingly painful lymphangitis and lymphadenitis, accompanied by fever and malaise. The infected nodes (bilateral in a third of cases) coalesce into a matted mass which may project outwards below or above the inguinal ligament to give the classical 'groove sign'. The nodes are liable to rupture, forming multiple sinuses. Untreated, the disease may cause extensive lymphatic damage, resulting in elephantiasis of the genitalia (Figure 21.16). The combination of elephantiasis with skin breakdown sometimes seen in late cases is referred to as esthiomène. An additional characteristic feature in long-standing cases is the development of fenestrations in the labia. In women and homosexual men the disease may present as an acute proctocolitis which, in a proportion of cases, leads much later to abscess formation, fibrosis, fistula and rectal stricture. In the Caribbean a high incidence of vulval carcinoma has been recorded among premenopausal women with scars of either LGV or donovanosis.[63] A substantial proportion of cases of rectal stricture may also develop carcinoma.

Diagnosis

The diagnosis of LGV can only be confirmed in specialist centres with facilities for the isolation and identification of *C. trachomatis* L1–3 strains, or the ability to perform the micro-immunofluorescence serological test.[64] Other serological tests show cross-reaction with other serovars of *C. trachomatis,* and with other species of *Chlamydia,*

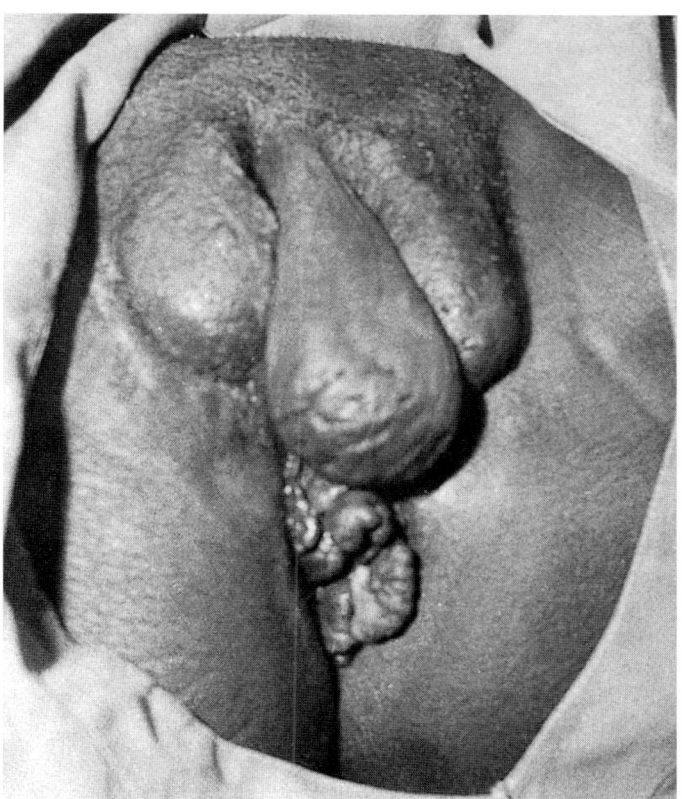

Figure 21.16: Lymphogranuloma venereum: elephantiasis in long-standing case. (Reproduced with permission of the publishers from Arya O P, Osoba A O & Bennett F J. *Tropical Venereology.* Edinburgh: Churchill Livingstone, 1980.)

e.g., the prevalent respiratory tract pathogen *C. pneumoniae.* The accepted criterion for a positive diagnosis is a micro-immunofluorescence titre of 1:512. The presence of stellate abscesses in biopsy material is suggestive of LGV. Direct fluorescent antibody (DFA) staining may be used to demonstrate chlamydial elementary bodies in tissue or discharge from buboes. Additional laboratory findings include leucocytosis, an elevated erythrocyte sedimentation rate and increases in IgG and cryoglobulins.

Treatment (Tables 21.5 and 21.6)

The drugs recommended for treatment of acute cases are of the tetracycline group or erythromycin, as for other chlamydial infections. Benefit in late cases, e.g., with rectal stricture, is slight. Plastic surgical operations may be of benefit in cases with extensive elephantiasis or deformity. Suspicious areas in healed scars should be biopsied for malignant change. Aspiration of buboes through adjacent healthy skin is usually advised.

Donovanosis

Synonyms: granuloma inguinale, granuloma venereum. It is important not to confuse this disease with *lymphogranuloma venereum* (see above) or to confuse Donovan bodies (see below) with Leishman–Donovan bodies (leishmaniasis). The disease was first recognized in India, where Donovan observed the bodies that bear his name in an oral lesion of the disease. Sir Patrick Manson did much to promote awareness of the disease by devoting a chapter to 'ulcerating granuloma of the pudenda' in the first edition of this textbook.

Epidemiology

Endemic areas are localized to a few specific areas of the tropics. The most important of these are currently India, Papua New Guinea (PNG), Brazil and eastern parts of South Africa. The disease is strongly associated with prostitution and low socio-economic status. Major epidemics of donovanosis have been reported from PNG but are unlikely to be seen again. Outside PNG the highest recently reported incidence of donovanosis has been in Durban, South Africa, where 16% of genital ulcers in men were due to donovanosis.[65] There is strong evidence that the disease is sexually transmitted in most patients, although some authors have put forward arguments for a non-sexual mode of transmission.[66] The risk of transmission to partners appears to be lower than for other STIs. Perinatal transmission is rare.

Aetiology

The disease is caused by a poorly characterized, encapsulated, Gram-negative coccobacillus, previously called *Calymmatobacterium granulomatis*, recently reclassified as a *Klebsiella* on the basis of ribosomal RNA sequences.[67] It is an intracellular parasite that can be grown in tissue culture.[68,69]

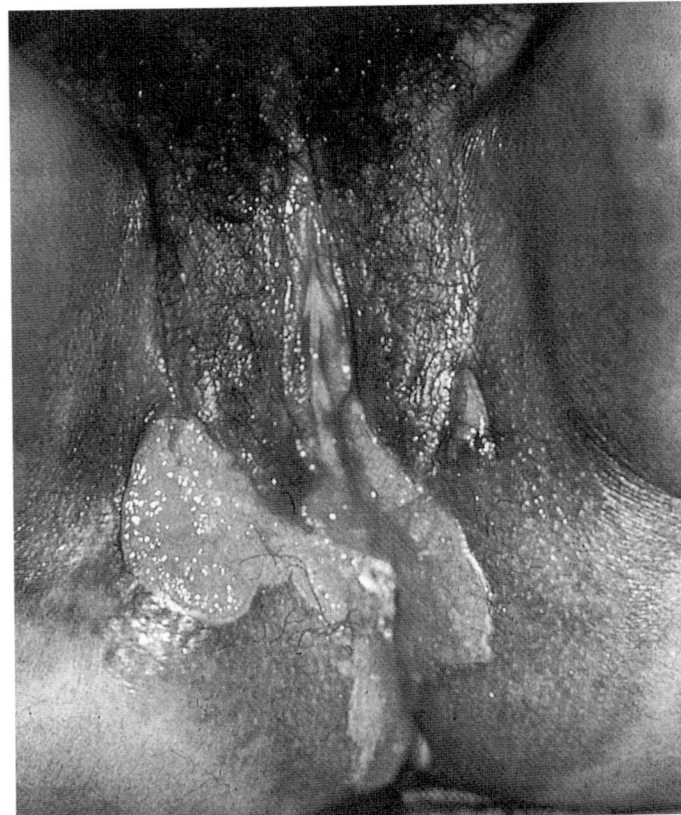

Figure 21.17: Donovanosis: slowly extending painless ulceration.

Pathology

The disease primarily attacks the skin. The bacteria are carried to inguinal nodes, where they occasionally cause a suppurating periadenitis ('pseudobubo') but more often they escape to produce ulcers in the overlying skin. The key histological features are (1) epithelial hyperplasia, (2) a dense dermal infiltrate of plasma cells, and (3) scattered large macrophages containing clusters of Donovan bodies. Donovan bodies stain poorly with haematoxylin and eosin but with Giemsa they typically display a capsule and bipolar densities which give a characteristic closed safety-pin appearance.

Clinical features

The first manifestation, appearing after a 3–40-day incubation period, is usually a small papule which ruptures to form a granulomatous lesion that is characteristically pain free, 'beefy-red' in colour, bleeds readily on contact and is often elevated above the level of the surrounding skin. The lesion has to be differentiated from other forms of genital ulcer. Most likely to cause confusion are chancroid,[70] condylomata lata, ulcerated warts and squamous carcinoma. Untreated, the ulcers slowly extend (Figure 21.17), particularly along skin folds towards the groins (Figure 21.18) and anus. Special features are extragenital lesions (mostly neck and mouth), cervical lesions (resemble carcinoma or tuberculous cervicitis), involvement of uterus, tubes and ovaries (hard masses, abscesses,

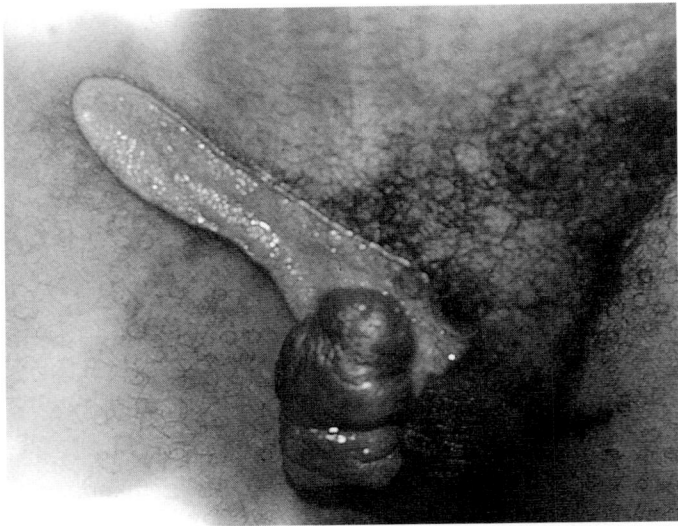

Figure 21.18: Donovanosis: lesion extending along inguinal fold.

'frozen pelvis', hydronephrosis) and rare cases of haematogenous dissemination to lung, liver, spleen and bone. Complications include rapid extension of lesions secondarily infected with fusospirochaetal organisms, scarring (in some populations very prominent), elephantiasis and the development of squamous carcinoma.

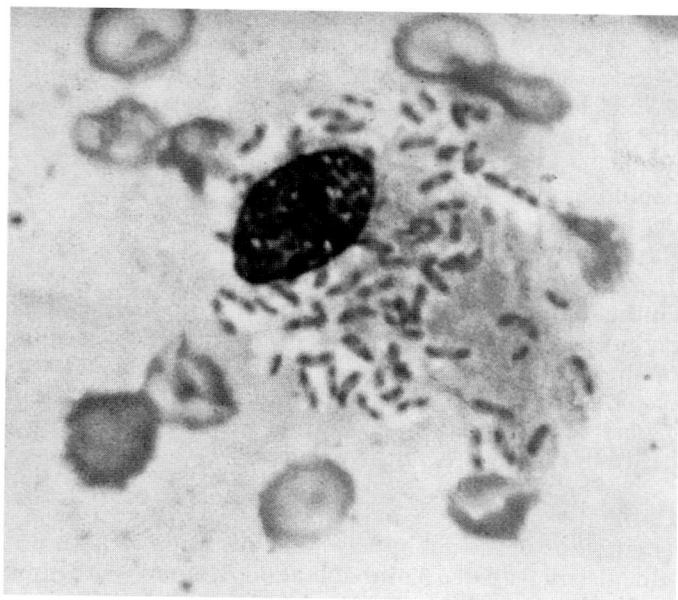

Figure 21.19: Donovan bodies: Giemsa-stained smear from genital ulcer demonstrating intracellular organisms with bipolar densities.

Diagnosis

The diagnosis requires the demonstration of *intracellular* Donovan bodies (Figure 21.19) in either biopsy material (best stained with silver stains or Giemsa) or smears taken from active areas which can be stained by Giemsa or Leishman stains. For collection of specimens, a recommended technique is to thoroughly clean the lesions of surface debris, detach one to three 3–5 mm pieces of tissue by punch or snip biopsy, and then prepare a smear from one piece, followed by air-drying and fixation in 95% ethanol and fixing the remaining tissue in 10% formalin for histology.[71]

Management (Tables 21.5 and 21.6)

The bacteria respond to many broad-spectrum antibiotics active against Gram-negative bacilli.[69] The most widely used in recent years have been tetracylines, chloramphenicol, co-trimoxazole and erythromycin. Thiamphenicol, lincomycin and norfloxacin have recently been shown to be of value, but studies in Australia have shown that azithromycin is the treatment of choice.[72] Treatment should be continued until lesions have resolved and, if possible, a little longer to reduce the risk of relapse. Plastic surgical procedures are required in some patients. Epidemiological treatment of contacts exposed within 40 days of the onset of symptoms in the index case may be recommended.

Genital herpes

Genital herpes is an ulcerative STI caused principally by herpes simplex virus type 2 (HSV-2) and to a lesser extent by herpes simplex virus type 1 (HSV-1), the usual cause of oral herpes. Genital herpes accounts for a much lower proportion of patients with genital ulcer in the tropics

than it does in developed countries, although this pattern is changing rapidly in areas with high HIV incidence. Recent studies in Africa have demonstrated that HSV seroconversion is an especially important risk factor for HIV acquisition.[73] Prior infection with HSV-1 infection, which is almost universal by the age of puberty in many developing countries, reduces the severity and frequency of clinical recurrences in HSV-2 infection.[74]

Clinical features

The clinical picture is highly characteristic in many cases, with its localized clusters of vesicles which break down to form ulcers (Figure 21.20), crust over and then resolve. Sites of involvement include the external genitalia, neighbouring skin, the urethra and cervix (both endocervix and ectocervix), pharynx and rectum. Tender lymphadenopathy may occur. During the primary attack the virus ascends the peripheral nerves to local ganglia, where a latency is established which is liable to be interrupted by periodic recurrences for the remainder of the patient's life. The primary attack is notably more severe than subsequent episodes, with lesions covering a wider and more symmetric area. HSV-2 causes substantially more severe primary disease than HSV-1 and is followed by more frequent relapse. The complications of genital herpes include a sacral radiculomyelopathy which may manifest with constipation and retention of urine as well as shooting pains down the legs. Other complications include aseptic meningitis, extragenital lesions and disseminated herpes. In pregnant women recurrences and dissemination are more frequent and premature delivery may complicate primary attacks. Severe and intractable ulceration due to HSV-2 occurs in patients immunosuppressed by HIV.

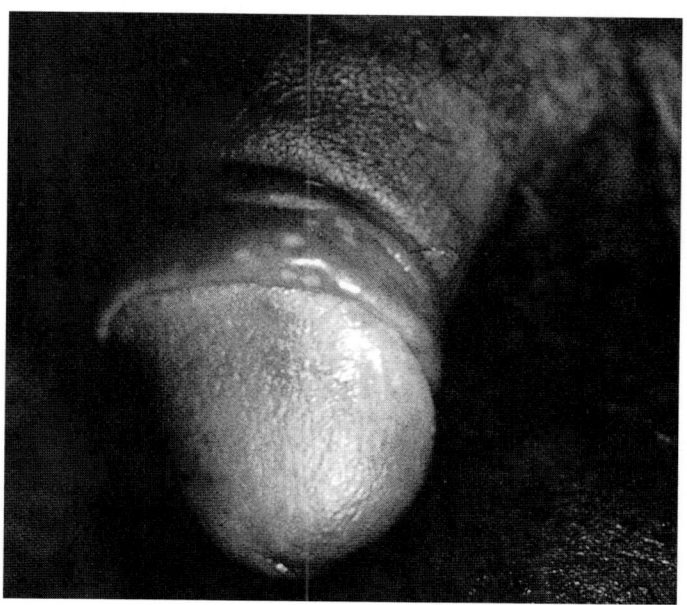

Figure 21.20: Recurrent genital herpes: cluster of small painful ulcers of corona.

Diagnosis

Clinical diagnosis alone is often sufficient. Genital herpes has to be distinguished from other STIs that cause painful genital ulcer and from non-infectious conditions such as Behçet's syndrome and Crohn's disease. The definitive diagnosis rests on viral isolation. Kits for antigen detection are available commercially, and DNA amplification tests have been successfully used to identify HSV-2 in symptomatic and asymptomatic shedders. Serological diagnosis is only of value in a primary attack.

Management (Tables 21. 5 and 21.6)

Specific treatment can rarely be offered in the tropics; nonetheless patients require explanation, reassurance and advice, just as elsewhere. Patients need to be instructed to keep the lesions clean and dry. They should be told that the disease is likely to recur and that they will transmit the infection to others if they have sexual intercourse while they have lesions. Acyclovir has been shown to be of value in ameliorating symptoms of the primary attack, treatment of infected neonates and adults with immunosuppression or disseminated disease. Continuous prophylactic therapy has been found useful in ameliorating and preventing recurrences in patients particularly troubled by recurrent disease. Recent studies have demonstrated that periods of asymptomatic shedding commonly occur and that this shedding can be suppressed by acyclovir.[75]

Herpes in pregnancy

Transmission from mother to child occurs in 50% of cases with a primary attack at term, is much lower in patients with recurrences (about 1%) and occasionally occurs as a result of asymptomatic viral shedding by the mother at term. Neonatal herpes carries a 60% mortality, which has changed little with the introduction of acyclovir. The presence of active herpetic lesions of the cervix at term is an indication for caesarean section, although this operation does not fully protect against infection developing in the neonate. Antenatal cultures for HSV in at-risk women are no longer recommended as they fail to identify neonates at risk. The use of acyclovir in late pregnancy is being investigated and it has been suggested that pregnant women at risk should be screened with specific HSV-2 serology.[76]

Genital warts

Epidemiology

In developed countries genital infection with the human papillomavirus (HPV) is the most common viral STI and is four times as frequent as genital herpes. Using the most sensitive diagnostic methods infection can be demonstrated in as many as 40% of sexually active women.[77] In the tropics HPV infections are common but are of relatively minor importance compared with the bacterial STIs.

Aetiology

Genital warts are caused by HPVs. The types most prevalent in genital lesions are designated HPV-6, -11 and -16. Of these, HPV-16 has been particularly associated with the development of cancer of the cervix, while HPV-6 and -11 have a lower potential for causing neoplasia and are more closely associated with exophytic (as opposed to flat) lesions and with the development of respiratory papillomas in children born to infected mothers.

Pathology

The virus infects the basal layer of differentiating squamous epithelium and produces a pathognomonic large, clear, perinuclear zone known as koilocytotic atypia. Full assembly of viral particles is confined to the more superficial layers of the epithelium. HPV is implicated in the causation of cancer of the cervix[78]—a cancer with a very high incidence in many parts of the tropics.

Clinical

The lesions produced by HPV vary from the well-known soft, fleshy, vascular condylomata acuminata with their frond-like appearance (Figure 21.21) to papular warts which resemble those seen on other parts of the body, pigmented and non-pigmented papules and leucoplakia. Warts may sometimes grow in the urethra. Recent research has shown that many patients have subclinical HPV infections that can only be visualized by colposcopy after application of 5% acetic acid or detected in tissue specimens by techniques such as PCR. In pregnancy, in

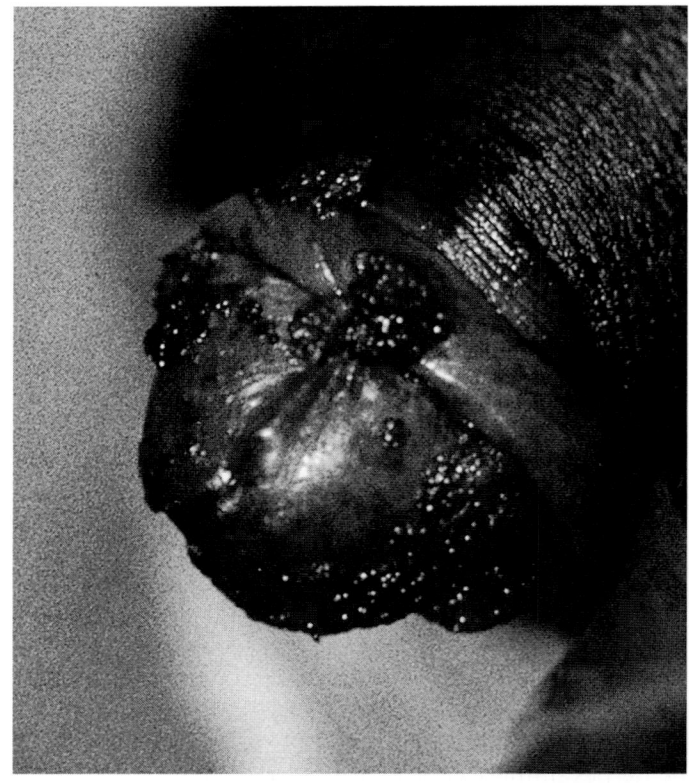

Figure 21.21: Genital warts: condylomata acuminata caused by human papillomavirus.

immunosuppressed patients and in the presence of genital discharges there is a tendency for warts to grow rapidly. The lesions showing the greatest similarity to genital warts are condylomata lata of secondary syphilis and, occasionally, verrucose forms of donovanosis.

Diagnosis and management

Biopsy confirmation of the diagnosis of condylomata acuminata warts is optional but cervical cytology, where available, is recommended for female patients and female contacts in order to detect progression of lesions to cervical intraepithelial neoplasia. Treatment is generally reserved for macroscopic lesions because subclinical infections show high spontaneous regression rates and also show a strong tendency to relapse with currently available forms of treatment. Specific treatment for warts includes treatment with trichloroacetic acid and the traditional application of 20% podophyllin (maximum 0.5 ml) once or twice weekly.[79] Cure rates with podophyllin, at <50%, are not very satisfactory. Care is needed to avoid burning normal skin, which can be protected with glycerine. Podophyllin should be washed off after 4 hours and is contraindicated in pregnant women. Larger warts can be removed with cryotherapy or diathermy. More modern treatments include the application of imiquimod or 5-fluorouracil cream, self-treatment with podophyllotoxin, and carbon dioxide laser treatment. Relapse rates of the order of 30% are seen with all forms of treatment.

The management of STI control programmes

The important components of an STI control programme are: (1) gathering of information, e.g., STI morbidity surveillance, special surveys on the aetiology of genital ulcer in a particular area, data on antibiotic sensitivities of local strains of *Neisseria gonorrhoea* and *Haemophilus ducreyi*; (2) provision of management guidelines; (3) training programmes; (4) provision of health care to patients with STIs wherever they may present; (5) coordinated programmes of education about STIs for patients and the general public; and (6) management and supervision of the programme. Each of these will be discussed in more detail.

Information gathering

Morbidity surveillance in the tropics is often incomplete and unreliable. Given the rudimentary facilities available in many centres, it is often best to record numbers of patients by syndrome (ulcer, discharge, etc.) rather than by specific diagnosis. Good reporting from a few representative sentinel sites may be more useful than unreliable reports collated from the whole country. When possible, special surveys should be undertaken periodically, such as studies of the prevalence of gonorrhoea, chlamydial infection and syphilis in antenatal mothers. Statistics on ophthalmia neonatorum, congenital syphilis, PID, ectopic pregnancy and infertility may be useful for impressing upon health planners the full extent of STI morbidity.

Standard management guidelines for STIs

When a reasonable amount of information is available about the picture of STIs in a country and the antibiotic sensitivity patterns of local isolates, it is possible to draw up rational guidelines for local use, based on those recommended by the WHO.[17] These guidelines can be tailored to different levels of the health system according to the availability of supporting laboratory tests and drugs. They can be conveniently set out as flow charts or algorithms in pocket manuals which are supplied to all health workers who need to manage STIs. In view of the constantly changing pattern of antibiotic sensitivities of *N. gonorrhoea* and *H. ducreyi*, it is important that guidelines are reviewed and revised at 3–4-yearly intervals.

Training

The high incidence of STIs in tropical populations makes it important for all health workers to acquire the basic skills to manage patients appropriately according to standard guidelines, to prevent ophthalmia neonatorum and congenital syphilis, and to promote the following health education messages which are important in STI prevention:

- Reduction of the number of sexual partners.
- Avoidance of sex with high-risk partners.
- Use of condoms for protection against STIs.
- Knowledge of the symptoms, sequelae and transmissibility of STIs.
- Avoidance of sexual contact when symptoms are present.
- Knowledge of what AIDS is and how HIV is transmitted.
- Obtaining proper treatment promptly for STI symptoms.
- Ensuring that the patients' contacts are treated whether they have symptoms or not.

Provision of services for patients with STIs

The aim should be to maximize coverage and access of STI services for men and women and to have a way of referring problem cases. Costs to patients should be kept as low as possible and confidentiality safeguarded. Specialist STI clinics are valuable where the volume of patients is high, but in general the provision of specialist clinics for the treatment of STIs, which has been successful in controlling these diseases in certain industrialized countries, is neither appropriate nor feasible in most developing countries, where patients with STIs should be managed at the primary health care level. Family planning and antenatal clinics provide opportunities for

STI control activities which tend to be underutilized at present.

Education programmes

The appropriate content for education messages has been described above. These messages must be expressed in a sensitive manner after widespread consultation and careful pretesting before they are disseminated by health workers, through posters and by the media. It is particularly important to target schoolchildren, sex workers and patients attending for treatment of STIs. Interest has recently focused on the use of peer educators to encourage people to listen to health messages. Condom promotion

is of particular importance and the social marketing of condoms has shown promise in some countries.

Supervision and management of STI control

It is important for programmes of STI and AIDS control to be fully integrated because of their many shared objectives. The delegation of much routine STI treatment and control to the primary health care level is unlikely to succeed unless the morale and commitment of health care workers responsible for treating patients with STIs are maintained by regular supportive visits by programme managers.

REFERENCES

1 Piot P & Hira S. Control and prevention of sexually transmitted diseases. In Lamptey P & Piot P (eds) *The Handbook for AIDS Prevention in Africa*. Durham, NC: Family Health International, 1990: 83–104.
2 De Schryver A & Meheus A. Epidemiology of sexually transmitted diseases: the global picture. *Bull World Health Organ* 1990; 68:639–654.
3 Mabey D C W, Lloyd-Evans N, Conteh S & Forsey T. Sexually transmitted diseases among randomly selected attenders at an antenatal clinic in The Gambia. *Br J Vener Dis* 1984; 60:331–336.
4 Laga M, Plummer F, Nsanze H et al. Epidemiology of ophthalmia neonatorum in Kenya. *Lancet* 1986; ii:1145–1148.
5 Meheus A, Friedman F, van Dyck E & Guyver T. Genital infections in prenatal and family planning attendants in Swaziland. *East Afr Med J* 1979; 57:212–217.
6 Hira S K. Sexually transmitted disease: a menace to mother and children. *World Health Forum* 1986; 7:243–247.
7 Bentsi C, Klufio C A, Perine P L et al. Genital infections with *Chlamydia trachomatis* and *Neisseria gonorrhoea* in Ghanaian women. *Genitourin Med* 1985; 61:48–50.
8 Wawer M J, Sewankambo N K, Serwadda D et al. Control of sexually transmitted diseases for AIDS prevention in Uganda: a randomised community trial. Rakai Project Study Group. *Lancet* 1999; 353:525–532.
9 Muir D G & Belsey M A. Pelvic inflammatory disease and its consequences in the developing world. *Am J Obstet Gynecol* 1980; 138:913–928.
10 Cates W, Farley T M M & Rowe P J. Worldwide patterns of infertility: is Africa different? *Lancet* 1985; ii:596–598.
11 Mabey D, Hanlon P, Hanlon L, Marsh V & Forsey T. Chlamydial and gonococcal ophthalmia neonatorum in The Gambia. *Ann Trop Paediatr* 1987; 7:177–180.
12 Hira S K, Ratnam A V, Sehgal D, Bhat G J, Chintu C & Mulenga R C. Congenital syphilis in Lusaka: incidence in a general nursery ward. *East Afr Med J* 1982; 59:241–246.
13 Fleming D T & Wasserheit J N. From epidemiological synergy to public health policy and practice: the contribution of other sexually transmitted diseases to sexual transmission of HIV infection. *Sex Transm Infect* 1999; 75:3–17.
14 Hayes R J, Schulz K F & Plummer F A. The cofactor effect of genital ulcers on the per-exposure risk of HIV transmission in sub-Saharan Africa. *J Trop Med Hyg* 1995; 98:1–8.
15 Cohen M S, Hoffman I F, Royce R A et al. Reduction of concentration of HIV-1 in semen after treatment of urethritis: implications for prevention of sexual transmission of HIV-1. *Lancet* 1997; 349:1868–1873.
16 Grosskurth H, Mosha F, Todd J et al. Impact of improved treatment of sexually transmitted diseases on HIV infection in rural Tanzania: randomised controlled trial. *Lancet* 1995; 346:530–536.
17 World Health Organization. *Guidelines for the Management of Sexually Transmitted Infections*. Geneva: World Health Organization, 2001.
18 Mayaud P & Mabey D C. Managing sexually transmitted diseases in the tropics: is a laboratory really needed? *Trop Doct* 2000; 30:42–46.
19 Grosskurth H, Mayaud P, Mosha F et al. Asymptomatic gonorrhoea and chlamydial infection in rural Tanzanian men. *BMJ* 1996; 312:277–278.
20 Pelouze P S. *Gonorrhoea in the Male and Female*. Philadelphia: W B Saunders, 1941.
21 Bewes P C. Urethral stricture. *Trop Doct* 1973; 3:77–81.
22 Osegbe D N & Amaku E O. Gonococcal strictures in young patients. *Urology* 1981; 18:37–41.
23 Collet M, Reniers S, Frost E et al. Infertility in Central Africa: infection is the cause. *Int J Gynaecol Obstet* 1988; 26:423–428.
24 Elliot B, Brunham R C, Laga M et al. Maternal gonococcal infection as a preventable risk factor for low birth weight. *J Infect Dis* 1990; 161:532–536.
25 Plummer F A, Laga M, Brunham R D et al. Postpartum upper genital tract infections in Nairobi, Kenya: epidemiology, etiology, and risk factors. *J Infect Dis* 1987; 156:92–98.
26 Stein C M & Hanly M G. Acute tropical polyarthritis in Zimbabwe: a prospective search for a gonococcal aetiology. *Ann Rheum Dis* 1987; 46:912–914.
27 Kestelyn P, Bogaerts J & Meheus A. Gonorrhoeal keratoconjunctivitis in African adults. *Sex Transm Dis* 1987; 14:191–194.
28 Laga M, Plummer F A, Piot P et al. Prophylaxis of gonococcal and chlamydial ophthalmia neonatorum: a comparison of silver nitrate and tetracycline. *N Engl J Med* 1988; 318:653–657.
29 Ison C A, Dillon J A & Tapsall J W. The epidemiology of global antibiotic resistance among *Neisseria gonorrhoea* and *Haemophilus ducreyi*. *Lancet* 1998; 351(Suppl. 3):8–11.
30 Isenberg S J, Apt L & Wood M. A controlled trial of povidone–iodine as prophylaxis against ophthalmia neonatorum. *N Engl J Med* 1995; 332:562–566.
31 Ison C A. Laboratory methods in genitourinary medicine: methods of diagnosing gonorrhoea. *Genitourin Med* 1990; 66:433–439.
32 Garnett G P & Bowden F J. Epidemiology and control and curable sexually transmitted diseases: opportunities and problems. *Sex Transm Dis* 2000; 27:588–599.

33 Peeling R W, Kimani J, Plummer F, Maclean I, Cheang M, Bwayo J & Brunham R C. Antibody to chlamydial hsp60 predicts an increased risk for chlamydial pelvic inflammatory disease. *J Infect Dis* 1997; 175:1153–1158.

34 Westrom L & Mårdh P-A. Chlamydial salpingitis. *Br Med Bull* 1983; 39:145–150.

35 Beem M O & Saxon E M. Respiratory tract colonisation and a distinctive pneumonia syndrome in infants infected with *Chlamydia trachomatis*. *N Engl J Med* 1977; 296:306–310.

36 Black C M. Current methods of laboratory diagnosis of *Chlamydia trachomatis* infections. *Clin Microbiol Rev* 1997; 10:160–184.

37 Steingrimmson O, Olaffson J H, Thorarinsson H et al. Azithromycin in the treatment of sexually transmitted disease. *J Antimicrob Chemother* 1990; 25(Suppl. A):109–114.

38 Watson-Jones D, Mugeye K, Mayaud P et al. High prevalence of trichomoniasis in rural men in Mwanza, Tanzania: results from a population based study. *Sex Transm Infect* 2000; 76:355–362.

39 Wolner-Hanssen P, Krieger J N, Stevens C E et al. Clinical manifestations of vaginal trichomoniasis. *JAMA* 1989; 261:571–576.

40 Hillier S L, Nugent R P, Eschenbach D A et al. Association between bacterial vaginosis and preterm delivery of a low-birth-weight infant. The Vaginal Infections and Prematurity Study Group. *N Engl J Med* 1995; 333:1737–1742.

41 Nugent R P, Krohn M A & Hillier S L. Reliability of diagnosing bacterial vaginosis is improved by a standardized method of gram stain interpretation. *J Clin Microbiol* 1991; 29:297–301.

42 Amsel R, Totten P A, Spiegel C A, Chen K C S, Eschenbach D & Holmes K K. Nonspecific vaginitis: diagnostic criteria and microbial and epidemiologic associations. *Am J Med* 1983; 74:14–22.

43 Hammond G W, Slutchuk M, Scatliff J et al. Clinical epidemiological, laboratory and therapeutic features of an urban outbreak of chancroid in North America. *Rev Infect Dis* 1980; 2:867–879.

44 Morse S A. Chancroid and *Haemophilus ducreyi*. *Clin Microbiol Rev* 1989; 2:137–157.

45 O'Farrell N. Increasing prevalence of genital herpes in developing countries: implications for heterosexual HIV transmission and STI control programmes. *Sex Transm Infect* 1999;75:377–384.

46 Plummer F A, D'Costa L J, Nsanze H et al. Epidemiology of chancroid and *Haemophilus ducreyi* in Nairobi. *Lancet* 1983; ii:1293–1295.

47 Hart G. Venereal disease in a war environment: incidence and management. *Med J Aust* 1975; 1:808–810.

48 Cameron D W, D'Costa L J, Gregory M M et al. Female to male transmission of human immunodeficiency virus type 1: risk factors for seroconversion in men. *Lancet* 1989; ii:403–407.

49 Plummer F A, Simonsen J N, Cameron D W et al. Co-factors in male to female transmission of HIV. *J Infect Dis* 1991; 163:233–239.

50 Al-Tawfiq J A, Thornton A C, Katz B P et al. Standardisation of the experimental model of *Haemophilus ducreyi* infection in human subjects. *J Infect Dis* 1998; 178:1684–1687.

51 Al-Tawfiq J A, Fortney K R, Katz B P, Hood A F, Elkins C & Spinola S M. An isogenic hemoglobin receptor-deficient mutant of *Haemophilus ducreyi* is attenuated in the human model of experimental infection. *J Infect Dis* 2000; 181:1049–1054.

52 Stevens M K, Latimer J L, Lumbley S R, Ward C K, Cope L D, Lagergard T & Hansen E J. Characterisation of a *Haemophilus ducreyi* mutant deficient in expression of cytolethal distending toxin. *Infect Immun* 1999; 67:3900–3908.

53 Fast M V, D'Costa L J, Nsanze H et al. The clinical diagnosis of genital ulcer disease in men in the tropics. *Sex Transm Dis* 1984; 11:72–76.

54 Hudson E H. *Non-venereal Syphilis*. Baltimore, MD: Williams & Wilkins, 1958.

55 Todd J, Munguti K, Grosskurth H et al. Risk factors for active syphilis and TPHA seroconversion in a rural African population. *Sex Transm Infect* 2001; 77(1):37–45.

56 Newell J, Senkoro K, Mosha F et al. A population-based study of syphilis and sexually transmitted disease syndromes in north-western Tanzania. 2. Risk factors and health seeking behaviour. *Genitourin Med* 1993; 69:421–426.

57 Gjestland T. The Oslo study of untreated syphilis. *Acta Derm Venereol Suppl (Stockh)* 1955; 35:1.

58 Ingraham N R. The value of penicillin alone in the prevention and treatment of congenital syphilis. *Acta Derm Venereol* 1951; 31(Suppl. 24):60.

59 Hira S K, Bhat G J, Patel J B et al. Early congenital syphilis: clinicoradiologic features in 202 patients. *Sex Transm Dis* 1985; 12:177–183.

60 Young H, Moyes A, Seagar L et al. Novel recombinant-antigen enzyme immunoassay for serological diagnosis of syphilis. *J Clin Microbiol* 1998; 36:913–917.

61 Young H. Guidelines for serological testing for syphilis. *Sex Transm Infect* 2000; 76:403-405.

62 Rolfs R T, Joesoef M R, Hendershot E F et al. for the Syphilis and HIV Study Group. A randomised trial of enhanced therapy for early syphilis in patients with and without human immunodeficiency virus infection. *N Engl J Med* 1997; 337:307–314.

63 Sengupta B S. Vulval cancer following or co-existing with chronic granulomatous diseases of the vulva. *Trop Doct* 1981; 11:110–114.

64 Perine P L, Andersen A J, Krause D W et al. Diagnosis and treatment of lymphogranuloma venereum in Ethiopia. In Nelson J D & Grassi C (eds) *Current Chemotherapy and Infectious Disease*. Washington, DC: American Society for Microbiology, 1980: 1280–1282.

65 O'Farrell N, Hoosen A A, Coetzee K D & Van den Ende J. Genital ulcer disease in men in Durban, South Africa. *Genitourin Med* 1991; 67:327–330.

66 Goldberg J. Studies on granuloma inguinale. VII. Some epidemiological considerations of the disease. *Br J Vener Dis* 1964; 40:140–145.

67 Carter J S, Bowden F J, Bastian I, Myers G M, Sriprakash K S & Kemp D J. Phylogenetic evidence for reclassification of *Calymmatobacterium granulomatis* as *Klebsiella granulomatis* comb. nov. *Int J Systemat Bact* 1999; 49:1695–1700.

68 Kharsany A B, Hoosen A A, Kiepiela P, Naicker T & Sturm A W. Growth and cultural characteristics of *Calymmatobacterium granulomatis*: the aetiological agent of granuloma inguinale (Donovanosis). *J Med Microbiol* 1997; 46:579–585.

69 Richens J. The diagnosis and treatment of donovanosis (granuloma inguinale). *Genitourin Med* 1991; 67:441–452.

70 Verdich J. *Haemophilus ducreyi* infection resembling granuloma inguinale. *Arch Derm Venereol* 1984; 64:452–455.

71 Bowden F. Donovanosis. In Holmes K K & Morse S (eds) *Atlas of Sexually Transmitted Infections* (in press).

72 Anonymous. National guideline for the management of donovanosis (granuloma inguinale). *Sex Transm Infect* 1999; 75(Suppl. 1):S38–39.

73 Pujades Rodriguez M, Obasi A, Mosha F et al. Herpes simplex virus type 2 infection increases HIV incidence: a propsective study in rural Tanzania. *AIDS* 2001 (in press).

74 Reeves W C, Corey L Adams H G et al. Risk of recurrence after first episodes of genital herpes: relation to HSV type and antibody response. *N Engl J Med* 1981; 305:315.

75 Wald A, Zeh J, Barnum G et al. Suppression of subclinical shedding of herpes simplex virus type 2 with acyclovir. *Ann Intern Med* 1996; 124:8–15.

76 Mercey D E & Mindel A. Preventing neonatal herpes? *Genitourin Med* 1991; 67:1–2.

77 Rando R F. Human papillomavirus: implications for clinical medicine. *Ann Intern Med* 1988; 108:628–631.

78 Munoz N, Bosch X & Kaldor J M. Does human papillomavirus cause cervical cancer? The state of the epidemiologic evidence. *Br J Cancer* 1988; 57:1–5.

79 Eskelinen A & Mashkilleyson N. Optimum treatment of genital warts. *Drugs* 1987; 34:599–603.

FURTHER READING

Holmes K K, Mårdh P A, Sparling P F et al. (eds). *Sexually Transmitted Diseases*, 3rd edn. New York: McGraw-Hill, 1999.

Schulz K F, Cates W Jr & O'Mara P R. Pregnancy loss, infant death, and suffering: legacy of syphilis and gonorrhoea in Africa. *Genitourin Med* 1987; 63:320–325.

1998 Guidelines for Treatment of Sexually Transmitted Diseases Treatment. *Morbidity and Mortality Weekly Report* 1998; 47:RR1–128.

Chapter 22
Musculoskeletal Diseases

A. O. Adebajo

Musculoskeletal disorders continue to be recognized as important but often neglected conditions in the tropics. These conditions are associated with considerable morbidity and even mortality in the tropics, much of which is preventable. The study of these conditions in the tropics may provide useful aetiopathogenetic clues.[1]

Musculoskeletal diseases are those disorders which affect muscles, tendons, ligaments, joints, the connective tissues and even bone. Not surprisingly many of these disorders in the tropics are of infectious origin (Table 22.1).

Table 22.1 Infectious agents particularly associated with rheumatic disorders in the tropics.

Viruses
O'nyong-nyong
Dengue
Chikungunya
Hepatitis B
Yellow fever
Human immunodeficiency virus (HIV)
Sandbis
Ross river
Spirochaetes
Yaws
Syphilis
Bacteria
Staphylococcus spp.
Salmonella spp.
Neisseria gonorrhoeae
Brucella spp.
Parasites
Malaria
Schistosomiasis
Dracontiasis
Filariasis
Amoebiasis
Fungi
Histoplasmosis
Madura foot

Diseases of skeletal muscle, tendons and ligaments

Primary diseases of skeletal muscle are uncommon in the tropics. Muscle disorders are more commonly seen in association with another pathology, such as prolonged corticosteroids given therapeutically, endocrine disorders such as thyrotoxicosis, and in association with neoplasms such as hepatoma. The low prevalence of polymyalgia rheumatica in the tropics is of interest and remains unexplained.[2]

Polymyositis

Although this inflammatory disorder is uncommon in the tropics it does occur.[2,3] Classical acute phase proteins, electromyographic and muscle biopsy changes are found. However, elevated serum creatinine kinase levels may occur in healthy black males[4] and must be interpreted with caution.

Infective pyomyositis

Pyomyositis is an acute inflammation of skeletal muscle mainly confined to the subtropics and tropics.[5–7] It occurs at any age but most frequently in children and young male adults. The initiating lesion may be a penetrating injury or crush injury or it may be secondary to staphylococcal arthritis. *Staphylococcus pyogenes* is the usual infecting organism. It is possible that pyomyositis arises when the staphylococcus reaches a muscle recently damaged by a viral myositis, but malnutrition and various parasitic infections have also been implicated.

Muscular pain is usually the first symptom, followed within the next week by fever, localized induration and oedema. Any muscle group may be affected but most commonly the proximal limb muscles (gluteal and quadriceps) are involved. The erector spinae and shoulder girdle muscles can also be affected. The clinical features are those of a localized abscess with mild to moderate systemic features. If untreated the condition will progress over the next 4 weeks until there is extensive muscle destruction. Pus can often be aspirated from 10 days onwards. Occasionally the systemic picture predominates and multiple muscle abscesses occur as a late finding. The more acute presentation and occurrence at peripheral sites make clinical differentiation from acute haematogenous osteomyelitis more difficult. There is often a minor degree of polymorphonuclear leucocytosis, and a moderate eosinophilia of about 10% is common.

Treatment involves the administration of an adequate dose of an appropriate antibiotic effective against penicillinase-producing organisms, given parenterally at least initially. Treatment for several weeks is often required and surgical drainage of fluctuant abscesses should be carried out. Despite the destruction of a large muscle bulk, functional and cosmetic recovery is usually remarkably good.

Parasitic pyomyositis

Several parasites can give rise to a myositis.[7] Trypanosomiasis causes an acute myositis, often with encephalomyelitis and myocarditis. The same is true of filariasis.

Soft tissue disorders

Diseases involving the musculoskeletal soft tissues (tendons and ligaments) present clinically in a manner identical to that found in the West. In contrast, however, patients with these problems in the tropics do not usually seek medical attention, as observed with shoulder lesions.[8] Similarly back pain is very prevalent in the tropics, often in association with manual work. The fact that health insurance schemes and compensation claims for injuries are uncommon in many tropical countries may be one reason why only a small proportion of back pain sufferers seek medical attention. These various reasons might also explain why chronic widespread soft tissue pain (fibromyalgia) is less common in the tropics than the West, even when the same ethnic group is compared.[9]

Hypermobility

Hypermobility is due to laxity of the ligaments surrounding a joint as a result of genetic and/or environmental causes (Figure 22.1). Studies on hypermobility indicate that African populations have a higher prevalence of hypermobility than Caucasians, although this prevalence may be lower than amongst populations from the Indian subcontinent.[10–12]

Diseases of joints

Diseases of joints form the bulk of the musculoskeletal disorders and particularly those seen in hospital clinics. Arthralgia refers to significant joint pain occurring in the total or virtual absence of any physical signs. Arthritis, on the other hand, refers to an inflammatory process of the joint lining, with the classical features of redness, warmth, swelling and limitation of function in addition to joint

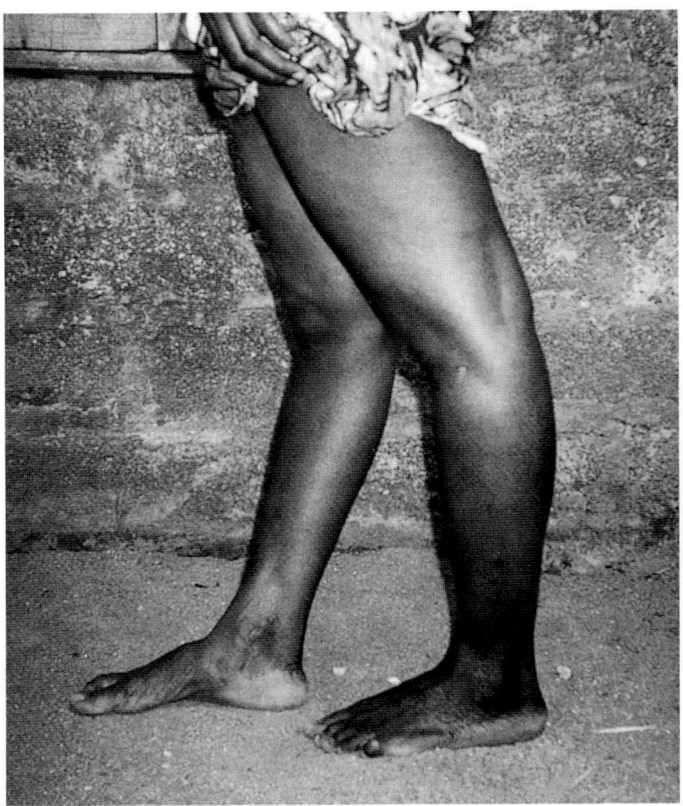

Figure 22.1: Hyperextensibility (hypermobility) of the knee in an African woman.

pain. Arthralgia occurs commonly in association with infectious diseases such as those due to arboviruses. Arthritis can be involved in a number of infective, immunological and metabolic conditions. Treatment usually involves the use of analgesics, non-steroidal anti-inflammatory drugs, physiotherapy and, where appropriate, second-line or disease-modifying drugs.

Rheumatoid arthritis

Rheumatoid arthritis is the most studied rheumatic disorder in the tropics. The disorder is a chronic inflammatory deforming and destructive polyarthritis usually affecting joints, often in a peripheral and symmetrical manner (Figure 22.2). In addition it is a systemic disease affecting various organs and body systems. Rheumatoid factor autoantibodies are frequently found on serological testing and erosive changes are the hallmark of rheumatoid arthritis radiologically. The disorder is a relatively recent condition on the African continent.[13] The cause of this disease is unknown but there is a strong genetic association with the DR4 haplotype. Environmental factors may also be important.[14,15] There is some evidence to suggest that the disease is more prevalent in urban than rural areas.[16,17] In South-East Asia and India the disease appears to be slightly less prevalent than in the West and to follow a milder course, with systemic manifestations

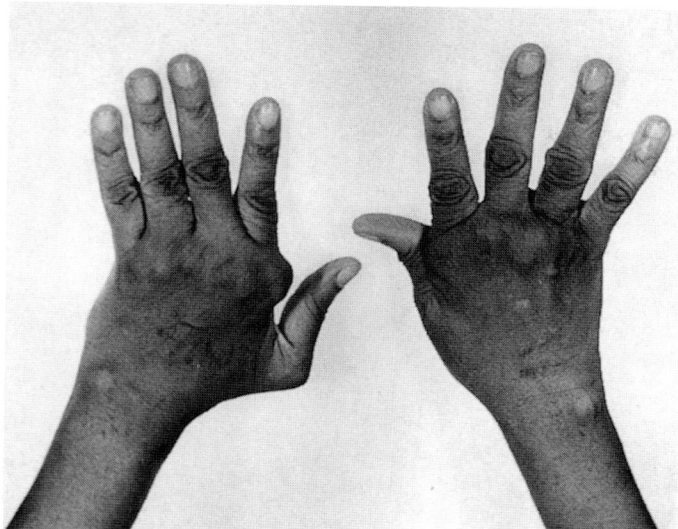

Figure 22.2: Hand deformity in an African woman with rheumatoid arthritis.

and subcutaneous nodules occurring rarely.[18] Interestingly, although the prevalence is seen to be less, morbidity and mortality are higher in South-East Asia, possibly due to socio-economic conditions. In Jamaica there is a high prevalence of the disease but it is mainly mild and rheumatoid factor seronegative.[19] In East Africa and among urban but not rural black South Africans rheumatoid arthritis has a similar pattern to that in Caucasian populations.[16,17,20,21] In West Africa, however, the disease is uncommon and mild.[22,23] A similar pattern has been found in some studies conducted in China.[24,25] In Malaysia rheumatoid nodules and other extra-articular features are uncommon.[26] The treatment of rheumatoid arthritis involves the use of second-line antirheumatoid drugs. Theoretical treatment problems in the tropics include the high prevalence of glucose-6-phosphate dehydrogenase deficiency (sulfasalazine), malaria drug resistance (choroquine and hydroxychloroquine), danger of complicating infections with regular injections (gold), infection due to immunosuppression (methotrexate) and drug costs (cyclosporin and leflunomide). The new antitumour necrosis factor drugs have the dual problems of high cost and risk of infection. Adequate monitoring of any of these second-line antirheumatoid drugs can be difficult in many parts of the tropics and low-dose oral steroids are often the most pragmatic form of treatment. The importance of a multidisciplinary approach to treatment involving physiotherapists, occupational therapists, nurses and others cannot be overemphasized.

Spondyloarthropathies

Spondyloarthropathies such as ankylosing spondylitis are uncommon in Africans[27] and in the Middle East,[28] in keeping with the low prevalence of HLA-B27 in these areas. Ankylosing spondylitis is less common in the Chinese than in white populations[29] but its prevalence

may be higher in rural parts of China.[24] Ankylosing spondylitis is characterized by limited spinal movement and sacroiliac joint tenderness. Peripheral joint involvement can also occur, particularly of lower limb joints. Radiologically, squaring of the vertebral bodies and ossification of the disc margins and longitudinal spinal ligaments resulting in a 'bamboo' spine as well as features of sacroiliitis are classically seen. Physiotherapy and non-steroidal anti-inflammatory drugs are the mainstay of treatment.

Reactive arthritis in general is common throughout the tropics and can be due to a number of organisms. It is commonly associated with *Chlamydia trachomatis* or enteric bacteria such as *Shigella*, *Yersinia* and *Salmonella*. By definition, the organism is not found in the joint in reactive arthritis, unlike septic arthritis. Recent molecular techniques such as polymerase chain reaction (PCR) are enabling particles from organisms to be identified even in reactive arthritis, thereby blurring the distinction between this and septic arthritis. Reiter's syndrome, comprising the triad of urethritis, conjunctivitis and arthritis, occurs predominantly after venereal disease in Africa and in Papua New Guinea.[30–32] Other seronegative arthropathies such as enteric associated arthritis (associated with Crohn's disease and ulcerative colitis), psoriatic arthritis and Behçet's disease are uncommon in the tropics.

Osteoarthritis

Osteoarthritis is a progressive joint disease characterized by destruction of articular cartilage and the generation of osteophytes. Osteoarthritis may be mono-, oligo- or poly-articular in joint distribution. Polyarticular disease is uncommon in many parts of the tropics.[33–35] Heberden's nodes (osteophytes involving the distal interphalangeal joints) are uncommon in Africans and Jamaicans.[36,37] Osteoarthritis of the hip joint is uncommon, in contrast with osteoarthritis of the knee (Table 22.2), among Chinese,[38,39] Africans,[40,41] Indians[42] and in the Middle East.[28] Various sociocultural activities including squatting and kneeling, either in prayer or as a form of greeting, have been suggested as influencing this distribution of osteoarthritis. Developmental knee abnormalities from rickets, trauma or parasitic infections and a low prevalence of congenital hip abnormalities in many parts of the tropics may also determine the joint distribution.

Table 22.2 Hip and knee joint involvement in Nigerian and British patients with osteoarthritis.

Patients	Hip (%)	Knee (%)
Nigerian (Adebajo, 1991)[34]	1.4	47.0
British	19.0	41.2

From Cushnaghan & Dieppe, Study of 500 patients with limb joint osteoarthritis. I. Analysis by age, sex and distribution of systemic joint sites. *Ann Rheum Dis* 1991; 50:8–13.[89]

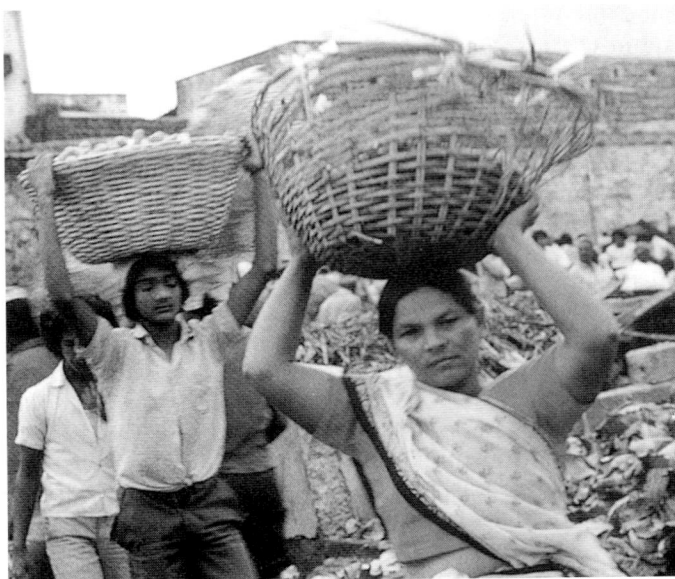

Figure 22.3: Carrying loads on the head is common in the tropics but is not associated with cervical spondylosis in the general population.

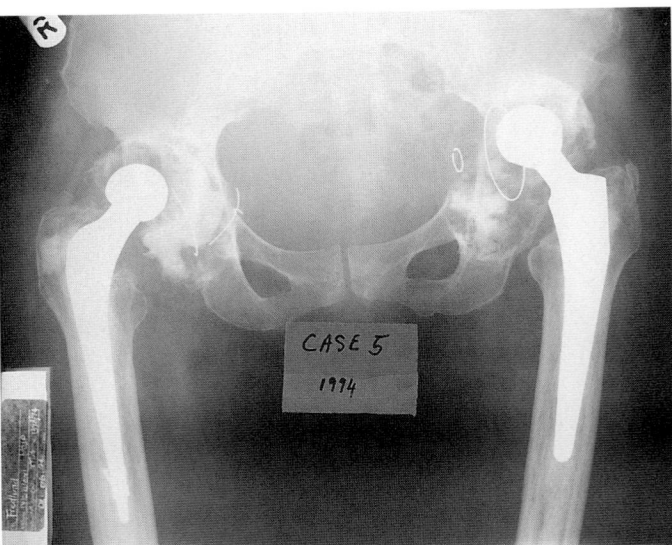

Figure 22.4: Hip joints of a gentleman with Mseleni's disease after joint replacement surgery.

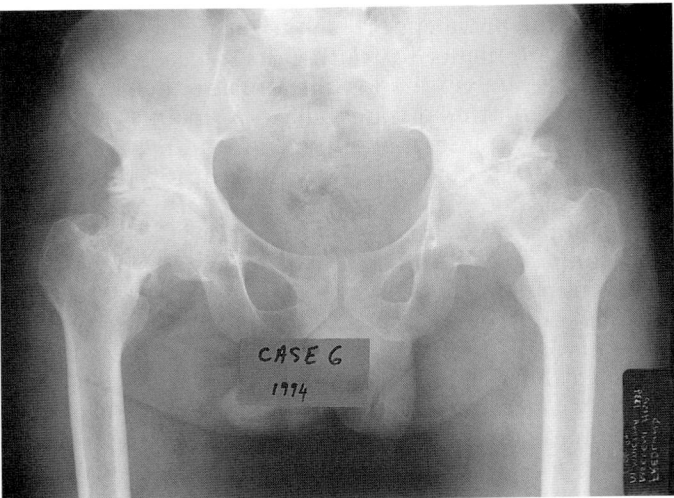

Figure 22.5: Hip joints of a gentleman with Mseleni's disease before joint replacement surgery.

Interestingly, the habit of carrying loads on the head by some populations does not seem to predispose to cervical spondylosis (Figure 22.3). Increasing life expectancy in many parts of the tropics appears to be associated with an increase in the prevalence of osteoarthritis, with a concomitant increased demand for joint replacement surgery. Although joint replacement surgery has been shown to significantly improve the quality of life for appropriate patients, there are still major difficulties of availability of joint prostheses, cost and postoperative care in the tropics.

An interesting degenerative arthropathy known as Mseleni's disease has been observed in southern Africa and was first described in 1970.[43,44] It is believed to be an unusual form of bone dysplasia and resembles dysplasia epiphysealis multiplex. A nutritional deficiency or toxin has been postulated to be the cause of this condition although no environmental factor has as yet been identified. The disorder commonly affects females before the age of 40 years and most frequently involves the hip joint, although other joints—particularly the knees and ankles—can be affected. Laboratory investigations are usually normal. Radiological changes resemble osteoarthritis and, in addition, protrusio acetabuli with deformity and medial subluxation of the femoral head may be seen in the hip joints (Figures 22.4 and 22.5). The clinical course is that of a slowly progressive disability and the treatment is as for osteoarthritis.

Arthritis of bacterial origin (septic arthritis)

Various organisms can give rise to septic arthritis. An acute pyogenic joint infection is one of the most common causes of joint disease in the tropics. It is commonly due to *Staphylococcus aureus*. The hip joints are most commonly affected in infants and the knee joint in older children and adults.[45]

Salmonella joint infections are also common, particularly in those with sickle cell disease. Meningococcal arthritis can occur either as a localized suppurative arthritis or as generalized polyarthritis. Occasionally, the synovial fluid of affected joints may be sterile, indicating that immune complexes could play a large part in the pathogenesis of the disease.[46] Treatment of septic arthritis is a medical emergency involving initially broad-spectrum antibiotics until the specific antibiotic to which the organism is sensitive is known. Where significant pus is present, surgical aspiration is recommended.

Gonococcal arthritis can occur following spread of *Neisseria gonorrhoea* from the urogenital tract. It may

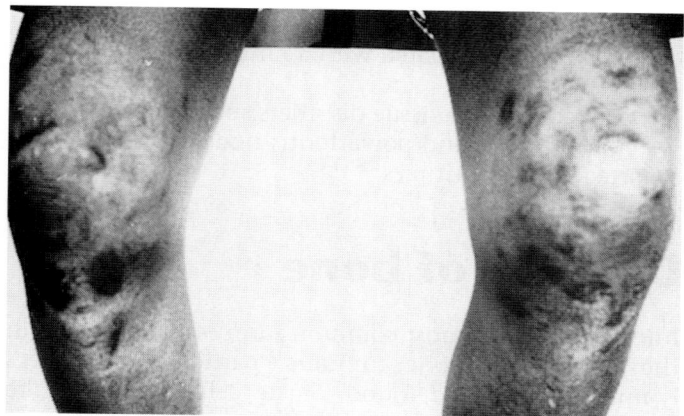

Figure 22.6: Left knee swelling in a young man with Reiter's syndrome.

mimic Reiter's syndrome (Figure 22.6) but, unlike the latter, the organism may be isolated from the synovial fluid on light microscopy and the condition responds to penicillin.

Tuberculosis may affect any joint, particularly the hip or the knee, but is usually monoarticular. There may also be other evidence of tuberculosis but diagnosis is often difficult and may require synovial biopsy. Once the diagnosis of tuberculosis has been made or there is a high index of suspicion, aggressive and appropriate antituberculosis therapy should be instituted. Surgical drainage and even excisional arthroplasty may be required.

Brucellosis occurs either as a local suppurative arthritis or a generalized non-suppurative polyarthritis in many parts of the tropics. Pastoral and nomadic populations are at particular risk.[47,48] As with spinal brucellosis and as with all forms of septic arthritis, treatment comprises appropriate antibiotics and adequate drainage.

Arthritis of viral origin

Arthralgia or arthritis can occur with most viral infections. In addition to such viruses as the hepatitis B virus, the arboviruses are particularly important as a cause of arthritis in the tropics. The arboviral infections include o'nyong-nyong, sindbis, chikungunya, dengue, mayaro and yellow fever amongst others.[49-53] In general, these infections cause fever, a maculopapular or erythematous rash as well as arthralgia or arthritis. Diagnosis is usually made by identifying raised viral titres. Although in a few cases chronic arthralgia or arthritis may persist, the prognosis is usually good and analgesics are the mainstay of treatment.

Arthritis of parasitic and fungal origin

Various parasitic infections may be associated with arthritis, or more commonly arthralgia. Malaria is one of the most common causes of polyarthralgia in the tropics.

Arthralgia and backache may occur as an extraintestinal symptom of amoebic dysentery and may even be a predominant symptom. Dracontiasis, schistosomiasis and filariasis have all been associated with joint problems. Usually there is arthralgia; however, arthritis may occur and the adult worm or larval form may be recovered from the joint fluid. Thus, in general, joint problems in association with these parasites may be due to several possibilities. The arthritis may be due to the invasion of the joint space by the parasite and in some cases discharge of larvae into the joint space, causing an inflammatory synovial fluid with microfilariae and eosinophilia. The arthritis may also be reactive, secondary to the localization of the parasite in surrounding tissues. Thirdly, septic arthritis can occur due to secondary bacterial infection, as can happen with *Staphylococcus* complicating Guinea worm infestation. Onchocerciasis can be associated with disabling back pain.

Fungal infection due to *Histoplasma duboisii* as well as Madura foot may be associated with a periarthritis and even erosive changes.

With all of these parasitic infections, treatment generally comprises symptomatic treatment with non-steroidal anti-inflammatory drugs and the use of the appropriate antiparasitic agent.

Acute tropical polyarthritis

Acute or idiopathic tropical polyarthritis is a condition which has generated considerable interest, as it is still uncertain as to whether it is a homogeneous entity. The declining frequency with which this diagnosis is being made would suggest that the entity is a diagnostic wastepaper basket for acute arthritis associated with unknown or undiagnosed tropical infections.[54-56] The condition appears to affect young adults of both sexes and usually involves large joints. Constitutional features including fever may be present and the erythrocyte sedimentation rate is raised. The white cell count, joint radiographs and synovial fluid analysis are normal. Spontaneous resolution of the condition commonly occurs and treatment is symptomatic.

Crystal arthropathies

Hyperuricaemia and gout are common in some Polynesian islands.[57] There is evidence that in some tropical countries gout is associated with urbanization, although both rich and poor may be affected.[58-60] Gout commonly affects the metatarsophalangeal joint of the large toe. Other joints that may be involved include the ankles, knees and small hand joints. Occasionally, polyarticular gout occurs which can mimic rheumatoid arthritis. Affected joints are acutely inflamed and very tender. Acute attacks may be precipitated by trauma or heavy drinking and thus may recur. Urate deposition into tissues leads to subcutaneous tophi, which is the hallmark of chronic gout. Other complications such as renal stones may also occur. In addition to these clinical features, the diagnosis is made by a raised serum uric acid level and evidence of uric acid crystals in synovial fluid. Radiographs may show areas of bone destruction around affected joints. Colchicine or non-steroidal anti-inflammatory drugs are useful for acute attacks, while xanthine oxidase inhibitors such as allopurinol, which reduce uric acid synthesis, are used to lower the serum uric acid level and thereby prevent further acute gouty attacks.

Chondrocalcinosis or pseudo-gout differs from gout in that calcium pyrophosphate crystals rather than uric acid crystals are deposited in the synovium and tissues. Pseudo-gout has been reported from the tropics.[61]

Connective tissue disorders

Connective tissue disorders such as systemic lupus erythematosus (a syndrome characterized by vasculitis, photosensitive skin rash, fever, nephritis and neuro-psychiatric disturbances, in association with antinuclear antibodies) are uncommon in Africa.[62,63] Systemic lupus erythematosus is, however, common in China,[29] Malaysia,[64] India,[65] Puerto Rico[66] and the West Indies.[67] In Malaysia those of Chinese ethnic origin seem to be more vulnerable to systemic lupus erythematosus than Malays or those of Indian origin.[64,68] It has been suggested that tropical infections such as malaria may protect Africans against connective tissue diseases,[69] perhaps mediated through tumour necrosis factor.[63,70] This hypothesis has recently been developed further through the theory that implicates nitric oxide, of which there are abnormally high levels in malaria-parasitized, asymptomatic individuals (malaria tolerant). Increased nitrous oxide is then protective by minimizing proliferation of autoreactive T cells. This is in contrast to Africans living in the West, who do not have parasite-induced nitrous oxide protection.[71] A simple alternative explanation is that systemic lupus erythematosus and other connective tissue diseases are still being underdiagnosed in the tropics, at least in part due to the immunodiagnostic tests required. Diseases like tuberculosis may also mimic some of these connective tissue disorders.[62] Another problem is that autoantibodies that are usually found in patients with systemic lupus erythematosus may also occur in associ-ation with various tropical infections.[72] Malaria, in particular, has been associated with a range of autoantibodies (Table 22.3).

Other connective tissue disorders such as scleroderma, systemic sclerosis and polyarteritis nodosa have all been reported from the tropics.[20,73–75]

Diseases of bone

Infections are the most common form of bone disease in the tropics but bone tumours, particularly Burkitt's lymphoma, are also found. Sickle cell disease can be complicated by bone lesions in those parts of the tropics where the disease occurs (mainly West Africa and the Caribbean). Rickets is still common in many parts of the tropics, but other metabolic bone diseases are less frequently seen. Congenital lesions of bone are rare.

Infective disease of bone

As with infective diseases of joints, many different organisms may be responsible. Acute osteomyelitis is commonly seen with or without any obvious focus of infection such as skin sepsis. In patients with sickle cell disease *Salmonella* organisms are common pathogens.[45] A chronic infection may develop with the formation of a sequestrum of dead bone, which can act as a nidus for the systemic spread of organisms. Acute infections are treated with antibiotics and drainage, while chronic infections often require prolonged antibiotics and excision of dead bone.

Tuberculosis can affect virtually any bone of the body. Tuberculosis of the vertebrae (Pott's disease) is a common problem in the tropics. The infection occurs most commonly in the thoracic spine, leading to vertebral collapse with a kyphosis. The spinal cord may be affected as a result of direct pressure of inflammatory tissue, or more commonly by occlusion of nutrient arteries. A para-vertebral abscess may track around the abdominal or thoracic wall or in front of the psoas muscle to point in the groin as a psoas abscess. Spinal tuberculosis can be treated on an outpatient basis with antituberculous chemotherapy and, for the few cases where indicated, anterior decompression and fusion.[76]

Osteoarticular brucellosis is a major health problem in South America, the Middle East and the Mediterranean, reflecting the continued existence of the natural reservoir in animals in these regions for the coccobacillus *Brucella*. Humans are secondarily infected through the consumption of contaminated milk. *Brucella* infection occurs most frequently in the lumbar spine but spinal cord damage is uncommon. Large peripheral joint articular pain, often with sterile effusions, is also frequently found. Radiographs show osteolytic lesions with new bone formation. Diagnosis is difficult but brucellosis should be considered in a patient with severe backache and radiological signs of bone destruction.[77] Treatment is with appropriate antibiotics, for example tetracycline or doxycycline for 6 weeks.

Table 22.3 Autoantibodies associated with malaria.

Autoantibody	Prevalence (%)
Rheumatoid factor	22
Antinuclear	30
Single-stranded DNA	10
Antiphospholipid	35
ANCA	< 5

From Adebajo et al., Autoantibodies in malaria, tuberculosis and hepatitis B in a West African population. *Clin Exp Immunol* 1993; 92:73–76.

Arthritis is a common feature of leprosy, with joint symptoms present in up to 75% of patients. Direct joint infection causes joint destruction, possibly worsened by coexisting peripheral neuropathy. Joint inflammation representing a reactive arthritis may occur with *Mycobacterium leprae* not being present in the joints. The polyarthritis can mimic erosive rheumatoid and can become chronic, with predilection for hands and wrists.[78]

Bone tumours

Primary tumours of bone are uncommon, although osteogenic sarcomas may mimic acute osteomyelitis. Secondary deposits often arise from lymphomas or hepatocellular carcinomas.

Metabolic bone disease

Rickets remains a common problem in the tropics and is sometimes related to a poor diet as well as the wearing of purdah by mothers, which may lead to calcium deficiency in their babies (Figures 22.7–22.9).

Blount's disease occurs in parts of the tropics, mainly amongst blacks,[79] and is an osteochondrosis affecting the medial tibial physis, causing tibia vara. Treatment is by tibial osteotomy.

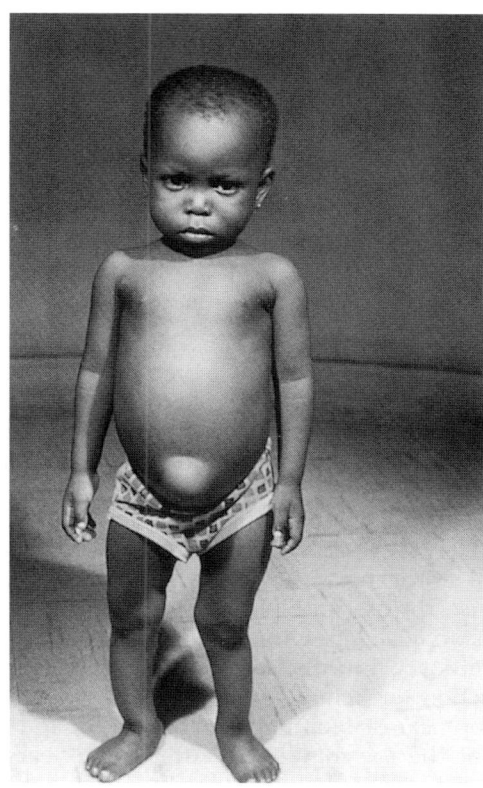

Figure 22.8: Child with rickets showing limb deformities.

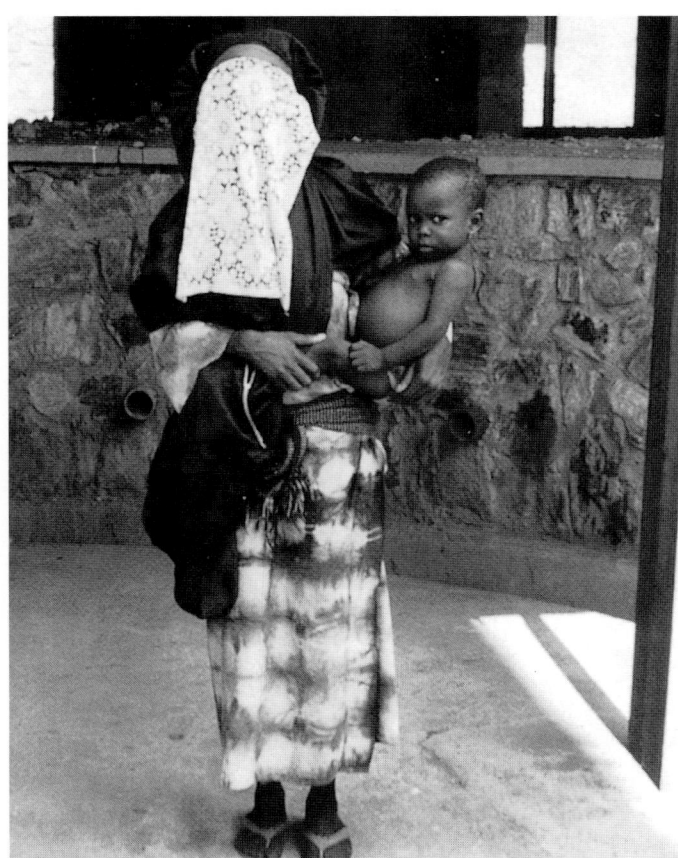

Figure 22.7: A mother in purdah; her child has rickets.

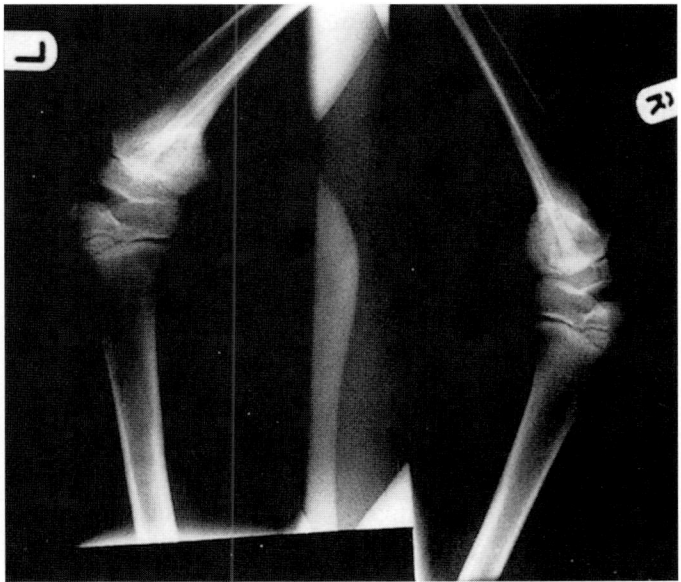

Figure 22.9: Radiograph of a child with rickets.

Osteoporosis is uncommon in many parts of the tropics;[80,81] this may be due to protection by sociocultural factors—in particular exercise.

Other metabolic bone diseases such as marble bone disease and Paget's disease appear to be uncommon in most parts of the tropics.

Haemoglobinopathies

Apart from osteomyelitis, bone lesions associated with haemoglobinopathies include bone crises as a result of infarction of bone(s), as well as bossing of the skull, biconcave vertebrae and dactylitis. Avascular necrosis of the femoral, or less commonly humeral, head is seen in patients with haemoglobin SC or SS disease.

Other bony lesions

Ainhum is a condition in which a stricture slowly develops between the fifth toe and the foot, leading to spontaneous amputation. It has its highest incidence in Africa, especially amongst women of the Transkei in South Africa,[82] but also occurs in people of African descent in the New World,[83] Polynesians[84] and Indians.[85] The aetiology is obscure and is considered as being due to abnormal fibrogenesis,[86] angiodysplasia[87] or a common toxic cause (possibly of plant origin) for both ainhum and phocomelia.[82] It is most common in people who walk barefoot. Clinically, there is a slow development of a constriction encircling the little toe at the level of the metatarsophalangeal joint(s). Pain may occur and the distal portion of the toe may swell. After some years the toe may remain attached to the foot by a fragile cutaneous pedicle only, and at this stage spontaneous or deliberate amputation usually occurs (Figures 22.10 and 22.11). There is no proven treatment for the condition but when troublesome the affected toe should be amputated.

Transkei foot is a disorder consisting of marked lateral deviation of the fifth toe; it has been described in the Xhosa population of the Transkei and is possibly of genetic origin.[88]

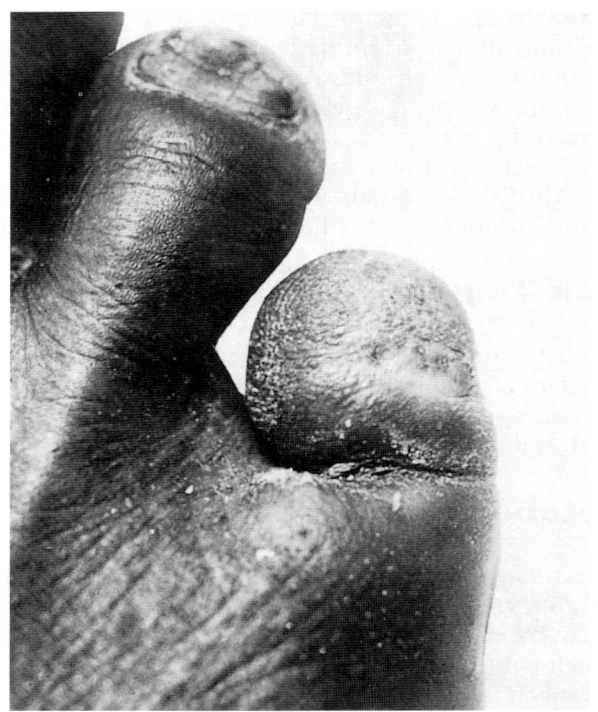

Figure 22.10: Ainhum at its height. (Courtesy of W. M. Meyers.)

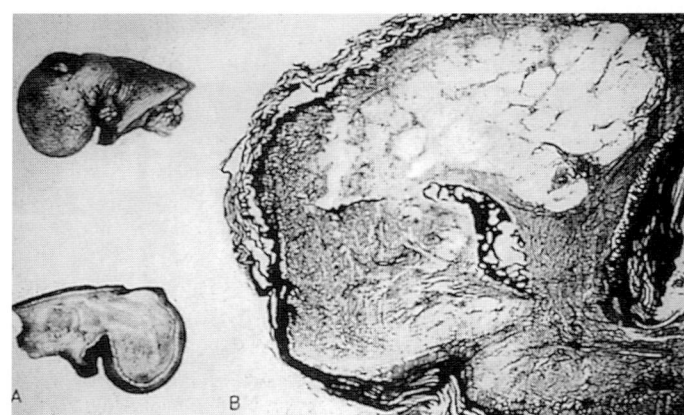

Figure 22.11: An amputated toe from a patient suffering from ainhum, showing constriction at the base. (Courtesy of B. H. Kean.)

REFERENCES

1 Muirden K D. What can be learned from Third World rheumatism. *Br J Rheumatol* 1987; 26:1–2.

2 Stein M & Davis P. Rheumatic disorders in Zimbabwe: a prospective analysis of patients attending a rheumatic diseases clinic. *Ann Rheum Dis* 1990; 40:400–402.

3 Gelfand M & Taube F. Polymyositis in the African. *J Trop Med Hyg* 1966; 69:232–235.

4 Worrall J G, Phongsathorn V, Hooper R J L & Paice E W. Racial variation in serum creatinine kinase unrelated to lean body mass. *Br J Rheumatol* 1990; 29:371–373.

5 Horn C V & Master S. Pyomyositis tropicans in Uganda. *East Afr Med J* 1968; 45:463–471.

6 Levin M J, Gardner P & Waldevogel F A. Tropical pyomyositis. *N Engl J Med* 1971; 284:196–198.

7 Chiedozi L C. Polymyositis: review of 205 cases in 112 patients. *Am J Surg* 1979; 137:255.

8 Adebajo A O & Hazleman B L. Soft tissue shoulder lesions in the African. *Br J Rheumatol* 1992; 31:275–276.

9 Njobvu P, Hunt I, Pope D & Macfarlane G. Pain among ethnic minority groups of Pakistani Muslim origin in the UK: a review. *Rheumatology* 1999; 38:1184–1187.

10 Beighton P, Solomon L & Seskilne C L. Articular mobility in an African population. *Ann Rheum Dis* 1973; 32:413–418.

11 Adebajo A O & Eastmond C J. Racial variation in lumbar spine flexion. *Br J Rheumatol* 1989; 28:13.

12 Birrell F, Adebajo A O, Hazleman B L & Silman A J. *Br J Rheumatol* 1994; 33:56–59.

13 Adebajo A O. Rheumatoid arthritis: a twentieth century disease in Africa. *Arthritis Rheum* 1991; 34:248.

14 Silman A J. Is rheumatoid arthritis an infectious disease? *BMJ* 1991; 303:200–201.

15 Adebajo A O. Is rheumatoid arthritis an infectious disease? *BMJ* 1991; 303:786.

16 Solomon L, Robin G & Valkenburg H A. Rheumatoid arthritis in an urban South African negro population. *Ann Rheum Dis* 1975; 34:128–135.

17 Beighton P, Solomon L & Valkenburg H A. Rheumatoid arthritis in a rural South African negro population. *Ann Rheum Dis* 1975; 34:136–141.

18 Chopra A, Raghunath D, Singh A & Subramain A R. The pattern of rheumatoid arthritis in the Indian population: a prospective study. *Br J Rheumatol* 1988; 27:454–456.

19 Lawrence J S, Brenner J M, Bull J A & Burch T. Rheumatoid arthritis in a subtropical population. *Ann Rheum Dis* 1966; 25:59–66.

20 Lutalo S K. Chronic inflammatory rheumatic diseases in black Zimbabweans. *Ann Rheum Dis* 1985; 44:121–125.

21 Bagg L R, Hansen D P, Mutibuko I K et al. Chronic polyarthritis at the Kenyatta National Hospital. *East Afr Med J* 1976; 53:567–572.

22 Greenwood B M. Polyarthritis in Western Nigeria. I. Rheumatoid arthritis. *Ann Rheum Dis* 1969; 28:488–496.

23 Adebajo A O & Reid D M. The pattern of rheumatoid arthritis in West Africa and comparison with a cohort of British patients. *Q J Med* 1991; 292:633–640.

24 Beasley P, Bennett P H & Lin C C. Low prevalence of rheumatoid arthritis in Chinese. *J Rheumatol* 1983; 10(Suppl.):11–15.

25 Moran H, Chen Shun-le, Muirden K D et al. A comparison of rheumatoid arthritis in Australia and China. *Ann Rheum Dis* 1986; 45:572–578.

26 Toy B H, Sengupta S, Ang A H, White J C & Lav K S. Pattern of rheumatoid arthritis in West Malaysia. *Ann Rheum Dis* 1973; 32:151–156.

27 Chalmers I M. Ankylosing spondylitis in African blacks. *Arthritis Rheum* 1980; 23:1366–1370.

28 Rajapakse C N. The spectrum of rheumatic diseases in Saudi Arabia. *Br J Rheumatol* 1987; 26:22–23.

29 Chang N C. Rheumatic diseases in China. *J Rheumatol* 1983; 10(Suppl.): 41–45.

30 Maddocks I. Reiter's syndrome in Port Moresby Papua. *Br J Vener Dis* 1967; 43:280–283.

31 Hall L. Polyarthritis in Kenya. *East Afr Med J* 1966; 43:161–170.

32 Csonka G W. The course of Reiter's syndrome. *BMJ* 1958; i:1088–1090.

33 Bremner J M, Lawrence J S & Miall W E. Degenerative joint disease in a Jamaican rural population. *Ann Rheum Dis* 1968; 27:326–332.

34 Brighton S W, de la Harper A L & van Staden D A. The prevalence of osteoarthrosis in a rural African community. *Br J Rheumatol* 1985; 24:321–325.

35 Adebajo A O. The pattern of osteoarthritis in a West African teaching hospital. *Ann Rheum Dis* 1991; 50:20–22.

36 Lawrence J S & Molyneux M. Degenerative joint disease among populations in Wensleydale, England and Jamaica. *Int J Biometeorol* 1968; 12:163–175.

37 Solomon L, Beighton P & Lawrence J S. Osteoarthrosis in a rural South African population. *Ann Rheum Dis* 1976; 35:274–278.

38 Hoagkund F T, Yau A & Wong W L. Osteoarthritis of the hip and other joints in Southern Chinese in Hong Kong: incidence and related factors. *J Bone Joint Surg (Am)* 1973; 55:545–547.

39 Gunn D R. Don't sit—squat! *Clin Orthop* 1974; 103:104–105.

40 Ebong W W & Lawson E A L. Pattern of osteoarthritis of the hip in Nigerians. *East Afr Med J* 1978; 55:81–84.

41 Solomon L. Pathogenesis of osteoarthritis. *Lancet* 1972; i:1072.

42 Mukhopadhaya B & Barooak B. Osteoarthritis of the hip in Indians: an anatomical and clinical study. *Indian J Orthop* 1967; 1:55–63.

43 Wittman W & Fellingham S A. Mseleni Unusual hip disease in remote parts of Zululand. *Lancet* 1970; 1:842–843.

44 Yach D & Botha J L. Mseleni joint disease in 1981: decreased prevalence rates, wider geographical location than before, and socioeconomic impact of an endemic osteoarthrosis in an underdeveloped community in South Africa. *Int J Epidemiol* 1985; 14:276–284.

45 Onyemelukwe G & Sturrock R D. Septic arthritis in Northern Nigeria. *Rheumatol Rehabil* 1979; 18:13–17.

46 Greenwood B M, Mohammed I & Whittle H C. Immune complexes and the pathogenesis of meningococcal arthritis. *Clin Exp Immunol* 1985; 59:513–519.

47 Manson-Bahr P E C. Clinical aspects of brucellosis in East Africa. *J Trop Med Hyg* 1955; 59:103–106.

48 Ali-Rawi Z S, Al-Khateeb N & Khalifa S J. Brucella arthritis among Iraqi patients. *Br J Rheumatol* 1987; 26:24–27.

49 Carey D E, Myers R M, De Ranitz C M, Jodhar M & Reuben R. The 1964 chikungunya virus infection in man in Thailand. *Trans R Soc Trop Med Hyg* 1969; 63:434–445.

50 Nimmannitya S, Halstead S B, Cohen S N & Margiotta M R. Dengue and chikungunya virus infection in man in Thailand. *Am J Trop Med* 1969; 17:107–111.

51 Adebajo A O. Dengue arthritis. *Br J Rheumatol* 1996; 35:909–910.

52 Haddow A J & Ellice J M. Studies on bush-babies (*Galago* spp) with special reference to the epidemiology of yellow fever. *Trans R Soc Trop Med Hyg* 1964; 58:521–538.

53 Causey O R, Madbouly H M, Kemp G E & Lee V H. Arbovirus surveillance in Nigeria, 1964–1967. *Bull Soc Pathol Exot* 1969; 62:249–259.

54 Editorial. Acute tropical polyarthropathy: homogeneous entity or diagnostic scrap heap? *Lancet* 1988; i:627–628.

55 Adebajo A O. Tropical polyarthritis. *Lancet* 1988; i:1103–1104.

56 Stein C M. Tropical polyarthritis. *Lancet* 1988; i:1103.

57 Prior I A M, Rose B S, Harvey H P B & Davidson F. Hyperuricaemia, gout and diabetic abnormality in Polynesian people. *Lancet* 1966; i:333–338.

58 Mongola E N & Odeny J W. Gouty arthritis. *Nairobi J Med* 1972; 5:6.

59 Fleischmann V & Adadevoh B K. Hyperuricaemia and gout in Nigerians. *Trop Geogr Med* 1973; 25:255–261.

60 Mody G M & Naidoo P D. Gout in South African Blacks. *Ann Rheum Dis* 1984; 43:394–397.

61 Ducloux M & Lartigau J. Un cas de chondrocalcinose articulaire diffuse chez le noir d'Afrique de l'Ouest. *Bull Soc Med Afr Noire* 1969; 14:451–456.

62 Taylor H G & Stein C M. Systemic lupus erythematosus in Zimbabwe. *Ann Rheum Dis* 1986; 45:645–648.

63 Adebajo A O. Does tumour necrosis factor protect against lupus in West Africans? *Arthritis Rheum* 1992; 35:839–840.

64 Frank A O. Apparent predisposition to systemic lupus erythematosus in Chinese patients in West Malaysia. *Ann Rheum Dis* 1980; 39:266–269.

65 Malaviya A, Misra R, Banerjee S et al. Systemic lupus erythematosus in Indian Asians: a prospective analysis of clinical and immunological features. *Rheumatol Int* 1986; 6:97–101.

66 Mendez-Bryan R, Gonsalez-Alcover R & Roger L. Rheumatoid arthritis: prevalence in a tropical area. *Arthritis Rheum* 1964; 7:171–176.

67 Harris E N, Williams E, Shah D J & De Ceular K. Mortality of Jamaican patients with systemic lupus erythematosus. *Br J Rheumatol* 1989; 28:113–117.

68 Veerapen K, Wong F, Bosco J & Manivasagar M. Systemic lupus erythematosus (SLE): a profile of 419 patients from Malaysia. *Br J Rheumatol* 1988; 27:40.

69 Greenwood B M, Herrick E M & Voller A. Can parasitic infection suppress autoimmune disease? *Proc Soc Med* 1970; 63:19–20.

70 Adebajo A O. Low frequency of autoimmune disease in tropical Africa. *Lancet* 1997; 349:361–362.

71 Clark I A, Al-Yaman F M, Cowden W B & Rockett K A. Does malaria tolerance, through nitric oxide explain the low incidence of autoimmune disease in Tropica Africa? *Lancet* 1996; 348:1492–1494.

72 Adebajo A O, Charles P, Maini R N & Hazleman B L. Autoantibodies in Malaria, tuberculosis and hepatitis B in a West African population. *Clin Exp Immunol* 1993; 92:73–76.

73 Buchanan W M & Gelfand M. Polyarteritis nodosa in the African. *Cent Afr J Med* 1970; 16:274–275.

74 Greenwood B M. Autoimmune disease and parasitic infections in Nigerians. *Lancet* 1968; ii:380–381.

75 Davis P, Stein M, Ley H & Johnston C. Serological profiles in connective tissue diseases in Zimbabwean patients. *Ann Rheum Dis* 1989; 48:73–76.

76 Louw J A. Spinal tuberculosis with neurological deficit: treatment with anterior vascularised rib grafts, posterior osteotomies and fusion. *J Bone Joint Surg* 1990; 72:686–693.

77 Rajapakse C N A, Al-Aska A K, Al Orainey I, Halim K & Arabi K. Spinal brucellosis. *Br J Rheumatol* 1987; 26:28–31.

78 Gibson T, Ahsan Q & Hussein K. Arthritis of leprosy. *Br J Rheumatol* 1994; 33:963–966.

79 Golding J S R & McNeil-Smith J D G. Observations on the etiology of tibia vara. *J Bone Joint Surg (Br)* 1963; 45:320–325.

80 Adebajo A O, Cooper C & Grimley Evans J. Fractures of the hip and distal forearm in West Africa and the United Kingdom. *Age Ageing* 1991; 20:435–438.

81 Solomon L. Osteoporosis and fracture of the femoral neck in the South African Bantu. *J Bone Joint Surg (Br)* 1968; 50:2–13.

82 Daynes W E S. Ainhum: its possible causation by ingestion of plants. *S Afr Med J* 1973; 47:320–321.

83 Kean B H, Tucker H A & Miller W C. Ainhum: clinical summary of 45 cases on Isthmus of Panama. *Trans R Soc Trop Med Hyg* 1946; 39:331–334.

84 Browne S G. Ainhum: a clinical and etiological study of 83 cases. *Ann Trop Med Parasitol* 1961; 55:314–320.

85 Aggarwal N D & Singh H. Ainhum: report of an atypical case. *J Bone Joint Surg (Br)* 1963; 45:376–378.

86 Browne S G. True ainhum: its distinctive and differentiating features. *J Bone Joint Surg (Br)* 1965; 47:52–55.

87 Dent D M, Fataar S & Rose A G. Ainhum and antiodysplasia. *Lancet* 1981; ii:396–397.

88 Schwartz P A, Shlugman D, Daynes G et al. Transkei foot. *S Afr Med J* 1974; 48:961–962.

89 Cushnaghan J & Dieppe P. Study of 500 patients with limb joint osteoarthritis. I. Analysis by age, sex and distribution of symptomatic joint sites. *Ann Rheum Dis* 1991; 50:8–13.

Section 4

Related Specialties in the Tropics

Tropical medicine has traditionally focused strictly on *medical* entities. However, 'medicine in the tropics' encompasses a far wider scenario; special problems arise in certain groups. A high proportion of the population of a developing country consists of infants and children; therefore, it is important that some of the major diseases affecting this group are emphasized and brought to the fore. Surgical conditions are also common, and all too frequently quality care is not available; as a consequence, many cases are not dealt with until the disease under consideration has reached an advanced stage. In addition, inadequate training and inept surgical practice all too frequently result in unfortunate consequences following an operative procedure. Obstetric problems abound; these too are frequently subject to all manner of complications that are often exceedingly difficult to manage with the limited facilities available.

Radiological and imaging services are essential for the proper functioning of health services, although the quality of service varies from country to country. Previous editions of 'Manson's' did not cover the subject of oral health. The importance of oral health as part of general health has now been recognized globally.

Travel medicine is expanding, largely due to the increased frequency of air travel. Disease does not respect international boundaries and travel-associated illnesses represent an enormous burden. The chapter on travel medicine covers the preventive aspects of travel to the tropics. It is essential, however, that the reader takes this section in conjunction with other components within the book where greater in-depth coverage of relevant disease entities—especially those with an infective basis—is to be found.

Chapter 23
Paediatrics in the Tropics

C. Luo, B. J. Brabin and J. Bunn

Children's lives in the tropics and subtropics continue to be threatened by endemic diseases, which in adults often present as mild illnesses. Compared to industrialized countries the under-five and infant mortality rates in developing countries remain high and, in 1998, were between 6 and 11 times higher than those in industrialized countries (Table 23.1). The most affected regions are sub-Saharan Africa and South Asia.

Both infant and under-five mortality rates require accurate recording of births and deaths. In many developing countries this does not happen, and population trends are difficult to follow.[1] The situation is compounded by political and economic instability.

The causes of this excess mortality rate in children from developing countries differ at different ages. In the early years they are greatly influenced by the health of the mother and events during pregnancy and labour. In children under five years of age, seven in ten child deaths are due to diarrhoea, pneumonia, measles, malaria, malnutrition and often a combination of these conditions. In addition to causing high mortality rates, these conditions are also the main reasons for seeking health care for at least three out of four sick children.

Neonatal deaths account for 65% of infant deaths in South Asia and approximately half of infant deaths in Africa, reflecting an urgent need for improvement in maternal health as well as health services and delivery systems. Perinatal mortality rates, i.e., late foetal deaths and postnatal deaths in the first week per thousand live births, are very high in areas where there are poor ante-natal services and deliveries are unsupervised. Maternal ill health, including malaria in pregnancy, other parasitic diseases, bacterial and viral infections including HIV, severe anaemia secondary to poor nutrition, sickle cell disease, rheumatic heart disease, severe malnutrition, hypertension in pregnancy and diabetes mellitus, contribute to still births, low birth weight, premature birth and poor neonatal and infant outcomes. Adolescent health in girls is a neglected area of concern. It is clear that a very high proportion of girls enter motherhood at a young age, undernourished, undersized, underprivileged and uneducated. To make things worse, health services are not sensitive or attractive to the adolescent.

Human immunodeficiency virus (HIV)/acquired immunodeficiency syndrome (AIDS) has, in recent years, emerged as a serious new problem in the tropics, especially in sub-Saharan Africa. Child mortality rates in Africa will progressively get worse due to the HIV/AIDS scourge. HIV infection in children is directly linked to the prevalence and incidence of the infection in women of the

Table 23.1 Regional summary of infant and under 5 mortality rates.

Region	Under 5 mortality rate (per 1000 live births)		Infant mortality rate (per 1000 live births)		Total population (1000s)	Annual births (1000s)
	1960	1998	1960	1998	1998	1998
Sub-Saharan Africa	261	173	156	107	580,939	23,671
Middle East/North Africa	241	66	153	51	324,970	9,227
South Asia	239	114	146	76	1,320,094	35,748
East Asia and Pacific	201	50	133	38	1,837,039	33,054
Latin America/Caribbean	154	39	102	32	498,220	11,441
CEE/CIS and Baltic states	101	35	76	29	475,350	6,413
Industrialized countries	37	6	31	6	847,998	9,830
Developing countries	216	95	138	64	4,702,849	116,297
Least developed countries	282	167	172	107	614,920	23,660
World	193	86	124	59	5,884,610	129,384

Source: The State of the World's Children 2000, UNICEF

Table 23.2 Infant and child mortality rates with/without AIDS by year 2010.

Country	Infant Mortality Rate (/1000 live births)		Child Mortality Rate (/1000 live births)	
	With AIDS	Without AIDS	With AIDS	Without AIDS
Kenya	55.9	32.9	110.3	45.4
Tanzania	90.9	65.2	166.1	95.8
Uganda	86.1	58.5	168.1	92.2
Botswana	66.1	26.3	147.5	38.3
Malawi	126.1	88.4	233.8	136
Zimbabwe	71.0	29.8	202.1	37.8
Zambia	97.0	58.4	152.9	96.9

Source: Stanecki and Way 1997[2]

reproductive age group. It is estimated that 2.4 million HIV-infected women deliver each year, resulting in approximately 600 000 new HIV infections in infants annually or 1600 infections each day.[1] Nearly 90% of children that are born with HIV or infected through breast-feeding are from sub-Saharan Africa, largely as a consequence of high fertility rates, high HIV infection rates in women of the reproductive age group, and limited resources for HIV interventions to prevent mother to child transmission.

It is projected that infant and child mortality rates will increase by the year 2010 due to AIDS, reversing the declines that were occurring in many countries over the past decade. HIV/AIDS is already affecting infant mortality rates.[2] For example, without HIV/AIDS, Kenya would have had an estimated infant mortality rate of 46.9 per 1000 live births in 1997, but the rate was 55.3. Likewise in Zambia and Zimbabwe, the infant mortality rates in 1997 were 25 percent higher than what they would have been without HIV/AIDS (Table 23.2). By the year 2010, the infant mortality rate will be more than 60% higher and in Zambia, nearly half of the childhood deaths will be due to AIDS.

Neonatal tetanus continues to be an important cause of neonatal mortality throughout the tropics. Only about half of pregnant women in developing countries are vaccinated against tetanus (UNICEF 2000), and evidence is accumulating that giving two tetanus vaccinations is not effective in preventing neonatal tetanus in high-risk groups. At-risk infants born in these situations will probably benefit from anti-tetanus serum and penicillin prophylaxis after birth.

Perinatal and neonatal health

Mortality and newborn care

A high proportion of babies die in their first month of life, and many die in the first week after birth. Deaths during the neonatal period account for two-thirds of all deaths in the first year of life, and 98% of these occur in developing countries. Many of these deaths are unrecognized, partly because they are so common. For this reason in some societies the baby is not given a name until it has survived a certain period.

In a typical sub-Saharan setting, about 1 out of every 20 families will be motherless because of pregnancy-related death and maternal deaths due to HIV infection. As a result there are many children from motherless families. These are often orphans of poor perinatal care.

Most mortality and morbidity events in the perinatal and neonatal period are preventable.[3] The causes can be classified as maternal, obstetric, foetal and neonatal. Direct causes of stillbirths include hypoxia during labour, perinatal asphyxia and congenital infections such as syphilis, bacterial sepsis, malaria and HIV. Common foetal neonatal infections include pneumonia, tetanus, sepsis and diarrhoea. Low birth weight (< 2500 g) is probably the most important indirect cause of early infant mortality. Other factors relate to poor maternal health care during pregnancy, inappropriate management of maternal complications or delivery, and lack of appropriate care for the newborn especially the resuscitation of mildly asphyxiated babies.

Improved perinatal and neonatal health will result from interventions starting with adolescent girls in order to improve the health of future mothers. These should aim to improve nutrition, discourage early marriage, improve female literacy and education and vaccinate girls against tetanus. Improved care of the pregnant woman is essential, including: reduction in anaemia, control of malaria in pregnancy and treatment of syphilis, treating pregnancy complications, e.g., pre-eclampsia, counselling on safe delivery and breast-feeding. The mother-baby package offers a minimum list of essential interventions (Table 23.3).[4] The emphasis for these is on the birth attendant who can ensure carefully monitored deliveries and life-saving interventions.[5] Low-cost technologies for the newborn are especially important in developing countries. One of the cheapest appropriate technologies for low birth weight babies is close skin-to-skin contact with the mother. This is the basis of the kangaroo method which can help in reducing perinatal mortality.

Table 23.3 Essential interventions for newborn care.

At birth	After birth
Safe and clean delivery (hand washing)	Exclusive breast-feeding
Clean cord cutting and tying	Maintain warmth
Dry, wrap and keep warm	Clean cord care
Early exclusive breast-feeding	Hand washing
Extra care if needed for resuscitation	Promote immunization and use of vitamin K
Prophylactic eye care	Recognize danger signs
Need to know resuscitation method	Treat infection early

Congenital syphilis (see also Chapter 15)

This is a resurgent problem in tropical countries. Suspicion may arise in high-risk pregnancies, e.g., drug abusers. Other clues include an unexplained large placenta, unexpected previous abortions and/or stillbirths, and ill-defined rashes or ulcerating lesions at unusual sites such as in the mouth, anus or breast. Most infants present at between one and three months with pallor due to haemolysis, hepatosplenomegaly and skin lesions. Such lesions include peeling and involvement of the palms and soles, condylomata lata and perinatal rashes which may resemble a persistent nappy rash. Other features are persistent nasal discharge ('snuffles'), failure to thrive, pseudoparesis of one or more limbs secondary to syphilitic epiphysitis, delayed closure of fontanelles and frontal bossing. Symptomatic newborns are often jaundiced.

The diagnosis of overt disease should not present a real diagnostic difficulty if syphilis is borne in mind. Positive serology in the presence of any of the classical clinical manifestations of congenital syphilis is diagnostic. Radiographic examination of the knees and legs will often reveal distinctive syphilitic pathology in children with indefinite clinical signs or who may be suspected on other grounds of having syphilis. This is particularly helpful when reliable serology is not easily or quickly available.

Where facilities permit, diagnosis should be firmly established by appropriate serological tests, but when diagnostic laboratory facilities are lacking, as is often the case in the tropics, proof of diagnosis relies on response to treatment. Definitive serological diagnosis is usually based on a positive Venereal Disease Research Laboratory (VDRL) test with persistently high or rising titres or a persistent positive fluorescent antibody absorption test (FTA-ABS).

Penicillin is the drug of choice and is recommended in a dose of 50 000 units/kg of aqueous procaine penicillin, by intramuscular injection, daily for 7–10 days. A large dose of a long-acting benzathine penicillin (at least 100 000 units/kg) given once, or preferably twice, a week apart, is recommended when daily treatment is not feasible

or patient compliance is suspect. All children with syphilis should be followed up to ensure control of all symptoms and to monitor serology. Persistence of positive serology six months after treatment is an indication for a further course of treatment.

Congenital parasitic infections

Congenital parasitic infections are unusual, except for congenital malaria. Malaria may be symptomatic or asymptomatic, and in a proportion of cases only cord parasitaemia occurs. The risk of congenital symptomatic malaria is low (< 1%) in babies born to women living under holoendemic conditions. If symptomatic at birth these babies present with anaemia, jaundice and splenomegaly. The diagnosis is frequently missed. Those with asymptomatic parasitaemia at birth may either suppress this spontaneously, or present with clinical symptoms in the late neonatal period.

Congenital infection with African trypanosomiasis has also been described. These infants may remain asymptomatic until the second year of life when they present with neurological sequelae and illness.[6] Congenital infection with South American trypanosomiasis ranges from 2% to 10% in some areas.

Childhood infections
Malaria (see also Chapter 71)

The estimated one to two million malaria deaths each year are mainly due to *Plasmodium falciparum* infections in children under 5 years of age. The clinical picture of malaria in children varies with the endemicity of the disease. Where malaria transmission is low or markedly seasonal, severe disease may occur at any age. Under conditions of persistent year-round transmission (stable or holoendemic malaria), severe disease occurs almost exclusively in very young children who, if they survive, develop a high degree of acquired immunity by 5–6 years of age which is sufficient to protect them thereafter from life-threatening malaria. In early infancy transplacentally acquired maternal malaria antibody provides passive immunity which suppresses, but does not prevent, malarial infection in the infant. Exclusive breast-feeding may protect in a similar way, i.e., not by preventing infection but by reducing parasite density.[7]

In some areas, *P. falciparum* prevalence approaches 100% by 12 months of age. There seems to be a persistent misapprehension that in such areas clinical manifestations of malaria tend to occur *after* 6 months of age. This is not true. Life-threatening malaria can occur in infants under 6 months. Cases may present as early as 6 weeks, the incidence increasing gradually thereafter to reach a peak sometime after 6 months. Fever (usually without rigors), cough, vomiting, pallor and convulsions are the well-known presenting symptoms in childhood. Acute haemolytic episodes causing jaundice are unusual. The serious complications seen when severe infections present late include coma, cardiac failure from severe anaemia, haemoglobinuria and its associated renal problems, circulatory collapse, metabolic acidosis, hypoglycaemia and rarely spontaneous bleeding.[8]

Cerebral malaria

The definition of cerebral malaria in children is the same as in adults: unrousable coma in *P. falciparum* malaria in the absence of an alternative or additional cause for altered consciousness. Peak prevalence occurs at 2–3 years and well-nourished children are more frequently and severely affected than malnourished. The condition is exceptionally rare in kwashiorkor. Clinical history is usually short, i.e., one to two days; convulsions preceded by alteration of consciousness and followed by coma is the most common mode of presentation. Headache and fever are common preceding complaints. The age incidence of 'febrile convulsions', which is 6 months to 5 years, overlaps precisely with the age incidence of cerebral malaria in holoendemic malarious areas, and this causes diagnostic difficulties in practice. Rapid recovery of full consciousness within half an hour of a convulsion virtually excludes cerebral malaria in childhood.

A common clinical finding is hepatosplenomegaly, but not infrequently neither organ is enlarged. Opisthotonos may occur and suggests the diagnosis of meningitis or tetanus. Hypoglycaemia occurs quite commonly in young children and may aggravate and prolong coma if unrecognized and uncorrected. In West Africa a popular traditional remedy for convulsions can cause hypoglycaemia and this is frequently given to children with cerebral malaria. The immediate administration of intravenous glucose is recommended for any child so treated who shows alteration of consciousness.

Case fatality is high (between 10 and 40%), with most deaths occurring within 24 hours. Time from starting of treatment to resolution of coma in children is short (one to two days). If the child recovers, neurological sequelae are few.

Malaria and anaemia

Anaemia is a very frequent and often serious complication of *P. falciparum* malaria in early childhood. There appears to be an inverse correlation between the degree of anaemia and cerebral involvement, i.e., the greater the degree of anaemia, the less the likelihood of cerebral malaria. The main cause of the anaemia appears to be dyserythropoeisis with a maturation arrest at the normoblast stage in bone marrow. Malarial anaemia responds very well to effective antimalarial treatment, but there is a lag period of four to five days before reticulocytosis occurs as a prelude to a rapid steady rise in haemoglobin concentration.

Quartan malaria

In terms of acute sickness, *P. malariae* quartan malaria is the most benign species of human malaria but it has the ability to compromise immune function(s). Quartan malarial nephrotic syndrome is the clinical expression of an immune complex nephritis caused by *P. malariae* which is arguably the most common cause of chronic parenchymatous renal disease in childhood in the tropics. Patients present with classic signs of nephrotic syndrome such as oedema, massive albuminuria, hypoproteinaemia and hypercholesterolaemia but, with few exceptions, do not show a satisfactory response to any form of treatment and eventually die from hypertension and renal failure.[9] The use of corticosteroids in these cases is fraught with danger and is only very rarely beneficial. A decision to try prednisolone in the management of this condition is only justified if the patient is under tight clinical control that enables early detection of adverse effects and withdrawal of treatment if it is harmful.

Management of severe malaria

The management is similar to that in adults.[8] If a child has a convulsion this is usually controlled with paraldehyde, 0.1–0.2 ml/kg body weight intramuscularly (given in a glass syringe), or a slow intravenous injection of diazepam, 0.15 mg/kg to a maximum of 10 mg. Diazepam, 0.5–1.0 mg/kg, can be given intrarectally if injection is not possible. The choice of antimalarial is the same as for adult malaria but weighing of children is mandatory and the dose of antimalarial should be calculated on a body weight basis.

If hypoglycaemia occurs it should be treated with an intravenous bolus injection of 50% glucose (up to 1.0 ml/kg body weight), followed by a slow intravenous infusion of 10% glucose to prevent recurrence of hypoglycaemia.

In children presenting with oliguria and dehydration, careful rehydration with isotonic saline is mandatory, with frequent re-examination of the jugular venous pressure and blood pressure.

Parasitic causes of fits

The main causes of childhood fits, other than malaria, are neurocystercosis and toxoplasmosis. Cysticercosis prevalence is probably grossly underestimated in children with epilepsy living in areas with a high pork consumption. Among 88 epileptic patients (> 15 years of age) in northern Togo (West Africa), 27 suffered from cysticercosis.

Convulsions, intracranial calcification and hydrocephalus in the newborn point to the diagnosis of toxoplasmosis. In later childhood, epilepsy, mental retardation, microcephalus and cranial nerve palsies are other sequelae.

Other parasitic causes of seizures include echinococcosis, cerebral paragonimiasis, African trypanosomiasis and *Schistosoma japonicum* infection.

Measles

Measles is now seldom seen in the Western world, where most children have now received measles vaccination, but it is still widespread in the tropics where vaccine coverage has been patchy and vaccine failures common. It is a disease of the under fives, with many cases in the first year of life and a peak incidence in 2–3 year-old children. The early phases of the disease are the same as classically described, but the rash is not easy to see in dark skins, especially in bad light. A haemorrhagic rash occasionally occurs. Misdiagnosed patients with measles are often admitted to general wards where the disease then spreads to non-immune children with other serious diseases.

In malnourished children, skin desquamation following the exanthem is usually extensive, severe and prolonged for several weeks (Figure 23.1). This is a period of debility and immunosuppression, with many infectious complications and when most deaths occur. Multiple complications are the rule rather than the exception; bronchopneumonia is the most frequent and most important cause of death from measles. Stomatitis and other oral lesions, including cancrum oris (noma), and chronic diarrhoea with fluid and electrolyte disturbances are important complications. Acute measles encephalitis occurs not infrequently and subacute sclerosing panencephalitis occasionally. Activation of primary tuberculosis and miliary or bronchogenic spread are constant risks following measles. Otitis media and skin sepsis are very common, but rarely fatal complications. Chronic otitis may lead to hearing impairment. A necrotizing laryngotracheitis may lead to stridor. Measles vaccination remains the only safeguard against the disease. Megadose vitamin A should be given to children with measles on admission to hospital in areas where vitamin A deficiency occurs, as this significantly reduces the mortality rate. Small frequent feeds are often required with good attention to oral hygiene to ensure nutrition is maintained. Use antibiotics for clear indications. The current Expanded Programme on Immunization rec-

ommendations for increasing coverage remains crucial to improve measles control.[10]

Tuberculosis (see Chapter 57)

In industrialized countries, tuberculosis in children has declined progressively over the decades, although it is still found in immigrants, minority groups and more recently in AIDS patients with immune suppression. This decline is mainly associated with improved living conditions and case management. In developing countries, tuberculosis is a common problem amongst adults and children. Infants, adolescents and pregnant women have heightened susceptibility to tuberculosis. Susceptibility is aggravated by protein energy or micronutrient malnutrition. Tuberculosis is a major problem in HIV-infected adults, but the association in children is unclear from existing literature. Some of the key cohort studies which have followed HIV-infected children for up to 5 years of age found tuberculosis to be uncommon.[11] The number of children seen beyond 2 years of age, however, were very few because of the high rate of early childhood mortality. In addition, the studies did not set out to make aetiological identification of tuberculosis. Autopsy studies have found that tuberculosis is an uncommon cause of death in this age group but only a few studies have been reported.[12,13]

Tuberculosis is discussed in detail elsewhere. This chapter highlights only issues relevant to children. Tuberculosis in children mainly results from primary infection presenting usually as focal pulmonary disease (primary focus) followed by involvement of lymph nodes (primary complex), although tuberculosis can infect virtually all parts of the body. In developing countries where mothers bring their children late to the hospital, children may present with progressive and post-primary disease. Commonly observed manifestations of primary disease include pleural effusion, segmental collapse with consolidation, bronchopneumonia and pericarditis in younger children, and meningitis and bone or joint tuberculosis in older children. Disseminated tuberculosis (miliary tuberculosis) and cavities are usually seen as complications in children with immunosuppression secondary to malnutrition or viral illness such as measles or chickenpox.

The diagnosis of primary tuberculosis is based on a positive tuberculin test and enlarged nodes on chest radiograph with or without pulmonary infiltrates. In older children and adults, a wheal less than 5 mm in diameter that appears after tuberculin challenge is regarded as insignificant, 6–9 mm is likely to be associated with non-tuberculous mycobacteria, and greater than 10 mm is indicative of infection with *Mycobacterium tuberculosis*. Widespread BCG vaccination in infancy creates problems in interpreting tuberculin test results in infancy. After BCG the tuberculin response is usually less than 10–15 mm. A stronger response is suggestive of sensitivity to *M. tuberculosis*. A negative tuberculin test in children,

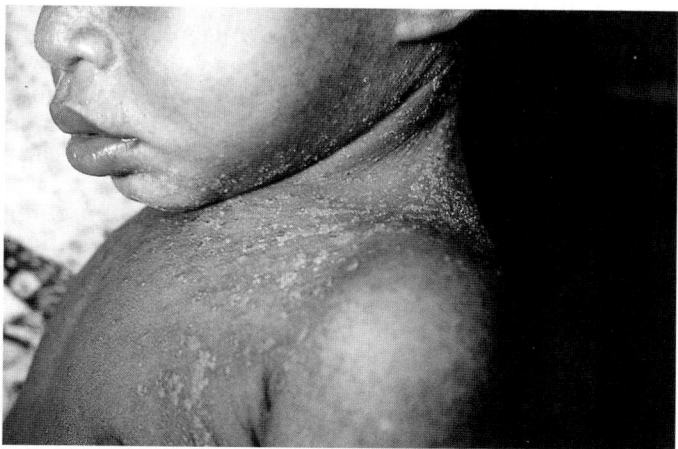

Figure 23.1: Measles desquamation in a Papua New Guinea child.

however, does not exclude tuberculosis. In developing countries the tuberculin response may be negative in malnutrition, miliary tuberculosis, following recent measles, chickenpox, pertussis, kala azar and HIV/AIDS. In infants and young children with clinical evidence of tuberculosis, those with malnutrition or in close contact with a case, an intermediate reaction of 6–9 mm may be significant. When the tuberculin response is negative in children with tuberculosis who are malnourished, it may become positive when the condition improves with therapy. In children with tuberculosis but negative to tuberculin, a BCG response in which local induration occurs within 48 hours followed by ulceration and scab formation has been observed. BCG therefore can be used for diagnosis of tuberculosis. This, however, has to be treated with caution in severely immune compromized children as disseminated BCGaemia may occur.

Specimens for microscopy and culture are usually obtained from gastric lavage, induced sputum or a laryngeal swab. The yield of *M. tuberculosis* from different sources of specimens has been variable. Gastric aspiration performed in the morning in a fasting child on three consecutive mornings is positive by culture in about 40–50% of children with pulmonary tuberculosis.[14] Sputum induction has yielded a positive smear or culture in 28% of patients. Studies comparing gastric lavage with laryngeal swabs have yielded variable results. In a series involving Ugandan children, laryngeal swab cultures were positive in 63% of cases compared to 28% for gastric aspirates. Changes secondary to tuberculosis on chest radiograph include hilar adenopathy, or collapse consolidation, or pleural effusion or miliary opacities. In children co-infected with HIV, radiograph changes may not be typical. For example, HIV-infected children with lymphocytic interstitial pneumonitis (LIP) have many features similar to tuberculosis, resulting in over-treatment.

The treatment of tuberculosis in children depends on the type and extent of the disease. The commonly used drugs are isoniazid (INH), rifampicin (RF) and pyrazinamide (PZA). Isoniazid kills about 90% of the bacillary population during the first few days of chemotherapy. Rifampicin is essential for short treatment (6 to 9 month schedules). Treatment schedules recommended are:

Asymptomatic primary infection: Positive tuberculin test in children under 5, normal chest radiograph – INH for 6 months or INH and RF for 3 months.
Symptomatic disease: Chest radiograph changes of tuberculosis and other supportive features – INH + RF + PZA for 2 months followed by INH + RF for 4 months. In severe disease, four drugs may be necessary. Thiacetazone can cause severe allergic reactions in HIV-infected children and should not be used in areas where HIV prevalence is high.
Tuberculous meningitis: Treatment should be longer. INH + RF + PZA for 2 months followed by INH + RF for 7 months. A fourth drug (ethambutol, ethionamide or streptomycin) can be added if the disease is severe or

the child is wasted. Corticosteroids are of benefit in tuberculous meningitis. Prednisolone or dexamethazone can be given for up to 4 weeks and then the dose can be tapered off over 4 to 8 weeks.

Human immunodeficiency virus

Human immunodeficiency virus infection is a major emerging problem in many paediatric care facilities in some tropical countries. In sub-Saharan Africa, for example, 50% of HIV infections are in women, and paediatric AIDS constitute 15–20% of AIDS cases compared with less than 4% in Europe. Children born from HIV-infected mothers may acquire HIV during pregnancy, labour or lactation. The HIV transmission rate from mother to infant without antenatal antiretroviral therapy has been estimated to be between 15 and 25% in industrialized countries and 20–45% in developing countries. The majority of infants acquire infection during labour.

Risk factors for transmission include high maternal viral load, low maternal CD4 cell count, maternal symptomatic HIV, newly acquired HIV infection, prematurity, vaginal delivery, prolonged rupture of membranes, chorioamnionitis and breast-feeding. Other factors with weaker evidence include viral characteristics, micronutrient deficiency and genetic factors. Risk factors for postnatal transmission during breast-feeding include newly acquired infection, sub-clinical or clinical mastitis, nipple disease including breast ulcers or abscess.

The natural course of HIV in children is bimodal. Some of the children develop HIV in the first year of life probably due to acquisition of infection during pregnancy. These children are known as rapid progressors. Other children survive several years before developing AIDS. Approximately a third will die by their first birthday, half by 24 months and about 80% by 5 years.[15] The diagnosis of paediatric HIV infection should begin with identification of maternal HIV infection during or before pregnancy as most (95%) paediatric HIV infections result from mother to child transmission (MTCT). This allows not only provision of preventive antiretroviral therapy in pregnancy and/or at delivery, but also early identification of at-risk babies for laboratory confirmation of HIV infection. Early diagnosis in the child will facilitate close clinical monitoring and, where possible, early preventive therapy for opportunistic infections and provision of antiretroviral therapy (ART) from early infancy.

In most tropical settings, HIV voluntary counselling and antibody testing (VCT) is not universal. In addition, paediatric infection cannot be confirmed using antibody tests alone under 18 months of age. A positive antibody test in this age group only confirms exposure to maternal infection, as maternal antibodies (IgG) persist for up to 15 to 18 months of age. The DNA polymerase chain reaction (PCR) test, recommended for early diagnosis of paediatric HIV, is not universally available in the tropics. It is expensive and requires both sophisticated equipment and experienced technologists, limited to tertiary facilities or in research settings.

The clinical presentation of paediatric HIV disease in children in the tropics often lacks specificity and usually mimics commonly observed clinical entities observed in children without HIV infection. Without specific clinical algorithms to aid front-line workers and with limited laboratory and other diagnostic facilities, arriving at a paediatric AIDS diagnosis is extremely difficult for most health care providers, especially in primary and secondary facilities, with most paediatric AIDS deaths occurring unconfirmed. The CDC classification was revised in 1994 and is most widely used for diagnosing paediatric HIV infection but is less appropriate for the tropics (Table 23.4). The classification uses CD4+ cell count or percentage as a marker of immune status according to the child's age (Table 23.5). CD4+ cell estimation requires complicated and expensive equipment which most settings in the tropics do not have.

HIV clinical entities observed in children in the tropics do not differ from those in industrialized countries (Table 23.6). For many children the diagnosis is missed, due to:

Lack of laboratory and other diagnostic facilities such as microbiology, virology, echocardiography and radiology.
Clinical entities such as pneumonia, diarrhoea, anaemia, wasting and meningitis are observed frequently in young African children without HIV infection.

For AIDS surveillance purposes the World Health Organization in 1985 defined clinical diagnostic criteria for settings with limited laboratory facilities (Table 23.7).[17] Confirmation of maternal HIV infection with antibody testing was included as a minor sign with the understanding that many health institutions would be unable to perform an HIV test. This definition has major limitations in many clinical settings.

In both definitions, paediatric AIDS is suspected in a child presenting with at least two major signs and two minor signs in the absence of known causes of immunosuppression.

Pneumocystis carinnii pneumonia (PCP) is the most frequent and severe cause of pneumonia affecting HIV-infected infants in industrialized countries.[18] It was earlier reported that PCP was less common in Africa than in industrialized countries. However, both autopsy and clinical studies have shown that the prevalence of PCP is common in sub-Saharan Africa.[19] Clinically, a diagnosis of PCP should be considered in an infant less than 6 months of age with severe pneumonia characterized by marked hypoxia who does not respond to standard antibiotics (ampicillin or chloramphenicol). Laboratory confirmation is difficult. Immunofluorescent techniques on nasopharyngeal aspirates may be useful, but probably underestimates the diagnosis.[19]

Children with HIV commonly present with chronic respiratory symptoms, the cause of which may be difficult to determine. Most of these children have HIV-related LIP, but the diagnosis may be confused with pulmonary tuberculosis because of radiological features of the interstitial infiltrates with hilar prominence. Other causes of chronic chest disease include Kaposi's sarcoma and bronchiectasis and less commonly cardiac disorders.

Rheumatic fever (see also Chapter 7)

Rheumatic fever occurs exclusively in human beings and there are no known animal reservoirs. The greatest

Table 23.4 Paediatric human immunodeficiency virus classification.

Immune category	Clinical Category			
	N: No signs/ Symptoms	A: Mild signs/ Symptoms	B: Moderate signs/ Symptoms	C: Severe signs/ Symptoms
1. No evidence of suppression	N1	A1	B1	C1
2. Evidence of moderate suppression	N2	A2	B2	C2
3. Severe suppression	N3	A3	B3	C3

Source: MMWR Morbidity Mortality Weekly Report 1994.[16]

Table 23.5 Immunological categories based on age specific CD4+ T lymphocyte counts and percent of total lymphocytes.

Immune status Immunological category	Age of the child					
	< 12 months		1–5 years		6–12 years	
	CD4+/mm³	%	CD4+/mm³	%	CD4+/mm³	%
No immunosuppression	≥ 1500	≥ 25	≥ 1000	≥ 25	≥ 500	≥ 25
Moderate immunosuppression	750–1499	15–24	500–999	15–24	200–499	15–24
Severe immunosuppression	< 750	< 15	< 500	< 15	< 200	15

Source: MMWR Morbidity Mortality Weekly Report 1994.[16]

Table 23.6 Clinical categories with human immunodeficiency virus infection.

Clinical category	Diagnosis
N	Asymptomatic or single category A event
A	Mildly symptomatic with two or more of the following: Lymphadenopathy Hepatomegaly Splenomegaly Dermatitis Parotitis Recurrent upper respiratory infection, sinusitis, otitis media
B	Moderately symptomatic but not limited to: Anaemia Neutropaenia Thrombocytopenia Cardiomyopathy CMV infection < 1 month of age Hepatitis Pneumonia Lymphoid interstitial pneumonia
C	Severely symptomatic: Multiple recurrent severe bacterial infection Oesophageal or pulmonary candiadiasis Disseminated coccidioidomycosis Extra pulmonary cryptococcosis Cryptosporidiosis or isosporiasis CMV infection > 1 month of age Disseminated histoplasmosis Kaposi's sarcoma Primary lymphoma of the brain Burkitt's or immunoblastic lymphoma Disseminated or extrapulmonary tuberculosis Disseminated other or unspecified mycobacteria sp. Disseminated *Mycobacteria avium* *Pneumocystis carinnii* pneumonia *Herpes simplex* virus infection > 1 month of age Progressive multi focal leucoencephalopathy Recurrent *Salmonella* (nontyphoidal) septicemia Toxoplasma of the brain (> 1 month of age) Wasting syndrome

Source: MMWR Morbidity Mortality Weekly Report 1994.[16]

Table 23.7 WHO case definition for paediatric AIDS.

Major signs	Minor signs
Weight loss or failure to thrive Chronic diarrhoea (> 1 month) Prolonged fever (> 1 month)	Generalised lymphadenopathy Oro-pharyngeal candidiasis Repeated common infections Generalized dermatitis Confirmed maternal HIV infection

secondary attacks can be prevented by the use of penicillin. The exact incidence is difficult to determine, since many cases may be subclinical. Disease results from auto-immunity as peptide sequences on the surface of the streptococcus are identical with that of collagen tissues in cardiac valves, joints and nervous tissue. Rheumatogenic streptococcal strains are associated with specific M-protein serotypes which can differ substantially in virulence. Clustering in families may reflect close contact and likelihood of spread, and this is one reason why the risk of rheumatic fever is higher in overcrowded conditions. Primary attacks of rheumatic fever are often not preceded by clinical pharyngitis and in about 20% there is no rise in the ASO titre. The site of infection in these children is unclear. The susceptibility of individuals relates to genetic factors and there is renewed interest in this area due to the recognition that gene products of the human major histocompatibility complex are associated with rheumatic fever. Nearly all cases of rheumatic fever possess B lymphocyte allo-antigens before disease onset, and these are normally present in peripheral blood in only 1 in 5 of a population.

In developing countries, improved socio-economic conditions and less overcrowding partly explain the dramatic decline in the incidence since the 1950s where incidence is low (0.2–05 per 100 000). In contrast, the incidence rate in developing countries is high, with rates reaching 10–20 per 1000 population. Recent outbreaks in prosperous communities in the USA in the mid-1980s suggested a change in pattern of streptococcal virulence amongst these communities. The outbreaks were atypical as there was a low rate of isolation of streptococci and outbreaks occurred in widely dispersed areas, in open middle-class communities with no overcrowding. Carditis occurred in almost 90% in one series.

Clinical signs of rheumatic fever are similar wherever in the world the disease is encountered. Mitral valve involvement is commonest with a predominance of mitral regurgitation, especially in younger children. Isolated mitral stenosis in children is well described and occurs at a younger age in children in developing countries. If recurrences are prevented, a large proportion of children with pure mitral incompetence will have no heart disease after a decade. With a first attack about 50% of children will have carditis detectable by auscultation.

susceptibility is after 5 years of age and in adolescents. Group A streptococcal infection always precedes rheumatic fever, and the most convincing evidence that this is the cause of the disease is that primary and

The risk of carditis with recurrent attacks is much higher (> 75%). In developing countries with inadequate prophylaxis, pure mitral regurgitation may progress to severe disease requiring cardiac surgery. These findings explain the high morbidity and mortality rates in less developed countries.

The prophylaxis of recurrent streptococci pharyngitis with penicillin V (125–250 mg orally twice daily) or benzathine penicillin G (0.6–1.2 million units intramuscularly every 3 or 4 weeks according to body weight) is highly effective and should be continued until 25 years of age. Patients with definite valvular disease will require life-time therapy.

Dengue haemorrhagic fever

Dengue virus infection in children may be asymptomatic, an undifferentiated virus illness, a febrile illness characterized as dengue, or the more serious dengue haemorrhagic fever and dengue shock syndrome. The presentation depends on age with overt clinical dengue fever (DF) mainly apparent in children over 5 years old. There is an incubation period of five to eight days following an infective mosquito bite. Clinical manifestations of DF include high continuous fever, headache, periorbital pain, myalgia, arthralgia, a maculopapular rash, leucopenia and occasionally haemorrhage.

The more severe dengue haemorrhagic fever (DHF) with plasma leakage and shock or haemorrhage occurs in individuals who have had previous infection with a different dengue serotype (of which there are four). This severe form therefore occurs mainly in areas where transmission of more than one serotype occurs, and commonly in children between 5 and 9 years of age. Clinical manifestations are the same as those of dengue fever, but in addition there may be evidence of plasma leakage (ascites and pleural effusion), a rising haematocrit hepatomegaly (with abnormal LFTs and clotting) and a low platelet count (<100 000/mm^3). Diagnosis is clinical and the tourniquet test can be helpful. The tourniquet test consists of applying an arm blood pressure cuff to the mean arterial pressure for five minutes, a positive test is more than 10 petechiae per square inch. Confirmation of dengue is usually by serology or positive viral culture.

The clinical course can be divided into a febrile phase (days 1–5), a haemorrhagic shock or toxic phase of one or two days duration (days 4–6), followed by a convalescent phase. The severity of the disease can be graded according to the presence of shock or bleeding.

Grade I: A febrile illness with non-specific constitutional symptoms and a positive tourniquet test.
Grade II: In addition to the above, there is haemorrhage in skin, gastrointestinal tract and other sites.
Grade III: Circulatory failure with rapid weak pulse, small pulse pressure, cold clammy extremities and hypotension.
Grade IV: Profound shock and moribund clinical state with undetectable pulse and blood pressure.

The management of DF and DHF is supportive, with antipyretics and analgesics. It is not advised to use non-steroidal anti-inflammatory drugs. Fluid management is critical to success in DHF, and should be titrated against the haematocrit and clinical condition, to maintain effective circulation during the 48 hour period of plasma leakage. The clinician walks a tightrope in managing DHF, as giving too much fluid may overload the circulation and can precipitate respiratory distress. Mortality rates of < 1% have been achieved in experienced centres, and recovery is almost always complete.

The increasing geographical distribution of dengue haemorrhagic fever has meant that DHF is being encountered by clinicians with no previous experience in its management, with poorer outcomes initially for a disease which can carry a mortality rate of up to 50%. Vector control is the only preventative measure in the absence of effective dengue virus vaccines, and recent outbreaks in South America and Cuba have been curtailed by these measures with variable success.

Acute respiratory infections

This section deals with the causes and management of acute respiratory infections (ARI) in low resource countries, and not the management of upper respiratory tract infections (URTIs).

Of the 10.5 million children aged less than 5 years who die every year, almost one-third of the deaths are due to pneumonia. Up to 50% of outpatient attendances are due to ARI of which two-thirds are URTIs. Some 30% of hospital admissions are for ARI, usually pneumonia. Outpatient management has been simplified through the development of a syndromic assessment strategy and standardized management protocols, which are now incorporated within the WHO Integrated Management of Childhood Illness (IMCI) programme.

Community-based studies from around the globe have shown a similar incidence of ARI with an average of six to eight episodes of ARI per year in urban areas. There is a much higher mortality rate from pneumonia in developing countries, with most deaths occurring in infants. Pneumonia not associated with measles accounted for 70% of the deaths due to ARI, followed by post-measles pneumonia (15%), pertussis (10%) and bronchiolitis and croup (5%) in 1983. This pattern has changed with improved immunization coverage for measles and pertussis, and as HIV-related pneumonia has become more common in certain regions.

Viruses are the primary cause of the majority of ARI, both of the upper and lower respiratory tract. Measles-related pneumonia carries a poor prognosis, and may be due to secondary staphylococcal infection. Respiratory syncytial virus (RSV) infection is seasonal worldwide; however, in most infants and children RSV bronchiolitis is a self-limiting illness. In some communities *Chlamydia trachomatis* is a common pathogen in infancy. The vast majority of bacterial pneumonia (diagnosed through lung aspiration research studies) is caused by *Streptococcus pneumoniae* or *Haemophilus influenzae*. In children around 5 years of age mycoplasma infections also occur. In HIV-infected infants *Pneumocystis carinii* infection is not uncommon, although most ARI remains due to organisms which normally cause community-acquired pneumonia. Children with severe malnutrition may also be infected with Gram-negative organisms such as *Salmonella, Pseudomonas, Klebsiella* and *Escherichia coli*. In infants under 2 months of age Gram-negative organisms are common. Factors that increase the incidence and severity of pneumonia include: young age, low birth weight, malnutrition, lack of breast-feeding, indoor smoke, and underlying disease.

The diagnosis of ARI and pneumonia is predominantly clinical, and with the promotion of IMCI, initiation of treatment on syndromic criteria is appropriate. Children usually present with cough and/or difficulty in breathing. Fever is common but not specific. It is important to identify the child with pneumonia who requires antibiotics and possibly hospital admission. A raised respiratory rate is consistently the most reliable clinical sign for pneumonia. More severe pneumonia is indicated by respiratory distress, with chest indrawing and possibly cyanosis or other 'danger signs'. These clinical signs of pneumonia have a lower predictive value in infants under 2 months, who may present with poor feeding, grunting, apnoea or hypothermia. Auscultation of the chest is often not helpful, especially in the young.

Chest radiographs are unreliable in differentiating viral from bacterial pneumonia, so do not generally help to determine specific treatment. They are best reserved for management failures and chronic cough. Blood cultures have a consistently low yield, and although nasopharyngeal culture may reflect the likely pathogen causing pneumonia in the community, it does not necessarily indicate the pathogen causing disease in an individual child. Lung aspiration remains a research tool.

Early treatment of pneumonia with appropriate antibiotics significantly reduces the morbidity and mortality rate attributed to ARI in developing countries. The choice of antibiotic for cases of pneumonia will depend on many factors, including drug availability, the likely aetiology, and the child's age and nutritional status. For children from 2 months up to 5 years of age, cotrimoxazole or amoxycillin are appropriate for the out-patient treatment of pneumonia, and for severe pneumonia parenteral benzylpenicillin (or ampicillin), changing to chloramphenicol if there is no improvement after 48 hours. Depending on the likely aetiology, a macrolide, cloxacillin, or for children under 2 months old or with malnutrition, gentamicin may be added. Oxygen concentrators (and pulse oximetry) are becoming more widely available, and oxygen should be given to children with severe indrawing, respiratory rates above 70/minute, or who are hypoxic.

Children with HIV should receive the same first-line antibiotics as above. For *Pneumocystis carinii* interstitial pneumonitis (PCP), which typically presents in the first 6 months of life with severe respiratory distress, severe persistent hypoxia, treatment should be with high-dose cotrimoxazole. The prognosis of PCP infection in HIV remains poor, particularly without intensive respiratory support.

Pertussis

Pertussis (whooping cough) occurs worldwide; the causative agent, *Bordetella pertussis,* is spread mainly by aerosol droplet. Infection with the related *B. parapertussis* and *B. bronchiseptica* cause a similar illness.

The typical illness occurs classically in three stages, commencing with a 1–2 week coryzal stage clinically indistinguishable from other URTIs. This is followed by a 2–4 week paroxysmal stage when paroxysms of coughing (up to ten staccato-like coughs) are followed by the characteristic high-pitched inspiratory whoop. Coughing may be followed by vomiting in younger children, cyanosis, apnoea and convulsions. With poor feeding and vomiting, rapid weight loss may be a problem, and rectal prolapse, subconjunctival haemorrhages and ulceration of the frenulum can occur. A convalescent stage usually of 1–2 weeks follows, but coughing can last for months and may be precipitated by intercurrent URTIs. The Chinese termed pertussis the '100 day cough'. In infants, classical disease is less common, and pertussis may present with apnoea, bradychardia, seizures or atypical cough with poor feeding.

Where available, a pernasal swab plated onto a Bordet-Gengou medium will confirm the diagnosis, but may not be positive in the paroxysmal stage of illness, when the clinical presentation is more helpful. The diagnosis is supported by finding blood lymphocytosis which occurs in the second to fifth weeks.

Management is mainly supportive, although erythromycin 50 mg/kg/day for 10–14 days if given during the catarrhal stage may shorten the clinical course. This is of most use in contacts that develop a coryzal illness. Prevention of paroxysms is best achieved by avoidance of the triggers and there is little benefit from cough suppressants or sedatives. Oxygen may be helpful and in infants may reduce apnoeic events. Maintenance of nutrition and hydration is important. Pneumonia is the commonest complication and may be from secondary bacterial infection or aspiration. Atelectesis due to obstruction of airways by tenacious secretions can occur and is often only apparent on radiography. Subsequent bronchiectasis may result. Encephalopathy is well recognized, and may be due to hypoxic brain injury, intracranial haemorrhage or toxin.

Treating cases with erythromycin and vaccinating unimmunized siblings may reduce transmission. Acellular and whole cell vaccines are both effective in preventing disease, with the more expensive acellular vaccine having fewer adverse reactions.

Diphtheria (see Chapter 65)

Diphtheria may occur as a mild or life-threatening illness

usually presenting in young children, and before vaccination was available had epidemic cycles with 2–4 year intervals. Epidemics still occur in parts of Africa, South-East Asia and the newly independent states of the former Soviet Union.

A child with early tonsilar diphtheria may not appear ill initially, but within a few days may become very toxic with extensive membrane formation. All children with diphtheria require management in hospital. Nasal diphtheria, commonest in infants, may initially resemble a common cold with nasal discharge slowly becoming serosanguinous and then mucopurulent. Tonsilar and pharyngeal diphtheria tend to be more severe forms of disease, and within 1–2 days a patch or patches of grey-yellow membrane may cover the tonsils and pharyngeal walls, which may then extend to the uvula, soft palate or larynx and trachea. Acute airways obstruction may resemble viral 'croup' in infants. Cervical lymphadenitis is variable and when associated with soft tissue oedema, gives the appearance of a 'bull neck'. Bleeding diatheses (usually nasal) is associated with a poorer prognosis.

Complete heart block and myocarditis are not uncommon, and develop after the first week of illness. Neuropathy occurs between two and ten weeks into the illness, often when the child is getting better, and is reversible. Soft palatal paralysis occurs most commonly. Paralysis of the diaphragm and a bilateral and usual motor peripheral neuropathy may also occur. Cutaneous diphtheria is not uncommon in warmer climates, and can lead to immunity in children, and is one of the causes of tropical ulcer.

Mortality from diphtheria increases with delayed administration of antitoxin, so treatment (following a test dose) should be started on clinical suspicion of disease. Penicillin or erythromycin will render most patients non-infectious within 24 hours, although resistance has been reported.

Prevention of diphtheria is by immunization, and although immunized persons can be infected by toxin-producing strains of diphtheria, systemic manifestations of diphtheria do not occur. Immunity may wane with time, particularly in communities where diphtheria is no longer present.

Common childhood disease entities in the tropics
Meningitis

Meningitis is discussed in more detail in chapter 56. This chapter will highlight some of the differences in children. Bacterial meningitis occurs at all ages in children but aetiological pathogens will depend on age. During the neonatal period the main pathogens are group B streptococcus, *E. coli*, *Streptococcus pneumoniae* and less commonly *Haemophilus influenzae* and *Listeria monocytogenes*. In early childhood (up to 5 years) *H. influenzae*

is the most common pathogen, but later *Neisseria meningitidis* predominates. In HIV/AIDS-affected children non-typhoidal *Salmonella* and tuberculous meningitis are becoming increasingly common, whereas cryptococcal meningitis which is commonly observed in adults, is rare.

Symptoms and signs of meningitis in children are also age specific. In young infants the symptoms do not differ from those of generalized illness. Early features consist of irritability, refusal of feeds, vomiting and convulsions. In less industrialized tropical countries mothers are likely to bring their young infants to the doctor late in the illness, with a high-pitched cry, neck stiffness and a bulging fontanelle. Older children present with headache, neckache, nausea, photophobia and projectile vomiting. Meningeal signs of neck stiffness (Kernigs) may be more prominent at an early stage in older children.

Meningitis should be confirmed by a lumbar puncture. The risk of coning is higher in children with repeated convulsions or papillodoema. In facilities with no microbiological facilities gram stain can still be very useful. The antibiotic regimen will depend on the age of the child, since aetiological pathogens are age specific. Penicillin will cover meningococcal and streptococcal infection; chloramphenicol will cover *H. influenzae* and ampicillin, *H. influenzae* and *L. monocytogene*. Third generation cephalosporins can be used if available. Dexamethasone is a recommended adjunct therapy for *H. influenzae* meningitis to dampen the inflammatory response and hence reduce neurological sequelae such as deafness.[20] There is no conclusive evidence of added benefit of dexamethasone treatment in meningococcal and pneumococcal meningitis.

The mortality rate is high in meningitis and it is mainly due to pneumococcal meningitis. In Africa, pneumococcal case fatality in 17 studies was 45%; 29% for *Haemophilus influenzae* meningitis in 20 studies; and 8% for meningococcal meningitis in 14 studies.[21] Sequalae to meningitis are frequent in the form of deafness (*H. influenzae*), hydrocephalus or cerebral palsy in infants, nerve palsies and blindness.

Diarrhoeal diseases

Acute gastroenteritis is a major cause of morbidity and mortality, with more than one billion cases and four million deaths annually in the developing world. Children in the tropics can have up to ten diarrhoeal episodes per year. Deaths in these children are usually due to dehydration, with most of these children reporting late to a health facility. There are many pathogens causing diarrhoea. The importance of the different viral, bacterial and protozoal enteropathogens differs according the age of the child, geographical location and whether the diarrhoea is acute or chronic. The type of pathogen isolated also depends on the timing and duration of the study as well as the sensitivity and spectrum of tests used for isolation.

The most frequent causes of diarrhoea in infants and children are viruses, with rotavirus as the most common. It is estimated that severe diarrhoea due to rotavirus is responsible for between 600 000 and 870 000 deaths in children under 5 years of age each year and accounts for 40% of all dehydrating diarrhoea. In tropical countries rotavirus produces epidemics in the hot dry seasons. The diarrhoea lasts for an average of six days, but duration can be longer.

Bacterial gastroenteritis is the second commonest cause of diarrhoea. *E. coli* is the mot important group, followed by *Campylobacter spp. Shigella* and *Salmonella* species. Enteropathogenic *E. coli* (EPEC) is associated with diarrhoea in infants, sometimes occurring in outbreaks, although infection may be asymptomatic. Enteroadherent *E. coli* causes persistent diarrhoea in malnourished children and enterotoxigenic *E. coli* (ETEC), travellers diarrhoea in the all age groups. Enterohaemorrhagic *E. coli* 0157 is well known for causing outbreaks associated with uncooked meat. It is associated with haemolytic uraemic syndrome in industrialized countries normally due to *Shigella dysentriae* type 1 in tropical countries. *Campylobacter jejuni* invades the ileum and large bowel and is often associated with abdominal pain and bloody diarrhoea. It is normally spread by chickens or dogs, and most children acquire immunity by the first year of life. *Salmonella* invade the ileum and may be associated with a secretory diarrhoea or dysentery like illness. In children bacteraemia may occur. *Vibrio* infection may be endemic or epidemic.

Giardia lamblia is a frequently isolated parasite. It is an important cause of diarrhoea in malnourished children, but its relative importance in well-nourished children or HIV-infected children is unclear. *Cryptosporidium parvum* is commonly seen in HIV-infected children with wasting disease and chronic diarrhoea.

Persistent diarrhoea (> 14 days) is associated with young infants especially under one year, poorly managed acute gastroenteritis, malnutrition, EPEC, cryptosporidium infection, micronutrient deficiency, lack of breast-feeding and lactose intolerance. It may be associated with infections such as tuberculosis, or measles.

Comprehensive stool microbiology is complex, expensive and unavailable in most clinical laboratories. Fortunately, an aetiologic diagnosis is not necessary for the management of most acute gastroenteritis, even though it might be important for epidemiologic or research purposes. Most diarrhoea will resolve without the use of antibiotics. The diarrhoeal diseases requiring antibiotics usually belong to the dysenteric group. Patients belonging to this group should have a stool culture where possible. Stool microscopy, which is more widely available, is necessary to identify intestinal parasites such as *G. lamblia* for which antimicrobial treatment is of benefit.

The approach to management in most cases is aimed at preventing and treating dehydration and malnutrition. The emphasis is on oral rehydration therapy (ORT) and continued feeding. Accurate assessment of hydration status is important, since most subsequent management is based on this parameter. Children with no signs of dehydration are managed at home with continuation of routine feedings and increased fluid intake. In this situation there is no preference for the fluids used, but in general those with increased sugar content should be avoided since they are likely to increase the severity and duration of diarrhoea. Children with some dehydration should receive 50–100 ml/kg body weight of oral re-hydration solution (ORS) at a health facility for 4–6 hours with periodic re-evaluation to assess response to treatment and amount of ongoing fluid losses. The use of intravenous fluids with Ringer's lactate should be reserved for children with severe dehydration.

Limitations for use of ORT include severe dehydration with shock, persistent vomiting that interferes with rehydration, high stool output, and abdominal distension. It should also be noted that recent studies indicated that reduced osmolarity rehydration solution is more effective than standard WHO rehydration solution. It has been shown to reduce the need for intravenous fluids, stool output and vomiting during rehydration. There is evidence to indicate that 80% of babies can tolerate full-strength lactose-containing formulas safely.[22] Caution should taken, however, for severely dehydrated children. Antidiarrhoeals such as opium and kaolin are of no value and may cause abdominal distension. Drugs such as loperamide are not recommended for children.

Nutritional deficiences

Anaemia

Iron-deficiency anaemia

Iron-deficiency anaemia continues to be the most common nutrient deficiency in the world, with peak prevalence at 6–24 months. Prevalence in young children in low socio-economic groups is frequently 50–70% of those examined. The main causes relate to poor dietary intake, low bio-availability of iron, blood loss caused by intestinal parasites and high requirements for iron in growing infants. Healthy breast-fed, normal birth weight babies are unlikely to become iron-deficient before 6 months of age. Iron stores at birth are reduced in premature babies and, because of their high growth rate, anaemia usually occurs as early as 1–3 months of age. Infants fed cow's milk from an early age are prone to anaemia as this is a poor source of iron and increases intestinal blood loss. Iron-deficiency in the first year of life delays psychomotor development and these deficits may persist into childhood. These findings are of importance because they indicate that behavioural deficit in children may relate to the early onset of iron-deficiency in infants.

Therapeutic doses of oral iron are usually given as 3 mg/kg/day in three divided doses and the importance of ensuring a response to treatment should be emphasised.[23] Clinical and dietary history and examination of the child, blood film and red cell indices should provide the diagnosis. If there is doubt, a therapeutic trial of iron should be given, together with dietary advice.

Folate-deficiency anaemia

Folate deficiency occurs much more frequently in children in tropical countries than elsewhere. It is a well-recognized complication of kwashiorkor, sickle cell anaemia and other inherited haemolytic anaemias, goat's milk feeding in infancy, and malabsorption from many causes. Low birth weight babies are very susceptible to folate deficiency, which should be suspected when these infants become anaemic and fail to thrive. Folate deficiency can cause persistent diarrhoea in infancy. Routine administration of folic acid, 400 µg daily, is recommended for the following conditions in childhood: sickle cell anaemia, thalassaemia and other inherited haemolytic anaemias; kwashiorkor; low birth weight babies; and children receiving long-term medication with drugs that have significant antifolate activity. Folate deficiency usually responds rapidly to treatment but megaloblastic anaemia in kwashiorkor may prove an exception.

Vitamin A deficiency

Deficiency of vitamin A is now widely recognized as a risk factor for child mortality in areas where xerophthalmia is a problem. This conclusion is based on the results of several intervention trials in which vitamin A was administered prophylactically to young children in doses of 200 000 IU every four to six months.[24] The severity of illness episodes, especially diarrhoeal disease, is reduced following such supplementation. In severe measles there is good evidence for a protective effect as children who received 400 000 IU recover more rapidly from pneumonia and diarrhoea. These benefits are also reported in children with measles who have subclinical deficiency of vitamin A.

Vitamin A supplementation is effective in preventing xerophthalmia. Xerophthalmia pre-eminently affects the young child (1–5 years), and not so much the infant, who may be partially protected by prolonged breast-feeding. The clinical classification of xerophthalmia is shown in Table 23.8 and a pigmented Bitot's spot and xerotic patch in Figure 23.2.

Table 23.8 Clinical classification of xerophthalmia.

Ocular sign	Classification
Night blindness	XN
Conjunctival xerosis	X1A
Bitot spot	X1B
Corneal xerosis	X2
Corneal ulcer/keratomalacia	X3
Corneal scar	XS
Xerophthalmia fundus	XF

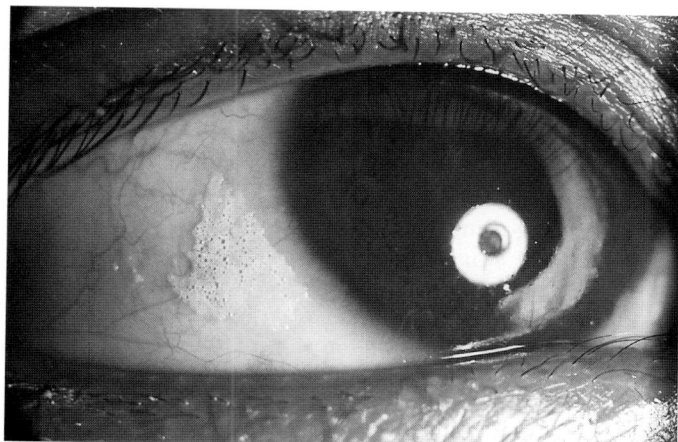

Figure 23.2: Pigmented Bitot spot.

Vitamin A is the treatment of choice for xerophthalmia, as recommended by the World Health Organization (WHO). It is usually prescribed in the form of retinyl palmitate or acetate in an oily solution, 200 000 IU orally immediately on diagnosis, repeated a day later and again four weeks later, or sooner if there is clinical deterioration. If there is vomiting or severe diarrhoea, 100 000 IU water-miscible vitamin A by intramuscular injection is preferred. In babies weighing under 8 kg and/or less than 1 year old, half of these doses should be given.

In discussing the prevention of nutritional blindness we have to be aware that the affection is easily curable without ophthalmological skills, that the survivor of the corneal stages, if untreated or if treated too late, will be blind, and that the medicinal cure is cheap. Promotional measures should encourage the use of green leafy vegetables which are an excellent underutilized, inexpensive source of vitamin A in food.

Micronutrient deficiencies

Rickets (see also Chapter 31)

Nutritional rickets occurs primarily in countries where for religious and/or social reasons, women and children are not exposed to the sun. It is quite common in Pakistan, Egypt, Somalia, Ethiopia the Middle East and West Africa, but is considered rare in East Africa, but is well described in Nigeria.

It commonly presents between 6 and 18 months of age and is increasingly recognized in very low birth weight babies. Rickets is a disease of growth and is infrequent therefore in severe PEM. Diagnosis is straightforward. The child may appear well nourished but restless and pale and a history of diarrhoea or respiratory infection may be given. Head sweating is common. Motor development is delayed, with poor linear growth. Infantile tetany may occur. Characteristic bony lesions in infancy include craniotabes, delayed closure of the fontanelles, delayed dentition, and epiphyseal enlargement best seen in the wrists and costochondral junctions. Bossing of the head, bow legs, knock knees and other limb deformities are common features in older children. Clinical diagnosis is confirmed by wrist radiographs and serum chemistry, which always shows raised alkaline phosphatase and depressed phosphate levels. Therapeutic vitamin D dose varies from 1500 to 5000 IU/day for 2–3 months, and the prophylactic dose is 400–600 IU/day. Where compliance with the long-term daily medication is poor and follow-up difficult, a single massive dose of vitamin D may be given by injection. This practice is quite common in the Middle East where the danger now exists that 'shopping around' for treatment may result in children receiving multiple doses of 100 000–200 000 IU of vitamin D. Breast milk may contain sufficient vitamin D to protect infants, but supplementation is required in high-risk infants, for those whose mothers keep them up out of the sun and for those whose diet is a poor source of calcium.[25]

Zinc deficiency

Zinc deficiency has a range of manifestations depending upon the severity of the restriction of the nutrient. Mild zinc deficiency would not be detected on clinical examination. Growth retardation and delayed development in children is one manifestation and it is recognized as having an important role in PEM, when it may contribute to frank failure to thrive. Zinc deficiency has dermatological manifestations ranging from mild generalized drying to a specific hyperkeratosis in the areas of pressure and stress points. Diarrhoea may be present. There is laboratory evidence of immunosuppression. Diets rich in fibre and phytate may contribute to a reduced zinc status in many rural tropical populations. The consumption of zinc from breast milk is below recommended intakes, but there is a high efficiency of absorption. Rich sources of zinc include whole grains, poultry, lamb, liver, leafy and root vegetables.

Selenium deficiency

Evidence that selenium deficiency was responsible for human disease was reported when its association with a cardiomyopathy in Chinese children and women of child-bearing age was described. Oral supplementation with selenium is of value in preventing the disease. It has been shown that myxoedematous cretinism, which occurs in regions of endemic goitre in tropical Africa, is related to a combined deficiency of selenium and iodine.

Interaction of nutrition and infection (see also Chapter 31)

Poor diets result in nutritional deficiencies associated with frequent infections and malnutrition. Malnutrition has a direct negative effect on the immune system leading to increased morbidity and mortality. Infection is a major force in the development of kwashiorkor. During weaning infections are more common, especially diarrhoea and respiratory infection and each infection results in growth faltering through energy depletion. Catch-up growth is usually incomplete and can lead through cumulative effects to severe malnutrition. The nutritional deficits from sequential infections accumulates, and a viscious cycle of infection-malnutrition results. These deficits are compounded by specific micronutrient and vitamin deficiencies. Nutrient supplementation of malnourished children may also alter infection risk. For example, iron supplementation may slightly increase the risk of malaria parasitaemia.[26]

Integrated management of childhood illnesses

In 1995, 11.6 million children under 5 years of age died in developing countries, with 70% of these deaths being due to ARI (mostly pneumonia), diarrhoea, measles, malaria or malnutrition, or a combination of these.[27] Most of these deaths would be averted if preventative measures and appropriate management were available at community level. At this level diagnostic support services such as radiology or laboratory services are minimal or not available, however despite this the majority of children can be allocated appropriate therapy using a syndromic approach to clinical assessment. For example, pneumonia requiring antibiotics or hospital admission can be identified with a high degree of sensitivity and reasonable specificity using a combination of a raised respiratory rate (age related), chest indrawing and the presence of 'danger signs'. Using this approach, children with fast breathing and fever may be allocated to receive both an anti-malarial and antibiotic, as for many sick children a single diagnosis may not be appropriate.

In 1997, the WHO initiated the 'Integrated Management of Childhood Illness' (IMCI), a strategy which combines the syndromic management of illness in the community with assessment and promotion of nutrition, immunization and other important factors influencing child health (see Table 23.9). By 2000 over 70 countries had embarked on introducing IMCI into their national programmes, which involves countries modifying the IMCI guidelines to their own situation and requirements. Through IMCI it is expected that death, and the frequency and severity of illness and disability will be reduced, and child growth and development will be improved.[28] Although IMCI focuses on the community care of children under 5 years, WHO has produced complementary materials[29] which give guidelines for hospital care of children at first referral level in developing countries, and are consistent with the IMCI strategy and management plans for sick children.

Immunization programmes

The Expanded Programme on Immunization (EPI) was launched in 1974 by the WHO at a time when less than 5% of the world's children were immunized during their first year in life against the initial six target diseases:

Table 23.9 Interventions currently included in the IMCI strategy.

	Promotion of growth Prevention of disease	Response to sickness ('curative care')
Home	• Community/home-based interventions to improve nutrition • Insecticide impregnated bednets	• Early case management • Appropriate careseeking • Compliance with treatment
Health Services	• Vaccinations • Complementary feeding and breast-feeding counselling • Micronutrient supplementation	• Case management of: ARI, diarrhoea, measles, malaria, malnutrition, other serious infection • Complementary feeding and breast-feeding counselling • Iron treatment • Anthelminthic treatment

Source: Reproduced from *IMCI Information* by permission of the World Health Organization, which retains copyright.

diphtheria, tetanus, whooping cough, polio, measles, and tuberculosis. Around 80% of children born each year are now immunized before their first birthday. This has been estimated to prevent the deaths of at least 3 million children a year with 750 000 fewer children blinded, crippled, mentally retarded, or otherwise disabled from these diseases. Tetanus immunization of women of child-bearing age will protect the neonate from tetanus, however in 1994 more than 50% of babies were born unprotected, resulting in almost 500 000 neonatal tetanus deaths. In 1993 it was suggested that the EPI package should also incorporate vaccines against hepatitis B and, where relevant, yellow fever, together with supplements of vitamin A and iodine. Hepatitis B is now included in the EPI programmes of over 100 countries.

At present five contacts are needed during the first year of life (at birth, 6 weeks, 10 weeks, 14 weeks, and at 9 months) and in most countries coverage rates decline progressively through this period (Table 23.10).

BCG (see Chapter 57)

Polio

Polio eradication is now within reach, with the Americas, China and much of Australasia certified as polio free in 2001. Transmission continues in the Indian subcontinent,

Table 23.10 The WHO recommended EPI schedule for infants.

Age	Vaccines	Hepatitis B vaccine	
		Scheme A	Scheme B
Birth	BCG, (OPV)	HB 1	
6 weeks	DPT 1, OPV 1	HB 2	HB 1
10 weeks	DPT 1, OPV 2		HB 2
14 weeks	DPT 3, OPV 3	HB 3	HB 3
9 months	Measles Yellow fever[1]		

[1]In countries where yellow fever poses a risk.

although at reduced levels, and many countries in Africa are now reporting no wild virus transmission.

The global eradication strategy is four-pronged: there is high routine immunization coverage with oral polio vaccine (OPV); supplementary immunization in the form of national immunization days (NIDs); effective surveillance for acute flaccid paralysis and wild poliovirus; and door-to-door immunization ('mopping up' campaigns).

While OPV vaccine is one of the safest vaccines available, one case of vaccine-associated polio occurs for every 2.5 million doses administered. In view of this some countries with no wild-type polio transmission have considered using inactivated poliovirus (IPV) in their EPI programmes. However, unlike OPV, IPV vaccine induces only very low levels of immunity to enteric poliovirus, and although providing protection against systemic disease, cannot prevent the spread of wild poliovirus. Use of OPV vaccines is central to the eradication of polio worldwide.

Measles

Globally, measles accounts for over 10% of deaths in children under 5 years of age, often through the complications of pneumonia, diarrhoea and malnutrition. Measles vaccines have lower efficacy before nine months of age as the vaccine may be neutralized by maternal antibodies acquired across the placenta. For children at high risk of measles exposure, e.g., children in refugee camps or in hospital, the WHO recommends an initial dose of measles vaccine at six months with a second dose at nine months.

Prevention of measles transmission in the Americas has been largely successful; however, measles remains a common problem in Africa. Where wild-type measles is not circulating, there is less boosting of antibody, and further doses of vaccine in later childhood have been introduced in some countries in response to this.

Diphtheria

With good coverage, diphtheria has become rare in the

industrialized world, and also in many developing countries. However, complacency has been tempered by recent outbreaks in the newly independent states of the former Soviet Union. With reduced boosting of immunity through natural exposure to diphtheria organisms, vaccine-induced immunity wanes over time, even in countries with consistently high levels of immunization coverage in infants. This allows groups of non-immune individuals to build up, creating the ideal conditions for epidemics, which may then occur if high coverage of infant immunization with diphtheria declines.

WHO recommends that at least 90% of children under the age of one are immunized with three doses of diphtheria vaccine, given as the combined DTP vaccine. In many developed countries a series of booster doses are also included in immunization schedules.

Pertussis

Loss of confidence in whole-cell pertussis vaccine due to a concern regarding vaccine-related encephalopathy in the 1970s reduced the uptake of this vaccine in a number of Western countries, resulting in a resurgence of infection, morbidity, and deaths. Although establishing a link between this adverse event and the vaccine proved difficult to confirm, the public perception of the vaccine was damaged. As a result a number of countries have incorporated the more expensive acellular vaccine in their immunization schedule, as this vaccine has a similar efficacy but fewer side effects such as local reactions and fever. This change is unlikely to be a priority for low-resource countries where uptake of the DPT vaccine remains good.

Hepatitis B

Hepatitis B infection is generally subclinical in infants and young children, and is predominantly acquired from mother to child, or by child to child transmission. The burden of disease develops in long-term carriers of Hepatitis B virus, and occurs in adult life as cirrhosis of the liver and liver cancer, which cause about a million deaths annually. This vaccine, now incorporated into the EPI schedule of over 100 countries, is unlikely to affect childhood morbidity, but it is expected to reduce one of the principal causes of cancer death in many parts of Africa, Asia, and the Pacific Basin. Where perinatal transmission of virus is common, e.g., in South-East Asia, immunization is recommended at birth, 6 and 14 weeks, whereas in sub-Saharan Africa it is recommended at 6, 10 and 14 weeks.

Yellow fever

A single dose of the safe and highly effective yellow fever vaccine protects against disease for at least ten years, and probably for life. It is therefore recommended to be included in the EPI schedules of those countries at risk of yellow fever transmission, and is given at 9 months alongside measles immunization. As a strategy, it is almost certainly cheaper to prevent disease through immunization, rather than responding to outbreaks when they occur.

Other vaccines relevant to EPI immunization programmes

A number of vaccines are available but not widely used in developing countries. These include a vaccine against Japanese encephalitis, which in Thailand has been added to the EPI schedule. Similarly *Haemophilus* B (HiB) conjugate vaccine has been included in the EPI programme in The Gambia, following trials that showed a reduction in invasive disease. The newly licensed seven valent pneumococcal conjugate vaccines are at present too expensive for developing countries to incorporate into EPI, and the antigens incorporated more suited to the serotypes prevalent in the USA. When conjugate pneumococcal vaccines appropriate for different regions become available, these are expected to offer protection against pneumonia and invasive pneumococcal disease, and significant reductions in childhood mortality. Similarly, rotavirus vaccines are also expected to have a significant impact on diarrhoeal deaths and malnutrition, but an initial vaccine introduced into the USA was subsequently withdrawn due to the rare adverse event of intusucception.

Other considerations

There are many constraints to the delivery of effective immunization to communities in low-resource countries. These include effective maintenance of the 'cold chain', missed opportunities for immunization because of inappropriate contraindications and fear of side effects, negative attitudes of health care workers, concerns about wastage of vaccine, and infrastructural difficulties in delivering vaccine at community level. HIV is not a contraindication to vaccination with the current EPI vaccines, apart from BCG which is only contraindicated in symptomatic children with AIDS, but should still be given to neonates born to HIV-positive mothers.

REFERENCES

1 Stanecki K A, Way P O. The demographic impacts of HIV/AIDS: Perspectives from the world population profile: 1996. International Programme Center, Population Division, US Bureau of the Census, Washington DC 20233.

2 World Health Organization. Report on the Global HIV/AIDS Epidemic. UNAIDS /WHO, Geneva, 1998.

3 Costello A M de L, Manandhar D S, (ed) *Improving Newborn Infant Health in Developing Countries*, London: Imperial College Press, 2000.

4 World Health Organization. *Mother-Baby Packages. Implementing Safe Motherhood in Developing Countries.* WHO/FHE/MSM/94.11 WHO, Geneva, 1994.

5 World Health Organization. *Postpartum Care of the Mother and Newborn: A Practical Guide.* WHO, Geneva, 1998.

6 Brabin L, Brabin B J. Parasitic infections in women and their consequences. *Advan Parasitol* 1992; 31:1–81.

7 Brabin B J. An analysis of malaria parasite rates in infants 40 years after Macdonald. *Trop Dis Bull* 1990; 87:1–21.

8 World Health Organization. *Management of Severe Malaria: A Practical Handbook*, second edit., WHO, Geneva, 2000.

9 Hendrickse R G, Adenige A. Quartan malarial nephrotic syndrome. *Kidney Int* 1979; 16:64–74.

10 Cutts G. *Measles Control in the 1990s: Principles for the Next Decade.* WHO/EPI, Geneva, 1990.

11 Spira R, Lepage P, Msellati P et al. Natural history of HIV type 1 infection in children: a five year prospective study in Rwanda. *Paediatrics* 1999; 104:1118–1119.

12 Abouya Y, Beaumel A, Lucas S et al. *Pneumocystis carinii* pneumonia. An uncommon cause of death in African children infected with HIV. J Am Med Assoc 1991; 265:1693–1697.

13 Lucas S B, Peacock C S, Hounnou A et al. Disease in children infected with HIV in Abidjan, Cote d'Ivoire. *Br Med J* 1996; 312:335–338.

14 Graham S M, Coulter J B S, Gilks C F. Pulmonary disease in HIV infected African children. *Int J TB Lung Dis* 2001; 5:12–23

15 Marun L H, Tindyebwa D, Gibb B. Care of children with HIV infections and AIDS in Africa. *AIDS* 1997; 11 (Suppl B): S125–S135.

16 Centers for Disease Control and Prevention Classification System for human immunodeficiency virus (HIV) infection in children under 13 years of age. *Morb Mortal Week Rep CDC Surv Sum* 1994; 43:1–17.

17 World Health Organization. Acquired immunodeficiency syndrome (AIDS). WHO/CDC case definition for AIDS. *Week Epidemiol Rec* 1985; 1:69–76.

18 Fleming A. Opportunistic infections in AIDS in developed and developing countries. *Trans R Soc Trop Med Hyg* 1990; 84:1–6.

19 Graham S M, Mtitimila E L, Kamanga H S et al. The clinical presentation and outcome of *pneumocystis carinii* pneumonia in Malawian children. Lancet 2000; 355: 369–373.

20 Lebel M H, Freij B J, Sirygiannopoulos A et al. Dexamethasone therapy for bacterial meningitis. New Engl J Med 1988; 319: 964–971.

21 Peltola, H. Burden of meningitis and other severe bacterial infections of children in Africa: Implications for prevention. Clin Infect Dis 2001; 31:64–75.

22 Brown K H, Peerson J M, Fontaine, O. Use of nonhuman milks in the dietary management of young children with acute diarrhoea: a meta-analysis of clinical trials. Paediatrics 1994; 93:17–27.

23 Stoltzfus R L, Dreyfuss M L. Guidelines for the use of iron supplements to prevent and treat iron deficiency anaemia. international nutrition anemia consultative group, World Health Organization, United Nations Childrens Fund, 1998.

24 McLaren D S A, Frigg M. Sight and life manual on vitamin A deficiency disorders. Task Force Sight and Life, Basel, Switzerland 1998.

25 Thacker T D, Fischer P R, Pettifor J M et al. A comparison of calcium, vitamin D, or both for nutritional rickets in Nigerian children. New Eng J Med 1999; 341:563–568.

26 INACG Consensus statement. Safety of iron supplementation programs in malaria-endemic regions. International Life Sciences Institute, Washington, USA, 1999.

27 World Health Organization Child and Adolescent Health and development Division. Integrated management of childhood illnesses information pack. WHO (chd@who.ch), Geneva, 1998.

28 World Health Organization. Integrated management of childhood illness: A WHO Initiative. Bull WHO 1997; 75 (Suppl).

29 World Health Organization. *Management of the Child with a Serious Infection or Severe Malnutrition. Guidelines for Care at the First Referral Level in Developing Countries.* Department of Child Health and Adolescent Health, Geneva, 2000, pp. 1–161.

Chapter 24
Surgery in the Tropics

J. E. Jellis

Introduction

There are some excellent centres of surgical expertise and technology within the tropics in which 'First World' surgery is practised. Research and teaching of the highest standards are to be found there and funding is available, as in the First World, for nearly all that is needed.

On the other hand, the tropics contain much of the two-thirds of the world's population that want for proper surgical care because of poverty, demography and lack of surgeons.[1] In these Third World countries, surgeons are concentrated in the cities, while doctors in the rural areas have to cope with very varied demands on their surgical skills. Patients are often divorced by distance and the cost of travel from the facilities of the central hospitals and less than 10% of referrals achieve their purpose.[2] More surgical operations are performed by doctors who are not qualified surgeons or by clinical officers or nurses than by surgeons themselves.[3]

Tropical medical schools exist in large (or overlarge) city hospitals which would aspire to the highest standards if funding allowed. They train doctors to improvise and seek more cost effective methods of treatment for the common surgical problems of their country.[4] More importantly, perhaps, effective non-operative methods of treatment, especially of trauma, have been developed and are employed.[5,6] It has been shown that relatively few of the surgical operations commonly performed actually need specialist expertise.[4]

Surgery is expensive and has a low priority in a poor nation's health budget, so only a small percentage of necessary operations are performed.[7] Since Noordberg's survey of 1984, the economies of many underdeveloped countries have deteriorated and the situation is now even worse.[8,9] The woman in obstructed labour, the man with a strangulated hernia, the patient with multiple injuries from a road traffic accident and the child with severe burns, have great difficulty in obtaining treatment. For such conditions, there are no effective traditional remedies either.

Human immunodeficiency virus (HIV) and acquired immunodeficiency syndrome (AIDS) are now widespread and have very marked effects on the surgical workload and practice in the tropics. Tuberculosis and sepsis have become even more common and management of many conditions has had to change. Books of surgical pathology written only a few years ago are already out of date. A considerable portion of this chapter, therefore, is devoted to the surgical aspects of HIV infection.

Trauma, often with delayed presentation, is a major problem for many doctors and surgeons working in the tropics. Appropriate management, dictated by cost, lack of expertise and of facilities, has to be very different from that of temperate regions.

Most surgical patients in the tropics are children and young adults. Their fitness to undergo major surgery is often influenced by concomitant 'tropical diseases'. In addition, there are many 'tropical' surgical pathologies, each needing special treatment. This chapter cannot be a textbook of 'tropical surgery' but attempts to direct the reader to successful management of the common surgical problems encountered.

The influence of HIV disease on surgery in the tropics

The HIV pandemic has radically altered the practice of surgery in most tropical countries. By 1998, it was estimated that there were 14 million people with HIV infection in Africa, 4 million in Asia and 2 million in South America.[10] In Zambia, HIV disease was first recognized in 1983.[11] By 1992, over 30% of adult patients admitted for trauma were HIV-positive[12] and some 40% of all surgical admissions were HIV-positive patients.[13]

A surgeon working in the tropics must be able to recognize HIV disease and the new HIV-related pathologies. He must know how other pathologies have been influenced by the disease and be able to assess the risks of surgical operations in such patients. Lastly, universal precautions against the risk of surgical staff contracting infection in the operating theatre must be adopted.

Recognition of HIV-positive patients

HIV-positive patients are not a homogeneous group. A positive serological test for HIV only records the presence of antibodies to HIV. It indicates an HIV infection, but tells the surgeon nothing about the patient's level of immune competence or fitness for surgery.

HIV disease is of insidious onset and progresses over a period, usually between five or ten years, to the full-blown syndrome of AIDS. At present, HIV disease is invariably fatal but there is some evidence that disease modifying drugs may extend life expectancy.[14]

Most HIV-positive patients admitted because of trauma or other unrelated pathology will have no physical signs of HIV disease.[12] It is impossible to test every patient, but by thorough clinical assessment the significant stages of HIV disease can be recognized and the patient's probable immune status assessed.

Every surgical patient should be examined undressed and in a good light, paying special attention to the mouth, axillary, epitrochlear and posterior cervical lymph nodes and skin signs.[13,15] The World Health Organization (WHO) proposed clinical classification (as modified in Table 24.1) should be used.[16] Stage 0 has been added to classify the serologically HIV-positive patient with no clinical symptoms or signs. A total lymphocyte count or CD4 lymphocyte count will indicate the degree of immune compromise (Table 24.2).[17,18]

In a series of 335 adults undergoing major orthopaedic surgery in Zambia between 1993 and 1995, 87 (26%) were HIV positive.[19] Of the HIV-positive patients, 49 had no symptoms or signs of HIV infection (stage 0), 16 were in

Table 24.1 Staging of HIV-positive patients. (Based on 'An interim proposal for a WHO staging system for HIV infection and disease[16] with modifications.)

Clinical stage 0
Serologically HIV-positive but no signs or symptoms related to HIV infection
Clinical stage 1
Asymptomatic
Persistent generalized lymphadenopathy
Clinical stage 2
Weight loss, < 10% of body weight
Minor mucocutaneous manifestations
Herpes zoster within the last five years
Recurrent upper respiratory tract infections
Clinical stage 3
Weight loss, > 10% body weight
Unexplained chronic diarrhoea, > 1 month
Unexplained prolonged fever, > 1 month
Oral candidiasis or hairy leucoplakia
Pulmonary tuberculosis, within the past year
Severe bacterial infections
Clinical stage 4
AIDS: the HIV wasting syndrome
Severe opportunistic infections
Extrapulmonary tuberculosis
Lymphoma or Kaposi's sarcoma
HIV encephalopathy

Table 24.2 Lymphocyte and CD4 cell counts in HIV disease. (Based on 'An interim proposal for a WHO staging system for HIV infection and disease[16] with modifications.) Each clinical stage can be subdivided on the absolute or CD4 lymphocyte counts to give further evidence of immune status.

Subdivision	Lymphocytes	CD4
(A)	> 2000	> 500
(B)	1000–2000	200–500
(C)	< 1000	< 200

stage I, 13 in stage II and only 9 were in stages III and IV of advanced HIV disease. As compared with that in HIV-negative patients, the rate of postoperative wound infection doubled in stage 0 patients and trebled in those with physical signs and symptoms of the disease (stages I-IV).[19] Most of the latter group were in stages I and II, so it is likely that the infection rate would be higher in those with more advanced disease. In a survey from America of HIV-positive haemophiliac patients with CD4 lymphocyte counts of 200/mm[3] or less,[20] the overall infection rate was 13.5% and that for joint arthroplasty was 45.9%.

Other postoperative complications such as chest infections, unexplained fevers, diarrhoea and urinary tract infections were all more common in patients with HIV disease. Necessary surgery should not be withheld from HIV-positive patients but the risks must be thoroughly assessed so that an appropriate operation can be planned and discussed with the patient.

Precautions against contracting HIV disease by inoculation while operating on HIV-positive patients

Any surgeon will damage his gloves and skin from sharp instruments, needles, wires and bone fragments. He should be immunized against hepatitis, but there is no immunization against HIV. The operating theatre staff should all take precautions to minimize the, admittedly small, risk of becoming infected with HIV.[21]

These precautions must be universally applied because it is impossible to know the HIV status of every patient. The most infectious patient is one in the viraemic phase of a recent infection who would test HIV negative. Most HIV-positive patients undergoing surgery, particularly for trauma or other conditions unrelated to HIV disease, will have no signs of HIV disease.[12]

Most precautions are simply common sense. If, as in operating on a ruptured spleen or performing a caesarean section, blood spillage is expected, boots and an apron beneath an impervious gown with gauntlets, double gloves and an eye shield would be ideal. Ideal, that is, apart from the discomfort in tropical heat and humidity.

If sharp bone fragments are likely to be handled or wires used, an armoured glove is useful or a sterilized cotton (dermatological) glove should be worn over the rubber glove. Dexterity is reduced but sharp fragments catch in the cotton glove rather than penetrating through to the skin. Eye protection is important, especially if an osteotome is in use, remembering that most fragments will fly towards the nurse or assistant. Power tools, which may produce an aerosol, should be used with great caution.

Large incisions should be made so that the surgeon operates by sight more than by feel and assistants' fingers should be kept well clear of the operative field. Any sharp instrument should be handed to the surgeon in a dish and the dish proffered by the nurse when returning the instrument. If a Mayo table is used, strict rules must be formulated to prevent the surgeons hands meeting those of the scrub nurse while placing sharp instruments on the table.

Any injury should be reported and HIV tests conducted on the patient and surgeon. Few hospitals have a policy of post-exposure prophylactic antiviral drug administration and doctors will have to obtain supplies if they want to adopt such a policy. Some may think that the risks of seroconversion are so low that antiviral prophylaxis is unwarranted.

Blood transfusion in the tropics

In recent years, it has become obvious that although blood transfusion may be life saving, it is also a dangerous procedure. Autologous blood floods the immune system with antigens and infections, such as HIV, hepatitis and malaria, are easily transmitted.[22] Even when every precaution is taken, viraemic HIV-negative donors may be bled or bottles mislabelled.[23]

The fear of HIV disease and its association with blood products, and perhaps the fear of having an HIV test, has reduced the intake of many blood banks in the tropics. It has become increasingly difficult to obtain donated blood and any stock should be reserved for emergency situations.

Patients can do well with haemoglobin levels well below the previously recommended minimum of 10 g/dl. A preoperative haemoglobin of 9 g/dl is acceptable for operations under tourniquet or when minimal blood loss is expected. After major surgery, haemoglobin levels down to 5 g/dl have been recorded without noticeably affecting respiration or wound healing.

Where major surgery is planned and time permits, a patient may donate several units of his own blood at weekly intervals but this has several disadvantages. If the patient is HIV-positive, the blood bank will refuse to store his donated blood. It is difficult to prevent any stored blood being used for other patients during life-threatening emergencies and all the usual technical problems and cost of blood storage apply.

Acute euvolaemic haemodilution[24,25] overcomes many of these problems. Immediately before surgery, several units of blood may be taken from the patient and stored in the theatre refrigerator to be infused during any intra-operative haemorrhage or given at the end of the operation. As each unit of blood is drawn, it is replaced by a double volume of intravenous saline. Each unit of blood taken will reduce the patient's haemoglobin by approximately 1g/dl and the preoperative haemoglobin should not be allowed to fall below 9 g/dl.

In Lusaka, acute euvolaemic haemodilution has been used in major orthopaedic surgery for the last five years with satisfactory results. Very rarely has additional banked blood been needed.

Pathologies associated with HIV disease
Tuberculosis

Tuberculosis is the commonest and most virulent of the opportunistic infections associated with HIV disease. HIV specifically inhibits and destroys the tissue macrophages and thymic lymphocytes that are the body's main defence against *Mycobacterium tuberculosis*.[26] In many tropical countries there is a dual epidemic of HIV disease and tuberculosis.[26] In Zambia, for example, over 60% of adult patients with pulmonary[27] and bone and joint tuberculosis[28] are HIV positive, as are 84% of those with tuberculous lymphadenitis.[29]

All extrapulmonary forms of tuberculosis have become more common, so the surgeon must be alert to unusual presentations.[30] Tuberculosis of the breast,[31] lymphadenopathy,[32] abdominal tuberculosis[33] and tuberculosis of the spine and major joints[28,34] are all common. HIV-associated tuberculosis does respond to standard antituberculous drug therapy, but the patient's prognosis depends more upon the stage of HIV disease rather than upon the extent of the tuberculous infection.

Lymphadenopathy

Although symmetrical chronic enlargement of the posterior cervical, axillary and epitrochlear lymph nodes is a sign of early HIV disease,[15] asymmetrical enlargement of nodes has become more common and still merits investigation.[29] The pathologies include the reactive hyperplasia of HIV disease itself, tuberculosis, HIV-associated Kaposi's sarcoma, lymphoma and other metastatic tumour deposits. Bem[29,32] has shown that the diagnosis can often be made on the naked eye appearance of a cut node rather than waiting for a histology report. Fine needle aspiration cytology and imprint cytology are also useful diagnostic tools.[35]

Empyema thoracis

Many HIV-positive patients, especially children under five years old and young adults, develop empyema and most have underlying tuberculosis.[36] Desai[37] has shown that if pus can easily be aspirated through a 21 French-gauge needle into a 10 ml syringe by one pull of the plunger, the empyema needs drainage through an intercostal tube and underwater-seal drain to prevent lung collapse. If the pus is too thick to aspirate easily, however, 7.5 cm sections of two adjacent ribs over the most dependent part of the empyema should be resected for open drainage. Drainage is encouraged by the patient sleeping on the affected side, blowing up balloons or old surgical gloves and irrigating the sinus with water. These patients can be discharged to home care within a week.

Adult haematogenous osteomyelitis

This was a rare condition before HIV disease existed. Now young adults often present with chronic haematogenous osteomyelitis of insidious onset.[38] The disease mainly affects the metaphyses of the tibia (Figure 24.1) and femur and may symmetrically affect both legs. The infections are often staphylococcal but salmonella and a variety

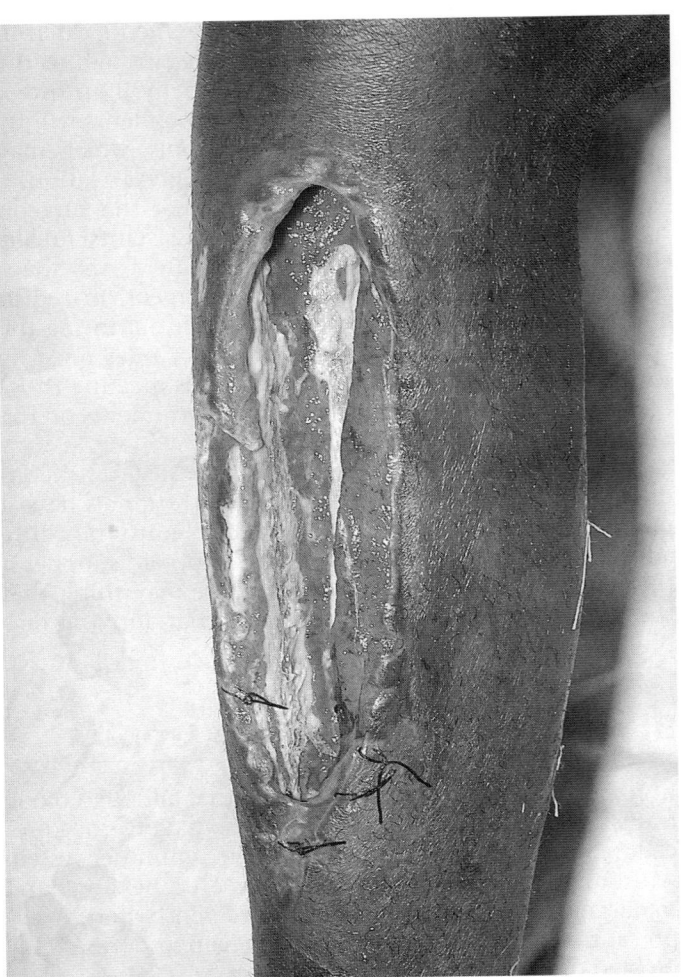

Figure 24.2: Non-healing wound after sequestrectomy for HIV-related haematogenous osteomyelitis of the tibia.

of other 'bowel' flora have been found. Mixed infections occur, even before there is an open wound.

Despite treatment by drainage, sequestrectomy and wide debridement, the infection often progresses in an inexorable manner causing much pain and suffering (Figure 24.2). On several occasions, amputation has been necessary for this condition. Above-knee amputations have healed well and have been followed by a worthwhile period of weight gain and better health for up to five years.[38] These patients are in stage III of HIV disease.

Similar haematogenous infections commonly occur around joint prostheses, Kuntscher nails and other implants, years after their insertion, in patients reaching advanced stages of HIV disease.[38] The infection may be controlled after removal of small implants, but it has proved impossible to eradicate after removal of Kuntscher nails and hip prostheses.

Tropical pyomyositis

Formerly a disease mainly of children,[38] it is now strongly associated with HIV disease in young adults.[39] In Uganda,

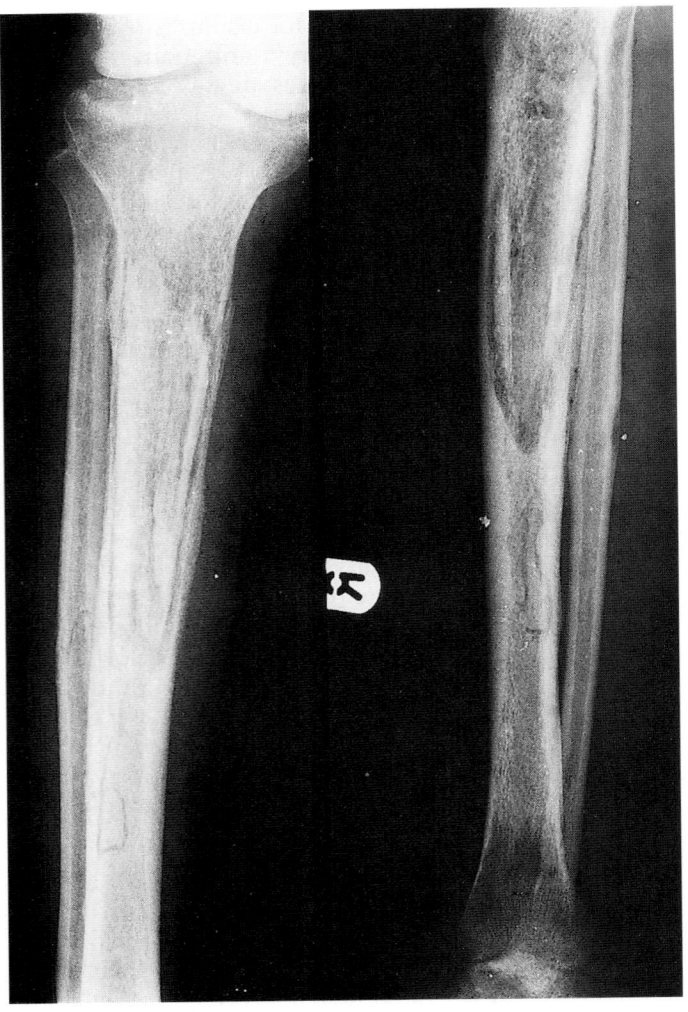

Figure 24.1: Radiograph of the tibia in a patient with HIV-related haematogenous osteomyelitis. There is bone destruction with very little new bone formation.

71% of sufferers of both sexes were HIV positive[40] and, if abscesses were multiple, the association was 81%. The abscesses are mainly in the large muscles of the trunk and proximal compartments of the limbs. *Staphylococcus aureus* is still the usual organism grown, but a variety of other organisms have been found in HIV-positive patients. Whether there is a primary lesion in the muscle that becomes secondarily infected is still debated.[41]

These debilitated patients need good supportive care and systemic antibiotic therapy if the large volumes of pus are to be safely drained. After incision, careful palpation of the abscess cavity will differentiate pyomyositis from haematogenous osteomyelitis, in which bare bone devoid of periosteum will be felt in the base of the cavity.

Other musculoskeletal pathology and rheumatoid disease

Many HIV-positive patients present with non-specific backache and tenderness of the thoracic or lumbar spine. Acute rheumatoid arthritis, reactive arthritis (especially of the knees and ankles), erosive arthritis and enthesitis (especially of the tendo Achilles and plantar fascia) are now commonly seen in HIV-positive patients.[42]

Neurological manifestations of HIV infection

At least 40% of patients with HIV infection develop neurological manifestations at some stage, and over 80% have neuropathological findings at autopsy.[10] The protean effects of HIV range from acute neuropathy, myelopathy or encephalitis within three months of infection, to the AIDS–dementia complex occurring in late HIV disease. Cryptococcal meningitis, tuberculoma and other cerebral space-occupying lesions and progressive multifocal leukoencephalopathy also occur later.[10,43]

Necrotizing fasciitis

Necrotizing fasciitis is a progressive, rapidly spreading synergistic infection with aerobic and anaerobic gas-forming organisms around the deep fascia. It has long been associated with diabetes mellitus, cancer, alcoholism and immunocompromized patients.[44] Now it is common in HIV-positive patients.

The disease carries a high mortality rate. Successful management demands early diagnosis, rapid resuscitation, aggressive surgical excision with frequent revision, coupled with high doses of broad-spectrum antibiotics.

Perianal infection

Even in the countries of southern Africa, where anal intercourse is rare, there is a strong association between HIV disease, fistula in ano and perianal abscess.[45,46]

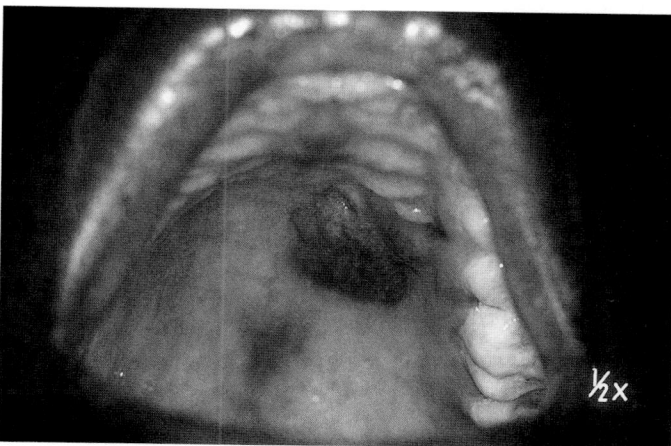

Figure 24.3: Purple plaque of Kaposi's sarcoma on the hard palate indicating gastrointestinal involvement.

Experienced surgeons consider that fistula in ano and haemorrhoids should be treated conservatively in HIV-positive patients because anal wounds heal poorly, and both anal dilatation and sphincterotomy impair continence for fluid diarrhoea.[13]

Kaposi's sarcoma

Endemic Kaposi's sarcoma is a rather benign vascular tumour occurring on the limbs of middle-aged and elderly men that is amenable to cytotoxic therapy. Atypical aggressive Kaposi's sarcoma is now common in HIV-positive children and young adults of both sexes.[11] It affects the skin, lymph nodes and gastrointestinal tract as well as other organs and responds poorly to cytotoxic drugs.[47] Surgery is rarely indicated except to amputate a painful useless hand, foot or limb. If there is gastrointestinal involvement, the purple Kaposi tissue may be seen on the hard palate (Figure 24.3). Plaques in the small bowel may give rise to intussusception.[48]

Trauma

A surgeon working in the tropics needs to be a good traumatologist capable of managing a very wide range of injuries with minimal equipment. In the First World, trauma services exist to provide first aid, resuscitation, life support and rapid transportation to hospital. Surgical intervention within hours of injury to repair soft tissue trauma and internally fix all skeletal injuries is the norm.

Such trauma services are expensive and are rare in the tropics. Great improvements could be made,[49] but currently many of the most severely injured die before reaching hospital[50] and delayed presentation is very frequent. Many arrive in hospital with wounds already infected. Of necessity, the management of neglected trauma is very different from the treatment appropriate soon after injury.[51]

In several East African countries, 60% of all patients in the surgical wards are trauma cases.[1] These patients have major fractures, head and spinal injuries, wounds and burns.

In urban areas and near major roads, most injuries result from road traffic accidents and interpersonal violence.[52] At the other extreme, in remote fishing communities, the major problems are horrendous injuries from crocodile[53,54] attacks. War has taken a great toll of both the civilian and military populations of many countries, and mutilating injuries are still seen from exploding landmines years after the conflicts have been resolved.

In Uganda in 1997, the road death toll was 8930 with a further 38 343 injured patients.[1] Of those injured in road traffic accidents, 80% are either passengers (in and on vehicles) or pedestrians.[52] The high incidence rate of accidents and the high death rate have been blamed on bad roads, poor driving skills, defective and overloaded vehicles and alcohol intoxication. Over one-third of road traffic accident victims in Uganda in 1996 were found to have blood alcohol levels of 50 mg/dl or more.[55] Preventive legislation exists in most countries but is ineffectively applied.

Dislocations

Dislocations are usually easily reduced when seen soon after injury, but can be very difficult several days later. Elbow dislocations may be reduced at up to two weeks,[51] but it needs prolonged steady stretching to do so. Closed reduction of late-presenting hip dislocations is also worth trying[56] because open reduction can be a very difficult procedure.

Fractures

Patterns of injury differ from those in the northern hemisphere, mainly because of the much younger population. Thus diaphyseal femoral fractures are much more common than those of the neck of femur. Because of the high cost and poor availability of implants, lack of orthopaedic surgeons and the prevalence of HIV disease, non-operative methods of management are appropriate in most situations.[1] Such methods have not advanced in the First World over many years, but the innovative use of traction, casting, cast-bracing and, for severe open injuries, external fixation, has advanced in the tropics. Perkin's traction (Figure 24.4) and 90/90 traction for femoral fractures[5] are good examples of this. The skills of fracture manipulation must be learnt and casts replaced to hold fractures as swelling diminishes.[57] Non-operative management is often more time consuming than internal fixation but very satisfactory end results can be obtained.

Wound management

It should be remembered that very few wounds need to

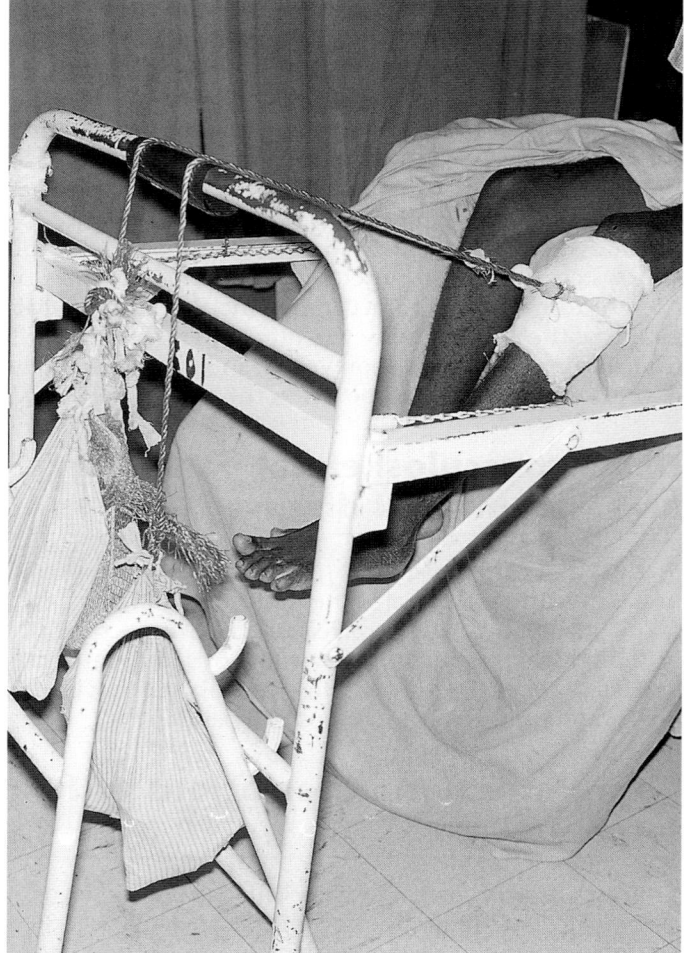

Figure 24.4: Patient exercising in Perkin's traction which encourages early union and prevents muscle wasting, knee stiffness and malrotation.

be closed primarily. Only cleanly incised wounds seen within a few hours of injury should be stitched. Wounds that have an element of crush injury, are contaminated or infected, or have presented late, should be debrided, cleaned and left open for suture or skin grafting several days later. Great savings on antibiotic usage can be made if such regimes are followed.[58]

Head injury and spinal injury

Many tropical countries do not have neurosurgical centres or they may be too distant for referral of injured patients. A good understanding of the principles of care for the unconscious or paraplegic patient will save many lives.[59,60] Burr holes or tracheostomy may be indicated early in head injury cases,[61] and should be done if the patient cannot reach specialist care within a very short time. Early operations on the spine are very rarely needed.[62-64] Cervical traction and reduction for neck fractures, positional reduction of others, two-hourly turning of the patient and intermittent catheterization are the best treatment for patients with spinal injury.[1,65] Indwelling catheters are a potent source of urinary tract infection and urethral stricture, and should not be used in spinal injuries. If intermittent catheterization is needed for long periods, the patient's relative may be taught to introduce the catheter. Later, clean self-catheterization should be taught to the patient. In this way much morbidity and possibly mortality may be avoided.

Burns

Severe burns are common in the tropics, especially in young children. In a survey from Uganda from 1992 to 1995, 56.5% of all burns admissions were children of under five years old.[66] Open fires are used for cooking and, especially on cold winter nights, become the focus of family life. Epileptic patients frequently fall into fires during their seizures. In many cultures they are thought to be spirit-possessed and will not be pulled clear until the fit has stopped.

Huts built of highly flammable material are often lit by primitive paraffin lamps which cause horrendous burns when they are knocked over or explode. In Malawi, during six months of 1998, 30 patients were seen with paraffin burns from lamp explosions.[67] These usually occurred when a hot lamp was being refilled. Eight patients had over 20% deep burns and ten out of the 30 died. Arson and burning as a reprisal and punishment are not uncommon[66] as is suicide by burning.[68,69]

Every hospital will have at least one patient with severe burn injury at any time.[1] Burn injuries increase in the cold season in higher areas and a heated burns ward may prevent deaths from hypothermia. A severe burn is any burn of over 10% body surface area in a child and over 15% in an adult. Prompt resuscitation with intravenous fluids as calculated by weight and age from the charts available in several books[70-72] should be monitored by urine output from an in-dwelling catheter.

A severely burnt patient not only loses his ability to regulate body temperature but also loses resistance to infection and may become severely anaemic from direct thermal damage and disseminated intravascular coagulopathy. These patients need very careful monitoring.[71] They have an increased metabolic rate and need extra food. Antibiotics and blood transfusion should be held in reserve for when signs of infection or anaemia appear. The burn wound should be treated with topical antibacterial agents such as silver sulphadiazine[71] or a mixture of honey and ghee both of which are inexpensive if made in the hospital.

Priority should be given to the treatment of the hands, neck, perineum and the flexor surfaces of joints where subsequent contracture will prove crippling. When not actively exercising, these areas should be splinted to prevent contracture. Deep circumferential limb and hand burns will need escharotomy to prevent distal ischaemic necrosis.[71] Very severe limb burns may require early amputation, and patients with deep burns of covering more than 50% of body surface area do not survive.

Using such treatment methods (Figure 24.5),[73] superficial and partial thickness burns should be healed within

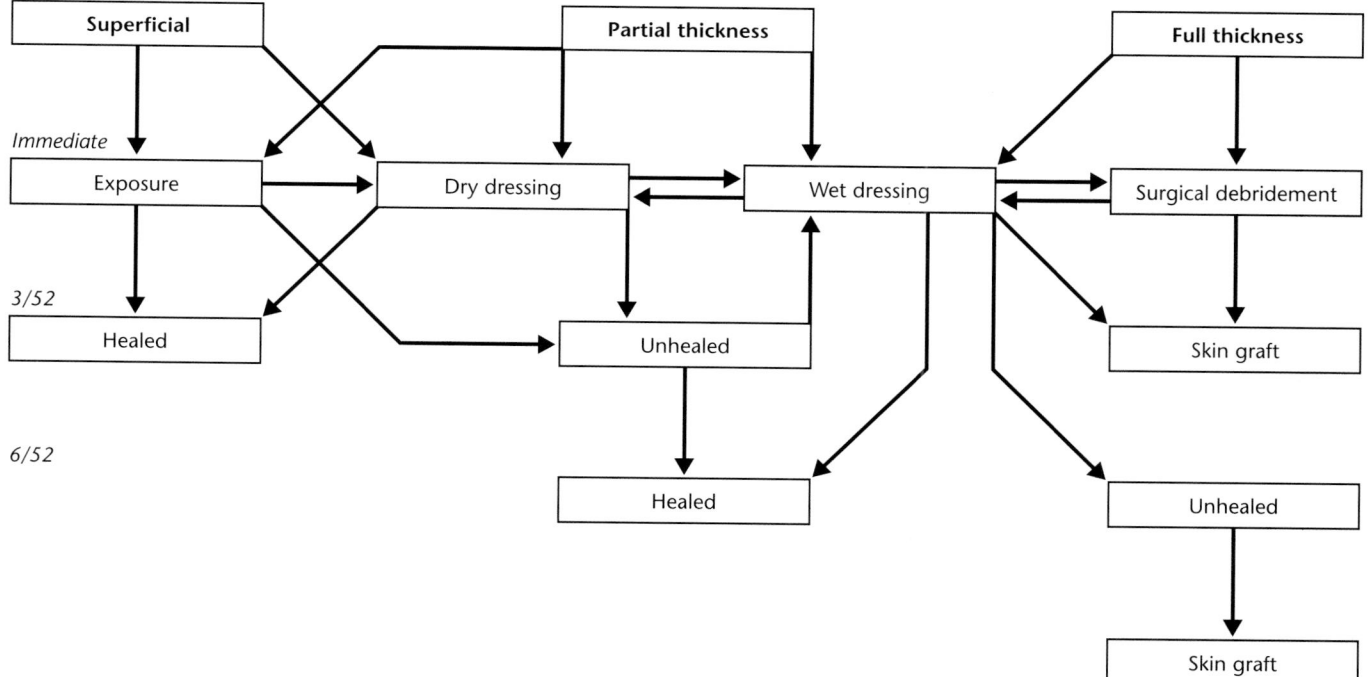

Figure 24.5: Scheme of burns management. (From James, J. Treatment of the burn wound. *East Cen Afr J Surg* 1999 5(1):61.)

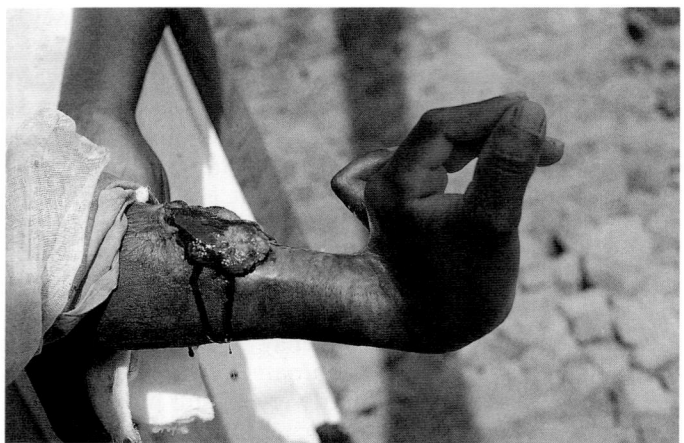

Figure 24.6: Squamous cell carcinoma in a burn contracture of the wrist.

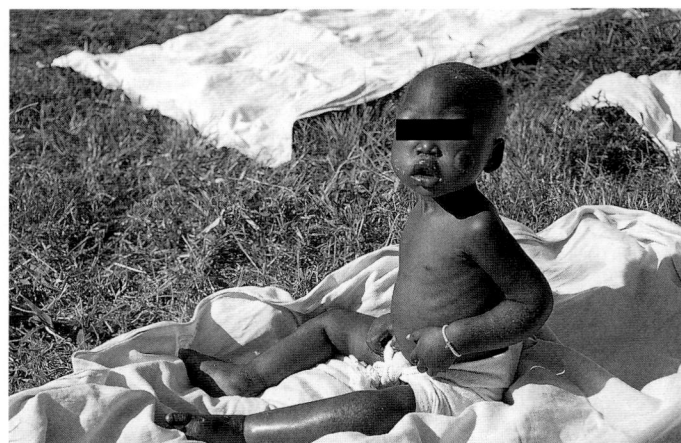

Figure 24.7: Kwashiorkor. The brown fine silky hair, distended abdomen and peripheral oedema are typical.

21 days. Unhealed areas should then treated by split skin grafting without further delay. In babies with severe burns, maternal split skin may be used as graft material and meshing of grafts extends the area of cover considerably. Split skin grafts themselves will contract in the first 12 weeks after application and splinting or plaster casts should be applied to prevent this as soon as the grafts are stable. It should be remembered that depigmented scar tissue, especially on areas of the body exposed to sunlight, carries a very high risk of malignant change with epithelioma (squamous cell carcinoma; Marjolin's ulcer) developing within 10 years (Figure 24.6).

The release of burns contracture and excision and grafting of depigmented scars occupies a large place in reconstructive and plastic surgical work in the tropics and can be very rewarding once the essential techniques have been mastered.[74]

As with other areas of trauma, prevention should take priority and several schemes are in place with measurable success.[66] All epileptic patients should be supplied with prophylactic anticonvulsants. In some countries these drugs are distributed by Psychiatric Clinical Officers and other health workers from government clinics. This simple measure will largely prevent repeated expensive hospital admissions for these dreadful injuries.

Factors affecting the safety of surgery

The outcome of any surgical operation may be adversely affected by the condition of the patient. In the First World, old age, obesity, hypertension, ischaemic heart disease, diabetes and chronic bronchitis are common. In the tropics these are overshadowed by starvation, malnutrition, anaemia, malaria, sickle cell disease and HIV disease. Apart from a good history and thorough examination, a haemoglobin determination and a blood slide for malaria are mandatory before surgery.

Starvation and malnutrition (see also Chapter 31)

Lack of food due to famine from natural catastrophes or displacement of populations by war occurs in many tropical countries. If surgery is needed, nutritional support will also be required.

Calorie/protein malnutrition or *kwashiorkor* can be recognized by the thin, sparse, silky brown hair, facial and peripheral oedema, pallor and swollen abdomen (Figure 24.7). Such children are often grossly anaemic, heavily parasitized and unfit for surgery. Preoperative transfusion, taking great care not to overload the circulation, will be necessary if emergency surgery is needed.

Anaemia (see also Chapter 13)

Average haemoglobin levels are lower in tropical countries and for practical purposes a haemoglobin of 9 g/dl is the lower limit acceptable for planned surgical operations. Of the many causes of anaemia, malnutrition, malaria and sickle cell disease are the most important. In adults, huge splenic enlargement (Figure 24.8) may cause chronic anaemia and thrombocytopenia. Splenectomy may be called for[75] but can be a hazardous undertaking.[76]

Sickle cell anaemia (see also Chapter 13)

In many sub-Saharan countries, up to 25% of the population carry the gene for sickle cell anaemia (HbS). Some offspring of these individuals will be afflicted with sickle cell disease (HbSS) and comprise about 1% of the population. They have a chronic haemolytic anaemia with periodic sickling crises characterized by severe anaemia, jaundice and painful infarcts in bone and other organs. Affected individuals are susceptible to infections such as otitis media, osteomyelitis and chest infections. In West Africa and Mediterranean countries, haemoglobin C

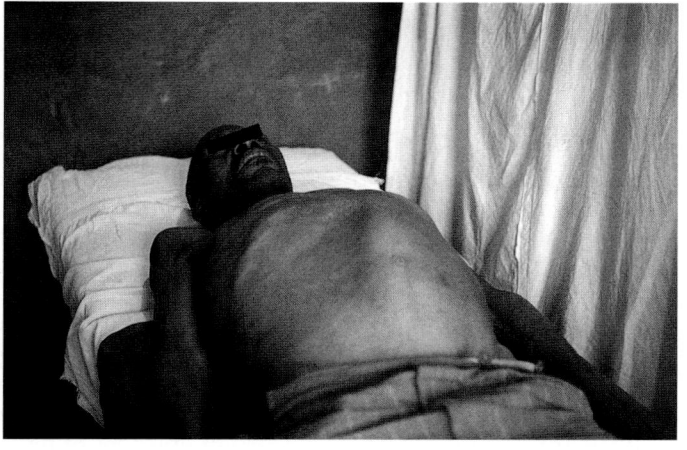

Figure 24.8: Patient with huge splenic enlargement. Splenectomy can be a formidable undertaking because of dense vascular adhesions.

disease and thalassaemia have similar, if less dramatic, effects. Those with the heterozygous condition (HbS) do not suffer from such problems.

In patients with sickle cell disease, the haemoglobin levels are usually between 5 g/dl and 8 g/dl but during a sickling crisis drop much lower. If major surgery is needed, preoperative transfusion to bring the haemoglobin to at least 8 g/dl should be given and blood should be available to maintain this level throughout surgery and the postoperative period.

One potent cause of sickling is hypoxia. High pO_2 levels should be maintained throughout the operation and postoperative period. A pulse oximeter is a convenient way of monitoring this, but good oxygenation during surgery and oxygen by mask for 24 hours after surgery should be given in every case. Local nerve block analgesia should be considered because drugs that cause somnolence or depress respiration should not be used. Sudden collapse and death some hours after operation are a consequence of not observing these precautions.

The use of a tourniquet is controversial in patients with sickle cell disease. If bleeding is likely to be excessive or would prolong an operation by obscuring the anatomy, it is probably better to use a tourniquet. The limb should be properly exsanguinated with an Esmarch bandage before the arterial tourniquet is inflated and high oxygen levels maintained when circulation to the limb is restored. The limb should be held elevated for at least five minutes after release of a tourniquet to prevent pooling of blood or reactive haemorrhage. Adverse effects or a marked drop in the monitored pO_2 during such manoeuvres have not been encountered.

Malaria (see also Chapter 71)

Malaria is a common endemic or epidemic problem in many areas of the tropics and, with the emergence of resistant strains, control is difficult. Many patients, especially children, may remain fit to work and play but carry malarial parasites in their blood. The stress of surgery commonly provokes a severe attack of malaria with marked haemolysis and possibly cerebral involvement. Fever within 48 hours of surgery is most likely due either to atelectasis and chest infection or to malaria.

For planned surgery, especially in children, a haemoglobin check and a blood slide for malarial parasites should be done before surgery. Any patient with a haemoglobin of below 9 g/dl needs investigation. Those in whom malarial parasites are found should have a course of antimalarial treatment and surgery should be delayed for several days. In an emergency situation, antimalarial drugs may be started soon after surgery.

Common 'tropical' conditions

Haematogenous osteomyelitis

Uncommon in temperate regions since the 1930s, haematogenous osteomyelitis is both a common and severe affliction of children in the tropics.[77] Many doctors find this a difficult pathology to understand and treat, so it is dealt with in some detail here.

Neonatal septic arthritis and osteomyelitis

Acute septic arthritis with adjacent osteomyelitis may develop within a few days of birth but the diagnosis, especially in the case of the hip joint, is often delayed. The neonatal response to severe infection is lethargy, failure to feed, subnormal temperatures and jaundice. Other causes of these symptoms, such as malaria and pneumonia, are often sought and treated until the mother reports that the child does not move one limb (pseudoparalysis) or gross swelling develops around a major joint. Aspiration of pus from the area will confirm septic arthritis and radiological changes of the adjacent bones are usually present by that time.

Treatment of this condition, with appropriate antibiotics, open drainage of the joint and splintage, is urgent if joint destruction is to be avoided. *S. aureus* and *Haemophilus influenzae* are both common organisms in this disease so a combination of cloxacillin and ampicillin or other broad-spectrum antibiotics should be given by intravenous infusion pending the results of cultures. Hips should be splinted in abduction to prevent dislocation, an affected knee kept straight and the arm rested in a sling for shoulder and elbow pathology.

Because of late diagnosis, hip dislocation, destruction of the femoral head and severe damage to other joints are commonly seen. Other causes of neonatal joint swelling, such as birth trauma and congenital syphilis (which is usually bilateral), should be excluded by radiographs and diagnostic aspiration.

Haematogenous osteomyelitis in childhood

This common and serious condition produces prolonged morbidity, occasional deaths and life-long crippling. Bacteria are carried to the metaphyses of long bones, especially those of the tibia, femur and humerus, in the blood stream. As blood flow slows in the medullary sinusoids, bacteria settle and produce acute inflammation. Intraosseous pressure rises, occluding the endosteal circulation and producing septic necrosis. The infection spreads to the diaphysis along the medullary cavity but the physeal plate usually prevents spread to the epiphysis. Pus eventually breaches the cortex, lifting the periosteum and depriving the bone of its remaining periosteal blood supply. The dead cortex becomes a sequestrum.

If the physeal plate is situated within the adjacent joint, as in the hip and elbow, infection will probably spread to the joint, producing septic arthritis. Eventually, pus will burst from beneath the periosteum into the soft tissues of the limb and through the skin to leave discharging sinuses. Recovery is by new periosteal bone forming an involucrum that eventually unites the unaffected regions of the bone but, while sequestra remain, discharging sinuses will persist.

In the acute phase, which lasts for only 48 to 72 hours, the child has a high fever and much pain. The affected area of bone is tender and very painful on light percussion but the leg is not swollen. This is the only stage where effective treatment may cure the infection and stop progression to chronic osteomyelitis. The acute stage, however, often passes before admission to hospital.

The diagnosis is entirely clinical, there being no easily recognizable radiological signs, though oedema of the periosteum may be confirmed by ultrasonography.

Treatment in the acute phase is pain relief, high doses of intravenous anti-staphylococcal antibiotics (e.g., cloxacillin 200 mg/kg/day), and decompression of the affected bone by drilling without periosteal stripping, followed by elevation and splintage of the limb. A radiograph at 14 to 21 days after onset will show the extent of disease. It may suggest resolution or show significant bone destruction.

Postacute haematogenous osteomyelitis

When pus tracks out of the bone and lifts the periosteum the intraosseous pressure is reduced. Although the leg now swells, the patient has less pain and the fever falls. This sign may erroneously suggest success of treatment rather than progression of the disease. Most children with osteomyelitis arrive at hospital at this postacute stage.

The same treatment is needed, but pus will be drained from the soft tissues rather than from the bone. The dead cortex (sequestrum) ensures that the disease will progress to chronic osteomyelitis. Radiographs will confirm death

and destruction of bone and the need for protection of the limb from stress until the involucrum is strong enough to bear weight.

Chronic osteomyelitis

This is characterized by the history and presence of a swollen limb with a palpably enlarged bone and discharging sinuses. Radiographs will show sequestra and involucrum or a Brodie's abscess. In principle, sequestrectomy should await the formation of enough involucrum to maintain integrity of the limb. A Brodie's abscess should be cleared by wide excision of the overlying cortex (saucerization). Antibiotics should be given at the time of surgery and for a week or so after sequestrectomy or until any cellulitis resolves. Recurrent episodes of fever indicate the need for further drainage of pus and sequestrectomy rather than for antibiotic therapy.

Haematogenous osteomyelitis in sickle cell disease

This infection probably develops in areas of bone infarction. Often polyostotic and affecting the upper limbs as commonly as the lower, the infection is frequently diffuse throughout a given bone. Salmonellae are as common as staphylococcal infections and the antibiotic therapy must be adjusted accordingly. In general, surgical treatment should be confined to drainage of pus and the removal of large discrete sequestra, being less radical than in other patients. Precautions (mentioned under sickle cell disease above) must be taken if surgery is performed.

Sigmoid volvulus

Sigmoid volvulus is occasionally seen in Europe and America in elderly or mentally ill patients. It is common in Africa especially among men of Bantu race.[78] A high bulk diet has been suggested as an aetiological factor but Gakwaya from Uganda has described 16 patients (sex ratio M:F;15:1) with a syndrome of symptomatic redundant sigmoid colon that he considers the precursor of sigmoid volvulus.[79] The patients gave an average six-year history of intermittent pain and diarrhoea alternating with constipation and of passing 'rabbit pellet' stools. Redundant sigmoid colon was demonstrated by barium enema, and at laparotomy all the patients had a narrow attachment of the sigmoid mesocolon with white scarring at the base. Two patients were lost to follow-up but 13 of the other 14 were cured of their symptoms by sigmoid colectomy. There was no operative morbidity or mortality.

By the time of complete colonic volvulus, the colon has become hypertrophied and thick walled with lateral stretching of the taenia coli. Strangulation is comparatively late and, if no signs of peritonitis are present, the volvulus can often be decompressed by passing a soft rubber flatus tube through the twist at sigmoidoscopy with the patient in the knee-elbow position.[80] Once deflated, the flatus tube should be left in situ for several days. Unfortunately, there is a very high incidence of recurrence and some form of sigmoid resection, or plication and fixation, is needed to prevent this.[80,81] Surgeons expert in large bowel surgery often perform primary sigmoidectomy.[82] They argue that many patients do not return for interval surgery. Patients, not realizing the seriousness of their condition, present even later with dehydration, biochemical imbalance and gangrenous bowel, when the volvulus recurs.

If signs of peritonitis exist, flatus tube decompression should not be attempted. After rapid correction of dehydration and electrolyte imbalance and having given high doses of broad-spectrum antibiotics and metronidazole, laparotomy should be performed. The gangrenous sigmoid colon should be resected. Whether to perform a primary colorectal anastomosis protected by a proximal colostomy or whether to leave the patient with an end colostomy and a closed rectal stump, will depend upon the condition of the patient and the experience of the operator.[80]

Small bowel volvulus

In Africa and India, primary small bowel volvulus is an uncommon cause of acute intestinal obstruction[83] and, in children, is associated with ascariasis[84] and recent treatment with vermicide.[85] In parts of Nepal, however, it is common in men, and associated with large bulky high fibre meals.[86] Adequate resuscitation of the patient before surgery will reduce the operative mortality.

Ileosigmoid knotting

This compound volvulus is not uncommon in the tropics and carries a high mortality rate.[87] The onset is acute, signs of peritonitis are already obvious at presentation and gangrenous small bowel is usually present. In a minority of early cases the small bowel can be unwound but usually both small and large bowel resections are necessary. Unless a referral centre is close by, such surgery should not be delayed by efforts at referral.

Helminthic intestinal obstruction

Infestation with the round worm, *Ascaris lumbricoides,* is a very common affliction of children in the tropics. A large mass of worms may block the ileum causing intestinal obstruction. In 80% of such cases, conservative management with nasogastric suction and intravenous infusion is successful.[88] After the child is passing flatus or faeces, a vermifuge (either piperazine or a benzimidazole compound) should be given. Close observation is mandatory and laparotomy undertaken if signs of peritonitis or volvulus develop.[84] Worms in viable segments of the ileum may be

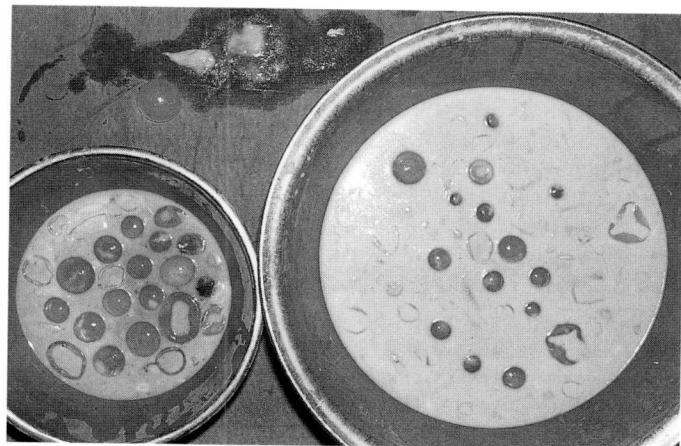

Figure 24.9: Pus and daughter cysts drained from an abdominal hydatid abscess

'milked' into the large intestine but resection of any gangrenous segments of small bowel with the contained worms and primary anastomosis is the treatment of choice.[89] These small children are often debilitated and postoperative complications are common. Ileal perforation, appendicitis and biliary ascariasis may also be encountered.[90]

Hydatid disease (see also Chapter 84)

Liver abscess[91,92] and hydatid disease of the lung are common and disease of the kidney,[93] brain,[94] bone[95] and other organs is not uncommon in many parts of the tropics where sheep and goats are the predominant livestock. The use of drugs such as albendazole and praziquantel and precautions against spillage of cyst contents (Figure 24.9) are the basis of successful treatment.

Overcoming isolation

Many tropical hospitals have only one doctor, others have only one surgeon. Communications by telephone are difficult and very slow by post. The district hospital may be 1000 km from the teaching hospital. How can the effects of such isolation be minimized?

First, assemble a reference library. The recommended surgical books are listed at the end of this chapter. To neglect such sources of wisdom and experience is to court disaster.[1] Many have cheap editions from TALC (PO Box 49, St Albans, Herts AL1 4AX, UK). IMPACT (impact@pavilion.co.uk) or local service clubs (Rotary, Lions or Round Table, etc) may help with book purchase and provide subscriptions to some of the relevant journals quoted in the references.

Some countries, such as Uganda, have continuing medical education (CME) programmes for up-country doctors which publish literature on clinical problems common to the area. In East Africa, the flying doctor service (AMREF) sends surgical teams to remote rural areas and similar, but smaller, outreach programmes exist in Zambia and elsewhere. An invitation to visit is the first step in developing a very useful network of contacts.

Information technology is getting cheaper. A computer with CD-ROM and modem will give wide access if a telephone exists. Satellite phones are still expensive but invaluable in really remote regions. Many specialists are willing to advise on clinical problems and acquisition of a simple digital camera makes the transmission of photographs and radiographs possible. Given project proposal, charitable organizations should think the price reasonable for breaking down a doctor's isolation.

RECOMMENDED REFERENCE BOOKS

Ansary M A, Hira S K, Bayley A C et al. *A Colour Atlas of AIDS in the Tropics*. London: Wolfe; 1989. ISBN 0-7234-1567-6.

British Medical Journal. *Appropriate technology* (collected articles published in the British Medical Journal). London: BMJ Books; 1985. ISBN 0-7279-0157-5.

Cook J, Sankaran B, Wasunna A. *General Surgery at the District Hospital*. Geneva: WHO:1988 ISBN 0-92-4-154235-7.

Dogson M. *Anaesthesia at the District Hospital*. Geneva: WHO; 1988 ISBN 0-92-4-154228-4.

King M. *Primary Anaesthesia*. Oxford: Oxford Medical; 1993 ISBN 0-19-261539-4

King M, Bewes P. *Primary Surgery vol.II - Trauma*. Oxford: Oxford Medical; 1987 ISBN 0-19-261599-8.

King M, Bewes P, Cairns J et al. *Primary Surgery vol. I - Non-trauma*. Oxford: Oxford Medical; 1990. ISBN 0-19-261694-3.

Rosenfield J V, Watters D A K. *Neurosurgery in the Tropics*. London: Macmillan; 2000. ISBN 0-333-68412-5.

Watters D A K, ed. 1988. Surgery in the Tropics. Bailliere's Clinical Tropical Medicine and Communicable Diseases, Vol 3 No 2 London: Bailiere; 1988. ISBN 0-7020-1309-9.

Watters D A K, Wilson I H, Leaver R J et al. *Care of the Critically Ill Patient in the Tropics and Sub-tropics*. Basingstoke: Macmillan; 1991. ISBN 0-33-353799-8.

REFERENCES

1 Bewes P C. Third World trauma. *Trauma* 1999; 1:341–350.

2 Wood A M. Surgery in East Africa: Technology and Training. Communications. *Proc Assoc Surg East Afr* 1981; 4:115–120.

3 Longombe A O. Surgical training of nurses for rural areas: necessity or aberration? *East Cen Afr J Surg* 1997; 3(1):43–48.

4 Watters D A K & Bayley A C. Training doctors and surgeons to meet the needs of Africa. *Br Med J* 1987; 295:761–763.

5 King M & Bewes P. Fractures of the shaft of the femur. In: King M, Bewes P, (eds.) *Primary surgery vol. II-trauma*. Oxford: Oxford Medical; 1987:313–321.

6 Jellis J E. Active conservative management of elbow injuries. *Proc Assoc Surg East Afr* 1991; 14:44–50.

7 Nordberg E. Incidence and estimated need of caesarean section, inguinal hernia repair and operation for strangulated hernia in rural Africa. *Br Med J* 1984; 289:92–93.

8 Fenton P M. The epidemiology of District Surgery in Malawi: a two-year study of surgical rates and indices in rural Africa. *East Cen Afr J Surg* 1997; 3(1):33–41.

9 Nordberg E, Holmberg S, Kiugu S. Output of major surgery in developing countries. *Trop Geograph Med* 1995; 47:206–211.

10 Rosenfield J V, Watters D A K. Neurological manifestations of HIV infection. In: *Neurosurgery in the Tropics*. London: Macmillan; 2000:256-259.

11 Bayley A C. Aggressive Kaposi's sarcoma in Zambia, 1983. *Lancet* 1984; i:1318.

12 Kehoe N S & Jellis J E. The incidence of human immunodeficiency virus infection in injured patients in Lusaka. *Injury* 1994; 25:375–378.

13 Bayley A C, Jellis J E, Watters D K. Surgery for HIV-infected patients. In: Leaper D J, Branicki F J, (eds.) *International Surgical Practice*. Oxford: Oxford Medical; 1992:65–93.

14 Rothenburg R, Woelfel M, Stoneburner R, et al. Survival with the acquired immune deficiency syndrome. Experience with 5833 Cases in New York City. *New Engl J Med* 1987; 317:1297–1302.

15 Ansary M A, Hira S K, Bayley A C et al. Cutaneous manifestations. In: *A Colour Atlas of AIDS in the Tropics*. London, Wolfe; 1989:28–54.

16 WHO AIDS: Interim proposal for a WHO staging system for HIV infection and disease. *Weekly Epidemiological Record* 1990; 65:221–228.

17 Rayer H D & Reinherz E L. Current concepts, T Lymphocytes: ontogeny, function and relevance to clinical disorders. *New Engl J Med* 1987; 317:1136–1142.

18 Creemers P C, O'Shaughnessy M, Bayko W T. Analysis of absolute T helper cell numbers and cellular immune defects in HIV antibody positive and negative homosexual men. *AIDS Res and Human Retroviruses* 1988; 4:268–278.

19 Jellis J E. HIV disease and the orthopaedic surgeon. *J Pakistan Orthop Assoc* 1997; 9(Suppl):45–48.

20 Ragni M V, Crossett L S, Herndon J H. Postoperative infection following orthopaedic surgery in HIV-infected haemophiliacs with CD4 counts < or = 200/mm^3. *J Arthroplasty* 1995; 10:716–721.

21 Association of Surgeons of East Africa. Guidelines for the management of HIV infection in East and Southern Africa. *East Cen Afr J Surg* 1995; 1(1):53–58.

22 Wake D J & Cutting W A M. Blood transfusions in developing countries: problems, priorities and practicalities. *Trop Doct* 1998; 28:4–8.

23 World Health Organisation, Global Programme on AIDS, Global Blood Safety Initiative. *Guidelines for the Appropriate Use of Blood*. WHO/GPA/Inf/89:18 Geneva:WHO, 1989.

24 Nielsen C H. Perioperative euvolaemic haemodilution. *East Cen Afr J Surg* 1997; 3(1):81–82.

25 Liaw Y, Boon P, Deshpande S. Haemodilution study in major orthopaedic surgery. *Aust NZ J Surg* 1994; 64:535–537.

26 Chretien J. Tuberculosis and HIV: the cursed duet. *Tuber Lung Dis* 1990; 65:25–32.

27 Elliot A M, Luo N, Tembo G et al. Impact of HIV on tuberculosis in Zambia: a cross sectional study. *Br Med J* 1990; 301:412–415.

28 Jellis J E. Orthopaedic surgery and HIV disease in Africa. *Internat Orthopaedics* (SICOT) 1996; 20:253–256

29 Bem C, Patil P S, Elliot A M et al. The pathology of lymphadenopathy in Lusaka. *Proc Assoc Surg East Afr* 1990; 13:62–65.

30 Dean G & Alderman P. An unusual presentation of tuberculosis. *Trop Doct* 1997; 27:185–186

31 Holcombe C, Weedon R, Llwin M. The differential diagnosis of breast lumps in the Tropics. *Trop Doct* 1999; 29:42–45.

32 Bem C. The value of naked eye examination of biopsied lymph nodes in the diagnosis of tuberculous lymphadenitis. *Trop Doct* 1996; 26:10–13.

33 Abdul-Ghaffar N U A M A, Ramadan I T, Marafie A A. Abdominal tuberculosis in Ahmadi, Kuwait: a clinico-pathological review. *Trop Doct* 1998; 28:137–139.

34 Govinder S, Annamalai K, Kumar KPS et al. Spinal tuberculosis in HIV positive and negative patients: immunological response and clinical outcome. *Int Orthop* (SICOT) 2000; 24:163–66

35 Dent A W, Seyfang M, Wallace S. Cytology and fine needle aspiration biopsy: appropriate technology, quick, safe and cheap. *Trop Doct* 1996; 37–39.

36 Desai G. Empyema thoracic in AIDS patients in the tropics. In: Zumla A, Johnson M A & Miller R F (eds). *AIDS and Respiratory Medicine*. London, Chapman & Hall; 1997:151–261.

37 Desai G & Mugala D D. Management of empyema thoracis at Lusaka, Zambia. *Br J Surg* 1992; 79:537–538.

38 Jellis J E. Orthopaedic infection associated with HIV disease. *Surgery* 1994; 12:175–177.

39 Sikasote C C & Erzingatsian K. Pyomyositis and HIV infection at the University Teaching Hospital. *East Cen Afr J Surg* 1998; 4(1):67.

40 Alidria-Ezati I. The association between pyomyositis and HIV infection in New Mulago Hospital. *Proc Assoc Surg East Afr* 1991; 14:91–94.

41 Ansaloni L. Tropical pyomyositis. *World J Surg* 1995; 20(5):613–617.

42 Njobvu P, McGill P, Kerr H et al. Spondyloarthropathy and human immunodeficiency virus infection in Zambia. *J Rheumatol* 1998; 25(8):1553–1559.

43 Adeloye A. Neurological and neurosurgical manifestations of human immunodeficiency virus (HIV) infections in Africa. *East Cen Afr J Surg* 2000; 5:49–54.

44 McGeehan D F. Necrotising fasciitis: a biological disaster. *Today's Emergency* 1999; 5:27–28.

45 Muthuuri J M. AIDS in general surgical practice. *East Cent Afr J Surg* 1997; 3:31–36

46 Bayley A C. Surgical pathology of HIV disease: Lessons from Africa. *Br J Surg* 1990; 863–866.

47 Bayley A C. Kaposi's sarcoma. *Bailliere's Clin Trop Medic Comm Dis* 1989; 311–327.

48 Korshid K A, Erzingatsian K, Watters D A K, et al. Intussusception due to Kaposi's sarcoma. *J Roy Coll Surg Edin* 1987; 32:339–341.

49 Bewes P C. Priorities in the management of trauma. *Bailliere's Clin Trop Med Comm Dis* 1988; 3:209–232.

50 Mbembati N A A, Museru L M, Lisokotala L, et al. The pattern of pre-hospital fatal injuries in Dar es Salaam. *East Cen Afr J Surg* 1999; 5:7–10.

51 Jellis J E. The management of neglected trauma. *East Cen Afr J Surg* 1999; 4:49–55.

52 Museru L M, Leshabari M T, Grob U et al. The pattern of injuries seen in patients in the orthopaedic/trauma wards of Muhimbili Medical Centre. *East Cen Afr J Surg* 1998; 4: 15–22.

53 Vanwersch K. Crocodile bite injury in Southern Malawi. *Trop Doct* 1998; 28:221–222.

54 Mekisic A P, Wardill J R. Crocodile attacks in the Northern Territory of Australia. *Med J Aust* 1992; 157:751–754.

55 Obote W W. Blood alcohol levels and injury severity in road traffic accident victims in Kampala. *East Cen Afr J Surg* 1996; 2:41–44.

56 Tepper M. Management of late traumatic posterior dislocation of the hip in developing countries. *East Cen Afr J Surg* 1999; 4:25–28.

57 Charnley Sir J. *The Closed Treatment of Common Fractures*, 3rd edn. Edinburgh: Churchill Livingstone, 1953.

58 Loefler I J P. Antibiotics and the surgeon. *East Cen Afr J Surg* 1999; 4:45–48.

59 Watters D A K. Coma & Head Injuries. In: Watters D A K, Wilson I H, Leaver R J, et al, (eds). *Care of the Critically Ill Patient in the Tropics and Sub-tropics*. Basingstoke: Macmillan; 1991:159–173, 175–184.

60 Watters D A K & Sinclaire J R. Outcome of head injuries in Central Africa. *J Roy Coll Surg Edin* 1988; 33:35–38.

61 Levy L F. The management of head injuries. *East Cen Afr J Surg* 1996; 2:49–62.

62 Rosenfield J V & Watters D A K. Head injury. In: *Neurosurgery in the Tropics*. London: Macmillan; 2000:52–89.

63 Newcombe R & Merry G. The management of acute neurotrauma in rural and remote locations. A set of guidelines for the management of head and spinal injuries. *J Clin Neurosci* 1999; 6:85–93.

64 Jaffrey D C. The orthopaedic management of spinal injuries. *East Cen Afr J Surg* 1996; 2:63–66

65 King M & Bewes P. The spine. In: *Primary surgery vol 2 Trauma*. Oxford: Oxford Medical; 1987:144–160.

66 Nzarubara G R. Risk factors for burns in Uganda and strategies for prevention. *East Cen Afr J Surg* 1999; 5:11–16.

67 Kumiponjera D. Burns caused by paraffin lamp explosion. *East Cen Afr J Surg* 2000; 5:82–83.

68 Cotton M H & Albertyn L. Self-immolation in Zimbabwe. *East Cen Afr J Surg* 1995; 1:43–47.

69 Barradas R. Suicide attempts by self immolation in Maputo. *Proc Assoc Surg East Afr* 1992; 15:70–75.

70 King M & Bewes P. Burns. In: *Primary surgery vol 2 Trauma*. Oxford: Oxford Medical; 1987:65–91.

71 Heywood A J. Burns. In: Watters D A K, Wilson I H, Leaver R J et al (eds). *Care of the Critically Ill Patient in the Tropics and Sub-tropics*. Basingstoke: Macmillan; 1991:213–231.

72 James J H. The treatment of burns in 1994. *East Cen Afr J Surg* 1995; 1:61–66

73 James J. Treatment of the burn wound. *East Cen Afr J Surg* 1999; 5:61.

74 Nath S, Erzingatsian K, Simonde S. Management of postburn contracture of the neck. *Burns* 1994; 20:438–441.

75 Jameson J S, Thomas W M, Dawson S, Wood J K et al. Splenectomy for haematological disease. *J Roy Coll Surg Edin* 1996; 41:307–311.

76 Erzingatsian K L. The enlarged spleen and early post-splenectomy complications. *East Cen Afr J Surg* 1996; 2:29–33.

77 Jellis J E. Haematogenous osteomyelitis. *Surgery* 1992; 10:145–148.

78 Loefler I J P. Bantu volvulus. *Surgery* 1990; 84:1196–1198.

79 Gakwaya A M. The diagnosis and treatment of symptomatic redundant sigmoid colon. *Proc Assoc Surg East Afr* 1991; 14:88–90.

80 King M, Bewes P C, Cairns J et al. Sigmoid volvulus. In: *Primary Surgery Vol 1 – Non-Trauma*. Oxford: Oxford Medical; 1993:161–167.

81 Mout P. Temporary colostomy as a permanent treatment for sigmoid volvulus: a simple and safe one-stage procedure. *Trop Doct* 1989; 19:20–30.

82 Erzingatsian K. One-stage sigmoid colectomy in patients with volvulus. *East Cen Afr J Surg* 1996; 2(2):25–28.

83 Duke J H Jr. Primary small bowel volvulus. *Arch Surg* 1997; 112:685–688.

84 Holcombe C. Surgical emergencies in tropical gastroenterology. *Gut* 1995; 36:9–11.

85 Wiermsa R & Hadley G P. Small bowel volvulus and intestinal ascariasis. *Br J Surg* 1988; 75:86–87.

86 Parkes G. Primary small bowel volvulus in rural Nepal. *Trop Doct* 1997; 27:156–158.

87 Oliver M J & Fleming A N M. Ileosigmoid knot at Mpilo Hospital *Proc Assoc Surg East Afr* 1988; 11:77–79.

88 Mokoena T & Luvuno F M. Conservative management of intestinal obstruction due to Ascaris worms in adult patients: a preliminary report. *J Roy Coll Surg Edin* 1988; 33:318–321.

89 Hyde G A Jr & Kyambi J M. Gangrenous intestinal obstruction in children due to *Ascaris lumbricoides*: surgical management. *East Cen Afr J Surg* 1996; 2(2):17–19.

90 Pandit S K & Zarger H U. Surgical ascariasis in children in Kashmir. *Trop Doct* 1997; 27:13–14.

91 Fenton-Lee D & Morris D L. The management of hydatid disease of the liver: part I. *Trop Doct* 1996; 26:173–176.

92 Fenton-Lee D & Morris D L. The management of hydatid disease of the liver: part 2. *Trop Doct* 1997; 27:87–88.

93 Mehdiratta N K, Gupta S C, Misra V et al. Renal hydatid disease. *Trop Doct* 1996; 26:33–34.

94 Rosenfeld J V, Clezy J K A, Watters D A K. Hydatid disease (cystic type). In: Rosenfeld J V & Watters D A K, eds. *Neurosurgery in the Tropics*. London: Macmillan; 2000:263–264.

95 Metcalfe J E & Grimer R J. Tackling osseous hydatidosis using orthopaedic oncology techniques. *Ann Roy Coll Surg Engl* 2000; 82:287–289.

Chapter 25
Obstetrics in the Tropics

Y. Ahmed

Maternal mortality: major causes and management

Complications of pregnancy and childbirth occur in all parts of the world and an estimated 15% of pregnant women may develop potentially life-threatening complications.[1] However, the outcome for both mother and fetus differs markedly across the world. Recent global estimates indicate that over half a million women die as a result of pregnancy complication each year and the vast majority occur in developing countries. Over half occur in Africa (273 000), about 42% (217 000) in Asia, about 4% (22 000) in Latin America and the Caribbean. Less than 1% (2800) occur in the more developed countries of the world.[2]

A maternal death is defined as the death of a woman while pregnant or within 42 days of delivery or the termination of a pregnancy, irrespective of the duration or the site of the pregnancy. The maternal mortality ratio (MMR) is expressed as the number of maternal deaths per 100 000 live births. Measuring maternal mortality can be difficult because of under-reporting and misclassification. There is wide variation in MMR within regions and even within countries. The highest estimates of MMR are for eastern and western Africa (1300 and 1100 per 100 000 live-births, respectively). This compares with low ratios of around 4–11 per 100 000 in Western Europe and North America.[2]

The levels of morbidity associated with pregnancy are even more difficult to calculate. It has been estimated that some 50 million women a year suffer complications as a result of pregnancy. These may produce long-term debilitating problems such as vesicovaginal fistula, infertility and chronic pelvic pain.[3] In addition to maternal mortality and morbidity, there are almost 8 million stillbirths and early neonatal deaths (within the first week of life) each year. These deaths are largely the result of the same factors that cause the death and disability of the mothers.

The main obstetric causes of maternal death include haemorrhage, infection and sepsis, hypertensive disorders of pregnancy including eclampsia, unsafe abortion and obstructed labour (Table 25.1). Strategies to prevent and reduce maternal deaths are discussed later in the chapter.

Table 25.1 Worldwide causes of maternal mortality[4]

Cause	Estimated percentage
Haemorrhage	24
Sepsis and infection	15
Hypertensive disorders and eclampsia	12
Unsafe abortion	13
Obstructed labour	8
Other direct*	8
Other indirect**	20

*Other direct causes include ectopic pregnancy.
**Indirect causes include anaemia, malaria, HIV and heart disease associated with pregnancy.

Haemorrhage

Haemorrhage is a major cause of maternal morbidity and mortality and of perinatal death. Anaemia is an important contributory problem and many women will be at substantial risk, as even a relatively small volume of blood loss before, during or after delivery can pose a major risk. Antepartum haemorrhage (APH) is defined as that occurring after 28 weeks gestation, although in the developed world 24 weeks is a more realistic figure. The two common causes of APH are abruptio placenta (premature separation of the placenta, which may be associated with pre-eclampsia) and placenta praevia (abnormally low placental implantation that partially or completely covers the internal cervical os).

A large retroplacental haemorrhage associated with separation of the placenta in abruptio placenta can lead to immediate fetal death and place the mother at risk due to hypotension, shock and possible disseminated intravascular coagulation (DIC). The signs of a tense, tender uterus, with the fetal parts difficult or impossible to palpate and the fetal heart absent may indicate abruptio placenta. Management includes prompt fluid replacement with plasma expanders or substitutes, if blood is not available. An artificial rupture of the membrane generally expedites delivery and reduces the risk of DIC in the mother. Intervention by caesarean section may be necessary, but is considered with extreme caution because of the complications of DIC. The priority is the survival of the mother.

In patients with placenta praevia the maternal and fetal condition may remain satisfactory until haemorrhage is considerable. A diagnosis of placenta praevia is considered in the presence of a high presenting fetal part, unstable or transverse lie, and would require prompt intervention by caesarean section.

Postpartum haemorrhage (PPH) often begins immediately after birth. It is primarily due to failure of the uterus to contract (uterine atony). This may be associated with retention of the placenta for more than 30 minutes after delivery. Vaginal and cervical lacerations cause less severe bleeding but require repair as soon as possible. The risks of PPH are higher in mothers who have had an APH during the pregnancy, those of high parity, multiple pregnancy and a previous history of PPH. In the management of PPH, 'rubbing up' or massaging the uterus per abdomen may be effective in contracting an atonic uterus. Prompt resuscitation with intravenous fluids, plasma substitutes and blood, if available, decreases the risk to the mother. Active management of the third stage of labour reduces the risk of PPH. This entails administration of an oxytocic to the mother after the birth of the anterior shoulder of the baby and delivery of the placenta by controlled cord traction, once it is evident that the uterus has contracted and signs of separation of the placenta are evident. Suitable oxytocics include: intramuscular or intravenous ergometrine, 0.5 mg, or ergometrine maleate with oxytocin ('Syntometrine') or 10 units of intravenous oxytocin.

Anaemia

Anaemia is defined as a haemoglobin concentration of less than 11 g/dl. However, in many communities it is common for women to have a haemoglobin level of <7 g/dl during pregnancy. As a consequence, anaemia can both be a cause of maternal death and contribute to the problems of haemorrhage and infection.

Anaemia is the end result of many factors in a woman's life. Poor nutrition in childhood may result in her starting her first pregnancy with low iron stores; repeated pregnancies too close together will deplete her iron, vitamin B_{12} and folate levels even further; and dietary traditions in pregnancy together with common infections such as hookworm and malaria compound the problem. Heavy periods prior to conceiving or intermittent blood loss during pregnancy may also be factors leading to anaemia.

Field workers should be trained to recognize the clinical signs of anaemia by examination of the mucous membranes of the eyelids and lips. Investigation can be limited to measuring the haemoglobin and also to exclude an underlying cause. In order for treatment of anaemia to be effective, women need to be registered for antenatal care at an early gestation, preferably in the second trimester, and their haemoglobin level checked at follow-up visits, typically at 30 and 36 weeks. Along with nutritional advice, a daily dose of 30–60 mg of elemental iron for women with a normal iron store and 120–240 mg for those women with low iron stores, accompanied by 0.4 mg of folate, is usually sufficient. A rise in the level of haemoglobin should be seen within a month of commencing treatment. If there is no response it may be due to an underlying disorder such as sickle cell disease or haemoglobinopathy, failure to comply with treatment or failure to absorb the oral therapy.

The problem of iron absorption may be overcome by the use of parenteral iron such as iron dextran given as a series of intramuscular injections or by total dose intravenous infusion. It is essential that the staff be trained to recognize and treat anaphylactic reactions, which may rarely occur with such administration. Between 0.5 and 1.0 ml of adrenaline 1:1000 should be given subcutaneously if an anaphylactic reaction occurs. It must be emphasized that parenteral iron does not increase the haemoglobin level any more quickly than oral therapy and should be reserved for those who cannot tolerate or absorb oral therapy.

For those patients who present in late pregnancy or in labour with a very low haemoglobin level, blood transfusion may be necessary, although in areas with endemic HIV infection this is an option that will be employed only as a last resort. Care must be taken to prevent cardiac failure when transfusing women with very low haemoglobin levels as the anaemia may lead to inefficient cardiac action and fluid overload. The use of packed cells and use of intravenous diuretics reduces the risk of cardiac failure due to fluid overload. In rare circumstances exchange transfusion may be employed.

Death due to cardiac failure may occur with haemoglobin levels below 4 g/dl. Women whose haemoglobin level is between 4 and 7 g/dl are also at greater risk of dying from infection due to poor resistance or from the effects of haemorrhage. Blood losses as low as 500 ml that may be easily tolerated by a woman with a normal haemoglobin level may be fatal in one with anaemia. Other effects of anaemia in pregnancy include stillbirth, intrauterine growth retardation and premature labour.

Prevention of anaemia is of the utmost importance. Much can be done by health workers in the promotion of a good diet, the composition of which will vary depending on the region but which should include green vegetables, staples, cereals and meat. Malaria prophylaxis is an important consideration in may parts of the world. Counselling on family planning would ensure adequate spacing to allow a woman to replenish her iron stores after pregnancy and breastfeeding.

Hypertensive disorders of pregnancy (see also Chapter 38)

Hypertensive disorders of pregnancy are common and complicate about 7–10% of all pregnancies. Almost 70% are due to pregnancy-induced hypertension (termed pre-eclampsia with the development of proteinuria and referred to as eclampsia when complicated by convulsions). Most of the other 30% are due to chronic hypertension, which is present before pregnancy or diagnosed early in pregnancy.

Pregnancy-induced hypertension (PIH) occurs worldwide and is predominantly a disease of young primigravidas in the second and third trimesters of pregnancy, although it can occur in any age group and also in subsequent pregnancies. PIH in older patients probably reflects undiagnosed chronic hypertension. Severe cases progress to eclampsia characterized by convulsions and coma and is associated with a high maternal mortality rate.

The aetiology of PIH is still unknown and this contributes to the problems in classification of the disease, its diagnosis and management. However, much more is known about the pathophysiology of PIH. Although the main feature of PIH is the development of hypertension (blood pressure greater than 140/90 mmHg), the disease affects multiple systems and is progressive in nature. PIH is associated with a mild degree of disseminated intravascular coagulation, which may worsen with increasing severity of disease. Renal perfusion decreases and this can lead to renal failure. A syndrome of haemolysis, elevated liver enzymes and low platelet count has been noted (HELLP) in severe pre-eclampsia. Cerebral haemorrhage often complicates eclampsia and uncontrolled hypertension, which may also lead to retinal detachment. Decreased uteroplacental flow due to the vasoconstrictive effects of pre-eclampsia leads to fetal growth restriction and fetal death. The perinatal mortality rate is increased in pre-eclampsia because of preterm delivery, uteroplacental insufficiency, abruptio placenta and unexplained fetal death. Preterm delivery is often necessitated by the fact that the definitive treatment of pre-eclampsia mandates termination of the pregnancy, regardless of the gestational age of the fetus.

Complications of the hypertensive disorders of pregnancy, including PIH, may be due to the disease itself, secondary to the convulsions in eclampsia or to the side effects of drugs or other treatment given. The main complications of treatment are related to respiratory depression and fluid overload. Regression of PIH only occurs after delivery of the fetus and placenta. The goals of management of a patient with PIH are to prevent deterioration to eclampsia, to prevent complications such as cardiovascular accidents, pulmonary edema, renal failure, abruptio placenta and fetal death, and the timely delivery of a surviving child with minimal trauma to the mother. Mild and moderate forms of the disease can only be detected by antenatal care, as the disease is symptomless at this stage other than the appearance of non-dependent oedema. The treatment of these patients is expectant, with admission to hospital if necessary. Labour can usually be induced without risk to the fetus after 37 weeks gestation. The objective of management prior to this time is to control blood pressure and monitor the maternal and fetal condition to ensure that deterioration does not occur. In the mild or moderate forms, treatment with antihypertensives under supervision may allow the pregnancy to be prolonged for a few weeks to allow for fetal maturation. Hypertension is just one sign of the multi-system disorder, and control of the blood pressure does not imply cure of the disease. Control of blood pressure can be achieved with any of the standard antihypertensive agents such as methyldopa, hydralazine, nifedipine or labetalol (see chapter 38). Beta-blockers such as propranolol are best avoided, as they tend to cause fetal bradycardia and hypoglycaemia in neonates.

The progress of PIH is extremely unpredictable. Some patients have only mild disease (with elevated blood pressure but no proteinuria) throughout the latter part of their pregnancy. Others progress rapidly within 24 hours from apparently mild disease to fulminating pre-eclampsia and eclampsia. Prior to the onset of convulsions in eclampsia, the woman may complain of frontal headaches, visual disturbances (particularly flashing lights), epigastric pain and vomiting. On examination, her reflexes tend to be exaggerated and urinary output decreased.

In areas with inadequate antenatal care provision or utilization, most women will present with severe pre-eclampsia or with eclampsia. Management in these circumstances is based on stabilizing the maternal condition and delivery of the fetus irrespective of gestation. Vaginal delivery may be possible following induction of labour by the use of prostaglandin analogues or rupturing the membranes and the judicious use of oxytocin. Careful monitoring of fluid intake and output is essential during this time as these patients are frequently oliguric and may develop pulmonary oedema. If the patient does not progress in labour, delivery by caesarean section may be necessary. Control of blood pressure is with intravenous antihypertensives, commonly hydrallazine given as 5 mg boluses intravenously.

Magnesium suphate (intravenously or intramuscular) is the drug of choice for treating convulsions in eclampsia and preventing their recurrence, although diazepam and phenytoin are also used. Diazepam may cause maternal and neonatal respiratory depression. Magnesium sulphate may also cause respiratory and cardiac arrest if plasma magnesium levels become too high. Suppression of the reflexes occurs prior to respiratory or cardiac arrest, and decreased urine output would exacerbate toxicity. Care must be taken, therefore, when using magnesium sulphate to check for adequate renal output and the presence of reflexes before giving a further dose. Its use in preventing eclampsia in patients with severe pre-eclampsia is still being evaluated. Phenytoin is less reliable in its action, is more expensive and requires close monitoring of the patient. Patients can be at risk of eclamptic fits for up to 48 hours after delivery. During this time they should therefore receive intensive nursing in a semi-prone position in a quiet room. Anti-hypertensive and prophylactic anti-convulsant therapy with magnesium sulphate should be continued.

Obstructed labour

Prolonged labour increases the likelihood of fetal hypoxia and may result in stillbirth or neonatal death. When associated with the prolonged labour, complications such as cephalopelvic disproportion, malpresentation (e.g., brow or shoulder presentation) and abnormal lie (e.g., transverse lie) will result in obstructed labour. In some cases vaginal delivery may still occur but at a cost not only of fetal death but also of serious maternal morbidity, such as vesicovaginal fistula due to pressure necrosis. In more extreme cases uterine rupture and subsequent maternal death will be the outcome.

The use of the partograph in the management of labour enables the health attendant to recognize when labour is not progressing normally, allowing for appropriate action to be taken.[5] Since a large number of deliveries are conducted by traditional birth attendants they should be taught to recognize the signs which precede obstructed labour and encouraged to refer to an appropriate centre where medical staff and facilities are available. Midwives and nurses are encouraged to use the partograph to monitor the progress of labour of mothers cared for and who have their babies delivered at primary health centres. This will enable them to identify when there is failure of progress of labour and to refer to a hospital for the judicious use of oxytocin to improve uterine contractions, providing cephalopelvic disproportion and malpresentation have been excluded. Further lack of progress requires intervention by Caesarean section that can then be performed early to ensure fetal survival and prevent maternal mortality and morbidity.

Puerperal sepsis

Following delivery or abortion, whether spontaneous or induced, the presence of a large denuded area of the uterus predisposes to the development of endometritis and subsequent ·puerperal sepsis. Sepsis may also occur secondary to laceration of the genital tract and in the presence of retained products of conception. Poor hygiene on the part of the birth attendant and poor sterilization of instruments inserted into the genital tract during delivery or abortion are a particular risk. The presence of a genital tract infection is suspected by the presence of foul-smelling lochia or discharge. Less specific symptoms include abdominal pain, vomiting, headache and loss of appetite. Examination reveals pyrexia and a tender bulky uterus. In more advanced stages of the disease tender masses in the adnexa or in the posterior fornix may be found, suggesting the presence of tubo-ovarian or Pouch of Douglas abscesses. Septicaemia may also occur.

Treatment in the early stages is by the use of broad-spectrum antibiotics followed by evacuation of the uterus after approximately 24 hours if retained products of conception are suspected. In more advanced cases, following the administration of intravenous antibiotics, laparotomy to drain the tubo-ovarian abscesses is necessary, and in extreme cases hysterectomy and pelvic clearance may be required. Abscesses in the Pouch of Douglas may be drained by colpotomy (via the vagina), but a significant proportion of such patients will subsequently require laparotomy.

Viral hepatitis (see also Chapter 40)

Pregnant mothers in developing countries are at greater risk of contracting hepatitis and have a higher mortality rate associated with the disease which is related to their poor nutritional status. Viral hepatitis could be due to hepatitis A (HAV), B (HBV), C (HCV), E (HEV). Fulminating hepatitis usually occurs during the third trimester. The early symptoms include nausea, malaise, fever, headache and joint pains. Later symptoms include epigastric pain and jaundice, with hepatic coma preceding death. Premature labour and postpartum haemorrhage are the common obstetric complications. Treatment is supportive and bed-rest is extremely important. A high carbohydrate diet is required, with intravenous glucose infusion in labour. Fresh blood should be transfused if a postpartum haemorrhage occurs.

Malaria in pregnancy (see also Chapter 71)

Malaria in general, and particularly infection with *Plasmodium falciparum*, is a major cause of morbidity and mortality in pregnancy, especially for the young primigravida. Pregnant women living in endemic areas tend to lose their immunity to malaria, particularly during the second trimester, and are at increased risk of infection that tends to be more severe in pregnancy. The most serious effect of malaria in pregnancy is the development of haemolytic anaemia that, if severe enough, can lead to hypoxia of both the mother and fetus. The hepatorenal syndrome and cerebral malaria is often the cause of death. Other sequelae of malaria include miscarriage, intrauterine fetal growth restriction, fetal death and premature labour. In areas where malaria is holoendemic, it is an important cause of anaemia. The presentation of malaria in pregnancy, however, may be atypical and its presence should be suspected in any pregnant woman in endemic areas with fever or jaundice.

Treatment is dependent on the geographical area and the local pattern of drug resistance. *P. falciparum* and *P. vivax* account for the majority of cases. It is essential to follow local, national and regional treatment guidelines. Chloroquine is the treatment of choice in chloroquine-sensitive areas. However, chloroquine resistance is widespread and oral sulfadoxine/pyrimethamine or quinine salt can be used instead. Where multi-drug resistant *P. falciparum* limits treatment options, artesunate is used instead.

In areas of mixed *falciparum-vivax* malaria, the proportions of malaria species and their drug sensitivity patterns vary, making reference to the local treatment guidelines even more important. Chloroquine alone is the treatment of choice during pregnancy in areas with chloroquine-sensitive *vivax* malaria and chloroquine-sensitive *falciparum* malaria. Where there is chloroquine-resistant *falciparum* malaria, it is managed as a mixed infection with the addition of sulfadoxine/pyrimethamine.

Routine chemoprophylaxis is advocated for pregnant women according to local guidelines. Regimens include weekly chloroquine (and daily proguanil) from 20 weeks gestation onwards. In areas of high transmission in sub-Saharan Africa, the current strategy for malaria prevention is presumptive intermittent treatment with sulfadoxine/pyrimethamine, once during the second trimester and once during the third trimester. In areas of high HIV prevalence, intermittent presumptive treatment with sulfadoxine/pyrimethamine every month beginning in the second trimester appears to be optimal.[6]

Tetanus (see also Chapter 62)

Maternal tetanus infection may occur as a result of abortion performed with improperly sterilized instruments or from delivery in unclean surroundings. Although maternal tetanus can occur as an ascending infection, neonatal tetanus is far more common. The neonate may get infected via the umbilicus. Traditions such as the application of cow dung to the umbilical stump predisposes the neonate to infections. Treatment is described in chapter 62, but mortality rates remain high. Training of birth attendants, particularly in the use of a clean delivery technique and use of sterilized equipment, would reduce the risk of infection. Antenatal programmes in developing countries now provide for tetanus immunization and aim to provide cover for the mother and also the neonate. To be effective, pregnant women need to receive two doses of tetanus toxoid 4 weeks apart and at least 4 weeks prior to giving birth. The first dose should ideally be given at the first clinic visit.

Post-abortion care

Spontaneous abortion (miscarriage) is a common problem all over the world and can occur in as many as 15% of pregnancies, usually in the first trimester. If untreated, incomplete abortion frequently leads to continued vaginal bleeding and consequent anaemia. The retained products may also give rise to uterine sepsis. In many countries, the common procedure is a sharp curettage of the uterine cavity, more frequently known as dilatation and curettage (D&C), which requires a physician, operating theatre, and general anaesthesia. Manual vacuum aspiration (MVA) using a plastic cannula and syringe to create a vacuum is the preferred procedure because of its lower risk of complications. It can be performed under local anaesthesia and a few countries have successfully trained midwives to conduct the procedure.[7]

Induced abortion is illegal in many countries, but even where it is legal this does not ensure access to quality services. Consequently, a high proportion of women presenting with incomplete abortion may have associated sepsis due to self-abortion or the procedure having been performed by unskilled or untrained personnel.

Post-abortion care services provide for emergency care of complications which includes resuscitation, use of antibiotics, and evacuation of the uterus using MVA if possible; counselling on symptoms and signs for the woman to look out for in the next few days; and also counselling and, if necessary, provision of other reproductive health services, especially family planning.

Ectopic pregnancy

Ectopic pregnancy can be a major life-threatening condition. The incidence has been reported as varying between 1 per 43 and 1 per 175 births. The main risk factors include age, previous pelvic inflammatory disease, use of an intrauterine contraceptive device, pelvic surgery, and induced abortion. Rupture of the ectopic pregnancy and subsequent intra-abdominal bleeding leads to the classical signs of acute lower abdominal pain and hypotension with signs of haemoperitoneum. Immediate intervention is by laparotomy with partial salpingectomy to control the bleeding. In many areas where there are no blood transfusion facilities, it is appropriate to carry out intraoperative auto-transfusion, with aspiration of blood from the peritoneal cavity into a sterile bottle containing 50 ml of citrate phosphate dextrose. The collected blood should then be filtered and can be transfused back into the patient. This can be done before dealing with the ectopic pregnancy and will reduce the risks to the patient.[8] In some cases the condition is chronic with slow leakage of blood into the peritoneal cavity, causing intermittent lower abdominal pain and pelvic tenderness or a pelvic mass. Anaemia usually develops in these situations. Laparoscopy, if available, will allow a positive diagnosis before appropriate intervention.

Strategies to reduce maternal mortality

Causes of maternal death are multi-factorial and have been conceptualized according to the 'four delays', which also allow potential interventions to be identified (Table 25.2).[9]

Health care providers and managers need to put measures in place that reduce the incidence of unwanted pregnancies through improving access to quality family planning and safe abortion (where it is legal); reduce the number and severity of obstetric complications through pre-pregnancy care, antenatal care (to prevent, identify and promptly treat complications), clean safe deliveries with skilled providers and quality postnatal care; and reduce the case fatality rate of complications through access to quality obstetrical and post-abortion services.

Essential and emergency obstetric care

As maternal emergencies are extremely difficult to predict, all women should have access to essential obstetric care (EOC). Interventions in EOC focus on health promotion during the pre-pregnancy period, antenatal care, labour/delivery and postpartum care as well as appropriate management of complications that directly focus on maternal mortality reduction. For the management of complications, EOC is required which focuses on interventions directed more towards reducing mortality. It is recommended that for every 500 000 people there should

Table 25.2 Causes of maternal death—the four delays

Delay in recognizing the need for medical care
These are related to problem recognition and the lack of information about complications or pregnancy and childbirth and danger signs. Interventions include health education for the women and health providers. Traditional birth attendants can be encouraged to seek prompt referrals to a health facility.
Delays in deciding to seek care
Related to socio-cultural/economic factors and can be addressed through: couple communication and educating key decision makers, encourage the use of a birth plan, encourage and motivate greater use of skilled providers (midwives, physicians) either at home or in health centres.
Delays in reaching the health facility
Related to the availability and access of services. Interventions include improving the transportation system by working with local communities; develop maternity waiting homes near the health facilities; improve the community's knowledge regarding the nearest health facility and how to access their services.
Delays in receiving treatment from the health facility
Related to the quality of care. Interventions include training of doctors and midwives in life saving skills; ensure that equipment is functional; proper infection control practices are utilised; an inventory control system is in place to maintain a sufficient stock of drugs and medical supplies on a regular basis; promote 'mother friendly' environments.

Adapted from Ross, 1998.[9]

Table 25.3 Essential obstetric care requirements

Comprehensive emergency obstetric care facilities (one facility per 500,000 people)
Perform surgery under general anaesthesia
Perform assisted removal of retained placenta (e.g., D&C or MVA)
Perform manual removal of retained placenta
Perform assisted vaginal delivery (e.g., vacuum extraction or forceps delivery)
Provide blood transfusion
Administer parenteral antibiotics
Administer parenteral sedatives (diazepam) and anticonvulsants (magnesium sulphate)
Administer parenteral oxytocics
Basic emergency obstetric care facilities (four facilities per 500,000 people)
Perform manual removal of retained placenta/pieces
Perform assisted vaginal delivery (e.g., vacuum extraction)
Administer antibiotics, sedatives, and oxytocin intramuscular or intravenously
Obstetric first aid in the community
Uterine massage or bimanual compression of the uterus to stop bleeding
Take measures to prevent a woman hurting herself in the event of eclamptic convulsions
In case of fever or prolonged rupture of membranes to administer antibiotics and antipyretics as a temporary measure.

be four facilities offering basic emergency obstetric care and one offering comprehensive emergency obstetric care (Table 25.3).[10]

HIV and pregnancy

Pregnant women who are HIV-1 infected are commonly encountered in some developing countries. This has important implications for the management of pregnancy and childbirth. Over 90% of HIV infections in children result from mother-to-child transmission. Although Africa has been the centre of the epidemic, a rapid rise in infection rates has been seen in South-East Asia, some Indian cities, Latin America and the Caribbean. UNAIDS estimates that 25.3 million of the 36.1 million people living with HIV by the end of 2000 were from sub-Saharan Africa. Women constituted 55% of those adults who were infected.[11] In several urban centres in eastern and southern Africa, HIV infection rates in pregnant women now exceed 25%. Of the two types of HIV, HIV-1 is the most common, though HIV-2 is found in parts of West Africa. The prevalence of HIV-2 has been stable and the clinical course is slower than that of HIV-1. Mother-to-child transmission occurs less frequently than with HIV-1. This section only deals with HIV-1.

Effect of pregnancy on the natural history of HIV infection

Pregnancy appears to have little effect on the progress of infection in asymptomatic HIV-positive women or in those in the early stages of infection. There may be a rapid progression in women with late-stage HIV infection.[12] African women, with additional factors of poor nutrition and repeated pregnancies, do not appear to experience more rapid progression of HIV infection during their pregnancies.[13] Nevertheless, in some African countries AIDS has become a common cause of maternal mortality.[14] This appears to be due to more women with advanced disease becoming pregnant.

Effect of HIV on pregnancy

HIV infection has been reported to have little effect on pregnancy in developed countries.[15] However, adverse outcomes including complications of early and late pregnancy, have been reported more commonly in a number of African studies. HIV may be the direct cause of complications, or a marker of interaction of related medical and social conditions that affect pregnancy. HIV has been linked to a higher rate of spontaneous abortion, preterm labour, preterm rupture of membranes, abruptio placenta and low birthweight. Although increased stillbirth rates have been reported in HIV-positive women, the risk appears to be lower in asymptomatic women and is independent for the presence of other sexually transmitted infections (STIs), including syphylis.[16]

Bacterial pneumonia, urinary tract infections and other infections are more common in HIV-positive women.[17] HIV-related opportunistic infections, particularly tuberculosis, are commonly found during pregnancy. Kaposi's sarcoma has been reported in pregnancy in HIV-positive women. Postnatal infectious complications are commoner in HIV-positive women particularly after caesarean section.[18]

Mother-to-child transmission of HIV

Timing and rate of mother-to-child transmission

In Europe and USA, rates of mother-to-child transmission (MTCT) of HIV in untreated non-breastfeeding populations has ranged from 14% to 32%. With the availability and use of routine antiretroviral therapy in many of these countries, dramatically lower transmission rates are being described. This is in contrast to rates of 25% to 48% among breastfeeding populations in African and Asian studies.[19] There are multiple reasons for higher rates in these developing countries, but near-universal breastfeeding is probably the most important.

Mother-to-child HIV transmission may occur in the intrauterine or intrapartum periods, or postnatally through breast milk. In the absence of breastfeeding, about 30% of infant HIV infections occur in utero and 70% during labor and delivery.[20] One-third to one-half, of perinatal HIV infections in African settings may be due to breastfeeding.[19]

Risk factors for transmission, include high maternal viral load, advanced maternal immune deficiency and prolonged rupture of membranes (>4 hours).[19,21] Risk factors for breast milk transmission include high viral load and subclinical mastitis.[22,23]

Interventions to prevent or reduce MTCT

The use of the antiretroviral drugs in pregnancy has been shown to reduce perinatal HIV transmission to the infant. Zidovudine given to the pregnant woman had been used either as a 'long course' through pregnancy, labour and for six weeks to the infant, or as a 'short course' from 36 weeks gestation onwards.[24,25] Several different short-course

antiretroviral regimens are efficacious in reducing mother-to-child transmission. Efficacy, measured at 3 to 6 months after delivery, is lower in breastfed than in non-breastfed infants. A simpler single-dose treatment with the antiretroviral nevirapine is a promising alternative. Nevirapine has a prolonged half-life, rapidly crosses the placenta, crosses into breast milk and is administered as a single dose to the mother at onset of labour and then to the neonate within 72 hours of birth.[26]

A randomized controlled trial of mode of delivery in Europe showed a dramatic decrease in transmission to the infant when delivered by caesarean section as opposed to a vaginal birth.[27] However, caesarean section in HIV-infected women must also take into account the possibility of maternal morbidity and mortality. Other considerations, particularly in developing countries include the availability of safe operating facilities, increased service commitments by overworked staff and the potential risks to future pregnancies due to ruptured uterus or repeat caesarean.[28]

The combination of antiretroviral use, caesarean section and the avoidance of breastfeeding with replacement feeding in developed countries has led to dramatic decreases in the rate of MTCT, although these treatments are not currently feasible in developing countries.[24,25,27] Low-cost preventive measures such as vaginal cleansing with chlorhexidine hydrochloride or maternal vitamin A supplementation have shown no overall efficacy in preventing MTCT.[29,30]

Modification of infant feeding practice

In resource-poor settings, alternatives to breastfeeding may not be feasible for financial, logistical and cultural reasons. Mothers should be given information on the advantages and disadvantages of breastfeeding and replacement feeding with regard to HIV infection and encouraged to make a fully informed decision about infant feeding.

Voluntary HIV counselling and testing in pregnancy

There are a number of advantages to a woman knowing her HIV status prior to, or during pregnancy. In the case of a woman found to be HIV positive, these include: facilitating early counselling and treatment; appropriate treatment and follow-up of the child; enables a woman to make a decision on continuation of the pregnancy and on future fertility; allows the implementation of strategies to attempt to prevent transmission to the child; enables the woman to take precautions to help prevent transmission to sexual partners; and enable sexual partners to be counselled and tested. If the test is negative, women can be guided in appropriate HIV prevention measures and risk-reduction behaviour. The possible disadvantages of HIV testing in pregnancy include reported increased risk of violence, stigmatization by community and health workers, higher levels of anxiety and psychological sequelae.

Management of HIV-positive pregnant women

Most HIV-positive women will be asymptomatic and have no major obstetrical problems during their pregnancies and can receive similar antenatal care to that given to HIV-negative women. If there are no complications of HIV infection, there is no need to increase the number of visits. Consideration could be given to assessment of fetal growth, whether by regular uterine fundal height measurements or, where available, by serial ultrasound assessments. Invasive diagnostic procedures, such as chorion villus biopsy sampling, amniocentesis or cordocentesis are best avoided where possible, due to a possible risk to the fetus. External cephalic version of a breech fetus may be associated with potential maternal-fetal circulation leaks.

At the first antenatal visit, a full physical examination of an HIV-positive woman is undertaken and particular attention paid to any signs of HIV related infections including tuberculosis, oral or vaginal thrush, or lymphadenopathy. Current herpes lesions and scars of herpes zoster is often an early sign of HIV infection. Clinical diagnosis of STIs, particularly gonorrhoea and syphilis, are undertaken. In subsequent visits, the pregnant woman is monitored for any signs of opportunistic infections and for intercurrent infections like urinary tract infections or respiratory infection. Maternal weight is monitored and nutritional supplements advised as appropriate.

Laboratory investigations would depend on availability of resources. A test for syphylis is undertaken at the first visit and followed up by a repeat test in late pregnancy. A haemoglobin estimation (and full count if feasible) is obtained and anaemia treated as necessary. T-cell subset investigations and viral load estimation are useful if they can be obtained and provide valuable prognostic indicators. A cervical smear is performed if a recent smear is not available.

Although vitamin A supplementation has not been proven to reduce transmission, together with the use of multivitamins, it has nutritional value. Mebendazole is given at the first visit in areas of high hookworm prevalence.

Malaria in pregnancy may be associated with increased risk of MTCT of HIV.[31] Intermittent treatment with an effective, preferably a single dose, anti-malarial drug should be made available to all primigravidae and secundigravidae in highly endemeic areas. This is started in the second trimester and given at monthly intervals.

Prophylaxis for opportunistic infections is given in pregnancy as indicated by the clinical stage and according to local policy. This includes prophylaxis and treatment for tuberculosis. Of the anti-tuberculosis drugs, streptomycin and pyrazinamide are not recommended during pregnancy. *Pneumocystis carinii* pneumonia (PCP) prophylaxis, if started, should continue during pregnancy with sulphametahxazole/trimethoprim (septrin) or pentamidine. The risk to the fetus is outweighed by the risk to the maternal health of PCP.

The use of antiretroviral therapy in pregnancy is considered for both the health of the mother and for prevention of transmission to the fetus. Pregnancy should not be a contraindication for antiretroviral therapy in the mother, if indicated. The use of zidovudine has been previously described for prevention of transmission, however this is sub-optimal adult retroviral therapy treatment and two antiretroviral drugs with the possible addition of a protease inhibitor is preferable. There is a theoretical risk to the fetus from combination therapy, although there is limited experience. Detailed recommendations have been released in the USA on combination therapy in pregnancy. If available, similar local guidelines should be referred to.[32] As many newer compounds do not have long-term safety data following use in pregnancy, this should be discussed with the patient.

Management of labour and delivery remains the same as that of HIV-negative women. Prolonged rutpture of membranes is avoided, as MTCT is increased where membranes are ruptured for more than four hours. The general rule is to avoid any procedure which breaks the baby's skin and/or increases the risk of contact with the mother's blood, such as scalp electrodes and fetal blood sampling. Episiotomy should not be a routine procedure, but should rather be reserved for those cases with an obstetrical indication. Caesarean section has been found to be associated with a decrease in prevention of HIV transmission to the infant, although there are considerations of maternal complications. Nevertheless, prophylactic antibiotics are recommended for both elective and emergency caesarian sections.[27] Babies of HIV-infected mothers should have maternal secretions and blood washed off as soon as possible, after which time they can be safely handled by mothers and health workers.

Postpartum care is similar to that for uninfected women. HIV-infected women are more prone to postpartum infections, including urinary tract infections; chest infections, episiotomy and caesarean section wound infections. Instructions are provided to women about early symptoms and also safe handling of lochia and bloodstained sanitary materials.

Counselling on breastfeeding includes discussing the risks and benefits of infant feeding choices. Mothers who chose to breastfeed are advised of the possible increased extra risk of transmission in the presence of cracked nipples, mastitis and breast abscess. Prevention of such problems can be achieved through adequate breastfeeding techniques. Reduced duration of breastfeeding and early cessation may be encouraged to reduce the risk of transmission if this can be safely achieved.[33]

Contraceptive advice is important when a mother chooses not to breastfeed because of the loss of the contraceptive effects of breastfeeding, and information on alternative methods should be provided.

REFERENCES

1   Mother Baby Package: Implementing Safe Motherhood in Countries. World Health Organization, Geneva, 1994. (See also: Care of the Mother and Baby at the Health Centre: a Practical Guide. WHO/FHE/MSM/94.2)

2   Maternal Mortality in 1995. Estimates developed by WHO, UNICEF and UNFPA (Statement). Global estimates of maternal mortality for 1995: Results of an in-depth review, analysis and estimation strategy. WHO web site. Available at http://www.who.int/reproductivehealth/index.htm. Accessed April 7th 2001. (See also : Revised 1990 Estimates of Maternal Mortality. A New Approach by WHO and UNICEF), 1996. WHO/FRH/MSM/96.11, UNICEF/PLN/96.1)

3   The Progress of Nations. UNICEF. New York, 1996.

4   Family Care International and Safe Motherhood Inter-Agency group. Safe Motherhood Fact Sheets; prepared from the Safe Motherhood Technical Consultation in Sri Lanka, 18–23 October 1997. Family Care International, 1997.

5   WHO. The Partograph: A Managerial Tool for the Prevention of Prolonged Labour. Section I: the principle and the strategy. WHO/MCH/88.3. Section II: a user's manual. WHO/MCH/88.4. Section III: facilitator's guide. WHO/MCH/89.1. Section IV: guidelines for operations research on the application of the partograph. WHO/MCH/89.2. Geneva: WHO, 1988.

6   Parise ME, Ayisi JG, Nahlen BL et al. Efficacy of sulfadoxine/pyrimethamine for prevention of placental malaria in an area of Kenya with a high prevalence of malaria and human immunodeficiency virus infection. *Am J Trop Med Hyg* 1998; 59:813–822.

7   Population Reports (September 1997). Care for Post-Abortion Complications: Saving Women's Lives, Series L, Number 10. World Health Organization, Geneva.

8   Laskey J, Wood PB. Ectopic pregnancies and intraoperative autotransfusion. *Trop Doc* 1991; 21:116–118.

9   Ross SR. Promoting Quality Maternal and Newborn Care: A Reference Manual for Program Managers. Care, Atlanta. 1998.

10 WHO/UNICEF/UNFPA. Guidelines for Monitoring the Availability and Use of Obstetric Services. UNICEF. 1997.

11 UNAIDS. Epidemic Update: December 2000. UNAIDS Web site. Available at: http://www.unaids.org/epidemic_update/report_dec00/index_dec.html. Accessed 27th April 2001

12 Johnstone FD. Pregnancy outcome and pregnancy management in HIV-infected women. In Johnson MA Johnstone FD (eds). *HIV Infection in Women*. Edinburgh: Churchill Livingstone, 1993:187–198.

13 Temmerman M, Nagelkerke N, Bwayo J et al. HIV-1 and immunological changes during pregnancy: a comparison between HIV-1-seropositive and HIV-1-seronegative women in Nairobi, Kenya. *AIDS* 1995; 9:1057-1060.

14 Taha TE, Miotti P, Liomba G et al. HIV, maternal death and child survival in Africa. *AIDS* 1996; 10:111–112.

15 Brocklehurst P, French R. The association between maternal HIV infection and perinatal outcome: a systematic review of the literature and meta-analysis. *Br J Obstet Gynaecol* 1998; 105:839–848.

16 Temmerman M, Plummer FA, Mirza NB et al. Infection with HIV as a risk factor for adverse obstetrical outcome. *AIDS* 1990; 4:1087–1093.

17 Minkoff HL, Willoughby A, Mendez H et al. Serious infections during pregnancy among women with advanced human immunodeficiency virus infection. *Am J Obstet Gynecol* 1990; 162:30–34.

18 Bergstrom S, Sonnerborg A, Osman NB Libombo A. HIV infection and maternal outcome of pregnancy in Mozambican women: a case-control study. *Genitourinary Med* 1995; 71:323–324.

19 Wiktor SZ, Ekpini E, Nduati RW. Prevention of mother-to-child transmission of HIV-1 in Africa. *AIDS* 1997; 11(suppl B):S79–S87.

20 Mock PA, Shaffer N, Bhadrakom C et al. Maternal viral load and timing of mother-to-child HIV transmission, Bangkok, Thailand. *AIDS* 1999;13:407–414.

21 UNAIDS,WHO. HIV in Pregnancy: A Review. WHO, Geneva, 1999. (UNAIDS/99.35E, WHO/CHS/RHR/99.15) p. 10.

22 Semba RD, Kumwenda N, Hoover DR et al. Human immunodeficiency virus load in breast milk, mastitis, and mother-to-child transmission of human immunodeficiency virus type 1. *J Infect Dis* 1999; 180:93–98.

23 UNAIDS, UNICEF, WHO. A Review of HIV Transmission through Breastfeeding. (WHO/FRH/NUT/CHD/98.3/UNAIDS 98.5)/UNICEF/PD/NUT/(J)98.1.

24 Connor EM, Sperling RS, Gelber R et al. Reduction of maternal-infant transmission of human immunodeficiency virus type 1 with zidovudine treatment. *N Engl J Med* 1994; 331:1173–1180.

25 Shaffer N, Chuachoowong R, Mock PA et al. Short-course zidovudine for perinatal HIV-1 transmission in Bangkok, Thailand: a randomised controlled trial. *Lancet* 1999; 353:773–780.

26 Guay LA, Musoke P, Fleming T et al. Intrapartum and neonatal single-dose nevirapine compared with zidovudine for prevention of mother-to-child transmission of HIV-1 in Kampala, Uganda: HIVNET 012 randomised trial. *Lancet* 1999; 354:795–802.

27 The European Mode of Delivery Collaboration. Elective Cesarean section versus vaginal delivery in prevention of vertical HIV-1 transmission: a randomised clinical trial. *Lancet* 1999, 353:1035–1039.

28 Bulterys M, Chao A, Dushimimana A Saah A. Fatal complications after Cesarian section in HIV-infected women. *AIDS* 1996; 10:923–924.

29 Taha TE, Biggar RJ, Broadhead RL et al. Effect of cleansing the birth canal with antiseptic solution on maternal and newborn morbidity and mortality in Malawi: clinical trial. *Br Med J* 1997;315:216–219.

30 Coutsoudis A, Pillay K, Spooner E et al. for the South African Vitamin A Study Group. Influence of infant-feeding patterns on early mother-to-child transmission of HIV-1 in Durban, South Africa: a prospective cohort study. *Lancet* 1999; 354:471–476.

31 Bloland PB, Wirima JJ, Steketee RW et al. Maternal HIV infection and infant mortality in Malawi: evidence for increased mortality due to placental malaria infection. *AIDS* 1995; 9:721–726.

32 Centers for Disease Control and Prevention. Public Health Service Task Force recommendations for the use of antiretroviral drugs in pregnant women infected with HIV-1 for maternal health and for reducing perinatal HIV-1 transmission in the United States. MMWR, 1998 47(Rr-2):1–30.

33 UNAIDS,WHO,UNICEF. HIV and Infant Feeding: A Guide for Health Care Managers and Supervisors. Geneva, 1998. (UNAIDS/98.4, WHO/FRH/NUT/CHD/98.2, UNICEF/PD/NUT(J)98.2)

Chapter 26
Radiology and Imaging Services in the Tropics

J. L. Richenberg and E. T. Tshibwabwa

Radiology is increasingly central to the investigation and treatment of patients in the developed world. The benefits that drive this shift in practice should be available to patients, and to planners of health care, in the tropics. Indeed, ironically, the benefits of minimally invasive therapy, as offered by interventional radiology, may be greater in the tropics where alternative treatments (long-term drug therapy, complex open surgery and so on) may not be available, or be prohibitively expensive.

While we should strive to place modern and dependable imaging ever more at the centre of provision of health care in the tropics, many practical considerations have to be tackled before this paradigm can be realized. In particular, we cannot simply translate from the model of radiology services in the developed world to the tropics. There are profound differences in the disease profiles between the two regions—infection and trauma account for much of the pathology in the tropics rather than ischaemic heart disease or cancer. Furthermore, the affluent areas in Europe and North America have comparatively large funds available to the provision of radiology equipment. Contrast this with the often impoverished regions in the tropics, which lack resources, equipment and personnel. The differential is exacerbated by a hostile topography and climate. Many areas are remote and sparsely populated, such that in many tropical countries resources are often concentrated in a few urbanized areas.[1-5]

Some principles in establishing a radiological service

The key to developing a sound radiological service is to match provision to demand. Most of the cities and rural areas in Africa are blighted by a common group of pathologies. HIV/AIDS and tuberculosis 'spearhead' the disease problem; and there are other prevalent infections including those due to amoebiasis or helminths. Trauma accounts for a second major drain on limited health care resources. Thus, tropical imaging should be geared up for managing trauma, investigating *and treating* infection (for example, percutaneous image-guided abscess drainage) and for obstetric care.

Plain radiography and ultrasound should form the core of any realistic imaging service.[3,5,6] Computed tomography (CT) has a limited role and magnetic resonance imaging (MRI) should be reserved for major centres alone.

All equipment should be reliable and durable and most should be portable. It needs to be user-friendly, cheap and uniform. There is increasing availability of such equipment, an evolution being driven by multinational companies not because they seek to assist the developing world, but rather in response to imaging demands of the armies of First World nations. Small portable machines are used in field hospitals, with rapid transmission of the images to large yet remote hospitals where interpretation is possible. The quality of the images generated by these machines is remarkably good. Alternatively, the World Health Organization (WHO) basic radiology system could often form a suitable basis for a simple but not rudimentary imaging service in the tropics.[1] The system comprises an X-ray unit together with clear instructions to enable technicians or physicians to use the equipment. Thought has gone in to allowing for the erratic and inconsistent power supply that dogs many underdeveloped countries. The control panel is intuitive and the design of the hardware means that it is very reliable.

A representative picture of radiological manpower and facilities has been built up for five sub-Saharan African countries. This confirms that there is a desperate shortage of radiologists, radiographers and equipment, with most of the services located in the capital cities and few at rural hospitals. Information pertaining to radiology utilization in other tropical settings has been outlined in several articles.[1-3,5] Only 40% of countries in the sub-Saharan region have any CT scanners or high-resolution ultrasound machines. This is in contrast to the situation in the northern African region and in the Republic of South Africa, where academic radiology departments as well as other private-owned departments are better equipped and serviced. At present, major South African cities have hospitals which provide such high-tech imaging and management to patients from the neighbouring countries, and even from as far as central and eastern Africa, where the few existing CT scanners cannot cope with the patient load. At the University Teaching Hospital (UTH) of Lusaka (Zambia), the CT scanner has only recently been installed but the facility is already being outstripped by increasing demand for neurological investigations. One question that remains is whether the facilities and radiology services in major conurbations will be adequate or not for the size of the population, which fluctuates significantly as large numbers of people daily migrate from rural areas to cities in search of work and sustenance.

Film consumption has been used to measure the relative use of radiological services in different countries and regions.[1] Unfortunately this data is difficult to determine at this time for all of these sub-Saharan countries. Not only is there a dearth of relevant national/provincial statistics, but there is also a tendency to record ultrasound findings on paper print rather than film. In this regard, the measurement of the number of examinations per thousand population in a year will serve as an indicator of radiological utilization. We estimate the annual frequency of both simple and special procedures for the year 2000 as approximately 10, 20, 24 and 31 per 1000 population for the war-torn Republic Democratic of Congo, Zambia, Ethiopia and Uganda, respectively. These countries have been classified as countries with health care level III.[2] These figures suggest that fewer examinations have been performed than expected for a country with a level III health care. By comparison, the annual frequency over 20 years in the UK and USA was 488 and 800, respectively.[1]

A shift in the practice of tropical medicine

The increasing availability of ultrasound machines, especially in tertiary hospitals such as UTH, or at competing private hospitals (and to a lesser extent at district hospitals), has led to an increase in the demand for ultrasound services. Supply, in other words, has fuelled demand. Of course, this is in part because ultrasound is so suited to the investigation of many abdominal, gynaecological and obstetrical conditions encountered in the tropics. Moreover, there is an increasing awareness that ultrasound examinations can clinch an early diagnosis of disease—specifically, when combined with ultrasound-guided intervention, such as aspiration of a collection. The wide range of ultrasound applications and the safety of this modality make it better suited to the budget of the tropical setting than any competing and more expensive high technology such as digital radiography, CT or MRI equipment. Naturally, the benefits are obtained only when the machines are properly serviced and appropriate probes are available. Rather ironically, increasing demand in 'high-tech' developed-world intensive care units has prompted the manufacture of the hardware that it is ideal for the rigours of the tropics: several high-quality yet small and affordable units are available which should function admirably in the intensive environments experienced in a tropical hospital.

In our experience of several departments in Africa, radiologists are fully responsible for daily diagnostic and interventional ultrasound, while residents carry out procedures under the supervision of a senior resident or staff radiologist. However, physicians, surgeons and radiographers who have been trained in ultrasound techniques (either from a local academic institution or abroad) and who have gained a satisfactory level in the practice of imaging and ultrasound-guided interventions are also a part of the radiological manpower outside university teaching hospitals. On the whole, the ultrasound service works, although there is a degree of concern from the established departments about users operating at private health centres that have not received adequate training. There is scope for misinterpretation which leads to inaccurate diagnosis. Another broad concern is that grey scale imaging is limited because limited resources prevent timely replacement of obsolete equipment. The inconsistency in operator and equipment and the consequent potential diagnostic errors become all the more worrying as the clinicians' reliance on ultrasound blossoms.

In this African setting, half of the patients referred for diagnostic ultrasound imaging present with large lesions. Patients may delay in seeking medical advice because of poverty, or because of traditional beliefs. However, the remaining half of the patients do present to the radiology department at an earlier stage of the disease, and benefit from rapid treatment made possible by the speed and accuracy of ultrasound diagnosis.

There follow a number of examples of lesions diagnosed by ultrasound in the setting of tropical clinical radiology (Figures 26.1–26.6). In all cases, diagnosis was achieved by ultrasound alone: no other further imaging was undertaken, with significant cost savings. (Ultrasound guided intervention proved to be the key in many of the examples.)

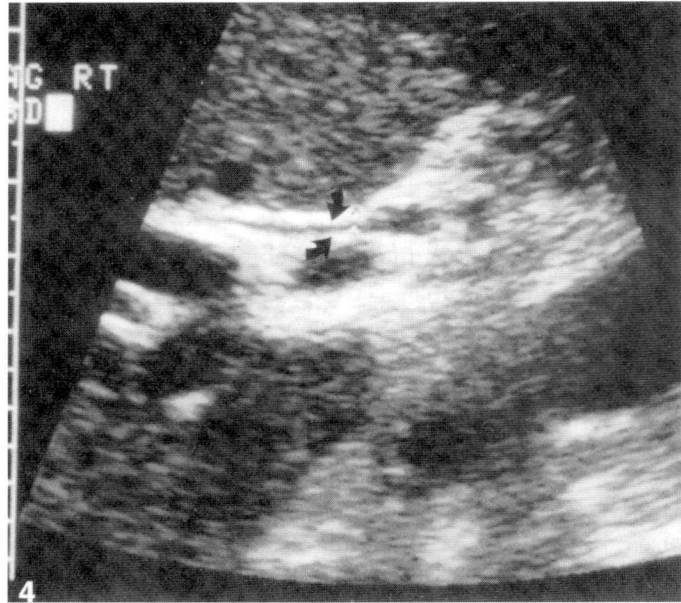

Figure 26.1: Cholangitis due to cryptosporidium infection. Arrows point to the infiltration of the distal common bile duct, which appears markedly thickened and echogenic. (Reproduced with permission from Tshibwabwa et al.[5])

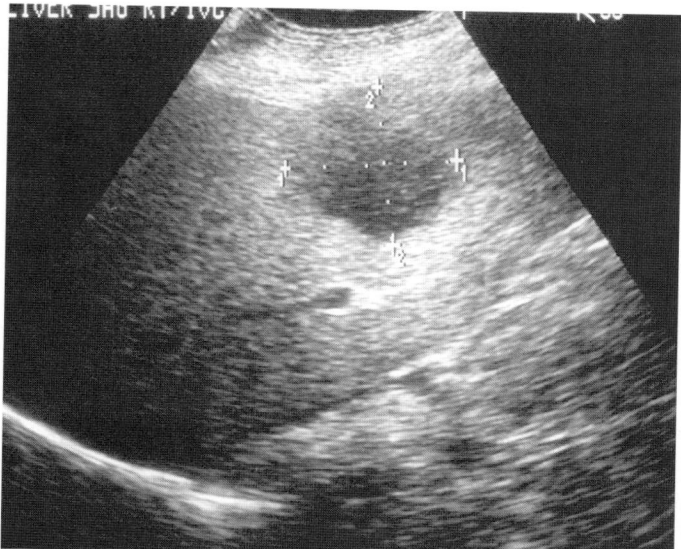

Figure 26.2: Hepatic abscess needle aspirate.

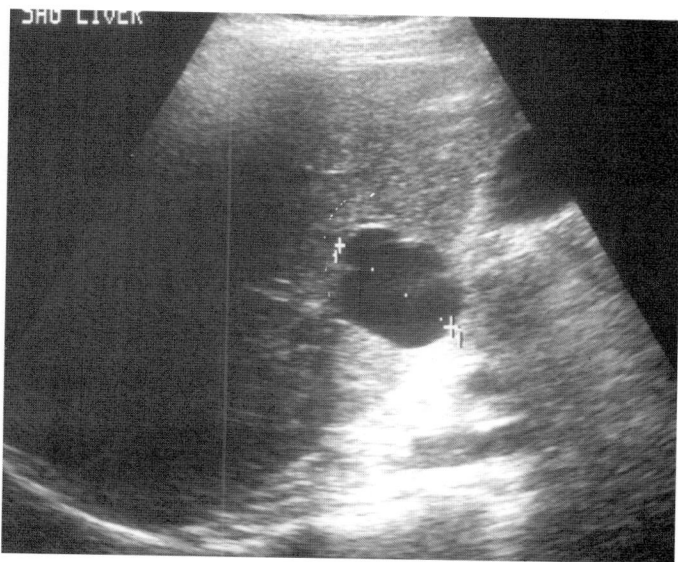

Figure 26.3: Echinococcus liver (ultrasound guided biopsy proven).

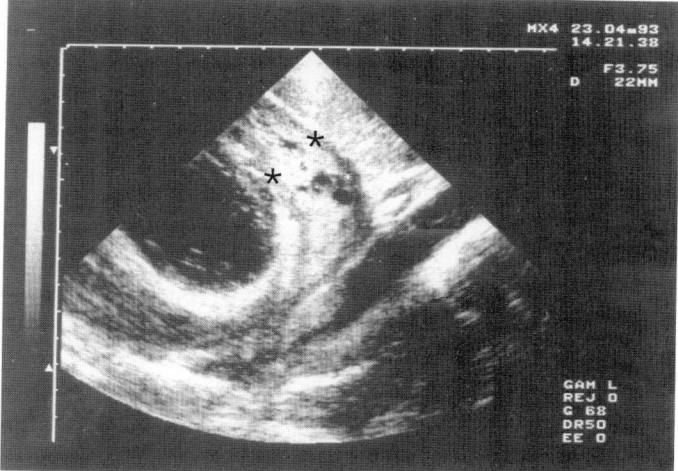

Figure 26.4: Large tuberculous proved pericarditis in AIDS patient. Note the thick fibrinous exudate in the pericardial sac (asterisks).

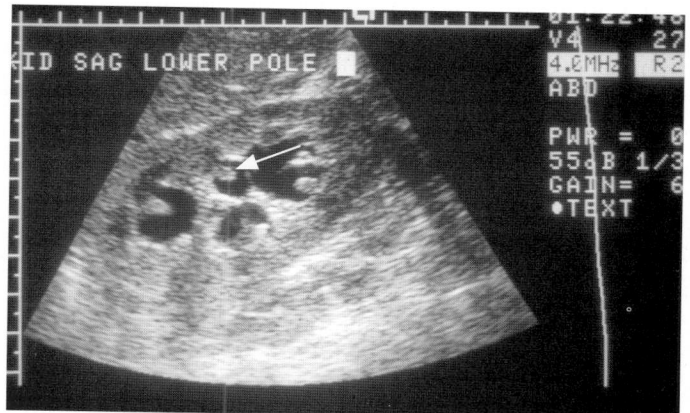

Figure 26.5: Papillary necrosis in a patient from Uganda with AS haemoglobin genotype. Arrow indicates damaged papillae.

Radiology in the wider context of health care

No amount of thought into the provision of the imaging equipment can on its own lead to a worthwhile imaging service. Imaging is only useful if it is coordinated with the clinical and pathological services within the hospital or within the region. There are two self-evident but nevertheless laudable statements which underpin this need for coordination: first, a radiographic study is only as good as the report it generates; and second, a report on its own is meaningless—it has worth only when it helps the physician managing the patient. In other words, a radiograph or ultrasound scan of the highest quality still needs intelligent and *clinically relevant* interpretation.[3,6]

We have to move away from the concept that this interpretation is to be provided at the site where the

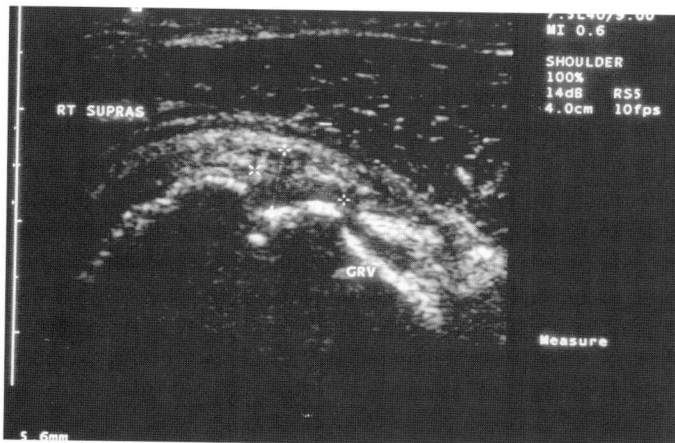

Figure 26.6: Rotator cuff lesions on a patient from Ethiopia who worked as manual labourer in a local farm.

images have been obtained. Dedicated landlines can be linked to inexpensive modems to permit transmission of digital ultrasound data across vast distances; on a more global scale, the World Wide Web offers potential for image transfer and storage. Telemedicine is coming of age: Several simple PC-based imaging software packages are available which allow Internet browsing of radiographs. The film or study, in other words, can be moved from the 'spoke' to a 'hub'. Once the film has been read by a trained radiologist at the hub the report can be sent back by a landline connection to the remote spoke. Such teleradiology is well established in parts of Scandinavia which are sparsely populated and isolated especially in winter.

Interventional radiology

Radiology has moved resolutely from merely a diagnostic service to one in which it is pivotal in the treatment of numerous conditions.[1,2,5,7] This has been possible because of developments in catheter, guide wire and needle design, because of phenomenal advances in the technology (which has allowed real-time imaging to become commonplace) and because of several visionaries who have been very active in the past quarter of the century. Radiologists are at the forefront of minimally invasive therapy, with percutaneous techniques being employed in genitourinary, biliary, gastrointestinal and vascular diseases. The more 'basic' techniques should certainly be available in the medium and larger centres within the tropics. Percutaneous drainage of abscesses and obstructed kidneys (renal stone disease is prevalent in hot countries) may be life-saving, and avoid the need for long-term antibiotic therapy. Many drains can be sited under ultrasound guidance as a 'single stick' procedure using only local anaesthetic and simple sedation.

The limiting factor, of course, in the provision of such a service would be trained personnel.[1,3,6] Here, as in many other aspects concerning the delivery of health care in the tropics, resourcefulness is crucial.[1–3,5] We must move away from the mindset that these procedures should only be undertaken by a trained radiologist. Under appropriate circumstances, they may even be offered by skilled technicians who are not formally medically qualified—after all, leg veins are harvested by nurse practitioners within several UK teaching hospitals as a prelude to coronary artery bypass grafting. Imaginative training and support for isolated units would help develop a cadre of technologists who could undertake these techniques. While this may seem heretical in the West, dedicated personnel who can perform simple image-guided drainage procedures are likely to save more lives than many doctors working in rarefied tertiary referral centres.

Techniques in fine needle aspiration and biopsy may be equally important in the management of patients in the tropics. Aspirants provide samples from which organisms can be isolated so that valuable antibiotics can be husbanded and only used where appropriate. After all, a liver abscess on ultrasound is simply that: aspirate obtained by inserting a needle under image guidance into the abscess may well reveal the pathogen.[7]

A tropical success story

In Kampala, the capital of Uganda, stands the Mulago University Teaching Hospital. Between 1998 and 1999 the Department of Radiology underwent major improvements with recruitment of appropriate staff at all levels and the establishment of high-resolution ultrasound, CT and gamma camera units. A retrospective analysis for the 2 years preceding (January 1997 to December 1998) and the 2 years following (January 1999 to December 2000) this transition reveals an average of 116 150 radiological examinations (simple and special procedures) during the first period and an average of 155 087 over the second period. The change represents 34% increase in the frequency of examinations.

There has been increasing reliance on diagnostic and interventional ultrasound. For the year 1999–2000 ultrasound comprised 29.4% of X-ray examinations performed, equivalent to 79.6% of all the special procedures. Intravenous urography decreased from three per day in the late 1980s to one per week now and at times none at all in the week.

In the same time period, and in comparison to the findings in the UTH Department of Radiology, the frequency of imaging examinations performed at a local major private hospital with similar imaging facilities remained almost static, probably due to both small workload and prohibitive costs of radiology services in a two-tier system.

While conceding that there is always a need to seek for improvement, the Mulago Hospital Department of Radiology is a model for delivery of imaging services in the tropics. The department succeeds because:

- It is committed to continuing professional development. This encompasses visiting professor exchanges, conferences, journals, libraries, a well thought out radiology residence programme, and intelligent medical school and school of radiographers curricula.
- X-ray equipment at the old Mulago Hospital has been modernized through a grant from the African Bank of Development. Further resources underwritten by the Uganda Ministry of Health have helped procure equipment for basic and high-tech radiological services (even though no MRI units are available). A radiologist, however skilled and versatile, can function only within the limits of the available equipment.
- There is a quality control policy for radiological equipment and images.
- The increasing reliance on ultrasound imaging and ultrasound-guided interventions has been anticipated and hence accommodated.

- Resourcefulness has overcome the constraints imposed by scarcity of equipment and personnel. In particular, there is a widespread use of telemedicine for the delivery of training and diagnostic ultrasound services. A telemedicine link to district hospitals facilitates the radiodiagnosis within the primary care level. After all, it deals with the same problems of abdominal/chest infections, trauma and obstetrics as those encountered at Mulago Hospital.

The imaging needs of the communities in Kampala city are identical to those elsewhere in Africa or the tropics. Therefore, the principles underpinning the performance of radiology services at this Ugandan hospital should be extrapolated to and adopted by other tertiary hospitals in the tropics. The paradigm of delivering a modern and dependable imaging service, at the centre of tropical health care, may then be realized in many regions of the world. How the restrictions imposed by the World Bank and International Monetary Fund on the fragile economies of the developing countries—the majority of them being located in the tropics—will impede the development of a robust modern service in diagnostic and interventional radiology remains to be seen.

Conclusion

We must aim for a first-class imaging service which is *global*, not least because modern radiology is increasingly central to the diagnosis and treatment of numerous conditions. The many obstacles to establishing this service in the tropics can be overcome with clear thinking, resourcefulness, determination and sage investment: the university teaching hospital in Kampala sets an example. As a first step, all tropical imaging services should concentrate on infectious diseases, trauma and obstetric care. To this end, plain radiography and ultrasound must be developed: this demands investment in suitable equipment and investment in training and supporting personnel, wherever they are based.

REFERENCES

1 Cockshott W P. Diagnostic radiology: geography of a high technology. *AJR* 1979; 132:339–344.

2 Schandorf C & Ketteh G K. Analysis of the status of X-ray diagnosis in Ghana. *BJR* 1998; 71:1040–1048.

3 Mindel S. Role of imager in the developing world. *Lancet* 1997; I:426–429.

4 Nadvi S S, Parboosing R & Van Dellen J R. Benefits to a regional neurosurgical unit following the introduction of a decentralised imaging facility. *SAMJ* 1997; 87:1669–1671.

5 Tshibwabwa E T, Mwaba P, Bogle-Taylor J & Zumla A. Four year study of abdominal ultrasound in 900 Central African adults with AIDS referred for diagnostic imaging. *Abdominal Imaging* 2000; 25:290–296.

6 Kurjak K & Kos M. Ultrasound screening for fetal anomalies in developing countries: wish or reality? *Ann NY Acad Sci* 1998; 847:233–237.

7 Klein J S & Sandhu J. Interventional procedures in the AIDS patient. *Radiol Clin North Am* 1997; 35:1223–1243.

Chapter 27
Tropical Oral Health
R. Bedi and C. Scully

Introduction

The importance of oral health as part of general health is now well established and this is true not only in industrialized countries but also tropical and subtropical climates. Oral health was notable by its absence in previous editions of *Manson's Tropical Diseases*, with the 20th edition limiting the section on the mouth per se to little more than half a page.[1] Therefore, the decision to develop a whole chapter to the subject testifies to the growing importance and awareness of the impact oral health and the delivery of dental services can have on those who live in tropical and subtropical areas. The term to be used in this chapter to cover such geographical areas will be 'developing countries', and, as is custom, to have this description also cover transition countries. It is also recognized that tropical dentistry is not just dentistry (oral health) in the tropics, but with migration and global travel oral diseases traditionally restricted in some developing countries have manifested themselves within all areas of the global community.

Dental caries

Together with the common cold, dental caries is perhaps the most prevalent disease of modern man, but unlike the cold, its effects, invariably, leave behind defects that are permanent.[2] The general consensus of international epidemiological studies is that non-milk extrinsic sugars are the most important dietary factor in the aetiology of dental caries. The role of nutrition during tooth development is now generally considered to be minimal in industrialized countries.[3,4] However, in tropical and subtropical areas where malnutrition is evident, delayed tooth eruption is observed, especially in the primary dentition,[5] but there is inconclusive evidence that malnutrition during tooth development can influence subsequent levels of dental caries.[6]

In the last few decades, there has been enormous progress in development. Since the 1960s life expectancy in developing countries has risen from 46 to 64 years, infant mortality rates have halved, there has been an increase of more than 80% in the proportion of children enrolled in primary school and there has been a doubling of access to safe drinking water and basic sanitation.[7]

Such development is all too often coupled with increasing access to sugars, commonly in the form of confectionery or carbonated drinks. The World Health Organization's global data bank on oral health was established in 1969 and continues to monitor dental caries levels across different countries. This valuable source demonstrates two clear trends: first the ongoing decline in dental caries for the industrialized world and, second, the increasing prevalence of caries in the developing world.[6]

The treatment of dental caries has not essentially changed over the past few decades, although tooth cavity design and filling materials have changed the practical approach to dental restorative treatment. The Atraumatic Restorative Technique (ART) has produced promising results in developing countries, especially those with a shortage of suitably qualified manpower.[8,9]

There has been a number of studies that have demonstrated significant caries reductions as a result of fluoride toothpaste.[10] The major barrier to the implementation of fluoride toothpaste to the developing world has been cost; however, the new WHO programmes to introduce locally produced affordable fluoridated toothpaste to many developing countries are producing encouraging results.[11]

Periodontal disease

There is no evidence that periodontal disease in developed and developing countries is in principle different.[12] There are indeed more similarities in periodontal conditions globally than differences.[12] Evidence shows that periodontal diseases are only more prevalent in developing countries in terms of poorer oral hygiene and greater calculus retention but not for periodontal destruction in adults.[12–15] Limited resources, in many developing countries, often inhibit the purchase of toothbrushes, and traditional cleaning materials such as the miswak chewing stick is still widely used.[16] The miswak are prepared from local tree roots or twigs, and are commonly used in several African and Asian countries and have been shown to be effective tooth-cleaning agents.[16]

Oral cancer

Most oral cancer is squamous cell carcinoma (SCC), and it is customary to include cancers of the lip (ICD 140), tongue (ICD 141), gum (ICD 143), floor of the mouth (ICD 144) and unspecified parts of the mouth (ICD 145).[17] There is clear inter-country variation in both the incidence and mortality from oral cancer and also ethnic differences. These are attributed mainly to specific risk factors such as alcohol and tobacco (smoking and smokeless) and sunlight exposure, in the case of lip cancer, but dietary factors as well as the existence of genetic predisposition may play a part.[18] Variations in accessing care services are also evident.[18]

The incidence of oral cancer varies widely between countries and geographical areas of the world and is generally most common in developing countries. These variations have traditionally been explained by the exposure of these groups to specific risk factors, e.g., tobacco and alcohol use. Mouth cancer worldwide is the 12th most common cancer but it is the eighth most common in males.[19] The gender ratio is 2:0 (M:F). Mouth cancer in men is most common in Western and Southern Europe, South Asia, Melanesia, southern Africa and Australia/NZ.[19] In females, it is most common in South-Central Asia, Melanesia and Australia/NZ. Lip cancer is particularly common in white Caucasians in the tropics and subtropics.[19]

The aetiology of oral cancer has been attributed to specific risk factors: tobacco[20] and/or alcohol in southern Africa, and betel quid in South-Central Asia and Melanesia.[21] Annually there are 197,000 deaths worldwide from cancer of the mouth and pharynx, with the highest mortality from mouth cancer in Melanesia and South-Central Asia.[19,22]

Oral cancer appears most prevalent in areas with a high Asian population. Chinese have a lower risk of oral cancer than Indians do in Malaysia and a later age of onset.

There is a plethora of studies linking specific behaviours such as tobacco and alcohol use to oral cancer.[21] Smokeless (chewing) tobacco use is an important factor for South Asian populations. The areca (betel) nut habit is important in the development of oral submucous fibrosis and of mouth cancer.[23] Some chew the nut only and others prefer 'paan', which includes tobacco, and sometimes lime and catechu. Studies from India have confirmed the association between 'paan' tobacco chewing and oral cancer, particularly cancer of the buccal and labial mucosa.

There is growing evidence associating increased alcohol consumption with risk of oral cancer. The role of alcohol drinking is observed in a negative social class gradient and for many countries follows a similar pattern to tobacco use.

There is a considerable body of evidence indicating a protective effect on oral cancer and pre-cancer, of diets rich in fresh fruits and vegetables and of vitamin A in particular.

The molecular changes found in oral carcinomas from Western countries (UK, USA, Australia), particularly p53 mutations, are infrequent in the East (India, South-East Asia), where the involvement of *ras* oncogenes, including mutation, loss of heterozygosity (H-*ras*) and amplification (K- and N-*ras*) are common, suggesting genetic differences.

It is also evident that there can be genetic differences in the metabolism of pro-carcinogens and carcinogens by xenometabolizing enzymes or ability to repair the DNA damage in different ethnic groups.

Carcinomas present anywhere in the oral cavity, commonly on the posterolateral margin of the tongue and floor of mouth—the 'coffin' or 'graveyard' area—and in the buccal mucosa in betel users. It is crucial, therefore, not only to examine visually and manually the whole oral cavity, but also to take particular care to inspect and palpate the posterolateral margins of the tongue and the floor of mouth (Figure 27.1). There is usually solitary chronic:

- ulceration;
- red lesion;
- white lesion;
- indurated lump;
- fissure;
- cervical lymph node enlargement.

Anterior cervical lymph node enlargement may be detectable by palpation. Thirty per cent of patients present with palpably enlarged nodes containing metastases and, of those who do not, a further 25% will go on to develop nodal metastases within 2 years.

Lip carcinoma presents with thickening, crusting or ulceration, usually of the lower lip.

Potentially malignant lesions or conditions may include some:

- erythroplasias;
- dysplastic leucoplakias (about 50% of oral carcinomas have associated leucoplakia);
- lichen planus;
- oral submucous fibrosis;
- chronic immunosuppression.

Diagnosis

Too many patients with oral SCC present or are detected late, with advanced disease and lymph node metastases. The earlier the tumour is detected and treated:

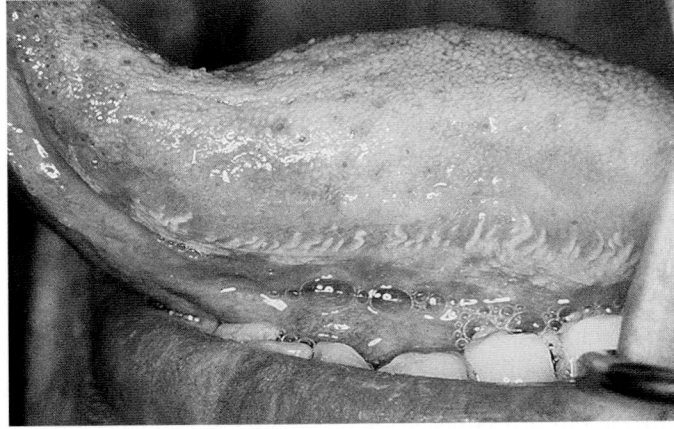

Figure 27.1: Hairy leucoplakia associated with HIV.

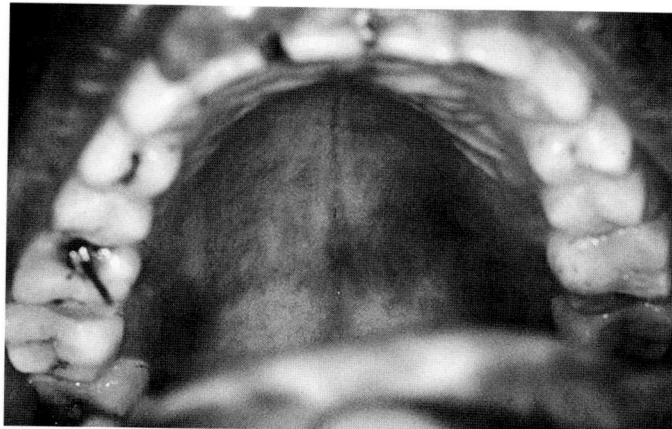

Figure 27.2: Kaposi's sarcoma associated with HIV.

- the less complicated is treatment;
- the better are the cosmetic and functional results;
- the greater is the improvement in survival.

There should be a high index of suspicion, especially of a solitary lesion present for over 3 weeks, particularly if it is indurated, there is cervical lymphadenopathy and the patient is in a high-risk group.

It is essential to confirm the diagnosis, and determine whether cervical lymph nodes are involved or there are other primary tumours, or metastases (Figure 27.2). Therefore almost invariably indicated are:

- lesional biopsy; an incisional biopsy is usually indicated but an oral brush biopsy is now available mainly for cases where there are widespread potentially malignant lesions, and for revealing malignancy in lesions of more benign appearance;
- jaw and chest radiography;
- endoscopy;
- full blood count and liver function tests.

Management

Oral cancer is now treated largely by surgery and/or irradiation, though there have been few unequivocal controlled trials of treatment modalities. Combined clinics, with surgeons, oncologists and support staff, usually have an agreed treatment policy and offer the best outcomes. However, mortality rates for oral cancer have substantially increased in many countries. Although the efficacy of screening for oral cancer to increase survival and reduce mortality remains unproven,[24,25] it is believed that Cuba's ongoing oral cancer screening programme has resulted in a higher proportion of cancers being localized at diagnosis and a comparatively high survival rate.[26] A reduced incidence of oral pre-cancerous lesions has been reported in a primary prevention trial.[27] In addition, the abstinence of tobacco for a 6-week period resulted in the reversal of potentially pre-cancerous oral lesions.[28]

The prognosis is very site-dependent. For:

- intra-oral carcinoma 5-year survival may be as low as 30% for posterior lesions presenting late, as they often do;
- lip carcinoma, there is often more than a 70% 5-year survival.

Erythroplasia (erythroplakia)

Erythroplasia is a rare, isolated, red, velvety lesion which affects patients mainly in the sixth and seventh decades. Erythroplasia usually involves the floor of the mouth, the ventrum of the tongue or the soft palate. This is one of the most important oral lesions because 75–90% of lesions prove to be carcinoma or carcinoma in situ, or are severely dysplastic. The incidence of malignant change is 17 times higher in erythroplasia than in leucoplakia. Erythroplasia should be excised and sent for histological examination.

Leucoplakia

All oral white lesions were formerly called leucoplakia and believed often to be potentially malignant. The term leucoplakia is now restricted to white lesions of unknown cause.

Most white lesions are innocuous keratoses caused by cheek biting, friction or tobacco, but:

- infections (e.g., candidosis, syphilis, and hairy leucoplakia);
- dermatoses (usually lichen planus);
- neoplastic disorders (e.g., leukoplakias and carcinomas);
- other conditions

must be excluded, usually by biopsy.

Keratoses are most commonly uniformly white plaques (homogeneous leucoplakia), prevalent in the buccal (cheek) mucosae, and are usually of low malignant potential. More serious are nodular and, especially, speckled leukoplakias, which consist of white patches or nodules in a red, often eroded, area of mucosa. The presence of severe epithelial dysplasia indicates a considerable risk of malignant development.

The overall prevalence of malignant change is 3–33% over 10 years, but a percentage (about 15%) regress clinically.

Diagnosis

It can be difficult to be certain of the precise diagnosis of a white patch, as even carcinoma can present as a white lesion. Incisional biopsy is indicated, sampling indurated, red, erosive or ulcerated areas rather than the more obvious whiter hyperkeratinized areas; staining with toluidine blue may help highlight the most appropriate area.

Management can be difficult, especially in extensive lesions of leucoplakia, and those with areas of erythroplasia. Obvious predisposing factors need to be reduced or eliminated. Some studies have shown regression of leucoplakia in over 50% of patients who stopped smoking for 1 year. Dysplastic lesions should certainly be excised and the patient should then be followed up regularly at intervals of 3–6 months. Unfortunately, more than one-third recur.

Oral submucous fibrosis

Oral submucous fibrosis (OSMF), though not regarded as a connective tissue disease, has pathological changes closely similar to those of scleroderma. Unlike the latter, which has severe effects on the skin but minimal effects on the oral mucosa, OSMF causes severe and often disabling fibrosis of the oral tissues alone.

OSMF affects virtually only those from the Indian subcontinent.[29,30] There is some evidence it is premalignant.[31] The condition appears to be related to the chewing of areca nut. Iron deficiency anaemia may be present but this is not uncommon in Asians in the absence of submucous fibrosis. No consistent specific immunological abnormalities appear to be associated, although there is a greater prevalence of connective tissue diseases and serum immunoglobulin IgG, IgA and IgM levels are raised.

Clinically, OSMF causes symmetrical fibrosis of such sites as the cheeks, soft palate or inner aspects of the lips. The fibrosis is often so severe that the affected area is almost white and so hard that it literally cannot be indented with the finger. Frequently the buccal fibrosis causes such severe restriction of opening that dental treatment becomes increasingly difficult and finally impossible. Ultimately tube feeding may become necessary.

Management

Intralesional corticosteroids and regular stretching of the oral soft tissues with an interdental screw or therabite may delay fixation in the closed position. Failing this, operative treatment may become necessary although some have found improvement with intralesional interferon α.

Infections

Bacterial

Acute necrotizing ulcerative gingivitis

Acute necrotizing ulcerative gingivitis (ANUG) is characterized by painful ulceration of the gum between the teeth (interdental papillae) (Figure 27.3), a pronounced

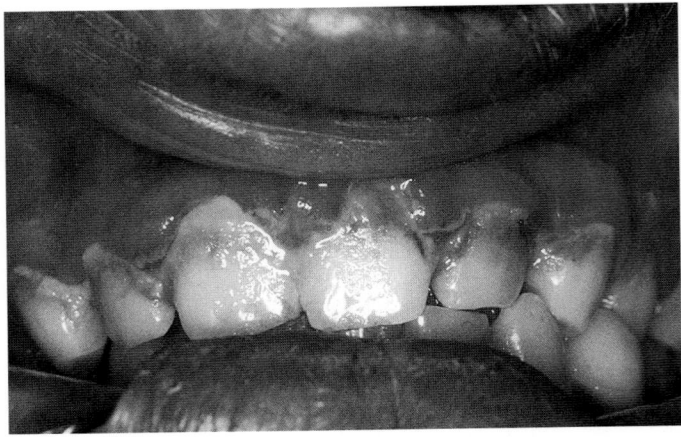

Figure 27.3: Acute necrotizing ulcerative gingivitis.

tendency to gingival bleeding and halitosis. Anaerobic fusiform bacteria and spirochaetes are implicated, predisposing factors including:

- poor oral hygiene;
- smoking;
- malnutrition;
- immune defects including HIV and other viral infections and leukaemias.

ANUG is a problem in certain populations, particularly in those who are encountering significant poverty and malnourishment. It also impacts upon patients who are immunocompromised. ANUG not infrequently follows a respiratory tract infection presumably being predisposed by the transient immune defect consequent upon some such infections, particularly viral. ANUG is increasingly seen in viral infections such as HIV disease; in some other persons with ANUG only more subtle immune defects, such as reduced salivary immunoglobulin A and neutrophil dysfunction, have been described. Worldwide the major cause of immunodeficiency is still malnutrition and ANUG is indeed seen in malnutrition. However, there are patients who suffer from ANUG in the absence of any clear immune defect, malnutrition or other systemic factor and, in these, poor oral hygiene and tobacco-smoking may be factors. It is seen primarily in early childhood, young adults and HIV disease.[32]

ANUG is typically seen where plaque control is poor. A mixed flora dominated by fusobacteria and spirochaetes such as *Treponema* species, *Bacteroides* (*Porphyromonas*) *melaninogenicus* species *intermedius*, *Fusobacterium* species, *Selenomonas* species and *Borrelia vincentii* is invariably present and the condition improves dramatically when treated with penicillin or metronidazole, suggesting a significant role for these bacteria. Viruses may play a role,[33] possibly also by inducing immune suppression.

Management includes:

- oral debridement and hygiene instruction;
- peroxide or perborate mouthwashes;
- metronidazole 200 mg t.d.s. for 3 days.

Gangrenous stomatitis (cancrum oris; noma)

Noma is derived from the Greek '*nomein*' which means to 'devour'; essentially it is a gangrenous stomatitis, which starts in the mouth as a benign oral lesion and rapidly destroys both the soft and hard tissues of the mouth and face (Figure 27.4).[34] Most noma suffers are under 6 years of age and it has been estimated that the case-fatality rate is probably between 70% and 90%. It is estimated that 100,000 African children under the age of 6 years contract noma every year.[34]

Noma is often an extension of an ANUG into the adjacent tissues, predominantly because of impaired host defences (Figure 27.5).[35] Other factors which predispose to the development of gangrenous stomatitis include protein–energy malnutrition and deficiencies of vitamins A, B, C, iron or magnesium. Therefore, poor living environment, exposure to debilitating childhood diseases, poor oral hygiene and malnutrition all appear to put children at risk for noma.[36]

The condition is seen especially in sub-Saharan Africa. Nigeria probably has the highest incidence, although The Gambia, Algeria, Uganda, Senegal, Madagascar, South Africa, Sudan and Egypt are also areas of high prevalence, as are Afghanistan, India, the Philippines, China, Vietnam, Papua New Guinea and South America.[36,37] In the developed world, gangrenous stomatitis is rare, and typically seen in immunocompromised persons such as HIV infection, leukaemia and diabetes.[38–45]

Clinical features

The presenting feature may be a painful red or purplish-red spot (an indurated papule), usually on the gingiva in the premolar–molar region, which enlarges and ulcerates rapidly and spreading to the labiogingival or mucobuccal fold, and exposing the underlying bone. There is pain

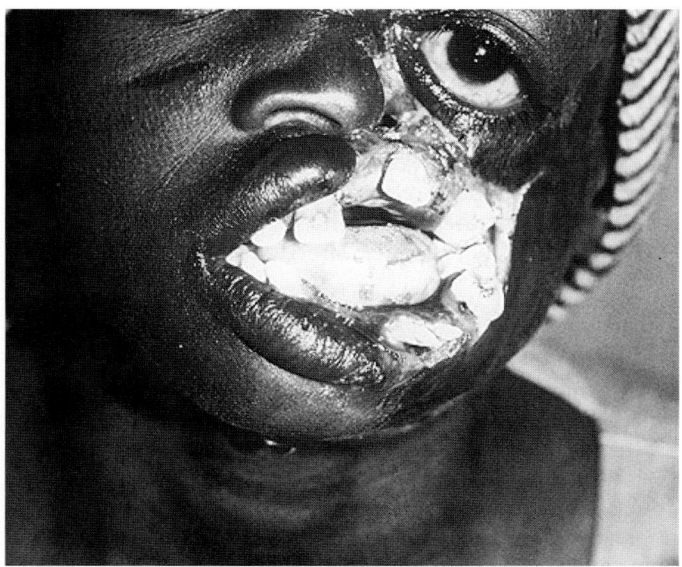

Figure 27.4: Noma.

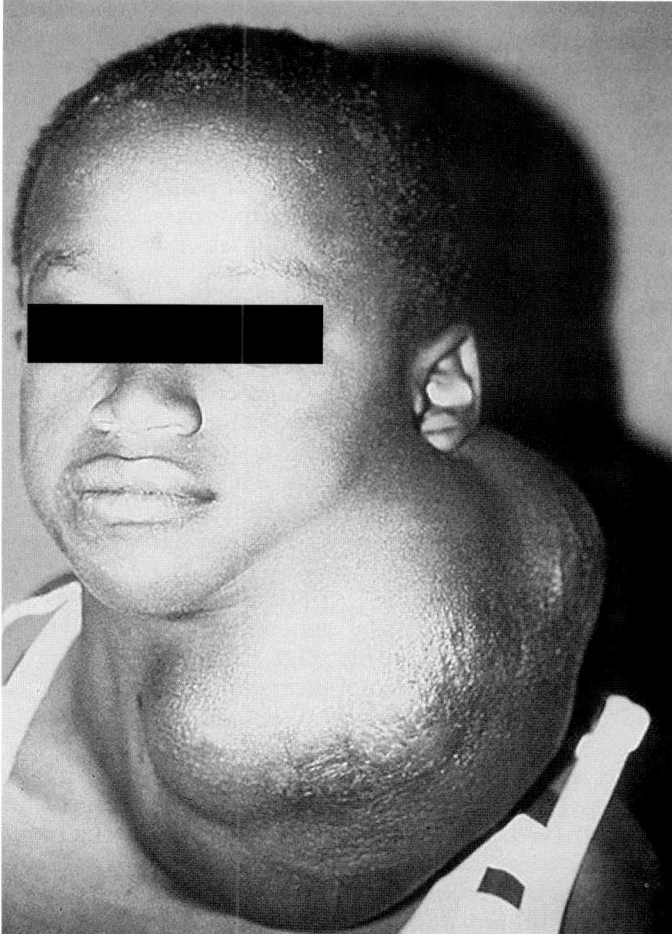

Figure 27.5: Burkitt's lymphoma.

and often fetor. A blue-black area of discoloration appears on the skin and leads to a perforating wound. Sequestration of the exposed bone and loss of teeth are rapid and then the wound heals slowly by secondary intention, often leaving a defect. In former times, noma was often a lethal condition.

Management

Gangrenous stomatitis does not respond readily to treatment unless the underlying disease is controlled, especially nutritional rehabilitation. The wound should be cleaned regularly with chlorhexidine and/or saline and/or hydrogen peroxide. A soft cotton gauze or tulle gras dressing may be used but changed frequently. Any loose slough, loose teeth and bony fragments should be removed. Parenteral fluids should be given to correct any dehydration and electrolyte imbalance. Penicillin is the antimicrobial of choice. Folic acid, iron, ascorbic acid and vitamin B complex may be required.

Syphilis (venereal treponematosis)

In 1995, it was estimated that there were approximately 12 million new cases of syphilis among adults worldwide, with the greatest number of cases occurring in South and South-East Asia, followed by sub-Saharan Africa.[46]

Oral lesions

The lip is the most common extragenital site of primary infection with *Treponema pallidum*. It causes a chancre (primary, hard or Hunterian chancre) which begins as a small, firm, pink macule, changes to a papule and then ulcerates to form a painless round ulcer with a raised margin and indurated base (Figure 27.6). About 60% of oral cases affect the lip or may present at the angles of the mouth.[47] Other oral sites affected may include the tongue and to a lesser extent the gingivae and fauces. Lymph nodes in the submaxillary, submental and cervical regions are usually enlarged. Chancres heal spontaneously within 3–8 weeks. Secondary syphilis follows the primary stage after 6–8 weeks but a healing chancre may still be present. As in the primary stage, the mucosal lesions are highly infectious. The typical signs and symptoms are fever, headache, malaise, a rash (characteristically symmetrically distributed coppery maculopapules or lesions on the palms) and generalized painless lymph node enlargement. It is this stage that classically causes oral lesions.[48,49] Painless oral ulcers (mucous patches and snailtrack ulcers) are the typical lesions and are slightly raised, greyish white, glistening patches seen on the fauces, soft palate, tongue, buccal mucosa and, rarely, gingivae.[50] Cervical nodes are enlarged and 'rubbery' in consistency. Latent syphilis follows secondary syphilis and persists until late syphilis (tertiary syphilis) develops. The characteristic lesion of tertiary syphilis is a localized midline granuloma ('gumma') varying in size from millimetres to several centimetres which breaks down to form a deep punched-out painless ulcer. The most common oral site for a gumma is the hard palate[51] although the soft palate, lips or tongue are commonly involved. The gumma starts as a small, pale, raised area which ulcerates and rapidly progresses to a large zone of necrosis with denudation of bone and, in the case of a palatal gumma, may eventually perforate into the nasal cavity.

Diagnosis

The presence of clinical manifestations together with a history of contact may suggest the diagnosis but sero-diagnostic tests, and sometimes dark-field microscopy are required for confirmation.

Oral management

There is no specific oral management except general palliative care if there is soreness of oral soft lesions, but the general management is straightforward: procaine penicillin intramuscularly for 10 days (erythromycin for 14 days) should be given.

Non-venereal treponematoses (endemic treponematoses): endemic syphilis (bejel)

The early stage of bejel may present with mucous patches in the oronasopharyngeal region, and angular stomatitis. Late- or tertiary-stage disease is mainly gummatous and can involve the oral mucous membranes or bones and can lead to gross facial deformity (rhinopharyngitis mutilans).[52]

Diagnosis

Dark-field microscopy and serology are needed to confirm the diagnosis but differentiation from the other treponematoses is difficult.

Management

Penicillin is the drug of choice; tetracycline and erythromycin are alternatives.

Pinta

The primary slowly developing subcutaneous granulomatous lesion may involve the face. Secondary lesions (pintides) are papules, which develop into plaques with scaly and centrally pigmented areas. Facial skin is extensively affected but there are no oral lesions described.

Yaws (framboesia; pian; bouba)

The primary papule may appear around the body orifices including the mouth (Figure 27.7).[53] Gummatous nodular ulcerative lesions may develop.[54] The other type of lesion seen involving facial structures is basically a destructive lesion starting either on the soft palate, uvula or hard palate, eventually destroying parts of the nose (gangosa) and causing a 'saddle-nose' defect. Bone involvement may result in thickening of the face on

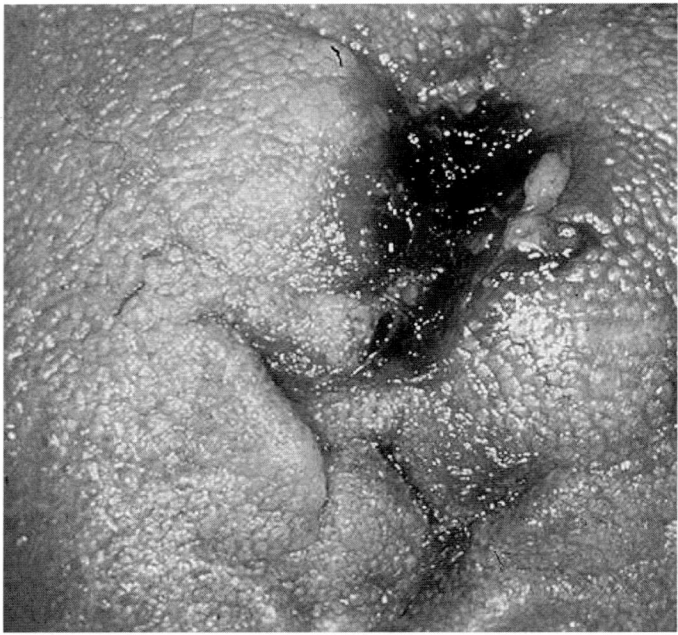

Figure 27.6: Oral lesion associated with syphilis.

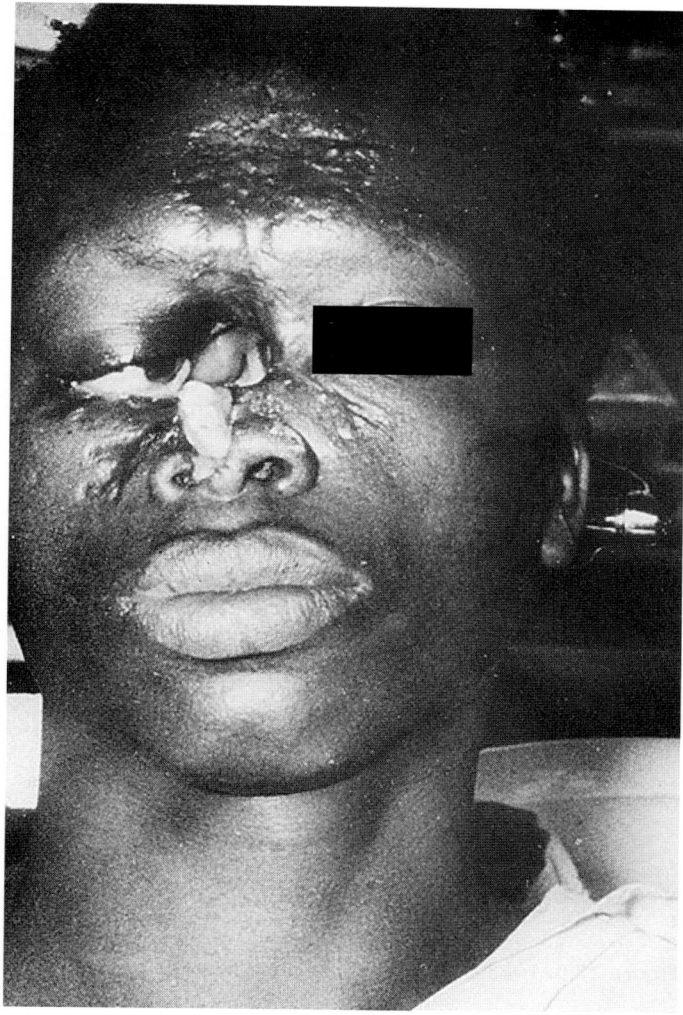

Figure 27.7: Yaws.

either side of the bridge of the nose, giving rise to the characteristic facial appearance of 'goundou'.[55]

Diagnosis

Clinical features supported by dark-field microscopy, biopsy and serology are useful.

Management

This is using penicillin, erythromycin or tetracycline.

Gonorrhoea

Oral, pharyngeal and tonsil involvement is being reported with increasing frequency particularly among homosexuals and heterosexuals practising oral sex. Infection of these sites is acquired primarily by fellatio and infrequently by cunnilingus. The tonsils become red and swollen with a greyish exudate and there is cervical lymphadenitis. Lesions in other parts of the mouth are described as showing fiery erythema and sometimes oedematous, perhaps with painful superficial ulceration of the tongue, gingiva, buccal mucosa, hard or soft palate. The inflamed mucosa may also be covered with a yellowish or greyish exudate, which when detached may leave a bleeding surface.

Diagnosis

A throat swab should be taken for Gram staining to show polymorphs containing Gram-negative diplococci. Confirmation is by culture and sugar fermentation to aid differentiation of species. Rapid identification of gonococci by fluorescent antibody techniques is possible.

Management

Penicillin is the drug of choice, given as 2 g ampicillin plus 1 g probenecid as a single oral dose. Patients hypersensitive to penicillin can be treated with co-trimoxazole. Many strains are resistant to penicillin in parts of Africa and the Far East. Tetracycline, or cefazolin–probenecid and streptomycin or spectinomycin may be used.

Granuloma inguinale (donovanosis)

A papule or nodule, usually in the inguinal or anogenital region, progresses to a destructive granulomatous ulcer. Most oral lesions are secondary to primary genital infection, can involve the periodontium, and are often misdiagnosed as actinomycosis.

Diagnosis

Direct examination of a piece of granulation tissue compressed between two slides and stained by Giemsa for the presence of Donovan bodies (clusters of bacilli lying within leucocytes) is the best method.

Management

Tetracycline, ampicillin or trimethoprim–sulfamethoxazole are first-line therapy.

Lymphogranuloma venereum

The tongue is the oral site most frequently affected in primary lymphogranuloma venereum (LGV) infections, usually with a painless vesicle. Lesions affecting the lips, cheeks, tongue, floor of mouth, uvula and pharynx but not gingivae have been described. As the disease progresses, the tongue enlarges with areas of scarring and deep grooves on the dorsum, which are intensely red with loss of superficial epithelium. Cervical lymphadenopathy is common sometimes with no clinical oral lesions of LGV.

Diagnosis

Laboratory confirmation of the diagnosis includes isolation of *Chlamydia trachomatis* and serological tests. *C. trachomatis* is isolated on cell cultures of the yolk sac of chicken embryos. A skin test (Frei test) is available but not specific.

Management

LGV is treated by sulfonamides, tetracycline, erythromycin or rifampicin.

Actinomycosis

A breach in the continuity of mucosa caused either by trauma or surgery is the prerequisite for the majority of actinomycotic infections. Cervicofacial actinomycosis occurs predominantly in adult males following trauma either accidentally or rarely from dental treatment such as exodontia or endodontics.[56–59] Rarely, a periodontal pocket with suitable anaerobic conditions predisposes to the disease.[60] The perimandibular area appears to be the commonest site. A relatively painless reddish-purple indurated mass appears at the angle of the jaw or in the vicinity of the parotid gland. It may drain through sinuses, the material containing the so-called sulfur granules. Actinomycosis may rarely involve the oral cavity, tongue, mandible, maxilla, paranasal sinuses, eye, ear, face, neck or salivary glands.

Diagnosis

Sulfur granules may be seen by direct vision or after staining with Gram stain. Actinomycosis should be confirmed by the isolation of *A. israelii* in anaerobic culture.

Management

Penicillin is the first-choice antimicrobial.[57] Alternatives include cephalosporin, clindamycin and lincomycin.

Nocardiosis

Nocardiosis caused by bacteria of the family Nocardiaceae, usually *Nocardia asteroides*, *N. brasiliensis* or *N. caviae* and is seen mainly in Latin America. Dissemination may lead to oral involvement; nocardiosis of the cheek[61] and gingivae[62] has been reported.

Diagnosis

Smears should be examined for Gram-positive rods of coccal forms but culture is more useful in the diagnosis.

Management

Surgical drainage and a sulfonamide such as co-trimoxazole should be used.

Tuberculosis

It is estimated that over 1.5 million tuberculosis cases per year occur in sub-Saharan Africa.[63] HIV and tuberculosis speed each other's progress, with the latter contributing about 15% of AIDS death worldwide.[63]

Oral lesions are seen mainly in pulmonary tuberculosis although systemic symptoms suggestive of lung disease are by no means always present.[64] Apart from pain, typically the main symptom of tuberculosis is chronic ulcers or granular masses. These are usually on the dorsum/base of the tongue,[64–68] gingivae (Figure 27.8)[64] or occasionally in the buccal mucosa, floor of the mouth, lips and the hard and soft palates.[69–72]

Primary oral lesions develop when bacilli are directly inoculated into the oral tissues of a person who has not

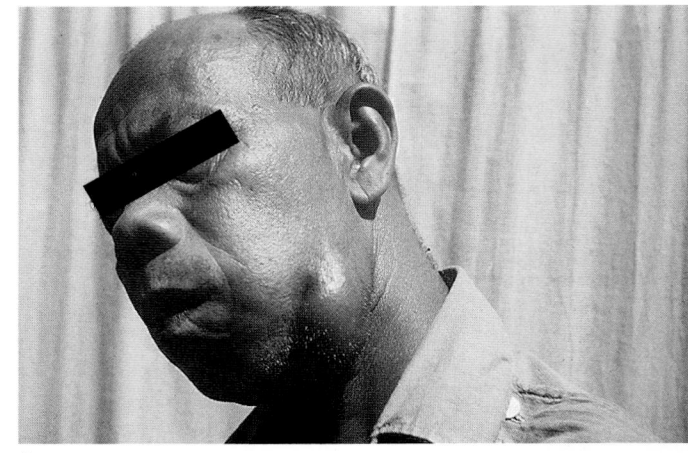

A

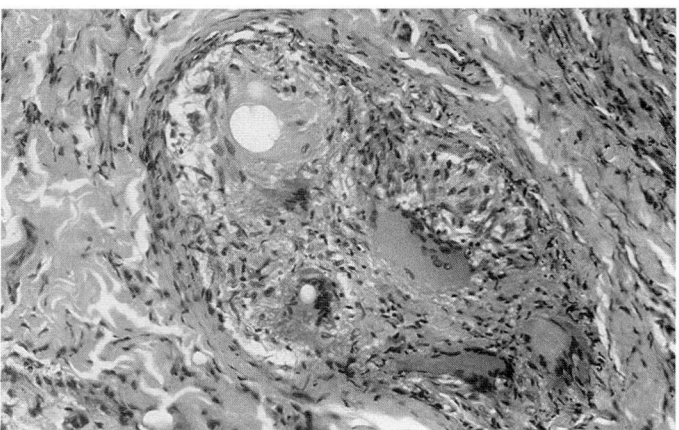

B

Figure 27.8: Head and neck swelling associated with tuberculosis.

acquired immunity. Primary tuberculosis of the mouth is more common in children and adolescents than adults. It usually presents as a single painless indolent ulcer commonly on the gingiva with enlarged cervical lymph nodes,[73] or the gingivae, tooth extraction sockets and the buccal folds.[74]

Occasional cases of primary jaw tuberculosis have been reported[75] usually resulting from extension of a gingival lesion, from an infected post-extraction socket, from an extension from a tuberculous granuloma at the apex of the tooth or haematogenous spread. Tuberculous osteomyelitis may involve the maxilla particularly, or the mandible. The same general pattern as seen in other affected bones is common, with a slow rarefying osteitis resulting in sequestration of bone.[76] Pain is not a prominent early feature but is seen later. Secondary infection may lead to difficulty in making a diagnosis. Tuberculous involvement of the mandible causes symptoms of pain, swelling, difficulty in eating, trismus, paraesthesia of the lower lip and enlargement of the regional lymph nodes.[75–81] The infection may spread throughout the jaw, producing multiple sinuses, which drain intra- or extra-orally.[82,83] The posterior mandible and ascending ramus are typically affected, and radiographical appearances include irregular linear calcifications along the lower border and irregular radiolucencies within the jawbone.[75] In the maxilla the infra-orbital region, particularly in the young, is the usual site affected. Typically, a cold abscess develops and may eventually drain through fistulae[84] but occasionally a firm intra-bony lesion may be present.[85]

Diagnosis

The diagnosis of pulmonary tuberculosis, suggested by a chronic cough, haemoptysis, loss of weight, night sweats and fever, is confirmed by physical examination, chest radiography, sputum smears and culture, and tuberculin testing (Mantoux or Heaf test). A lesional biopsy should be examined histologically, and with acid-fast stains and culture of the organism is the absolute proof of the disease.

Management

Conventional chemotherapy of tuberculosis consists of administering two or more active drugs for 18 months to 2 years. Isoniazid in combination with ethambutol, thiacetazone or para-aminosalicylic acid and, depending on the severity of the disease, streptomycin intramuscularly for a period of the first 2–3 months, may be necessary. Other available drugs include rifampin, pyrazinamide and ethionamide.

Non-tuberculous mycobacterial infections

Non-tuberculous (atypical) mycobacteria (NTM) include *Mycobacterium avium* and *M. intracellulare* (*M. avium-intracellulare* complex: MAC), *M. scrofulaceum* and *M. haemophilum*. Infections with NTM are being increasingly reported, especially in immunocompromised individuals.[86] Cervical lymphadenopathy is occasionally caused by NTM but oral lesions are rare.

Management

Atypical mycobacteria may be resistant to conventional antituberculous chemotherapy, although in children with cervical lymphadenitis caused by NTM conventional drug therapy alone[87] or cycloserine for very resistant cases may be effective, and only occasionally is surgical excision necessary.[88]

Leprosy

Accurate estimates of the number of cases of leprosy are difficult to obtain, but approximately 2.2 billion people live in areas where leprosy is an important problem, i.e., where the prevalence is such that the risk of contracting the disease is considered significant.[89]

Oral lesions are most commonly seen in *lepromatous* leprosy,[90–96] as nodules (lepromas) in the palate, tongue or elsewhere. These may eventually ulcerate and scar.[94,97–99] Lepromatous leprosy also affects nerves (eventually with hypoaesthesia), skin, lymph nodes and other tissues including bones, eyes, testes, kidneys and bone marrow.

Tuberculoid leprosy causes thickening of cutaneous nerves, flat and hypopigmented or raised and erythematous skin lesions and enlarged lymph nodes.

Diagnosis

The diagnosis is usually based on the presence of anaesthetic skin lesions and thickened peripheral nerves, confirmed by smears from an open lesion or biopsy. The lepromin test, a non-specific delayed type hypersensitivity skin test, is positive in many persons from endemic areas, whether leprotic or not.

Management

Dapsone is the standard treatment but clofazimine, rifampicin and prothionamide may be required if *M. leprae* is resistant.[100]

Fungal

Superficial mycoses
Candidosis

Candidosis (candidiasis) is the most common oral superficial mycosis. Caused mainly by *Candida albicans*, the condition typically reflects an underlying change in oral flora, depressed salivation, or immune defect. Increasingly, infections with variants of *C. albicans*, with other and sometimes new *Candida* species and of organisms resistant to antifungal agents, are now seen in immunocompromised persons especially.[101]

Pseudomembranous candidosis or thrush may be seen in neonates and among terminally ill patients, particularly in association with immunocompromising conditions (Figure 27.9). [102] Thrush is characterized by white patches on the surface of the oral mucosa, tongue, gingivae and elsewhere. The lesions form confluent plaques that resemble milk curds and can be wiped off the mucosa with a gauze. Oral candidosis in the form of thrush is classically an acute infection, but it may recur for many months or even years in patients using corticosteroids topically or by aerosol, in HIV-infected individuals and in other immunocompromised patients. The term chronic

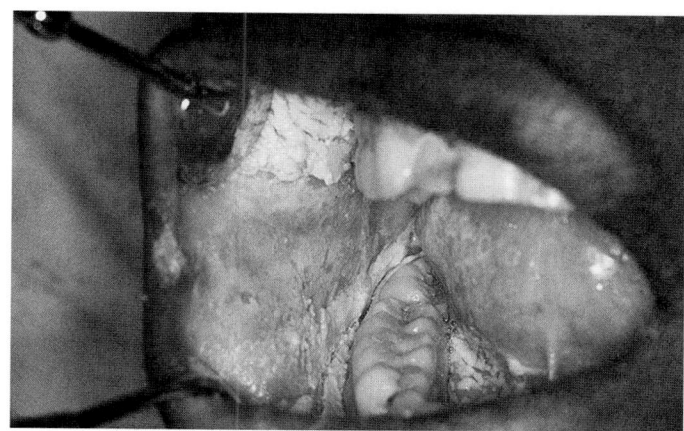

Figure 27.9: Thrush associated with HIV.

pseudomembranous candidosis has been used for chronic recurrence. *Erythematous or atrophic candidosis* is an uncommon and poorly understood condition. It may arise as a consequence of persistent acute pseudo-membranous candidosis, when the pseudomembranes are shed, or in HIV infection may precede pseudo-membranous candidosis. Erythematous areas are seen mainly on the dorsum of the tongue, palate, gingivae or buccal mucosa. Lesions on the dorsum of the tongue present as depapillated areas. Midline or median rhomboid glossitis, or glossal central papillary atrophy, is characterized by an area of papillary atrophy that is rhomboid in shape, symmetrically placed centrally at the midline of the tongue, anterior to the circumvallate papillae. Red areas are often seen in the palate in HIV disease. *Hyperplastic candidosis* (Candida leucoplakia) is typified by chronic, discrete raised lesions that are typically found at the commissures, rarely on the gingivae. *Angular stomatitis* (perlèche, angular cheilitis) is a clinical diagnosis of lesions that affect, and are restricted to, the angles of the mouth, characterized by soreness, erythema and fissuring, and is commonly associated with denture-induced stomatitis. Both yeasts and bacteria are involved, as interacting, predisposing factors. It is occasionally an isolated initial sign of anaemia or vitamin deficiency, and resolves when the underlying disease has been treated.[103] Angular stomatitis may also be seen in HIV disease and Crohn's disease.

Chronic multifocal oral candidosis is a term given when there are several lesions in the absence of predisposing drugs (except tobacco smoking) or medical conditions, typically angular stomatitis that is unilateral or bilateral, retrocommissural leucoplakia, which is the most con-stant component of the tetrad, median rhomboid glossitis, and palatal lesions where the lesions are of more than 1 month duration.

Diagnosis
Clinical diagnosis can be supported by culture from saliva or an oral rinse.

Oral management
Antifungal therapy is initially with topical agents, especially the polyenes (nystatin, amphotericin), except in immunocompromised persons in whom the azoles, especially fluconazole, may be required systemically.

Systemic (deep) mycoses
The systemic mycoses are potentially serious, sometimes lethal fungal infections seen mainly in the developing world, or in those who have visited endemic areas, and are increasingly seen in immunocompromised persons,[104,105] especially in HIV infection.[106]

In otherwise healthy persons, infection with these fungi is typically subclinical although some have pulmonary infection. The increase in mycoses in immunocompromised persons is accompanied by significant morbidity and mortality and 'new' opportunists are appearing.[107]

Orofacial lesions are mainly chronic ulcers or maxillary sinus infection, which are typically associated with respiratory lesions. Most of the mycoses are diagnosed on the basis of a history of travel to endemic areas, or an immunocompromising state, confirmed by taking a smear, biopsy or culture of the affected tissues. Sero-diagnosis, physical examination and chest radiograph may be indicated. Most systemic mycoses can be treated with systemic amphotericin or azoles.

Aspergillosis
Oral lesions are seen mainly in immunocompromised patients as invasive aspergillosis.[106] Yellow or black necrotic ulcers appear typically from antral invasion in the palate or occasionally are seen in the posterior tongue.[108–110]

Diagnosis
Diagnosis is confirmed by smear and lesional microscopy, staining with periodic acid–Schiff (PAS) or Gomori methenamine silver. Immunostains may help. Culture of tissue or fluids on Sabouraud's or mycosel agar may be positive but this is not invariable as the organisms are ubiquitous, so that isolation of *Aspergillus* is not proof of disease.

Oral management
Invasive aspergillosis should be treated with surgery and systemic antifungals.[111] Topical ketoconazole or clotrimazole may clear superficial infections, but if there is no resolution in 72 hours systemic amphotericin is needed.

Blastomycosis
Blastomycosis may disseminate to produce chronic proliferative mulberry-like ulcerated oral lesions.[112,113] The gingival or alveolar process are typical sites, but lesions are also seen particularly on the palate and lip.[112]

Diagnosis
Definitive diagnosis is based on smear or culture. Direct immuno-staining is the most useful confirmation. DNA probes can give an answer in 2 hours.

Oral management
Itraconazole is highly effective treatment as is amphotericin.

Coccidioidomycosis
Oral lesions are rare verrucous lesions sometimes with infection of the jaw, typically secondary to lung involve-ment.[104,105]

Diagnosis is supported by histology (DNA probes are now available), serology, and the spherulin or coccidioidin skin tests.

Oral management
Systemic amphotericin, sometimes supplemented with ketoconazole, itraconazole or fluconazole, is used.

Cryptococcosis

Oral *Cryptococcus* infection has presented mainly with non-healing extraction wounds, or chronic ulceration on the palate, gingivae or tongue[106] in disseminated disease. Wide dissemination is especially liable to occur in immunocompromised persons.[114] Most patients with disseminated cryptococcosis have cryptococcal meningo-encephalitis at the time of diagnosis and, untreated, this is fatal in over 70% of cases.

Diagnosis

Diagnosis is confirmed by microscopy, staining with periodic acid–Schiff, mucicarmine or methenamine silver. Culture may help the diagnosis.

Oral management

Systemic amphotericin is effective therapy. Ketoconazole or itraconazole may also be used.

Histoplasmosis

Oral lesions are usually ulcerative or nodular, on the tongue, palate, buccal mucosa or gingiva, and occasion-ally the mandible or the maxilla,[106] seen mainly in disseminated and potentially lethal histoplasmosis in immunocompromised persons (Figure 27.10).[115–117]

Diagnosis

Diagnosis of histoplasmosis is confirmed by microscopy. DNA probes are now available. Culture on Sabouraud's agar is also confirmatory. Complement fixation tests may be of value and several other serotests are available. The histoplasmin skin test is of little importance diagnostically.

Oral management

Amphotericin is given first for treatment followed by ketoconazole.

Mucormycosis (zygomycosis: phycomycosis)

Mucoraceae can commonly be cultured from the throat and mouth of many healthy individuals but infection is virtually unheard of in otherwise healthy individuals. Immunocompromising conditions typically underlie zygomycosis.[106,118] It usually commences in the nasal cavity or paranasal sinuses with pain and nasal discharge, and fever, and may then invade the palate to produce black necrotic oral ulcers.

Diagnosis is confirmed by smear or histology.

Oral management

Zygomycosis used to be almost uniformly fatal and still has a mortality approaching 20%. Control of underlying disease is essential if possible, together with systemic amphotericin and surgical debridement.

Paracoccidioidomycosis

Paracoccidioidomycosis caused by the dimorphic fungus *Paracoccidioides brasiliensis* is one of the most important systemic mycoses in Latin America (Figure 27.11).[119]

The disease causes cutaneous and/or respiratory tract mucosal lesions as well as lymph node enlargement. Involvement of the oral cavity and/or the nasopharynx/larynx, either alone or in association with the lungs, is one of the commonest clinical presentations.[119] Oral lesions are often granular, exophytic and ulcerated and often affect the gingivae.[112,113,120]

Diagnosis

Pus or scrapings from the lesion, examined in potassium hydroxide, may show the rounded refractile cells of *P. brasiliensis* which may show characteristic multiple budding. Biopsy may be required for definitive diagnosis. Smear or culture can also be diagnostically useful but *P. brasiliensis* grows only extremely slowly. Serology may be helpful.[121]

Oral management

Systemic amphotericin alone can be curative but with sulfamethoxypyridazine is more effective. Sulfadiazine plus trimethoprim may be useful. Ketoconazole and itraconazole are superior since they can be given orally, but are expensive.

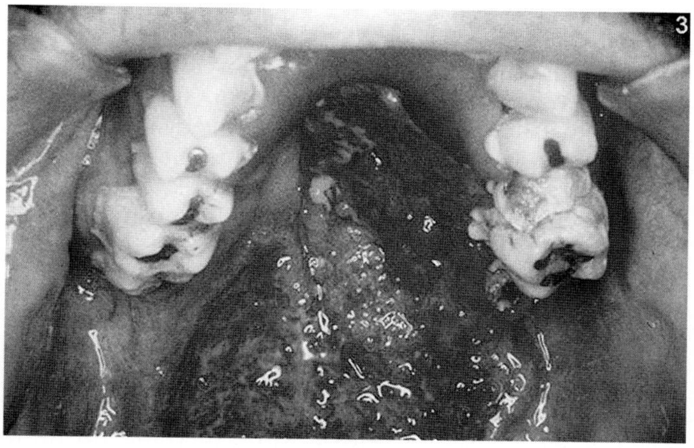

Figure 27.10: Histoplasmosis associated with HIV.

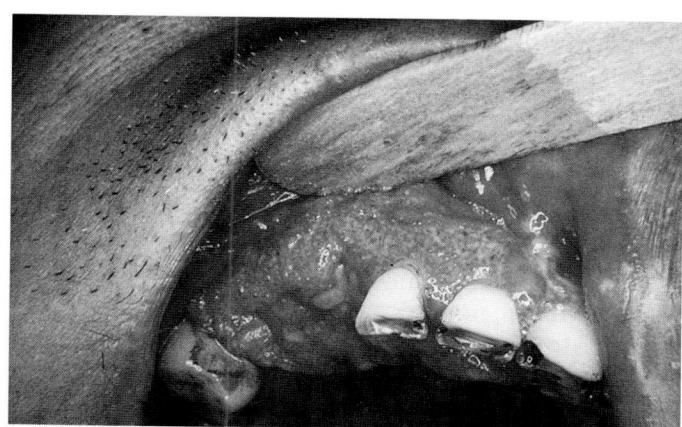

Figure 27.11: Paracoccidioidomycosis affecting the maxilla.

Rhinosporidiosis

Rhinosporidiosis, caused by *Rhinosporidium seeberi*, affects the nasal and other mucosae. Oral lesions are usually proliferative lumps on the palate.

Diagnosis is by biopsy.

Management is surgery.

Sporotrichosis

The primary lesion is a sporotrichotic chancre, which may ulcerate if in the mouth. Lesions may also then arise in lymphatics. Pulmonary and disseminated sporotrichosis is rare and of uncertain origin: antral and oral involvement has been described.

Diagnosis is confirmed by histology and culture.

Oral management

Potassium iodide is effective treatment for superficial sporotrichosis, itraconazole or amphotericin for other forms.

Parasitic infections

Malaria is the most important parasitic disease of man, and like many parasitic infestations has few oral complications. However, the lack of reporting of oral lesions in parasitic infestations may simply be a reflection of their under-diagnosis.

Toxoplasmosis

Toxoplasma gondii is an intracellular parasite that may cause a glandular fever type of illness with fever and lymphadenopathy, which often causes cervical lymphadenopathy, sometimes with fever, rash, hepatosplenomegaly, myalgia and other minor features. These general non-specific signs and symptoms and the fact that commonly there is submandibular lymphadenopathy makes the differential diagnosis of dental infections and toxoplasmosis a challenge. A number of cases have been reported in which children present to the dentist with apparent dental infection when the true problem is related to a parasitic infection.[122,123]

Diagnosis

The diagnosis of toxoplasmosis requires confirmation serologically by the Sabin–Feldman dye test, indirect fluorescent antibody test or indirect haemagglutination test. The organism may be demonstrable in tissue sections or smears.

Oral management

Treatment is not required for asymptomatic healthy persons who are not pregnant. For immunocompromised patients, treatment is a combination of pyrimethamine and sulfadiazine, together with folic acid, since pyrimethamine is a folate antagonist. Treatment may need to be carried on for at least 1 month after clinical resolution. Weekly full blood counts are essential.

Leishmaniasis

Transmitted by the bite of the infected female phlebotomine sandfly, the leishmaniases are a globally widespread group of parasitic diseases. Leishmaniasis presents itself in humans in four different forms; visceral, mucocutaneous, cutaneous and diffuse cutaneous. Oral lesions are most frequent in mucocutaneous leishmaniasis; up to two-thirds of patients have oral lesions.[124] The mouth may be involved by direct extension from cutaneous leishmaniasis (oriental sore or chiclero ulcer).[125,126] Cutaneous leishmaniasis may cause lip[127] or facial swelling.[128]

In oral leishmaniasis, the hard palate is typically involved (espundia) but lesions can spread to the soft palate, uvula and pharynx or, less commonly, to involve the gingivae and upper lip. A mid-facial granulomatous destructive lesion may result.

Oral lesions seen in Sudan are typically caused by *L. donovani*[129,130] and present as fungating lesions.

Oral symptoms in most patients centre upon pain or a sensation of a foreign body in the mouth, gingival bleeding or loosening of teeth.[129]

Leishmania/HIV co-infection is emerging as a serious and new disease.[131] Although people are bitten by sandflies that are infected with *Leishmania* protozoa, most do not develop the disease. However, among those who are immunosuppressed (e.g., HIV), cases can quickly evolve to a full clinical presentation of severe leishmaniasis. It is estimated that AIDS increases this risk by 100–1000 times in epidemic areas.[131]

In a similar way to HIV, leishmaniasis can be transmitted directly from person to person through the sharing of needles. This is important in developing countries where dental treatment is carried out by both trained and non-trained personnel, and where infection control procedures in the dental surgery can be variable.[132]

Diagnosis

There is no specific oral sign to help in the diagnosis of leishmaniases, and the approach to the clinical diagnosis is covered in the chapter dedicated to this disease.

Oral management

The management of lesions and symptoms is essentially palliative, and it is recognized that many mucocutaneous leishmaniasis oral lesions may heal spontaneously. Essentially, the clinical and parasitological cures are implemented and oral ulcerations are managed via a palliative approach by altering the diet (i.e., changing its consistency by making it more bland and consuming it at tepid temperatures).

Trichinosis

Trichinella spiralis occurs in two forms: the adult *T. spiralis*, which is a white worm barely visible to the naked eye: and the cystic form, which is formed by the larva encapsulated by the host tissue. Since its transmission is by mouth from eating undercooked meat, it is not surprising that trichinosis is the most frequent round-worm infestation to affect the oral tissues. As in other parts of the body, encystations are commonly in the striated muscle, and in the oral cavity this is predominantly in the tongue and masseter muscle. The usual cycle of events is that they invade the tongue and masseter muscle, where calcification will take place after about 6 months and lead to the death of the larva. The small intra-oral cyst-like lesions can commonly be confused as mucoceles; however, the latter are not associated with systemic symptoms. The cyst-like lesions become encapsulated and may calcify, at which time radiographically they appear as radiopaque nodules.[133]

Diagnosis is clinical, supported by investigations and a history of ingestion of poorly cooked meat, and by serology.

Oral management
There is no specific oral management and treatment is similar to that of a trichinosis infection elsewhere in the body, namely treatment directed against the larvae and the immune reaction, which they invoke. Prolonged oral high-dosage mebendazole or thiabendazole has been proved to be effective.

Echinococcosis (echinococciasis)
The larval stages of two small tapeworms, *Echinococcus granulosus* and *E. multilocularis*, cause the main forms of hydatid disease in man. In the oral tissues hydatid cysts are usually firm, round swellings of several months' duration, mainly in the tongue.[134]

Diagnosis
A history of possible exposure to infection may be elicited. A hydatid cyst may show a smooth round outline on radiography. Eosinophilia is merely suggestive of a parasitic disease and not specific. A definitive diagnosis is often made only by identifying the hydatid cyst at operation.

Oral management
As with the general management of this infection, high doses of mebendazole, albendazole or flubendazole interfere with growth of larvae but are not curative. The only curative treatment is surgery.

Cysticercosis
Cysticercosis is the infection by the small bladder-like larvae of the pork tapeworm, *Taenia solium*. Human cysticercoisis is essentially a faecal–oral infection, acquired by ingesting eggs excreted in the faeces of a human tapeworm carrier. Although cysticerci are not uncommon in the striated muscles in the tongue and neck and subcutaneous tissues, morbidity of cysticercosis is almost entirely due to the central nervous system disease. A number of cases of children presenting with oral lesions of cysticercosis have been reported.[135,136] Oral lesions are typically well circumscribed, nodular, soft,

elastic and fluctuant submucosal swellings situated in the dorsum of the tongue and buccal mucosa. Although such oral lesions may be present for a number of years, oral signs may be the first clinical sign of the infection.[136]

Diagnosis usually relies upon surgical removal of the parasite, the appearance of the translucent membrane with its central milky spot being characteristic.

Oral management
There is no reliable medical treatment but the general management approach is either albendazole or praziquantel (plus prednisolone can be curative).

Larva migrans
Oral lesions have been recorded in relation to various worms, including *Ancylostoma* and *Gongylonema* species.

Oral management
Local application of 10% thiabendazole, ethyl chloride, chloroform, electrocoagulation and cryotherapy have all been tried. If the lesions are multiple, particularly in the mouth, thiabendazole is indicated but can produce adverse effects such as anorexia, nausea and rashes. Albendazole or mebendazole are alternatives.

Filariasis
The filariases result from infection with vector-borne tissue-dwelling nematodes called filariae. In public health terms the two most important filariae are onchocerciasis and lymphatic filariasis.

Lymphatic filariasis, in humans, is estimated to infect 20% of the world's population and is the result of three species of filarial worms: *Wuchereria bancrofti*, *Brugia malayi* and *B. timori*.[137] It is fortunate that these species have rarely been found in the mouth.

Onchocerciasis (river blindness) is the result of infection with *Onchocerca volvulus*. The main clinical features of the infection are dermatitis, eye lesions and nodule formation. In Africa 80% of nodules occur on the body prominences of the pelvic girdle. However, in Central America nodules are commonly found in the head and neck region. It is thought that this reflects the biting habits of the vector flies.[138] Oral nodules are unusual, but when they occur they present as a rubbery nodule.

Diagnosis
The diagnosis is made by identifying the worm in biopsies.

Oral management
Nodulectomy has only limited use because many worms are present outside the nodules. However, it has been suggested that head nodules should be removed because their presence increases the risk of blindness.[138] The rationale for this procedure is that this will reduce the number of microfilariae which are produced. Nodulectomy campaigns have been attempted, but their impact has yet to be evaluated, but in Guatemala systematic campaigns were associated with decreased blindness.[138]

Gnathostomiasis

Gnathostomiasis may produce swellings in the skin or mouth, or occasionally bleeding. Skin tests and serodiagnosis help the diagnosis. Metronidazole may be of some benefit or the worm can be excised.

Myiasis

Myiasis is caused when fly maggots invade living tissue or when they are harboured in the intestine or bladder. In oral lesions they are seen mainly in the anterior maxillary or mandibular gingivae.[139–142] An opening burrow is usually patent, with induration of the marginal tissues and is raised, forming a dome-shaped 'warble', or an extraction wound may be effected. Often several larvae are present and there is severe inflammatory reaction in the surrounding tissues.

Diagnosis

Larvae can be seen with the naked eye.

Oral management

A few drops of turpentine oil or chloroform in light vegetable oil should be instilled in the lesion and the larvae removed with blunt tweezers. It may be prudent to give an antibiotic, as there is often a superimposed secondary infection.

REFERENCES

1   Cook G C. Tropical gastroenterological problems. In Cook G (ed.) *Manson's Tropical Diseases*, 20th edn. London: W B Saunders, 1998: 29–30.

2   Beighton D & Edgar W N. Dental Caries: aetiology and pathogenesis. In Arens U (ed.) *Oral Health: Diet and Other Factors*. Amsterdam: Elsevier, 1999.

3   Burt B A & Ismail A L. Diet, nutrition and food cariogenicity. *J Dent Res* 1986; 65:S1475–S1484.

4   Winter G B. Maternal nutritional requirements in relation to the subsequent development of teeth in children. *J Hum Nutr* 1976; 30:93–99.

5   Alvarez J O & Navia J M. Nutritional status, tooth eruption and dental caries: a review. *Am J Clin Nutr* 1989; 49:417–426.

6   Rugg-Gunn A J. *Nutrition and Dental Health*. Oxford: Oxford University Press, 1993.

7   Department for International Development. *Eliminating World Poverty: Making Globalisation Work for the Poor. White Paper on International Development*. London: Stationery Office, 2000.

8   Frencken J E, Pilot T, Songpaisan Y et al. Atraumatic restorative treatment (ART): rationale, technique and development. *J Public Health Dent* 1996; 56:135–140.

9   Holmgren C J, Lo E C M, Hu D Y et al. ART restorations and sealants placed in Chinese schoolchildren: results 3 years. *Community Dent Oral Epidemiol* 2000; 28:314–320.

10   Hansel-Petersson G & Bratthal D. The caries decline: a review of reviews. In *Dental Caries: Intervened—Interrupted—Interpreted. Suppl Eur J Oral Sci* 1996; 104:436–443.

11   Adyatmaka A, Sutopo U, Carlsson P et al. *School-Based Primary Preventive Programme of Children*. Geneva: World Health Organization, 1998.

12   Pilot T. The periodontal disease problem: a comparison between industrialised and developing countries. *Int Dent J* 1998 48(3, suppl. 1):221–232.

13   Ali R W, Johannessen A C, Dahlen G et al. Comparison of the subgingival microbiota of periodontally healthy and diseased adults in northern Cameroon. *J Clin Periodontol* 1997 24(11):830–835.

14   Cohen H D, Fisher R, Mann J et al. Periodontal treatment needs and oral hygiene among Ethiopian immigrants. *Int Dent J* 1995; 45(3):204–208.

15   Miyazaki H. A global overview of periodontal epidemiology. In Pack A R C & Newman H N (eds). *Periodontal Needs of Developing Nations. International Academy of Periodontology Symposium*, 4 June 1995. Northwood: Science Reviews, 1996: 1–7.

16   Darout I A, Albandar J M & Skaug N. Periodontal status of adult Sudanese habitual users of miswak chewing sticks or toothbrushes. *Acta Odontol Scand* 2000; 58(1):25–30.

17   World Health Organization. *Manual of the International Statistical Classification of Diseases, Injuries and Causes of Death* (based on the recommendations of the ninth revision conference). Geneva: WHO, 1977.

18   Scully C & Bedi R. Ethnicity and oral cancer. *Lancet Oncol* 2000: 1:37–42.

19   Parkin D M, Pisani P & Ferlay J. Estimates of the worldwide incidence of 25 major cancers in 1990. *Int J Cancer* 1999; 80:827–841.

20   International Agency for Research on Cancer. *IARC Monographs on the Evaluation of Carcinogenic Risks to Humans. Tobacco Smoking*, vol. 38. Lyon: International Agency for Research on Cancer, 1986.

21   International Agency for Research on Cancer. *IARC Monographs on the Evaluation of Carcinogenic Risks of Chemicals to Humans. Tobacco Habits Other than Smoking: Betel Quid and Areca Nut Chewing and some Related Nitrosamines*, Vol. 37. Lyon: International Agency for Research on Cancer, 1986.

22   Sankarnarayanan R, Black R J, Swaminathan R et al. An overview of cancer survival in developing countries. In Sankarnarayanan R, Black R J & Parkin D M (eds). *Cancer Survival in Developing Countries*. IARC Scientific Publication no. 145. Lyon: Oxford University Press; 1998, 135–157.

23   Van Wyk C W, Stander I, Padayachee A et al. The areca nut chewing habit and oral squamous cell carcinoma in South African Indians: a retrospective study. *S Afr Med J* 1993; 83:425–429.

24   Mathew B, Sankaranarayanan R, Sunilkumar K et al. Reproducibility and validity of oral visual inspection by trained health workers in the detection of oral cancer and precancer. *Br J Cancer* 1997; 76:390–394.

25   Sankaranarayanan R. Health care auxiliaries in the detection and prevention of oral cancer. *Oral Oncol Eur J Cancer* 1997; 33B:149–154.

26   Fernandez Garrote L, Sankaranarayanan R, Lence Anta J J et al. An evaluation of the oral cancer control program in Cuba. *Epidemiology* 1995; 6:428–431.

27   Gupta P C, Mehta F S, Pindborg J J et al. Primary prevention trial of oral cancer in India: a 10 year follow-up study. *J Oral Pathol Med* 1992; 21:433–439.

28   Martin G C, Brown J P, Eifler C W et al. Oral leukoplakia status six weeks after cessation of smokeless tobacco use. *J Am Dent Assoc* 1999; 130:945–954.

29   Bedi R. Betel-quid and tobacco chewing among the United Kingdom's Bangladeshi community. *Br J Cancer* 1996; 74(suppl. XXIX):S73–S77.

30   Bhonsle R B, Murti P R, Daftary D K et al. Regional variations in oral submucous fibrosis in India. *Commun Dent Oral*

Epidemiol 1987; 15:225–229.

31 Murti P R, Bhonsle R B, Pinborg J J et al. Malignant transformation rate in oral submucous fibrosis over a 17-year period. *Commun Dent Oral Epidemiol* 1985; 13:340–341.

32 Horning G M & Cohen M E. Necrotizing ulcerative gingivitis, periodontitis, and stomatitis: clinical staging and predisposing factors. *J Periodontol* 1995; 66:990–998.

33 Contreras A, Falkler W A, Enwonwu C O et al. Human Herpesviridae in acute necrotizing ulcerative gingivitis in children in Nigeria. *Oral Microbiol Immunol* 1997; 12:259–265.

34 World Health Organization. *Noma, the Face of Poverty.* WHO: Geneva, updated August 2000.

35 Costini B, Larroque G, Dubosco J C et al. Noma ou cancrum oris: aspects etiopathogeniques et nosologiques. *Med Trop* 1995; 55:263–273.

36 Idigbe E O, Enwonwu C O, Falker W A et al. Living conditions of children at risk for noma: Nigerian experience. *Oral Dis* 1999; 5(2):156–162.

37 Ndiaye F C, Bourgeois D, Leclercq M H et al. Noma: public health problem in Senegal and epidemiological surveillance. *Oral Dis* 1999; 5(2):163–166.

38 Akula S K, Chreticos C M & Weldon-Linne C M. Gangrenous stomatitis in AIDS. *Lancet* 1989; i:955.

39 Darie H, Veran Y, Dupin M et al. Noma d'adulte: maladie opportuniste du syndrome d'immunodéficience acquise? *Med Trop* 1994; 54:451–452.

40 Giovannini M, Zuccotti G V & Fiocchi A. Gangrenous stomatitis in a child with AIDS. *Lancet* 1989; ii:1400.

41 Limongelli W A, Clark M S & Williams A C. Noma-like lesion in a patient with chronic lymphocytic leukemia. *Oral Surg* 1976; 41:40–51.

42 Rotbart H A, Levin M J, Jones J F et al. Noma in children with severe combined immunodeficiency. *Pediatrics* 1986; 109;596–600.

43 Stassen L F, Batchelor A G, Rennie J S et al. Cancrum oris in an adult caucasian female. *Br J Oral Maxillofac Surg* 1989; 27:417–422.

44 Weinstein R A, Choukas N C & Wood W S. Cancrum oris-like lesions associated with acute myelogenous leukemia. *Oral Surg* 1974; 32:10.

45 Winkler J R, Murray P A & Hammerle C. Gangrenous stomatitis in AIDS. *Lancet* 1989; 2:108.

46 World Health Organization. *Young People and Sexually Transmitted Diseases.* Fact Sheet no. 186. WHO: Geneva, revised December 1997.

47 Fiumara N J & Berg M. Primary syphilis in the oral cavity. *Br J Vener Dis* 1974; 50:463–464.

48 Mani N J. Secondary syphilis initially diagnosed from oral lesions. *Oral Surg Oral Med Oral Pathol* 1984; 58:47–50.

49 Terezhalmy G T. Oral manifestations of sexually related diseases. *Ear Nose Throat J* 1983; 62:287–296.

50 Manton S L, Egglestone S I, Alexander I et al. Oral presentation of secondary syphilis. *Br Dent J* 1986; 160:237–238.

51 Meyer I & Shklar G. The oral manifestations of acquired syphilis. *Oral Surg Oral Med Oral Pathol* 1967; 23:45–48.

52 Erdelyi R L & Molla A A. Burned-out endemic syphilis (Bejel) facial deformities and defects in Saudi Arabia. *Plast Reconstr Surg* 1984; 74:589–602.

53 Furtado T & Almeida A F. A frambroesia tropica (Bouba) no nordeste de Minas Gerais. Analise de 5385 casos. *Anais Brasileiros Dermatol Sifilografia* 1954; 29:1.

54 Furtado T. Some problems of late yaws. *Int J Dermatol* 1973; 12:123–130.

55 Botreau-Roussel P. Goundou. In Simons R D G (ed.) *Handbook of Tropical Dermatology and Medical Mycology.* Amsterdam: Elsevier, 1952:6–76.

56 Holst E & Lund P. Cervicofacial actinomycosis: a retrospective study. *Int J Oral Surg* 1979; 8:194–198.

57 Hylton R P, Samuels H S & Oatis G W. Actinomycosis: it is really rare? *Oral Surg Oral Med Oral Pathol* 1970; 29:138–147.

58 Norman J E de B. Cervicofacial actinomycosis. *Oral Surg Oral Med Oral Pathol* 1970; 29:735–745.

59 Stenhouse D, MacDonald D G & MacFarlane T W. Cervicofacial and intraoral actinomycosis: a 5 year retrospective study. *Br J Oral Surg* 1975; 13:172–182.

60 Benoliel R & Asquith J. Actinomycosis of the jaws. *Int J Oral Surg* 1985; 14:195–199.

61 Roberts G D, Brewer W S & Hermans P E. Diagnosis of nocardiosis by blood culture. *Mayo Clin Proc* 1974; 49:293.

62 Rattner L J. Case of suspected oral nocardiosis. *Oral Surg Oral Med Oral Pathol* 1958; 11:441.

63 World Health Organization. *Tuberculosis.* Fact Sheet no. 104. WHO: Geneva, revised April 2000.

64 Eng H L, Lu S Y, Yang C H et al. Oral tuberculosis. *Oral Surg* 1994; 81:415–420.

65 Fujibayashi T, Takahasi Y Yoneda T et al. Tuberculosis of the tongue: a case report with immunologic study. *Oral Surg Oral Med Oral Pathol* 1979; 47:427–435.

66 Komet H, Scheffer R F & McHoney P L. Bilateral tuberculous granulomas of the tongue. *Arch Otolaryngol* 1965; 82:649–661.

67 Radden B G & Reade P C. Tuberculous ulceration of the mouth. *Aust Dent J* 1961; 6:105–106.

68 Yusuf H. Oral tuberculosis. *Br Dent J* 1975; 138:470–472.

69 McAndrew P G, Adekeye E O & Ajdukiewicz A B. Miliary tuberculosis presenting with multifocal oral lesions. *Br Med J* 1976; 1:1320.

70 Michaud M, Blancette G & Tomich C. Chronic ulceration of the hard palate: first clinical sign of undiagnosed pulmonary tuberculosis. *Oral Surg Oral Med Oral Pathol* 1984; 57:63–67.

71 Rao T V, Satyanarayana C V, Sundareshwar B et al. Unusual form of tuberculosis of lips. *J Oral Surg* 1977; 35:595–596.

72 Turbiner S, Giunta J & Maloney P L. Orofacial tuberculosis of the lip. *J Oral Surg* 1975; 33:443–447.

73 Agarwal M K, Gupta O P, Samant H C et al. Tuberculosis of the tongue. *Ann Acad Med Singapore* 1979; 8:217–219.

74 Boyes J, Jones J D T & Miller F J W. The recognition of primary tuberculous infection of the mouth. *Arch Dis Child* 1956; 31:81–86.

75 Taylor R G & Booth D F. Tuberculous osteomyelitis of the mandible. *Oral Surg Oral Med Oral Pathol* 1964; 18:7–13.

76 Thilander H & Wennstrom A. Tuberculosis of the mouth and the surrounding tissues. *Oral Surg Oral Med Oral Pathol* 1956; 9:858–870.

77 Foster C F & Young W B. Tuberculosis infection of a fractured mandible: report of a case. *J Oral Surg* 1970; 38:686.

78 Ratliff D P. Tuberculosis of the mandible. *Br Dent J* 1973; 35:595–596.

79 Sachs S A & Eisenbund L. Tuberculous osteomyelitis of the mandible. *Oral Surg Oral Med Oral Pathol* 1977; 44:425–429.

80 Shengold M A & Shengold H. Oral tuberculosis. *Oral Surg Oral Med Oral Pathol* 1951; 4:239–250.

81 Weidman G M & MacGregor A J. Tuberculous osteomyelitis of the mandible: report of a case. *Oral Surg Oral Med Oral Pathol* 1969; 28:632–635.

82 Bradnum P. Tuberculous sinus of the face associated with an abscessed lower third molar. *Dent Pract Dent Rec* 1961; 12:127–128.

83 Sowray J H. Tuberculous facial sinuses. *Br Dent J* 1967; 123:291–294.

84 Pratap V K, Samuel K C & Saxena H. Tuberculosis: manifestation at uncommon sites. *J Ind Med Assoc* 1972; 59:281–287.

85 Rosenquist J B & Beskow R. Tuberculosis of the maxilla: report case. *J Oral Surg* 1977; 35:309–310.

86   Waldman R H. Tuberculosis and the atypical mycobacteria. *Otolaryngol Clin North Am* 1982; 15:581–586.

87   Ord R J & Matz G J. Tuberculous cervical lymphadenitis. *Arch Otolaryngol* 1974; 99:327–329.

88   Salyer K E, Votteler T P & Dorman G W. Surgical management of cervical adenitis due to atypical mycobacteria in children. *JAMA* 1968; 204:103–106.

89   Noorden S K & Pannikar V K. Leprosy. In Cook G C (ed.) *Manson's Tropical Diseases* 20th edn. London: W B Saunders, 1996: 1016–1044.

90   Barton R P E. Lesions of the mouth, pharynx and larynx in lepromatous leprosy. *Leprosy India* 1974; 46:130–134.

91   Moller-Christensen V, Bakke S N, Melsum R S et al. Changes in the anterior nasal spine and the alveolar process of the maxillary bone in leprosy. *Int J Leprosy* 1952; 20:335–340.

92   Prahbu S R & Daftary D K. Atrophic lesions of the tongue in leprosy patients. *Odontostomatol Trop* 1982; V:75–85.

93   Reichart P. Facial and oral manifestations in leprosy. *Oral Surg Oral Med Oral Pathol* 1976; 41:385–399.

94   Reichart P. Pathologic changes in the soft palate in lepromatous leprosy. *Oral Surg Oral Med Oral Pathol* 1974; 38:898–904.

95   Scheepers A, Lemmer J & Lownie J F. Oral manifestations of Leprosy. *Leprosy Rev* 1993; 64(1):37–43.

96   Southam J C & Venkatraman B K. Oral manifestations of leprosy. *Br J Oral Surg* 1973; 10:272–274.

97   Girdhar B K & Desikan K V. A clinical study of the mouth in untreated lepromatous patients. *Leprosy Rev* 1979; 50:25–35.

98   Lighterman I, Watanabe Y & Hidaka T. Leprosy of the oral cavity and adnexa. *Oral Surg Oral Med Oral Pathol* 1962; 15:1178–1194.

99   Prabhu S R & Daftary D K. Clinical evaluation of orofacial lesions in leprosy. *Odontostomatol Trop* 1981; IV:83–95.

100 E-Silva R, Rebello P F. Leprosy: recognition and treatment. Am J Clin Dermatol 2001; 2(4):203–211.

101 Scully C, Monteil R & Sposto M R. Infectious and tropical diseases affecting the human mouth. In Scully C (ed.) *Oral Pathology and Medicine in Periodontics: Periodontology 2000*. Copenhagen: Munksgaard, 1998: 47–70.

102 Scully C. Infectious diseases. In Millard H D & Mason D K (eds) *1993 World Workshop on Oral Medicine*. Ann Arbor: University of Michigan, 1995.

103 Scully C & Cawson R A. *Medical Problems in Dentistry*. Bristol: Wright, 1987.

104 De Almeida O P & Scully C. Oral lesions in the systemic mycoses. *Curr Opin Dent* 1991; 1:423–428.

105 Scully C & De Almeida O P. Orofacial manifestations of the systemic mycoses. *J Oral Pathol Med* 1992; 21:289–294.

106 Scully C, De Almeida O P & Sposto M R. Deep mycoses in HIV infection. *Oral Dis* 1997; 3(suppl. 1):200–207.

107 Pfaller M & Wenzel R. Impact of the changing epidemiology of fungal infections in the 1990s. *Eur J Clin Microbiol Infect Dis* 1992; 11:287–291.

108 Napoli J A & Donegan J O. Aspergillosis and necrosis of the maxilla. *J Oral Maxillofac Surg* 1991; 49:532–534.

109 Rubin M M, Jui V & Sadoff R S. Oral aspergillosis in a patient with acquired immunodeficiency syndrome. *J Oral Maxillofac Surg* 1990; 48:997–999.

110 Shannon M T, Sclaroff A & Colm S J. Invasive aspergillosis of the maxilla in an immunocompromised patient. *Oral Surg Oral Med Oral Pathol* 1990; 70:425–427.

111 Denning D W & Stevens D A. Antifungal and surgical treatment of invasive aspergillosis: review of 2,121 published cases. *Rev Infect Dis* 1990; 12:1147–1201.

112 Sposto M R, Almeida O P D, Scully C, Jorge J, Graner E & Bozza L. Oral paracoccidioidomycosis: a study of 36 South American patients. *Oral Surg Oral Med Oral Pathol* 1993; 75:461–465.

113 Sposto M R, Mendes-Gianini M J, Moraes R A, Branco F C & Scully C. Paracoccidioidomycosis manifesting oral lesions: a clinical cytological and serological investigation. *J Oral Pathol Med* 1994; 23:85–87.

114 Schmidt-Westhausen A, Grunewald T, Reichart P A et al. Oral cryptococcosis in a patient with AIDS: a case report. *Oral Dis* 1995; 1(2):77–79.

115 Casariego Z, Kelly G R, Perez H et al. Disseminated histoplasmosis with orofacial involvement in HIV-1-infected patients with AIDS: manifestations and treatment. *Oral Dis* 1997; 3(3):184–187.

116 Nittayananta W & Chungpanich S. Oral lesions in a group of Thai people with AIDS. *Oral Dis* 1997; 3(suppl. 1):S41–45.

117 Warnakulasuriya K A, Harrison J D, Johnson N W et al. Localised oral histoplasmosis lesions associated with HIV infection. *J Oral Pathol Med* 1997; 26(6):294–296.

118 Jones A C, Bentsen T Y & Freedman P D. Mucormycosis of the oral cavity. *Oral Surg Oral Med Oral Pathol* 1993; 75(4):455–460.

119 De Castro C C, Bernard G, Ygaki Y et al. MRI of head and neck paracoccidioidomycosis. *Br J Radiol* 1999; 72(859):717–722.

120 De Almeida O P, Jacks J, Scully C et al. Orofacial manifestations of paracoccidioidomycosis (South American blastomycosis). *Oral Surg Oral Med Oral Pathol* 1991; 72:430–435.

121 Mendes-Giannini M J S. Serodiagnosis. In Franco M, da Silva Lacaz C, Restrepo-Moreno A & del Negro G (eds). *Paracoccidioidomycosis*. Boca Raton, FL: CRC Press, 1994: 345–357.

122 Azaz B, Milhem I, Hasson O et al. Acquired toxoplasmosis of a submandibular lymph node in 13-year-old boy: case report. *Paediatr Dent* 1994; 16(5):378–380.

123 Macey-Dare L V, Kocjan G & Goodman J R. Acquired toxoplasmosis of a submandibular lymph node in a nine-year-old boy diagnosed by fine-needle aspiration cytology. *Int J Paediatr Dent* 1996; 6(4):265–269.

124 Sithequee M A M, Qazi A A & Ahmed G A. Study into leishmaniasis. *Br J Oral Maxillofac Surg* 1990; 28:43–46.

125 Gombos F, Laino G & Femiano F. Leishmaniosi muco-cutanea e del cavo orale. *Arch Stomatol* 1984; 25:349–357.

126 Meyruey M, Benkiran D & Landon A. Leishmaniose stomato-pharyngo-laryngee observee au Maroc. *Bull Soc Pathol Exot* 1974; 67:625–632.

127 Sangueza O P, Sangueza J M, Stiller M et al. Mucocutaneous leishmaniasis: a clinicopathological classification. *J Am Acad Dermatol* 1993; 28:927–932.

128 Castling B, Layton S A & Pratt R J. Cutaneous leishmaniasis: an unusual cause of facial swelling. *Oral Surg* 1994; 78:91–92.

129 El-Hassan A M, Meredith S E, Yagi H I et al. Sudanese mucosal leishmaniasis: epidemiology, clinical features, diagnosis, immune responses and treatment. *Trans R Soc Trop Med Hyg* 1995; 89:647–652.

130 Goto H, Sotto M N, Corbett C E P et al. A case of multiple lesion mucocutaneous leishmaniasis caused by Leishmania (Viannia braziliensis) infection. *J Trop Med Hyg* 1990; 93:48–51.

131 World Health Organization. *The Leishmaniasis and Leishmania/HIV Co-infections*. Fact sheet no. 116. WHO: Geneva, revised May 2000.

132 Littleton P A Jr & Kohn W. Dental public health and infection control in industrialised and developing countries. *Int Dent J* 1991; 41(6):341–347.

133 Hansen L S and Allard R H. Encysted parasitic larvae in the mouth. *J Am Dent Assoc* 1984; 108(4):632–636.

134 Bouckaert M M, Raubenheimer E J & Jacobs F J. Maxillofacial hydatid cysts. *Oral Surg Oral Med Oral Pathol Oral Radiol Endod* 2000; 89(3):338–342.

135 Romero de Leon E, Aguirre A. Oral cysticercosis. *Oral Surg Oral Med Oral Pathol Oral Radiol Endod* 1995; 79(5):572–577.

136 Saran R K, Rattan V, Nijkawan R et al. Cysticercosis of the oral cavity: report of five cases and a review of literature. *Nt J Paediatr Dent* 1998; 8(4):273–278.

137 Nigam S, Singh T, Mishra A & Chaturvedi K U. Oral cysticercosis: reports of six cases. *Head and Neck* 2001; 23(6):497–499.

138 McMahon J E & Simonsen P E. Filariases. In Cook G C (ed.) *Manson's Tropical Diseases* 20th edn. London: W B Saunders, 1996: 1321–1368.

139 Al-Ismaily M I & Scully C. Oral myiasis: report of two cases. *Int J Paediatr Dent* 1985; 5:177–179.

140 Bozzo L, Almeida O D P & Scully C. Oral myiasis caused by sarcophagidae in an extraction wound. *Oral Surg Oral Med Oral Pathol* 1992; 74:733–735.

141 Erfan F. Gingival myiasis caused by Diptera (sarcophaga). *Oral Surg Oral Med Oral Pathol* 1980; 49:148–150.

142 Konstantinidis A B & Zamanis D. Gingival myiasis. *J Oral Med* 1987; 42:243–245.

Chapter 28
Travel Medicine

R. H. Behrens and R. Steffen

Travel, especially to developing countries, is associated with an increased risk of morbidity and mortality. Travel medicine has become increasingly important for the 50 million residents of industrialized nations who travel annually to developing countries. Between 80 and 95% of these travellers are short-term travellers. Some travellers who work abroad may either make repeated short visits (airline crews or business persons), or reside for prolonged periods (missionaries, volunteer workers). Health risks differ between these groups and, depending on the environment and their behaviour, may vary within a single group.

The aim of pre-travel health advice is to reduce these risks by increasing the awareness of travellers and by promoting the use of preventive measures. The choice of these measures is guided by balancing the risk of illness or death against the risks, costs, and benefits of prevention. Only frequent health risks will be considered for which epidemiological data are available. The reader should consult the specific topics for less common travel-related tropical infections such as leishmaniasis and schistosomiasis.

Measures must be tailor-made for each person, depending on the individual's lifestyle, itinerary, living conditions, allergies and other pre-existing medical conditions (Table 28.1).

An important prerequisite for accurately assessing risk and giving proper advice is up-to-date epidemiological data on travel mortality and morbidity (Figure 28.1), in addition to knowledge of geographical risk. Nearly two-thirds of travellers develop or report new symptoms during short-term visits to the tropics. If using malaria chemoprophylaxis, 20% of these symptoms may be attributable to their medication.[1] Over 95% of travel-associated morbidity is not vaccine preventable.

The travel medicine practitioner must balance the administration of prophylaxis with the realistic risk of acquiring infections, the adverse events to be expected from prophylaxis and the likely compliance of the patient. The highest priority must be given to health hazards that are common, treatable or avoidable, and those that are potentially fatal. These include illnesses such as malaria and hepatitis A, and hazards such as road traffic accidents or engaging in unprotected sex, or driving while intoxicated by drugs or alcohol. Health hazards that are rare, such as cholera or Japanese encephalitis, or those that have no effective prophylaxis, e.g., parasitic skin infections, have

Table 28.1 Essential questions to assess predisposing risks and host risk factors.

- What is your destination(s) state: countries, city/resort/off-the-tourist-trail, itinerary
- What is the purpose of your visit: tourism/business or other professional visit (specify)/visit (to relatives/expatriates), other reasons (military, airline crew, adoption, etc.)
- What standard of hygiene do you expect throughout your visit: high (e.g., five-star hotels)/low (e.g., low budget travel)
- Are you planning any special activities: e.g. high altitude trekking, diving, hunting, camping, etc.
- What is your planned date of departure?
- How long do you intend to stay abroad?

Potential travellers should also answer at least the following set of questions on their health status and medical history:

- Do you currently use any medication? If yes, which ones?
- Are you currently unwell?
- Do you feel feverish? If yes, do you know what your temperature is?
- Do you suffer from any chronic illnesses If yes, which ones?
- Are you allergic to eggs or medication? If yes, describe.
- Are you pregnant or breast-feeding? Provide details.
- Have you ever had seizures? Provide details.
- Have you ever had psychiatric or psychological problems? Provide details.
- Have you ever had jaundice or hepatitis? Provide details.
- Are you or anybody in your household infected by HIV? Do you have any other immunodeficiency illness? Provide details.

a lower priority. All travellers need to appreciate that any intervention is not 100% effective.

Pre-travel preparation is based on ensuring approriate behaviour to reduce risks; immunization, chemoprophylaxis, medication and the provision of advice for self-treatment of symptoms. Travel medicine is a multi-disciplinary subject and includes many other areas apart from tropical medicine. Knowledge of infectious disease, pharmacology,

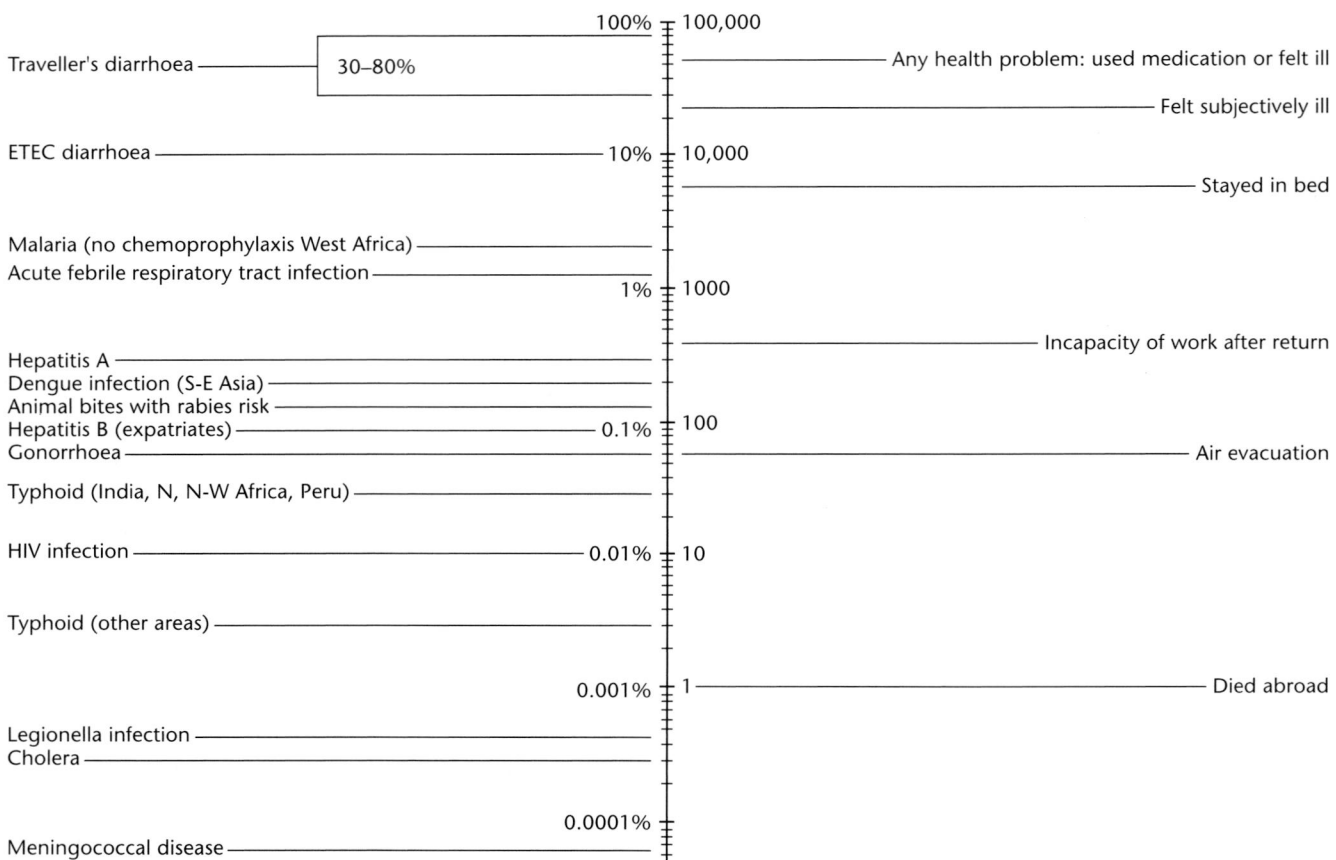

Figure 28.1: Monthly incidence rates of health problems. Estimated incidence per month of travel, of health problems calculated from a number of studies using a logarithmic scale.

public health, psychiatry, entomology, high-altitude physiology and behavioural sciences are all necessary to provide a complete service.

Consultation and risk assessment

In pre-travel consultations the prime consideration is to recognize that the potential traveller is not a patient. The collection of demographic information, including date of birth, is necessary at the start of a consultation. Medical details need to be obtained to assess, for example, the likely immune status of the person. The potential traveller should then describe in detail their travel plans.

With future use of anti-malarial drugs such as primaquine or its analogues, it may become necessary to question travellers about glucose-6-phospate dehydrogenase (G-6-PD) deficiency; this is currently not routinely done.

Usually, travellers are unable to recall information accurately about their immunization status; this is best discussed while reviewing the vaccination certificates. Travellers should be reminded to bring along to the consultation relevant records or documentation of previous immunizations. Whenever a medical problem is identified, the risk

of this condition and the planned journey should be carefully considered and assessed. A medical check-up or examination is not usually indicated unless the traveller plans to become a long-term resident abroad or particpate in extreme physical activity such as mountaineering at high altitudes. Psychological evaluation is also important in these circumstances.

Fatalities during travel

Accidents and cardiovascular events are the leading cause of death during intercontinental travel.[2] Fatalities due to injuries are two- to threefold higher in travellers aged between 15 and 44 years than in similar age groups living in industrialized countries. Fatal accidents are predominantly due to motor vehicle accidents, with fatality rates in Africa reported as high as 20–118 deaths per 10 000 motor vehicles and in Asia, 9–67 deaths per 10 000 motor vehicles. This compares to a fatality rate of 1.4 deaths per 10 000 motor vehicles in the UK[3] (Figure 28.2)

In one study tourists were found to be three times more likely than local drivers to be involved in a road traffic accident, and alcohol is often a frequent contributing factor.[4] Drowning is also an important cause of death and accounts for 16% of all deaths from injuries in

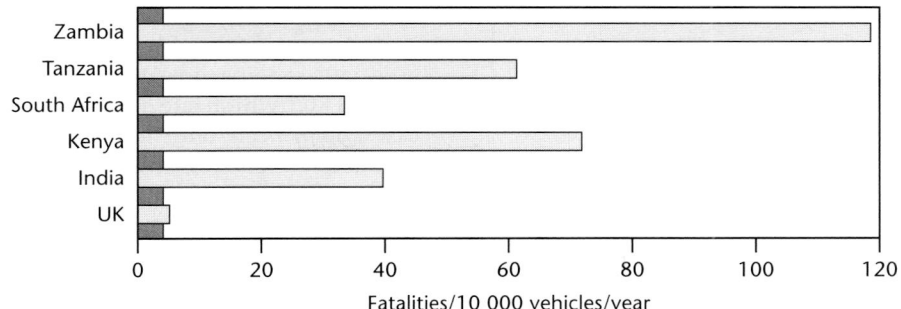

Figure 28.2: Road traffic fatalities per 104 vehicles/year in developing countries. *Fatalities per 10 000 vehicles from published data, with UK rates as a reference.*

US travellers. Half of the fatalities were associated with recently consumed alcohol.[5] Drowning in coastal resorts is often linked to swimming in unsupervised beaches where currents and undertows result in travellers being swept out to sea. Assaults or terrorism are infrequent causes of death. Trauma (traffic accidents or criminal attacks) is the main reason for aeromedical evacuation from Africa, Asia and Latin America.[2] Table 28.2 lists the strategies that have been proposed to prevent accidents.

Among deaths due to infectious disease, HIV has a prominent place although it does not appear in the usual statistics as it is a late consequence of infection abroad.[6]

Morbidity during travel

Studies of travellers describe that up to 62% of short-term travellers to malaria-endemic regions experience some new

Table 28.2 Strategies to reduce the risk of road traffic accidents.

> *Host/traveller factors:*
>
> *Advise travellers to:*
> - Avoid alcohol before driving, avoid alcohol and food before swimming
> - Use available safety equipment (seat belts, helmets, etc.)
>
> *Vehicle factors:*
>
> *Advise travellers to:*
> - Select safe cars—check availability of seat belts, good tyres
> - Rent larger vehicles where possible
> - Avoid using motorcycles and riding on the back of open trucks
> - Avoid small, non-scheduled aircraft
>
> *Environmental factors:*
>
> *Advise travellers to:*
> - Avoid travel at night
> - Employ a local driver who knows traffic and pedestrian patterns
> - Carefully select swimming areas
> - Know the local emergency medical system

symptoms or illness during travel, of which only 21% may be attributable to their chemoprophylaxis and the remainder relate to morbidity associated with travel. Of these self-reported health problems, 7% were considered severe, although 2% were probably related to the chemoprophylactic drugs being used.[7,8] The most common infectious health impairment of travellers results from traveller's diarrhoea, upper respiratory tract infections and skin sepsis which often follows an insect bite (Figure 28.3).

Traveller's diarrhoea
Epidemiology

There are three levels of risk for traveller's diarrhoea (TD): (i) travellers from industrialized countries spending two weeks in Canada, the United States, northern and central Europe or Australia and New Zealand have a low diarrhoeal incidence of up to 8%; (ii) an intermediate incidence (8–20%) is identified among travellers to destinations in the Caribbean, southern Europe, Israel, Japan and South Africa; and (iii) rates of TD during visits to developing

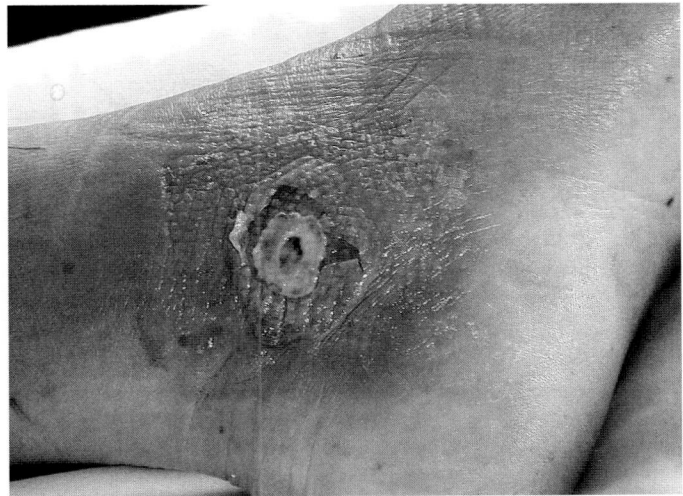

Figure 28.3: Skin sepsis following an insect bites. An insect bite on the ankle secondarily infected with streptococcus A and treated with oral antibiotic therapy in a returned traveller.

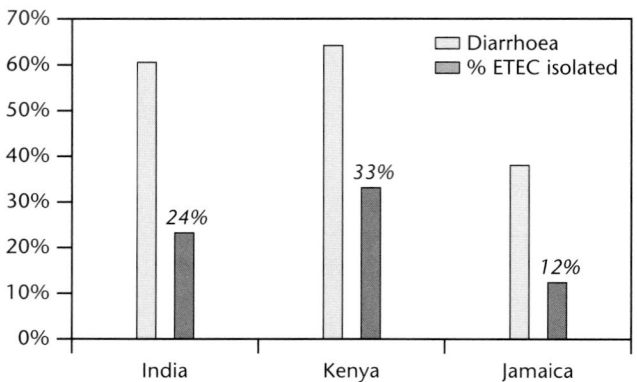

Figure 28.4: Diarrhoea rates in tourists from three different countries with the proprotions attributable to enterotoxigenic *E. coli*.

countries vary between 20 and 66% during the first two weeks of a stay[9] (Figure 28.4).

TD remains the most frequent infectious illness among travellers from industrialized countries visiting destinations in the developing world. Groups at particularly high risk of symptoms include infants, persons with an impaired gastric acid barrier and travellers with co-existing medical problems. TD may be particularly severe and long-lasting in small children.[10] The risk of illness is low in adults native to highly endemic areas because of naturally acquired immunity.

Classic TD is defined as three or more unformed stools per 24 hours with at least one accompanying symptom, but mild or moderate TD may also result in incapacitation.[11] The symptoms of TD in tourists frequently start on the third day of the stay abroad, with second episodes beginning about a week after arrival in 20% of the cases. Untreated, the mean duration of TD is four days (median two days), and in 1% of cases the symptoms may persist for more than a month. Twenty-two per cent of patients show signs of mucosal invasive disease with fever and/or blood in the stools.

TD is usually caused by faecal contamination of food and drink. Bacterial agents predominate (Table 28.3), especially enteroaggregative and enterotoxigenic *Escherichia coli* (ETEC) which are responsible for up to 60% of the cases. *Salmonella, Shigella, Campylobacter* and other species of bacterial pathogens, as well as *Giardia lamblia* and *Entamoeba histolytica*, each cause fewer than 5% of the cases.[12] Despite extensive microbiological assessment, approximately 20% of all cases remain of undetermined aetiology. Bacterial agents probably cause most of these cases because they can be prevented by use of antimicrobial agents.[13,14]

Prevention

There are various options to prevent TD. Parents with infants who intend to travel for pleasure to developing countries are advised to postpone their travel. Dietary restrictions using the rule of 'boil it, cook it, peel it, or forget it' may reduce the incidence of TD. These precautions are rarely complied with. One study which examined the impact of advice on behaviour revealed that the majority of tourists, despite advice to the contrary, still ate fresh salads, used ice cubes in their drinks and chose to eat raw oysters or uncooked meats.[15] Many drugs have been proposed to prevent TD, but only antimicrobial agents have been shown to have protective efficacies above 80%.[16] The drugs of choice for the prophylaxis of TD, unless they are contraindicated, are the quinolone antibiotics.[12] They are not indicated for all travellers as the risk of adverse reaction and costs restrict their widespread prescribing for chemoprophylaxis of TD. They should be considered for prophylaxis in certain circumstances (Table 28.4).

Effective polyvalent immunization against TD is not yet available, and current vaccines against typhoid or cholera do not prevent TD at an acceptable level.[17]

Self-therapy

Because of the limitations of preventative strategies against TD, travellers should be offered a means of

Table 28.3 Aetiology of traveller's diarrhoea.

Organism	Latin America (%)	Asia (%)	Africa (%)
Enterotoxigenic *E. coli* (ETEC)	17–70	6–37	8–42
Enteroinvasive *E. coli*	2–7	2–3	0–2
Shigella spp.	2–30	0–17	0–9
Salmonella spp.	1–16	1–33	4–25
Campylobacter jejuni	1–5	9–39	1–28
Other	0–4	0–25	0–6
Rotavirus	0–6	1–8	0–36
Parasitology	1–2	0–9	0–4
No pathogen identified	24–62	10–56	15–53

From Ericsson I. D. Clin N. America
Proportion varies by destination and season

Table 28.4 Indications for the chemoprophylaxis of traveller's diarrhoea.

- Persons with increased susceptibility
  - History of severe traveller's diarrhoea on each trip
  - Impaired gastric acid barrier, including patients taking H2 antagonists and PPI drugs, and post-gastric surgery
  - Immune deficiency, e.g., HIV, etc.
- Persons with increased risk of complications
  - By dehydration: patients after TIA, stroke, diabetes
  - By electrolyte imbalance: patients on digitalis, etc.
- VIPs who have to accept whatever food is offered

If chemoprophylaxis is indicated: quinolone best.

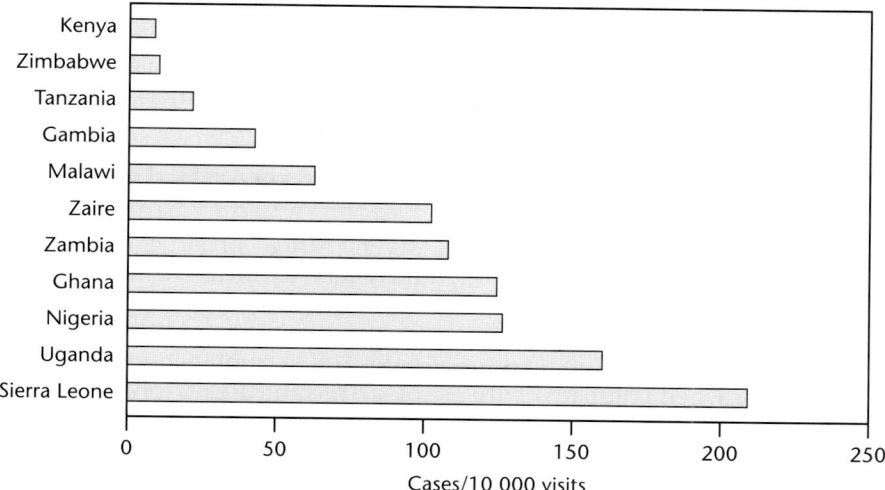

Figure 28.5: *P. falciparum* malaria rates in UK residents. Mean rates of 1989–1999. Rate of *P. falciparum* malaria per visit by UK residents, presented as a mean of the annual incidence. (Data by courtesy of the Malaria Reference Laboratory.)

self-treatment whilst travelling. One option is to wait for symptoms to resolve spontaneously whilst replacing fluid and electrolyte losses. Oral rehydration solution should always be used for infants, children and the older patient in whom dehydration can lead to serious complications. Adult travellers often request and benefit from early use curative, or suppressive therapy. Loperamide, an anti-secretory drug, is one of the fastest acting agents to bring symptomatic relief in non-invasive traveller's diarrhoea.[18] This may safely be used in mild to moderate, non-invasive illness. It is contraindicated in invasive disease where fever and/or blood are present in the stools as it may aggravate symptoms in patients with dysentery.[15]

For general treatment, quinolone administered as a single dose (or a three day course) has been shown to significantly reduce the duration of diarrhoeal symptoms.[19] A combination of loperamide and quinolone has not been found to add any benefit to quinolone used alone. Thus, both loperamide and a quinolone antibiotic can be recommended for inclusion in the travel kit. Bismuth subsalicylate[20] and non-absorbable antibiotics such as rifiximine[21] have also been found to reduce the duration of diarrhoeal symptoms.

Malaria in travellers

Malaria is transmitted in many tropical countries and is one of the most important causes of life-threatening morbidity in returning travellers. About 10 000 cases are reported annually in Europe, and there is an estimated 1.1% case fatality rate for those with *Plasmodium falciparum* malaria.[22]

Epidemiology

Using surveillance data and the numbers of travellers to the respective destinations, we can roughly estimate the risk of malaria in travellers visiting different countries (Figure 28.5).

Risk of infection

The risk of exposure to malaria depends on many factors relating to both vector and host behaviour. The selection of an appropriate anti-malarial chemoprophylaxis is based on the risk of infection during the specific journey, the probability of side effects and the health beliefs and compliance of the travellers. Generally, without prophylaxis risk of malaria is highest in sub-Saharan Africa, intermediate in South Asia and lowest in the Americas and South-East Asia, but it can be highly variable within countries. Any intervention that reduces the exposure to night-biting *Anopheles* mosquitoes, such as repellents and bed nets, will significantly reduce the risk of malaria. Other considerations include:

Type of travel—backpacking versus air conditioned, well screened urban hotels;
Travellers exposure to bites, compliance to prophylaxis;
Duration of stay—the cumulative risk of contracting malaria is proportional to the length of stay in the transmission area;
Region visited;
Altitude of destination—malaria is not transmitted above 2000 m; and
Season of travel—the rainy season is associated with higher transmission.

Malaria imported into Europe and the USA is predominantly *P. falciparum* (58–63%), and over a ten-year period an estimated 77 683 cases were reported in Europe.[22] Malaria rates in travellers to Kenya, a popular tropical destination, vary country by country. Malaria rates varied from 50–135 cases per 10 000 travellers. Mortality rates from malaria were also variable, with case fatality rates highest in Germany (3.6%) and lowest in the United Kingdom (0.65%). *P. falciparum* malaria rates in UK residents returning from visiting popular destinations in sub-Saharan Africa vary from 10–216 cases per 10 000 visits (Figure 28.5). It is often useful to advise travellers about risk using the entomological innoculation rate (EIR). This is the annual number of infective *P. falciparum* mosquito bites received per person. The EIR in east Thailand is around 0.91, which is roughly equivalent to one infective mosquito bite a year, whereas in rural Tanzania, a reported EIR of 667 is equivalent to two infective bites each night. In Kenya, the EIR ranges from 17 to 299.3[23] (one infective bite every three weeks to one bite a night). The transmission rates in coastal resorts appears to be lower when compared with inland data.

Prevention

Prevention of malaria is based on the acronym ABCD:

- Awareness: recognizing the risk;
- Bites by mosquitoes: prevent and avoid;
- Compliance with appropriate chemoprophylaxis; and
- Diagnose malaria swifty and treat promptly.

Appropriate health beliefs of travellers are important to ensure bite avoidance and compliance with advice and chemoprophylaxis. Educating travellers about the risk of malaria and how to recognize the symptoms is a priority in the travel consultation.

Anti-mosquito measures

Personal protection against *Anopheles* bites is based on the use of topical repellents during biting periods (dusk through to dawn) and the use of long clothing to reduce exposed skin. DEET-formulated repellents have variable activity depending on a number of factors. The repellent formulation is critical as it influences the duration of repellency. Extended duration formula can last for longer than eight hours.[24] Neat DEET (an organic solvent) evaporates relatively quickly and is effective at repelling for only a few hours. The concentration of DEET has marginal impact on duration of protection, and concentrations above 35% provide little added benefit.

Higher concentrations should not be used in infants and children.

Environmental measures include the use of insecticide sprays, vaporizers and nets. Sealed air conditioned rooms provide a closed environment into which insects cannot enter and therefore anti-mosquito measures other than spraying to clear the room are unnecessary. Heated vaporizer mats clear a room of insects in around 30 minutes and remain effective for over six hours. Burning pyrethroid-impregnated coils are less effective and cosmetically less acceptable. In non-airconditioned and poorly screened rooms, a pyrethroid-impregnated mosquito net is a very effective system for preventing bites. Limited compliance (35–70%) of travellers to one or more of these measures[25]

put many at risk of an infected bite. Optimal protection is provided when they are all used in combination. Oral Vitamin B6, garlic, and electric buzzers are of no proven value in bite prevention.

Chemoprophylaxis

Several drugs or drug combinations are available for travellers to areas with chloroquine-resistant malaria: mefloquine (Lariam®), doxycycline(Vibramycin®) or atovaquone proguanil (Malarone®). Chloroquine and proguanil in combination have a limited protective efficacy of < 70%[7] and are no longer considered adequate for areas of high transmission or resistance rates. The adverse event profile of chemoprophylactic regimens have a significant bearing on travellers acceptance and compliance with drugs. The reported adverse event rates of the differing regimens have varied depending on the study designs used. Blind control studies designed to identify adverse events in travellers have led to a more precise understanding of the tolerability and adverse event profiles of these drug regimens. (Figure 28.6). The incidence of the more severe reactions are detailed in Table 28.5.

Mefloquine

Mefloquine, which has been available for over 12 years, remains a highly effective drug with a protective efficacy of > 90% in sub-Saharan Africa. It has a weekly schedule and can be used in young and elderly people, and during most of pregnancy. Nineteen per cent of travellers using mefloquine reported a drug-associated neuropsychiatric problem, predominantly vivid or strange dreams, although a small number reported depression and anxiety. Minor gastrointestinal symptoms also occur. Neuropsychiatric problems are signifcantly more common among mefloquine users than among atovaquone + proguanil or chloroquine + proguanil users. Serious neuropsychiatric events (convulsions, psychosis, severe depression)

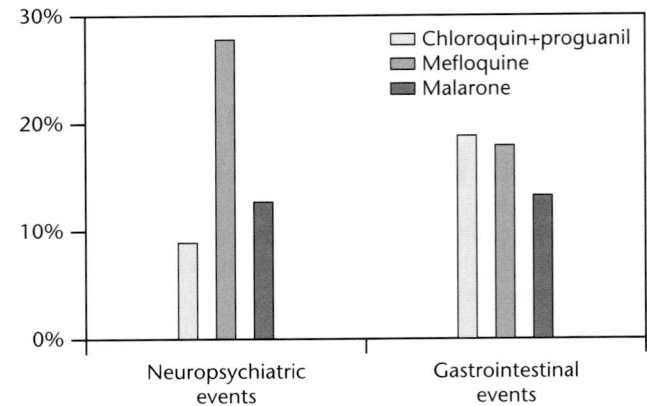

Figure 28.6: Frequency of prophylactic attributable adverse events by different regimens. Adapted from Hogh et al. *Lancet* 2000; 356:1888–1894 and Overbosch et al. *Clin Inf Dis.* 2001; 33:1015–1021.

Table 28.5 Adverse events attributed to chemoprophylaxis, resulting in stopping medication.[(7,8)]

Reported events	Atovaquone + proguanil	Chloroquine + proguanil	Mefloquine
Any treatment-limiting event (%)	1	2	5.5
Gastrointestinal (%)	0	2	1.5
Neuropsychiatric (%)	0.6	0	4

attributable to chemoprophylaxis regimens containing either chloroquine or mefloquine are similar at around 1 per 13 000 users.

Doxycycline

Doxycycline is an effective alternative for persons visiting areas of chloroquine or mefloquine resistance.[26] This drug is contraindicated for pregnant or breast-feeding women and children under 12 years of age. Side effects of doxycycline include monilial vaginitis, gastrointestinal symptoms in 3–7% of users (nausea or vomiting), and phototoxicity after sun exposure.[27,28]

Atovaquone and proguanil

Is manufactured in a fixed-dose combination (Malarone®) and has been shown to be effective in the treatment of malaria and, more recently, in the prophylaxis of malaria.[7,8,29] The combination of atovaquone and proguanil appears to have few side effects and, as yet, no resistance has been described. Cost may be a factor that will limit the wider use of this combination.

Chloroquine and proguanil

The combined use of chloroquine and proguanil has been widely used in sub-Saharan Africa for more than two decades. It has been shown to be safe in all age groups, during pregnancy and in long term (> 5 years) use. However, its protective efficacy has fallen in many parts of the world (Table 28.6), and breakthrough of *P. falciparum* malaria in compliant users is now a common problem. Adverse events associated with its use are predominately gastrointestinal.

Stand-by medication

Travellers to areas with a very low transmission rate of malaria may be advised to carry along a stand-by medication instead of using chemoprophylaxis.[30] With careful instructions they should be able to self-treat if symptoms associated with malaria develop. This strategy is not designed to replace professional medical care, but rather to supplement the management of the disease by local health providers. The self-treatment can also be used if no medical care can be obtained within 12–24 hours after the onset of illness. Persons using mefloquine or doxycycline for prophylaxis need not carry stand-by medication. There are various concerns about advocating stand-by medication. Malaria symptoms are difficult to explain to untrained persons and travellers do not always seek professional medical advice or utilize their stand-by

Table 28.6 Major drug regimens and estimated efficacy.

Drug regimen and schedule	Estimated prophylactic effectiveness (%)
Atovaquone & proguanil daily	> 90
Doxycycline daily	> 90
Mefloquine weekly	> 90
Chloroquine weekly & proguanil daily	< = 70
Chloroquine & proguanil daily (used in France only)	Unknown

treatment when they develop classical symptoms of malaria.[31] Prescribing should always be supported by advice that drugs should be supervised by a health professional and with a laboratory diagnosis of malaria wherever possible. Current drugs recommended for use as stand-by medication include Fansidar, Malarone® and the combination of Lumefantrine and Artemether (Riamet®). The indications for prescribing stand-by treatment include travel in regions of low transmission where chemoprophylaxis is not taken, or a long period of travel in a highly endemic area where chemoprophylaxis is not fully effective and where appropriate medical facilities are unavailable.

Self-administered diagnostic kits for malaria

Kits for self-diagnosis of *P. falciparum* malaria by travellers are on offer for use in remote areas where there is no access to diagnostic facilities (Figures 28.7 and 28.8). Histidine-rich protein (HRP2) or parasite lactose dehydrogenase (LDH) antigen-capture test-cards work reliably in the laboratory, and have been evaluated by infected travellers. One study found 32% of patients were unable to accurately perform the test,[32] whilst another study with simplified instructions found over 95% of sick patients successfully diagnosed their falciparum malaria.[33] The availability of these kits remains limited, but they could be of significant potential benefit to travellers prescribed stand-by malaria treatment.

Sexually transmitted diseases

Casual sexual contacts abroad play an important role in

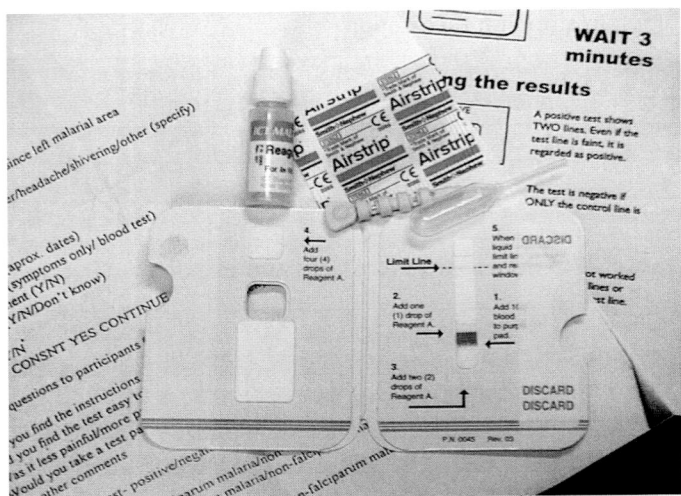

Figure 28.7: Immunochromatograpic self administered test kit for *P. falciparum*. A kit based on the HRP2 surface antigen of *P. falciparum* which requires a 10 ml capillary blood sample and three drops of reagent. The system takes around 8 to 10 minutes to complete.

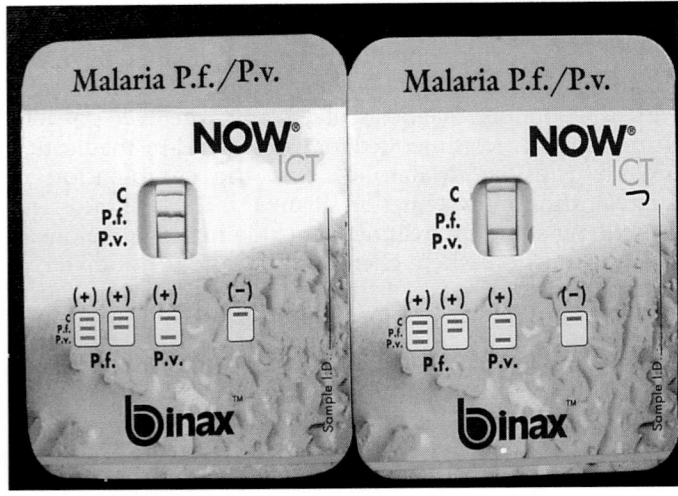

Figure 28.8: Positive antigen tests for malaria. Two positive test cards. The left-hand card revealing evidence of a *P. falciparum* and the right-hand card non-*falciparum* malaria (*P. vivax*). The appearance of a positive test with the control band confiirms the test has functioned. The system contains antigen to detects falicparum and non-falciparum species. The test may be positive for some weeks after all viable parasites have been cleared as antigen may continue to circulate.

the transmission of sexually transmitted disease (STD) infections.[34] Travel to tropical countries is an important factor in the spread of STDs. In spite of intensive anti-AIDS campaigns, some 5% of European or Canadian tourists have casual sexual contacts abroad. The prevalence of STDs is higher in tropical countries than in Western industrialized countries. More than 25% of cases of gonorrhoea treated in Switzerland from 1989–1991 were imported from abroad. The penicillin-producing *Neisseria gonorrhoea* strains (PPNG) isolated in Switzerland from 1989–1991 are mainly imported from abroad

(60%).[35] The typical 'imported STIs' in Switzerland are chancroid, lymphogranuloma venereum and donovanosis. The clinical manifestations, laboratory and special examinations, and treatment of these diseases are described elsewhere. The most frequent STI from the so-called 'imported tropical STIs' is chancroid, which is also a major risk factor associated with the transmission of HIV infection. Data on sexual behaviour of short-term tourists and of long-term overseas workers is of concern. Among young British travellers, 10% reported casual sex while travelling, and 25% did not use condoms. Men's use of condoms was no different to that which they practised at home. Patterns of condom use by women varied according to their partners' backgrounds.[36]

Long-term male expatriates and workers frequently have casual sex with a local woman or prostitutes.[37] Similar risk behaviour is described in Dutch expatriates working in sub-Saharan Africa where nearly one in three males had casual sexual contacts with the native population, and regular condom use was reported by less than one-quarter of them.[38] The WHO estimates that 75% of all HIV infections worldwide are sexually transmitted and that the efficiency of transmission per sexual contact ranges from 0.1 to 1%. The efficiency can be greatly increased by the presence of other STDs and genital lesions. In populations with a high prevalence rate of HIV and other STDs, as is often the case in female prostitutes in developing countries, the transmission probability of HIV is greatly enhanced. Studies indicate that the prevalence of HIV ranged from 0.4% in Dutch expatriates to 1.1% in Belgians and 8.6% in Danish volunteers. These rates are 100 to 500 times higher when compared to the ative population in these countries.[37]

Because of the risk of acquiring incurable viral STDs such as HIV, the emphasis should be on safe sex (i.e., always use a condom) for all those who travel and engage in casual sex. Other preventive measures include avoidance of inadequately screened blood. In some regions of West Africa, the risk of HIV infection per unit of blood transfused may be as high 1%.[39] The use of sterile needles and syringes should be encouraged and should be included in the travel kit.

Vaccine-preventable diseases
Epidemiology

No recent morbidity and mortality data exist on the most frequent vaccine preventable diseases (Figure 28.1), although there are indications that the incidence rate particularly of hepatitis A and typhoid fever are decreasing from rates identified in 1970s and 1980s.[40] Hepatitis A remains the most frequent vaccine-preventable disease. Typhoid rates are lower by a factor of 10–100 and cholera by a factor of 1000 in comparison to hepatitis

A. Polio is no longer reported in travellers. The risk factors for exposure to these pathogens includes duration of stay and hygiene associated with food and beverages (i.e., living with the local population or in high-class hotels). Previous immunity to hepatitis A can be predicted by the travellers age, history of previous stays or residence in highly endemic countries, history of jaundice and immunization status. There is a mortality risk associated with each of these diseases, but it is rarely above 1%. A major risk factor for typhoid fever is a visit to the Indian subcontinent, especially by ethnic traveller's when visiting friends and relatives (VFRs). Cholera may occur more frequently than reported[41] as it predominantly presents with typical symptoms of traveller's diarrhoea. It therefore poses no greater threat to travellers and responds to treatment with quinolone antibiotics. The last recorded case of polio in a traveller occurred in 1991; since then, global polio eradication has made further progress.

Hepatitis B is mostly diagnosed in expatriates in higly endemic countries, especially those in Asia. Tourists are rarely infected, despite deliberate or inadverent risk behaviour.[42] These risk factors include casual sexual contacts, tattooing, acupuncture, and occasionally medical and dental treatment in developing countries.

The risk of rabies exposure can be significant as shown in a study of contacts with dogs in Thailand. Nine per cent of respondents were licked and 2% bitten during an average 17-day visit to Thailand. The rate of exposure to animal bites is estimated to be 0.2–0.4% per month; in the majority of these incidents there was some concern about rabies infection.[43]

Yellow fever is extremely rare in travellers. Several cases in unvaccinated travellers have been reported in the last ten years, despite the fact these travellers should have been immunized.

There are various other vaccine-preventable diseases about which little epidemiological data in travellers exist, as only anecdotal cases have been reported. The incidence rate of vaccine-preventable disease overall is probably less than 1 per million travellers per month. Outbreaks of meningococcal disease have occurred in situations in which travellers lived in crowded conditions, such as after trekking or after the Hajj to Mecca.[44] Although an increased endemicity of Japanese encephalitis has lately been observed in the indigenous population in an area including all Asian countries east and northeast of India, less than 25 cases of Japanese encephalitis in civilian visitors have been recorded in the literature. Only two cases of plague have been reported in international travellers since 1966.[45] The risk of acquiring a *Mycobacterium tuberculosis* infection during travel was reported as around 2.8 per 1000 person-months of travel. Working in health care significantly increased the risk of tuberculosis infection,[46] but even transmission during air, train or bus travel have been reported.[47]

Influenza has resulted in outbreaks mainly on cruise ships. So far no seroepidemiological survey has established its role in individual travellers.[48]

Prevention

Immunizations required for international travel

According to the International Health Regulations, only yellow fever immunization may be required for international travel. Yellow fever vaccination is required for entry into many countries of tropical Africa or northern South America where the infection is endemic. In addition, some countries in Asia and in the Pacific require passengers that have transited through an infected or endemic area within the past ten days to show proof of vaccination. Some experts recommend yellow fever vaccination also for endemic areas in which no cases of the infection have been detected for decades, such as in East Africa, since the vector is present and epidemics may theoretically occur. Yellow fever vaccination must be performed in centres that are approved by the national authorities, and it must be documented on a Standard International Vaccination Certificate.

There is no valid indication for cholera vaccination, and even remote border posts have gradually realized that this can no longer be required. Saudi Arabia requires pilgrims to be immunized against meningococcal disease. Up-to-date information on mandatory immunizations can also be obtained from travel information manuals (e.g., TIM, TIMATIC) published by several airlines. However, the information regarding recommended immunizations published in these sources may be unreliable.

Routine immunizations

For reasons unrelated to travel, persons living in industrialized countries should be immune against poliomyelitis, tetanus and diphtheria, as well as against measles, mumps and rubella. As this applies even more for visits to the developing world, a medical consultation prior to departure makes it possible to administer the necessary booster doses, or sometimes to initiate vaccination against these infections.

Recommended immunizations

Hepatitis A immunization may be recommended to any non-immune traveller visiting developing countries, but seems to be unnecessary for visits to the Caribbean (except Haiti and the Dominican Republic) or to southern Europe or the western seaboard of the USA. The sero-prevalence of anti-HAV antibodies in Europeans is very low in those born after World War II, which makes pre-vaccination testing in this age group unnecessary.

Hepatitis B vaccination is indicated for residents and long-term or frequent travellers staying longer than one month in highly endemic countries.[30] It may also be considered for short-term visitors who intend to engage in high-risk sex, tattooing and ear piercing (although this still leaves them unprotected against HIV infection!).

Vaccination against typhoid fever is indicated for persons who eat and drink in poor hygienic conditions or who have a prolonged stay in developing countries. It is also recommended for all visits to the Indian subcontinent, North and West Africa (except Tunisia) and Peru.

Rabies vaccination should be considered for all long-term residents, particularly for those who will live in close contact with the local population and children.

Other special-risk vaccinations are those against meningococcal disease using quadrivalent vaccine for stays in the Sahel zone during the winter months, particularly where there is close contacts with the local population and children. Japanese encephalitis vaccine may be recommended for persons who will stay for at least four weeks in rural areas in endemic countries. There is no common policy on recommending immunization against tuberculosis to long-term residents abroad, which depends on local or national policy on the use of BCG.[49,50] Unless any primary vaccination is needed which requires several doses, most vaccines may be given simultaneously during one single consultation.

Conclusion

Every physician or nurse who counsels future travellers must tailor specific recommendations to travellers based on a balance of the health risks to be expected during travel with the benefits and tolerance of protective measures. One should not protect or advise travellers against rare risks while failing to advise them against more likely or severe health threats. Four strategies are available to reduce health risks of foreign travel: (i) appropriate behaviour can prevent STIs, reduce the risks of malaria and diarrhoea, and reduce the danger of injuries; (ii) prophylactic drug use can prevent malaria; (iii) drug therapy for traveller's diarrhoea can reduce duration and morbidity of the illness; (iv) immunization can prevent disease without requiring compliance from the traveller.

REFERENCES

1 Overbosch D, Miller G B, Schilthuis H et al. Travel-related adverse events in visitors to malaria-endemic countries. In Freedman D & Steffen R (eds) *Conference Proceedings CISTM7*, 27 May 2001.

2 Hargarten S W, Baker T D, Guptill K. Overseas fatalities of United States citizen travelers: an analysis of deaths related to international travel 2. *Ann Trav Med* 1991; 20:622–626.

3 Nordberg E. Injuries as a healh problem in Sub Saharan Africa: Epidemiology and prospects for control. *E Afr Med J* 2000; 77:S16–S38.

4 Petridou E, Askitopoulou H, Vourvahakis D et al. Epidemiology of road traffic accidents during pleasure travelling: the evidence from the island of Crete. *Accid Anal Prev* 1997; 29:687–693.

5 Alcohol use and aquatic activities—United States, 1991. *MMWR Morb Mortal Wkly Rep* 1993; 42:675, 681–3.

6 Hawkes S, Hart G J, Johnson A M et al. Risk behaviour and HIV prevalence in international travellers. *Aids* 1994; 8:247–252.

7 Hogh B, Clarke P D, Camus D et al. Atovaquone-proguanil versus chloroquine-proguanil for malaria prophylaxis in non-immune travellers: a randomised, double-blind study. Malarone International Study Team. *Lancet* 2000; 356:1888–1894.

8 Overbosch D, Schilthuis H, Bienzle U et al. Atovaquone/proguanil versus mefloquine for the malaria prophylaxis in non-immune travelers. Results from a randomised double-blind Study. *Clin Inf Dis* 2001; 33:1015–1021.

9 von Sonnenburg F, Tornieporth N, Waiyaki P et al. Risk and aetiology of diarrhoea at various tourist destinations. *Lancet* 2000; 356:133–134.

10 Pitzinger B, Steffen R, Tschopp A. Incidence and clinical features of travelers' diarrhea in infants and children. *Pediatr Infect Dis J* 1991; 10:719–723.

11 Steffen R, Collard F, Tornieporth N et al. Epidemiology, etiology, and impact of traveler's diarrhea in Jamaica. *J Am Med Assoc* 1999; 281:811–817.

12 Gomi H, Jiang Z, Adachi J et al. In vitro antimicrobial susceptibility testing among bacterial pathogens enteroptahogens causing travelers diarrhea in four areas of the world. *Antimicrob Angents Chemother* 2001; 45:212–216.

13 Jiang ZD, Steffen R, Tornieporth N. Prevalence of enteric pathogens among international travelers with diarrhoea acquired in Africa. 2001; in press.

14 Ericsson CD. Travellers' diarrhoea: epidemiology, prevention and self-treatment. *Infect Dis Clin N Am* 2000; 00:285–303.

15 Mattila L, Siitonen A, Kyronseppa H et al. Risk behavior for travelers' diarrhea among Finnish travelers. *J Travel Med* 1995; 2:77–84.

16 DuPont H L, Ericsson C D. Prevention and treatment of traveler's diarrhea. *N Engl J Med* 1993; 328:1821–1827.

17 Peltola H, Siitonen A, Kyronseppa H et al. Prevention of travellers' diarrhoea by oral B-subunit/whole-cell cholera vaccine. *Lancet* 1991; 338:1285–1289.

18 Wingate D, Phillips S F, Lewis S J et al. Guidelines for adults on self-medication for the treatment of acute diarrhoea. *Alimentary Pharmacol Ther* 2001; 15:773–782.

19 De Bruyn G, Hahn S, Borwick A. Antibiotic treatment for travellers' diarrhoea (Cochrane review). *Cochrane Database Syst Rev* 2000; 3:CD002242

20 Steffen R. Worldwide efficacy of bismuth subsalicylate in the treatment of travelers' diarrhea. *Rev Infect Dis* 1990; 12:S80–S86.

21 DuPont H L, Ericsson C D, Mathewson J J et al. Rifaximin: a nonabsorbed antimicrobial in the therapy of travelers' diarrhea. *Digestion* 1998; 59:708–714.

22 Muentener P, Schlagenhauf P, Steffen R. Imported malaria (1985–95): trends and perspectives. *Bull World Health Organ* 1999; 77:560–566.

23 Hay S I, Rogers D J, Toomer J F, Snow R W. Annual Plasmodium falciparum entomological inoculation rates (EIR) across Africa: literature survey, Internet access and review. *Trans R Soc Trop Med Hyg* 2000; 94:113–127.

24 Rutledge L C, Gupta R K, Mehr Z A et al. Evaluation of controlled-release mosquito repellent formulations. *J Am Mosq Control Assoc* 1996; 12:39–44.

25 Schoepke A, Steffen R, Gratz N. Effectiveness of personal protection measures against mosquito bites for malaria prophylaxis in travelers. *J Travel Med* 1998; 5:188–192.

26 Ohrt C, Richie T L, Widjaja H et al. Mefloquine compared with doxycycline for the prophylaxis of malaria in Indonesian soldiers. A randomized, double-blind, placebo-controlled trial. *Ann Intern Med* 1997; 126:963–972.

27 Frost P, Weinstein G D, Gomez E C. Phototoxic potential of minocycline and doxycycline. *Arch Dermatol* 1972; 105:681–683.

28 Schuhwerk M & Behrens R H. Doxycycline as first line malarial prophylaxis: how safe is it? *J Travel Med* 1998; 5:102.

29 Shanks D, Kremsner P T Y S et al. Atovaquone and proguanil for the chemoprophylaxis of malaria. *J Travel Med* 1999; 1:S21–S23.

30 WHO. International Travel and Health. World Health Organisation, 2001.

31 Schlagenhauf P, Steffen R, Tschopp A et al. Behavioural aspects of travellers in their use of malaria presumptive treatment. *Bull World Health Organ* 1995; 73:215–221.

32 Jelinek T, Amsler L, Grobusch M P, Nothdurft H D. Self-use of rapid tests for malaria diagnosis by tourists. *Lancet* 1999; 354:1609.

33 Whitty C, Armstrong M, Behrens R H. Self-testing for falciparum malaria with antigen-capture cards by travellers with symptoms of malaria. *Am J Trop Med Hyg.* 2001; in press.

34 Mulhall B P. Sex and travel: studies of sexual behaviour, disease and health promotion in international travellers—a global review. *Int J STD AIDS* 1996; 7:455–465.

35 Eichmann A. [Sexually transmissible diseases following travel in tropical countries]. *Schweiz Med Wochenschr* 1993; 123:1250–1255.

36 Bloor M, Thomas M, Hood K et al. Differences in sexual risk behaviour between young men and women travelling abroad from the UK. *Lancet* 1998; 352:1664–1668.

37 Bonneux L, Van der Stuyft P, Taelman H et al. Risk factors for infection with human immmunodeficiency virus among European expatriates in Africa. *Br Med J* 1988; 297:581–584.

38 de Graaf R, van Zessen G et al. Sexual risk of HIV infection among expatriates posted in AIDS endemic areas. *Aids* 1997; 11:1173–1181.

39 Savarit D, De Cock K M, Schutz R et al. Risk of HIV infection from transfusion with blood negative for HIV antibody in a west African city. *Br Med J* 1992; 305:498–502.

40 Behrens R H & Carroll B. The ten year trend of travel-associated infections (malaria, typhoid and hepatitis A) imported into the UK. In Freedman, D & Steffen R (eds), *Conference Proceedings CISTM7*, 27 May 2001.

41 Mahon B E, Mintz E D, Greene K D et al. Reported cholera in the United States, 1992–1994: a reflection of global changes in cholera epidemiology. *J Am Med Assoc* 1996; 276:307–312.

42 Zuckerman J N & Steffen R. Risks of hepatitis B in travelers as compared to immunization status. *J Travel Med* 2000; 7:170–174.

43 Bernard K W & Fishbein D B. Pre-exposure rabies prophylaxis for travellers: are the benefits worth the cost? *Vaccine* 1991; 9:833–836.

44 Taha M K, Achtman M, Alonso J M, Greenwood B, Ramsay M, Fox A et al. Serogroup W135 meningococcal disease in Hajj pilgrims. *Lancet* 2000; 356:2159.

45 Centers for Disease Control. Imported bubonic plague. *MMWR Morb Mortal Week Rep* 1990; 39:895–901.

46 Cobelens F G, van Deutekom H, Draayer-Jansen I W, et al. Risk of infection with *Mycobacterium tuberculosis* in travellers to areas of high tuberculosis endemicity. *Lancet* 2000; 356(9228):461–5.

47 Moore M, Valway S E, Ihle W, Onorato I M. A train passenger with pulmonary tuberculosis: evidence of limited transmission during travel. *Clin Infect Dis* 1999; 28:52–56.

48 Influenza activity—United States, 2000–01 season. *MMWR Morb Mortal Wkly Rep* 2001; 50:39–40.

49 Lifson A R. Mycobacterium tuberculosis infection in travellers: tuberculosis comes home. *Lancet* 2000; 356(9228):442–443.

50 Whitty C J, Macallan D C, Lewis D J. Use of BCG vaccination. *Lancet* 2000; 356:1609–1610.

Section 5

Environmental/Genetic Disorders

Classical 'tropical medicine' has been centred on a variety of 'exotic' infections—dominated by those of parasitic origin. In recent years a far greater emphasis has, quite rightly, been placed on disease entities that do not have an infective basis. Although these can be divided roughly into those with a predominantly environmental *or* genetic background, the majority (as with most disease entities in a non-tropical environment) fall somewhere within a grey area between these two poles; in fact, in many of them both genetic and environmental factors operate in conjunction. This section therefore focuses on a miscellaneous group of disorders.

Heat stress-associated illness and high altitude sickness have obvious associations with environmental phenomena. Nutrition-associated diseases—dominated by those precipitated by a deficiency of major and/or specific dietary ingredients, and 'toxicity' of animal and plant origin—are also clearly related to local environmental factors.

Areas of 'medicine in the tropics' that have hitherto been grossly underplayed in previous editions of 'Manson's'

are malignant disease and diseases commonly associated with an affluent environment: diabetes mellitus, hypertension, and lipid disorders (and resultant ischaemic cardiac disease). These already account for large numbers of cases in many of the more urbanized tropical areas. In each of them any attempt at dissecting genetic from environmental predisposing factors poses problems that are often seemingly insuperable.

Two other diseases which are covered in this section are podoconiosis and recurrent familial polyserositis (familial Mediterranean fever). The former has a relatively well-delineated geographical distribution and is confined to those areas where silica abounds and particles enter the lymphatics of the lower limbs via bare feet; the resultant clinical abnormality is barely distinguishable from lymphatic filariasis (elephantiasis). The latter is an under-recognized disease which usually (but not always) affects members of certain clearly defined ethnic groups; here, genetic factors which are beginning to be elucidated are clearly involved.

Chapter 29
Heat Stress and Associated Disorders

K. J. Collins

Heat-associated disorders appear most frequently when there is an unusual rise in heat stress, e.g., in heat waves, exertion in hot conditions and when newcomers are first exposed to the tropics. If the combination of environmental and metabolic heat exceeds the capacity of the thermoregulatory system to dissipate heat from the body, then a spectrum of symptom complexes may occur signifying heat illness. At one end of this spectrum is heatstroke, a life-threatening condition resulting from heat damage to tissues. Increased risk is associated with hard physical work in severe heat, existing disease, particularly cardiovascular, the elderly and young, medications, dehydration and lack of heat acclimatization.

Body temperature regulation

Constant internal body temperature is achieved by a process of heat exchange adjusting heat loss to heat gain. Heat balance is usually expressed in the form of an equation:

$$M \pm w = \pm R \pm C \pm k - E$$

where

M = the rate of metabolic heat production
w = the external work performed by or on the body
R = the loss or gain of radiant heat
C = the loss or gain of heat by convection
k = the conductive loss or gain of heat through body contact with objects
E = the evaporative heat loss by sweating and respiration.

Heat balance is maintained by the thermoregulatory system despite considerable heat loads imposed by heat stress from the environment and physical work.[1] Temperature homeostasis allows body temperature fluctuations, normally about ± 0.3°C diurnal change at rest in a neutral environment, to ± 2.0°C in more extreme ambient conditions and physical activity.

A rise in skin temperature and vasodilatation is an initial response to hot conditions brought about by vasomotor reflexes acting through the thermoregulatory centres in the brain and spinal cord and by the direct effects of heat on skin blood vessels. Much of the large increase in skin blood flow comes from opening of arteriovenous anastamoses deep to the skin capillaries. Dilatation of the large cutaneous vascular network causes a redistribution of blood from the body core to the skin and concomitant reduction in splanchnic blood flow. The compensatory fall in renal and hepatic blood flow produces oliguria in the heat and a reduced hepatic metabolic clearance. Skin temperature continues to rise and approaches 35°C over the whole body surface. At or near this point the deep body temperature is stabilized by the secretion of sweat. Sweating enhances body heat loss considerably, amounting to 670 watts for every litre of sweat evaporated. Sweat that is not evaporated when it drips from the body surface (as occurs in humid environments) does not contribute to the heat loss but adds to the loss of fluid. Up to 10 litres of hypotonic fluid in a day may be lost by profuse sweating, though this sweat rate is usually not maintained, and serious dehydration is therefore a possible outcome especially when water supplies are scarce. With fluid loss by sweating there is also a loss of salt, which may pose another potential problem. Salt concentration in sweat may vary from 1 g/litre in heat-acclimatized personnel to 3 g/litre in those who are not acclimatized. The rate of sweating, dietary intake of salt and endocrine balance are all variables that determine sweat salt concentration.

Cardiovascular strain develops with increasing demand for a higher cardiac output to transfer heat and water to vasodilated vascular beds. In resting conditions, extensive shunting of blood to the skin induces a fall in blood pressure and an increase in heart rate. With an adequate venous pressure, stroke volume is maintained and cardiac output increased. Dehydration as the result of excessive sweating, however, leads to a marked decrease in circulating blood volume, a reduction in stroke volume and an increased heart rate. Exercise in hot conditions presents a physiological dilemma when blood must be shunted to working muscles as well as to the skin for thermoregulation. In unacclimatized humans there is an initial period of cardiovascular instability characterized by increasing body temperature and heart rate and a decrease in stroke volume. Stability returns with acclimatization when plasma volume and stroke volume increase and heart rate decreases.[2] Several standard works describe these and other general thermoregulatory responses to heat in greater detail.[3–5] Thermoregulation during exposure to heat and exercise differs between children and adults, mainly due to a lower sweating capacity and to metabolic, circulatory and hormonal disparities.[6]

Thermoregulation is integrated by a controlling system in structures in the brain and spinal cord which respond to the heat content of tissues. Receptors sensitive to thermal information from the skin, deep tissues and in the central nervous system itself provide feedback signals to this system. Principal centres reside in the hypothalamus where the temperature of blood perfusing the hypothalamus is a major drive to temperature control. Ideas on the need for a hypothalamic 'set-point' have been developed in order to explain how body temperature is maintained at predetermined constant levels. The central thermoregulatory interface appears to consist essentially of two pathways from sensors with differing responses to thermal changes, and crossed inhibition between these two pathways. The effect may be to create a temperature null point or null zone.[7] Excessive increases in brain temperature are likely to affect the integrative function of central nervous structures and have profound deleterious consequences on the temperature control system. It has been postulated that some protection of the brain against hyperthermia may be provided by a countercurrent system in the blood supply of the face and head which permits selective cooling of the brain.[8] Unlike some desert-dwelling animals, humans do not have a carotid rete, and whether or not other mechanisms exist to minimize increases in brain temperature has been the subject of much conflicting research and discussion. Brain tissue appears to be highly susceptible to heat damage, as evidenced by observations on heatstroke patients.

Heat acclimatization and work performance

Writing more than 200 years ago on the heat hazard to newcomers to the tropics, Lind[9] pointed out that habituation to hot climates reduces the danger to health. The process of heat acclimatization was originally associated with an improved ability to perform work in the heat. In fact a useful degree of acclimatization to heat can be attained simply by hard physical training in a cool environment.[10] The immediate physiological responses to acute heat stress give way to reduced signs of heat strain after a few days of work in hot conditions. Heart rate and deep body temperature do not rise so high and the sweating mechanism becomes more efficient. Total sweat rates of 0.5–1 litre per hour may increase to 2 litres per hour or more in a fully acclimatized man, though such high rates cannot be maintained for many hours. A major part of the improvement in sweat output is due to increased cellular secretory capacity of the sweat glands brought about by sweat gland 'training'.[11] With the initial acclimatization process, the salt content of sweat is reduced in response to adrenal mineralocorticoids. Longer-term acclimatization to heat is associated with increments in blood volume, plasma volume, extra-

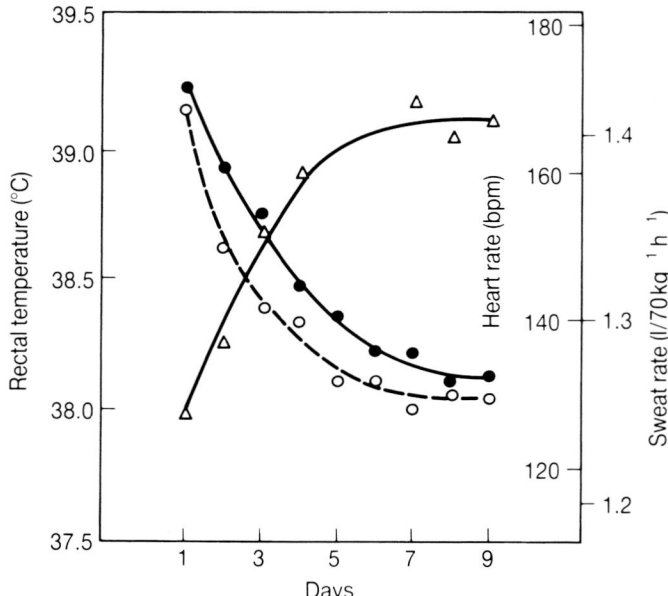

Figure 29.1: Typical mean rectal temperatures (●), heart rates (○) and sweat losses (△) in a group of men during the development of acclimatization to heat. (Adapted from Leithead & Lind.[20])

cellular fluid volume and total body water content. Endocrinological and metabolic responses to both acute and chronic heat exposures have been described.[12]

Heat tolerance can be achieved artificially by daily sessions of controlled hyperthermia or work–rest routines for 3–4 hours in a climatic chamber (acclimation) or normal daily physical work in the tropical environment (acclimatization). The adaptive process develops rapidly over the first 3 or 4 days and is virtually complete by 9 or 10 days (Figure 29.1). When exposure to heat and work ceases, the physiological adaptations are partly retained for up to 1 or 2 weeks but thereafter the benefits are rapidly lost. For healthy young adults, acclimation to heat has been shown to greatly reduce the incidence of heat disorders.

Part of the longer-term process of heat adaptation involves behavioural adjustments, such as resting during the hottest part of the day. This is intuitive to tropical indigenes who normally will seek to avoid the stresses of hyperthermia, and in consequence may often not be fully heat acclimatized. Data drawn from physiological and anthropometric investigations tend to support the view that adult body form varies among populations so as to confer some advantage in the environment inhabited.[13] The hot, dry climate that is the natural habitat of Nilotic people, for example, appears to confer morphological features of linearity and high surface area to body weight. A process of selection in favour of smaller body size appears as an adaptive response to a hot, humid environment in equatorial forests where heat loss through sweating is of little efficiency. Fitness and physical work capacity are regarded as fundamental determinants of human survival, and in many tropical populations agricultural work continues to underpin local economies.

The relationship between working capacity, heat acclimatization and avoidance of heat disorders plays an important role in human ability to exploit the tropical habitat.[14]

Heat stress

The heat stress of a given situation is measured by the combination of all those factors contributing to the heat gain of the body. Thus it is necessary to consider both climatic and non-climatic factors and to evaluate in some way their combined effects. Climatic factors include ambient temperature, humidity and air movement, and non-climatic variables such as physical activity and clothing. Assessment of the physiological strain in a person subjected to thermal stress is usually related to two measurements: the core temperature and the heart rate. Tolerance limits for work in adverse temperature conditions are commonly based on acceptable 'safe' levels of these two measurements, and in hot conditions the limits are usually 38.0°C core temperature and 180 beats per minute heart rate in normal healthy adults.

Heat stress indices provide a means of assessing hot environments and to predict their likely effect on people. Such indices provide the equivalence of various environmental factors,[15] usually with physical activity and clothing as independent variables. A number of different heat stress indices have been proposed which are divided broadly into those empirically derived and substantiated by the physiological effects on a test group of people, and those derived by theoretical consideration of the effects on the body's heat balance. No index or standard is universally applicable since all are affected to differing degrees by components of the thermal environment, clothing and metabolism.[16] The wet bulb globe temperature (WBGT) index calculated from 0.7 wet bulb + 0.2 globe (radiant) + 0.1 dry bulb temperature is probably most widely used for outdoor activities where solar radiation is a component of the heat stress.[17] It was used effectively to reduce the incidence of heat casualties in unacclimatized marine recruits in the 1950s. Safe physical activity schedules may be set according to the predicted environmental heat loads for the day, e.g., WBGT < 18°C (low risk), WBGT > 28°C (very high risk).[18] The increase in understanding of human thermoregulation and the processes of heat exchange have led to the development of mathematical models of human responses to hot environments, and the development of the digital computer has provided the opportunity for these relatively complex models to be conveniently used in practical applications.[19]

Heat disorders

The pathological conditions associated with the effects of heat arise from four main aetiologies :

1. Circulatory instability
   (a) Heat syncope
   (b) Heat oedema
2. Heat-induced skin disorders
   (a) Hidromeiosis
   (b) Prickly heat (miliaria rubra)
   (c) Anhidrotic heat exhaustion
3. Water and electrolyte imbalance
   (a) Heat cramps
   (b) Water-depletion heat exhaustion
   (c) Salt-depletion heat exhaustion
4. Hyperthermic failure of thermoregulation
   (a) Heatstroke

Another category of heat disorder is sometimes described under the general heading of psychological effects of heat.[20] The predominant effects are characterized by deterioration in performance and loss of efficiency, presenting as 'acute heat neurasthenia' or 'tropical fatigue'. Heat neurotic syndromes are ill defined and may not be attributable solely to the effects of heat.

Any factor that compromises the normal processes of thermoregulation may be implicated in the aetiology of heat disorders. Personnel most at risk have a history of heat intolerance, are overweight or physically unfit. There is sometimes failure on the part of the supervising authority, or the individuals themselves, to appreciate the potential dangers involved in exposure to severe heat stress.

Heat exposure may aggravate underlying pathology, especially cardiovascular disease, and in this respect the elderly are particularly at risk. Occult infections have been observed to cause transient anhidrosis, and the influence of endogenous pyrogens can raise the 'set-point' around which body temperature is regulated. Many heatstroke victims present with a previous history of infection or fever. Heat intolerance can also be extreme in cases of thyrotoxicosis, mucoviscidosis and congenital absence of sweat glands in ectodermal dysplasia.

Chemicals and medications may have direct effects on the control of body temperature, and some have indirect effects through induced toxicity reactions or drug interactions.[21] Special care is required in high temperature conditions with patients who have been prescribed diuretics, anticholinergics or central nervous stimulants or depressants.

It remains to say that there may be disorders other than those listed above which are causally related to heat stress. For example, it seems possible that environmental heat may be implicated in the pathogenesis of renal stones in hot countries where subclinical water depletion is commonplace.

Minor heat disorders

Heat oedema
Mild swelling of the feet and ankles may be experienced by unacclimatized people arriving in the tropics, which

with rest usually resolves within a few days. The aetiology is likely to be due to cutaneous vasodilatation and venous stasis in the legs. Mild oedema may also be a manifestation of an expansion of the extracellular space, influenced by aldosterone and antidiuretic hormone activity. Some newcomers to hot climates show their apprehension of the heat by overloading themselves with salt and water.

Heat syncope

It is common knowledge that fainting may follow prolonged standing, sudden postural changes or unaccustomed exercise, particularly in hot surroundings. Heat syncope occurs because of peripheral vascular pooling of blood and collapse of venomotor tone leading to hypotension and cerebral anoxia. The patient suddenly becomes pale with heart rate at first increasing and then slowing, and breathing is slow and sighing in nature. Consciousness is usually lost for a minute or so, but returns as cerebral circulation is restored when the patient is placed in the head-low position. Other causes of loss of consciousness must be excluded. Syncope may be the prelude to more serious heat disorders such as heat exhaustion or heatstroke.

Heat cramps

Heat-induced muscle cramps are probably due to a mild water intoxication or to salt depletion, occurring in people who are sweating profusely while at the same time drinking large amounts of unsalted fluids. Cramps may also be experienced by those who exercise regularly while adhering to a low-salt diet. The spasms usually last less than 1 minute, occasionally for 2 or 3 minutes, but they may recur every few minutes for several hours. Heat cramps must be distinguished from tetany, which may sometimes occur in individuals with raised body temperature who may hyperventilate sufficiently to develop acute respiratory alkalosis.

Intravenous normal saline (0.5–1 litre) can be given to treat severe cramps, or even a small quantity of 5% hypertonic saline. This should be followed by liberal quantities of salt in drinks until the urine contains at least 2–3 g chloride per litre. Prevention of heat cramps usually entails the provision of salted drinks at the place of work.

Skin disorders with sweat suppression

Hidromeiosis

The term hidromeiosis is applied to a particular type of reduction in sweating associated with wetting the skin,[11,15] previously thought to represent 'sweat gland fatigue'. Sweat evaporation may diminish when there is wetting of the skin in hot, humid climates. In this case, suppression of sweating is caused by obstruction of sweat glands by swelling of the keratin layer of the skin and closure of sweat pores when water is absorbed at high skin temperatures. The process can be readily reversed by moving into a dry environment. Hyperthermia develops more readily in hot humid conditions because of hidromeiosis and lack of effective evaporative cooling.

Prickly heat

This common skin complaint in hot climates causes considerable irritation and discomfort, also arising from prolonged wetting of the skin by sweat. Maceration of the stratum corneum causes acute (miliaria rubra) or chronic (miliaria profunda) blockage of the sweat ducts. The pathogenesis therefore resembles that of hidromeiosis, but the sweat glands become more permanently blocked by plugs of mucopolysaccharide debris and there is distension of the sweat ducts. The rash of miliaria rubra (prickly heat) is an erythematous epidermal vesicular eruption that is pruritic, and it is accompanied by a prickling or tingling sensation when sweating is provoked. Subsequently miliaria profunda may develop, characterized by dermal vesicles without erythema or pruritus, giving the affected skin area a gooseflesh appearance (Figure 29.2). Secondary bacterial and fungal infections may occur.

Treatment consists of removing the patient to cool quarters if possible to avoid sweating, and removing tight-fitting clothing. Prickling can be relieved by a cool shower, thorough drying of the skin and application of calamine lotion or zinc oxide powder. Mildly astringent lotions such as those containing mercuric chloride may be useful, as are topical antimicrobial agents.

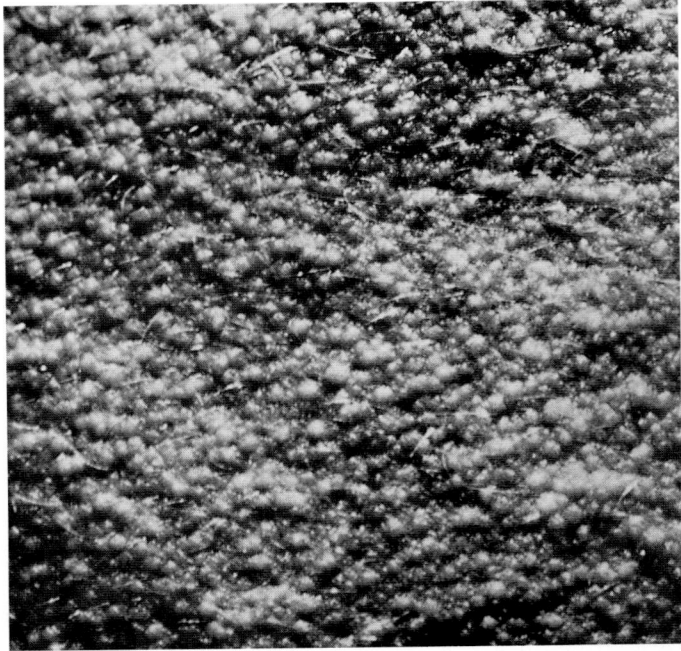

Figure 29.2: Miliaria profunda (mammillaria). Photographic enlargement of human skin. (From Horne and Mole.[22])

Anhidrotic heat exhaustion

Impairment of sweating by miliaria profunda or other skin disorders may lead to a state of heat exhaustion and heat intolerance, affecting personnel exposed for several months to a hot climate. Humid heat is responsible for most cases but the disorder may occur in desert climates. Dyshidrosis is probably a more accurate term to describe the sweat suppression since complete absence of sweating does not usually occur. Exfoliative dermatitis and other atrophic skin disorders are sometimes involved. Patients are unable to perform even limited amounts of physical work without suffering undue fatigue and discomfort in the heat. Attempts to do so may precipitate other heat disorders, including heatstroke.

Body fluid imbalance

Water-depletion heat exhaustion

People working in hot conditions frequently do not completely replace the volume of water lost by sweating (voluntary dehydration) and usually maintain a slight negative water balance averaging 1–2% of total body weight. This minor degree of dehydration is sufficient to impair maximum physical performance.[23] More serious degrees of dehydration develop when water supplies are scarce. Though water depletion is thought to cause mild reductions in thermal sweating, high sweat rates to defend body temperature appear to be possible during dehydration. The classic situations producing water-depletion heat exhaustion have been described among castaways at sea in the tropics, travellers stranded in the desert, labourers in hot mines[24] and in service personnel. An accessory factor is often the additional loss of fluid due to vomiting and diarrhoea.

Dehydration due predominantly to water depletion is characterized by intense thirst, fatigue, weakness, anxiety and impaired judgement. Irritability and syncope appear as water loss approaches 6% of body weight. Urine is scanty and concentrated. Extracellular fluid volume is diminished, with increasing osmolality, and water moves from the cells into the extracellular compartment. Haemoconcentration is marked and serum protein and sodium levels elevated.

It is important to decide whether heat exhaustion is due mainly to salt or water depletion, although there is usually a mixed depletion. The circumstances of onset are usually quite different. Sweat is hypotonic and a relatively far greater amount of water than salt is lost, so that progressive water depletion is always more rapid in development than salt depletion. Differential diagnosis may be established by the symptoms and signs shown in Table 29.1. In its most severe form, in individuals stranded in hot, dehydrating desert conditions without water, the situation may become rapidly fatal within a day. Studies of dehydration in the desert suggest that death is ultimately due to oligaemic shock and to heatstroke due to loss of thermoregulatory control.[20]

Table 29.1 Differential diagnosis of salt- and water-depletion heat exhaustion.

	Predominant salt depletion	Predominant water depletion
Duration of symptoms	3–5 days	Often less than 3–5 days
Thirst	Not prominent	Prominent
Fatigue	Marked	Less marked
Giddiness	Prominent	Less prominent
Muscle cramps	In most cases	Absent
Vomiting	In most cases	Usually absent
Thermal sweating	Usually unchanged	Diminished
Haemoconcentration	Early and marked	Slight until late
Urine chloride	Negligible	Normal
Blood sodium	Below average	Above average
Mode of death	Oligaemic shock	Oligaemic shock Heatstroke

From Leithead & Lind.[20]

Treatment consists of rest in cool surroundings with carefully controlled rehydration sufficient to ensure a net gain of 2–3 litres over the first 24 hours and 0.5–1 litre per day subsequently. Excessively rapid correction of hypernatraemia may cause cerebral oedema, convulsive seizures and possibly death due to uncal herniation. Unconscious patients will require intravenous fluid replacement, and if there is doubt whether the patient is predominantly water depleted or salt depleted isotonic saline should be given; otherwise the fluid of choice is 5% glucose solution. Recovery is indicated by increased urine output but it is essential to avoid fluid overload if renal damage has occurred.

Salt-depletion heat exhaustion

In unacclimatized personnel there is usually a high salt content in sweat, and enough salt may be lost to cause a negative salt balance during the first few days of heat exposure. Daily losses in 5 litres of sweat per day may amount to 15 g of salt and supplementation of dietary salt is required. Extra salt is usually unnecessary when heat acclimatization takes place since salt balance is restored after a few days by the salt-conserving action of aldosterone on the kidney and sweat glands.

Clinical findings in human salt deficiency include reduced plasma volume with haemoconcentration (Table 29.1). The concentration of sodium and chloride in urine is low. Extracellular fluid osmolality is reduced, causing hypovolaemia and a shift of fluid into the intracellular compartment. Plasma sodium concentration may sometimes be deceptively normal but the sodium and chloride content of whole blood is reduced. Fatigue, giddiness, nausea and muscle cramps are common clinical features.

Anorexia, diarrhoea and vomiting reduce the already inadequate intake of salt, establishing a vicious circle of events. Thirst is not a feature, unlike water depletion. In contrast to predominant water depletion, salt depletion does not generally predispose rapidly to heatstroke.

Treatment is usually easier than for water depletion and consists of bed rest in cool conditions with a high salt intake in the form of salted drinks. Salt should be added to cool fruit drinks (7 g/litre) and salty food encouraged to achieve an intake of up to 20 g daily. Complete clinical recovery occurs usually only after 5–7 days bed rest and salt replacement, and is accompanied by the consistent appearance of significant amounts of chloride in urine. For comatose patients, isotonic saline may be given intravenously at the rate of 2–4 litres over 12–24 hours. When extreme hyponatraemia causes symptoms of water intoxication, rarely is hypertonic saline indicated. It is important to examine neck veins and lung bases during treatment for signs of circulatory overloading.

Heatstroke

Heatstroke is caused by an excessive rise in deep body temperature due to thermoregulatory failure. It is characterized primarily by hyperthermia usually with core temperature above 40.6°C, central nervous system dysfunction resulting from tissue damage, and metabolic derangement and coma. Heatstroke is the least common but most serious of heat disorders and it carries a high mortality rate if effective treatment is not given immediately. In conditions in which heat disorders can be expected,[25] heat exhaustion syndromes usually occur up to 10 times more frequently than heatstroke in the population at risk.

Epidemiology

Heatstroke occurs during heat waves even in temperate regions. Infants, the elderly and patients with heart disease are most at risk in the community during hot weather.[26] Heatstroke also occurs in physically active people, e.g., service personnel, marathon runners during prolonged exercise or those engaged in hard work in hot conditions.[27] Each year, a mass of people, currently about two million, gather at Mecca for the seven-day pilgrimage, the Makkah Hajj. There is high radiant heat and ambient temperature, aggravated by many people assembled in a restricted area. Many of the pilgrims suffer from heat disorders and over 1000 may be treated for heatstroke in the hot seasons and some hundreds may die before reaching treatment centres.[25]

In many tropical countries precise statistics for morbidity and mortality are not available because of poor certification and the difficulty in defining the size and composition of the population at risk. In the South African gold mines, where the working population is homogeneous in its social background, heatstroke cases are reported at rates of 0.3 per 1000 per year in environments of 32°C wet bulb temperature and 4.0 per 1000 per year at 34.4°C wet bulb.[28] Reported mortality ratios for heatstroke varied considerably at treatment centres during the 1980–82 Makkah Pilgrimages, ranging from 5% to 80%,[25] but it is not always clear whether treated cases have been included.

Aetiology

Two types of heatstroke have been described: 'classical' heatstroke associated with intolerably hot conditions or heat waves but not involving significant exertion, and 'exertional' heatstroke generally observed in younger individuals, generating high metabolic loads by physical work in the heat. The main differences in presentation are given in Table 29.2, but there are common characteristics, e.g. hyperthermia, lack of heat acclimatization, dehydration, skin mottling and flushing, psychotic behaviour, convulsions, shock and coma.

Table 29.2 Presentation of 'classical' and 'exertional' heatstroke.

	'Classical'	'Exertional'
Age group	Infants, elderly	15–65 years old
Health status	Chronic illness	Usually healthy
History of febrile illness	Occasionally	Common
Activity	Sedentary	Usually highly active
Drug use	Diuretics, phenothiazines	Amphetamines, cocaine
Sweating	Usually absent	Usually present
Respiratory alkalosis	Dominant	Mild
Lactic acidosis	Absent or mild	Often marked
Rhabdomyolysis	Seldom severe	Severe
Creatinine phosphokinase/aldolase	Mildly elevated	Markedly elevated
Disseminated intravascular coagulation	Mild	Marked
Hypoglycaemia	Uncommon	Common

From Knochel.[34]

Malignant hyperthermia leading to heatstroke is a rare but often fatal complication of general anaesthesia.[27] In susceptible patients with a familial myopathy, certain anaesthetic agents such as halothane can produce sustained muscle contraction, resulting in a rapid rise in body temperature. The biochemical basis appears to involve an abnormally large release of calcium into the myoplasm.

Pathology

At about 42°C deep body temperature, hyperthermia causes denaturation of enzymes, liquefaction of membrane lipids, mitochondrial damage and destabilization of lipoproteins. The high temperature is primarily responsible for tissue damage, but cellular hypoxia, congestion, endotoxaemia and disseminated intravascular coagulation (DIC) are contributory.

Among the classically described anatomical changes found at autopsy are oedema of the brain and meninges, neuronal degeneration and petechial haemorrhages.[29] The predominance of changes in cerebellar structures corresponds to the clinical picture of central nervous damage in patients who survive heatstroke. These patients often show cerebellar ataxia with marked dysarthria, polyneuropathy or dysmetria. Haemorrhages are also observed in serous cavities and in the heart, kidney, liver and gastrointestinal mucosa. Myocardial damage is common and, characteristically, subendocardial haemorrhages occur beneath the left interventricular septum. Skeletal muscle may show necrosis if rhabdomyolysis has accompanied heatstroke.[30] Liver damage is one of the most prominent features, with centrilobular fatty changes, congestion and degenerating hepatocytes resembling Councilman bodies. The kidneys are damaged and show hyperaemia and petechial haemorrhages. Deleterious effects in the blood include haemolysis, thrombocytopenia, megakaryocyte damage, DIC and widespread fibrin deposition. DIC contributes to both the bleeding manifestations and shock syndrome.[25] As may be predicted, increased proinflammatory cytokine concentrations have been implicated in the pathogenesis of heatstroke.[31]

Clinical features

In most cases of heatstroke the onset of delirium or coma is sudden but, in some cases, several days of ill health precede the onset of coma and severe hyperthermia. With acute-onset heatstroke, prodromal symptoms lasting minutes or hours include headache, disorientation, stupor, emotional outbursts, dizziness, excessive thirst and locomotor changes.

Central nervous disturbances are typical presenting features. Often the patient is in coma with a rectal temperature of 40.6°C or more and there may be involuntary movements closely resembling epilepsy with tonic and clonic convulsions, and frequently urinary and faecal incontinence. Hyperpnoea with tetany[25] is sometimes observed. Sweating is present at the stage of collapse,

particularly in young active heatstroke casualties.[32] Anhidrosis with a hot, dry skin, thought to be a common feature of heatstroke cases, cannot therefore be regarded as pathognomic. On admission, the patient's pulse is thready and the face flushed or cyanotic. In some cases, blood pressure and pulse pressure may be increased, whereas in others there is profound hypotension and shock. The electrocardiogram often shows flattened or inverted T waves, transient conduction abnormalities and myocardial damage. Echocardiographic and Doppler studies reflect a hyperdynamic circulation with tachycardia and high cardiac output states in severe heat exposure.[33] Relative hypovolaemia and signs of peripheral vasoconstriction are more often present in heatstroke than in heat exhaustion. Gastrointestinal haemorrhage with haematemesis or melaena can sometimes occur as manifestations of coagulopathy.

Diagnosis

Heatstroke can be suspected in any patient who loses consciousness under conditions of heat stress. The diagnosis is highly probable if body temperature is above 40°C in the presence of clinical features described above. Measurement of rectal temperature is crucial but is often difficult in a struggling patient. High-reading, metal-cased thermometers or electronic probes should be made available where heatstroke is a known risk.

Cooling measures are urgently required, leaving little time for exploring alternative diagnoses. The possibility of high fevers from other causes must, however, be kept under consideration. In the tropics, malaria is the most important differential diagnosis. High fevers from other causes such as meningitis, salmonella and arbovirus infections, encephalitis, bacterial pneumonia, septicaemia, tetanus and cerebral (pontine) haemorrhage are also to be considered. It is important to examine the skull for signs of injury which may have occurred during convulsions.

Laboratory findings include leucocytosis and thrombocytopenia. Changes in plasma concentration of sodium, chloride and potassium are not consistent, though hypokalaemia has been frequently observed in heatstroke.[34] Serum glutamic oxaloacetic transaminase, glutamic pyruvic transaminase, lactic dehydrogenase and creatine phosphokinase are usually elevated within 24 hours of admission. The levels continue to rise for about 2 days and remain elevated for 12–14 days. Serum enzyme changes are of diagnostic and prognostic significance. Severe renal involvement with rising urea nitrogen is evident in many fatal cases.

Treatment

In the field situation, the patient should be placed in the shade, clothing removed and the skin kept wet and fanned. An effective degree of conductive cooling can be attained simply by immersing the patient in a bath of cold water, and the body and limbs massaged vigorously to promote skin circulation. In hospital, the patient may

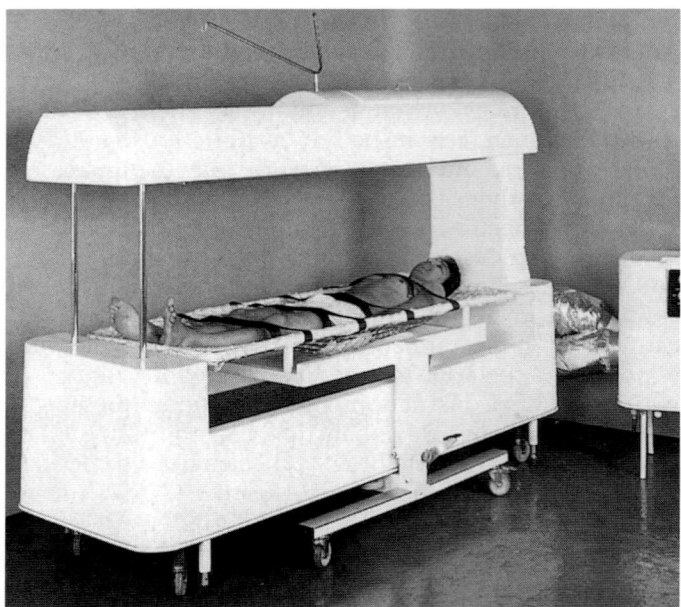

Figure 29.3: Body cooling unit for treatment of hyperthermia and heatstroke. (Photograph courtesy of Engments Ltd, Derby, UK)

be placed on a slatted trolley, exposing the skin to good air movement from an electric fan and a fine spray of water. Alternatively, the patient can be cooled by tepid water sponging or by wrapping in a wet sheet and fanning.

The need to avoid vasoconstriction during cooling and yet enable the management of a violent, delirious, incontinent and vomiting patient has led to the development of a body cooling unit (BCU) to treat heatstroke (Figure 29.3).[35] The method utilizes evaporative and convective cooling from sprays of atomized water at 20°C combined with a powerful flow of air at 45–50°C to maintain skin temperature above 31–32°C. The BCU has proved to be highly effective in the management of classical heatstroke patients among the Hajj pilgrims.[25]

Ice-water immersion is a simple and available form of treatment which has been advocated since the first edition of this textbook was published in 1898.[36] The method, however, appears to deny a critical principle of heat dissipation by preventing cutaneous vasodilatation. It has been suggested that the hydrostatic pressure of water during immersion increases venous return to the heart in hypotensive heatstroke patients, and that pathological rather than physiological vasomotor responses occur, such that the core-shell insulative barrier may not increase at the onset of heatstroke.[37] It is also reported that no deaths had occurred during the treatment by ice-water immersion in 252 heatstroke cases in Marine Corps recruits. A mean mortality of 12.1% using the BCU, on the other hand, was observed in Hajj pilgrims in 1982. However, there are obviously important differences between these two populations. The Marine Corps recruits were young, fit soldiers suffering from exertional heatstroke, all of whom were treated within

20 minutes of collapse. The Hajj pilgrims were often elderly or unfit, and were brought to treatment centres suffering from classical heatstroke at unknown periods after collapse.

With treatment, aspiration pneumonia must be avoided by keeping the airway clear and the patient nursed in a semi-lateral position. In addition to primary cooling procedures, intravenous chlorpromazine (20–50 mg) has been used to prevent shivering, though there is a danger that the drug may inhibit sweating.[25] To treat dehydration, 5% glucose in normal saline can be given intravenously, which should be done with care in order to avoid circulatory overloading. Oxygen should be given while danger to the central nervous system persists. DIC has been successfully treated with heparin, though fresh plasma provides a safer alternative. Dextran should be avoided since it may impair platelet function.

Prevention of heat disorders

Recognition and prevention of the ill effects of heat stress, for health workers in the tropics, in industry, in the services and other situations where the heat risk exists, requires a working knowledge of the techniques for measuring heat stress, e.g., the use of the WBGT index for assessing heat stress and heat tolerance times.[16] Migrants and individuals moving into hot regions or those working in hot industries require supervision and advice on the effects of high temperatures. Prevention of the ill effects broadly involves the control of human activities in outdoor heat and reduction of indoor heat loads by control measures so that temperatures are brought within recognized safety limits. It is essential to have a prepared treatment centre where cooling can be given at once.

Special care is required when conditions are hostile, when escape from hot conditions is difficult or when water is in short supply. Due attention must therefore be paid to the provision of adequate potable water supplies, suitable clothing and thermally comfortable quarters. Supplemental salt may be necessary, particularly for unacclimatized newcomers. Large, heavy meals and excess alcohol, especially during the hottest part of the day, are to be avoided. Successful prevention is often the result of careful selection and continuous screening of heat-exposed personnel and, if possible, artificial acclimatization to heat beforehand. Regular exercise helps to provide a degree of heat adaptation.

Climate change

An increase in the incidence of heat-associated disorders is likely to contribute to the potential health problems arising from climatic change. It is recognized that if global warming takes place, not all regions would be confronted by the same problems: extreme climatic events in different regions—heat waves, monsoons, droughts—may have a more profound impact than average climate change.[38] The direct effects of heat on individuals from increased heat stress in fact are likely to have less influence than indirect effects arising from complex changes in ecological infrastructure. Thus altered patterns of food production and the effects of inundation could lead to migration of large numbers of people into new zones. There are also likely to be changes in the distribution of vector-borne diseases in the tropics, sub-tropics and temperate climate zones. Since there are large areas of the world where water supplies and cooling systems are inadequate, in unusual heat wave conditions or prolonged periods of heat the availability of water may become the critical factor for survival.

Many scientists assert that global warming is now discernible, with forecasts of an increase in the average world temperature of 1.0–3.5°C over the present century.[39,40] Others, including some climatologists who believe that current climate models do not accurately portray the atmosphere–ocean system, maintain that the reality of global warming is still uncertain.[41]

Summer weather variability, rather than heat intensity, is regarded as the most important factor defining human vulnerability to heat.[42] People living in areas where summer climates are highly variable are poorly adapted to extreme heat, mainly because it occurs irregularly. There has, therefore, been a growing impetus to develop systems allowing urban health agencies to issue heat and health warnings taking into account climate, social structure and landscape. There are few paradigms useful for modelling the management of heat casualties occurring on a large scale. One, however, may be the programme adopted at the Hajj pilgrimage where up to 7000 cases of heat illness including heatstroke are treated each year.[25]

The human species has a marked capacity for adapting to temperature changes and to survive under widely different climatic conditions. In most regions, the predicted increase in average surface temperature may be easily tolerated, though much greater sustained rises of temperature in the higher latitudes may have more serious consequences for populations, including heat-associated disorders.

REFERENCES

1　Gagge A P & Gonzalez R R. Mechanisms of heat exchange: biophysics and physiology. In Fregly M J & Blatteis C M (eds). *Handbook of Physiology. Section 4. Environmental physiology*, vol. 1. New York: Oxford University Press, 1996: 45–84.

2　Rowell L B. Cardiovascular aspects of human thermoregulation. *Circ Res* 1983; 52:367–379.

3　Schonbaum E & Lomax P. Thermoregulation: physiology and biochemistry. Section 131, *International Encyclopedia of Pharmacology and Therapeutics*. New York: Pergamon, 1990.

4　Collins K J. Regulation of body temperature. In Tinker J & Zapol W M (eds). *Care of the Critically Ill Patient*, 2nd edn. Berlin: Springer, 1992: 155–173.

5　Blatteis C M. Proceedings of symposium on thermoregulation. *Ann NY Acad Sci* 1997; 813.

6　Falk B. Effects of thermal stress during rest and exercise in the paediatric population. *Sports Med* 1998; 25:221–240.

7　Bligh J. Mammalian homeothermy: an integrative thesis. *J Therm Biol* 1998; 23:143–258.

8　Cabanac M & Caputa M. Natural selective cooling of the human brain: evidence of its occurrence and magnitude. *J Physiol (Lond)* 1979; 286:255–264.

9　Lind J. *An Essay on Diseases Incidental to Europeans in Hot Climates*. London: T Becket, 1768.

10　Clark R P & Edholm O G. *Man and his Thermal Environment*. London: Edward Arnold, 1985.

11　Collins K J. Sweat glands: eccrine and apocrine. In Greaves M W & Shuster S (eds). *Pharmacology of the Skin I*. Berlin: Springer, 1989: 193–212.

12　Francesconi R P. Endocrinological and metabolic responses to acute and chronic heat responses. In Fregly M J & Blatteis C M (eds). *Handbook of Physiology. Section 4. Environmental Physiology*, vol. 1. New York: Oxford University Press, 1996: 245–260.

13　Collins K J. Physiological variation and adaptability in human populations. *Ann Hum Biol* 1999; 26:19–38.

14　Collins K J & Roberts D F. *Capacity for Work in the Tropics*. Cambridge, UK: Cambridge University Press, 1988.

15　Kerslake D McK. *The Stress of Hot Environments*. Cambridge, UK: Cambridge University Press, 1972. Reprinted Ann Arbor: University of Michigan Press, 2000.

16　British Occupational Hygiene Society. *The Thermal Environment*, 2nd edn. Technical guide No 12. Leeds: H & H Scientific Consultants, 1996.

17　International Standards Organization. Hot environments: estimation of heat stress on working man, based on the WBGT index (wet bulb globe temperature), ISO 7243. Geneva: ISO, 1989.

18　Shapiro Y & Saidman D S. Field and clinical observations of exertional heat stroke patients. *Med Sci Sports Exerc* 1990; 22:6–14.

19　Parsons K C. *Human Thermal Environments*. London: Taylor & Francis, 1993.

20　Leithead C S & Lind A R. *Heat Stress and Heat Disorders*. London: Cassell, 1964.

21　Schonbaum E & Lomax P. Thermoregulation: pathology, pharmacology and therapy. Section 132. *International Encyclopedia of Pharmacology and Therapeutics*. New York: Pergamon, 1991.

22　Horne G O & Mole R H. Mammillaria. *Trans R Soc Trop Med Hyg* 1951; 44:465–471.

23　Galloway S D. Dehydration, rehydration and exercise in the heat: rehydration strategies for athletic competition. *Can J Appl Physiol* 1999; 24:188–200.

24　Donoghue A M, Sinclair M J & Bates G P. Heat exhaustion in a deep underground metalliferous mine. *Occup Environ Med* 2000; 57:165–174.

25　Khogali M & Hales J R S. *Heat Stroke and Temperature Regulation*. New York: Academic Press, 1983.

26　Semenza J C, Rubin C H, Falter K H et al. Heat-related deaths during the July 1995 heat wave in Chicago. *N Engl J Med* 1996; 335:84–90.

27　Jardon O. Physiologic stress, heat stroke and malignant hyperthermia: a perspective. *Milit Med* 1982; 147:8–14.

28　Wyndham C H. A survey of the causal factors in heat stroke and their presentation in the gold mining industry. *J S Afr Inst Min Metall* 1965; 66:125–155.

29 Malamud N, Haymaker W & Cluster R P. Heat stroke: a clinico-pathological study of 125 fatal cases. *Milit Surg* 1946; 99:397–449.

30 Gardner J W & Kark J A. Fatal rhabdomyolysis presenting as mild heat illness in military training. *Milit Med* 1994; 159:160–163.

31 Hammami M M, Bouchama A, Al-Sedairy S et al. Concentrations of soluble tumor necrosis factor and interleukin-6 receptors in heatstroke and heat stress. *Crit Care Med* 1997; 25:1314–1319.

32 Hubbard R W. The role of exercise in the etiology of exertional heat stroke. *Med Sci Sports Exerc* 1990; 22:2–5.

33 Shahid M S, Hatle L, Mansour H & Mimish L. Echocardiographic and Doppler study of patients with heat stroke and heat exhaustion. *Intern J Cardiac Imaging* 1999; 15:279–285.

34 Knochel J P. Heat stroke and related heat disorders. *Dis Mon* 1989; 35:301–377.

35 Weiner J S & Khogali M. A physiological body cooling unit for treatment of heat stroke. *Lancet* 1980; i:507–508.

36 Manson P. *Tropical Diseases: A Manual of the Diseases of Warm Climates*. London: Cassell, 1898: 211–213.

37 Costrini A. Emergency treatment of exertional heat stroke and comparison with whole body cooling techniques. *Med Sci Sports Exerc* 1990; 22:15–18.

38 World Health Organization. *Potential Health Effects of Climatic Change: Report of a WHO Task Group*. Geneva: WHO, 1989.

39 Intergovernmental Panel on Climate Change (WG1). Houghton J T, Meira Filho L G, Callander B A et al (eds). *Climate Change 1995*. New York: Cambridge University Press, 1996.

40 McMichael A J & Haines A. Global climate change: the potential effects on health. *BMJ* 1997; 315:805–809.

41 Michaels P. Conspiracy, concensus or correlation? What scientists think about the 'popular vision' of global warming. *World Climate Rev* 1993; 1:11.

42 Kalkstein L S. Biometeorology: looking at the links between weather, climate and health. *Biometeorol Bull* 2000; 5:9–18.

Chapter 30
High-altitude Problems

J. S. Milledge

Introduction

In recent years more and more people are going to high altitude on trekking and climbing holidays. Access to high altitude has increased by both road and air so that tourists can and do reach significant altitudes in a very few days; thus they are exposed to the problems of mountain sickness very easily. There are millions of people who are resident at altitudes above 3000 m and others who have to commute to or visit high altitude in the course of their work and so are at risk of altitude illness. High-altitude problems are, therefore, of interest to all those involved in these activities and the doctors who have to advise them.

The physiology of high altitude

Barometric pressure falls with increasing altitude so, although the percentage of oxygen remains constant, the partial pressure (PO_2) falls. At 4000 m (the altitude of La Paz international airport) it is only 60% of the sea level value and on the summit of Mount Everest only one-third. A person exposed to this altitude acutely will become unconscious in about 2 minutes. However, acclimatized climbers can climb Everest without supplementary oxygen, though many have died in the attempt. That it can be done at all is due to the amazing way that the body can adapt to the low PO_2, given time. This process is termed altitude acclimatization and involves changes in a number of physiological systems.

Respiratory acclimatization

The most important aspect of acclimatization is respiratory. This results in an increase in ventilation and therefore in an increase in PaO_2 and a decrease in $PaCO_2$. Thus the decrease in inspired PO_2 is partially countered. This unconscious increase in breathing is brought about by changes in the control of ventilation involving the response to both carbon dioxide and hypoxia over the first few days at altitude. The increase in ventilation is seen at rest and even more on exercise and accounts for the breathlessness felt on even slight exertion at altitude.

Cardiovascular acclimatization

Heart rate

On exposure to hypoxia the heart rate is increased both at rest and during exercise. With acclimatization the resting heart rate falls. At altitudes below about 4500 m it falls to within the sea level range; above this altitude, resting heart rates remain modestly elevated.

Cardiac output and stroke volume

The early changes in cardiac output on exposure to hypoxia mirror the changes in heart rate and reflect sympathetic activity. After acclimatization the cardiac output is the same as at sea level for any given work rate in absolute terms.[1] It follows that after acclimatization the stroke volume is unchanged from that at sea level at moderate altitudes but reduced at altitudes where the heart rate is elevated.

Blood pressure, systemic and pulmonary

There is little or no change in systemic blood pressure after the first few days at altitude. The pulmonary blood pressure is increased. This hypoxic pulmonary pressor response is important in the fetus but at altitude is in no way beneficial. Indeed it merely puts strain on the right ventricle and is important in the genesis of acute pulmonary oedema of high altitude. It is of interest that the yak, an animal well adapted to high altitude, has little or no hypoxic pressor response, unlike lowland cattle, that have brisk responses.[2]

Haemoglobin and haematocrit

Probably the best-known effect of altitude is the increase in haemoglobin concentration [Hb] in the blood of people and animals at high altitude. The mechanism for this increase is the rise in erythropoietin levels triggered by hypoxia, which stimulates the bone marrow to produce more red cells. However, the rise in [Hb] in the first few days at altitude is due almost entirely to a reduction in plasma volume. Over weeks at altitude the red cell mass increases and the blood volume is restored.

The central nervous system and altitude

Acclimatized subjects seem to perform well mentally even at altitudes up to 6300 m. On the 1953 Everest expedition Bourdillon completed the *Times* crossword puzzle in the Western Cwm (6300 m). But climbers find that any task, mental or physical, requires a much greater effort of will to start and tests of psychomotor function can detect a diminution in function. Although simple well-learned tasks can be carried out quite well, tests of psychomotor function will bring out deficiencies in concentration, speed and dexterity.

Of equal interest to performance at altitude is the question of residual impairment after return to sea level. Anecdotally it has been pointed out that many of those pioneer climbers of pre-war Everest expeditions who climbed above 8000 m without oxygen went on to have distinguished careers afterwards and lived to a ripe old age, with mental faculties better than average. However, studies which have addressed this question rigorously have found some evidence of decrease in some aspects of psychomotor performance after return to sea level even 1 year later.[3]

Weight loss and anorexia

Anorexia and weight loss are features of life at high altitude. In the first few days at altitude anorexia, nausea and vomiting are likely to be part of the syndrome of acute mountain sickness. After a few days this passes and below about 4500 m appetite is regained and no further weight is lost. But above about 5500 m most people complain of anorexia, which gets worse the longer they spend at these altitudes. Above 6500 m anorexia is almost universal and weight loss common. No doubt reduced calorific intake plays a major part in the cause of this weight loss but there is evidence that there is malabsorption as well.[4]

Pathology at altitude

Acute mountain sickness

Acute mountain sickness (AMS) is a condition affecting previously healthy individuals who ascend rapidly to high altitude (Figure 30.1). There is a delay of a few hours to 2 days before symptoms develop. It is characterized by headache (usually frontal), nausea, vomiting, irritability, malaise, insomnia and poor climbing performance. The simple or benign form of the condition is self-limiting, lasting 3–5 days. After this time it does not recur at that given altitude though it may do so if the subject goes higher. The diagnosis of AMS relies on a history of the above symptoms, in the setting of recent ascent. There is a widely accepted scoring system, the Lake Louise system,[5] which allows comparison between research studies.

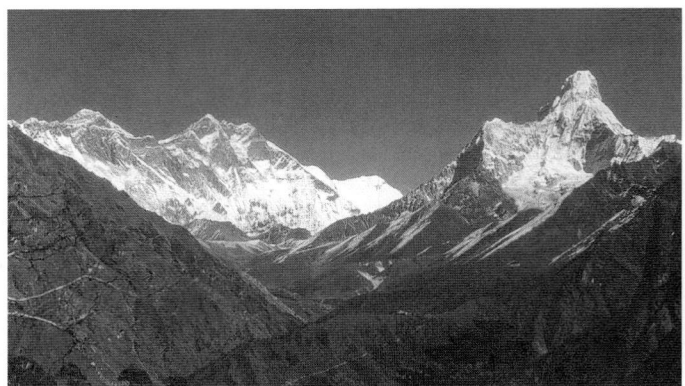

Figure 30.1: View of Everest, Lhotsi, Nupsi and Ama Dablam. The trail to Everest Base Camp can be seen going up the ridge to Tangboche Monastery (3800 m) in the centre of the picture. Many thousands of trekkers take this trail each season, 30–50% of whom will get acute mountain sickness.

Incidence of AMS

The incidence of AMS depends upon altitude and the rate of ascent. A survey in Alpine huts showed an incidence of 9% at 2850 m, 13% at 3050 m, 34% at 3650 m and 53% at 4559 m.[6] Among trekkers on the way to Everest base camp an incidence of 43% was found at 4300 m,[7] and was higher in those who had flown into an airstrip at 2800 m than in those who had walked all the way (49% vs. 31%).

Risk factors for AMS

Clearly hypoxia of more than a few hours' duration is required for the development of AMS and speed of ascent is important, but there is great variation in susceptibility. Amongst a group of people going together to high altitude there will be some unaffected, some mildly and some severely affected. At present there is no way to predict who is susceptible except that past performance at altitude is a guide.

Men, women and children seem to be equally affected but there is the impression that age reduces susceptibility. Fitness is no protection; indeed the fit are likely to ascend faster so they may be at greater risk. Any respiratory infection is probably a risk factor.

Mechanisms of AMS

Although hypoxia is obviously the starting point in the genesis of AMS it is not the immediate cause of the symptoms since these are delayed by several hours after arrival, whereas hypoxia is most severe in the first few minutes. It seems that hypoxia sets in train changes which, after a few hours, produce symptoms. The symptoms are similar to those associated with raised intracranial pressure as seen in neurosurgical patients and, at least in cases of high-altitude cerebral edema, there is good evidence of increased intracranial pressure. The most popular view is that even in simple AMS there develops a degree of cerebral oedema which causes the symptoms of AMS. Possibly there is some disturbance of fluid balance or capillary permeability throughout the body or there may be increased permeability of the blood–brain barrier resulting in cerebral oedema.

Prevention of AMS

A slow rate of ascent is the best way to prevent AMS. A suggested rule is that above 3000 m ascent should be not more than 300 m a day, with a 'rest' day, when no height gain is made, every 3 days. Even this rate will be too fast for some and unnecessarily slow for others. An added rule must be, 'If symptoms of AMS develop, go no higher. If they become severe, go down'.

Acetazolamide and dexamethasone

It is often not possible or practicable to plan for this rate of ascent, or a person may know that he is a poor acclimatizer. In such situations the use of acetazolamide (Diamox) can be considered. This drug, which is a carbonic acid anhydrase inhibitor, acts as a respiratory stimulant. There have been a number of good double-blind controlled trials which have shown that AMS is significantly reduced in those taking the drug.[8] The dose used in trials has usually been 250 mg 8 hourly but 250 mg or even 125 mg twice daily is usually recommended now. The drug is best started 24 hours before a major gain in altitude but has some effect even if started after early symptoms are felt. The side effects of the drug include a mild diuresis, which tends to diminish if the drug is continued, and paraesthesia of the fingers and toes, which is almost universal. Some subjects find this distressing. Beer and all fizzy drinks taste flat and metallic!

Dexamethasone has been shown to be an effective prophylactic drug but many would consider it unjustified to use it for this purpose.

Management

Simple or benign AMS is self-limiting and usually lasts about 3 days, so treatment is not essential; aspirin, paracetamol or ibuprofen can be used to relieve headache.

High-altitude pulmonary oedema

In the great majority of cases AMS is a minor affliction resolving in a few days. However, in a small proportion of people going to high altitude there develops the potentially lethal condition of acute pulmonary oedema (HAPE*) or cerebral oedema (HACE) or a mixture of these. The incidence will depend on the rate of ascent and the height reached. Figures of 0.5–2.0% of people going to altitude have been reported.[7] Individuals with a previous history of HAPE are at greater risk of subsequent problems.

Both lowlanders and high-altitude residents returning home after visits to low altitude are susceptible. Men and women of all ages can become victims and athletic fitness affords no protection.

---

*These are accepted abbreviations for these conditions from the US spelling of edema.

Clinical picture

The patient is typically a previously fit young man who has climbed rapidly to altitude and been very energetic on arrival. He becomes more breathless than his companions. A cough develops, dry at first then productive of frothy white sputum, later becoming blood tinged. He may complain of chest discomfort. Crackles will be heard at the lung bases and there will be increase in heart and respiratory rates. There may be peripheral oedema and raised jugular venous pressure. Over a few hours the patient's condition deteriorates; heart and respiration rates rise, breathing becomes 'bubbly' and cyanosis develops. Coma leads to death if no action is taken.

Investigations

The chest radiograph (Figure 30.2) typically shows asymmetric blotchy opacities. There is usually a mild pyrexia. Blood count usually shows neutrophil leucocytosis. Arterial oxygen saturation is low compared with fit individuals at the same altitude. The ECG shows tachycardia and changes suggestive of pulmonary hypertension. Cardiac catheter findings confirm the high pulmonary artery pressure but normal wedge pressure. The oedema fluid is found to have a high protein content, with concentrations approaching that of plasma.[9]

Mechanism of high-altitude pulmonary oedema

The mechanism of this condition is not clear. It is not that of acute left ventricular failure despite the clinical

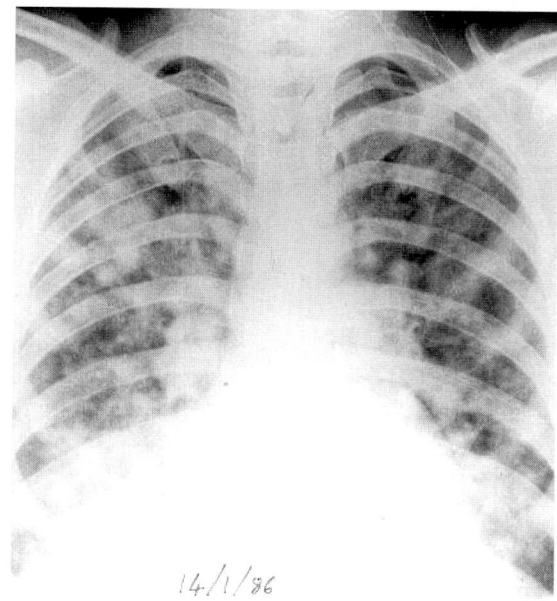

Figure 30.2: Chest radiograph of a patient with high-altitude pulmonary oedema. (Reproduced with permission from Dr T. Norboo of Leh, India.)

similarity. Catheter studies all show a normal wedge pressure. The most popular hypothesis, originally proposed by Hultgren et al.,[10] is that in susceptible subjects, who have been shown to have brisk hypoxic pulmonary artery pressor response,[11] the vasoconstriction is uneven. Those areas with greater vasoconstriction have reduced blood flow and are protected. Those areas with less constriction therefore have greatly increased blood flow. This torrential blood flow causes capillary damage by increased capillary pressure. West and colleagues have shown, in animals, that there is capillary stress failure at static pressures, which might easily obtain in HAPE patients.[12] Oedema then results. This accounts for the finding of pulmonary hypertension and the patchy nature of the oedema. Various kinins are found in the oedema fluid.[9] The release of these potent chemicals is likely to further increase permeability. However, recent studies suggest that the primary event in the genesis of HAPE is not inflammatory.[13]

Management

The most important measure in a case of HAPE is to evacuate the patient to lower altitude. A reduction in altitude of as little as 300 m may make all the difference. If this is not possible, or while awaiting evacuation, oxygen, if available, will help. Portable, lightweight, rubberized canvas hyperbaric chambers are now available (the Gamow or Certec bags, shown in Figure 30.3), into which the patient can be placed and the pressure increased by 2 psi using a foot pump. This has the effect of reducing the effective altitude by almost 2000 m. Trials have shown an improvement in the patient's condition following an hour's treatment. But the effect is lost over the next 6–12 hours[14] and it requires considerable effort to keep pumping if there is limited manpower available. However, the bag may be valuable in improving a patient sufficiently to be able to walk down unaided instead of having to be carried—an important consideration.

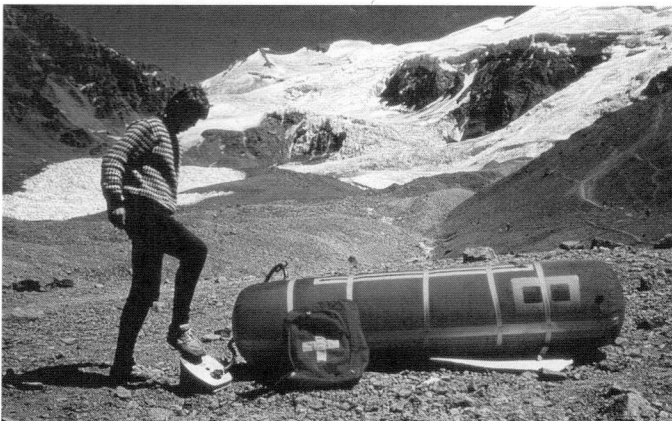

Figure 30.3: The Gamow bag. A rubberized canvas bag with window, into which the patient can be zipped. The bag is inflated using a foot pump to 2 psi, decreasing the effective altitude for the patient by almost 2000 m.

Since pulmonary vasoconstriction is thought to be important in the genesis of the condition, vasodilators have been tried; specifically the calcium channel blocker nifedipine has been shown to be beneficial.[15] A dose of 10 mg sublingually plus 20 mg slow release orally was used in this trial; however, since the sublingual drug can cause systemic hypotension it is probably best to use only the oral form unless the situation is critical.

Outcome

In fully established cases where evacuation is impossible or not carried out, the result is usually death within a few hours. In cases evacuated promptly, signs and symptoms are usually relieved within minutes or hours. Patients should be warned to be cautious in re-ascent to altitude but many have been able to go back to altitude with no recurrence.

High-altitude cerebral oedema

The other malignant form of AMS is HACE. In the early stages this is indistinguishable from simple AMS. When ataxia is added to the symptom cluster the line between simple AMS and HACE has been crossed. There may follow truncal ataxia, hallucinations, and clouding of consciousness with various neurological signs, including extensor plantar reflexes and papilloedema. There are often signs of pulmonary oedema as well. Finally the patient becomes unconscious and dies if not treated. The incidence is rather lower than acute pulmonary oedema.

The mechanism is presumably the same as simple AMS but it is not clear why a few individuals progress to this lethal complication whereas the majority suffer only a self-limiting reversible condition. As with HAPE, lowlanders and highlanders, men and women of any age can become victims.

Management

This is similar to that in acute pulmonary oedema. The most important measure is to get the patient down. While awaiting evacuation, oxygen breathing or use of a pressure bag helps but often not very quickly in more severe cases. Dexamethasone 4–8 mg intramuscularly in severe cases and orally in less severe cases will help reduce the cerebral oedema. The dose can be repeated at 4–6-hourly intervals until there is clear improvement.

Outcome

As in acute pulmonary oedema, descent often leads to rapid improvement. However, in some cases recovery is delayed for a number of days and there may even be permanent neurological defects, especially in cases where treatment has been delayed until coma is established.[16]

Subacute mountain sickness

Two forms of subacute mountain sickness have been

described: one in infants born at altitude taken to high altitude soon after birth[17] and the other in adults who have spent some months or more at extreme altitude.[18] In infants the presenting symptoms were commonly dyspnoea and cough, with often sleeplessness, irritability and signs of cyanosis, oedema of the face, oliguria, tachycardia, liver enlargement and fever. The majority of infants had been born at low altitude but two were born at high altitude, one of Han and one of Tibetan parents. The condition was usually fatal in a matter of weeks or months.

The adult form was described in soldiers who, after a full acclimatization period, had been posted to between 5800 m and 6700 m for several months (mean 1.8 years). They presented with dyspnoea, cough and effort angina and dependent oedema. They were treated at high altitude with diuretics with improvement. When they were evacuated to low altitude by aircraft they were found to have cardiomegaly with right ventricular enlargement and, in most cases, pericardial effusion. The pulmonary artery pressure was elevated and rose significantly on mild exercise. Recovery was rapid after descent from high altitude. The mechanism seems to be right heart failure due to chronic pulmonary hypertension.

Chronic mountain sickness

Chronic mountain sickness affects residents of high altitude and consists of extreme polycythaemia, with haemoglobin concentrations up to 23 g/dl. The victims become slow mentally and physically and complain of headaches, dizziness, somnolence, fatigue, difficulty in concentration etc. On going down to sea level symptoms clear and the polycythaemia disappears, only to recur on return to their high-altitude homes. Venesection helps to reduce symptoms. It is much more common in males and its incidence increases with age and time of residence at high altitude. It is more common in Andean highlanders than Tibetan and in Tibet it is more common in Han Chinese than in Tibetans. It is seen in Caucasians in altitude towns of Colorado, USA.

REFERENCES

1 Pugh L G C E. Cardiac output in muscular exercise at 5800 m (19000 ft.) *J Appl Physiol* 1964; 19:441–447.
2 Harris P. Evolution, hypoxia and high altitude. In Heath D (ed.) *Aspects of Hypoxia.* Liverpool: Liverpool University Press, 1986: 207–216.
3 Townes B D, Hornbein T F, Schoene R B, Sarnquist F H & Grant I. Human cerebral function at extreme altitude. In West J B & Lahiri S (eds) *High Altitude and Man.* Bethesda, MD: American Physiological Society, 1984: 32–36.
4 Ward M P, Milledge J S & West J B. *High Altitude Medicine and Physiology*, 3rd edn. London: Arnold, 2000: 168–177.
5 Roach R C, Bärtsch P, Hackett P H & Oelz O. The Lake Louise acute mountain sickness scoring system. In Sutton J R, Houston C S & Coates G (eds) *Hypoxia and Mountain Medicine.* Burlington, VA: Queen City Printers, 1993: 272–274.
6 Maggiorini M, Buhler B, Walter M & Oelz O. Prevalence of acute mountain sickness in the Swiss Alps. *BMJ* 1990; 301:853–855.
7 Hackett P H & Rennie D. The incidence, importance and prophylactics of acute mountain sickness. *Lancet*; 1979; ii:1449–1454.
8 Ward M P, Milledge J S & West J B. *High Altitude Medicine and Physiology*, 3rd edn. London: Arnold, 2000: 227.
9 Schoene R B, Swenson E R, Pizzo C J et al. The lung at high altitude: bronchoalveolar lavage in acute mountain sickness and pulmonary edema. *J Appl Physiol* 1988; 64:2605–2613.
10 Hultgren H N, Robison M C & Wuerflein R D. Over perfusion pulmonary edema. *Circulation* 1966; 34:132–133.
11 Yagi H, Yamada H, Kobayashi T & Sekiguchi M. Doppler assessment of pulmonary hypertension induced by hypoxic breathing in subjects susceptible to high altitude pulmonary edema. *Am Rev Respir Dis* 1990; 142:796–801.
12 West J B & Mathieu-Costello O. Stress failure of pulmonary capillaries in lung and heart disease. *Lancet* 1992; 340:862–867.
13 Swenson E R. The role of inflammation in the pathophysiology of HAPE. *High Altitude Med Biol* 2000; 1:267 (abstract).
14 Bärtsch P, Merki B, Hofstetter D, Maggiorini M, Kayser B & Oelz O. Treatment of acute mountain sickness by simulated descent: a randomised trial. *BMJ* 1993; 306:1098–1101.
15 Oelz O, Maggiorini M, Ritter M et al. Nifedipine for high altitude pulmonary oedema. *Lancet* 1989; ii:1241–1244.
16 Houston C S & Dickenson J. Cerebral form of high-altitude illness. *Lancet* 1975; ii:758–761.
17 Sui G I, Lui Y H, Cheng X S et al. Subacute infantile mountain sickness. *J Pathol* 1998; 57:71–76.
18 Anand I, Malhotra R M, Chandrashekhar Y et al. Adult subacute mountain sickness: a syndrome of congestive heart failure in man at very high altitude. *Lancet* 1990; 335:561–565.

Chapter 31
Nutrition-associated Disease

B. J. Brabin and J. B. S. Coulter

The inter-relationship between nutrition, health and disease has long been recognized as fundamental to medical care. Diets in the tropics are often unbalanced as well as being deficient in calories, and there is the added burden of bacterial and parasitic infections. These infections cause loss of appetite, maldigestion and malabsorption, which results in growth retardation, weight loss, micronutrient deficiencies and iron-deficiency anaemia. Seasonal and climatic variations have an enormous influence on disease transmission, agricultural potential and food security, which are all important factors affecting nutritional status. This concurrence can result in the 'hungry season' which describes the time between the exhaustion of the previous year's food stores and the new harvest. This generates a situation of nutritional stress in many developing countries. Traditional practices and cultural and religious food customs may lead to further dietary strictures.

Malnutrition in children

Malnutrition of variable degree is common in most developing countries. Over 50% of under five year old (under-fives) child deaths are associated with malnutrition. The interaction between infection and nutrition are key factors.[1–3]

Prevalence

The prevalence of malnutrition may be measured according to rates of stunting, underweight and wasting. Table 31.1 outlines the geographical distribution in developing countries. Approximately 38% of under-fives in developing countries are stunted.[4] Stunting is usually established by three years of age. Causes are multifactorial and reflect socio-economic, educational and health status, and development and wealth of society. Prenatal factors and low birth weight are also important causes. Approximately 31% of under-fives are underweight.[4] Catch-up growth resulting in normal weight for height ratios is possible, but adults are often stunted. Wasting (low weight for age or weight for height ratios) affects approximately 9% of children and usually occurs between six months to two years. Rates increase in times of famine, war, forced migration and depression of the

Table 31.1 Prevalence (%) of stunting, underweight and wasting for children under five years old in 1995 for UN regions.

	Stunting	Underweight	Wasting
Africa	38.6	28.4	8.0
Asia	41.0	35.0	10.3
Latin America and Caribbean	17.9	9.5	3.0
Oceania	31.4	22.8	5.0

Table 31.2 Socio-economical causes of malnutrition.

General	Food	Infection
Lack of education	Food insecurity	Poor hygiene
Poverty	• general	and sanitation
Frequent	• seasonal	HIV infection
pregnancies	Cultural	Failed measles
Low birth weight	practices and	immunization
Intrafamilial	taboos	
• divorce,	Maldistribution	
separation	within the family	
• working mothers		
• unemployment		
• sending a child		
away to be looked		
after by a relative		
Inadequate medical		
and nutritional		
support		

economy. Socio-economic causes of malnutrition vary geographically and are outlined in Table 31.2. Nutritional causes are difficult to assess. Wasting may be due more to deficient quantity and stunting to deficient quality of food.[1]

Severe malnutrition

Severe malnutrition is manifest by wasting and/or oedema. Major factors are *nutritional deficiency* and *recurrent infections,* both of which have underlying socio-economic causes, particularly poverty and lack of hygiene and education (Table 31.2). Inadequate infant feeding practices and weaning diets are compounded by infections associated with anorexia and increased metabolic demand. Many children with severe organic diseases, e.g., cardiac and renal disorders and mental and physical handicap, have variable degrees of malnutrition and are usually stunted and underweight. Neglect may also be an element in those who are disabled.

Measurement and classification

There are various methods of classifying malnutrition which depend on the type of information required and the prevalence of oedema; also the level of training of health workers undertaking measurements.

Weight for age

Weight for age as a percentage of the median standard is useful for assessment at child health clinics. Disadvantages include inaccuracy of age of the child for some uneducated mothers, and it also does not take into account lightness in weight due to stunting.

Mid upper arm circumference (MUAC)

This measurement is useful for screening children between one and five years of age, e.g., in large groups of refugees, and only requires a measuring tape. Standards: normal >14–16.5 cm; moderate 12.5–14 cm, severe malnutrition <12.5 cm. MUAC in relation to age may also be used.[5]

Weight for height

This is the most accurate for measuring acute malnutrition, but less 'user friendly' for health workers. It may be described as percentage of standard, standard deviations or standard deviation (or Z) scores.

Wellcome classification

This is very useful for areas such as sub-Saharan Africa, where oedematous malnutrition is common (Table 31.3).[6] The disadvantage is that it does not take stunting into account, e.g., low birth weight and stunted children may be classified as marasmic or marasmic kwashiorkor when weight for height is within normal limits.[7] The weight of children after loss of oedema provides a record of the degree of wasting.

Table 31.3 Wellcome classification.

Weight % of standard*	Oedema Present	Oedema Absent
60–80	Kwashiorkor	Underweight
< 60	Marasmic kwashiorkor	Marasmus

*Median of National Child Health Statistics (NCHS) or Harvard standards.[6]

Table 31.4 WHO classification of severe malnutrition.

Weight for height Standard deviation (or Z) score	Weight for height Percentage of median NCHS/WHO reference	Oedema
< –3	< 70%	Irrespective of weight or height

Adapted from *Management of severe malnutrition: a manual for physicians and other senior health workers.* Geneva WHO, 1999.

WHO classification

This uses weight for height and oedema measurements. Those with oedema are described as oedematous malnutrition irrespective of weight (Table 31.4).[8]

Aetiology
Nutrient deficiency

Breast feeding

Prolonged breast-feeding for one to two years or longer is common in many traditional societies. However, rarely is it exclusive; additional foods/fluids may be introduced as early as the first month of life. In poor societies, absence of breast-feeding or cessation before six months of age is associated with early onset of malnutrition, especially wasting, and high mortality rates. Prolonged breast-feeding provides important sources of energy and animal protein, and anti-infective factors, but if not supplemented by complementary feeds the child's weight becomes static or falls. In the latter situation, severe malnutrition may follow quickly upon stopping of breast-

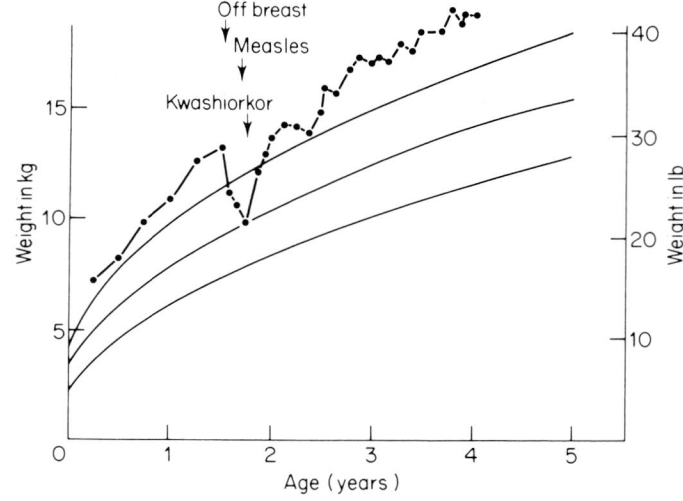

Figure 31.1: Effect of measles on weight gain. (From Morley, Prevention of protein-calorie deficiency syndromes. *Trans R Soc Trop Med Hyg* 1968; 62:200–208.)

feeding, commonly associated with recurrent infections, e.g., diarrhoea or measles (Figure 31.1).[9]

Weaning and infant diets

Diets often consist of single staples, e.g., millet, sorghum, maize or rice, which are usually bulky with high water content, low energy density and have high phytate levels (especially maize). High phytate concentrations reduce the bioavailability of nutrients such as zinc, iron and calcium. Contamination by pathogenic micro-organisms is common. Where the major component of diet is root crops, e.g., cassava, yams, potatoes or bananas, there is a low protein:energy ratio. Single-cereal diets may be deficient in a specific essential amino acids, e.g., tryptophan (maize) or lysine (cereals in general) and require to be balanced by a complementary plant protein source like legumes, e.g., beans, lentils, chickpeas and groundnuts, or even better, animal protein which has a high biological value, e.g., milk (human or animal), meat and eggs. Sick children require frequent meals during and for two weeks after the infection to assist catch-up growth.

Infection

Infection may cause severe weight loss through anorexia, catabolic loss and tissue depletion.[1,3] There are few prospective studies on the immunological effects of infection on growing children. Most studies are on hospitalized children with severe malnutrition. Of the latter, children with oedematous malnutrition tend to have more immune suppression than those with wasting only. Cell-mediated immunity is often severely depressed.[2] Their β lymphocytes and immunoglobulins are usually normal or raised due to recurrent infections (polyclonal stimulation), but the immune response to infections may be suboptimal. Complement is reduced. Activity of neutrophils in 'killing' ingested bacteria may also be depressed. An important factor in depression of the immune system associated with recurrent infections is failure of the system to recover because of nutrient deficiency, e.g., defective protein metabolism and micronutrient deficiency, especially zinc. Zinc is also important in promoting growth during rehabilitation[10] and in the prevention and management of persistent diarrhoea.[11]

Most children have a gut and/or respiratory infection and bacteraemia is common often due to Gram negative bacteria, including salmonellae. Urinary tract infection is not infrequent. Tuberculosis and HIV may be underlying factors. Infections may be difficult to diagnose clinically as the temperature may be normal (or subnormal), the pulse not increased nor the neutrophil count raised. Hydration may be difficult to assess and clinical signs of pneumonia may be minimal despite radiological changes.[7]

HIV infection

HIV-infected children are more likely to be marasmic and respond poorly to nutritional rehabilitation. Malnutrition occurs despite apparently reasonable breast milk intake. Chronic diarrhoea, persistent respiratory infections, tuberculosis and sometimes severe dermatological disorders are common. Their HIV-infected mothers may be symptomatic, depressed and have difficulty in coping.[7]

Epidemiology

The onset of frank malnutrition frequently dates from the time that breast-feeding stopped and/or of a severe infection. If the infant is bottle fed onset is usually in the first six months of life, usually with wasting. Artifical or cow's milk is often over diluted and infected. Otherwise, in breast fed children malnutrition usually presents in the second and third years. However, malnutrition may occur earlier in tuberculosis and HIV infection despite apparent adequate breast milk intake.

Geographical disposition

Kwashiorkor is associated with areas where staples have a low protein:energy ratio, e.g., root crops and bananas, or a maize diet (poor bioavailability of protein).[1] These foods may also be deficient in micronutrients. Kwashiorkor is not common in fish eating or cattle herding communities where diets are likely to be supplemented by animal protein. Comparison between village children in Keneba, The Gambia and the Baganda area of southern Uganda showed distinct differences in nutrition, growth and endocrine response.[12,13] In The Gambia, where the predominant type of malnutrition is marasmus, the main staple is a millet gruel which is low in energy. In the Baganda area of Uganda, kwashiorkor is the predominant type of malnutrition, the major staple is bananas (Matoke) and their diet has a lower protein:energy ratio than those in The Gambia. However, the energy intake was inadequate in both communities.

There are reports of kwashiorkor in middle-class American infants without significant infection, fed on low protein:energy ratio 'fad' diets.[14]

Season

In many parts of the world there is an increased rate of malnutrition in the wet (or hungry) season. There is deficiency of food as the previous year's crop has been consumed and families may have to survive on a meagre diet of fruits or vegetables while awaiting the harvest. Admissions for malnutrition often increase following an epidemic of measles. During the rains there is an increase in some infections, e.g., diarrhoea and malaria. The roads are often inaccessible and inhibit travel for medical care. Women are often busy working on the land and leave the younger children at home to be looked after and fed by siblings or relatives. They may only breast-feed at night or not at all.

Aetiology of kwashiorkor

The aetiology of hypoalbuminaemia and oedema in kwashiorkor has been debated since the 1930–50s when the simplistic theory of dietary protein deficiency was proposed by Cecily Williams who coined the name kwashiorkor.[15] Kwashiorkor is the name given by the Ga people in Ghana for 'the disease of the child displaced from the breast'. Recent theories include free radical generation[16-19] and aflatoxin toxicity.[20,21] Essentially, in malnutrition there is adaptation to an inadequate diet by a reduction in metabolic activity. This 'adaptation' is stressed and compromized by infection.

The cause of hypoalbuminaemia is generally considered to relate to failure of the liver to produce sufficient albumin. However, increased catabolic rate associated with infection may also be a factor.[22] Interleukin-1 and tumour necrosis factor released from macrophages depress albumin synthesis and divert amino acids to the production of acute phase reactants. There may be loss from a damaged gut and perhaps loss through capillary leak possibly associated with increased levels of leukotrienes.[23] In nutritionally vulnerable children a fall in serum albumin and lipoprotein levels commonly occurs in response to infections.[24]

Oedema occurs essentially due to retention of sodium and water. Capillary leak may also be a factor during the initial stages associated with inflammation and release of cytokines.[25] However, the cause of sodium and water retention in hypoalbuminaemic states, e.g., kwashiorkor, nephrotic syndrome, is still debated.[1,16,26-31]

In kwashiorkor, oedema may resolve during the initial stages of management on a low protein diet (0.6 g/kg) before serum albumin levels rise.[29] However, serum albumin may not reflect total vascular albumin mass or oncotic pressure.[27,31] Factors involved in clearance of established oedema may include restoration of homeostasis with stabilization of intracellular metabolism and cellular membranes of the kidney and other cells, and provision of energy and potassium. Experiments on red blood cells and leucocytes from kwashiorkor children suggest an increased permeability of the cell membranes associated with excess activity of the sodium pump, which, if operative in the kidney tubules, could result in excess fluid reabsorption.[26]

Free radicals

Free radicals (FR) are atoms or molecules containing unpaired electrons. They are unstable and highly reactive. Sepsis is particularly associated with increased generation of FR. In infection, there is a vigorous response to endotoxins by the immune system with release of cytokines, e.g., tumour necrosis factor and γ interferon which stimulates activation of polymorphonuclear cells that, in return, result in free radical generation. Antioxidants prevent either the initiation of the FR chain reaction or, once formed, their propagation. Superoxide

dismutase is a metalloenzyme containing zinc, copper, or manganese and is a major antioxidant. Selenium is the trace metal associated with glutathione peroxidase. Other antioxidants include vitamins, β carotene, E, C and riboflavin. Generally, kwashiorkor have lower levels of micronutrients than marasmus.[16] Whether this is due to deficient intake (suggesting differential diets between kwashiorkor and marasmus), reduced binding capacity of serum proteins, maldistribution because of the metabolic disorder, or increased loss, is not certain. Free iron can catalyse FR reactions and high levels of stored or free iron are detected in PEM.[16,30,32] Reduced glutathione and glutathione peroxidase are important intracellular compounds in protection against FR damage, and low levels are considered to be a marker of FR activity. Lower levels of reduced glutathione have been detected in red blood cells in kwashiorkor than marasmus and levels of thiobarbituric acid-reactive substances, a marker of lipid peroxidation, are raised in kwashiorkor.[16,17,33] These findings suggest there is more FR activity in kwashiorkor than marasmus. However, some studies have shown an overlap in reduced glutathione and glutathione peroxidase levels between kwashiorkor and marasmus.[17,18,32] In addition, there is a very slow restoration of reduced glutathione to normal levels despite a clinical response.[17] The low glutathione level could be partly due to dietary deficiency of sulphur-containing amino acids, e.g.—methionine, which are low in kwashiorkor.[34] Methionine is also essential for functions of the $Na^+/K^+/ATPase$ pump (sodium pump). Impaired sodium pump activity results in a large excess of intracellular sodium and a huge deficit in intracellular potassium. These intracellular electrolyte changes also occur in marasmus.

Increased FR activity appears to be established in children with severe malnutrition, especially those with oedema and kwashiorkor. Whether they are the cause or result of the condition, and whether any specific therapy would be effective at the advanced stage of disease at which these children are admitted remains to be seen. To date the main actions stemming from the above research is the provision of zinc and copper to solutions used during resuscitation and refeeding (see Table 31.6).

Aflatoxins

Aflatoxins are common contaminants of foods in tropical countries where the fungus *Aflatoxin flavus* thrives in the warm humid climate. Aflatoxins are commonly detected in urine of healthy adults and children in tropical countries, and they have also been detected in cord blood and breast milk.[20,21,35] Large doses administered to animals may be lethal and result in liver damage, profound metabolic disorders including hypoalbuminaemia and immunosuppression.

Studies in malnourished children in some (but not all) areas have demonstrated higher frequency and concentration of aflatoxins in blood of kwashiorkor than marasmus patients, and aflatoxical, a reversible derivative of aflatoxin B$_1$, has been detected in blood of kwashiorkor patients only.[20] Studies on autopsies[35] and biopsies[36] of livers from PEM children have demonstrated that aflatoxin detection is virtually confined to oedematous children. The above findings suggest there is a clear difference in liver metabolism of aflatoxins between kwashiorkor and marasmus. This is most likely due to liver dysfunction in kwashiorkor. However, in sick kwashiorkor children aflatoxin toxicity may be an additional aetiological factor in the metabolic disturbance.

Growth difference between kwashiorkor and marasmus patients

Kwashiorkor patients tend to be taller, heavier (more fat) and have larger head circumference, and less delayed milestones than marasmic children.[37] This may be due to the chronicity of disease, poorer socio-economic background and, in some cases, low birth weight in marasmus (and some marasmic kwashiorkor). However, the better growth of children predisposed to develop kwashiorkor may be a factor in aetiology by increasing the demand for energy, protein and micronutrients, thus making them more vulnerable when infection and acute deficits of nutrients occur.[13] Genetic factors may also be operative where the demand for nutrients may be higher in some children than others.[1]

Clinical features

In marasmus the main findings are growth failure with severe wasting of muscle and fat (Figure 31.2). There may be hair changes in longstanding cases. In kwashiorkor there is oedema, hair changes, skin changes (not always) and often an enlarged liver. Kwashiorkor tends to have an acute onset (Figure 31.3). Marasmic kwashiorkor has similar features to kwashiorkor, but there is more wasting and they are also more stunted and often have higher mortality rate. The main biochemical difference between marasmus and kwashiorkor is hypoalbuminaemia (present in kwashiorkor).

The following signs should be looked for:

Anaemia is common but is not usually severe, e.g., mean Hb 8 g/dl. It is due to a mixed deficiency of micronutrients, e.g., iron, folic acid and riboflavin and general depression of metabolism. An acute fall in haemoglobin may follow malaria or other infections. In older children hookworm may be a factor.

Oedema may vary from slight in the feet and legs with some swelling of the cheeks to marked and generalized. It can be exacerbated by giving excess oral rehydration fluid. Ascites is rare. Severe ileus may give an impression of ascites.

Hair changes, especially in colour, may antedate the florid appearance of malnutrition by some months. There may be dyspigmentation (change of colour to red or fair),

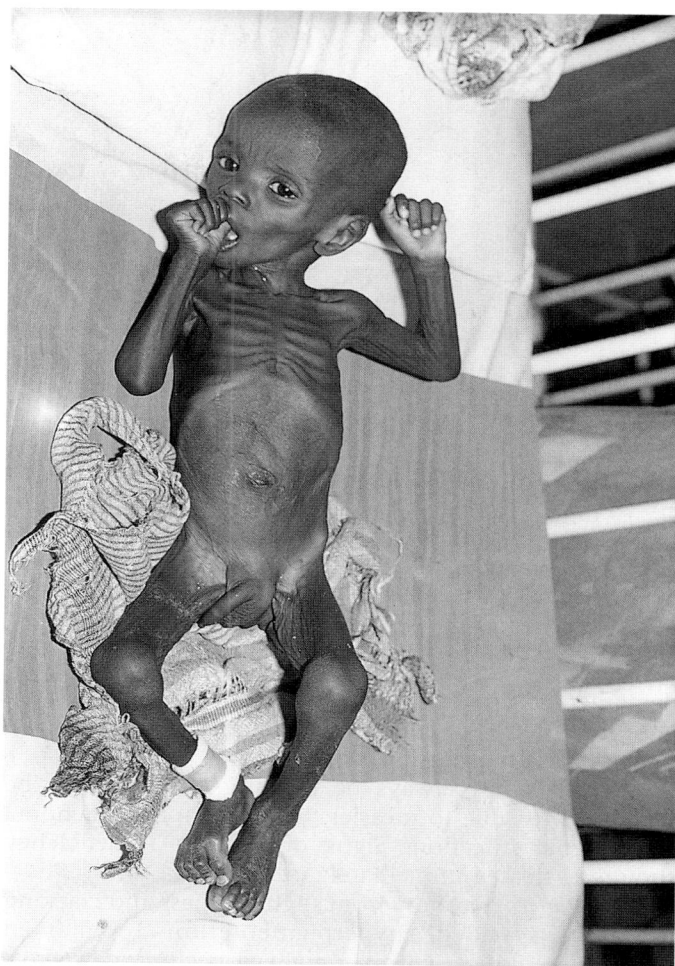

Figure 31.2: An 18-month-old Sudanese boy with marasmus. The mother has shaved his head because of hair changes.

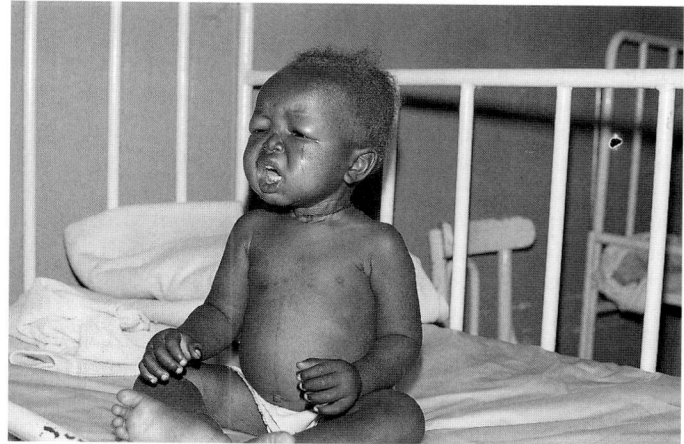

Figure 31.3: An 18-month-old Sudanese boy with acute kwashiorkor. Weight for age is above 80 per cent of standard. There is retention of fat and no skin changes.

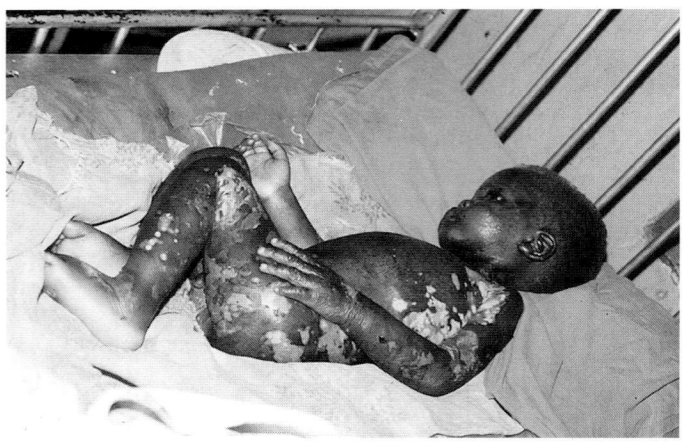

Figure 31.4: An 18-month-old apathetic Ugandan boy with kwashiorkor and persistent diarrhoea. There is widespread hyperpigmentated, flaky-paint skin changes with underlying hypopigmented areas. His hair is dyspigmented, sparse, straight and easily pluckable. The cheeks are puffy (moon facies).

sparseness (loss of hair), dry and thin hair fibres, loss of curls and easy-pluckability. The flag sign, alternating depigmented and normal hair, may be seen in children with long hair (not curly). Hair changes are common in longstanding malnutrition.

The *eyes* must always be examined. There may be conjunctivitis due to measles, herpes simplex, trachoma or bacterial infection. Signs of vitamin A deficiency should be treated immediately (see Table 31.8).

Skin changes may vary from slight dryness and cracking or mild 'speckled' hyperpigmentation to marked hyperpigmentation with generalized peeling, e.g., flaky paint dermatosis (Figure 31.4). Ulcers may develop in flexures and around the perineum. Purpura may occur. Peeling is usually only seen in those with oedema or with a history of oedema. There may be generalized loss of skin pigment or in areas where peeling has occurred, localized hypopigmentation. Consider HIV infection if there is severe ulceration and multiple infected areas.

Mucosal changes include angular stomatitis, cheilosis and glossitis (smooth red tongue). Angular stomatitis is an important cause of anorexia. Oral thrush is common.

Liver size may vary from impalpable to grossly enlarged. It is more likely to be enlarged in those with oedema. In kwashiorkor, the liver is usually fatty (whether enlarged or not). Fatty change is considered to be due to reduced lipoprotein production and thus inability to transport lipids (triglycerides) from the liver. Fat clears spontaneously with rehabilitation and there is no residual liver damage. Serum bilirubin and transaminases are usually normal except in severe or lethal cases.

Lymphadenopathy is uncommon except in cases of local infection, tuberculosis or HIV infection. Other lymphoid tissues, e.g., tonsils, are also small.

There may be a chronic enteropathy in the *gut*, with variable degrees of villous atrophy due to infection, nutrient deficiency and possibly bacterial overgrowth.

Protein loosing enteropathy may complicate measles and probably also persistent diarrhoea.

Brain: Mental changes vary from just irritability and lethargy to profound apathy (especially kwashiorkor) or semi-consciousness. Reversible shrinkage of cerebral tissue has been demonstrated on brain imaging in kwashiorkor and less frequently in marasmus. Long-term effects are related to age of onset, longevity of malnutrition, poverty and lack of education and intellectual stimulation in the child's home environment.[38]

Management[8]

The majority of deaths occur within the first week of admission (80%). To reduce the mortality rate, special care has to be given during this period. The basic principle is, after initial resuscitation, to give high energy feeds with increased protein so that the child regains weight as rapidly as possible compatible with safety. Measles vaccination should be given to children >6 months of age both on admission and discharge.

Resuscitation (first 1–7 days)

Avoid intravenous (IV) therapy if possible. Give modified WHO oral rehydration solution (ORS) (Table 31.5) over 4–10 hours, 5 ml/kg every 30 min for 2 hours then 6–10 ml/kg hourly for 4–10 hr. It has a lower sodium than standard ORS and additional potassium and minerals (Table 31.6). *Great care must be taken to prevent overhydration.* When hydrated (usually 4–6 hr) commence *phase I* formula (Table 31.7), 130 ml/kg/day (100 ml/kg/day for oedematous children) as per the *feeding regimen*. If IV therapy is required, give Ringer lactate with 5% dextrose 15 ml/kg over 1 hour, then 10 ml/kg/hour over next

Table 31.5 Modified WHO ORS solution: (low sodium).

Water	2 litres
WHO–ORS	1 packet
Sugar	50 g
Electrolyte/mineral solution (Table 6)	40 ml

If electrolyte/mineral solution is not available give additional potassium, 40 mmol/l

Table 31.6 Electrolyte/mineral solution*.

	grams	Molar content of 20 ml (mmol)
Potassium chloride	224	24
Tripotassium citrate	81	2
Magnesium chloride	76	3
Zinc acetate	8.2	300
Copper sulphate	1.4	45
Water:	to 2500 ml	–

*Available from Nutriset, Bois du Roule, BP 35, 76770 Malouney, France

Table 31.7 Phase I: Low protein milk formula.

	Milk (g)	Sugar* (g)	Vegetable oil (g)	Electrolyte/mineral mix (ml)	Water (ml)
Fresh cow's milk	300 (ml)	100	20	20	to 1000
Whole dried milk	35	100	20	20	to 1000
Dried skimmed milk	25	100	30	20	to 1000

Contains 0.9 g protein and 75 kcal/100 ml.
*A low osmolar feed can be prepared by replacing 30 g sugar with 35 g cereal/flour solution which is cooked for 4 minutes. Is useful for osmotic diarrhoea.

5 hours or so. Whole blood may be required for septic shock not responding to above.

Diarrhoea usually settles over 3–5 days. Lactose intolerance may be treated with yoghurt and/or a cereal/oil/sugar mix. In the rare situation where milk protein sensitivity is considered, alternative sources of protein include chicken, fish or soy protein. Give metronidazole if *Giardia lamblia* is detected or if treatment of anaerobic bacterial colonization of bowel is considered.

Hypothermia (rectal temp <35.5°C): Use low reading thermometer. Clothe child, including the head, and keep in warm room. Check for hypoglycaemia.

Hypoglycaemia (blood glucose <3 mmol/l): Use glucose test strip. If able to drink, give 50 ml of 10% glucose solution or sugared water (1 teaspoon sugar to 3½ tablespoons of water). If blood glucose remains low repeat glucose or sugar solution. If unconscious/convulsing, give 5 ml/kg 10% dextrose IV or 50 ml of 10% glucose by nasogastric tube.

Infection: For mildly sick children showing no signs of infection, give cotrimoxazole for 5 days. For ill children give ampicillin (parenterally for at least 2–3 days) + gentamicin for 7 days. If poor response by 48 hr, add chloramphenicol. Consider tuberculosis or HIV infection in children who fail to respond to nutritional rehabilitation.

Blood transfusion: 10 ml/kg whole blood should be given over 3 hours plus frusamide 1 mg/kg at commencement to anaemic children (Hb <4g/dl) who are sick. If heart failure is suspected, give 10 ml/kg of packed cells.

Electrolytes and minerals: Potassium 6–8 mmol/kg/day should be given for 1–2 weeks or so. When high protein and energy formula is given only 1–2 mmol potassium supplements are then required. Where possible magnesium 2–3 mmol/kg/day and other metals as per Table 31.6 should also be given. If this solution is unavailable, give zinc 2 mg/kg/day and one intramuscular injection of 50% magnesium sulphate 0.3 ml/kg (maximum 2 ml).

Table 31.8 Vitamin A supplements.

Age	
Infants <6 months	50,000 IU
Infants 6–11 months	100,000 IU
Children 12 months plus	200,000 IU

1 capsule = 50,000 IU vitamin A
If measles or xerophthalmia present repeat does next day. For xerophthalmia give third dose 4–5 weeks later.

Vitamin A: If vitamin A has not been given in the last month, give as capsules as per the doses listed in Table 31.8. If unable to take orally, give 100 000 units (55 mg) IM (water miscible). Additional doses are required for measles and xerophthalmia.

Anti-malarials: Administer in endemic areas as clinically indicated.

Intestinal parasites: Mebendazole (500 mg, single dose or 100 mg bid for 3 days) may be indicated in children older than 12 months in areas where parasites such as hookworm and *Ascaris lumbricoides* are prevalent.

Rehabilitation

This is the phase of gradual increase in energy and protein intake until values such as 150–220 kcalories/kg/day (normal requirement 100–110 kcalories) and protein 4–6 g/kg/day (normal 1.5–2 g/kg/day) are reached. To supply this amount of energy and protein without increasing the volume of fluid to excessive amounts, energy-rich food, such as vegetable oil and sugar are added to the energy/protein source, which is preferably milk (fresh or powder) (Tables 31.7 and 31.9).

Feeding regimen (phase I and II)

Phase I formula is given 2 hourly, including during the night. Unless the child is able to take all the milk by cup,

Table 31.9 Phase 2: High energy milk formula.

	Milk (g)	Sugar* (g)	Vegetable oil (g)	Electrolyte/mineral mix (ml)	Water (ml)
Fresh cow's milk	880 (ml)	75	20	20	to 1000
Whole dried milk	110	50	30	20	to 1000
Dried skimmed milk	80	50	60	20	to 1000

*Contains 2.9 g protein and 100 kcal/100 ml.

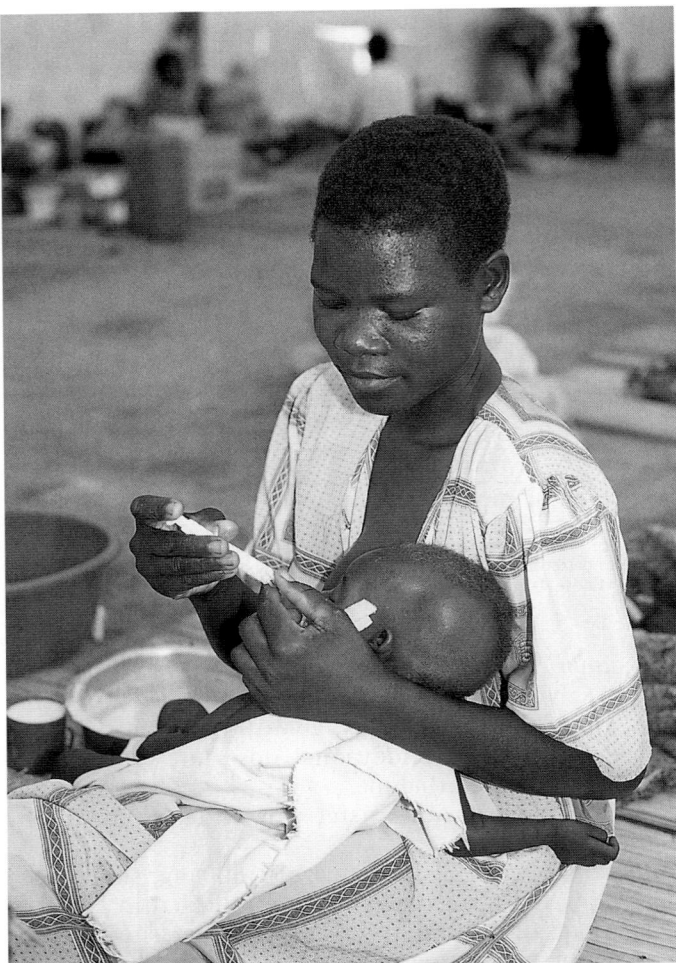

Figure 31.5: A mother tube feeding her malnourished child by syringe in a rehabilitation unit in northern Uganda.

it should be given wholly or partly by nasogastric tube. Frequency of feeds is increased to 3–4 hourly over the next week or so. Mothers should be taught to give milk by spoon/syringe (Figure 31.5). A gradual change-over from phase I to phase II should take approximately 3–4 days commencing after about a week. The volume of feed is gradually increased from 100 ml in phase I up to a maximum of around 200 ml/kg body weight in phase II.

As soon as the child wants food he is offered a normal diet in addition to his full requirement of phase II formula. Mothers should continue breast-feeding preferably after the formula feed.

The mother should receive advice on infant feeding and health education and should be encouraged to participate as much as possible in the feeding of her child.

Additional treatment

Folic acid 5mg on day 1 and 1 mg daily for 2–3 months. *Iron*—ferrous sulphate or gluconate 3 mg/kg/day for 3 months. Start iron 2 weeks after admission when the child starts to gain weight. *Multivitamin* solution should

also be administered. Extra vitamin K should be given if purpura or bleeding tendency is present.

Discharge

When the child has regained an appetite and is over 90% weight for height it is safe to discharge. This usually takes 4–6 weeks or more.[39] In busy, overcrowded units 80% weight for height may be acceptable. Relapse is less likely if follow-up is provided. Transfer to a nutritional rehabilitation unit when the child is able to take mixed diet may also help to reinforce education of the mother. Emotional (as well as medical) support for the child is essential during rehabilitation, especially in children of socially disrupted families. Encourage the family to stimulate and play with their child.

Milder cases and rehabilitated children are treated at a nutritional rehabilitation unit either on a daily basis (day-care centre) or through home visits. Very poor families may require food supplements, otherwise all children are given vitamin/mineral and iron/folic acid supplements.

Prognosis

Case fatality rates may range from 5 to 50% with a median of 20–30%.[40] The highest mortality rate occurs in oedematous malnutrition, especially marasmic kwashiorkor. The aim should be approximately 5–10% mortality rate. High mortality rates reflect both the severity of malnutrition on admission and management.

Mortality rates after discharge may be 10% or more. This depends on a number of factors including the condition of the child on discharge, the level of education of the mother, her ability to afford the necessary additional food and nutrients for catch-up growth, and facilities for, and compliance with follow-up.

Malnutrition in adults

The aetiology of malnutrition in adults is similar to children, although clinical manifestations may differ, e.g., effusions into serous cavities and ascites may be seen in adults.[1] The stresses that cause malnutrition may also differ, e.g., the necessity to continue manual work despite dietary inadequacy and/or infections; prison and concentration camps; famine, where adults may have to continue to use energy in obtaining food and caring for the young; psychiatric disorders and in postsurgical or secondary malnutrition. In areas where kwashiorkor in children is common and adults are subject to extreme dietary, physical and mental stress as in war, typical cases of kwashiorkor including skin changes, are seen in adolescents and adults.

A considerable amount of research has been undertaken on famine oedema in adults occurring during the First World War (1914–1918), the Second World War (1939–1945) in Europe and in Japanese prisoner camps and famines in Asia and Africa. The main controversy concerned the importance of hypoalbuminaemia.[1,16,41]

When serum albumin levels are borderline, a dilute, salted vegetable diet may precipitate oedema, as may excess ORS in children with marasmus. Hypo-albuminaemia was less common in studies of oedematous subjects after the Second World War in Europe than in famine oedema in Asia and Africa. This may have been due to more prolonged dietary protein and micronutrient deficiency in the latter.[41] Other causes of oedema in adults include dropsy caused by consumption of contaminated cottonseed or mustard oil and beriberi.

Iodine deficiency disorders

The term iodine deficiency disorders (IDD) replaces the terms 'endemic goitre' and 'cretinism' and emphasizes the wider spectrum of disorders which occurs as a result of iodine deficiency or the effect of goitrogens. The disorders include, apart from cretinism and varying degrees of brain damage, goitre and hypothyroidism in neonates, children and adults.

Epidemiology

Low iodine intake is related to lack of iodine in the environment. Areas of iodine deficiency are usually those far away from the sea, where iodine originally present in soil was leached by high rainfall and snow. The amount of iodine returned to the soil by rainwater is small and, as a result, many areas have insufficient iodine in the environment. The World Health Organization has estimated that in 1994 1.5 billion people were at risk in 118 countries, and 20 million people have varying degrees of preventable brain damage due to effects of iodine deficiency on fetal brain development. In the tropics it is found in Africa, Central and South America and in Asia and Papua New Guinea. Those exhibiting goitre are estimated at between 200 and 300 million. Goitre becomes endemic when the total goitre rate is 10% or more, or the visible goitre rate is 1% or more.

In western Africa nearly all countries are affected by IDD with an epicentre in Guinea.[42] It is a problem in the Atlas Mountains, Nile Valley, highland areas of Kenya, Tanzania, Rwanda, Burundi, Cameroon, and The Gambia. Central Africa contains some of the most severely affected populations in the world. In Central and South America, IDD occurs widely. Ecuador, Peru and Bolivia are particularly affected.The most affected populations in Asia are China, India, Indonesia, Nepal, Myanmar and Bangladesh.

Aetiology

Inadequate intake of iodine leads to reduced production of thyroid hormone and stimulation of thyroid-stimulating hormone (TSH) production. TSH increases thyroid hormone production resulting in the thyroid gland becoming hyperplastic and goitrous. The cause of endemic goitre is a failure of the thyroid gland to obtain adequate iodine to maintain its natural structure and function. Apart from iodine deficiency, other factors also influence iodine balance. Thiocyanate, a metabolic product of several factors, competitively inhibits active transport and is goitragenic. Dietary goitrogens are found in cassava, lime beans, sweet potatoes, cabbage and broccoli and certain types of millets. Cassava has been implicated as an important contributing factor in Zaire. Goitrogenic factors seem to be superimposed on primary iodine deficiency.

Pathology

In the later chronic stages when iodine stores are exhausted, the thyroid gland becomes soft and enlarged (goitre) with a large number of colloid follicles. Nodular formation takes place and haemorrhage and calcification may occur. The gland does not become 'toxic' and malignancy does not occur.

Iodine deficiency is the most common cause of preventable mental retardation in the world. The term 'endemic cretinism' refers to a combination of mental deficiency, deaf mutism and motor rigidity or, less commonly, to severe hypothyroidism. The two forms are often referred to as neurologic cretinism and hypothyroid cretinism, and can occur separately or together. They should be distinguished from 'sporadic cretinism' which results from congenital hypothyroidism and occurs worldwide. Endemic cretinism is associated with iodine deficiency that is sufficiently severe to cause goitre in 3% or more of the population, reaching 5–10% in areas with severe iodine deficiency. It appears that severe deficiency may be responsible for the impaired neurological development of the fetus from early in pregnancy.[43]

Clinical features

Goitre

Large goitres are easily recognized. Sizes are classified into three grades as shown below.[44] Tracheal pressure may interfere with the recurrent laryngeal nerve and produce hoarseness. Choking may occur with monstrous goitres. The patient is almost always euthyroid.

Classification of goitre:

0   No goitre
1A   Goitre detectable only by palpation
1B   Goitre palpable and visible when neck fully extended. Includes nodular glands if not goitrous
II   Goitre visible with neck in normal position
III   Very large goitre recognizable from a distance

Endemic cretinism

This includes severe mental deficiency and there is a characteristic facies. Neurological cretinism includes defects of hearing, speech, squint and spastic displagia of varying degrees. Myxoedematous cretinism includes the predominant feature of profound hypothyroidism and short stature. Neuromotor deficits are less profound than in the neurologic cretin and hearing is preserved.

Reproductive failure

There is higher risk of abortions, miscarriages, stillbirths, low birth weight and increased perinatal and infant mortality.

Diagnosis

Measurement of iodine in the urine is the most precise index of dietary iodine intake. Mild IDD occurs with iodine excretion ranging from 50–100 µg daily and in severe IDD the excretion is below 25 µg daily. In endemic goitre, serum T_4 levels are often low with a normal or slightly elevated serum T_3 and an increased TSH. In some countries newborns are screened for blood thyroxine and low levels identified which require immediate thyroxine replacement therapy.

Treatment

Cretinism with its associated mental deficiency cannot be reversed through treatment. For the myxodematous type thyroxine and iodine supplementation reduce the effects of hypothyroidism. Goitres in older children and adults may disappear completely following iodine administration. Beneficial results will be observed in 4–6 weeks. Advanced goitres must be treated surgically if causing symptoms.

Prevention

Fortification of salt for human and animal consumption is the method of choice for the prevention of IDD.[45] In Africa virtually all edible salt is iodized in several countries. The level of iodine in salt must be enough to meet the minimum daily iodine requirement of 150 µg per person. Iodination of irrigation water has also been used in China.[46] Iodinized oil is the major alternative and is the best option for severely afflicted areas. It is administered by intramuscular injection or the oral route. The recommended dose is 480 mg iodine (1 ml) for subjects 1 year or older and 240 mg iodine in infants. This is effective for at least one to two years.[47] Priority should be given to improving the iodine status of adolescent girls and young women before they begin pregnancy.

Scurvy

The disease is due to lack of vitamin C which is essential for collagen formation.

Epidemiology

Scurvy does not commonly affect any population as it did in the past, and therefore may be overlooked. Frank scurvy is uncommon and is most likely to occur in tropical areas where fresh fruit and vegetables are sparse. Babies are especially vulnerable when they are fed on dried cereals and boiled milk. Soldiers, prisoners and refugees in camps in dry desert areas are particularly vulnerable.[48] The possibility of widespread subclinical deficiency in these areas cannot be ruled out. A form of scurvy has been extensively studied in South Africa amongst Bantu male labourers who developed haemachromatosis attributed to drinking large quantities of beer. It was thought that vitamin C in the body was irreversibly oxidized by large deposits of ferric iron in tissues.

Pathology

Vitamin C is required for the formation of fibrous collagen in connective tissue and bone. This leads to extravasation of blood, loosening of teeth and easily fractured bones with subperiosteal haemorrhage. Autopsy shows extensive haemorrhage in internal organs.

Clinical features

Infantile scurvy

The majority of cases present in the second half of the first year, especially in premature and artificially fed infants. The three main features are: irritability, leg tenderness and pseudoparalysis. The baby lies in a characteristic position with legs partially flexed at the knees and hips and internally rotated due to pain from subperiosteal haemorrhages. This may be mistaken for rheumatic fever, polio or osteomyelitis because of pain. These extravasations may be palpable at the proximal end of the tibia and distal end of the femur. Costochondral beading (scorbutic rosary) is also usually palpable. The arms are rarely involved. There may be bleeding around erupting teeth. Scorbutic infants do not develop gingivitis (scorbutic buds). Bleeding into the skin is rarely a presenting sign. Hypochromic microcytic anaemia is commonly present. The anaemia may be megablastic due to accompanying folate deficiency resulting from lack of folate coenzymes associated with vitamin C. Pyrexia is frequent with associated infections, especially tuberculosis.

Adult scurvy

There is an insidious onset with weight loss, progressive weakness and aching in bones, joints and muscles especially at night and characteristic stiffness in the leg muscles or other muscles in extensive use. Haematomas form in calf and thigh muscles. Perifollicular haemorrhages occur with subcutaneous petechiae on the limbs and trunk producing scorbutic purpura. Haemorrhage into the myocardium may be life threatening. Splinter haemorrhages may form a crescent on the fingernails. In extreme deficiency the gums become affected with swelling and sponginess of the alveolar margin, which is friable and bleeds readily. Secondary infection, gangrene and loose teeth supervene. Wounds fail to heal and scars break down.

Diagnosis

The main differential diagnosis is from rickets which may coexist as 'scurvy rickets'. Radiography reveals a characteristic ground glass appearance due to generalized osteoporosis and atrophy of the trabeaulae. Epiphyseal ends are sharply outlined. Widening of the zone of provisional calcification causes a dense shadow at the end of the shaft (the white line of Frankel) and this is also seen at the periphery of ossification centres ('halo epiphysis' or pencilled effect). With treatment, even the grossest deformities resolve. The capillary permeability test of Hess using a sphygmomanometer to occlude venous return to the arm results in petechiae appearing. Laboratory tests on plasma or leucocyte levels of ascorbic are sensitive, although plasma levels are influenced by recent dietary intake.

Treatment

In infant scurvy ascorbic acid (50 mg four times daily) should be given for one week, followed by 50 mg twice daily for one month. In the adult the usual dose is 100 mg administered three to five times daily until 4 g has been administered. If the patient is critically ill 1 g can be given daily by intravenous infusion. Vitamin C may also be given as fresh daily orange juice. Severe weakness and bleeding rapidly resolve (48 hours) and haematomas heal within two weeks. Radiological evidence may persist for years.

Prevention

Foods steamed and cooked rapidly retain much of their vitamin C which is destroyed by prolonged cooking. Artificially fed infants require supplements (e.g., fresh orange juice).

Rickets and osteomalacia

Nutritional rickets is still a major problem in many developing countries and is common in North Africa and the Middle East. The term 'rickets' and 'osteomalacia' refer to the histological and radiological abnormalities seen in a variety of vitamin D deficiency conditions.

Aetiology

Vitamin D deficiency results from inadequate dietary intake and/or skin biosynthesis of vitamin D. Rickets describes the disordered growth and mineralization of the growth plate of the long bones. Osteomalacia describes abnormalities resulting from delayed and reduced mineralization of mature bone. Calcium deficiency has been implicated as a cause of rickets in African children with good exposure to sunlight.[49] After weaning, the staple food of many young African children is maize porridge which has low calcium and high fibre content. From 0 to 50 years an adequate vitamin D intake is 200 IU (5 µg) day.

Epidemiology

In the tropics rickets may occur where sunlight is reduced by urban high-rise buildings, and in crowded areas of cities where there are few play areas. It is described in higher socio-economic groups because these mothers tend to keep their babies indoors. Other factors are prolonged breast-feeding, weaning diets with inadequate vitamin D supplementation, high phytate diets, prematurity and low birth weight. Mothers with low sunshine exposure, vegetarians, dark-skinned mothers, cultural habits (e.g., purdah), and mothers with a low dietary intake of vitamin D whose breast-fed infants are at risk.

Pathology

Defective calcification of developing long bones results in slowing of calcium and phosphorus precipitation in the newly formed matrix. A mass of uncalcified osteoid tissue causes enlargement of the growing ends of bone and a softening of all bones in both rickets and osteomalacia.

Clinical features

Rickets

The onset during the first two years of life is later than that in scurvy. The child becomes ill, pale, flabby and irritable, and prone to tetany and laryngeal stridor. There is general physical and mental retardation and deformity of ribs ('rachitic rosary'), spine, pelvis and limbs (widening of wrists and ankles) and short stature (Figure 31.6). Craniotobes occurs due to thinning of the outer table of the skull. The muscles are poorly developed and lack tone. In calcium deficient rickets neither muscle hypotonia nor bone pain are features and cases tend to be older (4–16 years of age). As the child grows, the skeletal changes heal, but marked deformities remain, such as pigeon chest, spinal curvature, knock-knees, and bow legs (Figure 31.7). Clinical rickets is less common in malnourished children, probably because they have less demand for calcium and phosphorus due to slow growth.

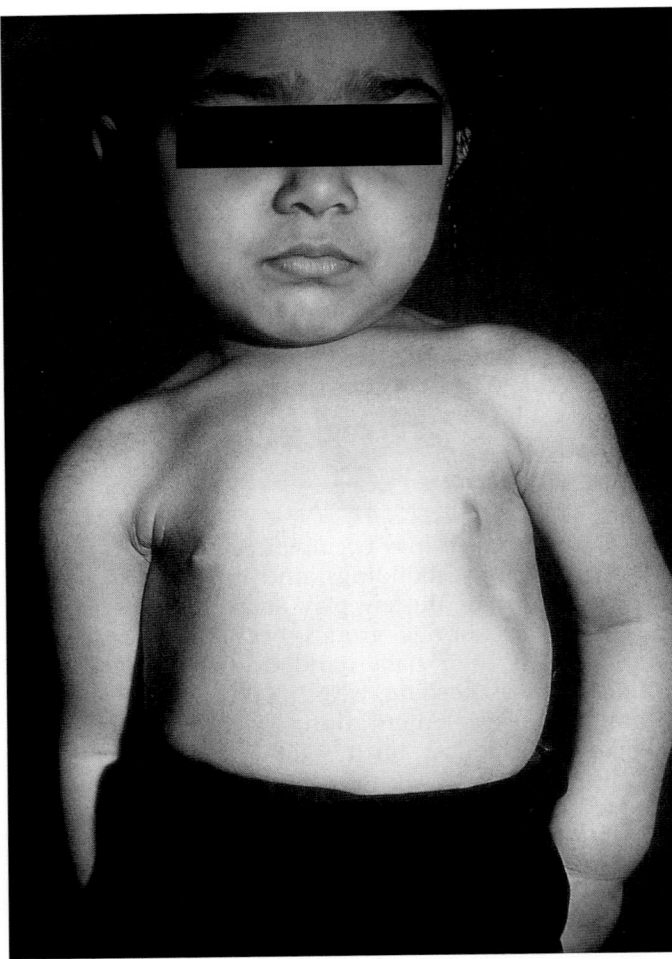

Figure 31.6: Rachitic rosary and chest deformity in a 2-year-old child.

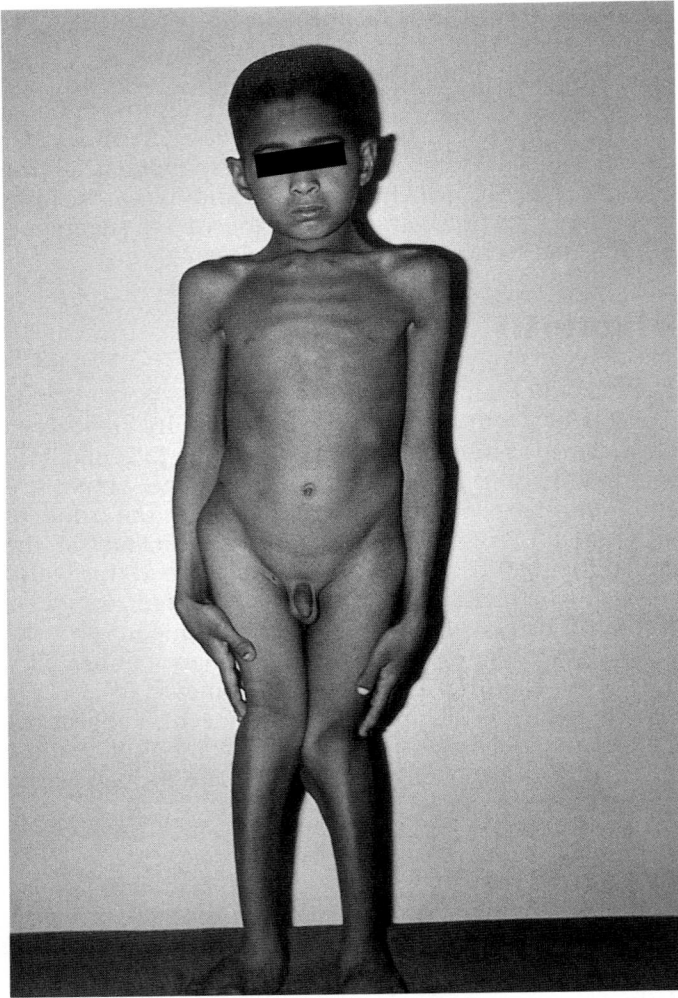

Figure 31.7: Stunting and limb deformity in a boy with ricketts from northern Pakistan.

Osteomalacia

This occurs in women of child-bearing age—usually in the first pregnancy. The bones of the pelvic girdle, ribs and femora become soft, painful and deformed. The gait is characteristic. Tetany is common. Anaemia is present and spontaneous fracture(s) occur. Fetal bones do not show signs of rickets.

Complications

Rickets may have severe consequences. It is strongly associated with pneumonia in young children in developing countries.[50] The relative risk of death for the children with rickets compared with those without was 1:7. Bony deformity of the pelvis in women leads to obstructed labour and increased perinatal morbidity and mortality rates.

Diagnosis

The distinction from infantile scurvy may be difficult, but rickets usually occurs in older infants and there are

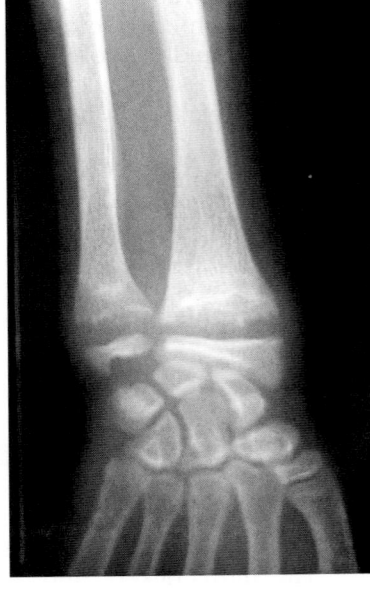

Figure 31.8: Radiological changes of rickets showing fraying, cupping and decreased density.

no subperiosteal haemorrhages; other possibilities are congenital syphilis, achondroplasia and osteogenesis imperfecta. Renal rickets does not respond to vitamin D. Radiographs show characteristic epiphyseal changes (cupping, fraying and decreased density; Figure 31.8). Early in vitamin D deficiency the following values are typically seen: a normal fasting serum calcium; low-normal to low phosphorus; low 25 (OH) D; elevated levels of PTH, 1,25 $(OH)_2D$ and alkaline phosphatase.

Treatment

Natural and artificial light are effective, but therapy is primarily based on providing an adequate calcium and vitamin D intake. The daily administration of 50–150 µg (2000–6000 IU) of vitamin D_3, or 0.5-2 µg of 1,25 $(OH)_2D$ will produce healing within 2–4 weeks. Calcium can be taken as milk, up to 500 ml daily. Administering 15 000 µg (600 000 IU) intravenously in a single dose may allow more rapid healing.

Vitamin B₁ deficiency (beriberi)
Epidemiology

Until recently, beriberi was common in many tropical and subtropical areas and was endemic in countries of Asia and the Far East, where highly milled rice was the staple cereal. It was the scourge of plantations in Malaysia, China and Indonesia and caused enormous mortality and morbidity rates. Outbreaks have occurred in ship's crews, mining communities, institutions such as mental homes and amongst prisoners of war in the Far East in the Second World War (1939–1945). Endemic beriberi can show a seasonal pattern with increasing incidence in the pre-harvest farming months, possibly related to physical exertion at this time. Incidence has decreased with improved eating habits, but the reappearance of thiamin deficiency has been reported in Japan, The Gambia and South Africa. It remains endemic in Thailand, China, Burma and Vietnam.[51] Cases of infantile beriberi have been frequently seen in refugee camps in Thailand.

Aetiology

Thiamin is present in the tissues in the phosphorylated form and a continuous supply is required to satisfy the body's relatively high turnover rate as little is stored. It acts as a co-enzyme for carbohydrate metabolism in the Krebs citric acid cycle and exerts a role in the oxidative breakdown of pyruvic acid. Since the brain nervous tissue and heart muscle use large amounts of glucose, it is in these tissues that carbohydrate metabolism is especially deranged in thiamin deficiency. Thiamin is also involved

in acetylcholine synthesis and in neurotransmission. Lactic acid accumulates with breakdown of the Krebs cycle, producing a metabolic acidosis.

The germ and bran portions of cereal grains contain the most thiamin. Highly milled rice is particularly low in thiamin (60 µg per 100 g), although parboiling, prior to milling, retains much of the thiamin. The discovery that milling of rice was an etiological factor was of great value in the prevention of beriberi. However, any factor leading to an increased thiamin demand may be etiological. For example young men are often affected possibly because they work hardest; onset may be associated with fever,[52] infections including dysentery, and HIV infection; other factors such as pregnancy, lactation and rapid growth may exacerbate sub-clinical deficiency. Thiamin levels in the milk secreted by thiamin-depleted mothers will be inadequate to prevent beriberi in the suckling infant. Antithiamin factors (thiaminases) occurring in foods can alter thiamin structure and reduce biological activity. Thiaminases are found in raw freshwater fish and shellfish, in several micro-organisms and in some vegetables, plants and tea.

True alcoholic beriberi is a form of oedematous cardiac disease with high output failure in severe alcoholics. It has been described as 'palm-wine tappers heart' in Gambia, as palm tappers work strenuously climbing trees and consume substantial quantities of fermenting sap. Drug-induced beriberi has been reported from the use of nitrofurazone (which interferes with pyruvate metabolism) in the treatment of trypanosomiasis.

Pathology

The pathological anatomy of beriberi involves changes in the nervous system, the heart and muscle fibres. Microscopically the nerve trunks show changes ranging from slight medullary degeneration to complete neural destruction (Wallerian degeneration). In Wernicke's encephalopathy foci of congestion and haemorrhage are scattered symmetrically in the grey matter of the brain stem, mamilliary bodies and hypothalamic regions. There are also numerous perivascular haemorrhages and widespread degenerative brain changes.

In the heart there is fatty degeneration of varying severity and loss of contractility due to water retention. The essential features of 'beriberi heart' are: a hyperkinetic circulation, peripheral vasodilation, right side enlargement and high output failure.[53] The cause of the hyperkinetic circulation deficiency is low peripheral arterial resistance from vasodilation due to loss of muscular arteriolar tone. Post-mortem appearances are those of severe right heart failure.

Clinical features

Beriberi assumes various clinical forms but can be grouped into five major types:[54]

1. Subacute cardiac (wet beriberi)
2. Acute fulminant

3. Neurological (dry beriberi)
4. Infantile
5. Wernicke's encephalopathy

The two main forms, dry and wet beriberi, constitute the same disease and a mixture of the two forms is usual. The onset is insidious, but may be acute with death within hours without nervous system symptoms occurring.

Subacute cardiac beriberi

Symptoms include anorexia, fatigue, irritability, depression and abdominal discomfort. These may be associated with fever. Cardiovascular features are prominent with warm extremities, tachycardia, palpitations and breathlessness. Oedema may occur at the end of a working day and calf muscles have a sensation of fullness.

Acute fulminant beriberi

When heart failure appears the hands may be cold. Blood pressure is low with a high pulse pressure producing a 'pistol shot' sound over larger arteries. There is cardiomegaly with right- and left-sided enlargement and a loud pansystolic murmur is audible over the pericardium. Atrial enlargement may cause paralysis of the recurrent laryngeal nerve. The liver is enlarged and tender. Pericardial effusion is unusual unless it is late-stage disease. Hydrothorax and ascites are frequent. The ECG shows inversion of T waves, a decreased P-R and increased Q-T interval, which rapidly revert to normal with treatment. Sudden cardiac failure is common. Death occurs from right heart failure and the patient usually dies fully conscious.

Neurological beriberi

The clinical features are those of a peripheral neuropathy of mixed motor and sensory type. There is peripheral neuritis with tingling, burning and paresthesias of the feet. Glove and stocking anaesthesia may spread from the feet to the thighs or from the tips of the fingers. There is loss of vibration sense and tenderness and cramping of the leg muscles. The gait becomes ataxic due to loss of postural sensation. The cranial nerves are not involved, although ptosis of the eyelids may occur. Motor signs include: flaccid weakness and wasting with foot, toe and wrist drop, difficulty in standing from the squatting position and loss of tendon reflexes and deep sensation. Paralytic symptoms are more common in adults than children.

Infantile beriberi

This occurs in breast-fed infants of thiamin-deficient mothers, especially in those babies receiving a high carbohydrate diet. Nearly all cases have infections before developing the symptoms of thiamin deficiency. These include pneumonia, diarrhoea, upper respiratory infections and cellulitis. The cases can be classified into three groups as: the cardiac form, the aphonic form and the

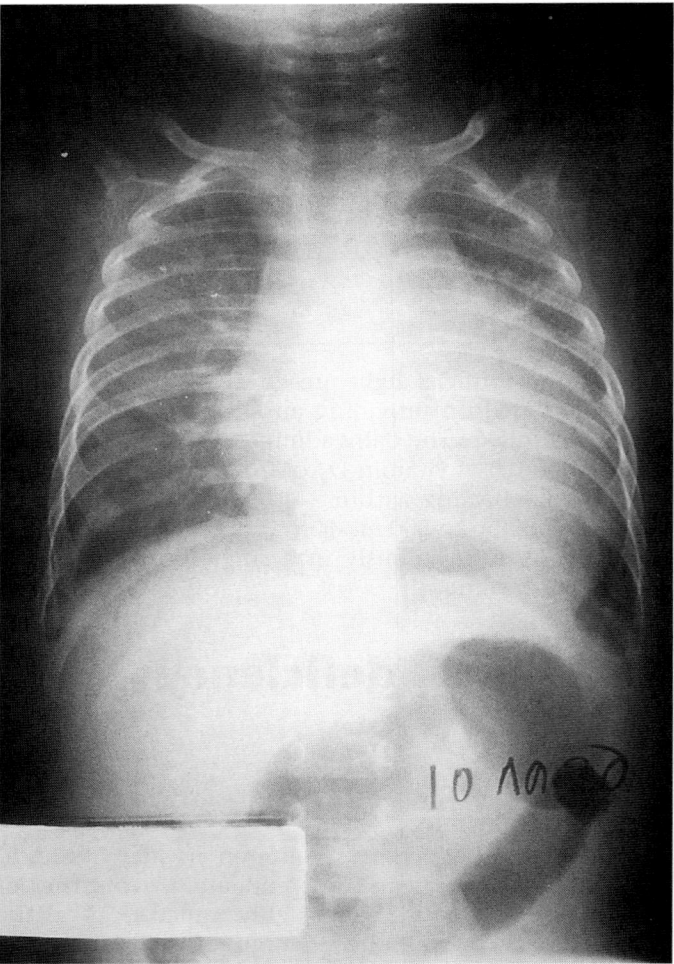

Figure 31.9: Chest radiograph showing cardiomegaly in an infant from Thailand.

pseudomeningitic form. It is not unusual to find features of two or three forms together. Characteristically, the cardiac form has its onset during the second or third month of life. The symptoms are dyspnoea, fever, cyanosis, vomiting and irritability with convulsions. The cardiorespiratory phase is most dramatic with rapid onset and physical examination reveals tachycardia, hepatomegaly and peripheral circulatory failure (Figure 31.9). Cardiac arrest may occur in a significant number of cases and infants may expire on the way to hospital. The overall mortality rate is between 5 and 20%. Blood chemistry shows metabolic acidosis. Survivors respond to parenteral thiamin within 24–48 hours. The aphonic form occurs in slightly older infants (4–6 months). There is anorexia, weight loss and constipation. Left recurrent laryngeal nerve involvement from left atrial pressure gives rise to a characteristic cry (crying but no sound is heard). This may last a few days before restlessness, oedema and dyspnoea develop. The pseudomeningeal form occurs in older infants (6–12 months). There is vomiting and irritability. The infant develops nystagmus, a bulging fontanelle, twitching of muscles and convulsions followed by unconsciousness. The illness resembles meningitis or encephalitis but the CSF is normal.

Wernicke's encephalopathy

This is characterized by cerebellar degeneration, peripheral and optic neuropathy and is caused primarily by thiamin deficiency in alcoholics by causing reduced absorption of the vitamin from the gastrointestinal tract. Outbreaks of this disease, unrelated to alcohol, occurred in the Far East during the Second World War (1939–1945). Diagnosis was established at autopsy by demonstration of mamillary body haemorrhages. Recent surveys suggest that the disease may have a prevalence of about 3% in all chronic alcoholics. Predisposing factors include diarrhoeal infections, sepsis and malaria. Clinical features of this syndrome include paralysis of one or more eye muscles, horizontal nystagmus, a wide gait, clouding of consciousness, insomnia, disorientation and semi-coma. Brain stem damage is associated with haemorrhage and necrosis and myelosis. Retinal haemorrhages occur. Wernicke's encephalopathy may be reversed with injection of thiamin, but the accompanying psychosis (Korsakoff's) is irreversible.

Laboratory diagnosis

The erythrocytes are among the first tissues affected in thiamin deficiency. The erythrocyte transketolase can be stimulated by TPP (thiamin pyrophosphate) and values >20% are found in deficient subjects. Urinary excretion of thiamin is low in subjects with thiamin deficiency but is not highly sensitive. The pyruvic acid concentration in blood is raised in acute beriberi and falls after thiamin administration.

Differential diagnosis

Wet beriberi must be must be distinguished from other causes of right heart failure with high output, e.g., severe anaemia and hookworm disease. Dry beriberi must be distinguished from other causes of flaccid paralysis and neuropathy: alcoholic, tabes dorsalis, chronic arsenic and lead poisoning, lathyrism, triorthocresyl phosphate paralysis in which there is a pure motor flaccid paralysis and nutritional neuropathies, e.g., vitamin B_{12} deficiency.

Treatment

In acute beriberi, patients may die without treatment. There is usually a dramatic improvement within hours of receiving parenteral thiamin (50 mg). In adult beriberi, oral treatment with 50 mg thiamin given three times daily should continue for some days followed by oral supplements of 10 mg/day for several weeks. In infants, 25 mg of thiamin should be given intravenously and a

further 25 mg intramuscularly once or twice daily until symptoms have improved when oral supplements (10 mg) can be given daily.[54] Breast-feeding mothers should also be treated with 50 mg daily for several days.

Prevention

Health education and improved milling methods in which the germ is retained have reduced incidence in some Middle Eastern countries. Hand pounding of rice would improve thiamin content, but this traditional practice is unpopular and many rice eaters have strong preferences for particular types of milled rice. A maternal diet containing adequate thiamin prevents deficiency in breast-fed infants. Thiamin requirements increase with a high carbohydrate diet. General dietary improvement may increase intake, but this is not easy to achieve in poor developing countries. Mixed diets with other sources of thiamin are important, e.g., with pulses, groundnuts, whole wheat, vegetables and fruits.

Pellagra

Pellagra is a nutritional disease caused by the combined deficiency of the vitamin niacin and the essential amino acid tryptophan.

Epidemiology

While pellagra has vanished from most parts of the world where it was formerly present, it continues to be a problem in southern and central Africa. Recent reports of outbreaks in refugee camps[55] highlight that its presence often follows social disturbances with the establishment of large camps.

Aetiology

The spread of pellagra largely followed the introduction of maize as a dietary staple. The reason maize predisposes to pellagra is that the proteins of maize are poor in tryptophan required for nicotinic acid (niacin) synthesis. Pellagra has never been a problem in Central America, the original home of maize, because in preparation, rather than milling, maize is soaked in lime water which hydrolyses nicotinoylesters releasing nicotinic acid. It is likely that other factors play a role: marginal intakes of other vitamins (B_2 and B_6) required for endogenous synthesis of nictotinamide from tryptophan; prolonged exposure to mycotoxins which can deplete the body of nicotinamide; dietary excess of leucine causing an amino acid intolerance; and the impairment of tryptophan metabolism by oestrogens and progesterone which may be sufficient to precipitate pellagra more commonly in women than men. Pellagra may occur due to malabsorption, inborn errors of metabolism, following prolonged isoniazid treatment for tuberculosis (due to inhibition of kynureninase) and with faddist diets. It may follow intestinal surgery and be associated with gastro-intestinal pathology, e.g., oesophageal stricture, carcinoma of the colon or stomach, Crohn's disease, chronic amoebiasis and tropical sprue). Alcoholic pellagra may complicate gastritis.

Pathology

The epidermis becomes hyperkeratotic and later becomes atrophic, and these changes are also present in the tongue, vagina and mucous membranes. The colonic mucous membrane is inflamed and pseudomembranes form; later, the mucosa atrophies. The viscera show fatty degeneration and a characteristic deep pigmentation. Haemorrhages may occur in the renal medulla. Nervous system changes occur late. Demyelination in the spinal cord may involve the posterior and lateral columns. Myelin degeneration in the peripheral nerves is common. Increased intracellular pigment is present in frontal lobes and basal ganglia.[56]

Clinical Features

The main features comprise the triad: 'diarrhoea, dermatitis and dementia'. Since it is also fatal, a fourth 'D' is death. The classic symptoms are usually less well developed in infants and children.

Pre-pellagrinous state

The early symptoms are vague: anorexia, lassitude, joint pains, dizziness and burning sensations which recur periodically for years. The complexion is 'muddy' with bluish leaden-coloured sclerae. The personality changes with irritability and character changes. There may be associated vitamin deficiencies and many people in endemic areas suffer from chronic ill health. In children with parasites or chronic disorders manifestations may be severe.

Dermatitis

The cause of the photosensitive dermatitis in pellagra is unknown, but it may relate to low histidine levels in skin. This amino acid may absorb ultraviolet light and minimize skin damage from sunlight. Dermatological lesions appear on sites exposed to sun and/or pressure. An erythema initially occurs which may develop suddenly or insidiously; it is symmetric and can resemble sunburn. Mild cases may escape recognition. The lesions are usually sharply demarcated and are often on the neck (Casal's necklace), backs of the hands and feet (pellagrinous glove or boot), and sometimes on the scrotum, female genitalia or anus (Figure 31.10). The affected area is swollen, pruritic with burning sensations which become acute on exposure to the sun. Petechia, bullae and vesicles (wet type) may develop. The skin then

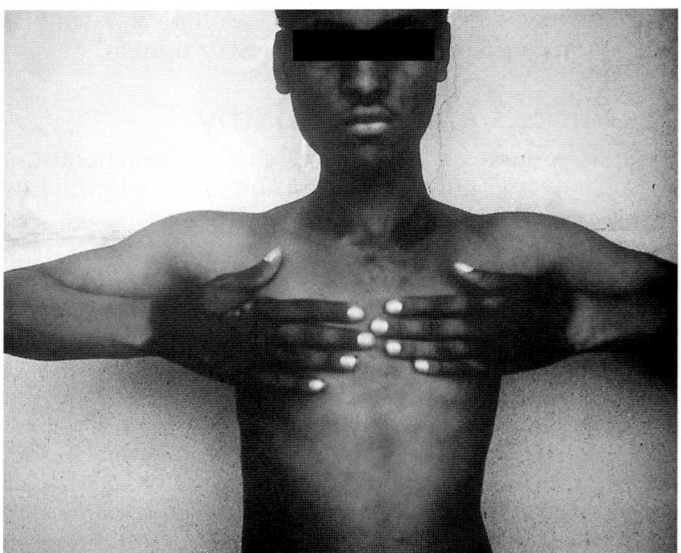

Figure 31.10: Pellagrinous 'glove' skin changes. Photo courtesy of the Liverpool School of Tropical Medicine.

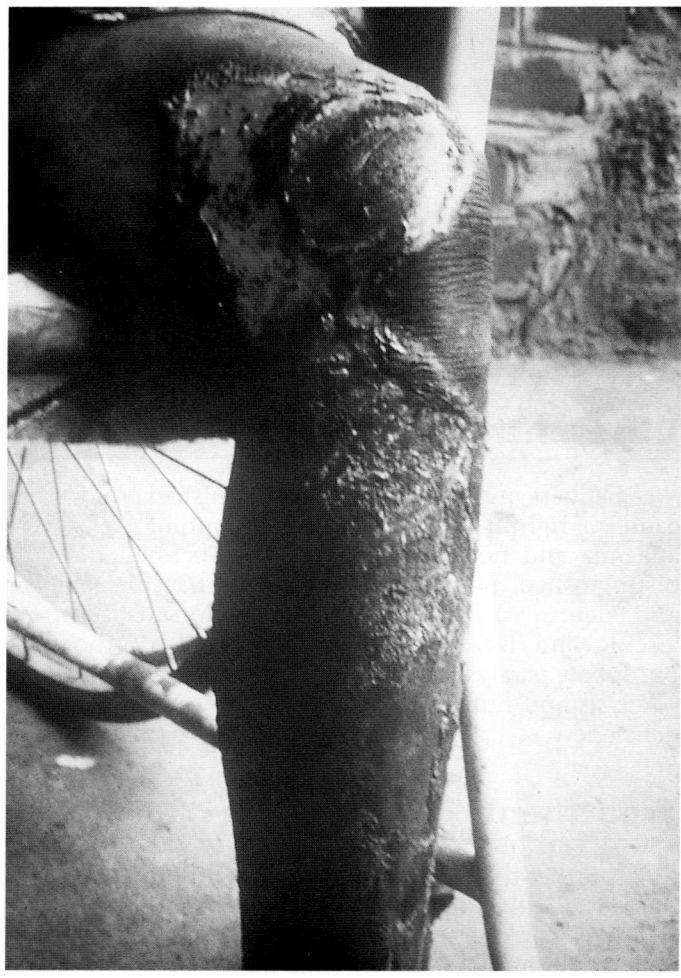

Figure 31.11: Limb dermatitis from pellagra.

becomes dry, rough, thickened, cracked with scaling a shiny surface and brown pigmentation (Figure 31.11). Erythema becomes blackish (or purplish) on black skin and is sepia in olive-skinned races. Hyperkeratosis may affect the malar or supraorbital regions and can involve the whole body. The cutaneous lesions are sometimes preceded by stomatitis, glossitis, vomiting, or diarrhoea. Swelling of the tongue may be followed by intense redness, ulceration, fissuring with atrophy of lingual papillae.

Diarrhoea

Diarrhoea is common in pellagrins, but is not a constant feature and in some cases there may be constipation. The cause is probably related to atrophy of intestinal mucosa. A characteristic symptom is pyrosis—a burning sensation in the oesophagus causing dysphagia. The stools are often pale, resembling those of tropical sprue.

Dementia

The psychiatric disturbances range from mild hallucinations with psychomotor retardation, insomnia, through confusion, to severe dementia, anxiety psychosis, intermittent stupor and possibly epileptiform convulsions and catatonia. Confusion and acute mania may herald death. The cause of the psychiatric disturbance is likely to be due to deficiency of tryptophan which is a precursor of the neurotransmitter serotonin. It has been estimated that 4–10% of patients with pellagra become permanently insane, and pellagrins were formerly numerous in lunatic asylums.[52]

The time of appearance of mental symptoms varies widely; they may be present from the start or occur during convalescence. In the later stages peripheral neuropathy, or ataxic or spastic paraplegia may develop. Tremors and rigidity (extra pyramidal) may occur. The cranial nerves may be involved (8th nerve deafness, retrobulbar neuritis, central scotomas). Some features of these late manifestations may be caused by vitamin B deficiencies. Corneal dystrophy and lens opacities may occur.

Acute encephalopathy is described to consist of cogwheel rigidity, clouding of consciousness, uncontrollable gasping and sucking. Stupor, delirium and acute psychotic symptoms may be present and a mild pellagrinous rash. These patients may respond dramatically to intravenous nicotinic acid.

Course

Symptoms may abate after two to three months although the skin remains dark and rough. It re-occurs the following year if the diet is similar. The eruption darkens and mental symptoms develop with melancholia, maniacal interludes and a suicidal tendency. The gait deteriorates and is of the paraplegic type. Body pains increase and may be acute with cramps, twitches and tremors. Symptoms may persist or deteriorate further unless treatment is given or the diet improved.

Diagnosis

This depends essentially on the history and physical examination. A rapid clinical response to niacin is an important confirming test. N-methylnicotinamide, a metabolite of niacin, is almost undetectable in urine in niacin deficiency (<0.5 mg/g creatinine).

Treatment

An adequate balanced diet is essentially supplemented with nictonic acid at 50–150 mg daily for two weeks. In a severe case or in cases of poor intestinal absorption, the dose can be doubled and 100 mg may be given intravenously. Administering large doses is usually followed within a half hour by sensations of local heat, flushing and burning of skin. Overdosage may cause numbness of the tongue and lower jaw. Intravenous nicotinic acid at high dose (1000 mg daily in divided doses) may produce rapid recovery in acute mania. Chronic psychotic and spinal symptoms respond poorly to nicotinic acid.

The diet should be supplemented with other vitamins especially riboflavin (1–3 mg daily). The diet of the cured pellalgrin should be continuously supervised to prevent recurrence. Isoleucine (5 g daily) can counteract the metabolic effect of leucine on the metabolism of tryptophan and nicotinic acid. Leucine is present in large quantities in maize and sorghum. Sun exposure should be avoided during the active phase and skin lesions covered with soothing applications.

Prevention

Pellagra may be prevented through improved socioeconomic conditions amongst populations dependent on subsistence agriculture. In institutions, the diet should not be confined to maize meal but must include fresh fruit and vegetables, milk and eggs. Hard physical labour should be avoided.

Ariboflavinosis
Epidemiology

Riboflavin deficiency without deficiencies of other vitamin B complex vitamins is rare. Deficiency is present in many developing countries and it was common in prisoner-of-war camps.

Aetiology

Riboflavin is not synthesized by higher animals and is therefore an absolute dietary requirement. The co-enzymes of flavin mono- and dinucleotide are synthesized from riboflavin, forming the prosthetic groups of several enzymes important in electron transport. Riboflavin is destroyed on exposure to light, and signs of deficiency occur if daily intake is less than 0.2–0.3 mg, although 2 mg is considered ideal for an adult. Riboflavin-poor staple diets, such as polished rice, are common in developing countries. Large amounts of riboflavin occur in liver, kidney, milk, cheese and eggs.

Clinical features

Cheilosis (sore red lips), vertical fissuring of lips (perlèche) and corners of the mouth (angular stomatitis), and a purplish raw, smooth tongue with loss of papillary structure are well-described features. Other features are scrotal dermatitis, keratitis, conjunctivitis, photophobia, corneal vasculation and seborrheic dermatitis. The skin has a roughened appearance due to hyperkeratosis (toad's skin or phrynoderma). Cheilosis epidemics occur in families and institutions on inadequate diets. A normocytic normochromic anaemia is common. Ariboflavinosis often complicates pellagra and PEM.

Diagnosis

Biochemical status estimates are based upon urinary excretion or measurements of erythrocyte glutathione reductase.

Treatment

Treatment consists of the oral administration of 3–10 mg of riboflavin daily. If no response occurs within a few days, intramuscular injections of 2 mg of riboflavin in saline may be used. A well-balanced diet should be given with increased intake of legumes, roots and proteins.

Vitamin A deficiency

(see Chapter 31)

Special groups

Pregnant women

In addition to the usual requirements, pregnancy incurs extra energy costs. It is, however, difficult to prescribe precise energy intakes for individual women as their metabolic and behavioural responses (activity and food intake) cannot be predicted. Inadequate pregnancy weight gains have been associated with lower birth-weights in undernourished women. It has long been recognized that pregnant and lactating women are especially vulnerable for mild xeropthalmia. Low vitamin A content of breast milk will also contribute to the increased susceptibility of the infant. A high proportion of pregnant women in developing countries are at risk of inadequate intakes of zinc, iron, vitamin B_{12}, folic acid and other micronutrients. Improving the diets of pregnant women and adolescent girls before their first pregnancy is therefore important for primary prevention of nutritional disorders.[57] Practical methods include modifying the diets to improve bioavailability, and provision of appropriate micronutrient supplements during pregnancy which may yield substantial benefits. Maternal arm circumference can be used as an indicator of risk in non-pregnant and pregnant women because of its high correlation with maternal weight for height. A suitable cut-off for assessing risk in developing countries is less than 21–23.5 cm.

Vegetarians

In poor populations of tropical countries the meat intake in the diet may be very low or absent. Despite this the macronutrient composition is unremarkable. Vegetarians are prone to iron deficiency due to low iron bioavailability. Combined deficiencies of vitamin B_{12} and folate can lead to megablastic anaemias. Consumption of unleavened breads such as chapattis, and brown rice may predispose to rickets and osteomalacia, particularly in Asian vegetarians. Leavening of bread with yeast destroys phytic acid which binds to calcium and this ameliorates this effect. Intake of high dietary fibre and phytates may modify zinc absorption. In general, vegetarians have lower rates of some cancers (mouth, prostate and possibly colon), but there is little evidence relating this to the absence of meat in the diet. The beneficial effects of a vegetarian diet may relate to cancer-preventive substances such as antioxidants and phytochemicals.

Refugees

Nutrition deficiencies in refugees and other uprooted people are well documented. Scurvy, xeropthalmia, anaemia, pellagra and beriberi are described in people dependent on refugee rations. Refugees are prone to anaemia because their food rations are often low in vitamin C which enhances iron absorption. Control of deficiency diseases amongst refugees has largely depended on the distribution of supplementary tablets and additional food, e.g., fruits, dried fish, meat. Nutrient fortification of bulk food to improve the quality of rations has been successfully exploited, e.g., micronutrients in cereals, vitamin A in oil and iron in sugar.

REFERENCES

1   Waterlow J C. *Protein-energy Malnutrition*. London: Edward Arnold, 1992.

2   Chandra R K. Nutrition and the immune system: an introduction. *Am J Clin Nutr* 1997; 66:460S–463S.

3   Scrimshaw N S & San Giovanni J P. Synergism of nutrition, infection and immunity: an overview. *Eur J Clin Nutr* 1997; 66:464S–477S.

4   de Onis M & Blossner M. WHO Global database on child growth and malnutrition. WHO/NUT/97.4. Geneva, Switzerland: Programme of Nutrition, World Health Organization, 1997.

5   de Onis M, Yip R, Mei Z. The development of MUAC-for-age reference data recommended by a WHO Expert Committee. *Bull Wld Hlth Org* 1997; 75:11–18.

6   Wellcome Trust Working Party. Classification of infantile malnutrition. *Lancet* 1970; 2:302–303.

7   Coulter J B S. Malnutrition related disease. *Curr Paediatr* 1999; 9:27–33.

8   World Health Organization. *Management of severe malnutrition: a manual for physicians and other senior health workers*. Geneva: World Health Organization, 1999.

9   Morley D. Prevention of protein-calorie deficiency syndromes. *Trans R Soc Trop Med Hyg* 1968; 62:200–208.

10 Golden M & Golden B. Effect of zinc supplementation on the dietary intake, rate of weight gain and energy cost of tissue deposition in children recovering from severe malnutrition. *Am J Clin Nutr* 1981; 34:900–908.

11 Roy S K, Tomkins A M, Mahalanabis D et al. Impact of zinc supplementation on persistent diarrhoea in malnourished Bangladeshi children. *Acta Paediatr* 1998; 87:1235–1239.

12 Whitehead R G, Coward W A, Lunn P G, Rutishauser I. A comparison of the pathogenesis of protein-energy malnutrition in Uganda and The Gambia. *Trans R Soc Trop Med Hyg* 1977; 71:189–195.

13 Lunn P G, Whitehead R G, Coward W A. Two pathways to kwashiorkor. *Trans R Soc Trop Med Hyg* 1979; 73:438–444.

14 Catto-Smith A G, Barr C, Fagan J E, Parsons H G. Non-dairy-creamer-induced kwashiorkor: 5 year follow-up. *J Pediatr Gastroenterol Nutr* 1991; 12:507–511.

15 Williams C D. Nutritional disease of childhood associated with a maize diet. *Arch Dis Child* 1933; 8:423–433.

16 Golden M H N. Oedematous malnutrition. *Brit Med Bull* 1998; 54:433–444.

17 Sive A A, Subotzky E F, Malan H, Dempster W S, Heese H De V. Red blood cell antioxidant enzyme concentrations in kwashiorkor and marasmus. *Ann Trop Paediatr* 1993; 13:33–38.

18 Becker K, Leichsenring M, Gana L, Bremer H J, Schirmer R H. Glutathione and associated antioxidant systems in protein energy malnutrition: results of a study in Nigeria. *Free Radical Biol Med* 1995; 18:257–263.

19 Manary M J, Leeuwenburgh C, Heinecke J W. Increased oxidative stress in kwashiorkor. *J Pediatr* 2000; 137:421–424.

20 Coulter J B S, Hendrickse R G, Lamplugh S M et al. Aflatoxins and kwashiorkor: clinical studies in Sudanese children. *Trans R Soc Trop Med Hyg* 1986; 80:945–951.

21 Hendrickse R G. Of sick turkeys, kwashiorkor, malaria, perinatal mortality, heroin addicts and food poisoning: research on the influence of aflatoxins on child health in the tropics. *Ann Trop Med Parsitol* 1997; 91:787–793.

22 Morlese J F, Forrester T, Badaloo A, Del Rosario M, Frazer M Jahoor F. Albumin kinetics in edematous and non-edematous protein-energy malnourished children. *Am J Clin Nutr* 1996; 64:952–959.

23 Mayatepek E, Becker K, Gana L, Hoffmann G F Leichsenring M. Leukotrienes in the pathophysiology of kwashiorkor. *Lancet* 1993; 342:958–960.

24 Frood J D L, Whitehead R G, Coward W A. Relationship between patterns of infection and development of hypoalbuminaemia and hypo-β-lipoproteinaemia in rural Ugandan children. *Lancet* 1971; ii:1047–1049.

25 Sauerwein T R W, Mulder J A, Mulder L et al. Inflammatory mediators in children with protein-energy malnutrition. *Am J Clin Nutr* 1997; 65:1534–1539.

26 Patrick J. Oedema in protein energy malnutrition: the role of the sodium pump. *Proc Nutr Soc* 1979; 38:61–67.

27 Fiorotto M & Coward W A. Albumin and nutritional oedema. *Lancet* 1980; i:430.

28 Annotation. Nutritional oedema, albumin and vanadate. *Lancet* 1981; ii:646–647.

29 Golden M H N. Protein deficiency, energy deficiency, and the oedema of malnutrition. *Lancet* 1982; i:1261–1265.

30 Sive A A, Dempster W S, Malan H, Rosseau S, Heese H de V. Plasma free iron: a possible cause of oedema in kwashiorkor. *Arch Dis Child* 1997; 76:54–56.

31 Orth S R & Ritz E. Nephrotic syndrome. *N Engl J Med* 1998; 338:1202–1211.

32 Ashour M N, Salem S I, El Gaban H M, Elwan N H, Basi T K. Antioxidant status in children with protein-energy malnutrition (PEM) living in Cairo, Egypt. *Eur J Clin Nutr* 1999; 53:669–613.

33 Jackson A A. Blood glutathione in severe malnutrition in childhood. *Trans R Soc Trop Med Hyg* 1986; 80:911–913.

34 Roediger W E W. New views on the pathogenesis of kwashiorkor: methionine and other amino acids. *J Pediatr Gastroenterol Nutr* 1995; 21:130–136.

35 Lamplugh S M. Investigations into the presence of aflatoxins in human body fluids in tissues in relation to child health in the tropics. *Ann Trop Paed* 1998; 18:S41–S46.

36 Coulter J B S, Suliman G I, Lamplugh S M et al. Aflatoxins in liver biopsies from Sudanese children. *Am J Trop Med Hyg* 1986; 35:360–365.

37 Coulter J B S, Suliman G I, Omer M I A et al. Protein energy malnutrition in northern Sudan: clinical studies. *Eur J Clin Nutr* 1988; 42:787–796.

38 Grantham-McGregor S, Powell C, Walker S et al. The long-term follow-up of severely malnourished children who participated in an intervention program. *Child Develop* 1994; 65:428–439.

39 Heikens G T, Schofield W N, Dawson S M, Waterlow J C. Long-stay versus short-stay hospital treatment of children suffering from severe protein-energy malnutrition. *Eur J Clin Nutr* 1994; 48:873–882.

40 Schofield C & Ashworth A. Why have mortaltiy rates for severe malnutrition remained so high? *Bull Wld Hlth Org* 1996; 74:223–229.

41 Waterlow J C. Protein-energy malnutrition: the nature and extent of the problem. *Clin Nutr* 1997; 16 (suppl 1):3–9.

42 Konde M, Ingelbleek Y, Daffe M et al. Goitrous endemic in Guinea. *Lancet* 1994; 344:1675–1678.

43 Xue-Yi C, Xin-Min J, Zhi-Hong D et al. Timing of vulnerability of the brain to iodine deficiency in endemic cretinism. *New Eng J Med* 1994; 331:1739–1744.

44 Dunn J T, Pretell E A, Daza C H & Viteri F. (eds) *Towards the Eradication of Endemic Goitre, Cretinism and Iodine Deficiency*. PAHO and WHO Scientific Publication No. 502. Geneva: WHO 1986.

45 WHO/UNICEF/ICCIDD. Indicators for assessing iodine deficiency disorders and their control through salt iodisation. WHO/NUT/94.6, Geneva: WHO, 1994.

46 Delong G R, Leslie P W, Wang S-H et al. Effect on infant mortality of iodination of irrigation water in a severely iodine-deficient area of China. *Lancet* 1997; 350:771–773.

47 Dunn J T & van der Haar F. A practical guide to the correction of iodine deficiency: technical manual no 3, ICCIDD-UNICEF-WHO. Wageningen, Netherlands: University of Wageningen, 1990.

48 Seaman J & Rivers J P W. Scurvy and anaemia in refugees. *Lancet* 1989; 336:1204.

49 Thacher T D, Fischer P R, Pettifor J M et al. A comparison of calcium, vitamin D, or both for nutritional rickets in Nigerian children. *New Eng J Med* 1999; 341:563–568.

50 Muhe L, Lulseged S, Mason K E, Simoes E A. Case-control study of the role of nutritional rickets in the risk of developing pneumonia in Ethiopian children. *Lancet* 1997; 349:1801–1804.

51 Krishna S, Taylor AM, Supanaranonad W et al. Thiamine deficiency and malaria in adults from southeast Asia. *Lancet* 1999; 353:546–549.

52 Cook G C. Nutrition-associated disease. In *Manson's Textbook of Tropical Diseases*, 20th edition. Ed. Cook G C. W.B. Saunders, London, 1996.

53 Cathcart A E, Thurnham D I. Beriberi. In *Encyclopaedia of Human Nutrition* (eds) Sadler M J, Strain J J & Cabalhero B. Academic Press, San Diego, 1999.

54 Di Rocco M, Patrini C, Rimini A Rindi G. A 6–month old girl with cardiomyopathy who nearly died. *Lancet* 1997; 349:616.

55 Malfait P, Moren A,. Dillon J C et al. An outbreak of pellagra related to changes in dietary niacin among Mozambican refugees in Malawi. *Int J Epid* 1993; 22:504–511.

56 Spillane J D (ed). *Tropical Neurology*. London, Oxford University Press, 1973.

57 Brabin L & Brabin B J. The cost of successful adolescent growth and development in girls in relation to iron and vitamin A status. *Am J Clin Nutr* 1992; 55:955–958.

Chapter 32
Animal Toxins

D. A. Warrell

Venomous bites and stings

Animal venoms are rarely single toxins, but are mixtures of proteins and other substances with toxic, irritant, allergic or unknown properties which are injected into prey or squirted at enemies. Possession of venom by an easily recognizable and often highly coloured reptile, amphibian or bird may confer protection both on its own species and on other harmless species which mimic its appearance or behaviour (Batesian or Müllerian mimicry). The venoms secreted on to the skin of some amphibians may protect their moist integument against infection as well as being distasteful, poisonous and therefore deterrent to predators. Animals have evolved various methods of injecting venom. Mammals (Insectivora and vampire bats), snakes, lizards, spiders, ticks, leeches and octopuses inject their venoms by biting with teeth, fangs, venom jaws, beaks or other hardened mouthparts; male duck-billed platypuses have a venom-injecting spur; fish, cnidarians (coelenterates), echinoderms, cone-shells, insects, centipedes and scorpions have various kinds of stinging apparatus. Some snakes, toads, scorpions and other arthropods can squirt their venom at enemies. Poisoning, which results from the ingestion of the flesh and viscera of aquatic animals, is discussed in the second part of this chapter. Allergic reactions to injected venoms (e.g. Hymenoptera— bee, wasp and ant venoms) and ingested poisons (e.g. ciguatera fish poisons) are in some cases far more dangerous than their direct toxic effects. This is a large subject in its own right; here it will be referred to only briefly.

Venomous mammals

The duck-billed platypus (*Ornithorhynchus anatinus*) is an aquatic egg-laying mammal of eastern Australia. Males have sharp spurs on their hindlimbs connected by a duct to crural venom glands. This venom apparatus is used aggressively in fights between males during the breeding season. Platypus venom contains four small molecular weight defensin-like peptides, a C-type natriuretic peptide and hyaluronidase. Each year at least one human is stung by a platypus in Victoria.[1] However, fewer than 20 cases have been reported. The venom can cause agonizing local pain—relieved only by regional nerve block—persistent local swelling and inflammation with regional lymphadenopathy. No local necrosis or cases of life-threatening envenoming have been reported. However, one patient experienced local weakness, stiffness and muscle wasting for at least 3 months after the sting. Experimentally, the venom is weakly haemolytic, coagulant and causes local haemorrhage, oedema and fatal hypotension in animals. Males of the echidna, another egg-laying mammal, also have a mildly venomous spur.

Several species of Insectivora produce a venomous secretion from enlarged, granular submaxillary salivary glands. These discharge at the base of the lower incisors, which may be grooved. Venom is conducted along the concave surfaces of these teeth and serves to immobilize amphibian and rodent prey and may be used, lethally, in internecine fights. Venomous species include the Haitian (*Solenodon paradoxus*) and Cuban (*S. (Atopogale) cubanus*) solenodons, the European water shrew (*Neomys fodiens*), Mediterranean shrew (*N. anomalous*) and the short-tailed shrew of the eastern USA and Canada (*Blarina brevicauda*). The venom of *B. brevicauda* is the most toxic and is probably a protein. It produces fatal cardiorespiratory and neurotoxic effects in rodents and lagomorphs. In humans, bites by these species occasionally cause local pain, swelling and inflammation. The saliva of vampire bats (Desmodontinae) increases capillary permeability and inhibits platelet aggregation. Draculin, a glycoprotein, inhibits activated factors X and IX. An activator of plasminogen (vPA) is being developed as a thrombolytic drug. These activities serve to promote blood flow while the bat is feeding.

Venomous snakes[2]

Taxonomy, identification and distribution

Of the 3000 species of snakes, about 500 belong to the three families of venomous snakes, Atractaspididae, Elapidae (including Hydrophiinae) and Viperidae. Only about 200 species have caused death or permanent disability by biting humans. Bites by more than 30 species of the large family Colubridae, once considered harmless, have produced signs of envenoming in man, while five of them have caused fatal envenoming.[3] Among non-venomous snakes, only the giant constrictors (family Boidae) are potentially dangerous to man. There have been a number of fatal attacks by these snakes reported from Africa (rock python, *Python sebae*), South-East Asia (especially Indonesia) (reticulated python, *Python reticulatus*) and South America (anaconda, *Eunectes murinus*). Some of the victims, even adults, were swallowed.

Snakes are classified morphologically by the arrangement of their scales (lepidosis), dentition, osteology, myology, sensory organs, the form of the hemipenes and increasingly by sequence analysis of DNA encoding important mitochondrial and other enzymes.[4]

Legless lizards, such as slow-worms, glass lizards (Anguidae), worm-like geckos (Pygopodidae) and legless skinks, may be distinguished from snakes by their eyelids, external ears, friable tails and by the lack of enlarged ventral scales. Some have vestigial limbs. Amphisbaenids have worm-like annular grooves along the length of their bodies and caecilians (legless amphibians) lack obvious eyes and scales. Eels and pipe-shaped fish are distinguished from snakes by their gills and fins.

All medically important species of snakes have one or more pairs of fangs in their upper jaw. These enlarged teeth have grooves or venom channels along which venom is injected through the skin of prey or human victims. Approximately 400 of the 2500 species of Colubridae have short, immobile opisthoglyphous fangs or enlarged solid aglyphous teeth at the posterior end of the maxilla (Figure 32.1). The African and Middle Eastern burrowing asps or stiletto snakes (genus *Atractaspis*, family Atractaspididae), also known as burrowing or mole vipers or adders, false vipers or side-stabbing snakes, have very long solenoglyphous front fangs on which they impale their victims by a side-swiping motion, the fang protruding from the corner of the partially closed mouth (Figure 32.2). The Natal black snake (*Macrelaps microlepidotus*) possesses two very large grooved opisthoglyphous fangs at the posterior ends of its maxillae. The Elapidae (cobras—*Naja*; kraits—*Bungarus*; mambas—*Dendroaspis*; shield-nosed snakes—*Aspidelaps*; Asian and American coral snakes—*Calliophis*, *Maticora*, *Micrurus*; African garter snakes—*Elapsoidea*; terrestrial venomous Australasian snake and sea snakes) have relatively short, fixed proteroglyphous front fangs (Figure 32.3). The

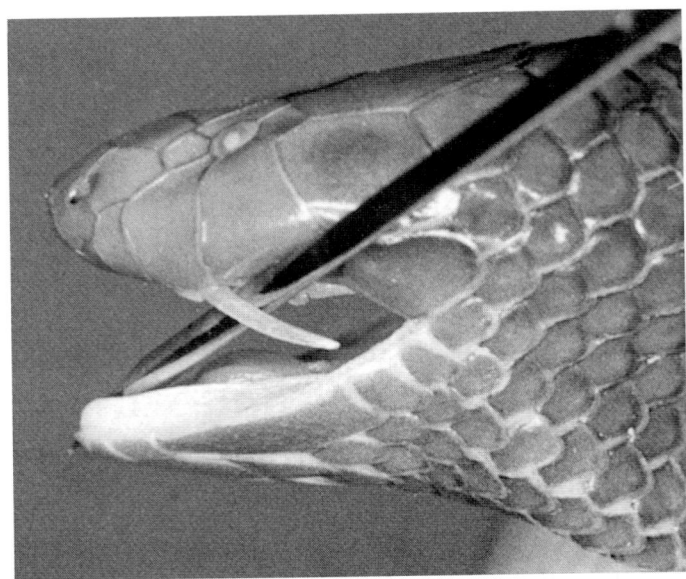

Figure 32.2: Very long front fang of a West African burrowing asp (*Atractaspis aterrima*: family Atractaspididae). (Copyright D. A. Warrell.)

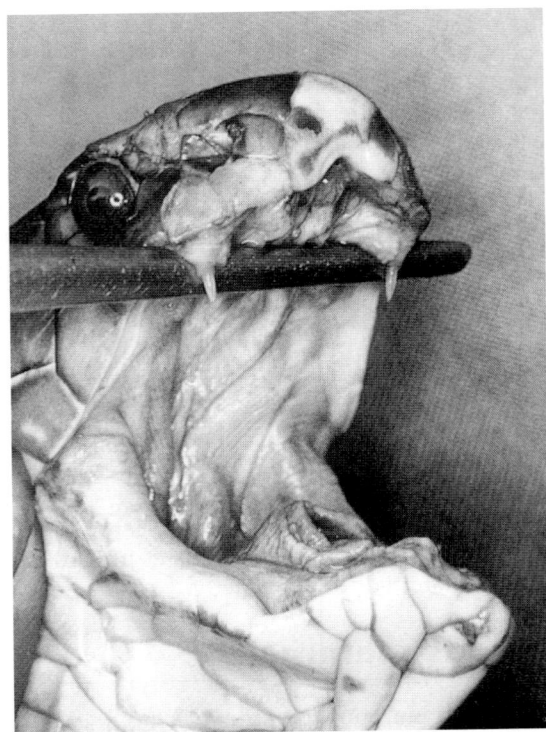

Figure 32.3: Short front fangs of the monocellate Thai cobra (*Naja kaouthia*: family Elapidae). (Copyright D. A. Warrell.)

Viperidae (vipers, adders, rattlesnakes, moccasins, lance-headed vipers and pit vipers) have highly evolved long, curved, hinged, solenoglyphous front fangs containing a closed venom channel, like hypodermic needles (Figure 32.4). The subfamily Crotalinae (pit vipers) includes rattlesnakes (genera *Crotalus* and *Sistrurus*), moccasins (*Agkistrodon*) and lance-headed vipers (genera *Bothrops*, *Bothriechis*, *Porthidium*, *Lachesis*, etc.) of the Americas and

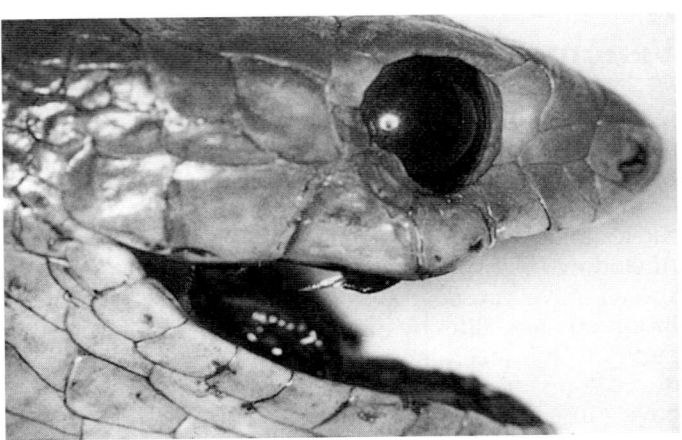

Figure 32.1: Rear fangs of the boomslang (*Dispholidus typus*), a dangerous African colubrid. (Copyright D. A. Warrell.)

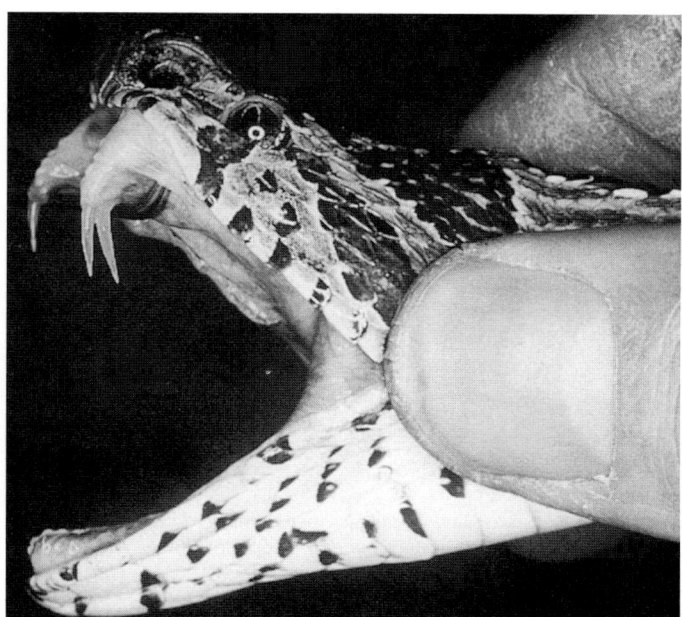

Figure 32.4: Long hinged front fangs, with reserve fang on its left side, enclosed in dental sheath, in a Thai Russell's viper (*Daboia russelii siamensis*: family Viperidae; subfamily Viperinae). (Copyright D.A. Warrell.)

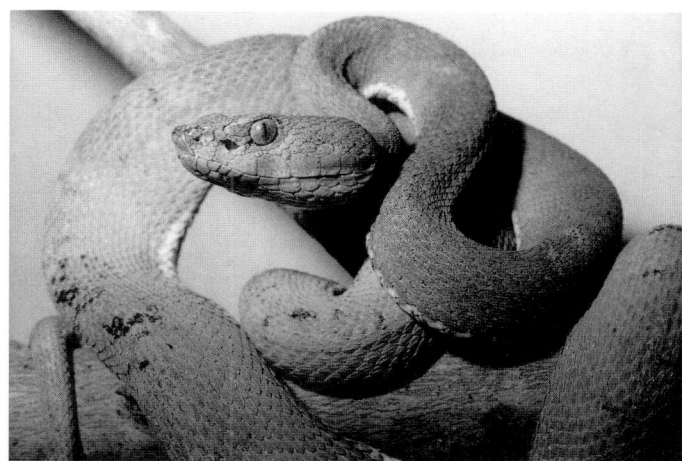

Figure 32.5: Amazonian green arboreal pit viper (*Bothrops bilineatus*: Family Viperidae; Subfamily Crotalinae) showing heat-sensitive pit organ between eye and nostril. (Copyright D. A. Warrell.)

the Asian pit vipers (genera *Gloydius/Agkistrodon, Deinagkistrodon, Calloselasma, Trimeresurus, Hypnale*, etc). The pit of crotaline snakes is a heat-sensitive organ, situated between the eye and nostril, which detects warm-blooded prey (Figure 32.5). Snakes of the subfamily Viperinae, the Old World vipers and adders lack this pit organ. The English words 'viper' and 'adder' have not been strictly applied to distinguish species which are ovoviviparous (produce live young) from those which lay eggs.

None of the care and skill lavished on the identification of parasites and their vectors is devoted by medical staff to the identification of venomous snakes. There is no simple and reliable method of distinguishing venomous from non-venomous snakes. The snake's upper jaw can be examined for the presence of fangs, but these may be very small in elapids, and folded back inside a sheath in vipers. However, the most dangerous species tend to be well known where they are important. The characteristic hood of cobras and some other elapids is evident only when the snake is rearing up in a defensive attitude (Figure 32.6). Vipers are often identifiable by their repeated and sometimes colourful dorsal pattern (Figure 32.7). Russell's viper (*Daboia russelii*) and puff adders (*Bitis arietans*) make a loud hissing sound by expelling air through their large nostrils, the saw-scaled or carpet vipers (genus *Echis*) produce a characteristic rasping sound by rubbing their coils together (Figure 32.8), rattlesnakes produce an unmistakable sound like castanets and king cobras (*Ophiophagus hannah*) 'growl'. Some harmless snakes are easily mistaken for venomous species that they mimic: for example *Telescopus* (cat snake) and *Dasypeltis* (egg-eating snake) with *Echis* (saw-scaled viper) species in Africa;

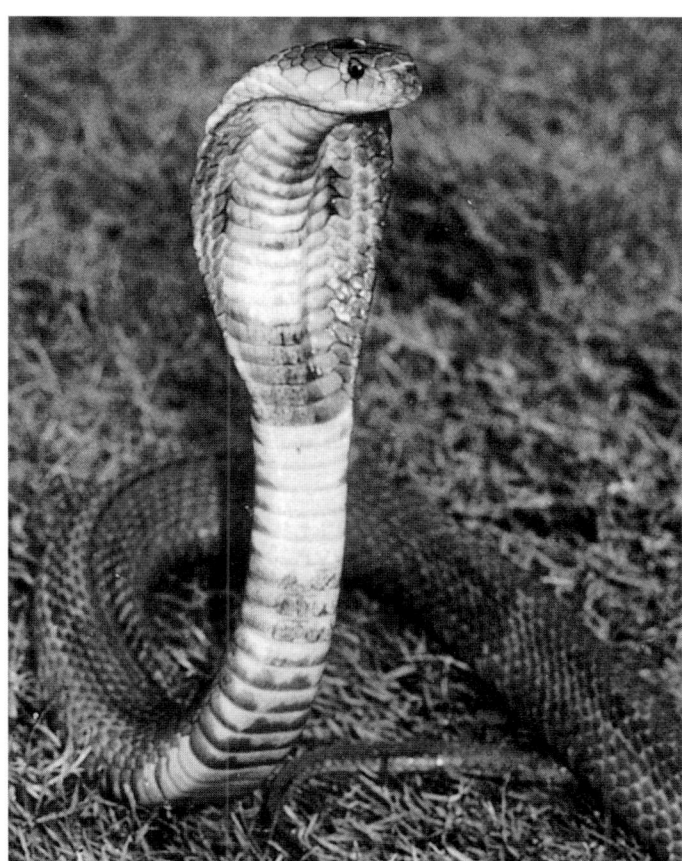

Figure 32.6: Thai spitting cobra, brown phase (*Naja siamensis*: family Elapidae) showing spread hood in threatening/defensive attitude. Specimen 1.3 m long from central Thailand. (Copyright D. A. Warrell.)

Boiga multomaculata with *Daboia russelii* in Thailand; various species of *Dryocalamus* and *Lycodon* with *Bungarus candidus* and *B. caeruleus* in South Asia; and *Xenodon severus* with *Bothrops brazili* and similar species in the Amazon region. Table 32.1 lists the species which, in each

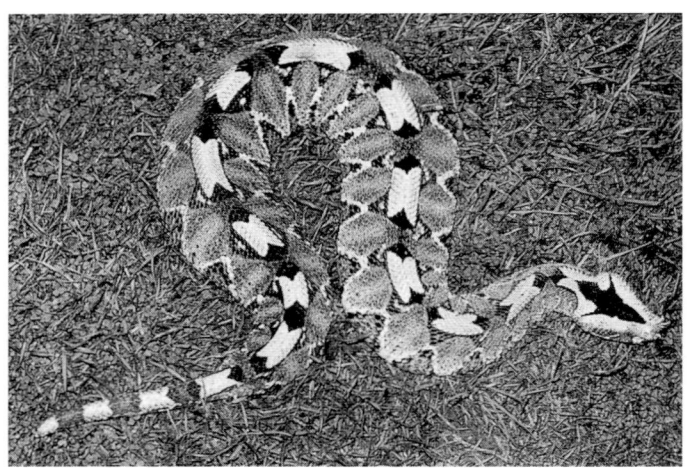

Figure 32.7: Rhinoceros or nose-horned viper of the African rain forest (*Bitis nasicornis*) showing distinctive repeated dorsal pattern. Specimen 90 cm long from Cameroon. (Copyright D. A. Warrell.)

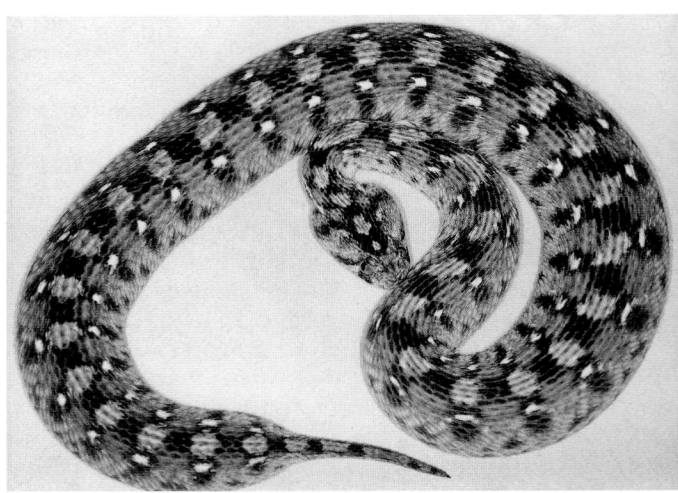

Figure 32.8: Saw-scaled or carpet viper (*Echis ocellatus*). Specimen 55 cm long from north-eastern Nigeria. (Copyright D. A. Warrell.)

Table 32.1 Species of snake probably responsible for most deaths and morbidity

Area	Scientific name	Common name
North America	*Crotalus adamanteus* *Crotalus atrox* *Crotalus viridis* ssp.	Eastern diamondback rattlesnake Western diamondback rattlesnake Western rattlesnakes
Central America	*Crotalus durissus* ssp. *Bothrops asper*	Central American rattlesnakes Terciopelo, caissaca
South America	*Bothrops atrox, B. asper* *Bothrops jararaca* *Crotalus durissus* ssp.	Fer-de-lance, barba amarilla Jararaca South American rattlesnakes, cascabel
Europe	*Vipera* spp. *V. ammodytes*	Vipers, adders Long-nosed viper
Africa	*Echis* sp. *Bitis arietans* *Naja nigricollis, N. mossambica*, etc. *Naja haje*	Saw-scaled or carpet vipers Puff adder African spitting cobras Egyptian cobra
Asia, Middle East	*Echis* sp. *Macrovipera lebetina* *Vipera palaestinae* *Naja oxiana*	Saw-scaled or carpet vipers Levantine viper Palestine viper Oxus cobra
Indian subcontinent and South-East Asia	*Naja naja, N. kaouthia, N. siamensis*, etc. *Bungarus* sp. *Daboia russelii* ssp. *Calloselasma rhodostoma* *Echis carinatus, E. sochureki*	Asian cobras Kraits Russell's vipers Malayan pit viper Saw-scaled or carpet vipers
Far East	*Naja atra* etc *Bungarus multicinctus* *Trimeresurus flavoviridis* *Trimeresurus mucrosquamatus* *Gloydius blomhoffii* ssp.	Asian cobras Chinese krait Japanese habu Chinese habu Mamushi
Australasia, New Guinea	*Acanthophis* sp. *Pseudonaja textilis* *Notechis scutatus* *Oxyuranus scutellatus* ssp.	Death adder Eastern brown snake Tiger snake Taipans

continent, are responsible for most snake bite deaths and severe morbidity. Some species, notorious for the potency of their venom (e.g. many species of sea snakes and Australasian elapids) or their great size (e.g. king cobra, *Ophiophagus hannah* and Gabon vipers *Bitis gabonica* and *B. rhinoceros*) rarely bite humans. The African night adders (genus *Causus*), Asian green pit vipers (genus *Trimeresurus*), North American copperheads (*Agkistrodon contortrix*) and Latin American hog-nosed vipers (e.g. *Porthidium nasutum*) bite many people but rarely cause severe envenoming. Illustrated books, papers and keys have been published for the identification of venomous snakes in most parts of the world and there are some useful websites.

Venomous snakes are widely distributed, up to altitudes of 4000 metres (*Gloydius/Agkistrodon himalayanus*), especially in tropical countries. One species (*Vipera berus*) is found within the Arctic Circle. There are no other venomous species in the Arctic, Antarctic, in North America (north of about latitude 51°N), Newfoundland, Nova Scotia, in most of the islands of the western Mediterranean, Atlantic and Caribbean (except in Martinique, Santa Lucia, Margarita, Trinidad and Aruba), in Madagascar and Chile (where there are mildly venomous colubrid snakes), New Caledonia, New Zealand, Hawaii and some other Pacific Islands, Crete, Ireland and Iceland. Sea snakes exist in the Indian and Pacific Oceans between latitudes 30°N and 30°S as far north as Siberia (*Pelamis platurus*), in estuaries, rivers and in some freshwater lakes (e.g. *Hydrophis semperi* in Lake Taal, Philippines; *Enhydrina schistosa* in Ton Ley Sap, Cambodia).

Epidemiology of snake bite

The determinants of incidence and severity of snake bite are summarized in Table 32.2. In the tropical countries where snake bite is most common there are few reliable data. Records of patients treated by traditional methods are lost to the official statistics. Hospital records, the sole source of most snake bite reporting, are likely to over-represent the more seriously envenomed patients, and depend on the enthusiasm and workload of hospital staff. Population surveys[5–8] give a more accurate picture of the incidence of snake bite. Certain hunter–gatherer tribes are at greatest risk from snake bite. Snakes were responsible for 2% of adult deaths among the Yanomamo of Venezuela, 5% among the Waorani of Ecuador and 24% among the Kaxinawa of Acré, Brazil.[9] An estimated

15 000–20 000 people die each year from snake bite in India. In Barddhaman (Burdwan) District, West Bengal, a field survey in randomly selected villages suggested that among the total population of nearly 5 million people nearly 8000 were bitten and 800 killed by snakes each year.[8] In the 1930s the annual snake bite mortality reported in Burma exceeded 2000 (15.4 per 100 000 population).[10] Thirty years later it was still estimated to exceed 1000 (3.3 per 100 000) per year and has been as high as the fifth most important cause of all deaths.[11] In 1984, about 900 snake bite deaths were recorded in Sri Lanka, an incidence of six per 100 000 per year. In the Amami and Okinawa Islands of Japan, there were 5488 bites by the habu (*Trimeresurus flavoviridis*) with 50 deaths during the 9 years from 1962 to 1970. The highest incidence of bites on one of the islands was 4.6 per 1000 population per year.[12] In the Benue Valley of north-eastern Nigeria the incidence of snake bite was found to be 497 per 100 000 population per year, with a mortality of 12.2%.[13] Snake bite is also common in Latin America. In Brazil, the case fatality of snake bites in the pre-antivenom era was thought to be about 25%, and the total number of bites 19 200 each year. By 1970, the estimated incidence was 51 026 bites and 1153 deaths per year, but recent figures indicate an average of 20 170 bites and 122 deaths per year. In the USA there are 7000 bites by venomous snakes each year with 12–15 deaths, and in Australia 1000–2000 bites per year with an average of three to four deaths per year. In Britain, there are more than 200 adder bites (*Vipera berus*) each year but there have been only 14 deaths during the last 100 years, the last in 1976. There were 44 deaths caused by this species in Sweden between 1911 and 1978, and in Finland 21 deaths in 25 years, with an annual incidence of almost 200 bites.

Snake bite as an occupational disease

In tropical countries snake bite is an occupational disease of farmers, plantation workers, herders and hunters. Rice farmers in Burma, Sri Lanka and central Thailand tread on Russell's vipers or inadvertently pick them up in a handful of paddy during the harvest[11] (Figure 32.9). In the savannah of West Africa farmers are bitten by *Echis* species as they dig the fields at the start of the rainy season.[13] Rubber-tappers in South-East Asia tread on Malayan pit vipers in the dark and are bitten as they make their early-morning rounds of the rubber trees, and

Table 32.2 Determinants of snake bite incidence and severity of envenoming

Incidence of bites	Severity of envenoming

1. Frequency of contact between snakes and humans, depends on:
  (a) Population densities
  (b) Diurnal and seasonal variations in activity
  (c) Types of behaviour (e.g. human agricultural activities)
2. Snakes' 'irritability'—readiness to strike when alarmed or provoked—varies with species
	1. Dose of venon injected—depends on mechanical efficiency of bite and species and size of snake
	2. Composition and hence potency of venom—depends on species and, within a species, the geographical location, season and age of the snake
	3. Health, age, size and (?) specific immunity of human victim
	4. Nature and timing of first aid and medical treatment

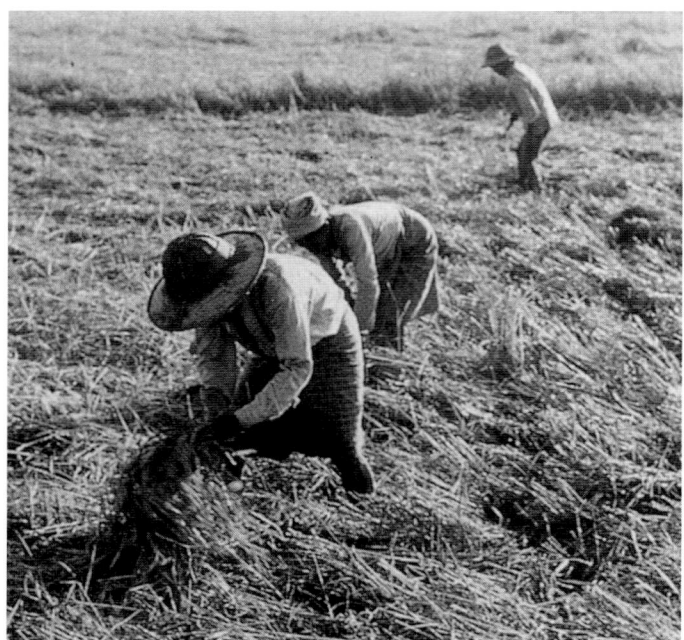

Figure 32.9: Burmese rice farmers harvesting the paddy, an occupation with a high risk of Russell's viper bite. (Copyright D. A. Warrell.)

in the jungles of western Brazil the collectors of natural rubber ('seringueiros') are bitten by *Bothrops atrox*.

Sea snake bites were an occupational hazard of fishermen in those parts of South-East Asia where hand nets were used. Records of 144 sea snake bites were collected in north-west Malaya in 1955–1956.[14] Mechanization of fishing methods in this region has resulted in a dramatic decrease in sea snake bites, but they still occur along the coast of South Vietnam.[15] The beaked sea snake (*Enhydrina schistosa*) has caused most bites and deaths. Other common and medically important species are *Hydrophis cyanocinctus*, *H. spiralis* and *Lapemis curtus*.

In the more industrialized countries venomous snakes are increasingly popular as pets. Many are held illegally. Most bites are inflicted on the hands when the snakes are picked up and in the USA 25% of bites resulted from snakes being attacked or handled. Unprovoked attacks are excessively rare, but snakes will bite if they are cornered or feel threatened. Some species, notably *Bungarus caeruleus* in India[16] and Sri Lanka, *B. candidus* in South-East Asia[17] and *Naja nigricollis* in West Africa,[18] enter human dwellings at night in pursuit of their prey (rodents, lizards, toads) and may strike at someone who moves in their sleep. Epidemics of snake bite have resulted from a sudden increase in snake population density, for example after flooding in Colombia, Pakistan, India, Bangladesh, Nepal and Burma. In Togo in the 1950s there was an unprecedented increase in *Echis ocellatus* and bites that remain unexplained.[13] Invasion of the snake's habitat by large numbers of people may also be followed by an increased incidence of snake bite. This has happened during the building of new roads through jungles in

South America and when farmers moved to areas in the former dry zone of Sri Lanka made newly fertile by the Mahaweli irrigation scheme.

Venom apparatus[19]
Colubridae
The most primitive method for injecting venom is found in the back-fanged Colubridae. The posterior part of the superior labial gland (Duvernoy's gland) drains into a periodontal fold of buccal mucosa. The venom tracks down grooves in the anterior surfaces of the several enlarged posteriorly situated fangs (see Figure 32.1). This arrangement is effective for envenoming the natural prey, for example a chameleon in the case of the boomslang, which is held in the snake's mouth until it is dead. Human envenoming is a very rare accident. The snake must seize and chew at the finger of its victim, usually a herpetologist.

Atractaspididae
The venom apparatus of Atractaspididae differs from all other venomous snakes in many respects and the homology of the venom glands is uncertain.[19] In *Atractaspis engaddensis* and *A. microlepidota*, as in some species of Elapidae (*Maticora*) and Viperidae (*Causus*), the venom glands are very long—perhaps one-sixth of the snake's total length. The fangs of Atractaspididae and their method of striking are also distinctive.

Elapidae (including Hydrophiinae) and Viperidae
In these families, the venom glands lie behind the eye. Compressor muscles, principally the adductor superficialis in Elapidae, and the compressor glandulae in Viperidae, squeeze venom out of the gland through the venom duct to the base of the fang. Venom is transmitted to the tip of the fang through a partially or completely closed canal in the case of the Viperidae. In several species of elapid, the African spitting cobras *Naja nigricollis*, *N. katiensis*, *N. pallida*, *N. nigricinctus* and *N. mossambica*, the South African ringhals or rinkals (*Hemachatus haemachatus*) and Asian spitting cobras (*N. sumatrana*, *N. siamensis*, *N. sputatrix* etc.), the fang is modified to allow the snake to eject a spray of venom for a metre or more into the eyes of an aggressor. Instead of opening downwards at the tip of the fang, the venom channel is angled forward at its point of exit in the anterior surface of the fang, a few millimetres above its tip.[20,21]

The performance of the venom apparatus has been studied in very few species. The Palestine viper (*Vipera palaestinae*) can inject doses of venom lethal to its natural prey at each of 10 or more consecutive strikes. When a snake bites two or more humans in rapid succession the second or third victims may, surprisingly, be more severely envenomed than the first. However, Russell's viper injects most of its available venom at the first strike.

Snake bite without envenoming ('dry bites')   Between about 10% (e.g. *Echis ocellatus*) and 80% (e.g. *Pseudonaja*

textilis) of people bitten by venomous snakes, with puncture marks to prove penetration of the fangs, develop no signs of envenoming. Perhaps snakes can bite defensively without injecting venom. However, there is little evidence that snakes can control their injection of venom or vary the amount according to the size of the prey: the strike is essentially a reflex 'all-or-nothing' action. The snake's venom apparatus has been evolved to deliver electively an effective bite to its natural prey, with injection of a supralethal dose of venom. However, when the snake lashes out reactively at a human foot or ankle after it has been trodden upon, it seems far less likely, for purely anatomical and mechanical reasons, that an effective strike with injection of venom will be achieved.

Venom composition[22]

Snakes have the most complex of all venoms. They may contain more than 20 components. More than 90% of the dry weight is protein, comprising a rich variety of enzymes, non-enzymatic polypeptide toxins and non-toxic proteins such as nerve growth factor. Non-protein ingredients of venom include carbohydrate and metals (often part of glycoprotein metalloprotein enzymes), lipids, free amino acids, nucleosides and biogenic amines such as serotonin and acetylcholine. Eighty to ninety per cent of viperid and 25–70% of elapid venom consists of enzymes, including digestive hydrolases, hyaluronidase and activators or inactivators of physiological processes. Most venoms contain L-amino acid oxidase, phosphomono- and di-esterases, 5'-nucleotidase, DNase, NAD-nucleosidase, phospholipase A_2 and peptidases. Elapid venoms, in addition, contain acetylcholinesterase, phospholipase B and glycerophosphatase, while viperid venoms have endopeptidase, arginine ester hydrolase, kininogenase, and thrombin-like, factor X and prothrombin activating enzymes. Phospholipase A_2 is the most widespread and extensively studied of all venom enzymes. Under experimental conditions it damages mitochondria, red blood cells, leucocytes, platelets, peripheral nerve endings, skeletal muscle, vascular endothelium and other membranes, and produces presynaptic neurotoxic activity, opiate-like sedative effects and the autopharmacological release of histamine. The acetylcholinesterase found in most elapid venoms is no longer thought to contribute to their neurotoxicity. Hyaluronidase promotes the spread of venom through tissues. Proteolytic enzymes (endopeptidases or hydrolases) are responsible for local changes in vascular permeability leading to oedema, blistering and bruising, and to necrosis. L-Amino acid oxidase, which gives yellow snake venoms their colour, may have a digestive function.

The polypeptide toxins, often called neurotoxins, are low molecular weight, non-enzymatic proteins found almost exclusively in elapid and hydrophiid venoms. Postsynaptic (α) neurotoxins such as α-bungarotoxin and cobrotoxin contain 60–70 amino acid residues and bind to acetylocholine receptors on the motor end-plate. Pre-synaptic (β) neurotoxins such as β-bungarotoxin,

crotoxin and taipoxin contain about 120–140 amino acid residues and a phospholipase A subunit. These release acetylcholine at the nerve endings at neuromuscular junctions and then damage the endings, preventing further release of transmitter. Biogenic amines such as histamine and 5-hydroxytryptamine, found particularly in viper venoms, may contribute to the local pain and permeability changes at the site of a snake bite.

Snake venom should not be regarded as a single toxin. The variation of venom composition from species to species and within a single species throughout its geographical distribution, at different seasons of the year and, as a result of ageing, explains the clinical diversity of snake bite.

Clinical features of envenoming[2]

Symptoms and signs in victims of snake bite are caused by fear, the direct action of the various venom components on tissues, indirect effects such as complement activation and autopharmacological release of endogenous vasoactive substances, effects of treatment and complications such as secondary infections.

Local swelling

In the bitten limb, increased vascular permeability leads to swelling and bruising. The factors responsible include endopeptidases, metalloproteinase haemorrhagins, membrane-damaging polypeptide toxins, phospholipases and endogenous autacoids released by the venom, such as histamine, 5-hydroxytryptamine and kinins. Venoms of some Viperidae, such as *Daboia russelii*, *Vipera berus* and *Crotalus* species, can produce a generalized increase in vascular permeability resulting in pulmonary oedema, serous effusions, conjunctival (Figure 32.23) and facial oedema and haemoconcentration.

Local tissue necrosis results from the direct action of myotoxins and cytotoxins, ischaemia caused by thrombosis, and compression of blood vessels by first-aid methods such as tight tourniquets, or by swollen muscle within a tight fascial compartment. Myotoxins are proteins that can damage the muscle cell plasma membrane directly. Most are phospholipases A_2, either enzymatically active (aspartate-49) or enzymatically inactive (lysine-49). Cobra cardiotoxins are low molecular weight polypeptides.

Hypotension and shock

Profound hypotension is part of the autopharmacological syndrome which may occur within minutes of bites by *Vipera palaestinae*, *V. berus*, *Daboia russelii*, *Bothrops*, *Lachesis* and *Actractaspis engaddensis*. Presumably this is caused by release of vasodilating autacoids. Oligopeptides in Viperidae venoms (e.g. *Bothrops* species) inhibit bradykinin-deactivating enzymes and angiotensin-converting enzymes (ACEs) and were the models for synthetic ACE inhibitors used to treat hypertension.[23] Snake handlers may become sensitized to snake venoms and can develop life-threatening anaphylactic reactions within minutes of being bitten. Leakage of plasma or blood into the bitten limb and elsewhere or massive gastrointestinal haemorrhage may cause hypovolaemia after viper bites. Vasodilatation, especially of splanchnic vessels, and a direct effect on the myocardium may contribute to hypotension after viper and rattlesnake bites.

Bleeding and clotting disturbances[24]

These are seen after bites by vipers, pit vipers, Australasian elapids and dangerously venomous colubrids. Snake venoms can cause haemostatic defects in a number of different ways: venom procoagulants can activate intravascular coagulation and produce consumption coagulopathy leading to incoagulable blood. For example, procoagulants in the venom of Colubridae, *Echis* species and *Notechis scutatus* activate prothrombin, *Daboia russelii* venom has procoagulants activating factors V and X, and many Crotalinae venoms have a direct thrombin-like action on fibrinogen. Some venoms, such as those of the rattlesnakes *Crotalus atrox* and *C. adamanteus*, cause defibrinogenation by activating the endogenous fibrinolytic system. Anticoagulant activity is attributable to venom phospholipases. Thrombocytopenia is a common accompaniment of systemic envenoming. Activators of platelet aggregation include botrocetin (*Bothrops jararaca*), mocarhagin (*Naja mossambica*) and alboaggregin B (*T. albolabris*) targeting GPIb-IX–V; many toxins targeting GPIIb–IIIa; convulxin (*Crotalus durissus*), trimucytin (*T. mucrosquamatus*) and alborhagin (*T. albolabris*) activating GPVI, and alboaggregin A (*T. albolabris*) activating both GPVI and GPIb-IX–V. Jararhagin (*B. jararaca*) and possibly rhodocytin (*Calloselasma rhodostoma*) inhibit platelet agglutination through integrin $\alpha_2\beta_1$. Few studies of platelet function have been attempted in envenomed humans. In patients bitten by Malayan pit vipers and green pit vipers (*T. albolabris*) there was initially inhibition of platelet agglutination followed by activation and the appearance of circulating clumps of platelets.[25] In the absence of trauma, defibrination induced by venom coagulants such as ancrod (Arvin, Arwin) from *C. rhodostoma* venom is a relatively benign state. Spontaneous systemic bleeding is attributable to distinct venom components, haemorrhagins, which damage vascular endothelium. These are zinc metallo-endopeptidases (reprolysins), some of which include disintegrin-like, cysteine-rich and lectin domains. The combination of incoagulable blood, thrombocytopenia and vessel wall damage will result in massive bleeding, a common cause of deaths from viper bites. This group of venom activities is often referred to, inappropriately, as 'vasculotoxic', 'haematotoxic' or even 'haemolytic'.

Intravascular haemolysis

Although most snake venoms are haemolytic in vitro, this effect is rarely of clinical significance. However, envenoming by some *Bothrops* species, Russell's viper (in India and Sri Lanka), some Australasian elapids and members of the colubrid genera *Dispholidus*, *Thelotornis* and *Rhabdophis* may be associated with massive intravascular haemolysis contributing to renal failure. Snake venom-induced disseminated intravascular coagulation (DIC) may result in deposition of fibrin on activated vascular endothelium producing microangiopathic haemolysis (schistocytes/helmet cells/fragmented erythrocytes), renal failure and a clinical picture reminiscent of haemolytic uraemic syndrome.

Complement activation[26]

Elapid and some colubrid venoms activate complement via the alternative pathway ('cobra venom factor' is cobra C3b), whereas some viperid venoms activate the classical pathway. Complement activation may in turn affect platelets, the blood coagulation system and other humoral mediators.[24]

Renal failure

Renal failure is a potential complication of severe envenoming, even by species which usually cause only mild envenoming such as *Trimeresurus albolabris*, the hump-nosed viper (*Hypnale hypnale*) and *Vipera berus*. However, it is a common event and cause of death following bites by Russell's vipers,[11] tropical rattlesnakes (*Crotalus durissus* subspecies) and sea snakes.[15] Possible mechanisms of acute tubular necrosis are prolonged hypotension and hypovolaemia, DIC, a direct toxic effect of the venom on the renal tubule, haemoglobinuria, myoglobinuria and hyperkalaemia. Russell's viper venom produces hypotension, DIC, direct nephrotoxicity[27] and, in Sri Lanka and India, intense intravascular haemolysis.[28] The mechanism of renal failure in victims of *C. durissus* is most likely to be generalized rhabdomyolysis, combined with hypotension in some cases.[29] A large variety of renal histological changes have been described after snake bite, including proliferative glomerulonephritis, toxic mesangiolysis with platelet agglutination, fibrin deposition, ischaemic changes, acute tubular necrosis, distal tubular damage ('lower nephron nephrosis') suggesting direct venom nephrotoxicity and bilateral renal cortical necrosis with subsequent calcification.[30] Pre-existing chronic renal disease and the effects of antivenom (serum sickness) may confuse interpretation.

Neurotoxicity

The neurotoxic polypeptides and phospholipases of snake venoms cause paralysis by blocking transmission at the neuromuscular junction. Paralytic symptoms are characteristic of envenoming by most elapids, such as kraits, coral snakes, mambas and cobras, but not of the African spitting cobras (*Naja nigricollis*, *N. pallida*, *N. mossambica*, etc.).[18] Venoms of terrestrial Australasian snakes, sea snakes and a few species of Viperidae, notably *Crotalus durissus terrificus*, Pallas' pit viper (*Gloydius/Agkistrodon blomhoffii brevicaudus*), Sri Lankan and South Indian *Daboia russelii*, the berg adder (*Bitis atropos*) and some other small *Bitis* species of southern Africa (*B. peringueyi*, *B. xeropaga*) are also neurotoxic in humans. Patients with paralysis of the bulbar muscles may die of upper airway obstruction or aspiration but the most common mode of death after neurotoxic envenoming is respiratory paralysis. Anticholinesterase drugs, by prolonging the activity of acetylcholine at neuromuscular junctions, may improve paralytic symptoms in patients bitten by snakes whose neurotoxins are predominantly postsynaptic in their action (e.g. Asian cobras; Australasian death adders, genus *Acanthophis*; Latin American coral snakes, genus *Micrurus*). Some patients bitten by elapids or vipers are unphysiologically drowsy in the absence of respiratory or circulatory failure. This is unlikely to be an effect of neurotoxic polypeptides, which do not cross the blood–brain barrier. It may be caused by endogenous opiates released by a venom component. Intracerebral injection of β-RTX (receptor-active protein) from *D. russelii* venom produced sedation in rats.

Rhabdomyolysis

Generalized rhabdomyolysis, with release into the bloodstream of myoglobin, muscle enzymes, uric acid, potassium and other muscle constituents, is an effect in man of presynaptic neurotoxins of most species of sea snakes,[15] many of the terrestrial Australasian elapids such as tiger snake (*Notechis scutatus* and *N. ater*), king brown or mulga snake (*Pseudechis australis*), taipan (*Oxyuranus scutellatus*), rough-scaled snake (*Tropidechis carinatus*), small-eyed snake (*Cryptophis nigrescens*) and several species of Viperidae; tropical rattlesnake (*Crotalus durissus terrificus*),[29] canebrake rattlesnake (*C. horridus atricaudatus*), Mojave rattlesnake (*C. scutulatus*) and Sri Lankan Russell's viper (*Daboia russelii russelii*).[28] Patients may die of bulbar and respiratory muscle weakness, from acute hyperkalaemia or later renal failure.

Venom ophthalmia[31]

Venoms of the spitting cobras and ringkals are intensely irritant and even destructive on contact with mucous membranes such as the conjunctiva and nasal cavity. Corneal erosions, anterior uveitis and secondary infections may result.

Envenoming by different families of venomous snakes

Colubridae (back-fanged snakes)[3]

Severe or fatal envenoming has been reported in patients bitten by several species of back-fanged colubrid snake: boomslang (*Dispholidus typus*) (see Figure 32.1); vine, twig, tree or bird snake (*Thelotornis kirtlandii* and *T. capensis*) of central and southern Africa; yamakagashi (*Rhabdophis tigrinus*) of Japan; red-necked keelback (*R. subminiatus*) of South-East Asia and green racer (*Philodryas olfersii*) of Brazil. Snakes of this family killed two outstanding herpetologists: Karl P. Schmidt (*Dispholidus typus*) and Robert Mertens (*Thelotornis kirtlandi*). Severe envenoming is possible if the snake is able to engage its rear fangs and chew for 15 seconds or longer. All the species give rise to similar symptoms, which may be delayed for many hours or even days after the bite. There is nausea, vomiting, colicky abdominal pain and headache. Bleeding develops from old and recent wounds such as venepunctures, and there is spontaneous gingival bleeding, epistaxis, haematemesis, melaena, subarachnoid or intracerebral haemorrhage, haematuria and extensive ecchymoses. Intravascular haemolysis and microangiopathic haemolysis have been described. Most of the fatal cases died of renal failure from acute tubular necrosis, many days after the bite. Local effects of the venom are usually trivial but several patients showed some local swelling and one bitten by *Dispholidus typus* had massive swelling with blood-filled bullae. Investigations reveal incoagulable blood, defibrination, elevated fibrin(ogen) degradation products (FDPs), severe thrombocytopenia and anaemia. These clinical features are explained by DIC triggered by a venom prothrombin activator.

Other potentially dangerous colubrids include Blanding's tree snake (*Toxicodryas/Boiga blandingi*), road guarder (*Conophis lineatus*) of Middle America and neotropical racers (*Alsophis* species and *Philodryas viridissimus*).

Atractaspididae (burrowing asps or stiletto snakes and Natal black snake)

Seventeen species of the genus *Atractaspis* and one species of *Macrelaps* have been described in Africa and the Middle East. All are venomous, but fatal envenoming has been described by only three species: *A. microlepidota*, *A. irregularis* and *A. engaddensis*. Local effects include pain, swelling, blistering, necrosis, tender enlargement of local lymph nodes, local numbness or paraesthesiae. The most common systemic symptom is fever. Most of the fatal cases died within 45 minutes of the bite after vomiting, producing profuse saliva and lapsing into coma.[32] Severe envenoming by *A. engaddensis* may produce violent autonomic symptoms (nausea, vomiting, abdominal pain, diarrhoea, sweating and profuse salivation) within minutes of the bite. One patient developed severe dyspnoea with acute respiratory failure, one had weakness, impaired consciousness and transient hypertension and in three there were electrocardiographic changes (ST–T changes and prolonged PR interval).[33] Mild abnormalities of blood coagulation and liver function have also been described. *Atractaspis* venom has very high lethal toxicity. The venom of *A. engaddensis* contains four 21-amino acid peptides—sarafotoxins, which show 60% sequence homology with endogenous endothelins. They cause coronary vasoconstriction and atrioventricular block. The venom also contains haemorrhagic and necrotic factors but no true neurotoxins. Bites by *Macrelaps microlepidotus* are said to have resulted in collapse and loss of consciousness.

Elapidae (cobras, kraits, mambas, coral snakes, sea kraits and true sea snakes)

Elapid venoms are best known for their neurotoxic effects. In the case of kraits, mambas, coral snakes, most of the Australasian elapids (see below), some of the cobras (e.g. Philippine cobra, *Naja philippinensis*; Cape cobra, *N. nivea*) and sea snakes, local effects are minimal. However, patients bitten by African spitting cobras (*N. nigricollis*, *N. pallida*, *N katiensis*, *N. mossambica* and *N. nigricinctus*) and Asian cobras (*N. naja*, *N. kaouthia*, *N. siamensis*, *N. sumatrana*, *N. sputatrix*, *N. atra*, etc.) commonly develop tender local swelling, which may be extensive, and regional lymphadenopathy. A characteristic lesion may appear within 24–48 hours. Blistering often surrounds a demarcated pale or blackened anaesthetic area of skin (Figure 32.10). The lesion smells putrid and eventually breaks down with loss of skin and subcutaneous tissue, which may be extensive (Figure 32.11). Skip lesions, separated by areas of apparently normal skin, may extend proximally up the limb. Prolonged morbidity may result and some patients may lose a digit or the affected limb if there is secondary infection. Severe envenoming by the king cobra (*Ophiophagus hannah*) results in swelling of the whole limb and formation of bullae at the site of the bite

but local necrosis is minimal or absent.[34] Rapidly developing neurotoxicity is the dominant clinical feature of envenoming by this species. Neurotoxic effects are also seen in patients envenomed by Asian cobras (it is the main feature in victims of *N. philippinensis*) and other elapids, but have not been documented in victims of African spitting cobras. The earliest symptom of systemic envenoming is repeated vomiting, but the use of emetic herbal medicines may confuse the interpretation of this symptom. Other early preparalytic symptoms include contraction of the frontalis (before there is demonstrable ptosis), blurred vision, paraesthesiae especially around the mouth, hyperacusis, loss of sense of smell and taste, headache, dizziness, vertigo and signs of autonomic nervous stimulation such as hypersalivation, congested conjunctivae and 'goose-flesh'. Paralysis is first detectable as ptosis and external ophthalmoplegia, as ocular muscles are most sensitive to neuromuscular blockade (Figure 32.12). These signs may appear as early as 15 minutes after the bite (cobras or mambas) but may be delayed for 10 hours

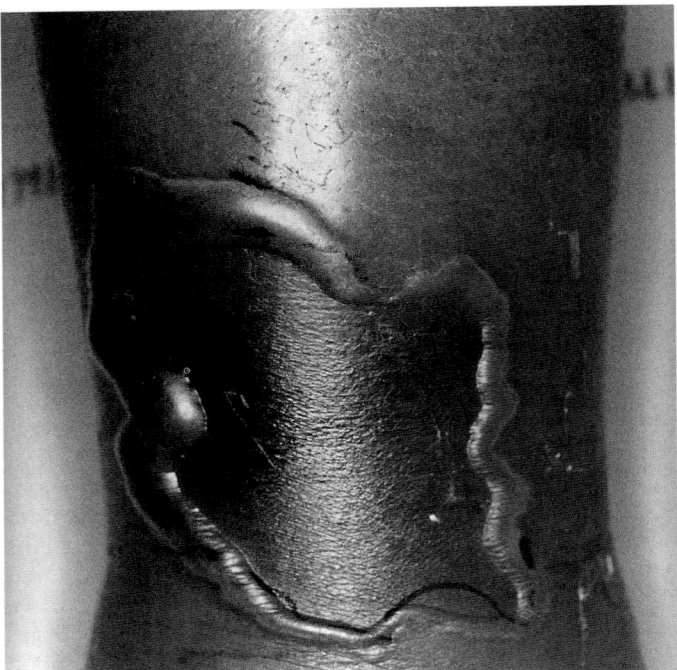

Figure 32.10: Characteristic local necrotic lesion produced by bites of African spitting cobras and Asian cobras. In this case, the patient was bitten by an Indo-Chinese spitting cobra (*Naja siamensis*). Thirty-six hours after the bite, there was a darkened anaesthetic area at the site of the bite, surrounded by a narrow blister. There was a characteristic smell of putrefaction. (Copyright R. E. Phillips.)

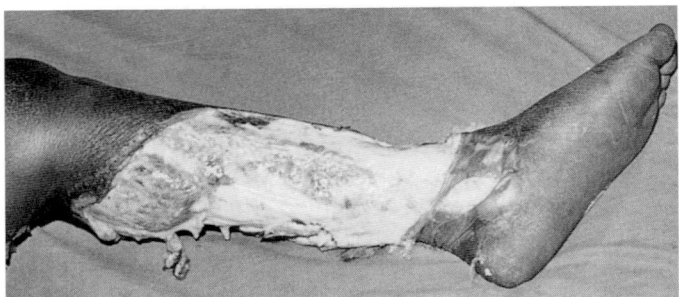

Figure 32.11: Extensive necrosis of skin and subcutaneous tissues in a Nigerian woman bitten 10 days earlier by a black-necked or spitting cobra (*Naja nigricollis*). (Copyright D. A. Warrell.)

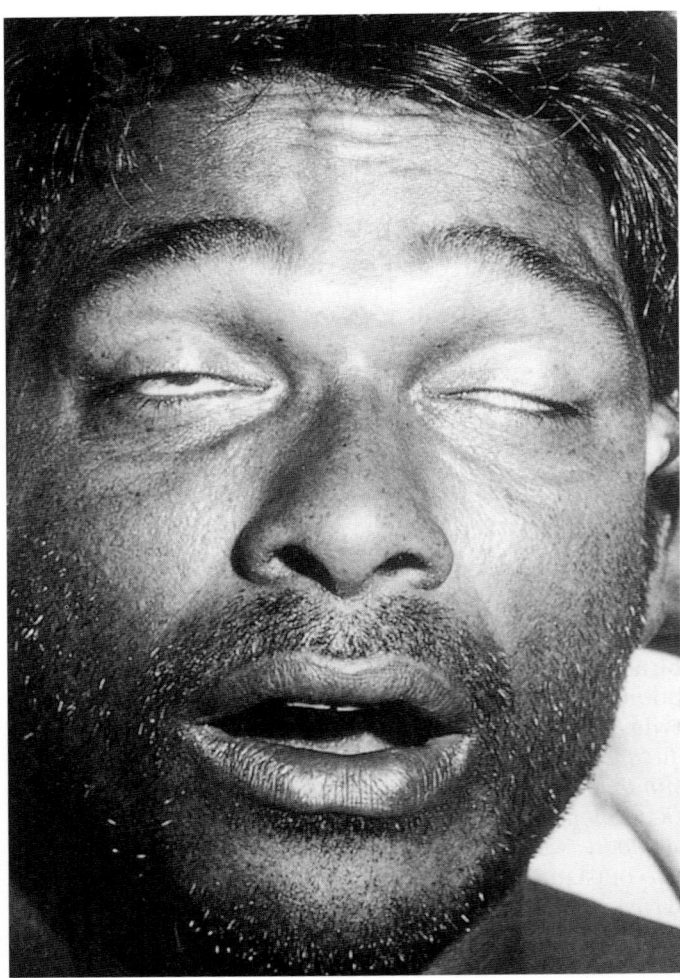

Figure 32.12: Severe ptosis, external ophthalmoplegia and inability to open the mouth, protrude the tongue or swallow in a Sri Lankan patient bitten by a common krait (*Bungarus caeruleus*). (Copyright D. A. Warrell.)

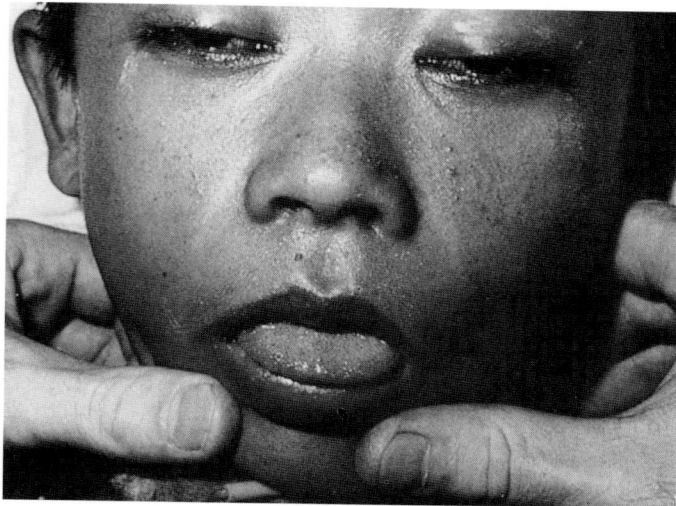

Figure 32.13: Ptosis and inability to open the mouth or protrude the tongue in a Thai patient bitten by a Malayan krait (*Bungarus candidus*). (Copyright D. A. Warrell.)

or more following krait bites. Later, the facial muscles, palate, jaws, tongue, vocal cords, neck muscles and muscles of deglutition may become paralysed (Figure 32.13). The pupils are dilated. Many patients are unable to open their mouths, but this can be overcome by force. In a minority, the jaw is said to hang open. Respiratory arrest may be precipitated by obstruction of the upper airway by the paralysed tongue or inhaled vomitus. Intercostal muscles are affected before the limbs, diaphragm and superficial muscles and, even in patients with generalized flaccid paralysis, slight movements of the digits may be possible, allowing the patients to signal. Loss of consciousness and generalized convulsions are usually explained by hypoxaemia in patients who have respiratory paralysis. However, drowsiness, before the development of significant paralysis, has often been described but remains unexplained. Drooping eyelids from tiredness may be misconstrued as ptosis, unless the extent of lid retraction with upward gaze is formally assessed. Patients with systemic envenoming suffer from headache, malaise and generalized myalgia. Intractable hypotension can occur in patients envenomed by Asian cobras, despite adequate respiratory support. Neurotoxic effects are completely reversible, either acutely in response to antivenom or (for example, in Asian cobra, South American coral snake and Australasian death adder bites) to anticholinesterases,[35] or they may slowly wear off spontaneously. In the absence of specific antivenom, patients supported by mechanical ventilators recover sufficient diaphragmatic movement to breathe adequately in 1–4 days. Ocular muscles recover in 2–4 days and there is usually full recovery of motor function in 3–7 days.

Bites by Australasian elapids[1,36,37]

Venoms of these snakes result in three main groups of symptoms: neurotoxicity similar to that seen with other elapid bites (Figure 32.14),[37,38] generalized rhabdomyolysis and haemostatic disturbances. Local signs are usually

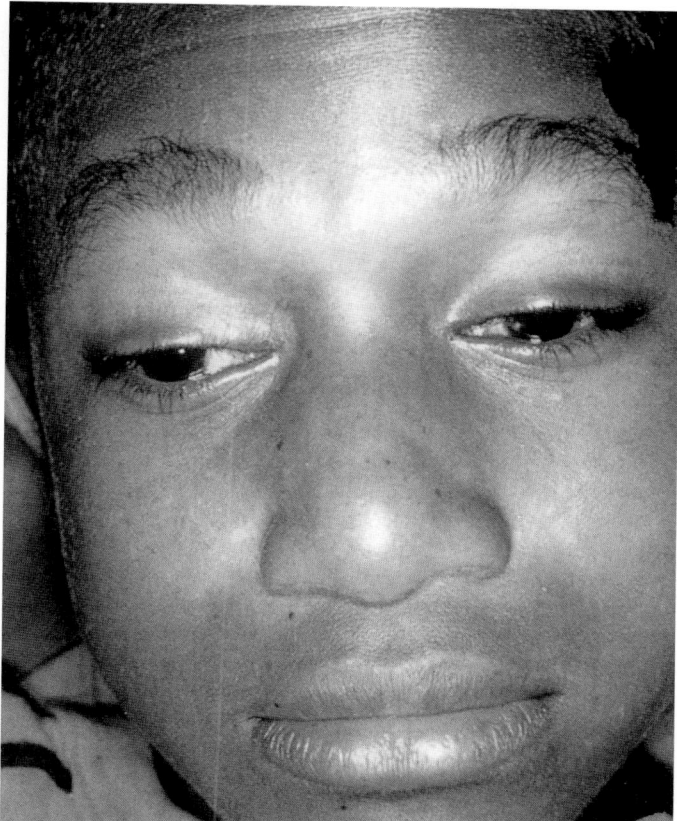

Figure 32.14: Ptosis, external ophthalmoplegia and facial paralysis in a Papua New Guinean boy bitten 24 hours previously by a taipan (*Oxyuranus scutellatus canni*). (Copyright D. A. Warrell.)

mild, but extensive local swelling and bruising with necrosis has been reported, especially after bites by the king brown or mulga snake (*Pseudechis australis*). Painful and tender local lymph nodes are a common feature in patients developing systemic envenoming. Early symptoms include vomiting, headache and syncopal attacks similar to those experienced after some viper bites. Electrocardiographic changes were common in patients envenomed by taipans (*Oxyuranus scutellatus canni*) in Papua New Guinea, but only a few had raised cardiac troponin-T levels suggesting myocardial damage. In dogs, common brown snake (*Pseudonaja textilis*) venom caused myocardial depression attributed to DIC and tiger snake (*Notechis scutatus*) venom caused formation of thrombi within the heart, leading to pulmonary and coronary artery thromboembolism.[1]

Persistent bleeding from wounds and spontaneous systemic bleeding from gums and gastrointestinal tract is found in association with incoagulable blood following bites by many Australasian species. Venoms of 15 out of 19 species exhibited procoagulant activity in vitro.[1] Some venoms (e.g. *Pseudonaja*, *Pseudechis* and *Micropechis ikaheka*, the New Guinean small-eyed snake) are anticoagulant. Haemostatic abnormalities are particularly frequent and serious in patients bitten by tiger snakes (*Notechis* species), taipans (*Oxyuranus* species) and brown snakes (*Pseudonaja* species), uncommon with bites by black snakes (*Pseudechis* species) and rare with bites by death adders (*Acanthophis* species).

In the past there has been some confusion between haemoglobinuria and myoglobinuria in patients passing dark urine. It is now clear, however, that haemoglobinaemia and haemoglobinuria can occur as a result of intravascular haemolysis (e.g. with envenoming by *Pseudechis australis*) but that myoglobinuria caused by generalized rhabdomyolysis is also a feature of envenoming by some species (e.g. *Notechis, Oxyuranus, Pseudechis australis*, etc.). Renal failure may result from haemoglobinuria or myoglobinuria.

Snake venom ophthalmia[5,31]

Venom ophthalmia results when venom of spitting elapids enters the eye. There is intense local pain, blepharospasm, palpebral oedema and leucorrhoea (Figure 32.15). Slit-lamp or fluorescein examination reveals corneal erosions in more than half the patients spat at by *Naja nigricollis*.[31] Secondary infection of the corneal lesions may result in permanent opacities, causing blindness or panophthalmitis, with destruction of the eye. Rarely venom is absorbed into the anterior chamber, causing hypopyon and anterior uveitis. Seventh (facial) cranial nerve paralysis is a rare complication.

Venom of other snakes, including Viperidae, may be forcibly ejected when striking, for example against the bars of a cage. There are reported cases of venom entering the eye under these circumstances and resulting in intense local pain and inflammation.

Bites by sea snakes[1,15,39]

The bite is usually painless and may not be noticed by the wader or swimmer. Teeth may be left in the wound. There is minimal or no local swelling and involvement of local

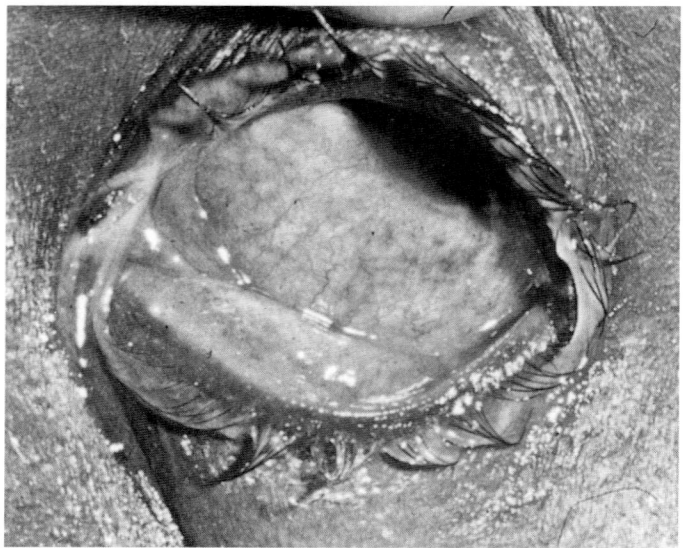

Figure 32.15: Intense conjunctivitis with leucorrhoea (and corneal erosions) in a patient 'spat' at 3 hours previously by an African black-necked or spitting cobra (*Naja nigricollis*). (Copyright D. A. Warrell.)

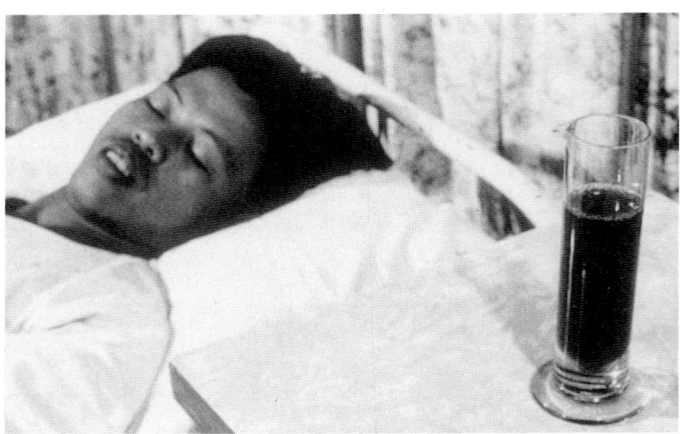

Figure 32.16: Myoglobinuria resulting from generalized rhabdomyolysis in a Malayan fisherman envenomed by a sea snake. (Courtesy of the late H. A. Reid.)

lymph nodes is unusual. Generalized rhabdomyolysis is the dominant effect of envenoming by these snakes. Early symptoms include headache, a thick feeling of the tongue, thirst, sweating and vomiting. Generalized aching, stiffness and tenderness of the muscles become noticeable between 30 minutes and 3½ hours after the bite. Trismus is common. Passive stretching of the muscles is painful. Later, there is progressive flaccid paralysis starting with ptosis, as in elapid envenoming. The patient remains conscious until the respiratory muscles are sufficiently affected to cause respiratory failure. Myoglobinaemia and myoglobinuria develop 3–8 hours after the bite (Figure 32.16). These are suspected when the serum/plasma appears brownish and the urine dark reddish-brown ('Coca-Cola-coloured'). 'Stix' tests will appear positive for haemoglobin/blood in urine containing myoglobin. Myoglobin and potassium released from damaged skeletal muscles may cause renal failure, while hyperkalaemia developing within 6–12 hours of the bite may precipitate cardiac arrest.

Viperidae (Old World vipers and adders, New World pit vipers, rattlesnakes, moccasins and lance-headed vipers, Asian pit vipers)

Venoms of vipers and pit vipers usually produce more local effects than other snake venoms. Swelling may appear within 15 minutes, but rarely is delayed for several hours. It spreads rapidly, sometimes to involve the whole limb and adjacent trunk. There is associated pain, tenderness and enlargement of regional lymph nodes. Bruising, especially along the path of superficial lymphatics and over regional lymph nodes, is common (Figure 32.17). There may be persistent bleeding from the fang marks. Swollen limbs can accommodate many litres of extravasated blood, leading to hypovolaemic shock. Blistering may appear at the bite site as early as 12 hours after the bite. Blisters contain clear or bloodstained fluid (Figure 32.18). Necrosis of skin, subcutaneous tissue and muscle (Figure 32.19) develops in up to 10% of hospitalized cases, especially following bites by North American rattlesnakes

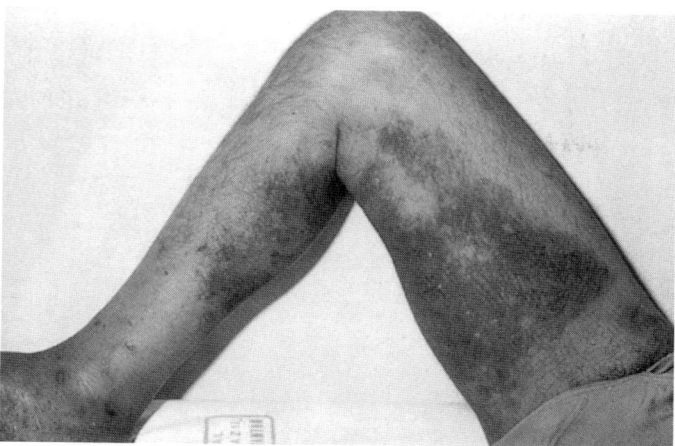

Figure 32.17: Extensive bruising in a Brazilian patient 36 hours after being bitten on the ankle by a jararaca (*Bothrops jararaca*). (Copyright D. A. Warrell.)

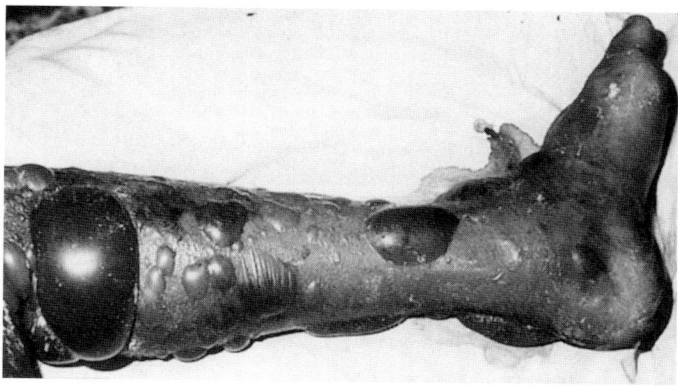

Figure 32.18: Massive swelling and bulla formation in a Thai patient 36 hours after being bitten by a Malayan pit viper (*Calloselasma rhodostoma*). (Copyright D. A. Warrell.)

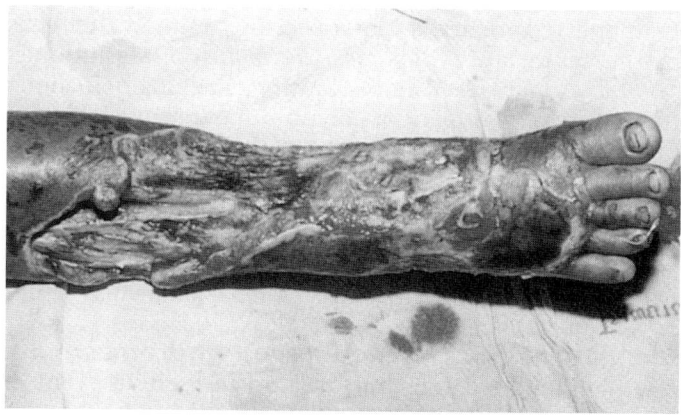

Figure 32.19: Extensive necrosis of the skin and muscle in a 5-year-old Thai child 10 days after being bitten by a Malayan pit viper (*Calloselasma rhodostoma*). (Courtesy of Sornchai Looareesuwan, Bangkok.)

(e.g. *Crotalus adamanteus*, *C. atrox*, *C. horridus* and *C. viridis*), South American lance-headed vipers (genus *Bothrops*), bushmasters (genus *Lachesis*) and Asian pit vipers (e.g. *Calloselasma rhodostoma*, *Deinagkistrodon acutus* and *Trimeresurus flavoviridis*), African vipers (genus *Bitis*), saw-scaled vipers (genus *Echis*) and Palestine viper (*Vipera palaestinae*). Bites on the digits and in areas draining into the tight fascial compartments, such as the anterior tibial compartment, are particularly likely to result in necrosis. High intracompartmental pressure may cause ischaemia which contributes, together with direct effects of the venom, to muscle necrosis. Severe pain associated with tense swelling, segmental anaesthesia and pain on stretching the intracompartmental muscles (e.g. dorsiflexion of the foot in the case of the anterior tibial compartment) should raise the possibility of raised intracompartmental pressure. Sudden severe pain, absence of arterial pulses and a demarcated cold segment of limb suggests thrombosis of a major artery. Deep venous thrombosis has been described surprisingly rarely.

The absence of detectable local swelling 2 hours after a viper bite usually means that no venom has been injected. However, there are important exceptions to this rule: fatal systemic envenoming by the tropical rattlesnake (*Crotalus durissus terrificus*), Mojave rattlesnake (*C. scutulatus*) and Burmese Russell's viper (*Daboia russelii siamensis*) may occur in the absence of local signs. Victims of *C. d. terrificus* may develop local erythema but rarely any swelling.[40]

Haemostatic abnormalities are characteristic of envenoming by Viperidae, but are usually absent in patients bitten by the smaller European vipers (*Vipera berus*, *V. aspis*, *V. ammodytes*, etc.) and some species of rattlesnakes. Persistent bleeding (> 10 minutes) from the fang puncture wounds and from new injuries such as venepuncture sites and old partially healed wounds is the first clinical evidence of consumption coagulopathy. Spontaneous systemic haemorrhage is most often detected in the gingival sulci (Figure 32.20). Bloodstaining of saliva and sputum usually reflects bleeding gums or epistaxis. True haemoptysis is rare. Haematuria may be detected a few hours after the bite. Other types of spontaneous bleeding are ecchymoses, intraocular and subconjunctival haemorrhages, bleeding into the floor of the mouth, tympanic membrane, and gastrointestinal and genitourinary tracts, petechiae and larger discoid and follicular haemorrhages (Figure 32.21). Bleeding into the anterior pituitary (resembling Sheehan's syndrome) may complicate envenoming by Russell's vipers in Burma and India and, rarely, by *Bothrops* species. Menorrhagia and antepartum and postpartum haemorrhage have been described after envenoming by vipers. Severe headache and meningism suggest subarachnoid haemorrhage, evidence of a developing central nervous system lesion (e.g. hemiplegia), irritability, loss of consciousness and convulsions suggest intracranial haemorrhage (Figure 32.22) or cerebral thrombosis. Abdominal distension, tenderness and peritonism with signs of haemorrhagic shock but no external blood loss (haematemesis or melaena) suggest retroperitoneal or intraperitoneal haemorrhage. Incoagulable blood resulting from defibrination or DIC is

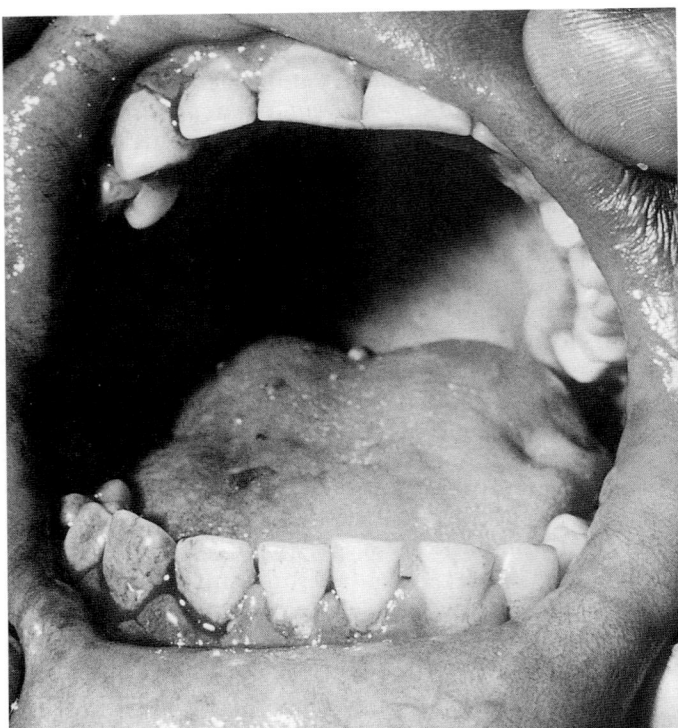

Figure 32.20: Bleeding from gingival sulci in a Nigerian patient bitten by a saw-scaled or carpet viper (*Echis ocellatus*). (Copyright D. A. Warrell.)

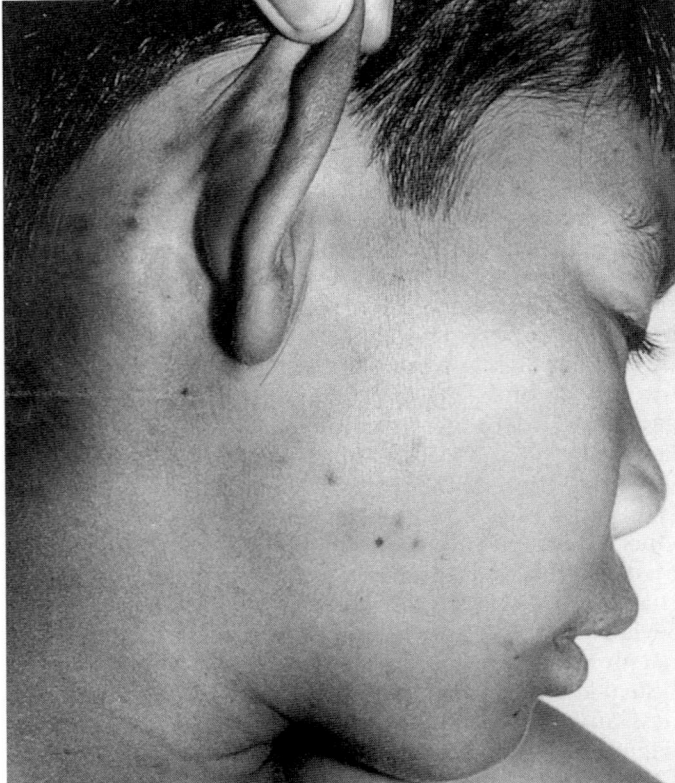

Figure 32.21: Discoid haemorrhages in a Thai boy 6 hours after being bitten by a Malayan pit viper (*Calloselasma rhodostoma*). (Copyright D.A. Warrell.)

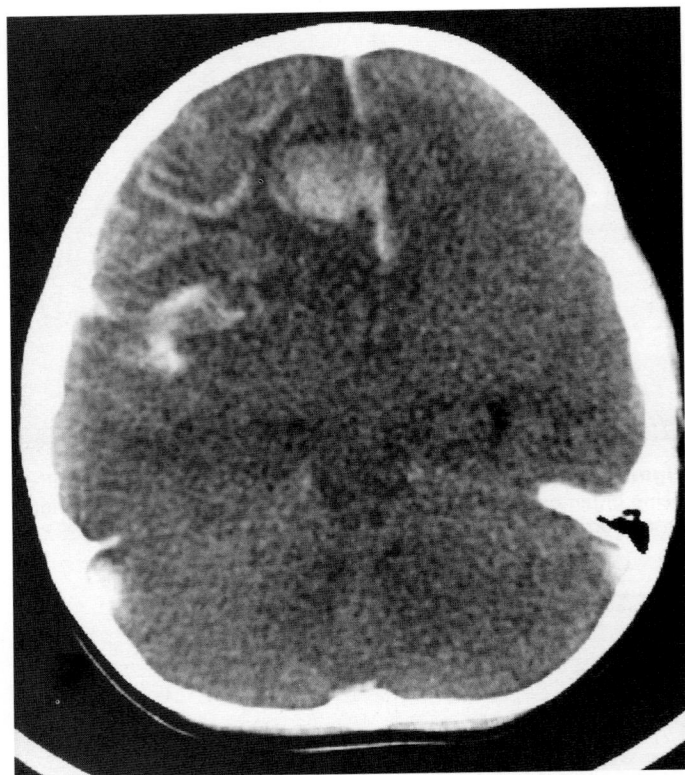

Figure 32.22: Cerebral CT scan of a 7-year-old Ecuadorian girl who had developed sudden headache followed by loss of consciousness 25 hours after being bitten by a *Bothrops atrox*. There is extensive intracranial haemorrhage with a fluid level indicating incoagulable blood. (Copyright D. A. Warrell.)

a common and important finding in patients systemically envenomed by members of the following genera: *Atheris, Daboia, Vipera, Echis, Lachesis, Agkistrodon, Gloydius, Bothrops, Calloselasma, Crotalus, Deinagkistrodon* and *Trimeresurus*. Thrombosis of major arteries (cerebral, pulmonary, coronary, etc.) is especially common after bites by the 'fer de lance' (*Bothrops lanceolatus*) of Martinique.

Intravascular haemolysis, causing haemoglobinaemia (pink plasma) and black or greyish urine (haemoglobinuria or methaemoglobinuria), has been convincingly described in patients bitten by Sri Lankan Russell's viper (*Daboia russelii russelii*),[28] desert horned viper (*Cerastes cerastes*) and South American *Bothrops* species. Features of micro-angiopathic haemolysis and haemolytic uraemic syndrome with progressive severe anaemia and renal failure may result.

Circulatory shock (hypotensive) syndromes

A fall in blood pressure is a common and serious event in patients bitten by vipers, especially in the case of some of the North American rattlesnakes (e.g. *Crotalus adamanteus, C. atrox* and *C. scutulatus*), South American Crotalinae (e.g. *Lachesis muta*) and Old World Viperinae (e.g. *Daboia russelii, Vipera palaestinae, V. berus, Bitis arietans, B. gabonica* and *B. rhinoceros*). Sinus tachycardia suggests hypo-volaemia resulting from external haemorrhage, blood loss into the tissues or local or generalized increase in capillary permeability. Patients envenomed by Burmese Russell's viper (*D. r. siamensis*) may develop conjunctival oedema (Figure 32.23), serous effusions, pulmonary oedema (Figure 32.24), haemoconcentration and a fall in serum albumin concentration—evidence of increased vascular permeability.[11] The pulse rate may be slow or irregular if the venom is affecting the heart directly or reflexly (e.g. *Vipera berus, Bitis arietans, Calloselasma rhodostoma*). Vasovagal syncope may be precipitated by fear and pain. Early, repeated and usually transient syncopal attacks with features of anaphylaxis develop in patients bitten by some Viperidae (e.g. *V. palaestinae,*

V. berus, V. aspis and *D. russelii*). Vomiting, sweating, colic, diarrhoea (with incontinence), shock, bronchospasm, urticaria and angio-oedema of face, lips, gums, tongue and throat may appear as early as 5 minutes or as late as many hours after the bite. Hypotension is an important feature of anaphylactic reactions to antivenom (see below). *Renal failure* can complicate severe envenoming by any species of snake, but it is common, and the most frequent cause of death in victims of Russell's viper, tropical rattlesnake (*Crotalus durissus* subspecies) and some species of *Bothrops*. Patients bitten by Russell's viper may become oliguric within a few hours of the bite. Loin pain and tenderness may be experienced within the first 24 hours and, in 3 or 4 days, the patient may become irritable, comatose or convulsive, with hypertension and evidence of metabolic acidosis. Neurotoxicity, attributable to venom phospholipases A_2, is a feature of envenoming by a few species of Viperidae (e.g. *C. d. terrificus, Gloydius blomhoffii, Vipera aspis, Bitis atropos* and other small South African *Bitis* species and Sri Lankan Russell's viper). The clinical features are the same as with elapid envenoming (Figure 32.25). Progression to respiratory or generalized

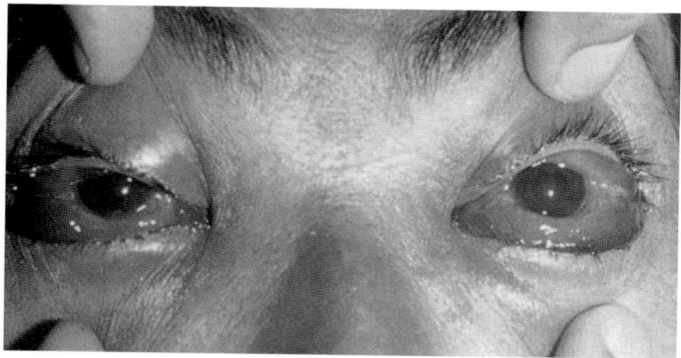

Figure 32.23: Intense bilateral conjunctival oedema (chemosis) in a Burmese man bitten 24 hours previously by a Russell's viper (*Daboia russelii siamensis*). (Copyright D. A. Warrell.)

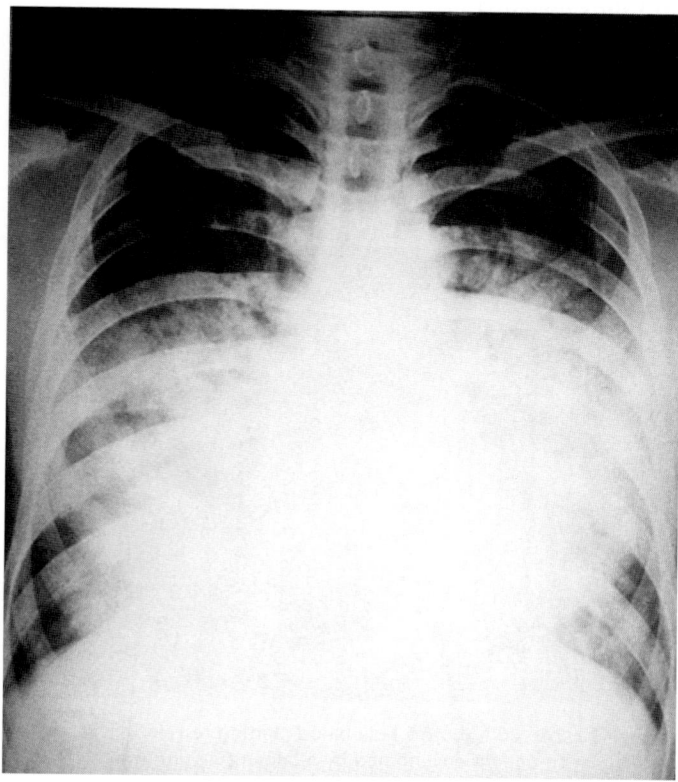

Figure 32.24: Chest radiograph of a Burmese man who developed pulmonary oedema after being bitten by a Russell's viper (*Daboia russelii siamensis*). (Copyright D. A. Warrell.)

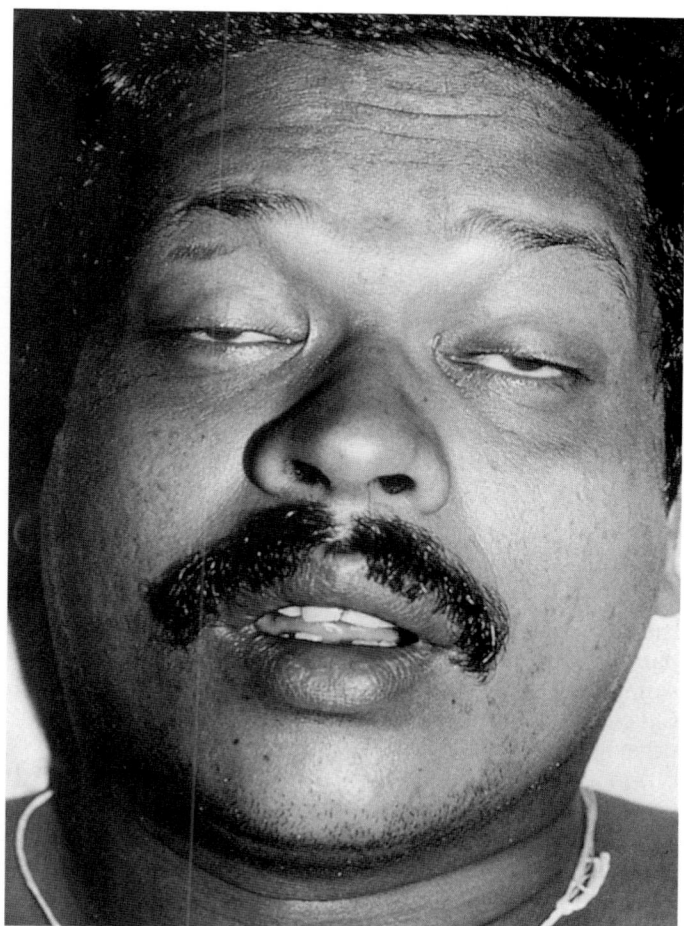

Figure 32.25: Sri Lankan man with neurotoxic envenoming by Russell's viper (*Daboia russelii russelii*). There is ptosis, ophthalmoplegia and inability to open the mouth and protrude the tongue. (Copyright D. A. Warrell.)

paralysis has been described. Associated generalized myalgia suggests the possibility of rhabdomyolysis. Pupillary dilatation, causing visual disturbance from loss of accommodation, is a feature of severe envenoming by tropical rattlesnakes and small *Bitis* species (e.g. *B. peringueyi*) and may be a permanent neurological sequel.

Clinical course and prognosis

Local swelling is usually evident within 2–4 hours of bites by vipers and cytotoxic cobras and may evolve very rapidly after rattlesnake bites. Swelling is maximal and most extensive on the second or third day after the bite. Resolution of swelling and restoration of normal function in the bitten limb may be delayed for months, especially in older people (e.g. after bites by the European adder *Vipera berus*). The earliest systemic symptoms such as vomiting and syncope may develop within minutes of the bite, but even in the case of rapidly absorbed elapid venoms patients rarely die less than an hour after the bite. Defibrination may be complete within 1–2 hours of the bite (e.g. saw-scaled or carpet viper *Echis ocellatus*).[41] Neurotoxic signs may progress to generalized flaccid paralysis and respiratory arrest within a few hours. If the venom is not neutralized by antivenom, these effects may be prolonged. Defibrination can persist for weeks (*Echis* species and *Calloselasma rhodostoma*). Patients with neurotoxic envenoming have recovered after being artificially ventilated for up to 10 weeks. Tissue necrosis usually declares itself within a week of the bite. Sloughing of necrotic tissue and secondary infections including osteomyelitis may occur during subsequent weeks or months. Deaths occurring from neurotoxic envenoming are caused by upper airway obstruction or respiratory paralysis, whereas later deaths may result from technical complications of mechanical ventilation or intractable hypotension. Late deaths, more than 5 days after the bite, are usually the result of renal failure. Delayed shock with recurrent spontaneous haemorrhage has been described in victims of Burmese Russell's viper: pituitary and other intracranial haemorrhages have been found at autopsy.

Risk of envenoming

Even when the fangs of a venomous snake have pierced the skin, envenoming is not inevitable. About 20% of patients bitten by North American rattlesnakes, Central American lance-headed vipers (mainly *Bothrops*), *Calloselasma rhodostoma* and *Daboia russelii* show absolutely no evidence of envenoming, and as many as 80% of those bitten by sea snakes and Australasian common brown snakes (*Pseudonaja textilis*) and 50% by *C. rhodostoma* or *D. russelii* have trivial or no envenoming. Untreated snake bite mortality is hard to assess, for hospital admissions include a disproportionate number of severe cases, and data for untreated snake bites is available only from the pre-antivenom era or from occasions when antivenom supply is limited, an antivenom of low potency is used[13] or when antivenom is withheld by doctors who doubt its efficacy. The untreated mortality of *Crotalus durissus*

terrificus is said to have been 74%, but has been reduced to 12% by antivenom, while the mortality of *Echis ocellatus* bites has been reduced from about 20% to 3% with antivenom. Prognosis appears to be worst in infants and in the elderly, but there is no convincing evidence that children have a worse prognosis than young adults, despite the larger dose of venom relative to their body weight.

Interval between bite and death

Death after snake bite may occur as rapidly as 'a few minutes' (reputedly after a bite by the king cobra *Ophiophagus hannah*) or as long as 41 days after a bite by the saw-scaled or carpet viper (*Echis carinatus*). The speed of killing has been exaggerated. Most elapid deaths occur within hours of the bite, most sea snake bite deaths between 12 and 24 hours and viper bite deaths within days.

Laboratory investigations

Systemic envenoming is usually associated with a neutrophil leucocytosis: counts above 20×10^9/litre indicate severe envenoming. Initially, haematocrit may be high from haemoconcentration when there is generalized increase in capillary permeability (e.g. *Crotalus* species, Burmese *Daboia russelii*). Later haematocrit falls because of bleeding into the bitten limb and elsewhere, and from intravascular haemolysis or microangiopathic haemolysis in patients with DIC. Thrombocytopenia is common (e.g. *D. russelii*, *Calloselasma rhodostoma*, *Crotalus viridis helleri* and *Bitis arietans*).

20-minute whole blood clotting test[41,42]
Incoagulable blood is a cardinal sign of systemic envenoming by most of the Viperidae, many of the Australasian elapids and the medically important Colubridae. For clinical purposes, a simple, bedside, all-or-nothing test of

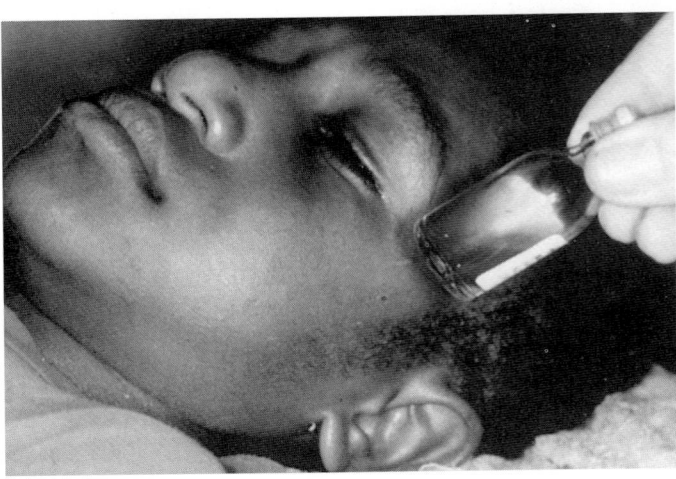

Figure 32.26: 20-Minute whole blood clotting test. In this Papua New Guinean patient envenomed by a taipan (*Oxyuranus scutellatus canni*) a few millilitres of venous blood were placed in the new, clean, dry, glass bottle and left to stand at room temperature for 20 minutes. At the end of this time the blood is still liquid, indicating defibrinogenation. (Copyright D. A. Warrell.)

blood coagulability is adequate. A few millilitres of blood taken by venepuncture is placed in a new, clean, dry, glass vessel; left undisturbed at room temperature for 20 minutes; then tipped once to see if there is clotting or not (Figure 32.26).

More sensitive tests which are rapid and relatively simple to perform are whole blood or plasma prothrombin times and detection of elevated concentrations of FDP by agglutination of sensitized latex particles or of D-dimer. Serum concentrations of creatine kinase, aspartate transferase and blood urea are commonly raised in patients with severe envenoming, because of local muscle damage at the site of the bite. Generalized rhabdomyolysis caused by sea snake, Australasian elapid, tropical rattlesnake and Sri Lankan Russell's viper bites causes a steep rise in serum creatine kinase and other muscle-derived enzymes, myoglobin and potassium concentrations. Plasma is stained brownish by myoglobin and pink by haemoglobin. Heparinized blood should be allowed to sediment spontaneously (without centrifugation) to reveal these pigments. Patients with intravascular haemolysis have black urine (as in malarial 'blackwater fever'). It is brownish, pinkish or reddish in those with haematuria or myoglobinuria. Blood urea or serum creatinine and potassium concentrations should be measured in patients who become oliguric, especially in cases with a high risk of renal failure (e.g. *Daboia russelli*, *Crotalus durissus terrificus*, *Bothrops* species, terrestrial Australasian snakes, sea snakes and Colubridae). Severely sick, hypotensive and shocked patients will develop lactic acidosis (suggested by an increased anion gap), those with renal failure will also develop a metabolic acidosis (decreased plasma pH and bicarbonate concentration, reduced arterial PCO_2), and patients with respiratory paralysis will develop respiratory acidosis (low pH, high arterial PCO_2, decreased PO_2) or respiratory alkalosis if they are mechanically overventilated.

All snake-bitten patients should be encouraged to empty their bladder on admission. Urine should be examined for blood/haemoglobin and protein (by 'Stix' test) and for microscopic haematuria and red cell casts.

Electrocardiographic abnormalities include sinus bradycardia, ST–T changes, various degrees of atrioventricular block and evidence of hyperkalaemia. Shock may induce myocardial ischaemia or infarction in patients with diseased coronary arteries.

Chest radiographs are useful for detecting pulmonary oedema (e.g. European *Vipera* and *Daboia russelii*; Figure 32.24), pulmonary haemorrhages and infarcts, pleural effusions and secondary bronchopneumonias (*D. russelii*).

Immunodiagnosis

Detection of venom antigens in body fluids of snake bite victims has improved diagnosis, understanding of pathophysiological mechanisms, assessment of first aid methods and control of antivenom treatment.[43,44] Enzyme immunoassay (EIA) has been the most widely used technique for research.[43,44] Venom detection kits are available commercially only in Australia from the Commonwealth Serum Laboratories.[1] They are highly sensitive but their specificity may be inadequate to distinguish between different species.

False-positive reactions are common, especially in the sera of rural populations in the tropics. Relatively high venom antigen concentrations (e.g. from wound swabs or aspirates) can be detected within 15–30 minutes. For retrospective diagnosis, including forensic cases, tissue around the fang punctures, wound and blister aspirate, serum and urine should be stored for EIA.

Management of snake bite[2,45]
First aid
First aid can be carried out only by bite victims themselves or bystanders, using materials that are immediately available.

1. Reassure the victim, who is usually terrified.
2. Do not tamper with the bite wound in any way, but immobilize the bitten limb using a splint or sling. If available, firm binding of the splint with a crepe bandage is the most effective form of immobilization.
3. Take the patient as quickly as possible to the nearest health clinic, dispensary or hospital where medical treatment can be given. Muscular contraction in the bitten limb will promote spread of venom, so this should be avoided as far as possible. Ideally, the patient should be transported by motor vehicle, bicycle (as a passenger), boat or on a stretcher.
4. Avoid harmful and time-wasting treatments.
5. Since species diagnosis is critically important, the snake should be taken along to hospital if it has already been killed. However, if the snake is still at large, do not risk further bites and waste time by searching for it. Even snakes which appear to be dead should not be touched with the bare hands but carried in a bag or dangling across a stick. Some species (e.g. *Hemachatus haemachatus*) sham death, and even a severed head can inject venom!

Rejected or controversial first aid methods Cauterization, incision or excision, amputation of the bitten digit, suction by mouth, vacuum pumps[46] or 'venom-ex' apparatus, instillation of chemical compounds such as potassium permanganate, application of ice packs (cryotherapy), 'snake stones' or electric shocks are absolutely contraindicated as they are harmful and have no proven benefit.[47] Incisions provoke uncontrolled bleeding when the blood is incoagulable, may damage nerves, blood vessels or tendons and introduce infection. Suction, chemicals and cryotherapy can cause tissue necrosis. The use of tourniquets, compression pads and crepe bandages to impede absorption of venom is controversial. Tight (arterial) tourniquets have been responsible for terrible morbidity and even mortality in snake bite victims and should not be used. The splinting and crepe bandaging method ('pressure immobilization') advocated by Sutherland in Australia proved effective in limiting the absorption of venom in restrained monkeys.[48] Crepe bandaging is thought to exert a pressure of about 55 mmHg—that of a venous tourniquet. In practice, it is difficult to judge how tightly to apply the crepe bandage and difficult for the patient to apply it unaided. External compression increases intracompartmental pressure and may accentuate the effects of some necrotic snake venoms.[49] Dangers of tourniquets are ischaemia and gangrene, if they are applied for more than about 2 hours, damage to peripheral nerves (especially the lateral popliteal nerve), increased fibrinolytic activity, congestion, swelling, increased bleeding, increased local effects of venom and shock or rapid development of life-threatening systemic envenoming after their release. However, if a patient is bitten by a dangerous neurotoxic elapid (such as a mamba, king cobra or taipan) or by a sea snake, there is a risk that respiratory paralysis might develop en route to hospital. In these cases it is recommended that a crepe bandage and splint be applied, as tightly as for a sprained ankle, but not so tightly as to obliterate the peripheral arterial pulse. Lymphoscintigraphy studies in simulated envenoming showed that excessive pressure (> 70 mmHg) and movement of the other limbs increased spread of venom.[50] The patient should lie down and remain as immobile as possible during the journey to hospital.

Treatment of early symptoms

Distressing and dangerous manifestations of envenoming may appear before the patient reaches hospital.

Local pain may be intense. Oral paracetamol is preferable to aspirin or non-steroidal anti-inflammatory agents, which carry the risk of gastric bleeding in patients with incoagulable blood. *Severe pain* should be treated with opiates.

Vomiting is a common early symptom of systemic envenoming. Patients should lie in the recovery position (on their left side) with their head down to avoid aspiration. Persistent vomiting can be treated with intravenous chlorpromazine (25–50 mg in adults, 1 mg/kg in children).*

Syncopal attacks and anaphylactic shock Patients who collapse within minutes of the bite may show features of either a vasovagal attack with profound bradycardia or of anaphylaxis with angio-oedema, urticaria, asthma, abdominal colic and diarrhoea. Anaphylaxis should be treated with adrenaline 0.1% (1 in 1000) (0.5 ml in adults, 0.01 ml/kg in children) by intramuscular injection, followed by a histamine H_1-blocker such as chlorpheniramine maleate (10 mg in adults, 0.2 mg/kg in children), which can be given by intravenous or intramuscular* injection.

Respiratory distress This may result from upper airway obstruction if the jaw, tongue and bulbar muscles are paralysed or from paralysis of the respiratory muscles. Patients should be placed in the recovery position, the airway cleared, if possible using a suction pump, an oral airway inserted and the jaw elevated. If the patient is cyanosed, or respiratory movements are very weak, oxygen should be given by any available means. If clearing the airway does not produce immediate relief, artificial ventilation must be initiated. In the absence of any equipment, mouth-to-mouth or mouth-to-nose ventilation can be life-saving. Manual ventilation by Ambu bag and anaesthetic mask is rarely effective. Ideally, a cuffed endotracheal tube should be introduced, using a laryngoscope, or a cuffed tracheostomy tube inserted. The patient can then be ventilated by Ambu bag. If no femoral or carotid pulse can be felt, external cardiac massage should be instituted.

Treatment at health clinic, dispensary or hospital by medically trained staff

Clinical assessment Snake bite is a medical emergency. The history, symptoms and signs must be assessed rapidly to direct urgent appropriate treatment. Three important preliminary questions are: Where (in which part of your body) were you bitten? How long ago were you bitten? Have you brought the snake or, if not, did you see what kind of snake it was? If the snake has been killed but not brought, someone should be despatched to collect it posthaste. Only if the snake can be diagnosed confidently as non-venomous can the patient can be discharged after a booster dose of tetanus toxoid. Patients should be asked whether they have taken any herbal or other treatment, whether they have vomited, fainted, or have noticed any bleeding or other ill-effects of the bite and whether they have passed urine since being bitten. Physical signs should be assessed before any compression bandage or tourniquet is removed. Fang marks are sometimes invisible and rarely help the diagnosis, although the discovery of only two or three discrete puncture marks suggests a bite by a venomous snake. Local swelling, tenderness and lymph node involvement are early signs of envenoming. The gingival sulci are usually the earliest site of detectable spontaneous bleeding. Bleeding from venepuncture sites, recent wounds and skin lesions suggests incoagulable blood. If the patient is shocked (collapsed, sweating, cold, cyanosed extremities, low blood pressure, tachycardia) the foot of the bed should be raised, and an intravenous infusion of a plasma expander such as fresh frozen plasma, dextran, Haemaccel, Gelofusine or fresh blood started immediately. The jugular or central venous pressure should be observed. The earliest symptom of neurotoxicity after elapid bites is often blurred vision, a feeling of heaviness in the eyelids and drowsiness. The earliest sign is contraction of the frontalis muscle (raised eyebrows and puckered forehead) even before true ptosis can be demonstrated. Signs of respiratory muscle paralysis (dyspnoea, 'paradoxical' abdominal respiration, contraction of intercostal muscles and cyanosis) are ominous. Patients with generalized rhabdomyolysis may have trismus and muscles that are stiff, tender and resistant to passive stretching. Urine output may dwindle very early in the course of Russell's viper bite. Black urine suggests myoglobinuria or haemoglobinuria.

---

*In patients with incoagulable blood, injections can cause haematomas. Pressure dressings should be applied to all injection sites to prevent oozing.

Even if there is no evidence of envenoming on presentation, patients should be admitted for observation, ideally for 24 hours. Every hour, symptoms, level of consciousness, ptosis, pulse rate and rhythm, blood pressure, respiratory rate, extent of local swelling and other new signs should be recorded. If there is any evidence of neurotoxicity, the ventilatory capacity or expiratory pressure should also be recorded every hour. Useful investigations include the 20-minute whole blood clotting test (or other tests of coagulation), peripheral leucocyte count, haematocrit, urine microscopy and 'Stix' testing and electrocardiography.

Antivenom (antivenin, antivenene, anti-snake bite serum)

Antivenom is the concentrated enzyme-refined immunoglobulin of animals, usually horses or sheep, which have been immunized with venom. It is the only specific treatment available and has proved effective against many of the lethal and damaging effects of venoms. In the management of snake bite, the most important clinical decision is whether or not to give antivenom, for only a minority of snake-bitten patients need it, it may produce severe reactions, and it is expensive and often in short supply.

Indications for antivenom

Systemic envenoming

1. Haemostatic abnormalities: spontaneous systemic bleeding, incoagulable blood or prolonged clotting time, elevated FDP, or D-dimer, thrombocytopenia.
2. Cardiovascular abnormalities: hypotension, shock, abnormal electrocardiogram, cardiac arrhythmia, cardiac failure, pulmonary oedema.
3. Neurotoxicity.
4. Generalized rhabdomyolysis.
5. In patients with definite signs of local envenoming, the following indicate significant systemic envenoming: neutrophil leucocytosis, elevated serum enzymes such as creatine kinase and aminotransferases, haemoconcentration, uraemia, hypercreatininaemia, oliguria, hypoxaemia, acidosis and vomiting in the absence of a history of ingesting emetic agents.

Severe local envenoming
In the absence of (1)–(4) above, an indication for antivenom is the development at any stage of local swelling involving more than half the bitten limb or extensive blistering or bruising, especially in patients showing the abnormalities listed above under (5) and in patients bitten by species known to cause local necrosis (e.g. Viperidae, Asian cobras, African spitting cobras, *Naja nigricollis*, *N. pallida*, *N. mossambica* and *N. nigricinctus*). Bites on the digits by these species carry a high risk of necrosis and so antivenom is also indicated in such cases.

Some wealthy countries can afford a wider range of indications for the use of antivenom. The following *additional* indications have been suggested:

- *United States and Canada*. Following bites by the most dangerous rattlesnakes (*Crotalus atrox*, *C. adamanteus*, *C. viridis*, *C. horridus* and *C. scutulatus*) antivenom therapy has been recommended if there is rapid spread of local swelling, even without evidence of systemic envenoming, and after bites by coral snakes (*Micruroides euryxanthus* and *Micrurus fulvius*) if there is immediate pain or any other symptom or sign of envenoming.
- *Australia*. Antivenom is recommended in any proved or suspected case of snake bite if there is any evidence of systemic spread of venom, including tender regional lymph nodes, and if there has been an effective bite by any identified highly venomous species.[1]
- *Europe*. To improve the rate of recovery of local swelling after bites by *Vipera berus*, antivenom has been recommended in adults with swelling extending up the forearm or leg within 2 hours of the bite.[51]

Contraindications Atopic patients and those who have had reactions to equine antiserum on previous occasions have an increased risk of developing severe antivenom reactions. In such cases antivenom should not be given unless there are definite signs of severe (potentially life-threatening) systemic envenoming. Pretreatment with adrenaline, antihistamine and corticosteroid is recommended. Rapid desensitization is not recommended.

Prediction of antivenom reactions Hypersensitivity testing by intradermal or subcutaneous injection or intraconjunctival instillation of diluted antivenom has been widely practised in the past. However, these tests delay the start of antivenom treatment, are not without risk, and have no predictive value for early (anaphylactic) or late (serum sickness type) antivenom reactions, which are usually not manifestations of IgE-mediated Type I hypersensitivity.[52]

Prevention of antivenom reactions Intramuscular promethazine is ineffective,[53] but in one trial subcutaneous adrenaline (epinephrine) (0.1%, adult dose 0.25 mg) reduced the incidence of early antivenom reactions.[54]

Administration of antivenom The range of venoms neutralized by an antivenom is usually stated in the package insert and is to be found in compendia of antivenoms.[55] If the biting species is known or can be deduced reliably, the appropriate monospecific antivenom should be used. In parts of the world where several species produce identical signs, patients who fail to bring the dead snake must be treated with polyspecific antivenom, which will contain a lower concentration of specific antibody to each species than the monospecific antivenom.

Manufacturers' expiry dates are often extremely conservative. Liquid lyophilized antivenoms stored at below 8°C usually retain most of their activity for 5 years or more.[56] Opaque solutions should not be given as precipitation of protein indicates loss of activity and an increased risk of reactions. Antivenom should be given as soon as it is indicated, but it is almost never too late to give it as long as signs of systemic envenoming persist (e.g. up to 2 days after a sea snake bite and many days or even weeks for prolonged defibrination following bites by Viperidae). In contrast, local effects of venoms are probably not reversible by antivenom delayed more than 1–2 hours after the bite. The intravenous route is the most effective. An infusion over 30–60 minutes of antivenom diluted in isotonic fluid may be easier to control than an intravenous 'push' injection of reconstituted but undiluted antivenom given over 10–20 minutes. There is no difference in the incidence of severity of antivenom reactions in patients treated by these two methods.[52] In the rural tropics the intravenous push method has the advantage that it involves less expensive equipment, is quicker to initiate and compels someone to remain with the patient at least while the injection is being given.

In the absence of anyone capable of giving an intravenous injection, antivenom may be given by deep intramuscular injection (e.g. at several sites into the anterolateral aspect of the thighs but not into the gluteal region) followed by massage to promote absorption. However, the volumes of antivenom normally required would make this route impracticable, as would the risk of haematoma

Table 32.3 Guide to initial dosage of some important antivenoms

Species			
Latin name	**English name**	**Manufacturer, antivenom**	**Approximate initial dose**
Acanthophis species	Death adder	CSL*, monospecific	3000–6000 units
Bitis arietans	Puff adder	Aventis-Pasteur ("Fav Afrique" & "FaviRept" polyspecific); SAIMR†; polyspecific	80 ml
Bothrops jararaca	Jararaca	Brazilian manufacturers, *Bothrops* polyspecific	20 ml
Bungarus caeruleus	Common krait	Indian manufacturers, polyspecific	100 ml
Calloselasma (Agkistrodon) rhodostoma	Malayan pit viper	Thai Red Cross Bangkok, monospecific	100 ml
Crotalus adamanteus	Eastern diamondback rattlesnakes	Protherics ("CroFab")	7–15 vials
Crotalus atrox	Western diaondback rattlesnakes		
Crotalus viridis subspecies	Western rattlesnakes		
Daboia (Vipera) russelii	Russell's vipers	Myanmar Pharmaceutical Industry, monospecific	40 ml
		Indian manufacturers, polyspecific	100 ml
		Thai Red Cross, monospecific	50 ml
Echis species	Saw-scaled or carpet vipers	SAIMR, *Echis*, monpsecific	20 ml
		Aventis-Pasteur ("Fav Afrique")	100 ml
Hydrophiinae	Sea snakes	CSL, sea snakes/tiger snake	1000 units
Naja kaouthia	Monocellate Thai cobra	Thai Red Cross, monospecific	100 ml
Naja naja	Indian cobra	Indian manufacturers, polyspecific	100 ml
Notechis scutatus	Tiger snake	CSL, monospecific	3000–6000 units
Pseudechis textilis	Eastern brown snake		
Oxyuranus scutellatus	Taipan	CSL, monospecific	12 000 units
Trimeresurus albolabris	Green pit viper	Thai Red Cross, monospecific	100 ml
Vipera berus	European adder	Immunoloski Zavod-Zagreb Vipera polyspecific	10 ml
		Protherics Fab monospecific "ViperaTAb"	100–200 mg
Vipera palaestinae	Palestine viper	Rogoff Medical Research Institute, Tel Aviv, Palestine viper monospecific	50–80 ml

* Commonwealth Serum Laboratories, Australia
† South African Institute for Medical Research

formation in patients with incoagulable blood. Local injection of antivenom, for example into the fang marks, seems rational but is difficult, painful and hazardous (especially when the bite is on a digit or other tight compartment) and has not proved effective in animal studies.

The average initial dose of antivenom required should be based on results of clinical studies, but these are rarely available. Most manufacturers base their recommendations on the mouse assay, which may not correlate with clinical findings.[57] Initial doses of some important antivenoms are given in Table 32.3. The apparent serum half-lives of antivenoms in envenomed patients range from 26 to 95 hours, depending on which IgG fragment they contain.[58,59] Systemic envenoming may recur several days after an initial good response to antivenom.[49] This is probably the result of continuing absorption of venom from the injection site after antivenom has been largely cleared from the circulation or perhaps by redistribution of venom from tissue in response to antivenom. The implication is that an initial dose of antivenom, however large, may not prevent late or recurrent envenoming. *Children must be given the same or larger doses of antivenom than adults.* The response to antivenom will determine whether further doses should be given. Neurotoxic signs may improve within 30 minutes of antivenom treatment but usually take several hours. Hypotension, sinus bradycardia and spontaneous systemic bleeding may respond within 10–20 minutes and blood coagulability is usually restored between 1 and 6 hours, provided sufficient antivenom has been given. A second dose of antivenom should be given if severe cardio-respiratory symptoms persist for more than about 30 minutes, and incoagulable blood persists for more than 6 hours, after the start of the first dose. Enormous doses of antivenom may be required to treat patients bitten by large species capable of injecting very large amounts of venom or extremely potent venom. Thus a patient bitten by the king cobra (*Ophiophagus hannah*) was given 1150 ml of specific antivenom and prolonged artificial ventilation.[34] Other exceptionally large species include bushmasters (genus *Lachesis*), diamondback rattlesnakes (*Crotalus adamanteus*, *C. atrox*), Gabon vipers (*Bitis gabonica*, *B. rhinoceros*) and black mamba (*Dendroaspis polylepis*).

Antivenom reactions   Antivenom treatment may be complicated by early (anaphylactic), pyrogenic or late (serum sickness-type) reactions.

Early antivenom reactions are not usually Type I IgE-mediated hypersensitivity reactions to equine serum proteins and are not predicted by hypersensitivity tests.[52] Antivenoms activate complement in vitro, while the clinically similar reactions to homologous serum are associated with complement activation and immune complex formation in vivo. The complement system is probably activated by aggregates of IgG. Reactions usually develop within 10–180 minutes of starting antivenom. There is itching, urticaria (Figure 32.27), fever, tachycardia, palpitations, cough, nausea and vomiting. The reported incidence, which varies from 3% to 84%, appears to increase

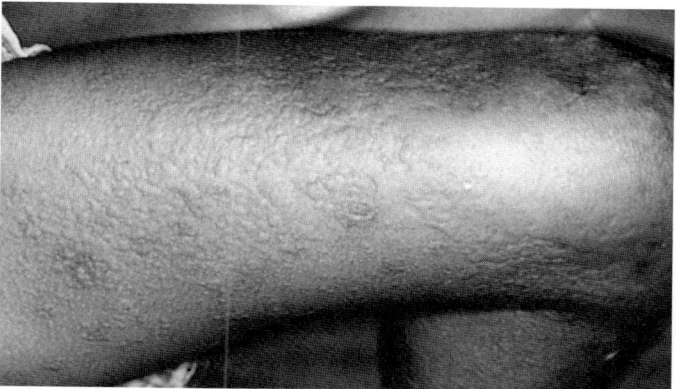

Figure 32.27: Urticaria of the thigh, coalescent over the knee, in a patient experiencing an early antivenom reaction 15 minutes after the start of treatment. (Copyright D. A. Warrell.)

with the dose and to decrease when refined antivenom is used and administration is by intramuscular rather than intravenous injection. Unless patients are watched carefully for 3 hours after treatment, mild reactions may be missed and deaths misattributed to the envenoming itself. Up to 40% of patients with early reactions show features of severe systemic anaphylaxis: bronchospasm, hypotension or angio-oedema, but deaths are rare. Early reactions respond readily to adrenaline given by intramuscular injection of between 0.5 and 1.0 ml of 0.1% (1:1000, 1 mg/ml) in adults (children 0.01 ml/kg) at the first sign of trouble. Antihistamines such as chlorpheniramine maleate (adult dose 10 mg, children 0.2 mg/kg) should be given by intravenous injection to combat the effects of histamine released during the reaction.

Pyrogenic reactions result from contamination of the antivenom by endotoxin-like compounds. High fever develops 1–2 hours after treatment and is associated with rigors, followed by vasodilatation and a fall in blood pressure. Febrile convulsions may be precipitated in children. Patients should be cooled and given antipyretic drugs such as paracetamol, by mouth, powdered and washed down a nasogastric tube (15 mg/kg) or by suppository.

Late (serum sickness-type) reactions develop 5–24 (mean 7) days after treatment. Their incidence and speed of development increase with the dose of antivenom. Symptoms include fever, itching, urticaria, arthralgia—which may involve the temporomandibular joint—lymphadenopathy, periarticular swellings, mononeuritis multiplex, albuminuria and rarely encephalopathy. This is an immune complex disease which responds to an antihistamine such as chlorpheniramine (adults 2 mg four times a day, children 0.25 mg/kg per day in divided doses) or, in more severe cases, to corticosteroid (prednisolone 5 mg four times a day for 5 days in adults, 0.7 mg/kg per day in divided doses for 5 days for children).

Supportive treatment (assuming that adequate doses of antivenom have been given)

Artificial ventilation was first suggested for neurotoxic envenoming more than 100 years ago but patients continue to die for lack of respiratory support. Neurotoxic effects are fully reversible with time: a patient bitten by *Bungarus multicinctus* in Canton recovered completely after being ventilated manually for 30 days, and a patient probably envenomed by *Tropidechis carinatus* recovered after 10 weeks mechanical ventilation in Queensland, Australia. Endotracheal intubation or tracheostomy, using cuffed tubes, is needed. The patient can be ventilated manually with an anaesthetic or Ambu bag or, preferably, with a mechanical ventilator (Figure 32.28).

Anticholinesterase drugs may produce a rapid, useful improvement in neuromuscular transmission in patients envenomed by some species of Asian and African cobras, mambas, death adders (*Acanthophis* species), coral snakes (*Micrurus* species) and kraits.[35] It is worth trying the 'Tensilon test' in all cases of severe neurotoxic envenoming, as with suspected myasthenia gravis. Glycopyrronium bromide (adults 200 µg, children 4 µg/kg) is given first by intravenous injection to block unpleasant muscarinic effects of acetylcholine (increased secretions, abdominal colic). Edrophonium chloride (Tensilon) is then given by slow intravenous injection in an adult dose of 10 mg, or 0.25 mg/kg for children. Patients who respond convincingly can be maintained on neostigmine methylsulphate, 50–100 µg/kg and glycopyrronium 4-hourly or by continuous infusion.

Hypotension and shock   These usually result from hypovolaemia and should be treated by infusing a plasma expander, preferably fresh whole blood or, failing that, fresh frozen plasma. Central venous pressure or pulmonary arterial catheter monitoring is the safest way to control volume replacement. Hypotensive patients envenomed by Burmese Russell's viper responded to dopamine, 2.5 µg/kg per minute by intravenous infusion; but methylprednisolone, 30 mg/kg, and naloxone were not effective.[11]

Renal failure[45]   If urine output drops below 400 ml/24 hours, urethral and central venous catheters should be inserted. If urine flow fails to increase after cautious rehydration, diuretics should be tried (e.g. frusemide by slow intravenous injection, 100 mg followed by 200 mg if urine output fails to increase, and then mannitol). If these measures fail to restore urine flow the patient should be placed on strict fluid balance. Peritoneal or haemodialysis will be required in most patients with established renal failure.

Local infection   Infection at the site of the bite should be prevented with penicillin, erythromycin or chloramphenicol (or by an antimicrobial effective against the bacterial flora of the buccal cavity and venoms of local snakes)[60] and a booster dose of tetanus toxoid should be given. An aminoglycoside such as gentamicin should be added for 48 hours if the wound has been tampered with or there is evidence of local necrosis. Bullae are best left alone. Snake-bitten limbs should not be elevated as this increases the risk of compartmental syndromes. *Necrotic tissue* should be debrided as soon as possible and the denuded area covered with split-skin grafts.

Intracompartmental syndromes   Swelling of muscles within tight fascial compartments may raise the tissue pressure to such an extent that perfusion is impaired and ischaemic damage is added to the effects of the venom. Risk factors include pressure bandaging and elevation of the limb. The signs of an intracompartmental syndrome include excessive pain, weakness of the compartmental muscles and pain when they are passively stretched, hypoaesthesia of areas of skin supplied by nerves running through the compartment and obvious tenseness of the compartment. Palpation of peripheral pulses or their detection by Doppler ultrasound does not exclude intracompartmental ischaemia. An intracompartmental pressure of more than 45 mmHg indicates a high risk of ischaemic necrosis. In these circumstances, fasciotomy may be justified to relieve the pressure in the compartment, but this treatment did not prove effective in saving envenomed muscle in animal experiments.[61] Necrosis

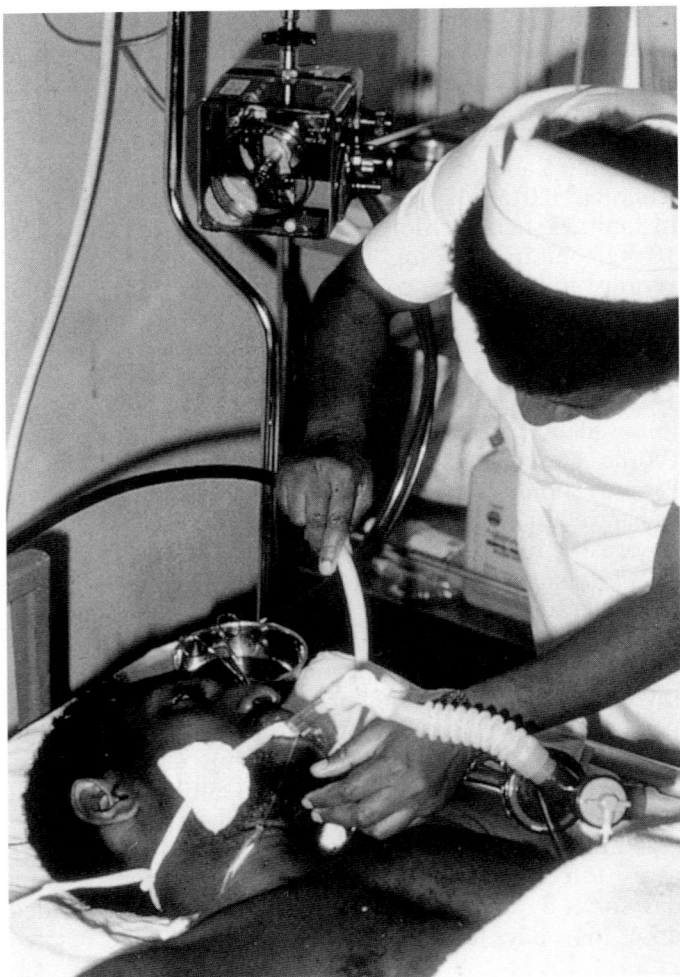

Figure 32.28: Artificial ventilation by Bird ventilator in a patient with complete flaccid paralysis following a bite by a taipan (*Oxyuranus scutellatus canni*) in Central Province, Papua New Guinea. (Copyright D. A. Warrell.)

occurs most frequently after digital bites. Fasciotomy must not be attempted until blood coagulability has been restored by adequate doses of specific antivenom, followed by the transfusion of fresh whole blood or clotting factors.

Corticosteroids, heparin, antifibrinolytic agents such as aprotinin (Trasylol) and ε-aminocaproic acid, antihistamine, trypsin and a variety of traditional herbal remedies have been used and advocated for snake bite. Most are potentially harmful and none has been proved to be effective.

Snake venom ophthalmia

The 'spat' venom should be washed from the eye or mucous membrane as soon as possible using large volumes of water or other bland fluid. Unless a corneal abrasion can be excluded by fluorescein staining or slit-lamp examination, a topical antimicrobial agent such as tetracycline or chloramphenicol should be applied, as with any other corneal injury.[31] Adrenaline eyedrops (0.1%) relieve the pain.

Prevention

Snake bites could be prevented by simple precautions. Unfortunately, these methods are impracticable for those, such as farmers, who have to do hard physical work in hot, snake-infested areas. Snakes should never be disturbed, attacked or handled unnecessarily even if they are thought to be harmless species or appear to be dead. Venomous species should never be kept as pets or as performing animals. Protective clothing—boots (not open sandals), socks, long trousers—should be worn when walking in undergrowth or deep sand and a light should always be carried at night. Particular care should be taken while collecting firewood, moving logs, boulders, boxes or debris likely to conceal a snake, and climbing rocks and trees covered with dense foliage or swimming in overgrown lakes and rivers. Wading in the sea, especially in sand or near coral reefs, is a dangerous pastime and should be avoided if possible. Shuffling is safer than a high-stepping gait. Divers should keep clear of sea snakes. Fishermen who catch sea snakes in nets or on lines should return them to their element without touching them.

Domestic animals such as chickens and rodent pests attract snakes into human dwellings. Snakes can be discouraged by rodent-proofing, by removing unnecessary junk and litter and by using solid building materials. Various toxic chemicals such as naphthalene, sulphur, insecticides (e.g. DDT, dieldrin and pyrethrins) and fumigants (e.g. methyl bromide, formaldehyde, tetrachloroethane) are lethal to snakes. No true repellents have been identified.

Prophylactic immunization against snake venoms

Venom toxoids (venoids) have been used to immunize farmers at high risk of habu bite (*Trimeresurus flavoviridis*) in the Ryukyu and Amami Islands in Japan but efficacy was not demonstrated.[62] To be effective, vaccination would have to stimulate sufficiently high and persisting levels of antibody to neutralize the venom injected at the time of the bite. Enhanced secondary antibody response, unlike in infectious diseases, would be too late to be helpful. For this reason, vaccination against snake bite is very unlikely to be useful.

Venomous lizards[63]

Two species of venomous lizard (genus *Heloderma*) are capable of envenoming humans. Venom from glands in the mandible is conducted along grooves in the lower teeth. The Gila monster (*H. suspectum*) is striped, with a short, thick tail, and grows up to 60 cm in length (Figure 32.29). It occurs in the south-western USA and the adjacent areas of Mexico. The Mexican beaded lizard or escorpión (*H. horridum*) is spotted, with a relatively long, thin tail, and reaches 80 cm in length. It is found in western Mexico and south to Guatemala. *Heloderma* venoms contain lethal glycoprotein toxins, gila and horridum toxins, phospholipase A_2 and five bioactive peptides of great interest. Helospectins I and II and helodermin are vasoactive intestinal peptide (VIP) analogues, while extendins-3 and -4 are glucagon-like peptide-1 (GLP-1) analogues.[64] Bites are rare. The lizard hangs on with its powerful jaws and is difficult to disengage. Radiolucent teeth may be left in the wound. There is immediate severe local pain with tender swelling and regional lymphadenopathy. Symptoms include weakness, dizziness, tachycardia, hypotension, syncope, angio-oedema, sweating, rigors, tinnitus, nausea and vomiting. There may be leucocytosis, coagulopathy, electrocardiographic changes, myocardial infarction and acute renal failure. No fatal cases have reliably been reported. Specific antivenom is not generally available. A powerful analgesic may be required. Hypotension should be treated with plasma expanders and perhaps adrenaline or a pressor agent such as dopamine.

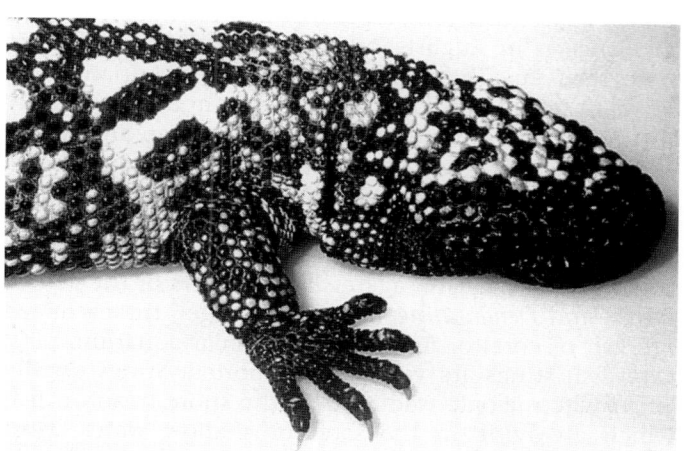

Figure 32.29: Gila monster (*Heloderma suspectum*), one of the two species of venomous lizards. (Copyright D. A. Warrell.)

Venomous fish[1,65,66]

Taxonomy

More than 100 species of fish, inhabiting temperate and tropical seas, possess a defensive venom-injecting apparatus which can inflict dangerous stings. Fatal stings have been reported from members of the orders Chondrichthyes (cartilagenous fish), Squaliformes (sharks and dogfish), Rajiformes (stingrays and mantas), Osteichthyes (bony fish), suborder Siluroidei (catfish) and families Trachinidae (weever fish), Scorpaenidae (scorpion fish, stonefish) and Uranoscopidae (stargazers or stone-lifters).

Venom apparatus

Venom is secreted around spines or barbs in front of the dorsal, anal or pectoral fins and tail and opercular spines in the gill covers. The venom gland in stingrays lies in a groove beneath a membrane covering the barbed precaudal spine up to 30 cm long. The most advanced venom apparatus is found in the genus *Synanceja* (stonefish): bulky venom glands drain through paired ducts to the tips of the short, thick spines.

Venom composition

Fish venoms are unstable at normal ambient temperatures and so have been difficult to study. Venoms of the North American round stingray (*Urolophus halleri*) and weever fish (*Trachinus*) were found to contain peptides, protein, enzymes and a variety of vasoactive compounds (kinins, serotonin, histamine, adrenaline and noradrenaline). Pharmacological effects include local necrosis, direct actions on cardiac, skeletal and smooth muscle, causing electrocardiographic changes, hypotension and paralysis, and central nervous system depression.

Incidence and epidemiology of fish stings

There are hundreds of weever fish stings around the British coast each year, especially in Cornwall. The peak incidence is in August and September. Fifty-eight cases were seen at a hospital in Pula on the Adriatic over 13 years. In the USA 1500 stings by rays and 300 stings by scorpion fish are thought to occur each year. Eighty-one cases of stonefish sting were seen over a 4-year period at a hospital in Pulau Bukom, an island near Singapore. Stings by venomous freshwater rays (*Potamotrygon* species) are common in the Amazon region. Ornate but highly venomous and aggressive members of the genera *Pterois* and *Dendrochirus* (zebra, lion, tiger, turkey or red fire fish or coral or fire cod) are popular aquarium pets. Fatal fish stings are very rarely reported. Stings usually occur when people wading near the shore tread on fish which are lying in the sand or shallow water. Most victims are stung on the sole of the foot, but stingrays lash their tails upwards and usually impale the ankle. Fishermen, scuba divers and aquarium enthusiasts are often stung on the fingers while carelessly handling or attempting to touch the fish.

Symptoms of envenoming

Immediate, sharp, agonizing pain is the dominant symptom. Even stoical adults may collapse screaming with pain. Bleeding may be seen from single or multiple puncture sites. Hot, erythematous swelling extends rapidly up the stung limb.

Stingrays

These fish are widely distributed in oceans and rivers.[67] The large barbed spine may cause severe lacerating injuries, usually to the lower part of the legs but occasionally penetrating the body cavities, heart and viscera when the swimmer falls or lies on the fish. Deaths from this mechanical trauma have been reported. The spine and fragments of its integument may remain in the wound. The venom produces local swelling and sometimes necrosis (Figure 32.30), with a high risk of secondary infection with unusual marine bacteria such as *Photobacterium* (*Vibrio*) *damsela*, *Vibrio vulnificus* and other *Vibrio* species, *Shewanella putrefaciens*, *Staphylococcus* and *Micrococcus* species and *Halomonas venusta*. The broken spine and other foreign material must be removed from the wound. Systemic effects include hypotension, cardiac arrhythmias, muscle spasms, generalized convulsions, vomiting, diarrhoea, sweating and hypersalivation.

Weevers[68]

Stings by Trachinidae produce intense local pain with slight swelling. Systemic symptoms are rare but some patients develop severe chest pain simulating myocardial ischaemia, cardiac arrhythmias and hypotension.

Scorpion fish and stonefish

The family Scorpaenidae comprises more than 350 species which are widely distributed in some temperate and all tropical seas and are especially abundant around the coral reefs of the Indo-Pacific region. The stonefish (genus *Synanceja*) are the most dangerous of venomous fish. They occur from East Africa, across the Indian Ocean, to the Pacific. Stings are excruciatingly painful and symptoms may persist for 2 days or more. There is local

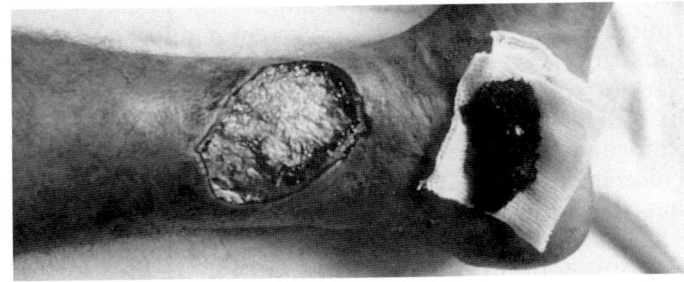

Figure 32.30: Sloughing of necrotic tissue 20 days after a sting by a freshwater ray (*Potamotrygon hystrix*) in the Amazon region of Brazil. (Courtesy of João Luiz Costa Cardoso, São Paulo.)

swelling, discoloration, sweating and paraesthesia and sometimes local lymphadenopathy. Systemic symptoms are more common than with other fish stings. They include nausea, vomiting, hypotension, cardiac arrhythmias, respiratory distress, neurological signs, convulsions and evidence of autonomic nervous system stimulation. Deaths within an hour of being stung by *S. verrucosa* are reported.

Management

The most effective treatment for pain is to immerse the stung limb in water that is uncomfortably hot but not scalding (i.e. just under 45°C). Temperature can be assessed with the unstung limb. It is not necessary to add magnesium sulphate to the water. Injection of local anaesthetic such as 1% lignocaine, for example as a ring block in the case of stung digits, is less effective. The spine, membrane and other foreign material must be removed from the wound. Prophylactic antibiotics and tetanus toxoid should be given to patients stung by rays or scorpion fish because of the size of wound and risk of necrosis, but these measures are not justified for weever fish stings. Local injection of potassium permanganate solution or acidifying solutions such as emetine hydrochloride were said to cure local pain, but they may promote local necrosis and are less effective than immersion in hot water. In patients with severe systemic envenoming, an adequate airway should be established and cardiorespiratory resuscitation instituted when necessary. Severe hypotension can be treated with adrenaline and bradycardia with atropine. The only anti-venom now available commercially is manufactured by the Commonwealth Serum Laboratories in Australia. It neutralizes the venoms of *Synanceja trachynis*, *S. verrucosa* and *S. horrida* and has paraspecific activity against venoms of the North American scorpion fish (*Scorpaena guttata*) and other members of the Scorpaenidae family. One 2 ml ampoule (2000 units) is given intravenously for each two puncture marks found at the site of the sting. The dose is increased in patients with severe symptoms.[1]

Prevention

Bathers and waders should adopt a shuffling gait to reduce the risk of stepping on a venomous fish skulking in sand or mud. Footwear protects against most species except stingrays.

Venomous marine invertebrates[1,65,66]

Cnidarians (coelenterates): hydroids, stinging corals, medusae, Portuguese men-o'-war or bluebottles, jellyfish, blubbers, box-jellies, stinging algae, sea anemones and sea pansies

The venom apparatus of the cnidarians is the stinging capsule or nematocyst which, when triggered by physical contact or chemicals, at enormous speed, acceleration and force, everts a thread-like tubule with sharpened tip which can penetrate the skin and inject toxin. The tentacles of cnidarians are armed with millions of these nematocysts, which produce lines of painful irritant wheals on the skin of swimmers unlucky enough to be embraced by them. Cnidarian venoms contain peptides together with vasoactive compounds such as serotonin, histamine, prostaglandins and kinins which cause immediate severe pain, inflammation and urticaria.

Epidemiology

The most dangerous cnidarian to man, the box-jellyfish (*Chironex fleckeri*), is found along the northern coast of Australia. It has been responsible for some 70 deaths since 1883. Most stings occur in December and January. Fatal jellyfish stings have also been reported from Bougainville Island in the east, to the west coast of India and north to the Philippines, where a similar species (*Chiropsalmus quadrigatus*) is common (Figure 32.31).

During a 3½-year period, 116 cases of marine stings were seen in Cairns, north Queensland.[69] Forty per cent of the patients had clinical features of 'Irukandji sting' caused by *Carukia barnesi*. Fatal stings by *Stomolophus nomurai* have been reported from China. Prodigious swarms of the scyphomedusa *Pelagia noctiluca* appeared along the northern Adriatic coast during the summers of 1977–1979. In 1978 it was estimated that 250 000

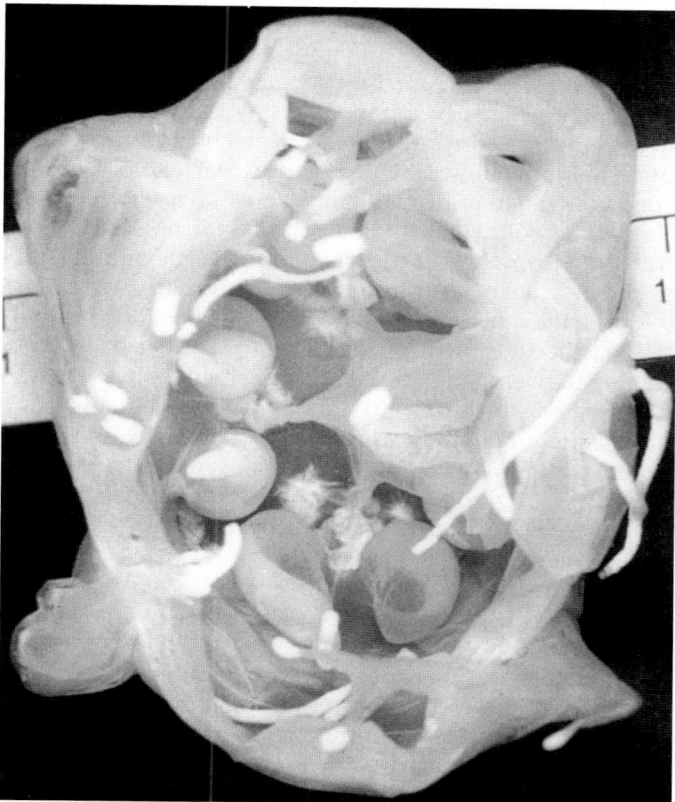

Figure 32.31: Underside of a box jellyfish from Sri Lanka (*Chiropsalmus buitendijki*). The bell is approximately 12 cm in diameter. (Copyright D. A. Warrell.)

swimmers had been stung. At Pula on the Adriatic coast, 55 patients stung by a sea anemone (*Anemonia sulcata*) were seen from 1965 to 1980. This cnidarian is widely distributed in the eastern Atlantic and Mediterranean. Cnidarian stings are common in most parts of the world but few reliable statistics are available.

Clinical features

The imprint of nematocyst stings on the skin may have a diagnostic pattern. *Chironex fleckeri* produces immediate brownish or purplish wheals 8–10 mm wide with cross-striations. More extensive swelling, erythema and vesiculation develop, with areas of necrosis and eventual healing with scar formation. *Carukia barnesi* produces an oval erythematous area about 7 cm in diameter and then transient papules with surrounding hyperhidrosis. Portuguese man-o'-war (*Physalia*) stings produce chains of oval wheals surrounded by erythema. These lesions persist for only about 24 hours. Histological sections of the skin lesions may reveal identifiable nematocysts, allowing differentiation between stings by different genera.

The dominant symptom of cnidarian stings is immediate severe pain coming in waves and sometimes becoming incapacitating in its intensity. Systemic symptoms are most severe following stings by cubomedusae (box-jellyfish), genera *Chironex* and *Chiropsalmus* (Figure 32.31). The victim, usually a child swimming in shallow water, suddenly screams with pain and within minutes becomes cyanosed, suffers generalized convulsions and is found to be pulseless. The whole jellyfish or a length of tentacles may still be adherent to the patient's skin. Autopsies reveal pulmonary oedema. Patients envenomed by *Carukia barnesi* develop severe systemic effects minutes to hours after the sting attributed to catecholamine- induced hypertension but with little or no local effect. Systemic effects of cnidarian stings include cough, nausea, vomiting, abdominal colic, diarrhoea, rigors, severe musculoskeletal pains, syncope and signs of autonomic nervous system stimulation such as profuse sweating. The Portuguese man-o'-war (*Physalia*) occasionally causes systemic symptoms and has been known to produce intravascular haemolysis leading to haemoglobinuria and renal failure. Rare fatalities have been attributed to *Physalia*. The sea anemone *Anemonia sulcata* produces painful local papules, erythema, oedema and vesiculation. Systemic symptoms such as sleepiness, dizziness, nausea, vomiting, myalgia and peri-orbital oedema are occasionally produced.

Management

First aid is all-important as patients may die within minutes of the sting. Lifeguards and others working on cnidarian-infested beaches should be trained to deal with jellyfish stings. The patient must be taken out of the water. The nematocysts in fragments of tentacles stuck to the skin must be inactivated to prevent further discharge and envenoming. For *Chironex* and other cubozoans, including Irukandji, commercial vinegar or 3–10% aqueous acetic acid is effective; but for *Chrysaora*, a widely distributed Atlantic genus, baking soda and water (50% w/v) proved effective. Vinegar may discharge *Physalia* nematocysts and is not recommended for treatment of stings by this genus or *Stomolophus*. Alcoholic solutions (methylated spirits, suntan lotion, aftershave, etc.) were advocated until recently, when it was shown that they cause massive discharge of nematocysts. Pressure immobilization with a crepe bandage may increase the amount of venom injected and is not recommended.[70] Application of ice packs relieves the intense pain. Mouth-to-mouth artificial ventilation has proved life-saving in several patients who developed severe respiratory depression with cyanosis, coma and pulselessness. If no pulse can be detected, external cardiac massage should be started. Experimentally, the venom of *Chironex* affects the heart directly and the central nervous system but, clinically, respiratory depression appears to be more important than cardiotoxicity. Treatment with verapamil is controversial and not currently recommended.

A specific 'sea wasp' antivenom is manufactured by the Commonwealth Serum Laboratories in Australia for *Chironex fleckeri* stings. The antivenom should be administered intravenously if symptoms of systemic envenoming persist after first aid treatment.

Prevention

People, and especially children, should keep out of the sea at times of the year when dangerous cnidarians are most prevalent and especially when they have been sighted and warning notices have been displayed on beaches. Wetsuits and other clothing, even fine-mesh nylon stockings, will protect against the stings.

Echinoderms (starfish and sea urchins)[1,65,66,71]

Echinoderms have hard protective exoskeletons. Starfish (Asteroidea) sprout numerous sharp spines which can penetrate human skin, releasing a violet-coloured liquid. *Acanthaster planci* of the Red Sea and Indian and Pacific Oceans is up to 60 cm in diameter and possesses venomous spines 6 cm long. The venom causes severe pain, redness, swelling, muscle weakness, hyper/hypoaesthesia, facial oedema, cardiac arrhythmias, vomiting and paralysis. Sea urchins (Echinoidea) (Figure 32.32), especially of the tropical families Diadematidae and Echinothuridae, have brittle, articulated spines (30 cm long in *Diadema*) and grapples (globiferous pedicellariae) (Figure 32.33). Both contain venom which is released when they are embedded in the skin. Severe pain, syncope, numbness, generalized paralysis, aphonia, respiratory distress and even death may result. The fragments of spines embedded in the skin may cause secondary infection, and granuloma formation several months later. Penetration of bones and joints may cause destructive changes.

Management

Spines and pedicellariae must be removed as soon as possible as they may continue to inject venom and give rise to later complications. The sites of penetration are

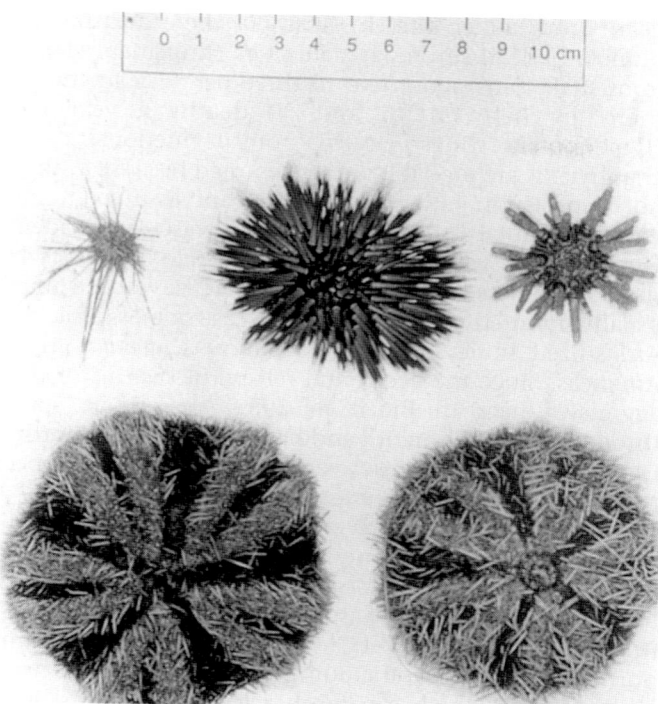

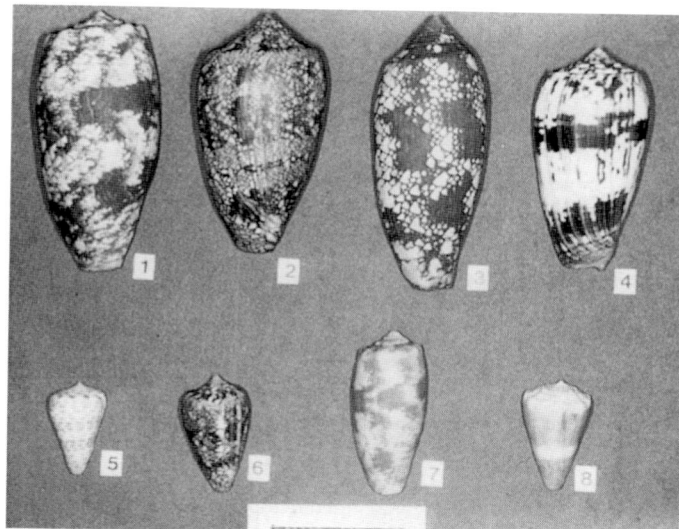

Figure 32.34: Venomous cone-shells, family Conidae, from Sri Lanka. 1, *Conus geographus*; 2, *C. textile*; 3, *C. aulicus*; 4, *C. striatus*; 5, *C. tessulatus*; 6, *C. abbas*; 7, *C. tulipa*; 8, *C. lividus*. (Scale in centimetres.) (Copyright D. A. Warrell.)

Figure 32.32: Sea urchins (Echinodermata) from Papua New Guinea. Above (left to right): *Diadema setorum, Echinometra methiae, Prioncidaris verticillata.* Below: *Tripeneuster gradua, T. gratilla.* (Copyright D. A. Warrell.)

usually on the soles of the feet. The superficial layer of thickened epidermis should be pared down and 2% salicylic acid ointment applied for 24–48 hours to soften the skin. Most spines can then be extruded, but deeply embedded ones may require surgical removal under local anaesthetic.[71]

Molluscs (cone-shells and octopuses)[1,65,66]

Cone-shells (family Conidae) (Figure 32.34), up to 20 cm

in length, are found in the Pacific and Indian Oceans. They kill their prey of small fish, polychaete worms, hemichordates and other molluscs, by harpooning them with a venom-filled radular tooth or dart carried on a proboscis. In humans the venom produces local paraesthesiae and numbness and paralysis, which progressed to fatal respiratory paralysis in eight out of the 30 reported cases. The venoms of cone-shells contain a vast array of neurotoxic peptides targeting Na^+, K^+ and Ca^{2+} ion channels and nicotinic, $5HT_3$, *N*-methyl-D-aspartate and vasopressin receptors.[72] No specific treatment is available. If respiratory paralysis develops, assisted ventilation may be needed.

Cephalopods (cuttlefish, squid and octopus) secrete toxic saliva which is inoculated by the sharp and powerful beak.[1] The venom contains tetrodotoxin-like activity,

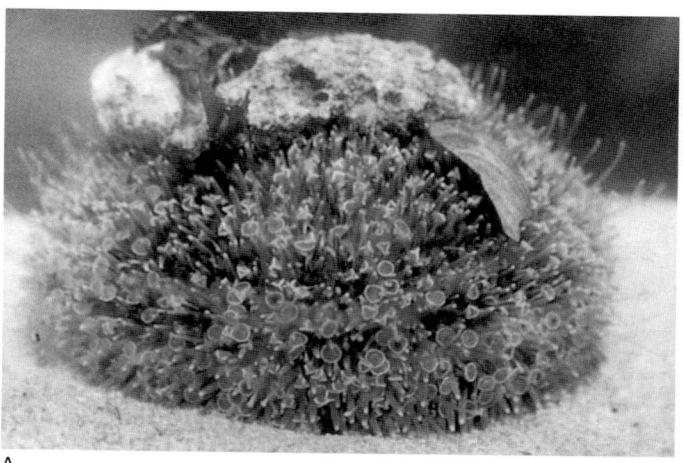

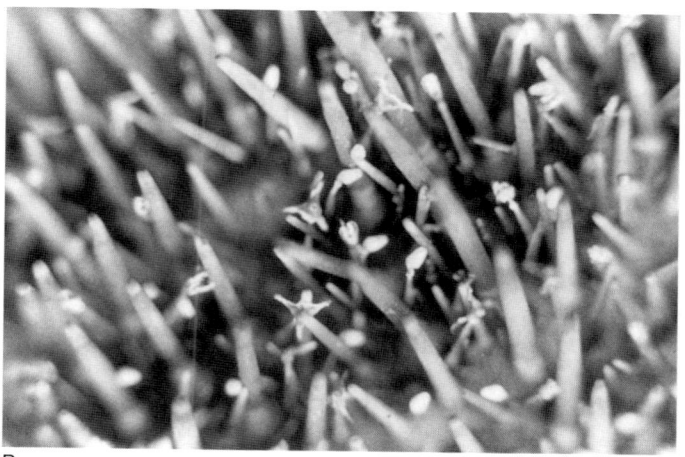

A   B

Figure 32.33: Flower or felt cap sea urchin (*Toxopneustes pileolus*) from Sri Lanka. (a) Whole animal. (b) Venom apparatus: pedecellariae. (Courtesy of Malik Fernando, Colombo, Sri Lanka.)

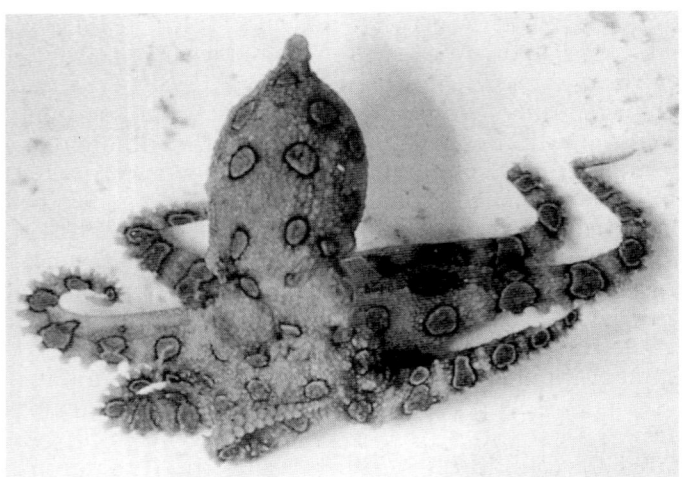

Figure 32.35: Spotted or blue-ringed octopus (*Octopus lunulatus*) from Madang, Papua New Guinea. (Copyright D. A. Warrell.)

other toxins, vasoactive amines and hyaluronidase. Cephalopod bites are usually painful and produce bleeding, swelling, redness, heat and irritation. Systemic symptoms include numbness of the mouth and tongue, blurring of vision, dysphonia, dysphagia and paralysis of the legs and arms. A number of severe cases including two fatalities have been reported from Australia; they were caused by small (20 cm long) octopuses, the southern blue-ringed or banded octopus (*Hapalochlaena maculosa*), the northern blue-ringed or spotted octopus (*H. lunulatus*) (Figure 32.35) and the blue-lined octopus (*H. fasciatus*). These species are abundant around the coast of Australia, especially in the south and frequent shallow water and rock pools. The two patients who died had handled octopuses while they were out of the water. They vomited soon after the bite, then developed respiratory paralysis and died 90 and 120 minutes later.

There is no specific treatment for octopus bites; the effects resemble rapidly developing tetrodotoxin poisoning. Mouth-to-mouth respiration combined with external cardiac massage (if the patient is pulseless) may be life-saving. An arterial tourniquet or crepe bandage and splint should be applied to delay absorption of the venom until the patient has reached hospital. Mechanical ventilation and other intensive care may be needed. It would be worth testing the response to anticholinesterase and treating bradycardia with atropine.

Insect stings

Hymenoptera stings (bees, wasps, yellow-jackets, hornets, fire ants)

In most temperate countries, anaphylactic reactions to Hymenoptera stings are a more common cause of death than direct effects of envenoming by any animal.[73] For example, between 1959 and 1972 there were 61 deaths from insect stings in England and Wales but only one death from adder bite. In Australia there are the same number of deaths from Hymenoptera sting anaphylaxis as from snake bite, about two to three per year. In the USA there are between 40 and 50 deaths a year from Hymenoptera stings. Deaths from Hymenoptera sting anaphylaxis are probably under-reported because a sting is not suspected in patients found dead and assumed to have had myocardial infarctions or cerebrovascular accidents. Hymenoptera venoms also have direct toxic effects but these are not seen in man unless there have been many, usually hundreds of stings, as in the case of mass attacks by Africanized honey-bees (*Apis mellifera scutellata*) in the Americas. Since the accidental release of swarms of these aggressive bees in Brazil in 1957, they have spread throughout Latin America and have reached as far north as Las Vegas in the USA. An average of 30 deaths have been reported each year from mass attacks by these insects.[74]

In other countries, Hymenoptera stings are usually caused by members of the Apidae (e.g. *Apis mellifera, A. cerania*, honey-bees; *A. dorsata, A. laboriosa*, giant honey-bees) and Vespidae (e.g. wasps such as *Paravespula vulgaris*), American yellow-jackets, genus *Dolichovespula*, and hornets, genus *Vespa*, including the enormous East Asian *V. mandarinia* which can reach a length of almost 4 cm and a weight of 3 g. In North America millions of stings each year are caused by imported fire ants (*Solenopsis*); hypersensitivity is common and there have been cases of fatal anaphylaxis.

Venom apparatus and composition[75,76]
Venoms are injected through a barbed sting. Bees inject approximately 50 µg of venom, the total capacity of the venom sac, and leave the stings embedded in the skin, but wasps and hornets can sting repeatedly. The venoms contain biogenic amines (histamine, serotonin and acetylcholine), enzymes such as phospholipase A and hyaluronidase and toxic peptides; kinins in the case of Vespidae; apamin, melittin and anti-inflammatory compounds such as mast cell degranulating peptide in Apidae.

Clinical features

Direct toxic effects in non-allergic subjects In people who are not allergic to the venom, single stings usually produce only local effects attributable to the injected biogenic amines, particularly serotonin. Pain, and an area of heat, redness, swelling and wealing, develop rapidly but rarely exceed 2–3 cm in diameter or last more than a few hours. Local effects are dangerous only if the airway is obstructed, for example following stings on the tongue.

In non-allergic subjects, fatal systemic toxicity can result from as few as 30 stings in children, while adults have survived more than 2000 stings by *Apis mellifera*. In some patients the clinical effects of massive envenoming resemble histamine overdose: vasodilatation, hypotension, vomiting, diarrhoea, throbbing headache and coma. However, mass attacks by Africanized bees in Latin America can cause intravascular haemolysis, generalized rhabdomyolysis (causing grossly elevated serum creatine phosphokinase, aminopeptidases and myoglobin), hyper-catecholinaemia (hypertension, pulmonary oedema, myocardial damage), bleeding, hepatic dysfunction and acute renal failure (Figure 32.36).[77] Hepatic dysfunction and rhabdomyolysis followed by myoglobinuria and renal failure can occur after multiple hornet stings (*Vespa affinis*). Intravascular haemolysis with haemoglobinuria (*Vespa orientalis*), thrombocytopenic purpura, myasthenia gravis (*Polistes* species) and various renal lesions, including nephrotic syndrome, have also been described.

Allergic effects   Three to four per cent of the population may be hypersensitive to Hymenoptera venoms. Clinical suspicion of venom hypersensitivity arises when systemic symptoms follow a sting. In England, sensitization to bee venom appears to require more stings (average 81 on 23 occasions) than sensitization to wasp venom (average four stings).[78] Most patients allergic to bee venom are bee-keepers or their relatives. Systemic symptoms include tingling scalp, flushing, dizziness, visual disturbances, syncope, wheezing, abdominal colic, diarrhoea and tachy-cardia developing within a few minutes of the sting. Over the next 15–20 minutes urticaria, angio-oedema, oedema of the glottis, profound hypotension and coma may develop. Patients may die within minutes of the sting. Raised serum concentrations of mast cell tryptase, which may persist for up to 6 hours, confirms the diagnosis of anaphylaxis. In a few cases, serum sickness develops a week or more after the sting. Atopy does not predispose to sting allergy but asthmatics who are allergic to venom are likely to suffer severe reactions. Reactions are enhanced by β-blockers. The diagnosis of venom hypersensitivity can be confirmed by intradermal skin testing with dialysed venoms, or by detecting specific IgE antibodies in serum by the radioallergosorbent test (RAST). Whole-body extracts of bees and wasps, traditionally used for skin testing, do not discriminate between hypersensitive patients and controls. A post-mortem diagnosis of insect sting ana-phylaxis can be supported by detecting specific IgE in the victim's serum. Pathological findings in cases of fatal systemic anaphylaxis include acute pulmonary hyper-inflation, laryngeal oedema, pulmonary oedema and intra-alveolar haemorrhage.

Management

The embedded bee sting should be removed as quickly as possible by any means. Domestic meat tenderizer (papain), diluted roughly 1 in 5 with tap water, is said to produce immediate relief of pain. Aspirin is an effective analgesic favoured from long experience by bee-keepers. Local antiseptics are acceptable but topical antihistamines should not be used as they promote sensitization.

Toxic effects

In cases of severe systemic envenoming, large doses of parenteral antihistamines and corticosteroids should be given and, if needed, bronchodilators and adrenaline. Bee antivenoms have been developed but none is com-mercially available. As in crush syndrome, renal damage by myoglobinuria or haemoglobinuria should be prevented by correcting hypovolaemia and giving mannitol and bicarbonate. Acute tubular necrosis will require treatment with haemofiltration or renal dialysis.

Allergic effects

The most effective treatment for sting anaphylaxis is 0.1% adrenaline in an adult dose of 0.5–1 ml, children 0.01 ml/kg, given by intramuscular injection. Patients known to be hypersensitive should wear an identifying tag (such as provided by Medic-Alert in Britain) as they may be discovered unconscious after a sting. They should be trained to give themselves adrenaline intramuscularly and should always carry a preloaded syringe of adrenaline for this purpose (eg "EpiPen" delivering 0.3 mg adult, or 0.15 mg child doses of 0.1% adrenaline). Adrenaline delivered by a pressurized inhaler (Medihaler-epi delivering 200 μg of adrenaline acid tartrate per puff) will relieve

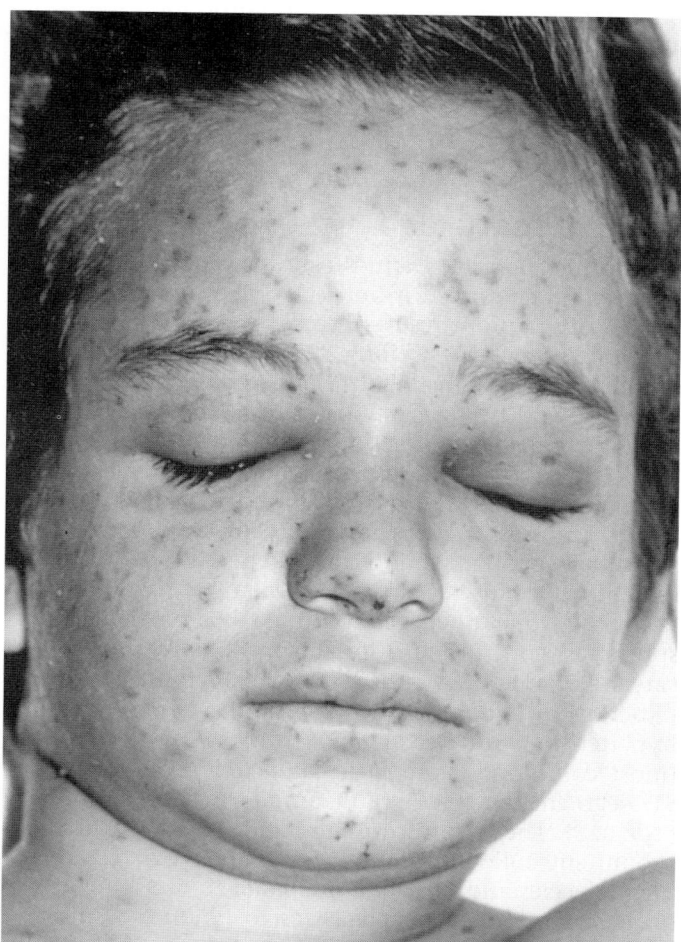

Figure 32.36: Multiple bee stings by Africanized honey-bees (*Apis mellifera scutellata*) causing severe envenoming in a 14-year-old Brazilian boy. (Copyright D. A. Warrell.)

bronchospasm, but about 20 consecutive puffs are needed to achieve blood concentrations similar to those produced by intramuscular injection, and the effect is more transient. Injection of an anti-H_1 antihistamine (e.g. chlorpheniramine maleate, 10 mg intravenously or intramuscularly) will alleviate the mild urticarial symptoms, and an antihistamine should be given for the next 24–48 hours to combat the effects of histamine released during the reaction. The role of anti-H_2 antihistamines (e.g. cimetidine) is uncertain. Corticosteroid may prevent recurrence of anaphylaxis, said to occur after about 6 hours in up to 10% of cases. Severe reactions may require cardiorespiratory resuscitation. Salbutamol is an effective bronchodilator and large doses of hydrocortisone may help the resolution of massive oedema. Respiratory tract obstruction is the main cause of death. Stings in the mouth may cause serious airway obstruction even in people who are not hypersensitive to venom.

Prevention of *Hymenoptera* sting anaphylaxis

In 1978, a controlled trial proved that hyposensitization using pure venom was effective in protecting allergic patients against anaphylactic reactions to sting challenge.[79] However, immunotherapy is probably only necessary in adult patients with histories of severe reactions and demonstrable venom-specific IgE. Most people are stung when they inadvertently crush the bee or wasp or interfere with their nests (i.e. bee-keepers). Wasps congregate where sweet things or meat are manufactured or consumed and in orchards and vineyards. Vespidae are attracted by brightly coloured floral patterns and perfumes. Some of the largest hornets (*Vespa veluntina* and *V. mandarinia*) are so aggressive that their territory cannot be cultivated until the nests have been destroyed.

Scorpion stings

Scorpions (order Scorpionida) capable of inflicting fatal stings in humans are all members of the families Buthidae and Scorpionidae.[75] Examples of the most deadly species are: *Androctonus australis* (North Africa and Middle East), *A. crassicauda* (Turkey, Middle East and North Africa), *Buthus occitanus* (countries bordering the Mediterranean and Middle East), *Leiurus quinquestriatus* (North Africa and Middle East), *Parabuthus* (South Africa), *Tityus trinitatis* (Trinidad and Venezuela), *T. serrulatus* (Figure 32.37) and *T. bahiensis* (Brazil, Argentina), *Centruroides sculpturatus* (California, New Mexico, Arizona and Baja California), *C. limpidus* and *C. suffusus* (Mexico) and *Mesobuthus tamulus* (India).

Epidemiology

Painful scorpion stings are a common event throughout the tropics; however, fatal envenoming is frequent only in parts of Latin America, North Africa, the Middle East and India. In southern Libya there were 900 stings with seven deaths per 100 000 population in 1979.[56] There has been no death from scorpion sting in the USA since 1968.

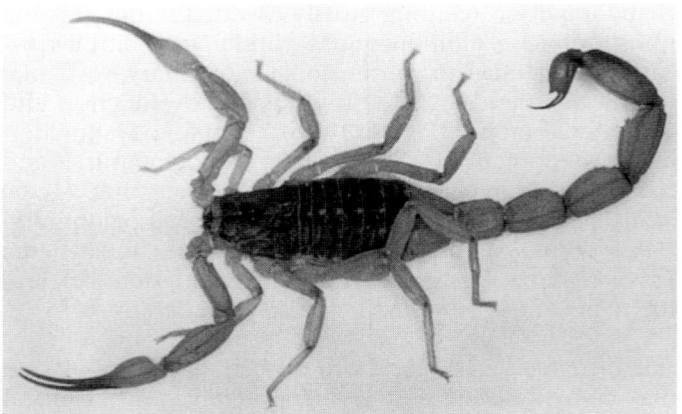

Figure 32.37: Brazilian scorpion (*Tityus serrulatus*; family Buthidae). (Scale in centimetres.) (Copyright D. A. Warrell.)

In Mexico there were between 1000 and 2000 deaths each year in the past, with an incidence of 84 deaths per 100 000 per year in Colima state and a mere three deaths per 100 000 per year in the infamous Durango state. Case mortality was about 50% in children up to 4 years old.[80] Much lower estimates of stings and deaths have been reported recently. In Brazil, mortality increases from around 1% in adults to 15–25% in children less than 6 years old. In Algeria there was an average of 1260 stings and 24 deaths per year. In India there are many cases of stings by the red scorpion (*Mesobuthus tamulus*), with fatalities in adults and children.

Clinical features

Rapidly developing, excruciating local pain is the most common symptom. It is not true that stings by different species of scorpions result in the same clinical syndrome. Local signs such as swelling, redness, heat and regional lymph node involvement are never extensive. Local blistering and necrosis is most unusual except following stings by *Hemiscorpius lepturus* (Scorpionidae) in Baluchistan, Iran, Iraq and Yemen. Systemic symptoms may develop within minutes, but may be delayed for as much as 24 hours. Features of autonomic nervous system excitation are initially cholinergic and later adrenergic. There is hypersalivation, profuse sweating, lacrimation, hyperthermia, vomiting, diarrhoea, abdominal distension, loss of sphincter control, and priapism. Massive release of catecholamines, as in phaeochromocytoma, produces piloerection ('gooseflesh'), tachycardia, hyperglycaemia, hypertension and toxic myocarditis with arrhythmias (most commonly sinus tachycardia), electrocardiographic ST segment changes, cardiac failure and pulmonary oedema.[81] These cardiovascular effects are particularly prominent following stings by *Leiurus quinquestriatus*, *Tityus* species and *Mesobuthus tamulus*.

Neurotoxic effects such as fasciculation, spasms and respiratory paralysis and convulsions are a particular feature of stings by *Centruroides sculpturatus*. *Parabuthus transvaalicus* envenoming is more likely to cause ptosis and dysphagia.

Hemiplegia and other neurological lesions have been attributed to fibrin deposition resulting from DIC, for example after stings by *Nebo hierichonticus*. Hyper-catecholaminaemia could explain hyperglycaemia and glycosuria but, in the case of stings by the black scorpion in Trinidad (*Tityus trinitatis*) there is acute pancreatitis. Fifteen to 120 minutes after the initial searing pain of the sting, patients stung by this species begin to salivate, feel nauseated and vomit persistently, producing coffee-grounds or frank haematemesis. Hyperglycaemia, glycosuria and sometimes albuminuria can be detected a few hours after the sting. There is abdominal pain with distension and rigidity. Electrocardiographic abnormalities (T wave inversion, QRS segment abnormalities and QTc pro-longation) are common and may last for 3–6 days. Other features include pyrexia, sweating, bradycardia, cardiac arrhythmias, hypotension and neuromuscular irritability. Acute oedematous or haemorrhagic pancreatitis with development of pancreatic pseudocysts has been demon-strated at autopsy or laparotomy.

Management

Pain may respond to local infiltration or ring block with local anaesthetic. Local injection of emetine is said to relieve the pain but may cause necrosis. Parenteral opiate analgesics such as pethidine and morphine may be required but are said to be dangerous in victims of *Centruroides sculpturatus*.

The use of antivenom is controversial, but is advocated by doctors in Central and South America, North Africa and parts of the Middle East. Antivenoms are manu-factured in many countries.[55] An antivenom has now been developed for the treatment of *Mesobuthus tamulus* stings in India.

Many accessory treatments have been suggested. There is some clinical evidence to support the use of the follow-ing treatments:

1. For patients with cardiovascular symptoms (hyper-tension, bradycardia and early pulmonary oedema) vasodilators such as prazosin are recommended.[82] The use of atropine (except in cases of life-threatening sinus bradycardia), cardiac glycosides and β-blockers is controversial.[83]
2. Anticonvulsants such as phenobarbital for neurotoxic symptoms (*Centruroides sculpturatus*).

In patients stung by *Mesobuthus tamulus* priapism, dilated pupils, sweating and bradycardia indicate a high risk of progression to pulmonary oedema. Early energetic treatment with an α-blocker may prevent this.

Prophylactic immunization with scorpion venom toxoid has been considered in Mexico.

Spider bites[84]

The spiders (Araneae) are an enormous group containing more than 30 000 known species. A single family, con-taining less than 1% of these species, is non-venomous.

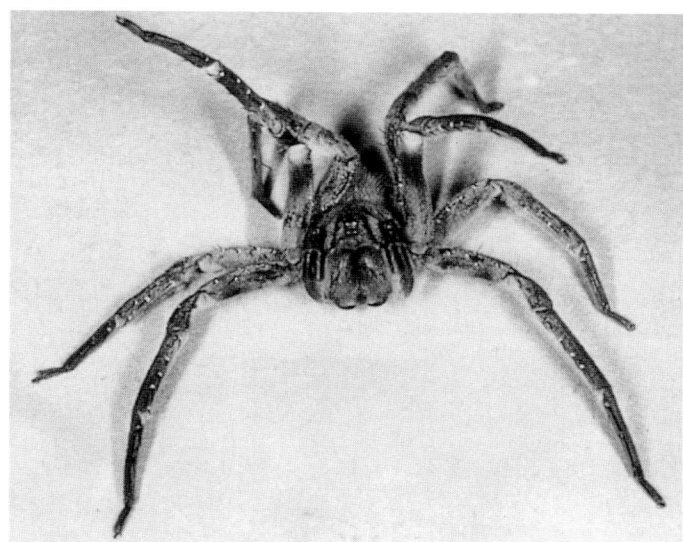

Figure 32.38: Threatening posture of a female Brazilian 'banana spider' (*Phoneutria keiserlingi*). Note venom jaws. (Copyright D. A. Warrell.)

Only about 20 species of spider are known to cause dangerous envenoming in humans, while another 20 are suspected of doing so. Spiders bite with a pair of fangs, the chelicerae (Figure 32.38), to which the venom glands are connected.[75] A central venom duct opens near the tip of the fang.

Clinical features

Two main clinical syndromes, 'necrotic' and 'neurotoxic', are caused by spider bite.

Necrotic araneism

Skin lesions, varying in severity from mild localized erythema and blistering to quite extensive tissue necrosis, have been attributed to a variety of species of spiders. The members of the genus *Loxosceles* (brown recluse spider) are the most important causes of the syndrome. Many of these spiders are extending their geographical ranges. *L. laeta* is widely distributed in Central and South America, especially in Chile. *L. reclusa*, the brown recluse or violin spider, has caused at least 200 bites with six deaths in the USA in the twentieth century. More than 60 cases were reported in Texas between 1959 and 1962. *L. rufescens* occurs in the Mediterranean region, North Africa, Israel and elsewhere.

Eighty per cent of patients are bitten indoors, usually in their bedrooms while asleep or dressing, and in the USA a number of men were bitten on their genitals while they sat on outdoor lavatories in which the spiders had spun their webs. The bite may be painless initially but a burning pain develops at the site over the next 12–36 hours with local oedema. An ischaemic lesion, coloured red (vasodilatation), white (vasoconstriction) and blue (prenecrotic cyanosis) appears (Figure 32.39) and over the course of a few days becomes a black eschar (Figure 32.40) which sloughs in a few weeks, sometimes leaving a necrotic

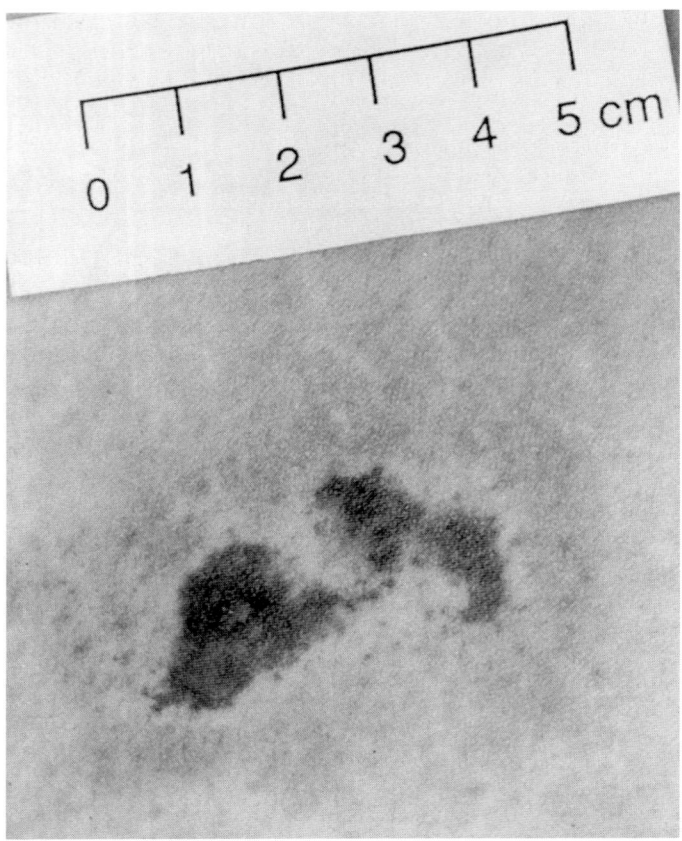

Figure 32.39: Early ischaemic lesion ('red, white and blue' sign) at the site of the bite of a Brazilian spider (*Loxosceles gaucho*). (Copyright D. A. Warrell.)

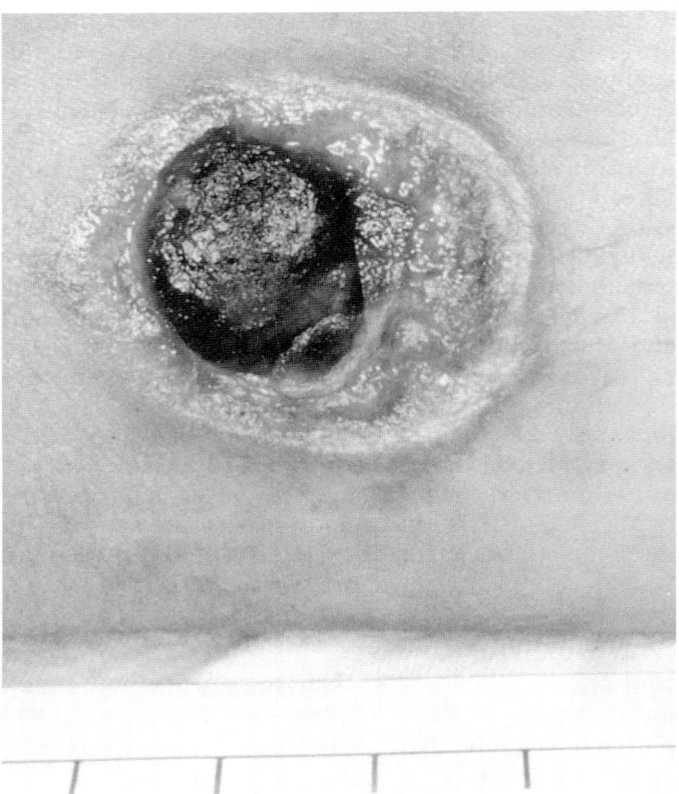

Figure 32.40: Necrotic eschar or slough at the site of a bite by a Brazilian spider (*Loxosceles gaucho*). (Scale in centimetres.) (Copyright D. A. Warrell.)

ulcer. Rarely, the necrotic area may cover an entire limb. In 12% of cases there are systemic effects including fever, methaemoglobinaemia, haemoglobinuria and jaundice resulting from haemolytic anaemia, scarlatiniform rash (Figure 32.41), respiratory distress, collapse and renal failure. The average case fatality is about 5%.

Neurotoxic araneism

Members of the genus *Latrodectus* (widow, hourglass, button or red-back spiders) are the most widespread and numerous of all venomous animals dangerous to man. *L mactans* (black widow spider) occurs in the Americas. Sixty-three deaths were attributed to this species in the USA from 1950 to 1959. *L. tredecimguttatus*, widely but incorrectly known as 'tarantula', lives in fields in the Mediterranean countries where it has been responsible for epidemics of bites. Nine hundred and forty-six cases were reported in Italy between 1946 and 1951. *L. hasselti*, the Australian and New Zealand red-back spider or 'katipo', causes up to 340 reported bites each year in Australia, where 20 deaths are known to have occurred. *L. mactans* and a related species *L. geometricus* also cause some bites in South and eastern Africa. *L. hasselti* bites produce local heat, swelling and redness, which is rarely extensive. Intense local pain develops in about 5 minutes; after 30 minutes there is pain in local lymph nodes and

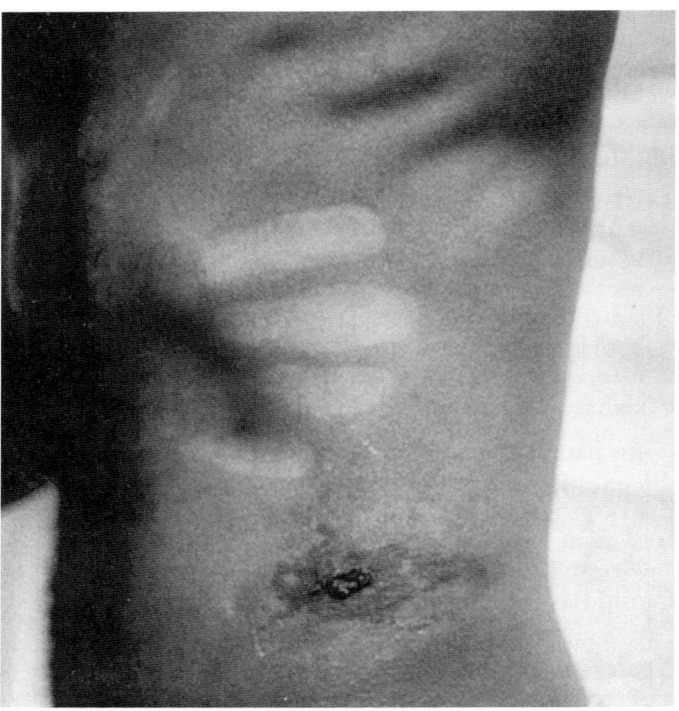

Figure 32.41: Scarlatiniform rash, blanching on pressure, associated with fever in a Brazilian patient bitten above the iliac crest 18 hours previously. (Courtesy of João Luiz Costa Cardoso, São Paulo.)

after about an hour headache, nausea, vomiting and sweating occur. Tachycardia and hypertension may follow and there are muscle tremors and spasms which may be severe enough to demand artificial ventilation.

L. mactans bites produce minimal local changes. Local dull aching or numbness may develop after 30–40 minutes. Painful muscle spasms and lymphadenopathy spread and increase in intensity during the next few hours until the trunk, abdomen and limbs are involved and respiration may be embarrassed. Other features include tachycardia, hypertension, irritability, psychosis, vomiting and priapism. Similar effects are produced by the Brazilian 'banana spider', *Phoneutria nigriventer* (Figure 32.38), which causes bites and deaths in South American countries. These spiders may be exported in bunches of bananas to temperate countries, where they have been responsible for a few bites and deaths.

Funnel-web spiders, genera *Atrax* and *Hadronyche*, are confined to south-eastern Australia, the Adelaide area and eastern Tasmania.[1] *A. robustus*, the Sydney funnel-web spider, occurs within a 160 km radius of Sydney. Unusually among spiders, the aggressive male is more dangerous to man than the larger female. The powerful chelicerae of this large spider produce a painful bite but with minimal local changes. Numbness around the mouth and spasm of the tongue may develop within 10 minutes, followed by nausea and vomiting, abdominal colic, profuse sweating, salivation and lacrimation, dyspnoea and coma. There are local or generalized muscle fasciculations and spasms, hypertension and in some of the fatal cases pulmonary oedema, thought to be neurogenic in origin. Thirteen deaths, occurring between 15 minutes and 6 days after the bite, were reported between 1927 and 1980.[1]

Management
First aid treatment
In the case of bites by spiders with rapidly active potent venom such as *A. robustus*, firm crepe bandaging and splinting of the bitten limb may delay venom spread until the patient reaches hospital.

Specific treatment
Antivenoms are manufactured in several countries.[55] Neurotoxic araneism seems more responsive to antivenom than does the necrotic type. *A. robustus* antivenom is effective against the venom of other *Atrax* and *Hadronyche* species.

Supportive treatment
Oral dapsone (100 mg twice a day) is said to reduce the extent of necrotic lesions by preventing neutrophil degranulation. Calcium gluconate (10 ml of a 10% solution given by slow intravenous injection) relieves the pain of muscle spasms caused by *Latrodectus* venom rapidly and more effectively than muscle relaxants such as diazepam or methocarbamol. Antihistamines, corticosteroids, β-blockers and atropine have also been advocated. Surgical

debridement for necrotic lesions caused by *Loxosceles* species is not recommended, and corticosteroids, antihistamines and hyperbaric oxygen have not proved helpful.

Tick bite paralysis[85–88]

Taxonomy and epidemiology
Ticks, with mites, form the order Acari of the class Arachnida. Adult females of about 30 species of hard tick (family Ixodidae) and immature specimens of six species of soft tick (family Argasidae) have been implicated in human tick paralysis.[86] The tick's saliva contains a neurotoxin which causes presynaptic neuromuscular block and decreased nerve conduction velocity. The tick embeds itself in the skin with its barbed hypostome, introducing the salivary toxin while it engorges with blood.

Although tick paralysis has been reported from all continents, most cases occur in western North America (*Dermacentor andersoni*), eastern USA (*D. variabilis*) and eastern Australia from north Queensland to Victoria (*Ixodes holocyclus*, known as the bush, scrub, paralysis or dog tick). In British Columbia there were 305 cases with 10% mortality between 1900 and 1968. About 120 cases have been reported in the USA, and in New South Wales there were at least 20 deaths between 1900 and 1945.

Clinical features
Ticks are picked up in the countryside or from domestic animals, particularly dogs, in the home. A majority of patients and almost all fatal cases are children. After the tick has been attached for about 5 or 6 days a progressive ascending, lower motor neurone paralysis develops with paraesthesiae. Often a child, who may have been irritable for the previous 24 hours, falls on getting out of bed first thing in the morning, and is found to be weak or ataxic. Paralysis increases over the next few days: death results from bulbar and respiratory paralysis and aspiration of stomach contents. Vomiting is a feature of the more acute course of *Ixodes holocyclus* envenoming.

This clinical picture is often misinterpreted as poliomyelitis. Other neurological conditions, including Guillain–Barré syndrome, paralytic rabies, Eaton–Lambert syndrome, myasthenia gravis or botulism, may also be suspected. Diagnosis depends on finding the tick, which is likely to be concealed in a crevice, orifice or hairy area of the body. The scalp is the most common place. Fatal tick paralysis has been caused by a tick attached to the tympanic membrane.

Management
The tick must be detached without being squeezed. It can be painted with ether, chloroform, paraffin, petrol or turpentine, or prised out between the partially separated tips of a pair of small curved forceps. Following removal of the tick there is usually rapid and complete recovery, but in Australia patients have died after the tick has been detached. An antivenom, raised in dogs, is available in

Australia and, recently, rabbits have been used to produce an antitoxin against *Ixodes holocyclus* saliva.[55] This is recommended for severely affected or very young patients; 20–30 ml are given intravenously.

Centipede and millipede bites[75]

Centipedes

Many species of centipede (Chilopoda) can inflict painful bites, producing local pain, swelling, inflammation and lymphangitis. Systemic effects such as vomiting, headache, cardiac arrhythmias and convulsions are extremely rare and the risk of mortality was probably greatly exaggerated in the older literature. The most important genus is *Scolopendra*, which is distributed throughout tropical countries. Local treatment is the same as for scorpion stings. No antivenom is available.

Millipedes (Diplopoda)[89]

Most species possess glands in each of their body segments which secrete, and in some cases squirt out, irritant liquids for defensive purposes. These contain hydrogen cyanide and a variety of aldehydes, esters, phenols and quinonoids. Members of at least eight genera of millipedes have proved injurious to man. Important genera are *Rhinocricus* (Caribbean), *Spirobolus* (Tanzania), *Spirostreptus* and *Iulus* (Indonesia) and *Polyceroconas* (Papua New Guinea). Children are particularly at risk when they handle or try to eat these large arthropods. When venom is squirted into the eye, intense conjunctivitis results and there may be corneal ulceration and even blindness. Skin lesions are initially stained brown or purple, blister after a few days, and then peel. First aid is generous irrigation with water. Eye injuries should be treated as for snake venom ophthalmia.

Poisoning by ingestion of marine animals[65]

A variety of illnesses, usually categorized as 'food poisoning', are caused by eating seafood. The most common are attributable to bacterial or viral infections. These include *Vibrio parahaemolyticus* (after eating crustaceans, especially shrimps), *V. cholerae* (crabs and molluscs), non-O1 *V. cholerae* (oysters), *V. vulnificus* (oysters), *Aeromonas hydrophila* (frozen oysters), *Plesiomonas shigelloides* (oysters, mussels, mackerel, cuttlefish), *Salmonella typhi* (molluscs), *Campylobacter jejuni* (clams), *Shigella* species (molluscs), hepatitis A virus (molluscs, especially clams and oysters), Norwalk virus (clams and oysters) and astro- and caliciviruses (cockles and other molluscs). Botulism has been reported in people eating smoked fish and canned salmon. Since 1953, approximately 100 000 Japanese are thought to have been affected by methyl mercury poisoning (Minamata disease) after eating fish and molluscs contaminated with methyl mercury derived from industrial waste dumped in Minamata Bay and at the mouth of the Agano River in Japan. The victims developed severe central nervous system damage, with a mortality of 33% in the initial outbreak. Pregnant women exposed to methyl mercury gave birth to infants who were mentally retarded and had cerebral palsy and convulsions.

A number of clinical syndromes have been recognized which are related to the presence in the ingested flesh or viscera of marine animals of toxins either derived ultimately from marine microalgae or bacteria (e.g. ciguatera, tetrodotoxic or paralytic shellfish poisoning) or resulting from bacterial decomposition of fish during storage (scombrotoxic fish poisoning).[90,91]

Gastrointestinal and neurotoxic syndromes

Nausea, vomiting, abdominal colic, tenesmus and watery diarrhoea may precede the development of neurotoxic symptoms. Paraesthesiae of the lips, buccal cavity and extremities are early symptoms. Other neurotoxic manifestations include a peculiar distortion of temperature perception so that cold objects feel hot (like dry ice) and vice versa, dizziness, myalgia, weakness starting with muscles of phonation and deglutition and progressing to respiratory paralysis and flaccid quadriplegia in some cases, ataxia, involuntary movements, convulsions, visual disturbances, hallucinations and psychoses, cranial nerve lesions and pupillary abnormalities. Cardiovascular abnormalities include hypotension and bradycardia and some patients develop florid cutaneous rashes.

Distinguishable within this general pattern of symptoms are a number of conditions related to the ingestion of a particular taxonomic group of animals. Some of the more important syndromes are described below.

Ciguatera fish poisoning

The word 'ciguatera' seems to derive from the Cuban word 'cigua' for a poisonous marine snail (*Livona pica*, the West Indian top-shell) which was coined by early Spanish settlers.[65] Ciguatera is now applied to an illness resulting from the ingestion of any one of more than 400 species of warm-water, shore or reef fish between latitudes 35°N and 34°S, especially in the South Pacific and Caribbean (including Florida). Overall, there must be more than 50,000 cases in the world each year with an incidence of up to 2% of the population each year and a case fatality of about 0.1%. The fish most often associated with ciguatera are from the families Serranidae (groupers), Lutjanidae (snappers), Scaridae (parrot fish) and Scombridae (mackerel). Other important groups are moray eels (Muraenidae), barracudas (Sphyraenidae) and jacks (Carangidae).

It is now known that the toxins responsible for ciguatera fish poisoning, the polyether ciguatoxins, maitotoxins and scaritoxins, originate from benthic dinoflagellates such as *Gambierdiscus toxicus* which are ingested by herbivorous fish. These in turn are the prey of the carnivorous fish which, when eaten by humans, may give rise to severe gastrointestinal, neurotoxic and cardiovascular symptoms. Ciguatoxins are concentrated in the intestine, gonads and viscera. The acquisition of toxin by fish cannot be predicted; there is no seasonal variation in its prevalence but the risk of poisoning is greater with some species, e.g. Moray eels, and definitely increases as the fish gets larger. Three toxins—ciguatoxin, maitotoxin and scaritoxin (from the parrot fish, *Scarus sordidus*)—have been identified. Ciguatoxins excite Na⁺ channels, while maitotoxin activates voltage-independent Ca^{2+} channels.

Clinical features

Exceptionally, symptoms first appear as early as minutes or as long as 30 hours after eating the poisoned fish; however, the usual interval is 1–6 hours. The earliest symptom is numbness or tingling of the lips, tongue, throat and extremities, a metallic taste and a dry mouth or hypersalivation. Reversed perception of heat and cold is a distinctive symptom. In many cases, especially with milder poisoning, the earliest symptoms are gastrointestinal: sudden abdominal colic, nausea, vomiting and watery diarrhoea. Myalgia, ataxia, vertigo, visual disturbances and pruritic skin eruptions develop later. In severely neurotoxic cases flaccid paralysis and respiratory arrest may develop. Gastrointestinal symptoms resolve within a few hours but paraesthesiae and myalgias may persist for a week, months or even years. Ciguatera poisoning from eating moray eels (*Gymnothorax* species) is particularly rapid and severe because of the high concentration of toxin in these animals.

Chelonitoxication results from the ingestion of marine turtles (Chelonia). Its clinical features resemble ciguatera poisoning. Most outbreaks have been in the Indo-Pacific area. The species usually implicated are green hawksbill and leathery turtles. The case fatality among reported cases is 28%.

Tetrodotoxic (puffer fish) poisoning

More than 50 species of tropical scaleless fish of the order Tetraodonitiformes have proved poisonous. They include porcupine fish (*Chilomycterus*), molas or sunfish (*Mola*) and puffer fish or toadfish (Tetraodontidae—genera *Arothron*, *Fugu*, *Lagocephalus*, etc.). The flesh of the puffer fish (Japanese fugu) is particularly relished in Japan where, despite the stringent regulations and skilful fugu cooks, there are cases of tetrodotoxin poisoning and about four deaths each year. Cases have been reported in Thailand and many other Indo-Pacific countries. Tetrodotoxin, an aminoperhydroquinazoline, is one of the most potent non-protein toxins known. It is concentrated in the fish's ovaries, viscera and skin. There is a definite seasonal variation in the toxin concentration which reaches a peak during the spawning season (May to June in Japan). Tetrodotoxin impairs nervous conduction by blocking the sodium ion flux without affecting

movement of potassium, producing neurotoxic and cardiotoxic effects. The origin of this toxin is unknown. It may be synthesized by *Pseudomonas* bacteria and acquired through the food chain. An identical toxin has been found in the skin of newts (genus *Taricha*), frogs (genus *Atelopus*) and salamanders, the saliva of octopuses (genus *Hapalochlaena*), in the digestive glands of several species of gastropod mollusc and in xanthid and horseshoe crabs, star fish, flatworms (*Planorbis*) and nemertine worms in Japan.

Clinical features

Paraesthesiae, dizziness and ataxia become noticeable within 10–45 minutes of eating the fish. Generalized numbness, hypersalivation, sweating and hypotension may develop. Some patients remain aware of their surroundings despite appearing comatose. Gastrointestinal symptoms may be completely absent. Death from respiratory paralysis usually occurs within the first 6 hours and is unusual more than 2 hours after eating the fish. Erythema, petechiae, blistering and desquamation may appear.

Paralytic shellfish poisoning

Bivalve molluscs, such as mussels, clams (*Saxidomus*), oysters, cockles and scallops may acquire neurotoxins such as saxitoxins from the dinoflagellates, *Alexandrium* species (formerly *Gymnodinium catenatum* and *Pyrodinium bahamense*), which occur between latitudes 30°N and 30°S. The dinoflagellates may be sufficiently abundant during the warmer months of May to October to produce a 'red tide'. The dangerous season is announced by the discovery of unusual numbers of dead fish and sea birds. Symptoms develop within 30 minutes of ingestion. They include perioral paraesthesia, gastrointestinal symptoms, ataxia, visual disturbances and pareses (progressing to respiratory paralysis within 12 hours) in 8% of cases. Milder gastrointestinal and neurotoxic symptoms without paralysis have been associated with ingestion of molluscs contaminated by neurotoxic brevetoxins from *Gymnodinium breve*, which act on sodium channels. These microalgae also produce a 'red tide'.

Histamine syndrome (scombrotoxic poisoning)

The red flesh of scombroid fish such as tuna, mackerel, bonito and skipjack, and of canned non-scombroid fish like sardines and pilchards, may be decomposed by the action of bacteria such as *Proteus morgani*, decarboxylating muscle histidine into histamine, saurine, cadaverine and perhaps other unidentified toxins. Toxic fish may produce a warning tingling or smarting sensation in the mouth when eaten. Between minutes and up to 24 hours after ingestion, flushing, burning, urticaria and pruritus of the skin, headache, abdominal colic, nausea, vomiting, diarrhoea, hypotensive shock and bronchial asthma may develop. Exogenous histamine may be detected in patients' plasma and urine and in the fish.[92] Identical symptoms have been described in Sri Lankan patients who ate fish while taking the antituberculosis drug isoniazid, which inhibits the enzyme normally responsible for inactivating histamine.

Poisoning by ingestion of carp's gallbladder

In parts of the Far East the raw bile and gallbladder of various species of freshwater carp (e.g. the grass carp *Ctenopharyngodon idellus*; 'plaa yeesok' *Probarbus jullienii*) are believed to have medicinal properties. Patients in China, Taiwan, Hong Kong, Japan, Thailand and elsewhere have developed acute abdominal pain, vomiting and watery diarrhoea 2–18 hours after drinking the raw bile or eating the raw gallbladder of these fish. One patient developed flushing and dizziness. Hepatic and renal damage may develop, progressing to hepatic failure and oliguric or non-oliguric acute renal failure (acute tubular necrosis).[93] The hepatonephrotoxin has not been identified, but is heat-stable and may be derived from the carp's diet.

Treatment of marine poisoning

The differential diagnosis includes bacterial and viral food poisoning and allergic reactions. No specific treatments or antidotes are available. Gastrointestinal contents should be eliminated by emetics and purges. Activated charcoal absorbs saxitoxin and other shellfish toxins. Atropine is said to improve gastrointestinal symptoms and sinus bradycardia in patients with gastrointestinal and neurotoxic poisoning. Oximes, such as pralidoxime and 2-pyridine aldoxime, have been claimed to benefit the anticholinesterase features of ciguatera poisoning but the evidence is not convincing. Calcium gluconate may relieve mild neuromuscular symptoms. In scombroid poisoning, anti-H_1 and anti-H_2 (e.g. cimetidine) antihistamines, corticosteroids and bronchodilators should be used. In cases of paralytic poisoning, endotracheal intubation and mechanical ventilation have proved lifesaving. Cardiac resuscitation may also be required. There is some evidence supporting the use of mannitol intravenously in acute ciguatera poisoning. In adults, 1 g/kg of 10% or 20% mannitol is given by intravenous infusion over 30 minutes as soon as possible after rehydration. Gabapentin has been suggested as a treatment for chronic persisting paraesthesiae after ciguatera poisoning.

Prevention of marine poisoning

Ciguatera, tetrodotoxin and histamine are heat-stable, so cooking does not prevent poisoning. In tropical areas the flesh of fish should be separated, as soon as possible, from the head, skin, intestines, gonads and other viscera which may have high concentrations of toxin. All scaleless fish should be regarded as potentially tetrodotoxic, while very large fish carry an increased risk of being ciguateratoxic. Moray eels should never be eaten. Some toxins are fairly water-soluble and may be leached out, so water in which fish are cooked should be thrown away. Scombroid poisoning can be prevented by prompt freezing or by eating the fish fresh. Shellfish should not be eaten during the dangerous season and when there are red tides.

REFERENCES

1　Sutherland S K & Tibballs J. *Australian Animal Toxins: The Creatures, their Toxins and Care of the Poisoned Patient*, 2nd edn. Melbourne: Oxford University Press, 2001.

2　Meier J & White J (eds). *Handbook of Clinical Toxicology of Animal Venoms and Poisons*. Boca Raton, FL: CRC Press, 1995.

3　Minton S A. Are there any non-venomous snakes? An update on colubrid envenoming. *Adv Herpetoculture* 1996; 127–134.

4　Knight A, Densmore L D & Rael E D. Molecular systematics of the Agkistrodon complex. In Campbell J A & Brodie E D (eds) *Biology of the Pit Vipers*. Tyler, TX: Selva, 1992: 49–69.

5　Pugh R N H, Theakston R D G, Reid H A & Briar I S. Malumfashi endemic diseases research project. XIII. Epidemiology of human encounters with the spitting cobra, *Naja nigricollis*, in the Malumfashi area of northern Nigeria. *Ann Trop Med Parasitol* 1980; 74:523–530.

6　Snow R W, Bronzan R, Rogues T, et al. The prevalence and morbidity of snake bite and treatment-seeking behaviour among a rural Kenyan population. *Ann Trop Med Parasitol* 1994; 88:665–671.

7　Trape J-F, Pison G, Guyavarch E, et al. High mortality from snake bite in south-eastern Senegal. *Trans R Soc Trop Med Hyg* (2001; 95:420–423).

8　Hati A K et al. Epidemiology of snake bite in the district of Burdwan, West Bengal. *J Indian Med Assoc* 1992; 90:145–147.

9　Pierini S V, Warrell D A, de Paulo A el Theakston R D G et al. High incidence of bites and stings by snakes and other animals among rubber tappers and Amazonian Indians of the Jurua Valley, Acré State, Brazil. *Toxicon* 1996; 34:225–236.

10　Swaroop S & Grab B. Snakebite mortality in the world. *Bull World Health Organ* 1954; 10:35–76.

11　Myint-Lwin, Warrell D A, Phillips R E, Tin-Nu-Swe, Tun-Pe & Maung-Maung Lay. Bites by Russell's viper (*Vipera russelli siamensis*) in Burma: haemostatic, vascular and renal disturbances and response to treatment. Lancet 1985; ii:1259–1264.

12　Sawai Y, Makino M, Kawa-Mura Y et al. Epidemiological study of habu bites on the Amami and Okinawa Islands of Japan. In Ohsaka A, Hayashi K & Sawai Y (eds) *Plant, Animal and Microbial Toxins*, vol. 2. New York: Plenum Press, 1976: 439–450.

13　Warrell D A & Arnett C. The importance of bites by the saw-scaled or carpet viper (*Echis carinatus*): epidemiological studies in Nigeria and a review of the world literature. *Acta Trop (Basel)* 1976; 33:307–341.

14　Reid H A & Lim K J. Sea-snake bite: a survey of fishing villages in northwest Malaya. *BMJ* 1957; ii:1266–1272.

15　Warrell D A. Sea snake bites in the Asia-Pacific region. In Gopalkrishnakone P (ed.) *Sea Snake Toxinology*. Singapore University Press, 1994: 1–36.

16　Saini R K, Singh S, Sharma S, et al. Snake bite poisoning presenting as early morning neuro-paralytic syndrome in jhuggi dwellers. *J Assoc Physicians India* 1986; 34:415–417.

17　Warrell D A, Looareesuwan S, White N J et al. Severe

neurotoxic envenoming by the Malayan krait Bungarus candidus (Linnaeus): response to antivenom and anticholinesterase. *BMJ* 1983; 286:678–680.

18 Warrell D A, Greenwood B M, Davidson N McD, Ormerod L D & Prentice C R M. Necrosis, haemorrhage and complement depletion following bites by the spitting cobra (*Naja nigricollis*). *Q J Med* 1976; 45:1–22.

19 Kochva E. Oral glands of the reptilia. In Gans C & Gans K A (eds) *Biology of the Reptilia*. London: Academic Press, 1978: 43–161.

20 Bogert C M. Dentitional phenomena in cobras and other Elapids with notes on adaptive modifications of fangs. *Bull Am Mus Nat Hist* 1943; 81:285–360.

21 Wüster W & Thorpe RS. Dentitional phenomena in cobras revisited: spitting and fang structure in the Asiatic species of Naja (Serpentes: Elapidae). *Herpetologica* 1992; 48:424–434.

22 Harvey A L (ed.). Snake toxins. *International Encyclopedia of Pharmacology and Therapeutics*, section 134. New York: Pergamon, 1991.

23 Douglas W W. Polypeptides: angiotensin, plasma kinins and others. In Goodman A G, Gilman L S, Rall T W & Murad F (eds) *The Pharmacological Basis of Therapeutics*. New York: Macmillan, 1985: 639–659.

24 Hutton R A & Warrell D A. Action of snake venom components on the haemostatic system. *Blood Rev* 1993; 7:176–189.

25 Hutton R A, Looareesuwan S, Ho M et al. Arboreal pit vipers (genus *Trimeresurus*) of Southeast Asia: bites by T. *albolabris* and T. macrops in Thailand and a review of the literature. *Trans R Soc Trop Med Hyg* 1990; 84:866–874.

26 Vogt W. Snake venom constituents affecting the complement system. In Stocker K F (ed) *Medical Use of Snake Venom Proteins*. Boca Raton, FL: CRC Press, 1990: 79–96.

27 Ratcliffe P J, Pukrittayakamee S, Ledingham J G G & Warrell D A. Direct nephrotoxicity of Russell's viper venom demonstrated in the isolated perfused rat kidney. *Am J Trop Med Hyg* 1989; 40:312–319.

28 Phillips R E, Theakston R D G, Warrell D A et al. Paralysis, rhabdomyolysis and haemolysis caused by bites of Russell's viper (*Vipera russelli pulchella*) in Sri Lanka: failure of Indian (Haffkine) antivenom. *Q J Med* 1988; 68:691–716.

29 Azevedo-Marques M M, Hering S E & Cupo P. Evidence that Crotalus durissus terrificus (South American rattlesnake) envenomation in humans causes myolysis rather than hemolysis. *Toxicon* 1987; 25:1163–1168.

30 Sitprija V & Chaiyabutr N. Nephrotoxicity in snake envenomation. *J Nat Toxins* 1999; 8:271–277.

31 Warrell D A & Ormerod L D. Snake venom ophthalmia and blindness caused by the spitting cobra (*Naja nigricollis*) in Nigeria. *Am J Trop Med Hyg* 1976; 25:525–529.

32 Warrell D A, Ormerod L D & Davidson N McD. Bites by the night adder (*Causus maculatus*) and burrowing vipers (*genus Atractaspis*) in Nigeria. *Am J Trop Med Hyg* 1976; 25: 517–524.

33 Kurnik D, Haviv Y, Kochva E. A snake bite by the burrowing asp, Atractaspis engaddensis. *Toxicon* 1999; 37:223–227.

34 Tin-Myint, Rai-Mra, Maung-Chit, Tun-Pe & Warrell D A. Bites by the king cobra (*Ophiophagus hannah*) in Myanmar: successful treatment of severe neurotoxic envenoming. *Q J Med* 1991; 80:751–762.

35 Watt G, Theakston R D G, Hayes C G et al. Positive response to edrophonium in patients with neurotoxic envenoming by cobras (*Naja naja philippinensis*): a placebo-controlled study. *N Engl J Med* 1986; 315:1444–1448.

36 Campbell C H. Symptomatology, pathology and treatment of the bites of elapid snakes. In Lee C Y (ed.) *Snake Venoms. Handbook of Experimental Pharmacology*. Berlin: Springer, 1979: 898–921.

37 Lalloo D G et al. Snake bites by the Papuan taipan (*Oxyuranus scutellatus canni*): paralysis, hemostatic and electrocardiographic abnormalities, and effects of antivenom. *Am J Trop Med Hyg* 1995; 52:525–531.

38 Connolly S et al. Neuromuscular effects of Papuan taipan snake venom. *Ann Neurol* 1995; 38:916–920.

39 Reid H A. Symptomatology, pathology and treatment of the bites of sea snakes. In Lee C Y (ed.) *Snake Venoms. Handbook of Experimental Pharmacology*. Berlin: Springer, 1979: 922–955.

40 Sano-Martins I S, et al. Coagulopathy following lethal and non-lethal envenoming of humans by the South American rattlesnake (*Crotalus dursis*) in Brazil. *Q J Med* 2001; 94:551–559.

41 Warrell D A, Davidson N McD, Greenwood B M et al. Poisoning by bites of the saw-scaled or carpet viper (*Echis carinatus*) in Nigeria. *Q J Med* 1977; 46:33–62.

42 Sano-Martins I S, Fan H W, Castro S C et al. Reliability of the simple 20 minute whole blood clotting test (WBCT20) as an indicator of low plasma fibrinogen concentration in patients envenomed by Bothrops snakes. *Toxicon* 1994; 32:1045–1050.

43 Theakston R D G, Lloyd-Jones M J & Reid H A. Micro-ELISA for detecting and assaying snake venom and venom-antibody. *Lancet* 1977; ii:639–641.

44 Ho M, Warrell M J, Warrell D A, Bidwell D & Voller A. A critical reappraisal of the use of enzyme-lined immunosorbent assays in the study of snake bite. *Toxicon* 1986; 24:211–221.

45 Warrell D A (ed.). WHO/SEARO Guidelines for the clinical management of snake bites in the South East Asian region. *SE Asian J Trop Med Publ Health* 1999; 30(suppl. 1):1–85.

46 Bush S P, Hegewald K G, Green S M, et al. Effects of a negative pressure venom extraction device (Extractor) on local tissue injury after artificial rattlesnake envenomation in a porcine model. *Wilderness Environ Med* 2000; 11:180–188.

47 Hardy D L. A review of first aid measures for pit viper bite in North America with an appraisal of Extractor™ suction and stun gun electroshock. In Campbell J A & Brodie E D (eds) *Biology of the Pit Vipers*. Tyler, TX: Selva, 1992: 405–414.

48 Sutherland S K, Coulter A R & Harris R D. Rationalisation of first-aid measures for elapid snake bite. *Lancet* 1979; i:183–186.

49 Warrell D A. The global problem of snake bite: its prevention and treatment. In Gopalakrishnakone P & Tan C K (eds) *Recent Advances in Toxinology Research*, vol. 1. National University of Singapore, 1992: 121–153.

50 Howarth D M, Southee A E, Whyte I M. Lymphatic flow rates and first-aid in simulated peripheral snake or spider envenomation. *Med J Aust* 1994; 161:695-700.

51 Reid H A. Adder bites in Britain. *BMJ* 1976; ii:153–156.

52 Malasit P, Warrell D A, Chanthavanich P et al. Prediction, prevention and mechanism of early (anaphylactic) antivenom reactions in victims of snake bites. *BMJ* 1986; 292:17–20.

53 Fan H W, Marcopito L F, Cardoso J L, et al. Sequential, randomised and double-blind trial of promethzine prophylaxis against early anaphylactic reactions to antivenom for Bothrops snake bites. *BMJ* 1999; 318:1451–1453.

54 Premawardhena A P, de Silva C E, Fonseka M M, et al. Low dose subcutaneous adrenaline to prevent acute adverse reactions to antivenom serum in people bitten by snakes: randomised, placebo-controlled trial. *BMJ* 1999; 318:1041–1043.

55 Theakston R D G & Warrell D A. Antivenoms: a list of hyperimmune sera currently available for the treatment of envenoming by bites and stings. *Toxicon* 1991; 29:1419–1470.

56 World Health Organization. Progress in the characterization of venoms and standardization of antivenoms. *WHO Offset Publ* 1981; No. 58.

57 Warrell D A, Warrell M J, Edgar W, Prentice C R M, Mathison J H & Mathison J. Comparison of Pasteur and Behringwerke antivenoms in envenoming by the carpet viper (*Echis carinatus*). *BMJ* 1980; 280:607–609.

58 Ho M, Silamut K, White N J et al. Pharmacokinetics of three commercial antivenoms in patients envenomed by the Malayan pit viper (*Calloselasma rhodostoma*) in Thailand. *Am J Trop Med Hyg* 1990; 42:260–266.

59 Theakston R D G, Fan H W, Warrell D A, Da Silva W D, Ward S A, Higashi H G & BIASG. Use of enzyme immunoassays to compare the efficacy and assess dosage regimens of three Brazilian Bothrops antivenoms. *Am J Trop Med Hyg* 1992; 47:593–604.

60 Theakston R D G, Phillips R E, Looareesuwan S, Echeverria P, Makin T & Warrell D A. Bacteriological studies of the venom and mouth cavities of wild Malayan pit vipers (*Calloselasma rhodostoma*) in southern Thailand. *Trans R Soc Trop Med Hyg* 1990; 84:875–879.

61 Garfin S R, Castilonia R R, Mubarak S J, Hargens A R, Russell F E & Akeson W H. Rattlesnake bites and surgical decompression: results using a laboratory model. *Toxicon* 1984; 22:177–182.

62 Sawai Y. Vaccination against snake bite poisoning. In Lee C Y (ed.) *Snake Venoms. Handbook of Experimental Pharmacology.* Berlin: Springer, 1979:881–897.

63 Russell F E & Bogert C M. Gila monster, venom and bite: a review. *Toxicon* 1981; 19:341–359.

64 Raufman J-P. Review. Bioactive peptides from lizard venoms. *Regul Peptides* 1996; 61:1–18.

65 Halstead B W. *Poisonous and Venomous Marine Animals of the World*, 2nd edn. Princeton New Jersey: Darwin Press, 1988.

66 Williamson J A, Fenner P J, Burnett J W & Rifkin J F (eds). *Venomous and Poisonous Marine Animals: A Medical and Biological Handbook.* Sydney: University of New South Wales Press, 1996.

67 Castex M N. Freshwater venomous rays. In Russell F E & Saunders P R (eds) *Animal Toxins.* Oxford: Pergamon Press, 1967: 167–176.

68 Maretic Z. Some epidemiological, clinical and therapeutic aspects of envenomation by weeverfish sting. In De Vries A & Kochva E (eds) *Toxins of Animals and Plant Origin*, vol. 3. New York: Gordon & Breach, 1973: 1055–1065.

69 Barnes J H. Observations on jellyfish stingings in North Queensland. *Med J Aust* 1960; 2:993–999.

70 Pereira P L, Carrette T, Cullen P, et al. Pressure immobilisation bandages in first-aid treatment of jelly fish envenomation: current recommendation reconsidered. *Med J Aust* 2000; 173:650–652.

71 Alender C B & Russell F E. Pharmacology. In Boolootian R A (ed.) *Physiology of Echinodermata.* New York: Interscience, 1966: 529–543.

72 Olivera B M & Cruz L J. Conotoxins, in retrospect. *Toxicon* 2001; 39:7–14.

73 Mueller U R. *Insect Sting Allergy: Clinical Picture, Diagnosis and Treatment.* Stuttgart: Gustav Fischer, 1990.

74 Winston M L. Killer Bees. *The Africanized Honey Bee in the Americas.* Cambridge, MA: Harvard University Press, 1992.

75 Bettini S (ed.). *Arthropod Venoms. Handbook of Experimental Pharmacology*, vol. 48. Berlin: Springer, 1978.

76 Piek T. *Venoms of the Hymenoptera: Biochemical, Pharmacological and Behavioural Aspects.* London: Academic Press, 1986.

77 França F O S, Benvenuti L A, Fan H W, et al. Severe and fatal mass attacks by 'killer' bees (Africanised honey bees—*Apis mellifera scutellata*) in Brazil: clinicopathological studies with measurement of serum venom concentrations. *Q J Med* 1994; 87:269–282.

78 Ewan P W. Allergy to insect stings: a review. *J R Soc Med* 1984; 78:234–239.

79 Hunt K J, Valentine M D, Sobotka A K, Benton A W, Amodio F J & Lichtenstein L M. A controlled trial of immunotherapy in insect hypersensitivity. *N Engl J Med* 1978; 299:157–161.

80 Mazzotti L & Bravo-Becherelle M A. Scorpionism in the Mexican Republic. In Keegan H L & Macfarlane W V (eds) *Venomous and Poisonous Animals and Noxious Plants of the Pacific Region.* Oxford: Pergamon Press, 1963: 111–131.

81 Bawaskar H S. Diagnostic cardiac premonitory signs and symptoms of red scorpion sting. *Lancet* 1982; i:552–554.

82 Bawaskar A S & Bawaskar P H. Severe envenoming by the Indian red scorpion (*Mesobuthus tamulus*): the use of prazosin therapy. *Q J Med* 1996; 89:701–704.

83 Freire-Maia L, Campos J A & Amaral C F S. Treatment of scorpion envenoming in Brazil. In Bon C & Goyffon M (eds) *Envenomings and their Treatments.* Lyon: Edition Fondation Marcel Mérieux, 1996: 301–310.

84 Maretic Z & Lebez D. *Araneism.* Pula, Italy: Novit, 1979.

85 Pearn J. The clinical features of tick bite. *Med J Aust* 1977; 2:313.

86 Murnaghan M F & O'Rourke F J. Tick paralysis. In Bettini S (ed.) *Handbook of Experimental Pharmacology*, vol. 48. Berlin: Springer, 1978: 419–464.

87 Gothe R, Kunze K & Hoogstraal H. The mechanism of pathogenicity in the tick paralyses. *J Med Entomol* 1979; 16:357–369.

88 Stone B F. Toxicoses induced by ticks and reptiles in domestic animals. In Harris J B (ed.) *Natural Toxins: Animal, Plant and Microbial.* Oxford: Clarendon Press, 1986: 56–71.

89 Radford A J. Millipede burns in man. *Trop Geogr Med* 1975; 27:279–287.

90 World Health Organization. Aquatic (marine and freshwater) biotoxins. *Environmental Health Criteria 37.* Geneva: WHO, 1984.

91 Daranas A H, Norte M & Fernández J J. Review: toxic marine micro-algae. *Toxicon* 2001; 39:1101–1132.

92 Morrow J D, Margolies G R, Rowland J & Roberts L J. Evidence that histamine is the causative toxin of scombroid-fish poisoning. *N Engl J Med* 1991; 324:716–720.

93 Lin Y F & Lin S H. Simultaneous acute renal and hepatic failure after ingesting raw carp gall bladder. *Nephrol Dial Transplantation* 1999; 14:2011–2012.

Chapter 33
Plant Poisons

J. K. Aronson

Since the earliest times people have used plants as sources of chemicals, for therapeutic, stimulant, and poisonous purposes. Curare (from *Chondodendron tomentosum*), used by South American Indians as an arrow poison (indeed the word toxin comes from a Greek word meaning a bow), is a good example of a poison that has been harnessed therapeutically. Its pharmacological action on skeletal muscle was demonstrated by Claude Bernard in 1856[1] and curare was introduced into anaesthetic practice in 1942.[2]

Many other plants that are regarded as poisonous have been used for their supposed therapeutic properties, but while many can still be found in herbals, not all have found their way into modern formularies. Some therapeutically useful chemicals found in plants are listed in Table 33.1. Relatively few of these drugs have been derived from tropical plants, and although ethnopharmacology aims

to remedy that, there are difficulties.[3] On the other hand, many tropical plants are used herbally.

The use of plants for stimulant (including aphrodisiac) or hallucinogenic effects is ancient.[4] Examples include absinthe (*Artemisia absinthium*), betel leaves (*Piper betle*) taken with areca (betel) nuts (*Areca catechu*), cannabis, cocaine, Jimson weed (*Datura stramonium*), kava (*Piper methysticum*), khat (*Catha edulis*), mescalin or peyotl (*Lophophora williamsii*), morning glory (*Ipomoea tricolori*), nicotine (from many plants, including *Nicotiana tabacum*), nutmeg (*Myristica fragrans*), ololiuqui (*Rivea corymbosa*), opioids and pituri (*Duboisia hopwoodii*). In contrast to many of the therapeutic plants listed in Table 33.1, many of these plants are native to the tropics.

Plants are also sometimes used for culinary purposes; examples include *Papaver rhoeas*, whose seeds are used to decorate bread and as a filling in the delicious Jewish pastry

Table 33.1 Some commonly used therapeutic agents that originally derived from plants (see also Table 33.2).

Drug	Example of medical use	Plant of origin
Artemether	Malaria	Qinghao (*Artemisia annua*)
Atropine	Anticholinergic	Deadly nightshade (*Atropa belladonna*)
Cannabinoids	Palliative care	Cannabis (*Cannabis sativa*)
Capsaicin	Painful neuropathies	Peppers (*Capsicum* spp.)
Cephaeline	Emetogenic	Ipecacuanha (*Cephaëlis ipecacuanha*)
Cocaine	Local anaesthetic	Coca (*Erythroxylon coca*)
Colchicine	Gout	Autumn crocus (*Colchicum autumnale*)
Curare	Anaesthesia	Pareira (*Chondrodendron tometosum*)
Digoxin/digitoxin	Atrial fibrillation and heart failure	Foxgloves (*Digitalis lanata/purpurea*)
Ephedrine	Sympathomimetic	Sea-grapes (*Ephedra sinica*)
Gamolenic acid	Mastodynia	Evening primrose (*Oenothera biennis*)
Hyosine	Anticholinergic	Thorn apple (*Datura stramonium*)
Ispaghula	Laxative	Ispaghula (*Plantago ovata*)
Opioid alkaloids	Analgesia	Poppies (*Papaver somniferum*)
Physostigmine	Myasthenia gravis	Calabar bean (*Physostigma venenosum*)
Pilocarpine	Glaucoma	Jaborandi (*Pilocarpus jaborandi*)
Quinine	Malaria	Cinchona (*Cinchona pubescens*)
Salicylates	Analgesics	Meadowsweet (*Spiraea ulmaria*)
		Willow (*Salix alba*)
		Wintergreen (*Gaultheria procumbens*)
Sennosides	Purgative	Senna (*Cassia acutifolia*)
Taxanes	Cytotoxic	Yew trees (*Taxus* spp.)
Theophylline	Asthma	Tea plant (*Camellia sinensis*)
Vinblastine	Cytotoxic	Madagascar periwinkle (*Catharanthus rosea*)

called Hamantaschen (Haman's ears), eaten in remembrance of the events in Persia recounted in the book of Esther; tansy (*Tanacetum vulgare*) used to make tansy cakes, for consumption at Easter time; cannabis in hashish fudge (a recipe for which can be found in *The Alice B. Toklas Cook Book*;[5] and a wealth of vegetables (such as cassava and yams) and culinary herbs and spices, too numerous to be listed.

And, of course, throughout the ages plants have been used as poisons. Socrates, for example, executed himself at the behest of the state using hemlock (*Conium maculatum*). We do not know what the hebenon was that Hamlet's uncle poured in the elder Hamlet's ear, but it may have been from henbane (*Hyoscyamus niger*) or some form of yew (*Taxus*; German *eibenbaum*) (Figure 33.1). The Bulgarian diplomat Georgi Markov was murdered when a tiny amount of what was probably ricin, a potent poison derived from the castor bean (*Ricinus communis*), was injected into his leg in a metal pellet via the medium of an umbrella tip.[6] And aconite (from *Aconitum napellus*) is a toxin that has been used as an arrow poison and was a favourite of professional poisoners in the Roman empire; it is still to be found in some Chinese herbs.[7]

Plant poisoning can occur as a result of accidental, unknowing or deliberate poisoning from contaminated foodstuffs or from toxic seeds and fruits; from the misuse of traditional or herbal medicines; or from the deliberate use of plants for their psychotropic properties. Contact dermatitis can occur from contact with irritant plants.[8]

Traditional medicines exist in many forms and lack standardization; very few have been rigorously tested for toxicity, especially for their long-term effects. They are prescribed by herbalists, usually as complex mixtures with uncertain pharmacology, or are prepared and taken by patients themselves. Poisoning occurs because the herb is itself toxic, has been mistaken for another plant, mislabelled, mixed accidentally or deliberately with other, poisonous, plants and medicines, contaminated with insecticides or herbicides, or, as in the Asian kushtays, mixed with appreciable amounts of heavy metals.[9] Herbal medicines are also used in combination with allopathic drugs and the often unpredictable effects of such combinations add to the hazards.[10]

The frequency of exposure to poisonous plants is difficult to assess; many reports are anecdotal. In one series of 912 534 plant exposures in the USA, *Philodendron* species were the most commonly implicated, followed by *Dieffenbachia*, *Euphorbia*, *Capsicum* and *Ilex*.[11]

Not all parts or constituents of a poisonous plant are poisonous. The stalks of rhubarb can be eaten but the leaves contain toxic oxalates; all parts of the yew are poisonous except the fleshy red aril. The purgative castor oil is expressed from the beans of *Ricinus communis*, but the beans also contain the highly toxic alkaloid ricin. Ackee fruit is poisonous only when unripe. Furthermore, the amount of toxic ingredient in a single part of a plant varies from season to season.

Nor are all poisonous plants poisonous to all species. Goats, for example, can eat foxgloves and nightshade with

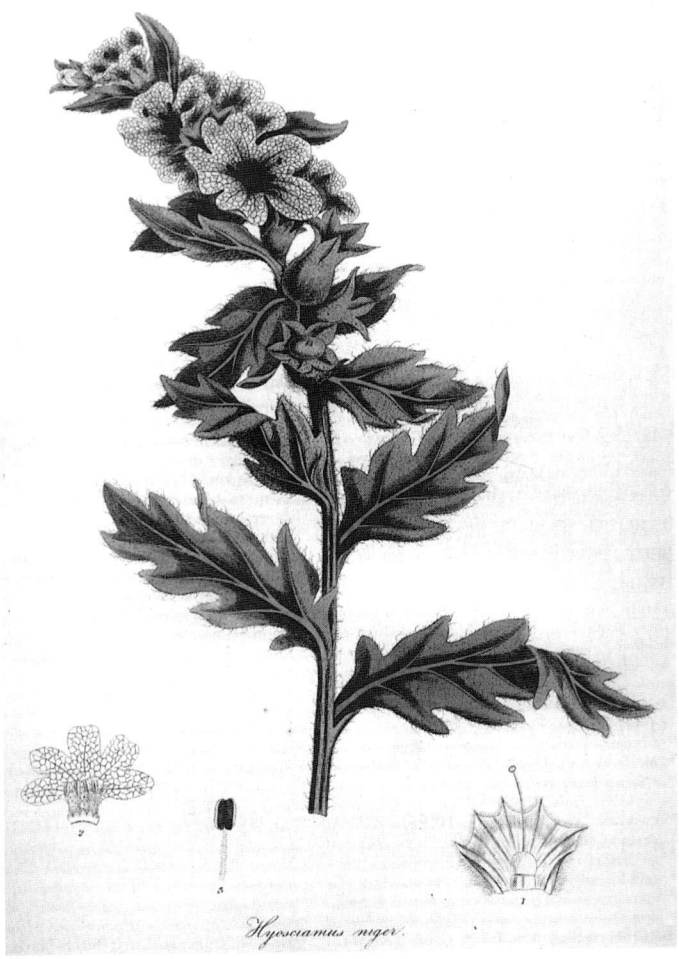

Hyosciamus niger.

Figure 33.1: Henbane (*Hyoscyamus niger*).

impunity, since they eliminate their toxic ingredients rapidly; bees can harvest pollen from poisonous plants, such as rhododendrons, which contain grayanotoxins, and the honey so produced may be poisonous to man.[12] One should not be misled by seeing an animal feed on a plant into thinking that it is safe for human consumption.

There is no simple way of classifying poisonous plants, other than by their scientific names, and even those change from time to time. Here I shall use headings that describe their pharmacological or clinical effects; when that is not possible I shall use the name of the plant or its chief constituent as a heading.

Cardiotoxic glycosides

The number of plants worldwide that contain cardiac glycosides (cardenolides or bufadienolides) is legion—the incomplete list given by Gibbs[13] runs to nearly 400 compounds and spans genera such as the Apocyanaceae, Asclepiadaceae, Cruciferae, Liliaceae, Moraceae, Ranunculaceae, and Scrophulariaceae. Some examples are given in Table 33.2.

Table 33.2 Some plants that contain cardiac glycosides.

Scientific name	Common name
Acokanthera ouabaio/ schimperi	Olmorijoi/Murichu
Adonis vernalis	False hellebore
Antiaris toxicaria	Upas tree
Apocynum cannabinum	Black Indian hemp
Asclepias curassavica	Redheaded cotton-bush
Asclepias fruiticosa	Balloon cotton
Asclepias syriaca	Milkweed
Calotropis procera	King's crown
Carissa acokanthera	Bushman's poison
Carissa spectabilis	Wintersweet
Cerbera manghas	Sea-mango
Cerbera odollum	Pong pong
Convallaria majalis	Lily of the valley
Cryptostegia grandiflora	Rubber vine
Digitalis lanata	Woolly foxglove
Digitalis purpurea	Purple foxglove
Gloriosa superba	Glory lily
Helleborus niger	Christmas rose
Nerium oleander	Oleander
Periploca sepium	Silkvine
Plumeria rubra	Frangipani
Scilla maritima	Squill
Strophanthus spp.	Various
Tanghinia venenifera	Ordeal tree
Thevetia peruviana	Yellow oleander
Urechites suberecta	Savannah flower
Uriginea maritima	Squill

Some cardenolides (such as digoxin and digitoxin, obtained from foxgloves) are used therapeutically, and even then toxicity readily occurs, because these drugs have a low therapeutic index.[14] Poisoning with plants containing cardenolides is not uncommon. In recent years there has been an epidemic of self-poisoning with the seeds of oleander trees in south India and Sri Lanka. In one series of 300 cases of self-poisoning with *Thevetia peruviana* (yellow oleander) (mostly women aged 11–20, of whom 97% took crushed seeds), the main symptoms were vomiting, palpitation, epigastric pain, a burning sensation in the abdomen, shortness of breath and diarrhoea; sinus bradycardia, sinus arrest, sinoatrial block and heart block were common.[15]

Other plants that have caused cardenolide poisoning include the pong pong (*Cerbera odollum*)[16] and the glory lily (*Gloriosa superba*).[17] In one series of 4556 cases of self-poisoning in Sri Lanka, 2.5% were caused by plants and mushrooms; *Gloriosa superba* was responsible for 44% of those (i.e., 50 cases).[18] The toxic effects of *Gloriosa* are due to both cardenolides and colchicine alkaloids. Plants containing cardenolides that have been used as arrow poisons include *Acokanthera schimperi* in Africa[19] and the upas tree (*Antiaris toxicaria*) in Malaysia and China.[20,21]

In Madagascar the ordeal tree (*Tanghinia venenifera*) was used to test the innocence or guilt of an accused person; death on eating it signified guilt.

Treatment of cardenolide poisoning is largely supportive (Table 33.3), but special attention should be paid to potassium balance, since cardenolides inhibit Na/K-ATPase (the Na/K pump), inhibiting the influx of potassium into cells; the severity of toxicity, and therefore the prognosis, is related to the degree of hyperkalaemia that results. Fab fragments of antidigoxin antibody are effective not only in poisoning with digoxin but with many other cardiac glycosides too;[22] they have been used in oleander poisoning.[23] Activated charcoal in repeated doses (50 g 4-hourly) may encourage the intestinal secretion of cardenolides; a trial of its efficacy in oleander poisoning is currently under way in Sri Lanka.

Cyanogenic glycosides

Several plants contain cyanogenic glycosides.[24] The best known of these is cassava (*Manihot esculenta*), a native of South America, which is widely grown in the tropics for the production of flour and tapioca. The grated roots must be thoroughly washed to remove the toxic material; badly prepared cassava causes signs of hydrocyanic acid poisoning: nausea, vomiting, abdominal distension and respiratory difficulty. Chronic cassava ingestion can cause an ataxic neuropathy, with bilateral primary optic atrophy, bilateral perceptive deafness, myelopathy and peripheral neuropathy.[25] Previous reports of goitre and pancreatitis as chronic effects have not been confirmed.

The broken kernels of *Prunus* species (plums, peaches, cherries, apricots, almonds) and of loquats (*Eriobotrya japonica*) also contain cyanogenic glycosides. The active principle, amygdalin (laetrile), has been used in patients with cancer; however, it is ineffective and adverse effects have not been uncommon.[26]

Yams are the tubers of *Dioscorea* of many varieties, including bitter toxic species, such as *D. dumetorum* and *D. hirsuta*, which contain cyanogenic glycoside, such as diosgenin. They can be steeped and washed in water and eaten sliced, but if badly prepared they are toxic. Bitter yams are sometimes interplanted with edible varieties in order to deter theft by strangers, and deaths have occurred from the consumption of bitter yams during food shortages.

Treatment of acute cyanide poisoning includes gastric lavage with 5% sodium thiosulfate within 1 h if possible; 300 ml of 25% sodium thiosulfate should be left in the stomach. Dicobalt edetate (dicobalt EDTA) should be given intravenously as soon as possible in all cases of poisoning in a dose of 600 mg in 40 ml over 1 minute. If recovery does not occur within a minute or two another 300 mg of dicobalt edetate should be given. Oxygen (100%) should also be given and acidosis should be corrected with sodium bicarbonate. If dicobalt edetate is not available give 10 ml of 3% sodium nitrite over 3 minutes intravenously, followed by 25 ml of 50% sodium thiosulfate over 10 minutes intravenously.

Dermatitis

Many tropical plants cause contact dermatitis, with erythema, vesiculation or urticaria.

Contact with the leaves of *Toxicodendron* (formerly *Rhus*) species (poison ivy, poison oak or poison sumach) causes intense irritation and inflammation (Figure 33.2).[27,28] In Japan severe dermatitis can follow contact with lacquer made from *Toxicodendron vernicifluum*.[29] Treatment consists of thorough washing of the skin with soap and water and removal of the poison from the clothes by soaking in 1% hypochlorite solution.

Dermatitis can be caused by pyrethrum in *Chrysanthemum* species.[30] Exposure to the leaves and flowers causes itching, usually beginning at the corners of the eyes, and lachrymation, followed by an irritating vesicular rash, peeling of the skin and the formation of painful fissures. Sweating and exposure to sunlight exacerbate the lesions. Urticaria and photosensitivity have also been reported.

Many plants and flowers, such as the euphorbias (which contain phorbol esters), orchids, primulas, lilies and mangos, can cause allergic dermatitis in sensitive people. The juice of some of the Umbelliferae contains photo-sensitizing furanocoumarin derivatives that on contact with the skin cause erythema and vesication after exposure to light.

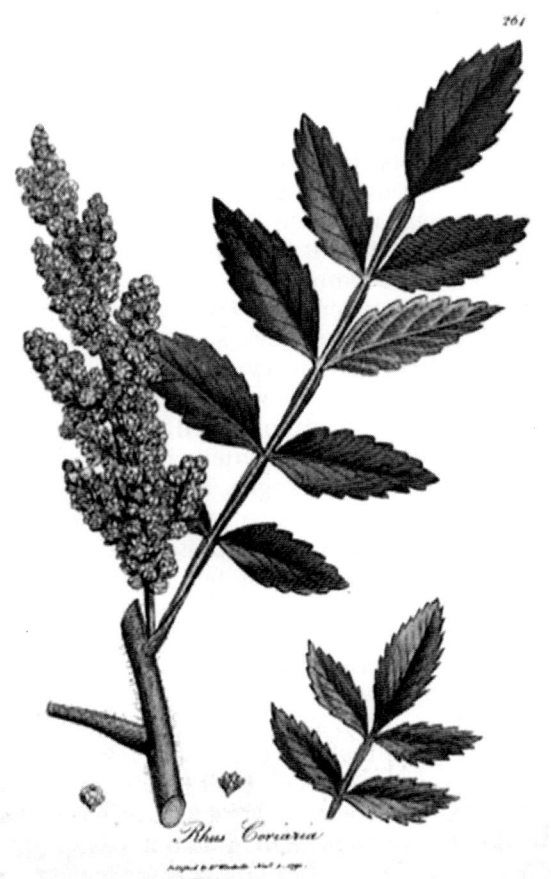

Figure 33.2: Poison oak (*Toxicodendron diversilobum (Rhus coriaria)*).

The manchineel, *Hippomane mancinella*, like many other members of the Euphorbiaceae, produces a highly irritant latex.[31] This small tree is common along the coastline of South and Central America, the West Indies and India. Both varieties, one with leaves like holly and the other like laurel, are poisonous. The attractive fruit resembles a crab-apple, and sensitive people who touch it develop erythema, bullae and vesiculation. The wood and even the sawdust are irritant and cause dermatitis, frequently of the genitalia and anus, with a vesiculopustular eruption, sometimes confined to the glans penis. In the eye the latex causes keratoconjunctivitis, with pain, photophobia and blepharospasm. If the fruit is eaten it causes vesiculation of the buccal mucosa with superinfection, bloody diarrhoea and sometimes death. Latex on the skin should be washed off at once; blisters should be protected against infection and, if extensive, treated like second-degree burns.

Seaweed dermatitis has been reported from Hawaii, probably as a result of contact with an alga, *Microcolus lyngbyaceus*, which produces a toxic rash in persons bathing in the sea off windward beaches.[32]

The dust from certain trees, such as iroko (African teak), pine, mahogany, satinwood and obeche, can cause skin irritation, facial oedema, blepharospasm, acute coryza and pharyngitis.[33] Asthma and rhinitis have also been reported.

Drugs acting on the parasympathetic nervous system
Anticholinergic compounds

Anticholinergic compounds, such as atropine, hyoscine (scopolamine) and semi-synthetic derivatives, are widely used therapeutically (for example, in Parkinson's disease and as adjuncts to anaesthesia). Poisoning causes tachycardia, a dry mouth and hot dry skin, dilated pupils (mydriasis), blurred vision and loss of accommodation, difficulty in micturition, confusion, an acute psychosis with hallucinations and convulsions; glaucoma can occur in elderly people, as can acute urinary retention in men with prostatic enlargement. Treatment of poisoning is symptomatic (Table 33.3); although physostigmine has been used,[34,35] it has a short duration of action, tolerance to its beneficial effects occurs and it has its own adverse effects—it should be reserved for life-threatening poisoning.[36]

The thorn apple or Jimson weed, *Datura stramonium* (Figure 33.3), grows in most parts of the world and is a frequent cause of poisoning in cereal crops. The seeds contain alkaloids of the tropane series, notably hyoscyamine. One outbreak of poisoning in Tanzania involved the consumption of porridge made from millet distributed by a local branch of the National Milling Corporation.[37] Jimson weed has also been used as a drug of abuse.[38]

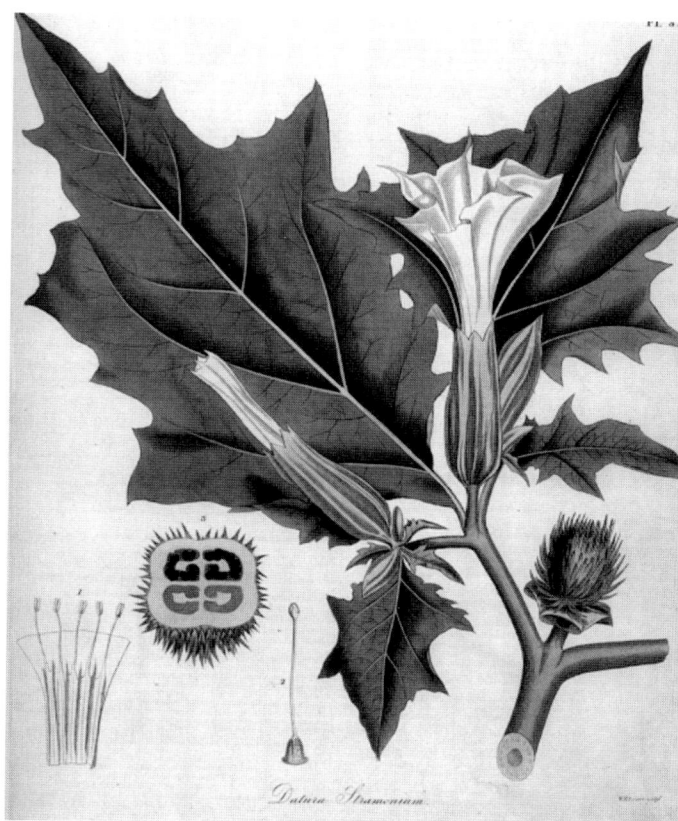

Figure 33.3: Thorn apple (*Datura stramonium*).

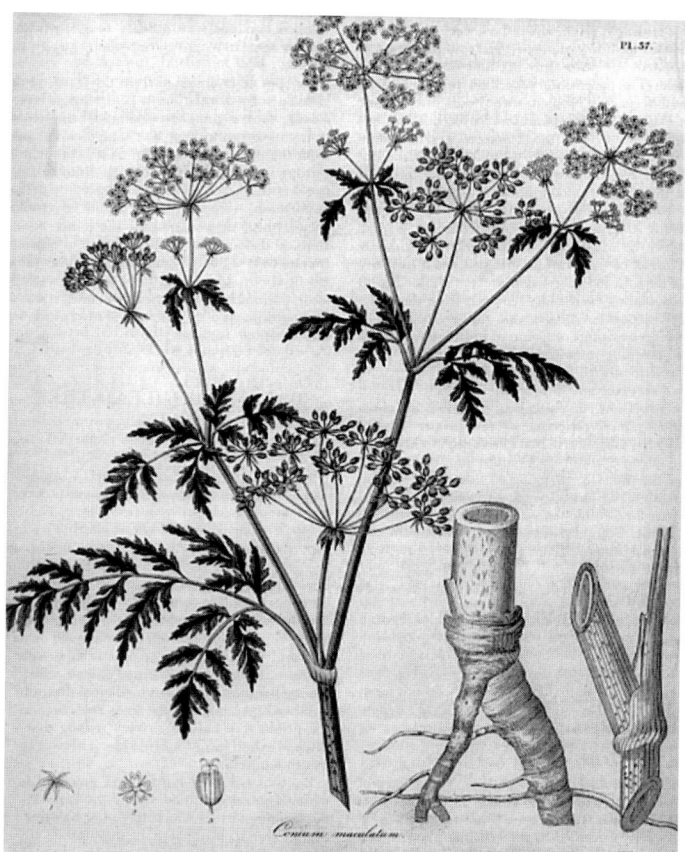

Figure 33.4: Poison hemlock (*Conium maculatum*).

Other plants that can cause anticholinergic poisoning include angel's trumpet (*Brugmansia* species, now called *Datura*),[39] found in Central and South America and prepared as a tea for its hallucinogenic effects, and jessamine (*Gelsemium sempervirens*),[40] which is native to North and Central America.

The seeds of various species of *Datura* have been used in cases of criminal poisoning in tropical countries. *D. fastuosa* was a favourite poison of practitioners of thagi in India, *D. sanguinea* is used in Colombia and Peru, *D. ferox* and *D. arborea* in Brazil, and the leaves of *Hyoscyamus fahezlez* by the Tuareg in the Sahara. The seeds of *D. stramonium* with *D. metel* have been used in East Africa for criminal purposes, as an inebriant to facilitate robbery, or to elicit confessions of witchcraft.[36]

Cholinergic compounds

Drugs can cause cholinergic effects either by stimulating acetylcholine receptors or by inhibiting acetylcholinesterase.

Drugs that stimulate acetylcholine receptors, of which nicotine and muscarine are the prototypes, are used therapeutically (for example, pilocarpine in glaucoma) and are found in a wide variety of plants. The effects of poisoning are constricted pupils (miosis); hypersalivation and sweating; nausea, vomiting, and diarrhoea; bradycardia; and headache, vertigo, confusion, delirium, hal-

lucinations, coma and convulsions. Bronchorrhoea, bronchospasm, and pulmonary oedema produce respiratory failure, the usual cause of death. Most cases of cholinergic poisoning with flowering plants have been reported with laburnum in temperate zones; other cases have been reported with hemlock (*Conium maculatum*) (Figure 33.4).[41]

Many fungi contain cholinergic compounds, and muscarinic poisoning can occur with, for example, jack o'lantern (*Omphalotus olearius*) and *Clitocybe* and *Inocybe* species. In severe cases of poisoning with *Amanita* species there may be cholinergic symptoms, but the main effects are due to the GABAergic compound muscimol.[42]

Anticholinesterases potentiate the actions of acetylcholine by inhibiting its breakdown. Solanine is one such compound, found in plants of the *Solanum* genus, including the unripe berries of the bittersweet nightshade (*S. dulcamara*) and greened tubers of potatoes (*S. tuberosum*). However, *S. dulcamara* poisoning can also present with anticholinergic effects.[43] Accidental or suicidal poisoning can occur with anticholinesterase organophosphorus insecticides;[44] treatment is with atropine[45] and cholinesterase reactivators, such as pralidoxime and obidoxime.[46]

Epidemic dropsy

Epidemic dropsy is caused by sanguinarine, an alkaloid

constituent of several plants, including the Mexican poppy, *Argemone mexicana*. The small, black, oily seeds of *Argemone* resemble those of mustard and can become mixed with them accidentally or by deliberate adulteration. Village boys in India can collect up to 8 kg of *Argemone* seeds a day in summer, and may sell them to unscrupulous dealers. As a contaminant of a widely used cooking oil derived from mustard seed, *Argemone* has led to outbreaks of so-called epidemic dropsy in many tropical countries. Sanguinarine is absorbed from the gut and through the skin if oil containing it is used for massage.[47] It causes capillary dilatation and increased permeability.

Epidemic dropsy is seen mostly in India,[48] but has also been reported in Mauritius, Fiji, South Africa and Nepal.[49] It presents with gastrointestinal symptoms a week or so before the onset of pitting oedema of the legs, fever and darkening of the skin, often with local erythema and tenderness. Perianal itching is common, and severe myocarditis and congestive cardiac failure can occur. Other features include anaemia, hepatomegaly, pneumonia, ascites, glaucoma, alopecia and sarcoid-like skin changes.

Ergot

Ergot (*Claviceps purpurea*) is a fungus whose sclerotia contain ergotoxine and related alkaloids that stimulate smooth muscle. It is harvested with the ears of rye and other grasses. Chronic consumption of small amounts causes uterine and vascular contraction, resulting in abortion, arterial occlusion and painful gangrene. In the Middle Ages this was called St Anthony's fire, because it was relieved by a pilgrimage to the shrine of St Anthony, in an area that was not affected by the fungus. Acute consumption of large amounts can cause headache, vertigo, hallucinations and convulsions; the Salem witches may have been victims of this. Ergot poisoning, although easy to prevent, still occurs from careless harvesting in times of food shortage; it can also occur with deliberate hallucinogenic or abortifacient use. Vasodilators, such as sodium nitroprusside, ease ischaemic pain and help to prevent gangrene.[50] Derivatives of ergot are used therapeutically (e.g., bromocriptine in Parkinson's disease) and as hallucinogens (e.g., LSD).

Gastroenteritis

Jequirity beans (*Abrus precatorius*) and castor oil beans (*Ricinus communis*) are bright and attractive and are sometimes made into necklaces (Figure 33.5). *Ricinus* is the source of the purgative castor oil and *Abrus* has been used to treat schistosomiasis. However, these beans contain poisons that, after a delay of 1–48 hours, can cause fatal gastroenteritis; their toxic principles, abrin and ricin, are among the most poisonous substances known;[51] one bean can kill a child. Acute poisoning is treated by gastric lavage, demulcents, and adjustment of fluid and electrolyte

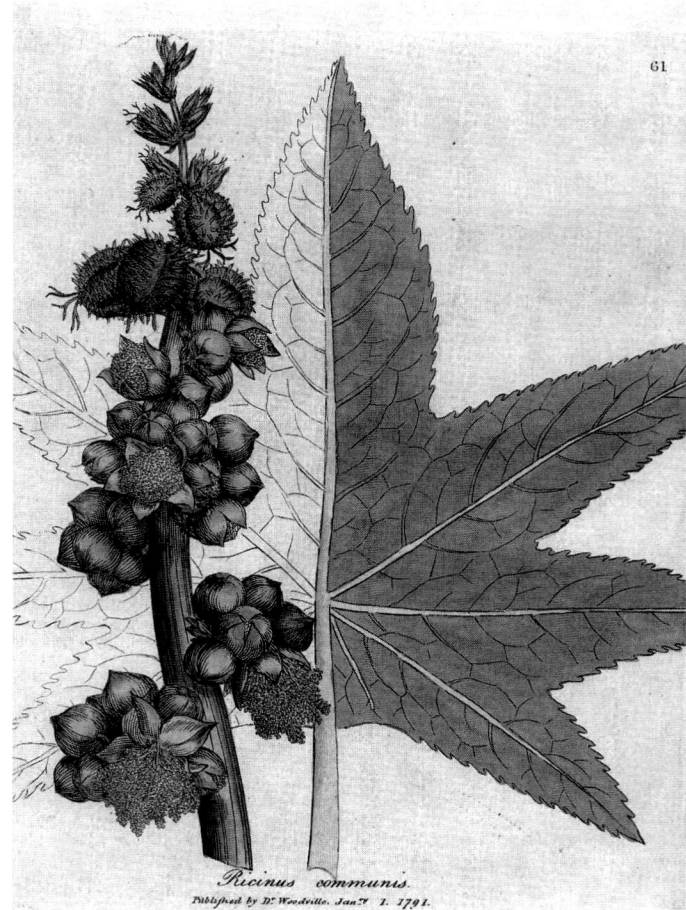

Figure 33.5: Castor oil plant (*Ricinus communis*).

balance. Abdominal pain may require analgesics. In serious cases ventilation or haemodialysis may be needed.

Many other plants can cause gastrointestinal disturbances, such as nausea, vomiting and diarrhoea. These include *Euphorbia* species, all plants that contain cardiac glycosides, and *Phytolacca americana*. Severe gastrointestinal toxicity can sometimes cause heart block, secondary to vagal stimulation.[52]

The leaves of *Dieffenbachia* species cause damage to the mucosa of the gastrointestinal tract if chewed or swallowed; this has been attributed to their oxalate content.[53] The sap can also cause corneal damage.

Lectins are phytohaemagglutinins that are resistant to digestion in the gut but are removed from food by proper cooking. They affect the integrity of the intestinal epithelium and the absorption of dietary antigens, and cause release of allergic mediators from mast cells in vitro. Many plants, such as *Jatropha macrorhiza* and *Euonymus europaeus*, contain lectins,[54] which, if not destroyed by cooking, can cause severe vomiting and bloody diarrhoea, in some cases followed by damage to the central nervous system, the cardiovascular system and the kidneys. Coral plants, *Jatropha curcas*, *J. glandulifera* and *J. multifida*, grow rapidly and are used as hedges in Africa and the West Indies. Their fruits, physic nuts, taste like sweet almonds but have been reported to cause colic, cramps, thirst and hypothermia. Another species, *J. gossypifolia*, is known in the West Indies as the bellyache bush.

Croton species, which are widespread in the tropics, cause violent purgation. They contain phorbol esters, which are carcinogenic.

The ackee, *Blighia sapida* (named after Captain Bligh of the *Bounty*), is a native of West Africa but is common in the West Indies and South America. The fruit has a large fleshy aril and is eaten when ripe; however, the unripe fruit is poisonous and has caused 'vomiting sickness' in Jamaica and other islands.[55] Unripe ackee fruits contain toxic hypoglycins: polypeptides that block gluconeogenesis in the liver and cause acute hypoglycaemia.[56] Anaphylaxis and cholestatic jaundice have also been reported. Typically, poisoning presents with abdominal discomfort and vomiting and, a few hours later, convulsions and coma. Extreme hypoglycaemia occurs, and unless glucose is given promptly death usually occurs within 12 hours of the initial vomiting. The liver shows fatty changes, with almost complete absence of glycogen.

Haemolysis in glucose-6-phosphate deficiency

Deficiency of the enzyme glucose-6-phosphate dehydrogenase (G6PD) in erythrocytes results in reduced production of NADPH. Consequently, oxidized glutathione (and to a lesser and insignificant extent methaemoglobin) accumulates. If the erythrocytes are then exposed to oxidizing agents haemolysis occurs, probably because of unopposed oxidation of sulfhydryl groups in the cell membrane, which are normally kept in reduced form by the continuous availability of reduced glutathione. The prevalence of this defect varies with race. It is rare among Caucasians and occurs most frequently among Sephardic Jews of Asiatic origin, of whom 50% or more are affected. It also occurs in about 10–20% of blacks. Inheritance of the defect is sex-linked but complex, the genetic basis for the abnormal enzyme being heterogeneous; most of the variations produce an unstable enzyme. In the variety that affects blacks (but is not confined to them) G6PD production is probably normal, but its degradation is accelerated, so that only erythrocytes older than about 55 days are affected; acute haemolysis occurs on first administration of the drug and lasts for only a few days, after which continued administration causes chronic mild haemolysis. In the Mediterranean variety the enzyme is abnormal, and both young and old erythrocytes are affected; in this form severe haemolysis occurs on first administration and is maintained with continued administration. The reaction is sometimes called favism, because it can result from eating broad beans (*Vicia faba*), which contain oxidant substances such as divicine and isouramil.[57] The condition is rare in Thailand, probably because the G6PD mutants that occur there are different.[58]

Hepatotoxicity
Hepatic carcinoma

Aspergillus flavus and *A. parasiticus* produce aflatoxins that are toxic to the liver and are carcinogenic;[59] for example, the consumption of contaminated groundnuts has been linked with hepatic carcinoma in Africa and Asia.

Veno-occlusive disease

Veno-occlusive disease, which occurs in the West Indies, East and West Africa, and India, is an acute, subacute or chronic condition that affects the central and sublobular hepatic veins. In the West Indies[60] it is related to the consumption of bush tea made from plants that contain toxic pyrrolizidine alkaloids, such as *Crotalaria* and *Senecio*.[61] Hepatotoxic compounds in *Crotalaria*, *Senecio*, *Heliotropium* and other composite plants can also enter the diet through contamination of cereals with weed seeds. For example, 28 of 67 patients died with veno-occlusive disease in central India after consuming a local cereal, gondli, contaminated with the seeds of *Crotalaria*.[62] *Heliotropium popovii* has been implicated in outbreaks in villages in north-western Afghanistan, with high mortality.[63]

The primary pathological change of hepatic veno-occlusive disease is subendothelial oedema, followed by intimal overgrowth of connective tissue, with narrowing and occlusion of the central and sublobular hepatic veins. Atrophy or necrosis of liver cells, with consequent fibrosis, leads to gross changes similar to those seen in cardiac cirrhosis; portal hypertension results.[64]

Nephrotoxicity

Djenkol beans (*Pithecolobium*) cause poisoning in Malaysia, Java and Thailand. Blood and casts appear in the urine, and the renal tract may be blocked, causing acute renal insufficiency;[65] crystals of djenkolic acid can form urinary calculi.[66] Treatment is by alkalinizing the urine (pH 8) by giving sodium bicarbonate by intravenous infusion (250 ml of a 3.5% solution four times in a single day for a 70 kg adult).

Aristolochia fangchi, and perhaps other constituents of Chinese herbal slimming remedies, can cause a nephropathy[67] through progressive interstitial fibrosis. It may also cause urothelial carcinoma.[68] Nephrotoxicity has been incorrectly attributed to *Stephania tetrandra* (Chinese: *fang-ji*) through confusion with *Aristolochia* (Chinese: *quang-fang-ji*).

Oxalate-rich foods (spinach, rhubarb, beets, nuts, chocolate, tea, wheat bran and strawberries) increase urinary oxalate excretion, predisposing to renal calculi.[69] Rarely acute oxalate toxicity can occur, for example due to ingestion of raw rhubarb stalks or leaves.[70]

Neurotoxicity

In some countries the root stocks of cycads (*Cycas* and *Zamia*) are used as foodstuffs. The seeds of *Cycas circinalis*, eaten by the Chamorro people of Guam and neighbouring islands,[71] contain a neurotoxic amino acid, β-*N*-methylamino-L-alanine, which is thought to cause amyotrophic lateral sclerosis, Parkinsonism and dementia.[72]

A related condition, lathyrism, is caused by *Lathyrus sativus*, the grass pea, which contains the neurotoxin β-*N*-oxalylamino-L-alanine.[71,73] It causes a symmetrical motor spastic paraparesis, with a pyramidal pattern and greatly increased tone in the leg muscles, causing sufferers to walk on the balls of their feet with a lurching gait. The arms can also be affected. Sensory signs are absent. Grass pea is a profitable cash crop that is used as a cheap adulterant in flour from other pulses; lathyrism is likely to occur in places remote from grass pea cultivation and follows food shortages in India and Africa. Attempts are being made to select strains with a low toxin content.[74]

The poison nut (*Strychnos nux-vomica*) is the source of poisonous alkaloids (strychnine, vomicine, icajine, brucine) (Figure 33.6). Strychnine is an antagonist of the actions of the inhibitory neurotransmitter glycine in the spinal cord and causes painful convulsions.[75]

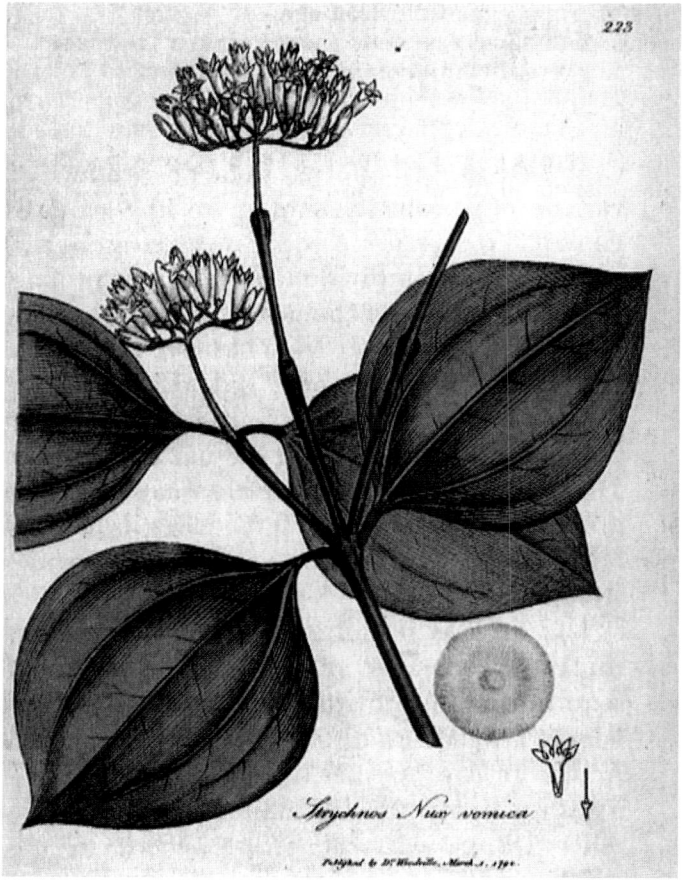

Figure 33.6: Nux vomica (*Strychnos nux-vomica*).

The fruit of *Diospyros mollis* (maklua) contains a derivative of hydroxynaphthalene and is used in Thailand for treating intestinal worms. It is oculotoxic[76] and has been reported to cause optic neuritis in children.

Psychotropic drugs
Alcohol

Rum (65–72% alcohol) is distilled from fermented molasses in the West Indies and South America; arrack or sake (50–60%) is manufactured in India, China, Java and Japan from fermented rice. Toddy, made from the sweet sap of various palms, such as coconut, is drunk in India, Sri Lanka and West Africa. A potent drink, pulque, is made in South America from the juice of agaves.

Alcohol causes three main medical and psychiatric problems:

- Acute alcohol intoxication.
- Alcohol withdrawal reactions (delirium tremens).
- Chronic alcoholism.

In the brain alcohol acts as a dose-dependent depressant, producing the well-known features of intoxication. At plasma concentrations of around 40 mg/dl (400 mg/l or 8.7 mmol/l) learned skills are impaired, including the ability to maintain self-restraint. Other early effects include loss of attentiveness, loss of concentration and impaired memory, and there may be lethargy. At progressively higher concentrations there are further changes in mood, behaviour, and a variety of sensory and motor functions. The effects on mood depend on the individual's personality, mental state and social environment. Commonly there is euphoria, but any kind of mood change can occur. Libido is often enhanced, but sexual performance impaired. Alcohol generally increases confidence, often resulting in aggressive or silly behaviour; loss of self-restraint leads to increased loquacity with immoderate speech content, such as swearing or the use of lewd language. Unsteadiness of gait, slurred speech and difficulty in carrying out even simple tasks, with impaired coordination, become obvious at plasma concentrations of about 80 mg/dl (the concentration above which driving is illegal in the UK and many other countries). Driving skills are therefore impaired, and are affected even at concentrations below 80 mg/dl. Recovery from dazzle is delayed, which may impair night-time driving. Visual acuity, peripheral vision, colour vision and visual tracking are impaired. Hearing and taste may also be impaired. The pain threshold is increased. At high concentrations there may be vertigo and nystagmus. Alcohol causes acute drowsiness and deep sleep, and in high concentrations causes coma and respiratory depression. In some individuals sleep may later be impaired. On waking there is the characteristic 'hangover', which usually consists of irritability, headache, thirst, abdominal cramps and bowel disturbance. The cause of hangover is not known.

Delirium tremens is an acute withdrawal reaction that can be fatal. The symptoms come on within a few hours after the last drink and mount over the next 2–3 days. At first there is anxiety, agitation, tremulousness and tachycardia. These are later accompanied by confusion, severe agitation and hallucinations (often visual). The patient is tremulous, sweating and tachypnoeic, and may be pyrexial, dehydrated, hypoglycaemic and vitamin deficient. The blood pressure may be high, low or normal. Nausea and vomiting are common. Seizures can occur and can be prolonged and potentially life-threatening.

The medical management of alcohol withdrawal (including delirium tremens) involves the maintenance of fluid and electrolyte balance, the administration of vitamins (particularly thiamine to prevent Wernicke's encephalopathy), a high-carbohydrate and high-calorie diet, and the use of sedating drugs to suppress symptoms and prevent seizures. Treatment is with a benzodiazepine (such as chlordiazepoxide) or clomethiazole.

For many years disulfiram (Antabuse®) and calcium carbamide have been prescribed in an attempt to prevent relapse in abstinent alcoholics. They act by inhibiting the enzyme aldehyde dehydrogenase, which results in a rapid build-up of blood acetaldehyde if the subject drinks. This produces severe vomiting and diarrhoea, along with potentially dangerous alterations in blood pressure. However, compliance is usually poor and the evidence of effectiveness probably does not justify the unpleasant adverse effects of these drugs.

Two newer drugs show some promise. Naltrexone is a μ-opioid receptor antagonist, whose use was suggested by demonstrated links between alcohol and opioid receptors. Small placebo-controlled trials have suggested that it significantly reduces the likelihood and severity of relapse in comparison with placebo. Acamprosate is derived from the amino acid taurine and has structural similarities to GABA. In the brain it reduces the effects of excitatory amino acids, such as glutamate, and alters GABA neurotransmission. Clinical trials have suggested that it is significantly better than placebo in preventing or delaying relapse, with a very low incidence of adverse effects. It can cause diarrhoea, nausea, vomiting or abdominal pain; occasionally it causes pruritus or a maculopapular rash.

Betel

Chewing betel, the leaves of *Piper betle*, together with lime and areca (betel) nuts (*Areca catechu*), is a common practice in India, Sri Lanka and other Eastern countries. It may act by inhibiting GABA uptake. The mouth, lips and cheeks are stained bright red and the face is flushed; there is euphoria, heightened alertness, sweating, salivation, a hot sensation in the body and an increased capacity to work; there are increases in heart rate, blood pressure, sweating and body temperature.[77]

Cannabis

Cannabis sativa, the hemp plant, yields marijuana and hashish. A cannabis smoker inhales at least 60 mind-altering chemicals, but the main psychoactive ingredient is Δ-9-tetrahydrocannabinol (Δ-9-THC), an antiemetic, antispasticity agent, appetite stimulant, analgesic, anxiolytic, hypnotic and antipyretic, which also lowers intraocular pressure. However, its beneficial effects in terminal disease are disappointing.

Marijuana ('grass', 'weed', 'bush', 'herb') is the dried mixture of crushed leaves and stalks of the plant. The flowering tops of the plant secrete a resin that can be compressed to form hashish ('hash', 'blow', 'puff', 'draw', 'ganja', 'dope', 'pot'), or dissolved into an oil or tincture. Marijuana is usually rolled in home-made cigarettes ('spliffs', 'joints' or, if enormous, 'blunts'), with or without tobacco. Hashish is heated and crumbled on to tobacco in spliffs or smoked in a wide variety of pipes. In many parts of the world cannabis is an ingredient of a range of culinary preparations.

Cannabis has physical and mental effects that begin within minutes. The physical effects include an increase in heart rate, peripheral vasodilatation, conjunctival suffusion, bronchodilatation, dryness of the mouth and, in large doses, tremor, ataxia, nystagmus, nausea and vomiting. The mental effects vary from person to person, depending on such variables as personality, mood, surroundings, expectations and previous cannabis experience. Generally there is a feeling of well-being, accompanied by feelings of enhanced sensory perception. There may be drowsiness or hyperactivity. Ideas flow rapidly and may be disconnected. Time seems to pass slowly. Motor performance may be altered, as it may be by any sedative drug, and driving skills may be impaired.

There may be mild tolerance and a mild withdrawal syndrome, rather like a mild benzodiazepine withdrawal syndrome. Physical dependence does not seem to be a big problem, but psychological dependence does occur.

Heavy use of marijuana is associated with social apathy, but this often precedes drug use and may not be an adverse effect. Adverse psychological effects include anxiety, acute panic reactions and paranoid ideas. Large doses can cause an acute toxic psychosis with confusion and hallucinations. There is controversy as to whether marijuana can produce a prolonged psychosis, but it can certainly aggravate pre-existing mental disease. Cannabis smoke contains more insoluble particulates and carcinogens than tobacco smoke, so lung and airways damage can be anticipated in heavy regular consumers. Birth defects occasionally follow use in pregnancy.

Coca

Erythroxylon coca is widely grown in South America and India. The leaves are dried in the sun and are chewed with lime or, in India, with betel. Cocaine powder can be sniffed, prepared as a solution for intravenous injection, or separated from its hydrochloride and smoked as the free base or as 'crack' (so called because of the popping and clicking of exploding impurities when it is burnt). Crack vaporizes at a much lower temperature than cocaine hydrochloride, so that the active ingredient escapes pyrolysis and reaches the lungs intact. Because the transfer from lung to brain is so fast, the impact of smoked cocaine gives a 'rush' comparable to that experienced after intravenous injection. However, the euphoriant effect also wears off quickly, producing a most unpleasant downswing of mood in many users, which they may attempt to fend off with repeatedly larger and larger doses.

The clinical effects of cocaine ('coke', 'snow', 'charlie' or 'crack') include euphoria, increased drive, increased confidence, increased sociability, loquacity and increased physical and mental capacities. After chewing there is loss of sensation in the tongue and lips.

The tendency to repeat administration to fend off rebound effects, and the rapid tolerance that occurs to the euphoriant effects of cocaine, combine to cause a typical pattern of escalating doses terminating in 'crash', characterized by exhausted sleep followed by depressed mood, which fuels the initiation of the next binge. Termination of a binge comes about either through physical or mental exhaustion, or lack of money or further drug supplies. Repeated sniffing can cause perforation of the nasal septum. The use of prolonged and high dosages can lead to a cocaine-induced psychosis, not dissimilar from acute paranoid schizophrenia. There are no major physiological withdrawal phenomena from cocaine, but troublesome dysphoria and craving can persist for months or even years. When it is taken during pregnancy, cocaine can cause constriction of the uterine and placental blood vessels and damage the fetus by depriving it of oxygen and other nutrients.

Kava

The powdered root of *Piper methysticum*, prepared as a beverage, is drunk on festive occasions throughout Polynesia.[78] Formerly the root was prepared by mastication by selected girls, a practice that caused the spread of tuberculosis. The actions of some of its constituents include altered activity at the $GABA_A$ receptor and inhibition of voltage-dependent sodium channels. Overindulgence in kava causes a state of hyperexcitement, with loss of power in the legs. Chronic intoxication leads to debility, with ataxia, visual and auditory defects, and a reversible ichthyosiform eruption (kava dermopathy).

Khat

Khat (cafta, miraa, muiragi) is derived from a small tree, *Catha edulis*, indigenous to North Africa.[79] The leaves and twigs are chewed, infused or smoked and are said to produce a happy, mellow sense of friendliness. The leaves contain cathinone, a phenylalkylamine derivative with effects similar to those of amphetamine; psychosis has been reported with heavy use. Chronic consumption may be genotoxic.

Nicotine

The leaves and flowers of *Nicotiana* species have been universally smoked, snuffed or chewed for their stimulant effects. Preparations of the leaves applied to the chest to relieve respiratory complaints have sometimes given rise to toxic effects by percutaneous absorption of nicotine. However, nicotine is much more widespread in plants, and occurs in such diverse species as *Acacia* species, *Aesculus hippocastanum*, *Asclepias* species, *Duboisia* species, *Echeviria* species, *Erythroxylon coca*, *Juglans regia*, *Mucuna pruriens*, *Prunus* species, *Sempervivum arachnoideum* and *Urtica dioica*. During the nineteenth and early part of the twentieth centuries Australian aborigines used pituri, a nicotine-containing preparation from the cured leaves of *Duboisia hopwoodii*.[80]

An unusual nostrum made by the Yoruba people of Nigeria is 'cow's urine mixture', which consists of green tobacco leaves, rock salt, citron (*Citrus medica*), the leaves of the bush basil, *Ocimum viride*, and cow's urine.[81] The remedy is swallowed or rubbed into the skin for the prevention and treatment of epileptic or eclamptic fits; the toxic effects are those of nicotine: central nervous excitation, with vomiting, diarrhoea, dehydration and hypoglycaemia, followed by depression and coma, sometimes with permanent neurological damage or death. Convulsions must be controlled and glucose given intravenously. The poison is removed by gastric lavage or cleansing of the skin; blood glucose, electrolytes and fluid balance should be monitored.

Opium alkaloids and their derivatives

Opioid dependence is a worldwide public health menace associated with a great deal of criminal activity. Heroin ('smack,' 'junk,' 'gear,' 'brown') is the opiate chosen by 75%, and heroin-related referrals are increasing by at least 15% per year. On initial use there may be nausea, vomiting and anxiety, but these symptoms disappear with subsequent use, and euphoria becomes predominant. As tolerance develops and the cost of the habit increases, the addict may switch to the intravenous route to maximize value for money. In an attempt to retain the euphoria (the 'rush') that results from rapidly increased concentrations of the drug in the brain, larger and larger doses will be used. Tolerance to constipation and pupillary constriction does not occur to any great extent. Eventually the addict becomes most concerned with combating withdrawal symptoms and must have a regular supply of the drug to avoid these.

Withdrawal symptoms begin at about 8 h after the last dose and reach a peak at about 36–72 h. Symptoms occur in the following order:

- Psychological symptoms: anxiety, depression, restlessness, irritability, drug craving.
- Lachrymation, rhinorrhoea, mydriasis, yawning, sweating, tachycardia and hypertension.

- Restless sleep, after which the above symptoms are accompanied by sneezing, anorexia, nausea, vomiting, abdominal cramps, diarrhoea, bone pain, muscle pain, tremor, weakness, chills and goose-flesh ('cold turkey'), twitching and jerking of the legs ('kicking the habit') and insomnia. Hypotension, cardiovascular collapse and convulsions occur rarely.

These symptoms gradually fade over about 5–10 days, during which time general malaise and abdominal cramps persist.

With methadone the onset of withdrawal symptoms is delayed for 24–48 h and peaks at 3–4 days; because of this slower effect, methadone is often used to help an addict withdraw, by substituting it for morphine or heroin.

Treatment of poisoning[82]

This is not the place for a thorough description of the treatment of poisoning, but a few simple principles are summarized in Table 33.3.

Drug interactions with plants

Drug interactions can occur between plant medicaments and allopathic medicines.[83–85] Some of these are summarized in Table 33.4. Many of these interactions are poorly

Table 33.3 A summary of the management of acute self-poisoning.[82]

Target	Therapeutic action
1. Respiratory function	Check gag reflex
	Remove dentures
	Clear out oropharyngeal obstructions, debris, secretions
	Lay on the left side with head down
	Insert oral airway or, if cough reflex lost, an endotracheal tube
	Give oxygen if hypoxic
	Assist respiration if required
2. Circulatory function	Check heart rate and blood pressure
	If systolic blood pressure below 80 mmHg (young patients) or 90 mmHg (old patients):
	Raise end of bed
	If ineffective, give volume expanders
	If fluid overload and oliguria:
	Give dopamine and/or dobutamine
3. Renal function	Monitor urine output
4. Consciousness	Assess level of consciousness (Glasgow coma scale):
	Grade 0: Fully conscious
	Grade 1: Drowsy, but responds to commands, or asleep but easily roused
	Grade 2: Unconscious, but responds to standard minimally painful stimuli
	Grade 3: Unconscious, but responds to standard maximally painful stimuli
	Grade 4: Unconscious, and does not respond to any stimuli
5. Temperature	Take temperature rectally; if below 36°C reheat slowly
	Warm all inspired air and i.v. fluids
6. Convulsions	Treat with diazepam, clomethiazole, phenytoin, or anaesthesia with assisted ventilation
7. Cardiac arrhythmias	Treat as required
8. Gastric lavage	Generally of no value after 1 h following poisoning
	Add non-specific or specific antidotes to lavage fluid or leave in stomach after lavage
9. Activated charcoal	A single dose after gastric lavage
	Repeated doses for some poisons
10. Fluid and electrolyte balance	Dehydration: oral fluids usually enough
	Unconscious patients: use i.v. fluids and insert a CVP line
	Treat hypokalaemia
11. Emergency measures	Specific to the poison
12. Chest radiography	In drowsy or comatose patients who vomit
	After endotracheal intubation
13. Collection of specimens	Gastric aspirate (drugs)
	Urine (drugs, renal function)
	Blood (drugs, arterial gases, electrolytes)

Table 33.4 Some reported drug interactions with plants and herbal products.

Precipitant plant(s)	Object drug(s)	Outcome
Areca nut (*Areca catechu*)	Neuroleptic drugs	Exacerbation of extrapyramidal effects
Berberine (*Berberis aristata*)	Tetracycline	Prolonged diarrhoea in cholera
Bran, ispaghula husk (*Plantago ovale*)	Digoxin, iron, lithium, lovastatin, tricyclic antidepressants	Reduced absorption
Gingko biloba	Thiazide diuretics	Hypertension
Ginseng (*Panax ginseng*)	Antidepressants	Risk of mania
	Cocaine	Tolerance inhibited
	Digoxin	Increased plasma digoxin concentration
	Methamphetamine	Tolerance inhibited
	Opioids	Reduced pharmacological effects of opioids (analgesia, tolerance, dependence)
	Phenelzine	Headache, tremulousness, hyperactivity
	Warfarin	Reduced anticoagulation
Grapefruit juice	Amiodarone	Risk of amiodarone toxity (e.g., cardiac arrhythmias)
	Antihistamines (astemizole, terfenadine)	Prolongation of QT_c interval; risk of ventricular tachycardia
	Cyclosporin	Risk of cyclosporin toxicity (immunosuppression)
	Benzodiazepines (alprazolam, diazepam, midazolam, triazolam)	Increased drowsiness; altered psychometric tests
	Calcium channel blockers (felodipine, nifedipine, nisoldipine)	Reduced blood pressure, increased heart rate, headaches, flushing, light-headedness
	Lovastatin	Risk of lovastatin toxicity (including rhabdomyolysis and renal insufficiency)
	Quinidine	Prolongation of QT_c interval; risk of ventricular tachycardia
	Saquinavir	Risk of saquinavir toxicity
	Sertraline	Risk of sertraline toxicity (serotonin syndrome)
Guar gum (*Cyanopsis tetragonolobus*)	Digoxin, glibenclamide, metformin, phenoxylmethylpenicillin	Reduced absorption
Liquorice (*Glycyrrhiza glabra*)	Corticosteroids	Increased risk of hypokalaemia
	Spironolactone	Reduced potassium-sparing effect
Saint John's wort (*Hypericum perforatum*)	Amitriptyline, cyclosporin, oral contraceptives, phenprocoumon theophylline, warfarin	Induction of metabolism by CYP3A4, causing reduced effects (e.g., increased risk of transplant rejection with ciclosporin, reduced anticoagulation with warfarin)
	Digoxin, indinavir	Induction of P glycoprotein, increasing clearance and reducing effects
	Serotonin reuptake inhibitors	Serotonin syndrome
Shankhapushpi (an Ayurvedic mixture of herbs)	Phenytoin	Decreased concentrations of phenytoin, leading to seizures
Siberian ginseng (*Eleutherococcus senticosus*)	Digoxin	Increased plasma digoxin concentration
Tamarind (*Tamarindus indica*)	Aspirin	Increased systemic availability of aspirin
Xaio chai hu tang (sho-salko-to)	Prednisolone	Reduced effect of prednisolone
Yohimbine (*Pausinystalia yohimbe*)	Tricyclic antidepressants	Increased risk of hypertension

attested, being anecdotal. However, interactions with grapefruit and St John's wort are well described and are dealt with below.

Pharmacodynamic interactions

If a herbal medicine shares a pharmacological action with an allopathic remedy, it may potentiate its therapeutic or adverse effects; the following are examples:

- Digitalis and heart remedies containing cardioactive glycosides (*Strophanthus, Convallaria, Cytisus, Scilla*).
- Antihypertensive drugs and hypotensive herbs (*Rauwolfia, Crataegus, Viscum*).
- Oral hypoglycaemic drugs and karela, the fruit of *Momordica charantia*; karela, which has a hypoglycaemic action,[86] is used in curries and is a traditional Indian remedy for diabetes.
- Antiasthma drugs and betel nut, which is thought to have a bronchoconstricting effect.
- ACE inhibitors and *Capsicum* species; ACE inhibitors increase the amount of bradykinin in the lung and enhance the cough response to capsaicin, which acts by depleting substance P from nerve endings; this is an example of an interaction enhancing an adverse rather than a therapeutic effect of a drug.

Anticoagulants

Table 33.4 is organized according to the plant product, but too many plants interact with oral anticoagulants (principally warfarin) to be included separately. The many plants and herbal products that have been reported to increase or reduce the actions of warfarin[87] include angelica root, anise, arnica flower, asafetida, bogbean, borage seed oil, bromelain, capsicum, celery, chamomile, clove, danshen (*Salvia miltiorrhiza*), devil's claw (*Harpagophytum procumbens*), dong quai (*Angelica sinensis*), fenugreek, feverfew, garlic, ginger, ginkgo, ginseng, green tea, horse chestnut, liquorice root, lovage root, meadowsweet, melilot, onion, papaya, parsley, passion-flower, poplar, quassia, red clover, rue, sweet clover (in which coumarin anticoagulants were originally discovered), sweet woodruff, tonka beans, turmeric, vitamin E and willow bark. The mechanisms vary: for example, garlic reduces platelet aggregation; some plants (e.g., dong quai) contain anticoagulant coumarins; and some (e.g., tonka beans) contain vitamin K, a natural antagonist of the actions of coumarin anticoagulants.

Citrus fruits

Various isoforms of the enzyme cytochrome P450 are responsible for the oxidative metabolism of many drugs.[88] One of these isoforms, CYP3A4, is responsible for the metabolism of several drugs in the gut wall while they are being absorbed after oral administration. Inhibition of the enzyme by something in grapefruits (*Citrus paradisi*) and Seville oranges (*Citrus bigaradia*) causes more of the drug to escape presystemic metabolism and enter the circulation unchanged, potentially leading to drug toxicity. The compounds in grapefruit juice and Seville oranges responsible for these interactions are not known. In some countries a drug label has been introduced, alerting patients to potential drug interactions with grapefruit.[89] In the UK in 1997 the antihistamine terfenadine was withdrawn from over-the-counter sales because of cardiac arrhythmias,[90] and a year later another antihistamine, astemizole, was withdrawn for similar reasons.[91] Drugs whose effects can be increased by grapefruit juice causing toxicity[92] are listed in Table 33.4.

Grapefruit juice probably also inhibits the P glycoprotein that is responsible for the intestinal secretion of many drugs,[93] and therefore other drug interactions are to be expected.

Ginseng

Reported drug interactions with ginseng (*Panax ginseng*) are listed in Table 33.4. The root has been used in China, Korea and Japan for centuries in the belief that it counters fatigue and stress and confers health, virility and longevity; it is supposed to enhance immunity and to combat the effects of oxidative free radicals that cause chronic diseases and ageing.[94] The pharmacological basis for its reputation is slender, but ginseng is now in fashion worldwide. It is often adulterated with *Eleutherococcus senticosus* (Siberian ginseng, Table 33.4), *Mandragora, Rauwolfia* and other roots of similar appearance. Ginseng contains a complex mixture of steroids and saponins; it can cause nervous excitation, tremor, hypertension and oestrogen-like effects. It may also increase the risk of gastric cancer.[95]

St John's wort[96]

As an antidepressant, St John's wort may enhance the effects of other antidepressants; since it is an inhibitor of 5-HT reuptake, combination with serotonin reuptake inhibitors can cause the serotonin syndrome. Hyperforin, an ingredient of St John's wort (*Hypericum perforatum*), is an enzyme inducer and increases the metabolism of certain drugs, reducing their effects. St John's wort also induces intestinal P glycoprotein, leading to increased clearance of some drugs by intestinal secretion. Examples of these pharmacokinetic interactions are listed in Table 33.4.

REFERENCES

1   Bernard C. Analyse physiologique des propriétés des systèmes musculaires et nervuex au moyen du curare. *CR Acad Sci (Paris)* 1856; 43:825–829.

2   Griffith HR & Johnson GE. The use of curare in general anesthesia. *Anesthesiology* 1942; 3:418–420.

3   Cox PA. The ethnobotanical approach to drug discovery: strengths and limitations. *Ciba Found Symp* 1994; 185:25–36.

4   Rudgley R. *The Alchemy of Culture: Intoxicants in Society.* London: British Museum Press, 1993.

5   Toklas AB. *The Alice B. Toklas Cook Book*, rev. edn. London: Brilliance Books, 1987.

6   Crompton R & Gall D. Georgi Markov: death in a pellet. *Med Leg J* 1980; 48:51–62.

7   Tai YT, But PP, Young K & Lau CP. Cardiotoxicity after accidental herb-induced aconite poisoning. *Lancet* 1992; 340:1254–1256.

8   De Groot AC. Dermatological drugs, topical agents and cosmetics. In Dukes MNG, Aronson JK (eds) *Meyler's Side Effects of Drugs*, 14th edn. Amsterdam: Elsevier, 2000: 447–480.

9   Garvey GJ, Hahn G, Lee RV & Harbison RD. Heavy metal hazards of Asian traditional remedies. *Int J Environ Health Res* 2001; 11:63–71.

10 Penn RG. Adverse reactions to herbal and other unorthodox medicines. In D'Arcy PF & Griffin JP (eds) *Iatrogenic Diseases*, 3rd edn. Oxford: Oxford University Press, 1985: 898–918.

11 Krenzelok EP & Jacobsen TD. Plant exposures: a national profile of the most common plant genera. *Vet Hum Toxicol* 1997; 39:248–249.

12 Von Malottki K & Wiechmann HW. Akute lebensbedrohliche Bradykardie: Nahrungsmittelintoxikation durch turkischen Waldhonig. *Dtsch Med Wochenschr* 1996; 121:936–938.

13 Gibbs RD. Chemotaxonomy of flowering plants. Montreal: McGill–Queen's University Press, 1974.

14 Aronson JK & Hardman M. ABC of monitoring drug therapy: digoxin. *Br Med J* 1992; 305:1149–1152.

15 Bose TK, Basu RK, Biswas B, De JN, Majumdar BC & Datta S. Cardiovascular effects of yellow oleander ingestion. *J Indian Med Assoc* 1999; 97:407–410.

16 Narendranathan M, Das KV & Vijayaraghavan G. Prognostic factors in *Cerbera odollum* poisoning. *Indian Heart J* 1975; 27:283–286.

17 Aleem HM. *Gloriosa superba* poisoning. *J Assoc Phys India* 1992; 40:541–542.

18 Fernando R & Fernando DN. Poisoning with plants and mushrooms in Sri Lanka: a retrospective hospital based study. *Vet Hum Toxicol* 1990; 32:579–581.

19 Cassels BK. Analysis of a Maasai arrow poison. *J Ethnopharmacol* 1985; 14:273–281.

20 Bisset NG. Arrow poisons in China. Part I. *J Ethnopharmacol* 1979; 1:325–384.

21 Kopp B, Bauer WP & Bernkop Schnurch A. Analysis of some Malaysian dart poisons. *J Ethnopharmacol* 1992; 36:57–62.

22 Aronson JK. Glycosides of plants and men. *Med J Aust* 1986; 144:505–506.

23 Eddleston M, Rajapakse S, Rajakanthan, Jayalath S, Sjostrom L, Santharaj W, Thenabadu PN, Sheriff MH & Warrell DA. Anti-digoxin Fab fragments in cardiotoxicity induced by ingestion of yellow oleander: a randomised controlled trial. *Lancet* 2000; 355:967–972.

24 Vetter J. Plant cyanogenic glycosides. *Toxicon* 2000; 38:11–36.

25 Njoh J. Tropical ataxic neuropathy in Liberians. *Trop Geogr Med* 1990; 42:92–94.

26 Anonymous. Unproven methods of cancer management: laetrile. *CA Cancer J Clin* 1991; 41:187–192.

27 Fisher AA. Poison ivy/oak dermatitis. Part I: Prevention—soap and water, topical barriers, hyposensitization. *Cutis* 1996; 57:384–386.

28 Fisher AA. Poison ivy/oak/sumac. Part II: Specific features. *Cutis* 1996; 58:22–24.

29 Park SD, Lee SW, Chun JH & Cha SH. Clinical features of 31 patients with systemic contact dermatitis due to the ingestion of *Rhus* (lacquer). *Br J Dermatol* 2000; 142:937–942.

30 Tanaka T, Moriwaki SI & Horio T. Occupational dermatitis with simultaneous immediate and delayed allergy to chrysanthemum. *Contact Dermatitis* 1987; 16:152–154.

31 Guillet G, Helenon R & Guillet MH. La dermite du mancenillier. *Ann Dermatol Venereol* 1985; 112:51–56.

32 Sims JK, Brock JA, Fujioka R, Killion L, Nakagawa L & Greco S. *Vibrio* in stinging seaweed: potential infection. *Hawaii Med J* 1993; 52:274–275.

33 Hinnen U, Willa-Craps C & Elsner P. Allergic contact dermatitis from iroko and pine wood dust. *Contact Dermatitis* 1995; 33:428.

34 Amlo H, Haugeng KL, Wickstrom E, Koss A, Husebye T & Jacobsen D. Forgiftning med piggeple. Fem tilfeller behandlet med fysostigmin. *Tidsskr Nor Laegeforen* 1997; 117:2610–2612.

35 Groszek B, Gawlikowski T & Szkolnicka B. Samozatrucie *Datura stramonium*. *Przegl Lek* 2000; 57:577–579.

36 Jones AL & Proudfoot AT. The features and management of poisoning with drugs used to treat Parkinson's disease. *Q J Med* 1997; 90:613–616.

37 Rwiza HT. Jimson weed poisoning: an epidemic at Usangi Rural Government Hospital. *Trop Geogr Med* 1991; 43:85–89.

38 Dewitt MS, Swain R & Gibson LB. The dangers of Jimson weed and its abuse by teenagers in the Kanawha Valley of West Virginia. *W Va Med J* 1997; 93:182–185.

39 Greene GS, Patterson SG & Warner E. Ingestion of angel's trumpet: an increasingly common source of toxicity. *South Med J* 1996; 89:365–369.

40 Blaw ME, Adkisson MA, Levin D, Garriott JC & Tindall RS. Poisoning with Carolina jessamine (*Gelsemium sempervirens* [L.] Ait.). *J Pediatr* 1979; 94:998–1001.

41 Frank BS, Michelson WB, Panter KE & Gardner DR. Ingestion of poison hemlock (*Conium maculatum*). *West J Med* 1995; 163:573–574.

42 Hanrahan JP & Gordon MA. Mushroom poisoning: case reports and a review of therapy. *J Am Med Assoc* 1984; 251:1057–1061.

43 Ceha LJ, Presperin C, Young E, Allswede M & Erickson T. Anticholinergic toxicity from nightshade berry poisoning responsive to physostigmine. *J Emerg Med* 1997; 15:65–69.

44 Martin-Rubi JC, Yelamos-Rodriguez F, Laynez-Bretones F et al. Intoxicaciones por insecticidas organofosforados. Estudio de 506 casos. *Rev Clin Esp* 1996; 196:145–149.

45 Fang Y, Pei ZI & Li Z. [Study on observation indexes of rational dosage of atropine in treatment of acute organophosphorus insecticides poisoning]. *Zhonghua Hu Li Za Zhi* 1997; 32:311–315.

46 Thiermann H, Mast U, Klimmek R et al. Cholinesterase status, pharmacokinetics and laboratory findings during obidoxime therapy in organophosphate poisoned patients. *Hum Exp Toxicol* 1997; 16:473–480.

47 Sood NN, Sachdev MS, Mohan M, Gupta SK & Sachdev HPS. Epidemic dropsy following transcutaneous absorption of *Argemone mexicana* oil. *Trans R Soc Trop Med Hyg* 1985; 79:510–512.

48 Singh NP, Anuradha S, Dhanwal D K et al. Epidemic dropsy: a clinical study of the Delhi outbreak. *J Assoc Phys India* 2000; 48:877–880.

49 Das M & Khanna SK. Clinicoepidemiological, toxicological, and safety evaluation studies on argemone oil. *Crit-Rev Toxicol* 1997; 27:273–297.

References **633**

50 Desjars P, Meignier M, Pinaud M, Tasseau F & Nicolas F. Place du nitroprussiate de sodium dans les accidents ischemiques de l'ergotisme aigu. *Nouv Presse Med* 1981; 10:2959–2961.

51 Kinamore PA, Jaeger R-W & De Castro FJ. *Abrus* and *Ricinus* ingestion: management of three cases. *Clin Toxicol* 1980; 17:401–405.

52 Hamilton RJ, Shih RD & Hoffman RS. Mobitz type I heart block after pokeweed ingestion. *Vet Hum Toxicol* 1995; 37:66–67.

53 Gardner DG. Injury to the oral mucous membranes caused by the common houseplant, *Dieffenbachia*: a review. *Oral Surg Oral Med Oral Pathol* 1994; 78:631–633.

54 Pusztai AJ. *Plant Lectins*. Cambridge: Cambridge University Press, 1991.

55 Addae JI & Melville GN. A re-examination of the mechanism of ackee-induced vomiting sickness. *West Indian Med J* 1988; 37:6–8.

56 Anonymous. Toxic hypoglycemic syndrome: Jamaica, 1989–1991. *MMWR* 1992; 41:53–55.

57 Morelli A, Grasso M, Meloni T, Forteleoni G, Zocchi E & De Flora A. Favism: impairment of proteolytic systems in red blood cells. *Blood* 1987; 69:1753–1758.

58 Kitayaporn D, Charoenlarp P, Pataroarechachai J & Pholpoti T. G6PD deficiency and fava bean consumption do not produce haemolysis in Thailand. *Southeast Asian J Trop Med Public Health* 1991; 22:176–181.

59 Kew MC. Hepatocellular cancer: a century of progress. *Clin Liver Dis* 2000; 4:257–268.

60 Williams NA, Lee MG, Hanchard B & Barrow KO. Hepatic cirrhosis in Jamaica. *West Indian Med J* 1997; 46:60–62.

61 McDermott WV & Ridker PM. The Budd–Chiari syndrome and hepatic veno-occlusive disease: recognition and treatment. *Arch Surg* 1990; 125:525–527.

62 Tandon BN, Tandon RK, Tandon HD, Narndranathan M & Joshi YK. An epidemic of veno-occlusive disease of liver in Central India. *Lancet* 1976; i:271–272.

63 Mohabat O, Srivastava RN, Younos MS, Mozad AA, Sediq GG & Aram GN. An outbreak of hepatic veno-occlusive disease in Northwestern Afghanistan. *Lancet* 1976; ii:269–271.

64 Stickel F, Seitz HK, Hahn EG & Schuppan D. Hepatotoxizität von Arzneimitteln pflanzlichen Ursprungs. *Z Gastroenterol* 2001; 39:225–232, 234–237.

65 Vachvanichsanong P & Lebel L. Djenkol beans as a cause of hematuria in children. *Nephron* 1997; 76:39–42.

66 Areekul S, Muangman V, Bohkerd C & Saenghirun C. Djenkol bean as a cause of urolithiasis. *Southeast Asian J Trop Med Public Health* 1978; 9:427–432.

67 Violon C. Belgian (Chinese herb) nephropathy: why? *J Pharm Belg* 1997; 52:7–27.

68 Nortier JL, Martinez MC, Schmeiser HH et al. Urothelial carcinoma associated with the use of a Chinese herb (*Aristolochia fangchi*). *N Engl J Med* 2000; 342:1686–1692.

69 Massey LK, Roman-Smith H & Sutton RA. Effect of dietary oxalate and calcium on urinary oxalate and risk of formation of calcium oxalate kidney stones. *J Am Diet Assoc* 1993; 93:901–906.

70 Sanz P & Reig R. Clinical and pathological findings in fatal plant oxalosis: a review. *Am J Forensic Med Pathol* 1992; 13:342–345.

71 Sacks O. Guam. In *The Island of the Colour-Blind*. London: Picador, 1996: 107–201.

72 Spencer PS, Hugon J, Ludolph A et al. Discovery and partial characterization of primate motor-system toxins. *Ciba Found Symp* 1987; 126:221–238.

73 Spencer PS, Ludolph AC & Kisby GE. Neurologic diseases associated with use of plant components with toxic potential. *Environ Res* 1993; 62:106–113.

74 Haimanot RT, Kidane Y, Wahib E et al. Lathyrism in rural Northwestern Ethiopia: a highly prevalent neurotoxic disorder. *Int J Epidemiol* 1990; 19:664–672.

75 Smith BA. Strychnine poisoning. *J Emerg Med* 1990; 8:321–325.

76 Pattanapanyasat K, Panyathanya R & Pairojkul C. A preliminary study on toxicity of diospyrol and oxidized diospyrol from *Diospyros mollis Griff.* (Maklua) in rabbits eyes. *J Med Assoc Thai* 1985; 68:60–65.

77 Chu NS. Effects of betel chewing on the central and autonomic nervous systems. *J Biomed Sci* 2001; 8:229–236.

78 Singh YN. Kava: an overview. *J Ethnopharmacol* 1992; 37:13–45.

79 Kalix P. *Catha edulis*, a plant that has amphetamine effects. *Pharm World Sci* 1996; 18:69–73.

80 Watson PL, Luanratana O & Griffin W J. The ethnopharmacology of pituri. *J Ethnopharmacol* 1983; 8:303–311.

81 Elegbe RA & Oyebola DDO. Cow's urine poisoning in Nigeria: cardiorespiratory effects of cow's urine in dogs. *Trans R Soc Trop Med Hyg* 1977; 71:127–132.

82 Grahame-Smith DG & Aronson JK. *The Oxford Textbook of Clinical Pharmacology and Drug Therapy*, 3rd edn. Oxford: Oxford University Press, 2002: Ch 35.

83 Griffin JP & D'Arcy PF. Drug interactions with remedies. In *A Manual of Drug Interactions*, 5th edn. Amsterdam: Elsevier, 1997: 537–548.

84 Fugh-Berman A. Herb–drug interactions. *Lancet* 2000; 355:134–138.

85 Gold JL, Laxer DA, Dergal JM, Lanctot KL & Rochon PA. Herbal–drug therapy interactions: a focus on dementia. *Curr Opin Clin Nutr Metab Care* 2001; 4:29–34.

86 Welihinda J, Karunanayake EH, Sheriff MH & Jayasinghe KS. Effect of *Momordica charantia* on the glucose tolerance in maturity onset diabetes. *J Ethnopharmacol* 1986; 17:277–282.

87 Heck AM, DeWitt BA & Lukes AL. Potential interactions between alternative therapies and warfarin. *Am J Health-Syst Pharm* 2000; 57:1221–1227.

88 Weber WW. *Pharmacogenetics*. New York: Oxford University Press, 1997.

89 Anonymous. Grapefruit warning label: now official in some countries. *Drugs Ther Perspect* 1998; 12:12–13.

90 Committee on Safety of Medicines, Medicines Control Agency. Terfenadine: now only available on prescription. *Curr Probl Pharmacovig* 1997; 23:9.

91 Committee on Safety of Medicines, Medicines Control Agency. Astemizole (Hismanal): only available on prescription. *Curr Probl Pharmacovig* 1999; 25:2.

92 Aronson JK. Forbidden fruit. *Nature Med* 2001; 7:7–8.

93 Ohnishi A, Matsuo H, Yamada S et al. Effect of furanocoumarin derivatives in grapefruit juice on the uptake of vinblastine by Caco-2 cells and on the activity of cytochrome P450 3A4. *Br J Pharmacol* 2000; 130:1369–1377.

94 Kitts D & Hu C. Efficacy and safety of ginseng. *Public Health Nutr* 2000; 3:473–485.

95 Ahn YO. Diet and stomach cancer in Korea. *Int J Cancer* 1997; Suppl: 10:7–9

96 Di Carlo G, Borrelli F, Izzo AA & Ernst E. St John's wort: Prozac from the plant kingdom. *Trends Pharmacol Sci* 2001; 22:292–297.

FURTHER READING

Burkill HM. *The Useful Plants of West Tropical Africa* (4 vols to date). London: Crown Agents for Overseas Governments and Administrations, 1985, 1994, 1995, 1997.

Chopra RN. *Poisonous Plants of India*. Calcutta: Government of India Press, 1940.

Chopra RN. *Indigenous Drugs of India*, 2nd edn. Calcutta: Dhat, 1958.

Duke, JA. *Amazonian Ethnobotanical Dictionary*. Boca Raton, FL: CRC Press, 1994.

Dukes MNG & Aronson JK (eds). *Meyler's Side Effects of Drugs*, 14th edn. Amsterdam: Elsevier, 2000.

Ellenhorn MJ, Schonwald S, Ordog G & Wasserberger J. *Ellenhorn's Medical Toxicology*, 2nd edn. Baltimore: Williams & Wilkins, 1997.

Everist SL. *Poisonous Plants of Australia*, 2nd edn. Sydney: Angus & Robertson, 1981.

Felter HW & Lloyd JU. King's American Dispensatory. http://www.ibiblio.org/herbmed/eclectic/kings/main.html.

Lampe KF & McCann MA. *AMA Handbook of Poisonous and Injurious Plants*. Chicago: American Medical Association, 1985.

Schmidt RJ. Botanical Dermatology Database. http://archive.uwcm.ac.uk/uwcm/dm/BoDD/index.html.

Sodt J. Ethnobotany Resources the Western Libraries. Western Washington University. http://www.library.wwu.edu/ref/subjguides/ethnobot.html.

Watt JM & Breyer-Brandwijk MG. *The Medicinal and Poisonous Plants of Southern and Eastern Africa*, 2nd edn. Edinburgh: E & S Livingstone, 1962.

Chapter 34
Podoconiosis (Non-filarial Elephantiasis)
G. C. Cook

Confusion has existed for many decades between elephantiasis caused by the lymphatic filariases (*Wuchereria bancrofti* and *Brugia malayi*) (Chapter 82) and endemic elephantiasis – which is *not* helminth related. This latter disease is caused by microparticles of silica and aluminosilicates which enter the lymphatics of the lower limbs through the soles of the feet. It is a disease mainly associated with rural communities (often known locally as 'big foot disease') and affects individuals not accustomed to footwear. The term podoconiosis (Greek: *podos*, of the foot; *konion*, dust) has recently gained widespread acceptance to describe the disease.[1]

History

Podoconiosis was probably described by the Latin philosopher Pliny, Augustine of Hippo (now Tunisia) and Isidore of Seville in Spain.[1] It was recognized as a 'specific' disease by the Persian physician Muhammed Ibn Zakariya (El Razi) in the tenth century AD; his original description in Arabic is (or was) housed at the Baghdad Medical School. He considered that 'if the disease is attended to at its onset and treated appropriately it can be cured or stopped and will not increase'; this differentiated it from filarial elephantiasis. Amongst early illustrations which probably depict podoconiosis is one in the thirteenth century *Mappa Mundi* (map of the world) preserved at Hereford Cathedral,[2] a carved oak pew-end in the church at Dennington, Suffolk, and in the sixteenth century *Cosmographia Universalis* of Munster.[1] Realization by Manson in the late nineteenth century that most cases of elephantiasis are associated with *W. bancrofti* (or *B. malayi*) infection[3,4] led to confusion regarding the aetiology of the disease, especially in parts of Africa where this helminthiasis seemed to be absent. In Guatemala there was apparently confusion with lepromatous leprosy.[1]

Epidemiology

In Africa, where most cases of the disease have been described, podoconiosis is most common in highland areas in east and central parts of the continent.[1,5] Here, the red clays are related to volcanism in prehistory.[6,7] In West Africa, highland areas are very limited involving only Cameroon,[8,9] part of Nigeria and the Island of Malabo, Gabon, and Equatorial Guinea;[10] although *Onchocerca volvulus* is present in some highland areas, *W. bancrofti* is invariably absent. The disease has also been recorded in several volcanic oceanic islands: the Cape Verde Islands, Canary Islands, and Malabo Island (formerly Fernando Po),[10] and more recently in Sao Tome and Principe.[11] There is also a report for the Mount Elgon area of Uganda.[12] It has also been recorded in Central America, from Mexico to Colombia and Ecuador. Other descriptions are from Guatemala, Costa Rica, Puerto Rico, Surinam, French Guiana and Brazil. Reports also exist from north-west India[13] and Sri Lanka.

Most affected individuals are from families of barefooted agriculturalists; the disease is less common in pastoral areas.[1] The altitudes, climates, soil composition and particle size in areas endemic for podoconiosis have been studied extensively.[14,15] The soil is invariably volcanic and of red clay, which becomes extremely slippery after rain.[1,13,16] Electron diffraction analysis shows this to consist of aluminosilicate kaolinite, with ultrafine particles of amorphous silica and iron oxides. Thermoluminescence and exoemission studies indicate that the dynamic surface properties of endemic soils are important criteria in cytoxicity.

In summary, the physical characterisitics of an endemic area are as follows:[1] (1) a temperate or near-temperate climate situated within the tropics at an altitude > 1500 m; (2) reddish-brown soil, of which approximately half (by weight) consists of microparticles < 10 μm in diameter and one-third < 2 μm; (3) microparticles with a predominance of silica in the 2–10 μm portion (silts), and of the aluminosilicate kaolinite in the < 2 μm portion (clay); (4) approximately half of the clay portion is < 0.4 μm and often 0.1 μm; this presupposes that the local population is agrarian and walks barefooted.

Pathogenesis

Podoconiosis consists of a slowly progressive obstructive lymphopathy caused by particles of optimal size (in suitable soil) having penetrated the soles of the feet. This has been confirmed by analysis of biopsy specimens from the dermis, lymphatic vessels, lymph glands (by elemental analysis of incinerated residues) and by electron microscopic microanalysis of particles in thin tissue sections.[17]

The initial pathogenetic event is, therefore, entry of toxic mineral microparticles into the dermis of the foot; the pathological consequences are dependent on particle size.[15,18] This takes place to a greater extent in the soft thin skin of young people, and by the age of 10–15 years a sufficient load of toxic material is present in the foot to produce clinical evidence of tissue damage.[1] The lymphatic vessels leading from the dermis become fibrosed and, in some cases, completely obstructed. Regional lymph node involvement (in the groin) occurs subsequently. These events are followed by fibrotic changes.

Pathology

Pathological features result from lymphatic obstruction and fibrosis. The anatomy and physiology of the lower limb lymphatics have been studied extensively. Associated lesions are 'pillowy' oedema, fibrous nodulation, hyperkeratosis, interdigital bacterial and fungal infection, tuberculous adenitis, and other changes which are a result of 'traditional' management.[1]

Clinical features

Podoconiosis commonly begins between the ages of 10 and 19 years in both sexes, but has been recorded as young as 5 and as late as 60 years of age.[1] A burning sensation of the sole following a long walk often heralds the disease; it may become worse in bed at night, after excessive alcohol intake, after prolonged exertion, during menstruation, and while standing in front of a fire. A local swelling of the foot, usually on the dorsum near the first toe cleft, slowly diminishes in size but recurs after further exertion. The lower part of the affected leg is progressively involved over a few months to several years, but the thigh is rarely affected. Both legs are, in fact, invariably affected, but the disease develops asymmetrically so that the swelling of one leg usually increases whilst the other remains constant. Femoral lymphadenitis is common and a cluster of nodes may reach 5 cm in length and weigh 5–6 g. Recurrent acute febrile episodes are a usual, but inconstant feature, and these lead progressively to lymphatic obstruction. The acute episodes are easily mistaken for a localized bacterial infection and in consequence an antibiotic is prescribed. After a varying period of time, lymphoedema (elephantiasis) becomes firmly established.

In an endemic area, early disease should be suspected in any young person complaining of discomfort in the lower legs and feet, especially in bed at night and after excessive exertion. Price[1] has summarized early signs indicating oedema of the dorsum of the foot and the plantar region: (1) increased skin markings and indentation on pressure; (2) a large second toe; (3) a splayed forefoot; (4) lymph dampness of the forefoot skin; (5) hyperkeratosis ('mossy foot'); (6) 'block toes' (early oedema of the forefoot causes the toes to appear rigid, as if they were wooden and were nailed to the forefoot); (7) plantar oedema; and (8) persistent itching of a lower part of one or other leg.

In a fully developed case of podoconiosis, appearances vary from lymphoedema to thickened, rough and leathery skin of the foot, i.e., traditional elephantiasis.[1] In most cases both features are present. In the oedematous form ('water bag' leg) the skin pits on pressure and can be pinched up with the fingers; it is smooth, with little hyperkeratotic change. There may be slight oozing of lymph, and skin hairs are usually lost. Secondary infection may supervene, and *Streptococcus* spp. lymphangitis may be a complication. In the fibrotic ('leathery' leg) form, the fibrotic dermis may be 3 cm or more in thickness and become fixed to the deep tissues; it does not pit and cannot be pinched up between the fingers. Hyprkeratosis is common and hyperpigmentation is present. Nodulation is common at the base of the toes or in front of the ankle. Inguinal nodes are usually prominent and tender, and abdominal nodes (sometimes tender) may be palpable on abdominal examination. In a minority of cases, the affected area may extend above the knee(s). Several conditions associated with prolonged lymphatic blockage (e.g., tuberculous adenitis) are described elsewhere in this book.

Management

Rhazes, writing in the ninth century AD, considered that 'This malady, if it takes hold, is incurable', but he continued 'if it is treated at the beginning it can be stopped with no further advances'.[1] Those observations remain valid today because the pathogenic effect of silica and aluminosilicate penetration into the tissues of the foot causes slowly progressive but irreversible pathological change. Individuals living in endemic areas have for many centuries recognized an association with the soil, and have also been aware that migration away from an area of high prevalence to one free of the disease arrests its progress, and vice versa. Sections of the community afflicted by this disorder usually originate in the lower strata of society in which financial resources for footwear, etc., are very limited.

Principles of management are as follows:[1] (1) the treatment of symptoms caused by early or established disease; (2) reduction of any additional load of silica particles in the dermis; and (3) either elevation of a limb and/or elastic stockings may help to assist in reducing the oedema. Obviously, use of footwear prevents further absorption of the responsible mineral particles. The use of matting to cover bare ground within residential huts should be encouraged. This controls the progress of early disease and prevents the mineral load reaching pathogenetic proportions in other (usually younger) members of the family. If possible, a young individual with early signs of the disease should be encouraged to take up residence in a non-endemic location, and may return to the site of high prevalence when footwear is available and is widely used. A change of occupation which reduces contact between the bare foot and soil is beneficial; home industries such as weaving and dressmaking may be encouraged. Oedema and fibrogenesis are interrelated; prolonged oedema produces fibrosis; similarly prolonged fibrosis predisposes to oedema. Oedema can be reduced by elevation of the limb or by compression with bandages or a stocking. A variety of drugs has been used with the object of reversing established fibrosis; in Africa, various traditional plant derivatives have also been used, but to no avail.

Surgical procedures are unlikely to provide satisfactory results, even when the uptake of mineral microparticles has been arrested. No method is available by which particles can be removed from the dermis, lymphatic tissues of the lower leg and regional lymph nodes. Surgery is indicated in the following situations:[1] (1) excision of 'nodules' on the foot; (2) removal of a femoral node which is subject to repeated attacks of adenitis; and (3) removal of superfluous skin, after the use of compression methods, in the lymphoedematous type of swelling.

Prevention

Podoconiosis is a *preventable* disease. With greater recognition of its prevalence geographically in the future, exposure to pathogenic particles should be avoided. However, prevention is also heavily dependent on the raising of socio-economic standards, and the provision of footwear.

REFERENCES

1 Price E W. *Podoconiosis: Non-Filarial Elephantiasis.* Oxford: Oxford University Press, 1990: 131.

2 Chancey M. *Mappa Mundi.* Hereford: Hereford Cathedral Publications, 1987.

3 Price E W. The elephantiasis story. *Trop Dis Bull* 1984; 81:R1-R12.

4 Cook G C. *From the Greenwich Hulks to Old St Pancras: A History of Tropical Disease in London.* London: Athlone Press, 1992: 332.

5 Price E W. Endemic elephantiasis of the lower legs in Rwanda and Burundi. *Trop Geogr Med* 1976; 28:283–290.

6 Oomen A P. Studies on elephantiasis of the legs in Ethiopia. *Trop Geogr Med* 1969; 21:236–253.

7 Price E W. Endemic elephantiasis of the lower legs in Ethiopia: an epidemiological survey. *Ethiop Med J* 1974;12:77–90.

8 Price E W & Henderson W J. Endemic elephantiasis of the lower legs in the United Cameroon Republic. *Trop Geogr Med* 1981; 33:23–29.

9 Price E W, McHardy W J & Pooley F D. Endemic elephantiasis of the lower legs as a health hazard of barefooted agriculturalists in Cameroon, West Africa. *Ann Occup Hyg* 1981; 24:1–8.

10 Corachan M, Tura J W, Campo E, Solely M & Traveria A. Podoconiosis in Equatorial Guinea: report of two cases from different geological environments. *Trop Geogr Med* 1988; 40:359–364.

11 Ruiz L, Campo E & Corachan M. Elephantiasis in Sao Tome and Principe. *Acta Tropica* 1994; 57:29–34.

12 Onapa A W, Simonsen P E & Pedersen E M. Non-filarial elephantiasis in the Mt. Elgon area (Kapehorwa District) of Uganda. *Acta Tropica* 2001; 78:171–176.

13 Kalra N L. Non-filarial elephantiasis in Bikaner, Rajasthan. *J Commun Dis* 1976; 8:337–340.

14 Hirsch A. *Handbook of Geographical and Historical Pathology.* London: New Sydenham Society, 1886; 3:712.

15 Price E W & Plant D A. The significance of particle size of soils as a risk factor in the etiology of podoconiosis. *Trans R Soc Trop Med Hyg* 1990; 84:885–886.

16 Price E W. The association of endemic filariasis of the lower legs in East Africa with soil derived from volcanic rocks. *Trans R Soc Trop Med Hyg* 1976; 70:288–295.

17 Heather C J & Price E W. Non-filarial elephantiasis in Ethiopia: analytical study of inorganic material in lymph nodes. *Trans R Soc Trop Med Hyg* 1972; 66:450–458.

18 Spooner N T & Davies J E. Possible role of soil particles in the aetiology of non-filarial (endemic) elephantiasis: a macrophage cytotoxicity assay. *Trans R Soc Trop Med Hyg* 1986; 80:222–225.

Chapter 35
Familial Mediterranean Fever

G. C. Cook

Familial Mediterranean fever is a clinical syndrome with a clear genetic basis which gives rise to recurrent febrile episodes associated with systemic manifestations, notably abdominal pain, pleurisy and arthropathy. It affects members of certain groups with an ethnic origin, usually but not always, from the Mediterranean littoral or the Middle East.[1,2] The major importance of this disease is that it forms an important differential diagnosis from other febrile illnesses. In addition, it gives rise to substantial morbidity (but not mortality) in those affected. In 1997, a new era opened up with cloning of the mutated gene (*MEFV*) responsible for this entity.[2]

History

The first description of a familial condition comprising 'recurring attacks of a peculiar nature' was made by Janeway and Mosenthal[3] in 1908: a 16-year-old Jewish schoolgirl 'without special neurotic inheritance' had suffered febrile bouts associated with abdominal pain, consisting of prodromal, crescendo and recovery phases, since the age of 2 weeks. Subsequent reports originated in the USA, and were dominated by accounts of individuals of Jewish origin.[4–6] Large series of cases were recorded involving Jewish residents of Israel,[7] Turks,[8] Armenians (most of them in the USA)[9,10] and 'fair-skinned' Arabs.[11] Many names have been applied to the syndrome, including:[1] benign paroxysmal peritonitis, periodic disease, periodic fever, periodic peritonitis, maladie dite périodique, épanalepsie méditerranéenne, familial paroxysmal polyserositis, recurrent polyserositis, paroxysmal peritonitis, familial Mediterranean fever (FMF), familial paroxysmal polyserositis, familial recurrent polyserositis and recurrent hereditary polyserositis. Renal amyloidosis was first demonstrated in this condition by Mamou and Cattan[12] in 1952 (see below). In 1972, colchicine was first used successfully in FMF by Goldfinger,[13] and the first clear evidence that its administration *prevents* renal amyloid deposition was provided by Zemer and her co-workers[14] in Jerusalem in 1986.

Epidemiology

One estimate is that 2 million people suffer, or have suffered from FMF, although the precise magnitude of the problem worldwide is impossible to ascertain. The major ethnic groups affected are Jews (both Sephardic, i.e., those descended from ancestors expelled from Spain in the fifteenth century, and Ashkenazi), Arabs, Armenians and Turks. In Sephardic and Iraqi Jews an estimated gene frequency of 1:45 with a prevalence of 1:2000 homozygous individuals has been calculated.[1] Corresponding figures for Armenians in Lebanon are put at 1:32 and 1:1000. Gene frequencies varying between 1:52 and 0.032, in non-Ashkenazi Jews and Armenians, respectively, have been suggested.[10] Sporadic cases (with no clear family history of the disorder) have been recorded from many countries, including the UK, Ireland, France, Germany, Sweden, the former USSR, Japan and India.[1] Occasional reports of a comparable syndrome have also been made in Maoris. In many, but not all of the reported series a significant male predominance has been recorded,[7,11] the mean ratio being of the order of 1.7:1. Most studies have indicated Mendelian recessive transmission,[1,10] although a dominant mode of inheritance has been claimed by some. Prevalence rates around 18% have been recorded when both parents are healthy, and 36% when only one is affected. In the presence of full penetrance, the likely figures would be 25% and 50%, respectively. In one study, the number of offspring affected was significantly lower than that anticipated.[15] Incomplete penetrance might be more common in females; late appearance of the syndrome in a minority of individuals has been suggested as an explanation for this inequality.

Aetiology and pathogenesis

Table 35.1 summarizes some of the numerous suggested aetiological and pathogenic bases for FMF.[2,5] Many investigators have concentrated on the likelihood of an immunological defect; suppressor T-cell activity and chemotaxis are decreased in untreated disease, and these abnormalities are corrected after colchicine administration. A C5a-inhibitor deficiency in joint and peritoneal fluids the acute inflammatory attacks.[16,17] However, none of these hypotheses has been confirmed.[2] Other suggested metabolic abnormalities include: a defect in one of the lipocortin proteins or a defect in the formation and elimination of circulating monohydroxy and dihydroxy fatty acids, and an inherited enzymatic error in catecholamine metabolism. There is no known relationship

Table 35.1 Some of the formerly suggested aetiological and pathogenic bases for FMF, together with a selection of known precipitating factors.[1]

Infective agent of unknown identity:
'Immune defect'
'Allergen'
Dietary 'allergy'
Angioneurotic oedema
'Autoimmune'
C5a-inhibitor deficiency (joint/peritoneal fluid)
Inborn error of metabolism
Lipocortin-protein defect
Abnormal catecholamine metabolism
Endocrine

Some *acknowledged* factors, in an *acute* attack:
Stress/anxiety
Cold
Physical exercise
Menstruation

Table 35.2 Clinical features of uncomplicated FMF.[1]

Abdominal pain (24–48 hours) + pyrexia (38–40°C) + tachycardia
Acute peritonitis (constipation common; diarrhoea unusual)
Pleurisy (+ effusion) (± 50%)
Arthropathy (large joints; symmetrical; usually non-destructive) (± 50%)
Dermotological lesions (usually resembling erysipelas) (10–70%)
Immune complex nephropathy

with another genetic marker; neither an ABO nor HLA link has been recorded. The fact remains, however, in the light of recent research that the disorder must possess a definite genetic basis.[2,18–21] There is a notable absence of descriptions of this syndrome in historical texts (including the Bible and the Koran);[1] involving affected groups this, therefore, leaves the possibility that a relatively recently introduced environmental factor (possibly dietary) might trigger the onset of the overt clinical syndrome.

Pathology

FMF is characterized by serosal inflammation and hyperaemic manifestations involving small blood vessels, venules and arterioles;[2,7] ultrastructural changes in the latter consist of basement membrane thickening, concentric layers being separated by ground substance. Serous membranes (precisely why they are the major targets of inflammation in FMF remains unexplained) exhibit both hyperaemia and an acute inflammatory exudate containing neutrophils, lymphocytes, monocytes, plasma cells and eosinophils. When present, adhesions are thin. Synovia are also affected. When present (see below), dermatological changes consist of mild acanthosis and hyperkeratosis with infiltration by neutrophils, lymphocytes and histiocytes around smaller blood vessels.

Clinical features

Approximately 50% of cases have an onset during the first decade of life; most present by the end of the second, and only about 1% at >40 years of age.[11] Table 35.2 summarizes the major clinical features of FMF. Vomiting in association with the abdominal pain is common, but

diarrhoea is unusual. A high percentage of affected individuals has undergone a previous abdominal operation (usually an appendicectomy). Prevalence of symptoms and signs varies in different series; arthropathy seems to be more severe in Sephardic Jews. Dermatological lesions consist most commonly of erysipelas-like lesions involving the legs, ankles and dorsum of the feet. Schönlein-Henoch purpura, urticaria, bullous lesions and vasculitis have also been recorded. Symptoms are frequently alleviated during pregnancy.[6,9] A classical presentation of an uncomplicated case is described below.

A 46-year-old Arab man, who was born in Jerusalem, was referred to a London hospital on account of irregular bouts (usually at intervals of about two months) of abdominal pain since the age of 18 years. A clinical diagnosis of Crohn's disease was made and sulphasalazine prescribed. Fifteen years earlier he had been subjected to appendicectomy on account of his recurrent abdominal pain. His mother's sister's son (i.e., his cousin) had experienced similar attacks. Extensive investigation between attacks proved negative: ESR 18 mm/h. Following initiation of colchicine chemotherapy (see below) he become totally asymptomatic, and has remained so after a follow-up period of several years.

Table 35.3 summarizes some less common *clinical* features of FMF, and Table 35.4 gives some differential diagnoses based on clinical criteria.[1,2]

Precise criteria for a *clinical* diagnosis of FMF are impossible to establish, but the following have been suggested: (1) >4 attacks (24–72 hours duration) of peritonitis and/or pleurisy in the presence of fever, and in many cases, arthropathy also; (2) absence of symptoms

Table 35.3 Some less common clinical features FMF.[1]

Severe headaches
Pharyngitis
Pericarditis[22]
Myocarditis
Myalgia[23]
Panniculitis
Ophthalmic problems: colloid bodies, episcleritis
Acute orchitis-infertility
Mollaret's meningitis
Childhood growth retardation

Table 35.4 Some clinical differential diagnoses of FMF.[1]

Pyrexia of undetermined origin
Other inherited periodic 'febrile' diseases (rare)
Abdominal infection
    Appendicitis
    Cholecystitis
    Perforated peptic ulcer
    Diverticulitis
Relapsing pancreatitis
Acute intermittent porphyria
Pulmonary embolism/atelectasis
Septic arthropathy
Juvenile rheumatoid arthritis
Tuberculous arthritis
Systemic lupus erythematosus
Other causes of amyloidosis

between attacks; and (3) lack of a known underlying aetiological and/or pathological factor. It is necessary to distinguish FMF from various rare clinical entities associated with recurrent febrile episodes.[2]

The most important complication of FMF is amyloid AA formation. The compound is deposited in many tissues, most importantly the kidneys (renal glomerulae),[12,24] but also involves the spleen, lung, heart, liver and intestine. This complication seems to be significantly more common in Sephardic Jews and Turks, although there might be selective errors in reporting.[25,26] Ashkenazi Jews, Armenians and Arabs are largely 'immune' from this complication. It seems possible that genetic mechanisms (as yet undefined) also protect some ethnic groups from amyloid formation.[25]

Investigations

Acute-phase reactants and ESR are elevated during an *acute* episode. However, this does not distinguish the syndrome from other conditions with an underlying inflammatory basis. Also, the polymorph leucocyte count is elevated. Transient haematuria may be present, and abnormalities can occur in both the electrocardiogram and electroencephalogram. Although initially considered to be of value, a metaraminol provocation test[27] and estimation of dopamine-β-hydroxylase concentration[28]

have not stood the test of time. In summary, none of the formerly used laboratory tests for FMF has proved satisfactory.[2] In affected individuals, rectal/gum biopsy demonstrates amyloid deposition. The presence of amyloid can be confirmed in a renal biopsy specimen; however, renal biopsy is not without risk as haemorrhage is a real possibility in the presence of amyloid deposition.

Since the cloning of MEFV, however, diagnosis of FMF has been revolutionized.[2,29–32] PCR primers can now be used to demonstrate the mutations responsible for the disease, three of which are present in 85% of FMF carrier chromosomes.

Management

Numerous therapeutic agents have been used historically in the management of FMF, those have included: *para*-aminobenzoic acid, chloroquine, corticosteroids, adrenaline, ephedrine, atropine, reserpine, nicotinic acid and tuberculin desensitization. In addition, numerous analgesics, narcotics, antiemetics and non-steroidal anti-inflammatory compounds have been used with limited degrees of success. In some studies, a low-fat diet has been claimed effective, and one low in tyrosine has also been advocated. Successful management was heralded by the introduction of colchicine in 1972 (see above). Although the mode of its action is unknown, 0.5–1.5 mg daily is usually adequate to prevent attacks.[13,33,34] Unfortunately, this agent has been associated with male infertility. Following widespread use of colchicine in the prevention of acute episodes, clear evidence later emerged that this form of management also prevents the onset of the amyloid nephropathy.[14] Therefore, in high-risk groups (for amyloid deposition) it is of paramount importance that regular colchicine administration be continued indefinitely.

Prognosis

This is entirely dependent on the presence or absence of amyloid AA deposition. Those in a low-risk group for this complication (Ashkenazi Jews and Armenians) and others successfully treated with colchicine should have a normal life expectancy.[1,2]

REFERENCES

1   Cook G C. Recurrent hereditary polyserositis or familial Mediterranean fever: an overview. *Ann Saudi Med* 1991; 11:576–584.

2   Ben-Chetrit E & Levy M. Familial Mediterranean fever. *Lancet* 1998; 351:659–664.

3   Janeway T C & Mosenthal H O. An unusual paroxysmal syndrome, probably allied to recurrent vomiting, with a study of the nitrogen metabolism. *Trans Assoc Am Phys* 1908; 23:504–518.

4   Alt H L & Barker M H. Fever of unknown origin. *J Am Med Assoc* 1930; 94:1459–1461.

5   Reimann H A. Periodic disease: periodic fever, periodic abdominalgia, cyclic neutropenia, intermittent arthralgia,

angioneurotic edema, anaphylactoid purpura and periodic paralysis. *J Am Med Assoc* 1949; 141:175–178.

6   Siegal S. Familial paroxysmal polyserositis: analysis of fifty cases. *Am J Med* 1964; 36:893–918.

7   Sohar E, Gafni J, Pras M & Heller H. Familial Mediterranean fever: a survey of 470 cases and review of the literature. *Am J Med* 1967; 43:227–253.

8   Ozedmir A I & Sokmen C. Familial Mediterranean fever among the Turkish people. *Am J Gastroenterol* 1969; 51:311–316.

9   Schwabe A D & Peters R S. Familial Mediterranean fever in Armenians: analysis of 100 cases. *Medicine (Baltimore)* 1974; 53:453–462.

10 Rogers D B, Shohat M, Petersen G M et al. Familial Mediterranean fever in Armenians: autosomal recessive inheritance with high gene frequency. *Am J Med Genet* 1989; 34:168–172.

11 Barakat M H, Karnik A M, Majeed H W A et al. Familial Mediterranean fever (recurrent hereditary polyserositis) in Arabs: a study of 175 patients and review of the literature. *Q J Med* 1986; 60:837–847.

12 Mamou H & Cattan R. La maladie périodique (sur 14 cas personnels dont 8 compliqués de nephropathies). *Sem Hôp Paris* 1952; 28:1062–1070.

13 Goldfinger S E. Colchicine for familial Mediterranean fever. *N Engl J Med* 1972; 287:1302.

14 Zemer D, Pras M, Sohar E et al. Colchicine in the prevention and treatment of the amyloidosis of familial Mediterranean fever. *N Engl J Med* 1986; 314:1001–1005.

15 Armenian H K. Genetic and environmental factors in the aetiology of familial paroxysmal polyserositis: an analysis of 150 cases from Lebanon. *Trop Geogr Med* 1982; 34:183–187.

16 Matzner Y & Brzezinski A. C5a-inhibitor deficiency in peritoneal fluids from patients with familial Mediterranean fever. *N Engl J Med* 1984; 311:287–290.

17 Schwabe A D & Lehman T J A. C5a-inhibitor deficiency: a role in familial Mediterranean fever? *N Engl J Med* 1984; 311:325–326.

18 Booth D R, Gillmore J D, Booth S E et al. Pyrin/marenostrin mutations in familial Mediterranean fever. *Q J Med* 1998; 91:603–606.

19 Ehrlich G E. Genetics of familial Mediterranean fever and its implications. *Ann Intern Med* 1998; 129:581–582.

20 Levin M. Genetics of familial Mediterranean fever. *Ann Intern Med* 1999; 130:780.

21 Booth D R, Gillmore J D, Lachmann H J et al. The genetic basis of autosomal dominant familial Mediterranean fever. *Q J Med* 2000; 93:217–221.

22 Odabas A R, Cetinkaya R, Selcuk Y & Kaya H. Severe and prolonged febrile myalgia in familial Mediterranean fever. *Scand J Rheumatol* 2000; 29:394–395.

23 Kees S, Langevitz P, Zemer D et al. Attacks of pericarditis as a manifestation of familial Mediterranean fever (FMF). *Q J Med* 1997; 90:643–647.

24 Mamou H. Maladie périodique amylogene. *Sem Hop Paris* 1955; 31:388–391.

25 Pras M, Bronshpigel N, Zemer D & Gafni J. Variable incidence of amyloidosis in familial Mediterranean fever among different ethnic groups. *Johns Hopkins Med J* 1982; 150:22–26.

26 Yalinkaya F, Tekin M, Cakar N et al. Familial Mediterranean fever and systemic amyloidosis in untreated Turkish patients. *Q J Med* 2000; 93:681–684.

27 Barakat M H, El-Khawad A O, Gumaa K A et al. Metaraminol provocative test: a specific diagnostic test for familial Mediterranean fever. *Lancet* 1984; i:656–657.

28 Barakat M H, Gumaa K A, Malhas L N et al. Plasma dopamine-beta-hydroxylase: rapid diagnostic test for recurrent hereditary polyserositis. *Lancet* 1988; ii:1280–1283.

29 Eisenberg S, Aksentijevich I, Deng Z et al. Diagnosis of familial Mediterranean fever by a molecular genetics method. *Ann Intern Med* 1998; 129:539–542.

30 Drenth J P & Van Der Meer J W. Periodic fevers enter the era of molecular diagnosis. *Br Med J* 2000; 320:1091–1092.

31 Grateau G, Pecheux C, Cazeneuve C, *et al*. Clinical versus genetic diagnosis of familial Mediterranean fever. *Q J Med* 2000 Apr; 93:223–229.

32 Nir-Paz R & Ben-Chetrit E. Molecular diagnosis of familial Mediterranean fever. *N Engl J Med* 2000; 342:60.

33 Dinarello C A, Wolff S M, Goldfinger S E et al. Colchicine therapy for familial Mediterranean fever: a double-blind trial. *N Engl J Med* 1974; 291:934–937.

34 Zemer D, Revach M, Pras M et al. A controlled trial of colchicine in preventing attacks of familial Mediterranean fever. *N Engl J Med* 1974; 291:932–934.

Chapter 36
Malignant Disease

C. L. M. Olweny

Any account of the problem of cancer must take into consideration several accepted generalizations. The term cancer is used to describe a group of diseases which are characterized by an abnormal, uncontrolled and purposeless proliferation of particular cells. Each tumour is classified according to its cell of origin, anatomical site and biological behaviour, and each is due to a specific factor or constellation of factors, the majority of which are determined by geographical, social, economic or cultural conditions, acting through physical, chemical or biological agents. Tumours due to direct genetic mechanisms are very rare, though genetic factors may render individuals or groups of people susceptible to particular environmental influences. The majority of tumours show an age-related incidence which reflects length of exposure to carcinogenic factor(s) in the environment.

Contrary to the common belief associating cancer with industrialization and urban lifestyle, cancer occurs very frequently in the developing world. Numerically, there are more cancer victims in developing countries than in the developed countries: of the estimated 9 million new cases diagnosed in 1985 globally, 5 million (56%) were in the developing countries, and of the estimated 5 million cancer deaths worldwide, 3 million (60%) were in the developing countries. The differences are likely to be more pronounced in years to come. Of the predicted 15 million new cancer cases in 2015, 10 million (67%) will likely occur in developing countries.

Global variations

There are global cancer incidence variations due to the fact that political boundaries rarely, if ever, comprise a population that is genetically, culturally and socio-economically homogeneous.[1] There is thus considerable variation of cancers observed in different regions of the world. Cancer of the cervix, for instance, the most common cancer in the developing countries, is the tenth most common in the developed countries. On the other hand, colorectal cancer, second only to lung cancer in the developed countries, is number eight in the developing countries (Table 36.1).[2] The variations occur not only in space, but in time as well. Kaposi's sarcoma (KS), which was relatively uncommon in most countries two decades ago, except for the endemic form in East and Central Africa and the sporadic form around the Mediterranean

Table 36.1 The 10 most common cancers globally.[2]

Developing countries	Developed countries
1. Uterine cervix	1. Lung
2. Stomach	2. Colorectal
3. Oropharynx	3. Breast
4. Oesophagus	4. Stomach
5. Breast	5. Prostate
6. Lung	6. Bladder
7. Liver	7. Lymphoma
8. Colorectal	8. Oropharynx
9. Lymphoma	9. Uterine body
10. Leukaemia	10. Uterine cervix

countries, is now the commonest male tumour in most of sub-Saharan Africa. While KS was extremely rare in females, it is now second only to cancer of the cervix in sub-Saharan Africa. This dramatic change is due to the emergence of the human immunodeficiency virus (HIV)/acquired immunodeficiency syndrome (AIDS) pandemic. These differences underscore the variations in health care priorities, as well as the need to revise these priorities from time to time.

Cancer in the tropics

During the first half of the twentieth century little was known or published about cancer in tropical countries and it was thought by many to be rare in the 'indigenous' populations of these regions. However, a few individuals recognized not only that cancer occurred, but also that the incidence and behaviour of some tumours was quite different from that seen in temperate climates. By the 1930s it was known that there was a high incidence of squamous cell carcinoma of the bladder in regions with a high prevalence of *Schistosoma haematobium* infection, such as the Nile Valley, of oral cancer in the Indian subcontinent and of nasopharyngeal carcinoma in the Far East. The first large series of histologically proven malignant tumours in Africans, published in 1934, showed several peculiar features, including descriptions of lymphosarcomas of the jaw, almost certainly Burkitt's lymphoma.

Although the incidence of stomach cancer is decreasing in many parts of the world, it remains an important cause of mortality in most Western countries and particularly in Japan. This tumour is relatively uncommon in most tropical regions such as Africa, the Indian subcontinent and much of the Far East. However, there are focal areas of high incidence such as that found around Mount Kilimanjaro in Tanzania and in the adjacent part of Kenya, near Lake Kivu in the Democratic Republic of Congo (former Zaire), and in the countries of Rwanda and Burundi. High rates are also found in the mountainous regions of Colombia and in Chile. Carcinoma of the pancreas, which is increasing in frequency in Western populations, is uncommon in most tropical countries.

Smoking and lung cancer

Unfortunately with the increasing adoption of a Western lifestyle, especially smoking, lung cancer incidence is expected to rise sharply in the developing countries. Such an increase has already been observed in Shanghai, China's largest city, in India and in Zimbabwe. The male lung cancer incidence recorded in Bulawayo, Zimbabwe, in 1968–1972 was 70.6/100 000 population. Such phenomenal increase calls for an urgent need to counteract the ruthless and sophisticated smoking campaign launched by the tobacco companies. More recent figures for the capital city of Harare show a decline. The age standardized rate (ASR) for lung cancer in Harare in 1990–1992 was 23.7/100 000 population, and the ASR for 1993–1995 was 14.1/100 000. The explanation for this downward trend is not immediately clear. It is not enough to merely persuade individuals to give up smoking or for governments to legislate against tobacco. There are powerful economic interests served by the production, promotion and sale of tobacco products, which seek to maximize consumption at all cost.[3] Tobacco is the major source of foreign exchange earnings in some countries. The most prominent cancer risk factor is cigarette smoking, associated primarily with lung cancer but contributing considerably to cancers of the oropharynx, oesophagus and urinary bladder. It has been suggested that tobacco smoking is the most deadly form of drug addiction, and that it is exacting a heavier toll in lives and dollars than cocaine, heroin, AIDS, traffic accidents, murder and terrorist attacks combined.[4] Lung cancer epidemic is threatening most developing countries. If we are to win the war against cancer, we must first win the battle against tobacco.[5]

Other causes of cancer

Genetic factors are known to play some role in the causation of certain cancers, notably increased incidence of skin cancers in individuals with defective capacity to repair DNA damage caused by ultraviolet light (xeroderma pigmentosa),[6,7] and the BRCA genes in breast cancer. BRCA1 cancer susceptibility gene was discovered in 1994.[8]

Table 36.2 Cancers associated with environmental factors.

Factors	Examples	Cancers
Physical	Ultraviolet light	Skin cancers,
	Ionizing radiation	e.g., melanoma
Chemicals	Aflatoxin	Liver
	Asbestosis	Mesothelioma
	Vinyl chloride	Liver
Biological: viruses	Hepatitis B virus	Liver
	Hepatitis C virus	Liver
	Human papilloma virus	Uterine cervix
	Human herpes simplex virus type 8	Kaposi's sarcoma
	Epstein–Barr virus	Nasopharynx Burkitt's lymphoma
Biological: parasites	*Schistosoma haematobium*	Bladder
	Clonorchis sinensis	Liver
Lifestyle	Smoking	Lung Oropharynx Bladder Oesophagus
	Diet	Colorectal Breast
	Alcohol	Liver Oesophagus
	Sunbathing	Skin cancers

A woman with a strong family history of breast cancer and/or ovarian cancer who carries the germ line mutation of BRCA1 faces an almost 85% lifetime risk of developing breast cancer, and a 60% chance of developing ovarian cancer.[9] In 1995, the discovery of BRCA2 gene was announced,[10] and both these genes account for most cases of familial breast cancer. It is, however, recognized that most cancers are due to factors in the environment (Table 36.2). These factors are physical, chemical, biological and, most importantly, lifestyle related.

Cancer registration

The establishment of medical schools in many former colonial countries of the tropics after the Second World War coincided with the extension of epidemiological interests and techniques in the field of non-infectious diseases, including cancer. During this period cancer registries were established in many tropical countries throughout the world, and these were able to obtain for the first time age-specific cancer rates in several localized areas, usually around teaching hospitals where diagnostic facilities were of a high quality and where there was an accurate census of the populations served. These incidence rate surveys were supplemented by proportional frequency studies (the frequency of individual tumours as a percentage of the whole) from different areas and tribal or ethnic groups in countries or regions.

These studies have shown not only that there are marked differences between the cancer pattern of tropical and of temperate countries, but also that there are large variations in frequency of specific cancers within regions and countries of the tropics. Some of the most important aetiological discoveries in the cancer field have stemmed from these geographical studies.

There are, however, few reliable estimates of cancer incidences in the tropics, especially in Africa. Some cancer registries, e.g., Kyadondo county in Uganda, record only histologically confirmed cases.[11] For others, though population based, e.g., Bamako in Mali,[12] the proportion of histologically confirmed cases is rather low by the accepted standards of developed countries. There are several possible reasons to account for this shortfall. First, the autopsy rates are low in some countries for religious and cultural reasons. Second, histopathological facilities are inadequate and are often located only in university teaching hospitals. Third, because of the costs incurred, most clinicians opt for simpler diagnostic techniques, e.g., α-fetoprotein (AFP) estimation for liver cancer. Fourth, most patients in the tropics present at an advanced stage of their illness, when therapeutic intervention is less important and histological diagnosis becomes an academic exercise. Lastly, for some tumours, such as liver cancer, therapeutic nihilism still prevails and once a clinical diagnosis is suspected the patient is not likely to be referred to a centre where the diagnosis will be confirmed and registered.

Cancer control and prevention

Cancer control is the application of existing knowledge covering the whole spectrum of approaches designed to actively prevent, cure or manage cancer. The aim of a national cancer control programme is to reduce morbidity and mortality due to cancer and to improve the quality of life of cancer patients. Treating cancer is an expensive, high-technology process that few tropical countries can afford.[3] Prevention must therefore be their primary focus. Fortunately in the tropics, a number of cancers are amenable to primary and secondary prevention. Liver cancer is mostly due to hepatitis B virus. An effective and affordable vaccine is available and is currently undergoing clinical trial in The Gambia to assess its efficacy in preventing chronic liver disease and hopefully primary liver cancer.[13] Given the fact that cancer of the uterine cervix is the most common cancer in the tropics, consideration must be given to prevention of this cancer by screening. The principles of screening are outlined on Table 36.3. Cancer of the cervix meets most of the required guidelines. It must, however, be stressed that there is no point setting up a screening programme unless there are facilities in place to diagnose and to treat cases identified through screening.

Table 36.3 Principles of screening.

1. The disease should be an important health problem
2. Its natural history should be well understood
3. It should be recognizable at an early stage
4. Early-stage treatment must be more beneficial than late-stage treatment
5. A suitable test exists to detect the disease at an early stage
6. The test should be acceptable to the general population
7. Adequate facilities must exist for diagnosis and treatment of cases identified
8. Benefit from screening must outweigh any possible physical or psychological harm
9. The benefits must clearly outweigh the costs involved

AIDS-associated tumours

The three malignancies that are currently AIDS defining are Kaposi's sarcoma, non-Hodgkin's lymphoma (NHL) and invasive cancer of the uterine cervix. The increased incidence of KS among homosexual men in the USA led to the recognition of AIDS, and KS became AIDS defining in 1981. Lymphoma is a relatively late manifestation and became AIDS defining in 1985. Cancer of the uterine cervix was added to the list of AIDS-defining conditions in 1993. With increased survival of AIDS patients, the incidence of malignancies can be expected to increase over time.

In tropical Africa the commonest HIV-associated cancers are KS, NHL, squamous cell carcinoma of the conjunctiva and possibly cancer of the uterine cervix. While the incidence of KS is on the decline in the industrialized countries, it continues to rise exponentially in tropical Africa. Even within the African tropical belt, the incidence of HIV-associated KS varies tremendously. The incidence of KS is relatively low in West Africa, while in East and Central Africa, by comparison, it is staggeringly high (Table 36.4). KS is now the commonest male tumour in East and Central Africa, and is second only to cancer of the cervix in females. KS is also the commonest childhood tumour in some African countries, notably Zimbabwe.[14] This is the result of the vertical HIV transmission from mother to child. In addition, children infected with HIV may have an increased risk of developing a variety of smooth muscle tumours that do not commonly arise in the setting of other immunodeficiency diseases.[15] Leiomyosaracoma[16] is particularly common and, given the low incidence of this tumour in the paediatric age group, its association with HIV is unlikely to be fortuitous. In Africa the increase in NHL has been modest. The ASR for NHL is 3.2/100 000 men and 2.6/100 000 women in Uganda. In Zimbabwe the corresponding figures for men and women are 4.5 and

Table 36.4 Age-standardized rates of Kaposi's sarcoma in some selected central, east and west African countries.

Registry source	Country	Year	Rates/100 000 population	
			Male	Female
Abidjan	Ivory Coast	1995–1997	2.2	0.7
Bamako	Mali	1987–1996	1.9	0.5
National	Gambia	1988–1997	0.4	0.1
Blantyre	Malawi	1994–1998	39.8	17.1
Kyadondo	Uganda	1991–1997	39.8	20.0
Harare	Zimbabwe	1990–1995	38.5	14.1

3.8/100 000 population, respectively.[14] HIV-associated NHL is of B cell origin in 80–90% of cases and is either intermediate grade, diffuse large cell, high-grade immunoblastic, or small non-cleaved NHL (Burkitt's or non-Burkitt's type). About 80% have systemic 'B' symptoms of fever, diaphoresis and cachexia and 60–90% have extranodal disease, while about 36% present with primary central nervous system involvement. Squamous cell carcinoma of the conjunctiva was rare in the pre-AIDS era. The risk has increased 10-fold in HIV-positive subjects. The ASR in Uganda in 1960–1971 was 0.2/100 000 men and 0/100 000 women. In 1995, the ASR for men was 2.1 and 2.3/100 000 women.[17] In Zimbabwe the ASR is 0.9/100 000 men and 1.5/100 000 women.[18]

While cancer of the uterine cervix remains the commonest cancer afflicting women in most of tropical Africa, there is as yet no evidence of increased incidence over time. However, since both cancer of the cervix and HIV are common, by coincidence alone a large number of women can be expected to have both afflictions concurrently.

The rest of this chapter will discuss only some of the common tumours encountered in the tropics. The choice for inclusion is based on the frequency, whether it is preventable and whether there is a lesson to learn from the tumour in question.

Cancer of the uterine cervix

(See also Chapter 25)

Cancer of the cervix is the most common cancer affecting women in the tropics. About 80% of the 500 000 cases diagnosed globally every year are in the developing countries.[19] In Latin America and the Caribbean, cancer of the cervix is considered to be the leading cause of death among women. It is estimated that approximately 1 in every 1000 women aged 30–55 years will develop cervical cancer every year. The rates are particularly high in Brazil, Columbia, Chile, Costa Rica and the Indian subcontinent, with rates ranging from 35.1 to 48.2/100 000.[20] Similar ASR are quoted for Africa, namely 53.8/100 000 in Harare, Zimbabwe (1993–1995), 43.6/100 000 in Kyadondo, Kampala, Uganda (1989–1991) and 46.0/100 000 in Guinea, Conakry (1992–1995).[14] In Africa the situation has generally

been described as tragic.[21] The disease affects young premenopausal women in over 50% of cases. More often than not there is considerable delay in diagnosis and most centres lack appropriate treatment facilities. Recent studies in Kenya,[22] Nigeria,[23] Tanzania[24] and Zimbabwe[25] all confirm these observations.

Aetiology

The relationship between cancer of the cervix and sexual behaviour is well established.[26] The most important factors are age at first intercourse and the number of sexual partners. Many studies show a two- to threefold increased risk in women with more than one partner.[27] Cancer of the cervix is far more common in married than unmarried women, and multiple live births seem to increase the risk. The role of the male partner is increasingly being recognized.[28,29] In addition, there are some non-sexual factors, notably smoking and oral contraceptive pill use, that seem to play an important role. The relative risk increases up to 13-fold in smokers when compared to non-smokers, even after correcting for sexual characteristics.[30] The exact role of smoking and oral contraceptives is still debatable[31,32] and this is particularly so in the tropics,[33] where female smoking and oral contraceptive use are recent introductions in lifestyle and behaviour. The observed increased incidence of cervical carcinoma in renal allograft recipients[34] and inpatients with Hodgkin's disease[35] suggests a potential role of immunosuppression. However, the role of HIV immunosuppression in the development of cervical intraepithelial neoplasia (CIN) and the role of HIV in invasive cancer of the cervix remains unclear. Although invasive squamous cell carcinoma of the cervix was added to the Centers for Disease Control (CDC) AIDS definition in 1993,[36] the situation in Africa is far from clear. In most developing countries, and especially in sub-Saharan Africa, both HIV and cancer of the cervix are very common and by coincidence alone up to 35% of patients can have both. However, in such situations cervical carcinoma tends to run a rapid downhill course.

Exposure to sexually transmitted agent or agents has been in the limelight for over three decades. Initial interest in the 1970s focused on herpes simplex virus type 2 (HSV-2). It was suggested that HSV-2 might be the initiating agent.[37] More recently human papilloma virus

(HPV) (especially HPV types 16 and 18) has emerged as the putative transmissible factor for cancer of the cervix.[38,39] HPV is a double-stranded DNA virus and is found in 95% of cervical condylomata acuminata. The evidence for incriminating HPV is based on clinical observations and molecular biological investigations.[40] Numerous studies have found HPV DNA in cervical cancer tissues. HPV is well known for its ability to immortalize cells in vitro. HPV-16/18 infection rates appear to be higher in Latin America (32%) than in Germany (2–13%) or Denmark (6–13%). A case–control study in Latin America revealed that cervical infection with HPV-16, -18 or both was strongly associated with cervical carcinoma. HPV DNA was detected by filter in situ hybridization in 62% of the cases, and 32% of age, sex and behavioral matched controls. The relative risk for cancer of the cervix in the presence of HPV DNA increases from twofold to almost 10-fold with increasing intensity of the hybridization reaction and this increase persists even after adjusting for other major risk factors. Latin America has the highest recorded incidence rates for cancer of the cervix. These and other observations provide circumstantial evidence for the hypothesis that HPV is an aetiological agent in cancer of the cervix.

Certain histological variants seem to be associated with specific HPV types. HPV-16 appears commonly in squamous cell carcinoma, while HPV-18 is seen frequently in adenocarcinomas.

Using Southern blot hybridization or the more sensitive polymerase chain reaction (PCR) techniques HPV DNA was detected in almost 85% of tumours. PCR is an in vitro DNA amplification technique capable of 100 000-fold amplification of specific DNA sequences using heat-stable DNA polymerase. In about 15% of cervical cancer cases HPV DNA sequences cannot be detected. There are several possible explanations. First, HPV may only play a role in the early intraepithelial stages of tumour development and the viral DNA sequences may get lost at later stages of disease progression.[41] Second, metastatic disease spread may also lead to loss of viral DNA sequences.[41,42] Third, it is possible some cervical cancers are associated with HPV types only remotely related to the known genital HPVs and are undetected by the currently available diagnostic methods. Lastly, a proportion of cancers may indeed develop independently of any HPV infection.

Staging

The staging system in wide use is the one recommended by the International Federation of Gynecology and Obstetrics (FIGO) (Table 36.5).

Pretreatment evaluation and assignment of stage, in addition to history and physical examination, must include pelvic examination under anaesthesia, chest X-ray, intravenous pyelography, barium enema, cystoscopy and/or sigmoidoscopy. The stage is determined clinically and does not change on the basis of surgical findings. A recent study using computed tomography (CT) and magnetic resonance imaging (MRI) to determine the utility of these imaging techniques in detecting local or regional metastasis concluded that the 60% accuracy was too low to warrant routine use of these tests for staging.[43] The majority of patients present with advanced disease

Table 36.5 FIGO staging of carcinoma of the uterine cervix: 1988 update.

Stage	Characteristics
0	*Carcinoma in situ, intraepithelial carcinoma* (cases of stage 0 should be included in statistics for invasive carcinoma)
I	*Carcinoma strictly confined to the cervix*
I-A1	Minimal, microscopically evident carcinoma of the cervix
I-A2	Lesion detected microscopically that can be measured. The lesion must invade less than 5 mm below the base of the surface or glandular epithelium and extend to no more than 7 mm in the horizontal plane
I-B	Lesions larger than stage I-A2. Preformed space involvement should not alter the staging but should be recorded
II	*Carcinoma extends beyond the cervix* but does not reach the pelvic wall. The carcinoma involves the vagina, but not the lower third
II-A	No obvious parametrical involvement
II-B	Obvious parametrical involvement
III	*Carcinoma extends to the pelvic wall.* On rectal examination there is no cancer-free space between the tumour and the pelvic wall. The tumour involves the lower third of the vagina. All cases with hydronephrosis or non-functional kidney should be included unless known to be due to other causes
III-A	No extension to the pelvic wall
III-B	Extension to the pelvic wall
IV	*Carcinoma extending beyond the true pelvis* or clinically involving the mucosa of the bladder or rectum
IV-A	Spread to adjacent organs
IV-B	Spread to distant organs

stage, with 80–90% being stages III and IV as observed in a number of African studies.[22–25] The full prestaging protocol proposed tends to be time consuming and expensive. A cost-effective protocol which omits some investigations without harming patients has been proposed for developing countries.[44]

Prognostic factors

The most reliable prognostic factors are stage at diagnosis, nodal status and size and grade of differentiation of primary tumour.[41] In addition HPV-negative tumours have a significantly worse overall recurrence rate (2.6 × higher risk of recurrence) than HPV-positive patients. Relapse-free survival at 24 months is of the order of 77% for HPV-positive patients and only 40% for the HPV-negative group. HPV-negative tumours have significantly (4.5 ×) higher risk of distant metastases than HPV-positive tumours. It would thus appear that HPV-negative cancers may represent a biologically distinct subset of tumours that are more aggressive and carry poorer prognosis than HPV-positive cancers.[41,45,46]

Prevention

Cancer of the cervix is a preventable disease. The process of carcinogenesis from induction to development of invasive cancer is approximately 10 years. Precancerous changes can be detected several years before the development of invasive cancer by a simple test, the Papanicolaou (Pap) test, named after its developer Dr George N. Papanicolaou. Early detection by Pap test (screening) if properly organized and executed has been shown to save lives.[47–49] The evidence in support of the beneficial effect of Pap screening is based on retrospective analysis. In the two Scandinavian countries of Sweden and Finland, which implemented country-wide screening with a coverage of >80% of the women, there was a significant reduction in the mortality and morbidity of cervical cancer. No such reduction was noted in Norway, which only covered about 5% of the population screened. Similar reduction in mortality and morbidity, as in Sweden and Finland, have been observed in Iceland and the Canadian Province of British Columbia, where country- or province-wide screening was undertaken. The test is reasonably sensitive but does occasionally produce abnormal results (false positive) in the absence of disease and normal findings (false negative) in women who subsequently are found to have disease. Furthermore, screening programmes tend to attract married healthy women, particularly those in the higher socio-economic groups, while the women most at risk are habitually missed. There is, in addition, lack of international agreement on the age range for screening and the frequency for such screening. The most cost-effective interval for Pap smear screening remains unknown. However, some groups, notably the American College of Obstetricians and Gynecologists and the American Cancer Society, recommend annual screening to begin either at 18 years

of age or when a woman becomes sexually active. If three or more consecutive such examinations are normal the interval can be lengthened. Considerable disquiet is growing in some circles about the possibility that cervical screening may actually cause psychological harm by engendering anxiety.[50]

It has also been suggested by others that cervical screening is not cost 'effective'.[51] Most of these observations do reflect Western culture where cancer of the cervix is not common and it would therefore cost exorbitant sums of money to identify one case. The situation in the tropics is clearly different, and although cost–benefit analyses have not been systematically undertaken the sheer numbers of victims would suggest that screening should be advocated. What is needed is proper education of the population in question and the installation of appropriate treatment facilities to handle the cases identified. It is, however, disheartening to observe that many cytological screening programmes set up in Africa have either collapsed or do not function properly. It is therefore imperative that any projected schemes undertake very careful study and analysis of current failures.

Management

Cervical screening, if successfully carried out, will reduce the incidence of clinically invasive squamous cell carcinoma and thus lower morbidity and mortality.[48]

Cancer in situ (stage 0) is best treated by abdominal hysterectomy, with or without vaginal cuff. If the patient wishes to retain fertility and she can be relied upon to return for regular review, then a cone biopsy may be adequate. The outcome for stage 0 is excellent, with less than 2% of patients developing recurrent cancer in situ or invasive carcinoma.[52] The treatment of stage I-A with minimal invasion is similar to that for stage 0. For stages I-B and II-A the treatment is either surgery (radical hysterectomy and pelvic lymphadenectomy) or radiotherapy, which consists of external beam irradiation and brachytherapy (temporary insertion of intrauterine and vaginal colpostats loaded with isotope, usually caesium-137). Surgery is the preferred approach for younger women who wish to retain ovarian function and avoid vaginal irradiation, which may result in stenosis. Radiotherapy is to be recommended for patients who are elderly and/or have surgical contraindications. The survival for the two approaches (radiation and surgery) is about equivalent, with survival at 5 years ranging from 80% to 90% under ideal conditions. Stages II-B and III patients are to be considered for radical hysterectomy and pelvic lymphadenectomy or external beam irradiation (4500–5500 cGy) followed by intracavitary brachytherapy. Patients with locally invasive stage IV-A or recurrence after radiotherapy may be considered for pelvic exenteration. Down-staging for patients with locally advanced disease is being advocated.

Role of chemotherapy

The main cause of death among women with cancer of

the cervix is uncontrolled disease within the pelvis. The use of chemotherapy has several theoretical advantages. Given in a neoadjuvant fashion, it may result in down-staging and may facilitate surgical resection or enhance the effect of radiation. Chemotherapy may also act as radiation sensitizer if used concurrently with radio-therapy. The possible mechanisms include: (a) the inhibition of repair of radiation-induced damage, (b) the promotion of synchronization of cells into radio-sensitive phase of the cell cycle, and (c) the reduction of the hypoxic cell fraction that is known to be radio-resistant.

A number of randomized phase III trials have recently been published which support the use of chemotherapy for various stages of locally advanced cervical carcinoma. In one study a group of patients with bulky (> 4 cm in diameter) node-negative, stage I-B were randomized to either receive radiation alone, or radiation together with 40 mg/m^2 of cisplatin given weekly for the 6 weeks of radiation. This phase was followed 3–6 weeks later by adjuvant hysterectomy. The relative risk of progression was 0.51 (95% confidence interval, 0.34–0.75) $p < 0.001$ and the overall survival was 0.54 (95% confidence interval, 0.34–0.86) $p = 0.008$, both favouring combined treat-ment. As expected, there were more transient grades 3 and 4 haematological toxicity (21% versus 2%), and more gastrointestinal effects (14% versus 5%) in the combined treatment arm.[53] Another study was reported by Rose et al.,[54] which included previously untreated invasive squa-mous, adenosquamous or adenocarcinoma stages II-B, III or IV-A without pelvic node involvement. Patients with adequate marrow reserve (WBC $> 3 \times 10^9$/litre, platelets $> 100 \times 10^9$/litre) and good renal function (creatinine < 177 µmol/litre) were randomized in addition to radiotherapy to receive one of three treatment arms as follows:

Group I: received cisplatin at 40 mg/m^2 weekly for 6 weeks;
Group II: received 50 mg/m^2 of cisplatin on days 1 and 29, plus 4 g/m^2 of 5-fluorouracil via a 96-hour infusion on days 1 and 29, plus 2 g/m^2 of hydroxyurea twice weekly for 6 weeks;
Group III: received 3 g/m^2 twice weekly of hydroxyurea for six weeks. After a median follow-up of 35 months, the cisplatin-containing regimens, namely Groups I and II, had significantly higher progression-free survival ($p < 0.001$) and overall survival than the hydroxyurea arm.[54]

The results of these and other studies led the United States National Cancer Institute to issue rare clinical announcements to the effect that 'strong considertion should be given to the inclusion of concurrent cisplatin-based chemotherapy with radiation therapy in women who require radiation therapy for treatment of cervical cancer'.[55]

The situation in Africa and most developing countries is such that the recommendations highlighted above may be inappropriate. Most patients present with disease at very advanced stage when even pelvic exenteration may not be possible. In many situations neither radio-therapy nor chemotherapy is available. Survival is diffi-cult to ascertain as default rate is high. Most patients request for discharge to try alternative forms of therapy.[23] Such pathetic situations underscore the need to develop comprehensive palliative care services, including pain control.

Hepatocellular carcinoma

(See also Chapters 10 and 40)

Primary liver cancer includes hepatocellular carcinoma (HCC), which is very common, cholangiocellular carci-noma, which is rare, and angiosarcoma of the liver, which is very rare. This discussion will concentrate on HCC only. HCC is among the 10 most common cancers worldwide.[2] It is estimated that there are at least 260 000 new cases every year; the majority of these are to be found in sub-Saharan Africa, South-East Asia and the western Pacific. In Shanghai the incidence rate is 34.4/100 000 males and 11.6/100 000 females. In the Philippines the figures quoted are 17.5/100 000 males and 7.1/100 000 females.[20] In sub-Saharan Africa, primary liver cancer has, until the emergence of AIDS-associated Kaposi's sarcoma, been the most common cancer affecting men. The highest recorded incidence rate is in Mozambique, among the Mozambican Shangaans, and HCC accounts for > 2/3 of all male and 1/3 of female tumours, with an incidence rate of over 100/100 000 population.[56] A more recent survey in Mozambique recorded incidence rates ranging from 9.3 to 60.7/100 000 males and from 3.7 to 13.0/100 000 females.[57] The striking feature was the high rates in the very young, with estimated crude rates for those aged 20–29 years being 82.2/100 000 and for those aged 30–39 being 85.8/100 000. The incidence rates for other African countries are shown in Table 36.6.[12]

By contrast, HCC is uncommon in northern India (1.4/100 000 annually in Bombay), although proportional frequencies suggest the tumour is more common in the

Table 36.6 Incidence rates of liver cancer in several African countries.[12]

Country	Years	Incidence per 100 000 Male	Female
Gambia	1986–88	33.1	12.6
Guinea (Conakry)	1992–95	32.8	12.5
Mali (Bamako)	1988–92	51.1	21.4
Nigeria (Ibadan)	1960–69	10.4	3.9
Uganda (Kampala)	1989–91	7.5	3.2
Senegal (Dakar)	1969–74	25.6	9.0
Swaziland	1979–83	10.5	3.0
Zimbabwe (Harare)	1993–95	30.2	12.3

southern part of the subcontinent. Rates intermediate between those of the Far East and those of Europe and North America are reported in countries of the Middle East, the Caribbean and parts of South America.

Aetiology

HCC is multifactorial in aetiology and causal factors differ in different parts of the world. Hepatitis B virus (HBV) is believed to play a causal role in about 80% of patients with HCC worldwide.[58] In low-risk populations about one-half of HCC cases in men and one-third in women can be attributed to a viral aetiology.[59] The non-viral aetiological factors associated with HCC are aflatoxin, cigarette smoking, oral contraceptives and alcohol ingestion.

Hepatitis B virus

About 80% of HCCs result from infection with HBV, a virus which causes other liver ailments as well, and is second only to tobacco as a known single cause of cancer. The evidence for its causal role in HCC is derived from epidemiological case–control and cohort studies, clinical data and laboratory investigations. Follow-up of patients with chronic liver disease associated with HBV markers indicate that hepatitis B surface antigen (HBsAg)-positive individuals with chronic hepatitis and/or cirrhosis have a greater risk of developing HCC. Retrospective investigations of HBV serum markers show a substantially higher rate in patients who subsequently develop HCC than in controls. The most convincing epidemiological evidence, however, comes from the prospective case–control surveillance of 22 000 middle-aged Chinese males in Taiwan observed for 75 000 man-years of follow-up. In the 15% who were HBsAg carriers there was a 223-fold excess risk of HCC over the non-carriers.[60] Molecular biology studies show HBV DNA integration in tissues of patients with chronic hepatitis and HCC. The process of integration makes the elimination of HBV DNA in chronic carriers impossible. Integration of HBV DNA into human hepatocytes was first detected in a continuous cell line expressing HBsAg derived from a male HBV carrier with HCC. HBV DNA is now known to be incorporated into the host genome of HCC patients whether they have evidence of viral infection or not.[61,62] However, the existence of low-incidence regions of HCC despite a high prevalence of HVB infection may indicate that HBV infection acting alone may have little carcinogenic effect and that it may need to be potentiated by another factor or factors.

Although HCC and HBV are closely associated, some patients with HCC have no serological evidence of past or active HBV infection. Tissue from 75–100% of patients with HCC who have no serological marker of HBV have no HBV DNA detected by hybridization studies and 50–90% have no HBV DNA detectable by PCR. In Japan and in Europe 54–69% of patients with HCC without serological markers for HBV have antibodies to hepatitis C virus (HCV). Seven well-documented cases have been reported in which chronic non-A, non-B hepatitis (HCV) had been prospectively followed and had progressed to HCC.[63] Cirrhosis is found in 86–100% of anti-HCV-positive HCC patients. The mechanism of oncogenesis for HCV is not clear as available data indicate lack of HCV integration in the host cell. Although it was previously felt that blood transfusion was the major mode of transmission, available evidence currently indicates that over 90% of anti-HCV-positive blood donors have no history of having received transfusions. It is currently estimated that over 50% of HCC diagnosed annually in Japan is probably HCV related.[62] The role of HCV in the tropics is entirely unknown but probably minimal.

Aflatoxin

Aflatoxin was first isolated in 1961 following an outbreak of fatal jaundice in turkeys. The 'turkey-X' disease was traced to poultry feed containing peanuts imported from Brazil contaminated with *Aspergillus flavus*. Subsequently aflatoxin B (so called because of its blue fluorescence) was found to be potently hepatotoxic and carcinogenic in a variety of animal species. Aflatoxins are a group of compounds produced by the mould *A. flavus*, which grows readily in warm, humid conditions. Although groundnuts are the substrate of choice for the mould, it can grow on other cereals, notably maize, millet, peas and sorghum.

People in some areas of the tropical world are frequently exposed to food contaminated with aflatoxin. In Mozambique 8% of prepared meal samples contain measurable aflatoxin. The average contamination level is 38.1 µg/kg wet food. The aflatoxin levels in food samples observed in Mozambique are the highest in the world.[57] In the Transkei the frequency of food sample contamination is much higher (25%) but the level of contamination is much lower than that in Mozambique.

The carcinogenic risk of aflatoxin has been evaluated and reported.[64] Laboratory research has demonstrated the hepatocarcinogenic properties of aflatoxin.[65,66] There is a clear correlation between HCC and the rate of aflatoxin ingestion (Table 36.7).[57,67,68] Further confirmation of an aetiological role for aflatoxin in HCC has come from a case–control study in the Philippines where the mean contamination level of different dietary items was established and individual levels of consumption determined retrospectively.[69] Studies in Kenya[70] and Thailand have more or less found similar results. In Egypt, a country with a very low level of aflatoxin contamination because the climate is hot and dry, the incidence of HCC is relatively low. In Botswana, which is very dry, and Greenland, which is very cold, the incidence of HCC is low and presumably *A. flavus* growth in such unfavourable climates is inhibited.

The mechanism of carcinogenesis is not well understood, but several plausible explanations have been suggested. Aflatoxin B is metabolized by a microsomal mixed function oxidase system to produce aflatoxin B-2,3-epoxide, which is believed to be the carcinogen.[71] It

Table 36.7 Aflatoxin ingestion and hepatocellular carcinoma in different countries.[57]

Country	Location	Aflatoxin B$_1$ ingestion (µg/kg)	HCC rate/100 000 per year
Kenya	High altitude	3.5	1.2
	Middle altitude	5.9	2.5
	Low altitude	10.0	4.0
Swaziland	High veld	5.1	2.2
	Middle veld	8.9	3.8
	Low veld	43.1	9.2
Mozambique	Inhambene	77.7	12.1
	Homoine-Maxixe	131.4	17.7
	Zavala	183.7	14.0

has also been suggested that aflatoxin may suppress cell-mediated immunity and facilitate persistent HBV infection and eventually HCC.[72] There is a suggestion that aflatoxin only accumulates in the liver after the liver's ability to degrade aflatoxin has been impaired by persistent HBV infection.[73]

Cigarette smoking

Cigarette smoking has only recently permeated rural developing countries. Its impact on HCC must therefore be minimal. Where studies have been done, as in South African blacks, the evidence supports the conclusion that cigarette smoking plays no aetiological role in HCC in South Africa.[74] In low-risk areas of the world, cigarette smoking is a significant risk factor with a relative risk ratio of greater than 2.[75]

Alcohol

It is estimated that heavy alcohol consumption is another risk factor, especially in the low incidence areas. HCC is almost fivefold as common in men who imbibe more than 80 g of ethanol per day than in non-drinkers.[75] However, in tropical countries most HCCs are associated with macronodular post-hepatitic rather than micronodular alcoholic cirrhosis.[76] There is very little evidence to implicate alcohol as playing a role in high-incidence areas of HCC. A case–control study in South Africa gave no indication that alcohol could be incriminated as a risk factor.[77]

Oral contraceptive use

The use of oral contraceptive pills has been shown to be significantly related to HCC in women, with a 5.5-fold increase in relative risk[75] in those women using it for over 5 years. Like cigarette smoking, the use of oral contraceptives is only beginning to take root in rural tropical areas and their impact on the incidence of HCC, though largely undetermined, must be minimal. Earlier reports suggested that oral contraceptives mostly caused liver adenomas, although some have transformed into carcinomas. The mechanism whereby oestrogens, including those used in oral contraceptive pills, cause cancer is not clearly understood, although it has been suggested that they may be powerful promoters of hepatocarcinogenesis in laboratory animals.[78]

Clinical features

HCC presents with right upper quadrant pain or discomfort, abdominal mass and distension. Physical examination reveals hepatomegaly in 90% of cases, wasting and ascites in 50%. Abdominal venous collaterals, if looked for, occur in 30% and icterus in 25%. A few patients may present with pathological fractures due to bone metastases. In Uganda, bone is the second most common site of metastases in HCC. Some patients have marked itching due to obstructive jaundice and about 10% may present with haematemesis and melaena following rupture of oesophageal varices in cases of advanced cirrhosis. Elevated alkaline phosphatase is detected in 75% of cases and AFP is above the normal level in 60%.

HCC affects young individuals, with remarkably high rates in the 10–29-year age group in Mozambique.[57] In Uganda the peak incidence is observed during the third and fourth decades. The male:female ratio is 2–4:1. The clinical diagnosis of HCC in the tropics is relatively simple. This is because other tumours likely to metastasize to the liver are relatively rare. Thus in the tropics any young adult male presenting with abdominal pain and mass and found to have hepatomegaly has HCC until otherwise proven. If alkaline phosphatase is elevated this raises the suspicion even further. A positive AFP almost certainly confirms the diagnosis. However, if an intervention is contemplated a needle biopsy is recommended. The most common differential diagnosis in the tropics is an amoebic liver abscess.

Prognosis

HCC in the tropics runs a fulminant downhill course. The mean interval from onset to death in South African patients was 11 weeks.[79] In a study which included Algerian and French patients, the mean survival time of untreated patients was 73 days, suggesting the natural history of French patients may be similar to African and Asian

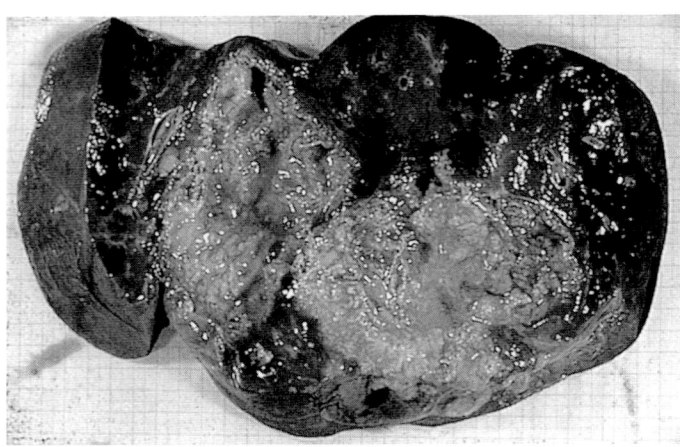

Figure 36.1: Hepatocellular carcinoma. Mass in liver.

patients with HCC.[80] Most patients present with a very advanced single massive tumour when first seen (Figure 36.1).

The fibrolamellar variant of HCC,[81] which occurs primarily in the young (peak in second to third decade), affects both male and female patients with non-cirrhotic livers and is rarely associated with positive AFP but has a good prognosis (average survival 44 months), is extremely rare in the tropics. No case of fibrolamellar HCC has been seen in South African blacks.[82]

Signs of poor prognosis include wasting, abdominal venous collaterals, ascites, elevated bilirubin and encephalopathy.[80,83–85]

Management

The treatment of HCC remains unsatisfactory. Surgical resection provides the only prospect for cure. However, less than 2% present at a stage when this approach is feasible. Even apparently early cases have advanced cirrhosis and recurrence in the remaining lobe after apparently curative resection is the rule rather than the exception.

The goal of treating most patients with HCC is palliation. Hepatic artery ligation is an effective way of relieving symptoms, especially pain and in individuals who have had spontaneous intraperitoneal rupture, a common complication.[86] The rationale is based on the observation that liver tumours (primary and secondary) derive their blood supply from the hepatic artery, while normal liver is supplied from both the hepatic artery and the portal vein. Before hepatic artery ligation can be recommended the patency of the portal vein must be established.

Radiation therapy is rarely recommended because liver tissue is extremely sensitive even to low-dose radiation. However, ^{90}Y-labelled microspheres are undergoing clinical trials.

Chemotherapy appears to be an effective form of palliation. The best single agent seems to be the anthracycline doxorubicin.[85,87] The overall response rate is of the order of about 40%. A recent multicentre study conducted under the auspices of the African Organization for Research and Training in Cancer (AORTIC) showed that epirubicin and doxorubicin were equally efficacious, although the latter was more toxic (C. F. Kiire, personal communications).

Several drug combinations have been tried, with disappointing results.[87,88] The combination of doxorubicin and cisplatin has been reported to result in a dramatic response, although it was complicated by the reactivation of hepatitis B infection.[89]

It should be stressed that in tropical areas the goal of treatment of HCC is to relieve symptoms and therefore the patient's quality of life is paramount. A recently completed quality of life-focused randomized clinical trial in Zimbabwe concluded that chemotherapy with doxorubicin, either at conventional monthly or weekly low doses, did not improve the quality of life or survival of patients so treated.[90]

Prevention

Since 80% of HCC is attributed to HBV infection and an effective vaccine against the virus is now available, the prospect for cancer prevention is certainly in sight.[91] A vaccination trial sponsored by the World Health Organization was started in 1986 in The Gambia, West Africa, to determine its efficacy in preventing chronic liver disease and HCC in particular.[13] As HBV transmission in Africa occurs by horizontal spread, with a second wave of infection occurring at the time of school entry (5–6 years), it is possible to include HBV vaccine in the expanded programme of immunization. A pilot study started in the villages of Keneba and Manduar in Gambia in 1984 revealed that the overall vaccine efficacies in 1993 against HBV infection was about 95%. Despite rapidly falling antibody concentration in vaccinated children and the presence of viral variants, the efficacy of HBV vaccination against HBV and HbsAg carrier was maintained.[92] In unvaccinated children in the Far East, early infection with HBV leading to a carrier state results from vertical perinatal transmission from replicative carrier mothers. To prevent this, the first dose of the vaccine must be given soon after birth. This approach has greatly reduced the carriage rate in Asian children.

Screening using modern imaging techniques, CT and ultrasonography, as well as serial AFP testing, has been tried[93] but this approach is clearly not cost effective in many tropical countries.

Cancer of the oesophagus

(See also Chapter 10)

Apart from the French provinces of Brittany and Normandy, which have incidence rates in excess of 80/100 000 population, cancer of the oesophagus is relatively rare in most of Europe. Outside Europe, high rates are recorded in Linxian in northern China, in the province of Mazandarin in Iran on the Caspian sea, in east, central and southern Africa, India and Central America. In Linxian province of the Peoples' Republic of China the incidence rate is 130/100 000 population and oesophageal cancer is second only to stomach cancer as the leading cause of cancer deaths in China, according to the 1974–1976 statistics.

In most tropical areas, cancer of the oesophagus has an uneven geographical distribution. Both rural and urban dwellers appear to be equally affected. In South Africa cancer of the oesophagus was a curiosity in the 1920s but it has now become one of the most common cancers affecting black males.[94,95] The highest rates are recorded in the Transkei: up to 63/100 000 males and 65/100 000 females. More recently, high rates have been recorded in Zimbabwe, Zambia, Malawi, parts of Tanzania and in the region around Kisumu in Kenya. By contrast oesophageal carcinoma appears to be rare in south-west Uganda, Democratic Republic of Congo and in West Africa. In all-high incidence areas there is a strong male dominance but in recent years the tumour has been increasing in frequency in women in South Africa.[96]

Aetiology

Alcohol and tobacco acting together have been established as the major cause of oesophageal cancer in the industrialized world. Epidemiological studies in France show that those who smoke or drink heavily run a 44 times greater risk of oesophageal cancer than light drinkers and smokers. It has been postulated that alcohol might act as a solvent facilitating the passage of carcinogens into the inner layers of the oesophagus. The role of alcohol in the causation of cancer of the oesophagus in developing countries is not clearly documented. In Iran, for instance, it is not the custom of Turkoman people to drink and very few of the oesophageal cancer victims smoke. In China, of 527 patients 83% reported that they did not drink alcohol, and those who drank did so only on rare occasions. In his study in South Africa, Oettle[97] concluded that smoking and alcohol use did not contribute as aetiological agents, and that the major factor appeared to be fortuitous, connected with a common African habit but not fundamental to it. In a more recent study, multiple logistic regression models identified four parameters which best discriminated cases from controls.[98] These were: smoking commercial cigarettes, smoking a pipe, eating bought (commercial) maize and eating butter or margarine. Earlier studies had indicated that 20–30% of oesophageal cancer patients had never smoked.[99] Even more at variance with the usual pattern of risk factors in the West is the apparent lack of appreciable effects of alcohol usage on the disease in Zulus. Observations in South Africa appear to lend support to nutritional predisposing factors to cancer of the oesophagus. Dietary staples appear to be low in vitamins and minerals.[100] In China and Iran oesophageal cancer may also be related to nutritional factors. It has been demonstrated that victims of oesophageal cancer are malnourished and get neither vitamin A nor riboflavine requirements. One study showed over 40% consumed less than 10% in winter and less than 20% in spring and autumn of vitamin A requirements. A deficiency of vitamin A has been shown to lead to carcinogenesis, while an adequate intake of vitamin C has been shown to have an anticarcinogenic effect. In China death from oesophageal cancer has been closely linked with ingestion of pickled vegetables.

In areas of Iran and China at high risk of oesophageal cancer precursor lesions of cancer of the oesophagus have been described as occurring prior to the development of invasive squamous cell carcinoma.[101,102] Unfortunately the addition of riboflavine, retinol and zinc had no effect on the high prevalence of precancerous oesophageal lesions.[103] There are several possible explanations for this negative result. First, the treatment may not have been given for a period long enough or the dosages were not large enough to effect change. Second, the precancerous oesophageal lesions, like gastritis, may be irreversible. Third, the hypothesis linking riboflavine/retinol deficiency with precancerous oesophageal lesions may not be correct.

Clinical features

In high-incidence areas cancer of the oesophagus may be seen in the fourth and fifth decades of life. Men are two to three times more commonly affected, except in northern Iran, where women predominate, and in South Africa, where the frequency in women is on the increase. The disease often becomes symptomatic, with progressive dysphagia and severe weight loss and wasting.

Staging

Pretreatment evaluation for accurate staging should include history, physical examination, barium swallow, upper gastrointestinal endoscopy and biopsy and a CT scan of the thorax and upper abdomen, and endoscopic ultrasound, if available. Direct laryngoscopy and bronchoscopy is advisable. Positron emission tomography (PET) scan has been shown to be a useful adjunct to conventional, non-invasive staging procedure. PET significantly improves the detection of stage IV disease and improves the diagnostic specificity for lymph nodes.[104] However, PET is not available as yet even in many developed country cancer centres. Staging recommended by the American Joint Committee on Cancer (AJCC), as shown in Table 36.8, applies the tumour, node and metastasis (TNM) system. A simplified staging with its TNM equivalent is shown in Table 36.9. The following clinical, radiographic and endoscopic evidence may suggest extension of the cancer outside the oesophagus: (1) recurrent laryngeal, phrenic or sympathetic nerve involvement; (2) fistula formation; (3) tracheal or bronchial tree involvement; (4) vena caval or azygos vein obstruction; and (5) malignant effusion.

Table 36.8 AJCC staging system for cancer of the oesophagus.

Stage	Description
T_x	Minimum requirement to assess primary tumour not met
T_0	No evidence of primary tumour
T_{is}	Cancer in situ
T_1	Involves 5 cm or less of oesophageal length, producing no obstruction and no circumferential involvement and no extraoesophageal spread
T_2	Greater than 5 cm of oesophageal length without extraoesophageal spread or tumour of any size that produces obstruction
T_3	Any tumour with extraoesophageal spread
N_x	Minimum requirement for nodal assessment not met
N_0	No clinically palpable or radiological evidence of nodal involvement
N_1	Movable unilateral palpable nodes or radiological evidence of 1 cm, 5 cm in length; unilateral or bilateral palpable movable nodes
N_2	Movable bilateral palpable or radiological evidence of > 1 cm, < 3 cm diameter nodes
N_3	Fixed palpable nodes > 3 cm on radiology
M_x	Minimum requirement to assess metastases not met
M_0	No evidence of distant metastases
M_1	Distant metastases present

Management

Treatment of patients with oesophageal cancer remains unsatisfactory. The goal of treatment is palliation. There are several possible approaches: surgery, radiotherapy, laser therapy, intubation and combined chemoradiotherapy. Surgical mortality has greatly improved,[105-107] with most series reporting 1–2% mortality. Following 'curative' resection, the 5-year survival ranges from 8% to 22%.[108,109] Improved outlook for surgically treated patients is the result of better preoperative and postoperative care, especially nutritional and respiratory support.

Improvements in the results of radiotherapy have been less impressive. Pearson's[110] results, with survival at 5 years of 25% for cervical, 16% for mid and 12% for lower oesophagus, remain unchallenged in Western countries. Controlled trials comparing radiotherapy with surgery are rare. Radiotherapy on its own or in addition to surgery has not altered prognosis.[111-113] Radiotherapy is frequently chosen as a means of palliation but its effectiveness may be marred by serious complications. These include fistula formation, if the tumour is adherent to the bronchus, and postirradiation stricture.

It is clear that late presentation is the limiting factor in improving results. Intubation should be reserved for patients with advanced disease and limited prognosis. Intubation provides poor palliation. Blockage of the tube is not infrequent and swallowing is far from optimal.

Given the limited usefulness of both surgery[111] and radiotherapy[112] and since systemic disease is a major factor in the failure pattern, there is growing interest in neoadjuvant trials (giving chemotherapy before definitive primary surgery).[114] Animal models have suggested the superiority of giving systemic therapy prior to surgery. In addition, preoperative chemotherapy allows an in vivo assessment of tumour sensitivity to the drugs.

More recently concurrent chemoradiotherapy is being advocated. This was based on promising observations of a similar approach for anal canal and rectal cancers. Preliminary observations reported greatly improved palliation as well as improved 12- and 24-month survival rates using preoperative chemoradiotherapy.[115] At Wayne State University the approach utilized 5-fluorouracil and mitomycin C, later changed to 5-fluorouracil and cisplatin (because of the unpredictable toxicity of mitomycin C), concurrently with radiotherapy.[116,117] The choice of 5-fluorouracil and cisplatin is based on their known antitumour activity in oesophageal cancer and because they are established radiation sensitizers.[118-120] Apart from possible radiosensitization of hypoxic cells, other mechanisms postulated include inhibition of repair of sublethal or potentially lethal damage, increased induction of chromosomal aberrations and binding to thiols. The pathological complete response is about 25–30%. Such combined chemoradiotherapy appears to provide excellent palliation but no studies have been done to assess the quality of life of patients undergoing such treatment. The toxicity encountered includes nausea, vomiting, oesophagitis, mucositis, stomatitis, leucopenia and thrombocytopenia.

Table 36.9 Simplified staging for oesophageal cancer.

Stage	TNM component	Description
0	T_{is}, N_0, M_0	Carcinoma in situ with no invasion or spread
I	T_1, N_0, M_0	Involves < 5 cm of oesophageal length with no spread or obstruction
II	T_1, N_1, M_2, M_0 T_2, N_0, N_2, M_0	Tumour causing obstruction or > 5 cm in length; unilateral or bilateral palpable movable nodes
III	T_3, and N_1, M_0 Any T_1, N_3, M_0	Extraoesophageal spread, fixed palpable nodes, no distant metastases
IV	Any T, and N_1, M_1	Distant metastases

A number of randomized clinical trials assessing the efficacy of preoperative chemoradiotherapy have recently been published. One study by Walsh et al. compared preoperative chemoradiotherapy to surgery alone in 113 patients with adenocarcinoma of the oesophagus.[121] They observed a significantly better median survival and survival at 3 years for the combined modality treatment. The European Organizations for Research and Training in Cancer (EORTC) enrolled 288 patients with squamous cell carcinoma of the oesophagus in a study comparing preoperative chemoradiotherapy to surgery alone.[122] No survival difference was noted. More recently, Urba et al. of the University of Michigan reported no differences in median survival or survival at 3 years.[123] Thus, it would seem the jury is still out for preoperative chemoradiotherapy in patients with oesophageal cancer and this approach remains experimental.

Malignant tumours of the skin (See also Chapter 19)

The skin is sometimes referred to as the window of human biology and pathology because many processes of life are reflected on the body surface. In addition, the skin is the largest organ of the body.

In light-pigmented people, i.e., inhabitants of Europe and North America, exposure to solar ultraviolet light is responsible for the very high incidence of skin cancers such as basal cell and squamous cell cancers and melanomas. Other factors which may influence the frequency and distribution of skin cancers include occupation, clothing, hairstyles and leisure habits, all of which determine the degree of exposure to the ultraviolet component of the sun.

Dark-skinned individuals appear to be well adjusted to the hot tropical environments. The protective and adaptive elements include the increased melanin and the large number of sweat glands. The dark pigment absorbs heat readily, such that 'sunbathing' is not a comfortable activity for dark-skinned people, contrary to the general belief that dark-skinned people enjoy heat! In any case, more suntan is not needed and not prized. Ultraviolet-related skin cancers are commonly observed in individuals with certain genetic abnormalities such as albinism, a group of inherited conditions in which there is a defect in melanin production and metabolism. Decreased pigmentation is particularly noticeable in the skin, hair and eyes. The skin becomes dry and wrinkled on exposure to sunlight. Albinos develop multiple skin tumours (basal cell and squamous cell), usually in the exposed areas of the body (head, neck, ears, conjunctiva and limbs). It is estimated that albinos are 1000 times more likely to develop basal cell cancers than pigmented people. Another genetic disorder associated with skin cancers is xeroderma pigmentosum, an inherited defect of DNA repair following ultraviolet-induced damage.[6,7]

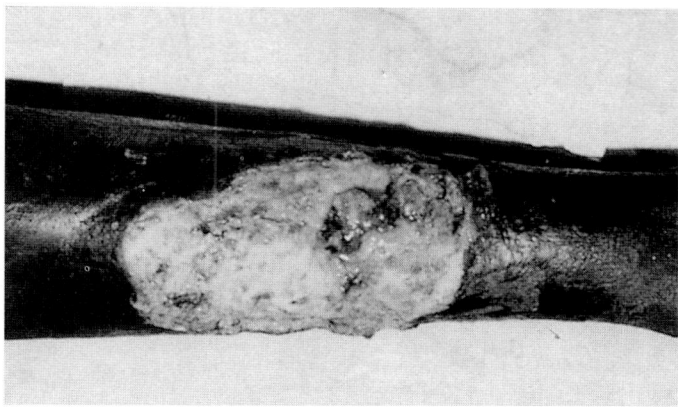

Figure 36.2: Squamous cell carcinoma in long-standing tropical ulcer. (Courtesy of E. H. Williams.)

Squamous cell cancer

Squamous cell cancer of the skin is common in some tropical populations, especially in poverty-stricken rural areas. In the tropics squamous cell cancers are clinically and aetiologically distinct from those seen in Europe. The majority arise in areas of damaged skin, most frequently in scars of long-standing tropical ulcers (Figure 36.2), old burns or epithelialized sinuses. In Uganda the annual incidence of squamous cell cancer is 1.70 men and 1.33 women per 100 000 population; it accounts for 12% of all malignancies. This relative frequency is similar to what has been observed in other tropical areas as far apart as Nigeria in West Africa and the Solomon Islands in the South Pacific. Squamous cell cancer may also occur as a result of certain cultural practices, such as the Kangri cancer of India.

Since about 80% of these cancers are superimposed upon or complicate long-standing tropical ulcers, the increased availability of clean water, soap and to a lesser extent antibiotics may lead to marked decline of these tumours in the tropics. However, once the tumour is established wide surgical excision of the localized lesion remains the treatment of choice. The role of radiotherapy and chemotherapy in the management of these tumours is not well documented.

Malignant melanoma

Malignant melanomas arise from the cells that produce skin pigmentation. Malignant melanomas of the skin occur most commonly in those areas of the world where light-skinned people, by default, live in an environment of abundant sunshine, e.g., Australia, Israel and South Africa. Sunbathing is a popular summer relaxation habit with light-skinned people. The incidence of malignant melanoma has increased 10-fold in the past three to four decades in Western countries, with a lifetime risk in the USA of 1:75, and in Australia of 1:25 individuals. In dark-skinned persons the primary site of malignant melanoma is on the non-pigmented sole of the foot (Figure 36.3) or

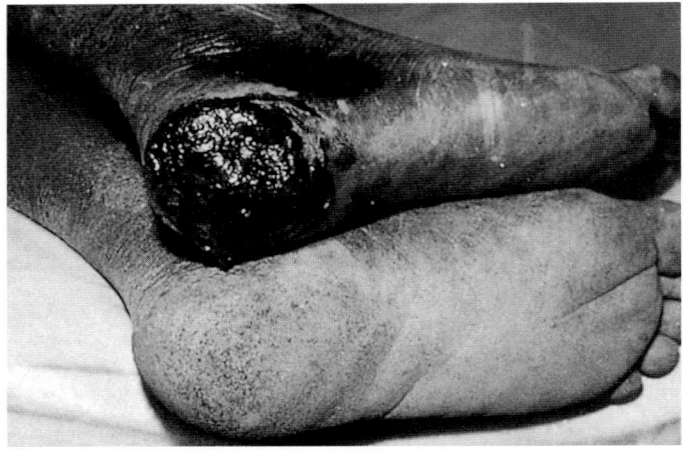

Figure 36.3: Malignant melanoma on sole of foot. (Courtesy of E. H. Williams.)

less commonly on the palmar side of the hands or fingers. It is extremely rare for dark-skinned people to develop melanoma in a pigmented site. If they do there is often preceding vitiligo. Vitiligous patches, if looked for, can often be found concurrently at other sites in dark-skinned patients with malignant melanoma.

It is probable that melanomas arise from pre-existing naevi, but because of the generally dark skin colour, events that predict malignant change may be difficult to observe and overlooked, especially if the primary lesion is located on the sole of the foot. Thus malignant melanoma tends to present at a very advanced stage as an exophytic fungating lesion with or without regional adenopathy. It has been suggested that trauma (physical, chemical or thermal) may play a role in the aetiology of these tumours in the tropics. There has, however, been no reduction of incidence observed among shoe-wearing urban dwellers in the tropics.

There is a clear relationship between thickness of the tumour and survival.[124] Early melanoma is potentially curable by wide excision. In the past the accepted surgical approach was a wide excision with a 5 cm margin. The current trend is towards a narrower margin tailoring to tumour thickness.[125] In general, for tumours less than 1 mm thickness a 1 cm margin is adequate, while 2–3 cm margins are recommended for thicker tumours.

Prognostic factors

The most important predictors of relapse and survival are Breslow's thickness of the primary melanoma, and whether the regional nodes are involved. Tumours with Breslow's thickness greater than 4 mm have 50% risk of recurrence, and individuals with positive nodes have a 60–85% risk of recurrence. A study done at the University of Pretoria in South Africa reveals four factors to be of prognostic importance for patients with metastatic melanoma in univariate analysis. These were performance status, dominant site, number of involved sites and treatment. On multivariate analysis only two (dominant site of disease and treatment) remained significant.[126]

Staging

The AJCC applies the TNM staging system.[127] In 1997 a modification was proposed to the AJCC staging system. T_1 is for 1 mm, T_2 for 2 mm, T_3 up to 4 mm, and T_4 > 4 mm thickness. Subcategory 'a' denotes absence and 'b' presence of ulceration. The proposed changes to the N refers to the number of involved nodes, rather than the diameter of nodes. In this proposal, N_1 refers to one positive node, N_2 for 2–4 nodes, and N_3 for > 4 nodes; subcategory 'a' for microscopic involvement and 'b' for macroscopic involvement; M_{1a} for favourable sites, e.g., skin, nodes, soft tissue, M_{1b} for pulmonary involvement and M_{1c} for patients with elevated LDH.[128]

Elective node dissection

Results of multicentre, randomized trials show no survival advantage for patients with intermediate-thickness melanoma (1–4 mm) undergoing elective node dissection when compared to observation without node dissection.[129] Only 20% of individuals who undergo an elective node dissection are found to have microscopic disease, making the procedure unnecessary in 80%. Sentinel node mapping accurately reflects the presence or absence of disease in 95% of patients. The use of intraoperative gamma probes leads to a high degree of accuracy in identifying sentinel nodes.[130] A negative sentinel node on biopsy is a reliable indicator that the nodal basin in not affected or involved by tumour.

Adjuvant therapy

Individuals often considered for adjuvant therapy are those at high risk of relapse and mortality, namely those with thick primary lesions and those with positive nodes. Several postsurgical adjuvant approaches in the past three decades, including chemotherapy, immune modulation with bacillus Calmette–Guéren (BCG), *Corynebacterium parvum*, levamisole and more recently the use of biological agents, notably interferons. Results were uniformly negative until the recent two large cooperative group trials, which published the results of high-dose interferon-α2b. The first Eastern Cooperative Oncology Group (ECOG) 1684 trial was activated in 1984 and accrued 280 assessable patients from 29 centres. Eligibility criteria included patients with T4 lesions, with or without involved regional nodes. One group received an induction therapy consisting of 20 million units/m^2 i.v. daily for 5 days for 4 weeks and then a maintenance phase of 10 million units/m^2 subcutaneously three times per week for 48 weeks. The control group was observed without active treatment. The median relapse-free survival for interferon-α2b was 1.72 years and was significantly better than 0.98 years for the observation group ($p = 0.0025$). The median survival for the treated group was 3.8 years and for the control group was 2.8 years. A subgroup analysis of node-positive subgroups showed a striking, enhanced effect with interferon resulting in a disease-free survival of 1.7 years, which was significantly better than 0.55 years for the observation group ($p = 0.0004$). The median time to death for the treated group was 3.8 years and 2.06 years for the observation group ($p = 0.0086$). The same impact from adjuvant treatment with interferon-α2b was not observed in the subset of node-negative patients. The toxicity was considerable. Constitutional flu-like symptoms were severe in 5 patients; 7 had severe neurological toxicities and there were 2 deaths from hepatic failure.[131] Based on the results of this study, the Food and Drug Administration (FDA) recommended approval for interferon-α2b for patients with melanomas > 4 mm thick with positive nodes.

In 1991, an intergroup study, E1690, was initiated to confirm the result of E1684, and to test the efficacy of low-dose interferon-α2b. Six hundred and eight eligible patients were randomized to receive either high-dose interferon alfa-2b, as in E1684 or low-dose interferon-α2b, 2 million units subcutaneously three times per week for 2 years, or observation only. After a median follow-up of 52 months, the estimated relapse-free survival at 5 years for high dose was 44%; 40% for low dose and 35% for observation only group. High-dose interferon resulted in significant impact on relapse-free survival, when compared with observation ($p = 0.03$), but there was no significant difference for low-dose interferon. Neither high dose nor low dose had any benefit on overall survival. Several factors may have confounded results of E1690 study. The median survival for the observation group for E1690 was 6 years, as compared to 2.8 years for E1684, so that there may have been a stage migration phenomenon. In trial 1690, lymphadenectomy was not required. Several relapsed patients on low dose or observation were placed on high-dose interferon.

A European study randomized 444 patients to low-dose interferon-α2a, 3 million units subcutaneously three times per week, or to observation for 3 years. There was no significant difference in disease-free survival or overall survival. This and E1690 study clearly indicated the lack of therapeutic advantage of low-dose interferon.

In the ECOG E1694 study 800 patients with resected high-risk melanoma were randomized to a vaccine given subcutaneously weekly for 1 month and then quarterly for 2 years, or high-dose interferon. An interim analysis in April 2000 revealed 151 had relapsed in the vaccine arm and 98 in the high-dose interferon arm. The relapse-free hazard ratio associated with high-dose interferon treatment was 1.47 ($p = 0.0015$). The hazard ratio for overall survival favouring interferon was 1.52 ($p = 0.009$). The data safety board recommended premature closure of the study.

Management of metastatic melanoma

Patients with metastatic disease have a median survival of 6–9 months with only 1–2% having long-term disease-free survival. The goal of treatment is palliative. Chemotherapeutic agents showing antitumour effects are imidazole carboxamide (DTIC), platinum analogues and nitrosoureas. DTIC is the best single agent, with response rates of 15–25%, and complete responses of 2–5% and response duration lasting 4–6 months, and has been the standard chemotherapeutic agent for melanoma.[132] Interferon-α2b leads to response rates of 10–20%. A study comparing DTIC with or without interferon-α2b at doses of 20 mg/m^2 i.v. for 5 days, every 28 days for DTIC, and 15 million units/m^2 i.v. for 5 days for 4 weeks, then 10 million units/m^2 subcutaneously 3 times per week, showed the combination to be significantly better in terms of response rates at 53% (95% CI, 26–72%) for the combination, as opposed to 20% (95% CI, 17–39%) for single agent ($p = 0.007$). Time to relapse was 2.53 months for single agent and 8.96 months for combination.[133] Temozolamide is a novel, oral alkylating agent with a broad spectrum of antitumor activity with relatively little toxicity. Both temozolamide and DTIC are pro-drugs of the active alkylating agent 5-(3-methyltriazen-1-yl) imidazole-4-caraboxamide (MTIC). Temozolamide offers an oral, less toxic alternative to DTIC.[134]

Kaposi's sarcoma (See also Chapter 20)

Kaposi's sarcoma (KS) is a tumour that commonly presents with skin involvement, although visceral and bone tumours are frequently observed. Epidemiologically KS can be classified into sporadic, endemic and epidemic forms (Table 36.10). The sporadic (classic) form represents what was originally described in 1872 by Moricz Kaposi. It is commonly seen in elderly males of Jewish, southern European and Mediterranean origin. The endemic form was described in sub-Saharan Africa, especially in eastern Zaire (now Democratic Republic of Congo) and western Uganda, with decreasing incidence from this 'epicentre'. The epidemic form was first described in the large North American cities of New York and Los Angeles, where the increased incidence of KS among homosexual men led to the recognition of AIDS, and KS became AIDS defining in 1981.

Aggressive forms of KS were observed in Uganda and Zambia at about the same time as the epidemic variety was described in North America. The distribution of AIDS in Africa corresponds closely to that of the endemic pre-epidemic KS. There is often confusion as to the nature of a particular case. In the USA the incidence of KS complicating AIDS is actually on the decline.[135] In most sub-Saharan Africa the incidence continues to rise exponentially. While the reported incidence of KS remains relatively low in West Africa, the incidence in East and Central Africa by comparison is staggeringly high (Table 36.4). In fact, KS is now the commonest male tumour in

Table 36.10 Clinico-epidemiological correlation of Kaposi's sarcoma.

Epidemiology	Clinical Form	Behaviour
Sporadic	Nodular	Indolent
Endemic	Nodular, plaque	Indolent
	Florid, infiltrative	Aggressive
Epidemic (HIV-associated)	Generalized	Fulminant

East and Central Africa, and is second only to cancer of the cervix in females. KS is also the commonest childhood tumour in some African countries, notably Zimbabwe.[14] This is the result of the vertical HIV transmission from mother to child.

Aetiology and pathogenesis

Kaposi's sarcoma is one of the tumours that is known to develop in iatrogenically immunosuppressed renal transplant recipients, where there is an observed 400–500-fold increase.[136,137] Anecdotal reports of spontaneous regression of KS in such patients upon discontinuation of immunosuppressive therapy support the relationship between the integrity of the immune system and the development of KS.[138,139] However, there have been cases of AIDS-related KS with no clinical or laboratory evidence of impaired immunity. Available data do suggest that activation of the immune system may play a role in the pathogenesis of AIDS-related KS.[140] In case of endemic African KS, multiple parasitic infestations, including malaria and bacterial and viral infections, could be the source of continuous activation. In classic KS high levels of anti-cytomegalovirus (CMV) antibodies were previously reported.

The multiple and disseminated nature of KS suggests a role of unique circulating transforming growth factors locally produced.[141] HIV-infected T cells, monocytes and transformed cells produce growth factors and viral regulatory protein (Tat protein) that result in autocrine and paracrine stimulation of host cell proliferation and viral expression.[142] Most of these cytokines (as growth factors are generally called) are angiogenesis factors which stimulate vascular endothelial cell proliferation and new blood vessel formation. Cytochemical and phenotypic marker studies have demonstrated KS cell to have features of vascular channel and endothelial cell lineage.[143]

Human herpes simplex virus, type 8 (HHV-8) has been identified as the putative agent for KS, and has been designated by some researchers as Kaposi's sarcoma-associated herpes virus (KSHV). The association between AIDS-associated KS and HHV-8 was originally described by Chang et al.[144] HHV-8 is detectable by PCR in all forms of KS and its seroprevalence correlates with the risk of developing KS. HHV-8 is closely related to the Epstein–Barr virus (human herpes virus 4) and infects CD_{19}-positive B cells, as well as the endothelial-derived spindle cells of KS.[145] HHV-8 not only causes KS, but is also known to cause primary effusion lymphomas. Unlike other herpes viruses, HHV-8 is not ubiquitous and is known to be rare in Asia. Recent studies have shown HHV-8 to be shed in oral cavity and saliva of some patients with KS, and less so in seminal fluid and rectum.[146] This may have a bearing on mechanisms of transmission.

Clinical features

There are features which distinguish epidemic AIDS-

Table 36.11 Clinical features of Kaposi's sarcoma.

Feature	Endemic	Epidemic
Age (years)	40–50	20–30
Gender M:F	12:1	2–3:1
Clinical course	Indolent Aggressive	Always aggressive
Treatment response	Excellent	Poor
Prognosis	Good–excellent	Poor

related KS from endemic African KS. These include peak age at presentation, sex distribution, clinical course and response to therapy (Table 36.11). In addition, opportunistic infections are commonly observed in epidemic KS. In the tropics tuberculosis is the most common infection related to HIV, while *Pneumocystis carinii* is rare.[147] 'Slim disease', a clinical syndrome dominated by chronic diarrhoea and weight loss, is a common presentation.[148] In some parts of Africa enteropathic AIDS (slim disease) accounts for over 70% of AIDS cases. The cause is as yet unknown, but the protozoa *Cryptosporidium parvum*, *Isospora belli* and *Enterozoa* are likely to be involved. In the tropics there are no real high-risk groups for HIV infection, as is the case in Europe and North America where homosexuality and intravenous drug abuse are high-risk behaviours. In the tropics HIV is spread by heterosexual contact. Blood screening is not universally practised and non-screened blood may be a common mechanism of spread as well.

Endemic KS presents mostly with unilateral limb oedema and skin nodules (Figure 36.4). Nodules may arise in the subcutaneous tissue (nodular form) (Figure 36.5) or from deeper than the deep fascia and may resemble granuloma pyogenicum (florid form) (Figure 36.6). Visceral involvement is frequent. The lymphadenopathic form of KS is rare in endemic form except in children[149] but is common in epidemic AIDS-related KS. Complications reported include haematemesis,[150] intestinal

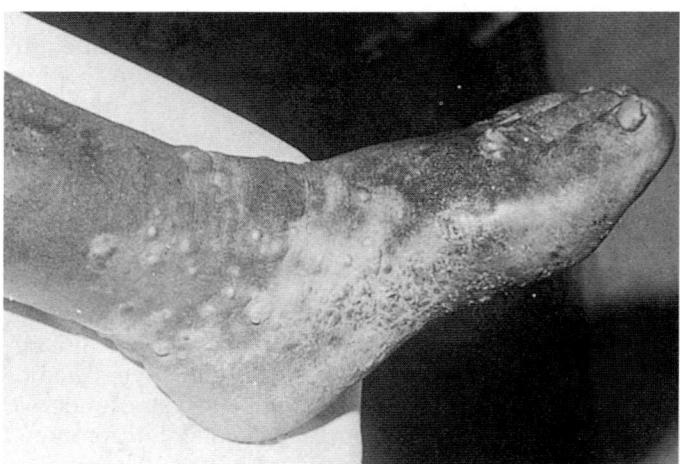

Figure 36.4: Endemic Kaposi's sarcoma. Nodular and plaque forms with oedema. (Courtesy of E. H. Williams.)

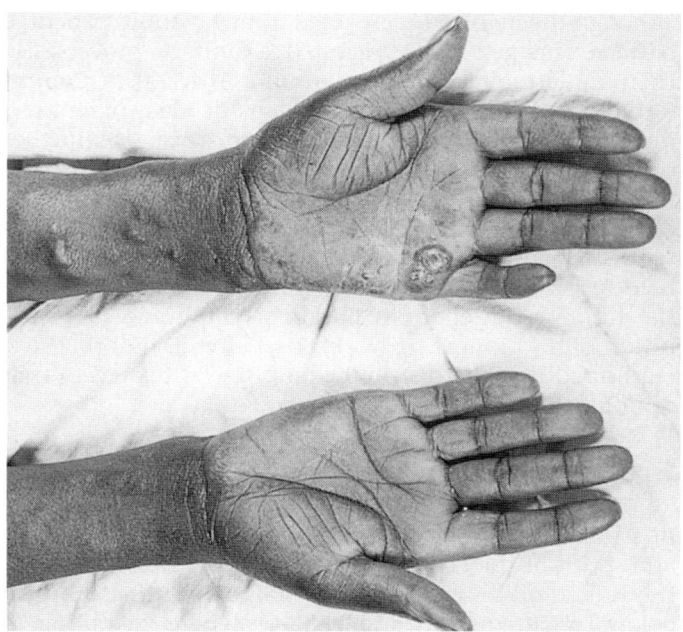

Figure 36.5: Endemic Kaposi's sarcoma. Nodular form. (Courtesy of E. H. Williams.)

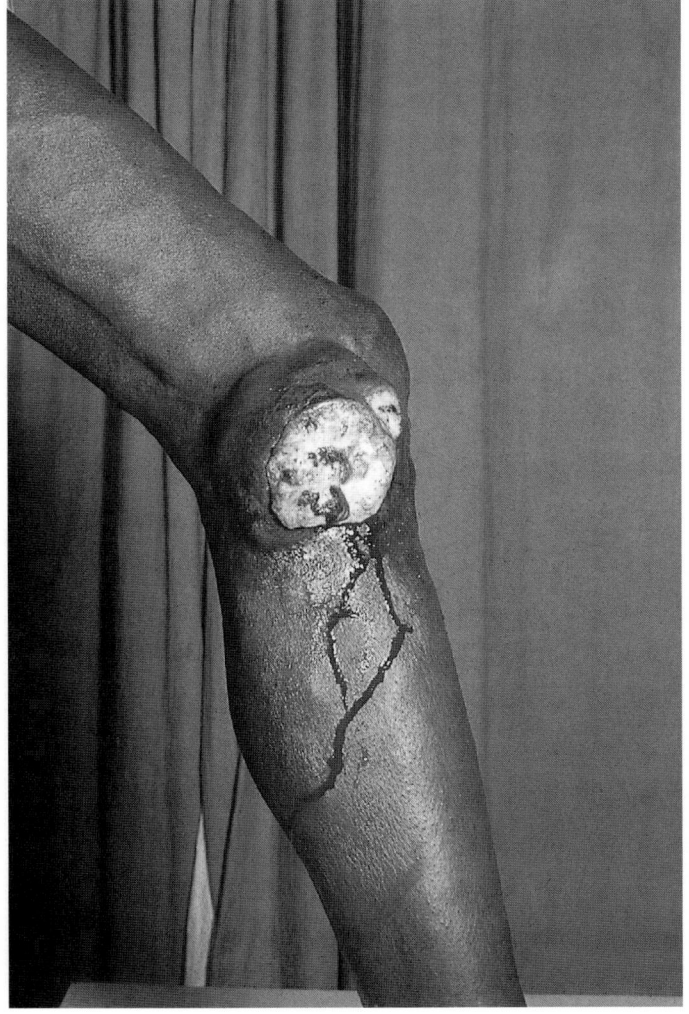

Figure 36.6: Endemic Kaposi's sarcoma. Florid variety.

obstruction,[151] perforation,[152] diarrhoea with protein-losing enteropathy[153] and intussusception.[154] Studies from East Africa have suggested that visceral involvement may occur frequently, despite a lack of abdominal or pulmonary symptoms and signs.[155,156] The epidemic AIDS-related KS presents with a combination of marked cachexia, skin hyperpigmentation (Figure 36.7) and oropharyngeal palatal and tongue involvement (Figure 36.8). The oropharynx may either exhibit purple KS nodules or ulcerations and plaques due to tumour or secondary fungal infections. Visceral involvement, especially pulmonary, is common. Systemic symptoms of fever, diaphoresis and weight loss are of prognostic significance.

Staging

Because of the multicentric nature of KS, staging has been difficult. The four-stage classification originally described by Krigel and co-workers[157] included epidemic as well as

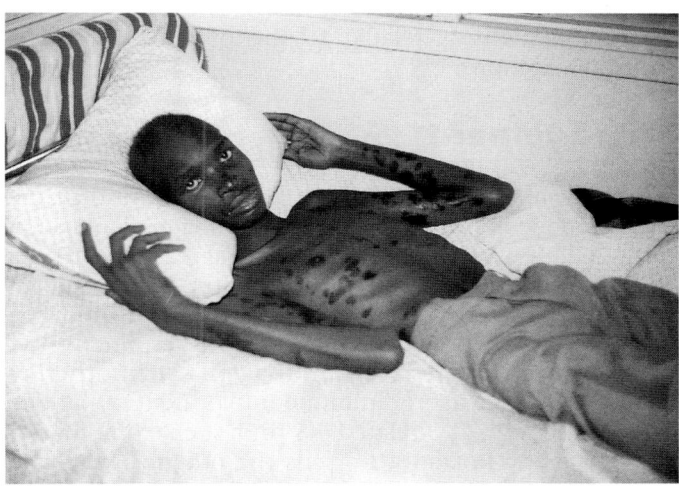

Figure 36.7: Epidemic AIDS-associated Kaposi's sarcoma. Note marked wasting and skin hyperpigmentation on chest wall, arms and face.

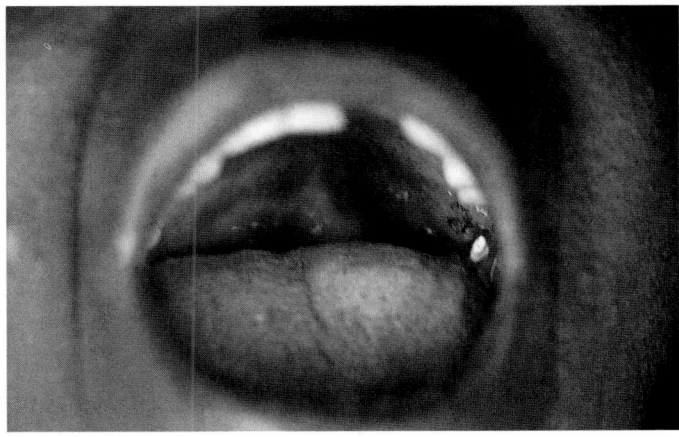

Figure 36.8: Epidemic AIDS-associated Kaposi's sarcoma. Note lesions on the hard palate.

Table 36.12 Suggested staging for epidemic Kaposi's sarcoma.

Stage	Characteristics
I	No prior or coexisting opportunistic infection. No systemic symptoms, $CD_4 > 300/\mu l$
II	No prior or coexisting opportunistic infection. No systemic symptoms, $CD_4 < 300/\mu l$
III	No prior to coexisting opportunistic infection. Systemic symptoms
IV	Prior or coexisting opportunistic infection

non-epidemic forms of disease. The staging system of Mitsuyasu and Groopman[158] was designed especially for classification of epidemic AIDS-related KS and takes into consideration the extent of tumour involvement, the presence of systemic symptoms and the presence of opportunistic infections (Table 36.12). Considerable data also support the use of immunological staging as a predictor of both survival and response to therapy. Patients with systemic symptoms are likely to have a low number of CD_4 cells and low $CD_4:CD_8$ ratios. The poor prognosis of such patients is related to the presence of opportunistic infections.[159]

Management

Studies from Uganda indicated that nodular and plaque forms of endemic KS respond to simple therapies, including oral alkylating agents.[160,161] The more aggressive endemic forms responded well to combination chemotherapy consisting of actinomycin D, vincristine and imidazole carboximide.[162] Localized endemic forms respond well to radiotherapy. Aggressive multi-agent chemotherapy exacerbates the existing immune impairment of patients with epidemic AIDS-related KS and such combination chemotherapy not only worsens the prognosis but may also increase mortality. A recently completed four-arm, randomized clinical trial of AIDS-associated KS in Zimbabwe suggests that, funds permitting, single-agent oral etoposide may be the most pragmatic approach and leads to less dramatic decline in quality of life than best supportive care, hemi-body radiotherapy, or three-drug combination.[163]

Burkitt's lymphoma (See also Chapter 44)

Burkitt's lymphoma (BL) is a malignant lymphoma of B cell origin. Dr Burkitt,[164] a British surgeon working in Kampala, Uganda, drew attention to the fact that some features of this disease occurred with certain repetitiveness. Other observers had noted similar tumours presenting at separate sites like jaws, orbits, ovaries, kidneys, adrenals, thyroid, testes and breasts and had concluded that they were all separate entities. Dr Burkitt felt that

although the involved sites varied from patient to patient, a pattern emerged that suggested a unitary process. He then undertook a journey around Africa (the famous 'tumour safari') and was able to map out the geographical distribution of this tumour within Africa. He further observed that the distribution was very similar to the malaria map and suggested that the tumour might be caused by an arthropod (mosquito)-borne virus. Subsequently, at a conference on lymphoreticular tumours held in Paris in 1963, it was unanimously agreed to give the tumour the eponym Burkitt's lymphoma in recognition of his pioneering work. Soon after, Dalldorf (1964) reaffirmed that the distribution of BL was related to that of holo- or hyperendemic malaria.

Epidemiology

BL is restricted to the geographical latitudes 10–15° north and south of the equator and to altitudes below 1500 m. It is rare in places where the diurnal temperature drops to below 16°C frequently and in places where the rainfall is less than 50 cm per annum. Outside tropical Africa BL is found in those areas of the tropical belt with the above climatic conditions, namely Papua New Guinea. In these endemic regions BL accounts for more than 50% of childhood tumours.

The highest incidence of BL is in the West Nile district of Uganda, where the number recorded approaches 13/100 000 population. It is in the same area where time–space clustering has been recorded.[165] A time trend has also been observed and over the last decade or so there has been a noticeable downward trend in the number of cases diagnosed both in Uganda and Tanzania. In Ibadan, Nigeria, it is estimated that the incidence is 15/100 000 children aged 5–9 years. Outside this endemic belt, sporadic cases of BL have been observed in the USA, Europe and the Middle East. More recently several cases have been noted in association with the AIDS epidemic.[166]

Table 36.13 Comparison between endemic and sporadic Burkitt's lymphoma.

Features	Endemic	Sporadic
Epidemiology	Related to climate	Unrelated to climate
	Very common in children	Rare in children
EBV association	> 95% are associated with EBV	Rarely associated with EBV
Chromosomal translocations	Invariably found	Invariably found
Clinical features	Presents commonly with jaw tumour Nodal disease rare	Presents commonly with abdominal, nodal and marrow

The clinical features of these non-endemic cases differ from those of the endemic forms (Table 36.13).

Aetiology

BL has provoked extensive tumour investigations because of its possible aetiological association with Epstein–Barr virus (EBV), the influence of malaria, the specific chromosomal abnormality, the role of oncogenes in lymphomagenesis, and the role of growth factors in tumorigenesis.

Epstein–Barr virus

EBV was initially discovered in 1964 in cells from endemic BL.[167] For a long time it has been a forerunner as a candidate for an oncogenic virus. For a virus to be considered oncogenic it has to fulfil certain criteria. These criteria (Henle–Koch's postulates) include:

- The ability of the candidate virus to transform in vitro.
- The finding of significant immune response to viral products in patients compared with controls.
- The detection of viral tumour markers, e.g., viral genomes, and viral products, e.g., antigens, in the tumour.
- The ability of the candidate virus to cause malignant tumours in vivo.

EBV is known to transform human B lymphocytes in vitro; patients with BL have a significantly higher EBV serological response (viral capsid antigen, VCA; early antigen, EA; EB-determined nuclear antigen, EBNA) than controls and Burkitt's tumours carry footprints of the virus (EBV genome), detected either as EBV DNA or EBNA.[168] In addition, EBV can transform B lymphocytes of some simian hosts, and these transformed cells can grow progressively and kill, after reimplantation into the original autochthonous host. In marmoset and owl monkeys EBV has direct oncogenic activity: it can induce lymphomas and these tumours carry the EBV genome.

In the large seroepidemiological study carried out in the West Nile district of Uganda, more than 40 000 children were bled and followed up for several years to determine the features of those that developed BL.[169] The hypotheses tested were that BL was due to delayed EBV infection, as in infectious mononucleosis, that EBV is a passenger virus and that BL developed in children heavily and chronically infected with EBV. During the follow-up period 14 children with previously stored sera developed BL. This and other studies led to the conclusion that BL was not due to delayed infection as patients developing BL seroconverted 6–24 months prior to BL becoming manifest. High VCA titre was not protective; on the contrary it favoured the development of BL. The failure to detect EBV genome in non-BL tumours, although these tumours came from individuals with positive EBV serology, negated the passenger hypothesis.[170]

Although EBV has more or less fulfilled Henle–Koch's postulates, there are still a number of features that do not fit. For instance, EBV is ubiquitous and yet BL is only found in restricted areas of the world. Even in the so-called endemic belt very few patients succumb to the disease. EBV DNA is only associated with endemic BL. The non-endemic, e.g. American, BL only very rarely contains EBV DNA. Even in Africa only 90% of BL tumours are EBV genome positive. Thus EBV is not absolutely necessary in the development of BL. The role of malaria in endemic BL may be to facilitate the development of lymphoma through either polyclonal B cell proliferation and/or T cell immunosuppression. Malaria prophylaxis was started in the North Mara province of Tanzania and this appeared to coincide with a downward trend. However, the curious geographical distribution of endemic BL in sub-Saharan Africa and in Papua New Guinea is best explained on the basis of malaria endemicity. In addition, recent studies in Uganda have suggested that other non-Burkitt, non-Hodgkin's lymphomas may also be related to malaria endemicity.[171]

Chromosomal abnormalities

Manolov and Manolova first reported a characteristic chromosome abnormality in BL in 1972. Part of the long arm of chromosome 8 was translocated to the long arm of chromosome 14.[172] Ninety per cent of BL tumours have this translocation, which always involved the same bands of the two chromosomes, namely band q24 of chromosome 8 and band q32 of chromosome 14. The remaining 10% of BL tumours exhibited two variant translocations: a reciprocal translocation involving q24 of 8 with either band p11 of chromosome 2 or band q11 of chromosome 22. These translocations were observed in all BL tumours irrespective of EBV genome status and whether they were endemic or non-endemic.

Human immunoglobulins

It was later discovered that the genes for human immunoglobulin heavy chains are located on band q32 of chromosome 14, whereas the genes for the κ and λ light chains are on band p11 of chromosome 2 and band q11 of chromosome 22 respectively. George Klein predicted that chromosome 8 probably carried an oncogene and the translocation was transferring this oncogene close to the immunoglobulin gene. His predictions have been borne out. The c-*myc* oncogene has been identified on band q24 of chromosome 8. It is believed it may have an immortalization function. In other words, while the translocation of the c-*myc* oncogene close to an immunoglobulin constant region is a constant feature, this, though necessary, is not sufficient to cause tumour. A second oncogene, B-*lym* of N-*ras*, appears to be needed to complete the neoplastic transformation.

Tumour suppressor gene p53

The p53 gene is a tumour suppressor gene located on 17p13 and is often inactivated by deletion and/or point

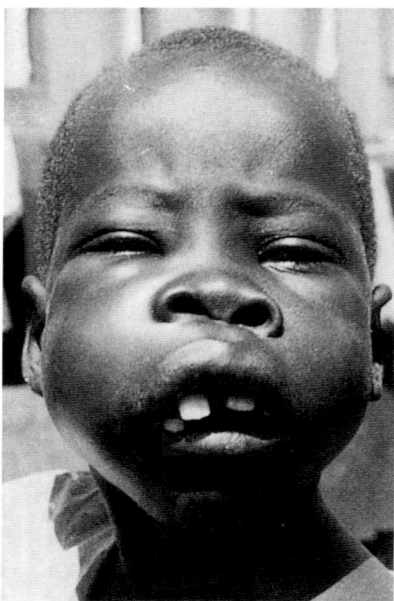

Figure 36.9: Burkitt's lymphoma. Jaw tumour.

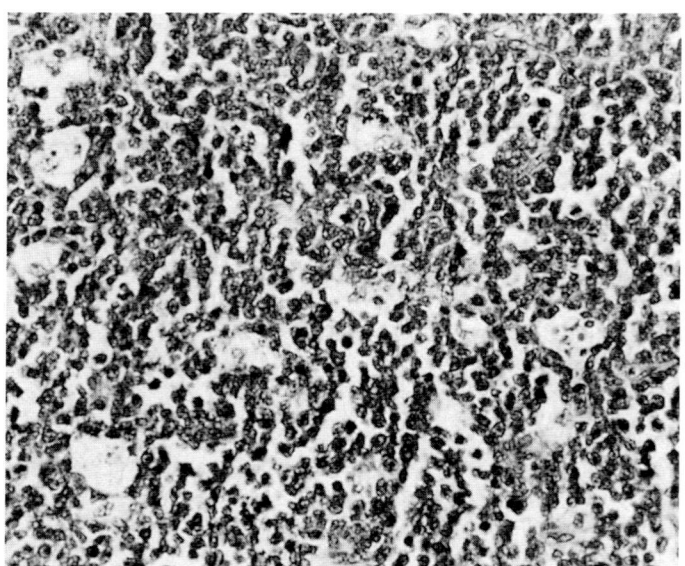

Figure 36.10: Burkitt's lymphoma. 'Starry sky' picture.

mutation in most solid tumours.[173,174] In endemic and sporadic BL as well as L$_3$ALL (Burkitt's acute lympho-blastic leukemia) p53 mutation has been identified in 20–40% of fresh tumour samples and in >70% of cell lines.[175]

Although p53 mutation is associated with features of poor prognosis, e.g., large tumour burden, low response to intensive chemotherapy and short survival in other haematological malignancies, notably acute myeloid leukaemia and myelodysplastic syndrome, this does not seem to be the case with either BL or L$_3$ALL.[176]

Clinical features

Endemic BL presents usually with jaw swelling (75%), abdominal swelling (60%) and central nervous system involvement (30%). Patients with jaw swellings generally present with maxillary involvement more commonly than mandibular tumour. Maxillary tumour often spreads upwards to involve the orbit (Figure 36.9). Bilateral maxillary tumour is common. Bilateral mandibular disease is rare unless all four quadrants are involved. Patients present complaining of loose teeth, and a lateral oblique radiograph of the jaw reveals loss of lamina dura. Abdominal swelling is a presenting feature in about 60% of patients, usually more so in females than in males. Almost any organ within the abdomen can and does get involved in the tumorous process and often malignant ascites is an accompanying feature. Central nervous system involvement is seen in about 30% of patients at presen-tation. This may be either as cranial nerve palsy (III, VI, VII commonly) or paraplegia or just malignant CSF pleocytosis alone. The peak age at presentation is 4–9 years. The tumour is unseen below 1 year, less than 1% under 2 years and peaks from 4 to 9 years, and then falls

off such that less than 5% of patients are over 15 years of age.

The diagnosis of BL is often evident because of the clinical presentation in a child from an endemic area. However, histological confirmation must always be sought as other tumours, notably embryonal rhabdomyosarcoma, neuroblastoma, lymphoblastic lymphoma and Wilms' tumour, may all mimic BL. Histologically the classical 'starry sky' picture (Figure 36.10) is suggestive of BL and is due to the presence of large numbers of phagocytic macrophages among tumour cells.

Staging

The staging system commonly applied to endemic BL was suggested by Ziegler and Magrath. It is based on the volume of tumour and reflects prognosis (Table 36.14).

Cell kinetics

BL is a very rapidly growing tumour. It is the fastest-growing tumour in man and has been referred to as the

Table 36.14 Staging of Burkitt's lymphoma.

Stage	Features
A	Solitary extra-abdominal site
AR	Resected intra-abdominal tumour
B	Multiple extra-abdominal sites
C	Intra-abdominal tumour
D	Abdominal tumour with sites of tumour other than facial

human equivalent of the L1210 mouse model. BL has a growth fraction of 100%, mean cell cycle time of 26 hours and observed volume doubling time of 2.8 days.

Management

Because of the peculiar cell kinetics BL is extremely responsive to drug therapy and is one of the early tumours noted to be curable by drugs alone. However, the management of this tumour requires a multidisciplinary approach. The role of surgery includes biopsy for diagnosis, spinal cord decompression and insertion of an Ommaya reservoir, but, most importantly, debulking. BL is one of the tumours where debulk surgery has been clearly shown to be beneficial.[177] An attempt should be made by the surgeon to remove as much tumour (> 90%) as possible. In case of bilateral ovarian involvement this means bilateral oophorectomy. Patients who have had more than 90% of their tumour taken out surgically have a survival advantage equal to those with early stage I or A disease. If the surgeon cannot remove sufficient tumour, removal of less tumour does not influence prognosis. BL is a radiosensitive tumour but because of its peculiar rapid growth conventional radiotherapy is ineffective as the tumour regrows between each day's therapy. This problem is circumvented by superfractionation of each day's dose of irradiation into three treatments given 4 hours apart. Such an approach is not practical in a busy radiotherapy department. However, prophylactic cranio-spinal irradiation failed to show any value in preventing or delaying central nervous system relapse.[178]

The treatment of choice for BL is chemotherapy. The single most effective agent is cyclophosphamide. Although single-agent cyclophosphamide is as effective as a three-drug combination consisting of cyclophosphamide, vincristine and methotrexate (COM), the combination is superior in preventing systemic relapse.[179] All in all about 80% of patients achieve complete tumour regression, 10% partial response. About 50% will relapse: those who relapse early, within 3 months, do poorly, while those who relapse late, after 3 months, respond well even to initial induction agents.[180] Patients remaining relapse-free after 1 year can be considered cured and the overall relapse-free survival at 10 years is 35–50%.[181]

Prevention

Dr Epstein[182,183] and his colleagues have developed an EB vaccine using the high molecular weight glycoprotein component of EBV membrane antigen. This vaccine conferred 100% protection against a lymphomagenic dose of EBV in the cotton-top tamarine (a South American marmoset). Preliminary safety studies are under way. It will be necessary to ascertain its efficacy in preventing infectious mononucleosis, and then BL and nasopharyngeal carcinoma.

Nasopharyngeal carcinoma

(See also Chapter 44)

Incidence and geographical distribution

Nasopharyngeal carcinoma (NPC) is an uncommon tumour in the white populations of Europe and North America, with an ASR of 1/100 000 population, but has long been recognized as an important problem in parts of the Far East, particularly southern China. In regions which have a high incidence the tumours are poorly differentiated, non-keratinizing squamous cell carcinomas and often show a heavy infiltration with lymphocytes and other inflammatory cells. This feature gave rise to the old term lymphoepithelioma. These tumours appear to be aetiologically distinct from the well-differentiated squamous cell carcinomas that may occur anywhere in old people. The highest incidence rates are found in the southern provinces of China, particularly around Guandong, and in Hong Kong and Singapore, where rates of between 12 and 26/100 000 are recorded. There is also a high incidence in the Chinese population of Malaysia, Thailand, Indonesia and Hawaii. NPC is some 20 times more common in the Chinese population of Malaysia than in Indians living there. The incidence of NPC in South-East Asia is directly related to the degree of inbreeding within the immigrant populations from southern China.

Regions of intermediate frequency (from 1.5 to 9/100 000 a year) are found in several parts of Africa; these include the highland areas of Kenya, and parts of the Sudan, Tunisia, Morocco and Algeria. In some of these countries the age distribution of the tumour shows two peaks, with the first occurring between 10 and 20 years.

Aetiology

The high incidence of NPC in peoples of southern Chinese descent who live in different environments, often contrasting with a low incidence in neighbouring ethnic groups, is suggestive of a genetic factor. HLA-typing has shown that Cantonese Chinese with A2, B17, BW46 haplotypes have an increased risk of developing NPC.

Epstein–Barr virus

Clinical disorders associated with EBV include infectious mononucleosis, endemic BL and NPC. In infectious mononucleosis both IgG and IgM antibodies directed at the VCA are detected. Nuclear antigen antibodies are absent as these develop 2–6 months after initial infection. The relationship between NPC and EBV was postulated on the basis of the finding of antibodies to EBV in the serum and the identification of viral genomes by in situ hybridization of epithelial tumour cells.[184] In NPC IgG

Table 36.15 World Health Organization classification of nasopharyngeal carcinoma and EBV antibodies.

Classification	Description	EBV antibodies	
		IgG EA (%)	IgA VCA (%)
Type I	Keratinizing squamous cell	35	16
Type II	Non-keratinizing squamous cell	94	84
Type III	Undifferentiated carcinoma	83	89

specific to EBV EA is often present as well as the IgA directed against VCA. These antibodies precede the appearance of the tumour and serve as a prognostic indicator of remission and relapse.[185] There is a correlation with the histological classification (Table 36.15), with the keratinizing squamous cell type (type I) having a much lower incidence of positive antibodies than the non-keratinizing or undifferentiated types.

Until recently EBV was considered to be exclusively a B-lymphotropic herpes virus and the observed presence of EBV in epithelial cells in NPC was difficult to explain. However, EBV receptors have now been demonstrated on, and virus binding to, the surface of epithelial cells. Regardless of whether a patient with NPC lives in an area of endemic or sporadic incidence, all the tumours contain EBV DNA.[186] Preinvasive lesions of NPC, including dysplasia and carcinoma in situ, are infected with EBV. The EBV is clonal, indicating that the lesions represent a focal cellular growth, which arose from a single cell infected with EBV. EBV infection appears to be an early and possibly an initiating event in the pathogenesis of NPC. The detection of EBV-transforming gene in all the neoplastic cells suggests that its expression is essential for the preinvasive epithelial proliferation associated with NPC.[187]

Dietary factors

It has been observed that ethnic differences in similar geographical regions (e.g. southern China) are associated with marked variations in the frequency of NPC and that these differences may be related to dietary habits. Evidence of the causative role of salted fish, especially if it is consumed early in life, has been postulated. Relatively high levels of nitrosamines have been identified in Cantonese salted fish and extracts have been shown to activate EBV in Raji cells (a BL cell line) in vitro.[188]

Clinical features

The diagnosis of NPC is often difficult because the nasopharynx is hard to visualize and the primary lesion tends to infiltrate submucosally and can easily be missed in a superficial biopsy.

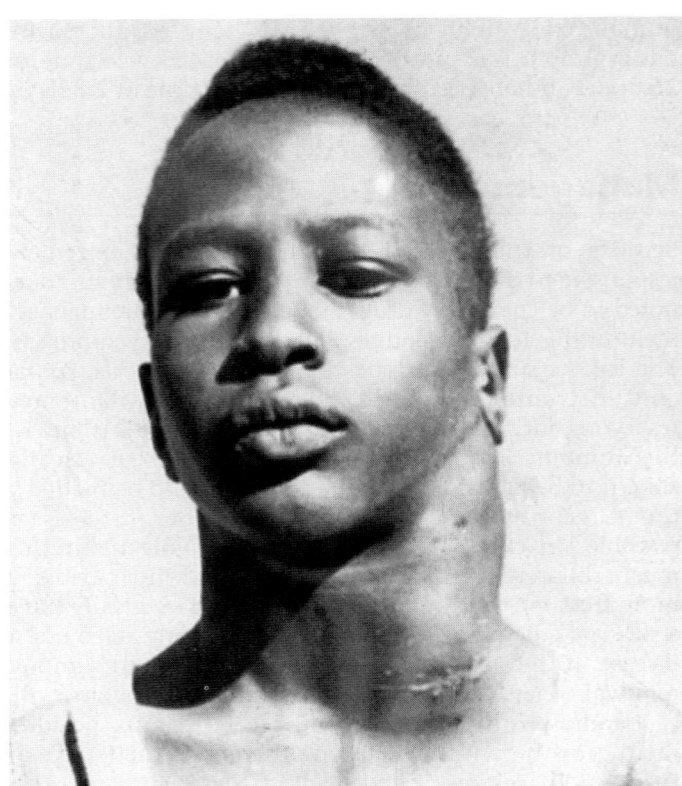

Figure 36.11: Nasopharyngeal carcinoma with massive cervical lymphadenopathy. (Courtesy of M. A. O. Malik.)

Many cases of NPC are diagnosed late or remain undiagnosed until they present with clinical nodes without an obvious primary site.[189] The majority of patients seen with NPC in East Africa present with enlarged, often massive, cervical lymph nodes which may be mistaken for tuberculosis or malignant lymphoma (Figure 36.11). In some instances lymphadenopathy is a late phenomenon and such patients have, in addition, multiple cranial nerve palsies and pain due to tumour extension through the base of the skull. A small percentage (about 5%) present only with cranial nerve palsies. Because of the location of the primary tumour patients may present with blockage of the Eustachian tube, causing otitis media. Thus any adult with persistent or recurrent otitis media should be suspected of having NPC. Less frequently patients may present with nasal blockage or epistaxis.

Management

Radiotherapy is the primary treatment of NPC regardless of the stage. The recommended dose is 6500–7000 cGy delivered to a port encompassing the nasopharynx as well as the base of the skull. Often a boost to the nasopharynx is considered, using intracavitary implants.[190] Surgery plays a limited role and is usually reserved for salvage therapy of residual cervical nodal disease. Several cytotoxic agents show activity in NPC. These include methotrexate, bleomycin, 5-fluorouracil, doxorubicin, cisplatin and vinblastine. Combination chemotherapy has often been given in sequential fashion with radiotherapy.[191] Concurrent chemoradiotherapy applying radiosensitizers, notably cisplatin, is undergoing clinical trial.

In most tropical areas mortality from NPC is high because patients present at a very advanced disease stage and most do not have access to radiotherapy facilities. Whenever possible focus should be placed on prevention.

Prevention

Because 10–20% of healthy donors may have false positive EBV antibodies, these may not be very useful for screening. However, some success using serological tests for EBV have been demonstrated in China.[192] In a study involving 67 891 healthy subjects, 9% were found to have elevation of IgA VCA (≥ 1:10). Of the 6102 with high titres, 48 (0.8%) were found on mirror examination to have obvious NPC. Endoscopic examination and blind biopsy of 130 randomly selected from the remaining 6054 individuals detected NPC in 5.4%.[192] Thus serological screening should be considered for high-risk populations.

Prevention should also focus on dietary education. The prospect for vaccination is in sight (see section on Burkitt's lymphoma, above). Such vaccines may be of value for high-risk groups.

Oral and oropharyngeal carcinoma

Incidence and geographical distribution

Mouth cancer is the most common cancer in South-East Asia, home of one-fifth of the world's population. Squamous cell carcinoma of the mucosa of the oral cavity and oropharynx is a tumour whose incidence is closely related to particular cultural habits. There is a high incidence in most of the populations of the Indian subcontinent and in peoples of Indian extraction living in other countries of the Far East such as Singapore, Sri Lanka, Thailand and Vietnam. These types of cancer account for nearly 50% of cancer patients registered at the Tata Memorial Hospital in Bombay, and incidence rates of over 20/100 000 have been recorded in some districts of India. In Malaysia these tumours account for 30% of all malignancies, and in Sri Lanka and India approximately 35–40% of all cancers occur in the oral cavity, compared with only 2–3% in the UK and USA.[193,194] Low rates are observed in Chinese and an intermediate pattern in Malaysia.

Aetiology

A high incidence of oropharyngeal tumour is related to the cultural practice of chewing betel quid and, less frequently, to smoking locally made cheroots called bidi. Betel quid consists of the young leaf of betel vine (*Piper betel*) mixed with slices of areca nut and varying quantities of slaked lime. Tobacco and spices are often added to this mixture. The resultant quid is held for long periods of time in the buccal sulcus. The development of squamous cell carcinoma is usually preceded by the development of precancerous leucoplastic changes in the oral epithelium. A high alcohol intake, vitamin A deficiency, dental caries and sepsis may be contributory factors in some patients. There is conflicting evidence as to the relative roles of tobacco and other constituents of the quid in the development of cancer.

Prevention and management

Oral precancer and cancer meet the essential requirements of a screening programme (Table 36.3). Up to 15 years may elapse before lesions in the mouth turn cancerous. Various studies in India have indicated a high prevalence of oral premalignant lesions.[195] These are leucoplakia and oral submucous fibrosis. If these lesions, which are the first signs of danger, are detected in sufficient time for treatment, the disease is curable through surgery and radiotherapy. Unfortunately, most patients seek medical attention only when they are in pain, which is a late symptom, and therefore too late for any therapy but pain relief.

In a study using primary health care workers in Sri Lanka it was demonstrated that the precancerous lesions can be detected by this category of workers.[196] This approach has been found to be reliable and pragmatic, and since these primary health care workers outnumber dentists by a ratio of 10 to 1, they may give a lead on how to approach other cancers in remote populous tropical environments. Any improvement in general nutrition, particularly an adequate intake of vitamins, trace elements and animal protein, is likely to reduce the incidence in high-risk populations. Reduction of alcohol intake, and particularly tobacco consumption, should also be encouraged.

Carcinoma of the bladder

(See also Chapter 15)

Incidence and geographical distribution

Bladder cancer is the sixth most common form of cancer in the developed world (see Table 36.1), with an age-standardized rate of approximately 25/100 000. The majority of tumours are transitional in histological type and over 75% occur in elderly men. Within most of the tropics the rates are low but in parts of east, central and southern Africa, Egypt and the Sudan and some regions of the Middle East rates are high. In Bulawayo, Zimbabwe, for example, they are 28.7 and 7.0/100 000 in men and women, respectively, and at the Cairo Cancer Institute bladder cancer accounts for 38.5% of all cancers in men and 11.3% in women. The tumours in these high-incidence regions are predominantly squamous in histological type.

Aetiology

The geographical distribution of high-incidence bladder cancer in the tropics parallels that of *Schistosoma haematobium*, an association that was first noted by Fergusson[197] in Egypt in 1911. Case–control studies in Zimbabwe, using bladder calcification as an index of infection, have shown a significantly higher rate of infection in patients than controls.[198] Estimated incidence rates in different districts and regions of east and central Africa show a close relationship between the prevalence and intensity of *S. haematobium* infection and high rates of bladder cancer.

The mechanisms of carcinogenesis are uncertain. Heavy, chronic infection with *S. haematobium* leads to inflammation, fibrosis and calcification of the bladder with impairment of function and inadequate emptying. This predisposes to recurrent, mixed bacterial infections. In such patients carcinogenic nitrosamines which are formed from excreted nitrates and nitrites have been detected.[199,200] It is thought that these substances acting on hyperplastic and metaplastic epithelium give rise to the characteristic squamous cell carcinomas.

Clinical features

Schistosomal bladder cancer occurs mostly in young individuals. It is commonly a well-differentiated squamous cell carcinoma and has less tendency to spread via the bloodstream and lymphatics. The mean age at presentation is about 45 years and in Egypt about 75% of the victims are under 50 years of age. It is rarely observed in the under-20 age group. This is in contradiction to non-schistosomal bladder cancer, where the mean age is about 65 years and less than 10% are under 50 years of age. The male:female ratio for schistosomal bladder cancer is 4–5:1. The male preponderance may be related to increased male exposure to schistosomal infection. Unfortunately the cardinal early sign of bladder cancer (painless haematuria) is often ignored in schistosomal endemic areas as most of the populace will have had haematuria since childhood. For this and other reasons the great majority of the cases present very late with symptoms of cystitis and obstructive uropathy. A plain radiograph of the abdomen may reveal a calcified outline of the urinary bladder. Cystoscopy and biopsy establishes the diagnosis. In centres such as the Cairo Cancer Institute, where investigators are experienced, urine cytology provides a fairly accurate diagnosis.[201] Biopsy is still necessary to confirm the diagnosis, although 'aggressive biopsy' to determine the depth of tumour muscle invasion may cause perforation because of the advanced nature of most cases. Prestaging work-up should include history and physical examination, urinalysis for cytology, looking for

Table 36.16 TNM staging of bladder carcinoma: UICC classification.

Stage	Description
T_{is}	Carcinoma in situ, 'flat tumour'
T_a	Non-invasive papillary carcinoma
T_1	Tumour invades subepithelial connective tissue
T_2	Tumour invades superficial muscle
T_3	Tumour invades deep muscle or perivesical fat
T_4	Tumour invades prostate, uterus, vagina, pelvic wall or abdominal wall
N_1	Metastasis in a single lymph node 2 cm or less in greatest dimension
N_2	Metastasis in a single lymph nodes, 2–5 cm in greatest dimension or multiple nodes ≤ 5 cm
N_3	Metastasis in node > 5 cm in greatest dimension
M_0	No distant metastasis

schistosomal eggs and for malignant cells, and a plain radiograph of the abdomen. Urography should be followed by an examination under anaesthesia. Cystoscopy to map out the location of bladder tumour and biopsy are essential. The currently recommended staging system is the TNM staging advocated by the International Union Against Cancer (UICC) (Table 36.16).

Management

Radical surgery is the only curative treatment modality. However, radical cystectomy is associated with postoperative morbidity and mortality as high as 15–30% in some series. Adjuvant radiotherapy has been used postoperatively to prevent or delay recurrence. Pre-operative radiotherapy has been tried in Cairo and the preliminary results are encouraging.[202] Radiotherapy as the sole treatment modality has been disappointing. This may be due to the massive tumour bulk associated with fibrosis and bacterial infection. Effective single cytotoxic agents include cisplatin, bleomycin, gemcitabine and methotrexate. The efficacy of combination chemotherapy or concurrent chemoradiotherapy has yet to be demonstrated. Unfortunately, most studies are patients with transitional cell carcinoma and the results cannot be extrapolated to include squamous cell carcinomas.

Prevention

The prevention of bladder cancer in those regions where schistosomiasis is endemic is dependent on effective schistosomal control (see Chapter 80). There is a minimum of 20 years lag period between infection and the development of bladder cancer. Schistosomal bladder cancer should therefore be amenable to screening. Screening has been advocated for high-risk populations in Egypt. Before such a practice is embarked upon on a wide scale, its cost-effectiveness needs to be carefully evaluated.

REFERENCES

1 Tomatis L. Environmental cancer risk factors: a review. *Acta Oncol* 1988; 27:465–472.

2 Parkin D M, Laara E & Muir C S. Estimates of the world wide frequency of sixteen major cancers in 1980. *Int J Cancer* 1988; 41:184–197.

3 Olweny C L M. Global inequalities in cancer care. *Trans R Soc Trop Med Hyg* 1991; 85:709–710.

4 Bailey B J. Tobaccoism is the disease—cancer is the sequela (editorial). *JAMA* 1986; 255:1923.

5 Olweny C L M. Goals and rationale of cancer treatment. *Med J Aust* 1991; 155:187–192.

6 Cleaver J R. Defective repair replication of DNA in xeroderma pigmentosum. *Nature* 1968; 218:652–656.

7 Takebe H, Nishigori C & Satoh Y. Genetics and skin cancer of xeroderma pigmentosum in Japan. *Jpn J Cancer Res* 1987; 78:1135–1143.

8 Miki Y, Swensen J, Shattuck-Eidens D et al. A strong candidate for the breast and ovarian cancer susceptibility gene BRCA1. *Science* 1994; 266:66–71.

9 Ford D, Easton D F, Bishop D T et al. Risk of cancer in BRCA1-mutation carriers. *Lancet* 1994; 343:692–695.

10 Wooster R, Bignell G, Lancaster J et al. Identification of the breast cancer susceptibility gene BRCA2. *Nature* 1995; 378:789–792.

11 Templeton A C, Buxton E & Bianchi A. Cancer in Kyadondo County, Uganda 1968–1970. *J Natl Cancer Inst* 1972; 48:865–874.

12 Bayo S, Parkin D M, Koumare A K et al. Cancer in Mali. *Int J Cancer* 1990; 45:679–684.

13 Whittle H C, Inskip H, Hall A J, Mendy M, Downer R & Hoare S. Vaccination against hepatitis B and protection against chronic viral carriage in the Gambia. *Lancet* 1991; 337:747–750.

14 Chokunonga E, Levy L M & Bassett M T. Cancer incidence in the African population of Harare, Zimbabwe: second results from the cancer registry 1993–1995. *Int J Cancer* 2000; 85:54–59.

15 Chadwick E G, Connor E J, Hanson C G et al. Tumours of smooth muscle origin in HIV-infected children. *JAMA* 1990; 263:3182–3184.

16 McLoughlin L C, Nord K S, Joshi V V et al. Disseminated leiomyosarcoma in a child with AIDS. *Cancer* 1991; 67:2618–2621.

17 Ateenyi-Agaba C. Conjunctival squamous cell carcinoma associated with HIV infection in Kampala, Uganda. *Lancet* 1995; 345: 695–696.

18 Newton R. A review of the aetiology of squamous cell carcinoma of the conjunctiva. *Br J Cancer* 1996; 74:1511–1513.

19 Parkin D M, Stjernsward J & Muir C. Estimates of worldwide frequency of 12 major cancers. *Bull World Health Organ* 1984; 62:163–182.

20 Whelan S L, Parkin D M & Masuyer E (eds). Patterns of cancer in five continents. *IARC Sci Publ* 1990; 102.

21 Grant M C. Cancer of the cervix: a tragic disease in South Africa. *S Afr Med J* 1982; 61:819–822.

22 Rogo K O, Omany J, Onyango J N, Ojwang S B & Stendahl U. Carcinoma of the cervix in the African setting. In *Human Papilloma Virus and Human Immunodeficiency Virus Infection in Relation to Cervical Cancer*. Umea University Medical Dissertations no. 293, part I, 1990: 1–22.

23 Briggs N D & Katchy K C. Pattern of primary gynaecological malignancies as seen in a tertiary hospital situated in the River State of Nigeria. *Int J Gynaecol Obstet* 1990; 31:157–161.

24 Mgaya H N & Mbura J S. The pattern of cervical cancer at Muhimbili Medical Centre, Dar-es-Salaam, Tanzania. *Tanzania Med J* 1985; 2:11–17.

25 Kasule J. The pattern of gynaecological malignancy in Zimbabwe. *East Afr Med J* 1989; 66:393–399.

26 Brinton L A & Fraumeni J F Jr. Epidemiology of uterine cervical cancer. *J Chronic Dis* 1986; 39:1051–1065.

27 Brinton L A, Hamman R F, Huggins G R et al. Sexual and reproductive risk factors for invasive squamous cell cervical cancer. *J Natl Cancer Inst* 1987; 79:23–30.

28 Skegg D C G, Corwin P A, Panel C & Doll R. Importance of the male factor in cancer of the cervix. *Lancet* 1982; ii:581–583.

29 Brinton L A, Reeves W C, Brenes M M et al. The male factor in the etiology of cervical cancer among sexually monogamous women. *Int J Cancer* 1989; 44:199–203.

30 Brinton L A, Schairer C, Haenzel W et al. Smoking and invasive cervical cancer. *JAMA* 1986; 255:3265–3269.

31 Layde P M. Smoking and cervical cancer: cause or coincidence? *JAMA* 1989; 261:1631–1632.

32 Piper J M. Oral contraceptives and cervical cancer. *Gynecol Oncol* 1985; 22:1–14.

33 Yach D & Townsend G S. Smoking and health in South Africa. *S Afr Med J* 1988; 73:391–399.

34 Halpert R, Fruchter R G, Sedlis A et al. Human papillomavirus and lower genital neoplasia in renal transplant patients. *Obstet Gynecol* 1986; 68:251–258.

35. Katz R L, Veanattukalathil S & Weiss K M. Human papilloma infection and neoplasia of the cervix and anogenital region in women with Hodgkin's disease. *Acta Cytol* 1983; 27:220–224.

36 Anonymous. Centers for Disease Control 1993 revised classification system for HIV-infections and expanded surveillance case definition for AIDS among adolescents and adults. *Morbid Mortal Wkly Rep* 1992; 41:1–19.

37 Zur Hausen H. Condylomata acumunata and human genital cancer. *Cancer Res* 1976; 36:794.

38 Meanwell C A, Cox M F, Blackledge G & Maitland N J. Human papilloma virus 16 DNA in normal and malignant cervical epithelium: implications for aetiology and behaviour of cervical neoplasia. *Lancet* 1987; i:703–707.

39 Wright T C Jr & Richart R M. Role of human papilloma virus in the pathogenesis of genital tract warts and cancer. *Gynecol Oncol* 1990; 37:151–164.

40 Reeves W C, Brinton L A, Garcia M et al. Human papilloma virus infection and cervical cancer in Latin America. *N Engl J Med* 1989; 320:1437–1441.

41 Riou G, Favre M, Jeannel D, Bourhis J, Le Dousaal V & Orth G. Association between poor prognosis in early-stage invasive cervical carcinoma and non-detection of HPV DNA. *Lancet* 1990; 335:1171–1174.

42 Fuchs P G, Girardi F & Pfister H. Human papilloma virus 16 DNA in cervical cancer and in lymph nodes of cervical cancer patients: a diagnostic marker for early metastases. *Int J Cancer* 1989; 43:41–44.

43 Brodman M, Friedman F, Dottino P et al. A comparative study of computerized tomography, magnetic resonance imaging and clinical staging for detection of early cervix cancer. *Gynecol Oncol* 1990; 36:409–412.

44 Du-Toit J P. A cost effective but safe protocol for the staging of invasive cervical cancer in a Third World country. *Int J Gynaecol Obstet* 1988; 26:261–264.

45 Kurman R J, Schiffman M H, Lancaster W D et al. Analysis of individual human papilloma virus types in cervical neoplasia: a possible role of type 18 in rapid progression. *Am J Obstet Gynecol* 1988; 159:293–296.

46 Barnes W, Delgado G, Kurman R J et al. Possible prognostic significance of human papilloma virus type in cervical cancer. *Gynecol Oncol* 1988; 29:267–273.

47 Day N E. Screening for cancer of the cervix. *J Epidemiol Community Health* 1989; 43:103–106.

48 Anderson G H, Boyes D A, Benedet J L et al. Organization and results of the cervical cytology screening programme in British Columbia. *BMJ* 1988; 296:975–978.

49 International Agency for Research on Cancer, Working Group on Evaluation of Cervical Cancer Screening Programmes. Screening for squamous cervical cancer; duration of risk after negative results of cervical cytology and implication for screening policies. *BMJ* 1990; 293:659–664.

50 Marteau T M. Ethics of clinical research. *BMJ* 1989; 299:513–514.

51 Raffle A E, Aldar B & MacKenzie E F D. Six years audit of laboratory workload and rates of referral for colposcopy in cervical screening programme in three districts. *BMJ* 1990; 301:907–911.

52 Van Nagell J R Jr, Hanson M B, Donaldson E S & Gallion H H. Treatment of cervical intraepithelial neoplasma III by hysterectomy without intervening conization in patients with adequate colposcopy. *Cancer* 1985; 56:2737–2739.

53 Keys H M, Bundy B N, Stehman F B et al. Cisplatin, radiation and adjuvant hysterectomy compared with radiation and adjuvant hysterectomy for bulky stage IB cervical carcinoma. *N Engl J Med* 1999; 340:1154–1161.

54 Rose P G, Bundy B N, Watkins E B et al. Concurrent cisplatin-based radiotherapy and chemotherapy for locally advanced cervical cancer. *N Engl J Med* 1999; 340:1144–1153.

55 National Cancer Institute. Concurrent chemoradiation for cervical cancer. Clinical announcement, Washington, DC, 22 February 1999.

56 Prates M D & Torres F O. A cancer survey in Lourenco Marques, Portuguese East Africa. *J Natl Cancer Inst* 1965; 35:729–757.

57 Van Rensburg S J, Cook-Mozaffari P, Van Schalkwyk D J, Van Der Watt J J, Vincent T J & Purchase I F. Hepatocellular carcinoma and dietary aflatoxin in Mozambique and Transkei. *Br J Cancer* 1985; 51:713–726.

58 Kew M C. The hepatitis B virus and hepatocellular carcinoma. *Semin Liver Dis* 1981; 1:59–67.

59 Yu M C, Tong M J, Coursaget P et al. Prevalence of hepatitis B and hepatitis C viral markers in black and white patients with hepatocellular carcinoma in the United States. *J Natl Cancer Inst* 1990; 82:1038–1041.

60 Beasley R P, Hwang L Y, Lin C C & Chien C S. Hepatocellular carcinoma and hepatitis B virus. *Lancet* 1981; ii:1129–1133.

61 Shafritz D A, Shouval D, Sherman N I, Hadziyannis S J & Kew M C. Integration of hepatitis B virus DNA into the genome of liver cells in chronic liver disease and hepatocellular carcinoma. *N Engl J Med* 1981; 305:1067–1073.

62 Brechot C, Nalpas B, Courouce A et al. Evidence that hepatitis B virus has a role in liver-cell carcinoma in alcoholic liver disease. *N Engl J Med* 1982; 306:1384–1387.

63 Tabor E, Kobayashi K. Hepatitis C virus, a causative infectious agent of non-A, non-B hepatitis: prevalence and structure. Summary of a conference of hepatitis C virus as a cause of hepatocellular carcinoma. *J Natl Cancer Inst* 1992; 84:86–90.

64 International Agency for Research on Cancer. Evaluation of carcinogenic risk of chemicals to man. *IARC Monogr* 1976; 10.

65 Newberne P M & Butler W H. Acute and chronic effects of aflatoxin on the liver of domestic and laboratory animals: a review. *Cancer Res* 1969; 29:230–235.

66 Carnaghan R B A. Hepatic tumours and chronic liver changes in rats following administration of aflatoxin. *Br J Cancer* 1967; 21:811–814.

67 Peers F, Bosch X, Kaldor J, Linsell A & Pluijmen M. Aflatoxin exposure, hepatitis B virus infection and liver cancer in Swaziland. *Int J Cancer* 1987; 39:545–553.

68 Peers F G, Gilman G A & Linsell C A. Dietary aflatoxin and human liver cancer: a study in Swaziland. *Int J Cancer* 1976; 17:167–176.

69 Bulatao J, Almero E M, Castro Jardeleza Ma T R & Salamat L A. A case–control dietary study of primary liver cancer from aflatoxin exposure. *Int J Epidemiol* 1982; 11:112–119.

70 Linsell C. Aflatoxin and liver cancer. *Trans R Soc Trop Med Hyg* 1977; 7:471–473.

71 Campbell T & Hayes J. Role of aflatoxin metabolism in its toxic lesion. *Toxicol Appl Pharmacol* 1976; 35:195–222.

72 Lutwik L. Relations between aflatoxin, hepatitis B virus and hepatocellular carcinoma. *Lancet* 1979; i:755–757.

73 Coady A. The aflatoxin–hepatoma hepatitis B surface antigen story. *BMJ* 1975; 3:592–593.

74 Kew M C, Dibisceglie A M & Paterson A. Smoking as a risk-factor in hepatocellular carcinoma: a case–control study in Southern African blacks. *Cancer* 1985; 56:2315–2317.

75 Yu M C & Tong M J. Non viral risk factors for hepatocellular carcinoma in low-risk population, the non-Asians of Los Angeles County, California. *J Natl Cancer Inst* 1991; 83:1820–1826.

76 Maynard E P, Sedikali F, Anthony P P & Barker L F. Hepatitis-associated antigen and cirrhosis in Uganda. *Lancet* 1970; ii:1326–1328.

77 Higginson J & Oettle A G. Cancer incidence in Bantu and 'Cape Colored' races of South Africa: report of a cancer survey in the Transvaal (1953–1955). *J Natl Cancer Inst* 1960; 24:589–671.

78 Li J J & Li S A. High incidence of hepatocellular carcinoma after synthetic oestrogen administration in Syrian golden hamsters fed alpha-naphthoflavine: a new tumour model. *J Natl Cancer Inst* 1984; 73:543–547.

79 Kew M C, Kassianides C, Hodkinson J, Coppon A & Paterson A C. Hepatocellular carcinoma in urban born blacks: frequency and relation to hepatitis B virus infection. *BMJ* 1986; 293:1339–1341.

80 Attali P, Prod'homme S, Pelletier G et al. Prognostic factors in patients with hepatocellular carcinoma. *Cancer* 1987; 59:2108–2111.

81 Sowl S H, Titelbaum D S, Gansler T S et al. The fibrolamellar variant of hepatocellular carcinoma: its association with focal nodular hyperplasia. *Cancer* 1987; 60:3049–3055.

82 Van Tonder S, Kew M C, Hodkinson J & Fernandes-Costa F. Serum vitamin B_{12} binders in Southern African blacks with hepatocellular carcinoma. *Cancer* 1985; 56:789–792.

83 Vogel C L & Linsell C A. International symposium on hepatocellular carcinoma, Kampala, Uganda. *J Natl Cancer Inst* 1972; 48:567–571.

84 Primack A, Vogel C L, Kyalwazi S K et al. A staging system for hepatocellular carcinoma: prognostic factors in Ugandan patients. *Cancer* 1975; 35:1357–1364.

85 Olweny C L M, Toya T, Katongole-Mbidde E, Mugerwa J, Kyalwazi S K & Cohen H. Treatment of hepatocellular carcinoma with adriamycin: preliminary communication. *Cancer* 1975; 36:1250–1257.

86 Chen M, Hwang T, Jeng L, Jan Y & Wang C. Surgical treatment for spontaneous rupture of hepatocellular carcinoma. *Surg Gynecol Obstet* 1988; 167:99–102.

87 Olweny C L M, Katongole-Mbidde E, Bahendeka S, Otim D, Mugerwa J & Kyalwazi S K. Further experience in treating patients with hepatocellular carcinoma in Uganda. *Cancer* 1980; 46:2717–2722.

88 Bezwoda W R, Weaving A, Kew M & Derman D P. Combination chemotherapy of hepatocellular cancer. *Oncology* 1987; 44:207–209.

89 Olweny C L M & Johnson R. Rapid response to cisplatin and doxorubicin in hepatitis B virus reactivation. *J Gastroenterol Hepatol* 1987; 2:533–537.

90 Olweny C, Hakim J, Gudza I et al. Manuscript submitted.

91 Prevention of hepatocellular carcinoma by immunization. *Bull World Health Organ* 1983; 61:731–744.

92 Whittle H C, Maine N, Pilkington J et al. Long-term efficacy of continuing hepatitis B vaccination in infancy in two Gambian villages. *Lancet* 1995; 345:1089–1092.

93 Kobayashi K, Sugimoto T, Makino H et al. Screening methods for early detection of hepatocellular carcinoma. *Hepatology* 1985; 5:1100–1105.

94 Rose E F. Oesophageal cancer in the Transkei: 1955–1969. *J Natl Cancer Inst* 1973; 51:7–16.

95 Cook P. Cancer of the oesophagus in Africa. *Br J Cancer* 1971; 25:853.

96 Van Rensburg S J, Benade A S, Rose E F & du Plessis J P. Nutritional status of African populations predisposed to oesophageal cancer. *Nutr Cancer* 1983; 4:206–216.

97 Oettle A G. *Cancer Research in Africa.* Johannesburg: Witwatersrand University Press, 1967.

98 Van Rensburg S J, Bradshaw E S, Bradshaw D & Rose E F. Oesophageal cancer in Zulu men, South Africa: a case–control study. *Br J Cancer* 1985; 51:399–405.

99 Bradshaw E & Schonland M. Smoking, drinking and oesophageal cancer in African males of Johannesburg, South Africa. *Br J Cancer* 1974; 30:157–163.

100 Van Rensburg S J. Epidemiologic and dietary evidence for a specific nutritional predisposition to esophageal cancer. *J Natl Cancer Inst* 1981; 67:243–251.

101 Crespi M, Munoz N, Grassi A et al. Oesophageal lesions in Northern Iran: a premalignant condition. *Lancet* 1979; i:217–221.

102 Munoz N, Crespi M, Grassi A et al. Precursor lesions of oesophageal cancer in high risk population in Iran and China. *Lancet* 1982; i:876–879.

103 Munoz N, Wanrendorf J, Bang L J et al. No effect of riboflavin, retinol and zinc on prevalence of precancerous lesions of oesophagus. *Lancet* 1985; ii:111–114.

104 Flemen P, Lerut A, Van Cutsem E et al. Utility of position emission tomography for the staging of patients with potentially operable oesophageal carcinoma. *J Clin Oncol* 2000; 18:3202–3210.

105 Ropp M B, Hawley D, Reising J et al. Improved survival in squamous oesophageal cancer, preoperative chemotherapy and irradiation. *Arch Surg* 1986; 121:1330–1335.

106 Ellis F H & Maggs P R. Surgery for carcinoma of the lower oesophagus and cardia. *World J Surg* 1981; 5:527–533.

107 Orringer M B. Technical aids in performing transhiatal esophagectomy without thoracotomy. *Ann Thorac Surg* 1984; 38:128–132.

108 Hennessy T P J. Choice of treatment in carcinoma of the oesophagus. *Br J Surg* 1988; 75:193–194.

109 Skinner D B. Surgical treatments for oesophageal carcinoma. *Semin Oncol* 1984; 11:135–143.

110 Pearson J G. The present and future potential of radiotherapy in the management of esophageal cancer. *Cancer* 1977; 39:882–890.

111 Earlam R & Cunha-Melo J R. Oesophageal squamous cell carcinoma: I. A critical review of surgery. *Br J Surg* 1980; 67:381–390.

112 Earlam R & Cunha-Melo J R. Oesophageal squamous cell carcinoma: II. A critical review of radiotherapy. *Br J Surg* 1980; 67:457–461.

113 Launois B, Delarne D, Campion J P et al. Preoperative radiotherapy for carcinoma of the oesophagus. *Surg Gynecol Obstet* 1981; 153:690–692.

114 Kelsen D. Multimodality therapy of oesophageal carcinoma: still an experimental approach. *J Clin Oncol* 1987; 5:530–531.

115 Steiger Z, Franklin R, Wilson R F et al. Complete eradication of squamous cell carcinoma of the oesophagus with combined chemoradiotherapy and radiotherapy. *Am J Surg* 1981; 47:95–98.

116 Leichman L, Steiger Z, Seydel H G et al. Combined preoperative chemotherapy and radiation therapy for cancer of the oesophagus. *Semin Oncol* 1984; 11:178–185.

117 Poplon E, Fleming T, Leichman L et al. Combined therapies for squamous cell carcinoma of the esophagus: a Southwest Oncology Group Study (SOGS-8037). *J Clin Oncol* 1987; 5:622–628.

118 Forastieve A A, Orringer M B, Perez-Tamayo C et al. Concurrent chemotherapy and radiotherapy followed by transhiatal esophagectomy for local regional cancer of the oesophagus. *J Clin Oncol* 1990; 8:119–127.

119 Dewit L. Combined treatment of radiation and cisdiamine dichlonoplatinum (II): a review of experimental and clinical data. *Int J Radiat Oncol Biol Phys* 1987; 13:402–426.

120 Pfeffer M R, Teicher B A, Holder S A, al-Achi A & Herman T S. The interaction of cisplatin plus etoposide with radiation +/– hyperthermia. *Int J Radiat Oncol Biol Phys* 1990; 19:1439–1447.

121 Walsh T N, Noonan N, Hollywood D et al. A comparison of multimodal therapy and surgery for oesophageal adenocarcinoma. *N Engl J Med* 1996; 335:462–467.

122 Bossett G F, Gignoux M, Tribulet J P et al. Chemoradiotherapy followed by surgery compared with surgery alone in squamous cell carcinoma of the oesophagus. *N Engl J Med* 1997; 337:161–167.

123 Urba S G, Orringer M B, Turrisi A et al. Randomized trial of pre-operative chemo-radiation versus surgery alone in patients with locoregional oesophageal carcinoma. *J Clin Oncol* 2001; 19:305–313.

124 Ho V C & Sober A J. Therapy of cutaneous melanoma: an update. *J Am Acad Dermatol* 1990; 22:159–176.

125 Balch C M. Excising melanoma: how wide is enough? And how to reconstruct? *J Surg Oncol* 1990; 44:135–138.

126 Falkson C I & Falkson H C. Prognostic factors in metastatic malignant melanoma. *Oncology* 1998; 55:59–64.

127 Beahrs O H, Henson D E, Hutter R V P & Myers M (eds). Manual for staging of cancer, 3rd edn. Philadelphia, J B Lippincott, 1988: 139–144.

128 Buzaid A C, Ross M I, Balch C M et al. Critical analysis of the current American Joint Committee on Cancer Staging system for cutaneous melanoma and proposal of a new staging system. *J Clin Oncol* 1997; 15:1039–1051.

129 Balch C M, soong S J, Bartolucci A A et al. Efficacy of an elective regional node dissection of 1–4 mm thick melanomas for patients 60 years of age and younger. *Ann Surg* 1996; 224:255–266.

130 Brady M S & Coit D E. Sentinel lymph node evaluation in melanoma. *Arch Dermatol* 1997; 133:1014–1020.

131 Kirkwood J M, Strawderman M H, Ernstoff M S et al. Interferon alfa-2b adjuvant therapy of high-risk resected cutaneous melanoma. The Eastern Cooperative Oncology Group Trial EST 1684. *J Clin Oncol* 1996; 14:7–17.

132 Lee S M, Betticher D C, Thatcher N. Melanoma: chemotherapy. *Br Med Bull* 1995; 51:609–630.

133 Falkson C I, Falkson G, Falkson H E. Improved results with the addition of interferon alfa-2b to decarbazine in the treatment of patients with metastatic malignant melanoma. *J Clin Oncol* 1991; 9:1403–1408.

134 Middleton M R, Grob J J, Aaronson N et al. Randomized phase III study of temozolamide versus dacarbazine in the treatment of patients with advanced metastatic malignant melanoma. *J Clin Oncol* 2000; 18:158–166.

135 Friedman-Kien A E & Saltzman B R. Clinical manifestations of classical, endemic African and epidemic AIDS-associated Kaposi's sarcoma. *J Am Acad Dermatol* 1990; 22:1237–1250.

136 Harwood A R, Osoba P, Hostader S W et al. Kaposi's sarcoma in recipients of renal transplants. *Am J Med* 1979; 67:759–765.

137 Penn I. The changing pattern of post transplant malignancies. *Transplant Proc* 1991; 23:1101–1103.

138 Stribling J, Weitzner S & Smith G U. Kaposi's sarcoma in renal allograft patients. *Cancer* 1978; 42:442–446.

139 Penn I. Kaposi's sarcoma in organ transplant recipients: report of 20 cases. *Transplantation* 1979; 27:8–11.

140 Safai B, Sarngadharan M G, Koziner B et al. Spectrum of Kaposi's sarcoma in the epidemic of acquired immunodeficiency syndrome. *Cancer Res* 1985; 45:4646–4648.

141 Ensoli B, Nakamura S, Salahuddin S Z et al. Acquired immunodeficiency syndrome Kaposi's sarcoma derived cells express cytokines with autocrine and paracrine growth effects. *Science* 1989; 243:223–226.

142 Ensoli B, Barillari G, Salahuddin S Z et al. Tat protein of HIV-1 stimulates growth of cells from Kaposi's sarcoma lesions of AIDS patients. *Nature* 1990; 345:84–86.

143 Salahuddin S Z, Nakamura S, Biberfield P et al. Angiogenic properties of Kaposi's sarcoma derived cells after long-term culture in vitro. *Science* 1988; 242:430–433.

144 Chang Y, Cesarman E, Pessin M S et al. Identification of herpes virus-like DNA sequences in AIDS-associated Kaposi's sarcoma. *Science* 1994; 266:1865–1869.

145 Antman K & Chang Y. Kaposi's sarcoma. *N Engl J Med* 2000; 342:1027–1038.

146 Pauk J, Huang M L, Brodie S J et al. Mucosal shedding of human herpes virus 8 in men. *N Engl J Med* 2000; 343:1369–1377.

147 Reeve P A. HIV infection in patients admitted to a general hospital in Malawi. *BMJ* 1989; 298:1567–1568.

148 Serwadda D, Mugerwa R D, Sewankambo N K et al. Slim disease: a new disease in Uganda and its association with HTLV III infection. *Lancet* 1985; ii:359–361.

149 Olweny C L M, Kaddu-Mukasa A, Atine I, Owor R, Magrath I & Ziegler J. Childhood Kaposi's sarcoma: clinical features and therapy. *Br J Cancer* 1976; 33:555–560.

150 Grore J H. Kaposi's disease: report of an unusual case. *Radiology* 1955; 65:236–239.

151 Coetzee T & LeRoux C G J. Kaposi's sarcoma presentation with intestinal obstruction. *S Afr Med J* 1967; 41:442–445.

152 Mitchell N & Feder A. Kaposi's sarcoma with secondary involvement of the jejunum, perforation and peritonitis. *Ann Intern Med* 1949; 31:324–329.

153 Novis B H, King N & Banks N. Kaposi's sarcoma presenting with diarrhoea and protein-losing enteropathy. *Gastroenterology* 1974; 67:996.

154 Khorshid K A, Erzingatsian K, Watters D A K & Bailey A C. Intussusception due to Kaposi's sarcoma. *J R Coll Surg Edinb* 1987; 32:339–341.

155 Cook J. The clinical features of Kaposi's sarcoma in the East African Bantu. *Acta Un Int Cancer* 1962; 18:388–398.

156 Slavin G, Cameron H McD, Forbes C et al. Kaposi's sarcoma in East African children: a report of 51 cases. *Pathology* 1970; 100:189–199.

157 Krigel R L, Laubenstein L J & Muggia F M. Kaposi's sarcoma: a new staging classification. *Cancer Treat Rep* 1983; 67:531–534.

158 Mitsuyasu R T & Groopman J E. Biology and therapy of Kaposi's sarcoma. *Semin Oncol* 1984; 11:53–59.

159 Taylor J, Afrasiabi R, Fahey J L et al. A prognostically significant classification of immune changes in AIDS with Kaposi's sarcoma. *Blood* 1986; 67:666–671.

160 Kyalwazi S K. Chemotherapy of Kaposi's sarcoma: experience with Trenimon. *East Afr Med J* 1968; 45:17–26.

161 Olweny C L M, Sikyewunda W & Otim D. Further experience with Razoxane (ICRF 159–NSC 129943) in treating Kaposi's sarcoma. *Oncology* 1980; 37:174–176.

162 Olweny C L M, Toya T, Katongole-Mbidde E et al. Treatment of Kaposi's sarcoma combination of actinomycin-D, vincristine and imidazole carboxamide (NSC 45388): results of a randomized clinical trial. *Int J Cancer* 1974; 14:649–656.

163 Olweny C, Borok M, Gudza I et al (manuscript submitted).

164 Burkitt D P. A sarcoma involving the jaws in African children. *Br J Surg* 1958; 197:218–223.

165 Pike M C, Williams E H & Wright D. Burkitt's tumour in the West Nile district of Uganda. *BMJ* 1967; ii:395–399.

166 Ziegler J L, Drew W L, Miner R C et al. Outbreak of Burkitt's-like lymphoma in homosexual men. *Lancet* 1982; ii:631–633.

167 Epstein M A, Achong B G & Barr Y M. Virus particles in cultured lymphoblasts from Burkitt's lymphoma. *Lancet* 1964; i:702–703.

168 Nonoyama M & Ragano J S. Homology between Epstein–Barr virus DNA and viral-DNA from Burkitt's lymphoma and nasopharyngeal carcinoma determined by DNA–DNA reassociation kinetics. *Nature* 1973; 242:44–47.

169 de-The G, Geser A, Day N E et al. Epidemiological evidence for a causal relationship between Epstein–Barr virus and Burkitt's lymphoma: results of the Ugandan prospective study. *Nature* 1978; 274:756–761.

170 Olweny C L M, Atine I, Kaddu-Mukasa A et al. Epstein–Barr virus genome studies in Burkitt and non-Burkitt lymphomas in Uganda. *J Natl Cancer Inst* 1977; 58:1191–1196.

171 Schmauz R, Mugerwa J W & Wright D H. The distribution on non-Burkitt, non-Hodgkin's lymphomas in Uganda in relation to malaria endemicity. *Int J Cancer* 1990; 45:650–653.

172 Zech L, Haglund U, Nilsson K et al. Characteristic chromosomal abnormalities in biopsies and lymphoid cell lines from patients with Burkitt and non-Burkitt lymphomas. *Int J Cancer* 1976; 17:47–56.

173 Levine A, Momand J & Finlay C. The p53 tumour suppressor gene. *Nature* 1991; 351:453–456.

174 Harris C C & Hollstein M. Clinical implications of the p53 tumour-suppressor gene. *N Engl J Med* 1993; 329:1318–1327.

175 Wiman K G, Magnusson K P, Ramquist T et al. Mutant p53 detected in a majority of Burkitt lymphoma cell lines by monoclonal antibody Pab240. *Oncogene* 1991; 6:1633–1639.

176 Preudhomme C, Dervite I, Wattel E et al. Clinical significance of p53 mutations in newly diagnosed Burkitt's lymphoma and acute lymphoblastic leukemia: A report of 48 cases. *J Clin Oncol* 1995; 13:812–820.

177 Magrath I T, Lwanga S, Carswell W & Harrison N. Surgical reduction of tumour bulk in the management of abdominal Burkitt's lymphoma. *BMJ* 1974; ii:308–312.

178 Olweny C L M, Atine I, Kaddu-Mukasa A et al. Cerebrospinal irradiation of Burkitt's lymphoma: failure in preventing central nervous system relapse. *Acta Radiol Ther Phys Biol* 1977; 16:225–231.

179 Olweny C L M, Katongole-Mbidde E, Kaddu-Mukasa A et al. Treatment of Burkitt's lymphoma: randomized clinical trial of single versus combination chemotherapy. *Int J Cancer* 1976; 17:436–440.

180 Ziegler J L, Bluming A Z, Fass L & Morrow R H. Relapse patterns in Burkitt's lymphoma. *Cancer Res* 1972; 32:1267–1272.

181 Olweny C L M, Katongole-Mbidde E, Otim D, Lwanga S K, Magrath I & Ziegler J L. Long-term experience with Burkitt's lymphoma in Uganda. *Int J Cancer* 1980; 26:261–266.

182 Epstein M A. Vaccination against Epstein–Barr virus: current progress and future strategies. *Lancet* 1986; i:1425–1427.

183 Epstein M A. Recent studies on a vaccine to prevent Epstein–Barr virus-associated cancers. *Br J Cancer* 1986; 54:1–5.

184 Wolf H, zur Hausen H & Becker V. Epstein–Barr virus genomes in epithelial nasopharyngeal cancer cells. *Nature (New Biol)* 1973; 244:245–247.

185 Henle G & Henle W. Epstein–Barr virus-specific IgA serum antibodies as an outstanding feature of nasopharyngeal carcinoma. *Int J Cancer* 1976; 17:1–7.

186 Desgranges C, Wolf H, De-Thé G et al. Nasopharyngeal carcinoma: presence of Epstein–Barr genomes in separated epithelial cells of tumours in patients from Singapore, Tunisia and Kenya. *Int J Cancer* 1975; 16:7–15.

187 Rathmanathan R, Prasad U, Sadler R et al. Clonal proliferations of cells infected with Epstein–Barr virus in pre-invasive lesions related to nasopharyngeal carcinoma. *N Engl J Med* 1995; 333:693–698.

188 Shao Y M, Poirier S, Ohshima H et al. Epstein–Barr virus activation in Raji cells by extracts of preserved food from high risk areas for nasopharyngeal carcinoma. *Carcinogenesis* 1988; 9:1455–1457.

189 Jesse R H, Perez C A & Fletcher G H. Cervical lymph node metastasis: unknown primary cancer. *Cancer* 1973; 31:854–859.

190 Ho J H. Nasopharyngeal carcinoma. *West J Med* 1985; 143:70–73.

191 Holoye P Y, Byers R M & Gard D A. Combination chemotherapy of head and neck cancer. *Cancer* 1978; 42:1661–1669.

192 Wei W I, Sham J S, Zong Y-S, Choy D & Ng M H. The efficacy of fibreoptic endoscopic examination and biopsy in the detection of early nasopharyngeal cancer. *Cancer* 1991; 67:3127–3130.

193 Binnie W H. Oral cancer. In Dolby A E (ed.) *Oral Mucosa in Health and Disease.* Oxford: Blackwell, 1975: 301–333.

194 Pindborg J J. Epidemiological studies of oral cancer. *Int Dent J* 1977; 27:172–178.

195 Mehta F S et al. *Oral Cancer and Precancerous Conditions in India.* Copenhagen: Munksgaard, 1971.

196 Warnakulasuriya K A A S, Ekanayake A N I, Sivayoham J et al. Utilization of primary health care workers for early detection of oral cancer and precancer cases in Sri Lanka. *Bull World Health Organ* 1984; 62:243–250.

197 Fergusson D R. Associated bilharziasis and primary malignant disease of the urinary bladder. *J Pathol Bacteriol* 1911; 16:76–79.

198 Gelfand M, Weinberg R W & Castle V M. Relation between carcinoma of the bladder and infestation with *Schistosoma haematobium. Lancet* 1967; i:1249–1251.

199 Hicks R M, Walters C L, el Sebai I et al. Demonstration of nitrosamines in human urine: preliminary observations on a possible etiology for bladder cancer associated with chronic urinary infection. *Proc R Soc Med* 1977; 70:413–417.

200 el Aaser A A & el Merzabani M M. Etiology of bladder cancer. In el-Sebai I & Hoogstraten B (eds) *Bladder Cancer,* vol. I (CRC Series on Experiences in Clinical Oncology). Boca Raton, FL: CRC Press, 1983: 39–58.

201 el-Bolkainy M N, Ghoneim M A, el-Morsey B A & Nasrs M. Cancer of bilharzial bladder: diagnostic value of urine cytology. *Urology* 1974; 3:319.

202 Awward H K, Abdel Baki H, el-Bolkainy M N et al. Preoperative irradiation of T_3 carcinoma in bilharzial bladder: a comparison between hyperfractionation and conventional fractionation. *Int J Radiat Oncol Biol Phys* 1979; 5:787.

Chapter 37
Diabetes Mellitus in the Tropics

T. I. L. Richardson, D. A. Cavan, and A. H. Barnett

Diabetes mellitus is a worldwide disease but varies greatly in prevalence. In temperate regions there are two common types, type I (insulin dependent) and type II (non-insulin dependent), accounting for about 15% and 85% of cases respectively. These diseases also occur in the tropics and, while the prevalence of type I diabetes is generally low, some discrete populations have very high incidences of type II diabetes.

A third type of disease is seen in tropical countries. This has been termed variously as J-type, Z-type, type III or tropical pancreatic diabetes. Such cases have been said to be associated with malnutrition and the general term malnutrition-related diabetes mellitus (MRDM) was coined by the World Health Organization (WHO) in 1985. Ongoing controversy within the field is leading to a change in nomenclature to *malnutrition-modulated diabetes mellitus (MMDM)*.[1] As discussed below, this shares features of both type I and type II diabetes.

The epidemiology and pathogenesis of each type of diabetes will be discussed separately, with particular emphasis on regional variations and the pattern of disease in tropical countries.

Type I diabetes mellitus

Type I diabetes is predominantly a Caucasoid disease[2] and the highest prevalence rates occur in northern European countries. Although only scanty data are available in some cases, evidence suggests that the prevalence is low in most other races, including Asian Indians,[3] Chinese,[4] Japanese[2] and black Africans[2] (Table 37.1). The prevalence of the disease in black Americans and Afro-Caribbeans is, however, intermediate between that seen in white Caucasians and black Africans.[5] This may result from admixture of Caucasian genes in the negroid genome (estimated to be around 21% in black Americans). Within Europe there is a north–south gradient of prevalence rates, which range from 2.2 per 1000 population in Finland[6] to 0.24 per 1000 in France.[7] Both genetic and environmental factors have been implicated to explain these differences.

Type I diabetes is characterized by T-cell-dependent destruction of pancreatic β cells.[8] This depends on activation of CD4$^+$ T cells following presentation of antigen bound to the human leucocyte antigen (HLA) molecule on the surface of antigen-presenting cells. Type

Table 37.1 Worldwide prevalence of type I diabetes.

Country	Prevalence per 1000
Finland	2.2
USA	1.0
UK	0.7
France	0.24
India	0.06–0.7*
China	0.09
Japan	0.03
Tropical Africa	0.03†

*The range given reflects regional differences in prevalence rates in India.
†Accurate prevalence figures not yet available for tropical Africa; the figure given is a realistic estimate based on available data.

I diabetes is associated with certain HLA types and antigen presentation, and hence disease susceptibility may be partly influenced by the nature of the HLA molecule(s). In Caucasians, 95% of affected subjects possess either HLA-DR3 or DR4[9] or both, while DR2 and DRw6 appear to be protective.[10] These antigens are encoded by the *DRB1* gene of the major histocompatibility complex (MHC) on chromosome 6 (Figure 37.1). The MHC genes exhibit much variation or polymorphism and there is strong linkage disequilibrium between specific variants (alleles) of the *DRB1* gene and those of the *DQA1* and *DQB1* genes. This implies that certain alleles will occur together at a frequency greater than expected by chance. Analysis of *DQA1* and *DQB1* genes in different ethnic groups has demonstrated that particular alleles show consistent disease associations in many races and may represent primary susceptibility determinants.[9] Furthermore, those races with low disease incidences have a reduced frequency of these susceptibility alleles (the DR4-related susceptibility allele is rare in Asians[11] and the DR3-related susceptibility allele is rare in Japanese[12]). A second important gene associated with susceptibility to type I diabetes has been mapped near the insulin (INS) gene on chromosome 11p. This has been identified as the INS VNTR (variable-number tandem repeat) locus and is said to account for around 10% of the genetic risk for developing type I diabetes.[13] Absence of these alleles or variations in the tandem repeat locus in a particular ethnic group may directly influence the prevalence of type I diabetes in that race.

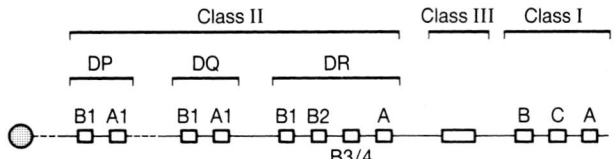

Figure 37.1: Simplified diagram of the HLA system on chromosome 6.

Despite the strong evidence for inherited susceptibility, studies of identical twins suggest that this accounts for only 30–40% of disease susceptibility.[14] Environmental factors must also play an important role. Seasonal variation in the onset of disease has been reported in many different populations, indicating a possible viral aetiology.[15] Migrants from low-risk to high-risk areas assume the higher risk of their host country, e.g., Japanese migrants to Hawaii and French migrants to Canada, suggesting that disease susceptibility may be influenced by the host environment.[16] Temporal changes in disease incidence have also occurred, with a doubling in incidence in 3 years in an area of western Poland.[17] These observations could be explained by viral infection triggering autoimmune β cell destruction. The nature of such infection remains elusive.

In summary, type I diabetes appears to be rare in the tropics. This may be due to the lack of one or more susceptibility genes or the absence of a disease-inducing environmental agent. The increased mortality from the disease in poor countries with limited health resources may also play a part in reducing the prevalence rates in these countries compared with developed nations. When it occurs, the disease is clinically indistinguishable from that seen in Caucasians.[2]

Type II diabetes mellitus

Type II diabetes is by far the more common of the two main types of the disease. It is characterized by the presence of residual endogenous insulin secretion and peripheral insulin resistance.[18] The latter has been suggested as the primary pathogenetic abnormality in type II diabetes as well as obesity and hypertension, with which it is often associated.[19] Insulitis does not occur but abnormal islet amyloid peptides have been demonstrated in some subjects, although their role, if any, in pathogenesis is unclear.[20]

Like type I diabetes, it shows a marked ethnic variation in prevalence (Table 37.2). In general, prevalence in developed nations lies between 1% and 4%, but is as high as 6% in Asian Indians, both in India[21] and in migrants to Africa,[22] whereas the prevalence in black Africans is low.[23] Asian migrants to South Africa[24] and the UK,[25] however, show a marked increase in disease prevalence. There are also discrete populations with very high disease rates, around 50% in Pima Indians in the United States[26] and in the Micronesians of Naura.[27] These ethnic variations suggest a genetic basis for type II diabetes. This

Table 37.2 Prevalence of type II diabetes in different populations.

Population	Prevalence (%)
White Caucasian	
Europe	2
USA	4
Asian	
South India	6
North India	1.2
UK	12
South Africa	20
Tanzania	7
Afro-Caribbean	
Tanzania	1.1
Nigeria	1.4
USA	5
Others	
Mauritius	10
Pima Indians (USA)	50
Micronesians (Naura)	50

is supported by the 90% disease concordance in identical twins.[13] Unlike type I diabetes, however, there has been little success in identifying possible susceptibility genes.

Apart from differences in prevalence, other racial differences also occur. Whereas onset is rare below the age of 40 years in Caucasians, the disease quite commonly appears in the third decade in Asian and, to a lesser extent, black subjects.[25] Such cases may need to be carefully evaluated to avoid unnecessary treatment with insulin: absence of ketosis, duration of presenting symptoms and the detection of plasma C peptide may help to distinguish this entity from type I diabetes.

Asian Indians with type II diabetes have a high prevalence of hypertension and coronary heart disease. One study demonstrated higher fasting insulin and triglyceride levels and higher blood pressure in Asian compared with European type II diabetic subjects.[28] This may indicate a greater role for insulin resistance in the disease in this race, which together with the early age of onset may account for the high prevalence of coronary heart disease.

Within the Asian Indian population, the prevalence amongst urban dwellers is up to four times that of rural communities.[29,30] This suggests that environmental as well as genetic factors are important in disease pathogenesis. Obesity is the most important nutritional factor in the aetiology of type II diabetes[31] and its rarity in rural workers may help explain their low prevalence of disease. Obesity is common, however, in the relatively wealthy urban dwellers who have access to plentiful food and who may take less exercise. This would explain the relative increase in prevalence in Asians in the UK compared with those in Tanzania, for example. Indeed many of the populations with very high incidences of type II diabetes have experienced a sudden increase in wealth over the last few decades associated with increasing urbanization and obesity. As well as the Pima Indians and Micronesians cited above, similar trends have been observed in black Americans[32] and some Arab populations.[33]

The high frequency in Asians compared with, for example, white Europeans, cannot, however, be explained by increased wealth and urbanization in the former. Available evidence points to a genetic predisposition to the disease in these populations, mostly within the tropics, which is manifest as type II diabetes with the adoption of a more 'Western' lifestyle. These observations led to the 'thrifty genotype' hypothesis first put forward nearly 30 years ago.[34] It was suggested that, in populations where famine alternated with periods of food abundance, individuals with a predisposition to type II diabetes used the limited food supply more efficiently and therefore had a selective advantage during famine. The 'progress' which has abolished famine in these populations has resulted in the expression of this genotype as type II diabetes and obesity.

This is supported by data from Tanzania which showed a low prevalence of type II diabetes (0.87%) in black Africans.[23] The prevalence of impaired glucose tolerance (defined as glucose tolerance between normal value(s) and frank diabetes, and may be associated with later development of type II diabetes), however, was similar to that of North Americans. This suggests that disease expression in rural Africans is inhibited by the absence of those environmental factors present in the US population.

This is an attractive hypothesis but cannot account for all cases of type II diabetes in tropical countries. Although rare, the disease does occur in rural Africans, many of whom (43% in one study) are underweight.[23] Another study of urban Kenyans showed a lower body mass index in diabetic than in control subjects.[35]

In summary, type II diabetes is very common in some Asian and other races but is relatively rare in much of tropical Africa. An urban lifestyle and increased wealth and availability of food correlate with increasing disease prevalence.

Malnutrition-related diabetes mellitus/ malnutrition-modulated diabetes mellitus

In 1955 the term J-type diabetes was used to describe those patients in Jamaica (around 6%) who could not be classified as having either type I or type II diabetes.[36] Despite an early age of onset, low body weight and the requirement for high doses of insulin, they were ketosis resistant. A condition termed Z-type or tropical pancreatic diabetes was reported from Indonesia in 1959.[37] In addition to the above features, this was characterized by a history of childhood malnutrition and pancreatic calcification and fibrosis. Both types have since been reported in most tropical countries, including India, Ethiopia, Nigeria, Uganda, Ghana, Tanzania, Malawi, Kenya, Zaire, Cameroon, Pakistan, India, Sri Lanka, Brazil, Madagascar, Zimbabwe, Singapore, Brunei and Papua New Guinea.[38]

The WHO proposed the term malnutrition-related diabetes mellitus (MRDM) to incorporate the above types of tropical diabetes and others which had been described since the early twentieth century.[39] It was thus implied that they constituted a single entity but this is doubted by some authors, as is the relationship with malnutrition: indeed in some cases malnutrition may result from the disease rather than be causative.

Under the WHO classification, MRDM is subdivided into protein-deficient pancreatic diabetes (PDPD) and fibrocalculous pancreatic diabetes (FCPD), which largely correspond to the J- and Z-types, respectively. FCPD implies the presence of pancreatic calcification and fibrosis, which result from a form of chronic pancreatitis known as tropical calcific pancreatitis (TCP).[38] Identification of MRDM as a distinct class of diabetes mellitus with FCPD and PDPD as specific subtypes has evoked controversy specifically with regard to the implied role of malnutrition in the pathogenesis of both types and to the distinctiveness of the two subclasses of MRDM.[40]

The diagnostic criteria for PDPD are: blood glucose greater than 11.1 mmol/litre, disease onset under the age of 30 years, body mass index less than 19 kg/m^2, absence of ketosis, poor socioeconomic status or history of childhood malnutrition and insulin requirement of more than 60 units per day.[41] Additional criteria for the diagnosis of FCPD include a history of recurrent abdominal pain from an early age and radiographic or ultrasonographic evidence of pancreatic calculi in the absence of alcoholism, gallstones or hyperparathyroidism.[42]

An alternative series of criteria which emphasize the presence of malnutrition has also been proposed: the two major criteria required for diagnosis are residence between the tropics of Cancer and Capricorn, and chronic low protein and calorie intake; in addition there are three supportive minor criteria (the presence of exocrine pancreatic disease, a requirement for insulin and early age of onset).[43]

Disease prevalence is often difficult to establish for the same logical reasons as with the other types of diabetes. These difficulties are compounded by a lack of consensus regarding diagnostic criteria and possible overlap with types I and II diabetes, especially in view of the young age of onset of the latter in many tropical countries. Thus one study from India which found that MRDM accounted for 23% of cases of diabetes[44] probably included cases of type II diabetes. Up to 80% of cases in Indonesia[37] and 50% of those under 20 years of age in Nigeria[45] are reported to have MRDM. Other reports, however, suggest much lower rates. FCPD was present in only 0.4% of 3100 cases in Madras, India;[46] a recent study from Nigeria found that only 6% of young patients could be classified as having MRDM[47] and it is absent from parts of Ethiopia.[48]

Pathology and pathogenesis

Available information on the pathological changes in MRDM is incomplete and largely confined to the FCPD variant. The hallmark is pancreatic fibrosis, which is much more marked in FCPD than PDPD. Pancreatic calcification and damage to exocrine tissue occur mainly in FCPD.[38] Islet tissue is affected to varying degrees but evidence of autoimmune damage has not been reported. In some cases the liver is involved and may show cirrhosis, fatty change or glycogen infiltration.[38]

The original concept of MRDM was that it resulted from malnutrition per se. Severe protein–energy malnutrition is associated with a diminished insulin response to oral glucose[49] and raised basal serum growth hormone: both factors may contribute to glucose intolerance. Resistance to ketosis may reflect impaired hepatic function and lack of non-esterified fatty acids in such patients.[38] Thus severe protein malnutrition could account for the typical findings, including absence of ketosis, in MRDM. Signs of malnutrition, hepatic dysfunction and fat malabsorption in the PDPD subtype of MRDM improved with insulin treatment and a nutritional diet in one study.[50] Subsequent withdrawal of insulin did not, however, correct the underlying glucose intolerance: all remained hyperglycaemic and some went on to become ketotic. Furthermore, a diminished glycaemic response to insulin has been demonstrated in several studies of MRDM, indicating insulin resistance.[38,44] It appears, therefore, that factors other than protein malnutrition may be involved in the aetiology of MRDM (Figure 37.2). Severe protein–calorie malnutrition occurs in many parts of the world where MRDM is unknown; conversely, many subjects with the disease show no signs of malnutrition.[43]

It has been suggested that cassava (tapioca) ingestion may trigger pancreatic dysfunction.[51] Cassava is the staple food in many areas where MRDM occurs, supplying perhaps up to three-quarters of total carbohydrate and one-half of protein intake. It contains the cyanogenic glycoside linamarin, which on hydrolysis releases hydrocyanic acid. This toxin is normally inactivated by conjugation with sulfhydryl groups derived from the amino acids methionine, cystine and cysteine to form thiocyanate. Deficiency of these amino acids in protein–calorie malnutrition may lead to accumulation of hydrocyanic acid, which may directly damage the pancreas.[38] This is an attractive, albeit unproven, hypothesis but cassava consumption itself does not adequately explain the distribution of MRDM. It is not consumed in two areas of India where MRDM is recognized (although another cyanide-containing food, ragi, is in regular use in these areas).[43] In addition, MRDM is not endemic in all cassava-consuming areas, although this may reflect differences in cooking habits.

A variant of the disease (previously termed K-type) is related to alcohol consumption.[51] This occurs in men aged over 30 years in Kenya, Uganda and South Africa. Kaffir beers in these areas are thought to be responsible and it has been suggested that these also contain small amounts of cyanide.[38,43]

The similarity of the clinical features of PDPD to type I diabetes has led to speculation that it is in fact a form of the latter, and that the observed weight loss is secondary to untreated diabetes.[53] There is some genetic data from Ethiopia in support of this hypothesis where HLA-DR3 was significantly positively associated and DR2 negatively associated both with PDPD and type I diabetes compared with controls.[54] Interestingly, however, DR4 was not associated with PDPD, although it was associated with type I diabetes. It has been suggested that DR3 is associated with a milder form of type I diabetes than DR4,[55] and PDPD may represent a variant of DR3-associated type I diabetes. This is an interesting observation and further genetic and histological evidence is required to substantiate it.

Tropical calcific pancreatitis and fibrocalculous pancreatic diabetes

(See also Chapter 10)

Although FCPD is thought to be secondary to TCP, not all cases of TCP develop frank diabetes: in some, glucose tolerance is impaired while in others it remains normal.[56] The latter tend to be younger, however, and longitudinal studies are required to ascertain whether all cases of TCP eventually become diabetic. The exocrine pancreatic dysfunction in FCPD has been shown to correlate directly with the extent of β cell loss: in one study plasma C peptide concentration (which reflects β cell function) was severely diminished (but detectable) in 75% and immunoreactive trypsin (a marker of exocrine function) almost undetectable in 66% of subjects with FCPD.[56] There was a significant correlation between these two parameters in all subjects with TCP, regardless of their glucose tolerance, indicating that both exocrine and endocrine function decrease occur concomitantly,

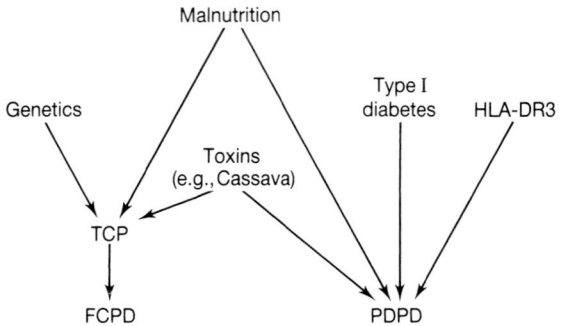

Figure 37.2: Possible factors in the aetiology of MRDM.

presumably as a result of the same pancreatic lesion. Most studies report residual insulin secretion, which would prevent the development of ketosis.[41,57]

The pancreatic lesion in TCP reflects chronic pancreatitis: the pancreas becomes shrunken, firm and fibrosed, with multiple stones in the major ducts.[38] The cause of pancreatitis is unclear and, while originally thought to result from malnutrition, other possibilities include toxic effects, particularly from cassava consumption, and genetic predisposition. Although most patients are underweight, evidence of malnutrition may be present in only 25%.[42] Plasma albumin has been shown to be normal in cases of TCP without diabetes and low only in those who had developed FCPD.[56] This suggests that protein malnutrition does not precede TCP and may result from it. Given the associated impairment of exocrine function (a third of one study group had steatorrhoea[42]), it could be expected that TCP itself may lead to malabsorption and weight loss.

Support for a genetic component to susceptibility in FCPD comes from the occurrence of familial aggregation of FCPD in south India.[58] Ten per cent of patients had a family member with pancreatic calculi or exocrine pancreatic pathology and there was a high prevalence of abnormalities of glucose tolerance.[59] Molecular genetic studies have shown associations of FCPD with a DQB restriction fragment length polymorphism (RFLP) similar to that found in type I diabetes, and a stronger association with the class 3 allele of the hypervariable region of the 5′ flanking region of the insulin gene, which was also associated with type II diabetes.[60]

In summary, MRDM is a geographically widespread condition which is still poorly understood. The FCPD subtype probably results from TCP which is of unknown aetiology and leads to pancreatic calcification and both endocrine and exocrine dysfunction. In PDPD only the endocrine pancreas is affected. The relative importance of malnutrition, toxin ingestion and genetic predisposition in the aetiology of both conditions remains to be elucidated.

Conclusions

Although the clinical picture of each type of disease is similar wherever it occurs, there is a wide geographical diversity in the rates of the different types of diabetes mellitus within the tropics. Increased awareness of the differences between the types of disease should result in more accurate diagnosis and better epidemiological data, which will be invaluable in further studies of the pathogenesis of this important and common condition.

REFERENCES

1 Consensus Statement. International Workshop on Types of Diabetes Peculiar to the Tropics, 1995, Cuttack, India.

2 Odugbesan O & Barnett A H. Racial differences. In Barnett A H (ed.) *Immunogenetics of Insulin Dependent Diabetes*. Lancaster: MTP Press, 1987: 91–101.

3 Vaishnava H, Bashin R C & Galati P O. Diabetes mellitus with onset under 40 years in North India. *J Assoc Physicians India* 1974; 22:879–888.

4 Shanghai Diabetes Research Cooperative Group. Diabetes mellitus survey in Shanghai. *Chin Med J* 1980; 93:663–667.

5 Lorenzi M, Cagliero E & Schmidt J J. Racial differences in incidence of juvenile onset type I diabetes: epidemiologic studies in southern California. *Diabetologia* 1985; 28:734–738.

6 Koivisto V A, Åkerblom H K & Wasz-Höckert O. The epidemiology of juvenile diabetes mellitus in northern Finland. *Nord Counc Arct Med Res* 1976; 15:58–65.

7 Lestradet H & Besse J. Prevalence and incidence of juvenile insulin-dependent diabetes in France. *Diabete Metab* 1977; 3:229–234.

8 Todd J A. Genetic control of autoimmunity in type I diabetes. *Immunol Today* 1990; 11:122–129.

9 Jenkins D, Mijovic C, Fletcher J A, Jacobs K H, Bradwell A R & Barnett A H. Identification of susceptibility loci for type I (insulin-dependent) diabetes by trans-racial gene mapping. *Diabetologia* 1990; 33:387–395.

10 Cavan D A, Penny M A Jacobs K H et al. Both DQA1 and DQB1 genes are implicated in HLA-associated protection from type 1 diabetes in a British Caucasian population. *Diabetologia* 1993; 36:252–257.

11 Jenkins D, Mijovic C, Jacobs K H, Penny M A, Fletcher J & Barnett A H. Allele-specific gene probing supports the DQ molecule as a determinant of inherited susceptibility to type I (insulin-dependent) diabetes mellitus. *Diabetologia* 1991; 34:109–113.

12 Jacobs K H, Jenkins D, Mijovic C H et al. An investigation of Japanese subjects maps susceptibility to type I (insulin-dependent) diabetes mellitus close to the DQA1 gene. *Hum Immunol* 1992; 33:24–28.

13 Bennett et al. Susceptibility to human type 1 diabetes at IDDM2 is determined by tandem repeat variation at the insulin gene mini-satellite locus. *Nat Genet* 1995; 9(3):284–292.

14 Barnett A H, Eff C, Leslie R D G & Pyke D A. Diabetes in identical twins: a study of 200 pairs. *Diabetologia* 1981; 20:87–93.

15 Gamble D R & Taylor K W. Seasonal incidence of diabetes mellitus. *BMJ* 1969; iii:631–633.

16 Diabetes Epidemiology Research International. Preventing insulin-dependent diabetes mellitus: the environmental challenge. *BMJ* 1987; 295:479–481.

17 Rewers M, LaPorte R E, Walczak M, Dmochowski K & Bogaczynska E. An apparent 'epidemic' of youth onset insulin-dependent diabetes mellitus in Western Poland. *Diabetes* 1987; 36:106–113.

18 Flier J S. Insulin receptors and insulin resistance. *Annu Rev Med* 1983; 34:145–160.

19 Reaven G M. Role of insulin resistance in human disease. *Diabetes* 1988; 37:1595–1607.

20 Cooper G J S, Willis A C, Clark A, Turner R C, Sim R B & Reid K B M. Purification and characterisation of a peptide from amyloid-rich pancreases of type 2 diabetic patients. *Proc Natl Acad Sci USA* 1987; 84:8628–8632.

21 Rao P V, Ushabala P, Seshiah V et al. The Eluru survey: prevalence of known diabetes in a rural Indian population. *Diabetes Res Clin Pract* 1989; 7:29–31.

22 Swai A B M, McLarty D G, Sherriff F et al. Diabetes and impaired glucose tolerance in an Asian community in Tanzania. *Diabetes Res Clin Pract* 1990; 8:227–234.

23 McLarty D G, Swai A B M, Kitange H M et al. The prevalence of diabetes and impaired glucose tolerance in rural Tanzania. *Lancet* 1989; i:871–875.

24 Jackson W P U. Epidemiology of diabetes in South Africa. *Adv Metab Disord* 1978; 9:111–146.

25 Mather H M & Keen H. The Southall diabetes survey: prevalence of known diabetes in Asians and Europeans. *BMJ* 1985; 291:1081–1084.

26 Knowler W C, Bennett P H, Hamman R F & Miller M. Diabetes incidence and prevalence in Pima Indians. *Am J Epidemiol* 1978; 108:497–505.

27 Zimmet P, Pinkstone G, Whitehouse S & Thomas K. The high incidence of diabetes mellitus in the Micronesian population of Naura. *Acta Diabetol Lat* 1982; 19:75–79.

28 McKeigue P M, Shah B & Marmot M G. Diabetes, insulin resistance and central obesity in South Asians and Europeans. *Diabetic Med* 1989; 6 (suppl. 1):A41–42.

29 Tripathy B B, Panda N C, Tej S C, Sahoo G N & Kar B K. Survey for detection of glycosuria, hyperglycaemia and diabetes mellitus in urban and rural areas of Cuttack district. *J Assoc Physicians India* 1971; 19:681–692.

30 Gupta O P, Joshi M H & Dave S K. Prevalence of diabetes in India. *Adv Metab Disord* 1978; 9:147–165.

31 World Health Organization Expert Committee on Diabetes Mellitus. Second Report. *WHO Tech Rep Ser* 1980; 646:1–80.

32 Bonham G S & Brock D B. *The Relationship of Diabetes with Race, Sex and Obesity.* America Statistical Association, Proceedings of the Social Statistics Section, 1982: 397–402.

33 Bacchus R A, Bell J L, MadKour M & Kilshaw B. The prevalence of diabetes mellitus in male Saudi Arabs. *Diabetologia* 1982; 20:87–93.

34 Neel J V. Diabetes mellitus: a 'thrifty' genotype rendered detrimental by 'progress'? *Am J Hum Genet* 1962; 14:353–362.

35 Obel A O K. Body mass index in non-insulin dependent diabetics in Kenya. *Trop Geogr Med* 1988; 40:93–96.

36 Hugh-Jones P. Diabetes in Jamaica. *Lancet* 1955; ii:891–897.

37 Zuidema P J. Cirrhosis and disseminated calcification of the pancreas in patients with malnutrition. *Trop Geogr Med* 1959; 11:70–74.

38 Abu-Bakare A, Taylor R, Gill G V & Alberti K G M M. Tropical or malnutrition-related diabetes: a real syndrome? *Lancet* 1986; i:1135–1138.

39 World Health Organization Study Group on Diabetes Mellitus. *WHO Tech Rep Ser* 1985; 727.

40 Tripathy B B & Samal K C. Overview and consensus statement on diabetes in tropical areas. *Diabetes Metab Rev* 1997; 13(1):63–76.

41 Ahuja M M. Diabetes: special problems in developing countries. *Bull Deliv Health Care Diabet Devel Countries* 1980; 1:5–6.

42 Mohan V, Mohan R, Sushjeela L et al. Tropical pancreatic diabetes in South India: heterogeneity in clinical and biochemical profile. *Diabetologia* 1985; 28:229–232.

43 McMillan D E. Tropical malnutrition diabetes. *Diabetologia* 1986; 29:127–128.

44 Tripathy B B & Kar B C. Observations on clinical patterns of diabetes mellitus in India. *Diabetes* 1965; 14:404–412.

45 Osuntokun B O, Akinkugbe F M, Francis T I, Reddy S, Osuntokun O & Taylor G O L. Diabetes mellitus in Nigerians: a study of 832 patients. *West Afr Med J* 1971; 20:295–312.

46 Viswanathan M, Mohamud U, Krishnamoorthy M & Balachandran P K. Diabetes in the young: a study of 166 cases. *Antiseptic* 1966; 63:741–745.

47 Akanji A O. Malnutrition-related diabetes mellitus in young adult diabetic patients attending a Nigerian diabetic clinic. *J Trop Med Hyg* 1990; 93:35–38.

48 Lester F T. A search for malnutrition diabetes in an Ethiopian diabetic clinic. *IDF Bull* 1984; 29:14–16.

49 Garg S K, Marwaha R K, Ganapathi V et al. Serum growth hormone, insulin and blood sugar responses to oral glucose in protein energy malnutrition. *Trop Geogr Med* 1989; 41:9–13.

50 Abdulkadir J, Mengesha B, Gebriel W et al. The clinical and hormonal (C-peptide and glucagon) profile and liability to ketoacidosis during nutritional rehabilitation in Ethiopian patients with malnutrition-related diabetes mellitus. *Diabetologia* 1990; 33:222–227.

51 McMillan D E & Geevarghese P J. Dietary cyanide and tropical malnutrition diabetes. *Diabetes Care* 1979; 2:202–208.

52 Mngola E N. Diabetes mellitus in the African environment: the dilemma. In Mngola E N (ed.) *Diabetes 1982*, Excerpta Med Int Congr Ser no. 600. Amsterdam: Excerpta Medica, 1983: 3–9.

53 Lester F T. Nutritional status of young adult Ethiopians before onset and after treatment of diabetes mellitus. *Ethiop Med J* 1990; 28:1–7.

54 Abdulkadir J, Worku Y, Schreuder G M T, D'Amaro J, de Vries R R P & Ottenhoff T M H. HLA-DR and DQ antigens in malnutrition-related diabetes mellitus in Ethiopians: a clue to its aetiology? *Tissue Antigens* 1989; 34:284–289.

55 Ludvigsson J, Samuelsson U, Baeufort C et al. HLA DR3 is associated with a more slowly progressive form of type I (insulin-dependent) diabetes. *Diabetologia* 1986; 29:207–210.

56 Yajnik C S, Shelgikar K M, Sahasrabudhe R A et al. The spectrum of pancreatic exocrine and endocrine (beta-cell) function in tropical calcific pancreatitis. *Diabetologia* 1990; 33:417–421.

57 Mohan V, Snehalatha C, Ramachandran A, Jayashree R & Viswanathan M. Pancreatic B-cell function in tropical pancreatic diabetes. *Metabolism* 1983; 32:1091–1092.

58 Pitchumoni C S. Familial pancreatitis. In Pai K N, Suman C R & Varghese R (eds) *Pancreatic Diabetes*. Trivandrum: Geo-Printers, 1980:46–48.

59 Mohan V, Chari S, Hitman G A et al. Familial aggregation in tropical fibrocalculous pancreatic diabetes. *Pancreas* 1989; 4:690–693.

60 Kambo P K, Hitman G A, Mohan V et al. The genetic predisposition to fibrocalculous pancreatic diabetes. *Diabetologia* 1989; 32:45–51.

Chapter 38
Hypertension in the Tropics

J. C. Mbanya, J. K. Cruickshank and D. B. Beevers

High blood pressure has only recently been regarded as an important health problem in the developing and developed countries of the tropics (see also Chapter 12). The quickening pace of change and increasing mass communication have put Western lifestyles within the immediate reach of the developing countries so that non-cardiovascular diseases, and particularly hypertension, have a sharply rising incidence, morbidity and mortality. As the main risk factors for cardiovascular disease are themselves treatable, it is to be hoped that they will not reach the epidemic proportions seen in the West. However, if cardiovascular disease prevention is to be achieved in tropical countries, major changes will be necessary in the methods of administering health care.

Hypertension is one of three major risk factors for the development of heart attack and stroke, renal failure, cardiac failure and peripheral vascular disease. The other factors, cigarette smoking and raised plasma lipid levels, should also be preventable.[1] These three risk factors themselves have a synergistic or multiplicative effect on each other in causing cardiovascular disease (Figure 38.1). More recently there has been an increasing awareness of the importance of type 2 diabetes mellitus as an independent cardiovascular risk factor and of the crucial role of blood pressure reduction in the management of diabetes (see also Chapter 26).

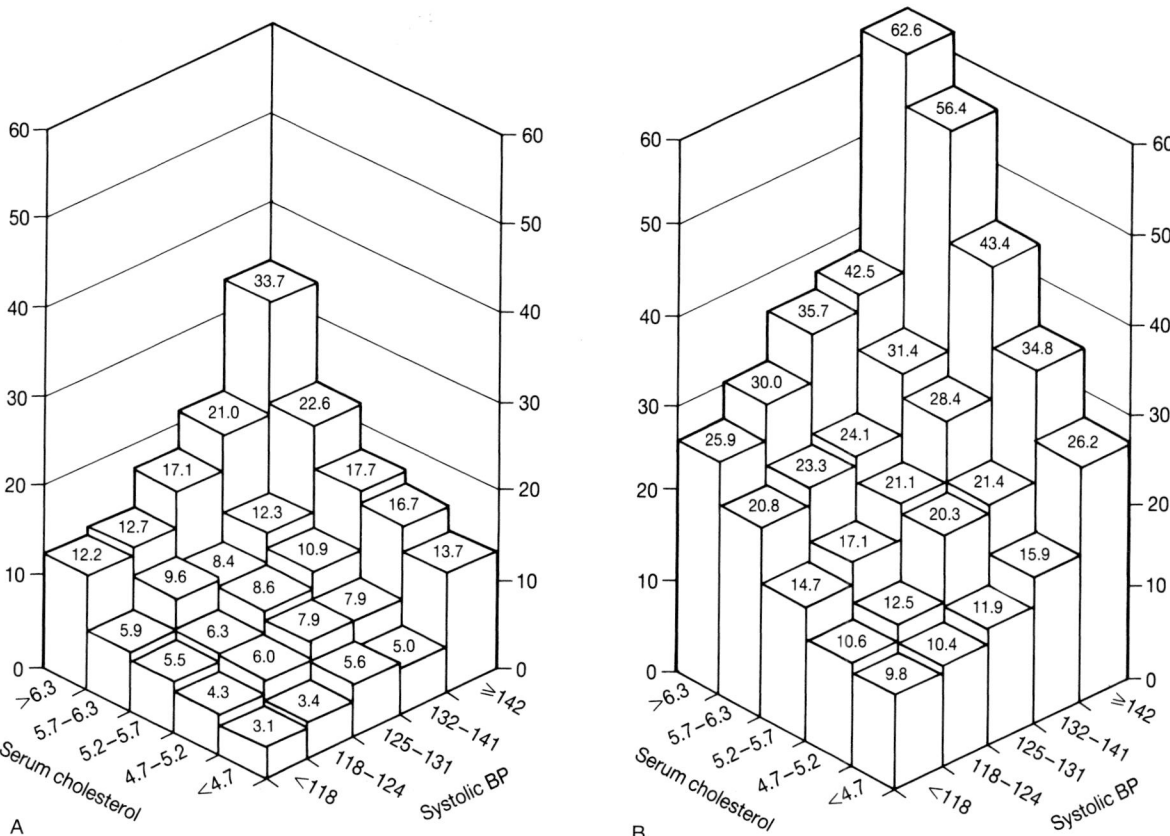

Figure 38.1: Coronary heart disease mortality per 10 000 person-years: (**A**) non-smokers; (**B**) smokers. (Adapted from Multiple Risk Factor Intervention Trial (MRFIT) examinees.[1])

Programmes to implement the control of high blood pressure are on the agenda of such bodies as the Pan American Health Organization, and the governments of countries in South-East Asia, India and many Pacific islands. In South America, major initiatives are taking place in Brazil. In tropical Africa, the Pan African Society of Cardiology is actively promoting initiatives to deal with hypertension even though funding is limited. An important factor that has encouraged these bodies is that programmes directed towards high blood pressure are applicable to other chronic conditions including diabetes mellitus and coronary heart disease.[2]

In urban Brazil and in the West Indies, as well as many parts of urban Africa, up to one-third of all outpatients and acute medical admissions are related to high blood pressure. In West Africa, hypertensive cardiac failure is now more common than rheumatic or other heart diseases. In parts of South Asia, diabetes mellitus and hypertension commonly coexist and predispose to the developing epidemic of coronary heart disease which has also struck migrant Indian origin people wherever they have settled. In South-East Asia, vascular diseases are now routine diagnoses, even if myocardial infarction remains relatively uncommon. In the West Indies and sub-Saharan Africa, hypertension, renal failure and stroke are common but again coronary heart disease remains relatively less common. A similar pattern is seen amongst the African-origin black communities in the UK and the USA.[3]

High blood pressure is also a major risk factor for perinatal and maternal mortality. Throughout the tropical world, eclampsia—which has many features akin to hypertensive encephalopathy—is thought to be killing over 50 000 women per year.

Much knowledge of hypertension and its consequences in tropical settings has come from studies of migrants. These include studies of migration in Africa from rural subsistence farming areas to the expanding cities and their associated shanty towns and surveys of African people and Indian subcontinental settlers in the West Indies, the USA and Britain. These studies assist our understanding of the relative roles of genetic versus environmental factors in the pathogenesis of hypertension.

The epidemiological transition

The transitions from traditional infective to chronic cardiovascular disease lead to the conclusion that attaining Westernized lifestyles, with all the social, financial, dietary and stress-related influences, as well as increasing tobacco and alcohol consumption, have profound long-term blood pressure-elevating effects. The observation that hypertension and its consequences are almost unheard of in remote tribal areas while reaching epidemic proportions in the cities implies that environmental factors are primarily responsible for hypertension (Figure 38.2). The emergence of the same problems in widely differing populations makes a major genetic basis for hypertension less likely.[4-7] It follows, therefore, that hypertension and its sequelae are generally preventable or reversible.

Definitions of hypertension

Blood pressure in any population is distributed in a 'normal' or Gaussian curve so that any definition of hypertension depends on arbitrary levels of blood pressure, above which individuals can be labelled as hypertensive (Table 38.1). Populations with a high

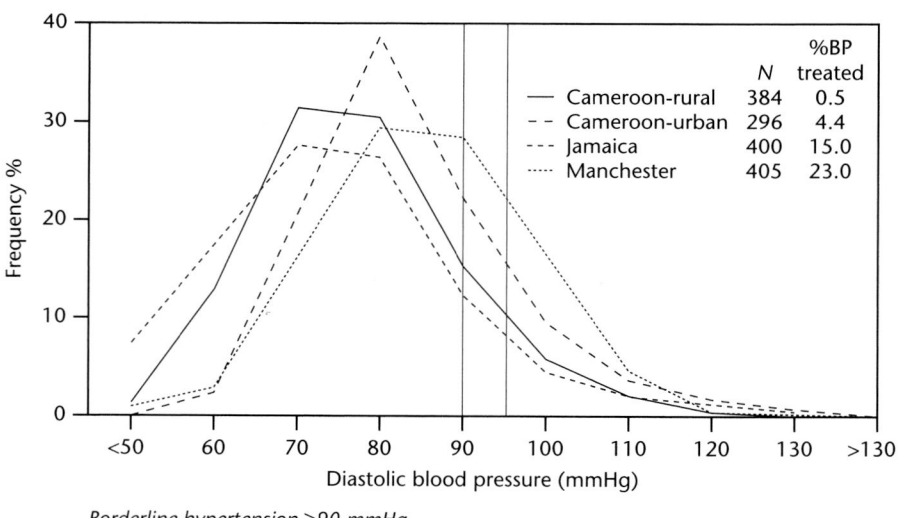

Borderline hypertension ≥90 mmHg
Hypertension ≥95 mmHg

Figure 38.2: Distribution and diastolic blood pressure in four different populations: rural Cameroon; urban Cameroon; Jamaica; Afro-Caribbeans in the UK. (From Cruickshank et al., *Int J Epidemiol* 2001; 30:111–117).

Table 38.1 Classification of blood pressure for adults aged 18 years and older.*

Category	Blood pressure (mmHg) Systolic		Diastolic
Optimal†	<120	and	<80
Notmal	<130	and	<85
High-normal	130–139	or	85–89
Hypertension‡			
Stage 1	140–159	or	90–99
Stage 2	160–179	or	100–109
Stage 3	≥180	or	N ≥ 110

*Not taking antihypertensive drugs and not acutely ill. When systolic and diastolic blood pressures fall into different categories, the higher category should be selected to classify the individual's blood pressure status. For example, 160/92 mmHg should be classified as stage 2 hypertension, and 174/120 mmHg should be classified as stage 3 hypertension. Isolated systolic hypertension is defined as systolic blood pressure 140 mmHg or greater and diastolic blood pressure less than 90 mmHg and staged appropriately (e.g., 170/82 mmHg is defined as stage 2 isolated systolic hypertension). In addition to classifying stages of hypertension on the basis of average blood pressure levels, clinicians should specify pressure levels or absence of target organ disease and additional risk factors. This specificity is important for risk classification and treatment.
†Optimal blood pressure with respect to cardiovascular risk is less than 120/80 mmHg. However, usually low readings should be evaluated for clinical significance.
‡Based on the average of two or more readings taken at each of two or more visits after an initial screening.
Reproduced with permission from the Sixth Report of the Joint National Committee on prevention, detection, evaluation and treatment of high blood pressure (JNC-VI). Arch Intern Med 1997; 157:2431–2446.

prevalence of hypertension are also those with higher average blood pressures. Thus, in a sense, the whole population could be regarded as hypertensive when compared with societies where hypertension is rare. The preventive solution to hypertension would, therefore, require a whole population strategy. From a clinical standpoint, the definition of hypertension must rely on the available evidence of the value of blood pressure reduction. Thus, a pragmatic definition of hypertension, taking into account the epidemiological principles and the current state of knowledge of the benefits of blood pressure reduction, is 'that level of blood pressure above which treatment does more good than harm'.[8] In the light of the recent trials, and the guidelines published by the American Joint National Committee in their sixth report[9] (JNC-VI) and the British Hypertension Society,[10] the threshold is around 160 mmHg systolic and/or 95–100 mmHg diastolic in low-risk individuals. In high-risk individuals (including all diabetics) the threshold is 140 mmHg systolic and/or 80 mmHg diastolic, irrespective of age.

Measurement

Important decisions are made on the basis of the height of blood pressure but sadly its measurement is often inaccurate. The standard mercury manometer, when used properly, is still the gold standard. Electronic automatic machinery should be treated with suspicion. The main problem with mercury manometers is related to their

incorrect use, and medical and related staff should ideally be retrained regularly. The British Hypertension Society[11] has provided guidelines on the measurement of blood pressure and these are briefly outlined here. The manometer should be well maintained with the mercury column vertical, and at rest the mercury should be at 0 mmHg. If the manometer is sloping away from the vertical, due to damaged hinges, this leads to overestimation of the pressure. The rubber bladder inside the arm cuff should encircle at least 80% of the upper arm. In order to achieve this, it is strongly recommended that the old 'adult cuff' with a bladder measuring 12.5 × 23 cm should be replaced by the 'alternative adult cuff' with a bladder measuring 12.5 × 33 cm. This cuff is applicable for individuals with arm circumferences of up to 43 cm. The use of too small a cuff leads to overestimation of blood pressure.

Blood pressures should normally be measured with the subject seated, with the cuff level with the heart. The arm should be slightly externally rotated and supported to avoid the isometric exercise required to hold the arm raised. The manometer cuff should be inflated to 15 mmHg above the level needed to occlude the brachial pulse and the stethoscope should be placed where the pulse was felt, on the medial side of the antecubital fossa. The column of mercury should be deflated slowly (2 mm/s). The systolic blood pressure is taken at the first appearance of Korotkoff sounds (phase I) and diastolic pressure at the final disappearance of sounds (phase V). Measurement of diastolic blood pressure at the phase of muffling of sounds (phase IV) is now obsolete. Blood pressures are measured to the nearest 2 mmHg.

On all occasions, blood pressure should be measured twice and decisions made on the basis of the second reading. In patients with mild hypertension, decisions on starting therapy should only be made after two readings on four separate occasions.

Failure to follow these simple guidelines will lead to overestimation of blood pressure and needless or excessive use of antihypertensive agents. Many people have blood pressures which are mildly elevated on first measurement but which settle on rechecking. These 'white coat hypertensives' may receive unnecessary drug therapy.

The careful training of observers, possibly with audiovisual aids, is important as the accurate assessment of hypertensive patients will differentiate between those requiring drug therapy, those requiring careful observation only and those who can be reassured. While many hypertensive patients remain undiagnosed, many are overtreated because of unreliable measurement.

Epidemiology

In developing countries where access to health care facilities is limited, the diagnosis of hypertension is often made only after complications have set in. Hypertension is not being diagnosed at the milder and presymptomatic stage when drug treatment is of proven value. The underdiagnosis of hypertension is a major problem in all countries and can only be solved when the routine screening of all apparently fit symptomless adults becomes an accepted part of medical care.

In most black populations, except those few remaining unexposed to 'development', hypertension is generally more common than in white or Indo-European communities. Hence, if health care facilities are limited, hypertension may appear to be more severe in blacks by giving rise to higher mortality rates at a younger age. However, the small number of follow-up studies of blacks does not support this view. For a given level of blood pressure, an individual black person has virtually the same prognosis as a white or Asian subject. This trend was found in studies in the USA, Jamaica and Trinidad.[12] The contention that black hypertensive patients have more severe hypertension than whites arises from the clinical fallacy of more people being at risk and thus being seen with the complications.

An important factor in the epidemiology of hypertension is that in all non-tribal societies average blood pressure rises with advancing age. Thus at the age of 70, about one-half of the population will have hypertension using JNC-VI criteria.[9] This rise in blood pressure with age is primarily due to environmental factors as it is not seen in genetically similar rural populations. There is evidence that the blood pressure age gradient is steeper in urban Africans than in the white communities of Europe and the USA. The consequences of raised blood pressure, and particularly stroke, thus become more common with advancing age in tropical countries. However, in all comparisons to date between African-origin and Western European (white) populations, there has been major confounding by socioeconomic factors. This was perhaps best illustrated in the follow-up of the 'MRFIT' Study, in which higher socioeconomic group black men had lower blood pressures and subsequent mortality than poorer white men.[13]

Prevalence

Blood pressures requiring drug therapy are seen in 5–10% of adult white populations in Europe and the USA, depending on the age distribution of the population, and are substantially more common in blacks. There is good evidence that these levels of blood pressure are also common in Africa, where the prevalence of hypertension may reach 20%, the highest figures being seen in the cities. In some regions, hypertension accounts for 10% and 5% of adult hospital morbidity and mortality, respectively. Untreated hypertension is associated with high rates of stroke that can account for as much as 5.5% of all deaths in the adult population in many sub-Saharan countries.[14]

There are few reliable data comparing blood pressures of black and white populations in Africa. Comparisons of studies in Africa with those in Europe or the USA tend to be confounded by lack of standardization of methods

and failure to take into account the effects of obesity and alcohol as well as the age distribution of the population(s). Another important consideration is the effect of ambient temperature (for a 1°C increase in temperature blood pressure falls by 1 mmHg). There is, however, evidence that hypertension is more common in black South Africans than in whites.[15] Urban/rural comparisons in several parts of Africa, including Cameroon, The Gambia, Ghana, Ivory Coast, Nigeria, South Africa and Kenya, report consistently higher rates (5–10%) in urban areas.[16,17] In Western countries, hypertension is more common in men until the age of about 50 years. At this stage, the difference between the genders lessens and hypertension eventually becomes more common in women, in part because of the impact of premature death in the men with higher blood pressures.

Risk factors for hypertension
Social gradient

An emerging phenomenon in tropical countries is that people of middle and upper socioeconomic class tend to have higher rates of hypertension than poorer groups. This excess is partly due to greater body mass but other factors, including physical inactivity and nutritional influences including alcohol consumption and a high-salt diet with a low intake of potassium-rich foods, may also be involved.[18] Studies in developed societies show the opposite phenomenon, with an inverse relationship between social class and blood pressure. As urbanization and development in the tropics settle down, this trend for hypertension and its complications to be more common in people of higher social class may reverse, as it did in the West about 50 years ago. Until then, hypertension is selectively killing off the more economically active members of the community.

Alcohol

Excess alcohol intake is a well-established risk factor for hypertension. It is of interest that the second ever study reporting a relationship between alcohol and blood pressure was conducted in Bombay.[19] While earlier reports suggest that the risk of hypertension appeared at the level of about five drinks per day, recent data suggest that there is a relationship even at lower alcohol levels.[18] Epidemiological and clinical studies show that the alcohol–blood pressure relationship is rapidly reversible with moderation or cessation of drinking.

Sodium and potassium

There is evidence from cross-sectional and longitudinal studies that a difference in mean sodium intake of

100 mmol/day is associated with a 7–10 mmHg difference in systolic blood pressure rise over 30 years. Furthermore, lower dietary potassium intakes are associated with an increased risk of hypertension. Both salt restriction and potassium supplementation can reduce blood pressure. The INTERSALT study, which was an international comparative study of hypertension in 32 countries, demonstrated that hypertension is most common in populations with the lowest potassium consumption and the highest 24-hour urinary sodium excretion.[18] Clinical studies in the USA show that black people are more sensitive to a given dietary salt load, exhibiting a greater rise in blood pressure and a delayed natriuresis when compared with whites.[20] Thus, black people may be more salt-sensitive even though they may consume similar amounts of salt. However, there is also evidence that a low salt diet is more effective at reducing blood pressure in black compared with white hypertensives.

Some of the electrolyte differences may be related to socioeconomic factors. Potassium-rich foods, which reduce blood pressure and hence strokes, are expensive and there is evidence, mainly from the USA, that their consumption in poor urban black communities is lower than in the rural populations and also lower than in white people.

Cation transport

Electrolyte membrane abnormalities may be associated with essential hypertension in man. Hypertensives have higher intracellular sodium levels compared with normotensives and the ouabain-sensitive sodium pump, responsible for extruding sodium from cells, is depressed and there is also raised intracellular calcium. A difference in sodium–potassium countertransport across cell membranes may be genetically determined, predisposing black more than white people to hypertension.[21] Higher intracellular sodium concentrations are found in both normotensive and hypertensive black people when compared with whites.

The renin–angiotensin system

Studies in North America, the UK and South Africa have consistently shown that adult black subjects have lower plasma renin and angiotensin II levels than whites.[22] Since this difference is not immediately related to a higher salt intake, these low renin levels may be genetically determined. It is possible, however, that genetic factors were originally less important as people living in tropical hunter-gatherer societies tended to die prematurely if they had higher renin levels and lacked the capacity to retain sodium. The low-renin/sodium-retaining people tended to survive. In the high-salt-consuming societies today, the capacity to retain sodium has become disadvantageous as it causes a rise in blood pressure.

Insulin metabolism

A series of abnormalities associated with insulin resistance, including hyperinsulinaemia, impaired glucose tolerance, obesity, increased plasma triglyceride levels, decreased high-density lipoprotein concentrations and high blood pressure, have been reported in studies in Britain and the USA (see also Chapter 39). Most of these factors are independently related to the development of ischaemic cardiac disease. Based on these considerations, it has been suggested that insulin resistance and hyperinsulinaemia may be involved in the aetiology of hypertension.[23] However, there is inconsistent evidence of a relationship between insulin resistance and hypertension in non-European populations. Since there is still a low incidence of ischaemic heart disease in hypertensive patients in Africa, it could be argued that insulin resistance and its effects on lipid metabolism are less important.

Animal fat intake in Africa is lower than in the West and this may explain the relative rarity of coronary heart disease, while hypertension-related strokes and renal failure are common. As in all populations, there is an excess of hypertension associated with diabetes mellitus. Community studies carried out in Cameroon and Madagascar put the association at between 20% and 30%. The association of raised blood pressure with non-insulin-dependent diabetes mellitus is associated with increased mortality rates from cardiovascular disease. Both risk factors are closely related to lifestyle so their rising prevalence should be preventable.

Underlying causes of hypertension

In a tiny minority of hypertensive patients, a treatable underlying disease may be found which is the cause of raised blood pressure and the reader is referred to the standard textbooks of hypertension.[24] Intrinsic renal diseases (glomerulonephritis and pyelonephritis) are more common in Africa but polycystic kidney disease, renal artery stenosis, endocrine diseases (Cushing's syndrome, primary aldosteronism, phaeochromocytoma and acromegaly) and coarctation of the aorta do not seem to occur with greater frequency. There is also an excess incidence of systemic lupus erythematosus in African-origin populations, which is an important cause of high blood pressure, especially in young women. Estimations of the prevalence of secondary hypertension are influenced by the availability of modern diagnostic facilities and this presents problems for most tropical countries. Extensive investigation reveals that between 10% and 20% of patients with hypertension presenting to hospital in some African countries have evidence of renal impairment but this kidney damage may be a consequence rather than a cause of the hypertension.

Hypertension in pregnancy (see also Chapter 25)

This is an important problem in the tropics and is associated with increased maternal and fetal mortality. Perinatal and maternal mortality rates are high in developing countries and about one-third of these deaths may be due to hypertension. The diagnosis of pre-eclampsia is made on the presence of proteinuria and elevation of the blood pressure. The drug treatment of more severe grades of hypertension at this stage of pregnancy is worthwhile. If the diastolic blood pressure remains consistently below 100 mmHg, drug treatment should not be given. Many mothers develop gestational or pregnancy-induced hypertension in which blood pressure rises in pregnancy and falls after pregnancy is over. Where this elevation of blood pressure is mild, and not associated with proteinuria, drug treatment should not be given.

Early life origins of high blood pressure: the Barker hypothesis

A watershed in understanding the development of hypertension has been the discovery of an inverse association between fetal growth and high blood pressure in later life.[25,26] The association is consistent and has been found in many settings; it implies a causal relationship although the mechanisms remain unclear. Disproportional impaired growth of the fetus and placenta appears to be a critical factor. Babies who were 'small for dates' are these most at risk. A recent meta-analysis estimated the impact as 1 mmHg increase in systolic pressure per 500 g decrease in birthweight.[26] It remains unclear whether maternal nutritional status, specific placental nutrient supply, poor placentation or placental function due to raised blood pressure underlies the association. Recently, both inadequate and excess 'catch-up' growth in childhood have been found to amplify the risk[27] although 'tracking' of blood pressure is generally characteristic: that is, the height of the blood pressure earlier determines its height later.

The association is particularly relevant to analysis of ethnic differences in high blood pressure because black populations, notably African Americans, continue to have average birthweights consistently some 200–300 g lighter than European Americans. The same applies to almost all other developing societies where hypertension and chronic disease epidemic has emerged. There is evidence that population average birthweights are socio-economically determined, with higher status African-origin women having heavier babies, making a genetic basis unlikely.[28] There are few studies of the birthweight–later blood pressure question in African Americans, but a clear link has been reported in Jamaica[29] and India where maternal undernutrition and low birthweight are common.

Hypercholesterolaemia and cigarette smoking

The presence of hypercholesterolaemia or cigarette smoking exerts a major influence on prognosis amongst hypertensive patients. Hypercholesterolaemia is not common in blacks in Africa or the Caribbean. By contrast, it has become a major problem in the Indian subcontinent and the Pacific islands and amongst Asians living the Caribbean[30] (see Chapter 39). The promotion of tobacco in the developing countries constitutes an international scandal. Neither of these risk factors themselves causes hypertension, but they increase the risk for any given level of pressure.

Symptoms and signs

Patients with mild to moderate hypertension rarely complain of symptoms. Dizziness, fatigue, headache and palpitations are more often due to anxiety or the side effects of antihypertensive drugs. Severely hypertensive patients may present for the first time with stroke or evidence of renal impairment or heart disease.

Clinical examination may reveal evidence of left ventricular enlargement. For a given level of blood pressure, if left ventricular hypertrophy is present the mortality is four times greater. Malignant hypertension is diagnosed if there are retinal haemorrhages and or exudates with or without papilloedema. In such cases, the diastolic blood pressure is usually more than 120 mmHg.

In the Indian subcontinent and in Asian populations in the West, coronary heart disease is a common complication of hypertension. Examination may reveal evidence of other arterial disease with absent peripheral pulses, as well as xanthelasmas, xanthomas, corneal arcus and femoral or carotid bruits. Clinical signs of heart failure may be due to coronary heart disease but severe hypertension alone can cause heart failure. Less commonly, heart failure may be due to cardiomyopathy or rheumatic heart disease.

Investigations

Investigation depends on the severity of the hypertension and availability of facilities. All patients receiving antihypertensive drug therapy should ideally have routine urine testing, and full biochemical profiling together with an ECG.

Haematuria and proteinuria may be due to hypertension or to underlying renal disease. For a given level of pressure, if there is proteinuria mortality is approximately doubled. Haematuria may also be due to neoplasm of the urinary tract. The measurement of microproteinuria (urine albumin below 300 mg/litre) is of value in diabetic hypertensives but its significance in other hypertensives is uncertain.

All patients should undergo at least one blood test to estimate plasma sodium and potassium levels. Serum potassium levels are low in both primary and secondary hyperaldosteronism, and if hypokalaemia is encountered this needs detailed investigation. The most common cause of hypokalaemia is diuretic therapy, which must be discontinued at least 4 weeks prior to testing. Serum urea or creatinine levels should be measured to obtain an estimate of renal function. The estimation of creatinine clearance is not valuable unless there is severe renal failure. Serum total and HDL cholesterol levels should be measured in the non-fasting state in populations where hypercholesterolaemia is common. If the ECG shows evidence of left ventricular hypertrophy, with the sum of the R wave in leads V_5 or V_6 and the S wave in V_1 amounting to more than 35 mm, then the prognosis is bad. Because left ventricular hypertrophy is such an important prognostic factor, a routine ECG in hypertensive patients is desirable.

Haematological profiling with estimations of plasma viscosity or erythrocyte sedimentation rate (ESR) may provide evidence of connective tissue diseases which may cause high blood pressure. In such cases, proteinuria may also be present.

If renal impairment is present or there is unexplained hypokalaemia, more detailed investigation with renal ultrasound scanning is necessary. If one or both kidneys are found to be small but with a smooth outline, then the possibility of correctable renal artery stenosis should be borne in mind and renal angiography is worth considering. If the kidneys are small with an irregular outline, pyelonephritis is more likely and investigations should be conducted to exclude obstructive uropathy with vesicoureteric reflux. If hypokalaemia is present, patients should undergo estimation of plasma renin and aldosterone levels. In primary hyperaldosteronism, plasma renin is low, while concurrent plasma aldosterone levels are high. If these features are found, patients should proceed to computed tomography to detect an adrenal adenoma. In Conn's syndrome, removal of the aldosterone-secreting adenoma may lead to cure of hypertension.

Patients with symptoms of a paroxysmal nature with sweating, blanching, tachycardia, weight loss, constipation and panic attacks should be investigated to exclude phaeochromocytoma. This requires a 24-hour urine test for catecholamines, metanephrines or 4-hydroxy-3-methoxymandelic acid.

Management

Effective management of hypertension reduces mortality and morbidity from stroke, heart attack and heart failure.[31,32] In developing countries, socioeconomic considerations dictate that costs should be kept to a minimum. For this reason, non-pharmacological methods of reducing blood pressure need to be applied even more rigorously. Dietary recommendations should emphasize the importance of the reduction of salt intake. Patients should be counselled on the avoidance of salty foods and told they should never add salt to food when cooking or at the table. An increase in potassium-rich foods, which can be achieved by increasing the consumption of fresh fruit and vegetables, will also help to lower blood pressure. Supplementation with potassium chloride tablets is not recommended.

All cigarette smokers should be instructed to stop. Smoking is an independent risk factor for heart attack and stroke but is not itself associated with hypertension.

A high alcohol intake is an established factor in hypertension. Males should consume no more than 21 units of alcohol per week and females no more than 14 units per week (one unit of alcohol is equivalent to half a pint (300 ml) of beer, or a single measure of spirits or a glass of wine). Enquiries about the amount of alcohol consumed is important but must be conducted with discretion.

Weight reduction in obese patients is important and where this can be achieved there will be a significant fall in both systolic and diastolic blood pressure of around 1 mmHg for each kilogram lost.

There is good evidence that regular physical exercise lowers blood pressure on a long-term basis, even though at the time of exercise pressure may rise acutely. A structured exercise programme should be encouraged, although in urban areas with limited facilities this may be difficult to achieve.

These recommendations are relevant to all people and not just those with raised blood pressure. Advice on achieving dietary goals should be administered by trained paramedical or nursing staff, who may be more aware of local food prices and availability. There is evidence that well-trained nurses can achieve better results when treating mild hypertension than their medical colleagues. Training programmes are necessary to provide nurses with the appropriate skills to manage chronic diseases like hypertension. Non-pharmacological methods of treating mild hypertension should be continued for at least 6 months. In severer cases, drug therapy will need to be initiated at an earlier stage but salt restriction is additive to most antihypertensive drugs.

Drug therapy

In many hypertensive patients, unfortunately, non-pharmacological methods are insufficient to reduce diastolic blood pressure below 140/80 mmHg. The recent Hypertension Optimal Treatment (HOT) trial clearly demonstrated that amongst treated hypertensives blood pressure should be reduced to this level, and in particular this target must be achieved in patients with diabetes mellitus or prior cardiovascular disease.[33] In such patients, antihypertensive drugs will be required (Figure 38.3) and there is a wide choice but many of the newer drugs are expensive.[10] Once drug treatment has been started, it is usually necessary to continue indefinitely or

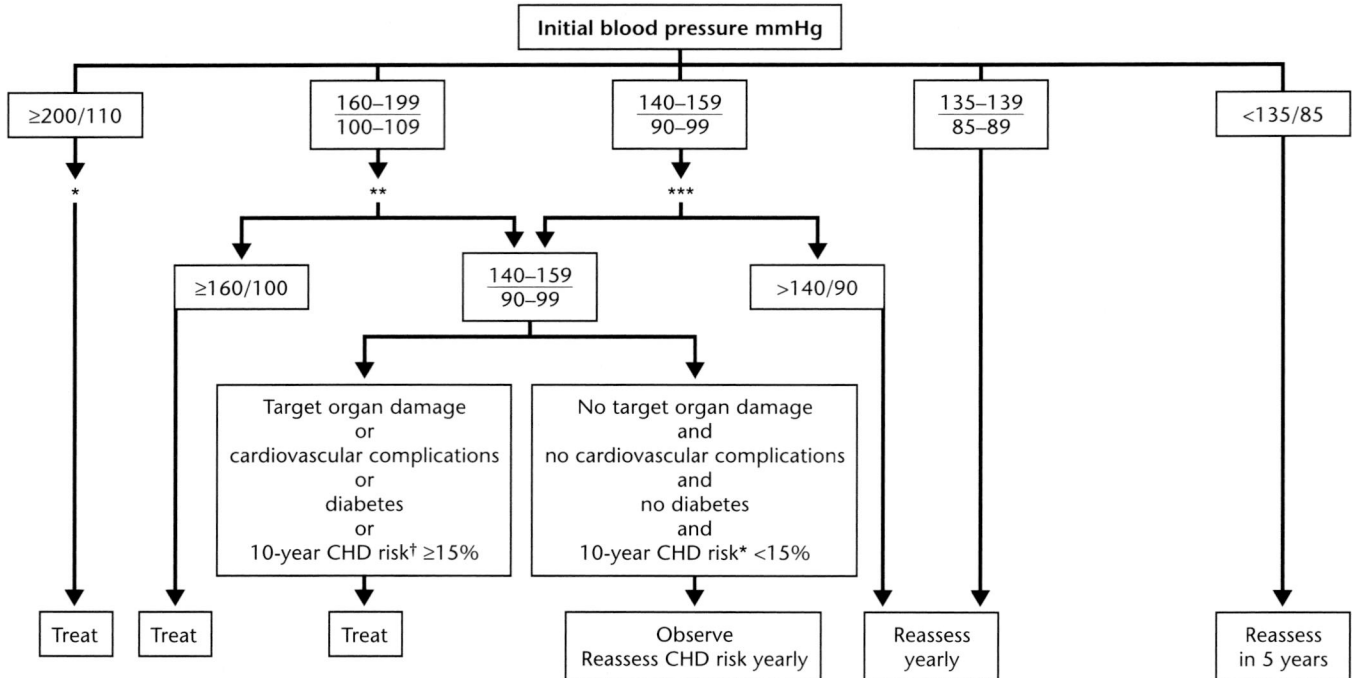

* *Unless malignant phase, or hypertensive emergency, confirm over 1–2 weeks, then treat.*
** *If cardiovascular complications, target organ damage, or diabetes is present, confirm over 3–4 weeks, then treat; if absent, remeasure weekly and treat if BP persists at these levels over 4–12 weeks.*
*** *If cardiovascular complications, target organ damage, or diabetes is present, confirm over 12 weeks, then treat; if absent, remeasure monthly and treat if these levels are maintained and if estimated 10-year CHD risk is ≥15%.*

† *Assessed with Cardiac Risk Assessor computer program or coronary heart disease risk chart.*

Figure 38.3: Blood pressure thresholds and drug treatment recommendations of the British Hypertension Society. (*J Human Hypertens* 1999; 13:569–592.)

at least until the age of 80. Compliance with long-term antihypertensive medication is often difficult to achieve and this problem may be compounded by limited or intermittent availability of antihypertensive drugs in some countries. Community studies done in general practice (primary care) have shown the much greater importance of achieved blood pressure on treatment rather than initial pressure.[34] Once-daily tablet regimens should be used routinely. Careful, sympathetic and systematic follow-up is necessary, preferably by suitably trained nurses or paramedical staff.

Antihypertensive drugs were first introduced in the 1950s and there are now seven different classes acting by various mechanisms. The drug treatment of hypertension can bring about approximately a 40% reduction in the incidence of stroke and a 20% reduction in coronary heart disease. Side effects can be kept to a minimum by employing the lowest possible doses in the first instance.

Tranquillizers and sedatives have no place in antihypertensive regimens and they should be reserved exclusively for patients with primary psychiatric ailments. There is no convincing evidence that any of the traditional or herbal remedies available in some countries have any useful effects on blood pressure and some of them may even be dangerous.

Treatment targets and reducing risk: the 'rule of halves'

The two interlinked components of managing hypertension are primary prevention for the whole population and secondary prevention for those needing treatment. Secondary prevention applies to only a small proportion (10–20% of most tropical societies), but effective implementation can be judged against the 'rule of halves'. As originally suggested, the 'rule' states that only 50% of those with 'hypertension' (however defined) are known, only half of those are treated and of those only half have their blood pressure adequately controlled (i.e., 12.5% of the total).

The 'rule' was recently examined in a careful international comparison between rural and urban Cameroon, Jamaica and in Caribbean migrants to Britain.[35] Age-adjusted prevalence rates in men rose from 5% to 17% in Cameroon and from 12% to 21% between Jamaica and Caribbeans in Britain. Rates in women were similar, except for Jamaica at 21% and 29% in Britain, as women were more overweight in both settings. Across the sites 28–67% of eligible people were treated and 4–59 had adequately controlled pressures (<140 and 90 mmHg). From these results, similar to those in other studies, we can estimate the likely burden of stroke and all-cause mortality. Some 15–45% of stroke mortality could be attributed to this deficit in treatment, as could 40% of strokes occurring while *on* treatment.

Drug choice

The choice of antihypertensive drugs depends on availability and cost as well as efficacy and side effects (Tables 38.2 and 38.3). Broadly speaking, all antihypertensive regimens are about equally effective. The central acting α-agonists and the β-blockers have the most side effects (sedation, lethargy, cold extremities, bradycardia and wheeze). Of the seven classes of blood pressure-lowering drugs only the thiazide diuretics, the β-blockers and calcium channel blockers have been demonstrated to prevent heart attacks or strokes and no agent has been shown convincingly to prevent renal failure. The angiotensin converting enzyme (ACE) inhibitors are particularly useful as they may be the most effective in reversing left ventricular hypertrophy and delaying renal failure in diabetic and non-diabetic hypertensives.

1. Centrally-acting α-agonists

This class includes methyldopa, clonidine and the reserpine group of drugs. Clonidine is generally regarded as being unacceptable because of side effects. The main problem with these drugs is that they cause lethargy and sometimes depression, and reserpine, when used in high doses, has been associated with suicide. In very low doses, these centrally acting drugs are effective and tolerable in mild hypertension and they are useful because they have the major advantage of being cheap.

2. Thiazide diuretics

These agents, which are also cheap, are still the mainstay of antihypertensive therapy for older patients. They should be prescribed only at the lowest possible dose, e.g., bendrofluazide 2.5 mg daily. Increased doses provide no further reduction of blood pressure but cause increased adverse side effects, including erectile impotence, glucose intolerance, elevation of plasma lipid levels, hyperuricaemia and hypokalaemia. Thiazides are best avoided in younger patients and particularly in sexually active men.

3. The β-blockers

These drugs, introduced in 1965, were rapidly shown to be effective, not only in treating hypertension but also in the management of angina and the secondary prevention of myocardial infarction. Their impact on primary coronary prevention has been disappointing. The hydrophilic β-blockers (e.g., atenolol) cause fewer central nervous system side effects (lethargy, sleep disturbance) than the lipophilic drugs like propranolol.

Table 38.2 Compelling and possible indications and contraindications for the major classes of antihypertensive drugs.

Class of drug	Indication		Contraindication	
	Compelling	Possible	Possible	Compelling
α-Blockers	Prostatism	Dyslipidaemia	Postural hypotension	Urinary incontinence
ACE inhibitors	Heart failure Left ventricular dysfunction Type I diabetic nephropathy	Chronic renal disease* Type II diabetic nephropathy	Renal impairment* Peripheral vascular disease†	Pregnancy
Angiotensin II receptor antagonists	Cough induced by ACE inhibitor‡	Heart failure Intolerance of other antihypertensive drugs	Peripheral vascular disease†	Pregnancy Renovascular disease
β-Blockers	Myocardial infarction, angina	Heart failure§	Heart failure§ Dyslipidaemia Peripheral vascular disease	Asthma or chronic obstructive pulmonary disease Heart block
Calcium antagonists (dihydropyridine)	Isolated systolic hypertension in elderly patients	Angina Elderly patients	–	–
Calcium antagonists (rate limiting)	Angina	Myocardial infarction	Combination with β-blocckade	Heart block Heart failure
Thiazides	Elderly patients	–	Dyslipidaemia	Gout

*Angiotensin converting enzyme (ACE) inhibitors may be beneficial in chronic renal failure but should be used with caution. Close supervision and specialist advice are needed when there is established and significant renal impairment.
†Caution with ACE inhibitors are angiotensin II receptor antagonists in peripheral vascular disease because of association with renovascular disease.
‡If ACE inhibitors indicated.
§β-Blockers may worsen heart failure, but in specialist hands may be used to treat heart failure.
Reproduced with permission from British Hypertension Society. *J. Hum Hypertens* 1999; 13:569–592.

Table 38.3 Check-list of common or important side effects with different classes of antihypertensive drugs.

Common side effect	Diuretic	β-Blocker	ACE inhibitor	Angiotensin receptor antagonist	Calcium antagonist	α-Blocker
Headache	–	–	–	–	+	–
Flushing	–	–	–	–	+	–
Dyspnoea	–	+	–	–	–	–
Lethargy	–	+	–	–	–	–
Impotence	+	+	–	–	–	–
Cough	–	–	+	–	–	–
Gout	+	–	–	–	–	–
Oedema	–	–	–	–	+	–
Postural hypotension	–	–	–	–	–	+
Cold hands and feet	–	+	–	–	–	–
Stress incontinence	–	–	–	–	-	+
Angioedema	–	–	+	+	–	–
Constipation	–	–	–	–	+	–

4. The α-blockers

The early α-blockers, indoramin and prazosin, have now largely fallen from use because of side effects and complexity of dosage. The recent introduction of doxazosin and terazosin has largely overcome these problems. These newer α-blockers are safe and may have beneficial effects on sexual function in men and also relieve prostatic symptoms but they can cause urinary incontinence in women. They also reduce plasma lipid levels slightly.

5. The direct-acting vasodilators

Hydralazine has been used mainly as an additive drug to control blood pressure where the thiazides and the β-blockers together have proved ineffective. Side effects include the drug-induced lupus phenomenon. Because hydralazine has to be given twice or thrice daily it has largely fallen from use. Minoxidil is a very powerful vasodilator which should only be used in the most resistant hypertensive patients in conjunction with β-blockers and a loop diuretic.

6. The angiotensin converting enzyme (ACE) inhibitors

These expensive drugs can cause over-rapid and dangerous falls in blood pressure if used in high doses in patients with renal impairment or those already receiving diuretic therapy. They are contraindicated in patients with renal artery stenosis. The ACE inhibitors are the only class of drug which has been convincingly shown to prolong life in patients with heart failure and should now be used in all such cases. They may also be specifically indicated in diabetic hypertensives as they have no adverse effects on insulin sensitivity or plasma lipid levels and they do preserve renal function in patients with hypertensive or diabetic nephrosclerosis. The main side effect is a dry, persistent, irritating cough in about 10% of patients. Life-threatening angioneurotic oedema is occasionally encountered, particularly in African-origin patients.

7. The angiotensin receptor antagonists (ARAs)

This class of antihypertensive therapy became available in 1995 and it rapidly became apparent that they were devoid of clinical side effects. Because they have only been available for a relatively short time, there is limited long-term data on their ability to prevent heart attacks, strokes and heart failure. They can be used as an alternative to an ACE inhibitor in heart failure. If long-term studies show that ARAs are as effective as ACE inhibitors and if they become cheap, they may replace the ACE inhibitors. At the moment they are only recommended in patients where ACE inhibitors have caused side effects.

8. The calcium channel blockers

This group can be subdivided into the dihydropyridines and the non-dihydropyridines (diltiazem and verapamil). The last two agents are effective at reducing blood pressure and are antianginal but, due to negative chronotropism and ionotropism, they are contraindicated in patients with heart failure and should not be used in conjunction with β-blockers. The dihydropyridines are very safe but cause headache, flushing and ankle oedema. They appear to be the least effective drugs in reducing left ventricular hypertrophy and are contraindicated after a myocardial infarction.

Individual variations of drug response

In general, if one antihypertensive drug is ineffective at its usual dose, it is best to change to a different class rather than to increase the dose. There are, however, some reasonably predictable differences in drug response which may influence the choice of first-line drug therapy. Drugs which work wholly or in part by blocking the renin–angiotensin system (i.e., the β-blockers, ACE inhibitors and ARAs) tend to be less effective when plasma renin levels are low. Low renin levels are encountered in older patients, patients of African origin and those with non-insulin-dependent diabetes. In such patients other agents may be more appropriate as first-line therapy.

Specific groups
Black hypertensives

Patients of black African origin, as stated earlier, have consistently lower plasma renin and angiotensin II levels than other ethnic groups.[28] The thiazide diuretics or the calcium channel blockers and the best first-line drugs although the other agents may need to be added in (Figure 38.4).

South Asians

The response of antihypertensive drugs in South Asians is broadly similar to that in whites. However, the high incidence of diabetes mellitus, glucose intolerance and hyperlipidaemia means that the thiazide, shown to be beneficial in diabetes, should only be used in low dose (e.g., bendrofluazide up to 2.5 mg/day, hydrochlorthiazide up to 25 mg/day). There is a very high incidence of coronary heart disease in people of Indian subcontinental origin and coronary preventive manoeuvres are particularly necessary.

Oriental patients

Hypertension is particularly common in people of oriental origin, especially the Japanese. This may, in part, be related to the very high salt intake in the North-West

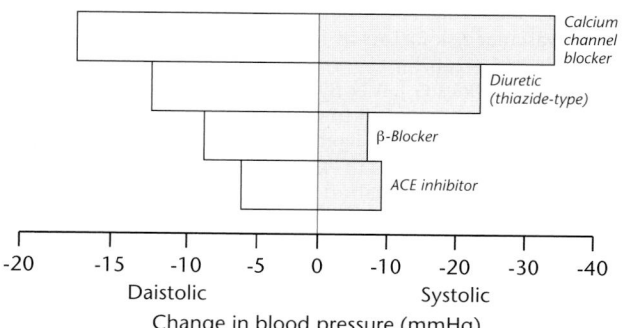

Figure 38.4: Average reduction in systolic and diastolic blood pressure in large clinical trials of monotherapy with four different classes of antihypertensive drug used for the treatment of mild-to-moderate essential hypertension in black men and women. (Reproduced from Hall W D. *Am J Hypertens* 1990; 3:336S–371S.)

Pacific rim. Salt restriction is effective in reducing the very high incidence of strokes in this area. Coronary heart disease is relatively uncommon but its incidence may be rising as dietary fat intake rises.

Pacific islanders

This group has a high incidence of extreme obesity, diabetes mellitus, hypertension, hyperuricaemia and alcohol excess. Non-pharmacological and pharmacological approaches to these problems are mandatory and the choice of antihypertensive drugs depends on the individual patient and the concurrent risk factors.

The Elderly

Antihypertensive drug therapy has been shown to be particularly useful in the elderly and is now indicated in hypertensive patients up to the age of about 80 years. Stroke and coronary prevention has been achieved with the use of the thiazide diuretics in low doses. β-blockers and ACE inhibitors are slightly less effective in reducing blood pressure in the elderly compared with younger patients, but the dihydropyridines can be used safely.

Resistant hypertension

The Hypertension Optimal Treatment (HOT) trial demonstrated that only above 25% of all hypertensives can achieve adequate blood pressure control with a single agent. Furthermore around 10% of patients have blood pressures which cannot be reduced despite the use of three antihypertensive drugs.[33] Some of these patients may be found to have a history of chronic alcohol abuse; many have long-standing hypertension with long interruptions of dietary and drug treatment. There are usually ECG changes of left ventricular hypertrophy.

All resistant hypertensives should undergo more detailed investigation to exclude any underlying cause for their high blood pressure. There are some antihypertensive regimens which are particularly effective and should be considered in such patients. These are the ACE inhibitors with the dihydropyridine calcium channel blockers, minoxidil with a β-blocker and a loop diuretic, and an ACE inhibitor with frusemide in high dosage.

Many apparently resistant hypertensives are, in fact, found not to comply with drug therapy. Compliance of therapy can be improved if drug regimens are simplified. Preferably, no antihypertensive regimen should require drugs to be taken more often than once daily.

Conclusions

Antihypertensive therapy has been validated. It prevents heart attacks and strokes and prolongs life by reducing death rates from these diseases. The dramatic decline in malignant hypertension and hypertensive cardiac failure in the Western world is closely related to the mass treatment of millions of hypertensive patients. The prognosis in hypertensive patients is more closely related to the accuracy of long-term blood pressure control than the severity of the hypertension when first diagnosed.

Much of the rising prevalence of hypertension in tropical countries is related to potentially reversible environmental factors and dietary habits. There is still time to bring about preventive measures in order to avoid a coronary 'epidemic', which has afflicted Western countries over the last 50 years. The principles of managing hypertension are similar in all communities, and intervention at an early, mild, presymptomatic stage is worthwhile. However, the health care facilities of many countries should be amended to take on this major but preventable hazard to health.

REFERENCES

1 Stamler J, Wentworth D & Neaton J D. Is the relationship between serum cholesterol and risk of premature death from coronary heart disease continuous or graded? *JAMA* 1986; 256:2823–2828.

2 Pobee J O M. Should hypertension control be considered a public health imperative in black Africa? *J Hum Hypertens* 1990; 4:199.

3 Cruickshank J K, Beevers D G, Osbourne V L, Haynes R A, Corlett J C K & Selby S. Heart attack, stroke, diabetes and hypertension in West Indian, Asians and Whites in Birmingham, England. *BMJ* 1980; 281:1108.

4 Sever P S, Gordon D, Peart W S & Beighton P. Blood pressure and its correlates in urban and tribal Africa. *Lancet* 1980; ii: 60–64.

5 Akinkugbe O O. World epidemiology of hypertension in blacks. In Hall W D, Saunders E & Shulman N B (eds) *Hypertension in Blacks*. Chicago: Year Book Medical Publishers, 1985: 3–16.

6 Shaper A G & Saxton G A. Blood pressure and body build in a rural community in Uganda. *East Afr Med J* 1969; 46:228–235.

7 Cruickshank J K et al. Sick genes, sick individuals or sick populations with chronic disease? The emergence of diabetes and high blood pressure in African-origin populations. *Int J Epidemiol* 2001; 30:111–117.

8 Evans J G & Rose G. Epidemiology of noncommunicable disease Hypertension. *Br Med Bull* 1971; 23:37–42.

9 Sixth report for a Joint National Committee on Detection Evaluation and Treatment of High Blood Pressure. *Arch Intern Med* 1997; 157:2413–2446.

10 Ramsay L E, Williams B, Johnston G D et al. British Hypertension Guidelines for hypertension management. *BMJ* 1999; 319:630–635.

11 British Hypertension Society. Recommendations on blood pressure measurement. *BMJ* 1986; 293:611.

12 Ashcroft M T & Desai P. Blood pressure and mortality in a rural Jamaican community. *Lancet* 1978; i:1167–1170.

13 Davey Smith G, Wentworth D, Neaton J, Stamler R & Stamler J. Socioeconomic differentials in mortality risk among men screened for the Multiple Risk Factor Intervention Trial: II. Black men. *Am J Public Health* 1996; 86:497–504.

14 Walker R W, McLarty D G, Kitange H M et al. Stroke mortality in urban and rural Tanzania. Adult morbidity and mortality project. *Lancet* 2000; 13;355:1684–1687.

15 Seedat Y K, Seedat M A & Hackland D B T. Prevalence of hypertension in the urban and rural Zulu. *J Epidemiol Community Health* 1982; 36:256–261.

16 Edwards R, Unwin N, Mugusi F et al. Hypertension prevalence and care in an urban and rural area of Tanzania. *J Hypertens* 2000; 18:145–152.

17 van Rooyen J M , Kruger H S, Huisman H W, Wissing M P, Margetts B M, Venter C S & Vorster H H. An epidemiological study of hypertension and its determinants in a population in transition: the THUSA study. *J Hum Hypertens* 2000; 14:779–787.

18 INTERSALT Cooperative Research Group. Intersalt: an international study of electrolyte excretion and blood pressure: results of 29 hour urinary sodium and potassium excretion. *BMJ* 1988; 297:319–328.

19 Shah W W & Kunjannam P V. The incidence of hypertension in liquor permit holders and teetotallers. *J Assoc Physicians India* 1959; 7:243–267.

20 Luft F C, Rankin L I, Bloch R et al. Cardiovascular and humoral responses to extremes of sodium intake in normal white and black men. *Circulation* 1979; 60:697–706.

21 Weissberg P L, Woods K L, West M J & Beevers D G. Genetic and ethnic influences on the distribution of sodium and potassium in normotensive and hypertensive subjects. *J Clin Hypertens* 1987; 3:20–25.

22 Freis E D, Materson B J & Flamenbaum V. Comparison of propranolol or hydrochlorothiazide alone for treatment of hypertension: III. Evaluation of the renin–angiotensin system. *Am J Med* 1983; 74:1029–1041.

23 Reaven G M. Role of insulin resistance in human disease. *Diabetes* 1988; 37:1595–1607.

24 Kaplan N M. *Clinical Hypertension*, 6th edn. Baltimore, MD: Williams & Wilkins.

25 Barker D J P. *Mothers, Babies and Health in Later Life*, 2nd edn. Edinburgh: Churchill Livingstone, 1998.

26 Huxley R, Shiell A W & Law C. The role of size at birth and postnatal catch-up growth in determining systolic blood pressure: a systematic review of the literature. *J Hypertens* 2000; 18:815–831.

27 Eriksson J G, Forsen T, Tuomilehto J, Winter P D, Osmond C & Barker D J. Catch-up growth in childhood and death from coronary heart disease: longitudinal study. *BMJ* 1999; 318:427–431.

28 David R J & Collins J W. Differing birthweight among infants of US-born blacks, African-born blacks, and US-born whites. *N Engl J Med* 1997; 337:1209–1213.

29 Forrester T E, Wilks R, Bennett F I et al. Fetal growth and cardiovascular risk factors in Jamaican schoolchildren. *BMJ* 1996; 312:156–160.

30 Miller G J, Beckles G L A & Byam N T A. Serum lipoprotein concentrations in relation to ethnic composition and urbanisation in men and women in Trinidad, West Indies. *Int J Epidemiol* 1984; 13:413–421.

31 Collins R, Peto R, MacMahon S et al. Blood pressure, stroke and coronary heart disease. Part 2: Short-term reductions in blood pressure: overview of randomised drug trials in their epidemiological context. *Lancet* 1990; 335:827–838.

32 Hall W D. Pathophysiology of hypertension in blacks. *Am J Hypertens* 1990; 3:366S–371S.

33 Hansson L, Zanchetti A, Caruthers S G et al. Effects of intensive blood pressure lowering and low-dose aspirin in patients with hypertension: principal results of the Hypertension Optimal Treatment (HOT) randomised trial. *Lancet* 1998; 351:1755–1762.

34 Du X, Cruickshank J K, McNamee R et al. Case–control study of stroke and the quality of hypertension control in north west England. *BMJ* 1997; 314:272–276.

35 Cruickshank J K, Mbanya J C, Wilks R et al. Hypertension in 4 African-origin populations: current 'Rule of Halves', quality of blood pressure control and attributable risk (fraction) for cardiovascular disease. *J Hypertens* 2001; 19:41–46.

Chapter 39
Ischaemic Heart Disease

N. Unwin and K. G. M. M. Alberti

Introduction

Ischaemic heart disease (IHD) is the single largest cause of death worldwide and, with the exception of sub-Saharan Africa, is estimated to be responsible for around 1 in 10 or more of all deaths in all world regions.[1] As populations age and lifestyles change, this burden will grow. This chapter aims to provide a description of the global distribution, risk factors, pathogenesis and clinical manifestations of this disease. It is beyond the scope of the chapter to describe its diagnosis or treatment.

Definition

Ischaemia refers to the situation where the oxygen supply to a tissue or organ is inadequate for its needs. IHD is the disturbance of cardiac function due to inadequate oxygen supply. Most commonly this is due to narrowing or complete occlusion of the coronary arteries caused by coronary atherosclerosis and associated thrombosis, and this chapter is concerned largely with ischaemia of atherosclerotic origin. There are, of course, many other causes of ischaemia related to either increased oxygen demand from the heart or decreased oxygen-carrying capacity of the blood. For example, ischaemia may also arise in severe ventricular hypertrophy due to hypertension or aortic stenosis, or in extremely severe anaemia. Quite commonly two or more causes of ischaemia will coexist, such as coronary atherosclerosis with increased oxygen demand due to the ventricular hypertrophy of hypertension.

Global distribution of ischaemic heart disease and recent trends
Framework of the epidemiological transition

Diseases of the cardiovascular system are found in populations at all stages of economic development. They are a significant contributor to morbidity and mortality in populations as diverse as those of rural Africa and North America. However, the types of cardiovascular disease that predominate differ with the level of economic development.[2] This changing pattern of cardiovascular diseases with economic development is part of a broader picture known as the 'epidemiological transition'.[3] This provides a useful framework for considering the inter-relationships between demography, disease patterns, and social and economic conditions. The nature of the epidemiological transition and the relationships between these various factors are summarized in Figure 39.1. The figure illustrates the change from high fertility and high mortality, largely from infectious diseases that particularly afflict infants and children, to low fertility and low mortality, largely from chronic non-infectious diseases that particularly afflict adults and the elderly. The pace and details of change can and do vary greatly between populations and between subgroups, such as the rich and poor, within populations. The falling mortality and fertility is

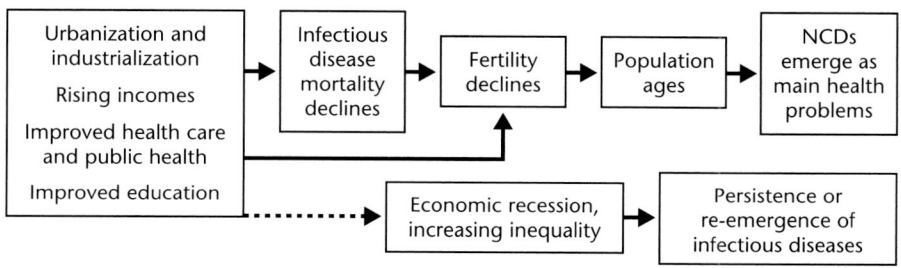

Figure 39.1: Representation of the epidemiological transition. The dashed line represents a protracted and polarized transition, where persistent or new infectious diseases (such as HIV) are found alongside rising levels of non-communicable diseases (NCDs). This is the case in many of the world's poorest countries.

associated with huge changes in population age structure, from a very young age structure to that found in Western industrialized countries today. Four stages can be identified within this process according to the predominant disease patterns and life expectancy. Table 39.1 lists the predominant causes of death from cardiovascular disease at each of these stages. The table illustrates the fact that IHD becomes a predominant contributor to mortality only in the later stages of the transition.

Global distribution of ischaemic heart disease

IHD is estimated to be the single largest cause of death worldwide.[1,4] A little over 1 in 7 of all deaths in the year 2000 were estimated to be due to IHD. However, 6 out of 10 deaths from IHD occur in developing countries, partly reflecting the fact that 8 of 10 of all deaths worldwide occur in developing countries.

There is marked regional variation in the importance of IHD as a cause of death (Figure 39.2). Thus, in 'developed regions' (established market economies and former socialist economies) around 23–28% of all deaths are due to IHD. In 'developing regions' (all other regions) the proportion varies from the lowest of 3% (sub-Saharan Africa) to the highest of just under 17% (Middle Eastern Crescent and India). Broadly, these differences represent different stages of the epidemiological transition described above. When the proportion of deaths due IHD is examined by age group, in some developing regions, notably India and the Middle Eastern Crescent, IHD is found to contribute a similar, or in some age groups a greater, proportion of deaths than in developed regions. Estimates of age-specific death rates from IHD (Figure 39.3) also suggest that these are higher in India and the Middle Eastern Crescent than in

Table 39.1 Deaths from cardiovascular disease by stage of epidemiological transition

Stage of transition	% Deaths from CVD	Main CVDs	Examples
Pestilence and famine	5–10	Rheumatic fever, infectious and nutritional cardiomyopathies	Sub-Saharan Africa, Rural India
Receding pandemics	10–35	As above + hypertensive heart disease and haemorrhagic stroke	China
Degenerative and human-made diseases	35–55	All stroke, IHD at relatively young ages	Urban India
Delayed degenerative diseases	< 50	Ischaemic stroke and IHD at older ages	Western Europe, USA

From Howson C, Reddy S, Ryan T & Bale J (eds) *Control of Cardiovascular Diseases in Developing Countries. Research, Development and Institutional Strengthening.* Washington, DC: National Academy Press, 1998.

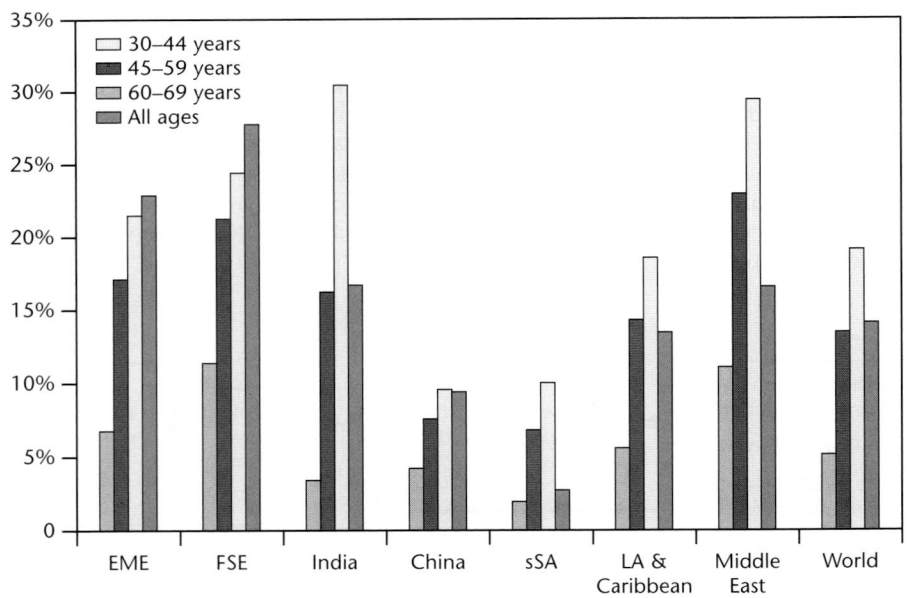

Figure 39.2: Estimated percentage of deaths due to ischaemic heart disease in 2000 for men and women in different regions of the world. EME, established market economies; FSE, former socialist economies; sSA, sub-Saharan Africa; LA & Carib, Latin America and the Caribbean. Data from Murray C & Lopez A (eds). *The Global Burden of Disease: A Comprehensive Assessment of Mortality and Disability from Diseases, Injuries, and Risk Factors in 1990 and Projected to 2020.* Geneva: World Health Organization, 1996.

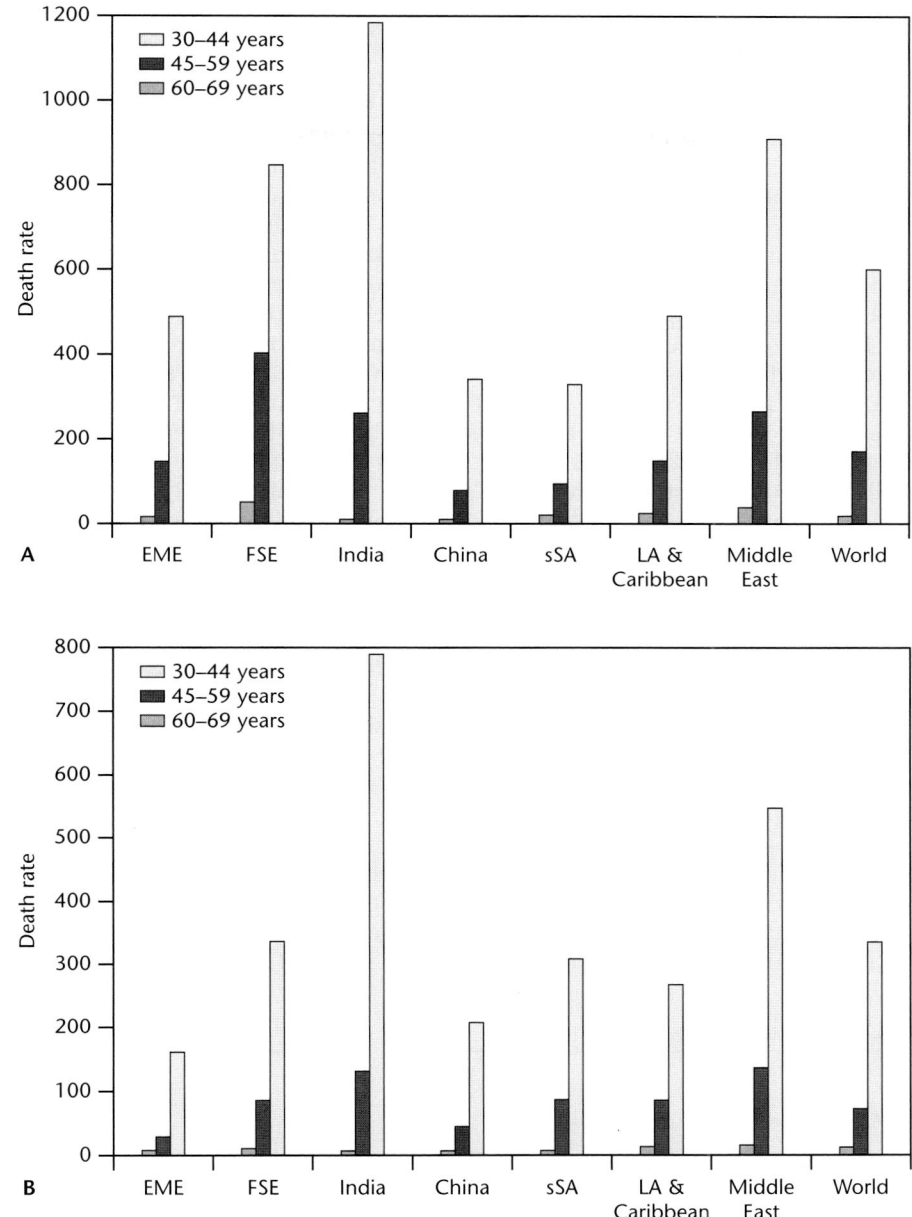

Figure 39.3: Estimated annual age-specific death rates from ischaemic heart disease in (**A**) men and (**B**) women per 100 000 population in different world regions in 2000. EME, established market economies; FSE, former socialist economies; sSA, sub-Saharan Africa; LA & Carib, Latin America and the Caribbean. Data from Murray C & Lopez A (eds). *The Global Burden of Disease: A Comprehensive Assessment of Mortality and Disability from Diseases, Injuries, and Risk Factors in 1990 and Projected to 2020.* Geneva: World Health Organization, 1996.

established market economies. In summary, most IHD deaths occur in developing countries and in some developing countries IHD is now a more important contributor to mortality in adults than in developed regions.

Trends in 'developed' regions

The beginning of the twentieth century witnessed the start of an epidemic of IHD in most industrialized countries, particularly those of northern Europe, North America,

Australia and New Zealand. This epidemic was most pronounced in men, in whom, even allowing for the contribution of artefact such as changes in diagnostic practice, there was a very substantial rise in age-specific mortality rates from IHD over the first half of the twentieth century.[5] In women, for reasons not fully understood, increases in age-specific death rates were much less marked.[6] The evidence suggests that early in the epidemic, rates of IHD were highest in the socioeconomically better off but moved across socioeconomic groups to produce the current picture, where the least well off have the highest rates.[7]

In Western industrialized countries, age-specific mortality rates from IHD began to fall from around 1970. Declines of between 20% and 50% occurred between 1965 and 1990. The precise reasons for these declines remain the subject of debate, but are likely to represent a combination of falls in levels of risk factors and improvements in clinical care. Most estimates suggest that half or a little more of the decline can be attributed to trends in the major risk factors (smoking, dyslipidaemia and high blood pressure), and most of the rest to improvements in clinical care.[8-10]

In the former socialist economies of Russia and Eastern Europe, recent trends have been somewhat different, with rising age-specific death rates from these and other conditions in adults during the 1980s.[11] This rise seemed to coincide with the end of the socialist system in these countries and may be related to increases in excessive alcohol consumption, falls in the consumption of fresh fruit and vegetables, and widening inequalities in income.[12]

Trends in 'developing' regions

The lack of good quality data means that trends in developing regions are often based on the earlier experience of developed regions. It is a safe prediction that crude IHD rates (e.g., per 1000 total population per year) will increase substantially over the coming years as the population age structure of developing regions grows older.[4] It also seems a safe prediction that in many—probably most—developing nations age-specific IHD rates will increase as the proportion of the population living in urban rather than rural areas increases. There are data from several developing regions, including India[4] and sub-Saharan Africa,[13] that demonstrate marked differences in IHD risk factor levels between rural and urban populations. Thus traditional rural lifestyles in developing countries tend to be associated with low levels of IHD risk factors (see below), with high complex carbohydrate diets, high levels of physical activity, and low levels dyslipidaemia, obesity, hypertension and diabetes. In contrast, urban living is associated with high rates of obesity, physical inactivity, saturated fat intake, smoking, alcohol intake, dyslipidaemia, hypertension and diabetes. Contrary to popular perception, high levels of these risk factors are not limited to the urban wealthy. For example, in a middle-income area of Dar es Salaam one in five adults was hypertensive and one in twenty had diabetes.[14] The global burden of disease study estimates that between the year 2000 and 2020 the crude death rates from IHD will increase by 9% for the world as a whole, but with more substantial increases in all developing regions except for sub-Saharan Africa (Figure 39.4).[1]

Risk factors for ischaemic heart disease

A risk factor for ischaemic heart disease is simply an attribute or exposure that is associated with an increased probability of either having or developing the disease. More than 250 possible cardiovascular risk factors have been identified. However, a much smaller number has been shown consistently to be important (Figure 39.5).[15-18] These include unmodifiable personal characteristics, such as age and sex; modifiable behaviours such as diet, smoking and physical inactivity; and intervening physiological

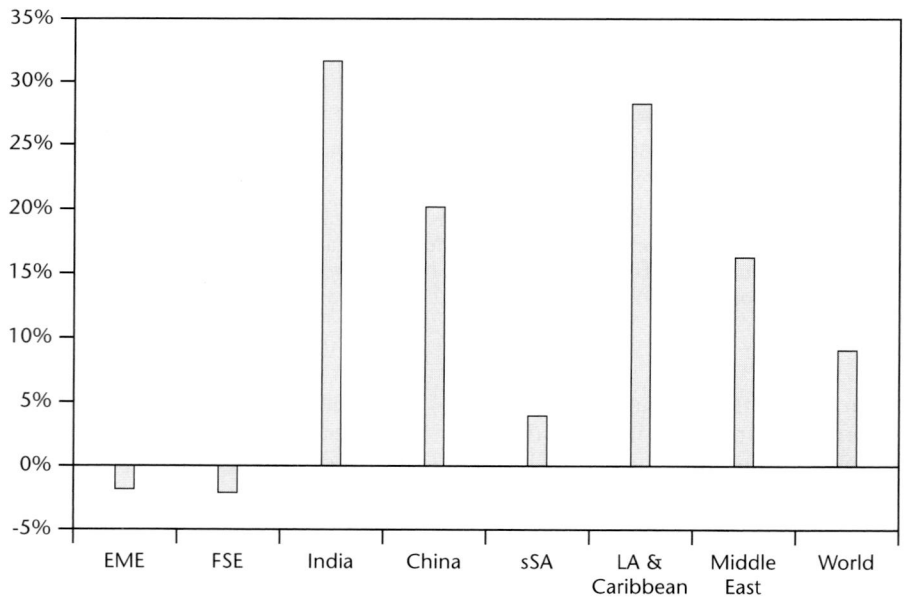

Figure 39.4: Estimated percentage change in number of deaths from ischaemic heart disease per 1000 total population between 2000 and 2020. EME, established market economies; FSE, former socialist economies; sSA, sub-Saharan Africa; LA & Carib, Latin America and the Caribbean. Data from Murray C & Lopez A (eds). *The Global Burden of Disease: A Comprehensive Assessment of Mortality and Disability from Diseases, Injuries, and Risk Factors in 1990 and Projected to 2020.* Geneva: World Health Organization, 1996.

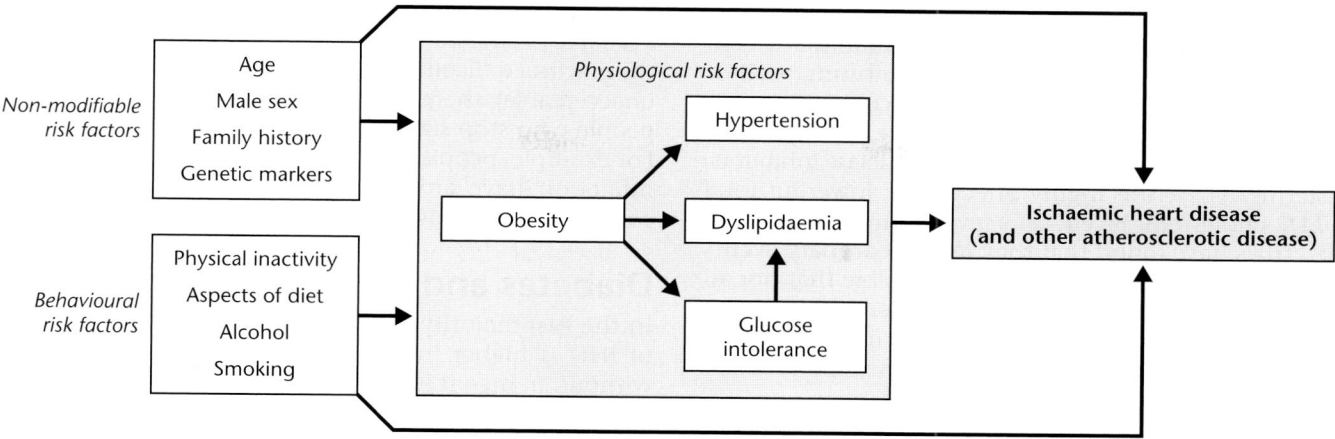

Figure 39.5: Established risk factors for ischaemic heart disease and their interrelationships. See main text for details. Modifed from Howson et al. Control of cardiovascular diseases in developing countries. Research, developmental and institutional strengthening. Washington DC: National Academy Press; 1998.

variables such as obesity, blood pressure and lipid levels. Risk factors are often grouped simply into those that cannot be changed (unmodifiable) and those that can be changed (modifiable), and are thus of potential importance for the prevention of IHD.

Unmodifiable risk factors

Unmodifiable risk factors include increasing age, male sex, strong family history of IHD and genetic markers.

Age and sex

Death rates from IHD tend to increase exponentially with age in populations with both low and high rates of IHD. Rates are higher in men than in women in all populations. Below the age of 50 years, rates tend to be 4–5-fold higher in men compared with women. With increasing age above 50 years, rates in women approach but never reach those of men. This pattern of male to female rates is thought by most researchers to reflect premenopausal protective effects of oestrogen, mediated at least partly through higher levels of high density lipoprotein (HDL) cholesterol (see below), and the loss of these effects following the menopause.

Family history and genetic markers

A strong family history of IHD, often measured as a history of IHD in a first-degree relative below the age of 60 years, is associated with an increased risk over and above the effect of shared risk factors between family members. In the Framingham study, for example, such a family history was associated with a 30% increased risk independent of other risk factors.[18] At the time of writing, a limited number of genetic markers has been associated with an increased risk of IHD and it seems likely that the number will increase as further work is undertaken. In a disease as complex as IHD it is likely that a large number of genetic markers, for

example reflecting aspects of such areas as lipid metabolism, blood pressure control and endothelial function, will be identified. Examples of current candidates that may contribute to variation in the risk of IHD between individuals and populations include genes for apolipoproteins (e.g, ApoE) and the angiotensin-converting enzyme gene.[19]

Modifiable risk factors

High total or low density lipoprotein (LDL) cholesterol (particularly when associated with low HDL cholesterol), high blood pressure and smoking have been shown to be the most important modifiable risk factors in most populations. Diabetes and lesser forms of glucose intolerance are also discussed here.

Dyslipidaemia

Total serum cholesterol concentration is strongly related to differences in IHD rates between and within populations. There is a strong and continuous relationship, for example, between the average serum cholesterol level in a population and that population's rate of IHD.[20] Within a population there is a strong and continuous relationship between an individual's cholesterol level and their risk of developing IHD. Total cholesterol is made up of several components, the most important of which are LDL and HDL cholesterol. The main atherogenic component of total cholesterol is LDL cholesterol, which is made particularly atherogenic through oxidation (see the section on pathogenesis). HDL cholesterol is independently related to a reduced risk of IHD. This is thought to be through its role in removing cholesterol from the tissues, including the arterial wall, and returning it to the liver. The single most predictive measures of dyslipidaemia that were found in the Framingham study are the ratios of LDL cholesterol: HDL cholesterol or of total cholesterol: HDL cholesterol. For example, a total: HDL cholesterol ratio of 9.6 is associated with double the rate of IHD compared with a ratio of 5.0, which is associated with double the rate compared with a ratio of 3.4.[18] There is now substantial randomized controlled trial evidence of the benefits of lowering total or LDL cholesterol levels by means of pharmacological agents. The strongest evidence is for the use of hydroxy-methylglutaryl coenzyme A (HMGCoA) reductase inhibitors, the statins. These are highly effective at lowering total and LDL cholesterol levels, and several randomized controlled trials have found that they reduce coronary events by around one-third.[21] However, it is possible that not all of this effect is due to lowering LDL cholesterol levels, as intermediates of cholesterol synthesis are involved in the regulation of several functions, including the inflammatory response, which may also be important.[22]

Blood pressure

Raised blood pressure is a strong and independent risk factor for IHD. Prospective data on over 350 000 men in the United States, screened as part of the Multiple Risk Factor Intervention Trial (MRFIT),[23] demonstrated a continuous positive relationship between diastolic blood pressure from a level of 75 mmHg. With systolic blood pressure there was evidence of a plateau below 120 mmHg and a continuous positive relationship with IHD incidence above this. These and similar data suggest that a 5–6 mmHg reduction in diastolic blood pressure should lead to a 20–25% reduction in IHD events. A meta-analysis of 14 randomized controlled trials of blood pressure lowering, involving 37 000 individuals with diastolic hypertension, demonstrated a significant reduction in IHD events of around 14% in those receiving treatment.[24] The difference between this and the predicted value may reflect some unwanted effects of antihypertensive agents on lipid and glucose metabolism.

Left ventricular hypertrophy, often a consequence of prolonged hypertension, is also a risk factor for IHD events. Left ventricular hypertrophy is also associated with diabetes and obesity, and participants in the Framingham study with either electrocardiographic or echocardiographic evidence of this condition were at two to three times the risk of IHD.[18]

Smoking

There is overwhelming evidence for a causal role of cigarette smoking in IHD. Both the duration of smoking and the amount of tobacco smoked daily are directly related to the risk of IHD events. The relative risk associated with smoking varies by age, being highest in younger adults. For example, in a study of over 30 000 male British physicians, the risk of IHD death in those smoking 25 or more cigarettes a day was 15 times higher than in non-smokers. However, the risk was twice as high in those aged 55–64 years. Across all age groups, smokers of more than 25 cigarettes a day were 40% more likely to die from IHD than non-smokers.[25] Because smoking is common it contributes substantially to IHD event rates. For example, smoking is estimated to be responsible for between one-sixth and one-fifth of all IHD deaths in North America and Britain.[26]

Although randomized controlled trial evidence is not available on the benefits of smoking cessation (apart from the practical difficulties, such a study would now be ethically unacceptable), there are many 'natural experiments' where people who stop smoking have been followed over time. For example, people who stop smoking after a myocardial infarction have around a 50% reduction in death rate compared with those who continue smoking.[27]

Diabetes and glucose intolerance

In the vast majority of populations studied the incidence of IHD is higher in people with diabetes than in those without. In men it is roughly twice as high, and in women three times as high at all ages. The relative advantage in IHD rates that women have over men is lost in people with diabetes.[28] Some, but not all,[29] of the excess IHD incidence in people with diabetes is accounted for by higher levels of other risk factors, particularly dyslipidaemia and high blood pressure. Lesser forms of glucose intolerance, such as impaired glucose tolerance, are also associated with higher rates of IHD. Pooled prospective data from Europe with over 20 000 participants demonstrate that impaired glucose tolerance predicts IHD mortality independently of other major cardiovascular risk factors.[30]

Obesity, aspects of lifestyle and cardiovascular risk

Obesity and certain aspects of lifestyle, such as physical inactivity, alcohol consumption and aspects of diet, are risk factors for cardiovascular disease. Much of the effect of these is through their influence on the risk factors described above. For example, obesity is related to dyslipidaemia, particularly low HDL cholesterol and raised triglyceride levels, glucose intolerance, raised blood pressure and insulin resistance (a group of disorders referred to as the 'metabolic syndrome').[31] Physical inactivity is related to a similar group of disorders.[32] At a population level, the saturated fat content of the diet is the most important determinant of mean population total and LDL cholesterol levels. In individuals the relationship between saturated fat content and cholesterol concentration is less clear. This is probably because at the individual level dietary intake interacts with several different genetic factors to determine cholesterol level. There is evidence that other aspects of diet, such as fresh fruit and vegetable content, are also likely to be important in determining the risk of IHD. Likely mechanisms include the role of antioxidants in protecting against the oxidation of LDL cholesterol (see the section on pathogenesis below) and the beneficial effects of potassium, and the detrimental effects of sodium, on blood pressure. The protective effects of moderate alcohol consumption, around 2 units per day, on IHD in populations at high risk of the condition are well documented. At least part of this benefit is through the effect of alcohol on raising HDL cholesterol levels. An important caveat to the protective effects of alcohol is that these are associated with regular drinking, and that heavy binge drinking may have quite the opposite impact on cardio-vascular outcomes.[33]

The interactive nature of risk factors

As would be expected, the greater the number of risk factors an individual possesses the higher is the probability of an IHD event, such as sudden death, myocardial infarction or the development of angina. The risk associated with a combination of risk factors is often greater than simply adding the risk associated with the individual risk factors together: it tends to be multiplicative. This is illustrated in Figure 39.6, which is based on a risk prediction formula from the Framingham study.[18] The figure shows how the risk of developing IHD in a 50-year-old man currently without IHD varies over 7-fold with different levels of the three main modifiable risk factors. Several scoring systems have been derived to provide an estimate of the risk of IHD within individuals based on their risk factor levels. Factors that are usually taken into account include age, sex, presence or absence of diabetes, blood pressure level, smoking status, and total: HDL cholesterol ratio. Such scoring systems are being promoted as aids to decision making, for example to help determine who should receive lipid- or blood pressure-lowering medication. A major limitation of these systems is that they tend to be based on data from high-risk populations of European origin (the majority are based on data from one study, the Framingham study). There is evidence that the level of risk associated with both individual factors and combinations of factors varies between populations, depending both on their overall level of risk and the influence of less well understood IHD risk factors.[34,35]

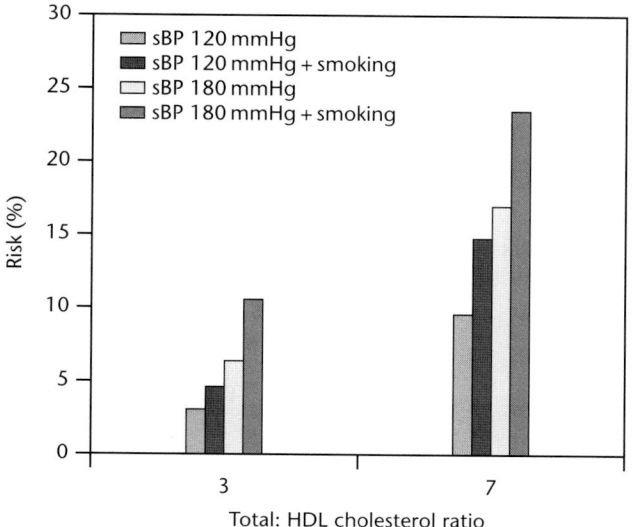

Figure 39.6: Risk of ischaemic heart disease over 10 years in a 50-year-old man with different levels of total : high density lipoprotein (HDL) cholesterol ratio, systolic blood pressure (sBP) and smoking status.

The 'only 50%' explanatory power of the major IHD risk factors

It is commonly stated that the major IHD risk factors described above can explain only about half the variation in IHD incidence.[5] In other words, within a population only about half the cases of IHD can be predicted by the above risk factors. Or, when comparing populations with different IHD rates, such as different socioeconomic groups, only about half the difference in rates appears to be due to differences in smoking, lipid levels, blood pressure and diabetes. The 'only 50%' explanatory power has recently been challenged by results from a very large cohort study in the United States. This found that non-smoking individuals with low blood pressure and low total cholesterol level had one-fifth or less the incidence of IHD compared with the rest.[36] Nonetheless, the apparent inability of the major risk factors to explain much more than 50% of variation in IHD incidence has led to a huge research effort to identify other risk factors that will improve our ability to predict IHD. There is a very long list of putative risk factors under investigation.[15,37] The list includes new putative atherogenic factors, such as homocysteine. Clinical homocysteinuria is associated with very premature IHD, but epidemiological evidence suggests that levels of homocysteine within the general population are also related to increased risk of IHD, and that this risk is reduced by intake of vitamin B_{12} and folate, vitamins that promote the metabolism of homocysteine. Thrombogenic risk markers under investigation include fibrinogen, factor VII and plasminogen activator inhibitor. Markers and promoters of inflammation are also of interest and include C-reactive protein and interleukin 6, with the possibility that certain infections, such as *Chlamydia pneumoniae*, may increase the risk of atherosclerosis. Finally, a quite different category of risk markers that are being investigated are psychosocial stressors, such as psychological traits, working environment and social support. There is good observational evidence that some of these are associated with IHD risk,[38] although the biological mechanisms for such effects remain to be elucidated.

Ethnic group differences in IHD risk factors

The associations between IHD and the major modifiable risk factors described above have been demonstrated in a wide variety of populations, whether defined by ethnic group or by geography. In this respect the evidence suggests that ethnic groups are much more alike than different in terms of the causes of IHD. Analyses of the predictive power of risk factors have found some differences between groups, for example between southern and northern European populations,[34] or between Japanese and white populations in the United States. Thus, for example, a recent analysis suggested that the risk prediction formula used to produce Figure 39.6 applies equally well to African and white Americans. However, some modification is needed to account for underlying differences in the prevalence of risk factors and the overall IHD rates before the formula can be applied to Japanese and native American groups.[35] The reasons for differences between ethnic groups are likely to be complex. Possible explanations include differences in exposures to lifestyle and environmental factors mediated by geography, socioeconomic status and culture. Differences in genetic background leading to differences in gene–environment interactions may also be important.

Migrant populations whose ancestral origins are from the Indian subcontinent suffer from particularly high rates of IHD compared with indigenous populations.[39] As with other groups, the major modifiable risk factors are important, but they do not appear to account for the higher rates of IHD,[40] and other factors have been suggested, including a higher prevalence of insulin resistance and metabolic syndrome.[41]

Pathogenesis of atherosclerosis and ischaemic heart disease

Atherosclerosis is a patchy, nodular type of arteriosclerosis (thickening and hardening of the arterial wall) that occurs mainly in large and medium-sized elastic and muscular arteries. It is characterized by lipid accumulation, hyperplasia and scarring in the arterial intima. These are reflected in the derivation of the term atherosclerosis, which comes from the Greek words *athero* (meaning gruel or paste) and *sclerosis* (hardness).

Atherosclerosis underlies the vast majority of ischaemic vascular disease, including IHD. Its major complications are myocardial, cerebral and peripheral (particularly lower limb) ischaemia and infarction. A broad spectrum of clinical disease is associated with atherosclerotic lesions in the coronary arteries. For example, atherosclerotic lesions may be silent and not give rise to any symptoms or signs. They may gradually lead to narrowing of a coronary artery giving rise to stable angina, or their surface may be disrupted leading to thrombus formation and the acute coronary syndromes of unstable angina and myocardial infarction. The evolution and behaviour of atherosclerotic lesions and their relationship to clinical disease are considered below.

Morphology and classification of atherosclerotic lesions

At the beginning of the twentieth century two types of intimal lesion were recognized and associated with atherosclerosis. These were the fatty streak (a thin lipid deposit in the intima in children) and the fibrous plaque (a thick lipid and fibrous lesion in adults). At this time it

was not universally accepted that these two lesions were the early and advanced expressions of a single disease. By the 1950s, however, a classification that consisted of the sequence fatty streak, fibrous plaque and complicated lesion was widely used. The term 'complicated lesion' was used for a fibrous plaque that contained a haemorrhage or had ulcerated or fissured with associated thrombosis. The World Health Organization's classification, published in 1958, added the term 'atheroma' to these three terms.[42] This was added to distinguish advanced lesions with a predominantly lipid component (atheroma) from those with a predominantly collagenous component (fibrous plaque). More recently, the American Heart Association (AHA) reviewed the classification of lesions and using the latest available histological evidence proposed a classification based on six main types of lesion.[43,44] The classification essentially incorporates both the type and sequence of lesions described in previous classifications (Figure 39.7). Types I and II are early lesions and include the fatty streak. Types IV–VI are advanced lesions and include atheroma through to complicated lesions. Type III represents the transitory phase between early and advanced lesions.

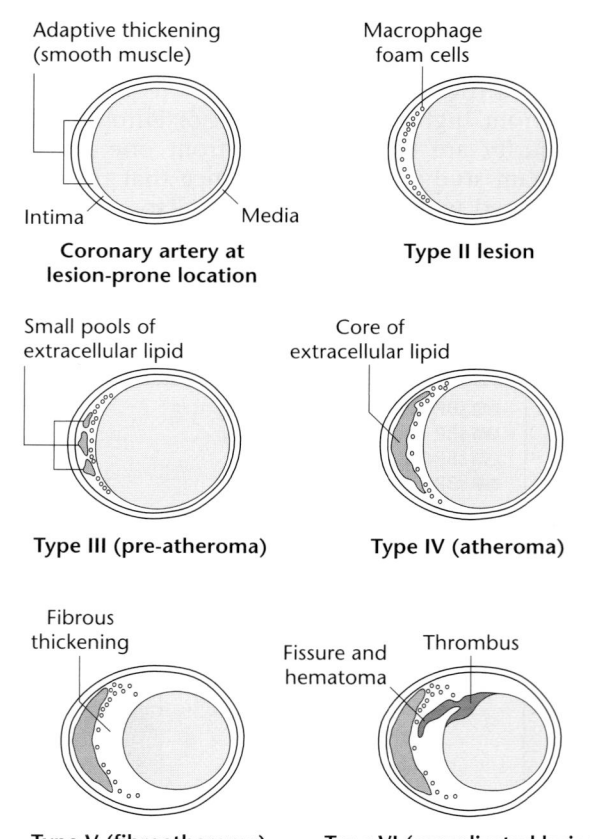

Figure 39.7: Types of atherosclerotic lesion. From Stary et al. A definition of initial, fatty streak, and intermediate lesions of atherosclerosis. A report from the Committee on Vascular Lesions of the Council on Arteriosclerosis, American Heart Association. *Circulation* 1994; 89:2462-2478. © 1994, American Heart Association.

Pathogenesis of atherosclerotic lesions

Exactly how atherosclerosis begins and evolves, and what factors drive and determine the direction of this whole process, is not fully known. However, any description of its pathogenesis must be able to account for the fact that lesions are not uniformly distributed throughout the arterial tree. Whether in human populations with a high or low incidence of atherosclerotic disease, or in animal models of atherosclerosis, the distribution of lesions is highly characteristic. They occur predominantly at bifurcation points and bends of the arteries. The 'response to injury hypothesis' suggests that endothelial and other cells within the arterial wall actively respond to a range of potential insults in a way that initiates and may promote the atherosclerotic process. One source of 'injury' is haemodynamic forces, and at arterial bifurcation points and bends there are low shear forces and turbulent blood flow. In such regions there is increased residence time for circulating blood constituents, some of which may also be causes of injury.[45] In these regions endothelial cells alter their normal homeostatic properties leading to increased adhesiveness for monocytes, T lymphocytes and platelets, and increased permeability to lipids. Their responses include the formation of vasoactive molecules, adhesion molecules, cytokines and growth factors. Such responses will be increased and sustained by the presence of other causes of injury and insult to the endothelium. These may include raised and modified LDL cholesterol levels, free radicals caused by cigarette smoking, hypertension and diabetes mellitus, raised plasma homocysteine concentrations and infectious micro-organisms such as herpes viruses or *Chlamydia pnuemoniae*.

Type 1 and type 2 atherosclerotic lesions (Figure 39.7) occur in all human populations studied, including those with a low incidence of IHD. These lesions, therefore, appear to represent a controlled, limited and universal inflammatory response to certain haemodynamic forces. The development of more advanced lesions seems to be dependent upon greater and continuing stimulation of this response.[46] Particularly central to this is the accumulation, within the arterial intima, of LDL cholesterol that has been mildly oxidized (oxLDL) when crossing the endothelial cell, and may be further modified within the intima. Accumulation of oxLDL acts as an attractant for monocytes and promotes their conversion to macrophages. Macrophages ingesting large amounts of oxLDL become foam cells. In addition, continuing inflammation sees migration, probably from the arterial media, and proliferation of smooth muscle cells. Smooth muscle cells are found in two main phenotypes: those of the contractile type, which are rich in myofilaments, and those of the synthetic type (derived from the contractile type in response to stimuli associated with injury), which are rich in rough endoplasmic reticulum. The synthetic phenotype of smooth muscle cells responds to various growth factors and secretes extracellular matrix components including collagen.

The lipid core of type IV lesions contains cholesterol and its esters,[44] some in crystalline form, and includes debris from macrophage and foam cell death. The lipid core is surrounded by macrophages. These are highly activated inflammatory cells, producing cell mediators such as tumour necrosis factor α, interleukins and metalloproteinases (connective tissue matrix degrading enzymes).[46] The connective tissue capsule surrounding the lipid core consists of collagen and matrix synthesized by smooth muscle cells, and as the size of the capsule increases and a fibrous cap clearly develops the lesion can be classified as a type V lesion.

Ulceration or fissuring of the fibrous cap is the precursor of complicated (type VI) lesions in which thrombus formation occurs (Figure 39.7). Highly activated macrophages are involved in both ulceration and fissuring. Ulceration is due to endothelial denudation exposing subendothelial connective tissue on which thrombus forms. Fissuring exposes the highly thrombogenic lipid core of the plaque. Thrombus forms initially within the plaque and may then extend into the arterial lumen.[47]

Relationship between coronary atherosclerosis and presentation of IHD

Clinically overt IHD is largely associated with type IV–type VI lesions.[44] Reduction in the diameter of the coronary artery by an atherosclerotic lesion can lead to ischaemia when the demands for blood supply through that artery are increased (e.g., by physical activity or emotion). Chronic stable angina and stable silent ischaemia (ischaemia without classical symptoms and detected through electrocardiography) are the clinical outcomes of this situation. Interestingly even large stable atherosclerotic lesions may not lead to symptoms. This is because much of the initial growth of the lesion occurs outwards, producing a bulging and remodelling of the arterial wall and leaving the cross-sectional area of the lumen untouched. Narrowing of the lumen starts to occur only when the lesion occupies more than 40% of the circumference.[48] Even then, the narrowing needs to be 50% or more before blood flow starts to decrease. One of the implications of these facts is that a coronary artery that appears normal on coronary arteriography may nonetheless be substantially diseased and, although not currently producing symptoms, may threaten an acute coronary syndrome (myocardial infarction or unstable angina).

Myocardial infarction and unstable angina arise from complicated (type VI) lesions. Thrombus formation, in response to plaque rupture or erosion of its surface, may occlude the lumen of the artery and thus lead to infarction of the heart muscle supplied by that artery. Unstable angina is associated with thrombus formation that neither fully occludes the artery nor fully resolves.[47] The thrombus thus severely restricts blood flow, producing symptoms without causing infarction.

Clinical syndromes of ischaemic heart disease

Classification and presentation of IHD

IHD can present in several ways. Figure 39.8 provides a classification based on how people with IHD may first come to the attention of clinicians. It is important to note that the categories are not mutually exclusive. For example, someone may present with the symptoms of myocardial infarction and cardiac insufficiency, and be subject to dysrrhythmias. Similarly, once IHD has become manifest, an individual may through the course of the disease experience several of the categories shown in Figure 39.8. For example, they may be diagnosed with angina, suffer from episodes of silent ischaemia, be prone to dysrrhythmias because of ischaemic damage to the conducting system of the heart, and develop cardiac insufficiency (heart failure) through accumulated ischaemic damage to the cardiac muscle.

Figure 39.9 shows the presentation of new cases of IHD in the Framingham study.[49] In this cohort the first indication of IHD in around 15% of men and women was death as a result of the condition, with two-thirds of these deaths occurring within 1 hour of the onset of symptoms (the definition of 'sudden death'). Women more commonly presented with angina than men, with a small proportion presenting with unstable rather stable angina. One-third of myocardial infarctions in men, and almost half in women, were unrecognized at the time (many presumably because they were painless) and picked up later by electrocardiographic changes.

Stable or classical angina pectoris

The pain of stable angina pectoris is brought on by an increase in cardiac workload. Examples of activities that can result in angina include physical exertion, such as walking up hill, carrying a heavy load, emotion, eating a heavy meal or cold weather. The site of pain of angina pectoris is typically mid-sternal with radiation to the left arm. It may also radiate to the angle of the jaw and through to the back. It is usually described as a 'gripping' or 'tight' pain. Patients may describe it as like having a tight band around their chest. However, in some cases the pain is little more than a dull ache, and this may be felt only in the arm or jaw and not necessarily in the chest.

The pain of angina is typically relieved rapidly by rest. Thus, usually within 2 minutes or so of stopping exertion, the pain has gone. Another factor that should lead to

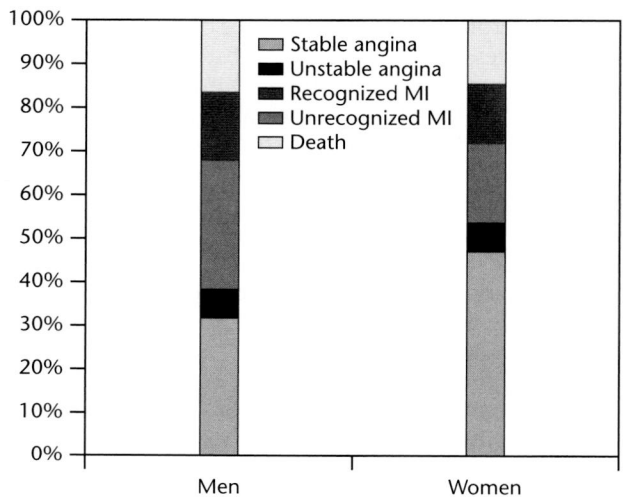

Figure 39.9: Presentation of new cases of ischaemic heart disease in men and women in the Framingham study. Based on data from Murabito J M, Evans J C, Larson M G & Levy D. Prognosis after the onset of coronary heart disease. An investigation of differences in outcome between the sexes according to initial coronary disease presentation. *Circulation* 1993; 88(6):2548–2555.

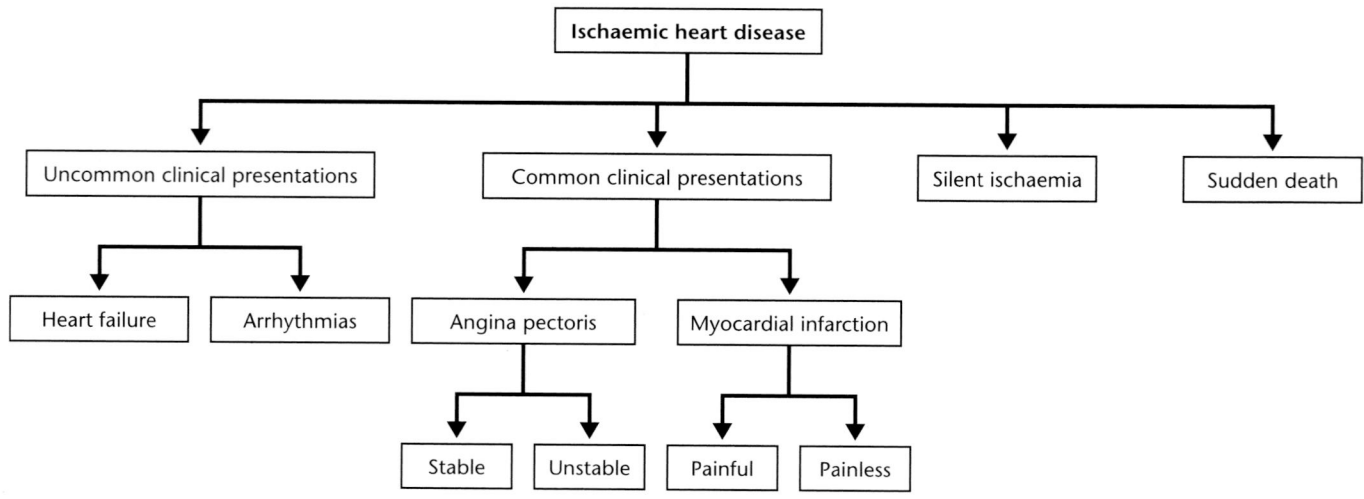

Figure 39.8: Classification of ischaemic heart disease based on clinical presentation.

rapid relief of the pain is the use of nitroglycerine tablets or spray (applied under the tongue). Indeed nitroglycerine is sometimes used to assist with diagnosis and to help distinguish angina pectoris from other causes of chest pain.

Unstable angina pectoris

Unstable angina is often also called 'angina at rest'. This is anginal chest pain that is not associated with exertion and which can come on suddenly while the patient is at rest. It may range from brief single episodes to prolonged and repeated episodes. Clinically it may be difficult to distinguish from a myocardial infarction, requiring further investigations such as electrocardiography and measurement of cardiac enzymes to determine whether the pain represents 'unstable angina' or 'myocardial infarction'. Indeed, unstable angina often signifies advanced disease and impending infarction.

Myocardial infarction

The pain of myocardial infarction is similar in distribution to that of angina, but is typically much more severe, lasts from 30 minutes to several hours, and is not relieved by rest or nitroglycerine. Patients often describe it as a crushing pain, as though a heavy weight or person was sitting on their chest. Nausea, vomiting and sweating may be present, especially at the start of the pain. With large infarcts, breathlessness may be present from left ventricular failure.

Although myocardial infarction is usually painful, it is painless in a substantial proportion (possibly more than one-fifth) of cases. Painless myocardial infarction is commoner in people with diabetes and increases with age.[50] The patient may present with non-specific complaints such as transient loss of consciousness, acute confusion, a sense of weakness or nausea. Other painless signs include the appearance of an arrhythmia (such as atrial fibrillation of heart block) or an unexplained drop in blood pressure. Thus a high degree of suspicion is necessary, particularly in the elderly and in people with diabetes, in order to detect such cases.

The most immediate life-threatening complication of myocardial infarction comes from arrhythmias, particularly ventricular fibrillation. Around 25–30% of people suffering a myocardial infarction die before they reach hospital, largely from ventricular fibrillation. This knowledge has led to great efforts in many countries both to reduce the time between the onset of symptoms and admission to hospital, and to make resuscitation equipment and people trained to use it more widely available in public places. Heart failure and clinical shock may ensue in the hours and days after large infarcts, with low blood pressure, low cardiac output and poor oxygenation of the blood. Other potential complications in the first few days include myocardial rupture, rupture of the interventricular septum, mitral regurgitation following damage to the papillary muscle, and systemic and pulmonary embolism. Typically a quarter of patients admitted to hospital with myocardial infarction die before discharge, although modern intensive therapy can reduce the mortality rate substantially.

Sudden cardiac death

By definition, 'sudden cardiac death' occurs within 1 hour of the onset of symptoms. Sudden cardiac death is often associated with myocardial infarction leading to ventricular fibrillation, as described above. However, fatal arrhythmias may also occur in the absence of recent myocardial infarction, with a poorly functioning ventricle damaged by previous ischaemia being susceptible to arrhythmias including ventricular fibrillation.

Silent ischaemia

The widespread use of electrocardiography (ECG), including exercise ECG and continuous ambulatory monitoring, has identified people who have ECG evidence of ischaemia (S-T depression) on exertion but no symptoms. Such individuals are at an increased risk of coronary events, such as sudden death, myocardial infarction and clinical angina. Silent ischaemia is commoner in people with diabetes.

Conclusions and challenges

This chapter has aimed to provide a description of IHD, from its epidemiology to its pathogenesis. It has not aimed to cover treatment or prevention, although within these lie immense challenges, particularly in low- and middle-income countries. Much of the treatment given for IHD in developed countries is beyond the resources of low- and middle-income countries for all but the most privileged few of their population. Yet inexpensive and effective treatments do exist, such as the use of aspirin in those with IHD, and the use of inexpensive blood pressure-lowering agents for those with hypertension. One of the challenges is to ensure that such treatments are delivered in the most clinically and cost-effective way.[13] However, it is clear that the greatest emphasis should be on prevention.

Primary prevention of IHD is possible.[51] The major modifiable risk factors of tobacco smoking, high blood pressure, dyslipidaemia and glucose intolerance are consistent across different populations. The last three of these arise from the common soil of an atherogenic diet (high in saturated fat and salt, low in fresh fruit and vegetables), physical inactivity and obesity. The evidence from some developed countries suggests that much of the decline in IHD mortality has come from identifying and treating high-risk individuals (those with established risk factors). This approach is unlikely to be affordable or cost-effective in many low- and middle-income countries and the emphasis should be either on preventing the emergence of the 'common soil' of lifestyle risk factors or on reducing their prevalence where they exist. Methods appropriate to the cultural, social and economic contexts within each population will need to be developed and evaluated. Lessons should be learnt from the experience of population-based preventive measures in developed regions.[52,53] Approaches likely to be cost-effective in most contexts include broad-based policy and fiscal measures, particularly supporting tobacco control and the control of certain food products.[54,55]

REFERENCES

1   Murray C & Lopez A (eds). The Global Burden of Disease: A Comprehensive Assessment of Mortality and Disability from Diseases, Injuries, and Risk Factors in 1990 and Projected to 2020. Geneva: World Health Organization, 1996.

2   Howson C, Reddy S, Ryan T & Bale J (eds) Control of Cardiovascular Diseases in Developing Countries. Research, Development and Institutional Strengthening. Washington, DC: National Academy Press, 1998.

3   Omran AR. The epidemiologic transition. A theory of the epidemiology of population change. *Milbank Memorial Fund Quarterly* 1971; 49(4):509–538.

4   Reddy KS & Yusuf S. Emerging epidemic of cardiovascular disease in developing countries. *Circulation* 1998; 97(6):596–601.

5   Nieto FJ. Cardiovascular disease and risk factor epidemiology: a look back at the epidemic of the 20th century. *Am J Publ Health* 1999; 89(3):292–294.

6   Lawlor D, Ebrahim S & Davey Smith G. Sex matters: secular and geographical trends in sex differences in coronary heart disease mortality. *BMJ* 2001; 323:541–545.

7   Marmot M. Coronary heart disease: the rise and fall of a modern epidemic. In Marmot M & Elliott P (eds) *Coronary Heart Disease Epidemiology: From Aetiology to Public Health.* Oxford: Oxford University Press, 1992: 3–19.

8   Capewell S, Morrison CE & McMurray JJ. Contribution of modern cardiovascular treatment and risk factor changes to the decline in coronary heart disease mortality in Scotland between 1975 and 1994. *Heart* 1999; 81(4):380–386.

9   Hunink MGM, Goldman L, Tosteson ANA et al. The recent decline in mortality from coronary heart disease, 1980–1990. The effect of secular trends in risk factors and treatment. *JAMA* 1997; 277:535–542.

10 Vartiainen E, Puska P, Pekkanen J, Tuomilehto J & Jousilahti P. Changes in risk factors explain changes in mortality from ischaemic heart disease in Finland. *BMJ* 1994; 309:23–27.

11 Chenet L, McKee M, Fulop N et al. Changing life expectancy in central Europe: is there a single reason? *J Public Health Med* 1996; 18(3):329–336.

12 Ginter E. Cardiovascular risk factors in the former communist countries. Analysis of 40 European MONICA populations. *Eur J Epidemiol* 1995; 11(2):199–205.

13 Unwin N, Setel P, Rashid S et al. Non-communicable diseases in sub-Saharan Africa: where do they feature in the health research agenda? *Bull World Health Organ* 2001; 79(10):947–953.

14 Aspray TJ, Mugusi F, Rashid S et al. Rural and urban differences in diabetes prevalence in Tanzania: the role of obesity, physical inactivity and urban living. *Trans R Soc Trop Med Hyg* 2000; 94(6):637–644.

15 Wood D, Joint European Societies Task Force. Established and emerging cardiovascular risk factors. *Am Heart J* 2001; 141(2 Supplement):S49–S57.

16 Gensini GF, Comeglio M & Colella A. Classical risk factors and emerging elements in the risk profile for coronary artery disease. *Eur Heart J* 1998;19 (Supplement A):A53–A61.

17 Braunwald E. Shattuck lecture—cardiovascular medicine at the turn of the millennium: triumphs, concerns, and opportunities. *N Engl J Med* 1997; 337(19):1360–1369.

18 Kannel WB & Wilson PW. An update on coronary risk factors. *Med Clin North Am* 1995; 79(5):951–971.

19 Winkelmann BR, Hager J, Kraus WE et al. Genetics of coronary heart disease: current knowledge and research principles. *Am Heart J* 2000; 140(4):S11–S26.

20 Simons LA. Interrelations of lipids and lipoproteins with coronary artery disease mortality in 19 countries. *Am J Cardiol* 1986; 57(14):5–10G.

21 LaRosa JC, He J & Vupputuri S. Effect of statins on risk of coronary disease. a meta-analysis of randomized controlled trials. *JAMA* 1999; 282:2340–2346.

22 Bellosta S, Ferri N, Bernini F, Paoletti R & Corsini A. Non-lipid-related effects of statins. *Ann Med* 2000; 32(3):164–176.

23 Neaton JD & Wentworth D. Serum cholesterol, blood pressure, cigarette smoking, and death from coronary heart disease. Overall findings and differences by age for 316 099 white men. Multiple Risk Factor Intervention Trial Research Group. Arch Intern Med 1992; 152(1):56–64.

24 Collins R, Peto R, MacMahon S et al. Blood pressure, stroke, and coronary heart disease. Part 2: Short-term reductions in blood pressure: overview of randomised drug trials in their epidemiological context. *Lancet* 1990; 335(8693):827–838.

25 Doll R & Peto R. Mortality in relation to smoking: 20 years' observations on male British doctors. *BMJ* 1976; ii(6051):1525–1536.

26 Walters R & Whent H. *Health Update: Smoking.* London: Health Education Authority, 1996.

27 Wilhelmsen L. Coronary heart disease: epidemiology of smoking and intervention studies of smoking. *Am Heart J* 1988; 115(1):242–249.

28 Barrett-Connor EL, Cohn B A, Wingard DL & Edelstein SL. Why is diabetes mellitus a stronger risk factor for fatal ischemic heart disease in women than in men? *JAMA* 1991; 265(5):627–630.

29 Haffner SM, Lehto S, Ronnemaa T, Pyorala K & Laakso M. Mortality from coronary heart disease in subjects with type 2 diabetes and in nondiabetic subjects with and without prior myocardial infarction. *N Engl J Med* 1998; 339:229–234.

30 DECODE Study Group, European Diabetes Epidemiology Group. Glucose tolerance and mortality: comparison of WHO and American Diabetes Association diagnostic criteria. Diabetes epidemiology: collaborative analysis of diagnostic criteria in Europe. *Lancet* 1999; 354(9179):617–621.

31 Abate N. Obesity and cardiovascular disease—pathogenetic role of the metabolic syndrome and therapeutic implications. *J Diabet Complications* 2000; 14(3):154–174.

32 Whaley MH, Kampert JB, Kohl HW III & Blair SN. Physical fitness and clustering of risk factors associated with the metabolic syndrome. *Med Sci Sports Exerc* 1999; 31(2): 287–293.

33 Britton A & McKee M. The relation between alcohol and cardiovascular disease in Eastern Europe: explaining the paradox. *J Epidemiol Community Health* 2000; 54(5):328–332.

34 Menotti A, Lanti M, Puddu PE & Kromhout D. Coronary heart disease incidence in northern and southern European populations: a reanalysis of the seven countries study for a European coronary risk chart. *Heart* 2000; 84(3):238–244.

35 D'Agostino RB, Grundy S, Sullivan LM, Wilson P, CHD Risk Prediction Group. Validation of the Framingham coronary heart disease prediction scores: results of a multiple ethnic groups investigation. *JAMA* 2001; 286(2):180–187.

36 Stamler J, Stamler R, Neaton J et al. Low risk-factor profile and long-term cardiovascular and noncardiovascular mortality and life expectancy: findings for five large cohorts of young adult and middle-aged men and women. *JAMA* 1999; 282(21):2012–2018.

37 Ridker PM. Novel risk factors and markers for coronary disease. *Adv Intern Med* 2000; 45:391–418.

38 Hemingway H & Marmot M. Psychosocial factors in the aetiology and prognosis of coronary heart disease: systematic review of prospective cohort studies. *BMJ* 1999; 318:1460–1467.

39 McKeigue PM, Miller GJ & Marmot MG. Coronary heart disease in south Asians overseas: a review. *J Clin Epidemiol* 1989; 42(7):597–609.

40 Lee J, Heng D, Chia KS, Chew SK, Tan BY & Hughes K. Risk factors and incident coronary heart disease in Chinese, Malay and Asian Indian males: the Singapore Cardiovascular Cohort Study. *Int J Epidemiol* 2001; 30:983–988.

41 McKeigue PM, Shah B & Marmot MG. Relation of central obesity and insulin resistance with high diabetes prevalence and cardiovascular risk in south asians. *Lancet* 1991; 337:382–386.

42 World Health Organization. Classification of Atherosclerotic Lesions: Report of a Study Group. WHO Technical Report Series. Geneva: WHO, 1958.

43 Stary HC, Chandler AB, Glagov S et al. A definition of initial, fatty streak, and intermediate lesions of atherosclerosis. A report from the Committee on Vascular Lesions of the Council on Arteriosclerosis, American Heart Association. *Circulation* 1994; 89(5):2462–2478.

44 Stary HC, Chandler AB, Dinsmore RE et al. A definition of advanced types of atherosclerotic lesions and a histological classification of atherosclerosis. A report from the Committee on Vascular Lesions of the Council on Arteriosclerosis, American Heart Association. *Circulation* 1995; 92(5):1355–1374.

45 Gimbrone MA Jr. Vascular endothelium, hemodynamic forces, and atherogenesis. *Am J Pathol* 1999; 155(1):1–5.

46 Ross R. Atherosclerosis—an inflammatory disease. *N Engl J Med* 1999; 340(2):115–126.

47 Davies MJ. The pathophysiology of acute coronary syndromes. *Heart* 2000; 83(3):361–366.

48 Glagov S, Weisenberg E, Zarins CK, Stankunavicius R & Kolettis GJ. Compensatory enlargement of human atherosclerotic coronary arteries. *N Engl J Med* 1987; 316(22):1371–1375.

49 Murabito JM, Evans JC, Larson MG & Levy D. Prognosis after the onset of coronary heart disease. An investigation of differences in outcome between the sexes according to initial coronary disease presentation. *Circulation* 1993; 88(6):2548–2555.

50 Vokonas PS & Kannel WB. Diabetes mellitus and coronary heart disease in the elderly. *Clin Geriatr Med* 1996; 12(1):69–78.

51 Lenfant C. Can we prevent cardiovascular diseases in low and middle income countries. Bull World Health Organ 2001; 79:980–987.

52 Nissinen A, Berrios X & Puska P. Community-based noncommunicable disease interventions: lessons from developed countries for developing ones. *Bull World Health Organ* 2001; 10:963–970.

53 Ebrahim S & Davey Smith G. Exporting failure? Coronary heart disease and stroke in developing countries. *Int J Epidemiol* 2001; 30:201–205.

54 World Bank. Curbing the Epidemic: Governments and the Economics of Tobacco Control. Washington, DC: International Bank for Reconstruction and Development/World Bank, 1999.

55 Guo X, Popkin BM, Mroz T A & Zhai F. Food price policy can favorably alter macronutrient intake in China. *J Nutr* 1999; 129(5):994–1001.

Section 6

Viral Infections

When the first edition of this text was written in 1898, the discipline *virology* was as yet unborn; the vast range of tropical 'fevers' (after *Plasmodium* spp. had been excluded) remained without a delineated aetiological agent. Since then, viruses—some commonplace and widely distributed, and others rare and with a localized geographical distribution—have been implicated in a high proportion of febrile illnesses in many tropical countries; although not exhaustive, this section covers many of them.

Dengue accounts for much morbidity, but rarely mortality, in tropical countries, whilst its major clinical manifestation *dengue haemorrhagic fever* is the cause of serious illness and mortality in children—especially in South-East Asia. The cosmopolitan Epstein–Barr virus (EBV) causes an acute illness (infectious mononucleosis) the world over, but its role in the causation of Burkitt's lymphoma and nasopharyngeal carcinoma in several tropical locations is rapidly becoming clearer and is the subject of a great deal of current research. Of the more exotic viruses, some of those causally related to the viral haemorrhagic fevers periodically hit the media headlines—for example, Lassa fever and Ebola disease—an outbreak of which in Zaire in 1995 attracted widespread attention. But there can be no doubt that the 'tropical' virus (most likely derived from a sub-human primate arising in Africa) that has really shaken the world (medicine and politics included) is the human immunodeficiency virus (HIV).

Viral hepatitis accounts for a vast amount of morbidity and mortality in tropical countries. Previous editions of Manson's have paid less attention to the pathogens responsible for this group of infections than they clearly warranted; hopefully this deficiency has been rectified in this edition. The role of gastrointestinal viruses, for example, rotavirus, in tropical paediatrics rapidly becomes clearer. Also, the viruses responsible for respiratory tract disease, and those causing measles and other childhood maladies are gaining their rightful place in 'medicine in the tropics'. A short time ago the mere mention of rabies caused alarm and denoted an automatic death sentence. Research into preventive strategies for this disease has progressed at a remarkable pace, and the spectacular advances surrounding this viral infection are summarized in this section.

It is perhaps of interest that the first human infection to have been swept out from the face of the globe—variola (smallpox)—was caused by a virus. As 'tropical medicine' was in its formative years dominated by advances in protozoology and helminthology—with virology a distant 'dream'—this might seem surprising. But it should be recalled that almost two centuries before, Edward Jenner—a Gloucestershire general practitioner—had introduced the appropriate preventive strategy that ultimately dealt a lethal blow (as Jenner envisaged) to this devastating worldwide disease, the last naturally occurring case of which arose in October 1977. Unfortunately, the threat of global biological warfare has brought renewed attention on this potentially lethal infection.

Chapter 40
Viral Hepatitis

J. N. Zuckerman and A. J. Zuckerman

Since the 1970s there has been an explosion in knowledge of viral hepatitis, a major public health problem throughout the world affecting several hundreds of millions of people. Viral hepatitis is a cause of considerable morbidity and mortality in the human population, from both acute infection and chronic sequelae which include, with hepatitis B and hepatitis C infection, chronic active hepatitis, cirrhosis and primary liver cancer.

The hepatitis viruses include a range of unrelated and often unusual human pathogens:

- *Hepatitis A virus (HAV)*: a small unenveloped symmetrical RNA virus, which shares many of the characteristics of the picornavirus family. This virus has been classified in the hepatovirus genus, and is the cause of infectious or epidemic hepatitis transmitted by the faecal–oral route.
- *Hepatitis B virus (HBV)*: a member of the hepadnavirus group double-stranded DNA viruses which replicate by reverse transcription. Hepatitis B virus is endemic in the human population and hyperendemic in many parts of the world.
- *Hepatitis C virus (HCV)*: an enveloped single-stranded RNA virus which appears to be distantly related (possibly in its evolution) to flaviviruses, although hepatitis C is not transmitted by arthropod vectors. Infection with this virus is common in many countries, and it is associated with chronic liver disease and also with primary liver cancer.
- *Hepatitis D virus (HDV)*: an unusual single-stranded circular RNA virus with a number of similarities to certain plant viral satellites and viroids. This virus requires hepadnavirus helper functions for propagation in hepatocytes, and is an important cause of acute and severe chronic liver damage in some regions of the world.
- *Hepatitis E virus (HEV)*: an enterically transmitted non-enveloped, single-stranded RNA virus which shares many biophysical and biochemical features with caliciviruses. Hepatitis E virus is an important cause of large epidemics of acute hepatitis in the subcontinent of India, central and South-East Asia, the Middle East, parts of Africa and elsewhere; this virus is responsible for high mortality during the third trimester of pregnancy.

Hepatitis A

Outbreaks of jaundice have been described for many centuries and the term 'infectious hepatitis' was coined in 1912 to describe the epidemic form of the disease. HAV is spread by the faecal–oral route and is endemic throughout the world and hyperendemic in areas with poor standards of sanitation and hygiene. Common-source outbreaks are initiated most frequently by faecal contamination of food and water. The seroprevalence of antibodies to HAV has declined since the Second World War in many industrialized countries. The exact incidence is difficult to estimate because of the high proportion of subclinical infections and infections without jaundice, differences in surveillance and differing patterns of disease. The extent of under-reporting is very high.

The incubation period of hepatitis A is about 28 days. The virus replicates in the liver. Very large amounts of virus are shed in the faeces during the incubation period, before the onset of clinical symptoms and a brief period of viraemia occurs (Figure 40.1). The severity of illness ranges from asymptomatic to anicteric or icteric hepatitis

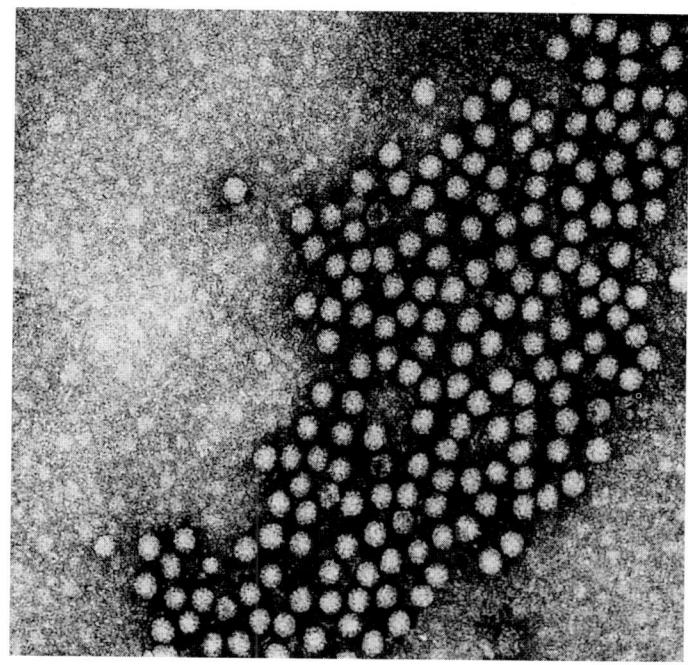

Figure 40.1: Electron micrograph showing the large number of hepatitis A virus particles in faeces during the incubation period of the infection. (Reduced from 120 000 ×. From a series by Anthea Thornton and A. J. Zuckerman.)

and rarely fulminant hepatitis. The virus is non-cytopathic when grown in cell culture. Its pathogenicity in vivo, which involves necrosis of parenchymal cells and histiocytic periportal inflammation, may be mediated via the cellular immune response. By the time of onset of symptoms, excretion of virus in the faeces has declined and may have ceased and anti-HAV IgM, which is diagnostic of acute infection and appears late during the incubation period, increases in titre. Anti-HAV IgG may be detected 1–2 weeks later and persists for years. The virus does not persist and chronic excretion of HAV does not occur. There is no evidence of progression to chronic liver disease.[1]

Classification

Examination by electron microscopy of concentrates of filtered faecal extracts from patients during the incubation period reveals 27 nm unenveloped spherical particles typical of the Picornaviridae. The entire nucleotide sequence of the viral genome has been determined.

Comparison with other picornavirus sequences revealed limited homology to the enteroviruses or, indeed, the rhinoviruses; however, the structure and genome organization are typical of the Picornaviridae. HAV is now considered as a separate genus (*Hepatovirus*) within the Picornaviridae as are the cardioviruses (of mice) and apthoviruses (foot and mouth disease viruses).

Organization of the HAV genome

The HAV genome comprises about 7500 nucleotides (nt) of positive sense RNA which is polyadenylated at the 3′ end and has a polypeptide (VPg) attached to the 5′ end. A single, large open reading frame (ORF) occupies most of the genome and encodes a large polyprotein.

The viral polyprotein is processed to yield the structural (located at the amino terminal end) and non-structural viral polypeptides. Many of the features of replication of the picornaviruses have been deduced from studies of prototype enteroviruses and rhinoviruses, in particular poliovirus type 1. The virus replicates in the cytoplasm of hepatocytes.

Prevention and control of hepatitis A

Passive immunization

Control of hepatitis A infection is difficult. Since faecal shedding of the virus is at its highest during the late incubation period and the prodromal phase of the illness, strict isolation of cases is not a useful control measure. Spread of hepatitis A is reduced by simple hygienic measures and the sanitary disposal of excreta.

Normal human immunoglobulin, containing at least 100 iu/ml of anti-hepatitis A antibody, given intramuscularly before exposure to the virus or early during the incubation period, will prevent or attenuate a clinical illness. The dosage should be at least 2 iu anti-hepatitis A antibody/kg body weight, but in special cases, such as pregnancy or in patients with liver disease, that dosage may be doubled. Immunoglobulin does not always prevent infection and excretion of HAV, and inapparent or subclinical hepatitis may develop. The efficacy of passive immunization is based on the presence of hepatitis A antibody in the immunoglobulin, but the minimum titre of antibody required for protection has not yet been established. Immunoglobulin is used most commonly for close personal contacts of patients with hepatitis A and for those exposed to contaminated food. Immunoglobulin has also been used effectively for controlling outbreaks in institutions such as homes for the mentally handicapped and in nursery schools. Prophylaxis with immunoglobulin is recommended for persons without hepatitis A antibody visiting highly endemic areas. After a period of 6 months the administration of immunoglobulin for travellers should be repeated, unless it has been demonstrated that the recipient has developed his or her own hepatitis A antibodies. Active immunization (see below) is strongly recommended.

Hepatitis A vaccines

In areas of high prevalence most children have antibodies to HAV by the age of 3 years and such infections are generally asymptomatic. Infections acquired later in life are of increasing clinical severity. Less than 10% of cases of acute hepatitis A in children up to the age of 6 years are icteric but this increases to 40–50% in the 6–14 age group and to 70–80% in adults. Of 115 551 cases of hepatitis A in the USA between 1983 and 1987, only 9% of the cases, but more than 70% of the fatalities, were in those aged over 49. It is important, therefore, to protect those at risk because of personal contact with infected individuals or because of travel to highly endemic areas. Other groups at risk of hepatitis A infection include staff and residents of institutions for the mentally handicapped, day care centres for children, sexually active male homosexuals, intravenous narcotic drug abusers, sewage workers, health care workers, military personnel and members of certain low socio-economic groups in defined community settings. Active immunization for travellers is strongly recommended. It is also recommended that food handlers should be immunized. In some developing countries the incidence of clinical hepatitis A is increasing as improvements in socio-economic conditions result in infection later in life and strategies for immunization are yet to be agreed.

Killed hepatitis A vaccines

The foundations for a hepatitis A vaccine were laid in 1975 by the demonstration that formalin-inactivated virus extracted from the liver of experimentally infected marmosets induced protective antibodies in susceptible marmosets on challenge with live virus. Subsequently

HAV was cultivated, after serial passage in marmosets, in a cloned line of fetal rhesus monkey kidney cells (FRhK6), thereby opening the way to the production of hepatitis A vaccines. Later it was demonstrated that prior adaptation in marmosets was not a prerequisite to growth of the virus in cell cultures and various strains of virus have been isolated directly from clinical material using several cell lines, including human diploid fibroblasts, and various techniques have been employed to increase the yield of virus in cell culture. The vaccines are highly immunogenic and provide long-term protection against infection. Combined preparations of killed hepatitis A vaccines with hepatitis B vaccine and other vaccines are available or are under clinical trial.

Live attenuated hepatitis A vaccines

The major advantages of live attenuated vaccines, such as the Sabin type of oral poliomyelitis vaccines, include the ease of administration on a large scale by the oral route, relatively low cost and the fact that, since the virus vaccine strain replicates in the gut, the production of both local immunity in the gut and humoral immunity thereby mimicking natural infection, antibodies tend to persist longer. Disadvantages include the potential of reversion towards virulence, interference with the vaccine strain by other viruses in the gut, relative instability of the vaccine and shedding of the virus strain in the faeces for prolonged periods and the potential of spread to contacts.

The most extensively studied live attenuated hepatitis A vaccines are based on the CR326 and HM175 strains of the virus attenuated by prolonged passage in cell culture.

Two variants of the CR326 strain have been investigated after passage in marmoset liver in FRhK6, MRC5 and WI-38 cells. Inoculation of susceptible marmosets demonstrated seroconversion, and protection on challenge. Biochemical evidence of liver damage did not occur in susceptible chimpanzees, although a number had histological evidence of mild hepatitis with the F variant and the vaccine virus was shed in the faeces for about 12 weeks prior to seroconversion. There was no evidence of reversion towards virulence. Studies in human volunteers indicated incomplete attenuation of the F variant, but better results were obtained with the F[1] variant without elevation of liver enzymes.

Studies with the HM175 strain, which was isolated and passaged in African green monkey kidney cells, showed that this strain was not fully attenuated for marmosets, although it did not induce liver damage on challenge. Further passages and adaptation of HM175 revealed some evidence of virus replication in the liver of chimpanzees and minimal shedding of the virus into faeces. Other studies are in progress in non-human primates.

Markers of attenuation of HAV have not been identified and reversion to virulence may occur. On the other hand, there is also concern that 'over-attenuated' viruses may not be sufficiently immunogenic. Current candidate live attenuated hepatitis A vaccines require administration by injection. Preparations which may be suitable for oral administration are not presently available.

Hepatitis E

Retrospective testing of serum samples from patients involved in various epidemics of hepatitis associated with contamination of water supplies with human faeces led to the conclusion that an agent other than hepatitis A or hepatitis B was involved. Epidemics of enterically transmitted non-A, non-B hepatitis in the Indian subcontinent were the first to be reported, in 1980, but outbreaks involving tens of thousands of cases have also been documented in the former USSR, South-East Asia, northern Africa and Mexico. The average incubation period is longer than that for hepatitis A, with a mean of 6 weeks. The highest attack rates are found in young adults, and high mortality rates (up to 20%) have been reported in women in the third trimester of pregnancy.

Virus-like particles measuring 28–34 nm in diameter have been detected in faecal extracts of infected individuals by immune electron microscopy using convalescent serum. However, such studies have often proved inconclusive because a large proportion of the excreted virus may be degraded during passage through the gut. Cross-reaction studies between sera and virus in faeces associated with a variety of epidemics and other viral isolates in several different countries indicate that there are at least four major genotypes and phylogenetic and sequence analyses define at least nine different groups.

Studies on HEV have progressed following transmission to susceptible non-human primates. HEV was first transmitted to cynomolgus macaques, and a number of other species of monkey, including chimpanzees, have also been infected. There are reports of transmission to pigs and rodents, and virus has been isolated from domestic farm animals, particularly swine. Reports on replication of the virus in cell culture have thus far not been confirmed.

The problem of degradation of HEV in the gut was circumvented when the bile of infected monkeys was found to be a rich source of virus. This material permitted the molecular cloning of DNA complementary to the HEV (RNA) genome and the entire 7.5 kb sequence was determined. The organization of the genome is distinct from the Picornaviridae and the non-structural and structural polypeptides are encoded respectively at the 5' and 3' ends. HEV resembles the caliciviruses in the size and organization of its genome as well as in the size and morphology of the virion.

Laboratory tests

Sequencing of the HEV genome has resulted in the development of a number of specific diagnostic tests. For example, HEV RNA was detected, using the polymerase chain reaction (PCR), in faecal samples. An enzyme-linked immunosorbent assay (ELISA), which detects both IgG and IgM anti-HEV, has been developed using a recombinant HEV–glutathione-S-transferase fusion protein and used to detect antibodies in sporadic cases of infection in children and adults and during a number of epidemics. Epidemics are usually associated with warm weather and poor sanitation leading to faecal contamination of drinking water. Sporadic cases occur where HEV is endemic and also in Western countries in individuals without a history of travel to endemic countries.[2]

Hepatitis B

HBV was originally recognized as the cause of 'serum hepatitis', the most common form of parenterally transmitted viral hepatitis, and an important cause of acute and chronic infection of the liver. The incubation period of hepatitis B is variable, with a range of between 1 and 6 months. The clinical features of acute infection resemble those of the other viral hepatitides. Frequently, acute hepatitis B is anicteric and asymptomatic, although a severe illness with jaundice can occur and acute liver failure may develop. The virus persists in about 10% of infected immunocompetent adults and in as many as 90% of infants infected perinatally, depending on the ethnic group of the mother. About 350 million people worldwide are persistent carriers of hepatitis B. Liver damage is mediated by the responses of the cellular immune response of the host to the infected hepatocytes. Approximately 25% of all patients with chronic hepatitis will progress to cirrhosis and about 20% of those with cirrhosis will develop hepatocellular carcinoma. Hepatocellular carcinoma is one of the most common cancers worldwide.[3]

During the first phase of chronicity, virus replication continues in the liver and replicative intermediates of the viral genome may be detected in DNA extracted from liver biopsies. Markers of virus replication in serum include HBV DNA, the pre-S1 proteins (see below) and a soluble antigen, hepatitis B e antigen (HBeAg), which is secreted by productively infected hepatocytes. In those infected at a very young age this phase may persist for life but, more usually, virus levels decline over time. Eventually in most individuals there is immune clearance of infected hepatocytes associated with seroconversion from HBeAg to anti-HBe. During the period of replication the viral genome may integrate into the chromosomal DNA of some hepatocytes and these cells may persist and expand clonally. Rarely, seroconversion to anti-HBs follows clearance of virus replication but, more frequently, the surface antigen (HBsAg) persists during a second phase of chronicity as a result of the expression of integrated viral DNA.

Structure of the virus

The hepatitis B virion is a 42 nm particle comprising an electron-dense nucleocapsid or core, 27 nm in diameter,

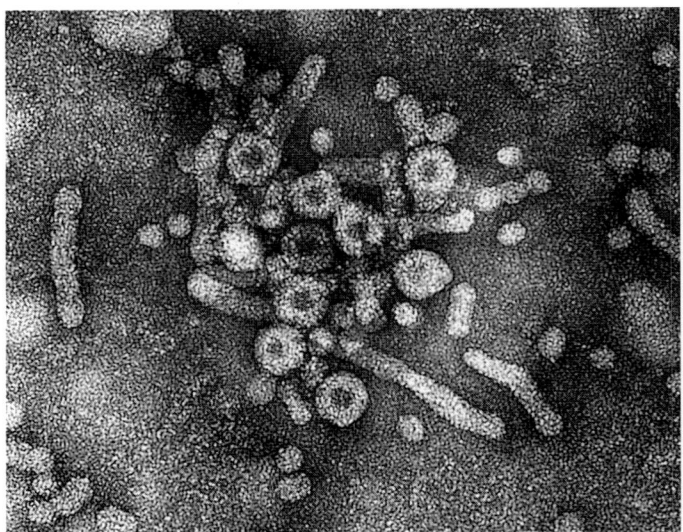

Figure 40.2: Hepatitis B virus. (Reduced from 250 000 ×. From a series by A. J. Zuckerman et al.)

surrounded by an outer envelope of the surface protein (HBsAg) embedded in membranous lipoprotein derived from the host cell (Figure 40.2). The surface antigen is produced in excess by the infected hepatocytes and is secreted in the form of 22 nm particles (initially referred to as Australia antigen) and tubular structures with the same diameter.

The 22 nm particles are composed of the major surface protein in both non-glycosylated (p24) and glycosylated (gp27) form in approximately equimolar amounts, together with a minority component of the so-called middle proteins (gp33 and gp36) which contain the pre-S2 domain, a glycosylated 55 amino acid N-terminal extension. The surface of the virion has a similar composition but also contains the large surface proteins (p39 and gp42) which include both the pre-S1 and pre-S2 regions. These large surface proteins are not found in the 22 nm spherical particles (but may be present in the tubular forms in highly viraemic individuals) and their detection in serum correlates with viraemia. The domain which binds to the specific HBV receptor on the hepatocyte resides within the pre-S1 region.

The nucleocapsid of the virion consists of the viral genome surrounded by the core antigen (HBcAg). The carboxy terminus of the core protein is arginine rich and this highly basic domain is believed to interact with the genome. The genome, which is approximately 3.2 kb in length, has an unusual structure and is composed of two linear strands of DNA held in a circular configuration by base pairing at the 5' end. One of the strands is incomplete and the 3' end is associated with a DNA polymerase molecule which is able to complete that strand when supplied with deoxynucleoside triphosphates. In the past, this endogenous DNA polymerase reaction was used as a serological assay for the hepatitis B virion but this has now been superseded by DNA–DNA hybridization and PCR. The 5' ends of both strands of the genome are modified. The 5′ end of the complete strand is covalently linked to a protein and the 5′ end of the incomplete strand is an oligoribonucleotide. In both cases these moieties seem to be primers for the synthesis of the respective strands during the genome replication. A motif of 12 base pairs is directly repeated in the genome near to the 5′ ends of the two strands (DR1 and DR2, respectively) and these sequences play an important role in replication.

Organization of the HBV genome

To date, the genomes of more than a dozen isolates of HBV have been cloned and the complete nucleotide sequences determined. Analysis of the coding potential of the genome reveals four ORFs which are conserved between all of these isolates (Figure 40.3), but there is some variation of sequence of up to 12% of nucleotides. These have the same polarity as the incomplete strand of genomic DNA, which therefore has been designated the plus strand.

The first ORF encodes the various forms of the surface protein and contains three in-frame methionine codons which are used for initiation of translation. Both the middle (gp33 and gp36) and major (p24 and gp27) proteins are translated from a family of 2.1 kb mRNAs transcribed from a promoter located in the pre-S1 region and polyadenylated in response to a signal sequence located just downstream from the start of the core ORF.

A second promoter is located upstream of the pre-S1 initiation codon. This directs the synthesis of a 2.4 kb mRNA which is co-terminal with the other surface messages and is translated to yield the large (pre-S1) surface proteins. This promoter seems to be weak (or may be down-regulated) so that the message is of low abundance and relatively little of the large surface proteins is synthesized. Unlike the middle and major surface proteins, the large surface region is not secreted from the cell. In fact its synthesis inhibits the secretion of the smaller proteins and may be a signal for virus assembly.

The core ORF also has two in-phase initiation codons. The 'precore' region is highly conserved, has the properties of a signal sequence and is responsible for the secretion of HBeAg.

The third ORF, which is the largest and overlaps the other three, encodes the viral polymerase. The fourth ORF was designated 'x', identified recently as a transcriptional transactivator, and may be an 'early' gene product which functions to up-regulate the viral promoters.

Replication of the HBV genome

Following infection of a hepatocyte the single-stranded region of the virion DNA is repaired by the endogenous polymerase and the genome appears on a covalently closed, circular form in the nucleus. This DNA is the template for the transcription of all of the viral RNAs. Synthesis of minus strand DNA is primed by a protein,

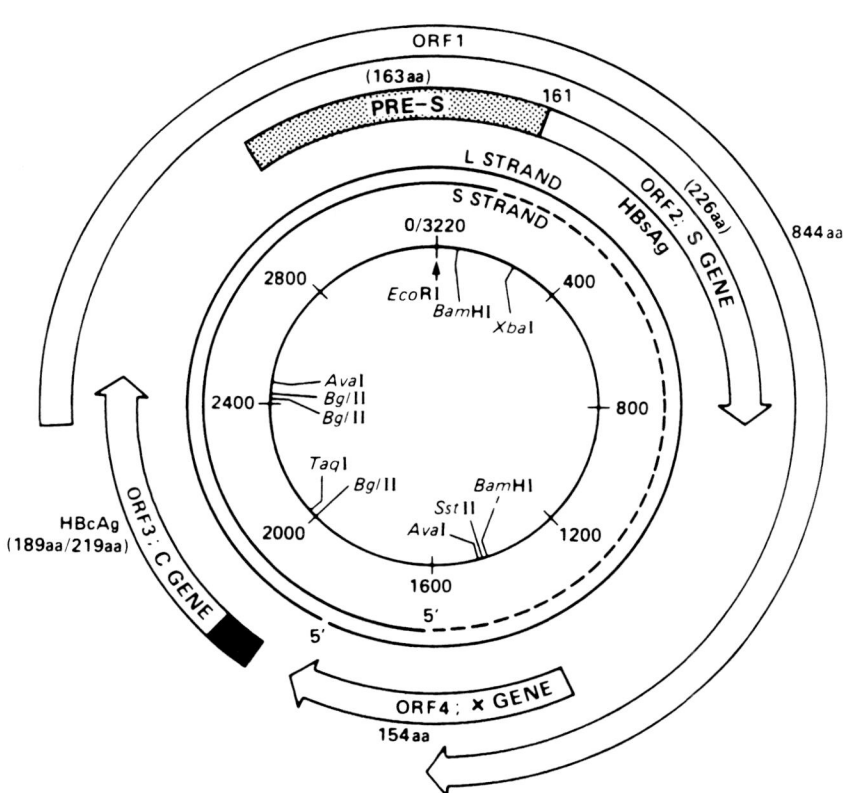

Figure 40.3: Organization of the genome of hepatitis B virus.

now believed to be the amino terminal domain of the polymerase, and proceeds with the concomitant degradation of the RNA template by the RNAase H activity. There is no semi-conservative replication of the covalently closed circular DNA in the nucleus and a pool of up to 30 copies of template DNA initially is built up by transfer of some of the progeny DNA from the cytoplasm to the nucleus. The mode of replication of the viral genome resembles those of the phylogenetically related retroviruses and, more closely, a family of plant viruses (the caulimoviruses).

Mode of spread of hepatitis B virus

Specific laboratory tests for hepatitis B confirmed the importance of the parenteral routes of transmission and blood-to-blood contact, and infectivity appears to be especially related to blood. However, the infection is not spread exclusively by blood and blood products. There are observations that under certain experimental circumstances the virus is infective by mouth and the infection may be endemic in closed and semi-closed institutions and in institutions for the mentally handicapped. It is more prevalent in adults in urban communities and among those living in poor socio-economic conditions. Considerable differences in prevalence of the infection and of the carrier state exist in different geographical regions and between different ethnic and socio-economic groups.

There is much evidence for the transmission of hepatitis B by intimate contact and by the sexual route. The sexually promiscuous, particularly active male homosexuals who change partners frequently, are at very high risk of infection with HBV. Hepatitis B surface antigen has been found in blood and in various body fluids such as saliva, menstrual and vaginal discharges, seminal fluid, colostrum and breast milk and serous exudates, and these have been implicated as vehicles of transmission of infection. Contact-associated hepatitis is thus of major importance. Transmission of infection may result from accidental inoculation of minute amounts of blood or body fluids contaminated with blood, such as may occur during medical, surgical and dental procedures, immunization with inadequately sterilized syringes and needles, intravenous and percutaneous drug abuse; tattooing, ear-piercing and nose-piercing, and acupuncture with non-sterile equipment; laboratory accidents and accidental inoculation with razors, shared toothbrushes, bath brushes, towels and similar objects which have been contaminated with blood. Additional factors may be important for the transmission of hepatitis B infection in the tropics and in warm-climate countries. These include traditional tattooing and scarification, blood-letting, ritual circumcision and repeated biting by blood-sucking arthropod vectors. Results of investigations into the role which biting insects may play in the spread of hepatitis B are conflicting. Hepatitis B surface antigen has been detected in several species of mosquito and in bedbugs

which have either been trapped in the wild or fed experimentally on infected blood, but no convincing evidence for replication of HBV in insects has been obtained, and there is no epidemiological evidence of mechanical transmission of the infection by insects.

The presence of hepatitis B surface antigen has been reported in faeces, bile and urine, usually as a result of contamination with blood. Hepatitis B is not transmitted by the faecal–oral route and urine is not infectious unless contaminated with blood. There is no evidence that airborne infections occur. Clustering of hepatitis B also occurs within family groups, but it is not related to genetic factors and does not reflect maternal or venereal transmission. The mechanisms of intrafamilial spread of hepatitis B infection remain to be established.

Mother-to-infant transmission

Transmission of hepatitis B from carrier mothers to their babies can occur during the perinatal period and appears to be the single most important factor in determining the prevalence of the infection in some regions, particularly in China and South-East Asia. The risk of infection in the infant may reach 90% and appears to be related to ethnic groups. Infection of infants is especially important because a large proportion of these infants will become carriers. Infectivity is directly related to the presence of high titres of hepatitis B surface antigen and/or hepatitis B e antigen in the mother's circulation. When e antigen is present, as many as 95% of their newborn children are infected, usually in the perinatal period. The prevalence of e antigen among surface antigen maternal carriers, and thus the infectivity of mothers for their infants, varies markedly in different geographical areas and in different ethnic groups.

In some parts of Asia, particularly in South-East Asia, 30–50% of surface antigen carrier women of childbearing age also carry e antigen in their blood, and perinatal infections may account for about half the carriers in the population. Perinatal transmission is of intermediate frequency in mothers of west Asian or Afro-Caribbean origin. In contrast, the carrier state and perinatal transmission are uncommon in Caucasian mothers. The pattern of mother-to-infant transmission and establishment of the carrier state is different in Africa, where e antigen is less frequent in carrier mothers and infection of infants occurs most commonly during the first 5 years of life as a result of horizontal transmission. Another mode of transmission of hepatitis B is infection of children of non-carrier mothers by contact with children who had been infected by their carrier mothers.

There is a substantial risk of perinatal infection if the mother has acute hepatitis B, particularly during the third trimester of pregnancy or within 2 months after delivery. Intrauterine infections are uncommon, since the virus does not cross the intact placenta and the few infections which occur in utero are probably the result of a leakage of maternal blood into the fetal circulation associated with a tear in the placenta.

Finally, the precise mechanism of perinatal infection is uncertain but it probably occurs during or shortly after birth as a result of a leak of maternal blood into the baby's circulation or its ingestion or inadvertent inoculation. Most of the children infected during the perinatal period become persistent carriers.

The carrier state

The carrier state is defined on the basis of longitudinal studies as persistence of the hepatitis B surface antigen in the circulation for more than 6 months. The carrier state may be life-long and may be associated with liver damage varying from minor changes in the nuclei of hepatocytes to persistent hepatitis, chronic active hepatitis, cirrhosis and hepatocellular carcinoma. In carriers of hepatitis B virus with or without histological evidence of liver disease, integration of the viral DNA may be at many sites or at a unique site in the host genome. Most of these carriers have circulating surface antigen with or without other viral markers such as e antigen or e antibody, DNA polymerase and HBV DNA, and it has been suggested that the continued expression of the surface antigen in patients may result from integrated viral DNA. Some carriers, however, may have hepatitis B viral DNA in their liver without expression of the surface antigen (latent viral infection).

Several risk factors have been identified in relation to the development of the carrier state. It is commoner in males, more likely to follow infections acquired in childhood, as described above, than those acquired in adult life and more likely to occur in patients with natural or acquired immune deficiencies. A carrier state becomes established in approximately 5–10% of infected adults.

The prevalence of carriers among apparently healthy adults, particularly among blood donors, who have been studied most intensively, varies geographically. The world can be divided broadly into three zones according to the prevalence of infection with HBV:

- Hyperendemic regions where the infection is almost universal includes many countries in South-East Asia (including China), the Western Pacific and sub-Saharan Africa. Carrier rates in these populations vary from more than 5% to 20%. In most of these countries infection in early life is very common.
- Intermediate endemic regions in which the overall prevalence of infection as judged by serological markers of HBV such as HBsAg, anti-HBs and anti-HBc range from 20% to 50% and carriers of HBsAg from 1% to 5% of the general population. These include countries of north Africa, the Middle East, parts of southern and eastern Europe and South America.
- Low-prevalence areas include northern Europe, most western European countries, the United States, Canada, Australia and New Zealand. In these countries less than 10% of the population have serological evidence of infection with HBV and a carrier rate of 0.1% or less. However, even in these countries the prevalence of

infection and carriers may vary considerably within different groups of the population including the distribution of ethnic groups.

Age distribution and the prevalence of infection

Two different patterns of age distribution of infection are recognized. In populations with a high prevalence of hepatitis B virus, infection is usually acquired early in the life, and the highest infection and carrier rates are seen amongst children and young adults, with lower prevalence among older age groups. The e antigen has been found more commonly in young than in adult carriers, while the prevalence of e antibody is higher in older age groups. These findings suggest that young carriers could be the most infective.

In countries in which infection with hepatitis B virus is relatively uncommon, the highest prevalence of hepatitis B surface antigen is found in the 20–40 age group. The highest rates of infection are found among groups who have an increased risk of contact with blood or blood products, as outlined above, including health care personnel, certain categories of patients, intravenous drug abusers and male homosexuals who change partners frequently.

It should be noted that the prevalence of HBV infection and the age distribution of infection and the carrier rate are changing, and in some countries changing dramatically, with the implementation of a strategy of universal immunization against hepatitis B.

Prevention and control of hepatitis B

Hepatitis B virus has been classified into six genotypes designated A–F based on phylogenetic analysis of complete viral genomes. Genotypes A and D are disseminated widely throughout the Old World, while genotypes B and C are confined to the East Asian populations, and genotype E to sub-Saharan Africa. Genotype F is more divergent from the other genotypes and is found in aboriginal American populations. All six genotypes share a common immunodominant region on the surface antigen, termed the *a* determinant, which spans amino acids 124–147. The *a* determinant is hydrophilic and is believed to be in a form of two major and one minor loops with cysteine disulphide bonds. Neutralizing antibodies induced by immunization are targeted principally to the conformational epitopes of the *a* determinant, and evidence is reviewed below that amino acid substitutions within this region of the surface antigen can allow replication of HBV in vaccinated persons since antibodies induced by current vaccine do not recognize critical changes in the surface antigen domain.

The major response to immunization with the current hepatitis B vaccines is to the common *a* epitope with consequent protection against all subtypes of the virus.

Passive immunization

Hepatitis B immunoglobulin (HBIG) is prepared from pooled plasma with high titre of hepatitis B surface antibody (anti-HBs) and may confer temporary passive immunity under certain defined conditions. The major indication for the administration of HBIG is a single acute exposure to HBV, such as occurs when blood containing surface antigen is inoculated, ingested or splashed on to mucous membranes and conjunctivae. The optimal dose has not been established but doses in the range of 250–500 iu have been used effectively. It should be administered as early as possible after exposure and preferably within 48 hours, usually 3 ml (containing 200 iu of anti-HBs per ml) in adults. It should not be administered 7 days following exposure. It is generally recommended that two doses of HBIG should be given 30 days apart.

Results with the use of HBIG for prophylaxis in babies at risk of infection with HBV are encouraging if the immunoglobulin is given as soon as possible after birth or within 12 hours of birth, and the chance of the baby developing the persistent carrier state is reduced by about 70%. More recent studies using combined passive and active immunization indicate an efficacy approaching 90%. The dose of HBIG recommended in the newborn is 1–2 ml (200 iu of anti-HBs per ml).

Active immunization

Immunization against hepatitis B is required for groups which are at an increased risk of acquiring this infection. These groups include individuals requiring repeated transfusions of blood or blood products, prolonged inpatient treatment, patients who require frequent tissue penetration or need repeated access to the circulation, patients with natural or acquired immune deficiency and patients with malignant diseases. Viral hepatitis is an occupational hazard among health care personnel and the staff of institutions for the mentally handicapped and in some semi-closed institutions. High rates of infection with hepatitis B occur in narcotic drug addicts and drug abusers, male homosexuals who change partners frequently and prostitutes. Individuals working in high endemic areas are also at increased risk of infection. Women in areas of the world where the carrier state in that group is high are another segment of the population requiring immunization in view of the increased risk of transmission of the infections to their offspring. Young infants, children and susceptible persons living in certain tropical and subtropical areas where present socio-economic conditions are poor and the prevalence of hepatitis B is high should also be immunized.

The failure to grow HBV in tissue culture has directed attention to the use of other preparations for active immunization. Since immunization with HBsAg leads to the production of protective surface antibody, purified 22 mm spherical surface antigen particles have been developed as vaccines. These vaccines have been prepared from the plasma of symptomless carriers. Trials on protective efficacy in high-risk groups have demonstrated the value of the vaccines and their safety. There is no risk of transmission of the acquired immune deficiency syndrome (AIDS) or any other infection by vaccines derived from plasma which meet the World Health Organization requirements of 1981, 1983 and 1987. Local reactions reported after immunization have been minor, occurring in less than 20% of immunized individuals, and consist of slight swelling and reddening at the site of inoculation. Temperature elevations of up to 38°C were observed in only a few individuals.

Site of injection for vaccination

Hepatitis B vaccination should be given intramuscularly in the upper arm or the anterolateral aspect of the thigh and *not* in the buttock. There are over 100 reports of unexpectedly low antibody seroconversion rates after hepatitis B vaccination using injection into the buttock. In one centre in the USA a low antibody response was noted in 54% of healthy adult health care personnel. Many studies have since shown that the antibody response rate was significantly higher in centres using deltoid injection than centres using the buttock. On the basis of antibody tests after vaccination, the Advisory Committee on Immunization Practices of the Centers for Disease Control, USA, recommended that the arm be used as the site for hepatitis B vaccination in adults, as have the Departments of Health in the UK.

A comprehensive study in the USA by Shaw et al.[4] showed that participants who received the vaccine in the deltoid had antibody titres that were up to 17 times higher than those of subjects who received the injections into the buttock. Furthermore, those who were injected in the buttock were two to four times more likely to fail to reach a minimum antibody level of 10 miu/ml after vaccination. (Recent reports have also implicated buttock injection as a possible factor in a failure of rabies postexposure prophylaxis using a human diploid cell rabies vaccine.)

The injection of vaccine into deep fat in the buttocks is likely with needles shorter than 5 cm, and there is a lack of phagocytic or antigen presenting cells in layers of fat. Another factor may involve the rapidity with which antigen becomes available to the circulation from deposition in fat, leading to delay in processing by macrophages and eventually presentation to T and B cells. An additional factor may be denaturation by enzymes of antigen which has remained in fat for hours or days. The importance of these factors is supported by a finding at the Royal Free Hospital, London, and elsewhere that thicker skin fold was associated with a lowered antibody response.

These observations have important public health implications, well illustrated by the estimate that about 20% of subjects immunized against hepatitis B via the buttock in the USA by March 1985 (about 60 000 people) failed to attain a minimum level of antibody of 10 miu/ml and were therefore not protected.

Hepatitis B surface antibody titres should be measured in all individuals who have been immunized against hepatitis B by injection into the buttocks, and when this is not possible a complete course of three injections of vaccine should be administered into the deltoid muscle or the anterolateral aspect of the thigh—the only acceptable sites for hepatitis B immunization.

Intradermal immunization

The high cost of hepatitis B vaccines is a serious economic obstacle to extensive immunization against hepatitis B, which is needed in many countries in Africa and Asia. The possibility of reducing the amount of antigen required for immunization by reducing the dose of vaccine or by using the intradermal route has been explored. Presentation of antigen to the immune system intradermally results in a macrophage-dependent T lymphocyte response via specific epidermal cells, and the intradermal route has been used for immunization against tuberculosis, diphtheria, typhoid, cholera, influenza, rabies and other infections. A second reason for attempting to use hepatitis B vaccine intradermally is to accelerate the immune response in persons who suddenly experience a high risk of infection—for example, after accidental exposure to hepatitis B or infants born to carrier mothers.

A review of reports on the intradermal administration of hepatitis B vaccines raises several important and unresolved issues:

1. The immunogenicity of the plasma-derived vaccine given intradermally in doses of 0.1 ml (2.0 μg of antigen protein) has been clearly demonstrated. However, although the antibody titres after two intradermal or intramuscular doses given 1 month apart were similar, the booster injection at 6 months resulted in anti-HBs levels which were 10 times higher after intramuscular than intradermal inoculation.
2. Multi-site intradermal inoculation of a single reduced dose of rabies vaccine resulted in rapid seroconversion and antibody levels similar to those obtained with the extended intramuscular immunization route. However, after multi-site intradermal inoculation of a single reduced dose of hepatitis B vaccine, seroconversion was slower than that with intramuscular injection, and the antibody titres after the booster injection were also lower after intradermal than after intramuscular injections.
3. Intradermal inoculation requires skill, and subcutaneous injection into fat will result in a poor immune response.
4. Although adverse reactions after intradermal injection were not marked, local reactions at the site of administration of the vaccine (which contains aluminium hydroxide as adjuvant) frequently included the development of an erythematous macule 5–10 mm in diameter after 24–48 hours; the lesion would subside after days or weeks, leaving a small pigmented macule, occasionally overlying a small palpable nodule.
5. The use of jet injectors for inoculation of hepatitis B vaccine has been considered. Current advice is that until further studies clarify the risk of transmission of infection (such as hepatitis B and the human immuno-deficiency virus) by different types of jet injectors their use should be restricted to special situations where large numbers of persons need to be immunized within a short time. The use of jet injectors in the UK has been generally discouraged (although this does not apply to the use of jet injectors by individuals for self-administration of insulin or low-dose heparin).

Trials of intradermal hepatitis B vaccines in Gambian children illustrate many of the problems reviewed above. In the first trial 1 μg of a plasma-derived vaccine was given to neonates intradermally in the same syringe with BCG followed by two further doses of 1 μg of intradermal HBV vaccine. The trial was considered a failure because 19 of 32 neonates (59.4%) had a low response of less than 10 miu/ml of anti-HBs compared with two of the 33 neonates who received the vaccine intramuscularly ($p <$ 0.01). In the second trial in young children, two different regimens were used: two doses of 2 μg of the vaccine were given intradermally after a 20 μg intramuscular dose or three doses of 2 μg were given intradermally. In both cases the geometric mean antibody responses were significantly lower than in the control group who were given 20 μg intramuscularly followed by two 10 μg doses intramuscularly. Vaccine failures, defined as the presence of surface antigen or core antibody or the absence of surface antibody, were also significantly higher in the intradermal groups. In the third trial, 4 μg of vaccine were given intradermally with a multiple-orifice puncture gun to 20 young children and all had a good surface antibody response. It was pointed out, however, that this was a large dose, 40% of the recommended intramuscular dose, and might have been just as successful if it had been given intramuscularly. It was concluded that in an endemic area people soon become infected with hepatitis B virus and that at present the conventional intramuscular regimens using relatively large doses of vaccine are to be preferred, despite their considerable costs.[5] The overriding consideration is efficacy of protection. In most of the studies reported to date, those who received hepatitis B vaccine intradermally were young healthy subjects, in whom the antibody response is known to be good, and the vaccine was given by experienced staff under ideal conditions. There are no data on the longer-term duration of anti-HBs, on the subclass(es) of the antibody induced, or on antibody specificity and affinity. Furthermore, protective efficacy studies of intradermal immunization against hepatitis B have not been reported so far.

International and national requirements for vaccine manufacture and licence require assurance on safety, immunogenicity and protective efficacy of the recommended dosage and schedule of administration. It seems imprudent to ignore these requirements and recommendations. Careful evaluation and review of the intradermal route (and indeed of low-dose schedules) are essential, especially in countries where circumstances are not ideal either for storage or for accurate intradermal administration of a vaccine.

Immunization strategies and the kinetics of antibody production

Immunization strategies

Immunization against hepatitis B is now recognized as a high priority in all countries, and strategies for immunization are being revised. Universal vaccination of infants and adolescents is recommended, and more than 110 countries now offer hepatitis B vaccine to all children, including the USA, Canada and most western European countries (but not the UK).

There are three main approaches to developing new hepatitis B immunization strategies:

1. The introduction of universal antenatal screening to identify hepatitis B carrier mothers and vaccination of their babies. It is important that any other strategies do not interfere with the delivery of vaccine to this group. Immunization of this group will have the greatest impact in reducing the number of new hepatitis B carriers. For children outside this group it is difficult to estimate the lifetime risk of acquiring a hepatitis infection.
2. Vaccinate all infants.
3. Vaccinate all adolescents. This approach delivers vaccination at a time close to the time when 'risk behaviour' would expose adolescents to infection. Vaccination could be delivered as part of a wider package on health education in general, to include sex education, the risk of AIDS, the dangers of drug abuse and smoking, and the benefits of a healthy diet and lifestyle.

The problems with this approach are as follows:

- Persuading parents to accept vaccination of the children against a sexually transmitted disease, a problem they may not wish to address at that time.
- Ensuring that a full course of three doses is given.
- Evaluating and monitoring vaccine coverage. The systems for monitoring uptake of vaccine in this age group may not operate efficiently.

The advantages of vaccinating infants are as follows:

- It is now known that effective hepatitis B vaccination can be delivered to babies.
- Parents will accept vaccination against hepatitis B along with other childhood vaccinations, without reference to sexual behaviour.

The disadvantages are:

- It is not known whether immunity will last until exposure in later life (but see below). This may become less of a problem as more people are vaccinated and the chance of exposure to infection thereby reduced.
- The introduction of another childhood vaccination may reduce the uptake of existing childhood vaccinations. The problem would be avoided if hepatitis B could be delivered in a combined vaccine containing DPT (diphtheria, polio, tetanus), and such preparations have been developed.

Vaccination of infants is preferable to vaccination of adolescents, as there are sufficient mechanisms to ensure, monitor and evaluate cover. A booster dose could be given in early adolescence, combined with a health education package. A rolling programme could be introduced, giving priority to urban areas.

It should also be stressed that in 31% of acute hepatitis B in the USA the mode of infection is not known (Centers for Disease Control, Atlanta, Georgia, 1992–1993) and this is therefore a powerful argument for universal immunization against hepatitis B.

Finally, travellers constitute an important group which is often overlooked. Susceptible adults and younger persons who have not been immunized are at risk of hepatitis B when travelling, particularly to areas where socio-economic conditions are poor and the prevalence of hepatitis B is high, should be immunized. A combined vaccine with hepatitis A is recommended.

The kinetics of anti-HBs response

The titre of vaccine-induced anti-HBs declines, often rapidly, during the months and years following immunization. The highest anti-HBs titres are generally observed 1 month after booster vaccination followed by rapid decline during the next 12 months and thereafter more slowly. Mathematical models have been designed and an equation was derived consisting of several exponential terms with different half-life periods. It is considered by some researchers that the decline of anti-HBs concentration in the serum of an immunized subject can be predicted accurately by such antibody kinetics and recommendations made on booster vaccination (reviewed by Zuckerman[6] and the European Consensus Group[7]). If the minimum protective level of anti-HBs is accepted at 10 iu/litre, which is being debated, consideration should be given to the diversity of the individual immune response and the decrease in levels of anti-HBs as well as to possible errors in quantitative anti-HBs determinations. It would then be reasonable to define a level of >10 iu/l and <100 iu/l as an indication for booster immunization, particularly in certain risk groups (but see below). It has been demonstrated that a booster inoculation results in a rapid increase in anti-HBs titres within 4 days. However, even this time delay might permit infection of hepatocytes.

Several options should therefore be considered for maintaining protective immunity against hepatitis B infection:

1. Relying upon immunological memory to protect against clinical infection and its complications—a view which is supported by in vitro studies showing immunological memory for HBsAg in B cells derived from vaccinated subjects who have lost their anti-HBs but not in B cells from non-responders and by clinical data.
2. Providing booster vaccination to all vaccinated subjects at regular intervals without determination of anti-HBs. This option is not supported by a number of investigators because non-responders must be detected.

In addition, while an anti-HBs titre of about 10 iu/l may in theory be protective, this level is not protective from a laboratory point of view since many serum samples may give non-specific reactions at this antibody level.

3. Testing anti-HBs levels after the first booster and administering the next booster before the minimum protective level is reached. A protective level of 100 iu/l seems to be appropriate.

The European Consensus Group,[7] however, concluded that long-term protection against clinically significant breakthrough hepatitis B infection and persistent carriage of the virus depends on immunological memory, which lasts for at least 15 years in the immunocompetent, allowing for a rapid and protective anamnestic antibody response, and therefore there is no need to administer booster doses of hepatitis B vaccine after the primary course of immunization had been completed. Groups at risk of hepatitis B infection need to be considered separately and several countries have a policy of administering booster doses. Boosters are required for immunocompromised patients, particularly when the antibody titre falls below 10 iu/l, and boosters may be used to provide reassurance of protective immunity, for example in health care workers undertaking invasive procedures. The group also concluded that long-term follow-up studies should continue to monitor groups of immunized individuals to determine if breakthrough infections occur or whether a carrier state develops.

Production of hepatitis B vaccines by recombinant DNA techniques

Recombinant DNA techniques have been used for expressing HBsAg and HBcAg in prokaryotic cells (*Escherichia coli* and *Bacillus subtilis*) and in eukaryotic cells, such as mutant mouse LM cells, HeLa cells, COS cells, CHO cells and yeast cells (*Saccharomyces cerevisiae*).

Recombinant yeast hepatitis B vaccines have undergone extensive evaluation in clinical trials. The results have indicated that this vaccine is safe, antigenic and free from side effects (apart from minor local reactions in a proportion of recipients). The immunogenicity is similar, in general terms, to that of the plasma-derived vaccine. Recombinant yeast hepatitis B vaccines are now being used in many countries. A vaccine based on HBsAg expressed in mammalian (CHO) cells is in use in the Peoples' Republic of China.

Mutations of hepatitis B surface antigen

The emergence of variants of hepatitis B virus, possibly due to selection pressure associated with extensive immunization in an endemic area, was suggested by the findings of hepatitis B infection in individuals immunized successfully.[8] These studies were extended subsequently by the finding of non-complexed HBsAg and anti-HBs

and other markers of hepatitis B infection in 32 of 44 vaccinated subjects, and sequence analysis from one of these cases (AS) revealed a mutation in the nucleotide encoding the *a* determinant, the consequence of which was a substitution from glycine to arginine at amino acid position 145 (G145R).[9]

Various mutations and variants of HBsAg have since been reported from many countries including Italy, the UK, Holland, Germany, the USA, Brazil, Singapore, Taiwan, China, Japan, Thailand, India, west and South Africa and elsewhere. However, the most frequent and stable mutation was reported in the G145R variant. A large study in Singapore of 345 infants born to carrier mothers with HBsAg and HBeAg who received hepatitis B immunoglobulin at birth and plasma-derived hepatitis B vaccine within 24 hours of birth and then 1 month and 2 months later revealed 41 breakthrough infections with HBV despite the presence of anti-HBs. There was no evidence of infection among 670 immunized children born to carrier mothers with HBsAg and anti-HBe, nor in any of 107 immunized infants born to mothers without HBsAg.[10] The most frequent variant was a virus with the G145R mutation in the *a* determinant. Another study in the USA of serum samples collected between 1981 and 1993 showed that 94 (8.6%) of 1092 infants born to carrier mothers became HBsAg positive despite postexposure prophylaxis with hepatitis B immunoglobulin and hepatitis B vaccine. Following amplification of HBV DNA, 22 children were found with mutations of the surface antigen, most being in amino acids 142–145; five had a mixture of wild-type HBV and variants, and 17 had only the 145 variant.[11]

The recent report from Taiwan[12] of the increase in immunized children in the prevalence of mutants of the *a* determinant of HBV over a period of 10 years, from 8 of 103 (7.8%) in 1984 to 10 of 51 (19.6%) in 1989, and 9 of 32 (28.1%) in 1994, is of particular concern. The prevalence of HBsAg mutants among those fully immunized was higher than among those not vaccinated (12/33 vs. 15/153, *p* = 0.0003). In all 27 children with detectable mutants, the mean age of those vaccinated was lower than of those not vaccinated, and mutation occurred in a region with greatest hydrophilicity of the surface antigen (amino acids 140–149) and more frequently among those vaccinated than among those not vaccinated. More mutations to the neutralizing epitopes were found in the 1994 survey in Taiwan.

Another important aspect of the identification of surface antigen variants is the evidence that HBsAg mutants may not be detected by all of the blood donor screening tests and by existing diagnostic reagents. Such variants may therefore enter the blood supply or spread by other means. This is emphasized by the finding in Singapore, between 1990 and 1992, of 0.8% of carriers of HBV variants in a random population survey of 2001 people. These findings add to the concern expressed in a study of mathematical models of HBV vaccination, which predict, on the assumption of no cross-immunity against the variant by current vaccines, that the variant will not become dominant over the wild-type virus for at least 50 years—but the G145R mutant may emerge as the common HBV in 100 or more years time.[13]

It is important therefore to institute epidemiological monitoring of HBV surface mutants employing test reagents which have been validated for detection of the predominant mutations; and consideration should be given to incorporating into current hepatitis B vaccines of antigenic components which will confer protection against infection by the predominant mutant(s).

HBV precore mutants

When DNA–DNA hybridization replaced the less sensitive assay of the endogenous DNA polymerase activity as a method for detecting hepatitis B virions in serum, it became clear that some patients with anti-HBe were seropositive for virus. These and other early reports suggested that this finding was more common in Greece and other Mediterranean regions than elsewhere, raising the possibility of the involvement of a variant form(s) of HBV.

Vaudin et al.[14] reported the nucleotide sequence of the genome of a strain of HBV cloned from the serum of a naturally infected chimpanzee. A surprising feature was a point mutation in the penultimate codon of the precore region which changed the tryptophan codon (TGG) to an amber termination codon (TAG). The nucleotide sequence of the HBV precore region from a number of anti-HBe-positive Greek patients was investigated by direct sequencing PCR-amplified HBV DNA from serum.[15] An identical mutation of the penultimate codon of the precore region to a termination codon was found in seven of eight anti-HBe-positive patients who were positive for HBV DNA in serum by hybridization. In most cases there was an additional mutation in the preceding codon. Similar variants were found in an Italian study by amplification of HBV DNA from serum from a further seven anti-HBe-positive patients, one of whom seemed to be coinfected with wild-type virus. These variants are not confined to the Mediterranean region; the same nonsense mutation (without a second mutation in the adjacent codon) has been observed in patients from Japan and elsewhere, as well as rarer examples of defective precore regions caused by frameshifts or loss of the initiation codon for the precore region.

Patients without HBeAg with high levels of HBV replication from various geographical areas may be infected frequently by viruses with variant precore regions. Presumably these can replicate without secretion of HBeAg. The majority of patients who are infected with these variants are anti-HBe positive, implying past infection with non-defective HBV. It is not clear whether these patients were infected originally with a mixture of wild-type and mutant viruses or whether the variants arose throughout the course of natural infection. The process of seroconversion from HBeAg to anti-HBe seems to select the variant viruses and this may be related to the expression of HBeAg on the surface of hepatocytes infected by the wild-type virus.

In many cases precore variants have been described in patients with severe chronic liver disease and who may have failed to respond to therapy with interferon. This observation raises the question of whether they are more pathogenic than the wild-type virus. For example, a nosocomial outbreak of fatal fulminant hepatitis B in Israel was associated with transmission of mutant HBV from a common source to five individuals; and in a study of British patients with fulminant hepatitis B, precore mutants were found in eight of nine HBeAg-negative patients but in none of six who were HBeAg positive on presentation.

HBV and hepatocellular carcinoma

Regions of the world where persistent carriage of HBV is common have been found to coincide with a high prevalence of primary liver cancer. Furthermore, in these areas patients with the tumour are almost invariably seropositive for HBsAg. In a prospective study in Taiwan, 184 cases of hepatocellular carcinoma occurred in 3454 carriers of HBsAg at the start of the study, but only 10 such tumours occurred in 19 253 control males who were HBsAg negative.[16]

Southern hybridization of tumour DNA yields evidence of chromosomal integration of viral sequences in at least 80% of hepatocellular carcinomas from HBsAg carriers. There is no similarity in the pattern of integration between different tumours, and variation is seen both in the integration site(s) and in the number of copies or partial copies of the viral genome. Sequence analysis of the integrants reveals that the direct repeats in the viral genome often lie close to the virus–cell junctions, suggesting that sequences around the ends of the viral genome may be involved in recombination with host DNA. Integration seems to involve microdeletion of host sequences, and rearrangements and deletions of part of the viral genome may also occur. When an intact surface gene is present, the tumour cells may produce and secrete HBsAg in the form of 22 nm particles. Production of HBcAg by tumours is rare, however, and the core ORF is often incomplete and modifications such as methylation may also modulate its expression.

Cytotoxic T cell targeted against core gene products on the hepatocyte surface seems to be the major mechanism of clearance of infected cells from the liver, and cells with integrated viral DNA which are capable of expressing these proteins may also be lysed. Thus there may be immune selection of cells with integrated viral DNA which are incapable of expressing HBcAg.

The mechanism(s) of oncogenesis by HBV remains obscure. HBV may act non-specifically by stimulating active regeneration and cirrhosis, which may be associated with long-term chronicity. However, HBV-associated tumours occur occasionally in the absence of cirrhosis and it is difficult to explain the frequent finding of integrated viral DNA in tumours. In rare instances the viral genome has been found to be integrated into cellular genes such as cyclin A and a retinoic acid receptor. Translocations and other chromosomal rearrangements also have been observed. Although insertional mutagenesis of HBV remains an attractive explanation for oncogenicity, supportive evidence is lacking. In contrast to these findings in human hepatocellular carcinoma, liver cancer in woodchucks associated with persistent infection with the woodchuck hepatitis virus frequently involves integration of the viral genome in or near to cellular *myc* genes.

An alternative possibility is that tumour formation is associated with a viral gene product. The product of the x gene is known to be a transactivator of transcription and so may cause inappropriate upregulation of cellular genes. Truncated forms of HBsAg, which may be produced from incomplete surface ORFs integrated in tumour cells, can also have transactivating activity, perhaps through interaction with receptors in the cell membrane. Like many other cancers, the development of hepatocellular carcinoma is likely to be a multifactorial process. The clonal expansion of cells with integrated viral DNA seems to be an early stage in this process and such clones may accumulate in the liver throughout the period of active viral replication. In areas where the prevalence of primary liver cancer is high, virus infection usually occurs at an early age and virus replication may be prolonged, although the peak incidence of tumour is many years after the initial infection.

Hepatitis D

Delta hepatitis was first recognized following the detection of a novel protein, delta antigen (HDAg), by immunofluorescent staining in the nuclei of hepatocytes from patients with chronic active hepatitis B. Hepatitis delta virus (HDV) requires a helper function of HBV for its replication. HDV is coated with HBsAg, which is needed for release from the host hepatocyte and for entry in the next round of infection.

Two forms of delta hepatitis infection are known. In the first, a susceptible individual is coinfected with HBV and HDV, often leading to a more severe form of acute hepatitis caused by HBV. Vaccination against HBV also prevents coinfection. In the second, an individual chronically infected with HBV becomes superinfected with HDV. This may accelerate the course of the chronic liver disease and cause overt disease in asymptomatic HBsAg carriers. HDV itself appears to be cytopathic and HDAg may be directly cytotoxic.

Delta hepatitis is common in some areas of the world with a high prevalence of hepatitis B infection, particularly the Mediterranean region, parts of eastern Europe, the Middle East, Africa and South America. It has been estimated that 5% of HBsAg carriers worldwide (approximately 15 million people) are infected with HDV. In areas of low prevalence for hepatitis B, those at risk of hepatitis B infection—particularly intravenous drug abusers—are also at risk of HDV infection.[17]

Structure and replication of HDV

The HDV particle is approximately 36 nm in diameter and is composed of an RNA genome associated with HDAg, surrounded by an envelope of HBsAg. The virus reaches higher concentrations in the circulation than HBV—up to 10^{12} particles per millilitre have been recorded. The HDV genome is a closed circular RNA molecule of 1679 nucleotides with extensive sequence complementarily that permits pairing of approximately 70% of the bases to form an unbranched rod structure. The genome thus resembles those of the satellite viroids and virusoids of plants, and similarly seems to be replicated by the host RNA polymerase II with autocatalytic cleavage and circularization of the progeny genomes via *trans*-esterification reactions (ribozyme activity). Consensus sequences of viroids which are believed to be involved in these processes are also conserved in the delta virus.

Unlike the plant viroids, however, HDV codes for a protein, HDAg. This antigen, which contains a nuclear localization signal, was originally detected in the nuclei of infected hepatocytes and may be detected in serum only after removing the outer envelope of the virus with detergent.

Prevention and control of HDV are similar to those for hepatitis B. Immunization against hepatitis B protects against HDV. The problem is protection against HDV superinfection of established carriers of hepatitis B. Specific HDV immunization based on HDV antigens is under development.

Hepatitis C

Before the identification of hepatitis C virus (HCV), transmission studies in chimpanzees established that the main agent of parenterally acquired non-A, non-B hepatitis was likely to be an enveloped virus some 30–60 nm in diameter. The studies by Bradley et al.[18] provided a pool of plasma that contained a relatively high titre of the agent. In order to clone the genome, the virus was pelleted from the plasma. Because it was not known whether the genome was DNA or RNA, a denaturation step was included prior to the synthesis of cDNA so that either DNA or RNA could serve as a template. The resultant cDNA was then inserted into the bacteriophage expression vector λ gt11 and the libraries screened using serum from a patient with chronic non-A, non-B hepatitis.[19] This approach led to the detection of a clone (designated 5-1-1) which was found to bind to antibodies present in the sera of several patients with non-A, non-B hepatitis. This clone was used as a probe to detect a larger, overlapping clone in the same library. It was possible to demonstrate that these sequences hybridized to a positive-sense RNA molecule of around 10 000 nt which was present in the livers of infected chimpanzees but not in uninfected controls. By employing a 'walking' technique it was possible to use newly detected overlapping clones as hybridization probes in turn to detect further virus-specific clones in the library. Thus clones covering the entire viral genome were assembled and the complete nucleotide sequence determined. The organization of the genome closely resembles those of the pestiviruses and flaviviruses.

Detection of HCV infection

Since the 5-1-1 antigen was originally detected by antibodies in the serum of an infected patient it was an obvious antigen for the basis of an ELISA to detect anti-HCV antibodies. A larger clone, C100, was assembled from a number of overlapping clones and expressed in yeast as a fusion protein using human superoxide dismutase sequences to facilitate expression. This fusion protein formed the basis of first-generation tests for HCV infection. The 5-1-1 antigen comprises amino acid sequences from the non-structural, NS4, region of the genome and C100 contains both NS3 and NS4 sequences. It is now known that antibodies to C100 are detected relatively late following an acute infection. Furthermore, the first generation ELISAs were associated with a high rate of false positivity when applied to low-incidence populations and there were further problems with some retrospective studies on stored sera. Data based on this test alone should, therefore, be interpreted with caution.

Second and subsequent generation tests include antigens from the nucleocapsid and further non-structural regions of the genome. The former (C22) is particularly useful, and antibodies to the HCV core protein seem to appear relatively early in infection. These second-generation tests confirmed that HCV is the major cause of parenterally transmitted non-A, non-B hepatitis. Routine testing of blood donations is now in place in many countries and prevalence rates vary from 0.2–0.5% in northern Europe to 1.2–1.5% in southern Europe and Japan. Most of those with antibody have a history of parenteral risk, such as a history of transfusion or administration of blood products or of intravenous drug abuse. There is little evidence for sexual or perinatal transmission of HCV and the natural routes of transmission have yet to be identified.

The availability of the nucleotide sequence of HCV made the use of PCR possible as a direct test for the genome of the virus itself. The first step is the synthesis of a cDNA copy of the target region of the RNA genome using reverse transcriptase (primed by the antigenomic PCR primer or, better, by random hexamers) and the product of this reaction is then a suitable target for amplification. The concentration of virus in serum samples is often very low, so that the mass of product(s) from the PCR reaction is insufficient for visualization on a stained gel. Thus either a second round of amplification (with nested primers) or detection of the primary product by southern hybridization is required. There is considerable variation in nucleotide sequences among different isolates

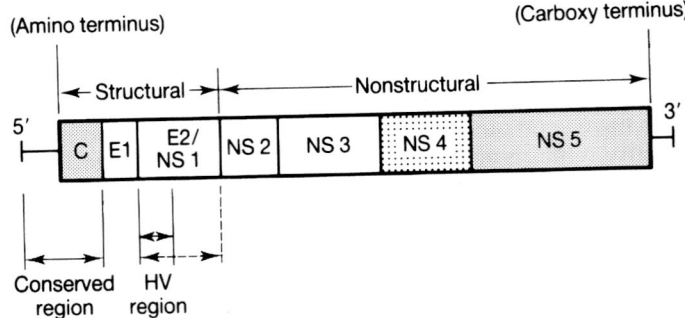

Figure 40.4: Hepatitis C viral genome. HV, hypervariable.

of HCV, and the 5' non-coding region, which seems to be highly conserved, is the preferred target for the PCR.

Organization of the HCV genome

The genome of HCV (Figure 40.4) resembles those of the pestiviruses and flaviviruses in that it comprises around 10 000 nt of positive-sense RNA, lacks a 3' poly A tract and has a similar gene organization. It has been proposed that HCV should be the prototype of a third genus in the family Flaviviridae. All of these genomes contain a single large ORF which is translated to yield a polyprotein from which the viral proteins are derived by post-translational cleavage and other modifications.

There is a short, untranslated region at the 5' end of the genomic RNA and a further untranslated region at the 3' end, the large ORF accounting for over 95% of the sequence. The structural proteins are located forwards at the 5' end and the non-structural proteins towards the 3' end. The first product of the polyprotein is the non-glycosylated capsid protein, C, which complexes with the genomic RNA to form the nucleocapsid. As with the flaviviruses, a hydrophobic domain may anchor the growing polypeptide in the endoplasmic reticulum and facilitate cleavage by a cellular signalase, releasing the nucleocapsid precursor (anchored C). The amino acid sequence of the nucleocapsid protein seems to be highly conserved among different isolates of HCV.

The next domain in the polyprotein also has a signal sequence at its carboxy terminus and may be processed in a similar fashion. The product is a glycoprotein which is probably found in the viral envelope and is referred to as E1/S or gp35. The third domain may be cleaved by a protease within the viral polyprotein to yield what is probably a second surface glycoprotein, E2/NS1 or gp70. These proteins are of considerable interest because of their potential use in tests for the direct detection of viral proteins and for HCV vaccines. Nucleotide sequencing studies reveal that both domains contain hypervariable regions. It is possible that this divergence has been driven by antibody pressure and that these regions specify important immunogenic epitopes.

The non-structural region of the HCV genome is divided into regions NS2–NS5. In the flaviviruses, NS3 has two functional domains: a protease which is involved in cleavage of the non-structural region of the polyprotein and a helicase which is presumably involved in RNA replication. Motifs within this region of the HCV genome have homology to the appropriate consensus sequences, suggesting similar functions. NS5 seems to be the replicase and contains the gly-asp-asp motif common to viral RNA-dependent RNA polymerases.

Epidemiology and clinical features

Infection with HCV occurs throughout the world. Many of the seroprevalence data are based on blood donors, who represent a selected population. The prevalence of antibodies to HCV in blood donors varies from 0.02% to 1.25% in different countries. Higher rates have been found in southern Italy, Spain, central Europe, Japan and parts of the Middle East, with as many as 19% in Egyptian blood donors. Until screening of blood donors was introduced, hepatitis C accounted for the vast majority of non-A, non-B post-transfusion hepatitis. However, it is clear that, while blood transfusion and the transfusion of blood products are efficient routes of transmission of HCV, these account for a small proportion of cases of acute clinical hepatitis in a number of countries (with the exception of patients with haemophilia). Current data indicate that in 30% or more of patients in industrialized countries the source of infection cannot be identified; although transmission by contact with blood and contaminated materials is likely to be important, 35% of patients have a history of intravenous drug misuse; household contact and sexual exposure do not appear to be major factors in the epidemiology of this common infection (6–8%); and occupational exposure in the health care setting accounts for about 2% of cases. Transmission of HCV from mother to infant occurs in about 10% of viraemic mothers and the risk appears to be related to the level of viraemia. It should be noted, however, that information on the natural history of hepatitis C is limited because the onset of the infection is often unrecognized and the early course of the disease is indolent and protracted in most patients.

Most acute infections are asymptomatic: less than 30% of patients with acute infections have non-specific symptoms and some develop mild jaundice. Fulminant hepatitis has been described. Extrahepatic manifestations include mixed cryoglobulinaemia, membranous proliferative glomerulonephritis and porphyria cutanea tarda.

Between 50% and 80% of patients do not clear the virus by 6 months and develop chronic hepatitis. The majority have fluctuating abnormal alanine transaminase levels, but some 30% have normal levels. Histological examination of liver biopsies from asymptomatic HCV carriers (blood donors) reveals that none has normal histology and that up to 70% have chronic active hepatitis and/or cirrhosis. The rate of progression of chronic hepatitis is highly variable. The presence of antibodies to specific antigen components is variable and may or may not reflect viraemia, and in the case of interferon treatment there is a correlation between response and loss of specific antibodies to the E2 component.

Detection and monitoring of viraemia are important for management and treatment and sensitive techniques are available for the measurement of HCV RNA. The identification of specific types and subtypes is important, with observations suggesting an association between response to interferon and particular genotypes.

Chronic hepatitis C infection leads to cirrhosis within two decades of the onset of infection in at least 20% of patients. Chronic infection is also associated with an increased risk of hepatocellular carcinoma, which occurs on a background of inflammation and regeneration related to chronic hepatitis over three or more decades. The risk of developing hepatocellular carcinoma (HCC) is estimated at 1–5% after 20 years, but this varies considerably in different areas of the world. It develops more commonly in men than in women.[20]

A vaccine against HCV is not available.

There is evidence that alcohol and hepatitis C may aggravate synergistically hepatic damage. Alcohol restriction is essential and abstinence from alcohol is strongly recommended.

Antiviral therapy for HCV infection is described below.

Management of acute viral hepatitis

There is no specific treatment. General measures include bed-rest and a generally nutritious diet. Patients should be encouraged to exercise regularly if they feel well. Consumption of alcohol should be avoided during the acute phase and continue to be modest after convalescence.

Corticosteroids and non-steroidal anti-inflammatory drugs are *not* indicated and should not be used.

Treatment of chronic hepatitis B infection

Specific treatment is now available following the demonstration that interferon α inhibits replication of HBV, and that prolonged treatment can lead to remission of the disease.

Antiviral therapy is aimed at patients with active disease and viral replication, preferably at a stage before signs and symptoms of cirrhosis or significant injury have occurred. Eradication of the disease is possible in only a minority of patients. Permanent loss of HBV DNA and HBeAg results in an improvement in necro-inflammatory change(s), and reduced infectivity. It is possible that the accompanying histological improvement reduces the risk of cirrhosis and hepatocellular carcinoma.

Unfortunately, treatment of chronic hepatitis with interferon is effective in less than half of those treated. It is relatively expensive, requires administration by injection and is not free of side effects. Nonetheless, recombinant interferon α has been licensed for treatment of chronic hepatitis B in the UK and several European countries.

The interferons act by interaction with specific membrane receptors, thereby inducing a number of enzymes and proteins, the best characterized of which are the 2',5'-oligoadenylate synthetases (2',5'- A synthetases) and protein kinases. The expression of the class I major histo-compatibility antigen (MHC) genes is activated by all interferons, and those of class II by interferon γ, to increase the expression of MHC at the cell surface, and thereby amplify viral antigen recognition and display. Interferons also modify the cellular and humoral immune response.

Three preparations of interferon α are currently available, two of which are recombinant preparations and one of which is prepared from a lymphoblastoid cell line. Approximately 40% of patients respond. Highest response rates are usually seen in carriers with higher baseline serum aminotransferase levels, lower levels of HBV DNA and without AIDS. Although these factors provide some predictive information, none of these criteria is absolute, and individual carriers, for example ethnic Chinese, with active disease or those patients with anti-HIV antibodies but normal CD4 lymphocyte counts may respond, making the prediction of treatment outcome somewhat difficult. The appropriate dose of interferon is not yet established, but 5–10 mu three times weekly for 3–4 months is currently prescribed.

The subclinical exacerbation of the hepatitis frequently seen in responders suggests that interferon acts by augmenting the immune response to HBV, perhaps triggered by the inhibition of viral replication as well as the effects of interferon on cytotoxic T cells. Although residual HBV DNA can be detected by PCR, the disease appears to be ameliorated. Approximately 20% of patients who respond to treatment with clearance of HBeAg will also clear HBsAg within a year of treatment, and up to 65% may later clear HBsAg after 6 years of follow-up.

Pulsed corticosteroid treatment and interferon may also be of benefit in patients without elevated serum aminotransferases. This treatment regimen should be used with caution in those patients with decompensated hepatitis B because of the risk of inducing severe hepatic necrosis.

The major early side effects of interferon include an influenza-like illness. Later side effects include malaise, muscle aches, headaches, poor appetite, weight loss, increased need for sleep, irritability, anxiety and depression, hair loss, thrombocytopenia and leucopenia. Unusual or severe side effects include seizures, acute psychosis, bacterial infections, autoimmune reactions, thyroid disease, proteinuria, cardiomyopathy, skin rashes and interferon antibodies.

Other antiviral drugs

A number of other agents have been used for the treatment of hepatitis B. These include interferon γ, acyclovir (acycloguanosine), 6-deoxyacyclovir, ganciclovir, foscarnet (trisodium phosphonoformate), azido-3'-deoxythymidine triphosphate, 2',3'-dideoxycytidine and 2',3'-dideoxyinosine, adenine arabinoside 5'-monophosphate (ara-AMP), phyllanthrus amarus, interleukin 2, isoprinosine, thymosin, tumour necrosis factor, transfer factor, adenine arabinoside 5'-monophosphate conjugated with lactosaminated albumin, interferon γ plus α, interferon γ plus β, and acyclovir plus interferon. Few of these agents are useful clinically.

Lamivudine, a second-generation nucleoside analogue, inhibits both HBV DNA-dependent and RNA-dependent DNA polymerase activity. This may cause suppression of HBV DNA replication at four sites, and also has the indirect effect of restoring T cell hyporesponsiveness. The decline in viral titre is rapid and dose related, and maximum inhibition is observed with treatment with 100 mg by mouth once daily. While production of virus is inhibited rapidly, production of viral protein which is dependent on the presence of the RNA pregenome is unaffected by lamivudine. Reduction of viral protein concentrations depends on the destruction of infected liver cells, and with immune control of HBV replication viral protein production also declines.

Approximately 20% of patients clear HBeAg and HBV DNA within 1 year of starting treatment with lamivudine. Long-term therapy may be required, and extended therapy is feasible as, in contrast to interferon α, lamivudine can be taken orally and is associated with a lower incidence of adverse events. Extended therapy with lamivudine has also been found to produce significant improvements in liver histology and increasing levels of seroconversion. In one cohort about 40% of patients seroconverted after 3 years. Seroconversion rates are likely to be enhanced if patients with alanine aminotransferase (ALT) elevations are selected (i.e., ALT levels > 2× the upper limit of normal).

As with all antiviral agents, prolonged treatment with lamivudine is associated with a risk of HBV variants (mutants). The key variant with lamivudine therapy involves the highly conserved tyr-met-asp-asp (YMDD) motif, which forms part of the active site of the polymerase. Although experimental studies have shown that such YMDD variants confer resistance of lamivudine in vitro, they also have reduced replication competence both in vitro and in the clinical setting. As such their emergence is not a signal to stop treatment with lamivudine. In patients with HBeAg, 14% of patients developed the variant. While this was associated in one study with elevation of HBV DNA and ALT, these had not reached baseline levels by week 52, and the variant was not associated with any reduction in the histological response. The YMDD variants also emerged in anti-HBe patients, and while 40% of such patients have lost HBV DNA by 52 weeks, about 25% have the variant. In either case, the emergence of the variants is not a signal to stop treatment with lamivudine. Indeed, HBeAg seroconversion can still occur in patients with the YMDD variant.[21,22]

Nevertheless, in considering treatment options in the future for those who develop YMDD variants, other antiviral agents that do not share cross-resistance with lamivudine may be added. In vitro data suggest that lamivudine-resistant and famciclovir-resistant variants remain sensitive for example to adefovir, but combination therapy is yet to be evaluated clinically.

The introduction of lamivudine has made transplantation feasible in patients with decompensated liver disease with HBV DNA. It may also be of benefit in suppression of replication in non-decompensated patients prior to transplantation, and in post-transplant patients. The combination of lamivudine and hepatitis B immunoglobulin is an effective prophylaxis against recurrent hepatitis B after transplantation, leading to improved graft and patient survival. Lamivudine is effective for the treatment of recurrent HBV infection after transplantation.

Other antiviral agents are also under evaluation including BMS 200, 475, ganciclovir, famciclovir and adefovir dipivoxil. Combination therapy will probably be required in the longer term.

The development of specific antiviral therapies offers a new opportunity to treat chronic carriers of hepatitis B virus, and while there is a need to define more precisely the indications for treatment, the costs of treatment and the logistics of screening for asymptomatic hepatitis B infection and assessment of active replicative HBV infection are substantial and constitute a major challenge particularly in countries where HBV is hyperendemic.[23]

Several newer nucleoside analogues suppress hepatitis B in vitro, and these drugs are at present undergoing clinical trial in humans.

Treatment of chronic hepatitis C infections

Interferon α treatment is indicated for patients with well-documented chronic hepatitis C in whom other causes of chronic hepatitis have been excluded, and who have at least a twofold elevation of serum alanine aminotransferase. Interferon α ameliorates disease activity in approximately 50% of patients with hepatitis C after short courses (6 months) of treatment. Liver biopsy histology provides useful information regarding the extent of liver damage. Treatment should be started at a dose of 3×10^6 units, three times weekly, and administered subcutaneously for 6 months. Treatment can be discontinued after 3 months if no response has occurred. However, approximately 50% of responders relapse when treatment is stopped. Almost all of these relapses tend to re-respond to retreatment.

Ribavirin, a nucleoside analogue which is taken orally, has also been shown to inhibit HCV. This drug may be a better choice for patients with cirrhosis, who respond poorly to interferon, or it can be used in combination with interferon. The major side effect of ribavirin is haemolysis, and the drug is still under study.

REFERENCES

1   Koff R S. Hepatitis A. *Lancet* 1998; 351:1643–1649.
2   Tam A W, Bradley D W, Krawczynski K et al. Hepatitis E virus. In Zuckerman A J & Howard H C (eds) *Viral Hepatitis* 2nd edn. Edinburgh: Churchill Livingstone, 1998: 395–416.
3   Zuckerman A J (ed.). *Hepatitis B in the Asian-Pacific Region*, vols 1–3. London: Royal College of Physicians, 1997, 1998, 1999.
4   Shaw F E Jr, Guess I J A, Roets J M et al. Effect of anatomic site, age and smoking on the immune response to hepatitis B vaccination. *Vaccine* 1989; 7:425–430.
5   Whittle H C, Lamb W H & Ryder R W. Trials of intradermal hepatitis B vaccines in Gambian children. *Ann Trop Paediatr* 1987; 7:6–9.
6   Zuckerman J N. Nonresponse to hepatitis B vaccines and the kinetics of anti-HBs production. *J Med Virol* 1996; 50:283–288.
7   European Consensus Group on Hepatitis B Immunity. Are booster immunisations needed for lifelong hepatitis B immunity? *Lancet* 2000; 355:561–565.
8   Zanetti A R, Tanzi E, Manzillo G et al. Hepatitis B variant in Europe. *Lancet* 1988; 2:1132–1133.
9   Carman W F, Zanetti A R, Karayiannis P et al. Vaccine-induced escape mutant of hepatitis B virus. *Lancet* 1990; 336:325–329.
10 Oon C-J, Lim G-K, Zhao Y et al. Molecular epidemiology of hepatitis B virus vaccine variants in Singapore. *Vaccine* 1995; 13:699–702.
11 Nainan O V, Stevens C E, Taylor P E et al. Hepatitis B virus (HBV) antibody resistant mutants among mothers and infants with chronic HBV infection. In Rizzetto M, Purcell R H, Gerin J L & Verme G (eds) *Viral Hepatitis and Liver Disease*. Torino: Minerva Medica, 1997: 132–134.
12 Hsu H Y, Chang M H, Liaw S H et al. Changes of hepatitis B surface antigen variants in carrier children before and after universal vaccination in Taiwan. *Hepatology* 1999; 30:1312–1317.
13 Wilson J N, Nokes D J & Carman W F. The predicted pattern of emergence of vaccine-resistant hepatitis B: a cause for concern? *Vaccine* 1999; 17:973–978.
14 Vaudin M, Wolstenholme A J, Tsiquaye K N et al. The complete nucleotide sequence of the genome of a hepatitis B virus isolated from a naturally infected chimpanzee. *J Gen Virol* 1988; 69:1383–1389.
15 Carman W F, Jacyna M R, Hadziyannis S et al. Mutation preventing formation of hepatitis B e antigen in patients with chronic hepatitis B infection. *Lancet* 1989; 2:588–591.
16 Beasley R P & Hwang L-Y. Overview of the epidemiology of hepatocellular carcinoma. In Hollinger F B, Lemon S M & Margolis H S (eds) *Viral Hepatitis and Liver Disease*. Baltimore: Williams & Wilkins, 1991: 532–535.
17 Verme G, Bonino F & Rizzetto M (eds). *Viral Hepatitis and Delta Infection*. New York: Alan R Liss, 1983: 1–421.
18 Bradley D W, McCaustland K A, Cook E H et al. Post-transfusion non-A, non-B hepatitis in chimpanzees: physicochemical evidence that the tubule-forming agent is a small, enveloped virus. *Gastroenterology* 1985; 88:773–779.
19 Choo Q L, Kuo G, Weiner A J et al. Isolation of a cDNA clone derived from a blood-borne non-A, non-B viral hepatitis genome. *Science* 1989; 244:359–362.
20 Report of a WHO Consultation. Global surveillance and control of hepatitis C. *J Viral Hepatitis* 1999; 6:35–47.
21 Lai C L & Yuen M F. Profound suppression of hepatitis B virus replication with lamivudine. *J Med Virol* 2000; 61:367–373.
22 Schiff E R. Lamivudine for hepatitis B in clinical practice. *J Med Virol* 2000; 61:386–391.
23 Zuckerman A J & Lavancy D. Treatment options for chronic hepatitis: antivirals look promising. *Br Med J* 1999; 319:799–800.

Chapter 41
Arbovirus Infections

A. K. Broom, D. W. Smith, R. A. Hall, C. A. Johansen and J. S. Mackenzie

Arboviruses (arthropod-borne viruses) are a diverse group of viruses that survive in nature by transmission from infected to susceptible hosts by certain species of mosquitoes, ticks, sand flies or biting midges.[1,2] These viruses multiply within the tissues of the arthropod to produce a high-titre viraemia (extrinsic incubation period) and are then passed on to humans or other vertebrates by the bites of the insect. Most diseases caused by arboviruses are zoonoses, that is they are primarily infections of vertebrates other than humans; however, a number of these viruses can cause incidental infections in humans. Two major exceptions to this are o'nyong-nyong and dengue viruses, whose only known vertebrate host is the human. However, for dengue virus, monkeys have been implicated as an alternative vertebrate host to man in rural settings. Some viruses are classed as arboviruses even though they have not been associated with an arthropod vector.

The names by which these viruses are known are of mixed origin. Some are dialect names for the illnesses they cause (chikungunya, o'nyong-nyong), some are place names (West Nile, Bwamba) and some derive from clinical characteristics (Western equine encephalitis, yellow fever).[1,2]

In this chapter we will concentrate on the medically important arboviruses. For more detailed information about the viruses and the diseases they cause, a number of major reviews of specific viruses are cited at the beginning of each section.

Aetiology

There are over 500 arboviruses recognized worldwide[2] but only some are implicated in human disease. Some infect humans only occasionally or caused only mild illness, whereas others are of great medical importance and can cause large epidemics with considerable mortality (Table 41.1).

In this chapter viruses are classified according to the seventh report of the International Committee on Taxonomy of Viruses.[3] Arboviruses belong to three major families: Togaviridae, Flaviviridae and Bunyaviridae. The alphaviruses and flaviviruses are enveloped, single-stranded, positive-sense RNA viruses. They are spherical particles, measuring from 40 to 70 nm.[4,5] The bunyaviruses are enveloped, negative-strand RNA viruses. They are generally spherical and measure 80–120 nm in diameter.

The flaviviruses are the most important group medically and three infections cuased by viruses in this group, yellow fever, dengue and Japanese encephalitis, are sufficiently prevalent to be of global concern.[6] Others, including tick-borne encephalitis, VEE, SLE and West Nile fever, are usually restricted to specific regions. However, the spread of these viruses to several regions may cause international health problems.[1] This has occurred recently with West Nile virus moving from Africa into North America, RVF moving from Africa to the Middle East, and Japanese encephalitis moving into the Australasian region. The major reasons for virus movement will be discussed later in the chapter.

Epidemiology

For effective arbovirus transmission to occur, three components are necessary: the vector (mosquito, tick, sandfly, biting midge), the vertebrate host(s) and suitable environmental conditions. Transmission cycles range from simple (involving one vector and one host) to the highly complex involving multiple vectors and hosts. The epidemiology of arboviral diseases usually involves one of two transmission cycles. In the jungle or sylvatic cycle, an infected arthropod bites either a human or domestic animal that has strayed into the ecological niche of the virus/vector. This mode of infection results in small clusters of cases initiated at the same site. The second is the urban cycle where a person or domestic animal, infected via the sylvatic mode, acts as an amplifier host in the transfer of the virus to other persons or domestic animals in the community. These cases occur as epidemics or epizootics in nature.[2] The vector species involved in the urban cycle may be the same or different to that in the sylvatic cycle. Yellow fever is a good example of an arbovirus that undergoes both modes of transmission.[7]

Figure 41.1 shows examples of the types of transmission cycles that can occur in nature.

The interactions of the vectors, hosts and environmental conditions that are necessary for virus transmission to occur will now be discussed briefly.

Vertebrate hosts

The major hosts for arboviruses are mammals and birds.[1] The potential for virus dispersal is dependent on the type

Table 41.1 Arboviruses

Virus[†]	Geographical distribution	Transmission	Fever	Clinical form	Rash
TOGAVIRIDAE					
Alphaviruses					
Babanki	Africa	Mosquito			
*Barmah Forest (BF)	Australia	Mosquito	+	A	+
*Chikungunya (CHIK)	Africa, India, South-East Asia	Mosquito	+	H/A	+
Getah (GET)	Asia, Australasia	Mosquito	+		
*Mayaro (Uruma) (MAY)	South America	Mosquito	+		+
*O'nyong-nyong (ONN)	Africa	Mosquito	+	A	+
*Ross River (RR)	Australia, South Pacific	Mosquito	+	A	+
*Sindbis (SIN)	Africa, Asia, Europe, Australia	Mosquito	+	A	+ (Africa only)
Mucambo (MUC)	Brazil	Mosquito	+		
Semliki Forest (SF)	Africa, Russia	Mosquito	+		
Ockelbo (OCK)	Europe	Mosquito	+	A	+
*Eastern equine encephalitis (EEE)	North and South America	Mosquito	+	E	
*Western equine encephalitis (WEE)	North and South America	Mosquito	+	E	
*Venezuelan equine encephalitis (VEE)	North and South America	Mosquito	+	E	
Flaviviruses					
Mosquito-borne					
Banzi (BAN)	Southern Africa	Mosquito	+		
Bussuquara (BSQ)	Central and South America	Mosquito	+	A	
*Dengue-type 1–4	Asia, America, the Caribbean and Pacific Islands, China, Taiwan, Indonesia, Australia	Mosquito	+	H	+
Edge Hill (EH)	Australia	Mosquito	+	A	
Ilhéus (ILH)	South and North America	Mosquito	+	E	
*Japanese encephalitis (JE)	Asia, Australia	Mosquito	+	E	
Kokobera (KOK)	Australia, New Guinea	Mosquito	+	A	+
Koutango (KOU)	Senegal	Tick	+	A	+
Kunjin (KUN)	Australia, Indonesia, Malaysia	Mosquito	+	A/E	+
*Murray Valley encephalitis (MVE)	Australia, New Guinea	Mosquito	+	E	
Negishi (NEG)	Japan, China	Tick/mosquito	+	E	
*Rocio (ROC)	Brazil	Mosquito	+	E	
Sepik (SEP)	New Guinea	Mosquito	+		
Spondweni (SPO)	South Africa	Mosquito	+	A	
*St Louis encephalitis (SLE)	Americas	Mosquito	+	E	
Tyuleniy (TYU)	??	Tick	+	A	
Usutu (USU)	Sub-Saharan Africa	Mosquito	+		+
Wesselsbron (WSL)	Africa, Asia	Mosquito	+	E	+
*West Nile (WN)	Africa, India, Europe, North America	Mosquito	+	E	+
*Yellow fever (F)	Africa, South and Central America	Mosquito	+	H	
Zika (ZIK)	Africa	Mosquito	+		+
Tick-borne					
*Kyasanur Forest disease (KFD)	India	Ixodid tick	+	H/E	+
Kumlinge (KUM)	Finland	Tick	+	E	+
Langat (LAN)	Malaysia, Asia, Japan	Ixodid tick	+	E	
Louping ill (LI)	Britain	Ixodid tick	+	E	

Table 41.1 (*Cont'd*)

Virus[†]	Geographical distribution	Transmission	Fever	Clinical form	Rash
*Omsk haemorrhagic fever (OHF)	Former USSR	Ixodid tick	+	H	+
*Powassan (POW)	Canada, USA, USSR	Ixodid tick	+	E	
*Tick-borne encephalitis (TBE)					
Eastern subtype TBE (RSSE)	Former USSR, Asia	Ixodid tick	+	E	
Western subtype TBE	Europe and Scandinavia	ixodid tick	+	E	
Negishi (NEG)	Japan	Tick/mosquito	+	E	
Other vectors					
Rio Bravo (RB)	USA, Trinidad	?Bat saliva	+	E, meningitis	
BUNYAVIRIDAE					
Bunyamwera group					
Bunyamwera (BUN)	Africa	Mosquito	+		
Germiston (GER)	Africa	Mosquito	+		
Guaroa (GRO)	South and Central America	Mosquito	+		
Ilesha (ILE)	Africa	Mosquito	+		
Tensaw (TEN)	North America	Mosquito	+	E	
Maguari (MAG)	South America	Mosquito	+		
Bwamba group					
Bwamba (BWA)	Africa	Mosquito	+		
C group					
Apeu (APEU)	South America	Mosquito	+		
Caraparu (CAR)	South America	Mosquito	+		
Itaqui (ITQ)	South America	Mosquito	+		
Marituba (MTB)	South America	Mosquito	+		
Murutuca (MUR)	South America	Mosquito	+		
Oriboca (ORI)	South America	Mosquito	+		
Ossa (OSSA)	Panama	Mosquito	+		
Restan (RES)	Trinidad	Mosquito	+		
Nepuyo (NEP)	Central America	Mosquito	+		
California group					
*California encephalitis (CE)	USA, Canada	Mosquito	+	E	
Inkoo (INK)	Finland	Mosquito	+	Meningism	
*La Crosse (LAC)	USA, Canada	Mosquito	+	E	
*Tahyna (Lumbo) (TAH)	Europe, Africa	Mosquito	+		
Trivattatus (TVT)	USA	Mosquito	+		
Simbu group					
*Oropouche (ORO)	South America	Mosquito	+	E/A	
Guama group					
Guama (GMA)	South America	Mosquito	+		
Catu (CATU)	South America	Mosquito	+		
Other Bunyaviridae					
Bhanja (BHA)	India, southern Europe	Tick	+		
Tataguine (TAT)	Nigeria	Mosquito	+		

Table 41.1 (*Cont'd*)

Virus[†]	Geographical distribution	Transmission	Fever	Clinical form	Rash
Nairoviruses					
Crimean–Congo group					
*Crimean–Congo haemorrhagic fever (C-CHF)	Europe, Africa, Middle East, central Asia, Pakistan	Ixodid tick	+	H	+
Hazara (HAZ)	Pakistan	Ixodid tick		H	
Nairobi sheep disease group					
Dugbe (DUG)	Africa	Ixodid tick	+		
Nairobi sheep disease (NSD)	Africa, India	Ixodid tick	+	A	
Phleboviruses					
*Sandfly fever (Naples, SFN; Sicily, SFS)	Africa, Asia, central Europe	Phlebotomines/ sandflies	+		
Toscana (TOS)	Italy, Portugal, Cyprus	Sandflies		E, meningitis	
*Rift Valley fever (RVF)	Africa, Middle East	Mosquito	+	H/E	
Candiru (CDU)	Brazil	?	+		
Chagres (CHG)	Panama	?Phlebotomines/ mosquito	+		
ORBIVIRIDAE					
Coltivirus					
*Colorado tick fever (CTF)	North America	Tick	+	H/E (in children)	+
Orungo (ORU)	Africa	Mosquito	+		

H, haemorrhagic; E, encephalitis; A, arthralgia.
*Of clinical importance.
†Classification of viruses according to virus taxonomy: 7th Report of the International Committee on Taxonomy of Viruses (2000).[3]
For a complete list of mosquito vectors and the arboviruses they transmit, see Appendix IV.

of vertebrate host involved. Birds can facilitate virus movement over large distances whereas most animal hosts are more sedentary and virus activity tends to be restricted to a particular region. These were reviewed elsewhere[8] and are summarized below.

Reservoir hosts

These include hosts that have previously been referred to elsewhere as either maintenance or amplifier hosts. These hosts are responsible for virus transmission and are 'essential for the continued existence of the virus'. The immune status of the host species will affect the rates of transmission of arboviruses. Reservoir hosts become infected by the virus and produce high-titre viraemias to allow virus transmission to occur; however, they are generally not susceptible to disease. Arboviruses may have more than one host species involved in transmission cycles. An example of this is the flavivirus JE, for which birds (particularly herons) are considered to be the major maintenance hosts in natural cycles. However, in Asia pigs are often kept in close proximity to human dwellings and it has been shown that these animals amplify the virus to high titres and therefore can readily infect mosquitoes, which can then transmit the virus to humans. This was thought to have occurred in

the Torres Strait (Australia) in 1995, when JE virus was detected in the region for the first time.

Incidental hosts

These become infected but transmission does not occur with sufficient regularity for stable maintenance. Humans are usually an incidental host, often, but not always being a dead end in the chain. Incidental hosts may or may not show symptoms.

Disseminating hosts

These host species may move virus from an area of active transmission to another location. Movement by viraemic waterbirds has been suggested as a mechanism of movement for a number of arboviruses including MVE, JE, WN and EEE. Arboviruses can also be introduced into new areas by the movement of humans. For example, humans infected with dengue viruses who travel on jet aircraft are the main means by which this virus is spread among continents.

Dead-end hosts

These species can become infected by the virus but do not transmit to other vectors. Humans are thought to be a dead-end host for many arboviruses.

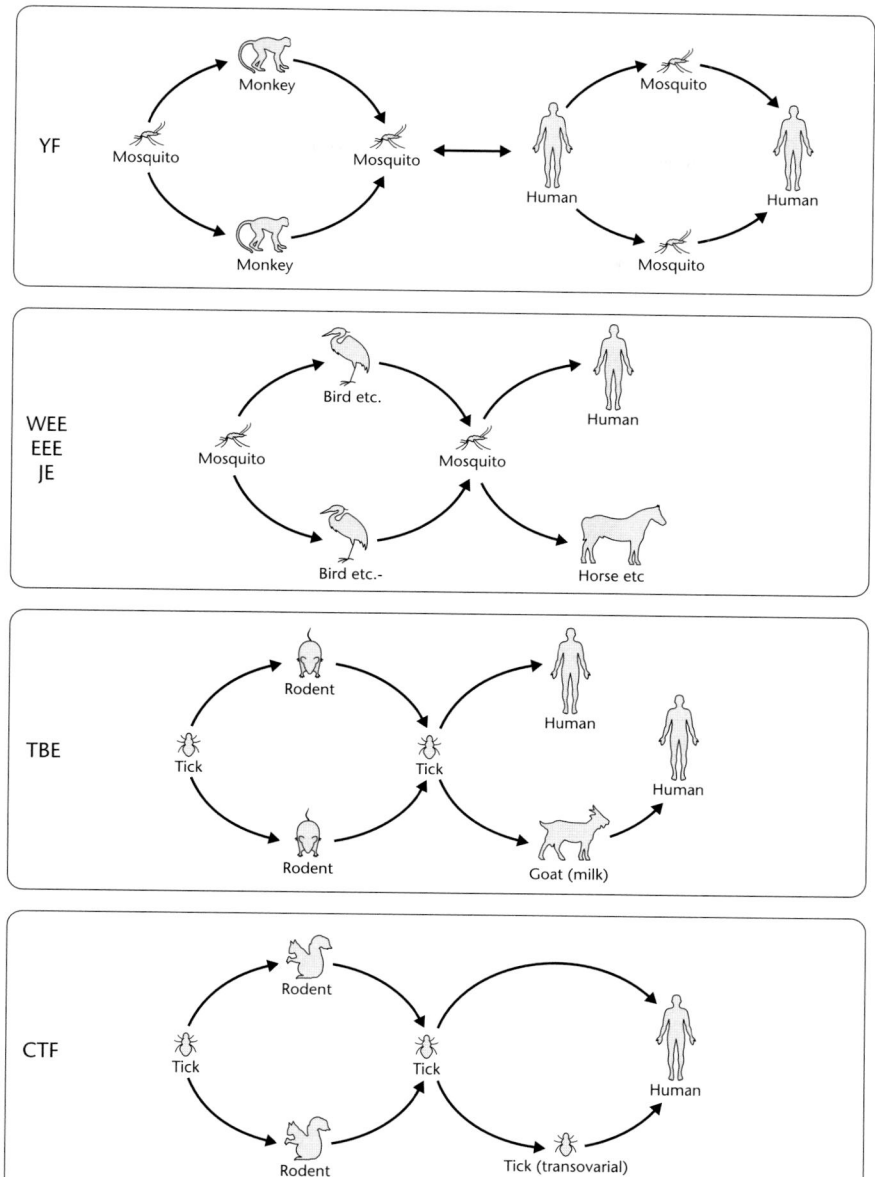

Figure 41.1: Transmission of some arboviruses. CTF, Colorado tick fever; EEE, Eastern equine encephalitis; JE, Japanese encephalitis; TBE, tick-borne encephalitis; WEE, Western equine encephalitis; YF, yellow fever.

A wide variety of host species have been implicated in arbovirus diseases. These include birds, mammals (including primates), rodents, marsupials and bats. The host species associated with the major human and animal pathogens described in this chapter are included in the sections on the specific viruses.

Vectors/invertebrate hosts

Arthropod-borne viruses are distinguished from other animal viruses because of their ability to infect both vertebrate and invertebrate hosts. The virus is replicated within the cells of the arthropod vector before being transferred to a susceptible host.[9] Arthropods may also transmit viruses by mechanical transmission whereby the vector simply transfers the virus from an infected to a susceptible host.

Invertebrate hosts include mosquitoes, sandflies, ticks and culicoides (biting midges). Most arboviruses have been recovered from mosquitoes; a list of the vectors is given in Table 41.1 and Appendix IV. Ixodid ticks are involved in transmission of a closely interrelated sub-group of the flaviviruses and also in some of the other groups. Genera of ticks involved in arbovirus transmission include *Haemaphysalis*, *Ixodes* and *Dermacentor* (see also Appendix IV). Recent changes in mosquito taxonomy have lead to the reclassification of numerous *Aedes* subgenera to the new genus *Ochlerotatus*. Previous nomenclature has been retained in this chapter.

Transmission

Transmission by arthropods involves several processes:

- Ingestion by the arthropods of virus in the blood (usually) or tissue fluids of the vertebrate hosts.
- Penetration of the viruses into the tissue of the arthropods, in the gut wall, or elsewhere after passing through the gut wall ('gut barrier').
- Multiplication of the viruses in the arthropod cells, including those of the salivary glands.[10]

The time interval between the ingestion of a viraemic blood meal and the ability of a vector to transmit the virus is known as the extrinsic incubation period of the disease. In mosquitoes this period is short: 10 days at 30°C (ambient temperature) and longer at lower temperatures. The quantity of blood, and therefore the amount of virus ingested, also affects the length of the extrinsic incubation period. This threshold phenomenon is extremely important in determining the efficiency of a vector and may also vitally affect the course of an epidemic. Mosquitoes remain infective for life without any apparent ill-effects, and their effectiveness as transmitters depends upon longevity and the frequency with which they bite. Different species of female mosquitoes vary in their ability to transmit different arboviruses. Thus, one mosquito species may be a competent vector of one virus but be unable to vector another virus. In contrast, some mosquito species may be competent vectors for many arboviruses (e.g., *Culex tarsalis* vectors both WEE and SLE, *Cx. annulirostris* vectors MVE, JE, Kunjin, RR and BF viruses).

Viruses have been reported to persist in overwintering mosquitoes and this could be an important factor in virus survival. This has been shown to occur in *Cx. tritaeniorhynchus* infected with JE and in *Cx. tarsalis* infected with WEE (infective by bite up to 8 months). Transovarial or vertical transmission from one generation to the next via the desiccation-resistant eggs of some *Aedes* species has also been suggested as a possible mechanism of persistence for some arboviruses. However, Turell[11] suggests that other methods, including reintroduction of virus by migratory birds or survival in other vectors, may be more important in the long-term persistence of these viruses. Trans-stadial persistence of virus is normal in ticks and transovarial passage has been observed in some species; both are of great epidemiological importance.

Important factors in transmission by arthropods

- Susceptibility of the arthropods to infection and ability to transmit it. There is wide variation in this.
- Breeding habits of the arthropods and preferred habitats, whether near humans and other hosts of the virus.
- Biting habits of the arthropods—in mosquitoes whether they are anthropophilic (attracted to humans) or zoophilic (attracted to animals), exophilic (feeds outdoors) or endophilic (feeds inside).
- Longevity of the arthropods, which depends to a great extent on temperature, humidity and (especially in ticks) the availability of hosts to feed on. Persistence of the virus by overwintering in adult mosquitoes or vertical transmission between generations may carry virus from one year to the next.
- Abundance of the arthropods. An efficient vector may have a wide range of animals on which to feed, but if the arthropod species is abundant and, even if it bites humans only infrequently in the presence of other (and preferred) animals, the large numbers enable it to maintain transmission to man. For instance, *Cx. tritaeniorhynchus*, which bites mostly birds, cattle, dogs and especially porcines, and only to a limited extent humans, can maintain transmission of JE from pigs to humans by sheer numbers.
- Migratory birds can help by spreading virus that is circulating in their blood or by carrying infected ticks.
- Interactions in ecological systems are of primary importance in transmission. A good example of this is the circulation of YF virus in East Africa among forest monkeys and tree-living mosquitoes. Monkeys often leave the forests and raid banana plantations. Hence, YF virus can then infect mosquitoes in these locations and from there can be transmitted to humans. Similarly, humans becomes infected with KFD when they enter the domain of infected monkeys and pick up infected ticks. Other mosquito-borne and tick-borne infections are variations on the same theme.

Although transmission of arboviruses usually takes place through the bites of arthropods, it is important to remember that some of the viruses can, in some instances, be transmitted in other ways. European TBE can be acquired by drinking the milk of infected goats, VEE (in cotton rats) apparently via urine or faeces infecting the nasopharynx, WEE possibly through aerosol from a patient and EEE (in pheasants) by one bird pecking another. Laboratory infections have been reported with Kunjin virus in Australia and CTF virus is reported to have been transmitted by blood transfusion.

Humans are usually only an incidental host in arbovirus infections. However, it is their behaviour as well as environmental factors that determine the activity and spread of these viruses.[1] Many human activities encourage transmission of these animal viruses to people. The construction of dams and extensive areas of irrigation often promotes the breeding of enormous numbers of mosquitoes. For instance, the development of rice fields encourages *Cx. tritaeniorhynchus* in Sarawak, spreading JE, and *Mansonia uniformis* and *Anopheles gambiae* in Kenya spreading chikungunya, ONN, possibly WN and Sindbis. The seasonal cutting of old vegetation in Sarawak produces heavily polluted pools which support massive populations of culicines. The keeping of cattle driven into marginal forest areas in India promotes the growth and transport of ticks, and the intrusion of people into forest areas lays them open to infection with YF and the tick-borne diseases. In many countries the practice of using large containers for water storage has helped to increase the *Aedes aegypti* populations and hence has increased the transmission of dengue, chikungunya and other viruses vectored by this species.[12]

For a fuller discussion of the effect of human-related behaviour on arbovirus transmission, other reviews should be consulted.[13]

Environmental conditions

Environmental conditions, particularly rainfall, temperature and humidity, play an important role in arbovirus transmission cycles. Arbovirus activity is generally seasonal. For example, the alphaviruses transmitted by mosquitoes in temperate regions cause disease in summer during periods of increased vector activity.[14] In tropical areas human infections caused by arboviruses usually occur during the wet season, with increased virus activity again coinciding with periods of high vector numbers.

Rainfall

Mosquito larvae and pupae are aquatic and hence require water for breeding.[15] The abundance of arthropod vectors is directly affected by the amount of rainfall and flooding in a particular region. Rainfall can also affect the spread of some bird-borne arboviruses as the birds move to breed in areas where high rainfall has occurred. For example, extensive rainfall and flooding occurred in northern Australia during the 2000 wet season. This resulted in the unprecedented southerly spread of MVE activity from areas of the tropical north of Western Australia to subtropical and temperate regions. High tides can also lead to increased mosquito breeding and hence increased activity of viruses that are vectored by salt-marsh mosquitoes.

Temperature

High external temperatures may have an adverse effect on vector survival. In addition, some mosquito species are temperature limited in their breeding. For example, *Cx. annulirostris*, the major vector of MVE, RR, JE viruses in Australia, will not breed when the daily temperatures fall below 17.5°C.[16] Temperature can also affect the length of the extrinsic incubation period and most studies have shown that the extrinsic incubation period for mosquitoes is shorter at 30°C than at lower temperatures.[10] Hence the mosquito will become 'infectious' in a shorter time at higher temperatures.

Humidity

Increased humidity facilitates increased survival of mosquitoes.

Climate change

It is predicted that future climate changes such as those associated with global warming may affect arbovirus transmission cycles throughout the world. It has been suggested that global warming will affect the amount and extent of rainfall, frequency of high tides and actual tide heights, and temperature. The extent of these environmental changes is unknown but, because of the complex interactions between these viruses, their hosts and vectors and the environment, it seems likely that even minor changes will affect arbovirus activity in different regions. This may result in an increased number of cases or a greater geographical spread of these viruses.[15]

Immunity[17,18]

After inoculation of an arbovirus into the skin of a vertebrate by the arthropod vector, the virus probably multiplies first in local tissues and regional lymph nodes where the earliest immune responses occur. As with most viral infections, non-specific innate responses occur during the first few days. These include the antiviral effects of macrophages, natural killer cells and virus-induced interferon. However, within 4–7 days after infection, the specific actions of the humoral (antibody) and cell-mediated (T cell) immune responses come in to play. Initially, immunoglobulin IgM antibodies are produced to the virus, but within a few weeks are replaced by a predominantly IgG response. Therefore the presence of IgM antibodies in serum is a useful marker of a recent infection, and because IgM tends to be more specific than the long-lasting IgG it is diagnostically important. These antibodies can be detected in a variety of assays including immunofluorescence (IFA), haemagglutination inhibition (HI) and virus neutralization (N). However, most current diagnostic methods use rapid formats such as enzyme-linked immunosorbent assay (ELISA). In general, antibody responses to arbovirus infections appear early and are long lasting; however, some viruses do not produce high antibody titres in humans while others produce short-lived or late responses.

A person who recovers from an arbovirus infection such as yellow fever or Japanese encephalitis, generally possesses life-long immunity against reinfection with the homologous virus. Neutralizing antibodies can be found as early as a few days after the beginning of the disease and are found constantly for many years in the serum of these individuals. This persistence of immunity does not depend upon re-exposure to the virus and the mechanism by which this immunological memory is maintained is not clear. While neutralizing antibodies are a good indication of protective immunity, antibodies that do not neutralize virus in vitro may also provide protection in vivo via other immune mechanisms such as complement-mediated cytolysis (CMC) or antibody-dependent cell-mediated cytotoxicity (ADCC).

Arboviruses are often grouped together according to antigenic similarity. For example, JE, MVE and West Nile virus are all members of a single antigenic complex within the *Flavivirus* genus, while the four serotypes of dengue represent another. Inoculation of one virus of the group into a naive animal produces antibody that is reactive not only to the homologous virus, but also to heterologous viruses of the same antigenic group. Indeed, recovery from an infection by one member of the group may provide a degree of resistance to a subsequent infection by another member of the same group; for instance, immunity to MVE virus may provide subsequent protection against JE virus, and vice versa. This protection against infection with related viruses probably results in reduced clinical disease rather than prevention of infection. One notable exception to this trend is the scenario of serial infection with heterologous dengue serotypes. While infection with one serotype may provide short-lived protection against heterologous serotypes, once antibody titres have waned pre-existing antibody to the initial infecting serotype may serve to enhance the infection with a second. This phenomenon is known as antibody-dependent enhancement of infection and is believed to be the mechanism by which most cases of dengue haemorrhagic fever (DHF) and dengue shock syndrome (DSS) (more severe manifestations of dengue infection) are induced.

While the action of antibody in protective immunity to arbovirus infection has been clearly demonstrated, the role of T cell-mediated immunity is not as clear. Broadly, cross-reactive CD8[+] cytotoxic T cells are induced by infection with flaviviruses and alphaviruses but their importance for protective immunological memory is doubtful. Indeed the inflammatory responses and cytolysis effected by virus-specific T cells may contribute to the pathology of some arbovirus infections.

Infant rhesus monkeys and human infants born of mothers immune to YF have protective antibodies in their serum at birth, which persist for several months. These antibodies are probably transmitted via the placenta rather than in the mother's milk, because they disappear from infant serum while the child is still suckling. Passive immunity induced by injection of immune gamma-globulin has also been used for protection against TBE in circumstances of special risk. Passive transfer of antibody to MVE virus has also been used to protect individuals after accidental laboratory infection and has been assessed in an animal model for use as a prophylaxis for infants living in MVE-endemic areas who are most likely to contract the disease.[19]

Clinical features in general

Arbovirus infections are distributed throughout most of the world, and in areas with endemic or regular epidemic activity infection rates are quite high within the human populations. However, the vast majority of infected individuals will have had either an asymptomatic or non-specific mild illness, and only a handful of those infected will develop one of the recognizable clinical syndromes.

The case:infection ratio is usually low (e.g., around 1:300 for encephalitis due to JE) but varies depending on the virus. It may be higher during epidemic (rather than endemic) disease activity, and will be modified by host susceptibility factors. In particular, the major burden of disease is felt at the extremes of life—the very young and the elderly. If clinical manifestations arise after infection they do so after an intrinsic incubation period lasting from a few days to a week or more. During that time the virus replicates at the site of inoculation, then further amplifies within the reticuloendothelial system before it becomes viraemic and spreads to its target organs.

The most important clues to a possible arbovirus infection lie in a detailed travel and exposure history, coupled with a current knowledge of the viruses circulating in the potential area of exposure. That can be particularly difficult if the patient is a returned traveller. Information can be obtained from travel health websites such as those of the World Health Organization or the Centers for Disease Control in Atlanta, Georgia, USA, or from software programs such as GIDEON (Global Infectious Diseases EpidemiOlogy Network). However, it may also be necessary to seek the advice of local experts to get the full picture in difficult cases.

The major clinical syndromes may be grouped as follows:

1. Systemic febrile disease.
2. Arboviral haemorrhagic fever.
3. Encephalitides.
4. Polyarthralgic illness.

Systemic febrile disease

All of the arbovirus infections will produce a systemic febrile illness as their most common clinical manifestation. This illness may be completely non-specific or even suggest another viral illness, including gastro-intestinal and respiratory infections, particularly in the early stages of illness. There are some clinical features that are more characteristic of arbovirus infections. Headache is common and may be severe and accompanied by meningism. Joint aches are also common, especially with alphavirus infections. Rash may be present and is usually generalized and maculopapular, although occasionally it is vesicular. Petechial rashes are less common and may be an early indicator of the haemorrhagic fevers. In the vast majority of cases the febrile illness is followed by recovery. In the remainder the illness progresses to one of the more serious forms of disease, sometimes following a few days of remission. Occasionally the infections have a fulminant course, particularly in young children, where the initial febrile illness is short and advances rapidly to severe illness.

The notable exception to the generally benign nature of the febrile illnesses is YF. This virus produces sufficient liver damage to cause clinical jaundice and a resulting severe febrile illness, even without progressing to haemorrhagic disease.

Haemorrhagic fever[20]

Most commonly caused by:

- Flaviviruses: DEN, YF, KFD, OHF
- Phleboviruses: RVF

These are the most serious manifestations of arbovirus infection. Haemorrhagic disease most often manifests as bleeding from the gums or gastrointestinal haemorrhage (haematemesis and melaena) and cutaneous petechiae and purpura. The pathogenesis is complex and poorly understood for most. Yellow fever produces sufficient liver dysfunction to cause a reduction of the coagulation factors produced in that organ. However, in severe YF, there is also a consumptive coagulopathy (disseminated intravascular coagulopathy; DIC) due to complement and cytokine activation, resulting in a reduction of most coagulation factors and a rise in the levels of fibrin degradation products. There may also be platelet dysfunction.

DHF is associated with a marked thrombocytopenia and platelet dysfunction, and DIC may develop in severe disease. Complement activation is likely to be important in the induction of the coagulopathy, as is cytokine release from mononuclear cells. However, the major problem in DHF relates to endothelial cell damage and increased vascular permeability resulting in loss of fluid from the intravascular into the extravascular spaces.

There is little information about KFD, OHD and RVF, but DIC seems to be an important component of the haemorrhagic disease.

Treatment is directed mainly at control of the haemorrhage, maintenance of intravascular fluid volumes to prevent hypotension, and management of complications such as pneumonia and renal failure. Fluid loss in DHF can initally be replaced with 5% dextrose in saline, Ringer's lactate or similar, but if this fails then plasma, plasma substitutes or colloidal solutions may be needed. If the haemoglobin level is falling, blood transfusion is needed.

Fresh frozen plasma may be used to provide coagulation factors, although they need to be used with caution owing to the potential for worsening DIC. In the early stages of YF when there is a selective decline in the hepatic coagulation factors, these can be replaced selectively. Vitamin K has also been suggested, but it is doubtful that the liver will be able to respond to this.

If significant bleeding is occurring as a result of thrombocytopenia, platelet transfusions may be necessary, but they should be used with caution when DIC is established.

There is some experimental evidence that ribavirin may be useful for RVF, but clinical data are lacking.

Encephalitis

Most commonly caused by:

- Alphaviruses: EE, WEE, VEE
- Flaviviruses: JE, MVE, WN, KUN, SLE, TBE, LI, KFD
- Phleboviruses: RVF

Many of the arboviruses are capable of infecting the central nervous system. It is assumed that they enter across the blood–brain barrier after the viraemic phase of infection. However, this has not yet been established and there is some evidence that entry via the olfactory bulb may be important. In either event, the resulting encephalitis has a fairly characteristic pattern of involvement. The major effects are seen within the central cerebral structures including the midbrain, basal ganglia and brainstem. The cerebellum and upper spinal cord are also often affected, particularly the anterior horn cells of the latter. As a result of the involvement of essential structures, encephalitis may result in coma, respiratory failure and flaccid paralysis. Milder manifestations include cranial nerve palsies, tremor, cogwheel rigidity, cerebellar ataxia and upper limb weakness. The differential diagnosis in the early stages includes herpes simplex encephalitis, early bacterial cerebritis and tuberculous meningitis. Once signs of involvement of central cerebral structures appear, then it is more characteristic of arboviral encephalitis. Occasionally herpes simplex, postinfectious encephalitis, acute cerebral vasculitis and others may produce a similar picture.

The frequency and nature of sequelae varies with the virus, the severity of the initial illness and the age of the patient. Many survivors are left with mild residua and a few unfortunate ones with major intellectual and physical disabilities. Late neuropsychiatric manifestations are also prominent with the arboviral encephalitides, while other patients develop Parkinsonian-type features.

During the acute illness the CSF usually shows a mild to moderate lymphocyte pleocytosis (although a neutrophil predominance may be seen in early illness), accompanied by some increase in the levels of protein but a normal glucose concentration. Samples of serum and CSF should be collected for IgM testing as early as possible. If available, virus isolation and/or RNA detection by reverse transcriptase–polymerase chain reaction (RT-PCR) should also be performed on these samples. Computed tomography (CT) may show changes in the affected central structures, but magnetic resonance imaging (MRI) is more sensitive. Late scans in those with chronic disease show destructive changes in the thalamus and other central structures.

Limited data are available on treatment of arboviral encephalitis and no specific antiviral agents are currently available. Steroids have been shown to be ineffective in JE, but interferon α may be beneficial. In view of the similarity of the different forms of arbovirus encephalitis, it seems likely that the same will apply to other flavivirus infections. The successful use of hyperimmune globulin for the Western subtype of TBE suggests that corresponding preparations for other flaviviruses may also work. However, treatment of these conditions is largely supportive in order to ensure that the patient does not succumb to respiratory failure or haemodynamic instability, or die from complications such as pneumonia that may arise with any serious illness.

Polyarthralgic illness

Most commonly caused by:

- Alphaviruses: CHIK, RR, BF, SIN, ONN, OCK
- Flaviviruses: KUN, KOK
- Bunyaviruses: ORO
- Phleboviruses: Sandfly fever

A number of the alphavirus infections have polyarthralgia as a common and prominent component of the presenting illness. Typically, the small joints of the hands and feet, the wrists, elbows and knees are involved. Symptoms may consist just of joint pain, but often there is evidence of true arthritis manifesting as joint swelling and morning stiffness. The tenderness and swelling are largely due to synovitis rather than effusions. Occasionally back, neck or jaw pain may occur. Arthralgia is usually accompanied by myalgia and fatigue. Tendonitis and fasciitis may also be clinically evident. Flaviviruses less commonly produce polyarthralgia, with the exception of dengue. The alphavirus infections are prone to cause prolonged arthralgia and arthritis, with up to 25% or more having symptoms that persist for months or years. The pathogenesis of this ongoing arthritis has not been determined.

The acute polyarthritis has a wide differential diagnosis. In some areas more than one arbovirus will be potentially responsible for the illness. In addition there are a number of other causes of polyarthritis with or without rash, including rubella, acute hepatitis B, parvovirus B19 (erythema infectiosum), human immunodeficiency virus (HIV) seroconversion illness, Henoch–Schoenlein purpura, drug-related serum sickness, and the acute onset of other non-infectious arthritides. Subacute or chronic disease following RR virus or BF virus infection may be confused with rubella or parvovirus B19 arthritis, as well as other chronic arthritides including rheumatoid arthritis, systemic lupus erythematosus and adult Still's disease.

Treatment is symptomatic with rest, gentle exercise, analgesics, and non-steroidal anti-inflammatory drugs. Steroids should be avoided owing to the uncertainty about the pathogenesis and their efficacy. Also, if steroids are commenced, they may need to be maintained for long periods with all the associated problems of long-term steroid use.

Diagnosis
Virus detection

Viraemia lasts for a few days after the onset of illness and virus can be isolated from blood at that time. However, as it is technically demanding, limited in availability and often fails to yield a positive result, virus cultures are rarely undertaken as a part of routine diagnosis. They should be reserved for unusual cases or rare pathogens. In cases of meningitis or encephalitis, culture from the CSF may also be undertaken, but with the same constraints as above. Where culture is attempted, blood and/or CSF should be collected as early as possible in the course of illness. Post-mortem tissue may yield virus in the later stages of illness. Many will grow in a variety of cell lines, but maximum sensitivity for the mosquito-borne alphaviruses and flaviviruses is achieved by initially inoculating the sample on to a mosquito cell line (e.g., C6/36, AP-61 or TRA-284) and incubating for 3–4 days at 28°C. In order to obtain a cytopathic effect, this must be blind passaged to Vero, BHK, PS, chick embryo or various other cell lines and incubated at 37°C for a few days. Virus can also be isolated by inoculation of specimen into suckling mouse brain or intrathoracic inoculation in appropriate mosquito species. Virus growth in mice manifests as paralysis and death after a few days, and is confirmed by identification of the virus in the brain. For the Bunyaviridae, suckling mouse brain inoculation or culture in mosquito cells (C6/36 or AP-61) are suitable. Coltiviruses grow in suckling mouse brain or in Vero or BHK-21 cell lines.

When an arbovirus is isolated in cell culture, it is most easily identified by the monoclonal antibody binding in IFA or enzyme immunoassay (EIA) formats. Neutralization with antisera or complement fixation (CF) assays are used less commonly. Specific RT-PCR assays may also be used for identification, and sequencing of the product can provide detailed genetic mapping.

A variety of antigen detection methods has been described, either by IFA or antigen capture EIA. They have been used for blood, CSF and tissues.

Virus may also be detected by amplification of viral RNA by RT-PCR. Methods have been described for most of the flaviviruses and some of the alphaviruses. They are more sensitive and quicker to perform than virus culture, but are largely confined to specialized laboratories. Like culture, they can be performed on blood, CSF or tissues, and should be done as early as possible in the course of illness.

Post-mortem tissues can be used for virus detection if available. The preferred site for sampling is dictated by the major sites of involvement. RT-PCR can be performed on fixed tissues, even if paraffin embedded, but the sensitivity of detection for these samples is uncertain.

Serological diagnosis

This is the main routine diagnostic method for arboviral infections. Antibody may be detected by EIA, IFA, HI, N or CF assays. Most diagnosis is based on EIA and HI tests, with some use of IFA. The EIA and IFA tests can be formatted to detect either IgG or IgM, or both in the case of competitive EIA formats. HI will detect both IgG and

IgM, and differentiation between them requires separation of the antibody classes by sucrose density centrifugation or in chromatography columns. N assays are regarded as the most specific of the tests, but are confined to specialized laboratories that are able to culture the viruses.

Recent infection is best diagnosed by an increase in antibody levels between acute and convalescent samples tested in parallel, but it may take 2–4 weeks before a diagnostic rise is detected. Detection of IgM is helpful in making an earlier diagnosis. IgM usually appears within a few days after onset of illness. A negative IgM using a sensitive test such as EIA or IFA in a sample collected a week or more into the illness makes recent infection very unlikely. For samples collected earlier in the illness or where there is a strong clinical suspicion despite the negative IgM finding, a second sample at least 2 weeks after onset is recommended. As IgM often persists for weeks or months, it is not sufficient to diagnose recent rather than past infection. False-positive IgM results may also occur occasionally. Therefore diagnosis of recent infection based on detection of IgM alone requires a clinically consistent illness and a suitable exposure history.

Cross-reactivity between antibodies within the major subgroups of arboviruses is a problem and may result in a misleading diagnosis. Alphavirus antibodies show limited cross-reactivity and standard tests are usually sufficient to identify the infecting virus, although it does depend on the particular alphaviruses circulating within that region. However, antibodies to the different flaviviruses generally cross-react widely, so that detection of IgM and/or IgG to one of these viruses in the routine tests is not definite evidence of infection due to that virus rather than another flavivirus. The clinical and epidemiological circumstances may indicate that only one flavivirus is possible, for example detection of dengue antibody in a person with clinical dengue during a known epidemic. Otherwise specific serological tests, such as N or epitope-blocking EIA, are needed to identify the antibody. The latter has been applied to MVE and KUN diagnosis and uses monoclonal antibodies to species-specific epitopes to inhibit the binding of patient serum. If inhibition occurs then there is a significant amount of specific antibody in the patient's serum.

Diagnosis may be further complicated by the phenomenon of 'original antigenic sin'. This occurs in people who have had previous flavivirus infection, and who have a new infection with a different flavivirus. Owing to the antigenic similarities, they may mount a vigorous anamnestic antibody response to the original virus before they develop specific antibody to the new virus. As a result, serological tests may initially suggest recent infection with their previous virus. Late convalescent sera may clarify the situation, but sometimes it is not possible determine the infecting virus. Occasionally a similar phenomenon is seen with closely related alphavirus such as CHIK and ONN.

A detailed travel and exposure history is important for the accurate interpretation of arbovirus serology.

Management

There are no specific antiviral agents currently in use for the treatment of arboviral infections, nor are these likely in the near future. Treatment is supportive and symptomatic. Limited data on steroids and interferon is discussed under the relevant viruses.

Immunization[17,18]

Highly effective vaccines have been developed against several arboviruses of public health significance. However, only vaccines against YF, JE and TBE are licensed for use in the wider community.

The YF 17D vaccine is one of the safest and most successful viral vaccines ever produced. This live vaccine was derived from a highly virulent strain of YF virus (Asibi) that has been attenuated by in vitro serial passage in mouse embryonic tissue and chick embryo cells. After prolonged propagation in this medium, it was found that neurotropism and viscerotropism were both greatly reduced, but the virus retained its antigenic properties. The 17D vaccine is still widely used and highly effective, giving protection for at least 10 years, and probably longer. Less than 10% of vaccinees experience headache and malaise, while allergic reactions, liver function abnormalities and neurological complications are extremely uncommon. Nevertheless recent reports of 17D vaccination-related morbidity and mortality have prompted calls for a review of the safety of the vaccine.[21] The vaccine is contraindicated for infants under 6 months of age for whom the frequency of neurological accidents is significantly increased. Depending on the relative risk of natural infection, immunization should also be avoided in pregnant women. Immunization against YF is required by law before travellers are allowed into certain countries either for their protection or to prevent the importation of the disease to areas where *Ae. aegypti* is present.

Formalin-inactivated vaccines against JE are licensed for use in several countries and immunization is recommended for individuals living in endemic areas, or for travellers visiting regions that are experiencing current outbreaks. This vaccine is also used to immunize military personnel and laboratory workers who may be exposed to the virus. At least three doses of the vaccine at 7–14-day intervals are required to achieve more than 90% seroconversion, with booster doses recommended after 12 months. Minor side effects such as local tenderness and mild systemic symptoms occur in 10–30% of vaccines, although more serious neurological complications are rare. Allergic responses, particularly in Western travellers, are not uncommon, with up to 1% of vaccinees experiencing reactions within 7 days of inoculation. A live attenuated JE vaccine (SA14-14-2) has also been developed and is used extensively in China. Evaluation studies indicate the vaccine is both effective and safe. Several genetically engineered JE vaccines are also being tested for clinical use.

Inactivated vaccines against TBE virus are used widely in several European countries. The highly purified Austrian vaccine induces seroconversion rates of more than 97% in the field with negligible side effects. Immunization may be warranted for people living in endemic areas or those involved in high-risk activities, such as laboratory workers, military personnel, foresters, farmers or campers. Passive immunization with TBE immunoglobulin is also used for before or after exposure to tick bite in some European countries.

To protect personnel who work with RVF virus in the laboratory, or troops who may be exposed to this virus, an inactivated vaccine given as three subcutaneous doses (at 0, 7 and 28 days) induces a greater than 90% sero-conversion rate in recipients. Military trials indicate that the vaccine is safe and provides good long-term immunity in humans when boosted after 12 months.[22]

Although no alphavirus vaccines have been licensed for widespread human use, several preparations have been used to protect laboratory workers or livestock. Inactivated EEE and WEE virus and EEE whole-virus vaccines are available for restricted human use and have a veterinary application in horses. An inactivated vaccine for RR virus in humans is undergoing clinical trials, while live attenuated vaccines for CHIK and VEE have been tested in a limited number of volunteers and laboratory workers. More recently, several experimental recombinant and genetically engineered vaccines have also been developed and may prove useful in the future.

Currently there is an urgent need for an effective and safe vaccine against dengue. However, to avoid vaccine-induced antibody-dependent enhancement of infection with heterologous serotypes, the vaccine must be delivered as a multivalent preparation so that immunization against each of the four serotypes is concurrent. A live attenuated tetravalent vaccine is currently undergoing clinical trials.

Control
Vector control

Vector control has been successful in some circumstances, for instance during the construction of the Panama Canal when, by strict discipline, all collections of water capable of breeding *Ae. aegypti* (and vectors of malaria) were eliminated from the area. Similar methods have been applied to cities and towns in South America under the threat of YF. When DDT was introduced, extensive use in Guyana and elsewhere soon eradicated *Ae. aegypti* and with it the threat of urban YF. In Africa, however, *Ae. aegypti* has shown resistance to DDT, and in some areas it is exophilic in habit, so that spraying dwellings with insecticide is ineffective. Forest mosquitoes, of course, are not susceptible to ordinary methods of spraying. Tick control by residual insecticides has, however, achieved some success in the former USSR. However, the problems of vector control, especially in rural areas, are formidable.

Medically important arboviruses

The remaining sections describe the distribution, aetiology, transmission cycles, clinical features, diagnosis, treatment, control and epidemiology of individual medically important arboviruses in more detail.

Alphaviruses
Barmah Forest virus (BF)[23]

Geographical distribution
BF virus is confined to the Australian mainland. Human infections have been described in all mainland states, but most disease occurs in the tropical north and the temperate coastal region of the south-west and northern half of the east coast.

Aetiology
BF virus is an alphavirus that occupies its own antigenic group.

Transmission
Transmission is similar to that of RR virus.

Clinical features
Natural history
The *incubation period* is probably 7–9 days. Clinical illness is similar to the more common Ross River virus infection, although joint pain is slightly less common (about 85%) and joint swelling or stiffness occurs in only about 30% of cases. Skin rash is more common, occurring in 90% of patients. It is usually maculopapular, but may be urticarial or vesicular. BF virus disease occurs mainly between the ages of 20 and 60 years of age. Clinical illness appears to be uncommon in children.

Diagnosis
The diagnostic methods used are similar to those described for RR virus. IgM may persist for many months following acute infection.

Management
In the absence of any controlled data, the infection is usually managed symptomatically, as recommended for RR virus disease.

Epidemiology
BF virus is found only on the Australian mainland and has an epidemiology similar to that of RR virus, although it is much less common. Activity requires the same

environmental conditions as RR virus, but does not necessarily occur at the same time. There has been a gradual southward movement of this virus within Australia, with a pattern of small epidemics as it enters a new area, with low level seasonal epidemics following that.

Chikungunya (CHIK)[14,17,24–27]

Geographical distribution

Chikungunya virus was first isolated from patients in Tanzania during an epidemic in 1952–1953. Its name is a local word meaning 'that which contorts or bends up'. Infection and human disease are widespread in Africa, and CHIK is also present in Saudi Arabia, India (Calcutta and southern India), Thailand, Cambodia, Burma, Vietnam, Malaysia, Borneo, Indonesia and the Philippines (Figure 41.2). Large outbreaks have occurred in urban settings in many parts of Africa and Asia, and these may extend over several years.

Aetiology

CHIK virus is an alphavirus in the Semliki Forest complex, and is most closely related to ONN virus.

Transmission

The main vector to humans is *Ae. aegypti,* although a number of other species can transmit infection. In Africa, the virus appears to be maintained in forest and savannahs in a cycle involving non-human primates and a variety of *Aedes* species and *Mansonia africana.* In Asia, *Ae. aegypti* is responsible for urban epidemics (see Table 41.1 and Appendix IV).

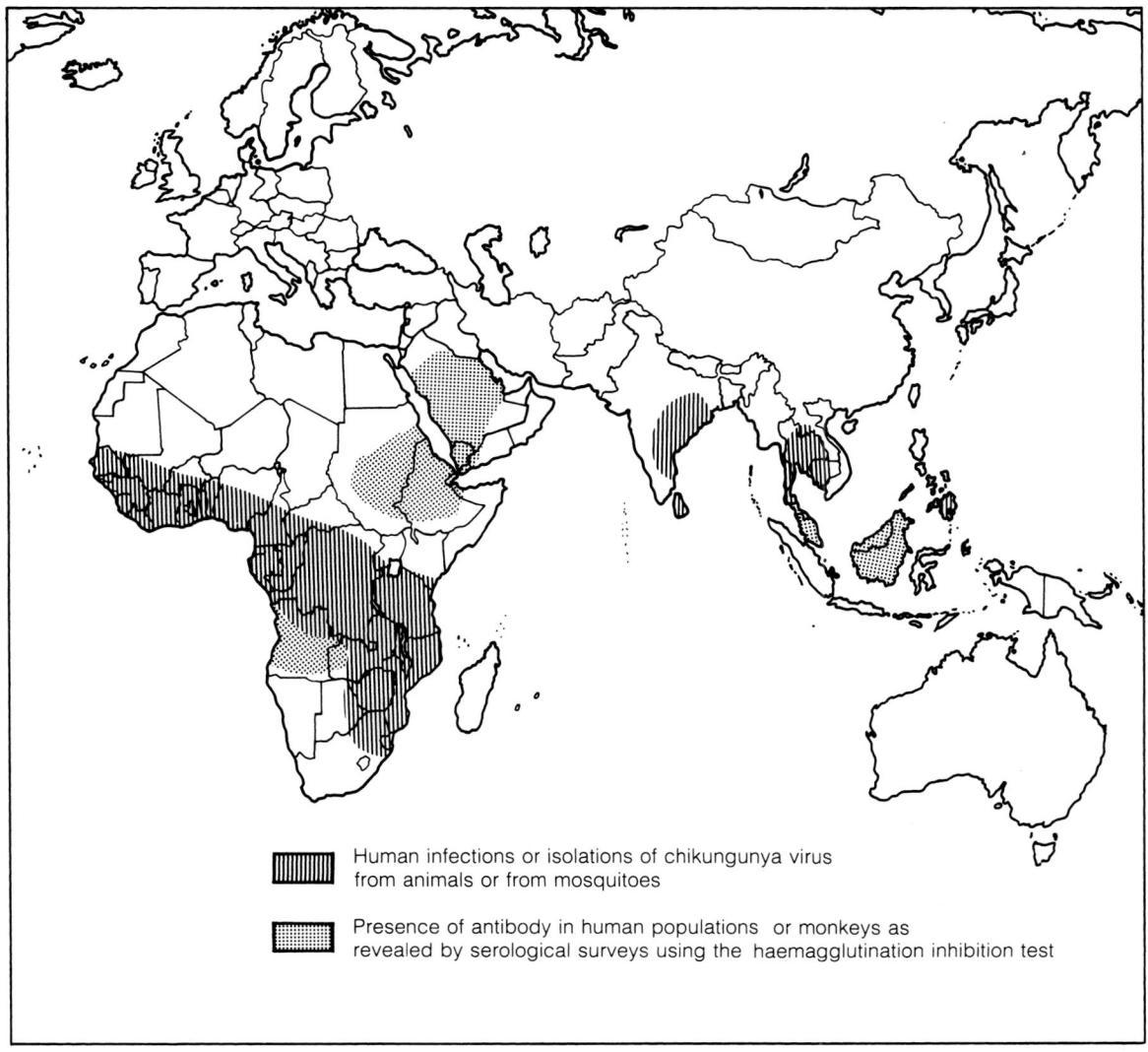

Figure 41.2: Geographical distribution of chikungunya virus. (Courtesy of the Department of Entomology, London School of Hygiene and Tropical Medicine.)

Pathology

The pathology is not known, but is probably the same as for dengue.

Clinical features

Natural history

The *incubation period* is 1–12 days, with an average of 2–3 days. Classical illness begins with the rapid onset of severe arthralgia. Back pain may be prominent. There is associated myalgia, high fever and conjunctivitis. This usually improves after 2–3 days and is followed by the onset of a generalized maculopapular rash. Fever may recur after a break of 1–2 days. Petechiae, bleeding from the gums and a positive tourniquet test have been seen in many patients and may lead to the infection being mistaken for dengue. The joint pains, myalgia, conjunctivitis and maculopapular rash are the most important distinguishing features. Some patients develop a febrile illness without rash or arthralgia. Most patients recover fully over a few weeks, although 5–10% experience chronic joint symptoms including pain, stiffness and swelling that may persist for years. The erythrocyte sedimentation rate is often mildly raised in acute and chronic disease.

Children who are infected are less likely to develop the characteristic clinical illness.

Diagnosis

Virus can be isolated from serum in the first 3–4 days of illness. IgM can be detected by IFA or EIA in acute sera and persists for weeks or months. Acute infection can be confirmed by HI and N titres on paired sera for antibodies. There are cross-reactions with other alphaviruses, especially SFV, ONN and RR viruses, although they are less frequent with IgM than with IgG. This may pose difficulties in Africa where SFV and ONN are also found, but in Asia the other viruses are not known to be present. In areas where both ONN and CHIK co-circulate, patients may have had previous infection with one of these. In that situation, recent infection with one may result in a misleading rise of specific antibody to the previous infecting virus.

Epidemiology

There is a forest cycle involving monkeys (vervets and baboons) transmitted by *Ae. africanus* and other mosquitoes. Rodents may also be hosts as they show a transient viraemia on being inoculated with virus, whereas monkeys show a high viraemia.

Equine encephalitides

Western equine encephalitis (WEE)[14,17,28]

Geographical distribution (Figure 41.3)

WEE is found in North America in Texas, Colorado and Saskatchewan, and in Argentina, Brazil, Mexico and Guyana, where human infections are unknown but equine epizootics occur.[28]

Aetiology

WEE is an alphavirus that is in the same group as SIN virus. It has several antigenic variants, particularly among the South American strains.

Transmission

Transmission is by mosquitoes. *Cx. tarsalis*, which feeds readily on birds, transmits the infection in the western USA, and *Culiseta malanura* in areas where *Cx. tarsalis* does not occur (eastern USA) (see Appendix IV).

Immunity

Immunity is antibody mediated and protects against second attacks. Serological surveys show inapparent infections, and children are most affected in epidemics.

Pathology

The CNS shows extensive changes with neuronal necrosis, perivascular inflammatory changes and meningeal inflammation. These are found in the cerebral cortex, striatum, thalamus and pons.

Clinical features

Natural history

The majority of infections are asymptomatic or non-specific. Encephalitis occurs in about 1 in 1000 adults, but about 1 in 50 children, especially infants. The case fatality rate is 3–7% and is highest in the elderly. Severe sequelae are largely confined to infants.

Symptoms and signs

The *incubation period* is 5–10 days.

The onset in older children and adults is gradual, with mild fever, malaise, headache, photophobia, nausea, vomiting and sore throat, sometimes with meningism and drowsiness. In the minority who progress to encephalitis, the fever and headache increases, with deterioration of conscious state, possibly with flaccid or spastic paralysis. Infants have a much more rapid course with fever, convulsions and coma. There is a peripheral leucocytosis in the early stages and the CSF shows a pleocytosis with increased protein levels in those with CNS involvement. Most adults recover fully, although this may take months. Some have residual paralysis, intellectual disability, epilepsy or neuropsychiatric disease. High rates of residual paralysis and severe intellectual impairment are seen in infants, especially those under 3 months.

Diagnosis

The virus may be isolated from serum early in illness, but this is unusual. It can be isolated from post-mortem brain and has been detected in the CSF in some cases. Recent infection can be diagnosed by the detection of rising titres in HI or N tests. IgM detection by EIA is usually positive in the serum at the time of presentation.

Epidemiology

WEE virus circulates in more than 75 species of wild birds and some domestic ones. The basic transmission cycle is between *Cx. tarsalis* and birds in the summer. Over-wintering of the virus may occur in hibernating mammals but more likely in overwintering mosquitoes. Epizootics in horses acting as amplifying hosts precede human epidemics. In humans, the highest attack rates are in infants and young males in a rural environment.

Control

Anti-mosquito measures are difficult in rural areas, but where small towns are involved 'fogging' with insecticide may terminate an epidemic. A non-neurotropic strain of virus isolated from birds has been used successfully as a vaccine, but only experimentally.

Eastern equine encephalitis (EEE)[14,17,29,30]

Geographical distribution (Figure 41.3)

EEE is found in the eastern USA (where epizootics occur in horses but human cases are rare), Mexico, Panama, Brazil, Argentina and Guyana. Two small human outbreaks have occurred in Dominica and Jamaica, and in 1962 there was a major epidemic of 6762 cases in Venezuela; 0.6% were fatal.

Aetiology

EEE virus is an alphavirus that occupies its own antigenic group. There are two major variants: North American (including Caribbean strains) and South American.

Transmission

Transmission is by mosquitoes; *Culiseta melanura* and *Cs. morsitans*, *Ae. sollicitans* and *Ae. taeniorhynchus* are the main vectors but isolations of virus have been made from other mosquitoes in the field (see Table 41.1 and Appendix IV).

Immunity

Immunity is antibody mediated and affords protection against second attacks.

Pathology

The CNS shows extensive changes with neuronal necrosis, perivascular inflammatory changes and meningeal inflammation. These are found in the cerebral cortex, hippocampus and pons, and more severely in the thalamus and basal ganglia. There is little involvement of the cerebellum and spinal cord.

Clinical features
Natural history

This is the most severe arboviral encephalitis of humans. While most infections are asymptomatic or mild, the rate of encephalitic disease is very high, being 5% or more. The mortality rate for encephalitis is 50–75%, with most survivors having severe sequelae. Outcomes are worst in children.

Signs and symptoms

The *incubation period* is 7–10 days.

The illness begins as a febrile illness lasting up to 11 days. In most this resolves, but in about 2% of adults and 6% of children there is sudden onset of encephalitis. Headache, meningism and reduction of conscious state develop. This progresses to coma and convulsions, with most dying in the first few days. There is a peripheral leucocytosis in the early stages, and the CSF usually shows an early polymorph pleocytosis, with a mildly to moderately raised protein level. Those who recover usually have intellectual disability, neuropsychiatric illness and possibly paralysis.

Diagnosis

It is possible to isolate the virus from patients in the prodromal period, but this is rarely achieved in practice. The virus can be isolated from post-mortem brain. Recent infection can be diagnosed by the detection of rising titres in HI or N tests. IgM detection by EIA is usually positive in the serum at the time of presentation.

Management

There is no specific treatment for this virus. High-level supportive therapy is required for patients with encephalitis.

Epidemiology

Transmission is maintained by birds and mosquitoes in an extensive geographical area. Infection of horses and humans is accidental, and in the centre of the area serological evidence of inapparent human infection can be found. EEE may cause a high mortality rate in birds, both wild and domestic. Infection in horses is severe, most dying within a few days.

Control

Mosquito control is the only method. Vaccination is not yet available.

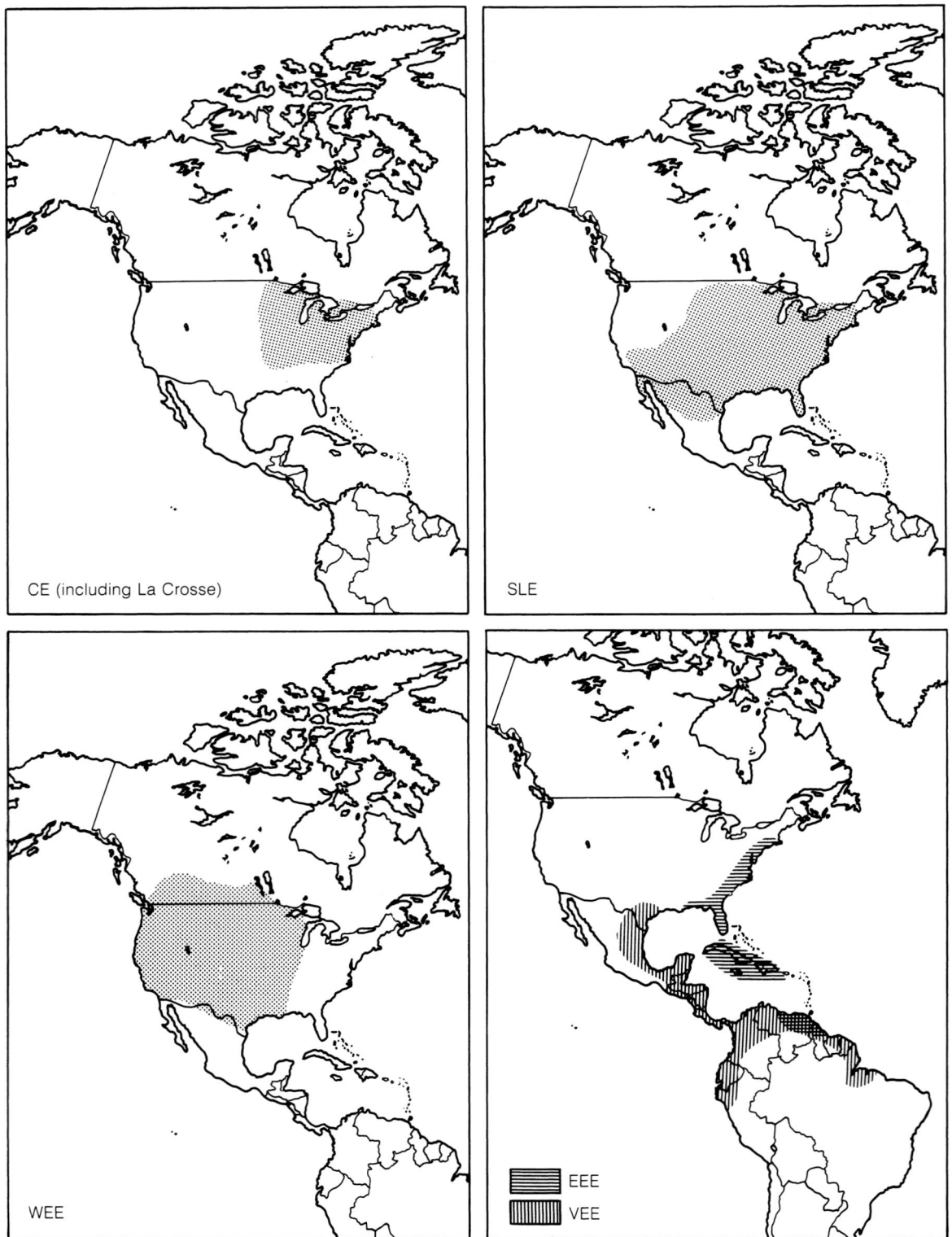

Figure 41.3: Geographical distribution of mosquito-borne encephalitis in the New World. CE, California encephalitis; SLE, St Louis encephalitis; WEE, Western equine encephalitis; EEE, Eastern equine encephalitis; VEE, Venezuelan equine encephalitis. (Courtesy of the Department of Entomology, London School of Hygiene and Tropical Medicine.)

Venezuelan equine encephalitis (VEE)[14,17,31,32]

Geographical distribution (Figure 41.3)

Extensive outbreaks with human cases have occurred in Venezuela (100 000 cases in 1962—almost wiping out the equine population), Trinidad, Colombia, Brazil and Panama. The virus is now extending its area and evidence of human infection has been found in Florida.

Aetiology

VEE virus is an alphavirus with a number of antigenic subtypes. The IABC subtypes cause epizootic disease, with associated epidemics of human infection. The other subtypes circulate enzootically and cause occasional human infections.

Transmission

The main vectors are *Ae. serratus* and *Ae. taeniorhynchus* and *Culex* species including *Cx. quinquefasciatus*. Isolations have been made from about 40 other species (see Table 41.1 and Appendix IV). *Simulium* spp. may transmit infections and there is a possibility of person-to-person spread by droplet infection; spread among horses can occur without an insect vector.

Immunity

Immunity is antibody mediated and provides protection against second attacks. It therefore takes about 10 years to build up a susceptible population of humans and equines to sustain a new epidemic.

Clinical features

Natural history

Most infections are inapparent and the majority of the overt infections are mild and transient, although virulence may vary in epidemics.

Signs and symptoms

The *incubation period* is 2–5 days.

The onset is sudden, with fevers, rigors, headache and myalgia. A sore throat and upper respiratory symptoms are a feature, as are vomiting and conjunctivitis. Some also have diarrhoea. In some cases, and in about 4% of children under 15 years of age, symptoms progress with involvement of the CNS. Neck stiffness, convulsions, coma, and flaccid or spastic paralysis may develop. There is an initial leucopenia and sometimes thrombocytopenia, with pleocytosis and raised protein levels in the CSF. Long-term sequelae seem to be uncommon, and mental depression is common.

Aerial spread can occur, so appropriate precautions should be instituted in the hospital to protect staff, visitors and other patients.

Diagnosis

Virus may be isolated from the blood in the acute phase, especially within 48 hours of onset, and also from the throat. Recently a RT-PCR-based method has shown good results for detection of virus in the serum. Recent infection can be diagnosed by the detection of rising titres in HI or N tests. IgM detection by EIA is usually positive in the serum within 1 week of onset.

Aerosol spread can occur and laboratory-acquired infections are well documented. The virus and samples likely to contain virus should be handled with extreme caution, and people working with the virus should be vaccinated.

Management

There is no specific treatment for this virus. High-level supportive therapy is required for encephalitis cases.

Vaccination

A live attenuated vaccine (TC-83) is available for primary immunization against the epidemic strains. It does not elicit good responses in people with previous alphavirus infections, nor is it very effective as a booster. An inactivated vaccine (C-84) seems to be better for these applications.

Epidemiology

VEE virus circulates silently in small mammals and, with a high rainfall and an increase in the number of mosquitoes and their biting, horses become infected, acting as amplifying hosts. Equine cases precede human cases, most commonly children in whom the disease is more severe. A high proportion of equines develop immunity so that 10 years is necessary to build up another susceptible population.

Control

Mosquito control is difficult in rural conditions.

Mayaro[33]

Mayaro virus is an alphavirus found initially in Trinidad and has since been recognized in Central and South America. It is transmitted by *Haemagogus* mosquitoes, and primates may serve as the animal hosts. Human disease resembles CHIK and some develop persisting arthralgias (see Table 41.1 and Appendix IV).

Ockelbo

Ockelbo virus is closely related to SIN virus and causes a very similar disease. It is responsible for summer outbreaks in Sweden, Finland and Russia.

O'nyong-nyong (ONN)[14,17,34,35]

Geographical distribution

ONN is present in Uganda, Kenya, Tanzania and southern Sudan (Figure 41.4).

Aetiology

ONN virus is an alphavirus closely related to CHIK.

Transmission

Anopheles funestus is the major vector but *An. gambiae* is also involved (see Appendix IV).

Clinical features

The clinical illness is very similar to CHIK, with the exception that generalized lymphadenopathy is common, while fever is less prominent.

Epidemiology

There is no animal reservoir and the cycle is purely from person to person. Large epidemics occur when there are enough susceptible subjects, in which 70% of the population may be attacked, with all the age groups affected.

Control

Wearing of mosquito nets and anti-*An. funestus* measures will control the epidemics.

Ross River virus disease (epidemic polyarthritis)[14,17,23,36]

Geographical distribution

RR virus disease occurs annually in epidemics in northern and eastern Australia, and epidemically in Fiji, American Samoa, Cook Islands and New Caledonia. Antibody

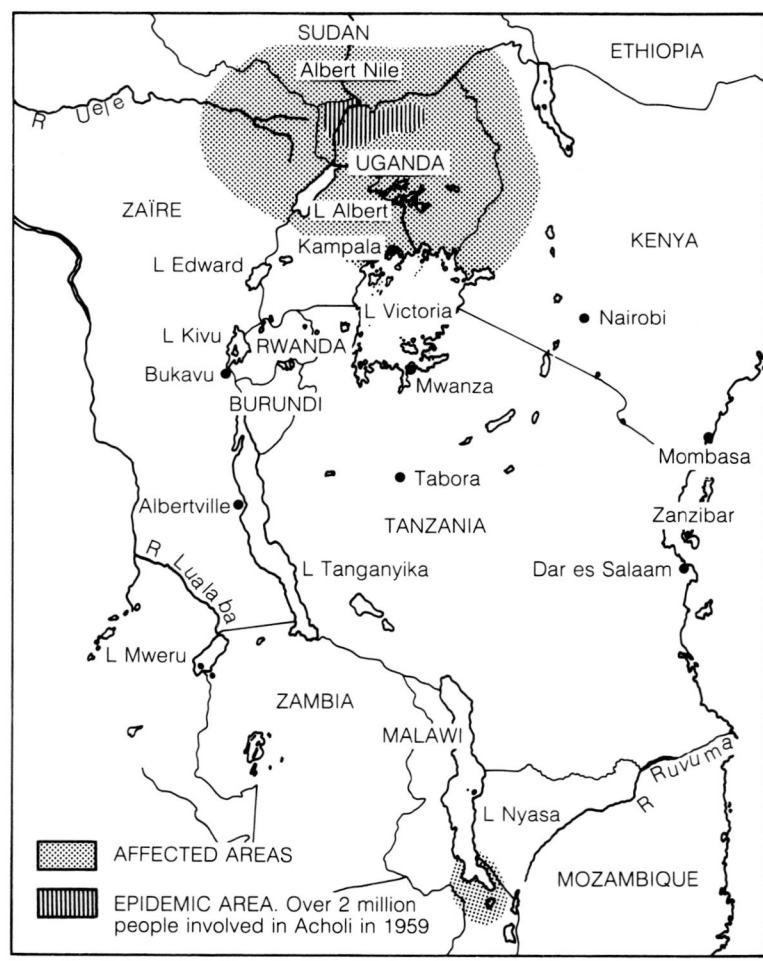

Figure 41.4: Geographical distribution of o'nyong-nyong fever. (Courtesy of the Department of Entomology, London School of Hygiene and Tropical Medicine.)

studies have shown infection to be present in New Guinea, Solomon Islands, the Moluccas and Vietnam.

Transmission

Transmission is by *Ae. vigilax*, *Ae. camptorhynchus* and *Cx. annulirostris* in Australia[37] and *Ae. polynesiensis* in the Cook Islands.[38] *Ae. aegypti* and *Ae. albopictus* are efficient experimental vectors (see Table 41.1 and Appendix IV).

Pathology

Observation based on examinations of joint fluids suggests that the virus multiplies in synovial cells in early arthritis and it may possibly persist within joint macrophages. However, the pathogenesis of acute and chronic disease is not well understood.

Clinical features
Natural history
The *incubation period* for RR virus disease is usually 7–9 days but may vary from 5 to 21 days.

Illness usually begins as joint pains (in a distribution typical of alphavirus arthritis) and myalgia, accompanied by lethargy in most patients and fever in about half. A generalized maculopapular rash occurs in 50%, usually after the onset of joint pains but sometimes preceding it. The rash is occasionally vesicular. Headache, photophobia, sore throat and lymphadenopathy may accompany the acute illness. Overall joint pains, swelling and stiffness develop in 80–90% of individuals. The swelling is largely due to synovitis without effusion. The lethargy may be profound and debilitating. The acute illness may resolve over weeks to months, but about 25% will have joint pains, lethargy and myalgia persisting for over a year, and for several years in some. The chronic illness often follows a relapsing and remitting course.

Diagnosis

Viraemia lasts only a few days and infection is rarely diagnosed by virus isolation. IgG and IgM can be detected by HI, EIA or IFA. There is some cross-reaction with antibody to other alphavirus such as BF, SIN and CHIK, but IgM reactions are usually limited to the infecting virus. If necessary, specific antibody may be identified by N titres. IgM persists for many months after infection and is therefore only a presumptive indicator of recent infection. Demonstration of seroconversion or a significant rise in IgG levels is required to confirm recent infection.

Management

Treatment is symptomatic, with judicious use of non-steroidal anti-inflammatory agents and simple analgesics for the relief of joint and muscle pains. Physiotherapy and graduated exercise programmes help some people. The use of steroids should be avoided until there is a better understanding of the pathogenesis of this disease and their value is proven.

Epidemiology

Macropods (kangaroos and wallabies) are thought to be the natural vertebrae hosts, but in epidemics the virus can spread from person to person. In Australia cases occur annually between summer and autumn. Explosive epidemics have occurred in Fiji, Samoa and the Cook Islands when the disease encountered a fresh non-immune population. Infection rates were 90%, with 40% of the population showing clinical attacks.

Sindbis[14,17]

Geographical distribution
SIN infection occurs in Europe, Africa, Asia and Australia, and the virus appears to be widespread in these regions.

Aetiology

SIN is an alphavirus in the Western equine encephalitis serogroup. There are two antigenic lineages: the Oriental/Australian and the Palearctic/Ethiopian.

Transmission

Transmission to birds is via various *Culex* species, including *Cx. univittatus* and *Cx. pipiens*. *Aedes* species probably transmit infection to humans.

Clinical features
Natural history
There has been only a small number of documented human cases. The *incubation period* is up to 1 week. Onset is usually joint pains typical of alphavirus infection, usually accompanied by a rash, malaise and fatigue. Fever is mild or absent. The rash is initially widespread and maculopapular, with a tendency to develop vesicles on the extremities. True arthritis may be uncommon, but tendonitis is common. The illness duration and chronicity are similar to that seen with CHIK and RR viruses.

Diagnosis

HI antibody can be detected but does cross-react with other alphaviruses. IgM can be detected by EIA, IFA, as well as HI.

Management

Treatment is symptomatic, as for other alphavirus arthritides.

Epidemiology

SIN virus is maintained primarily in a mosquito–bird cycle. Birds develop a prolonged viraemia, and infected migratory birds may be responsible for spread of the virus.

Flaviviruses

Dengue (see also Chapter 42)[20,29,39,40–42]

Geographical distribution

Dengue has a worldwide tropical and subtropical distribution between 30°N and 40°S (Figure 41.5). It is endemic in South-East Asia, the Pacific, West Africa, East Africa, the Caribbean and the Americas. Occasional epidemics occur owing to periodic reintroduction in north-eastern Australia. There has been a worldwide resurgence of dengue virus in the past 50 years. The virus has spread and the number of epidemics has increased, often with multiple serotypes circulating simultaneously. Accompanying this has been the emergence of epidemic dengue haemorrhagic fever (DHF). Epidemic DHF is a perennial problem in South-East Asia, where it is a major cause of child morbidity and mortality. It has gradually spread west to India, Sri Lanka, Pakistan and the Maldives, as well as east to China and into the islands of south and central Pacific. Following the elimination of most *Ae. aegypti* from Central and South America, dengue became uncommon in the Americas. However, after a large epidemic in Cuba in the early 1980s and the spread of *Ae. aegypti*, dengue has been re-established in Central America, much of South America and the south-east of the USA, with the appearance of epidemic DHF in some areas. Sporadic DHF does occur in Africa, but epidemic disease has not yet been described.

Aetiology

Dengue is an RNA virus in the flavivirus group. It is 17–25 nm in diameter and can be grown in a variety of mosquitoes and tissue cultures. It possesses antigens that overlap with YF, JE and WN viruses, and there are four serotypes (1, 2, 3 and 4), all of which can be involved in both classical dengue and dengue haemorrhagic fever. Dengue virus can be passed vertically in *Aedes* experimentally; however, the epidemiological significance of this is uncertain.

Transmission

Dengue is transmitted by mosquitoes (see Table 41.1 and Appendix IV). The classical type is transmitted worldwide by *Ae. aegypti* and *Ae. albopictus* (Asia, Philippines and Japan); *Ae. polynesiensis*, *Ae. scutellaris* and *Ae. pseudoscutellaris* (Pacific islands and New Guinea); *Ae. polynesiensis* (Society Islands); and *Ae. niveus* (Philippines). Mosquitoes can be infected from the onset until the fourth day of illness and become infective from 8 to 11 days after feeding, remaining infective for life. In nature, transovarial transmission of dengue types 2 and 4 by *Ae. aegypti* has been demonstrated.

Pathology

After inoculation the virus rapidly spreads to regional lymph nodes and then more widely through the reticuloendothelial system. It appears to replicate

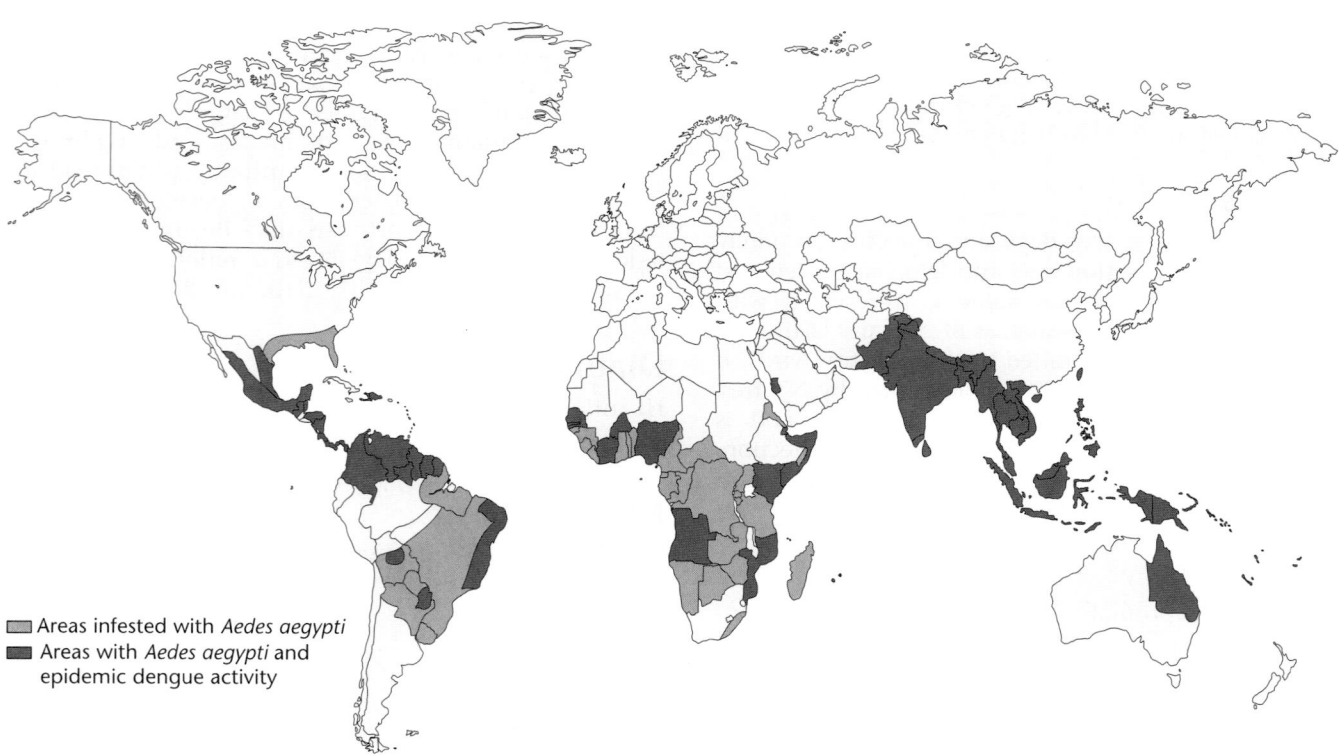

Areas infested with *Aedes aegypti*
Areas with *Aedes aegypti* and epidemic dengue activity

Figure 41.5: Geographical distribution of dengue and *Aedes aegypti*. (Courtesy of the Centers for Disease Control, Fort Collins, Colorado, USA.)

primarily in phagocytic macrophages and monocytes, but possibly in various lymphocyte populations as well. Viraemia begins 3–7 days after infection. Virus persists in the infected mononuclear cells after clearance of viraemia. The speed and extent of viral spread appears to be much higher in secondary infections compared with primary ones. With onset of effective antibody responses there is normally resolution of viraemia and recovery. However, this is also the period in which progression to DHF may occur, especially in those with secondary dengue infections. There is considerable evidence that DHF is largely a result of enhanced viral replication due to the presence of heterotypic non-neutralizing antibody. Consistent with this is that virtually all cases occur in patients with secondary dengue infection. However, the likelihood of developing DHF may also be modified by other factors such as the age of the patient and the combination of serotypes responsible for primary and secondary infection. In DHF there is widespread dissemination of virus into a large number of organs, including the liver, spleen, heart, bone marrow and, rarely, the brain. Haemorrhages may occur due to thrombocytopenia and platelet dysfunction. More severe cases have a general coagulopathy. There is also a generalized abnormality of the vascular endothelium resulting in extensive leakage of fluid from the intravascular compartment.

Dengue replicates in the liver and increased levels of liver enzymes are common. Necrotic changes may occur and rarely result in fulminant hepatic failure. Hepatomegaly due to fluid leakage from the intravascular space is seen in DHF. The *kidneys* rarely show glomerulonephritis, probably due to immune complexes. There is *reticuloendothelial* reaction (proliferation of lymphocytes, plasmacytoid cells and increase in phagocytosis), maturation arrest of *megakaryocytes* and hypocellularity of the bone marrow. Capillary damage results in leakage of fluid, plasma and erythrocytes into interstitial spaces and serous cavities, causing pleural and peritoneal effusions, and retroperitoneal oedema. Haemorrhages are not generally severe but major gastrointestinal bleeding is found in most fatal cases.

Immunity

Immunity is antibody mediated and after recovery there is a long-standing immunity to the homologous strain but none to other serotypes or other flaviviruses. In fact, it appears that infection with one serotype increases the risk of more severe disease if there is a subsequent infection with another serotype. It is likely that the cross-reacting antibody binds to the new serotype but does not neutralize it. There is then enhanced uptake of the antibody-coated virus into macrophages and other mononuclear cells, leading to accelerated viral replication. A similar phenomenon may occur in infants who have circulating maternal antibody.

Clinical features

The *incubation period* is 2–7 days.

Natural history

Classical dengue is a short-lived infection with complete recovery and is not usually fatal, but under certain circumstances it may cause a severe haemorrhagic fever which can be fatal. DHF had a mortality rate of 10% in the past, but with good supportive care this can be reduced to less than 1%.

Symptoms and signs
Classical dengue
Classical dengue occurs in older children and adults. The onset is sudden with high fever (40°C), severe muscle pains ('break bone fever'), headache and prostration, often accompanied by flushing of the face, retro-orbital discomfort and conjunctival inflammation. An early transient erythematous rash occurs in about half of cases. The fever continues for 4–6 days with anorexia, constipation and restlessness. The tourniquet test may show capillary fragility, and mild haemorrhagic manifestations (epistaxis, petechiae and purpura) may appear. The platelet count usually remains above 100 000/mm³ but occasionally drops much lower. Leucopenia may also occur. Resolution of fever is rapid and often followed by appearance of a morbilliform or scarlatiniform rash, beginning on the extremities, accompanied by generalized lymphadenopathy. Petechiae may be present, especially on the legs. Abnormalities of liver enzymes are common, but hepatomegaly is unusual unless the patient progresses to more severe disease. The second febrile phase lasts 2–3 days and the rash then desquamates. Convalescence is long and may be accompanied by general debility and depression. Classical dengue is seldom fatal.

Infection in young children is usually milder and less characteristic. They often present with fever, malaise, cough, vomiting, headache and/or abdominal pain. The physical findings and investigations may be similar to those above, but abnormalities are fewer and less severe.

Dengue haemorrhagic fever
DHF is defined by the World Health Organization as dengue accompanied by minor or major haemorrhagic manifestations (or a positive tourniquet test), thrombocytopenia (< 100 000/ml), and objective evidence of increased capillary permeability such as haemoconcentration (haematocrit increased by ≤ 20%), pleural effusion on chest radiography or other imaging methods, ascites or hypoproteinaemia. If there is also hypotension or narrow pulse pressure (≤ 20 mmHg), then the condition meets the criteria for dengue shock syndrome (DSS). Most cases occur in children.

On days 2–5 of classical dengue illness at the end of the first phase, the patient deteriorates rapidly, with development of the shock syndrome. Restlessness, sweating and hypotension appear, coincident with a positive tourniquet test, petechiae, purpura and spontaneous haemorrhages from the gums and gastrointestinal tract. There is tender enlargement of the liver in some cases, with hypoproteinaemia, hyponatraemia and a mild increase in the levels of the liver enzymes.

Thrombocytopenia may be profound (< 10 000/ml) and there may be a dysfunction of the remaining platelets. The presence of disseminated intravascular coagulation is shown by the alteration in clotting factors and reduced fibrinogen levels. Leucopenia may occur, but is usually not severe or prolonged. The clinical illness and progress are largely determined by the degree of haemorrhage and hypotension. Respiratory failure due to fluid accumulation and alveolar haemorrhage is common in severe cases. Renal failure may develop secondary to hypotension and possibly immune complex deposition. Encephalopathy occurs uncommonly and, at least in some cases, is due to a true dengue encephalitis.

Diagnosis

Virus detection

This is not usually undertaken as a routine diagnostic test. Virus may be isolated from serum or tissues in the early stages of illness. The sample is cultured by inoculation on to cell cultures: LLC-MK2 or Vero cells, cells of *Ae. albopictus*, *Ae. pseudoscutellaris*, or *Toxorhynchites amboinensis* and examined after 7–14 days by IFA. Dengue viruses can also be cultured by intrathoracic inoculation of live mosquitoes belonging to the *Toxorhynchites* genus. N tests or IFA with type-specific monoclonal antibodies can be used for typing. RNA detection by PCR has been found to be quicker and easier than culture. It is particularly useful in early infection before the appearance of antibody, and for severe cases where confirmation of the diagnosis is particularly important. It can be performed on CSF and on postmortem tissues. Virus can be typed with specific primers or by sequencing or probing of the product. The early stages of the febrile illness must be distinguished from malaria, typhoid and hepatitis. Chikungunya, sandfly fever and RVF can closely resemble dengue.

Serological diagnosis

The HI test, EIA or IFA performed on acute stage serum taken in the first 4 days and convalescent serum taken 2–3 weeks later will show a 4-fold increase to one or more of the four serotype antigens. Antibody responses are more rapid and reach higher titres in secondary infections. IgM can be detected in serum of nearly all cases within a few days of onset. Although not specific in itself, determination of IgM is sufficient to diagnose dengue within the appropriate clinical and epidemiological setting. Otherwise, characterization of IgG by N tests or other specific tests is needed to confirm dengue antibody. IgM may persist for weeks or months in the serum. Testing of CSF may be undertaken in suspected dengue encephalitis.

Identification of the infecting serotype requires N tests against the four serotypes. These may be misleading in secondary dengue when the antibody to the previous infecting serotype may rise more rapidly.

Management

There is no specific treatment available for dengue. Mild dengue resolves with symptomatic care. In view of the coagulation problems, paracetamol is the preferred analgesic/antipyretic rather than aspirin. Management of DHF is complex owing to the potential severity of the illness and the multiple organ systems involved. Adequate fluid replacement is essential, although overload will worsen the fluid accumulation in the tissues. Fluid loss in DHF can initially be replaced with 5% dextrose in saline, Ringer's lactate or similar, but if this fails then plasma, plasma substitutes or colloidal solutions may be needed. If the haemoglobin concentration is falling, blood transfusion is needed. Respiratory and renal support are used as required. Transfusion of fresh human platelet concentrates may be required in severe thrombocytopenia, although in late stages with established DIC, platelets may worsen the disease. Management of DIC requires a delicate balance of fluid replacement, anticoagulants and coagulation factors.

Isolation of the patient is not necessary, except that mosquitoes should be excluded by mosquito nets or screens in situations where they may gain access to the patient.

Epidemiology

A jungle cycle of dengue involving forest mosquitoes and wild monkeys has been postulated in Malaya and West Africa where antibodies have been found in monkeys, the significance of which is not clear.

Dengue fever epidemics involve many thousands of cases, with attack rates of 75–80%, completely disrupting the life of communities. These epidemics result from the introduction of a new serotype or the availability of a susceptible population (immigrants and young persons born since the last epidemic). These epidemics have swept up the Caribbean and eastern seaboard of the Americas and up the eastern shores of East Africa, involving the islands. More recently, dengue has caused vast epidemics in South-East Asia.

Most cases of DHF occur in children less than 16 years old. As discussed above, the recent decades have seen the emergence and spread of epidemic DHF, reflecting the resurgence of dengue and the presence of multiple serotypes during epidemics.

Control

Control of dengue rests upon vector control, mainly the domestic breeding of *Ae. aegypti* in domestic water containers. The *Aedes* index can be used to monitor populations of mosquitoes and hence foresee outbreaks and institute proper vector control. Control measures for DHF are those applied to classical dengue fever. A satisfactory vaccine has yet to be developed. However, immunization with vaccines presents a problem because an individual with antibodies to one serotype runs the danger of developing DHF when infected with another serotype. Therefore vaccine development is aimed at tetravalent vaccines that elicit good neutralizing antibody to all serotypes.

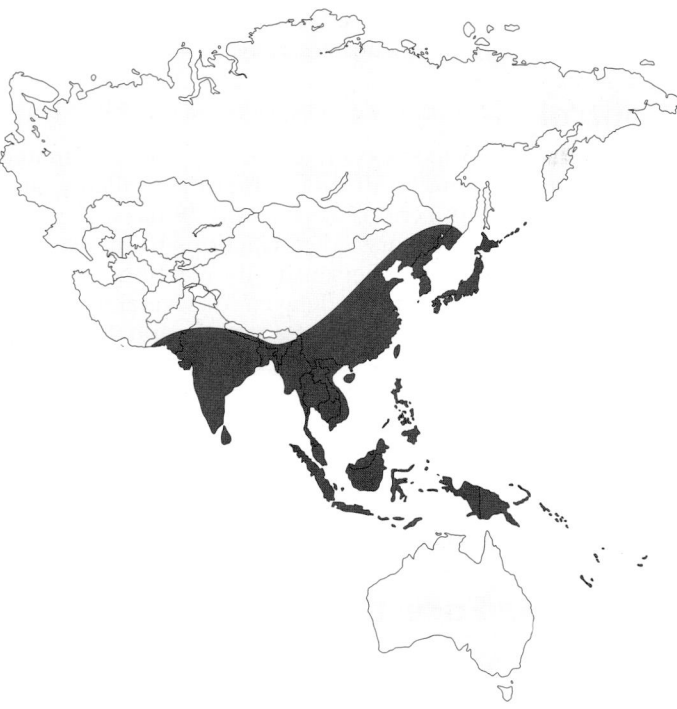

Figure 41.6: Geographical distribution of Japanese encephalitis virus.

Japanese encephalitis (JE)[43–48]

Geographical distribution

The geographical range of JE now extends from Japan, maritime Siberia and Korea in the north, through all except two provinces of China to the Philippines in the east and through South-East and southern Asia to Sri Lanka, India and Nepal in the west (Figure 41.6). More recently, JE has spread to Pakistan and India in the west, and to the Torres Strait and has been detected once in far north Queensland in Australia.

Aetiology

JE virus is 50 nm in diameter and shares antigens with SLE and MVE.

Transmission

Culex tritaeniorhynchus, a rice-field breeding mosquito, is the main vector in north Asia and Japan. Other vectors include *Cx. annulirostris* in Guam and northern Australia, *Cx. gelidus* and *Cx. fusocephala* in India, Malaysia and Thailand, and *Cx. vishnui* in India (see Table 41.1 and Appendix IV). Vertical transmission of JE in both *Culex* and *Aedes* mosquitoes has been demonstrated.

Pathology

After inoculation, the virus may replicate in the lymphatic tissues and possibly other organs before invading the CNS. In the brain there are areas of necrosis with small haemorrhages and perivascular cuffing in the grey matter of the cerebral cortex and in the thalamus, midbrain, cerebellum, brainstem and anterior horns of the spinal cord.

Immunity

An antibody-mediated immunity protects against second attacks and builds up resistance in the population.

Clinical features

Natural history

Many infections are asymptomatic or non-specific, with encephalitis estimated to occur in only 1 in 300 infections. Encephalitis has a mortality rate of 10–25%, but rises to 40–50% for comatosed patients.

The *incubation period* is 6–16 days.

The onset is sudden, although it may be preceded by gastrointestinal disturbance, especially in children. Fever, headache, altered mental state and convulsions are the main presenting features. Patients may show generalized weakness or paralysis, cranial nerve palsies and a coarse tremor. A characteristic attitude with head retracted, arms and knees bent, and shoulders pressed to the chest has been described (Figure 41.7). Some patients make a rapid and complete recovery, but generally severe depression of conscious state and/or evidence of respiratory paralysis are poor prognostic signs. If the acute stage is survived, recovery is slow and 25–50% will have neurological residua. These include paralysis, ataxia, Parkinsonism, mental deterioration, psychiatric disorders and speech difficulties.

The CSF usually shows a lymphocytic pleocytosis and the protein concentration is normal or moderately raised. Electroencephalography (EEG) and CT findings are usually non-specific, but MRI has proven more useful in showing changes.

A variety of psychiatric disturbances has been described in patients several months after recovering from the acute infection.

Diagnosis

The virus has occasionally been cultured from human material, mainly CSF in severe cases. The viraemia is

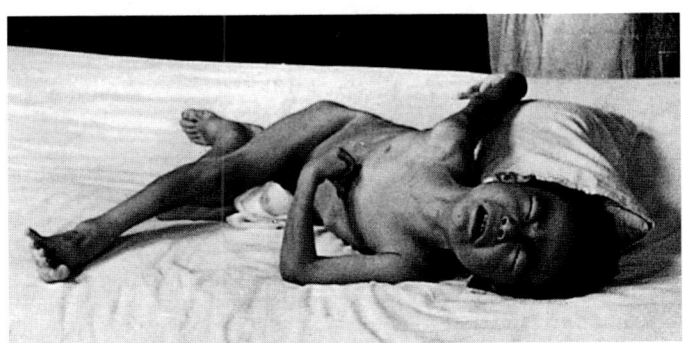

Figure 41.7: A 5-year-old boy with Japanese encephalitis.

likely to be short lived and samples should be collected early in infection. JE virus will grow in mosquito cell lines, some other cell lines and suckling mouse brain. A RT-PCR method has been described and should be useful for virus detection in serum, CSF and brain. Antigen detection methods have also been used for virus detection in brain.

Paired sera taken in the first few days after onset and 2–3 weeks later will show rising antibody levels by HI test, EIA or IFA. IgM is usually detected by EIA or IFA and is present in the serum in the early stages of illness in 80% of cases. IgM may persist for weeks or months in the serum. Antibody will cross-react broadly with other flaviviruses. The specificity of antibody can be determined by N tests.

Management

Treatment is supportive, and access to high-level support is important in the survival of severe cases. Dexamethasone has not been shown to influence the outcome and is not recommended unless needed to reduce intracranial pressure. There are preliminary data on the possible effectiveness of α-interferon for treatment of JE.

Epidemiology

The main source of infection is the rice fields where the vector *Cx. tritaeniorhynchus* breeds, becoming infected from pigs or birds. Three weeks after mosquito breeding begins in the spring, virus can be found in birds and pigs, but humans are not involved until there is a high density of mosquitoes. The infection is amplified by pigs and conveyed to humans. Birds (night herons and egrets) carry the infection from rural to urban areas. There is a seasonal summer incidence, with epidemics every year in Japan. Most cases are in children and elderly people, although visitors of any age are affected.

Control

An inactivated vaccine derived from the attenuated Nakayama strain grown in mouse brain is available, and is given in three injections at 0, 7 and 28 days. Boosters are required every 3 years. Local reactions to the vaccine are common. Serious hypersensitivity reactions occur in 1 in 200 people, and may be delayed for several days after administration. Several cases of acute encephalomyelitis have been reported following vaccination, but it is not yet certain that these are due to the vaccine. Two other vaccines are currently used extensively in China, including the live SA14/14/2 attenuated vaccine. Vector control using chemical larvicides and adulticides has been successful in many areas, although there are increasing problems with insecticide resistance.

Kyasanur Forest disease (KFD)[49–51]

Local synonym: 'Monkey disease'

Geographical distribution (Figure 41.8)

KFD was first described in 1957 in the Kyasanur Forest of Mysore (now Karnataka) in southwestern India, but has been gradually spreading from there.

Aetiology

KFD virus is a flavivirus (see Table 41.1) antigenically related to TBE, OHF and WN viruses, but there is no cross-immunity.

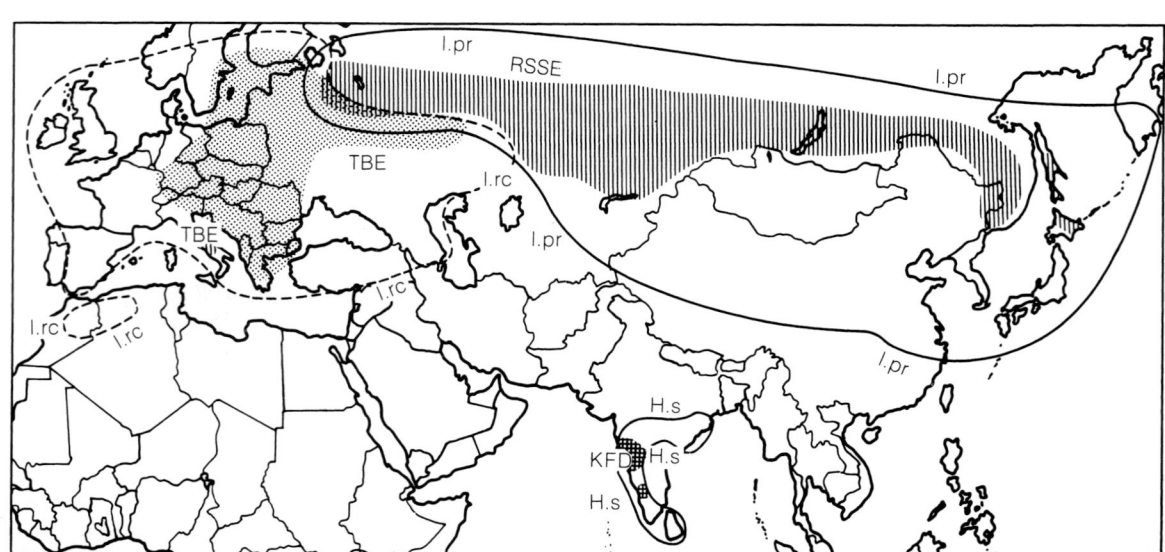

Figure 41.8: Geographical distribution of tick-borne encephalitis—RSSE, Russian spring–summer encephalitis (Eastern subtype TBE); TBE, European tick-borne encephalitis (Western subtype TBE); KFD, Kyasanur Forest disease—and the main vectors. I.pr, *Ixodes persulcatus*; I.rc, *Ixodes ricinus*; H.s, *Haemophysalis spinigera*. (Courtesy of the Department of Entomology, London School of Hygiene and Tropical Medicine.)

Transmission

KFD virus is transmitted by the nymphal stages of ticks that have been infected in the larval stage from a rodent or monkey. The ticks are *Haemaphysalis spinigera, H. turturis* and *H. papuana (kinneari)*. KFD virus is also carried by *Ixodes petauristae* and *I. ceylonensis*, and has been recovered from *Dermacentor* nymphs. KFD is not normally transmitted from person to person, but the blood is potentially infective until the 12th day (see Table 41.1 and Appendix IV).

Pathology

There are degenerative changes in the large organs. The spleen shows reduction of malpighian corpuscles and erythrophagocytosis. There is focal haemorrhagic bronchopneumonia with focal necrosis of the liver and gastrointestinal tract. The kidneys show acute degeneration of the proximal and collecting tubules. There is no encephalitis (monkeys show encephalitis and anterior horn cell damage).

Immunity

Immunity is antibody mediated. Little is known about immunity to second attacks, but monkeys that recover are immune. There is no cross-immunity to other flaviviruses.

Clinical features

Natural history

KFD is mainly a severe febrile illness with complete recovery following a prolonged convalescence. However, meningoencephalitis and/or haemorrhagic disease may develop in a small proportion of cases. The mortality rate is 3–5%, and no sequelae have been reported in survivors.

Signs and symptoms

The *incubation period* is 3–8 days after the infective tick bite. In about 20% of cases the disease is biphasic.

The onset is sudden with fever, headache, myalgia, cough, vomiting, diarrhoea, dehydration, hypotension and bradycardia. In the majority of cases there are no haemorrhages, but gastrointestinal bleeding and haemoptysis may occur. After 10 days the illness subsides. In 20% of cases, the fever returns 1–2 weeks after the first phase, lasting 1–7 days. There may then be symptoms of meningoencephalitis, with neck stiffness, mental disturbance, tremors and giddiness, lasting until the fever subsides. After recovery there is a prolonged convalescence, the patient remaining weak for some time. There is a marked leucopenia and a heavy albuminuria with casts in the urine. The CSF is normal in the first phase, but shows increased levels of protein but without cells in the second phase.

Diagnosis

Virus can be isolated from the blood up until the 12th day in suckling mice, hamster or monkey kidney cells or HeLa cells with cytopathic effect. Serological diagnosis can be made with rising antibody (IFA, HI and N) titres in acute and convalescent sera, as well as by EIA tests.

Management

Treatment is supportive. Care must be taken in the first 12 days to avoid contamination of medical and nursing staff with blood.

Epidemiology

KFD virus circulates in forest rodents, especially the shrew (*Suncus murinus*) but also *Rattus wroughtoni, R. blandfordi* and a squirrel (*Funambulus tristriatus*), maintained mainly by larval ticks of *H. spinigera, H. turturis* and *H. papuana (kinneari)*.

Langur monkeys (*Presbytes entellus*) and bonnet macaques (*Macaca radiata*) acquire larval ticks when foraging on the ground and become infected. Many die, but some recover and are immune for life. When infected, the monkeys show a heavy viraemia. The larvae emerge from the ground as nymphs and come into contact with humans, to whom they transmit the infection as a dead-end infection.

Birds (grey jungle fowl and golden-backed woodpecker) are important because they carry adult ticks around and can therefore spread the infection; although antibodies have been found in some, they are not thought to play a role in maintaining the infection in nature.

Amplifying mechanism

Under natural conditions the contact of humans and monkeys with ticks is low, and to raise the number of ticks to epizootic levels it is necessary to increase their numbers and the rate of infection. Monkeys provide an efficient source of infection because of their heavy viraemia, and the number of ticks is increased by human activity in bringing cattle into the forest where they provide a good source of food for *Haemaphysalis* ticks, thus increasing their numbers. The monkeys move around the forest, forming foci of infection. KFD has spread since humans invaded the forest for rice cultivation, timber extraction and cattle ranching. The cut-down forest forms an interface of lantana thicket in which many species of birds nest and which is crossed by innumerable trails used by cattle, deer, ground birds and small mammals. Infection of humans is basically an occupational disease contracted by people who enter the forest, and is preceded by illness and death in langur and macaque monkeys.

Control

Control is essentially a breaking of the tick–human contact. Alteration of the environment and keeping cattle out of the forest are important. Personal protection involves regular (daily) de-ticking of the body and the use of repellents and protective clothing. A formalin-inactivated vaccine produced in chick embryo fibroblasts is now used in the endemic areas.

Kunjin (KUN)[52]

KUN is a flavivirus in the JE antigenic group. It is now considered to be a subtype of WN virus. Human infection and disease have been demonstrated only in Australia, although the virus has been isolated from mosquitoes in South-East Asia. The distribution, reservoirs and transmission seem to be the same as for MVE. Most infections are asymptomatic, although some produce a febrile illness with headache, with or without arthralgia, myalgia, fatigue and a maculopapular rash. Rare encephalitis cases occur that are clinically identical to MVE.

Louping ill (LI)[53]

Louping ill is a sheep virus transmitted by *Ixodes ricinus* and found in the UK and parts of southern Europe. It causes an illness very similar to the Western subtype TBE, and the vaccine for that virus will also protect against LI.

Murray Valley encephalitis (MVE)[52,54–57]

Geographical distribution

MVE is found in Australia and New Guinea. Human disease has been identified mainly in the tropical northern areas of Australia, particularly the western and central areas of the north. Epidemic activity occasionally occurs outside these regions, and rarely it extends to the south-eastern corner of the mainland.

Aetiology

MVE is a flavivirus that lies in the JE antigenic group.

Transmission

Cx. annulirostris is the major mosquito vector. MVE has also been isolated from a number of *Aedes* species and vertical transmission in these mosquitoes is proposed as a mechanism of persistence in many arid areas.

Pathology

The pathology of MVE is similar to that of JE, with perivascular cuffing in the grey matter, most marked in the thalamus and substantia nigra. These may extend into cerebral white matter, cerebellum and spinal cord. In more advanced disease there is neuronal loss and areas of focal necrosis in the basal ganglia and thalamus. In severe residual disease these changes are more marked and thalamic necrosis may be seen.

Clinical features

The majority of infections are asymptomatic or non-specific. Only about 1 in 500 to 1 in 1000 develop encephalitis.

The *incubation period* is not well established, but is in the range of 1–3 weeks.

Non-encephalitis illness consists of fever and headache, with or without arthralgia. It settles over 1–2 weeks, although full recovery may take some time. Encephalitic illness in children presents as fever of 1–2 days' duration, almost always with convulsions. Reduction of mental state and respiratory failure may follow. Some patients recover rapidly, whereas others progress to more severe disease characterized by involvement of central brain structures, brain stem and possibly the spinal cord. In adults, the encephalitic illness begins with headache, fever and altered mental state. Tremor may be apparent on examination and cranial nerve palsies may develop. The course may then vary from rapid recovery to a prolonged illness with respiratory paralysis or even death. The mortality rate is around 25%, and about 50% of survivors have neurological residua varying from mild cranial nerve palsy to spastic quadraparesis. Death and severe residua are much more likely in the elderly and in infants.

In encephalitis cases the CT findings are usually unremarkable or show non-specific cerebral oedema, and the EEG show non-specific changes. MRI in late disease has been reported to show thalamic destruction. The CSF shows a variable leucocyte pleocytosis, usually with lymphocyte predominance and raised protein levels.

Diagnosis

The virus has rarely been cultured from human material, and the viraemia is likely to be short lived. It will grow in mosquito cell lines and suckling mouse brain. RT-PCR has been used to detect virus in the serum and CSF in the first few days of infection. Paired sera taken in the first few days after onset and 2–3 weeks later will show rising antibody by HI, EIA or IFA, although the HI test is the least sensitive and levels may rise late or not at all. IgM is nearly always present in the serum in the early stages of illness, and can also be detected in about 75% of CSF samples in suspected encephalitis. IgM may persist for weeks or months in the serum. Antibody will cross-react with other flaviviruses, particularly KUN and JE, which may also cause encephalitis in the same geographical area. The specificity of antibody can be determined by N tests or epitope-blocking EIA, although misleading results may occur in patients who have had a previous flavivirus infection.

Management

Treatment is supportive, and access to respiratory support is important in the survival of severe cases. Based on the experience with JE, steroids are not recommended, although dexamethasone may be used to reduce intra-cranial pressure if needed. In contrast, preliminary data on the possible effectiveness of α-interferon for JE suggests that this may be useful.

Epidemiology

The virus is maintained in a cycle involving water birds and mosquitoes. The vector *Cx. annulirostris* becomes infected with MVE virus after feeding on birds, which can carry the infection widely by migration. There is also evidence for vertical transmission. A variety of wild and domesticated animals can be infected, but their role in the natural history is unclear (see Table 41.1 and Appendix IV).

Immunization

There is no specific vaccine for MVE. There are data from a mouse model that antibody induced by the inactivated JE vaccine may enhance disease; this is a cause for concern in areas where both viruses may circulate.

Omsk haemorrhagic fever (OHF)[49]

Geographical distribution

OHF occurs in the Omsk area of Siberia and possibly other areas of western Siberia.

Aetiology

The virus OHF is a flavivirus (see Table 41.1) separated into two subgroups: (1) isolated from human blood, and (2) isolated from *Dermacentor marginatus*. The virus can be grown in HeLa cells or chick embryos.

Transmission

The virus is harboured by ticks—*Dermacentor pictus (reticulatus)* and *D. marginatus*—with trans-stadial and transovarial transmission. The ticks transmit the infection to humans from rodents, mainly muskrats (see Table 41.1 and Appendix IV). The mechanism of inter-rodent transmission in nature is not known, but mites may transmit the infection between muskrats and other rodents. Infection by direct contact with muskrat carcasses and pelts is common, and inter-human transmission occurs. There is some evidence of infection by the respiratory route.

Pathology

The pathology of fatal cases is that of haemorrhagic fevers with haemorrhage in tissues and necrotic areas in the liver. Immunity is antibody mediated; little is known about second attacks.

Clinical features

OHF is essentially a self-limiting acute infection in the majority of cases, although a small proportion develop haemorrhagic disease. The mortality rate is 1–3%.

The *incubation period* is 3–7 days.

Symptoms and signs

The illness is very similar to KFD. Complete recovery is usual, although it may take several weeks. There is no CNS involvement.

Diagnosis

Virus can be isolated from the blood in the febrile period. Serological diagnosis is made by the CF, HI and N tests, and differentiation needs to be made with TBE antibody.

Epidemiology and control

The reservoir of infection is the muskrat and ticks. Human infection depends upon muskrat–human contact, which may be via ticks or the handling of muskrat carcasses and pelts. When there is a great mortality of muskrats then contact is greater and outbreaks occur. TBE vaccine may offer cross-protection against this virus.

Powassan encephalitis[49]

Geographical distribution

Powassan virus is found in Russia, the USA and Canada, and has been isolated from several tick species, including *Ixodes* species and *Dermacentor andersoni*. The natural hosts are mainly squirrels and groundhogs. Human infections are probably largely asymptomatic. However, some infected individuals develop a non-specific febrile illness that progresses to meningoencephalitis. The disease may resemble acute herpes simplex encephalitis, while others are similar to the eastern subtype of TBE, with upper limb paralysis.

Rocio virus (ROC)[58,59]

Rocio virus emerged as a cause of outbreaks of encephalitis in Brazil in 1975–1976. It is probably carried by wild birds and transmitted by *Psorophora ferox* mosquitoes (see Table 41.1). It has an *incubation period* of 7–14 days, and illness begins with headache, fever, nausea and vomiting, sometimes with pharyngitis and conjunctivitis. Meningitis or encephalitis follows in many, with altered mental state and cerebellar tremor. Convulsions are uncommon. The mortality rate is about 5% with good medical care, and death occurs in patients of all ages. Gait disturbances may appear in survivors. There is no specific therapy or vaccine.

St Louis encephalitis (SLE)[59–62]

Geographical distribution (see Figure 41.3)

This is the most important arbovirus in the USA. It is widespread throughout North America but has also occurred in Jamaica, and evidence of infection in birds is found in Central America, Brazil and Argentina.

Aetiology

SLE virus is 30–40 nm in diameter; it is best grown in newborn white mice, but also grows in hamster and chicken kidney cell cultures. It shares antigens with JE and WN viruses.

Transmission

The basic transmission cycle is between birds and several culicine mosquitoes. After the winter the virus is introduced by migrant birds or long-term infection of bats. The main vector to humans is *Cx. quinquefasciatus* in the eastern USA and *Cx. tarsalis* in the western USA. Transovarial transmission is usual (see Table 41.1 and Appendix IV).

Clinical features

Natural history

The vast majority of infections are asymptomatic or non-specific. When clinically apparent, infection most often manifests as encephalitis, and less frequently as meningitis or as fever with severe headache. Children are less likely to develop symptomatic disease and it is usually mild. The overall mortality rate is 7%, but is age dependent with most deaths being in the elderly.

The *incubation period* is 6–16 days.

Onset is sudden, with fever and severe headache. Neck stiffness and photophobia may occur. Progression to CNS involvement is shown by drowsiness and confusion. Cerebellar ataxia and cranial nerve palsies, and cogwheel rigidity, may develop. About 60% have intention tremor. Upper limb paralysis may occur. Convulsions are more common in children and, if severe and prolonged, are a poor prognostic sign. The CSF usually shows a mild to moderate lymphocyte pleocytosis and a raised protein concentration. Following recovery from the acute encephalitis, mild to serious sequelae may be found, particularly in the elderly. Parkinsonism, paralysis, tremor, confusion, gait disturbances and more general declines in cerebral function are seen. Neuropsychiatric disease is a relatively common late effect.

Diagnosis

Virus may be isolated from CSF in the early stages of the illness, but rarely from acute blood. Antigen may be detected by immunofluorescence in brain tissue or CSF mononuclear cells. Serological diagnosis is achieved by showing rising antibody by HI, CF or N tests, and IgM detection by EIA helps to diagnose early infection. Detection of IgM in the CSF is a reliable indicator of encephalitis. IgM is relatively specific for the infecting virus, but persists in serum for several months after acute illness. To confirm the identity of the antibody, N tests are required to differentiate it from antibody to other flaviviruses such as WN.

Epidemiology

Cx. quinquefasciatus, being an urban mosquito, is responsible for urban outbreaks, while *Cx. tarsalis* in the western USA is responsible for rural outbreaks. In urban areas both children and adults are affected equally, but elderly people are most affected. In rural areas males are affected more than females. Epidemics occur in the late summer and early autumn.

Treatment

Treatment is largely supportive, the level depending on the severity of disease. Interferon-α improves survival in a mouse model and should be considered in severe cases. There is some evidence of clinical efficacy for another flavivirus encephalitis, JE.

Control

Environmental sanitation to control *Cx. quinquefasciatus* in urban areas is essential. 'Fogging' with insecticides may be necessary during epidemics.

Tick-borne encephalitis (TBE)[49,63,64]

This tick-borne flavivirus has two subtypes: the Eastern, found mainly in the Asian part of the former USSR, and the Western in Europe, although there is considerable overlap. Other names include Russian epidemic encephalitis, Russian Far-East encephalitis, Russian spring–summer, central European encephalitis and others.

Geographical distribution (Figure 41.8)

The Eastern subtype is seasonally epidemic in scattered foci in the far eastern part of the former USSR and extending across into China. The Western subtype occurs in European Russia, Austria, Hungary, the Balkans, Czech Republic, Slovakia and Scandinavia.

Aetiology

The virus is spherical, 20–30 nm in diameter, with a dense centre and surface membrane. It shares antigens with the viruses causing LI, OHF and KFD, but not JE.

Transmission (see also Table 41.1 and

Appendix IV)

The vectors are *Ixodes persulcatus* for the Eastern subtype and *Ix. ricinus* for the Western. Viral infection is maintained by transovarial transmission. People may also become infected from drinking infected goat's milk and less commonly by entry through injured skin or mucosa, such as crushing an infected tick on the skin. Rare aerosol transmission may occur.

Pathology

The virus enters via a tick bite, ingestion of infected milk or, rarely, through injured skin or mucosa or by inhalation. After multiplying at the site of injection it spreads through the reticuloendothelial system where it is further amplified. In some cases it then invades the CNS. It causes neuronal destruction in the cerebral cortex, basal ganglia, cerebellar cortex, brainstem and anterior horns of the spinal cord.

Clinical features

Natural history

The infection is often inapparent but when overt is severe, the Eastern subtype (mortality rate 20%) being more severe than the Western subtype (mortality rate 1–2%).

The *incubation period* is 3–7 days. The Western subtype begins as an influenza-like illness that lasts a few days and may lead to a full recovery. In about one-third of cases a second phase begins several days later, and progresses to a mild meningoencephalitis. Some have more severe disease resembling the Eastern subtype. Some 10–20% have residual neurological disease.

The Eastern subtype has a sudden onset with severe headache, fever, nausea and photophobia. In mild cases the fever subsides after a few days and the patient recovers. In others, the disease progresses to meningoencephalitis with headache, neck stiffness, photophobia, and convulsions or altered mental state. Sometimes the fever has a biphasic pattern. Localizing signs, especially flaccid paralysis of the neck and upper limbs, can appear early with the Eastern subtype but uncommonly with the Western subtype. The CSF shows a lymphocytic pleocytosis with raised levels of protein. About 30–40% of survivors have significant neurological sequelae, particularly residual paralysis involving the upper extremities and shoulder girdle.

Diagnosis

Virus can be isolated from the blood in the first week, but this is rarely done in practice. RT-PCR has been used for virus detection also. Paired acute and convalescent sera will show rising IgG levels by HI, CF, IFA, EIA or N tests. IgM can be detected in acute serum and possibly the CSF. Specific antibody can also be detected by N tests.

Treatment

Hyperimmune serum may be used in the first week, preferably within the first 3 days of onset of the initial illness. It is of no use once meningoencephalitis has set in. Otherwise, treatment is supportive.

Epidemiology

The virus circulates in small wild animals, chiefly rodents, and is transmitted by larval and nymphal ticks which, when they mature, feed on larger mammals, including humans. The incidence of the disease is seasonal—spring and early summer—occurring in small epidemics in the eastern part of the former USSR, where it is a disease of the forest and the taiga. In Europe it is a forest disease and occurs from late spring until early autumn, and outbreaks often follow a period when voles are numerous.

Control

Tick repellents and protective clothing may be of help. Pesticide treatment of large areas or restriction of access has been used.

Immunization

A formalin-inactivated vaccine grown in chick embryo cells is commercially available for the Western subtype. The initial vaccine had a high rate of reactions, but current purified vaccines do not have that problem. It is 97–98% effective and has been used for mass vaccination in Austria. It is also recommended for people going to work in or visiting high-risk areas, and for laboratory personnel working with the virus. Hyperimmune globulin can also be used as prophylaxis before and after exposure.

Formalin-inactivated vaccines made from infected mouse brain and later from chick embryo cells have also been produced for the Eastern subtype.

West Nile (WN) fever[18,65]

Geographical distribution

Serological surveys, virus isolations and reports of disease outbreaks in humans and animals indicate that WN virus is widely spread throughout Africa, the Middle East, southern Europe, Russia, southern India, parts of South-East Asia, and more recently North America (Figure 41.9). In addition, the Australian virus Kunjin has now been recognized as a subtype of WN.[66]

Virus morphology

WN virus is a member of the JE antigenic complex within the *Flavivirus* genus. Similar to other flaviviruses, the virion is roughly spherical and approximately 40–50 nm in diameter. A lipid envelope encloses a nucleocapsid that contains the single-stranded, positive-sense RNA genome.

Transmission

Culex mosquitoes, particularly those that feed on birds, play a major role in the transmission of WN virus. The virus has also been isolated from mosquitoes of other genera, including *Aedes* and *Mansonia*, which may also serve as natural vectors. WN virus has also been isolated from several species of ticks, some of which have been shown to transmit the virus under laboratory conditions. These long-lived vectors may play an important role in the dispersal and overwintering of the virus.

Pathology

In a small proportion of cases, especially in elderly patients, the first phase may be followed by the development

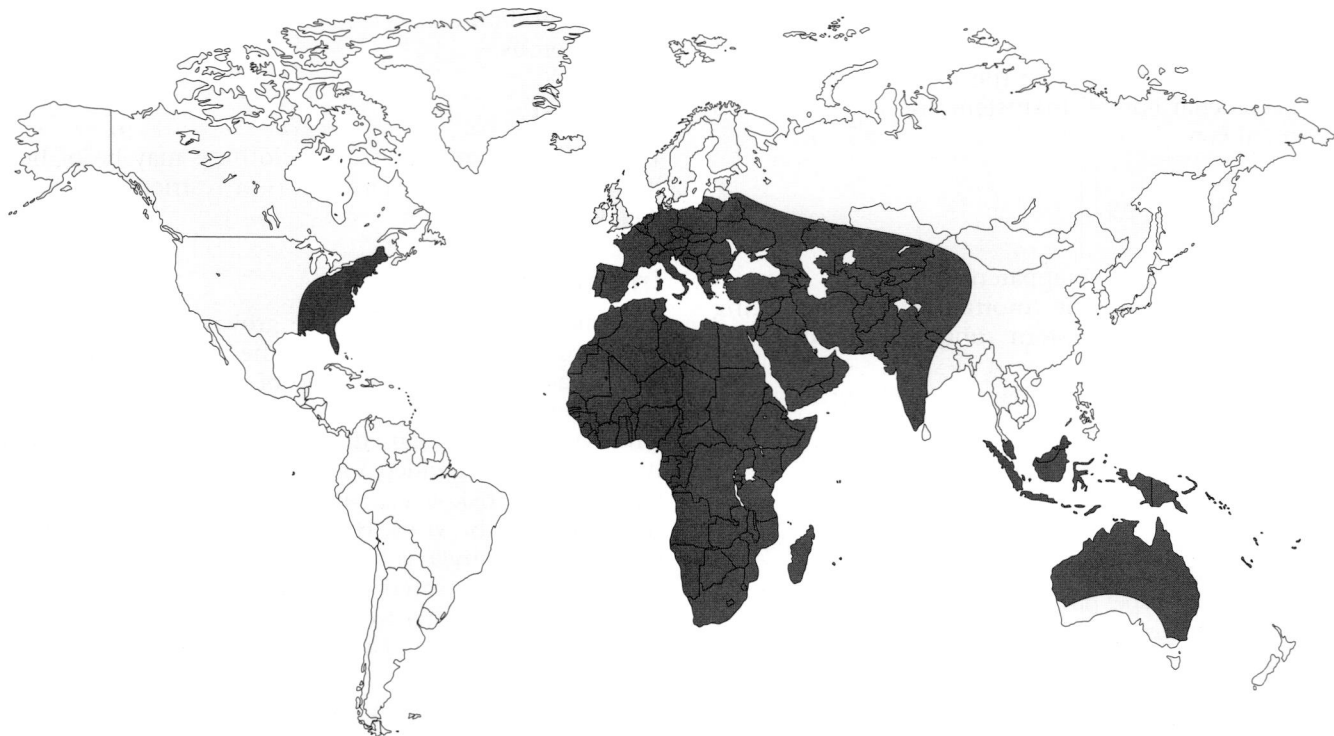

Figure 41.9: Geographical distribution of West Nile and Kunjin viruses.

of a meningoencephalitis. Histopathological examination of four fatal cases from the 1999 New York outbreak 'showed varying degrees of neuronal necrosis in the gray matter, with infiltrates of microglia and polymorphonuclear leukocytes, perivascular cuffing, neuronal degeneration, and neuronophagia. Immunohistochemical staining demonstrated viral antigens in neurons, neuronal processes, and areas of necrosis. No immunostaining was seen in other major organs, including lung, liver, spleen, and kidney. The histopathologic lesions and immunostaining were more prominent in the brain stem and spinal cord, which may explain the clinical manifestation of muscle weakness in some patients.'[67]

Clinical features

Natural history

In the great majority of cases WN virus causes an inapparent infection; in others there is an acute dengue-like fever (for which it has often been mistaken) followed by recovery, but a few patients develop meningo-encephalitis. Encephalitis is much more likely in adults than in children, and disease is more severe in older adults. The mortality rate from encephalitis is 15–40%.

The *incubation period* is 1–6 days. Historically the disease has been typically mild, with fever, headache, myalgia, backache and anorexia. Generalized lymphadenopathy, maculopapular rash and nausea are also commonly reported. Where progression to CNS involvement occurs, the patient develops severe headache, confusion and depression of conscious state, neck stiffness, cranial nerve palsies and generalized weakness. The CSF shows a mild pleocytosis with a raised protein level. CT is usually not helpful in early disease and the EEG shows non-specific changes. Most survivors have significant neurological residua.

Diagnosis

Virus may be detected in clinical samples by isolation or RNA detection by PCR.[68] Detection of WN virus-specific IgM in acute-phase serum of patients provides reliable evidence of recent infection; however, it is wise to also test for antibody to other members of the JE antigenic complex to exclude serological cross-reaction. Indeed, the initial diagnosis of index cases of WN in New York in 1999 were confounded by cross-reactions of WN IgM with SLE virus. Detection of IgM in CSF is a good indicator of encephalitis, but is absent in many cases.

Epidemiology

WN virus is maintained in nature primarily in bird–mosquito cycles. Several species, including crows and pigeons, develop high titres of virus in the blood and provide an infectious blood meal for competent mosquito vectors. Although humans and horses exhibit clinical disease, they are probably dead-end hosts. WN virus may be widely dispersed by migration of infected birds.

Early serological studies in Egypt and the Sudan revealed that human infections with WN virus were extremely common, indicating the virus was endemic in parts of Africa. However, the disease has historically manifested as a febrile illness in that continent, with rare incidents of CNS involvement. In more recent times, there have been several outbreaks of WN encephalitis in Europe, Russia, North America and Israel. Relatively high proportions (5–14%) of these cases were fatal. Molecular analysis of the virus strains causing these outbreaks has revealed that WN virus exists as two main genetic lineages (I and II). While the latter appears to be restricted to Africa and has been associated with febrile illness, virus strains of lineage I have been found on several continents and have been associated with all outbreaks of WN encephalitis.

While a neurological disease of horses has been associated with WN virus infection for many years, recent WN outbreaks in North America and Israel have also revealed high levels of morbidity and mortality in several species of birds.

Yellow fever (YF) (see also Chapter 10)[7,69,70]

Geographical distribution

Yellow fever is found in the tropical forest areas of Africa and South America (Figure 41.10) and until early in this century caused large epidemics in the Caribbean and the subtropical and temperate regions of North America as far north as Baltimore and Philadelphia. 'Jungle' YF still occurs in Brazil and there was an outbreak in Trinidad in 1978–1979, with 18 cases and eight deaths. Many other epidemics have occurred in South America, and a large epidemic in Ethiopia was responsible for many deaths in 1960–1962, and in Senegal in 1965–1966. YF has caused fatalities in tourists, especially in West Africa, who have not been vaccinated.

West Africa was probably the original home of YF, which may have been transported to the Americas by ships carrying infected mosquitoes in the post-Columbian period. YF has never been established in Europe, Asia or Australasia although potential vectors (*Ae. aegypti* in South-East Asia) abound, so that if it were introduced into Asia catastrophic epidemics could occur.

Aetiology

YF is a flavivirus (see Table 41.1) 25–65 nm in size, which can survive at 4°C for a month and freeze-dried for many years. It can be grown on a variety of vertebrate cell cultures, chick or mouse embryo, PS or HeLa cell cultures with a cytopathic effect. There are several strains that can infect humans. Freshly isolated strains that are pantropic lose viscerotropism in the chick embryo. African strains of YF possess an antigen absent from American strains. The 17D strain, which is used so successfully as a live vaccine, has acquired an antigen absent from the original 'Asibi' strain from which it was developed.

Transmission

Mosquitoes (see Table 41.1 and Appendix IV)
In nature mosquitoes of several genera transmit YF. In the

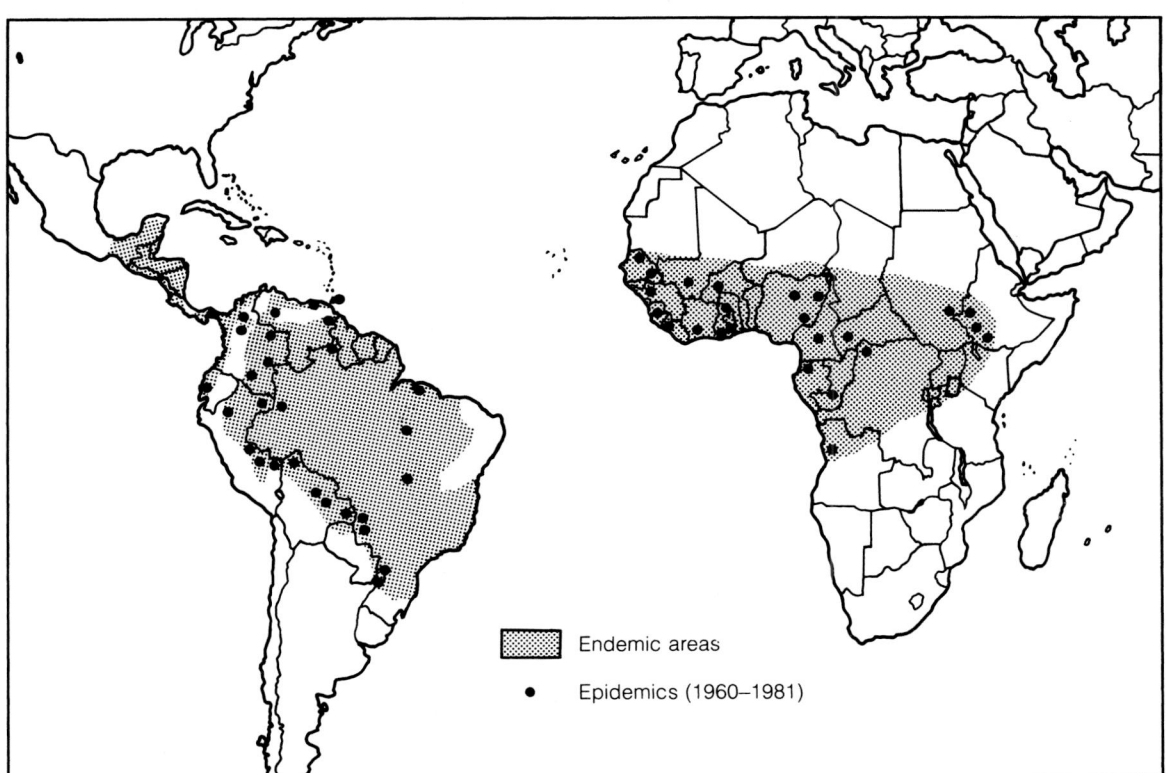

Figure 41.10: Geographical distribution of yellow fever.

Americas the forest cycle is maintained by mosquitoes belonging to the genera *Haemagogus* and *Sabethes*. *Ae. aegypti* is responsible for urban outbreaks. Virus has also been isolated from *Ae. fulvus* in Brazil. In Africa, *Ae. africanus* maintains the monkey–mosquito–monkey cycle in the forest, while *Ae. simpsoni,* which breeds close to humans in the axils of banana plants, becomes infected from monkeys raiding the plantations, and transmits YF to people. Other *Aedes* involved in the forest cycle include *Ae. luteocephalus*, *Ae. opok*, *Ae. furcifer* and *Ae. taylori*. Vertical transmission of YF virus from one generation to another in mosquitoes is thought to be important for virus survival during the dry season. In Africa the urban cycle is maintained by *Ae. aegypti*.

Mosquitoes become infected from the first to third day of fever. The intrinsic cycle in the mosquito is 4 days at 37°C and 18 days at 18°C. Mosquitoes remain infected for life, about 2–4 months. The possibility of transovarial transmission has already been mentioned.

Ticks

YF virus has been isolated from *Amblyomma variegatum* in Brazil and trans-stadial transmission was demonstrated by infecting nymphs and passing on the infection to uninfected monkeys at the adult stage. The epidemiological significance of this is not clear.

Other methods of transmission

Human blood is infective in the first 3 days of illness and handling of infected monkeys in the early stages of viraemia could cause infection. Interhuman transmission is unimportant but laboratory work with infected monkeys and mosquitoes can be dangerous.

Pathology

There is no evidence of any immune reactions influencing the pathogenesis of YF. The virus affects highly specialized epithelial or myocardial cells only; stroma cells are not involved. The changes are toxic, beginning with cloudy swelling and going on to degenerative fatty changes and coagulative necrosis. There is no inflammatory response.

Liver

Typical lesions may not be found in biopsy specimens from patients who later recover and serological evidence is necessary for diagnosis in such cases. In fatal cases, however, the liver is not shrunken; it may be reddish-yellow and feels greasy. The typical lesions form a characteristic triad: microglobular fatty degeneration of epithelial liver cells throughout the hepatic lobule; dissociation of the hepatic lobule, most marked in the mid-zone (but some normal liver cells always remain around the central zone); and coagulative necrosis of the epithelial liver cells, mainly affecting the mid-zone (Figure 41.11). The nuclei of the liver cells are pyknotic

and the coagulated contents of the cells stain deeply with eosin, the Councilman bodies resulting from this degeneration taking on a salmon-pink colour (Figure 41.12). Under low power a stained section looks as though red pepper has been scattered on it.

Other organs

The lesions are variable: some degree of nephritis or nephrosis (with transient proteinuria in mild cases), adrenal lesions, lesions of the heart (fatty changes, even in the sinoatrial node and the bundle of His, corresponding with the clinical bradycardia) and lesions of the brain (perivascular haemorrhages). In the kidneys there are fatty changes with necrosis of tubular epithelium and casts in both cortex and medulla. Encephalitis was not formerly thought to be part of the picture of naturally occurring YF, but meningoencephalitis was a dominant feature of an epidemic in the Sudan and Ethiopia in 1960. Severe haemorrhages may take place in the digestive system, the internal cavities, the lungs (common), liver,

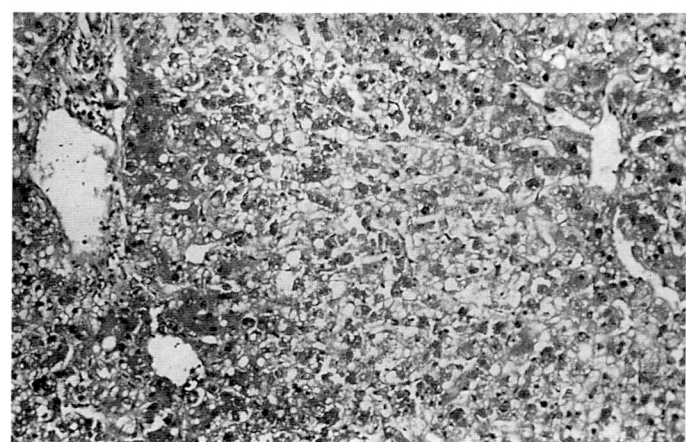

Figure 41.11: Post-mortem appearance of the liver of a rhesus monkey with yellow fever, showing well marked mid-zonal necrosis and minimal inflammatory changes.

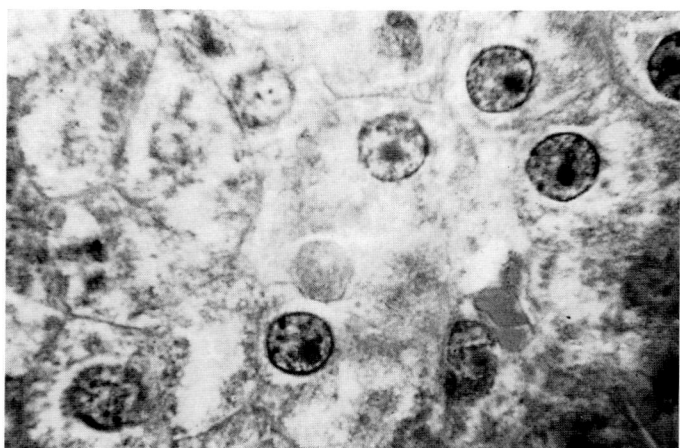

Figure 41.12: Councilman body in the liver cell of a rhesus monkey affected with yellow fever.

spleen and kidneys. Death results from failure of the liver or kidneys or both, although cardiac damage may contribute. Patients who recover show complete replacement of lost tissue by direct regeneration and hypertrophy of surviving cells.

Immunity

Immunity is antibody mediated, and lifelong immunity follows infection with YF virus. In many endemic areas where contact with virus-carrying mosquitoes is constant (i.e., near the forest), infection is common in childhood, leading to a solid immunity. The immunity is antibody mediated, HF and N antibodies being found from the end of the first week of infection.

Clinical features
Natural history
Inapparent infections, especially in endemic areas, are common, leading to high levels of immunity within indigenous populations. When disease occurs in endemic areas it is generally mild with a mortality rate of 5–10%. During epidemics the mortality rate is several magnitudes higher, but the exact figure is unclear.

Symptoms and signs
The *incubation period* is 3–6 days. Most infections are asymptomatic or mild, with only a small proportion progressing to severe classical YF. The mild form is an acute febrile illness with sudden onset of fever and headache without other symptoms, lasting 48 hours or less. In some other patients the headache is more severe, accompanied by myalgia, low back pain and slight proteinuria. The characteristic bradycardia in relation to temperature is present and the illness may last several days with recovery.

In severe illness the onset is abrupt with higher fever, severe headache, nausea, vomiting, abdominal pain and distressing pain in the back, loins and limbs. The patient is dehydrated with a dry tongue and foul breath. Early signs of jaundice may appear in the conjunctivae and skin, and minor bleeding from the gums and nose may be noted. This is called the 'period of infection' corresponding with the viraemia. It lasts about 3 days, and the patient may recover spontaneously after this. If they progress, there may be a 24-hour period of apparent improvement, followed by rapid deterioration. Jaundice worsens and there is frank haemorrhaging from the gastrointestinal tract and other sites. Epigastric pain and vomiting develop and there is a deterioration of renal function and albuminuria. There can be hypotension and heart failure, with a characteristic prolongation of the PR and QT intervals on electrocardiography. The patient may recover rapidly after a period of 3–4 days, or recovery may take over 2 weeks. Death occurs on the seventh to tenth day of illness. Bad prognostic signs are increasing proteinuria, haemorrhages, a rising pulse, hypotension, oliguria and azotaemia. Suppurative parotitis and bacterial pneumonia may complicate the disease.

If the patient recovers from a severe attack, convalescence tends to be long but usually without sequelae. Late deaths after convalescence are very rare and are related to myocardial damage, cardiac arrhythmia or cardiac failure.

Disease in children is usually milder and dominated by jaundice.

Diagnosis

Virus can be isolated from the blood in the first 3 days of from autopsy samples. Antigen-capture EIA has also been described. RNA detection by RT-PCR appears to be more sensitive and easier than these other techniques. Virus may be detectable in liver biopsy by IFA, probe hybridization or RT-PCR.

Serological diagnosis
IFA, HI and N antibodies appear within 1 week of onset and CF antibodies later. Paired acute and convalescent sera showing a rising titre are diagnostic. There are cross-reactions with other flaviviruses but N antibodies are specific. IgM can be detected during the acute phase by EIA, IFA or HI following IgM separation.

Management

There is no specific therapy and treatment is supportive and similar to the management of other haemorrhagic fevers such as DHF. The patient does not need to be isolated, but should be screened from mosquitoes if being nursed in an area that has potential vector species.

Epidemiology

There are two cycles: the forest cycle (jungle yellow fever) and the urban cycle (urban yellow fever).

Forest cycle (jungle yellow fever)
America
YF virus is maintained in rainforests in a cycle involving monkeys and marmosets and *Haemagogus* (tree-hole breeding) mosquitoes. Recurrent epizootics occur in howler (*Alouatta*) monkeys who die in large numbers, starting in Panama and spreading up the east coast of Central America to Guatemala, confirming the belief recorded by Balfour in 1914 that a 'silent forest' where all the howler monkeys had died denoted the presence of YF.

Africa
In the forests of West, Central and East Africa, a jungle cycle exists as an apparent infection in monkeys, mainly *Cercopithecus* (vervet) monkeys. Other susceptible primates with inapparent infections include colobus (important in Ethiopia), mangabeys (*Cercocebus*) and baboons (*Papio*). In East Africa some species of bushbaby (*Galago*), which are susceptible to the virus, have been shown to have high levels of YF antibodies and may be involved in transmission cycles. Several different *Aedes* spp. are important vectors of YF in Africa (see the section on YF transmission).

Human infection

Human infection occurs because of ecological changes created by humans—in Africa, by cutting down the forest and planting banana plantations, bringing monkeys into contact with *Ae. simpsoni*, a plant axil breeder which passes the infection on to humans. In the Americas, humans contract the disease by engaging in wood-cutting, and *Haemagogus* mosquitoes bite in and around houses in forest clearings. *Sabethes* (a drought-resistant mosquito) transmits infection during the dry season (see Appendix IV).

An endemic area population will show a rising percentage of positive antibody tests with age, whereas an epidemic situation will be shown by antibodies in the older age and none in the younger age groups.

Urban cycle (urban yellow fever)

When there is a high population of *Ae. aegypti*, intense transmission among humans occurs, with large epidemics where there are enough non-immunes in the population, which can be brought about by immigration, or a rising number of people born since the last epidemic. In the early years of the twentieth century huge epidemics of this nature frequently spread throughout the Caribbean and up the east coast of North America. These epidemics of 'yellow jack' terrified the inhabitants. Similar epidemics occurred in the 'White Man's Grave' in West Africa. Once *Ae. aegypti* was controlled, these epidemics became a thing of the past and no urban cases of YF have been described from the Americas for the past 40 years.

However, *Ae. simpsoni* spreading up wooded valleys in an otherwise deforested environment can come into contact with humans, with resulting epidemics. In the Nuba mountains of southern Sudan in 1940 there was an epidemic (17 000 cases; mortality rate 10%) and in south-western Ethiopia along the Omo River in 1960–1962 (15 000–30 000 deaths; mortality rate up to 85%). In 1965–1966 in Senegal there was an epidemic mainly affecting children under 10 years with a mortality rate of 15%. Mass vaccination has been suspended since 1960.

Control

Urban cycle (urban yellow fever)

Eradication and control of *Ae. aegypti* is the key to the prevention of urban YF. This includes an attack on the breeding sites in water containers and tanks, and a monitoring system that gives an *Aedes* index of the numbers of *Aedes* mosquitoes. When this reaches a certain level an epidemic may result. In the presence of an epidemic, adult control by 'fogging' of towns and cities with insecticide will bring the epidemic to a halt. *Ae. aegypti* had been eradicated from the USA but has now returned to Louisiana, once a hotbed of YF, in its previous numbers.

Vaccination

Yellow fever 17D is a safe, live, attenuated vaccine providing a long-lasting immunity. For purposes of certification, 10 years is considered the limit but immunity after 40 years has been documented and it may be life-long. Vaccination to YF is imperative for travellers to endemic areas and certificates are demanded for travellers from endemic areas to non-infected tropical areas. Immunity develops within 10 days of vaccination. Serious complications are rare. No consequences for the fetus have been recorded but pregnant women should avoid vaccination unless the risk from YF is considered great. Vaccination is not recommended for children under 6 months of age, and especially children aged less than 4 months, because of an increased risk of encephalitis. It should also be avoided in immunosuppressed patients. The vaccine is prepared in chick embryos and people sensitive to egg protein may have reactions. Serious side effects are rare with the 17D vaccine. Encephalitis, classical YF and severe multisystem illness have been reported.

Bunyaviruses

California encephalitis (CE)

CE was the first identified member of the California serogroup of bunyaviruses. It was identified as a cause of encephalitis in California in the 1940s, but rarely causes human infection (see Figure 41.3). It infects rabbits and rodents, and is transmitted by *Aedes* species.

Oropouche virus (ORO)[71]

ORO virus is a member of the Simbu group of bunyaviruses (see Table 41.1) and is a major cause of disease in the Amazon region of Brazil. It is transmitted by the midge *Culicoides paraensis* and some mosquito species. It is maintained in a jungle cycle involving sloths and monkeys. Disease onset is sudden, with fever, chills, headache, myalgia, arthralgia and photophobia being most common. The illness lasts 1–2 weeks and patients make a full recovery. Diagnosis is usually by serology.

Rift Valley fever (RVF)[71–74]

Geographical distribution

RVF was first recognized in Kenya in 1931 as causing a disease in sheep and humans. Until 1977 it was restricted to humans and domestic animals in sub-Saharan Africa, with epizootics in Kenya, South Africa, Zimbabwe, Sudan, Egypt, Uganda, Tanzania and Zambia. A similar virus (Zinga virus) was found to be present in West Africa (Mali, Nigeria and Zaire) and in Botswana and Mozambique, but without epizootics. In 1977 RVF spread to Egypt where it caused massive epidemics and epizootics, and showed a capability to spread beyond sub-Saharan Africa (Figure 41.13). The Egyptian episode was centred largely in the Nile delta where approximately 600 human deaths are

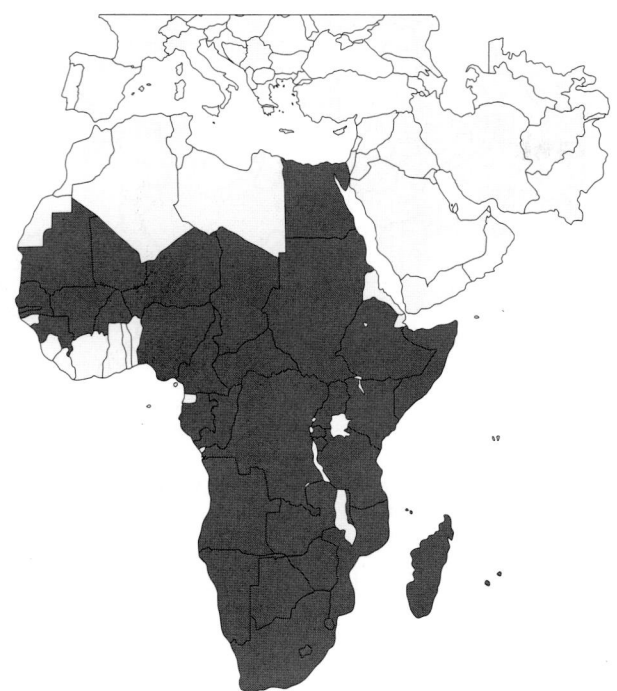

Figure 41.13: Geographical distribution of Rift Valley fever.

thought to have occurred. This was probably preceded by a massive epizootic along the Nile bank from Aswan in the south to Cairo in the north. RVF occurred again in Aswan in 1993 and several cases with ophthalmic complications have been seen in the Nile delta.

Aetiology

RFV is a member of the genus *Phlebovirus* in the Bunyaviridae family (see Table 41.1).

Pathology

The pathogenesis of RVF appears to be similar to that of YF, with initial spread to lymphatic tissue and then to the liver, with necrotic change in the latter. In a small proportion this is followed by haemorrhage. Cerebral invasion with encephalitis may occur, as may retinal involvement.

Transmission

The virus infects a large range of domestic animals. Transmission between the zoonotic hosts is by mosquitoes of the *Eretmapodites*, *Coquillettidia*, *Mansonia*, *Aedes* and *Culex* groups (see Table 41.1 and Appendix IV), and possibly to humans by *Ae. caballus* and *Cx. theileri* in South Africa and *Cx. pipiens* in Egypt. Direct transmission, especially during epidemics, is by the aerosol route from infected animal tissues. Person-to-person transmission does not occur but acute-phase blood and infected animal tissues are highly infectious, especially in abattoirs. Laboratory-acquired infections have been

described and the virus should be handled with extreme caution.

Immunity
Active immunity
Immunity is antibody mediated and there is prolonged immunity to reinfection with homologous strains after recovery. Antibodies formed are of the usual viral response (HI, CF and N). HI and CF antibodies are used in diagnosis, whereas N antibodies give specificity.

Passive immunity
A passive immunity can be transferred via the placenta to the child and lasts for several months; the possession of antibodies, especially N antibodies, can be used in treatment using convalescent sera.

Clinical features
Natural history
RVF is a self-limiting disease in the great majority of infections, with a short, acute, febrile phase and complete recovery. However, in less than 5% of cases, encephalitis, retinal lesions, haemorrhage and hepatic disease develop.

Symptoms and signs
The *incubation period* is 2–6 days. The onset is abrupt with fever, headache, joint and muscle pains, conjunctivitis and photophobia. In the majority of cases this is followed by complete recovery. In a few cases there may be recrudescence of symptoms after the initial short illness and convalescence may be prolonged. Retinal disease develops in 5–10% of cases, between 1 and 3 weeks after the febrile illness, with macular exudates and, in some instances, retinal haemorrhages and vasculitis. About half of the patients are left with permanent impairment of vision. In a further 5%, encephalitis develops, but is rarely fatal. Haemorrhagic disease occurs in approximately 1% of cases and is very similar to YF. Mortality rates are in the region of 10%, but deaths are nearly always found in those with more severe forms of the disease.

Diagnosis

Isolation of virus within the first 7 days from the blood can be done by intracerebral inoculation into baby mice, and most kinds of cell culture. Virus may also be detected in blood by RT-PCR and by antigen detection methods. Standard serological diagnosis is by the HI test on paired sera, using a standard antigen from the World Health Organization. EIA has also been used for IgG and IgM detection, and the latter can assist early diagnosis. The N tests can be used to show RVF-specific antibody.

Management

High-level supportive care may be needed for the more serious cases. Ribavirin has activity against this virus in animal models and it may be considered in the treatment of human disease. Immune serum, if available, may also be tried for severe cases.

Epidemiology

RVF is maintained in the forest in an enzootic fashion between vertebrates and the vector mosquito species. Spectacular epizootics in domestic animals are the result of large numbers of susceptible (European) breeds of cattle and sheep, high arthropod densities, and spillover from the forest cycle. Originally restricted to domestic animals and humans in sub-Saharan Africa, since 1997 it has spread to Egypt, causing explosive epidemics in humans and domestic animals. The spread was possibly by camels from the Sudan carrying infection or arthropods, establishing new enzootic foci in the changing arthropod and vertebrate population after the construction of the Aswan High Dam.

Control

Quarantine is not effective, but movements of animals should be controlled and sick animals should be allowed to die or recover, and not be slaughtered, to avoid spreading the infection in abattoirs. Control of abattoirs and vaccination of workers should be enforced.

Immunization

Vaccination of exposed laboratory workers and veterinary staff using a formalin-inactivated cell culture vaccine (expensive) should be performed.

Veterinary vaccines are the first line of defence against the spread of RVF. Both live and inactivated vaccines have been used to control the spread in animals, with some success.

Sandfly fever (phlebotomus fever)[71,75,76]

Geographical distribution

Sandfly fever is widespread throughout the Mediterranean and Middle East, Malta, Aegean Islands, Egypt and Iran, North Africa, Red Sea and Arabian Gulf; and in Asia in the Caucasus and Himalayas up to 4000 feet (Figure 41.14).

Aetiology

The virus causing sandfly fever is a phlebovirus with eight antigenically distinct strains, only two of which, Sicilian and Neapolitan, cause disease. The others have been isolated from insects and animals.

Transmission

The sandfly responsible for transmission, *Phlebotomus papatsii*, becomes infective 6 days after feeding and remains infective for life. Transovarial transmission occurs so that newly emerged sandflies are capable of transmitting

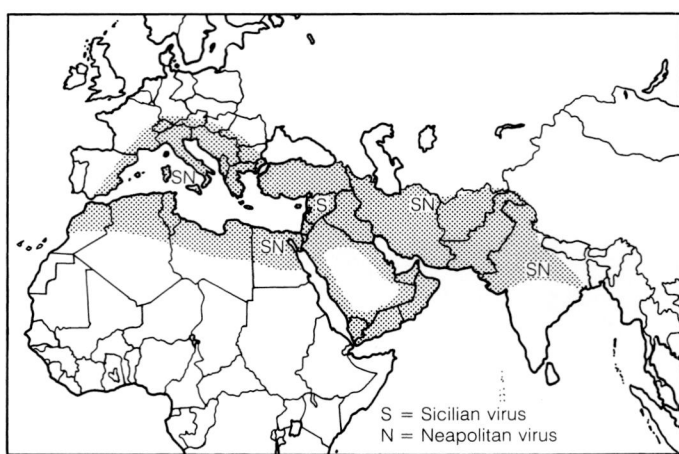

Figure 41.14: Endemic areas of sandfly fever viruses. (Courtesy of the Wellcome Tropical Institute.)

infection. It is possible that a parasitic mite of the sandflies acts as a reservoir.

Clinical features
Natural history
Sandfly fever is an acute self-limiting disease lasting 2–4 days, with complete recovery and immunity to further attacks, and no mortality.

The *incubation period* is 3–6 days.

Symptoms and signs
The onset is abrupt, with high fever, headache, myalgia, arthralgia and neck stiffness. After 3 (range 2–8) days the fever settles. Retro-orbital pain may be prominent and persist after resolution of fever. Mild neck stiffness develops in some patients. Occasionally there is a recrudescence (saddle back fever) lasting for 1–2 days.

Diagnosis

The viraemia lasts for only 24–36 hours, so attempts at virus isolation from serum are unlikely to be successful. Paired sera for HI and N antibody tests are required.

Management

There is no specific treatment.

Epidemiology

There are no animal reservoirs. In endemic areas transmission lasts from April to October. Epidemics occur among non-immune entrants to the community, especially military forces.

Tahyna

Tahyna virus is a bunyavirus transmitted by *Aedes* species and causing occasional outbreaks of an influenza-like illness in central Europe (see Table 41.1 and Appendix IV).

Toscana[77,78]

Toscana virus is a phlebovirus currently recognized as a member of the sandfly fever Naples virus serological complex. It is found in Italy, Portugal and Cyprus. It is transmitted by Phlebotomus papatsii and P. perfiliewi and causes a benign meningitis and occasional meningo-encephalitis, with full recovery. Diagnosis is usually by serology, but virus can be detected in the CSF by culture and by RT-PCR.

Coltiviruses
Colorado tick fever (CTF)[79]

CTF is caused by a coltivirus, and is a member of the Reoviridae. It is found in the mountain regions of western USA and Canada, especially in the Rocky Mountain area in Colorado. Clinical illness consists of headache, fever, myalgia, arthralgia, retro-orbital pain, photophobia and neck stiffness, accompanied by a macular, maculopapular or petechial rash in about 10% of cases. It is biphasic in about half the patients, characterized by 2–3 days of illness, then 2 days of remission, followed by 2–3 days' more illness. Children may develop encephalitis. The most important hosts are the chipmunk and the golden-mantled ground squirrel, which infect immature ticks (Dermacentor andersoni). Other species of rodents may act as alternative secondary hosts of the virus.

Miscellaneous arboviruses

There are a large number of other arthropod viruses that only rarely cause human infection or where their role in human disease is uncertain.

Alphaviruses

Babanki virus
Babanki is related to SIN and has been found in West and Central Africa, and Madagascar. It has been isolated from humans, but its role as a cause of disease is uncertain.

Getah virus
This mosquito-borne virus is closely related to RR virus. It is distributed widely through Asia, South-East Asia and Australia. Human infection is rare and it is not clearly associated with any disease.

Semliki Forest virus[80]
This virus is transmitted by various mosquito species in sub-Saharan Africa. Its role in human disease has not been established, but a laboratory-acquired case of fatal encephalitis has been reported.

Flaviviruses

Banzi virus
Banzi virus is a rodent virus found in southern Africa and transmitted by Culex species. Febrile illness has been reported.

Bussuquara virus
This is a Central and South American rodent virus transmitted by Culex species; it causes fever with arthralgia.

Edge Hill virus
Edge Hill virus has been isolated from Ae. vigilax and Cx. annulirostris mosquitoes and is widely distributed in Australia. Human infection occurs and a single possible case of polyarthralgic illness has been described.

Ilheus virus
This virus is found in Aedes and Psorophora mosquitoes in Brazil. Rare cases of fever with headache, and a case of encephalitis, have been documented.

Kokobera virus
Kokobera virus is found in Australia and New Guinea and is transmitted by Ae. vigilax and Cx. annulirostris mosquitoes. Human infections on the east coast have been documented in serosurveys. Kokobera virus can cause a polyarthralgic illness, sometimes with rash.

Koutango virus
Koutango virus is a tick-borne virus found in Senegal. Natural human infection is not known to occur, but one laboratory-acquired infection caused fever, headache, arthralgia and rash.

Negishi virus
This virus is closely related to TBE, but is mosquito transmitted as well as tick transmitted. Human infection has been found in Japan and China, and the virus has been found in Russia. Clinical disease resembling JE has been described.

Rio Bravo virus
This is a flavivirus, but is not arthropod-borne. It is transmitted directly from bats to humans, with one case of febrile illness being reported.

Sepik virus
Sepik virus has been found in a variety of mosquito species in Papua New Guinea and has caused a case of fever plus headache.

Spondweni virus
Spondweni virus is transmitted by several mosquito species in South Africa. It may cause fever, headache and arthralgia.

Usutu virus
This virus is found in sub-Saharan Africa and is a rodent

virus transmitted by several mosquito species, causing fever and rash.

Tyuleniy virus

Tyuleniy virus is a tick-borne virus, reported to have caused a single human infection with arthralgia and skin haemorrhages.

Wesselsbron virus

Wesselsbron virus is found in sub-Saharan Africa and Thailand. It is transmitted by several mosquito species. Human illness is characterised by fever, hepatosplenomegaly, rash and sometimes encephalitis, with full recovery.

Zika virus

This virus is transmitted by *Aedes* species in East and West Africa, and maintained in a cycle similar to that of YF. It causes fever, headache and rash.

Bunyavirus family[81]

There is a large number of bunyaviruses that have been implicated in rare and mild human infection.

Nairoviruses
Congo–Crimean haemorrhagic fever (C-CHF)

While this virus has been isolated from various species of ticks, there is no evidence that these arthropods are responsible for its transmission to humans. This serious infection is discussed in Chapter 43 with the non-arthropod-borne viral haemorrhagic fevers.

Dugbe virus

This virus was found to cause a mild febrile illness in Nigeria and Central African Republic, with rare meningitis.

Nairobi sheep disease

Nairobi sheep disease virus infects sheep and goats and is transmitted by a number of tick species. Human infection has been reported from East Africa and India, consisting of a fever and arthralgia. The illness is mild and recovery is full.

Orbiviruses

Kemerovo complex

This is a complex of a large number of viruses found in the former USSR and central Europe. They are tick-borne, and cause illnesses varying from fever to meningoencephalitis.

Orungo virus

Orungo virus is found in West and Central Africa and may be transmitted by a number of mosquito species. It causes fever and headache, with rare cases of encephalitis.

REFERENCES

1 World Health Organization. Arthropod-borne and rodent-borne viral diseases. Report of a WHO Scientific Group. *Wld Hlth Org Tech Rep Ser* 1985; 719:1–114.

2 Bres P. Impact of arboviruses on human and animal health. In Monath T P (ed.) *The Arboviruses: Epidemiology and Ecology*, vol. I. Florida: CRC Press, 1988:1–18.

3 van Regenmortel M H V, Fauquet C M, Bishop D H L et al. (eds) *Virus Taxonomy: 7th Report of the International Committee on Taxonomy of Viruses.* San Diego: Academic Press, 2000.

4 Harrison S C & Skehel J J. Virus structure. In Fields D C, Knipe B N & Howley D M (eds) *Fields Virology,* vol. 1, 3rd edn. Philadelphia: Lippincott-Raven, 1996:59–100.

5 Calisher C H & Karabatsos N. Arbovirus serogroups: definition and geographic distribution. In Monath T P (ed.) *The Arboviruses: Epidemiology and Ecology*, vol. I. Florida: CRC Press, 1988:19–58.

6 Monath T P. Pathobiology of the flaviviruses. In Schlesinger S & Schlesinger M J (eds) *The Togaviridae and the Flaviviridae.* New York: Plenum Press, 1986:375–440.

7 Monath T P. Yellow fever. In Monath T P (ed.) *The Arboviruses: Epidemiology and Ecology*, vol. V. Florida: CRC Press, 1988:139–231.

8 Scott T W. Vertebrate host ecology. In Monath T P (ed.) *The Arboviruses: Epidemiology and Ecology*, vol. I. Florida: CRC Press, 1988:257–280.

9 Porterfield J S. Comparative and historical aspects of the Togaviridae and Flaviviridae. In Schlesinger S & Schlesinger M J (eds) *The Togaviridae and the Flaviviridae.* New York: Plenum Press, 1986:1–19.

10 Hardy J L. Susceptibility and resistance of vector mosquitoes. In Monath T P (ed.) *The Arboviruses: Epidemiology and Ecology*, vol. 1. Florida: CRC Press, 1988:87–126.

11 Turell M J. Horizontal and vertical transmission of viruses by insect and tick vectors. In Monath T P (ed.) *The Arboviruses: Epidemiology and Ecology*, vol. I. Florida: CRC Press, 1988:127–152.

12 Simpson D I H. Arbovirus diseases. *Br Med Bull* 1972; 28(1);10–15.

13 Dunn F L. Human factors in arbovirus ecology and control. In Monath T P (ed.) *The Arboviruses: Epidemiology and Ecology*, vol. I. Florida: CRC Press, 1988: 281–290.

14 Calisher C H. Alphavirus infections (family Togaviridae). In Porterfield J S (ed.) *Kass Handbook of Infectious Diseases: Exotic Viral Infections.* London: Chapman & Hall, 1995:1–18.

15 Mackenzie J S, Lindsay M & Daniels P. The effect of climate change on the incidence of vector-borne viral diseases in Australia: the potential value of seasonal forecasting. In Hammer G L (ed.) *The Australian Experience.* Dordrecht: Kluwer Academic, 2000:429–452.

16 Kay B H & Aaskov J G. Ross River virus (epidemic polyarthritis). In Monath T P (ed.) *The Arboviruses: Epidemiology and Ecology*, vol. III. Florida: CRC Press, 1988:93–112.

17 Johnson R E & Peters C J. Alphaviruses. In Fields B N, Knipe D M & Howley P M (eds) *Fields Virology*, 3rd edn, vol. 1. Philadelphia: Lippincott-Raven, 1996:843–898.

18 Monath T P & Heinz F X. Flaviviruses. In Fields B N, Knipe D M & Howley P M (eds) *Fields Virology*, 3rd ed, vol. 1. Philadelphia: Lippincott-Raven, 1996:961–1034.

19 Broom A K, Wallace M J, Mackenzie J S et al. Immunization with gamma globulin to Murray Valley encephalitis virus and with an inactivated Japanese encephalitis virus vaccine as a prophylaxis against Australian encephalitis: evaluation in a mouse model. *J Med Virol* 2000; 61:259–265.

20 World Health Organization. *Dengue Haemorrhagic Fever: Diagnosis, Treatment, Prevention and Control*, 2nd edn. Geneva: World Health Organization, 1977.

21 Martin M, Tsai T F, Cropp B et al. Fever and multisystem organ failure associated with yellow fever vaccination: a report of four cases. *Lancet* 2001; 358:98–104.

22 Pittman P R, Liu C T, Cannon T L et al. Immunogenicity of an inactivated Rift Valley fever vaccine in humans: a 12-year experience. *Vaccine* 1999; 18:181–189.

23 Flexman A W, Smith D W, Mackenzie J S et al. A comparison of the diseases caused by Ross River virus and Barmah Forest virus. *Med J Aust* 1998; 169:159–163.

24 Brighton A W, Prozesky O W & De La Harpe A D. Chikungunya virus infection. A retrospective study of 107 cases. *S Afr Med J* 1983; 63:313–315.

25 Nimmannitya S, Halstead S B, Cohen S N et al. Dengue and chikungunya virus infections in man in Thailand, 1962–1964. I. Observations on hospitalized patients with hemorrhagic fevers. *Am J Trop Med Hyg* 1969; 18:954–971.

26 Halstead S B, Nimmannitya S & Margiotta M R. Dengue and chikungunya virus infections in man in Thailand, 1962–1964. II. Observations on dengue in outpatients. *Am J Trop Med Hyg* 1969; 18:972–983.

27 Jupp P G, McIntosh B M. Chikungunya virus disease. In Monath T P (ed.) *The Arboviruses: Epidemiology and Ecology*, vol. II. Florida: CRC Press, 1988:137–158.

28 Reisen W K & Monath T P. Western equine encephalomyelitis. In Monath T P (ed.) *The Arboviruses: Epidemiology and Ecology*, vol. I. Florida: CRC Press, 1988:89–138.

29 Morris C D. Eastern equine encephalomyelitis. In Monath T P (ed.) *The Arboviruses: Epidemiology and Ecology*, vol. III. Florida: CRC Press, 1988:1–20.

30 Deresiewicz R L, Thaler S J, Hsu L et al. Clinical and neuroradiographic manifestations of eastern equine encephalitis. *N Engl J Med* 1997; 336:1867–1874.

31 Walton T E & Grayson M. Venezualan equine encephalomyelitis. In Monath T P (ed.) *The Arboviruses: Epidemiology and Ecology*, vol. IV. Florida: CRC Press, 1988:203–231.

32 Linssen B, Kinney R M, Aguilar P et al. Development of reverse transcription-PCR assays for specific detection of equine encephalitic viruses. *J Clin Microbiol* 2000; 38:1527–1535.

33 Pinheiro F P, Freitas R B, Travassos Da Rosa J F et al. An outbreak of Mayaro virus disease in Belterra, Brazil. I. Clinical and virological findings. *Am J Trop Med Hyg* 1981; 30:674–681.

34 Johnson B K. O'nyong nyong virus disease. In Monath T P (ed.) *The Arboviruses: Epidemiology and Ecology*, vol. III. Florida: CRC Press, 1988: 217–223.

35 Shore H. O'nyong-nyong fever: an epidemic virus disease in East Africa. III. Some clinical and epidemiological observations in the northern province of Uganda. *Trans R Soc Trop Med Hyg* 1961; 55:361–373.

36 Mackenzie J S & Smith D W. Mosquito-borne viruses and epidemic polyarthritis. *Med J Aust* 1996; 164:90–92.

37 Russell R C. Vectors vs humans – who is on top down under? An update on vector-borne disease and research on vectors in Australia. *J Vector Ecol* 1998; 23(1):1–46.

38 Rosen L, Gubler D J & Bennett P H. Epidemic polyarthritis (Ross River) virus infection in the Cook Islands. *Am J Trop Med Hyg* 1981; 30:1294–1302.

39 Gubler D J. Dengue. In Monath T P (ed.) *The Arboviruses: Epidemiology and Ecology*, vol. II. Florida: CRC Press, 1988:223–260.

40 Gubler D. Dengue and dengue haemorrhagic fever. *Clin Microbiol Rev* 1998; 11:480–496.

41 Lum L D, Lam S K, Choy Y S et al. Dengue encephalitis: a true entity? *Am J Trop Med Hyg* 1996; 54:256–259.

42 Pinheiro F & Corber S J. Global situation of dengue and dengue haemorrhagic fever, and its emergence in the Americas. *World Health Stat Q* 1997; 50:161–168.

43 Burke D S & Leake C J. Japanese encephalitis. In Monath T P (ed.) *The Arboviruses: Epidemiology and Ecology*, vol. III. Florida: CRC Press, 1988:63–92.

44 Solomon T & Vaughn D W. Pathogenesis and clinical features of Japanese encephalitis and West Nile virus infections. In Mackenzie J S, Barrett A D T & Deubel V (eds) *Japanese Encephalitis and West Nile Viruses. Current Topics in Microbiology and Immunology* 2002 (in press).

45 Vaughn D W & Hoke C H. The epidemiology of Japanese encephalitis: prospects for prevention. *Epidemiol Rev* 1992; 14:197–221.

46 Harinasatu C, Nimmanitya S, Titsa U et al. A clinical trial of interferon-alpha on Japanese encephalitis in Thailand. *Southeast Asian J Trop Med Public Health* 1989; 20:656–657.

47 Kalita J & Misra U K. Comparison of CT scan and MRI findings in the diagnosis of Japanese encephalitis. *J Neurol Sci* 2000; 17:3–8.

48 Gajanana A, Samuel P P, Thenmozhi V et al. An appraisal of some recent diagnostic assays for Japanese encephalitis. *Southeast Asian J Trop Med Public Health* 1996; 27:673–679.

49 Gaidamovich S. Tick-borne *Flavivirus* infection. In Porterfield J S (ed.) *Kass Handbook of Infectious Diseases: Exotic Viral Infections*. London: Chapman & Hall, 1995:203–222.

50 Pavri K. Clinical, clinicopathologic and hematologic features of Kyasanur Forest disease. *Rev Infect Dis* 1989; 11(Supplement 4):S854–S859.

51 Boshell J. Kyasanur forest disease: ecologic considerations. *Am J Trop Med Hyg* 1969; 18:67–80.

52 Marshall I D. Murray Valley and Kunjin encephalitis. In Monath T P (ed.) *The Arboviruses: Epidemiology and Ecology*, vol. III. Florida: CRC Press, 1988:151–190.

53 Davidson M M, Williams H & Macleod J A. Louping ill in man: a forgotten disease. *J Infect* 1991; 23:241–249.

54 Mackenzie J S, Smith D W, Broom A K et al. Australian encephalitis in Western Australia, 1978–1991. *Med J Aust* 1993; 158:591–595.

55 Burrow J N, Whelan P I, Kilburn C J et al. Australian encephalitis in the Northern Territory: clinical and epidemiological features, 1987–1996. *Aust N Z J Med* 1998; 28:590–596.

56 Cordova S P, Smith D W, Broom A K et al. Murray Valley encephalitis in Western Australia in 2000, with evidence of southerly spread. *Comm Dis Intell (Aust)* 2000; 24:368–372.

57 Hall R A, Broom A K, Hartnett A C et al. Immunodominant epitopes on the NS1 protein of MVE and KUN viruses serve as targets for a blocking ELISA to detect virus-specific antibody in sentinel animal serum. *J Virol Methods* 1995; 51:201–210.

58 Figueiredo L T M. The Brazilian flaviviruses. *Microbes Infect* 2000; 2:1643–1649.

59 Luby J P. St. Louis encephalitis, Rocio encephalitis and West Nile fever. In Porterfield J S (ed.) *Kass Handbook of Infectious Diseases: Exotic Viral Infections*. London: Chapman & Hall, 1995:183–202.

60 Tsai T F & Mitchell C J. St Louis encephalitis. In Monath T P (ed.) *The Arboviruses: Epidemiology and Ecology*, vol. IV. Florida: CRC Press, 1988:113–144.

61 Brooks T J & Phillpotts R J. Interferon-alpha protects mice against lethal infection with St Louis encephalitis virus delivered by the aerosol and subcutaneous routes. *Antiviral Res* 1999; 41:57–64.

62 Southern P M, Smith J W, Luby J P et al. Clinical and laboratory features of epidemic St Louis encephalitis. *Ann Intern Med* 1969; 71:681–689.

63 Greskova M & Calisher C H. Tick-borne encephalitis. In Monath T P (ed.) *The Arboviruses: Epidemiology and Ecology*, vol. IV. Florida: CRC Press, 1988:177–202.

64 Dumpis U, Crook D & Oksi J. Tick-borne encephalitis. *Clin Infect Dis* 1999; 28:882–890.

65 Peterson L R & Roehrig J T. West Nile virus: a reemerging global pathogen. *Emerg Infect Dis* 2001; 7:611–614.

66 Hall R A. The emergence of West Nile virus: the Australian connection. *Viral Immunol* 2000; 13:447–461.

67 Shieh W J, Guarner J, Layton M et al. The role of pathology in an investigation of an outbreak of West Nile encephalitis in New York, 1999. *Emerg Infect Dis* 2000; 6:370–372.

68 Lanciotti R S, Kerst A J, Nasci R S et al. Rapid detection of West Nile virus from human clinical specimens, field-collected mosquitoes, and avian samples by a TaqMan reverse transcriptase-PCR assay. *J Clin Microbiol* 2000; 38:4066–4071.

69 Digoutte J, Cornet M, Deubel V et al. Yellow fever. In Porterfield J S (ed.) *Kass Handbook of Infectious Diseases: Exotic Viral Infections*. London: Chapman & Hall, 1995:67–98.

70 Marianneau P, Georges-Courbot M-C & Duebel V. Rarity of adverse events after 17D yellow fever vaccination. *Lancet* 2001; 358:84–85.

71 Gonzalez-Scarano F & Nathanson N. *Bunyaviridae*. In Fields D C, Knipe B N & Howley D M (eds) *Fields Virology*, vol. 1, 3rd edn. Philadelphia: Lippincott-Raven, 1996:1473–1504.

72 Meegan J M & Bailey C L. Rift Valley fever. In Monath T P (ed.) *The Arboviruses: Epidemiology and Ecology*, vol. IV. Florida: CRC Press, 1988:51–76.

73 Jouan A, Le Guenno B, Digoutte, J P et al. A RVF epidemic in Mauritania. *Ann Inst Pasteur/Voirol* 1998; 139:307–308.

74 World Health Organization. The use of veterinary vaccines for prevention and control of Rift Valley fever: memorandum from a WHO/FAO meeting. *Bull World Health Organ* 1983; 61:261–268.

75 Verani P & Nicoletti L. *Phlebovirus* infections. In Porterfield J S (ed.) *Kass Handbook of Infectious Diseases: Exotic Viral Infections*. London: Chapman & Hall, 1995:295–318.

76 Tesh R B. *Phlebotomus* fevers. In Monath T P (ed.) *The Arboviruses: Epidemiology and Ecology*, vol. IV. Florida: CRC Press, 1988:15–28.

77 Braito A, Corbisiero R, Corradini S et al. Toscana virus infections of the central nervous system in children: a report of 14 cases. *J Pediatr* 1998; 132:144–148.

78 Braito A, Ciufolini M G, Pippi L et al. Phlebotomus-transmitted Toscana virus infections of the central nervous system: a seven year experience in Tuscany. *Scand J Infect Dis* 1998; 30:505–508.

79 Brown S E & Knudson D L. *Coltivirus* infections. In Porterfield J S (ed.) *Exotic Viral Infections*. London: Chapman & Hall, 1995:329–342.

80 Willems W R, Kaluza G, Boschek C B et al. Semliki forest virus: cause of a fatal case of human encephalitis. *Science* 1979; 201:1127–1129.

81 Calisher C H & Nathanson N. Bunyavirus infections. In Porterfield J S (ed.) *Exotic Viral Infections*. London: Chapman & Hall, 1995:247–260.

Chapter 42
Dengue and Dengue Haemorrhagic Fever

S. Nimmannitya

Dengue infections caused by the four antigenically distinct dengue virus serotypes (DEN1, DEN2, DEN3, DEN4) of the family Flaviviridae are the most important arbovirus diseases in humans, both in terms of morbidity and mortality. The infection is transmitted from person to person by *Aedes* mosquitoes. Dengue infections may be asymptomatic or may lead to an undifferentiated fever (or viral syndrome), dengue fever or dengue haemorrhagic fever (DHF).[1]

Dengue fever

Geographical distribution

Dengue is a worldwide condition spread throughout the tropical and subtropical zones between 30°N and 40°S, where environmental conditions are optimal for dengue virus transmission by *Aedes* mosquitoes. It is endemic in South-East Asia (types 1–4), the Pacific (types 1–4), East and West Africa (types 1–4), the Caribbean (types 1–4) and the Americas (types 1–4).[2,3]

Aetiology

The dengue virus, a member of the flavivirus group in the family Flaviviridae, is a single-stranded enveloped RNA virus, 30 nm in diameter, which can grow in a variety of mosquitoes and tissue cultures. There are four distinct but closely related serotypes (DEN1–4). They possess antigens that cross-react with yellow fever, Japanese encephalitis and West Nile viruses. Although the four dengue serotypes are antigenically distinct, there is some evidence that serological subcomplexes may exist within the group. DEN1 and DEN3 have been shown to share some antigenic determinants by neutralization tests and by immuno-fluorescence using monoclonal antibodies. A close genetic relationship has been demonstrated between DEN1 and DEN4 using cDNA hybridization probes. DEN2 appears to be quite distinct from the others as it shows low sequence homology with all other serotypes.[4]

There is evidence from field and laboratory studies to suggest that there are distinct strain differences between dengue viruses. Recent developments in molecular virology provided further proof for strain variation. Multiple genetic topotypes have been identified by RNA oligonucleotide fingerprinting for DEN1, DEN2 and DEN3 serotypes. The data suggest that most dengue viruses circulating in a particular geographic area are similar to each other, while viruses from different geographic areas show some biological and antigenic differences.[5,6] However, this is not always the case; in the Caribbean basin countries two topotypes of DEN2 have been documented.[2] Marked differences were also observed between DEN2 viruses isolated from forest mosquitoes and those isolated from human or from *Ae. aegypti* mosquitoes in an urban setting in West Africa, suggesting that enzootic strains of dengue virus in West Africa are genetically distinct from epidemic or endemic strains.[6]

Transmission

Dengue virus is transmitted from human to human by mosquito bites. Man is the main reservoir of the virus, though studies have shown that the monkey is the jungle reservoir in Malaysia and Africa.[2]

Ae. aegypti is the most efficient of the mosquito vectors because of its domestic habit. The female mosquito bites humans during the day. After feeding on a person whose blood contains the virus, the female *Ae. aegypti* can transmit dengue, either immediately by a change of host when its feeding is interrupted, or after an incubation period of 8–10 days during which time the virus multiplies in the salivary glands. Once infected, the mosquito host remains infective for life.

Other *Aedes* mosquitoes capable of transmitting dengue include *Ae. albopictus*, *Ae. polynesiensis* and several species of the *Ae. scutellaris* complex. Each of these species has its own particular geographic distribution and they are in general less efficient vectors than *Ae. aegypti*.

Transovarian transmission of dengue viruses has been documented but its epidemiological importance has not been established.[2]

Pathology

From experimental studies in rhesus monkeys after inoculation the virus reaches the regional lymph nodes and disseminates to the reticuloendothelial system, in which it multiplies and from which it enters the blood.[7] Skin lesions in non-fatal, uncomplicated dengue fever seen in human volunteers were studied by biopsy. The chief abnormality occurred in and around small blood vessels and consisted of endothelial swelling, perivascular oedema and infiltration with mononuclear cells. Extensive extravasation of blood without appreciable inflammatory reaction was observed in the petechial lesions.[8]

Immunity

Immunity is antibody mediated. After an acute phase of infection by a particular dengue serotype there is an antibody response to all four dengue serotypes. There is a long-lasting immunity to the homologous serotype of the infecting strain. A cross-reactive heterotypic immunity has been reported by Sabin[8] to last for about 2 months in experimental human volunteers, while another community study reported a period of up to 1 year.[9] After infection by one serotype, the individual concerned will be immune to other serotypes for 2–12 months and become susceptible thereafter. A second attack of dengue has been reported.[10] The waning cross-reactive heterotypic antibody is implicated in the occurrence of DHF.[11]

Clinical features

The clinical features of dengue fever are age dependent: infants and children infected with dengue virus for the first time (i.e. primary dengue infection) usually develop a simple fever or undifferentiated febrile illness; dengue fever is most common in adults and older children and may be benign or may be a classical incapacitating disease (classical dengue fever) with severe muscle, joint and bone pain (break bone fever).[1]

Typically, after an incubation period of 5–8 days following an infective mosquito bite, the disease in adults begins with a sudden onset of fever with severe headache, and any of the following: chilliness, pain behind the eyes—particularly on eye movement or eye pressure—photophobia, backache, and pain in the muscles, bone and joints of the extremities.

The temperature is usually high (39–40°C); the fever may be sustained for 5–6 days and may occasionally have a biphasic course. As the disease progresses the patient becomes anorexic and may show marked weakness and prostration. Other common symptoms include sore throat, altered taste sensation, colicky pain and abdominal tenderness, constipation, dragging pain in the inguinal region and general depression. A relative bradycardia is common during the febrile phase. Symptoms vary in severity and usually persist for several days.

Several types of skin rash have been described. Initially, diffuse flushing, mottling or fleeting pinpoint eruptions may be observed on the face, neck and chest. These are transient in nature. A second type of skin rash is a conspicuous rash that may be maculopapular or scarlatiniform and appears on approximately the third or fourth day. This rash starts on the chest and trunk and spreads to the extremities and face and may be accompanied by itching and dermal hyperaesthesia.

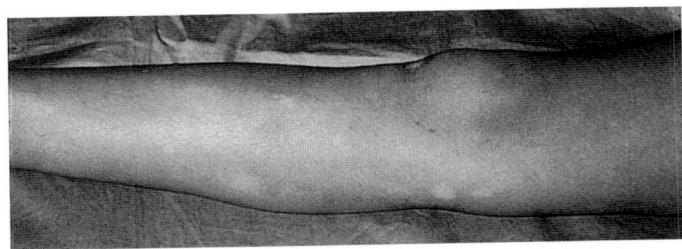

Figure 42.1: Dengue fever: convalescent rash-confluent petechial rash.

There is generalized enlargement of the lymph nodes but the liver and spleen are not usually palpable. A positive tourniquet test and petechiae on extremities are not uncommon.

Towards the end of the febrile period or immediately after defervescence the generalized rash fades and localized clusters of petechiae may appear over the dorsum of the feet and on the legs, hands and arms. This confluent petechial rash is characterized by a scattered pale round area of normal skin (Figure 42.1).

Convalescence may be abrupt and uneventful but is often prolonged in adults, sometimes taking several weeks, and may be accompanied by pronounced asthenia and depression. Bradycardia is common during this period. Loss of hair has been reported during convalescence.

Haemorrhagic complications such as epistaxis, gum bleeding, gastrointestinal haemorrhage, haematuria and hypermenorrhoea have been reported in many epidemics of dengue fever, and on rare occasions severe bleeding has caused deaths in some epidemics.[8,10]

Dengue fever with encephalitic signs but with normal cerebrospinal fluid has been reported in some epidemics.[10] Reye's syndrome associated with dengue infection is not uncommon.[12] Recently there has been an increase in reported cases of dengue encephalitis which was confirmed either by demonstration of virus, antigen or anti-dengue IgM antibody in cerebrospinal fluid.[13]

The most significant laboratory findings during the acute illness is leucopenia, which is usually noted 2–3 days after onset and lasts throughout the febrile phase. Mild to moderate thrombocytopenia is occasionally observed.[14]

Diagnosis

It is not possible to make a diagnosis of mild dengue or classical dengue fever from the clinical features as they resemble those of many other diseases, particularly chikungunya infection. Differential diagnosis includes malaria, leptospirosis and other viral, bacterial and rickettsial diseases. The presence of flushed face, a positive tourniquet test and leucopenia are helpful in differentiating dengue from other diseases. The diagnosis is best accomplished by serological tests for antibodies and virus isolation, or detection of dengue antigen by polymerase chain reaction (PCR).[1]

Virological diagnosis

See DHF below.

Management

This is entirely symptomatic and supportive.

Epidemiology

The first reported epidemics of dengue or dengue-like disease occurred in 1779 and 1780 in Egypt and Indonesia and in 1780 in the USA (Philadelphia).[10] It is clear that dengue and other arboviruses with similar ecology had a widespread distribution in the tropics as long as 200 years ago. Historically, Asia has been the area of highest endemicity, with all four dengue serotypes circulating in the large urban centres in most countries.[2,3]

During and after the Second World War, *Ae. aegypti* became more widespread in Asia and with an increased facility of communication and travel of susceptible foreigners into the endemic areas, together with the subsequent urbanization that occurred in most countries, the incidence of dengue infection increased dramatically. These changes coincided with the emergence of a newly described DHF in the 1950s. The advent of commercial jet air transport in the 1960s promoted the ideal mechanism for the carriage of dengue virus by persons who had visited endemic areas and were travelling during the incubation period. A trend of increased spread of dengue throughout the world has since developed. Increased epidemic activity was observed in the Pacific Islands and the Caribbean basin in the 1970s and epidemics of all four dengue serotypes were documented in both regions. In the American region, all four viruses are probably now endemic.[2,3]

In the 1980s increased dengue activity was observed in Africa, and all four dengue serotypes have now been documented in Africa.[2,3]

The incidence of dengue infection has increased markedly since the 1960s, first in Asia then in the Pacific and Americas and finally in Africa. It appears that most of the tropical world, with an estimated population of 2.5 billion, is at risk of infection with dengue.

Dengue transmission occurs throughout the year in endemic tropical areas; however, in most countries there is a distinct seasonal pattern, with increased transmission usually associated with the rainy season. While in some areas increases in dengue transmission coincide with periods of increased rainfall, the interactions between temperature and rainfall or variation in daily microclimates may be important determinants of dengue transmission.[2]

In dengue endemic areas with multiple serotypes children become infected early in childhood. Classical dengue fever is rare among indigenous people as most of the adults are immune. In these areas both mild dengue illness and DHF occur mainly in children.

Control

See DHF below.

Dengue haemorrhagic fever

(See also Chapters 23 and 41)

Geographical distribution

DHF is widespread in the South-East Asian and Western Pacific regions. It is now occurring in most countries in tropical Asia, with the exception of Bangladesh and Pakistan. DHF has also appeared in Cuba, the Caribbean, the Pacific islands, Venezuela and Brazil. During the past 10 years, DHF has been reported in 17 countries in Central and South America. To date DHF has not been reported in Africa or the Middle East.[2,3]

Aetiology

All four dengue serotypes are capable of causing dengue fever or DHF, depending on the immune status and probably age of the host as DHF occurs almost exclusively in children under the age of 16 years and is associated with secondary dengue infection. A strong association between DHF and secondary dengue infection has led to the proposed concept of two sequential infections by Halstead. Based on his in vitro and monkey studies, an antibody-dependent immune enhancement theory has been hypothesized by Halstead:[11] it is suggested that during the second infection with a heterotypic dengue virus which differs from the first one, pre-existing antibody from the first infection fails to neutralize and may instead enhance viral uptake and replication in the mononuclear phagocytes. Such infected cells may then become the target of an immune elimination mechanism which can trigger the production of mediators with activation of complement and the clotting cascade and eventually produce DHF.[11]

In Thailand, studies over the last 40 years have demonstrated transmission of all four dengue serotypes, with dengue type 2 as the predominating serotype.[15] The studies and experience in Thailand, as well as in Cuba, confirm the two sequential infections in the pathogenesis of DHF and led to a suggestion that the interval between the two dengue infections (probably 1–5 years) and the sequences of infecting dengue serotypes, i.e. secondary infection with DEN2 following DEN1 infection may be important factors in determining the occurrence and severity of DHF.[11,16] A recent study by Vaughn et al. reveals that increased dengue disease severity (dengue fever vs. DHF) correlated with high viraemia titre, secondary dengue virus infection and DEN2 virus type.[17]

Other theories involving a virulent strain of dengue virus[18] and the genetic difference in the hosts[19,20] have been proposed. The association of the introduction of a specific (South-East Asian) genotype of DEN2 and the appearance of DHF in America suggested that a certain genotype has potential to cause severe dengue (DHF). The finding that the same DEN2 genotype may cause dengue fever or DHF in Thailand suggested that both virus genotype and secondary infection are important contributing factors in the pathogenesis of DHF.[21]

Pathophysiology and pathology

The pathophysiological hallmarks of DHF are leakage of plasma and abnormal haemostasis. Evidence supporting plasma leakage includes a rapid rise in haematocrit, pleural effusion and ascites, hypoproteinaemia and reduced plasma volume. A significant loss of plasma leads to hypovolaemic shock and death. The acute onset of shock and the rapid and often dramatic clinical recovery when the patient is treated properly, together with the absence of inflammatory vascular lesions, suggest a transient functional increase in vascular permeability that results in plasma leakage.

A disorder in haemostasis involves all three major factors: vascular change(s), a positive tourniquet test and easy bruisability, thrombocytopenia and coagulopathy. Acute-type disseminated intravascular clotting is documented in severe cases with shock and is responsible for the severe bleeding. Bone marrow studies show depression of all marrow elements, with maturation arrest of megakaryocytes during the early phase of the illness, which is readily reversed when the fever subsides and during the stage of shock. Moderate to marked leucopenia as a result of bone marrow suppression is common as in dengue fever.[14]

Kidney studies in non-fatal cases show changes similar to glomerulonephritis but these are usually mild and transient.[1,22]

Postmortem studies show that serous effusions with high protein content and widespread petechial haemorrhages in many organs are constant findings.[22]

Histological changes[1,22]

Significant changes are found in major organ systems:

- Vascular changes include vasodilatation, congestion, perivascular haemorrhage and oedema of arterial walls.
- Proliferation of reticuloendothelial cells with accelerated phagocytic activity is observed frequently.
- The lymphoid tissues show increasing activity of the B lymphocyte system with active proliferation of plasma cells and lymphoblastoid cells.
- In the liver there is focal necrosis of the hepatic and Kupffer cells, with formation of Councilman-like bodies.

Dengue virus antigen is found predominantly in cells of the spleen, thymus and lymph nodes, in Kupffer cells and in the sinusoidal lining cells of liver and alveolar lining cells of the lung.

The pathogenetic mechanism of DHF is presumed to be immunological, involving both humoral and cell-mediated immune modulation. A constant finding in DHF is activation of the complement system with profound depression of C3 and C5 levels.[1] Immune complexes have been described in DHF cases associated with secondary infection, and they may contribute to complement activation. The C3a and C5a anaphylatoxins are released and their association with the time of leakage, shock and disease severity has been demonstrated.[23] They are the most likely vascular permeability-increasing mediators among the other yet unidentified agents.

Immunity

The immune status of the host appears to be the important component that determines the development of DHF as the disease occurs with high frequency in two immunologically defined groups: (1) children who have experienced a previous dengue infection; and (2) infants with waning levels of maternal dengue antibody. The acute phase of infection by a particular dengue serotype is believed to provoke long-lasting homotypic immunity. A cross-reactive heterotypic immunity has been reported to last about 2 months in one study of experimental infection,[8,10] while another community study presented epidemiological data suggesting that this cross-reactive heterotypic immunity might last up to 1 year.[9] It is hypothesized that this cross-heterotypic antibody, when weak and failing to neutralize the infecting dengue virus during the second infection, can enhance virus multiplication in the mononuclear phagocyte and trigger immune modulation and eventually produce DHF.[11] Passive IgG dengue antibody from the mothers of infants under the age of 1 year has been shown to be capable of enhancing virus replication when falling to below the neutralization level and produce DHF during primary infection.[11,24]

A study of the cell-mediated immune response revealed that during a secondary dengue infection serotype cross-reactive dengue-specific T lymphocytes are activated and proliferate with production of lymphokines and monokines. It is suggested that this response, while contributing to recovery from infection, may also in some circumstances play a role in the immunopathogenesis of DHF.[25] Recently it has been shown that cytokines, including tumour necrosis factor α (TNFα) interleukin 2 (IL-2), IL-6, IL-8 and interferons IFNα and IFNγ, were released into the circulation during the early phase of DHF and there levels correlated well with disease severity.[26]

A second attack of DHF is very rare: it has been shown to occur in about 0.5% of cases in a study over a 16-year period at the Children's Hospital in Bangkok.[27]

Clinical features (Figure 42.2)

DHF is a severe form of dengue infection that is accompanied by haemorrhage and a tendency to develop fatal shock (dengue shock syndrome: DSS) as a consequence

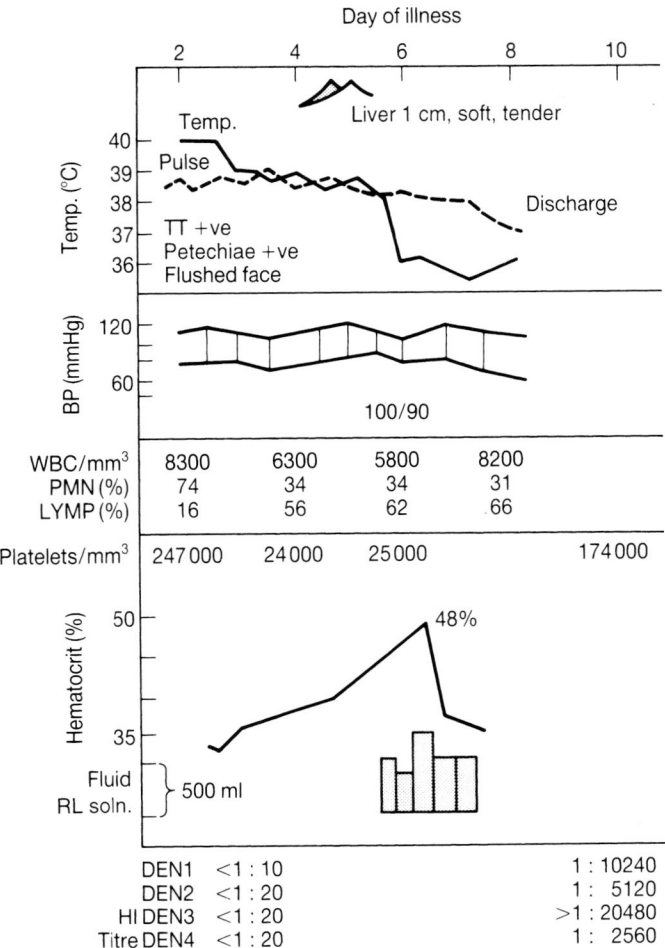

Figure 42.2: Dengue haemorrhagic fever: typical clinical course in a 9-year-old girl (with secondary dengue infection). TT, tourniquet test; PMN, polymorphonuclear leucocytes; LYMP, lymphocyte; RL, Ringer's lactate; HI, haemagglutination inhibition (antibody test by HI titres).

of plasma leakage. The clinical course could be divided into febrile, critical and convalescence phases.

Typically the disease begins with the febrile phase with an abrupt onset of high fever, accompanied by facial flush and headache. Some patients with an infected pharynx may complain of sore throat but rarely have rhinitis or cough. Anorexia, vomiting and abdominal pain are common. During the first few days of the febrile phase, which usually lasts for 2–7 days, the illness resembles dengue fever in many respects but a maculopapular rash and myalgia are less common. Occasionally the body temperature may be as high as 40–41°C and febrile convulsions may occur.

A haemorrhagic diathesis commonly presents in the febrile phase as scattered petechiae on extremities, axillae, trunk and face. A positive tourniquet test and/or tendency to bruise at venepuncture sites are invariably present. Bleeding from the nose, gums and gastrointestinal tract are less common. Haematuria is extremely rare.

The liver is often enlarged, soft and tender but jaundice is not observed. Splenomegaly is rarely observed in small

infants. Generalized lymphadenopathy is noted in about half of the cases.

The critical stage, which is the period of plasma leakage, is reached near 0 by the time the fever subsides. Accompanying, or shortly after, a rapid drop in the temperature there are varying degrees of circulatory disturbance. The child is often sweating and restless and has cool extremities. In less severe cases the changes in vital signs are minimal and transient; the patient recovers spontaneously or after a brief period of therapy. In more severe cases shock ensues. The skin is cold and clammy and the pulse pressure is narrow (≤ 20 mmHg). The course of shock is brief and stormy. If no treatment is given the patient deteriorates rapidly into the stage of profound shock with an imperceptible pulse and blood pressure and dies within 12–24 hours. Prolonged shock is often complicated by metabolic acidosis and severe bleeding, which indicates a poor prognosis. However, if the patient is properly treated before irreversible shock has developed, rapid, often dramatic recovery is the rule. Infrequently encephalitic signs associated with metabolic disturbances, intracranial haemorrhage or hepatic failure (a form of Reye's-like syndrome) occur and give rise to a more complicated course and grave prognosis.[12] The critical phase usually last 24–48 hours.

The convalescence phase is usually short and uneventful. Sinus bradycardia is common. A characteristic confluent petechial rash with scattered round areas of pale skin, as described in dengue fever, is frequently observed on the lower extremities. The course of the illness is about 7–10 days in most uncomplicated cases.

A normal white blood count or leucopenia is common and neutrophils may predominate initially. Towards the end of febrile phase there is a reduction in the number of total leucocytes and neutrophils shortly before or simultaneously with a relative increase in lymphocytes with the presence of atypical lymphocytes. The leucopenia usually reaches a nadir shortly before the platelets drop. This observation is valuable in predicting the end of the febrile period and the beginning of the critical phase. Thrombocytopenia and haemoconcentration are constant findings. The platelet count drops shortly before or simultaneously with the haematocrit rise and both changes occur before the subsidence of fever and before onset of shock. Clotting abnormalities are usually found. Other changes include hypoproteinaemia, hypoalbuminaemia, hyponatraemia and mildly elevated alanine aminotransferase/aspartate aminotransferase levels.[1,14]

Disease severity is arbitrarily classified as 'non-shock' cases (grades I and II—grade II is more severe than grade I with the presence of spontaneous haemorrhage) and 'shock' cases (grades III and IV—the latter is a profound shock with imperceptible pulse and/or blood pressure).[1,28]

Diagnosis

The clinical features of DHF are rather stereotyped; thus it is possible to make a correct clinical diagnosis based on the major characteristic manifestations as described. The World Health Organization established criteria for clinical diagnosis:[1,28] high continuous fever for 2–7 days; a haemorrhagic diathesis; hepatomegaly and shock; together with two laboratory changes: thrombocytopenia ($\leq 100\,000/mm^3$) with concurrent haemoconcentration (haematocrit elevation of 20% or more). The time course relationship between the drop in platelet count and a rapid rise in haematocrit appears to be unique in DHF. These changes, which represent the major pathophysiological hallmarks of DHF, i.e. abnormal haemostasis and plasma leakage, clearly distinguish DHF from dengue fever and other diseases. A normal or low erythrocyte sedimentation rate (ESR) observed in DHF and DSS helps in differentiating DSS from septic shock.[29]

Virological diagnosis

Aetiological diagnosis can be confirmed by serological testing and virus isolation from the blood during the early febrile phase. Antibodies to dengue virus antigens increase rapidly in patients with secondary dengue infection. A diagnostic (fourfold) increase in dengue antibody by the haemagglutination inhibition test can usually be demonstrated from paired sera obtained early in the febrile phase or on admission, and 3–5 days later. A third specimen 2–3 weeks after onset is, however, required to confirm diagnosis of primary dengue infection.[1]

Serological diagnosis by detection of anti-dengue IgM and IgG by enzyme-linked immunosorbent assay (ELISA) is now widely used to document primary and secondary infection. IgM antibody capture (MAC)-ELISA is a relatively new test. It is specific in distinguishing dengue from other flavivirus infections and has the advantage over the haemagglutination test in that a definite diagnosis can be made from an acute blood specimen alone, with a sensitivity of about 78%; when convalescent sera are tested the sensitivity is > 97%.[30]

Management

The management of DHF is entirely symptomatic and supportive and is principally aimed towards replacement of plasma loss during the period of active leakage of about 24–48 hours. Prognosis depends on early clinical recognition and frequent monitoring for a drop in platelet count and rise in haematocrit. Early volume replacement when the haematocrit rises sharply as plasma leaks out can modify severity and prevent shock.

The management of DHF during the febrile phase is similar to that of dengue fever. Antipyretics may be needed to control the high fever; aspirin must not be used (to avoid gastric irritation and bleeding and as a precaution to prevent Reye's syndrome associated with dengue). Oral fluid and electrolyte therapy are recommended for patients who have anorexia and vomiting.

The critical period when plasma leakage and shock may develop is at the transition from the febrile to the afebrile phase, which is from the third day. A drop in the platelet count to 100 000/mm³ or less usually precedes a rise in haematocrit. A rise in haematocrit of 20% (e.g. from 35% to 42% or more) indicates significant plasma loss and intravenous fluid therapy is indicated. In mild to moderately severe cases (grades I and II) fluid therapy can be given for a period of 12–24 hours at an outpatient clinic. Patients who are restless and have cool extremities, acute abdominal pain and oliguria should be admitted to hospital.

The fluid used for volume replacement in DHF should be an isotonic solution that has an electrolyte composition similar to plasma. The total volume needed is usually approximately maintenance plus 5–6% deficit (similar to mild or moderate dehydration). The rate of intravenous fluid infusion must be adjusted according to the rate of plasma leakage, which is more rapid during the first 6 hours of the critical phase. The need for intravenous therapy usually lasts for no more than 48 hours in uncomplicated cases.

When shock has developed, satisfactory results have been obtained with the following regimen:

1. Immediately and rapidly correct hypovolaemia from plasma loss with isotonic salt solution (5% dextrose in saline, Ringer lactate or acetate solution) and colloid (plasma or plasma expander) in cases of profound shock at the rate of 10–20 ml/kg per hour until improvement in vital signs is apparent.
2. Continue to replace further plasma losses to maintain effective circulation for a period of 24–48 hours. The rate of infusion should be reduced and adjusted according to rate of plasma leakage after initial resuscitation.
3. Correct metabolic and electrolyte disturbances (acidosis and hyponatraemia).
4. Give fresh blood transfusions and occasionally platelet-rich plasma in cases of significant bleeding.

It is important to adjust the rate of intravenous infusion according to the extent of leakage, as guided by the haematocrit level, vital signs and urine output, to avoid excessive fluid replacement. It must be emphasized that the total volume of fluid replacement should be just sufficient to maintain effective circulation during the period of leakage. Fluid replacement must be stopped when haematocrit and vital signs return to normal and become stable and a diuresis ensues. If further fluid replacement is given at this stage it can cause cardiac failure and/or acute pulmonary oedema when extravasated plasma is reabsorbed.

With this regimen the fatality rate of DHF cases at the Children's Hospital in Bangkok has fallen to below 1%. There is no evidence that corticosteroids are of benefit in reducing the fatality rate or reducing the disease severity.[31,32] The efficacy of heparin in the treatment of cases with severe bleeding from disseminated intravascular coagulation has not been proved.[14]

Good nursing care with close observation 24 hours a day is essential for management of patients with DHF/DSS.

Epidemiology

Since it was first recognized in the Philippines in 1954, DHF has occurred in Thailand, Malaysia, Singapore, Sri Lanka, Vietnam, India, Myanmar and Malaysia, several Pacific islands, China, Laos and Kampuchea. Between 1956 and 1990, there were 3 071 245 cases with 51 087 deaths reported from 12 Asian countries, the Pacific Islands, Cuba and Venezuela. The first outbreak of DHF to occur outside the South-East Asian and Western Pacific regions was in Cuba in 1981. Since then sporadic cases of DHF have been reported from the Caribbean and small outbreaks occurred in Venezuela in 1989 and Rio de Janeiro in 1991.[33] Between 1991 and 1995, DHF has emerged to become a major public health problem in 17 countries in tropical America; there were 34 739 reported cases of DHF with 514 deaths. More adult cases were observed in these areas.[3,34] Recent outbreaks of DHF in adults who had DEN2 in 1997 following primary DEN1 infection in 1977 or 1981 in Cuba confirmed the role of secondary infection and sequence of DEN1–DEN2 infections as risk factors for the occurrence of DHF. It is noteworthy that DEN2 involved in the outbreak both in 1981 and 1997 in Cuba was of South-East Asian genotype.[34]

Outbreaks occur most frequently in areas where most environmental conditions are optimal for dengue transmission and multiple types of dengue virus are simultaneously endemic or sequentially epidemic, and infections with heterologous types are frequent. In endemic areas where dengue infection is frequently asymptomatic and occurs in early childhood, classical dengue fever is rarely a recognizable disease among indigenous people. DHF occurs most frequently in children aged between 2 and 15 years. Older and many of the younger inhabitants are usually immune and escape DHF. However, cases in infants as young as 2 months and in young as well as aged adults have been reported. DHF is usually associated with secondary dengue infection but can appear during a primary infection, especially in infants under the age of 1 year, all of whom possess maternal IgG dengue antibody.[11] With increasing reports of dengue in adults, neonatal dengue cases including DHF as a result of vertical transmission have been reported.[35]

A seasonal incidence pattern usually coincides with the rainy season in many countries in tropical zones.

Prevention and control

The control of dengue depends on control of the vector, particularly *Ae. aegypti*, an anthropophilic domestic mosquito which lives intimately with its human host(s). These mosquitoes breed primarily in man-made containers such as those used for water storage, flower vases, old jars, tin cans and used tyres in and around human dwellings. Elimination of these breeding sites is an effective and definitive method of controlling the vector and preventing dengue transmission. The use of larvicides and insecticides during outbreaks has some limitations. Efforts are now focusing on health education and community participation in an attempt to control the vector(s) by eliminating or reducing the breeding sites.[1]

There is no dengue vaccine available for public health use at present. Research is in progress to develop an effective and safe tetravalent dengue vaccine. Many candidate dengue vaccines, e.g. live attenuated, inactivated whole virus, and recombinant vaccines are in the process of development. Some have been in phase 2 field trials.[36] In the absence of a dengue vaccine for public health use at present, prevention and containment of dengue outbreaks will require an effective long-term vector control and aggressive epidemiological surveillance.

REFERENCES

1 World Health Organization. Dengue *Hemorrhagic Fever: Diagnosis, Treatment and Control.* Geneva: WHO, 1997.

2 Gubler D J. Dengue. In Monath T P (ed.) *The Arboviruses: Epidemiology and Ecology.* Boca Raton, FL: CRC Press, 1988: 223–260.

3 Gubler D J. Dengue and dengue hemorrhagic fever: its history and resurgence as a global public health problem. In Gubler D J & Kuno G (eds) *Dengue and Dengue Hemorrhagic Fever.* Willingford, UK: CAB International, 1997: 1–22.

4 Henchal E A & Putrak J R. The dengue viruses. *Clin Microbiol Rev* 1990; 3:376–396.

5 Trent D W, Grant J A, Rosen L & Monath T P. Genetic variation among dengue 2 virus of different geographic areas. *Virology* 1983; 128:271–284.

6 Kerschner J H, Vorndam A V, Monath T P & Trent D W. Genetic and epidemiologic studies of dengue type 2 virus by hybridization using synthetic deoxyoligonucleotides as probe. *J Gen Virol* 1986; 67:2645–2661.

7 Marchette N J, Halstead S B, Falker W A Jr, Stenhouse A & Nash D. Studies on the pathogenesis of dengue infection in monkeys III: sequential distribution of virus in primary and heterologous infections. *J Infect Dis* 1973; 128:28–30.

8 Sabin A B. Dengue. In Rivers T M & Horsfall F L (eds) *Viral and Rickettsial Infections of Man.* Philadelphia: Lippincott, 1959: 361–373.

9 Winter P E, Nantapanich S & Nisalak A. Recurrence of epidemic dengue hemorrhagic fever in an insular setting. *Am J Trop Med Hyg* 1969; 18:573–579.

10 Schlesinger R W. *Dengue Viruses.* New York: Springer, 1977: 90–91.

11 Halstead S B. The pathogenesis of dengue: the Alexander D Langmuir Lecture. *Am J Trop Med Hyg* 1981; 114:632–648.

12 Nimmannitya S, Thisyakon U & Hemserchart V. Dengue hemorrhagic fever with unusual manifestation. *Southeast Asian J Trop Med Public Health* 1987; 18:398–406.

13 George, R & Lum L C S. Clinical spectrum of dengue infection. In Gubler D J & Juno G (eds) *Dengue and Dengue Hemorrhagic Fever.* Wallingford, UK: CAB International, 1997: 89–113.

14 Srickaikul T & Nimmannitya S. Haematology in dengue and dengue haemorrhagic fever. *Baillière's Clin Haematol* 2000:261–273.

15 Hoke C H, Nimmannitya S, Nisalak A & Burke D S. Studies on dengue hemorrrhagic fever at Bangkok Children's Hospital

1962–1984. In Pang T & Pathmanathan R (eds) *Proc Int Conf Dengue/DHF*. University of Malaysia Press, 1984.

16 Sangkawibha N, Rojanasuphots S, Ahandrik S et al. Risk factors in dengue shock syndrome: a prospective epidemiological study in Rayong, Thailand. *Am J Epidemiol* 1984; 120:653–669.

17 Vaughn D W, Green S, Kalayanarooj S et al. Dengue viremia titer, antibody response pattern, and virus serotype correlate with disease severity. *J Infect Dis* 2000; 181:2–9.

18 Rosen L. The Emperor's New Clothes revisited, or reflections on the pathogenesis of dengue hemorrhagic fever. *Am J Trop Med Hyg* 1977; 26:337–343.

19 Chiewsilp P, Scott R M, Bhamarapravati N et al. Histocompatibility antigens and dengue hemorrhagic fever. *Am J Trop Med Hyg* 1981; 30:1100–1105.

20 Guzman M G, Kouri G P, Bravo J, Soler M, Vazquez S & Morier L. Dengue hemorrhagic fever in Cuba, 1981; a retrospective seroepidemiologic study. *Am J Trop Med Hyg* 1990; 42:179–184.

21 Rico-Hesse R, Harrson L M, Nisalak A et al. Molecular evolution of dengue type 2 virus in Thailand. *Am J Trop Med Hyg* 1998; 58(1):96–101.

22 Bhamarapravati N, Tuchinda P & Boonyapaknavik V. Pathology of Thai haemorrhagic fever: a study of 100 autopsy cases. *Ann Trop Med Parasitol* 1967; 61:500–510.

23 Malasit P. Complement and dengue hemorrhagic fever/shock syndrome. *Southeast Asian J Trop Med Public Health* 1987; 18:316–320.

24 Klick S C, Nimmannitya S, Nisalak A & Burke D S. Evidence that maternal dengue antibodies are important in the development of dengue hemorrhagic fever in infants. *Am J Trop Med Hyg* 1988; 38:411–419.

25 Kurane I, Innis B L, Nimmannitya S et al. Activation of T lymphocytes in dengue virus infections: high levels of soluble interleukin 2 receptor, soluble CD4, soluble CD8, interleukin 2, and interferon γ in sera of children with dengue. *J Clin Invest* 1991; 88:1473–1480.

26 Green S, Vaughn DW, Kalayanarooj S et al. Early immune activation in acute dengue illness is related to development of plasma leakage and disease severity. *J Infect Dis* 1999; 179:755–762.

27 Nimmannitya S, Kalayanarooj S, Nisalak A & Innis B L. Second attack of dengue hemorrhagic fever. *Proceedings of the International Symposium on Dengue and DHF*, 1–3 October 1990, Bangkok.

28 Nimmannitya S. Clinical manifestations of dengue/dengue hemorrhagic fever. In Thongcharoen P (ed.) *Monograph on dengue/dengue hemorrhagic fever WHO/SEARO No 22*. New Delhi, 1993: 48–54.

29 Kalayanarooj S & Nimmannitya S. A study of erythrocyte sedimentation rate in dengue hemorrhagic fever. *Southeast Asian J Trop Med Public Health* 1989; 20:325–330.

30 Innis B L, Nisalak A, Nimmannitya S et al. An enzyme linked immunosorbent assay to characterize dengue infections where dengue and Japanese encephalitis co-circulate. *Am J Trop Med Hyg* 1989; 40:418–427.

31 Sumarmo, Talogo W, Asrin A, Isnuhandojo B & Sahudi A. Failure of hydrocortisone to affect outcome in dengue shock syndrome. *Pediatrics* 1982; 69:45–49.

32 Nimmannitya S. Clinical spectrum and management of dengue hemorrhagic fever. *Southeast Asian J Trop Med Public Health* 1987; 18:392–397.

33 *Dengue Newsletter*, Vol 17. WHO, 1992.

34 Guzman M G, Kouri G, Vazquez, S, Rosario, D, Bravo J, & Valdes L. DHF epidemics in Cuba in 1981 and 1997: some interesting observations. *Dengue Bull* 1999; 23:39–43.

35 Chye J K, Lim C T, Ng K B. Vertical transmission of dengue. *Clin Infect Dis* 1997; 25:1374–1377.

36 Bhamarapravati N & Yoksan S. Live attenuated tetravalent dengue vaccine. In Gubler D J & Kuno G (eds) *Dengue and Dengue Hemorrhagic Fever*. Wallingford, UK: CAB International, 1997: 367–377.

Chapter 43
Viral Haemorrhagic Fevers

T. Solomon

Few diseases create such fear among the general public and health care community as the viral haemorrhagic fevers (VHFs). Although, in terms of the actual risks, this fear is often unfounded, there are many questions relating to the origin, pathogenesis, treatment and control of VHFs that remain to be answered.

Epidemiology

The haemorrhagic fever viruses form a diverse group of viruses from four viral families—the *Arenaviridae*, *Filoviridae*, *Bunyaviridae* and *Flaviviridae*—which are considered together because of the similarity of the clinical syndrome they produce (Table 43.1). They have important differences in their natural cycles, geographical distributions and potential for nosocomial transmission, which can be confusing. The epidemiology may be simplified by considering three questions (Figure 43.1):

- How is the virus transmitted in its natural cycle—via arthropods, directly or unknown?
- How do human index cases become infected—via insects, directly or unknown?
- Is there nosocomial transmission from the human index case to secondary cases?

Most haemorrhagic fever viruses exist in enzootic (animal) cycles, causing little harm in their natural hosts. Humans become infected by these viruses coincidentally when they encroach upon this enzootic cycle. (Dengue is an important exception because humans *are* one of the natural hosts.) The viruses are transmitted naturally between host animals either via biting arthropods (insects or ticks), or directly via excretions such as urine.[1] Those that are transmitted by arthropods—dengue, yellow fever, Crimean–Congo haemorrhagic fever (CCHF) and Rift Valley fever (RVF)—are labelled with the ecological term arboviruses (arthropod-borne viruses; see Chapter 41). Viruses transmitted naturally via animal excreta include Lassa and Hantaan, the cause of haemorrhagic fever with renal syndrome (HFRS).

Some VHF viruses are particularly important because of their potential for direct transmission from one human to another in blood and other secretions. This group includes Lassa fever, CCHF, and Ebola and Marburg, whose natural cycle remains unknown.

Pathogenesis

Although different pathophysiological processes occur in different VHFs, the following are common:

- Vascular damage, which may be due to direct viral invasion of endothelial cells, complement and cytokine activation and immune complex deposition.
- Disorders of coagulation, which may be due to thrombocytopenia (caused by bone marrow suppression and increased consumption), abnormal platelet function, impaired production of clotting factors by the liver, and disseminated intravascular coagulation (DIC).
- Immunological impairment, which inhibits the immune response and allows uncontrolled viral replication.
- End-organ damage, which is most often due to direct viral cytopathology (e.g., hepatic damage in yellow fever), or in some cases due to the host inflammatory response (e.g., nephritis in HFRS).

Clinical features

The clinical manifestations that may result from these pathophysiological processes include:

1. Increased vascular permeability which allows leakage of plasma from the vessels into the tissue and leads to two problems:
   (a) low blood pressure, which may manifest with cold, clammy and sweaty skin, irritability, drowsiness, and in children a prolonged capillary refilling time and a narrow pulse pressure (i.e., the difference between systolic and diastolic blood pressure is less than 20 mmHg). If uncorrected, secondary complications of hypovolaemic shock occur, such as acidosis, renal failure, and other metabolic complications.[2]
   (b) pulmonary oedema, pleural effusions, oedema of the face and neck (which can all contribute to respiratory failure); in some VHFs pericardial and retroperitoneal effusions.
2. Haemorrhagic manifestations are sometimes relatively minor (e.g., skin petechiae, bruising, oozing from venepuncture sites, gum or nose bleeding). More serious manifestations include gastrointestinal bleeding.

Table 43.1 Overview of the major viral haemorrhagic fevers.

Family	Genus	Virus	Disease	Geographical area	Natural cycle	Human disease
Arenaviridae	Arenavirus	Lassa	Lassa fever	Western Africa	Mastomys rodent	Direct transmission from rodent excreta and human to human spread. Mortality rate 2–15%. Treat with ribavirin
		Junin, Machupo, Guanarito	Argentine, Bolivian, Venezuelan haemorrhagic fevers	Localized areas in South America	Calomys and other rodents	Direct transmission from rodent excreta and human to human spread. Mortality rate 15–30%. Treat with ribavirin
Filoviridae	Filovirus	Ebola and Marburg	Ebola and Marburg haemorrhagic fevers	Sub-Saharan Africa	Unknown	Nosocomial spread common. Mortality rate 25–90%. No antiviral treatment
Bunyaviridae	Hantavirus	Hantaan, Dobrava, Seoul, Puumala	Haemorrhagic fever with renal syndrome	Far East, Europe	Various rural rodents	Direct transmission from rodent excreta. No human to human spread. Mortality rate 1–15%, depending on virus. Treat severe disease with ribavirin
	Nairovirus	Crimean–Congo haemorrhagic fever	Crimean–Congo haemorrhagic fever	Eastern Europe, Asia, Africa	Hyalomma ticks and livestock	Mosquito bites and direct transmission from blood of infected animals. Human-to-human spread. Mortality rate 15–30%. Treat with ribavirin
	Phlebovirus	Rift Valley fever	Rift Valley fever	Africa, Middle East	Aedes and other mosquitoes, and livestock	Tick bites and direct transmission from blood of infected animals. Human-to-human spread not documented, but possible. Most natural infections asymptomatic. Mortality rate 50% for VHF. Treat with ribavirin
Flaviviridae	Flavivirus	Dengue	Dengue fever, dengue haemorrhagic fever	Tropics and subtropics worldwide	Aedes mosquitoes and humans	Transmission from mosquito bites. No direct transmission. Mortality rate < 1% with adequate fluid treatment. No antivirals
		Yellow fever	Yellow fever	Africa, South America	Various mosquitoes and monkeys	Transmission from mosquito bites. No direct transmission. Mortality rate 20–50%. No antivirals
		Omsk haemorrhagic fever	Omsk haemorrhagic fever	Western Siberia	Muskrats, other rodents, Dermacentor ticks	Direct contact with muskrats, and tick bites. Mortality rate 1–10%. No antivirals
		Kyasanur Forest disease	Kyasanur Forest disease	South-western India	Haemaphysalis ticks	Tick bites, no antivirals

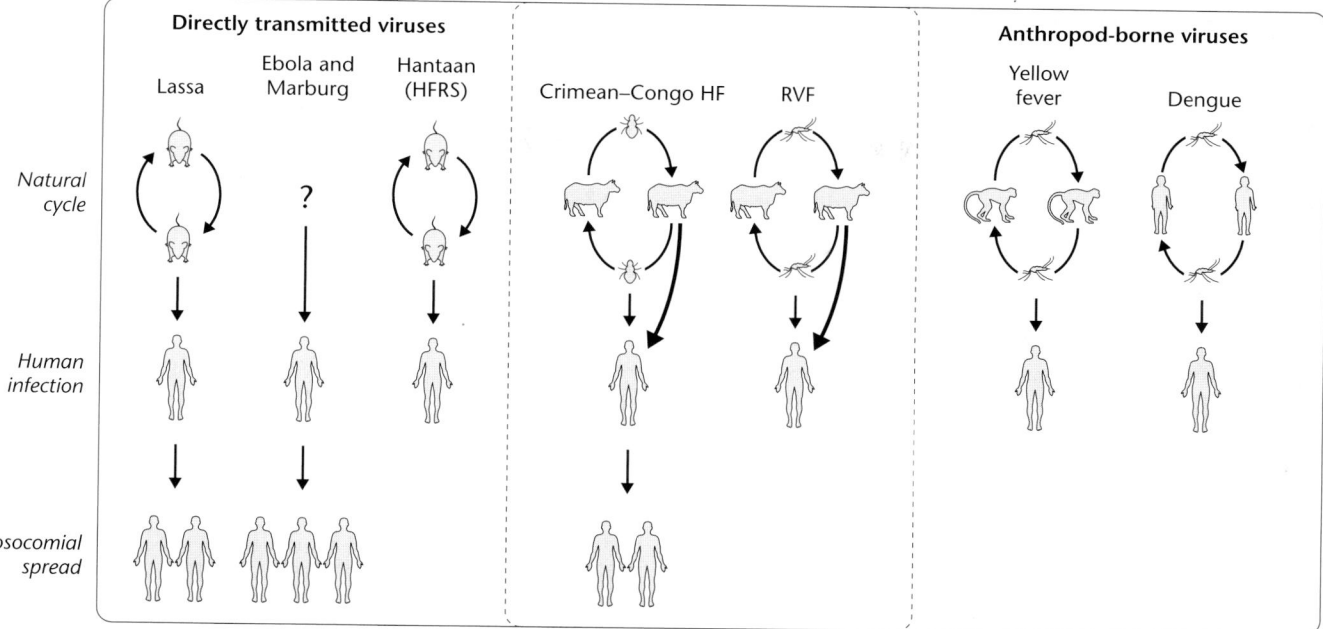

Figure 43.1: Ecological overview of viral haemorrhagic fevers showing natural cycle, transmission to humans and potential for nosocomial spread. Note the distinction between directly transmissible viruses, arthropod-borne viruses and viruses transmitted by both routes (CCHF and RVF). HF, haemorrhagic fever; HFRS, haemorrhagic fever with renal syndrome; RVF, Rift Valley fever.

However, for most VHFs, when shock occurs it is a result of vascular leakage and other factors, not haemorrhage.

3. Increased capillary fragility, determined by a positive tourniquet test (Figure 43.2).
4. Hepatic failure, including mild hepatitis and jaundice or fulminant hepatic failure.
5. Renal failure, which may be a consequence of hypovolaemia, or in HFRS, direct renal damage.
6. Encephalopathy, which may be secondary to the severe metabolic disturbances or, for some VHFs, caused by virus invading the central nervous system (CNS).[3]

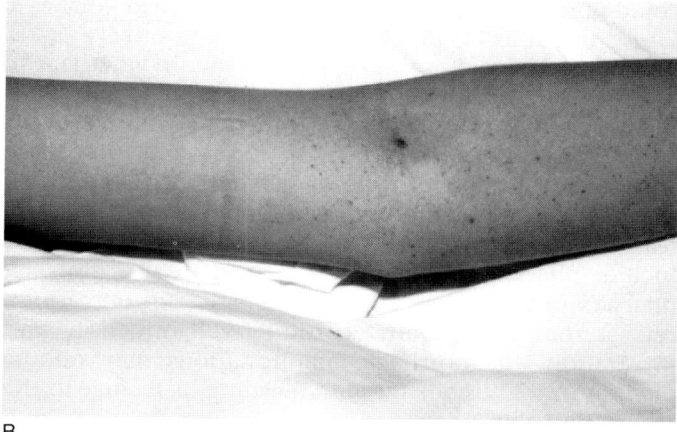

B

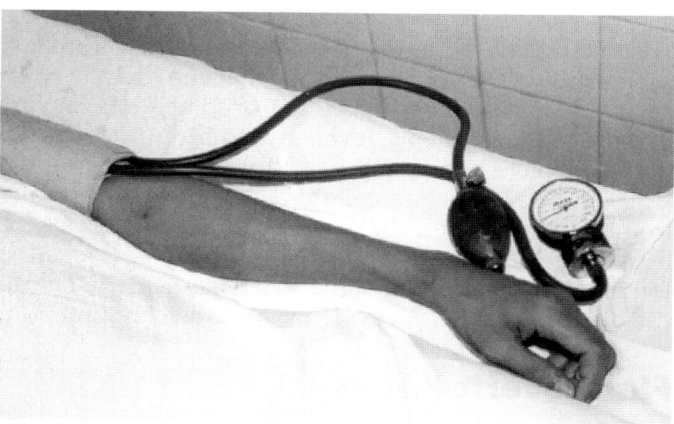

A

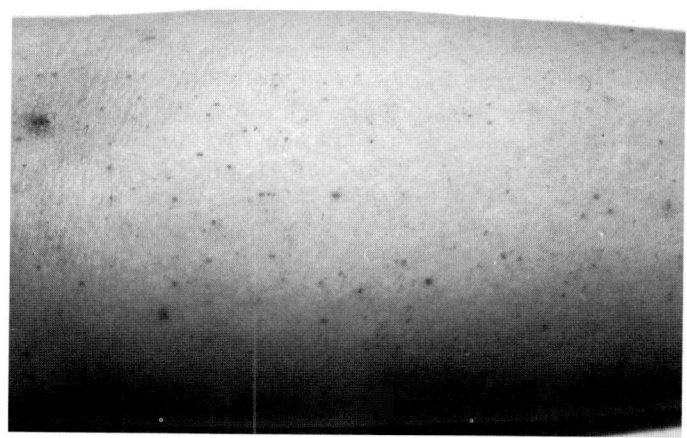

C

Figure 43.2: The tourniquet test of capillary fragility. A blood pressure cuff inflated to half-way between systolic and diastolic pressure for 5 minutes (**A**) causes more than 20 petechaie in a 2.5-cm square over the forearm (**B, C**). Note also bruising around a venepuncture site in the antecubital fossa. (Photo: Tom Solomon.)

Management of VHF

Although the general principles are the same, the practicalities of managing a suspected case of VHF in a traveller returning from the tropics are different to those of managing a patient locally during a known epidemic. Specific issues for each disease are addressed later in the chapter. In general, management incorporates:

- Identifying, diagnosing and treating a patient with suspected VHF.
- For the directly transmissible VHFs, limiting any further spread.
- Identifying others who may have been infected.

Identifying VHF cases

Most patients with suspected viral haemorrhagic fever turn out to have malaria, typhoid, gastroenteritis or another non-transmissible disease. A travel history should include details not only of the countries visited, but also the regions of the country. Under natural circumstances the directly transmissible VHFs are most often acquired in rural rather than urban areas. Because their importance may not be realized by the patient, specific questions should be asked about activities that could potentially have allowed exposure to haemorrhagic viruses, such as caving and exposure to monkeys or rat urine. In addition it is important to ascertain whether the person was in contact with any sick individuals, their tissues, or even those of sick animals.

An interval of 3 weeks between the last possible exposure and onset of illness rules out the diagnosis of VHF. Many early symptoms are non-specific but certain features should ring alarm bells (Figure 43.3). These include pharyngitis, (especially if there are ulcers on the pharynx or it is severe enough to cause pain on eating), retrosternal chest pain, conjunctival injection and prostration. Haemorrhagic manifestations may not be obvious initially. Look for gum bleeding, petechiae in the axillae and skin folds, and microscopic haematuria, and perform a tourniquet test (see Figure 43.2). Vascular leakage may also not be apparent immediately. Ask relatives if they think the patient's face looks puffy around the eyes. A decubitus chest radiograph may reveal a small pleural effusion. Laboratory investigations that may suggest a VHF include a rising haematocrit (a consequence of increased vascular permeability, which is easily measured and a useful early marker of impending shock), leucopenia, thrombocytopenia, raised levels of transaminases, prolonged clotting times and proteinuria.

Differential diagnosis of VHF

The differential diagnosis of VHF includes many causes of fever in the tropics (Table 43.2). Repeated blood film examination by an experienced technician may be needed to exclude malaria, especially if the patient had prophylaxis, or partial treatment. Blood cultures should be performed, and presumptive treatment will often be started before a diagnosis of VHF is considered.[4]

Diagnosis

Extreme care must be taken in obtaining specimens, which must be labelled so that their infectivity is clear. Serum, throat swabs, urine and, where appropriate, cerebrospinal fluid (CSF) samples should be sent to laboratories with biosafety level (BSL) 4 facilities. VHFs are diagnosed by virus isolation, reverse transcriptase– polymerase chain reaction (RT-PCR) or antigen detection early in the disease, or by antibody detection later in the illness. Antigen detection enzyme-linked immunosorbent assays (ELISAs) have the advantage that they can be performed on clinical samples that have been rendered non-infectious by γ irradiation. The traditional serological method used to diagnose many VHFs—the indirect fluorescent antibody test—has been replaced by IgM and IgG capture ELISAs.

Management

The antiviral drug ribavirin (a guanosine analogue) is effective in Lassa fever, CCHF and, based on laboratory data and limited clinical data, should also be used in severe RVF and HFRS and the South American haemorrhagic fevers. An intravenous (i.v.) loading dose of 30 mg/kg should be followed by 16 mg/kg i.v. every 6 hours for 4 days, then 8 mg/kg i.v. every 8 hours for 6 days.[2] All patients with VHF should be given oxygen, pain relief and gentle sedation if necessary, and supportive treatment for the complications of infection, as described below.

Hypovolaemic shock

This occurs as a consequence of increased capillary permeability. Patients need to be rehydrated with intravenous colloid or crystalloid. For some VHFs, such as dengue haemorrhagic fever in children, treatment protocols have been published.[5] Intravenous crystalloid is recommended before colloid, although recent studies from Vietnam suggest that earlier use of a colloid may be beneficial in patients who are severely shocked.[6,7] Ionotropes are useful in some VHFs, particularly late in the disease or if there is evidence of cardiac dysfunction.

Fluid overload

Fluid overload is common, especially as in some VHFs the vascular permeability can return to normal rapidly. The rate of fluid infusion needs to be carefully tailored according to the vital signs, haematocrit and urine output. Even cautious treatment may precipitate fluid

	Directly transmissible VHF(a)						Non-directly transmissible VHF		
	Ebola/ Marburg	Lassa	South American VHFs	CCHF	RVF(b)		HFRS	DHF	Yellow fever

1. Obtain a travel history:

	Ebola/Marburg	Lassa	South American VHFs	CCHF	RVF(b)		HFRS	DHF	Yellow fever
Africa	+	+		+	+				+
Middle East				+	+			+	
Asian subcontinent				+				+	
Europe				+			+		
Far East							+		
Americas			+					+	+

2. Ask about activities that may have caused exposure to virus:

	Directly transmissible VHF					Non-directly transmissible VHF		
Exposure to human cases	Recent contact (< 3 weeks) with any sick individual with unexplained fever and bleeding					–	–	–
Exposure to animal reservoir	?Monkeys ?Bats	Rodent excreta (urban) (rural)		Livestock		Rodent excreta	–	Monkeys
Activities undertaken	Jungle visits, caving	Cleaning basements, etc.	Farming, harvesting	Farming, abattoir work, rural activities		Rural, agricultural work	Urban mosquito exposure	Jungle mosquito exposure

3. Look for suggestive clinical features:

Early features	Pharyngitis	Rash	Facial oedema
	Conjunctival injection	Venepuncture oozing	Small pleural effusions
	Retrosternal chest pain	Petechial haemorrhages	Abdominal pain
	Prostration	Mucosal bleeding	Tender hepatomegaly
Late features	Shock	Haematemesis	Renal failure
	Pleural effusions	DIC	Encephalopathy
	Ascites	Hepatic failure	Acidosis
	Pericardial effusions		

4. Consider investigative findings common in VHFs:

Leucopenia	Proteinuria	Prolonged TT, APTT
Thrombocytopenia	Haematuria	Raised transaminase levels
Rising haematocrit	Renal impairment	

5. If malaria film and other tests negative and patient deteriorating despite presumptive treatment, suspect VHF:

For a directly transmissible VHF, begin isolation procedure; alert medical, nursing, laboratory, cleaning and laundry staff and public health officials	For non-transmissible VHF, ensure standard safe practices are being followed; inform public health authorities

6. Start intravenous ribavirin if likely to respond:

–	+	+	+	+		+	–	–
Ebola/ Marburg	Lassa	South American VHFs	CCHF	RVFb		HFRS	DHF	YF
Directly transmissible VHF						Non-directly transmissible VHF		

Notes:
a Directly transmissible between humans.
b Patients with VHF due to RVF should be treated as infectious, although direct transmission between humans has not yet been shown.

Figure 43.3: Algorithm for suspected viral haemorrhagic fever (VHF) in a febrile patient. APTT, activated partial thromboplastin time; CCHF, Crimean–Congo haemorrhagic fever; DHF, dengue haemorrhagic fever; DIC, disseminated intravascular coagulation; HFRS, haemorrhagic fever with renal syndrome; RVF, Rift Valley fever; TT, thromboplastin time.

Table 43.2 Differential Diagnoses of viral haemorrhagic fever.

Viral haemorrhagic fevers (in order of incidence)
Dengue haemorrhagic fever
Haemorrhagic fever with renal syndrome
Yellow fever
Lassa fever
Crimean–Congo haemorrhagic fever
Argentine, Bolivia, and Venezuelan haemorrhagic fevers
Rift Valley fever
Kyasanur Forest disease and Omsk haemorrhagic fever
Ebola and Marburg haemorrhagic fevers
	Fever with rash due to arboviruses
	Alphaviruses
	  Barmah Forest
	  Chikungunya
	  O'nyong nyong
	  Mayaro
	  Ross River
	  Sindbis
	Bunyaviruses
	  Oropouche
	Coltiviruses
	  Colorado tick fever

Fever with rash/haemorrhage due to parasites/bacteria
Parasites
  Malaria
Bacteria
  Meningococcus
  Typhoid
  Septicaemic plague
  Shigella
  Any severe sepsis with DIC
Rickettsia
  Tick and epidemic typhus
  Rocky mountain spotted fever
Spirochaetes
  Leptospirosis
  Borrelia
	Fever with rash due to non-arthropod-bourne viruses
	Enteroviruses
	  Coxsackieviruses
	  Echoviruses
	  Enteroviruses 68–71
	Paramyxoviruses
	  Measles
	Herpesviruses
	  Herpes zoster virus,
	  Humanherpesvirus 6 and 7
	Orthomyxoviruses
	  Influenza A and B
	Rubiviruses
	  Rubella

Fulminant hepatic failure Hepatitis viruses A–E Paracetamol and other drugs Reye syndrome Alcohol	**Miscellaneous** Drug reactions Toxins Acute surgical emergencies (upper gastrointestinal bleeding)

overload. Central venous pressure monitoring using a line inserted via a compressible site, such as the internal jugular or femoral veins, or measurement of pulmonary capillary wedge pressure with a Swan–Ganz catheter, is helpful if it is possible. Diuretics and ventilatory support are sometimes needed.

Respiratory failure

This may occur secondary to swelling of the neck and larynx, pulmonary oedema or effusions.

Bleeding diatheses

In many patients this presents as minor bleeding. Blood transfusions are therefore not required in most patients. Fresh frozen plasma is used in severely ill patients with deranged clotting. Although thrombocytopenia is common, it is not normally severe enough to require platelet transfusions. Intramuscular injections should be avoided, as should aspirin because of its antiplatelet effects and

potential to cause further damage of the liver in a Reye-like syndrome.

Other

Acid–base imbalance, renal failure, liver failure and encephalopathies are managed along standard lines.

Prevention of nosocomial spread

Patients with suspected, directly transmissible VHF should be isolated from other patients and strict barrier nursing techniques practised. The risk of person-to-person transmission is highest during the later stages of the disease. Hospital staff who come into contact with patients should wear gowns, gloves, goggles and masks, which must not be reused unless disinfected. The patient should use a chemical toilet. The risks of respiratory spread of VHFs between humans is low (possibly documented once only for Lassa fever[8]), but in the West patients are transferred to specialized isolation units with negative pressure or a tent facility.

Laboratory staff processing samples for routine investigations and performing tests to rule out other causes (e.g., full blood count and blood film) must also be warned about the nature of the specimens. Particular attention should be paid to the disposal of clinical waste and sharps. Patients who die from the disease should be promptly buried or cremated by specialist teams trained to avoid the risk of further contamination.[9] In African settings where directly transmissible VHFs may occur, advance planning, which includes training staff in VHF procedures and identifying a VHF coordinator, may save many lives in the event of an outbreak. Comprehensive manuals are available to facilitate such planning.[4]

Contact tracing

Contact tracing requires the identification of hospital personnel, family members and others who may have had contact with the patient (usually before the diagnosis was suspected). 'High risk' contacts who were exposed to blood, secretions or body fluids, or had close physical contact with the patient, should have their body temperature checked twice daily for 3 weeks after their last contact. Any in whom the temperature rises above 38.5°C should be immediately hospitalized, isolated and started on ribavirin if appropriate. Casual contacts who are at only low risk should be warned of their low risk of exposure and asked to report any fever.

The presence of VHFs in the community causes much fear and alarm. In the African setting identifying community leaders and other resources to help educate about the risks of transmission can be very important. When VHF cases occur in the West, dealing with the media is one important and time-consuming aspect of the care.

Arenaviruses

Arenaviruses cause chronic infections of rodents indigenous to Europe, Africa, America and possibly other continents. They are transmitted between rodents via their urine, and humans become infected when they come into contact with excreted viruses. For some there may then be secondary nosocomial transmission. Lymphocytic choriomeningitis virus (LCMV), the first arenavirus isolated, was discovered during a study of a St Louis encephalitis epidemic in 1933. It has received most attention as a model of viral immunology, being instrumental in developing concepts of immune tolerance, immune complex disease, and cytotoxic T-cell function.[10] LCMV is not typical of other arenaviruses in that, in humans, it causes occasional CNS, rather than haemorrhagic, disease. It is transmitted by the house mouse (*Mus* complex) and is widely distributed. Sero-surveys have shown an antibody prevalence of 10% in parts of Europe and America.[11]

The first haemorrhagic arenaviruses isolated were Junin virus, which causes Argentine haemorrhagic fever, and then Machupo virus, which causes Bolivian haemorrhagic fever.[12] Lassa virus, the arenavirus most important to humans, was recognized in Africa in 1969.[13] In total, seven arenaviruses cause significant disease in humans and at least 11 others have been isolated (Table 43.3; Figures 43.4 and 43.5). The New World arenaviruses are each associated primarily with a single rodent host, and are focal in their geographical distribution. Phylogenetics studies have shown that they are closely related to one another, and group separately from the Old World arenaviruses.[14]

Table 43.3 Arenaviruses pathogenic for humans[a]

Virus	Disease	Natural host	Geographical distribution
Old World Arenaviruses			
Lassa	Lassa fever	*Mastomys* species	West Africa
Lymphocytic choriomeningitis	Aseptic meningitis	*Mus domesticus, Mus muluscus*	Europe, Americas, ?elsewhere
New World Arenaviruses			
Junin	Argentine haemorrhagic fever	*Calomys musculinus*	Argentine pampas
Machupo	Bolivian haemorrhagic fever	*Calomys callosus*	Beni region of Bolivia
Guanarito	Venezuelan haemorrhagic fever	*Zygodontomys brevicauda*	Plains of Venezuela
Sabia	Not yet named	Unknown	San Paulo, Brazil
Whitewater Arroyo	Not yet named	*Neotoma albigula*	Southern USA

[a]Arenaviruses isolated that are not significant pathogens for humans include the Old World viruses, Mopeia, Mobala and Ippy, and the New World viruses, Tacaribe, Amapari, Parana, Tamiami, Pichinde, Latino, and Flexel virus, which has causesd two symptomatic laboratory infections.

Virology

Arenaviruses (genus *Arenavirus*, family *Arenaviridae*) are small single-stranded RNA viruses, usually 100–130 nm in diameter (but ranging from 50 to 500 nm), with a lipid membranous envelope that contains projections on the surface. Within the virion are cellular ribosomes which resemble grains of sand on electron microscopy (*arena* = Latin for sand) and two circular nucleocapsid segments. The genome comprises two linear segments of single-stranded RNA: a long (L) segment, which encodes the viral RNA polymerase (L) and a zinc binding protein, and a small (S) segment, encoding the nucleoprotein (NP) and two glycoproteins (GP-1 and GP-2). Most of the genome is negative sense, but a small portion is positive sense, making it an *ambisense* virus.

Pathogenesis of arenavirus infections

Following aerosol inhalation, arenaviruses are believed to replicate initially in the lung and hilar lymph nodes before disseminating.[14] The reticuloendothelial system, and particularly the macrophages, are major sites of replication throughout infection. Immunosupression facilitates chronic infections in rodents, and probably contributes to the pathogenesis in humans. The exact mechanisms leading to haemorrhage and vascular leakage are incompletely understood, but pathological

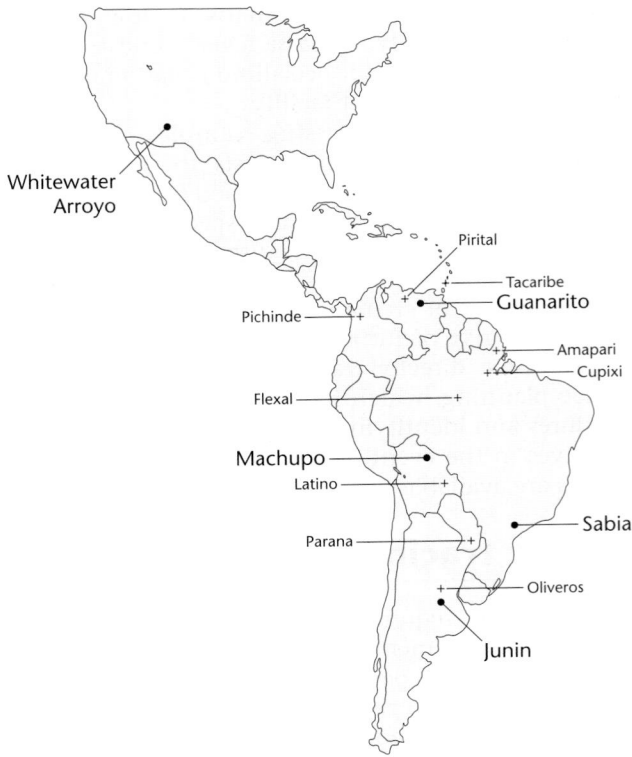

Figure 43.5: Geographical location of New World arenaviruses, including those that cause disease in humans (●), and those that are not significant human pathogens (+).[14]

changes in the host tissues are relatively minor, and inflammatory cells are minimal or absent.[15] Direct viral invasion of vascular endothelium has been demonstrated in vitro and to a lesser extent in vivo.[16] Cytokines secreted from infected macrophages are thought to be responsible for many of the circulatory changes seen and are associated with a worse prognosis. Unlike other viral haemorrhagic fevers, activation of complement or coagulation pathways does not appear to be important in the pathogenesis. Immunological recovery from arenavirus infections is now thought to to mediated mostly by cellular immunity. Production of neutralizing antibodies in Lassa fever is late, and inefficient, but may be more important for other arenaviruses.[15]

Pathology of arenavirus infection

At autopsy of the liver there is a focal eosinophilic necrosis of hepatic cells with the presence of eosinophilic bodies resembling Councilman bodies (seen in yellow fever). The extent of necrosis is not thought to be sufficient to explain the observed hepatic insufficiency,[17] but animal models show that histologically normal hepatocytes are also infected. The spleen shows lymphoid depletion with areas of eosinophilic necrosis; the lungs show pleural and peritoneal effusions and focal patches of pneumonitis; and the kidneys show focal necrosis of renal tubules. There are interstitial

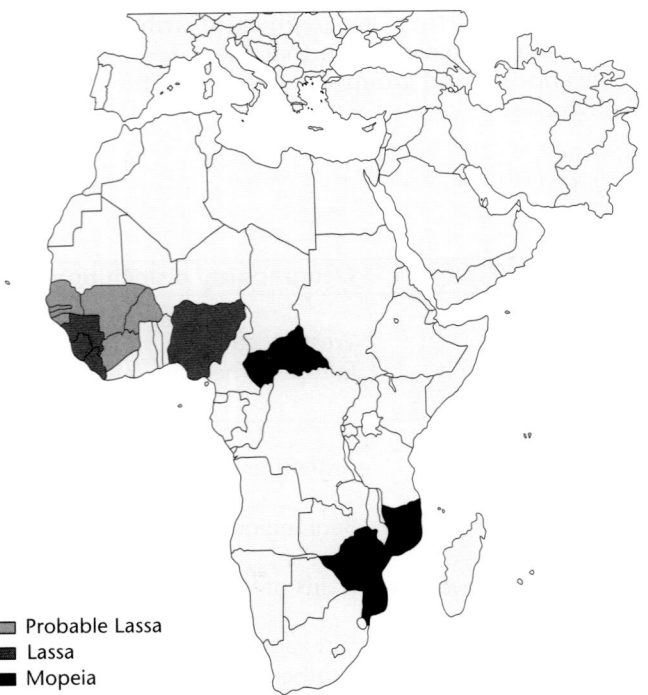

Probable Lassa
Lassa
Mopeia

Figure 43.4: Geographical location of Lassa virus and the related Old World arenavirus, Mopeia.

haemorrhages in other organs. The CNS shows meningo-encephalitis with oedema, congestion, neuronophagia and perivascular cuffing.

Lassa fever

In 1969 a nurse in a mission hospital in Lassa, Nigeria, developed a febrile illness with haemorrhage, and died. Two other nurses became ill, and a new arenavirus was isolated from one of them, by arbovirologists at Yale University, after she had been evacuated to New York, by arbovirologists at Yale University.[13] It has since been shown that Lassa virus is common in West Africa and, although Lassa fever can be fatal, and person-to-person transmission is a risk, neither the lethality nor the contagiousness is as pronounced as was initially suspected.

Epidemiology

Lassa virus is enzootic in the West African multimammate mouse *Mastomys natalensis*, in which it causes a chronic asymptomatic infection with constant excretion of virus in the urine and saliva. This peridomestic rodent lives in or near human dwellings, breeds year round, and is widely distributed across Africa. The virus is stable and infectious in aerosols, and is transmitted horizontally between rodents, as well as vertically to their offspring. Humans are thought to be infected by inhalation of the virus. In addition, excreta containing virus may be ingested with food, or enter through cuts. Secondary cases of Lassa fever occur by nosocomial spread, which in one situation was suspected to be by aerosol,[8] but tertiary cases are rare. Because of the high prevalence of Lassa virus, and its relatively long incubation period, it is the most common directly transmissible VHF of international travellers. Cases have occurred in the United States, the Netherlands, Japan, Israel, Germany and the UK, including one recent case.[18]

Geographical distribution

Lassa fever is confined to West Africa, although related arenaviruses (not pathogenic for humans) occur in other parts of Africa (Figure 43.4). The virus has caused major outbreaks in Nigeria, Guinea, Liberia and Sierra Leone. In addition, antibody surveys and occasional confirmed cases implicate the Ivory Coast, Mali, Burkina Faso and Senegal. Serological surveys indicate that millions of West Africans have antibody. In most cases the infection causes a minor illness or inapparent infection. Estimates suggest that there are 100 000 cases annually, with 5000 fatalities.[19] Cases peak in the dry season, but outbreaks occur when human exposure to *Mastomys* increases. For example, major outbreaks were associated with the migration of nearly 100 000 people to the surface diamond mines in Sierra Leone.[20] More recently armed conflicts in Sierra Leone and Liberia have created the circumstances for enhanced transmission to humans.

Clinical features

Patients typically present 7–14 days after exposure to the virus, although the incubation period may range from 5 days to 3 weeks. There is a gradual onset of non-specific fever with malaise and myalgia, followed by conjunctival injection, sore throat, cough, chest and abdominal pain with vomiting and diarrhoea.[21] The pharynx is often inflamed with characteristic white or yellow patches on the tonsils, and sometimes ulcers. In patients with mild disease these features resolve within 10 days. However, in a proportion there is a rapid progression with facial and laryngeal oedema (which causes stridor and respiratory distress), central cyanosis, a mild bleeding diathesis and shock. Pleural and pericardial effusions are common, and there may be bradycardia. There is often mild thrombocytopenia. Neurological complications include confusion, tremors, convulsions and coma, and carry a poor prognosis. Sensorineural deafness occurs as a late complication in 30% of patients, is thought to be immune mediated, and is often permanent.[22] Like other arenaviruses, Lassa crosses the placenta into the fetus, causing abortion and maternal death (particularly in the third trimester). The virus has also been isolated from milk, and may be a risk to breast-feeding infants.

Investigations reveal that the platelets are often reduced and have been shown in vitro to have dysfunction. The leucocyte count may be normal, low or even moderately raised. The plasma aspartate amino transferase (AST) level is usually increased, and albuminuria is common.

Prognostic indicators

Approximately 15% of hospitalized patients die. A prospective clinical study found patients with vomiting, sore throat, tachpynoea, bleeding, diarrhoea or pyrexia (≥ 39°C) were more likely to die. The combination of fever, sore throat and vomiting was associated with five times the risk of death.[21] Other poor prognostic indicators include the peak viraemia, peak Lassa virus antigen level, and an increase in the plasma AST level, to above 150 IU/ml.[23]

Differential diagnosis

The most important conditions in the differential include falciparum malaria, typhoid, other VHFs, meningococcaemia and septicaemia. (see Table 43.2). In an endemic area of Sierre Leone, the combination of fever, exudative pharyngitis, retrosternal pain and proteinuria was able to distinguish Lassa fever from other febrile illness with a positive predictive value of 80%.[21]

Laboratory diagnosis

Lassa fever is confirmed by isolating virus from blood, throat swabs or urine in a BSL-4 laboratory, or by demonstrating antibody to the virus. Viraemia persists into the second week, and virus can also be isolated from urine and semen for 2–3 months (hence precautions must be taken in convalescence). A new ELISA that detects Lassa virus antigen and RT-PCR allow more rapid diagnosis. The traditional technique for detecting antibodies, the indirect fluorescent antibody test, lacked specificity. It is being replaced by a new IgM ELISA, which has high sensitivity and specificity for acute infection, and an IgG ELISA that may be used to diagnose recent infection.[24]

Management

As with other VHFs, the issues in management are to treat the patient, identify others who may have been infected, and limit any further spread. High-dose intravenous ribavirin administered during the first 6 days reduces the mortality rate significantly.[25] Ribavirin has been used principally in patients with a poor prognosis (i.e., those with an AST level > 150 IU). Oral ribavirin also has some effect, and has been used as prophylaxis for close contacts, or given at the first sign of fever. Immune convalescent serum with high antibody content has also been used, with apparent success. The development of standardized monoclonal antibody directed against specific Lassa virus epitopes offers a possible future therapeutic approach. In the vast majority of cases Lassa virus is not transmitted from a patient to secondary cases. Early in the disease and in mild cases, the risks of transmission are thought to be minimal. Nosocomial outbreaks and infection of multiple contacts is more likely for patients who are severely ill.

Control

Although complete control of the rodent reservoir, *Mastomys*, is not possible, reducing their numbers (by trapping, poisoning and using cats) and their contact with humans may have some effect. An inactivated vaccine, despite producing high titres of antibody against all viral proteins, does not prevent virus replication and death in experimental animals, probably reflecting the importance of T-cell immunity in controlling infection. Vaccination of macaque monkeys with vaccinia virus expressing Lassa virus structural nucleoproteins and glycoproteins protects against Lassa virus and offers hope for the development of a human vaccine.[26]

Argentine haemorrhagic fever

Argentine haemorrhagic fever was first recognized in the 1950s. The arenavirus responsible, Junin virus, was isolated in 1958.[14]

Epidemiology

The virus is enzootic in *Calomys* voles (particularly *Calomys musculinus*) which inhabit the maize fields of the pampas (Figure 43.1). Agricultural workers are exposed to the virus by contact with the rodent and its excretions, particularly at harvest times. At its peak, between 100 and 800 cases were diagnosed annually.

Clinical features

Patients present with a non-specific febrile illness. Within 3–4 days they may be prostrated and have signs of vascular damage, which include conjunctival injection, facial and neck flushing, mild hypotension and petechiae in the axilla, soft palate and gingival margin.[12] Neurological signs are more common than in Lassa fever, and include irritability, lethargy, hyporeflexia, and tremor of the tongue and hands. In severe cases there is bleeding of the mucous membranes, haemorrhage, shock, anuria, coma and convulsions. Untreated, approximately 15–30% of hospitalized patients die.

Diagnosis

The diagnosis is confirmed in the first few days of illness by isolation of Junin virus from blood (in a BSL-4 laboratory) or antigen ELISA. Subsequently IgM and then IgG antibodies are detected by ELISA.

Management

Immune treatment with convalescent plasma from patients who have recovered reduced the mortality rate of Argentine haemorrhagic fever from 15–30% to 1–2%. However, it is associated with a late neurological syndrome in 10% of patients. Preliminary studies with ribavirin have also been promising.[14]

Prevention and control

Control of the rural rodent *Calomys* is not practical. A live attenuated Junin vaccine is effective[27] and has been used widely among men, and more recently in women and children. Its use in pregnant women should be avoided because of the risk to the fetus.[14]

Bolivian haemorrhagic fever

Bolivian haemorrhagic fever is caused by the arenavirus Machupo virus, which appears to be confined to the Beni, an isolated agricultural region in north-east Bolivia. The clinical features are similar to those of Argentine haemorrhagic fever. The natural host is the rodent *Calomys callosus*, which lives in the grasslands and invades houses in villages and small towns. Urban cases have been reduced by means of rodent trapping, but rural cases continue. One of these was recently followed by six fatal secondary cases in family members.[14]

Venezuelan haemorrhagic fever

Guanarito virus was discovered in 1990 during investigations of VHF cases that followed the clearing of forests in the municipality of Guanarito on the plains of Venezuela (Figure 43.5). The cane mouse *Zygodontomys brevicauda* is thought to be the main natural host. Clinically, Venezuelan haemorrhagic fever is similar to

Argentine haemorrhagic fever, with thrombocytopenia, bleeding and, in some cases, neurological involvement.[28]

Sabia virus infection

This arenavirus was isolated from a patient with a fatal viral haemorrhagic fever, who was from Sabia, outside San Paulo, Brazil, in 1990. There was extensive liver necrosis and yellow fever was initially suspected. Later a laboratory worker and a virologist became infected. The latter was successfully treated with ribavirin.[29] The natural host of Sabia virus, presumed to be a rodent localized to this part of Brazil, has yet to be identified.

Whitewater Arroyo virus

This virus is a newly recognized North American arenavirus. It was first isolated from the white-throated woodrats (*Neotoma albigula*) collected from north-western New Mexico, but is widely distributed throughout the south-western United States.[30] To date, two human cases of VHF have had evidence of acute Whitewater Arroyo virus infection.

Filoviruses

In 1967 an outbreak of haemorrhagic fever occurred among employees of a viral laboratory in Marburg, and spread to medical personnel and their relatives. The outbreak was traced to African green (Vervet) monkeys imported from Uganda. A long filamentous virus was isolated from both humans and monkeys, and named Marburg virus[31]. Nine years later, two further epidemics of haemorrhagic fever occurred simultaneously in Africa (Table 43.4). One originated in villages near the Ebola River in the rainforests of the Democratic Republic of Congo (then known as Zaire), the other 600 km away in southern Sudan (Figure 43.7). Secondary nosocomial spread was an important feature of both outbreaks. A virus, morphologically identical to but antigenically distinct from Marburg, was isolated from both sites and named Ebola.[32] Subsequently the two distinct biotypes were designated Ebola Zaire and Ebola Sudan, and two further subtypes have been isolated since then, including one originating in the Philippines (see below) (Table 43.4). The natural host and ecology of the viruses have remained elusive despite extensive investigation. However, procedures for controlling outbreaks have been devised, and shown to be effective.[33]

Virology

Filoviruses (genus *Filovirus*, family Filoviridae; *filo* = thread in Latin) appear as long filamentous U-, branch, or S-shaped rods, or more compact convoluted forms (Figure 43.6). They are composed of a lipid bilayer envelope with glycoprotein spikes surrounding a helically wound nucleocapsid.[34] The virions are 80 nm in diameter, and may be as long as 14 000 nm. Within the nucleocapsid is a single strand of negative-sense RNA encoding seven structural proteins: NP, VP35, VP40, GP, VP30, VP24 and L.

Pathogenesis and pathology of filovirus infections

The pathogenesis of filovirus disease appears to be a combination of direct viral cytopathology, cytokine-mediated vascular leakage, and an impairment of the host immune response (including an inflammatory response) that inhibits clearance of the virus.

Macrophages and monocytes are thought to be infected early, impairing the immune response and disseminating the virus around the body. Viral particles are found in endothelial cells, macrophages and the parenchymal cells of almost all organs in the body.[35] The

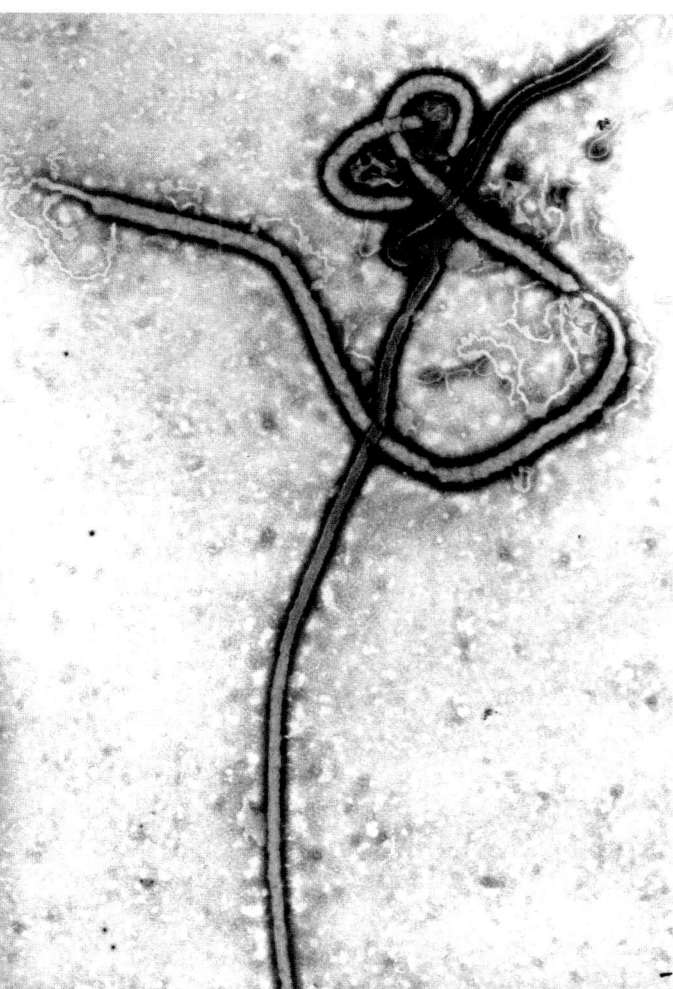

Figure 43.6: Electronmicrograph of Ebola virus showing the long filamentous forms. (Courtesy of Centers for Disease Control and Prevention.)

increased vascular permeability is thought to be a result of direct infection with virus and the effects of raised levels of cytokines. Levels of tumour necrosis factor (TNF) α, interleukin (IL) 2, IL-10, interferon (IFN) β and IFNγ are all raised in filovirus infections.[36] In vitro studies suggest the GP protein on the outer coat of the virus may have a major role by inhibiting T-cell proliferation and causing loss of endothelial cell adhesion.[37] In most fatal cases, no antibodies are detected. In prolonged cases and survivors,

a delayed humoral response occurs, although a vigorous cell-mediated immune response is thought to be the major mechanism of viral clearance.[38]

Pathologically there is extensive necrosis in the parenchymal cells of many organs, particularly the liver, spleen and kidneys, without much inflammatory infiltration. In the liver, intracytoplasmic inclusion bodies (aggregates of viral nucleocapsid material) are seen in intact hepatocytes.

Table 43.4 Outbreaks and cases of filovirus disease.

Virus and subtype	Year	Location	No. of cases	Mortality rate (%)	Source and spread
Marburg virus					
Marburg	1967	Germany (Marburg and Hamburg), Yugoslavia (Belgrade)	32	23	First ever cases, from Vervet monkeys imported from Uganda
Marburg	1975	South Africa (Johannesburg)	3	33	Index cases infected in Zimbabwe, travelled to South Africa; secondary cases in companion and nurse
Marburg	1980	Western Kenya (Nzoia) then Nairobi	2	50	Index case in Mount Elgin region; secondary case was in infected doctor who survived
Marburg	1987	Western Kenya (Kisumu)	1	100	Visited bat-infested cave in Mount Elgon region
Marburg	1999	DRC (Yambuku)	86	57	Community outbreak
Ebola virus					
Ebola Zaire	1976	DRC (Yambuku)	318	88	Unknown origin, nosocomial spread
Ebola Sudan	1976	Southern Sudan (Maridi)	284	53	Origin in a bat-infested cotton factory; nosocomial spread
Ebola Zaire	1977	Zaire (Tandala)	1	100	Sporadic case
Ebola Sudan	1979	Southern Sudan (Nzara and Yambio)	34	65	Site close to 1976 outbreak
Ebola Reston	1989	USA (Reston, Virginia)	4	0	Disease in monkeys imported from Philippines; humans asymptomatic
Ebola Reston	1990	USA (Reston, Virginia, and Texas)	0	0	Monkeys imported from Philippines only
Ebola Reston	1992	Italy (Sienna)	0	0	Monkeys imported from Philippines
Ebola Zaire	1994	Gabon (Minkouka)	44	63	Origin unknown; outbreak identified retrospectively in 1995
Ebola Côte d'Ivoire	1994	Ivory Coast (Tai Forest)	1	0	Conducted autopsy on dead chimpanzee, evacuated to Switzerland
Ebola Côte d'Ivoire	1994	Liberia	1	0	Serological diagnosis only
Ebola Zaire	1995	DRC (Kikwit)	315	77	Source unknown; secondary nosocomial and family cases
Ebola Zaire	1996	Gabon (Mayibout)	31	68	Contact with dead monkeys; secondary family cases
Ebola Zaire	1996	Gabon (Booué)	60	75	Index case a hunter; secondary nosocomial cases included doctor transferred to South Africa, and nurse infected there
Ebola Reston	1996	USA (Alice, Texas)	0	0	Monkeys imported from Philippines
Ebola Sudan	2000	Uganda (Gulu)	425	53	Community and nosocomial cases

DRC, Democratic Republic of Congo (formerly Zaire).

The search for the filovirus reservoir

The natural reservoir of Ebola and Marburg viruses remains unknown. Primary infection in humans has always occurred in rural areas (sometimes bat infested) or following contact with non-human primates. However, primates are unlikely to be the natural hosts, given that the virus causes disease in them, and they do not have latent infections. Studies in South Africa have shown that following inoculation bats have a prolonged asymptomatic viraemia, which would be expected for a natural host.[39] Similar experiments have failed to show filovirus replication in insects, reptiles or plants. However, attempts to find evidence of natural infection have so far proved negative in more than 3000 vertebrates (including 500 bats) and 30 000 arthropods.[40] Recently, however, Ebola virus RNA has been detected in a small number of rodents and shrews from the Central African Republic, suggesting they have been exposed to the virus, even if they are not the natural reservoir.[41]

Transmission to humans

Secondary human cases of filovirus infection occur among those who come into contact with patients, their blood or other secretions. In the early outbreaks, the reuse of unsterilized needles and lack of barrier nursing led to rapid nosocomial spread. Family members who have contact with body fluids are also at risk. Occasionally those who have just touched the skin have become infected (e.g., mourners at a burial service).[42] This may be explained by histological studies showing virus in the skin and sweat glands. The exact route of entry is unknown for secondary cases, but based on animal models is thought to be via cuts in the skin and contact with the conjunctivae. There is no firm evidence for aerosol spread in humans, although it has been shown in animals. Marburg virus has been isolated from semen, and sexual transmission has been documented. Serological surveys using ELISAs have revealed an antibody prevalence of around 10% among gold panners in Gabon and rural villagers in the Democratic Republic of Congo.

Ebola haemorrhagic fever

Epidemiology and geographic distribution

The first outbreaks of Ebola haemorrhagic fever occurred in 1976, simultaneously in northern Democratic Republic of Congo (then Zaire) and southern Sudan[32] (Figure 43.7). No clear index case was identified in the Congo outbreak, but in the Sudan outbreak the first patients came from a bat-infested cotton-weaving factory. In both outbreaks subsequent spread to relatives, hospital staff and other patients occurred. In 1989, another Ebola subtype (Ebola Reston) was isolated from sick cynomoglus monkeys that had been imported to the United States from

the Philippines and were being kept at a holding facility in Reston, Virginia. There were no human cases but serological evidence showed that humans had had asymptomatic infection with Ebola Reston. On subsequent occasions, the same virus has been isolated from sick monkeys imported to the USA and Italy, which always originated from the same export facility in the Philippines. How the virus arrived at this facility is uncertain. In 1994 an ethnologist became sick after performing a necropsy on a chimpanzee in the Ivory Coast. She was evacuated to Switzerland, and the fourth Ebola species, Ebola Côte d'Ivoire, was isolated. Ebola Zaire caused a large outbreak around Kikwit in the Democratic Republic of Congo in 1995, with 325 cases (81% fatal), and in 2000–2001 there were 425 cases (53% fatal) of Ebola Sudan in Uganda. In December 2001 a new outbreak of Ebola haemorrhagic fever was confirmed in Gabon. As this volume goes to press (May 2002) 60 cases were confirmed in Gabon (50 fatal) and 32 cases in neighbouring Democratic Republic of Congo (19 fatal).

Clinical features

After an incubation period of 4–10 days, patients present with an abrupt onset of fever, severe headache, myalgia, abdominal pain, diarrhoea and sore throat, with herpetic lesions on the mouth and pharynx.[43] There is severe conjunctival injection and gingival haemorrhages. A maculopapular rash may be evident (especially on white skin). This is followed by bleeding with petechiae,

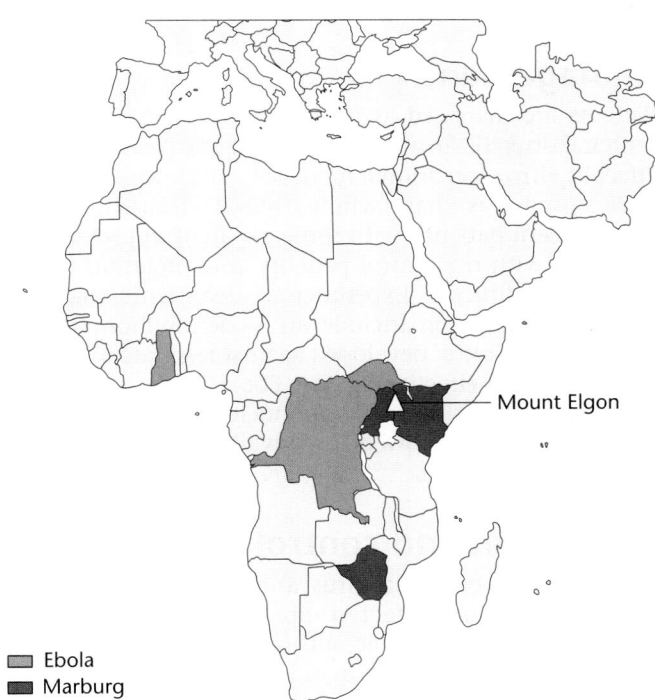

Ebola
Marburg

Figure 43.7: Location of outbreaks or isolated cases of Ebola and Marburg haemorrhagic fevers in Africa (Ebola subtype Reston has been isolated in monkeys from the Philippines).

echymosis, oozing from venepuncture sites, mucosal haemorrhage, haematemesis and bloody diarrhoea. Neurological manifestations (hemiplegia, psychosis, coma, convulsions) are common. Later complications include shock, severe metabolic changes and a diffuse coagulopathy. Death occurs most commonly around day 10. Mortality rates are higher for Ebola Zaire (60–90%) than for Ebola Sudan (50–60%), and higher among patients who were infected by injection.[33,43]

Laboratory investigations reveal an initial leucopenia and lymphopenia, with a later increase in neutrophils and the appearance of large abnormal lymphocytes with dark cytoplasm (virocytes). There is a marked thrombocytopenia, and experiments in non-human primates have shown abnormal platelet function. Serum transaminase levels are raised, whereas alakaline phosphatase and bilirubin concentrations are normal or only mildly increased.

Differential diagnosis

The differential diagnosis for Ebola infection is broad. In patients with appropriate risk factors (travel to endemic areas, or potential contact with infected people or animals), the presence of fever, abdominal pain and bloody diarrhoea should arouse suspicion in the physician.

Laboratory diagnosis

Ebola infection is diagnosed early in the disease by virus isolation in Vero cells, RT-PCR or antigen-capture ELISAs. In those who survive long enough, IgM and then IgG antibodies can be detected by ELISA.[44]

Management

Patients are managed as for other VHFs, and there is no antiviral drug. IFNα, although used in one patient, has little effect in vitro or in animal models. Convalescent serum has been used, as has whole blood transfused from convalescent patients, with some apparent improvement.[45] However, with no control patients, interpretation of these findings is difficult. Experimental treatments that merit further investigation include an S-adenosylhomocysteine hydrolase inhibitor, developed against respiratory syncytial virus, which is effective against Ebola in vitro and in the mouse model, and a human monoclonal antibody derived from the bone marrow of a convalescent patient, which protected guinea-pigs.

Prevention and control

As the source of Ebola virus and the means by which humans become infected are not known, primary prevention is not possible, although contact with sick or dead primates should be avoided. Control measures are therefore focused on limiting the spread from primary to secondary cases. This comprises containment of suspected cases and contact tracing to identify further possible cases. In recent outbreaks there has been less nosocomial spread,

probably because of better implementation of these practices. For example, in Zaire in 1995 nearly 30% of cases occurred in medical personnel, compared with less than 7% in Uganda in 2000.[33,43]

Marburg haemorrhagic fever

Epidemiology

Marburg virus was the first filovirus identified, when in 1967 it caused an outbreak of haemorrhagic fever in a polio vaccine laboratory in Marburg, Germany. It affected laboratory staff who handled blood tissue or cell cultures from African green monkeys. Secondary cases occurred in Marburg, Frankfurt and Belgrade.[31] There were 31 cases with seven deaths. The monkeys had been imported from the Kyoga region of Uganda, in a shipment that included sick monkeys. Excess deaths had also been seen among monkey colonies near Lake Kyoga to the east of Mount Elgin in Kenya (Figure 43.7). A few sporadic cases occurred in 1975 and 1987 (Table 43.4), and then in 1999 there was a large community outbreak in the Democratic Republic of Congo. This started among gold-mine workers in Durba and affected around 100 people, with 60% mortality rate.[46]

Clinical features

The clinical features are similar to those of Ebola virus infection, but the mortality rate is around 25–30%. Uveitis complicated one case,[47] and virus was isolated from the anterior chamber of the eye 80 days after onset. In one laboratory infection, the illness was mild and recovery complete after a long convalescence.

Diagnosis

Like Ebola virus, Marburg virus infection is diagnosed during the acute stage by virus isolation, PCR or antigen detection. Virus has been isolated from semen up to 3 months after the initial infection. In survivors, levels of IgM and then IgG antibodies are subsequently raised.

Control

Secondary control of Marburg infection is the same as that of Ebola: barrier nursing to prevent spread, and tracing and monitoring of contacts.

Bunyaviridae

The family *Bunyaviridae* consists of five genera:

1. The *Hantavirus* genus includes Hantaan virus, the cause of haemorrhagic fever with renal syndrome (HFRS).
2. The *Nairvovirus* genus includes Crimean–Congo haemorrhagic fever virus.
3. The *Phlebovirus* genus includes Rift Valley fever virus.

4. The *Bunyavirus* genus contains viruses that cause fever with rash (e.g., Oropouche) or CNS disease (e.g., La Crosse encephalitis), but not VHF, and so are not discussed further in this chapter.

5. The *Tospovirus* genus includes plant viruses, but has no human pathogens.

Virological properties

All members of the family Bunyaviridae are spherical virions, 90–100 nm in diameter, with a lipid envelope that contains glycoprotein peplomers and encloses three circular nucleocapsids. The genome consists of three linear segments of single-stranded RNA, designated L (large), M (medium) and S (small), which code for a transcriptase (L), a nucleocapsid protein (N), and two glycoproteins (G1 and G2). Most have negative-sense genomes, but the S segment of phleboviruses is ambisense.

Haemorrhagic fever with renal syndrome (HFRS)

During the Korean war of 1950–1952, more than 3000 United Nations troops developed a disease characterized by fever, haemorrhagic manifestations, acute renal failure and shock, with a mortlaity rate of up to 10%, which was originally named Korean or epidemic haemorrhagic fever. In 1978 the causative virus was isolated from the fieldmouse (*Apodemus agrarius*)[49] and named Hantaan virus after the river where the original cases occurred. Similar diseases with different names had been recognized earlier in China and the former Soviet Union. Later, three other hantaviruses were isolated and shown to be associated with similar clinical syndromes elsewhere: Dobrava virus causes a severe haemorrhagic fever syndrome in the Balkans, Seoul virus causes a milder syndrome in the Far East, and Puumala virus causes 'nephropathia epidemica' in Scandanavia (Table 43.5,

Figure 43.8). Subsequently these disease have all been grouped together as haemorrhagic fever with renal syndrome (HFRS). In 1993, a new syndrome of fever, non-cardiogenic pulmonary oedema and shock was described in North America (hantavirus pulmonary syndrome; HPS). It is caused by Sin Nombre virus, transmitted by the common deer mouse (*Peromyscus maniculatus*). Related hantaviruses transmitted by different rodents cause HPS throughout much of North and South America.

Epidemiology and geographical distribution

After infection, rodents excrete hantaviruses in urine, faeces and saliva for several months. Transmission among rodents is thought to occur primarily by biting and scratching. Humans become infected following inhalation of infectious virus in rodent excretions.[50] There is no evidence of human-to-human transmission. Most cases of hantavirus disease are sporadic, but epidemics do occur (see below). Each hantavirus is associated with a unique rodent host, and its epidemiology and geographical distribution reflect that natural reservoir.

Hantaan virus causes epidemic HFRS in Korea, eastern China and far eastern Rusia. Because it is transmitted by a fieldmouse (*Apodemus agrarius*), agricultural workers are at greatest risk of infection. Most cases of HFRS occur in men, and peak in the autumn, possibly because virus-infected mice are abundant at this time, and exposure is increased during the harvest. Approximately 100 000 cases are reported annually from China, and up to 1000 in Korea.

Dobrava virus is transmitted by the rural *Apodemus flavicollis* and causes a similar severe HFRS in the Balkans and possibly in other parts of Europe. Approximately 200 cases are seen annually. Epidemics have been seen in times of conflict, when rodent populations are high, and the number of troops and civilians living outside is increased.

Table 43.5 Summary of major hantaviruses causing disease in humans.

Virus	Disease	Natural host	Geographical distribution
Causing HFRS			
Hantaan	HFRS (previously known as Korean or epidemic haemorrhagic fever)	*Apodemus agrarius*	Asia, Far East, Russia
Dobrava	Severe HFRS	*Apodemus flavicollis*	Balkans, Europe
Seoul	Mild HFRS	*Rattus norvegicus, R. rattus*	Worldwide
Puumala	HFRS with predominant renal disease: 'nephropathia epidemica'	*Clethrionomys glareolus*	Beni region of Bolivia
Causing HPS			
Sin Nombre	HPS	*Peromyscus maniculatus*	North America
Andes	HPS	*Oligoryzomys longicaudatus*	Argentina and Chile

HFRS, haemorrhagic fever with renal syndrome.
HPS, hantavirus pulmonary syndrome. At least 16 other hantaviruses, each associated with its own host in the Sigmodontinae rodent subfamily, have been isolated in the Americas; many of these viruses cause HPS.

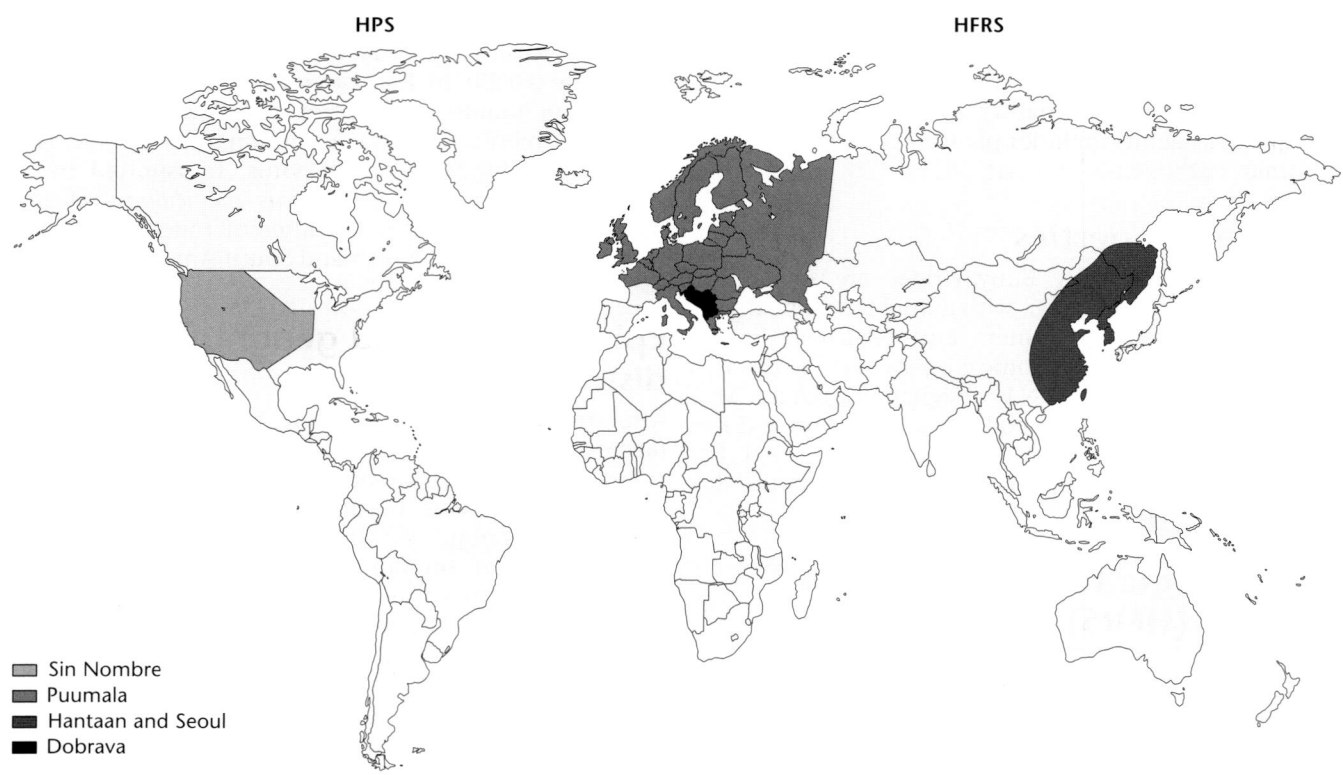

Figure 43.8: Location of major hantaviruses causing haemorrhagic fever with renal syndrome (HFRS) and hantavirus pulmonary syndrome (HPS).

Seoul virus is transmitted by the domestic rat (*Rattus norvegicus* and *R. rattus*) and causes mild HFRS in urban areas. Although this rodent and the virus are found worldwide, for reasons that are unclear Seoul virus-related HFRS is rare outside China, Korea and laboratory institutions that house rats. Cases of HFRS due to Seoul virus peak in the spring and early summer, and are frequently related to cleaning barns or basements, or other activities that result in human exposure to rodent excreta.

Puumala virus causes *nephropathia epidemica*, which is a milder disease transmitted by the bank vole *Clethrionomys glareolus*) across Scandinavia and northern Europe, including the UK.

Pathogenesis and pathology

Hantaviruses are thought to infect humans primarily via the respiratory mucosa, entry into cells being mediated by cell surface integrens. Viral DNA is detectable in the patient's blood early in the disease. Viral antigens are subsequently found in endothelial cells throughout the body, particularly in the kidney in HFRS[51] and the lung in HPS. However, there are no viral cytopathic effects associated with these infected cells and, unlike with most VHFs, the damage is thought to be mediated by the host immune response. In HFRS renal biopsies show acute tubulointerstitial nephritis, with a moderate inflammatory infiltrate, increased expression of cytokines (TNFα, TGFβ, platelet-derived growth factor), upregulation of endothelial adhesion molecules (CD54, CD106, vascular cell adhesion molecule (VCAM), CD31) and deposition of immune complexes. Similar changes are seen in the lung in HPS. As with other VHFs, the bleeding manifestations are thought to be a combination of increased vascular permeability (caused by a combination of viral infection, complement activation, the cytokine cascade and immune complex deposition) and a reduced number of functionally impaired platelets. There is some evidence that certain human leucocyte antigen (HLA) haplotypes (HLA-B8 DRB1*301) are associated with more severe disease.

Clinical features

Classically, patients infected with Hantaan or Dobrava virus go through five phases. After an incubation period that is relatively long for VHFs (usually 2–3 weeks, but ranging from 2 days to 2 months), patients present with an acute influenza-like illness. There is flushing of the face and neck, with conjunctival and pharyngeal injection, which are thought to reflect capillary dilatation. Lower back pain caused by retroperitoneal oedema is also common. The febrile phase is followed by a hypotensive phase, with mild shock lasting for 1–2 days and haemorrhagic manifestations. These range from a mild petechial rash to major gastrointestinal bleeding, are associated with marked thrombocytopenia, and in some patients a low-grade DIC. An oliguric phase associated with hypertension and biochemical renal failure follows, contributing to about half the deaths if untreated.[48] At this stage there may also be pulmonary oedema and CNS signs. Patients who survive then have a diuretic phase which may last for several months, followed by a convalescent phase. The mortality rate of patients with these classical features is 5–15%, although many patients with milder disease are probably not recognized. Laboratory findings include leucocytosis, thrombocytopenia, a rising haematocrit, deranged clotting and increasing proteinuria.

Patients infected with Seoul virus tend to have milder HFRS, typically with just febrile and mild haemorrhagic manifestations. Hepatomegaly and hepatic impairment with mildly raised serum transaminase levels is common. Puumala infection results in the mildest form of HFRS with fever, mild hypotension and petechiae, rather than haemorrhage. Around the sixth day there is oliguria or renal failure, and this is often the cause of hospital admission (hence the pseudonym nephropathica epidemica). About 10% of patients require renal dialysis, and about one-fifth of patients have mild transient neurological features (e.g., confusion, dizziness).

Differential diagnosis

In endemic parts of Asia and northern Europe, any febrile patient with thrombocytopenia and renal impairment should be questioned about possible rodent exposure and investigated for hantavirus infection. The differential includes leptospirosis, typhus, pyelonephritis, post-streptococcal glomerulonephritis, an acute abdomen and other haemorrhagic fevers.

Diagnosis

As antibodies are almost always in evidence at presentation, hantavirus infections are diagnosed serologically. The indirect fluorescent antibody test has been replaced by IgM capture ELISAs which use infected cell preparations or recombinant nucleocapsid proteins as antigen. Attempts to isolate virus are usually negative (presumably because of the strong host immune response), but RT-PCR has been used.

Management

In a double-blind placebo-controlled trial, ribavirin was shown to reduce the mortality and morbidity rates associated with HFRS in China.[52] Supportive treatment is similar to that for other VHFs, paying particular attention to fluid balance and the risk of renal failure. In the febrile phase, overhydration should be avoided; during the hypotensive phase, salt-poor plasma expanders and ionotropes should be used; during the oliguric phase, electrolyte balance and acid–base status should be carefully monitored. Severe hyperkalaemia, or fluid overload causing pulmonary oedema, should be treated with haemodialysis or peritoneal dialysis.

Prevention and control

Measures to minimize human exposure to rodent excreta include trapping rodents, rodent-proofing homes, correctly storing food, airing closed cabins and removing rodent droppings. Several formalin-inactivated vaccines for Hantaan and Seoul viruses are used in Asia, and recombinant DNA vaccines are in development.[53]

Crimean–Congo haemorrhagic fever (CCHF)

CCHF is an arboviral infection, transmitted by ticks, which causes a severe viral haemorrhagic fever associated with a high mortality rate and the potential for secondary nosocomial spread. Crimean haemorrhagic fever was first described in people bitten by ticks while harvesting crops in the Crimean peninsula in 1944, although descriptions of a compatible disease have existed since antiquity.[54] After the virus was isolated in 1967, it was shown to be identical to Congo virus, which had been isolated from a febrile child in 1956 in the Belgian Congo (now the Democratic Republic of Congo),[55] and the combined name has been used since. CCHF virus is a member of the *Nairovirus* genus (family *Bunyaviridae*), which contains at least 32 principally tick-borne viruses, although a few isolates have been made from culicoides flies and mosquitoes. The genus is named after the prototype Nairobi sheep disease virus, which was isolated from sheep in 1910. This virus, along with Dugbe virus, causes occasional mild febrile disease in humans.

Epidemiology and geographical distribution

CCHF virus is maintained in nature in ixodid ticks, which are field-dwelling three-host ticks. Virus is transmitted vertically to the tick's offspring (via transovarial and trans-stadial transmission), venereally from males to females for some species, and horizontally to vertebrate hosts, when the ticks take a blood meal. Ticks of the genus *Hyalomma* appear to the most important vectors for transmitting CCHF virus to vertebtrates. The wide geographical distribution of CCHF in Eastern Europe, Asia and Africa coincides with the distribution of Hyolamma ticks (Figure 43.9). Small mammals such as hares are the preferred host for immature ticks, while adults prefer large herbivorous species including sheep, goats, cattle and ostriches. Infection is usually inapparent in these animals.

Humans become infected with CCHF after being bitten by, or crushing, infected ticks, or by contact with blood from infected livestock, or patients.[56] Direct transmission is thought to occur through contact of viraemic blood or other fluids with broken skin. Most patients are farmers, veterinarians or slaughter workers, but CCHF also occurs in town dwellers visiting the country, and in health staff. The disease tends to occur sporadically in endemic countries, but in recent years there have been outbreaks in Afghanistan, Pakistan, the Russian Federation and South Africa.

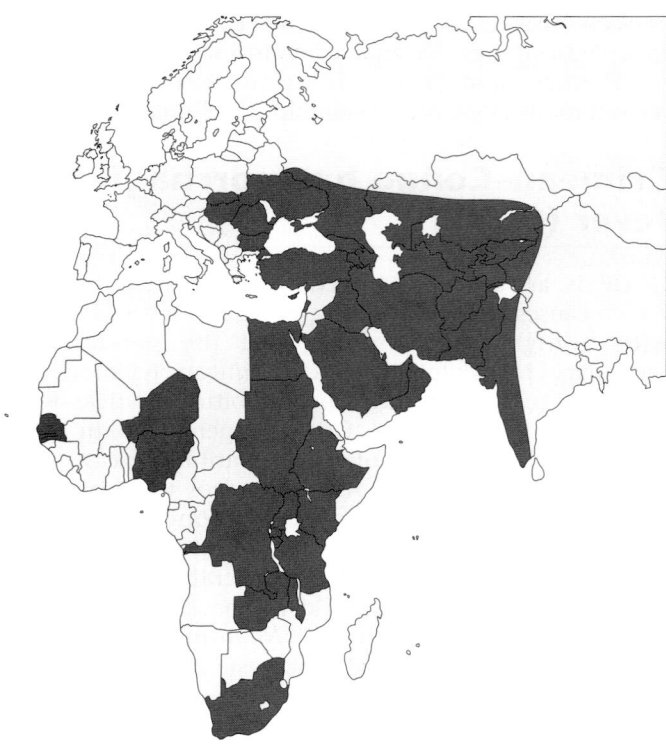

Figure 43.9: Distribution of Crimean–Congo haemorrhagic fever.

Clinical features

Unlike many other arboviruses, most infections with CCHF virus appear to cause symptoms. The incubation period is 1–3 days following a tick bite, or 5–6 days following exposure to infected blood. Patients present with a sudden onset of febrile illness with chills, headache, dizziness, neck pain and myalgia. Lymphadenopathy and tender hepatomegaly is common. This is followed by facial flushing and haemorrhage, which is often major and, unlike other VHFs, more important than vascular leakage. Gastrointestinal bleeding may be profuse and confused with surgical causes of bleeding. Laboratory abnormalities include thrombocytopenia, leucopenia and raised transaminase levels. Severely ill patients develop DIC, hepatic, renal and pulmonary failure, and coma. Approximately 30% of patients die.

Diagnosis

CCHF should be suspected in patients with an acute febrile illness and known exposure to tick bites or contact with livestock or their fresh products. The diagnosis is confirmed by virus isolation or antigen detection ELISA, under BSL-4 conditions. Antibody may be detected by IgM ELISAs in patients who ultimately survive, but is rare in fatal cases.

Management

Ribavirin is effective against CCHF virus in vitro and in the mouse model. Oral ribavirin has been used successfully in Pakistan when surgeons were infected nosocomially while operating on a patient whose gastrointestinal bleeding turned out to be due to CCHF virus.[57] This remarkable paper includes the surgeons' personal accounts of their illness.

Prevention and control

Exposure to tick bites is minimized by those in the agricultural and related industries treating their clothing with pyrethroid preparations and using insect repellents containing DEET on their skin. Workers in the livestock industry should wear appropriate clothing to reduce their exposure to potentially infected blood and tissue products. Patients with suspected CCHF should be barrier-nursed, and measures taken as for other directly transmissible VHFs. Formalin-inactivated vaccines have been developed in Eastern Europe, but have not been used widely.

Rift Valley fever (RVF)

RVF virus is an arbovirus transmitted by a range of mosquitoes that is genetically related to the sandfly fever viruses (and hence a member of the *Phlebovirus* genus of the *Bunyaviridae* family). It is zoonotic in livestock, in which it causes abortions. Originally found in the Rift Valley of Kenya, the virus is distributed across sub-Saharan Africa, Egypt, Saudi Arabia and the Yemen.[58] Disease in animals follows the explosive increases in mosquito populations caused by heavy rains or new irrigation projects. Humans become infected by mosquitoes or contact with animal blood or other products. Although direct transmission between humans has never been documented, patients should be managed as for other directly transmissible VHFs. Most human infections cause a non-specific febrile illness, but about 2% cause retinitis, 1% cause CNS disease and 1% result in VHF.[59] This is associated with hepatitis and has a high mortality rate. Ribavirin treatment is probably effective, based on laboratory studies. Control measures include vaccination of livestock (with a live attenuated or inactivated vaccine), mosquito control, and personal protection of workers in the livestock industry.

Flaviviruses[60]

The VHFs caused by flaviviruses all are transmitted by mosquitoes or ticks, with no risk of nosocomial spread, and thus are discussed in detail in Chapter 41. The genus *Flavivirus* (family *Flaviviridae*) is named after the prototype yellow fever virus (*flavus* = yellow in Latin). Its members include important causes of CNS disease, such as Japanese encephalitis virus,[61] as well as major causes of VHF.

Dengue haemorrhagic fever (DHF)

This is the most common VHF worldwide, and the one most likely to be seen in returning travellers. It is unusual among VHF viruses in that humans are the natural hosts. There are an estimated 100 million cases per year and 2.5 billion people at risk. Dengue has spread dramatically since the end of World War II, linked to a resurgence of the principal vector *Aedes aegypti*. Virtually every country between the tropics of Capricorn and Cancer is now affected. Infection with one of the four serotypes of dengue virus can lead to a non-specific febrile illness, dengue fever (a fever-arthralgia-rash syndrome) or DHF.[60]

DHF is charicterized by a massive increase in vascular permeability which leads to plasma leakage, a raised haematocrit, oedema and effusions.[62] In addition there is thrombocytopenia and haemorrhagic manifestations (which may range from a few petechiae to frank bleeding). When the leakage is sufficient to cause shock, this is known as dengue shock syndrome. There is often also tender hepatomegaly and sometimes neurological disease.[3] Diagnosis of DHF has been facilitated by new rapid diagnostic kits.[63] With early recognition and careful fluid management, the mortality rate of DHF has been reduced from around 30% to less than 0.02 %. Control of *Aedes* mosquitoes is the main preventive measure. Tetravalent vaccines are currently undergoing clinical trials.

Yellow fever

Yellow fever virus is transmitted by mosquitoes between non-human primates in sylvatic cycles in South America and Africa. Humans become infected by entering this cycle, and may then carry the virus to populated areas. Here *A. aegypti* spreads the disease causing 'urban yellow fever'. In the savannah of Africa, smaller epidemics are known as 'intermediate yellow fever'. After a short incubation there is an acute febrile illness, sometimes associated with a paradoxical slowing of the pulse (Faget's sign, suggesting viral cardiac damage). After a brief period of remission about 15% of patients develop VHF with mild jaundice (due to hepatitis) and impaired renal function. The mortality rate is 20–50%. The diagnosis is confirmed by ELISA, virus isolation or, in fatal cases, post-mortem liver biopsy. There is no antiviral treatment, but a live attenuated vaccine has been available for many years; it is one of the safest vaccines known, despite recently documented adverse events.[64]

Omsk haemorrhagic fever (OHF)

OHF virus is unusual among flaviviruses in that the vectors, *Dermacentor* ticks, are important reservoirs of the virus. It is found in the Omsk area of Siberia,[65] and causes disease in many of the small mammals (including muskrats) to which it is transmitted. Muskrat hunters become infected by direct contact with infected carcasses, or from tick bites. Most infections are asymptomatic, but there may be a papulovesicular eruption on the soft palate, and mucosal and gastrointestinal bleeding.

Kyasanur Forest disease

Kyasanur Forest disease is caused by a closely related tick-borne flavivirus found in forest rodents in south-western India. It is transmitted by *Haemaphysalis* ticks and causes annual outbreaks of febrile or haemorrhagic disease in monkeys and humans. A formalin-inactivated vaccine appears to be effective.[66] Other preventive measures include the treatment of cows with acaricides to reduce the tick population and the personal use of insect repellents.

Acknowledgement

Some of the work described in this chapter was funded by the Wellcome Trust of Great Britain. I thank C J Peters and Robert Swanepoel for helpful comments.

REFERENCES

1   Solomon T. Emerging viral diseases. *Medicine* 2001; 29(5):6–7.
2   Anonymous. Management of patients with suspected viral hemorrhagic fever. *MMWR Morb Mortal Wkly Rep* 1988; 37(S3):1–16.
3   Solomon T, Dung N M, Vaughn D W et al. Neurological manifestations of dengue infection. *Lancet* 2000; 355:1053–1059.
4   Centers for Disease Control and Prevention and World Health Organization. *Infection Control for Viral Haemorrhagic Fevers in the African Health Care Setting*. Atlanta: Centers for Disease Control and Prevention, 1998.
5   World Health Organization. *Dengue Haemorrhagic Fever: Diagnosis, Treatment and Control*, 2nd edn. Geneva: WHO, 1997.
6   Dung N M, Day N P, Tam D T et al. Fluid replacement in dengue shock syndrome: a randomized, double-blind comparison of four intravenous-fluid regimens. *Clin Infect Dis* 1999; 28:787–794.
7   Nhan N T, Phuong C X T, Kneen R et al. Acute management of dengue shock syndrome: a randomised double blind comparison of four intravenous fluid regimens in the first hour. *Clin Infect Dis* 2001; 32:204–213.
8   Carey D E, Kemp G E, White H A et al. Lassa fever. Epidemiological aspects of the 1970 epidemic, Jos, Nigeria. *Trans R Soc Trop Med Hyg* 1972; 66:402–408.
9   Lloyd E S, Zaki S R, Rollin P E et al. Long-term disease surveillance in Bandundu region, Democratic Republic of the Congo: a model for early detection and prevention of Ebola hemorrhagic fever. *J Infect Dis* 1999; 179 (Supplement 1):S274–S280.
10   Buchmeier M, et al. The virology and immunobiology of lymphocytic choriomeningitis virus infection. *Adv Immunol* 1980; 30:275–331.
11   Ambrosio A M, Feuillade M R, Gamboa G S & Maiztegui J I. Prevalence of lymphocytic choriomeningitis virus infection in a human population of Argentina. *Am J Trop Med Hyg* 1994; 50:381–386.

12 Harrison L H, Halsey N A, McKee K T Jr et al. Clinical case definitions for Argentine hemorrhagic fever. *Clin Infect Dis* 1999; 28:1091–1094.

13 Frame J D, Baldwin J M Jr, Gocke D J & Troup J M. Lassa fever, a new virus disease of man from West Africa. I. Clinical description and pathological findings. *Am J Trop Med Hyg* 1970; 19:670–676.

14 Buchmeier M J, Bowen M D & Peters C J. Arenaviridae: the viruses and their replication. In Fields B N, Knipe D M & Howley P M (eds) *Fields Virology*, 4th edn. Philadelphia: Lippincott Williams & Wilkins, 2001:1635–1668.

15 Peters C J, Jahrling P B, Liu C T, Kenyon R H, McKee K T Jr & Barrera Oro J G. Experimental studies of arenaviral hemorrhagic fevers. *Curr Top Microbiol Immunol* 1987; 134:5–68.

16 Jahrling P, Smith S, Hesse R A & Rhoderick J B. Pathogenesis of Lassa virus infection in guinea pigs. *Infect Immun* 1982; 37:771–778.

17 Walker D H, McCormick J B, Johnson K M et al. Pathologic and virologic study of fatal Lassa fever in man. *Am J Pathol* 1982; 107:349–356.

18 Anonymous. Lassa fever imported to England. *Commun Dis Rep CDR Wkly* 2000; 10:99.

19 Clegg J C. Possible approaches to a vaccine against Lassa fever. *Trans R Soc Trop Med Hyg* 1984; 78:307–310.

20 Fraser D W, Campbell C C, Monath T P, Goff P A & Gregg M B. Lassa fever in the Eastern Province of Sierra Leone, 1970–1972. I. Epidemiologic studies. *Am J Trop Med Hyg* 1974; 23:1131–1139.

21 McCormick J B, King I J, Webb P A et al. A case–control study of the clinical diagnosis and course of Lassa fever. *J Infect Dis* 1987; 155:455–455.

22 Cummins D, McCormick J B, Bennett D et al. Acute sensorineural deafness in Lassa fever. *JAMA* 1990; 264:2093–2096.

23 Johnson K M, McCormick J B, Webb P A, Smith E S, Elliott L H & King I J. Clinical virology of Lassa fever in hospitalized patients. *J Infect Dis* 1987; 155:456–464.

24 Bausch D G, Rollin P E, Demby A H et al. Diagnosis and clinical virology of Lassa fever as evaluated by enzyme-linked immunosorbent assay, indirect fluorescent-antibody test, and virus isolation. *J Clin Microbiol* 2000; 38:2670–2677.

25 McCormick J B, King I J & Webb P A. Lassa fever. Effective therapy with ribavirin. *N Engl J Med* 1986; 314:20–26.

26 Fisher-Hoch S P & McCormick J B. Towards a human Lassa fever vaccine. *Rev Med Virol* 2001; 11:331–341.

27 Maiztegui J I, McKee K T Jr, Barrera Oro J G et al. Protective efficacy of a live attenuated vaccine against Argentine hemorrhagic fever. AHF Study Group. *J Infect Dis* 1998; 177:277–283.

28 de Manzione N, Salas R A, Paredes H et al. Venezuelan hemorrhagic fever: clinical and epidemiological studies of 165 cases. *Clin Infect Dis* 1998; 26:308–313.

29 Barry M, Russi M, Armstrong L et al. Treatment of a laboratory-acquired Sabiá virus infection. *N Engl J Med* 1995; 333:294–296.

30 Fulhorst C F, Bowen M D, Ksiazek T G et al. Isolation and characterization of Whitewater Arroyo virus, a novel North American arenavirus. *Virology* 1996; 224:114–120.

31 Kissling R E, Robinson R Q, Murphy F A & Whitfield S G. Agent of disease contracted from green monkeys. *Science* 1968; 160:888–890.

32 Johnson K M, Lange J V, Webb P A & Murphy F A. Isolation and partial characterisation of a new virus causing acute haemorrhagic fever in Zaire. *Lancet* 1977; i:569–571.

33 Anonymous. Outbreak of Ebola haemorrhagic fever, Uganda, August 2000–January 2001. 2001.

34 McCormick J B & Fisher-Hoch S P. Filovirus infections. In Porterfield J S (ed.) *Exotic Viral Infections*. London: Chapman & Hall, 1995:319–328.

35 Sanchez A, Khan A, Zaki S R, Nabel G J, Ksiazek T G & Peters C J. Filoviridae: Marburg and Ebola viruses. In Fields B N, Knipe D M & Howley P M (eds) *Fields Virology*. Philadelphia: Lippincott Williams & Wilkins, 2001:1279–1304.

36 Villinger F, Rollin P E, Brar S S et al. Markedly elevated levels of interferon (IFN)-gamma, IFN-alpha, interleukin (IL)-2, IL-10, and tumor necrosis factor-alpha associated with fatal Ebola virus infection. *J Infect Dis* 1999; 179 (Supplement 1):S188–S191.

37 Yang Z Y, Duckers H J, Sullivan N J, Sanchez A, Nabel E G & Nabel G J. Identification of the Ebola virus glycoprotein as the main viral determinant of vascular cell cytotoxicity and injury. *Nature Med* 2000; 6:886–889.

38 Nabel G J. Surviving Ebola virus infection. *Nature Med* 1999; 5:373–374.

39 Swanepoel R, Leman P A, Burt F J et al. Experimental inoculation of plants and animals with Ebola virus. *Emerg Infect Dis* 1996; 2:321–325.

40 Leirs H, Mills J N, Krebs J W et al. Search for the Ebola virus reservoir in Kikwit, Democratic Republic of the Congo: reflections on a vertebrate collection. *J Infect Dis* 1999; 179 (Supplement 1):S155–S163.

41 Morvan J M, Deubel V, Gounon P et al. Identification of Ebola virus sequences present as RNA or DNA in organs of terrestrial small mammals of the Central African Republic. *Microbes Infect* 1999; 1:1193–1201.

42 Roels T H, Bloom A S, Buffingto N J et al. Ebola hemorrhagic fever, Kikwit, Democratic Republic of the Congo, 1995: risk factors for patients without a reported exposure. *J Infect Dis* 1999; 179 (Supplement 1):S92–S97.

43 Ndambi R, Akamituna P, Bonnet M J, Tukadila A M, Muyembe-Tamfum J J & Colebunders R. Epidemiologic and clinical aspects of the Ebola virus epidemic in Mosango, Democratic Republic of the Congo, 1995. *J Infect Dis* 1999; 179 (Supplement 1):S8–S10.

44 Saijo M, Niikura M, Morikawa S et al. Enzyme-linked immunosorbent assays for detection of antibodies to Ebola and Marburg viruses using recombinant nucleoproteins. *J Clin Microbiol* 2001; 39:1–7.

45 Mupapa K, Massamba M, Kibadi K et al. Treatment of Ebola hemorrhagic fever with blood transfusions from convalescent patients. International Scientific and Technical Committee. *J Infect Dis* 1999; 179 (Supplement 1):S18–S23.

46 Anonymous. Marburg fever, Democratic Republic of the Congo. *Wkly Epidemiol Rec* 1999; 74:145.

47 Gear J J S, Cassel G A, Gear A J et al. Outbreak of Marburg virus disease in Johannesburg. *BMJ* 1975; iv:489–493.

48 Earle D P. Symposium on epidemic hemorrhagic fever. *Am J Med* 1954; 16:617–709.

49 Lee H W, Lee P W & Johnson K M. Isolation of the etiologic agent of Korean hemorrhagic fever. *J Infect Dis* 1978; 137:298–308.

50 Tsai T F. Hemorrhagic fever with renal syndrome: mode of transmission to humans. *Lab Anim Sci* 1987; 37:428–430.

51 Hung T, Zhou J Y, Tang Y M, Zhao T X, Baek L J & Lee H W. Identification of Hantaan virus-related structures in kidneys of cadavers with haemorrhagic fever with renal syndrome. *Arch Virol* 1992; 122:187–199.

52 Huggins J W, Hsiang C M, Cosgriff T M et al. Prospective, double-blind, concurrent, placebo-controlled clinical trial of intravenous ribavirin therapy of haemorrhagic fever with renal syndrome. *J Infect Dis* 1991; 164:1119–1127.

53 Hooper J W & Li D. Vaccines against hantaviruses. *Curr Top Microbiol Immunol* 2001; 256:171–191.

54 Hoogstraal H. The epidemiology of tick-borne Crimean–Congo hemorrhagic fever in Asia, Europe, and Africa. *J Med Entomol* 1979; 15:307–417.

55 Simpson D I, Knight E M, Courtois G, Williams M C, Weinbren M P & Kibukamusoke J W. Congo virus: a hitherto undescribed virus occurring in Africa. I. Human isolations—clinical notes. *East Afr Med J* 1967; 44:86–92.

56 Fisher-Hoch S P, McCormick J B, Swanepoel R, Van Middlekoop A, Harvey S & Kustner H G. Risk of human infections with Crimean–Congo hemorrhagic fever virus in a South African rural community. *Am J Trop Med Hyg* 1992; 47:337–344.

57 Fisher-Hoch S P, Khan J A, Rehman S et al. Crimean-Congo haemorrhagic fever treated with oral ribavirin. *Lancet* 1995; 346:472–475.

58 Anonymous. Outbreak of Rift Valley fever—Yemen. *MMWR Morb Mortal Wkly Rep* 2000; 49:1065–1066.

59 Laughlin L W, Meegan J M, Strausbaugh L J, Morens D M & Watten R H. Epidemic Rift Valley fever in Egypt: observations of the spectrum of human illness. *Trans R Soc Trop Med Hyg* 1979; 73:630–633.

60 Solomon T & Mallewa M J. Dengue and other emerging flaviviruses. *J Infect* 2001; 42:104–115.

61 Solomon T. Japanese encephalitis. In Gilman S, Goldstein G W & Waxman S G (eds) *Neurobase*. San Diego: Medlink, 2000.

62 Bethell D B, Gamble J, Pham P L et al. Noninvasive measurement of microvascular leakage in patients with dengue hemorrhagic fever. *Clin Infect Dis* 2001; 32:243–253.

63 Vaughn D W, Nisalak A, Solomon T et al. Rapid serological diagnosis of dengue virus infection using a commercial capture ELISA that distinguishes primary and secondary infections. *Am J Trop Med Hyg* 1999; 60:693–698.

64 Vasconcelos P F, Luna E J, Galler R et al. Serious adverse events associated with yellow fever 17DD vaccine in Brazil: a report of two cases. *Lancet* 2001; 358:91–97.

65 Gaidamovich S Y. Tick-borne flavivirus infections. In Porterfield J S (ed.) *Exotic Viral Infections*. London: Chapman & Hall, 1995:203–221.

66 Upadhyaya S, Dandwate C N & Banerjee K. Surveillance of formolized KFD vaccine administration in Sagar-Sorab Talukas district. *Indian J Med Res* 1979; 69:714–719.

Chapter 44
Epstein–Barr Virus and Associated Diseases

H. Williams and D. H. Crawford

Epstein–Barr virus (EBV) was first isolated from cultures of Burkitt's lymphoma (BL) biopsy material and was rapidly shown to be a unique herpesvirus.[1] EBV is a ubiquitous human virus, infecting over 90% of the human population globally. This large DNA virus is normally transmitted via saliva; EBV is present in the oral secretions of most infected individuals and a naive host becomes infected through contact with infectious virus shed in saliva.[2] Most people undergo subclinical infection as infants; however, in the West delayed primary infection as a young adult may result in infectious mononucleosis (IM). After primary infection the virus persists for life; EBV infects memory B lymphocytes and these cells are the site of the long-term viral reservoir (latent infection).[3]

In the vast majority of healthy carriers EBV does not cause disease. This is because a delicate balance is maintained between the host immune system, which limits production of new virus, and the virus, which persists and is successfully transmitted in the face of host antiviral immunity. Disruption of this balance, due to primary or acquired abnormalities of the host's immune system, may lead to the development of EBV associated disease.

EBV plays a central role in the development of a number of lymphoid and epithelial cell-derived cancers. Viral-driven cell proliferation is thought to be key to the development of both BL and nasopharyngeal carcinoma (NPC), and, like other cancers driven by an infectious agent, these cancers are more common in the developing world than the West. Overall, infectious agents are responsible for 21% of all tumours in the developing world and 9% in the West. NPC comprises 0.7% of new tumours occurring on a worldwide basis each year.[4] The global HIV pandemic has caused significant changes in the profile of EBV-related conditions. Most crucially EBV is associated with many non-Hodgkin's lymphomas and with oral hairy leucoplakia in HIV-positive individuals. Lymphocytic interstitial pneumonia may also be linked to EBV infection.

Infection in healthy individuals

Primary infection with EBV is commonly subclinical, occurs predominantly in early childhood, and gives rise to a lifelong carrier state.[5] In most populations sero-positivity increases with age, and over 90% of adults have persistent infection. However, the rate of seroconversion varies according to economic status, such that over 90% of children over the age of 2 years in developing countries have evidence of persistent infection,[6] whereas seroconversion may be delayed until adolescence in high socio-economic groups of industrialized countries. It is thought that close family contact is the main route of spread in young infants, and that large family size and close proximity of living conditions are likely to aid spread. In the West 5–10% of people remain EBV negative for life, whereas in Africa over 97% of the population carry the virus.[7] Most normal hosts carry only one of the two major virus subtypes of EBV, A or B (also called 1 and 2),[8] which have 70–80% sequence homology.[9] Type A is most common throughout the world; type B is rare, but is more prevalent in Africa and the Far East than the West.[10,11] In addition to EBV subtypes, minor sequence variants are classified as strains and are usually unique to one individual. There is no evidence that variation of either strain or type affects clinical pathogenesis.

In healthy adults 1–50 B cells per million in peripheral blood are latently infected.[12] Significant numbers of these B cells can be identified in tonsils, where activation of virus-infected cells may lead to virus production (lytic infection) and continuous or intermittent low-level shedding of free virus in the oral cavity.[13] Infectious virus has also been recovered from male and female genital secretions (see later).

Infectious mononucleosis

Infectious mononucleosis (IM) is an acute febrile illness, caused by primary infection with EBV, which presents with sore throat, fever, lymph node enlargement and severe fatigue.

Epidemiology

IM mainly affects affluent groups in the West, and is the commonest cause of prolonged illness in young army recruits in the USA.[14] In a recent study in the UK up to 25% of students entering university were seronegative for EBV (personal communication), but the vast majority of individuals seroconvert by their middle twenties. Approximately 45–65% who seroconvert at this age develop IM; the remaining infections are asymptomatic or non-specific, as in primary infection in young children.[15,16] It is not clear what environmental or genetic risk factors predispose to the development of clinical illness. However, it is likely that milder forms of the disease occur without detection, and a spectrum of clinical features exists ranging from mild sore throat to full-blown IM. Rare cases of IM have also been documented in children, middle-aged adults and the elderly.[17]

Transmission

IM is colloquially known as the 'kissing disease', and it is presumed that the initiation of sexual activity in adolescence places seronegative individuals at risk of contact with infectious virus in saliva. However, infectious virus is present in both male and female genital secretions of asymptomatic carriers[18,19] and recent evidence suggests that IM often results from spread during sexual intercourse (personal communication).

Pathogenesis and EBV

Primary infection occurs when virus particles infect B lymphocytes in the oropharynx (or possibly the genital tract) of EBV-negative individuals. It was originally thought that the initial site of infection was oropharyngeal squamous epithelial cells. However, it has not proved possible to identify EBV-infected epithelial cells in tonsils taken from patients with IM, although latent and lytic infection in B cells can be seen. Therefore, the consensus of opinion now is that the B cell is the site of both viral replication and persistence. The EBV major viral envelope glycoprotein (gp 350) binds to the CD21 receptor (also called complement receptor (CR) 2) on resting B cells, followed by fusion of the viral envelope with the cell membrane and release of the capsid into the cell. Once a cell is infected, the virus may replicate (lytic infection) with new virus production and cell death, or lie dormant in B cells (latent infection). During IM lytic infection predominates in the oropharynx, with large amounts of new virus produced and excreted into saliva. In lytic infection nearly 100 viral proteins are transcribed which are important in modulating the host immune response, replicating viral DNA and forming the structural components of new virions.[20]

One of the ways the virus attenuates the host immune system is by producing virally encoded cytokines. The EBV BCRF1 protein has 70% homology with human interleukin 10.[21] This inhibits the production of interferon γ (IFNγ), which is key to the host's response to early viral infection.

Neutralizing antibody to gp 350, the main viral envelope glycoprotein, is produced during primary infection, and there is increasing evidence that innate immune mechan-isms, particularly natural killer cells, are important in controlling the early events in primary infection.[22]

The prolonged systemic symptoms of IM are thought to be caused by a dramatic cellular immune response to EBV-infected B cells, with large expansions of characteristic 'atypical' lymphocytes. These are predominantly, but not exclusively, CD8-positive cytotoxic effector cells. Large amounts of TH-2 cytokines are released; IFNγ, tumour necrosis factor α (TNFα) and TNFβ have all been identified in IM tonsils.[23] Analysis of CD8 T cell antigen specificities from patients with acute IM patients has revealed that up to 50% of the total T cell numbers in peripheral blood are directed against single viral epitopes.[24] These virus-specific activated lymphocytes are thought to be essential in limiting virus spread to uninfected B cells.

After acute infection a state of viral persistence is established with long-term cellular immunity provided by EBV-specific CD8 positive cytotoxic T lymphocytes. These cells can be detected in the circulation in all normal seropositive individuals.

Clinical features

It is estimated that IM occurs 30–50 days after exposure to the virus. The majority of patients experience fever, lymphadenopathy, sore throat and fatigue. Examination normally reveals marked tonsillar enlargement, sometimes with associated exudate and petechia, lymphadenopathy (which may be generalized or restricted to the cervical region) and splenomegaly. A degree of hepatomegaly and mildly abnormal liver function tests are also common, but jaundice is rare (< 10%). Urticarial skin rashes can occur, most commonly associated with the use of ampicillin. Rare complications include acute liver necrosis, splenic rupture, pharyngeal or tracheal obstruction, and haematological disorders, including autoimmune thrombocytopenia and haemolytic anaemia.[25]

In the vast majority of cases IM is a benign and self-limiting disease with prolonged fatigue being the most disabling symptom, and full recovery after 6–8 weeks is the norm. Treatment is supportive, with advice to avoid both alcohol (particularly if hepatitis is present) and vigorous exercise, the latter because of the risk of splenic rupture. Steroids are reserved for serious complications and, if required, a short reducing course is usually adequate. Acyclovir inhibits viral replication but is ineffective in altering the clinical course of IM, since symptoms are not due to viraemia, but to the marked immune response to EBV, which is well established by the time of clinical presentation.

Relapses can occur in the first 6–12 months following infection, and IM may be a risk factor, in the short term, for the development of a prolonged fatigue syndrome and depression.[26] However, there is no evidence that the chronic fatigue syndrome is caused by an abnormal immunological response to EBV.[27]

X-linked lymphoproliferative syndrome is a rare familial condition, in which primary infection with EBV leads to uncontrolled lymphoproliferation and usually death from subsequent hepatic or bone marrow failure. A few individuals survive primary infection, but later develop fatal EBV-driven lymphomas. The defect on the X chromosome underlying this disorder has recently been identified as mutations in SAP (signalling lymphocyte activation molecule (SLAM) associated protein).[28,29]

Chronic active EBV infection is another rare, but non-familial, disorder that again presents with inability to control primary EBV infection. Most identified cases have been in the Far East, and some of those affected develop severe EBV-linked organ failure or lymphoma. Treatment options are improving with introduction of use of etoposide and adoptive transfer of EBV-specific cytotoxic T lymphocytes.[30]

Laboratory diagnosis

The majority of individuals with IM have a profound lymphocytosis, with 'atypical' lymphocytes (activated T cells) in the peripheral blood. The presence of these cells is not diagnostic of IM because they are also found to a lesser extent in other infections, including HIV sero-conversion illness, cytomegalovirus infection, viral hepatitis, toxoplasmosis, rubella, mumps and roseola.[31]

In the early stages of infection serum antibodies appear to a variety of viral antigens (Figure 44.1), but the gold standard for the diagnosis of IM is detection of IgM antibodies to viral capsid antigen (VCA). Most laboratories use an enzyme-linked immunosorbent assay (ELISA) as a screening method, but may supplement this with an indirect immunofluorescence assay as a more sensitive test.

Infection and activation of B cells by EBV results in polyclonal antibody production, leading to elevated titres of heterophile antibodies, which form the basis for the rapid monospot test used for diagnostic screening. This is positive in 85% of acute IM cases (Figure 44.1). On occasions auto-antibodies such as cold agglutinins, cryoglobulins, antinuclear antibodies or rheumatoid factor arise.

EBV-associated malignancies

EBV infection is increasingly linked to a diverse group of lymphoid and epithelial cell-derived malignancies. Experimental infection of cotton-topped tamarins rapidly leads to lymphoid tumour development[32] and this, combined with EBV's ability to transform cultured B cells to continuously proliferating long-lived lymphoblastoid cell lines, has confirmed its oncogenic potential.[33] A limited set of viral gene products are expressed by these transformed B cells, and identification of their function, both in laboratory models and EBV-associated tumours, has been key to the understanding of viral driven oncogenesis. However, we will only know how fundamental EBV infection is to tumour development if vaccination leads to a reduction in EBV-linked tumours.[34]

EBV-associated lymphoid malignancies

EBV DNA is present in approximately 95% of endemic Burkitt's lymphoma, and this was the first malignancy to be linked to EBV.[35] It is now recognized that EBV is linked to three groups of lymphoid tumours: non-Hodgkin's lymphoma (NHL), including Burkitt's lymphoma and AIDS-related NHL, Hodgkin's disease, and lympho-proliferative disease in the immunocompromised host. AIDS-related tumours will be discussed in the section on EBV and HIV.

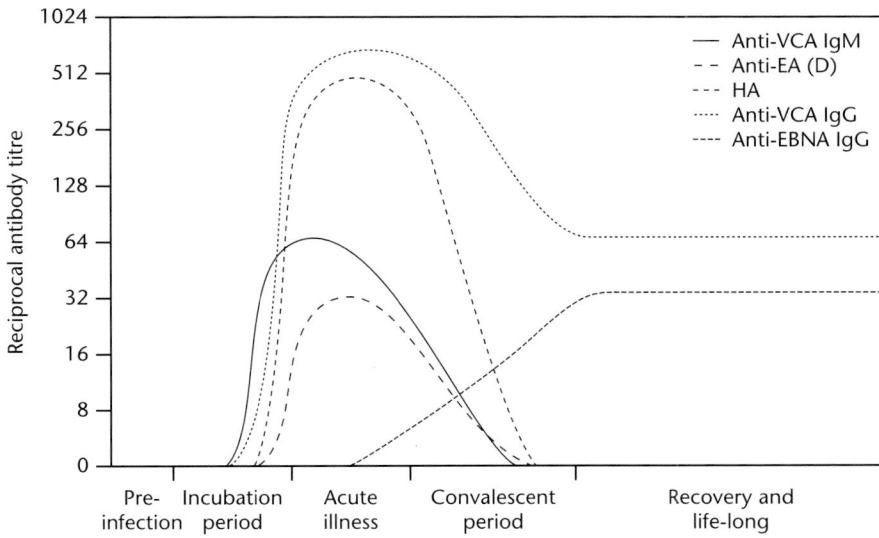

Figure 44.1: Profile of serum antibodies to EB virus-associated antigens before, during and after primary infection. EA(D), diffuse form of early antigen; VCA, viral capsid antigen; HA, heterophile antigen; EBNA, EB virus nuclear antigen.

Burkitt's lymphoma

Burkitt's lymphoma (BL) is a high-grade B cell NHL which commonly occurs in children.

Epidemiology (endemic, sporadic and intermediate)

The incidence of BL is categorized as high (endemic), low (sporadic) and intermediate.

Endemic BL is the most common childhood cancer in parts of equatorial Africa and Papua New Guinea (Figure 44.2A), with an annual incidence in Africa of 15–20 cases per 100 000 population.[36] Endemic BL occurs between the ages of 3 and 15 years, with a peak incidence at 5–7 years and a male predominance. The endemic areas, though geographically separate, have climatic features ideal for holoendemic malaria. These include an annual rainfall above 55 cm and a minimum temperature above 16.5°C.[37] In the Ivory Coast, West Africa, it has also been noted that the majority of children with BL live in rural communities, more often coming from forested areas (where tumour incidence is 5:100 000) than the savannah (where the incidence is less than 1:100 000).[38]

BL is not unique to endemic regions; the disease exists throughout the world at low incidence, and several areas of intermediate incidence have recently been recognized. In a series of children treated for NHL in north-east Brazil, 92 of 98 tumours were classified as being of Burkitt subtype, with 8 out of 11 cases studied being EBV-positive.[39] This area of tropical Brazil has a similar pattern of communicable disease and poverty to Africa.[40] Small studies of childhood lymphoma have also identified several other areas of intermediate incidence such as temperate South America, including Chile and Argentina, and Turkey. A review of cases in Turkey found that affected children were often from low socio-economic groups.[41]

Childhood tumours with BL-like characteristics also occur in the West, but this sporadic form has an incidence which is 50–100 times lower than the endemic form, and an EBV association of 10–25%.[35] Further work

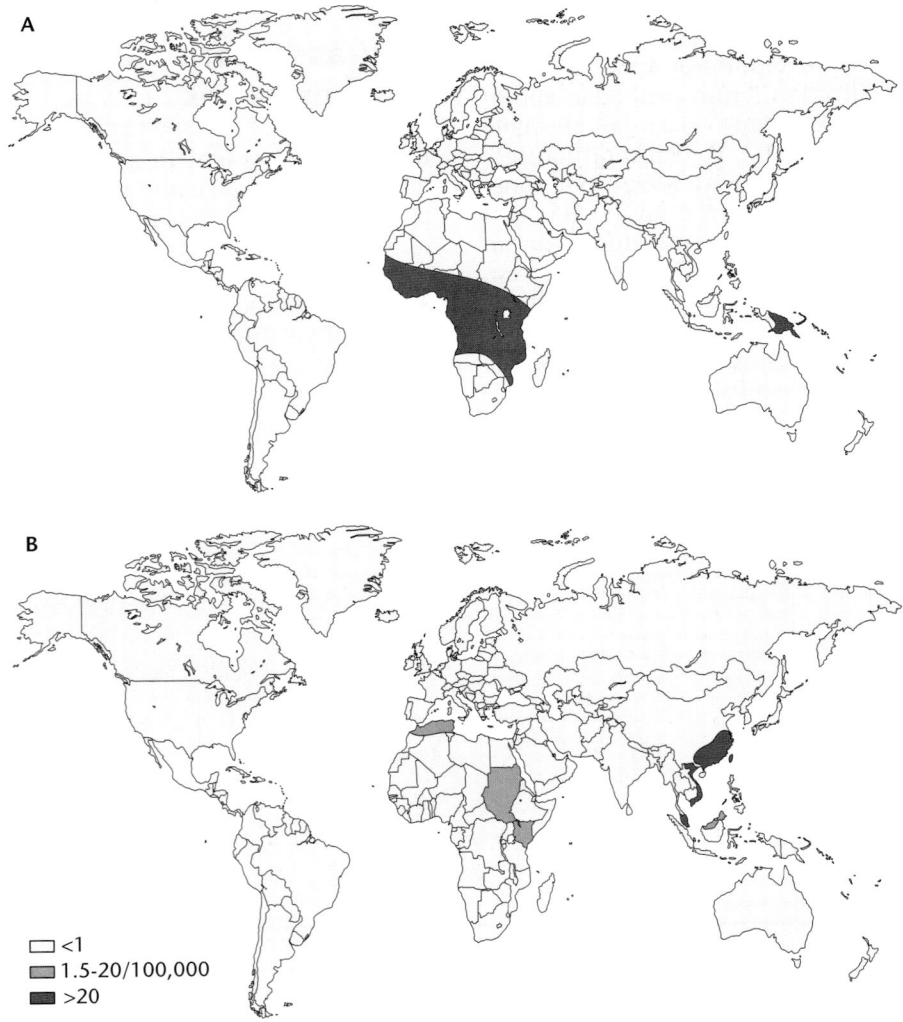

<<1
1.5-20/100,000
>20

Figure 44.2: Worldwide distribution of incidence to EB virus-associated tumours: (**A**) Burkitt's lymphoma, and (**B**) nasopharyngeal carcinoma.

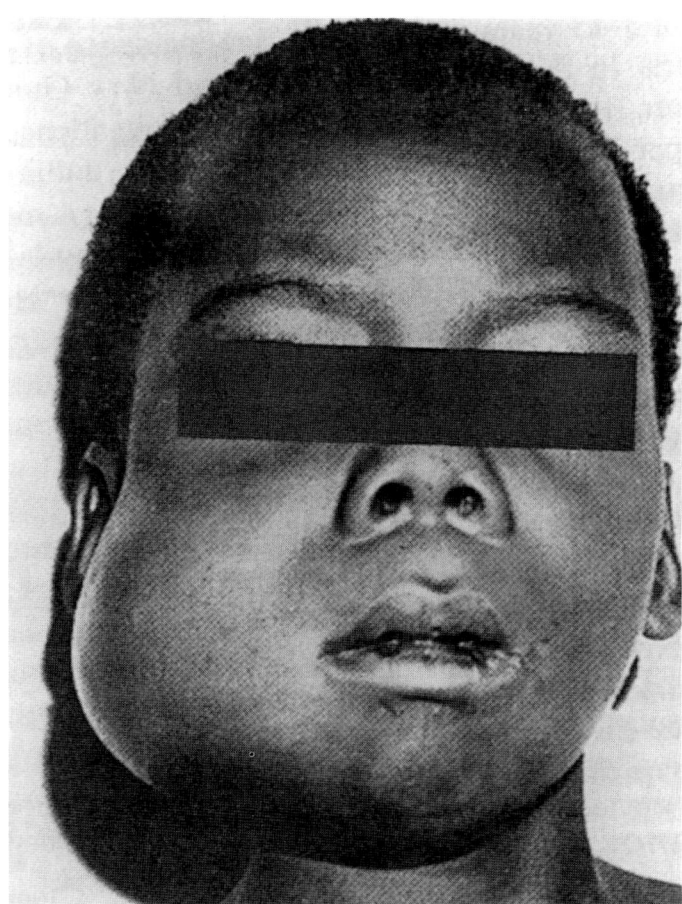

Figure 44.3: An African male child with Burkitt's lymphoma of the jaws.

is needed to clarify the epidemiology and patterns of disease in these different geographical areas. Of particular interest will be incidence in other countries where EBV-related tumours are common, e.g., China.

Pathogenesis and EBV

The transformation of a normal B lymphocyte to a malignant BL cell is a complex multi-step process, in which early childhood infection with EBV, chronic malaria infection and chromosomal translocation have all been identified as important contributory factors.

A constant feature of BL is the presence of a reciprocal chromosomal translocation between the *c-myc* oncogene on chromosome 8 and the immunoglobulin (Ig) heavy chain locus on chromosome 14 or, more rarely, the light chain loci on either 2 or 22.[42] This translocation event in B cells leads to deregulation of *c-myc*, a gene which normally drives cell proliferation, and this predisposes to lymphoma development. Mutations in the tumour suppressor gene p53 have also been identified in BL tumour cells, although these are thought to occur late in tumorogenesis.[43]

EBV DNA is present in up to 95% of tumours from endemic areas. The viral genome is clonal, indicating that virus infection was present in the initial tumour cell. Nearly all children in endemic areas are likely to have encountered EBV in early childhood. However, a prospective study of 42 000 children in Uganda found that those children who subsequently developed BL had a 10 times higher geometric mean IgG antibody titres to EB VCA than matched controls.[44] A similar pattern has been seen in more recent studies in Turkey.[45] In BL cells the only EBV protein expressed is EBNA-1, which is required for viral replication and EBV genome maintenance. The classic EBV oncogenes, latent membrane protein (LMP)1, EB viral nuclear antigen (EBNA)2 are not expressed, and the role of the virus in BL is therefore unclear. However, it is thought that this limited viral gene expression reduces recognition by the host immune system.[46]

At present it is not clear how early EBV infection, chronic parasitaemia and *c-myc* deregulation are linked in tumour pathogenesis. It is postulated that chronic parasite infection, be it malaria or other agents, leads to immunosuppression, altered cytokine profiles and polyclonal B cell stimulation. The increased turnover of B cells resulting from polyclonal activation increases the chance of a *c-myc* translocation occurring during Ig gene rearrangement, whereas the immunosuppression reduces EBV-specific cytotoxic T cell activity and allows a correspondingly higher number of circulating EBV-infected B cells to survive. This expanded pool of infected B cells also increases the chance of a translocation event occurring in a cell infected with EBV.

Further evidence for the role of malaria in BL is provided by the falling incidence of BL in areas of malaria eradication.[47] It has been postulated that sickle cell trait may reduce the risk of BL development as a consequence of its protection from malaria; however, epidemiological investigations have not reached statistical significance.[48] Though holoendemic malaria is thought to be an important co-factor in African BL, in other areas where a high rate of EBV-associated BL has been identified, there is little *Plasmodium falciparum* malaria. In tropical Brazil young children commonly suffer from other infections such as schistosomiasis and leishmaniasis, in which chronic parasitaemia also leads to polyclonal B cell stimulation, and immunosuppression. Recent reports from Brazil have identified cases of BL in close association with schistosomiasis granuloma, and it is postulated that this chronic parasite infection predisposes to BL by inducing a change in local cytokine expression and a reduction in local immune surveillance.[40] This hypothesis requires further investigation.

Clinical features

BL is a very fast-growing tumour which in endemic areas classically presents in the jaw, possibly in association with molar tooth development (Figure 44.3). At diagnosis the tumour is often multifocal, with other common sites being the testis, ovary, breast (in pubertal girls), liver, stomach and intestine. Intra-abdominal lesions are being recognized more frequently with increased availability of ultrasound imaging. Lymph nodes and spleen are rarely involved, and bone marrow invasion only occurs during the terminal phase of the disease. The tumours cause little constitutional disturbance, and this, combined with the low socio-economic status of the children, means presentation is often late.[38] Neurological complications such as facial palsy carry a poor prognosis (clinical management reviewed by Magrath[50]).

Outside endemic areas the clinical presentation is more variable. In some areas of intermediate incidence an abdominal mass is a common mode of presentation and in the USA the primary lesion is rarely in the jaw. It is not clear whether these differences in presentation reflect distinctive biological patterns of disease.[49]

The diagnosis of BL is made on clinical and histological grounds. Histopathological examination reveals a small, non-cleaved cell lymphoma, typically infiltrated with large pale-staining histiocytes giving a classical 'starry sky' pattern (Figure 44.4). Once the lesion is identified, treatment should not be delayed, as the disease may advance very rapidly. Chemotherapy is the mainstay of treatment, with surgical debulking only required when there is no access to chemotherapy. The regime normally includes cyclophosphamide, vincristine, prednisolone and doxorubucin. Because of the large tumour burden and extreme sensitivity to chemotherapy, therapy carries a significant risk of renal and metabolic complications.[50]

With adequate access to health care, the prognosis in children is excellent; survival rates are of 80–90%. However, the outcome in resource-poor countries where the majority of cases occur is poor. A review of 18 years' experience from the Côte d'Ivoire identified 433 BL patients, of whom only 219 completed systemic chemotherapy. Of these, 117 achieved complete remission, 40 achieved partial remission, 21 died during chemotherapy, and 41 were lost to follow-up. The 2-year survival rate was 70% of those that achieved complete remission.[38]

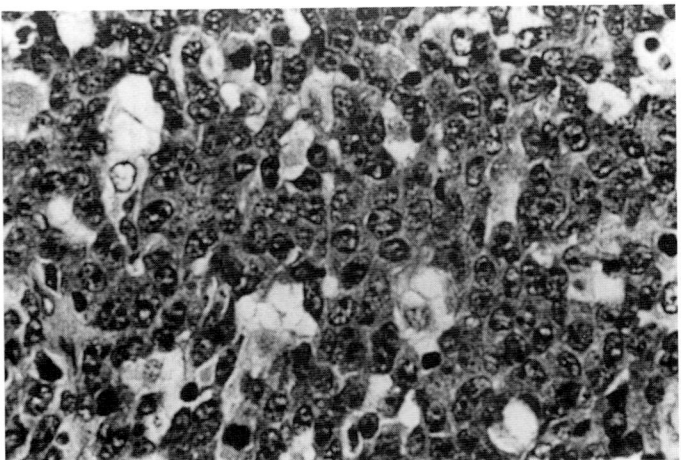

Figure 44.4: Histological section of Burkitt's lymphoma showing monomorphic lymphoid cells with histocytic infiltration. (H & E, 800 ×; courtesy of P. Isaacson, University College Hospital, London.)

Survival was linked not only to availability of expensive chemotherapy, but the ability to manage common complications such as secondary infection and uricosaemic renal failure. Ultimately, the outcome of BL is linked to socio-economic status.

Hodgkin's disease

Hodgkin's disease is a lymphoid tumour which is characterized by the presence of large malignant multinucleate Reed–Sternberg cells, in a reactive background of lymphocytes, eosinophils and fibrous tissue.

Epidemiology

Hodgkin's disease is the most common lymphoma in young people in the West, but in the developing world NHL occurs more frequently. The link between Hodgkin's disease and EBV is well established; studies in South America have found that up to 79% of tumours harbour EBV, whereas in the USA and UK the association is between 40% and 60%. The presence of EBV in Hodgkin's disease varies with age and tumour type.[51]

Pathogenesis and EBV

The link between EBV and Hodgkin's disease was first suggested by the clinical observation of a threefold increased risk of Hodgkin's disease in the 5 years following IM. Further serological investigations revealed that abnormal antibody profiles to EBV antigens occur prior to tumour development.[52] More direct evidence of the role of EBV in pathogenesis has come from detailed studies of the virus in tumour sections, including detection of EBV DNA and latent gene expression in the Reed–Sternberg cell. The demonstration of viral clonality indicates that infection was present at the time of malignant transformation, suggesting that the virus contributes to the initial transformation event.[53] Extensive laboratory studies have identified expression of a number of key genes in EBV replication and oncogenesis. Of these EBNA1, which is vital to replication, and LMP1, which is a viral oncogene, have both been identified in Hodgkin's disease.[54,55] As in other EBV-linked tumours, the restricted number of EBV genes expressed probably limits the ability of the immune system to identify aberrant malignant cells.

Another important clinical insight into the role of EBV in the disease is the increased incidence of Hodgkin's in those with HIV, and the link with EBV is stronger in the immunosupressed than the immunocompetent.[56]

Clinical features

Hodgkin's disease classically presents with lymph node enlargement and is treated with a combination of chemotherapy and radiotherapy. Prognosis is linked to stage at presentation, but the overall 10-year survival is approximately 60%. Early evidence from the UK, India and South Africa suggests that individuals with

EBV-associated tumours have a better response to therapy, but it is not yet clear whether overall survival rates are also improved.[57–59] In the search for new treatment strategies, the presence of EBV in the tumour may be exploited to develop immunotherapy targeted at viral antigens.[60]

Post-transplant lymphoproliferative disease

Solid organ transplant recipients require long-term immunosuppression to prevent organ rejection. This places the recipient at risk of loss of immune control of persistent viruses as well as infection with new or unusual agents. EBV infection in this context, either as primary infection in children, or increased viral replication in adults, can predispose to the development of clonal B cell expansions and B cell lymphoma, collectively known as B cell lymphoproliferative disease (BLPD).[61] Between 1% and 10% of solid organ transplant recipients develop BLPD; the tumours are nearly always associated with EBV and usually follow an aggressive course. First-line treatment for BLPD is reduction of immunosuppression; however, recurrences often occur, and mortality remains high. Novel immunotherapies are currently being developed,[61] which may be extended for use in AIDS-related lymphoma and Hodgkin's disease.[60]

Epithelial cell tumours and EBV

Although there is no direct evidence of EBV infection of epithelial cells in the healthy host, EBV is able to infect epithelial cells in a number of pathological situations, both benign and malignant, oral hairy leucoplakia being an example of the former and nasopharyngeal carcinoma of the latter.[62,63]

Nasopharyngeal carcinoma

Nasopharyngeal carcinoma (NPC) is the most common of all the EBV-associated malignancies on a worldwide basis, and is the most consistently linked with EBV. NPC arises from squamous epithelial cells in the postnasal space, and histopathologically it is subdivided into three categories: WHO I, II, III. WHO I is a keratinizing squamous carcinoma, WHO II is a non-keratinizing epidermoid type, and WHO III is undifferentiated or anaplastic (Figure 44.5). WHO III is invariably linked to EBV and is the most common type.[64]

Epidemiology

NPC has a distinct geographic pattern (Figure 44.2B): 44% of all NPC cases occur in China and 23% in South-East Asia. Endemic areas include southern China (Guangdong, Guanxi, Hunan and Fujian), where it is the most common tumour in men and the second commonest in women, and additionally Hong Kong, Thailand and Vietnam.[4] Outside Asia the incidence is lower, the only other high-risk population being the Inuit in Alaska and Greenland. The incidence is moderate in Morocco, Algeria, Sudan, Kenya and the Mediterranean basin, but NPC is rare in the rest of the world. In emigrés from endemic areas the incidence falls in one or two generations, but remains above that of low-risk populations.[65]

Pathogenesis and EBV

The presence of EBV DNA in malignant cells from nearly every case of undifferentiated NPC strongly suggests the virus has an essential role in oncogenesis. The events leading to malignant transformation are yet to be fully identified, but a number of important observations

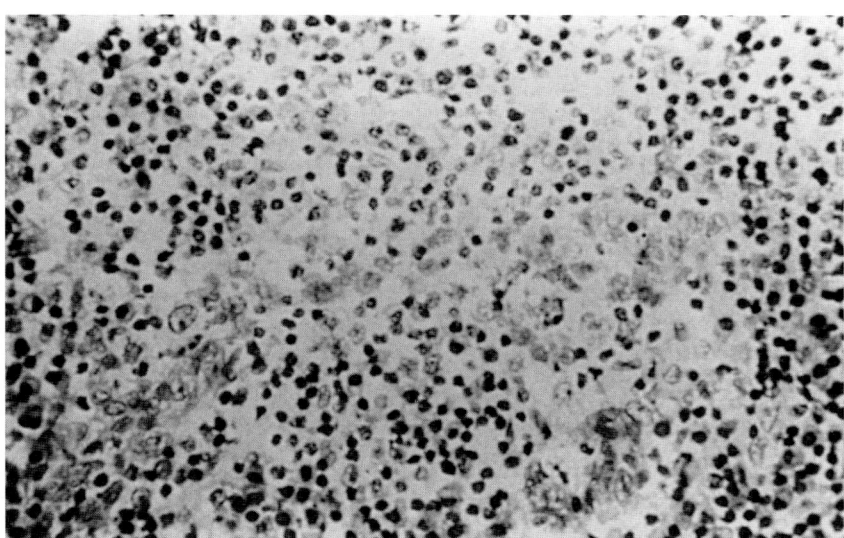

Figure 44.5: Histological section of undifferentiated nasopharyngeal carcinoma showing scattered malignant epithelial cells with heavy infiltrate of small lymphocytes. (H & E, 400 ×.)

support a central role for the virus in the malignant process. Clonal EBV DNA has been identified in pre-invasive NPC lesions, indicating that infection is a premalignant event.[66] The EBV oncogene LMP-1 is expressed in the malignant epithelial cells. Patients with NPC have abnormal EBV serology, typically with raised titres of IgA antibody against EBV early antigen (EA) and VCA which correlate with tumour burden.[64] Environmental and genetic co-factors are thought to be important in tumour development. The restricted geographical pattern of disease suggests that a genetic predisposition is important, and linkage to a HLA locus has been identified in Chinese populations at risk of NPC.[67] Childhood consumption of chemical carcinogens in preserved food has been suggested as a further risk factor in diverse geographical groups, including the Cantonese, Tunisians and Eskimos.[68]

Clinical features

NPC commonly occurs in the postnasal space and may present with non-specific symptoms such as nose bleeds or prolonged otitis media. However, the disease is often not symptomatic until spread to cervical lymph nodes or invasion of cranial nerves has occurred. The mainstay of treatment is radiotherapy, and 5-year survival rates following treatment are 80% for tumours limited to one site, but this is reduced to 20% for those with metastatic disease. Early detection is the best way to improve survival, and studies of EBV antigen-specific IgA in serum and saliva have proved useful for screening high-risk groups in southern China.[69] Rising antibody titres following treatment may herald a recurrence of disease; low or declining titres are indicative of a good prognosis.

Despite this clinical experience, a large population-based evaluation of screening strategies is warranted to establish the optimal panel of antibodies, as well as the sensitivity, specificity, cost effectiveness and timing of screening. The majority of survival data comes from countries with adequate access to health care, with limited data from resource-poor countries. In one series of 150 patients in India the 5-year survival was only 13%.[70]

EBV and other cancers

EBV is associated with 4–18% of all stomach cancers on a worldwide basis. In tumours positive for the virus, EBV infection can be identified in every malignant cell and the DNA is clonal. These facts, as well as the identification of EBV in premalignant gastric lesions, suggest that EBV infection has a role in tumour pathogenesis.[71] EBV DNA has also been identified in a small percentage of breast cancers. However, it is not clear at present whether this is a bystander infection or whether EBV contributes to tumour formation.[72,73] Other malignancies which have been linked to EBV include nasal T cell lymphoma, smooth muscle tumours in transplant recipients and salivary gland tumours.

EBV and HIV

The immunodeficiency of HIV disturbs the tight control the host immune system has over quiescent persistent viral infections such as EBV, Kaposi's sarcoma-associated herpes virus, human papilloma virus and hepatitis C. Those with advancing HIV disease have decreased EBV-specific cytotoxic T cell activity, which allows increased viral replication and increased numbers of infected B cells, and results in high EBV loads in both blood and oropharyngeal secretions.[74,75] Immunocompromised individuals, either from HIV or immunosuppressive drugs, may harbour more than one EBV type and strain, whereas this rarely occurs in healthy individuals.[76] Diseases which occur in HIV have become some of the most common clinical problems associated with EBV.

Oral hairy leucoplakia

Oral hairy leucoplakia (OHL) is common in HIV-infected individuals throughout the world; in South Africa as many as 20% of those infected with HIV have evidence of OHL.[77] OHL presents as a white plaque with a characteristic ribbed appearance, typically on the lateral border of the tongue. It may occur as part of a seroconversion illness or as an early sign of progressive HIV disease.

Multiple strains of EBV infect the superficial layers of the squamous epithelium, resulting in epithelial cell hyperproliferation. In OHL the infected epithelial cells contain actively replicating virus, but there is no evidence that infection leads to malignant transformation.[62]

The lesions respond to a 2–3-week course of high-dose acyclovir, or to topical application of acyclovir cream or retinoic acid gel.

Lymphocytic interstitial pneumonitis

In lymphocytic interstitial pneumonitis (LIP) the lung alveolar septa are infiltrated mononuclear cells leading to expansion of the lung interstitium. LIP is a common manifestation of HIV in children, particularly in Africa.[78] Like other opportunistic infections, the incidence of LIP has fallen in the West since the introduction of highly active antiretroviral therapy. LIP also occurs in those affected by autoimmune disease or treated with immunosuppressive therapies. Children usually present with hypoxia and the chest radiograph typically shows bilateral diffuse reticular–nodular shadowing. Ideally, the diagnosis is confirmed by lung biopsy.

LIP in children has been linked to primary EBV infection, or may reflect increased viral replication due to reduced immune function. Examination of lung biopsy material has identified expansions of foci of B cells infected with EBV.[79] Further studies are warranted to clarify the role of EBV in the disease process.

EBV and AIDS-related cancers

Non Hodgkin's lymphoma and EBV

AIDS–NHL are commonly aggressive high-grade B cell tumours, and are classified as an AIDS-defining illness. 'AIDS-related BL' and 'Burkitt-like lymphoma' (BLL) both have different epidemiological and biological characteristics from endemic childhood BL. BLL has morphological features intermediate between BL and large cell lymphoma, and commonly occurs in HIV, though not exclusively so.[80] Other AIDS-related NHL include AIDS-related primary central nervous system lymphoma (PCNSL) and AIDS-related diffuse large cell lymphoma (DLCL).

Epidemiology

NHL is the second commonest cancer in HIV-infected individuals, Kaposi's sarcoma being the most common,[81] and the aetiology of both cancers is linked to latent herpes virus infections. It is well established in the West that HIV-infected individuals have a much higher incidence of NHL, the risk of developing NHL being 60 times the risk of the general population.[82] In Africa, now that the median survival with HIV has increased to around 10 years,[83] the burden of AIDS-associated cancers has become apparent. In Uganda significant increases in incidence of NHL, including BL in children, have been identified.[84] In the West the incidence of NHL has fallen following the introduction of highly active antiretroviral therapy. All types of AIDS-related NHL are linked to EBV, but the percentage of tumours in which EBV DNA can be identified varies with tumour type.[85] PCNSL is invariably linked with EBV, whereas 80% of DLCL are EBV positive and BL is only linked in around 50% of cases in the West.[53] At present there is no evidence of increase in EBV-related epithelial cell-derived tumours in HIV-positive individuals.

Pathogenesis and EBV

As in BL, the development of NHL in AIDS is a complex multi-step process, in which EBV infection may be one significant event. As already noted, HIV-infected individuals have impaired immune surveillance of EBV, and the combination of decreased cytotoxic T cells against EBV and increased viral load have been correlated with increased risk of AIDS DLCL. Persistent generalized lymphadenopathy (PGL) has long been recognized as being a common feature of HIV infection, and is caused by chronic B cell stimulation and expansion. The identification of EBV infection in PGL tissue may be a predisposing factor for the evolution of lymphoma.[86]

Clinical Features

BL tends to occur quite early in the course of HIV, when the immune system is still relatively intact, and it typically occurs in young adults. It is not clear if the clinical course of BL in African children has changed in the context of marked immunosuppression.

In contrast to BL, primary cerebral NHL usually occurs with a CD4 count less than 50×10^6 and has a particularly poor prognosis. The majority of patients present with systemic features of weight loss, night sweats and fevers, combined with extranodal disease. Diagnosis is usually confirmed by biopsy. When brain biopsy is not appropriate, the identification of EBV in the cerebrospinal fluid of a patient with a cranial mass may help confirm the diagnosis of cerebral lymphoma.[87]

Primary effusion lymphoma is a rare variant of HIV-associated lymphoma in which there is no solid mass, but effusions in serosal cavities; both EBV and Kaposi's sarcoma-associated herpes virus can be readily identified in the malignant cells.

The outcome for AIDS-related NHL remains poor, with the prognosis most critically linked to the degree of immunosuppression. Ideally, combination chemotherapy should be offered to those in the better prognostic groups. However, median survival even in the West is only 7–9 months, though outcomes have improved since the introduction of highly active antiviral therapy.[88]

Vaccine development

Both primary and persistent EBV infections are associated with significant pathology and this has led to interest in the development of an EBV vaccine. An ideal vaccine would prevent the main complication of late primary infection, IM, and prevent viral persistence, thereby potentially eradicating EBV-driven cancers. At present there are two main approaches to vaccine development.

First, induction of neutralizing antibody to gp 350 should prevent virus binding to CD21, the key B cell receptor, and thus prevent infection. Gp 350 vaccines are under trial, but it is not clear yet whether induction of an antibody response, possibly with induction of cytotoxic T cells to the same viral epitope, will provide sterile immunity.[89]

The second approach to vaccination is the induction of cytotoxic T cells specific to EBV by vaccination with synthetic peptides. As cytotoxic T cells are critical to controlling primary infection, this mechanism may limit early viral replication. This may significantly attenuate the immune response to primary infection, and the associated clinical features of IM, but probably would not prevent establishment of viral persistence.[90] This type of vaccine may be exploited as a therapeutic vaccine against EBV epitopes in tumours.

REFERENCES

1   Epstein M A, Achong B G & Barr Y M. Virus particles in cultured lymphoblasts from Burkitt's lymphoma. *Lancet* 1964: 702–703.

2   Gerber P, Lucas S, Nonoyama M, Perlin E & Goldstein L I. Oral excretion of Epstein–Barr virus by healthy subjects and patients with infectious mononucleosis. *Lancet* 1972; 11(2):988–999.

3   Lewin N et al. Characterization of EBV-carrying B-cell populations in healthy seropositive individuals with regard to density, release of transforming virus and spontaneous outgrowth. *Int J Cancer* 1987; 39(4):472–476.

4   Pisani P et al. Cancer and infection: estimates of the attributable fraction in 1990. *Cancer Epidemiol Biomarkers Prev* 1997; 6(6):387–400.

5   Henle W, Henle G & Lennette E T. The Epstein–Barr virus. *Sci Am* 1979; 241(1):48–59.

6   Haque T et al. Seroepidemiological study of Epstein–Barr virus infection in Bangladesh. *J Med Virol* 1996; 48(1):17–21.

7   Essers S et al. Seroepidemiological correlations of antibodies to human herpesviruses and human immunodeficiency virus type 1 in African patients. *Eur J Epidemiol* 1991; 7(6):658–664.

8   Dambaugh T et al. Epstein–Barr virus (B95-8) DNA VII: molecular cloning and detailed mapping. *Proc Natl Acad Sci USA* 1980; 77(5):2999–3003.

9   Sample J et al. Epstein–Barr virus types 1 and 2 differ in their EBNA-3A, EBNA-3B, and EBNA-3C genes. *J Virol* 1990; 64(9):4084–4092.

10 Zimber U et al. Geographical prevalence of two types of Epstein–Barr virus. *Virology* 1986; 154(1):56–66.

11 Sculley T B et al. Coinfection with A- and B-type: Epstein–Barr virus in human immunodeficiency virus-positive subjects. *J Infect Dis* 1990; 162(3):643–648.

12 Miyashita E M et al. Identification of the site of Epstein–Barr virus persistence in vivo as a resting B cell. *J Virol* 1997; 71(7):4882–4891.

13 Ikeda T et al. Detection of lymphocytes productively infected with Epstein–Barr virus in non-neoplastic tonsils. *J Gen Virol* 2000; 81(5):1211–1216.

14 Nikoskelainen J et al. Epstein–Barr virus (EBV) infections in army recruits. *Acta Med Scand* 1974; 196(5):439–443.

15 Sawyer R N et al. Prospective studies of a group of Yale University freshmen. I. Occurrence of infectious mononucleosis. *J Infect Dis* 1971; 123(3):263–270.

16 Hallee T J et al. Infectious mononucleosis at the United States Military Academy: a prospective study of a single class over four years. *Yale J Biol Med* 1974; 47(3):182–195.

17 Auwaerter P G. Infectious mononucleosis in middle age (clinical conference). JAMA 1999; 281(5):454–459.

18 Israele V, Shirley P & Sixbey J W. Excretion of the Epstein–Barr virus from the genital tract of men. *J Infect Dis* 1991; 163(6):1341–1343.

19 Sixbey J W, Lemon S M & Pagano J S. A second site for Epstein–Barr virus shedding: the uterine cervix. *Lancet* 1986; ii(8516):1122–1124.

20 Cohen J I. Epstein–Barr virus infection. *N Engl J Med* 2000; 343(7):481–492.

21 Taga H et al. Human and viral interleukin-10 in acute Epstein–Barr virus-induced infectious mononucleosis. *J Infect Dis* 1995; 171(5):1347–1350.

22 Parolini S et al. X-linked lymphoproliferative disease: 2B4 molecules displaying inhibitory rather than activating function are responsible for the inability of natural killer cells to kill Epstein–Barr virus-infected cells. *J Exp Med* 2000; 192(3):337–346.

23 Foss H D et al. Patterns of cytokine gene expression in infectious mononucleosis. *Blood* 1994; 83(3):707–712.

24 Callan M F et al. Large clonal expansions of CD8+ T cells in acute infectious mononucleosis. *Nat Med* 1996; 2(8):906–911.

25 Epstein M A & Crawford D H. The Epstein–Barr virus. In Weatherall D J, Ledingham J G G & Warrell D A (eds) *Oxford Textbook of Medicine*. Oxford: Oxford University Press, 1996: 352–356.

26 White P D et al. Incidence, risk and prognosis of acute and chronic fatigue syndromes and psychiatric disorders after glandular fever. *Br J Psychiatry* 1998; 173:475–481.

27 Swanink C M et al. Epstein–Barr virus (EBV) and the chronic fatigue syndrome: normal virus load in blood and normal immunologic reactivity in the EBV regression assay. *Clin Infect Dis* 1995; 20(5):1390–1392.

28 Coffey A J et al. Host response to EBV infection in X-linked lymphoproliferative disease results from mutations in an SH2-domain encoding gene. *Nat Genet* 1998; 20(2):129–135.

29 Sayos J et al. The X-linked lymphoproliferative-disease gene product SAP regulates signals induced through the co-receptor SLAM. *Nature* 1998; 395(6701):462–469.

30 Maia D M & Peace-Brewer A L. Chronic, active Epstein–Barr virus infection. *Curr Opin Hematol* 2000; 7(1):59–63.

31 Klein G et al. Search for tumour-specific immune reactions in Burkitt lymphoma patients by the membrane immunofluorescence reaction. *Natl Acad Sci USA* 1968; 55:1628–1635.

32 Miller G et al. Lymphoma in cotton-top marmosets after inoculation with Epstein–Barr virus: tumor incidence, histologic spectrum antibody responses, demonstration of viral DNA, and characterization of viruses. *J Exp Med* 1977; 145(4):948–967.

33 Pope J H, Horne M K & Scott W. Transformation of foetal human leukocytes in vitro by filtrates of a human leukaemic cell line containing herpes-like virus. *Int J Cancer* 1968; 3(6):857–866.

34 Rickinson A B. Epstein–Barr virus in action in vivo. *N Engl J Med* 1998; 338(20):1461–1463.

35 Ziegler J L et al. Detection of Epstein–Barr virus DNA in American Burkitt's lymphoma. *Int J Cancer* 1976; 17(6):701–706.

36 Williams E H et al. Space-time clustering of Burkitt's lymphoma in the West Nile district of Uganda: 1961–1975. *Br J Cancer* 1978; 37(1):109–122.

37 Burkitt D P & Wright D H. *Geographical Distribution of Burkitt's Lymphoma*. Edinburgh: E & S Livingstone, 1970: 186–197.

38 Plo K J. Burkitt lymphoma in the Côte d'Ivoire from 1966 to 1995: a progress report. *Med Pediatr Oncol* 2000; 34(3):206–209.

39 Sandlund J T et al. Predominance and characteristics of Burkitt lymphoma among children with non-Hodgkin lymphoma in northeastern Brazil. *Leukemia* 1997; 11(5):743–746.

40 Araujo I et al. Expression of Epstein–Barr virus-gene products in Burkitt's lymphoma in Northeast Brazil. *Blood* 1996; 87(12):5279–5286.

41 Ertem U et al. Burkitt's lymphoma in 63 Turkish children diagnosed over a 10 year period. *Pediatr Hematol Oncol* 1996; 13(2):123–134.

42 Klein G. In defense of the 'old' Burkitt lymphoma scenario. Series title: *Advances in Viral Oncology*. New York: Raven Press, 1987: 207–211.

43 Gaidano G et al. p53 mutations in human lymphoid malignancies: association with Burkitt lymphoma and chronic lymphocytic leukemia. *Proc Natl Acad Sci USA* 1991; 88(12):5413–5417.

44 de Thé G et al. Epidemiological evidence for causal relationship between Epstein–Barr virus and Burkitt's lymphoma from Ugandan prospective study. *Nature* 1978; 274(5673):756–761.

45 Cavdar A O et al. Burkitt's lymphoma between African and American types in Turkish children: clinical, viral (EBV), and molecular studies. *Med Pediatr Oncol* 1993; 21(1):36–42.

46 Epstein M A & Crawford D H. Gammaherpesviruses: Epstein–Barr virus. In Mahy B W J & Collier L (eds) *Topley and Wilson's Microbiology and Microbial Infections*, vol. 1. London: Arnold, 1998: 351–366.

47 Geser A, Brubaker G & Draper C C. Effect of a malaria suppression program on the incidence of African Burkitt's lymphoma. *Am J Epidemiol* 1989; 129(4):740–752.

48 Proceedings of the IARC Working Group on the Evaluation of Carcinogenic Risks to Humans. Epstein–Barr Virus and Kaposi's Sarcoma Herpesvirus/Human Herpesvirus 8. Lyon: France, 17–24 June 1997. *IARC Monogr Eval Carcinog Risks Hum* 1997; 70:1–492.

49 Magrath I, Jain V & Bhatia K. Epstein–Barr virus and Burkitt's lymphoma. *Semin Cancer Biol* 1992; 3(5):285–295.

50 Magrath I T. Management of high-grade lymphomas. *Oncology* 1998; 12(10, Suppl 8):40–48.

51 Chapman A L & Rickinson A B. Epstein–Barr virus in Hodgkin's disease. *Ann Oncol* 1998; 9(suppl. 5):S5–S16.

52 Mueller N et al. Hodgkin's disease and Epstein–Barr virus: altered antibody pattern before diagnosis. *N Engl J Med* 1989; 320(11):689–695.

53 Weiss L M et al. Detection of Epstein–Barr viral genomes in Reed–Sternberg cells of Hodgkin's disease. *N Engl J Med* 1989; 320(8):502–506.

54 Pallesen G et al. Expression of Epstein–Barr virus latent gene products in tumour cells of Hodgkin's disease. *Lancet* 1991; 337(8737):320–322.

55 Murray P G et al. Immunohistochemical demonstration of the Epstein–Barr virus-encoded latent membrane protein in paraffin sections of Hodgkin's disease. *J Pathol* 1992; 166(1):1–5.

56 Carbone A et al. Human immunodeficiency virus-associated Hodgkin's disease derives from post-germinal center B cells. *Blood* 1999; 93(7):2319–2326.

57 Murray P G et al. Effect of Epstein–Barr virus infection on response to chemotherapy and survival in Hodgkin's disease. *Blood* 1999; 94(2):442–447.

58 Naresh K N et al. Epstein–Barr virus association in classical Hodgkin's disease provides survival advantage to patients and correlates with higher expression of proliferation markers in Reed–Sternberg cells. *Ann Oncol* 2000; 11(1):91–96.

59 Engel M et al. Improved prognosis of Epstein–Barr virus associated childhood Hodgkin's lymphoma: study of 47 South African cases. *J Clin Pathol* 2000; 53(3):182–186.

60 Rooney C M et al. Treatment of relapsed Hodgkin's disease using EBV-specific cytotoxic T cells. *Ann Oncol* 1998; 9(suppl. 5):S129–S132.

61 Haque T & Crawford D H. The role of adoptive immunotherapy in the prevention and treatment of lymphoproliferative disease following transplantation. *Br J Haematol* 1999; 106(2):309–316.

62 Greenspan J S et al. Replication of Epstein–Barr virus within the epithelial cells of oral 'hairy' leukoplakia, an AIDS-associated lesion. *N Engl J Med* 1985; 313(25):1564–1571.

63 zur Hausen H et al. EBV DNA in biopsies of Burkitt tumours and anaplastic carcinomas of the nasopharynx. *Nature* 1970; 228(276):1056–1058.

64 Vokes E E, Liebowitz D N & Weichselbaum R R. Nasopharyngeal carcinoma. *Lancet* 1997; 350(9084):1087–1091.

65 Pagano P S. The Epstein–Barr virus and nasopharyngeal carcinoma. *Cancer* 1994; 74(9):2414–2424.

66 Raab-Traub N. Epstein–Barr virus and nasopharyngeal carcinoma. *Semin Cancer Biol* 1992; 3(5):297–307.

67 Simons M J et al. Immunogenetic aspects of nasopharyngeal carcinoma. IV. Increased risk in Chinese of nasopharyngeal carcinoma associated with a Chinese-related HLA profile (A2, Singapore 2). *J Natl Cancer Inst* 1976; 57(5):977–980.

68 West S, Hildesheim A & Dosemeci M. Non-viral risk factors for nasopharyngeal carcinoma in the Philippines: results from a case–control study. *Int J Cancer* 1993; 55(5):722–727.

69 Chen H H, Prevost T C & Duffy S W. Evaluation of screening for nasopharyngeal carcinoma: trial design using Markov chain models. *Br J Cancer* 1999; 79(11–12):1894–1900.

70 Koppikar S B et al. Nasopharyngeal carcinoma in India: end-result analysis (1980–1984). *J Surg Oncol* 1988; 39(3):179–182.

71 Yanai H et al. Epstein–Barr virus infection in non-carcinomatous gastric epithelium. *J Pathol* 1997; 183(3):293–298.

72 Glaser S L et al. Absence of Epstein–Barr virus EBER-1 transcripts in an epidemiologically diverse group of breast cancers. *Int J Cancer* 1998; 75(4):555–558.

73 Bonnet M et al. Detection of Epstein–Barr virus in invasive breast cancers. *J Natl Cancer Inst* 1999; 91(16):1376–1381.

74 Birx D L, Redfield R R & Tosato G. Defective regulation of Epstein–Barr virus infection in patients with acquired immunodeficiency syndrome (AIDS) or AIDS-related disorders. *N Engl J Med* 1986; 314(14):874–879.

75 Kersten M J et al. Epstein–Barr virus-specific cytotoxic T cell responses in HIV-1 infection: different kinetics in patients progressing to opportunistic infection or non-Hodgkin's lymphoma. *J Clin Invest* 1997; 99(7):1525–1533.

76 Yao Q Y et al. Frequency of multiple Epstein–Barr virus infections in T-cell-immunocompromised individuals. *J Virol* 1996; 70(8):4884–4894.

77 Arendorf T M et al. Oral manifestations of HIV infection in 600 South African patients. *J Oral Pathol Med* 1998; 27(4):176–179.

78 Jeena P M et al. Persistent and chronic lung disease in HIV-1 infected and uninfected African children. *AIDS* 1998; 12(10):1185–1193.

79 Brodie S J et al. Pediatric AIDS-associated lymphocytic interstitial pneumonia and pulmonary arterio-occlusive disease: role of VCAM-1/VLA-4 adhesion pathway and human herpesviruses. *Am J Pathol* 1999; 154(5):1453–1464.

80 Davi F et al. Burkitt-like lymphomas in AIDS patients: characterization within a series of 103 human immunodeficiency virus-associated non-Hodgkin's lymphomas. Burkitt's Lymphoma Study Group. *J Clin Oncol* 1998; 16(12):3788–3795.

81 Highly active antiretroviral therapy and incidence of cancer in human immunodeficiency virus-infected adults. *J Natl Cancer Inst* 2000; 92(22):1823–1830.

82 Beral V et al. AIDS-associated non-Hodgkin lymphoma. *Lancet* 1991; 337(8745):805–809.

83 Morgan D & Whitworth J. The natural history of HIV-1 infection in Africa. *Nat Med* 2001; 7(2):143–145.

84 Wabinga H R et al. Trends in cancer incidence in Kyadondo County, Uganda, 1960–1997. *Br J Cancer* 2000; 82(9):1585–1592.

85 Gaidano G, Capello D & Carbone A. The molecular basis of acquired immunodeficiency syndrome-related lymphomagenesis. *Semin Oncol* 2000; 27(4):431–441.

86 Shibata D et al. Epstein–Barr virus in benign lymph node biopsies from individuals infected with the human immunodeficiency virus is associated with concurrent or subsequent development of non-Hodgkin's lymphoma. *Blood* 1991; 77(7):1527–1533.

87 Bower M & Fife K. In Gazzard B (ed.) *Chelsea and Westminster Hospital AIDS Care Handbook*. London: Mediscript, 1999: 102–110.

88 Vaccher E et al. Concomitant cyclophosphamide, doxorubicin, vincristine, and prednisone chemotherapy plus highly active antiretroviral therapy in patients with human

immunodeficiency virus-related, non-Hodgkin lymphoma. *Cancer* 2001; 91(1):155–163.

89 Jackman W T et al. Expression of Epstein–Barr virus gp350 as a single chain glycoprotein for an EBV subunit vaccine. *Vaccine* 1999; 17(7–8):660–668.

90 Khanna R, Moss D J & Burrows S R. Vaccine strategies against Epstein–Barr virus-associated diseases: lessons from studies on cytotoxic T-cell-mediated immune regulation. *Immunol Rev* 1999; 170:49–64.

Chapter 45
Rabies

M. J. Warrell

Rabies is a widespread infection of certain animal species which is occasionally transmitted to man. Rabies is also known as hydrophobia, *la rage* in French, *la rabbia* in Italian, *la rabia* in Spanish and, in German, *die Tollwut*.

History

Transmission of the infection from dogs' saliva was known to the Egyptians at the time of the Pharaohs, and suggested methods of treatment are found in Chinese manuscripts from the fifth century BC.[1] Animal rabies was described by Aristotle in the fourth century BC, and the Roman, Celsus, wrote of the human illness in the first century AD, when knowledge and fear of the disease were widespread. A sixteenth-century Italian physician, Fracastoro, described the clinical features of rabies.[2]

John Hunter initiated a scientific approach to rabies in 1793 and experiments on transmission of the infection were carried out in Germany by Zinke, and in France by Magendie early in the nineteenth century. Louis Pasteur's work in the 1880s demonstrated that rabies was an infection of the central nervous system. He repeatedly passaged virulent 'street' virus in rabbits, attenuating it to a 'fixed' laboratory strain, used to make the first rabies vaccine.[2]

Growth of the virus in tissue culture was achieved in the 1930s and the virus was first visualized by electron microscopy in the early 1960s.[3]

Virus

Rabies virus is a species of the genus *Lyssavirus* (Greek *lyssa*, rage/frenzy) of the large family of Rhabdoviridae (Gk *rhabdos*, rod). Seven lyssaviruses are now recognized:[4,5] rabies, and six rabies-related viruses, five of which have caused fatal infection in man (see below). Other rhabdoviruses which very rarely cause disease in humans are: the vesicular stomatitis viruses, Chandipura, Piry and Le Dantec viruses.[6]

The bullet-shaped rabies virion (Figure 45.1) measures approximately 180 × 75 nm, and contains a single strand

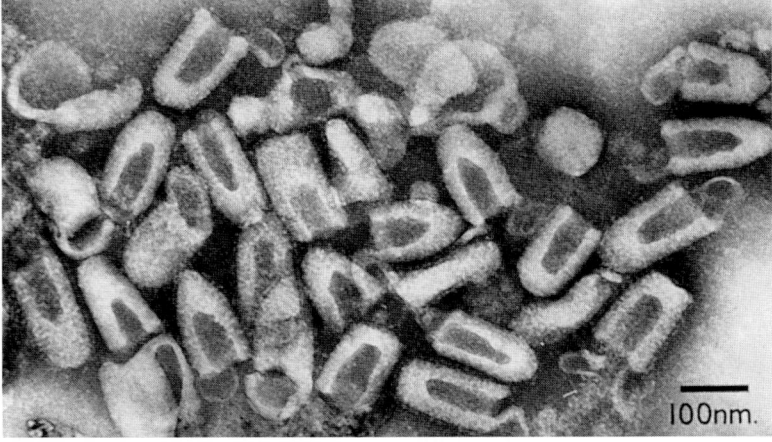
100nm.

A

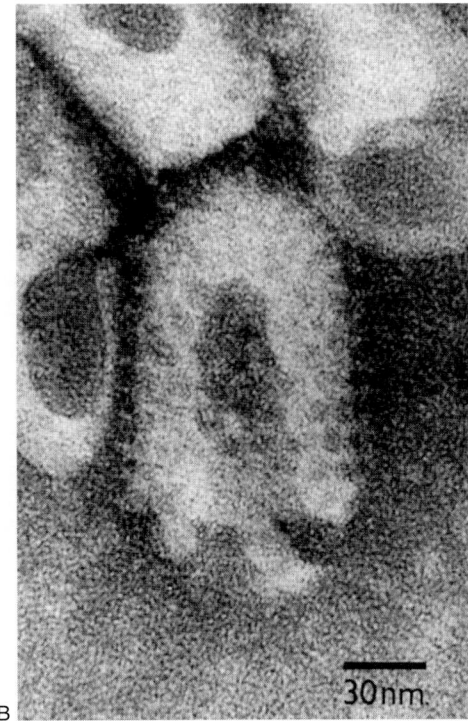
30nm.

B

Figure 45.1: (A) and (B) Negatively stained electron micrographs of bullet-shaped rabies virions; (B) shows projections on the surface of the glycoprotein coat, covering all but the blunt end of the virion. (Courtesy of C. J. Smale and Joan Crick.)

of RNA of negative polarity. This combines with a nucleo-protein, a phosphoprotein and RNA polymerase to form a helical coil. This core of the virus is the ribonucleoprotein complex. It is covered by a matrix protein and then by a glycoprotein bearing club-shaped spikes (Figure 45.1b) which project outward through a host cell-derived lipid bilayer.[7]

Inactivation

Rabies virus is rapidly inactivated by heat. At 56°C the half-life is less than a minute, but at 37°C it is prolonged to several hours in moist conditions. At 4°C there is little loss after 2 weeks.[8]

The lipid coat is disrupted by detergents or a simple 1% soap solution. Other virucidal agents include 45% ethanol, iodine solutions (1:10 000 available iodine) and 1% benzalkonium chloride, but phenol is not so effective.

Geographical distribution

Rabies is a widespread zoonosis, occurring in separate cycles within dogs and wild mammal vector species. The infection sometimes spills over to non-vector species such as humans. Strains of virus from different species can be identified by genetic sequence analysis or by antigenic typing using a panel of monoclonal antibodies. The *urban* enzootic in domestic dogs is of most importance to man, and is the cause of more than 90% of human rabies cases (Figure 45.2). Dogs also frequently infect cats and other domestic mammals. The pattern of *sylvatic* (wildlife) rabies shows great geographical variation, and knowledge of local current epizootics is important in the prevention of human rabies fatalities (Figures 45.3 and 45.4). The distribution of dominant vector species is summarized [9–19] in Table 45.1.

Areas of the world which have recently been reported to be free of rabies include: New Zealand; Papua New

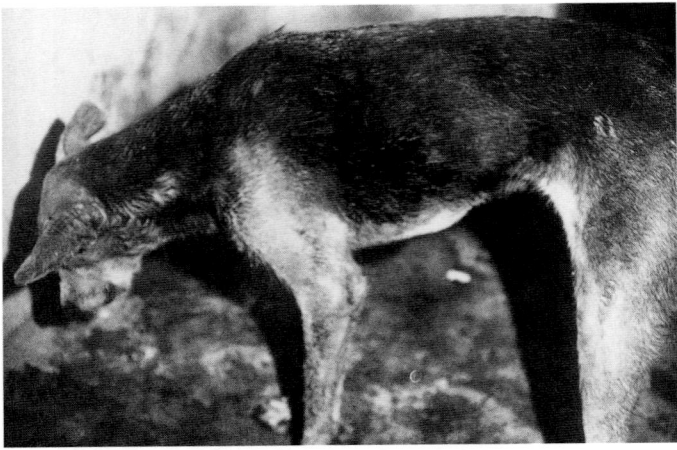

Figure 45.2: Domestic dog with paralytic rabies in Nigeria. Note paralysis of limbs and drooling of saliva. (Copyright D. A. Warrell.)

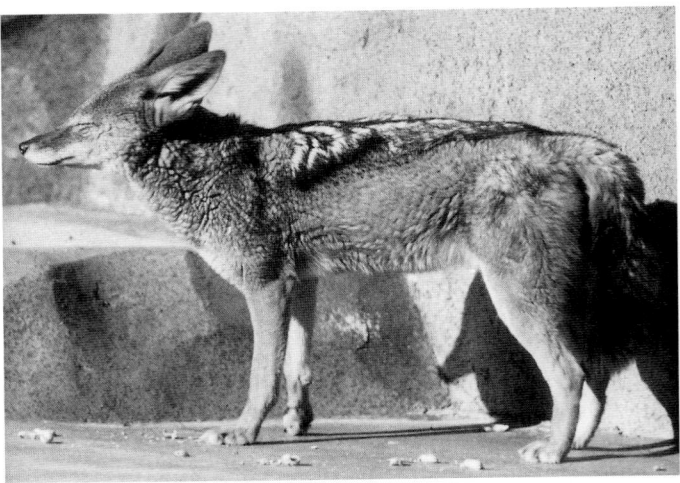

Figure 45.3: Black-backed jackal (*Canis mesomelas*), an important vector/reservoir of sylvatic rabies in Zambia, Zimbabwe and Namibia. (Copyright D. A. Warrell.)

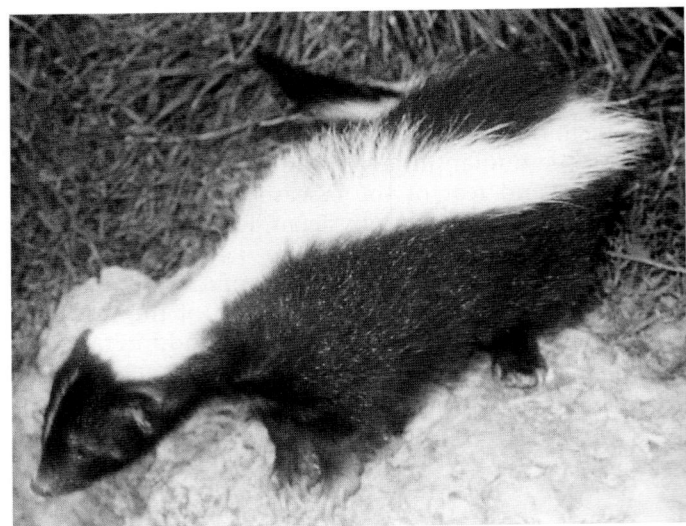

Figure 45.4: Striped skunk (*Mephitis mephitis*), an important vector/reservoir of sylvatic rabies in North America. (Copyright D. A. Warrell.)

Guinea; Japan; Taiwan; Hong Kong Islands; Singapore; Sabah, Sarawak, some islands of Indonesia (e.g. Bali), and in the Indian Ocean; many Pacific islands, e.g. Solomon Islands, Fiji, Samoa and Cook Islands; Uruguay, UK, Ireland, Iceland, Finland, Sweden, Norway, Switzerland, Portugal, Italy, Greece, the Mediterranean islands; some Caribbean islands (e.g. Barbados, Bahamas, Jamaica and Antigua); and Antarctica.

Although some countries have no urban or sylvatic rabies, infected wild animals cross land borders. Imported rabies is a universal risk.

Incidence

In endemic tropical areas, especially where dogs are the

Table 45.1 Distribution of important rabies vector species

Species	Distribution
Africa[9,10]	
Domestic dog[11]	Widespread dominant vector
Black-backed jackals (Canis mesomelas)*	Zambia, Zimbabwe, Namibia
Yellow mongoose (Cynicitis penicillata)	South Africa
Americas[12]	
Arctic fox (Alopex lagopus)	North-west Canada, Alaska
Striped skunk (Mephitis mephitis)†	Central Canada and USA, California
Raccoon (Procyon lotor)	Mid-Atlantic states and south-east USA
Fox	Arizona, Texas and north-eastern USA, Canada
Coyote (Canis latrans)	Southern Texas
Insectivorous bats[12,13]	USA and South America
Domestic dog	Widespread Mexico, Central and parts of South America
Vampire bat[14] (Desmodontidae)	Southern Texas, Mexico, Trinidad and Tobago, Central and South America south to Argentina and Chile
Mongoose[15] (Herpestes species)	Puerto Rico, Grenada, Cuba, Dominican Republic
Asia[9]	
Domestic dog	Widespread dominant vector
Wolf	Iran, Iraq, Afghanistan
Europe	
Fox[16]	Widespread from France east to Russia
Arctic fox[9] (Alopex lagopus)	Northern Russia
Raccoon dog[17] (Nycterentes procyonoides)	Baltic states, Russia, Poland, Ukraine
Wolf[17]	Russia
Dog	Turkey, southern Russian states
Insectivorous bats[18]	Germany, Denmark, Netherlands, Russia, Poland, Spain, France, Czech Republic, Switzerland, Hungary
Australia[14,19]	
Fruit bats (flying foxes) (Pteropus spp.)	Northern & eastern coastal regions

* See Figure 45.3
† See Figure 45.4

dominant vector, the true incidence of human rabies is unknown because of under-reporting or lack of published figures. In India 30 000 (3/10⁵ population) deaths were reported to the WHO in 1998;[20] in Bangladesh the estimate was 2000 cases (1.6/10⁵ population). In 1999 in Sri Lanka 110 rabies deaths were reported (0.6/10⁵ population); in Nepal 155 (0.66/10⁵); in Vietnam 119 (0.15/10⁵) and in the Philippines 398 (0.5/10⁵). In the whole of Africa 204 cases were reported in 1998, 43 of these from Ethiopia alone. Gross under-reporting is suspected. In the Americas, the highest mortalities are in Brazil, Mexico, Ecuador and El Salvador.

In the USA, where sylvatic rabies is endemic, there have been 32 deaths over 10 years since 1990. Twenty-four (75%) of these were due to bat rabies viruses, and only two reported a bat bite, although half had had some contact with a bat.[21]

Rabies-related virus infections

The *Lyssavirus* genus comprises rabies genotype 1, and rabies-related viruses genotypes 2–7. They have all been found to be human pathogens except for genotype 2: Lagos bat virus. Genotype 3, Mokola virus in shrews and cats, and genotype 4 Duvenhage virus in bats, are occasionally found only in Africa. Mokola virus caused fatal encephalitis in a Nigerian child, while another recovered from pharyngitis and probably a febrile convulsion.[10,22,23] A laboratory worker recovered from an accidental infection.[24] Duvenhage virus is named after a patient who had rabies-like encephalitis caused by the virus.[10,25]

European insectivorous bats harbour European bat lyssavirus genotypes 5 and 6, and each is subdivided into subtypes a and b.[18] Genotype 5 viruses are found predominantly in *Eptesicus serotinus* species in Denmark, Germany, the Netherlands, Russia, Poland, Spain, France, the Czech Republic and Hungary. Two Russian girls died of rabies following bat bites.[26,27] Genotype 6 occurs in *Myotis* bat species in the Netherlands and Switzerland, and it was identified in a bat in a British port in 1996, presumed to have been imported. In Finland in 1985, a Swiss zoologist bitten by a bat from an unknown source died of furious rabies-like encephalitis, due to this genotype.[28]

In Australia in 1996, flying foxes (fruit bats, genus *Pteropus*) were discovered to harbour the Australian bat lyssavirus (genotype 7), which has caused a rabies-like fatal illness in two women. [5,19]

Transmission of infection

Animal contact

Inoculation of rabies virus into a wound or on to a mucous membrane may result in infection. This includes contamination of an unhealed lesion. Intact skin is a barrier against viral entry. Humans are usually infected by virus-laden saliva, inoculated during the bite of a rabid dog. The chance of developing rabies following exposure is revealed by data from the prevaccine era (see below: Efficacy of postexposure prophylaxis).

Human-to-human

There are old anecdotal reports of infections from contact with human saliva, kissing, biting, sexual intercourse, breast-feeding and eating infected meat, but these routes remain unproven in man.[29] Viraemia has not been detected.[29]

Transmission has occurred through *grafting of infected corneas*. Six virologically proven cases followed transplants from donors with unsuspected rabies. Another patient who received a cornea from an infected donor survived following treatment with high-dose postexposure therapy including interferon.[30]

Transplacental infection occurs in animals and a Turkish woman and her 2-day-old infant died of virologically confirmed rabies.[31] This is exceptional. Many mothers with rabies have been delivered of healthy babies.

Other routes

Inhalation of rabies virus in aerosols infected two people in bat-infested caves.[32] Two more inhaled aerosols of 'fixed' virus in laboratory accidents.[33,34]

Pathogenesis[35,36]

The extraordinary journey of rabies virions along nerves up to the brain, and then outward to many organs, is poorly understood. It usually begins with the bite of a rabid animal inoculating virus-laden saliva through the skin, often into muscle. Experiments show viral replication occurring locally in striated muscle or mucous membrane, or directly invading a nerve cell. The virus can attach to several types of cell receptors. One important site of attachment is the nicotinic acetylcholine receptor at neuromuscular junctions,[37] where binding is competitive, not only with cholinergic ligands, but also with a snake venom neurotoxin, α-bungarotoxin, which has a homologous sequence with rabies glycoprotein.[38]

Once inside a neurone the virus moves centripetally, but it has not been observed in peripheral axons. Virions or perhaps naked nucleocapsids are probably carried passively by retrograde axonal transport, at a rate of 3 mm/h experimentally. Its progress can be halted by sectioning nerves or by inhibitors, such as colchicine. Rabies ascends through ganglia, eventually reaching the brain, where intraneuronal replication occurs on a massive scale. Viral proteins accumulate in the cytoplasm, appearing as inclusions—the classical Negri bodies. Virions are now visible by EM in neurones and the infection spreads transsynaptically. Involvement of the limbic system causes aggressive behaviour and enables transmission from a vector species to another host. The often minimal histopathological changes do not account for the gross neuronal dysfunction, but there is evidence of altered neurotransmitter activity.

The rabies virus remains virtually confined to neurones as centrifugal dissemination then progresses via autonomic and peripheral nerves. Virus has been isolated from human skeletal and cardiac muscle, skin, lung, kidney, adrenal, lacrimal and, of course, salivary glands.[29,39]

In contrast to events in neurones, virus replication in acinar cells of the salivary glands produces large amounts of extracellular virus. Although there is no evidence of viraemia, rabies virus is shed in human lacrimal and respiratory tract secretions and possibly in urine[29] and in milk.

Rabies virus evades recognition by the immune system until a late stage of the disease. At the site of inoculation, some virus is briefly exposed, but once within the CNS virions and their antigens are hidden from immune surveillance. During the final centrifugal phase of infection, when extracellular virus is produced, rabies antigens are expressed on cell membranes but the immune response is too late to combat the overwhelming infection.

Pathology

Cerebral congestion and a few petechial haemorrhages are usual findings in rabies encephalitis, but not gross cerebral oedema.[40,41] A lymphocytic perivenous infiltrate is common, and neutrophils are occasionally seen, perhaps only early in the disease. Eosinophilic cytoplasmic inclusions (Negri bodies) are found in 75% of cases, most frequently in large neurones of the hippocampus, Purkinje cells of the cerebellum and medulla.[42] Negri bodies contain eosinophilic rabies nucleoprotein matrix, occasional virions and small basophilic masses, probably fragments of host cell organelles, mechanically trapped during fusion of smaller inclusions.[3] Neuronophagia, microglial reaction, foci of demyelination and perineural infiltration (Babès' nodules) also occur.[42] The brain stem and spinal cord are predominantly affected, but changes are often widespread. A meningeal reaction is common in children, and in paralytic disease the spinal cord is most severely affected. The extent of the histopathological change varies from complete disruption of neuronal structure and axonal degeneration of peripheral nerves following intensive care,[43] to an absence of any inflammation or degeneration.[40,41,44]

Extraneural pathology includes focal degeneration of salivary glands, liver, pancreas, adrenal medulla and lymph nodes,[45] and also interstitial myocarditis.[46]

Immunity

Response to infection

Following a rabid bite, no immune response is detectable in unvaccinated subjects before encephalitis has developed. Rabies antibody is first found in serum, then in cerebrospinal fluid (CSF) about a week after the onset.[47,48] Neutralizing antibody may rise to a high level if life is prolonged. Specific rabies IgM antibody is occasionally found, but is unhelpful in diagnosis as it does not appear early and can also be present in postvaccinal encephalitis.[49]

There is little evidence of lymphocyte-mediated responses to encephalitis in man. Pleocytosis is observed in only 60% of patients, with a mean leucocyte count of 75/mm^3.[47] Peripheral blood lymphocyte transformation has been shown in a few cases of furious rabies.[50] Very low levels of interferon have been found in the serum and CSF of about 30% of patients with rabies encephalitis.[51] Viral clearance from the brain of lethally infected rats has been achieved by treatment with a particular monoclonal antibody.[52] No such treatment is available for man. Rabies nucleoprotein acts as a superantigen, but the effect on human disease is unknown.[53]

Response to vaccine

The best available measure of immunity after vaccine treatment is the level of neutralizing antibody,[54] which usually appears 7–14 days after starting a primary vaccine course. The amount of antibody needed for protection against rabies in man cannot be determined, but the World Health Organization (WHO) recommends that a minimum neutralizing antibody level of 0.5 IU/ml should be attained to demonstrate unequivocal seroconversion.[55]

The degree of protection from vaccine and the production of antibody in animals are genetically controlled although unlinked traits. In man there is an apparent genetic link with production of neutralizing antibody following rabies vaccine. A relatively delayed, lower level of response occurred in about 10% of vaccinees.[56] Increasing age (over 50 years) also impairs antibody production.[57]

The viral glycoprotein coat bears the antigens capable of stimulating the protective neutralizing antibody and T lymphocyte activation. In animals, injections of purified core ribonucleoprotein also induce protective immunity, in association with non-neutralizing antibody, helper T lymphocyte activity and interferon-γ induction.[58] This protection is effective against a variety of rabies and rabies-related strains,[59] unlike the more specific glycoprotein-mediated immunity. The role of helper T lymphocytes and the cytotoxic T cell response in protection against disease is not clear.

A small amount of interferon may be induced briefly following a first dose of rabies vaccine,[60] but it is very unlikely to afford significant protection in man.[54]

Clinical features

Incubation period

The interval between inoculation and the onset of symptoms is between 20 and 90 days in at least 60% of cases, but it has varied from 4 days to 19 years.[61,62] Short incubation periods have been reported from Thailand, where 42% of patients develop symptoms after 10–20 days.[63] In general, the nearer the bite is to the head, the shorter the incubation period,[64] but this correlation cannot be relied upon in individual cases.

Prodromal symptoms

Itching or paraesthesiae at the site of the healed bite wound are the only specific prodromal symptoms, occurring in about 40% of patients (Figure 45.5).[65] The wide range of non-specific features include fever, headache, myalgia, fatigue, sore throat, gastrointestinal symptoms, irritability, anxiety and insomnia. The disease progresses

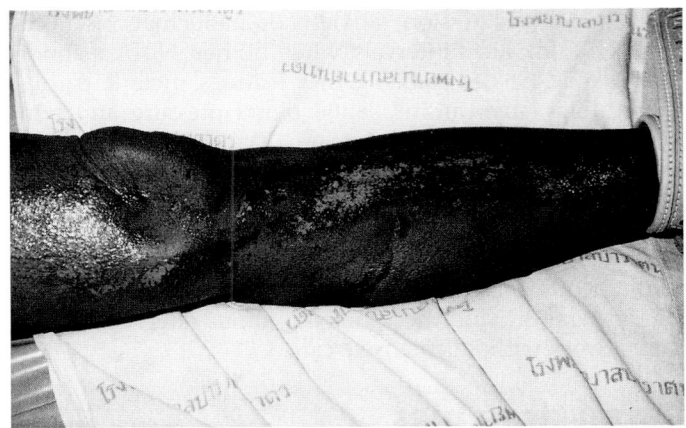

Figure 45.5: Intense itching of the bitten limb provoking scratching and excoriation, a common prodromal symptom of rabies encephalitis. (Copyright D. A. Warrell.)

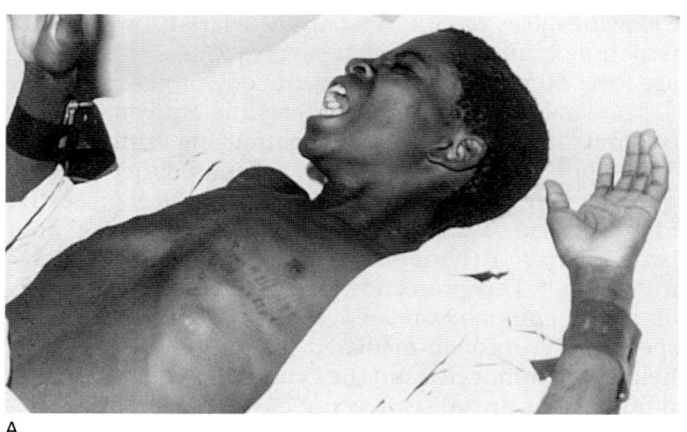
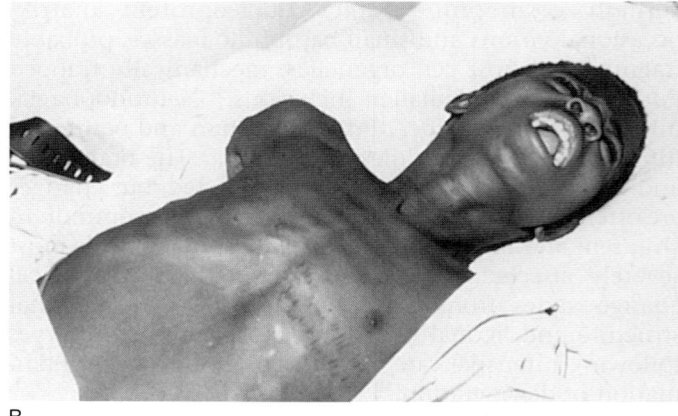

A   B

Figure 45.6: Progression of a hydrophobic spasm associated with terror in a Nigerian boy with furious rabies. (A) Note the powerful contraction of the diaphragm (depressing the xiphisternum) and sternocleidomastoid muscles. (B) The episode terminates in opisthotonos. (Copyright D. A. Warrell.)

to either furious or paralytic rabies encephalitis, usually within a week.[66]

Furious rabies

This well-known form is probably the more common. Malfunction of the brain stem, limbic system and higher centres results in the characteristic hydrophobic spasms. This is a reflex contraction of inspiratory muscles provoked by attempts to drink water, and later even the sound or mention of water, and also sometimes by draughts of air (aerophobia), touching the palate, bright lights or loud noises.

Intense thirst forces patients to try to drink. They may have a tight feeling in the throat, the arm trembles, and jerky spasms of the sternomastoids, diaphragm and other inspiratory muscles lead to a generalized extension, sometimes with convulsions and opisthotonos (Figure 45.6).[66] There is an associated inexplicable feeling of terror which occurs during the first episode, and is not a learned response.[67] Respiratory or cardiac arrest following a hydrophobic spasm is fatal in one-third of cases.

Excitation, aggression, anxiety or hallucinations occur between calm, lucid intervals, when no neurological abnormality may be detectable. Other features include cardiac arrhythmias, myocarditis, labile blood pressure and temperature, respiratory disturbances (e.g. cluster breathing), meningism, lesions of cranial nerves III, VII and IX, abnormal pupillary function, muscle fasciculation,[66] autonomic stimulation with lacrimation and salivation (Figure 45.7) and rarely increased libido, priapism and spontaneous orgasms.[68,69] Coma eventually ensues, with flaccid paralysis, and the agonizing illness rarely lasts more than a week without intensive care.

Paralytic rabies

Less common than furious rabies, paralytic or 'dumb' rabies may be missed unless there is a high level of

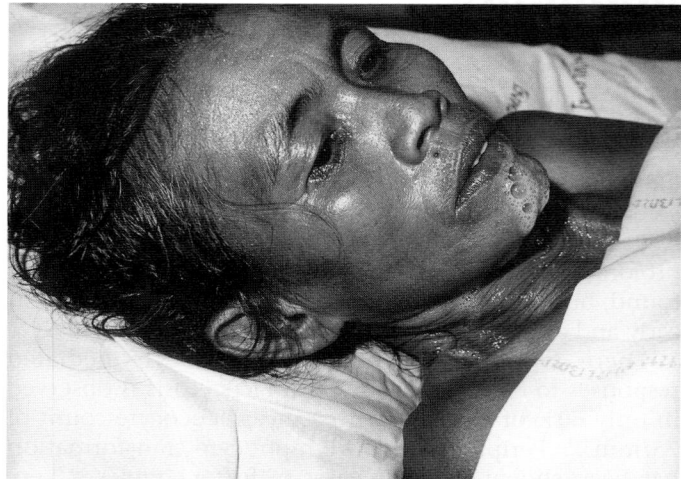

Figure 45.7: Hypersalivation and sweating in a Thai woman with furious rabies. (Copyright D. A. Warrell.)

suspicion. Paralytic disease is characteristic of vampire bat-transmitted rabies[70] and it is more common following infections by attenuated viruses,[33,34,71] and perhaps after postexposure vaccination.[48]

Prodromal symptoms are followed by paraesthesiae or hypotonic weakness, commonly starting near the site of the bite and spreading cranially. Fasciculation, myoedema or piloerection may be seen. The ascending paralysis results in constipation, urinary retention, respiratory failure and inability to swallow. Flaccid paralysis, especially of proximal muscles, is associated with loss of tendon and plantar reflexes, but sensation is often normal. Hydrophobic spasms may occur in the terminal phase and death ensues after 1–3 weeks.[66]

Management and complications

All rabies patients should be admitted to hospital and sedated heavily to relieve their agonizing symptoms. It remains a fatal infection, although rare recoveries have been reported (see below). Intensive care therapy can prolong life for 3–4 weeks, occasionally for months[34,72] and exceptionally for years[73,74] (see below).

During this time complications arise in every system. Cardiac arrhythmias are controlled by pacing, and respiratory failure requires ventilation. Full barrier nursing of the unconscious patient is needed, with specific treatment for likely complications such as convulsions, fluctuating blood pressure, pneumonia, pneumothorax, cerebral oedema, hyper- or hypopyrexia, inappropriate antidiuretic hormone secretion (diabetes insipidus) and haematemesis from stress ulceration.[66]

Treatment with hyperimmune serum and several antiviral agents, including intrathecal tribavirin (ribavirin) and interferon-α, have not been effective.[6,51,75]

Recovery from rabies

Two patients are claimed to have recovered completely from rabies encephalitis. They had been given post-exposure prophylaxis with nervous tissue vaccines and then intensive care.[76,77] Three further patients, given pre- or postexposure tissue culture vaccines, survived months or years with profound neurological impairment: a microbiologist who inhaled fixed rabies virus,[34] and two boys in Mexico.[73,74] All the diagnoses were based on high rabies neutralizing antibody levels in the serum and CSF. No virus or antigen was identified.

Differential diagnosis

Rabies should be suspected if inexplicable neurological, psychiatric or laryngopharyngeal symptoms occur in those who have been to an endemic area. The animal contact may have been forgotten. The differential diagnoses include the following:[66]

- *Tetanus*, another wound infection, has a short incubation period, usually less than 15 days. The muscle rigidity is constant, without relaxation between spasms. The CSF is always normal.
- *Intoxications* with drugs acting on the CNS, poisons and even delirium tremens could be confused with rabies.
- *Rabies phobia* is a hysterical response, usually very soon after a bite, with aggressive behaviour and an excellent prognosis.
- *Guillain–Barré syndrome* may present as paralytic rabies, and very rarely follows rabies tissue culture vaccine treatment.
- *Postvaccinal encephalitis* (see below), an allergic response to nervous tissue-containing rabies vaccine, can be clinically indistinguishable from paralytic rabies.
- *Other viral encephalitides*, including Japanese encephalitis, poliomyelitis and treatable herpes simiae B, from a monkey bite, should be considered.

Diagnosis
Intravitam diagnosis of human rabies encephalitis

The diagnosis of rabies can be confirmed by virus isolation, rapid identification of antigen or, in unvaccinated people, antibody detection.[78]

Isolation of rabies virus

Culture of the virus is most successful during the first week of illness—from saliva, throat, tracheal or eye swabs, brain biopsy samples, CSF and possibly urine.[47] The method of inoculation of suckling mice yields results in 1–3 weeks, but tissue culture isolation in murine neuroblastoma cells takes 1 or 2 days.[79,80]

Antigen detection[78,80]

Rapid rabies diagnosis by polymerase chain reaction (PCR) tests on saliva, CSF[81] and skin biopsy are available in a few reference laboratories. A direct immunofluorescent antibody (IFA) test also rapidly identifies antigen in frozen sections of skin biopsies taken from a hairy area, usually the nape of the neck (Figure 45.8). Rabies-specific immunofluorescence appears in nerve twiglets around the base of hair follicles (Figure 45.9).[82] Careful controls of specificity are needed, but this method is 60–100% sensitive.[49,83] False positives have not been reported.

The corneal smear test is too insensitive to be useful and false positives have occurred.[47,49,81]

Antibody detection

In unvaccinated patients, rabies seroconversion often occurs during the second week of illness and is diagnostic,[47] but

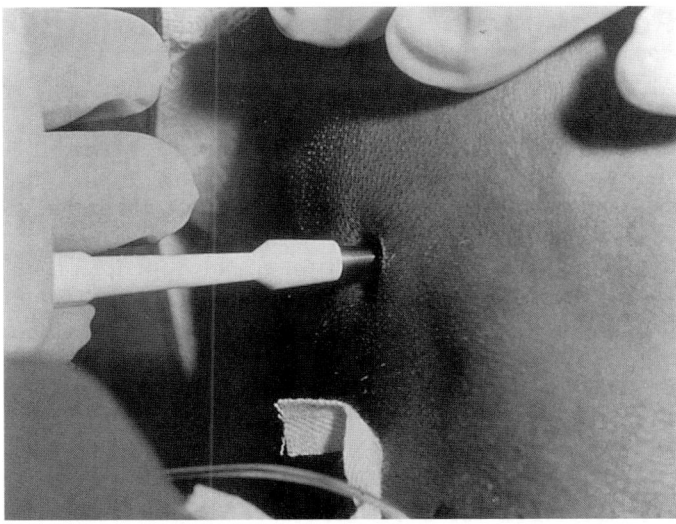

Figure 45.8: Punch biopsy of skin in the hairy nuchal region for rabies antigen detection in a patient with suspected rabies encephalitis. (Copyright D. A. Warrell.)

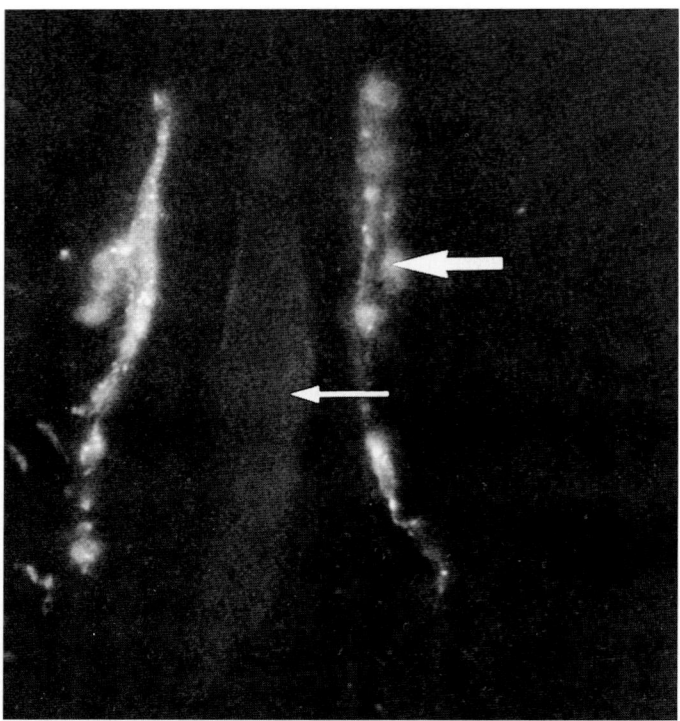

Figure 45.9: Diagnosis of rabies during life from a skin biopsy. Vertical section through a hair follicle. The small arrow shows the hair shaft. The bright fluorescence (large arrow) indicates rabies antigen in nerve cells around the follicle. (Copyright M. J. Warrell.)

absence of antibody up to 24 days after the onset of symptoms has been observed, possibly related to interferon therapy.[84]

In vaccinated people, very high levels of antibody in the serum, and especially in the CSF, are needed to suggest the diagnosis.[77]

Postmortem diagnosis in humans

Although virus isolation from secretions is usually unsuccessful after 2 weeks of illness, culture of brain tissue should be possible post mortem, even if the IFA staining is negative. Samples can be obtained without a full postmortem examination. Brain necropsies are taken with a Vim–Silverman or other long biopsy needle via the medial canthus of the eye, through the superior orbital fissure or an occipital approach through the foramen magnum.

Retrospective diagnosis using formalin-fixed brain specimens is possible by trypsin digestion and labelled antibody staining with immunofluorescent[85] or enzymatic[86] techniques.

Diagnosis in the biting mammal

If laboratory facilities are available, suspect rabid animals should be killed immediately and their brains tested for rabies infection.[87] Observation in captivity is potentially dangerous and uncertain.[62] Ideally, samples of hippocampus, brain stem and cerebellum should be tested, but brain specimens can be obtained from dogs without craniotomy via the occipital foramen.[88] IFA staining of acetone-fixed impression smears takes a few hours[80] and is the usual method of diagnosis. It is about 98% sensitive compared with viral culture by the mouse inoculation test. The IFA test is unreliable in detecting rabies-related viruses.[10] If fluorescence microscopy is not available, a rapid enzyme immunodiagnostic kit will test for antigen in brain tissue suspensions, but this is 3% less sensitive than the IFA test.[78,80]

No single test should be relied upon to make this important diagnosis. Virus isolation should be attempted on all IFA test-negative samples, by inoculation of suckling mice or tissue culture.

Strains of street rabies, or rabies-related viruses from different vector species or geographical areas, can be differentiated by genetic sequence analysis[89] or monoclonal antibody typing.[80]

Control of animal rabies

The optimum method of protecting man from rabies infection or economic loss due to rabies varies greatly in different endemic areas. The species of vector, its prevalence and interaction with man dictate whether elimination or vaccination of animals is appropriate and economically feasible.

Urban rabies

The control of endemic rabies in urban areas, where dogs are the dominant vectors, requires: epidemiological surveillance; laboratory diagnostic facilities; education to avoid unnecessary contact with animals, especially stray dogs; and vaccination of dogs, cats and humans.

The size of a population of stray dogs depends on available food and shelter. Attempts at control by killing dogs result in an increased reproduction rate and rapid restoration of numbers. There has been an impressive reduction in the number of local human cases following vector control campaigns, including dog vaccination and population control. Mass vaccination campaigns, aimed at immunizing 80% of dogs, have eliminated canine rabies in Japan and Taiwan, and from densely populated urban areas of Argentina, Brazil and Peru.[90] Despite localized successes, there has been no evidence of a significant change in the overall incidence of animal rabies in most tropical endemic areas of Africa and Asia for decades.

Efficient postexposure vaccine treatment of dog-bite victims should be ensured. This includes a rapid diagnostic service and adequate supplies of vaccine and immune serum.

Sylvatic (wildlife) rabies

For some vector species active control is not attempted, owing to the low rate of transmission to other species and lack of effective methods. Insectivorous bats in North America and Europe are examples and simple measures are used to prevent contact with man. In contrast, where infection of domestic animals and humans is likely, as with fox rabies in Europe, campaigns for population control and vaccination have been mounted.

Trapping, gassing, poisoning and hunting are generally inefficient means of population reduction. Oral fox vaccine campaigns have been used to great effect. Live attenuated rabies virus vaccine or a live vaccinia recombinant vaccine expressing rabies glycoprotein[91] disguised in baits has been distributed by aircraft over areas of Canada and many European countries including Germany, Belgium, Switzerland, Austria, France, Italy and Hungary. As a result, Switzerland and large parts of other countries are now free of rabies. The recombinant vaccine is also effective in the control of rabies in racoons, coyotes and skunks in North America.[91]

In Latin America vampire bat rabies[14] is a major cause of death in cattle, with disastrous economic consequences. Specific control methods include vaccination or treatment with anticoagulants, diphenadione or warfarin, to which bats, but not cattle, are highly sensitive.

Postexposure prophylaxis

This treatment is aimed at killing or neutralizing rabies virus in a wound before any virions enter a nerve ending. Once within the nervous system, the immune response is thought to be incapable of preventing disease. Postexposure treatment is needed after possible contact with rabies virus through an open wound or mucous membrane (Figure 45.10). Intact skin is a barrier against infection.

Assessing the risk of rabies infection

Knowledge of the local epidemiology of rabies vectors,

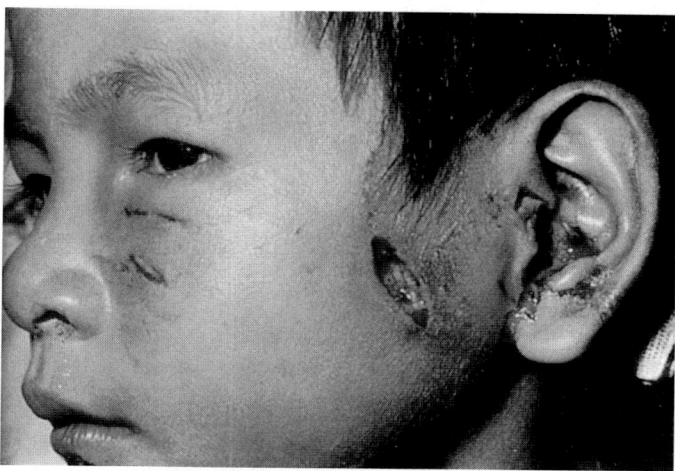

Figure 45.10: Facial bites inflicted by a rabid dog in Thailand. (Copyright D. A. Warrell.)

the circumstances of the animal bite or contact, and the health and behaviour of the animal all contribute to assessment of the risk of exposure to rabies. An unprovoked attack by an unvaccinated sick animal indicates a high risk, but so does contact with a paralysed or unusually tame wild mammal. Vaccinated animals have also transmitted rabies. In endemic areas, strenuous efforts should be made to have the biting animal put down and its brain examined for rabies.[87] If the animal has escaped or there is any doubt, postexposure prophylaxis should be given, irrespective of the length of time since the bite. The official WHO recommendations are summarized in Table 45.2.

Postexposure treatment has three components: wound treatment, active immunization and passive immunization with rabies immune globulin.

Wound treatment

Immediate cleaning of the wound or site of contact with a rabid animal is imperative (Figure 45.11) by thorough scrubbing with concentrated soap solution or detergent. If possible, swab with a virucidal agent: iodine solutions or 40–70% alcohol.[92] Quaternary ammonium compounds

Table 45.2 Specific postexposure prophylaxis for use in a rabies endemic area (following contact with a domestic or wild rabies vector species, whether or not the animal is available for observation or diagnostic tests)*

Exposure	Treatment
Minor (including licks of broken skin, scratches or abrasions without bleeding)	• Start vaccine administration immediately • Stop treatment if animal remains healthy for 10 days • Stop treatment if animal's brain proves negative for rabies by appropriate laboratory tests
Major (including licks of mucosa, minor bites or major bites—multiple or on face, head, fingers or neck)	• Immediate rabies immune globulin and vaccine • Stop treatment if domestic cat or dog remains healthy for 10 days • Stop treatment if animal's brain proves negative for rabies by appropriate laboratory tests

*This scheme is a simplification of the WHO recommendations (1997).[87]

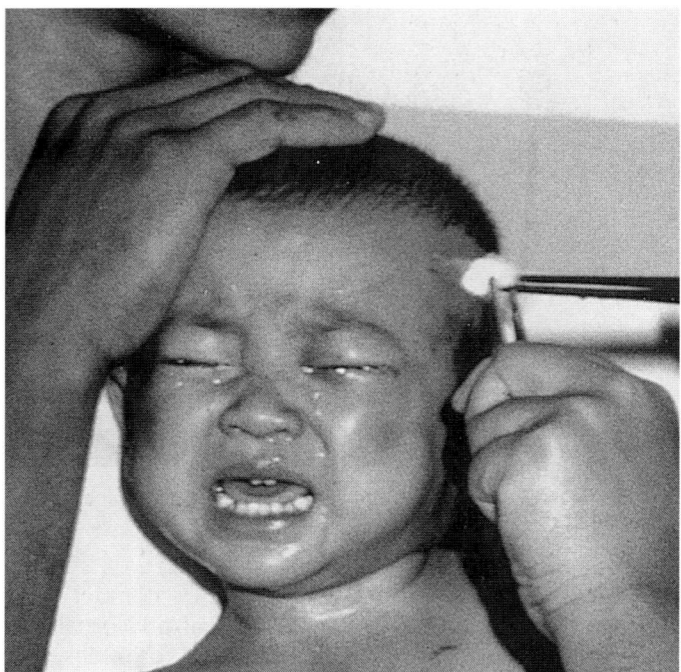

Figure 45.11: Thorough wound cleaning following an attack by a rabid dog (as in this Thai boy) is an essential part of postexposure prophylaxis. (Copyright D. A. Warrell.)

are neutralized by soap and are not generally recommended.[93] Energetic wound cleaning may require local or even general anaesthesia. Suturing should be delayed or avoided to prevent inoculation of virus deeper into the tissues.[87]

Tetanus prophylaxis may be required, and other bacterial infections associated with mammal bites may be treated with antibiotics; for example, *Pasteurella multocida* is usually sensitive to ampicillin, tetracycline and co-trimoxazole.

Active immunization: postexposure vaccine treatment

All human rabies vaccines currently produced contain inactivated whole virus which has been grown on a variety of substrates.

Modern rabies vaccines

Tissue culture vaccine was introduced about 25 years ago in Europe and North America, and since then it has been replaced in other countries including China, Japan,

Russia, Sri Lanka and Thailand.

The original human diploid cell vaccine (HDCV) is produced in slow-growing fibroblast monolayer cultures. It is too expensive for widespread use so several other cell lines are now employed to manufacture cheaper products. Two widely exported vaccines are a German purified chick embryo cell vaccine (PCEC) and a French purified vero cell vaccine (PVRV). Tissue culture vaccines are also made, mainly for local use, in China, Japan, the Russian Federation and the USA.[94,95]

These three well-tested vaccines are currently recommended by the WHO (Table 45.3).

Tissue culture vaccine regimens[87,96,97]

The WHO recommends that PCEC, PVRV, HDCV and PDEV are used with the following three postexposure regimens:

The standard *intramuscular (i.m.) regimen* is a 1.0 ml dose (or for PVRV the dose is 0.5 ml) i.m. into the deltoid (or anterolateral thigh in children, but never the buttock) on days 0, 3, 7, 14 and 28.[97] This is too expensive for worldwide use,[63] so economical intradermal (i.d.) schemes have been devised. Two multisite i.d. regimens have been approved by the WHO: an eight-site regimen and a two-site regimen.

The *eight-site intradermal postexposure regimen* has been tested in patients bitten by proven rabid animals, and only those with severe bites (see below) also received immune globulin, as is common in tropical areas. This method for use with PCEC,[98] and HDCV (whose i.m. dose is 1 ml) has a wide margin of safety, and consists of:[99]

Day 0:	0.1 ml injected i.d. at eight sites (right and left deltoid, suprascapular, thigh and lower lateral abdominal areas) using up the whole 1.0 ml ampoule.
Day 7:	0.1 ml i.d. at four sites (deltoids and thighs).
Days 28 and 91:	0.1 ml i.d. at one site (deltoid).

The distribution of sites is designed to stimulate many different groups of lymph nodes. Neutralizing antibody induction is fast: 88% are positive by day 7, and antibody is detectable a year later, whether or not immune globulin was also given.[99] Less than two ampoules of vaccine are needed—a 60% reduction of the i.m. regimen. Only four visits to the clinic are required, which reduces the cost of travel and time off work for patients. Sharing of ampoules of vaccine needs great care. Opened ampoules must be kept in the refrigerator and used within 24 hours. A *separate syringe and needle* must be used for every patient to prevent viral cross-infection.[100]

Table 45.3 WHO recommended rabies vaccines for humans

Vaccine	Abbreviation	Virus	Origin	Licensed
Human diploid cell vaccine	HDCV	PM1503	France	1974
Purified vero cell rabies vaccine	PVRV	PM1503	France	1984
Purified chick embryo cell	PCEC	LEP	Germany	1984
Purified duck embryo vaccine	PDEV	PM	Switzerland	1985

The *two-site intradermal postexposure regimen* has been tested post exposure, with immune globulin in every case.[101] It was designed for use with PVRV (0.5 ml/ampoule) with an i.d. dose of 0.1 ml per i.d. site. If the other, 1.0 ml, vaccines are used each i.d. dose must be 0.2 ml:

Days 0, 3 and 7:   0.1 ml i.d. at two sites (deltoids).
Days 28 and 91:   0.1 ml i.d. at one site (deltoid).

The two i.d. regimens use the same amount of vaccine, and the above precautions are needed when sharing ampoules of vaccine. Comparative studies of these i.d. regimens show that the eight-site method induces neutralizing antibody more rapidly and to higher levels than the two-site regimen.[102] Therefore the eight-site method is preferable, but it has not been used with PVRV, when the dose would be 0.05 ml per site. If an economical regimen is required with PVRV and no immune globulin is available, the two-site method can be used with a double dose (0.1 ml in four sites using the whole ampoule) on the first day of treatment.

The manufacturer's instructions should be followed for all other vaccines.

Postexposure treatment for those who have had previous vaccination

Wound care and booster doses of vaccine are still vital and urgent. Provided that a full pre- or postexposure course of one of the four recommended vaccines (Table 45.3) has been given, or if at least 0.5 IU/ml of rabies neutralizing antibody has been documented following any other treatment, a short course of two doses of vaccine given i.m. on days 0 and 3 is recommended.[87] Passive immunization is not required. Otherwise a full course of vaccine and rabies immune globulin are needed.

Nervous tissue vaccines

These are inactivated homogenates of infected animal brains and they are still produced in many countries in Asia, Africa and South America. Sheep brain Semple vaccine was first produced in 1911 and is still widely used in Pakistan and India.[20] Fourteen or 21 daily injections are given subcutaneously over the anterior abdominal wall, a large area able to accommodate the 2 to 5 ml doses of vaccine. The potency of Semple vaccine is variable, and 7% of 707 Thai patients with rabies had had a full course of vaccine.[63] Fuenzalida's suckling mouse brain vaccine is used in South America and parts of Asia and Africa. Although post-vaccinal encephalitis is a serious complication (see below), postexposure treatment is urgent, so if it is the only vaccine available, treatment can be started and changed to tissue culture vaccine at any time.

Side effects of tissue culture vaccines

Minor local reactions occur in 2–74% of vaccinees, and include pain, erythema, swelling, aching and paraesthesia. Multiple-site i.d. injections cause local itching in 7–64% in different studies. Mild systemic reactions, reported by 3–40% of vaccinees, consist of influenza-like symptoms, headache, fever, malaise, myalgia, nausea, dizziness or a rash.[87]

Booster doses of HDCV, usually about a year after previous treatment, have caused systemic allergic reactions in 6% of American vaccinees. After 3–13 days, urticaria, rash, angio-oedema and arthralgia appear, but always respond promptly to symptomatic treatment.[103] This is possibly an IgE-mediated response to non-viral vaccine constituents—for example, human serum albumin rendered immunogenic by reaction with β-propiolactone, a virus inactivator.[104] Highly purified vaccines may not have this complication.

Extremely rare neurological illness following HDCV[97] is either Guillain–Barré-like (in four patients) or local limb weakness (in two patients).[105] These syndromes are no more frequent after rabies than after other commonly used viral vaccines. Recovery is usually rapid, and none has been fatal.

Rabies vaccines have been used widely in pregnancy without problems.

Postvaccinal encephalomyelitis following nervous tissue vaccines

This is an inflammatory, demyelinating, autoimmune response due to sensitization by myelin and other neural antigens contained in the vaccine.[106] Estimates of its incidence vary with different products, but the frequency is up to 1:220 recipients of Semple vaccine, with a mortality rate of 3%.[107] Symptoms usually appear within 2 weeks of starting the course, but may not appear until 2 months later.[6] Suckling mouse brain vaccines have a lower complication rate (1:8000[108] to 1:27 000[109]) but peripheral nervous system signs, such as Guillain–Barré-like syndrome, frequently predominate and are fatal in 22% of cases.[108]

A wide variety of neurological signs include polyneuritis often involving limbs, transverse myelitis, ascending paralysis and meningoencephalitis.[110,111] Corticosteroid therapy (e.g. prednisolone 40–60 mg/day) is conventional, and cyclophosphamide in addition has been suggested.[110] Recovery often occurs within 2 weeks[111] and is usually complete, but residual neurological deficits can ensue.

Postvaccinial encephalitis can be clinically identical to paralytic rabies, and the diagnosis must be made by exclusion. The skin biopsy technique of rabies antigen detection has proved a useful rapid method.[49] No further nervous tissue vaccine must be given, but the course completed with a tissue culture vaccine.

Passive immunization

Rabies immune globulin (RIG) provides passive protection during the first 7–10 days of a primary postexposure course of vaccine, when no neutralizing antibody is detectable. This not only neutralizes virus in the wound, but also may enhance the presentation of vaccine antigens to T lymphocytes.[112]

The efficacy of RIG treatment combined with rabies vaccine has been proved by many animal studies and natural experiments when wolves have bitten large numbers of people in Iran[113] and China.[114] The mortality from head wounds was reduced fivefold by the addition of immune serum to vaccine treatment.[115]

A dose of 40 IU/kg of equine RIG or 20 IU/kg of human RIG should ideally accompany every primary post-exposure vaccine course, but it is essential following severe bites: that is, on the head, neck or fingers and multiple or deep bites.[87] RIG is infiltrated around the wound if anatomically possible, and any remaining injected i.m. at a site remote from the vaccine. RIG given days or even hours before the vaccine is started impairs the immune response.[116] The dose must not be exceeded because RIG may reduce the immunogenicity of the vaccine.

RIG is prohibitively expensive for Third World use. Human RIG costs at least US $300, and equine RIG US $30 per person.[63] They are unavailable in large areas of Asia and Africa, including some whole countries.

The incidence of serum sickness following equine RIG varies between 1% and 6%, depending on which product is used.[117] An intradermal skin test does not predict most reactions[118] and RIG should be given despite a positive result. The test should be abandoned. Adrenaline should always be at hand in case of anaphylaxis. Human RIG has not been associated with serum sickness.

Efficacy of postexposure prophylaxis

The untreated mortality from rabid animal bites depends on the part of the body affected and the severity of the bite. Data from the prevaccine era give an estimate of the chance of infection from suspect rabid dogs. The mortality from multiple bites on the head was 60–80%, from a single facial bite 30%, and from bites on the hand 15–67%.[119,120] In India the overall mortality from proven rabid dog bites was 35–57%.[121,122] Regrettably, no information on wound treatment is given in these studies.

If wound treatment, tissue culture vaccine and RIG, are given on the day of the bite in the correct manner, prophylaxis is virtually 100% effective. Nevertheless, patients are known to have died of rabies after receiving these vaccines.[123] This mortality has been attributed to human or circumstantial failure to deliver optimum treatment, and not to reduced antigen content or other failure of the vaccine.

Possible reasons for failure of postexposure prophylaxis are as follows:

1. Any delay in starting vaccine increases the chance of rabies virus entering neurones before the immune response is generated. The mortality following head wounds from Iranian rabid wolves doubled if vaccine was delayed beyond 8 days.[115] Treatment is urgent, and it is never too late to begin. Vaccine and RIG should both be used even if the bite occurred months before.

2. Failure to give rabies immune globulin or to infiltrate the wound, especially with severe exposure.
3. Injecting vaccine into the buttock instead of the deltoid, which can impair antibody production.[124]
4. Inability of the patient to mount an immune response due to chronic disease (e.g. HIV infection, cirrhosis) or immunosuppressive drugs (e.g. steroids).[123]

Street rabies virus strains show a high degree of homology with the strains used in vaccine production, but there is great antigenic diversity among the rabies-related viruses. Protection against Australian bat lyssavirus is effective,[19] but the protection afforded against infection by European bat lyssaviruses and Duvenhage virus is less efficient than that against street rabies virus strains,[18] and there is little if any protection against Mokola virus.

If a reduced or delayed immune response to treatment is predicted for any of these reasons, an attempt can be made to increase the immune stimulus, either by doubling the initial dose of vaccine (one intramuscular dose in each deltoid) or by dividing the first dose between eight sites intradermally, as for the eight-site i.d. postexposure regimen (see above).

Pre-exposure prophylaxis

No deaths from rabies have been reported in anyone who has had pre-exposure treatment and booster injections after exposure. Pre-exposure prophylaxis is advisable for anyone likely to be in contact with a rabid animal. This may include veterinarians, animal handlers, laboratory staff, zoologists, wildlife enthusiasts, health workers, travellers and residents in endemic areas where dogs are the dominant vector species.

A pre-exposure vaccine course is three doses of one of the recommended vaccines (Table 45.3), given intramuscularly on days 0, 3 and 28 (or 21). An economical alternative is i.d. injections of 0.1 ml at the same intervals.[87,97] A separate syringe must be used for each patient. Chloroquine taken as malaria prophylaxis can suppress the antibody response to i.d. primary pre-exposure treatment,[124] so the vaccine must be given i.m. to those taking the drug.

A booster dose 1 to 2 years after the primary course increases the persistence of antibody to 10 years in 96% of people in a study of i.m. treatment.[125] Although the titre of antibody falls more rapidly after i.d. than i.m. inoculation, the response to a booster dose is dramatic whatever the original route. Confirmation of seroconversion is unnecessary unless immunosuppression is suspected.[97]

Booster doses may be given intradermally or intramuscularly at intervals depending on the risk of infection.[126] Laboratory staff handling rabies virus should either check that their neutralizing antibody level is at least 0.5 IU/ml, or have a booster injection every 6 months,[87,97] but others may require booster doses after 2–10 years according to their risk of exposure. Repeated booster injections should only be given when necessary because of the risk of hypersensitivity reactions.[103]

REFERENCES

1 Théordoidès J. *Histoire de la Rage, Cave Canem*. Paris: Masson, 1986.

2 Wilkinson L. The development of the virus concept as reflected in corpora of studies on individual pathogens. 4. Rabies: two millennia of ideas and conjecture on the aetiology of a virus disease. *Med Hist* 1977; 21:15–31.

3 Matsumoto S. Rabies virus. *Adv Virus Res* 1970; 16: 257–301.

4 Bourhy H, Kissi B & Tordo N. Molecular diversity of the *Lyssavirus* genus. *Virology* 1993; 194:70–81.

5 Gould AR, Hyatt AD, Lunt R et al. Characterization of a novel Lyssavirus isolated frim Pteropid bats in Australia. *Virus Res* 1998; 54:165–187.

6 Warrell M J & Warrell D A. Rhabdovirus infections of man. In Porterfield J S & Tyrrell D A J (eds) *Handbook of Infectious Diseases*, vol. 3. Exotic viral infections. London: Chapman & Hall, 1995: 343–383.

7 Gosztonyi G. Reproduction of Lyssaviruses: ultrastructure composition of lyssavirus and functional aspects of pathogenisis. In Rupprecht C E, Dietzschold B & Koprowski H (eds) *Lyssaviruses*. Berlin: Springer, 1994: 43–68.

8 Michalski F, Parks N F, Soko F & Clark H. F. Thermal inactivation of rabies and other rhabdoviruses: stabilization by the chelating agent EDTA at physiological temperatures. *Infect Immun* 1976; 14:135–143.

9 Blancou J. Epizootiology of rabies: Eurasia and Africa.. In Campbell J B & Charlton K M (eds) *Rabies*. Boston: Kluwer, 1988: 243–265.

10 Swanepoel R, Barnard B J H, Meredith C D et al. Rabies in southern Africa. *Onderstepoort J Vet Res* 1993; 60:325–346.

11 Bingham J, Foggin C M, Wandeler A I & Hill F W G. The epidemiology of rabies in Zimbabwe. 1. Rabies in dogs (*Canis familiaris*). *Onderstepoort J Vet Res* 1999; 66:1–10.

12 Smith J S. Molecular epidemiology of rabies in the United States. *Sem Virol* 1995; 6:387–400.

13 Dreesen D W, Orciari L A & Rupprecht C E. The epidemiology of bat rabies in the United States: with emphasis on *Lasionycteris noctivagans*, the silver-haired bat. *Soc Vet Epidemiol Prevent Med Proc* 1998; 48–54.

14 McColl K A, Tordo N & Aguilar Setién A. Bat lyssavirus infections. *Rev Sci Tech Off Int Epiz* 2000; 19:177–196.

15 Everard C O R & Everard J D. Mongoose rabies. *Rev Inf Dis* 1988; 10:S610–S614.

16 Bourhy H, Kissi B, Audry L et al. Ecology and evolution of rabies virus in Europe. *J Gen Virol* 1999; 80:2545–2557.

17 Cherkasskiy B L. Roles of the wolf and the raccoon dog in the ecology and epidemiology of rabies in the USSR. *Rev Infect Dis* 1988; 10:S634–S636.

18 Amengual B, Whitby J E, King A, Cobo J S & Bourhy H. Evolution of European bat lyssaviruses. *J Gen Virol* 1997; 78:2319–2328.

19 Hooper P T, Lunt R A & Gould A R. A new lyssaviris: the first endemic rabies-related virus recognized in Australia. *Bull Inst Pasteur* 1997; 95:209–218.

20 World Health Organization. World Survey of Rabies No 34 for year 1998. WHO/CDS/CSR/APH/99.6. World Health Organization, 2000.

21 Centers for Disease Control. Human rabies: California, Georgia, Minnesota, New York, and Wisconsin, 2000. *MMWR* 2000; 49:1111–1115.

22 Familusi J B & Moore D L. Isolation of a rabies related virus from the CSF of a child with 'aseptic meningitis'. *Afr J Med Sci* 1972; 3:93–96.

23 Familusi J B, Osunkoya B O, Moore D L et al. A fatal human infection with Mokola virus. *Am J Trop Med Hyg* 1972; 21:959–963.

24 Crick J. Rabies. In Gibbs E P J (ed.) *Virus Diseases of Food Animals*, vol. II. London: Academic Press, 1981: 469–516.

25 Meredith C D, Rossouw A P & van Praag Koch H. An unusual case of human rabies thought to be of chiropteran origin. *S Afr Med J* 1971; 45:767–769.

26 Selimov M A, Tatarov A G, Botvinkin A D et al. Rabies related Yulivirus: identification with a panel of monoclonal antibodies. *Acta Virol (Praha)* 1989; 33:542–546.

27 King A & Crick J. Rabies-related viruses. In Campbell J B & Charlton K M (eds) *Rabies*. Boston: Kluwer, 1988: 177–199.

28 Lumio J, Hillbom M, Roine R et al. Human rabies of bat origin in Europe. *Lancet* 1986; i:378.

29 Helmick C G, Tauxe R V & Vernon A A. Is there a risk to contacts of patients with rabies? *Rev Infect Dis* 1987; 9:511–518.

30 Sureau P, Portnoi D, Rollin P et al. Prévention de la transmission inter-humaine de la rage après greffe de cornée. *C R Acad Sci* 1981; 293:689–692.

31 Sipahioglu U & Alpaut S. Transplacental rabies in humans. *Mikrobiyol Bül* 1985; 19:95–99.

32 Winkler W G. Airborne rabies. In Baer G M (ed.) *The Natural History of Rabies*, vol. II. New York: Academic Press, 1975: 115–121.

33 Winkler W G, Fashinell T R, Leffingwell L et al. Airborne rabies transmission in a laboratory worker. *JAMA* 1973; 226:1219–1221.

34 Centers for Disease Control. Rabies in a laboratory worker: New York. *MMWR* 1977; 26:183–184.

35 Tsiang H. Pathophysiology of rabies virus infection of the nervous system. *Adv Virus Res* 1993; 42:375–412.

36 Charlton K M. The pathogenisis of rabies and other lyssaviral infections: recent studies. In Rupprecht C E, Dietzschold B & Koprowski H (eds) *Lyssaviruses*. Berlin: Springer, 1994: 95–119.

37 Lewis P, Fu Y & Lentz T L. Rabies virus entry at the neuromuscular junction in nerve–muscle cocultures. *Muscle Nerve* 2000; 23:720–730.

38 Lentz T L. Rabies virus binding to an acetylcholine receptor alpha-subunit peptide. *J Mol Recognit* 1990; 3:82–88.

39 Dueñas A, Belsey M A, Escobar J et al. Isolation of rabies virus outside the human central nervous system. *J Infect Dis* 1973; 127:702–704.

40 Tangchai P, Yenbutr D & Vejjajiva A. Central nervous system lesions in human rabies: a study of twenty-four cases. *J Med Assoc Thai* 1970; 53:471–486.

41 Dupont J R & Earle K M. Human rabies encephalitis: a study of forty-nine fatal cases with a review of the literature. *Neurology* 1966; 15:1023–1034.

42 Perl D P. The pathology of rabies in the central nervous system. In Baer G M (ed.) *The Natural History of Rabies*, vol. I. New York: Academic Press, 1975: 235–272.

43 Maton P N, Pollard J D & Newsom-Davies J. Human rabies encephalomyelitis. *BMJ* 1976; i:1038–1040.

44 Iwasaki Y, Liu D-S, Yamamoto T & Konno H. On the replication and spread of rabies virus in the human central nervous system. *J Neuropathol Exp Neurol* 1985; 44:185–195.

45 Sandhyamani S, Roy S, Gode G R & Kalla G N. Pathology of rabies: a light and electronmicroscopical study with particular reference to the changes in cases with prolonged survival. *Acta Neuropathol (Berl)* 1981; 54:247–251.

46 Metze K & Feiden W. Rabies ribonucleoprotein in the heart. *N Engl J Med* 1991; 324:1814–1815.

47 Anderson L J, Nicholson K G, Tauxe R V & Winkler W G. Human rabies in the United States, 1960 to 1979: epidemiology, diagnosis and prevention. *Ann Intern Med* 1984; 100:728–735.

48 Hattwick M A W. Human rabies. *Public Health Rev* 1974; 3:229–274.

49 Warrell M J, Looareesuwan S, Manatsathit S et al. Rapid diagnosis of rabies and post-vaccinal encephalitides. *Clin Exp Immunol* 1988; 71:229–234.

50 Hemachudha T, Phanuphak P, Sriwanthana B et al. Immunologic study of human encephalitic and paralytic rabies: preliminary report of 16 patients. *Am J Med* 1988; 84:673–677.

51 Merigan T C, Baer G M, Winkler W G et al. Human leucocyte interferon administration to patients with symptomatic and suspected rabies. *Ann Neurol* 1984; 16:82–87.

52 Dietschold B, Kao M, Zheng Y M et al. Delineation of putative mechanisms involved in antibody-mediated clearance of rabies virus from the central nervous system. *Proc Natl Acad Sci USA* 1992; 89:7252–7256.

53 Lafon M, Thoulouze M-I, Astoul E & Lafage M. Rabies virus and immunopotentiation. In Cunningham M W & Fujinami R S (eds) *Effects of Microbes on the Immune System.* Philadelphia: Lippincott, Williams & Wilkins, 2000: 631–642.

54 Turner G S. Immune response after rabies vaccination: basic aspects. *Ann Inst Pasteur Virol* 1985; 126E:453–460.

55 World Health Organization, Working Group II. Vaccine potency requirements for reduced immunization schedules and pre-exposure treatment. *Dev Biol Stand* 1978; 40:268–270.

56 Kuwert E K, Barsenbach C, Werner J et al. Early/high and late/low responders among HDCS vaccinees? In Kuwert E K, Wiktor T J & Koprowski H (eds) *Cell Culture Rabies Vaccines and their Protective Effect in Man.* Geneva: International Green Cross, 1981: 160–167.

57 Anderson L J, Winkler W G, Smith J S et al. Post-exposure rabies prophylaxis with 5 doses of a tri-*N*-butyl phosphate inactivated human diploid cell vaccine. In Kuwert E K, Wiktor T J & Koprowski H (eds) *Cell Culture Rabies Vaccines and their Protective Effect in Man.* Geneva: International Green Cross, 1981: 300–306.

58 Dietzschold B & Ertl H C J. New developments in the pre- and post-exposure treatment of rabies. *Immunology* 1991; 10:427–439.

59 Celis E, Ou D, Dietzschold B & Koprowski H. Recognition of rabies and rabies-related viruses by T-cells derived from human vaccine recipients. *J Virol* 1988; 62:3128–3134.

60 Nicholson K G, Kuwert E K, Werner J & Harrison P. Interferon response to human diploid cell strain rabies vaccines in man. *Arch Virol* 1979; 61:35–39.

61 Smith J S, Fishbein D B, Rupprecht C E & Clark K. Unexplained rabies in three immigrants in the United States: a virological investigation. *N Engl J Med* 1991; 324: 205–211.

62 Editorial. Human rabies: strain identification reveals lengthy incubation. *Lancet* 1991; 337:822–823.

63 Wilde H, Chutivongse S, Tepsumethanon W et al. Rabies in Thailand: 1990. *Rev Infect Dis* 1991; 13:644–652.

64 Wang S P. Statistical studies of human rabies in Taiwan. *J Formosan Med Assoc* 1956; 55:548–555.

65 Vibulbandhitkij S. Data of rabies patients from Bhamrasnaradura Hospital between 1971–1977. In Tongcharoen P (ed.) *Rabies* Bangkok: Aksornsamai Press, 1980.

66 Warrell D A. The clinical picture of rabies in man. *Trans R Soc Trop Med Hyg* 1976; 70:188–195.

67 Warrell D A, Davidson N Mc D, Pope H M et al. Pathophysiologic studies in human rabies. *Am J Med* 1976; 60:180–190.

68 Talaulicar P M. Persistent priapism in rabies. *Br J Urol* 1977; 49:462.

69 Udwadia Z F, Udwadia F E, Rao P P & Kapadia F. Penile hyperexcitability with recurrent ejaculations as the presenting manifestation of a case of rabies. *Postgrad Med J* 1988; 64:85–86.

70 Hurst E W & Pawan J L. An outbreak of rabies in Trinidad, without history of bites, and with the symptoms of acute ascending myelitis. *Lancet* 1931; ii:622–628.

71 Pará M. An outbreak of post-vaccinal rabies (rage de laboratoire) in Fortaleza, Brazil in 1960: resistant fixed virus as the etiological agent. *Bull World Health Organ* 1965; 33:172–182.

72 Emmons R W, Leonard L L, De Genaro F et al. A case of human rabies with prolonged survival. *Intervirology* 1973; 1:60–72.

73 Alvarez L, Fajardo R, Lopez E et al. Partial recovery from rabies in a nine-year-old boy. *Pediatr Inf Dis J* 1994; 13:1154–1155.

74 Alvarez L, Lomeli H M M B, Baer G M et al. Human rabies: partial recovery in two Mexican children. *Abstr 7th Int Cong Inf Dis*, Hong Kong, 1996; No. 59.002.

75 Warrell M J, White N J, Looareesuwan S et al. Failure of interferon alfa and tribavirin in rabies encephalitis. *BMJ* 1989; 299:830–833.

76 Porras C, Barboza J J, Fuenzalida E et al. Recovery from rabies in man. *Ann Intern Med* 1976; 85:44–48.

77 Hattwick M A W, Weis T T, Stechschulte C J, Baer G M & Gregg M B. Recovery from rabies: a case report. *Ann Intern Med* 1972; 76:931–942.

78 Bourhy H. Lyssaviruses: special emphasis on rabies virus. In Stephenson J R & Warnes A (eds) *Methods in Molecular Medicine, vol. 12: Diagnostic Virology Protocols.* Totowa, NJ: Humana, 1998: 129–142.

79 Rudd R J & Trimarchi C V. Development and evaluation of an in vitro virus isolation procedure as a replacement for the mouse inoculation test in rabies diagnosis. *J Clin Microbiol* 1989; 27:2522–2528.

80 Bourhy H & Sureau P. *Laboratory Methods for Rabies Diagnosis.* Paris: Institut Pasteur, 1990.

81 Crepin P, Audry L, Rotivel Y et al. Intravitam diagnosis of human rabies by PCR using saliva and cerebrospinal fluid. *J Clin Microbiol* 1998; 36:1117–121.

82 Bryceson A D M, Greenwood B M, Warrell D A et al. Demonstration during life of rabies antigen in humans. *J Infect Dis* 1975; 131:71–74.

83 Blenden D C, Creech W & Torres-Anjel M J. Use of immunofluorescence examination to detect rabies virus antigen in the skin of humans with clinical encephalitis. *J Infect Dis* 1986; 154:698–701.

84 Centers for Disease Control. Human rabies acquired outside the United States from a dog bite. *MMWR* 1981; 30:537–540.

85 Swoveland P T & Johnson K P. Identification of rabies antigens in human and animal tissues. *Ann NY Acad Sci* 1983; 420:185–191.

86 Fekadu M, Greer P W, Chandler F W & Sanderlin D W. Use of the avidin–biotin peroxidase system to detect rabies antigen in formalin-fixed paraffin-embedded tissues. *J Virol Methods* 1988; 19:91–96.

87 World Health Organization. WHO recommendations on rabies post-exposure treatment and the correct technique of intradermal immunization against rabies. 1997: WHO/EMC/ZOO.96.6

88 Hirose J A, Bourhy H & Sureau P. Retro-orbital route for brain specimen collection for rabies diagnosis. *Vet Rec* 1991; 129:291–292.

89 Smith J S, Orciari L A, Yager P A, Seidel H D & Warner C K. Epidemiologic and historical relationships among 87 rabies virus isolates as determined by limited sequence analysis. *J Infect Dis* 1992; 166:296–307.

90 Larghi O P, Arrosi J C, Nakajata-a J & Villa-Nova A. Control of urban rabies. In Campbell J B & Charlton K M (eds) *Rabies.* Boston: Kluwer, 1988: 407–422.

91 Brochier B, Aubert MFA, Pastoret P-P et al. Field use of a vaccinia–rabies recombinant vaccine for the control of sylvatic rabies in Europe and North America. *Rev Sci Tech Off Int Epiz* 1996; 15:947–970.

92 Kaplan M M & Cohen D. Studies on the local treatment of wounds for the prevention of rabies. *Bull World Health Organ* 1962; 26:765–775.

93 Anderson L J & Winkler W G. Aqueous quaternary ammonium compounds and rabies treatment. *J Infect Dis* 1979; 139:494–495.

94 Roumiantzeff M, Ajjan N, Montagnon B & Vincent-Falquet J C. Rabies vaccines produced in cell culture. *Ann Inst Pasteur Virol* 1985; 136E:413–424.

95 Centers for Disease Control. Rabies vaccine, adsorbed: a new rabies vaccine for use in humans. *MMWR* 1988; 37:217–218, 223.

96 Warrell M J. Multi-site intradermal regimens: safe, economical post-exposure treatment for developing countries. In Dodet B & Meslin F-X (eds) *Rabies Control in Asia*. Paris: John Libbey Eurotext 2001; pp 51–57.

97 Centers for Disease Control. Human rabies prevention—United States, 1999: Recommendations of the Immunization Practices Advisory Committee (ACIP). *MMWR* 1991; 48:RR-1.

98 Suntharasamai P, Warrell M J, Viravan C et al. Purified chick embryo cell rabies vaccine: economical multisite intradermal regimen for post-exposure prophylaxis. *Epidem Infect* 1987; 99:453–458.

99 Warrell M J, Nicholson K G, Warrell D A et al. Economical multiple site intradermal immunisation with human diploid-cell-strain vaccine is effective for post-exposure rabies prophylaxis. *Lancet* 1985; i:1059–1062.

100 Koepke J W, Reller L B, Masters H A & Selner J C. Viral contamination of intradermal syringes. *Ann Allergy* 1985; 55:776–778.

101 Chutivongse S, Wilde H, Supich C et al. Post-exposure prophylaxis for rabies with antiserum and intradermal vaccination. *Lancet* 1990; 335:896–898.

102 Madhusudana S N, Anand N P, Shamsundar R. Evaluation of two intradermal vaccination regimens using purified chick embryo cell vaccine for post-exposure prophylaxis of rabies. *Natl Med J India* 2001; 14:145–147.

103 Dreesen D W, Bernard K W, Parker R A et al. Immune complex-like disease in 23 persons following a booster dose of rabies human diploid cell vaccine. *Vaccine* 1986; 4:45–49.

104 Swanson M C, Rosanoff E, Gurwith M et al. IgE and IgG antibodies to β-propiolactone and human serum albumin associated with urticarial reactions to rabies vaccine. *J Infect Dis* 1987; 155:909–913.

105 Gardner S D. Prevention of rabies in man in England and Wales. In Pattison J R (ed.) *Rabies: A Growing Threat*. Wokingham: Van Nostrand Reinhold, 1983: 39–49.

106 Piyasirisilp S, Hemachudha T & Griffin D E. B-cell responses to myelin basic protein and its epitopes in autoimmune encephalomelitis induced by Semple rabies vaccine. *J Neuroimmunol* 1999; 98:96–104.

107 Swaddiwuthipong W, Prayoonwiwat N, Kunasol P & Choomkasien P. A high incidence of neurological complications following Semple anti-rabies vaccine. *Southeast Asian J Trop Med Public Health* 1987; 18:526–531.

108 Held J R & Lopez Adaros H. Neurological disease in man following administration of suckling mouse brain antirabies vaccine. *Bull World Health Organ* 1972; 46:321–327.

109 Larghi O P. Improvement of post- and pre-exposure immunization in Latin America. In Kuwert E K, Wiktor T J & Koprowski H (eds) *Cell Culture Rabies Vaccines and their Protective Effect in Man*. Geneva: International Green Cross, 1981: 283–287.

110 Swamy H S, Shankar S K, Chandra P S et al. Neurological complications due to beta-propiolactone (BPL)-inactivated antirabies vaccination. *J Neurol Sci* 1984; 63:111–128.

111 Applebaum E & Greenberg M. Neurological complications following antirabies vaccination. *J Am Med Ass* 1953; 151: 188–191.

112 Celis E, Wiktor T J, Dietzschold B & Koprowski H. Amplification of rabies-virus induced stimulation of human T-cell lines and clones by antigen-specific antibodies. *J Virol* 1985; 56:426–433.

113 Baltazard M & Bahmanyar M. Practical trial of antirabies serum in people bitten by rabid wolves. *Bull World Health Organ* 1955; 13:747–772.

114 Fang-tao L, Shu-beng C, Guan-Fu W et al. Study of the protective effect of the primary hamster kidney cell rabies vaccine. *J Infect Dis* 1986; 154:1047–1048.

115 Fathi M, Sabeti A & Bahmanyar M. Séroprophylaxie antirabique chez les sujets mordus par loups enragés en Iran. *Acta Med Iran* 1970; 13:5–9.

116 Wiktor T J, Lerner R A & Koprowski H. Inhibitory effect of passive antibody on active immunity induced against rabies by vaccination. *Bull World Health Organ* 1971; 45:747–753.

117 Wilde H, Chomchey P, Prakongsri S et al. Adverse effects of equine rabies immune globulin. *Vaccine* 1989; 7:10–11.

118 Wilde H, Chomchey P, Prakongsri S & Punyaratabandhu P. Safety of equine rabies immune globulin. *Lancet* 1987; ii:1275.

119 Babès V. *Traité de la Rage*. Paris: Baillière, 1912.

120 Suzor R. *Hydrophobia*. An account of M Pasteur's system containing a translation of all his communications on the subject, the techniques of his method, and the latest statistical results. London: Chatto & Windrush, 1887.

121 Cornwall J W. Statistics of antirabic inoculations in India. *BMJ* 1923; 298.

122 Veeraraghavan N. Annual report of the Director 1969 and scientific report 1970. Coonoor: Pasteur Institute of Southern India, 1971.

123 Editorial. Rabies vaccine failures. *Lancet* 1988; i:917–918.

124 Fishbein D B & Weir E H. Administration of human diploid-cell rabies vaccine in the gluteal area. *N Engl J Med* 1988; 318:214–215.

125 Pappaioanou M, Fishbein D B, Dreesen D W et al. Antibody response to pre-exposure human diploid-cell rabies vaccine given concurrently with chloroquine. *N Engl J Med* 1986; 314:280–284.

126 Strady A, Lang J, Lienard et al. Antibody persistence following preexposure regimens of cell-culture rabies vaccines: 10-year follow-up and proposal for a new booster policy. *J Infect Dis* 1998; 177: 1290–1295.

Chapter 46
Diarrhoea Caused by Viruses

C. A. Hart, N. A. Cunliffe and J. S. Bresee

A variety of viruses can be found in the gastrointestinal tract. These include non-pathogenic (at least for humans) bacteriophages and human viruses that use the gastrointestinal tract as a portal of entry such as enteroviruses, hepatovirus and some adenoviruses (non-group F). The latter group rarely if ever cause diarrhoeal disease. In contrast there is an increasing list of viral enteropathogens. In general viral enteropathogens affect the duodenum and upper jejunum, causing a non-inflammatory diarrhoea, and are the major causes of diarrhoeal disease in children. The relative importance of the different viral enteropathogens in children hospitalized with diarrhoea is shown in Table 46.1.

Rotavirus

Human rotavirus (HRV) was first described as a pathogen in 1973 on thin-section electron microscopy of duodenal biopsies and called duovirus. The same investigators subsequently demonstrated that the virus was shed in large numbers in faeces and could be detected by direct negative-stain electron microscopy.[1] It was subsequently renamed rotavirus because of its characteristic wheel-shaped morphology.

Geographical distribution

Rotavirus infection is found as frequently in developed as

Table 46.1 The relative contributions of viral enteropathogens to childhood gastroenteritis

	% of cases Community-based	% of cases Hospital-based
Rotavirus	5–40	25–65
Calicivirus[1,2]	10–25	20–30
Adenovirus 40/41	10–15	5–12
Astrovirus[1]	10–25	5–10
Coronavirus	1–3	1–2
Breadavirus	?	< 1
Torovirus	?	0–3.5
Picobirnavirus	?	< 1

1. Can cause food-borne epidemics
2. Includes both Norwalk-like and Sapporo-like viruses

in developing countries. It is, however, more likely to produce life-threatening diarrhoea in developing countries,[2,3] and most of the mortality is in children in developing countries (Figure 46.1).

Epidemiology

HRV is a major cause of gastroenteritis among infants and young children and is the most common cause of severe dehydrating diarrhoea in this age group. In hospital-based surveys it is found to be responsible for 25–65% of cases, while in community-based surveys rotavirus is detected in 5–40% of cases. The peak of infection in most parts of the world occurs from 4 months to 3 years of age, although most will have been infected by 2 years. There is a difference in the peak ages of infection between developed and developing countries. The median age of children hospitalized with rotavirus gastroenteritis in Africa was 6 months and 81% were under 1 year,[3] whereas in developed countries the median age is over 11 months. Adults can be infected and epidemics of infection can occur when antigenically different strains of rotavirus emerge.[4,5] Recent estimates of disease burden indicate that in developed countries hospitalization rates are between 2.5 and 5 per 1000 in children under 5 years,[6] whereas in Venezuela it may be as high as 30 per 1000.[7] Rotavirus is estimated to cause 20% of childhood deaths—a total of approximately 870,000 each year,[8] with 170,000–210,000 in Africa,[3] or an annual death rate there of 3.4 per 1000 infants.[9]

In temperate countries infections peak in the winter months, with low numbers of cases at other times. In tropical countries, although more cases of infection occur in cooler drier months, infection is highly prevalent throughout the year.[3,7,11]

Virology

Rotavirus is a member of the family Reoviridae. It has a characteristic double-shelled capsid which gives it the wheel-shaped (rota is Latin for a wheel) morphology on electron microscopy (Figure 46.2). It is approximately 75 nm in diameter and has a genome of 11 double-stranded RNA segments. Each segment encodes one or more polypeptides (Table 46.2). VP (virus proteins) 1, 2 and 3 form the core of the virion and are involved in

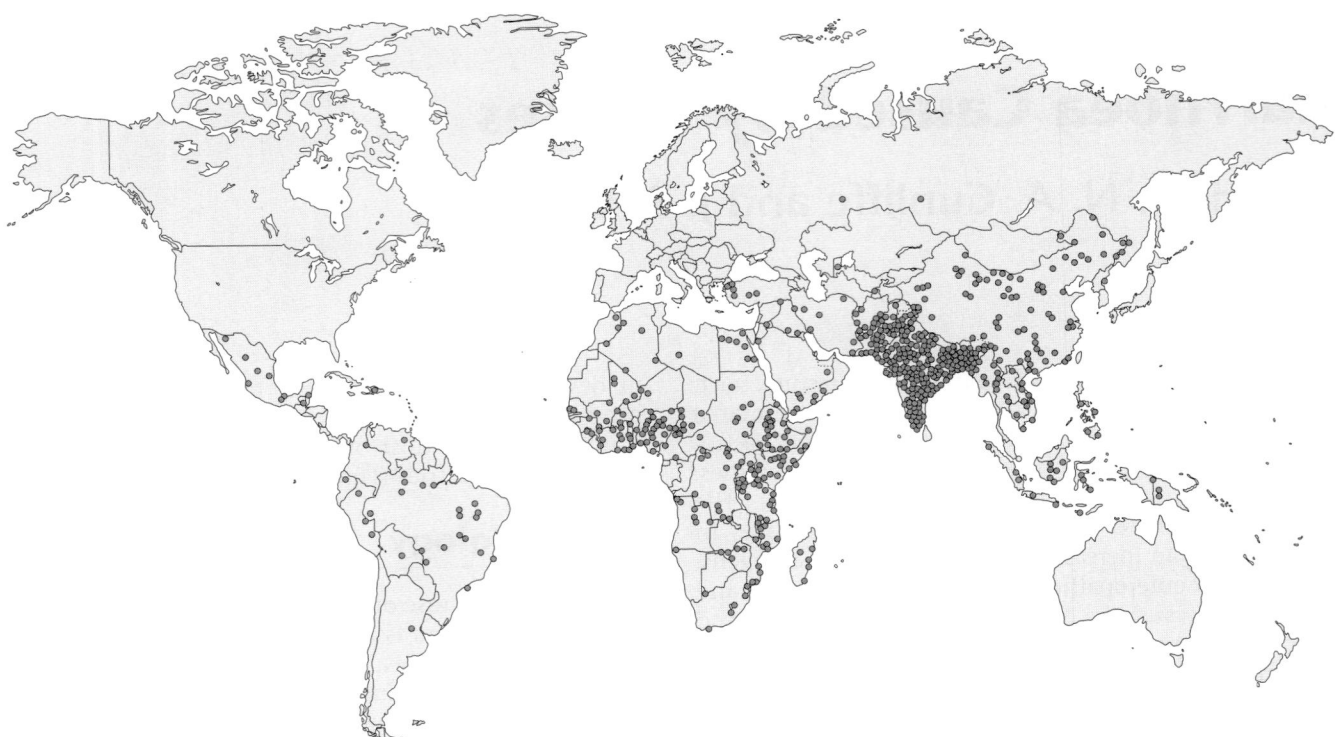

Figure 46.1: Estimated global distribution of the annual deaths caused by rotavirus diarrhoea (*n* = 600 000). (Reprinted from Parashar et al.[10])

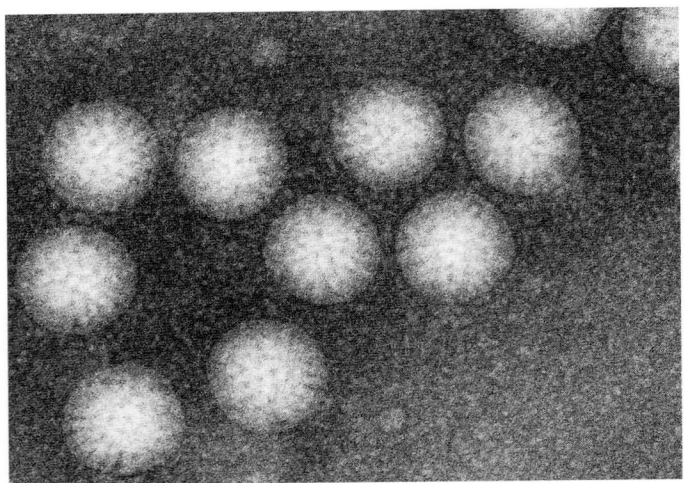

Figure 46.2: Negative-stain electrograph of rotavirus. (× 200 000.)

genome replication and packaging. VP6 forms the inner capsid and is the most abundant viral protein. VP4 is a protein that is present in the outer capsid. To be fully infective VP4 must be cleaved by intestinal proteolytic enzymes into VP5* and VP8*. These are involved in viral attachment and penetration into host cells. VP7 is another outer capsid glycoprotein and may be involved in viral attachment. There are five non-structural proteins (NSP1–5) that are present in the infected cell but not the mature virion. They are all involved in viral replication and one of them, NSP4, is the first viral enterotoxin to be described.[12]

Rotaviruses are classified by group, subgroup, serotype and electropherotype. Group (A–G) and subgroup (I, II, I and II or neither) specificities are present on the inner capsid protein (VP6). Thus far humans have been found to be infectable by groups A, B and C rotaviruses (Table 46.3) but infections with these groups also occur in other animals. The majority of human infections are with group A rotaviruses. Group B rotavirus infections appear to be uncommon but have been associated with large outbreaks of infection in China and India.[4,5] Up to a third of adult humans have serological evidence of infection with group C rotavirus.[13] Serotype specificities are arguably more important as antibodies to serotype antigens are neutralizing in vitro and protective in vivo. The P (or protease) type is located on VP4 and so-called because VP4 is proteolytically digested for full infectivity. There are a total of 20 different P types but P[4], P[6] and P[8] are most frequently implicated in human infection. The other major neutralizing antigen is carried on VP7 and defines the G (or glycoprotein) type. There are 14 different G types. Four G types (1, 2, 3 and 4) account for up to 80% of human infections.[14] However, recently other G types have emerged. For example, in Malawi G8 was the commonest type detected over a 2-year period[15] and G9 has emerged as a global serotype.[16,17] Although particular P and G combinations are found frequently (e.g. P[8], G1), because rotavirus has a segmented genome when two different rotaviruses infect the same cell, reassortment is possible (equivalent to antigenic shift in influenza A virus). Infection of humans with two rotaviruses simultaneously is not rare.[15,18] Furthermore it is also clear

Table 46.2 Rotavirus genome and gene products

Genome segment	Molecular size (bp)	Gene product	Molecular weight (kDa)	Location in virion	Function
1	3302	VP1	125	Core	RNA polymerase
2	2690	VP2	94	Core	RNA binding
3	2591	VP3	88	Core	Guanylytransferase
4	2362 (VP5* + VP8*)	VP4	88	Outer capsid	Cell attachment and penetration; haemagglutin; neutralizing antigen (P-serotype)
5	1581	NSP1	53	Non-structural	RNA binding (zinc finger)
6	1356	VP6	41	Inner capsid	Group and subgroup antigen
7	1104	NSP3	34	Non-structural	RNA binding
8	1059	NSP2	35	Non-structural	RNA binding
9	1062	VP7	38	Outer capsid	Neutralizing antigen (G-serotype)
10	751	NSP4	28	Non-structural	Virus assembly; enterotoxin
11	667	NSP5	26	Non-structural	RNA binding

*Virus protein (VP)4 must be cleaved by proteolysis for full infectivity.

Table 46.3 Reservoirs in which infection has been detected

Group	Reservoirs in which infection has been detected
A	Man, primates, horse, sheep, pig, cattle, dog, cat, turkey, chicken, mice
B	Man, pigs, cattle, sheep, rats
C	Man, pigs, cattle, ferret
D	Chicken, turkey
E	Pigs
F	Chicken
G	Chicken

that the rotavirus genome is also subject to mutational change (antigenic drift). Thus rotavirus appears to be in a process of constant change.[19] Finally rotaviruses can be subdivided into two major patterns (long and short) according to the mobility of their 11dsRNA segments on polyacrylamide gel electrophoresis.

Pathogenesis

Large amounts of rotavirus, (up to 10^{12} virions per gram) are excreted in faeces during acute infection. The infective dose is low (10^2–10^3 virus particles) and although person-to-person spread by the faeco-oral route is the most likely, the possibility of aerosol spread by the airborne route is not inconceivable. Rotaviruses are quite hardy and waterborne outbreaks are also possible. The incubation period is usually 1–3 days. Rotavirus infects the mature villous enterocytes of the upper small intestine. It is unable to infect the immature villous crypt cells or colonic enterocytes. VP4 seems to be the major ligand binding HRV to cells but the nature of the receptor is

unclear. HRV enters the cell by endocytosis or by direct penetration if VP4 has been cleaved to VP5* and VP8*. Three mechanisms have been described for the pathogenesis of rotavirus diarrhoea. In the first 12–24 hours post infection enterocytes are intact but levels of the brush border disaccharides (sucrose, maltose, lactase) are greatly decreased.[20] This is apparently due to interference with transport of the enzymes to the brush border.[21] The result of this is that disaccharides in the diet cannot be hydrolysed to monosaccharides and thus cannot be absorbed, producing an osmotic diarrhoea. Secondly, NSP4, which is involved in rotavirus assembly, has a collateral effect in opening calcium channels in the enterocyte. This causes an efflux of sodium and water and thus a secretory diarrhoea.[12] Finally, the raised intra-enterocyte calcium concentration causes them to die by oncosis.[22] The rate of death of the villous body enterocytes exceeds the rate of production of new enterocytes in the crypts and villous blunting occurs and thus malabsorption. Infection resolves both as the virus runs out of susceptible mature enterocytes and an immune response is generated. Virus continues to be excreted for up to 2 weeks after cessation of diarrhoea but excretion for up to 57 days has been detected after severe disease.[23] It appears that individuals are repeatedly infected with rotavirus throughout their lives. However, it is only on the first two or three occasions that disease occurs,[24] unless infection is with different serogroups[4,5] or novel serotypes.[15–17]

Immunity

In general, one episode of rotavirus diarrhoea confers good protection against subsequent symptomatic infection. Children who have experienced one, two or three episodes of rotavirus disease have adjusted relative risks of experiencing a further attack of rotavirus diarrhoea of

0.23, 0.27 and 0.08 respectively but of asymptomatic rotavirus infection of 0.62, 0.40 and 0.34 respectively.[24] Subsequent infections are decreasingly severe and likely to be due to a different G type. Heterotypic protection between different G types is less good.[25] It is not entirely clear what the relative contributions of the humoral and cell-mediated arms of the immune system are. Infection with HRV elicits both mucosal and serum antibody responses.[26,27] In challenge experiments only serum IgG but not serum neutralizing antibody correlated with protection from infection and only jejunal neutralizing antibody but not serum IgG was associated with protection from clinical infection.[26] Following natural infection high serum IgA anti-HRV was associated with a lower risk of both rotavirus infection and diarrhoea and provided protection against severe disease.[28] In contrast, high serum IgG anti-HRV protected against rotavirus infection but not diarrhoea. Protective titres were achieved after two symptomatic infections. Cytotoxic T cell responses appear to be important in resolution of rotavirus infection and appear to be cross-protective for the different G serotypes.[29]

Protection of neonates against rotavirus infection appears to be by both transplacentally acquired maternal antibody[30,31] and by antibodies and other factors in breast milk.[32] Interestingly HRV in neonates does not usually produce diarrhoea unless novel serotypes emerge,[31] and may circulate silently in neonatal units. Neonatal HRV infection induces immunity to subsequent HRV gastroenteritis[33] raising the possibility of the use of neonatal strains as vaccine candidates.

Clinical features

The outcome of HRV infection varies from asymptomatic,[24] through mild short-lived watery diarrhoea to an overwhelming gastroenteritis with dehydration leading to death. Severe disease and death are more common in children who are already malnourished or have measles. Vomiting is often a part of HRV gastroenteritis and usually precedes diarrhoea. Infantile diarrhoea due to HRV tends to be more severe than that due to other enteropathogens[34] but co-infection with another pathogen does not increase disease severity.[35] Respiratory signs are often found during HRV gastroenteritis. How these occur is not clear since HRV has not been demonstrated in the respiratory mucosa. Extra-intestinal HRV infections have been described including acute myositis, haemophagocytic lymphohistiocytosis, polio-like paralysis and encephalitis.[35]

It is not possible to distinguish HRV gastroenteritis from other viral causes or non-inflammatory diarrhoeas on clinical grounds. The stools are usually pale and watery or loose and are said to have a characteristic milky odour. In hospitalized patients the duration of diarrhoea is from 2 to 23 days with a median of 6 days.[36] Patients continue to excrete virus for extended periods of time[23,37] and may thus be a reservoir for infecting others.

The cause of death is dehydration, which can be hypo- or hypernatraemic and is often associated with a metabolic acidosis.

Diagnosis

Rotavirus was first discovered using negative-stain electron microscopy of faeces.[1] This is still a valuable diagnostic tool since it is a 'catch-all' technique that will also detect other potential viral enteropathogens. However, the equipment is expensive to buy and maintain and requires a skilled operator. A variety of simpler, cheaper diagnostic tests are available which will only detect rotavirus.

Antigen detection tests include enzyme-linked immunosorbent assay (ELISA) and latex particle agglutination (LPA).[38] The sensitivity and specificity of these tests are generally high (90–95%) but can be relatively costly. LPA is useful for a 'one-off' test and ELISA for batches of samples. Surprisingly, rotavirus can also be detected by polyacrylamide gel electrophoresis of RNA extracted directly from faeces. This technique is relatively simple with good specificity (100%) and sensitivity (80–90%), and can be performed in tropical countries relatively cheaply.[38] It has the added advantage of providing epidemiological information because the electrophoretic pattern of the 11dsRNA segments varies between HRV strains. Detection of viral genome by the reverse transcriptase polymerase chain reaction is a research tool which provides information on the genotype and duration of shedding of HRV.[14–18,23,37]

Although HRV can be cultured this is not a useful diagnostic test. Similarly, antibody detection can be undertaken but this is of little value diagnostically.

In addition to the specific diagnostic tests, measurement of serum electrolytes, urea and bicarbonate will help greatly in the management of dehydration.

Management

The mainstay of management is assessment and replacement of fluid loss. In the majority of cases this can be accomplished using oral rehydration therapy. The major limiting factors are severe dehydration with shock or the high rate of vomiting that can occur early in HRV infection. In such circumstances intravenous rehydration will be needed.

There is no specific antiviral chemotherapy for rotavirus but human or bovine colostrum and hyperimmune human serum immunoglobulin have been used to manage chronic rotavirus infection. Administration of probiotics such as *Lactobacillus casei* GG appears beneficial.

Prevention and control

Rotavirus infection is highly prevalent in both developed and developing countries so it would seem unlikely that improving public and family hygiene could prevent infection. The infective dose of HRV is low and infected individuals excrete virus in massive quantities.

A number of different vaccines have been investigated for prevention of HRV. A quadrivalent reassortant rhesus rotavirus vaccine has been derived from rhesus rotavirus (10 of its genomic segments) in which the genomic segment encoding VP7 has been replaced by human rotavirus VP7 genes encoding G1–G4 specificities. This proved highly effective in trials in developed and developing countries.[2,6,36] It was approved for use in US infants in a three-dose schedule at 2, 4 and 6 months in 1998 and it is estimated that some 1.5 million doses of vaccine were given to 800,000 infants. However, the vaccine was withdrawn from use less than a year later following reports of intussusception among vaccine recipients. It was estimated that one case of intussusception occurred for every 4670–9474 infants immunized.[39] Unfortunately this means that children in developing countries have no access to vaccine where it would have had a major impact on mortality.[40]

Adenovirus 40/41

Adenoviruses are unenveloped DNA viruses with an icosahedral capsid 70–75 nm in diameter (Figure 46.3). Their genomes are double-stranded linear DNA comprising 33–45 kilobase pairs. Human adenoviruses belong to the genus Mastadenovirinae and are subdivided into six subgenera (A–F), which contain a total of 49 serotypes. Only serotypes 40 and 41 (subgenus F) have been clearly associated with diarrhoeal disease. In most surveys they are second in importance to rotaviruses in causing gastroenteritis, being responsible for 0.9–11% of cases in hospitalized children. Similarly in community-based studies adenoviruses have been shown to be important causes of childhood diarrhoea.[41] Most infections occur in children under 2 years.[42] There is no apparent seasonality to infection. Enteric adenoviruses are spread from person to person by the faeco-oral route; foodborne and waterborne spread has not been described.

The clinical features of adenovirus 40/41 gastro-enteritis do not differ greatly from those of rotavirus but tend to be less severe. Some studies have reported a longer duration of diarrhoea with adenovirus.[43,44] Electron microscopy cannot distinguish adenovirus 40/41 from other adenoviruses but immuno-electron microscopy can. There are now a number of antigen detection kits including ELISA and LPA, which are highly sensitive and specific. Genomic detection is also possible by DNA hybridization or polymerase chain reaction (PCR).

Treatment of adenovirus diarrhoea is by managing dehydration. There are no specific therapeutic interventions, nor is there a vaccine.

Astrovirus

Astrovirus was first described in 1975. It is a small (28 nm) round unenveloped virus with a star shape 'stamped' on its surface (*astron* is Greek for a star) (Figure 46.4). It has a positive-sense single-stranded RNA genome which encodes an RNA polymerase, a serine proteinase and a capsid protein. There are at least eight human astrovirus serotypes (HastV 1–8) but serotype 1 is most commonly detected.[45] However, other serotypes can be responsible for outbreaks of foodborne infection[46] and there appears to be a greater diversity of serotypes in developing countries.[47] The burden of disease attributable to astrovirus is only recently being recognized with the development of improved highly sensitive diagnostic tests. Like rotavirus and enteric adenovirus infections, astrovirus infections predominate in young children both in developed and developing countries, where they are responsible for between 2% and 10% of cases of childhood gastroenteritis. It tends to be associated with milder diarrhoea and thus appears more frequently in community-based studies.[48] A community-based cohort study from Mexico has estimated the astrovirus disease incidence rate to be 0.1 episodes per child per year.[49] Sero-epidemiological studies have demonstrated that over 90% of children in the USA will have been infected by

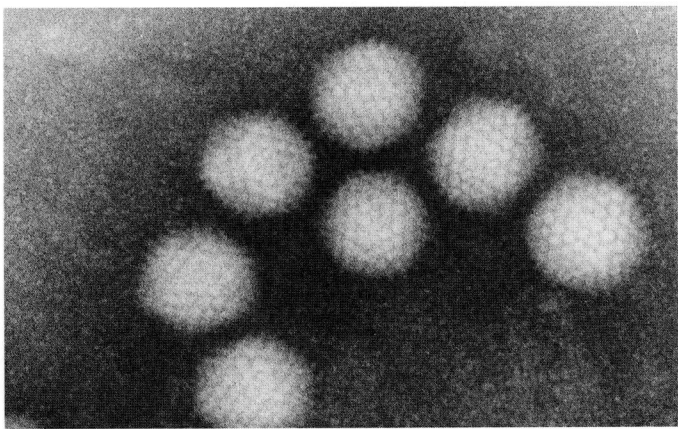

Figure 46.3: Negative-stain electron micrograph of adenovirus. (× 200 000.)

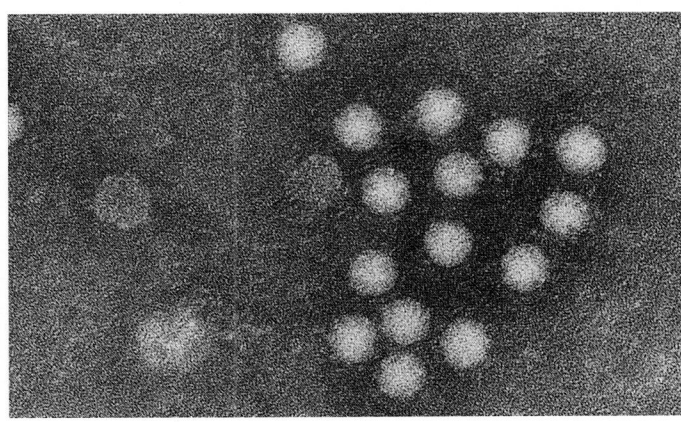

Figure 46.4: Negative-stain electron micrograph of astrovirus. (× 200 000.)

HastV by 6–9 years of age.[50] There are no similar data from developing countries. Astrovirus has been detected in all countries where sufficiently sensitive detection methods have been used, including Malawi,[51] Mexico,[49] South Africa[52] and Egypt.[53] In temperate countries it shows a similar seasonal distribution to rotavirus but with peaks a month earlier.

Infection is transmitted faeco-orally either directly or as a foodborne illness. The infective dose is not established. Astrovirus infects the upper small intestine but how it causes diarrhoea is not known. The illness is less severe than with rotavirus but with similar features and lasting on average 4–5 days. In Bangladesh astrovirus was found to be associated with prolonged diarrhoea.[47]

Although electron microscopy was the method used first to detect astrovirus[54] it is less sensitive than commercially available ELISAs or RT-PCR. The treatment involves assessing the degree of dehydration and correcting it. There is no vaccine available for its prevention and little is known of immunity to infection other than that children with immunodeficiency excrete the virus for long periods.[55]

Caliciviruses

Viral enteropathogens were first delineated by their appearance on electron microscopy and a number of small round viruses (SRVs) (c. 20–40 nm) were described. These SRVs were subdivided into those with distinctive surface structures (astrovirus and calicivirus) and those with an amorphous surface structure, which were called small round structured viruses (SRSVs). With the advent of genomic analysis it became clear that the SRSVs and enteric caliciviruses were related, whereas the astroviruses were distinct. Thus the enteric caliciviruses (Figure 46.5) and SRSVs (Figure 46.6) are included within the family Caliciviridae (the other human pathogen in this family is hepatitis E virus).

The viruses are 27–30 nm in diameter with a positive-sense single-stranded RNA genome varying from 7.5 to

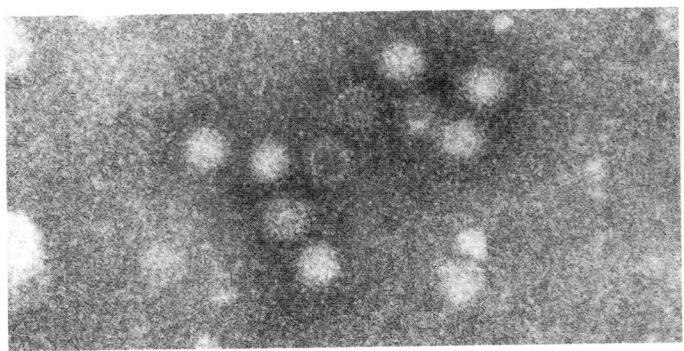

Figure 46.6: Negative-stain electron micrograph of a small round structured virus (SRSV) with a feathery-ragged outline. (× 200 000.)

7.7 kb, and no envelope.[56] The human enteric caliciviruses have a characteristic shape of a central stain-filled cup (calyx is Greek for cup), surrounded by six peripheral cup-shaped depressions, giving it the appearance of a 'Star of David' (Figure 46.5). In contrast, the SRSVs have a characteristic feathery-ragged outline (Figure 46.6). The SRSVs are usually referred to as Norwalk-like viruses (NLVs) after the town in the USA in which the first cases were diagnosed.[57,58] The more classical enteric caliciviruses are usually referred to as Sapporo-like viruses (SLVs). The NLVs are further divided into two genogroups (Table 46.4).

Caliciviruses have a worldwide distribution and some global NLV strains have been found over the same time period in eight countries on five continents.[59] Infection can occur as point source foodborne epidemics or sporadically. Illness due to SLVs tends to predominate in young children, while all age groups appear to be at risk of NLV infection. No particular seasonal distribution is evident for SLVs but outbreaks due to NLV are more common in temperate countries. Spread is faeco-orally directly or indirectly in food such as seafood or vegetables.[60] However, it does appear that transmission occurs readily and

Table 46.4 The Human Caliciviruses

	Representative strains	
Norwalk-life Viruses		
Genogroup I	Norwalk Southampton Desert Shield Cruise Ship	
Genogroup II	Snow Mountain Hawaii Mexico Toronto Lorsdale Grimsby	Gwynedd White River Melksham Camberwell Bristol
Sapporo-like viruses	Sapporo Manchester Parkville London	

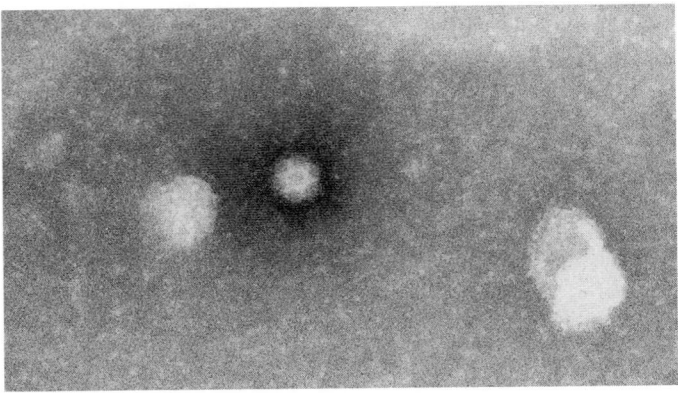

Figure 46.5: Negative-stain electron micrograph of a human enteric calicivirus with the classical 'Star of David' morphology. (× 200 000.)

it is possible that infection could be spread via saliva or even the airborne route.[61] In a study in Finnish children NLVs were responsible for 20% of cases of gastroenteritis and SLVs for 9%.[62] For comparison, astroviruses were detected in 10%, enteric adenoviruses in 6% and rotavirus in 31% of cases.

The incubation period in short (1–2 days) and in general NLVs produce profuse vomiting in most with diarrhoea in above a third of cases, while SLVs produce predominantly diarrhoea with vomiting in some cases. The illness is usually short-lived (2–3 days) but in volunteer studies excretion of NLVs continued for up to 13 days after challenge and excretion was longer in those who had more severe disease.[63]

Electron microscopy is relatively insensitive for detection of calicivirus infection except in the first days of illness. Antigen detection kits are available but separate tests may be required for SLVs and the two NLV genogroups or even individual viruses.[56] The most sensitive detection is by RT-PCR but this is not yet available in kit form. Recombinant antigens can be used for sero-epidemiological surveys. Following infection patients produce serum and faecal antibody to viral capsid proteins[56,63] but their role in immunity is not fully defined. There is no specific therapy nor are vaccines available.

Other viruses

A number of other viruses including within the Corona-viridae coronavirus[64] (Figure 46.7), and torovirus,[65] picobirnaviruses[66] and pestiviruses,[67] have been found to be associated with diarrhoeal disease. Their relative importance seems to be small and most are not well studied.

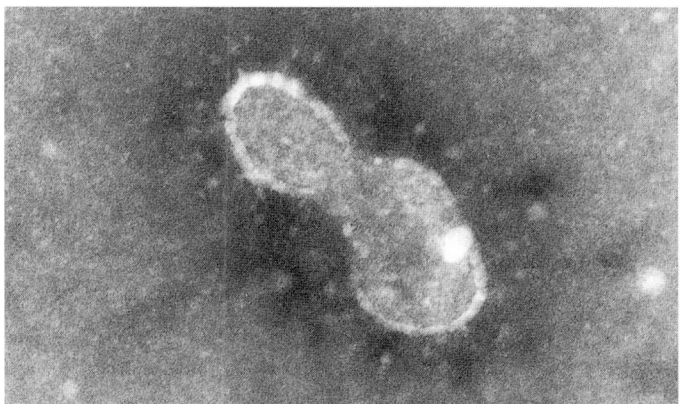

Figure 46.7: Negative-stain electron micrograph of a coronavirus. (×200 000.)

REFERENCES

1 Bishop R F, Davidson G P, Holmes I H & Ruck B J. Detection of a new virus by electronmicroscopy of faecal extracts from children with acute gastroenteritis. *Lancet* 1974; i:149–151.

2 Miller M A & McCann L. Policy analysis of the use of hepatitis B, *Haemophilus influenzae* type b; *Streptococcus pneumoniae*—conjugate and rotavirus vaccines in national immunization schedules. *Health Economics* 2000; 9:19–36.

3 Cunliffe N A, Kilgore P E, Bresee J S et al. Epidemiology of rotavirus diarrhoea in Africa: a review to assess the need for rotavirus immunization. *Bull World Health Organ* 1998; 76:525–537.

4 Hung T, Chen G, Zhaoying F et al. Waterborne outbreak of rotavirus diarrhoea in adults in China caused by a novel rotavirus. *Lancet* 1984; i:1139–1142.

5 Krishnan T, Sen A, Choudhury T S et al. Emergence of adult diarrhoea rotavirus in Calcutta, India. *Lancet* 1999; 353:380–381.

6 Lynch M, Bresee J S, Gentsch J R & Glass R I. Rotavirus vaccines. *Curr Opin Infect Dis* 2000; 13:495–502.

7 Perez-Schael I. The impact of rotavirus disease in Venezuela. *J Infect Dis* 1996; 174(Suppl 1): S19–S21.

8 Institute of Medicine. The prospect of immunizing against rotavirus. In *New Vaccine Development: Diseases of Importance in Developing Countries*, vol. 2. Washington, DC: National Academy Press, 1986: D13.1–D13.12.

9. Molbak K, Fischer Perch T K & Mikkelsen C S. The estimation of mortality due to rotavirus infection in sub-Saharan Africa. *Vaccine* 2001; 19:393–395.

10 Parashar U D, Bresee J S, Gentsch J R et al. Rotavirus. *Emerg Infect Dis* 1998; 4:1–12.

11 Bingnan F, Unicomb L, Rahim Z et al. Rotavirus-associated diarrhea in rural Bangladesh: two year study of incidence and serotype distribution. *J Clin Microbiol* 1991; 29:1359–1363.

12 Ball J M, Tian P, Zeng C Q-Y et al. Age dependent diarrhea induced by a rotaviral non-structural protein. *Science* 1996; 272:101–104.

13 Riepenhaff-Talty S M, Morse K, Wang C H et al. Epidemiology of group C rotavirus infection in western New York women of child-bearing age. *J Clin Microbiol* 1997; 35:486–488.

14 Gentsch J R, Woods P A, Ramachandran M et al. Review of G and P typing results from a global collection of rotavirus strains: implications for vaccine development. *J Infect Dis* 1996; 174(Suppl 1):S30–S36.

15 Cunliffe N A, Gondwe J S, Graham S M et al. Rotavirus strain diversity in Blantyre, Malawi from 1997 to 1999. *J Clin Microbiol* 2001; 39:836–843.

16 Ramachandran M, Kirkwood C D, Unicomb L et al. Molecular characterization of serotype G9 strains from a global collection. *Virology* 2000; 278:436–444.

17 Cunliffe N A, Dove W, Bunn J E G et al. Expanding global distribution of rotavirus serotype G9: detection in Libya, Kenya and Cuba. *Emerg Infect Dis* 2001; 7:890–892.

18 Tabassum S, Shears P & Hart C A. Genomic characterization of rotavirus strains obtained from hospitalized children with diarrhoea in Bangladesh. *J Med Virol* 1994; 43:50–56.

19 Editorial. Puzzling diversty of rotavirus. *Lancet* 1990; 355:573–575.

20 Batt R M, Embaye H, Van der Waal S et al. Application of organ culture of small intestine to the investigation of enterocyte damage by equine rotavirus infection in foals. *J Pediatr Gastroenterol Nutr* 1995; 20:326–332.

21 Jourdan N, Brunet J P, Sapia C et al. Rotavirus infection reduces sucrase-isomaltase expression in human intestinal epithelial cells by perturbing protein targeting and organization of microvillar cytoskeleton. *J Virol* 1998; 72:7228–7236.

22. Perez J F, Chemello M C, Liprandi F et al. Oncosis in MA104 cells is induced by rotavirus infection through an increase in intracellular Ca^{2+} concentrations. *Virology* 1998; 252:17–27.

23 Richardson S, Grimwood K, Gorrell R et al. Extended excretion of rotavirus after severe diarrhoea in young children. *Lancet* 1998; 351:1844–1848.

24 Velazquez F R, Matson D O, Calva J J et al. Rotavirus infection in infants as protection against subsequent infections. *N Engl J Med* 1996; 355:1022–1028.

25 Moulton C H, Staat M, Santosham M & Ward R L. The protective effectiveness of natural rotavirus infection in an American Indian population. *J Infect Dis* 1998; 178:1562–1566.

26 Ward R C, Bernstein D I, Shukla R et al. Effects of antibody to rotavirus on protection of adults challenged with a human rotavirus. *J Infect Dis* 1989; 159:79–88.

27 Aiyar J, Bhan M K, Bhandari N et al. Rotavirus-specific antibody response in saliva of infants with rotavirus diarrhoea. *J Infect Dis* 1990; 162:1383–1384.

28 Velazquez F R, Matson D O, Guerrero M L et al. Serum antibody is a marker of protection against natural rotavirus infection and disease. *J Infect Dis* 2000; 182:1602–1609.

29 Heath R R, Stagg S, Xu F & McCrae N A. Mapping of the target antigens of the rotavirus-specific T-cell response. *J Gen Virol* 1997; 78:1065–1075.

30 Ramachandran M, Vij A, Kumar R et al. Lack of maternal antibodies to P-serotypes may predispose neonates to infection with unusual rotavirus strains. *Clin Diagn Lab Immunol* 1998; 5:527–530.

31 Widdowson M A, van Doornum G J J, Van der Poel W H M et al. Emerging group A rotavirus and a nosocomial outbreak of diarrhoea. *Lancet* 2000; 356:1161–1162.

32 Jayashree S, Bhan M K, Kumar R et al. Protection against neonatal rotavirus infection by breast milk antibodies and trypsin inhibitors. *J Med Virol* 1988; 26:333–338.

33 Bishop R F, Barnes G L, Cipriani F & Lund J J. Clinical immunity after neonatal rotavirus infection. *N Engl J Med* 1983; 309:72–76.

34 Perez-Schael I, Garcia D, Gonzalez M et al. Prospective study of diarrhoeal diseases in Venezuelan children to evaluate the efficacy of rhesus rotavirus vaccine. *J Med Virol* 1990; 30:219–229.

35 Unicomb L E, Faruque S M, Malek M A et al. Demonstration of a lack of synergistic effect on rotavirus with other diarrheal pathogens on severity of diarrhea in children. *J Clin Microbiol* 1996; 34:1340–1342.

36 Hart C A & Cunliffe N A. Viral gastroenteritis. *Curr Opin Infect Dis* 1999; 12:447–457.

37 Wilde J, Yolken R, Willoughby R & Eiden J. Improved detection of rotavirus shedding by polymerase chain reaction. *Lancet* 1991; 337:323–326.

38 Ibrahim O S, Sunderland D & Hart C A. Comparison of four methods for detection of rotavirus in faeces. *Trop Doctor* 1990; 20:30–32.

39 Murphy T V, Garguillo P M, Massoudi M S et al. Intussusception among infants given an oral rotavirus vaccine. *N Engl J Med* 2001; 334:564–572.

40 Weijer C. The future of research in rotavirus vaccine. *Br Med J* 2000; 321:525–526.

41 Cruz J R, Caceres P, Cane F et al. Adenovirus types 40 and 41 and rotaviruses associated with diarrhea in children from Guatemala. *J Clin Microbiol* 1990; 28:1780–1784.

42 Barnes G L, Uren E, Stevens K B & Bishop R F. Etiology of acute gastroenteritis in hospitalized children in Melbourne, Australia from April 1990 to March 1993. *J Clin Microbiol* 1998; 36:133–138.

43 Yolken R H, Lawrence F, Leister F et al. Gastroenteritis associated with enteric type adenovirus in hospitalized infants. *J Pediatr* 1982; 101:21–26.

44 Kotloff K L, Losonsky G A, Morris J G et al. Enteric adenovirus infection and childhood diarrhea: an epidemiologic study in

45 Shi M, Sikotra S, Lee T et al. Use of a nested PCR method for the detection of astrovirus serotype 1 in human faecal material. *Molec Cell Probes* 1994; 8:481–486.

46 Belliot G, Laveran H & Monroe S S. Outbreak of gastroenteritis in military recruits associated with serotype 3 astrovirus infection. *J Med Virol* 1997; 51:101–106.

47 Unicomb L E, Banu N N, Azim T et al. Astrovirus infection in association with acute, persistent and nosocomial diarrhea in Bangladesh. *Pediatr Infect Dis J* 1998; 17:611–614.

48 Maldonaldo Y, Cantwell M, Old M et al. Population based prevalence of symptomatic and asymptomatic astrovirus in rural Mayan infants. *J Infect Dis* 1998; 178:334–339.

49 Guerrerro M L, Noel N S, Mitchell K D et al. A prospective study of astrovirus diarrhea of infancy in Mexico City. *Pediatr Infect Dis J* 1998 17:723–727.

50 Mitchell D K, Matson D O, Cubitt W D et al. Prevalence of antibodies to astrovirus types 1 and 3 in children and adolescents in Norfolk, Virginia. *Pediatr Infect Dis J* 1999; 18:249–254.

51 Pavone R, Schinaia N, Hart C A et al. Viral gastroenteritis in children in Malawi. *Ann Trop Paediatr* 1990; 10:15–20.

52 Steele A D, Basetse H R, Blacklow N R et al. Astrovirus infection in South Africa: a pilot study. *Ann Trop Paediatr* 1998; 18:315–319.

53 Naficy A B, Rao M R, Holmes J L et al. Astrovirus diarrhea in Egyptian children. *J Infect Dis* 2000; 182:685–690.

54 Madeley C R & Cosgrove B P. 28 nm particles in faeces in infantile gastroenteritis. *Lancet* 1975; ii:451–452.

55 Cox G J, Matsui S M, Lo R S et al. Etiology and outcome of diarrhea after marrow transplantation: a prospective study. *Gastroenterology* 1994; 107:1398–1407.

56 Atmar R L & Estes M K. Diagnosis of the noncultivable gastroenteritis viruses, the human calicivirues. *Clin Microbiol Rev* 2001; 14:15–37.

57 Adler J L & Zickl L R. Winter vomiting disease. *J Infect Dis* 1969; 119:668–673.

58 Dolin R, Blacklow N R, Dupont H et al. Transmission of acute infectious non-bacterial gastroenteritis to volunteers by oral administration of stool filtrates. *J Infect Dis* 1971; 123:307–312.

59 Noel J S, Fankhauser R L, Ando T et al. Identification of a distinct common strain of 'Norwalk-like viruses' having a global distribution. *J Infect Dis* 1999; 179:1334–1344.

60 O'Ryan M L, Vial P A, Mamani N et al. Seroprevalence of Norwalk virus and Mexico virus in Chilean individuals: assessment of independent risk factors for antibody acquisition. *Clin Infect Dis* 1998; 27:789–795.

61 Becker K M, Moe C L, Southwick K L et al. Transmission of Norwalk virus during a football game. *N Engl J Med* 2000; 343:1223–1227.

62 Pang X-L, Honma S, Nakata S et al. Human caliciviruses in acute gastroenteritis of young children in the community. *J Infect Dis* 2000; 181(Suppl 2):S288–S294.

63 Okhuysen P C, Jiang X, Ye L et al. Viral shedding and fecal IgA response after Norwalk virus infection. *J Infect Dis* 1995; 171:566–569.

64 Zhang X M, Herbst W, Kousoulas K G et al. Biological and genetic characterization of a haemagglutinating coronavirus isolated from a diarrhoeic child. *J Med Virol* 1994; 44:152–161.

65 Jamieson F B, Wang E L, Bain C et al. Human torovirus: a new nosocomial gastrointestinal pathogen. *J Infect Dis* 1998; 178:1263–1269.

66 Ludert J E & Liprandi F. Identification of viruses with bi- and tri-segmented double stranded RNA genomes in faeces of children with gastroenteritis. *Res Virol* 1993; 144:213–244.

67 Yolken R, Dubovi E, Leister F et al. Infantile gastroenteritis with excretion of pestivirus antigens. *Lancet* 1989; i:517–520.

Chapter 47
Respiratory Viruses

J. S. M. Peiris and C. R. Madeley

No individual can survive without a functioning respiratory tract. It is frequently invaded by infective agents of all kinds, including viruses and bacteria. The consequences depend not only on the particular agent but also on the individual patient. Pre-existing impairment of the tract by congenital malformations or damage from previous episodes of infection, as well as the circumstances of the individual as a whole (malnutrition, poverty, overcrowding, sanitation, etc.), will profoundly affect the outcome. This chapter primarily concerns viruses but other micro-organisms may be involved, alone or in combination. The respiratory tract may also be involved in part of a more extensive disease process which may itself be due to a virus. Infection of one part of the respiratory tract should therefore not be seen in isolation; the wider implications must be considered.

Acute respiratory infections are estimated to cause 4.5 million childhood deaths annually. The overwhelming majority occur in developing countries and they account for one-third of all deaths in childhood. Bacterial infections in general have a higher case fatality than acute viral infections, but viruses are far more common causes of acute respiratory infection. Overall they contribute to at least one-third of the deaths caused by acute respiratory infection in the developing world.

Clinical picture (See also Chapter 11)

The respiratory tract can be divided into an upper and a lower part, with the boundary at the lower end of the larynx. Viral infections confined to the upper part (upper respiratory tract infection, URTI) are rarely life threatening, with the exception of croup in the tropics. They can be uncomfortable but do not usually call the individual's future into question. These infections do not automatically spread to the lower respiratory tract, but where the lower respiratory tract is involved the process is extensive and rarely confined to one lobe or even one lung. This is in contrast to pneumococcal pneumonia, which is typically confined to one lobe of one lung.

Although widespread, the process of viral infection is usually less intense than that seen in bacterial pneumonia; otherwise such infections would be much more lethal. The most common manifestations of a lower respiratory tract infection (LRTI) are bronchiolitis (in infants) or an atypical pneumonia. When an LRTI occurs, the upper tract is also involved and the causative virus can usually be isolated from it. The main exception is cytomegalovirus pneumonitis in the immunocompromised patient, where the presence or absence of the virus may not be directly related to the pathology in the lung.

There are no clear-cut differences between the clinical presentation(s) of any viruses in the respiratory tract. For example, although respiratory syncytial virus (RSV) is the most common cause of bronchiolitis in the world, this clinical condition may also be caused by parainfluenzaviruses, influenzaviruses, adenoviruses or rhinoviruses. Consequently, it must not be assumed that two patients with similar clinical illnesses will have been infected by the same virus. This is particularly so in babies and young children.

The viruses

Table 47.1 lists those viruses generally associated with the respiratory tract. Nevertheless, other viruses may be present as part of a generalized process in which the respiratory component is only a (small) part.

Table 47.1 is divided into two sections. Section A lists those viruses usually associated with respiratory tract disease. Confirming their presence will usually identify the cause of the illness, although dual and even triple infections can occur, particularly in the compromised host. The viruses are listed in approximately descending order of importance in terms of numbers of cases annually and their potential severity. By almost any criterion RSV would head the list but the others could be ranked in a different order, depending on the age, time of year and geographic location of the population. This is discussed further under Epidemiology, below.

Section B lists three viruses which may be found in the respiratory tract of clinically normal individuals, especially children. Herpes simplex virus may cause no overt lesions in the respiratory tract, although its presence indicates a potential to cause damage if the opportunity occurs—particularly in compromised patients. Enteroviruses and reoviruses are not proven pathogens in the respiratory tract, although the former are frequently isolated from the throats of children.

Important features of each virus are discussed below.

Table 47.1 Viruses infecting the respiratory tract

Virus	No. of serotypes	Group antigen?	Common disease presentation[a]
A. Usually pathogenic in the respiratory tract			
RSV	1 (2 subtypes: A and B)	Yes[b]	Bronchiolitis in < 2 years (also URTI, failure to thrive, febrile fits)
Influenza A	Genetically unstable → sequential variants[c]	Yes	URTI, influenza
Influenza B	Genetically unstable → sequential variants[c]	Yes	URTI, influenza, may include abdominal pain
Parainfluenza	1–4a,b	No	URTI, croup, bronchiolitis
Adenovirus	47[d]	Yes	URTI, acute respiratory disease
Rhinovirus	>100	No	URTI ('common cold')
Coronavirus	Several[e]	No	URTI ('common cold')
Epstein–Barr virus	1	Yes[b]	Glandular fever
Cytomegalovirus	1	Yes[b]	Various (in the immunocompromised only)[f]
Measles	1	Yes[b]	Measles[g]
Hantaviruses	Several	No	Hantavirus pulmonary syndrome
B. May be recovered from the respiratory tract but role in respiratory disease uncertain			
Herpes simplex (hominis)	1	Yes[b]	–[h]
Enteroviruses	68	No	–
Reovirus	3	No	–[i]

[a] Although this column lists the more common presentations, there is considerable overlap in clinical signs and symptoms between respiratory viruses.
[b] There is only one serotype. This is used as a group antigen for diagnostic purposes.
[c] The RNA of influenza A and B viruses is constantly undergoing mutation which is reflected antigenically, causing 'drift' in both influenza A and B and 'shift' in influenza A.
[d] Most respiratory infections are due to types 1–7.
[e] The total is not known.
[f] Usually no overt illness in the immunocompetent, except congenital damage and for some examples of glandular fever.
[g] Rash may be absent in the immunocompromised.
[h] Causes stomatitis and may be a cause of pneumonitis in compromised patients.
[i] No identified disease in man.

Respiratory syncytial virus (RSV)

This virus is distributed worldwide and is found wherever it has been sought. It is frequently associated with bronchiolitis in babies—with a peak incidence at about 6 months—and is the most common virus detected, especially in children infections under 1 year of age hospitalized with respiratory (see below). Large epidemics occur annually at the same season. The starting date and extent of the epidemic may vary a little but the annual epidemic is reliable. For diagnostic purposes there is only one serotype. Two subtypes (A and B) have been described and they may co-circulate, with one usually predominating in any given year. No obvious differences in disease severity or pathogenesis have been documented.

More recently, it is becoming clear that RSV causes significant morbidity in the elderly as well as in infants.[1]

Influenza A and B viruses

Antigenically, these are the most variable of the respiratory viruses. Both exhibit antigenic *drift*, in which the surface antigens of the virus change gradually in the face of immunological pressure from the host species. One or two variants predominate at a given time. In this progressively evolving change, they are unique among respiratory viruses. Influenza A, but *not* influenza B, also shows occasional major antigenic *shift* changes as a result of genetic reassortment with animal strains, which introduces new viral surface antigens to which the human population is immunologically naïve. The timing, extent and direction of either *drift* or *shift* have so far been completely unpredictable. However, when viruses with antigenic shift appear in the human population, a worldwide pandemic of influenza A is a possibility, with memorable examples in 1918 ('Spanish flu'), 1957 ('Asian flu') and 1968 ('Hong Kong flu'). With no animal reservoirs to provide new strains, shift does not occur in influenza B.

Influenza epidemics associated with antigenic drift contribute to mortality in the elderly and those with pre-existing conditions such as chronic cardiopulmonary or renal disease, diabetes, immunosuppression or severe anaemia. The risk of Reye's syndrome is increased following influenza in children on long-term aspirin therapy. While the morbidity and excess mortality associated with influenza in temperate regions are well documented, there is a paucity of information on its impact in the tropics. The more diffuse seasonality (see Epidemiology) obscures the disease burden due to influenza in the tropics. However, lack of evidence should not be taken for evidence of a lack of impact.

In 1997, a purely avian influenza virus (H5N1) was transmitted from chickens to man, with fatal results in 6 of the 18 patients who were found to be infected.[2] The disease was unusual in that previously healthy young adults were those most severely ill. The outbreak was controlled by the slaughter of all chickens in the 'live-poultry' retail markets and no further cases have occurred since. The following year, another avian influenza virus (H9N2) was isolated from two cases of mild influenza in children.[3] Neither virus became established in man, but their emergence is a reminder of the zoonotic nature of influenza virus and of what might happen.

Parainfluenzavirus

There are four serotypes of parainfluenza, with type 4 possessing two subtypes: 4a and 4b. Types 1 and 2 typically cause croup, a high-pitched barking cough in children which is profoundly irritating to their parents. Type 3 can cause bronchiolitis or pneumonia and, less often, croup. In temperate countries types 1 and 2 (together with RSV) are more prevalent in the winter months, whereas type 3 is unusual (among respiratory viruses) in occurring more often in spring and early summer. This dissociation between the peaks of activity of parainfluenza type 3 and RSV has also been observed in tropical regions.[4,5]

Adenovirus

There are 47 different serotypes but the majority of respiratory infections involve types 1–7. Types 1, 2, 5 and 6 are usually associated with endemic disease in temperate regions, and types 3, 4 and 7 with epidemics. The higher-numbered serotypes appear in the respiratory tract from time to time but the majority of them have been found only in the gut.

Adenoviruses are unusual in that prolonged carriage (up to 2 years in some cases) may occur in the tonsils of children, often with no continuing illness. The clinical significance of adenoviruses isolated from the throat of children must therefore be interpreted cautiously. However, they may cause a primary and severe pneumonia in debilitated children, in whom it may be rapidly fatal.

The use of disabled adenoviruses as vectors for gene therapy and targeted anticancer drug treatment is now being explored.[6] How useful these initiatives may be in the future is unclear at present but, if used widely, markers of adenovirus activity may become more common but without extra episodes of disease.

Rhinovirus

These are frequent causes of the common cold, itself a common winter and summer illness in temperate countries. Information on the seasonality of rhinoviruses in the tropics is scanty. They can be difficult to grow in culture (the only practical way to confirm infection) and are very under-reported, mainly because diagnosis is not attempted. Although the infection is usually uncomfortable and significant in the number of workdays lost, it is not usually severe. Nevertheless, rhinoviruses are now recognized to be a significant precipitating factor in exacerbations of asthma and chronic obstructive airways disease, and they have occasionally been the sole pathogens present in the lungs of immunocompromised patients dying with respiratory signs and symptoms.

Coronavirus

These viruses are the second main cause of the common cold. Little is known about them, other than their existence and that there may be over 30 serotypes. They require specialist techniques for diagnosis that are not widely available, and most laboratories (even in research studies) do not attempt to document their role.

Measles (See also Chapters 23 and 48)

Measles is often not recognized as a major cause of LRTI morbidity or mortality, and there are a number of factors that may account for this underassessment.[7] Children with measles may not always be admitted to a general paediatric ward, the aetiology may be attributed to a superinfecting pathogen rather than to measles, and some patients with measles (especially when immunocompromised as a result of malnutrition, cytotoxic drug treatment or for other reasons) will fail to develop the typical rash. In patients who do not manifest typical clinical features, both clinical and laboratory diagnosis of measles is difficult, even in the developed world, because the virus is not isolated readily and good antisera for reliable immunofluorescence are not commercially available. Where the diagnosis has been actively sought in developing countries, measles is found to be a major cause of LRTI, accounting for 6–21% of morbidity and 8–50% of the mortality attributed to LRTI. The effects of the virus on the respiratory tract can be direct (giant cell pneumonitis) or indirect. The latter includes the depressive effects of the virus on the host immune system, stores of vitamin A and overall nutritional status. All of these can lead to an increased risk of superinfection with other viral or bacterial pathogens.

Cytomegalovirus

This is an opportunist pathogen in immunocompromised patients, in whom it can cause respiratory complications. Perinatal cytomegalovirus infection may occasionally present as pneumonitis in the newborn and (together with chlamydiae) must be considered in the differential diagnosis.

Apart than such occasional illnesses most cytomegalovirus infections are clinically silent, although serological surveys have shown positivity rates approaching 100% in some overcrowded populations.

New viruses

Recently, viruses infecting fruit bats in Australia (Hendra)[8] and flying foxes in Malaysia (Nipah)[9] have been transmitted to horses and pigs respectively, and from them to man. Hendra caused a fatal respiratory infection in man, and Nipah an encephalitis. The place of neither virus as causes of human disease has been established and they are mentioned here for completeness.

Of possibly greater significance is the hantavirus pulmonary syndrome (HPS). In May 1993 there was an outbreak of a severe, and frequently fatal, respiratory disease in the area in the United States where the four states Arizona, Colorado, New Mexico and Utah abut. The causative agent was found to be a hantavirus, later called Sin Nombre virus. The natural host was found to be the deer mouse, *Peromyscus maniculatus*, the local population of which had recently increased rapidly, bringing them more into contact with humans and allowing the virus to cross the species gap. Related viruses causing a similar disease syndrome have since been isolated in North (e.g. New York, Bayou, Black Creek Canal viruses) and South (e.g. Andes virus) Americas.[10] All these viruses belong to the same hantavirus genus as those causing haemorrhagic fever with renal syndrome (HFRS) in the Old World: Hantaan, Seoul and Puumala viruses. Both HFRS and HPS have a similar febrile prodrome with thrombocytopenia and leucocytosis. In HPS, the key differences are that the capillary leakage which follows is localized to the lungs and that, with Sin Nombre virus, renal dysfunction is minimal. Humans acquire infection by Sin Nombre virus from rodents and there was no evidence of human-to-human transmission. However, there is early evidence that some of the South American hantaviruses causing HPS may be transmitted between humans in a nosocomial setting.

Other agents

The diagnosis of several other agents has been undertaken in virus laboratories because these agents cause respiratory infections which overlap clinically with those due to viruses, and they are diagnosed serologically (see below). They include psittacosis, Q fever and mycoplasmosis, and isolation of the causative organism is either difficult or dangerous. They also include *Chlamydia pneumoniae* (TWAR), which is recognized as a cause of community-acquired pneumonia although diagnostic tests are not yet widely available.

The activities of these agents are under-recorded in most parts of the world. Since they are amenable to antibiotic therapy, it is important that they are diagnosed.

Epidemiology

The aetiology and epidemiology of acute respiratory infections have been intensively studied in the temperate areas of the world. Information from tropical regions is more scanty, but what evidence there is suggests that the viruses responsible for respiratory disease in the tropics are no different from those found in temperate zones.[11-15] However, the severity of illness and its sequelae, as well as their seasonality, may be markedly different from those in the developing world. Although there are a large number of viruses indigenous to the tropics (most notably a large number of insect-transmitted viruses), there is no evidence that they contribute significantly to respiratory tract disease.

The data on respiratory infections obtained by Jacob John and his colleagues[5] in Vellore, India, and shown in Tables 47.2 and 47.3, confirm a pattern of activity familiar to workers elsewhere. RSV is the predominant virus in

Table 47.2 Frequency of virus detection, by age, in 809 subjects with acute respiratory of infection*

No. of children of indicated age in whom virus detected					
	< 1 year	1 year	2 years	3 years	≥ 4 years
Virus	(n = 359)	(n = 226)	(n = 92)	(n = 74)	(n = 58)
RSV	108	32	16	6	1
Influenza A	6	3	2	4	1
Influenza B	3	2	3	2	4
Parainfluenza 1	9	7	4	3	2
Parainfluenza 2	1	4	0	2	0
Parainfluenza 3	29	18	7	4	4
Adenovirus	9	13	1	6	2
Other viruses positive[†]	23	10	12	3	1
Total no. (%)	177 (49)	79 (35)	42 (46)	29 (39)	15 (26)

*Reproduced with permission from Jacob John et al. Etiology of acute respiratory infections in children in tropical Southern India. *Rev Infect Dis* 1991; 13:S463–S469.
[†] Two different viruses were isolated in 11, 10, 3 and 1 children of < 1, 2, and 3 years of age, respectively.

Table 47.3 Frequency of virus detection, by syndrome, in 331 children with lower respiratory tract infection (LRTI)*

Type of LRTI	No. of children	No. (%) positive for virus	No. in whom virus was detected				
			RSV	Influenza	Parainfluenza	Adenovirus	Other[†]
Pneumonia	178	65 (37)	34	3	15	6	11
Bronchiolitis	116	83 (72)	67	1	13	4	3
Tracheobronchitis	14	7 (50)	2	1	2	2	0
Croup	8	4 (50)	0	0	5	0	1
Other[†]	15	4 (27)	3	0	1	0	0
Total	331	163 (49)	106	5	36	12	15

*Reproduced with permission from Jacob John et al. Etiology of acute respiratory infections in children in tropical Southern India. *Rev Infect Dis* 1991; 13:S463–S469. Two viruses were detected in four children with pneumonia, five with bronchiolitis, two with croup.
[†] Enterovirus (21 children), herpes simplex (13), measles virus (7), mumps virus (1), unidentified virus (7).
[†] Acute exacerbation of bronchial asthma (8), tropical pulmonary eosinophilia (2), tuberculosis (2), foreign body aspiration (2) and membranous tracheitis (1).

young children under 2 years of age and accounts for 163 out of 367 (44%) of the viruses detected. Parainfluenza type 3 was the second most common virus and, other than RSV, is probably more predictable in its epidemiology than any of the others listed.

In temperate regions, respiratory infections have generally been shown to increase in the autumn and winter, although the exact mechanisms are still not fully understood. A similar periodicity is shown in tropical regions but this may be related to fluctuations in rainfall or humidity rather than temperature. In contrast to temperate regions, influenza in the tropics may occur in the summer months or all year round, and RSV in Hong Kong is a summer disease.

The activities of influenza A and B remain impossible to predict and can fluctuate greatly from year to year. The appearance of a 'new' strain of either A or B can be associated with an epidemic the size of which is likely to be greater as the size of the antigenic change increases, although other, so far unidentified, virulence factors may be even more influential. With no shift changes in influenza B, major epidemics are less common.

Even where high-quality, competent diagnostic services are available, not every clinical respiratory disease yields unequivocal evidence of infection by a virus or other micro-organism. The proportion in which a positive diagnosis is made varies from a quarter to a half, depending on laboratory, area, population and time of year.

Hospitalized versus community patients

Berman[16] has summarized the data from developing countries and found that the percentage of hospitalized patients who were virus positive was about twice the figure found in those attending as outpatients. This difference is not surprising and probably reflects both the greater opportunity to make a specific diagnosis in the hospitalized patient and the severity of their disease. The majority of trivial episodes (head colds and increased nasal secretions) are not subjected to virus diagnosis and the causative viruses are unconfirmed.

It could be argued that infections too trivial to require hospital admission can be mostly ignored—a dismissal even more appropriate for those who remain at home. This argument, however, is flawed for two reasons. First, human viruses are caught from other humans, although the severity varies. Hence most respiratory viral transmission occurs within the community. Second, patients may become too ill to attend a hospital, a situation exacerbated by other contributing factors such as poverty and lack of facilities.

Other factors

As with most other diseases, respiratory infections are made worse by other components of the patient's environment. Poverty, malnutrition, pollution and overcrowding (common in urban environments everywhere in the world) are well recognized to contribute to the frequency and severity of respiratory illness. The effects may be direct or indirect through the presence of other disease, poor sanitation and poor personal hygiene (Figure 47.1).

Nevertheless, although a poor, malnourished child in a densely populated inner city slum will have many respiratory illnesses, viruses are no respecters of persons and his or her better-off cousin in a wealthy environment may also have a considerable number of infections. Where the difference lies is that the latter will cope better and will have fewer longer-term sequelae, which include chronic respiratory impairment, wheezing, asthma, bronchitis and bronchiectasis.

Laboratory diagnosis

There are three main reasons for providing a laboratory diagnosis of viral respiratory infections: to tell the clinician what is causing the illness (individual diagnosis); to monitor routine virus activity in the community (epidemiology); or research investigations.

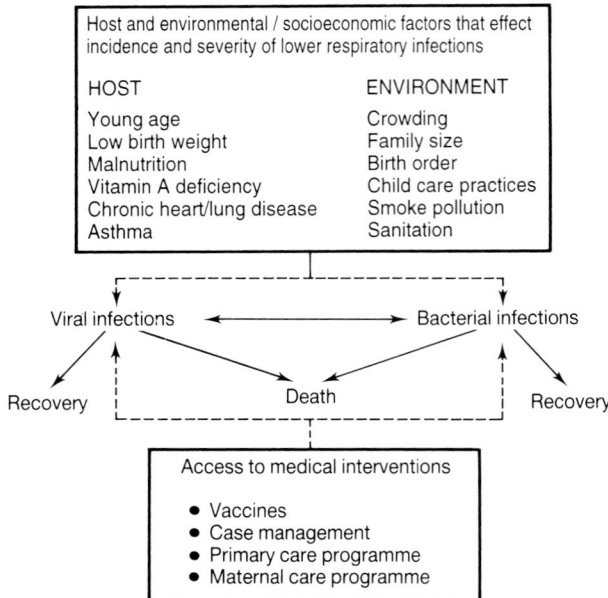

Figure 47.1: Aetiology and epidemiology of lower respiratory tract infections in developing countries. (Reproduced with permission from Berman, Epidemiology of acute respiratory infections in children of developing countries, *Rev Infect Dis* 1991; 13:S454-S462.[16])

Rapid diagnosis of viral respiratory infections (i.e. in less than 3 hours) has been shown to reduce antibiotic use and to be cost-effective.[17] In addition, such confirmation of the cause is useful in hospital infection control (e.g. in cohorting similar cases) and, occasionally, in deciding whether to use antiviral drugs in selected high-risk patients (see below). The new antineuraminidase drugs for treating influenza provide an additional incentive for making a rapid diagnosis, although their cost may yet deter their widespread use.

It is self-evident that individual diagnosis must be quick if it is to influence clinical management. Rapidity of diagnosis is also important in epidemiological studies because the clinician will lose interest in sending specimens if there is no equally rapid feedback on the cause of the patient's illness. It is not surprising that the epidemiological data are patchy, but they can reflect year-by-year variations if the population on which the studies are performed remains approximately constant.

Diagnosis of respiratory infection is achievable within 2–3 hours using techniques such as antigen detection[18–20] (see below). However, these techniques are not universally available, even in hospitals in the developed world, mainly because they are labour intensive and are perceived as being expensive. In the developing world this is compounded by a shortage of staff experienced in the use of such techniques, but these objections are surmountable.[16] While availability of viral diagnosis is not likely to be widespread in the tropics, there is a sound argument for ensuring availability of competent diagnostic facilities in a few centres, at least, to provide continuing epidemiological data and to underpin clinical training.

Methods of viral diagnosis

Laboratory diagnosis of respiratory virus infections depends on the demonstration of *either* virus or viral components in the patient at the acute stage of the illness, *or* subsequently an immune (serological) response to the virus.

Demonstration of virus

There are several approaches to this. They include demonstration of: (1) viral antigens by immunofluorescence[18,19] or enzyme immunoassays;[20] (2) viral infectivity by growth in cell culture; or (3) viral nucleic acid by various techniques. Details of the techniques are not given here, but the advantages and disadvantages of each are indicated in Table 47.4. Before setting up a diagnostic laboratory the aims of the operation should be clearly thought out. If the catchment population is very large, the number of specimens may also be large and the advantages of automation (e.g. in machine-based enzyme immunoassays) may be decisive. However, this level of abundance is rare and the number of available specimens may be too few. Automation may then be less advantageous and is often minimal except in serology (see below). Except for special studies, most of the specimens will come from hospitalized patients because of the practical difficulties of collecting specimens in the community. In any case, virology specimens are perishable and must be delivered to the laboratory without delay.

Demonstration of immune response

This, at present, means demonstrating an antibody response in the serum to the stimulus provided by the virus. Seeking responses in cellular immunity or antibody in other body fluids remain research techniques only.

For a valid diagnosis, a convalescent specimen of serum (taken after enough time for a response has elapsed) is needed but may be difficult to collect 2 weeks after the onset from patients who may by then be totally recovered and unwilling to oblige the investigator's interest! This is particularly true with children. Nevertheless, unless an antibody response can be demonstrated (seroconversion or a rising titre) some uncertainty over the validity of the result will remain. The alternative is demonstration of an IgM-class response but this suffers from the twin disadvantages that such tests are not available for all viruses and the sample (to be reliably positive) may have to be taken after the illness is over, with the problem(s) already mentioned.

Serology remains the routine choice for some respiratory agents which, although not viral in nature, are traditionally diagnosed by virus laboratories. These include: psittacosis, Q fever and *Mycoplasma pneumoniae* infection. All cause an illness with an insidious onset and are difficult and/or dangerous to isolate. Since all, therefore, are susceptible to antibiotics, a diagnosis is important and can be life-saving. The role of *Chlamydia pneumoniae* is poorly documented at present in the absence of an easily used test.

Table 47.4 Advantages and disadvantages of various techniques of virus diagnosis

Technique	Advantages	Disadvantages
Immunofluorescence	• Rapid, i.e. same day • Allows assessment of specimen quality • Sensitive and specific in experienced hands	• Labour-intensive • Requires experienced observer(s) • Requires high-quality reagents • Obtaining good specimens requires skill and determination
Enzyme immunoassay	• Relatively rapid • Suitable for large numbers • Can be semiautomated • Detects incomplete virus particles	• No feedback on specimen quality • Requires high-quality reagents • Automated equipment expensive • Difficult to assess results at threshold of positivity
Culture	• Provides more virus for further analysis • Confirms presence of infective virus • Generally regarded as the gold standard • Only currently feasible method for some viruses (e.g. rhinoviruses and enteroviruses)	• Expensive and a continuing expense • Labour-intensive • Some viruses difficult to isolate • Mixed infections pose problems • Requires high-quality reagents to identify isolates
Detection of nucleic acid by polymerase chain reaction (PCR)	• Can be made both very sensitive and specific • Can detect virus in the presence of antibody	• Expensive • Requires constant vigilance against cross-contamination • Unsuitable for large numbers • Labour and skill intensive

Infections in the immunocompromised host

(See also Chapter 20)

A detailed analysis of the respiratory complications of the immunocompromised patient (oncology, leukaemia, transplantation) is outside the compass of this book but some mention is necessary of opportunistic infections in patients who have been immunodepressed by the human immunodeficiency virus (HIV) or who have the acquired immune deficiency syndrome (AIDS). They are likely to contract any of the viruses already mentioned and may have difficulty in eradicating them due to the lack of functioning cellular immunity. However, viral respiratory infections are not in themselves a life-threatening problem in patients with AIDS, with three exceptions: measles, varicella-zoster and cytomegalovirus.

Giant cell pneumonitis due to measles can be fatal, and may occur even in patients who have past immunity (naturally derived or vaccine induced). Chickenpox is usually trivial in school-age children but may be severe and include respiratory complications in adults. Cyto-megalovirus pneumonitis (although less commonly seen than in other groups of immunocompromised patients) can also be fatal.

The diagnosis of chickenpox is usually clinically obvious, but measles may present problems because the skin rash is often absent in the immunocompromised patient. Immunofluorescent examination of naso-pharyngeal secretions for measles-infected cells provides a rapid diagnosis, but this is unlikely to be widely available. Cytomegalovirus can be cultured from the sputum (voluntary or induced) or detected in bronchoalveolar lavage/lung biopsy specimens, if available.

Nosocomial infection

RSV and influenza viruses are particularly highly infectious, and are notorious causes of cross-infection in hospitals. This may pose particular hazards to patients at higher risk, such as those with underlying heart or lung disease (e.g. congenital heart damage or bronchopulmonary dysplasia). Transmission of RSV (as with most other respiratory viruses) is by direct contact or via infected surfaces or fomites. Influenza A, on the other hand, is efficiently spread by aerosols.

Precautions that may help reduce the risk of cross-infection include the isolation or cohort nursing of infected patients and scrupulous care in hand-washing between patients. It is essential to remember that viruses can also infect medical and other hospital staff (RSV may be asymptomatic or cause a 'common cold' in adults) and be transmitted by and through them.

Prevention and treatment

With the cells of the target organ immediately accessible

to viruses, it is proving difficult to produce effective vaccines to respiratory tract viruses. Other than in measles, which has a systemic phase, vaccines have had only limited success. In the tropics, even the measles vaccine has limitations because much of the impact of this virus on morbidity and mortality is during infancy, and existing measles vaccines are not effective at inducing immunity in the presence of passive maternal antibody. Newer vaccines, including one using canarypox virus as a vector, have been explored but not yet adopted. A second dose of conventional vaccine has also been suggested but cost may make this impractical in many countries.

Influenza vaccine is used for persons at high risk (e.g. patients with underlying heart, respiratory or immuno-compromising diseases, patients on dialysis, the elderly) and contains antigens from both influenza A and B. The constituents are modified as the prevalent strains alter but, inevitably, they will always lag behind the emerging wild strains. In addition, it is not yet known how to induce the long-term secretory IgA mucosal antibody that is probably necessary for protection. Within these limitations the vaccine, usually formalin-killed egg-grown virus, has provided useful protection, particularly in the elderly and those with pre-existing lung damage in whom even minimal protection may be enough to prevent death. An alternative approach of a live attenuated vaccine containing cold-adapted influenza strains has been used widely in Russia, particularly in schools, but has yet to be adopted elsewhere to any great extent.

An experimental enteric coated vaccine to adenovirus 14 was developed for use in the US Army to combat epidemics in recruit camps but has found no application elsewhere.

There is evidence that humanized mouse antibodies or hyperimmune γ-globulin may give some protection from, or reduce the severity or duration of, RSV infections in the more vulnerable (e.g. premature) babies, but these preparations are very expensive and their use should be confined to those in whom infection will be life-threatening on standard management.[21]

Prevention of severe measles and varicella in susceptible (immunocompromised or severely malnourished) contacts may also be achieved by passive immunization. Normal human γ-globulin is effective in preventing/attenuating measles if administered within 3 days of contact. For the prophylaxis of varicella, high-titre varicella-zoster human immune globulin (ZIG) must be used. Maximum protection (from severe disease, but not from infection) follows administration within 48 hours of contact, but some benefit may accrue if given within 10 days.

Amantadine, and its alternative rimantadine, have been shown to provide protection against influenza A (but not influenza B) but to be of little use in treatment. Its main use has been to give short-term passive protection to limit spread of influenza A in closed communities or in vulnerable patients (see above).

With the start of the twenty-first century, drugs such as zanamivir and oseltamivir, which inhibit the influenza A and B viral enzyme neuraminidase (concerned with release of the virus from infected cells) have been assessed in clinical trials.[22] To be effective, they have to be given within 48 hours of onset. They are expensive and are best used on those most at risk of serious illness—those at the extremes of life. These drugs are not active on other viruses, even those with viral neuraminidases.

Generally, the management of viral respiratory infections is essentially symptomatic and is dealt with elsewhere (Chapter 11). Antibiotics are not routinely indicated for viral respiratory infections unless secondary bacterial superinfection occurs. The 'atypical' bacterial infections mentioned above (Q fever, mycoplasmosis and chlamydiosis) are amenable to antibiotic therapy. (T)ribavirin given as an aerosol inhalation is claimed to reduce the severity of RSV infection in infants, but this remains controversial. It is a very expensive drug, but may be life-saving in those with congenital heart and/or lung damage for whom RSV infection may be the final insult which pushes them into heart or lung failure. (T)ribavirin may have some effect in influenza but the evidence is minimal.

Acyclovir (given intravenously) is effective in the treatment of varicella or herpes simplex infections in the immunocompromised patient. It should also be used in an immunocompetent patient (usually an adult) with varicella pneumonia. Ganciclovir and foscarnet are useful in cytomegalovirus infection in the immunosuppressed, but a detailed discussion of this problem is beyond the scope of this book.

Summary

Respiratory infections are very common throughout the world and are worse where social conditions are inadequate. Much childhood respiratory tract disease is either totally due to viruses or is virus-initiated and the same viruses appear to be involved in all regions, tropical or temperate. Epidemiological data are incomplete everywhere (but more so for the poorer parts of the world) and come mostly from hospitalized patients.

Nevertheless, RSV is a universal childhood pathogen, found everywhere it has been sought. The number of virologically confirmed diagnoses each year (most them in patients in hospital) in the Newcastle and Tyneside area in the UK (population about 1 million) and from Hong Kong island (population about 0.7 million) are remarkably similar: 500–600 and 500–700 cases respectively. There are likely to be many more in the crowded cities of India, China, the Philippines, Brazil and elsewhere. The effects of RSV (and other viruses) are exacerbated by overcrowding, malnutrition, air pollution, poor sanitation, minimal medical care, etc. Respiratory disease, like diarrhoea, results in significant morbidity and mortality in the developing world, has significant economic consequences and will require an enormous commitment of resources to abate. Viruses and bacteria are both involved and there are few effective vaccines at present.

REFERENCES

1 Falsey A R, Cunningham C K, Barker W H et al. Respiratory syncytial virus and influenza A infections in the hospitalised elderly. *J Infect Dis* 1995; 172:389–394.

2 Yuen K Y, Chan P K S, Peiris M et al. Clinical features and rapid viral diagnosis of human disease associated with avian influenza A H5N1. *Lancet* 1998; 351:467–471.

3 Peiris M, Yam W C, Chan K H et al. Influenza A H9N2: aspects of laboratory diagnosis. *J Clin Microbiol* 1999; 37:3426–3427.

4 Suwanjutha S, Chantarojanasiri T, Watthana-Kasetr S et al. A study of nonbacterial agents of acute lower respiratory tract infection in Thai children. *Rev Infect Dis* 1990; 12(Suppl 8):S923–S928.

5 Jacob John T, Cherian T, Steinhoff M C, Simoes E A F & John M. Etiology of acute respiratory infections in children in tropical Southern India. *Rev Infect Dis* 1991; 13(Suppl 6):S463–S469.

6 Alemany R, Balagué C & Curiel D T. Replicative adenoviruses for cancer therapy. *Nature Biotechnol* 2000; 18:723–727.

7 Markowitz L E & Nieburg P. The burden of acute respiratory infection due to measles in developing countries and the potential impact of measles vaccine. *Rev Infect Dis* 1991; 13(Suppl 6):S555–S561.

8 Mackenzie J S. Emerging viral diseases: An Australian perspective. *Emerg Inf Dis* 1999; 5:1–8.

9 Chua K B, Bellini W J, Rota P A et al. Nipah virus: a recently emergent deadly paramyxovirus. *Science* 2000; 288:1432–1435.

10 Schmaljohn C & Hjelle B. Hantaviruses: a global disease problem. *Emerg Inf Dis* 1997; 3:95–103.

11 Bale J R (ed.). Symposium on etiology and epidemiology of acute respiratory tract infection in children in developing countries. *Rev Infect Dis* 1990; 12(Suppl 8):S861–S1083.

12 Steinhoff M C (ed.). Bellagio conference on the pathogenesis and prevention of pneumonia in children in developing regions. *Rev Infect Dis* 1991; 13(Suppl 6):S451–S580.

13 Assaad F & Cockburn W C. A seven year study of WHO virus laboratory reports on respiratory viruses. *Bull World Health Organ* 1974; 51:437–445.

14 Forgie I M, Campbell H, Lloyd-Evans N et al. Etiology of acute lower respiratory tract infections in children in a rural community in The Gambia. *Paediatr Infect Dis J* 1992; 11:466–473.

15 McIntosh K, Halonen P & Ruuskanen O. Report of a workshop on respiratory viral infections: epidemiology, diagnosis, treatment and preventions. *Clin Infect Dis* 1993; 16:151–164.

16 Berman S. Epidemiology of acute respiratory infections in children of developing countries. *Rev Infect Dis* 1991; 13(Suppl 6): S454–S462.

17 Woo P C Y, Chiu S S, Seto W H, Peiris J S M. Cost-effectiveness of rapid virus diagnosis of viral respiratory tract infections in pediatric patients. *J Clin Microbiol* 1997; 35:1579–1582.

18 Gardner P S & McQuillin J. *Rapid Virus Diagnosis: Application of Immunofluorescence*. London: Butterworth, 1980, 2nd edition.

19 Madeley C R. Respiratory viruses. In Caul E O (ed.) *Immunofluorescence Antigen Detection Techniques in Diagnostic Microbiology*. London: Public Health Laboratory Service, 1992: 33–48.

20 Arstila P P & Halonen P. Direct antigen detection. In Lennette E H, Halonen P & Murphy F A (eds) *Laboratory Diagnosis of Infectious Diseases: Principles and Practice*, vol. II. New York: Springer, 1988: 60–75.

21 Anonymous. Prevention of respiratory syncytial virus infections: indications for use of palivizumab and update on the use of RSV-IGIV. American Academy of Pediatrics Committee on Infectious Diseases and Committee of Fetus and Newborn. *Pediatrics* 1994; 102:1211–1262.

22 Gubareva L V, Kaiser L & Hayden F G. Influenza virus neuraminidase inhibitors. *Lancet* 2000; 355:827–835.

Chapter 48
Cutaneous Viral Diseases

G. C. Cook and A. Zumla

The skin is a common site of lesions resulting from systemic diseases as well as localized skin infections. Tables 48.1 and 48.2 summarise medically important RNA and DNA viral infections of the skin in adults and children and the diseases they cause. With the advent of the human immunodeficiency virus (HIV) pandemic, the incidence, severity and clinical presentations of cutaneous viral infections have changed over the past two decades. Cutaneous manifestations of these viral diseases often lead to a diagnosis of HIV or the underlying immuno-suppressive disease.

RNA viruses causing cutaneous disease

A large number of RNA viruses cause skin manifestations in humans (Table 48.1). This section considers only measles and rubella. Diseases due to other RNA viruses are dealt with elsewhere in this book with in Section 6/Viral Infections.

Measles

Geographical distribution

Measles has a worldwide distribution.[1] It is one of the most prevalent infectious diseases of the tropics, and certainly one of the most serious of the acute childhood communicable illnesses.[2] Its introduction to many countries that had previously been free, such as Fiji, Tasmania, Greenland, and many tropical areas where there were isolated people without previous contact with the disease, frequently had disastrous results.

Aetiology

The causative agent, which is closely related to rinderpest and canine distemper, is a single-stranded RNA virus with a pleomorphic appearance on electron microscopy (120–250 nm in size); it consists of two components, an outer envelope with short projections and an inner nucleocapsid of RNA and a glycoprotein. There is only one strain and no known antigenic variation; alterations in virulence worldwide is due to underlying host and environmental factors. The virus grows slowly in human and monkey cell cultures. Viraemia occurs 4–5 days before the appearance of the rash, and abates within 24–48 hours. The virus can also be isolated from the throat in the coryzal stage.

Transmission

Measles is one of the most contagious of infections; approximately 90% of susceptible individuals will

Table 48.1 Aetiology and cutaneous manifestation of disease due to RNA viruses.

Family	Virus	Cutaneous disease
Paramyxovirus	Respiratory syncitial virus (RSV) Measles virus Mumps virus Retroviruses HIV-1, HIV-2	Skin rash Measles (rubeola) Mumps AIDS; dermatitis

Picornavirus	Enterovirus
	    Coxsackie
	    ECHO virus
		Herpangina; hand, foot and mouth disease
		Exanthem

Togavirus	Rubivirus Group A arboviruses	Rubella (German measles) Haemorrhagic fevers
Flavivirus	Group B arboviruses	Haemorrhagic fevers
Arenaviruses	Machupo virus Junin virus Lassa virus	Haemorrhagic fevers

HIV, human immunodeficiency virus; AIDS, acquired immunodeficiency syndrome.

Table 48.2 Aetiology and cutaneous manifestation of disease due to DNA viruses.

Family	Virus	Cutaneous disease
Pox viruses	Variola	Smallpox
		Monkeypox
		Orf
		Cowpox
		Tanapox
	Molluscum	Molluscum contagiosum
Herpesviruses	Herpes simplex virus (HSV) type 1	Orofacial herpes
	Herpes simplex virus (HSV) type 2	Genital herpes
	Varicella–zoster virus (VZV)	Chickenpox; shingles
	Cytomegalovirus (CMV)	Ulcers, exanthem
	Epstein–Barr virus (EBV)	Infectious mononucleosis
	Human herpesvirus (HHV)	
	HHV-6	Exanthema subitum
	HHV-7	Roseola infantum or 'sixth disease'
	HHV-8 (KSAHV)	Kaposi's sarcoma
Adenoviruses	Adenovirus	Adenovirus dermatitis in the immunosuppressed
Papovavirus	Human papilloma virus (HPV)	Warts
Parvoviruses	Parvovirus B19	Erythema infectiosum (fifth disease)
Hepadnaviruses	Hepatitis B virus	Macular skin rash

KSAHV, Kaposi's sarcoma-associated herpesvirus.

contract the disease after contact with a case. Transmission is direct—from secretions from the respiratory tract—by droplet spread. Cases are infectious only in the early stages, when virus can be isolated from the throat. Transplacental spread does not seem to occur and, although it is possible that fetal damage may follow measles contracted during pregnancy, this is not proven.

Pathology

Infection begins in the nose and throat from which, following limited multiplication, the virus spreads (via leucocytes) to the cells of the reticuloendothelial system; here it attacks the lymphocytes of the immune system. Further multiplication precedes the viraemic phase; epithelial cells are affected and the clinical signs and symptoms of measles develop after an incubation period of 10–14 days. Virus multiplication occurs in the reticuloendothelial system, in which it produces the appearance of large multinucleate giant cells. Target organs affected are the skin, conjunctivae, mouth, larynx, bronchial tree, and gastrointestinal tract. The essential lesion is 'catarrhal' inflammation of the respiratory and gastrointestinal tracts, the initial inflammation of epithelial cells being rapidly followed by fatty degeneration and exfoliation of dead cells. Complete resolution with recovery is the rule, although widespread denudation of epithelium in the gastrointestinal tract may result in significant enteropathy (see Chapter 10).

Immunity

Immunity to measles is both antibody and cell mediated;

following an acute attack this is lifelong. Antibodies appear simultaneously with the rash and IgM concentration peaks at 10 days, disappearing after 1 month; a resulting increased IgG concentration decreases slowly over 6 months. Passive immunity (transferred from mother to infant transplacentally) lasts for the first few months of life and evidence of inapparent infection during months of declining maternal antibody can be found in one-quarter of older children. Cell-mediated immunity plays an important role in virus elimination. Resultant on its action on the cells of the reticuloendothelial system, measles depresses cell-mediated immunity, which can also be reduced simultaneously by malnutrition. This accounts for the severity of the disease in many tropical countries. Depressed cell-mediated immunity also reactivates tuberculosis and allows secondary infections, which are common in patients with measles, to develop.

Clinical features
Natural history

Measles consists of an acute self-limiting infection; recovery occurs in the majority of cases. In tropical populations it may be complicated by severe bronchopneumonia, diarrhoea, malabsorption, malnutrition, severe conjunctivitis and blindness, gangrene of limbs and death.[1,2] The case mortality rate in the tropics is estimated to be about 5% (sometimes reaching 10% in rural areas).[3,4] In some village epidemics, 40% of children have died as a result of infection; a combination of pertussis and measles is particularly dangerous.

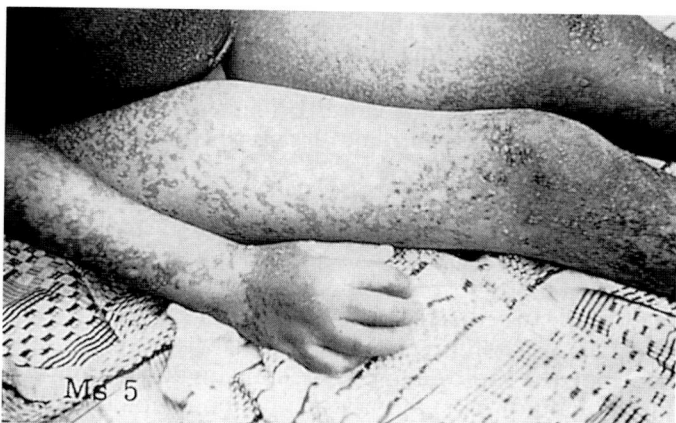

Figure 48.1: Measles rash near the knee in an African child. In a pigmented skin the rash has a deep bluish colour. (Courtesy of David Morley.)

Symptoms and signs

The incubation period is 10–14 days. Onset is gradual; prodromal fever and coryzal symptoms appear within 24 hours. Severe conjunctivitis and cough follow; this prodromal phase lasts for 3–4 days. Within 3 days of onset (and 24 hours before the rash) Koplik's spots can be visualized as blobs of bright red with a small bluish-white centre on the buccal mucous membrane. The exanthem (Figure 48.1) appears 24 hours later, first on the forehead and neck, spreading to invade the trunk over 3–4 days. The lesions are at first reddish and maculopapular, later becoming brown, and in dark skin appearing totally different to lesions in pale skins, with a diffuse deep red or purple rash followed by severe desquamation 2–4 days later. This may lead to patchy depigmentation and, occasionally, boils. Haemorrhagic measles with a purpuric rash and accompanied by bleeding from mucous membranes is rare; it carries a high mortality rate.

Other systems

The mouth becomes sore, interfering with sucking and eating; this can lead to malnutrition and cancrum oris. Laryngitis is common; this is followed by bronchopneumonia—which carries a high mortality rate. Diarrhoea, sometimes accompanied by tenesmus and blood and mucus in the stool, leads to dehydration; parenteral replacement may be necessary to prevent death.

Central nervous system

The most common manifestation is a short, generalized convulsion early in the course of infection, from which recovery is complete.

Encephalitis

Measles encephalitis is associated with generalized convulsions—the risk increasing with age; the course is variable. Onset is usually 4–7 days after appearance of the rash (48 hours to 2 weeks after onset) and is characterized by fever, irritability, meningism and coma. The cerebrospinal fluid shows moderate pleocytosis and an increase

in protein concentration. The mortality rate can be as high as 10–15%; one-quarter of affected children are left with a permanent neurological deficit. This phenomenon probably has an immunological basis, as shown by the histological changes, perivascular cuffing, demyelination and gliosis.

Subacute sclerosing panencephalitis

This complication is caused by a persistent viral infection within the brain. It usually manifests 5–10 years after infection, and pursues a slow degenerative course, starting with personality change(s) and deterioration of intellect (with signs of mental deterioration), and progressing to a state of decerebrate rigidity. Very high levels of antibody to measles virus are present in cerebrospinal fluid.

Complications

Depression of cell-mediated immunity can give rise to giant cell pneumonia, also seen in patients with defective cell-mediated immunity. Severe ulcerative herpes of the mouth and eye result from cell-mediated immune depression. Severe conjunctivitis, often associated with vitamin A deficiency,[5–7] causes corneal perforation and blindness. Respiratory complications are common and sometimes fatal. Bronchitis, bronchioloitis, croup and giant cell bronchopneumonia occur. Measles is one of the most common causes of blindness in the tropics (see Chapter 18). Gangrene of the extremities may develop. Malnutrition associated with measles can precipitate kwashiorkor and marasmus. Otitis media leads to mastoiditis and a hearing deficit. Measles exerts a major impact on infant and child development.

Diagnosis

The association of fever, cough, conjunctivitis, coryza, Koplik's spots in the mouth, and a morbilliform rash is usually diagnostic, but other conditions with dermatological manifestations have often been mistaken for measles; tick-borne and louse-borne typhus, meningococcaemia, scarlet fever and infectious mononucleosis are also associated with morbilliform rashes. There is a leucocytosis in the early stage(s), followed by an increase in lymphocytes—some of the Turk type.

During the prodromal phase large multinucleate (giant) cells can be visualized in stained smears of sputum or urine, or of Koplik's spots on the buccal mucosa. Serological tests on acute (IgM measles antibody) and convalescent sera reveal haemagglutination-inhibiting (HI) and neutralizing (N) antibodies, with a fourfold rise in titre following the initial infection. Immunoflourescent staining of cells may demonstrate measles antigen in smears from the nasopharynx or Koplik's spots.

Management

No chemotherapeutic agent influences the course of the viraemia. Food and fluid intake should be maintained, and rehydration undertaken.[8] Antibiotics are essential when otitis media, bacterial pneumonia and skin infections are present. Temperature control may lead to a reduction in febrile convulsions.

Epidemiology

Homo sapiens is the sole reservoir of infection. The incidence of measles worldwide is diminishing in developed countries, where the mean age of onset is now over 5 years. As infant immunization becomes more widely practised, the mean age of infection is rising; consequently, unprotected individuals and visitors to developing countries that have no immunization programme are at increased risk.

In developing countries, children generally develop the disease at 18–30 months; epidemics occur during the dry season when festivals and concourses of people take place. In isolated populations (e.g., nomadic ones) measles may occur at any age if the last exposure was many years previously. In large cities measles is endemic throughout the year; in smaller towns childhood epidemics occur every 2–3 years and infection spreads to the villages.

Control

Both passive immunization with human immunoglobulin and active immunization with a live attenuated vaccine are highly successful.[9–13]

Passive immunization

Passive immunization (human gammaglobulin 0.25 mg/kg) is effective if given within 5 days of exposure. In one study, passive immunization of children on admission to hospital gave complete protection—which was immediate.

Active immunization

A live attenuated strain of the virus is used; this gives a 98% seroconversion rate under ideal conditions. Fever of moderate severity and a mild rash occur rarely. Encephalitis is a rare complication. Immunization programmes now incorporate this vaccine into a triple vaccine containing live attenuated mumps, measles and rubella (MMR). MMR is given to all children in the second year of life with a booster at school entry. Immunity appears long lasting but the effects of immunizing HIV-positive children is not yet known. A high uptake of the vaccine may lead to increased herd immunity to the level where few susceptible hosts remain for the three viruses to survive in the community.

Contraindications to measles immunization include pregnancy, immunodeficiency states and hypersensitivity to eggs.

Maternal antibody is transferred transplacentally and this inhibits vaccine efficacy up to the age of 6 months. Normally, vaccination is aimed at children of 9 months of age,[14] but vaccination at 6 months, despite a lower seroconversion rate, is used in areas of high risk, sometimes in conjunction with a booster dose 1 year later. In order to eradicate the disease, immunization uptake rates of 90–95% are required.[15]

A 49% reduction in mortality rate in African children hospitalized with pneumonia and gastroenteritis has been recorded when measles vaccine was given as a routine admission procedure. Human immunoglobulin should be combined with measles vaccine in malnourished children.

Live vaccines are rapidly inactivated at room temperature, and the difficulty of maintaining the 'cold chain' is a major handicap to its use in most tropical countries. Monitoring of seroconversion rates should be a feature of all anti-measles campaigns.

An aerosol-administered vaccine has been successfully developed; it can be administered by anyone (with minimum qualifications) by hand pump, and should prove a great advance compared with previous methods of mass immunization. A heat-stable vaccine is under development. A major problem is that measles vaccination campaigns have to be repeated regularly; it is essential that measles vaccine is incorporated into the regular health-care system for rural areas, together with other immunizations.

Rubella (German measles)

Rubella is a mild systemic viral infection, with skin rashes as the cutaneous manifestation. The clinical importance of rubella lies in the potentially disastrous consequences of the infection in early pregnancy leading to severe congenital malformations.

Epidemiology

Rubella is less infectious than measles, and transmission occurs via the airborne route by person to person contact. The incubation period from exposure to development of fever is 14–21 days. A person with rubella remains infectious from 7 days before the onset of rash to 4–5 days afterwards.

Clinical features

After an incubation of 2–3 weeks, the patient may develop a mild pharyngitis, a gritty feeling in the eyes due to mild conjunctivitis, and fever. A macular skin rash appears on the second or third day; petechiae or papules are not common. The rash spreads down the face and behind the ears. A skin rash may not be present in all cases and thus the diagnosis may be difficult. The macules diffuse into one another, forming a generalized 'blush' by 2 days, and fading without desquamation in 4–5 days. Painful joints of the hands and feet are common in young adults, and suboccipital and posterior cervical lymphadenopathy are common. Differential diagnosis of a rubelliform skin rash includes:

Parvovirus infection.
Measles.
Enterovirus infection.
Scarlet fever.
Toxic shock syndrome.

Complications

Complications of rubella include: (a) idiopathic thrombo-cytopenic purpura, (b) encephalitis and (c) arthralgia. The thrombocytopenia is transient, lasting from 1 to 3 weeks. If the case is severe, intravenous immunoglobulin and steroids may be required. Encephailitis occurs in 1 in 5000 cases and is variable in severity.

Diagnosis

The following laboratory investigations are important in the diagnosis of rubella:

1. Serology. Two serological tests have been used widely:
   (a) detection of rubella-specific IgM by enzyme-linked immunosorbent assay (ELISA) or particle agglutination.
   (b) fourfold rise in haemagglutinin inhibition antibodies in paired sera.
2. Viral culture.
3. Detection of rubella-specific RNA fragments using polymerase chain reaction (PCR).

Other tests used for detection of immunity (before infection or post-vaccination immunity) in pregnant women include: (a) single radial haemolysis test and (b) passive haemagglutination test.

Prevention

Rubella vaccine is a live attenuated preparation of the virus. Live rubella vaccine is contraindicated in people with immunosuppression and in pregnancy. Rubella is a notifiable disease. Children should be excluded from school for at least 7 days after onset of the rash. Contact with pregnant women should be avoided and, where contact occurs during the first trimester of pregnancy, serological testing of the mother should be carried out to determine previous immunity to rubella.

Congenital rubella

Rubella is potentially teratogenic if contracted by the pregnant mother in the first 16 weeks of pregnancy. The main defects caused by rubella in the fetus are a triad of: (a) cataract, (b) nerve deafness and (c) heart abnormalities (e.g. patent ductus arteriosus, ventricular septal defect (VSD), pulmonary artery stenosis, Fallot's tetralogy). Affected infants also have a generalized infection which, together with the congenital defects, is called the rubella syndrome. The physical signs may include: (a) hepato-splenomegaly; thrombocytopenic purpura, low birth weight, intellectual impairment, jaundice, anaemia, and lesions in the metaphysis of long bones.

Diagnosis of maternal rubella

Recent infection is diagnosed by detection of rubella-specific IgM antibodies via ELISA or immunoflourescence. PCR may detect rubella-sepcific RNA fragments.

Management

Antenatal mothers less than 16 weeks' pregnant with rubella are best advised to terminate the pregnancy. Those who find this unacceptable may be given passive immunization with immunoglobulin, which may have some attenuating or prophylactic effect.

DNA viruses that cause cutaneous disease

Table 48.2 lists DNA viruses that cause cutaneous disease in humans.

Diseases due to pox viruses

Orthopox viruses

Poxviruses are DNA viruses that are especially adapted to epidermal cells. The orthopox viruses are DNA double-stranded viruses, brick or ovoid shaped, and 200–250 nm in size; they are all antigenically related and include cowpox, ectromelia (mice), monkeypox, Turkmenia rodent pox and vaccinia. The only members of the group that have infected humans are variola (smallpox), vaccinia (see Chapters 9 and 23), monkeypox and cowpox. Tanapox, although not an orthopox virus, is closely related.

Smallpox

Smallpox was formerly a devastating, severe, febrile illness characterized by an extensive, profuse, vesicular rash and a high mortality rate. Survivors were left with severe disfiguring facial scars. The human smallpox virus was one of the most fatal of all viral infections and it is probably the only infectious disease that has been eradicated globally. The success of this eradication programme was based on several factors:

1. Human beings were the only hosts.
2. An effective vaccine inducing solid immunity was available.
3. Governments were committed to the vaccination programmes. This was backed up the World Health Organization's 'search and containment' campaigns where cases were isolated and contacts traced and vaccinated.

The world has been free from smallpox for the past two decades and the eradication campaign is heralded as one of the most successful carried out by the WHO.

Monkeypox
Geographical distribution
This disease is confined to tropical Africa (Figure 48.2). Although monkeypox has been recorded since 1958 in captive monkeys, the first human case was recognized in Zaire in 1970;[16,17] since then more than 200 cases have

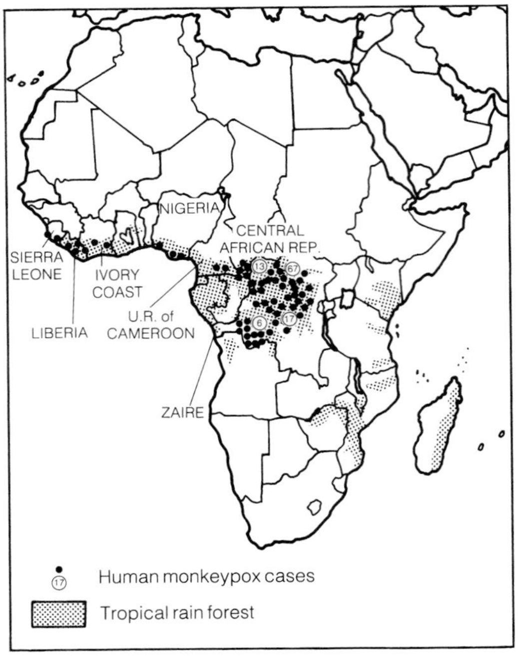

Figure 48.2: Geographical distribution of human monkeypox showing number of cases reported from 1970 to 1984. (Courtesy of the World Health Organization.)

been reported, mainly in Zaire, but also in Liberia, Nigeria, Ivory Coast, Cameroon and Sierra Leone. Monkeypox has been reported only rarely outside these areas of tropical rainforest.

Aetiology

The causative agent is a 'brick-shaped' orthopox virus (200–250 nm in size) which forms cytoplasmic inclusions and is morphologically indistinguishable from variola. It can be readily distinguished in culture because the pocks on chick chorio-allantoic membrane are slightly larger and more haemorrhagic than those caused by variola. Unlike variola, monkeypox virus is pathological in rabbits, and has a higher temperature ceiling for growth. It grows readily in the green monkey and rodent cell cultures. Four strains of poxviruses have been isolated from monkey kidney cells and from rodents; these differ from monkeypox, but are closely related to variola, from which they can be distinguished by DNA analysis. These are known as 'whitepox' viruses; their relation to human infection is unknown.

Transmission

The usual mode of transmission from monkey to humans is unclear, but infection is sometimes direct, resulting from handling dead monkeys for eating, or by droplet spread via the respiratory tract.[16] Transmission by a chimpanzee bite has also been recorded. The disease is not readily transmitted from person to person, but secondary cases have been recorded. Little tertiary spread occurs, and epidemic spread is not a feature.

Pathology

Few individuals are known to have died from monkeypox; no autopsies have been performed, and therefore histopathological information is not available. It seems likely that pathological changes resemble those previously attributable to smallpox.

Immunity

There is well defined immunity to reinfection, and complete cross-immunity with variola and vaccinia. Monkeypox has never been recorded in an individual vaccinated for smallpox.[16]

Natural history

Monkeypox infection in humans is a dead-end infection, manifesting itself as a typical smallpox-like illness. It possesses a 2–3-day prodromal period, and the smallpox-like rash evolves over 2–4 days. The illness is usually mild, and is followed by complete recovery. When death has occurred, it has usually been in children.

Clinical features

The incubation period is 5–17 days. The onset is abrupt with fever and a prodromal illness lasting 2–3 days.[16] On the third day a rash appears; this consists of a single crop of discrete papules, more abundant on the face and extremities than on the trunk. The soles of the feet and palms are involved. The papules form pustules which become umbilicated and are covered with crusts which separate after about 10 days, leaving small scars. Marked lymphadenopathy may occur (Figure 48.3). Mild atypical cases occur in which there may be fewer than ten lesions, separation of the crusts occurring by the fifth day. There have not been any recorded complications.

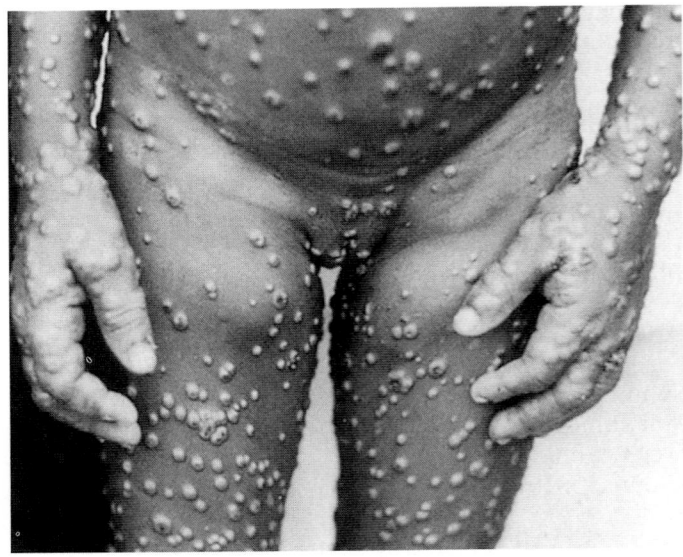

Figure 48.3: Monkeypox, showing characteristic inguinal and femoral lymphadenopathy. (Reproduced with permission from Breman J G, Kalisa-Ruti, Steniowski M V et al. *Bull World Health Org* 1980; 58: 849–868.)

Diagnosis

The differential diagnosis was formerly from smallpox; diagnosis is based on epidemiology and a history of contact with monkeys.[16] Lymphadenopathy was an important distinguishing feature. Isolation of the virus, together with its cultural characteristics and antigenic structure, provide the definitive diagnosis.

Management

Treatment is symptomatic and supportive.

Epidemiology

It is not known whether the primary maintenance hosts are chimpanzees, other primates or small mammals. Most patients give a clear account of contact with monkeys which they have caught and/or eaten.[16,17] Most cases occur during the dry season. Children are affected more than adults. The attack rate is 10% in susceptible individuals in close contact with a primary case, in contrast to smallpox infection in which it was 20%. Secondary spread occurs amongst families, but tertiary transmission is rare and epidemics are not a feature. Now that vaccination level in communities has fallen dramatically, human monkeypox may become more common.

Tanapox

Tanapox[18] was first described in 1957 and 1962 in epidemics in the lower Tana River of Kenya. Serological surveys have shown continuing transmission along the lower Tana River. Human infections have since been recorded in the forest area of Zaire. A closely related virus has been isolated from outbreaks in primate colonies in the USA, and in contacts of human cases.

Aetiology

Tanapox virus is not an orthopox virus; with the Yabapox virus it forms a distinct subgroup of poxviruses. It cannot be cultured on chick chorio-allantoic membrane, but grows well on green monkey kidney cell and Vero cell cultures.

Transmission

Epidemiological studies suggest that the virus is transmitted from monkeys to humans by mosquitoes; outbreaks in humans have occurred in low-lying country near the Tana River after floods had isolated wild animals, humans and their domestic animals on islands in the flood water, on which *Mansonia uniformis* and *M. africanus* had proliferated in immense numbers. There is no evidence of direct person-to-person spread.

Pathology

Pathology is limited to the epidermis—where the pock forms. There are few or no destructive changes. Hypertrophied epidermal cells containing acidophilic inclusion bodies predominate; cellular infiltration is mild, and the dermis escapes intact.

Immunity

Virtually nothing is known about second attacks. Antibodies that develop in infected individuals and monkeys persist for some years. There is no cross-immunity with vaccinia; recently vaccinated people can develop the disease.

Clinical features

The infection is usually mild; fever heralds the appearance of one or two pock-like lesions. Complete recovery follows.

Symptoms and signs

The incubation period is unknown. Onset is abrupt with fever lasting 3–4 days, accompanied in some cases by severe headache and prostration. Severity is open to doubt because histories have usually been recorded retrospectively, long after the event—in the major published studies. During the febrile episode one or two (but never more) pock-like lesions appear on the skin, resembling those formerly caused by smallpox. Lesions become umbilicated; they never proceed to pustule formation, but form firm cheesy centres instead (Figure 48.4). The pocks occur mainly on the exposed surfaces: upper arms, face, neck and trunk, but never on the hands, legs or feet. Recovery takes place rapidly; no scars are left and there are no residual complications.

Diagnosis

Tanapox had formerly to be distinguished from modified smallpox in a vaccinated person; the character of the

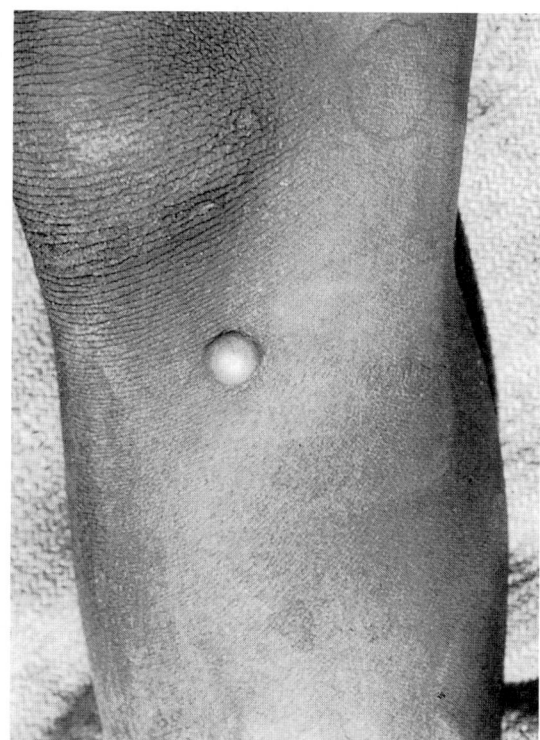

Figure 48.4: Tanapox. Solid pock containing firm cheesy material.

pock (which at first looks like smallpox) differs in its larger size, firm, solid nature and absence of pustulation. Electron microscopical appearances are similar to those previously associated with smallpox. Virus can be isolated by culture in green monkey kidney or Vero cells, and is clearly distinguished by antigenic structure from orthopox viruses. Serum antibodies develop slowly, but complement fixation and neutralizing tests on both human and monkey sera show antibody at low titre; this persists for some years and can be used for a retrospective diagnosis.

Management
Treatment is not required and patients make a complete recovery.

Epidemiology
The epidemiology is poorly understood. The primary maintenance hosts are unknown; many monkeys, especially vervet (*Cercopithecus aethiops*) are susceptible, and are common in endemic area(s). Small outbreaks have occurred after flooding, but transmission was shown to be continuing along the lower Tana River in serological surveys carried out in 1971 and 1976; infection has persisted since 1962. Antibodies were detected in 9.2% of the population, and in children between the ages of 2 and 12 years. There is no evidence of direct person-to-person transmission.

Molluscum contagiosum

Molluscum contagiosum (MC) causes a wart-like skin condition and is produced by a poxvirus infection of the prickle cell layer of the skin.[19] Infection is transmitted by contact. The infected cells proliferate, vacuolate, enlarge and protrude above the skin surface as pearly, *umbilicated* lesions. The central cavity of the lesion contains white, pulpy material with infectious vacuolated cells. Accumulation of the molluscum bodies in the cytoplasm causes compression of the nucleus to the periphery of the cell, leading to rupture of the cell and thus infecting adjacent cells.

The lesions occur in groups, on the face, arms or near genitals, and their appearance is diagnostic. The number of lesions in HIV-positive individuals can exceed 100 (Figure 48.5), leading to coalescence of lesions forming large plaques with many smaller lesions ('agminate form'). In some cases, MC infection can induce a localized dermatitis known as *molluscum dermatitis*.

In immunocompetent individuals the lesions are self-limiting and regress spontaneously with time (6–12 weeks). Lesions in HIV-positive individuals do not usually resolve spontaneously-persisting for months or even years, although marked improvements in MC are now being observed in patients receiving highly active antiretroviral therapy (HAART).

Diagnosis
The diagnosis of MC is usually on clinical grounds; however, HIV-positive patients may have other lesions of

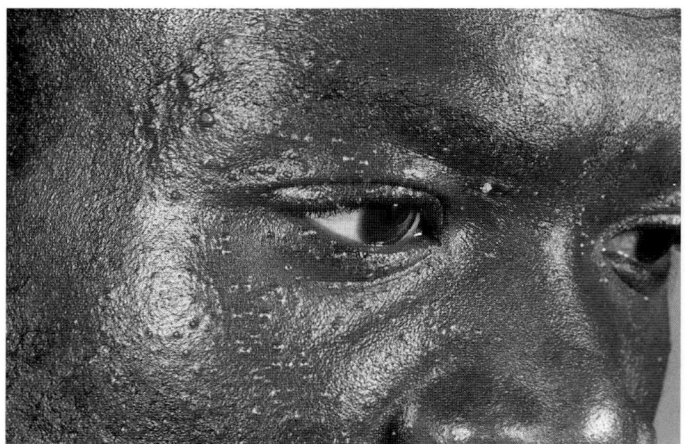

Figure 48.5: Molluscum contagiosum—multiple facial lesions.

similar appearance, such as those caused by cryptococcosis, cutaneous pneumocystosis and other infectious disorders. Solitary MC lesions may resemble other entities (e.g., pyogenic granuloma, keratoacanthoma and basal cell carcinoma). A biopsy can be taken to exclude more serious conditions.

Management
Treatment of persisting lesions is by physical means, including cryotherapy, electrosurgery, topical keratolytic preparations, cantharidin and curettage. These methods may be effective; however, they can be very painful and may lead to scarring and discoloration of the skin. An orange stick dipped in 80% phenol solution is sometimes used to pierce the umbilicated centre. This must not be used on the face or near the genitalia. Other treatment modalities that have been used with moderate success include wax stripping and application of salicylic acid pastes.

Human herpesviruses

The human herpesvirus family[20] includes eight viruses that cause disease *Homo sapiens* (Table 48.3). All herpesviruses are enveloped double-stranded DNA viruses that have the property of remaining latent in viable form within host cells after primary infection. The herpesviruses can reactivate from time to time from the latent

Table 48.3 Human herpesviruses.

HHV-1	Herpes simplex virus (HSV) type 1
HHV-2	Herpes simplex virus (HSV) type 2
HHV-3	Varicella–zoster virus (VZV)
HHV-4	Epstein–Barr virus (EBV)
HHV-5	Cytomegalovirus (CMV)
HHV-6	Human herpesvirus 6
HHV-7	Human herpesvirus 7
HHV-8	Human herpesvirus 8 (KSAHV)

state to produce recurrent clinical lesions, many of which have cutaneous manifestations.

Herpes simplex viruses

Herpes simplex viruses[21] are unusual among viruses in causing a wide variety of clinical syndromes. Two types of herpes simplex virus cause human disease:

1. Herpes simplex virus type 1 (HSV-1).
2. Herpes simplex virus Type 2 (HSV-2).

The basic pathological lesions are cutaneous or muco-cutaneous vesicles, and transmission of HSV involves direct contact with either active lesions on skin or mucous membranes, or areas of asymptomatic viral shedding from saliva, semen or cervical secretions. Diseases due to herpes simplex viruses can be grouped into two categories:

1. Primary disease.
2. Reactivation disease.

Primary HSV infections

Primary clinical disease occurs when the virus is first encountered. Transmission is by contact (kissing or touching). Most primary infections are asymptomatic. When primary infection causes disease, a range of clinical manifestations can occur. HSV-1 mainly causes lesions affecting the orofacial region, whereas HSV-2 mainly causes lesions affecting the anogenital region; HSV-1 can, in a small proportion of cases, cause anogenital lesions while HSV type 2 can cause orofacial lesions.

Clinical syndromes due to HSV type 1 (orofacial)

1. Gingivostomatitis (vesicles or ulcers in and around gums and mouth) (Figure 48.6).
2. Ocular herpes: keratoconjunctivitis (vesicles or ulcers on eyelids, conjunctiva, cornea) (Figure 48.7).
3. Meningoencephalitis.

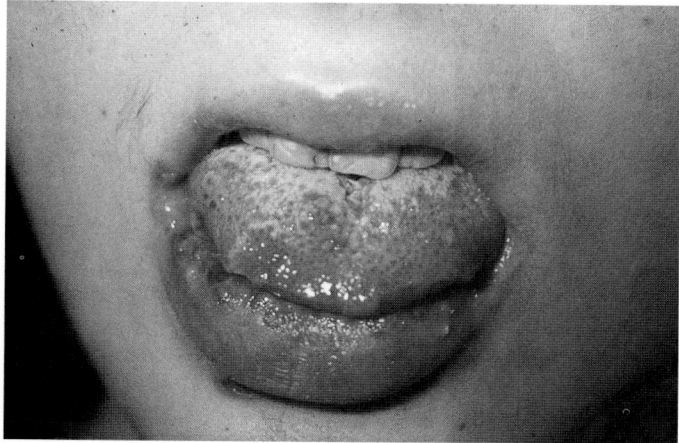

Figure 48.6: Herpes simplex lesions around the mouth (gingivostomatitis).

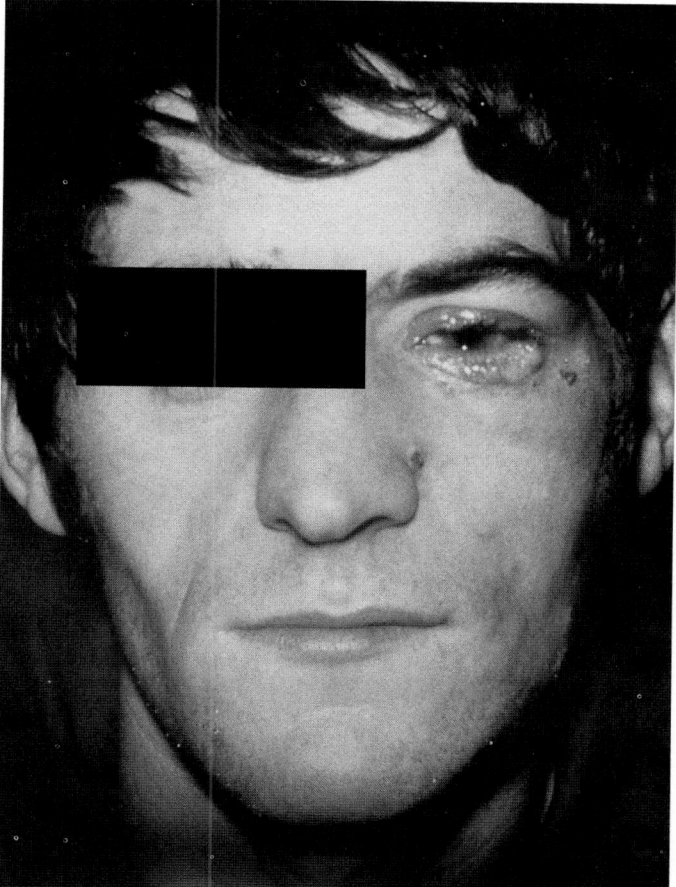

Figure 48.7: Herpes simplex virus ocular lesions (keratoconjunctivitis).

Clinical syndromes due to HSV type 2 (anogenital)

1. Balanoposthitis (vesicles or ulcers on prepuce and glans penis).
2. Vulvovaginitis (vesicles or ulcers on vulva and vaginal mucosa).
3. Anoproctitis (vesicles or ulcers around the anal skin and in the anus).

Other clinical cutaneous syndromes due to herpes simplex

1. *Herpetic whitlow* is the term given to herpes simplex vesicles on fingertips. This is an occupational hazard of doctors, nurses and anaesthetists who deal with unconscious patients; herpes infection is acquired through fingertip contamination. The lesion looks similar to a staphylococcal whitlow, but the exudate is serous rather than purulent.
2. *Kaposi's varicelliform eruption.* This is a superinfection by herpes simplex of eczematous skin, seen mainly in young children. It may progress to a serious disease with a significant mortality rate.
3. *Neonatal infection.* Primary genital infection in the mother (HSV-2) can give rise to severe generalized

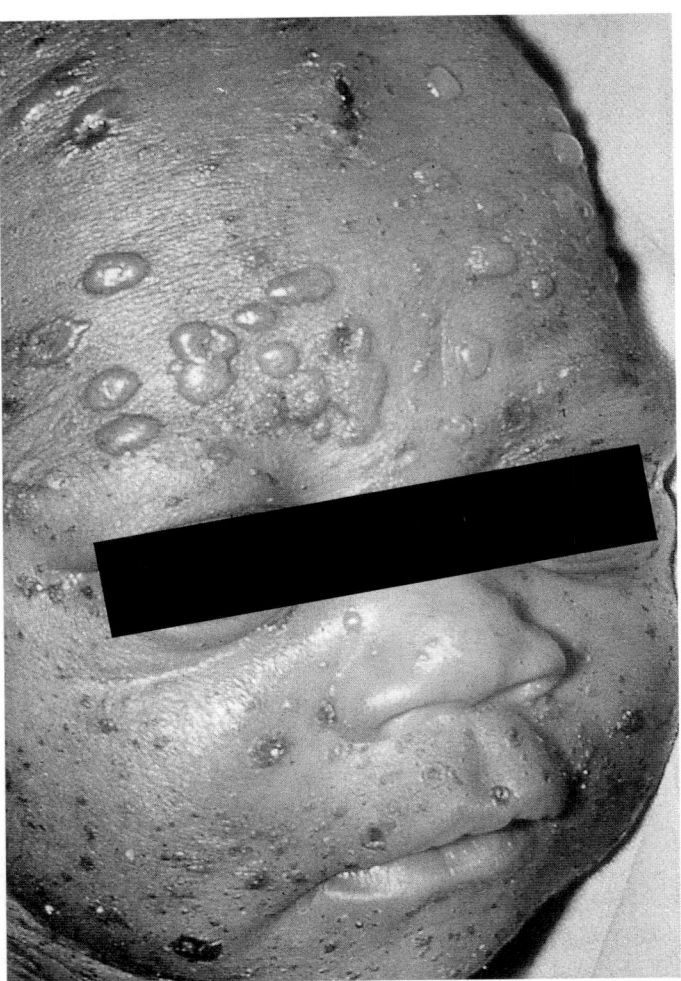

Figure 48.8: Generalized herpes simplex vesicular skin lesions.

infection in neonates (Figure 48.8). Affected children may have jaundice, hepatosplenomegaly, thrombocytopenia and large vesicular lesions on the skin. There is a high case fatality rate.

Latency

After a primary mucocutaneous infection, HSV enters nerve endings underlying the skin lesion and travels up the peripheral nerve to nerve cell bodies in the dorsal root ganglion (DRG). HSV then enters a latency stage in the DRG for days to years. Reactivation can occur as a result of immunosuppression, physical or emotional stress, fever (e.g., orofacial herpes is common in patients with lobar pneumonia and malaria), skin damage, menstruation, fatigue or ultra-violet light. During reactivation, HSV is transmitted back to the primary mucocutaneous site via efferent nerves. Reactivation may recur sporadically throughout life.

Primary HSV infections in HIV-infected individuals

Up to half of HIV-positive patients have clinical

manifestations of a herpesvirus infection in the course of the disease, and these tend to be more severe and persistent than recurrences in normal host individuals.[19,22] In HIV-positive individuals, primary infections may be so severe that they are life threatening, or may manifest as chronic ulcerative mucocutaneous lesions, verrucous plaques or hyperplastic nodules. Painful and often deep, these chronic ulcers usually present around the perianal area, penis and lips.[23] HSV can affect other areas in HIV-positive patients, such as the cornea, tracheobronchial tree, oesophagus, lung, pericardium, liver and brain.

As one of the leading causes of genital ulcers, HSV may enhance acquisition of HIV via reduced epithelial barriers and by localizing CD4+ cells, the primary target of HIV, to the ulcers. It is hypothesized that antigenic stimulation of mucosal sites by reactivation of HSV can potentially increase HIV-1 replication on mucosal surfaces.

The differential diagnosis of HSV includes all causes of ulceration. Ulcerated lesions can mimic: (a) aphthous ulcers, (b) cytomegalovirus (CMV) ulcers, (c) drug reactions, (d) opportunistic atypical mycobacterial infections, (e) fungal infections and (f) traumatic ulcers. Verrucous-appearing lesions can mimic such entities as warts and epithelial neoplasms.

Diagnosis of HSV infections

Confirmation can be made from: (1) smears of lesions, (2) vesicular fluid (can be obtained by placing a small needle into vesicle and aspirating) and (3) tissue biopsy to several laboratory investigations. These include: (a) culture of virus, (b) electron microscopic visualization, (c) serology (complement fixation test; immunfluorescence for antigen and antibody detection; ELISA for anti-HSV IgM antibodies) and (d) DNA amplification tests (e.g., PCR).[24]

Treatment of HSV infections

Antiviral drugs are rarely required in primary infections in an immunocompetent individual. Topical acylcovir preparations may provide relief from tingling senstation and shorten the duration of lesions. Treatment of HSV infections in immunocompromised individuals is described below.

Varicella–zoster virus infections

Varicella (chickenpox) and zoster (shingles or herpes zoster) are different diseases caused by the same virus. Varicella is a primary illness, whereas zoster is a reactivation disease.

Varicella (chickenpox)

Chickenpox is a systemic viral infection with a characteristic cutaneous vesicular rash. The primary infection usually occurs in young children and is always symptomatic; in the majority of cases recovery is complete. The disease may be severe and fatal in infants aged less than 2 weeks, in adults and in the immunosuppressed.

Incubation period and transmission

The incubation period for chickenpox is 12–24 days, averaging 15–18 days. Chickenpox is transmitted by person-to-person contact, or by airborne spread of respiratory secretions or vesicular fluid. The infectious period is usually 1–2 days before and up to 6 days after appearance of the rash. This may be prolonged in the presence of immunodeficiency.

Clinical features

Children rarely have prodromal symptoms, whereas adults may experience fever, headache and myalgia. The appearance of a skin rash on the trunk is often the first sign of disease. The macule rapidly progresses to a papule and forms a clear vesicle; vesicles are oval, with their long axis along creases of skin. These evolve to opaque pustules and may become umbilicated as they dry to crusts. New waves of lesions occur as the older ones evolve (cropping). Successive crops of lesions are smaller and eventually fail to develop. Lesions appear most densely on the trunk and face; the hands and feet are relatively spared. Lesions may affect the conjunctivae, buccal mucosa, intestinal mucosa, and lungs.

In immunosuppressed patients (post-transplantation, corticosteroid therapy, HIV/AIDS), primary chickenpox infection may cause a serious clinical disease with extensive cutaneous and systemic manifestations[25] (Figure 48.9). Treatment is with intravenous antiviral agents.

Complications

Systemic involvement: Widespread systemic involvement may sometimes occur. Chickenpox pneumonia, disseminated intravascular coagulation, and abnormal renal and hepatic function may result in a life-threatening illness. Patients with chickenpox pneumonia may have secondary bacterial infections. Those who survive chickenpox pneumonia may have calcified lesions on chest radiography. Post-chickenpox encephalitis can occur, and is mild and self-limiting leading to a complete recovery in most cases. Patients may present with a cerebellar disturbance (ataxia, nystagmus). Thrombocytopenia may occur, manifesting clinically as purpura and haematuria, and the rash may appear haemorrhagic (Figure 48.10).

Secondary bacterial infections: As the skin vesicles burst leaving an itchy surface, secondary infection with *Staphylococcus aureus* or *Streptococcus pyogenes* may occur. These may sometimes progress to toxic shock syndrome, scarlet fever or erysipelas.

Diagnosis of chickenpox

Diagnosis of chickenpox is usually obvious on clinical examination. Confirmation can be made by subjecting smears of vesicular lesions, vesicular fluid (can be obtained by placing a small needle into a vesicle and aspirating) and tissue biopsy to several laboratory investigations: (a) culture of virus, (b) electron microscopic visualization, (c)

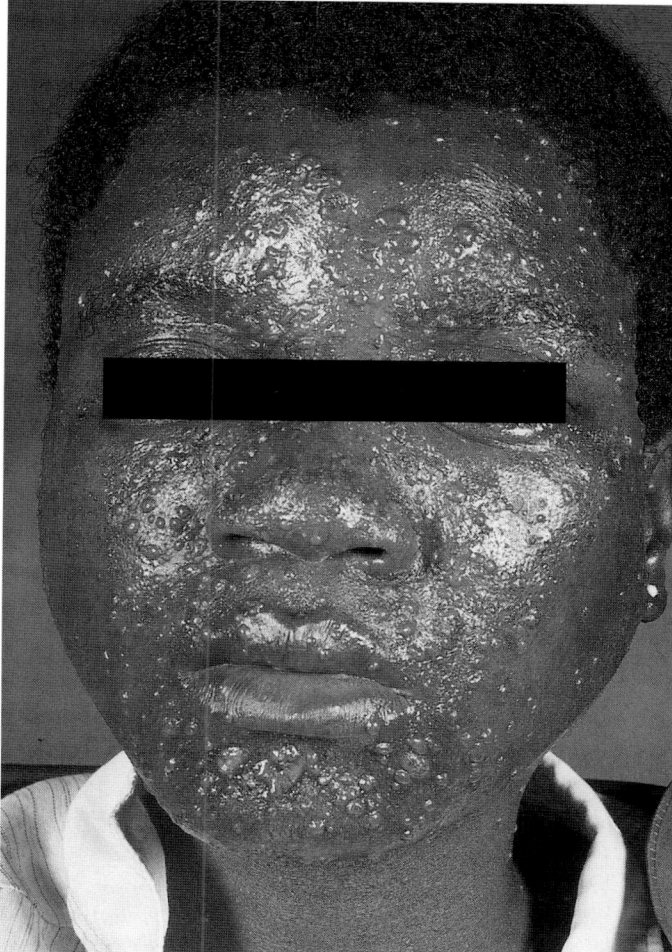

Figure 48.9: Severe chickenpox lesions in an immunosuppressed patient.

serology (complement fixation test; immunfluorescence for antigen and antibody detection; ELISA) and (d) DNA amplification tests (e.g., PCR).

Management

Most patients recover without specific treatment. Pruritus may be reduced by antihistamines. Oral acclover (10 mg/kg five times a day for 5 days) reduces the duration of fever and active rash (from 6.5 to 5.7 days). Aspirin (acetylsalicylic acid) should not be used for reduction of fever or analgesia because of the association with Reye's syndrome.

Treatment of chickenpox pneumonia requires early infusion with acclover (10 mg/kg 8 hourly intravenously), infusion being given slowly over 1 hour to avoid nephrotoxicity, which is related to peak levels. Urea, creatinine and electrolytes must be monitored during therapy. Secondary bacterial infections are common and thus broad-spectrum antibiotics with antistaphylococcal activity must be used. Arterial oxygen saturation must be monitored where possible; patients with falling oxygen saturations may require assisted ventilation. Newer antiviral agents effective against all herpesviruses are described below (see

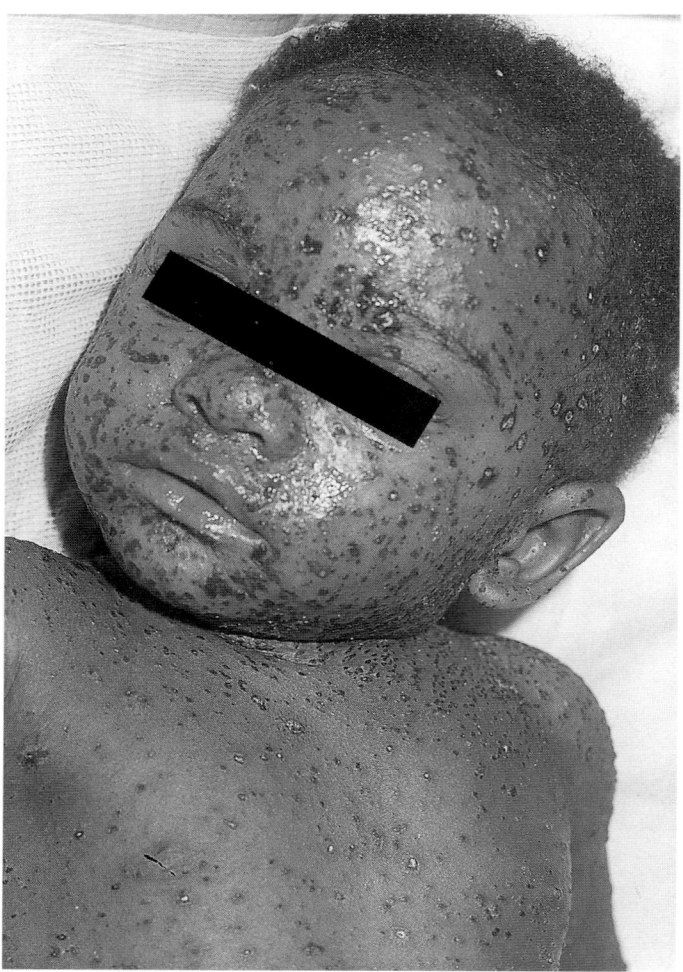

Figure 48.10: Haemorrhagic chickenpox in a child.

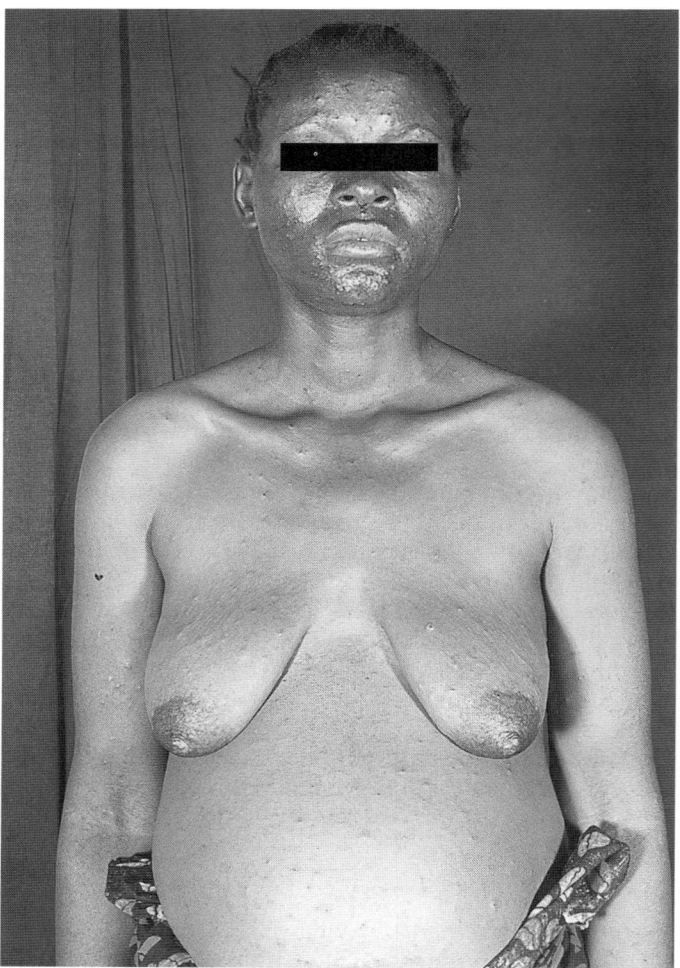

Figure 48.11: Chickenpox in a pregnant woman.

section on treatment of herpes viruses). Thrombocytopenia can be managed by a short course of corticosteroids and/or immunoglobulin. Platelet transfusion should be given, depending on the platelet count.

Prevention and control
Live varicella vaccines have been developed and shown to be highly effective.[26]

Passive immunization using varicella–zoster immunoglobulin (VZIG) is indicated for use in: (a) leukaemic and other immunosuppressed patients who do not have a previous history of chickenpox, and have been in contact with patients with chickenpox or zoster; (b) neonates whose mothers develop chickenpox (Figure 48.11) 7 days before or after delivery; and (c) non-immune pregnant contacts.

Children with chickenpox should be excluded from school for 1 week after the appearance of the rash. Patients are no longer infectious when the lesions are dry and scabbed. In hospital, because of the risk to other susceptible patients, all patients with zoster and chickenpox should be isolated.

Shingles or zoster
Varicella zoster virus produces lifelong latency and may reactivate later in life causing the clinical entity 'shingles'. The varicella–zoster virus (VZV) remains dormant in the dorsal root ganglia until reactivation, at which time it travels down the nerve to manifest the typical cutaneous lesions of zoster (shingles), which presents as a vesicular eruption along the distribution of one or two dermatomes served by a dorsal root ganglia (Figure 48.12). The mechanism of reactivation is unclear, although it is related clinically to stress, ageing, underlying malignancy and immunosuppression.

Clinical features
Patients with herpes zoster typically experience a prodromal phase which may manifest as pain, numbness, tingling and/or itching in a specific dermatomal distribution on any part of the body. This is commonly followed by an eruption of vesicles in the dermatomal distribution, on an erythematous base. Often the prodromal pain can be so severe as to lead to a misdiagnosis of myocardial infarction or an abdominal

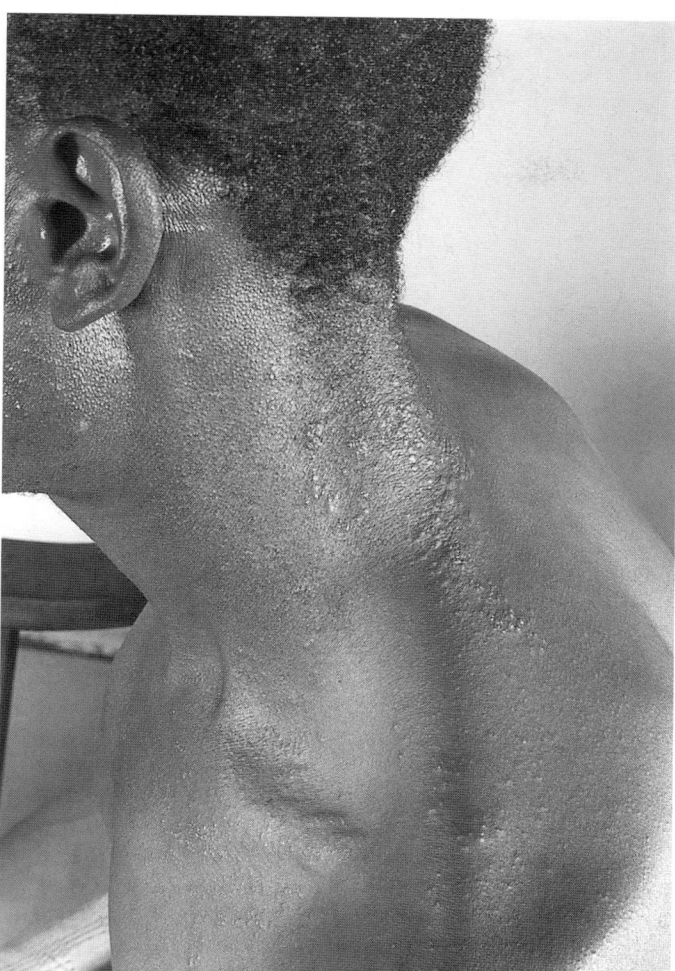

Figure 48.12: Herpes zoster (shingles) affecting a single dermatome.

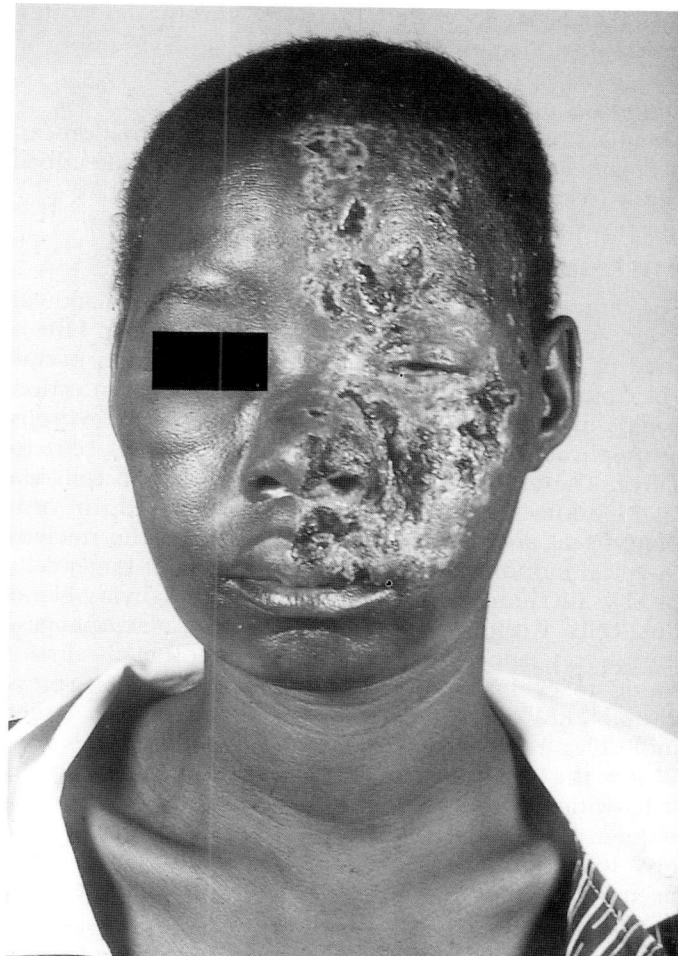

Figure 48.13: Multidermatomal herpes zoster in a patient with AIDS.

emergency. The usual dermatomal distribution is unilateral in appearance; however, a large number of cases of multidermatomal zoster[27] (Figure 48.13) are being seen in patients infected with HIV infection. Zoster generally appears within 2–7 years of HIV seroconversion, most commonly during the asymptomatic phase. In these cases zoster is more severe, more intense and more difficult to treat, leaving serious scarring. Shingles is now being seen frequently in HIV-positive children (Figure 48.14).

Complications

Ophthalmic zoster must be treated aggressively and watched carefully because there is a high likelihood of eye involvement resulting in conjunctivitis and blindness. The risk of postherpetic neuralgia tends to increase with age but not with immunosuppression, and pain may continue for months or even years (postherpetic neuralgia).

Complications of zoster in immunocompromized individuals include dissemination over large areas of the skin with possible secondary infection, potentially fatal pulmonary involvement, and encephalitis. Zoster also tends to have a higher rate of recurrence (5–23%) in HIV-

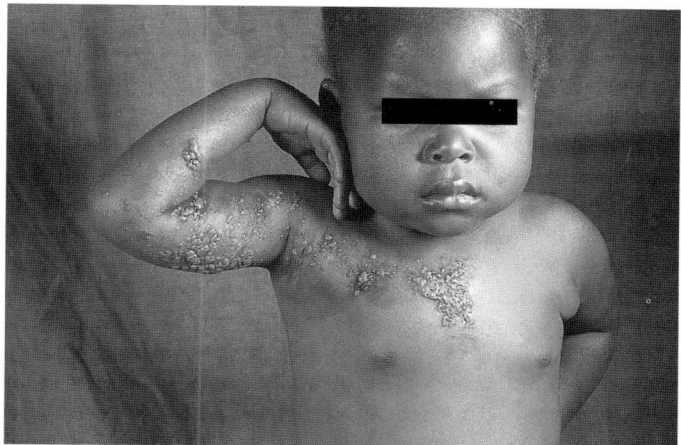

Figure 48.14: Herpes zoster in an HIV-positive child.

infected individuals, compared with a rate of less than 5% in normal hosts. In addition to the severe pain experienced by patients with postherpetic neuralgia, crusted, punched-out ulcerations that leave painful atrophic scars (Figure 48.13) may also occur. Verrucous plaques can also occur in zoster; these are chronic and often resistant to therapy with acclovir.

Diagnosis of zoster

The diagnosis is usually a clinical one. Confirmation can be made using the laboratory investigations described below (see section on diagnosis of herpesvirus).

Epstein–Barr virus

The clinical disease 'infectious mononucleosis' or 'glandular fever' is caused by the Epstein–Barr virus (EBV). EBV is shed in pharyngeal secretions, and transmission occurs via close contact (e.g., kissing). Primary EBV infection begins in oropharyngeal epithelium, where EBV virions are replicated and released from the epithelial cells to saliva. The virions carrying gp350/220 infect B cells via CD21 molecules, or receptors for the C3d in oropharyngeal areas, and form an episome in the nucleus (atypical mononuclear cells). Although major target cells of EBV are human B cells, epithelial cells, salivary gland duct cells, T cells, natural killer (NK) cells, macrophages/monocytes, smooth muscle cells and endothelial cells are found to be infected. The EBV-infected B cells express various EBV-associated antigens that are the target molecules recognized by the host immune response. When the immune surveillance system breaks down, reactivation of EBV-infected B cells occurs with subsequent polyclonal proliferation and dissemination of EBV to other tissues. Over 50% of healthy adults have been previously infected with EBV or human herpesvirus 4, which usually remains in a latent phase.

Clinical features

In primary infection the virus selectively infects B lymphocytes as well as certain types of squamous epithelia; this manifests as infectious mononucleosis. The virus replicates primarily in the oropharyngeal epithelium, followed by entry into the B-cell system, where it remains latent until reactivation or dissemination to other sites. In HIV-infected individuals with severe immunodeficiency, viral replication leads to the clinical manifestations of: hairy leucoplakia, Burkitt's lymphoma or EBV-associated large cell lymphoma (Chapter 36).

Cutaneous manifestations of EBV infection

In immunocompetent patients the cutaneous manifestations of infectious mononucleosis may include a petechial skin rash (due to thrombocytopenia) or a macular skin one due to use of ampicillin. The mucocutaneous manifestations of EBV in HIV-infected patients[28] include oral hairy leucoplakia (OHL),[29] correlating with moderate to advanced immunodeficiency. As with zoster, OHL has also been linked with advance from HIV infection to AIDS, and manifests as whitish plaques on the inferolateral margins of the tongue (Figure 48.15). The surface of the plaques may be smooth, corrugated or folded with thick hair-like projections. Lesions of OHL can mimic other mucous membrane lesions such as tobacco-associated

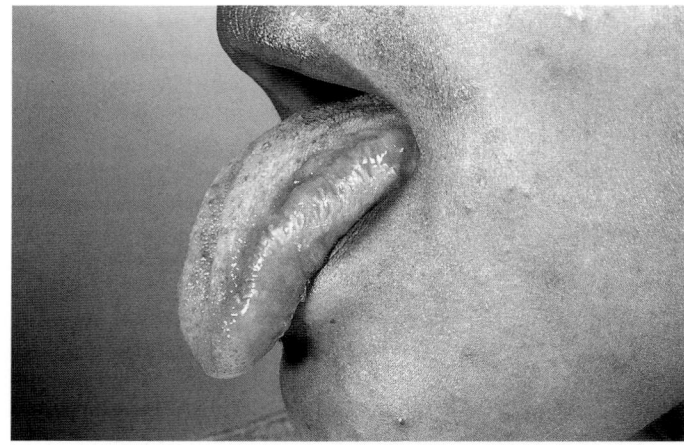

Figure 48.15: Hairy leucoplakia of the tongue.

leucoplakia and candidiasis. Lesions caused by OHL cannot be dislodged by a tongue depressor. They are asymptomatic and cause few problems; however, they occasionally become verrucous and may lead to dysphagia.

Differential diagnosis

OHL must be distinguished from candidiasis by the absence of hyphae in a microscopic examination of scrapings. Lesions caused by OHL can also mimic tobacco-associated leucoplakia, squamous cell carcinoma, condyloma acuminatum, lichen planus, white sponge naevus, leucokeratosis oris, mucous patches of syphilis and aphthous ulcers.

EBV and human cancer

EBV has been linked epidemiologically with two human cancers: (a) Burkitt's lymphoma and (b) nasopharyngeal carcinoma (see Chapter 36).

Diagnosis

Diagnosis is made by detection of viral capsid antigen (VCA) and anti-IgM anti-EBV capsid antibody. A monospot (Paul Bunnell) test to detect heterophile antibodies may be useful in diagnosing glandular fever. Molecular methods using PCR may detect EBV DNA in peripheral blood mononuclear cells.

Management

Treatment is palliative: no specific treatment is available.

Cytomegalovirus

Human cytomegalovirus (CMV or human herpesvirus (HHV-5) is a ubiquitous member of the herpes family of viruses.[30] More than 80% of healthy adults are seropositive for CMV, indicating previous exposure. After primary infection, usually asymptomatic, CMV, like other herpes viruses, undergoes latency, persisting in the infected individual. It is not clear which types of cell can harbour the virus and support an on-going infection, nor is it clear whether leucocytes behave as specific carriers of the virus during a systemic infection, or represent a reservoir of replicating virus or a possible site of latency. The mechanism of reactivation is unknown. Although dermatologists are generally familiar with cutaneous manifestations of infection with herpes simplex virus and varicella–zoster virus, CMV infection has seldom been discussed.

CMV rarely causes symptomatic disease in the immunocompetent individual. It became a significant clinical problem after the introduction of transplantation and associated immunosuppressive therapy. Nowadays, about 90% of patients with AIDS develop acute active CMV infection at some point during their illness; it is one of the most common opportunistic viral infection in patients with AIDS.[31,32] About 95% of HIV-positive patients with a CD4 count of less than 100 cells/mm^3 have clinical manifestations of CMV.

Clinical features

A typical CMV viraemia is found as basophilic intranuclear inclusions, or 'owl's eyes' (Figure 48.16), in urine, tears, breast milk, faeces, semen, cervical secretions, blood, bronchoalveolar lavage specimens and saliva. This viraemia is usually followed by infection of the vascular endothelium of every organ, skin rash, vasculitis and ulceration of mucosal surfaces.

Cutaneous lesions of CMV can have a varied presentation, including:

1. Localized and diffuse ulceration.
2. Keratotic verrucous lesions.
3. Palpable purpuric papules.
4. Vesicular, bullous and generalized morbilliform eruptions.
5. Hyperpigmented indurated plaques.
6. Generalized bullous toxic epidermal necrolysis-like eruption associated with CMV hepatitis.

Other clinical manifestations of a CMV infection include retinitis and gastroenteritis in about 50% of all patients with AIDS. Up to 10% of patients have serious CMV

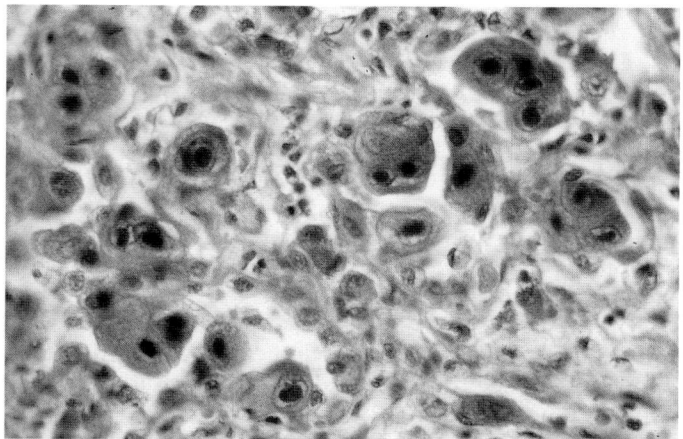

Figure 48.16: Intranuclear inclusions in a CMV infection.

pneumonia, CMV retinitis (increasing to 30% at autopsy), oesophagitis, colitis and proctocolitis causing perianal ulceration,[26] which is believed to be a contiguous spread to the skin from the gastrointestinal tract. Lesions caused by CMV can also appear ulcerated, and must be distinguished from other ulcerated lesions as described for HSV.

Diagnosis

Cutaneous manifestations of CMV infection are not sufficiently distinctive to allow the diagnosis to be made on *clinical* findings alone. The diagnosis of cutaneous CMV involvement has usually been established by microscopic examination. Cytomegalic inclusions, CMV antigens or CMV DNA detected in skin biopsy specimens have been considered a significant sign to diagnose cutaneous CMV infection. However, whether CMV detected in skin biopsy specimens is responsible for the pathogenesis of cutaneous manifestations is still controversial, because the characteristic cytomegalic cells in biopsy specimens taken from uninvolved skin in a patient with AIDS have been detected.

There are no laboratory assays that are diagnostic of recent infection. Standard methods applied to all herpes viruses are used in the diagnosis of CMV.

Microscopy: Historically, the detection of characteristic intranuclear inclusions known as 'owl's eye' has been considered to be an indicator of active CMV disease. However, the detection of inclusions by microscopic examination may be an inadequate method for establishing the diagnosis, because intranuclear inclusions can also be caused by other viruses.

Viral culture: Routine cell culture of samples obtained from body fluids takes a long time to confirm characteristic cytopathic effects, because of the slow growth of this virus.

Serological diagnosis: Serological diagnosis, by use of complement fixation test, and detection of IgM and IgG antibodies may be helpful—they are widely used to determine previous infection. The demonstration of a fourfold rise in IgM antibody titres in the serum of ill patients could be interpreted as an indication of a primary infection with CMV. Useful findings for acute CMV infection in normal adults are: culture of blood and tissue biopsies for CMV and CMV-specific IgG seroconversion. Nevertheless, it is difficult to distinguish between primary infection and reactivation.

Immunohistology: Immunohistochemical study of samples with antibodies against specific viral antigens of CMV may reveal cell-inclusions. Although the DNA hybridization assay was expected to be useful for the diagnosis of CMV infection, because of the insensitivity of hybridization, this assay has failed to achieve widespread use.

Molecular methods: Recent developments in the fields of CMV diagnosis are exciting. Molecular amplification methods such as the PCR have been utilized to study CMV infection with samples such as urine, leucocytes, plasma, serum and paraffin-embedded sections. This method has been used with nearly uniform success in almost all clinical settings. Nevertheless, positive results in PCR studies should be viewed with caution, because such a sensitive procedure may demonstrate the presence of viruses totally unrelated to the aetiology of diseases. Precautions also have to be adopted to avoid contaminations that may yield false-positive results.

The most rapid available approach to the diagnosis of CMV infection is the direct detection of CMV antigen in nuclei of peripheral blood leucocytes, an assay known as the pp65 direct antigenaemia test. Monoclonal antibodies directed against the CMV lower matrix protein pp65 (UL83) are used for the direct detection of CMV in circulating polymorphonuclear leucocytes by use of immunoperoxidase techniques. The predictive value of this test rests on the capacity to quantify the number of pp65-positive cells, thus providing an estimate of viral burden. This assay is one of the most rapid and reliable tests for the diagnosis of CMV disease in both patients with AIDS and organ transplant recipients.

Management

The most common treatment for clinical disease caused by CMV is intravenous ganciclovir (dihydroxypropylguanine; DHPG). Cidofovir, foscarnet and fomivirsen are also approved for the treatment of CMV retinitis in patients with AIDS.

Human herpesviruses 6 and 7

HHV-6 and HHV-7 are relatively recently discovered viruses and are prevalent in humans with a tropism for CD4+ lymphocytes.[33] Primary infection with HHV-6 has been associated with exanthema subitum (roseola or sixth disease) in children and febrile illnesses with seizures. Other clinical associations made with this virus include: (a) multiple sclerosis, (b) infectious mononucleosis-like illness and (c) drug-induced hypersensitivity syndrome. More recently, HHV-6 has been recognized as an opportunistic pathogen in patients with HIV infection and in transplant recipients, causing fever, skin rash and malaise.

The clinical characteristics of HHV-7 are not well defined, although some cases of exanthema subitum have been linked with this virus.

Human herpesvirus 8

This herpesvirus was first discovered in 1994 and was named Kaposi's sarcoma-associated herpesvirus (KSAHV) because it was found in almost 100% of Kaposi's sarcomas (KS) from patients with AIDS.[34] This virus is now commonly referred as human herpesvirus 8 (HHV-8) and has subsequently been found in peripheral blood mononuclear cells of patients with KS, in body cavity-based lymphomas in HIV-positive patients without KS, in classical KS and in other forms of KS. HHV-8 DNA has also been found in patients with pemphigus vulgaris, pemphigus foliaceus, carcinoma and lymphoma.

Diagnosis of herpesvirus infections

Usually, diagnosis of herpesvirus infections is made on clinical grounds. However, because of the varied appearance of lesions in HIV-positive individuals, laboratory investigations may aid in diagnosis. The main laboratory analyses of patient samples for the diagnosis of herpesviruses include:

1. Electron microscopy.
2. Viral culture ('gold standard').
3. Immunofluorescence (antigen detection).
4. Histopathological examination of biopsied lesions (Tzanck smear with the presence of multinucleated giant cells can help diagnose HSV or VZV but cannot distinguish between HSV-1, HSV-2 and VZV).
5. In situ hybridization of biopsied lesions.
6. Immunoperoxidase stains of biopsied lesions for EBV, CMV, HSV.
7. PCR for detecting viral DNA.
8. ELISA to detect virus-specific IgM (acute) and IgG (chronic) antibodies.

Management of herpesvirus infections

Several antiviral drugs and immunomodulatory agents are now available for treating herpesvirus infections.[35–38]

Aciclovir (ACV): ACV is the most widely used medication for herpesvirus infections. It is a safe, systemic antiviral agent.

Oral ACV stimulates herpesvirus-infected cells to produce thymidine kinase (TK), an enzyme that sequentially phosphorylates ACV to an active triphosphate form which inhibits viral DNA polymerase, resulting in chain termination. First-episode genital herpes requires a 200-mg dose of ACV given orally five times a day for 10 days. Recurrent herpes requires 200 mg of ACV five times per day for a period of 5 days or longer depending on the clinical response. ACV has an intracellular half life of 1 hour, so frequent dosing is necessary. Greater convenience can be achieved by dosing ACV at a dose of 400 mg given three times daily instead of five times daily.

Acute herpes zoster requires a dosage of ACV 800 mg given orally five times per day for 7–10 days. This dosing regimen reduces the duration of postherpetic neuralgia symptoms from 62 to 20 days for immunocompetent patients treated with placebo versus ACV, respectively.

Topical ACV is also available; however, it is not commonly used because of its low efficacy, although it does appear to reduce the pain and tingling sensation if used early.

Dosing of ACV in HIV-infected patients is similar to the dosing schedule described above; however, variations occur. Because of the low bioavailability of ACV in the oral form, patients with HIV and extensive HSV disease may require the intravenous (i.v.) form, especially when both dissemination and visceral organ involvement occur.

Ophthalmic preparations including idoxuridine, trifluridine and vidarabine are used for herpes keratitis and keratoconjunctivitis.

Two new agents, valaciclovir and famciclovir, have been approved for treatment of herpes in order to provide both easier convenience and higher bioavailability.

Valaciclovir (VACV): VACV is the valyl ester of ACV with a five times greater bioavailability (54%) than oral ACV, reaching plasma levels of ACV similar to the level attained with intravenous ACV. First-episode genital herpes is usually treated with 500 mg of VACV given twice daily for 10 days. Recurrent episodes of genital herpes are treated with 500 mg of VACV twice daily for 5 days. VACV can be used at a dose of 500 mg once daily for suppression of recurrent genital herpes in immuno-competent individuals with fewer than 10 episodes per year. It has been approved for the treatment of acute herpes zoster at a dose of 1000 mg given three times daily for 7 days. This therapy is as safe as oral ACV.

VACV has been safe and well tolerated for both short- and long-term use in immunocompromised patients, including HIV-positive patients. The dose schedule for HIV-positive patients is similar to that described above; however, patients may require 500 mg of VACV twice daily, or 1000 mg once daily for suppression of chronic recurrent genital herpes.

Famciclovir (FCV): FCV is the oral prodrug form of the nucleoside penciclovir. As with ACV, FCV must be phosphorylated to a triphosphate form in order to be active. As with VACV, FCV has greater bioavailability (77%) than ACV. It is approved for the episodic treatment of recurrent genital herpes at a dose of 125 mg twice daily for 5 days.

FCV can be used for first-episode genital herpes at a dose of 250 mg three times per day for 10 days. Recently, approval was granted by the US Food and Drug Administration (FDA) for FCV at a dose of 250 mg twice daily for recurrent genital herpes suppression. Also, FCV can be used for acute herpes zoster infection at a dose of 500 mg three times daily for 7 days. At this dose, it has been shown to decrease the healing time of cutaneous manifestations of herpes zoster, and significantly reduce the duration of postherpetic neuralgia (PHN).

FCV can also be used in immunocompromised individuals including those infected with HIV. In HIV-infected patients, FCV is effective for the suppression of symptomatic as well as asymptomatic HSV reactivation; duration of symptoms is decreased by 65% and there is an 81% reduction in viral shedding. Suppressive dosing of FCV (500 mg twice daily) has the same effectiveness as ACV (400 mg five times a day) for recurrent genital herpes in HIV-infected individuals at a more convenient dosing regimen.

Evidence for resistance to ACV in HIV-infected individuals has recently emerged. Most ACV-resistant HSV isolates can be treated and are susceptible to certain other antivirals not requiring thymidine kinase activation.

Foscarnet: Foscarnet is an FDA-approved pyrophosphate analogue that directly inhibits HSV DNA polymerase without activation; it is typically given for treatment of ACV-resistant HSV at a dose of 40 mg/kg intravenously every 8 hours. Its use is limited owing to significant renal toxicity.

Cidofovir(CDV): CDV is a nucleotide analogue of deoxycytidine monophosphate that requires phosphorylation to an active metabolite by host cellular enzymes, rather than the virus-specific enzymes used by the other antivirals. This agent has broad-spectrum anti-DNA virus activity. The gel formulation has been evaluated for treatment of ACV-resistant mucocutaneous HSV infection in patients with AIDS and significant benefits in lesion healing, pain reduction and virological effects has been demonstrated.

Postherpetic neuralgia: PHN can be treated symptomatically with topical analgesic agents such as capsaicin, which may be helpful in some cases. Other modalities of treating PHN that have been shown to be effective include: (a) amitriptyline, (b) carbamazepine, (c) nerve blocks, (d) Triavil, (e) lidocaine (lignocaine) and (f) fentanyl patches.

Oral hairy leucoplakia: Often OHL requires no treatment; however, several therapeutic agents have been tried, including: ACV, topical podophyllin resin, topical isotretinoin, as well as local destructive measures.

Papovaviruses

Human papillomavirus

Human papillomavirus (HPV) causes cutaneous warts at any site on the body.[39] HPV is transmitted by contact and is an asymptomatic infection in the majority of immuno-competant people who acquire the infection. In a small proportion of individuals, HPV causes warts, which vary in size and number. The warts are in most cases self-limiting.

Various causes of immunodeficiency are associated with an increased incidence of HPV infection.[33] Penile and perianal warts are twice as common in HIV-seropositive men than in individuals with a normal immune system. Depressed cell-mediated immunity in HIV-seropositive persons is associated with an increased prevalence of HPV infection. The incidence of genital warts in HIV-seropositive women has been reported to be increased by as much as 10-fold. Extensive HPV infections involving multiple portions of the anogenital area are common in HIV-seropositive persons. The cutaneous lesions are increased in number and severity, and are difficult to treat. Many recurr after treatment.

Invasive cervical cancer, which is closely associated with oncogenic HPV, is considered an AIDS-defining illness in HIV-seropositive women.[40] Cervical cancer is the second most common cancer killer of women worldwide. The high prevalence of HIV in Third-World women and the increasing incidence in women in industralized countries are adding to the cervical cancer epidemic.[34]

Anogenital warts in people with a normal immune system usually do not contain oncogenic HPV and are thus not considered to be premalignant. In HIV-seropositive persons, however, anogenital warts often harbour multiple HPV types including some considered to be oncogenic.

Management

Depending on the size, extent and location, warts can be treated by topical agents (podophyllin; imiquimod), surgery (excision or cautery) or cryotherapy using a cryoprobe.

Surgical therapy of HPV-related lesions in HIV-seropositive patients carries the risk of transmission of HIV to the surgeon. Laser surgery and electrosurgery carry a risk of transmission of both HIV and HPV from the aerosolized wart tissue. There are high recurrence rates of warts in HIV-positive patients receiving surgical therapy.

Experimental cytokine therapy for warts

Interferon (IFN) α was the first FDA-approved antiviral agent for genital warts, and has also been reported as useful adjunction treatment for HIV.[41,42] Because of systemic side effects (i.e., influenza-like syndrome) of IFN, the need for multiple intralesional injections, high cost and relatively slow rate of lesion resolution, exogenous IFN therapy has been used in combination with other methods.

Imiquimod[43] can be used as a topical (5% cream) self-applied therapy for condyloma acuminatum. Imiquimod acts by inducing endogenous production of IFNα and a spectrum of other cytokines. Thus, imiquimod is an immunomodulatory agent that also acts via antiviral mechanisms. It has proved safe and efficacious in the treatment of condyloma acuminatum in otherwise healthy persons when used overnight on alternating nights, three times a week for up to 16 weeks.

Parvovirus infections

Human parvovirus B19

The cutaneous manifestations of human parvovirus B19 infection include a petechial eruption in a 'glove and stocking' distribution, reticular truncal erythema and the 'slapped cheek sign'.[44] The dermatopathology of B19 infection suggests that tissue injury is mediated by delayed-type hypersensitivity, antibody-dependent cellular immunity directed at microbial antigenic targets in the epidermis and endothelium, and by circulating immune complexes in the setting of leucocytoclastic vasculitis. These findings appear to generate a picture of connective tissue disease.

REFERENCES

1 Katz S L & Gellin B G (eds) Measles control—resetting the agenda: a report of the Children's Vaccine Initiative ad hoc Committee on an investment strategy for measles control. *J Infect Dis* 1994; 170 (Supplement 1):S1–S66.

2 Egunjobi L. Spatial distribution of mortality from leading notifiable diseases in Nigeria. *Soc Sci Med* 1993; 36:1267–1272.

3 Aaby P, Andersen M & Knudsen K. Excess mortality after early exposure to measles. *Int J Epidemiol* 1993; 22:156–162.

4 Uyirwoth G P. Measles in Mashonaland Central Province: Zimbabwe. *East Afr Med J* 1993; 70:455–459.

5 Hussey G D & Klein M. Routine high-dose vitamin A therapy for children hospitalized with measles. *J Trop Pediatr* 1993; 9:342–345.

6 Latham M C. Vitamin A and childhood mortality. *Lancet* 1993; 342:549.

7 Ross D A. Vitamin A and childhood mortality. Ghana Vitamin A Supplementation Trials Study Team. *Lancet* 1993; 342:861.

8 Foster S O, Spiegel R A & Mokdad A. Immunization, oral rehydration therapy and malaria chemotherapy among children under 5 in Bomi and Grand Cape Mount counties, Liberia, 1984 and 1988. *Int J Epidemiol* 1993; 22 (Supplement 1):S50–S55.

9 Garenne M, Leroy O, Beau J P & Sene I. Efficacy of measles vaccine after controlling for exposure. *Am J Epidemiol* 1993; 138:182–195.

10 Longini I M Jr, Halloran M E, Haber M & Chen R T. Measuring vaccine efficacy from epidemics of acute infectious agents. *Stat Med* 1993; 12:249–263.

11 Nokes D J & Cutts F T. Immunization in the developing world: strategic challenges. *Trans R Soc Trop Med Hyg* 1993; 87:353–354, 398.

12 Tulchinsky T H, Ginsberg G M, Abed Y, Angeles M T, Akukwe C & Bonn J. Measles control in developing and developed countries: the case for a two-dose policy. *Bull World Health Organ* 1993; 71:93–103.

13 Orenstein W A, Markowits L E, Atkinson W L & Hinman A R. Worldwide measles prevention. *Isr J Med Sci* 1994; 30:469–481.

14 Aaby P, Andersen M, Sodemann M, Jakobsen M, Gomes J & Fernandes M. Reduced childhood mortality after standard measles vaccination at 4–8 months compared with 9–11 months of age. *BMJ* 1993; 307:1308–1311.

15 Burstrom B, Aaby P & Mutie D M. Child mortality impact of a measles outbreak in a partially vaccinated rural African community. *Scand J Infect Dis* 1993; 25:763–769.

16 Diven D G. An overview of poxviruses. *J Am Acad Dermatol* 2001; 44:1–16.

17 Cook G C. Human monkeypox: a viral disease with an uncertain future in Africa. *Trop Dis Bull* 1988; 85:R1–R16.

18 Knight J C, Novembre F J & Brown D R. Studies on Tanapox viruses. *Virology* 1989; 172:116–124.

19 Yen-Moore A, Straten M V, Carrasco D et al. Cutaneous viral infections in HIV-infected individuals. *Clin Dermatol* 2000; 18(4):423–432.

20 Roizman B. Herpesviridae. In Fileds B N, Knipe D M & Howley R M (eds) *Field's Virology*, 3rd edn. Philadelphia, PA: Lippincott-Raven, 1996: 2221–2230.

21 Corey L. Herpes simplex virus. In Mandell G L, Bennett J E & Dolin R (eds) *Principles and Practice of Infectious Diseases*,

5th edn. Philadelphia, PA: Churchill Livingstone, 2000: 1564–1580.

22 Safran S, Ashley R, Houlihan C et al. Clinical and serological features of herpes simplex virus infection in patients with AIDS. *AIDS* 1991; 5:1107–1110.

23 Siegal F P, Lopez C, Hammer G F et al. Severe acquired immunodeficiency in male homosexuals manifested by chronic perianal ulcerative herpes simplex lesions. *N Engl J Med* 1981; 305:1439-1444.

24 Jain S, Wyatt D, McCaughey C, O'Neill H J & Coyle P V. Nested multiplex PCR for the diagnosis of cutaneous hepres simplex and herpes zoster infections and a comparison with electronmicroscopy. *J Med Virol* 2001; 63(1):52–56.

25 Jura E, Chadwick E G, Josephs H S et al. Varicella zoster virus infections in children infected with human immunodeficiency virus. *Pediatr Infect Dis J* 1989; 8:856–890.

26 Arvin A M. Varicella vaccine—the first six years. *N Engl J Med* 2001; 344:1007–1009.

27 Magro C M, Dawood M R & Crowson A N. The cutaneous manifestations of human parvovirus B19 infection. *Hum Pathol* 2000; 31(4):488–497.

28 Iwatsuki K, Xu Z, Ohtsuka M & Kaneko F. Cutaneous lymphoproliferative disorders associated with Epstein–Barr virus infection: a clinical overview. *J Dermatol Sci* 2000; 22:181–195.

29 Reichart P S, Langford A, Gelderblom H R et al. Oral hairy leukoplakia: observations in 95 cases and review of the literature. *J Oral Pathol Med* 1989; 18:410–415.

30 Drago F, Aragone M G & Rebora A. Cytomegalovirus infection in normal and immunocompromised humans: a review. *Dermatology* 2000; 200:189–195.

31 Nico M M, Cymbalista N C, Hurtado Y C & Borges L H. Perinal cytomegalovirus ulcer in an HIV infected patient: case report and review of literature. *J Dermatol* 2000; 27:99–105.

32 Kano Y & Shiohara T. Current understanding of cytomegalovirus infection in immunocompetant individuals. *J Dermaol Sci* 2000; 22:196–204.

33 Kosuge H. HHV-6, 7 and their related diseases. *J Dermatol Sci* 2000; 22:205–212.

34 Chang Y, Cesarman E, Pessin M S et al. Identification of herpesvirus-like DNA sequences in AIDS-associated Kaposi's sarcoma. *Science* 1994; 266:1865–1869.

35 Herne K, Cirelli R, Lee P et al. Advances in antiviral therapy. *Curr Opin Dermatol* 1996; 3:195–201.

36 Tyring S, Barbarash R A, Nahlik J et al. Famciclovir for the treatment of acute herpes zoster: Effects on acute disease and postherpetic neuralgia. *Ann Intern Med* 1995; 123:89-96.

37 Lalezari J P, Stagg R J, Jaffe H S et al. A preclinical and clinical overview of the nucleotide-based antiviral agent cidofovir (HPMPC). In Mills J & Corey L (eds) *Antiviral Chemotherapy*. New York: Plenum, 1996.

38 Conant A. Immunomodulatory therapy in the management of viral infections in patients with HIV infection. *J Am Acad Dermatol* 2000; 43:S27–S30.

39 Tyring S K. Human papillomavirus infections: epidemiology, pathogenesis and host immune response. *J Am Acad Dermatol* 2000; 43:S18–S26.

40 Palefsky J. Human papillomavirus-associated malignancies in HIV-positive men and women. *Curr Opin Oncol* 1995; 7:437–441.

41 Semprini A E, Stillo A, Marcozi S et al. Treatment with interferon for genital HPV in HIV-positive and HIV-negative women. *Eur J Obstet Gynecol Reprod Biol* 1994; 53:135–137.

42 Rockley P F & Tyring S K. Interferons alpha, beta, and gamma therapy of anogenital human papillomavirus infections. *Pharmacol Ther* 1995; 65:265-287.

43 Edwards L, Ferenczy A, Eron L et al. Self-administered topical 5% imiquimod cream for external anogenital warts. *Arch Dermatol* 1998; 134:25-30.

44 Drago F, Aragone M G, Lugani C & Rebora A. Cytomegalovirus infection in normal and immunocompromised humans: a review. *Dermatology* 2000; 200:189–195.

Chapter 49

Virus Infections of the Central Nervous System

S. Amor

Although virus infections of the central nervous system (CNS) are rare, they are responsible for some of the most devastating and diverse effects of disease in humans and animals. While prion diseases are not strictly 'viral', a short section is also dedicated to these diseases.

CNS viral infections were first reported in Babylonian times, and trepanning in early times was possibly the earliest treatment for such diseases. However, with the explosion in advances in the fields of virus isolation techniques, immunology and molecular biology in addition to detailed knowledge of viral replication have enabled the control by prophylactics such as immunization and vector control, or following pharmacological intervention.

The broad spectrum of clinical manifestations of CNS infections poses the clinician not only a problem of prompt diagnosis but also that of treatment and aggressive management to allow recovery with little chance of sequelae. The major clinical manifestations resulting from viral infections of the CNS are outlined in Table 49.1.

Viral spread to the CNS

Consideration of how viruses may enter the CNS is paramount in determining the methods by which such potential infections may be avoided or controlled. Space does not allow detail on entry of viruses and the reader is referred to Johnson[1] and Fields et al.[2] Although the skin is the most extensive barrier to the entry of viruses, once broached viruses may rapidly invade. Likewise the respiratory, gut and genitourinary tracts, which form the most formidable barrier due to mucous film and secretory immunoglobulin, may nevertheless be permeable to acid-resistant viruses such as the enteroviruses. The major portals of entry of viruses causing human CNS infections are summarized in Table 49.2.

Following entry into the host, viruses must disseminate and enter the CNS either through the neural route and be transported via axonal transport, through

Table 49.1 Clinical manifestations of viral infections of the CNS.

Disease	Duration	Clinical signs	Examples
Acute meningitis	Days	Rapid onset of high fever, stiff neck, altered mental state, photophobia, raised intracranial pressure	Viral meningitis
Chronic meningitis	Months	Gradual onset of signs associated with the above	Enteroviruses
Acute encephalitis	Days	Association with systemic illness, nausea, vomiting, seizures. Specific signs associated with tropism of virus, e.g., temporal lobe lesions following HSV infection	Measles, herpes simplex
Chronic encephalitis	Months to years	Gradual onset of signs as above, progressing to severe disability and death. General debility and dementia may develop	SSPE, HIV encephalitis
Postinfectious	Days to weeks	Onset of signs following recovery from viral infection. Such signs include the development of chronic fatigue syndrome or Guillain–Barré syndrome	Postinfectious encephalomyelitis
Slow viruses	Months to years	Progressive signs of neuronal destruction. Observed following immunosuppressive therapy	PML
Prion diseases	Months to years	Progressive signs of neurological dysfunction. Not associated with conventional virus	Creutzfeldt–Jakob disease, Kuru

HSV, herpes simplex virus; SSPE. subacute sclerosing panencephalitis; HIV, human immunodeficiency virus; PML, progressive multifocal leucoencephalopathy.

Table 49.2 Routes of entry of neurotropic viruses.

Route of entry	Example
Inoculation	
Arthropod bite	Arboviruses
Animal bite	Rabies
Blood transfusion	Cytomegalovirus
Transplantation	Creutzfeldt–Jakob disease
Respiratory	Influenza
Enteric	Polio
Venereal	HIV
Transplacental	Cytomegalovirus

the olfactory route, or via the blood across the blood–brain barrier (BBB).

Neural route

Retrograde transmission along the axon is a well recognized route for rabies virus and the site of entry determines the incubation period. The importance of this route of entry for rabies is demonstrated by the prevention of experimental infection when the infected nerve is severed. Likewise, neural spread of poliomyelitis, varicella zoster and herpes simplex virus (HSV) has also been shown experimentally. Both retrograde and anterograde transneuronal and nonneuronal (ependymal cells and cerebrospinal fluid) pathways are utilized by vesicular virus (VSV) within the CNS.

Olfactory route

Experimental intranasal infection with HSV and some togaviruses shows that virus is spread to the CNS via the olfactory route, resulting in an early infection of the CNS with histological changes in the olfactory tracts. In contrast to rabies virus and HSV-1, VSV does not use the trigeminal nerve for entry into the brain, as the trigeminal ganglion remains virus free following intranasal infection. These results indicate that VSV has a tropism for olfactory receptor cells, using them for entry into the CNS.

Haematogenous route

The majority of viruses that induce CNS infection are acquired from the blood. The presence of a BBB was based on the finding that following peripheral dye injection in small animals all tissues were stained with the exception of the brain.[3] Conversely, injection of dye into the cerebrospinal fluid (CSF) stained the brain but not peripheral tissues. The morphological BBB is represented by the cerebral endothelial cells, which lack fenestrations but are joined by tight junctions, and pericytes that form a discontinuous layer around the endothelial cells with which they share a common basement membrane. Discontinuities in the basement membrane allow the endothelial cells direct contact with the pericytes. Astrocytic foot processes surround the pericytes. A diagrammatic representation of the BBB is shown in Figure 49.1.

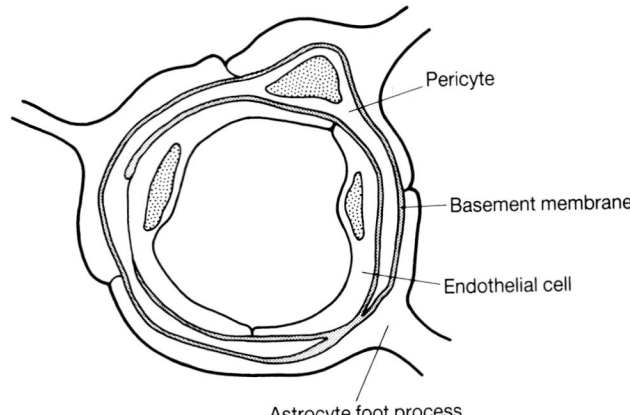

Figure 49.1: The blood–brain barrier.

In general the physical and chemical nature of the molecule determines its ability to cross the BBB and, thus, whereas lipid-soluble molecules are readily transferred across the BBB, charged non-lipid-soluble molecules are less effective. The BBB also forms a barrier for the entry of viruses; nevertheless most viruses invade the CNS. Transfer of viruses across the BBB may take place either after infection of leucocytes, as is observed for measles and mumps virus, or following adherence of virus to erythrocytes, as is seen with togaviruses and paramyxoviruses. The infected cells may then migrate across the BBB during infection due to the upregulation of cellular adhesion molecules.[4] Such traffic is limited in the normal situation, although it may be extensive

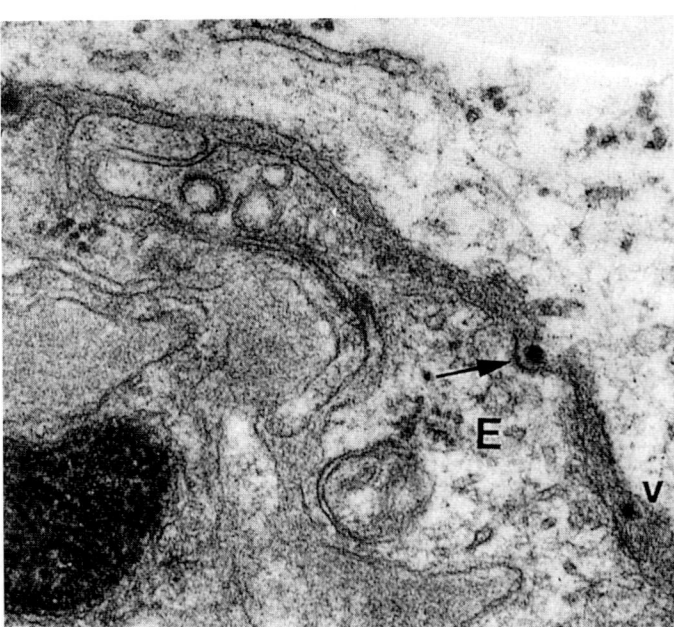

Figure 49.2: Brain capillary endothelial cell (E) showing the formation of coated vesicle containing mature virus (arrow). Mature virus (V) also present in the basement membrane. Semliki Forest virus × 60 000. (Kindly provided by L Pathak, St Thomas' Hospital.)

during injury or infection. Alternatively viruses may be taken up by receptors, induce the formation of pynocytotic vesicles on the endothelial cells and be actively transported, as in Semliki Forest virus infection (Figure 49.2).

Spread within the nervous system

Whether viruses reach the CNS via the haematogenous, olfactory or neural route, the progression of clinical signs is dependent on the subsequent spread of virus within the tissue. Additionally the tropism of viruses for different cells determines the characteristic clinical signs and manifestation of disease associated with specific viruses (see Table 49.1). For example, the spread of HSV within the temporal lobes leads to temporal lobe seizures, whereas infection of oligodendrocytes by JC papovavirus induces lesions of demyelination.

Attachment of viruses to cells prior to entry is obviously important in the development of disease, and binding domains or receptors for numerous viruses have been identified, such as the β-adrenergic receptor for reoviruses. The utilization of neurotransmitter receptors by viruses and interference in the functioning of specific neurones may explain why viruses have been implicated in chronic fatigue syndrome.[5] Other receptors include the CD4 receptor for the human immunodeficiency virus (HIV), acetylcholine receptor for rabies virus, and fibroblast growth factor receptor for HSV-1.

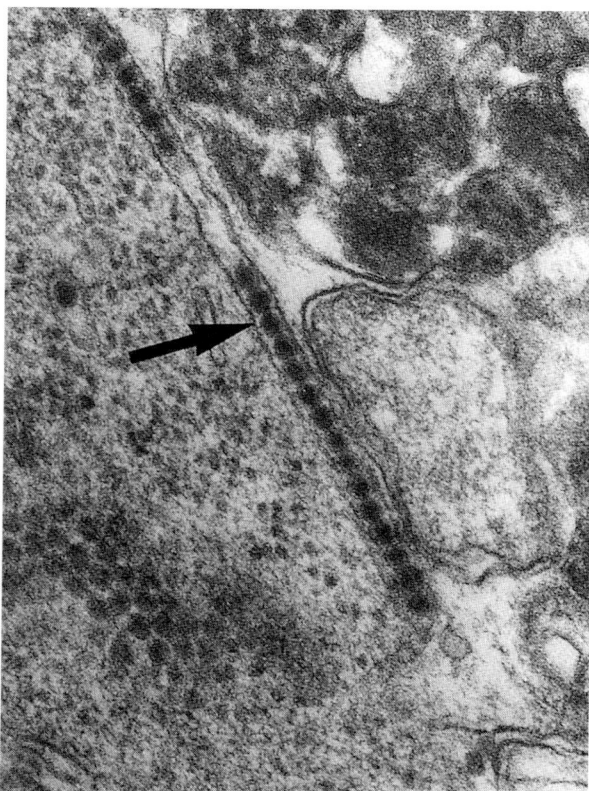

Figure 49.3: Langat virus (family *Flaviviridae*) (arrow) within the extracellular space of CNS tissue.

Once the virus has gained entry into the cell, replication and dissemination are necessary for progression of disease. Although cell-to-cell spread is the most obvious, there is little evidence for any virus that this occurs. Viruses have been observed in the extracellular spaces (Figure 49.3) and reduction of togavirus titres by specific antibody[6] suggests that extracellular movement must occur. Alternatively transport via glial cells and axons has been suggested.[7]

As with entry of viruses into the CNS, the infiltrating leucocytes may be important in the spread of virus within the tissue. This is observed in human herpes viruses and especially with cytomegalovirus (CMV). Additionally the role of the immune response in the progression of the disease must be considered since autoimmune responses initiated by viruses are an important phenomenon.[8]

Arboviruses (see also Chapter 41)

The vast majority of CNS infections are due to viruses transmitted by arthropod vectors, such as mosquitoes or ticks, and are termed arboviruses (*ar*thropod-*bo*rne viruses). The arbovirus group, which includes approximately

Table 49.3 Arthropod-borne viruses responsible for CNS diseases.

Arbovirus	Genus	Family
California encephalitis	*Bunyavirus*	Bunyaviridae
La Crosse	*Bunyavirus*	Bunyaviridae
Crimean haemorrhagic fever	*Nairovirus*	Bunyaviridae
Tensaw	Bunyamwera group	Bunyaviridae
Rift Valley fever	*Phlebovirus*	Bunyaviridae
Dengue		Flaviviridae
Ilheus		Flaviviridae
Japanese B		Flaviviridae
Kumlinge		Flaviviridae
Murray Valley encephalitis		Flaviviridae
Negishi		Flaviviridae
Powassan		Flaviviridae
Russian spring–summer encephalitis		Flaviviridae
Rocio		Flaviviridae
St Louis encephalitis		Flaviviridae
West Nile		Flaviviridae
Yellow fever		Flaviviridae
Colorado tick fever	*Orbivirus*	Reoviridae
Chikungunya	*Alphavirus*	Togaviridae
Eastern equine encephalitis	*Alphavirus*	Togaviridae
O'nyong-nyong	*Alphavirus*	Togaviridae
Semliki Forest	*Alphavirus*	Togaviridae
Venezuelan equine encephalitis	*Alphavirus*	Togaviridae
Western equine encephalitis	*Alphavirus*	Togaviridae
Thogoto	Ungrouped	

500 viruses, spans several families: i.e., Bunyaviridae, Togaviridae, Flaviviridae, Reoviridae and Rhabdoviridae (Table 49.3). These arboviruses and viruses of other families implicated in CNS disorders are discussed under the virus family heading(s).

Arenaviridae

The name is derived from the Latin *arena*, meaning sand, to describe the granules observed inside the virions. The two major groups within this family are the lympho-cytic choriomeningitis (LCM) group and the Tacaribe complex, which are distinguished on the basis of antigenic reactivity. These viruses are single-stranded RNA viruses of various sizes.

LCM complex is comprised of LCM and Lassa in which aseptic meningitis, encephalomyelitis and meningo-encephalomyelitis have been described. LCM virus (LCMV) was the first virus isolated from aseptic meningitis in humans. The other members of this complex, namely Ippy, Mopeia and Mobala, are not associated with human disease.

Epidemiology

LCMV, although now rarely identified in humans, is transmitted by rodents to humans via exposure of open wounds or contamination of food by infected animal excrement. Human-to-human contact has not been reported and, due to the nature of transmission, animal handlers or those living in impoverished conditions are at higher risk. Although LCMV infections of humans have not been documented for several years, the seroprevalence is thought to be less than 0.1%.[9] LCMV infection in humans ranges from asymptomatic infection, mild systemic illness to CNS involvement. The severity of the illness may depend on dose, route of infection and host immunogenetic background. Early fetal or transovarian infection in mice does not induce a sufficient immunological response to clear the virus and gives rise to a persistent infection in which virus is secreted in respiratory droplets, faeces and urine. Experimentally, infection of mice induces severe encephalitis, and damage within the CNS is primarily due to the immunopathological effect.

Clinical features

The typical disease begins with fever, malaise, weakness, headache and myalgia, which is most severe in the lumbar region. Anorexia, nausea and dizziness are also common and the patients may have any combination of sore throat, vomiting and arthralgia with chest pain and pneumonitis. The incubation period is 6–13 days and in some cases haematological disturbances such as leucopenia are observed. Neurological complications signified by headache, stiff neck and typical signs of encephalitis have been reported in approximately 15% of infections, of which some are severe encephalitis. Fatal cases have also been reported.[10] The white blood cell count is often 3000/mm^3 or less with a mild thrombocytopenia. CSF from patients with meningeal signs contains several hundred white cells, predominantly lymphocytes (> 80%), with increased protein and occasionally low sugar levels. Virus is often found in the spinal fluid during acute disease.[11] Convalescence is prolonged, with persistent fatigue and dizziness.

Lassa fever
Epidemiology
Lassa fever was first described in West Africa in the 1950s, although the virus was not isolated until 1969. The only known reservoir of Lassa fever virus in West Africa is *Mastomys natalensis*, one of the most commonly occurring rodents in Africa. The virus is rapidly spread from person to person, giving rise to a mortality rate of 30–66%, and consequently knowledge of the pathological features is limited. Rates of seroconversion to Lassa virus range from 5 to 20% in populations of Sierra Leone villages.[12] The highest rates are in crowded, highly mobile, populations. Clinically, infection gives rise to haemorrhage, nephropathy, myocarditis and encephalitis.

Clinical diagnosis
Lassa fever begins 7–18 days after primary infection, leading to onset of fever, headache and malaise. Patients with Lassa fever show features of anxiety and there is a raised respiratory rate. In 15–20% of patients, bleeding occurs from gums and nose. Oedema of the face and neck are commonly seen in severe cases. Important clinical events in fatal disease are intractable hypovolaemic shock and/or severe CNS involvement, bleeding and oedema of the face. There is also endothelial and platelet dysfunction and mild thrombocytopenia.

Pathogenesis and pathology
The most common and consistently observed lesions in fatal human Lassa fever are focal necroses of the liver, adrenal glands and spleen.[13] Although high virus titres occur in other organs, such as the brain, ovary, pancreas, uterus and placenta, no lesions have been reported in humans, while infected monkeys have been reported to have CNS lesions.

Prevention and control
The ideal method of prevention is to prevent contact between rodents and humans. This can be achieved by improving the housing and food storage, which might reduce the domestic rodent population. There are two vaccines for arenaviral diseases. A live attenuated vaccine has been used extensively. A second vaccine has been made by cloning and expressing the Lassa virus glycoprotein gene into vaccine virus. This vaccine has proven highly successful in preventing severe disease and death in challenged monkeys and may be relevant for treating humans.[15]

Management
Ribavirin can prevent death in Lassa fever when given at

Table 49.4 Genera and serogroups within the family Bunyaviridae.

Genus	Serogroups
Bunyavirus	Anopheles A, Anopheles B, Bunyamwera, Bwamba, California, Capim, Gamboa, Guama, Koongol, Olifantsvlei, Patois, Simbu, Teteu, Turlock
Nairovirus	Crimean–Congo, Dera Gharzi Khan, Hughes, Nairobi SD, Qalyub, Sakhalin
Phlebovirus	Phlebotomus, Rift Valley fever
Uukuvirus	Uukuniemi
Hantavirus	Hantaan

any point in the illness, but is more effective when given early and administered intravenously.[16]

Bunyaviridae

The Bunyaviridae family is divided into five genera (*Bunyavirus, Nairovirus, Phlebovirus, Uukuvirus, Hantavirus*) and comprises over 250 members (Table 49.4). The viruses are between 80 and 120 nm in size and have a lipid envelope derived from the host cell membranes during maturation. The structure and replication of bunyaviruses are excellently covered in *Fields' Virology*.[17]

This section will concentrate on those viruses within the genera that are important with respect to causing significant human disease.

Bunyaviruses

The most important serogroup with respect to induction of human diseases is the California (CAL) group which include California encephalitis and La Crosse (LAC) viruses. This group of viruses has 14 serotypes, the prototype virus being La Crosse virus, first isolated from a child in La Crosse, Wisconsin, in 1960.[18]

Epidemiology
Members of the California encephalitis virus serogroup have been isolated in Canada, the USA, Trinidad, Europe, Africa and Finland,[19] although each has a very narrow host range and geographical distribution. Animals such as chipmunks and squirrels are commonly involved. La Crosse virus, the prototype virus, is transmitted by the mosquito *Aedes triseriatus*, which is the most important vector in California, although other *Aedes* species may be involved. Children and young adults aged 1–19 years are at greatest risk of exposure to this vector, which is a woodland mosquito, during activities such as camping and hiking.

La Crosse infection is the second most prevalent mosquito-borne viral infection in the USA and accounts

for approximately 75 definite cases a year, although seroprevalence may reach 20% in older persons. La Crosse virus is transmitted mainly by *Ae. triseriatus*, a treehole-breeding woodland mosquito that frequently feeds on small mammals, particularly chipmunks and squirrels.[20] An alternative mosquito habitat is provided by discarded tyres, which hold rainwater on which egg rafts may be laid. This virus produces acute encephalitis in children. The acute illness lasts 10 days or less in most cases. The first symptoms are non-specific and last for 1–3 days, followed by involvement of the CNS. The symptoms include stiff neck, lethargy and seizures. Earlier examination shows high counts of both polymorphonuclear neutrophil leucocytes and mononuclear cells in about 65% of patients. The most important sequelae of La Crosse encephalitis is epilepsy, which occurs in about 10% of the children. A few patients (2%) have persistent paresis. Learning disabilities and other objective cognitive deficits have been reported in a small proportion of patients. Tahyna virus, a bunyavirus related to California virus, has been associated with mild encephalitis in Slovakia.

Pathology
The lesions induced by bunyaviruses are typical of acute viral encephalitis. Examination of the CNS reveals perivascular cuffing of mononuclear cells and, in severe cases, necrotic areas. Histopathologically the lesions, which consist of scattered glial nodules, perivascular cuffs, mild leptomeningitis and occasional areas of focal necrosis, are found more often in the cerebral cortex and to a lesser extent in the brain stem and medulla.

Clinical features
Following an incubation period of 3–7 days, features associated with acute encephalitis are observed. Brief 'flu-like' symptoms and primary viraemia, which follows the arthropod bite, are observed. The secondary phase is marked by fever and a secondary viraemia coinciding with CNS involvement. Clinical expression includes headache, fever and meningoencephalitis, with upper motor neuronal signs and occasionally chorea. Neurological sequelae may occur, in which persistent seizures are observed. Onset of seizures may be rapid with no other signs of disease. Acute arthritis is observed with Tahyna virus, whereas respiratory system involvement is more commonly seen in Jamestown Canyon virus infections.

Diagnosis
Clinical diagnosis of La Crosse virus may be made as a result of localization of neurological lesions. Specific diagnosis is based on complement fixation (CF) or haemagglutination inhibition (HI) assays, although neutralization tests (NTs) are also used. Artsob[21] has described an enzyme-linked immunosorbent assay (ELISA) for serotyping. Isolations in suckling mice and Vero cells have been used for virus typing.

Prevention and control

To date, no specific treatment for the California serogroup virus infections is available and anticonvulsants are used to control seizures. Recently reports in mice have suggested that plasmid DNAs, encoding either of the virus surface glycoproteins G1 and G2 or they efficiently blocked the spread of virus from the primary replication site to the brain, suggesting that such approaches may be beneficial in patients.

Phleboviruses

Rift Valley fever

Rift Valley fever (RVF) virus is the most notable virus in the genus *Phlebovirus*. An epidemic outbreak of fever and myalgia in which a few people developed encephalitis was reported in Egypt in 1979.[22] Additional outbreaks have been observed throughout Africa, including Nigeria, Egypt, Sudan and Kenya. More than 20 species of mosquitoes have been implicated as possible vectors. *Culex pipiens, Cx. theileri, Ae. caballus* and other mosquitoes of the *Culex* and *Aedes* group may be involved. The major sources of reservoirs are animals such as sheep, cattle and goats, although camels and antelopes can be infected. Transmission of the virus from animal to animal during epidemics may result from biting flies.

Clinical features

RVF illness is biphasic. The primary phase is associated with fever, back and joint pains, and headaches that last about 1 week. After 1–2 days' remission, the second phase consists of similar symptoms for 1–2 days, with nausea and sometimes a haemorrhagic diathesis with evidence of liver and renal damage. Occasionally disturbed vision, with evidence of a retinitis and cotton-wool exudates in the region of the macula, is observed. Altered levels of consciousness are observed with, in some cases, persistent fever. Meningeal irritation occurs, with focal motor signs and hallucinations.[23]

Diagnosis

Identification of increasing levels of IgM-specific antibodies in the CSF is used for the specific diagnosis.

Management

No specific treatment exists for Rift Valley fever, although a formalin-inactivated vaccine may be of use for laboratory workers and troops who may be exposed to this virus. More recently an inactivated RVF vaccine TSI-GSD-200 has been found beneficial.

Coronaviridae

Members of the Coronaviridae family are pleomorphic RNA viruses, 80–130 nm in diameter, which replicate within the cytoplasm. The family includes several animal viruses, including murine hepatitis virus known to induce demyelination in the CNS of infected mice and several human serotypes implicated in chronic bronchitis in adults.

The neurotropic strain of mouse hepatitis virus, JHM, was first isolated from a spontaneously paralysed mouse. The virus induces lesions of acute demyelination in the brain and spinal cord.[24] Virions are observed within the neurones. The relevance of this infection to human disease is the finding of coronaviruses in the brains of patients with multiple sclerosis.[25] Thus coronaviruses may be involved in the pathogenesis and aetiology of this human demyelinating disease.

Flaviviridae

Formerly classified as Group B arboviruses, the Flaviviridae were reclassified as an independent family by Westaway et al.[26] This family comprises the largest group of viruses known to induce CNS diseases and contains the yellow fever virus which, although not implicated in CNS disease, is the prototype virus (L. *flavus* = yellow). Flaviviruses are small icosahedral enveloped viruses that replicate and mature cytoplasmically, deriving the lipid envelope from the internal membrane of the host cell. Flaviviruses may be subdivided depending on the mode of transmission, i.e., mosquitoes or ticks (Table 49.5) and consist of approximately 66 viruses. Further serological subgroups may be distinguished on the basis of reactivity in HI and neutralization assays.

To date, unfortunately, no specific antiviral therapy is available for the treatment or prevention of infection with viruses of the Flaviviridae. Ongoing research has identified possible targets for inhibition, including binding and uptake of the virus to cells together with the viral proteases and some factors governing replication, and these may be useful in the future development of antiviral therapeutic strategies. Preliminary studies in mice using DNA-based vaccine or passive transfer of immunoglulin have been shown to be effective.

Table 49.5 Insect vector and examples of viruses in the family Flaviviridae.

Insect vector	Virus
Mosquito	Japanese B encephalitis (JE)
	West Nile (WN)
	St Louis encephalitis (SLE)
	Murray Valley encephalitis (MVE)
	Rocio virus
Tick	Tick–borne encephalitis (TBE), e.g.,
	Russian spring–summer encephalitis (RSSE)
	Powassan encephalitis
	Louping ill
	Negishi

Japanese encephalitis

A disease resembling Japanese encephalitis (JE) was recorded as early as 1871. In 1935, an infectious agent was recovered from the brain of a person in Tokyo and was virologically and serologically established as the prototype (Nakayama) strain. JE virus is the prototype of the JE antigenic complex. The complete nucleotide sequence of the JE viral genome has been determined. Antibody adsorption HI, CF, kinetic neutralization, agar gel diffusion and monoclonal antibody analysis have demonstarted antigenic variations. At least two immuno-types have been identified: Nakayama and JaGAr-01 (isolated from *Culex* mosquitoes). The virus replicates in a number of primary and continuous cell cultures of hamster, porcine, monkey, Vero and mosquito. JE virus produces lethal encephalitis in infant mice by any route, whereas weanling mice succumb to intracerebral virus inoculation. Hamsters and monkeys die after intra-cerebral inoculation but develop asymptomatic viraemia after intraperitoneal inoculation. JE virus does not cause death in rabbits and guinea pigs after inoculation by any route.

Epidemiology

JE continues to be the major type of encephalitis in eastern, south-eastern and southern Asia including Japan, the Far East, Guam, the former USSR, Malaysia, India and western Pacific island areas. In endemic areas, children are affected most, with attack rates in the 3–15 years age group 5–10 times higher than those in older people because of the higher incidence of protective immunity in older age groups. Among factors that influence mortality are age, different virus strains and cross-protective immunity to other flaviviruses, especially dengue. The *Cx. tritaeniorhynchus* and *Cx. vishnui* mosquitoes are the most important vectors.[26,27] Other species of *Culex*, *Aedes*, *Anopheles* and *Mansonia* have been implicated. Pigs and many birds, including herons and egrets, may be the chief source of virus. Other domestic animals can become infected and humans may play a part in epidemics.

Clinical illness

Clinical illness is characterized by headache, fever and other signs of meningitis. Convulsions occur in children. Upper motor neurone involvement with extrapyramidal disturbances is a feature of this disease. The mortality rate of those with meningoencephalitis is around 20% in children and up to 50% in those over 50 years of age. Motor and psychological disturbances are common sequelae.[28]

Pathogenesis and pathology

Pathogenicity in mice varies with different strains of JE virus. During the acute stage oedema and small haemorrhages are found in the brain. Destruction of cerebellar Purkinje cells may occur. Lesions include neuronal degeneration and necrosis, glial nodules and perivascular inflammation. These changes occur mainly in grey matter and predominantly affect diencephalic, mesencephalic and brain stem structures. In the extra-neural tissue a variety of pathological features, including hyperplasia of germinal centres of lymph nodes, enlargement of malpighian bodies in the spleen, interstitial myocarditis and focal haemorrhages in the kidneys, are seen. Transplacental infection in swine results in abortion and stillbirth. Pregnant mice inoculated intraperitoneally also transmit JE virus to the fetus, with subsequent abortion.[29]

Diagnosis

The IgM-capture ELISA is especially well suited for diagnosis by detection of locally synthesized antibody in the CSF. The HI, CF assays and NT are applicable. More recently the potential application of JE non-structural protein (NS) 1-specific indirect ELISA to differentiate infection from vaccination has been described.

Prevention and control

Formalin-inactivated vaccines for use in humans are prepared from infected adult mouse brains or infected primary hamster kidney cell cultures in Japan and China, respectively.[30–32] Primary immunization requires two doses at a 7–14-day interval. Booster vaccinations are given during the first year after primary immunization and then at 3–4-year intervals. A bivalent vaccine has been developed incorporating Nakayama and JaGAr-01 (the two subtypes of JE virus). This vaccine has also proved to be effective. Vaccination of horses with formalin-inactivated vaccines has been successful. Use of pesticides in rice-growing areas has reduced populations of *Cx. tritaeniorhynchus*. Spraying of residual insecticides in livestock pens has reduced the case incidence in China.[32] Treatment consists of good general management and nursing care, especially in the semicomatose and comatose patient. Hyponatraemia secondary to inappropriate antidiuretic hormone secretion is managed with water restriction. Increased intracranial pressure should be considered in severely ill patients with deepening coma and loss of brain stem reflexes. Anti-convulsant therapy may be required.

West Nile virus

This virus is distributed in Africa, Europe and Asia.[33] It has a mosquito as a vector. *Culex* species and other ornithophilic mosquitoes are involved. Birds, including domestic poultry, are the reservoirs. An outbreak of West Nile meningoencephalitis in New York City in 1999 was the first time this virus has been detected in the Western hemisphere. Given the subsequent rapid spread of the virus, which led to the hospitalization of 59 patients, of whom 37 (63%) had clinical signs of encephalitis and seven (12%) died, this infection should be now considered as a serious threat.

Clinical illness

The symptoms presenting include fever, headaches, retrobulbar and muscular pain, sore throat, nausea and vomiting. Development of a maculopapular rash on the trunk, face and limbs may be seen. Occasionally arthralgia may occur. The disease is usually mild in the young, but in older age groups a second phase with mild meningoencephalitis may develop with no sequelae.

St Louis encephalitis virus

St Louis encephalitis (SLE) virus was first identified in Illinois in 1932 and associated with human disease. The virus was later isolated from monkeys previously infected with human brain tissue. SLE virus is transmitted by the mosquitoes *Cx. tarsalis* and *Cx. pipiens*, giving rise to one of the most common and important epidemic arbovirus infections in the USA. Since the 1930s numerous outbreaks have been described in Texas, Ohio and Florida.

Epidemiology

SLE in central USA is commonly dependent on *Cx. pipiens* and *Cx. quinquefasciatus*, whereas in Florida *Cx. nigripalpus* is the principal vector. In western USA *Cx. tarsalis* is the major vector. Epidemic outbreaks appear every 10 years and appear to be dependent on the breeding of *Cx. pipiens*. Disease occurs in late summer and early autumn, and the number of affected humans ranges from 0.1 to 8%.

Clinical illness

SLE induces febrile headache, aseptic meningitis and encephalitis. Although persons of all ages are affected, morbidity and mortality is seen more commonly in the elderly. Following a 3–4-day incubation a generalized illness is observed, with malaise, fever, myalgia, headache and vomiting.[34] After a similar period the symptoms may resolve or progress to clinical findings indicative of neurological involvement. Of patients with neurological signs, 50% die within 7 days of exhibiting signs and a further 30% succumb in the second week. Many patients who survive neurological involvement have persistent headaches and memory loss, and others have overt neurological sequelae such as speech or sensory disturbances.

Diagnosis

Patients exhibiting signs of encephalitis in SLE endemic areas, particularly in late summer and early autumn, should be investigated for SLE. Virus isolation from biological specimens such as blood and urine may be difficult, although virus has been isolated from brain tissue. Confirmation of SLE infection is made by HI or CF tests. IgM-capture ELISA is useful for diagnosis.

Prevention and control

There is no specific treatment or vaccine for SLE. Education of individuals within infected areas and vector control has been shown to be useful following detection of SLE virus activity.

Murray Valley encephalitis

In 1917 and 1918 an infectious agent was isolated following inoculation of monkeys. In 1951 Murray Valley encephalitis (MVE) virus was first isolated from human brain following an outbreak of disease and referred to as Australian X disease. MVE virus is a member of the JE antigenic complex. This virus can be propagated in various cell lines, including primary chick embryo and continuous lines of pig kidney, monkey kidney and hamster kidney cells. Immune enhancement of virus growth has been shown in primary chick embryo fibroblast cultures mediated by a subpopulation of macrophages with Fc receptors.[35] The host range of MVE is wide. Monkeys, horses, sheep and some birds develop encephalitis after intracerebral inoculation. Pigeons and chickens infected subcutaneously develop viraemic infections without clinical illness.

Epidemiology

MVE virus is found in Australia and Papua New Guinea. *Cx. annulirostris* is the major mosquito vector. *Ae. normanensis* may be involved. Birds, including herons, cormorants and other water birds, are the major reservoir of this virus.

Clinical illness

Onset is sudden with headaches, fever and symptoms of a meningoencephalitis. Paresis of both upper and lower motor neurones may occur and breathing and swallowing may become impaired. With modern intensive care the fatality rate has been reduced dramatically to 20%. However, as a result of the increased survival rate, the number of people with both upper and lower motor neurone and psychiatric sequelae has increased.[36]

Prevention and control

No specific treatment for MVE exists. Vector control is as with other members of this family, and massive insecticide programmes are deployed when vector breeding is increased.

Rocio encephalitis

Rocio (ROC) virus is typical of flaviviruses, being spherically shaped with a diameter of 43 nm and cross-reacting with other members of the group (i.e., SLE, Ilheus, JE and MVE virus). Infection of mice, either intraperitoneally or intracerebrally in hamsters induces encephalitis and death. In March 1975 an outbreak of encephalitis was recorded in São Paulo, south-east Brazil, from which an epidemic spread; between March and June 1975, 465 cases with 61 deaths were recorded.[37] The majority of those affected were workers who frequented the forest areas; this was suggestive of an arbovirus infection. In 1975 an unknown arbovirus was isolated from the cerebellum and spinal cord of a 39-year-old farmer and referred to as Rocio virus. Further analysis identified 47 arbovirus isolates in an area previously unknown for arbovirus infections.

Epidemiology

Outbreaks in neighbouring areas followed the 1975–1976 epidemic which affected 18 counties. The disease spread south in 1977. The epidemic peaks followed seasonal parameters that favoured the increased population of mosquitoes.

Pathogenesis

The pathology has been detailed by Rosenberg.[38] Interstitial mononuclear infiltration, microglial proliferation and perivascular cuffing are observed. In acute disease neuronophagia is evident with a distinctive topographical pattern in which the dentate nucleus is more susceptible and the brain stem less so.

Clinical diagnosis

In humans the incubation period is between 7 and 14 days. The clinical features include headache, fever, vomiting, anorexia and nausea, hyperaemia of the oropharynx and conjunctivae, and photophobia. Involvement of the CNS includes meningeal irritation, alteration in consciousness, motor abnormalities and abnormalities in cranial nerve function.

Diagnosis

Epidemiological background and clinical history is paramount. Diagnosis is by cytochemical analysis of the CSF and isolation of the virus in 2-day-old mice from infected tissue. Haemagglutination, CF and plaque reduction techniques in Vero cells, IgM antibody-capture ELISA and ultimately histological examination confirm infection.

Prevention and control

The use of larvicides in ditches and flooded areas, and sanitary measures to drain stagnant waters, have decreased the incidence of infection. Formalin-treated extract of infected mouse brain is used as a vaccine.

Tick-borne encephalitis

The tick-borne encephalitis (TBE) virus complex consists of 14 antigenically closely related viruses, eight of which cause human disease. Russian spring–summer encephalitis (RSSE) and central European encephalitis virus (CEE) are very closely related antigenically and are considered to be subtypes of the same virus. They are separated on the basis of kinetic HI and CF tests and at the molecular level. Peptide maps of both the E and the largest non-structural protein (NS-5) of the two subtypes show some differences.

TBE complex viruses grow in a variety of cell cultures, including pig, bovine and chick embryo, HeLa, human amnion, Hep2, Vero, and primary reptilian and amphibian cells.[39] Cytopathic effect and plaquing are variable. TBE viruses cause encephalitis in rats, guinea pigs, sheep, monkeys and swine after intracerebral inoculation. Infant and weanling mice develop fatal encephalitis by all routes of inoculation. Experimental inoculation of wild vertebrate species, including rodents, foxes, birds,

hares and bats, results in viraemia and antibody formation. Cows, goats and sheep infected by inoculation or tick bite develop viraemia and secrete virus in their milk. The Far Eastern virus type (RSSE) is more virulent for sheep and monkeys inoculated intracerebrally than the Western (CEE) virus.

Epidemiology

TBE encompasses a wide area including Siberia across to Scandinavia, through Vienna into Belgium, to Scotland and Northern Ireland, across Canada, the USA and Japan. The disease occurs in areas that are favourable for ticks. The virus is maintained in nature in a cycle involving ticks and wild vertebrate hosts. Small rodents such as shrews, moles and hedgehogs are believed to be important reservoirs. Large mammals, such as goats, sheep and cattle, serve as host for adult *Ixodes* ticks. *I. ricinus* and *I. persulcatus* are responsible for transmission in Europe and the former Soviet Union, respectively.[40] Other tick species, of the genera *Dermacentor* and *Haemaphysalis*, have been implicated in transmission, especially in areas that do not support *Ixodes* ticks. Transmission to humans occurs mainly in adults over 20 years old who come in contact with infected animals. The disease occurs in two peaks (May–June and September–October) coinciding with the activity of adult *Ixodes* ticks. Small outbreaks involving all age groups result from consumption of raw sheep or goat's milk or cheese.

Pathogenesis and pathology

In monkeys the anterior horn cells of the spinal cord and cerebellar cortex appear to be more affected than other neuronal cells. Members of the TBE complex cause persistent infection in experimental animals. For instance, CEE virus has been isolated from monkey tissues by co-cultivation and explant techniques long after infection. Mice infected with Kyasanur Forest virus are shown to survive for months, with paralysis, low titres of virus in the brain and absence of detectable neutralizing antibodies.[41] Monkeys infected with TBE complex develop chronic encephalitis with degenerative spongiform lesions and astrocytic proliferation. Chronic progressive human encephalitis and seizure disorders have been associated with RSSE virus.

Histopathological findings consist of meningeal and perivascular inflammation, neuronal degeneration and necrosis, and glial nodule formation in areas such as cerebellar cortex, brain stem, basal ganglia, cerebrum and spinal cord. The anterior horn cells of the cervical cord are especially vulnerable, which may result in the lower motor neurone paralysis seen in many cases.

Clinical features

The clinical characteristics of TBE infection in humans have been described by Radsel-Medvescek et al.[42] Most of the tick-borne viruses have been associated with human disease, but there is a gradation of virulence. The Far Eastern (Siberian) strains (formerly called RSSE virus) cause severe encephalitis, often with bulbar and cervical cord involvement, a high fatality rate and frequent sequelae. The disease seen in central Europe is frequently biphasic, with influenza-like symptoms and signs of mild encephalitis. The strains found in Scotland and Northern Ireland cause a sheep disease called louping ill, which is characterized by cerebellar ataxia.

Diagnosis

Definitive diagnosis depends on virus isolation or serology. The virus may be isolated from the blood during the first phase of illness and from brain tissue of patients dying early in the infection. Suckling mice, embryonated eggs and chick embryo cell cultures (with detection of virus by interference assay or immunofluorescence) have been used for virus isolation. Serological diagnosis including HI, CF, single radial haemolysis and NT have been used. Diagnosis by estimation of IgM antibodies is valuable for rapid diagnosis and is applicable to both serum and CSF.

Prevention and control

In the former USSR, formalin-inactivated mouse brain vaccines were used before World War II (1939–1945). Recently vaccines have been produced in embryonated eggs or chick embryo cell cultures. However, the most effective vaccine is derived from chick embryo cell culture-grown virus which is highly purified and inactivated by formalin.[43] The vaccine produces serological conversions in over 95% of recipients and has provided 99% protection in field trials. Preventive measures include pasteurization or boiling of raw milk, avoidance of tick bite by use of repellents and protective clothing. More recently, as with other viral therapeutic strategies, DNA vaccine encoding TB viral components have been shown to be effective in mice and offers the possibility of rational therapy in humans.

Herpetoviridae

Herpesviruses are double-stranded DNA viruses approximately 100–110 nm in diameter and able to establish latency and reactivation. Of the nearly 100 herpesviruses that have been characterized at least partially, the following have been isolated from humans and associated with CNS infections particularly in patients with acquired immune deficiency syndrome (AIDS):

- Herpes simplex virus 1 (HSV-1)
- Herpes simplex virus 2 (HSV-2)
- Human cytomegalovirus (HCMV)
- Varicella-zoster virus (VZV)
- Epstein–Barr virus (EBV)
- Human herpesvirus 6 (HHV-6)
- Human herpesvirus 7 (HHV-7)
- Human herpesvirus 8 (HHV-8)

The simian herpesvirus, B virus (*Crypotetia crypta*), is also known to result in CNS disturbances in humans. For further details the reader is referred to Roizman[44] and Whitley and Schlitt.[45]

Herpes simplex virus

Infections caused by HSV have been known since the time of ancient Greece, where the name herpes was used to mean 'creep' or 'crawl' and probably described the spreading nature of some of the skin lesions resulting from infections. Mouth ulcers and lip vesicles associated with fever were referred to as *herpes febralis* by the Roman scholar Herodotus. It was only later that herpetic lesions and genital infections were associated and by the late nineteenth century the vesicular nature of the lesions was characterized. Histological descriptions of herpes infections were identified in the early twentieth century. The infectious nature of herpesvirus was shown by Lowenstein in 1919: lesions on the rabbit cornea were induced by extracts obtained from a human with herpes simplex. Furthermore such experiments also showed that material from the lesions of herpes could induce encephalitis. The recurrent nature of HSV was first described in the 1930s, and Nahmias and Dowdle[46] identified two antigenic types of HSV, which were later referred to as HSV-1, pertaining to infections 'above the belt', and HSV-2 to those 'below the belt' (i.e., genital infections). Major advancess in antiviral therapy and molecular biology have allowed the rapid elucidation of the replication of these viruses and the subsequent control of infection.

Epidemiology

Herpes simplex viruses are distributed worldwide and, because animal vectors have not been described, humans are deemed to be the sole reservoir for transmission from individuals to susceptible hosts during close personal contact. There is no seasonal variation in infections and, because of the nature of infection, it is estimated that more than one-third of the world's population is infected. Antibody prevalence studies have demonstrated that geographical location, socioeconomic status and age influence the frequency of infection.

Pathogenesis

The pathogenesis of both HSV types is unclear, although it is apparent that both primary and recurrent HSV infection may result in CNS disease. Experiment has shown that HSV gains entry to the CNS via the olfactory and trigeminal nerves,[47] although whether this occurs in humans is unknown. Whether HSV is reactivated within the CNS to result in recurrent disease episodes is also unknown.

Pathology

Acute necrotizing encephalitis is the most common type of acute encephalitis and is observed in all age groups, with the exception of young children. The gross appearance of the brain in adults shows acute inflammation, congestion and softening of the brain. The necrosis is widespread and asymmetrical, associated predominantly with the temporal lobes. The necrotic tissue is sometimes haemorrhagic. In patients who survive for more than several weeks, the tissue starts to disintegrate. Severe microglial reactivity is observed and in cases of disseminated HSV infection mononuclear infiltrates and perivascular cuffing are observed. Viral inclusion bodies may be detected in the nuclei of neurones and to a lesser extent in oligodendrocytes and astrocytes.

Clinical features

The effects of HSV encephalitis on the CNS vary with the type of infection. Patients present with the sudden onset of an acute febrile encephalitic illness characterized by headaches, confusion and meningeal irritation. This is rapidly followed by deterioration in consciousness and may include focal epilepsy and focal motor neurological signs. Disseminated HSV infection is commonly observed in neonates and is related to HSV-2.

Diagnosis

Patients presenting with neurological involvement and suspected herpes simplex encephalitis may be evaluated by scanning procedures such as computed tomography or magnetic resonance imaging, together with CSF analysis. Imaging often shows evidence of oedema and a midline shift in cortical structures. However, virus isolation remains the definitive diagnosis for HSV and allows for typing of the virus. In patients with encephalitis a brain biopsy is necessary to establish diagnosis and eliminate conditions that mimic HSV encephalitis. The most commonly used tests are CF, NT and ELISA.[47] The development of DNA amplification assays will be of value in that non-invasive diagnostic procedures may be carried out on CSF samples to avoid biopsy.

Management

Owing to the high risk of infection during birth in women with active genital HSV, infants born to such mothers should be isolated and cultures obtained after birth and repeated at intervals to exclude infection; otherwise therapy should be administered.

Prevention and control

HSV infections may be controlled by avoidance of infectious secretions, vaccination or antiviral therapy. Patients thus presenting with obvious HSV sores should avoid contact with persons at risk, particularly neonates. The antiviral agents vidarabine and acyclovir have proved useful in the therapy of HSV encephalitis, although the outcome is dependent on factors of age, level of consciousness and disease duration. Such agents have also been suggested to be of use prophylactically for the newborn and for women at the onset of labour. Vaccination remains the preferred method for the prevention of virus infection, although recurrent episodes of infection occur in the presence of antibody and this introduces problems. However, protection from life-threatening infections has been achieved in experimental animal models.[48]

Varicella-zoster virus
History

VZV causes two distinct diseases: chickenpox and 'shingles'. Chickenpox (varicella) is the primary disease, generally of children, and results in a highly contagious, generalized exanthem which occurs in epidemics. (The disease should not be confused with smallpox (variola) with which there is no relation.) The name 'chickenpox' is thought to be derived from the French *chich* (chickpea), referring to the appearance of the vesicle or pox. Shingles (herpes zoster) is a less common disease that occurs in immunocompromised or older individuals and is characterized by dermatomal vesicular rashes. *Herpes zoster* is regarded as a secondary infection associated with the reactivation of VZV that has remained latent since an earlier attack of varicella. The name 'shingles' is derived from the Latin *cingulum*, meaning girdle, which is the appearance of the lesions on the dermatome.

The association between varicella and zoster was described in 1888 by von Bókay, who noted the appearance of chickenpox in a family after exposure to zoster. Furthermore, serological testing could not distinguish between the viruses and the ultimate confirmation came from studies by Weller and Stoddard,[49] who isolated virus from varicella lesions and zoster lesions, and determined that the recovered viruses were identical.

Epidemiology

Varicella is endemic in the population and becomes epidemic during late winter and early spring. The disease affects 90% of children under the age of 10 years. Intimate contact is necessary for infection. In contrast zoster infections are a consequence of reactivation of VZV. Patients at greatest risk are those with Hodgkin's and non-Hodgkin's lymphoma and immunosuppressive conditions such as AIDS. The incidence of CNS complications following varicella is unknown but has been reported as between 0.1 and 0.75%.[50] In contrast, the incidence of encephalitis following zoster is much higher, particularly in immunosuppressed patients.

Pathogenesis

Primary infection with VZV results from respiratory droplet transmission. The virus enters the mucosa of the upper respiratory tract, and to a lesser extent the conjunctiva, and disseminates via the blood. Cycles of replication occur, giving rise to a secondary viraemia from which the virus becomes widespread before the formation of cutaneous lesions. The complications of neurological involvement following varicella infection are classified into: (1) cerebellar ataxia, (2) generalized meningo-encephalitis, (3) transverse myelitis, and (4) aseptic meningitis. The pathogenesis of these conditions is unknown, although immunological mechanisms of tissue damage, as a result of infection, have been suggested.[51] In general the CNS involvement following zoster infections is associated with higher mortality rates than varicella. Complications following infection include encephalitis, ophthalmic zoster, myelitis, multifocal leucoencephalopathy, Guillain–Barré syndrome, and cranial and peripheral nerve palsies. VZV has been isolated from several patients with zoster encephalitis, and inclusions have been found in the glial cells and neurones. Antiviral antibodies have been demonstrated in the CSF of such patients.

Pathology

The neuropathological changes observed in varicella or zoster virus infections depend on the complication induced. In fatal varicella encephalitis, mononuclear infiltration and demyelination have been reported.[52] More detailed pathological findings have been reported for zoster complications because of the higher incidence of death. Zoster meningoencephalitis includes mononuclear infiltration of the meninges, necrosis and axonal degeneration. Degeneration may also involve the posterior columns where neurophagia is observed.

Clinical features

The incubation period for varicella in children is between 14 and 15 days, and is associated with malaise and mild fever. Anorexia and a sore throat are additional clinical features of adult varicella infection. The rash proceeds to the characteristic vesicles that crust. CNS involvement occurs more often in children who present with cerebellar ataxia a few days after the onset of the rash.[50]

The rash of zoster is preceded by pain in the dermatome affected. The lesions, which resemble varicella, appear unilaterally and generally do not cross the midline. Crusts appear up to 1 week after eruption and last for approximately 2 weeks. Neurological complications of zoster may precede the appearance of the rash or appear as late as 10 months afterwards.[53] Further complications are observed in immunosuppressed patients as a result of persistence of virus within the CNS.

Diagnosis

The onset of neurological signs concomitant with appearance of varicella or zoster rash would suggest such infection of the CNS. However, infection is not usually verified by virus isolation from the brain tissue, the exception being at necropsy. Serological assessment utilizes CF, immunofluorescence, ELISA and radioimmunoassays.

Prevention and control

There is generally no specific treatment, apart from antipyretics (not aspirin), for varicella in the immunocompetent host. Neurological complications of varicella, particularly in the immunocompromised host, are important because of the high morbidity and mortality rates. Although α-interferon is effective, two nucleoside analogues, vidarabine and acyclovir, are also employed, although side effects have been reported. The possibility that immune-mediated reactions contribute to the CNS manifestations has given rise to the use of corticosteroids as a treatment of CNS involvement. In contrast, as

evidence suggests active viral replication within the CNS, it would appear that antiviral agents should be employed.

Epstein–Barr virus (see also Chapter 44)

EBV infections are known to give rise to several CNS complications, such as meningoencephalomyelitis, encephalitis and neuropsychiatric syndromes, although the frequency of such manifestations is extremely low. The more usual association is that of Guillian–Barré syndrome. The CSF of patients with CNS disorders following EBV infection shows an increased protein level. In patients dying from EBV infection, the CNS is more often affected and shows perivascular cuffing, oedema and demyelination.

Cercopithecine herpesvirus 1 (B virus)

The non-human primate cercopithecine herpesvirus 1 (B virus) is highly pathogenic to humans. Originally transmitted by the bite of rhesus or macaque monkeys, the virus is now thought to be transmitted from person to person.

History

In 1932, following the bite from a monkey, a physician developed a localized reaction, lymphangitis, lymphadenitis and transverse myelitis, and died. The virus was subsequently recovered from the CNS of the patient and found to be lethal to rabbits following injection.

Epidemiology

The B virus is indigenous to Old World monkeys. Although B virus has been reported in only 22 human cases and is generally transmitted via a bite, individuals in Florida have been affected (two fatally), suggesting person-to-person spread of the virus.[54] Virus is secreted in the saliva and stools of infected animals and these must therefore be considered as potential sources of infection for humans.

Pathogenesis

After the bite a local reaction occurs, followed by lymph node involvement. The course of the disease is dependent on the route of inoculation (as determined from animal studies), although transverse myelitis is a prominent neurological finding before invasion of the CNS. As with other herpesviruses, the B virus becomes latent and may be reactivated under certain conditions.[55] Virus spread to the brain is suggested to occur via the neural routes, as with HSV.

Pathology

All regions of the brain may be infected by B virus and show haemorrhagic foci, necrosis and inflammation in the form of perivascular cuffing of mononuclear cells. Motor neurones are affected and show degeneration. Astrocytosis is observed, with gliosis.

Clinical features

Incubation of B virus varies from 2–3 to 24 days. The neurological involvement is observed 3–7 days after the appearance of the vesicular rash. Death may ensue within 10–14 days, although the progression of the disease depends on the age, site of bite and immunological status of the patient. Clinically the patients present with a localized inflammatory reaction at the site of the bite, or with a respiratory illness, such responses have been described in two individuals.

Diagnosis
Although serological tests demonstrate the presence of B virus, a significant problem is the cross-reactivity with HSV antigens. Diagnosis is therefore dependent on the isolation of virus, particularly from the CSF of humans suspected of being infected, and the use of cell lines susceptible to B virus infection. These include rabbit kidney cells or cell lines such as BSC or LLC-RK1. Definitive diagnosis may be made using molecular methods and neutralization of isolates in serological assays.

Prevention and management
Procedures that limit the transmission of the virus should be adhered to. These include limited contact with macaque monkeys and the routine screening of such animals. The use of hyperimmune serum has not proved effective in controlling human infection, although some success has been achieved in experimental infections.[56] Antiviral therapy has concentrated on the nucleoside analogues: vidarabine, acyclovir and ganciclovir. The use of acyclovir in humans has been reported to slow the infection.[57]

Orthomyxoviridae

Orthomyxoviruses are large enveloped RNA viruses and consist of the influenza viruses which infect swine, horses, seals and a large variety of birds as well as humans. Genetic reassortment produces subtypes that give rise to epidemics of highly contagious, acute respiratory illness afflicting humans.

Epidemiology
Influenza viruses are unique among the respiratory tract viruses in that they undergo significant antigenic variation. Antigenic drift involves minor antigenic changes in haemagglutinin and neuraminidase.

Pathogenesis and pathology
A wide spectrum of CNS involvement has been shown during influenza A virus infection in humans ranging from irritability, drowsiness and confusion to more serious manifestations of psychosis and coma. There are two specific CNS syndromes: influenza encephalopathy and postinfluenza encephalitis. Encephalopathy occurs at the height of the influenza illness and may progress to death.[58] Histological changes are minimal. The CSF is usually normal and the brain shows severe congestion at autopsy. The postencephalitis syndrome is extremely rare and occurs 2–3 weeks after recovery from influenza. The CSF findings suggest that inflammatory changes have

occurred. Influenza A virus has only rarely been isolated from the brain or CSF. It has been suggested that the syndrome of encephalitis lethargica followed by postencephalitic Parkinson's disease was associated with the influenza epidemics of 1918.[59]

Clinical features
Influenza A virus infections in avian species vary with the strain of the virus. Infection with most strains of influenza virus are asymptomatic. However, some strains cause chronic respiratory infections and a minority lead to a rapidly fatal infection accompanied by CNS involvement, with death occurring within 1 week. Febrile convulsion may occur in children with and without underlying CNS abnormalities. Pregnant women in the second or third trimester also have an increased risk of developing fatal influenza disease,[60] and increased incidences of congenital abnormalities and haematological malignancies have been reported following influenza virus infection in pregnancy.[61] Toxic shock syndrome has been seen during influenza virus infection in humans and is believed to be the consequence of bacterial exotoxin secreted by a colonizing *Staphylococcus aureus* strain.[62]

Prevention and control
Antiviral drugs
There are several antiviral drugs that are effective against influenza virus. Amantadine hydrochloride, which has a tricyclic structure, has antiviral properties against all subtypes of influenza A virus but not against influenza B or C viruses.[63,64] The antiviral activity of this drug is exerted after adsorption of the virus to cells but before primary transcription. Amantadine and rimantadine, an analogue of amantadine, are useful for prophylaxis against H1N1, H2N2 and H3N2 influenza A virus infections in adults and children.[65] Ribavirin has an antiviral activity against influenza A and B viruses in tissue cultures and in mice, but not in humans. The antiviral activity is exerted after adsorption, penetration and uncoating have taken place.[66] Interferon induces resistance to influenza infection in mice but has no effect in humans. Preliminary studies with recombinant α-interferon indicate slight protection against illness and virus shedding. Zanamivir is the first widely approved neuraminidase inhibitor for the treatment of influenza. It is delivered directly to the primary site of viral replication, the respiratory tract, and is well tolerated and effective in the treatment of both influenza A and B.

Vaccines
Inactivated influenza A and B virus vaccines are commonly used. The vaccines are designated either whole virus (WV) or split product (SP). The WV vaccines contain intact formalin-treated virus, whereas SP vaccines contain purified formalin-treated virus disrupted with chemicals that solubilize the lipid-containing viral envelope. In addition, experimental vaccines containing the isolated haemagglutinin (HA) and neuraminidase (NA) surface proteins are called subunit vaccines. Other

types of vaccine are those that contain a monovalent influenza A H1N1 virus of a mixture of H1N1, H3N2 and B viruses.

Papovaviridae

The family Papovaviridae is divided into the two subfamilies—polyomaviruses and papillomaviruses—which, although they share several properties, are not related immunologically or genetically.

Polyomaviruses

History
The first human disease associated with a polyomavirus was a rare demyelinating disease of the CNS called progressive multifocal leucoencephalopathy (PML). The disease is observed in immunodeficient individuals and was suggested, in 1961, to be due to a common virus which in the immunocompromised host runs an atypical course of infection. In 1971 two viruses implicated in PML were isolated from the brain (JC virus) of a patient with PML and the urine (BK virus) of a renal transplant patient.[67] JC and BK viruses are contracted in early childhood, persist in the host and are reactivated in cases of immunocompromise, such as in AIDS.

Epidemiology
Polyomaviruses are widely distributed in many species of animals, although they are generally species specific. BK and JC viruses do not naturally infect species other than humans. Antibody titres to BK virus are acquired by 50% of children by 3 years of age and against JC virus by 50% at 6 years of age.[68] PML is worldwide in distribution and occurs as a complication in lymphoproliferative disorders, and chronic disease such as sarcoidosis, in immunodeficiency diseases and in patients on long-term immunosuppressive therapy. Reactivation of both JC and BK viruses is also known to occur in pregnancy, diabetes, chronic disorders and old age. Approximately 20% of patients with PML have AIDS, whereas PML is reported to occur in as many as 3.8% of patients with AIDS presenting with neurological disorders.[69]

Pathogenesis
Primary JC infections of healthy individuals are not associated with illness, although BK virus has been linked with mild respiratory illness. The mode of transmission of BK and JC viruses is unknown, although the rapid acquisition of antibodies has been suggested to be consistent with respiratory disorders. Following primary infection the virus remains latent in the kidney and is reactivated under immunosuppression.

Pathology
The PML brain is characterized by foci of demyelination that are widespread and vary in size. In advanced cases the areas may be necrotic. The lesions occur in the absence of inflammatory cells and are more frequent in the white matter of the cerebrum. Nuclear changes in the oligodendrocytes at the edge of the demyelinated plaques are associated with the presence of JC virus. The lesions are also marked with bizarre giant astrocytes and oligodendrocytes with enlarged nuclei which, at light microscopical level, are deeply basophilic and may contain inclusion bodies. Neurones are unaffected.

Clinical features
Symptoms of a multifocal brain disease without signs of raised intracranial pressure in an immunocompromised host suggest the diagnosis of PML.

Diagnosis
Computed tomography or magnetic resonance imaging of the brain will detect lesions of demyelination. Verification of PML may be carried out following examination of brain tissue in which JC virus may be identified by electronmicroscopy, immunohistological identification as well as in CNS sections, cultivation of the virus in fetal glial cells and characterization of viral DNA by in situ hybridization and PCR.[70]

Management and control
There is no certain treatment for PML, although the accepted regimen is to discontinue the immunosuppressive therapy in combination with the use of antiviral drugs. Attempts at treatment with nucleic acid-based analogues have been reported. See also under HIV infections, as PML is more prevalent in patients with AIDS.

Paramyxoviridae

The Paramyxoviridae family consists of negative-stranded enveloped RNA viruses. These viruses are classified into the three genera, *Paramyxovirus*, *Morbillivirus* and *Pneumovirus*, and include four important human pathogens: measles, mumps, parainfluenza (types 1–4) and respiratory syncytial viruses.

Morbilliviruses

The *Morbillivirus* genus is important in that it contains the human neurotropic virus measles and the canine distemper virus.

Measles (see also Chapter 48)
History
Measles as a disease was first described by Sydenham in the early seventeenth century and the implication that this was a virus infection was established in the 1920s. The disease is generally a childhood illness and is not fatal, although it may be serious in the very young or elderly. Great epidemics of measles have been described, such as the 'black measles' of the eighteenth century.

Waves of measles infection are occasionally observed, with the greatest incidence between November and March.

Epidemiology

In the less developed countries, measles is the most important cause of death between the ages 1 and 5 years. Death occurs predominantly from respiratory and CNS complications. Measles does not have animal reservoirs and no vectors are involved. The principal mode of transmission is via droplets of infected respiratory tract secretions inhaled as a consequence of face-to-face exposure. However, air-borne transmission may be important in certain settings, including schools, hospitals and other institutions.

Virus is present in respiratory secretions and in the conjunctivae during the latter part of the incubation period. Viraemia is also present during this time. Virus is present in the urine for 4 or more days after the onset of rash. Patients are considered infectious from the onset of symptoms through the fourth day of rash.[71] Maternal antibodies provide protection during the first 6 months of life and often longer. Cell-mediated immunity is required to clear measles virus infection, although both humoral and cell-mediated immunity appear to be capable of preventing infection in normal individuals infected with the virus. The slow infection of measles in humans (i.e., subacute sclerosing panencephalitis (SSPE)) is a rare disease in which virus persists in the CNS. The incidence of SSPE is more common in males than females, and is more prevalent in rural areas. The average age of onset is between 5 and 15 years, and infection with measles before the age of 15 years increases the risk of developing SSPE. In the USA the mean annual incidence rate of SSPE was estimated at 0.06 cases per million (aged under 20 years) in 1980.

Clinical features

Measles begins, after an incubation period of 8–12 days, with fever, malaise and anorexia followed by conjunctivitis and cough. The infection then spreads to the epithelial surfaces of the mouth, vasopharynx, respiratory tract and gastrointestinal tract. Two to three days before the onset of the rash, Koplik's spots appear on the buccal mucosa. Koplik's spots are small (1–3 mm), irregular, bright red spots, each of which has a minute bluish-white speck at its centre. The temperature reaches 39.4–40.6°C at the height of the eruption on the fifth day of the illness. The rash starts around day 3 or 4 of prodromal symptoms and spreads downward over the face, neck and trunk, continuing downwards until it reaches the feet by the third day. Cough and coryza follow as a result of an intense inflammatory reaction that involves the mucosa throughout the respiratory tract. The most common complications involve the middle ear, CNS, eyes and skin.[72]

There are three forms of measles encephalitis. Acute postinfectious measles encephalitis is the most common neurological complication of measles. Children under the age of 2 years are rarely affected but it occurs in older children in the ratio of 1 in 1000. It appears a short time after the rash. Between 10 and 20% die and the majority of the survivors have some neurological sequelae. Histopathological examination shows perivascular inflammatory changes and demyelination.

A second form of measles encephalitis, acute progressive infectious encephalitis, occurs in immunosuppressed patients following exposure to measles.[73] Seizures, motor and sensory deficits, and lethargy occur. In the absence of normal cell-mediated immunity, unrestricted cytolytic replication of the virus occurs.

The third form of measles encephalitis is a rare late complication of measles. The symptoms develop over months reflecting loss of cerebral cortical function.[74] In the early stage subtle mental changes and diminishing intellectual capacity are seen. Later, myoclonic jerks occur and progress to chorioathetosis, ataxia and finally coma. Focal retinitis occurs in the majority of the cases, leading to blindness.

Pathogenesis and pathology

Measles virus replicates initially in the respiratory mucosa and spreads, perhaps carried intracellularly in pulmonary macrophages and other cells, to draining lymph nodes where further replication occurs. Virus then enters the bloodstream and from here dissemination of the virus throughout the reticuloendothelial system takes place. This results in a secondary viraemia that disseminates the infection to tissues throughout the body. The most striking feature of measles virus infection in vivo and in vitro is the formation of multinucleated giant cells which result from the fusion of infected cells with the adjacent cells.[75] In tissue culture these giant cells contain eosinophilic cytoplasmic inclusion bodies and their nuclei show condensation of chromatin at the nuclear membrane. The CNS of patients with SSPE shows inflammation of the meninges and perivascular cuffing in both grey and white matter. In the later stages of disease, demyelination and gliosis are observed. Although the mechanisms of myelin damage are unknown, it may be a result of either neural damage or the involvement of an autoimmune response, as T-lymphocyte reactivity to the myelin constituent, myelin basic protein, has been observed.[76]

Diagnosis

Most measles infections are easily recognizable by the distinctive Koplik's spots, rash and catarrhal symptoms. Effective tests for laboratory diagnosis are available and include virus isolation in primary human or monkey cells and antibody determination by simple HI test and by ELISA.[77] Serological tests are effective in identifying cases of SSPE. Patients with this disease have increased serum antibody titres which are 10–100 times higher than those seen in late convalescent-phase sera. There is also a pronounced local production of oligoclonal measles virus antibodies in the CNS.[78] Viral antigen can be identified by immunofluorescence.

Management

No effective treatment is available, although in vitro measles virus replication is sensitive to interferon and ribavirin treatment.

Prevention and control

No treatment is presently available but pooled immunoglobulin can be administered for postexposure prophylaxis up to 5 days after exposure. Live attenuated vaccines are widely used. The rate of seroconversion after vaccination exceeds 90%. Vaccine complications are very rare. Encephalitis occurs at the same rate as in non-vaccinated individuals and the frequency of occurrence of SSPE is reduced by a factor of at least 10 in vaccinated persons.[79] Recently, early administration with intrathecal high-dose interferon-α and intravenous ribavirin has been shown to be effective in the treatment of SSPE.

Canine distemper virus

Canine distemper virus (CDV) deserves mention in this chapter because of its relationship with measles virus and implication in the human neurological disease, multiple sclerosis. This virus gives rise to a chronic relapsing disease of dogs in which demyelination lesions are observed.[80] Furthermore, several studies have suggested associations between the incidence of multiple sclerosis and canine distemper in the dog population.[81]

Paramyxoviruses

Mumps

Mumps has been recognized from the fifth century BC when Hippocrates described the disease as one of swellings behind the ears accompanied by swelling of the testes. However, the first description of neurological involvement was that by Hamilton[82] in the eighteenth century. Transfer of disease from filtered secretions of an affected patient into experimental animals suggested the disease had a viral aetiology.

Epidemiology

Mumps infection increases in the winter months. Immunity to mumps is usually acquired between the ages of 5 and 14 years, with maximal humoral antibody occurring between 4 and 7 years of age.[83] Mortality from mumps is related primarily to the complications of meningitis/encephalitis and orchitis. These occur as age- and sex-specific hazards, with a peak risk in postpubertal males. The incidence of CSF pleocytosis is reported in 30% of patients with mumps parotitis, whereas encephalitis occurs in as many as 35% of cases.[84]

Clinical features

The most characteristic feature of mumps is the swelling of the salivary glands which occurs in up to 95% of all symptomatic cases. The parotid glands are often involved. A moderate febrile response is present at the time of the disease onset. A wide variety of other organs have been involved and include the testes, CNS, epididymis, prostate, ovaries, liver, pancreas, spleen, thyroid, kidneys, eyes, thymus, heart and joints. The onset of mumps meningitis is marked by fever, with vomiting, neck stiffness, headache and lethargy. Seizures occur in 21–30% of patients with CNS symptoms. In cases of CNS involvement about one-third of all patients have evidence of intrathecal IgG synthesis and the presence of oligoclonal immunoglobulins during the first week of CNS symptoms. Examination of the CSF shows abnormalities in the vast majority of the cases. The protein content in the CSF is markedly increased in 60–70% of all cases. This may be due to a damaged BBB, as indicated by high albumin indices that do not normalize for several weeks to months after the onset of the CNS symptoms. The CSF glucose content is depressed to 17–41% of the serum value in 6–29% of all cases.[85]

Pathogenesis and pathology

It has been suggested that the natural infection is initiated by droplet spread with primary viral replication in nasal mucosa or upper respiratory mucosal epithelium. The incubation period from exposure to first clinical symptoms is about 18 days. Virus is actively shed in saliva for as long as 6 days before the onset of symptoms. During this time it is likely that the virus multiplies in the upper respiratory mucosa and spreads to draining lymph nodes with subsequent transient plasma viraemia. Plasma viraemia is terminated by the developing humoral antibodies as early as 11 days after experimental infections of humans. Mumps virus has been shown to infect human lymphocytes in vitro and appears preferentially to infect activated cells of the T-lymphocyte subset. This could imply that cell-associated viraemia may be another mode of virus dissemination. Viral replication in the parotid glands is accompanied by periductal interstitial oedema and a local inflammatory reaction involving lymphocytes and macrophages. Once within neurones, virus is able to distribute widely along neuronal pathways.

Viral invasion of the CNS occurs across the choroid plexus, although rarely is mumps meningoencephalitis fatal. CNS pathology is restricted to perivascular infiltration with mononuclear cells, scattered foci of neuronophagia and microglial proliferation.[86] Perivascular demyelination also occurs; this may be the result of an autoimmune attack on the brain tissue. Persistence of mumps virus has been suggested within the CNS of humans. Deafness is probably the result of direct damage to the cochlea and, to a lesser extent, cochlear neurones.[87] Most cases of mumps meningitis resolve without sequelae. However, ataxia and behavioural disturbances may be slow to resolve following mumps meningoencephalitis.[88,89]

Diagnosis

The clinical diagnosis of mumps is seldom problematic in the presence of parotitis. Laboratory diagnosis includes determination of virus-specific IgM and IgG levels.

Mumps meningitis can be confirmed on the basis of a raised CSF serum antibody ratio.

Management and control

Hyperimmune γ-globulin to modify the course of mumps is used in selected cases. Two general types of vaccine have been used. Recently controversy over the links with autism and measles–mumps–rubella (MMR) vaccination has led to the idea of single vaccines. However, the most widely used are the live attenuated mumps virus preparations given as the triple MMR vaccine; killed mumps virus antigens have a more restricted use.[90]

Parvoviridae

To date parvoviruses have not been implicated in human CNS disease although infections of experimental animals with parvoviruses are known to induce cerebellar ataxia[91] and affect the development of the cerebellum during the perinatal period.

Picornaviridae

The Picornaviridae family consists of small RNA viruses and comprises four genera: *Enterovirus, Rhinovirus, Aphthovirus* and *Cardiovirus.* Those involved in neurological disease are listed in Table 49.6.

Enteroviruses

Enteroviruses multiply throughout the alimentary tract and tend to be resistant to known antibiotics and chemotherapeutic agents. The host range of the enteroviruses is varied and may be readily induced to yield variants, which has led to the development of attenuated polio vaccine strains. The viruses of this genus, which are important CNS pathogens of humans, are the polioviruses and coxsackieviruses. For more detailed studies on enteroviruses, the reader is referred to Melnick.[92]

Poliovirus (see also Chapter 16)

The disease poliomyelitis has existed since ancient times, although the fact that the causative agent was a virus was first demonstrated only in 1909 by Landsteiner and Popper.[93] Studies in monkeys and the adaptation to tissue culture resulted in the development of methods of purification and the production of reliable vaccines through which infection can now be controlled. Poliomyelitis may be caused by one of three strains of virus: polio types 1, 2 or 3. Three forms of clinical disease have been recognized: paralysis, aseptic meningitis and minor febrile illness.

Epidemiology

Poliovirus was, until very recently, endemic worldwide, infecting susceptible infants and producing paralytic poliomyelitis in those who were not protected by maternal antibody. In 1916 80% of cases were in those under 5 years of age. The changes in sanitation and hygiene in the late nineteenth century, with industrialization in the north of Britain, decreased the incidence in infants but resulted in a higher incidence of paralytic poliomyelitis in later childhood due to delay in exposure to the virus. In the epidemics of 1950 the peak age was 5–9 years, although about one-third of cases and two-thirds of deaths were in those over 15 years.[92] Since 1985, most of the cases of polio worldwide have been in developing countries, although the number of deaths due to other diseases may mask the true incidence of infantile paralysis.

Pathogenesis

Following ingestion, poliovirus replicates in the pharynx and intestines, from which it is excreted. Transmission is by the faecal–oral route and thus the necessity for hygiene is paramount. After initial replication in the lymphoid tissue of the pharynx and gut, which leads to viraemia, the virus infects the CNS via the blood. Neural spread has been demonstrated in children following tonsillectomy.[92]

Pathology

The anterior horn cells of the spinal cord are susceptible to infection with poliovirus and are damaged or, in severe cases, completely destroyed.[94] The lesions observed in the CNS may extend to the hypothalamus and thalamus. Neuronophagia is commonly observed, with inflammation being secondary to neuronal attack. In less severe cases oedema, which results in temporary disturbance of neural functions, subsides and the cells recover completely.

Table 49.6 Picornaviruses implicated in human neurological disease.

Genus	Virus	Disease
Enterovirus	Human polio	Paralysis, aseptic meningitis, febrile illness, aseptic meningitis, paralysis
	Human coxsackie (groups A and B)	Aseptic meningitis, paralysis, meningoencephalomyelitis
	Echoviruses	Aseptic meningitis, paralysis, encephalitis, ataxia, or Guillain–Barré syndrome
	Enterovirus (types 70, 71)	Paralysis, meningoencephalitis
Cardiovirus		Encephalomyocarditis

Clinical features

Following infection approximately 1% of patients present with clinical disease. Abortive poliomyelitis is the most common form of the disease in which fever, malaise, drowsiness, headache and sore throat are experienced to varying degrees. The signs abate within a few days. Stiffness and pain in the back of the neck may also be experienced, in which case non-paralytic poliomyelitis, or aseptic meningitis, is diagnosed. The disease may become biphasic, whereby a minor illness is followed by a remission, but which subsequently develops into a major severe illness.

Diagnosis

Antibodies are usually present by the time paralysis occurs and a viraemia may be detected and used to determine the subtype using serological techniques. More recently molecular biological techniques have been used to demonstrate poliovirus in CSF.

Prevention

In the early 1950s Jonas Salk calculated the inactivation kinetics of formalin on poliovirus grown in monkey kidney cells.[95] A vaccine was developed that was licensed in the USA in 1955, the aim of which was to induce protection by way of stimulating antibody production. Using the formalin-inactivated vaccine it was necessary to reimmunize at 1 and 6 months with successive boosters. The advance of cell culture techniques has enabled the production of large batches of virus and more effective vaccines. In contrast, oral polio vaccines were developed using live attenuated virus which today consists of a mixture of three strains. The oral vaccine protects by producing both systemic antibody and local secretory IgA which would block virulent virus, preventing spread from the gut. These vaccines have the advantages over killed preparations of ease of administration and long-lasting immunity, although they have the 'disadvantage' of being excreted and thus have the potential to spread to non-vaccinated persons.[96]

Coxsackie and echoviruses

Of the non-polio enterovirus infections, echovirus 9 is the most frequent cause of enterovirus disease and the most common virus to be isolated in epidemics.

The chief viruses implicated in CNS disease are coxsackie B1-6, A7 and A9, although many echoviruses have been associated with meningitis, as has enterovirus type 70. Severe CNS disease has been observed in enterovirus 71 infections, particularly in the severe epidemic of 1975 in Bulgaria.[97] Antibodies to enterovirus 71 were detected in 72% of patients presenting with paralysis and virus isolations were made from numerous tissues including the CNS. Of the seven reported epidemics with enterovirus 71, all reported evidence of CNS involvement.[98]

Poxviridae

Neurological complications of poxvirus infections are generally associated with vaccination, namely *postvaccinial encephalitis*. The pathogenesis and pathology resemble other postinfectious encephalitides and include perivascular cuffing, mononuclear infiltration and demyelination.

Prion diseases

Several so-called 'slow virus infections' of the CNS that are not a result of conventional virus infection, although transmissible, are classified as prion diseases or subacute spongiform encephalopathies. They are listed in Table 49.7.

These transmissible agents are thought to have a unique characteristic in being devoid of nucleic acid and yet able to transfer disease. Transmission of disease does not occur if the agents are treated with proteases. Additionally, attempts at molecular cloning are negative and nucleic acid antagonists have been shown to be ineffective. The name of the so-called infectious agents, termed *prions*, is derived from *pro*tein and infec*tion*, meaning that the infectious agent is protein devoid of nucleic acid. This 'protein only' hypothesis is still under debate.

Of particular importance is the presence of a normal form of the protein found on all cells, particularly neurones. The two forms of prion proteins (PrP) (normal and infectious) are identical in terms of amino acid sequences but differ in their conformations. Furthermore the normal protein is broken down by enzymes, whereas the abnormal prion protein (PrP^{sc}) is resistant to attack by enzymes and found in the CNS only during disease where the protein accumulates in the cell.

Kuru

Kuru was restricted to the population of villages in the highland of Papua New Guinea. The disease, which means shaking or shivering in the Fore language, is characterized by tremors that progress to lack of motor control and complete cerebellar ataxia. The clinical course of the disease generally results in death within 1 year of onset, although prolonged disease has been reported. Kuru was described by Gajdusek.[99] The disease was more

Table 49.7 Prion diseases of humans and animals.

Host	Disease
Human	Kuru
	Creutzfeldt–Jakob disease
	Gerstmann–Sträussler–Scheinker syndrome
Animals	Scrapie
	Transmissible mink encephalopathy
	Chronic wasting disease of mule deer and elk
	Bovine spongiform encephalopathy

common in children and females than in males, and was thought to be due to the practice of certain tribal rituals. The changes in ritual cannibalism and treatment of corpses have halted the contact of persons with infected brain tissue, resulting in a virtual cessation in the incidence of disease.

The pathological picture is restricted to the CNS and is characterized by diffuse neuronal degeneration and astrocytic hypertrophy. The term 'spongiform encephalopathy' is derived from the large vacuolation of the large neurones of the striatum. In many cases amyloid-containing plaques are observed and electron microscopy reveals scrapie-associated fibrils common to other diseases in this group.

Creutzfeldt–Jakob disease and Gerstmann–Sträussler–Scheinker syndrome

Patients with Creutzfeldt–Jakob disease (CJD) present with rapidly progressive dementia and motor dysfunction; like Kuru, it is usually fatal within 1–2 years following onset. The incidence of CJD is low (prevalence of 1 per million) and is generally sporadic, although there is evidence for a familial trait in 10% of all cases. Furthermore, rare mutations in the natural PrP segregate with disease, which may be linked with genetic predisposition.[100] The disease is transmissible experimentally, as shown in laboratory animals,[101] or as a result of 'accidental transmission' to humans following surgery.[102] Although the average age of CJD onset is in middle to late life, the disease has been described in young (4–19 years) patients undergoing growth hormone therapy. In these transmissions the disease resembled Kuru rather than typical CJD, suggesting that Kuru may have originated in New Guinea as a result of contamination of tissue from a patient with CJD.

Gerstmann–Sträussler–Scheinker syndrome (GSS) is a variant of CJD in which patients present with progressive cerebellar ataxia, giving rise to a longer period from onset to death compared with CJD. Again several mutations in the PrP have been described and the disease is transmissible to laboratory animals.

Prevention and control

The resistance of the CJD/GSS prion to common sterilization procedures, such as boiling or the use of ultraviolet light, has resulted in a change in operating procedures and the use of hypochlorate and sodium hydroxide for sterilization.[103] To date, no treatment for the human diseases has been effective. Future therapeutic regimens will possibly include drugs that interfere with the PrPsc, preventing it from accumulating in the cell, or gene therapy to switch off production of the protein.

More recently, studies directed towards blocking infective prion protein migration have been to be dependent on B-cells. In addition, therapeutic strategies using antibodies directed against the conformational forms of PrP are currently under investigation.

Animal prion diseases

Scrapie was observed in the 1930s following the use of louping ill virus vaccine produced in scrapie-contaminated brain tissue, although the disease has been recognized in sheep breeders for more than two centuries. The disease is a chronic disease in which affected animals present with progressive ataxia tremor and wasting. The name 'scrapie' is derived from the necessity of animals to rub or scrape themselves as a result of the disease. Susceptibility to scrapie is dependent on the strain of sheep and is linked to polymorphisms in ovine PrP.

The disease, like the human prion infections, is characterized histologically by the presence of vacuolated neurones and spongiform changes, and may be induced experimentally in laboratory mice and guinea pigs. The use of transgenic mice, in which mutations in the PrP are deliberately introduced with resulting neurological defect, supports the role of this protein in initiating disease. Furthermore, transgenic mice lacking the gene that codes for the natural PrP are resistant to infection with the scrapie PrP.[104] The use of experimental prion disease has allowed the investigation of potential therapies and, although no effective treatment is available, the use of amphotericin B has been shown to reduce the concentration of scrapie PrP during the preclinical phase and to prolong the incubation period of the disease.[105]

Transmissible mink encephalopathy, which is very similar to scrapie, is spread through mink colonies as a result of fighting and cannibalism, and is thought to have originated from contaminated food derived from cattle. Infected tissue can transfer disease. Likewise bovine spongiform encephalopathy, first described in England in 1986, is possibly a result of feeding scrapie-contaminated food.[106]

Reoviridae

The family Reoviridae contains three genera: *Reovirus*, *Rotavirus* and *Orbivirus*. To date, the first two are not known to be implicated in human neurological diseases.

Orbiviruses

Many of the viruses of this genus are important in veterinary disease and produce illness in a wide variety of animals, including horse sickness and blue-tongue disease.[107] The exception is the dengue-like illness of humans, Colorado tick fever.

Colorado tick fever

Colorado tick fever (CTF) was first described in the mid-nineteenth century in the Rocky Mountain states. Bowen et al.[108] isolated the virus from human blood and later demonstrated that CTF virus could be isolated from the tick *Dermacentor andersoni*.

Epidemiology

This disease is confined to the geographical distribution of the adult *Dermacentor andersoni* tick in the Rocky Mountain states and in parts of north-western Canada; it is a common infection in hikers and foresters during May and June.

Pathogenesis

Infection with CTF virus gives rise to little or no disease in the natural host and induces a prolonged or persistent viraemia in vertebrate hosts such as ground squirrels and chipmunks that serve as amplificatory rodents. CTF virus is involved in bone marrow precursor cells and its presence in erythrocyte precursors renders the host susceptible to haemorrhagic disorders.[109] The onset of disease occurs 3–6 days after the tick bite.

Pathology

CTF virus infections do not generally result in death and thus pathological features are not well described. However, following experimental infections of mice, the cerebellum shows widespread necrosis and cellular infiltration.

Clinical features

A febrile illness develops, with headache and myalgia. A maculopapular rash is seen in about 50% of patients. Colorado tick fever is a benign disease but in very rare cases a bleeding diathesis may develop and, particularly in children, there may be a typical meningoencephalitic illness. Resolution of the acute phase may take 5–10 days. Infection in the CNS may be observed as a mild meningeal reaction to severe encephalitis. The frequency of CNS involvement ranges from 1 to 10%.[110]

Diagnosis

Abnormalities include leucopenia and thrombocytopenia; virus may be isolated from the blood owing to its persistence in the erythrocytes. Some time after disease onset, CF and neutralizing antibodies may be detected in the blood. CSF findings are typical of encephalitis.

Prevention

At present there is no treatment for CTF, although health awareness when hiking in the affected areas may help to limit exposure to tick bites.

Retroviridae

Several features of retroviruses, such as their unique replication cycle, oncogenic ability and the wide variety of interactions with the host, including their ability to remain latent, have led to the intense scientific attention these viruses have received. Retroviruses are classified into the three subfamilies: Oncovirinae, Lentivirinae—lentiviruses (e.g., maedi-visna, which results in chronic inflammation of the CNS) and human immunodeficiency viruses which result neurologically in AIDS dementia and demyelination—and Spumavirinae.

Lentiviruses

In contrast to viruses that cause acute disease and where virus is finally eliminated, the lentiviruses include those that are able to escape such elimination and persist in the host. These include the maedi-visna of sheep which give rise to chronic neurological disorders, and human immunodeficiency viruses in which neurological damage has been recognized.

Maedi-visna

Maedi-visna (*maedi* = laboured breathing, *visna* = wasting and paralysis—Icelandic translations) is the prototype lentivirus in which the slow onset of clinical disease resulting from prolonged incubation of the virus is very similar to the prion disease of sheep (scrapie).

Epidemiology

The disease was first recognized in Iceland[111] but is observed in most countries with large sheep populations. Early transmission studies in Iceland showed that the disease could be transmitted from infected sheep to naive sheep by intracerebral inoculation. Many strains of visna have been obtained which vary in their ability to, for example, be propagated in tissue culture.

Pathogenesis

Virus is isolated from many tissues, particularly the lymphatics, spleen and peripheral blood leucocytes. Higher titres are isolated from the brain and lung. Conversion of the maedi illness to visna may occur as a result of infected peripheral blood leucocytes crossing the BBB and subsequently infecting the CNS.

Pathology

Following experimental infection, severe meningitis and encephalitis are observed, coinciding with perivascular lesions of inflammatory cells. The inflammatory cells observed in the CNS consist of monocytes/macrophages, plasma cells and T lymphocytes. Depending on the duration of the disease, the brain may show large areas of focal demyelination. Additionally, inflammatory lesions and/or demyelination may occur in the presence of areas of necrosis and gliosis.[112]

Clinical features

Clinical disease is observed as lymphadenopathy, pneumonia and CNS involvement. The sheep appear dyspnoeic with loss of flesh. The appearance of clinical disease is dependent on the strain of animal and dose of inoculation.[113]

Prevention and control

Due to the expense of developing vaccines for animals, very few studies on controlling infection have been attempted. However, sheep hyperimmunized with disrupted virus are known to develop neutralizing antibodies which were able to confer some protection against homologous virus infection.[113]

Human immunodeficiency virus (see also Chapter 20)

The human immunodeficiency viruses consist of HIV-1 and HIV-2 and are typical lentiviruses (see Chapter 20). This chapter will concentrate only on the CNS disease in HIV infections. Details of other features are to be found elsewhere in this book and in other comprehensive articles.[114]

CNS disorders associated with HIV infection are import-ant because they are commonly seen during all stages of the disease and contribute to the outcome of the disease. The variations in clinical manifestation are dependent on both the stage of HIV disease and opportunistic infections, whether viral, such as JC infection giving rise to PML, or bacterial (e.g., *Listeria monocytogenes* meningitis).

The gross clinical features observed in neurological complications of HIV infections have been outlined by Price et al.[114] and are classified by the neuroanatomical localization, i.e., whether the brain or cord is involved and whether the lesions are focal or non-focal. With regard to the neurological complications, these may be categorized depending on the stage of the disease: (1) during acute HIV infection of the CNS; (2) asymptomatic infection; (3) aseptic meningitis and headache; and (4) AIDS dementia complex (ADC). CNS syndromes of children give rise to a fifth syndrome resulting in abnormal neurological develop-ment and arrested intellectual and motor function.

HIV infection of the CNS

HIV may enter the brain across the BBB or by infecting monocytes (macrophages and microglia) which are productively infected by virtue of having surface CD4 molecules. Such macrophages may then cross the BBB, thus allowing the HIV access to the CNS. During the asymptomatic phase CNS involvement is common and at least 40% of all persons with HIV have abnormal CSF, with increased cell counts and protein levels. Anti-HIV antibodies are detectable in the CSF and in some patients oligoclonal bands are observed. It has been suggested that aseptic meningitis and headache, AIDS dementia complex and progressive encephalopathy of children are due to the direct effects of HIV infection.[115]

Aseptic meningitis

The common neurological symptoms of early or primary HIV-1 infection are headaches and photophobia, which may be either acute or chronic.[116] Although the cause of such clinical symptoms is not known in all patients, headaches have been related to systemic disease such as *Pneumocystis carinii* infection. Such features may subside or progress to encephalitis, meningitis or ataxia. Aseptic meningitis affects 5–10% of HIV-infected patients; HIV may be diagnosed by positive virus culture or p24 antigen in the serum or CSF.

AIDS dementia complex

ADC is commonly observed in the later stages of HIV-1 infection in relation to major systemic infections, although in a small group of patients ADC occurs in the absence of opportunistic infections and may be related to HIV-1 infection of the brain. Infection and disease are not synonymous. ADC may be classified into five major stages ranging from stage 0, which encompasses normal mental and motor functions, to stage 4, in which the patient demonstrates rudimentary levels of intellectual and social comprehension and is paraparetic or paraplegic.[114]

Epidemiology

The progression of HIV-1 infection to ADC is related, in general, to the level of immunosuppression in the patient. In early disease with opportunistic infections approxi-mately 10–30% of patients exhibit ADC stage 1, while 5–15% exhibit severe neurological disturbances (stage 2–3). In contrast, in the late stages of infection the majority of patients with AIDS show severe disability (stage 4).[115]

Pathology

Pathological changes in the CNS of patients with ADC are most prominent in the subcortical regions, correlating with the observed subcortical clinical abnormalities. The most common changes include: (1) pallor of the white matter and demyelination; (2) gliosis, necrosis and mild neuronal loss; (3) multinucleated giant cells, which may be observed in the later stages of disease; and (4) spongiform changes, which are related to severity of dementia.[116]

Clinical features

Patients with ADC show distinct cognitive changes associated with subcortical, as opposed to cortical, changes. There is general mental slowing, including apathy, impaired concentration and features associated more with depression than CNS infection. Confusion, halluci-nations, impaired memory and problem-solving deficiencies are common prior to obvious dementia. ADC may progress in steps or with sudden deterioration associated with systemic infection.

Diagnosis

In patients with ADC, computed tomography and magnetic resonance imaging show cerebral atrophy, although such a finding is non-specific. The CSF of ADC patients contains HIV-specific cytotoxic T cells, increased protein, oligoclonal bands and soluble intercellular adhesion molecule 1 (ICAM-1), which may serve as a marker for disease.[117]

Prevention and control

Zidovudine (formerly AZT) has been shown to improve neuropsychological performance and reduce the incidence of ADC, as has the anti-inflammatory alkaloid cepharanthine.[118] Psychiatric disorders such as mania may be treated with lithium, as in non-infected patients.

CNS syndromes in children

Mother-to-child transmission accounts for 80% of HIV infections in children. Infected children present with encephalopathy, either progressive or static, and may be seen from the age of 2 months. The children with progressive encephalopathy become inactive and may develop paralysis and, if untreated, die within 1 year. The CSF may show an increased protein concentration and high levels of HIV-specific antibodies. Antibody levels in the serum (as a means of diagnosis) may be difficult to interpret owing to the presence of transplacental maternal antibodies. The brains of HIV-infected children are atrophic and contain perivascular inflammation, and the small vessels show calcification.

Opportunistic viral infections of the CNS

Although a variety of opportunistic CNS infections occur with HIV infection, only viral infections will be considered in this section. The major infections are observed with JC virus that gives rise to PML (see under Papoviruses) and cytomegalovirus (CMV). PML occurs in 2–5% of patients with AIDS; its effects are observed as dementia and/or focal neurological signs. Herpesvirus infections, in the form of CMV, VZV and HSV-1 and -2, give rise to 'secondary viral encephalomeningitides'. CMV may result in encephalitis and retinal infiltration, which is observed in approximately 20% of patients with AIDS. As a result of immunosuppression VZV may be reactivated, giving rise to neurological syndromes such as hydrocephalus or ventriculitis. Like VZV, HCMV causes disease after both primary and recurrent infections. The former is more serious, particularly in pregnant women, who may transmit the virus to their offspring, with a high risk of intellectual impairment and deafness. Various experimental vaccines are in development, ranging from live, attenuated HCMV, subunit envelope glycoprotein, poxvirus vectors with CMV genes inserted, and plasmid DNA.

Rhabdoviridae

The family Rhabdoviridae is divided into the genera *Lyssavirus*, which contains rabies virus, and *Vesiculovirus*, containing vesicular virus (VSV). The name Rhabdoviridae is derived from the Greek *rhabdos*, meaning rod. The viruses in this family are rod or bullet–shaped and infect a wide variety of species.

Lyssaviruses (see also Chapter 45)

The name of this genus is derived from the Greek *lyssa*, meaning rage or frenzy, and includes rabies virus. The Duvenhage and Mokola viruses of this genus are also associated with human disease.

The rabies virus is a 180 × 75-nm helical nucleocapsid with a lipid bilayer from which protrude 10-nm protein spikes. Of the five proteins identified, those designated G and N have been characterized most extensively. The G protein is the only viral protein that induces virus-neutralizing antibody and is also a target for T-helper and

T-cytotoxic lymphocyte reactivity. The importance of such antigenic determination offers an approach for the development of vaccines. For further literature on rabies virus the reader is referred to the excellent reviews of Whitley and Middlebrooks[119] and Fields' *Virology*.[120]

History

Literary references to rabies infections have been recorded since before 2000 BC and they have been mentioned in a number of historical documents, including those of Democritis, Aristaeus and Artemis. There have been six important events in the history of rabies since the 1880s, including the application of the human rabies vaccine (1885) and the finding of the pathognomonic Negri bodies for diagnosis (1903). In the 1940s a mass application of potent rabies vaccine for dogs was introduced which greatly diminished the spread of disease. More recently the introduction of oral vaccination of foxes has resulted in the virtual elimination of rabies from Switzerland. Rabies hyperimmune antiserum was used in addition to the human vaccine regimen (1954) and the adaptation of rabies virus to cell culture and the development of a fluorescent antibody test for diagnosing infected animal brains (1958) has resulted in a dramatic improvement in the control of the disease.[121]

Epidemiology

Rabies virus is capable of infecting all warm-blooded animals, but there is a hierarchy for susceptibility.[122] Most susceptible are foxes, coyotes, jackals and wolves. The opossum is the least susceptible species. Moderately susceptible animals include dogs, the most frequent vector for transmission to humans, as well as cats, racoons and skunks. An increasing source of rabies is observed in bat populations[123] and accounts for approximately 10% of rabies-infected animals in the USA. The epidemiology of human rabies parallels that in the animal population. A higher incidence is observed in areas where public health programmes are not implemented, such as in India and Mexico where the incidence is 3.3 cases per 100 000.

Pathogenesis

The major route of infection is invariably via the bite from a rabid animal, although transmission by aerosols and as a result of corneal grafts must be taken into account. Once introduced, rabies virus is quickly sequestered. It was thought that the virus stayed in the nervous tissue close to the wound site, although studies by Murphy et al.[124] indicated that the virus replicates in muscle tissue before progressing to the peripheral nervous tissue via the neuromuscular connections. That rabies virus travels to the central nervous tissue via the nerves has been demonstrated experimentally: when the sciatic nerve was severed prior to injection of rabies virus in the foot of an animal, disease was prevented.

The incubation period of the disease varies and may be as short as 2 weeks but is more commonly 1–3 months, and in a few cases more than 1 year. Although it is widely accepted that the incubation period is related to the distance between the site of the bite and proximity to the CNS, a study by Dupont and Earle[125] did not support this view.

Pathology

Human rabies pathology, apart from the pathognomonic Negri body, consists of perivascular cuffing, some neuronophagia and limited neuronal necrosis. The limited pathology does not match the marked symptoms of hydrophobia, aerophobia, excitation and coma. There is pathology in other organs, and Negri bodies have been found in the cornea and adrenal glands.

Clinical features

Development of infection depends on the severity of the exposure, the site of the bite and possibly other factors. Neurological findings may be classified as either 'furious' or 'paralytic' and are not exclusive. Furious rabies is far more common and is characterized by spasms in response to tactile, auditory, visual and olfactory stimuli (e.g., aerophobia and hydrophobia). Such symptoms alternate with periods of lucidity, agitation, confusion and autonomic dysfunction. The alternative form of paralytic rabies ranges from paralysis of one limb to quadriplegia. Disease progresses to coma with neurological complications associated with abnormal hormonal homeostasis, alterations in temperature and inability to control blood pressure.

Diagnosis

Clinical diagnosis of rabies may be difficult in patients presenting with a paralytic or Guillain–Barré-like syndrome, and the World Health Organization (WHO) Committee on Rabies[126] has emphasized that rabies must be included in the differential diagnosis of all persons presenting with neurological involvement.

The laboratory diagnosis of rabies may be performed by fluorescent antibody techniques, on smears or frozen sections, and by the use of ELISA. A rapid rabies enzyme immunodiagnosis assay allows the antigen to be visualized by the naked eye and is thus a test that can be carried out in the field (with a special test kit). Molecular tests, such as the polymerized chain reaction, are available. Virus isolation can be performed using a murine neuroblastoma cell line (NAC1300), which reduces the time taken for diagnosis by 2 days.

Prevention and control

Rabies mortality can be reduced by preventing exposure to the virus, aborting infection and thereby preventing illness, or curing clinical disease.

The WHO committee has stressed the importance of the adoption and establishment of international and regional surveillance systems in combination with dog control. In over 80 countries rabies is prevalent in dogs, which appear to be the most dangerous reservoir. Each year approximately 4 million people in these areas receive treatment after exposure to rabies and in 99% of all human cases the virus is transmitted by dogs. Furthermore 90% of people who receive post-exposure treatment live in areas of canine rabies.

Vaccination

The control of rabies is through oral immunization of domestic and, more recently, wild animals. Recombinant vaccines that make use of poxvirus, baculovirus and adenoviruses are possible. The vaccines available for human immunization are: (1) brain tissue vaccine (possible side effects of autoreactivity to brain tissue); (2) purified duck embryo vaccine inactivated with β-propriolactone; and (3) tissue culture vaccines. For animal vaccination, nervous tissue-derived virus has been shown to be effective in mass vaccination of the canine population in North Africa. In contrast, cell culture-derived virus (either inactivated or modified live virus) for canine rabies has been used in a combined vaccination programme with distemper, hepatitis, parvo and leptospirosis vaccines. Combined vaccines with foot and mouth vaccine are used for cattle, sheep and goats. For feline control the rabies vaccine is combined with panleucopenia virus, feline calicivirus and feline parvovirus vaccines.

The 1992 WHO report[126] describes the use of post-exposure treatment for humans. This makes use of three vaccine doses applied in the deltoid muscle of the right and left arm at day 0 and a further dose on day 7. The results show an increase in both the cellular and humoral response. Such treatment has also been combined with antirabies immunoglobulin.

Monoclonal antibodies

Postexposure treatment with murine monoclonal antibodies, and more recently murine–human chimeric antibodies and humanization of monoclonal antibodies, offers a more specific treatment regimen.

Interferon and interferon inducers

Administration of recombinant α-interferon with vaccines decreases rabies virus in subhuman primates. Exogenous interferon has already been shown to be effective in a patient given a corneal transplant from a patient with rabies.

Togaviridae

The family Togaviridae originally contained the genera of alphaviruses, flaviviruses and rubiviruses, based on various characteristics such as size, mode of replication and transmission by mosquitoes. The name is derived from the structure of the virus which consists of a ribonucleic acid within a lipid envelope (L. *toga* = coat). With advances in virology, the structure of the genomes and replication strategies of the genera have become more distinct and the flaviviruses are now classified as a separate family. Detailed studies of togaviruses and flaviviruses may be found in an excellent review by Schlesinger and Schlesinger.[127]

The togaviruses are now divided into the alphaviruses, rubiviruses and pestiviruses.

Alphaviruses (see also Chapter 41)

The knowledge of the structure and replication of alphaviruses has been based on Sindbis (SIN) and Semliki Forest viruses (SFV), which provide valuable models for study. Of the alphaviruses that are important encephalitogenic agents, eastern equine encephalitis (EEE), Venezuelan equine encephalitis (VEE) and western equine encephalitis (WEE) viruses are the most important, although chikungunya virus (CHIK) infection is also known to induce neurological complications.

Chikungunya
History
The word *chikungunya*, meaning 'to contort or bend', was used by a tribe in Tanzania to describe the clinical manifestations of a virus epidemic of 1952–1953. Because this virus invariably results in crippling arthritis, CHIK infection was probably responsible for the epidemic in 1779 in Indonesia.

Epidemiology
CHIK is found in Africa, including Tanzania, Zimbabwe, Transvaal, Zambia and the Congo, and India, Sri Lanka and South-East Asia, including Vietnam and Thailand.[128] The disease is transmissible by mosquitoes. *Ae. aegypti* and various *Culex* species are the vectors in urban epidemics in Asia. In Africa, the vector involved in forest areas is *Ae. africanus* and in Sudan *Ae. leuteocephalus*.

Clinical illness
The disease is biphasic. In the first phase, symptoms include fever and severe joint, limb, and spine pains. This phase can last 6–10 days. The second phase occurs after a febrile period of 2–3 days and is associated with an irritating maculopapular rash over the body, particularly on the extensor surface of the limbs. Joint pains may persist occasionally, without fever, for up to 4 months. In some cases myocarditis and peripheral circulatory failure have been seen. In this second phase, encephalitis and manifestations of neurological involvement are occasionally observed.[129] The mortality rate is estimated at 0.4%, but in patients under 1 year old it may be as high as 2.8% and similarly in those aged over 50 years the death rate may increase.

Diagnosis
Definitive diagnosis is by specific serological analysis such as HI, CF and ELISA, although the combination of febrile illness and rheumatic manifestations in a patient returning from sub-Saharan Africa or parts of Asia are characteristic features of CHIK infection.

Management and control
Supportive care for patients with CHIK infections are important with respect to the arthralgia. In severe cases chlorquine phosphate may be administered. Inactivated virus vaccines have been shown to be effective but vaccination is restricted to laboratory workers, although a live attenuated virus is undergoing trials in experimental animals. The live CHIK vaccine TSI-GSD-218 has been reported to be promising in humans.

Eastern equine encephalitis
History
EEE was first isolated in 1933[130] and retrospective studies of epidemics are suggestive of EEE as early as 1931.

Epidemiology
EEE virus is endemic along the eastern coast of the USA, Canada, Trinidad, Guyana, Mexico, Panama, Brazil, Peru, Columbia and Argentina. In most areas the virus is transmitted between marsh birds and *Culiseta melanura* mosquitoes, which do not feed on large vertebrates. With alterations in the conditions of the marshes or swamps, the virus is transmitted to other host mosquitoes that feed on small rodents, reptiles and amphibians. *Culex* species are considered to be the vectors for transmission of EEE virus in South America.[131] Human and equine cases are seen only when the spread becomes endemic.

Pathogenesis and pathology
Viraemia occurs soon after infection and may be accompanied by a febrile prodrome. Virus gains access to the nervous system and results in severe encephalitis. HI and neutralizing antibody is present in samples taken during the first 3–5 days of encephalitis.[132] However, this effective humoral immune response does not eradicate the virus from the brain, and neural destruction continues through direct cytopathic effect, inflammatory damage and vasculitis. The primary pathological features of EEE are confined to the CNS.[133] Lesions are scattered throughout the cortex and are particularly severe in basal ganglia and the brain stem; the cerebellum and spinal cord are minimally involved. There is extensive neuronal damage as well as thrombosis of arterioles and venules. Inflammatory cells are widespread in lesions, perivascular areas and meninges. The cells are predominantly polymorphonuclear in the first week, but later mononuclear cells may predominate. Virions are present in oligodendrocytes.

Clinical illness
Human infections are rare but when they occur the ratio of inapparent to apparent infection is remarkably low. In children the ratio is estimated to be from 2:1 to 8:1; in adults it is from 4:1 to 50:1. In severe cases the onset is abrupt, with high fever followed by all the features of meningitis, including coma, convulsions and neurological damage. Age is not a major factor in mortality but severe sequelae are more pronounced in children under 10 years of age.[134]

Diagnosis and investigation

The abrupt onset of a severe febrile CNS illness is suggestive of this disease, and death in horses—associated with hot, wet summers and the proximity of salt marshes—gives further credence to EEE infection.

The virus may be isolated from serum during the initial infection but most cases are diagnosed by testing paired sera in conventional HI or NT. Very high CF titres occur in most people convalescing from EEE. IgM antibodies are readily detected in acute sera by ELISA.[135] Virus may be isolated at autopsy.

Prevention and control

A vaccine inactivated by formalin treatment is available for use in laboratory workers or others at high risk of exposure.[136] The same vaccine is used to protect endangered whooping cranes, which are susceptible to lethal visceral infection.

Venezuelan equine encephalitis

This virus was first isolated by Beck and Wyckoff[137] from equine encephalitis epizootics in Venezuela. Viral strains belonging to the VEE IABC group are pathogenic for horses and have been involved in human infections. In contrast, other VEE strains (ID-F, II, III, IV, V, VI) are not known to be virulent in horses.

Epidemiology

VEE is endemic in Central and South America and parts of North America, and has occurred particularly in Venezuela, Colombia, Equador, Panama, Brazil, Mexico, Florida, Texas and Trinidad. Mosquitoes of both the *Aedes* and *Culex* genera are involved. *Cx. melanoconion* and *Deinocereites* species are the main vectors in rodent-to-rodent transmission. Horses are a major reservoir of infection and transmission of the virus can occur from horse to horse as well as transplacentally. More than 150 different animal species, including domestic and wild dogs and pigs, have been found to be infected with this virus. Birds have low viraemias but could infect mosquitoes, which may spread the disease and cause new epidemics.

Pathogenesis

Conventional serological methods show that the viruses grouped into the VEE complex are all closely related. The viruses in this group were further divided into subtypes and variants by Young et al.[138] using the HI test, and it seems that these minor distinctions are responsible for the fundamental differences in pathogenicity and biochemical significance.

The earliest humoral immune response appears around day 5 in hamsters and is directed to virion surface component.[139] An epitope on E2 is shown to produce the most dominant protective neutralizing antibodies. In the mouse model, cell transfer experiments suggest that T-helper lymphocyte activity is important in protection.

Clinical illness

The clinical disease in humans resembles an influenza-like syndrome, with fever lasting for 1–4 days. Occasionally this is complicated by shock and coma, in which case there appears to be widespread destruction of lymphoid tissues. Meningoencephalitis can occur, particularly in children, but is much less common in adults. Deaths may occur in undernourished populations and in the absence of medical care.

Diagnosis

VEE should be suspected in any person suffering from febrile myalgic illness 6 days after being exposed to an enzootic biotope. Vaccinia virus recombinants containing genes encoding the VEE virus structural gene regions (C-E3-E2-6 K-E1) protect mice against virulent VEEV, but provide only partial protection against airborne challenge. VV recombinants encoding the structural genes E3-E2-6 K-E1, E3-E2-6 K or 6 K-E1 also demonstrate the importance of E2 in protection.

Western equine encephalitis
Epidemiology

WEE virus is found in the USA but human infections are limited to the western two-thirds of the country. It is also found in Canada, particularly Manitoba, Saskatchewan, Alberta and British Columbia, and in South America. The disease is transmitted by various species of mosquito vectors. These include *Cx. tarsalis*, *Culiseta melanura* and other mosquitoes of these two genera. *Aedes* and *Anopheles* species may be slightly involved. The natural cycle is between *Cx. tarsalis* mosquitoes and wild birds. *Culex* mosquitoes readily feed on large vertebrates, so equine and human cases occur annually. The number of cases is dependent on rainfall because mosquito breeding is largely in ground pools.

Pathogenesis and pathology

The pathogenesis of WEE in humans resembles that of EEE. However, WEE is less neuroinvasive and neuro-virulent, in both humans and laboratory animals. In the CNS the pathology consists of multiple foci of necrosis, often without cellular infiltrate, found predominantly in areas such as the striatum, globus pallidus, cerebral cortex, thalamus and pons. In some areas polymorphonuclear infiltrates occur. There is widespread perivascular cuffing and meningeal reaction. The pathogenesis in rodents is similar to that of other alphaviruses.[140]

Clinical illness

WEE is characterized by sudden onset of fever, headache and general symptoms of meningoencephalitis which can be clinically severe but rarely fatal. Neurological and psychological sequelae are seen primarily in children under 2 years of age. The ratio of inapparent to apparent clinical infection is estimated at 50:1–8:1 in children and more than 1000:1 in adults.

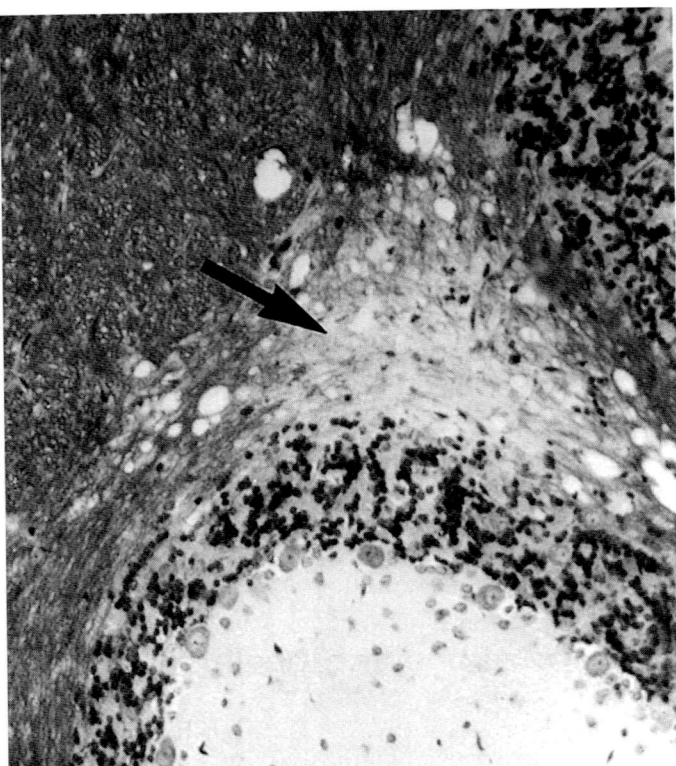

Figure 49.4: Demyelination (arrow) within the cerebellum of a mouse infected with Semliki Forest virus.

Prevention and control

Social activities such as screening of windows and doors and avoiding external pursuits are necessary to avoid infection. An inactivated vaccine is available for workers at risk from infection.

Semliki Forest virus

Although SFV has been assumed not to infect humans, the death of a scientist from whom SFV was isolated may suggest otherwise. More recently mild febrile illness has been reported in humans in Africa and was suggested to be due to SFV. The fact that SFV is known to induce neurological disease in experimental animals, with perivascular infiltrates and demyelination (Figure 49.4), warrants mention of this virus in this chapter. SFV was originally isolated in Uganda in 1944. Experimentally the virus induces encephalitis in a variety of laboratory rodents. Infection of mice with the A7 or M9 strains of SFV gives rise to lesions of demyelination in the CNS.[8]

Rubiviruses

History

The sole member of the rubivirus genus, rubella virus, was initially described in the early 1800s.[141] Although it is primarily a childhood illness, the disease is endemic worldwide and serious complications such as encephalomyelitis and postinfectious encephalopathy have been reported in adults and children. The large number of studies by German scientists have given rubella virus the synonym 'German measles', although the organism is unrelated to measles virus.

Epidemiology

Unlike most other togaviruses, rubella has no known vertebrate host and the only natural reservoir is humans. Rubella virus infections are found worldwide and in the temperate regions the epidemics occur in late winter and early spring. Periods of increased incidence every 6–9 years occur, with major epidemics every 10–30 years.[142] Such epidemics are related to the susceptibility of individuals and factors that increase the transmission. Infection is generally acquired in childhood and approximately 60% of the population have antibodies by the age of 14 years. With the introduction of the rubella vaccine in 1969,[143] the incidence of rubella has decreased, although the seroprevalence rates approach 90–95%. The incidence of infection is higher in the tropics. Post-infectious encephalopathy or encephalomyelitis is estimated to occur in 1 in 6000 cases of natural rubella.

Pathogenesis and pathology

The pathology resulting from rubella infection is dependent on the mode of infection, i.e., whether it is due to maternal–fetal transmission or is acquired postnatally. The effect on the fetus depends on the gestation period. In the first trimester there is a high risk of infection and developmental growth is arrested, although the mechanism of damage is unknown. Maternal infection after the first trimester does not appear to damage the fetus, although the risk of congenital disease is known to increase before birth. Delayed neurological disease has been reported following late-onset rubella infection and may be associated with either congenital rubella or a rare complication of natural rubella acquired in childhood.

The pathological features of CNS involvement, particularly in the adult, include perivascular lesions of mononuclear cells and demyelination. In childhood encephalopathy, neural degeneration is more apparent than in the adult, whereas perivascular infiltrates and demyelination are less common. The suggestion that autoreactivity may play a role in the pathology of late-onset rubella encephalitis, often referred to as progressive rubella panencephalitis, chronic progressive panencephalitis or non-congenital rubella, comes from studies in which lymphocytes proliferate in response to CNS proteins such as myelin basic protein.[144]

Clinical features

Rubella infection in early childhood or adult life is usually mild and asymptomatic. Symptoms of post-infectious rubella encephalopathy are observed shortly after the onset of the rash of typical rubella. The clinical features of encephalitis are similar to those of other forms of encephalitis, including headache, vomiting, stiff neck, fevers and convulsions, and altered levels of consciousness. The mortality rate is approximately 20%, with death occurring within a few days of the onset of symptoms. The late-onset rubella encephalitis is similar to other slow virus infections of the CNS. Following a prolonged asymptomatic period, neural degeneration is observed, usually in the second decade of life. Symptoms include behavioural changes, ataxia and seizures. Death usually results within 8 years of onset.

Diagnosis

The common symptoms of rubella, such as low-grade fever and maculopapular rash, should not be confused with other such infections. Confirmation of rubella may be made following isolation of the virus or by specific serological assays such as ELISA. The CSF cell count of patients with rubella encephalitis is high (50 per mm^3); the majority of the cells are lymphocytes. The electro-encephalogram is abnormal, oligoclonal bands are observed in the CSF[145] and rubella virus may be isolated.[146]

Management and prevention

Treatment of rubella encephalitis with corticosteroids has been reported.[147] Rubella vaccines, developed in the 1960s, have been used to vaccinate both school-aged children (USA) and women of childbearing age (UK) in an attempt to decrease the incidence of congenital rubella infection. The attenuated viruses used are capable of infecting the fetus and thus vaccination of pregnant women is not recommended. More recently the policy of including the combined MMR vaccination procedure for all schoolchildren has been implemented in the UK. Future development of subviral vaccines may be necessary to counter the side effects of vaccination using attenuated virus.

REFERENCES

1. Johnson R T. *Viral Infections of the Nervous System*. New York: Raven Press, 1982.

2. Fields B N, Knipe D M, Chanock R M et al. *Virology*, 2nd edn. New York: Raven Press, 1990.

3. Goldmann E E. Vitalfarbung am Zentralnervensystem. *Abh Preuss Akad Wiss, Phys-Math* 1913; 1(1):1–60.

4. Male D & Rezaie P. Colonisation of the human central nervous system by microglia: the roles of chemokines and vascular adhesion molecules. *Prog Brain Res* 2001; 132:81–93.

5. Webb H E & Parsons L M. Treatment of the postviral fatigue syndrome—rationale for the use of antidepressants. In Jenkins R & Mowbray J (eds) *Post Viral Fatigue Syndrome*. New York: Wiley, 1991:297–303.

6. Levine B, Hardwick J M, Trapp B D, Crawford T O, Bollinger R C & Griffin D E. Antibody-mediated clearance of alphavirus infection from neurons. *Science* 1991; 254:856–860.

7. Mazarakis N D, Azzouz M, Rohll J B et al. Rabies virus glycoprotein pseudotyping of lentiviral vectors enables retrograde axonal transport and access to the nervous system after peripheral delivery. *Hum Mol Genet* 2001; 10:2109–2121.

8. Amor S, Scallan M F, Morris M M, Dyson H & Fazakerley J K. Role of immune responses in protection and pathogenesis during Semliki Forest virus encephalitis. *J Gen Virol* 1996; 77:281–291.

9. McCormick J B & Johnson K M. Lassa fever: historical review and contemporary investigation. In Pattyn S R (ed.) *Ebola Virus Haemorrhagic Fever*. Amsterdam: Elsevier–North Holland, 1978:279–292.

10. Warkel R L, Rinaldi D F, Bancroft W H, Cardiff R D, Holmes G E & Wilsnack R E. Fatal acute meningoencephalitis due to lymphocytic choriomeningitis virus. *Neurology* 1973; 23:198–203.

11. Vanzee B E, Douglas R G Jr, Betts R F, Bauman A W, Frazer D W & Hinman A R. Lymphocytic choriomeningitis virus in university hospital personnel. Clinical features. *Am J Med* 1975; 58:803–809.

12. McCormick J B, Webb P A, Krebbs J W, Johnson K M & Smith E S. A prospective study of the epidemiology and ecology of Lassa fever. *J Infect Dis* 1987; 155:437–444.

13. Monath T P & Casals J. Diagnosis of Lassa fever and the isolation and management of patients. *Bull World Health Organ* 1975; 52:707–715.

14. Walker D H, McCormick J B, Johnson K M et al. Pathologic and virologic study of fatal Lassa fever in man. *Am J Pathol* 1982; 107:349–356.

15. Fisher-Hoch S P & McCormick J B. Towards a human Lassa fever vaccine. *Rev Med Virol* 2001; 11:331–341.

16. McCormick J B, King I J, Webb P A et al. Lassa fever. Effective therapy with ribavirin. *N Engl J Med* 1986; 314:20–26.

17. Gonzalez-Scarano F & Nathanson N. Bunyaviruses. In Fields B N, Knipe D M, Chanock R M et al. (eds) *Virology*, 2nd edn. New York: Raven Press, 1990:1195–1228.

18. Thompson W H, Kalfayan B & Anslow R O. Isolation of Californian encephalitis group virus from a fatal human illness. *Am J Epidemiol* 1965; 81:245–253.

19. Calisher C H. Toxonomy, classification and geographical distribution of Californian serogroup bunyaviruses. In Calisher C H & Thompson W H (eds) *Californian Serogroup Viruses*. New York: Alan R Liss, 1983:1–16.

20. Grimstad P R, Craig G B, Ross Q E & Yuill T M. *Aedes triseriatus* and La Crosse virus: geographical variation in vector susceptibility and ability to transmit. *Am J Trop Med Hyg* 1977; 26:990–996.

21. Artsob H. Distribution of California serogroups and virus infection in Canada. In Calisher C H & Thompson W H (eds) *California Serogroup Viruses*. New York: Alan R Liss, 1983:277–292.

22. Meegan J M. The Rift Valley fever epizootic in Egypt 1977–1978. 1. Description of the epizootic and virological studies. *Trans R Soc Trop Med Hyg* 1979; 73:618–623.

23. Maar S A, Swanepoel R & Gelfand M. Rift Valley fever encephalitis. A description of a case. *Cent Afr J Med* 1979; 25:8–11.

24. Lampert P W, Sims J K & Kniazeff A J. Mechanism of demyelination in JHM virus encephalomyelitis. Electron microscopic studies. *Acta Neuropathol (Berl)* 1973; 24:76–85.

25. Burks J S, De Vald L D, Jankcvsky L D & Gerdes J C. Two coronaviruses isolated from the central nervous system tissue of two multiple sclerosis patients. *Science* 1980; 209:933–934.

26. Westaway E G, Brinton M A, Gaidamovich S Y et al. Flaviviridae. *Intervirology* 1985; 24:183–192.

27. Gressler I, Hardy J L, Hu S M K & Scherer W F. Factors influencing transmission of Japanese B encephalitis virus by a colonized strain of *Culex tritaeniorhynchus* Giles, from infected pigs and chicks to susceptible pigs and birds. *Am J Trop Med Hyg* 1958; 7:365–370.

28. Weaver O M, Haymaker W, Pieper S & Kurland R. Sequelae of the arthropod-borne encephalitides. V. Japanese encephalitis.

Neurology 1958; 8:887–890.

29 Mathur A, Arora K L & Chaturvedi U C. Transplacental Japanese encephalitis virus (JEV) infection in mice during consecutive pregnancies. *J Gen Virol* 1982; 59:213–217.

30 Hsu T C & Hsu S T. Supplementary report. Effectiveness of Japanese encephalitis vaccine. Study in the second year following immunisation. In Hammon W McD, Kitaoka M & Downs W G (eds) *Immunisation for Japanese Encephalitis.* Baltimore, MD: Williams & Williams, 1971:266–267.

31 Srivastava A K, Putnak J R, Lee S H et al. A purified inactivated Japanese encephalitis virus vaccine made in Vero cells. *Vaccine* 2001; 19:4557–4565.

32 Huang C H. Studies of Japanese encephalitis in China. *Adv Virus Res* 1982; 27:71–101.

33 Chamberlain R W. Epidemiology of arthropodborne togaviruses: the role of arthropods as hosts and vectors and of vertebrate hosts in natural transmission cycles. In Schlesinger R W (ed.) *The Togaviruses: Biology, Structure, Replication.* New York: Academic Press, 1980:175–227.

34 Finley K & Riggs N. Convalescence and sequelae. In Monath T P (ed.) *St Louis Encephalitis.* Washington, DC: APHA, 1980: 535–550.

35 Kliks S C & Halstead S B. An explanation for enhanced virus plaque formation in chick embryo cells. *Nature* 1980; 285:504–505.

36 Cordova S P, Smith D W, Broom A K, Lindsay M D, Dowse G K & Beers M Y. Murray Valley encephalitis in Western Australia in 2000, with evidence of southerly spread. *Commun Dis Intell* 2000; 24:368–372.

37 de Souza Lopes O, de Abreu Sacchetta L, Coimbra T L, Pinto G H & Glasser C M. Emergence of a new arbovirus disease in Brasil. II. Epidemiological studies on 1975 epidemic. *Am J Epidemiol* 1978; 108:394–401.

38 Rosenberg S. Neuropathology of Sao Paulo south coast epidemic encephalitis (Rocio encephalitis). *J Neurol Sci* 1980; 45:1–12.

39 Pudney M & Varma M G R. The growth of some tick-borne arboviruses in cell cultures derived from tadpoles of the common frog, *Rana temporaria. J Gen Virol* 1971; 10:131–138.

40 Shope R E. Medical significance of togaviruses: an overview of diseases caused by togaviruses in man and in domestic and wild vertebrate animals. In Schlesinger R W (ed.) *The Togaviruses: Biology, Structure, Replication.* New York: Academic Press, 1980:47–82.

41 Chiba N, Iwasaki T, Mizutani T, Kariwa H, Kurata T & Takashima I. Pathogenicity of tick-borne encephalitis virus isolated in Hokkaido, Japan in mouse model. *Vaccine* 1999; 17:779–787.

42 Radsel-Medvescek A, Marolt-Gomiscek M & Gajsek-Zima M. Clinical characteristics of patients with TBE treated at the university medical centre hospital for infectious diseases in Ljubljana during the years 1974–1977. *Zentralbl Bakteriol (Suppl)* 1980; 9:277–280.

43 Kunz C, Heinz F X & Hofmann H. Immunoreactivity and reactigenicity of a highly purified vaccine against tick-borne encephalitis. *J Med Virol* 1980; 6:103–109.

44 Roizman B. Herpesviridae: a brief introduction. In Fields B N, Knipe D M, Chanock R M et al. (eds) *Virology*, 2nd edn. New York: Raven Press, 1990:1787–1793.

45 Whitley R J & Schlitt M. Encephalitis caused by herpesviruses, including B virus. In Scheld W M, Whitley R J & Durack J T (eds) *Infections of the CNS.* New York: Raven Press, 1991:41–46.

46 Nahmais A J & Dowdle B. Infection with herpes simplex viruses 1 and 2. *N Engl J Med* 1973; 289:667–781.

47 Whitley R J. Herpes simplex viruses. In Fields B N, Knipe D M, Chanock R M et al. (eds) *Virology*, 2nd edn. New York: Raven Press, 1990:1843–1887.

48 Mohamedi S A, Heath A W & Jennings R. A comparison of oral and parenteral routes for therapeutic vaccination with HSV-2 ISCOMs in mice; cytokine profiles, antibody responses and protection. *Antiviral Res* 2001; 49:83–99.

49 Weller T H & Stoddard M B. Intranuclear inclusion bodies in cultures of human tissue inoculated with varicella vesicle fluid. *J Immunol* 1952; 68:311–319.

50 Johnson R & Milborne P E. Central nervous system manifestations of chickenpox. *Can Med Assoc J* 1970; 102:831–834.

51 Applebaum E, Rachelson M H & Dolgopol V B. Varicella encephalitis. *Am J Med* 1953; 15:223–230.

52 Heppleston J D, Paerch K M & Yates P O. Varicella encephalitis. *Arch Dis Child* 1959; 34:318–321.

53 Gelb L D. Varicella-zoster virus. In Fields B N, Knipe D M, Chanock R M et al. (eds) *Virology*, 2nd edn. New York: Raven Press, 1990:2011–2054.

54 Centers for Disease Control. Herpes B encephalitis— California. *MMWR Morb Mortal Wkly Rep* 1973; 22(40):333–334.

55 Vizoso A D. Latency of herpes simiae (B virus) in rabbits. *Br J Exp Pathol* 1975; 56:489–494.

56 Buthala D A. Hyperimmunised horse anti-B virus globulin: preparation and effectiveness. *J Infect Dis* 1962; 111:101–106.

57 Boulter E A, Thornton B, Bauer E J & Bye A. Successful treatment of experimental B virus (herpesvirus simiae) infection with acyclovir. *BMJ* 1980; 280:681–683.

58 Delorme L & Middleton P J. Influenza A virus associated with acute encephalopathy. *Am J Dis Child* 1979; 133:822–824.

59 Ravenholt R T & Foege W H. Before our time. 1918 influenza, encephalitis lethargica, parkinsonism. *Lancet* 1982; ii:860–864.

60 McKinney W P, Volkert P & Kaufman J. Fatal swine influenza pneumonia during late pregnancy. *Arch Intern Med* 1990; 150:213–215.

61 Randolph V L & Heath C W Jr. Influenza during pregnancy in relation to subsequent childhood leukemia and lymphoma. *Am J Epidemiol* 1974; 100:399–409.

62 MacDonald K L, Osterholm M T, Hedberg C W, Schrock C G & Peterson G F. Toxic shock syndrome: a newly recognised complication of influenza and influenza-like illness. *JAMA* 1987; 257:1053–1058.

63 Consensus Development Conference at National Institutes of Health. Amantidine: does it have a role in the prevention and treatment of influenza? *Ann Intern Med* 1980; 92:256–258.

64 Zlydnikov D M, Kubar O I, Kovaleva T P & Kamforin L E. Study of rimantadine in the USSR: a review of the literature. *Rev Infect Dis* 1981; 3:408–421.

65 Dolin R, Reichman R C, Madore H P, Maynard R, Linton P N & Webber-Jones J. A controlled trial of amantadine and rimantadine in the prophylaxis of influenza A infection. *N Engl J Med* 1982; 307:580–584.

66 Oxford J S. Inhibition of the replication of influenza A and B viruses by a nucleoside analogue (ribavirin). *J Gen Virol* 1975; 28:409–414.

67 Gardner S. The new human papovaviruses: their nature and significance. In Waterson A P (ed.) *Recent Advances in Clinical Virology.* New York: Livingstone, 1977:93–115.

68 Taguchi F, Kajioka J & Miyamura T. Prevalence rate and age of acquisition of antibodies against JC and BK virus in human sera. *Microbiol Immunol* 1982; 26:1057–1064.

69 Berger J R, Kaszovita B, Donavan Post J & Dickinson G. Progressive multifocal leukoencephalopathy associated with human immunodeficiency virus infection. *Ann Intern Med* 1987; 107:78–87.

70 Flaegstad T, Sundsfjord A, Arthur A A, Pedersen M, Traavik T & Subraman S. Amplification and sequencing of the control

regions of BK and JC virus from human urine by polymerase chain reaction. *Virology* 1991; 180:553–560.

71 Lee M S, Nokes D J, Hsu H M & Lu C F. Protective titres of measles neutralising antibody. *J Med Virol* 2000; 62:511–517.

72 Krugman S, Katz S L, Gershon A A & Wilfert C M. Measles (rubeola). In Mosby C V (ed.) *Infectious Diseases of Children*. St Louis: Mosby 1985:152–166.

73 Markowitz L E, Chandler F W, Roldan E O et al. Fatal measles pneumonia without rash in a child with AIDS. *J Infect Dis* 1988; 158:480–483.

74 Font R L, Jenis E H & Tuck K D. Measles maculopathy associated with subacute sclerosing panencephalitis. *Arch Pathol* 1973; 96:168–174.

75 Pinkerton H, Smiley W L & Anderson W A D. Giant cell pneumonia with inclusions: lesion common to Hecht's disease, distemper and measles. *Am J Pathol* 1945; 21:1–23.

76 Fleischer B & Kreth H W. Clonal expansion and functional analysis of virus-specific T lymphocytes from cerebrospinal fluid in measles encephalitis. *Hum Immunol* 1983; 7:239.

77 Kleiman B M, Blackburn L K, Zimmerman E S & French V L M. Comparison of enzyme linked immunosorbent assay for acute measles with hemagglutination inhibition, complement fixation and fluorescent antibody methods. *J Clin Microbiol* 1981; 14:147–152.

78 Vandvik B & Norrby E. Oligoclonal IgG antibody response in the central nervous system to different measles virus antigens in subacute sclerosing panencephalitis. *Proc Natl Acad Sci USA* 1973; 70:1060–1063.

79 Modlin J F, Jabbour J T, Witte J J & Halsey N A. Epidemiologic studies of measles vaccine and subacute sclerosing panencephalitis. *Pediatrics* 1977; 59:505–513.

80 Raine C S. On the development of CNS lesions in natural canine distemper encephalomyelitis. *J Neurol Sci* 1976; 30:13–28.

81 Cook S D, Dowling P C & Russell W C. Neutralising antibody to canine distemper and measles virus in multiple sclerosis. *J Neurol Sci* 1979; 41:61–70.

82 Hamilton R. An account of a distemper, by the common people in England, vulgarly called the mumps. *London Med J* 1790; 11:190–211.

83 Anderson R M, Cromble J A & Grenfell B T. The epidemiology of mumps in the UK: a preliminary study of virus transmission, herd immunity and the potential impact of immunization. *Epidemiol Infect* 1987; 99:65–84.

84 Koskiniemi M, Donner M, Pettay O. Clinical appearance and outcome in mumps encephalitis in children. *Acta Paediatr Scand* 1983; 72:603–609.

85 Wilfert C M. Mumps meningoencephalomyelitis with low cerebrospinal-fluid glucose, prolonged pleocytosis and elevation of protein. *N Engl J Med* 1969; 280:855–859.

86 Taylor F B & Toreson W E. Primary mumps meningoencephalitis. *Arch Intern Med* 1963; 112:114–119.

87 Lindsay J R, Davey P R & Ward P H. Inner ear pathology in deafness due to mumps. *Ann Otol Rhinol Laryngol* 1960; 69:918–935.

88 Spataro R F, Lin S R, Horner F A, Hall C B & McDonald J V. Aqueductal stenosis and hydrocephalus: rare sequelae of mumps virus infection. *Neuroradiology* 1976; 12:11–13.

89 Thompson J A. Mumps: a case of acquired aqueductal stenosis. *J Paediatr* 1979; 94:923–924.

90 Brunell P A, Brickman A & Steinberg S. Evaluation of a live attenuated mumps vaccine Jeryl Lynn: with observations on the optimal tissue for testing serologic responses. *Am J Dis Child* 1969; 118:435–440.

91 Kilham L & Margolis G. Cerebellar ataxia in hamsters inoculated with rat virus. *Science* 1964; 143:1047–1048.

92 Melnick J L. Enteroviruses: polioviruses, coxsackieviruses, echoviruses and newer enteroviruses. In Fields B N, Knipe D M, Chanock R M et al. (eds) *Virology*, 2nd edn. New York: Raven Press, 1990:549–605.

93 Landsteiner K & Popper E. Ubertragung der Poliomyelitis acuta auf Affen. *Z Immunitatsforsch Orig* 1909; 2:377–390.

94 Melnick J L. Current status of poliovirus infections. *Clin Microbiol Rev* 1996; 9:293–300.

95 Salk J & Salk D. Control of influenza and poliomyelitis with killed virus vaccines. *Science* 1977; 195:834–837.

96 Benyesh-Melnick M, Melnick J L, Rawls W E et al. Studies on the immunogenicity, communicability and genetic stability of oral poliovaccine administered during the winter. *Am J Epidemiol* 1967; 86:112–136.

97 Shindarov L M, Chumakov M P, Voroshilova M K et al. Epidemiological, clinical and pathomorphological characteristics of epidemic poliomyelitis-like disease caused by enterovirus 71. *J Hyg Epidemiol Microbiol Immunol* 1979; 23:284–295.

98 Melnick J L. Enterovirus type 71 infections: a varied clinical pattern sometimes mimicking paralytic poliomyelitis. *Rev Infect Dis* 1984; 6:387–390.

99 Gajdusek D C. Kuru. *Trans R Soc Trop Med Hyg* 1963; 57:151–169.

100 Goldgaber D, Goldfarb L G, Brown P et al. Mutations in familial Creutzfeldt–Jakob disease and Gerstmann–Sträussler's syndrome. *Exp Neurol* 1989; 106:204–206.

101 Gajdusek D C & Gibbs C J Jr. Transmission of two subacute spongiform encephalopathies of man (kuru and Creuzfeldt–Jakob disease) to New World monkeys. *Nature* 1971; 230:588–591.

102 Anonymous. Rapidly progressive dementia in a patient who received cadavaric dura mater graft. *MMWR Morb Mortal Wkly Rep* 1987; 36:49–50.

103 Brown P, Rohwer R G & Gajdusek D C. Sodium hydroxide decontamination of Creutzfeldt–Jakob disease virus. *N Engl J Med* 1984; 310:727.

104 Weissmann C, Bueler H, Fischer M, Sauer A & Aguet M. Susceptibility to scrapie in mice is dependent on PrPC. *Philos Trans R Soc Lond [Biol]* 1994; 343:431–433.

105 Amor S & Mehta S. Prions, viruses and antiviral drugs. *Lancet* 1993; 342:545.

106 Ferguson-Smith M A. BSE and variant CJD. Assumption that BSE originated from scrapie in sheep led to misjudgment. *BMJ* 2001; 322:1544–1545.

107 Howell P G & Verweord D W. Bluetongue virus. In Gard S, Hallauer C & Meyer K F (eds) *Virology Monographs*, vol. 9. New York: Springer, 1971:37–74.

108 Bowen G S, McLean R G, Shriner R B et al. The ecology of Colorado tick fever in Rocky Mountain National Park in 1974. II. Infection in small mammals. *Am J Trop Med Hyg* 1981; 30:490–496.

109 Ater J L, Overall J, Yeh T & O'Brien A. Circulating interferon and clinical symptoms in Colorado tick fever. *J Infect Dis* 1985; 151:966–968.

110 Calisher C H. Medically important arboviruses of the United States and Canada. *Clin Microbiol Rev* 1994; 7:89–116.

111 Sigurdsson B. Observations on three slow infections of sheep, maedi, paratuberculosis, rida, a slow encephalitis of sheep with general remarks on infections which develop slowly and some of their special characteristics. *Br Vet J* 1954; 110:255–270.

112 Nathanson N, Georgsson G, Lutley R, Palsson P A & Petursson G L. Pathogenesis of visna in Icelandic sheep: demyelinating lesions and antigenic drift. In Mims C A, Cuzner M L & Kelly R E (eds) *Viruses and Demyelinating Diseases*. London: Academic Press, 1983:111–124.

113 Narayan O & Clements J E. Lentiviruses. Bunyaviruses. In Fields B N, Knipe D M, Chanock R M et al. (eds) *Virology*, 2nd edn. New York: Raven Press, 1990:1571–1589.

114 Price R W, Brew B J & Roke M. Central and peripheral nervous system complications of HIV-1 infection and AIDS. In Devita V, Hellman S & Rosenberg S (eds) *AIDS: Etiology, Diagnosis, Treatment and Prevention.* Philadephia: J B Lippincott, 1992:ch. 14.

115 Evans B K, Donley D K & Whitaker J N. Neurological manifestations of infection with the human immunodeficiency viruses. In Scheld W M, Whitley R J & Durak D T (eds) *Infections of the Central Nervous System.* New York: Raven Press, 1991:201–232.

116 Carne C A, Tedder R S, Smith A et al. Acute encephalopathy coincident with seroconversion for anti-HTLV-III. *Lancet* 1985; ii:1206–1208.

117 Heidenrich F, Arendt G, Jander S, Jablonowski H & Stoll G. Serum and cerebrospinal fluid levels of soluble intercellular adhesion molecule 1 (sICAM) in patients with HIV associated neurological diseases. *J Neuroimmunol* 1994; 52:117–126.

118 Okamoto M, Ono M & Baba M. Suppression of cytokine production and neural cell death by the anti-inflammatory alkaloid cepharanthine: a potential agent against HIV-1 encephalopathy. *Biochem Pharmacol* 2001; 62:747–753.

119 Whitley R J & Middlebrooks M. Rabies. In Scheld W M, Whitley R J & Durack D T (eds) *Infections of the Central Nervous System.* New York: Raven Press, 1991:127–144.

120 Baer G M, Bellini W J & Fishbein D B. Rhabdoviruses. In Fields B N, Knipe D M, Chanock R M et al. (eds) *Virology,* 2nd edn. New York: Raven Press, 1990:883–930.

121 Goldwasser R A & Kissling R E. Fluorescent antibody staining of street and fixed rabies virus antigens. *Proc Soc Exp Biol Med* 1958; 98:219–233.

122 World Health Organization. Sixth report of the expert committee on rabies. *WHO Tech Rep Ser* 1973:523.

123 Graubelle P C, Baagoe H J, Fekadu M, Westergaard J & Zoffman N. Bat rabies in Denmark. *Lancet* 1987; i:379–380.

124 Murphy F A, Harrison A K, Winn W C & Bauer S P. Comparative pathogenesis of rabies and rabies-like viruses. Infection of the CNS and centrifugal spread of virus to peripheral tissues. *Lab Invest* 1973; 28:361–376.

125 Dupont J R & Earle K M. Human rabies encephalitis: a study of forty-nine cases with a review of the literature. *Neurology* 1966; 15:1023–1034.

126 WHO Expert Committee on Rabies. *WHO Tech Rep Ser* 1992; 824:1–84.

127 Schlesinger S & Schlesinger M J. *The Togaviridae and Flaviviridae.* New York: Plenum Press, 1986.

128 Halstead S B, Nimmannitya S & Margiotta M R. Dengue and chickungunya virus infection in man in Thailand 1962–1964. Observations on disease in out-patients. *Am J Trop Med Hyg* 1969; 18:972–978.

129 Brighton S W, Prozesky O W & de la Harpe A L. Chikungunya virus infection. A retrospective study of 107 cases. *S Afr Med J* 1983; 63:313–315.

130 Hayes R O. Eastern and western encephalitis. In Steele J H & Beran G W (eds) *Handbook Series in Zoonoses, Section B: Viral Zoonoses,* vol. 1. Boca Raton, FL: CRC Press, 1981:29–57.

131 Downs W G, Aitkin T H G & Spence L. Eastern equine encephalitis virus isolated from *Culex nigripalpus* in Trinidad. *Science* 1959; 130:1471.

132 Goldfield M, Taylor B F & Welsh J N. The 1959 outbreak of eastern encephalitis in New Jersey. 3. Serological studies of clinical cases. *Am J Epidemiol* 1968; 87:18–22.

133 Bastain F O, Wende R D, Singer D B & Zeller R S. Eastern equine encephalitis. Histopathological and ultrastructural changes with isolation of the virus in a human case. *Am J Clin Pathol* 1975; 64:10–13.

134 Goldfield M, Taylor B F & Welsh J N. The 1959 outbreak of eastern encephalitis in New Jersey. 6. The frequency of prior infection. *Am J Epidemiol* 1968; 87:39–49.

135 Calisher C H, El-Kafrawi A O, Al-Deen Mahmud M I & Travassos da Rosa A P. Complex-specific immunoglobulin M antibody patterns in humans infected with alphaviruses. *J Clin Microbiol* 1986; 23:155–159.

136 Cole F E Jr. Inactivated eastern equine encephalomyelitis vaccine propagated in rolling-bottle cultures of chick embryo cells. *Appl Microbiol* 1971; 22:842–845.

137 Beck C E & Wyckoff R W G. Venezuelan equine encephalomyelitis. *Science* 1938; 88:530.

138 Young N A, Johnson K M & Gauld L W. Viruses of the Venezuelan equine encephalomyelitis complex. *Am J Trop Med Hyg* 1969; 18:290–296.

139 Jahrling P B, Hesse R A, Anderson A O & Gangemi J D. Opsonization of alphaviruses in hamsters. *J Med Virol* 1983; 12:1–16.

140 Griffin D E. Alphavirus pathogenesis and immunity. In Schlesinger S & Schlesinger M J (eds) *The Togaviridae and Flaviviridae.* New York: Plenum Press, 1986:209–249.

141 Wesselhoeft C. Rubella (German measles). *N Engl J Med* 1947; 236:943–950.

142 Witte J J, Karchmer A W, Case G et al. Epidemiology of rubella. *Am J Dis Child* 1969; 118:107–111.

143 Polk B F, Modlin J F & White J A. A controlled comparison of joint reactions among women receiving one of two rubella vaccines. *Am J Epidemiol* 1982; 115:19–25.

144 Johnson R T, Griffin D E, Hirsch R L et al. Measles encephalomyelitis—clinical and immunological studies. *N Engl J Med* 1984; 310:137–141.

145 Vandvik B, Weil M L, Grandien M & Norrby E. Progressive rubella panencephalitis: synthesis of oligoclonal virus-specific IgC antibodies and homogenous free light chains in the central nervous system. *Acta Neurol Scand* 1978; 57:53–64.

146 Squadrini F, Taparelli F, DeRienzo B, Giovannini G & Pagani C. Rubella virus isolation from cerebrospinal fluid in postnatal rubella encephalitis. *BMJ* 1977; ii:1329–1330.

147 Neveh Y & Friedman A. Rubella panencephalitis successfully treated with corticosteroids. *Clin Pediatr* 1975; 22:143–148.

Section 7

Rickettsial Infections

The first reports of typhus, derived from the ancient Greek word meaning 'fever with stupor', began in 430BC. The genus rickettsia is transmitted to humans by insects and are the responsible species are divided into three main groups: (a) the typhus group; (b) the spotted fever group; and (c) scrub typhus. These organisms have been responsible for major epidemics throughout history. This section stands alone and includes a comprehensive chapter on rickettsial infections.

Chapter 50
Rickettsial Infections

G. O. Cowan

The typhus and 'spotted' fevers are caused by bacteria of the family Rickettsiaceae, which are obligate, intracellular, Gram-negative, non-flagellate small pleomorphic coccobacilli (0.3–0.6 × 0.8–2.0 μm), which are often carried to humans by insects from reservoirs in animals or in the insects themselves, in which they may be maintained transovarially.

The species of the genus *Rickettsia* are divided into:

- The *typhus group*, containing *R. prowazekii*, the agent of classical epidemic typhus transmitted by the human body louse, and *R. typhi (mooseri)*, the cause of endemic murine typhus carried by the rat flea.
- The *'spotted fever' group* (SFGR), containing a large number of species (*R. rickettsii*, *R. conorii*, etc.) transmitted from rodents and other animals by ticks (except *R. akari*).
- *Scrub typhus*, caused by *Orientia tsutsugamushi* and transmitted by larval trombiculid mites.

The genus previously named *Rochalimaea* has been reclassified in the family *Bartonellaceae* and contains the closely related species *Bartonella quintana*, the cause of *trench fever* in humans, *Bartonella vinsoni*, which occurs in voles, and also *Bartonella henselae*, the agent of cat-scratch fever. (South American bartonellosis is described in Chapter 61).

Coxiella burnetii, the only species of its genus, causes Q fever.

The tribe Ehrlichieae comprises *Ehrlichia sennetsu, E. canis, E. chaffeensis* and *E. ewingii*, which can cause fever in humans and in several equine and canine species, *Cowdria ruminantium*, the cause of 'heartwater' in cattle and other domestic animals in Africa, and *Neorickettsia helminthoeca*, which causes illness in North American canines eating salmonid fish infected with flukes containing the bacterium.

History

'*Typhus*' is derived from *τυφos*, the ancient Greek word for 'fever with stupor' or 'smoke' cognate with the Sanskrit word for 'smoke', *dhupa*.

The earliest reference to epidemic typhus is in the account by Thucydides of the Great Plague of Athens in 430 BC in the second year of the Pelopennesian war. The historical centres of the disease were in the Middle East, North Africa and the eastern shores of the Mediterranean Sea. In the eleventh century AD, epidemics occurred in Sicily and Bohemia, but it was not until siege warfare on a large scale became common in the late fifteenth century that epidemics spread through armies to the civilian population (e.g., Granada 1459, Naples 1528 and Metz 1552).

The earliest medical accounts of typhus were written by Cardano[1] (1536) and Fracastoro[2] (1546) from Venice. Coyttarus[3] (1578) first suggested that typhoid and typhus were different diseases, a distinction that took three centuries to resolve. Cober[4] (1685) proposed that the body louse was involved in the spread of typhus.

Epidemics were common in the latter half of the sixteenth century in the Italian cities, Hungary, Germany, the Netherlands and England, and flourished in the armies of the Thirty Years' War (1618–1648) and the English Civil War. In the eighteenth century fevers were classified as 'continued', 'putrid', 'malignant' or 'spotted'; physicians recognized that armies, ships and prisons were fertile sources of 'spotted' fever.

Damaging outbreaks of typhus occurred in the British Government army in Scotland in 1746,[5] on both sides in the American War of Independence in 1776, in the British army after the retreat from Corunna in 1809, and in Napoleon's Grand Army in Russia in 1812. The first modern clinical description was given by von Hildenbrand[6] from Vienna in 1810 and led to the eponymous title of the disease. Typhus was common in the tenements of Edinburgh in the early nineteenth century, and epidemics occurred in Ireland in the potato blight famines of 1816–1817 and 1846–1847, with migration carrying the disease to Liverpool, Glasgow and the USA. The Reverend Patrick Brontë's two oldest daughters, Maria and Elizabeth, died from typhus in an epidemic of 45 cases at their boarding school in west Lancashire in 1826, an episode described by Charlotte in her novel *Jane Eyre*.

Gerhard in 1832 in Philadelphia first described the pathological differences between typhus and typhoid fevers, and was soon followed by Perry (1836), Stewart (1840) and Ritchie (1846), who first coined the phrase 'enteric fever'. Sir William Jenner expanded on the differences in his Goulstonian Lectures of 1853, but the Registrar-General of England and Wales did not separate the two diseases statistically until 1869. To this day in Germany, typhoid fever is known as *typhus abdominalis* and typhus as *typhus exanthematicus*, and this confusing terminology is still used for typhoid fever in Medline.

Nicolle[7] in 1910 in Algeria proved that typhus is carried by the body louse; da Rocha Lima[8] (1916) described the organism and proposed the name *Rickettsia prowazekii* to honour Howard Taylor Ricketts and Stanislaus von Prowazek, who had both recently died from typhus acquired in their research laboratories.

Louse-borne typhus caused large epidemics in the First World War in Serbia, Poland, eastern Germany and Mesopotamia, and in the Second World War in the Balkans, Naples, Russia and Germany, especially in the concentration camps at Belsen, Auschwitz and Buchenwald.

Flea-borne (murine) typhus had been described in Mexico in 1570 by Bravo,[9] and the complicating myocarditis was to kill Ricketts there in 1910. It was described clinically in grain silo workers in South Australia by Hone in 1923, but the final bacteriological separation from *R. prowazekii* did not occur until studies by Maxcy[10] (1926) and Mooser[11] (1928), the organism being named *R. mooseri* or *R. typhi*.

Earlier work by Ricketts was on Rocky Mountain spotted fever (RMSF), which had first been described in 1872 in the Bitter Root Valley of western Montana and on the Snake River in Idaho in the USA.[12] He identified the causative organism in 1906, and demonstrated that ticks were its vector,[13] the first bacterial disease proved to be transmitted by an insect. The organism was named *R. rickettsii*.

Old World tick-borne typhus was not described until 1910 by Conor and Bruch[14] in Tunisia as *fièvre éruptive*—transmitted by ticks, and by Megaw in 1916 in the Himalayan foothills. The species was named *R. conorii*.

Scrub typhus, or Japanese river fever, was known in Japanese folklore to be associated with the jungle mite or chigger, which was named 'dangerous bug' (*tsutsu ga mushi*). The illness was described by Hashimoto in 1810 and again in 1878 by Palm, a missionary at Nagaoka, and in 1879 by Baelz and Kawakami.[15] Dowden (1915) and Fletcher and Lesslar[16] in 1925 reported the disease in Malaya, and Ogata[17] in 1931 isolated the organism and named it *R. tsutsugamushi*.

Trench fever was first described by Graham[18] and Hunt and Rankin[19] in 1915 in soldiers on the Western Front, and by His[20] in 1916 in the Volhynia region of Poland. Töpfer[21] (1916) isolated the organism from body lice. It was named *Rochalimaea quintana*.

Rickettsial pox was described in the Kew Gardens district of the borough of Queens, New York, by Sussman[22] in 1946 and the organism was named *R. akari*.

Q fever (query fever) was reported by Derrick[23] in abattoir workers in Brisbane, Australia, in 1937, and the organism subsequently named *Coxiella burnetii*.

The earliest crude vaccine was made by Weigl in 1924 and used widely until a purified version devised by Cox and Bell[24] in 1940 superseded it for use against epidemic and endemic typhus. Fulton and Joyner[25] in 1945 developed a vaccine for scrub typhus from the lungs of infected cotton rats, but the vaccines were largely superceded in 1947 by the introduction of chlor-amphenicol for treatment and prophylaxis, initially for scrub typhus in Malaya by Smadel et al.,[26] and soon for all types of typhus with the tetracyclines, which remain in use today.

Serological diagnosis was pioneered in 1916 by Weil and Felix,[27] who described heterophile antibody agglutination of the OX-2 and OX-19 strains of *Proteus mirabilis* by typhus sera; this was extended to scrub typhus in 1926 by Fletcher and Lesslar,[28] who named an agglutinated variant strain OX-K in honour of their colleague Kingsbury.

Rickettsiae grow in guinea-pigs injected with infected human blood; *R. tsutsugamushi* and *R. akari* also grow in mice. Only *C. burnetii* and *Bartonella quintana* can be cultured in vitro.

Pathogenesis

The rickettsial diseases consist of acute fevers accompanied by general constitutional symptoms and especially by headache and, in severe cases, neurological disturbances, and often by a skin rash, either macular or haemorrhagic. In some types of typhus fever the site of inoculation may form a characteristic skin ulcer with a black crust (eschar).

The early part of the febrile illness represents a period of proliferation of rickettsiae in the blood and on the endothelial surface of small blood vessels. Toxins are produced which damage endothelial cell integrity, leading to leakage of fluid into tissues and to platelet aggregation and proliferation of polymorphonuclear leucocytes and monocytes within the vessel wall and in the perivascular spaces. This results in a focal occlusive end-angiitis of small venules and arterioles leading to microinfarction, producing the characteristic histological appearances of the 'typhus nodule' described by Fränkel and Wohlbach[29] (Figure 50.1).

All body tissues may be involved in this process, with important effects especially in the brain, cardiac and skeletal muscles, the skin, lungs, kidneys and the retina; in severe cases the end-angiitis causes venous thrombosis

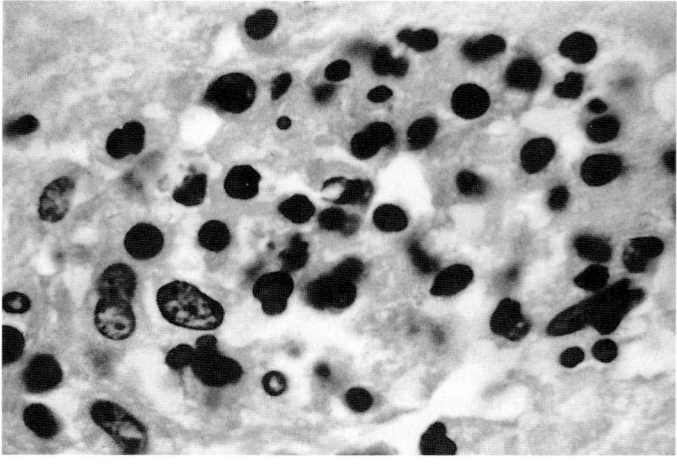

Figure 50.1: Typhus, or Wohlbach's nodule.

and peripheral gangrene. In the latter part of the fever, if significant rickettsaemia persists, excessive immune complex deposition may occur within the skin, kidneys and other tissues. Convalescent patients exhibit delayed hypersensitivity reactions to injected rickettsial antigens which may perpetuate the endangiitis.

Epidemic louse-borne typhus

Epidemiology

R. prowazekii is transmitted by the human body or clothing louse *Pediculus humanus* from person to person. There is no evidence that head lice act as vectors of this infection. Rickettsiae from the blood of a human case are ingested by the biting louse and multiply in the gut of the insect so that its faeces are heavily infected. Scratching of a subsequent bite inoculates the organisms, which can also enter the body through rubbing into the conjunctival membrane. Infected lice may die from the disease but can transmit the rickettsiae to other lice through ingestion of faeces. Transovarial vertical transmission does not occur in lice. Air-borne infection may occur in crowded conditions by the inhalation of dried louse faeces. Blood transfusion has rarely transmitted the disease. Laboratory infection is a major risk. Specimens suspected of containing rickettsiae must be treated as for a 'dangerous pathogen'. In the USA *R. prowazekii* has also been isolated from flying squirrels (*Glaucomys volans*) and is transmitted between them by their lice and fleas; the significance of this finding in transmission to humans is uncertain.

The genome of *R. prowazekii* has recently been sequenced, providing new and fascinating evidence of an evolutionary relationship between rickettsiae and intracellular mitochondria in general.[30]

Foci of endemic human infection from which epidemic spread can occur in times of famine, war, migration and overcrowding exist mainly in the cooler mountainous regions of tropical countries, such as Rwanda, Burundi, Uganda, Ethiopia, Lesotho, Transkei, Ciskei, Transvaal, Namibia, Nigeria, Kurdistan, northern India and Pakistan, China, Papua New Guinea, the Andes Mountains, Guatemala, Mexico, and Serbia and Greece (Figure 50.2).

Typical cicumstances prevailed in the Burundi epidemic of 1995, which began with cases in a prison and spread to the malnourished inmates of refugee camps in the central highlands, causing over 50 000 cases with a mortality rate of 2.6%.[31,32]

Chronic human carriage of *R. prowazekii* may result in later relapses of typhus fever, a phenomenon first

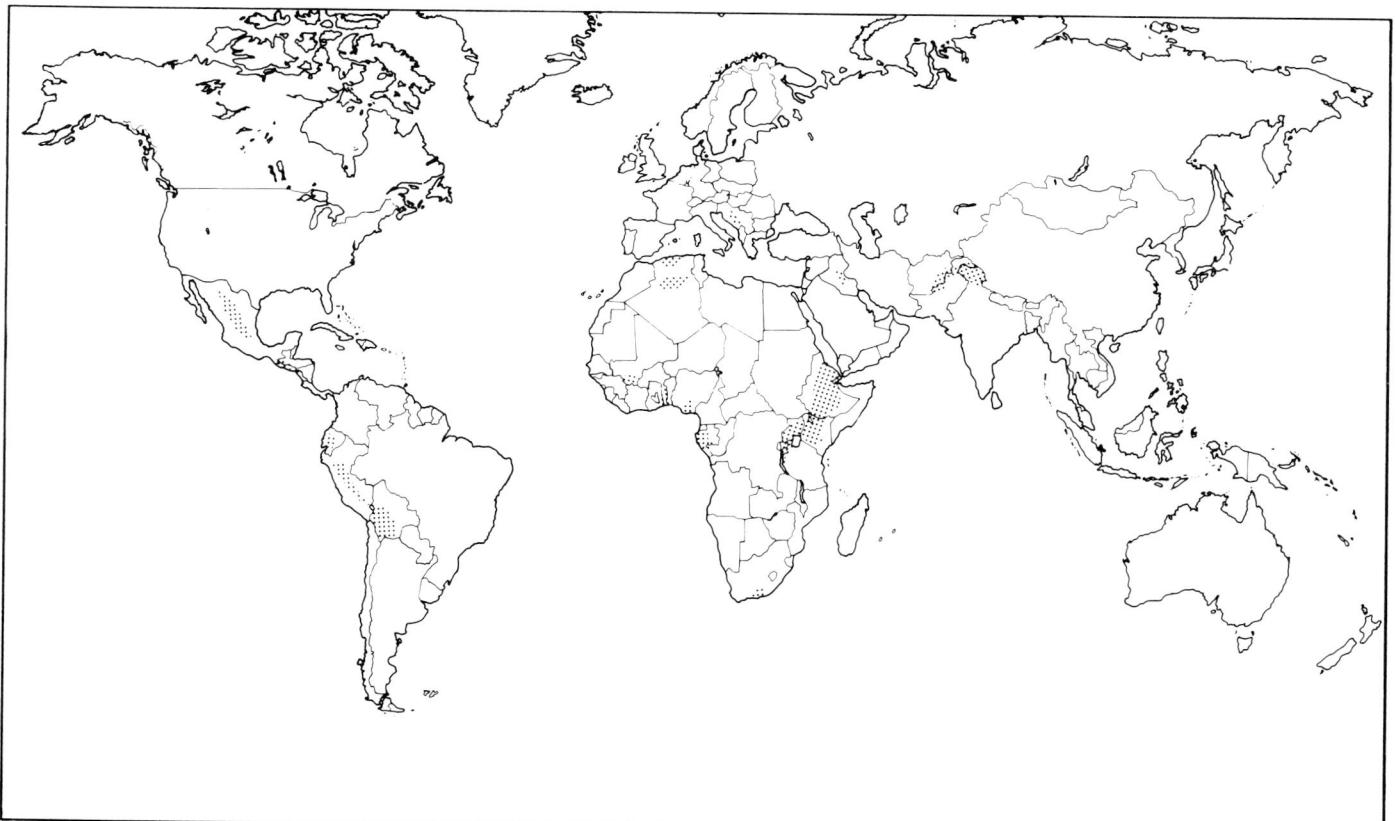

Figure 50.2: Present-day endemic foci of louse-borne typhus (*R. prowazekii*). (Courtesy of the Department of Entomology, London School of Hygiene and Tropical Medicine.)

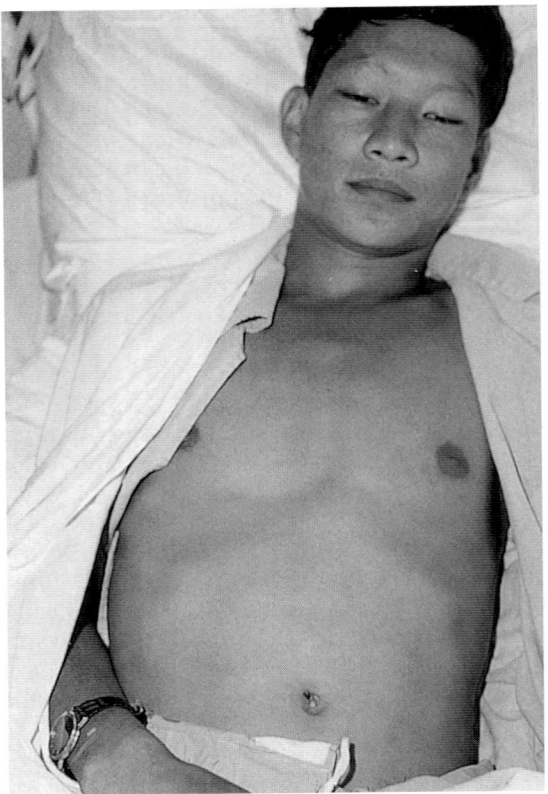

Figure 50.3: A patient with mild typhus encephalitis.

Clinical description

In the populations at risk of epidemic typhus fever, nutrition and general immunity to infection are inadequate, so that the illness is often severe, with a mortality rate of up to 20% overall, and greater than 50% in the weak and aged. The incubation period averages 12 days. There is an abrupt onset of fever, prostration and severe headache, with pain in the limbs, especially the shins, and nausea and vomiting. Fever rises rapidly to 39–40°C, and remains high until death or resolution by 'crisis' towards the end of the second week, if untreated. The conjunctivae are suffused, the face congested, and the patient looks vacant and depressed as if drugged or drunk (Figure 50.3). Delirium may ensue and a mid-brain ischaemic syndrome of akinetic mutism can occur. There is fetor oris, and epistaxis and a dry cough are common. Splenomegaly is usual. The typhus rash appears on the second to fourth day of fever, mainly on the trunk and proximal limbs (Figure 50.4). It consists of small irregular pink macules which rapidly darken to a mulberry or purple colour, and rarely become frankly petechial (Figure 50.5). Coalescence to a generalized patchy purple mottling under the skin may occur a few days later. There is no eschar at the site of inoculation. Patients are said to smell of mice, boot polish or rifle-barrel washings. Constipation is usual, and paralytic ileus may occur.

In up to 50% of severe cases a meningoencephalitis ensues with meningism, tinnitus and hyperacusis followed by deafness, dysphagia, dysphoria, agitated delirium and coma. Survivors may suffer transverse myelitis, hemiparesis, peripheral neuropathy with hyperaesthesia, and prolonged psychiatric disturbances.

Other possible complications include secondary infection leading to bronchopneumonia, suppurative parotitis or otitis media, and peripheral blood vessel occlusion resulting in leg vein thrombosis and peripheral gangrene,

described by Brill[33] in 1910 in Jewish migrants from the Balkans to New York, and subsequently confirmed by Zinsser[34] (Brill–Zinsser disease). Such patients are thought to form a source of potential infection when louse infestation becomes common in prisons and refugee camps or in insanitary crowded conditions.

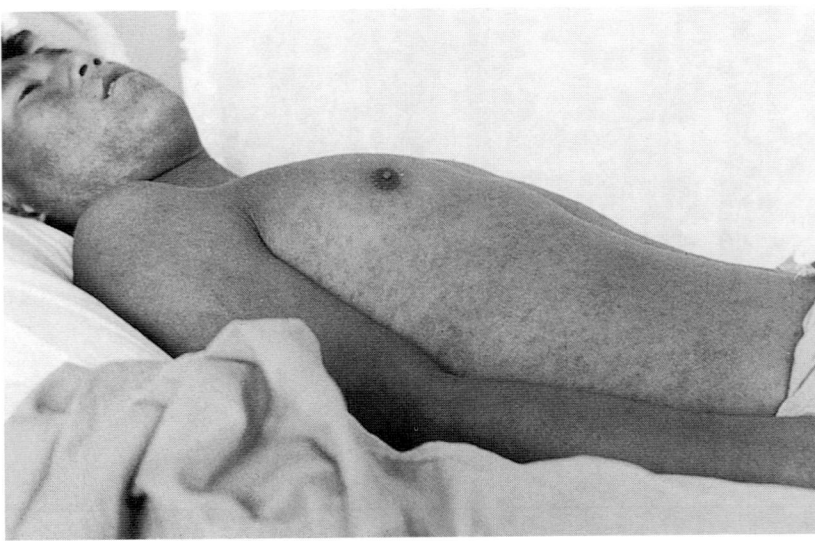

Figure 50.4: The rash of typhus fever. (Courtesy of G. W. Brown.)

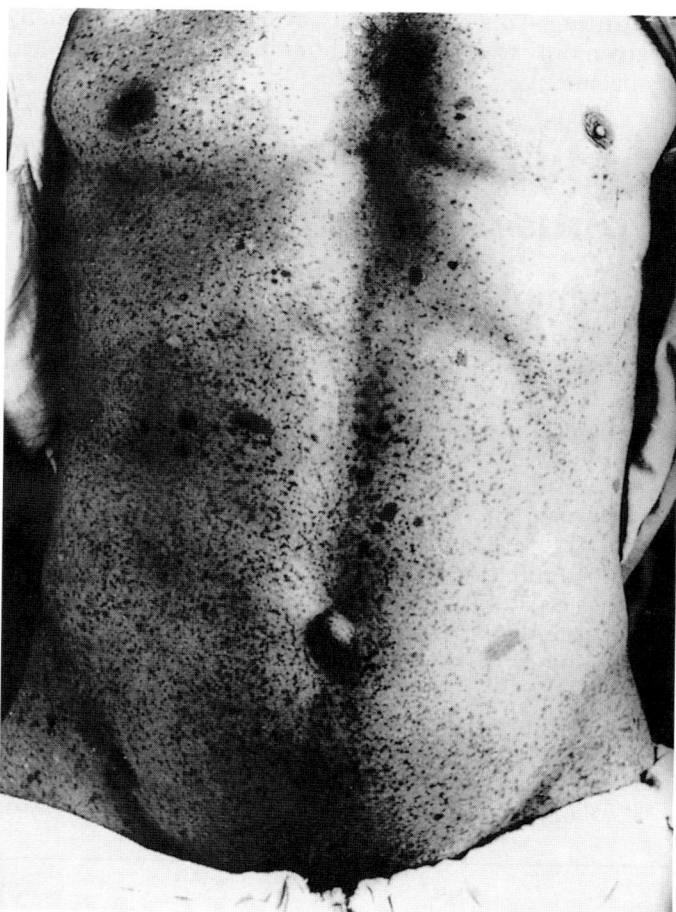

Figure 50.5: Typhus rash in the second week showing the typical distribution. The dark-coloured areas are petechial; the lighter-coloured, discrete areas disappear on pressure.

for instance of digits. An important further complication is myocarditis, which can occur during recovery with or without specific treatment. This presents with hypotension, tachycardia and low-output cardiac failure or sudden arrhythmic collapse.

Differential diagnosis

The differential diagnosis of epidemic typhus includes:

- Typhoid fever. This may be clinically very similar and should be excluded by blood or bone marrow culture(s) for *Salmonella typhi*.
- Measles, especially if haemorrhagic. The rash of measles affects the face severely, unlike that of typhus.
- Viral haemorrhagic fevers (e.g., dengue, Rift Valley fever, Congo–Crimea haemorrhagic fever and yellow fever). These may require to be excluded serologically.
- Meningococcal septicaemia, which can be excluded by culture of blood or cerebrospinal fluid (CSF).
- Louse-borne relapsing fever. This may be very similar clinically, but with a haemorrhagic rash. Blood cultures should be performed.
- Leptospirosis. This may be clinically similar in the

early stages of the illness. Distinguishing features include marked skeletal muscle tenderness and peripheral blood polymorphonuclear leucocytosis.
- *Plasmodium falciparum* malaria, especially if cerebral involvement has occurred. Blood films should be stained to exclude this, although rashes and skin haemorrhage are rare in malaria.

Diagnosis

Routine blood investigations in typhus are unhelpful, with a normal total and relative white blood cell count. More severe cases have reduced serum levels of sodium, chloride and albumin, and features diagnostic of diffuse intravascular coagulation. CSF may be at increased pressure, with modest rises in protein and monocyte count, but normal glucose content.

Specific diagnosis may be made:

- On clinical grounds, in an epidemic situation, confirmed by rapid response to specific treatment.
- Serologically by the demonstration of heterophile antibodies to *Proteus mirabilis* OX-19 and OX-2 strains in the Weil–Felix test.

It may also be made, in specialized laboratories only:

- By isolation of rickettsiae by inoculation of blood into guinea-pigs or fertile duck eggs.
- Serologically by a group-specific microagglutination test (MAT) or species-specific immunofluorescence antibody test (IFAT) or enzyme-linked immunosorbent assay (ELISA). IFAT can be modified for use without a fluorescence microscope in the indirect immuno-peroxidase reaction, and the ELISA test can also be modified for field use by application to filter paper.
- By detection of the organism by polymerase chain reaction (PCR),[35] by gas–liquid chromatography of acute serum, and by antigen detection by immuno-fluorescence on skin biopsy.

Management

General medical and nursing care is important, with attention to fluid balance, mouth toilet, avoidance of bed sores, adequate analgesia, treatment of agitation with judicious doses of diazepam, appropriate antibiotics (e.g., amoxicillin) for secondary lung and middle ear infection and, in severe cases, the prescription of oral prednisolone 40 mg initially and 20 mg daily for several days, followed by reducing doses. Oliguria and anuria may require peritoneal or haemodialysis.

Specific chemotherapy should be with:

- *Chloramphenicol* in an adult dose of 500 mg 6 hourly, orally or intravenously for 7 days, or in children at 75 mg per kg per day, divided 6 hourly, for 7 days; or
- *Tetracycline* at an adult dose of 500 mg 6hourly, orally or intravenously for 7 days, or in children at 50 mg per kg per day, divided 6 hourly for 7 days; or
- *Doxycycline* (Vibramycin) in a single oral dose of 200 mg for adults or 100 mg for children, repeated

once later if necessary, or in a short course of 100–200 mg daily for 3 days.[36]

Rickettsiae are also sensitive to rifampicin and quinolones, but these agents are expensive and unnecessary, except in special circumstances in scrub typhus (see below).

Rapid defervescence should be anticipated within 48 hours if the diagnosis is correct.

Measures directed against the louse vector are essential. On admission, patients should be stripped of clothing and washed thoroughly with soap and water. Clothing should be incinerated or autoclaved. Delousing powder (1% malathion) can be applied to hospital clothing and bed sheets. Treatment of medical and nursing attendants with delousing powder once weekly is also desirable.

Prevention and control

Epidemic typhus should be controlled by:

1. Delousing of patients and all members of closed communities (e.g., refugee camps, prisons) where infection occurs—using 1% malathion powder.
2. Consideration of doxycycline single-dose treatment (200 mg) of all contacts and residents of infected areas, and medical and nursing attendants.
3. Use of a formalinized purified vaccine from chick embryo culture, made by the Swiss Serum and Vaccine Institute. This is not widely available and is normally given only to workers in laboratories handling infected specimens.

Murine, endemic, 'shop' typhus

Epidemiology

Murine typhus is caused by *R. typhi (R. mooseri)* which is transmitted to humans by *Xenopsylla cheopis* fleas living on *Rattus rattus* (the black rat), *Rattus norvegicus* (the brown rat) and various species of mouse, and between rats by the louse *Polyplax spinulosa* and the mite *Liponyssus bacoti*. Flea faeces infected with rickettsiae contaminate the flea bite, which is then scratched, so inoculating the infection, or may be inhaled when dried or rubbed into the conjunctival membrane. Rodents with rickettsaemia of this type do not suffer serious illness and so act as a reservoir of infection. Humans are infected by close contact with rodents and their fleas in granaries, breweries, shops and food stores, and domestically in developing countries. Garbage workers are at special risk. Human disease is known to occur in the USA, Mexico, northern South America, Israel, Pakistan, India, South-East Asia, China and Australia[37] and Spain[38] (Figure 50.6).

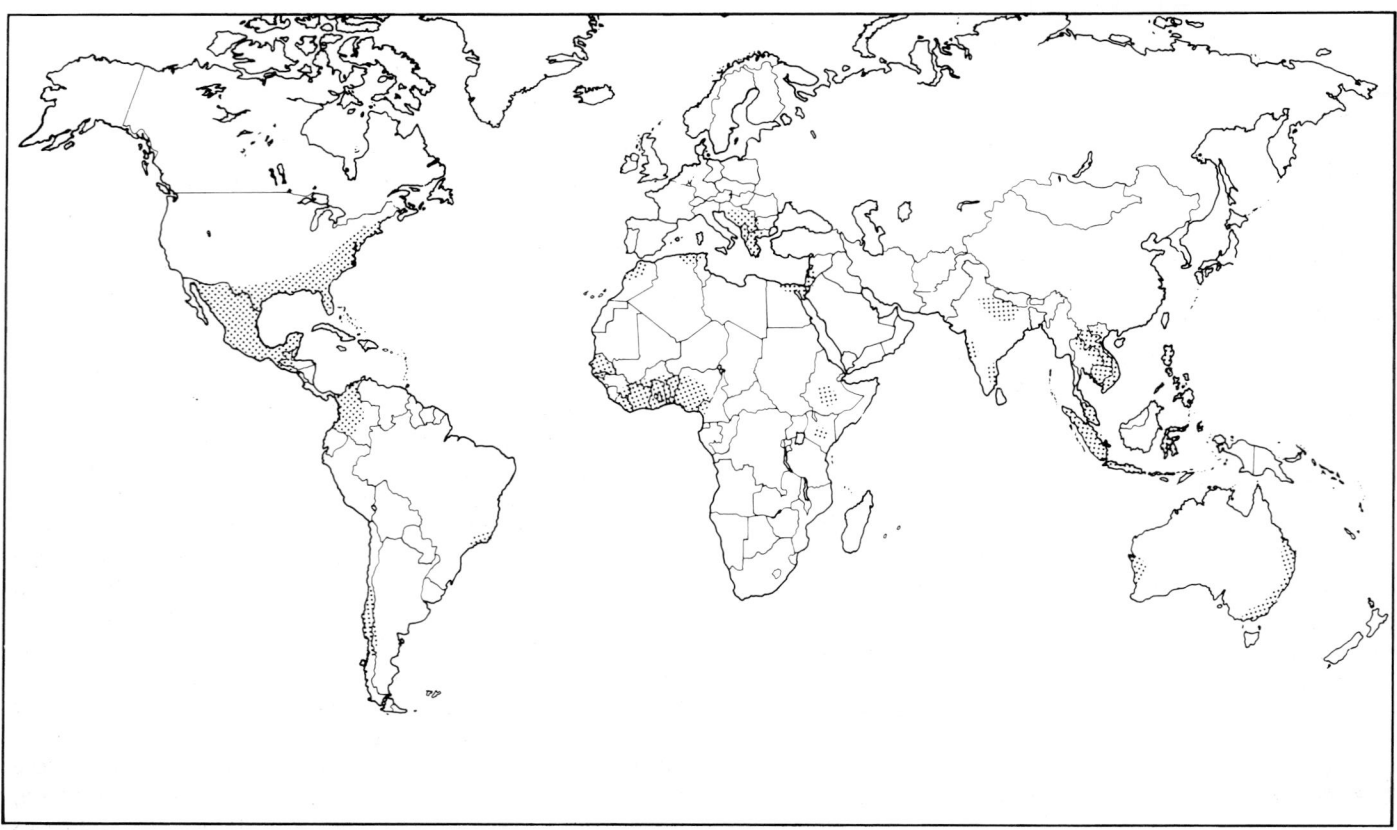

Figure 50.6: Geographical distribution of flea-borne (murine) typhus (*R. mooseri*). (Courtesy of the Department of Entomology, London School of Hygiene and Tropical Medicine.)

It is an important cause of fever in Khmer refugees in Thailand.[39]

Clinical description

The incubation period is similar to that of louse-borne typhus, and the illness is also similar, but generally much less severe, with a mortality rate of only 1–2%. Headache and muscular pains are the predominant symptoms. There is no eschar at the site of inoculation, and the rash of fine red macules is less extensive than in epidemic typhus. Serious neurological, renal and other complications are unusual.

Differential diagnosis

The differential diagnosis of murine typhus includes:

- Typhoid fever—excluded by blood or bone marrow culture.
- Louse-borne and scrub typhus—distinguished only by specific serological tests, and treated identically anyway.
- Arbovirus infections with a macular rash (e.g., dengue and chikungunya)—distinguished serologically.
- Relapsing fever, transmitted by lice or ticks, distinguished by blood culture.
- Leptospirosis—distinguished by exquisite muscle tenderness and polymorphonuclear leucocytosis.
- Malaria—excluded by stained blood films.
- Other causes of fever with macular rash (e.g., Epstein–Barr virus, human immunodeficiency virus (HIV) seroconversion illness)—distinguished serologically.

Diagnosis

The diagnosis is made by the same method(s) as in louse-borne typhus. The Weil–Felix reaction may be positive to OX-19 and OX-2 strains, but less strongly so. Group-specific serology is not helpful in differentiation from *R. prowazekii*, but a specific ELISA will distinguish *R. mooseri* antibodies.

Management

The general and specific treatment of murine typhus is the same as for louse-borne typhus. Steroid treatment is needed only exceptionally.

Prevention and control

The prevention of murine typhus has to depend on reducing human contact with rodents and their fleas by:

1. Urban and domestic rodent control using warfarin.
2. Proofing of grain and other food stores against rodents.
3. Residual insecticide spraying of rat runs in stores and breweries.
4. The wearing of protective clothing by garbage workers.

Rickettsial spotted fevers

These infections are caused by a large number of rickettsial species, all of which, except *R. akari*, are transmitted to humans by the bite of animal ticks (Table 50.1) or by inoculation of tick faeces or body fluids if the attached tick is crushed. Many other species of tick-borne rickettsiae exist (in animal reservoirs) that have yet to be characterized or identified.

Rocky Mountain spotted fever

Rocky Mountain spotted fever (RMSF), due to *R. rickettsii*, is a potentially life-threatening infection. Following its original description in the mountain states of north-west USA in the late nineteenth century and the demonstration of the organism in its tick vector by Ricketts in 1906, RMSF has since been recognized as an important cause of illness throughout the USA, especially now in the south-eastern states and on the eastern seaboard. In all, some 700 cases are reported annually in the USA (Figure 50.7). It also occurs in Canada, Mexico, Colombia and Brazil, especially in the area of São Paulo.

The ixodid tick vectors are:

- *Dermacentor andersoni* (wood tick)—western USA.
- *Dermacentor variabilis* (dog tick)—western USA.
- *Amblyomma americanum* (lone-star tick)—south and south-eastern USA.
- *Amblyomma cajennense*—Brazil and Colombia.
- *Haemaphysalis leporispalustris*—this rabbit tick does not bite humans but transmits the infection between rabbits, which act as a reservoir for transmission to human-biting ticks (Figure 50.8).

Transovarial transmission of rickettsiae occurs in ixodid hard ticks, which are thus the main reservoir of infection.

Dermacentor andersoni ticks normally live on goats, sheep, badgers, lynx and black bears, and their larvae on squirrels. *Dermacentor variabilis* and *Amblyomma* ticks live on domestic dogs, rabbits, foxes, opossums, gophers and racoons, and their larvae on field mice.

Clinical description

Surprisingly, in RMSF there is rarely an eschar at the site of the tick bite. After an inoculation period of 6–10 days there is an abrupt onset of fever with severe headaches and muscle pains, and a dry cough. After 2–3 days the typhus rash of fine pink macules develops (Figure 50.9), which in this disease is most marked on the soles of the feet, wrists and forearms. In more severe infections the rash quickly spreads and becomes petechial with large ecchymoses and the potential for gangrene of digits and pressure areas. The overall mortality rate is 7–10%, and in young children and elderly adults the rate is up to 25%. Meningoencephalitis is common in severe cases and, as the illness progresses, the stuporose or comatose patient will become hypotensive, oliguric or anuric, and uraemic. Other complications are similar to those seen in severe louse-borne typhus and include bronchopneumonia, otitis media, parotitis and intestinal ileus. In severe cases disseminated intravascular coagulation is a common accompaniment.

Table 50.1 Rickettsial spotted fevers.

Disease	Agent	Vector reservoir	Mammals also involved	Geographical location
Rocky Mountain spotted fever (RMSF) (Brazilian spotted fever)	R. rickettsii	Ticks	Rodents Dogs Rabbits Opossums	USA South America Canada
Boutonneuse fever (tick typhus)	R. conorii	Ticks	Dogs	Africa Mediterranean Middle East India
South African tick typhus	R. conorii R. africae	Ticks	Cattle Hippopotamus Rhinoceros	Zimbabwe South Africa
Israeli tick typhus	R. sharoni	Ticks	Rodents Deer Cattle Horses	Israel
Siberian tick typhus	R. sibirica	Ticks	Rodents	Armenia Kazakhstan Kirghizia East Asia Central Europe
Japanese tick typhus	R. japonica	Ticks	Rodents Dogs	Japan
Queensland tick typhus	R. australis	Ticks	Rodents	Australia South-East Asia
Flinders Island fever	R. houei	Ticks	Marsupials(?)	South-East Australia
Other rickettsiae in ticks and animals not proved to cause human disease:				
	R. montana	Ticks	Rodents, birds	North America
	R. parkeri	Ticks	Rodents, birds	North America
	R. rhipicephalus	Ticks	Dogs	North America
	R. helvetica	Ticks	Rodents	Europe
	R. heilongjangi	Ticks	Rodents	China
	R. belli	Ticks	Rodents, dogs	North America
	R. canada	Ticks	Rabbits, hares	Ontario, Canada California
and others as yet untyped in Thailand, Brunei, Sicily, Pakistan, etc.				

Differential diagnosis

RMSF should be distinguished from:

- Meningococcal septicaemia—by blood and CSF culture.
- Tick-borne relapsing fever—by blood culture.
- Haemorrhagic measles—by serological methods.
- Tularaemia—by blood culture.
- Lyme disease—by serological methods.

Diagnosis

The diagnosis of RMSF is based on similar methods to those used in epidemic typhus. The Weil–Felix reaction may be positive for OX-19 antibodies but specific IFAT or immunoperoxidase methods should be used if available.

Management

Treatment with chloramphenicol, tetracycline or doxycycline is the same as for louse-borne typhus. Intensive supportive management may be needed for uraemia and diffuse intravascular coagulation, as appropriate, and patients with a severe case should receive large doses of corticosteroids initially.

Prevention and control

It is not possible to eradicate the infection in ticks and animals, but the number of human cases can be reduced by:

1. The wearing of stout boots and outer garments during hunting and rambling expeditions in forests; clothing may be impregnated, for instance with permethrin, to reduce tick bites.

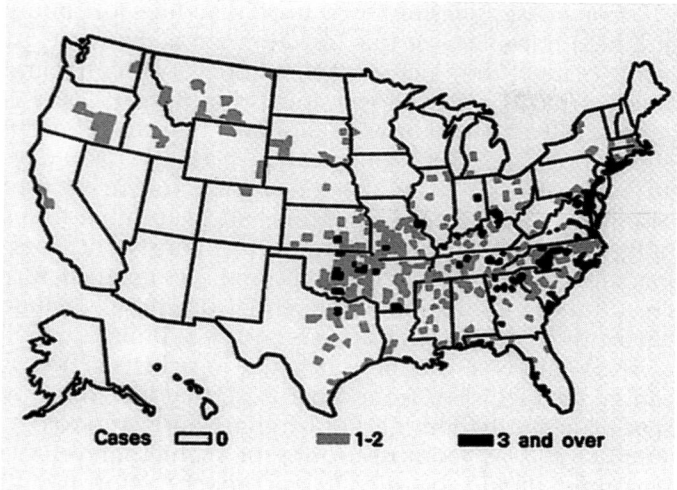

Figure 50.7: Typhus fever—tick-borne (Rocky Mountain spotted fever). Reported cases by country—USA, 1988.

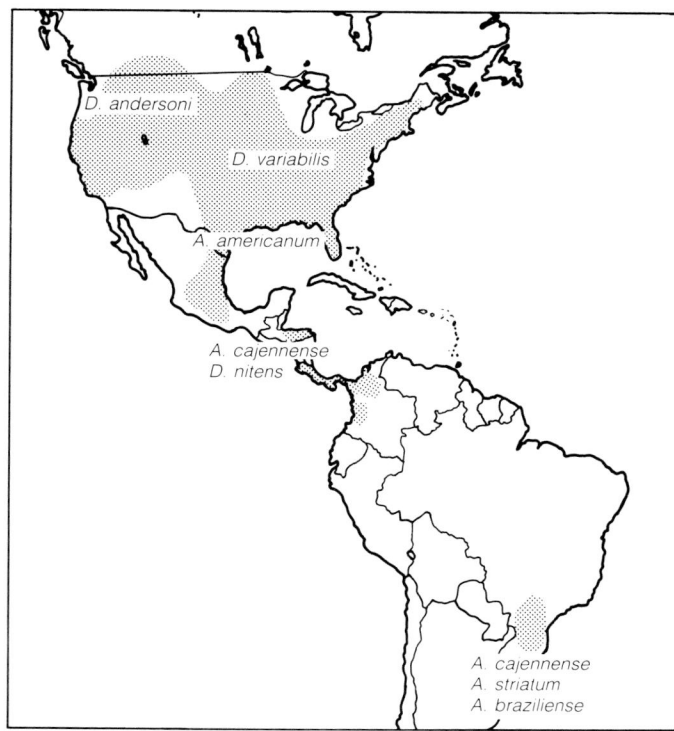

Figure 50.8: Geographical distribution of Rocky Mountain spotted fever (*R. rickettsii*). (Courtesy of the Department of Entomology, London School of Hygiene and Tropical Medicine.)

2. Surveillance for tick attachment after episodes of exposure to animal contact and forest habitats; ticks still attached should be treated with absolute alcohol and then removed gently with tweezers, taking care to remove the head.
3. Residual insecticide spraying of established woodland tracks.
4. Surveillance of domestic dogs for ticks, with use of insecticide powders and impregnated collars.

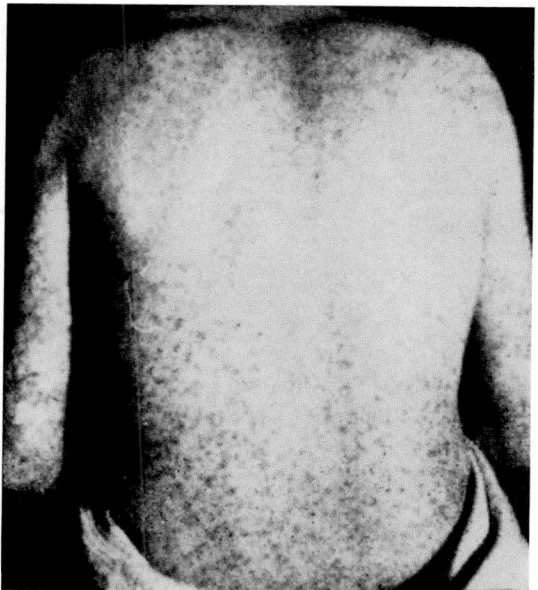

Figure 50.9: The rash of Rocky Mountain spotted fever.

There is no useful vaccine available for the prevention of RMSF.

Brazilian spotted fever is caused by *R. rickettsii* with *Amblyomma cajennense* as the vector tick. An eschar at the site of the tick bite is usual; the illness is otherwise similar to RMSF.

Mediterranean tick typhus (fièvre boutonneuse) occurs throughout the coastal countries of the Mediterranean and is increasingly recognized in France and Spain.[40] *R. conorii* is transmitted by the dog tick *Rhipicephalus sanguineus*, and the main reservoir of infection is in domestic dogs, rabbits and rodents. The illness is similar to RMSF, with the possibility of a haemorrhagic rash and renal and cerebral involvement, but in most cases it is less severe.

There is almost always an eschar (*tache noire*) at the site of the tick bite, with regional adenitis (Figure 50.10).

The differential diagnoses include typhoid, meningococcal septicaemia and measles. Specific serological tests are similar to those for other forms of typhus. The Weil–Felix reaction produces positive results at low titres for OX-19 and OX-K. Management is as for other forms of typhus. Prevention depends on methods similar to those for RMSF to reduce tick bites. There is no vaccine.

Israeli tick typhus, which is caused by a variant organism, *R. sharoni*, is transmitted by *Rhipicephalus* dog ticks, but eschar formation is unusual.

African tick typhus, due to *R. conorii*, is reported from most African countries, including South Africa. Various dog and other animal ticks act as vectors and main reservoirs. Savanna and veld are the main areas of risk, travellers

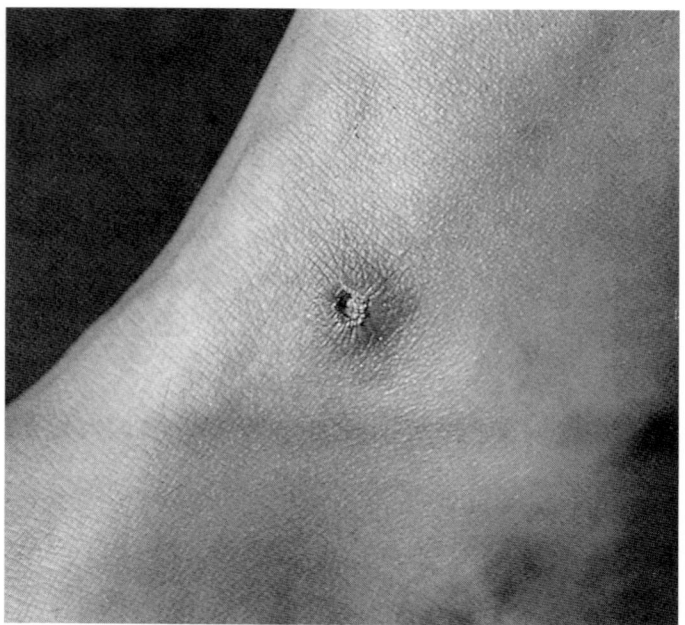

Figure 50.10: A primary eschar of African tick typhus.

being exposed on safari holidays. The illness closely resembles Mediterranean tick typhus. A variant form in Zimbabwe is due to a separate rickettsial species, *R. africae*, which has a reservoir in domestic cattle and probably also in hippo and rhino.[41] The differential diagnoses in Africa included tick-borne relapsing fever, typhoid, meningococcal septicaemia, measles and viral haemorrhagic fevers. Another new species, *R. honei*, named after the Adelaide physician who first described murine typhus in grain silo workers, has recently been found on Flinders Island, off Tasmania.[42] Treatment is as for other forms of typhus.

Other forms of tick typhus

Tick-borne typhus occurs in the mountainous northern fringes of the Indian subcontinent and as far west as Astrakhan, where it is caused by *R. conorii*. The Siberian form is due to a separate type, *R. sibirica*, which also infects birds and domestic animals, and occurs in Siberia, Kirghizia, Kazakhstan, Armenia and eastern Europe.

Separate species have also been found in Japan (*R. japonica*)[43] and Australia (*R. australis, R. honei*[44]), and suspected in Thailand. As yet untyped rickettsial species probably exist in nature for potential transmission to humans by ticks. In general these illnesses resemble Mediterranean tick typhus, and there is an eschar in over 75% of cases. Specific serological diagnosis should be attempted if possible. Antibiotic treatment is as for other forms of typhus.

Rickettsial pox is a spotted fever that produces a distinctive rash and is caused by *R. akari*, which is transmitted by *Allodermanyssus sanguineus*, a mite that lives on house and field mice. Foci of this infection are known to exist in the eastern USA, including New York City, Central and South Africa, Crimea, Korea and Costa Rica. *R. akari* is serologically more akin to *R. austrialis* than to *R. conorii* and *R. rickettsii*. After an incubation period of 7–10 days an eschar is present at the inoculation site in 90% of cases. Fever and general symptoms are as in other forms of typhus. The rash appears rapidly and consists of sparse macules and papules that become vesicular before crusting and fading. The differential diagnoses include chickenpox, monkeypox and secondary syphilis.

The Weil–Felix reaction is negative in rickettsial pox. It can be distinguished from other rickettsial infections by specific agglutination but not by group antigen serology. Treatment is as for other forms of typhus. Preventive measures should be directed at rodent control and efficient garbage clearance.

Scrub typhus
Epidemiology

Scrub typhus is a significant and widespread disease in Asia. It is due to *Orientia tsutsugamushi*,[44] previously known as *R. orientalis* or *R. tsutsugamushi*, of which at least six distinct serological strains (Gilliam, Karp, Kato, Shimokoshi, Kawasaki, Kuroki) can be detected by immunoperoxidase reactions.[45] It occurs in Japan (some 900 cases annually), South Korea, Taiwan, the Philippines, southern China (including Hong Kong and Hainan islands), East and West Malaysia, Thailand, Cambodia, Vietnam, Laos, Myanmar, Sri Lanka, India, Nepal, northern Pakistan, the islands of the Indian Ocean, Indonesia, Papua New Guinea and its neighbouring islands, Queensland[46] and northern New South Wales (Figure 50.11).

A recent study in Malaysia of 'pyrexia of unknown origin' has shown antibodies to spotted fever group rickettsiae in 42.5% of patients, *R. typhi* in 28% and *O. tsutsugamushi* in 25%.[47]

The vector insect to humans is the larva of a number of trombiculid mites in which transovarial transmission maintains the infection in nature. There is also a wild rodent reservoir, and the infection characteristically occurs in discrete foci ('mite islands') where infected mites live on the jungle grass *Imperata cylindrica*, known as *lalang* (Malaysia, Indonesia), *illuk* (Philippines) or *kunai* (Papua New Guinea, Australia), which grows only where primary jungle has been cleared for cultivation or to build villages (Figure 50.12). Human cases occur when workers in oil palm and rubber estates, and police officers and soldiers, traverse this habitat, brushing against the sharp stiff blades of waist-high *Imperata* grass, allowing the larval mites access. It is an important military disease, many thousands of cases having occurred in the Far East theatre in the Second World War.[39]

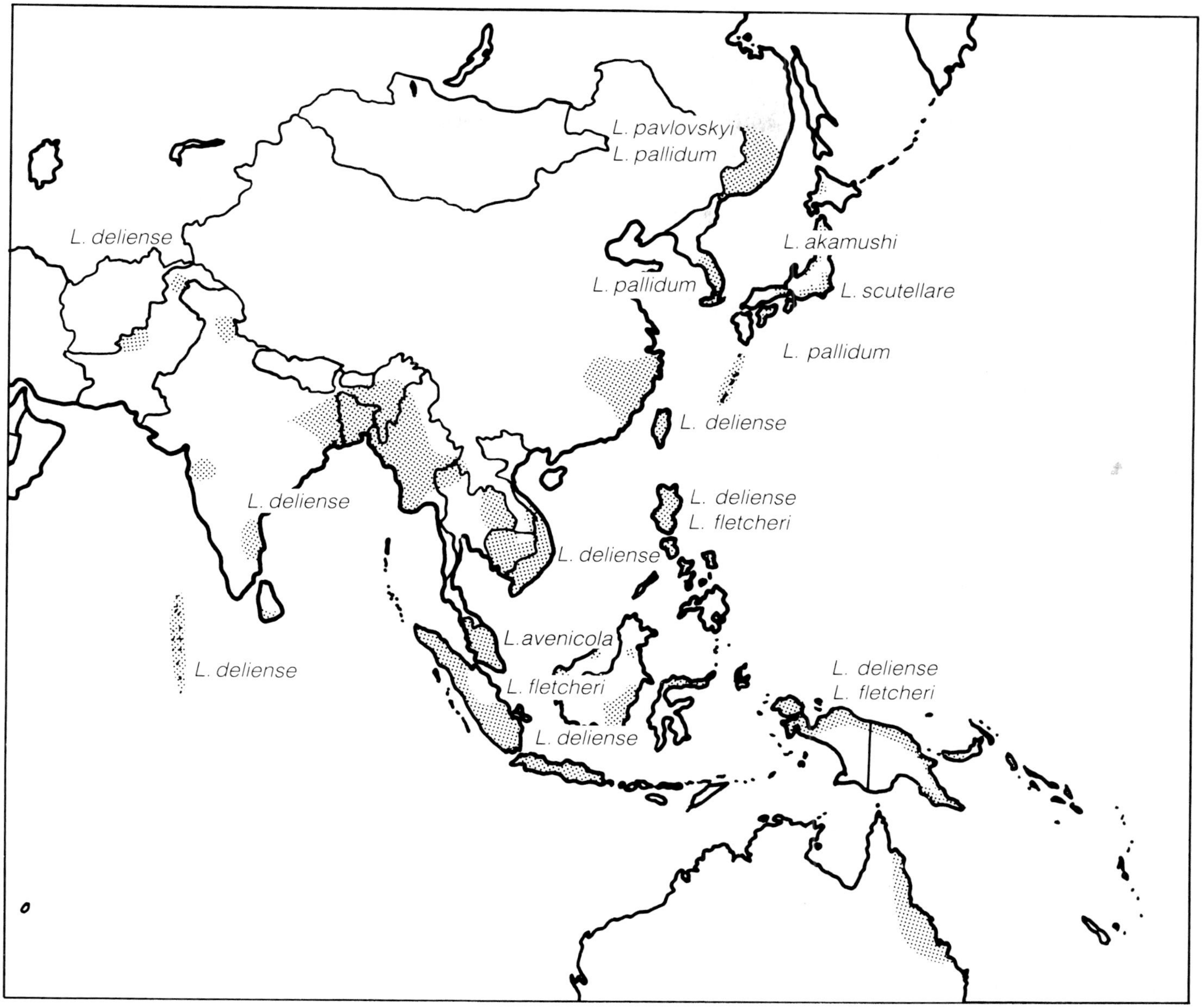

Figure 50.11: Geographical distribution of scrub (mite-borne) typhus (*R. tsutsugamushi* (*orientalis*)). (Courtesy of the Department of Entomology, London School of Hygiene and Tropical Medicine.)

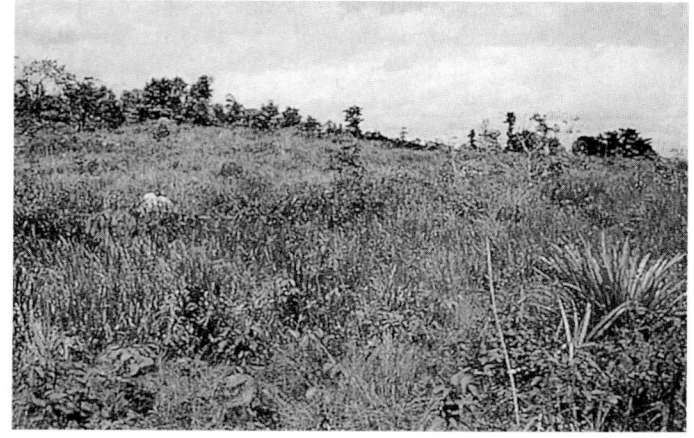

Figure 50.12: Typical scrub typhus country. (Courtesy of G. W. Brown.)

Clinical description

The incubation period is 5–10 days. The mite bite has usually passed unnoticed, but the patient may be aware, as the febrile illness begins, of painful axillary or inguinal lymph nodes. Careful examination will reveal an adjacent eschar, especially on the scrotum (Figure 50.13) or in the axilla, in 50–80% of cases. This is a firm adherent black scab, 3–6 mm in diameter, with a fine red margin, which is painless (Figure 50.14). Multiple eschars can occur, for instance under a trouser belt. The fever starts abruptly and has the usual typhus accompaniments of suffused conjunctivae and face, severe headache, drowsiness, apathy, pain in the shins and other muscles, and, more characteristically, generalized

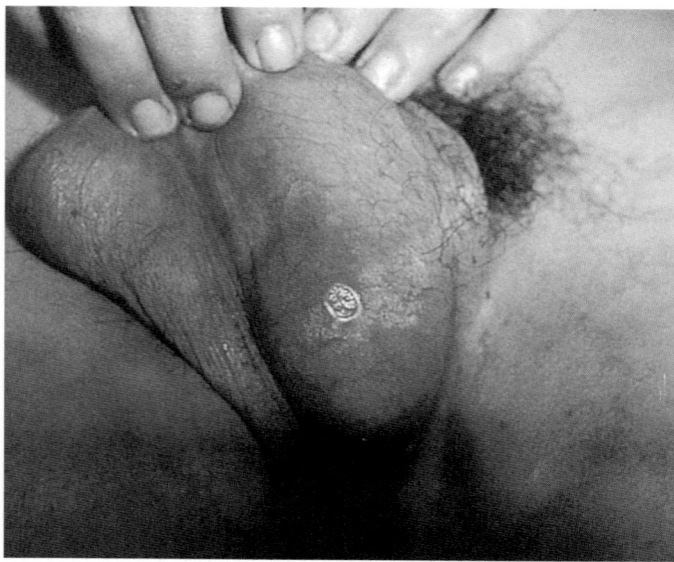

Figure 50.13: The eschar of scrub typhus. (Courtesy of G. W. Brown.)

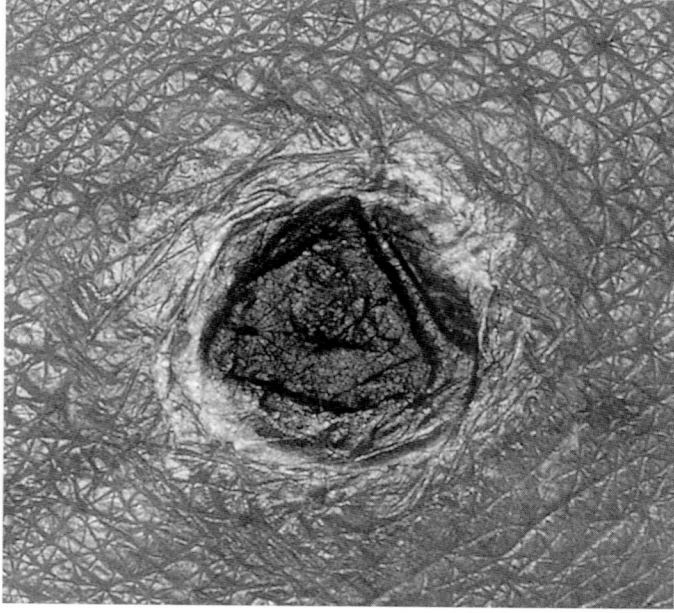

Figure 50.14: The eschar of scrub typhus, close-up view. (Courtesy of G. W. Brown.)

lymphadenopathy and hepatosplenomegaly. Other symptoms may include nausea and vomiting, tinnitus and hyperacusis followed by deafness, constipation, epistaxis and a dry cough.

The rash is similar to that of louse-borne typhus and occurs mainly on the arms, thighs and trunk. In severe cases, meningoencephalitis ensues with neck stiffness, delirium, focal signs, papilloedema and coma. Myocarditis may complicate this phase, and oliguria with uraemia is common in severe cases. Adult respiratory distress syndrome (ARDS) and septic shock have also been reported.[48]

Indigenous peoples of areas endemic for scrub typhus commonly have a less severe illness, often without any rash or eschar. This is one of the most common causes of 'pyrexia of unknown origin' in such areas,[49] after malaria is excluded, but severe pneumonia has also been described.[50]

Immunity to scrub typhus following an attack is remarkably short-lived, lasting only a few months, and is specific to each strain of the organism, so that further attacks are common.

Patients who are HIV positive and then contract scrub typhus show a curious phenomenon of a fall in their HIV viral load, which is so far unexplained.[51]

Differential diagnosis

Scrub typhus should be distinguished from:

- Malaria—by stained blood films.
- Arbovirus infections (e.g., dengue)—by serological methods. The macular rash of dengue fever is much finer and often accompanied by marked thrombocytopenia
- Leptospirosis—by blood cultures and serology.
- Meningococcal disease—by blood and CSF cultures.
- Typhoid—by blood and bone marrow cultures.
- Infectious mononucleosis and HIV seroconversion illness—by serological methods.

Diagnosis

As in other forms of typhus, routine blood examinations are unhelpful. The Weil–Felix reaction of specific agglutination of *Proteus* OX-K is positive in only 50% of cases, and positive titres may be delayed for up to 3 weeks. Specific immunoperoxidase or PCR serology should be sought where available. Commonly, the clinical diagnosis is based on the geographical history and physical signs, and confirmed by the rapid response to specific chemotherapy. The occurrence of a Jarisch–Herxheimer reaction after the institution of treatment with tetracycline suggests that leptospirosis was either the primary diagnosis, or coexisted.

Management

The treatment of scrub typhus is now most commonly with a single oral 200-mg dose of doxycycline for adults, and 100 mg for children. In the small proportion of patients in whom the usual rapid defervescence is followed by a relapse of fever 5–7 days later, an identical second dose is given. Alternatively, a short course of doxycycline, 200 mg daily (for adults) for 3 days has been reported as useful.[52] Continuous chloramphenicol or tetracycline therapy can be given for 7 days, as in louse-borne typhus, but in all forms of typhus tetracycline should not be given to oliguric or anuric patients; doxycycline is safe in such circumstances.

O. tsutsugamushi is so far the only member of the Rickettsiae tribe that has been shown to have developed antibiotic resistance, to chloramphenicol and tetracycline, and only in northern Thailand.[55] Both are bacteriostaic agents, so that patients with infection acquired there should be treated with rifampicin or a quinolone (e.g., ciprofloxacin).

Prevention and control

Scrub typhus can be partly prevented or controlled by:

1 The wearing of stout boots with trousers well tucked in or strapped at the ankle with gaiters or *puttees* in those likely to be occupationally exposed to infection.
2 Impregnation of clothing with permethrin in those at occupational risk.
3 Avoidance of cleared jungle areas known to contain infected 'mite islands'.
4 Clearance by burning of *lalang* grass in peridomestic settings (e.g., refugee camps, *kampongs*, military camps).
5 Consideration of use of chemoprophylaxis with doxycycline 200 mg weekly by those at high occupational risk, such as soldiers on field operations.
6 Use of cotton-rat lung vaccine; this is not now generally available.

Trench fever

Epidemiology

Trench fever (His–Werner disease, Wolhynia fever) was first described as an epidemic disease in the First World War—in 1915 on the Western Front and in 1916 in Poland. It is still known to occur in Mexico, Canada, Ethiopia, Burundi, China and Japan. The causative organism, *Bartonella quintana*, is closely related to the rickettsiae but is not an obligate intracellular parasite and can thus be cultured on blood agar. It is transmitted by the human body louse, *Pediculus humanus*. It is thought that wild voles and other rodents may act as a reservoir, although the organism in voles, *Bartonella vinsoni*, is subtly different serologically. *Bartonella henselae* infection has recently been found in HIV-positive patients with fever, with peliosis hepatis, and with bacillary angiomatosis,[56] but there is no evidence implicating such an infection in the aetiology of Kaposi's sarcoma. Bacterial endocarditis is now a recognized complication.

Clinical description

The illness is usually fairly mild, with fever, headache, lumbar muscle pains, dizziness, nausea and vomiting. There is usually a sparse macular rash, but no eschar. The patient may have a single episode of fever lasting a few days, or suffer recurrent fever at intervals of about 5 days (quintan fever), or a more prolonged 'typhoidal' fever. Full recovery is usual and the mortality rate negligible, although some patients suffer prolonged debility with dyspnoea on exertion, but without objective evidence of myocarditis.

Differential diagnosis

Trench fever should be distinguished from:

- Louse-borne typhus, although the treatment is identical.
- Louse-borne relapsing fever—by blood cultures and serology.
- Typhoid—by blood and bone marrow cultures.
- Brucellosis—by serological methods.
- Q fever—by serological methods.

Diagnosis

Bartonella quintana can be isolated from blood by culture on blood agar in a carbon dioxide-enriched environment. A specific serological agglutination test is also possible.

Management

Trench fever is treated with doxycycline or other tetracyclines—as for scrub typhus—but other *Bartonella* species may respond better to aminoglycosides.

Prevention and control

Outbreaks of trench fever require that cases should be treated, and patients and attendants deloused—as in epidemic typhus.

Q fever

Epidemiology

Q fever was so named by Derrick in 1937 as 'query fever' before the causative organism was discovered, and not after Queensland where he discovered it. The strange name has persisted, despite the discovery and naming of the causative agent as *Coxiella burnetii*. The disease has also been known as 'Balkan grippe', 'Red River fever' (Zaire) and 'Nine Mile fever' (from a creek in the Rocky Mountains). *C. burnetii* is a very small (0.2×1.5 μm) rickettsia-like organism that is particularly resistant to heat and drying. It can be cultured in yolk sacs or minced chicken embryo cell cultures. It exists in nature as a zoonosis of rodents, rabbits and birds; it is transmitted to domestic goats and cattle by ticks and thence to humans, not usually by insects but by direct infection through milk, placental products and dried faeces in dust, although rarely sheep and cattle ticks transmit it to humans. It has a worldwide geographical distribution (Figure 50.15) and is an important cause of abortion in domestic goats and cattle.

C. burnetii produces is an intracytoplasmic infection in which the organism multiplies, especially in splenic histiocytes and the Kupffer cells of the liver, where it elicits a granulomatous response.[58]

Clinical description

The clinical course of Q fever may vary from an inapparent infection with seroconversion through a mild

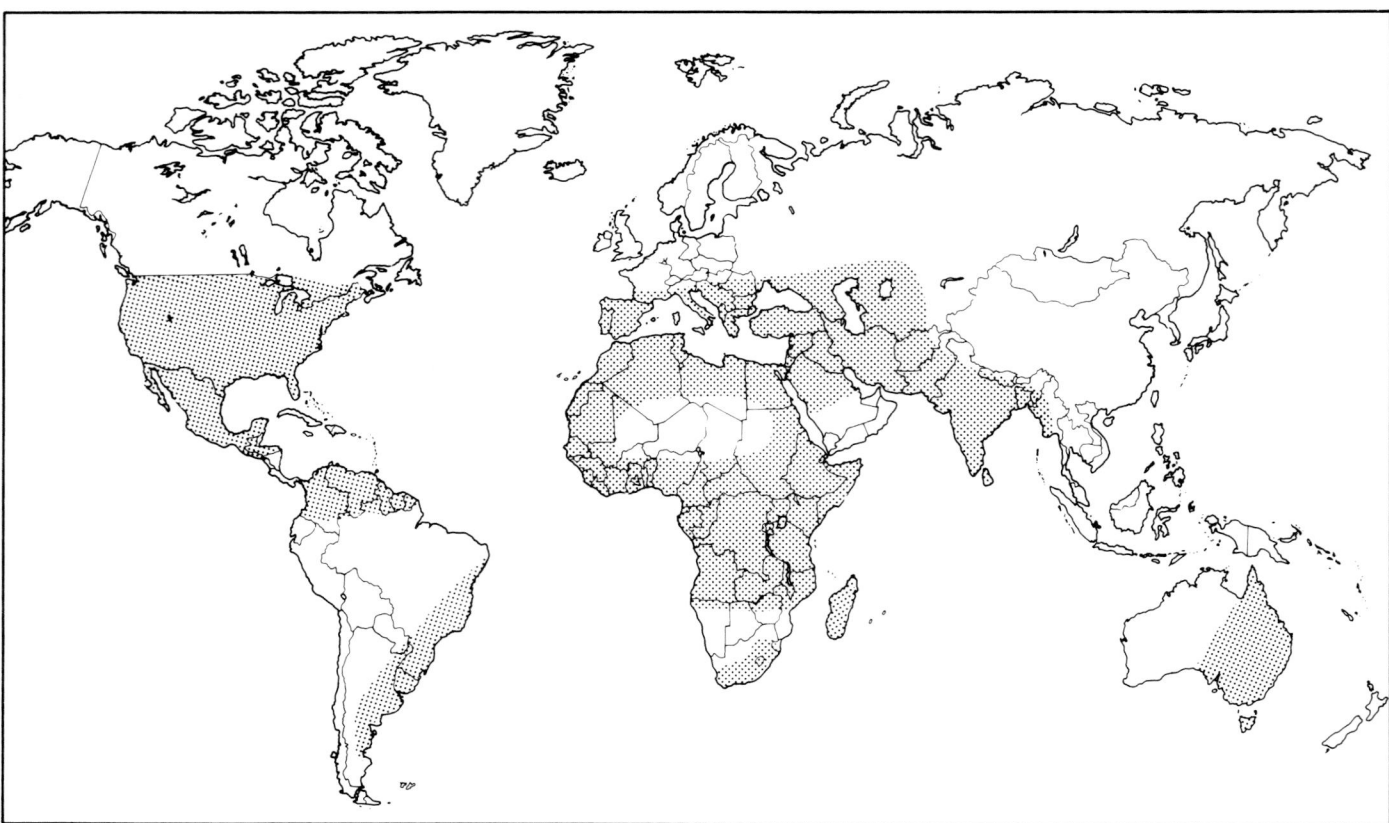

Figure 50.15: Geographical distribution of Q fever.

brief fever, to a chronic debilitating febrile illness with hepatitis, pneumonitis, pericarditis and a later risk of destructive valvular endocarditis.[57] The initial illness may resemble the typhus fevers, but without a rash, although many patients present with 'atypical pneumonia' with clinical and radiological evidence of patchy pneumonitis. Hepatomegaly with biochemical evidence of hepatitis occurs in up to 30% of cases, but marked jaundice is unusual. Splenomegaly and generalized lymphadenopathy may resemble that present in Epstein–Barr virus infection. The acute illness may subside spontaneously and complicating endocarditis may not be apparent from the usual clinical features until many months have elapsed. Cardiac involvement may occur in up to 10% of cases. The destruction of a previously healthy or congenitally abnormal valve usually involves the aortic valve, and often necessitates operative valve replacement; subsequent reinfection of a prosthetic valve can occur, indicating that the infection is difficult to eradicate.

Differential diagnosis

Q fever should be distinguished from:

- Typhoid—by blood and bone marrow culture.
- Other causes of atypical pneumonia (e.g., viruses, *Mycoplasma pneumoniae*, ornithosis)—by appropriate serological methods.

- Toxoplasmosis—by serology.
- Virus infections such as Epstein–Barr, HIV, cytomegalovirus—by appropriate serology.
- Viral hepatitis—by serology.
- Miliary tuberculosis—by chest radiography and tuberculin testing.
- Syphilis—by serology.
- Other causes of bacterial endocarditis—by blood cultures; and Lyme disease—by serology.

Diagnosis

The diagnosis of Q fever is best made serologically by a fourfold rise in antibody titre in two complement fixation tests separated by 10–14 days.

ELISA and IFAT serological tests are also available. Liver biopsy shows a granulomatous hepatitis, but this has many other possible causes.

Management

The treatment for early uncomplicated Q fever is as for typhus fever—with tetracycline, doxycycline or chloramphenicol.

In endocarditis, combination chemotherapy for many months is required with rifampicin and co-trimoxazole, or tetracycline and co-trimoxazole. Quinolone antibiotics may also be effective. Cardiac surgical treatment may be required.

Prevention and control

Aerosol dissemination of *C. burnetii* is very difficult to prevent because control of the disease in domestic animals is difficult. Milk should be pasteurized, and slightly higher temperatures may be needed for milk from herds known to be infected.

A formalinized vaccine is available for the protection of abattoir workers, farmers and herdspeople, and laboratory workers; this is used widely in Australia.

Ehrlichiosis

Ehrlichia sennetsu, an intraleucocytic bacterium closely related to the Rickettsiae, was first isolated in Japan in 1954 from a patient with an illness similar to infectious mononucleosis,[59] and named accordingly—*sennetsu* being the Japanese name for glandular fever. Similar cases have been reported in Japan, Malaysia and the Philippines. No insect vector has yet been implicated in its transmission. Tetracyclines are successful in treatment.

E. canis has been known since 1935 to be the cause of tropical canine pancytopenia, transmitted by *Rhipicephalus sanguineus*, the brown dog tick. Dogs suffer an acute illness with fever, lymphadenopathy and thrombocytopenia, which passes into a chronic phase with bone marrow hypoplasia—which may prove fatal.[60] This disease is known to occur in the USA and South-East Asia, and probably exists worldwide.

Human infection with *E. canis*, transmitted by dog and deer ticks, was not reported until 1986 in the USA,[61] where cases were described of a febrile illness following a tick bite similar to RMSF. Intraleucocytic organisms were detected, and antibodies against *E. canis* found at high titre. Features of the illness included a macular rash, encephalopathy, renal insufficiency, joint pains and thrombocytopenia. The response to treatment with chloramphenicol, doxycycline and corticosteroids, with haemodialysis, was satisfactory. A few patients with acquired immune deficiency syndrome (AIDS) have also been reported as having *E. canis* infection.

The human infection has since been separately characterized as caused by *E. chaffeensis*.[62,63]

In Hong Kong an illness very similar to scrub typhus, but with negative specific serological tests for *O. tsutsugamushi*, has been described and named 'Lion Rock fever' after a geographical feature overlooking the area where cases have been reported.[64] It is possible that this is also a form of ehrlichiosis, although an unknown rickettsia could be responsible. These illnesses respond dramatically to doxycycline.

A closely related organism, *E. ewingii*, previously known only in dogs, has recently been shown to cause fever in immunocompromised patients in the USA.[65]

REFERENCES

1 Cardano G. *De malo recentiorum medicorum medendi usu libellus.* Venetiis, apud O. Scotum, 1536.

2 Fracastoro G. *De sympathia et antipathia rerum liber unus. De contagione et contagiosis morbis et curatione.* Venetiis, apud heredes L. Iuntae, 1546.

3 Coyttarus J. *De febre purpura epidemiali et contagiosa libri duo.* Parisiis, apud M. Juevenem, 1578.

4 Cober T. *Observationum medicorum Castrensium Hungaricarum Helmstadii.* F. Linderwald, 1685.

5 Pringle J. *Observations on the Nature and Cure of Hospital and Jayl-Fevers.* London: Millar & Wilson, 1750.

6 von Hildenbrand J V. *Ueber den Ansteckenden Typhus.* Wein, 1810.

7 Nicolle C J H. Recherches experimentales sur le typhus exanthematique. *Ann Inst Pasteur* 1910; 24:243–275; 1911; 25:97–144; 1912; 26:250–280, 332–350.

8 da Rocha-Lima H. Zür Aetiologie des Fleckfiebers. *Berl Klin Wochenschr* 1916; 53:567–569.

9 Bravo F. *Opera Medicinalia.* Mexico: Ocharte, 1570, 1–90.

10 Maxcy K F. Clinical observations on endemic typhus in southern United States. *Public Health Rep* 1926; 41:1213–1220, 2967–2995.

11 Mooser H. Experiments relating to the pathology and etiology of Mexican typhus (tabardillo). *J Infect Dis* 1928; 43:241–272.

12 Maxey E E. Some observations on the so-called spotted fever of Idaho. *Med Sentinel* (Portland, OR) 1899; 7:433–438.

13 Ricketts H T. The transmission of Rocky Mountain spotted fever by the bite of the wood tick (*Dermacentor occidentalis*). *JAMA* 1906; 47:358.

14 Conor A L J & Bruch A. Un fièvre éruptive. *Bull Soc Pathol Exot* 1910; 3:45–96.

15 Baelz E & Kawakami K. Das japanische Fluss-oder-Ueberschwemmungs-fieber, eine acute Infections-Krankheit.

Virchows Arch [Pathol Anat] 1879; 78:373–420, 528–530.

16 Fletcher W & Lesslar J E. *Tropical Typhus in the Federated Malay States, with a Compilation on Epidemic Typhus.* London: John Bale, 1925.

17 Ogata N. Aetiologie der Tsutsugamushi-Krankheit; Rickettsia tsutsugamushi. *Zentralbl Bakteriol* (Abt Orig) 1931; 122:249–253.

18 Graham J H P. A note on a relapsing febrile illness of unknown origin. Lancet 1915; ii:703–704.

19 Hunt G H & Rankin A C. Intermittent fever of obscure origin occurring among British soldiers in France. Lancet 1915; ii:1133–1136.

20 His W. Ueber eine neue periodische fieberkrankung (Febris Wolhynica). *Berl Klin Wochenschr* 1916; 53:322–323.

21 Töpfer H W. Zür Ursache und Uebertragung des Wolhynischen fiebers. *Munch Med Wochenschr* 1916; 63:1495–1496.

22 Sussman L N. Kew Gardens spotted fever. *N Y Med* 1946; 2(15):27–28.

23 Derrick E H. Q fever, a new fever entity; clinical features and laboratory investigations. *Med J Aust* 1937; 2:281–299.

24 Cox H R & Bell E J. Epidemic and endemic typhus. Protective value for guinea-pigs of vaccines prepared from infected tissues of the developing chick embryo. *Public Health Rep* 1940; 55:110–115.

25 Fulton F & Joyner L. Cultivation of *Rickettsia tsutsugamushi* in lungs of rodents. Preparation of a scrub typhus vaccine. Lancet 1945; ii:729–734.

26 Smadel, J E, Woodward T E, Ley H L et al. Chloramphenicol (chloromycetin) in the treatment of tsutsugamushi disease (scrub typhus). *J Clin Invest* 1949; 28:1196–1215.

27 Weil E & Felix A. Zür seroligischen Diagnose des Fleckfiebers. *Wein Klin Wochenschr* 1916; 29:33–35.

28 Fletcher W & Lesslar J E. *The Weil–Felix Reaction in Sporadic Tropical Typhus.* London: John Bale, 1926.

29 Wohlbach S B. *The Aetiology and Pathology of Typhus.* Cambridge, MA; Harvard University Press, 1922.

30 Anderson S G E, Zomorodipour A, Anderson J O et al. The genome sequence of *Rickettsia prowazekii* and the origin of mitochondria. Nature 1998; 396:133–140.

31 Raoult D, Ndihokubwayo J B, Tissot-Dupont H et al. Outbreak of epidemic typhus associated with trench fever in Burundi. Lancet 1998; 348:86–89.

32 Ndihokubwayo J B & Raoult D. Epidemic typhus in Africa—a review. *Med Trop (Mars)* 1999; 59(2):181–192.

33 Brill N E. An acute infectious disease of unknown origin. A clinical study based on 221 cases. *Am J Med Sci* 1910; 139:484–502.

34 Zinsser H. Varieties of typhus vaccine and the epidemiology of the American form of European typhus fever (Brill's disease). *Am J Hyg* 1934; 20:513–532.

35 Carl M, Tibbs C W, Dobson M E et al. Diagnosis of acute typhus infection using the polymerase chain reaction. *J Infect Dis* 1990; 161:791–793.

36 Huys J, Freyens P, Kahiyigi J & Van den Berghe G. Treatment of epidemic typhus. *Trans R Soc Trop Med Hyg* 1973; 67:718–721.

37 O'Connor L F, Kelly H A, Lubich J M et al. A cluster of murine typhus cases in Western Australia. *Med J Aust* 1996; 165(1):24–26.

38 Bernaben-Wittel M, Pachon J, Alarcon A et al. Flea-borne typhus in Spain. *Arch Intern Med* 1999; 170(2):872–876.

39 Duffy P E, Le Guillozic H, Gass R F & Innis B L. Murine typhus identified as a major cause of febrile illness in a camp for displaced Khmers in Thailand. *Am J Trop Med Hyg* 1990; 43:520–526.

40 Rauolt D, Weiller P J, Chagnon A et al. Mediterranean spotted fever: clinical, laboratory and epidemiological features of 199 cases. *Am J Trop Med Hyg* 1986; 35:845–850.

41 Kelly P J, Mason H R, Matthewman L A & Rauolt D. Sero-epidemiology of spotted fever group rickettsial infections in humans in Zimbabwe. *J Trop Med Hyg* 1991; 94:304–309.

42 Kelly P J, Beati L, Matthewman L A et al. A new pathogenic spotted fever group rickettsia from Africa. *J Trop Med Hyg* 1994; 97:129–137.

43 Uchida T, Yu X, Uchiyama T & Walker D M. Identification of a unique spotted fever group rickettsia from humans in Japan. *J Infect Dis* 1989; 159:1122–1125.

44 Stenos J, Roux V, Walker D & Rauolt D. *Rickettsia honei* sp. nov.—the agent of Flinders Island spotted fever. *Int J Syst Microbiol* 1998; 48:1399–1404.

45 Tamura A, Ohashi N, Urakami H et al. Classification of *Rickettsia tsutsugamushi* in a new genus *Orientia* gen. nov. as *Orientia tsutsugamushi* comb. nov. *Int J Syst Microbiol* 1995; 45:589–591.

46 Tange Y, Kanemitsu N & Kobayashi Y. Analysis of immunological characteristics of newly isolated strains of *Rickettsia tsutsugamushi* using monoclonal antibodies. *Am J Trop Med Hyg* 1991; 44:371–381.

47 McBride W J, Taylor C T, Pryor J A & Simpson J D. Scrub typhus in Northern Queensland still occurs. *Med J Aust* 1999; 170(7):318–320.

48 Tay S T, Ho T M, Rohani M Y & Devi S. Antibodies to *Orientiae tsutsugamushi*, *Rickettsia typhi* and spotted fever group rickettsiae among febrile patients in rural areas of Malaysia. *Trans R Soc Trop Med Hyg* 2000; 94:280–284.

49 Sayers M H P & Hill I G W. The occurrence and identification of the typhus group of fevers in South East Asia Command. *J R Army Med Corps* 1948; 90:6–22.

50 Tsay R W & Chang F Y. Serious complications in scrub typhus. *J Microbiol Immunol Infect* 1998; 31(4):240–244.

51 Brown G W, Shirai A, Jegathesan M et al. Febrile illness in Malaysia—an analysis of 1629 hospitalised patients. *Am J Trop Med Hyg* 1984; 33:311–315.

52 Chayakul P, Panich V & Silpapojakul K. Scrub typhus pneumonitis: an entity which is frequently missed. *Q J Med* 1988; 68:595–602.

53 Watt G, Kantipong P, de Souza M et al. HIV-1 suppression during acute scrub typhus infection. Lancet 2000; 356:475–479.

54 Song J-H, Lee C, Chang W H et al. Short course doxycycline treatment versus conventional tetracycline therapy for scrub typhus; a multicenter randomized trial. *Clin Infect Dis* 1995; 21:506–510.

55 Watt G, Chouriyagune C, Ruangweerayand R et al. Scrub typhus infections poorly responsive to antibiotics in northern Thailand. Lancet 1996; 348:86–89.

56 Relman D A, Loutit J S, Schmidt T M et al. The agent of bacillary angiomatosis. *N Engl J Med* 1990; 323:1573–1580.

57 Whittick J W. Necropsy findings in a case of Q fever in Britain. *BMJ* 1950; i:979–980.

58 Turck W P G, Howitt G, Turnberg L A et al. Chronic Q fever. *Q J Med* 1976; 45:193–217.

59 Misao T & Kobayashi Y. Studies on infectious mononucleosis (glandular fever). I. Isolation of etiologic agent from blood, bone marrow and lymph nodes from a patient with infectious mononucleosis by using mice. *Kyushu J Med Sci* 1955; 6:146–152.

60 Huxsoll D L, Bildebrandt P K, Nims R M & Walker J S. Tropical canine pancytopenia. *J Am Vet Med Assoc* 1970; 157:1627–1632.

61 Maeda K, Markowitz N, Hawley R C et al. Human infection with *Ehrlichia canis*, a leukocytic rickettsia. *N Engl J Med* 1987; 316:853–856.

62 Taylor J P, Betz T G, fishbein D B et al. Serological evidence of possible human infection with *Ehrlichia* in Texas. *J Infect Dis* 1988; 158:217–220.

63 Dawson J E, Anderson B, fishbein D B et al. Isolation and characterization of an *Ehrlichia* sp. from a patient diagnosed with human ehrlichiosis. *J Clin Microbiol* 1991; 29:2741–2745.

64 Cohen M A H, Li P K T, Cheng A F B et al. A fatal case of rickettsial spotted fever in Hong Kong—Lion Rock Fever. *J H K Med Assoc* 1989; 41:185–186.

65 Buller R S, Arens M, Hmiel S P et al. *Ehrlichia ewingii*, a newly recognised agent of human ehrlichiosis. *N Engl J Med* 1999; 341:148–155.

Section 8

Bacterial Infections

The emergence of successive generations of antibiotics and of anti-mycobacterial drugs during the last few decades has engendered much false optimism regarding control of bacterial disease in tropical and subtropical countries. However, the present situation remains a problem of enormous significance; in fact, in 2002 this disease probably accounts for, on a global basis, a greater degree of morbidity and mortality than any other single bacterial infection, despite the fact that streptomycin was first introduced into clinical medicine in 1944 and cheap, effective combination chemotherapy has been available since the 1960s! A further problem of vast magnitude has resulted from the fact that *Mycobacterium* spp. infections are of major significance as opportunistic infections in the context of the human immunodeficiency virus (HIV) and the acquired immune deficiency syndrome—a problem that will inevitably continue to escalate during the years ahead. A new chapter on pneumococcal infections has been introduced, since the responsible pathogen is of major importance in HIV-infected patients, especially in Africa. Resistance to antituberculous agents (MDRTB) and antibiotics (e.g., MRSA, VRE, penicillin-resistant pneumococci) is now also of major importance.

Intestinal infections are rapidly becoming exceedingly difficult to treat: bacterial resistance has, for example, become a major problem in *Salmonella* spp. and *Shigella* spp. infections. Numerically, the archetypal small-intestinal infection *Vibrio cholerae* has, far from being brought under control, expanded its boundaries to much of southern America and also Africa. A further problem of great topicality is that the non-O1 variant (to which classical *V. cholerae* renders no immunological protection) is becoming commonplace in southern Asia.

Of the more exotic infections, plague is again proving a major problem in many developing countries; this 'historical' disease has been responsible for many of the pestilences of the past and has exerted a major influence on human civilization, probably for many millennia.

Many of these infections described in this section are especially lethal in those under 5 years old. This applies especially to intestinal infections—in which a vicious cycle with malnutrition results in failure to thrive and a great deal of mortality. Although in many cases appropriate antibacterial agents are available, the cost to the health budgets of developing countries is frequently insuperably high, putting them quite out of reach. Thus, to most of the world's populations, such agents might just as well not exist!

Overall, therefore, although the antibiotic era has led to a sharp decline in bacterial infections in the developed world, this certainly does not apply to those vast areas of the globe situated in the tropics and subtropics. Many of these infections are reviewed in this section.

Chapter 51
Introduction to Acute Infective Diarrhoea

C. A. Hart

Diarrhoeal disease is a major cause of morbidity and mortality worldwide. In a global estimate of causes of death in 1990, diarrhoeal disease was the fourth commonest after ischaemic heart disease (6.25 million deaths), cardiovascular disease (4.4 million) and respiratory tract infections (4.3 million).[1] It was responsible for approximately 3 million of the total 50.5 million deaths.

Although the burden of diarrhoeal disease is greatest in children under 5 years, and especially in developing countries, there are approximately 2 million deaths per annum worldwide;[2] adults and especially the elderly are also at risk. In general, viral enteropathogens are more important in childhood gastroenteritis in developed and developing countries alike, whereas bacterial and protozoal enteropathogens predominate in adults.[3]

In developing countries estimates of the annual incidence of diarrhoea in children vary from 3.3 episodes,[4] to 7.9 episodes,[5] to 10 episodes per year in urban Lima, Peru.[6] In contrast the incidence is much lower in children in developed countries; for example, children in Winnipeg, Canada, were reported to experience 0.8 diarrhoeal episodes per year,[7] and the overall incidence for all ages in Holland was 0.8 per annum.[8] The contrast between paediatric diarrhoea in developed and developing countries is shown in Table 51.1. The relative importance of the various viruses, bacteria and protozoa in developing and developed countries is shown in Table 51.2. However, it must be remembered that the relative importance of the various enteropathogens will depend on a variety of factors including the pathogens sought and the sensitivity and

Table 51.1 Paediatric diarrhoea in developed and developing countries (after Kumate and Isibasi[9]).

Feature	Developed countries	Developing countries
Episodes per annum	< 1	3–10
Seasonality	Winter	None
Severe dehydration	Rare	Frequent
Nutritional sequelae	Rare	Usual
Measles associated	Non-existent	15–63%
Epidemic	Rare	Frequent
Polymicrobial	Unusual	> 20%
Case fatality rate	< 0.01%	0.6%

Table 51.2 Relative importance of enteropathogens in childhood diarrhoeal disease.

	Mexico[10]	Multicentre[11]	China[12]	Philippines[13]	Malawi[14]	Canada[15]	Chile[16]	Australia[17]
No. of subjects	271	3640	186	236	168	206	90	4637
Duration of survey	4.5 months	24 months	22 months	25 months	2 months	24 months	12 months	13 years
Setting	Community	Outpatient	Inpatient	Inpatient	Outpatient	Inpatient	Outpatient	Inpatient
Percentage positive								
Rotavirus	3.7	16	56	65	42	3.9	1.1	39.6
Astrovirus	61	NT	8.5	0.4	1.2		5.6	NT
Adenovirus 40/41	12.9	4	2.5	0.4	4.2	3.9	1.1	6
Caliciviruses[a]	NT	3	7.6	0.4	1.2		NT	NT
Toroviruses	NT	NT	NT	0	0	3.5	NT	NT
Total viruses	77.6	23	74.6	66.2	48.6	42.8	7.8	45.6
Total bacteria	20.3	51	NT	23.4	NT	NT	32.2	9.2
Total protozoa	NT	3.3	NT	2.1	4.2	NT	3.3	NT
Mixed infection	7.4[b]	0	0	7[b]	0	NT	30[b]	0
No pathogen detected	NA	22.7	25.4	1.2	NA	NA	42	43.5

NT, not tested; NA, not applicable.
[a]Includes classical calicivirus and Norwalk-like viruses.
[b]Predominantly viruses.

specificity of the diagnostic tools used, the age group studied, the duration and season of study, geographical location and whether the survey is hospital or community based. For example, improved diagnostic methods have increased the detection rates of astrovirus and caliciviruses, and in community-based studies astrovirus, which causes a milder diarrhoea, assumes greater importance than rotavirus,[10] whereas the converse is found in hospital-based studies. In addition to the morbidity and mortality associated with diarrhoeal disease, it is also a major drain on health resources in developing countries. For example, in Indonesia it was estimated that US $2.50 was spent per annum per child on diarrhoeal disease, against a yearly per capita health budget of US $5.41, at 1990 costs.

There are over 40 different enteropathogens able to cause gastroenteritis and even in the best-funded laboratories not all are sought. To arrive at an aetiological diagnosis in all cases is neither possible nor necessary, except for epidemiological purposes, for example when a vaccine has been introduced or when large epidemics occur. However, it is possible to subdivide diarrhoeal disease into two major categories, inflammatory and non-inflammatory. There are, of course, areas of overlap but this classification does provide a framework for discussing diarrhoeal disease (Table 51.3). In addition to the enteropathogens listed in Table 51.4, there are those that produce vomiting with no or very little diarrhoea. This usually results from ingestion of emetic toxins liberated by certain strains of *Staphylococcus aureus* or *Bacillus cereus*.

Non-inflammatory diarrhoea

The pathogens causing non-inflammatory diarrhoea are

Table 51.3 Cinical features of inflammatory and non-inflammatory diarrhoea.

	Non-inflammatory	Inflammatory
Symptoms	Nausea, vomiting; abdominal pain and fever not major features	Abdominal pain, tenesmus, fever
Stool	Voluminous, watery	Frequent, small volume; blood-stained, pus cells present, mucus
Site	Proximal small intestine	Distal ileum, colon
Mechanism	Osmotic or secretory	Invasion of enterocytes leading to mucosal cell death and inflammatory response

shown in Table 51.4. For the majority of these, their principal site of action is the upper small intestine. As the transit time is so rapid through the small intestine, an important pathogenic factor is the ability to adhere to the small intestinal mucosa. The mechanisms most commonly employed in producing diarrhoea are osmotic and secretory. In the former there is an inability to degrade, for example, disaccharides to monosaccharides. Because only monosaccharides can be absorbed by enterocytes, the disaccharides pass down the intestine taking water

Table 51.4 Pathogens in inflammatory and non-inflammatory diarrhoea.

	Inflammatory	Non-inflammatory
Viruses (see Chapter 46)	Nil	Rotavirus Adenovirus 40/41 Astrovirus Norwalk agent Calicivirus Small round structureless virus Coronavirus Torovirus Bredavirus Picobirnavirus
Bacteria (see Chapter 52)	Enteroinvasive *E. coli* (EIEC) Entero haemorrhagic *E. coli* (EHEC) (e.g. O157) Enteroaggregative *E. coli* (EAggEC) *Aeromonas hydrophila* *Campylobacter* spp. *Salmonella* spp. *Shigella* spp. *Yersinia enterocolitica* *Clostridium difficile*	Enterotoxigenic *E. coli* (ETEC) Enteropathogenic *E. coli* (EPEC) *Vibrio cholerae* *Vibrio parahaemolyticus* *Campylobacter* spp. *Salmonella* spp. *Plesiomonas shigelliodes* *Bacillus cereus* *Clostridium perfringens*
Protozoa (see Chapter 77)	*Entamoeba histolytica* *Balantidium coli*	*Cryptosporidium parvum* *Giardia intestinalis (lamblia)* *Cyclospora cayetanensis* *Blastocystis hominis* *Isospora belli* *Enterocytozoon bieneusi* (microsporidia)

with them. In secretory diarrhoea the enterocyte is stimulated to secrete fluid into the gut lumen.

Inflammatory diarrhoea

Although there is some overlap (e.g., *Salmonella* spp. and *Campylobacter* spp. can cause non-inflammatory diarrhoea), the pathogens causing inflammatory diarrhoea form a distinct group (Table 51.4). Their site of action is usually the distal ileum and colon, and they produce disease by destroying parts of the enteric mucous membranes, leading to an inflammatory response. This in turn leads to the excretion of neutrophils and erythrocytes in faeces, which can be detected by simple wet film microscopy or myeloperoxidase by enzyme-linked immunosorbent assay (ELISA).

Epidemiological aspects

The prevalence of different enteropathogens varies with the age of the individual, how the diarrhoea is acquired (e.g., food poisoning or traveller's diarrhoea), between acute and chronic diarrhoea, and with the state of the host's immunity (see Table 51.2).

Age

In general, paediatric diarrhoea is most often due to viral enteropathogens (see Chapter 46). Up to 60% of cases in most hospital-based surveys are due to viruses, with rotavirus accounting for a large proportion of cases, followed by adenovirus 40/41 and then astrovirus. Bacterial enteropathogens such as enteropathogenic *Escherichia coli* (EPEC), enteroinvasive *E. coli* (EIEC), enterotoxigenic *E.coli* (ETEC), enteroaggregative *E. coli* (EAggEC), salmonellae, *Campylobacter jejuni* and shigellae, and the protozoan *Cryptosporidium parvum* are responsible for the majority of the remaining cases where a pathogen is found.

In adults, bacteria assume greater importance, although viral gastroenteritis does occur, for example as a result of unusual serogroups of rotavirus or astrovirus.[18,19] For example, it is estimated that *C. jejuni* is responsible for 17–20% of episodes of adult diarrhoea.

Environmental factors

In temperate countries viruses, except for calicivirus, produce peaks of disease in the cold dry weather of winter,[20] whereas in tropical Africa the seasonality is blurred but with a upsurge in cases in the dry season.[21] In contrast, bacterial and protozoal diarrhoeas tend to occur in the wetter seasons in the tropics and summer in temperate countries. In temperate countries cryptosporidiosis peaks in spring with an lesser peak in autumn, but, for example, in Gaza most cases occur in the hottest and driest parts of the year, perhaps when water availability and quality may be compromised.[22] On a more global scale during the 1997–1998 El Niño, when mean ambient temperatures are 5°C higher than normal in Peru, the number of daily hospital admissions with gastroenteritis is doubled.[23]

Food poisoning

Diarrhoeal disease following ingestion of food or water contaminated by bacteria, toxins or protozoa is still an important problem in both developed and developing countries. Although high-intensity animal rearing is important in the maintenance of human enteropathogens in developed countries, in developing countries human-derived enteric pathogens such as *Salmonella* spp. and *C. jejuni* and enterohaemorrhagic *E. coli* (EHEC) may still be implicated in outbreaks of food poisoning. Recently, water-borne outbreaks of *C. parvum* have been assuming greater importance.

Traveller's diarrhoea (turista, Aztec two-step, Montezuma's revenge, Delhi belly, etc.)

It is estimated that every year approximately 16 million people will travel from their domicile in industrialized countries to less developed countries. Approximately one-third of these will develop diarrhoeal disease and in the majority of cases this will be due to an infective agent.[24] A large number of different enteropathogens has been implicated, but in most surveys ETEC is the predominant pathogen (Table 51.5), followed by *C. jejuni* and *Shigella* and *Salmonella* spp. The aetiological agents vary considerably according to the country visited; for example, *C. parvum* has recently been shown to be important in visitors to the Caribbean[25] and Africa.[26] Viral enteropathogens can cause traveller's diarrhoea but have, for example, been more frequently associated with

Table 51.5 Enteropathogens in traveller's diarrhoea.

Pathogen	Prevalence (%)
Enterotoxigenic *E. coli*	30–80
Campylobacter jejuni	*c.* 20
Shigella spp.	5–15
Salmonella spp.	3–15
Giardia lamblia	0–3
Cryptosporidium parvum	?
Entamoeba histolytica	0–3
Rotavirus	10
Astrovirus	1
Norwalk agent	1
Unknown	10–15

shipboard epidemics in which astrovirus and calicivirus have been implicated.

Immunocompromised host

In tropical countries the immune compromise due to malnutrition and human immunodeficiency virus (HIV) are of major importance; both affect the frequency and severity of diarrhoeal disease. With the appearance of acquired immune deficiency syndrome (AIDS), diarrhoeal disease due to previously unrecognized pathogens, such as *C. parvum*, *Isospora belli*, *Enterocytozoon bieneusi* and *Mycobacterium avium intracellulare*, has assumed increasing importance, albeit more often causing chronic diarrhoea.[27] Interestingly there is little information on the role of rotavirus—the major cause of infantile gastroenteritis—in HIV-infected children.

Management of acute diarrhoea

The mainstay of management of diarrhoeal disease is the assessment of dehydration (Figure 51.1) and the appropriate replacement of fluid and electrolytes.[28] Although diarrhoeal disease can produce dehydration at any age, its impact is greatest in those under 5 years of age. This is because, as a result of their relatively greater surface area

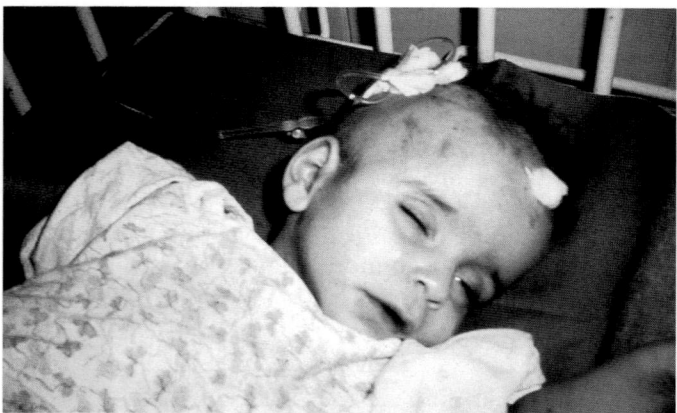

Figure 51.1: A child with severe dehydration being rehydrated intravenously.

and thus greater fluid loss through skin, infants require 2.5 times more water per kilogram of body weight than older individuals. Fluid and electrolyte loss is also greatly exacerbated by vomiting. Both the initial degree of dehydration and the response to rehydration therapy should be monitored clinically (Table 51.6).

Originally, rehydration was exclusively intravenous. This resulted in a tremendous drop in fatality rates, for example from 40% to less than 1% when properly administered in patients with cholera. A major advance was made when an effective oral rehydration regimen was devised.

Oral rehydration therapy

Early oral rehydration solutions (ORSs) contained only electrolytes and water, and it was not until it was realized that glucose or sucrose was required to enhance sodium absorption that effective oral rehydration therapy became available. Glucose and sodium transport into enterocytes is coupled. Sucrose, a dimer of glucose and fructose, must be cleaved by brush border sucrase for it to be absorbed. Nevertheless, glucose and sucrose seem to be equally effective in ORSs,[29] although there may be minor advantages with glucose.[30]

There is also some debate over the use of bicarbonate or citrate to correct acidosis. Both are equally effective but citrate is more stable, and has replaced bicarbonate in World Health Organization solutions. A further modification has been the incorporation of glycine, which is taken into the enterocyte by a specific amino acid transport system. Glycine, when present in ORS at a concentration of 111 mmol/l, was found to decrease both duration of diarrhoea and stool volume.[31] The composition of various ORSs is shown in Table 51.7. ORS can be obtained in packets from UNICEF or can be made up locally. The solution should contain sodium chloride (3.5 g), potassium chloride (1.5 g), glucose monohydrate (22 g) made up to 1 litre with potable water (sucrose (40 g) may replace glucose, and trisodium citrate dehydrate (2.9 g) may replace sodium bicarbonate). To be fully effective, ORSs should be available at the village level so that therapy can be initiated as rapidly as possible. This will require the solution(s) to be available, either prepacked or in bulk, with appropriate measuring spoons, a method of providing the correct volume of potable water and instructions on use, including the need to discard unused

Table 51.6 Clinical assessment of rehydration.

Severity	Body weight loss (%)	Clinical state	Signs
Mild	< 5	Not unwell	Thirsty, mucous membranes dry
Moderate	5–10	Apathetic	Sunken eyes, sunken fontanelle, tachypnoea, oliguria, loss of skin turgor
Severe	10–15	Shocked	Hypotensive, peripheral circulatory failure
Critical	> 15	Moribund	Severely shocked, comastose

Table 51.7 Composition of oral rehydration solutions.

Component	Concentration (mmol/l water)		
	Citrate ORS	bicarbonate ORS	Glycine ORS[a]
Sodium	90	90	90
Potassium	20	20	20
Chloride	80	80	80
Citrate	10	–	–
Bicarbonate	–	30	30
Glucose	111	111	111
Glycine	–	–	111

[a]May contain either bicarbonate or citrate.

solution within 24 hours. Studies have shown that, when properly instructed, 98% of mothers can prepare ORS with a sodium range of 30–110 mmol/l.[32]

Recently, rice powder-based ORSs have been investigated, because these are more readily available. Rice powder at 30–50 g/l is an effective substitute for glucose. It tastes better than simple electrolyte–glucose ORS and is thus more acceptable to children. A recent meta-analysis of 13 randomized trials of rice-based versus glucose-based oral rehydration therapy demonstrated the superiority of the rice-based solution in cholera diarrhoea, although the benefit was considerably less for children with acute non-cholera diarrhoea.[33] During the initial phase of oral rehydration therapy, while the patient is dehydrated, adults can consume 750 ml/h and children up to 300 ml/h. Maintenance therapy of 20 ml solution per kg body weight should be started as soon as signs of dehydration have gone. ORSs are suitable for rehydration of all except severely dehydrated infants and those with shock (Table 51.8).

Intravenous rehydration

Approximately 98% of children will respond to oral rehydration therapy. The remainder are generally infants with severe dehydration or those with profuse vomiting or a high purging rate. These will require rehydration by the intravenous route. Suitable solutions include: Ringer's lactate (Hartman's), consisting of NaCl 6.2 g, KCl 0.4 g, sodium lactate 2.3 g and 2 ml 50% glucose in 1 litre of solution; Dhaka solution (NaCl 5 g, NaHCO$_3$ 4 g, KCl 1 g

and 50% glucose per litre); or acetate solution (NaCl 5 g, KCl 1 g, sodium acetate 6.5 g and 2 ml 50% glucose per litre of solution). Oral rehydration therapy should be started as soon as possible following institution of intravenous rehydration, but if signs of severe dehydration persist it may be necessary to continue using Ringer's lactate at 100 ml per kg body weight per 4 hours.

Adjunctive therapy

Other potential therapeutic interventions include antimicrobial agents, antimotility drugs and antisecretory drugs. These have varying degrees of efficacy and some are absolutely contraindicated for certain conditions.

Antimicrobial drugs

In general, infants with acute watery diarrhoea are best managed without recourse to antibiotics. However, if there is evidence of systemic spread, cholera or dysentery, then antimicrobials will shorten the course of diarrhoea and ameliorate its effects. With the advent of the fluoroquinolones such as ciprofloxacin and ofloxacin, the debate on the use of antimicrobials has been reopened. First, there is no doubt that the widespread indiscriminate use of antimicrobials, often in subtherapeutic regimens, encourages resistance in both pathogens and normal enteric flora.[34] On the other hand, even with ETEC early treatment with co-trimoxazole[35] or ciprofloxacin can decrease the severity of diarrhoea. This is preferred to the widespread prophylactic use of these antimicrobials—which will certainly produce resistant bacteria.

In cholera, tetracycline or ciprofloxacin decreases the duration of diarrhoea and shedding of bacteria. In countries where dysentery caused by *Shigella* spp. is endemic or when epidemics occur, antimicrobials are of benefit but development of resistance during the course of epidemics occurs with monotonous regularity.[34] Metronidazole (or tinidazole) is valuable in the treatment of giardiasis or amoebic dysentery.

Antimotility drugs

These should be avoided.

Antisecretory drugs

These will, of course, be effective only if there is a secretory component to the diarrhoea. The value of loperamide as

Table 51.8 Guidelines for rehydration.

Degree	Age group	Type of fluid	Volume (ml/kg body weight	Timing
Mild	All	ORS	50	Every 4 hours
Moderate	All	ORS	100	Every 4 hours
Severe	Infants	i.v. (Hartman's)	70	Every 4 hours
Severe and shock	All	i.v. (Hartman's)	70–100	Every 4 hours

an adjunct in treating diarrhoea in well nourished children has been demonstrated,[36] but these authors warned against its use in malnourished children.

Compounds such as kaolin or charcoal which, it is postulated, act by absorbing toxins have had little effect in controlled trials.

Nutritional supplements

Micronutrient deficencies have been associated with increased incidence, severity and duration of diarrhoeal and other diseases. Micronutrient supplementation trials have yielded varying results. For example, a trial of vitamin A supplementation in Haiti demonstrated an increased 2-week prevalence of diarrhoea following supplementation,[37] whereas a trial of zinc supplementation in India demonstrated an clinically important decrease in the severity and duration of diarrhoea.[38]

There is increasing interest in the value of administering commensal bacteria (probiotics) to ameliorate diarrhoeal disease.[39] In trials in Pakistan and Thailand, the administration of one such probiotic, *Lactobacillus casei* GG, was shown to result in a decrease in the duration of diarrhoea and a reduction in stool frequency in patients with acute watery diarrhoea.[40,41]

Control of diarrhoeal disease

In industrialized countries it has been the separation of human and animal excreta from potable water and foodstuffs that has contributed to the great decline in the incidence of diarrhoeal disease. In addition, improvement in facilities for personal hygiene within the home have decreased the intrafamilial spread of enteropathogens. To implement these measures in developing countries, a massive input from industrialized countries will be needed. Other simpler and more locally applicable measures to prevent diarrhoeal disease include the development of

technologies and practices that interrupt disease transmission by muscid flies.[42,43] Recently it was shown that exposure of drinking water (in plastic bottles) to tropical sunlight decreased diarrhoeal disease in Maasai children in Kenya.[44]

There is little doubt that measles and malnutrition increase the morbidity and mortality associated with diarrhoeal disease, and control of measles by immunization should be possible. Finally, it is unlikely that spread of some enteric pathogens, such as the rotavirus, may be prevented completely by public health and good hygiene. A safe and effective vaccine would be of major benefit.

Conclusion

Diarrhoeal disease is still a major cause of death, even though it has been shown that the introduction of oral rehydration therapy can decrease the mortality rate to less than 0.5% in defined study areas.

Morbidity

Malnutrition greatly affects immunity[45,46] and the incidence and severity of diarrhoeal disease. Similarly, diarrhoeal disease will greatly exacerbate malnutrition, thus creating an inexorable downward spiral. Acute diarrhoeal disease may become chronic, and chronic diarrhoea, for example that due to *C. parvum*, can become greatly prolonged.[47] Disaccharide (principally lactose) intolerance following certain types of diarrhoea has been a source of great controversy. Certain pathogens, such as rotavirus or EPEC, produce a great decrease in disaccharidase levels in the small intestine. Some consider that infants should not be given their normal diet because of the problem of disaccharide intolerance. Most evidence now suggests that infants should return to their normal diet within 24 hours of the onset of diarrhoea unless there are specific contraindications.[48]

REFERENCES

1   Murray C J L & Lopez A D. Mortality by cause for eight regions of the world: global burden of disease study. *Lancet* 1997; 349:1269–1276.

2   Bern C, Martines J, de Zoysa I & Glass R I. The magnitude of the global problem of diarrheoal disease: a ten year update. *Bull WHO* 1992; 70:705–714.

3   Hart C A & Cunliffe N A. Diagnosis and causes of viral gastroenteritis. *Curr Opin Infect Dis* 1996; 9:333–339.

4   WHO/CDD/VID/84.4 *Diarrhoeal Disease Control Programme. Report of the Third Meeting of the Scientific Working Group on Viral Diarrhoeas. Microbiology, Epidemiology, Immunology and Vaccine Development.* Geneva: WHO, 1984:8–14.

5   Mata L, Simhon A, Urrutia J, Kronmal R, Fernandez R & Craraia B. Epidemiology of rotavirus in cohort of 45 Guatemalan Mayan Indian children from birth to age 3 year. *J Infect Dis* 1984; 148:452–461.

6   Black R C, Lopez de Romana G, Brown K H, Bravo N, Bazalar O G & Kanashiro H C. Incidence and etiology of infantile diarrhea and major routes of transmission in Huascar, Peru. *Am J Epidemiol* 1989; 129:785–799.

7   Gurwith M, Wenman W, Hinde D, Feltham S & Greenberg H. A prospective study of rotavirus infection in infants and young children. *J Infect Dis* 1981; 144:218–224.

8   de Wit M A S, Koopmans M P G, Kortbeek L A et al. Gastroenteritis in sentinal practices, The Netherlands. *Emerg Infect Dis* 2001; 7:82–91.

9   Kumate J & Isibasi A. Pediatric diarrheal diseases: a global perspective. *Pediatr Infect Dis J* 1986; S1:21–28.

10 Maldonaldo Y, Cantwell M, Old M et al. Population-based prevalence of symptomatic and asymptomatic astrovirus infection in rural Mayan infants. *J Infect Dis* 1998; 178:834–839.

11 Hulian S, Zhen L G, Mathan M M et al. Etiology of acute diarrhoea among children in developing countries: a multicentre study in five countries. *Bull WHO* 1992; 69:549–555.

12 Qiao H P, Nilsson M, Abreu E R et al. Viral diarrhea in children in Beijing, China. *J Med Virol* 1999; 5:390–396.

13 Pajé-Vilar E, Co B G, Caradang E H et al. Non-bacterial diarrhoea in children in the Philippines. *Ann Trop Med Parasitol* 1994; 88:53–58.

14 Pavone R, Schinaia N, Hart C A et al. Viral gastroenteritis in children in Malawi. *Ann Trop Paediatr* 1990;10:15–20.

15 Jamieson F B, Wang E L, Bain C et al. Human torovirus: a new nosocomial gastrointestinal pathogen. *J Infect Dis* 1998; 178:1263–1269.

16 Gaggero A, O'Ryan M, Noel J S et al. Prevalence of astrovirus infection among Chilean children with acute gastroenteritis. *J Clin Microbiol* 1998; 36:3691–3693.

17 Barnes G L, Uren E, Stevens K B et al. Etiology of acute gastroenteritis in hospitalized children in Melbourne, Australia from April 1980 to March 1993. *J Clin Microbiol* 1998; 36:133–138.

18 Krishnan T, Sen A, Choudhury J S et al. Emergence of adult diarrhoea rotavirus in Calcutta, India. *Lancet* 1999, 353:380–381.

19 Glass R I, Noel J, Mitchell D et al. The changing epidemiology of astrovirus-associated gastroenteritis: a review. *Arch Virol* 1996; 12 (Supplement):287–300.

20 Hart C A & Cunliffe N A. Viral gastroenteritis. *Curr Opin Infect Dis* 1999; 12:447–457.

21 Cunliffe N A, Kilgore P E, Bresee J S et al. Epidemiology of rotavirus diarrhoea in Africa: a review to assess the need for rotavirus immunization. *Bull WHO* 1998; 76:525–537.

22 Sallon S, El Showaa R, El Masri M et al. Cryptosporidiosis in children in Gaza. *Ann Trop Paediatr* 1990; 11:277–281.

23 Checkley W, Epstein L D, Gilman R H et al. Effects of El Niño and ambient temperature on hospital admissions for diarrhoeal diseases in Peruvian children. *Lancet* 2000; 355:442–450.

24 Steffan R, van der Linde F, Gyre K et al. Epidemiology of diarrhea in travellers. *JAMA* 1983; 249:1176–1180.

25 Ma P, Kaufman D C, Helmick C G, D'Souza A J & Navin T R. *Cryptosporidium* in tourists returning from the Caribbean. *N Engl J Med* 1985; 312:647–648.

26 Soave R & Ma P. *Cryptosporidium*: traveller's diarrhea in two families. *Arch Intern Med* 1985; 145:70–72.

27 Smith P D. Gastrointestinal infections in AIDS. *Ann Intern Med* 1992; 116:63–77.

28 Cash R A. Oral rehydration therapy. In Farthing M J G & Keusch G T (eds) *Enteric Infection*. London: Chapman & Hall,1989:441–451.

29 Sack D A, Chowdhury A M A K, Eusof A et al. Oral rehydration in rotavirus diarrhoea: a double blind comparison of sucrose with glucose electrolyte solution. *Lancet* 1978; ii:280–283.

30 Nalin D R, Levine M M, Mata L et al. Comparison of sucrose with glucose in oral therapy of infant diarrhoea. *Lancet* 1978; ii:277–279.

31 Mahalanabis D & Patra F C. In seach of a super oral rehydration solution: can optimum use of organic solute medicated transport lead to the development of an absorption promoting drug? *J Diarrhoeal Dis Res* 1982; 2:76–81.

32 Bhatia S, Cash R A & Cornaz I. Evaluation of the oral therapy expansion program (OTEP) of the Bangladesh rural advancement committee (BRAC). *Swiss Development Cooperation and Humanitarian Aid* 1983: January 24–February 12.

33 Gore S M, Fontaine O & Pierce N F. Impact of rice based oral rehydration solution on stool output and duration of diarrhoea: meta-analysis of 13 clinical trials. *BMJ* 1992; 304:287–291.

34 Shears P. A review of bacterial resistance to antimicrobial agents in the tropics. *Ann Trop Paediatr* 1993; 13:219–226.

35 DuPont H R, Randall R R, Galindo E, Sullivan P S, Wood L V & Mendiola J G. Treatment of traveller's diarrhea with trimethoprim/sulfamethoxazole and with trimethoprim alone. *N Engl J Med* 1982; 307:841–844.

36 Diarrhoeal Diseases Study Group (UK). Loperamide in acute diarrhoea in childhood: results of a double blind placebo controlled multicentre clinical trial. *BMJ* 1984; 298:1263–1267.

37 Stansfield S K, Muller P-L, Lerebours G & Augustin A. Vitamin A supplementation and increased prevalence of childhood diarrhoea and acute respiratory infections. *Lancet* 1993; 342:578–582.

38 Sazawal S, Black R E, Bhan M K et al. Zinc supplementation in young children with acute diarrhea in India. *N Engl J Med* 1995; 333:839–844.

39 MacFarlane G T & Cummings J H. Probiotics and prebiotics: can regulating the activities of intestinal bacteria benefit health? *BMJ* 1999; 318:999–1003.

40 Raza S, Graham S M, Allen S J et al. *Lactobacillus* GG promotes recovery from acute non-bloody diarrhea in Pakistan. *Pediatr Infect Dis J* 1995; 14:107–111.

41 Pant A R, Graham S M, Allen S J et al. *Lactobacillus* GG and acute diarrhoea in young children in the tropics. *J Trop Pediatr* 1996; 42:162–165.

42 Chavasse D C, Shier R P, Murphy O A et al. Impact of fly control on childhood diarrhoea in Pakistan: community randomised trial. *Lancet* 1999; 353:22–25.

43 Emerson P M, Lindsay S W, Walraven G E L et al. Effect of the fly control on trachoma and diarrhoea. *Lancet* 1999; 353:1401–1403.

44 Conroy R M, Elmore-Meegan M, Joyce T et al. Solar disinfection of drinking water and diarrhoea in Maasai children: a controlled field trial. *Lancet* 1996; 348:1695–1696.

45 Chandra R K. Nutrition, immunity and infection: present knowledge and future directions. *Lancet* 1983; i:688–691.

46 Dowd P & Heatly R. The influence of undernutrition on immunity. *Clin Sci* 1984; 66:241–248.

47 Sallon S, Deckelbaum R J, Schmid II et al. *Cryptosporidium*, malnutrition and chronic diarrhea in children. *Am J Dis Child* 1988; 142:312–315.

48 Committee on Nutrition. Use of oral fluid therapy and posttreatment feeding following enteritis in children in a developed country. *Pediatrics* 1985; 75:358–361.

Chapter 52
Gastrointestinal Bacteria

C. A. Hart and P. Shears

The adult human comprises some 10^{14} cells but only 10% of these are mammalian. The remaining 9×10^{13} consists of the bacteria, fungi, protozoa and even multicellular parasites that make up normal flora. The gastrointestinal tract is the major reservoir for these flora. Although bacteria can be found in the stomach and small intestine, they are present in low numbers (10^2–10^4 colony forming units (c.f.u.) per ml) and are usually transient(s). In contrast, the lower ileum and colon contain large numbers of bacteria (approximately 10^{12} c.f.u./ml) and half the weight of faeces is made up of bacteria. To detect small numbers of pathogens in this mass of normal flora can therefore be problematic and has led to the formulation of selective media that work with varying degrees of success.

Helicobacter pylori

Since the beginning of the 20th century histopathologists have described spiral bacteria in the stomach. It was not until 1983 that a bacterium was grown, rather serendipitously.[1] This micro-organism was originally named *Campylobacter pyloridis,* renamed *C. pylori* for grammatical reasons, and was finally designated *Helicobacter pylori.*[2,3] It is now accepted that *H. pylori* causes acute and chronic non-autoimmune gastritis and is probably the commonest bacterial infection of humankind. It is responsible for up to 80% of gastric and 95% of duodenal ulcers (odds ratio 3–12). In 1994 *H. pylori* was classified as a grade 1 carcinogen by the International Agency for Research on Cancer—the only bacterium to be so classified. It causes gastric carcinoma (odds ratio 2–12) and is estimated to be involved in up to 60% of gastric carcinomas, but only after long-term infection (30–40 years). It is also associated with intestinal mucosal associated lymphoid tumours (MALTomas) (odds ratio > 10).

Epidemiology

Infection with *H. pylori* is present in all areas of the world surveyed.[2,3] In developed countries approximately 10% of healthy individuals under 30 years of age have serological evidence of infection and this rises to 60% in those over 60 years of age. In developing countries infection is highly prevalent and develops at a younger age. For example, in The Gambia 15% of infants aged under 20 months and 46% of those under 5 years have antibodies to *H. pylori;*[4] in Peru 48% of children aged from 2 months to 12 years have evidence of infection.[5] In most developing countries virtually 100% of individuals are seropositive by early childhood.[6] It is accepted that infection is usually acquired in the first 5 years of life but that improving hygienic and socio-economic conditions in developed and some developing countries has led to a decreased rate of acquisition and an apparent birth cohort effect. Humans appear to be the major reservoir for *H. pylori*, which been grown (or its genome has been detected) in saliva, dental plaque, vomitus, gastric juice and faeces.[7]

How *H. pylori* is transmitted is unclear. Person-to-person spread via endoscopes, pH electrodes or nasogastric feeding tubes[3,7] has been documented, but this is unlikely to be a major mode of transmission. Close contact promotes spread; for example, families of infected children have a higher incidence of infection, as have gastroenterologists who are endoscopists.[8,9] Family clusters of infection are related to socio-economic status,[10] and infection is most readily transmitted between siblings, especially if their age gap is small.[11] The faecal–oral route is the most likely mode of spread, and *H. pylori* DNA has been detected in faeces. However, others have suggested that interoral spread is most important and some have suggested that the oral cavity is a permanent reservoir of *H. pylori*.[12] The domestic fly (*Musca domestica*) can become colonized by *H. pylori*, and *H. pylori* DNA has been detected in houseflies from three continents.[13] This raises the possibility of fly contamination of food leading to food-borne infection. *H. pylori* does not grow in foods but does survive, provided it is kept cool, moist and is not too acid. Waterborne spread has also been suggested as a major factor in developing countries.[5] Finally, some animal species, including the macaque, sheep and pig, have been shown to harbour *H. pylori*, suggesting the possibility of zoonotic spread.[7] *H. pylori* has even been detected in sheep's milk.

A number of other *Helicobacter* species have been detected in a variety of animals but of these only *H. heilmanii* is found in the human stomach.

Microbiology

H. pylori is a sinusoidal Gram-negative bacterium approximately $3.5\,\mu m$ long and 0.5–$1\,\mu m$ in diameter (Figure 52.1). It has a smooth surface and four to six sheathed flagella with terminal bulbs (unlike *Campylobacter* spp). The bacterium produces a powerful urease and

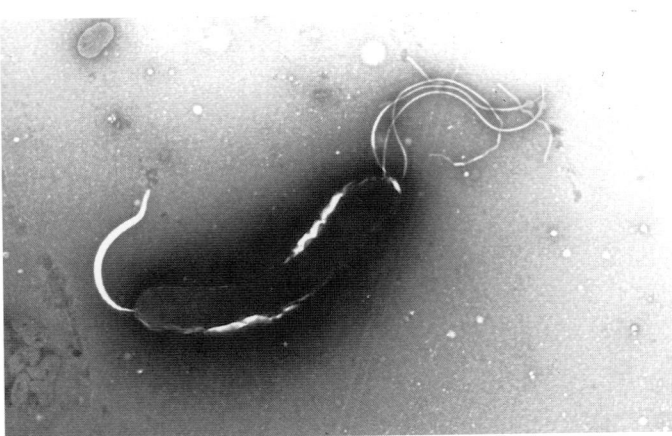

Figure 52.1: Negatively stained electronmicrograph of *Helicobacter pylori* showing sheathed flagella with a terminal bulb.

seems well adapted to living beneath the mucous layer attached to the surface of gastric enterocytes. *H. pylori* is fastidious and slow growing. It requires enriched selective media for isolation from clinical specimens. Growth is optimal at 37°C under humidified microaerophilic conditions in 10% carbon dioxide and takes 4–6 days.

Pathogenesis

Koch's postulates have been largely accepted for an association of *H. pylori* caused antral non-autoimmune (type B) gastritis in both adults and children.[2,3,14,15] There is also a strong association between *H. pylori* and peptic ulceration.[2] In feeding experiments doses of between 10^5 and 10^9 c.f.u. have established infection but the minimum dose has not been determined. *H. pylori* appears to be able to survive an acidic gastric pH to penetrate the mucus covering the gastric epithelial cells. It has been postulated that the bacterium's spiral morphology and flagella are important in this aspect of pathogenesis.[9] The bacteria can exist free in the mucous layer or firmly attached to the epithelial cells (Figure 52.2). *H. pylori* then

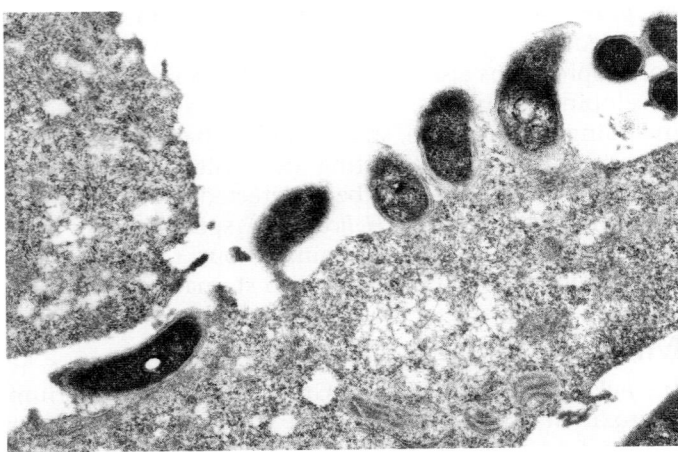

Figure 52.2: Thin-section electronmicrograph of *H. pylori* intimately attached to a gastric enterocyte.

elaborates a powerful urease which helps to neutralize the acidic pH, a cytotoxin that causes vacuolation (VacA), a protease that hydrolyses mucus, and other factors that stimulate gastric acid secretion.

Recently it has been found that certain strains of *H. pylori* are more likely to produce inflammation. These tend to possess a 40-kb pathogenicity island (a region of chromosomal DNA acquired by horizontal transmission) called the *cag* pathogenicity island (PAI). This region encodes a secretion system (type IV) that transports a protein, cag, across both bacterial membranes and injects it into host cells. Cag is also encoded in the PAI and once inside the gastric enterocyte induces the secretion of proinflammatory cytokines including interleukin 8.[16]

The pathogenesis of MALToma production appears to involve chronic antigenic stimulation, and elimination of *H. pylori* is associated with cure of the lymphomas. Infected individuals mount a systemic and local humoral immune response to the bacterium. *H. pylori*-specific secretory immunoglobulin (IgA) can be detected in both saliva and gastric juice. What role this plays in immunity is unclear because antibody is detectable in patients who are colonized or infected.

Pathology

H. pylori is strongly associated with chronic antral gastritis and with its active phase. Although macroscopic inflammation is usually not present, examination of biopsies reveals *H. pylori* in close apposition to the gastric mucosa which shows an infiltrate with mono- and polymorphonuclear leucocytes. *H. pylori* and evidence of inflammation may also be found in areas of gastric metaplasia in the oesophagus (Barrett's oesophagus) or duodenum.

Clinical features

Chronic epigastric pain is very common in the populations of many developing and developed countries. In sub-Saharan Africa non-ulcerous dyspepsia and duodenal ulcer are the most common causes of epigastric pain.[17,18] Infection with *H. pylori* was found in 141 (88%) of adult Malawians undergoing gastroscopy for chronic epigastric pain.[18] Other features associated with *H. pylori* gastritis include nausea, vomiting and flatulence. Similar features may also be seen in children with *H. pylori* infection.[15] The clinical features of gastritis relapse and remit, thus it is possible to detect *H. pylori* infection in individuals who have histological evidence of gastritis but no signs or symptoms.

Duodenal ulceration is associated with chronic antral gastritis. *H. pylori* can be detected in both antrum and duodenal ulcer tissue, but it will not colonize the duodenum except in areas of duodenal metaplasia.[19]

Diagnosis

Specific diagnosis may be reached by invasive or non-invasive techniques (Table 52.1).

Table 52.1 Invasive and non-invasive tests for the diagnosis of *Helicobacter pylori* infection.

Test	Sensitivity (%)	Specificity (%)	Cost	Comment
Non-invasive				
Antibody detection—ELISA	84–95	80–95	+	Can be used for proof of cure
Antibody detection—rapid	60–75	88–92	+	Can be used for proof of cure
Stool antigen detection	90–100	92–95	++	Becomes negative rapidly after therapy
^{13}C breath test	90–96	99	+++	Needs specialized equipment
^{14}C breath test	90–96	99	+++	Needs specialized equipment
Invasive				
Histology	80–90	93–100	+++	Takes time
Culture	75–90	100	+	Takes 3–4 days
Urease	85–95	99	+	Rapid test
Gram or other stain	75–90	80–90	+	Rapid but not ideal
PCR	95–100	95–99	+++	Very sensitive, takes 4–5 hours

Invasive techniques

Gastroscopic biopsies from the antrum, duodenal ulcer(s) or other areas of potential colonization are examined by culture and histological methods, and for urease activity. Two biopsy specimens from the antrum are sufficient to detect *H. pylori*.[18] Histological samples may be stained by Giemsa, silver impregnation or acridine orange for detection of *H. pylori*. This is more sensitive than culture in most surveys.

For culture, biopsy specimens are either rolled on the surface of an appropriate culture medium (e.g., brain–heart infusion-enriched Columbia blood agar incorporating Skirrow's antibiotics) or homogenized and similarly applied. In tropical countries it is advisable to incorporate an antifungal agent such as amphotericin B into the medium. A '1 minute' urease test in which the biopsy is immersed in a urea (10% de-ionized water) solution containing a pH indicator (phenol red) has proved highly sensitive and specific.[18]

Non-invasive techniques

Detection of antibody to *H. pylori* in serum or saliva is possible using an enzyme-linked immunosorbent assay (ELISA). Such tests have proved highly sensitive[14,15] but the specificity is variable as it is possible to detect antibody in those who are no longer infected.[18]

Breath tests that, for example, involve administering [^{13}C]urea and measuring the release of the isotope in the patient's breath have proved useful in developed and developing countries.[5] They depend upon the presence of *H. pylori* urease which hydrolyses the urea with release of $^{13}CO_2$.

Recently an antigen-capture ELISA has been developed for the detection of *H. pylori* in stool. It has proved sensitive and specific[20] and is useful as a test of cure. This test is rapid and easy to carry out. It currently costs £14 per test,[21] which is about half the cost of a breath test but still unaffordable in most developing countries.

Management

Often non-ulcer dyspepsia is not treated other than by symptomatic management. *H. pylori* is susceptible in vitro to a wide range of antimicrobials, including ampicillin, quinolones, cephalosporins, nitroimidazoles and macrolides, but all fail as monotherapy in vivo. Combinations of tripotassium dicitratobismuthate and ampicillin or metronidazole achieve 40% and 80% eradication rates, respectively,[22] but require 2–4 weeks of administration. Unfortunately resistance of *H. pylori* to metronidazole is high in African countries.[18]

Although treatment with H_2-blockers heals most duodenal ulcers, the majority (70–80%) relapse within 12 months. A combination of bismuth salts with amoxicillin and metronidazole with or without H_2-blockers is associated with ulcer healing, eradication of *H. pylori* and a greatly decreased relapse rate.[22,23] Current optimal regimens are based on the macrolide clarithromycin combined with proton pump inhibitors or ranitidine bismuth citrate with or without amoxicillin.[24] However, these regimens need to be evaluated locally.

Complications

In Gambian children an association between *H. pylori* and chronic diarrhoea and malnutrition has been described.[4] *H. pylori* gastritis was associated with protein-losing enteropathy in South African children.[25] Coinfection with *H. pylori* and *Vibrio cholerae* 01 was found frequently in Peruvian children and elderly adults, suggesting that hypochlorhydria induced by acute and chronic *H. pylori* infection might increase susceptibility to cholera.[26] Finally epidemiological studies have suggested a link between current infection with *H. pylori* and atherothrombogenesis.[27]

Prevention and control

Infection with *H. pylori* is ubiquitous throughout the world but highly localized in individuals. Until more is known about the mode of spread, pathogenesis and immunity, prevention and control are impossible. However, the decrease in infection in children in developed countries suggests that improving socio-economic and hygiene conditions should help.

Escherichia coli

Escherichia coli is the major aerobic component of the normal intestinal flora (approximately 10^7 c.f.u./ml) but is also a major cause of diarrhoeal disease. In some surveys it is estimated that *E. coli* is responsible for up to 30% of cases of gastroenteritis.[28] The strains of *E. coli* causing diarrhoea were originally termed enteropathogenic *E. coli* (EPEC) but as the different mechanisms of pathogenicity were determined, EPEC came to be used to described one particular mechanism. To date, five different mechanisms have been described: EPEC, enterotoxigenic *E. coli* (ETEC), enteroinvasive *E. coli* (EIEC), enterohaemorrhagic *E. coli* (EHEC) and enteroaggregative *E. coli* (EAggEC).

E. coli was first described as a cause of gastroenteritis by its association with outbreaks of diarrhoea in infants.[29,30] This was done by showing that all infants were excreting strains of *E. coli* with the same O or somatic antigen. Different O antigens were associated with the different enteropathic mechanisms of *E. coli* (Table 52.2). However, these are associations, and to test for O serogroup is not sufficiently specific to ascribe pathogenicity to a particular strain of *E. coli*. To do this, the specific pathogenicity genes (or their gene products) must be sought.

Enterotoxigenic *E. coli* (ETEC)

Epidemiology

ETEC have a worldwide distribution and are a major health hazard in adults and children in developing countries. In addition, they are a major cause of traveller's diarrhoea. In community-based studies in developing countries, ETEC are responsible for 15–20% of cases of diarrhoea.[31,32] In most hospital-based studies ETEC are second only to rotavirus as a cause of gastroenteritis. ETEC infections occur throughout the year but are most common in the wet season.[32] Spread is by the faecal–oral route either directly or indirectly via food or water. Infants are at particular risk at weaning. The infective dose is high in the normal host (10^6–10^{10} c.f.u.).

Pathogenesis

To produce disease, ETEC must be able to colonize the small intestine and elaborate one or both of heat-labile toxin (LT) and heat-stable toxin (ST). ETEC colonize the small intestine by means of protein spikes (colonization factor antigen; CFA) called fimbriae or pili (Figure 52.3), which bind to specific receptors on the enterocyte surface. The bacteria then release their toxins.

LT is a subunit toxin with a structure and mode of action similar to those of cholera toxin. Subunit B, the toxophore, binds to ganglioside M_1 (GM_1) on the enterocyte surface and allows subunit A to activate adenylate cyclase inside the enterocyte. The raised intracellular cyclic adenosine monophosphate (cAMP) concentration causes an efflux of Cl^-, Na^+ and water from

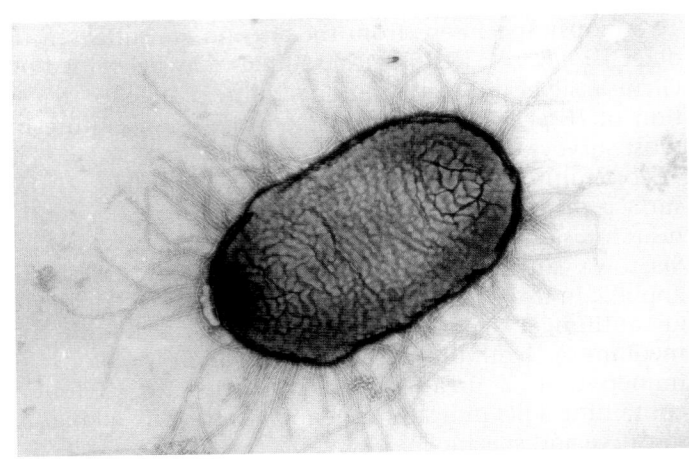

Figure 52.3: Negatively stained electronmicrograph of an enterotoxigenic *E. coli* covered with fimbriae.

Table 52.2 *Escherichia coli* and gastroenteritis.

Pathogenicity type	Site of action	Associated serogroups	Pathogenicity genes/products	Acute or chronic diarrhoea	Antibiotic therapy needed
ETEC	Small bowel (secretory)	O6, O8, O15, O2O, O25, O128 O139, O148, O153, O159	CFA, LT, ST	Acute	No
EIEC	Large bowel (inflammatory)	O28, O29, O124, O136, O143	*Ipa, ial*, EIEC	Acute	Not usually
EPEC	Small bowel (osmotic)	O55, O86, O111, O119, O125, O126, O127, O128, O142	LEE (EspA, Intimin, Tir)	Chronic	Yes
EHEC	Large bowel (inflammatory)	O26, O111, O118, O138, O157	LEE, EHEC, VT1, VT2	Acute	No
EAggEC	Large bowel (inflammatory)	O44, O111, O126 but most are non-groupable	EAggEC adhesin, EAST-1	Acute and chronic	Yes

CFA, colonization factor antigen; LT, heat-labile toxin; ST, heat-stable toxin; *Ipa* and *ial*, invasion-associated loci; Lee, locus of enterocyte effacement; VT, vero (or shiga-like) toxin; EAST, EAggEC heat-stable toxin.

villous crypt cells and has an antiabsorptive effect on villus tip cells. The net effect is that a large fluid load enters the colon and a voluminous watery stool is produced.

ST is a low molecular weight protein that activates guanylate cyclase. This results in secretion of fluid and electrolytes into the intestinal lumen. There are no specific histopathological changes to be seen in the small intestinal mucosa, and no evidence of inflammation.

The genes encoding fimbriae, LT and antibiotic resistance can be carried on plasmids in ETEC.

Clinical features

The incubation period is 1–2 days with anorexia, vomiting and abdominal cramps in 25% of patients. The diarrhoea is explosive, voluminous and watery, occurring up to 10 times a day. The illness is self-limiting and usually lasts for 1–5 days in well nourished individuals, but for up to 3 weeks in malnourished children. Dehydration is the major complication which, in a study in Bangladesh, was seen in 46% of adults and 16% of children.[32]

Diagnosis

Specific diagnosis depends upon culture of *E. coli* from faeces and detection of pathogenicity genes (CFA, LT, ST) by polymerase chain reaction (PCR), or of their gene products by ELISA, immunoprecipitation or bio-assay. To rely on O serogrouping is not sufficiently sensitive or specific, except in epidemics.

Management

The mainstay of treatment is the assessment of dehydration and replacement of fluid and electrolytes. Administration of antibiotics has been shown to shorten the course of illness and duration of excretion of ETEC in adults in endemic areas[33] and in those with traveller's diarrhoea.[34] The antibiotic used depends upon susceptibility patterns in the particular geographical region. Currently trimethoprim or fluoroquinolones such as ciprofloxacin are most likely to be effective.

Prevention

Although a B-subunit/whole-cell cholera vaccine provided 86% protection in Bangladeshi mothers and children, it was short lived (less than 3 months). A similar preparation was 52% effective in preventing ETEC diarrhoea in tourists.[35]

Enteroinvasive *E. coli* (EIEC)

This is a small group of *E. coli* that produce inflammatory diarrhoea by invading and killing colonic enterocytes (Figure 52.4). The organisms resemble shigellae in O antigens and in being non-motile, and have similar pathogenicity genes on a large plasmid that encode

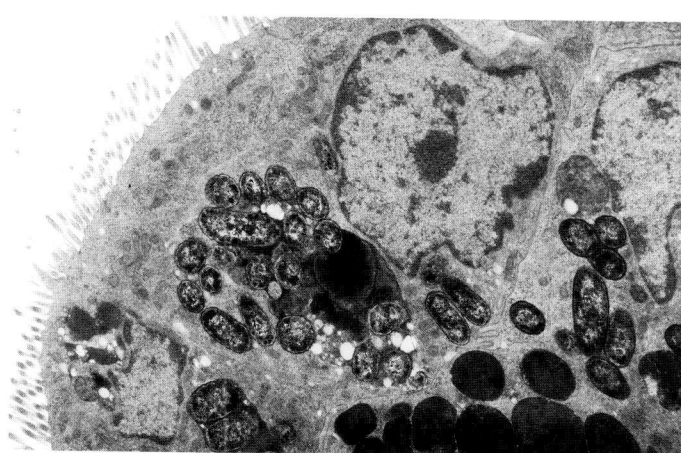

Figure 52.4: Thin-section electronmicrograph of colonic enterocytes showing enteroinvasive *E. coli* that have invaded into the cells.

surface proteins mediating invasion into cells. Infection is less common than that due to shigellae. For example, EIEC were responsible for 4.2% of episodes of endemic diarrhoea in children in Thailand and shigellae for 23%.[36] Infection is uncommon in children under 1 year of age but may be a cause of traveller's diarrhoea.

The clinical features of EIEC infection are similar to those of shigellae but the latter often produce more severe diarrhoea. Diagnosis is by stool culture and detection of EIEC pathogenicity genes by DNA hybridization[36] or PCR, or of gene products by ELISA.[37] Antimicrobial chemotherapy is usually not indicated and no vaccine is currently available for prevention.

Enteropathogenic *E. coli* (EPEC)

In the early 1970s when the pathogenesis of ETEC and EIEC had been defined, it became apparent that a large number of the classical O serogroups did not elaborate LT or ST, nor were they invasive. However, they were able to produce diarrhoea in volunteers.[38] As these were the original classical O serogroups that caused outbreaks of infantile diarrhoea, they were termed enteropathogenic *E. coli*.

Epidemiology

The first infections with EPEC were described in the UK and the USA in the 1940s and 1950s in epidemics of infantile diarrhoea.[29,30] Nowadays they are a cause of sporadic disease. In developing countries EPEC are still a major cause of infantile diarrhoea.[39–41] In Thailand 11% of children under 1 year of age with diarrhoea in a refugee camp were infected with EPEC,[28] and in an outbreak in pre-term neonates in Kenya 13 of 30 were infected with EPEC, three of whom died.[41] EPEC has also been associated with traveller's diarrhoea. Transmission is by the faecal–oral route, either directly or in food or water. The infective dose appears to be low (less than 10^4 c.f.u.).

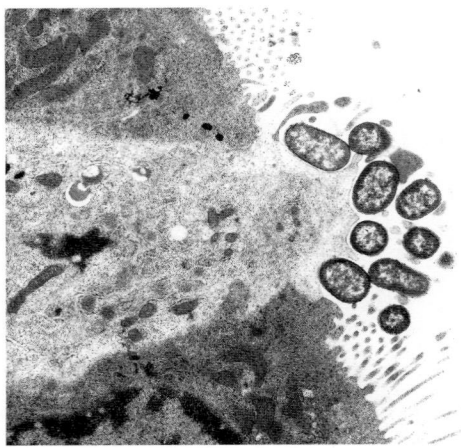

Figure 52.5: Thin-section electronmicrograph of duodenal mucosa showing loss of brush border and intimately attached enteropathogenic *E. coli* (attaching/effacement).

Pathogenesis

The ingested EPEC adhere to the mucus overlying the small intestinal enterocytes using fimbriae. On contact with enterocytes, pathogenicity island (called the locus of enterocyte effacement; LEE) associated genes are activated. This induces the formation of a type III secretion system that delivers effector molecules across both bacterial membranes and through a pilus-like structure into the enterocyte.[42] Secreted effectors include Tir (translocatable intimin receptor), which becomes inserted in the enterocyte membrane. This has affinity for intimin, a surface protein on the EPEC. Thus EPEC are unique in synthesizing, secreting and inserting their own receptor into host cell membranes. This then mediates the intimate attachment of EPEC to the enterocyte surface.[43] Then the brush border is lost by a process of vesiculation.[43] This process is termed 'attaching effacement' (Figure 52.5). Although the process is maximal in the small intestine, it can occur throughout the gastrointestinal tract.[43] The net result is that large areas for absorption of nutrients are lost. In addition, because the disaccharidase enzymes are integral proteins in the microvillous membrane, levels of these enzymes are markedly depressed.[44,45] The disaccharides sucrose, lactose and maltose in the diet must be hydrolysed to monosaccharides to be absorbed. Because of loss of the brush border, the disaccharides cannot be cleaved and are thus not absorbed. They pass to the colon and cause a non-inflammatory osmotic diarrhoea, although in some cases there also appears to be a secretory component.[38]

Clinical features

EPEC tend to produce more severe and prolonged diarrhoea, which may remit and relapse. There is initially vomiting, with fever and profuse diarrhoea with mucus but no blood. Fatality rates in epidemics range from 30 to 50%, but with oral rehydration and antibiotic therapy mortality rates have decreased to less than 8%.[46,47]

Management and prevention

The initial treatment should be to rehydrate. Because the diarrhoea can be prolonged, enteral or parenteral nutrition and antibiotics may be indicated. Ampicillin is unlikely to be effective even if the EPEC are sensitive. Administration of oral non-absorbable antibiotics such as neomycin or polymyxin B is effective. Oral absorbable antibiotics such as fluoroquinolones or trimethoprim may also be of benefit. However, antibiotic resistance to most antibiotics has been observed in EPEC.

A vaccine is not available for prevention of infection.

Enterohaemorrhagic *E. coli* (EHEC)

EHEC were first described in Canada in 1983 when they were linked to cases of haemorrhagic colitis[48] and haemolytic–uraemic syndrome.[49] Infections were caused by a newly emerged (in the late 1970s) bacterium, *E. coli* O157. Subsequently a number of other *E. coli* O serogroups and other coliforms (*Enterobacter cloacae* and *Citrobacter freundii*) have caused disease in humans.

Epidemiology

Infections with EHEC were initially described in industrialized countries. Here they tend to cause outbreaks of infection, usually as the result of the consumption of incompletely cooked beef or pork.[50] EHEC can be part of the normal enteric flora of cattle, pigs, sheep, goats, cats and dogs in which they cause no disease.

An initial survey of adults in Thailand with diarrhoea showed that 2% of 458 patients were infected by EHEC.[51] There have recently been large outbreaks of haemorrhagic colitis, including in southern Africa,[52] apparently associated with cooked market foods and due to EHEC, and more recently in Cameroon.[53] However, because the infective dose is low (less than 10^2 c.f.u.), person-to-person spread also occurs.

Pathogenesis

EHEC produce attaching effacement, limited to the terminal ileum and colon, and have most of the genes in the LEE pathogenicity island of EPEC. In addition they release one or both of the toxins, verocytotoxin (VT) 1 or 2. These toxins are also called shiga-like toxins (SLT) 1 and 2; they inhibit protein synthesis and are cytotoxic.[54] They are subunit toxins that bind to globoside receptors (the P blood group antigen) on cells. The receptors are more densely expressed on renal endothelial cells and in children. In the colon they kill enterocytes, leading to an inflammatory haemorrhagic colitis. If they enter the systemic circulation they can damage renal endothelial cells and precipitate the haemolytic–uraemic syndrome.[50]

Clinical features

Haemorrhagic colitis presents with abdominal cramps and watery diarrhoea that is followed by a haemorrhagic discharge resembling a colonic bleed. There is rarely an accompanying fever. Haemolytic–uraemic syndrome is one, if not the most common, cause of acute renal failure in childhood in industrialized countries. In an Indian study, EHEC were implicated in 19 of 28 cases of haemolytic–uraemic syndrome and *Shigella* spp. in only six.[55] Haemolytic–uraemic syndrome presents with acute renal failure, thrombocytopenia, coagulopathy and evidence of microangiopathic haemolytic anaemia. With peritoneal dialysis the outlook is good, with the fatality rate falling from 50% to less than 10%.

Diagnosis

The first strains of *E. coli* associated with haemorrhagic colitis and haemolytic–uraemic syndrome were of serogroup O157 and sorbitol non-fermenters. Thus serogrouping and sorbitol MacConkey agar are used to diagnose infections. However, other serogroups (Table 52.1) are also implicated. The toxins VT1 and 2 are transferable between bacteria on promiscuous bacteriophages. Thus specific diagnosis depends upon detection of VT or its genes (by DNA hybridization or PCR) or of EHEC plasmid-encoded fimbrial adhesin genes.[51] Excretion of EHEC beyond the period of diarrhoea is short lived. For retrospective diagnosis it is possible to detect serum antibody to VT.[56]

Management and prevention

The treatment of haemorrhagic colitis is essentially treatment of dehydration. Antibiotics have no role and in some cases (as with *Shigella dysenteriae* 1) may increase the risk of complications.[57] For haemolytic–uraemic syndrome, peritoneal dialysis is the most important intervention. No vaccine is currently available.

Enteroaggregative *E. coli* (EAggEC)

EAggEC are the most recently discovered pathogenic group.[58] They are named for their characteristic pattern of adherence to tissue culture cells—in large aggregates.

EAggEC can cause both acute and persistent diarrhoea. In a survey of EAggEC infection in India the most notable clinical features were fever, vomiting, overt blood in the stool and a mean duration of diarrhoea of 17 days.[59] How diarrhoea is produced is not known but intestinal inflammation appears to be linked to stimulation of interleukin 8 secretion.[60]

Diagnosis is by culture of *E. coli* that produce a distinctive aggregative pattern on cultured cells and that contain EAggEC pathogenicity genes detectable by PCR.[61]

Campylobacter jejuni

The genus *Campylobacter* is a major cause of gastroenteritis in both developed and developing countries. Although *C. fetus* was recognized as an opportunist pathogen as early as 1947, the full role of *Campylobacter* spp. as major enteric pathogens was not realized until appropriate selective media were devised.[62,63]

Epidemiology

The major enteric pathogens in the genus are *C. jejuni* (I and II), *C. coli* and *C. lari*, although *C. upsaliensis* is incresingly recognized. Of these, *C. jejuni* is the most common cause of gastroenteritis. All can be normally present in the gastrointestinal tract of domestic and wild animals and birds, which act as the major reservoir for infection. *C. lari*, in particular, may be part of the normal intestinal flora of birds. Campylobacters can survive for 2–5 weeks in cow's milk or water kept at 4°C but they do not multiply. Infection is spread faeco-orally, human to human or animal to human (there have even been cases of human-to-animal spread), either directly or indirectly in food and water.

Animal to human. Close contact with animals, such as that in villages in developing countries where poultry, goats, cattle and dogs roam freely, increases the risk of infection.

Human to human. Transmission may occur from infected individuals or from convalescent carriers, especially young children. Epidemics of infection can occur in nurseries or paediatric wards.

Food. Contamination may occur during preparation of food from the animal's intestinal content(s) or by incomplete cooking.

Milk. Consumption of raw unpasteurized milk is strongly associated with illness,[64,65] as is contamination of bottled milk following attack by birds.[66]

Water. Excreta from wild and domesticated animals can contaminate surface water; water-borne transmission is important in developing countries.

The incubation period is 2–5 days[65] with an infective dose of 500 c.f.u. The median duration of excretion of *C. jejuni* following cessation of diarrhoea is 2–3 weeks.

Infection is most common in those under 1 year of age, with a decrease in attack rate with increasing age. *C. jejuni* is isolated in from 5–10% of children with gastroenteritis in developing countries, but it may be isolated as frequently from children without diarrhoea.[67]

Bacteriology

Campylobacters are Gram-negative bacteria with a single polar flagellum (Figure 52.6). They are spiral or bent rods 0.2–0.5 μm in diameter and 1.5–3.5 μm long. They are themophilic and will grow at 42°C but prefer a microaerophilic atmosphere. *C. jejuni* can hydrolyse hippurate, which distinguishes it from *C. coli* and *C. lari*. *C. coli* is sensitive to nalidixic acid but *C. lari* is resistant. All can be cultivated on simple media.

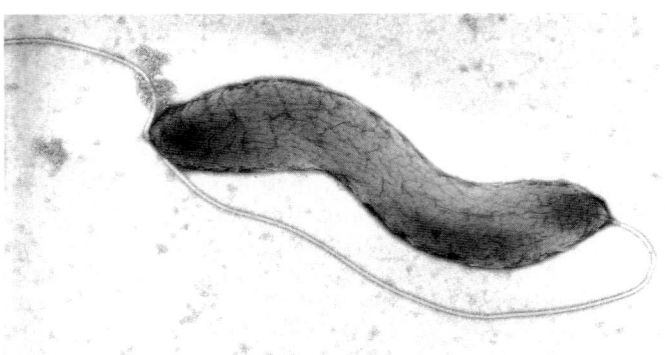

Figure 52.6: Negatively stained electronmicrograph of *Campylobacter jejuni*.

Pathogenesis

Campylobacters can produce both an inflammatory and a non-inflammatory diarrhoea. How campylobacters cause diarrhoea is unclear but it does involve attachment to the intestinal mucosa, and is also dependent of motility by means of flagella.[68] Other factors include iron acquision, invasion of enterocytes and possibly toxin production.

Immunity to infection is acquired after one or more infective episodes but duration of immunity is unknown. Following infection, serum and secretory antibodies to *Campylobacter* flagella, enterotoxin, lipolysaccharide and other surface antigens that are involved in attachment are produced. In developing countries antibodies are acquired in early life[69,70]—perhaps because of continuous exposure from animals. This may account for the lower prevalence of infection in adults in developing countries compared with developed countries, and the higher prevalence of asymptomatic infection in the former. It is probable that the presence of secretory IgA against *Campylobacter* spp. is the main determinant of immunity.

In a small proportion of those infected, usually the immunoincompetent, bacteria translocate from the intestinal lumen, causing bacteraemia.

Pathology

In the dysentery-like illness, inflammatory infiltrates into the lamina propria and crypt abscesses can be seen in the rectal, colonic and terminal ileal mucosa. This is a similar finding to that seen in *Shigella* or *Salmonella* infections, Crohn's disease or ulcerative colitis.

Clinical features

In developing countries *Campylobacter* spp. enteritis is generally less severe than that in developed countries. It is more likely to be of the non-inflammatory type, without fever or bloody diarrhoea.[70] However, severe bloody diarrhoea resembling bacillary dysentery can occur and will also occur in travellers acquiring infection in developing countries. In general the diarrhoea is self-limiting and resolves in 2–7 days.

Disseminated infection can occur; predisposing factors include malnutrition, hepatic dysfunction, malignancy, diabetes mellitus, renal failure and immunosuppression. Extraintestinal and rare forms of infection include: asymptomatic bacteraemia, meningitis, deep abscesses and cholecystitis. Reactive arthritis may follow *Campylobacter* spp. enteritis in genetically susceptible individuals (HLA-B27). Campylobacter enteritis is one of the commonest precipitating causes of Guillain–Barré syndrome resulting from antigenic cross-reactivity between the bacterial surface and neuronal glycolipids.

Diagnosis

The features of *Campylobacter* infection are not sufficiently distinct to make a clinical diagnosis. Examination of faecal smears by Gram stain or dark field microscopy can provide a rapid presumptive diagnosis. Where laboratory facilities are not optimal, this may be the best diagnostic tool. However, the basis of specific diagnosis is isolation of the bacteria from faeces. *Campylobacter* spp. will grow on most basal media, especially if lysed blood is incorporated. In order to make the media selective, antibiotics such as trimethoprim are incorporated.[71] Culture is usually at 42°C (to inhibit gut commensals) and in a microaerophilic atmosphere. Culture plates and swabs should be kept out of the light before use because *Campylobacter* spp. are rapidly killed by free radicals generated by ultra-violet irradiation.

Management

Patients with severe watery diarrhoea will need adequate rehydration. Those with severe dysentery or disseminated infection will require antimicrobial chemotherapy. *C. jejuni* is usually sensitive to erythromycin, but *C. coli* may occasionally be resistant. Nevertheless, erythromycin remains the best choice.

Prevention and control

There is no vaccine for prevention of infection; thus non-specific methods for prevention such as improvements in sanitation, provision of clean potable water and good food hygiene are important.

Yersinia enterocolitica

The genus *Yersinia* comprises *Y. pestis*, the cause of plague, *Y. pseudotuberculosis* and *Y. enterocolitica*. Of these, *Y. enterocolitica* is the only important cause of diarrhoea.[72]

Epidemiology

Although *Yersinia* spp. infection is said to have a worldwide distribution, it is found much more commonly in temperate zones than in the tropics. Even in temperate countries infection is more prevalent in colder climates and is more common in winter.[72] In most surveys of acute diarrhoeal disease where *Y. enterocolitica* was sought, it was either absent or present in less than 1% of cases.[73] However, cases of generalized infection have been recorded in South Africa[74] and serological evidence of infection has been found in Nigeria.[75]

The reservoir for *Y. enterocolitica* is a variety of animal species, including birds, frogs, fish, snails, oysters and most mammals. The organism is excreted in faeces from pigs and cattle, and can persist in lakes, streams, soil and vegetables. Patient-to-patient spread is rare except by blood transfusion. The incubation period is 1–11 days and bacteria are excreted for 14–97 (mean 42) days.

Bacteriology

Y. enterocolitica is a small Gram-negative rod with peritrichous flagellae. It will grow on simple media and is lactose non-fermenting on MacConkey agar. It is psychrophilic, and isolation from clinical samples often involves a cold enrichment step. O serogrouping is used to subdivide strains.

Pathogenesis

Pathogenic strains of *Y. enterocolitica* carry a large plasmid which encodes surface proteins and lipopolysaccharides mediating cell attachment, resistance to phagocytosis and serum resistance. Chromosomal genes (*inv, ail*: attaching invasion locus) encode the ability to invade epithelial cells. Although *Y. enterocolitica* produces a toxin similar to LT, its role in pathogenesis is unclear. *Y. enterocolitica* invades ileal enterocytes and M cells in Peyer's patches, where it multiplies. This produces a inflammatory diarrhoea. Bacteria may pass to local lymph nodes, thence to produce systemic disease.

In addition to disease produced directly by *Y. enterocolitica* there are a number of autoimmune phenomena that present in a proportion of patients after initial infection. These include: erythema nodosum, reactive arthropathy, Reiter's syndrome and glomerulonephritis. In addition there is a linkage with thyroid disorders, in that patients with Hashimoto's thyroiditis have high titres of *Y. enterocolitica* agglutinating antibodies. It is noteworthy that the surface of *Y. enterocolitica* has receptors for thyroid stimulating hormone.

Clinical features

Most symptomatic infections are in children under 5 years of age.[72] Characteristically, clinical features consist of diarrhoea, low-grade fever and abdominal pain. The diarrhoeic stool will be frankly blood stained in a quarter of cases. Nausea, vomiting, headache and pharyngitis are minority presentations. The abdominal pain may be present alone or with mild diarrhoea, and is often termed the pseudoappendicular syndrome. Infection may spread elsewhere to produce bacteraemia, peritonitis, hepatic, renal and splenic abscesses, pyomyositis and osteomyelitis.[72,74] These are more likely to occur in patients who are immunocompromised or who have iron overload, as in haemochromatosis.[74] The extraintestinal manifestations are more likely to occur in adults, as are the autoimmune phenomena. Of those with reactive arthritis, 80% are of HLA-B27 histoincompatibility type.

Diagnosis

Y. enterocolitica can be isolated from stool, appendix, mesenteric lymph nodes, blood and other focal sites of infection using simple media. Strategies for isolation include MacConkey agar incubated at 25–30°C for 48 hours or selective media such as cefsulodin–irgasan–novobiocin (CIN) agar at 37°C. For isolation from food or water, cold enrichment in phosphate-buffered saline for up to 4 weeks at 4°C prior to plating on to CIN agar greatly increases the yield of both pathogenic and non-pathogenic *Yersinia* spp. Speciation is obtained by biochemical tests and it is noteworthy that all non-pathogenic *Y. enterocolitica* have pyrizinamidase activity. Pathogenic *Y. enterocolitica* all possess the virulence plasmid. For retrospective diagnosis, serology using ELISA, whole cell agglutination or complement fixation tests can be performed. They may be difficult to interpret and cross-reactions (e.g., *Y. enterocolitica* 0:9 with *Brucella abortus*, *E. coli*, *Morganella morganii* and *Salmonella* spp.) do occur. The specificity of the test can be improved by detecting a greater than fourfold increase in titre between acute and convalescent sera.

Management and control

In children with uncomplicated diarrhoea, antimicrobial treatment is of little benefit.[76] In complicated infection co-trimoxazole, tetracycline or chloramphenicol should be effective. Although natural infection with *Y. enterocolitica* produces immunity, no vaccine is available.

Clostridium spp.

Clostridia are anaerobic sporing Gram-positive rods (Figure 52.7). Two species *C. perfringens* and *C. difficile* are associated with diarrhoeal disease.

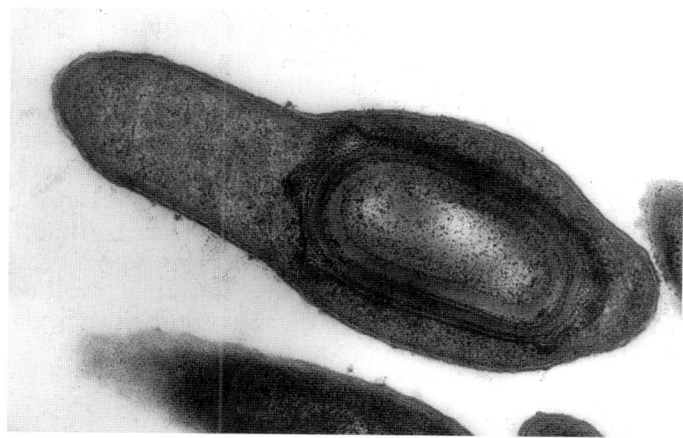

Figure 52.7: Thin-section electronmicrograph of *Clostridium perfringens* showing its endospore.

Clostridium perfringens

Two forms of diarrhoeal disease are associated with *C. perfringens* (formerly *welchii*). The first is a food-poisoning illness due to ingestion of *C. perfringens* type A or the α-toxin (enterotoxin) it produces. Although this is a common cause of food poisoning in industrialized countries, it produces mild, short-lived disease and is extremely uncommon in the tropics.

C. perfringens type C, in contrast, is common in certain areas of the tropics and produces a severe necrotic enteritis.

Epidemiology

C. perfringens type C has been implicated in enteritis necroticans (Darmbrand) seen in malnourished individuals in northern Europe after World War II[77] and 'pigbel' in the highlands of Papua New Guinea.[78] A similar disease has been described in Uganda,[79] Malaysia, Thailand, Indonesia, China[80] and, more recently, in India.[81]

Infection may occur sporadically[79,80] but also in epidemics.[77,78] It occurs at any age but is more likely to present as acute toxic or acute surgical problems in children under 10 years of age.[78,80] In Papua New Guinea, pigbel is associated with large 'pig feasts' that occur every 3–10 years. Infection is more common in males than females; whether this represents a true difference in susceptibility or male greed is unclear. *C. perfringens* type C can be found in the human normal intestinal flora, in pig excreta and in soil.

Microbiology

C. perfringens type C produces both α- and β-toxins which, it is presumed, are responsible for disease manifestations.

Pathogenesis

Since *C. perfringens* type C can be found as part of the normal intestinal flora, it is considered that host-dependent factors are also involved. First, the bulk of the normal anaerobic flora is found in the large bowel and one hypothesis is that overgrowth of *C. perfringens* type C in the jejunum might be related to development of disease. A more attractive hypothesis links malnutrition and type of diet with disease. β-Toxin is readily inactivated by intestinal proteases. Protein deficiency decreases intestinal protease levels; in addition, the sweet potato, which is a staple diet in highland Papua New Guinea, contains heat-stable trypsin inhibitors. Thus consumption of meat contaminated by *C. perfringens* type C or its β-toxin in an individual with low intestinal protease activity due to malnutrition or dietary protease inhibitors would allow the toxin to produce intestinal damage.[80,82]

Pathology

Gross pathology shows patchy segmental acute ulcerative necrosis of the jejunum, and to a lesser extent of the ileum, caecum and colon. This may progress rapidly to segmental gangrene with gas in the mucosa, mesentery or lymph nodes. Microscopically the intestinal wall shows separation of the mucosa from the submucosa, with large denuded areas covered with a pseudomembrane of dead enterocytes and infiltrating neutrophils and red blood cells. Healing occurs with fibrosis, and strictures and adhesions may form later.

Clinical features

Pigbel varies in severity from mild diarrhoea to a rapidly fatal necrotizing enteritis, with a high mortality rate (up to 85%). The incubation period is approximately 48 hours after the feast but may vary from 24 hours to up to 1 week.

Disease has been classified into four main presentations:[79,78]

Type I (acute toxic) presents with fulminant toxaemia and shock.

Type II (acute surgical) presents as mechanical and paralytic ileus, acute strangulation, perforation and peritonitis.

Type III (subacute surgical) presents later with complications of mild type II.

Type IV (mild or trivial) presents with mild diarrhoea but may rarely progress to type III.

Type I disease occurs most commonly in young children and has the highest mortality rate (85%). Type II disease has a 42% mortality rate, type III 44%, and type IV is never fatal. In type II and type III disease a palpable segment of thickened intestine may be found. The stool will contain blood and pus cells, and there is a neutrophilic leucocytosis in peripheral blood. The differential diagnosis includes acute causes of inflammatory diarrhoea, peritonitis, acute abdominal obstruction, acute pancreatitis, acute amoebic colitis and sickle cell crisis.

Diagnosis

C. perfringens can be cultured from faeces, peritoneal fluid or other infected sites by plating on to neomycin blood agar and incubating anaerobically. *C. perfringens* type C is differentiated from other *C. perfringens* by serological techniques, including immunofluorescence and type C antibody-coated silica beads.[83] Interpretation of results may be difficult because *C. perfringens* type C is also found in normal individuals. Detection of antibodies to the toxin can be useful in reaching a diagnosis in survivors.[78]

Management

Acute resuscitation is by fluid and electrolytes intravenously, together with bowel decompression by restricting oral intake and nasogastric intubation. Antibiotics will be needed if there is extraintestinal spread of the organism (e.g., peritonitis); metronidazole, ampicillin, chloramphenicol or penicillin should be of value. Administration of *C. perfringens* type C antiserum is also beneficial.[78] Surgical intervention will be necessary if there is persisting obstruction, increasing signs of toxaemia, or signs of peritonitis or strangulation. There is some evidence that early surgical intervention may decrease the mortality rate.[78]

Prevention

Active immunization with a toxoid prepared from *C. perfringens* type C toxins has decreased the incidence of pigbel in children.[84]

Clostridium difficile

C. difficile is the cause of antibiotic-associated colitis and of pseudomembranous colitis. The organism and toxin can be detected in asymptomatic infants but their finding in older individuals is related to disease. Although the bacterium can be found worldwide it is probably an unusual cause of diarrhoeal disease in developing countries.[85]

Aeromonas and *Plesiomonas*

These two genera within the Vibrionaceae family are both aquatic micro-organisms and can be readily isolated from fresh and salt water, fish, soil and food.

Aeromonas hydrophila

Epidemiology

A. hydrophila has been associated with gastroenteritis in many countries throughout the world.[86] In tropical countries it can be isolated from healthy as well as diarrhoeic individuals. In Thailand, *Aeromonas* spp. were isolated from 9% of patients with gastroenteritis and were second in importance only to ETEC.[87]

Microbiology

The genus *Aeromonas* encompasses three motile species: *A. hydrophila*, *A. caviae* and *A. sobria*. A fourth non-motile species, *A. salmonicida*, is a fish pathogen and does not grow above 30°C. These organisms are oxidase positive and will grow on most simple media. *Aeromonas* produces a wide range of extracellular factors including proteases, elastases, esterases, DNase, haemolysins, cytotoxins and enterotoxins.

Pathogenesis

Aeromonas is associated with both inflammatory and non-inflammatory diarrhoea. It possesses fimbrial and non-fimbrial adhesins for attachment to the intestinal mucosa. It produces an enterotoxin that has a similar mode of action to *E. coli* LT but uses a different receptor.

The haemolysins of *Aeromonas* are also cytotoxic for cultured cells. Finally, *Aeromonas* can invade cells in vitro and in vivo, and this property might be related to production of inflammatory diarrhoea.

Clinical features

Gastroenteritis associated with *Aeromonas* spp. can vary from acute watery diarrhoea with fever, to chronic dysentery with fever and abdominal cramps.

Diagnosis

Aeromonas can be isolated from faeces using selective media such as ampicillin blood agar. Prior enrichment in alkaline peptone water increases the sensitivity of isolation. Since *Aeromonas* spp. can be isolated from normal individuals, isolation does not prove causation. For the future, it may be necessary to detect pathogenicity factors (toxins, adhesins or invasiveness) to link isolation with the disease in a particular patient.

Management

Rehydration is usually the only intervention needed. If infection becomes disseminated or there is chronic dysentery, antimicrobials such as fluorinated quinolones might be of benefit.

Plesiomonas shigelloides

This micro-organism has been isolated from patients with food-borne (usually fish) gastroenteritis in Mali and India,[88,89] and there has even been a case of snake-to-human transmission.[90]

Shigellosis (bacillary dysentery)

Dysentery has been a disease of poor and crowded communities throughout history, and continues to be a major cause of morbidity and mortality in the tropics. Dysentery bacilli were first demonstrated by Shiga in 1898, and subsequent studies showed that four species, *Shigella dysenteriae*, *Sh. flexneri*, *Sh. boydii* and *Sh. sonnei*, were responsible for the disease described as bacillary dysentery. *Sh. dysenteriae* and *Sh. flexneri* are responsible for most infections in the tropics, with case fatality rates of up to 20%.[91] Shigellosis occurs both endemically and as epidemics. In many tropical countries, endemic infection is largely due to *Sh. flexneri* and is more commonly a disease of children. Studies in Thailand[92] and Bangladesh[93] have shown *Shigella* spp. to be isolated from up to 50% of children presenting with bloody diarrhoea. Case fatality rates among children with shigellosis may be as high as 30% in those with severe complications, particularly the haemolytic–uraemic syndrome.[94]

Table 52.3 Classification of *Shigella* serotypes.

Species	No. of serotypes	Glucose	Mannitol (fermentation)	Lactose
Sh. dysenteriae	10	+	–	–
Sh. flexneri	6	+	+	–
Sh. boydii	15	+	+	–
Sh. sonnei	1	+	+	Late

Bacteriology

Shigella spp. are members of the Enterobacteriaceae and are aerobic, Gram-negative, non-motile bacilli. They are typically non-lactose fermenting, lysine decarboxylase-negative and do not produce gas from glucose. The exceptions are *Sh. sonnei*, which ferments lactose slowly, and *Sh. flexneri* 6 and *Sh. boydii* 13, which produce gas from glucose. *Sh. dysenteriae*, *Sh. flexneri* and *Sh. boydii* are each divided into a number of serotypes (Table 52.3).

Serotype (O) antigens are located on the outer polysaccharide chains of the lipopolysaccharide component of the cell wall. *Shigella* spp. are non-motile and do not possess H antigens.

For epidemiological studies, serotypes may be subdivided by molecular methods such as plasmid and chromosomal DNA restriction endonuclease digests.[95]

In pure growth, *Shigella* spp. are readily cultured on non-selective media, but for isolation from clinical specimens, selective media such as MacConkey and xylose lysine deoxycholate (XLD) are necessary.

Pathogenesis

Shigella dysentery is characterized by invasion of the colonic mucosa, local spread of the infecting organism and death of intestinal epithelial cells. In a proportion of cases, extraintestinal complications occur, including seizures, hyponatraemia and hypoglycaemia, septicaemia, Reiter's syndrome, encephalopathy and the haemolytic–uraemic syndrome. A number of pathogenicity factors and their genetic determinants have been described. Invasion is associated with specific outer membrane proteins that are encoded on plasmid (extrachromosomal) DNA of size 220 kilobases (kb). Strains not containing these plasmids have been shown to be non-virulent. The lipopolysaccharide component of the cell membrane, which includes the polysaccharide side chains specific to different O antigenic types, is a further virulence factor.[96] The lipid A component has endotoxic activity and contributes to the systemic effects of infection. The O-antigen polysaccharides provide the bacteria with resistance to host defence mechanisms including opsonization, phagocytosis and intracellular killing. O-polysaccharide genes are generally chromosomally encoded. However, in *Sh. sonnei* the genes are present on a 180-kb plasmid, and in *Sh. dysenteriae* 1 a 9-kb plasmid, in conjunction with chromosomal genes, is associated with O-antigen synthesis. Genes responsible for invasion (*ipa* genes), intracellular spread (*ics* gene) and virulence regulation (*vir*R genes) have been described, and increasing understanding of their role

may contribute to vaccine development. In addition to these virulence factors, *Sh. dysenteriae* 1 produces a toxin, shiga or vero toxin (Stx). Stx inactivates ribosomal RNA, inhibiting protein synthesis and leads to cell death. Stx is composed of A and B subunits, the genes being chromosomally located, and is the same as VT1 produced by EHEC. The cytotoxic effects of shiga toxin are involved both in the haemorrhagic intestinal manifestations and the haemolytic–uraemic syndrome.

Pathology and immunology

The characteristic pathology is an acute, locally invasive colitis, ranging from mild inflammation of the mucous membranes of the distal colon to severe necrosis of much of the large bowel. Sigmoidoscopy reveals a red, bleeding mucosa with patches of necrotic membrane, which may separate to leave ulcerated areas. The inflammatory process may extend through the submucosa to the muscle layer. In severe cases, complete healing may not occur, resulting in fibrous tissue formation and persistent ulceration. Bacteraemia is uncommon in *Shigella* infection, but is a probable risk factor for increased mortality.[97] Circulating endotoxin is likely to play an important role in the systemic manifestations of *Shigella* infection. In *Sh. dysenteriae* 1 infections, shiga toxin exerts both enterotoxic effects, through specific glycolipid binding sites, and is responsible for the haemolytic–uraemic syndrome. Infection with *Shigella* spp. leads to both local (gut) immunity and the production of circulating antibodies. Circulating antibodies are directed against the O (lipopolysaccharide) antigens and have been shown to be serotype specific.

Epidemiology

Humans are the only natural host for infection by *Shigella* spp. Infection is by ingestion, the infective dose being as low as 10–100 bacteria for *Sh. dysenteriae*. The incubation period is 1–5 days. Shigellosis occurs as an endemic disease in conditions of crowding, poor sanitation and inadequate water supply, and is primarily a disease of poor disadvantaged communities in the tropics.

Endemic shigellosis is largely a paediatric disease, most cases occurring in children below 10 years of age. Routes of infection include direct person-to-person transmission (from cases or asymptomatic excreters) and transmission via contaminated water or food. The evidence for person-to-person transmission in endemic areas of the tropics comes from a number of community studies that show a high frequency of secondary household cases in the family of an index case, but no differences between families with cases, and control families in relation to water or food supply.[98] In epidemics of *Sh. dysenteriae* 1, person-to-person transmission is also more common than point-source food or water outbreaks. Although occasional water-borne epidemics have been described, a seasonal pattern of shigellosis is seen in most endemic areas. In Bangladesh, peak transmission rates occur at the beginning of the monsoon season, with a second—lower—peak in the winter season.[99]

The epidemiology of *Shigella* infections in endemic areas of the tropics is complicated by the wide range of serotypes isolated. Studies in Ethiopia have shown shigellae of all main serotypes in community studies in Addis Ababa.[100] In epidemics of *Sh. dysenteriae* 1 a single strain is most commonly responsible. Very extensive outbreaks have occurred among displaced communities in recent African crises. A *Shigella* dysentery outbreak that followed a cholera epidemic in the refugee camps in Goma, eastern Democratic Republic of Congo (former Zaire), resulted in considerable mortality, particularly among malnourished children.[101] Outbreaks have continued in neighbouring areas of central Africa and in southern Africa.[102,103]

Clinical features

Shigellosis may vary from relatively mild watery diarrhoea to severe dysentery with intestinal and extra-intestinal complications. In severe cases, the onset is abrupt, with tenesmus, fever and frequent passage of bloody, mucoid stools. The degree of dehydration may be considerably less than in other diarrhoeas, although stool frequency may be as high as 30 times per day. Diarrhoea is often accompanied by fever, headache and malaise. Intestinal complications include toxic megacolon, perforation and a protein-losing enteropathy. Electrolyte imbalance may arise, in particular prolonged hypo-natraemia. *Sh. dysenteriae* and *Sh. flexneri* infections may result in a number of extraintestinal complications. Haemolytic–uraemic syndrome occurs particularly with *Sh. dysenteriae* 1 and may develop 7–10 days after the onset of disease. Convulsions may occur with infections caused by all species of *Shigella*, particularly in children. They may occur before diarrhoea begins, and are usually accompanied by a rising fever. Encephalopathy and hemiplegia have been reported.[104]

Diagnosis

In many parts of the tropical world, the diagnosis and subsequent management of *Shigella* infections occur in the absence of laboratory facilities. While clinical algorithms (Figure 52.8) have been used to aid in the differential diagnosis of dysentery symptoms, the more general case definition of 'acute diarrhoea with visible blood in the stools' is the clinical case definition recommended for surveillance.[105] Laboratory isolation and identification of *Shigella* spp. is necessary to confirm the diagnosis and to enable antimicrobial sensitivities to be determined.

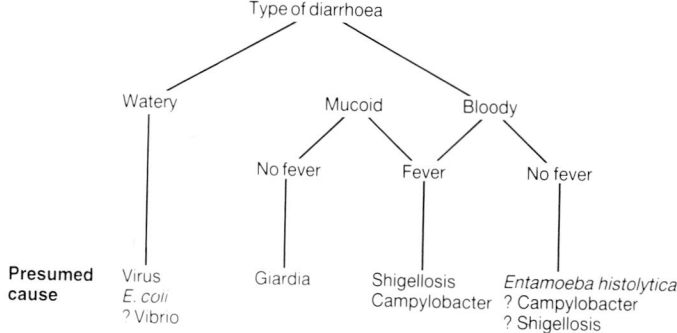

Figure 52.8: Clinical algorithm in the differential diagnosis of diarrhoea.

Shigellae survive poorly in ambient temperatures in the tropics, and if the stool specimen cannot be cultured within a few hours of collection it should be placed in transport medium and stored at +4°C. Cary–Blair medium and buffered glycerol saline (BGS) are the recommended transport media. In the investigation of epidemics, it is more useful to collect specimens from a small number of patients who fit the clinical case definition, and to ensure that these specimens are transported and processed appropriately.

Figure 52.9 shows the World Health Organization (WHO) guidelines for the culture of specimens for isolation and identification of *Shigella* spp. Faecal

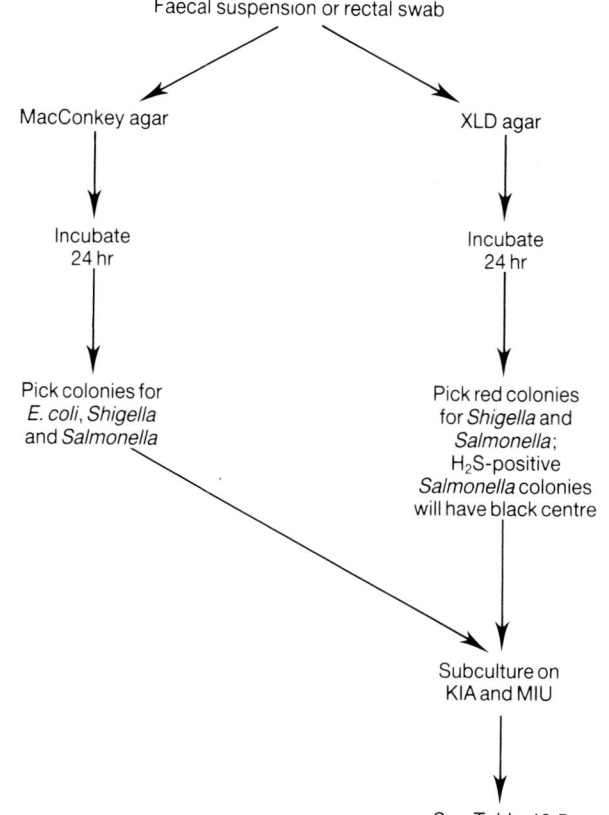

Figure 52.9: Culture protocol for isolation of *Shigella* spp.

Table 52.4 Reactions of *Shigella* spp. on Kligler iron agar (KIA) and motility indole urea (MIU) medium.

Bacterium	Urea	Slant	Butt	H₂S	Gas	Motility	Indole
E. coli	–	A	A	–	+	(+)	d
Sh. dysenteriae	–	K	A	–	–	–	d
Sh. flexneri	–	K	A	–	–[a]	–	d
Sh. boydii	–	K	A	–	–[b]	–	d
Sh. sonnei	–	K	A	–	–	–	–

K, alkaline (red) reaction; A, acid (yellow) reaction; +, positive reaction; –, negative reaction; d, different biochemical types.
[a]Some *Sh. flexneri* serotypes 6 gas (+).
[b]Serotypes 13 and 14 gas (+).

specimens or rectal swabs should be cultured overnight on MacConkey medium and a more selective medium such as xylose–lysine–deoxycholate agar (XLD). Shigellae appear as pale, non-lactose-fermenting colonies on MacConkey medium and as pink colonies on XLD. Suspect colonies are incubated overnight on Kligler iron agar (KIA) and motility indole urea (MIU) medium. Table 52.4 shows the typical reactions of *Shigella* spp. in these composite media. Positive isolates may be typed by slide agglutination using the appropriate *Shigella* antisera. Antimicrobial sensitivities should be determined using a disc diffusion method. It is essential that a standardized technique is used, and the Kirby Bauer-based NCCLS methodology is recommended.[106]

Management

The management of cases of shigellosis requires appropriate rehydration and electrolyte therapy, antimicrobial treatment, and the management of complications. Dehydration is rarely severe; oral rehydration is usually sufficient to restore water and electrolyte imbalances. High-risk patients include children aged less than 5 years, patients who are dehydrated or seriously ill when first seen, and older children and adults who are malnourished. Effective antimicrobial therapy will shorten the duration of illness and is particularly necessary in severe cases. Resistance of *Shigella* spp. to commonly used antimicrobial agents is an increasing problem in many tropical countries and data on local sensitivities are essential if effective treatment is to be implemented.

Resistance of *Sh. dysenteriae* to ampicillin, co-trimoxazole and chloramphenicol is now widespread, and nalidixic acid is the first-line drug of choice in most areas. Treatment should be given for 5 days. Resistance to nalidixic acid is increasing in some areas, leaving only fluoroquinolones such as ciprofloxacin and ofloxacin, and pivmecillinam as effective oral therapies. Several clinical trials have demonstrated the efficacy of short courses of fluoroquinolones, two doses of ofloxacin (total of 15 mg/kg in one study) being effective.[107] Unresolved issues remain over the use of fluoroquinolones in children. While fluoroquinolones may be required in some areas, in most regions the majority of strains remain sensitive to nalidixic acid, and the importance of local sensitivity data cannot be overemphasized.

Maintaining adequate levels of nutrition in patients is an essential component of management, particularly in children, who may already be malnourished. Studies in Bangladesh have shown the value of supportive nutrition in the outcome of children with shigellosis.

Prevention and control

Shigellosis is primarily a disease of crowded and usually poor communities, living in an environment characterized by inadequate sanitation and often polluted water. In the long term, the incidence of shigellosis will be reduced only by improved public health and the alleviation of poverty.

As most transmission is from person to person, improvements in water supply quality alone may have little impact. Most studies show that increased water quantity, and allowing general improvement in the level of hygiene, do reduce the incidence of diarrhoeal disease. Improvement in hygiene at the household level, particularly through the provision of soap for hand washing, has been shown to reduce the transmission of shigellosis.

In epidemics of shigellosis coordinated action will be necessary at the local and regional level in diagnosis, local public health interventions and possibly restrictions on population movements, markets, religious gatherings, etc.

While no effective vaccines to prevent shigellosis are currently available, a number of potential vaccines are under development.[108] Attenuated strains of *Sh. dysenteriae* 1 and *Sh. flexneri* 2a have been developed as candidate oral vaccines, which result in production of antibodies to surface antigens, and recombinant vaccines that express modified shiga toxin determinants are being developed to stimulate specific antitoxin antibodies. For the foreseeable future, however, prevention of morbidity and mortality caused by shigellosis will depend on public health interventions and effective and timely case management.

Cholera

Cholera occurs endemically in many areas of the tropics, particularly in South and South-East Asia and Africa. In 1991, cholera appeared in Latin America for the first time

Table 52.5 The first six cholera pandemics.

Pandemic	Date	Indian subcontinent	South-East Asia	Middle East	Europe	North Africa	East Africa	America
First	1817–1823	+	+	+	–	–	+	–
Second	1826–1837	+	+	+	+	+	+	+
Third	1842–1862	+	+	+	+	+	+	+
Fourth	1865–1875	+	+	+	+	+	+	+
Fifth	1881–1896	+	+	+	+	+	+	+
Sixth	1899–1923	+	+	+	+	–	+	–

in the twentieth century. A cholera-like disease was described by early Indian, Greek and Chinese writers, but it is uncertain whether the disease had spread beyond the Indian subcontinent before the nineteenth century. From 1817 to 1923 there were six pandemics of cholera, spreading extensively from its natural home in the Ganges plain and delta (Table 52.5). The seventh pandemic of cholera, which began in 1961, is described under Epidemiology (see below).

Bacteriology

In 1883, Koch demonstrated the bacterial cause of cholera during a visit to Egypt, and subsequent work defined the species *Vibrio cholerae*. Vibrios are comma-shaped, aerobic, Gram-negative bacteria which have a characteristic darting movement (Figure 52.10). They are oxidase positive, and ferment sucrose and glucose but not lactose. Vibrios possess both flagellar and somatic antigens. The species *V. cholerae* is divided into many serovars according to somatic antigens. Until the appearance of *V. cholerae* serotype O139 in 1992, *V. cholerae* O1 was the only serotype responsible for cholera. Other serovars with different O antigens may cause a diarrhoea-like illness, but are not associated with epidemic cholera. There are two biotypes of *V. cholerae* O1: classical and El Tor. Table 52.6 summarizes their characteristic properties. *V. cholerae* El Tor was first isolated from pilgrims at the El Tor quarantine station in

Sinai in 1906. Until 1961, the El Tor biotype was isolated only in Sulawesi, Indonesia, and had caused four localized epidemics between 1937 and 1958. The classical and El Tor biotypes are each divided into three serotypes: Ogawa, Inaba and Hikojima. *V. cholerae* O139 is related to the El Tor biotype.

V. cholerae does not form spores, is killed by heating at 55°C for 15 minutes and by phenolic and hypochlorite disinfectants. It can survive in saline conditions at low temperatures for up to 60 days, and may survive in aquatic environments for extended periods in a 'dormant state'. Excluding seafoods, *V. cholerae* survives for only a limited time on foodstuffs, although contaminated food may act as a vehicle for transmission. In fish and shellfish, *V. cholerae* may survive from 2 to 5 days at ambient temperatures—a property often associated with food-related outbreaks.

Pathogenesis and immunity

Cholera is characterized by severe watery diarrhoea leading to dehydration, electrolyte imbalance and hypovolaemia, with a mortality rate ranging from less than 1 to 40%.

There is a wide spectrum of severity, and mild and asymptomatic cases may occur. *V. cholerae* is non-invasive; pathogenesis is due to an enterotoxin that causes excessive fluid and electrolyte loss. The initial step in pathogenesis is adherence of the vibrios to the mucosa of the small intestine. Adherence is due to both outer membrane protein and flagellar adhesins. Cholera toxin comprises two subunits: B (binding) and A (active). The B subunit comprises five polypeptides, each of molecular weight 11 500, and binds to specific monosialosyl ganglioside, GM_1 receptors on small intestinal epithelial cells. The A subunit is then able to migrate through the epithelial cell membrane. This subunit has adenosine diphosphate (ADP) ribosyltransferase activity and causes the transfer of ADP ribose from nicotinamide–adenine

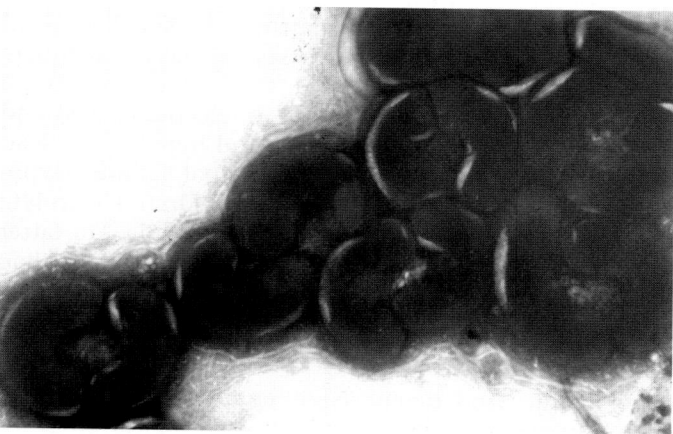

Figure 52.10: Negatively stained electronmicrograph showing numerous 'comma shaped' *Vibrio cholerae*.

Table 52.6 Differentiating properties of classical and El Tor biotypes of *Vibrio cholerae* O1.

	Classical	El Tor
Chicken cell haemagglutination	–	+
Voges–Proskauer test	–	+
Polymyxin B sensitivity	Sensitive	Resistant

dinucleotide (NAD) to a guanosine triphosphate (GTP) binding protein that regulates adenylate cyclase activity. There is a resulting increase in cAMP production which, by inhibiting sodium chloride absorption and stimulating chloride excretion, results in a net loss of water, sodium chloride, potassium and bicarbonate. Additional toxins and other factors are now known to be involved in cholera pathogenesis. Zonula occludens toxin (Zot) increases the permeability of the small intestinal mucosa by affecting the structure of the intercellular tight junctions.[109] Accessory cholera exotoxin (Ace) was described in 1993, and increases transmembrane ion transport. Colonization factors, particularly the pilus colonization factor TCP, are necessary for the adherence of *V. cholerae* to intestinal epithelial cells.

Immunity to both cholera toxin and bacterial surface antigens follows natural infection. Most studies of immune response have measured serum bactericidal antibodies, although protection in vivo is more likely to be mediated by secretory IgA.

Epidemiology

Humans are the only known natural hosts of *V. cholerae*. Transmission is by ingestion, through contaminated water or food. The infective dose is high, up to 10^{11} bacteria being required. The incubation period ranges from a few hours to 5 days.

Serological studies have shown that, in both endemic areas and during outbreaks, for each symptomatic case there may be 5–40 infected but asymptomatic or mildly symptomatic cases. Contamination of water or food may thus occur from symptomatic cases or asymptomatic, transient carriers. Most are free from infection within 2–3 weeks, and there have been few examples of persistent carriage.

V. cholerae O1 can survive for weeks to months in the natural aquatic environment, but there is uncertainty whether this occurs only in relation to frequent contamination by infected persons, or whether *V. cholerae* O1 truly survives as an environmental bacterium. Recent studies have described the occurrence of 'non-culturable' dormant strains, which may persist for long periods in natural aquatic environments.[110] Change from the dormant to a culturable form may be influenced by environmental factors influencing toxin regulatory genes.

There are important epidemiological differences between classical and El Tor *V. cholerae*. For El Tor, the ratio of carriers to cases may range from 30 : 1 to 50 : 1, compared with 5 : 1 for classical infection. El Tor can also survive for longer periods in the environment. These factors give El Tor an epidemiological advantage in the spread of the disease, which has occurred in the seventh pandemic and has contributed to the displacement of the classical type by El Tor. Only in parts of southern Bangladesh has the classical biotype persisted.[111]

The seventh pandemic of cholera began in 1961, originating on the island of Sulawesi in Indonesia. The pandemic strain was *V. cholerae* O1 El Tor, and it spread rapidly to countries of South-East Asia. Between 1963 and 1969 the pandemic spread to the Indian subcontinent, displacing the classical biotype, and by 1970 had reached the Middle East. The pandemic entered Africa by two routes, in West Africa probably by a returning traveller, and from the Arabian peninsula, through Djibouti into East Africa. By 1978, most countries of central and southern Africa were affected. The final stage of the pandemic was the arrival of cholera in the South American continent in January 1991, the first time that cholera had entered the continent since the fifth pandemic in the 1880s.

V. cholerae O139 was first isolated in south India in 1992. It was designated O139 as it did not agglutinate with O1 antisera, nor with antisera to any of the 137 other known non-cholera-producing serotypes of *V. cholerae*. During 1992–1994 *V. cholerae* O139 spread to Bangladesh, where for some time it was the dominant serotype, and now both serotypes coexist.

The largest epidemics of cholera since the middle 1990s have been in Africa, partly associated with mass refugee movements in central Africa, but also in eastern and southern regions. In 1994, the largest proportion of all cholera cases globally, and 42% of all cholera deaths were in Africa. This was largely due to the explosive epidemic in Rwandan refugees displaced to the eastern region of the Democratic Republic of the Congo (DRC; formerly Zaire), where over a 6-week period there were an estimated 70 000 cases and up to 12 000 deaths.[112] A pandemic has continued in this central area of Africa, with localized epidemics in DRC, Burundi, Tanzania and Congo Brazzaville. In East Africa, excessive rains and flooding in 1997 were followed by extensive outbreaks of cholera in Somalia and northern Kenya. Beginning in August 2000 there has been an extensive outbreak in Kwazulu-Natal in South Africa, with over 75 000 cases reported by March 2001.

Clinical features

The clinical picture of infection with *V. cholerae* O1 may range from mild diarrhoea to severe dehydration with death occurring within hours. In most cases there is progress from the onset of diarrhoea to shock in 4–12 hours, with death following in several days if adequate management is not instituted. The symptoms are a reflection of the severe dehydration, electrolyte loss and metabolic acidosis. Hypovolaemia and hypotension lead to impaired consciousness and to renal failure. Hypoglycaemia may occur, particularly in children. Electrolyte loss leads to hyponatraemia and hypokalaemia. The latter may result in ileus, muscle weakness and cardiac arrhythmias.

Diagnosis

In epidemics the diagnosis of cholera may be made presumptively on clinical and epidemiological grounds. The WHO clinical case definition for suspected cholera or 'acute watery diarrhoea' is 'a patient 5 years of age or older, who develops acute watery diarrhoea with or without vomiting', with the caveat that it is in an area where cholera is likely to occur. Laboratory diagnosis may be required when sporadic cases occur, and when an extensive outbreak requires confirmation and typing of the aetiological agent. Dark-field microscopy of faecal specimens may show the characteristic darting movement of the vibrios. Inhibition of movement by addition of diluted O1 antisera to the slide will provide strong evidence that *V. cholerae* O1 is the causative agent. To confirm the diagnosis, specimens need to be cultured on a selective medium, such as thiosulphate citrate bile salt sucrose (TCBS) agar. Specimens should be transported from the field in alkaline peptone water or Cary–Blair transport medium and kept cool. *V. cholerae* O1 yields yellow oxidase-positive colonies after overnight incubation on TCBS, which may be confirmed by slide agglutination specific with antiserum. In outbreak investigations, isolates should be sent to a reference laboratory for biotyping and serotyping. Sensitivity to tetracycline and other antimicrobial agents should be performed on a selected number of isolates. Where detailed epidemiological data are required, molecular methods have been used to distinguish different strains.[113]

Case management

The successful management of cholera cases relies on adequate and appropriate rehydration and restoration of electrolyte balance. Except in the most severe cases, oral replacement solutions may be used. Oral solutions are based on the role of glucose enhancing the active uptake of sodium and water. As glucose is rarely available in rural areas, sucrose and rice water-based solutions have been used with success.[114] The volume of replacement will depend on the degree of dehydration and the rate of continuing fluid loss. The composition of oral and intravenous rehydration solutions are given in Table 52.7. WHO guidelines[113] provide detailed protocols for rehydration and fluid maintenance. Severe dehydration is characterised by 10% or more loss of body weight, lethargy or impaired consciousness, hypovolaemic shock and acidosis. In such patients rapid intravenous rehydration is necessary, using a large-bore needle and multiple sites if necessary, aiming to restore normal hydration and acid–base balance within 2–3 hours. Fifty per cent losses should be replaced in the first 30–45 minutes, at a rate of 30 ml/kg, requiring 1–2 litres in adults. Rehydration should then be slowed to 1 litre per 30–45 minutes until normal hydration is achieved.

Once rehydration is achieved, the maintenance phase requires the replacement of continuing stool losses. In the severely ill patient this may require continuing intravenous therapy for some time, but in most cases oral rehydration using WHO or other rehydration solution is appropriate. Fluid replacement should be in the ratio of 1.5 volumes of oral fluid for each volume of stool, usually 100–200 ml in children, and for adults fluid intake should be encouraged as required. Moderate dehydration, characterized by 5% loss of body weight, clinical dehydration (poor skin turgor, etc.) but no acidosis or shock requires oral or intravenous rehydration initially, followed by oral maintenance. In adults 2–4 litres of ORS may be required in the first 4 hours to ensure rehydration.

Potential complications in severely ill patients on presentation and during intravenous therapy include renal failure, hypoglycaemia, particularly in children and in prolonged dehydration, hypokalaemia and ileus, and pulmonary oedema during rapid intravenous therapy when the metabolic acidosis has not been corrected, which is more likely when normal saline alone is used for rehydration. Hypokalaemia may occur during the maintenance phase, but should be uncommon if potassium-containing oral fluids are used.

Antimicrobial agents have been shown to shorten the period of diarrhoea and the amount of fluid loss. Tetracycline or doxycycline is the drug of choice in adults where strains are sensitive, but the increasing occurrence of resistant strains limits their usefulness. Co-trimoxazole and furazolidone have been used, but antibiotics are secondary to the importance of early rehydration.

Prevention and control

Cholera is transmitted by the faecal–oral route through the contamination of water or food, hence public health measures to improve water and sanitation are essential for long-term control. The management of outbreaks is based on interrupting transmission, appropriate control and management of cases and contacts, and effective surveillance. In most cholera outbreaks the source and routes of transmission are not obvious and general sanitary measures will need to be imposed. These may include chlorination of water supplies, the boiling of water at household level, and construction and maintenance of temporary latrines. Action will need to be taken to control the cleanliness of markets, and to postpone festivals and gatherings. Adequate, although basic, sanitation facilities must be made for disposal of faeces from cases during treatment.

Table 52.7 Composition of rehydration solutions.

	Composition (mmol/l)				
	Na	Cl	K	Bicarbonate	Glucose
Ringer's	130	109	4	28	0
Dhaka	133	98	13	48	0
WHO ORS	90	80	20	30	111

The most appropriate group for chemoprophylaxis are household contacts of cases. The relatively high carriage rate of *V. cholerae* in this group has been described previously. Assuming strains are sensitive, tetracycline or doxycycline may be used in adults. For doxycycline a single oral dose of 300 mg is adequate.

The formerly used killed whole-cell vaccines, given parenterally, have no useful role to play in the management or prevention of cholera: individual protection does not exceed 50–60%; vaccination does not reduce excretion of vibrios and is likely to give a false sense of security to both the affected population and the authorities during outbreaks.

Effective surveillance is an essential component of cholera control. Active reporting of suspected cases in areas previously uninfected, with appropriate bacteriological confirmation, will allow the early introduction of the control measures described above. At the international level, systematic reporting of cases to the WHO and its collaborative bodies will help to coordinate the international response and limit spread between countries.

Cholera vaccines

While the formerly used killed whole-cell vaccine given parenterally was of only limited efficacy, new oral vaccines are being developed. The principle of these vaccines is to give an oral vaccine providing both somatic (O antigen) and B-subunit toxin immunity in the gut. Two main strategies have been used. The killed whole-cell/B-subunit vaccine (WC/BS) is a two-dose oral vaccine given 1 week apart. Studies in Bangladesh and South America[115] have demonstrated its safety and efficacy

against both classical and El Tor *V. cholerae* O1. The second strategy has been to develop a genetically modified *V. cholerae* strain, deficient in the gene for the A-subunit of cholera toxin, CVD-103 HgR. There have been only limited field studies with this vaccine. The WC/BS vaccine is used in some cases for travellers but is unlikely to have a role as a public health intervention in cholera-endemic areas. Trials of a locally produced killed whole-cell vaccine, containing both O1 and O139 *V. cholerae*, have been implemented in Vietnam.[116] Results suggest that in selected areas such a strategy may be beneficial. Recent recommendations[117] have suggested there may be role for the WC/BS vaccine among refugee and displaced populations in areas at risk for cholera, although as a preventive rather than a control measure.

Non-cholera vibrios

Vibrio species other than *V. cholerae* O1 and O139 may cause diarrhoeal diseases in the tropics but are rarely associated with extensive outbreaks. Five species have been associated with diarrhoeal diseases: *V. cholerae* non-O1, *V. parahaemolyticus*, *V. fluvialis*, *V. hollisae* and *V. mimicus*. Among *V. cholerae* O1 strains, some have been isolated that are non-toxigenic but cause diarrhoea. They have been isolated from 1–3% of patients admitted to the cholera hospital in Dhaka, Bangladesh. *V. parahaemolyticus* is principally associated with seafoods. *V. fluvialis* has been implicated in an outbreak of diarrhoeal disease in Bangladesh. Few data are currently available on the prevalence of these vibrios in most tropical countries.

REFERENCES

1   Marshall B J, Royce H & Annear D I. Original isolation of *Campylobacter pyloridis* from human gastric mucosa. *Microbiol Lett* 1985; 25:83–88.

2   Peterson W I. *Helicobacter pylori* and peptic ulcer disease. *N Engl J Med* 1991; 321:1043–1048.

3   Hart C A, Murray A E & Walker S J. *Helicobacter pylori* and gastritis. *Postgrad Doctor* 1990; 6:60–66.

4   Sullivan P B, Thomas J E, Wight D G D et al. *Helicobacter pylori* in Gambian children with chronic diarrhoea and malnutrition. *Arch Dis Child* 1990; 65:189–191.

5   Klein P D, Graham D Y, Gaillour A, Opekun A R & O'Brien Smith E. Water source as risk factor for *Helicobacter pylori* infection in Peruvian children. *Lancet* 1991; 337:1503–1506.

6   Megraud F, Brassen-Rabbe M P, Denis F, Belbouri A & Hoa D Q. Seroepidemiology of *Campylobacter pylori* infections in various populations. *J Clin Microbiol* 1989; 27:1870–1873.

7   Brown L M. *Helicobacter pylori*: epidemiology and routes of transmission. *Epidemiol Rev* 2000; 22:283–297.

8   Hildebrand P, Meyer-Wyss B M, Mossi S & Bellinger C. Risk among gastroenterologists of acquiring *Helicobacter pylori* infection: a case–control study. *BMJ* 2000; 321:149.

9   Lee A, Fox J G, Otto G et al. Transmission of *Helicobacter* spp. A challenge to the dogma of faecal–oral spread. *Epidemiol Infect* 1991; 107:99–109.

10 Dominici P, Bellentani S, Di Biase A R et al. Familial clustering of *Helicobacter pylori* infection: population based study. *BMJ* 1999; 319:537–541.

11 Goodman K J & Correa P. Transmission of *Helicobacter pylori* among siblings. *Lancet* 2000; 355:358–362.

12 Song Q, Spahr A, Schmid R M et al. *Helicobacter pylori* in the oral cavity: high prevalence and great DNA diversity. *Dig Dis Sci* 2000; 45:2162–2167.

13 Grubel P, Huang L, Masubuchi N et al. Detection of *Helicobacter pylori* DNA in houseflies (*Musca domestica*) on three continents. *Lancet* 1998; 352:788–789.

14 Blaser M J. *Helicobacter pylori* and the pathogenesis of gastroduodenal inflammation. *J Infect Dis* 1990; 161:626–633.

15 Drumm B. *Helicobacter pylori*. *Arch Dis Child* 1990; 65:1278–1282.

16 Peek R M. Microbes and microbial toxins IV. *Helicobacter pylori* strain specific activation of signal transduction cascades related to gastric inflammation. *Am J Physiol Gastrointest Liver Physiol* 2001; 280:G525–G530.

17 Rouvroy D, Bogaerts J, Nsengiumwa O et al. *Campylobacter pylori* gastritis and peptic ulcer disease in central Africa. *BMJ* 1987; 295:1174.

18 Harries A D, Stewart M, Deegan M K et al. *Helicobacter pylori* in Malawi, Central Africa. *J Infect* 1992; 24:269–276.

19 Wyatt J I, Rathbone B J, Sobala G M et al. Gastric epithelium in the duodenum. Its association with *Helicobacter pylori* and inflammation. *J Clin Pathol* 1990; 43:981–986.

20 Vaira D, Malfertheiner P, Megraud F et al. Diagnosis of *Helicobacter pylori* infection with a new non-invasive antigen-based assay. *Lancet* 1999; 354:30–33.

21 Oderda G, Rapa A, Ronchi B et al. Detection of *Helicobacter pylori* in stool specimens by non-invasive antigen enzyme immunoassay in children: multicentre Italian study. *BMJ* 2000; 320:347–348.

22 McKinlay A W. Antibiotics in the treatment of peptic ulcer disease. *J Antimicrob Chemother* 1992: 29:92–96.

23 Rauws E A J & Tytgat G N J. Care of duodenal ulcer associated with eradication of *Helicobacter pylori*. *Lancet* 1990; 335:1233–1235.

24 de Boer W A & Tytgat G N J. Treatment of *Helicobacter pylori* infection. *BMJ* 2000; 320:31–34.

25 Hill I D, Sinclair-Smith C, Lastovica A J et al. Transient protein-losing enteropathy associated with acute gastritis and *Campylobacter pylori*. *Arch Dis Child* 1987; 62:1215–1219.

26 Shahinian M, Passaro D J, Swerdlow D L et al. *Helicobacter pylori* and epidemic *Vibrio cholerae* 01 infection in Peru. *Lancet* 2000; 355:377–378.

27 Hoffmeister A, Rothenbacher D, Bode G et al. Current infection with *Helicobacter pylori* but not seropositivity to *Chlamydia pneumoniae* or cytomegalovirus is associated with an atherogenic, modified lipid profile. *Arterioscler Thromb Vasc Biol* 2001; 21:427–432.

28 Moyenuddin M, Rahman K M & Sack D A. The aetiology of diarrhoea in children at an urban hospital in Bangladesh. *Trans R Soc Trop Med Hyg* 1987; 81:299–302.

29 Bray J & Beavan T E D. Slide agglutination of *Bact. coli* neapolitanum in summer diarrhoea. *J Pathol* 1948; 60:395–401.

30 Neter E. Enteritis due to enteropathogenic *Escherichia coli*. Present day status and unsolved problems. *J Pediatr* 1959; 55:223–239.

31 Guerrant R C, Kirchhoff L V, Nations M K et al. Prospective study of diarrhoeal illness in north eastern Brazil. *J Infect Dis* 1983; 148:986–987.

32 Black R E, Merson M H, Rahman A S M M et al. A two year study of bacterial viral and parasitic agents associated with diarrhoea in rural Bangladesh. *J Infect Dis* 1980; 142:660–665.

33 Merson M H, Sack R B, Islam S et al. Disease due to enterotoxigenic *E. coli* in Bangladesh adults. Clinical aspects and a controlled trial of tetracycline. *J Infect Dis* 1980; 141:702–711.

34 DuPont H L, Reves R R, Galindo E et al. Treatment of traveller's diarrhoea with trimethoprim/sulfamethoxazole and trimethoprim alone. *N Engl J Med* 1982; 307:841–844.

35 Peltola H, Siitonen A, Kryonseppa H et al. Prevention of traveller's diarrhoea by oral B-subunit/whole cell cholera vaccine. *Lancet* 1991; 338:1258–1289.

36 Taylor D N, Echeverria P, Sethabutr O et al. Clinical and microbiologic features of *Shigella* and enteroinvasive *Escherichia coli* infections detected by DNA hybridization. *J Clin Microbiol* 1988; 26:1362–1366.

37 Pal T, Pasca S, Emody L & Voros S. Antigenic relationship among virulent enteroinvasive *Escherichia coli*, *Shigella flexneri* and *Shigella sonnei* detected by ELISA. *Lancet* 1983; ii:102.

38 Levine M M, Berquist E J, Nalin D R et al. *Escherichia coli* strains that cause diarrhoea but do not produce heat-labile or heat-stable enterotoxins and are non-invasive. *Lancet* 1978; i:1119–1122.

39 Edelman R & Levine M M. Summary of a workshop on enteropathogenic *Escherichia coli*. *J Infect Dis* 1983; 147:1108–1118.

40 Echeverria P, Taylor D N, Bettelheim K A et al. HeLa cell-adherent enteropathogenic *Escherichia coli* in children under 1 year of age in Thailand. *J Clin Microbiol* 1987; 25:1472–1475.

41 Senerwa D, Olsvik O, Mutanda L N et al. Enteropathogenic *Escherichia coli* serotype O111:HNT isolated from preterm neonates in Nairobi Kenya. *J Clin Microbiol* 1989; 27:1307–1311.

42 Vallance B A & Finlay B B. Exploitation of host cells by enteropathogenic *Escherichia coli*. *Proc Natl Acad Sci USA* 2000; 97:8799–8806.

43 Embaye H, Batt R M, Saunders J R et al. Interaction of enteropathogenic *Escherichia coli*: O111 with rabbit intestinal mucosa in vitro. *Gastroenterology* 1989; 96:1079–1086.

44 Embaye H, Hart C A, Getty B et al. Effects of enteropathogenic *Escherichia coli* on microvillar membrane proteins during organ culture of rabbit intestinal mucosa. *Gut* 1992; 33:1184–1189.

45 Taylor C J, Hart C A, Batt R M et al. Ultrastructural and biochemical changes in human jejunal mucosa associated with enteropathogenic *Escherichia coli* (O111) infection. *J Pediatr Gastroenterol Nutr* 1986; 5:70–73.

46 Rothbaum R, McAdams A J, Giannella R & Partin J C. A clinicopathologic study of enterocyte-adherent *Escherichia coli*: a cause of protracted diarrhoea in infants. *Gastroenterology* 1982; 83:441–454.

47 Jerse A E, Yu J, Tall B D & Kaper J B. A genetic locus of enteropathogenic *Escherichia coli* necessary for the production of attaching and effacing lesions on tissue culture cells. *Proc Natl Acad Sci USA* 1990; 87:7839–7843.

48 Riley L W, Remis R J, Helgerson S D et al. Hemorrhagic colitis associated with a rare *Escherichia coli* serotype. *N Engl J Med* 1983; 308:681–685.

49 Karmali M A, Steele B T, Petric M & Lim C. Sporadic cases of haemolytic uraemic syndrome associated with faecal cytoxin-producing *Escherichia coli*. *Lancet* 1983; i:619–620.

50 Karmali M A. Infection by verocytoxin-producing *Escherichia coli*. *Clin Microbiol Rev* 1989; 2:15–38.

51 Bettelheim K A, Brown J E, Lolekha S & Echeverria P. Serotype of *Escherichia coli* that hybridized with DNA probes for genes encoding shiga-like toxin I, shiga-like toxin II and serogroup O157 enterohaemorrhagic *E. coli* fimbriae isolated from adults with diarrhoea in Thailand. *J Clin Microbiol* 1990; 28:293–295.

52 Isaacsons M, Canter P H, Effler P et al. Haemorrhagic colitis epidemic in Africa. *Lancet* 1993; 341:961.

53 Cunin P, Tedjouka E, Germani Y et al. An epidemic of bloody diarrhea: *Escherichia coli* emerging in Cameroon. *Emerg Infect Dis* 1999; 5:285–290.

54 Roe A J & Gally D J. Enteropathogenic and enterohaemorrhagic *Escherichia coli* and diarrhoea. *Curr Opin Infect Dis* 2000; 13:511–517.

55 Kishore K, Rattan A, Bagga A et al. Serum antibodies to verotoxin-producing *Escherichia coli* (VTEC) strains in patients with haemolytic uraemic syndrome. *J Med Microbiol* 1993; 37:364–367.

56 Chart H, Smith H R, Scotland S M et al. Serological identification of *Escherichia coli* O157: H7 infection in haemolytic uraemic syndrome. *Lancet* 1991; 337:138–140.

57 Kimmitt P T, Harwood C R & Barer M R. Toxin gene expression by shiga toxin-producing *Escherichia coli*: the role of antibiotics and the bacterial SOS response. *Emerg Infect Dis* 2000; 6:458–465.

58 Nataro J P, Steiner T & Guerrant R L. Enteroaggregative *Escherichia coli*. *Emerg Infect Dis* 1998; 4:251–261.

59 Bhan M K, Raj P, Levine M M et al. Enteroaggregative *Escherichia coli* associated with persistent diarrhoea in a cohort of rural children in India. *J Infect Dis* 1989; 159:1062–1064.

60 Steiner T S, Lima A A M, Nataro J P et al. Enteroaggregative *Escherichia coli* produce intestinal inflammation and growth impairment and cause interleukin-8 release from intestinal epithelial cells. *J Infect* 1998; 177:88–96.

61 Dutta S, Pal S, Chakrabarti S et al. Use of PCR to identify enteroaggregative *Escherichia coli* as an important cause of acute diarrhoea among children living in Calcutta, India. *J Med Microbiol* 1999; 48:1011–1016.

62 Butzler J P, Dekeyser P, Detrain M & Dehaen F. Related vibrio in stools. *J Pediatr* 1973; 82:493–496.

63 Skirrow M B. *Campylobacter* enteritis: a 'new' disease. *BMJ* 1977; ii:9–11.

64 Potter M E, Blaser M J, Sikes R K et al. Human *Campylobacter* infection associated with certified raw milk. *Am J Epidemiol* 1983; 117:475–483.

65 Korlath J A, Osterholm M T, Judy L A et al. A point source outbreak of campylobacteriosis associated with consumption of raw milk. *J Infect Dis* 1985; 152:592–596.

66 Southern J P, Smith R M M & Palmer S R. Bird attack on milk bottles: possible mode of transmission of *Campylobacter jejuni* to man. *Lancet* 1990; 336:1425–1427.

67 Rajan D P & Mathan V I. Prevalence of *Campylobacter fetus* subsp. *jejuni* in healthy populations in India. *J Clin Microbiol* 1982; 15:729–751.

68 Altekruse S F, Stern N J, Fields P J et al. *Campylobacter jejuni* – an emerging foodborne pathogen. *Emerg Infect Dis* 1999; 5:28–35.

69 Glass R I, Stoll B J, Juq M I et al. Epidemiologic and clinical features of endemic *Campylobacter jejuni* infection in Bangladesh. *J Infect Dis* 1983; 148:292–296.

70 Black R F, Levine M M, Brown K H et al. Immunity to *Campylobacter jejuni* in man. In Pearson D A, Skirrow M B, Lior H & Rowe B (eds) *Campylobacter III*. London: Public Health Laboratory Service, 1985:129.

71 Butzler J P & Skirrow M B. *Campylobacter* enteritis. *Clin Gastroenterol* 1979; 8:737–765.

72 Cover T L & Aber R C. *Yersinia enterocolitica*. *N Engl J Med* 1989; 321:16–24.

73 Gomes T A T, Rassi V, MacDonald K C et al. Enteropathogens associated with acute diarrhoeal disease in urban infants in Sao Paulo, Brazil. *J Infect Dis* 1991; 164:331–337.

74 Rabson A R, Hallett A F & Koornhof H J. Generalized *Yersinia enterocolitica* infection. *J Infect Dis* 1975; 131:447–451.

75 Awunor-Renner C & Lawande R V. *Yersinia* and chronic glomerulopathy in the savannah region of Nigeria. *BMJ* 1982; 285:1464–1465.

76 Pai C H, Gillis F, Tuomanen E & Marks M I. Placebo-controlled doubled-blind evaluation of trimethoprim sulfamethoxazole treatment of *Yersinia enterocolitica* gastroenteritis. *J Pediatr* 1984; 104:308–311.

77 Jeckeln E. Uber 'Darmbrand': das pathologisch antatomische Bild des Darmbrandes. *Dtsch Med Wochenschr* 1947; 11:105.

78 Murrell T G C, Roth L, Egerton J, Samels J & Walker P D. Pigbel: enteritis necroticans. A study in diagnosis and management. *Lancet* 1966; i:217–222.

79 Foster W D. The bacteriology of necrotising jejunitis in Uganda. *East Afr Med J* 1966; 45:550.

80 Shann F, Lawrence G & Jun-Bi P. Enteritis necroticans in China. *Lancet* 1979; i:1083–1084.

81 Gupta S C, Mishra V, Mishra S P et al. Necrotizing enteritis stimulating pig-bel disease in northern India. *Indian J Gastroenterol* 1994; 13:109–111.

82 Lawrence G & Walker P D. Pathogenesis of enteritis necroticans in Papua New Guinea. *Lancet* 1976; i:125–126.

83 Lawrence G, Brown R, Baters J et al. An affinity technique for isolation of *Clostridium perfringens* type C from man and pigs in Papua New Guinea. *J Appl Bacteriol* 1984; 57:333–338.

84 Lawrence G, Shann F, Freestone D S & Walker P D. Prevention of necrotising enteritis in Papua New Guinea by active immunization. *Lancet* 1979; i:227–230.

85 Griffin G E. *Clostridium difficile*. In Farthing M J G & Keusch G T (eds) *Enteric Infections*. London: Chapman & Hall, 1989: 327–336.

86 Ljungh A & Wadstrom T. *Aeromonas* and *Plesiomonas*. In Farthing M J G & Keusch G (eds) *Enteric infections*. London: Chapman & Hall, 1989: 169–181.

87 Echeverria P, Seriwatana, J, Taylor D N et al. A comparative study of enterotoxigenic *Escherichia coli*, *Shigella*, *Aeromonas* and *Vibrios* as etiologies of diarrhoea in north eastern Thailand. *Am J Trop Med Hyg* 1985; 34:547–554.

88 Vandepitte J, VanDamme L, Fofana Y & Desmyter J. *Edwardsiella tarda* et *Plesiomonas shigelloides*: leur rôle comme agents de diarrhées et leur épidémiologie. *Bull Soc Pathol Exot* 1980; 73:139–149.

89 Sakazaki R, Tamura K, Prescott L M et al. Bacteriological examination of diarrhoeal stools in Calcutta. *Indian J Med Res* 1971; 59:1025–1034.

90 Davis W A, Chretien J H, Gargarusi V F & Goldstein M A. Snake to human transmission of *Aeromonas (Pl.) shigelloides* resulting in gastroenteritis. *South Med J* 1978; 71:474–476.

91 Bennish M L. Potential lethal complications of shigellosis. *Rev Infect Dis* 1991; 13 (Supplement 4):S319–324.

92 Taylor D N, Bodhidatta L & Echeverria P. Epidemiological aspects of shigellosis and other causes of dysentery in Thailand. *Rev Infect Dis* 1991; 13 (Supplement 4):S231–237.

93 Ahmed F, Clemens J D, Rao M R et al. Epidemiology of shigellosis among children exposed to cases of *Shigella* dysentery: a multivariate analysis. *Am J Trop Med Hyg* 1997; 56:258–264.

94 Nathoo K J, Porteous J E, Siziya S et al. Predictors of mortality in children hospitalized with dysentery in Harare, Zimbabwe. *Cent Afr J Med* 1998;44:272–276.

95 Litwin C M, Stom A L, Chipowsky S & Ryan K J. Molecular epidemiology of *Shigella* infections: plasmid profiles, serotype correlation, and restriction endonuclease analysis. *J Clin Microbiol* 1991; 29:104–108.

96 Lindberg A A, Karnell A & Weibtraub A. The lipopolysaccharide of *Shigella* bacteria as a virulence factor. *Rev Infect Dis* 1991; 13 (Supplement 4):S279–284.

97 Usman J, Aziz S, Karamat K A & Butt T. *Shigella* septicaemia in an infant. *J Pak Med Assoc* 1997; 47:150–151.

98 Boyce J M, Hughes J M, Alim A R et al. Patterns of *Shigella* infections in families in rural Bangladesh. *Am J Trop Med Hyg* 1982; 31:1015–1020.

99 Hassain M A, Albert J M & Hassan K Z. Epidemiology of shigellosis in Teknaf, a coastal region of Bangladesh: a 10 year survey. *Epidemiol Infect* 1990; 105:41–49.

100 Mache A, Mengistu Y & Cowley C. *Shigella* serogroups identified from adult diarrhoeal patients in Addis Ababa: antibiotic resistance and plasmid profile analysis. *East Afr Med J* 1997; 74:179–182.

101 Milleliri J M, Soares J L, Signoret J et al. Epidemic of bacillary dysentery in the Rwanda refugee camps of the Goma region (Zaire, North Kivu) in August 1994. *Ann Soc Belg Med Trop* 1995; 75:201–210.

102 Ries A A, Wells J G, Olivola D et al. Epidemic *Shigella dysenteriae* type 1 in Burundi: panresistance and implications for prevention. *J Infect Dis* 1994; 169:1035–1041.

103 Karas J A, Pillay D G, Naicker T & Sturm A W. Laboratory surveillance of *Shigella dysenteriae* type 1 in KwaZulu-Natal. *S Afr Med J* 1999; 89:59–63.

104 Bhimma R, Rollins N C, Coovadia H M & Adhikari M. Post dysenteric haemolytic uraemic syndrome in children during an epidemic of *Shigella* dysentery in KwaZulu-Natal. *Paediatr Nephrol* 1997; 11:560–564.

105 World Health Organization. *Recommended surveillance standards*. WHO/CDS/CDR/ISR 99.2. Geneva: WHO, 1999.

106 National Committee for Clinical Laboratory Standards. *Performance standards for antimicrobial disc susceptibility tests*, 6th edn. NCCLS document M2-A6,1997. Wayne, PA: NCCLS.

107 Vinh H, Wain J, Chinh M T et al. Treatment of bacillary dysentery in Vietnamese children: two doses of ofloxacin versus 5-days nalidixic acid. *Trans R Soc Trop Med Hyg* 2000; 94:323–326.

108 Weekly Epidemiological Record. Vaccine research and development. New strategies for accelerating *Shigella* vaccine development. *Wkly Epidemiol Rec* 1997; 72:73–79.

109 Colombo M M, Mastrandrea S, Santoni A et al. Distribution of ace zot and ctx-a toxin genes in clinical and environmental *Vibrio cholerae*. *J Infect Dis* 1994; 88:298–299.

110 Islam M S, Miah M A , Hassan M K et al. Detection of non-culturable *Vibrio cholerae* 01 associated with a cyanobacterium from an aquatic environment in Bangladesh. *Trans R Soc Trop Med Hyg* 1994; 88:298–299.

111 Siddique A K, Baqui A H, Eusof A et al. Survival of classic cholera in Bangladesh. *Lancet* 1991; i:1125–1127.

112 Goma Epidemiology Group. Public health impact of Rwandan refugee crisis: what happened in Goma, Zaire in July 1994. *Lancet* 1995; i :339–344.

113 World Health Organization. *Guidelines for Cholera Control.* WHO/CDD/SER/80.4. Geneva: WHO, 1993.

114 Patra F C, Mahalanbis D, Jalan K V et al. Is oral rice-water electrolyte solution superior to glucose electrolyte solution in infantile diarrhoea? *Arch Dis Child* 1982; 57:910–912.

115 Clemens J D, Sack D A, Harris J R et al. Field trial of oral cholera vaccines in Bangladesh: results of a three year follow up. *Lancet* 1990; 335:270–273.

116 Trach D D, Clemens J D, Ke N T et al. Field trial of a locally produced, killed oral cholera vaccine in Viet Nam. *Lancet* 1997; 349:231–235.

117 World Health Organization. *Potential use of oral cholera vaccines in emergency situations. Report of a WHO meeting.* WHO/CDS/CSR/EDC/99.4. Geneva: WHO, 1999.

Chapter 53
Salmonella Infections

S. Gillespie

Bacteriology

The genus *Salmonella* is part of the family of Enterobacteacieae (see Chapter 10). There is only a single species in the genus *Salmonella enterica* of which there are seven subtypes: *enterica, salamae, arizonae, diarizonae, houtenae,* and *Salmonella bongori*.[1-4] Serovars are given names that are often written as if they are different species, e.g., *Salmonella typhimurium* when strictly speaking they should be described as *Salmonella enterica* subsp. *enterica* serotype Typhimurium. There are more than 2000 different serovars and these include organisms that typically cause localized enteritis and organisms such as *S. enterica* subsp. *enterica* serotype Typhi that causes the systemic infectious disease. The serotypes are defined on the basis of the somatic O—the lipopolysaccharide and flagellar H antigens (see below).

The serotypes of *enterica* subspecies account for most human and warmblooded animal infections. These serotypes are grouped on the basis of sharing of a common O antigen (Kaufmann–White scheme).[2] Examples of commonly occurring groups of *enterica* subspecies serotypes are given in Table 53.1. In this chapter the familiar (although taxonomically outdated approach to naming) will be used.

Table 53.1 Some examples of commonly occuring *Salmonella* serotypes and the groups to which they belong

Group	Serotype
A	*S. parartyphi* A
B	*S. paratyphi* B
	S. stanley
	S. saintpaul
	S. agona
	S. typhimurium
C	*S. paratyphi* C
	S. cholerae-suis
	S. virchow
	S. thompson
D	*S. typhi*
	S. enteritidis
	S. dublin
	S. gallinarum

Further differentiation of strains within individual serotypes by bacteriophage typing and DNA fingerprinting helps epidemiological investigations.

On the basis of host preference and disease manifestations in man, the salmonellae can be conveniently placed into two broad categories:

- *S. typhi, S. paratyphi* A, *S. paratyphi* B and *S. paratyphi* C. These serotypes are primarily host-adapted to man and cause a bacteraemic illness also known as enteric fever in which diarrhoea rarely plays a major role.
- Other serotypes. These are host-adapted to animals, and infection in man is usually confined to the bowel and presents as acute diarrhoea, but sometimes causes life-threatening bacteraemia.

Typhoid and paratyphoid fevers or enteric fever

Typhoid fever was so named because its symptoms and signs resembled typhus. The confusion between the two was resolved only with the publication in 1850 of William Jenner's book *On the Identity and Non-Identity of Typhoid and Typhus Fevers*.[5]

Epidemiology

Typhoid and paratyphoid fevers are endemic in the Indian subcontinent, South-East and Far-East Asia, the Middle East, Africa, Central and South America. A low level of endemicity also exists for paratyphoid B infections in the southern and eastern parts of Europe. In the rest of Europe, North America and Australasia enteric fevers occur almost exclusively as imported infections. Paratyphoid C is rare, with occasional cases in Guyana and eastern Europe.[6]

Transmission

Typhoid is an exclusively human disease and the organisms that are responsible for infection are transmitted through food or water contaminated with faeces or urine of a patient or carrier. Paratyphoid infections are less often water-borne because they need a higher infective dose which is unlikely to be found in water as multiplication does not occur. Raw fruit and vegetables are important vehicles in some countries where human faeces are used as a fertilizer or where contaminated water is used to make fruit look attractive in the market. Shellfish harvested in coastal water polluted by raw sewage may cause outbreaks.[3,6]

Pathogenesis

Natural infection in enteric fever is by ingestion, followed by penetration through the intestinal mucosa. Disease production is dependent on several factors: number of organisms swallowed; state of gastric acidity; and possession of Vi antigen by the organisms. The infecting dose of *S. typhi* needs to be large to produce illness in healthy individuals. In volunteers, a dose of 10^9 organisms induced disease in most (95%) but a dose of 10^3 rarely did so. Some 25% of the volunteers became ill after ingesting 10^5 organisms.[7] Possession of Vi antigen is linked with increased infectivity: Vi antigen-positive strains caused illness more commonly than non-Vi variants in healthy volunteers.[7] Gastric acidity is an important defence against enteric infections, and gastric hypoacidity from any cause (e.g., antacids, H2 antagonists) will allow a greater number of organisms to enter the small intestine.[8] Also the infective dose is reduced if it comes in food where the organisms are protected from gastric acid. Once in the small intestine, the organisms penetrate rapidly through the intestinal mucosa, and this process is described in more detail below. Organisms multiply in the lumen for a short period and stools can be culture positive during the first 4 days of the incubation period.[3,6,7]

From the submucosa, the organisms travel to mesenteric lymph nodes. After a brief period of multiplication here the organisms enter the bloodstream via the thoracic duct (transient primary bacteraemia) and are transported to the liver and spleen. After a period of further multiplication at these sites huge numbers of organisms enter the bloodstream, marking the onset of clinical illness (secondary bacteraemia). During this secondary bacteraemia, which continues for the greater part of the illness, very few organs escape invasion but the involvement of the gallbladder and Peyer's patches in the lower small intestine have important clinical significance. The gallbladder is probably infected via the liver and the resultant cholecystitis is usually sub-clinical. The infected bile renders stool cultures positive. Pre-existing gallbladder disease predisposes to chronic biliary infection, leading to chronic faecal carriage.

Invasion of the Peyer's patches occurs either during the primary intestinal infection or during the secondary bacteraemia, and further seeding occurs through infected bile. The Peyer's patches become hyperplastic, with infiltration of chronic inflammatory cells. Later, necrosis of the superficial layer leads to formation of irregular, ovoid ulcers along the long axis of the gut, so that stricture formation does not occur after healing (Figure 53.1).

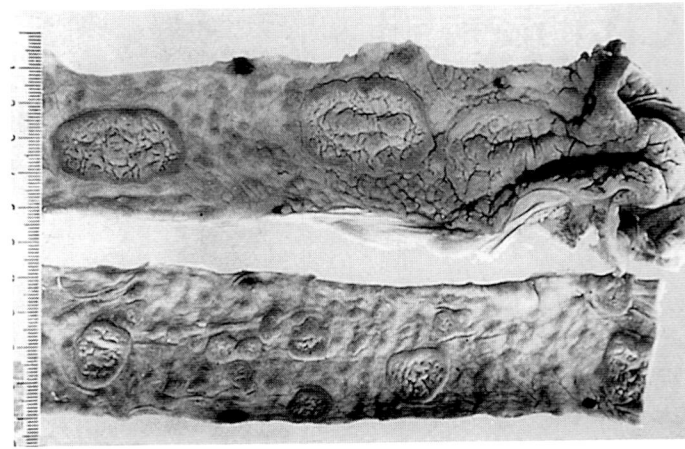

Figure 53.1: Typhoid ulceration of the small intestine. (Courtesy of the Wellcome Tropical Institute Museum (WTIM).)

When an ulcer erodes into a blood vessel, severe haemorrhage results and transmural perforation leads to peritonitis.

Molecular basis of pathogenesis

To be effective pathogens, salmonella must be able to invade epithelial cells and for organisms to cause enteric fever they have to be adapted to survive inside cells of the reticulo-endothelial system.

Epithelial invasion

The target of *Salmonella* invasion is the M cell but must cross the epithelial later to achieve this.[8] *Salmonella* invade the intestinal epithelial cells by a complex mechanism which includes triggering active rearrangements, formation of pseudopodia and phagocytosis of the bacterium into the cells. Membrane ruffling then returns to normal after the bacterium has invaded. The ruffling-internalization process is controlled by a type III secretion system encoded by genes found in the *inv* locus (containing genes *inv A-H*).[9] These genes are located on a pathogenicity island SPI-1 (*Salmonella* pathogenicity island 1) which encodes all of the genes necessary for the invasion of intestinal epithelial cells and the induction of intestinal secretory and inflammatory responses.[10,11] This gene cluster has considerable sequence homology with the *yops* locus of *Yersinia* and the G+C percentage of the *inv* locus is much closer to the overall G+C percentage of *Yersinia*, suggesting that these genes were acquired by lateral gene transfer.

Intra-cellular survival

For *Salmonella* serotypes that cause enteric fever they must be able to survive and replicate within the host macrophage system so that they may establish a systemic infection. Once inside these locations they are shielded from the effect of human immunity, but to do this they must overcome the nutrient-poor environment within the macrophage and defeat its bactericidal mechanisms. *Salmonella* genes necessary for survival inside macrophages are constituents of a two-component response regulator termed *phoP/phoQ*. Genes activated by this phoP/phoQ are known as *pag* genes of which *pag* A–C have been characterized. The *pag* genes are expressed within the macrophage phagosome and are required for survival within it.[12,13] Conversely, the phoP repressed genes switch off in the phagosome and include components of the SPI-1. Mutants that are phoP null or with constitutive expression of phoP are avirulent suggesting that proper timing of switching on and off of these mechanisms is critical in ensuring successful invasion and survival.

More recently, a second type-three secretion mechanism necessary for survival inside macrophages has been described in a second pathogenicity island SPI-2. This system activates within the phagosome and translocates bacterial effector proteins from the phagosome into the macrophage cytosol.[14]

Mechanism of immunity

Production of humoral antibody appears to play little role in recovery from acute infection as the patient often continues to deteriorate despite the appearance of O, H and Vi antibodies. Cell-mediated immunity is probably the key factor in recovery. The ability of Vi antibody to prevent infection is demonstrated by the efficiency of Vi antigen vaccine.[15] However, protection afforded by phenolized-killed vaccine, which does not contain Vi antigen, indicates a role for other antibodies. Local gut immunity is probably important in preventing reinfection. Specific secretory IgG and IgA antibodies have been demonstrated in gut.[16]

In the endemic countries, enteric fevers have the highest prevalence in the young, adults having acquired substantial immunity through previous exposure(s).

Clinical manifestations

The incubation period of typhoid fever varies with the size of the infecting dose[5,7] and averages from 10 to 20 (range 3–56) days. In paratyphoid fever it ranges from 1 to 10 days.

The duration of illness in untreated cases of average severity is usually 4 weeks. In the first week the features are non-specific, with headache, malaise and a rising remittent fever. Constipation and a mild non-productive cough are common. During the second week the patient looks toxic and apathetic with sustained high temperature. The abdomen is slightly distended and splenomegaly is common. In about 50% of cases, crops of 2–4 mm diameter pink papules (rose spots), which fade on pressure, develop on the upper abdomen and lower chest, between the 7th and 12th days. They are difficult to detect in dark-skinned individuals. Rose spots may also occur in invasive salmonellosis[17] and shigellosis.[18] The

spots are caused by bacterial embolization and rose spot cultures may be positive. Relative bradycardia, a pulse lower than anticipated in a febrile patient, is common during the first 2 weeks.

With the onset of the third week the patient becomes more toxic and ill. Continuous high fever persists and a delirious confusional state sets in (typhoid state). Abdominal distension becomes pronounced, with scanty bowel sounds. Diarrhoea is common, with liquid, foul green-yellow stools. The patient is weak with a feeble pulse and rapid breathing; crackles may develop over the lung bases. Death may occur at this stage from overwhelming toxaemia, myocarditis, intestinal haemorrhage or perforation. Considerable weight loss is common. In patients who survive into the fourth week, the fever, mental state and abdominal distension slowly improve over a few days but intestinal complications may still occur. Convalescence is usually a slow process.

Variation in the clinical picture is common. Mild and inapparent infections are frequent. Diarrhoea may occur even during the first week[19] and children may present with a high fever and febrile convulsion(s). Chronic or recurrent fever with bacteraemia may occur in association with concurrent schistosomiasis, as salmonellae are able to survive within the parasites protected from the body's defences.[20,21]

Relapse

Between 10 and 20% of patients treated with antibiotics suffer a relapse after initial recovery, whereas in the pre-antibiotic era the incidence used to be somewhat lower (8–12%). A relapse typically occurs a week or so after stoppage of therapy but occurrence after 70 days has been reported. The blood culture is again positive, even in the presence of high serum levels of H, O and Vi antibodies, and rose spots may reappear. A relapse is generally milder and shorter than the initial illness.

Rarely, second or even third relapses may occur. It is noteworthy that the relapse rate is much lower following treatment with the new quinolone drugs which have effective intracellular penetration.[22]

Complications
Intestinal

The two most serious complications of enteric fever are intestinal haemorrhage and perforation, which usually occur when the sloughs overlying the Peyer's patches separate during the late second or early third week of the illness. Signs of haemorrhage are a sharp fall in body temperature and blood pressure, and sudden tachycardia. The blood passed per rectum is usually bright red but may be altered if intestinal stasis is present. Sometimes there may not be any passage of blood—when frank ileus is present.

Management of haemorrhage is conservative, with sedation and transfusion unless there is evidence of perforation, when surgery is indicated.

Unlike other causes of intestinal perforation, typhoid perforation occurs in a patient who already had a vaguely tender distended abdomen with scanty bowel sounds. Therefore, recognition of perforation can be difficult.[23, 24] Usually pain and tenderness worsen, the pulse rises and the temperature falls suddenly. However, abdominal rigidity may not be a prominent sign and bowel sounds may not disappear altogether. The discovery of free fluid in the abdomen may be the only sign of perforation. Demonstration of gas under the diaphragm is a valuable aid to diagnosis.

The treatment of choice for typhoid perforation is surgical intervention, although conservative management with nasogastric suction, antibiotic therapy, directed against anaerobes and Enterobacteriacae, and general supportive care will reduce the mortality to 30%.[25,26] Most surgeons prefer simple closure of perforation with drainage of the peritoneum, and reserve small bowel resection for patients with multiple perforations. Early diagnosis, energetic resuscitation and rapid, simple surgery are the key to lower mortality. The prognosis is clearly related to the time elapsed between perforation and surgery.

Liver, gallbladder and pancreas
Mild jaundice may occur in enteric fever and may be due to hepatitis, cholangitis, cholecystitis or haemolysis. Biochemical changes indicative of hepatitis are common during the acute stage.[27] Liver biopsy in such cases often shows cloudy swelling, balloon degeneration with vacuolation of hepatocytes, moderate fatty change and focal collection of mononuclear cells—'typhoid nodules' (Figure 53.2). Intact typhoid bacilli can be seen at these sites.[28] Pancreatitis has also been reported.[29]

Cardiorespiratory
Toxic myocarditis is a significant cause of death in endemic countries.[30] It occurs in severely ill toxaemic patients and is characterized by tachycardia, weak pulse and heart sounds, hypotension and electrocardiographic abnor-malities. Mild bronchitis is common and broncho-pneumonia or lobar consolidation may develop rarely.

Nervous system
A toxic confusional state, characterized by disorientation, delirium and restlessness, is characteristic of late-stage typhoid but occasionally these and other neuropsychiatric features may dominate the clinical picture from an early stage.[31] Facial twitching or convulsion(s) may be the presenting features; sometimes paranoid psychosis or catatonia may develop during convalescence.[32] Meningism is not uncommon but bacterial meningitis caused by *S. typhi* is a rare, but recognized complication. Encephalo-myelitis may develop and the underlying pathology may be that of demyelinating leucoencephalopathy.[33] Rarely, transverse myelitis, polyneuropathy or cranial mono-neuropathy may develop.

Haematological and renal
Subclinical disseminated intravascular coagulation occurs commonly in typhoid fever; this rarely manifests as haemolytic–uraemic syndrome.[34] Haemolysis may also be associated with glucose 6-phosphate dehydro-genase (G6PD) deficiency. Immune complex glomerulitis has been reported and IgM immunoglobulin, C3 and *S. typhi* antigen can be demonstrated in the glomerular capillary wall.[35] Nephrotic syndrome may complicate chronic *S. typhi* bacteraemia associated with urinary schistosomiasis.[36]

Musculoskeletal and other systems
Skeletal muscle characteristically shows Zenker's degeneration (a hyaline degeneration of muscle fibres), particularly affecting the abdominal wall and thigh muscles; clinically evident polymyositis may occur.[37]

Localization may occur in almost any organ/system and involvement of bones, joints, meninges, endocardium, spleen and ovary have all been reported but such cases are rare.[38]

Comparison of typhoid fever and paratyphoid fever
In general, the illness in paratyphoid B infection is milder and of shorter duration than in typhoid fever and complications are less frequent.[39] It can also present as acute gastroenteritis. Paratyphoid A and C fall between typhoid and paratyphoid B fevers in severity.

Laboratory findings

Mild leucocytosis may develop initially but, with disease progression, leucopenia and neutropenia commonly develop. Even in uncomplicated cases, low grade normocytic anaemia, mild thrombocytopenia, modestly elevated serum transaminases and mild proteinuria are common.

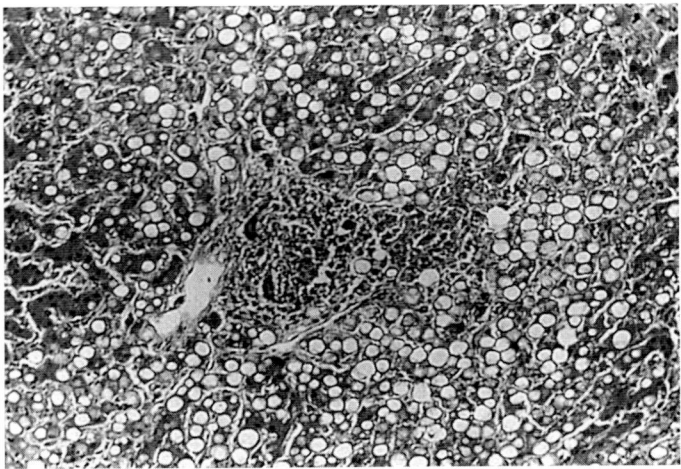

Figure 53.2: Typhoid nodule in portal tract of liver. (Courtesy of WTIM.)

Diagnosis

The definitive diagnosis of enteric fever requires isolation of the organism from blood or bone marrow.[3] Isolation from stool or urine provides strong presumptive evidence only in the presence of a characteristic clinical picture.

Blood and bone marrow culture

The definitive diagnosis of typhoid is by the isolation of the organism from a sterile site. Isolation of the organism from the stool is useful information but may be a false positive due to long-term carriage. Thus, in patients suspected with typhoid blood or bone marrow cultures should be performed. Modern automated systems rapidly detect the presence of the organism, but conventional non-automated methods also have a high diagnostic yield.

In the untreated, blood cultures are usually positive in about 80% during the first week, declining to 20–30% later in the course of the disease.[40] A success rate of about 90% is obtained from bone-marrow culture.[41] Prior antibiotic therapy makes positive blood culture less likely but the bone-marrow culture often remains positive in the face of antibiotic therapy.[41] A high yield (60%) has also been reported from rose spot cultures in such a situation.[41]

Faecal and urine cultures

With modern techniques faecal cultures are often positive even during the first week, though the percentage positivity rises steadily thereafter. Urine cultures are positive less often.

Serology

The traditional Widal test measures antibodies against flagellar (H) and somatic (O) antigens of the causative organism. In acute infection, O antibody appears first, rising progressively, later falling and often disappearing within a few months. H antibody appears a little later but persists for longer. Rising or high O antibody titre generally indicates acute infection, whereas raised H antibody helps to identify the type of enteric fever. However, the Widal test has many limitations. Raised antibodies may have resulted from previous typhoid immunization or earlier infection(s) with salmonellae sharing common O antigens with *S. typhi* or *S. paratyphi*. In endemic countries, patients have higher H antibody titres. This is a particular problem in developing countries where background antibiodies mean that the Widal test lacks sensitivity. Some patients show a poor or negligible antibody response to active infection. Vi antibody is often raised during acute infection and persists afterwards during chronic carriage. However, its use as a screening test for the carrier state is limited because of the frequency of false positives and false negatives.[42]

Newer diagnostic methods

Detection of IgG and IgM antibodies to LPS have proved to provide improved diagnosis compared to Widal. Also detection of antibodies to flagellin, and a set of outer membrane proteins have proved valuable in field studies. Some of these tests have been adapted to a simple dipstick technique using whole bacteria antigens to detect IgM antibody are beneficial in situations where a laboratory is not available.[43–45]

Carrier state in enteric fever

Faecal carrier

After clinical recovery, faecal cultures remain positive in a high proportion of patients during the immediate convalescent period but stools rapidly become negative although up to 3% of patients will still be positive by the end of the third month. Between 1 and 3% will continue to excrete organisms in their stools for more than a year and will be designated as chronic carriers—they are likely to remain so for the rest of their lives. The incidence of chronic carriage is higher in women and in the elderly. A similar situation exists with paratyphoid infections.

Urinary carrier

In the absence of urinary tract pathology, persisting urinary carriage is rare after the third month, but it is common in countries where urinary schistosomiasis is endemic.

Treatment

Patients should be managed under strict enteric precautions, with attention to adequate hand washing and safe disposal of faeces and urine. Antibiotic therapy is essential and should begin empirically if the clinical suspicion of an enteric fever is strong.

Choice of antimicrobial agents in enteric fever

Ciprofloxacin and other 4-quinolone drugs

Ciprofloxacin has proved to be highly effective in the treatment of typhoid and paratyphoid fevers. Defervescence occurs in 3–5 days; convalescent carriage and relapses are rare.[46,47] Other 4-quinolone drugs such as ofloxacin, norfloxacin and pefloxacin are equally effective.[22,48] Ciprofloxacin is usually given orally 500 mg twice daily for 14 days, but there are reports that courses of seven days may be adequate.[49] If vomiting or diarrhoea is present, the drug should be given intravenously, 200–400 mg twice daily. The 4-quinolone drugs are highly effective against multi-resistant strains and trials have shown this in comparison with parenteral and oral ceftriaxone and cefixime.[48,22] Quinolone-resistant strains are now emerging as a clinical problem.

The 4-quinolone drugs are not currently recommended for use in children and pregnant women because of their observed potential for causing cartilage damage in growing animals. However, arthropathy has not been reported in children following the use of nalidixic acid—an earlier quinolone known to produce similar joint damage in young animals, or in children with cystic fibrosis despite high-dose ciprofloxacin treatment. For children with severe infection with a strain that is likely to be multiple drug resistant the balance of risk shifts towards treatment with quinolones.[50]

Third generation cephalosporins

Cefotaxime, ceftriaxone and cefoperazone have excellent in vitro activity against *S. typhi* and other salmonellae and have acceptable efficacy in the treatment of typhoid fever.[51] Only intravenous formulations are available. Cefotaxime is given 1g three times daily (in children: 200 mg/kg daily in divided doses) for 14 days. Ceftriaxone has an advantage of only requiring a single dose daily. The cephalosporins are not active against many MDR strains and this limits its use in empirical treatment when resistant typhoid is likely.

Chloramphenicol

Since its introduction in 1948, chloramphenicol has proved to be remarkably effective in the treatment of enteric fever worldwide. It produces a rapid improvement in the patient's general condition, followed by defervescence in 3–5 days. The recommended adult dose is 500 mg every 4 hours till defervescence, then 6-hourly for a total course of 14 days. The drug is given orally unless the patient is nauseous or having diarrhoea, when the intravenous route should be used initially. The intramuscular route should be avoided as this gives unsatisfactory blood levels and may delay defervescence. The disadvantages of chloramphenicol are: rare marrow toxicity and aplastic anaemia; higher relapse rate following its use; and emergence of resistant strains of *S. typhi*. *S. typhi* strains with plasmid-mediated resistance to chloramphenicol began to appear in the 1960s and later became widespread in many of the endemic countries of the Americas and South-East Asia, highlighting the need for alternative therapeutic agents.

Ampicillin and amoxycillin

Although ampicillin is distinctly inferior to chloramphenicol, its close relative amoxycillin is at least as effective as chloramphenicol in respect of defervescence and relapse rate, and convalescence carriage occurs perhaps less commonly. It is usually given orally four times daily for 14 days.

Co-trimoxazole

This combination of trimethoprim and a sulphonamide amide is also as effective as chloramphenicol in terms of defervescence and relapse rate, and is given orally 960 mg twice daily but can be given parenterally if necessary.

Azithromycin

Azithromycin is a macrolide antibiotic which produces high tissue concentrations, but low serum concentrations because of its unique pharmacokinetic properties. The antibiotic is concentrated within cells, making it ideal for the treatment of infection by an organism with an intracellular lifestyle. Animal models have shown that azithromycin is highly effective against *Salmonella typhi* and non-typhoid *Salmonella*. It has now been shown to be effective in a series of open and randomized control trials. Oral administration is an aid to administration and the results of clinical studies demonstrate that it is as effective as chloramphenicol, cefriaxone and as ciprofloxacin. It was also effective in cases of MDR typhoid. This provides a useful alternative for the management of children with uncomplicated typhoid in developing countries.[52–54]

Emergence of multi-resistant typhoid fever

Since 1989 there has been a rapid emergence and spread of *S. typhi* strains with simultaneous plasmid-mediated resistance to chloramphenicol, ampicillin and co-trimoxazole in the Indian subcontinent and parts of South-East Asia (see also Chapter 54). Quinolones and azithromycin are possible alternatives for treatment of infection with these organisms.

Current therapeutic strategy

Because of the efficacy and low relapse and carrier rates associated with their use, the 4-quinolone drugs are now the drugs of choice in the treatment of adult typhoid, certainly in areas where multi-resistant typhoid fever has been reported.[46,55] However, because of its cheapness, choramphenicol will continue to be used in other areas where the local strains are sensitive, although azithromycin may in the future be a useful alternative especially in children.

In children with possible multi-resistant typhoid, a third generation cephalosporin, e.g., cefotaxime, will be the preferred drug if 4-quinolone drugs are to be avoided. However, their cost and the need for intravenous administration are significant disadvantages, particularly in the developing countries, and ciprofloxacin is being used increasingly in children with typhoid. Azithromycin is another potential alternative that combines oral availability with intracellular penetration and activity against the pathogen.

Corticosteroid therapy

High-dose dexamethasone (initially 3 mg/kg body weight, followed by eight doses of 1 mg/kg 6-hourly) reduces mortality in severely ill patients with depressed levels of consciousness or shock.[56]

In the non-endemic countries, patients should be kept under bacteriological surveillance after clinical recovery until six consecutive negative faecal and urine cultures are obtained.

Management of chronic carriers

Prolonged courses of amoxycillin or co-trimoxazole may be effective, but the failure rate is high if there is chronic gallbladder disease. Ciprofloxacin (750 mg twice daily) and norfloxacin (400 mg twice daily) have been much more effective, with cure rates of 78 and 83%, respectively.

Cholecystectomy is not always successful because of persisting hepatic infection. It is a major operation which should be performed only if strictly indicated for the patient's gallbladder disease, but not for the sole purpose of eradicating the carrier state.

Chronic urinary carriers should be investigated for urinary tract abnormalities, including schistosomiasis.

Prognosis

Early antibiotic therapy has transformed a previously life-threatening illness of several weeks duration with a mortality rate approaching 20% into a short-lasting febrile illness with negligible mortality. The high mortality rates which continue to be reported from some endemic countries are undoubtedly related to delayed diagnosis and/or inappropriate treatment.

Prevention

In the endemic countries the most cost-effective strategy for reducing the incidence of enteric fever is the institution of public health measures to ensure safe drinking water and sanitary disposal of excreta. The effects of these measures are long lasting and will also reduce the incidence of other enteric infections which are a major cause of morbidity and mortality in those areas. In the absence of such a strategy, mass immunization with typhoid vaccines at regular intervals will also reduce the incidence of infectións considerably.[57]

No effective paratyphoid vaccines are available. Two types of typhoid vaccine are currently in use.

1. Vi capsular polysaccharide antigen vaccine

This is a single parenteral dose vaccine from the Merieux Institute. Observed overall protection rates of 75% in Nepal[58] and 64% in South Africa[59] compare favourably with the efficacy of the killed vaccine and it has the advantage of minimal side effects. Booster doses are necessary every 3 years to maintain protection. It is not suitable for children under 18 months of age as polysaccharide antigens evoke a weak antibody response.

2. Live-attenuated oral vaccines

An oral vaccine containing live attenuated *S. typhi* Ty21a strains in an enteric-coated capsule is now commercially available and has given a 67% protection rate in Chile lasting for 3 years after three doses given on alternate days. A four-dose schedule, which appears to give better

protection[60] is preferred in the USA. However, only 42% efficacy was recorded in Indonesia, suggesting that the vaccine may not be as effective in areas where exposure is intense.[61]

Typhoid vaccination is recommended for travellers to highly endemic areas in Asia, Africa and the Americas. However, the protection is partial and travellers should be made aware of this and encouraged to pay close attention to personal, food and water hygiene.

Other salmonella infections (Salmonellosis)

Although human salmonellosis occurs worldwide, it has become a major public health problem in developed countries. Individual cases and outbreaks in community and institutions are common. Of the large number of *Salmonella* serotypes, only a few account for the vast majority of human infections. Worldwide, examples of common human isolates are: *S. enteritidis*, *S. typhimurium*, *S. virchow*, *S. newport*, *S. hadar*, *S. heidelberg*, *S. agona* and *S. indiana*, the order of prevalence is variable according to geography and time.[3,4]

Epidemiology

The organisms are widely distributed in the animal kingdom. Domestic animals, notably cattle, pigs and poultry are frequent excretors and many wild animals are also infected. Household pets such as dogs, cats, birds and turtles are all potential, albeit rare, sources of human infection. Human cases and convalescent carriers are also important sources. Transmission is faecal–oral, usually through ingestion of contaminated foods such as improperly prepared poultry, meat and egg. The carcass of an animal harbouring *Salmonella* in its gut becomes contaminated during evisceration and infection spreads to other non-infected carcasses during large-scale storage. Thus, inadequately cooked meat or precooked food contaminated from raw meat in the kitchen are important vehicles of transmission. *Salmonella* may survive deep freezing, and adequate thawing is essential before cooking. In recent years, fresh shell hen eggs infected through vertical transmission have emerged as an important source of *S. enteritidis* infection in both Europe and the USA.[62]

The factors that are responsible for the dramatic rise of *Salmonella* infections in developed countries in recent years are the adoption of large-scale intensive farming methods for rearing food animals and the use of bulk-imported infected animal feeds, both of which create conditions suitable for rapid spread of infection among the animals. The rising incidence of drug-resistant salmonellae has been linked to the extensive and poorly controlled use of antimicrobials in farm animals.[63]

Transmission from a human source is infrequent; convalescent excretors with adequate standards of personal hygiene rarely transmit infection once their stools are formed. However, infected asymptomatic food-handlers have caused a number of restaurant-associated outbreaks. Institutional outbreaks are usually food related, but outbreaks in maternity, neonatal and geriatric units have followed admission of patients with an undiagnosed *Salmonella* infection.

Unpasteurized milk is a recognized source in some countries. Unusual sources include pharmaceutical or diagnostic products of animal origin. In the developing countries, the epidemiological pattern is different as large-scale rearing of food animals is not common and methods of cooking are different. Salmonellosis is uncommon in adults. However, it is an important cause of childhood infection, often contracted in hospitals through cross-infection, and there is some evidence that the hospitals are acting as a reservoir for maintaining infection in the community.[64]

Infection is more common and may be more severe in those that are predisposed to infection. This includes patients with reduced gastric acid or who have been prescribed antibiotic agents. Immunocompromise, most notably with HIV, predisposes to salmonellosis. Splenectomy and sickle cell disease also predispose to invasive salmonellosis.

Pathogenesis

Site of invasion

Most of our understanding about the mechanisms of disease production by salmonella infection in man have come from work in animals and are described in detail above.

Mechanism of diarrhoea production

The exact mechanisms responsible for diarrhoea are unclear. Mucosal invasion and inflammation are clearly important, at least accounting for the bloody, mucoid type of stools which occur commonly, but do not explain the copious watery stools in the early stages. Observations in experimental animals of an enteropathy with water and electrolyte transport defects suggests the existence of secretory mechanisms.[65] Production of prostaglandin-like secretagogues and other mediators by the inflammatory tissues[66,67] and toxin production by the organisms[68] have been suggested. Salmonellae produce an enterotoxin and a cytotoxin. The enterotoxin activates adenylate cyclase and has some physicochemical characteristics in common with cholera toxin but limited antigenic homology.

Infecting dose

The size of the infecting dose is important to the outcome of a *Salmonella* infection. The rarity of water-borne outbreaks of salmonellosis suggests the necessity of a large infecting dose that can usually be found only in

food following multiplication. Limited experimental evidence in volunteers suggests an infecting dose of 10^5 in the production of clinical illness.[4] However, very small infecting doses, possibly as low as 17 organisms, have caused outbreaks. The size of the infecting dose is clearly influenced by the infectivity of the organism and host factors such as age, immune status, underlying debilitating disease or stress factors, and the physiological state of the stomach and upper small intestine at the precise time of intake of the organism. Gastric acidity is a significant barrier to enteric infection, and hypoacidity or increased transit time increase the susceptibility to infection.

Virulence of the organism

The serotypes vary greatly in their potential to produce invasive illness outside the gastrointestinal tract. Although any serotype can cause invasive disease, some are more invasive than others. *S. cholerae-suis* regularly produces septicaemic or metastatic illnesses, and less commonly gastroenteritis. Other serotypes with increased invasiveness are *S. virchow* and *S. dublin*.[69] The multi-resistant *S. typhimurium* strains which have caused large outbreaks in Africa, India and the Middle East produce a high incidence of septicaemia and metastatic organ involvement.[64] What governs this virulence potential is unclear, but in animal models serotypes bearing high molecular weight plasmids (virulence plasmids) have the ability to spread beyond the initial site of infection in the intestine.[70] Virulence plasmids may be important in the pathogenesis of bacteraemia in humans.[71]

Clinical manifestations

There is wide variation in both the severity and the nature of manifestations of salmonellosis. Two often overlapping clinical syndromes are seen: acute enterocolitis (most common) and invasive salmonellosis with septicaemia or metastatic extraintestinal localization of infection. The incubation period is usually between 12 and 48 hours but longer incubation periods of up to 72 days have been reported.[72]

Acute enterocolitis

This is the preferred term to describe the acute diarrhoea of salmonellosis because both small and large intestines are involved in the disease process. The illness begins with nausea and vomiting, often associated with malaise, headache and fever. Very soon, cramp-like abdominal pains and diarrhoea supervene. Initially the stools are of large volume and watery without visible blood or mucus; later, the volume may decrease as blood and mucus appear, indicating development of colitis. This may be associated with localization of pain over the left iliac fossa and some degree of rebound tenderness may develop. The severity of diarrhoea is quite variable, from a mild attack of several loose stools for a day to voluminous watery stools every half-hour or so over several days—

leading to dehydration. The elderly, particularly those with debilitating illnesses, and individuals with gastric hypoacidity are prone to develop severe diarrhoea; this may have a cholera-like intensity in patients with a partial gastrectomy.

Occasionally, *colitis* may dominate the clinical picture with the passage of frankly bloodstained stools containing pus. Toxic dilatation may complicate the picture. Sigmoidoscopy shows mucosal oedema, hyperaemia, petechial haemorrhages and, in severe cases, friable mucosa with ulcerations. Histological features include dilatation and congestion of capillaries in the mucosa

and submucosa with focal collections of polymorphonuclear leucocytes in the lamina propria (Figure 53.3A). In others there may also be a diffuse increase in chronic inflammatory cells in the lamina propria (Figure 53.3B). Crypt abscesses may be seen, but crypt architecture is usually normal with a normal goblet cell population; however, but in severe cases crypt distortion with mucus depletion may occur and distinction from inflammatory bowel disease is difficult (Figure 53.3C). Barium enema usually shows features of diffuse colitis but segmental involvement may occur, mimicking Crohn's disease.

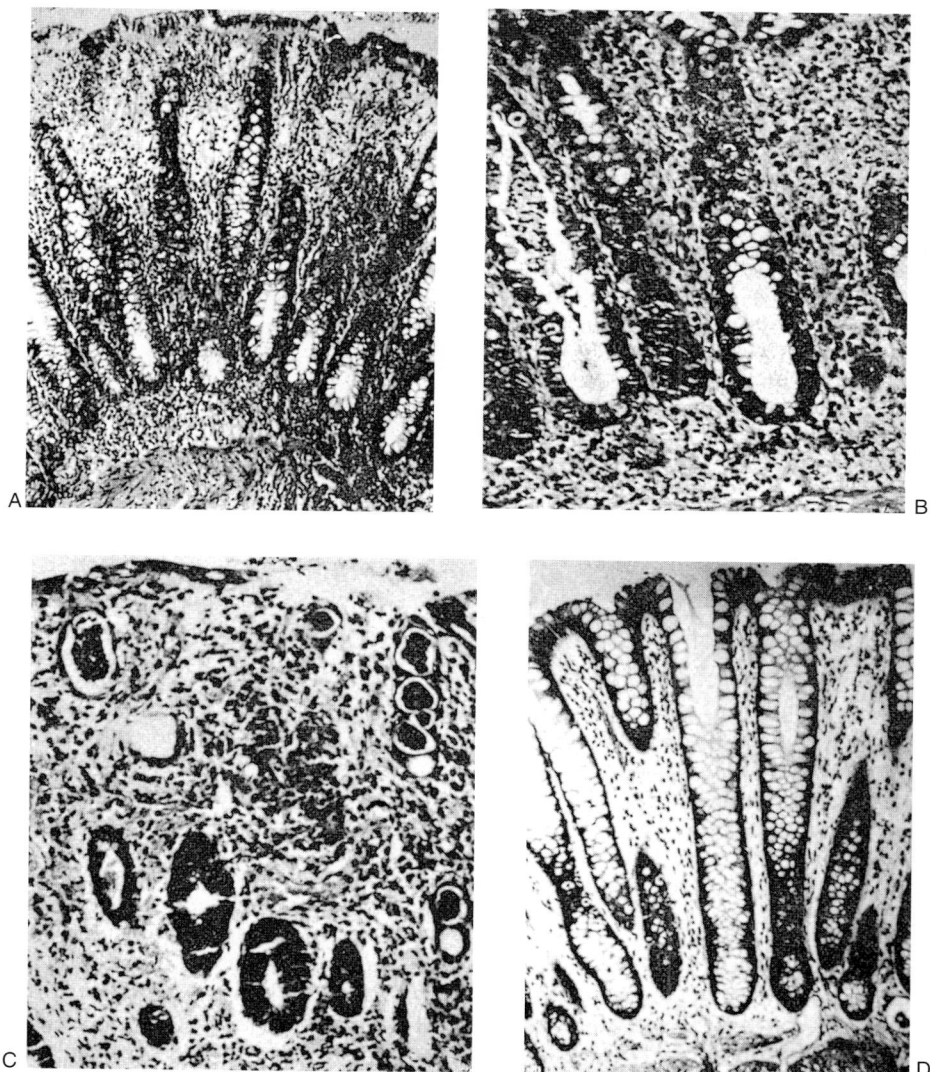

Figure 53.3: (**A**), (**B**) and (**C**) are from rectal biopsies from patients with *Salmonella* spp. infection. (**A**) Milder lesions: focal inflammation of mucosa with polymorphonuclear leucocytes in the lamina propria and mucosal capillaries, but no increase in chronic inflammatory cells. (H & E, 80 ×.) (**B**) More severe lesions: severe acute inflammation with polymorphs in the lamina propria infiltrating the crypt epithelium and present on the mucosal surface. There is an increase in chronic inflammatory cells but the goblet cell population is well preserved. (H & E, 135 ×.) (**C**) Severe focal abscesses tending to be localized in the crypt: there is marked depletion of mucus but crypt architecture is not distorted. The surface epithelium is flattened. (H & E, 150 ×.) (**D**) Normal mucosa. (H & E, 120 ×.) (**A**), (**B**) and (**C**) are reproduced from Day et al. The rectal biopsy appearances in *Salmonella* colitis. *Histopathology* 1978; 2:117–131, with permission of the authors and the editor of *Histopathology*, (**D**) is reproduced by courtesy of B. C. Morson. (Reproduced with permission from P.C.B. Turnbull. Food poisoning with special reference to salmonella: its epidemiology, pathogenesis and control. *Clin Gastroenterol* 1979; 8(3).)

Alternatively, ileal involvement may be the predominant feature, with pain and tenderness localized over the right lower abdomen; this may be misdiagnosed as appendicitis.

Invasive salmonellosis

Bacteraemia is not uncommon in *Salmonella* infection, even in previously healthy individuals, and its frequency depends on the serotype of the organism and host factors. Overall, bacteraemia rates of 8% have been observed, with higher rates for some serotypes, e.g., *S. cholerae-suis*, *S. virchow* and *S. dublin*, and in the very young. Apart from age, other host factors are: immune suppression, malignancy, gastric hypoacidity, debilitating disease, bartonellosis and sickle cell disease.

In previously healthy individuals, bacteraemia is usually a transient event but in a minority of patients, particularly those with the risk factors outlined, bacteraemia may be significant and characterized by either a septicaemic illness (swinging fever, rigors and general toxicity complicating the diarrhoeal illness) or a typhoid-like illness (sustained fever, splenomegaly and even rose spots but minimal diarrhoea) or evidence of metastatic localization in the meninges, bone and joints, lungs, endocardium and arteries, liver, spleen, ovary and kidneys.[38] Soft tissue localization can also occur. Metastatic infections may be unassociated with a diarrhoeal illness, as in *S. cholerae-suis* infections. Meningitis occurs almost exclusively in neonates and children under 2 years of age and reports of high incidence have come from a number of the developing countries.[64] *Salmonella* infection accounts for most cases of aortic and other vascular infections in the elderly. Atherosclerotic aneurysms of the abdominal aorta or iliac vessels, or prosthetic valves and grafts may all be infected. Normal arteries are affected very rarely. Children with sickle cell disease are particularly prone to developing osteomyelitis. Patients with chronic schistosomiasis are prone to suffer from recurrent bacteraemia from salmonella organisms living within the helminth.[73] HIV infection is an important predisposition to invasive *Salmonella* infections especially in sub-Saharan Africa where the HIV epidemic coincides with conditions of poor sanitation. Infection is associated with prolonged excretion of the organisms and an enhanced risk of invasive disease. In adults with documented bacteraemia *Salmonella* was identified in 35%.[74-76]

Reactive arthritis

Sterile synovitis may follow salmonella infection, particularly in HLA-B27-positive individuals. The symptoms usually develop 1–2 weeks after the acute infection. Any joint may be affected, although the knees and ankles are most frequently involved. Occasionally, there is migratory polyarthritis, resembling acute rheumatic fever, or bilateral proximal interphalangeal joint involvement, as in rheumatoid arthritis. Acute iridocyclitis may complicate the picture. Deposition of salmonella polysaccharide in the synovial cells may be an important factor in the pathogenesis of reactive arthropathy.

Carrier state

Adults recovering from salmonellosis usually continue to excrete the organism(s) for 4–8 weeks; infants and the elderly excrete for longer periods. Chronic carriage beyond 1 year occurs in far fewer than 1% of cases.

Diagnosis

Definitive diagnosis of salmonella enterocolitis requires positive faecal isolation. Blood cultures should be done in all severely ill patients. Coincidental inflammatory bowel disease should be suspected if bloody diarrhoea persists beyond 2 weeks despite the use of an appropriate antibiotic (e.g., ciprofloxacin). Sigmoidoscopic and barium contrast study findings are not discriminatory at this stage, but rectal biopsy is often helpful as crypt distortion and prominent goblet cell depletion are features of ulcerative colitis and are very rarely present in severe primary salmonella colitis. When such a distinction is not possible, the patient should be treated with prednisolone and antibiotics continued. In those who respond promptly the diagnostic dilemma can be resolved only by a repeat biopsy after 6 weeks. In primary salmonella colitis the rectal biopsy histology usually returns to normal by this time, but this is quite uncommon in ulcerative colitis.

Treatment

Most patients with salmonella enterocolitis have a short-lasting, self-limiting illness and require only increased fluid intake.

Antibiotics such as neomycin, colistin, ampicillin, chloramphenicol and co-trimoxazole do not influence the clinical illness and may prolong the duration of intestinal carriage. However, the 4-quinolone drugs (e.g., ciprofloxacin 500 mg twice daily for 5 days) have been shown to shorten the duration of the illness and should be used in patients who are at high risk of developing severe enterocolitis and/or invasive illness, i.e., the elderly, patients who are immunocompromised or have gastric hypoacidity, aortic aneurysm, vascular graft(s), valve prosthesis or debilitating diseases. Antibiotics are definitely indicated in patients with suspected or confirmed septicaemia and/or metastatic infection(s). Severe colitis is another indication for therapy.

Chloramphenicol, co-trimoxazole and amoxycillin are also effective against invasive disease if the infective organism is sensitive. However, the incidence of infection due to salmonella organisms resistant to one or more of these drugs has increased in many parts of the world, including the UK and the USA. There is much geographical variation in the prevalence of the resistant strains and local knowledge of it is essential if these drugs are to be used (see Chapter 54).

Third generation cephalosporins (e.g., cefotaxime, ceftriaxone and cefoperazone) are highly effective and resistance to these drugs is rare. They are particularly suitable for use in children if 4-quinolone drugs are to be avoided.

The complication of colonic dilatation usually resolves without surgery. Aortic salmonellosis generally requires surgical intervention.

Ciprofloxacin is also useful in eradicating persisting faecal carriage and should be given to food handlers.

Antibiotic resistance

There is increasing incidence of multiple drug resistance in *Salmonella* with reports of *S. typhimurium* with resistance to ampicillin, chloramphenicol, trimethoprim-sulphamethazole, streptomycin and tetracycline. More recently there are reports of reduced susceptibility to ciprofloxacin. Much of the resistant in non-typhoidal *Salmonella* is due to the use of antibiotics in animal husbandry. For example enrofloxacin is a quinolone antibiotic used in veterinary medicine that may be related to the increased incidence of quinolone resistance. Resistance to extended spectrum cephalosporins has now also been reported narrowing the options when antibiotic therapy is indicated.

Prevention

The main control measures are directed at maintaining high standards of hygiene in slaughterhouses and all areas of food preparation and distribution—both commercial and private. Raw meat and cooked food must be stored and handled separately. Thorough cooking of raw meat after adequate thawing is essential. Eggs should be boiled for 5 minutes and liquid egg for commercial use should be pasteurized. In the developing countries, adequate infection control procedures are essential in paediatric hospitals if the problem of endemic *Salmonella* spp. cross-infection is to be controlled.

Control of infection in the animal reservoir is a much more difficult problem. However, heat treatment of animal feeds, better standards of animal care and hygiene on the farm, and raising of infection-free flocks are some of the measures which will lower the contamination rates of flesh foods destined for human consumption.

Asymptomatic excretors who are handlers of unwrapped food meant for consumption without further cooking or reheating should be free of infection before returning to work. Others may do so or return to school once their diarrhoea has settled, provided their hygienic standards are adequate.

REFERENCES

1   Le Minor L & Popoff M Y. Request for an opinion. Designation of *Salmonella enterica* sp.nov, nom.rev, as the type and only species of the genus *Salmonella*. *Int J Syst Bacteriol* 1987; 37:465–468.
2   Brenner FW, Villar RG, Angulo FJ, Tauxe R & Swaminathan B. *Salmonella* nomenclature. *J Clin Microbiol* 2000; 38:2465–2467.
3   Gillespie SH. Salmonella. In: Emmerson AM, Hawkey PM, Gillespie SH, eds. *Principles and Practice of Clinical Bacteriology*, 1st edn. Chichester: Wiley, 1997:399–412.
4   Hohmann EL. Nontyphoidal salmonellosis. *Clin Infect Dis* 2001; 32:263-269.
5   Christie AB. *Infectious Diseases: Epidemiology and Clinical Practice*, 3rd edn. Edinburgh: Churchill Livingstone, 1980.
6   Ivanoff B, Levine MM & Lambert PH. Vaccination against typhoid fever: present status. *Bull World Health Organ* 1994; 72:957–971.
7   Hornick R B, Greiseman S E, Woodward T E et al. Typhoid fever: pathogenesis and immunological control. *N Engl J Med* 1970; 283:686–691.
8   Jones BD, Ghori N & Falkow S. *Salmonella typhimurium* initiates murine infection by penetrating and destroying the specialized epithelial M cells of the Peyer's patches. *J Exp Med* 1994; 180:15–23.
9   Collazo CM & Galan JE. The invasion-associated type-III protein secretion system in Salmonella — a review. *Gene* 1997; 192:51–59.
10   Altmeyer RM, McNern JK, Bossio JC et al. Cloning and molecular characterization of a gene involved in Salmonella adherence and invasion of cultured epithelial cells. *Mol Microbiol* 1993; 7:89–98.
11   Galan JE. Salmonella interactions with host cells: type III secretion at work. *Ann Rev Cell Dev Biol* 2001; 17:53–86.
12   Pegues DA, Hantman MJ, Behlau I, Miller SI. PhoP/PhoQ transcriptional repression of *Salmonella typhimurium* invasion genes: evidence for a role in protein secretion. *Mol Microbiol* 1995; 17:169–181.
13   Behlau I & Miller SI. A PhoP-repressed gene promotes *Salmonella typhimurium* invasion of epithelial cells. *J Bacteriol* 1993; 175:4475–4484.
14   Ohl ME & Miller SI. *Salmonella*: a model for bacterial pathogenesis. *Annu Rev Med* 2001; 52:259–274.
15   lugman K P, Gilberton I T, Koornhof H J et al. Vaccination advisory committee: protective activity of Vi capsular polysaccharide vaccine against typhoid fever. *Lancet* 1987; ii:1165–1169.
16   Sarasombath S, Banchuin N, Sukusol T, Rungpitarangsi B & Manasatif S. Systemic and intestinal immunities after natural typhoid infection. *J Clin Microbiol* 1987; 25:1088–1093.
17   Mani V, Brennand J & Mandal B K. Invasive illness with *Salmonella virchow* infection. *Br Med J* 1974; ii:143–144.
18   Rahaman M M & Alam A K M J. Rose spots in shigellosis caused by *Shigella dysenteriae* type I infection. *Br Med J* 1977; ii:1123–1124.
19   Roy S K, Speelman P, Butler T et al. Diarrhoea associated with typhoid fever. *J Infect Dis* 1985; 151:1138–1143.
20   Teixeira R. Typhoid fever of protracted course. *Rev Inst Med Trop São Paulo* 1960; 2:65–70. Quoted by Prata A. Schistosomiasis. *Clin Gastroenterol* 1978; 7:49–75.
21   Farid Z, Bassily S, Kent D C et al. Chronic urinary *Salmonella* carriers with intermittent bacteraemia. *J Trop Med Hyg* 1970; 73:153–156.
22   Cao XT, Kneen R, Nguyen TA, Truong DL, White NJ & Parry CM. A comparative study of ofloxacin and cefixime for treatment of typhoid fever in children. The Dong Nai Pediatric Center Typhoid Study Group. *Pediatr Infect Dis J* 1999; 18:245–248.
23   Archampong E Q. Operative treatment of typhoid perforation of the bowel. *Br Med J* 1969; iii:273–276.
24   Angorn I B, Pillay S P, Hegarty M & Baker L W. Typhoid perforation of the ileum: a therapeutic dilemma. *S Afr Med J* 1975; 49:782–784.

25 Huckstep R L. Recent advances in the surgery of typhoid fever. *Ann R Coll Surg Engl* 1960; 26:207–230.

26 Gibney J. Typhoid perforation. *Br J Surg* 1989; 76:887–889.

27 Khosla S N. Typhoid hepatitis. *Postgrad Med J* 1990; 66:923–925.

28 Calva J J & Ruiz-Palacios G M. Salmonella hepatitis: detection of salmonella antigens in the liver of patients with typhoid fever. *J Infect Dis* 1986; 154:373–374.

29 Hermans P, Gerard M, Laethem Y V et al. Pancreatic disturbances and typhoid fever. *Scand J Infect Dis* 1991; 23:201–205.

30 Gupta F P, Gupta M S, Bhardwaj S & Chugh T D. Current clinical patterns of typhoid fever: a prospective study. *J Trop Med Hyg* 1985; 88:377–381.

31 Osuntoken B O, Bademosi O, Ogunremi K & Wright S G. Neuropsychiatric manifestations of typhoid fever in 959 patients. *Arch Neurol* 1972; 27:7–13.

32 Breaky W R & Kala A K. Typhoid catatonia responsive to ECT. *Br Med J* 1977; ii:357–359.

33 Ramachandran S, Wickremesinghe H R & Perera M V F. Acute disseminated encephalomyelitis in typhoid fever. *Br Med J* 1975; i:494–495.

34 Baker N M, Mills A E & Rachman I. Haemolytic uraemic syndrome in typhoid fever. *Br Med J* 1974; ii:84–87.

35 Sitprija V, Pipatanagul V, Boonpucknavig V & Boonpucknavig S. Glomerulitis in typhoid fever. *Ann Intern Med* 1974; 81:210–213.

36 Farid Z, Higashi G I, Bassily S & Milner W F. Immune-complex disease in typhoid and paratyphoid fevers. *Ann Intern Med* 1975; 83:432.

37 Naidoo P N & Yan C C. Typhoid polymyositis. *S Afr Med J* 1975; 49:1975–1976.

38 Cohen J I, Bartlett J A & Corey G R. Extra-intestinal manifestations of *Salmonella* infections. *Medicine* 1987; 66:349–388.

39 Gadeholt H & Madsen S T. Clinical course complications and mortality in typhoid fever as compared with paratyphoid B. A survey of 2647 cases. *Acta Med Scand* 1963; 174:753.

40 Stuart B M & Pullen R L. Typhoid: clinical analysis of two hundred and sixty cases. *Arch Intern Med* 1946; 78:629–661.

41 Gilman R H, Terminel M, Levine M M, Hernandez-Mendoza P & Hornick R B. Relative efficacy of blood, urine, rectal swab, bone-marrow and rose-spot cultures for recovery of *Salmonella typhi* in typhoid fever. *Lancet* 1975; i:1211–1213.

42 Parry CM, Hoa NT, Diep TS, Wain J, Chinh NT, Vinh H et al. Value of a single-tube Widal test in diagnosis of typhoid fever in Vietnam. *J Clin Microbiol* 1999; 37:2882–2886.

43 Choo KE, Davis TM, Ismail A, Tuan Ibrahim TA, Ghazali WN. Rapid and reliable serological diagnosis of enteric fever: comparative sensitivity and specificity of Typhidot and Typhidot-M tests in febrile Malaysian children. *Acta Trop* 1999; 72:175–183.

44 Handojo I & Dewi R. The diagnostic value of the ELISA-Ty test for the detection of typhoid fever in children. *SE Asian J Trop Med Public Health* 2000; 31:702–707.

45 House D, Wain J, Ho VA et al. Serology of typhoid fever in an area of endemicity and its relevance to diagnosis. *J Clin Microbiol* 2001; 39:1002–1007.

46 DuPont HL. Quinolones in *Salmonella typhi* infection. *Drugs* 1993; 45(Suppl 3):119–124.

47 Wallace MR, Yousif AA, Mahroos GA et al. Ciprofloxacin versus ceftriaxone in the treatment of multiresistant typhoid fever. *Eur J Clin Microbiol Infect Dis* 1993; 12:907–910.

48 Arnold K, Hong CS, Nelwan R et al. Randomized comparative study of fleroxacin and chloramphenicol in typhoid fever. *Am J Med* 1993; 94:195S–200S.

49 Alam MN, Haq SA, Das KK et al. Efficacy of ciprofloxacin in enteric fever: comparison of treatment duration in sensitive and multidrug-resistant *Salmonella*. *Am J Trop Med Hyg* 1995; 53:306–311.

50 Dutta P, Rasaily R, Saha MR et al. Ciprofloxacin for treatment of severe typhoid fever in children. *Antimicrob Agents Chemother* 1993; 37:1197–1199.

51 Soe G B & Overturf G D. Treatment of typhoid fever and other systemic salmonellosis with cefotaxime, ceftriaxone, cefoperazone and other newer cephalosporins. *Rev Infect Dis* 1987; 9:719–736.

52 Butler T, Sridhar CB, Daga MK et al. Treatment of typhoid fever with azithromycin versus chloramphenicol in a randomized multicentre trial in India. *J Antimicrob Chemother* 1999; 44:243–250.

53 Frenck RW, Jr, Nakhla I, Sultan Y et al. Azithromycin versus ceftriaxone for the treatment of uncomplicated typhoid fever in children. *Clin Infect Dis* 2000; 31:1134–1138.

54 Girgis NI, Butler T, Frenck RW et al. Azithromycin versus ciprofloxacin for treatment of uncomplicated typhoid fever in a randomized trial in Egypt that included patients with multidrug resistance. *Antimicrob Agents Chemother* 1999; 43:1441–1444.

55 Ferreccio C, Morris JG Jr, Valdivieso C et al. Efficacy of ciprofloxacin in the treatment of chronic typhoid carriers. *J Infect Dis* 1988; 157:1235–1239.

56 Hoffman S L, Punjabi N H, Kumala S et al. Reduction of mortality in chloramphenicol treated severe typhoid fever by high dose dixamethasone. *N Engl Med J* 1984; 310:82–87.

57 Bodhidatt L, Taylor D N, Thisyakorn U & Echeverria P. Control of typhoid fever in Bangkok, Thailand, by annual immunization of school children with parenteral typhoid vaccine. *Rev Infect Dis* 1987; 9:841–845.

58 Acharya I L, Lowe C U, Thapa R et al. Prevention of typhoid fever in Nepal with the Vi capsular polysaccharide of *Salmonella typhi*: a preliminary report. *N Engl J Med* 1987; 317:1101–1104.

59 Levine M M, Ferreccio C, Black R E, Germanier R and the Chilean Typhoid Committee. Large scale field trial of Ty21a live oral typhoid vaccine in enteric-coated capsules: a field trial in an endemic area. *Lancet* 1987; i:1049–1052.

60 Ferreccio C, Levine M M, Rodriguea H, Contreras R and the Chilean Typhoid Committee. Comparative efficacy of two, three or four doses of Ty21a live oral typhoid vaccine in enteric-coated capsules: a field trial in an endemic area. *J Infect Dis* 1989; 159:766–769.

61 Simanjuntak C H, Paleologo F P, Punjabi N H et al. Oral immunisation against typhoid fever in Indonesia with Ty21a vaccine. *Lancet* 1991; 338:1055–1059.

62 Cowden J M. Salmonellosis and egg: public health, food poisoning and food hygiene. *Curr Opin Infect Dis* 1990; 3:246–249.

63 Rowe B & Threlfall E J. Antibiotic resistance in salmonella. *Microbiol Dig* 1986;3:2–5 (Salmonella special March 1987 revision).

64 Mandal B K. Typhoid fever and other salmonellae. *Curr Opin Gastroenterol* 1986; 2:109–112.

65 Rout W R, Formal S B, Dammin G J & Giannella R A. Pathophysiology of *Salmonella* diarrhoea in the rhesus monkey: intestinal transport, morphological and bacteriological studies. *Gastroenterology* 1974; 67: 59–70.

66 Gianella R A, Rout W R & Formal S B. Effect of indomethacin on intestinal water transport in salmonella-infected rhesus monkeys. *Infect Immun* 1977; 17:136–139.

67 Gianella R A. Importance of the intestinal inflammatory reaction in salmonella mediated intestinal secretion. *Infect Immun* 1979; 23:140–145.

68 Acheson D W K. Enterotoxins in acute infective diarrhoea. *J Infect* 1992; 24:225–245.

69   Mandal B K & Brennand J. Bacteraemia in salmonellosis: a 15 year retrospective study from a regional infectious diseases unit. *Br Med J* 1988; 297:1242–1243.

70   Gulig P A. Virulence plasmids of *Salmonella typhimurium* and other salmonellae. Mini-review. *Microb Pathog* 1990; 8:3–11.

71   Fierer J, Krause M, Tauxe R & Guiney D. *Salmonella typhimurium* bacteraemia: association with the virulence plasmid. *J Infect Dis* 1992; 166:639–642.

72   Cowden J M, O'Mahoney M, Bartlett C L R et al. A national outbreak of *Salmonella typhimurium* DT 124 caused by contaminated salami sticks. *Epidemiol Infect* 1989; 103:219–225.

73   Young S W, Higashi G, Kamel R et al. Interactions of salmonellae and schistosomes in host–parasite relations. *Trans R Soc Trop Med Hyg* 1973; 67:797–802.

74   Arthur G, Nduba VN et al. Trends in bloodstream infections among human immunodeficiency virus-infected adults admitted to a hospital in Nairobi, Kenya, during the last decade. *Clin Infect Dis* 2001; 33:248–256.

75   Gilks CF. Acute bacterial infections and HIV disease. *Br Med Bull* 1998; 54:383–393.

76   Graham SM, Molyneux EM, Walsh AL et al. Nontyphoidal Salmonella infections of children in tropical Africa. *Pediatr Infect Dis J* 2000; 19:1189–1196.

Chapter 54
Resistant Gut Bacteria

E. J. Threlfall

Resistance to antimicrobial drugs, and particularly multiple resistance, is now a major problem in bacterial enteric pathogens in both developing and developed countries throughout the world. The problem affects *Salmonella enterica*, including not only *S. enterica* serotype Typhi and Paratyphi, but also a range of other serovars, notably Typhimurium and Wien in developing countries and Typhimurium, Virchow and Hadar in developed countries. Multiple resistance is also an increasing problem in *Shigella*, especially *Sh. dysenteriae* 1 (Shiga's bacillus), but also in *Sh. flexneri* and *Sh. boydii*, *Vibrio cholerae* O1, O139 and non-O1, non-O139 strains, and to a lesser extent, *Escherichia coli*. Since the early 1990s resistance to key antimicrobials has also been reported in *Campylobacter* spp., and in this organism the development of resistance has been linked to the use of antimicrobials in animal husbandry.

Salmonellas

The occurrence of resistance is of particular concern in *S. typhi* and *S. paratyphi* where treatment with an appropriate antibiotic is essential in the treatment of infections caused by these organisms, and should commence as soon as clinical diagnosis is made. However, the increasing occurrence of multiple resistance in serotypes other than Typhi has also had a profound effect, particularly in developing countries in the treatment of salmonella septicaemia in infants and young children, where since 1980 multiply resistant strains have been implicated in numerous outbreaks in hospital paediatric units.

Salmonella typhi and *paratyphi*

Salmonella enterica serotype Typhi remains endemic in developing countries in Africa, South and Central America, and the Indian subcontinent, with an estimated incidence of 33 million cases each year.[1] In contrast, in developed countries such as the UK or the USA the incidence of *S. typhi* is much lower, and the majority of cases are in travellers returning from endemic areas. For example, in the UK between 150 and 300 cases occur each year with at least 70% of cases in patients with a history of recent foreign travel.[2] Similarly in the USA 293

infections were reported in the 12-month period from 1 June 1996 to 31 May 1997, of which 81% were recorded in patients who had travelled abroad.[3]

For patients with typhoid fever, the administration of an effective antibiotic is essential. Ideally treatment should commence as soon as clinical diagnosis is made without recourse to the results of antimicrobial sensitivity tests. From 1948 to the mid-1970s chloramphenicol was the first-line drug of choice and in developed countries the use of chloramphenicol resulted in a reduction in the mortality rate from 10% to less than 2%. Following the occurrence of extensive outbreaks of typhoid fever in Mexico and India in the early and mid-1970s, in which the epidemic strains were resistant to chloramphenicol,[4,5] there were fears that the efficacy of this antimicrobial had been seriously jeopardized.[6]

Developing countries: the current situation

Alternative drugs that have been used for typhoid fever are ampicillin and trimethoprim. However, since 1989 chloramphenicol-resistant *S. typhi* with additional resistance to ampicillin and trimethoprim (= MR) have been isolated with increasing frequency in several countries. In India several outbreaks caused by MR strains, predominantly of Vi-phage type E1, have been reported[7] and such strains have been isolated in Chandigarh in the north,[8] Calcutta in the east,[9] Kerala in the south-west,[10] Dindigul in the south-east,[11] and also in Vellore[12] and Delhi.[13] In Pakistan from 1989 to 1992 the predominant multiresistant Vi-phage type was M1[14] and over this period there was an extensive outbreak in Rawalpindi caused by strains of this phage type.[15] MR strains of Vi-phage types E1 and M1 linked to immigrant workers from the Indian subcontinent have also been isolated in several countries in the Arabian Gulf.[16]

In addition, multiresistant strains of different phage types have been isolated in Egypt,[17] Canada,[18] South Africa,[19] Kuala Lumpar,[20] the Philippines[21] and Vietnam[22] (Table 54.1). Since 1997 MR strains of *S. typhi* have also become increasingly common in Africa, with isolations reported from countries as far apart as Nigeria[23] and Kenya.[24] Strains from these countries have been resistant to chloramphenicol, ampicillin and co-trimoxazole, with a significant proportion of isolates from Nigeria also

Table 54.1 Outbreaks of multiresistant *Salmonella* Typhi, 1989–2000.

Year	Country or area	Phage type	R-type	Plasmid
1989	Pakistan	M1	ACSSuTTm	H$_1$
1990–1995	India	E1, 51, O	ACSSuTTm	H$_1$
1990–1995	Arabian Gulf	E1, 51, O	ACSSuTTm	H$_1$
1990–1993	Kuala Lumpur	E1	ACSSuTTm	H$_1$
1991	UK	M1	CSTTm	H$_1$
1991	South Africa	A	ACKSSuT	H$_1$
1991–1992	Egypt	E2, C1, D1-N	ACSSuTTm	H$_1$
1992–1994	Vietnam	?	ACSSuTTm	H$_1$
1993–1994	Philippines	?	CKSSuTTm	?
1994, 1998	Bangladesh	E1	ACSSuTTm	H$_1$
1994–1998	Pakistan	E1	ACSSuTTm	H$_1$
1993–1998	Vietnam	?	ACSSuTTm (Cp$_L$)	H$_1$
1997–1999	Kenya	?	ACSSuTTm	?
1997–1998	Nigeria	?	ACSSuTTm	?
1998–1999	Tajikistan	UVS	ACSSuTTmCp$_L$	H$_1$

Resistance symbols: a, ampicillin; C, chloramphenicol; K, kanamycin; S. streptomycin; Su, sulphonamides; T, tetracyclines; Tm, trimethoprim; Cp$_L$, ciprofloxacin (MIC 0.25–1.0 mg/l); ?, not known; UVS, untypable Vi-strain.

showing resistance to nalidixic acid.[23] Examples of outbreaks caused by multiresistant strains that have occurred since 1989 are shown in Table 54.1.

UK isolates

In the UK between 1978 and 1985 resistance to chloramphenicol was identified in only a very small proportion (0.47%) of strains studied.[25] From 1986 to 1989 the occurrence of chloramphenicol resistance increased threefold, but in 1990 there was a dramatic change, with 20% of isolates resistant to chloramphenicol of which most were also resistant to ampicillin and trimethoprim.[26] Because of the substantial increase in the occurrence of strains resistant to chloramphenicol, in 1991 ciprofloxacin was recommended as an alternative to chloramphenicol for patients with a history of recent return from epidemic areas.[27–29]

Between 1990 and 1999 the number of patients per annum with typhoid fever in the UK ranged from 151 to 291 (mean 210). During this period the incidence of multiple drug resistance to chloramphenicol, ampicillin and trimethoprim (MR strains) increased from 21% in 1991 to 36% in 1994, declining to 13% in 1997 but increasing to 26% in 1999.[30] Over 90% of patients infected with MR strains provided a history of recent return from the Indian subcontinent, particularly Pakistan and India. The most common MR phage types have been M1 and E1. The majority of patients infected with MR strains of phage type M1 had acquired their infections in Pakistan. However, strains of phage types E1 have been isolated from patients infected in both Pakistan and India. Infections have also been recorded in patients returning from Bangladesh, Sri Lanka and Afghanistan. Irrespective of phage type or country of origin, in all MR strains resistance to chloramphenicol, ampicillin and trimethoprim has been encoded by plasmids of approximately 100 MDa belonging to the H$_1$ incompatibility group (*inc* H$_1$).[30]

Decreased susceptibility to fluoroquinolone antimicrobials

In 1991 a strain of *S. typhi* with plasmid-encoded resistance to chloramphenicol, ampicillin and trimethoprim and with chromosomally encoded resistance to nalidixic acid (minimum inhibitory concentration (MIC) 512 mg/l) was isolated from a 1-year-old child who had recently returned to the UK from India. The strain also showed a marked decrease in sensitivity to ciprofloxacin (MIC 0.6 mg/l).[31] In 1995 3% of 291 isolations showed decreased sensitivity to ciprofloxacin (MIC 0.38–0.75 mg/l), of which five were also resistant to chloramphenicol, ampicillin and trimethoprim. In 1998, 21% of 151 strains exhibited decreased susceptibility to ciprofloxacin. Several treatment failures have been reported. One patient infected with a strain with a MIC to ciprofloxacin of 1.0 mg/l failed to respond to twice-daily treatment with ciprofloxacin 400 mg intravenously. Following treatment with ceftriaxone her condition improved dramatically and after a further 5 days she was apyrexial.[32]

The occurrence in the UK of *S. typhi* with decreased susceptibility to ciprofloxacin increased to 23% in 1999.[30] All strains with decreased sensitivity to ciprofloxacin have also been resistant to nalidixic acid (MIC 512 mg/l). The majority of patients had recently returned from India or Pakistan. However, in both 1998 and 1999 strains with decreased susceptibility to ciprofloxacin were isolated from travellers returning from Sri Lanka, Nepal, Bangladesh and Thailand. Furthermore, in both years over 50% of isolates with decreased susceptibility to ciprofloxacin were also MR. At least 10 patients infected with strains with decreased susceptibility to ciprofloxacin did not respond to treatment with fluoroquinolone antimicrobials. In such cases ceftriaxone was the most frequently used alternative antimicrobial.[30] In contrast to resistance to chloramphenicol, ampicillin and trimethoprim, resistance to ciprofloxacin has been chromosomally encoded in all isolates with decreased sensitivity to this antimicrobial.

Since 1993 strains of *S. typhi* with decreased susceptibility to ciprofloxacin have been isolated with increasing frequency in Vietnam.[22] In 1997 there were over 6000 recorded cases in an extensive epidemic in Tajikistan of nalidixic acid-resistant *S. typhi* with decreased susceptibility to ciprofloxacin.[33] In both Vietnam and Tajikistan treatment failures with fluoroquinolone antibiotics have been noted. Despite the low level of resistance, treatment failures are increasingly being noted. In such cases possible alternatives such as ceftriaxone or cefotaxime could be considered. In this respect it is reassuring that all strains of *S. typhi* so far tested have been sensitive to these antimicrobials.[30]

S. paratyphi

Decreased susceptibility to ciprofloxacin has also been reported in an increasing number of strains of *S. paratyphi A* isolated in India since 1998.[34] Such resistance has been attributed to the widespread use of ciprofloxacin and ciprofloxacin derivatives to treat many human infections irrespective of prescription. To maintain the efficacy of fluoroquinolones it is essential that such antimicrobials are reserved for the treatment of invasive diseases and are not used for prophylaxis or for the treatment of uncomplicated gastroenteritis.

Other salmonella serovars

In developed countries such as the UK, the majority of countries in western Europe and the USA, salmonella infections excluding those with *S. typhi* and *S. paratyphi* are primarily zoonoses. When resistance is present, in the majority of instances it has been acquired prior to transmission of the organism through the food chain to humans. Such resistance acquisition has been related to the use of antimicrobials in animal husbandry.[35] The most important serotypes in the UK, Europe and the USA are Enteritidis, Typhimurium and Virchow, and the main method of spread is through contaminated food. In general, person-to-person transmission is not of major importance in the spread of these serotypes. In most cases the clinical presentation is that of mild to moderate enteritis, the disease is usually self-limiting and antimicrobial therapy is seldom required. In contrast, in developing countries, particularly in the Indian subcontinent, South-East Asia, South and Central America and Africa, serotypes such as Typhimurium, Wien, Johannesburg and Oranienburg have undergone changes in both their epidemiology and their clinical disease. An additional feature of these strains has been the possession of plasmid-mediated multiple drug resistance, often with resistance to seven or more antimicrobial agents.

Developing countries

Since 1970, multiply resistant salmonellas have caused extensive outbreaks in many developing countries. The common pattern has been for several hospitals, often situated many miles apart, to be involved. The majority of outbreaks have occurred in neonatal and paediatric wards, but community outbreaks in villages and small towns have also been reported. The clinical disease has been severe with enteritis frequently accompanied by septicaemia and in several outbreaks a mortality rate of up to 30% has been reported. Serotypes involved include, notably, Typhimurium in the Middle East[36] and the Indian subcontinent,[37] and Wien in southern Europe, north Africa and India,[38-40] although infections caused by multiply resistant strains belonging to several other serotypes have also been reported.[40] Strains have been resistant to up to 10 antimicrobials. Examples of such outbreaks are shown in Table 54.2. A disturbing development in recent years has been an increase in developing countries in the incidence of strains of multiresistant non-typhoidal salmonellas with high-level resistance to nalidixic acid (MIC > 100 mg/l) and with reduced

Table 54.2 Examples of outbreaks of multiresistant non-typhoidal *Salmonella enterica* in developing countries, 1969–2000.

Year	Country or area	Serotype	Phage type	R-type	Plasmid
1969–1972	North Africa, Southern Europe, India	Wien	–	ACSSuT	FI*me*
1972–1980	Middle East	Typhimurium	208, UT	ACSSuT, ACGKSSuT	FI*me*
1979–1990	India	Typhimurium	66/122	ACSSuT, ACGKSSuTTmNx	FI*me*
1976–1980	Kenya	Typhimurium	NC	ACSSuT	FI*me*
1974–1996	Turkey	Typhimurium	UT	ACGKSSuTTm	FI*me*
1974–1978	South Africa	Johannesburg	–	ACKSSuT	FI*me*
1990–1999	Albania, Italy	Typhimurium	?	ACKSSuTTm	FI*me*
1990–2000	India	Senftenberg	–	ACGKSSuTTmNx	FI*me*

Resistance symbols: see Table 54.1; also, G, gentamicin; Nx, nalidixic acid; –, not applicable; ?, not known; Nc, non-conforming; UT, untypable.

susceptibility to ciprofloxacin (MIC 0.1 versus 0.0075 mg/l for nalidixic acid-sensitive strains). This has been particularly evident in countries such as India,[41] particularly for *S. typhimurium*[41] but also for *S. senftenberg*.[42]

A particular feature of infections with multiresistant nontyphoidal salmonellas in developing countries has been the lack of involvement of food animal reservoirs. Spread has been by person-to-person contact and antibiotic resistance has developed as a result of the use of antibiotics in human medicine, particularly in those countries where there is little control over the use of antibiotics. An example of the type of epidemic caused by multiresistant salmonellas is that which has occurred throughout India since 1977.[37,40] The serotype involved was Typhimurium and strains have belonged to closely related phage types. Outbreaks occurred in both communities and in hospitals, particularly amongst neonates, although older children and adults have also been affected. The most common presentation has been severe enteritis and cases of septicaemia have also been reported. Mortality was high in at least five outbreaks. The majority of strains have been characterized by plasmid-mediated resistance to at least seven antimicrobials, including ampicillin, chloramphenicol, gentamicin, kanamycin, streptomycin, sulphonamides, tetracyclines and trimethoprim. Chromosomally mediated resistance to furazolidone and nalidixic acid, accompanied by decreased susceptibility to ciprofloxacin, has also been common.

Plasmids

With the exception of resistance to furazolidone and nalidixic acid/ciprofloxacin, all resistances have been plasmid mediated and have been encoded by high molecular mass, transmissible plasmid belonging to incompatibility group FI*me* (*inc* FI*me*). Such plasmids have also been identified in unrelated phage types of *S. typhimurium* which have caused similar outbreaks throughout the Middle East, in several countries in Africa,[40] and in multiresistant strains of *S. Wien* responsible for outbreaks in Europe, North Africa and India between 1978 and 1990.[39,40] These plasmids have also recently been identified in strains of *S. typhimurium* isolated in Italy and originating in Albania.[43–45] In addition to coding for multiple drug resistance, such plasmids also carry genes coding for the production of the hydroxamate siderophore aerobactin, which is a known virulence factor for some enteric and urinary tract pathogens.[43] Recent studies have demonstrated that in these strains the resistance genes are incorporated into integrons, which are themselves highly mobile genetic elements capable of horizontal transfer between different bacterial strains.[45]

Antimicrobial therapy

Antimicrobial therapy is often essential for the treatment of infections caused by these multiresistant strains, particularly when such strains cause extraintestinal infections. As yet, patients infected with these strains appear to be responding to treatment with ciprofloxacin and some of the newer fluoroquinolone antibiotics, although decreased susceptibility in strains isolated in India has been reported (see above). In some cases alternative antimicrobials such as ceftriaxone have been used for individual patients. However, isolates of *S. typhimurium* of diverse resistance phenotypes with plasmid-mediated resistance to extended-spectrum β-lactamases have recently been reported in outbreaks of infection in Turkey[46] and the USA,[47] and the efficacy of such antimicrobials for the treatment of serious disease is already being eroded.

Developed countries

In contrast to the situation in developing countries, in developed countries such as England and Wales salmonella septicaemia is rare in other than a few serotypes of limited epidemiological importance. Indeed, over the 10-year period from 1981 to 1990 the occurrence of bloodstream invasion for the two most common serovars, Enteritidis and Typhimurium, was less than 2%.[48] A similar situation was observed in strains isolated in England and Wales in the 3-year period from 1995 to 1997.[49] However, salmonella septicaemia can be a life-threatening disease and resistance of strains to drugs of therapeutic importance may limit the choice of antimicrobials available for therapy.[50] Also in contrast to developing countries, in developed countries the use of antibiotics in food-producing animals has been an important factor in the development of multiple resistance in salmonellas isolated from cases of human infection.

In the 10-year period from 1990 to 1999, *S. enteritidis*, *S. typhimurium* and *S. virchow* comprised over 70% of all human salmonella isolations identified in England and Wales, with Enteritidis and Typhimurium comprising 60% of strains. From 1990 to 1996 the overall incidence of drug resistance remained constant at about 10% for *S. enteritidis* and 76% for *S. virchow*, but increased from 53% to 90% for *S. typhimurium*. However, over this period multiple resistance (to four or more antimicrobials) increased from 19% to 90% in *S. typhimurium* and from less than 1% to 19% for *S. virchow*.[51,52] In contrast the incidence of multiple resistance for *S. enteritidis* has remained at less than 1%. Although multiple resistance in *S. typhimurium* and *S. virchow* has subsequently fallen slightly, in 1999 59% of isolates of *S. typhimurium* and 14% of isolates of *S. virchow* were multiply resistant.[53] Since the early 1980s multiple resistance has been particularly common in *S. typhimurium* in three definitive phage types (DTs), DT 204c, 193 and 104. In DT 204c multiple resistance, including resistance to ampicillin, chloramphenicol and trimethoprim, has been plasmid mediated, and multiresistant strains possess at least three independent resistance plasmids;[54] in DT 193 multiple resistance to ampicillin, streptomycin, sulphonamides and tetracyclines is also plasmid mediated and has become integrated into the *S. typhimurium* serovar-specific mouse virulence plasmid.[55] In contrast, in DT 104 multiple resistance (to ampicillin, chloramphenicol, streptomycin, sulphonamides and tetracyclines) (= MR *S. typhimurium* DT 104) is chromosomally integrated[56] and is encoded by a sequence of approximately 14 kilobases (kb).[57,58]

MR *S. typhimurium* DT 104

MR *S. typhimurium* DT 104 became widely distributed in bovine animals in the UK in the late 1980s and early 1990s, and soon became transmitted to humans through the food chain. In England and Wales isolations of MR DT 104 from humans increased from about 200 in 1990 to over 4000 in 1996.[58] MR DT 104 has also become common in poultry, particularly turkeys, pigs and sheep.[59] Human infection with MR DT 104 has been associated with the consumption of chicken, beef, pork sausages and meat paste, and to a lesser extent with occupational contact with infected cattle.[58] Over the last 4 years this particular clone has caused outbreaks of infection in food animals and humans in numerous European countries including the Irish Republic, Denmark, Germany, Austria, France, Israel, the Czech Republic, Italy and Sweden. Infections in humans have also been recognized in Trinidad, South Africa, the Netherlands, Northern Ireland, the United Arab Emirates, the Philippines,[58] and more recently in Japan.[60] In 1996 infections with MR DT 104 were recognized in cattle and humans in North America, in both Canada and the USA. Of particular concern has been the resistance of the organism to a wide range of therapeutic antimicrobials. Furthermore, in some countries there have been reports of an apparent predilection of the organism to cause serious disease.[50]

Since 1992 a disturbing feature of infections with MR DT 104 has been the appearance of additional resistance to trimethoprim and decreased susceptability to ciprofloxacin. In 1998 13% of MR DT 104 in England and Wales were additionally resistant to trimethoprim and 16% also showed decreased susceptibility to ciprofloxacin with a MIC ranging from 0.5 to 1.0 mg/l. Some 2% of isolates were additionally resistant to both trimethoprim and ciprofloxacin.

In isolates with decreased susceptibility to cipro-floxacin it has been suggested that the emergence of resistance to this antimicrobial is related to the use of the related fluoroquinolone antibiotic enrofloxacin in cattle and poultry, which was licensed for veterinary use in the UK in November 1993. Recently, the use of the fluoroquinolone antimicrobial marbofloxacin in cattle has been linked to the emergence of a strain of MR *S. typhimurium* DT 104 with decreased susceptibility to ciprofloxacin. This strain was responsible for an extensive outbreak in humans in the north-west of England in 1998.[61] For humans, the clinical significance of decreased susceptibility to ciprofloxacin is controversial. However, in an outbreak in Denmark in the summer of 1998 four hospitalized patients did not respond to treatment with ciprofloxacin and there were two deaths.[50] This outbreak clearly demonstrates the potential of MR DT 104 for causing serious disease and the clinical consequences of decreased susceptibility to ciprofloxacin in this epidemic strain.

Of note in strains isolated in England and Wales in 1999 was the increasing incidence of decreased susceptibility to fluoroquinolone drugs in *S. virchow*.[53] This is particularly concerning because of the invasive propensity of this organism, as ciprofloxacin is now the therapeutic agent of choice for severe salmonella infections.

It should be realized that multiple resistance in salmonellas in developed countries is not confined to *S. typhimurium* DT 104 and related strains. In Spain, emergent multiresistant strains of *S. enterica* serotype [4,5,12:i:-] have been associated with an increasing number of human infections since the mid-1990s.[62] Such strains have also caused infection in humans in the UK[63] and Denmark. Similarly in Greece, multiresistant strains of *S. Blockley* have caused numerous infections in humans since 1996.[64] It should be emphasized that, although the most common presentation has been gastroenteritis in infections caused by both *S. enterica* serotype [4,5,12:i:-] and *S. Blockley*, in some cases patients have not responded to antimicrobial treatment, possibly as a consequence of the wide resistance spectrum of the organisms concerned.

Shigellas

Developing countries

Since 1969 multiresistant strains of *Shigella* spp., and in particular *Sh. dysenteriae* (Shiga's bacillus), have caused extensive outbreaks in many countries in Central America, Africa and the Indian subcontinent. The first major outbreak was that which occurred in Central America from 1969 to 1972 and the strain was resistant to chloramphenicol, streptomycin, sulphonamides and tetracyclines (R-type CSSuT). More than 10 000 deaths were reported. In the 1970s a series of outbreaks, although not of the same scale as the Central American outbreak but caused by strains with the same resistance pattern, were reported in several countries in the Indian subcontinent (for a review see Rowe and Threlfall[40]). In all these outbreaks resistance to chloramphenicol, streptomycin, sulphonamides and tetracyclines was invariably plasmid mediated and encoded by a plasmid of the *inc* B group.

The second major international outbreak occurred in central Africa (Zaire, Rwanda, Burundi) from 1979 to 1982. Over 13 000 cases were reported in eastern Zaire between 1981 and 1982, with over 1700 deaths. The strain was of R-type ACSSuT (A, ampicillin) and, although resistances were plasmid encoded, the plasmids were of different incompatibility groups to that identified in the Central American and Indian strains.[65] Following the discontinuation of the use of tetracyclines and the introduction of co-trimoxazole early in 1981, plasmid-mediated resistance to the latter antimicrobial soon emerged.[66] Nalidixic acid was subsequently introduced in Zaire in November 1981 for the treatment of Shiga dysentery, and the use of this antimicrobial resulted in a drop in the case fatality rate from 4.6% to 2.0%.[66] Subsequent to these outbreaks in the 1980s, serious epidemics of multiresistant *Sh. dysenteriae* 1 have been reported in the 1990s in Zimbabwe[67] and Zambia.[68] The causative strains were resistant to a wide range of antimicrobials including ampicillin, chloramphenicol, tetracyclines and trimethoprim.[67]

Since 1984 there have been reports of epidemics and outbreaks in several states in India of bacillary dysentery caused by multiresistant *Sh. dysenteriae* type 1. Of particular note was that which occurred in West Bengal in 1984,[69] in which the strains were resistant to ampicillin, chloramphenicol, tetracyclines and co-trimoxazole. Because of the appearance in such strains of resistance to ampicillin and co-trimoxazole—at that time the drugs of choice for first-line treatment of bacillary dysentery in India—nalidixic acid became the first-line alternative treatment in the 1980s[70] and has subsequently been used extensively throughout India for this purpose. However, strains with resistance to nalidixic acid have now emerged in the Indian subcontinent,[71] thus undermining the efficacy of this antimicrobial for the treatment of bacillary dysentery in that area. Although resistant to nalidixic acid, strains of *Sh. dysenteriae* type 1 isolated in India have been found to be highly susceptible to the newer fluoroquinolones, and for adults a single dose (1 g) of ciprofloxacin coupled with standard rehydration therapy has been reported to be highly effective.[70] Outbreaks of multiresistant *Sh. dysenteriae* 1 have also been reported in Burma (1985)[72] and Bangladesh (1988).[72] In the Bangladesh outbreak the strains were additionally resistant to nalidixic acid.[72]

Strains of multiresistant *Sh. dysenteriae* 1 are now becoming commonplace in other developing countries, not only in Central America, India and Africa but also in the Middle East. For example, in the 5-year period comprising 1990–1993 and 1996, *Sh. dysenteriae* accounted for 5% of *Shigella* strains isolated in Kuwait.[73] All isolates were multiresistant. Once more, because of multiresistance the therapeutic options for oral therapy were severely restricted.[73] Details of outbreaks caused by multiresistant *Sh. dysenteriae* 1 are summarized in Table 54.3.

An increasing problem in many developing countries in recent years has been the appearance and spread of multiresistant strains of *Sh. flexneri*. Outbreaks with such strains have been reported in many countries in South-East Asia and the Indian subcontinent,[74,75] and treatment problems have been recorded in infections in Kuwait,[72] Israel,[76] Turkey,[77] Italy,[78] Tanzania[79] and the UK.[80] Strains have often been resistant to at least five antimicrobials, including ampicillin, chloramphenicol and trimethoprim, with an increasing number of strains from the Indian subcontinent showing resistance to nalidixic acid.[71] In strains from Tanzania resistance to ampicillin has been related to integron-mediated OXA-1 and TEM-1 β-lactamases.[79]

Table 54.3 Outbreaks of multiresistant *Shigella dysenteriae* 1, 1969–1994.

Year	Country or area	Drug resistance	Plasmid
1969–1972	Central America	CSSuT	B
1979–1982	Zaire, Rwanda, Burundi	ACSSuT	X
1984	India	ACSSuTTm	B
1985	Burma	CSSuT	B
1988	Bangladesh	ACSTTmNx	?
1992–1994	Zimbabwe	ACSSuTTm	?
1992–1994	Zambia	ACSSuTTm	?

Resistance symbols: see Tables 54.1 and 54.2; ? unknown.

Britain

Between 1983 and 1987 the incidence of resistance to ampicillin in *Sh. dysenteriae*, *Sh. flexneri* and *Sh. boydii* infections in England and Wales increased from 42% to 65% and the incidence of resistance to trimethoprim from 6% to 64%.[81] Furthermore, of 1524 strains tested in 1995–1996, 46% were resistant to both these antimicrobials.[80] Resistance to nalidixic acid was uncommon and only a very small number of strains were resistant to ciprofloxacin. On the basis of these observations it was concluded that, if it should be necessary to commence treatment before the results of laboratory-based sensitivity tests were available, the best options would be to use nalidixic acid for children and a fluoroquinolone antibiotic such as ciprofloxacin for adults.[80]

It is important to note that *Sh. dysenteriae*, *Sh. flexneri* and *Sh. boydii* are not indigenous in England and Wales, and the majority of infections have been identified in patients either with a history of recent foreign travel, particularly to the Indian subcontinent, or who have had contact with recent travellers. Thus, resistance in these serotypes does not reflect the use of antibiotics for the treatment of shigellosis in Britain.

Shigella sonnei

For *Sh. sonnei*, which is indigenous to Britain and the USA, a different picture has emerged. In Britain multiple resistance declined from 38% in 1972 to 8% in 1977,[81] but increased to 45% in 1995–1996.[80] In the USA, strains of *Sh. sonnei* have developed resistance to trimethoprim–sulfamethoxazole in response to antimicrobial therapy during the course of outbreaks,[82] and in 1987 a large outbreak of shigellosis possibly affecting over 6000 people was caused by a strain of *Sh. sonnei* resistant to ampicillin, tetracyclines, streptomycin and trimethoprim–sulfamethoxazole.[83] However, since antimicrobial susceptibility testing of *Shigella* isolates is not routinely done in the USA, the overall occurrence and persistence of such resistant strains is unknown.

Recommendations for therapy

Until 1984 ampicillin was widely regarded as the drug of choice for the treatment of severe bacillary dysentery, with trimethoprim the drug of choice for patients infected with ampicillin-resistant strains.[84] More recently, because of the increased prevalence of strains resistant to ampicillin and trimethoprim, nalidixic acid has been used increasingly in developing countries as a primary alternative.[70] However, if *Sh. dysenteriae* type 1 infection is suspected or nalidixic acid-resistant strains of *Shigella* have been identified, treatment with pivmecillinam has been recommended. For children, treatment with pivmecillinam or ceftriaxone has been suggested, although reservations have been expressed both about the cost of these antibiotics and about the non-availability of an oral formulation of ceftriaxone.[85] It has also been recommended that in developing countries the newer quinolone drugs should be held in reserve for the treatment of strains resistant to nalidixic acid and pivmecillinam. For developed countries where resistance to ampicillin and co-trimoxazole is less common, it has been recommended that, if antibiotic therapy is indicated, children should continue to be treated with ampicillin or trimethoprim–sulfamethoxazole, and that adults should be treated with one of the new quinolone drugs.[85] However, because of the rapidly increasing range of resistance in *Shigella* strains, it has been strongly recommended that, whenever possible, antibiotic sensitivities should be determined before commencing treatment, as the choice of antibiotic for initial treatment is becoming increasingly limited.[80] This is particularly the case in Britain (see above), where it has been recommended that the best options would be to use nalidixic acid for children and a fluoroquinolone antibiotic such as ciprofloxacin for adults until the results of laboratory-based sensitivity tests are available.[80]

Vibrio cholerae

Vibrio cholerae O1

The first protracted outbreak of *Vibrio cholerae* O1 with multiple drug resistance was that which occurred in Tanzania in 1977.[86] The strains were of R-type ACKSSuT (K, kanamycin) and the appearance of resistance was attributed to the extensive use of tetracyclines for cholera prophylaxis in Tanzania. Outbreaks caused by drug-resistant strains of *V. cholerae* O1 have subsequently been reported in Bangladesh in 1979–1980 and 1981, in Zaire in 1982–1983 and in Tanzania in 1983.[40] A variety of R-types has been identified and, in addition to the resistances listed above, strains with resistance to gentamicin and trimethoprim have been identified in Bangladesh and Zaire. In 1993 strains of *V. cholerae* O1 with resistance to ampicillin, chloramphenicol, kanamycin, sulphonamides, tetracyclines and trimethoprim were identified in epidemic cholera in Ecuador, South America,[87] and it has been subsequently reported that up to 36% of strains from this epidemic were multiresistant.[88] In 1995 multiresistant strains of *V. cholerae* O1 were reported to have caused outbreaks in the horn of Africa (Ethiopia and Somalia) in epidemics in the 1980s,[89] and multiresistant strains of have subsequently been reported in Uganda,[90] Albania and Italy,[91] India[92] and Guinea-Bissau.[93]

In all multiresistant strains of *V. cholerae* O1 from outbreaks in Africa, the Indian subcontinent and South America, the complete spectrum of resistance has been encoded by plasmids of the *inc* C group.[87] It would therefore appear that plasmids of this incompatibility group have an affinity for *V. cholerae* similar to that shown by *inc* H[1] plasmids for *S. typhi* (see above). However, it is noteworthy that in these *inc* C plasmids resistance to trimethoprim and aminoglycosides is contained within class I integrons.[91,93] Such integrons are similar to those identified in multiresistant *S. typhimurium* DT 104 and *Sh. flexneri* (see above). Thus it is possible that resistance genes contained on these *inc* C cholera plasmids may have originated in other pathogenic Gram-negative bacteria.

Although the therapy of choice for cholera is oral rehydration, when antimicrobial therapy is indicated doxycycline, a long-acting form of tetracycline, is recommended for adults and co-trimoxazole for children, with furazolidone, erythromycin and chloramphenicol considered to be effective alternatives.[94] The appearance in countries with low standards of hygiene of strains with resistance to three of the drugs of choice for the treatment of cholera is of some concern, and reappraisal of the use of antimicrobials in some outbreak situations may now be necessary. Indeed, because of the development of resistance to tetracyclines in epidemic strains, in some developing countries fluoroquinolone drugs have been used in combination with oral rehydration therapy. However, the emergence of resistance to norfloxacin in an outbreak in Malda, West Bengal, in 1997[95] suggests that the efficacy of such antimicrobials for *V. cholerae* has already been jeopardized.

Vibrio cholerae O139

Since early 1993 there have been reports of outbreaks of cholera caused by *V. cholerae* O139 in the Indian subcontinent.[96] A limited study of strains isolated in the UK from travellers known to have returned recently from the Indian subcontinent demonstrated that these strains were resistant to streptomycin, sulphonamides and trimethoprim.[97] As with infections caused by *V. cholerae* O1, the therapy of choice for infections caused by non-O1 *V. cholerae* is oral rehydration, and the occurrence of resistance to streptomycin, sulphonamides and trimethoprim should have little effect on treatment regimens.

Escherichia coli

The occurrence of antibiotic resistance in pathogenic *E. coli* responsible for gastrointestinal illness has been documented elsewhere[40] and will not be discussed at length in this chapter. Plasmids have been identified that code for antibiotic resistance and the production of both heat-stable (ST) and heat-labile (LT) toxin,[98] and in a study of drug resistance among toxin-producing strains isolated in the Far East 72% of strains were reported to be drug resistant and 44% multiresistant.[99]

For Vero cytotoxin-producing *E. coli* O157 (VTEC O157) 23% of 1087 isolates from people in England and Wales were drug resistant but only 2% were multiresistant; the most common resistance patterns were streptomycin, sulphonamides and tetracyclines, and sulphonamides and tetracyclines.[100,101] Until 1999, resistance to fluoroquinolone antibiotics had not been identified in VTEC O157 from humans in infections associated with foods or food animals in the UK. However, it should be realized that, in general, antimicrobials are not recommended for the treatment of VTEC O157 infections in humans. Indeed, the use of quinolone antibiotics may stimulate the production of toxin-encoding bacteriophages from strains of Shiga-toxin producing *E. coli* and thereby potentially exacerbate the disease syndrome in humans.[102]

The use of antibiotics for the treatment of *E. coli* gut infections is also a contentious issue. There is little doubt that a number of antibiotics reduce the incidence and duration of diarrhoea in travellers,[103] and both ciprofloxacin[104] and norfloxacin[105] have been reported to be particularly effective. However, concern has been expressed that the widespread use of these antimicrobials for prophylaxis may in the long term reduce their efficacy.[106]

Although antibiotics are not recommended for the treatment of uncomplicated enteritis caused by pathogenic strains of *E. coli*, as with *Salmonella*, should such strains spread extraintestinally then treatment with an appropriate antibiotic could be life saving. In such circumstances ciprofloxacin is often the drug of choice. It is therefore concerning that, in England and Wales in 1996, 6% of isolates of pathogenic *E. coli* from cases of extraintestinal infections were resistant to ciprofloxacin with MICs well in excess of anticipated serum levels following treatment at recommended doses.[107] Similarly for *E. coli* from blood and cerebrospinal fluid in 1996, 6% of isolates showed decreased susceptibility to ciprofloxacin.[108] These findings suggest that the efficacy of ciprofloxacin for the treatment of serious infections with *E. coli* is being eroded.

Campylobacter spp.

Campylobacter jejuni is now recognized as the most common cause of bacterial gastroenteritis in many developed countries.[109,110] Because *Campylobacter* enteritis is usually a self-limiting disease, antibiotics are not usually administered except to septicaemic patients and those with other underlying complications. However, when antibiotics have been indicated for the treatment of *Campylobacter* gastroenteritis, until the mid-1990s erythromycin has been the drug of choice.[111,112] Gentamicin, tetracyclines, chloramphenicol and furazolidone were also used with some success, and gentamicin and chloramphenicol have been recommended for the treatment of patients with erythromycin-resistant strains.[113] In studies of the occurrence of resistance to different antimicrobials, only 0.5% of strains isolated in 1978 in a targeted study in the UK were resistant to erythromycin[114] but, in contrast, 10% of strains isolated in Sweden[115] and 9% of strains isolated in Belgium in 1978[116] were erythromycin resistant. In contrast, in a study of strains isolated in north-west England and Wales in 1997, less than 1% were resistant to erthromycin.[117]

The use of fluoroquinolone drugs for the treatment of a variety of acute diarrhoeal diseases including *Campylobacter* enteritis has recently been advocated.[118–121] Therefore, of potential importance for therapy was a reported increase of up to 11% in the incidence of fluoroquinolone resistance in campylobacters isolated from humans in the Netherlands in 1990 following the extensive use of enrofloxacin in the poultry industry in that country.[122] Similarly in England and Wales in 1997, 11% of 5400 isolates were resistant to ciprofloxacin at greater than 8 mg/l.[117] More recently quinolone-resistant strains of *C. jejuni* isolated from patients in the USA were shown by molecular methods to be indistinguishable from similar strains isolated from poultry.[123] These findings have given rise to concern that the injudicious use of fluoroquinolone-containing products in the poultry industry in Europe, and more recently in the USA, has resulted in the emergence of strains of *Campylobacter* spp. with resistance to ciprofloxacin. However, in this respect it is important not to overlook the role of foreign travel, as in the USA study quoted above a substantial number of quinolone-resistant isolates were associated with patients with a recent history of foreign travel, particularly to Mexico.[123]

Conclusion

Multiple drug resistance is now common in pathogenic gut bacteria in both developing and developed countries throughout the world. The rapid emergence of resistance to the drugs of choice for diseases such as typhoid fever, bacillary dysentery and cholera is of particular concern. Although for the most part such resistance is plasmid mediated, a recent development is the emergence of strains with chromosomal resistance, not only to antibiotics such as chloramphenicol, ampicillin and trimethoprim, but also to nalidixic acid and some of the newer fluoroquinolone drugs such as ciprofloxacin, which are now the first-line choice for the treatment of invasive disease. To preserve the efficacy of such drugs for the treatment of life-threatening infections, it is essential that their usage be strictly regulated. Thus, whenever possible, drugs such as ciprofloxacin should be reserved for the treatment of severe infections that do not respond to more conventional antimicrobials. In developed countries, where resistance is often associated with the use of antimicrobials in food-producing animals, such usage should be strictly regulated and the unnecessary prophylactic use of antimicrobials avoided wherever possible.

REFERENCES

1   Ivanoff B. Typhoid fever: global situation and WHO recommendations. *Southeast Asian J Trop Med Publ Health* 1995; 26 (Supplement 2):1–6.

2   Anonymous. Typhoid and paratyphoid fevers. OPCS Monitor 1985; MB2 85/2:9–11C.

3   Ackers M L, Puhr N D, Tauxe R V & Mintz E D. Laboratory-based surveillance of *Salmonella* serotype Typhi infections in the United States: antimicrobial resistance on the increase. *JAMA* 2000; 283:2668–2673.

4   Anonymous. Typhoid fever—Mexico. *MMWR* 1972; 21:177–178.

5   Paniker C K J & Vilma K N. Transferable chloramphenicol resistance in *Salmonella typhi*. *Nature* 1972; 239:109–110.

6   Anonymous. Chloramphenicol resistance in typhoid. *Lancet* 1973; ii:1008–1009.

7   Prakash K & Pillai P K. Multidrug-resistant *Salmonella typhi* in India. *APUA Newslett* 1992; 1:1–3.

8   Panigrahi D, Roy P & Sehgal R. Ciprofloxacin for typhoid fever. *Lancet* 1991; 338:601.

9   Anand A C, Kataria V K, Singh W et al. Epidemic multiresistant enteric fever in Eastern India. *Lancet* 1990; 335:352.

10 Kumar P D. Ciprofloxacin for typhoid fever. *Lancet* 1991; 338:1143.

11 Threlfall E J, Ward L R, Rowe B et al. Widespread occurence of multiple drug-resistant *Salmonella typhi* in India. *Eur J Clin Microbiol Infect Dis* 1992; 11:990–993.

12 Jesudasan M V & John T J. Multiresistant *Salmonella typhi* in India. *Lancet* 1990; 36:256.

13 Gupta B L, Bhujwala R A & Shrinwas. Multiresistant *Salmonella typhi* in India. *Lancet* 1990; 336:252.

14 Rowe B, Threlfall E J & Ward L R. Spread of multiresistant *Salmonella typhi*. *Lancet* 1990; 336:1065.

15 Karamat K A. Multiple drug resistant *Salmonella typhi* and ciprofloxacin. In *Proceedings of the Second Western Pacific Conference on Infectious Diseases and Chemotherapy*, Thailand: Infectious Disease Association of Thailand, Western Pacific Society of Chemotherapy, 1990:480.

16 Wallace M & Yousif A A. Spread of multiresistant *Salmonella typhi*. *Lancet* 1990; 336:1065–1066.

17 Mourad A S, Metwally M, Nour El Deen A et al. Multiple-drug-resistant *Salmonella typhi*. *Clin Infect Dis* 1993; 17:135–136.

18 Hartnett N, McLeod S, AuYong Y et al. Emergence in Ontario, Canada, of multiresistant *Salmonella typhi* from South Asia. *Lancet* 1992; 340:177.

19 Coovadia Y M, Gathiram V, Bhamjee A et al. An outbreak of multiresistant *Salmonella typhi* in South Africa. *Q J Med* 1992; 82:91–100.

20 Rowe B, Ward L R. & Threlfall E J. Multiresistant *Salmonella typhi*—a world-wide epidemic. *Clin Infect Dis* 1997; 24 (Supplement 1):S106–S109.

21 Superable J F T, Castillo M T G, Magboo F P et al. Multiresistant *Salmonella typhi* outbreak in Metro Manilla, Philippines. In *Proceedings of the Second Asia Pacific Symposium on Typhoid Fever and Other Salmonellosis*. Bangkok: Infectious Disease Association of Thailand, 1994:76.

22 Parry C, Wain J, Chinh N T et al Quinolone-resistant *Salmonella typhi* in Vietnam. *Lancet* 1998; 351:1289.

23 Akinyemi K O, Coker A O, Olukoya D K et al. Prevalence of multi-drug resistant *Salmonella typhi* among clinically diagnosed typhoid fever patients in Lagos, Nigeria. *Z Naturforsch* 2000; 55:489–493.

24 Kariuki S, Gilks C, Revathi G & Hart C A. Genotypic analysis of multidrug-resistant *Salmonella enterica* serovar Typhi, Kenya. *Emerg Infect Dis* 2000; 6:649–651.

25 Rowe B, Threlfall E J & Ward L R. Does chloramphenicol remain the drug of choice for typhoid? *Epidemiol Infect* 1987; 98:379–383.

26 Threlfall E J, Rowe B & Ward L R. Occurence and treatment of multi-resistant *Salmonella typhi* in the UK. *PHLS Microbiol Digest* 1992; 8:56–59.

27 Rowe B, Ward L R & Threlfall E J. Treatment of multiresistant typhoid fever. *Lancet* 1991; 337:1422.

28 Rowe B, Ward L R & Threlfall E J. Ciprofloxacin and typhoid fever. *Lancet* 1992; 339:740.

29 Mandal B K. Modern treatment of typhoid fever. *J Infect* 1991; 22:1–4.

30 Threlfall E J & Ward L R. Decreased susceptibility to ciprofloxacin in *Salmonella enterica* serotype Typhi, United Kingdom. *Emerg Infect Dis* 2001; 7:448–450.

31 Umasankar S, Wall R A & Berger J. A case of ciprofloxacin-resistant typhoid fever. *CDR Rev* 1992; 2:R139–R140.

32 Threlfall E J, Ward L R, Skinner J A et al. Ciprofloxacin-resistant *Salmonella typhi* and treatment failure. *Lancet* 1999; 353:1590–1591.

33 Murdoch D A, Banatvala N A, Bone A et al. Epidemic ciprofloxacin-resistant *Salmonella typhi* in Tajikistan. *Lancet* 1998; 351:339.

34 Chandel D S, Chaudhry R, Dhawan B et al Drug resistant *Salmonella enterica* serotype Paratyphi A in India. *Emerg Infect Dis* 2000; 6:420–421.

35 Advisory Committee on the Microbiological Safety of Food. *Report on Microbial Antibiotic Resistance in Relation to Food Safety*. London: The Stationery Office, 1999.

36 Anderson E S, Threlfall E J, Carr J M et al. Clonal distribution of resistance plasmid-carrying *Salmonella typhimurium*, mainly in the Middle East. *J Hyg (Camb)* 1977; 79:429–448.

37 Rowe B, Frost J A & Threlfall E J. Spread of a multiresistant clone of *Salmonella typhimurium* phage type 66/122 in South-East Asia and the Middle East. *Lancet* 1980; i:1070–1071.

38 Le Minor S. Apparition en France d'une épidémie à *Salmonella wien*. *Med Mal Infect* 1972; 2:441–448.

39 McConnell M M, Smith H R, Leonardopoulos J & Anderson E S. The value of plasmid studies in the epidemiology of infections due to drug-resistant *Salmonella wien*. *J Infect Dis* 1979; 139:178–190.

40 Rowe B & Threlfall E J. Drug resistance in Gram-negative aerobic bacilli. *Br Med Bull* 1984; 40:68–76.

41 Lewin C S, Nandivada L S & Amyes S G B. Multiresistant salmonellae and fluoroquinolones. *J Antimicrob Chemother* 1991; 27:147–149.

42 Gupta V, Ray P & Sharma M. Ciprofloxacin-resistant *Salmonella senftenberg* in north India. *Indian J Gastroenterol* 1999; 18:42.

43 Colonna B, Nicoletti M, Visca P et al. Composite IS1 elements

encoding hydroxamate-mediated iron uptake in FI*me* plasmids from epidemic *Salmonella* spp. *J Bacteriol* 1985; 162:307–316.

44 Carattoli A, Tosini, F & Visca P. Multidrug-resistant *Salmonella enterica* serotype Typhimurium infections. *N Engl J Med* 1998; 338:1333–1338.

45 Tosini F, Visca P, Luzzi I et al. Class I integron-borne multiple antibiotic resistance carried on IncFI and IncL/M plasmids in *Salmonella enterica* serotype Typhimurium. *Antimicrob Agents Chemother* 1998; 42:3053–3058.

46 Vahaboglu H, Fuzi M, Cetin S et al. Characterisation of extended-spectrum beta-lactamase (TEM-52)-producing strains of *Salmonella enterica* serovar typhimurium with diverse resistance phenotypes. *J Clin Microbiol* 2001; 39:791–793.

47 Fey P D, Safranek T J, Rupp M E et al. Ceftriaxone-resistant *Salmonella* infection acquired by a child from cattle. *N Engl J Med* 2000; 342:1242–1249.

48 Threlfall E J, Hall M L M & Rowe B. Salmonella bacteraemia in England and Wales, 1981–1990. *J Clin Pathol* 1992; 45:34–36.

49 Threlfall E J, Ward L R & Rowe B. Multiresistant *Salmonella typhimurium* DT 104 and salmonella bacteraemia. *Lancet* 1998; 352:287–288.

50 Mølbak K, Baggesen D L, Aarestrup F M et al. An outbreak of multidrug-resistant, quinolone-resistant *Salmonella enterica* serotype Typhimurium DT 104. *N Engl J Med* 2000; 4:1420–1425.

51 Ward L R, Threlfall E J & Rowe B. Multiple drug resistance in salmonellas isolated from humans in England and Wales: a comparison of 1981 with 1988. *J Clin Pathol* 1990; 43:563–566.

52 Threlfall E J, Ward L R, Skinner J A & Rowe B. Increase in multiple drug resistance in non-typhoidal salmonellas from humans in England and Wales: a comparison of data for 1994 and 1996. *Microb Drug Resist* 1997; 3:263–266.

53 Threlfall E J, Ward L R, Skinner J A & Graham A. Antimicrobial drug resistance in non-typhoidal salmonellas from humans in England and Wales in 1999: decrease in multiple resistance in *Salmonella enterica* serotypes Typhimurium, Virchow and Hadar. *Microb Drug Resist* 2000; 4:319–325.

54 Threlfall E J, Rowe B, Ferguson J L & Ward LR. Characterization of plasmids conferring resistance to gentamicin and apramycin in strains of *Salmonella typhimurium* phage type 204c isolated in Britain. *J Hyg (Camb)* 1986; 97:419–426.

55 Threlfall E J, Hampton M D, Chart H & Rowe B. Identification of a conjugative plasmid carrying antibiotic resistance and salmonella plasmid virulence (*spv*) genes in epidemic strains of *Salmonella typhimurium*. *Lett Appl Microbiol* 1994; 18:82–88.

56 Threlfall E J, Frost J A, Ward L R & Rowe B. Epidemic in cattle of S typhimurium DT 104 with chromosomally-integrated multiple drug resistance. *Vet Rec* 1994; 134:577.

57 Ridley A & Threlfall E J. Molecular epidemiology of antibiotic resistance genes in multiresistant *Salmonella typhimurium* DT 104. *Microb Drug Resist* 1998; 2:113–118.

58 Threlfall E J. Multiresistant *Salmonella typhimurium* DT 104: a truly international multiresistant clone. *J Antimicrob Chemother* 2000; 46:7–10.

59 Ministry of Agriculture, Fisheries and Food; Welsh Office Agriculture Department; Scottish Office, Agriculture and Fisheries Department. *Salmonella in Livestock Production, 1997*. Central Veterinary Laboratory, 1998.

60 Matsomuto M, Suzuki M. Hiramatsu R et al. An increase in multi-drug-resistant isolates of *Salmonella typhimurium* from healthy carriers in Aichi, Japan. *Jpn J Infect Dis* 2000; 53:164–165.

61 Walker R A, Lawson A J, Lindsay E A et al. Decreased susceptibility to ciprofloxacin in outbreak-associated multiresistant *Salmonella typhimurium* DT104. *Vet Rec* 2000; 14:395–396.

62 Guerra B, Laconcha I, Soto S M et al. Molecular characterisation of emergent multiresistant *Salmonella enterica* serotype [4,5,12:i:-] organisms causing human salmonellosis. *FEMS Microb Lett* 2000; 190:341–347.

63 Walker R A, Lindsay E, Woodward M J et al. Variation in clonality and antibiotic resistance genes among multiresistant *Salmonella enterica* serotype Typhimurium phage type U302 (MR U302) from humans, animals and foods. *Microb Drug Resist* 2001; 7:13–21.

64 Tassios P T, Chadjihristodoulou C, Lambiri M et al. Molecular typing of multidrug-resistant *Salmonella blockley* outbreak isolates from Greece. *Emerg Infect Dis* 2000; 6:60–64.

65 Frost J A, Rowe B, Vandepitte J & Threlfall E J. Plasmid characterisation in the investigation of an epidemic caused by multiply-resistant *Shigella dysenteriae* type 1 in Central Africa. *Lancet* 1981; ii:1074–1076.

66 Frost J A, Rowe B & Vandepitte J. Acquisition of trimethoprim resistance in epidemic strains of *Shigella dysenteriae* type 1 from Zaire. *Lancet* 1982; i:963.

67 Mason P R, Nathoo K J, Wellington M & Mason E. Antimicrobial susceptibilities of *Shigella dysenteriae* type 1 in Zimbwabe—implications for the management of dysentery. *Cent Afr J Med* 1995; 41:132–137.

68 Tuttle J, Ries A A, Chimba R M et al. Antimicrobial resistant epidemic *Shigella dysenteriae* type 1 in Zambia; modes of transmission. *J Infect Dis* 1995; 171:371–375.

69 Pal S C. Epidemic bacillary dysentery in West Bengal, India. *Lancet* 1984; i:1462.

70 Bhattacharya S K, Battacharya M K, Dutta D et al. Single dose ciprofloxacin for shigellosis in adults. *J Infect* 1992; 25:117–119.

71 Sen D, Dutta P, Deb B C & Pal S C. Nalidixic acid-resistant *Shigella dysenteriae* type 1 in Eastern India. *Lancet* 1988; ii:911.

72 Shears P & Hart C A. Gastrointestinal bacteria. In Cook G C (ed.) *Manson's Tropical Diseases*, 20th edn. London: W B Saunders, 1996: 824–848.

73 Jamal W Y, Rotimi V O, Chugh T D & Pal T. Prevalence and susceptibility of *Shigella* species to 11 antibiotics in a Kuwait teaching hospital. *J Chemother* 1998; 10:285–290.

74 Sohail M & Sultana K. Antibiotic susceptibilities and plasmid profiles of *Shigella flexneri* isolates from children with diarrhoea in Islamabad, Pakistan. *J Antimicrob Chemother* 1998; 42:838–839.

75 Agarwal S K, Tewari M & Banerjee G. A study on transferable R-plasmids among *Shigella* species at Luknow. *J Commun Dis* 1997; 29:351–354.

76 Ashkenazi S, May-Zahav M, Sulkes J et al. Increasing antimicrobial resistance of *Shigella* isolates in Israel during the period 1984 to 1992. *Antimicrob Agents Chemother* 1995; 39:819–823.

77 Asev A D & Guriz H. Drug resistance of *Shigella* strains isolated in Ankara, Turkey in 1996. *Scand J Infect Dis* 1998; 30:351–353.

78 Agodi A, Marranzano M, Jones C S & Threlfall E J. Molecular characterization of trimethoprim resistance in salmonellas isolated in Sicily, 1985–1988. *Eur J Epidemiol* 1995; 11:33–38.

79 Navia M M, Capitano L, Ruiz J et al. Typing and characterisation of mechanisms of resistance of *Shigella* spp. isolated from feces of children under 5 years of age from Ifakara, Tanzania. *J Clin Microbiol* 1999; 37:3113–3117.

80 Cheasty T, Skinner J A, Rowe B & Threlfall E J. Increasing incidence of antibiotic resistance in shigellas from humans in England and Wales: recommendations for therapy. *Microb Drug Resist* 1998; 4:57–60.

81 Gross R J, Threlfall E J, Ward L R & Rowe B. Drug resistance in *Shigella dysenteriae*, *Sh. flexneri* and *Sh. boydii* in England and Wales: increasing incidence of resistance to trimethoprim. *BMJ* 1984; 288:784–786.

82 Centers for Disease Control. Multistate outbreak of *Shigella*

sonnei gastroenteritis—United States. *MMWR Morb Mortal Wkly Rep* 1987; 36:440–442, 448–449.

83 Wharton M, Spiegal R A, Horan J M et al. A large outbreak of antibiotic-resistant shigellosis at a mass gathering. *J Infect Dis* 1990; 162:1324–1328.

84 Gross R J, Rowe B, Cheasty T & Thomas L V. Increase in drug resistance in *Shigella dysenteriae, Sh. flexneri* and *Sh. boydii* isolated in England and Wales. *BMJ* 1981; 283:575.

85 Bennish M L & Salam M A. Rethinking options for the treatment of shigellosis. *J Antimicrob Chemother* 1992; 30:243–247.

86 Mhalu M S, Mmari P W & Ijumba J. Rapid emergence of El Tor *Vibrio cholerae* resistant to antimicrobial agents during first month of fourth cholera epidemic in Tanzania. *Lancet* 1979; i:345–347.

87 Threlfall E J, Said B, Rowe B & Dávalos-Pérez A. Emergence of multiple drug resistance in *Vibrio cholerae* El Tor from Ecuador. *Lancet* 1993; 342:1173.

88 Weber J T, Mintz E D, Canizares R et al. Epidemic cholera in Ecuador: multidrug-resistance and transmission by water and seafood. *Epidemiol Infect* 1994; 112:1–11.

89 Coppo A, Columbo M, Pazzani C et al. *Vibrio cholerae* in the horn of Africa: epidemiology, plasmid mediated tetracycline resistance gene amplification, and comparison between O1 and non-O1 strains. *Am J Trop Med Hyg* 1995; 53:351–359.

90 Kruse H, Sörum H, Tenover F C & Olsvik O. A transferable multiple drug resistance plasmid from *Vibrio cholerae* O1. *Microb Drug Resist* 1995; 1:203–210.

91 Falbo V, Carattoli A, Tosini F et al. Antibiotic resistance conferred by a conjugative plasmid and class I integron in *Vibrio cholerae* O1 El Tor strains isolated in Albania and Italy. *Antimicrob Agents Chemother* 1999; 43:693–696.

92 Garg P, Chakraborty S, Basu I et al. Expanding multiple antibiotic resistance among clinical strains of *Vibrio cholerae* isolated from 1992–7 in Calcutta, India. *Epidemiol Infect* 2000; 124:393–399.

93 Dalsgaard A, Forslund A, Peterson A et al. Class 1 integron-borne multiple-antibiotic resistance encoded by a 150-kilobase conjugative plasmid in epidemic *Vibrio cholerae* strains isolated in Guinea-Bissau. *J Clin Microbiol* 2000; 38:3774–3779.

94 World Health Organization. *Guidelines for Cholera Control.* Geneva: WHO, 1993.

95 Bhattacharya M K, Ghosh S, Mukhopadhyay A K et al. Outbreak of cholera caused by *Vibrio cholerae* O1 intermediately resistant to norfloxacin in Malda, West Bengal. *J Indian Med Assoc* 2000; 98:389–390.

96 Basu A, Garg P, Datta S et al. *Vibrio cholerae* O139 in Calcutta, 1992–1998: incidence, antibiograms, and genotypes. *Emerg Infect Dis* 2000; 6:139–147.

97 Cheasty T, Rowe B, Said B & Frost J A. *Vibrio cholerae* serogroup O139 in England and Wales. *Lancet* 1993; 307:1007.

98 McConnell M M, Willshaw G A, Smith H R et al. Transposition of ampicillin resistance to an enterotoxin plasmid in an *Escherichia coli* strain of human origin. *J Bacteriol* 1979; 139:346–355.

99 Echeverria P, Verhaert L, Ulangco C V et al. Antimicrobial resistance and enterotoxin production among isolates of *Escherichia coli* in the Far East. *Lancet* 1978; ii:589–592.

100 Willshaw G A, Cheasty T, Frost J A et al. Antimicrobial resistance of O157 VTEC in England and Wales. *Notiziario dell' Istituto Superiore di Sanita.* 1996; 9 (Supplement 3) EVC news 5:3–4.

101 Threlfall E J, Ward L R, Frost J A & Willshaw G A. The emergence and spread of antibiotic resistance in food-borne bacteria. *Int J Food Microbiol* 2000; 62:1–5.

102 Zhang X, McDaniel A D, Wolf L E et al. Quinolone antibiotics induce Shiga toxin-encoding bacteriophages, toxin production, and death in mice. *J Infect Dis* 2000;181:664–670.

103 Gross R J. *Escherichia coli* diarrhoea. In Smith G (ed.) *Topley and Wilson's Principles of Bacteriology, Virology and Immunity,* 8th edn, vol. 3. London: Edward Arnold, 1990: 470–487.

104 Ericsson C D, Johnson P C, DuPont H L et al. Ciprofloxacin or trimethoprim–sulfamethoxazole as initial therapy for travellers' diarrhoea. A placebo-controlled, randomized trial. *Ann Intern Med* 1987; 106:216–220.

105 Wistrom J, Jertborn M, Hedstrom S A et al. Short-term self-treatment of travellers' diarrhoea with norfloxacin: a placebo-controlled study. *J Antimicrob Chemother* 1989; 23:905–913.

106 Wood M J. The use of antibiotics in infections due to *Escherichia coli* O157:H7. *PHLS Microbiol Digest* 1991; 8:18–21.

107 Threlfall E J, Graham A, Cheasty T et al. Resistance to pathogenic Enterobacteriaceae in England and Wales in 1996. *J Clin Pathol* 1997; 50:1027–1028.

108 Threlfall E J, Cheasty T, Graham A & Rowe B. Antibiotic resistance in *Escherichia coli* isolated from blood and cerebrospinal fluid: a 6-year study of isolates from patients in England and Wales. *Int J Antimicrob Agents* 1998; 9:201–205.

109 Frost J A. Current epidemiological issues in human campylobacteriosis. *J Appl Microbiol* 2001; 90 (in press).

110 Tauxe R T. Epidemiology of *Campylobacter jejuni* infections in the United States and other industrialized nations. In Nachamikin I, Blaser M J & Tomkins L S (eds) Campylobacter jejuni: *current status and future trends.* Washington, DC: American Society for Microbiology, 1992: 9–19.

111 McNulty C A M. The treatment of campylobacter infections in man. *J Antimicrob Chemother* 1987; 19:281–284.

112 Bibhat K, Mandal P, De Mol P & Butzler J-P. Clinical aspects of *Campylobacter* infection in humans. In Butzler J-P (ed.) Campylobacter *Infection in Man and Animals.* Boca Raton, FL: CRC Press, 1984: 22–30.

113 Rowe B & Gross R J. Salmonellosis, *Campylobacter* enteritis and *Shigella* dysentery. In Goodwin C S (ed.) *Microbes and Infections of the Gut.* Oxford: Blackwell 1984: 47–77.

114 Brunton W A T, Wilson A M M & MacRae R M. Erythromycin-resistant campylobacters. *Lancet* 1978; ii:1385.

115 Walder M & Fosgren A. Erythromycin-resistant campylobacters. *Lancet* 1978; ii:1201.

116 Vanhoof R, Vanderlinden N P, Dierickz R et al. Susceptibility of *Campylobacter fetus* subsp. *jejuni* to 29 antimicrobial agents. *Antimicrob Ag Chemother* 1978; 14:553–556.

117 Thwaites R T & Frost J A. Drug resistance in *Campylobacter jejuni, C. coli* and *C. lari* isolated from humans in North west England and Wales, 1997. *J Clin PathOL* 1999; 52:812–814.

118 Dupont H L, Corrado M & Sabbaj J. Use of norfloxacin in the treatment of acute diarrheal disease. *Am J Med* 1987; 82 (supplement 6B):79–83.

119 Pichler H E T, Stickler D G & Wolf D. Clinical efficacy of ciprofloxacin compared to placebo in bacterial diarrhea. *Am J Med* 1987; 82 (supplement 4A); 329–332.

120 Anonymous. The choice of antibacterial drugs. *Med Lett Drugs Ther* 1998; 40:33–42.

121 Blaser M J. *Campylobacter* and related species. In Mandell G L, Bennett J E & Dolin R (eds) *Mandell, Douglas and Bennett's Principles and Practice of Infectious Diseases*, 4th edn. New York: Churchill Livingstone, 1995: 1948–1956.

122 Endtz H P, Ruijs G J, van Klingeren B et al. Quinolone resistance in campylobacter isolated from man and poultry following the introduction of fluoroquinolones in veterinary medicine. *J Antimicrob Chemother* 1991; 27:199–208.

123 Smith K E, Besser J M, Hedberg C W et al. Quinolone-resistant *Campylobacter jejuni* infections in Minnesota, 1992–1998. *N Engl J Med* 1999; 20:1525–1532.

Chapter 55
Pneumococcal Disease

N. French and C. Gilks

Streptococcus pneumoniae, the pneumococcus, is a ubiquitous human respiratory bacterial pathogen, well known for its association with pneumonia, sinusitis, otitis and meningitis. It causes disease in all age groups but particularly at the extremes of infancy and old age. Although ubiquitous in distribution, during the past decade there has been an increased awareness of the importance of the pneumococcus as a cause of morbidity and mortality in the tropics. The promotion of the syndromic management of respiratory infections in children is centred on the importance of pneumococcal (along with *Haemophilus influenzae*) infections in this age group. The World Health Organization (WHO) global health burden estimated acute respiratory infection as the leading cause of disability-adjusted life-years (DALYs) in 2000, the pneumococcus being the primary cause of respiratory infection.[1] In addition, the epidemiology of pneumococcal infection in many regions of the tropics has been profoundly altered by the interaction of the pneumococcus with the human immunodeficiency virus (HIV). Perhaps of greatest concern is the rise of antibiotic resistance amongst pneumococci. The continued global expansion of resistance to penicillin threatens to undermine the basic principles of affordable management.

Set against these concerns has been a renewed interest in prevention of pneumococcal disease, driven by the developments in conjugate vaccine technology. The first trials of a pneumococcal polysaccharide-based vaccine were undertaken in South African goldminers during the early twentieth century, and it is perhaps fitting that South Africa will be the first developing nation to report the outcome of trials of polyvalent polysaccharide–protein conjugate vaccines in children. However, widespread vaccine-based control of pneumococcal disease is not an immediate prospect and the pneumococcus will continue to be a leading and evolving pathogen.

Epidemiology

No significant animal reservoir of infection exists and pneumococcal transmission is a consequence of human contact. Indeed, exposure to and colonization with pneumococci is an inescapable fact of human life. The overwhelming majority of human–bacteria encounters will result in asymptomatic nasopharyngeal carriage, which will persist for days or months. In only a few of these human–bacteria interactions will clinical disease develop—by local mucosal spread to the sinuses, middle ear or bronchial tree. Rarely the bacteria will invade tissue to produce bacteraemia, meningitis and other metastatic infections.

Young children and elderly adults are typically at greatest risk of serious pneumococcal infection. However, in regions of high HIV prevalence invasive disease has become a feature of young adults. Males have higher rates of disease than females at all ages and this is a consistent phenomenon in geographically and historically diverse reports. The mechanism underlying this excess risk is unknown, but is unlikely to be explained by environmental factors or reporting bias. Pneumococcal infections also show seasonality. In the temperate regions of the globe, infection rates increase during the winter months and decline in the summer. In the tropics, rates of disease rise at the end of the rainy season and tend to persist through the cooler dry periods.[2]

Pneumococci can be subtyped by determining the seroreactivity of their bacterial capsule against a set of standard antisera—so-called serotypes. In excess of 80 serotypes have been identified and serotyping has been used as a tool for epidemiological surveillance. The predominant serotypes causing disease vary by age and by region[3,4] with some notable for causing serious disease in children (serotype 1) and in adults (serotype 3), whereas other serotypes are associated with multiple antibiotic resistance (6B, 19F and 23F). More sophisticated molecular epidemiology tools have been developed and provide greater discriminatory power than serotyping.[5] These have been used to map the global spread of antibiotic-resistant bacterial clones and to demonstrate the ability of pneumococci to change their capsular structure and consequently their serotype.[6]

Epidemiology of carriage

Nasopharyngeal carriage is critical to the maintenance and spread of pneumococci. Evidence from several sites in the tropics suggests that early colonization is more intense than that found in developed countries. Point prevalence studies in infants and children throughout the tropics have recorded high rates of carriage, typically 60–80% and very often with multiple serotypes.[2] These rates fall in older children and adults, in whom 20% carriage rates are more typical. Nevertheless these rates are still higher than those found in age-matched populations in the developed world. Defects in the mucosal immune response may contribute to these higher rates of carriage, but a more likely explanation is continued high exposure to pneumococci at all stages of life. Carried serotypes tend to be those associated with lower virulence, but are often the serotypes implicated in mucosal disease in children. Carriage may be increased in adults with underlying HIV disease: carriage point prevalence was 50% greater (29% versus 19%) in HIV-infected age-matched adults in two separate studies in Nairobi and Entebbe (C. Gilks and N. French, unpublished results). There are no data from the tropics describing carriage rates in the elderly.

Childhood epidemiology

Serious manifestations of pneumococcal disease are highly prevalent in paediatric populations across the tropics. *S. pneumoniae* is a leading blood culture isolate from most reported bacteraemia studies in infants and children globally.[7,8] Community-based incidence data are more limited; nevertheless reports from Soweto in South Africa[9] and from a rural region of The Gambia[10] measured rates of invasive disease in children aged under 5 years of 130 and 240 per 100 000 child-years respectively, rates several fold higher than those in the developed world (compare with a rate of 20 per 100 000 child-years in the UK in under-fives).[11] Peak rates are found in those aged less than 1 year, and in The Gambia exceeded 500 per 100 000 child-years. Moreover, rates of pneumococcal pneumonia are almost certainly significantly higher and may contribute between 40% and 60% of all cases of childhood pneumonia.[12,13] Meningitis is the most lethal of the clinical syndromes associated with pneumococcal infection. Outside the meningococcal epidemics of the central African meningitis belt, the pneumococcus is the leading cause of meningitis in children and a significant contributor to neonatal meningitis. Between 5% and 25% of all invasive disease is accounted for by meningitis.[2]

The explanation for these high rates of disease is undoubtedly multifactorial. Low birth weight, poor nutrition, micronutrient and vitamin deficiencies, and increased pneumococcal exposure have all been suggested. In a formal case–control study in The Gambia overcrowding, parental education and occupation showed no clear association with risk but passive smoking, cooking indoors and preceding illness were significant risk factors.[14]

Acute otitis media is the most common manifestation of pneumococcal disease in children in the developed world but little is known about its epidemiology in the developing world. Hearing impairment and chronic suppurative ear problems are a frequent finding in children in the tropics[15] and the long-term consequences of this in terms of failure of language skills and education are poorly understood. The pneumococcus-attributable contribution to acute and subsequent chronic ear disease remains to be established. Prevention of acute pneumococcal otitis media is not currently a priority for pneumococcal vaccine strategies in the developing world. With more data on disease burden, priorities may change.

Adult epidemiology

Limited community-based incidence rates of pneumococcal disease exist for adult populations in the tropics. Little of this is properly stratified by age and the additional disease burden in the elderly is not well characterized. The best available estimates would suggest rates of between 20 to 300 cases of invasive (bacteraemia and/or meningitis) pneumococcal disease per 100 000 adult-years.[16,17] The lower-level estimates are similar to the rates of invasive disease in elderly populations in the UK.[11] In otherwise healthy adults, bacteraemia complicates pneumonia in about one-quarter of cases; thus the rates of pneumococcal pneumonia may be four times greater. Pneumonia is invariably a leading cause of admission to hospital in reported series[18–20] and the pneumococcus is responsible for between 46% and 80% of cases.[21–23] As in children the pneumococcus is the leading cause of bacterial meningitis in adults outside the central African meningitis belt, although meningitis accounts for a smaller proportion of invasive disease in adults than in children.

The high rates of pneumococcal infection in otherwise fit and well adults in the tropics, and particularly in sub-Saharan Africa, compared with adults in the developed world is incompletely understood. Environmental and social factors are believed to play a leading part and it is perhaps important to note the similarities in rates of disease today in the tropics to those measured in the industrialized world in the pre-penicillin era of the 1920s and 1930s.[24] Host genetic factors are also believed to be important. Studies in the USA have found rates of pneumococcal infection to be higher amongst African Americans than in European Americans, a finding that is incompletely accounted for by social and environmental confounding.[25] The dynamics of carriage and the intensity of exposure to serotypes not previously encountered may also contribute to disease rates. Pneumococcal disease is more likely to occur when an individual is exposed to a new pneumococcal serotype, and this will happen more frequently in an environment of intense transmission. This was an important factor in the epidemics of pneumococcal disease in South African goldminers, which drove the initial studies of pneumococcal vaccination. More recently similar epidemics have occurred in army barracks and prisons.[26] However, the role of epidemic spread of pneumococci in the community setting and its association with disease are less clearly defined.

The use of tobacco in the developing world, a predisposing factor for invasive pneumococcal disease in the industrialized world, is on the increase.[27] There is every reason to suspect that this adverse effect of smoking will also contribute to an increased burden of disease as smoking rates rise. However, of greatest importance as a risk factor for developing pneumococcal disease is HIV infection.

HIV-associated pneumococcal disease

HIV is now widespread in the tropics and increases the risk of pneumococcal pneumonia by 6–20-fold.[16,17,28] Bacteraemia complicates pneumonia in 80% of cases. Thus rates of invasive disease are 10–100 times more frequent in age-matched HIV-infected adults than the HIV uninfected. Community-based incidence data from East Africa have recorded rates of invasive disease in HIV-infected adults of 1700–4200 per 100 000 person-years.[16,29] Rates of disease show a strong association with HIV-related immunosuppression: higher rates at lower CD4+ T cell counts.[29] Furthermore reinfection rates are extremely high: 25 000 per 100 000 person-years.[16,29] In the Queen Elizabeth Central Hospital in Blantyre, HIV was associated with 95% of admissions with invasive pneumococcal disease during 1997–1998.[30] The underlying rate of adult HIV seroprevalence in this region is estimated at 20%. Within this series there was also a high proportion of meningitis cases, which may also be a feature of the HIV–pneumococcal interaction in the tropics. The impact of HIV on pneumococcal disease in children in the tropics is not well described, but there appears a similar amplifying effect on risk, as in adults.[17]

Microbiology

S. pneumoniae is a Gram-positive bacterium, which grows in chains in liquid media, but is more characteristically seen as pairs in clinical specimens. The term lanceolate is used to describe this paired appearance, the organisms appearing egg shaped with their flatter ends opposed. A source of H_2O_2 is required for growth and consequently pneumococci grow better in the presence of catalase. In the diagnostic laboratory this is usually achieved by growing the organism in the presence of blood on a blood agar or heated blood agar (chocolate agar) plate. They grow best at 37°C (growth range 25–40°C) in the presence of 5–10% CO_2, conditions that can be achieved in a candle extinction jar. Horse blood is typically used in media preparation. When this is not readily available sheep or goat blood provides a suitable alternative. Human or cow blood is best avoided, not only for the infection risks associated with handling human blood products, but because they both contain inhibitory factors that interfere with the growth of pneumococci. Liquid media appropriate for use in manual blood culture systems to recover pneumococci are nutrient broth, tryptone soya broth and brain heart infusion broth. Further information on media and reagent preparation relevant to laboratory practice in the developing world is available in Cheesborough.[31]

On a blood agar plate, pneumococci form colonies that are usually opaque, 1–2 mm in diameter with central umbilication, and surrounded by a characteristic green zone as a result of the action of an exotoxin, pneumolysin, which produces a pigment from haemoglobin. This is referred to as α-haemolysis. Production of a polysaccharide capsule by the bacteria is responsible for the opaque appearance. Colonies may appear mucoid if the bacteria produce large quantities of capsule. Failure to produce a significant capsule leads to the growth of transparent colonies. These phenotypic characteristics may be important in pathogenesis (see below). Pneumococci readily undergo autolysis and death, and this explains the umbilicated characteristics of the colonies, with the centre of the colony collapsing. This characteristic may occasionally hinder diagnosis. Pneumococci grown in liquid media will produce turbidity that may then clear on further culture in as little as 16 hours. Although not a problem with modern, continually monitored, blood culturing systems, laboratories using manual systems need to time visual inspections and subculturing to avoid this pitfall. A zone of 'haemolysis' above the sedimented red cells in a manual system will provide additional evidence of bacterial growth.

Pneumococci must be differentiated from other α-haemolytic streptococci by demonstrating sensitivity to optochin (ethyl hydrocupreine, a quinine derivative once used for therapy but withdrawn because of toxicity) and solubility when cultured after exposure to bile salts. Sensitivity testing using a Kirkby–Bauer or modified Stokes method and an appropriate buffered agar should be performed, with available antibiotics. Penicillin sensitivity is best assessed with a 1-µg oxacillin disc. Not only is oxacillin more stable and storage-friendly than low-strength penicillin discs, it is relatively precise in predicting reduced susceptibility to penicillin (zone diameter ≤ 19 mm). Accurate determination of the susceptibility characteristics of pneumococci will require measurement of the minimal inhibitory concentration (MIC) by a broth or agar dilution method or the use of a graduated antibiotic-impregnated plastic strip, E-test® (AB Biodisk, Sweden). Serotyping of pneumococci is unnecessary for routine clinical diagnostic work, but may be performed for epidemiological surveillance. Although several techniques are available, the Quellung reaction remains the standard. A suspension of pneumococci in saline is incubated with capsular-type-specific antiserum and methylene blue for 10 minutes. If there is recognition of the capsule by the antiserum present, the resultant capsular–antibody complex leads to a change in the refractive index of the capsule that stands out and contrasts (often referred to as swelling) against the methylene blue-stained intracellular contents.

Bacterial anatomy and physiology

The membranous and external structures of the pneumococci are made up of a triple-layered cell membrane, cell wall and a polysaccharide capsule (Figure 55.1). These

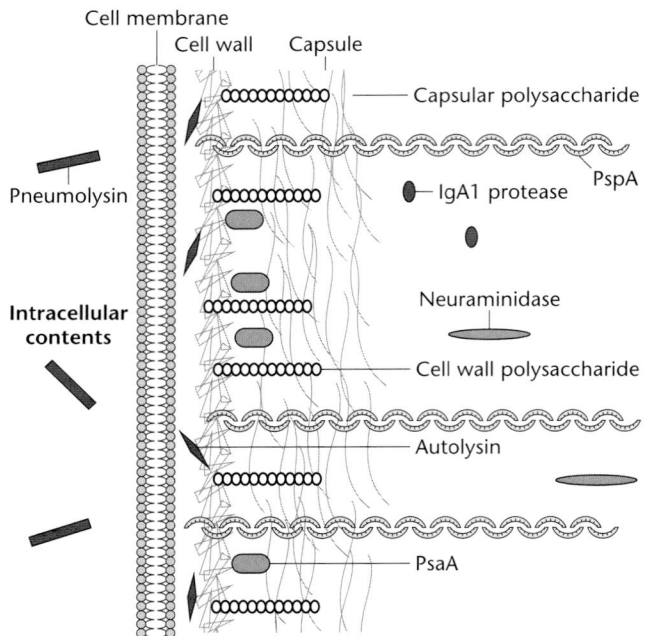

Figure 55.1: Schematic structure of pneumococcal cell membrane, wall and capsule. Pneumococcal surface protein A (Psp A) protrudes through the capsule and may act to stabilize the capsular structure. Psp A is highly variable with over 40 serotypes recognized and marked genetic heterogeneity but with a number of stable immunologically cross-reactive molecular epitopes. Psa A is genetically and antigenically conserved across most capsular serotypes. Its anatomical localization within the surface components is unclear. Cell wall polysaccharide consists of teichoic acid, peptidoglycan and phosphorylcholine. When bound to a lipid molecule it is able to extend into the lipid-rich cell membrane, and is then known as the Forsmann or F-antigen.

structures confer the principal mechanisms underlying the pathogenicity and virulence of the bacteria. In addition the antigenic characteristics of the capsule have been used as the principal typing method for pneumococci. Exotoxin production is more limited than in other streptococcal species, and tissue damage as a consequence of pneumococcal infection is primarily the consequence of the inflammatory response triggered by cell wall and capsular components.

The cell wall is made up of a combination of peptidoglycan bound covalently to teichoic acid which protrudes deep into the capsule. These cell wall constituents are known as the C-polysaccharide and are unique (with the exception of a few Viridans streptococci) to the pneumococcus. C-polysaccharide activates complement by either the alternative or the classical pathway in the presence of anti-C-polysaccharide antibody, and also leads to the production of inflammatory cytokines.

The pneumococcal capsule is formed from the polymerization of oligosaccharides, which are transported to the outer surface of the cell wall and anchored by covalent binding to the cell wall constituents. Permutations in the monosaccharides used in the production of the oligosaccharide macromolecules leads to antigenic diversity. Genetic control of capsule production

is incompletely understood. The process appears to depend on the use of several genes combined into a single translational unit,[32] but importantly bacteria may possess or acquire additional capsule-related genes and thus be able to change their capsular characteristics. In vivo capsular switching has been described in human nasopharyngeal isolates as a spontaneous phenomenon,[33] and may occur following conjugate polysaccharide vaccination (see below). Alterations in mucosal immune pressure are the presumed stimulation for this.

The polysaccharide capsule is critical to the organism's virulence and in the absence of type-specific opsonizing antibody the capsule blocks phagocytosis. The mechanism by which the capsule does this is not clear. It is probably in part related to its ability to cover and hide cell wall-bound complement and immunoglobulin, which would otherwise act as opsonins. The consequence of failed phagocytosis is uncontrolled replication of pneumococci, deleterious inflammatory responses and death of the host.

Other cell surface components have been identified and are likely to play a role in pathogenesis. Pneumococcal surface protein A (Psp A) and pneumococcal surface adhesin A (Psa A, although not physiologically an adhesion molecule) are the two best described members of a family of choline-binding proteins. They are anchored to the cell wall and protrude through the capsule. Experiments in mice using mutant pneumococci with selective deletions of these proteins have shown decreased virulence and mucosal surface binding. The specific interest in these proteins comes from their possible use as a vaccine or vaccine component.

Pneumolysin and autolysin are exotoxins that contribute to virulence. Pneumolysin is a member of a group of cholesterol-binding cytolytic bacterial toxins found in several other Gram-positive organisms. It is cytotoxic for phagocytic and respiratory epithelial cells and is proinflammatory by activating complement. Pneumolysin injected into lung tissue leads to the histological characteristics of acute pneumonia. Pneumolysin-deficient pneumococci show reduced virulence in animal models. Autolysin is a peptide responsible for bacterial cell wall remodelling, and the reason for the in vitro culture characteristics of autolysis described above. In disease, autolysin may contribute to virulence by liberating cell wall polysaccharides that in turn will intensify the host inflammatory response. Other bacterial components (e.g., neuraminidase and hyaluronidase) may also contribute to virulence and pathogenicity, but their role in human disease awaits clarification.

Host susceptibility

For pneumococcal disease to develop, several critical events must take place. The bacteria must gain entry to the nasopharynx (or rarely to the female genital tract) and adhere to the epithelial cells. Subsequently they must spread to susceptible anatomical sites, such as sinuses, middle ear and bronchial tree (peritoneum), reproduce freely and finally may breach endothelial surfaces and invade the bloodstream and other distant sites. In broad terms, the host defends itself against pneumococcal mucosal infection by preventing mucosal attachment and spread, using the mucociliary system that lines the respiratory tract and adaptive mucosal immune responses. Defence against invasive disease is critically dependent on the presence of opsonizing anticapsular antibodies and a functioning phagocytic system. A list of conditions predisposing to pneumococcal infection is shown in Table 55.1.

Anatomical defences

The immature development of the Eustachian tube and the inability to clear secretions and bacteria from the middle ear are believed to underlie the susceptibility of young children to otitis. Similarly other factors that interfere with mucociliary function will predispose to infection, such as cigarette smoking, smoke inhalation from poorly ventilated fires, and preceding viral infection leading to direct destruction of ciliated epithelium in the upper respiratory mucosa. In addition viral infections may upregulate the mucosal expression of ligands for the choline-binding proteins on the surface of the pneumococci, improving mucosal attachment. This may be particularly relevant for allowing access of more virulent pneumococcal serotypes, which may have a decreased capacity for carriage but a high propensity for invasion once attached. Pneumococci of the transparent phenotype (see above) produce little capsule but have a phosphatidylcholine-rich cell wall and are believed to bind upper respiratory epithelium more effectively than their capsulate counterparts. They are never found as invasive isolates, the presence of a capsule being essential for this characteristic. Furthermore, inflammatory changes, mucus hypersecretion and the subsequent postnasal drip that often accompanies 'colds and flu' will predispose to the aspiration of pneumococci through the larynx and into the bronchial tree.

Mucosal immune response

Innate and adaptive immune system responses contribute to prevention of carriage or spread of pneumococci across mucosal surfaces. Lactoferrin, lysozyme, lactoperoxidase and mannose binding protein (MBP) are components of the innate immune system and act by binding and opsonizing pneumococci for clearance by mucosally associated phagocytes. C-reactive protein (CRP), another agent of the innate immune response, also acts in a similar way, but during systemic infection. Polymorphisms in the genes encoding MBP and CRP are associated with invasive pneumococcal disease and have begun to be described in African populations.[34] It has been postulated that the evolutionary persistence of CRP is a direct consequence of its ability to protect against pneumococcal disease.

Secretory IgA, the predominant human immunoglobulin at mucosal surfaces, has the ability to prevent the binding of pneumococci (and possibly neutralize pneumolysin) and to opsonize bacteria for phagocyte recognition. Of the two IgA isotypes IgA2 is the more important because it is resistant to an IgA protease secreted by the pneumococcus that is able to disrupt IgA1. Animal studies have confirmed the defensive properties of IgA; however, the importance of IgA in the overall scheme of protection against pneumococci in humans remains unclear. Selective deficiencies of IgA are not clearly associated with pneumococcal infection and are believed to be uncommon in non-caucasian populations.

The principal (and most studied) phagocyte in the respiratory tract is the human alveolar macrophage. These cells are able rapidly to destroy pneumococci following phagocytosis. The pneumococcus, unlike *Mycobacterium tuberculosis* for instance, possesses little in its armamentarium to prevent phagolysosomal digestion. Central to the competent functioning of the macrophage is appropriate activation of the cell and opsonization of the pneumococcal target.[35] Failure of the macrophage to respond to chemokine and cytokine signals may compromise effective phagocytic function. Similar to the IgA story, however, alveolar macrophages appear to be central to defence against pneumococci, but much remains to be understood.

Systemic immune response

Critical to protection against invasive disease is the presence of capsule-specific opsonizing antibodies and an intact phagocytic cell system in the liver and particularly the spleen.

The central role of serum in protection was identified in the late nineteenth century. It was shown that protection could be achieved in animal models by the infusion of immune serum. In the 1920s further discoveries led to the realization that the antibody conferring protection was directed against the pneumococcal capsule. Subsequently, passive vaccination or serum therapy using serotype-specific antisera formed the basis of early therapeutic successes in treating pneumococcal disease. Recent studies have confirmed the association between low levels or decreased activity of capsule-specific IgG and the risk of disease.[29,36] Unfortunately the absolute level of capsule-specific immunoglobulin in isolation is not a reliable predictor of protection or susceptibility. This is in part due to the measurement of low-affinity or cross-reactive antibodies. Measurement of the functional activity of anticapsular antibodies is believed (although by no means proven) to be a more accurate measure of immunity. These techniques assess the ability of antibodies to opsonize bacteria and stimulate phagocytosis by a standardized phagocytic cell, and therefore should directly reflect the function of these antibodies in vivo.[37]

Table 55.1 Conditions that predispose to pneumococcal infection in the tropics by mechanism of susceptibility.

	Decreased antibody	Reduced mucosal clearance[a]	Anatomical defects	Complement deficiency	Increased exposure	Phagocyte dysfunction	Comment
Important							**Common condition**
HIV infection	✓	✓				✓	Debility interferes with respiratory secretion clearance in late stages
Sickle cell disease	✓			✓		✓	
Infancy and ageing	✓		✓		✓		High carriage rates in siblings of infants leads to increased exposure
Alcoholism		✓				✓	
Chronic chest disease		✓	✓			✓	Tuberculosis, asthma and bronchiectasis
Malnutrition	✓	✓				✓	
Diabetes						✓	
Smoking		✓					Mucociliary interference and direct toxicity on alveolar macrophages
Poverty			✓		✓		Overcrowding and usually co-existent nutritional deficiencies
Less important							**Less common condition**
Kidney disease	✓			✓		✓	
Liver cirrhosis				✓		✓	
Lymphoproliferative disease	✓						
Visceral leishmaniasis (and other parasitic infections[b])	✓						Complex immune defects and abnormalities of splenic function

[a]By virtue of immobility, bedridden or defective mucociliary action.
[b]Malaria and invasive nematode and trematode infections, although association unclear.

Diseases that lead to underproduction of immuno-globulins are associated with an increased risk of pneumococcal disease. This is perhaps most dramatic in the primary and acquired hypogammaglobulinaemias, in which repeated episodes of otitis, sinusitis, pneumonia and invasive disease occur. The high rates of invasive pneumococcal disease in early childhood are in part related to underproduction of an IgG isotype, IgG2, the principal isotype contributing to anticapsular antibodies in adults. A powerful IgG2 response is produced when derivatives of the complement factor C3, which is an important opsonin of pneumococcal polysaccharide, binds a co-receptor on the B cell (complement receptor 2 CD21) in association with B-cell receptors binding polysaccharide. Importantly, children under 2 years of age do not adequately express complement receptor 2 on B cells,[38] and consequently little IgG produced is of the IgG2 isotype.

Deficient capsule-specific IgG production underpins the increased susceptibility of HIV-infected individuals to pneumococcal disease. Massive and progressive B-cell destruction is a feature of uncontrolled HIV infection. The envelope glycopeptide gp120 of the HIV virus acts as a B-cell superantigen, binding the variable region of the heavy chain of the B-cell receptor, but at a site distinct from that for antigen-specific binding.[39] The effect is massive polyclonal expansion and the subsequent rapid death of the B cell by apoptosis. This in turn leads to steady and progressive erosion of the B-cell population. Gp120 specifically binds B-cell receptors using heavy-chain variable regions derived from the VH3 family of heavy-chain genes. In healthy adults it is antibodies of the VH3 idiotype that make up the majority of those active against pneumococci; thus HIV preferentially destroys the humoral immune response responsible for protecting against pneumococcal infection.

Malnutrition, old age, chronic liver disease including alcohol-related disease, and renal failure are associated with pneumococcal disease. Although impaired immuno-globulin production to a greater or lesser extent is a feature of these conditions, other factors play a part in increasing susceptibility (e.g., overcrowding, impaired cough reflex, immobility, phagocyte defects, presence of ascites and orthostasis).

In addition to immunoglobulin, complement also possesses opsonic activity against pneumococci. In vitro studies confirm the value of complement in stimulating phagocytosis of pneumococci and, as mentioned above, complement is able to modulate B-cell responses to poly-saccharides. Gram-positive organisms are able to resist the effects of the terminal membrane attack complex (C5–C9); consequently it is the early complement factors that are implicated in defence. Perhaps surprisingly, there are few reports of specific complement deficiency states associated with pneumococcal infection, although the increased risk of disease in nephrotic syndrome is believed to be due to hypocomplementaemia as a con-sequence of deposition and consumption of the early complement factors in the kidneys.

Once opsonized, pneumococci must be removed from circulation and killed by phagocytes. Polymorphonuclear leucocytes and macrophages in the liver and spleen under-take this task. Surprisingly, primary defective functioning of phagocytes by either chemotaxis or impaired oxidative killing is not associated with increased rates and severity of pneumococcal disease, although neutropenic indi-viduals are at greater risk. Individuals who lack a spleen (following splenectomy) or who are functionally asplenic (homozygous sickle cell disease) suffer high rates of pneumococcal disease, which is in large part due to the reduction in phagocytic function, although other factors including abnormal antibody production contribute to increased susceptibility. Other phagocytic defects occur as a result of variation in phagocyte-expressed Fc recep-tors, particularly FcγRIIa.[40] These have been associated with increased susceptibility to respiratory infections in children. However, the importance of polymorphisms in these receptors and risk of pneumococcal disease in African or Asian populations remains to be established.

Clinical syndromes

Pneumonia

Pneumonia is the most important presentation of pneumococcal disease by virtue of its frequency—accounting for 80–90% of all pneumococcal disease in adults—and its significant mortality. In the pre-antibiotic era, the case fatality rate was 40–50%, and even now rates of 10% are seen with antibiotic therapy.[23,29] Delayed disease presentation with compromised health-seeking behaviour through poverty or lack of access to health services markedly influences the case fatality rate. Mortality rates in children were similarly high, but early access to antibiotic therapy dramatically improves out-come from pneumococcal pneumonia, and mortality rates of 1–2% are achievable.[10,41] A clear understanding of the presentation, management and expected outcome of pneumonia is essential knowledge for basic health care provision in the tropics.

Clinical presentation

This is typically acute with a 2–3-day history of cough, fever, dyspnoea and purulent sputum production. A more prolonged presentation may occur if the pneumonia has been partially treated or if there is underlying chronic chest disease, in particular tuberculosis. Other symptoms that may be prominent include: haemoptysis—the classical 'rusty sputum' is characteristic when present (the pigmentary effect of exotoxins on haemoglobin), but infrequent; pleuritic chest pain; headache, often severe and associated with meningism without confirmed meningitis; and diarrhoea, which may occasionally be the primary presenting complaint and lead to confusion with acute gastroenteritis.

Patients appear unwell and may be tachycardic and tachypnoeic. Cyanosis, if present, indicates more severe disease but is difficult to assess in individuals with black skin. Chest signs of consolidation (dullness to percussion, bronchial breathing and aegophony) or more commonly coarse inspiratory crackles consistent with retained secretions are usually heard on auscultation. A pleural rub may also be present and does not necessarily predict complicated pleural disease. Diagnostic confusion may occur if the presentation is hyperacute with abrupt onset of rigors, when malaria, other bacterial septicaemic illness or fulminant viral illness may then head the list of differential diagnoses. Presentations with acute psychosis,

confusion, hypothermia, jaundice[42] and abdominal pain may also mislead the unwary.

The presentation, recognition and assessment of pneumonia in children are detailed in Chapter 23.

Investigations

Confirmation of pneumonia is achieved by finding confluent consolidation in a lobar, segmental or subsegmental distribution on chest radiography. Chest radiography will often resolve diagnostic confusion (Figure

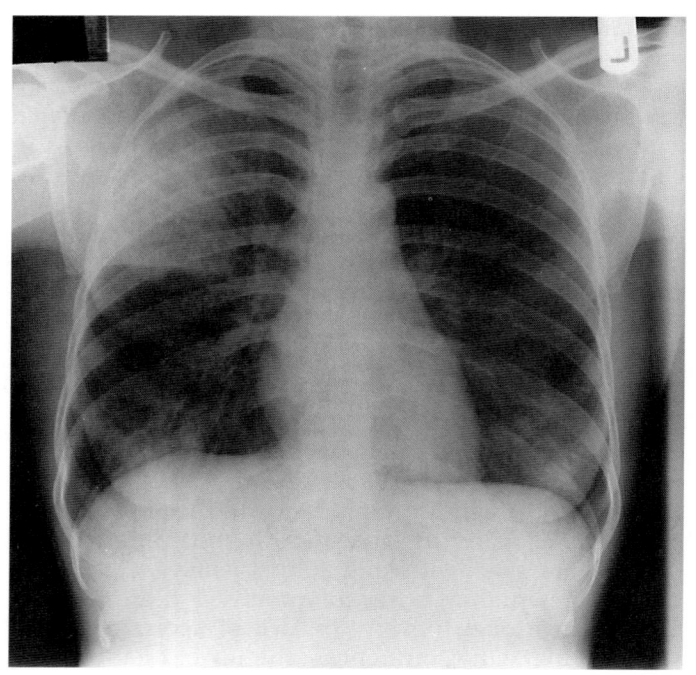

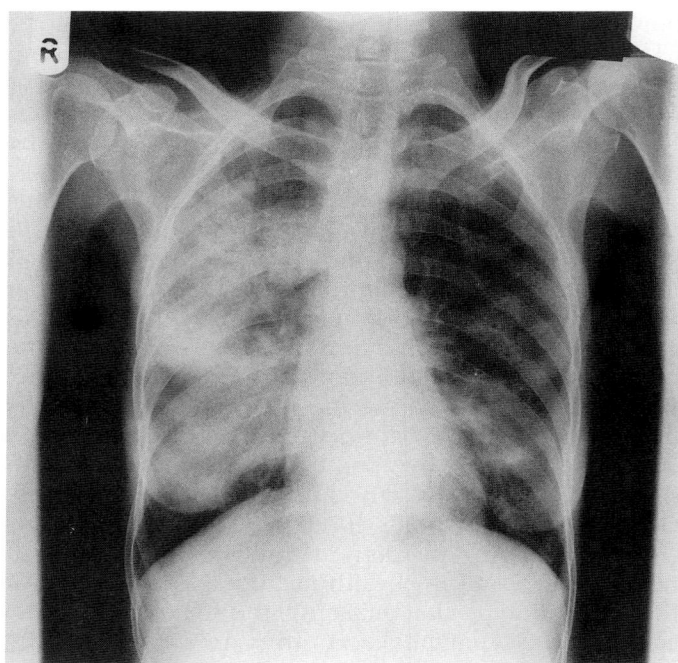

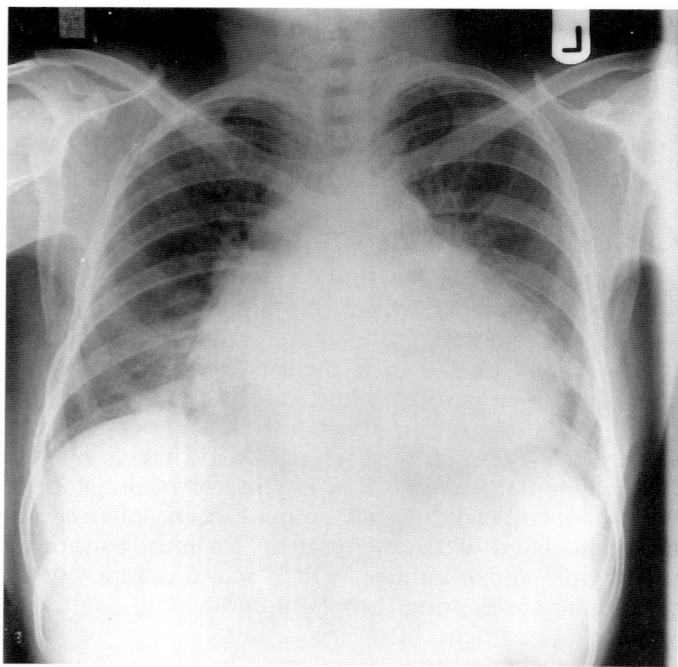

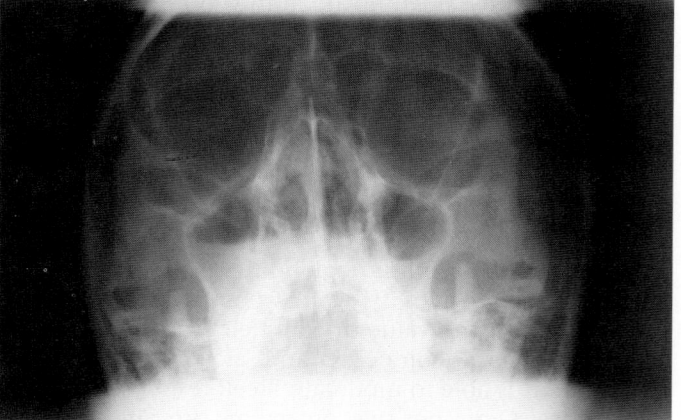

Figure 55.2: Radiographic appearances of pneumococcal disease: (**A**) Classical right upper lobe pneumococcal pneumonia in a 32-year-old HIV-infected Kenyan woman; (**B**) bilateral pulmonary consolidation, particularly in the right lung, as a consequence of a *S. pneumoniae–M. tuberculosis* coinfection in a 26-year-old HIV-infected Kenyan woman; (**C**) pneumococcal pericarditis and pericardial effusion in a 34-year-old Ugandan male of uncertain HIV status; (**D**) bilateral maxillary sinus fluid levels in a 28-year-old HIV-infected Kenyan with pneumococcal bacteraemia and no pulmonary focus.

55.2). Confirmation of a pneumococcal aetiology can be made definitively by the recovery of pneumococci from blood culture or from a transthoracic needle lung aspirate. This latter technique has proved a safe and valid technique when aspiration is performed on consolidated pulmonary tissue using a small-gauge needle. Sputum is often the most readily available clinical specimen and most commonly used for diagnosis. Interpretation of Gram stain examination and culture results require some caution. Pneumococci carried in the nasopharynx may contaminate expectorated sputum specimens and lead to a false-positive diagnosis. Adhering to the criteria in Figure 55.3 can increase specificity. Examination of the sputum for acid- and alcohol-fast bacilli should be performed because of the frequent coexistence of tuberculosis with pneumococcal pneumonia. Commercial kits for the identification of pneumococcal capsular polysaccharide in blood or urine are available but have variable sensitivity and are usually an unjustifiable cost for basic diagnostic laboratories. Likewise serological tests based on pneumolysin–immune complexes or rising antibody titres to Psa A do not have a place in routine clinical practice at present.

Subsidiary investigations including white cell count, arterial blood gases, electrolyte measurements and liver function tests are not helpful in establishing a diagnosis, but may be used as measures of severity.[23,43]

Differential diagnosis

When respiratory symptoms and signs are lacking, pneumococcal pneumonia may need to be differentiated from a wide range of febrile conditions. When a diagnosis of pneumonia is established, the primary differential is from other bacterial pneumonias, and occasionally typhoid or amoebic liver abscess (right-sided effusion). *Haemophilus influenzae* and less frequently other Gram-negative bacteria are the aetiological agent in up to 10% of cases of adult community-acquired pneumonia (CAP) in sub-Saharan Africa.[22,23] Making a definitive diagnosis of these infections is in many ways more difficult than diagnosing pneumococcal disease. They may coinfect with the pneumococcus, and diagnosis is usually presumptive based on failure of penicillin therapy and successful treatment with an aminoglycoside. Tuberculosis is the most critical differential diagnosis to consider. It may present as an acute pneumonic illness or as a coinfection with the pneumococcus. *Mycobacterium tuberculosis* may be implicated in 5–15% of adult cases of CAP in sub-Saharan Africa,[22] the association being

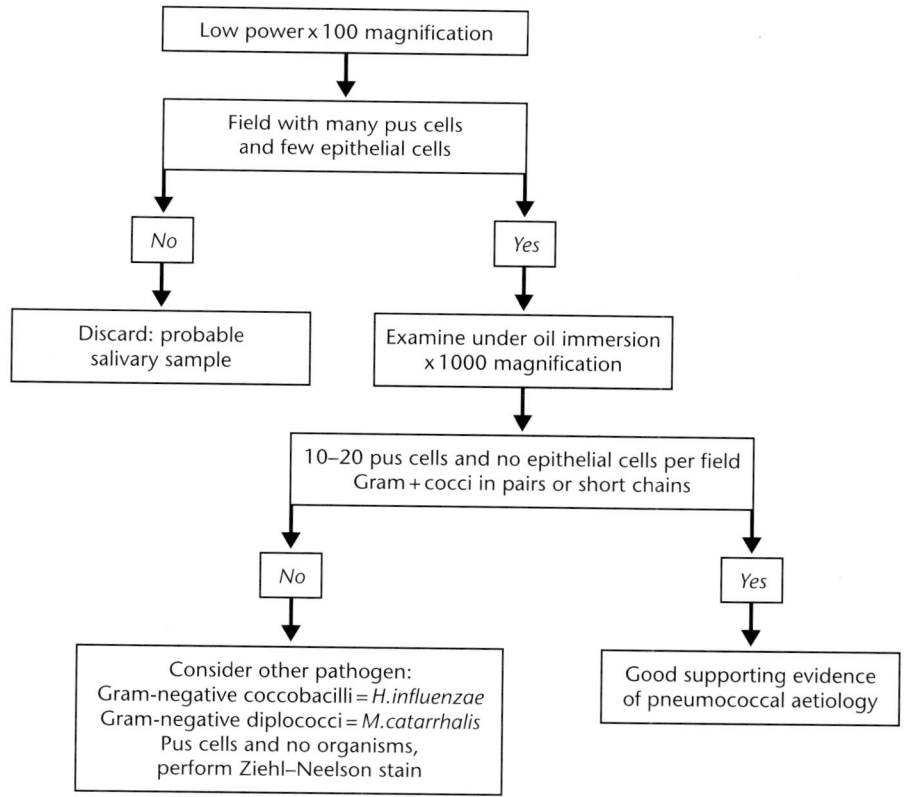

Figure 55.3: Criteria for the interpretation of sputum microscopy in the presence of appropriate clinical signs of pneumonia.

particularly important in HIV-infected adults.[23] Ziehl–Neelsen staining of sputum samples will help in making the diagnosis; however, in up to one half of the cases of *M. tuberculosis* infection reported in a series of CAP from the Kenyan coast, culture for mycobacteria was required to establish a diagnosis. It is also important to note that many of these patients had shown an initial response to antipneumococcal therapy as a consequence of pneumococcal coinfection.[23] Poor response to antibiotics, pleural effusions, cavitation of lung lesions, cervical or axillary lymphadenopathy or incomplete resolution of pneumonia at follow-up should raise the suspicion of *M. tuberculosis* infection.

Management and therapy

With overcrowded inpatient facilities, the threshold for admission to hospital may be more severe in tropical regions, and an assessment to differentiate suitability for outpatient oral therapy or the need for inpatient parenteral therapy is required. Indicators of poor outcome are listed in Table 55.2. Further indicators of the suitability of oral therapy involve an assessment of gastrointestinal symptoms and microbial factors.

Table 55.2 Associations of severe disease and poor outcome in pneumonia.

	Severity grading
Demographic features	
Age > 55 years	A
Use of traditional healer	A
Increasing distance from health centre	B
Recent migration or refugee camp	B
Clinical features	
Confusion	B
Diastolic blood pressure < 60 mmHg	A
Respiratory rate > 30 breaths/min	A
Pulse rate > 120 beats/min	A
Cyanosis	B
Extrapulmonary infection	B
Jaundice	B
Reduced body mass index or wasted	B
Investigations: available at initial assessment	
Multilobar disease	B
White cell count < 4000 cells/μl	A
White cell count > 18 000 cells/μl	B
Investigations: available during therapy	
Penicillin-resistant pneumococcus	B
Coinfection with tuberculosis	B
Pneumococcal bacteraemia	B

The table represents a summary of information from several sources.[22,23,44,45,69] A, factor strongly associated with severe disease and death (five times or greater risk of death if present); B, moderately associated (less than five times or poorly quantified increased risk of death). No validated scheme to determine hospital admission or use of parenteral antibiotics exists; however, the presence of two or more grade A factors or three or more grade B factors should lead to hospital admission, if possible. Such an approach will be sensitive for identifying severe disease but will lack specificity.

Vomiting or profuse diarrhoea are relative contraindications to oral therapy as antibiotic absorption may be impaired. Confirmation or suspicion of a penicillin-resistant pneumococcus should also lead to a reconsideration of dose and route of antibiotic administration (see below).

In addition to antimicrobial therapy, other supportive treatment should be initiated. If available, supplemental oxygen, preferably monitored with blood gases or peripheral saturation measurements, should be provided when hypoxia is present. Clearance of respiratory secretions by changing posture, suctioning and provision of moist air may also be necessary. Maintenance of appropriate hydration (with intravenous fluids if necessary) and nebulized saline may be particularly helpful at preventing desiccation of respiratory and pharyngeal secretions, and may assist expectoration. Assisted ventilation, when available, will be necessary in some cases when respiratory muscle fatigue develops, heralded by a rising partial pressure of CO_2 and more latterly altered level of consciousness blood pressure instability and decreasing respiratory effort. However, few centres in the tropics have the resources, capacity and budget to deliver these ancillary therapies regularly.

Complications

Pneumococcal pneumonia may be further complicated by metastatic spread of infection and empyema. Osteomyelitis, arthritis, endocarditis, suppurative pericarditis and other localized infections are unusual. Meningitis was found in association with 15% of fatal cases of pneumonia in an early post-mortem study from Kenya.[44] Empyema complicates 2–3% of pneumonic episodes.[21,22,44] Inadequate or subtherapeutic antibiotic therapy may predispose to this complication. Management of pleural effusions and empyema should be aggressive from the outset to avoid the late sequelae of chronic empyema. Sampling of fluid with a needle and syringe should be performed on all effusions detected by clinical examination, with the intention of removing as much fluid as possible if purulence is detected. Use of a large bore chest drain is desirable to achieve this.

Meningitis

Meningitis is the most lethal syndrome associated with pneumococcal infection and high rates of serious complications are present in survivors. A case fatality rate in children has been measured in excess of 60% and similar rates have been recorded in adults.[2,45] These rates are substantially higher than those seen in the developed world. The reason for this mortality difference is uncertain. It is unlikely that the difference is wholly down to therapy. Even in study settings, where access to therapy was good, high case fatality rates were recorded.[47] Meningitis occurs after haematogenous seeding of the central nervous system and it may be that meningitis reflects the consequence of late presentation of a bacteraemic illness.

Clinical presentation

Pneumococcal meningitis in adults follows the typical pattern of headache and fever in association with neck stiffness, progressive alteration in level of consciousness and features of disseminated sepsis, with symptoms evolving over 12–48 hours. Preceding or superimposed pneumonia is also common. Difficulties in diagnosis arise when neck stiffness is absent, which may be associated with advanced disease, infancy, old age and immuno-suppression, and the diagnosis may be missed or confused with cerebral malaria.

Investigations

Examination of cerebrospinal fluid (CSF) is important to confirm a diagnosis. CSF findings will show the characteristics of a bacterial infection, polymorphonuclear leucocyte pleocytosis, raised protein concentration, low sugar level and a Gram stain demonstrating Gram-positive lanceolate diplococci. In the absence of a confirmatory Gram stain or following antibiotic therapy, it may be possible to detect pneumococcal antigen in the CSF to provide a rapid diagnosis. Definitive proof of pneumococcal aetiology relies on culture and laboratory characterization. In the absence of evidence of pneumococcal aetiology, empirical therapy should always include an agent effective against pneumococci. In laboratories able to perform sensitivity testing, this should be performed on all isolates from CSF as reduced susceptibility to penicillin is important in determining therapy for meningitis (see below).

The risks of performing a lumbar puncture must be balanced against the value of the information obtained. However, only basic laboratory equipment is required to perform a CSF examination (microscope, counting chamber, slides, Gram stain) and this will often rapidly establish an aetiological diagnosis. The presence of a focal neurological deficit (present in 20% of cases of bacterial meningitis), altered consciousness level (in more than 60% of cases), papilloedema (less than 1% of cases), seizures (30% of cases) and suppurative ear disease should necessitate a reconsideration of the need for lumbar puncture, but these are not absolute contraindications.

Differential diagnosis

This includes: other bacterial meningitis (see Chapter 56), the meningococcus being the most important; falciparum malaria; rickettsial infections; relapsing fever; viral meningoencephalitis; and cryptococcal meningitis, although the latter tends to run a characteristically sub-acute course. Tetanus, hypertensive crisis, poisoning, subarachnoid haemorrhage and bilateral sinusitis (with underlying HIV infection) may also need to be considered. Differentiation relies on CSF examination. Blood cultures should also be performed on all cases of suspected meningitis when available. Bacterial growth will occur within 24 hours and this is a particularly valuable investigation when lumbar puncture is contraindicated. Antibiotic therapy instituted before carrying out a blood culture will dramatically reduce sensitivity.

Management and therapy

Therapy for meningitis should be given as soon as a diagnosis is considered but after blood cultures have been taken. Parenteral therapy is considered obligatory. In addition to antimicrobial agents (see below), other supportive therapy is needed. This is aimed at treating the complications of bacteraemia with intravenous fluids and supplemental oxygen if available, preventing the complications of immobility by good nursing care, and minimizing the rise in intracranial pressure by nursing in a head-up position. High-dose corticosteroids have been advocated for control of intracranial pressure, but no efficacy data exist to support their use in pneumococcal meningitis.

Complications

Outcome following pneumococcal meningitis is poor. In survivors convalescence may be prolonged and residual neurological deficit and disability is common, notably deafness, stroke and blindness.

Other syndromes

The pneumococcus is associated with several other common syndromes, notably sinusitis, otitis media and conjunctivitis.

Sinusitis is characterized by fever, facial pain and tenderness, and a unilateral bloody nasal discharge. Disease is usually uncomplicated, but can rarely lead to osteomyelitis of the facial bones or cavernous sinus thrombosis. In the immunocompromised the sinuses may act as a source of bacteraemia and meningitis. Therapy should include antibiotics and decongestants along with appropriate analgesia.

Acute otitis media is predominantly a complication of children, for anatomical and other reasons outlined above in the section on susceptibility. A diagnosis of otitis media is usually based on the presence of an inflamed and bulging or ruptured tympanic membrane. Confirmation of pneumococcal aetiology will depend on culture of the bacteria from middle ear fluid, obtained either after rupture or from needle puncture (tympanocentesis). It is likely that much acute otitis media in the tropics passes unnoticed—otoscopic examination is rarely performed in the febrile irritable child who receives antimalarials and improves spontaneously. Therapy of otitis media with antibiotics is probably unnecessary in the majority of cases, and can be reserved for complicated disease (i.e., perforation of typanum or symptom duration of over 72 hours).

S. pneumoniae may cause a purulent conjunctivitis; the condition is usually unilateral and responds quickly to topical chloramphenicol, but variably to aminoglycosides. The condition is notable as acapsulate strains

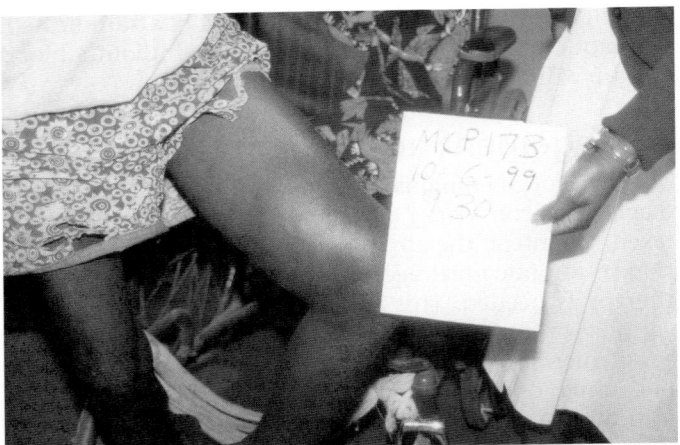

Figure 55.4: Spontaneous pneumococcal pyomyositis of the thigh in a 28-year-old HIV-infected Malawian woman, successfully treated with surgical drainage and penicillin. Courtesy of Miss Maria Callaghan, Specialist Surgical Registrar, Mersey Deanery; Lecturer, College of Medicine, Malawi.

of pneumococci have been implicated in its causation, perhaps due to their greater ability to bind the conjunctival surface, without requiring the defensive capsule that typifies other pathogenic *S. pneumoniae*.

Pneumococci have been implicated in numerous other uncommon presentations: pericarditis, arthritis, osteomyelitis, mediastinitis, endocarditis, brain abscess and peritonitis (particularly in young women and alcoholics). Pyomyositis is the development of pus-forming infection in the body of one of the larger skeletal muscles. A rare condition elsewhere in the world, it has been regularly reported from sub-Saharan Africa. Historically, *S. pneumoniae* has been reported as an unusual cause of this syndrome (in only 5% of cases), with *Staphylococcus aureus* responsible for the majority. This may be changing, however, with the increasing importance of HIV in this region. Management of pyomyositis requires drainage and antimicrobial therapy (Figure 55.4).

Special situations

Human immunodeficiency virus

HIV infection dramatically increases susceptibility to pneumococcal infection and particularly invasive disease. It is consistently reported as one of the leading causes of bloodstream infection in both adults and children with HIV.[48,49] Moreover, underlying HIV infection should be considered in any individual suffering an invasive pneumococcal event. The risk of developing pneumococcal disease increases as clinical stage or CD4 T cell count deteriorates. Pneumonia continues to be the most frequent presentation. Although bacteraemic in up to 80% of cases, the clinical and radiological presenting features are consistent with cases seen in HIV-uninfected individuals.[28,50] Case fatality is independent of HIV status if there is early access to appropriate therapy, but delayed presentation and remoteness from health care services

are associated with increased mortality. In addition bacteraemia may occur as a complication of sinusitis or as a primary occult phenomenon, a presentation that would otherwise be extremely rare in adults.[16,51] Clinical presentation of diseases in HIV-infected adults is more akin to a paediatric spectrum of disease. Increased susceptibility to meningitis has been suggested, but may be a function of the increased rate of invasive disease combined with late presentation. General management of pneumococcal disease should be unaffected by HIV status. The presence of diarrhoea, a common HIV-associated problem, will interfere with antibiotic absorption, and parenteral therapy may be required. HIV infection may also be associated with a broader range of infecting serotypes and as a consequence an increased risk of infection with penicillin-resistant pneumococci in sub-Saharan Africa. This may need to be considered when choosing therapy.[17,28]

Sickle cell disease

Fulminant pneumococcal sepsis is a feature of sickle cell disease and equal to malaria as a cause of death in this population.[52] The most serious infections occur in the under-fives and commonly present as a septicaemic illness. The features of infarction that will accompany the infective episode may confuse presentation. Presumptive therapy of a sick sickle cell child with infection should include antipneumococcal therapy as a priority. Adrenal failure (Waterhouse–Friderichsen syndrome) is a recognized complication and steroid support may also be necessary. Despite the relative frequency of osteomyelitis with sickle cell disease, the pneumococcus is an infrequent cause, the majority of cases due to salmonella species, other Gram-negative organisms and staphylococci.

Antimicrobial therapy

Antibiotic therapy is considered obligatory in the treatment of invasive pneumococcal disease and pneumococcal pneumonia. Penicillins continue to be the agents of choice for managing pneumococcal disease (Table 55.3). However, the expanding problem of pneumococci with reduced susceptibility and resistance to penicillin is beginning to threaten the simplicity of this approach.

In 1973 pneumococci with a reduced susceptibility to penicillin were first reported from South Africa. During the 1990s increasing resistance to penicillin amongst pneumococci has been steadily emerging and continues to evolve throughout most parts of the globe. Pneumococci that need a concentration of penicillin between 0.1 and 1 mg/l to inhibit growth (minimal inhibitory concentration; MIC) may be referred to as pneumococci with reduced susceptibility whereas pneumococci that have a MIC of 2 mg/l or more are referred to as resistant. Some authors consider all pneumococci with a MIC of 0.1 mg/l or greater as resistant. This classification is helpful to the clinician as penicillin-resistant pneumococcal pneumonia

Table 55.3 Antimicrobial therapy for pneumococcal infections.

	Penicillin sensitive		Penicillin resistant	
	Adult	Child	Adult	Child
Pneumonia and/or bacteraemia				
Parenteral	BZP 0.6–1.2 g 6 hourly	BZP 50–100 mg/kg/day[a]	BZP 1.2–2.4 g 4 hourly	BZP 100–300 mg/kg/day
Oral	AXL[b] 250–500 mg 8 hourly	AXL 125–250 mg 8 hourly	AXL 1 g 6–8 hourly	AXL 90 mg/kg/day
Meningitis[c]				
Parenteral	BZP 1.8 g 4–6 hourly	BZP 100–300 mg/kg/day	CFX[d] 2 g 6 hourly *or* CHL 1 g 6 hourly	CFX 200 mg/kg/day *or* CHL 50–100 mg/kg/day
Sinusitis and otitis media				
Oral	AXL 250–500 mg 8 hourly	AXL 125–250 mg 8 hourly	AXL 1 g 6–8 hourly	AXL 90 mg/kg/day

The decision to treat an infection as penicillin resistant may be based on known sensitivity testing or local knowledge and suspicion. Failure of response to first-line therapy over 48 hours should stimulate a reconsideration of the diagnosis, a search for localized infection or abscess, and the possibility of antimicrobial resistance. Parenteral therapy may be discontinued after 48 hours in the presence of a response. Continuation therapy should continue for at least 3 days after cessation of fever. Meningitis should be treated with parenteral therapy for a minimum of 10 days. In the event of penicillin allergy, a third-generation cephalosporin (10% cross-sensitivity) or chloramphenicol should be used as a parenteral alternative. Erythromycin, co-trimoxazole and chloramphenicol offer oral alternatives.
BZP, benzylpenicillin; AXL, amoxicillin; CFX, cefotaxime; CHL, chloramphenicol.
[a]In neonates, two divided doses; in infants 1–4 weeks, three divided doses; other children, four to six divided doses.
[b]Ampicillin may be substituted, given 6 hourly.
[c]Dosages used for meningitis are appropriate for managing peritonitis, pericarditis, arthritis and other body cavity infections combined with suitable drainage of pus.
[d]Other third-generation cephalosporins may be substituted (e.g. ceftriaxone 2 g 12 hourly).

and bacteraemia may be treated successfully with penicillin, but penicillin is inadequate treatment for pneumococcal meningitis even with reduced susceptibility. Penicillin penetration into the CSF (an active process across the blood–brain barrier) is poor, leading to concentrations of penicillin below those required to achieve effective bacterial clearance, and clinical failure is now well described.[53,54]

Penicillin exerts its antibacterial action by covalently binding and inhibiting enzymes (penicillin-binding proteins-PBPs) involved in the production of cell wall peptidoglycans. Six enzymes with decreased affinity for binding penicillin have been identified. Altered PBPs in pneumococci result predominantly from transformational changes after acquisition of genetic material from other streptococcal species carried in the nasopharynx and further subsequent rearrangements of the DNA.[55] The consequences of these alterations is a graduated increase in the concentration of penicillin required to achieve inhibition of growth or killing of the bacteria and a selective growth advantage over other pneumococci when exposed to β-lactam antibiotics. With the widespread and often unregulated use of antibiotics, penicillin-resistant pneumococcal clones have become widespread. Indeed, some identified clones have been so successful that their spread has been pandemic: the 'Spanish' 23F clone has been identified in Asia, Africa, Europe and North America.[56] Penicillin-resistant pneumococci are frequently multidrug resistant. Penicillin, co-trimoxazole, macrolide and chloramphenicol resistance is commonly found in the same pneumococcal clone, genetic material conferring resistance to these other agents being found in the same translational elements encoding for the altered PBPs.

The scale of antibiotic resistance in pneumococci in the tropics is unclear, and is based on information from only a few centres. Penicillin resistance appears at its greatest in South-East Asia where up to 60% of clinically relevant pneumococci are resistant, with 80% of these isolates having a MIC greater than 2 mg/l.[57] In South Africa and Brazil is similar, with 20–30% resistance is reported, but this is mostly of the reduced susceptibility type and these values are more typical of other reports from Africa and Asia.[58,59] Organisms with a MIC for penicillin in excess of 16 mg/l have not yet been described.

For uncomplicated bloodstream infections and pneumonia, penicillin remains the antimicrobial drug of choice. A single intravenous bolus of 5 megaunits (MU) of penicillin (3.0 g benzylpenicillin) will achieve a serum and pulmonary concentration of penicillin above 4 mg/l for 4–5 hours after the dose in an adult.[60] Thus four daily doses of 5 MU penicillin will provide effective coverage of all but the most resistant pneumococci. Moreover, a 4-MU bolus followed by a continuous infusion of 24 MU penicillin over 24 hours will achieve a steady serum concentration of 20 mg/l—a concentration in excess of the highest MIC yet reported for pneumococci. Thus the approach to the management of pulmonary and bloodstream infections in regions where penicillin resistance is recognized should be an increase in the dose of penicillin and/or an adjustment in the dosing schedule. This principle can also be applied to oral penicillin dosing when oral therapy is appropriate. Amoxicillin given as 1 g three times daily in an adult (90 mg/kg in a child) with normal gastrointestinal function will achieve serum and pulmonary concentrations well above the MIC of all but the most resistant strains. The principal limitation to increased oral dosing is gastrointestinal intolerance.

The principal impact of penicillin resistance is its effect on therapy for meningitis and other body cavity infections where antibiotic penetration is decreased. Increased penicillin dosing cannot be used in the treatment of meningitis caused by PSRP or PRP. CSF concentrations of penicillin are usually between 1% and 5% of serum levels, and maintaining a concentration above the MIC for at least 40% of the dosing interval (a figure required for therapeutic success with β-lactams in animal studies) is unachievable. Where resources are available, a third-generation cephalosporin should be used as the initial therapy of meningitis, and modified on the basis of sensitivity testing. In the absence of cephalosporins, chloramphenicol may be appropriate. However, the association of chloramphenicol with penicillin resistance may make this approach inappropriate.[53] Local sensitivity knowledge will assist with these decisions, but in the absence of laboratory information the combination of penicillin and chloramphenicol represents the most pragmatic approach. Other agents with antipneumococcal activity, which have been used to treat penicillin-resistant pneumococcal meningitis, include carbapenems (e.g., meropenem), glycopeptides (e.g., vancomycin), oxazoladinones (e.g., linezolid) and rifampicin. These agents are expensive and less readily available than cephalosporins and, with the exception of rifampicin, none is included in the WHO essential drugs list. Rifampicin is widely available as a combination tablet with other antituberculous therapy, but is more difficult to find as a single agent and resistance rapidly develops when used alone. The aminoglycosides gentamicin and streptomycin should not be used as single agents as achievable tissue concentrations are below the MIC of even the most sensitive organisms. The use of these antibiotics in synergy with a β-lactam has been suggested for penicillin-resistant pneumococcal infections, but this approach has no role in meningitis because of the minimal CSF penetration of aminoglycosides.

Prevention

At present there is little structured approach to the prevention of pneumococcal disease in the tropics, despite its clear importance as a public health and clinical problem. This is in large part due to the failure of the currently available polysaccharide vaccines to protect young children. Several newer vaccines based on conjugation of pneumococcal polysaccharides to a protein have proved far more immunogenic and protective against invasive disease in North American children.[61] Efficacy trials of these vaccines are under way in South Africa, the Philippines and The Gambia, and their results are awaited.

Polysaccharide vaccine

Two 23-valent polysaccharide vaccines are presently available commercially (Pnu-immune®, Wyeth-Ayerst Pharmaceuticals, Philadelphia, USA; Pneumovax®, Aventis Pasteur, Lyon, France) and are presumed to be equipotent. They contain capsular polysaccharide from the 23 commonest disease-causing pneumococcal serotypes. Depending on geography and the prevalent disease causing serotypes, they will provide potential coverage against 85–95% of invasive pneumococcal disease events. Vaccination is given as a single intramuscular injection, with repeat doses recommended every 5–10 years, or 3 years in asplenia. Side effects other than injection site discomfort are unusual.

The vaccine has no role in the protection of children under the age of 2 years. Antenatal vaccination of women is being investigated as a means of protecting children in the neonatal period and during breast-feeding from passive transfer of maternal antibodies transplacentally and in breast milk. The effectiveness of this approach is as yet unproven. Vaccination is recommended for children over 2 years of age and adults at increased risk of pneumococcal disease. This includes children with sickle cell disease and adults with chronic health problems including cardiorespiratory illness, diabetes, asplenia and HIV infection. Unfortunately evidence to support these recommendations is weak. Trials carried out in otherwise fit and well South African goldminers living in barrack-style accommodation in the early 1970s showed 6 and 13 valent vaccine to be effective in reducing high rates of definitive pneumococcal pneumonia, with 63% efficacy.[62] A separate study carried out amongst highlanders in Papua New Guinea also reported a decrease in respiratory illness associated with vaccine use.[63] However, subsequent prospective studies carried out in the developed world have failed to show a convincing benefit of vaccination in adult risk groups and most recently a trial of 23 valent polysaccharide vaccine in HIV-infected Ugandan adults showed no benefits associated with vaccination.[29]

The uncertainty over the vaccine's effectiveness and its unsuitability as a component of the childhood extended programme of immunization (EPI) has led to the 23-valent polysaccharide vaccine being unavailable in much of the tropics.

Protein conjugate pneumococcal vaccine

The failure of pure polysaccharide vaccines to protect young children led to the development of the protein conjugate vaccines. This was first achieved successfully with *Haemophilus influenzae* type b, whereby the capsular polysaccharide was covalently bound to a polypeptide 'carrier'. The peptide carrier, unlike the polysaccharide, is recognized and bound by T-cell lymphocytes which are then able to present the polysaccharide to B lymphocytes in association with major histocompatibillity complex (MHC) class II molecules. These T cell-dependent responses are present from birth, unlike the responses to pure polysaccharide, which rely on B-cell responses alone and are independent of T cells. The result of T-cell involvement is the production of functionally competent antibodies and the creation of long-lived memory B lymphocytes.

A single pneumococcal conjugate vaccine is currently commercially available (Prevenar®, Wyeth). This is based on the covalent binding of seven serotypically distinct pneumococcal polysaccharides to a mutant diphtheria toxin-based protein carrier. Several other manufacturers have similar products close to licensing, based on other protein carriers such as tetanus toxoid, diphtheria toxoid and meningococcal outer membrane protein. Evidence to date from trials in North America and Europe shows these vaccines to be safe and highly effective at preventing invasive disease and pneumonia caused by vaccine-specific pneumococcal serotypes. Results of studies in paediatric populations in South Africa, The Gambia and the Philippines are awaited and it is hoped that these studies will help to delineate the role and impact of these vaccines amongst children in the developing world. The role of these vaccines in adult populations and in HIV-related immunosuppression is uncertain, although studies to investigate their efficacy are under way.

The principal drawback to the widespread use of these vaccines—if they prove effective in the developing world—will be their high cost. In addition, several further concerns have been identified. The limited number of serotypes in these vaccines may provide inadequate coverage in regions where a significant burden of pneumococcal disease is caused by non-vaccine serotypes.[3] Increasing the valency of these vaccines to achieve broader coverage will inevitably increase costs. Furthermore, immunological pressure created by the use of these vaccines may lead to changes in the prevalent disease-causing pneumococcal serotypes by both serotype replacement and/or capsular transformation amongst pneumococci, limiting the vaccine's long-term efficacy.[64,65]

Other vaccine candidates

Concerns over the high production costs of conjugate vaccines and their serotype-specific limitations have led to the search for other vaccine candidates.[66] Pneumolysin and pneumococcal surface adhesin A (Psa A) are at present the most likely alternatives. They are attractive because they provide a relatively homogeneous antigenic structure and are independent of capsular serotype, and may be significantly easier to produce with modern cloning technology. Although early work in animal models is encouraging, phase 3 efficacy trials in humans are several years off.

Chemoprophylaxis

The use of penicillin prophylaxis (oral phenoxymethyl penicillin 125–250 mg twice daily or intramuscular benzathine penicillin 1.2 MU 4 weekly) is recommended for the prevention of pneumococcal disease in sickle cell disease sufferers and in individuals without a spleen. Prophylaxis should continue at least until the age of 5 years in sickle cell disease and for a minimum of 5 years following splenectomy. More prolonged prophylaxis may be beneficial as the true morbidity and mortality of late pneumococcal sepsis in these conditions is uncertain. The increasing prevalence of penicillin-resistant pneumococci may decrease the value of this approach in the future.

Once-daily co-trimoxazole (480 mg) has been recommended by UNAIDS for HIV-infected individuals with symptomatic disease. This recommendation is distinct from its use as an agent to prevent *Pneumocystis carinii* pneumonia. Two studies from Côte d'Ivoire showed the benefits of this approach at reducing several morbid end-points including pneumonia.[67,68] Confirmation of the effectiveness of this approach outside of West Africa is, however, awaited. High rates of co-trimoxazole resistance in pneumococci found in East and southern Africa and South-East Asia may limit the impact of this approach on pneumococcal and respiratory disease in HIV-infected populations in these regions.

REFERENCES

1 World Health Organization/Organisation Mondiale de la Santé. *World Health Report 2000*. Geneva:WHO, 2000.

2 Greenwood B. The epidemiology of pneumococcal infection in children in the developing world. *Philos Trans R Soc Lond [Biol]* 1999; 354:777–785.

3 Hausdorff W P, Bryant J, Paradiso P R & Siber G R. Which pneumococcal serogroups cause the most invasive disease: implications for conjugate vaccine formulation and use, part I. *Clin Infect Dis* 2000; 30:100–121.

4 Scott J A, Hall A J, Dagan R et al. Serogroup-specific epidemiology of *Streptococcus pneumoniae*: associations with age, sex, and geography in 7000 episodes of invasive disease. *Clin Infect Dis* 1996; 22:973–981.

5 Henrichsen J. Typing of *Streptococcus pneumoniae*: past, present, and future. *Am J Med* 1999; 107:50S–54S.

6 Barnes D M, Whittier S, Gilligan P H, Soares S, Tomasz A & Henderson F W. Transmission of multidrug-resistant serotype

23F *Streptococcus pneumoniae* in group day care: evidence suggesting capsular transformation of the resistant strain in vivo. *J Infect Dis* 1995; 171:890–896.

7 Cotton M F, Burger P J & Bodenstein W J. Bacteraemia in children in the south-western Cape. A hospital-based survey. *S Afr Med J* 1992; 81:87–90.

8 Nathoo K J, Chigonde S, Nhembe M, Ali M H & Mason P R. Community-acquired bacteremia in human immunodeficiency virus-infected children in Harare, Zimbabwe. *Pediatr Infect Dis J* 1996; 15:1092–1097.

9 Karstaedt A S, Khoosal M & Crewe-Brown H H. Pneumococcal bacteremia during a decade in children in Soweto, South Africa. *Pediatr Infect Dis J* 2000; 19:454–457.

10 O'Dempsey T J, Mcardle T F, Lloyd-Evans N et al. Pneumococcal disease among children in a rural area of west Africa. *Pediatr Infect Dis J* 1996; 15:431–437.

11 Sleeman K, Knox K, George R et al. Invasive pneumococcal

disease in England and Wales: vaccination implications. *J Infect Dis* 2001; 183:239–246.

12 Shann F, Gratten M, Germer S, Linnemann V, Hazlett D & Payne R. Aetiology of pneumonia in children in Goroka Hospital, Papua New Guinea. *Lancet* 1984; ii:537–541.

13 Wall R A, Corrah P T, Mabey D C & Greenwood B M. The etiology of lobar pneumonia in the Gambia. *BullWHO* 1986; 64:553–558.

14 O'Dempsey T J, Mcardle T F, Morris J et al. A study of risk factors for pneumococcal disease among children in a rural area of west Africa. *Int J Epidemiol* 1996; 25:885–893.

15 Hatcher J, Smith A, Mackenzie I et al. A prevalence study of ear problems in school children in Kiambu district, Kenya, May 1992. *Int J Pediatr Otorhinolaryngol* 1995; 33:197–205.

16 Gilks C F, Ojoo S A, Ojoo J C et al. Invasive pneumococcal disease in a cohort of predominantly HIV-1 infected female sex-workers in Nairobi, Kenya. *Lancet* 1996; 347:718–723.

17 Jones N, Huebner R, Khoosal M, Crewe-Brown H & Klugman K. The impact of HIV on *Streptococcus pneumoniae* bacteraemia in a South African population. *AIDS* 1998; 12:2177–2184.

18 Williams E H, Hayes R J & Smith P G. Admissions to a rural hospital in the West Nile District of Uganda over a 27 year period. *J Trop Med Hyg* 1986; 89:193–211.

19 Harries A D, Speare R & Wirima J J. Medical admissions to Kamuzu Central Hospital, Lilongwe, Malawi in 1986: comparison with admissions to Queen Elizabeth Central Hospital, Blantyre in 1973. *Trop Geogr Med* 1990; 42:274–279.

20 Petit P L & van Ginneken J K. Analysis of hospital records in four African countries, 1975–1990, with emphasis on infectious diseases. *J Trop Med Hyg* 1995; 98:217–227.

21 Roe P. Lobar and segmental pneumonia in Busoga. *East Afr Med J* 1968; 45:619–624.

22 Allen S C. Lobar pneumonia in northern Zambia: clinical study of 502 adult patients. *Thorax* 1984; 39:612–616.

23 Scott J A, Hall A J, Muyodi C et al. Aetiology, outcome, and risk factors for mortality among adults with acute pneumonia in Kenya. *Lancet* 2000; 355:1225–1230.

24 Heffron R. *Pneumonia with Special Reference to Pneumococcus Lobar Pneumonia*. Cambridge, Massachusetts: Harvard University Press, 1939.

25 Robinson K A, Baughman W, Rothrock G et al. Epidemiology of invasive *Streptococcus pneumoniae* infections in the United States, 1995–1998: opportunities for prevention in the conjugate vaccine era. *JAMA* 2001; 285:1729–1735.

26 Hoge C W, Reichler M R, Dominguez E A et al. An epidemic of pneumococcal disease in an overcrowded, inadequately ventilated jail. *N Engl J Med* 1994; 331:643–648.

27 Nuorti J P, Butler J C, Farley M M et al. Cigarette smoking and invasive pneumococcal disease. Active Bacterial Core Surveillance Team. *N Engl J Med* 2000; 342:681–689.

28 Gilks C F. Royal Society of Tropical Medicine and Hygiene meeting at Manson House, London, 12 December 1996. HIV and pneumococcal infection in Africa. Clinical, epidemiological and preventative aspects. *Trans R Soc Trop Med Hyg* 1997; 91:627–631.

29 French N, Nakiyingi J, Carpenter L M et al. 23-Valent pneumococcal polysaccharide vaccine in HIV-1-infected Ugandan adults: double-blind, randomised and placebo controlled trial. *Lancet* 2000; 355:2106–2111.

30 Gordon M A, Walsh A L, Chaponda M et al. Bacteraemia and mortality among adult medical admissions in Malawi—predominance of non-typhi salmonellae and *Streptococcus pneumoniae*. *J Infec.* 2001; 42:44–49.

31 Cheesbrough M. *Medical Laboratory Manual for Tropical Countries*. Butterworth-Heinemann and Tropical Health Technology, 1992.

32 Morona J K, Morona R & Paton J C. Molecular and genetic characterization of the capsule biosynthesis locus of *Streptococcus pneumoniae* type 19B. *J Bacteriol* 1997; 179:4953–4958.

33 Nesin M, Ramirez M & Tomasz A. Capsular transformation of a multidrug-resistant *Streptococcus pneumoniae* in vivo. *J Infect Dis* 1998; 177:707–713.

34 Lipscombe R J, Sumiya M, Hill A V et al. High frequencies in African and non-African populations of independent mutations in the mannose binding protein gene. *Hum Mol Genet* 1992; 1:709–715.

35 Gordon S B, Irving G R, Lawson R A, Lee M E & Read R C. Intracellular trafficking and killing of *Streptococcus pneumoniae* by human alveolar macrophages are influenced by opsonins. *Infect Immun* 2000; 68:2286–2293.

36 Musher D M, Phan H M, Watson D A & Baughn R E. Antibody to capsular polysaccharide of *Streptococcus pneumoniae* at the time of hospital admission for Pneumococcal pneumonia. *J Infect Dis* 2000; 182:158–167.

37 Jansen W T, Vakevainen-Anttila M, Kayhty H et al. Comparison of a classical phagocytosis assay and a flow cytometry assay for assessment of the phagocytic capacity of sera from adults vaccinated with a pneumococcal conjugate vaccine. *Clin Diagn Lab Immunol* 2001; 8:245–250.

38 Timens W, Boes A, Rozeboom-Uiterwijk T & Poppema S. Immaturity of the human splenic marginal zone in infancy. Possible contribution to the deficient infant immune response. *J Immunol* 1989; 143:3200–3206.

39 Berberian L, Goodglick L, Kipps T J & Braun J. Immunoglobulin VH3 gene products: natural ligands for HIV gp120. *Science* 1993; 261:1588–1591.

40 Sanders L A, van de Winkel J G, Rijkers G T et al. Fc gamma receptor IIa (CD32) heterogeneity in patients with recurrent bacterial respiratory tract infections. *J Infect Dis* 1994; 170:854–861.

41 Usen S, Adegbola R, Mulholland K et al. Epidemiology of invasive pneumococcal disease in the Western Region, The Gambia. *Pediatr Infect Dis J* 1998; 17:23–28.

42 Hall E W & Parry E H O. Lobar pneumonia with jaundice in adult Nigerians. *Trans R Soc Trop Med Hyg* 1963; 57:206.

43 British Thoracic Society and the Public Health Laboratory Service. Community-acquired pneumonia in adults in British hospitals in 1982–1983: a survey of aetiology, mortality, prognostic factors and outcome. *Q J Med* 1987; 62:195–220.

44 Trowell H C. A clinical study of pneumonia among Africans in Nairobi. *East Afr Med J* 1932; 9:258–268.

45 Sofowora E O & Onadeko B O. Complications and prognostic factors in pneumonia among Nigerians. *Niger Med J* 1973; 3:144–145.

46 Gordon S B, Walsh A L, Chaponda M et al. Bacterial meningitis in Malawian adults: pneumococcal disease is common, severe, and seasonal. *Clin Infect Dis* 2000; 31:53–57.

47 Goetghebuer T, West T E, Wermenbol V et al. Outcome of meningitis caused by *Streptococcus pneumoniae* and *Haemophilus influenzae* type b in children in The Gambia. *Trop Med Int Health* 2000; 5:207–213.

48 Arthur G, Naluba V N, Kariyuki S et al. Trends in bloodstream infections among human immunodeficiency virus-infected adults admitted to a hospital in Nairobi, Kenya, during the last decade. *Clin Infect Dis* 2001; 33:248–256.

49 Ssali F N, Kamya M R, Wabwire-Mangen F et al. A prospective study of community-acquired bloodstream infections among febrile adults admitted to Mulago Hospital in Kampala, Uganda. *J Acquir Immune Defic Syndr Human Retrovirol* 1998; 19:484–489.

50 Feldman C, Glatthaar M, Morar R et al. Bacteremic pneumococcal pneumonia in HIV-seropositive and HIV-seronegative adults. *Chest* 1999; 116:107–114.

51 Austrian R. Untreated pneumococcal bacteraemia of cryptic origin in the human adult with spontaneous recovery. *S Afr Med J* 1986; Supplement:46–49.

52 Fleming A F. The presentation, management and prevention of crisis in sickle cell disease in Africa. *Blood Rev* 1989; 3:18–28.

53 Friedland I R & Klugman K P. Failure of chloramphenicol therapy in penicillin-resistant pneumococcal meningitis. *Lancet* 1992; 339:405–408.

54 Muhe L & Klugman K P. Pneumococcal and *Haemophilus influenzae* meningitis in a children's hospital in Ethiopia: serotypes and susceptibility patterns. *Trop Med Int Health* 1999; 4:421–427.

55 Dowson C G, Coffey T J & Spratt B G. Origin and molecular epidemiology of penicillin-binding-protein-mediated resistance to beta-lactam antibiotics. *Trends Microbiol* 1994; 2:361–366.

56 Munoz R, Coffey T J, Daniels M et al. Intercontinental spread of a multiresistant clone of serotype 23F *Streptococcus pneumoniae*. *J Infect Dis* 1991; 164:302–306.

57 Parry C M, Diep T S, Wain J et al. Nasal carriage in Vietnamese children of *Streptococcus pneumoniae* resistant to multiple antimicrobial agents. *Antimicrob Agents Chemother* 2000; 44:484–488.

58 Felmingham D & Gruneberg R N. The Alexander Project 1996–1997: latest susceptibility data from this international study of bacterial pathogens from community-acquired lower respiratory tract infections. *J Antimicrob Chemother* 2000; 45:191–203.

59 Paul J, Bates J, Kimari J & Gilks C. Serotypes and antibiotic susceptibilities of *Streptococcus pneumoniae* in Nairobi, Kenya. *J Infect* 1996; 32:139–142.

60 Bryan C S, Talwani R & Stinson MS. Penicillin dosing for pneumococcal pneumonia. *Chest* 1997; 112:1657–1664.

61 Black S, Shinefield H, Fireman B et al. Efficacy, safety and immunogenicity of heptavalent pneumococcal conjugate vaccine in children. Northern California Kaiser Permanente Vaccine Study Center Group. *Pediatr Infect Dis J* 2000; 19:187–195.

62 Austrian R, Douglas R M, Schiffman G et al. Prevention of pneumococcal pneumonia by vaccination. *Trans Assoc Am Physicians* 1976; 89:184–194.

63 Riley I D, Tarr P I, Andrews M et al. Immunisation with a polyvalent pneumococcal vaccine. Reduction of adult respiratory mortality in a New Guinea Highlands community. *Lancet* 1977; i:1338–1341.

64 Mbelle N, Huebner R E, Wasas A D, Kimura A, Chang I & Klugman K P. Immunogenicity and impact on nasopharyngeal carriage of a nonavalent pneumococcal conjugate vaccine. *J Infect Dis* 1999; 180:1171–1176.

65 Obaro S K. Confronting the pneumococcus: a target shift or bullet change? *Vaccine* 2000; 19:1211–1217.

66 Briles D E, Hollingshead S, Brooks-Walter A et al. The potential to use PspA and other pneumococcal proteins to elicit protection against pneumococcal infection. *Vaccine* 2000; 18:1707–1711.

67 Anglaret X, Chene G, Attia A et al. Early chemoprophylaxis with trimethoprim–sulphamethoxazole for HIV-1-infected adults in Abidjan, Cote d'Ivoire: a randomised trial. Cotrimo-CI Study Group. *Lancet* 1999; 353:1463–1468.

68 Wiktor S Z, Sassan-Morokro M, Grant A D et al. Efficacy of trimethoprim–sulphamethoxazole prophylaxis to decrease morbidity and mortality in HIV-1-infected patients with tuberculosis in Abidjan, Cote d'Ivoire: a randomised controlled trial. *Lancet* 1999; 353:1469–1475.

69 Grumwade K & Gilks C F. Cotrimoxayole prophylaxis in adults infected with HIV in low income countries. *Curr Opin Infect Dis* 2001; 14:507–512.

Chapter 56
Bacterial Meningitis

C. A. Hart and L. E. Cuevas

Bacterial meningitis is a medical emergency and is common in many areas of the tropics. It has a significant mortality rate, especially in children (see also Chapter 16). The bacteria causing meningitis vary with geographical and climatic conditions, with immunosuppression, with age, availability and usage of vaccines, and whether the illness is chronic or acute (Tables 56.1 and 56.2). Outside the neonatal period the three major pathogens are: *Streptococcus pneumoniae*, *Haemophilus influenzae* and *Neisseria meningitidis*. Neonatal meningitis may also be caused by these organisms,[1] but other bacteria such as *Escherichia coli*, *Str. agalactiae* (group B streptococcus) and *Klebsiella pneumoniae* tend to predominate. The relative importance of *H. influenzae*, pneumococci and meningococci outside the neonatal period varies according to country; for example, in humid low-lying regions *Str. pneumoniae* and *H. influenzae* predominate, whereas in dryer regions, for example the meningitis belt of sub-Saharan Africa, the meningococcus causes vast spreading epidemics.[2] *H. influenzae* meningitis is rare in individuals over 7 years of age. In addition to a high mortality rate, bacterial meningitis carries a high risk of neurological sequelae.

Neonatal meningitis

With improvements in, and the more widespread availability of, neonatal intensive care, neonates of increasing prematurity have a chance of survival. The premature neonate is not only immature in terms of pulmonary, alimentary and renal function but is also an immune-compromised host. This means that the neonate, and especially the premature neonate, is at increased risk of infection. Early bacterial meningitis is usually part of a syndrome of sepsis neonatorum with few specific signs in the premature neonate.[3] Once infection is established, convulsions, bulging fontanelle and neck stiffness may be detected.

Geographical aspects

Although some geographical variations in the incidence and microbiology of neonatal meningitis are reported, the variability relates more to the presence of neonatal

Table 56.1 Aetiology of acute meningitis.

Purulent	Lymphocytic
Neonatal	
Group B streptococcus	Herpes simplex virus
Listeria monocytogenes	Enteroviruses
Escherichia coli and other coliforms	
Salmonella spp.	
Pseudomonas aeruginosa	
Candida albicans	
Older individuals	
Neisseria meningitidis	*Mycobacterium tuberculosis*
Haemophilus influenzae	*Leptospira* spp.
Streptococcus pneumoniae	*Treponema pallidum*
Salmonella spp.	*Borrelia* spp.
L. monotyogenes	Enteroviruses
Burkholderia pseudomallei	Mumps virus
Naegleria fowleri	Arthropod-borne
Anaerobes such as	Togaviruses
Fusobacterium necrophorum	Adenovirus
	Lymphocytic chroriomeningitis virus
	Human immunodeficiency virus

Table 56.2 Aetiology of chronic meningitis.

Bacteria	Fungi	Parasites
Mycobacterium tuberculosis	*Cryptococcus neoformans*	*Toxoplasma gondii*
Brucella spp.	*Histoplasma capsulatum*	Cysticercosis
Treponema pallidum	*Coccidiodes immitis*	
Borrelia burgdorferi	*Candida albicans*	
Neisseria meningitidis	*Actinomyces israelii*	

Table 56.3 Bacterial pathogens in neonatal meningitis.

Location	Year	No. studied	Group B streptococci	E. coli	Salmonellae	Klebsiellae	S. aureus	Other	Reference
					% Due To				
England and Wales	1996–97	144	48	18	0.7	0	0.7	33*[a]	1
Taiwan	1984–97	85	32	20	0	3.5	0	44*[b]	8
Ethiopia	1987–96	30	0	23	7	30	7	33[c]	9
South Africa	1981–92	87	32	23	0	15	0	32[d]	7
Malawi	1996–97	37	38	19	24	0	0	19[e]	10

Other bacteria include:
[a]*Str. pneumoniae, H. influenzae, N. meningitidis, L. monocytogenes, Staph. epidermidis.*
[b]*Proteus mirabilis, Enterobacter cloacae, Str. pneumoniae, Chryseobacterium meningosepticum* and enterococci.
[c]*Str. pneumoniae,* GpA streptococci, *H. influenzae, Enterobacter* spp. and *Staph. epidermidis.*
[d]*N. meningitidis, H. influenzae, Listeria monocytogenes.*
[e]*Str. pneumoniae, H. influenzae, N. meningitidis.*

intensive care units and thus whether the infection is hospital or community acquired. For example, in Nigeria, *Salmonella* spp. and *Staphylococcus aureus* are the major pathogens,[4,5] whereas in neonatal intensive care units in South Africa group B streptococci, *Klebsiella* spp. and *E. coli* predominate[6,7] (Table 56.3).

Epidemiology

The incidence of neonatal meningitis varies according to the degree of prematurity and in some areas appears to be decreasing. In Durban the incidence was 2.27 per 1000 live births in 1981 and had fallen to 0.22 per 1000 live births in 1987.[6] Over the period 1981–1992, the overall incidence of neonatal meningitis was 0.72 per 1000 live births, but for low birth weight neonates (< 2500 g) was 1.69 per 1000 in another part of South Africa.[7] A survey in Oman has revealed an incidence of 1 per 1000 live births.[11] In Ethiopia an incidence of 0.97 per 1000 live births was found in term neonates, but in pre-term neonates the incidence was 3.66 per 1000.[9]

Bacteriology

The bacteria causing neonatal sepsis have altered considerably over the past 60 years.[12] This change reflects, in part, the changes in neonatal intensive care and in the availability of antibiotics of increasing potency and breadth of spectrum. In the first part of the twentieth century, group A β-haemolytic streptococci, followed by *Staph. aureus*, were the major pathogens. After the introduction of penicillins, Gram-negative bacteria such as *E. coli* and *Klebsiella* spp. emerged as significant pathogens. Then, in the 1970s, the importance of the group B streptococcus (*Str. agalactiae*) was realized and antibiotic-resistant coliforms emerged. Latterly, low-virulence pathogens such as *Staph. epidermidis* have been shown to be capable of causing septicaemia and meningitis.[3] In tropical countries this evolution has been apparent only in centres with neonatal intensive care units. Elsewhere primary pathogens such as *Salmonella* spp., *Str. agalactiae* and *Listeria monocytogenes* are more important. For example, in Malawi non-typhoidal salmonellae (NTS) account for 33% of cases of neonatal meningitis.[13] It must not be forgotten that the classical bacterial pathogens, *Str. pneumoniae, H. influenzae* and *N. meningitidis*, can also cause neonatal meningitis (Table 56.3). Finally, in endemic areas unusual pathogens such as *Burkholderia pseudomallei* may cause meningitis.[14]

Pathogenesis

In most cases the neonate first becomes colonized by the pathogen, which then translocates to produce bacteraemia. Bacteria may then lodge in the meninges to produce infection. In cases where infection presents within the first 48 hours of life, the bacteria have been acquired from the birth canal or maternal perineum. Bacteria that cause early overt infection include *Str. agalactiae, E. coli, L. monocyogenes* and *Salmonella* spp. These same bacteria may also cause meningitis occurring later in the neonatal period, but often bacteria such as *Pseudomonas aeruginosa* and *Klebsiella* spp. are commonly encountered.

The premature neonate has defects in both humoral and cell-mediated immunity that predispose it to serious infection. For example, the neonate's phagocytes do not work efficiently and the activity of the complement cascade is only 50% of that of the adult. At birth the neonate's own IgM production is 20% of adult levels, IgG is 5% of adult levels and IgA production begins at birth. Thus the neonate also has defects in humoral immunity, and especially in the tropics where placental malaria, human immunodeficiency virus (HIV) infection and maternal hypergammaglobulinaemia independently impair transplacental transfer of antibody.[15]

Clinical features

The early signs of meningitis in premature neonates are often indistinguishable from those of septicaemia. The signs of septicaemia in premature neonates are not specific to infections; for example, in one series of 139 episodes of septicaemia, pyrexia was present in only six episodes.[3] Signs that suggest neonatal meningitis, such as bulging fontanelle, stiff neck, convulsions or opisthotonos, are uncommon. For example, 17% of neonates with meningitis present with a bulging fontanelle, 33% with opisthotonos, 23% with neck stiffness and 12% with convulsions.[7–10,16–18] Thus, the diagnosis of neonatal meningitis requires a high index of suspicion, and part of the investigation of suspected neonatal septicaemia should include examination and culture of cerebrospinal fluid (CSF).

The results of infection can be dire. The mortality rate associated with neonatal meningitis varies according to the gestational age. Thus meningitis in neonates of extremely low birth weight (< 1000 g) is associated with mortality rates of up to 80%, and that in neonates of very low birth weight (< 1500 g) is 20–30% in developed countries. In less well developed countries the mortality rate varies with gestational age from 46 to 90%.[6–10] The mortality rate is also greater if the meningitis is due to Gram-negative bacilli.[6,19] Other acute complications include hydrocephalus, subdural effusions, deafness and blindness. Ventriculitis complicates Gram-negative bacillary meningitis in particular (70% of cases) and can make therapy very difficult. *Citrobacter koseri* (formerly *diversus*), in particular, causes central nervous system (CNS) abscesses following initial neonatal meningitis.[20] In long-term follow-up, 5–10% of neonates with meningitis have severe neurological deficit.

Diagnosis

The definitive diagnosis depends on examination of CSF taken by either lumbar or ventricular puncture. The interpretation of the findings depends upon a knowledge of what is normal in neonatal CSF. For example, in the first days of life 'normal' neonatal CSF may contain up to 30 white blood cells per cubic millimetre (60% polymorphs), up to 170 mg/dl protein and a raised glucose concentration. Unfortunately, for certain bacteria, the early cellular and biochemical findings overlap with the 'normal' cellular response.[21] In contrast, most (96%) of those with Gram-negative bacillary meningitis have abnormal CSF findings. It follows that rapid detection of bacteria in CSF is of prime importance in diagnosing neonatal meningitis. Examination of Gram-stained smears will detect up to 80% of cases and provide information on the aetiology. Tests for the detection of bacterial antigens are available for some pathogens. Both countercurrent immuno-electrophoresis and latex particle agglutination tests are available for detection of *Str. agalactiae*, *Str. pneumoniae*, *N. meningitidis*, *H. influenzae* and *E. coli* K1 antigens. In general, the latter is more sensitive and convenient than the former, but countercurrent immunoelectrophoresis may be less expensive.

Culture is the 'gold standard', but takes 18–24 hours. It also has the advantage that it will provide information on the antimicrobial susceptibility of the pathogen.

Management

Neonates with meningitis may require elective ventilation and circulatory support, but the mainstay of therapy is the administration of antibiotics that achieve therapeutic levels in CSF. Because there is a large range of potential pathogens, blind initial therapy must cover as wide a spectrum as possible. Most neonatal intensive care units employ a combination of ampicillin and gentamicin. This, however, does have some drawbacks, especially in treating Gram-negative bacteria which may be resistant to ampicillin and the CSF penetration of gentamicin, even through inflamed meninges, is not good.[22] Penicillin or ampicillin is sufficient for treating *Str. agalactiae* or *L. monocytogenes* meningitis, and little resistance has developed. The susceptibility of Gram-negative bacilli to antibiotics is less predictable and varies from unit to unit and with time. A third-generation cephalosporin such as ceftazidime or cefotaxime may prove useful.[6] Chloramphenicol, although effective against Gram-negative bacilli in vitro, is not uniformly effective in vivo because it is not bactericidal. Instillation of gentamicin directly into the ventricles is not recommended for therapy of neonatal bacterial meningitis.[21] Corticosteroids appear not to have a role in managing neonatal meningitis.[23]

Prevention

Prevention of neonatal meningitis can be difficult, first because so many different pathogens may be involved and, second, the premature neonate is an immuno-incompetent host. For prevention of *Str agalactiae* sepsis, two strategies are being investigated. Following the successful immunoprophylaxis of neonatal tetanus by actively immunizing the mother in the last trimester, a similar intervention is being pursued using the group B streptococcal capsular polysaccharide, but this may be compromised by poor transplacental transfer of maternal antibodies.[15] Vaginal irrigation with chlorhexidine before delivery has been shown to decrease the incidence of neonatal group B streptococcal sepsis in Sweden,[24] and in Malawi a similar strategy decreased neonatal sepsis (including meningitis) and mortality due to sepsis.[25]

Meningitis in older individuals

Outside the neonatal period, *N. meningitidis*, *Str. pneumoniae* and *H. influenzae* are responsible for over 90% of cases of acute bacterial meningitis. The remaining cases are due to a variety of bacteria, including both *Salmonella typhi* and non-typhoidal salmonellae. The latter can produce meningitis in the immunocompetent, but may occur more commonly in the malnourished or in patients with sickle cell disease.[26]

History

The history of meningitis covers only epidemics of 'cerebrospinal fever' with or without 'malignant purpuric fever', and this probably refers only to meningococcal disease. The meningococcus was first isolated in 1887 at autopsy, and in 1896 in life. Thereafter, the individual pathogens were gradually isolated and the disease more clearly defined.

Geographical aspects

Acute bacterial meningitis is found throughout the world but the relative contribution of the three main pathogens varies considerably. The reasons for this variation are still unclear. In the meningitis belt of sub-Saharan Africa (Figure 56.1), epidemics of meningococcal meningitis occur with 8–14-year cycles. During epidemics the incidence rises to over 400 cases per 100 000 population per year, but even between epidemics the hyperendemic rate is often more than 40 cases per 100 000 per year.[27] These cases are most often due to group A meningococci, but occasionally group C meningococci may cause an epidemic. In recent years the classical meningitis belt has expanded to include Tunisia and Algeria to the north and Kenya, Tanzania, Zambia, Uganda and Rwanda to the south.[2] Over the last 10 years epidemics have also been reported from Angola, Namibia, Mozambique, the south of the Democratic Republic of Congo (DRC, previously Zaire) and Botswana (Figure 56.2). A common feature for the occurrence of epidemics is the 300–1100 mm mean annual rainfall isohyets. Thus climatic changes may govern

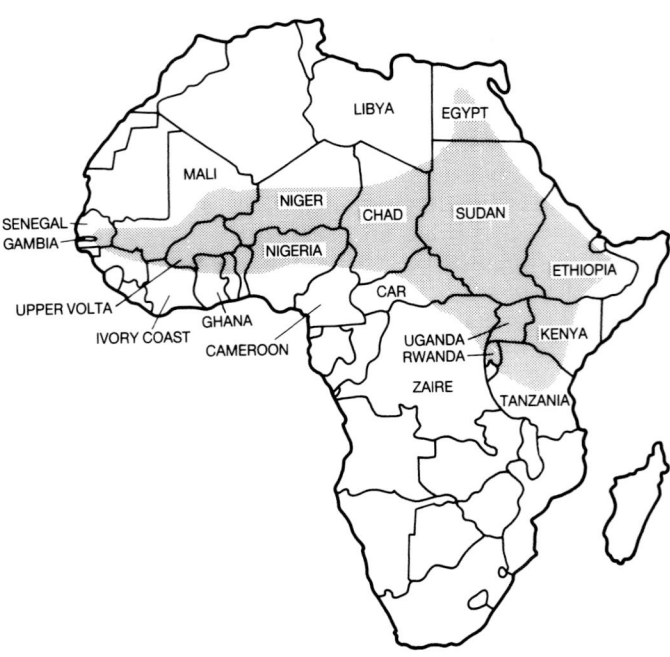

Figure 56.1: The 'classical meningitis belt' of sub-Saharan Africa where epidemics occur in 8–14-year cycles.

the distribution of the meningitis belt. In contrast, in certain parts of Africa such as in the Congo basin of DRC (Table 56.4) and in temperate industrialized countries epidemics with group A meningococci are rarely reported. In low-lying regions such as DRC, pneumococci are the major meningeal pathogens in all age groups.[32] *H. influenzae* is responsible for cases of meningitis in

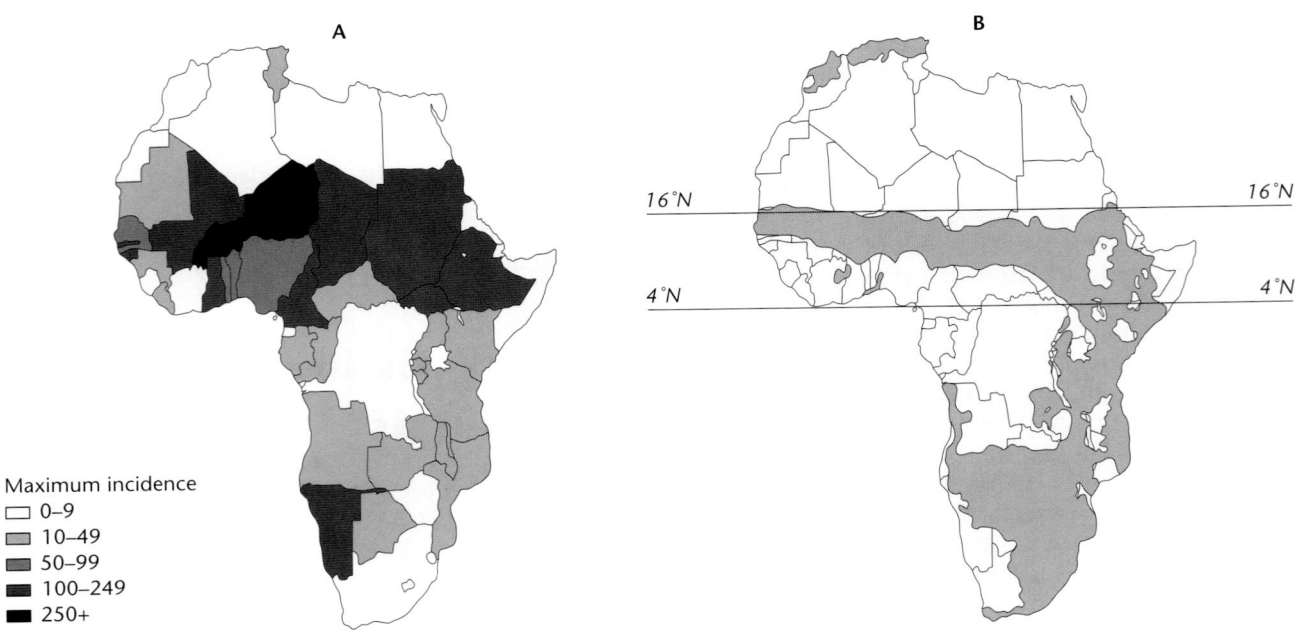

Maximum incidence
- ☐ 0–9
- 10–49
- 50–99
- 100–249
- ■ 250+

Figure 56.2: (**A**) Incidence of meningococcal meningitis in Africa (no. of cases per 100 000 population) reported to the World Health Organization, 1980–1999. (**B**) Areas with 300–1100 mm annual rainfall.

Table 56.4 Relative importance of meningeal pathogens.

	N. meningitidis	S. pneumoniae	H. influenzae	Population	Year	Reference
Cases of meningitis (%)*						
Africa						
South Africa	31	22	16	M	1980–82	28
Malawi	4	54	38	C	1983	29
Malawi	47	42	11	M	1983–89	30
Zambia	23	38	6.3	M	1978–81	31
Zaire	1.6	33	46	C	1958–77	32
Nigeria	16	39	28	C	1976–79	33
Ivory Coast	6.4	39	17	M	1971–75	34
Libya	10	18	27	C	1981–84	35
Senegal	11	29	20	M	1970–79	36
Algeria	30	11	19	M	1969	37
Asia						
India	0	61	7	M	1972–80	38
Malaysia	5.6	24	54	C	1985–87	39
Thailand	5.6	47	39	C	1967–68	40
Australia						
Papua New Guinea	36	59	4	A	1974–79	41
Vanuatu	35	33	23	C	1983–88	42
Caribbean						
Jamaica	4.1	38	30	M	1965–80	43
Puerto Rico	1.4	10	74	C	1976–82	44
America						
Brazil	40	21	28	A	1973–82	45
Chile	8.6	33	58	C	1972–81	46
Panama	14	14	0	A	1975–82	47
Europe						
UK (Merseyside)	57	14	30	C	1981–90	
Denmark	41	19	8	A	1966–76	48

A, adults; C, children; M, children and adults.
*Percentage of bacteriologically proven cases.

children under 5 years old in all regions of the world where the conjugate vaccine is not used routinely.

Epidemiology

For each of the three main pathogens spread is by droplet or exchange of saliva. Spread is facilitated by close contact. For example, household contacts of a person with meningococcal disease run a risk of developing infection that is 1245 times greater than that for the general population.[49] In most cases colonization of the nasopharynx precedes invasive disease. The incubation period may be as short as 2–3 days, but secondary cases of meningococcal disease have been reported as long as 4 months after contact. However, in studies of secondary cases in households with an index case of meningococcal disease, 70% of secondary cases occur within the first week of contact, 13% in the second week, 6% in the third week and the remaining 11% from the fourth to tenth weeks.[49]

Although the incidence of pneumococcal and *H. influenzae* meningitis remains relatively constant, *N.* *meningitidis* is able to produce epidemics spreading through many parts of the world.[2,27] For example, a clone of group A *N. meningitidis* (III-1) produced an epidemic of disease in China in the 1970s that spread to Nepal and India in 1982, causing an epidemic in 1983–1984. The same clone was responsible for epidemics in New Delhi (1985) and Pakistan (1985). It was then brought by hadjis to Mecca in (1987) (Figure 56.3). Clone III-1 was then disseminated throughout the world by hadjis returning home. In the African meningitis belt it initiated the 1988 epidemic, but in other areas such as Europe and USA, despite up to 11% of returning pilgrims being carriers, it did not spread. However, recent epidemics have been due to serogroup W135 and, with this, secondary cases did occur when pilgrims returned to Europe.[50]

Although in Africa epidemic meningococcal disease occurs in the dry season, this is not the sole determinant. Person-to-person spread of the meningococcus occurs as readily throughout the year, and the seasonality of disease is thought to be related to increased invasiveness. This may reflect an effect of the dust storms, extreme dryness and heat on the host's mucosal defences.[2,27]

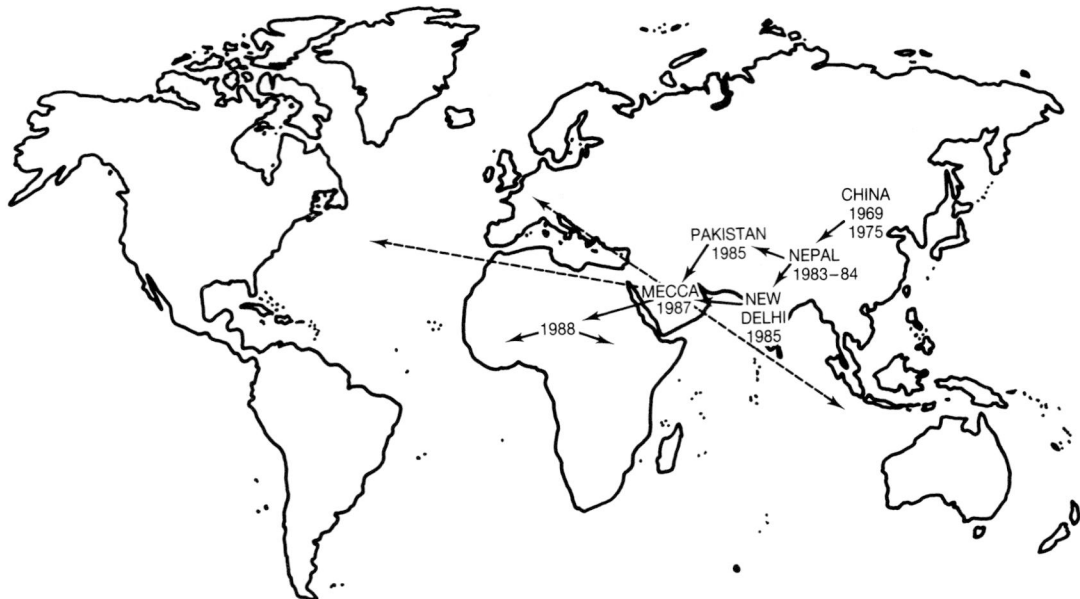

Figure 56.3: Intercontinental spread of clone III-1 of group A *Neisseria meningitidis*.

Bacteriology

Neisseria meningitidis

Meningococci are small (0.8×0.6 μm) non-motile Gram-negative cocci arranged in pairs with contiguous sides flattened.

Optimal growth of meningococci is achieved on enriched media (blood or chocolatized agar) in carbon dioxide (10%) in air at 37°C. Small convex greyish mucoid colonies are produced after 18–24 hours of incubation. All pathogenic meningococci are piliated (protein spikes for attachment to epithelial and endothelial cells) and capsulate. The capsules are acidic polysaccharides that allow the bacteria to evade phagocytic killing. There are at least nine different capsular serogroups (A, B, C, D, X, Y, Z, W135 and 29E). Groups A, B and C are associated with most cases of meningitis. Groups A and C are associated with epidemics, and group B with sporadic endemic disease. Groups B and C may be further subdivided on the basis of outer membrane proteins to provide further epidemiological information. Group A meningococci may be further subdivided by means of multilocus enzyme electrophoresis,[51] and more recently by multilocus sequence typing.[52]

Haemophilus influenzae

This is a small pleomorphic (1.5×0.4 μm) non-motile Gram-negative coccobacillus. It requires chocolatized blood agar and an atmosphere of carbon dioxide (10%) in air for growth, and produces small convex greyish mucoid colonies after 18–24 hours. Only one of the capsulate strains of *H. influenzae* is able to produce invasive disease in the immunocompetent host. This is *H. influenzae* (b),

which possesses a polyribitol phosphate capsule. Although *H. influenzae* meningitis is rare in those over 5–7 years of age, it can still occur in adults.[31,35,38]

Streptococcus pneumoniae

These are lanceolate Gram-positive cocci (0.8×1.0 μm), usually arranged in pairs. They grow best on blood agar in carbon dioxide (10%) in air, where they produce either small draughtsman-like colonies or large transparent mucoid (like drops of water) α-haemolytic colonies. The latter are the more virulent strains. Pneumococci are sensitive to optochin, which differentiates them from other α-haemolytic streptococci. There are more than 80 different capsular types, but the 23 included in the current capsular vaccine are responsible for 90–95% of cases of invasive disease. Pneumococci also produce an exotoxin: pneumolysin.

Pathogenesis

Each of the three main pathogens is able to colonize the naropharynx. There is evidence to suggest that the risk of disease is greatest in the period immediately after colonization. Bacteria in the nasopharynx then translocate to enter the circulation. How this occurs is not clear, but for the meningococcus there is an association between respiratory tract infection with viruses or mycoplasma and meningitis.[53] The bacteria localize in the pia and arachnoid maters, and set up an inflammatory response in the meninges and CSF. The presence of capsule allows bacteria to survive longer in the circulation and meninges. Various components of the bacterial cell surface, such as teichoic acid in pneumococci, lipopolysaccharide (endotoxin) in meningococci and *H. influenzae*, and peptidoglycan in all of them, induce secretion of a variety of factors such as tumour necrosis factor (TNF), interleukin (IL) 1 and IL-6, eicosanoids, and platelet activating factor (PAF). This results in potentiation of inflammation, further activation of neutrophils, further complement activation and increased permeability of the blood–brain barrier. This can then produce cerebral vessel thrombosis and vasculitis, cerebral oedema, intracranial hypertension and cerebral infarction. Finally the activated neutrophils consume large amounts of glucose and oxygen, and deprive neuronal tissues of these essential components, driving the brain into anaerobic respiration and production of lactate, which is also neurotoxic.

Pathology

The pathological features of acute bacterial meningitis are similar for each of the pathogens and have been well reviewed.[54] The principal feature is of a purulent exudate in the subarachnoid space which often damages the pia mater and the underlying superficial cortex. There is cerebral vessel vasculitis and thrombosis with neuronal damage and superficial encephalitis. There may also be damage to cranial and spinal nerves as they traverse the subarachnoid space.

Clinical features

The signs and symptoms of bacterial meningitis are those of infection and of inflammation of the meninges. The onset is sudden with fever in most cases, but is often preceded by symptoms of upper respiratory tract infection. Meningeal irritation will become manifest by nausea, vomiting, headache, irritability, confusion, back pain and neck stiffness. In addition it may be possible to elicit Kernig's (pain on attempting to extend the knee with the hips flexed) or Brudzinski's (neck flexion producing flexion of the hips and knees) sign. It is unusual for all of these features to be present at once, especially in young patients or in the early stages of disease. For example, in a review of over 1000 children with meningitis, 1.5% showed no signs of meningeal irritation throughout the infection.[55]

Even early in infection there may be some evidence of mental dysfunction, ranging from drowsiness and lethargy to coma in fulminant infection. Convulsions may occur, especially in children. These are reported in up to 20% of children prior to admission and in 26–30% overall. There may be signs of raised intracranial pressure reflected by headache, and in infants by bulging fontanelle or even diastasis of sutures. Papilloedema is not common in children. Finally, inappropriate secretion of antidiuretic hormone is a common occurrence (in up to 80% of cases) in childhood meningitis. This leads to water retention and may result in a further rise in intracranial pressure.

Pneumococcal meningitis in particular is more likely to be associated with focal signs on admission.

Differential diagnosis

Meningitis can be missed in its early stages, especially in children in whom there may be only subtle signs of meningism. It should be considered in any child with febrile convulsions or in patients who suddenly become confused. Similar clinical features may be seen in cerebral malaria, typhus, relapsing fever and cerebral tumours. Viral, fungal or tuberculous meningitis may also present in a similar fashion. Examination of CSF will help to differentiate bacterial meningitis from the rest.

Complications

The mortality rates associated with bacterial meningitis vary according to the age of the patient and the infecting micro-organisms. For example, in one survey in Brazil the overall mortality rate in non-neonatal meningitis was 32% but rose to 48% in those aged 2–6 months and to 40% in those aged from 6 months to 2 years.[45] The mortality rate from pneumococcal meningitis is highest (57%), followed by *H. influenzae* meningitis (38%), with meningococcal meningitis having the lowest mortality rate (14%). Overall mortality rates were much lower (19%) in a series reported from Malaysia.[39]

The acute and later sequelae of *H. influenzae* meningitis are shown in Table 56.5. Unfortunately, there are few long-term follow-up studies of bacterial meningitis in the tropics and most of the information has been extrapolated from temperate zones. However, in one study in Malaysia, 47% of children attending follow-up at least once had neurological sequelae.[39] The incidence of sequelae in *H. influenzae* and pneumococcal meningitis is similar, and higher than that encountered in meningococcal meningitis. A proportion of children with *H. influenzae* meningitis redevelop pyrexia at day 5 or 6 of therapy. This can represent the formation of subdural effusion or abscesses, but most often no reason is found.

Table 56.5 Complications of *H. influenzae* meningitis.

Complication	Cases (%)
Early	
Recurrent or persistent pyrexia	35-40
Subdural effusions	33
Inappropriate antidiuretic hormone secretion	50–80
Paralysis	16
Late	
Persistent paralysis	2–3
Relapse of meningitis	4
Visual impairment	2–3
Hearing deficit	10–15
Hypertension	2–3
Hydrocephalus	<1
Epileptic fits	7

Meningococcal disease

Although the mortality rate from meningococcal meningitis is relatively low, if infection is complicated by septicaemia it may prove rapidly fatal. The meningococcus continuously blebs off part of its outer membrane (Figure 56.4). Approximately 25% of the lipid in the outer membrane is lipo-oligosaccharide (LOS). This is a powerful endotoxin, and release of endotoxin produces activation of clotting and complement factors, activation of neutrophils and macrophages, with release of IL-1 (endogenous pyrogen) and TNF vasculitis. This may result in profound shock and bleeding from capillaries. On the skin this produces petechiae, purpura and ecchymoses which, together with adrenal haemorrhage, constitute the Waterhouse–Friedrichsen syndrome. The onset of disease is sudden with fever and progression through shock, purpura and coma, and death may be rapid (as fast as 2 hours). It is important to distinguish meningococcal meningitis from meningococcal meningitis with septicaemia or septicaemia alone,[56] because the management and progression of the two differ. Defects in the terminal components of the complement cascade (C6–9) and properdin predispose to the development of fulminant meningococcal septicaemia. The proportion of cases of meningococcal disease with a septicaemic component appears to be significantly lower in the meningitis belt. For example, only 4 of 112 (4%) of cases of meningococcal disease had septicaemia in one study in Sudan,[57] and the present authors have observed only 11 cases of septicaemia out of 329 cases (3%) of meningococcal disease in Malawi.[2] A similarly low incidence of meningococcal septicaemia (5%) was observed in Nigeria.[58] In contrast, only 19% of cases of meningococcal disease on Merseyside had no septicaemic component.[56] Whether this difference represents a true difference in susceptibility to meningococcal septicaemia, or is a reflection of the difficulties of recognizing a petechial rash on a dark skin (Figure 56.5), or patients in Africa with septicaemia are dying before reaching hospital, is unclear. However, the former seems more likely.[2]

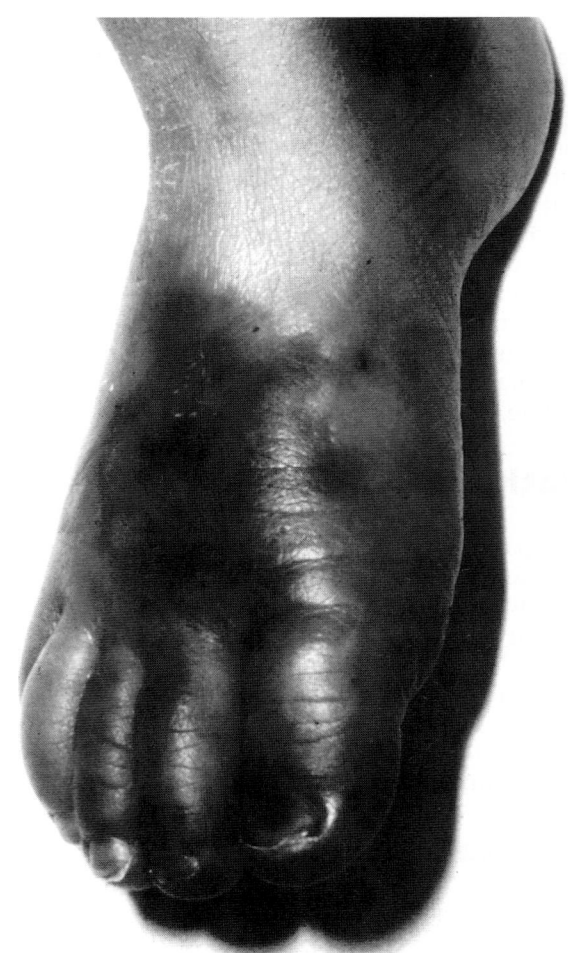

Figure 56.5: An African child with meningococcal septicaemia.

Complications of meningococcal septicaemia include gangrene of the skin and extremities, and arthritis, which can be purulent or immunologically mediated. There is also evidence of some neurological deficit.[59]

Diagnosis

The definitive diagnosis of bacterial meningitis depends upon examination of CSF (Table 56.6). The CSF is usually turbid because of the presence of large numbers of neutrophils. However, in early infection low cell counts (200/mm^3) may cause the CSF to appear clear. A high CSF neutrophil count and protein concentration and low CSF glucose level reflect the extent of inflammation and indicate a poorer prognosis. A specific aetiological diagnosis can be obtained rapidly by examining a Gram-stained smear of centrifuged CSF deposits. This will provide a specific diagnosis in 80–85% of cases. A useful, if expensive, adjunct to diagnosis is detection of bacterial capsular antigens (acidic polysaccharides). Countercurrent immuno-electrophoresis is less sensitive than latex particle agglutination, which has a sensitivity and specificity of

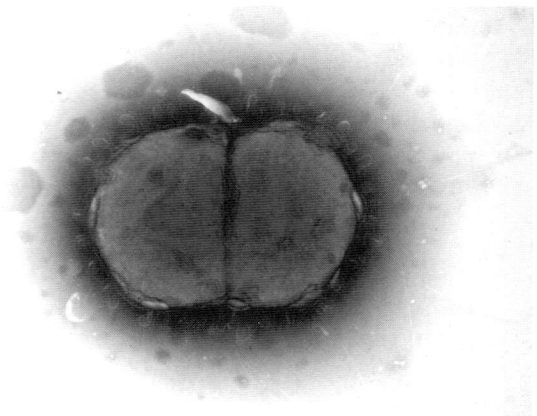

Figure 56.4: Transmission electronmicrograph of *N. meningitidis* showing pili and loss of the outer membrane by 'blebbing'.

Table 56.6 Cerebrospinal fluid in meningitis.

	Normal	Bacterial Meningitis	Aseptic Meningitis
Volume (ml)	40–120	–	–
Appearance	Clear	Turbid	Clear to opalescent
Pressure (mmH$_2$O)	<180–200	Raised	Normal
Protein (g/l)	0.15–0.4	0.5–6.0	0.5–1.0[†]
Mononuclear cells ($\times 10^6$/l)	0–5	Can be raised	15–500
Neutrophils ($\times 10^6$/l)	0	100–6000	<15
Glucose (mmol)*	2.2–3.3	0–2.2	2.2–3.3[†]

*Must be compared with blood glucose (should be 50–60% of blood glucose level).
[†]In tuberculous meningitis the CSF protein is often high and glucose low.

Table 56.7 Penetration of antibiotics into cerebrospinal fluid.

Antibiotic	Serum level in CSF (%)	Therapeutic Level
Penicillins		
Penicillin	2–6	+
Ampicillin	10	+
Cephalosporins		
Cephalothin	1–5	±
Cefuroxime	5–10	+
Cefotaxime	10–25	+
Ceftazidime	20	+
Ceftriaxone	5–10	+
Aminoglycosides		
Gentamicin	10–30	–
Netilmicin	20–25	–
Other		
Sulfadiazine	50–80	+
Sulfamethoxazole	25–30	±
Trimethoprim	30–50	+*
Tetracycline	25	+
Chloramphenicol	90	+
Ciprofloxacin	5–20	+[†]

*Not effective against *N. meningitidis*.
[†]Not effective against *Str. pneumoniae*.

85–100% and 96–100%, respectively, for detection of the appropriate micro-organism.[60,61]

CSF culture takes 18–24 hours but has the advantage of being relatively cheap and providing data on the antimicrobial susceptibility of the bacterium. Blood culture, if facilities are available, is a useful adjunct to diagnosis. Detection of antigen in urine or serum may also be of value for diagnosis of pneumococcal or *H. influenzae* meningitis, but is less useful in meningococcal meningitis.[61] However, a recent study from Kenya estimated that the diagnosis of acute childhood bacterial meningitis is likely to be missed in about one-third of cases in the absence of adequate and reliable laboratory support.[62]

Management

Patients with meningitis should, where possible, be managed in hospital. Blood pressure and respiratory and pulse rates should be monitored regularly. The unconscious patient should be nursed so as to maintain an open airway. Fluid intake should be monitored to prevent dehydration (due to fever and poor fluid intake) or overhydration (due to inappropriate antidiuretic hormone secretion). If fits occur, appropriate anticonvulsants should be administered, bearing in mind that hepatic microsomal enzyme inducers such as phenobarbital or phenytoin might increase the rate of conjugation of chloramphenicol and decrease blood levels. In studies in the USA and Europe, high-dose intravenous dexamethasone (0.15 mg/kg 6 hourly for children, or 12 g every 12 h for adults) has been shown to decrease mortality in pneumococcal meningitis[63] and to reduce the neurological sequelae and inflammation in *H. influenzae* meningitis.[63] However, results of trials of dexamethasone in developing countries have not been uniformly positive.[63–67] For example, in one study in Pakistan there was a mortality rate of 25% in children receiving dexamethasone, compared with 12% in those receiving placebo.[64]

The efficacy of antimicrobial themotherapy depends upon the penetration of the antibiotic into CSF (Table 56.7) and the susceptibility of the infecting micro-organism.

For blind initial therapy, chloramphenicol has been shown to be as effective as a chloramphenicol–penicillin combination,[68] and a long-acting oily suspension of chloramphenicol as effective as ampicillin.[69] The oily suspension has the benefit of providing treatment even for those who abscond from hospital and is particularly useful in epidemics of meningococcal meningitis.[70] However, the availability of high-quality oily chloramphenicol has been problematic.[70] Early antibiotic treatment even prior to hospital admission has been shown to improve outcome in bacterial meningitis.[71]

Meningococcal neningitis

Benzylpenicillin (300 000 units/kg per day) should be given intravenously or intramuscularly 6 hourly for up to 7 days. Chloramphenicol (75–100 mg/kg per day) is a useful alternative, given 6 hourly orally or intramuscularly. There are sporadic reports of penicillin-insusceptible meningococci,[72] but most are still exquisitely sensitive.

Pneumococcal meningitis

Benzylpenicillin (400 000 units/kg per day) is given 6 hourly intravenously or intramuscularly, usually for 10 days. Chloramphenicol can also be used in a regimen, as for meningococcal meningitis. The emergence of penicillin-resistant pneumococci is an increasing problem worldwide.[73-75] Meningitis due to such strains is unlikely to be treatable successfully by penicillin. In some cases these penicillin-resistant pneumococci, although susceptible to chloramphenicol in vitro, are not eradicated by chloramphenicol in vivo.[74]

H. influenzae meningitis

Chloramphenicol (75–100 mg/kg per day) should be given every 6 hours parenterally and subsequently may be given orally. Treatment is usually continued for 10 days. Ampicillin (200 mg/kg per day) is an alternative, although this may be associated with higher morbidity rates. Strains of H. influenzae (b) resistant to ampicillin (5–10%) or chloramphenicol (5%), and even to both antibiotics,[76] are emerging.

Although penicillin and chloramphenicol have the advantage of cheapness and ready availability in tropical countries, a recent randomized open study in Finland demonstrated that cephalosporins such as cefotaxime or ceftriaxone had a clear advantage over chloramphenicol.[77] However, these cephalosporins are expensive and none of the antibiotics was associated with a 100% cure rate.

Meningococcal septicaemia

The treatment of fulminant meningococcal septicaemia is difficult and requires intensive management. Clinical scoring systems such as the Glasgow Meningococcal Septicaemia Prognostic Score[78] are of value in assessing the severity of disease and identifying those at greatest risk of dying (Table 56.8). Its use has also been validated in a tropical setting.[79] If possible, patients should be artificially ventilated electively and given plasma and inotropes such as dobutamine as well as penicillin. Dexamethasone does not alter the course of endotoxic shock.

Table 56.8 Glasgow Meningococcal Septicaemia Prognostic Score (GMSPS).

	Points[†]
Blood pressure	3
<75 mmHg systolic <4 years	
<85 mmHg systolic >4 years	
Skin/rectal temperature difference	
>3°C	3
Modified coma scale score[*] <8 *or*	3
deterioration of >3 points in 1 h	
Deterioration in hour prior to scoring	2
Absence of meningism	2
Extending purpuric rash *or* widespread	
ecchymoses	1
Base deficit (capillary or arterial) >8.0	1

[*]Modified coma score. (1) *Eyes open*: spontaneously, 4; to speech, 3; to pain, 2; none, 1. (2) *Best verbal response*: oriented, 6; words, 4; vocal sounds, 3; cries, 2; none, 1. (3) *Best motor response*: obeys commands, 6; localized pain, 4; moves to pain, 1; none, 1. Add scores in (1), (2) and (3) to obtain coma score.
[†]AGMSPS >8 predicts mortality with a sensitivity of 100% and a specificity of 95%.

Prevention

Chemoprophylaxis

Chemoprophylaxis is used to prevent secondary cases of meningococcal and *H. influenzae* meningitis in household contacts of an index case. There is no evidence that it is beneficial in pneumococcal meningitis. Most trials of chemoprophylaxis use eradication of nasopharyngeal carriage of meningococci or *H. influenzae* as their endpoint and there are no data that demonstrate the efficacy of chemoprophylaxis in preventing infection in the community.[80]

N. meningitidis

Reports from the USA before the availability of vaccination and chemoprophylaxis showed that secondary attack rates of 4–10% within households were common.[81] More recently it has been shown that 10% of patients presenting with meningococcal meningitis in Nigeria were secondary cases.[82] Two strategies are employed. In the first phenoxymethyl-penicillin or amoxicillin is given as pre-emptive therapy for 7 days. The rationale for this is that most secondary cases occur in the first week after contact.[49] This will not affect nasopharyngeal carriage, nor will it prevent secondary cases after therapy has ceased.

The second strategy aims to eradicate nasopharyngeal carriage. Antibiotics that are effective in eradicating susceptible nasopharyngeal meningococci include sulfadiazine, minocycline, rifampicin, ciprofloxacin or ceftriaxone.[80,83] Resistance to sulphonamides limits the value of these agents and minocycline has a high incidence of side effects and cannot be used in children, pregnancy or lactation.

Rifampicin has been used in Africa[84] and does eradicate carriage. It is given as a 2-day regimen orally (600 mg twice daily for adults, 10 mg/kg per day for children aged 1–12 years and 5 mg/kg per day for children under 1 year). Disadvantages include the emergence of resistant meningococci during treatment[83] and the possibility of compromising the use of rifampicin as a first-line drug in tuberculosis. Ciprofloxacin (500–700 mg orally) or ceftriaxone (125 mg intramuscularly) are given as single-dose regimens and are as effective as rifampicin in eradicating carriage.[80] Unless sulphonamides are used, chemoprophylaxis is expensive. To use vaccines would be much more cost effective; however, vaccines are of no value in the immediate protection of household contacts because it will take 2 weeks or more to develop protective antibody levels.

H. influenzae

In the USA secondary attack rates in households by invasive *H. influenzae* in children under 5 years are 500–800 times greater than the endemic rate.[85] Chemoprophylaxis is by means of a 4-day regimen of rifampicin (20 mg/kg per day once daily). This is given to all household members where there is an index case and a child under 3 years, except for pregnant or lactating women and those with severe hepatic impairment.

Vaccination

The acidic capsular polysaccharides of each of the three bacteria are highly immunogenic and vaccines are available for all of them. The problem in using polysaccharide antigens is that they are T cell-independent antigens, which means that the antibody response is predominantly IgM and IgG$_2$ and immunological memory is poor.

The immunogenicity of such vaccines is particularly poor in infants and young children. For example, in children under 4 years of age the group A meningococcal polysaccharide vaccine had produced persistent protective antibody 1 year after immunization in 100%, in 52% after 2 years and in 0% after 3 years, whereas in children of 4 years or older the corresponding values were 85%, 75% and 67% respectively.[86] This, however, was with only one dose of vaccine and there is evidence that for group A vaccine two or more doses are better.[87]

H. influenzae (b)

The capsular polysaccharide of *H. influenzae* (b) (Hib) is polyribitol phosphate. The problem of poor immunogenicity of the capsular antigen has been overcome by conjugating it to a protein (diphtheria or tetanus toxoid). This significantly improves the quantity and duration of antibody response, even in those under 2 years of age.[88] The Hib vaccine can be given together with the triple (diphtheria, pertussis, tetanus) vaccine with no deleterious effects. Hib vaccine has been shown to have 74% efficacy in preventing invasive Hib infection and 76% efficacy in preventing Hib meningitis in children aged 18–59 months.[89] It also eliminates oropharyngeal carriage and thus provides herd immunity.

N. meningitidis

A meningococcal vaccine incorporating groups A and C capsular polysaccharides (as well as Y and W135) is available. Its use has proved effective in controlling epidemics of meningococcal disease in Asia, Africa and Latin America. Protective antibodies persist for up to 5 years in adults but for only 1–2 years in children under 4 years old when given as a single-dose regimen. The vaccine does not affect nasopharyngeal carriage[90] and thus does not provide herd immunity.

Recently both conjugate group A and conjugate group C meningococcal vaccines have been introduced, which induce long-term immunological memory when given to infants.[91] The conjugate group C meningococcal vaccine was introduced into routine use in the UK and has been shown to have 92% and 97% protective efficacy in infants and adolescents, respectively.[92] Unfortunately the conjugate polysaccharide vaccines are much more expensive than the polysaccharide alone. Whether a conjugate group A vaccine is needed has been questioned,[87]

especially as in outbreaks in the meningitis belt adolescents and young adults represent the peak of the age spectrum. How the vaccine should be used in the meningitis belt is also an area of intense discussion. Ideally vaccine, probably conjugate, would be given to all infants to give life-long immunity.[93] However, this is not possible at present and mass emergency immunization with the non-conjugate polysaccharide vaccine at the start of an epidemic is current World Health Organization policy.[94] This policy requires good surveillance, which is not always available, and sets thresholds for interventions. In populations of more than 30 000 people, an incidence of five cases per 100 000 population per week is an alert threshold when investigation and confirmation of cases is required, and surveillance should be enhanced. If there have been no epidemics in the region, and vaccine coverage is less than 80% or it is the dry season, then mass immunization is introduced when the incidence reaches 10 cases per 100 000 per week; otherwise the vaccination threshold is 15 cases per 100 000 per week. For populations of less than 30 000 the alert is two cases per week, and the vaccination threshold is five cases per week. The introduction of mass immunization is a major undertaking, requiring the transport of vaccine, needles and syringes to the epidemic area, mobilization of large numbers of health care workers, and gaining access to the population. If the thresholds are too high then the mass vaccination campaign may not begin until the epidemic has passed its peak; if too low there may be false alarms. Others have concluded that an alert threshold of five cases per 100 000 population per week allows time to prepare for an epidemic, and 10 cases per 100 000 per week should signal mass vaccination.[95]

The group B meningococcal capsule is a homopolymer of *N*-acetylneuraminic acid (as is the *E. coli* K1 capsule) and is a self-antigen, being found on human neuronal glycoproteins and glycolipids. Thus there is no group B capsular vaccine. Vaccines incorporating group B meningococcal outer membrane proteins have worked well in Cuba[96] but less well in Chile or Norway.[97]

Str. pneumoniae

The pneumococcal polysaccharide vaccine incorporates 23 of the 84 pneumococcal capsular polysaccharides. These 23 serogroups are responsible for 90–95% of invasive pneumococcal disease. The vaccine is not widely used and suffers from the same problems as other polysaccharide vaccines. Its use is confined to those who are about to have splenectomy and patients with sickle cell disease. Seven-valent and nine-valent polysaccharide conjugate vaccines have been developed which incorporate serogroups important in invasive disease and otitis media in developed countries, some of which are also important in the tropics.[98] Clinical trials so far have been directed towards the prevention of otitis media and bacteraemia, and there are no data on the prevention of pneumococcal meningitis in the tropics.

REFERENCES

1   Holt D E, Halket S, de Louvois J & Harvey D. Neonatal meningitis in England and Wales: 10 years on. *Arch Dis Child Fetal Neonatal Ed* 2001; 84:F85–F89.

2   Hart C A & Cuevas L E. Meningococcal disease in Africa. *Ann Trop Med Parasitol* 1997; 91:777–785.

3   Hensey O J, Hart C A & Cooke R W I. Serious infection in a neonatal intensive care unit. *J Hyg* 1985; 95:289–297.

4   Barcley B. High frequency of *Salmonella* species as a cause of neonatal meningitis in Ibadan, Nigeria. *Acta Paediatr Scand* 1971; 60:540–544.

5   Longe A C, Omene J A & Okolo A A. Neonatal meningitis in Nigerian infants. *Acta Paediatr Scand* 1984; 74:477–481.

6   Coovadia Y M, Mayosi B, Adhikari M, Solwa Z & van den Ende J. Hospital acquired neonatal meningitis: the impacts of cefotaxime usage on mortality and of amikacin usage on incidence. *Ann Trop Paediatr* 1989; 9:233–239.

7   Nel E. Neonatal meningitis: mortality, cerebrospinal fluid, and microbiological findings. *J Trop Pediatr* 2000; 46:237–239.

8   Chang Chien H Y, Chiu N C, Li W C & Huang F Y. Characteristics of neonatal bacterial meningitis in a teaching hospital in Taiwan from 1984–1997. *J Microbiol Immunol Infect* 2000; 33:100–104.

9   Gebremariam A. Neonatal meningitis in Addis Ababa: a ten year review. *Ann Trop Paediatr* 1998; 18:279–283.

10 Molyneux E, Walsh A, Phiri A & Molyneux M. Acute bacterial meningitis in children admitted to the Queen Elizabeth Central Hospital, Blantyre, Malawi in 1996–1997. *Trop Med Int Health* 1998; 3:610–618.

11 Rajab A & de Louvois J. Survey of infection in babies at the Khoula Hospital, Oman. *Ann Trop Paediatr* 1990; 10:39–43.

12 Freedman R M, Ingram D L, Gross I, Ehrenkranz R A, Warkshaw J B & Baltimore R S. A half century of neonatal sepsis at Yale: 1928 to 1978. *Am J Dis Child* 1981; 135:140–144.

13 Molyneux E M, Walsh A L, Malenga G, Rogerson S & Molyneux M E. *Salmonella* meningitis in children in Blantyre, Malawi, 1996–1999. *Ann Trop Paediatr* 2000; 20:41–44.

14 Halder D, Zainal N, Wah C M & Haq J A. Neonatal meningitis and septicaemia caused by *Burkholderia pseudomallei*. *Ann Trop Paediatr* 1998; 18:161–164.

15 De Moraes Pinto M I, Verhoeff F, Milligan P et al. Placental antibody transfer: influence of maternal HIV-infection and placental malaria. *Arch Dis Child Fetal Neonatal Ed* 1998; 79:F202–F205.

16 Overall J C. Neonatal bacterial meningitis: analysis of predisposing factors and outcome compared with matched control subjects. *J Pediatr* 1970; 76:499–508.

17 Berman P H & Bank B Q. Neonatal meningitis: a clinical and pathological study of 29 cases. *Pediatrics* 1996; 38:6–18.

18 McCracken G H & Shinefield H R. Changes in the pattern of neonatal septicaemia and meningitis. *Am J Dis Child* 1966; 112:33–41.

19 McCracken G H & Mize S G. A controlled study of intrathecal antibiotic therapy in Gram negative enteric meningitis of infancy. *J Pediatr* 1976; 89:66–74.

20 Doran T I. The role of *Citrobacter* in clinical disease of children: review. *Clin Infect Dis* 1999; 28:384–394.

21 Sarff L D, Platt L H & McCracken G H. Cerebrospinal fluid evaluation in neonates. Comparison of high risk infants with and without meningitis. *J Pediatr* 1976; 88:473–479.

22 McCracken G H, Mize S G & Threlkeld N. Intraventricular gentamicin therapy in Gram negative bacillary meningitis of infancy. *Lancet* 1980; i:787–791.

23 Daoud A S, Batieha A, Al-Sheyyab M et al. Lack of effectiveness of dexamethazone in neonatal bacterial meningitis. *Eur J Pediatr* 1999; 158:230–233.

24 Burman L G, Christensen P, Christensen K et al. Prevention of excess neonatal morbidity associated with group B streptococci by vaginal chlorhexidine disinfection during labour. *Lancet* 1992; 340:65–69.

25 Taha T E, Biggar R J, Broadhead R L et al. Effect of cleansing the birth canal with antiseptic solution on maternal and new-born morbidity and mortality in Malawi: clinical trial. *BMJ* 1997; 315:216–220.

26 Webb D K H & Serjeant G R. Systemic *Salmonella* infections in sickle cell anaemia. *Ann Trop Pediatr* 1989; 3:169–172.

27 Moore P S. Meningococcal meningitis in sub-Saharan Africa: a model for the epidemic process. *Clin Infect Dis* 1992; 14:515–525.

28 Liebowitz L D, Koornhof H J, Barrett M et al. Bacterial meningitis in Johannesburg—1980–1982. *S Afr Med J* 1984; 66:677–679.

29 Borgstein A. Pyogenic meningitis in children at Queen Elizabeth Central Hospital Blantyre. *Malawi Med Quart J* 1984; 17:26–27.

30 Cuevas L E & Hart C A. Acute bacterial meningitis in Malawi. *Malawi Med J* 1991; 7:2–6.

31 Dube S D & Shenderov B A. Incidence and pattern of bacterial meningitis in Lusaka. *Cent Afr J Med* 1983; 29:100–103.

32 Omanga U, Nethihinyurwa M, Shako D et al. Aspectes étiologiques et évolutifs des méningites purulentes de l'enfant à Kinshasa: analyse de 471 cases. *Méd d'Afrique Noire* 1980; 27:25–34.

33 Babalola A A & Coker A O. Pyogenic meningitis among Lagos children: causative organisms, age, sex and seasonal incidence. *Cent Afr J Med* 1982; 28:14–18.

34 Couprie F & Chippaux-Hyppolite C. Les méningites purulentes á Abidjan. *Méd Armées* 1977; 5:823–828.

35 Elzouki A Y & Vesikari T. First international conference on infections in children in Arab countries. *Pediatr Infect Dis* 1985; 4:527–531.

36 Cadoz M, Denis F & Diop Mar I. Etude épidémiologiques des cas de méningites purulentes hospitalisés à Dakar pendant la décennie 1970–79. *Bull World Health Organ* 1981; 59:575–584.

37 Behhassine M & Mered B. Les méningites purulentes en Algérie: étude bactériologique de 133 cas. *Arch Inst Pasteur Algér* 1969; 47:13–26.

38 Bhat B V, Verma I C, Puri R K, Srinivasan S & Nalini P. Prognostic indicators in pyogenic meningitis. *Indian Pediatr* 1987; 24:977–983.

39 Choo K F, Ariffin W A, Ahmad T, Lim W L & Gururaj A K. Pyogenic meningitis in hospitalized children in Kelantan Malaysia. *Ann Trop Paediatr* 1990; 10:89–98.

40 Sunakorn P, Lexomboon U & Sindhurat S. Acute bacterial meningitis at the children's hospital Bangkok. *J Med Assoc Thai* 1969; 52:1001–1011.

41 Naraqi S. Aetiology of acute bacterial meningitis in the highlands and islands of Papua New Guinea. *Papua New Guinea Med J* 1980; 23:108–110.

42 McKay T. Experience of changing antibiotic protocol in childhood bacterial meningitis in Vanuatu. *Trop Doct* 1989; 19:158–159.

43 Sharma A, Sharma D & Prabhakar P. Infectious meningitis at the university hospital of the West Indies. Review of clinical and laboratory findings (1965–1980). *West Indian Med J* 1984; 33:14–30.

44 Munoz A I. Bacterial meningitis in pediatric patients: a five year experience. *Bol Asoc Med P R* 1982; 74:62–65.

45 Bryan J P, de Silva H R, Ravares A, Rocha H & Scheld W M. Etiology and mortality of bacterial meningitis in north eastern Brazil. *Rev Infect Dis* 1990; 12:128–135.

46 Juliet C, Rodriguez G, Marti A & Burgos O V. Meningitis bacteriana en el nino: experiencia con 441 casos. *Rev Med Chil* 1983; 111:690–698.

47 Cherigo-Quiros E Z & Rodriguez-French A. Meningitis bacteriana en Hospital Santo Tomas (1975–1982). *Rev Med Panama* 1984; 9:35–44.

48 Bohr V, Hansen B, Jessen O et al. Eight hundred and seventy five cases of bacterial meningitis. I: Clinical data, prognosis and the role of specialized hospital department. *J Infect* 1983; 7:21–30.

49 De Wals P, Hertoghe L, Boree-Grimee I et al. Meningococcal disease in Belgium. Secondary attack rate among household, day-care nursery and pre-elementary school contacts. *J Infect* 1981; 3 (Supplement I):53–61.

50 Taha M K, Achtman M, Alonso J M et al. Serogoup W135 in meningococcal disease in Hajj pilgrims. *Lancet* 2000; 356:2159.

51 Caugant D A, Froholm L O, Bovre K et al. Intercontinental spread of a genetically distinctive complex of clones of *Neisseria meningitidis* causing epidemic disease. *Proc Natl Acad Sci USA* 1986; 83:4927–4931.

52 Maiden M C J, Bygraves J A, Feil E et al. Multilocus sequence typing: a portable approach to the identification of clones within populations of pathogenic microorganisms. *Proc Natl Acad Sci USA* 1998; 95:3140–3145.

53 Moore P S, Hierholzer J, De Witt W et al. Respiratory viruses and mycoplasma as cofactors for epidemic group A meningococcal meningitis. *JAMA* 1990; 264:1271–1275.

54 Adams R D, Kubik C S & Bonner F J. The clinical and pathological aspects of influenzal meningitis. *Arch Pediatr* 1948; 65:354–376.

55 Geisler P J & Nelson K E. Bacterial meningitis without clinical signs of meningeal irritation. *South Med J* 1982; 75:448–450.

56 Riordan F A I, Marzouk O, Thomson A P J, Sills JA & Hart C A. Changing presentation of meningococcal disease. *Eur J Pediatr* 1995; 154:472–474.

57 Salih M A M, Ahmed H S, Karrar Z A et al. Features of a large epidemic of group A meningococcal meningitis in Khartoum, Sudan in 1988. *Scand J Infect Dis* 1990; 22:161–170.

58 Whittle H C & Greenwood B M. Meningococcal meningitis in the northern savanna of Africa. *Trop Doct* 1976; 6:99–104.

59 Fellick J M, Sills J A, Marzouk O et al. Neurodevelopmental outcome in meningococcal disease: a case–control study. *Arch Dis Child* 2001; 85:6–11.

60 Cuevas L E, Hart C A & Mughogho G. Latex particle agglutination tests as an adjunct to the diagnosis of bacterial meningitis: a study from Malawi. *Ann Trop Med Parasitol* 1989; 83:375–379.

61 Holland S J, Marzouk O, Thomson A P J, Sills J A & Hart C A. Sensitivity and specificity of serum antigen detection for diagnosis of meningococcal disease in children. *Serodiagn Immunother Infect Dis* 1990; 4:345–349.

62 Berkley J A, Mwangi I, Ngetsa C J et al. Diagnosis of acute bacterial meningitis in children at a district hospital in sub-Saharan Africa. *Lancet* 2001; 357:1753–1757.

63 McIntyre P B, Berkey C S, King S M et al. Dexamethasone as adjunctive therapy in bacterial meningitis. A meta-analysis of randomized clinical trials since 1988. *JAMA* 1997; 278:925–931.

64 Girgis N I, Farid Z, Mikhail I A et al. Dexamethasone treatment for bacterial meningitis in children and adults. *Pediatr Infect Dis J* 1989; 8:848–851.

65 Qazi S A, Khan M A, Mughal N et al. Dexamethasone and bacterial meningitis in Pakistan. *Arch Dis Child* 1996; 75:482–488.

66 Macaluso A, Pivetta S, Maggi R S, Tamburlini G & Cattaneo A. Dexamethasone adjuctive therapy for bacterial meningitis in children: a retrospective study in Brazil. *Ann Trop Paediatr* 1996; 16:193–198.

67 Shembesh N M, Elbargathy S M, Kashbur I M, Rao B N & Mahmoud K S. Dexamethasone as adjuctive treatment of

bacterial meningitis. *Ind J Pediatr* 1997; 64:517–522.

68 Shann F, Barker J & Poore P. Chloramphenicol alone versus chloramphenicol plus penicillin for bacterial meningitis in children. *Lancet* 1985; ii:681–701.

69 Pecoul B, Varine F, Keita M et al. Long acting chloramphenicol versus intravenous ampicillin for treatment of bacterial meningitis. *Lancet* 1991; 388:862–866.

70 Lewis R F, Dorlencourt F & Pinel J. Long-acting oily chloramphenicol for meningococcal meningitis. *Lancet* 1998; 352:823.

71 Gedde-Dahl T W, Hoiby E A & Eskerud J. Unbiased evidence on early treatment of suspected meningococcal disease. *Rev Infect Dis* 1990; 12:973–992.

72 Esso D V, Fontanals D & Uriz S. *Neisseria meningitidis* strains with decreased susceptibility to penicillin. *Pediatr Infect Dis* 1987; 6:438–439.

73 Allen K D. Penicillin-resistant pneumococci. *J Hosp Infect* 1991; 17:3–13.

74 Friedland I R & Klugman K P. Failure of chloromphenicol therapy in penicillin-resistant pneumococcal meningitis. *Lancet* 1992; 339:405–408.

75 Yomo A, Subramanyam V R, Fudzulani R et al. Carriage of penicillin-resistant pneumococci in Malawian children. *Ann Trop Paediatr* 1997; 17:239–243.

76 Coovadia Y M, Coovadia H M & van den Ende J. Meningitis due to beta-lactamase producing, chloramphenicol resistant *Haemophilus influenzae* type b in South Africa. *J Infect* 1986; 12:247–249.

77 Peltola H, Anttila M & Renkonen OK. Randomized comparison of chloramphenicol, ampicillin, cefotaxime and ceftriaxone for childhood bacterial meningitis. *Lancet* 1989; i:1281–1287.

78 Thomson A P J, Sills J A & Hart C A. Validation of the Glasgow Meningococcal Septicaemia Prognostic Score. A ten year retrospective survey. *Crit Care Med* 1991; 19:26–30.

79 Silva P S L, Fonseca M C M, Iglesias S B O et al. Comparison of two different severity scores (Paediatric Risk of Mortality [PRISM] and the Glasgow Meningococcal Prognostic Score [GMSPS]) in meningococcal disease. *Ann Trop Paediatr* 2001; 21:135–140.

80 Hart C A. Meningococcal disease. *Clinical Evidence* 2001; 5:520–527.

81 French M R. Epidemiological study of 383 cases of meningococcal meningitis in the city of Milwaukee, 1927, 1928 and 1929. *Am J Public Health* 1931; 21:130–138.

82 Greenwood B M, Bradley A K & Cleland P G. An epidemic of meningococcal meningitis at Zaria, northern Nigeria. *Trans R Soc Trop Med Hyg* 1979; 73:557–573.

83 Cuevas L E & Hart C A. Chemoprophylaxis of bacterial meningitis. *J Antimicrob Chemother* 1993; 31:79–91.

84 Blakebrough I S & Gilles H M. The effect of rifampicin on meningococcal carriage in family contacts in northern Nigeria. *J Infect* 1980; 2:137–143.

85 Glode M P, Daum R S, Goldmann D A, Leclair J & Smith A. *Haemophilus influenzae* type b meningitis: a contagious disease in children. *BMJ* 1980; i:899–901.

86 Reingold A C, Broome C V, Hightower A W et al. Age specific differences in duration of clinical protection after vaccination with meningococcal polysaccharide A vaccine. *Lancet* 1985; ii:114–118.

87 Robbins J B, Schneerson R & Gotschlich E C. A rebuttal: epidemic and endemic meningococcal meningitis in sub-Saharan Africa can be prevented now by routine immunization with group A meningococcal capsular polysaccharide vaccine. *Pediatr Infect Dis J* 2000; 19:945–953.

88 Booy R & Moxon E R. Immunization of infants against *Haemophilus influenzae* type b in the UK. *Arch Dis Child* 1991; 66:1251–1254.

89 Wenger J D, Pierce R, Deaver K A et al. Efficacy of *Haemophilus influenzae* type (b) polysaccharide–diphtheria toxoid conjugate vaccine in US children aged 18–59 months. *Lancet* 1991; 338:395–398.

90 Blakebrough I S, Greenwood B M, Whittle H C, Bradley A K & Gilles H M. Failure of meningococcal vaccination to stop the transmission of meningococci in Nigerian schoolboys. *Ann Trop Med Parasitol* 1983; 77:175–178.

91 MacLennan J, Obaro S, Deeks J et al. Immunologic memory 5 years after meningococcal A/C conjugate vaccination in infancy. *J Infect Dis* 2001; 183:97–104.

92 Ramsay M E, Andrews J, Kaczmarski E B & Miller E. Efficacy of meningococcal serogroup C conjugate vacine in teenagers and toddlers in England. *Lancet* 2001; 357:195–196.

93 Peltola H. Emergency or routine vaccination against meningococcal disease in Africa. *Lancet* 2000; 355:3.

94 World Health Organization. Detecting meningococcal meningitis epidemics in highly-endemic African countries. *Wkly Epidemiol Rec* 2000; 75:306–309.

95 Lewis R, Nathan N, Diarra L, Balanger F & Paquet C. Timely detection of meningococcal meningitis epidemics in Africa. *Lancet* 2001; 358:287–293.

96 Sierra G V G, Campa H C, Varacel N M et al. Vaccination against group B *Neisseria meningitidis*: protection trial and mass vaccination results in Cuba. *NIPH Ann* 1991; 14:195–210.

97 Bjune G, Hoiby E A, Gronnesby J K et al. Effect of outer membrane vesicle vaccine against group B meningococcal disease in Norway. *Lancet* 1991; 338:1093–1096.

98 Choo S & Finn A. New pneumococcal vaccines for children. *Arch Dis Child* 2001; 84:289–294.

Chapter 57
Tuberculosis

J. M. Grange and A. Zumla

Tuberculosis has been, and continues to be, one of the most significant infections causing human disease. So worried were The World health Organization (WHO) about the relentless spread of tuberculosis throughout the world that it declared tuberculosis a 'Global Emergency' in 1993. Tuberculosis has afflicted the human race since the dawn of recorded history and several historical descriptions of the disease exist. Many names have been given to this disease and some are still in use today (Table 57.1). Skeletal changes typical of tuberculosis have been seen in Egyptian mummies and in Neolithic skeletons in Europe and there is compelling evidence that the disease occurred in the indigenous populations of the American continent long before the arrival of European explorers and settlers. Among the infectious diseases, tuberculosis remains a leading cause of illness and death, particularly in tropical countries. Owing to increased poverty in an overpopulated world, lack of attention to tuberculosis services and the impact of the HIV/AIDS pandemic, there are more cases of tuberculosis today than at any previous time in human history. The WHO has estimated that, unless tuberculosis control is strengthened, between the years 2000 and 2020 nearly one billion people will be infected with the tubercle bacillus, 200 million people will develop clinical tuberculosis and 35 million will die from it. Although the incidence of tuberculosis declined greatly during the twentieth century in the industrially developed nations, these nations are now experiencing an upsurge of tuberculosis. Multi-drug resistant tuberculosis (MDRTB) has become a major problem in several countries in Europe, Africa and Asia and threatens the rest of the world.

Aetiology of tuberculosis

The causative organism of tuberculosis, the tubercle bacillus, was isolated and described by Robert Koch in 1882 (Figure 57.1). It was subsequently included in the genus *Mycobacterium* and named *Mycobacterium tuberculosis*. A closely related species isolated from cattle which is also able to cause human tuberculosis is termed *M. bovis*. Mycobacterial strains with rather variable properties

Table 57.1 Historical clinical descriptions of tuberculosis

Description	Clinical type of tuberculosis
Consumption	Pulmonary
Pthisis	Pulmonary
Tabes pulmonalis	Pulmonary
Tissic	Pulmonary
Hectic fever	Pulmonary
Asthenia	Pulmonary
Galloping consumption	Pulmonary
Scrofula	Cervical lymphadenitis
Struma	Cervical
King's evil	Cervical
Hydrocephalus (acute or infantile)	Tuberculous meningitis
Pott's disease	Spinal/vertebral tuberculosis
Tuberculous chancre	Skin
Scrofuloderma	Skin
Lupus vulgaris	Skin

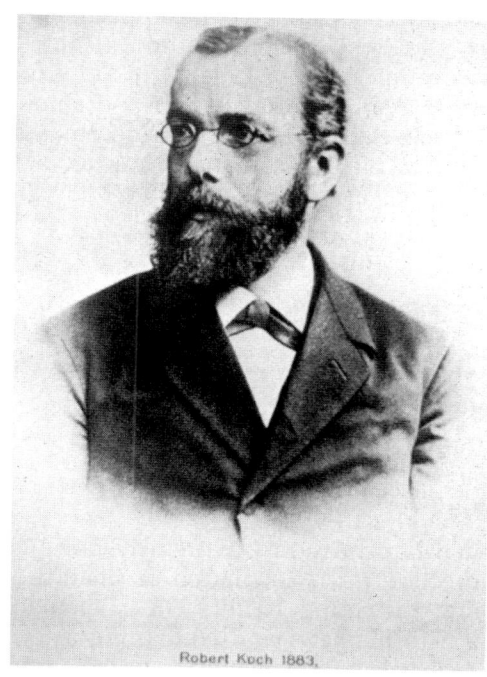

Robert Koch 1883.

Figure 57.1: Professor Robert Koch, discoverer of *Mycobacterium tuberculosis*.

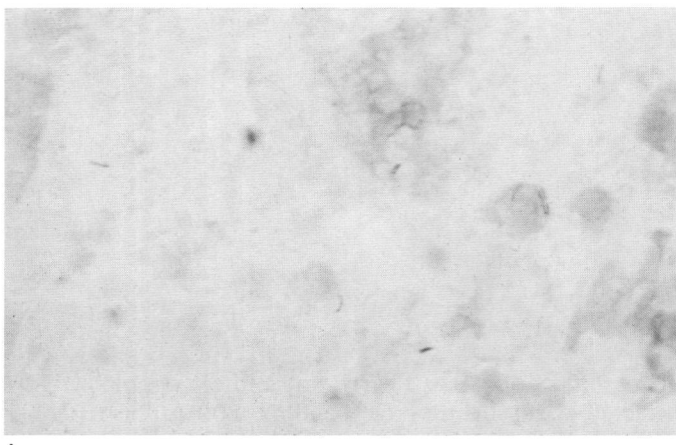

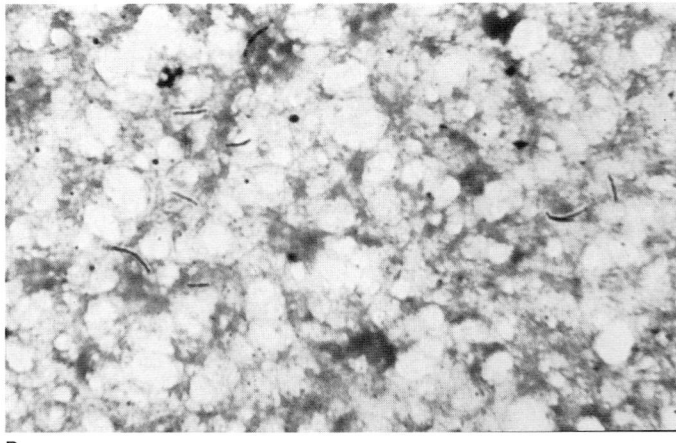

A   B

Figure 57.2: (**A**) Ziehl–Neelsen staining of a sputum sample and (**B**) a bronchoalveolar lavage washing showing acid-fast bacilli.

principally encountered in Equatorial Africa are collectively termed *M. africanum*. In addition, a rarely encountered type forming unusual smooth colonies on solid culture media has been named *M. canettii*. *M. microti*, a rare cause of tuberculosis in small mammals but of very low virulence in humans, is also closely related. Strictly speaking, these bacilli are all members of a single species which is usually termed the *Mycobacterium tuberculosis* complex. Members of this complex are obligate pathogens and thus distinct from almost all other mycobacteria, of which there are over 80 named species.

Tubercle bacilli are aerobic, non-motile, non-sporing, often slightly curved rods 2–4 μm in length and 0.3–0.5 μm in diameter. In common with other mycobacteria, they retain arylmethane dyes on treatment with mineral acids, a property termed acid-fastness. This property is widely used to detect mycobacteria in clinical specimens by light microscopy (the Ziehl–Neelsen method) (Figure 57.2) or by fluorescence microscopy. Tubercle bacilli grow slowly on conventional solid culture media and colonies take from 2 to 6 weeks to appear. More rapid automated culture systems are becoming available and nucleic acid-based detection systems using molecular methods are being developed.

Pathogenesis

Infection of humans with *M. tuberculosis* can occur via several routes:

1. Inhalation
2. Ingestion
3. Inoculation

Congenital transmission is extremely rare. The usual route of infection is via inhalation of small droplets of cough spray containing bacilli. These spray particles, around 5 μm in diameter and containing a few bacilli, lodge in the alveolae or small airways, usually in the lower regions of the lung. The usual sources of such infectious particles are other human beings with open pulmonary

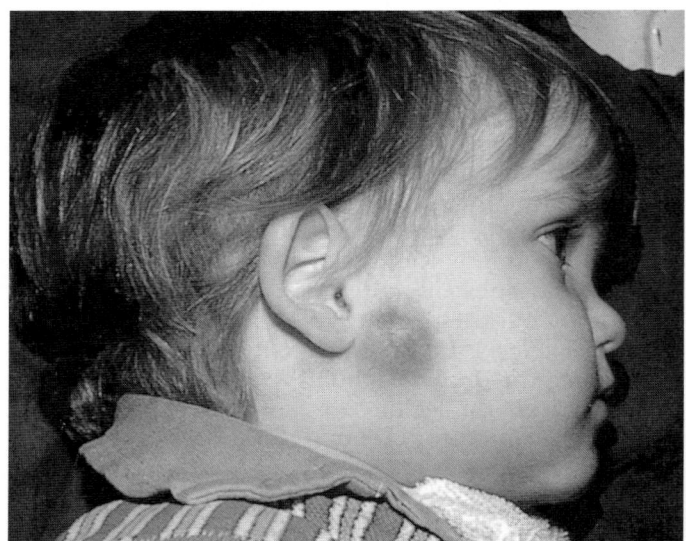

Figure 57.3: Primary tuberculous lesion of the skin.

tuberculosis but agricultural workers may be infected by *M. bovis* in the cough spray of diseased cattle. A less frequent mode of infection is consumption of milk or food contaminated by *M. bovis*, in which case the bacilli often lodge in the tonsil or intestinal wall. Rarely, tubercle bacilli enter the skin through cuts and abrasions (Figure 57.3) and tuberculosis was an occupational hazard of butchers, anatomists and pathologists. The French physician Laenecc, the inventor of the stethoscope, contracted tuberculosis by injuring his left forefinger while sawing through the vertebrae of a patient who had died of spinal tuberculosis.

Traditionally, tuberculosis has been divided into two forms:

1. Primary tuberculosis
2. Post-primary tuberculosis

It was usually assumed that post-primary tuberculosis was the result of endogenous reactivation of latent or

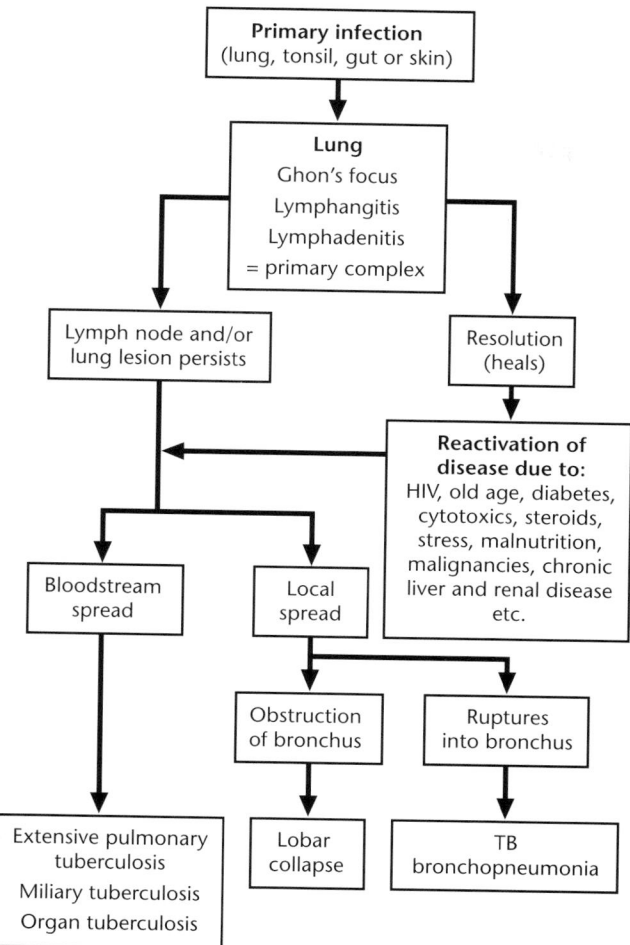

Figure 57.4: Natural history and sequelae of tuberculosis infection.

primary focus is in the lung) where secondary lesions develop. The combination of the tuberculosis primary focus, with lymphangitis and lymphadenitis, is termed the *primary complex* (Figure 57.5). Some bacilli may subsequently enter the bloodstream and lodge in various organs of the body and cause the various non-pulmonary forms of primary tuberculosis.

In the majority of cases, the immune response enables the primary complex to contain the infection; the lesions

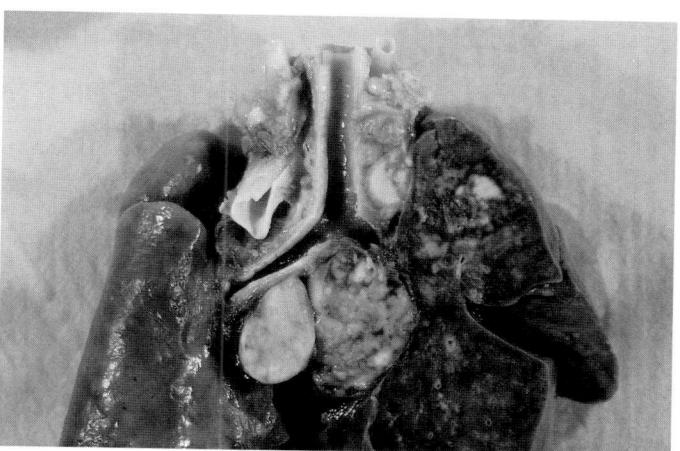

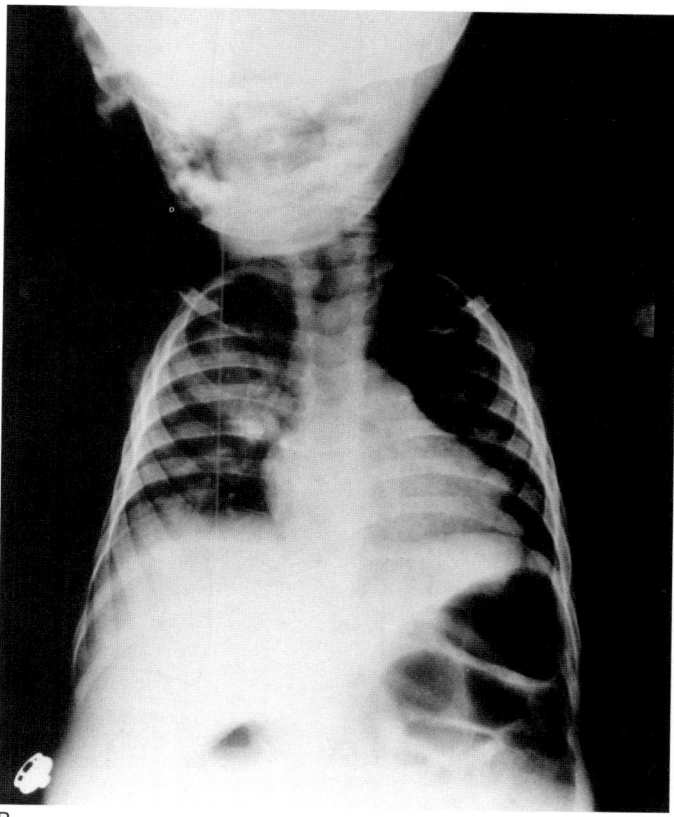

Figure 57.5: (**A**) Post-mortem lung specimen showing the 'primary complex': caseating primary lesion (Ghon's focus) with regional lymphadenitis. (**B**) Chest X-ray of an infant with primary tuberculosis showing right hilar node involvement.

dormant primary lesions but DNA fingerprinting has shown that many cases, particularly among immuno-suppressed persons, are due to exogenous reinfection.[1]

The natural history of infection with *M. tuberculosis* and its sequelae are shown in Figure 57.4. The majority of people infected by tubercle bacilli do not develop clinically evident tuberculosis and the primary infection may go unnoticed. Their bodies mount an effective immune response that encapsulates the organism and contains it for the rest of their lives. As a general rule around 2–5% of persons infected develop clinically evident primary tuberculosis and a further 2–5% subsequently develop post-primary disease. Little is known of the early events following initial infection and our limited understanding derives principally from experimental observations in animals. In the case of pulmonary infection, the bacilli are initially engulfed by alveolar macrophages in which they multiply, eventually killing the cell. Additional blood-borne phagocytic cells, both macrophages and polymorphonuclear leucocytes, aggregate around the focus of infection and form a foreign body granuloma termed the *primary focus*. Some bacilli are transported to the regional lymph nodes (the mediastinal, paratracheal and, occasionally, the supraclavicular nodes when the

A **Focus and complications**

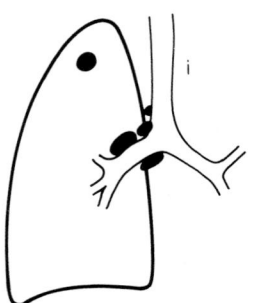 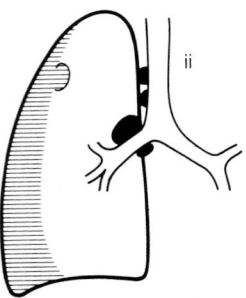 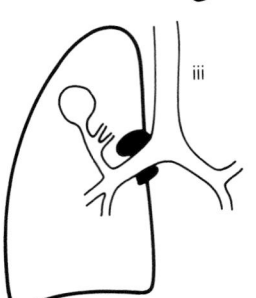 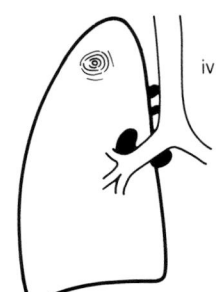

Caseous nodes

Primary complex.
Focus and regional glands

Rupture of focus into pleural
space with effusion; serous
occasionally purulent

Rupture of focus into
bronchus: cavitation

Enlarged focus sometimes
laminated 'round' or 'coin'
shadow

B **Mediastinal (regional) nodes and complications**

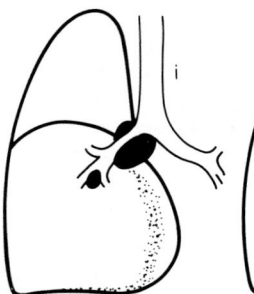 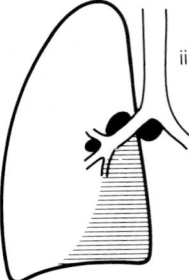 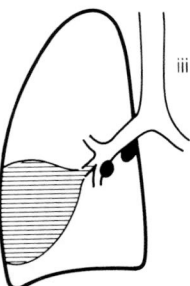 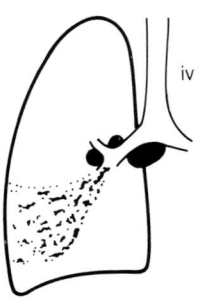 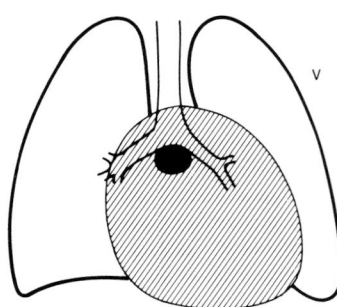

Incomplete
bronchial obstruction
(ball valve)
Inflation of middle
and lower lobes

Collapsed
lower lobe after
complete bronchial
obstruction without
consolidation

Collapse after
partial
consolidation
segmental
lesion

Erosion into
bronchus
inhalation and
areas of tuberculous
bronchopneumonia

Pericardial effusion post-rupture
of node through pericardium

C **Sequelae of bronchial complications**

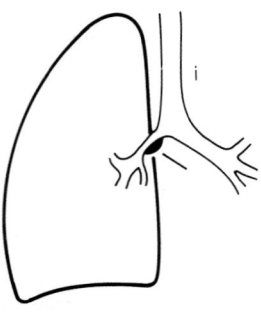 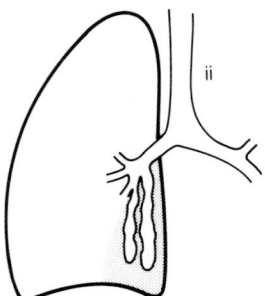 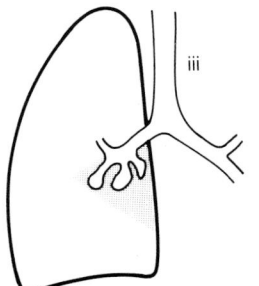 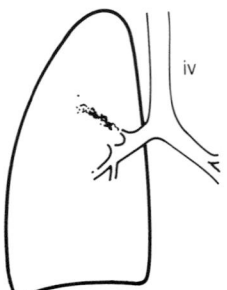

Structure of
bronchus

Cylindrical
bronchiectasis in
area of old collapse

Wedge shadow with
fibrosis and
bronchiectasis
following contracture
of segmental lesion

Linear scar of fibrosis
following segmental
lesion

Figure 57.6: The complications and sequelae of primary pulmonary tuberculous lesions. (Reproduced with permission from Miller F.J.W. *Tuberculosis in Children*. Edinburgh: Churchill Livingstone. © 1982.)

become fibrotic and may subsequently become calcified but tubercle bacilli may persist within these dormant lesions for years or decades. Bacilli may also persist outside lesions as in situ nucleic acid amplification techniques have revealed the presence of DNA specific for the *M. tuberculosis* complex in various cells in normal lung tissue derived post-mortem from persons in areas with a high incidence of tuberculosis. The nature and form of these 'persisters' have generated much speculation. Some researchers postulate that they are truly dormant and that their reactivation involves a 'wake-up gene' producing a resuscitation-promoting cytokine/factor (*Rpf*), while others suggest that they replicate, albeit slowly, but are destroyed by immune mechanisms at roughly the same rate.

Primary infection is often self-limiting and resolves in a large majority of cases but in a minority of cases it manifests as clinical disease in a number of ways[2] (Figure 57.6) and local or systemic spread may occur. The primary foci at the periphery of the lung may rupture into the pleural cavity, causing a self-limiting pleural effusion or a much more serious empyema. Diseased mediastinal lymph nodes may rupture into the pericardial cavity, causing tuberculous pericarditis, or into a bronchus, causing a spreading endobronchial infection and broncho-pneumonia. Enlarged mediastinal lymph nodes may press on the major bronchi, causing partial or total obstruction and pulmonary collapse (Figure 57.7). The primary lesion may progress to tuberculous pneumonia with tissue destruction, especially when immunity is compromised. Alternatively, the primary lesion may gradually enlarge to form a circular 'coin lesion' which may progress to a characteristic post-primary lesion or may heal with calcification. Concentric rings of calcifi-

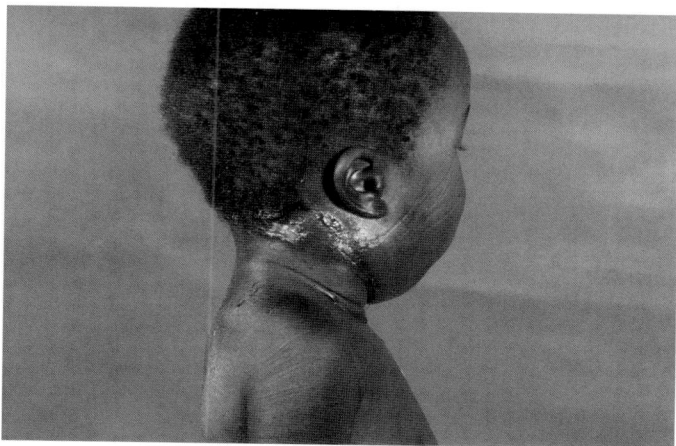

Figure 57.8: Caseating cervical lymph nodes in child with tuberculosis.

cation, resulting from alternating periods of progression and healing, may be seen. Primary lesions in the tonsils may spread to cervical nodes (Figure 57.8), from which local and systemic spread may occur.

Haematogenous dissemination following infection leads to serious, often fatal, non-pulmonary disease, principally involving the central nervous system, bones and kidneys. Observations in the pre-chemotherapy era, notably by Wallgren,[3] revealed a sequence of events, or 'timetable', of primary tuberculosis, as shown in Table 57.2. This is only a rough guide and many individual variations occur. Young children are very prone to overt disease following infection but those between the age of 5 years and the onset of puberty appear to be relatively protected—the 'safe school age'.

Within 3–8 weeks of initial infection conversion to dermal reactivity to tuberculin occurs. Since the description of the tuberculin skin test by the Austrian physician Clemens von Pirquet in the early 1900s, there has been considerable speculation as to the nature and significance of the positive tuberculin test, particularly its relevance to protective immunity. It now appears that the dermal induration seen in a positive tuberculin reaction is due to tissue oedema resulting from a number of immune processes, some associated with protection and some not. Thus a positive test is an indicator of recent or past infection by a tubercle bacillus or BCG vaccination but not of the immune status of the infected person.

Post-primary tuberculosis differs from primary disease in several important features. It may develop directly from a primary lesion—*progressive primary tuberculosis*—but more often there is a latent phase of several years or even decades before the disease becomes apparent. As mentioned above, post-primary tuberculosis may be the result of endogenous reactivation of latent foci of infection or to exogenous reinfection. In the case of the lung, post-primary lesions often develop, for poorly understood reasons, in the upper regions of the lung. The characteristic feature of post-primary pulmonary tuberculosis is gross tissue necrosis which is attributable to cytokines,

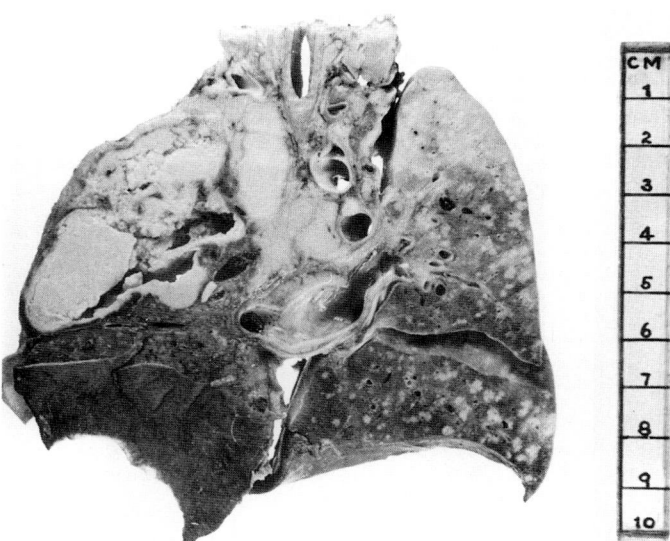

Figure 57.7: Progressive primary tuberculosis. Postmortem specimen of the lungs of a 6-month-old child showing extensive caseous necrosis, enlarged hilar lymph nodes and numerous tuberculous lesions throughout the lung fields.

Table 57.2 The 'timetable' of primary tuberculosis*

Stage	Duration	Features
1	3–8 weeks	The primary complex develops. Conversion to tuberculin positivity occurs.
2	About 3 months	Life threatening forms of disease due to haematogenous dissemination occur, i.e. tuberculous meningitis and miliary tuberculosis.
3	3–4 months	Tuberculous pleurisy may be the result of either haematogenous spread or direct spread from an enlarging primary focus.
4	Up to 3 years	This stage lasts until the primary complex resolves. More slowly developing extrapulmonary lesions, particularly in the bones and joints, may appear.
5	Up to 12 years	Genitourinary tuberculosis may occur as a late manifestation of primary tuberculosis.

*adapted from Wallgren and Ustvedt.[3,49]

thought to be secreted by Th2 helper T cells, which render infected tissue very susceptible to killing' by tumour necrosis factor.[4] As a result, large lesions containing abundant caseous necrotic tissue develop and, as they radiologically resemble tumours, they are termed tuberculomas. The centre of the tuberculoma is anoxic and acidic and is a hostile environment to tubercle bacilli, so that relatively few viable bacilli are present. The caseous material is softened and eventually liquefied by proteases secreted by activated macrophages. The enlarging tuberculoma may eventually erode into a bronchus so that the softened or liquefied caseous material is discharged into the bronchial tree and a cavity—a characteristic feature of post-primary pulmonary tuberculosis—is formed. The environment of the cavity is quite different from that of the closed tuberculoma. Air enriched with carbon dioxide enters the cavity, providing oxygen

for the bacilli and neutralizing the acidity. The tubercle bacilli are then able to replicate freely and huge numbers line the cavity wall. These bacilli gain access to the bronchi and are expectorated in the sputum, the patient becomes infectious and is said to have open tuberculosis.

Bacilli escaping from the cavities also infect other parts of the same, and often the other, lung via the bronchial tree. A typical radiological appearance of post-primary pulmonary tuberculosis is of one or more apical cavities and numerous smaller lesions in the other lung fields (Figure 57.9). Bacilli in the sputum may also lodge in the larynx, causing tuberculous laryngitis, or may be swallowed and cause indurating ulcers in the intestinal tract and, rarely, anal fistulae. In contrast to primary tuberculosis, the post-primary lesions are usually so walled off by fibrosis that lymphatic and haematogenous dissemination of disease is unusual. Both cavity

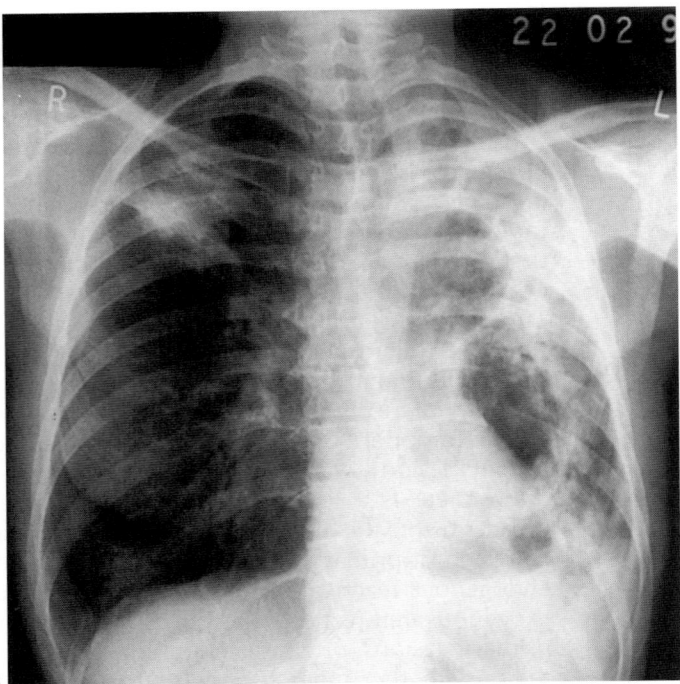
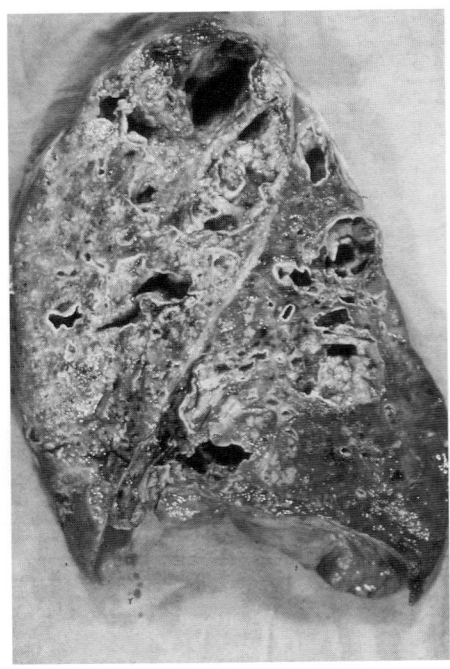

Figure 57.9: (**A**) Extensive pulmonary tuberculosis with cavitation. (**B**) Post-mortem lung showing several cavities and extensive lung involvement due to tuberculosis.

formation and the localization of disease are due to immune processes and, as described below, are compromised in immunosuppressed patients.

Pathology of tuberculosis

A wide spectrum of pathological manifestations is seen in tuberculosis.[5,6] The initial host response to infection with *M. tuberculosis* consists of an acute inflammatory reaction with an influx of polymorphonuclear neutrophil leucocytes. This acute inflammatory response is unable to limit the infectious process and is followed by a progressive infiltration with macrophages. The macrophages have a pale eosinophilic cytoplasm, nuclei become elongated and vesicular, and as these cells resemble epithelial cells they are called epithelioid cells. Some macrophages fuse to form larger 'Langhans giant cells'. A zone of lymphocytes surrounds this mass of cells and fibroblasts grows

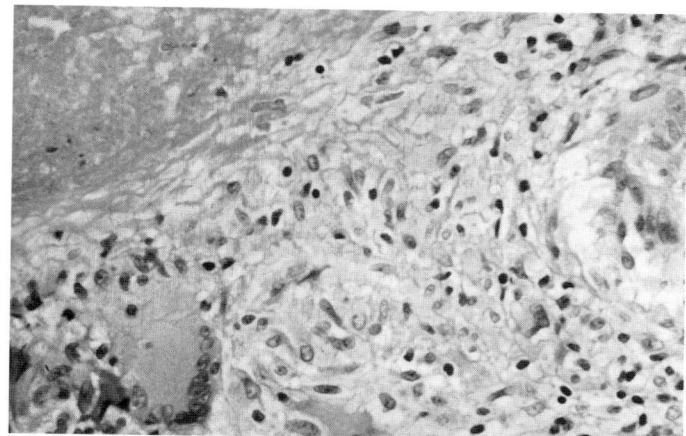

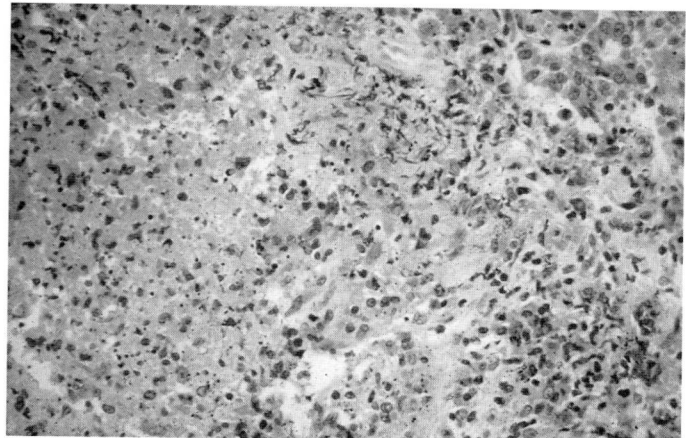

Figure 57.10: (**A**) Classical caseating granuloma due to *M. tuberculosis*. Note the central area of caseous necrosis surrounded by a rim of epithelioid cells, Langhans giant cells and lymphocytic infiltrate. (**B**) Lung histopathology illustrating an 'anergic response' to infection with *M. tuberculosis* in a lung of a patient with AIDS. There is widespread granular necrosis and a non-reactive 'anergic' cellular response with a few lymphocytes and epithelioid cells and no Langhans giant cells.

alongside. Within 2 weeks a firm, coagulative necrosis begins in the centre. Histologically the necrosis is structureless and eosinophilic. In the older literature this type of appearance was called a '*productive*' or '*proliferative*' reaction because it is dominated by cells rather than fluid. The characteristic pathological feature of tuberculosis is the epithelioid cell caseous granuloma (Figure 57.10A) often called a 'tubercle' because it can resembles a potato tuber when visible to the naked eye. While this is characteristic of tuberculosis, it may also occur in deep-seated fungal infections (e.g. *Histoplasma capsulatum*) and thus a specific diagnosis based on the determination of the aetiological agent is important. The tuberculous process may involve serous cavities, usually the pleural cavities but sometimes the pericardial cavity. Such involvement appears to be primarily due to a hypersensitivity reaction to antigens of the tubercle bacillus and is characterized by an outpouring of an inflammatory, fibrin-rich exudate which is infiltrated with lymphocytes and polymorphonuclear leucocytes. Epithelioid and Langhans giant cells are scanty. In the older literature this was termed the '*exudative*' reaction.

The tuberculous lesion may cease to progress with time, being restricted by the immune response, and may heal by fibrosis and eventually calcify. Alternately, it may soften and enlarge with individual necrotic foci tending to coalesce, resulting in large areas of necrotic debris. The surrounding granulomatous reaction and associated scarring assist in localization of the infection. On the basis of these tissue reactions, three principal pathological forms of pulmonary tuberculosis can be identified:

1. *Acute caseous tuberculosis.* This produces confluent caseation of much of the lung lobe (caseous bronchopneumonia). Large amounts of caseous debris in large bronchi occur.
2. *Chronic tuberculosis.* Caseous destruction occurs side by side with some healing by fibrosis. Depending on the ratio of caseous necrosis and fibrosis, radiological lesions are termed caseous, fibro-caseous and fibrotic. Bronchiectasis is a frequent complication of this type of tuberculosis.
3. *Non-reactive or anergic tuberculosis.* Extensive foci of necrosis teeming with mycobacteria occur without any significant cellular reaction around them being seen (Figure 57.10B). This type of pathology is seen in the elderly and in persons with malnutrition, malignancies and immunosuppression. The spectrum of pathological changes seen in persons infected with HIV is described below.

Expression of clinical disease

The variety of clinical presentation of pulmonary tuberculosis seen in clinical practice appears to be associated with a complex series of interactions between mycobacteria, immunocompetent cells and their secreted cytokines. Mild disease is associated with preserved cellular immune responses whereas advanced disease is accompanied by impaired cell-mediated immune responses and augmented humoral responses. The pathogenesis of tuberculosis should be viewed as an interplay between the macrophage-activating cellular Th1 type immune response and the mechanisms that lead to tissue damage. Despite an enormous literature on the subject, neither the various immune processes seen in tuberculosis nor the relationship between them is fully understood.

Host immune responses to *M. tuberculosis*

An enormous literature exists on the immunology of tuberculosis[7] but despite that the exact mechanism of protective immunity to tuberculosis remains unknown. The immunological response to initial infection with *M. tuberculosis* may restrict its replication and spread in the majority of people who are infected with it. If these mycobacteria continue to replicate, local dissemination via lymphatics and systemic spread throughout the body may occur via the bloodstream, creating new foci of infection. Many factors including host genetics, microbial virulence and disturbances in host immunity (Table 57.3)

Table 57.3 Factors affecting susceptibility to tuberculosis*

Age	Extremes of age: below the age of 5 years and old age
Geographical origin	Asians, Africans, North American Indians
Immune suppression	HIV infection Protein-calorie malnutrition Steroid therapy Cytotoxic drugs Congenital immunodeficiencies Vitamin D deficiency
Medical conditions	Liver failure Cancer Diabetes mellitus Smoking-related lung damage Industrial dust disease of the lungs, e.g. silicosis, asbestosis Renal failure Measles Schistosomiasis Gastrectomy
Genetic factors	HLA-DR allele, NRAMP gene, vitamin D receptors
Stress	Excess corticosteroid production
Environmental factors	Exposure to populations of environmental mycobacteria
Mycobacterial factors	Strain variation in virulence

*adapted from Zumla A, Mwaba P, Rook G, Lucas S. Tuberculosis. In James DG, Zumla A, eds. The Granulomatous disorders, Cambridge: Cambridge University Press. 1999: 132–160, with modifications.

determine whether infection by *M. tuberculosis* is contained or progresses to overt disease. There is a constant battle between the mycobacterium and the host; the outcome is dependent on many factors and the pathogen has developed mechanisms for evading the host immune responses. The reasons why the immune system in most people is capable of preventing active disease but is not capable of clearing the infection are not fully understood. Many basic questions remain unanswered regarding the host–organism interactions:

1. What are the mechanisms of protective immunity to *M. tuberculosis*?
2. Why do only a fraction of people who are infected go on to develop clinical disease?
3. In those who develop disease, why does tuberculosis present as a spectrum of clinical manifestations?
4. Why can mycobacteria survive for such long periods of time?
5. Why do some patients with apparently normal immune systems go on to develop disease?

Both non-specific and specific effector mechanisms appear to play a role in protective immunity to tuberculosis.

Non-specific immune effector mechanisms

When *M. tuberculosis* bacilli are inhaled they pass through the upper and lower respiratory tract and reach the alveoli, where initial infection occurs. The mycobacteria are phagocytosed by alveolar macrophages, phagocytosis being facilitated by surfactant apoprotein A. This initial interaction can result in destruction of the organism or persistence and replication of the organism within the macrophage.

Protective T cell-mediated immunity

It is now recognized that killing of mycobacteria in humans is a manifestation of acquired resistance. Much immunological research has focused on the role of T lymphocytes. Two observations have suggested that CD4+ lymphocytes may play a central role in immunity to tuberculosis. First, T cell responsiveness correlates inversely with disease progression in terms of low blastogenic responses to mycobacterial antigens in vitro, and reduced/absent skin tuberculin hypersensitivity is seen in patients with advanced or uncontrolled disease. Secondly, persons infected with the human immunodeficiency virus (HIV) are extremely susceptible to tuberculosis. Among this population tuberculosis may occur even before severe depletion of CD4+ lymphocytes occurs, suggesting that slight reductions in CD4+ lymphocytes may predispose to developing disease. How CD4+ lymphocytes control disease activity is the subject of intense research activity. In mouse models of tuberculosis, immunity to the disease appears to correlate with a Th1 type response. Indeed, if mice are pre-immunized so that they have a mixed response that is mostly Th1, but includes a minor Th2 component, they are more susceptible to the disease than are non-immunized controls. Thus a Th2 response may actually be harmful. In vivo, Th1 or Th2 cells appear to act in concert with CD8+ cells as well as with numerous other cell types including macrophages, B cells and some stromal cells. Collectively, these cellular interactions give rise to two patterns of cytokine release often known as Type 1 (dominated by the interleukins IL-2, IL-12 and interferon γ—IFNγ) and Type 2 (dominated by IL-4, 5, 6, 10 and 13). The term 'Type 1' is used in preference to Th1 when it is intended to refer to the overall pattern of cytokine release by all cell types in the infected site, rather than merely that produced by the CD4+ helper T cells.

Immunity does not entirely depend only on CD4+ Th1 cells. Mice with defective β_2-microglobulin genes, and thereby rendered unable to express normal quantities of Class I MHC products, are very susceptible to tuberculosis. This may imply a role for CD8+ cytotoxic T cells because such cytotoxicity could release organisms from macrophages that were failing to kill them and enable their up-take by fresh activated cells. There is also a large proportion of human peripheral blood γ/δ T cells that proliferate in response to mycobacterial infection but their protective function, if any, is not yet known.

Antibody responses

Antibody responses to *M. tuberculosis* antigens occur but the role of these in protective immunity is unclear at present. Despite numerous attempts, no clinically useful serodiagnostic tests for tuberculosis have been developed.

Role of macrophages

Although it is likely that most mycobacteria are ultimately killed by cytokine-activated macrophages, the final effector pathway is not known. In the mouse IFNγ activates macrophages so that they express enhanced capacity for production of oxygen reduction products such as super-oxide anion and hydrogen peroxide, and also increased expression of the inducible form of nitric oxide synthase (iNOS; also known as Type II NOS). The trigger that then causes nitric oxide (NO) production may be tumour necrosis factor α (TNFα). It has been suggested that high-output NO production is a property of alveolar macrophages from patients with tuberculosis.

The NO released may have some intrinsic anti-mycobacterial activity but the final effector molecules may be peroxynitrites produced by the interaction of NO and oxygen reduction products.

Recently an entirely different type of antimycobacterial mechanism has been suggested. Certain signals that induce apoptosis of infected macrophages can lead to death of some of the contained mycobacteria.

Mycobacterial factors

Mycobacteria have evolved various strategies for avoiding killing by phagocytes (Figure 57.11).[4] They inhibit acidification of the phagosome, modify intracellular trafficking of vesicles, and cause lipoarabinomannan (LAM) to insert into the glycosylphosphatidylinositol (GPI)-rich domains in the cell membrane. LAM is itself a GPI of unusual glycan structure, with the ability to modify numerous macrophage functions including the ability to respond to IFNγ and to present antigen. The last point may explain the apparent inability of macrophages containing mycobacteria to present antigen to CD4+ T cells.

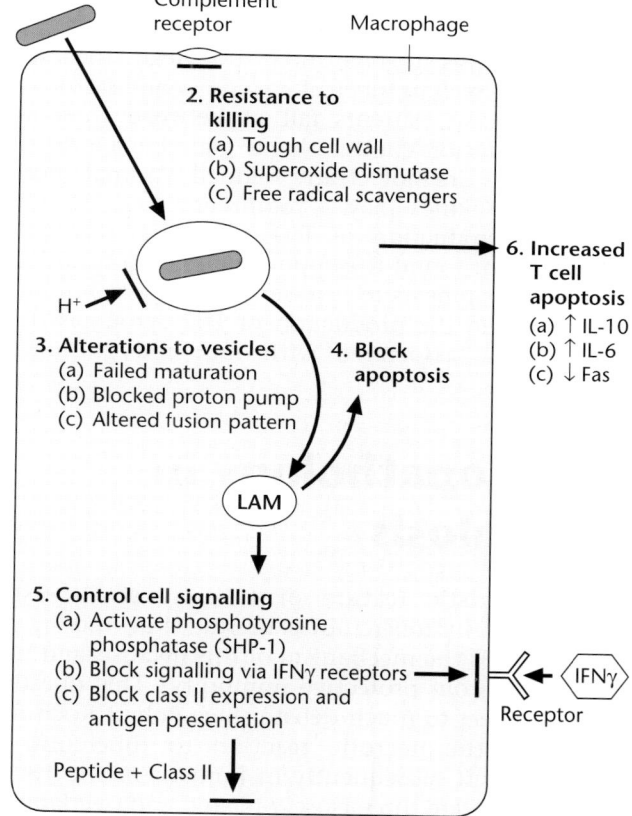

Figure 57.11: Mechanisms of survival of *Mycobacterium tuberculosis* in macrophages. *M. tuberculosis* avoids the killing mechanisms in macrophages and blocks apoptosis of macrophages, presumably because apoptosis also can lead to death of the contained bacteria. *Bad* is a pro-apoptotic protein, inactivated when phosphorylated. LAM has multiple roles, including activation of SHP-1, a phosphotyrosine phosphatase intimately involved in cell signalling pathways. Down-regulation of *Fas*, together with increased expression of Fas ligand may lead the macrophage to signal apoptosis to Fas-positive T cells. Short thick lines indicate blocked pathways. IFN, interferon; IL, interleukin; LAM, liporabinomannan; TGF, transforming growth factor; TNFr2, tumor necrosis factor receptor-2.

Granulomas and cytokine patterns in tuberculosis

Granuloma formation is an important event in the immune response against *M. tuberculosis*. While the granuloma is formed primarily to restrict the spread the infection, the physiological process of granuloma formation can also contribute to destruction of surrounding normal tissues. Granulomas are dynamic structures characterized by the accumulation of activated macrophages and an infiltration of T lymphocytes. Both the extent of granuloma formation and the morphological features are subject to considerable variation from person to person. In tuberculosis, a wide spectrum of granulomatous reactions are seen. At one end of this spectrum, persons with compromised immune responses show poor granuloma formation and extensive areas of tissue necrosis containing large numbers of mycobacteria. At the other end of the spectrum, some immunocompetent patients show indolent non-caseating granulomas containing few organisms. This is typically seen in chronic skin tuberculosis (lupus vulgaris) and histologically the lesions resemble those seen in tuberculoid leprosy and sarcoidosis. Most tuberculosis patients fall in between these two extremes. The factors contributing to granuloma formation in tuberculosis are not clearly defined. Animal models show that cytokines play a prominent role. In tuberculosis, the production of Th1 cytokines (IL-2, IFNγ, TNFβ) has been found to support granuloma formation, and TNFα also appears to be essential, whereas immunosuppression and the production of Th2 cytokines (IL-4, IL-5, IL-10) is associated with impaired granuloma formation.

Immunopathology in tuberculosis

The characteristic feature of tuberculosis is tissue necrosis, both in tuberculin skin test sites and in the lesions. What is the mechanism of this necrosis and how does it differ from protective immunity? This question has been subject to much debate since Robert Koch first documented the necrotic reaction to tuberculin in guinea-pigs, and subsequently in humans in the 1890s. Currently there are three closely related and overlapping hypotheses as to the nature of the immunopathology (Koch phenomenon). Some authors suggest that there is a lack of balance between the cytokines involved in the immune process. Thus too much TNFα could account for symptoms of tuberculosis, such as fever, weight loss and tissue damage. Evidence that these symptoms may indeed depend on TNFα in human tuberculosis has come from the experimental use of thalidomide, which decreases the half-life of the mRNA for this cytokine. Patients treated with thalidomide show rapid symptomatic relief and weight gain. We are therefore faced with a paradox: TNFα is essential for immunity, but may also be responsible for pathology.

The second hypothesis also holds that TNFα is a mediator of the tissue damage, not because there is too much of it but because it is being released into sites that contain a mixture of Th1 and Th2 cytokines. Although immunity to tuberculosis requires a Type 1 response, there is clear evidence in tuberculous mice that Type 2 cytokines are also expressed. The same is true in humans, although this is less striking. While the Th1 component remains dominant the data indicate the presence of an inappropriate Th2 component in disease. Even a small Th2 component leads to greatly enhanced susceptibility to tuberculosis and to TNFα toxicity in mice.

The third hypothesis emphasizes the potential role of transforming growth factor β (TGFβ), which can cause tissue damage and fibrosis, and can also inactivate the antimycobacterial functions of macrophages. These three hypotheses are not mutually exclusive, and they are probably all important components of immunopathology.

Hormonal factors in tuberculosis

There has been speculation about the possibility of changes in the function of the adrenal glands or of the hypothalamo-pituitary–adrenal axis in tuberculosis, but the data are conflicting. Recent studies show a striking shift in the balance of metabolites of cortisol to metabolites of cortisone, with an abnormal proportion of the daily output of glucocorticoid being excreted in the urine as derivatives of cortisol. There may be inappropriate recruitment of circulating cortisone to provide cortisol in the infected tissues and this may contribute to deactivation of macrophages, and to the induction of the small but important Th2 component.

Before the age of 5 years, children are susceptible to tuberculosis but they tend to develop consolidation and pneumonia, without cavitation or caseous necrosis. Between the ages of 5 and 10 (i.e. during adrenarche) children appear to be resistant to the disease in spite of an increasing incidence of tuberculin test positivity indicative of continuing exposure to infection in this age group. This interval between the ages of 5 and 10 was known as the 'safe school age' in nineteenth-century Europe, and the phenomenon is re-emerging in high-incidence areas such as Cape Town, South Africa. Finally, susceptibility returns at puberty, but the type of disease now resembles that seen in adults, with typical cavitation and necrosis. Clearly these changes suggest an underlying endocrinological cause. A reasonable hypothesis, for which there is supportive animal data, is that the three periods correspond to age-related changes in the ratio of cortisol to the antiglucocorticoid hormone, dehydroepiandrosterone (DHEA).

Epidemiology of tuberculosis

As discussed above, not all those infected by the tubercle bacillus develop overt tuberculosis, and the interval between infection and disease may be years or decades. On the basis of skin-testing surveys, the WHO has estimated that in the year 2000 one-third of the world's human population, around 2000 million people, were infected by tubercle bacilli.[8] Almost 1% of the world's population is newly infected each year. The percentage of the population infected varies from region to region: in Europe, around 11% are infected, mostly elderly persons, while in tropical countries over half may be infected, with a much higher proportion of younger people being infected.

Infection is spread predominantly by those with 'open', cavitating, post-primary pulmonary tuberculosis. Thus those positive on microscopy are much more likely to be infectious than those who are negative. Children are rarely infectious, though exceptions occur. The number of persons infected by a source case is termed the *contagion parameter*. On average, an untreated source case infects between 10 and 15 people every year but the actual number varies greatly and is affected by many factors including crowding and ventilation.

In the year 2000, around 8 million new cases of tuberculosis arose from the infected pool, 95% of them in the developing nations. Around 1.5 million cases occurred in sub-Saharan Africa, nearly 3 million in South-East Asia and over a quarter of a million in Eastern Europe. Figure 57.12(A) illustrates the estimated rates of tuberculosis incidence by continent and Figure 57.12(B) shows the HIV-positive rates in patients with tuberculosis. Owing to the chronic nature of the disease and the limited resources for effective diagnosis and treatment in many countries, there are at any given time around 20 million people with active tuberculosis. Around half of these have infectious forms of the disease and infect some 100 million people annually. Between 2 and 3 million people, principally young adults, die of tuberculosis each year, with 98% of deaths occurring in the developing nations.

Molecular epidemiology of tuberculosis

Until about a decade ago, the only markers available to study the epidemiology of tuberculosis were drug susceptibility profiles and phage types. In recent years, a large number of DNA fingerprinting methods have become available to type mycobacterial isolates.[9,10] DNA fingerprinting is performed most commonly by using restriction fragment length polymorphism (RFLP) analysis. RFLP analysis is based on the fact that there are repetitive insertion elements throughout the genome of *M. tuberculosis*. IS*6110* is the most commonly used insertion sequence that is specific for *M. tuberculosis* and is usually found in 5–25 copies throughout the chromosome. IS*6110* belongs to the IS3 family of insertion sequences and is present in almost all strains of the *M. tuberculosis* complex. Up to 25 copies of IS*6110* can be found in one strain. The mycobacterial DNA is extracted and then cleaved with restriction endonucleases, and subsequent electrophoresis and probing/hybridization with IS*6110* fragment result in a series of bands of various lengths. The variability in band number and position distinguishes between different strains. IS*6110* typing is based on the assumption that the distribution pattern of IS*6110* in related clinical isolates is identical or similar, whereas the distribution pattern in unrelated species is varied. Other potentially useful insertion sequences that have been found in *Mycobacterium tuberculosis* include IS*1081*, IS*1547* and the IS-like element.

This technique has been used to study what is now termed the molecular epidemiology of tuberculosis. There have been several applications of this method: (a) to identify cases of transmission which are part of a cluster during an outbreak of tuberculosis within a community; (b) to understand the dynamics of specific outbreaks of tuberculosis; (c) to determine whether new cases of tuberculosis are due to reactivation or reinfection; (d) to study the characteristics of MDRTB outbreaks by using RFLP and resistance screening in combination; (e) to detect multiple infections. IS*6110* RFLP is recognized as the standard typing method for *M. tuberculosis*. The technical process is, however, laborious and requires large quantities of high-quality genomic DNA. An alternative method is to detect strain-to-strain variations in the structure of short sequences of DNA found in the region of the insertion sequences. This technique, spacer oligonucleotide typing (spoligotyping), is PCR based and is therefore rapid and easier to perform. Spoligotyping can be performed on non-viable organisms or directly on clinical samples.

Impact of the HIV/AIDS epidemic

In recent years, the epidemiological trends of tuberculosis have been adversely affected by the HIV/AIDS pandemic, as infection by HIV is now the most important predisposing factor for the development of active tuberculosis.[6,11] While, as described above, a non-immunocompromised person who has overcome the primary infection has about a 5% chance of developing post-primary tuberculosis later in life, the chance rises to 50% in an HIV-positive person. The annual risk of a person co-infected with the tubercle bacillus and HIV developing tuberculosis is around 8%— over 20 times higher than in an HIV-negative person. The chance of an HIV-positive person developing tuberculosis following either primary infection or reinfection is very

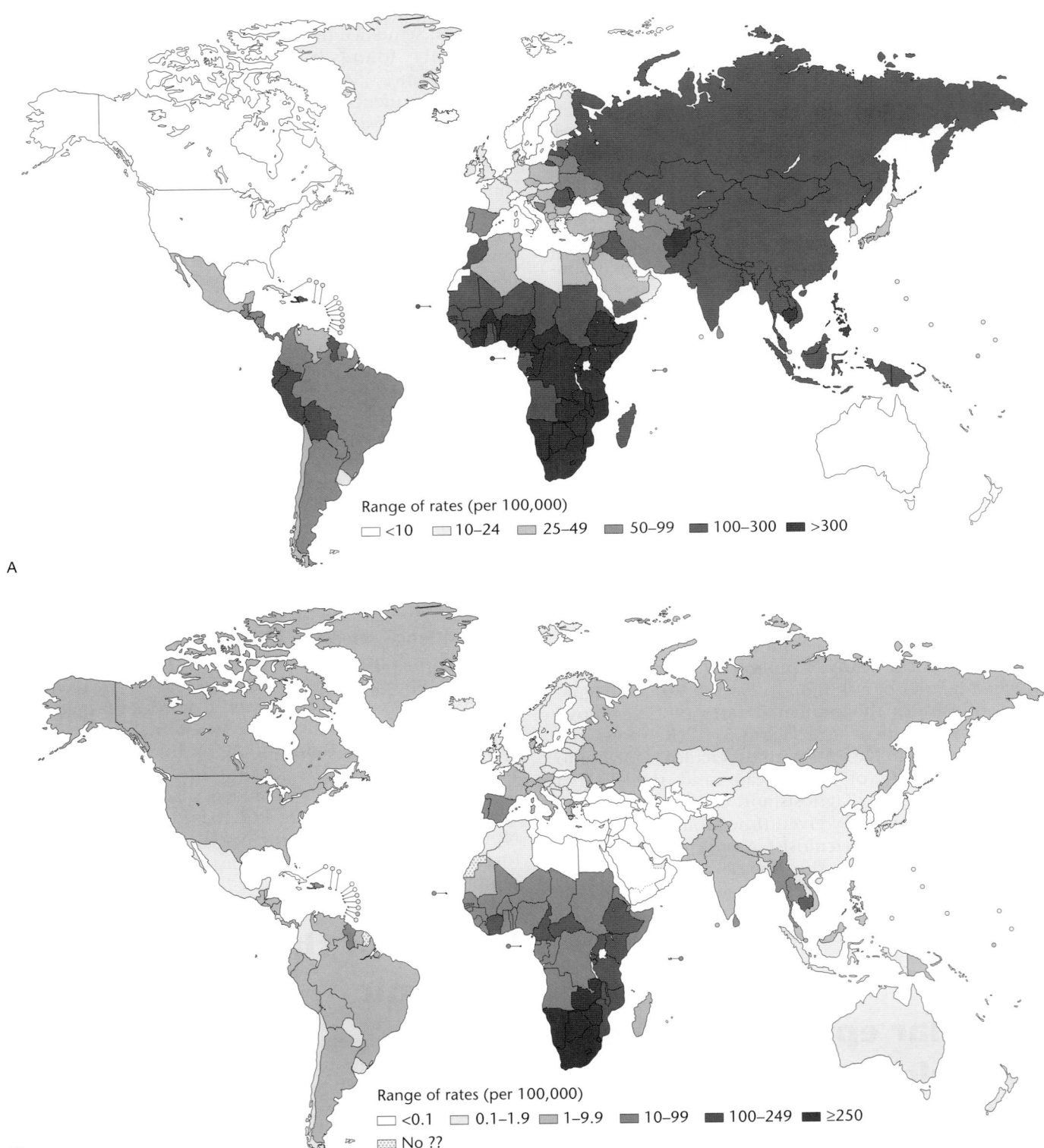

Figure 57.12: (**A**) Estimated TB incidence rates, 1999 (all forms). (**B**) Incidence rate of HIV-positive cases, 1999. (From WHO Global TB Report, © 2001.)

high, especially in those with AIDS. In addition, the progression from infection to overt disease is very rapid, the time-scale being 'telescoped' from several years to a few months. These factors have led to a number of explosive mini-epidemics of tuberculosis in centres caring for AIDS patients.

In the year 2000 there were an estimated 35 million HIV-positive persons worldwide. As one-third of these were co-infected with tubercle bacilli and therefore had an 8% chance of developing overt tuberculosis annually, an additional million cases of this disease would have occurred in that year as a result of HIV infection. Tuberculosis is a common cause of death in those with AIDS and accounted for 30% of the estimated 3 million AIDS-related deaths in 2000. At present, the greatest impact of HIV-related tuberculosis is felt in sub-Saharan Africa, where 70% of the world's cases occur and where the disease is having a devastating effect on health services and on societal structure in this region. In Zambia, for example, one in four pregnant women is infected with HIV and tuberculosis is now among the top non-obstetric causes of maternal death in that country.[12] Two-thirds of Zambian children and adults with tuberculosis are co-infected with HIV.[13,14] Tragically, HIV infection is spreading rapidly in the Indian subcontinent and in South-East Asia where, owing to the huge population, most of the world's cases of tuberculosis occur. Thus, unless the spread of HIV is checked by public health measures or by the advent of effective vaccination or therapeutic strategies, the problems currently facing Africa, Asia, Eastern Europe and South America will be experienced on a much greater scale in those regions.

Impact of drug and multi-drug resistance

Effective control of tuberculosis is threatened by the emergence of strains of *M. tuberculosis* resistant to one or more of the standard antituberculosis agents[15] (Table 57.4). Such resistance occurs by bacterial mutation in patients treated with inadequate or inappropriate drug regimens or poorly formulated combination drugs and in those whose therapy is suboptimal. Such resistance is termed secondary or acquired resistance whereas a person who is infected by a strain already resistant is said to have initial or primary resistance.

The contributing factors to acquired resistance include:

- Poor compliance in taking therapy.
- Irregular supplies of drugs.
- Addition of single drugs to failing regimens in the absence of bacteriological control.
- Unacceptably high cost to the patient in respect to the drugs and thus intermittent medication.
- Travel to the clinic and time off work leading to irregular intake.
- Use of time-expired, or impure or mishandled drugs.
- Use of poorly formulated combination preparations.
- Prescription of inappropriate drug regimens.
- Unregulated over-the-counter sale of drugs, including cough mixtures containing isoniazid.

It should be noted that even combination preparations of antituberculosis drugs, which ensure that the patients

Table 57.4 Prevalence of combined primary and acquired drug resistance, as percentage of tested isolates, by country or region, 1996–1999.*

Country or region	Any form of resistance	Poly-resistance (2 or more drugs)	Multidrug resistance
Uruguay	4.6	0.4	0.2
Venezuela	4.7	1.9	0.4
Malaysia	5.1	0.6	0.1
Nepal	6.4	1.4	1.4
Botswana	7.7	2.5	2.0
Cuba	8.3	1.5	0.9
South Africa	10.2	3.5	2.5
Central African Republic	10.5	3.8	1.1
Guinea	15.9	6.0	1.5
Peru	18.4	7.1	4.3
Mexico	20.6	9.1	7.3
Uganda	22.1	8.1	0.8
Mozambique	23.1	10.0	3.5
India (Tamil Nadu State)	24.1	13.4	7.1
Sierra Leone	27.7	8.7	2.6
Estonia	40.8	26.8	15.1

*Data from WHO/IUATLD 2000.[19]

receive all drugs in the preparation, can lead to drug or multi-drug resistance if taken irregularly.[16] In addition, it is important to obtain combination preparations from WHO-approved manufacturers as poorly formulated preparations can reduce the bioavailability of the component drugs.[17]

By definition, strains resistant to rifampicin and isoniazid, irrespective of other resistances, are termed multi-drug resistant (MDR).[18] Patients with MDRTB do not respond to standard short-course therapeutic regimens and must be treated with more costly, less effective and more toxic drugs for extended periods. Under ideal conditions, a high proportion of patients with MDRTB are curable but the cost of managing such a case is 100 times that of a case of drug-susceptible disease. As a consequence, cases largely go untreated in the developing nations and pass the infection on to others.

The World Health Organization and the International Union Against Tuberculosis and Lung Disease have undertaken surveys of the prevalence of drug resistance in the world.[19] These surveys showed that acquired resistance is commoner than primary resistance and that the relative prevalence of both varies enormously from region to region. Examples are given in Table 57.4. A number of 'hot-spots' of very high prevalence of drug resistance have been found,[20] notably prisons within countries of the former Soviet Union.[21]

Factors affecting dynamics of tuberculosis in populations

An epidemic wave of tuberculosis in England began in the sixteenth century and reached its peak around 1780, at the time of the Industrial Revolution. Similar peaks were seen in Western Europe in the early 1800s and in Eastern Europe around 80 years later. This wave pattern has led some workers to propose that the disease rapidly rises to epidemic proportions in genetically susceptible populations and declines as a more resistant population develops by natural selection. In fact, there is very little hard evidence for such a selection. Although a number of genetic factors affecting resistance to tuberculosis have been described, such factors appear much less important than environmental ones in determining the prevalence of the disease in a community.[22] The decline in the incidence of tuberculosis in the industrially developed nations may as likely have been due to socio-economic factors as to evolutionary selection. In this context, however, the inverse relationship between the incidence of tuberculosis and the improvement of social conditions is by no means straightforward. Thus some workers hold that the decline in the incidence of tuberculosis is a natural and predictable consequence of better nutrition and living and working conditions but others argue that the decline is the cumulative result of many specific public health measures introduced only after intense political lobbying. The distinction is a crucial one as proponents of the first view claim that tuberculosis will decline as socio-economic conditions increase worldwide while those holding the second view stress the need for specific tuberculosis control measures and health advocacy.

Risk factors for tuberculosis

The principal factors predisposing to tuberculosis are listed in Table 57.3. In recent years, HIV infection has, as described above, emerged as the most important and widespread risk factor for the development of active tuberculosis. Other infections such as measles and whooping cough and chronic malaria and causes of lung damage, particularly smoking and exposure to silicon and other industrial dusts, are also risk factors. Other predisposing conditions are those that compromise immune responsiveness and include malnutrition, alcoholism and other substance abuse, diabetes, renal failure (particularly if haemodialysis is required), treatment with immunosuppressive drugs and steroids (see below), liver failure and cancers, especially haematological malignancies. Transmission of infection is facilitated by overcrowding, poor ventilation and low levels of ultra-violet light—conditions frequently linked to poverty.

Tuberculin reactivity
Tuberculin reactivity is a risk factor for the development of tuberculosis as it is usually indicative of past infection by the tubercle bacillus, but the relation between such reactivity and risk of disease is not straightforward. In general, small reactions imply no increased risk, or even a degree of protection, and large reactions imply increased risk, but considerable regional variations in the risk in relation to reaction size occur.[23]

Immunosuppressive drugs and steroids
Patients receiving post-transplant or other immuno-suppressive therapy are prone to develop tuberculosis which is often insidious in onset, and miliary or cryptic disseminated forms of the disease are common. Prophylaxis against tuberculosis should be considered, particularly for tuberculin negative patients who receive an organ from a tuberculin positive donor.[24] Disease due to environmental mycobacteria is also common in these patients and poses diagnostic difficulties.[25] There is a widespread belief that treatment with steroids predisposes to tuberculosis although the evidence for this is weak. Nevertheless, the American Thoracic Society recommends that those on long-term corticosteroid therapy and with healed pulmonary tuberculous lesions should receive isoniazid chemoprophylaxis for 1 year.[26] Others advocate prophylaxis for patients on long-term steroid therapy with one or more of the following: a history of inadequately treated tuberculosis, an abnormal chest radiograph, a tuberculin reaction of 10 mm or more in diameter and recent exposure to a tuberculosis patient.[25]

Age and sex

As outlined above, children up to the age of 3 years are highly susceptible to tuberculosis, especially miliary tuberculosis and tuberculous meningitis, but those aged 3–15 appear relatively resistant. In developing countries the vast majority of cases occur between the ages of 15 and 59 years. Surveys in several countries show that more males than females are diagnosed with tuberculosis but it is not clear whether this is affected by gender-related differences in access to health services. Studies on the effect of pregnancy on tuberculosis are confusing.[27] Some suggest a protective effect, some a worsening of the disease and others no effect. Yet others suggest protection during pregnancy but an exacerbation after delivery—a phenomenon observed in leprosy. This subject is in urgent need of investigation as tuberculosis is a major cause of death of pregnant women in sub-Saharan Africa, being responsible for more loss of life than obstetric complications.[12] The added impact of HIV infection on pregnancy-related mortality due to tuberculosis is also poorly understood.

Contact tracing and examination

Most tuberculosis is spread within households, although 'mini-epidemics' occur in schools, prisons, hospitals and other situations where people at risk are crowded together. Household contacts of smear-positive patients should be examined: screening of casual contacts only yields a further 1% of cases and is usually not justified. Although children with primary tuberculosis are rarely infectious, household screening will often reveal a sputum-positive source case. Procedures for contact tracing vary according to local facilities and the prevalence of tuberculosis in the community. Tuberculin testing is useful in young children and, where indicated, a chest radiograph should be obtained.

Diagnosis of tuberculosis

The success of tuberculosis control programmes depends critically on the quality of diagnostic services. Detailed accounts of the establishment and management of tuberculosis laboratories, the collection of specimens and subsequent laboratory procedures are available.[28,29]

Diagnosis in a community may either be active—involving a deliberate search for cases—or passive, relying on patients with symptoms presenting for treatment. The latter approach requires much less investment in time and personnel but its success depends on public education and the availability of user-friendly facilities.

Diagnosis of tuberculosis is based on a high index of clinical suspicion (described in relevant sections below)

Table 57.5 Clinical specimens which can be examined for *Mycobacterium tuberculosis*

	ZN stain	Culture	Histology	PCR
Fluids, pus, swabs, excreta				
1. Sputum (spot specimen or induced)	+	+	−	+
2. Laryngeal swab	+	+	−	+
3. Bronchoalveolar lavage specimen	+	+	+	+
4. Effusions (pleural, pericardial or ascites)	+	+	−	+
5. Gastric aspirate	+	+	−	+
6. Urine (early morning sample)	+	+	−	+
7. Cerebrospinal fluid	+	+	−	+
8. Pus (cold abscess or pus from sinuses)	+	+	−	+
9. Blood culture	+	+	−	+
10. Faeces	+	+	−	−
11. Fine needle aspirate (lymph node or bone)	+	+	−	+
Tissue samples				
1. Pleural biopsy	+	+	+	+
2. Lung biopsy	+	+	+	+
3. Lymph node biopsy	+	+	+	+
4. Liver biopsy	+	+	+	+
5. Bone marrow	+	+	+	+
6. Skin biopsy	+	+	+	+
7. Intestinal biopsy	+	+	+	+
8. Biopsy of brain lesion	+	+	+	+
9. Uterine cervix curetings	+	+	+	+
10. Autopsy tissue samples	+	+	+	+

and several clinical samples can be subject to laboratory investigations (Table 57.5). The following investigations help to confirm the diagnosis and monitor treatment:

1. *Bacteriology* (identification of *M. tuberculosis* by microscopy and through culture of the organism from various clinical samples such as sputum, pleural fluid, blood, caseous exudates, bone marrow, lymph node aspirate, cerebrospinal fluid—CSF).
2. *Imaging techniques* including radiology, ultrasound, computed axial tomography (CAT) scanning, magnetic resonance imaging (MRI) and radioisotope scans.
3. *Tissue biopsy* and processing the tissue for histopathology (granuloma formation and identification of acid-fast bacilli in specimen), bacteriology (culture), and for molecular identification of mycobacterial DNA.
4. *Molecular techniques* utilizing nucleic acid amplification systems such as polymerase chain reaction (PCR) or ligase chain reaction (LCR) have been applied to clinical specimens to identify mycobacterial DNA in biological samples.
5. *Haematology and biochemistry* (haematological investigations such as haemoglobin, erythrocyte sedimentation rate (ESR), C-reactive protein and liver function tests and urea and elctrolytes).
6. *Serology*.
7. *Tuberculin skin test*.

Obviously, in resource-poor settings, clinical acumen and simple microscopy are the mainstay of diagnosis. In many cases treatment has to be started on clinical suspicion only where a trial of therapy is given.

Bacteriological identification

Microscopy

Several clinical specimens can be examined by light microscopy for acid-fast bacilli after staining with the Ziehl–Neelsen stain: sputum, bronchoalveolar lavage, gastric washings, CSF, pleural aspirates, lymph node aspirates, bone marrow and tissue biopsies. Three sputum specimens collected on successive days should be examined. In children this may not be possible and gastric aspirates may be useful. Laryngeal swabs are less sensitive than sputum or gastric washings. Differentiation of species is not possible on light microscopy.

Microscopy, usually applied to sputum, has the great advantage of speed, enabling a diagnosis to be made at the time of the patient's first attendance. It is, however, not very sensitive although it detects those who are the most infectious and thus in need of urgent management. For a standard examination of Ziehl–Neelsen-stained smears to be positive, there must be at least 5000 acid-fast bacilli in 1 ml of sputum. Fluorescence microscopy, where the more expensive equipment is available and adequately maintained, is more sensitive as larger areas of the smear can be scanned at low-power magnification.

Many patients will present with a productive cough and a 'spot' specimen of sputum should be obtained. Ideally, a further two sputum samples should be examined as this improves the chance of detecting tubercle microscopically by around 10%. If tuberculosis is suspected but no sputum is produced, physiotherapy and the inhalation of nebulized twice-normal (hypertonic) saline may yield sputum suitable for examination. If indicated, such induction of sputum should be conducted well away from other patients, especially those who are immunosuppressed as mini-epidemics of tuberculosis have followed such practices on open wards.

Laryngeal swabs provide material suitable for culture but not for direct microscopy. Swabs should only be taken by staff experienced in visualizing the vocal cords and, as patients usually cough violently during the procedure, the operator should wear a gown and a full face visor. Gastric aspiration after overnight fasting to harvest any swallowed tubercle bacilli is useful in children who rarely produce sputum. Aspirated material must be either neutralized immediately or transported to the laboratory without delay. Where facilities permit, fibreoptic bronchoscopy is an excellent means of obtaining bronchial washings and brushings and transbronchial biopsies.[30]

Pleural, pericardial and peritoneal fluids are obtained by aspiration and CSF by lumbar puncture. For culture, portions of these fluids may be added directly to double-strength liquid media supplemented with suitable antibiotics to suppress the growth of micro-organisms other than mycobacteria.

In some cases, needle or open biopsies of various organs and tissues are required. Peritoneal biopsies obtained laparoscopically are preferable to aspirated peritoneal fluid for the diagnosis of abdominal tuberculosis.

Culture

Isolation of *M. tuberculosis* in culture from the clinical specimen provides a definitive diagnosis. Cultivation, usually on solid media, is more sensitive than microscopy and increases the diagnostic yield by up to 50%. Its disadvantage is the delay, usually 3–6 weeks, between receipt of the specimen and the emergence of visible growth.

For culture of mycobacteria, a range of media have been described. Commonly used media are the solid egg-based Löwenstein–Jensen (LJ) medium or Kirschner broth containing a mixture of antibiotics to prevent overgrowth of other bacteria and fungi. Modifications of LJ and other egg-based media include Stonebrink, the American Thoracic Society and the International Union Against Tuberculosis media. Liquid media such as Kirschner's allow a large inoculum to be used, thereby enhancing the likelihood of obtaining a positive result. Other methods such as BACTEC 460 radiometric system and Roche MB check system rely on the growth of bacilli in a Middlebrook broth. The BACTEC system incorporates a ^{14}C-labelled substrate and during metabolism ^{14}C-labelled carbon dioxide is produced and is monitored by the machine. Using these systems, mycobacterial growth is detected about 9 days quicker than by use of LJ slopes. Radiometry indicates the presence of tubercle bacilli within 2–12 days but the equipment is costly and requires facilities for the disposal of radioactive waste. The latter problem has been resolved by the more recent development of equally rapid automated non-radiometric systems in which bacterial growth is indicated by changes in the colour or fluorescence of dyes. In one system, the mycobacterial growth indicator tube (MGIT), the results can be read by holding the tube over a source of ultraviolet light, thereby avoiding the cost of the automated reading system.[31]

Radiological imaging (See also Chapter 26)

The advantage of a chest X-ray in the diagnosis of tuberculosis is that of speed, but the equipment is expensive to obtain, maintain and operate. Experienced radiologists are required in order to interpret the often rather non-specific radiological signs increasingly being seen in patients with HIV/AIDS. Ideally, full-size anteroposterior radiographs should be obtained but miniature radiography may be useful under some circumstances, such as for the screening of refugees, residents of hostels for the homeless and other high-risk populations. Mass miniature radiography is, on grounds of effectiveness and cost-effectiveness, rarely used for routine screening of the general population. Fluoroscopy is of very limited diagnostic value and poses a serious radiation hazard to the operator and should therefore be abandoned.

Radiology is very sensitive although, exceptionally, the radiograph may appear normal in patients with smear-positive pulmonary tuberculosis. On the other hand, radiology is not specific since a wide spectrum of radiological changes is seen and all the changes associated with tuberculosis occur in other respiratory conditions.

Chest X-rays: Features highly suggestive of post-primary pulmonary tuberculosis are unilateral or bilateral patchy shadows in the upper zone, single or multiple cavities and calcification. Conditions mimicking tuberculosis include unresolved pneumonias, atypical pneumonia, carcinoma, sarcoidosis, Kaposi's sarcoma and mycetoma.

CT scans: High-resolution CT scanning, where available, may be required to distinguish these conditions. Even when CAT scanning is performed the diagnosis may be difficult and bronchoscopy may be required to obtain lung samples for analyses.

Radioisotope scans may be helpful in detecting extent of disease or relapses, especially in cryptic areas such as bones and lymph nodes.

MRI with appropriate contrast enhancement may be useful in diagnosis and management of space-occupying lesions in cerebral tuberculosis.

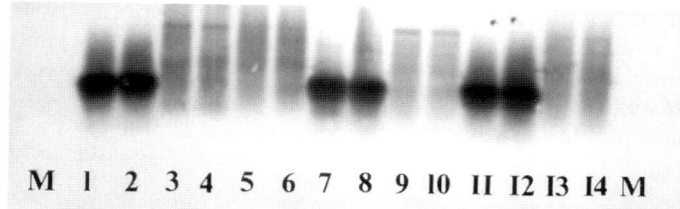

Figure 57.13: Diagnosis of tuberculosis by molecular methods: a Southern blot of PCR products. M, pGem molecular weight markers; lanes 1–10, clinical specimens from patients (lanes 1, 2, 7 and 8 are positive for mycobacterial DNA); lanes 11 and 12 are positive controls and lanes 13 and 14 are negative DNA controls.

Molecular methods for diagnosis of tuberculosis

Although the gold standard for identification of *M. tuberculosis* is still culture this is laborious in terms of both time and space. In view of the problems of sensitivity and speed of the conventional bacteriological diagnostic systems, much effort has been put into developing novel methods for the amplification of species-specific nucleic acid sequences, such as PCR or, more recently LCR[32,33] (Figure 57.13). These are proving rapid, sensitive and specific in most circumstances, with sensitivities approaching 100% and specificities from 85% in non-pulmonary samples to 95% for sputum, and kits are now available commercially. The American Food and Drug Administration (FDA) has approved two nucleic acid amplification (NAA) tests for the direct detection of *Mycobacterium tuberculosis* from clinical specimens: the enhanced *M. tuberculosis* Direct Test (E-MTD; Gen-Probe, San Diego, California) and the Amplicor *M. tuberculosis* Test (Amplicor, Roche Diagnostic Systems, Inc., Branchburg, New Jersey). The use of such systems is largely restricted to major reference centres in the industrially developed nations or at major reference centres in tropical countries.

Haematological and biochemical examination

Haematological and biochemical changes in tuberculosis are rather non-specific. Blood examination may reveal a raised lymphocyte count, a raised ESR, elevated C-reactive protein levels and a mild anaemia. These changes resolve on effective treatment. Serum albumin levels are sometimes low and there may be mild abnormalities of liver function. Elevations in the levels of various enzymes in cerebrospinal, pleural, pericardial and peritoneal fluids have been described but their diagnostic significance has not been clearly established.

Serological tests

There have been numerous reports of elevated levels of antibodies to a range of antigens of the tubercle bacillus in tuberculosis but the low sensitivity and specificity of serodiagnostic tests limit their usefulness. Despite several descriptions of enzyme-linked immunosorbent assay tests for tuberculosis, no universally applicable test with acceptable sensitivity and specificity is available.

Tuberculin test

This is usually positive in patients with tuberculosis although, due to genetic factors, a minority (up to 8% in some regions) fail to respond.[34] The test does not clearly distinguish between active tuberculosis, past infection by the tubercle bacillus and BCG vaccination. In some regions sensitization by environmental mycobacteria induces low levels of tuberculin cross-reactivity. The dermal response is suppressed to a varying extent in malnourished persons and those suffering from advanced tuberculosis, sarcoidosis, chronic renal failure, cancer and viral infections including HIV, measles, chickenpox and glandular fever. It is also suppressed in those receiving anticancer chemotherapy, immunosuppressive drugs and high doses of corticosteroids. False negative results may be due to faulty storage of the material or poor technique. The usual form of tuberculin employed in epidemiological and diagnostic work is purified protein derivative of tuberculin (PPD), the strength of which is expressed in international units (IU). The principal forms of the test are the Mantoux, Heaf and tine tests.

Mantoux test

An intracutaneous injection of 0.1 ml of tuberculin is given on the dorsal aspect of the forearm. After 48 or 72 hours, the transverse diameter of any palpable induration, but not the erythema, is measured. In both epidemiological and diagnostic work the criteria for a positive reaction will be determined by the national tuberculosis programme, taking into account the type and concentration of PPD used and the degree of sensitization by environmental mycobacteria. In the UK and USA responses of 5 mm or more to 1 IU and of 10 mm or more to 5 IU are, respectively, regarded as positive. In diagnostic work, smaller reactions are usually regarded as negative, although they do not exclude tuberculosis because of the conditions mentioned above which suppress the response and the small number of people who never react. Conversely, a positive reaction, for the reasons discussed above, does not necessarily indicate active disease. Reactions may be due to prior BCG vaccination but a reaction of 15 mm or more in diameter in a vaccinated child is a very likely indication of infection by the tubercle bacillus.

Heaf test

This method employs a spring-loaded 'gun' which drives six needles into the skin of the dorsal aspect of the forearm through a drop of undiluted PPD. The method is technically easy but it is necessary to autoclave the gun

Table 57.6 The grades of reactions of the Heaf test

Grade 0	No reaction
Grade I	At least four discrete papules
Grade II	Confluent papules forming a ring
Grade III	A disc of induration
Grade IV	A disc of induration greater than 10 mm in diameter or vesiculation of the disc

between use in order to avoid transmission of HIV and other viruses. Some guns have detachable magnetic heads which can be autoclaved separately. The practice of dipping the head in alcohol and flaming it is unsafe. The test is read at 48–72 hours (although a strong reaction will still be visible at 7 days) and the reaction is scored as shown in Table 57.6.

Grades III and IV correspond to a Mantoux reaction of 15 mm or more and are regarded as definite evidence of infection by the tubercle bacillus. Grade II corresponds to a Mantoux reaction of 10–14 mm and indicates probable infection.

Tine test

This is similar, except that PPD is dried onto four spikes (tines) on a small, single-use, disposable unit. The device is pressed firmly onto the skin so that the tines penetrate the skin and held in place for 10 seconds so that the dried PPD dissolves in the tissue fluids. Results are more variable than with the other test methods but it has some advantages when very few people are tested.

Tuberculosis in children

(See also Chapter 23)

There are many differences between the pathological, clinical, radiological and epidemiological features of tuberculosis in children and adults and several reviews of the disease in children are available.[35,36] Children are usually infected by the aerogenous route and develop primary pulmonary complexes as described below. The most usual source is an adult with tuberculosis in the family. Less frequently they are infected by drinking milk containing *M. bovis*, usually with implantation of the bacilli in the tonsil or intestinal wall. Primary inoculation lesions due to infection of cuts and abrasions and congenital tuberculosis resulting from intrauterine infection are rarely encountered.

Clinical presentations of tuberculosis in children

Many children with primary tuberculosis have no obvious symptoms or signs and may go unnoticed for a while.

A

PATIENT'S DETAILS	HOSPITAL OR PHC LOCATION
Name Age yrs (d.o.b. / /) Sex MF Weight kg BCG scars 0/1/2/3	Date Scored by: Nurse/Health Ass/Doctor

SCORE CHART   (Circle box and write in score)

Children suspected of having tuberculosis

FEATURE	0	1	3	
LENGTH OF ILLNESS	LESS THAN 2 WEEKS	2–4 WEEKS	MORE THAN 4 WEEKS	
NUTRITION (WEIGHT)	ABOVE 80% FOR AGE	BETWEEN 60% AND 80%	LESS THAN 60%	
FAMILY TUBERCULOSIS PAST OR PRESENT	NONE	REPORTED BY FAMILY	PROVED SPUTUM POSITIVE	

SCORE FOR OTHER FEATURES IF PRESENT

Positive tuberculin test	3
Large painless lymph nodes; firm, soft, sinus in neck, axilla, groin	3
Unexplained fever, night sweats, no response to malaria treatment	2
Malnutrition, not improving after 4 weeks	3
Angle deformity of spine	4
Joint swelling, bone swelling or sinuses	3
Unexplained abdominal mass or ascites	3
CNS: change in temperament fits or coma (send to hospital if possible)	3

TOTAL SCORE

When score is 7 or more treat for tuberculosis – see notes.

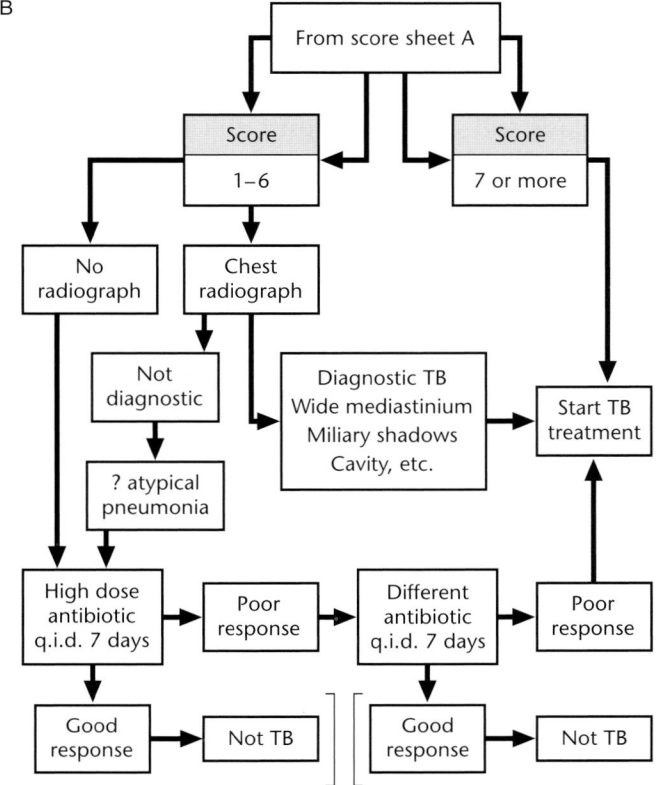

Figure 57.14: Paediatric tuberculosis management flow chart.

Thus a high index of suspicion is essential throughout the tropical countries and other regions where tuberculosis is common. Bacteriological investigations are of limited use for the diagnosis of pulmonary tuberculosis in children since obtaining sputum samples is more difficult than in adults and as tubercle bacilli are only demonstrable in a minority of cases. On the other hand, one study showed that where facilities for extensive investigation exist bacteriological investigations were positive in 78% of infants aged under 1 year.[37] Bacteriological investigations are essential and valuable in the diagnosis of non-pulmonary disease, especially tuberculous meningitis. In view of the diagnostic difficulties, clinical algorithms have been developed,[38] and a flow diagram that has been in use for some time for diagnosis is shown in Figure 57.14.

Primary pulmonary tuberculosis

Clinical features are usually non-specific and include a failure to gain weight or loss of weight, a lack of energy, a persistent cough and/or wheeze and an unexplained fever for more than a week. The tuberculin test is usually positive and the primary focus and/or enlarged intrathoracic lymph nodes may be seen on X-ray. It is not uncommon, however, for children with primary pulmonary tuberculosis to have normal chest X-rays, although in one study computed tomography (CT) revealed enlarged mediastinal nodes in 60% of such radiologically normal children.[39]

Gross enlargement of the intrathoracic lymph nodes or spread of the disease process from lymph nodes to the bronchi causes obstruction of the bronchi and the children present with cough and wheezing. Partial blockage of a major bronchus may limit exhalation, resulting in hyperinflation of the lung and clinically detectable mediastinal shift. Involvement of paratracheal nodes may cause stridor, sometimes requiring emergency tracheostomy.

Endobronchial spread of the disease process results in a range of clinical and radiological changes including pulmonary collapse, consolidation and hyperinflation and, in severe cases, widespread bronchopneumonia. particularly in younger children. In most cases, the lesions resolve clinically and radiologically on effective treatment although a few are left with residual bronchiectasis.

Extrapulmonary tuberculosis

These manifestations are described elsewhere in the chapter.

Congenital tuberculosis

This is a very rare condition and the mother always has tuberculosis, although sometimes in a form that is not clinically or radiologically obvious, such as renal tuberculosis.[40] There are two main types resulting from, respectively, transplacental infection and aspiration or inhalation of infected amniotic fluid.

Transplacental infection causes primary hepatic lesions and the infant presents with hepatic enlargement, fever and failure of weight gain. Jaundice is common. Respiratory infection leads to extensive lung involvement resulting in respiratory distress and cyanosis and diffuse nodular opacities on chest X-ray. Intrathoracic lymphadenopathy, sometimes extensive enough to cause respiratory obstruction, and miliary disease are common.

The tuberculin test is often negative but there are numerous tubercle bacilli in the lungs and/or liver which are usually demonstrable by examination of tracheal or gastric aspirates or fine-needle liver biopsies. Mortality is high, as many as one-half die, and therapy should be commenced on suspicion of the disease. Treatment with corticosteroids may be life-saving in seriously ill children.

Hypersensitivity reactions

Primary tuberculosis in childhood is sometimes associated with hypersensitivity reactions: phlyctenular conjunctivitis and erythema nodosum (Figure 57.15).

Phlyctenular conjunctivitis is characterized by conjunctival itching or pain, lacrimation and photophobia, usually in one eye. Small, grey, translucent nodules are seen near the limbus of the cornea and the blood vessels in the adjacent conjunctiva are dilated. A leash of small blood vessels extends to the edge of the conjunctival sac. Occasionally corneal ulceration occurs. More usually, the condition regresses over several days but recurrent attacks may occur. The condition occurs most frequently in children aged between 5 and 10 years; it is much more frequent in girls than in boys and is most common in the spring. Some cases have followed BCG vaccination and streptococcal infection. It usually occurs soon after primary infection but a few cases have been reported in children with calcified primary complexes.

Erythema nodosum also usually occurs in association with primary tuberculosis and affects a similar age group as phlyctenular conjunctivitis. It is more common in girls and in those with fair skin. It is characterized by erythematous, indurated, painful plaques or nodules, usually on the lower limbs, and may be accompanied by fever and joint pain. The ESR is raised and, if the cause is tuberculosis, the tuberculin test is strongly positive.

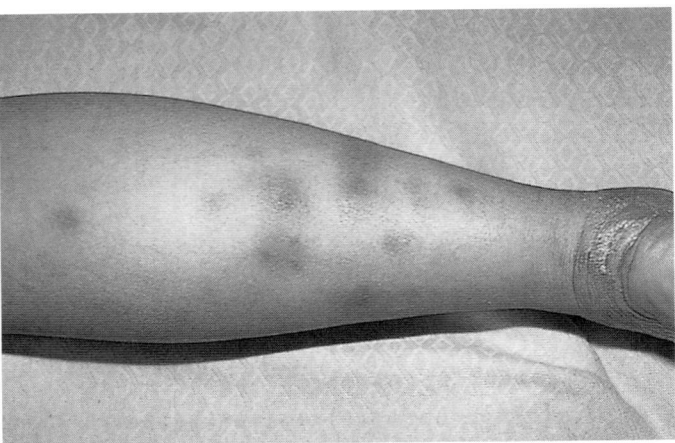

Figure 57.15: Erythema nososum due to tuberculosis.

Resolution usually occurs within 2 weeks although the skin may remain discoloured for several weeks. Treatment, other than that of the underlying condition, is unnecessary, although corticosteroids may be given if joint pain is severe. The condition is not unique to tuberculosis as it also occurs in streptococcal infections, sarcoidosis, leprosy, systemic fungal infections, lymphoproliferative disorders and after treatment with certain drugs.

Tuberculosis in HIV-infected children

HIV infection is increasingly encountered in children as the risk of an HIV-positive mother transmitting the virus to her child during pregnancy or at birth is between 24% and 40%, and even higher if the mother has AIDS. In sub-Saharan Africa a serious epidemic of tuberculosis closely linked to HIV infection has broken out in children. The HIV seroprevalence rates[13] in Zambian children with tuberculosis have risen from 24% in 1989 to 70% in 1998. Such dually infected children are highly susceptible to tuberculosis and forms such as tuberculous meningitis, miliary tuberculosis and widespread lymphadenopathy are frequently seen. The diagnosis of tuberculosis in children remains difficult, even in the best centres. Pulmonary tuberculosis is very common in the tropics and diagnosis is difficult as both the specific and the non-specific symptoms, such as weight loss and fever, as well as clinical and radiological signs, are similar to those seen in several common respiratory illnesses and in HIV-related opportunistic infections such as *Pneumocystis carinii* pneumonia (PCP). The tuberculin test is often negative. In the absence of sophisticated diagnostic facilities, therapy is based on clinical suspicion and many children with tuberculosis will be misdiagnosed and receive no anti-tuberculosis therapy.

Post-primary pulmonary tuberculosis

Sometimes called 'adult-type' tuberculosis, this is the most common form of the disease seen worldwide. In the industrially developed countries, most cases occurred in the elderly but this pattern has changed in recent times and is now seen throughout the tropics in young adults.

Clinical features

Non-specific constitutional symptoms of anorexia, weight loss, night sweats and malaise are present. Symptoms related to the lung include cough, mucoid or purulent sputum, haemoptysis, breathlessness and chest wall pain. More general symptoms include fever and sweating (particularly at night), weight loss, lassitude and anorexia. None of these symptoms are specific for tuberculosis and some patients, even those with quite extensive disease, may have no apparent symptoms at all. Physical chest signs may be absent or limited to fine apical crackles. In more advanced cases there may be areas of dullness on percussion or localized wheezing. Clubbing of the finger is rare but is sometimes seen in severe cases of advanced disease with bronchiectasis. In general, clinical signs are less obvious than would be expected from the radiological picture.

Diagnosis

Diagnosis is usually made by examination of sputum smears by microscopy and, where facilities are available, bacteriological culture and radiological examination (Figures 57.16–57.20). Advanced imaging techniques where available are useful in localizing pathology in cryptic sites (Figure 57.21–57.23).

Complications

The complications of post-primary pulmonary tuberculosis include pleural effusion and empyema, pneumothorax or pyopneumothorax due to formation of a bronchopleural fistula, tuberculous laryngitis and indurated intestinal ulcers due to implantation of tubercle bacilli in swallowed sputum. Occasionally an empyema on an intercostal node ruptures into the chest wall to form a cold abscess. Spread to other organs by the haematogenous or lymphatic route is uncommon when patients are relatively immunocompetent, but it is seen in many patients infected with HIV or with other conditions compromising their

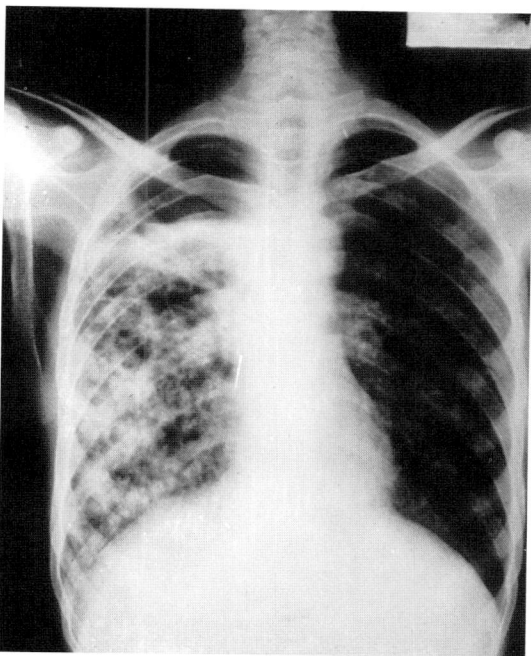

Figure 57.17: Chest X-ray with extensive patchy consolidation in the right lung fields. Sputum examination revealed acid-fast organisms confirmed on culture to be *M. tuberculosis*.

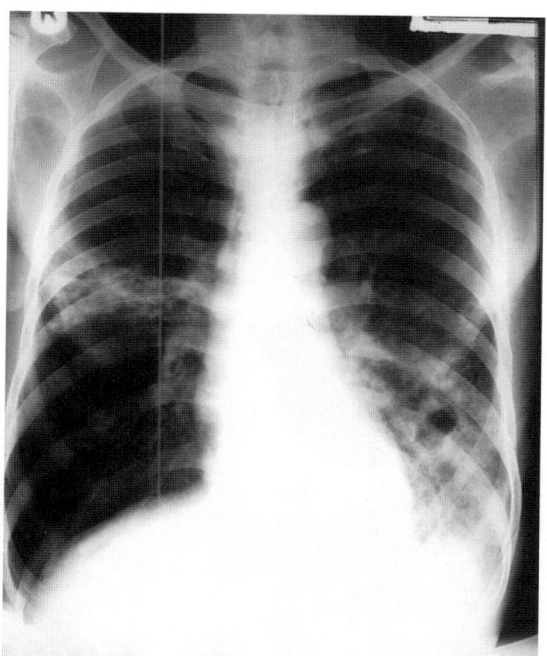

Figure 57.18: Chest X-ray of an HIV-positive patient with cavitating tuberculous consolidation in the right middle and left lower lung fields.

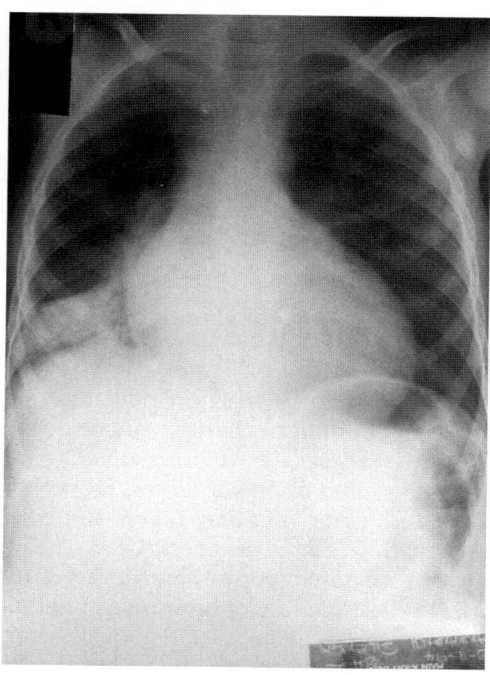

Figure 57.16: Chest X-ray showing right lower lobe consolidation due to tuberculosis.

immunity. A late complication is chronic obstructive airways disease and cor pulmonale secondary to extensive pulmonary fibrosis. Other, much rarer, late complications include amyloidosis and aspergillomas developing in healed cavities (Figure 57.24).

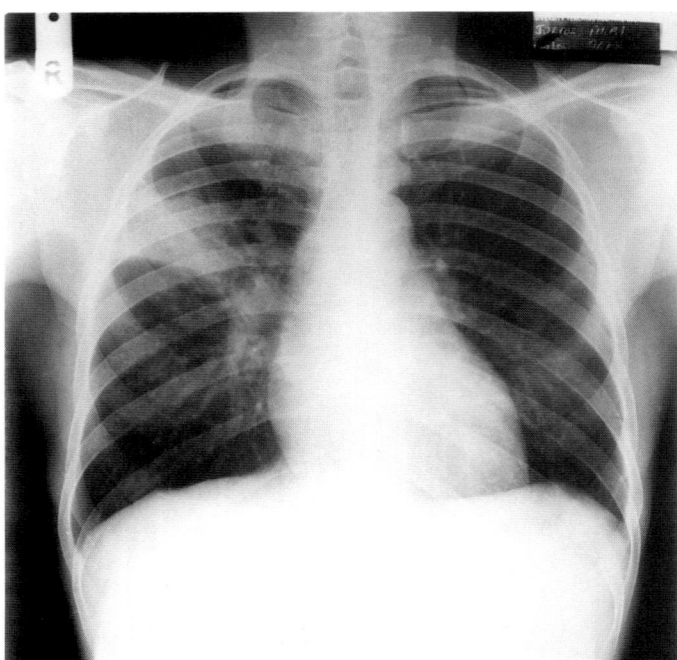

Figure 57.19: Post-primary tuberculous. Right upper lobe tuberculous consolidation in a 15-year-old HIV-positive patient.

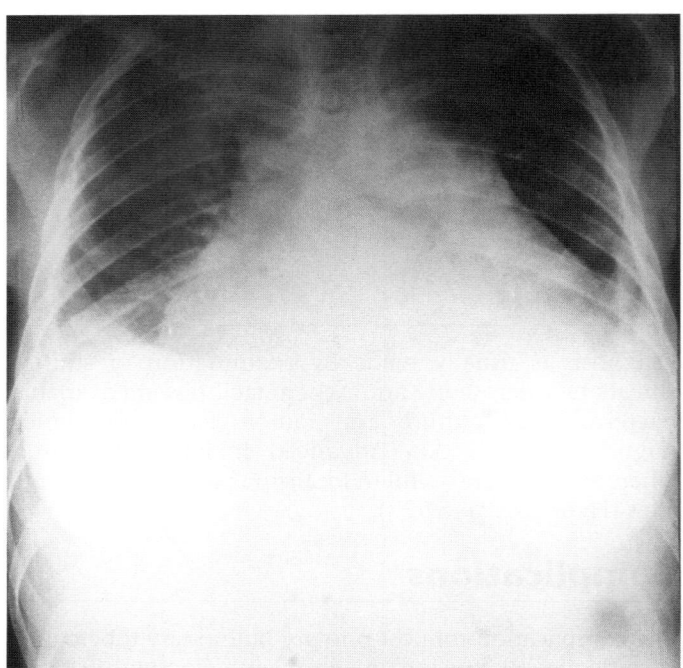

Figure 57.20: Post-primary tuberculous. Pleural and pericardial effusions in a 44-year-old HIV-positive patient. *M. tuberculosis* was isolated from pleural fluid.

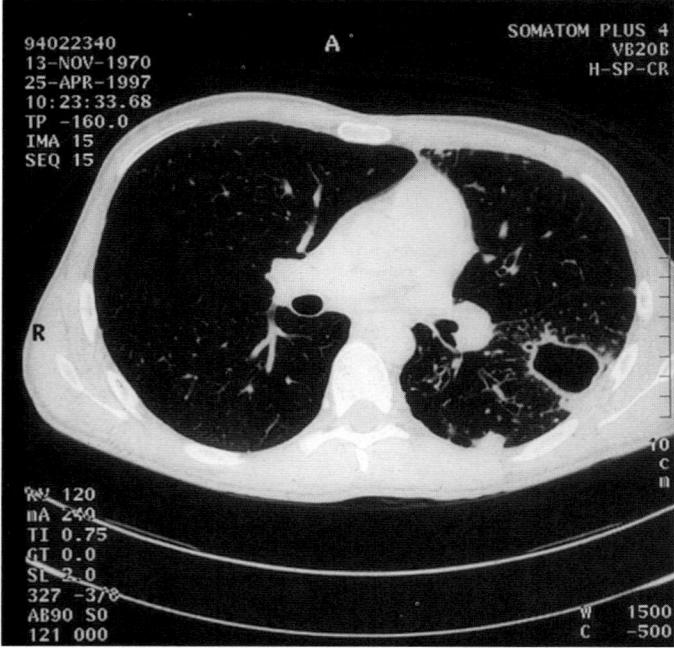

Figure 57.21: CT of the chest showing tuberculous cavity.

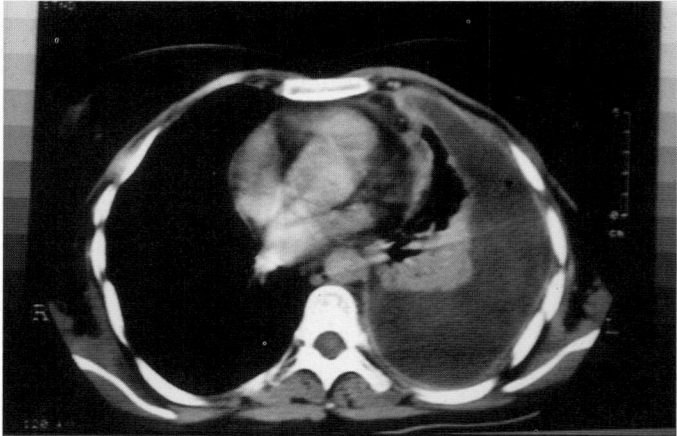

Figure 57.22: CT scan of the chest showing pleural effusion.

Differential diagnosis

The principal conditions with which pulmonary tuberculosis may be confused are community acquired pneumonias, carcinoma of the lung, unresolved pneumonias, Kaposi's sarcoma, helminth infections of the lung (hydatid, schistosomiasis, paragonimiasis), pulmonary fibrotic lung disease secondary to sarcoidosis or industrial dust disease and pulmonary infarct. Lung cancers, pulmonary amoebiasis and abscesses of unresolved pneumonia, especially when caused by *Staphylococcus aureus* or *Klebsiella pneumoniae*, and cysts of *Paragonimus westermanii* may appear as cavitating lesions on chest X-ray. The absence of acid-fast bacilli on microscopy may suggest one of these other causes and, in the case of unresolved pneumonia, the causative organisms may be isolated by the appropriate bacteriological examinations. A therapeutic trial with a suitable antibiotic(s) may also differentiate tuberculosis from atypical pneumonia and pulmonary abscesses. The cachexia

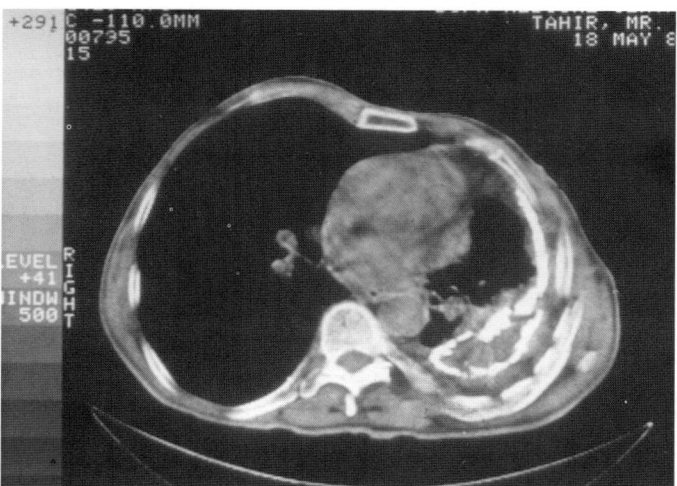

Figure 57.23: CT scan of the chest showing calcified empyema of 'old' treated tuberculosis.

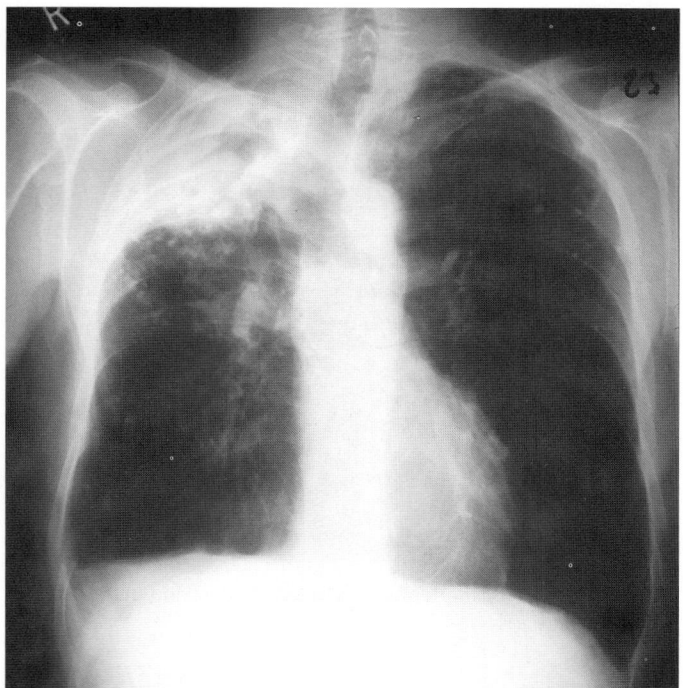

Figure 57.24: Chest X-ray showing a fungal (*Aspergillus*) ball in a tuberculous cavity.

and malaise of advanced tuberculosis resemble that seen in AIDS, disseminated cancer and diabetes mellitus.

Management

The management of pulmonary tuberculosis involves: (a) prescription of standard antituberculosis drug treatment; (b) management of complications, (c) patient follow-up until end of therapy and (d) active contact tracing.

Tuberculous pleural effusion and empyema

Pleural effusions occur in both primary and post-primary tuberculosis and are due to spread of the disease process from a lesion in the periphery of the lung or, occasionally, from an intercostal node into the pleural space. Effusions may be small and transitory and due, in part, to a hypersensitivity reaction to antigens of the tubercle bacillus. In other cases, particularly in older patients, an empyema develops.

Clinical features

The main clinical features, in addition to those of the underlying pulmonary disease, are chest pain accentuated by breathing, a dull ache over the lower chest and breathlessness on exertion. There is 'stony' dullness on percussion over the lower chest and diminished air entry on the affected side and, if the effusion is large, the mediastinum may be shifted to the opposite side.

Diagnosis

On chest X-ray, a small effusion (about 100 ml) causes a blunting of the costophrenic angle, while larger ones are denser at the base, tailing up into the axilla (Figures 57.18 and 57.21). Fluid levels are seen in cases where there is a bronchopleural fistula. The diagnosis of tuberculosis is made by aspiration of pleural fluid from the pleural space and subjecting it to bacteriological examination, or by pleural biopsy histopathology. Where facilities for bacteriological culture exist, some of the pleural fluid should be added to an equal volume of double-strength liquid culture medium at the bedside. Large effusions should be aspirated slowly as rapid expansion of the lung may cause coughing, breathlessness and, occasionally, pulmonary oedema. Histopathological examination of pleural biopsies may show tuberculous granulomas or the presence of acid-fast bacilli. Mycobacterial DNA can be detected in pleural fluid and biopsy samples by PCR.

Differential diagnosis

Tuberculous pleural effusions must be differentiated from those secondary to pneumonia, cardiac failure, malignancy, pulmonary embolism and infarction and amoebiasis.

Management

Management involves: (a) prescription of standard antituberculosis drug treatment, (b) management of complications, (c) patient follow-up until end of therapy and (d) active contact tracing. Small effusions usually resolve on antituberculosis chemotherapy but larger ones may require needle aspiration. Corticosteroid treatment prevents recurrence of large effusions and subsequent constrictive fibrosis which may affect pulmonary function. Thick empyema fluid may be difficult to aspirate through a needle and surgical drainage is required. Surgical removal of the pleura (decortication) may be required to prevent or relieve gross constrictive scarring.

Disseminated Tuberculosis

This form of tuberculosis was described in the year 1620 by Sylvius, who wrote 'I came moreover constantly upon various traces of glands small and almost invisible to the eyes, except occasionally, when they were unnaturally larger and I have seen them distributed throughout the viscera and flesh of our entire body.'

The clinical and histopathological features of disseminated tuberculosis are determined by the immune status of the patient. In cases in which the immune responses are intact, the disease is characterized by the formation of widespread, multiple, discrete granulomas macroscopically resembling millet seeds (Latin: *milium*, a millet seed), hence the name miliary tuberculosis.

Miliary tuberculosis

Classically, this was a disease of young children but nowadays it occurs in those of all ages. The symptoms are non-specific and include fever, malaise and weight loss. Meningeal involvement may cause headache. On chest X-ray the numerous minute lesions produce a characteristic

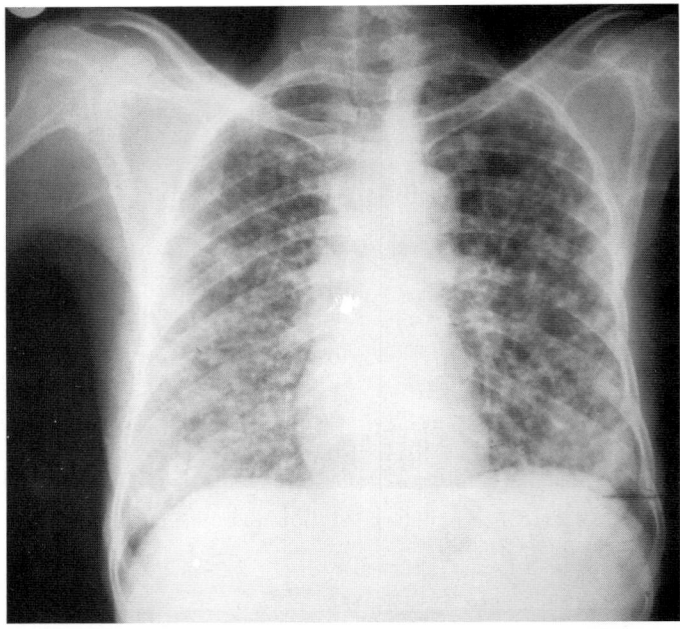

Figure 57.26: Miliary tuberculosis. Chest X-ray of an HIV-positive patient showing extensive bilateral shadowing.

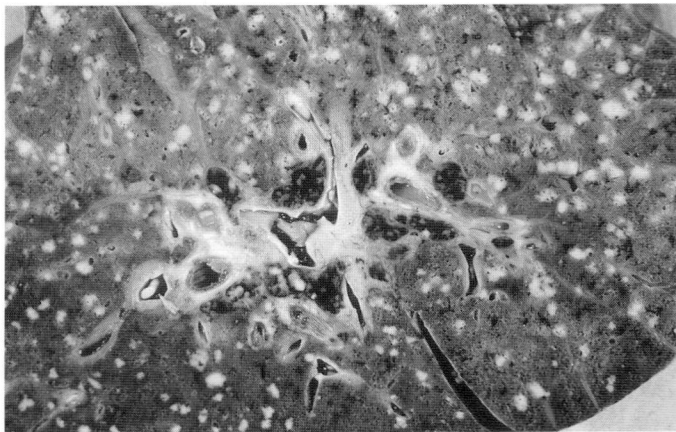

Figure 57.27: Post-mortem kidney specimen showing miliary tuberculosis.

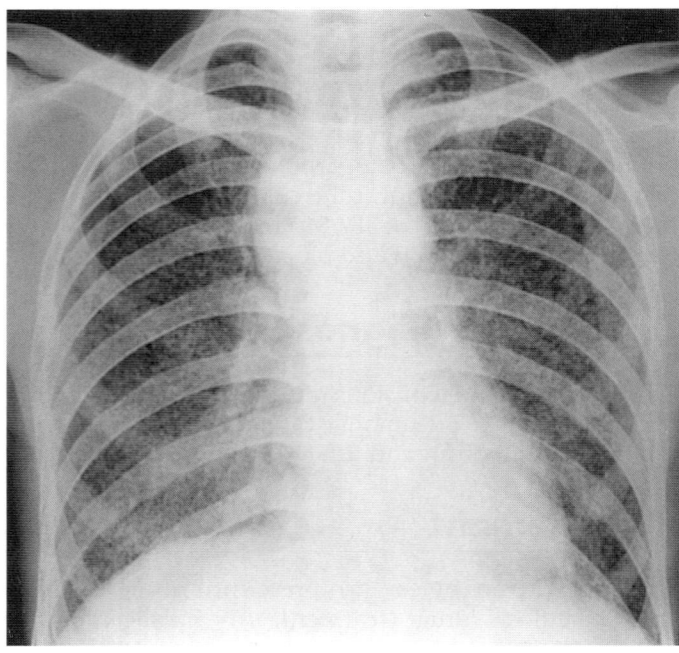

Figure 57.25: Chest X-ray-miliary tuberculosis. Note enlarged paratracheal nodes.

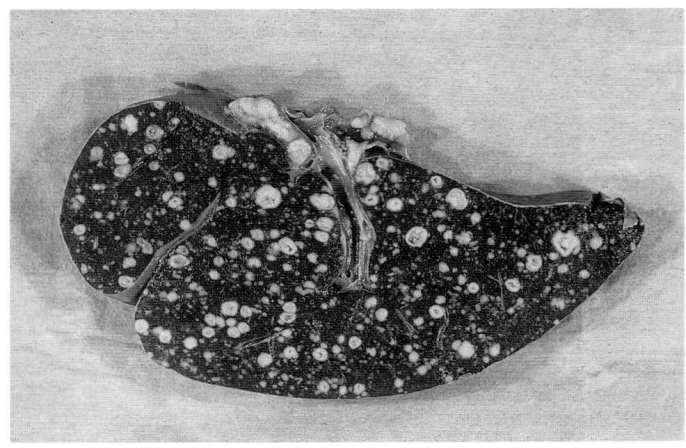

Figure 57.28: Miliary tuberculosis involving the spleen.

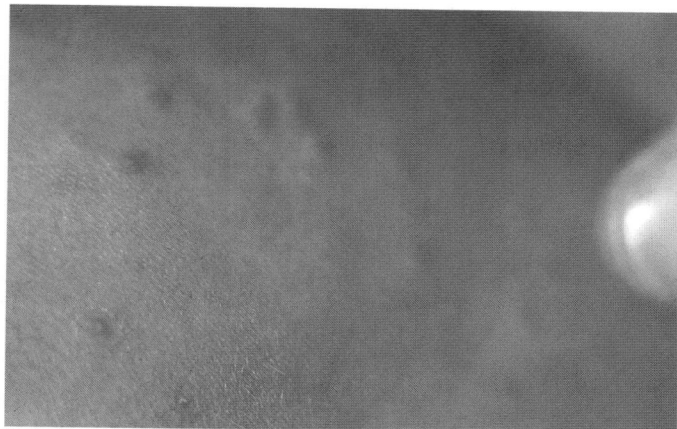

Figure 57.29: Grouped erythematous papules on the skin of the face in miliary tuberculosis.

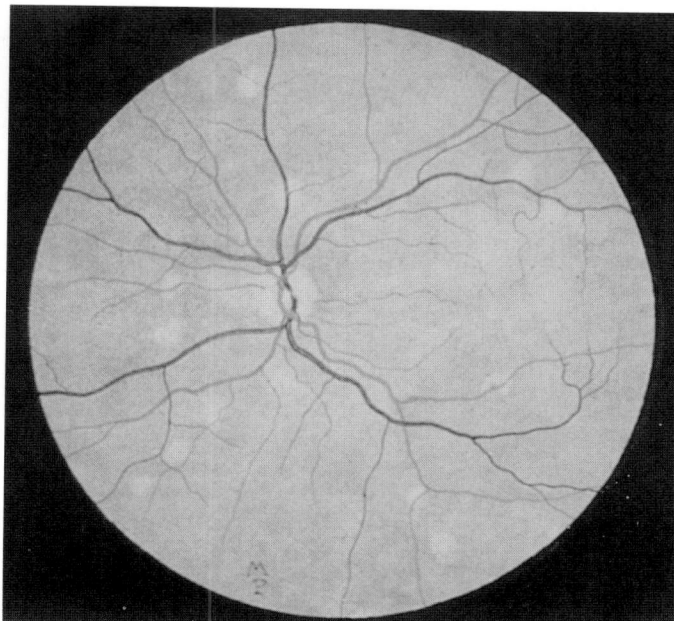

Figure 57.30: Choroidal tubercles.

'snowstorm' appearance (Figures 57.25 and 57.26). Apart from miliary lesions in the lung, lesions also occur in the kidney (Figure 57.27), spleen (Figure 57.28) and tubercle bacilli are found in the urine of about 25% of patients with miliary disease. The disease may be acute, and rapidly progressive and fatal if untreated, but in other cases it is surprisingly chronic and insidious. Pleural involvement with small effusions may occur, the meninges are affected in about 10% of cases, hepatosplenomegaly is detectable in 20–30% of cases and, rarely, papular or macular miliary lesions of the skin are seen (Figure 57.29).

Acid-fast bacilli are demonstrable in sputum in about half the cases and in liver biopsies in about a quarter of cases. Probably the best diagnostic procedure, if facilities are available, is transbronchial biopsy through a fibre-optic bronchoscope. The tuberculin test is usually positive in early cases but becomes negative as the disease advances.

Characteristic single or multiple tubercles, greyish-white or yellowish in colour and 0.5–3 mm in diameter (Figure 57.30) may be seen on the choroid of the eye. Although not present in all cases, this is a very useful diagnostic sign and a very careful examination by ophthalmoscopy should always be undertaken in cases of suspected miliary tuberculosis and, indeed, in anyone with an unexplained fever. The differential diagnosis includes viral or mycoplasmal pneumonia, histoplasmosis and coccidioidomycosis in cryptic miliary disease.

Miliary tuberculosis responds well to chemotherapy but corticosteroid therapy may be life-saving in seriously ill patients.

Cryptic disseminated tuberculosis

In cases in which immune responses are suppressed, or weakened due to old age, the widespread lesions show very little cellular infiltration but consist of minute necrotic foci teeming with acid-fast bacilli. The lesions are usually too small to be visible on chest X-ray and this form of the disease has been termed cryptic disseminated tuberculosis.[41] The diagnosis is often missed as patients present with non-specific features such as fever, weight loss and anaemia, the tuberculin test is almost always negative and the chest X-ray may be deceptively normal. In many cases the patients are extremely ill on presentation and, without therapy, rapidly die. Diagnosis is easily missed and many cases are only detected at autopsy. Biopsy of the lung, liver or bone marrow may provide the diagnosis after staining for acid-fast mycobacteria, culture for *M. tuberculosis* or identification of myco-bacterial DNA by PCR. This form of tuberculosis is common in HIV-positive children and adults, particularly in the more profoundly immunosuppressed.

Bone and joint tuberculosis

This form of tuberculosis is the result of haematogenous dissemination of bacilli from a primary focus and, in the tropics, it is a common manifestation of tuberculosis in children. Most cases present 6 months to 3 years after the initial infection. Any bone or joint may be affected but the most frequent site is the spine, involved in half the cases, followed in frequency by the large joints of the lower limb (hip, knee and ankle) and then the large joints of the upper limb (shoulder, elbow and wrist). Multiple lesions, often cystic, may occur in disseminated tuberculosis and are easily mistaken for metastatic carcinoma.[42]

Spinal tuberculosis, also termed Pott's disease, after Sir Percival Pott (1713–1788), a surgeon at St Bartholomew's Hospital, London, is a cause of severe deformity and handicap. Although any part of the spine may be affected, lesions most often occur at or near the 10th thoracic vertebra. The disease process usually begins in an inter-vertebral disc and subsequently involves the anterior parts of the adjacent vertebrae (Figure 57.31). Erosion of

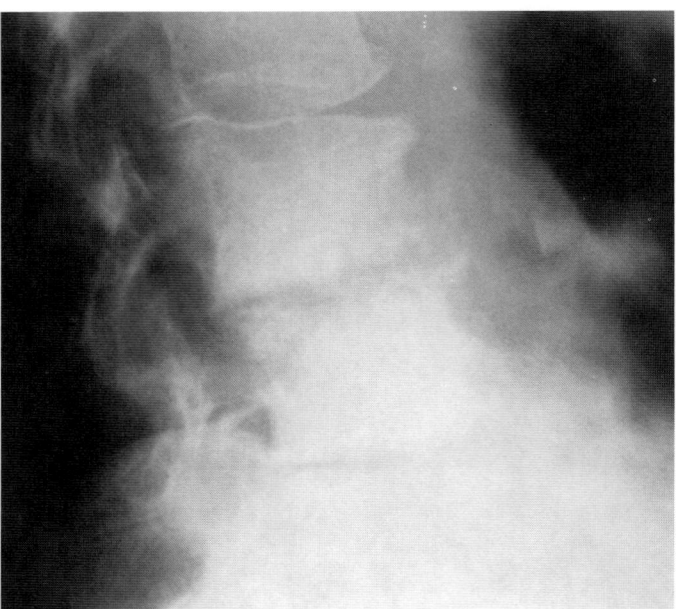

Figure 57.31: Spinal tuberculosis. Note involvement of two adjacent vertebrae and loss of joint space.

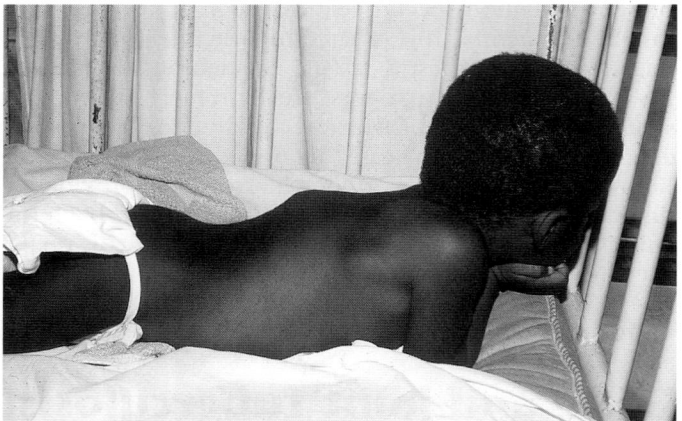

Figure 57.32: Pott's disease of the spine: spinal tuberculosis in a child showing a visible, palpable lump (gibbus) over the spine. The nappy was being used for urinary incontinence caused by spinal cord involvement.

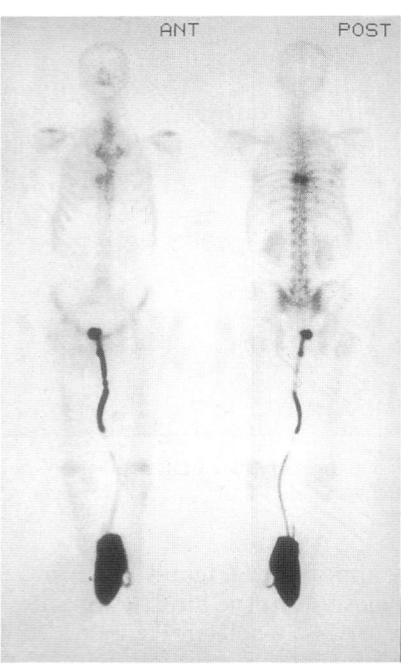

Figure 57.33: Tuberculous osteomyelitis. Radionuclide bone scan shows abnormal, increased tracer uptake in D7. The vertebra has collapsed, with spinal cord compression resulting in paraplegia. The excreted activity is seen in the urinary catheter.

the bone due to osteomyelitis causes vertebral collapse with anterior wedging and, in severe cases, the characteristic angular spinal deformity or 'gibbus' (Figure 57.32). 'Cold' abscesses are common and may track along fascial planes and emerge at the skin surface well away from the site of disease. Thus psoas abscesses secondary to disease in the lumbar vertebrae may emerge in the thigh below the inguinal ligament. Tuberculosis of the cervical spine may present as a retropharyngeal abscess.

The usual presenting feature is chronic back pain, often with stiffness and limitation of movement. An unwillingness to pick something off the floor is a characteristic sign. Clinical features may, however, be minimal and non-specific and diagnosis is often delayed. Neurological

signs due to pressure on, or vasculitis of, the spinal cord occur in about half the cases and paraplegia develops in severe cases. Clinical examination may reveal muscular spasm and rigidity, cold abscesses, sinuses and spinal deformity. Radiological signs may be minimal and give an underestimate of the extent of the disease. Where available, CT, MRI or radionuclide bone scan (Figure 57.33) may permit a more accurate assessment of the extent of the disease. Biopsies or fine-needle aspirates, conducted by those with adequate experience, may establish or confirm the diagnosis. Histological as well as bacteriological examination is essential as there may be too few acid-fast bacilli in the biopsy material for them to be detectable microscopically. The tuberculin test is usually positive although it may be negative in malnourished or immunosuppressed patients.

The differential diagnosis includes bacterial osteomyelitis (due to *Staphylococcus*, *Brucella* and *Salmonella* species) and primary or secondary (lung, breast, prostate, kidney or thyroid) tumours. Blood tests for staphylococcal and streptococcal infections and for typhoid, paratyphoid and brucellosis may help to rule out the latter. Care should be taken not to confuse the combination of opacities on chest X-ray and osteolytic lesions of the spine with metastatic lung cancer.

Treatment is by administering a standard course of antituberculosis chemotherapy. The need for surgical intervention depends on the presence and extent of spinal deformity and neurological signs. In the absence of such complications, ambulant treatment is usually effective. The most effective form of surgery for correction of deformity and relief or prevention of paraplegia is radical excision of diseased tissue and anterior spinal fusion—the so-called 'Hong Kong operation'. This, however, calls for surgical skills and resources that are not widely available.

Tuberculosis of other bones and joints

This mimics a wide range of other conditions, especially the various forms of arthritis, and diagnosis is not easy. Disseminated lesions in many bones may mimic metastatic carcinoma. Tuberculosis of the skull usually presents with fluctuant abscesses (Figure 57.34), sometimes with sinus formation, and underlying osteolytic lesions—a condition sometimes termed 'Pott's puffy tumour'. Osteitis is a rare complication of BCG vaccination in neonates and young children. Diagnosis may require bacteriological examination of biopsies of bone or synovium or of aspirated synovial fluid.

Unless prevented by pain, joint mobility should be maintained during chemotherapy. Arthroplasty or other orthopaedic procedures may be required if there is residual immobility or deformity. Poncet's disease and hypertrophic osteoarthropathy are rare conditions affecting bones and joints in patients with tuberculosis but are thought to be due to metabolic or immunological factors rather than the direct result of bacillary invasion. Poncet's disease is a form of polyarthritis which resolves on treatment of the underlying disease.[43] Hypertrophic osteoarthropathy is characterized by periosteal inflammation and subperiosteal new bone formation.[44] It occasionally occurs in both humans and animals with pulmonary tuberculosis although it is more usually associated with lung cancer.

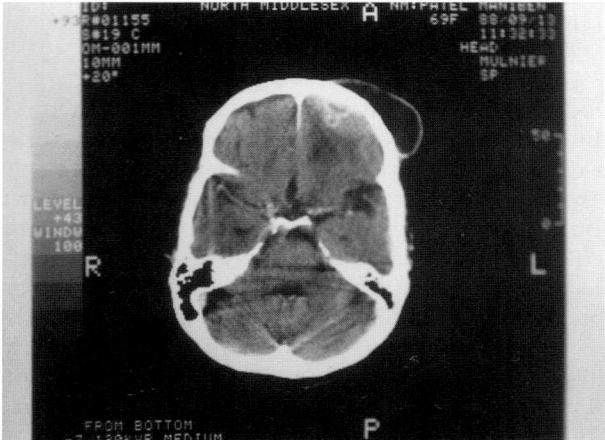

Figure 57.34: CT scan of the head showing a brain tuberculoma exuding its contents through the skull into scalp soft tissues: 'collar stud abscess'.

Tuberculosis of the central nervous system

Tuberculosis of the central nervous system can present as serious and life-threatening conditions and three main types are encountered in clinical practice:[45]

1. Tuberculous meningitis.
2. Solitary space-occupying lesions in the brain or spinal cord.
3. Disseminated miliary lesions.

Tuberculosis presenting as meningitis is the most common form of CNS tuberculosis and constitutes a medical emergency as a diagnostic and therapeutic delay may have very serious consequences. Nearly 50% of patients with advanced CNS disease fail to survive and there is a high incidence of serious neurological complications in those who survive.

Tuberculous meningitis

This is most often seen in infants but it may occur at any age.[45] It is usually a manifestation of primary tuberculosis and there may be radiological evidence of a primary pulmonary complex. The disease commences with the rupture of a meningeal or subcortical lesion with liberation of tubercle bacilli into the CSF and the development of many tubercles on the meninges. The ensuing meningeal inflammation, particularly at the base of the brain, leads to the secretion of a thick exudate which may lead to strangulation of the cranial nerves, especially the optic and auditory nerves, at the base of the brain and to raised intracranial pressure due to obstruction to the flow of CSF. Raised intracranial pressure is a major complication of tuberculous meningitis and some degree of hydrocephalus occurs in 80–90% of children with stage 2 or 3 disease as defined below. An inflammatory endarteritis may lead to thrombosis of the cerebral blood vessels causing cerebral infarction with convulsions or paralysis.

Clinically, cases are classified into three stages:

Stage 1. The patient is fully conscious and rational with non-specific symptoms such as general malaise, low-grade fever, apathy, irritability, personality changes, depression and intermittent headache but with no focal signs and little or no evidence of meningitis. Symptoms may be limited or even absent in immunosuppressed patients, including those who are HIV-positive.
Stage 2. The patient is mentally confused and/or has focal neurological signs such as cranial nerve palsies. Other symptoms include more severe and persistent headache and vomiting and some degree of photophobia.
Stage 3. The patient is deeply stuporose or comatose and/or has complete hemiplegia, paraplegia or quadriplegia.

Examination of CSF is essential although this should be performed carefully after ruling out raised intracranial pressure. This may reveal lymphocytes, a raised protein level and decreased glucose level, but these parameters may be normal. In some cases there is a high polymorph count, which suggests tuberculous meningitis of rapid onset or a non-acid-fast bacterial infection. A chest X-ray may be helpful as pulmonary tuberculous lesions are evident in about half the patients. The diagnosis is confirmed by the microscopical detection of acid-fast bacilli in centrifuged samples of CSF, although a very thorough search only detects such bacilli in 10–30% of cases. Where a CSF 'clot' of fibrin is present, acid-fast bacilli may be seen in it. Culture of CSF is far too slow, even with the use of automated systems but, where facilities are available, PCR and related nucleic acid amplification techniques may be useful.[45] If in any doubt as to the diagnosis, antituberculosis therapy should be commenced immediately. CT and MRI, where available, are of value in the investigation of tuberculous meningitis as they detect cryptic lesions, raised intracranial pressure, hydrocephalus and cerebral infarctions.

Tuberculomas of the brain and spinal cord

These usually manifest as space-occupying lesions.[46] CT and MRI, where available, are very helpful as the lesions often have a characteristic appearance (Figures 57.33–57.38).

Treatment

Standard short-course antituberculosis chemotherapy is effective although many physicians extend the duration of therapy to 9 or 12 months to minimize the risk of relapse. Both isoniazid and pyrazinamide readily cross

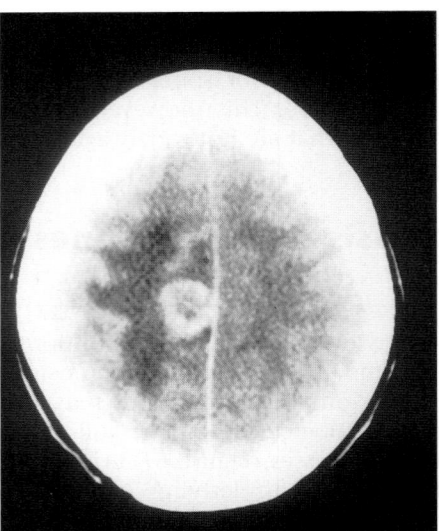

Figure 57.36: Post-contrast enhanced cranial CT. See also Figure 57.35.

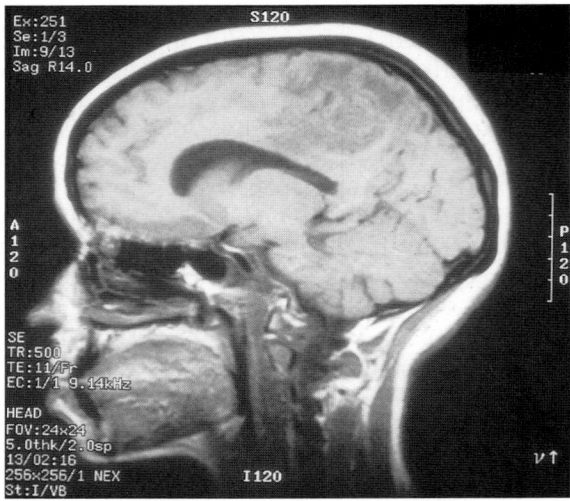

Figure 57.37: T1-weighted MRI, pre-contrast. Multiplanar reformation (coronal, left column, sagittal, right column) is 'as routine as' conventional axial images. Enhancement patterns mirror those of CT scan. The patient has cerebral tuberculosis.

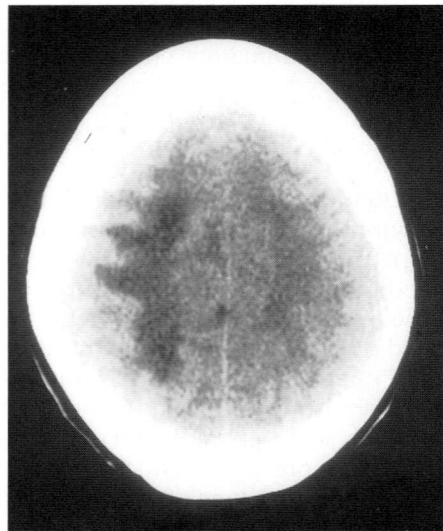

Figure 57.35: Pre-contrast enhanced cranial CT. The parafalcine ring-enhancing lesion exerts mass effect. Its appearance is non-specific, in this case being an example of an intracranial abscess due to *M. tuberculosis*.

the blood–brain barrier but rifampicin does not penetrate so readily and therefore higher doses, but not exceeding 600 mg daily, may be given. Some authorities recommend giving pyrazinamide throughout the course of treatment. Ethambutol enters the CSF when the meninges are inflamed but ocular complications may occur in children. Intrathecal administration of drugs is not generally recommended. In a major centre in South Africa only one relapse was seen in a series of over 200 children with tuberculous meningitis receiving a 6-month course of daily isoniazid (20 mg/kg), rifampicin (20 mg/kg), ethionamide (20 mg/kg) and pyrazinamide (40 mg/kg).

The use of steroids has been a source of controversy as, although steroids suppress hypersensitivity reactions and the formation of basal exudates, some workers claimed

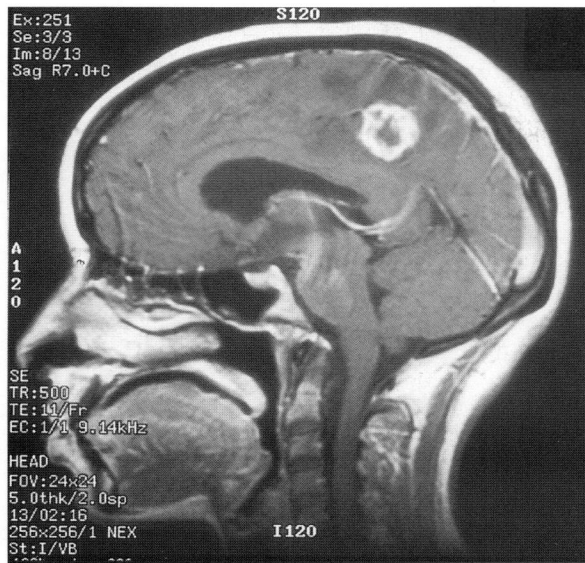

Figure 57.38: T1-weighted MRI, post-contrast. See also Figure 57.37.

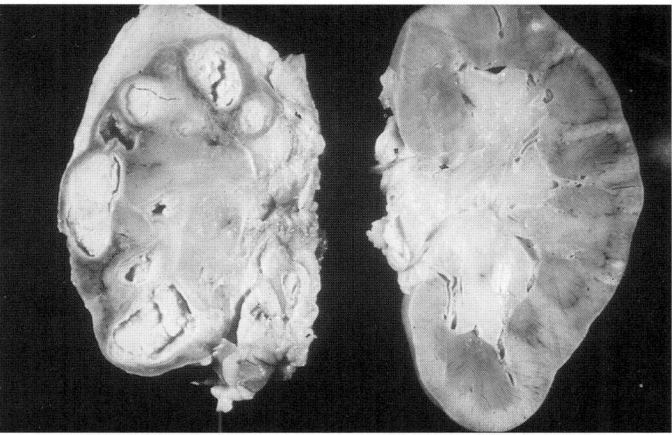

Figure 57.39: Post-mortem kidney specimens showing caseating tuberculous lesions.

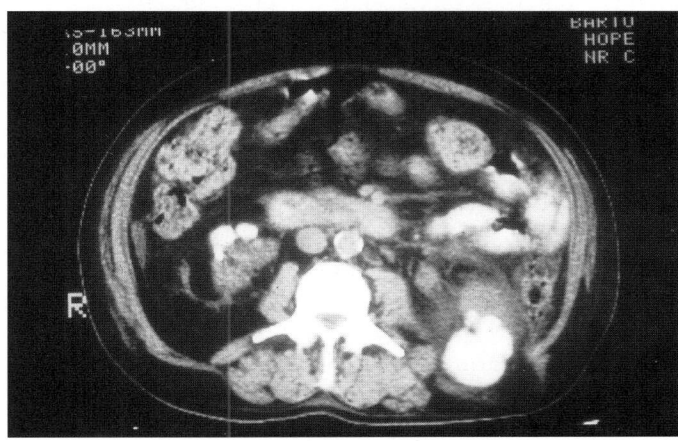

Figure 57.40: Non-enhanced CT scan through the lower abdomen. Large parenchymal deposits of calcification involving both kidneys as a result of earlier tuberculous infection.

that, while they lowered mortality, they allowed more very seriously disabled children to survive. In a more recent study, prednisolone 4 mg/kg daily for 1 month reduced both mortality and morbidity but did not lower raised intracranial pressure.

Raised intracranial pressure may resolve in many cases on treatment with acetazolamide (100 mg/kg per day) or frusemide (1 mg/kg per day) given in divided doses at 6- or 8-hour intervals for 1 month. Dehydration must be prevented, especially in children who are vomiting. Children who fail to respond require the insertion of ventriculoperitoneal shunts.

Small solid lesions in the brain and spinal cord often resolve with medical treatment alone,[47] but surgery is required for larger lesions, especially if sight is threatened or, in the case of the spinal cord, if there is paralysis.

Urinary and genital tracts

Tuberculosis of the kidney is a common form of extra-pulmonary tuberculosis. Autopsy studies indicate that it is commoner than expected in AIDS patients.[48] Renal tuberculosis is usually a late manifestation of haematogenous spread from a primary focus of tuberculosis, presenting 6–15 years after the initial infection.[49] The disease, which may be unilateral or bilateral, usually commences in the renal cortex and progresses towards the medulla (Figures 57.39 and 57.40). Lesions may eventually rupture into the renal pelvis with release of tubercle bacilli into the urine, causing secondary lesions in the ureters and bladder and, in males, in the epididymis, testis, seminal vesicles and prostate.[50] Although usually secondary to tuberculosis of the kidney, some cases of tuberculous epididymitis appear to be due to direct haematogenous spread from primary foci of disease.

Symptoms include frequency, dysuria, nocturia, suprapubic pain and haematuria, resembling symptoms of non-acid-fast bacterial cystitis.[51,52] In other cases, symptoms are of a vague 'orthopaedic' nature. Renal colic is uncommon, occurring in less than 10% of patients and constitutional symptoms are also uncommon. Secondary infection of the kidney, with renal pain and fever, may develop or if, as is often the case, diagnosis is delayed, ureteric obstruction, shrinkage and fibrosis of the bladder and even renal failure may develop. About 40% of patients have subclinical impairment of renal function indicated by raised serum creatinine levels and about 10% have mild hypertension which resolves on antituberculosis therapy. A male patient may present with a swollen epididymis or testis or with infertility.

An insidious form of renal tuberculosis termed tuberculous interstitial nephritis may lead to advanced renal failure without the usual tissue destruction and anatomical distortion.[53] Renal biopsies reveal an interstitial granulomatous infiltrate with limited caseation and scanty acid-fast bacilli. Diagnosis is not easy as it is unusual

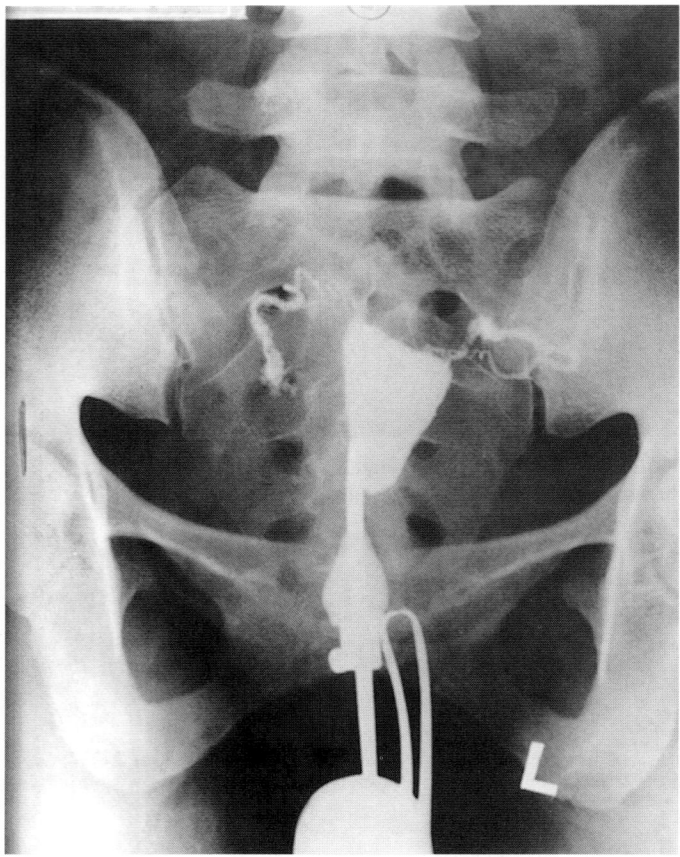

Figure 57.41: Hysterosalpingogram showing distortion of Fallopian tubes due to chronic tuberculous salpinigitis.

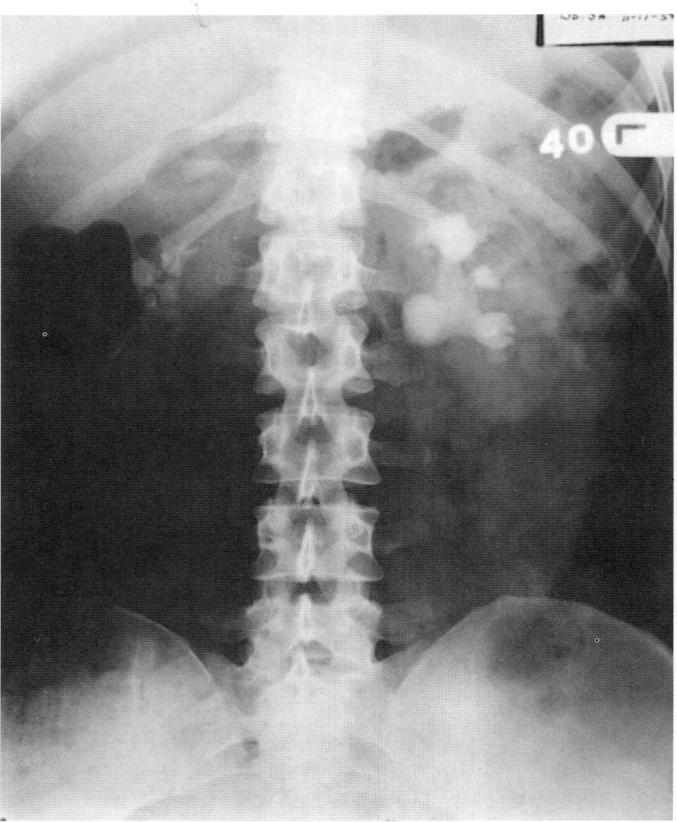

Figure 57.42: Renal tuberculosis. Note loss of calyceal architecture and ureteric obstruction.

to find acid-fast bacilli in the urine. As tuberculosis is common in the tropics, it should be considered in all cases of renal failure when there are no other obvious causes.[54]

Tuberculosis of the female genital tract is, in contrast to the disease in males, almost always the direct result of haematogenous dissemination from the primary focus. Sexually transmitted tuberculosis has been reported but is exceedingly rare. The disease usually commences in the epithelium of the Fallopian tubes (Figure 57.41) and spreads to the endometrium or to the peritoneal cavity, causing tuberculous peritonitis. Presenting features include infertility, pelvic pain and either excessive menstrual bleeding or amenorrhoea.

Diagnosis

Examination of the urine may reveal a few white cells, red cells and protein. Care is required in the interpretation of acid-fast bacilli seen in urine as various environmental mycobacteria occur as contaminants of the lower urethra and external genitalia. Diagnosis is confirmed by cultivation of tubercle bacilli in urine, for which purpose up to six specimens, preferably taken in the early morning, should be examined.

Radiology of the urinary tract (Figure 57.42) is useful for the detection of urinary obstruction and other forms of gross tissue damage. Being a late manifestation of primary tuberculosis, appearances suggestive of pulmonary tuberculosis are only seen in 5% of cases but patients may give a history of tuberculosis. Ultrasonography may reveal renal calyceal dilatation and more overt evidence of obstruction. Between 50% and 75% of males with genital tuberculosis have radiological abnormalities in the urinary tract, so the appropriate radiological investigations should be undertaken.

Diagnosis of tuberculosis of the female genital tract is made by histological and bacteriological examination of endometrial biopsies and culture of cervical secretions and menstrual blood.

Management

Treatment of all forms of genitourinary tuberculosis is by standard short-course antituberculosis chemotherapy. Surgical intervention may be required for relief of ureteric or urethral obstruction,[55] shrunken bladders or, rarely, for the removal of grossly damaged and non-functioning kidneys in the presence of symptoms. Ureteric obstruction may respond to treatment with steroids.

A

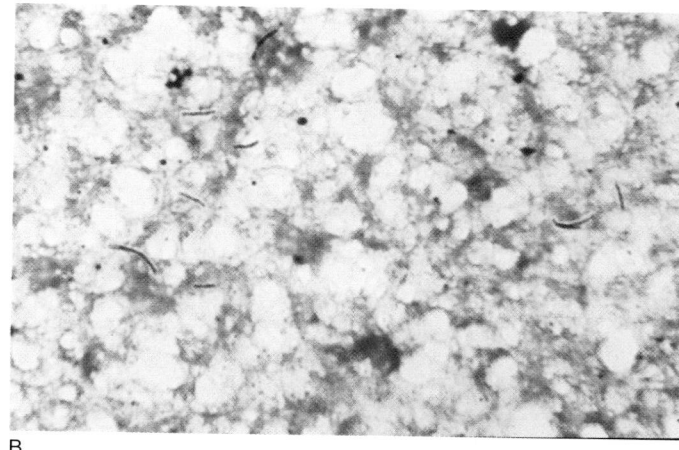

B

Plate 57.2: (**A**) Ziehl–Neelsen staining of a sputum sample and (**B**) a bronchoalveolar lavage washing showing acid-fast bacilli.

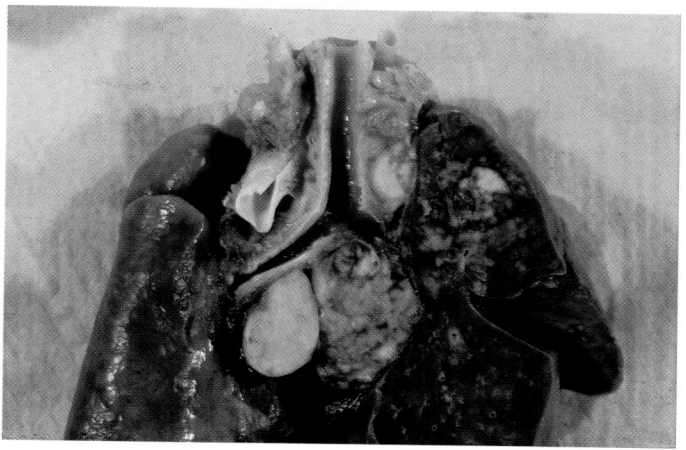

A

Plate 57.5: (**A**) Post-mortem lung specimen showing the 'primary complex': caseating primary lesion (Ghon's focus) with regional lymphadenitis.

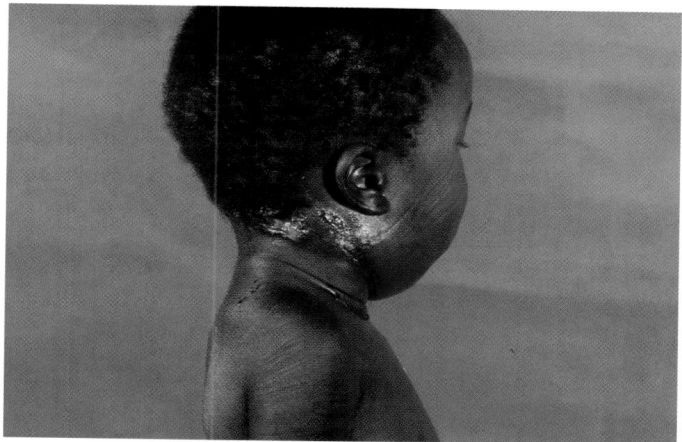

Plate 57.8: Caseating cervical lymph nodes in child with tuberculosis.

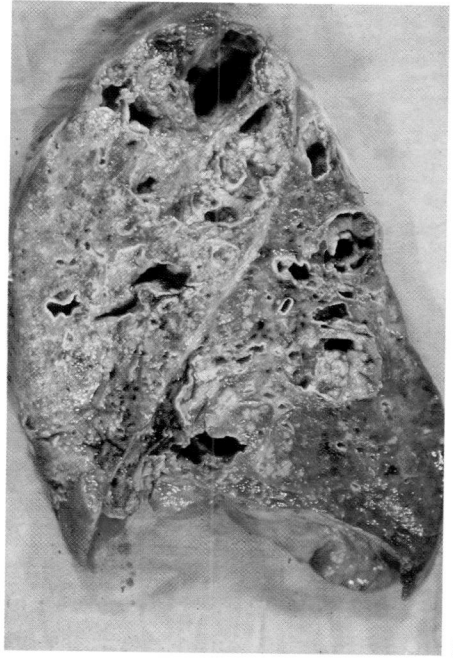

B

Plate 57.9: (**B**) Post-mortem lung showing several cavities and extensive lung involvement due to tuberculosis.

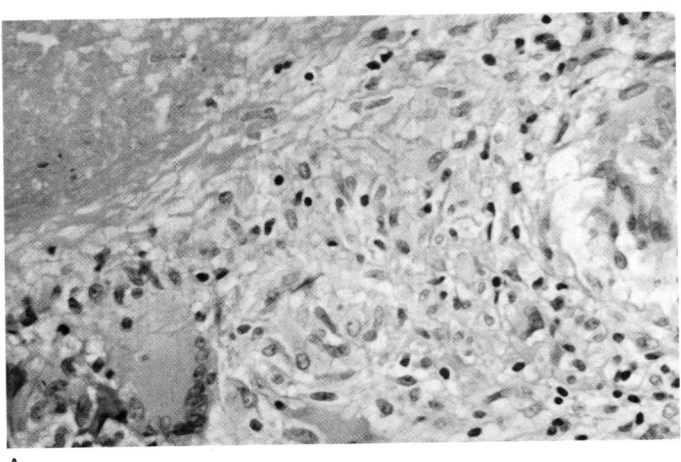

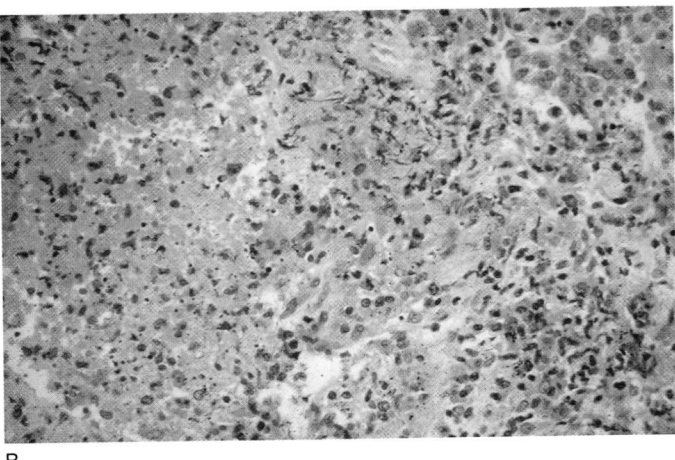

A

B

Plate 57.10: (**A**) Classical caseating granuloma due to *M. tuberculosis*. Note the central area of caseous necrosis surrounded by a rim of epithelioid cells, Langhans giant cells and lymphocytic infiltrate. (**B**) Lung histopathology illustrating an 'anergic response' to infection with *M. tuberculosis* in a lung of a patient with AIDS. There is widespread granular necrosis and a non-reactive 'anergic' cellular response with a few lymphocytes and epithelioid cells and no Langhans giant cells.

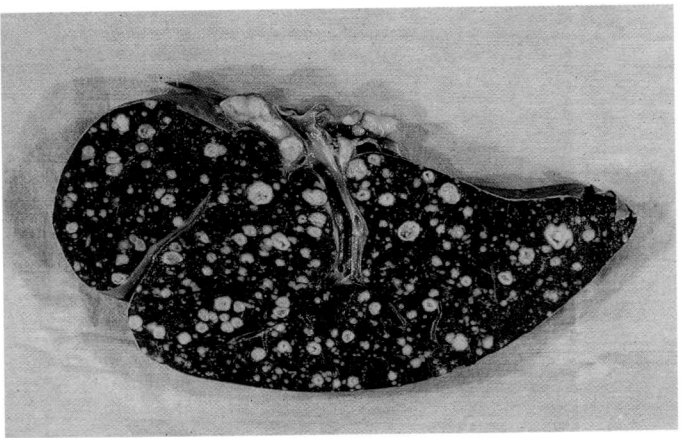

Plate 57.28: Miliary tuberculosis involving the spleen.

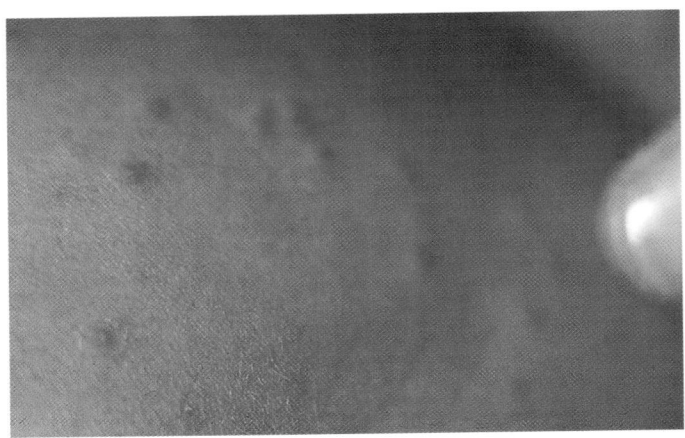

Plate 57.29: Grouped erythematous papules on the skin of the face in miliary tuberculosis.

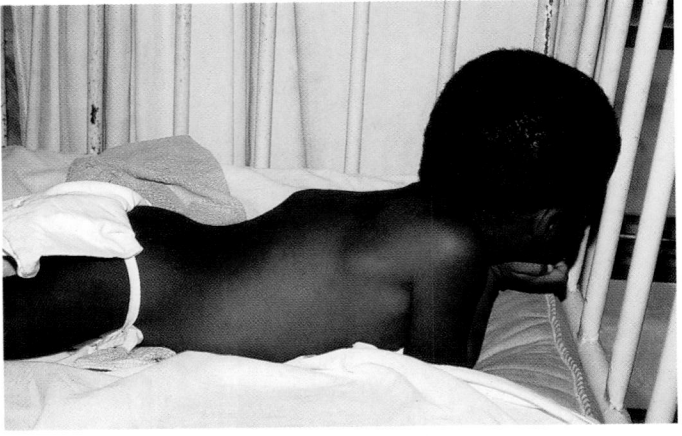

Plate 57.32: Pott's disease of the spine: spinal tuberculosis in a child showing a visible, palpable lump (gibbus) over the spine. The nappy was being used for urinary incontinence caused by spinal cord involvement.

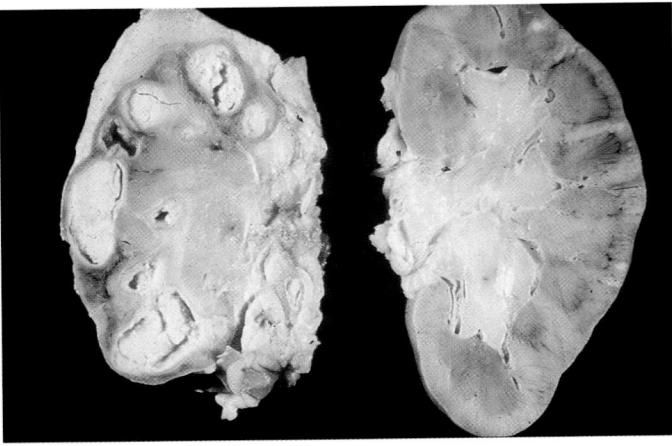

Plate 57.39: Post-mortem kidney specimens showing caseating tuberculosis lesions.

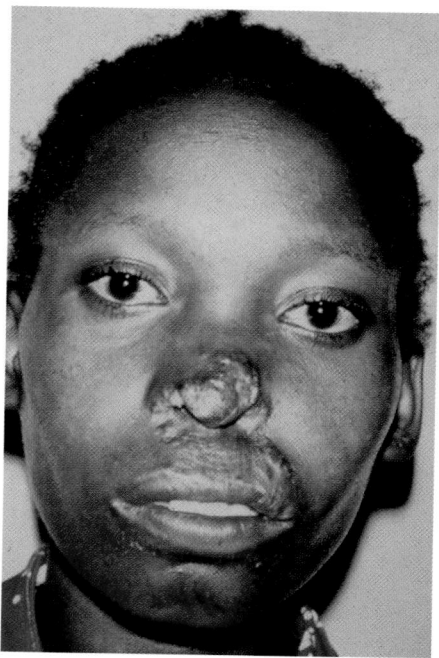

Plate 57.47: Chronic granulomatous skin lesions due to
M. tuberculosis on the nose and around the mouth (lupus vulgaris).

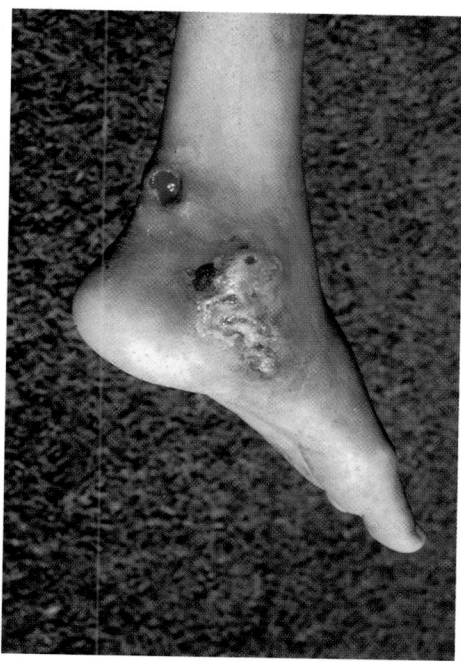

Plate 57.48: Verrucous plaque, chronic granulomatous reaction and
superficial ulceration of the foot due to skin tuberculosis: 'tuberculosis
verrucosa cutis'.

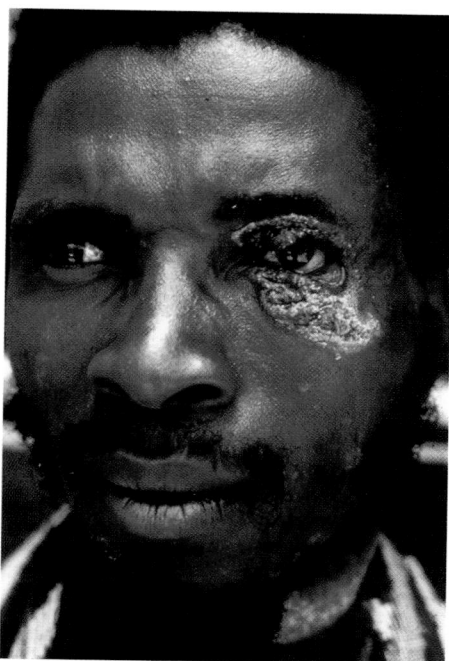

Plate 57.52: Chronic granulomatous skin lesions on the face due to
M. tuberculosis (lupus vulgaris).

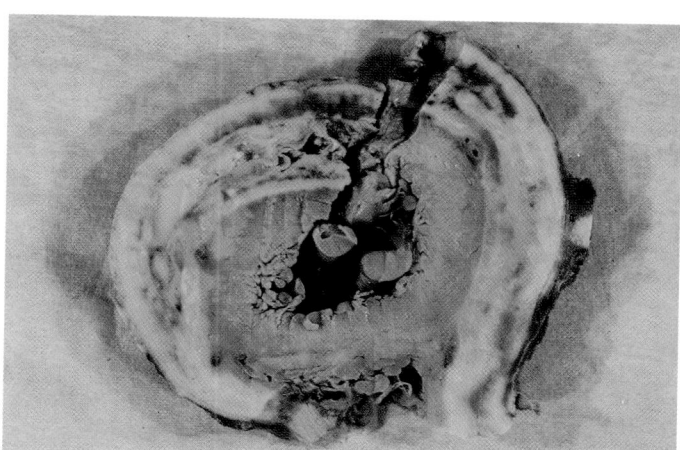

Plate 57.58: Section of the heart showing chronic tuberculous
pericarditis. Note the 2 cm thick band of tuberculous caseation.

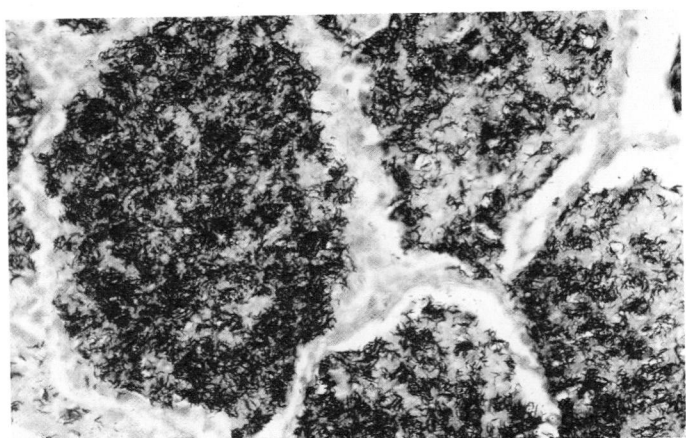

Plate 57.60: Lung histopathology of an AIDS patient who died of tuberculosis. Note the vast number of acid-fast tubercle bacilli in the alveolar necrotic exudate.

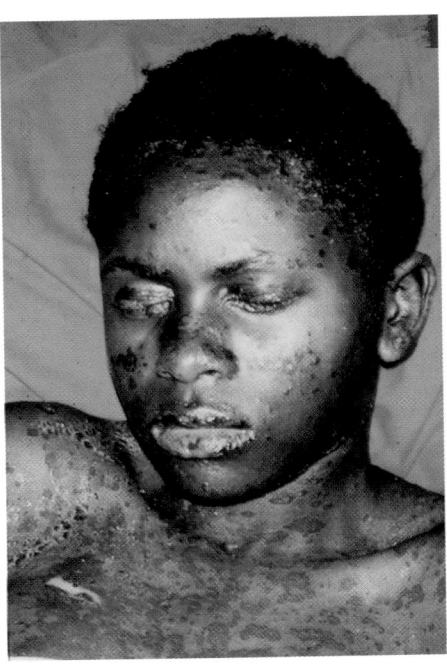

Plate 57.62: Stevens-Johnson syndrome due to thiacetazone.

Abdominal tuberculosis

This is divisible into intestinal and peritoneal disease. The former is due to primary infection, usually due to drinking milk containing *M. bovis* or as a manifestation of post-primary disease as a result of swallowing sputum containing tubercle bacilli. The latter is the result of lymphatic or haematogenous dissemination from a primary focus, usually pulmonary, or to spread from an infected intra-abdominal organ such as the intestine or a Fallopian tube.

Primary intestinal tuberculosis usually involves the ileocaecal region and results in mucosal hypertrophy which, together with enlarged lymph nodes, presents as a tender mass in the right iliac fossa. Complications include malabsorption, intestinal obstruction, fistulae, peritonitis and, rarely, massive rectal bleeding which may be life-threatening.

The stomach and small intestine are the usual sites of post-primary lesions and ulceration, rather than hypertrophy, is characteristic, with a risk of intestinal perforation leading to peritonitis. Symptoms include loss of weight, anorexia, diarrhoea, fever and night sweats. A mass, usually in the right iliac fossa, may be palpable. Some patients present with intestinal strictures causing subacute obstruction, suggesting carcinoma. Swallowed tubercle bacilli may enter anal fissures and lead to local granulomatous lesions and fistula formation.

The principal groups of patients developing tuberculous peritonitis are young women and older alcoholic men. It is a common cause of ascites: in a study in Lesotho it was found to account for 42% of all cases of ascites.[56] Diagnosis is difficult, especially in elderly alcoholics, as the symptoms and signs are non-specific. The 'doughy abdomen' cited in many textbooks as a classical sign is an uncommon manifestation of advanced disease.

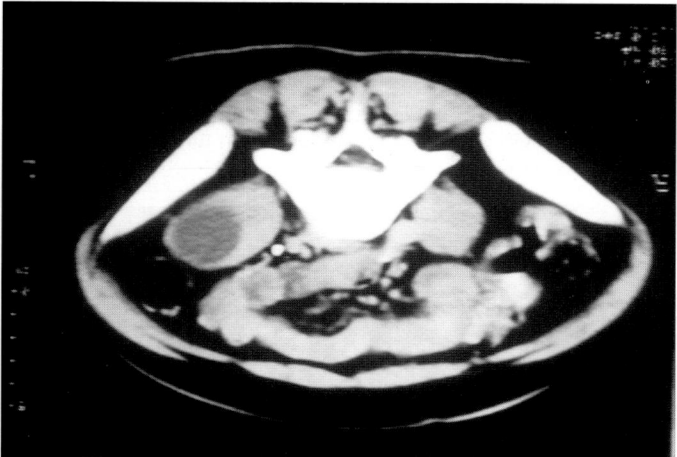

Figure 57.43: Abdominal CT scan. Left psoas abscess. Pus aspirate grew *M. tuberculosis*.

Diagnosis of abdominal tuberculosis

Where available, ultrasonography may demonstrate ascites, thickened intestinal walls and enlarged mesenteric lymph nodes.[57] Colonoscopy enables biopsies to be obtained from the caecal region, which is commonly involved in primary disease. Diagnosis of tuberculous peritonitis is made by examination of peritoneal biopsies obtained by laparoscopy or through a 3–4 cm midline abdominal incision under local anaesthetic.[58] Aspirated peritoneal fluid is usually negative on examination. Other viscera in the abdominal cavity may be affected by tuberculosis and tuberculosis lesions in the psoas muscle (Figure 57.43), para-aortic nodes (Figures 57.44 and 57.45) and spleen (Figure 57.28) are illustrated.

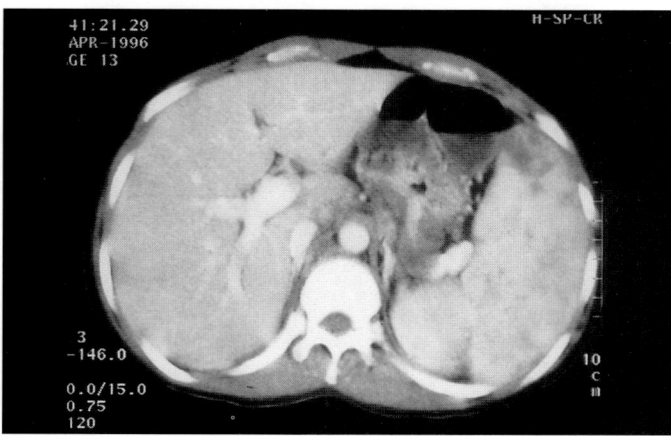

Figure 57.44: Abdominal CT, post-contrast, at level of splenic hilum.

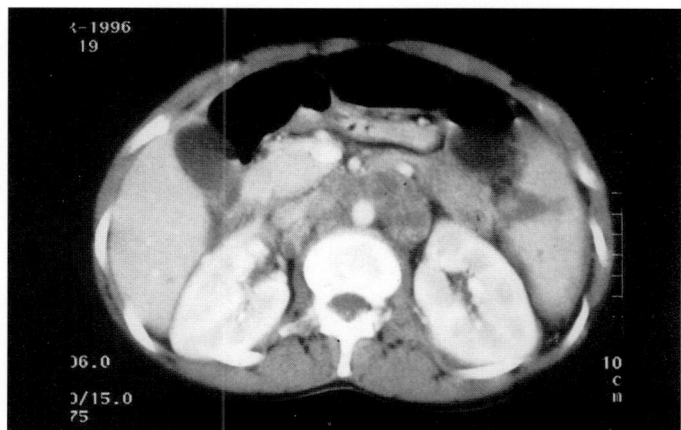

Figure 57.45: Hypo-attenuating lesions in the spleen and associated para-aortic lymph nodes. The main differential lies between lymphoma and tuberculosis. The cystic change in the lymph nodes on the lower cuts, with strongly enhancing periphery, favours tuberculosis.

Management

Treatment is by standard chemotherapy although the mortality among elderly alcoholics is high: 26% in a study in Lesotho. Subacute obstruction may be relieved by steroid therapy. Surgery is required for the rare cases of massive rectal bleeding.

Skin tuberculosis

Skin tuberculosis can manifest in several ways (Figures 57.46–57.52). This form of tuberculosis has accumulated a large number of quaint and outmoded names which confuse the description of the disease. There are four main categories of skin tuberculosis:

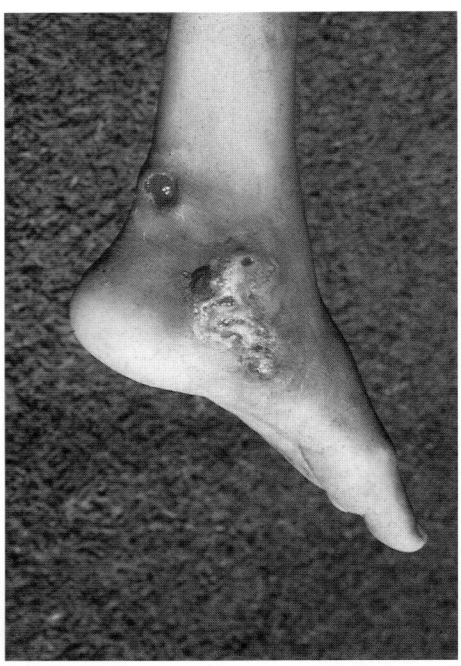

Figure 57.48: Verrucous plaque, chronic granulomatous reaction and superficial ulceration of the foot due to skin tuberculosis: 'tuberculosis verrucosa cutis'.

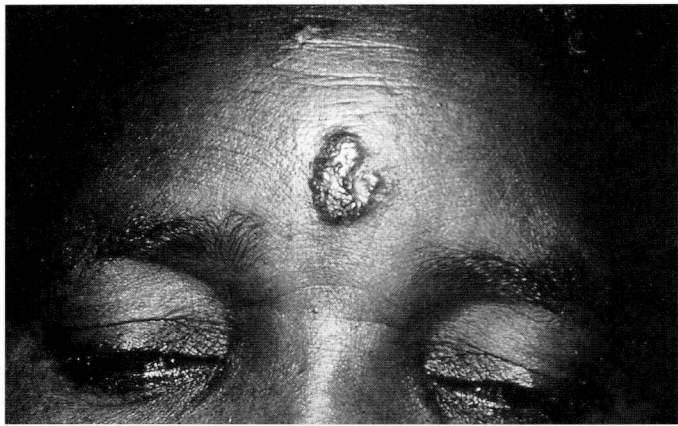

Figure 57.46: Chronic skin lesion on forehead due to *M. tuberculosis*.

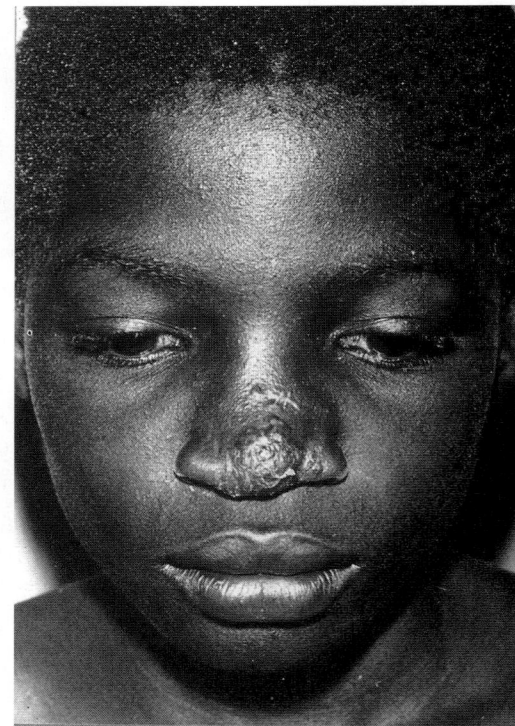

Figure 57.49: Lupus vulgaris of the face. Chronic ulcerating granulomatous lesion due to *M. tuberculosis*.

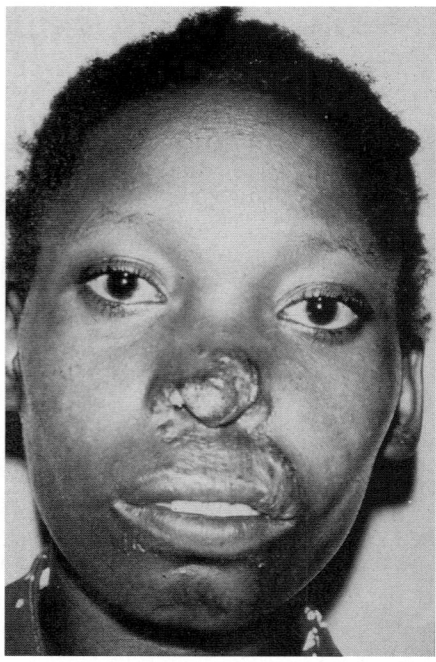

Figure 57.47: Chronic granulomatous skin lesions due to *M. tuberculosis* on the nose and around the mouth (lupus vulgaris).

- Inoculation into skin injuries: this may be due either to primary exogenous infection or autoinoculation by contaminated sputum in patients with post-primary pulmonary tuberculosis (tuberculosis orificialis cutis).

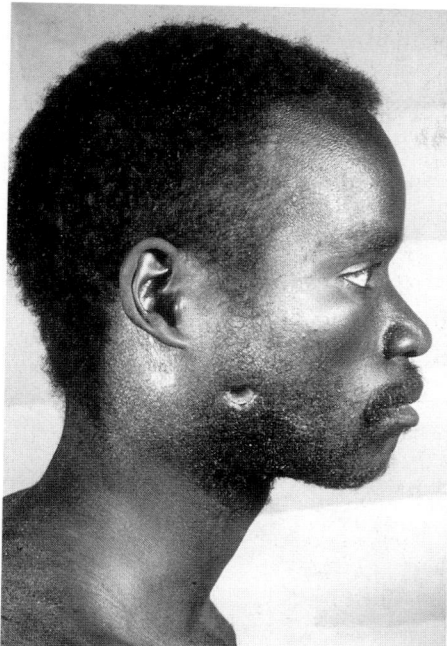

Figure 57.50: Chronic ulcerating lesion with parotid fistula due to parotid gland tuberculosis.

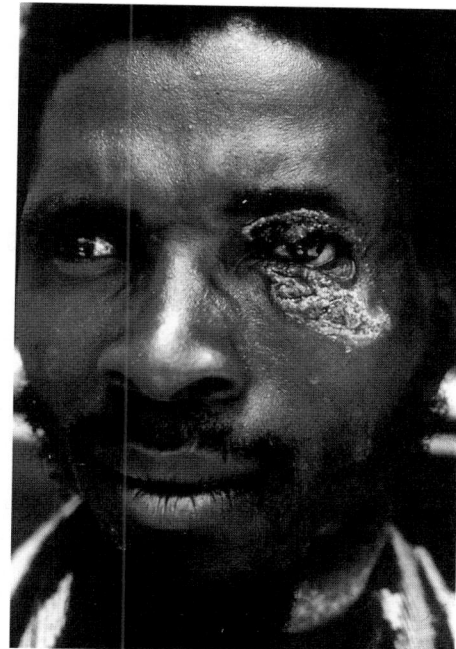

Figure 57.52: Chronic granulomatous skin lesions on the face due to *M. tuberculosis* (lupus vulgaris).

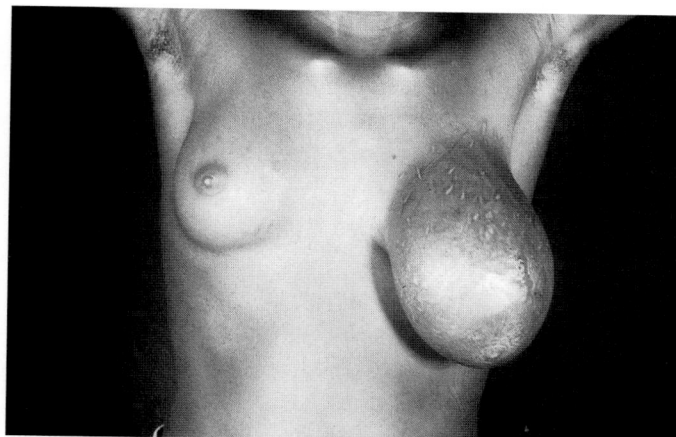

Figure 57.51: Tuberculous mastitis affecting the left breast.

The latter may occur on or near the mouth, and also on the anus as a result of implantation of swallowed sputum containing tubercle bacilli.
- Lesions resulting from direct extension of disease from underlying organs or tissues such as lymph nodes, bones or the thoracic cage.
- Lesions resulting from haematogenous dissemination from an internal organ.
- A range of skin lesions of uncertain pathogenesis termed tuberculides.

Primary inoculation tuberculosis is an occupational hazard of butchers and pathologists and an old name for it is 'prosector's or butcher's wart'.[59] Occasional cases occur in medical laboratory workers and in children exposed to sources of infection. Warty lesions develop at the inoculation site and there may be secondary lesions along the draining lymphatics and regional lymphadenopathy. It is, in common with other forms of primary tuberculosis, often self-limiting.

Extension of disease from underlying structures results in sinus formation. The usual cause is a spread from an underlying tuberculous lymph node: a condition termed 'scrofuloderma'.

Lupus vulgaris is a very slowly progressive and chronic form of skin tuberculosis that usually occurs on the nose, cheeks or neck and, if untreated, may cause severe disfigurement (Figures 57.47, 57.49 and 57.52). It is characterized by red-brown semi-translucent nodules which may subsequently coalesce and ulcerate. When compressed with a glass slide the nodules often have an opalescent 'apple jelly' appearance. It is due either to haematogenous dissemination of tubercle bacilli from internal organs or to secondary spread from scrofuloderma. There is some evidence to suggest that lupus vulgaris is more likely to be caused by *M. bovis* than *M. tuberculosis*. Several small skin papules may be seen in cases of miliary tuberculosis (Figure 57.29).

The tuberculides are uncommon and poorly understood skin lesions associated with tuberculosis.[60] Two main types have been described: lichen scrofulosorum and papulonecrotic tuberculide. These are characterized, respectively, by non-necrotic dermal granulomas with epithelioid and giant cells and by tissue necrosis, sometimes extensive, due to an obliterative vasculitis. The aetiology of the tuberculides is unknown but it has been suggested that they are due to hypersensitivity reactions to blood-borne whole tubercle bacilli, bacillary debris or antigens. The rarely encountered erythema induratum (Bazin's disease) and tuberculosis-associated idiopathic gangrene of the extremities may be due to similar necrotic hypersensitivity reactions in larger blood vessels. Lupus vulgaris occasionally develops at the site of a tuberculide, indicating the presence of viable tubercle bacilli.

Superficial lymph nodes

Tuberculous lymphadenitis is well documented in early literature in which it is referred, for unknown reasons, as scrofula (Figures 57.8, 57.53–57.57). The usual site is the neck and two main types have been described: that due to primary inoculation of bacilli, usually milk-borne *M. bovis*, into the pharynx and that secondary to intrathoracic primary complexes. Lymphadenopathy also occurs as a component of disseminated tuberculosis in HIV-positive patients. Lymphadenopathy in children aged 5 years or below is occasionally caused by other mycobacterial species.

Lymphadenopathy associated with a primary pharyngeal lesion usually affects the tonsillar and pre-auricular nodes, while the supraclavicular nodes are involved when the disease is due to an upward extension of an intrathoracic primary complex. The latter is more common in females than males. In early disease, affected nodes are discrete, rubbery in texture and usually painless. Constitutional symptoms occur in less than half the patients. Subsequently, the affected glands may undergo necrosis and become fluctuant, and the disease may invade the surrounding tissues and ultimately the skin with the formation of sinuses. The disease process may then spread into the surrounding skin—a condition termed 'scrofuloderma'. There are relatively few tubercle bacilli in the affected lymph nodes: much of the enlargement is due to the

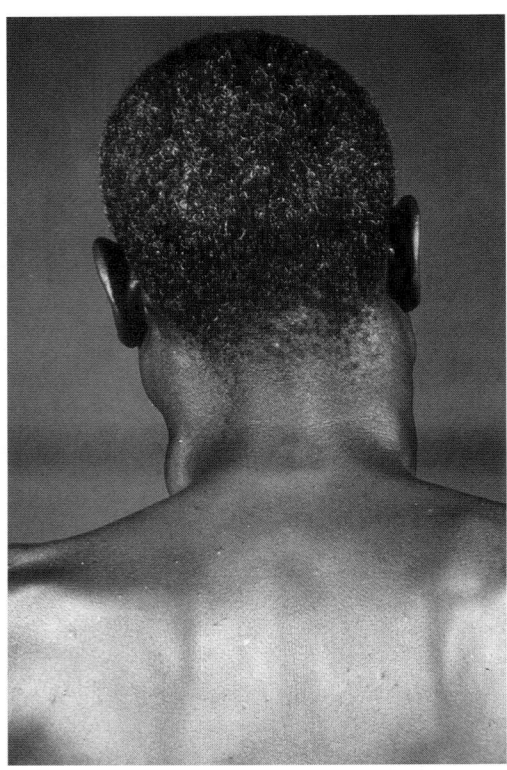

Figure 57.54: Cervical lymphadenopathy due to tuberculosis in an HIV-positive Zambian adult.

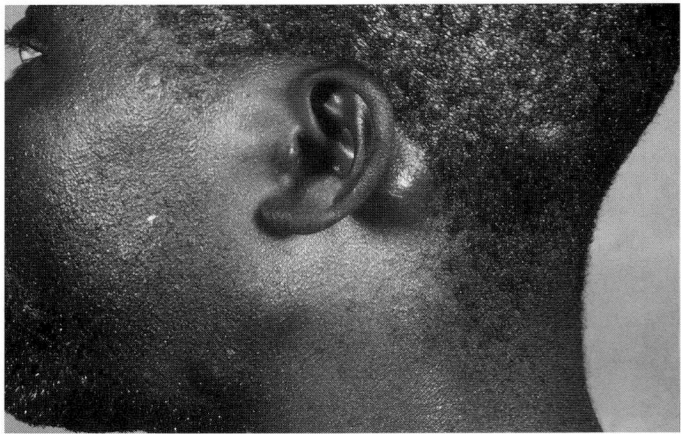

Figure 57.55: Enlarged posterior auricular lymph node in an HIV-positive adult. *M. tuberculosis* was isolated from a lymph node aspirate.

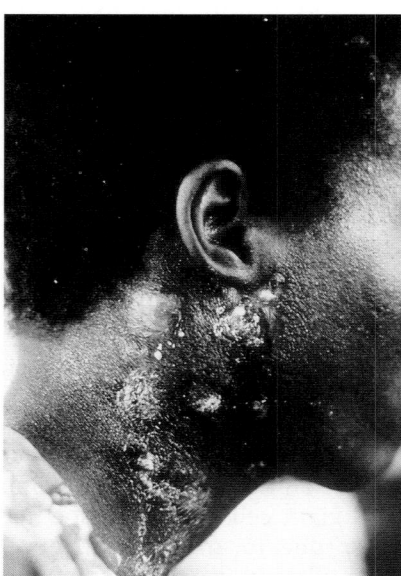

Figure 57.53: Enlarged tuberculous cervical lymph nodes exuding caseous material ('open tuberculosis').

immune response. Microscopy is positive for acid-fast bacilli in less than half the cases and cultures are positive in only 60–70%. Diagnosis is thus often based on histological examination of biopsies or cytological examination of fine-needle aspirates which, in trained hands, establishes the diagnosis in 80% of cases.[61] The tuberculin test is usually positive and a chest X-ray often reveals lesions of pulmonary tuberculosis. Tuberculous lymphadenopathy must be differentiated from other infections, lymphomas and other neoplasms, sarcoidosis and branchial cysts.

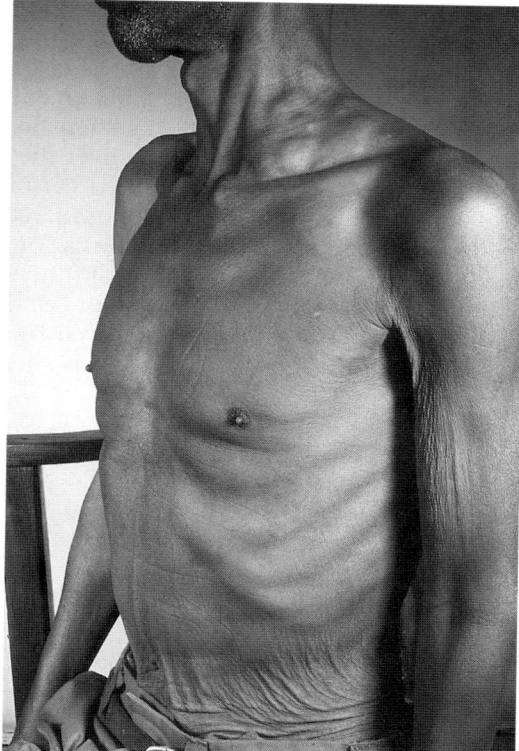

Figure 57.56: Enlarged cervical and supraclavicular lymph nodes in an HIV-positive Zambian patient. *M. tuberculosis* was isolated from lymph node aspirates. Note the generalized muscle wasting.

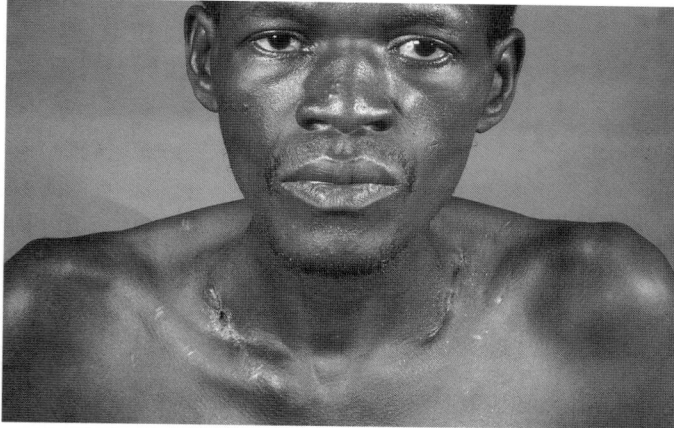

Figure 57.57: Supraclavicular lymphadenopathy due to *M. tuberculosis*.

Tuberculous lymphadenopathy responds to standard short-course chemotherapy. Nodes may undergo enlargement, sometimes quite extensive and with sinus formation, during the course of therapy but this is due to hypersensitivity reactions and usually responds to steroid therapy. Surgical intervention is seldom indicated.

Tuberculosis at other sites

Tuberculous lesions may develop in any site of the body although muscles are rarely involved, except in widespread disseminated disease.

Tuberculous pericarditis

This occurs either as a manifestation of miliary disease or secondary to the rupture of an involved mediastinal lymph node into the pericardial sac. Although uncommon, a high incidence of tuberculous pericarditis occurs, for unknown reasons, in certain regions such as the Transkei, where it has been termed the 'Transkei heart'.[62] Exudates cause distension of the pericardium, exerting pressure on the heart (cardiac tamponade) which may be sufficient to cause heart failure and requiring urgent aspiration of the fluid. Clinical findings include chest pain, fever, breathlessness, low blood pressure, a rapid pulse and a raised jugular venous pressure. Hepatomegaly and ascites may be detected in severe cases. An enlarged heart shadow is visible on chest X-ray and the presence of pericardial fluid is confirmed by ultrasonography. T wave changes may be seen on electrocardiography. Diagnosis is confirmed by bacteriological examination of the effusion or pericardial biopsies. The case fatality is very high (Figure 57.58).

High-dose corticosteroid therapy, such as prednisolone 80 mg daily for 1 week and then progressively reduced over the ensuing 6–8 weeks reduces the size of the effusion and associated mortality and also the incidence of constrictive sequelae. Healing with fibrosis and calcification may result in chronic constriction of the heart, requiring surgical relief (Figure 57.59). Tuberculous myocardial lesions are very rare but are a cause of fatal heart block.

Tuberculosis of upper respiratory tract

Tuberculous laryngitis is usually due to the implantation of tubercle bacilli from sputum. The principal clinical feature is pain, which may be severe enough to prevent eating. Speech is often affected. The disease may occur in

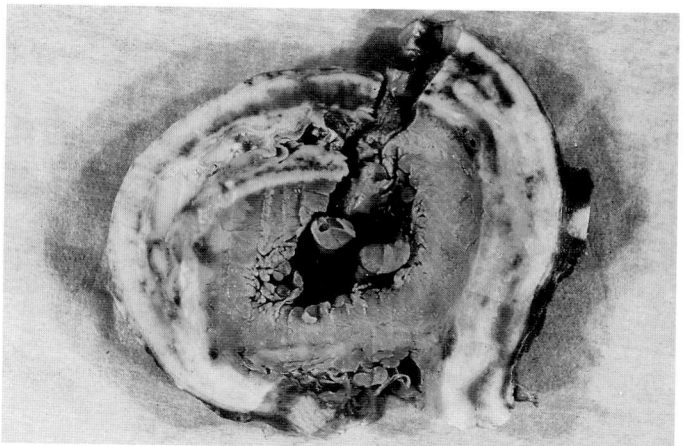

Figure 57.58: Section of the heart showing chronic tuberculous pericarditis. Note the 2 cm thick band of tuberculous caseation.

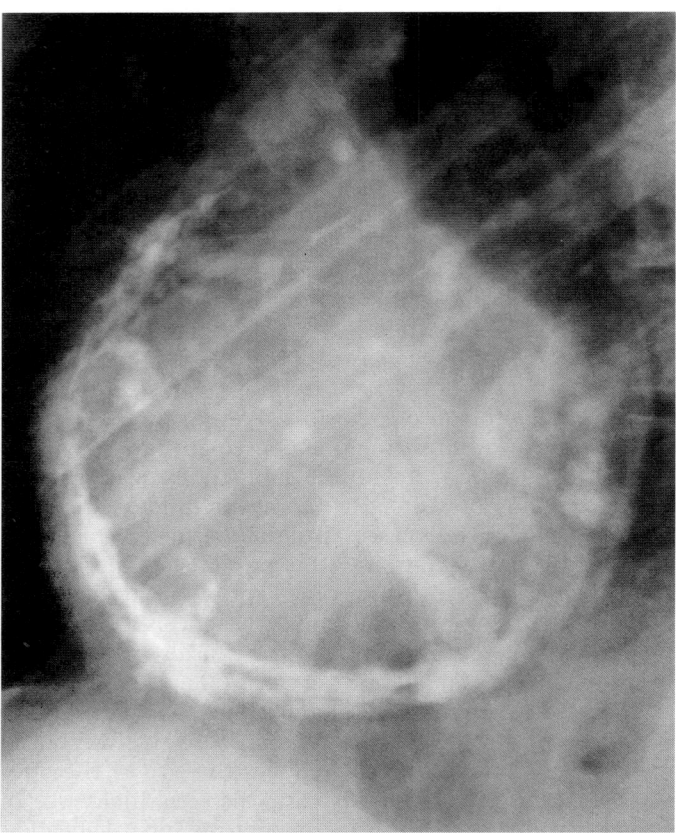

Figure 57.59: Constrictive tuberculous pericarditis: X-ray shows pericardial calcification.

the absence of radiological evidence of pulmonary tuberculosis, especially in older patients, and may thus be misdiagnosed as cancer. Diagnosis is made by histological examination of biopsy. Pain responds rapidly to corticosteroid therapy.

Primary tuberculous lesions occasionally occur in the nose, pharynx, epiglottis and Eustachian tubes or on the gums. The presenting feature may be an enlarged cervical lymph node. Lesions in the Eustachian tube may spread to the middle ear and mastoid.

Ocular tuberculosis

The eye may be involved in disseminated tuberculosis as, for example, choroidal lesions in miliary tuberculosis or by direct invasion from surrounding skin in lupus vulgaris (Figure 57.49).[63–65] Primary lesions under the eyelids rarely occur in young children exposed to source cases. The eyelids are swollen, the eye becomes irritable and the disease may spread to the pre-auricular lymph nodes.

The optic nerve may be damaged in tuberculous meningitis, sometimes leading to blindness.

Adrenal gland

Tuberculosis is a well-recognized but uncommon cause of hypoadrenalism or Addison's disease and is the result of haematogenous spread of tubercle bacilli to the adrenal gland. The clinical features of Addison's disease include weakness, weight loss, low blood pressure, amenorrhoea and gastrointestinal symptoms. A characteristic hyperpigmentation of the skin, most notably over the elbows and the lower back, occurs in fair-skinned persons. Pigmented patches also occur in the mouth, a useful sign in dark-skinned patients. Diagnosis of hypoadrenalism is confirmed by tests of adrenal function and tuberculosis is suggested by the presence of calcification in the adrenals visible on abdominal X-rays. Hormonal replacement, in addition to antituberculosis therapy, is required.

Other manifestations of tuberculosis

Tuberculosis of the breast presents as a painless mastitis which is easily confused with cancer (Figure 57.52). Tuberculous breast abscesses may follow rupture of involved intercostal lymph nodes through the chest wall. Tuberculous nodules or abscesses may occur in the thyroid.

Discrete hepatic tuberculous lesions are a very rare cause of hepatomegaly but the liver is frequently involved in disseminated tuberculosis. The liver is also usually involved in congenital tuberculosis due to infection via the umbilical artery.

Tuberculosis in HIV-infected persons

Infection with HIV appears to be the highest risk factor for reactivation of tuberculosis in populations who are dually infected with *M. tuberculosis* and HIV. In 1997, approximately 11 million people were thought to be dually infected with the two organisms. The strongest association between HIV and tuberculosis has been recorded in sub-Saharan Africa. HIV seropositivity rates among adults and children with tuberculosis range from 20% to 70%, and there are some countries such as Malawi and Zambia where HIV seroprevalence rates are consistently above 50%. In Zambia and Côte d'Ivoire,[13,66] HIV seroprevalence rates in children with tuberculosis aged 1 month to 14 years are between 10% and 40%, with the highest overall age-specific HIV seroprevalence being found in children aged 1–4 years. Molecular studies from the USA using DNA fingerprinting techniques have shown that, in almost two-thirds of HIV-infected persons, tuberculosis is due to recent infection rather than reactivation of latent infection. Similarly, recent work from sub-Saharan Africa has shown that a significant number of new cases of tuberculosis, and recurrent cases of tuberculosis, also result from recent transmission.

Effects of tuberculosis on HIV

It is recognized that HIV infection worsens the risk and clinical course of tuberculosis. Conversely, co-infection with *M. tuberculosis* accelerates progression of disease caused by HIV-1 infection. It is now well known that tuberculous infection enhances local HIV-1 replication in vivo, although the exact mechanisms operating are not known. Cytokines produced during infection with *M. tuberculosis* may result in activation of latently HIV-infected cells with virus expression and induction of virus replication. Recent studies have demonstrated marked increases in plasma viral load in tuberculosis. Increased IL-2, IL-6 and TNFα (Th-2 type cytokines) generated by infection with *M. tuberculosis* may be responsible for these increases in HIV viral load.

Pathology of tuberculosis in HIV infection

Autopsy studies in Africa showed that 38% of all HIV-positive cadavers and 43–54% of those dying with AIDS-defining pathology had active tuberculosis.[67,68] Autopsy studies in HIV-positive patients with tuberculosis show fibrous and calcified lesions of tuberculosis adjacent to recent active lesions with bacilli. These new lesions may be due to reactivation of primary complex lesions but they could also be due to reinfection. Relapse has been observed with different genotypes of *M. tuberculosis*, suggesting reinfection. The suggested mechanism of reactivation or increase in susceptibility to mycobacterial infections is the HIV-related depletion of CD4+ lymphocytes and macrophages, although tuberculosis has been seen in patients with a range of CD4+ lymphocyte counts. Quantitative and qualitative defects of these cells lead to impaired granuloma formation. In patients infected with HIV, the progressive decline of CD4+ lymphocytes provides a suitable model for the study of the role of the interaction between the mononuclear cells and formation of epithelioid granulomas. In non-HIV infected patients with tuberculosis, without any obvious evidence of immunodeficiency, granuloma formation and progression of human monocytes through stages of differentiation are well characterized and are typical of cell-mediated immune responses found in other granulomatous disorders. The monocytes differentiate through young macrophages and mature macrophages to epithelioid cells and finally to giant cells of the Langhans type. In HIV-infected patients a range of histological features are seen. Those persons with a well preserved CD4+ lymphocyte count show well-formed epithelioid granuloma formation, while poor epithelioid cell formation and 'sick' macrophages occur in patients with more severe forms of immunodeficiency.

Histopathological features of tuberculosis in HIV-infected persons

There are three identifiable histological stages of cellular immune responses which correlate well with the stage of HIV infection:[6] granulomatous response, hyporeactive response and anergic response.

Granulomatous response

These patients have relatively intact cellular immune responses, including a typical granulomatous response. Epithelioid macrophages and Langhans giant cells are abundant, the numbers of mycobacteria are low and there are clusters of CD4+ T cells around epithelioid macrophages and Langhans giant cells. The majority of macrophages have abundant cytoplasm and stain intensely with KP-1 (CD68) macrophage markers.

Hyporeactive response

With progressive immunosuppression and decline of CD4+ T cell counts, loss of Langhans giant cells and, subsequently, epithelioid cells occurs. The proportion of macrophages with abundant cytoplasm is also decreased. Intracellular killing of mycobacteria is compromised and therefore the number of mycobacteria increase. The caseous centres enlarge centrifugally and lesions coalesce. A mixture of suppurative and caseous necrosis is seen.

Anergic response

In the late stages of AIDS, disseminated anergic tuberculosis develops and is often first detected at autopsy. While no relative decrease in number of macrophages in the tuberculous lesion is seen, there is decreased intensity of staining with CD68. Epithelioid cells are scanty, Langhans giant cells are absent and granuloma formation is not

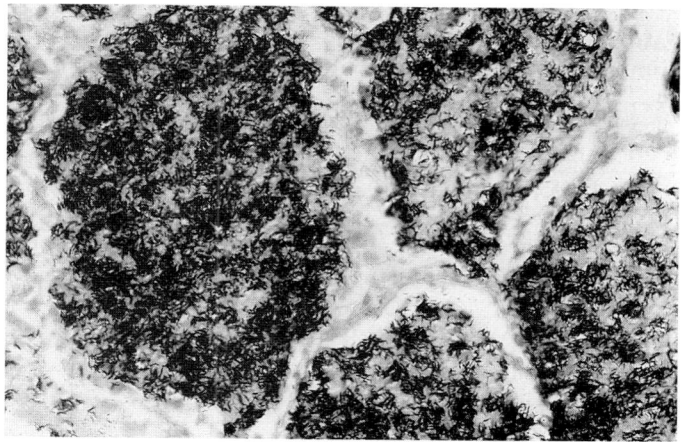

Figure 57.60: Lung histopathology of an AIDS patient who died of tuberculosis. Note the vast number of acid-fast tubercle bacilli in the alveolar necrotic exudate.

seen (Figures 57.10A and B). There are few CD4+ T cells in the lesions. Caseous necrosis is replaced by suppuration, coagulative necrosis and large amounts of apoptotic debris. Large numbers of mycobacteria are present within macrophages and in the necrotic areas (Figure 57.60).

Clinical manifestations of HIV-related tuberculosis

Pulmonary tuberculosis occurs in patients with a wide spectrum of immunodeficiency and is not entirely dependent on the degree of depletion of CD4+ lymphocytes. The clinical manifestations of tuberculosis are related to the extent of immunodeficiency. Around 30% of cases of tuberculosis in HIV-positive patients are extrapulmonary. If tuberculosis occurs in the early stages of HIV infection when immunity is only partially compromised, the features are characteristic of those which occur in post-primary tuberculosis in HIV-negative persons. Tuberculosis is localized to the apices of the lungs; there is lung destruction and cavitation and abundant acid-fast bacilli are seen on sputum microscopy. HIV-positive patients with more advanced immunodeficiency present with atypical pulmonary disease characterized by extensive pulmonary infiltrates with limited or no cavitation, involvement of the lower lobes of the lung, enlargement of the lymph glands around the hilar region and sputum smears which show no acid-fast bacilli. Dissemination of the disease beyond the lung is common.

Diagnosis of pulmonary tuberculosis in HIV-positive adults

The proportion of patients with smear-negative pulmonary tuberculosis is greater in those with HIV infection than in those who are HIV-negative. The diagnosis of tuberculosis in an HIV-positive patient with a chronic cough, night sweats, weight loss but negative sputum smears for acid-fast bacilli is a diagnostic challenge for the clinician. In studies in HIV-positive African patients with respiratory illness and negative sputum smears, about one-third have M. tuberculosis confirmed using bronchoscopy with bronchoalveolar lavage or induced sputum. Another third have other pathogens or diseases such as PCP, bacterial pneumonia due to a wide range of pathogens, Kaposi's sarcoma, nocardiosis and fungal infections. Even where facilities exist for more extensive investigations (e.g. bronchoscopy with bronchoalveolar lavage and biopsy, sputum culture and molecular methods) the identification of the M. tuberculosis may be difficult. In most developing country health centres, the diagnosis of pulmonary tuberculosis is based on simple techniques only: sputum smear microscopy and chest radiography, when available.

On radiological examination, the lesions may resemble those of typical pulmonary tuberculosis but atypical appearances are common, notably in the more profoundly immunosuppressed. These include vague, spreading opacities suggestive of pneumonia, predominantly lower lobe disease, pleural effusions, air–fluid levels and intrathoracic lymphadenopathy. It is important to note that many HIV-positive tuberculosis patients in the tropics have a different pattern of chest X-ray changes from HIV-negative patients.[69] A significantly increased incidence of lymphadenopathy, pleural effusions, parenchymal changes, consolidation and miliary disease, but significantly less cavitating disease and atelectasis, is seen in HIV-infected adults. These radiological features may change rapidly in appearance. Studies from the USA and sub-Saharan Africa have found that the chest radiograph becomes more atypical (with lower lobe infiltrates, no cavities, intrathoracic adenopathy) as immunosuppression becomes pronounced, and in a significant proportion of patients the chest radiograph can be normal. Classical miliary lesions are seen in a minority of HIV-positive patients with disseminated disease; in most cases the formation of the characteristic miliary granuloma is suppressed and the X-rays may appear deceptively normal. The atypical clinical and radiological features seen in the more profoundly immunosuppressed patients are summarized in

Table 57.7 Comparison of the clinical and radiological characteristics of postprimary tuberculosis in non-immunosuppressed and immunosuppressed persons

Characteristic	Non-immunosuppressed	Immunosuppressed
Pulmonary cavitation	Prominent	Diminished or absent
Localization by fibrosis	Marked	Limited
Intrathoracic lymphadenopathy	Uncommon	Common
Pleural effusions	Present	Very common
Miliary disease	Uncommon	Common
Atelectasis	Uncommon	Common
Lymphatic and haematogenous dissemination	Uncommon	Common
Adverse drug reactions	Uncommon	Common
Tuberculin test	Positive	Small reaction or negative
Relapse following therapy	Uncommon	Frequent
Mortality rate	Low	Increased

Table 57.7. Further details on the clinical aspects of HIV-related tuberculosis are available from the World Health Organization.[70]

Extrapulmonary tuberculosis in HIV-positive adults

Frequent manifestations of extrapulmonary tuberculosis seen in HIV-infected persons in sub-Saharan Africa include pleural disease, lymphadenopathy (usually asymmetrical), miliary disease and pericardial disease. Tuberculosis affecting the CNS, genitourinary tract and bone marrow is, in contrast to the industrialized countries, infrequently reported but this probably reflects patient selection and differences in the availability of diagnostic facilities. Patients usually present with non-specific constitutional symptoms (fever, night sweats and weight loss) and local symptoms and signs related to the site of disease. Lymphadenopathy is a frequent manifestation of tuberculosis in HIV-infected persons and can present in a variety of ways. While usually chronic and cryptic, it may also occasionally be acute and resemble an acute pyogenic infection. Diagnosis of lymph node tuberculosis can be made using simple techniques such as needle aspiration and staining for acid-fast bacilli; naked eye inspection of biopsied lymph nodes for macroscopic caseation; and microscopy of smears from the cut surface of a lymph node. The CSF may be normal or near-normal in HIV-infected patients with tuberculous meningitis and can easily be confused with cryptococcal meningitis (a common presenting feature of HIV infection), making the diagnosis very difficult. Empirical treatment may have to be given on clinical suspicion alone.

Management considerations in HIV-positive persons

There are several specific management issues which arise in the treatment of HIV-infected persons with tuberculosis. These patients overall tend to have:

1. Increased morbidity rates.
2. Increased mortality rates.
3. Increased number of drug side effects.
4. Serious interactions between antiretroviral drugs and antituberculosis drugs.
5. Immune reconstitution syndrome.
6. Increased recurrence rates after completion of treatment.

Increased morbidity rates
Clinical response to antituberculosis treatment, clearing of chest X-ray abnormalities and sputum conversion rates occur at the same rates during treatment in both HIV-positive and HIV-negative patients with tuberculosis. On the other hand, HIV-positive patients on treatment for tuberculosis often have other opportunistic infections and tumours and thus commonly suffer from recurrent fever, chest infections, recurrent diarrhoea, oral candidiasis, bacteraemia, cryptococcosis and Kaposi's sarcoma. This increased morbidity calls for increased prescriptions for antibiotics, antifungal agents, antidiarrhoeal agents and analgesics, rendering the care more expensive than is the case with HIV-negative patients. There is also evidence that delay in the diagnosis and treatment of tuberculosis may compromise the chances of individual cure in HIV-positive patients. Untreated tuberculosis in HIV-infected persons may accelerate the decline in immunocompetence and the progression to severe immunodeficiency.

Increased mortality rates
HIV-positive patients not receiving antiretroviral therapy have a much higher mortality during and after antituberculosis treatment compared with HIV-negative patients. In sub-Saharan Africa, approximately 30% of HIV-positive smear-positive tuberculosis patients die within 12 months of commencing treatment, and about 25% of those who survive die during the subsequent 12 months. The introduction of highly active antiretroviral treatment has dramatically reduced mortality rates in HIV-infected patients in the USA and in Europe. Efforts are being made to make HAART (highly active antiretroviral therapy) available to all HIV-infected patients in developing countries, although the likelihood of this becoming a reality is small. Since opportunistic infections are a cause of mortality in HIV-positive persons with tuberculosis, alternative interventions with prophylactic antibiotics may be useful. A placebo-controlled clinical trial using co-trimoxazole prophylaxis in Côte d'Ivoire in HIV-positive smear-positive pulmonary tuberculosis patients showed a 50% reduction in mortality in those receiving co-trimoxazole.[71] On the basis of these data, UNAIDS has suggested that all tuberculosis programmes in sub-Saharan Africa should consider using co-trimoxazole prophylaxis as an intervention strategy in an attempt to reduce mortality. By contrast, a study from Senegal revealed no advantage in using co-trimoxazole prophylaxis and this suggests that use of such prophylaxis may not be universally applicable.[72] The antibiotic susceptibility patterns of local pathogens and also the costs, cost–benefit and consequences of introduction of prophylactic regimens require careful consideration.

Increased drug side effects
Adverse reactions to antituberculosis drugs are more frequent in HIV-positive patients, leading to interruption of treatment and occasional fatalities. In HIV-positive patients who were given the old treatment regimens in the mid-1980s (streptomycin, isoniazid and thiacetazone), adverse cutaneous reactions occurred in 15–20%, and up to 6% of these reactions were severe, including cases of Stevens–Johnson syndrome (Figure 57.61) and toxic epidermal necrolysis. Cutaneous hypersensitivity reactions were particularly common in HIV-positive children, and severe reactions were frequently associated with death.[73] Thiacetazone, which was a useful and cheap antituberculosis drug in the pre-HIV era, was the main cause

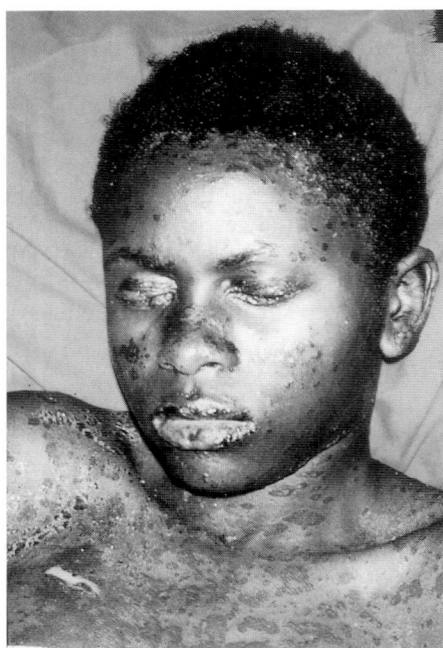

Figure 57.61: Stevens–Johnson syndrome due to thiacetazone.

of adverse cutaneous reactions. For this reason, usage of this drug has now been abandoned in favour of ethambutol. In HIV-positive patients given short-course regimens containing rifampicin, isoniazid and pyrazinamide adverse reactions to antituberculosis drugs appear to be infrequent although side effects to these drugs do occur.

Interactions between antiretroviral drugs and antituberculosis drugs

Serious interactions between antiretroviral and antituberculosis drugs can occur. Protease inhibitors and non-nucleoside reverse transcriptase inhibitors interfere with the metabolism of rifampicin, the most potent of the antituberculosis drugs. Rifampicin is a potent liver cytochrome p450 inducer and thus may enhance the metabolism of protease inhibitors and non-nucleoside reverse transcriptase inhibitors, causing serum levels to be decreased to sub-therapeutic levels.

Immune reconstitution syndrome

The use of antiretroviral therapy and subsequent improvement in immunological parameters may actually make some patients feel worse—a paradoxical response, due to immune reactivation. Patients may develop ascites, lymphadenopathy, fever, increase in size of cerebral lesions and pleural effusions. Clinicians treating tuberculosis in HIV-positive patients receiving antiretroviral therapy need to be aware of this phenomenon.

Drug resistance

Several outbreaks of MDRTB have been reported from industrialized countries among patients infected with HIV.[74] HIV infection itself does not induce MDRTB, but it

fuels the spread of this dangerous condition by increasing susceptibility to infection and accelerating transmission between persons, especially in closed confined spaces such as prisons. Recent data collated from the WHO[75] have shown that MDRTB is highest in India, Eastern Europe, China and South-East Asia, and lowest in sub-Saharan Africa. However, given the problems faced by many tuberculosis programmes in sub-Saharan Africa and the virtual absence of second-line antituberculosis drugs in these countries, MDRTB is a real and potential threat to tuberculosis control in this region. The advent of HIV with large increases in tuberculosis cases has threatened to overwhelm National Tuberculosis Control Programmes in sub-Saharan Africa.

Quality of health care

The capacity and quality of health care provided by the local health service and the health status of the staff (clinical officers, clinicians, nurses, technical personnel) available to care for patients influence the outcome of tuberculosis treatment. The health staff in many African countries have the same HIV-seroprevalence rates as the general adult population, and in some urban areas this approaches 30% or more. High absentee rates from work due to illness or attending funerals, and high death rates of the health care staff due to AIDS, threaten the capacity of many developing countries to deliver good and effective health care. Tuberculosis programmes are no exception to this serious threat.

Recurrence after treatment

Recurrence rates of tuberculosis (defined as return of clinical features of active tuberculosis, positive sputum smears for acid-fast bacilli or positive sputum cultures for *M. tuberculosis*) after completion of antituberculosis therapy are increased in HIV-positive patients. Recurrence rates have been observed at between 18 and 22 per 100 person-years of observation. It is not known to what extent endogenous reactivation or exogenous reinfection contributes to the recurrence of tuberculosis in HIV-infected patients in sub-Saharan Africa. Information on this issue would be of value in determining strategies, such as isoniazid prophylaxis, to prevent recurrence of tuberculosis. Patients who relapse with smear-positive pulmonary tuberculosis are treated with the WHO-recommended retreatment regimen—a regimen based on five drugs on account of the risk of acquired resistance to isoniazid and streptomycin.[76]

Preventive therapy

Preventive treatment with isoniazid for 6–12 months provides significant protection against tuberculosis in HIV-infected adults, at least in the short to medium term.[74,75] Protection seems to be greatest in those with a positive tuberculin skin test, in whom death is also less frequent. Feasibility studies with tuberculosis preventive therapy in sub-Saharan Africa have been disappointing, and no country in the region has yet adopted chemo-prophylaxis as a strategy for tuberculosis control in HIV-positive persons. While it may be difficult to implement chemoprophylaxis as a country-wide control strategy, it could be used safely and selectively in certain situations such as in occupational health services for private businesses and factories, for personnel working in international agencies and missions, and among high-risk groups such as health care workers and prisoners. Isoniazid chemoprophylaxis may be useful in selected groups of people, and it may also be useful to prevent disease recurrence after an episode of tuberculosis has been successfully treated. Chemoprophylaxis is unlikely to have a major impact on tuberculosis control because of the difficulties of country-wide implementation.

Issues relating to control of tuberculosis and HIV

The best way of controlling tuberculosis in high HIV-prevalent countries in sub-Saharan Africa appears to be the WHO directly observed therapy, short course (DOTS) strategy.[77] Countries need to be helped in implementing this strategy, with particular emphasis on diagnosis based on high-quality microscopy, health education, un-interrupted drug supplies and follow-up care. The DOTS strategy must be adaptable to the challenges posed by the HIV epidemic if credibility is to be maintained, and operational research may be very useful in this setting. Botswana is described as a country with a good DOTS programme with high cure rates and very low levels of drug resistance. However, Botswana has experienced a massive rise in the prevalence of HIV infection over the last 5–10 years and this has been associated with an escalating incidence of tuberculosis. It is clear from the experience in Botswana that DOTS alone may not be sufficient to control tuberculosis in areas with epidemic HIV infection, and additional strategies may be needed for tuberculosis control. Tuberculosis programmes should integrate more with AIDS control programmes, because it is now apparent that HIV/AIDS control is an essential component of tuberculosis control.

Human tuberculosis of bovine origin

This a neglected area of interest. Human tuberculosis due to *M. bovis* was a major problem in the industrially developed countries before the completion of bovine tuberculosis eradication programmes in the middle of the twentieth century but is now very uncommon. Tuberculosis is known to occur in cattle in many tropical countries, although little has been done to survey the extent of the problem and even less to control it.[78] The number of tropical countries reporting bovine tuberculosis and the number that have adopted the test and slaughter control strategy are shown in Table 57.8.

Owing to a lack of laboratory facilities in many regions, the prevalence of human tuberculosis due to *M. bovis* in most tropical countries is likewise unknown. One reason for the lack of concern is that early reports indicated that, even in rural communities where cattle disease was common, transmission to humans was rare. In addition, it has been generally but rather dogmatically assumed that *M. bovis* is less virulent than *M. tuberculosis* in humans and is rarely transmitted from person to person. All these assumptions have been seriously questioned by recent surveys undertaken by the WHO and human tuberculosis due to *M. bovis* has been found in many regions where it has been actively sought.[79] Thus further surveys are required to determine the magnitude of the problem in both cattle and humans and to determine the cost-effectiveness of eradication programmes.

The clinical presentation of tuberculosis due to *M. bovis* depends on the route of infection. Oral infection acquired by drinking milk from diseased cattle usually leads to cervical or mesenteric lymphadenopathy (Figures 57.62 and 57.63) and other forms of non-pulmonary disease. Aerogenous infection from cattle or humans leads to pulmonary tuberculosis indistinguishable from that caused by *M. tuberculosis*. The treatment is as for disease due to *M. tuberculosis*, although as *M. bovis* is naturally resistant to pyrazinamide this agent may be omitted.

Infection by HIV increases the risk of human disease following infection by *M. bovis* and a number of examples

Table 57.8 Reports of the prevalence of bovine tuberculosis and use of the test and slaughter policy in countries within the WHO regions*

Region	Number of countries reporting				Number of countries with test and slaughter policy
	Enzootic or high prevalence	Sporadic or low prevalence	Not reported	No data	
Africa	55	8	25	18	7
Asia	36	1	16	9	7
Latin America and Caribbean	34	8	12	2	12

*Data from Cosivi et al.[78]

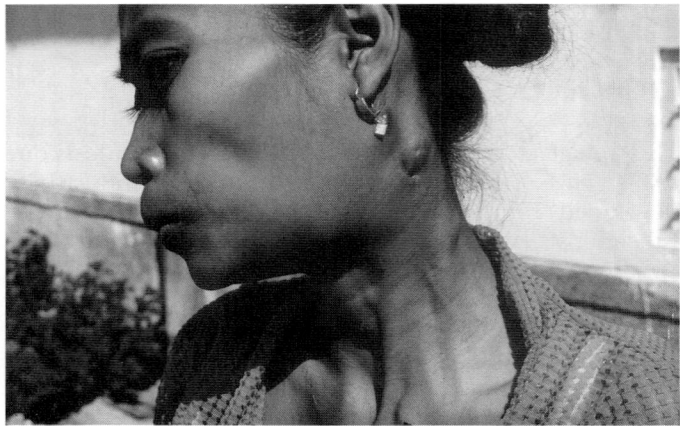

Figure 57.62: Lymphadenopathy (tonsillar node) with sinus formation in tuberculosis due to *M. bovis*.

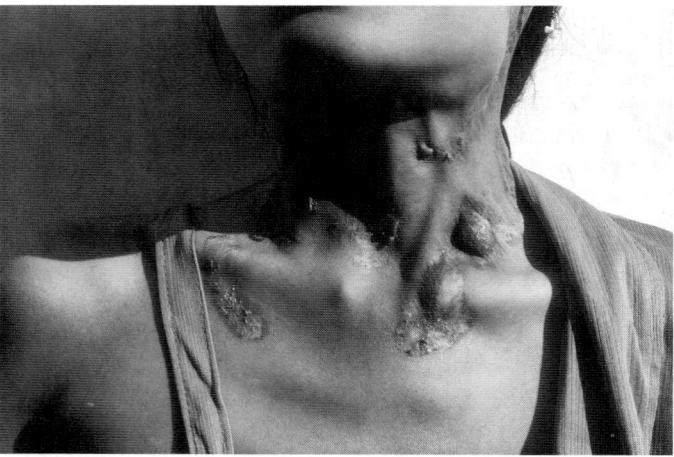

Figure 57.63: Chronic skin tuberculosis due to *M. tuberculosis* (secondary to tracking and sinus formation from lymph node involement).

of human-to-human transmission of disease have been reported. Thus HIV infection could exacerbate the risk of human disease following infection from cattle as well as human sources and this is therefore another incentive to consider the institution of bovine tuberculosis eradication programmes.

Treatment of tuberculosis

Highly effective drug treatments for tuberculosis have been available for half a century. These treatments, when used within the WHO DOTS strategy, form the basis of the modern management of tuberculosis.

Chemotherapy

The three aims of antituberculosis chemotherapy are:

1. To cure the patient.
2. To render the patient rapidly non-infectious.
3. To prevent the emergence of drug resistance.

From the point of view of therapy, the tubercle bacilli may be thought of as being in three different 'compartments': those replicating rapidly on the walls of the cavities, those replicating less rapidly in anoxic and acidic solid lesions and those in a dormant or near dormant state within dense lesions or macrophages.[80] It is important to kill all bacilli as the immune responses cannot be relied on to deal with any remaining bacilli.

Effective cure of the patient is ensured by using agents able to kill bacilli in all three physiological compartments. In those with open or infectious pulmonary tuberculosis, the great majority of bacilli are freely replicating in the cavity walls and are rapidly killed by isoniazid, thereby rendering the patient non-infectious. Isoniazid is less active against slowly replicating bacilli in closed, acidic lesions but rifampicin and pyrazinamide are effective against this population. There are two phases in the drug treatment of tuberculosis:

1. *An initial phase* lasting for 2 months where three (rifampicin, isoniazid, pyrazinamide) or four (plus ethambutol) antituberculosis drugs are given. This intense attack reduces the load of mycobacteria and allows sensitivity patterns to be established.
2. *A continuation phase* during which rifampicin and isoniazid are continued for a further 4 months at least. There are other continuation regimens recommended by the WHO in use in low-income countries.

If the patient regularly receives at least two drugs to which the bacilli are susceptible, the chance of the emergence of drug resistance is very small. In view of the increasing prevalence of resistance to one or two drugs, a fourth drug, usually ethambutol, is now routinely given in the intensive phase of treatment. An alternative to ethambutol is streptomycin but, as this must be given by intramuscular injection, there is a risk of transmitting HIV and other viruses by use of inadequately sterilized needles.

The best drug for the destruction of near-dormant persisting bacilli is rifampicin, which is therefore given during the continuation phase. Although isoniazid has little activity against near-dormant bacilli, it is included in the continuation phase to destroy any rifampicin-resistant mutants that commence active replication.

Modern short-course regimens have the added advantages of low toxicity and low cost. In most regimens, all the drugs are given orally. As four drugs are used in the intensive phase, resistance to one of the drugs used does not render the regimen ineffective. Combination tablets are available, usually isoniazid + rifampicin or isoniazid + rifampicin + pyrazinamide. The WHO recommends that only those combination tablets that have been shown in human studies to yield bactericidal levels of the constituent drugs should be used.

Drugs and regimens

The selection of the drug regimen depends on the nature and extent of the disease. The WHO divides patients into

Table 57.9 The WHO-recommended short-course antituberculosis drug regimens in four categories of patients

Treatment category	Definition	Initial intensive phase (daily or three times each week)	Continuation phase*
I	New smear-positive pulmonary TB; new smear negative pulmonary TB with extensive lung involvement; new severe forms of extrapulmonary TB	2 EHRZ (SHRZ) 2 EHRZ (SHRZ) 2 EHRZ (SHRZ)	6 HE 4 HR 4 H_3R_3
II	Smear-positive pulmonary TB: relapse, treatment failure or treatment after interruption	2 SHRZE/1 HRZE 2 SHRZE/1 HRZE	5 HRE 5 H_3R3E_3
III	New smear-negative pulmonary TB (other than Category I; new less severe forms of extrapulmonary TB	2 HRZ 2 HRZ 2 HRZ	6 HE 4 HR 4 H_3R_3
IV	Chronic cases, i.e. still bacteriologically positive after supervised re-treatment.	Second line drugs required according to WHO guidelines in specialised centres	

*The subscripted figure 3 indicates thrice weekly intermittent dosing.
E, ethambutol; H, Isoniazid; R, rifampicin; Z, pyrazinamide; S, streptomycin.

four groups, with regimens suitable for each, as shown in Table 57.9. Ideally, drugs are administered daily, but for ease of supervision they may be given thrice weekly during the continuation phase or, in some cases, throughout. Alternative drug regimens are still in use in some regions. Some of these omit rifampicin on cost grounds, but this is a false economy as the much lower relapse rates obtained with the rifampicin-based regimens more than justify the slightly greater cost. Thus, these other regimens should be abandoned in favour of those recommended by the WHO,[76] and they are not therefore reviewed here.

Supervision of therapy is considered essential for the cure of the patient, the prevention of relapse and of the emergence of drug resistance. Thus, directly observed therapy (DOT) is strongly advocated by the WHO. DOT should not be confused with DOTS, which is a five-point strategy for the control of tuberculosis discussed on p. 1045.

Short-course chemotherapy is suitable for all forms of tuberculosis although in some cases, notably HIV-related or meningitis, therapy is continued for longer, usually 8–12 months.

Drugs used in chemotherapy

As referred to above, the antituberculosis drugs used in the WHO-recommended short-course regimens (the first-line drugs) include isoniazid, rifampicin, pyrazinamide and either ethambutol or, in some cases, streptomycin. Other drugs are available for the treatment of disease resistant to the first-line drugs. These include ethionamide and the closely related prothionamide, thiacetazone, cycloserine, capreomycin, p-aminosalicylic acid, fluoroquinolones such as ofloxacin and sparfloxacin and the newer macrolides including clarithromycin and azithromycin. Limited evidence indicates that the antileprosy drug clofazimine and combinations of aminopenicillins and β-lactamase inhibitors, such as amoxycillin

with sulbactam, are also of use. These drugs are generally more toxic, more expensive and less active than the first-line drugs and treatment is often prolonged and therefore very costly.

Isoniazid

This has a powerful bactericidal activity against replicating tubercle bacilli but little or no activity against near-dormant bacilli. It is cheap, has few serious side effects and cross-resistance with other drugs does not occur. Effective concentrations of the drug are obtained in all tissues and the CSF. Isoniazid is converted to an inactive form by the process of acetylation which is under genetic control, with some people being rapid acetylators and others slow acetylators. About 50% of Caucasians and Africans and 80–90% of Chinese and Japanese are rapid acetylators. The elimination half-lives in slow and rapid acetylators are, respectively, 2–4 and 0.5–1.5 hours. Acetylation status does not affect the efficacy of standard short-course antituberculosis therapy but adverse side effects and interactions with other drugs are more pronounced in slow acetylators. The rate of acetylation is reduced in renal failure. Adverse side effects of isoniazid are uncommon and are mostly neurological, including restlessness, insomnia, muscle twitching and difficulty in starting micturition. Dermatological side effects have been observed in HIV-positive patients (Figure 57.64). More serious but rare side effects include peripheral neuropathy, optic neuritis, encephalopathy and psychiatric disorders including anxiety states, confusion, depression and paranoia. The risk of neurological side effects is greatly reduced by giving pyridoxine (vitamin B_6) 10 mg/day and this has become standard practice in most countries. Some national programmes recommend the routine prescription of pyridoxine to patients with liver disease, renal failure requiring dialysis, pregnant women, alcoholics, HIV-positive patients, the malnourished and the elderly.

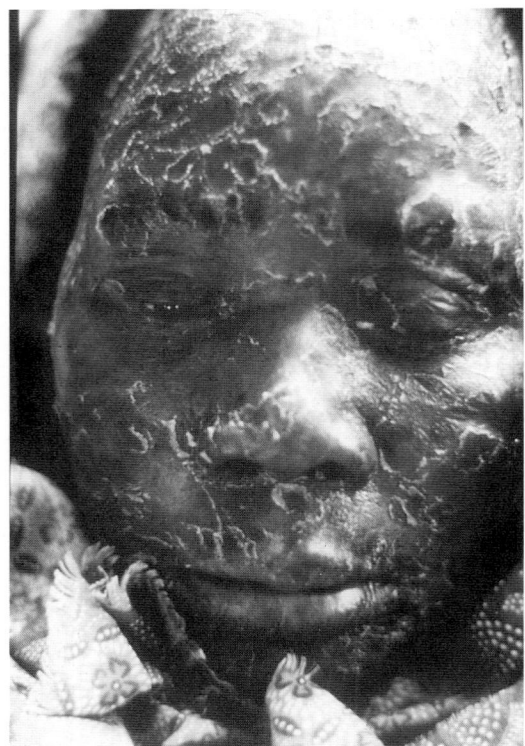

Figure 57.64: Extensive skin reaction due to isoniazid.

Rifampicin (rifampin in the USA)

This is readily absorbed from the gastrointestinal tract and effective concentrations are obtained in all tissues, with moderate levels in the CSF. Cross-resistance to other antituberculosis drugs does not occur. It is red coloured and patients should be warned that it imparts this colour to urine, tears and sweat.

Adverse reactions include mild and usually self-limiting erythema and itchiness of the skin and, rarely, a skin rash (Figure 57.65). Gastrointestinal upsets occur in some patients and are reduced by giving rifampicin with food. Impairment of liver function may be seen in

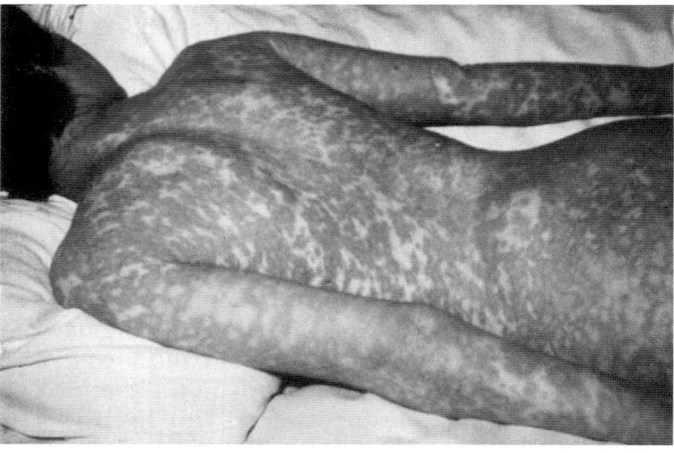

Figure 57.65: Erythema multiforme skin reaction due to rifampicin.

patients with pre-existing liver disease and a history of alcoholism and, if possible, assay of serum bilirubin and other liver function tests should be done monthly on such patients.

Some adverse effects are very rarely seen in patients given rifampicin daily but, for unknown reasons, may occur in those on intermittent treatment. The most frequently seen is the 'flu syndrome', characterized by fever, chills and headache, aching bones and, in some cases, a mild thrombocytopenic purpura.

Much rarer, but serious, adverse events usually associated with intermittent dosing include respiratory shock syndrome, thrombocytopenic purpura with a very low platelet count and haemorrhages, haemolytic anaemia and renal failure. Rifampicin must be stopped immediately if one of these serious adverse reactions develops and must never be given again. Corticosteroid therapy may be required for the respiratory shock syndrome.

Ethambutol

This has limited bactericidal activity in the early, intensive, phase of treatment. There is some evidence that ethambutol enhances the activity of other antituberculosis agents by increasing mycobacterial cell wall permeability. Resistance is uncommon. It is concentrated in the alveolar macrophages. It does not diffuse through healthy meninges but CSF levels of 25–40% of the plasma concentration, with considerable variation between patients, are achieved in tuberculous meningitis.

The most important side effect is optic neuritis, which may become irreversible and lead to blindness. This is a rare occurrence if no more than 25 mg/kg is given daily for a maximum of 2 months. National codes of practice for detection and prevention of ocular toxicity should be followed. Patients should be instructed to stop therapy and to seek medical advice if they notice any change in visual acuity, peripheral vision or perception of colour. Ethambutol should not be given to young children and others unable to comply with this advice. Other adverse effects include peripheral neuritis, joint pain due, in some cases, to hyperuricaemia, rashes and, rarely, thrombocytopenia and jaundice.

Pyrazinamide

Pyrazinamide is only active in acidic environments and is therefore principally active against intracellular tubercle bacilli and those in acidic, anoxic inflammatory lesions. It freely enters the CSF, where levels achieved are similar to those in the plasma. Resistance is uncommon.

Despite early reports of hepatotoxicity, pyrazinamide is usually well tolerated and skin rashes occur rarely (Figure 57.66). Although moderate elevations of serum transaminases occur early in treatment, severe hepatotoxicity is uncommon except in patients with pre-existing liver disease. Its principal metabolite, pyrazinoic acid, inhibits renal excretion of uric acid, occasionally

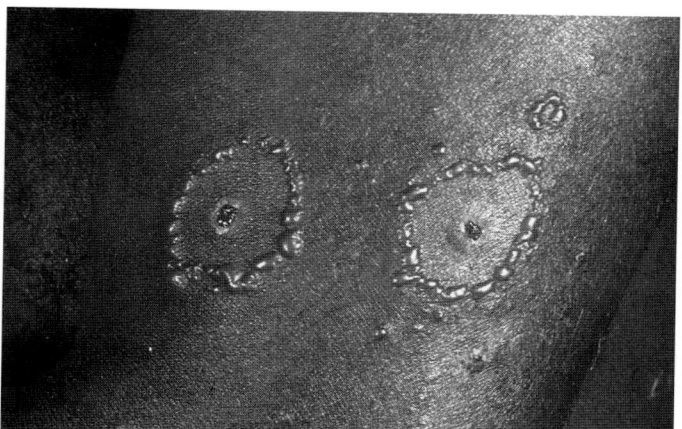

Figure 57.66: Reaction to antituberculosis drugs: 'Target lesions' due to pyrazinamide.

resulting in gout requiring treatment with allopurinol. An unrelated arthralgia, notably of the shoulders and responsive to analgesics, also occurs. Other side effects include anorexia, nausea and photosensitization of the skin.

Streptomycin

This is occasionally used as an alternative to ethambutol in short-course regimens but it has the disadvantage that, as it is not absorbed from the intestine, it must therefore be given by intramuscular injection. This raises the associated danger of transmission of HIV and other viruses by contaminated needles. The principal side effects involve the vestibular apparatus of the inner ear and manifest as unsteadiness and vertigo. This complication is more likely in older patients and the damage may be permanent if the drug is not stopped immediately the symptoms commence. Deafness occasionally occurs and, if given during pregnancy, can lead to impaired hearing in the child. A further uncommon complication is anaphylaxis.

Second-line drugs

These are indicated in cases of drug resistance and, very occasionally, when the use of a first-line drug is prevented by adverse drug reactions. In general, they are less effective, more toxic and more expensive than the first-line drugs. p-Aminosalicylic acid and viomycin are now unobtainable in a number of countries.

Ethionamide and prothionamide

These bacteriostatic drugs are useful in drug-resistant tuberculosis. Although these closely related drugs are similar in structure and mode of action to isoniazid, no cross-resistance occurs. Their use is restricted by a high incidence of gastric irritation, although this undesirable effect is reduced by commencing with a low dose and gradually increasing to the full dose and by taking the drugs at bedtime.

Aminoglycosides

In addition to streptomycin, the principal aminoglycosides active against tubercle bacilli are kanamycin and amikacin. As with all aminoglycosides, they must be given by intramuscular injection and are ototoxic and nephrotoxic.

Capreomycin and viomycin

These are of limited availability and their use is limited to cases of multi-drug resistant tuberculosis. In common with the aminoglycosides, they must be given by intramuscular injection and are ototoxic and nephrotoxic. They show partial cross-resistance with the aminoglycosides.

p-Aminosalicylic acid

This was one of the early antituberculosis drugs but is now rarely used as it has only bacteriostatic activity, commonly causes gastrointestinal upsets and is of limited availability.

Thiacetazone

This weak drug was once widely used, principally on account of its cheapness. Many strains of M. tuberculosis isolated in East Africa, India and Hong Kong are more resistant to thiacetazone than strains from Europe and acquired resistance is prevalent in the developing countries. The principal adverse side effects are skin rashes, which occur frequently in 2–4% of African patients but much more frequently in patients of Chinese ethnic origin. More severe skin reactions, including exfoliative dermatitis, erythema multiforme (Figure 57.65) and Stevens–Johnson syndrome (Figure 57.61), occur in less than 0.5% of patients, but there is a 10-fold increase of these reactions in HIV-positive patients, proving fatal in up to 3% of such patients. For these reasons and its poor activity its use should be avoided, especially in regions with a high incidence of HIV infection, and it should never be knowingly given to an HIV-positive person. Thiacetazone causes similar reactions in HIV-positive children, who should likewise not receive this agent.[73]

Cycloserine

This is a bacteriostatic drug which has unpleasant side effects including headache, dizziness, depression, confusion. It tends to be one of the last drugs of choice.

Other, including experimental, agents

There is limited but increasing evidence that the fluoroquinolones such as ciprofloxacin, ofloxacin and sparfloxacin,[81] and newer macrolides including azithromycin and clarithromycin,[82] are of value in the treatment of multi-drug resistant tuberculosis and various other mycobacterial diseases. Among the rifamycins, rifabutin is used as an alternative to rifampicin in HIV-positive patients receiving antiretroviral therapy and there is some evidence that rifapentine may permit the frequency of dosing to be reduced. There is anecdotal evidence for efficacy of the antileprosy drug clofazimine and of amidopenicillins in combination with β-lactamase inhibitors, such as amoxycillin with sulbactam.

More detailed accounts of the antituberculosis drugs are available in other texts.[83-86]

Immunotherapy

The use of immunotherapy is a subject of growing interest. Agents under investigation include cytokines such as IFNγ and a heat-killed preparation of an environmental mycobacterium, *M. vaccae*. A clinical trial of a single dose of the latter as an adjunct to standard antituberculosis therapy in South Africa showed no beneficial effect,[87] but another in Uganda showed that it hastened clearance of acid-fast bacilli from the sputum and resolution of lesions seen radiologically.[88]

Adverse drug reactions and interactions

Adverse reactions are discussed in the descriptions of the individual drugs above and summarized in Table 57.10.

Drug interactions require careful attention, notably in HIV-positive patients, in whom such interactions may be accentuated and who may be taking a number of drugs, such as antiretroviral combinations and/or antibiotics for the treatment or prevention of opportunistic infections, with which antituberculosis agents are likely to interact. Care must therefore be taken in prescribing concurrent antituberculosis therapy and, in cases where drug interactions are known, changes to therapy may be required.

The principal interactions between the antituberculosis agents and other drugs are listed in Table 57.11. Most drug interactions encountered in antituberculosis therapy are associated with the rifamycins (rifampicin, rifabutin and rifapentine), which induce hepatic cytochrome enzymes, notably cytochrome p450 isoenzyme 3A4 (CYP3A4), involved in the metabolism of many drugs. Rifabutin is less enzyme-inducing than rifampicin. Cytochrome induction by antituberculosis agents affects some antiretroviral agents, notably the protease inhibitors such as saquinavir, indinavir, nelfinavir and ritonavir, and thus could result in significantly reduced levels and promote the development of viral resistance. Conversely, co-administration of ritonavir or indinavir with rifamycins inhibits their metabolism and dose adjustments may be required. Thus the concomitant administration of antituberculosis drugs and antiretroviral agents poses serious problems as described below.

Table 57.10 Adverse reactions (side effects) of the antituberculosis agents

Agent	Adverse reactions
Isoniazid	
Common	Anorexia, nausea, vomiting, fever, skin rashes, peripheral neuropathy
Rare	Vertigo, convulsions, optic neuritis and atrophy, psychiatric disturbance, haemolytic anaemia, aplastic anaemia, dermal reactions including pellagra, purpura and lupoid syndrome, gynaecomastia, hyperglycaemia, arthralgia
Rifampicin	
Common	Orange-red discolouration of urine, anorexia, nausea, vomiting, diarrhoea, skin rashes
Rare (usually associated with intermittent therapy)	Dyspnoea, hypotension with or without shock, Addisonian crisis, haemolytic anaemia, acute renal failure, thrombocytopenia with or without purpura, transient leucopenia or eosinophilia, menstrual disturbances, muscular weakness, pseudomembranous colitis
Pyrazinamide	
Common	Anorexia, fever, nausea, vomiting
Uncommon	Hepatitis, nausea and vomiting, urticaria, skin rash, nausea, arthralgia
Rare	Sideroblastic anaemia, photosensitization, gout, dysuria, aggravation of peptic ulcer
Ethambutol	
Uncommon	Optic neuritis, arthralgia
Rare	Hepatitis, cutaneous hypersensitivity including pruritis and urticaria, photosensitive lichenoid eruptions, parasthesia of the extremities, interstitial nephritis
Streptomycin	
Uncommon	Vertigo, ataxia, deafness, tinnitus, cutaneous hypersensitivity
Rare	Renal damage, aplastic anaemia, agranulocytosis, peripheral neuropathy, optic neuritis with scotoma, severe bleeding due to antagonism of Factor V, neuromuscular blockade in patients receiving muscle relaxants or with myaesthenia gravis

Table 57.10 (*Cont'd*) Adverse reactions (side effects) of the antituberculosis agents

Agent	Adverse reactions
Other aminoglycosides	
Uncommon	Cutaneous hypersensitivity, vertigo, deafness
Rare	Renal damage, hypoglycaemia, hypokalaemia
Thiacetazone	
Common	Gastrointestinal upsets, cutaneous hypersensitivity, vertigo, conjunctivitis
Uncommon*	Hepatitis, erythema multiforme, exfoliative dermatitis, Stevens–Johnson syndrome, haemolytic anaemia
Rare	Agranulocytosis
p-Aminosalicylic acid	
Common	Gastrointestinal upsets
Uncommon	Cutaneous hypersensitivity, hepatitis, hypokalaemia
Rare	Acute renal failure, haemolytic anaemia, thrombocytopenia, hypothyroidism
Ethionamide/Prothionamide	
Common	Gastrointestinal upsets, salivation, metallic taste
Uncommon	Cutaneous hypersensitivity, hepatitis
Rare	Alopecia, convulsions, deafness, diplopia, gynaecomastia, hypotension, impotence, psychiatric disturbance, menstrual irregularity, hypoglycaemia, peripheral neuropathy
Capreomycin and viomycin	
Common	Eosinophilia (with capreomycin), pain and induration at injection site
Uncommon	Loss of hearing, vertigo, tinnitus, electrolyte disturbances including hypokalaemia, leucopenia or leucocytosis
Rare	Renal impairment, hepatitis, thrombocytopenia
Clofazimine	
Common	Discolouration of skin and body fluids, nausea, vomiting, abdominal pain, diarrhoea
Uncommon	Dryness of skin, ichthyosis, photosensitivity
Rare	Intestinal obstruction
Cycloserine	
Common (especially with daily doses exceeding 500 mg)	Drowsiness, sleep disturbance, headache, tremor, vertigo, confusion, irritability, aggression and other personality changes, psychosis (sometimes with suicidal tendencies)
Uncommon	Convulsions, cutaneous hypersensitivity, hepatitis, megaloblastic anaemia
Rare	Congestive heart failure
Ofloxacin	
Uncommon	Gastrointestinal upsets, headache, dizziness, insomnia, cutaneous hypersensitivity reactions
Rare	Restlessness, convulsions, psychiatric disturbances including psychotic reactions and hallucinations, oedema of face, tongue and epiglottis, disturbance of taste and smell, anaphylactoid reactions

*Severe thiacetazone-induced skin reactions are common in HIV-positive persons.

It is important to note that rifamycins enhance the metabolism of oral contraceptives and alternative means of contraception should therefore be used during therapy. Rifamycins also reduce the therapeutic levels of azoles such as ketoconazole and fluconazole. In patients taking dapsone prophylaxis for PCP, there are seven- to ten-fold reductions in dapsone levels.

Absorption of rifampicin is significantly reduced by the co-administration of antacids such as aluminium hydroxide and magnesium trisilicate due to an increased gastric pH. Aluminium may also form chelates with rifampicin which are less soluble and less well absorbed.

Isoniazid may produce significant increases in the area under the curve of warfarin, carbamazepin and phenytoin. Isoniazid induces the metabolism of the azoles and reduces their plasma levels.

Table 57.11 Interactions between antituberculosis drugs and other therapeutic agents

Drugs whose effects are opposed by rifampicin	Antiretroviral agents Azathioprine Corticosteroids Cyclosporin Diazepam Digoxin Haloperidol Imidazoles	Opioids Oral contraceptives Phenytoin Propranolol Quinidine Theophylline Tolbutamide Warfarin
Drug potentiating the effects of rifampicin	Trimethoprim–sulfamethoxazole (Cotrimoxazole)	
Drug whose effects are opposed by isoniazid	Enflurane	
Drugs whose effects are potentiated by isoniazid	Phenytoin	Carbamezapine
Drug potentiating the effects of isoniazid	Insulin	
Drugs opposing the effects of isoniazid	Prednisolone	Antacids (inhibit absorption)
Drugs whose effects are potentiated by streptomycin	Neuromuscular blocking agents	
Drug potentiating the effects of quinolones	Cimetidine	
Drugs whose effects are potentiated by quinolones	Aminophylline	Theophylline
Drugs opposing the effects of quinolones	Antacids, iron preparations, sucralfate, didanosine (all inhibit absorption)	

Treatment of tuberculosis in patients receiving antiretroviral agents

Although patients with HIV-related tuberculosis can be prescribed concomitant therapy such as antiretroviral agents, careful management through frequent follow-up is required. The subject of antiretroviral therapy is a rapidly changing one as new agents and regimens are constantly being introduced. Drug interactions are therefore being reported with increased frequency and the literature on the subject rapidly becomes out of date.

Detailed discussion on interactions between antituberculosis drugs and antiretroviral agents, and on optimal antituberculosis drug regimens for patients receiving antiretroviral agents, is beyond the scope of this book. The clinician is therefore advised to seek specialist help or refer to the latest guidelines issued by the Centres for Disease Control, Atlanta, Georgia, or the WHO. Currently

Table 57.12 Antituberculosis drug regimens with concomitant antiretroviral regimens

Antituberculosis regimen	Months of therapy	Antiretroviral therapy
Rifampicin	1–6	Triple non-nucleoside
Isoniazid	1–6	reverse transcriptase
Pyrazinamide	1–2	inhibitors (NRTI)
Ethambutol	1–2	
Rifabutin	1–6	Nelfinavir, indinavir,
Isoniazid	1–6	amprenavir, efavirenz
Pyrazinamide	1–2	or nevirapine
Ethambutol		

acceptable regimens are summarized in Table 57.12. The basic principle to follow in the treatment of tuberculosis in HIV-positive patients in the tropics is to give priority to the treatment of tuberculosis. It is preferable to defer treatment with antiretroviral agents until after completion of the course of antituberculosis therapy. If antiretroviral therapy is then required, this should commence 3 weeks after completion of the course of antituberculosis therapy to allow the plasma drug levels to clear.

Hypersensitivity reactions to antituberculosis drugs and their management

These are uncommon in the first week of treatment and are mostly seen in the second to fourth weeks. The reactions are graded as follows:

- *Mild*: itching of the skin only.
- *Moderate*: fever and a rash which may be mistaken for measles or scarlet fever. Blistering may be seen.
- *Severe*: in addition to fever and rash there may be hypotension, generalized swelling of lymph nodes, enlargement of liver and spleen, swelling round the eyes and swelling of the mucous membranes of the mouth and lips. Stevens–Johnson syndrome (a generalized and severe exfoliative rash and ulceration of the mucous membranes of the mouth, genitals and eyes) may occur, particularly in HIV-positive persons and those receiving thiacetazone.

Mild itching is often transitory and relieved by antihistamines but if the patient is receiving thiacetazone and could be HIV-positive, this drug should be withdrawn and never given again. If the moderate or severe signs and symptoms listed above develop, antituberculosis

Table 57.13 Sequence of reintroduction and challenge doses for restarting therapy

Agent	Likelihood of the drug causing a reaction and sequence of reintroduction	Challenge dose Day 1	Day 2	Day 3
Isoniazid	Least/first	50 mg	300 mg	300 mg
Rifampicin		75 mg	300 mg	Full dose
Pyrazinamide		250 mg	1 g	Full dose
Ethambutol		100 mg	500 mg	Full dose
Streptomycin	Greatest/last	125 mg	500 mg	Full dose

therapy must be stopped immediately. If the patient is seriously ill, corticosteroids should be administered. If the patient is able to swallow, prednisolone 15 mg three times a day is given until improvement occurs and the dose is than reduced gradually every 2 days according to the patient's response. If the patient is unable to swallow, a suitable regimen consists of hydrocortisone 200 mg i.v. or i.m. followed by dexamethasone 4 mg i.v. or i.m. until the patient can swallow, when it is replaced by prednisolone 15 mg three times a day. When clinical improvement occurs, the oral dose is reduced as above. Intravenous fluid replacement is required if the patient is unable to swallow.

When the hypersensitivity reaction has subsided, antituberculosis therapy should be recommenced with other drugs. Alternatively, challenge doses of the first-line drugs (but never thiacetazone) may be given in order to determine which drug was responsible. The challenges should commence with the drug least likely to have caused the reaction and with the doses shown in Table 57.13. The patient must remain under close observation during administration of challenge doses.

Desensitization may be carried out if the patient is hypersensitive to isoniazid or rifampicin. Desensitization to other drugs is rarely required and must never be attempted outside specialist centres. Desensitization to any antituberculosis agent must never be attempted in HIV-positive patients. The usual method is to give the patient one-tenth of the standard dose of the drug and to increase this by one-tenth each day until the standard dose is reached. As with challenge testing, the patient must remain under close observation during the procedure. During desensitization the patient should be given two antituberculosis drugs that he or she has not received before.

Special treatment situations
Renal insufficiency
Rifampicin, isoniazid, pyrazinamide, ethionamide and prothionamide are either fully metabolized or eliminated in the bile and may be used safely at the normal doses in patients with renal impairment. Ethambutol is mainly eliminated by the kidney but may be used in reduced doses in patients with impaired renal function. As streptomycin and other aminoglycosides are eliminated entirely by the kidney and are nephrotoxic their use

should be avoided whenever possible. Encephalopathy is an uncommon but serious complication of isoniazid therapy in patients with renal failure and in those on dialysis but is preventable in most cases by giving pyridoxine.

Impaired liver function
Patients with impaired liver function may be treated safely with isoniazid, ethambutol and, if required, streptomycin. It is usually advised that pyrazinamide should be avoided although there is no clear evidence that it is any more toxic in patients with impaired hepatic function. Rifampicin should be used with caution: doses should be reduced in patients with bilirubin concentrations exceeding 50 mmol/l. Liver function should be regularly monitored, where possible, in alcoholics, the elderly, malnourished children and children under 2 years of age.

If jaundice develops during antituberculosis therapy, treatment should be stopped until the jaundice resolves. In many cases resumption of treatment does not cause a recurrence of the jaundice. If the patient is seriously ill with tuberculosis, he or she may be treated with streptomycin and ethambutol even in the presence of jaundice.

Pregnancy
Streptomycin, other aminoglycosides, capreomycin and viomycin should be avoided as they may damage the inner ear of the foetus, leading to impairment of hearing. Ethionamide and prothionamide should also be avoided as they have been shown to be teratogenic. Despite early controversy, rifampicin and pyrazinamide appear to be safe in pregnancy. Thus, standard short-course regimens may be used but pyridoxine 10 mg daily prevents damage of foetal nerves by isoniazid.

Management of patients with drug- and multi-drug resistant organisms

Patients with organisms resistant to one of the first-line drugs usually respond to modern short-course therapy. Resistance to isoniazid and rifampicin (multi-drug resistance) is much more serious as patients with such resistance do not respond to standard regimens. Indeed, there is a risk that such treatment will result in the development of resistance to the other agents in the regimen, usually pyrazinamide and ethambutol.

Treatment of MDRTB is based on the second-line drugs, which are more toxic, more costly and less effective than the first-line drugs. Therapy must often be continued for much longer than standard regimens—for at least 12 months after the sputum becomes bacteriologically negative—and, even in the best hands, the mortality is high. Strict supervision of therapy is essential to prevent emergence of organisms resistant to almost all known antituberculosis agents. Guidelines for the management of MDRTB have been published by the WHO.[89–91]

In view of the growing problem of MDRTB in several regions, the 'DOTS-plus' strategy has been advocated.[92] In principle, all possible steps should be taken to link the tuberculosis control programmes in which MDRTB is encountered with a reference laboratory where drug susceptibility testing can be carried out. The alternative is to develop empirical regimens for the treatment of MDRTB based on a knowledge of the patterns of drug resistance in a given region.

In the absence of good-quality laboratory services, treatment should be based on drugs which the patient has not received before. Unfortunately it is often far from easy to ascertain which drugs a patient has previously received.

The 'golden rule' of empirical therapy is that a single drug must never be given to a patient whose therapy is failing. This is a certain way of generating further drug resistance.

The difficulties in the management of MDRTB cannot be overestimated. Practical advice has been published by the WHO and, whenever possible, expert advice should be obtained. Inadequate therapy will be of no benefit to the patient and will only exacerbate the growing problem of resistance.

The role of corticosteroids in tuberculosis

Corticosteroids play no part in the treatment of uncomplicated pulmonary tuberculosis. Although some studies indicate that they relieve symptoms, they may well suppress protective immune responses. Their use may prevent sequelae due to scarring in some forms of extrapulmonary tuberculosis and in some cases their use may be life-saving.[93] They should never be administered unless the patient is receiving supervised antituberculosis therapy. Their use is discussed under the various headings of extrapulmonary tuberculosis above and is briefly summarized here:

- *Hypersensitivity reactions* to drugs, particularly if they are life-threatening.
- *Life-threatening tuberculosis.* Some physicians consider that steroids reduce mortality in those very seriously ill with tuberculosis, but there is no firm evidence. Notwithstanding, nothing is to be lost and there may be some gain in giving steroids under these

circumstances. There are limited reports of clinical benefits of steroid therapy in HIV-positive patients with serious progressive tuberculosis, even though such therapy is likely to further reduce immune function.

- *Pleural, pericardial and peritoneal tuberculosis.* Corticosteroids reduce the effusion, and enhance its clearance and subsequent restrictive scarring.
- *Tuberculous meningitis.* Despite earlier controversy, there is evidence that corticosteroids increase survival and reduce long-term adverse sequelae in this condition.
- *Genitourinary tuberculosis.* Corticosteroids relieve ureteric obstruction and prevent further obstructive scarring and shrinkage of the bladder.
- *Lymph node tuberculosis.* Corticosteroids are indicated when massive enlargement of a lymph node causes respiratory distress. The use of steroids in cases with non-life-threatening enlargement of lymph nodes due to hypersensitivity reactions during therapy is controversial, although skin necrosis, sinus formation and scarring may be prevented in cases of extensive enlargement.
- *Other indications.* Steroid therapy is indicated in destructive ocular lesions to preserve sight, in laryngeal lesions to ameliorate pain, for hormone replacement therapy in Addison's disease and, extremely rarely, in life-threatening generalized hypersensitivity reactions to tuberculin.

Dosage

There are no absolute guidelines but the following have been recommended. When the patient is not seriously ill and when the risk of sequelae due to fibrous scarring is low, 10 mg of prednisolone twice daily for 4–6 weeks, followed by a reduction of the daily dose by 5 mg each week, is usually adequate.

For more serious conditions, including tuberculous meningitis and pericarditis, 30 mg of prednisolone twice daily for 4 weeks should be administered, or longer if indicated, followed by a tailing off as above. Pleural effusions usually respond to 20 mg twice daily for 2 weeks.

The dose in children, depending on severity, is 1–3 mg/kg body weight daily. It is important to note that rifampicin leads to a more rapid metabolism of steroids and the dose should therefore be increased by a half for up to 4 weeks in patients receiving this agent.

The use of steroids in the treatment of severe drug reactions is described on p. 1040.

Chemoprophylaxis

Few areas of tuberculosis control have generated as much controversy as chemoprophylaxis. Strictly speaking, the term should be applied to the prevention of tuberculosis in uninfected persons at a high risk of being infected and developing the disease, such as a young child exposed to a source case in the home. More usually, the term refers to treatment of latent infection in order to prevent the emergence of active tuberculosis. Thus, in some countries such as the USA, where tuberculosis is very uncommon in most states and where BCG vaccination is no longer used, chemoprophylaxis is given to tuberculin reactors. In such circumstances, isoniazid monotherapy, usually for 1 year, is given on the assumption that very few viable bacilli are present and the chance of mutation to isoniazid resistance is therefore very small. Such therapy has been shown, under these circumstances, to be effective and, as the chance of reinfection is very low, protection is long-lasting. The major problems encountered in the use of isoniazid monotherapy are those of ensuring compliance and the occurrence of hepatic complications. On account of the latter, some authorities recommend that only those under 35 years of age should receive chemoprophylaxis.[94] Another problem is the high incidence of multi-drug resistant tuberculosis in some regions, against which isoniazid monotherapy would afford no protection. It is understandable that health care staff are anxious about the risk to their health if reliance is placed on chemoprophylaxis rather than BCG vaccination.

In general, the role of chemoprophylaxis in tuberculosis control in high-incidence regions has, in view of problems of compliance and organization, not played a major role in tuberculosis control.[74,75,95,96] The advent of the HIV/AIDS pandemic has led to a reappraisal of chemoprophylaxis as the chance of a dually infected person developing overt tuberculosis is very high. Several placebo-controlled studies of isoniazid monotherapy in patients co-infected with *M. tuberculosis* and HIV have shown that such chemoprophylaxis is effective. Unfortunately, however, the preventive effect is short-lived in HIV-positive persons and rapidly declines after completion of the course of chemoprophylaxis. Indeed, in one study no protection was apparent after 18 months. Thus, repeated courses of chemoprophylaxis or even lifetime medication may be required. The preventive effect is greatest in those who are tuberculin-positive and who have a relatively high lymphocyte count. For this reason, and on account of the difficulty of diagnosing infection by *M. tuberculosis* in tuberculin-negative persons, the WHO recommends that chemoprophylaxis should be restricted to HIV-positive persons who are tuberculin-positive.

Isoniazid monotherapy for 9 months is suitable for chemoprophylaxis in HIV-positive persons: continuation of therapy to 12 months adds very little. Rifampicin monotherapy for 4 months or rifampicin with pyrazinamide for 2 months have been evaluated but the only clear advantage over isoniazid monotherapy is the shorter duration of treatment.

It is very important to ensure that HIV-positive persons receiving chemoprophylaxis do not have active tuberculosis or there is a strong risk of masking the disease and encouraging the emergence of drug resistance. It is also necessary to supervise the therapy and this adds another burden to stretched tuberculosis control services.

Policies for the use of chemoprophylaxis vary from country to country. National guidelines should be consulted for indications for chemoprophylaxis and for the recommended drug regimens.

Surgical treatment

In general, surgery plays a minor role in the treatment of pulmonary tuberculosis, although resection of localized lesions caused by multi-drug resistant tubercle bacilli is undertaken in some centres. Other indications include life-threatening haemoptysis, mycetomas forming in old tuberculous cavities, empyema and respiratory distress due to grossly enlarged mediastinal lymph nodes. Surgery has also been used in cases of localized pulmonary disease due to environmental mycobacteria but the availability of more effective therapeutic regimens is reducing the need for surgical resection.

Surgical treatment for extrapulmonary disease is discussed under the appropriate headings.

Tuberculosis control programmes

These should be based on the WHO five-point DOTS strategy,[77,97] of which the elements are:

- Government commitment to tuberculosis control.
- An uninterrupted supply of good-quality drugs, free at the point of delivery to the patient.
- Facilities for diagnosis by microscopy.
- Directly observed administration of the drugs.
- Evaluation of the efficiency of the control programme.

Case finding

This may be active, involving a deliberate enquiry of symptoms, usually a history of a cough for more than 3 weeks duration, sometimes by means of door-to-door surveys. Passive case finding relies on patients with symptoms presenting at a clinic. The efficiency of the latter approach critically depends on public health education, the proximity of the clinic from the patients' homes and the reputation of the clinic in the region. In some regions, poor people prefer attending private practitioners even though they can ill afford them, as the state-sponsored centres have a poor reputation for caring and competence.

Diagnosis

This is usually based on sputum microscopy. As case holding is of key importance, the number of times that a patient has to attend a clinic should be kept to a minimum. Thus, ideally, a diagnosis will be made on a sputum sample produced by the patient on his or her first visit and treatment commenced immediately. The chance of diagnosis is improved by examining three, preferably early-morning, sputum samples and the patient with suspected tuberculosis should be requested to provide these if the 'spot' specimen is negative.

The efficiency and accuracy of sputum microscopy critically depend on the skill and dedication of the microscopist. Such microscopy is tedious; it is important to give laboratory staff a variety of examinations to undertake and no technician should examine more than 20 sputum smears each day. Quality control, training and attention to job satisfaction are important factors to be attended to in the management of microscopy services. The organization and practice of microscopy and other aspects of the tuberculosis laboratory are discussed in detail elsewhere.[28]

Supply of drugs

It is essential that a regular supply of good-quality drugs is maintained and that these are available to the patients at no cost to them. Intermittent supplies of drugs are a major cause of treatment failure, the emergence of drug resistance and a loss of public confidence in the treatment services. Combination preparations, containing two or three antituberculosis drugs, must only be purchased from WHO-recommended manufacturers as poorly formulated preparations may not allow adequate levels of the drugs to be absorbed, with a risk of treatment failure and the development of drug resistance.

Supervision of therapy

As a result of the effectiveness of modern short-course therapy, and the rapid loss of infectiousness, patients with no complicating factors can be treated as outpatients and pursue normal occupational and social activities. As hospitalization is thus the exception rather than the rule in many regions, the question of supervision of therapy must be addressed. This is, however, the most controversial of the five points of the WHO DOTS strategy.[98] While non-compliance with therapy is one of the major reasons for the global failure to control tuberculosis, dogmatic assertions on the need for every dose to be taken in the presence of a qualified health worker may well add to the problems. In some countries, patients accept a restrictive discipline of attending regularly for their medicine but in others this may prove counterproductive. Good results have been obtained by the use of volunteer supervisors chosen from the local community as this encourages a relationship between equals—concordance rather than compliance with 'authority'. Various incentives may enhance adherence to therapy. In one successful programme, patients pay a nominal fee at the commencement of therapy which is reimbursed, with interest, on successful completion of therapy.[99,100] Supervision strategies must be 'user-friendly', and must respect the dignity and human rights of the patient. In this respect, it is important to organize services on the basis of local attitudes and related factors and not on dogma.[101–105] Tuberculosis, especially HIV-related tuberculosis, carries a definite stigma which may hinder treatment-seeking and adherence, and should be addressed in health education activities.[106,107]

Monitoring of tuberculosis control services

This is essential to ascertain whether the above strategies are effective and cost-effective in a given circumstance. For this purpose, record-keeping is essential and patients reaching the end of therapy should be followed up to detect early bacteriological relapse due to inadequate supervision of therapy.

Traditionally, tuberculosis control has been organized on a 'vertical' basis, with a central administrative office, often combined with teaching facilities and a reference laboratory. The central facility had direct responsibility for regional and local treatment centres and would ensure regular supplies of drugs, laboratory equipment and reagents, and would conduct epidemiological studies and run training courses.

In many countries, so-called 'health sector reforms' are being imposed by the World Bank and other international agencies as part of the structural adjustment required for financial aid and have caused some concern.

Among the imposed structural adjustments are the sector-wide approaches (SWAPS) to funding which have led to shift from support of specific projects to what has been termed 'basket funding'. In principle, by establishing a central fund for health services, this should lead to an equitable service that meets the needs of all of the population. In practice, 'horizontal' general primary health services may replace well-established and effective disease-specific 'vertical' programmes before the former can take over the functions of the latter. Furthermore, funding bodies dedicated to certain health issues, such as tuberculosis, may withdraw financial support if no guarantee is given as to its specific use. In addition, tuberculosis is a disease that particularly affects the very poor and some aspects of health sector reform, such as the introduction of user fees, and the development of the private health sector adversely affects those who, on account of poverty, are in greatest need of health services.

Guidelines for the control of tuberculosis in the developing countries are available from the International Union Against Tuberculosis and Lung Disease.[29]

Bacille Calmette–Guérin vaccination

The only vaccine against tuberculosis is Bacille Calmette–Guérin (BCG), named after Albert Calmette and Camille Guérin, the French investigators who developed the vaccine by attenuating a strain of M. bovis early in the twentieth century. The vaccine was intended for oral administration in neonates to mimic protection conferred by milk-borne M. bovis infection that did not progress to disease. Following a tragedy at the German city of Lübeck in 1930, when children were accidentally vaccinated with a virulent strain of M. tuberculosis with the death of over 70, the vaccine was prepared in central facilities and freeze-dried for intradermal use.

Table 57.14 The results of nine major BCG vaccine trials

Region	Year of commencement	Age range	Protection afforded (%)
North America[1]	1935	0–20 years	80
Chicago, USA	1937	3 months	75
Great Britain	1950	14–15 years	78
Puerto Rico	1949	1–18 years	31
South India	1950	All ages	31
Georgia, USA	1950	5 years	14
Illinois, USA	1948	Young adults	0
South India[2]	1968	All ages	0
Malawi	1978	All ages	0

[1]Amerindian population.
[2]A later follow-up revealed some protection in those vaccinated in infancy.

The mode of action of BCG vaccination is poorly understood. It prevents disseminated forms of primary tuberculosis, such as tuberculous meningitis, in children but its impact on post-primary, infectious, pulmonary tuberculosis is minimal. It is therefore of limited value in the global control of the incidence of tuberculosis. A major problem in its use is that, as shown in Table 57.14, its efficacy has been found to vary from region to region, from around 80% to no protection at all.[108] Indeed, in some studies, it appears to have a small adverse effect, in rendering vaccinated subjects more susceptible to clinical tuberculosis. The reason for this variation in efficacy appears to be related to prior exposure to various mycobacterial species in the environment. Some such exposure induces immune responses that appear to antagonize the ability of BCG to afford protection. Neonatal BCG vaccination, however, induces Th1 responses and affords some degree of protection in infants and small children against disseminated forms of the disease even in regions where no protection is seen in older children and adults. For this reason BCG remains a part of the vaccination programme in most countries.

Many questions remain over the use of BCG vaccine. There is very little information on the relative efficacy of the numerous daughter strains in the human population, the added benefits of revaccination and the duration of conferred protective immunity. Tuberculin reactivity following vaccination is not a correlate of protective immunity and a diminution or loss of such reactivity is not a reliable indication of loss of protection.

BCG is living attenuated vaccine which is given by intradermal injection or, in neonates, percutaneously by means of multi-puncture devices. Vaccine for intradermal use is usually supplied in 10-dose ampoules which are reconstituted with 1 ml of distilled water and 0.1 ml (0.05 ml in neonates) is administered. Complications have followed the accidental administration of the entire contents of the 10-dose ampoule by deep cutaneous or intramuscular injection and by the intradermal injection of vaccine prepared for percutaneous use, which contains many more bacilli than the preparations for intradermal use. Vaccines should be used within 4 hours of reconstitution and must be protected from sunlight.

BCG vaccination causes a small papule to develop within a week or so and in some cases a shallow ulcer forms but usually heals within 6–12 weeks. At least 3 weeks should elapse between BCG vaccination and administration of yellow fever, measles, rubella, mumps and smallpox vaccines and no vaccination should be given in the same arm for 4 months.

Complications of BCG vaccination

If properly given, complications are very uncommon. Local adverse reactions usually occur at a rate of 0.1–0.5 per 1000 vaccinations and serious, disseminated complications occur at a rate of less than one in a million vaccinations. Local complications include necrotic lesions due to excessive delayed hypersensitivity reactions, subcutaneous abscesses, lymphadenopathy, mostly axillary, and keloid formation. Hypersensitivity reactions usually occur within a few days of vaccination and are more frequent in revaccinated subjects and in those who are tuberculin-positive. Local abscesses usually appear between 1 and 5 months after vaccination or even later. Lymphadenopathy occurs in the drainage area of the vaccinated site, usually the axilla, although cervical lymphadenopathy may occur if the vaccine is given in the upper deltoid region. Some degree of transient lymphadenopathy is not uncommon after percutaneous vaccination of neonates. The risk of keloid scarring is reduced by giving the injection in the skin overlying the insertion of the deltoid muscle. Injections higher up the arm are much more likely to lead to keloid scaring.

Osteitis is a rare complication of neonatal BCG vaccination. A relatively high incidence in Scandinavia ceased when the BCG daughter strain was changed. Disseminated disease ('BCG-osis') is a very rare complication of BCG vaccination and the mortality rate is high. Some cases have occurred in HIV-positive persons and others in children with various forms of congenital immunodeficiency.

Local hypersensitivity reactions resolve spontaneously; topical steroids are often prescribed but there is no firm evidence that they are effective. Local abscesses may resolve after aspiration but if the abscess recurs isoniazid, 6 mg/kg body weight daily to a maximum of 300 mg, or erythromycin, 250 mg four times daily, each for 1 month, is usually curative. Local lymphadenitis usually resolves spontaneously, antimicrobial therapy has little effect and surgery should only be used if the nodes are grossly enlarged or if there is suppuration and sinus formation. More serious disease, such as osteitis and disseminated infection, requires treatment with standard antituberculosis therapy, although pyrazinamide can be omitted as BCG, in common with *M. bovis*, is naturally resistant to this agent.

Vaccination strategies

These vary from region to region, and are influenced by the incidence of tuberculosis and information on the efficacy of the vaccine in a given region. The WHO recommends that BCG should be given to all neonates in high-prevalence regions and communities. In view of the risk of BCG-related complications, there has been debate as to whether the vaccine should be used in regions where there is a high incidence of HIV infection.[109,110] A literature review revealed that there is a small increase in the incidence of adverse effects of BCG in children born to HIV-infected women but almost all are mild and in regions with a high incidence of tuberculosis the benefits of vaccination greatly outweigh any disadvantages. Accordingly the WHO advises vaccination of all children according to national policies unless they have symptoms indicative of HIV/AIDS. In low-incidence regions, vaccination should be withheld from children and adults suspected of being infected with HIV.

Development of new vaccines

Since no disease has ever been eradicated with drug treatment alone, the current tools available for tuberculosis control will be insufficient to achieve total eradication of tuberculosis worldwide. A new vaccine will eventually be required and several alternatives are under development.[111] The complete sequencing of the genome of *M. tuberculosis* will enable identification of antigens that confer protective immunity and lead to candidate vaccines. Since little is known about the immune mechanisms that confer resistance to tuberculosis, there is a need to pursue different vaccine candidates. The development of DNA vaccines appears to be a novel way forward. This involves taking a gene encoding a protective antigen, inserting it into an expression plasmid, and the plasmid DNA is amplified in transformed bacteria. The plasmid DNA encoding the mycobacterial antigen is then injected into the host. The plasmid directly infects a living host cell, leading to the host being immunized against a heterologous protein provided by its own cells. While mouse models show that this can induce specific T cell responses that restrict tuberculosis infection, the duration of the effect is

unknown. Safety and ethical issues will also be paramount to the use of such vaccines. As efforts to find effective vaccines continue, existing WHO recommendations for the diagnosis, management and control of tuberculosis must continue.

Conclusions

There can be no doubt that tuberculosis ranks among the leading causes of morbidity and mortality in the tropics.[112] This is a tragedy as the therapy for tuberculosis is among the most effective and cost-effective of all treatments for life-threatening conditions. The incidence of the disease declined rapidly in the industrially developed countries during the late nineteenth and twentieth centuries and this led to the false assumption that it would do likewise in other parts of the world.[113] Too much emphasis was, however, placed on the concept of the development of population immunity—a very dubious proposition—and the very many public health innovations, often introduced only after intense advocacy, that contributed to the decline of tuberculosis in the industrially developed countries.[114] Tuberculosis is a disease of poverty,[115] and the fact that it is both preventable and treatable attests to the fact that a rectification of the gross inequities and injustices that deny the poor ready access to treatment will play a crucial role in the eventual conquest of this affliction.[116]

There is, perhaps, cause for optimism that changes are underway. In the era of globalization, it has become abundantly clear that global health is a local issue and that, in the face of infectious disease, 'no one is safe until all are safe'. It is also clear that the epidemic of 'new tuberculosis, fuelled by HIV and multi-drug resistance, could have the most catastrophic social and economic impacts from which no part of the globe will be immune. Urgent action is required, not just to facilitate the WHO DOTS strategy worldwide but to develop novel drugs, immunotherapeutic agents and vaccines. In October 2000 the Global Alliance for Tuberculosis Drug Development was launched at the International Conference on Health Research for Development in Bangkok. The aim of this alliance, which includes governments, non-governmental organizations, pharmaceutical companies and funding agencies, is to facilitate the application of recent scientific advances to the development of new cost-effective antituberculosis drugs that will shorten the duration of treatment or otherwise simplify its completion, that will improve the treatment of latent infection by the tubercle bacillus and will also be effective against multi-drug resistant tuberculosis.

In addition, the alleviation of poverty as the key component of the eventual eradication of tuberculosis and other preventable infectious diseases is being placed high on the agenda of the global community. This concern led to the foundation of the Advocacy Forum for Massive Effort Against Diseases of Poverty, sponsored by the WHO and UNAIDS, in October 2000 in Winterthur, Switzerland. The statement on the Advocacy Forum's website is impressive: 'This year—at the start of a new millennium—a movement is building that has the power to break the vicious cycle of poverty and disease. For the first time in history, the international community has the financial means, the medications, and the know-how to take a stand against a small number of diseases that cause tremendous suffering and economic loss. This massive effort against the diseases of poverty, which unites partners in unique ways, is moving the world from words to action—action that can facilitate sustainable development, stimulate economic growth, ensure greater global public health security and, most importantly, save human lives.'

This call for action is echoed by the International Union Against Tuberculosis and Lung Disease, the US National Institutes of Health and the WHO through its 'Stop TB' initiative which, in March 2001, launched its Global Tuberculosis Drug Facility, which will purchase high-quality antituberculosis drugs for countries with a high burden of the disease. The aim of the Global Tuberculosis Drug Facility is to provide drugs for 10 million tuberculosis patients over the next 5 years and 45 million patients over a 10-year period. Also, in the year 2000, the Ministers of Health and Finance of the 20 countries with the greatest burden of tuberculosis, in what has been termed the Amsterdam Declaration, have pledged support of the WHO's 'Stop TB' initiative.[117]

The major problem of HIV-related tuberculosis is being addressed by the forging of stronger links between the WHO and UNAIDS for the development of evidence-based approaches to this issue,[118] and pilot projects to evaluate the DOTS-Plus strategy for the management of multi-drug resistant tuberculosis are being developed.[119]

Notwithstanding these encouraging recent developments, it is the responsibility of all those involved in the global campaign against tuberculosis to be relentless in their advocacy efforts to ensure that declarations, initiatives and intentions are translated into sustained and effective action.

Acknowledgements

We would like to thank the following for use of their illustrations: Professor Sebastian Lucas (pathology), Dr Jonathan Richenberg (radiology) and Dr Peter Mwaba (clinical). Cambridge University Press kindly gave permission to reproduce some illustrations.

REFERENCES

1   van Rie A, Warren R, Richardson M et al. Exogenous reinfection as a cause of recurrent tuberculosis after curative treatment. *N Engl J Med* 1999; 341:1174–1179.

2   Milburn H J. Primary tuberculosis. *Curr Opin Pulmon Med* 2001; 7:133–141.

3   Wallgren A. The timetable of tuberculosis. *Tubercle* 1948; 29:245–251.

4   Rook G A W & Zumla A. Advances in the immunopathogenesis of pulmonary tuberculosis. *Curr Opin Pulmon Med* 2001; 7:116–123.

5   Zumla A, Lucas S, Mwaba P & Rook G. Tuberculosis. In James D G & Zumla A (eds) *Granulomatous Disorders*. Cambridge, UK: Cambridge University Press, 2000: 132–160.

6   Lucas S. Pathology of tuberculosis. In Davies P D O (ed.) *Clinical Tuberculosis*. London: Chapman & Hall, 1998: 113–127.

7   Flynn J L & Chan J. Immunology of tuberculosis. *Annu Rev Immunol* 2001; 19:93–129.

8   World Health Organization. *Global Tuberculosis Control*. Geneva: WHO, 2000.

9   Van Soolingen D. Molecular epidemiology of tuberculosis and other mycobacterial infections: main methodologies and achievements. *J Int Med* 2001; 249:1–26.

10 Fletcher H. Molecular epidmiology of tuberculosis: recent development and applications. *Curr Opin Pulmon Med* 2001; 7:154–159.

11 Zumla A, Malon P, Henderson J et al. The impact of the human immunodeficiency virus (HIV) infection epidemic on tuberculosis. *Postgrad Med J* 2000; 76:259–268.

12 Ahmed Y, Mwaba P, Chintu C et al. A study of maternal mortality at University Teaching Hospital, Lusaka, Zambia: the emergence of tuberculosis as a major non-obstetric cause of maternal death. *Int J Tuberc Lung Dis* 1999; 3:675–681.

13 Chintu C, Luo C, Bhat G et al. Seroprevalence of HIV-1 infection in Zambian children with tuberculosis. *Paediatr Infect Dis J* 1993; 12:499–504.

14 Chintu C, Malek A, Nyumbu M et al. Case definition for paediatric AIDS: the Zambian experience. *Int J STD AIDS* 1993; 4:83–85.

15 Espinal M A, Laszlo A, Simonsen L et al. Global trends in resistance to antituberculosis drugs. *N Engl J Med* 2001; 344:1294–1303.

16 Mitchison D A. How drug resistance emerges as a result of poor compliance during short course chemotherapy of tuberculosis. *Int J Tuberc Lung Dis* 1998; 2:10–15.

17 Fox W. Drug combinations and the bioavailability of rifampicin. *Tubercle* 1990; 71:241–245.

18 Kochi A, Vareldzis B & Styblo K. Multidrug-resistant tuberculosis and its control. *Res Microbiol* 1993; 144:104–110.

19 World Health Organization. Anti-tuberculosis drug resistance in the world. *Report no. 2. The WHO/IUATLD Project on Antituberculosis Drug Resistance Surveillance*. Geneva: WHO, 2000.

20 Becerra M C, Bayona J, Freeman J et al. Redefining MDR-TB 'hot spots'. *Int J Tuberc Lung Dis* 2000; 4:387–394.

21 Perelman M I. Tuberculosis in Russia. *Int J Tuberc Lung Dis* 2000; 4:1097–1103.

22 Davies R P O, Tocque K, Bellis M A et al. Historical declines in tuberculosis in England and Wales: improving social conditions or natural selection? *Int J Tuberc Lung Dis* 1999; 3:1051–1054.

23 Watkins R E, Brennan R & Plant A J. Tuberculin reactivity and the risk of tuberculosis: a review. *Int J Tuberc Lung Dis* 2000; 4:895–903.

24 Woeltje K F, Mathew A, Rothstein M et al. Tuberculosis infection and anergy in hemodialysis patients. *Am J Kidney Dis* 1998; 31:848–852.

25 Qunibi W Y, Al-Sibai M B, Taher S et al. Mycobacterial infection after renal transplantation: a report of 14 cases and a review of the literature. *Q J Med* 1990; 77:1039–1060.

26 American Thoracic Society, Centers for Disease Control. Treatment of tuberculosis and tuberculosis infection in adults and children. *Am J Respir Crit Care Med* 1994; 149:1359–1374.

27 Grange J M, Ustianowski A & Zumla A. Tuberculosis and pregnancy. In Diwan V, Thorson A & Winkvist A (eds) *Gender and Tuberculosis*. Göteborg: Nordic School of Public Health, 1998: 77–88.

28 Collins C H, Grange J M & Yates M D. *Tuberculosis Bacteriology: Organization and Practice*, 2nd edn. London: Butterworth-Heinemann, 1997.

29 International Union Against Tuberculosis and Lung Disease. *Management of Tuberculosis: A Guide for Low Income Countries*, 5th edn. Paris: IUATLD, 2000.

30 Funahashi A, Lohaus G H, Poliotis J et al. Role of fibreoptic bronchoscopy in the diagnosis of mycobacterial disease. *Thorax* 1983; 38:267–270.

31 Chien H P, Yu M C, Wu M H et al. Comparision of the BACTEC MGIT 960 with Löwenstein–Jensen medium for recovery of mycobacteria from clinical specimens. *Int J Tuberc Lung Dis* 2000; 4:866–870.

32 Foulds J & O'Brien R. New tools for the diagnosis of tuberculosis: the perspective of developing countries. *Int J Tuberc Lung Dis* 1999; 2:778–783.

33 Soini H & Musser J M. Molecular diagnosis of mycobacteria. *Clin Chem* 2001; 47:809–814.

34 Davies P D O & Leitch G. Practical problems of the tuberculin test. In Davies PDO (ed.) *Clinical Tuberculosis*. London: Chapman & Hall, 1994: 345–349.

35 Donald P R, Fourie P B & Grange J M. *Tuberculosis in Childhood*. Pretoria: van Schaik, 1999.

36 Milburn H. Primary tuberculosis. *Curr Opin Pulmon Med* 2001; 7(3):133–141.

37 Maltezou H C, Spyridis P & Kafetzis D A. Tuberculosis during infancy. *Int J Tuberc Lung Dis* 2000; 4:414–419.

38 Fourie P B, Becker P J, Festenstein F et al. Procedures for developing a simple scoring method based on unsophisticated criteria for screening children for tuberculosis. *Int J Tuberc Lung Dis* 1998; 2:116–123.

39 Delacourt C, Mani T M, Bonnerot V et al. Computed tomography with normal chest radiograph in tuberculous infection. *Arch Dis Child* 1993; 69:430–432.

40 Snider D E & Bloch A B. Congenital tuberculosis. *Tubercle* 1984; 65:81–82.

41 Proudfoot A T. Cryptic disseminated tuberculosis. *Br J Hosp Med* 1971; 5:773–780.

42 Ormerod L P, Grundy M & Rathman M A. Multiple tuberculous bone lesions resembling metastatic disease. *Tubercle* 1989; 70:305–307.

43 Wilkinson A G & Roy S. Two cases of Poncet's disease. *Tubercle* 1984; 65:301–303.

44 Webb J G & Thomas P. Hypertrophic osteoarthropathy and pulmonary tuberculosis. *Tubercle* 1986; 67:225–228.

45 Thwaites G, Chan T T, Mai N T, Drobniewski F, McAdam K & Farar J. Tuberculous meningitis. *J Neurol Neurosurg Psychiatry* 2000; 68:289–299.

46 Labhard N, Nicod L & Zellweger J P. Cerebral tuberculosis in the immunocompetent host: 8 cases observed in Switzerland. *Tuberc Lung Dis* 1994; 75:454–459.

47 Tandon P N & Bhargava S. Effect of medical treatment on intracranial tuberculoma: a CT study. *Tubercle* 1985; 66:85–89.

48 Lanjewar D N, Ansari M A, Shetty C R et al. Renal lesions associated with AIDS: an autopsy study. *Ind J Pathol Microbiol* 1999; 42:63–68.

49 Ustvedt H J. The relationship between renal tuberculosis and primary infection. *Tubercle* 1947; 28:22–25.

50 Petersen L, Mommsen S & Pallisgaard G. Male genitourinary tuberculosis: report of 12 cases and review of the literature. *Scand J Urol Nephrol* 1993; 27:425–428.

51 Eastwood J B, Corbishley C M & Grange J M. Tuberculosis and the kidney. *Nephrology* 2001; 12:1307–1314.

52 Gow J G & Barbos A S. Genitourinary tuberculosis: a study of 1117 cases over a period of 34 years. *Br J Urol* 1984; 56:449–455.

53 Morgan S H, Eastwood J B & Baker L R I. Tuberculous interstitial nephritis: the tip of an iceberg. *Tubercle* 1991; 71:5–6.

54 Eastwood J B, Zaidi M, Maxwell J D et al. Tuberculosis as primary renal diagnosis in end-stage uraemia. *J Nephrol* 1994; 7:290–293.

55 Ramanathan R, Kumar A, Kapoor R et al. Relief of urinary tract obstruction in tuberculosis to improve renal function: analysis of predictive factors. *Br J Urol* 1998; 81:199–205.

56 Menzies R I, Alsen H, Fitzgerald J M et al. Tuberculous peritonitis in Lesotho. *Tubercle* 1986; 67:47–54.

57 Tshibwabwa-Tumba E, Mwaba P, Bogle-Taylor J et al. Four year study of abdominal ultrasound in 900 Central African adults with AIDS referred for diagnostic imaging. *Abdom Imaging* 2000; 25:290–296.

58 Falkner M J, Reeve P A & Locket S. The diagnosis of tuberculous ascites in a rural African community. *Tubercle* 1985; 66:55–59.

59 Grange J M, Noble W C, Yates M D & Collins C H. Inoculation mycobacterioses. *Clin Exp Dermatol* 1988; 13:211–220.

60 Morrison J G L & Fourie E D. The papulonecrotic tuberculide from Arthus reaction to lupus vulgaris. *Br J Dermatol* 1974; 91:273–277.

61 Lau S K, Wei W I, Hsu C et al. Efficacy of fine needle aspiration in the diagnosis of tuberculous cervical lymphadenopathy. *J Laryngol Otol* 1990; 104:24–27.

62 Strang J I. Tuberculous pericarditis in Transkei. *Clin Cardiol* 1984; 7:667–670.

63 Dinning W J & Marston S. Cutaneous and ocular tuberculosis: a review. *J R Soc Med* 1985; 78:576–581.

64 Khooshabeh R, Grange J M, Yates M D et al. A case report of Mycobacterium chelonae keratitis and a review of mycobacterial infections of the eye. *Tubercle Lung Dis* 1994; 75:377–382.

65 Rosen P H, Spalton D J & Graham E M. Intraocular tuberculosis. *Eye* 1990; 4:486–492.

66 Lucas S B, Peacock C S, Hounnou A et al. Disease in children infected with HIV in Abidjan, Cote-d'Ivoire. *Br Med J* 1996; 312:335–338.

67 Lucas S & Nelson A M. Pathogenesis of tuberculosis in human immunodeficiancy virus-infected people. In Bloom B (ed.) *Tuberculosis: Pathogenesis, Protection and Control*. Washington, DC: ASM Press, 1994: 503–513.

68 Lucas S, Sewankumbo N, Nambuya A, et al. The morbid anatomy of African AIDS. In *AIDS and Associated Cancers in Africa*. International symposium, Naples. Basel: Karger, 1988: 124–133.

69 Tshibwabwa-Tumba E, Mwinga A, Pobee J O M et al. Radiological features of pulmonary tuberculosis in 963 HIV-infected adults at three Central African hospitals. *Clin Radiol* 1997; 52:837–841.

70 World Health Organization. *TB/HIV: A Clinical Manual*. Geneva: WHO, 1996.

71 Wiktor S Z, Sassan-Morokro M, Grant A D et al. Efficacy of trimethoprim–sulphamethoxazole prophylaxis to decrease morbidity and mortality in HIV-1 infected patients with tuberculosis in Abidjan, Cote d'Ivoire: a randomised controlled trial. *Lancet* 1999; 353:1469–1475.

72 Maynart M, Lievre L, Sow P S et al. Primary prevention with co-trimoxazole for HIV-1-infected adults: results of a pilot study in Dakar, Senegal. *J Acquir Immune Defic Syndr* 2001; 26:130–136.

73 Chintu C, Luo C, Bhat G et al. Cutaneous hypersensitivity reactions due to thiacetazone in Zambian children infected with tuberculosis and the human immunodeficiency virus. *Arch Dis Child* 1993; 68:331–334.

74 Centers for Disease Control and Prevention. Prevention and treatment of tuberculosis among patients infected with human

immunodeficiency virus: principles of therapy and revised recommendations. *Morb Mortal Wkly Rep* 1998; 47(RR-20):1–58.

75 World Health Organization Global Tuberculosis Programme and UNAIDS. *Policy Statement on Preventive Therapy Against Tuberculosis in People Living with HIV.* Geneva: WHO, 1998.

76 World Health Organization. *Treatment of Tuberculosis: Guidelines for National Programmes.* Geneva: WHO, 1997.

77 World Health Organization. *What is DOTS? A Guide to Understanding the WHO-Recommended TB Control Strategy Known as DOTS.* Geneva: WHO, 1999.

78 Cosivi O, Grange J M, Daborn C J et al. Zoonotic tuberculosis due to Mycobacterium bovis in developing countries. *Emerg Infect Dis* 1998; 4:59–70.

79 Kazwala R R, Daborn C J, Sharp J M et al. Isolation of Mycobacterium bovis from human cases of cervical adenitis in Tanzania: a cause for concern? *Int J Tuberc Lung Dis* 2001; 5:87–91.

80 Mitchison D A. The role of individual drugs in the chemotherapy of tuberculosis. *Int J Tuberc Lung Disease* 2000; 4:796–806.

81 Gillespie S H & Kennedy N. Fluoroquinolones: a new treatment for tuberculosis? *Int J Tuberc Lung Dis* 1998; 2:265–271.

82 Luna-Herrera J, Reddy M V, Danneluzzi D et al. Anti-tuberculosis activity of clarithromycin. *Antimicrob Agents Chemother* 1995; 39:2692–2695.

83 Winstanley P A. Clinical pharmacology of antituberculosis drugs. In Davies P D O (ed.) *Clinical tuberculosis*, 2nd edn. London: Chapman & Hall; 1998: 225–242.

84 Grange J M & Zumla A. Anti-tuberculosis agents. In Armstrong D & Cohen J (eds). *Infectious Diseases*, vol. 2. London: Mosby International, 1999: 7:13.1–7:13.14.

85 Grange J M, Winstanley P A & Davies P D O. Clinically significant drug interactions with antituberculosis agents. *Drug Safety* 1994; 11:242–251.

86 Grange J M. Antimycobacterial agents. In O'Grady F, Lambert H P, Finch R G & Greenwood D (eds). *Antibiotic and Chemotherapy*, 7th edn. Edinburgh: Churchill Livingstone, 1997:499–512.

87 Durban Immunotherapy trial group. Immunotherapy with *Mycobacterium vaccae* in patients with newly diagnosed pulmonary tuberculosis: a randomised control trial. *Lancet* 1999; 354:116–119.

88 Johnson J L, Kamya R M, Okwera A et al. Randomized controlled trial of *Mycobacterium vaccae* immunotherapy in non-human immunodeficiency virus-infected Ugandan adults with newly diagnosed pulmonary tuberculosis. *J Infect Dis* 2000; 181:1304–1312.

89 World Health Organization. *Multidrug Resistant Tuberculosis (MDRTB): Basis for the Development of an Evidence-Based Case-Management Strategy for MDRTB within the WHO's DOTS Strategy.* Geneva: WHO, 1999.

90 World Health Organization. *Guidelines for the Management of Drug-Resistant Tuberculosis.* Geneva: WHO, 1997.

91 Crofton J, Chaulet P & Maher D. Guidelines for management of drug-resistant tuberculosis. Geneva: WHO, 1997.

92 Farmer P & Kim J Y. Community based approaches to the control of multidrug resistant tuberculosis: introducing 'DOTS-plus'. *Br Med J* 1998; 317:671–674.

93 Alzeer A H & FitzGerald J M. Corticosteroids and tuberculosis: risks and use as adjunct therapy. *Tubercle Lung Dis* 1993; 74:6–11.

94 Israel H L. Chemoprophylaxis for tuberculosis. *Respir Med* 1993; 87:81–83.

95 Hawken M P & Muhindi D W. Tuberculosis preventive therapy in HIV-infected persons: feasibility issues in developing countries. *Int J Tuberc Lung Dis* 1999; 3:646–650.

96 Wilkinson D, Squire S B & Garner P. Effect of preventive treatment for tuberculosis in adults infected with HIV: systematic review of randomised placebo controlled trials. *Br Med J* 1998; 317:625–629.

97 Bleed D, Dye C & Raviglione M C. Dynamics and control of the global tuberculosis epidemic. *Curr Opin Pulmonary Med* 2000, 6:174–179.

98 Grange J & Zumla A. Making DOTS succeed. *Lancet* 1997; 350:157.

99 Chowdhury A M R, Chowdhury S A, Islam M N et al. Control of tuberculosis through community health workers in Bangladesh. *Lancet* 1997; 350:160–172.

100 Chowdhury A M R, Vaughan J P, Chowdhury S et al. Demystifying the control of tuberculosis in rural Bangladesh. In Porter J D H & Grange J M (eds) *Tuberculosis: An Interdisciplinary Perspective.* London: Imperial College Press, 1999: 379–396.

101 Porter J D H & Grange J M (eds). *Tuberculosis: An Interdisciplinary Perspective.* London: Imperial College Press, 1999.

102 Volmink J & Garner P. Interventions for promoting adherence to tuberculosis management (Cochrane Review CD-ROM). *Cochrane Database Syst Rev* 2000, 4:CD000010.

103 Grange J M. DOTS and beyond: towards a holistic approach to the conquest of tuberculosis. *Int J Tuberc Lung Dis* 1997; 1:293–296.

104 Weil D E. Advancing tuberculosis control within reforming health systems. *Int J Tuberc Lung Dis* 2000, 4:597–605.

105 Ogden J. The resurgence of tuberculosis in the tropics: improving tuberculosis control—social science inputs. *Trans R Soc Trop Med Hyg* 2000; 94:135–140.

106 Kelly P. Isolation and stigma: the experience of patients with active tuberculosis. *J Commun Health Nurs* 1999, 16:233–241.

107 Ngamvithayapong J, Winkvist A & Diwan V. High AIDS awareness may cause tuberculosis patient delay: results from an HIV epidemic area, Thailand. *AIDS* 2000; 14:1413–1419.

108 Fine P E M. Variation in protection by BCG: implications of and for heterologous immunity. *Lancet* 1995; 346:1339–1345.

109 Besnard M, Sauvion S, Offredo C et al. Bacillus Calmette–Guérin infection after vaccination of human immunodeficiency virus-infected children. *Pediatr Infect Dis* 1993; 12:993–997.

110 Bhat G J, Diwan V K, Chintu C et al. HIV, BCG and TB in children: a case control study in Lusaka, Zambia. *J Trop Paediatr* 1993; 39:219–223.

111 Doherty M & Andersen P. Tuberculosis vaccines: developmental work and the future. *Curr Opin Pulmonary Med* 2000; 6:203–208.

112 Zumla A, Squire S B, Chintu C et al. The tuberculosis pandemic: implications for health in the tropics. *Trans R Soc Trop Med Hyg* 1999; 93:113–117.

113 Lauzardo M & Ashkin D. Phthisiology at the dawn of the new century: a review of tuberculosis and prospects for its elimination. *Chest* 2000;117:1455–1473.

114 Grange J M, Gandy M, Farmer P et al. Historical declines in tuberculosis: nature, nurture and the biosocial model. *Int J Tuberc Lung Dis* 2001; 5:208–212.

115 Grange J M & Zumla A. Tuberculosis and the poverty–disease cycle. *J R Soc Med* 1999; 92:105–107.

116 Grange J M & Zumla A. Tuberculosis: an epidemic of injustice. *J R Coll Physicians Lond* 1997; 31:637–640.

117 World Health Organization. *Report of the Ministerial Conference on TB and Sustainable Development*, Amsterdam. Geneva: WHO, 2000.

118 World Health Organization. *An Evidence-Based Approach to Developing a New WHO/UNAIDS Strategy for TB/HIV.* Geneva: WHO, 2001.

119 World Health Organization. *Guidelines for Establishing DOTS plus Pilot Projects for the Management of Multi-Drug Resistant Tuberculosis.* Geneva: WHO, 2000.

GENERAL READING

Crofton J, Horne N & Miller F. *Clinical Tuberculosis*, 2nd edn. London: Macmillan, 1999.

Davies P D O (ed.). *Clinical Tuberculosis*, 2nd edn. London: Chapman & Hall, 1998.

Donald P R, Fourie P B & Grange J M. *Tuberculosis in Childhood*. Pretoria: van Schaik; 1999.

Interactive tutorial on CD-ROM. *Tuberculosis*. Topics in International Health. London: Wellcome Trust, 1999.

International Union Against Tuberculosis and Lung Disease. *Management of Tuberculosis: A Guide for Low Income Countries*, 5th edn. Paris: IUATLD, 2000.

Iseman M D. *A Clinican's Guide to Tuberculosis*. Philadelphia: Lippincott Williams, 2000

Chapter 58

Human Disease due to Environmental Mycobacteria

J. M. Grange and A. Zumla

In addition to the obligate mycobacterial pathogens of humans, the *Mycobacterium tuberculosis* complex and *M. leprae*, the genus contains around 100 named species that are usually encountered as environmental saprophytes.[1] They are therefore termed environmental mycobacteria (EM) but are also known, particularly in the USA, as non-tuberculous mycobacteria (NTM) or mycobacteria other than typical tubercle (MOTT) bacilli, while in the older literature they are termed atypical mycobacteria. They commonly occur in watery environments such as marshes, ponds, lakes and rivers. Some species colonize industrial and domestic water pipes.[2,3] Human contact with them by drinking water, inhalation of aerosols or by inoculation into skin wounds is a common and regular event. This contact may, in some regions, be sufficient to induce tuberculin cross-reactivity and to affect, sometimes adversely, protection against tuberculosis afforded by BCG vaccine. Although they are much less virulent than members of the *M. tuberculosis* complex, some of the EM can cause human disease.

Being common in nature, EM may contaminate containers and equipment used to collect clinical specimens. The use of inadequately sterilized containers for the collection or transport of sputum or urine has resulted in a number of 'pseudo-epidemics' of disease.[4] Unlike the obligate pathogens, EM may occur as transient commensals on the skin and external genitalia and in the pharynx, gastrointestinal tract and the lower urethra. They may also colonize diseased tissues, such as damaged lung tissue in children with cystic fibrosis or bronchiectasis. Therefore, in contrast to *M. tuberculosis*, isolation of EM from clinical specimens does not necessarily mean that they are causing the disease. As described below, great care is required in determining whether EM isolated from clinical specimens, especially sputum and urine, are primary pathogens rather than contaminants, colonizers or commensals.

Microbiology

Some species of EM were described soon after the discovery of the tubercle bacillus but little serious interest in them was evident until the middle of the twentieth century when Runyon divided isolates from clinical specimens into four groups according to their rate of growth and their ability to synthesize yellow or orange pigments, as shown in Table 58.1.[5] Those species producing visible growth on standard egg-based media within a week *on subculture* are regarded as rapid growers: paradoxically, some rapid growers grow very slowly on primary isolation from clinical material. The slowly and rapidly growing species differ in many properties, including antigenic structure and DNA relatedness, and some workers consider them to be distinct subgenera, with the latter more closely related to the genus *Nocardia*.

Subsequently, species were identified according to a range of cultural and biochemical properties and by more specialized techniques including analysis of their cell wall lipids by thin-layer chromatography, gas chromatography or mass spectroscopy and antigenic analysis by immuno-diffusion in gel or agglutination serology.[6] At the present time there is increasing use of nucleic acid-based techniques, including the use of specific DNA probes (which are commercially available for a limited number of species) and the sequencing of ribosomal RNA ('ribotyping').[7]

Table 58.1 The Runyon classification of the environmental mycobacteria

Group		Characteristics	Examples
I	Photochromogens	Producing pigment only on or after exposure to light	*M. kansasii*, *M. marinum*
II	Scotochromogens	Producing pigment in the dark	*M. scrofulaceum*, *M. gordonae*
III	Nonchromogens	Producing no pigment	*M. avium* complex, *M. malmoense*, *M. nonchromogenicum*
IV	Rapid growers*	Rapid growth and any of the above pigment types	*M. chelonae*, *M. fortuitum*, *M. vaccae*

*Most isolates from cases of human disease, on which the classification was based, are non-pigmented. Environmental isolates, e.g. *M. vaccae*, are mostly chromogenic.

Mycobacteria may be directly detected and, in many cases, identified at species level by amplification of DNA or RNA in clinical specimens by the polymerase chain reaction (PCR) in certain specialized reference centres.

The EM most frequently associated with human disease are listed in Table 58.2. The most common causes of disease are the closely related slow-growing species *M. avium* and *M. intracellulare*, which are usually grouped together as the *M. avium* complex (MAC). This complex was originally subdivided by serotyping, which yielded serotypes 1, 2 and 3 corresponding to *M. avium* and serotypes 4–27 corresponding to *M. intracellulare*. More recent typing based on DNA homology shows that serotypes 1–6, 8–12 and 21 correspond to *M. avium* and the other serotypes to *M. intracellulare*, although there is considerable genetic diversity within some serotypes.[8] For reasons that are not understood, clinically significant isolates of MAC from HIV-positive patients usually belong to the group defined by DNA analysis as *M. avium*, whereas a broader distribution of types is found in HIV-negative patients and in the environment.[9,10]

Some species of EM grow very poorly, or not at all, on standard culture media and some require nutritional supplements for growth. Thus, *M. paratuberculosis*, the cause of chronic hypertrophic enteritis or Johne's disease in cattle and some strains of MAC, require the addition of mycobactin, a lipid iron-chelating agent found in the cell walls of most mycobacteria, and *M. haemophilum* requires the addition of haem or other sources of iron to the culture medium.

Very few of the rapid-growing species cause human disease: the two species most usually encountered are *M. chelonae* and *M. fortuitum*. Some workers, rather confusingly, divide *M. chelonae* into two separate species, *M. chelonae* and *M. abscessus*, and likewise divide *M. fortuitum* into *M. fortuitum* and *M. peregrinum*. In this chapter, the original nomenclature will be used.

Very little is known about the determinants of virulence of the EM causing human disease. One species, *M. ulcerans*, produces a toxin, as described below. In the case of MAC, there is evidence that the more hydrophobic strains are more likely to contain additional genetic elements called plasmids and also to cause disease,[11] but this may simply reflect the ease with which these strains enter aerosols as a means of transmission to humans.

Epidemiology and predisposing factors

Except, perhaps, in extreme environments such as deserts and the polar regions, the human population is regularly exposed to EM, yet disease resulting from such contact is very uncommon. On the other hand, EM may cause 'silent' non-progressive lesions that may induce immune responses that affect the efficacy of BCG vaccination and the outcome of infection by the tubercle and leprosy bacilli. Such 'immunologically effective contact' with EM is the most plausible explanation for the wide geographical variations in the efficacy of BCG vaccination.[12,13]

Patients with pulmonary and disseminated disease due to EM often have an underlying predisposing condition such as cystic fibrosis, cancer (including lymphoproliferative disorders such as Hodgkin's disease and hairy cell leukaemia), autoimmune disease, renal failure, post-transplant immunosuppressive therapy, high-dose corticosteroid therapy, overt congenital immunodeficiencies and the acquired immune deficiency syndrome (AIDS). As mentioned above AIDS patients are, for reasons that are not understood, particularly susceptible to disease due to a restricted range of genotypes of the MAC. A small proportion of cases of pulmonary disease due to EM occur in patients who are apparently otherwise healthy although there is evidence that many such patients have low levels of cytokines involved in protective immunity to mycobacterial disease.[14]

Most children with cervical lymphadenopathy due to EM appear to be otherwise healthy but a few have various forms of congenital immune defects and are prone to develop disseminated mycobacterial disease.

The risk of disease due to EM depends on the opportunities for exposure to them, the number and types of EM in the environment and the immune status of those in

Table 58.2 The usual environmental mycobacteria causing human disease according to category of disease

Disease	Causative agent
Lymphadenopathy	*M. avium* complex[1]
	M. scrofulaceum
Skin lesions	
Post-trauma abscesses	*M. chelonae*[2]
	M. fortuitum[3]
	M. terrae group[4]
Swimming pool granuloma	*M. marinum*
Buruli ulcer	*M. ulcerans*[5]
Pulmonary disease	*M. avium* complex
	M. celatum
	M. gordonae
	M. kansasii
	M. malmoense
	M. simiae
	M. szulgai
	M. xenopi
Disseminated disease	
AIDS related	*M. avium* complex
	M. genevense
Non-AIDS related	*M. avium* complex
	M. chelonae
	M. haemophilum[6]

[1]Human pathogens in this group are *M. avium* and *M. intracellulare*.
[2]Includes strains named *M. abscessus*.
[3]Includes strains name *M. peregrinum*.
[4]Includes *M. terrae*, *M. nonchromogenicum* and *M. triviale*.
[5]Includes strains named *M. shinshuense*.
[6]A rare cause of skin lesions in renal transplant patients and lymphadenopathy in children.

contact with them. Some species of EM causing disease, such as the MAC, are found worldwide while others, such as *M. xenopi*, *M. malmoense* and *M. ulcerans*, are more restricted in their geographical distribution. Infection is directly from the environment: human-to-human transmission leading to disease, if it occurs at all, is extremely rare and the few reported clusters of cases probably resulted from exposure to a common environmental source. Thus the incidence of disease due to EM in a given region is independent of that of tuberculosis, which is spread principally by human-to-human transmission. Accordingly, EM are responsible for only a small minority of cases of mycobacterial disease where tuberculosis is common but are the cause of a relatively much higher proportion of cases where tuberculosis is a rare disease. There has, however, been a recent increase in the absolute prevalence of disease due to EM in some regions as a result of AIDS and other forms of immune suppression. An increase in prevalence of disease due to EM has also been observed in non-HIV infected persons in some regions but it is not clear whether this is a real increase or merely the result of improvements in microbiological technique. One particular disease, Buruli ulcer (see below), has certainly increased in prevalence in parts of Africa and this increase appears to be associated with environmental changes. On the other hand, AIDS-related MAC disease was common in Europe before the introduction of highly active antiretroviral therapy (HAART) but, although the organisms are present in the African environment, such disease is rare in that continent where HAART is, at present, rarely available.

The incidence of disease due to EM may to some extent be affected by BCG vaccination. Thus a substantial increase in the incidence of lymphadenopathy due to EM in children coincided with the termination of neonatal BCG vaccination in Scandinavia and Czechoslovakia.[15,16]

Diagnosis

The only disease due to EM with clear-cut pathognomonic features is Buruli ulcer. The other dermatological, pulmonary and disseminated manifestations of EM disease are non-specific and require differentiation from tuberculosis and a range of other infectious and non-infectious conditions with which they may easily be confused. The diagnosis is usually based on isolation and identification of the causative organism although, as mentioned above, EM are ubiquitous in nature and their isolation from a clinical specimen does not per se indicate that they are causing disease.

It is not unusual to obtain single isolates of EM from sputum and, more especially, from urine.[17] Thus, as a general rule, several cultures of an EM from sputum—at least two, but preferably three or four, cultures yielding a heavy growth at least 1 week apart—with compatible clinical features in whom other causes, including tuberculosis, are carefully excluded, are required for diagnosis of pulmonary disease.[18] As the external genitalia and lower urethra are frequently contaminated by EM, and as

renal disease due to them is very rare, even stricter criteria for diagnosis are required, including histological demonstration of granulomas in, and isolation of the EM from, the lesion itself.[19]

It is very important that all specimens are collected directly into sterile containers as false diagnoses resulting from the use of unsterile containers is not uncommon.[4] Where available, fibreoptic bronchoscopy is a useful technique for obtaining aspirates or biopsies directly from suspicious pulmonary lesions,[20] but false diagnoses have resulted from the use of inadequately sterilized endoscopes.[21]

Once isolated, the mycobacteria can be identified at reference laboratories on the basis of a battery of tests including speed and temperature range of growth, pigment production, biochemical reactions, susceptibility to antimicrobial agents and demonstration of patterns of cell wall lipids by thin-layer chromatography. Several newer tests based on molecular biological techniques such as DNA hybridization using gene probes, PCR followed by hybridization, and other nucleic acid amplification techniques have been developed.

The use of reagents prepared from *M. tuberculosis* and a range of EM have been used in differential skin testing for the diagnosis of lymphadenitis and pulmonary disease due to EM, notably the *M. avium* complex.[22,23] The British Thoracic Society concludes, however, that more research is needed before this diagnostic method can be recommended.[24]

Clinical manifestations of disease due to environmental mycobacteria

There are four principal groups of human disease due to EM: (1) postinoculation; (2) pulmonary; (3) lymphadenitis; and (4) disseminated.

Postinoculation disease

Postinoculation disease includes two specifically named entities —(a) Buruli ulcer caused by *M. ulcerans* and (b) swimming pool (or fish tank) granuloma caused by *M. marinum*—as well as (c) non-specific postinoculation lesions, principally caused by the rapidly growing species *M. chelonae* and *M. fortuitum*.

Buruli ulcer

This disease was first reported in the Bairnsdale district of Australia in 1948.[25] The causative organism, named *M. ulcerans*, grows very slowly on conventional bacteriological media and has a very narrow temperature range of growth: around 33°C. Some years later, a large outbreak of a very

Table 58.3 Countries in which Buruli ulcer has been reported*

Africa	Angola, Benin, Burkina Faso, Cameroon, Congo, Democratic Republic of Congo, Côte d'Ivoire, Gabon, Ghana, Guinea, Liberia, Nigeria, Sierra Leone, Sudan, Togo, Uganda
Western Pacific	Australia, Papua New Guinea
Asia	China, India, Indonesia, Japan, Malaysia
Americas	Bolivia, French Guiana, Mexico, Peru, Surinam

*Data adapted from the World Health Organization.[36]

similar disease occurred in the Buruli district of Uganda. The disease was called Buruli ulcer and the organism was named *M. buruli*, until it was found to be identical to the previously described *M. ulcerans*. The disease has also been reported in Mexico, Malaysia, Papua New Guinea and several African countries including the Congo (previously Zaire), Ghana,[26] Benin,[27,28] Côte d'Ivoire,[29] Togo[30] and Angola.[31] An organism termed *M. shinshuense* has been isolated from rare cases of ulcerative skin lesions in Japan and China and has been shown to be a variant of *M. ulcerans*.[32] The countries in which Buruli ulcer has been reported are listed in Table 58.3.

Buruli ulcer is emerging as the third most prevalent mycobacterial disease in the world,[33] and is posing a severe economic burden on the communities affected by it, both in terms of cost of management and in residual disability in the patients after recovery.[34,35] There has, in recent years, been a marked increase in the prevalence of Buruli ulcer in some parts of West Africa: the disease was almost unknown in the Côte d'Ivoire before 1978, but 10,000 cases were reported between 1988 and 1997 and in some villages up to 16% of the population are affected.[29] The reason for this increase is unknown, but several workers have observed that outbreaks of Buruli ulcer tend to follow environmental upheavals that lead to flooding and swamp formation.[36] This, and other, epidemiological characteristics of the disease suggest that the causative organism lives in the environment and enters the skin through injuries.[37] Although prickly vegetation including tall grasses may cause many such injuries, cases have followed gunshot wounds and scorpion and snake bites.[38,39] The possibility of transmission by biting insects,[35] and aerosols of contaminated water,[40] has been raised.

Pathogenesis and clinical features
Four stages of the disease have been described:[27]

I. Subcutaneous nodule.
II. Vasculitis and spreading cellulitis.
III. Ulceration.
IV. Healing with gross fibrosis.

The first sign of the disease is a firm and sometimes itchy skin nodule which may resolve spontaneously or enlarge with an intense vasculitis and necrosis of the subdermal tissue and overlying firm oedema (Figure 58.1). The vasculitis and necrosis are, at least in part, due to bacterial toxins, especially a macrolide termed mycolactone,[41] but there is probably also an immunological basis.[42] Secondary necrosis of the overlying skin due to anoxia results in deeply undermined ulcers (Figure 58.2). During Stage III, the ulcers grow in size, often becoming enormous, and numerous mycobacteria are present in the lesions (Figures 58.3 and 58.4). There appears to be some degree of suppression of immune reactivity to mycobacteria in this stage as patients are negative on skin testing with tuberculin and also Burulin—a reagent

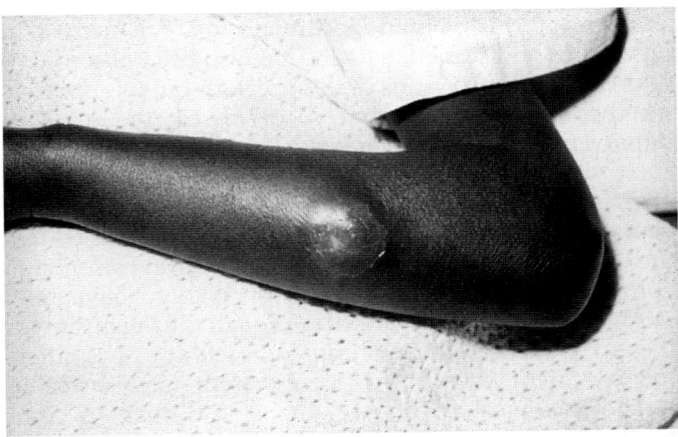

Figure 58.1: *Buruli ulcer:* pre-ulcerative lesion on the forearm.

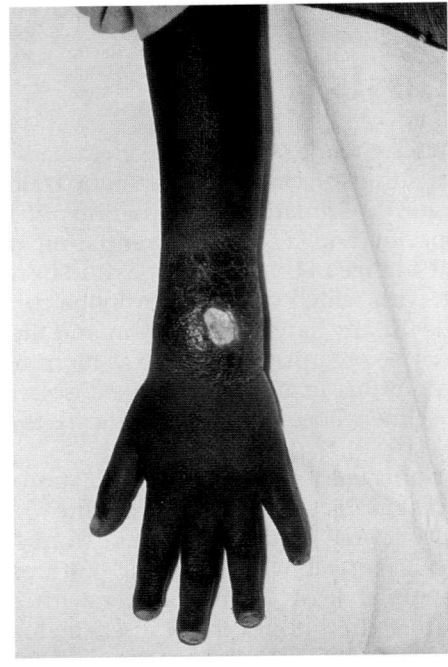

Figure 58.2: *Buruli ulcer:* early ulcerative lesion with skin changes around the ulcer.

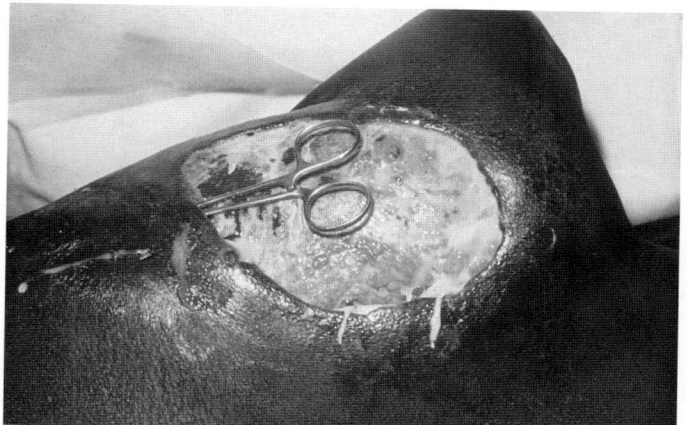

Figure 58.3: *Buruli ulcer*: large and deeply undermined ulcer overlying the left shoulder. The inserted 'Spencer Wells' forceps illustrates the extensive undermining of the ulcer.

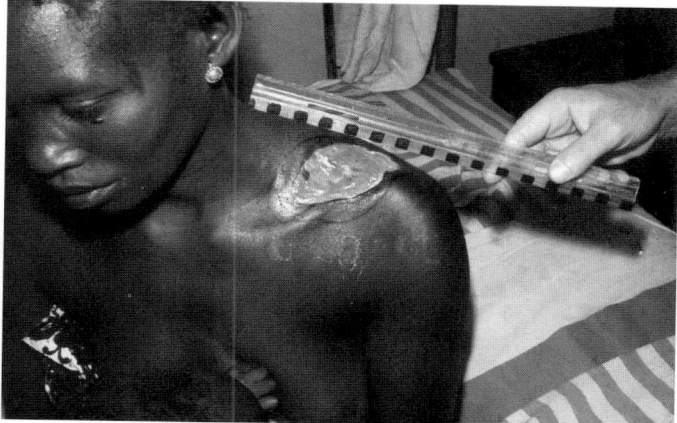

Figure 58.5: *Buruli ulcer*: a resolving ulcer on the left shoulder. Note the granulating base and absence of trophic changes in the surrounding skin.

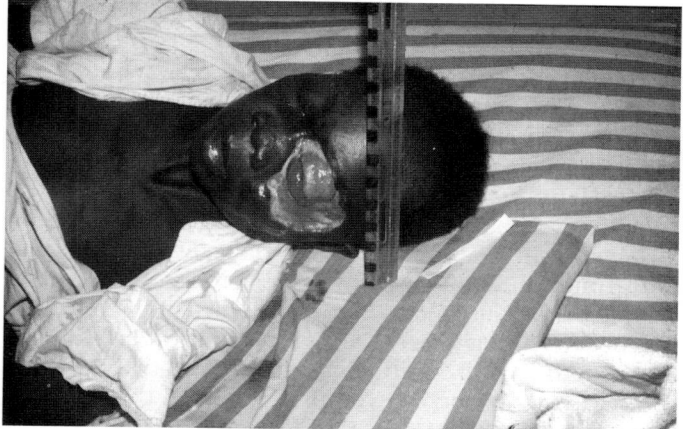

Figure 58.4: *Buruli ulcer*: lesion involving the left eye and orbit. The lesion eventually resolved, unfortunately with loss of vision in the eye.

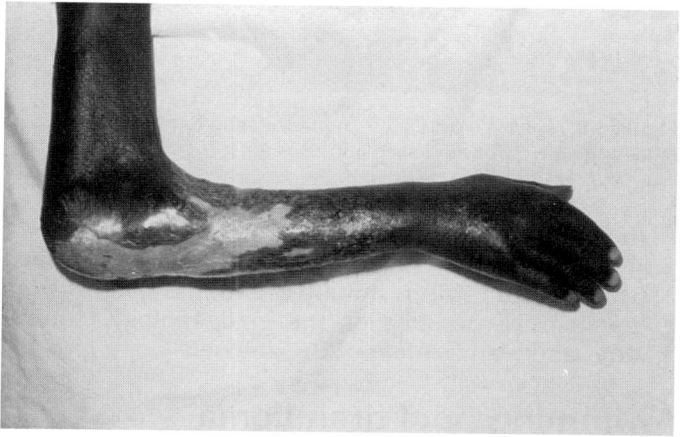

Figure 58.6: *Buruli ulcer*: healed lesion with extensive scarring leading to a fixed elbow joint. The skin is thin and easily traumatized. Note the oedematous hand due to a compromised lymphatic drainage.

prepared from *M. ulcerans*.[43] It has been postulated that the toxins of *M. ulcerans* have immunosuppressive properties.[44] Death may occur in this stage from sepsis or tetanus.[35]

Lesions occur on any part of the body but particularly on exposed parts, as determined by local dress customs. Males and females are equally affected and no age group is exempt, although most cases occur in children. In Ghana, for example, the disease was most common in the first decade of life, after which the numbers declined with age.[26]

An unusual and unexplained characteristic is that, after 2 or 3 years of active and progressive disease, many patients enter Stage IV, in which the lesions regress (Figure 58.5) and eventually heal, though often with gross and disfiguring and deforming scarring (Figure 58.6).[35,36] This healing appears to be the result of a switch to immune reactivity as the patients become positive on skin testing with tuberculin and Burulin, granulomas appear in the lesion and the acid-fast bacilli disappear. Occasionally, progression and healing occur simul-

taneously in different ulcers, or even in different parts of the same ulcer.

Although usually confined to the skin, the bones in the region of the lesions may be involved with necrosis and sinus formation, and cases of disseminated osteomyelitis have been reported.[39] A diffuse non-ulcerative form of the disease has been reported in Benin[45] and observed in the Congo (Figure 58.7). Draining lymph nodes may contain acid-fast bacilli but clinically evident lymphadenopathy is uncommon.

The clinical features of Buruli ulcer are usually characteristic but conditions likely to cause diagnostic confusion include tropical ulcers, cutaneous diphtheria, actinomycosis, cancrum oris, bacterial abscesses, skin tuberculosis and cutaneous leishmaniasis.[36] Diagnosis is made on clinical features, demonstration of acid-fast bacilli in smears from the bases of progressive ulcers, biopsy and demonstration of *M. ulcerans* by conventional culture or, where available, PCR.[46]

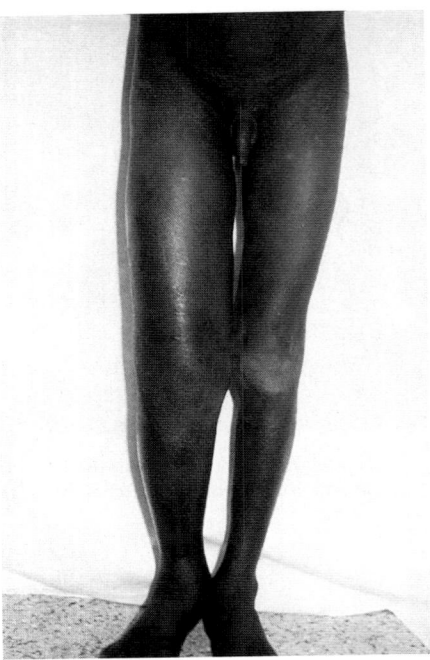

Figure 58.7: *Buruli ulcer:* Diffuse, non-ulcerating form of the disease in a Congolese child with lower limb swelling.

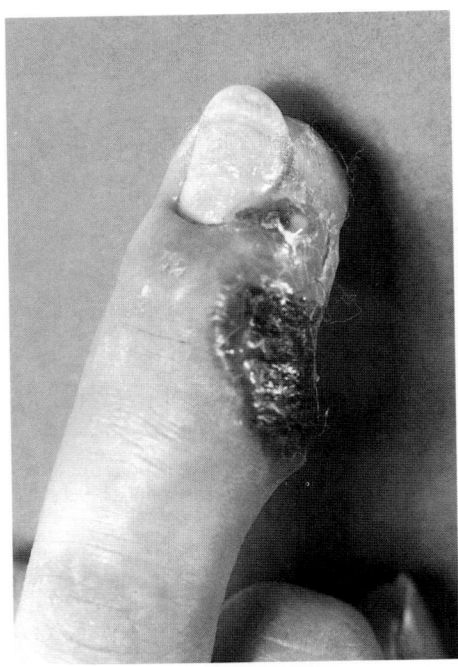

Figure 58.8: 'Fish tank granuloma' due to *M. marinum* infection.

In view of the increasing seriousness of the burden of Buruli ulcer in many countries, the WHO has established a Global Buruli Ulcer Initiative and has published a comprehensive account of the epidemiology, clinical features and management of the disease.[36]

Swimming pool granuloma

Also called fish tank granuloma, this disease is caused by *M. marinum*, a water-borne EM that enters cuts and abrasions acquired while swimming or handling tropical fish tanks.[47] Cases have also occurred among fishermen. The disease was initially described in Sweden in 1954 following an outbreak of lesions among users of a swimming pool.[48] The condition is characterized by the development of warty skin lesions resembling those of skin tuberculosis at the site of inoculation (Figure 58.8). Secondary lesions often develop along the draining lymphatics, resembling those seen in the fungal disease sporotrichosis and thus termed sporotrichoid spread. Rare complications include carpal tunnel syndrome, osteomyelitis and disseminated disease. Uncomplicated lesions usually heal spontaneously after a few months but treatment (described below) accelerates resolution.

Other postinjection and post-traumatic EM disease

Three main types of lesion are encountered: (i) superficial warty lesions similar to those of swimming pool granuloma; (ii) localized postinjection abscesses; and (iii) deeper lesions following more serious penetrating injuries or surgical procedures.

Superficial warty lesions

Sometimes with sporotrichoid spread, these have occasionally been caused by *M. kansasii*, *M. szulgai*, *M. chelonae* and unidentified slow-growing scotochromogens.[47,49] Outbreaks of skin ulcers associated with non-cultivable mycobacteria have been reported on the USA/Canada border and in Brazil and are termed Feldman–Hershfield ulcers, after the workers who first described them.[50]

Postinjection abscesses

These are caused principally by the rapid-growing species *M. chelonae* and *M. fortuitum*. These abscesses may occur sporadically, especially when dirty needles are used, and are a cause of 'sterile' postinjection abscesses, so called because cultivation on standard media yields no bacterial growth. There have also been instances of small outbreaks of abscesses after injection of contaminated material from multi-dose containers. Examples include a histamine solution used for challenge tests for atopy[51] and a batch of triple vaccine.[52] Abscesses develop 1–12 months after the injection and may reach an enormous size, up to 8 cm in diameter. Many abscesses remain localized and resolve after surgical drainage, curettage or excision but a spreading cellulitis requiring chemotherapy may develop, especially in insulin-dependent diabetic and immuno-suppressed persons.[53] Corneal ulcers and abscesses due to *M. chelonae* or *M. fortuitum* have followed abrasions or penetrating injuries of the cornea (Figure 58.9).[54]

Deeper lesions

Serious and life-threatening post-traumatic lesions due to *M. chelonae* or *M. fortuitum* have followed cardiac surgery involving the insertion of bioprosthetic heart valves.[55]

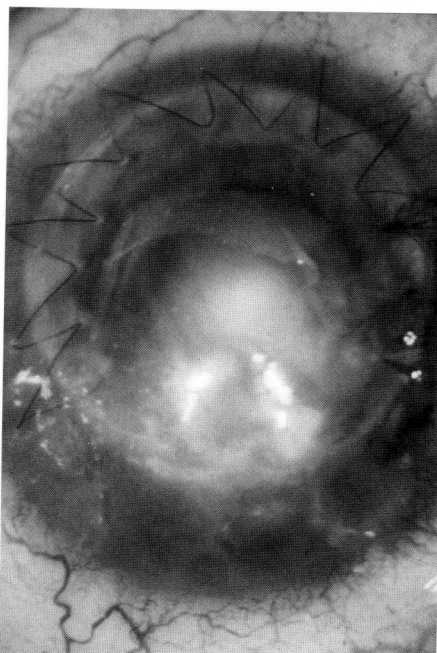

Figure 58.9: Chronic keratitis due to recurrence of *M. chelonae*. Note the characteristic 'cracked windscreen' appearance.

Meningitis and hepatitis due to *M. gordonae* ('*M. aquae*') has followed the insertion of a ventriculo-atrial shunt for the relief of hydrocephalus in a child,[56] and peritonitis due to the accidental introduction of EM has occurred in patients on intermittent peritoneal dialysis.[17,57]

Pulmonary disease

Most cases occur in middle-aged or elderly men who often have a history of smoking, bronchiectasis, silicosis, healed tuberculosis or exposure to industrial dusts, but cases also occur in otherwise healthy persons although, as mentioned above, some may have low levels of certain cytokines. A number of cases have been reported in elderly, non-smoking women with no other evidence of lung disease—the 'Lady Windermere syndrome'.[58] If the disease continues undetected for years, cavities develop in the lung and respiratory failure may ensue. The causative organisms include MAC and *M. kansasii* and, less frequently, *M. xenopi*, *M. scrofulaceum*, *M. szulgai*, *M. malmoense*, *M. simiae*, *M. celatum* and *M. chelonae*. Although rare in childhood, a few cases caused by *M. chelonae* and *M. fortuitum* have been reported in children with cystic fibrosis. Diagnosis is made by bacteriological examination but it is important to distinguish true disease from mere contamination of sputum by these ubiquitous organisms, as described under Diagnosis.

Although some differences in radiological features between tuberculosis and disease due to EM, and even between different species of EM, have been described, there is so much overlap in these features that a radiological determination of cause is not possible in the individual patient.[59] Some patients, notably non-smokers with no other evidence of lung disease, tend to have nodular lesions localized to the middle lobe or the lingula.[60] When MAC causes chest disease in immunocompetent individuals, there are three categories of chest X-ray patterns which are seen in clinical practice:

- The most common appearance is similar to that of apical post-primary tuberculosis, with or without cavities. It is not possible to differentiate this from tuberculosis although the cavities have been described as being thinner and smaller.
- Patchy, nodular opacities in any zone of the lung which, on computed tomography (CT) scanning, are shown to be associated with local bronchiectasis.
- Least common is the isolated pulmonary nodule. Mediastinal lymphadenopathy and pleural effusion are also rare.

Bizarre and rapidly changing radiological appearances are seen in those with AIDS and other immunosuppressive disorders and the chest X-ray may appear normal in up to a third of AIDS patients with EM pulmonary disease.

Lymphadenitis

Most cases occur during the first 5 years of life, with cases being rare in the first year of life and most common in the second.[61,62] In most cases a single cervical or preauricular node is involved: such nodes are usually painless and not tender on palpation, although there may be reddening of the overlying skin. Characteristic features of the lesions are demonstrable by CT or magnetic resonance scanning.[63] Total excision, when technically possible, is usually curative. Lymphadenitis in older patients, involving more than one node or involving other sites, should arouse suspicion of immunodeficiency, notably HIV infection. Nodes should not be merely incised and drained as this predisposes to chronic sinus formation. Most affected children are otherwise healthy and, in the absence of immunosuppression, dissemination of the disease is rare. Opinions differ on the need for routine antimicrobial therapy.

Several species of EM cause lymphadenitis, the most common being MAC, but other species, depending on the geographical region, include *M. malmoense*, *M. scrofulaceum*, *M. kansasii*, *M. fortuitum* and *M. chelonae*.[64] Rarer causes in apparently healthy children include *M. haemophilum*[65] and *M. interjectum*.[66,67]

The pathogenesis of mycobacterial lymphadenitis is poorly understood but it is likely that the affected lymph nodes are secondary to a primary tonsillar lesion. There is evidence that EM may colonize the tonsil, with seasonal variation. Although most affected children appear healthy, the possibility of minor defects in cytokine production or function must be considered. As mentioned above, neonatal BCG vaccination protects against lymphadenitis due to EM in childhood.

Disseminated EM disease

Cases of isolated non-pulmonary lesions in the bones and joints,[68] and the genitourinary system,[17] have been reported but these are extremely rare. More widespread disseminated disease was very rare before the advent of the HIV pandemic, the very few cases being described in young people with congenital immune deficiencies and in organ transplant recipients. Serious, recurrent and often fatal disseminated infections due to EM during childhood have been reported in some families as a result of inherited abnormalities in gamma interferon receptors on macrophages, thereby compromising the immune activation of these cells.[69,70]

The usual cause of non-HIV related disseminated disease is MAC but cases due to *M. haemophilum*, *M. chelonae* and *M. fortuitum* have been described. In some children with congenital immunodeficiencies there is bacillary infiltration of tissues and organs but in others osteolytic skeletal lesions occur, particularly involving the cranium and orbit.[71–73] Disseminated disease due to *M. chelonae* and *M. haemophilum* may present with multiple skin abscesses and ulcers in children with congenital immune defects, transplant recipients and patients with lymphoma.[74,75]

Disseminated mycobacterial disease became a frequent complication of AIDS, notably in the USA and Europe, although it was (and still is) infrequently reported in Africa.[76] The great majority of cases, 90% or more, are caused by the MAC although cases due to other species including *M. genevense* also occur.[77,78] The latter is a very slow-growing mycobacterium which has also been isolated from pet birds.[79]

Disseminated disease due to MAC and other EM in HIV-positive persons almost always occurs in the profoundly immunosuppressed, usually after the onset of other AIDS-defining conditions. The risk factors include a low CD4 count (of under 50/µl), the wasting syndrome and *Pneumocystis carinii* pneumonia.[80] The clinical features of patients with MAC infection are many and varied. Patients may remain asymptomatic for several months and are often not acutely ill and thus the diagnosis can easily be missed. Symptoms include weight loss, anorexia, abdominal discomfort, general malaise, haemoptysis, night sweats, diarrhoea, nausea and vomiting, but these symptoms are also frequently encountered in other AIDS-related opportunist infections. Infiltration of bone occasionally results in pathological fractures. Large numbers of acid-fast bacilli are present in many organs, especially the lung, liver and intestine (Figures 58.10 and 58.11). Multiple skin lesions, hepatomegaly, generalized lymphadenopathy, arthritis and various haematological abnormalities may occur, but these may also be caused by other AIDS-related opportunist pathogens. Bone marrow infiltration leads to anaemia and leucopenia and infiltration of the intestinal wall is a cause of vomiting, abdominal discomfort and severe diarrhoea.

Diagnosis of MAC infection is made by detection of the bacilli by microscopy or culture of biopsies of affected tissues including the rectal mucosa and intestinal

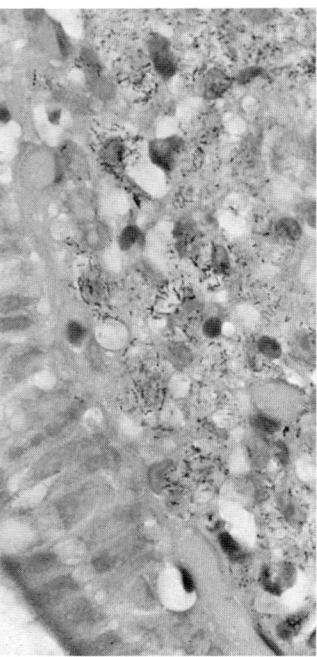

Figure 58.10: Liver biopsy from an AIDS patients stained with Ziehl–Neelsen stain showing numerous acid-fast bacillli (*M. avium* complex).

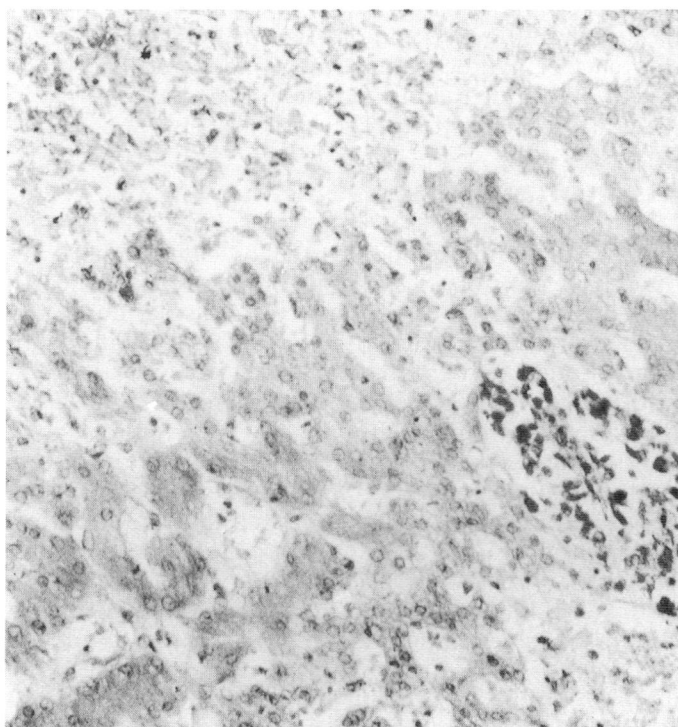

Figure 58.11: Ziehl–Neelsen stain of a small bowel biopsy showing a large infiltrate of acid-fast bacilli (*M. avium* complex) in a patient with AIDS.

biopsies (Figure 58.11) and bone marrow and by blood culture, preferably by radiometric or other automated systems or by a lysis–centrifugation system.[81] The presence of acid-fast bacilli in clinical specimens in severely immunocompromised HIV-positive individuals poses management dilemmas for the clinician who has to decide whether the isolated acid-fast bacillus is clinically significant and, if so, whether to start conventional antituberculosis therapy or to give the combination of drugs described below for the more resistant MAC to cover the period before culture results are available.

The incidence of AIDS-related disease due to MAC and other EM has declined considerably in the industrially developed nations since the introduction of HAART which, regrettably, is rarely available in the poorer countries. HAART leads to a fivefold reduction in the risk of first occurrence of disseminated MAC disease and most cases that occur do so during the first 2 months of HAART.[82]

Diseases of possible mycobacterial aetiology

Several authors have postulated that certain chronic granulomatous diseases of unknown aetiology, notably sarcoidosis and Crohn's disease, are caused by EM, possibly in unusual morphological or physiological forms. Although DNA specific for *M. paratuberculosis*, the cause of chronic hypertrophic enteritis (Johne's disease) in cattle, has been detected by PCR in intestinal biopsies of a proportion of patients with Crohn's disease in some regions,[83] serious questions of cause and effect remain. It is thus possible that *M. paratuberculosis* detected in some cases is a secondary saprophyte of diseased tissue rather than a primary pathogen. Although a fascinating and important topic, much more research is required before a definitive conclusion can be reached.

Therapy of disease due to EM

Very few controlled clinical trials into the therapy of disease due to EM have been conducted. Although guidelines have been published, these by their own admission are largely based on small uncontrolled studies or accumulated anecdotal evidence.[18,24] Thus only general indications of therapeutic experience can be given and this is a subject that is likely to evolve and change rapidly. Likewise there is hardly any useful information on the duration of therapy, which must be determined on the basis of the clinical course of the individual patient. As a general rule, disease due to EM does not respond to standard antituberculosis therapy and in vitro drug susceptibility testing is of limited value in predicting in vivo responses to treatment. If drug susceptibility tests are performed, it is important to use standardized methods.[84]

Buruli ulcer

The treatment of Buruli ulcer depends on the stage of the disease. Despite in vitro susceptibility to some agents including rifampicin, amikacin and clarithromycin,[85] chemotherapy is generally ineffective. Treatment is therefore surgical, ranging from simple excision of Stage I lesions to radical excision, often requiring extensive skin grafting, for Stage II and III lesions.[35] This poses serious problems in rural hospitals with limited facilities and, in high-prevalence areas, the local population should be encouraged to attend for treatment before the disease has progressed beyond the first stage. Stage IV lesions require less extensive surgery, but excision of scar tissue and skin grafting may be required for the prevention of contractures and disfigurement. An exception to the general experience that chemotherapy is ineffective was the single case in China caused by *M. ulcerans* subspecies *shinshuense* which responded to treatment with clarithromycin and rifabutin.[86]

Swimming pool granuloma

Lesions due to *M. marinum* usually resolve spontaneously but resolution is accelerated by systemic treatment with minocycline, trimethoprim with sulfamethoxazole (co-trimoxazole) or a combination of rifampicin and ethambutol. Clarithromycin with ethambutol also seems to be efficient.[87] Small lesions may also be cured by surgical excision.[88]

Post-injection and post-traumatic lesions

Localized postinjection abscesses usually respond to excision, curettage or drainage, but multiple abscesses or spreading cellulitis, as are sometimes seen in insulin-dependent diabetics and immunocompromised persons, require chemotherapy. Most lesions are caused by the rapid growers *M. chelonae* (including *M. abscessus*) and *M. fortuitum*. Information on treatment is derived from anecdotal experience, which indicates that useful agents for localized disease include erythromycin with trimethoprim and/or doxycycline, and those for spreading or disseminated disease include amikacin, gentamicin, cephalosporins, clarithromycin, imipenem and quinolones such as ciprofloxacin. The outcome of therapy is very unpredictable and no guidelines on length of therapy can usefully be given.

Lymphadenopathy

Involvement of a single lymph node in an otherwise healthy child is usually curable by excision if that can be achieved without damaging the facial nerve or other important structures.[89] If total excision is not possible, chemotherapy is required and clarithromycin in combination with either ethambutol or rifampicin has been found to be effective for disease due to MAC.[61,90]

Pulmonary disease

Disease due to MAC, *M. xenopi* or *M. malmoense* in non-immunocompromised patients responds in 80% of cases to a combination of rifampicin and ethambutol for 18 or 24 months. Some workers add isoniazid to this regimen although there is no reliable evidence that it improves the outcome. In one of the very few controlled clinical trials of therapy for disease caused by EM, a 9-month course of rifampicin and ethambutol has been shown to be sufficient in most cases of pulmonary disease due to *M. kansasii*.[91] The results of formal trials of quinolones and newer macrolides conducted by the British Thoracic Society are expected by the end of the year 2001, but anecdotal experience indicates a useful role for these therapies and the present body of experience justifies the addition of clarithromycin to the regimens.[90] Surgery is used for localized lesions that fail to respond to chemotherapy.

Pulmonary disease due to *M. fortuitum* or *M. chelonae*, as occurs for example in children with cystic fibrosis, responds in a very unpredictable manner to therapy, which is based on the drugs described above (Postinjection and post-traumatic lesions).

Disseminated disease

The most effective agents for the treatment of disseminated disease, usually due to the *M. avium* complex, in AIDS patients are the newer macrolides clarithromycin and azithromycin.[92] One of these should be given with at least one companion drug, selected when possible on the basis of in vitro drug susceptibility tests from rifabutin (preferably), a quinolone and ethambutol. Serious cases with high fever may require treatment with intravenous amikacin. The duration of therapy depends on the clinical response. Disease due to the less common mycobacteria must be treated empirically; for example, *M. genevense* infections are treated with the drug combinations used for MAC.

The same regimens are recommended for disseminated disease due to other slow-growing species. The very rare cases due to *M. fortuitum* or *M. chelonae* in both HIV and non-HIV infected persons should be treated empirically as described above for serious wound infections due to these species.

As in the case of tuberculosis (Chapter 57), care must be taken when giving rifamycins to patients receiving HAART. In general, HAART appears to be more important in the treatment of AIDS-related EM disease than specific antimycobacterial therapy and should not therefore be withdrawn. Rifabutin causes less drug interaction than rifampicin but, if problems are encountered, patients should be treated with macrolides and ethambutol. Some patients receiving HAART and antimycobacterial therapy may develop immune phenomena, such as a painful lymphadenitis, which usually respond to corticosteroid therapy.

Conclusions

Relative to tuberculosis, disease due to EM is uncommon, although in some countries, notably in West Africa, Buruli ulcer is becoming a major health problem. Although many cases are associated with various forms of immunosuppression, some forms of EM disease such as post-inoculation lesions and lymphadenitis in children occur in otherwise healthy persons. Diagnosis is usually made by bacteriological techniques. There are relatively few firm guidelines to therapy, although several clinical trials are underway. If control measures succeed in reducing the prevalence in tuberculosis worldwide, disease due to EM, which is acquired by environmental exposure rather than human-to-human spread, will continue as a challenge to the physician.

REFERENCES

1 Holland S M. Nontuberculous mycobacteria. *Am J Med Sci* 2001; 321:49–55.

2 Schulze-Röbbecke R, Janning B, Fischeder R et al. Occurrence of mycobacteria in biofilm samples. *Tubercle Lung Dis* 1992; 73:141–144.

3 von Reyn C F, Maslow J N, Barber T W et al. Persistent colonisation of potable water as a source of *Mycobacterium avium* infection in AIDS. *Lancet* 1994; 343:1137–1141.

4 Collins C H, Grange J M & Yates M D. Mycobacteria in water. *J Appl Bacteriol* 1984; 57:193–211.

5 Runyon E H. Anonymous mycobacteria in pulmonary disease. *Med Clin North Am* 1959; 43:273–290.

6 Collins C H, Grange J M & Yates M D. *Tuberculosis Bacteriology: Organization and Practice*, 2nd edn. London: Butterworth-Heinemann, 1997.

7 Kirschner P, Springer B, Vogel U et al. Genotypic identification of mycobacteria by nucleic acid sequence determination: report of a 2-year experience in a clinical laboratory. *J Clin Microbiol* 1993; 31:2882–2889.

8 Arbeit R D, Slutsky A, Barber T W et al. Genetic diversity of *Mycobacterium avium* strains causing monoclonal and polyclonal bacteremia in patients with the acquired immunodeficiency syndrome (AIDS). *J Infect Dis* 1993; 167:1384–1390.

9 Guthertz L S, Damsker B, Bottone E J et al. *Mycobacterium avium* and *Mycobacterium intracellulare* infections in patients with and without AIDS. *J Infect Dis* 1989; 160:1037–1041.

10 Portaels F. Epidemiology of mycobacterial diseases. *Clin Dermatol* 1995; 13:207–222.

11 Meissner P S & Falkingham J O. Plasmid DNA profiles as epidemic markers for clinical and environmental isolates of *Mycobacterium avium*, *Mycobacterium intracellulare* and *Mycobacterium scrofulaceum*. *J Infect Dis* 1986; 153:325–331.

12 Stanford J L, Shield M J, Rook G A W. How environmental mycobacteria may predetermine the protective efficacy of BCG. *Tubercle* 1981; 62:55–62.

13 Fine P E M. Variation in protection by BCG: implications of and for heterologous immunity. *Lancet* 1995; 346:1339–1345.

14 Greinert U, Schlaak M, Rüsch-Gerdes S et al. Low in vitro production of interferon-γ and tumour necrosis factor-α in HIV-seronegative patients with pulmonary disease caused by non-tuberculous mycobacteria. *J Clin Immunol* 2000; 20:445–452.

15 Romanus V, Halalander H O, Wahlen P et al. Atypical mycobacteria in extrapulmonary disease among children: incidence in Sweden from 1969 to 1990, related to changing BCG-vaccination coverage. *Tubercle Lung Dis* 1995; 76:300–310.

16 Trnka L, Dankova D & Svandova E. Six years' experience with the discontinuation of BCG vaccination. 4. Protective effect of BCG vaccination against the *Mycobacterium avium intracellulare* complex. *Tubercle Lung Dis* 1994; 75:348–352.

17 Eastwood J B, Dilly S A & Grange J M. Tuberculosis, leprosy and other mycobacterial diseases. In Cattell W R (ed.) *Infections of the Kidney and Urinary Tract.* Oxford: Oxford University Press, 1996: 291–318.

18 Official Statement of the American Thoracic Society. Diagnosis and treatment of disease caused by nontuberculous mycobacteria. *Am J Respir Crit Care Med* 1997; 156(Suppl.): S1–S25.

19 Brooker W J & Aufderheide A C. Genitourinary infections due to atypical mycobacteria. *J Urol* 1980; 124:242–244.

20 Funahashi A, Lohaus G H, Poliotis J et al. Role of fibreoptic bronchoscopy in the diagnosis of mycobacterial disease. *Thorax* 1983; 38:267–270.

21 Gubler J G H, Salfinger M & von Graevenitz A. Pseudoepidemic of non-tuberculous mycobacteria due to a contaminated bronchoscope washing machine: report of an outbreak and a review of the literature. *Chest* 1992; 101:1245–1249.

22 Colville A. Retrospective review of culture-positive mycobacterial lymphadenitis cases in children in Nottingham, 1979–1990. *Eur J Clin Microbiol Infect Dis* 1993; 12:192–195.

23 von Reyn C F, Williams D E, Horsburgh C R et al. Dual skin testing with *Mycobacterium avium* sensitin and purified protein derivative to discriminate pulmonary disease due to *M. avium* complex from pulmonary disease due to *Mycobacterium tuberculosis. J Infect Dis* 1998; 177:730–736.

24 Subcommittee of the Joint Tuberculosis Committee of the British Thoracic Society. Management of opportunist mycobacterial infections: Joint Tuberculosis Committee guidelines 1999. *Thorax* 2000; 55:210–218.

25 MacCallum P, Tolhurst J C, Buckle C et al. A new mycobacterial infection in man. *J Pathol Bacteriol* 1948; 60:93–122.

26 van der Werf T S, van der Graaf W T A, Groothuis D G et al. *Mycobacterium ulcerans* infection in Ashanti region, Ghana. *Trans R Soc Trop Med Hyg* 1989; 83:410–413.

27 Muelder K & Nourou A. Buruli ulcer in Benin. *Lancet* 1990; 336:1109–1111.

28 Josse R, Guédénon A, Darie H et al. Les infections cutanées à *Mycobacterium ulcerans*: ulcères de Buruli. *Méd Trop* 1996; 55:363–373.

29 Marston B J, Diallo M O, Horsburgh C R et al. Emergence of Buruli ulcer disease in the Daloa region of Côte d'Ivoire. *Am J Trop Med Hyg* 1995; 52:219–224.

30 Meyers W M, Tignokpa N, Priuli G B et al. *Mycobacterium ulcerans* infection (Buruli ulcer): first reported patients in Togo. Identification of the etiologic agent by DNA sequencing. *Br J Dermatol* 1996; 134:1116–1121.

31 Bar W, Rusch-Gerdes S, Richter E et al. *Mycobacterium ulcerans* infection in a child from Angola: diagnosis by direct detection and culture. *Trop Med Int Health* 1998; 3:189–196.

32 Portaels F, Fonteyne P-A, De Beenhouwer H et al. Variability in the 3' end of 16S rRNA sequence of *Mycobacterium ulcerans* is related to geographic origin of isolates. *J Clin Microbiol* 1996; 34:962–965.

33 Dobos K M, Quinn F D, Ashford D A et al. Emergence of a unique group of necrotising mycobacterial diseases. *Emerg Infect Dis* 1999; 5:367–378.

34 Asiedu K & Etuaful S. Socioeconomic implications of Buruli ulcer in Ghana: a three-year review. *Am J Trop Med Hyg* 1998; 59:1015–1022.

35 van der Werf T S, van der Graaf W T, Tappero J W et al. *Mycobacterium ulcerans* infection. *Lancet* 1999; 354:1013–1018.

36 Asiedu K, Scherpbier R & Raviglione M. Buruli ulcer: *Mycobacterium ulcerans* infection. Geneva: WHO Global Buruli Ulcer Initiative, 2000.

37 Barker D J P. Epidemiology of *Mycobacterium ulcerans* infection. *Trans R Soc Trop Med Hyg* 1973; 67:43–50.

38 Meyers W M, Shelly W M, Connor D H et al. Human *Mycobacterium ulcerans* infections developing at sites of trauma to skin. *Am J Trop Med Hyg* 1974; 23:919–923.

39 Hofer M, Hirschel B, Kirschner P et al. Disseminated osteomyelitis from *Mycobacterium ulcerans* after a snake bite. *N Engl J Med* 1993; 328:1007–1009.

40 Veitch M G, Johnson P D & Flood PE. A large localized outbreak of *Mycobacterium ulcerans* infection on a temperate southern Australian island. *Epidemiol Infect* 1997; 119:313–318.

41 George K M, Chatterjee D, Gunawardana G et al. Mycolactone: a polyketide toxin from *Mycobacterium ulcerans* required for virulence. *Science* 1999; 283:854–857.

42 Burchard G D & Bierther M. Buruli ulcer: a clinical pathological study of 23 patients in Lambarene, Gabon. *Trop Med Parasitol* 1986; 37:1–8.

43 Stanford J L, Revill W D L, Gunthorpe W J et al. The production and preliminary investigation of Burulin, a new skin test reagent for *Mycobacterium ulcerans* infection. *J Hygiene* 1975; 74:7–16.

44 Pimsler M, Sponsler T A & Meyers W M. Immunosuppressive properties of the soluble toxin from *Mycobacterium ulcerans. J Infect Dis* 1988; 157:577–580.

45 Abalos F M, Aguiar J, Guedenon A et al. *Mycobacterium ulcerans* infection (Buruli ulcer): a case report of the disseminated nonulcerative form. *Ann Diagn Pathol* 2000; 4:386–390.

46 Guimaraes-Peres A, Portaels F, de Rijk P et al. Comparison of two PCRs for detection of *Mycobacterium ulcerans. J Clin Microbiol* 1999; 37:206–208.

47 Collins C H, Grange J M, Noble W C et al. *Mycobacterium marinum* infections in man. *J Hyg (Camb)* 1985; 94:135–149.

48 Linell F & Norden A. *Mycobacterium balnei*: a new acid-fast bacillus occurring in swimming pools and capable of producing skin lesions in humans. *Acta Tuberc Scand* 1954; 33(Suppl.):1–84.

49 Grange J M, Noble W C, Yates M D et al. Inoculation mycobacterioses. *Clin Exp Dermatol* 1988; 13:211–220.

50 Feldman R A & Hershfield E. Mycobacterial skin infections by an unidentified species: a report of 29 patients. *Ann Intern Med* 1974; 80:445–452.

51 Inman P M, Beck A, Brown A E et al. Outbreaks of injection abscesses due to *Mycobacterium abscessus. Arch Dermatol* 1969; 100:141–147.

52 Borghans J G & Stanford J L. *Mycobacterium chelonei* in abscesses after injection of diptheria–pertussis–tetanus–polio vaccine. *Am Rev Respir Dis* 1973; 107:1–8.

53 Jackson P G, Keen H, Noble C J & Simmons N A. Injection abscesses due to *Mycobacterium chelonei* occurring in a diabetic patient. *Tubercle* 1981; 62:277–279.

54 Khooshabeh R, Grange J M, Yates M D et al. A case report of *Mycobacterium chelonae* keratitis and a review of mycobacterial infections of the eye. *Tubercle Lung Dis* 1994; 75:377–382.

55 Grange J M. Mycobacterial infections following heart valve replacement. *J Heart Valve Dis* 1992; 1:102–109.

56 Gonzalez E P, Crosby R M N & Walker S H. *Mycobacterium aquae* infection in a hydrocephalic child (*Mycobacterium aquae* meningitis). *Paediatrics* 1971; 48:974–977.

57 White R, Abreo K, Flanagan R et al. Non-tuberculous mycobacterial infections in continuous ambulatory peritoneal dialysis patients. *Am J Kidney Dis* 1993; 22:581–587.

58 Reich J M & Johnson R E. *Mycobacterium avium* complex pulmonary disease presenting as an isolated lingular or middle lobe pattern: the Lady Windermere syndrome. *Chest* 1992; 101:1605–1609.

59 Cook P L, Riddell R W & Simon G. Bacteriological and radiographic features of lung infection by opportunist mycobacteria. *Tubercle* 1971; 52:232–241.

60 Erasmus J J, McAdams H P, Farrell M A et al. Pulmonary non-tuberculous mycobacterial infection: radiologic manifestations. *Radiographics* 1999; 19:1487–1505.

61 Green P A, von Reyn C F & Smith RP. *Mycobacterium avium* complex parotid lymphadenitis: successful therapy with clarithromycin and ethambutol. *Pediatr Infect Dis J* 1993; 12:615–617.

62 Grange J M, Yates M D & Pozniak A. Bacteriologically confirmed non-tuberculous mycobacterial lymphadenitis in South east England: a recent increase in the number of cases. *Arch Dis Child* 1995; 72:516–517.

63 Robson C D, Hazra R, Barnes P D et al. Nontuberculous mycobacterial infection of the head and neck in immunocompetent children: CT and MR findings. *Am J Neuroradiol* 1999; 20:1829–1835.

64 Wolinsky E. Mycobacterial lymphadenitis in children: a prospective study of 105 nontuberculous cases with long term follow up. *Clin Infect Dis* 1995; 20:954–963.

65 Dawson D J, Blacklock Z M & Kane D W. *Mycobacterium haemophilum* causing lymphadenitis in an otherwise healthy child. *Med J Austr* 1981; 2:289–290.

66 Haas W H, Kirschner P, Ziesing S et al. Cervical lymphadenitis in a child caused by a previously unknown mycobacterium. *J Infect Dis* 1993; 167:237–240.

67 Springer B, Kirschner P, Rost-Meyer G et al. *Mycobacterium interjectum*, a new species isolated from a patient with chronic lymphadenitis. *J Clin Microbiol* 1993; 31:3083–3089.

68 Prosser A. Spinal infection with *Mycobacterium xenopi*. *Tubercle* 1986; 67:229–232.

69 Levin M, Newport M J, D'Souza S et al. Familial disseminated atypical mycobacterial infection in childhood: a human mycobacterial susceptibility gene? *Lancet* 1995; 345:79–83.

70 de Groot R, van Dongen J J M, Neijens H J et al. Familial disseminated atypical mycobacterial infection in childhood. *Lancet* 1995; 345:993.

71 Levine R A. Infection of the orbit by an atypical mycobacterium. *Arch Ophthalmol* 1969; 82:608–610.

72 van der Hoeman L H, Rutter F J & van der Sar A. An unusual acid-fast bacillus causing systemic disease and death in a child. *Am J Clin Pathol* 1958; 29:433–445.

73 Yakovac W C, Baker R, Sweigert C et al. Fatal disseminated osteomyelitis due to an anonymous mycobacterium. *J Pediatr* 1961; 59:909–914.

74 Azadian B S, Beck A, Curtis J R et al. Disseminated infection with *Mycobacterium chelonei* in a haemodialysis patient. *Tubercle* 1981; 62:281–284.

75 Moulsdale M T, Harper J M, Thatcher G N et al. Infection by *Mycobacterium haemophilum*, a metabolically fastidious acid-fast bacillus. *Tubercle* 1983; 64:29–36.

76 Horsburgh C R. *Mycobacterium avium* complex infection in the acquired immunodeficiency syndrome. *N Engl J Med* 1991; 324:1332–1338.

77 Böttger E C, Teske A, Kirschner P et al. Disseminated '*Mycobacterium genavense*' infection in patients with AIDS. *Lancet* 1992; 340:76–80.

78 Nadal D, Caduff R, Kraft R et al. Invasive infection with *Mycobacterium genavense* in three children with the acquired immunodeficiency syndrome. *Eur J Clin Microbiol Infect Dis* 1993; 12:37–43.

79 Hoop R K, Böttger E C, Ossent P et al. Mycobacteriosis due to *Mycobacterium genavense* in six pet birds. *J Clin Microbiol* 1993; 31:990–993.

80 Arasteh K N, Cordes C, Ewers M et al. HIV-related nontuberculous mycobacterial infection: incidence, survival analysis and associated risk factors. *Eur J Med Res* 2000; 5:424–430.

81 Kiehn T E & Cammarata R. Comparative recoveries of *Mycobacterium avium–M. intracellulare* from isolator lysis–centrifugation and BACTEC 13A blood culture systems. *J Clin Microbiol* 1988; 26:760–761.

82 Baril L, Jouan M, Agher R et al. Impact of highly active antiretroviral therapy on onset of *Mycobacterium avium* complex infection and cytomegalovirus disease in patients with AIDS. *AIDS* 2000; 14:2593–2596.

83 Selby W. Pathogenesis and therapeutic aspects of Crohn's disease. *Vet Microbiol* 2000; 77:505–511.

84 Woods G L. Susceptibility testing for mycobacteria. *Clin Infect Dis* 2000; 31:1209–1215.

85 Portaels F, Traore H, De Ridder K et al. In vitro susceptibility of *Mycobacterium ulcerans* to clarithromycin. *Antimicrob Agents Chemother* 1998; 42:2070–2073.

86 Faber W R, Arias-Bouda L M, Zeegelaar J E et al. First reported case of *Mycobacterium ulcerans* infection in a patient from China. *Trans R Soc Trop Med Hyg* 2000; 94:277–279.

87 Bonnet E, Debat-Zoguereh, Petit N et al. Clarithromycin: a potent agent against infections due to *Mycobacterium marinum*. *Clin Infect Dis* 1994; 18:664–666.

88 Gluckman S J. *Mycobacterium marinum*. *Clin Dermatol* 1995; 13:273–276.

89 Kuypers F Y, Zwiertstra R P & de Langen Z J. De chirurgische behandling van lymfadenitis door niet-tuberculeuze mycobacteriën bij kinderen. *Ned Tijdschr Geneeskd* 1995; 139:2036–2039.

90 Campbell I A, Jenkins P A & Wallace R J. Chemotherapy of nontuberculous mycobacterial disease. In Gangadharam P R J & Jenkins P A (eds) *Mycobacteria*, vol. 2. London: Chapman & Hall; 1997: 145–177.

91 Research Committee, British Thoracic Society. *Mycobacterium kansasii* pulmonary infection: a prospective study of the results of 9 months treatment with rifampicin and ethambutol. *Thorax* 1994; 49:442–445.

92 Dunne M, Fessel J, Kumar P et al. A randomized, double-blind trial comparing azithromycin and clarithromycin in the treatment of disseminated *Mycobacterium avium* infection in patients with human immunodeficiency virus. *Clin Infect Dis* 2000; 31:1245–1252.

Chapter 59
Leprosy

Leprosy Group, WHO

Among communicable diseases, leprosy is one of the leading causes of permanent physical disabilities in the world. The disease and its visible deformities contribute to intense social stigma resulting in discrimination of patients and their families. In addition, as leprosy commonly afflicts individuals in their most productive stage of life, it imposes a significant burden on society. Early detection and cure through treatment with multi-drug therapy (MDT) are the key elements of the strategy to eliminate leprosy as a public health problem (defined as a prevalence rate of less than 1 case per 10 000 population). In addition to reducing the prevalence of the disease to very low levels, this strategy aims at bringing about 'cure without disabilities', and thus is the most effective way of reducing the social and economic burden caused by the disease.

Global situation

Leprosy currently affects about 1 million people in Africa, Asia, South America and the Pacific. The WHO estimates that between 2 and 3 million individuals are permanently disabled because of leprosy.[1] For many of these individuals the programme failed to reach them in time with MDT and its services.

There had been a very steady increase in the number of registered cases between 1966 and 1985; 2.8 million for 1966, 3.6 million for 1976, and 5.4 million for 1985. The last figure represented an increase of 49.1% over 1976, and 89.6% over 1966. The prevalence of registered cases had correspondingly increased from 8.4 cases per 10 000 population in 1966 to 8.8 in 1976, and 12.0 in 1985.[2] However, since 1985 there has been a steady decline so that by the beginning of 2000 the total number of registered cases was 0.75 million, with a prevalence rate of 1.25 per 10 000 population. This represents globally a reduction in the prevalence rate of about 89.6% since 1985.[3]

As shown in Table 59.1, at the beginning of 2000, 753 263 leprosy cases were registered for treatment, with a prevalence rate of 1.25 per 10 000 population. Out of 122 countries where leprosy was considered a public health problem in 1985, so far 98 countries have reached the elimination target. Almost all leprosy patients registered for treatment are being treated with MDT, even in countries facing difficult problems. During 1999, 738 284 new cases were detected with a detection rate of 12.3 per 100 000 population.[3] Over the last few years, the detection of new cases continued to increase, mainly due to improved and intensified efforts in all endemic countries. This also underlines the importance of the 'hidden' backlog cases remaining in the community for various reasons, the main being the stigma attached to the disease and limited health infrastructure to provide adequate services in most of the endemic countries.

Leprosy still remains a public health problem in 24 countries, situated mainly in the inter-tropical belt of the world. About 673 000 registered cases and 677 000 new cases are found in the top 11 endemic countries, which represent 90% of prevalence and detection globally. As shown in Table 59.2, the prevalence rate is still 4.1 per 10 000 population in these countries.

The significant achievements made towards eliminating leprosy over the last two decades is the result of two important events in the history of the fight against leprosy. The first event took place in 1981, when a WHO Study Group on Chemotherapy of Leprosy recommended the

Table 59.1 Prevalence and detection of leprosy by WHO region

WHO Region	Registered cases at the beginning of 2000 (rate per 10 000)	New cases detected during 1999 (rate per 100 000)
Africa	64 490 (1.0)	55 635 (8.6)
Americas	90 447 (1.1)	45 599 (5.7)
South-East Asia	574 924 (3.8)	621 620 (41.3)
Eastern Mediterranean	8 785 (0.2)	5 757 (1.2)
Western Pacific	13 771 (0.1)	9 501 (0.6)
Europe	846 (–)	172 (–)
Total	753 263 (1.25)	738 284 (12.3)

Table 59.2 Registered prevalence and detection of leprosy in the top 11 countries

Country	Registered cases at the beginning of 2000	Prevalence per 10 000	New cases detected during 1999	Detection rate per 100 000
India	495 073	5.0	537 956	54.3
Brazil	78 068	4.3	42 055	25.9
Myanmar	28 404	5.9	30 479	62.9
Indonesia	23 156	1.1	17 477	8.3
Nepal	13 572	5.7	18 693	78.7
Madagascar	7 865	4.7	8 704	51.6
Ethiopia	7 764	1.3	4 457	7.4
Mozambique	7 403	3.9	5 488	28.7
D.R. Congo	5 031	1.0	4 221	8.6
Tanzania	4 701	1.4	5 081	15.4
Guinea	1 559	2.0	2 475	32.0
Total	672 596	4.1	677 086	41.7

The top endemic countries included in the table have the following characteristics: (1) they have a prevalence of more than 1 in 10 000 population; and (2) the number of prevalent leprosy cases is more than 5000, *or* the number of newly detected cases is more than 2000. Ranking of countries is based on the number of registered cases.

use of MDT as the standard treatment for leprosy.[4] The success of MDT led to the second event in 1991, when the 44th World Health Assembly passed the resolution to eliminate leprosy as a public health problem (prevalence at the global level less than 1 case per 10 000 population) by end of the year 2000.

The causative organism

The aetiological agent in leprosy is *Mycobacterium leprae*. The organism was discovered by G. H. Armauer Hansen in Norway in 1873, making it the first bacterium to be identified as causing disease in man.[5] It is a strongly acid-fast, rod-shaped organism with parallel sides and rounded ends. In size and shape it closely resembles the tubercle bacillus. It occurs in large numbers in the lesions of lepromatous leprosy, chiefly in masses within macrophages, often grouped together like bundles of cigars or arranged in a palisade. Most striking are the intracellular and extra-cellular masses, known as globi, which consist of clumps of bacilli in capsular material.

Under the electron microscope the bacillus appears to have a great variety of forms. The most common is a slightly curved rod-shaped organism with parallel sides and rounded ends, 1–8 μm long and 0.3 μm in diameter. It is believed that only leprosy bacilli that stain with carbol-fuchsin as solid acid-fast rods are viable and that bacilli that stain irregularly are probably dead and degenerating. The differences are valuable pointers in biopsy specimens to the effects of treatment. In patients receiving standard MDT, a very high proportion of bacilli are killed within days, which suggests that many of the manifestations of leprosy, including reactions of the erythema nodosum type—which follow initial treatment—are probably due in part to antigens from dead organisms rather than living bacilli.

Portal of exit of *M. leprae*

The two portals of exit of *M. leprae* often described are the skin and the nasal mucosa. However, the relative importance of these two portals is not clear. It is true that the lepromatous cases show large numbers of organisms deep down in the dermis. However, whether they reach the skin surface in sufficient numbers is doubtful. Although there are reports of acid-fast bacilli being found in the desquamating epithelium of the skin, Weddell et al.[6] have reported that they could not find any acid-fast bacilli in the epidermis, even after examining a very large number of specimens from patients and contacts. In a recent study, Job et al.[7] found fairly large numbers of *M. leprae* in the superficial keratin layer of the skin of lepromatous leprosy patients, suggesting that the organism could exit along with the sebaceous secretions.

Regarding the nasal mucosa, its importance was recognized as early as 1898 by Schäffer,[8] particularly that of the ulcerated mucosa. The quantity of bacilli from nasal mucosal lesions in lepromatous leprosy was demonstrated by Shepard[9] as large, with counts ranging from 10 000 to 10 000 000. Pedley[10] reported that the majority of lepromatous patients showed leprosy bacilli in their nasal secretions as collected through blowing the nose. Davey and Rees[11] indicated that nasal secretions from lepromatous patients could yield as many as 10 million viable organisms per day.

Viability of *M. leprae* outside the human host

The possibility of discharge of *M. leprae* from the nasal mucosa raises the question of survival of the discharged organisms outside the human host. Davey and Rees[11] reported that *M. leprae* from the nasal secretions can survive up to 36 hours or more. Desikan[12] reported on the survival of *M. leprae* in nasal secretions under tropical conditions for up to 9 days. Such survival of the organisms suggests the possibility of contaminated clothing and other fomites acting as sources of infection.

Portal of entry of *M. leprae*

The portal of entry of *M. leprae* into the human body is not definitely known. However, the two portals of entry seriously considered are the skin and the upper respiratory tract. With regard to the respiratory route of entry of *M. leprae*, the evidence in its favour is on the increase in spite of the long-held belief that the skin was the exclusive portal of entry. Rees and McDougall[13] succeeded in the experimental transmission of leprosy through aerosols containing *M. leprae* in immune-suppressed mice, suggesting a similar possibility in humans. Successful results have also been reported on experiments with nude mice when *M. leprae* was introduced into the nasal cavity by topical application.[14]

In summary, entry through the respiratory route appears most probable, although other routes, particularly broken skin, cannot be ruled out.

Culture in vitro

Claims of successful culture have been made in the past but none has been substantiated and *M. leprae* has not yet been successfully cultured in vitro. There have been many reports of cultivation in artificial media of acid-fast bacilli from the skin or other tissues of leprosy patients and many authors have claimed such bacilli to be true leprosy bacilli, but no satisfactory evidence of this has been produced. Most of the organisms isolated in culture from lepromatous tissues appear to be mycobacteria related to the *M. avium* complex.

Culture in vivo

Normal mice

The mouse footpad inoculation method developed by Shepard is still the chief method of culture in vivo. Inoculation of 10^4 bacilli into the hind footpads yields 10^6 bacilli after 5–6 months, although no clinical disease develops. During the logarithmic phase the mean generation time is about 14 days, which is consistent with the natural history of disease in man and is responsible for the long time of several months taken to measure multiplication in the footpad test.[15] No subsequent local increase in bacterial numbers takes place and the bacilli slowly degenerate.

The mouse footpad has been used to test the minimum concentration of drugs necessary and the sensitivity of the bacilli to new drugs. It is a valuable tool for measuring drug resistance in patients.

Immunologically deficient mice

Rees et al.[16] have developed an experimental lepromatous leprosy model in animals by inoculating thymectomized irradiated (TR) mice. The generation time remained unchanged but the bacilli continued to multiply until 10^8–10^9 bacilli per footpad were obtained after 9–12 months. The histological picture is that of lepromatous leprosy, and numerous bacilli can be found in the liver and spleen, although the main spread is to the nose, tail, front paws and ears. The TR mouse has been used to detect small numbers of viable organisms.

The nine-banded armadillo (*Dasypus novemcinctus*)

An important development has been the discovery that the nine-banded armadillo can be infected with *M. leprae*[17] and this animal has become the main source of *M. leprae* for biochemical and immunological research. The armadillo has a primitive immunological system and a low body temperature. Intravenous inoculation produces widespread disseminated disease, with yields from the liver and spleen reaching 10^{12} organisms per gram of tissue.

M. leprae genome

M. leprae has the longest doubling time of all known bacteria and has thwarted every effort at culture in the laboratory. Comparing the genome sequence of *M. leprae* with that of *M. tuberculosis* provides clear explanations for these properties and reveals an extreme case of reductive evolution. Less than half of the genome contains functional genes. Gene deletion and decay appear to have eliminated many important metabolic activities, including siderophore production, part of the oxidative and most of the micro-aerophilic and anaerobic respiratory chains, and numerous catabolic systems and their regulatory circuits.[18]

The genome sequence of a strain of *M. leprae*, originally isolated in Tamil Nadu and designated 'TN', has been completed recently. The sequence was obtained by a combined approach, employing automated DNA sequence analysis of selected cosmids and whole-genome 'shotgun' clones. After the finishing process, the genome sequence was found to contain 3 268 203 base-pairs (bp), and to have an average G + C content of 57.8%, values much lower than the corresponding values for *M. tuberculosis*, which are 4 441 529 bp and 65.6% G + C. There are 1500 genes which are common to both *M. leprae* and *M. tuberculosis*. The comparative analysis suggests that both mycobacteria derived from a common ancestor and, at one stage, had gene pools of similar size. Downsizing from a genome of 4.42 Mb, such as that of *M. tuberculosis*, to one of 3.27 Mb would account for the loss of some 1200 protein coding sequences. There is evidence that many of the genes that were present in the genome of *M. leprae* have truly been lost.[19] Information from the completed genome can be useful to develop diagnostic skin tests, understanding the mechanism of nerve damage and drug resistance and to identify novel drug targets for rational design of new therapeutic regimens and drugs to treat leprosy and its complications.

Epidemiology
Method of transmission

The exact mechanism of transmission of leprosy is not known. The most widely held belief is that the disease was transmitted by contact between persons with leprosy and healthy persons. In general, closeness of contact is related to the dose of infection, which in turn is related to the occurrence of disease. Of the various situations that promote close contact, contact within the household is the only one that is easily identified. The actual incidence among contacts and the relative risk for them appear to vary considerably in different studies. Attack rates for contacts of lepromatous leprosy have varied from 6.2 per 1000 per year in Cebu[20] to 55.8 per 1000 per year in a part of South India.[21]

The possibility of transmission of leprosy through the respiratory route has gained increasing attention in recent years. It is based on (1) the inability to find organisms on the surface of the skin; (2) the demonstration of a large number of organisms in the nasal discharge; (3) the high proportion of morphologically intact bacilli in the nasal secretions; (4) the evidence that *M. leprae* could survive outside the human host for several hours or days; and (5) the ability to infect experimental animals through the nasal route.

There is evidence that not all people who are infected with *M. leprae* develop leprosy. The factors that determine clinical expression after infection appear to be as important as the factors that determine infection after exposure. Genetic factors have been considered for a long time in leprosy. This is largely due to the observation of clustering of leprosy around certain families, and the failure to understand why certain individuals develop lepromatous leprosy while others develop other types of leprosy. Admittedly, it is the host factors that play a key role. However, what is not clear is the role of genetics vis-à-vis other factors in determining this clinical expression.

Studies by Shepard et al.[22] in the mouse footpad model suggest that the route of entry of the organism may, to some extent, determine the occurrence of leprosy. This is based on the observation that, while intradermal administration of killed *M. leprae* sensitizes the animal, intravenous administration of killed *M. leprae* tends to tolerize the animal, as studied through skin test reactivity. This also raises the possibility of tuberculoid and lepromatous leprosy being the result of different routes of entry of the organisms. In addition, malnutrition and possible prior exposure to other environmental mycobacteria may play a role in development of the overt disease.

Age at onset

Leprosy mainly affects young adults in their most productive period of life. The youngest age reported for the occurrence of leprosy is 3 weeks in Martinique.[23] Occurrence of leprosy, presumably for the first time, is not uncommon even after the age of 70 years. There is a recent report from Nepal describing leprosy in a 141-year-old individual.[24]

Sex distribution

Although leprosy affects both sexes, in most parts of the world males are affected more frequently than females, often in the ratio of 2:1. This preponderance of males is observed in as diverse geographic situations as India, the Philippines, Hawaii, Venezuela and Cameroon. Doull et al.,[20] from their studies in the Philippines, have also pointed out that the difference is a true difference due to higher incidence among males, and not due to differing duration of disease for the two sexes. It should be pointed out that the male preponderance in leprosy is not universal and there are several areas, particularly in Africa, where there is either equal occurrence of leprosy in the two sexes or occasionally even a higher prevalence among females. Such situations have been observed in Uganda, Nigeria, Malawi, Gambia, Burkina Faso, Zambia, Thailand and Japan.

Incubation period

In leprosy both the reference points for measuring the incubation period and the times of infection and onset of disease are difficult to define; the former because of the lack of adequate immunological tools and the latter because of the insidious nature of the onset of leprosy. Even so, several investigators have attempted to measure the incubation period for leprosy. The minimum incubation period reported is as short as a few weeks and this is based on the very occasional occurrence of leprosy among young infants.[23] The maximum incubation period reported is as long as 30 years, or over, as observed among war veterans known to have been exposed for short periods in endemic areas but otherwise living in non-endemic areas. It is generally agreed that the average incubation period is between 3 and 5 years.

Prevalence

The point prevalence rate is defined as the number of cases registered for chemotherapy at a given point in time among the population in which the cases have occurred.[25] This indicator reflects the magnitude of the problem and helps in planning and monitoring elimination activities. The use of prevalence to monitor elimination is based on MDT rendering patients non-infective after only a few doses and completely curing the disease after completion of the full course of treatment. Since leprosy patients are assumed to be the sole source of infection, intensified case finding and treatment with MDT of all patients should reduce the reservoir of infection in the community and interrupt its transmission.

Case detection and incidence

The detection rate is defined by the number of newly detected cases, previously untreated, during a year divided by the population in which the cases have occurred. This usually includes cases with onset of disease in the year in question (true incidence) and a large proportion of cases with onset in previous years (backlog prevalence). Although the number of new cases with established disabilities might give some indication of backlog prevalence, determination of time of onset is generally unreliable, is labour-intensive and is seldom done in recording these statistics. Annual incidence rates are important as a measure of transmission of leprosy; however, it is difficult to measure owing to long incubation period, delays in diagnosis after onset of the disease and lack of laboratory tools to detect leprosy in very early stages.

Subclinical infection

Subclinical infection with *M. leprae* is far more common than is indicated by cases of overt disease. Factors that influence the occurrence of disease among individuals infected with *M. leprae* may differ from those that influence the occurrence of infection itself. Availability of specific and reliable tests for detecting infection and the occurrence of disease among infected individuals would permit more accurate assessment of the risk factors for infection and disease.

Contact examination

Household contacts of leprosy patients are at significantly greater risk of developing leprosy than non-household contacts. Household contacts, however, contribute only a limited proportion of all new cases. Thus, on detection of a new case, his or her household contacts should be examined for evidence of leprosy. They should then be educated on the early signs of the disease and their significance, and requested to return if any suspect skin, motor or sensory lesions occur.

Extra-human reservoirs

While the human being is considered the major host and reservoir of the leprosy bacillus, other sources, including the armadillo, chimpanzee and mangabey monkey, have also been incriminated as reservoirs of infection.[26, 27] The epidemiological significance of these findings is unknown but is likely to be very limited.

Impact of HIV epidemic

Unlike in tuberculosis, there is no evidence suggesting an association between HIV infection and leprosy.[28, 29] One explanation is that the HIV-positive subjects do not survive long enough in a state of severe immunosuppression to allow the development of leprosy. Although most investigators believe that the clinical manifestations and the frequency of relapses do not differ significantly between HIV-negative and HIV-positive leprosy patients, additional information is needed as there are reports which suggest an increase of type 1 reaction and neuritis among HIV-positive MB leprosy cases.

Impact of BCG vaccination

Protection against leprosy by BCG vaccination was demonstrated in five large field trials conducted in India, Malawi, Myanmar, Papua New Guinea and Uganda, although the protective effect varied from 20–30% in Myanmar and India to 80% in Uganda. The observed protective effect of BCG was significantly greater among individuals vaccinated at below 15 years of age in some studies. While most investigators think that the effect was primarily against paucibacillary leprosy, more detailed analysis suggested that the protection against multibacillary leprosy was similar.[30] The results of vaccine trials conducted in India, Malawi and Venezuela demonstrated a protective effect of around 50% against leprosy by BCG and second or repeated doses of BCG offered additional protection.[31–33] However, the addition of killed *M. leprae* did not improve the protection afforded by BCG vaccination.

The widespread application of BCG is therefore likely to be a factor contributing to the decline in leprosy incidence observed in certain populations. Repeated doses of BCG to prevent leprosy are not recommended on the grounds of poor cost-effectiveness, lack of acceptability to recipients, operational difficulties, and the fact that it is contraindicated in symptomatic HIV individuals.

Disability burden

It is estimated, using information from national leprosy elimination programmes, that the current prevalence of people with disability due to leprosy is around 2 million. Most studies show the risk of disability is higher for men and for multibacillary patients, and the risk increases with age and duration of the disease. The risk of disability has been significantly reduced following the implementation of MDT[1] due to early case detection, efficacy of MDT, reduced frequency and severity of leprosy reactions, and such operational factors as improved management of cases.

Lepromin

The lepromin reaction is still used in several countries. It is held to be an indicator of the ability of the host to mount a cell-mediated response to *M. leprae*. However, its usefulness in diagnosis, classification and as a marker of protective immunity to identify at-risk individuals is very limited. The use of lepromin is restricted to research purposes only.

Cure of disease

With the availability of effective treatment, cure after completion of treatment with MDT is now an important mode of elimination of cases from the prevalence pool.

Mortality in leprosy

Mortality in leprosy is often not considered important because the disease is rarely an immediate cause of death. However, leprosy patients are exposed to increased mortality risks due to its indirect effects. In studies in the Philippines[34] and India[35] it was found that the mortality rate for lepromatous patients was four times that of the general population, and that the non-lepromatous patients themselves have a mortality risk, which was twice that of the general population.

Clinical features
Natural history

The natural history of leprosy is very variable. The majority of people who come into contact with untreated lepromatous patients develop no symptoms or signs of infection, although the lymphocyte transformation test shows that a majority will have experienced infection, which they overcome. The majority of those who experience clinical effects mount a strong cell-mediated immune response and develop tuberculoid leprosy. A minority who mount a weak cell-mediated immune response or none at all develop lepromatous leprosy, a chronic progressive disseminated infection. A proportion of cases mount varying degrees of cell-mediated immune response and develop borderline or indeterminate leprosy, and may then swing one way or the other on the pendulum, downgrading or upgrading, depending upon changes in the immunological response.

Symptoms and signs

The mode of onset is very variable. An early lesion may occur as a vague ill-defined hypopigmented or erythematous patch with anaesthesia. The disease can also occur with multiple infiltrated patches or just diffuse skin infiltration. In certain instances leprosy can manifest itself as areas of anaesthesia in the skin with no skin patches.

Spontaneous healing may take place in a very high proportion of early lesions of childhood and this is quite common in some communities; however, a definite diagnosis is an indication for treatment.

As compared with tuberculosis, one of the chief characteristics of leprosy is the absence of toxicity; enormous numbers of bacilli may be present in the body with few signs. The local inflammatory reactions to lepra bacilli vary within wide limits. Thus, in one patient the disease may be so localized that it affects one small skin area or its main nerve supply. There may be acute inflammatory swelling, local pain and trophic, sensory and other disturbances. In contrast, some cases show involvement of almost the whole body, so that a preparation taken from any part of the skin may reveal numerous bacilli, although the patient is not acutely ill and is able to go about and work normally. The nerves are not noticeably thickened and superficially the skin appears normal. At any stage during invasion sudden exanthematous reactions may appear, accompanied by fever and general symptoms.

The *chronic onset* is so gradual and insidious that the disease has advanced to a considerable extent before any abnormality is evident. There may be tenderness, tingling or thickening of a nerve, an area of anaesthesia, with some change in the appearance of the skin, insensitiveness to burning, formication, tingling or numbness of extremities. Discoloured skin patches may be mistaken for eczema or ringworm; these may at first be small, gradually increasing in size. In *acute onset*, which is much less common, there are occasionally multiple lesions with less diffused margins, which tend to spread rapidly and which contain very numerous bacilli. The first noticeable sign may be an evanescent rash. The onset may be determined by occurrence of some other acute disease or physiological change or stress, e.g. extra strain imposed on the body during puberty, parturition and the menopause.

Definition of a case of leprosy

A case of leprosy is a person having one or more of the following features, and who has yet to complete a full course of treatment:[36]

- Hypopigmented or reddish skin lesion(s) with definite loss of sensation.
- Involvement of the peripheral nerves, as demonstrated by loss of sensation and weakness of the muscles of hands, feet or face.
- Skin smear positive for acid-fast bacilli.

Diagnosis of leprosy

The diagnosis of leprosy is most commonly based on clinical signs and symptoms. These are easy to observe and elicit by any health worker after a short period of training. In practice, people with such complaints usually report on their own to a health centre. Only in rare instances is there a need to use laboratory and other investigations to confirm a diagnosis of leprosy.

The skin lesions can be single or multiple, usually less pigmented than the surrounding normal skin. Sometimes the lesion is reddish or copper-coloured. A variety of skin lesions may be seen but macules, papules or nodules are common.

Sensory loss is a typical feature of leprosy. The skin lesion shows loss of sensation to pin prick and/or light touch.

Nerve damage, mainly to peripheral nerve trunks, constitute another important feature of leprosy. There may be loss of sensation in the skin and weakness of muscles supplied by the affected nerve. In the absence of these signs, nerve thickening by itself, without sensory loss and/or muscle weakness, is not a reliable sign of leprosy.

In a small proportion of patients, rod-shaped, red-stained leprosy bacilli may be seen in smears taken from the affected skin and examined under the microscope after appropriate staining.

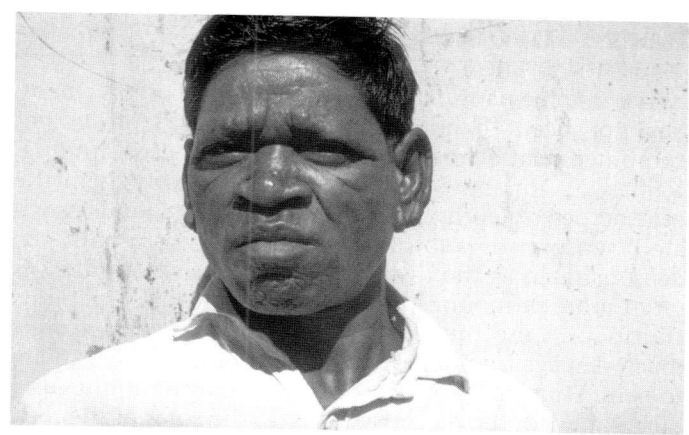

Figure 59.1: Multibacillary leprosy.

Lepromatous leprosy

This is the type of leprosy seen in persons with a negligible resistance; leprosy bacilli are widely disseminated throughout the skin, nerves and reticuloendothelial system. In addition, there may be bacillary invasion of eyes, testes, bones and mucous membranes of mouth, nose, pharynx, larynx and trachea.

Skin lesions

These are multiple, small and symmetrically distributed; they take the form of macules, infiltrations (plaques), papules and nodules, all of which may be present in the same patient at the same time once the disease has become well established.

The earliest skin lesions are macules; they are level with the skin and therefore cannot be palpated. They are small, circular or elliptical; they are erythematous in light skins, sometimes with a coppery or purple hue, and coppery in dark skins, sometimes with a faintly hypopigmented background. They have a smooth and shiny surface; their edges are indistinct. Owing to the fact that these macules are often difficult to see and are not associated with itching or definite anaesthesia, they may be ignored by the patient. They may be situated on any part of the body, but are unusual in the axillae, groin, perineum, on the external genitalia or on the scalp. They are most commonly found on the face, buttocks and extremities; on the limbs the flexor surfaces may be involved as well as the extensor, and the palms and soles as well as the backs of hands and feet.

Infiltrated lesions are raised above the level of the skin and give a sensation of thickening when gripped between finger and thumb. Their distribution and colouring are the same as those of lepromatous macules, except that they do not appear on palms and soles because of the thickness and tightness of the skin. They are raised in the centre and slope away peripherally to merge imperceptibly with the surrounding skin, have a smooth and shiny surface, and do not exhibit sensory loss, unless situated in a region of skin which is already anaesthetic as a result of peripheral nerve damage. Papules and nodules make their appearance as the disease advances and particularly favour the face, ears and buttocks. Ears should always be carefully examined, for the lobes are more constantly affected than any other part and appear thickened quite early in the course of the disease, such thickening being readily confirmed by palpation with finger and thumb. Advanced infiltration and nodulation of the face give rise to leontiasis or 'leonine facies', in which the normal wrinkles on the forehead and cheeks have become deep furrows. Nodules and infiltrations may undergo superficial necrosis and ulceration and large ulcers may form on the lower legs when leprous infiltration of the skin is associated with chronic bilateral lymphoedema, secondary to massive bacillary invasion of the lymphatics. Thinning of the eyebrows is common, commencing in the lateral half and sometimes progressing to complete loss of eyebrows and eyelashes (superciliary and ciliary madarosis; Figure 59.1).

One particular variety of skin infiltration requires separate mention, namely the pure diffuse type described by Lucio and Alvarado in Mexico in 1852 and later by Latapi in 1938. The skin of the whole body becomes diffusely infiltrated (no macular stage being observed), rendering it stiff and smooth, as in scleroderma. There is no obvious disfigurement, apart from loss of eyebrows and eyelashes, which always occurs, but there may be widespread small telangiectases; nasal destruction may develop and sometimes there is alopecia and loss of body hair. Laryngeal ulceration has been recorded but cutaneous nodules and ocular involvement are absent. Mexican physicians have described, in these patients, a unique form of lepra reaction known as 'Lucio's phenomenon', in which painful, purpuric, ulcerating patches appear on the skin, becoming crusted and leaving scars.[37] This may be differentiated from the erythema nodosum leprosum (ENL) reaction by the absence of fever and leucocytosis, absence of tender lesions and a good response to anti-leprosy drugs. It may also be distinguished histologically.[38,39]

Nerve involvement

Nerve involvement, in the absence of skin involvement, has not been described in lepromatous leprosy, but combined dermal and neural changes are a usual finding. Nerves do not show signs of damage as early as in the other types of leprosy, but nerve thickening and associated sensory or motor dysfunction can usually be demonstrated as the disease advances. As sensory loss is often more pronounced than muscular wasting, patients continue to use the affected limbs and the skin suffers much damage from repeated trauma owing to insensitivity to pain. Thus the hands become scarred from injuries and burns and trophic ulcers develop on the soles of the feet. Nerve thickening, like skin involvement, tends to be bilateral and symmetrical. It is found in those peripheral nerves which are superficial in some part of their course, e.g. the great auricular nerves in the neck (Figure 59.2), the supraclavicular nerves as they cross the clavicles, the ulnar nerves just above the elbows, the antebrachial cutaneous nerves in the forearms, the radial and median nerves at the wrists, the femoral cutaneous nerves, the common peroneals as they wind round the necks of the fibulae, the superficial peroneals in front of the ankles and the posterior tibial nerves immediately below the internal malleoli.

The earliest sensory disturbances may take the form of paraesthesia, hyperaesthesiae and hyperalgesia, to be followed later by impairment of light touch, temperature or pain sensation. All three modalities should be tested when examining a patient, as sometimes only one is affected (dissociated anaesthesia); in such a case it is usually the ability to differentiate between hot and cold which is lost first. Loss of position sense, vibration sense and tendon reflexes may occur, but not commonly. Muscle wasting may produce deformities such as claw hand (ulnar nerve), main-en-griffe (combined ulnar and median nerves), drop foot (common peroneal nerve) and facial palsy (facial nerve), but careful examination of muscles will show evidence of weakness long before paralysis occurs.

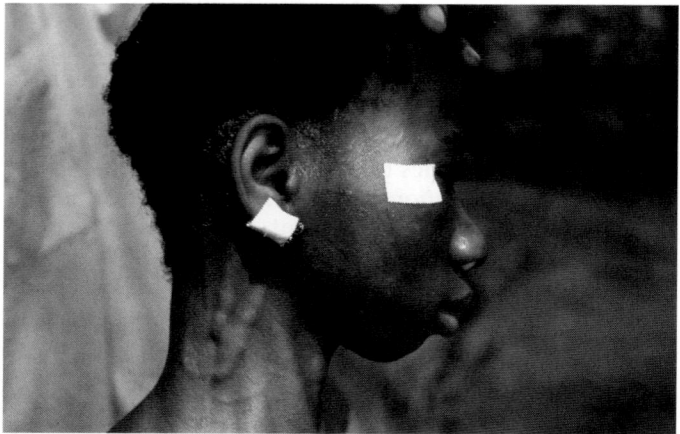

Figure 59.2: Leprosy patient with enlarged superficial nerves.

Involvement of autonomic nerves manifests itself in the early stages by slight oedema of the hands or feet; more marked vasomotor disturbance develops later, causing the skin of hands and feet to be puffy and cyanosed.

Other tissues involved in lepromatous leprosy

Nails of fingers and toes

These are affected when trophic changes take place in digits, and appear dry, lustreless, narrowed and longitudinally ridged.

Mucous membranes

The patient may complain of nasal discharge, possibly blood-stained, and of blocking of the airway; examination reveals hyperaemia and swelling of the mucosa, together with nodules or ulcers on the nasal septum. Ulceration leads to septal perforation and later to cartilage destruction and consequent 'saddle-nose' deformity. Nodules may also form on the lips, tongue, palate and larynx, leading to ulceration. Laryngeal involvement gives rise to hoarse cough, husky voice and stridor. Oedema of the glottis, occurring as part of a reactional state, used to be a dreaded complication in the presulphone era, calling for immediate tracheotomy.

Eye

Visual impairment and blindness occur frequently in those with advanced lepromatous leprosy. Leprosy is the third leading cause of blindness worldwide. The major complications leading to blindness from leprosy are the following:

- Corneal changes are exposure keratitis due to lagophthalmos, and reduced or absent corneal sensation, both predisposing to corneal ulceration and scarring. The early stages can be recognized by fine punctate superficial spots on the cornea. Secondary bacterial infection or a foreign body may subsequently cause a corneal ulcer.
- Iris involvement may be either in the acute form of iridocyclitis, which occurs as part of the ENL reaction, or a chronic process. The acute form causes pain, photophobia and pericorneal redness. If acute iritis is untreated it may smoulder on as a chronic iritis, with posterior synechiae formation and small irregular pupil. A chronic insidious form of iridocyclitis frequently occurs in lepromatous leprosy. Early in the disease process, 'flare' (cloudiness of aqueous fluid) and cells can be detected in the anterior chamber, if examined with a slit lamp. This form of chronic iridocyclitis will tend to lead to iris atrophy and a regular pinpoint pupil without posterior synechiae formation.
- Cataract may be caused by or made worse by iridocyclitis or the use of systemic steroids in reaction, and intraocular invasion with bacilli.

Bones

Changes in bones in lepromatous leprosy are confined to the skull and limbs. In the limbs the changes are almost solely concentrated in the hands and feet and are due to a combination of factors, which include: (1) deposition of bacilli; (2) neurotrophic atrophy; (3) repeated trauma resulting from analgesia; (4) disuse owing to paralysis and contractures; (5) secondary infection from trophic ulceration; and (6) generalized osteoporosis of hormonal origin. Deposition of bacilli in the medullary cavities, the periosteum and the nutrient vessels gives rise to bone cysts, enlarged nutrient foramina, aseptic necrosis and spindle-shaped leprous dactylitis closely simulating that of tuberculosis or syphilis. Leprous periostitis of the tibia, fibula and ulna has been described. Neurotrophic atrophy affecting the hands is localized to the phalanges. Metacarpals and carpal bones are spared. In the feet the atrophic changes are localized to the metatarsals and phalanges, commencing in the proximal phalanges or in the heads of the metatarsals. In the proximal phalanges the diaphyses become gradually thinned by rarefying osteitis, known as 'concentric bone atrophy', so that eventually there is but a fine needle of bone left. This may be followed by disappearance of the affected bones and the shortened toes are connected to the foot by soft tissue only. In the metatarsals absorption begins at the distal ends, which become thinned and pointed—the 'sucked candystick' appearance.

Sensory loss results in repeated trauma, both major and minor, and this is an important contributory factor to the production of bone atrophy and absorption[40] which may lead to the development of Charcot joints in the fingers, toes, wrists or ankles.

Muscle paralysis can lead to disuse and, in neglected cases, to fibrous or bony ankylosis of the interphalangeal, metacarpophalangeal and metatarsophalangeal joints. Disuse also results in osteoporosis due to decreased osteoblastic activity.

Secondary infection commonly follows neglected trophic ulceration of feet or hands and can result in pyogenic osteomyelitis.

Generalized osteoporosis may follow defective production of testosterone as a result of testicular damage.

Changes in the skull in lepromatous leprosy consist of atrophy of the anterior nasal spine and the maxillary alveolar process, probably caused by a combination of aseptic necrosis, due to leprous endarteritis, and pyogenic osteomyelitis, due to gross ulceration in the nose. In advanced, untreated cases, these changes may lead to nasal collapse, loss of incisor teeth and sometimes perforation of the palate.

Reticuloendothelial system

Lymph glands may be enlarged and painless, with the consistency of soft rubber, particularly the femoral, inguinal and epitrochlear glands, but occasionally one or more glands become very swollen and tender as part of a reactional state. The reticuloendothelial elements of the abdominal viscera are invaded by bacilli, especially in the spleen and liver, and the red marrow is similarly invaded. Lymphoedema of the lower legs may occur, giving rise to elephantiasis in neglected cases.

Testes

Testicular atrophy may occur, resulting in sterility and gynaecomastia.

Kidneys

Glomerulonephritis, interstitial nephritis and pyelonephritis may occur. Renal amyloidosis is a prevalent complication in some geographical areas but is uncommon in others; it appears to be related to the severity and frequency of type 2 lepra reactions (ENL).

Tuberculoid leprosy

This is the type of leprosy seen in persons with a good resistance and may be purely neural or combined neural and dermal. The infection is never widespread but is localized to one area or to a few areas asymmetrically. Affected nerves are thickened, sometimes irregularly, and there are associated sensory or motor changes depending on the type of nerve involved. If the patient complains of sensory disturbance, such as paraesthesiae or anaesthesia, a search must be made for palpable thickening of the nerve responsible for the sensation of that area, e.g. face (trigeminal nerve), neck (great auricular nerve), forearm (antebrachial cutaneous nerve), little and ring finger (ulnar nerve), hand (median nerve at the wrist), thigh (femoral cutaneous nerve), lower leg (common peroneal nerve at the neck of the fibula), dorsum of foot (superficial peroneal nerve) and sole of foot (posterior tibial nerve just below the internal malleolus).

Motor changes are shown by muscle weakness or wasting and must be sought in the face, the intrinsic muscles of the hand and the dorsiflexors of the foot. It is extremely rare for the dorsiflexors of the wrist to be affected, owing to the fact that the radial nerve in the arm and forearm follows a deep course among the muscles and is therefore rarely involved. Abscesses in the course of affected nerves are not uncommon in tuberculoid leprosy.

Skin lesions take the form of macules or infiltrations (plaques; Figure 59.3). A tuberculoid macule is erythematous on fair skins and hypopigmented (not depigmented) on dark ones, has a dry and rather rough surface, its edges are well defined, and it is anaesthetic and anhidrotic. Infiltrated lesions are erythematous, sometimes with a coppery, brownish or purple hue, have a dry and rather rough surface, which may be irregular or pebbled, are sometimes scaly, have well-marked sensory loss and have edges which are raised and clear-cut, while the centres show variable flattening. Central healing and peripheral extension give rise to annular lesions in which the *outer*

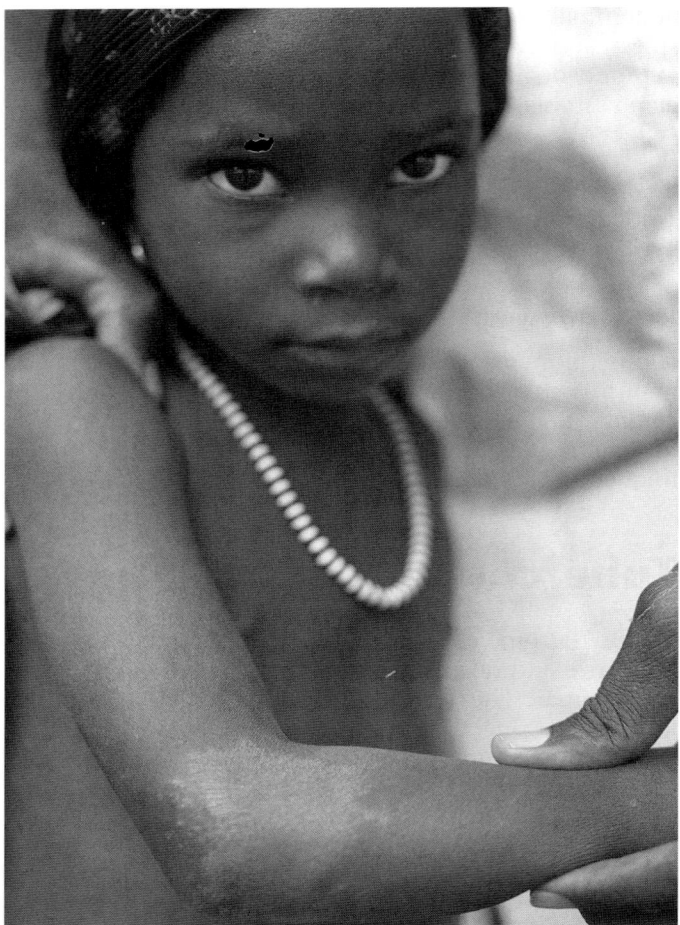

Figure 59.3: Child with paucibacillary leprosy.

edges are raised and well defined and the *inner* ones are flattened and indistinct.

Lesions of tuberculoid leprosy are usually few, large and asymmetrically situated; they favour the face, extensor surfaces of limbs, back and buttocks. Sometimes one or two small 'satellite' lesions are seen in the vicinity of a large plaque. Thickened cutaneous nerves may be palpated in the vicinity of the lesions, but tissues other than skin and nerves are not involved directly. The eye may suffer indirectly from corneal ulceration when there is damage to the facial nerve (exposure keratitis) and also when there is damage to the trigeminal nerve (neuropathic keratitis).

Bone changes in hands or feet are less common than in the lepromatous type as leprosy bacilli are not deposited in the bones or their nutrient arteries. The early development of muscle wasting and paralysis results in disuse. However, neuropathic atrophy may occur in the phalanges of fingers or in the metatarsals and phalanges of feet but, unlike the changes in lepromatous leprosy, they are never bilateral and symmetrical. Bone changes secondary to disuse, to loss of sensation and to trophic ulceration may occur as described under lepromatous leprosy. Trophic ulcers of the feet are common.

Borderline leprosy

This is the type of leprosy seen in persons with a limited or variable resistance and usually presents with skin and nerve involvement. The infection is neither as strictly localized as in tuberculoid leprosy nor as widespread as in the lepromatous type.

Skin lesions are macular, infiltrated or both, the earliest lesions being macules which are erythematous or hypopigmented. In number and character they are intermediate between the two polar types (lepromatous and tuberculoid). Careful testing will reveal impairment of sensation in some if not all of the macules.

Infiltrated lesions have their own distinctive features in which the characteristics of the two polar types are merged. They are moderate in number, asymmetrical in distribution, their erythema has an admixture of purple or brown, their surface is smooth and often shiny and they slope away peripherally from raised centres. The edges are well defined in places and indefinite in others.

Some of these infiltrations may take the form of bands, annular lesions and small nodules. Annular lesions have a characteristic form in which an oval area of normal looking but anaesthetic skin is surrounded by a band of infiltrated tissue of varying width, the *inner* edge being raised and clear-cut (giving the oval area a punched-out appearance), the *outer* merging imperceptibly with the surrounding skin. Sometimes there is an oval band of infiltrated tissue, even in width, and more raised in the central part of the band, which has well-defined outer and inner edges. Infiltrated lesions are invariably anaesthetic and may be found on any part of the body, with the exception of axillae, groin, perineum and scalp, but favour the limbs and buttocks (Figure 59.4).

Nerve involvement can always be demonstrated in borderline leprosy, and neurological symptoms such as paraesthesiae and hyperalgesia often precede the onset of skin manifestations. Nerves are involved asymmetrically and show palpable thickening and impaired function

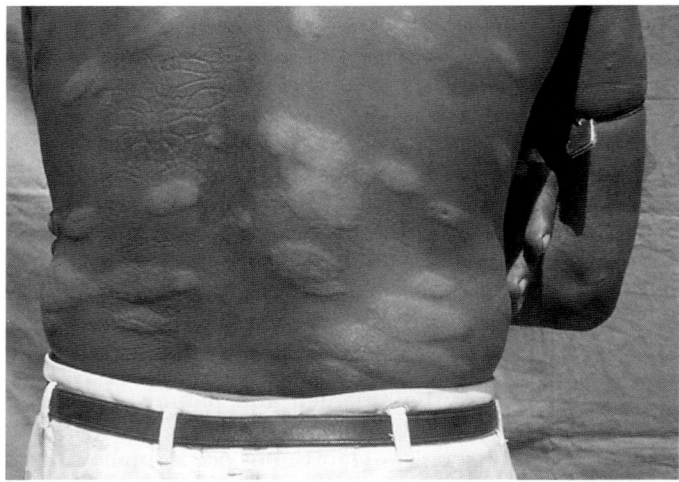

Figure 59.4: Multiple lesions of multibacillary leprosy.

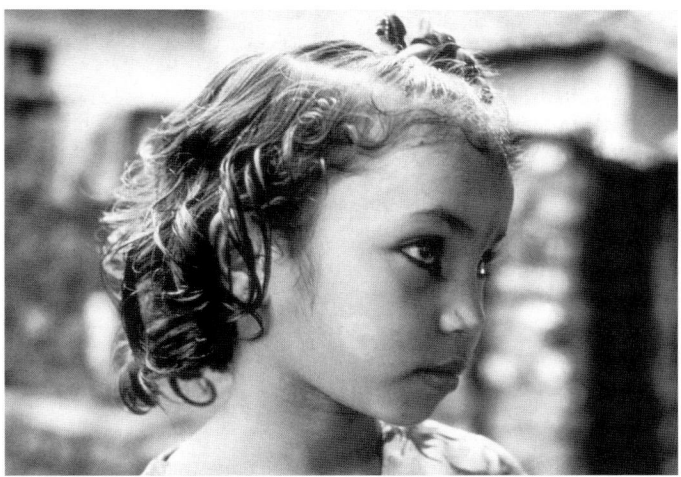

Figure 59.5: Early single lesion of paucibacillary leprosy.

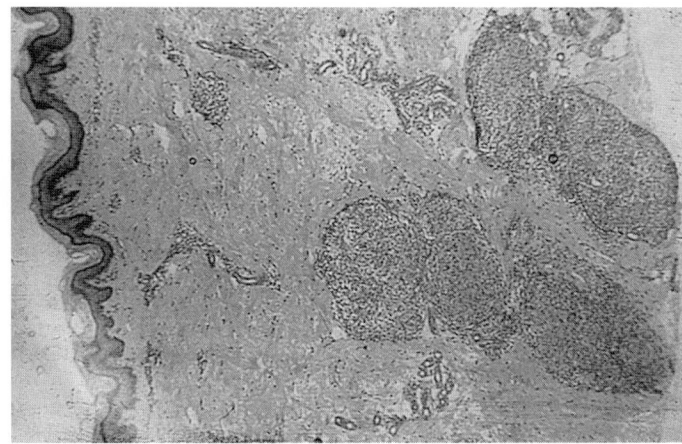

Figure 59.6: Skin lesions of tuberculoid leprosy (high power). (Courtesy of the late S. G. Browne.)

(sensory, motor or both). Other tissues are not affected directly but only indirectly, as in the tuberculoid type.

Indeterminate leprosy

This is an early phase in the natural history of leprosy. At this stage the disease has not yet determined into which type it is going to evolve. It usually presents as a single macule with uncharacteristic histology and absence of bacilli (Figure 59.5).

Pathological changes

In very early infection the acid-fast bacilli proliferate in the fixed cells of the dermis and thereafter monocytes from the blood migrate towards the bacilli, engulfing and disintegrating them. Leprosy bacilli may also enter nerves, causing focal damage related to the blood vessels near their site of entry into the nerves. They spread along the fine fibres of cutaneous nerve twigs and are carried centripetally, multiplying within Shwann cells and bursting into the endoneural spaces, where they are phagocytosed by histiocytes. If a skin lesion develops, a biopsy specimen at this stage shows foci of inflammatory cellular exudate, mainly around the finest nerve fibres in plexuses in the dermis. The exudate is determined by the ability of the host to react immunologically and it consists of lympho-cytes, histiocytes and other cells; clinically it is marked on the skin by wheal-like papules or pink or pale macules. This is the *indeterminate* stage of infection, which usually occurs in children in whom resistance has not been determined and which may last for months, or resolve, or progress to *tuberculoid*, *borderline* or *lepromatous* leprosy, depending on the immunological response of the body.

In persons whose resistance is poor, the histiocytes gradually change into lepra cells, which in more severe cases become foamy; the ingested bacilli are not destroyed. In persons whose resistance is good, the histiocytes change into epithelioid cells after ingesting the bacilli, which they destroy.

Although the manner of evolution of these cells contain-ing *M. leprae* is important, the mediators of immunity are the lymphocytes, and although the lymphocytes in skin lesions are not all immunologically active, the numbers present in tuberculoid and borderline lesions are significant indications of the degree of resistance to the infection.

Tuberculoid leprosy

The change from indeterminate to tuberculoid leprosy involves the appearance of groups of epithelioid cells (derived from histiocytes) inside fine nerve twigs and the formation of sharply circumscribed foci of these cells in the dermis, often surrounded by a zone of lymphocytes, which are fairly numerous. The epithelioid cells often coalesce to form giant cells. The epidermis is thinner than normal and there are foci of inflammatory cells reaching the epidermis without a clear space. In the dermis the granulomatous cords follow the lines of neurovascular bundles (Figure 59.6). The nerve bundles in the skin are swollen by proliferation of Schwann cells, which develop into epithelioid cells. The nerves become difficult to recognize; they occasionally undergo caseation, which does not occur in leprosy except in nerves.

The most consistent feature of tuberculoid leprosy is the early involvement of peripheral nerves. In the upper extremity this often goes on to weakness and paralysis of the intrinsic muscles of the hand (main-en-griffe) and in the leg to drop foot. Damage to the sympathetic nerves leads to slow atrophy and absorption (osteoporosis) of the small bones of the hands and feet through interference with vasodilatation.

Borderline leprosy

The histological picture shows features intermediate

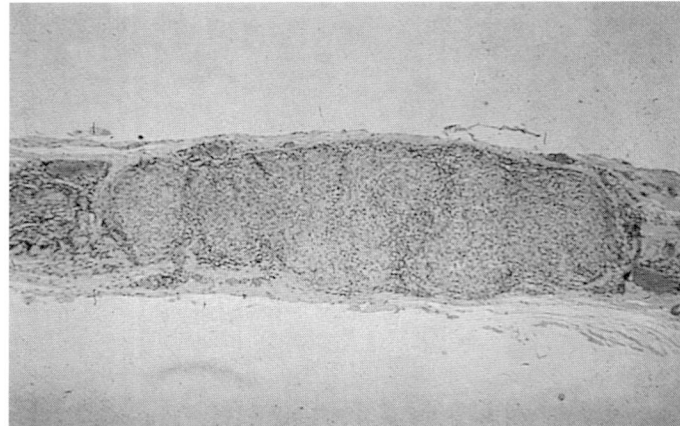

Figure 59.7: Nerve lesions (low power) of tuberculoid leprosy. (Courtesy of the late S. G. Browne.)

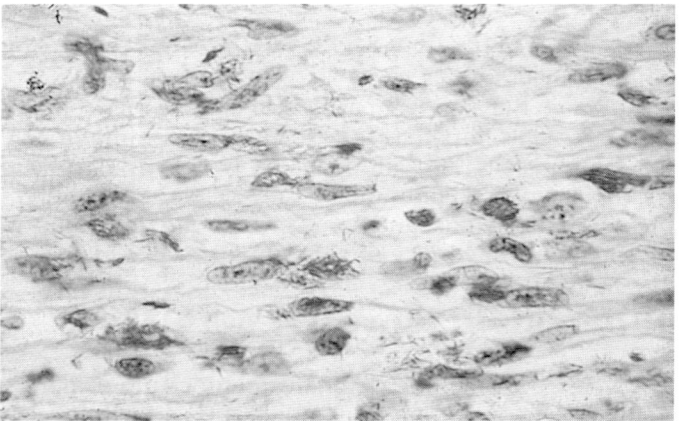

Figure 59.8: Nerve lesions (high power) of lepromatous leprosy. (Courtesy of the late S. G. Browne.)

between those of lepromatous and tuberculoid lesions. There is an inflammatory reaction with cellular exudate in the superficial layers of the dermis; it consists of small round cells, histiocytes and clumps of epithelioid cells but no giant cells. Nerves may show large numbers of bacilli and round cells or epithelioid cells with few bacilli; i.e. they may resemble nerves in lepromatous or tuberculoid disease (Figures 59.7 and 59.8). This borderline leprosy is unstable and tends to progress to the lepromatous form if not treated.

Lepromatous leprosy

In fully developed lepromatous disease large areas of the dermis are converted into continuous sheets of chronic inflammatory tissue containing enormous numbers of bacilli in slabs of lepra (Virchow) cells (derived from histiocytes) (Figure 59.9), interspersed with groups of mononuclear and plasma cells. Lymphocytes are scanty. The subepidermal zone of the dermis is clear of infiltrate. The disease is now systemic, the bacilli being transported by blood or lymph nodes, liver, spleen and bone marrow,

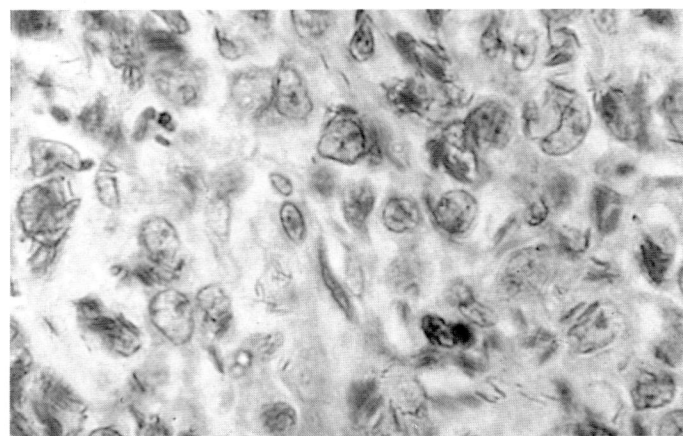

Figure 59.9: Skin lesions of lepromatous leprosy (high power) showing the lepra cellular tissue. (Courtesy of the late S. G. Browne.)

where miliary lepromas and even large lepromas may be found and subcutaneous veins may be involved.

The mucous membrane of the upper respiratory tract from the nose to the larynx, including the root of the tongue and the peritonsillar tissues, is heavily infiltrated in advanced lepromatous leprosy. It is oedematous, thickened and ulcerated and the nasal cartilages may be perforated. If the disease regresses as a result of treatment, the skin lesions heal in a remarkable manner.

Immunity

Protective immune response in leprosy is based on cellular immune mechanisms and leprosy bacilli are killed or eliminated only by this mechanism. Although not killed by humoral antibodies, leprosy bacilli stimulate the production of humoral antibodies against various constituent antigens. The type of leprosy produced depends on the ability to produce and develop cell-mediated immunity (CMI). CMI (mediated by lymphocytes) is strong in tuberculoid leprosy but weak or absent in lepromatous leprosy.[41] However, antibodies are produced plentifully in lepromatous leprosy but their immunological role is unclear. Tuberculoid leprosy patients give a positive lepromin test showing the immune response to *M. leprae*. The histological picture shows numerous lymphocytes and epithelioid cells, whereas lepromatous patients show little cellular reaction. The inability of a small proportion of individuals to mount an effective CMI response to *M. leprae* may be due to genetic factors, as shown by some that HLA types do play a part in the process.[42,43] Leprosy patients can resist other infections so that the anergy is specific, as demonstrated in lymphocyte transformation tests using *M. leprae* as antigen.[44]

Studies on T lymphocyte subpopulations have shown that the distribution of T helper and T suppressor cells varies in the different types of leprosy and that the distribution of helper and suppressor cells in tuberculoid leprosy resembles that found in sarcoidosis.[45] Whereas macrophage function in lepromatous leprosy is satisfactory, there is a deficiency in lymphokines.[46] *M. leprae* possesses a number of antigens which are specific[47] but they have a wide variation in sensitivity in immunological tests. In tuberculoid leprosy CMI is intact but aberrant, resulting from delayed recognition of *M. leprae* antigens.

Bacteriological examination

This consists in carrying out a series of smears from the lesions. The slit-scrape method is recommended. By this method acid-fast bacilli will always be found in lepromatous leprosy and frequently in the borderline form, but will usually be absent in the tuberculoid type and in the indeterminate group. In routine practice, bacteriological examination is rarely necessary, as most leprosy cases can be easily diagnosed and classified by clinical findings.

Skin biopsy

Biopsy of the skin or nerve is sometimes necessary when the diagnosis is doubtful or there is atypical presentation. In carrying out a biopsy the most active part of the lesion must be chosen. Paraffin sections are stained with haematoxylin and eosin to show the histological changes and, with the Ziehl–Neelsen method, to demonstrate acid-fast bacilli. A nerve biopsy will be necessary in a purely neural case or where a skin biopsy has not given sufficient information; a thickened sensory nerve is chosen, such as the great auricular in the neck, the antebrachial cutaneous in the forearm, the radial at the lateral aspect of the wrist, the femoral cutaneous in the thigh, the sural in the leg or the superficial peroneal on the dorsum of the foot.

Differential diagnosis

The characteristic marks of leprosy are sufficiently distinctive, but they have to be differentiated from psoriasis, seborrhoeic dermatitis, scars from burns or other injuries, various forms of tinea, eczema, lichen planus, pellagra and filarial disease. Blastomycosis produces skin lesions reminiscent of leprosy. Differentiation from syphilis and yaws may not always be so easy. Syphilitic and yaws skin lesions may often closely resemble the maculae of leprosy but the absence of sensory changes and reaction to treatment are sufficiently distinctive. The VDRL reaction alone cannot always be depended upon in differential diagnosis as a false positive reaction is not uncommon in lepromatous leprosy.

The early lesions of mycosis fungoides might possibly be mistaken for early nodular leprosy, and leucoderma is frequently associated with leprosy in the popular mind. Depigmentation in leucoderma, however, is more complete and sensory changes are absent. Lupus vulgaris and other tuberculides are very likely to be mistaken for leprosy

lesions and in both diseases acid-fast bacilli are difficult to demonstrate. Lupus evinces a greater tendency to scar formation and there are no sensory changes.

Cutaneous leishmaniasis and, in South America, espundia may be mistaken for leprosy. The lesions on the skin of the face tend to concentrate round the mouth and nose and form a more raised margin than those in leprosy. Demonstration of the Leishman–Donovan body will always settle the matter but leishmanial lupus-like lesions on the ears may cause difficulty. Burns and other injuries may leave behind anaesthetic scars.

Polyneuritic leprosy affecting the hands has to be differentiated from syringomyelia, in which analgesia and loss of heat sense are accompanied by retention of sense of touch and normal sweat function. The absence of nerve swelling and tenderness is important. The nerve injuries caused by trauma of the ulnar nerve or by cervical rib may possibly be called into question, but can be settled by X-ray examination. Meralgia paraesthetica (Bernhardt's syndrome) may cause anaesthesia of the anterolateral region of the thigh and Raynaud's disease can cause trophic changes in the extremities. Familial hypertrophic interstitial neuritis (Déjérine–Scottas disease) may cause confusion because of the characteristic thickening of peripheral nerves, together with sensory and motor changes in the limbs. Anaesthesia of the feet, leading to trophic ulceration and mutilation, can occur in diabetes, tabes, familial sensory radicular neuropathy and primary amyloidosis involving peripheral nerves. Von Recklinghausen's disease (neurofibromas) may sometimes resemble leprosy. Scarring and anaesthesia caused by extensive herpes zoster on the chest may give rise to difficulty. Scleroderma, localized or diffuse, may be confused with lepromatous leprosy but madarosis is not present, nerves are not thickened, acid-fast bacilli are absent from smear and skin biopsy is diagnostic. The absence of fever and the presence of neural signs should differentiate tuberculoid leprosy in reaction from erysipelas. Erythema nodosum leprosum may be mistaken for other forms of erythema nodosum or for the Weber–Christian syndrome (a relapsing, febrile, non-suppurative, nodular panniculitis). Sarcoidosis can resemble tuberculoid leprosy but there is no sensory loss and no nerve thickening. Granuloma annulare may simulate tuberculoid leprosy but there is no sensory loss or nerve thickening and the histological appearances are different. Granuloma multiforme may resemble tuberculoid leprosy; it appears to be localized to Nigeria. There is no sensory loss or nerve thickening and the histological appearances are different.

Clinical classification for control programmes

In 1981, the WHO Study Group on Chemotherapy of Leprosy for Control Programmes classified leprosy as multibacillary (MB) and paucibacillary (PB) according to the degree of skin-smear positivity.[4] It was essentially an

Table 59.3 A guide for clinical classification

	Paucibacillary leprosy (PB)	Multibacillary leprosy (MB)
Skin lesions (includes macules: flat lesions; papules: raised lesions and nodules)	– Up to 5 lesions – Hypopigmented or erythematous – Asymmetrically distributed – Definite loss of sensation	– More than 5 lesions – Distribution more symmetricall – Loss of sensation
Nerve damage (resulting in loss of sensation or weakness of muscles supplied by the affected nerve)	– Only one nerve trunk	– Many nerve trunks

Any patient showing a positive skin smear, irrespective of the clinical classification, should be treated with the MDT regimen for MB leprosy.

operational classification to serve as a basis for chemotherapy. MB leprosy included polar lepromatous (LL), borderline lepromatous (BL), and mid-borderline (BB) cases in the Ridley–Jopling classificadin, with a bacteriological index of 2 or more at any site in the initial skin smears. PB leprosy included indeterminate (I), polar tuberculoid (TT) and borderline tuberculoid (BT) in the Ridley– Jopling classification, with a bacteriological index of < 2 at all sites in the initial skin smears. In 1987, the Expert Committee on Leprosy at its sixth meeting endorsed the principles upon which this classification is based, with the modification that all smear-positive cases should be classified as MB leprosy for the purpose of MDT programmes.[48] In 1993, the Second WHO Study Group on Chemotherapy of Leprosy concluded that approaches based on clinical classification may be required where reliable facilities for the bacteriological examination of skin smears are not available, and it recommended that, when classification is in doubt, the patient should be treated as having MB leprosy (see Table 59.3).[49]

Because skin smear services are not always available, and also because their reliability is often doubtful, more and more programmes base their classification on clinical criteria. The essential feature is based on the number of lesions, especially the skin lesions.[35] The assumption is that the protective immunity is inversely correlated with the number of lesions and, therefore, the MB cases have a significantly greater number of lesions or number of body areas affected than the PB cases.

Management

Antileprosy drugs for standard multi-drug therapy

Currently three antileprosy drugs are recommended for use in the standard MDT regimens of limited duration. It is recommended that none of these should be used as monotherapy.

Rifampicin (rifampin, rifadin, rimactane)

Rifampicin is a semi-synthetic derivative of rifamycin that inhibits ribonucleic acid synthesis in a broad range of microbial pathogens. Rifampicin is by far the most effective bactericidal drug against *M. leprae*. Rifampicin given as a monthly dose of 600 mg is highly bactericidal and is almost as effective as daily rifampicin. The standard dose of 600 mg monthly in MDT regimens has proved relatively non-toxic, although occasional cases of renal failure, thrombocytopenia, influenza-like syndrome and hepatitis have been reported. Rifampicin may produce a reddish-brown colour in urine, sputum and sweat. It should be noted that the effects of steroids are reduced by rifampicin and the drug also impairs the effectiveness of oral contraceptives. In patients given rifampicin as monotherapy cases of rifampicin resistance have been reported.

Clofazimine (Lamprene, B663, G30320)

This is a rimino compound derived from phenazine dye. It is well absorbed when formulated in a microcrystalline oil–wax base. It is bactericidal against *M. leprae* and also exhibits anti-inflammatory activity. In the dosage employed in the MDT regimen for MB leprosy, clofazimine is virtually non-toxic. Pigmentation of the skin, particularly within skin lesions, is common but it clears completely within 6–12 months after treatment is discontinued. The higher dose (200–300 mg daily) of clofazimine is used for the control of leprosy reactions, particularly for patients who cannot take corticosteroids due to dependence, toxicity or other contraindications. In higher doses it may occasionally produce severe gastrointestinal side effects. So far no confirmed case of clofazimine resistance has been reported.

Dapsone (DDS, 4,4′-diaminodiphenylsulfone)

Dapsone acts as a synthetase inhibitor in the folate-synthesizing enzyme system of *M. leprae*. Dapsone is inexpensive and relatively non-toxic in the doses used, although occasional cases of delayed hypersensitivity reactions and less commonly agranulocytosis have been reported. Mild haemolytic anaemia is common following treatment with the drug, but severe haemolytic anaemia

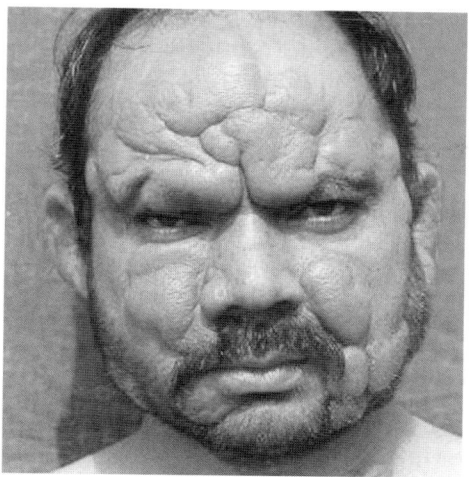

Figure 59.10: Multibacillary leprosy before MDT treatment.

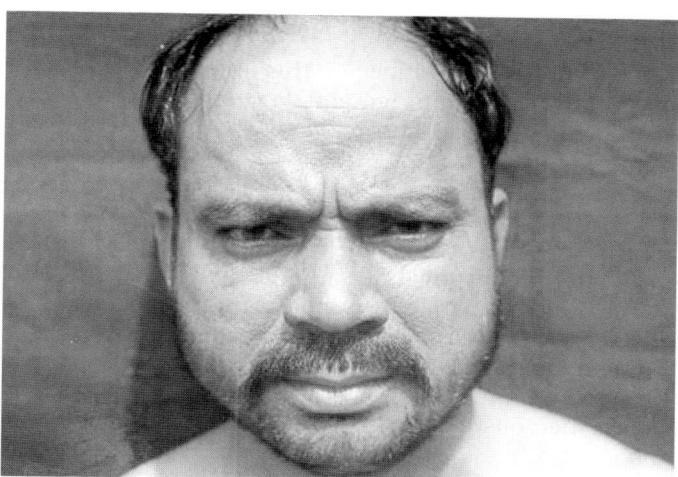

Figure 59.11: Same person cured with MDT.

is rare except in patients with glucose-6-phosphate dehydrogenase deficiency. When given in a dosage of 100 mg daily, dapsone is weakly bactericidal against *M. leprae*. Dapsone when used as monotherapy had limited effectiveness and resulted in widespread emergence of dapsone resistance.

Standard MDT regimens

Multibacillary leprosy

For adults, the recommended standard regimen is:

Rifampicin: 600mg once a month, supervised.
Dapsone: 100 mg daily, self-administered.
Clofazimine: 300 mg once a month, supervised, and 50 mg daily, self-administered.

Duration: 12 months (Figures 59.10 and 59.11).

Paucibacillary leprosy

For adults, the recommended standard regimen is:

Rifampicin: 600 mg once a month, supervised.
Dapsone: 100 mg daily, self-administered.

Duration: 6 months.
(Children should receive appropriately reduced doses of the above drugs.)

Management of leprosy during pregnancy and lactation

Leprosy is exacerbated during pregnancy, so it is important that the standard MDT be continued unchanged during pregnancy. Some small quantities of antileprosy drugs are excreted through breast milk but there is no report of adverse effects as a result of this except for mild discoloration of the infant due to clofazimine.

Management of patients with HIV infection or tuberculosis

HIV infection is a significant problem in many countries where leprosy is endemic. As yet, leprosy has not been found to be more common in such areas, but occasionally patients may be encountered who both are HIV-positive and have active leprosy. The information available indicates that the response of such patients to the standard MDT is similar to that of other leprosy patients and does not require modification. Patients suffering from both leprosy and tuberculosis will also occasionally be encountered. They require standard antituberculosis therapy in addition to MDT for their leprosy. At present only rifampicin will be common to the two regimens and it must be given in the doses required for tuberculosis.

Antileprosy drugs for special situations

Currently three additional drugs are available for treatment of leprosy under special situations. It is recommended that none of these should be used as monotherapy.

Ofloxacin

Ofloxacin, one of the fluoroquinolones, interferes with bacterial DNA replication by inhibiting the A subunit of the enzyme DNA gyrase. The results of clinical trials have indicated that the optimal dosage for the treatment of leprosy is 400 mg daily. While a single dose of ofloxacin displayed a modest bactericidal effect against *M. leprae*, 22 doses killed 99.99% of the viable *M. leprae* in patients with advanced MB leprosy. Side effects include nausea, diarrhoea and other gastrointestinal complaints, and a variety of central nervous system complaints including insomnia, headaches, dizziness, nervousness and hallucinations.

Minocycline

Minocycline is a member of the tetracycline group of antibiotics. It inhibits protein synthesis via a reversible binding at the 30S ribosomal subunit, thereby blocking the binding of aminoacyl transfer RNA to the messenger RNA ribosomal complex. Its bactericidal activity against *M. leprae* is greater than that of clarithromycin, but much less than that of rifampicin. The standard dose of 100 mg daily has been shown to be effective clinically when administered to patients with advanced MB leprosy. Side effects include discoloration of teeth in infants and children, occasional pigmentation of the skin and mucous membranes, and various gastrointestinal symptoms and central nervous system complaints, including dizziness and unsteadiness. It should therefore not be given to children and pregnant women.

Clarithromycin

Clarithromycin is a member of the macrolide group of antibiotics and displays significant bactericidal activity against *M. leprae*. The drug inhibits bacterial protein synthesis by linking to the 50S ribosomal subunit, thereby preventing elongation of the protein chain. It is readily absorbed from the gastrointestinal tract and converted to its active metabolite, 14-hydroxyclarithromycin. In patients with advanced MB leprosy, daily administration of 500 mg of clarithromycin killed 99% of viable *M. leprae* within 28 days, and >99.9% by 56 days. Side effects include nausea, vomiting and diarrhoea.

Special treatment regimens

Regimen for single-lesion paucibacillary leprosy

There is evidence to suggest that single-lesion leprosy can be cured by a limited amount of chemotherapy. The efficacy of a single dose of a drug combination consisting of 600 mg of rifampicin, 400 mg of ofloxacin and 100 mg of minocycline (ROM) for the treatment of single-lesion PB leprosy has been proved in a multicentre, double-blind field trial. A single dose of ROM was marginally less effective, in terms of clinical improvement, than the standard MDT regimen for PB leprosy. However, in some specialized programmes where a significant number of new patients are classified as having single-lesion PB leprosy, a single dose of ROM is an acceptable and cost-effective alternative regimen for the treatment of patients belonging to this category.

Patient who cannot take rifampicin

Special treatment regimens are required for individual patients who cannot take rifampicin because of side effects or intercurrent diseases, such as chronic hepatitis, or who have been infected with rifampicin-resistant *M. leprae*.

The following 24-month regimen is recommended: daily administration of 50 mg clofazimine, together with two of the following drugs—400 mg ofloxacin, 100 mg minocycline or 500 mg clarithromycin—for 6 months; followed by daily administration of 50 mg clofazimine, together with 100 mg minocycline or 400 mg ofloxacin for an additional 18 months.

Patient who refuses to take clofazimine

MB patients who refuse to take clofazimine because of skin discoloration also need a safe and effective alternative treatment. In such patients, clofazimine in the normal 12-month MDT for MB patients may be replaced by ofloxacin, 400 mg daily, or by minocycline, 100 mg daily for 12 months.

In 1997, the WHO Expert Committee on Leprosy[50] also recommended the following alternative 24-month (ROM) regimen for MB adult patients who refuse to take clofazimine: rifampicin, 600 mg once a month, ofloxacin, 400 mg once a month, and minocycline, 100 mg once a month for 24 months.

Patient who cannot take dapsone

If dapsone produces severe toxic effects in any leprosy patient, either PB or MB leprosy, dapsone must be immediately stopped. No further modification of the regimen is required for patients with MB leprosy. However, clofazimine in the dosage employed in the standard MDT for MB leprosy should be substituted for dapsone in the regimen for PB leprosy for a period of 6 months.

Management of lepra reactions, neuritis and other complications

Lepra reactions

During the course of leprosy, immunologically mediated episodes of acute or subacute inflammation known as lepra reactions occur in about 5% of PB and about 20% of MB patients. Because peripheral nerve trunks are often involved, unless reactions are promptly and adequately treated such episodes can result in permanent disabilities. Most reactions belong to one of two major types: reversal (type 1) reaction or erythema nodosum leprosum (ENL or type 2) reaction. Reversal reaction occurs in both PB and MB leprosy, while ENL reaction occurs exclusively in patients with advanced MB leprosy. In general, ENL reactions appear to be less common among patients treated with MDT than those treated with dapsone monotherapy, probably owing to the anti-inflammatory activity of clofazimine.

Because of the high risk of permanent damage to the peripheral nerve trunks, particularly associated with reversal reactions, such episodes should be diagnosed early and treated adequately (Figure 59.12). The drug of choice is prednisolone, the cheapest and most widely available corticosteroid. The usual course begins with 40–60 mg daily (up to a maximum of 1 mg/kg body weight),

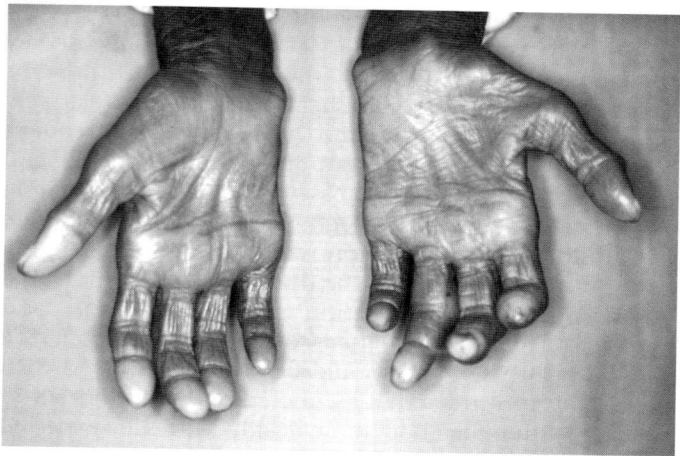

Figure 59.12: Typical hand deformities due to leprosy.

and the reaction is generally controlled within a few days. The dose is then gradually reduced weekly or fortnightly and eventually stopped. Most reversal reactions and neuritis can be treated successfully under field conditions with a standard 12-week course of prednisolone.

ENL varies in severity, duration and organ involvement. Mild ENL can be treated with analgesic or antipyretic drugs such as aspirin, while severe ENL, often accompanied by neuritis, should be treated with prednisolone, as for reversal reaction. Clofazimine is also effective for ENL but is less potent than corticosteroids and often takes 4–6 weeks to develop its full effects, so it should never be started as the sole agent for the treatment of severe ENL. However, clofazimine may be extremely useful for reducing or withdrawing corticosteroids in patients who have become dependent on steroids. The dose required in such cases is 300 mg daily, which may be given in three divided daily doses to minimize the gastrointestinal side effects; the total duration of high-dose clofazimine therapy should not exceed 12 months.

The crucial elements in the management of leprosy reactions and, thereby, the prevention of disabilities are early diagnosis of reactions together with prompt and adequate treatment. Therefore, leprosy programmes should ensure that:

- Patients are taught to recognize the early signs/symptoms of reactions and to report promptly for treatment.
- Health workers are able to diagnose and treat reactions and to refer patients when necessary.
- Adequate stocks of prednisolone are maintained at the peripheral level.
- During a lepra reaction the appropriate leprosy MDT is continued without any interruption.

Management of eye complications

The eye may be damaged by direct bacillary invasion or by nerve damage. Leprosy patients may develop ocular complications, such as corneal ulceration, iridocyclitis and lagophthalmos. Corneal ulceration may result from corneal anaesthesia or from paralysis of the eyelids. Iridocyclitis is one of the most important causes of blindness in leprosy and therefore should be treated promptly with mydriatics and anti-inflammatory drugs. Protection must be afforded to those patients with lagophthalmos by use of goggles or sunglasses. Frequent use of artificial teardrops during the day and ointments or oily drops at night is advocated.

Prevention and management of disabilities

The common paralytic disabilities in leprosy are claw hand, footdrop, lagophthalmos and wristdrop. Sensory loss over the extremities leads to misuse of the affected limb, with resultant ulceration, infection and, ultimately, severe deformities and disabilities. Most of the disabilities occur before a patient is diagnosed. Therefore, the most cost-effective method to prevent disabilities is early detection and prompt treatment with MDT, including proper management of neuritis associated with lepra reactions.

Drug resistance and relapse

MDT was developed mainly because of the widespread emergence of dapsone resistance, and the regimens were designed on the principle that they would effectively prevent development of resistance to any single drug used in the combination. Results obtained from several leprosy programmes and research projects indicated that after completion of MDT the overall relapse rates are about 0.1%, which is less than one-tenth of the rate observed in the past, when patients were treated with dapsone alone.[51] All *M. leprae* from patients who relapse remain susceptible to rifampicin and clofazimine and respond favourably to a second course of MDT.

Strategy for eliminating leprosy as a public health problem

The strategy[52] for the elimination of leprosy as a public health problem is based on early case detection and cure with MDT. The target, defined as reducing the global prevalence to less than one case per 10 000 population, is not only aspirational but also managerial. However, the strategy involves certain assumptions and these need to be understood. These assumptions are as follows:

- Treatment with MDT, together with early case-finding, is the best way of dealing with the problem of leprosy and its consequences.
- The major objective is to reduce the disease burden in terms of prevalence to very low levels, and the reduction of disease prevalence will lead, in the course of time, to a reduction in transmission of infection and reduction of disease incidence.
- With leprosy having a chronic and insidious onset, and a very strong self-healing component, it is not

possible to measure incidence from routine information systems.

- Until a steady state is reached, when there are no more 'hidden' cases and when geographic and MDT coverage are universal, case detection figures will reflect essentially the operational performance and not incidence.
- Experience over the past 15 years has established that these assumptions are largely valid. It is important to realize, however, that the elimination of leprosy as a public health problem is a more modest goal than eradication, as eradication means zero disease and zero transmission, for which we have no tools as yet.

Main achievements over the last 15 years

- By the beginning of 2000, more than 10 million cases had been cured.
- Currently almost 100% of registered cases are receiving MDT.
- The numbers of relapses remain low, at about 0.1% person years.
- Drug resistance following MDT has not been reported.
- The number of countries showing prevalence rates above 1 per 10 000 population has been reduced from 122 in 1985 to 24 at the beginning of 2000.

Elements of the intensified strategy

Ensuring that MDT services are available and readily accessible to patients at the nearest health facility is the most critical element in the elimination strategy, without which all the efforts of case-finding, diagnosis, classification and drug supply are rendered meaningless. The revised strategy aims at focusing activities at the district level in countries at risk of not achieving elimination.

Identification of endemic districts

The situation at the district level in most countries remains unclear. Endemic countries naturally exhibit regional differences in terms of the disease burden, health service coverage and efficiency of the programme. There are many reasons for this, including the availability of trained health staff, difficult terrain or poor security, lack of logistic support for distribution of MDT drugs, and limited participation of the general health services and community in the programme activities. For similar reasons, there can also be wide disparities within individual regions of endemic countries. In order to fully interpret and manage both these inter-regional and intra-regional disparities, countries where leprosy is still endemic should implement an information system focused at a more micro-level than is generally used at present.

MDT services integrated into general health facilities

It is important that MDT services should be available and accessible at the nearest health centre so that patients can get their treatment easily. The integration of MDT services within the general health services is regarded as the key to achieving elimination. The rationale behind this approach is that the general health services are relatively more widely distributed, and have close and frequent contact with the local community. Involving the general health services will improve case-finding and case-holding activities, as well as cost-effectiveness of the programme. In addition, such integration will help to reduce stigma and increase awareness of the disease in the community.

The process of integration should be simple and practical. The tasks assigned to the workers from the general health services should be clear and in line with their daily routine activities, including the information systems. With integration, more health centres are expected to be providing treatment, and the case-load in each centre will be relatively low in comparison to the attendance at leprosy clinics opened by the specialized/vertical programmes. Integration will help in maintaining MDT services at the peripheral level, especially in areas where prevalence is declining. Several national programmes, even in countries with very high prevalence, have integrated leprosy services, mainly because of the urgent need to expand MDT coverage. However, it is important to have an element of a specialized programme in all endemic countries, either at the central level or—in some large countries—at an intermediate level. This specialized element for leprosy will be needed for providing technical guidance, monitoring and evaluating the progress of elimination, training and for research purposes. Referral centres will also support the general health services in diagnosing difficult cases and in providing certain specialized care to patients with complications.

Monitoring elimination at the district level

Most endemic countries are currently using well-standardized leprosy information systems. The essential indicators used for monitoring progress towards the elimination of leprosy are prevalence, case detection, coverage with MDT, patients cured with MDT, relapses and newly detected cases with grade 2 disabilities and impairments. These indicators should be analysed at the district level through the development of an integrated district-level database for other activities related to health. The internal validity of the indicators should be continuously assessed by independent monitors in collaboration with the national programme. The main objective of such monitoring will be to collect indicators that reflect the performance of MDT services, especially the availability of drugs, cure rates and the quality of patient care at the district level.

Promoting community action

The participation of the community in the elimination activities needs to be increased in order to positively change the image of leprosy and reduce the stigma attached to the disease. This will require identifying obstacles to community participation and developing strategies for promoting community action. The main difficulties are ignorance about the symptoms/signs and curability of the disease. The local community and its leaders should play a key role in improving public awareness of the disease and the availability of free and effective treatment. In some situations, they may be the only option in supporting MDT services in case-finding and ensuring that patients complete their treatment, particularly in areas where routine general health services either are not available or do not function properly. The elimination strategy cannot depend on the health services alone and therefore the involvement of other sectors in this process will be crucial to achieving the goal.

Social marketing/advocacy

Leprosy has always had certain very special features, as a disease affecting mainly under-served populations and generating intense emotions linked with the age-old stigma against those affected by it. As a result, the fight against leprosy has traditionally been undertaken by a relatively small group of people, highly dedicated but often reluctant to share the responsibility for the disease and its control with a wider audience. This phenomenon is encountered at various levels, notably among expert groups, programme managers and charitable agencies raising funds in the name of leprosy. This explains to some extent why the tremendous achievements in leprosy control during the last half of the twentieth century are not well known, or are even underplayed. Today we know leprosy to be curable, but making it interesting to the public, the scientific community, decision-makers and politicians is not easy. The major approaches to creating awareness and support in the community are through information, education and communication. The mass media can be very helpful in improving community awareness, but may also have a negative impact through biased stories. The issues here are how to improve communication and collaboration for advocacy between the programme and the media, how to make leprosy elimination attractive to the public and how to generate support for the activities.

Remotivating the research community

It is clear that in some endemic countries the period of time required to reach elimination may not be easy to estimate, particularly in areas with high new case detection rates. In view of these uncertainties and possible difficulties, and taking into account that our arsenal against leprosy is limited, it appears fully justified to revitalize leprosy research activities, in order to develop new diagnostic, prophylactic and even therapeutic tools. In addition, there is a particular need to encourage and strengthen the capacity for epidemiological and operational research.

Close collaboration between basic research and clinical research groups should be encouraged. Studies are needed to identify alternative drugs that are highly effective and less toxic for the management of reactions. Optimal methods for the early detection and treatment of reactions and neuritis need to be developed and approach to their prevention explored. A common regimen for both MB and PB leprosy would be an advantage. These regimens would make chemotherapy simpler, particularly after the goal of elimination has been reached. The most promising avenues for vaccine development are probably genomic research and research on the development of vaccines for other mycobacterial diseases.

Prevention of disabilities and rehabilitation

There is a need for incorporating simple disability prevention and management components within leprosy elimination programmes. The most cost-effective approach will be to strengthen collaboration with other relevant services and organizations working in this field, starting with a good assessment of the problem, and implementation of integrated projects. It will facilitate the development of national integrated projects for rehabilitation of individuals with severe physical disabilities due to various causes in the community.

Future challenges

Although significant progress has been made towards eliminating leprosy as a public health problem, at the end of 2000 six countries had not reached the elimination target at the national level (Brazil, India, Madagascar, Mozambique, Myanmar and Nepal). In countries that have reached the target at the national level, there is a need to reach elimination at the sub-national level and to sustain elimination activities for a number of years.

It is evident that, due to improved disease control activities, the detection of new cases has increased over the last few years. This does not mean that transmission is on the increase or is not interrupted. This status simply reflects the inadequacy and inefficiency of some of the programmes which were relying (and some are still continuing) on keeping the ownership of leprosy elimination with the highly specialized leprosy services. This approach has not only harmed the control of the disease but has also perpetuated and even increased the negative image of leprosy in the community.

The occurrence of disabilities is the main reason why leprosy is such a fearsome disease. There is very limited progress in addressing the issue of prevention of disabilities and rehabilitation of the affected. There are several reasons for this: inadequate efforts to develop effective tools and failure to address the issue through integrated services for all disabled in the community are probably the most important ones. The problem, in socio-economic and human terms, is enormous and we will need many partners to solve this, including the affected communities in the endemic countries. In the meantime, early detection and treatment with MDT will remain the best strategy for preventing the occurrence of disabilities.

The image of leprosy is still unchanged from what it was thousands of years ago, mainly due to poor advocacy and lack of sensitivity to understand the impact of negative messages being directed towards the community in the name of information, education and communication.

Many excellent institutions have contributed immensely towards improving care through research and training in this long battle against leprosy. They will be needed now to further simplify case management, improve surveillance, strengthen socio-economic rehabilitation services and remain alert to counter any unforeseen challenges in the path towards ultimate eradication of this disease during the twenty-first century.

In the new millennium, the priorities and commitments are likely to change. Other diseases like malaria, tuberculosis and AIDS, which are on the increase, will divert all resources available for health. This is totally justified. However, within this context it will be important to ensure that leprosy is kept on the health agenda and the opportunity for its elimination is not lost. All organizations involved in this effort will be called to revise their agenda and roles to meet the challenging task of eliminating leprosy as a public health problem.

REFERENCES

1. World Health Organization. Leprosy disabilities: magnitude of the problem. *Weekly Epidemiol Rec* 1995; 70:269–275.
2. Noordeen S K & Lopez Bravo L. *World Health Stat Q* 1986; 39:122–128.
3. World Health Organization. Leprosy: global situation. *Weekly Epidemiol Rec* 2000; 75:226–231.
4. World Health Organization. *WHO Tech Rep Ser* 1982; 675.
5. Hansen G A. *Norsk Magazin for Laegevidenskaben* 1874; 4:76.
6. Weddell A G M, Palmer E & Rees R J W. *Lepr Rev* 1963; 34:156–158.
7. Job C K, Jayakumar J & Aschhoff M. *Int J Lepr* 1999; 67:164–167.
8. Schäffer I. *Arch Dermato Syphilis* 1898; 44:159–174.
9. Shepard C C. *Am J Hyg* 1960; 71:147–157.
10. Pedley J C. *Lepr Rev* 1973; 44:33–35.
11. Davey T F & Rees R J W. *Lepr Rev* 1974; 45:121–134.
12. Desikan K V. *Lepr Rev* 1977; 48:231–235.
13. Rees R J W & McDougall A C. *J Med Microbiol* 1977; 10:63–68.
14. Chehl S, Job C K & Hastings R C. *Am J Trop Med Hyg* 1985; 34:1161–1166.
15. Rees R J W. *Trans R Soc Trop Med Hyg* 1967; 61:581.
16. Rees R J W, Waters M F R, Weddell A G M et al. *Nature* 1967; 215:599–602.
17. Kirchheimer W F, Storrs E E & Binford C H. *Int J Lepr* 1972; 40:229.
18. Cole S T, Brosch R, Parkhill J et al. *Nature* 1998; 393:537–544.
19. Cole S T, Eiglmeier K, Parkhill J et al. *Nature* 2001; 409: 1007–1011.
20. Doull J A, Guinto R S, Rodriguez J N et al. *Int J Lepr* 1942; 10:107–131.
21. Noordeen S K & Neelan P N. *Indian J Med Res* 1978; 67:515–527.
22. Shepard C C, Walker L L, Van Landingham R M et al. *Infect Immun* 1982; 38:673–680.
23. Montestruc E & Berdonneau R. *Bull Soc Pathol Exot Filiales* 1954; 47:781–783.
24. Agrawal S, Joshi A, Jacob M et al. *Int J Lepr* 1999; 67: 471–473.
25. World Health Organization. Report of a study group. *WHO Tech Rep Ser* 1985; 716.
26. Walsh G P, Meyers W M, Binford C H et al. *Lepr Rev* 1981; 52(Suppl. 1):77–83.
27. Gormus B J, Xu K, Baskin J B et al. *Lepr Rev* 1995; 66:96–104.
28. World Health Organization. Report of a meeting on HIV infection in leprosy. 1993; WHO/CTD/LEP/93.3.
29. Lucas S. *Lepr Rev* 1993; 64:97–103.
30. Fine P E M. *Int J Lepr* 1992; 60:71–80.
31. Karonga Prevention Trial Group. *Lancet* 1996; 348:17–24.
32. Convit J et al. *Lancet* 1992; 339:446–450.
33. Gupte M D, Vallishayee R S, Anantharaman D S et al. *Indian J Lepr* 1998; 70:369–388.
34. Guinto R S, Doull J A, de Guia L et al. *Int J Lepr* 1954; 22:273–284.
35. Noordeen S K. *Indian J Med Res* 1972; 60:439–445.
36. World Health Organization. A guide to eliminating leprosy as a public health problem. 1997; WHO/LEP/97.7.
37. Jopling W H. *Handbook of Leprosy*, 2nd edn. London: Heinemann, 1978.
38. Rea T H & Levan N E. *Arch Dermatol* 1978; 114:1023.
39. Rea T H & Ridley D S. *Int J Lepr* 1979; 47:161.
40. Brand P. *Insensitive Feet: A Practical Handbook on Foot Problems in Leprosy*. London: Leprosy Mission, 1966.
41. Turk J L. *Immunology in Clinical Practice*. London: Heinemann, 1969.
42. Eden W, Van Vries R R P, Mehra N K et al. *J Infect Dis* 1980; 141:693–701.
43. Eden W, Van Vries R R P, de Marao J D et al. *Hum Immun* 1982; 4:343–350.
44. Godal T, Lofgren M & Negassi K. *Int J Lepr* 1972; 40:243–250.
45. Narayanan R B, Bhutani L K, Sharma A K et al. *Clin Exp Immunol* 1983; 51:421–430.
46. Haregewoin A, Godal R, Mustafa A S et al. *Nature* 1983; 303:542–544.
47. Harboe M. *Int J Lepr* 1982; 50:342–350.
48. World Health Organization. WHO Expert Committee on Leprosy. Sixth Report. *WHO Tech Rep Ser* 1988; 768.
49. World Health Organization. Report of a WHO Study Group. *Tech Rep Ser* 1994; 847.
50. World Health Organization. WHO Expert Committee on Leprosy. Seventh Report. *WHO Tech Rep Ser* 1998; 874.
51. World Health Organization. Risk of relapse in leprosy. 1994; WHO/CTD/LEP/94.1.
52. World Health Organization. The final push towards elimination of leprosy: Strategic Plan 2000–2005. 2000; WHO/CDS/CPE/200.1.

Chapter 60
Brucellosis

S. G. Wright

Brucellosis is a zoonotic infection due to infection with one of three species of the genus *Brucella: B. melitensis, B. abortus* and *B. suis*.[1] *B. canis, B. ovis* and *B. neotomae* are also recognized but human infection with the latter two does not occur and with the former, *B canis*, is rare. The infection has a worldwide distribution, predominantly in rural areas among pastoralist peoples. It also occurs in urban settings when small numbers of animals are kept in and around houses. Eradication campaigns have been successful in a number of areas, such as the United Kingdom, but these have required much effort and considerable expense.

Bacteriology
Characteristics and growth

Brucellae are aerobic, Gram-negative bacilli or coccobacilli. They are non-motile and non-spore forming and grow slowly in vitro on enriched media, such as serum dextrose agar, optimally at 37°C. *B. abortus* and *B. ovis* grow better in the presence of added CO_2. Slow growth in vitro requires cultures to be maintained and subcultured blindly for up to 6 weeks before discarding clinical samples for culture. Isolates from clinical material have a smooth appearance to the colonies; this becomes rough after a time in culture. Catalase production is uniformly present and oxidase production is a common feature. For a detailed description of microbiological features see Corbel.[1]

Laboratory infections

Laboratory transmission of *Brucella* species is a well-recognized occurrence and in endemic areas staff are well aware of this. An organism identified as *Moraxella phenylpyruvica* with a probability of 90.5% using the API20NE microbiological test strip was subsequently found to be *B. melitensis* using agglutinating sera.[2] Laboratories in countries where *Brucella* species isolates are uncommon should be aware of this potential problem.

Taxonomy

Several biovars are recognized for each of the three main pathogens: *melitensis* (three biovars), *abortus* (nine) and *suis* (five). These species and biovars represent the presently accepted taxonomy for the genus but DNA homology studies have shown greater than 95% homology such that revision of the present taxonomic divisions has been suggested to yield a single-species genus, *B. melitensis*, with a number of biovars. As yet there has been no move to institute this change. There is evidence for relationships between *Brucella* and *Agrobacterium, Bartonella, Mycoplana, Ochrobactrum, Phyllobacterium* and *Rhizobium*.

Antigens and cross-reactions

In agglutination reactions two antigens of the smooth lipopolysaccharide surface antigen, designated A and M, have been defined. These are the most studied of a wide range of brucella antigens. A antigen predominates in *abortus* and *suis*, while M is the major antigen in *melitensis*.[1] Antigenic cross-reactivity exists between brucellae and a number of other Gram-negative species including *Escherichia coli* O116, *Francisella tularensis, Pseudomonas maltophila, Vibrio cholerae, Yersinia enterocolitica* serogroup O9 and *Salmonella urbana*.

Epidemiology
Animal infections

The three main pathogenic species are fairly restricted in their host specificities, with bovines harbouring *abortus*, goats, camels and sheep infected with *melitensis* and pigs with *suis*. Cross-infection among these animals can occur but the resulting infections are short lived. Infection in utero or early in life usually results in lifelong infection.

Infection in animals often causes abortion soon after acquisition of the organism, and thereafter latent infection recrudesces with subsequent pregnancy, causing congenital infection or milk-borne infection in the offspring. This pattern is similar for cattle, goats and sheep. Among pigs the boar transmits infection to sows through semen. Brucellosis causes considerable economic losses through reduced fecundity, fetal loss and diminished milk production.

Transmission

Several routes of transmission of infection to man are possible. Ingestion of infected, unpasteurized milk is most readily thought of and, as brucellae are very acid sensitive, it is convenient to think of milk neutralizing gastric acid, allowing organisms to survive transit through the stomach to the duodenum, where they enter the mucosa. It has been suggested that persons taking antacid medications or H_2-receptor antagonists have an increased risk of infection. Soft cheeses and similar products made from unpasteurized milk also transmit infection because the shorter time for preparation does not allow the pH to fall sufficiently to kill the organisms. It is also likely that organisms can enter through the epithelium overlying lymphoid tissue in the nasopharynx.

Aerosols occurring in laboratories or through splashing of amniotic fluid or milk may be infective through inhalation or contact with conjunctiva or nasopharynx. Semen may also be a route of transmission between humans, as may blood transfusion and organ transplantation. Brucellae may be introduced through cuts and abrasions on the hands when slaughtering infected animals in either commercial or domestic settings. Congenital infection is also reported, as is infection through human breast milk. Vaccine strains used in animals are not attenuated for humans and may cause human disease from accidental inoculation. Brucellae are capable of surviving for prolonged periods in the environment and so inhalation of contaminated dusts in hot, dry countries may be a source of infection.

Distribution and incidence

The disease occurs in all areas of the world, with few countries spared. As it is frequently present in rural communities the infection may well go unrecognized. The frequency of animal infections is a useful guide to the likely occurrence in man. Human brucellosis is present in the countries of southern Europe. For example, in France the incidence varies between 1.07 and 18.4 per 100 000 of the populations of different regions. Brucellosis due to *B. melitensis* was particularly common in the Arabian peninsula and the Middle East from the 1980s; in Kuwait the incidence increased from 1.15 to 42.8 per 100 000 over the decade to 1984. As with many infectious diseases the true incidence of brucellosis is several times greater than the reported incidence.

Because of the animal origin of infection there is a strong occupational predisposition to infection among those having close contact with animals or their infected milk or tissues. Shepherds, cowherds, swineherds, veterinarians and their assistants, abattoir workers and those handling meat, etc. in kitchens are all at risk. In many communities humans and animals live in close proximity and so the occupational exposure is associated with increased consumption of infected milk products. Laboratory infections with brucella are a particular concern and must be borne in mind when assessing infections in veterinary or hospital laboratory workers.

Both sexes and all age groups are susceptible to infection. Infections among children represent the minority of cases. There is evidence of an increased occurrence among males compared with females, although a study from Saudi Arabia[3] showed a higher incidence among females than males at all age groups between 15 and 64 years. Over 65 years the incidence was higher in males.

Pathogenesis and pathology

Brucellae are facultatitive intracellular pathogens. Within the body they are phagocytosed by neutrophils which kill *B. abortus* and avirulent, but not virulent, *B. melitensis*.[4] Smooth lipopolysaccharide is the main determinant of virulence in the organism. Complement enhances phagocytosis. Macrophages subsequently become parasitized by the organisms.

Phylogenetic relationships were noted above between *Brucella* and *Rhizobium*. The latter is capable of establishing chronic infections in the roots of leguminous plants. The *bacA* gene is thought to be important in this and *Brucella* has a similar gene showing considerable sequence homology.[5] In in vitro and animal studies introduction of a modified *bacA* gene into *B. abortus* produced a significant decline in survival of *Brucellae* in macrophages and of *Brucellae* in mice. In addition there are interactions between the organism and the mechanisms responsible for killing in phagolysosomes. These are inhibited by virulent brucellae.

In mice, numbers of organisms in liver and spleen macrophages rise progressively during the first 14 days of infection and then decline dramatically with the development of T cell reactivity. The T cells concerned have a suppressor–cytotoxic phenotype. In mice that have apparently contained the infection small numbers of persisting organisms can be isolated and it seems possible that these persisting organisms may give rise to the relapses that occur in brucellosis. This persistence phenomenon is perhaps explained by the *bacA* gene noted above.

Antibody responses to brucellae are capable of affecting the progression of infection in mice receiving antilipopolysaccharide or antipeptidoglycan antibodies prior to inoculation of organisms. Their contribution to controlling infection in man is uncertain.

The pathological feature in affected tissues is granuloma formation. As the organism is widely distributed through the bloodstream these are found in many tissues. There are no characteristic features of the granuloma and the differential diagnosis of febrile illnesses associated with granuloma formation is considerable, with tuberculosis being a particularly important alternative cause to consider as the two infections can produce very similar clinical syndromes. There may be progression to microabscess formation around these granulomas. Clinically apparent abscess formation is not uncommon and may occur in a range of tissues, including the vertebrae and the psoas muscle.

Clinical features

The incubation period is about 2–4 weeks. This has been

gauged most accurately in instances of laboratory infection resulting from a broken culture flask. The initial illness is non-specific, with fevers, lethargy, anorexia and night sweats. This illness, while causing marked symptoms, is often not troublesome enough to bring the patient to seek medical advice and often it is the appearance of localized disease that brings this about. In this early phase enlargement of liver and spleen, present in 27% of a large series of cases, with perhaps lymph node enlargement may be the only clinical evidence.[6]

One of the names given to this infection was 'undulant fever', so called because of the waxing and waning of fever in a cycle lasting 2–4 weeks. This is not usually seen currently because the diagnosis is made before a sufficient time has passed to see the undulations but it was apparent to physicians in the pre-antibiotic era. The *Lancet* for 9 September 1899 carried an article describing several cases, including that of Almroth Wright who had injected himself with a living culture of brucellae to test the efficacy of a killed vaccine he had previously received. He became ill 16 days later with a fever showing an undulant pattern with a cycle of 4 weeks between the first two peaks. Other cases described show a range of periodicity to the undulations. These and other reports show that, while spontaneous resolution after weeks or months of clinical illness occurs, there was a mortality associated with brucellosis, estimated at up to 7%.

Skeletal disease

Bone and joint involvement is a particularly common feature, certainly in *B. melitensis* infections, which have been the subject of study in large series of cases reported in recent years.[6,7] Where peripheral joints are involved it is usually a large weight-bearing joint such as the hip or knee. Pain is severe and the patient may not be able to walk. Sacroiliitis is also common. Often the organisms cannot be isolated from joint fluid but this may relate to numbers of organisms in the tissues and difficulties experienced with culture. Arthritis in the knee may cause posterior rupture of the joint capsule, giving the appearance of a ruptured Baker's cyst. Any joint may be affected; examples are the sternoclavicular joint and costochondral junctions.

Involvement of the axial skeleton is common.[8] This may present with sciatica in young adults, most likely the result of inflammation and swelling of the affected intervertebral disc(s). Infection of adjacent vertebral bodies may lead to abscess formation and may present with a psoas abscess. Any part of the spine may be affected, but the lumbar region is an area of predilection. The clinical presentation is very similar to that of tuberculosis, particularly when brucella causes paravertebral or psoas abscess, and careful distinction of the two conditions is necessary.

Localization to other sites

Epididymo-orchitis is frequent, occurring in about 7% of cases. Renal involvement occurs and brucellae can be cultured from the urine. Pulmonary disease is not common. Endocarditis is one of the most serious complications affecting either a normal valve, the aortic, or a previously diseased valve, usually the mitral.

Neurological disease is infrequent but can cause a wide range of manifestations, including meningitis, papilloedema, cranial neuritis, focal or diffuse cerebritis, encehalopathy, meningoencephalitis, Parkinsonian syndromes, transient ischaemic episodes and vasculitis. The changes in cerebrospinal fluid mimic those of tuberculous meningitis with a lymphocytic pleocytosis, raised protein, reduced sugar and no growth within 48 hours. Spinal involvement may present with cord compression due to vertebral abscess, a cauda equina syndrome, myelitis and myelopathy; peripheral nerve involvement can cause sensory and/or motor abnormalities affecting either single or multiple nerve roots.

Rashes have been described, as has ocular infection. Brucellosis can cause abortion but this may be an effect of the febrile illness rather than a specific feature of this infection, as is seen for example in cattle with *B. abortus*.

Chronic brucellosis

Chronic infection is a feature that has long been associated with brucellosis, causing both protracted fever and recrudescent infection over many years with symptom-free periods intervening. Ten per cent of a series of cases from Kuwait had symptoms for more than 1 year. In individual cases it can be difficult to assess, requiring careful clinical assessment and serological testing with the use of more invasive procedures such as bone marrow examination and liver biopsy, as indicated clinically. The association between brucellosis and depression is one that is widely held, though the evidence for it is far from clear.

Laboratory investigations
Culture

Isolation and identification of the organism prove the diagnosis.[1] Blood is most often taken for culture and in standard media with blind subculture every 5 days it commonly takes 12 days, even with automated culture systems, before isolation and may take up to 6 weeks. Positive results are obtained in 14–50% of cases. Prior use of antibiotics interferes with growth of *Brucella*. Culture of bone marrow aspirate may give higher yields, for example a positive culture on 90% of samples from a series of cases of acute infection in Chile.[9] Pus or tissue obtained at biopsy should also be cultured in the investigation of febrile patients.

Serology

While a single high titre in agglutination tests in the

appropriate clinical setting may be diagnostic, serological testing alone may not be diagnostic and the result or a series of results obtained over a period must be considered in relation to the case under investigation.[10] Occasionally, entirely paradoxical results are obtained; for example, negative agglutination tests when the organism has been isolated in culture. While this apparently does occur, a more common explanation is the presence of blocking antibodies which bind but do not agglutinate. These account for the prozone phenomenon, which causes negative agglutination reactions at low dilutions of the test sera. As the blocking antibodies are present at low titre their effects are readily diluted out and testing at high dilution will give a positive agglutination. Smooth strains of brucellae should be used as antigen. Antigen detection in brucellosis is possible but gave results equal to good culture results.[11]

Agglutination reactions

These are carried out by incubating a standard suspension of brucellae with test sera and assessing the highest dilution at which agglutination can be seen. In general a titre of 1:160 or over is associated with infection, though it must be stated that a titre below this level does not exclude infection. The value of the method is extended by treating the test sera with 2-mercaptoethanol (2-me) before retesting as this destroys IgM.

If an initial high-titre positive test is reduced to a low-titre positive this suggests that IgM is the major antibody class producing the effect and that the infection is recent, while a titre that is not affected by 2-me is due to IgG antibody and the infection is more long standing. Predominantly 2-melabile responses suggest a low chance of relapse after treatment. IgG agglutinins disappear over a period of up to 30 months after treatment.

For many countries this method of measuring brucella antibody responses will remain the standard for some time to come because of the relative ease with which the test can be performed and the absence of specialized laboratory equipment needed to do it.

Antiglobulin test

This is a Coombs' test in which non-agglutinating antibody is detected by adding an antihuman globulin after thorough washing of the non-agglutinated antigen. It gives higher yields of positivity in chronic infections.

Enzyme-linked immunosorbent assays

These tests are in the process of being developed and offer the chance to use more specifically defined subcellular antigens.[12] Antibody classes may be more readily identified. Internationally agreed standardization of these procedures is awaited.

Polymerase chain reaction

This technique, which produces the multiplication of predetermined specific nucleotide sequences, offers great potential for the microbiological diagnosis of brucellosis because brucellae tend to be difficult to isolate by standard culture methods and the laboratory risks of handling this organism are considerable. The method has been applied successfully using a range of primers that allow genus-specific and species recognition. As yet they are not in routine use.[13]

Other investigations

Normochromic normocytic anaemia with a white count in the normal range showing more or less equal numbers of lymphocytes and granulocytes are usual findings in the peripheral blood. Liver function tests show elevation of the alkaline phosphatase associated with granulomatous inflammation in the liver. There may be some elevation of transaminases. Globulins increase and albumin levels decline—non-specific effects of inflammation.

Radiological changes accompany skeletal involvement. Abnormal technetium bone scans may indicate brucella-induced inflammation before there is radiographic evidence of damage to bones and joints. In the vertebrae there may be swelling of intervertebral discs, demonstrable on computed tomography or magnetic resonance imaging. Bone destruction is usually evident on plain radiographs, with destruction of anterior superior margins of vertebrae. With increasing duration of untreated infection osteophyte and later syndesmophyte formation will appear in addition to destruction. Soft tissue swelling may be visible around the affected area. Madkour and Sharif[14] have reviewed the radiological changes.

Management

There have been several prospective randomized studies of the treatment of brucellosis. Overall these have shown that probably the best results are obtained by the use of streptomycin 1 g intramuscularly daily for 14–21 days, together with doxycycline 200 mg daily for 6–12 weeks. Treatment should be prolonged for 12 weeks or more when there is evidence of joint, neurological or other localized organ involvement. The better results with streptomycin plus doxycycline in comparison with doxycycline with rifampicin,[15] which has the appeal of oral medication and the known activity of rifampicin against a range of intracellular bacteria, are not yet explained but there is the possibility that hepatic enzyme induction by rifampicin may reduce doxycycline levels in plamsa. Meta-analysis of published trials has borne out these better results. Endocarditis is a particular problem and long-term antibiotic treatment with three drugs including a cephalosporin usually has to be combined with valve replacement. Many authors recommend use of three drugs when there is neurological involvement. Surgical drainage of abscesses may be needed although the need for open exploration for diagnostic purposes is not so frequent where there are adequate imaging facilities to allow needle aspiration.

Children under the age of 8 years cannot be given tetracyclines; co-trimoxazole together with an aminoglycoside or rifampicin should be given in appropriate doses for the same periods.[16] Co-trimoxazole should not be given alone as it is associated with an unacceptably high relapse rate. In pregnancy, rifampicin should be given.

Alternatives to streptomycin have been tried because of their greater in vitro activity against brucellae. Gentamicin or netilmicin in single daily doses can be used. The fluorinated quinolones have not proved effective in brucellosis.

Relapse of brucellosis has always been a source of concern in the antibiotic era and genetic clues to the reasons for this were mentioned above. In any prolonged course of treatment lack of compliance may be a factor in apparent failure of a regimen. Solera studied factors that predicted the chance of relapse and found three that were valuable: temperature of 38.3°C or over in the presenting illness, positive blood culture and 10 days or more of symptoms before treatment.[17]

Prevention

For individuals in endemic areas the boiling of milk before drinking it or using it to make other products is protective. However, this commonly requires a change in behaviour which is not easy to bring about. When commercial dairy enterprises are set up they should ideally be stocked with brucella-free cattle and kept free of infection with regular serological testing. Pasteurization of milk by commercial dairies prevents infection. Brucella eradication schemes using the attenuated Rev-1 (*B. melitensis*) or S19 (*B. abortus*) vaccines to protect animals who show no seroreactivity to agglutination tests and, ideally, destruction of reactors, will ultimately lead to control and eradication of this zoonosis but continued surveillance is necessary to ensure that reinfection does not occur. Eradication has been successful in a number of European countries but the costs have been high due to surveillance and vaccine activities and the compensation payments. However, these costs have to be set against the economic benefits among human and animal populations resulting from eradication. As yet there is no vaccine that can be used in man.

REFERENCES

1   Corbel M J. Microbiological aspects. In Madkour M M (ed.) *Brucellosis*. Berlin: Springer, 2001: 51–64.

2   Microbiological test strip (API20NE) identifies *Brucella melitensis* as *Moraxella phenylpyruvica. Commun Dis Rep* 1991; 1:165.

3   Cooper C W. The epidemiology of human brucellosis in a well defined urban population in Saudi Arabia. *J Trop Med Hyg* 1991; 94:416–422.

4   Young E J, Borchert M, Kretzer F L et al. Phagocytosis and killing of *Brucella* by human polymorphonuclear leukocytes. *J Infect Dis* 1985; 151:682–690.

5   LeVier K, Phillips R W, Grippe V K, Roop II R M & Walker G C. Similar requirements of a plant symbiont and a mammalian pathogen for prolonged intracellular survival. *Science* 287:2492–2493.

6   Lulu A R, Araj G F, Khateeb M I et al. Human brucellosis in Kuwait: a prospective study of 400 cases. *Q J Med* 1986; 66:39–54.

7   Madkour M M, Rahman A, Talukder M A & Kudwah A. Brucellosis in Saudi Arabia. *Saudi Med J* 1985; 6:324–332.

8   Ariza J, Gudiol F, Valverde J et al. Brucella spondylitis: a detailed analysis based on current findings. *Rev Infect Dis* 1985; 7:656–664.

9   Gotuzzo E, Carrillo C, Guerra J & Llosa L. An evaluation of diagnostic methods for brucellosis: the value of bone marrow culture. *J Infect Dis* 1986; 153:122–125.

10 Young E J. Serologic diagnosis of human brucellosis: analysis of 214 cases by agglutination tests and review of the literature. *Rev Infect Dis* 1991; 13:359–372.

11 Araj G F & Kaufmann A F. Determination by enzyme linked immunosorbent assay of immunoglobulin G (IgG), IgM and IgA to *Brucella melitensis* with major outer membrane proteins and whole-cell heat-killed antigens. *J Clin Microbiol* 1989; 27:837–842.

12 Al Shamahy H & Wright S G. Enzyme linked immunosorbent assay for brucella antigen detection. *J Med Microbiol* 1998; 47:169–172.

13 Romero C, Gamazo C, Pard M & Lopez-Goni I. Specific detection of brucella DNA by PCR. *J Clin Microbiol* 1995; 33:616–617.

14 Madkour M M & Sharif H. Bone and joint imaging. In Madkour M M (ed.) *Brucellosis*. London: Butterworth, 1989: 90–104.

15 Solera J, Rodrguez Z M, Geijo P et al. Doxycycline–rifampicin versus doxycycline–streptomycin in treatment of human brucellosis due to Brucella melitensis. *Antimicrob Agents Chemother* 1995; 39:2061–2067.

16 Lubani M M, Dudin K I, Sharda D C et al. A multi-centre therapeutic study of 1100 children with brucellosis. *Pediatr Infect Dis J* 1987 8:75–78.

17 Solera J, Rodriguez-Zapata M, Geijo P et al. Multivariate model for predicting relapse in human brucellosis *J Infect* 1998 36:85–92.

Chapter 61A
Actinomycosis

G. Scott

Actinomycosis is characterized by indolent abscesses that cross fascial planes, forming chronic sinuses that discharge pus containing (in 40% of cases) 'sulphur granules'.[1] The causative organisms are mouth flora, so the jaw is a characteristic site for infection; other sites include the appendix, lung and uterus, but any organ may be infected.

Geographical distribution

Because the organisms are part of the normal buccal flora, the infection may occur in any part of the world.

Aetiology

The primary causative agents are Gram-positive anaerobic (or rarely facultatively aerobic), branching bacteria of the genera *Actinomyces* and *Arachnia*. These organisms used to be thought of as fungi because they branched and formed aerial mycelia. However, they are clearly bacteria, by being prokaryocytic, by the absence of typical fungal carbohydrates (e.g., chitin) in the cell wall and by their method of reproduction. The term is derived from *aktino* (Greek: ray), suggested by the spikes radiating from the edge of the sulphur granules. The first species described (*Actinomyces bovis*) from tumours of the jaws of cattle does not cause disease in humans. However, one or more of a number of species (*A. israelii* (the most important species named after the pioneering microbiologist Israel who first described sulphur granules from a human lesion in 1878), *A. naeslundii, A. meyeri, A. viscosus, A. odontolyticus* and *Arachnia propionica*[2]) may cause human disease. These bacteria are rarely found alone in clinical specimens but are intimately associated with Gram-negative bacteria such as *Actinobacillus actinomycetemcomitans* and *Haemophilus aphrophilus* (both well known for causing endocarditis). Separating and identifying these bacteria is difficult even in the specialized laboratory.

Clinical presentation

Head and neck actinomycosis is unlikely to be recognized specifically when it presents early. If associated with local invasion from the mouth, there will be soft, relatively non-tender, swellings which grow insidiously and then break down and discharge to the outside. Some report that the abscesses look blue. Because the infection can spread unhindered by fascial planes, the abscesses may discharge anywhere in the region of the head and neck, including the tongue, palate or even scalp. Direct extension of the abscess may lead to invasion of the central nervous system. Infection in the thyroid has been recorded. Occasionally an actinomycetoma will develop more rapidly than usual but it will still be 'cold'.

When the patient presents, it may well be possible to elicit a history of predisposing dental work or it may be quite obvious that the patient has very poor dentition with extensive caries. Sometimes the infection is precipitated by trauma, such as dental extraction or even an external blow. Human bites or trauma to the fist from front teeth in a fight may cause local inoculation and infection.

Infection in the lungs spreads locally through to pleura, chest wall or mediastinum, and presumably follows the inhalation of a foreign body colonized with mouth flora. The presentation is one of constitutional upset associated with some symptoms referable to the chest (even haemoptysis) with an abnormal radiographic finding. Rare fatal disease is usually associated with invasion of the myopericardium.

Dissemination

Bloodstream spread of the organism occurs most commonly from established chronic infections at any site. This may lead to miliary multifocal infection and skin lesions. Extensive spread has been documented in association with malignant disease.

Abdominal

One-quarter to one-half of all cases of actinomycosis involve an abdominal organ. There may be a precipitating event such as abdominal surgery, or internal (e.g., foreign body) or external trauma. The most usual antecedent surgery is for acute appendicitis and it is no surprise, therefore, that the most common site for infection is the ileocaecal region. The infection spreads gradually from the primary site, is very difficult to diagnose and may become obvious only when the infection points and discharges characteristic pus. Even then, a small discharging sinus may go unrecognized for years. Spread through the portal system leads to liver abscess, which may spread insidiously through chest wall or diaphragm.

Pelvic or endometrial actinomycosis is rare but some cases have been recognized in patients using intrauterine contraceptive devices. This is rather uncommon—beware the cytopathologist's report of the Papanicolaou stain of cervical smear suggesting that *Actinomyces* spp. are present.[3] This is not a sensitive or specific way of making the diagnosis. However, it is worth considering the diagnosis if patient with an intrauterine contraceptive device does develop indolent uterine or parauterine disease, which is often initially considered to be a malignant tumour.

Differential diagnosis

In extensive late disease, where sinuses are discharging pus with characteristic sulphur granules, the diagnosis should be obvious and can easily be confirmed in the laboratory. Sulphur granules may also be demonstrated in section by the histologist searching for presumed tumour: the organism will not be seen on haematoxylin and eosin staining but will require a silver or Gram stain (Figures 61A.1 and 61A.2). Several other organisms yield sulphur granules from pus but rarely are they as characteristically gritty, with the stellate radiations seen in *Actinomyces*. They include *Nocardia* spp. (which produce almost indistinguishable disease, more often in immunosuppressed patients, but which demands rather different antimicrobial therapy): the sulphur granules in nocardiasis are grey and smooth. *Staphylococcus aureus* may cause chronic abscesses which discharge rather soft, irregular, yellow granules—a condition known as botriomycosis. Various fungi (e.g., *Streptomyces* spp.) may cause granules, and it is not unusual for these to be discharged from *Madurella* mycetoma, without any hint of *Actinomyces* spp. on culture.

Pulmonary disease will most often be diagnosed initially as tuberculosis or tumour. *Nocardia* and fungi are more

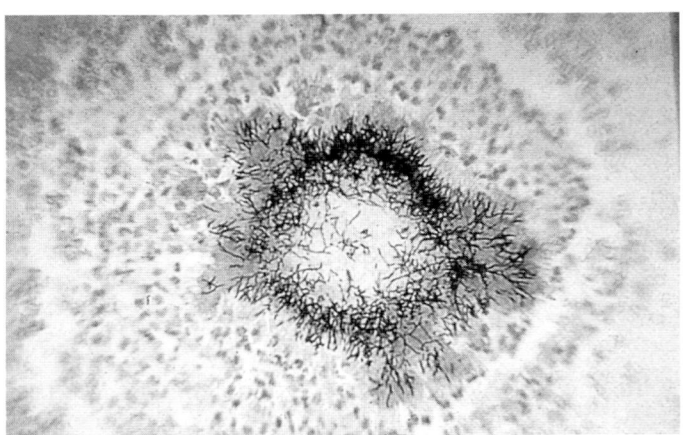

Figure 61A.2: Sulphur granule stained with Gram stain, revealing typical central Gram-positive branching bacteria.

important opportunistic pulmonary pathogens than *Actinomyces*, which most often affects otherwise healthy people. Abdominal disease may be misdiagnosed as appendix mass, Crohn's disease or ileocaecal tuberculosis.

Uterine disease, if not diagnosed early, may present with a massive tumour in a fixed pelvis, which will inevitably first be diagnosed as malignancy.

Diagnosis

The diagnosis is by macroscopic and microscopic examination of pus and granules and culture—preferably prolonged, in anaerobic conditions at 37°C. Whereas most strains have classical branching bacillary morphology, some appear as pleomorphic coccobacilli. Pus should be cultured in thioglycollate broth with added rabbit serum or brain–heart infusion broth or trypticase soy agar. Complex semisynthetic media may be more successful. Some species grow aerobically in carbon dioxide after a while, but this is not reliable. Under optimal conditions, a fine aerial mycelium is seen at day 1, then the colony grows into a solid white block which collapses centrally over a period of 7–14 days, known (most appropriately) as a 'molar tooth'.

Most microbiologists will not bother to speciate the strain, although this can be done by chemical tests provided the bacterium can be separated from the concomitant Gram-negative organisms. Another method is to use species-specific conjugated antibody either on the original specimen or the cultured organism.[4,5] *Arachnia propionica* forms smaller, smoother colonies than *A. israelii*, and they are not molar-tooth shaped; the organism produces propionic acid which can be detected by gas–liquid chromatography.

Management

Actinomyces spp. are sensitive to a wide variety of antimicrobials, including penicillin, which remains the

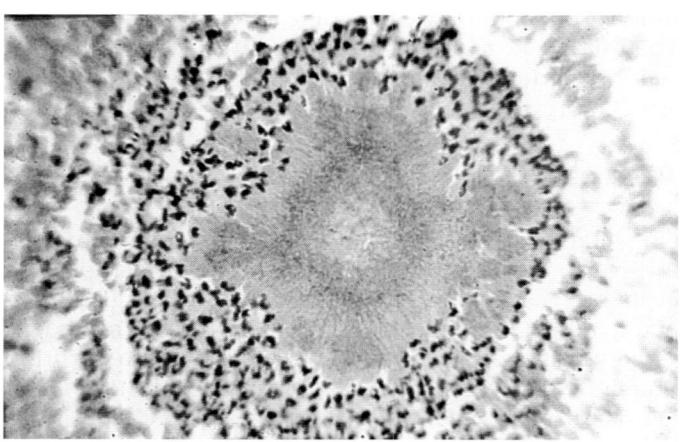

Figure 61A.1: Sulphur granule stained with haematoxylin and eosin.

drug of choice. Unfortunately, penicillin V is not well absorbed so is not suitable for initial therapy, and amoxicillin is more suitable. High and prolonged dosage is indicated together with appropriate surgical drainage and debridement. The level of amoxicillin can be enhanced by concomitant administration of probenecid. Virtually every other simple antibiotic can be used as an alternative—sulphonamide, erythromycin, chloramphenicol and tetracycline being effective. There is little correlation between in vitro sensitivity tests and clinical results. Drugs relatively ineffective in vitro are often very effective. However, metronidazole is inactive. Clindamycin seems a logical choice, being active in vitro, well absorbed and penetrating into tissues and bone well, and might be the drug of choice when bone is involved.

Prevention

Actinomycosis is rare. Disease associated with poor dentition can be prevented naturally by improving dental hygiene. The association with intrauterine contraceptive devices is sufficiently rare that it should not be considered a contraindication to this method of contraception.

REFERENCES

1 Weese W C & Smith J M. A study of 57 cases of actinomycosis over a 36 year period. *Arch Intern Med* 1975; 135:1562–1568.
2 Brock D W, Georg L K, Brown J M et al. Actinomycosis caused by *Arachnia propionica*. Report of 11 cases. *Am J Clin Pathol* 1973; 59:66–77.
3 Spence M R, Gupta P K, Frost J K & King T M. Cytologic detection and chemical significance of *Actinomyces israelii* in women using intrauterine contraceptive devices. *Am J Obstet Gynecol* 1978; 131:295–298.
4 Slack J M & Gerencser M A. Two new serological groups of *Actinomyces*. *J Bacteriol* 1970; 103:265–266.
5 Slack J M, Landfried S & Gerencser M A. Identification of *Actinomyces* and related bacteria in dental calculus by the fluorescent antibody technique. *J Dent Res* 1971; 50:78–82.

Chapter 61B
Bartonellosis, Cat-scratch Disease, Trench Fever, Human Erlichiosis, Whipple Disease

G. M. Scott and S. A. Wyllie

The genus *Bartonella*

Bartonella resemble *Rickettsia*: both are minute, pleomorphic, Gram-negative and, although found intracellularly in vivo, are able to grow on solid media.[1,2] Recent work has shown a link between *Bartonella bacilliformis* (the type species, the cause of Oroya fever and verruga peruana) and organisms variously thought to cause cat-scratch disease or bacillary angiomatosis (*Bartonella henselae*). *B. bacilliformis* is closely related to *Bartonella* (formerly *Rochilimaea*) *quintana*[3] by 16S DNA hybridization[2] and to *Brucella abortus*, but a probe to detect a conserved region of *B. bacilliformis* by polymerase chain reaction from clinical specimens failed to recognize *Brucella abortus*.[3] Bartonellae are sufficiently removed from the *Brucella* and *Rickettsia* to be considered a separate genus. When *Bartonella quintana* is transmitted by body louse (*Pediculus humanis corporis*) it causes trench fever; *B. quintana* and *B. henselae* transmitted by cat scratch or fleas cause cat-scratch disease in healthy subjects or bacillary angiomatosis, peliosis hepatis and disseminated infections in patients with acquired immune deficiency syndrome (AIDS).[4–6] As yet, the term bartonellosis is applied to infections caused by *B. bacilliformis*. Molecular techniques are appropriately being applied to differentiate species[7,8] and have shown that *B. henselae* has two distinct genotypes.[9] Other species whose importance is yet to be established in human disease include *B. elizabethiae* (from rats and causing diseases like trench fever),[10] *B.* (formerly *Rochilimaea*) *vinsonii* (from dogs and voles), *B. clarridgeiae*, *B. grahamii* (formerly *Grahamella,* a genus of bacteria infecting the red blood cells of birds and fish, although not of humans), found in an immunocompromised patient with retinitis,[11] and *B. koehlerae* from cats.[12] *Bartonella*-like infections associated with febrile anaemia or dermal nodules have been reported from Thailand, Sudan, Niger, Pakistan and the eastern USA but their relationship to *B. bacilliformis* is not clear. *Bartonella*-like (*Haemobartonella muris*) bodies are found in the blood of healthy mice and certain rodents; they cannot be cultured and exist as a latent infection. They are transmitted by rat lice and after splenectomy cause an acute fatal anaemia resembling Oroya fever. A similar anaemia occurs in the dog after splenectomy when infected with *B. canis*. It is likely that many species-specific members of the genus separable genotypically will be discovered in time.

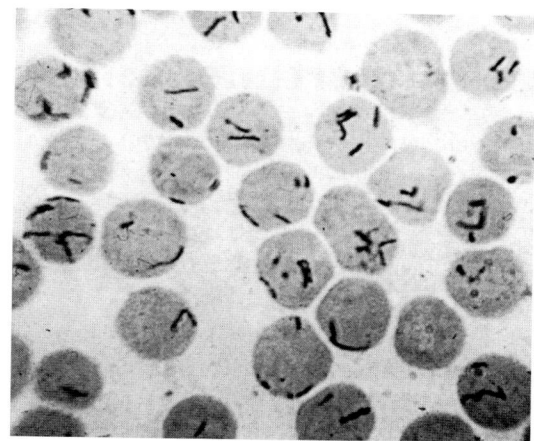

Figure 61B.1: Bartonella bacilliformis in blood.

B. bacilliformis, the cause of definitive bartonellosis, infects the red cells of humans. It occurs in two forms. One is a rod-shaped, slightly curved, Gram-negative bacillus, $2 \times 0.5\,\mu m$, staining well with Giemsa, often in branching rods and chains but never crossed, which occurs in a large proportion of the red cells (Figure 61B.1) during Oroya fever. V- and Y-shaped forms probably represent dividing organisms. The other form is coccoid, about $1\,\mu m$ or less in diameter, oval or pear shaped, and contains chromatin granules. They occur singly or end-to-end in pairs or chains.

Although aggressively motile, *B. bacilliformis* is difficult to detect in fresh blood. When dried films are 'shadowed' with palladium and examined by bright-field microscopy, it is found that the organisms lie in depressions in red cells; by electron microscopy polar flagellae, 20 nm in diameter, in bundles of up to 10 are visible. Other species do not tend to be associated with human red cells in the same way.

Cultural characteristics

Bartonella was first seen by Barton in 1909, then cultured on solid media from citrated blood of patients with Carrión's disease by Noguchi and Battistini in 1926. It is an obligate aerobe and grows best at 25–28°C on blood agar. Battistini's method of culture is simple: a small drop of blood from the finger of the patient is withdrawn into serum agar or Noguchi's *Leptospira* medium, the vial sealed and incubated at 28°C. Colonies are visible in 5–6 days. *B. bacilliformis* is also readily cultivated in the allantoic fluid of the developing chick embryo at 25–28°C. The growth is rapid and abundant, and the cultivated bodies are 0.6–1.6 μm in length. Zinsser's agar slant method for cultivation of rickettsiae may also be used.[13]

Various bartonellae can be isolated in conventional blood cultures. DNA amplification methods are much more sensitive than classical culture[14] and sensitivity of this can approach 90% when using serology plus histology as the gold standard for diagnosis.

Classical bartonellosis

Alternative names: Oroya fever, Guaitara fever, Carrión's disease, verruga peruana.

Introduction

Carrión, a medical student, infected himself with tissue from verruga peruana in 1885, a cutaneous eruption of haemangioma-like growths. He developed Oroya fever, an acute febrile haemolytic illness, and died, thus establishing the intimate link between these two disparate clinical conditions.[15]

Geographical distribution

Classical bartonellosis has a remarkable focal distribution, occurring between latitudes N05 and S16, between altitudes 800 and 3000 m on the western slopes of the Andes in Columbia, Peru and Ecuador.[16,17] Furthermore, the infection tends to cause outbreaks only in narrow valleys (quebradas) where the vector proliferates.

Experimental transmission: bartonellosis as a zoonosis?

Intravenous injection of *B. bacilliformis* into macaque monkeys causes irregular fever and anaemia, while the organisms can be demonstrated in the blood cells. The monkeys are often asymptomatic unless splenectomized, and then the blood from a patient with Oroya fever is fatal.[13] Intradermal inoculation into the supraorbital tissues gives rise to verrugous nodules. After inoculation of grey squirrels (*Citellus tridecemlineatus*) the organism could be recovered only for the first 24–48 hours, and the animals were asymptomatic. Verruga can be conveyed by inoculation to puppies and rabbits, and *B. vinsonii* occurs as a natural infection in native American Indian dogs. It is possible that human infection is a zoonotic disease depending on a natural animal reservoir, although in the case of Oroya fever this has not been established with certainty.

Human reservoir

It is likely that the main reservoir consists of asymptomatic human cases. *Bartonella* was cultured from seven of 81 students and three of these seven were asymptomatic. In the verruga zone, 10–15% of people have been shown to be chronic carriers with positive blood cultures.[13,18] *B. bacilliformis* can be seen in the endothelial cells of cutaneous verruga nodules, suggesting that they could act as a source of continuing infection to sandflies.

Sandfly transmission

The only proven vectors in humans are New World sandflies, *Lutzomyia* spp.: *L. verrucarum* is the definitive vector.[19] Evidence incriminating *L. noguchii* (and *L. verrucarum*) was obtained when insects were collected in a verruga district of Peru and sent to New York, where they were ground up in saline and injected intradermally into monkeys.[20] An outbreak of Oroya fever in the Mantaro valley of Peru occurred in the absence of *L. verrucarum*, but *L. pescei* (rare below 2400 m) and *L. bicornutus* (rare above 2600 m) were identified as being prevalent in the area of the epidemic. The former species was thought to be more likely to be responsible for the outbreak because the cases occurred at higher altitudes.[21] In the Narino department of south-western Colombia, the habits of *L. colombianus* are so like those of *L. verrucarum* that it may be a vector in this area. *L. noguchii* and *L. peruensis* are also suspected vectors.

The organisms adhere to the midgut of the sandfly in moderate numbers after feeding on infected patients and have been found occasionally on the proboscis of wild-caught sandflies, suggesting that transmission may be by mechanical inoculation during biting.

Pathology

Red blood cells

The organisms bind to multiple surface glycoproteins of erythrocyte membranes.[22] They invade erythrocytes, in which they multiply, causing destruction of the cells.[23] In severe cases, the blood count may drop in 3 or 4 weeks to 500 000/mm^3. There is an associated polymorphonuclear leucocytosis, but without eosinophilia. The anaemia is typically normocytic and hypochromic but may be macrocytic because of reticulocytosis or if there is associated dietary folate deficiency.[24] Destruction of the red cells is due to intravascular haemolysis; 50% of labelled erythrocytes have a half-life of 6 days (normal median survival 120 days). However, those red cells that survive this period have a normal survival rate. Normal erythrocytes injected into patients in the febrile anaemic phase behaved similarly, but red cells from a patient with verruga peruana survived normally, suggesting that the patient had acquired resistance to the haemolytic process after cessation of the febrile stage.

Reticuloendothelial system

The organism invade the cells of the reticuloendothelial system causing hyperplasia in the lymph glands, with proliferation of Kupffer cells of the liver and histiocytes in the spleen, bone marrow, kidneys, adrenals, pancreas, thyroid and testes. They also parasitize the endothelial lining cells of the blood and lymph vessels, which may be so distended by closely packed masses of the bacteria that infected cells can be detected on low-power microscopic examination of lymph glands, spleen, liver and intestine.[21] Marked changes are present in the liver, spleen and bone marrow. In the liver, areas of degenerative and central necrosis are found around the hepatic veins. In the centre of the necrotic areas, a yellow pigment resembling haemosiderin is present in abundance. The spleen is invariably enlarged and contains necrotic areas with pigment. The lymph glands contain large macrophage endothelial cells studded with bacteria. The bone marrow shows proliferation, necrosis and marked phagocytosis of the large endothelial cells. The malpighian bodies are not affected.

Verruga stage

The verrugous eruption is a sequela to the lesions in the reticuloendothelial system.[25] There is proliferation of the endothelium of the lymphatic channels which become obstructed by plasma cells and fibroblasts, but the structure is much more vascular than that of yaws, which it otherwise resembles. The capillary blood vessels become dilated so that the granulomatous tumours are vascular, almost cavernous, and apt to bleed profusely. Nodules of angioblasts around the blood vessels are characteristic of the disease. *B. bacilliformis* is seen in considerable numbers in the endothelial cells of cutaneous verruga nodules, but distension of the cells is less than that seen in cases of Oroya fever. Scanty bacteria may be found in blood corpuscles.

Immunity

Recovery from the disease in any of its forms confers lasting immunity but this is not solely dependent on the presence of specific agglutinins in the blood.[26] Passage from Oroya fever to the verruga stage, which is a change in the host–parasite relationship resulting from the development of immunity, is accompanied by a diminution of symptoms. It was shown that graduated inoculation of verrugous material induces an artificial immunity.[21] In monkeys infected with verruga tissue, splenectomy reverses the process and produces Oroya fever.

Serum antibodies that agglutinate the organism in titres from 10 to 80 have been found in patients in both the Oroya fever and verruga stages.[26,27] Cross-reactions occur with *Proteus* sp. OX19, OXK and OX2 (another tenuous link with rickettsiae). A strong agglutinating serum can be prepared for laboratory identification of *B. bacilliformis*.

Prophylactic inoculation with a formalinized suspension of *B. bacilliformis* resulted in partial immunity so that subsequent attacks of Oroya fever were modified.[26]

Clinical features[16]

Natural history

The spectrum of disease ranges from common asymptomatic carriage, to the severe and often fatal Oroya fever and on to verruga peruana.

Symptoms and signs
Oroya fever

The incubation period of Oroya fever is about 3 weeks.[16,28] Onset of the fever is insidious, and marked by malaise, soon followed by a rapidly developing anaemia and an irregular remittent pyrexia, associated with very severe pains in the head, joints and long bones. The bone pains are probably connected with disturbances in the haemopoietic system. The initial fever is like that of malaria, and the most severe illness resembles fulminant typhus and is known as the 'severe fever of Carrión'. The liver, spleen and lymph nodes are enlarged and tender.

A characteristic anaemia develops with a tendency to macrocytosis with nucleated red cells and a high reticulocytosis. In the febrile phase, most of the red cells contain numerous bacilliform organisms and there is a polymorphonuclear leucocytosis.

The death rate varies from 10 to 40%, death coming within 2–3 weeks of the onset of the disease. A terminal delirium is often noted. In cases that proceed to the verruga stage, the fever may have lasted for 3–4 months. Superinfection with *Salmonella typhimurium* may prove fatal.[29]

Verruga peruana stage (localized bartonellosis or eruptive stage)

The latent interval subsequent to the development of Oroya fever is 30–40 days. Although verruga is usually a sequel of Oroya fever, it may arise spontaneously as long as 2 months after exposure. The initial stages are characterized by rheumatic-like pains together with fever, the pains being like those of yaws only more severe. As in yaws, the constitutional symptoms subside on the appearance of the skin lesions. The eruption may be sparse or abundant, discrete or confluent. Some granulomas fail to erupt, others subside rapidly, and others may continue to increase and then, after remaining stationary for a time, gradually wither, shrink and drop off without leaving a scar.

Two types of eruption are seen. The miliary eruption (Figure 61B.2), not exceeding the size of a small pea, is found most abundantly on the face and extensor aspects of the extremities, less commonly on the trunk. A pink macule first appears, later darkening and becoming nodular. The verruga artificially produced in monkeys by injection of *Bartonella* bodies is bright cherry-pink. The nodules, which are flat or somewhat pedunculated, are vascular and may develop on mucous surfaces in the

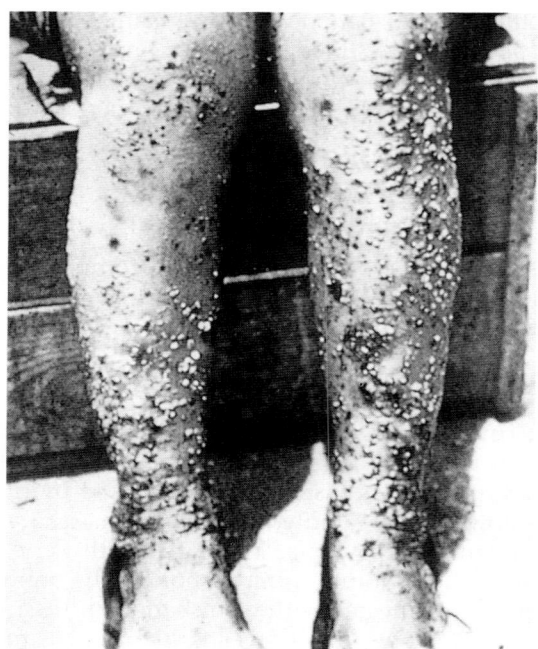

Figure 61B.2: Verruga-like eruption in bartonellosis. (Courtesy of P. D. Marsden.)

mouth, oesophagus, stomach, intestine, bladder, uterus and vagina; hence dysphagia is a common symptom, with occasional haematemesis, melaena, haematuria and bleeding from the vagina.

The Oroya and verruga stages frequently coexist and relapses of both the fever and the eruption may occur.

The nodular eruption (Figure 61B.3) is rarer but more chronic than the miliary form. Individual lesions can grow to the size of a pigeon's egg and may become strangulated and a source of danger as a result of haemorrhage. This type does not invade the mucous membranes and is usually confined to the regions of the knees and elbows. It appears in crops and lasts 2–3 months. The mortality rate from verruga is practically nil.

Neurobartonellosis

Bartonella may invade the brain in large numbers in parasitized red cells.[30] The pathological changes are found in the ependyma and choroid plexus, the vessels of the meninges and in the neurones. Vascular changes include venous thrombosis, adventitious haemorrhage and characteristic glioepithelial verrucomas.

Clinically, nervous system involvement occurs during the haemolytic phase; the cerebral form presents as meningoencephalitis with or without convulsions and has a high mortality rate. The spinal form, which is less common, presents as spastic or flaccid paralysis which may leave permanent disability, and the neuronal forms appear during the verruga stage arising from granulomas in the spinal or cranial nerves; these resolve with little or no disability. The cerebrospinal fluid shows a raised protein concentration, with a pleocytosis and numerous intracellular *Bartonella*. Treatment is that of the systemic disease.

Diagnosis

B. bacilliformis can be seen in the red cells on blood examination in the acute febrile stage(s) and in smears from verruga. The organisms can be cultured from the blood on appropriate special media. Serology is of no practical use except perhaps in travellers who pass transiently through an endemic area.[27]

Management

Chloramphenicol (4.0 g daily in divided doses) is the antibiotic of choice. The fever subsides in 48 hours and there is a rapid return of the blood to normal.[31] Other effective antibiotics include tetracycline, streptomycin and co-trimoxazole.

Complications

Salmonellosis is the most frequent complication, occurring in 40–50% of cases of Oroya fever. *Salmonella* infection is shown by a worsening of the patient's condition and a recurrence of fever with gastrointestinal symptoms.

Other complications are thromboses, pleurisy, parotitis and meningoencephalitis; transitory arthralgia may precede the eruption.

Differential diagnosis

The Oroya fever stage must be distinguished from other acute fevers such as malaria, typhus, typhoid and acute haemolytic anaemia. The verruga stage may resemble yaws, secondary syphilis or Kaposi's sarcoma. A single lesion may resemble a fibrosarcoma or angioma.

Epidemiology

History

It is probable that this disease existed in certain Andean

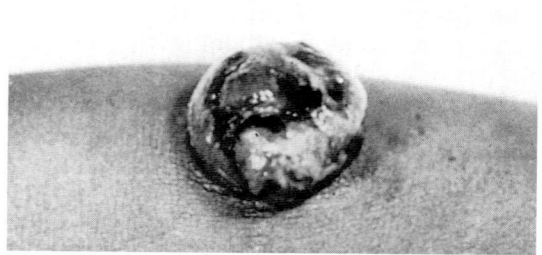

Figure 61B.3: Giant nodule on the arm caused by bartonellosis. (Courtesy of P. D. Marsden.)

valleys in north-west South America in pre-Columbian days. Many thousands died during the reign of the Inca Huayna Capac and it is possible that Pizarro's men also suffered from it. The earliest account was that of Gago de Vadilla in 1630. In the 1870s, when the central railway was being constructed from Lima to Oroya in Peru, a severe epidemic broke out among the construction workers, resulting in 7000 deaths. In 1906, of 2000 men employed on tunnel work, 200 perished. In 1885, the eponymous Carrión inoculated himself with blood from a verruga nodule and died from Oroya fever, from which experiment Peruvian physicians deduced that verruga and Oroya fever were different stages of the same disease.[15]

Present status

A considerable outbreak occurred in the Guaitara valley in southern Colombia near the Ecuador boundary in 1936, mainly in the valleys of the Mayo, Sambingo, Pacual and Juanambu tributaries of the Rio Patia. An outbreak with 200 deaths occurred in 1959 between January and April in the city of Anco which lies 2400 m above sea level in the valley of the Mantaro River in the Peruvian Andes.[20] Another outbreak with 28 symptomatic individuals (14 deaths) occurred between February and October 1987 in Shuapillar, also in Peru.[32] It is thought that Oroya fever has again become a serious problem in Peru following the cessation of spraying which was part of the malaria eradication programme. In a recent outbreak in Peru 123 (14% of the exposed population) developed Oroya fever; 18% developed verruga peruana. More than half of the seropositive patients had been asymptomatic.[33] Some 22 patients in the Urumba region of Peru were involved in an outbreak in 1998.[10]

The range of the infection is singularly limited and is confined to certain narrow valleys and ravines, the inhabitants of neighbouring places being exempt. The disease is acquired only at night and a single night's residence in an endemic area may be sufficient. During the outbreak in the 1870s on the central railway in Peru, infection could be avoided by leaving the endemic area before nightfall. The disease is most prevalent from January to April when streams are in flood, the air hot, still and moist, malaria epidemic and insect life abundant.

Control

Control of the vector sandflies is easily obtained with DDT, and sandflies have been eradicated from human habitations.[34]

Cat-scratch disease and disseminated disease
Introduction

Classically, this is a mild self-limiting zoonosis characterized by unilateral lymphadenitis in nodes draining the sites of minor trauma from cat bites or scratches or flea (*Ctenocephalides*) bites or, more rarely, disseminated infection. Patients with AIDS or alcoholism develop larger skin lesions at the primary site of inoculation and disseminated cutaneous and systemic disease.

Aetiology

Cat-scratch fever is caused by *Bartonella henselae*,[9] sometimes by *B. quintana*[35] and, much more rarely, by *Afipia felis*,[36,37] which is probably an environmental saprophyte living like *Legionella* with amoebae,[38] and *B. vinsonii* subsp. *berkhoffii* and possibly related species such as *B. clarridgeiae*.[39] The likely definitive host is the cat or, more rarely, the dog.[40] Serodiagnosis suggests that exposure to the agent(s) is much more common than classical overt disease and there are protean manifestations.

Epidemiology

From small studies from around the world, the organisms involved are probably holoendemic, although molecular epidemiology of the genus *Bartonella* is in its infancy. Because *B. henselae* was recognized only recently as a cause of non-specific febrile illness other than classical cat-scratch fever, epidemiological studies are sparse and cross-reacting antibodies may confound which species have been involved in past infection.[41] Some 15% of cats in Germany have antibodies to *Bartonella* spp., but none to *A. felis*.[42] It is likely also that the latter organism is a very rare cause of human disease. Antibodies are more common in feral cats. Seroprevalence studies show that colonization by related agents may be very common in ruminants in some areas[43] and in ticks.[44] Most classical human infections arise by scratches and bites of domestic cats and their fleas, and, less commonly, dogs. *B. vinsonii* subsp.*berkhoffii* is isolated from domestic and wild dogs,[45] and probably causes some human disease.[46] Dogs develop myocarditis and endocarditis with this agent.

Clinical presentation

Classical cat-scratch disease involves prominent enlargement of lymph nodes draining an area that has been bitten or scratched. There is often a small papule after 3–10 days at the site of the scratch or flea bite. However, the rash may occasionally become much more extensive. Enlargement of the nodes draining the site of the bite may be delayed for a few weeks. A third of patients have low-grade fever and malaise. The lymph nodes resolve spontaneously over several months.

In patients with AIDS and those immunosuppressed by alcohol, cancer or chemotherapy, both *B. henselae* and *B. quintana* (and probably other zoonotic species) cause bacillary angiomatosis and peliosis.[4,5,47,48] Bacillary angiomatosis presents as multiple red skin papules or nodules with minor symptoms of fever, headache, anorexia and weight loss. Dissemination may affect respiratory and gastrointestinal mucosae, the heart, bone marrow, liver, spleen and bone. Fever, nausea, vomiting, diarrhoea and abdominal distension are features of peliosis hepatis. The treatment of choice is erythromycin.

Interest in the cutaneous and diffuse systemic disease induced by *B. henselae* in patients with AIDS has allowed the recognition of similar syndromes in immunocompetent individuals, especially children.[49] In those with AIDS, the systemic symptoms are more pronounced, the local lesion develops into bacillary angiomatosis with focal cutaneous lesions and involvement of any internal organs (e.g., peliosis hepatis). Disseminated skin lesions are seen, some nodular and angiomatous, some erythematous papules, or a mixture of these.

Disseminated infection with *B. henselae* may occur in immunocompetent people. The patient may present simply with persistent pyrexia of unknown origin[50] or erythema nodosum. Other forms, particularly in healthy children, include infectious mononucleosis-like syndrome in a third of cases,[51] with a paradoxically raised neutrophil count and hepatosplenomegaly, seronegative for Epstein–Barr virus, toxoplasmosis and cytomegalovirus.

Ocular and neurological involvement may occur. Patients may present with conjunctivitis, oculoglandular syndrome[52] (like that caused by *M. avium* in children) or disciform keratitis,[53] neuroretinitis with facial palsy,[54,55] and optic neuritis.[56] An encephalitis, demyelination or transverse myelitis may precede or occur without lymph node involvement.[57,58]

Rarely recognized presentations of disseminated bartonellosis include 'gastroenteritis'[59] or mesenteric adenitis with acute ileitis.[60] Spread to the liver and spleen via the portal system leads to hepatosplenic syndrome,[61] granulomatous hepatitis[62] and splenic abscess.[63,64] Infections may simulate pyogenic conditions such as osteomyelitis,[65,66] parotitis,[67] breast mass[68] or even bacillary angiomatosis on an area of burned skin.[69]

Differential diagnosis

Local lymphadenitis is usually considered at first to be due to tuberculosis, and the nodular skin lesions in patients with AIDS are usually confused with Kaposi's sarcoma. A history of animal contact is valuable. The differential diagnosis of fever with disseminated lymphadenopathy is so wide that serology must simply be borne in mind. Granuloma formation may occasionally lead to hypercalcaemia, as in sarcoid. Biopsy of persistently enlarged nodes and masses involving other organs is therefore essential to differentiate these diseases, and the histological findings are likely to be a surprise. It is wise to keep some biopsy material fresh and unfixed, preferably frozen, so that appropriate cultures and DNA studies can be set up once histological examination is completed.

Beyond classical cat-scratch disease, the manifestations of infection with *B. henselae* are so diverse and the differ-ential disease is so wide that patients are often thought to have serious disease, including malignancy[70] or tuberculosis, and the diagnosis is usually delayed.

Diagnosis

Diagnosis may be made serologically[71] and the histopathological changes are characteristic although not pathognomonic. Serological kits are available.[72] Culture in the conditions suggested above for bartonellosis may be positive but caution has to taken if reliance is placed on binding to polyclonal antiserum which may react with *Chlamydia* spp.[73] Differentiation of *B. henselae* from *B. quintana* may be made with specific monoclonal antibodies[9,74,75] with polymerase chain reaction- restriction fragment length polymorphism (PCR-RFLP) and then using appropriate restriction endonucleases.[76] DNA amplification methods are likely to be the method of diagnosis of choice in the future.[77,78] A skin test preparation has been described but is not properly validated and not available commercially.

Pathology

B. henselae does not bind to human red cells like *B. bacilliformis*, but intraerythrocyte growth in cat red cells occurs. Both *B. henselae* and *B. quintana* grow in human epithelial cells and stimulate the proliferation of endothelial cells.[79] Cat-scratch disease is characterized by a necrotizing and coalescent granulomatous reaction to the infection.[63] This differs from other granulomas in having some neutrophil infiltration and clumps of bacteria. Bacillary angiomatosis is a proliferation of new vessels lined with cuboidal epithelium and a neutrophil infiltrate (Figure 61B.4). Microcolonies of bacteria can be seen by Giemsa or silver stain, or on electron microscopy. Bacillary peliosis is characterized by blood-filled lacunae up to several millimetres in size, lined with discontinuous endothelial cells lying in a stroma loaded with clumps of

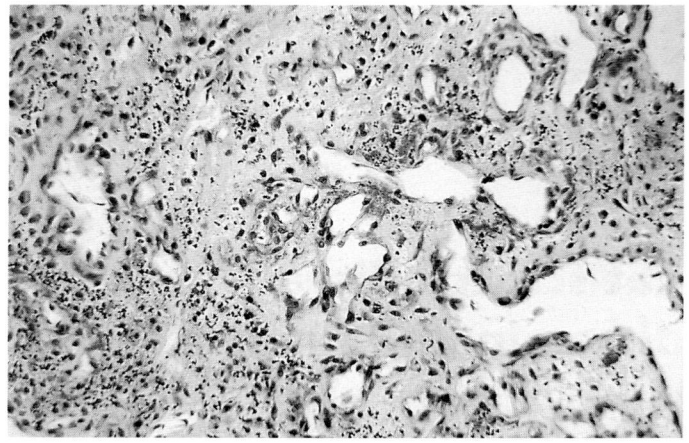

Figure 61B.4: Histological appearance of cutaneous angiomatosis (haematoxylin and eosin stain). (Courtesy of S. Lucas.)

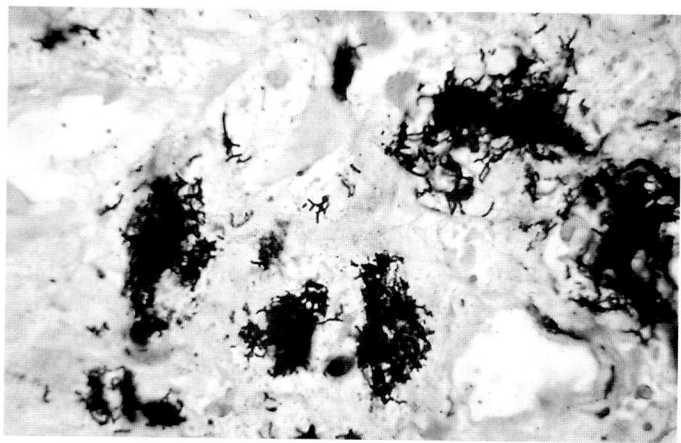

Figure 61B.5: Peliosis hepatitis (silver stain). (Courtesy of S. Lucas.)

bacteria (Figure 61B.5), with inflammatory cells and capillaries. Although generally recognized in the liver, they may be seen in other organs of infected patients with AIDS. The organism will grow on special media, provided enough time is allowed, which probably accounts for low yields from routine methods.

Management

Bartonellae are sensitive to many antimicrobials in vitro, including penicillins and cephalosporins, co-trimoxazole, tetracyclines, rifampicin and fluoroquinolones. Spontaneous resolution is the norm but one placebo-controlled trial with azithromycin showed more rapid resolution of large lymph nodes.[80]

Trench fever

'...*my servant and one other, are the only non-verminous bodies in the platoon; not to say licentious*' (**Wilfred Owen, letters, 1917**)

Introduction

Louse-borne bartonellosis is caused predominantly by *B. quintana*. This disease was described in the First World War. Chronic carriage is possible and some patients develop endocarditis.

History

The term trench fever was coined by Hunt and Rankin,[81] who described 30 cases. In 1916, His and Werner described the disease in German troops on the Eastern front, calling it Wolhnyian fever, and McNee et al.[82] wrote a detailed description from the Western Front. Gratzer, an experienced army physician, said it had been endemic in Eastern Front troops since 1914. It was the cause of 20–30% of troop wastage on both sides in the Great War.[83] The disease is found in patients infested with body lice, although not head lice, even though the latter have been shown to support the organism. The aetiology was established by experimental transmission of the aetiological agent (now named *B. quintana*).[84]

Clinical presentation

In experimental trench fever, the incubation period is usually 7–9 days but it may be much longer, depending on the inoculum—whether whole blood, the red cell fraction or extracts of infected lice or louse faeces. Although biting by lice may cause disease, this is less efficient than rubbing louse faeces into scarified skin. Classically the patient develops sudden-onset general influenza-like illness with a high fever (> 39°C), retro-orbital headache and lower limb pain. Severe and persistent anterior tibial pain is a classical, although unexplained, feature. Hyperaesthesia of thoracic and lumbar dermatomes and an analogy to tabes dorsalis, with a lack of periosteal or muscle inflammation, suggest that the pain is neurological in origin. Patients often have a transient erythematous rash. Splenomegaly is not unusual. The fever lasts a matter of 2–8 days, resolves suddenly with all symptoms, but classically relapses after a few more days. The height of the fever in the relapse may be the same as that in the presenting phase but is often less marked and may become chronic. Some patients have a prolonged relapsing–remitting fever and convalescence may be prolonged. Patients returned to base hospitals from the front were unfit for duty for an average of 60–70 days, and some 10% of these became semi-permanent invalids. Blood remains infectious to volunteers and positive on culture for many weeks. However, the disease is rarely fatal.

Many carriers are asymptomatic. Alcoholics with bacteraemia are likely to have headaches, severe leg pain, pruritic lesions and reduced platelet counts.[85] *B. quintana* may cause retinal artery occlusion and peripapillary angiomata with severe loss of vision.[86]

Endocarditis

B. quintana is now recognized as an important cause of 'culture negative' endocarditis.[87–90] Duke criteria may not be fulfilled.[91] Serological studies and special attention to the blood cultures are essential when preliminary investigations prove negative. A history of urban homelessness and likely exposure to lice is very important.[87]

Differential diagnosis

When the disease was first recognized, it was quite clear to experienced physicians that this was something different from rheumatic fever (which was surprisingly rare in the troops), enteric and typhus fevers, and influenza.

Most cases were initially called suspected typhoid fever, a diagnosis not confirmed on blood culture. The characteristics of the remitting fever with severe limb pain were quite unlike typhoid. Patients with typhus were severely ill with a high mortality rate, and tended to have a purpuric rash.

Management

There is a dirth of information about antimicrobial treatment and its effects. The organism is sensitive to many antibiotics in vitro. Patients who have endocarditis should probably be treated by valve replacement.[90]

Diagnosis

The diagnosis may be made serologically, by culture and histologically with specific PCR on infected tissues such as heart valve. Blood culture is slow. The organism can be seen by acridine orange staining of cultured blood, and the DNA can be amplified from a positive culture.[92]

Transmission

There is no known animal reservoir. Early attempts to infect common laboratory animals failed, although there were some reports of severe infections in cats and mice. The organism may pass transovarially in the louse, although this was not apparent in early clinical experiments.[93]

Epidemiology

The worldwide risk of being infested by body lice is increasing as a result of a decrease in living standards, continuing conflicts and major refugee problems globally. Examination of lice themselves from different parts of the world can be used to estimate the risk of acquisition of *B. quintana*, *R. prowazeki* and *Borrelia recurrentis* in different countries.[94,95] In the West, trench fever is an urban disease of alcoholic street dwellers and other socially deprived people. Control is achieved by delousing.

Human erlichiosis

Animal ehrlichiosis has been recognized in veterinary medicine for almost a century. *Ehrlichia sennetsu* was the first ehrlichial pathogen to be identified in humans in the early 1950s.[96] It caused an infectious mononucleosis-like disease characterized by fever, lymphadenopathy, asthenia, anorexia and mononucleosis in Western Japan. In 1986, a new type of human ehrlichial disease caused by *E. chaffeensis* was recognized in Arkansas, USA.[97] Since then, *E. phagocytophilia* and *E ewingii* have been described.[98,99] *E. phagocytophilia* is homologous to *E. equi*.[100] *Ehrlichia* are small obligate intracellular bacteria that predominantly infect white cells. They are transmitted by ticks from animal reservoirs. Infection is characterized by transient pleomorphic rash and systemic involvement.[101] There is a low but significant mortality rate.

Aetiology

Erlichia chaffeensis infects cells of the monocyte/macrophage and *E. (formerly Anaplasma) equi/E. phagocytophilia* and *E. ewingii* infect cells of granulocytic lineage. The diseases are named human monocytic (HME) and granulocytic (HE) erlichiosis, respectively. The organisms are clearly seen in inclusions in the white cells. Gene sequences resemble those in bartonellae, but are distinct from rickettsiae to which they are closely related. The organisms can be passaged in tissue culture but have not yet been cultivated on conventional media.

Geographical distribution and epidemiology

The diseases are recognized in areas where there are high concentrations of deer, such as north-east and mid-west USA and California,[101] and northern and eastern Europe.[102,103] Most tick bites are acquired close to home and there are reports of suburban erlichiosis,[104] which reflect the recent increase in deer populations and their encroachment into towns. The risk is greater when families have a domestic dog. Rates of infection in endemic areas are around 50–60 per 100 000 per annum, and peaks of disease coincide with peaks of tick activity (early summer and early autumn). Males are affected three or four times more commonly than females. Various species of deer and small mammals act as a reservoir for erlichiosis and there is likely to be an enzootic cycle.[105] Antibodies to *Erhlichia* spp. in animals are found to be widespread in Africa and Eurasia but do not differentiate species.

Natural transmission

Various species of *Ixodes* ticks are involved (e.g., *I. Ricinus*, *I. spinipalpis*). and *E. ewingii* is transmitted by *Amblyoma americanum* in the USA. The organism is passed trans-stadially but not transovarially. Ticks are often co-infected with *Erlichia* spp. and *Borrelia burgdorferi*.[106]

Pathology

The organisms reside in intracytoplasmic inclusions and resist phagolysosome fusion.[107] Control of the intracellular infection depends on cytokines such as interferon-γ produced by lymphocytes which are activated either directly or by chemokines secreted by infected neutrophils.[108]

Clinical presentation

About 1 week after the exposure, patients develop a sudden high fever with a transient rash (10%) with systemic symptoms such as fever, nausea, vomiting and central nervous system involvement (rarely with a cerebrospinal fluid pleocytosis). Some 80% of patients give a history of tick bite. The rash may be erythematous, maculopapular or even vesicular, and usually, although not always, spares the palms and soles. There may be some confusion because of co-infection with *Borrelia burgdorferi*.[109] The clues to the diagnosis of erlichiosis will be unexpected thrombocytopenia with leucopenia in either or both the mononuclear and polymorphonuclear series. Inclusions may be seen in neutrophils or mononuclear cells depending on the infecting species. Most illnesses are short lived and resolve rapidly without treatment. In some series, around 15% of patients with overt infection have severe manifestations such as septic shock, adult respiratory distress, various demyelinating neuropathies, or myolysis of striated or cardiac muscle. Older patients with diabetes are more prone to severe disease. The mortality rate is around 3–5% in those who are recognized as having erlichiosis, and probably slightly higher with the monocytic than with the granulocytic forms. Monocytic erlichiosis has been described as causing overwhelming infection in the immunosuppressed, particularly in patients with AIDS, but also in transplant recipients and those treated for cancer.[110]

Diagnosis

The diagnosis is usually made serologically, but about half of patients have antibodies to both agents and it may be impossible to differentiate an individual cause. Occasionally, antibodies cross-react with *Coxiella* and *Rickettsia*.[111] DNA amplification methods are performed in specialist centres.[112]

Differential diagnosis

If a history of tick bite is obtained, the infection may be confused with Rocky Mountain spotted fever, especially if there is a rash. However, the rash is predominantly macular and not petechial, and the changes in haematological indices are characteristic. Patients may be co-infected with *Borrelia burgdorferi*, leading to considerable diagnostic confusion.

Management

The treatment of choice is doxycycline, which should be given empirically before the diagnosis is confirmed. Chloramphenicol is the reserve choice but the quinolones and co-trimoxazole are ineffective. Rifampicin has been used successfully in pregnancy.

Whipple disease

Whipple disease is a systemic bacterial infection classically causing 'intestinal lipodystrophy', as first described by George Hoyt Whipple in 1907.[113] Clinical presentation is characteristically dominated by weight loss, diarrhoea and malabsorption.[114] Musculoskeletal, neurological, cardiac, pulmonary and dermatological manifestations also occur and may precede digestive symptoms, thereby leading to diagnostic delay.[115] A diagnosis of Whipple disease was traditionally made on the basis of a characteristic history and histological examination of a small bowel biopsy. More recently, the polymerase chain reaction (PCR) has become an important diagnostic method.[116] The causative bacterium has been named as *Tropheryma whippelii* (*trophe* for 'nourishment' and *eryma* for 'barrier').[117] The first successful culture of *T. whippelii* has stimulated renewed interest in Whipple disease.[118]

Epidemiology

Whipple disease is rare. It predominantly affects white male Caucasians and presents clinically around the end of the fourth decade.[115,119] There are only a few case reports of Whipple disease in children.

Aetiology

Whipple originally described rod-shaped structures on silver staining of an intestinal biopsy.[117] A bacterial aetiology, however, was not formally suggested until 1961 when 'bacillary' or 'bacilliform' bodies were demonstrated by electron microscopic examination of intestinal biopsies from patients with clinical Whipple disease.[120,121] Electron microscopic studies have shown the *T. whippelii* to be 1–2 μm in length and to have a trilaminar appearance. The bacterium is seen intracellularly within a wide variety of cells, as well as extracellularly. Amplification and sequencing of bacterial 16S ribosomal RNA retrieved from intestinal lesions has phylogenetically classified the bacterium within the Actinomycetes.[122]

T. whippelii was first isolated in human macrophages inactivated by interleukin 4 from two patients with culture-negative endocarditis.[123] This isolate has not been successfully subcultured. In 2000, Raoult and collegues reported the successful isolation and subsequent establishment of a strain of *T. whippelii* from the mitral valve of a 42-year-old Canadian man with culture-negative endocarditis.[118] *T. whippelii* has since been isolated from the duodenum of a patient with relapsed Whipple disease.[124] To date, molecular studies have revealed six genotypes (numbered 1–6) of *T. whippelii* based on sequence variation within the inter 16S–23S ribosomal DNA spacer (ITS)[125,126] and two genotypes (named A and B) based on sequence variation within the 23S ribosomal RNA gene.[127] It is remains to be determined whether these genetically different types of *T. whippelii* cause the various systemic pathologies seen in clinical Whipple's disease.

Pathogenesis

A predisposition in males, association with HLA-B27,[128] and persistence of the organism in affected tissues despite prolonged antibiotic therapy, suggest that an immunological host factor plays a role in pathogenesis. Studies of patients with Whipple disease have demonstrated altered T-cell populations and altered T-cell function.[129,130] B cells, immunoglobulin levels and macrophages may also be abnormal.[131,132] A recent study reported successful treatment of refractory Whipple disease using a combination of antimicrobials and recombinant interferon γ.[133] This report provides supportive evidence for the pathogenic relevance of impaired cellular immunity. It is not yet known whether these immunological defects are primary, thereby predisposing the individual to Whipple disease, or secondary, due to infection with *T. whippelii*.

T. whippelii is believed to be an environmental organism[134] and presumably invades via the gastrointestinal system. Genetic material from the bacterium has been demonstrated in the saliva, gastric juice, and duodenal biopsies and monocytes,[135] and in synovial tissue of individuals with and without clinical or histological evidence of Whipple disease.[136,137] These findings are disputed.[138] The conflicting data highlight the problems inherent in using genetic amplification as a diagnostic method, especially if the organism occurs naturally in the environment.

Clinical presentation

The clinical manifestations of Whipple disease are multiple and non-specific. The classical triad of weight loss, diarrhoea and malabsorption may or may not be present. Patients are often non-specifically unwell with low-grade fever and lymphadenopathy. Laboratory investigations usually reveal malabsorption with a raised erythrocyte sedimentation rate.[114,115] Apart from the classical changes in the bowel, patients may have seronegative arthralgia and uveitis. Synovium may be positive for *T. whippelii*.[139,140] The cardiovascular and central nervous systems may be involved. Heart valves and coronary arteries may be involved, and rarely a patient may have myocarditis.[141] Whipple disease is a rare cause of non-specific global encephalopathy[142] and may be diagnosed by brain biopsy or PCR on cerebrospinal fluid.

Diagnosis

Classical disease is diagnosed by histopathological examination of intestinal biopsies, which reveal heavy deposits of periodic acid–Schiff (PAS)-positive material. Sampling error may lead to failure to identify abnormalities, although tissues are still positive by molecular methods.[143] Histopathologists should perform PAS staining for the bacteria when confronted by non-specific granulomatous inflammation. Bacteria similar to those seen in the intestine can be found in the coronary arteries of patients who have died with classical Whipple disease.[144] Clumps of bacteria, some intracellular, have been associated with the arterial media and atheroma, sometimes, although not always, with evidence of local inflammation. Changes such as sarcoidosis have been seen in affected lymph nodes positive for *T. whippelii* 16S RNA.[145] Serodiagnosis is not applicable. Molecular diagnosis of tissues in reference centres is likely to be the diagnosis of choice.

Management

The treatment of choice is at present—based on empirical tests—co-trimoxazole, which should be continued for at least 1 year. However, breakthrough infections have been described.[146]

REFERENCES

1. Peters D & Weigand R. Bartonellaceae. *Bacteriol Rev* 1955; 19:150–159.
2. Brenner D J, O'Connor S P, Hollis D G, Weaver R E & Steigerwalt A G. Molecular characterization and proposal of a neotype strain for *Bartonella bacilliformis*. *J Clin Microbiol* 1991; 29:1299–1302.
3. Brenner D J, O'Connor S P, Winkler H H & Steigerwalt A G. Proposals to unify the genera *Bartonella* and *Rochalimaea*. *Int J Syst Bacteriol* 1993; 43:777–786.
4. Koehler J E, Sanchez M A, Garrido C S et al. Molecular epidemiology of *Bartonella* infections in patients with bacillary angiomatosis-peliosis. *N Engl J Med* 1997; 337:1876–1883.
5. Adal K A, Cockerell C J & Petri W A Jr. Cat scratch disease, bacillary angiomatosis and other infections due to Rochalimaea. *N Engl J Med* 1994; 330:1509–1515.
6. Cockerell C J. *Rochalimaea* infections. *Curr Opin Infect Dis* 1995; 8:130–136.
7. Jensen W A, Fall M Z, Rooney J, Kordick D L & Breitschwerdt E B. Rapid identification and differentiation of *Bartonella* species using a single-step PCR assay. *J Clin Microbiol* 2000; 38:1717–1722.
8. Handley S A & Regnery R L. Differentiation of pathogenic *Bartonella* species by infrequent restriction site PCR. *J Clin Microbiol* 2000; 38:3010–3015.
9. Sander A, Posselt M, Bohm N, Ruess M & Altwegg M. Detection of *Bartonella henselae* by two different PCR assays and determination of the genotypes of strains involved in histologically defined cat scratch disease. *J Clin Microbiol* 1999; 37:993–997.
10. Ellis B A, Regnery R L, Beati L et al. Rats of the genus *Rattus* are reservoir hosts for the pathogenic *Bartonella* species: an Old World origin for a New World disease. *J Infect Dis* 1999; 180:220–224.
11. Kerkhoff F T, Ossewaarde J M, de Loos W S & Rothova A. Presumed ocular bartonellosis. *Br J Ophthalmol* 1999; 83:270–275.
12. Droz S, Chi B, Horn E, Steigerwalt A G, Whitney A M & Brenner D J. *Bartonella koehlerae* sp. nov. isolated from cats. *J Clin Microbiol* 1999; 37:1117–1122.

13 Weinman D J & Pinkerton H. Carrión's disease. Experimental production in animals. Natural sources of *Bartonella* in the endemic zone. Studies on *Phlebotomus* as the possible vector. *Proc Soc Exp Biol Med* 1938; 37:594–600.

14 La Scola B & Raoult D. Culture of *Bartonella quintana* and *Bartonella henselae* from human samples: a 5-year experience (1993–1998). *J Clin Microbiol* 1999; 37:1899–1905.

15 Schultz M G. Daniel Carrión's experiment. *N Engl J Med* 1968; 278:1323–1326.

16 Ricketts W E. Clinical manifestations of Carrión's disease. *Arch Intern Med* 1949; 84:751–781.

17 Dooley J R. Haemotropic bacteria in man. *Lancet* 1980; ii:1237–1239.

18 Herrer A. Carrión's disease. Presence of *Bartonella bacilliformis* in the peripheral blood of patients with the benign form. *Am J Trop Med Hyg* 1953; 2:645–649.

19 Townsend C H T. The transmission of verruga by *Phlebotomus. JAMA* 1913; 61:1717–1718.

20 Herrer A & Blancas F. Estudios sobre la enfermedad de Carrión en el valle interandino del Matyjaro I. Observaciones entomologicas. *Rev Med Exp* 1959; 13:27–45.

21 Pinkerton H & Weinman D J. Carrión's disease. Behaviour of the etiological agent within cells growing or surviving in vitro. Comparative morphology of the etiological agent in Oroya fever and verruga peruana. *Proc Soc Exp Biol Med* 1937; 37:587–593.

22 Buckles E L & McGinnis Hill E. Interaction of *Bartonella bacilliformis* with human erythrocyte membrane proteins. *Microb Pathog* 2000; 29:165-174.

23 Benson L A, Kar S, McLaughlin G & Ihler G M. Entry of *Bartonella bacilliformis* into erythrocytes. *Infect Immun* 1986; 54:347–353.

24 Reynafarje C & Ramos J. The haemolytic anaemia of human bartonellosis. *Blood* 1961; 17:562–578.

25 Arias-Stella J, Lieberman P H, Erlandson R A & Arias-Stella J Jr. Histology, immunohistochemistry and ultrastructure of the verruga in Carrión's disease. *Am J Surg Pathol* 1986; 10:595–610.

26 Howe C. Carrión's disease. Immunologic studies. *Arch Intern Med* 1943; 72:147–167.

27 Knobloch J, Solano L, Alvarez O et al. Antibodies to *Bartonella bacilliformis* as determined by fluorescent antibody test, indirect haemagglutination and ELISA. *Trop Med Parasitol* 1985; 36:183–185.

28 Ricketts W E. Carrión's disease. A study of the incubation period in thirteen cases. *Am J Trop Med* 1947; 27:657–659.

29 Cuardra M. Salmonellosis complication in human bartonellosis. *Tex Rep Biol Med* 1956; 14:97–113.

30 Trelles J O. In Spillane J D (ed.) *Tropical Neurology.* Oxford: Oxford Medical Publications, 1973:387

31 Urteaga B O & Payne E H. Treatment of the acute febrile phase of Carrión's disease with chloramphenicol. *Am J Trop Med Hyg* 1955; 4:507–511.

32 Gray G C, Johnson A A, Thornton S A et al. An epidemic of Oroya fever in the Peruvian Andes. *Am J Trop Med Hyg* 1990; 42:215–221.

33 Kosek M, Lavarello R, Gilman R H et al. Natural history of infection with *Bartonella bacilliformis* in a nonendemic population. *J Infect Dis* 2000; 182:865-872.

34 Hertig M & Fairchild G B. Control of *Phlebotomus* in Peru with DDT. *Am J Trop Med* 1948; 28:207–230.

35 English C K, Wear D J, Margileth A M, Lissner C R & Walsh G P. Cat-scratch disease: isolation and culture of the bacterial agent. *JAMA* 1988; 259:1347–1352.

36 Gerber M A, Sedgwick A K, MacAlister T J, Gustafson K B, Ballow M & Tilton R C. The aetiological agent of cat scratch disease. *Lancet* 1985; i:1236–1240.

37 Giladi M, Avidor B, Kletter Y et al. Cat scratch disease: the rare role of *Afipia felis. J Clin Microbiol* 1998; 36:2499–2502.

38 La Scola B & Praoult D. *Afipia felis* in hospital water supply in association with free-living amoebae. *Lancet* 1999; 353:1330.

39 Sander A, Zagosek A, Bredt W et al. Characterization of *Bartonella clarridgeiae* flagellin (FlaA) and detection of antiflagellin antibodies in patients with lymphadenopathy. *J Clin Microbiol* 2000; 38:2943–2948.

40 Tsukahara M, Tsuneoka H, Iino H, Ohno K & Murano I. *Bartonella henselae* infection from a dog. *Lancet* 1998; 21:1682–1683.

41 Del Prete R, Fumaola D, Fumarola L, Basile V, Mosca A & Miragliotta G. Prevalence of antibodies to *Bartonella henselae* in patients with suspected cat scratch disease (CSD) in Italy. *Eur J Epidemiol* 1999; 15:583–587.

42 Arvand M, Klose A J, Schwartz-Porsche D, Hahn H & Wend C. Genetic variability and prevalence of *Bartonella henselae* in cats in Berlin, Germany, and analysis of its genetic relatedness to a strain from Berlin that is pathogenic for humans. *J Clin Microbiol* 2001; 39:743–746.

43 Chang C C, Chomel B B, Kasten R W et al. *Bartonella* spp. isolated from wild and domestic ruminants in North America. *Emerg Infect Dis* 2000; 6:306–311.

44 Schouls L M, Van de Pol I, Rijpkema S G & Schot C S. Detection and identification of *Erlichia, Borrelia burgdorferi* sensu lato, and *Bartonella* species in Dutch *Ixodes ricinus* ticks. *J Clin Microbiol* 1999; 37:2215–2222.

45 Chang C, Yamamoto K, Chimel B B et al. Seroepidemiology of *Bartonella vinsonii* subsp. *Berkhoffii* infection in California coyotes, 1994–1998. *Emerg Infect Dis* 1999; 5:711–715.

46 Roux V, Eykyn S J, Wyllie S & Raoult D. *Bartonella vinsonii* subsp. *bekhoffii* as an agent of febrile blood culture-negative endocarditis in a human. *J Clin Microbiol* 2000; 38:1698–1700.

47 DeBoit P E, Berger T G, Egbert B M et al. Epithelioid haemangioma-like vascular proliferation in AIDS: manifestation of cat scratch disease bacillus infection? *Lancet* 1988; i:960–964.

48 Plettenberg A, Lorenzen T, Burtsche B T et al. Bacillary angiomatosis in HIV-infected patients-an epidemiolological and clinical study. *Dermatology* 2000; 201:326–331.

49 Massei F, Messina F, Talini I et al. Widening of the clinical spectrum of *Bartonella henselae* infection as recognized through serodiagnostics. *Eur J Pediatr* 2000; 15:416–419.

50 Tsukahara M, Tsuneoka H, Iino H, Murano I, Takahashi H & Uchida I. *Bartonella henselae* infection as a cause of fever of unknown origin. *J Clin Microbiol* 2000; 38:1990–1991.

51 Massei F, Messina F, Massmetti M, Macchia P & Maggiore G. Pseudoinfectious mononucleosis: a presentation of *Bartonella henselae* infection. *Arch Dis Child* 2000; 33:443–444.

52 Grando D, Sullivan L J, Flexman J P, Watson M W & Andrew J H. *Bartonella henselae* associated with Parinaud's oculoglandular syndrome. *Clin Infect Dis* 1999; 28:1156–1158.

53 Lohmann C P, Gabler B, Kroher G, Spiegel D, Linde H J & Reischl U. Disciform keratitis caused by *Bartonella henselae*: an unusual ocular complication in cat scratch disease. *Eur J Ophthalmol* 2000; 10:257–258.

54 Thompson P K, Vaphiades M S & Saccente M. Cat-scratch disease presenting as neuroretinitis and peripheral facial palsy. *J Neuroophthalmol* 1999; 19:240–241.

55 Rosen B S, Barry C J, Nicoll A M & Constable I J. Conservative management of documented neuroretinitis in cat scratch disease associated with *Bartonella henselae* infection. *Aust N Z Ophthalmol* 1999; 27:153–156.

56 Ormerod L D & Dailey J P. Ocular manifestations of cat-scratch disease. *Curr Opin Ophthalmol* 1999; 10:209–216.

57 Salgado C D & Weisse M E. Transverse myelitis associated with probable cat-scratch disease in a previously healthy pediatric patient. *Clin Infect Dis* 2000; 31:609–611.

58 McNeill P M, Verrips A, Mullaart R, Gabreels F J, Gabreels-Festen A W & Knibbeler J G. Chronic inflammatory demyelinating polyneuropathy as a complication of cat scratch disease. *J Neurol Neurosurg Psychiatry* 2000; 68:797.

59 Liapi-Adamidou G, Tsolia M, Magiakou A M, Zeis P M, Theodoropoulos V & Karpathios T. Cat scratch disease in two siblings presenting as acute gastroenteritis. *Scand J Infect Dis* 2000; 32:317–319.

60 Massei F, Massimetti M, Messina F, Macchia P & Maggiore G. *Bartonella henselae* and inflammatory bowel disease. *Lancet* 2000; 356:1245–1246.

61 Arisoy E S, Correa A G, Wagner M L & Kaplan S L. Hepatosplenic cat-scratch disease in children: selected clinical features and treatment. *Clin Infect* Dis 1999; 28:778–784.

62 Lenoir A A, Storch G A, Deshryver-Kecskemeti K et al. Granulomatous hepatitis associated with cat scratch disease. *Lancet* 1988; i:1132–1136.

63 Ventura A, Massei F, Not T, Massimetti M, Bussani R & Maggiore G. Systemic *Bartonella henselae* infection with hepatosplenic involvement. *J Pediatr Gastroenterol Nutr* 1999; 29:52–56.

64 Mehanna D, Peck N, Arnot R, Solano T & Sheldon D. Cat scratch disease presenting as splenic abscess. *Aust N Z J Surg* 2000; 70:622–624.

65 Krause R, Wenisch C, Pladerer P, Daxbock F, Krejs G J & Reisinger E C. Osteomyelitis of the hip joint associated with systemic cat-scratch disease in an adult. *Eur J Clin Microbiol Infect Dis* 2000; 19:781–783.

66 Ruess M, Sander A, Brandis M & Berner R. Portal vein and bone involvement in disseminated cat-scratch disease: report of two cases. *Clin Infect Dis* 2000; 31:818–821.

67 Malatskey S, Fradis M, Ben-David J & Podoshin L. Cat-scratch disease of the parotid gland: an often mis-diagnosed entity. *Ann Otol Rhinol Laryngol* 2000; 109:679–682.

68 Fortune S M, Kaelin C M, Gulizia J M & Daily J P. Cat scratch disease presenting as a breast mass. *Obstet Gynecol* 2000; 95:1027.

69 Karakas M, Baba M, Aksungur V L, Homan S, Memisoglu H R & Uguz A. Bacillary angiomatosis on a region of burned skin in an immunocompetent patient. *Br J Dermatol* 2000; 143:609–611.

70 Millot F, Tailboux L, Paccalin M et al. Cat-scratch disease simulating a malignant process of the chest wall. *Eur J Pediatr* 1999; 158:403–405.

71 Cimolai N, Benoit L, Hill A & Lyons C. *Bartonella henselae* infection in British Columbia: evidence for an endemic disease among humans. *Can J Microbiol* 2000; 46:908–912.

72 Harrison T G & Doshi N. Serological evidence of *Bartonella* spp. infection in the UK. *Epidemiol Infect* 1999; 123:233–240.

73 Maurin M & Raoult D. Isolation in endothelial cell cultures of *Chlamydia trachomatis* LGV (serovar L2) from a lymph node of a patient with suspected cat scratch disease. *J Clin Microbiol* 2000; 38:2062–2064.

74 Sander A & Penno S. Semiquantitative species detection of *Bartonella henselae* and *Bartonella quintana* by PCR-enzyme immunoassay. *J Clin Microbiol* 1999; 37:3097–3101.

75 Liang Z & Raoult D. Species-specific monoclonal antibodies for rapid identification of *Bartonella quintana*. *Clin Diagn Lab Immunol* 2000; 7:21–24.

76 Matar G M, Koehler J E, Malcolm G et al. Identification of *Bartonella* species directly in clinical specimens by PCR-restriction fragment length polymorphism analysis of a 16S rRNA gene fragment. *J Clin Microbiol* 1999; 37:4045–4047.

77 Del Prete R, Fumarola D, Ungari S, Fumarola L & Miragliotta G. Polymerase chain reaction detection of *Bartonella henselae* bacteraemia in an immunocompetent child with cat scratch disease. *Eur J Pediatr* 2000; 159:356–359.

78 Maas M, Schreiber M & Knobloch J. Detection of *Bartonella bacilliformis* in cultures, blood and formalin preserved skin biopsies by use of the polymerase chain reaction. *Trop Med Parasitol* 1992; 43:191–194.

79 Maeno N, Oda H, Yoshiie K, Wahid M R, Fujimura T & Matayoshi S. Live *Bartonella henselae* enhances endothelial proliferation without direct contact. *Microb Pathog* 1999; 27:419–427.

80 Conrad D A. Treatment of cat-scratch disease. *Curr Opin Pediatr Dis* 2001; 13:56–59.

81 Hunt G H & Rankin A C. Intermittent fever of obscure origin, occurring among British soldiers in France: the so-called 'trench fever'. *Lancet* 1915; ii:1133–1136.

82 McNee J W, Renshaw A & Brunt E H. Trench fever: a relapsing fever occurring with the British forces in France. *BMJ* 1916; i:225–234.

83 Swift H F. Trench fever. *Arch Intern Med* 1920; 26:76–98.

84 Vinson J W, Varela G & Molina-Pasquel C. Trench fever 3: Induction of clinical disease in volunteers inoculated with *Rickettsia quintana* propagated on blood agar. *Am J Trop Med Hyg* 1969; 18:713–722.

85 Brouqui P, Lascola L, Roux V & Raoult D. Chronic *Bartonella quintana* bacteremia in homeless patients. *N Engl J Med* 1999; 340:184–189.

86 Gray A V, Reed J B, Wendel R T & Morse L S. *Bartonella henselae* infection associated with peripapillary angioma, branch retinal artery occlusion and severe vision loss. *Am J Ophthalmol* 1999; 127:223–224.

87 Drancourt M, Mainardi J L, Brouqui P et al. *Bartonella (Rochalimaea) quintana* endocarditis in three homeless men. *N Engl J Med* 1995; 332:419–423.

88 Barbe K P, Jaeggi E, Ninet B et al. *Bartonella quintana* endocarditis in a child. *N Engl J Med* 2000; 342:1841–1842.

89 Ohl M E & Spach D H. *Bartonella quintana* and urban trench fever. *Clin Infect Dis* 2000; 31:131–135.

90 James E A, Hill J, Uppal R & Prentice M B. *Bartonella* infection: a significant cause of native valve endocarditis necessitating surgical management. *J Thorac Cardiovasc Surg* 2000; 119:171–172.

91 Simon-Vermont I, Altwegg M, Zimmerli W & Fluckiger U. Duke criteria-negative endocarditis caused by *Bartonella quintana*. *Infection* 1999; 27:283–285.

92 Patel R, Newell J O, Procop G W & Persing D H. Use of polymerase chain reaction for citrate synthase gene to diagnose *Bartonella quintana*. *Am J Clin Pathol* 1999; 119:36–40.

93 Azad A F, Sacci J B Jr, Nelson W M, Dasch G A, Schmidtmann E T & Carl M. Genetic characterization and transovarial transmission of a typhus-like rickettsia found in cat fleas. *Proc Natl Acad Sci USA* 1992; 89:43–46.

94 Roux V & Raoult D. Body lice as tools for diagnosis and surveillance of reemerging diseases. *J Clin Microbiol* 1999; 37:596–599.

95 Raoult D, Birtles R J, Montoya M et al. Survey of three bacterial louse-associated diseases among rural Andean communities in Peru: prevalence of epidemic typhus, trench fever and relapsing fever. *Clin Infect Dis* 1999; 29:434–436.

96 Fukuda T, Kitao T, Keida Y. Studies on the causative agent of "hyuganetsu" disease. I. Isolation of the agent and its inoculation trial in human beings. *Med Biol* 1954; 32:200–209.

97 Maeda K, Markowicz N, Hawley R C, Ristic M, Cox D & McDade J E. Human infection with *Erlichia canis*, a leukocytic rickettsia. *N Engl J Med* 1987; 316:853–856.

98 Dawson J E, Anderson B E, Fishbein D B et al. Isolation and characterization of an *Erlichia* sp. from a patient with human erlichiosis. *J Clin Microbiol* 1991; 29:2741–2745.

99 Buller R S, Arens M, Hamiel S P et al. *Erlichia ewingii*, a newly recognised agent of human erlichiosis. *N Engl J Med* 1999; 341:195–197.

100 Chen S-M, Dumler J S, Bakken J S & Walker D H. Identification of a granulocytotropic *Erlichia* species as the etiologic agent of human disease. *J Clin Microbiol* 1994; 32:589–595.

101 Fishbein D B, Dawson J E & Robinson L E. Human erlichiosis in the United States, 1985–1990. *Ann Intern Med* 1994; 120:736–743.

102 Lotrick-Furlan S, Petrovec M, Avsic-Zupanc T et al. Human erlichiosis in central Europe. *Wien Klin Wochenschr* 1998; 110:894–897.

103 Bjoersdorff A, Berglund J, Kristiansen B E, Soderstrom C & Eliasson I. Varying clinical picture and course of human granulocytic erlichiosis. Twelve Scandinavian cases of the new tick-borne zoonosis are presented. *Lakartidningen* 1999; 96:4200–4204.

104 Aguero-Rosenfeld M, Horowitz H W, Wormser G P et al. Human granulocytic erlichiosis (HE): a series from a single medical center in New York State. *Ann Intern Med* 1996; 125:904–908.

105 Telford S R, Dawson J E, Katavolos P, Warner C K, Kolbert C P & Persing D H. Perpetuation of the agent of human granulocytic erhlichiosis in a deer tick-rodent cycle. *Proc Natl Acad Sci USA* 1996; 93:6209–6214.

106 Thompson C, Spielman A, Krause PJ. Coinfecting deer-associated zoonoses: Lyma disease, Babesiosis and Ehrlichiosis. *Clin Infect Dis* 2001; 33:676–685.

107 Rikihasa Y. Clinical and biological aspects of infection caused by *Erlichia chaffeensis*. *Microbes Infect* 1999; 1:367–376.

108 Klein M B, Hu S, Chao C C & Goodman J L. The agent of human granulocytic ehrlichiosis induces the production of myelosuppressing chemokines without induction of pro-inflammatory cytokines. *J Infect Dis* 2000; 182:200–205.

109 Belongia E A, Reed K D, Mitchell P D et al. Clinical and epidemiological features of early Lyme disease and human granulocytic ehrlichiosis in Wisconsin. *Clin Infect Dis* 1999; 29:1472–1477.

110 Martin G S, Christman B W & Standaert S M. Rapidly fatal infection with *Erlichia chaffeensis*. *N Engl J Med* 1999; 341:763–764.

111 Comer J A, Nicholson W L, Olson J G & Childs J E. Serologic testing for human granulocytic erlichiosis at a national referral center. *J Clin Microbiol* 1999; 37:558–564.

112 Horowicz H W, Aguero-Rosenfeld M E, McKenna D F et al. The clinical and laboratory spectrum of culture proven human granulocytic erlichiosis: comparison with culture negative cases. *Clin Infect Dis* 1998; 27:1314–1317.

113 Whipple G H. A hitherto undescribed disease characterised anatomically by deposits of fat and fatty acids in the intestinal and mesenteric lymphatic tissues. *Bull Johns Hopkins Hosp* 1907; 18:382–391.

114 Maizel H, Ruffin J M & Dobbins W O III. Whipple's disease. A review of 19 patients from one hospital and review of the literature since 1950. *Medicine (Baltimore)* 1970; 49:175–205.

115 Vitel-Durand D, Lecomte C, Cathebras P, Rousset H & Godeau P. Whipple disease: clinical review of 52 cases. *Medicine (Baltimore)* 1997; 76:170–184.

116 Razman N N, Loftus E Jr, Burgart L J et al. Diagnosis and monitoring of Whipple disease by polymerase chain reaction. *Ann Intern Med* 1997; 126:520–527.

117 Relman D A, Schmidt T M, MacDermott R P & Falkow S. Identification of the uncultured bacillus of Whipple's disease. *N Engl J Med* 1992; 327:293–301.

118 Raoult D, Birg M L, La Scola B et al. Cultivation of the bacillus of Whipple's disease. *N Engl J Med* 2000; 342:620–625.

119 Dobbins W O III. *Whipple's Disease*. Springfield, Illinois: Charles C Thomas, 1987.

120 Yardley J H & Hendrix T R. Combined electron and light microscopy in Whipple's disease. Demonstration of 'bacillary bodies' in the intestine. *Bull Johns Hopkins Hosp* 1961; 109:80–98.

121 Chears W C & Ashworth C T. Electron microscopy study of the intestinal mucosa in Whipple's disease. Demonstration of encapsulated bacilliform bodies in the lesion. *Gastroenterology* 1961; 41:129–138.

122 Wilson K H, Blitchington R, Frothingham R & Wilson J A. Phylogeny of the Whipple's disease-associated bacterium. *Lancet* 1991; 338:474–475.

123 Schoedon G, Goldenberger D, Forrer R et al. Deactivation of macrophages with interleukin-4 is the key to the isolation of *Tropheryma whippelii*. *J Infect Dis* 1997; 176:672–677.

124 Raoult D, La Scola B, Lecocq P, Lepidi H & Fournier P-E. Culture and immunological detection of *Tropheryma whippelii* from the duodenum of a patient with Whipple disease. *JAMA* 2001; 285:1039–1043.

125 Maiwald M, Von Herbay A, Lepp P W & Relman D A. Organisation, structure, and variability of the rRNA operon of the Whipple's disease bacterium (*Tropheryma whippelii*). *J Bacteriol* 2000; 182:3292–3297.

126 Hinrikson H P, Dutly F, Nair S & Altwegg M. Detection of three different types of *Tropheryma whippelii* directly from clinical specimens by sequencing, single-strand conformation polymorphism (SSCP) analysis and type-specific PCR of their 16S–23S ribosomal intergenic spacer region. *Int J Syst Bacteriol* 1999; 49:1701–1706.

127 Hinrikson H P, Dutly F & Altwegg M. Evaluation of a specific nested PCR targeting domain III of the 23S rRNA gene of 'Tropheryma whippelii' and proposal of a classification system for its molecular variants. *J Clin Microbiol* 2000; 38:595–599.

128 Feule G E, Dorken B, Schopf E et al. HLA-B27 and defects in the T-cell system in Whipple's disease. *Eur J Clin Invest* 1979; 9:385–389.

129 Ectors N, Geboes K, De Vos R et al. Whipple's disease: a histological, immunocytochemical and electron microscopic study of the immune response in the small intestinal mucosa. *Histopathology* 1992; 21:1–12.

130 Marth T, Roux M, von Herbay A et al. Persistent reduction of complement receptor 3 alpha-chain expressing mononuclear blood cells and transient inhibitory serum factors in Whipple's disease. *Clin Immunol Immunopathol* 1994; 72:217–226.

131 Dobbins W O III. Is there an immune deficit in Whipple's disease? *Dig Dis Sci* 1981; 26:247–252.

132 Bjerkness R, Odegaard S, Bjerkvig R et al. Demonstration of a persisting monocyte and macrophage dysfunction. *Scan J Gastroenterol* 1988; 23:611–619.

133 Schneider T, Stallmach A, von Herbay A et al. Treatment of refractory Whipple's disease with interferon-gamma. *Ann Intern Med* 1998; 129:875–877.

134 Maiwald M, Schuhmacher F, Ditton H J & von Herbay A. Environmental occurrence of the Whipple's disease bacterium (*Tropheryma whippelii*). *Appl Environ Microbiol* 1998; 64:760–762.

135 Raoult D, Lepidi H & Harle JR. *Tropheryma whippelii* circulating in blood monocytes. *N Engl J Med* 2001; 345:548.

136 Ehrbar H U, Bauerfeind P, Dutly F, Koelz H R & Altwegg M. PCR-positive tests for *Tropheryma whippelii* in patients without Whipple's disease. *Lancet* 1999; 353:2214.

137 Street S, Donoghue H D & Neild G H. *Tropheryma whippelii* DNA in saliva of healthy people. *Lancet* 1999; 354:1178–1179.

138 Maiwald M, von Herbay A, Persing D H et al. *Tropheryma whippelii* DNA is rare in the intestinal mucosa of patients without other evidence of Whipple disease. *Ann Intern Med* 2001; 134:115–119.

139 Puechal X, Saad R & Poveda J D. *Tropheryma whippelii* in synovial tissue and blood. *Ann Intern Med* 1999; 131:795–796.

140 Schilling D, Adamek H E, Kaufmann V, Maier M & Riemann J F. Arthralgia as an extraintestinal symptom of Whipple's disease. Report of five cases. *J Clin Gastroenterol* 1997; 24:18–20.

141 McGettigan P, Mooney E E, Sinnott M, Sweeney E C & Feely J. Sudden death in Whipple's disease. *Postgrad Med* 1997; 73:509–511.

142 Anderson M. Neurology of Whipple's disease. *J Neurol Neurosurg Psychiatry* 2000; 68:2–5.

143 Lynch T, Odel J, Fredericks D N et al. Polymerase chain reaction-based detection of *Tropheryma whippelii* in central nervous system Whipple's disease. *Ann Neurol* 1997; 42:120–124.

144 James T N. On the wide spectrum of abnormalities in the coronary arteries of Whipple's disease. *Coron Art Dis* 2001; 12:115–125.

145 Gras E, Matias-Guiu X, Garcia A et al. PCR analysis in the pathological diagnosis of Whipple's disease: emphasis on the extraintestinal involvement or atypical morphological features. *J Pathol* 1999; 188:318–321.

146 Garas G, Cheng W S, Abrugiato R & Forbes G M. Clinical relapse in Whipple's disease despite maintenance therapy. *J Gastroenterol Hepatol* 2000; 15:1223–1226.

Chapter 61C
Tularaemia

G. Scott

Tularaemia is an acute febrile zoonotic infection. The causative organism is distinguished from other parvo-bacteria and has been named *Francisella tularensis* after Edward Francis (born 1872), an American bacteriologist who studied the agent and pathogenesis.

Tularaemia is an infectious disease of rodents caused by *F. tularensis*, which is transmitted from these animals to humans by the bite of infected blood-sucking insects, by handling infected animals, by the ingestion of infected meat or water, or by the inhalation of contaminated aerosols or dust. It is also known locally as deer-fly fever, Pahvant Valley plague, rabbit fever, Ohara disease, yato-byo (Japan) or lemming fever.

Geographical distribution

Human tularaemia has been recognized in relatively restricted geographical environments in North America (about 200 cases per annum), Europe and the former Soviet Republics, and also to a lesser extent in Japan.[1,2] A recent outbreak was reported from Spain.[3]

Aetiology

F. tularensis is a small, non-motile, aerobic, Gram-negative coccobacillus measuring $0.2 \times 0.2{-}0.7$ μm. Some of the organisms pass through coarser bacterial filters. Possession of a capsule confers virulence and is seen consistently in isolates from human infections. The organisms stain in tissue preparation with Giemsa, but stain poorly with Gram; in smears from cultures they show up well with aniline gentian violet. Immuno-fluorescent techniques can be used specifically to identify the organisms in clinical material.[4]

The organism is not difficult to culture on chocolated blood agar rich in cystine, aerobically at 37°C, but it does not grow well on ordinary blood or nutrient agar. Most blood culture media support growth, but animal blood or spleen can be inoculated directly on to media enriched with cystine and thiamine with satisfactory results. Cystine agar consists of beef infusion agar (pH 7.6), to which 0.02% of cystine is added. Growth appears on about the third day and flourishes luxuriantly in sub-cultures without the addition of fresh animal tissue. The organism causes green staining of blood and brown staining of chocolated blood. To ensure the primary growth, it is necessary that a piece of animal tissue be added to the medium. Tissue should be rubbed into agar and then left on the medium. Fermentation of glucose, laevulose, maltose and glycerine occurs with acid formation. Intraperitoneal injection of fresh capsulate isolates causes death in guinea pigs in 5–10 days. Cultures of *F. tularensis* are very infectious to the microbiology staff and should be handled with great care.

There are two broad types of infection in humans: one is associated with a rabbit reservoir and a tick vector, with a mortality rate of 5–7%, and the other, which is less virulent, is associated with rodents. Four subspecies of *F. tularensis* and various biovars are recognized: ssp. *tularensis* (causing type A, the more serious infection) and *palaearctica* (*holarctica*) biovars I and II (causing type B or milder disease).[5] Type A is almost exclusive to North America, although there has been one recent report of an isolate with very similar characteristics to ssp. *tularensis* from central Europe.[6,7] Type B is found in Europe and Japan, and also in North America. Subspecies *mediasiatica* has been found in central Asia and a part of the former Soviet Union. The fourth subspecies is *novicida*, found in water in Utah in 1950 but rarely associated with human disease. The subspecies are differentiated by fermentation of glycerol, presence of citrulline ureidase and sensitivity to erythromycin, but it is not easy to separate the biovars in the laboratory. DNA amplification methods of various repetitive genes characteristic for Enterobacteriaceae have been developed recently for identification and typing.[7,8]

Transmission

F. tularensis is transmitted in nature by a wide variety of routes but the three main ones appear to be: (1) between rodents in water and by close contact; (2) to carnivores by consumption of infected rodents; and (3) to birds and larger animals by ticks, biting flies and mosquitoes. Humans acquire the infection by direct contact from skinning rabbits, by eating them as food, and from tick, horsefly and mosquito bites. Outbreaks may be associated with inhaled dust in rural areas, particularly where the rodent population increases and then becomes epizootically infected. *F. tularensis* can also be acquired easily in the laboratory.

Water-borne infection

The infection is maintained among rodents mainly in water. The water is contaminated by dead animals[9] and excreta, and large numbers of rodents may be infected and die in this way.

Ingestion

Carnivores are infected chiefly from the consumption of sick, infected rodents which are easy to catch. Domestic cats may become infected in this way and then transmit the organisms to humans by biting.[10–12]

Insect vectors

A wide variety of ticks can act as vectors. The nymph stages feed on small rodents and adults feed on larger mammals, including humans. The infection persists during the development of the tick, but infection is also transmitted transovarially. By this method infection can be maintained through the winter.

Dermacentor andersoni (wood tick), *D. variabilis*, *D. occidentalis*, *D. reticulates*, *Ixodes ricinus* and *Haemaphysalis leporispalustris* (rabbit tick) can all transmit the infection. *D. andersoni* is particularly important in the USA and *F. tularensis* is found in the intestinal lumen, in the cells of the gut wall, in the body fluids and in the faeces. The organism can also be transmitted by biting fleas, the deer-fly (*Chrysops discalis*) as well as the stable fly (*Stomoxys calcitrans*), the squirrel flea (*Ceratophyllus acutus*), the rabbit louse (*Haemodipus ventricosus*) and the mouse louse (*Polyplax serratus*). The bacteria may be found in bed bugs or mites, but it is not certain how important these are in transmission. *Aedes* and *Theobaldia* spp. mosquitoes have been shown to transmit *F. tularensis* under experimental conditions, and in Sweden *Aedes cinereus* does so in nature. Mosquitoes transmit the infection to and between birds.

Pathology

As the disease is rarely fatal in humans, the pathology is best seen in infected animals. The pathological appearances of infected guinea pigs and rabbits at autopsy resemble those of plague. In an experimentally infected guinea pig there is haemorrhagic oedema at the site of inoculation, blood-stained peritoneal exudate and a diffusely enlarged spleen with characteristic small necrotic foci. Similar lesions may be detected in the liver. On microscopic section of these organs, a dense infiltration with polymorphonuclear cells can be found, but the organisms can be detected only with difficulty. In the spleen of the mouse, on the other hand, little or no leucocytic response occurs and *F. tularensis* can be demonstrated in large numbers. In the few recorded autopsies in humans, nodules have been found in the lung and spleen.

Immunity

There is a great deal of interest in the immunopathology of tularensis, a typical intracellular infection where cell-mediated immunity plays an important part in response to infection.[13–16] Non-immune mice given neutralizing antibodies to tumour necrosis factor α (TNFα) and interferon γ (IFNγ) are rendered defenceless against sublethal doses of *F. tularensis*.[17] Virulent strains with capsules consume complement, leading to resistance to the bactericidal activity of serum.[18] Infection induces long-lasting immunity in humans and there is no record of a second generalized attack. However, local reinfection may occur and persistent infection in those treated with bacteriostatic antibiotics is not infrequent. Agglutinating antibodies appear in the serum in the second week and reach a maximum level between the fourth and eighth weeks, after which there is a gradual fall, but they may persist for as long as 11 years. Serum antibodies can be used in diagnosis, but cross-reactions occur with *Brucella melitensis* and *B. abortus* (23% of tularaemia sera cross-react with *B. melitensis* and *B. abortus*, and 35% of *B. melitensis* and *B. abortus* with tularaemia). In 13% of cases of tularaemia, the serum agglutinates *Proteus* OX19 at a titre of 80 or over.

Type IV hypersensitivity can be demonstrated by an intradermal test employing a suspension of killed organisms, and peripheral lymphocytes proliferate in response to *F. tularensis* antigens[19] and heat-shock protein chaperone 60.[20]

Clinical features

Subclinical infections

Seroprevalence surveys during outbreaks and in areas of hyperendemicity reveal that the majority acquire *F. tularensis* asymptomatically or without a characteristic infection. In Sweden, up to 23% of a population studied had been infected, the infection being subclinical in one-third of those with positive reactions. The disease presents in a number of ways, depending on the route of infection. The incubation period is 1–10 days.

Cutaneous (ulceroglandular) form (approximately 60% of cases)[21]

Local cutaneous disease results from the bite of an infected tick or fly, or an animal,[10–12] or from direct contact of the broken skin with an infected source. An inflamed papule develops at the site of infection, which becomes pustular with a necrotic centre. This separates, leaving a punched-out ulcer (Figure 61C.1), which is replaced by a scar on healing. Small sores on the hands are usually not diagnosed as tularaemia. Often, however, there is painful enlargement of the local lymph glands

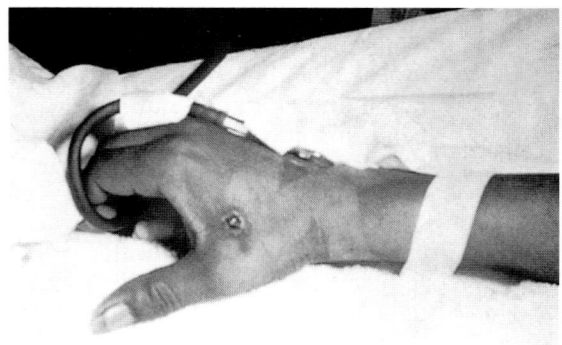

Figure 61C.1: An ulcer on the hand of a patient with tularaemia. (Courtesy of Tropical Resources Unit.)

which may suppurate after 1–2 months and may remain enlarged for 2–3 months. A glandular form of the disease may be seen (in about 15% of cases) without any sore. Sometimes the local lesion is associated with general signs of infection such as fever and prostration.

Ophthalmic (oculoglandular) form (1% of cases)

The site of entry of infection is the conjunctival sac, which is usually involved unilaterally. The patient may have rubbed the eyes while handling infected material or have been bitten on the eyelid by an infected insect. There is itching, lacrimation, photophobia and pain in the eye with swelling of the preauricular, parotid, submaxillary and cervical lymph glands. The eyelids become swollen and the conjunctiva red and covered with small discrete nodules and grey exudate. Punched-out ulcers develop and last for 2–3 weeks. Suppuration of the glands is common. Dacryocystitis and corneal ulcers occur, and permanent impairment of vision may follow.

Oral and abdominal form

This follows ingestion of infected meat or other food or water contaminated by rodent excreta. There is a necrotizing pharyngitis with abscesses on the roof of the mouth, fever, enlargement of local lymph glands and sometimes abdominal pain, vomiting and diarrhoea. Peritonitis may develop with persistent ascites, appendicitis or intestinal haemorrhage.

Pneumonic and typhoidal (septicaemic) forms

These forms may arise primarily from infection via the respiratory route or as a late result of dissemination from a local infection. The onset is sudden with severe headache, vomiting, chills and fever. Myalgia and arthralgia are common. The initial rise in temperature is above 40°C, with generalized weakness, aching, prostration,

sweats and loss of weight. The fever may show an initial rise followed by remission and a secondary rise or a continuous course lasting usually for 10–15 days, and rarely 3–4 weeks. Petechial, roseolar, papular and pustular rashes are seen. A slightly tender enlargement of the spleen is found in one-third of cases. There may be a moderate polymorphonuclear leucocytosis of $12–15 \times 10^9/l$ but more often in this infection the white count is normal.

In one-half of the cases (some 10–20% of the total in the USA[22]), pulmonary symptoms develop, particularly dyspnoea and pleuritic pain. Milder forms resemble atypical pneumonia but may last for a month and there may be a solitary pulmonary nodule. There may be pleurisy, effusion, pneumonic consolidation or lobular bronchopneumonia with abscess and cavitation in severe cases and occasionally pericarditis. The effusion mimics that seen in tuberculosis.[23] There is an associated enlargement of the bronchial and mediastinal glands.

Dissemination may lead to meningitis, which mimics tuberculous meningitis, or osteomyelitis or even endocarditis on native[24] or prosthetic material.[25] The disease may present with lone neurological symptoms suggestive of encephalitis.[26] These presentations are all rare.[27]

Course

The infection is rarely fatal but in a series of severe untreated cases there was a mortality rate of 62% in pulmonary and 20% in typhoidal forms of the disease. The mean duration of fever in untreated cases is 26 days and adenopathy may last for 3–4 months. In one-third of cases, recovery is slow, the debilitating effect being very marked and lassitude persisting for months. *F. tularensis* may remain dormant intracellularly for years.

Diagnosis

The diagnosis is suspected only by a keen clinical awareness of behavioural risk in the patient and local geographical pathology. The differential diagnosis of the local form must be made from anthrax, plague, tick typhus and rat bite fever.[27] The organism is isolated from an ulcer or lymph node aspirate on enriched agar or broth or by inoculation into guinea pigs, mice or rabbits, from whose tissues the organism may be isolated on special media as described. The organisms are rarely present in the blood[28] but may be isolated from sputum.[29] A serological diagnosis may be attempted using agglutination tests with cultures of *F. tularensis* from the spleens of infected mice in a formalinized citrate suspension, but cross-reactions with undulant and typhus fevers may occur. Half of patients with culture-proven tularaemia are seronegative. Recently, diagnostic polymerase chain reaction (PCR) has been tried with limited success (sensitivity 73%) from the ulcers of patients with serologically proven tularaemia.[30] From other specimens, PCR has roughly the same sensitivity as culture.[31]

The differential diagnosis of the pulmonary form of tularaemia[32] includes all the causes of atypical pneumonia, including legionellosis, psittacosis, Q fever, *Mycoplasma pneumoniae* and *Chlamydophila pneumoniae*.

Treatment

Streptomycin is extremely effective: 1 g intramuscularly daily for 7 days will terminate the infection. Gentamicin is a suitable, less toxic, alternative. The patient should be kept in bed for a time after subsidence of the fever and convalescence should be prolonged. More recently, tetracycline (250 mg four times daily for 2 weeks) has been preferred, but there may be a relapse. Although erythromycin may be selected empirically to treat atypical pneumonia, and has been successful in tularaemia,[33] it is worth noting that some strains are constitutively resistant. Doxycycline and ciprofloxacin were both effective in an animal model of virulent tularaemia.[34] The fluoroquinolones are very active in vitro[35] and have been successful in treating the few cases where they have been tried.[12,36–40]

Epidemiology

Tularaemia in humans is essentially a rural infection and has a varying epidemiology according to the area in which it occurs and the method of transmission. Several important methods of acquisition have been identified:

1. Vector-borne: by ticks, tabanid flies and mosquitoes.
2. Trapping: from the skins of infected rodents, muskrats and rabbits.
3. Hunting: from the consumption of rabbit meat.
4. Water-borne: from the water of streams infected by dead rats; well water infected by mice and field voles.
5. Agricultural: from working in haystacks contaminated by field voles and mice; processing of agricultural products; airborne transmission by contaminated dust.
6. Domestic: use of grain and other products contaminated by mice; from bites by domestic cats.
7. Laboratory infections: presumably by the aerosol route or by accidental ingestion.
8. Wartime: trench and foxhole outbreaks.

Outbreaks in humans invariably follow natural epizootics of different species of wild mammals.

USA: Wandering shrew, grey fox, dog, cat, various ground squirrels (Pirote, Wyoming, Beechey's and Columbian), chipmunk, beaver, wood rat, white-footed mouse, meadow mouse and varieties (Sawatch and Tule) of muskrat and brown rat (*Rattus norvegicus*), varying hare, jack rabbit, black-tailed jack rabbit, cotton-tail rabbit, sheep, calves, ruffed grouse, sharp-tailed grouse, bobwhite quail and horned owl.

Canada: Richardson's ground squirrel, Osgood's white-footed mouse, Drummond meadow mouse, varying hare, white-tailed jack rabbit and Franklin's gull.
Sweden: Lemming and varying hare.
Central Europe: Rabbit and hare.
USSR (former): Introduced muskrat, little ground squirrel, steppe lemming, water rat, continental vole, large water vole, house mouse, long-tailed field mouse and hamster.
Asia Minor: Continental vole, house and harvest mouse.
Japan: Local rabbit.

Natural infections

F. tularensis occurs as a natural infection of wild rodents, especially rats, field mice, hares and rabbits. It has an extremely wide host range and many other species of animals as well as birds can be infected.[41]

North America

In North America the most important reservoirs of infection are the jack rabbit, hare and their relatives. The infection is found in Wyoming and Montana in streams contaminated by dead beavers, which have been found in large numbers. Humans acquire the infection from skinning infected animals after hunting, and preparing carcasses for cooking, and also after tick and deer fly (*Chrysops discalis*) bites. Occasionally contact with sheep is a source of infection. The disease is most prevalent during the months of June, July and August.[42]

Europe

In Sweden, the lemming and varying hare are the main reservoirs and tularaemia is known as 'lemming fever'; it is caused by contact with infected water contaminated by the bodies and excreta of infected lemmings. Outbreaks have occurred in peasant women who go barefoot in summer and are bitten by numerous mosquitoes (*Aedes cinereus*). A very large outbreak involving 676 identified cases occurred in Sweden in the winter of 1966, in which the likely source was airborne dust from hay contaminated by vole faeces.[43] In Austria, the Czech and Slovak Republics, and in Poland, the rabbit and hare are the main reservoirs. In France, the infection has become much more common since the introduction of hares from central Europe for sporting purposes. In northern Europe, cases occur from July to October and in southern Europe from June to August.

The former USSR

In Russia, the water rat and introduced muskrat, which spread widely in the Ukraine after the disturbance caused by the great tank battles of the Second World War (1939–1945), are the main reservoirs. There was a great increase in the number of human infections after the Second World War (1945 onwards). In central Asia, *Microtus* and *Arvicola* are the predominant rat hosts.

Prevention

Prevention depends upon avoidance of the circumstances leading to infection in the various endemic areas. Rabbits should not be skinned without gloves, and sick rabbits should not be eaten. However, proper cooking destroys the organism, as does prolonged freezing. Experimental work with *F. tularensis* in the laboratory must be undertaken with great caution, and staff in routine laboratories are discouraged from handling the organism. Killed and live attenuated vaccine strains have been used in the former Soviet Republics for years. Live attenuated vaccines are much more effective than killed ones; they induce cell-mediated immunity[19,44] and protective antibodies against lipopolysaccharide.[45] They do not reduce the risk of ulceroglandular disease but simply the danger from bacteraemia.

REFERENCES

1   Ohara Y, Sato T & Homma M. Arhtropod-borne tularaemia in Japan: clinical analysis of 1374 cases observed between 1924 and 1996. *J Med Entomol* 1998; 35:471–473.

2   Ohara Y, Sato T & Homma M. Epidemiological analysis of tularaemia in Japan (yato-byo). *FEMS Immunol Med Microbiol* 1996; 13:185–189.

3   Bellido-Casado J, Perez-Casrillon J L, Bachiller-Luque P et al. Report on five cases of tularaemic pneumonia in a tularaemic outbreak in Spain. *Eur J Clin Microbiol Infect Dis* 2000; 19:218–220.

4   Eigelsbach H T & McGann V G. Genus *Francisella*. In Krieg NR & Holt JG (eds) *Bergey's Manual of Systemic Bacteriology*, vol. 1. Baltimore, MD: Williams & Wilkins, 1984: 394–399.

5   Uhari M, Syrjala H & Salminen A. Tularaemia in children caused by *Francisella tularensis* biovar *palaearctica*. *Pediatr Infect Dis J* 1990; 9:80–83.

6   Gurycova D. First isolation of *Francisella tularensis* subsp *tularensis* in Europe. *Eur J Epidemiol* 1998; 14:797–802.

7   Johansson A, Ibrahim A, Goransson I et al. Evaluation of PCR-based methods for discrimination of *Francisella* species and subspecies and development of a specific PCR that distinguishes the two major subspecies of *Francisella tularensis*. *J Clin Microbiol* 2000; 38:4180–4185.

8   de la Puente-Redondo V A, del Blanco N G, Gutierrez-Martin C B, Garcia-Pena F J & Rodriguez Ferri E F. Comparison of different PCR approaches for typing of *Francisella tularensis* strains. *J Clin Microbiol* 2000; 38:1016–1022.

9   Berdal B P, Mahl R, Haaheim H, Loksa M et al. Field detection of *Francisella tularensis*. *Scand J Infect Dis* 2000; 32:287–291.

10   Liles W C & Burger R J. Tularaemia from domestic cats. *West J Med* 1993; 158:619–622.

11   Cappelan J & Fong I W. Tularaemia from a cat bite: case report and a review of feline-associated tularaemia. *Clin Infect Dis* 1993; 16:472–475.

12   Arav-Boger R. Cat-bite tularaemia in a seventeen-year-old girl treated with ciprofloxacin. *Paediatr Inf Dis J* 2000; 19:583–584.

13   Tarnvik A. Nature of protective immunity to *Francisella tularensis*. *Rev Infect Dis* 1989; 11:440–451.

14   Surcel H M. Diversity of *Francisella tularensis* antigens recognised by human T lymphocytes. *Infect Immun* 1990; 58:2664–2668.

15   Karttunen R, Surcel H M, Andersson G, Eicre H P & Herve E. *Francisella tularensis*-induced in vitro gamma interferon, tumor necrosis factor alpha, and interleukin 2 responses appear within two weeks of tularaemia vaccination in human beings. *J Clin Microbiol* 1991; 29:753–756.

16   Tarnvok A, Ericsson M, Golovliov I, Sandstrom G & Sjostedt A. Orchestration of the protective immune response to intracellular bacteria; *Francisella tularensis*. *FEMS Immunol Med Microbiol* 1996; 13:221–225.

17   Sjostedt A, North R J & Conlan J W. The requirement of tumour necrosis factor-alpha and interferon-gamma for the expression of protective immunity to secondary murine tularaemia depends on the size of the challenge inoculum. *Microbiology* 1996; 142:1369–1374.

18   Sorokin V M, Pavlovich N V & Prozorova L A. *Francisella tularensis* resistance to bactericidal action of normal human serum. *FEMS Immunol Med Microbiol* 1996; 13:249–252.

19   Waag D, Galloway A & Sandstrom G et al. Cell mediated and humoral responses induced by scarification vaccination of human volunteers with a new lot of the live vaccine strain of *Francisella tularensis*. *J Clin Microbiol* 1992; 30:2256–2264.

20   Ericsson M, Golovliov I, Sandsrom G, Tarnvik A & Sjostedt A. Characterisation of the nucleotide sequence of the *groE* operon encoding heat shock proteins chaperone-60 and -10 of *Francisella tularensis* and determination of the T-cell response to the proteins in individuals vaccinated with *F. tularensis*. *Infect Immun* 1997; 65:1824–1829.

21   Rohrbach B W, Westerman E & Istre G R. Epidemiology and clinical characteristics of tularaemia in Oklahoma, 1979–1985. *South Med J* 1991; 84:1091–1096.

22   Gill V & Cunha B A. Tularaemia pneumonia. *Semin Respir Infect* 1997; 12:61–67.

23   Pettersson T, Nyberg P, Nordstrom D & Riska H. Similar pleural fluid findings in pleuropulmonary tularaemia and tuberculous pleurisy. *Chest* 1996; 109:572–575.

24   Tancik C A & Dillaha J A. *Francisella tularensis* endocarditis. *Clin Infect Dis* 2000; 30:399–400.

25   Cooper C L, Van Caeseele P, Canvin J & Nicolle L E. Chronic prosthetic device infection with *Francisella tularensis*. *Clin Infect Dis* 1999; 29:1589–1591.

26   Le Doux M S. Tularaemia presenting with ataxia. *Clin Infect Dis* 2000; 30:211–212.

27   Kostman J R & DiNubile M J. Nodular lymphangitis: a distinctive but often unrecognised syndrome. *Ann Intern Med* 1993; 118:883–888.

28   Hoel T, Scheel O, Nordahl S H & Sandvik T. Water- and airborne-*Francisella tularensis* biovar *palaearctica* isolated from human blood. *Infection* 1991; 19:348–350.

29   Fredricks D N & Remington J S. Tularaemia presenting a community-acquired pneumonia. Implications in the era of managed care. *Arch Intern Med* 1996; 156:2137–2140.

30   Sjostedt A, Eriksson U, Berglund L & Tarnvick A. Detection of *Francisella tularensis* in ulcers of patients with tularaemia by PCR. *J Clin Microbiol* 1997; 35:1045–1048.

31   Johansson A, Berglund L, Eriksson U, Goransson I et al. Comparative analysis of PCR versus culture for diagnosis of ulceroglandular tularaemia. *J Clin Microbiol* 2000; 38:22–26.

32   Scofield R H, Lopez E J & McNabb S J. Tularaemia pneumonia in Oklahoma 1982–1987. *J Okla State Med Assoc* 1992; 85:165–170.

33   Harrell R E Jr & Simmons H F. Pleuropulmonary tularaemia: successful treatment with erythromycin. *South Med J* 1990; 83:1363–1364.

34 Russell P, Eley S M, Fulop M J, Bell D L & Titball R W. The efficacy of ciprofloxacin and doxycycline against experimental tularaemia. *J Antimicrob Chemother* 1998; 41:461–465.

35 Ikaheimo I, Syrjala H, Karhukorpi J, Schildt R & Koskela M. In vitro antibiotic susceptibility of *Francisella tularensis* isolated from humans and animals. *J Antimicrob Chemother* 2000; 46:287–290.

36 Syrjala H, Schildt R & Raisaninen S. In vitro susceptibility of *Francisella tularensis* to fluoroquinolones and treatment of tularaemia with norfloxacin and ciprofloxacin. *Eur J Clin Microbiol Infect Dis* 1991; 10:68–70.

37 Scheel O, Hoel T, Sandvik T & Berdal B. Susceptibility pattern of Scandinavian *Francisella tularensis* isolates with regard to oral and parenteral antimicrobial agents. *Acta Pathol Microbiol Immunol Scand* 1993; 101:33–36.

38 Chocarro A, Gonzalez A & Garcia I. Treatment of tularaemia with ciprofloxacin. *Clin Infect Dis* 2000; 31:623.

39 Johansson A, Berglund L, Gothefors L, Sjostedt A & Tarnvik A. Ciprofloxacin for treatment of tularaemia in children. *Pediatr Infect Dis J* 2000; 19:449–453.

40 Limaye A P & Hooper C J. Treatment of tularaemia with fluoroquinolones: two cases and a review. *Clin Infect Dis* 1999; 29:922–924.

41 Burrough A L, Holdenreid R, Longanecker D S & Meyer K F. A field study of latent tularaemia in rodents with a list of all known naturally infected vertebrates. *J Infect Dis* 1945; 76:115–119.

42 Cumming H S. La tularémie aux Etats-Unis. *Bull Off Int Hyg Publique* 1937; 29:2532–2535.

43 Dahlstrand S, Ringertz O & Zetterburg B. Airborne tularaemia in Sweden. *Scan J Infect Dis* 1971; 3:7–16.

44 Fortier A H, Slayter M V, Ziemba R, Meltzer M S & Nacy C A. Live vaccine strain of *Francisella tularensis*: infection and immunity in mice. *Infect Immun* 1991; 59:2922–2928.

45 Waag D M, Sandstrom G, England M J & Williams J C. Immunogenicity of a new lot of *Francisella tularensis* live vaccine strain in human volunteers. *FEMS Immunol Med Microbiol* 1996; 13:205–209.

FURTHER READING

Proceedings of the First International Conference on Tularaemia, Sweden, 1995. *FEMS Immunol Med Microbiol* 1996; 13:179–260.

Chapter 61D
Anthrax

G. Scott

Anthrax (Greek: black) is a disease of domestic herbivores caused by the bacterium *Bacillus anthracis*, which lives in topsoil and is ingested by the animals when grazing. Infection in humans is rare considering the potential exposure to the organism, and it presents as a local cutaneous lesion, gastrointestinal infection or with overwhelming pneumonia and disseminated disease.

Geographical distribution

Anthrax occurs worldwide but is 'endemic' in herbivorous livestock in certain regions. Domestic carnivores (dogs and cats) may be infected by eating contaminated carcasses. Human disease is most likely to occur in endemic regions (Iran,[1] central Africa, South America, Russia) by direct contact with infected carcasses. Industrial cases may occur anywhere and reflect exposure to imported animal carcass products such as bone meal (which used to be used for making glues) or hides.

Aetiology

B. anthracis is a large, non-motile, brick-shaped, aerobic, Gram-positive rod which has the capacity to make heat- and dry-resistant spores under adverse conditions. The spore is central and does not expand the bacterium. Spores may survive for decades in topsoil and resist high temperatures (e.g., 140°C in dry heat for 3 hours, and 100°C in moist heat for 10 minutes). The organism may be provisionally identified by Gram staining of pus aspirated from a lesion and will grow in air within 24 hours to give large irregular colonies on simple media. The edge of the colony is sometimes likened to Medusa's head, and the colony has a ground-glass appearance and adheres to the loop. The organism is then distinguished from other *Bacillus* spp. on chemical grounds and non-motility. Virulence is conferred by a capsule (which develops soon after germination in vivo and inhibits phagocytosis) and a complex exotoxin, which is plasmid determined. The exotoxin is released by germinating spores and replicating organisms, and consists of 'oedema' and 'lethal' factors together with a 'protective antigen' determinant.

Epidemiology and transmission

The sequence of events leading to the manifestation of anthrax in animals (and, usually subsequently, in humans) is complex and not completely understood. In areas of endemicity, the soil may be heavily contaminated by spores. These spores originated from vast numbers of organisms shed from animals who died from the disease. The bacteria have to compete with other soil bacteria, and rapid sporulation encouraged at high ambient temperature is critical to their survival. Vegetative forms die. Germination of spores occurs in conditions of high humidity, again encouraged by high temperature. In temperate conditions, although very humid, the temperature is rarely high enough to encourage either sporulation or germination, so it is rare for the topsoil to become significantly contaminated. Most new veterinary infection is imported with animal foodstuffs. The organism may be transmitted by insects, including house flies.[2,3]

If the summers are hot and dry, germination never occurs but the spores remain viable. If germination does occur after a period of rain followed by drought, animals will crop the grass down to the soil and be more likely to eat soil contaminated by the organisms. Humans will then tend to become infected during the dry season.[4] Infection of the animal is not well understood but it is thought that minor trauma from rough vegetation and soil itself in the mouth may cause a sufficient portal of entry. An infected animal that dies is loaded with vast numbers of bacteria.

Humans acquire infection by direct inoculation of spores through breaks in the skin, by inhalation of spores or by ingestion of contaminated meat. There may be some indirect person-to-person spread in peculiar circumstances: for example, an outbreak in The Gambia was in part traced to the use of communal loofahs when bathing,[4] and in the UK and Russia shaving brushes have been a source. In some areas, cutaneous disease is prevalent,[3,4] but in others the intestinal form is much more common,[5] a difference that has not been fully explained.

Clinical presentation

Cutaneous

After an incubation period of 2–3 days there is a small papule in the skin, perhaps with a central vesicle at the site of inoculation. A bacteriological diagnosis can be made from this point onwards. The next day, there are vesicles around the central lesion, which ulcerates and then dries leaving a black eschar. Atypically, there may be no vesicles. The eschar spreads to involve the vesicles as these dry up. There is no pain or even discomfort. The lesion does not discharge pus, but by the third day considerable local oedema has developed and the local lymph nodes are swollen. Anthrax lesions are common on the head and neck and exposed arms, but rarely on the hands. If lesions of the neck are associated with massive oedema, they may cause respiratory obstruction (Figure 61D.1). The lesion always resolves slowly, over a period of 2–6 weeks, despite appropriate antimicrobial treatment. The peripheral white cell count is usually normal.

Pulmonary

Classically, the patient inhales spores from contaminated hides. Wool sorters must be generally very resistant to disease because in factory conditions, when opening bales, they would be expected to inhale about 1000 spores during an 8-hour shift, yet rarely contract the disease. It appears that workers who are continuously exposed become relatively resistant to infection. However, there have been occasional unexplained outbreaks, possibly associated with a very large inoculum.

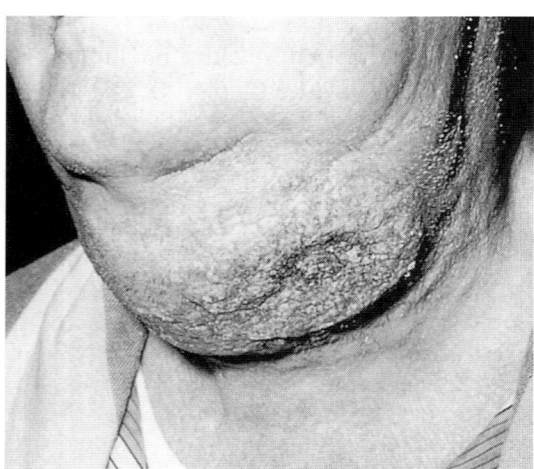

Figure 61D.1: Anthrax pustule on the jaw.

After a short incubation period, pulmonary anthrax starts with fever and chills, and the patient rapidly becomes cyanotic and short of breath. The lungs fill with interstitial fluid and the illness progresses inexorably to death over some days. The diagnosis is rarely made before death unless the history reveals occupational risk or doctors are alert to an outbreak.

Intestinal

Common in Africa[5] but very rare elsewhere in the world, this is thought to arise as a result of the consumption of contaminated meat. The presentation is non-specific with vomiting, diarrhoea and fever, occasionally with haematemesis and dysenteric stools. In autopsy cases an eschar may be found in the gut, but most patients recover spontaneously.

Other sites

Local lesions in the oropharynx may occur after eating contaminated meat—local severe oedema is again a prominent and life-threatening effect.[6] Bacteraemia may lead to infection at any site and will usually be fatal. Meningeal anthrax secondary to bacteraemia has been described.

Pathology

The organism is found in the capillaries. The malignant pustule is an area of local necrosis of the skin. In the lung, pulmonary oedema, haemorrhage, pleural effusion and mediastinitis are found but there is no single lesion. Generalized petechiae reflect vasculitis secondary to bloodstream spread. Often the spleen is enlarged and infected in fatal cases. Patients make antibody to the organism after natural infection, but the persistence of this antibody is very variable.

Differential diagnosis

A typical cutaneous malignant pustule is easy to recognize. Other local lesions that may cause confusion include tick bites with local rickettsia infection, orf, tularaemia, cutaneous diphtheria and plague. A scraping must be done and examined microscopically, a common alternative cause for the lesion being *Streptococcus pyogenes* with *Staphylococcus aureus*. In the early stages the lesion is just a small spot with a vesicle and is unlikely to present to a doctor. Oropharyngeal anthrax may be confused with diphtheria. Anthrax must be a very rare cause of overwhelming pneumonitis, for which the differential diagnosis is huge. A diagnosis of anthrax would be entertained only in someone with occupational or terrorist exposure.

Diagnosis

The organism is seen on direct scraping and aspiration—little pus is obtained—and will grow rapidly on simple media. Blood cultures are also useful.

Management

Penicillin remains the proven drug of choice and is best given intravenously in high doses to sick patients. Otherwise intramuscular penicillin (short and long acting) or oral amoxicillin appears to be satisfactory—the vast majority of patients with mild infection will to recover anyway. Co-trimoxazole seems to be a useful alternative, but the organism tends to be resistant to chloramphenicol. The clinical course of the severe illness is not materially modified by antibiotics. Strains resistant to penicillin will tend to be used in germ warfare, and the consensus view as to the drug of choice in this situation is ciprofloxacin.

Prevention

The population should be encouraged not to eat the meat of animals that become ill or die.[7,8] The spread of the disease from animals that have died from anthrax can be reduced by burying their carcasses in lime. Hides should be disinfected before export and occupational exposure reduced as far as possible by simple, sensible measures. There is no longer any place for the hyperimmune serum that used to be popular. However, a vaccine may be obtained for those at special risk of exposure[9] and live attenuated strains are under evaluation.[10] The protective antigen gene has recently been cloned into vaccinia and baculovirus vectors.[11]

Bioterrorism

Bacillus anthracis is perhaps the most suitable of all potential agents for germ warfare.[12] It is easy to grow in bulk, survives well in spore form and can be delivered as a powder on fomites and by the airborne route. Inhalational anthrax is almost always rapidly fatal. A cloud of spores released from a faulty plant in Sverdlovsk in the former USSR in 1979 caused many deaths in villagers downwind from the plant.[13] Construction of antibiotic-resistant mutants has been achieved.

REFERENCES

1 Amidi S, Dutz W, Kohout E & Ronaghy A. Human anthrax in Iran. Report of 300 cases and review of the literature. *Z Tropenmed Parasitol* 1974; 25:96–104.
2 McKendrick D R A. Anthrax and its transmission in humans. *Cent Afr J Med* 1980; 26:126–129.
3 Turner M. Anthrax in humans in Zimbabwe. *Cent Afr J Med* 1980; 26:160–161.
4 Heyworth B, Ropp M E, Meinel H & Darlow H M. Anthrax in the Gambia: an epidemiological study. *Br Med J* 1975; iv:79–82.
5 Fendall N R E & Grounds J G. The incidence and epidemiology of disease in Kenya. I. Some diseases of social significance. *J Trop Med Hyg* 1965; 68:77–84.
6 Sirisanthana T, Navachareon N, Tharavichitkul P, Sirisanthana V & Brown A E. Outbreak of oral–oropharyngeal anthrax: an unusual manifestation of human infection with *Bacillus anthracis*. *Am J Trop Med Hyg* 1984; 33:144–150.
7 Kunanusont C, Limpakarnjanarat K & Foy H M. Outbreak of anthrax in Thailand. *Ann Trop Med Parasitol* 1990; 84:507–512.
8 Sekhar P C, Singh R S, Sridhar M S, Bhaskar C J & Rao Y S. Outbreak of human anthrax in Ramabhadrapuram village of Chittar district of Andhra Pradesh. *Indian J Med Res* 1990; 91:448–452.
9 Turnbull P C. Anthrax vaccines: past, present and future. *Vaccine* 1991; 9:533–539.
10 Ivins B E, Welkos S L, Knudson G B & Little S F. Immunization against anthrax with aromatic compound-dependent (Aro-) mutants of *Bacillus anthracis* and with recombinant strains of *Bacillus subtilis* that produce anthrax protective antigen. *Infect Immun* 1990; 58:303–308.
11 Iacono-Connors L C, Welkos S L, Ivins B E & Dalrymple J M. Protection against anthrax with recombinant virus-expressed protective antigen in experimental animals. *Infect Immun* 1991; 59:1961–1965.
12 Klietmann WF, Ruoff KL. Bioterrorism: implications for the clinical microbiologist. *Clin Microbiol Rev* 2001; 14:364–381.
13 Meselson M, Guillemin J, Hugh-Jones M et al. The Sverdlovsk anthrax outbreak of 1979. *Science* 1994; 266:1202–1208.

Chapter 62
Tetanus

C. L. Thwaites, N. T. N. Nga and M. D. Smith

Tetanus is a disease characterized by muscle rigidity and spasms. It derives its name from the Greek word 'tetanos' meaning 'to contract'. Despite the World Health Organization's efforts to eradicate the disease by 1995, tetanus remains one of the world's major preventable causes of death, estimated to cause up to 1 million deaths a year.[1]

People have recognized the association between wounds and subsequent rigidity, spasms and death since ancient times. The Edwin Smith papyrus (1000 BC) outlines the case of a man with a scalp wound who developed trismus and muscle rigidity. Hippocrates (400 BC) describes a similar case of a man who, having sustained a penetrating wound to the back, experienced trismus and muscle spasms then died on the second day of the illness.[2] However, it was not until 1880 that Nicolaier demonstrated that soil contamination of wounds resulted in tetanus. Nicolaier also discovered identical bacilli in the wounds, but it was Kitasato who isolated the first pure culture of *Clostridium tetani* 9 years later. In 1890, Faber discovered tetanus toxin, the same year as von Berhring and Kitasato produced the first antitoxin. Then, using formaldehyde, Ramon succeeded in detoxifying tetanus toxin, yet still preserving its antigenicity. In 1926 he performed the first successful vaccination of humans.[2]

The availability of a tetanus vaccine has enabled developed countries to virtually eliminate the disease. However *C. tetani* will never be eradicated from the soil and so wherever vaccination programmes are ineffective or inadequate, tetanus will continue to occur.

Epidemiology

C. tetani is a ubiquitous organism, present in the soil and in human and animal faeces. The disease it causes is now primarily confined to developing countries where immunization is either not available or vaccine supplies are of poor quality, often as a consequence of substandard preparation and storage procedures.[1] Eighty per cent of tetanus cases occur in Africa and South-East Asia. In these countries tetanus remains one the most common infectious causes of death, particularly of neonates but also of children and young adults. In the developed world tetanus is rare: in 1998 there were seven cases in the UK and 41 in the USA (including one neonate). Most of these cases occurred in the elderly—a group at increased risk due to declining protective antibody levels.[3]

Neonatal tetanus is one of the world's most under-reported notifiable diseases (in some countries only 4% of cases are reported by routine surveillance systems). In 1993 an estimated 515 000 neonatal deaths occurred worldwide—giving a global mortality of 4.1 per 1000 live births.[4] The disease usually arises from contamination of the umbilical stump. Infection is linked to traditional midwifery practices such as cutting the umbilical cord with bamboo and applying soil, cow dung, clarified butter or even engine oil to the umbilical stump. Ritual surgery such as ear-piercing or circumcision may also cause infection.[5] Even after maternal immunization, the infant is still at risk in many countries as malaria and HIV reduce placental transfer of protective antibody.[6, 7]

In children and adults, lacerations to feet and hands are common injuries associated with tetanus. Otitis media is an important portal for the disease in children. Tetanus arising from intramuscular injections carries an especially poor prognosis and in particular following intramuscular injection of quinine, when it is almost always fatal.[8] Quinine causes local necrosis, creating a particularly favourable environment for *C. tetani* multiplication. The usual quinine preparation is acidic and low pH is known to facilitate toxin entry into nerves in vitro.

Quinine has also been implicated as the cause of high mortality in intravenous drug abusers, another group with a poor prognosis. A fulminating form of the disease was described in the 1940s in New York drug addicts.[9] At the time quinine was 'cut' with the narcotics as its bitter taste was similar to that of heroin. Drug abusers continue to exhibit a rapidly progressing severe form of the disease for unclear reasons. Their prognosis remains poor despite modern intensive care facilities.[10]

Bacteriology

C. tetani is a strictly anaerobic Gram-positive bacillus is found in soil and animal faeces. When subjected to adverse conditions rounded terminal spores are formed: this gives the classical 'drumstick' appearance to the bacillus, although this is not always seen. *C. tetani* is described as Gram positive, but from cultures more than 24 hours old it is readily decolourized and thus can appear to be Gram negative. It is motile by means of numerous flagella and when cultured on blood agar this results in swarming, giving a film with a feathery margin on the surface of the agar. Increasing the concentration of agar in the medium will inhibit swarming. Discrete colonies are flat, translucent and show a narrow zone of haemolysis.

The biochemical activity of *C. tetani* is limited. In general it does not ferment sugars, although some strains will ferment glucose. Gelatin is slowly hydrolysed but other proteins used in laboratory tests are not digested. Indole is produced slowly, but not hydrogen sulphide. Neither lecithinase nor lipase are produced. Gas–liquid chromatography of broth culture extracts reveals the major bacterial products to be acetic, butyric and proprionic acids.

Antibiotics to which the bacilli of *C. tetani* are susceptible include penicillin, erythromycin, clindamycin, tetracycline, chloramphenicol and metronidazole. The spores are very resistant to many physical and chemical agents. Spores may survive in boiling water for several minutes or longer (although they are destroyed by autoclaving at 121°C for 15–20 minutes), and they can survive desiccation, most household disinfectants and marked changes in pH. Spores are commonly found in soil from all areas of the world, and the organism may be found in animal and human faeces although isolation rates have varied widely.[11]

Pathogenesis

C. tetani requires low oxygen tensions for germination and multiplication. In well-oxygenated healthy tissue germination does not occur and spores are removed by phagocytes. However, if spores are inoculated into damaged tissue, along with adjuvants such as soil, faeces, chemical substances or other bacteria, local oxygen tensions are lowered and favourable conditions are created for germination and vegetative growth.[12]

Tetanus is a toxin-mediated disease and only toxin-producing strains of *C. tetani* are capable of causing disease. Tetanus toxin is a potent neurotoxin. It is encoded on a 75 KB plasmid, and produced as a single chain (molecular mass 150 kDa) which undergoes post-translational cleavage to form one heavy and one light chain linked by a disulphide bond.[13] The entire amino acid sequence has been determined and is similar to that of the botulinum toxins.[14] Botulinum toxins are also potent neurotoxins but, unlike tetanus toxin, are not transported into the central nervous system, and consequently produce a flaccid paralysis by presynaptic inhibition of neurotransmitter release.[15]

Tetanus toxin enters the nervous system from adjacent muscle. It may also be disseminated to distant sites via the lymphatics and the blood. It is unlikely that it penetrates the blood–brain barrier directly; instead it undergoes internalization, retrograde axonal transport from the periphery, then trans-synaptic transition to presynaptic nerves, where it exerts its effects.[16] Internalization results from binding of the carboxy terminal of the heavy chain to gangliosides GT_{1b} and GD_{1b}. These gangliosides are predominantly neuronal and hence the neurospecificity of the toxin. The toxin light chain is a zinc-dependent metalloprotease which cleaves the vesicle-associated membrane protein 2, VAMP-2 (or Synaptobrevin).[17] This protein is a key component of the SNARE (soluble *N*-ethylmalemide-sensitive factor attachment protein receptors) complex responsible for endocytosis and release of neurotransmitter. By this mechanism, tetanus toxin blocks the release of neurotransmitter. The toxin acts as a presynaptic inhibitor at many neuronal sites including the neuromuscular junction, but its principal effect is on the γ-aminobutyric acid (GABA) inhibitory interneurones, normally responsible for inhibition of α motor neurones. Reduced inhibition at this site results in disinhibited motor neurone discharge which gives rise to characteristic features of muscle rigidity and spasms. Muscle groups with the shortest neuronal pathways are affected first—hence trismus and dysphagia are common early symptoms.

Disinhibition of the autonomic nervous system also occurs and results in uncontrolled sympathetic and parasympathetic discharge. Tetanus toxin is able to enter adjacent neurones and spread within the CNS. Animal experiments with radiolabelled toxin show transportation of toxin within the brain stem.[18] The effects of toxin here may explain the cardiovascular, respiratory and temperature disturbances seen in severe cases of the disease.

Clinical picture

Tetanus is characterized by muscular rigidity and spasms. It is sometimes confined to muscles adjacent to the site of the wound (local or cephalic tetanus) but usually involves the whole body (generalized tetanus).

Following wound contamination with *C. tetani*, there is a period of a few days or weeks before symptoms occur. This is termed the 'incubation period'. The first symptom is usually trismus, or 'lockjaw', as a result of rigidity of the masseter muscles. As the disease progresses, rigidity spreads to all muscle groups, usually in a descending fashion. Admission data from 500 consecutive patients admitted to the Centre for Tropical Diseases, Ho Chi Minh City, Vietnam, revealed that lockjaw, muscle stiffness and backache are almost universal presenting complaints.[19]

In very mild forms of tetanus rigidity may be the only symptom. However, most patients will progress to experience spasms. Spasms are phasic amplifications in muscle tone, varying in intensity and duration from brief twitches to prolonged contractions. They are most pronounced during the first 2 weeks of the disease. Spasms occur spontaneously or as a result of stimuli such as loud noises, bright lights or physical manipulation. Spasms can be strong enough to cause vertebral fractures or tendon avulsions and are excruciatingly painful.[20] The latter may be partly due to disinhibition of pain pathways within the spinal cord. Facial muscle involvement results in the characteristic facial appearance of the 'risus sardonicus' or 'sardonic smile' (Figure 62.1). Involvement of muscles of the back and neck produces opisthotonos accompanied by head retraction. Particularly serious are

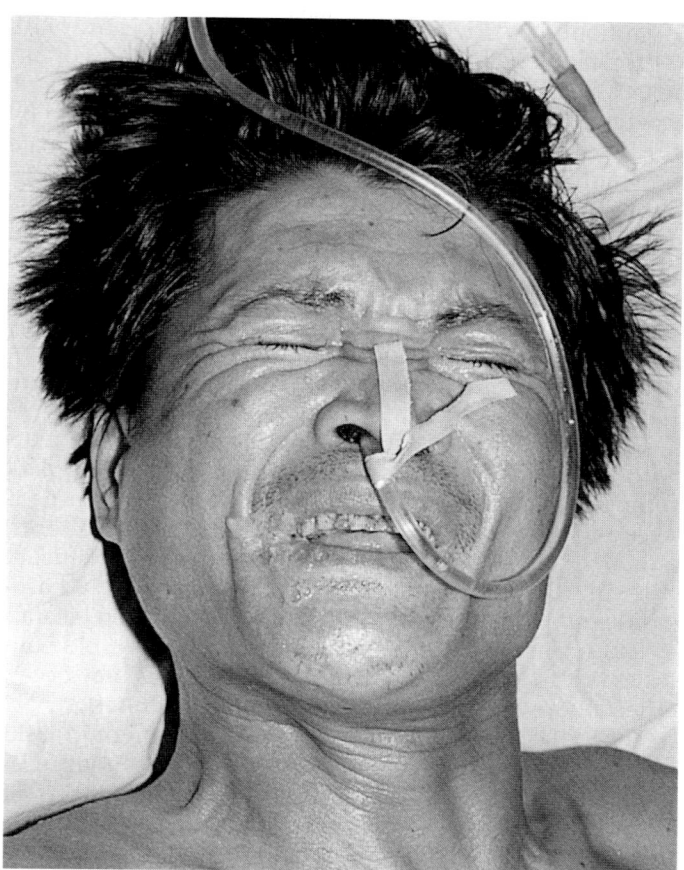

Figure 62.1: Tetanus: risus sardonicus with profuse salivation.

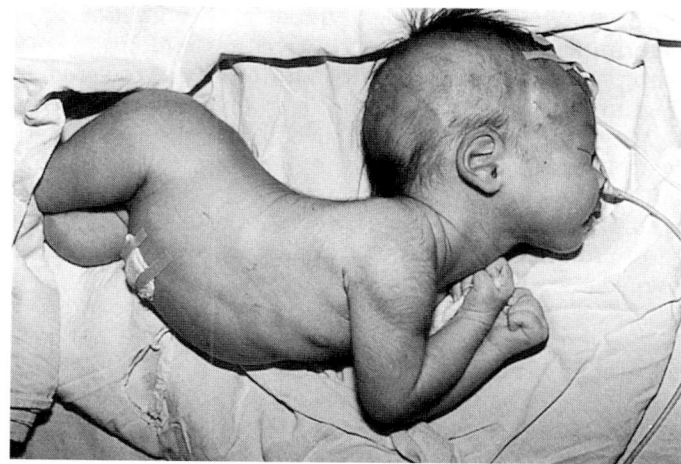

Figure 62.2: Neonatal tetanus: typical features of generalized tetanus resulting from an infected umbilical stump.

spasms involving the respiratory muscles which, if frequent or prolonged, may result in death due to asphyxia. Laryngeal spasm involving the vocal cords usually occurs without warning relatively early in the course of the disease and can result in acute airway obstruction. Aspiration is a particular problem in tetanus, occurring as a consequence of the combination of excessive secretions and inability to swallow due to pharyngeal muscle rigidity. Together these factors explain why hypoxia is a common feature in those presenting with moderate to severe tetanus.[21]

The advent of mechanical ventilation has led to a reduction in mortality from respiratory failure, but in doing so has unmasked another major cause of mortality: the syndrome of autonomic overactivity. This usually becomes apparent during the second week of the illness and typically takes the form of sustained labile hypertension and tachycardia, accompanied by pyrexia and profuse sweating. The peripheries remain cool to the touch.[22] The variation in blood pressure is primarily due to changes in systemic vascular resistance, with little change in the cardiac index.[23] Circulating catecholamines are raised, sometimes up to levels seen in phaeochromocytoma,[24] and may cause direct myocardial toxicity.[25] Occasionally, the opposite occurs: bradyarrhythmias, refractory hypotension and even cardiac arrest. This is usually a preterminal event.

Autonomic system dysfunction commonly affects the gastrointestinal system, resulting in excessive production of secretions, gastric stasis or diarrhoea. The syndrome is also associated with acute renal failure. This occurs in the absence of rhabdomyolysis and is characteristically non-oliguric.[26]

Severe tetanus often requires 3–4 weeks of intensive care treatment. As a consequence, the various problems of prolonged hospitalization become apparent after the second week of the illness: nosocomial infections are common, as are gastrointestinal bleeding and pressure sores.

The clinical features of neonatal tetanus are similar to those in older people. Figure 62.2 illustrates the characteristic appearance. Infants usually present between 5 and 28 days of age. Those whose mothers have received prior vaccination experience milder disease. Infants present with stiffness, inability to feed and spasms. The ability to cry signifies a good prognosis as it indicates the respiratory muscles and vocal cords are functioning. Aspiration is common and one-third of infants have concomitant septicaemia.[27] The organisms responsible are mainly coliforms and *Staphylococcus aureus*.

Prognosis in all patients depends upon the severity of the disease, occurrence of complications and the setting. With modern intensive care facilities mortality rates of less than 10% have been reported. However, without such facilities mortality figures of greater than 45% (and higher in neonates) are common.[5] A short incubation period (time from injury to first symptom) of 4 days or less generally indicates severe disease. The period between the first symptom and the development of muscular spasms is termed the period of onset. Shorter periods of onset, particularly less than 48 hours, are again associated with more severe forms of tetanus. Several authors have a produced prognostic scoring systems. The two most popular are Dakar and Phillips.[28,29] These take into account the incubation period, clinical signs, the state of immune protection and the nature of the injury.

For those who survive, residual effects include limb deformities due to residual contractures which improve with physiotherapy, and chest deformities due to vertebral fractures. Rehabilitation is hindered by persisting muscle rigidity which may last for several months. Temporary neurological sequelae following tetanus include irritability, sleep disturbance, fits and myoclonus.[30] Neonatal tetanus may have more lasting sequelae, especially in those infants who experienced prolonged periods of hypoxia.

Diagnosis

The diagnosis of tetanus is clinical, based on the history and examination findings. For an experienced clinician there is little difficulty in making the diagnosis. There are no confirmatory tests, although some may help exclude other diseases. There may be no obvious site of entry and isolation of *C. tetani* from a wound is not diagnostic without the characteristic clinical picture. A definite history of immunization would argue against a diagnosis of tetanus, although tetanus has been reported in patients with conventionally 'protective' levels of antibody. The spatula test is useful in distinguishing tetanus from other causes of masseter spasm. Sudden depression of the tongue with a spatula produces a reflex spasms of masseter muscles causing the patient to bite down strongly on the spatula.

The differential diagnosis includes strychnine poisoning, which may closely mimic tetanus. Strychnine is a competitive antagonist of the inhibitory neurotransmitter glycine, which results in presynaptic disinhibition, leading to hyperreflexia, severe muscle spasms and convulsions. There is usually a history of ingestion and symptoms may begin within 30 minutes; toxicological tests of urine, serum or gastric contents can confirm the diagnosis.

Dystonic reactions to phenothiazines may simulate trismus and may cause spasms of the back resembling opisthotonos. However, the abnormality rapidly disappears after administration of anticholinergic agents.

Management

Management of tetanus is essentially supportive. It involves three main strategies: to prevent further toxin release, to neutralize any unbound toxin and to minimize effects of already-bound toxin while maintaining the airway and adequate respiration.

Prompt debridement of the wound is essential to prevent further multiplication and toxin release of *C. tetani*. Metronidazole is the antibiotic of choice, although penicillin is still widely used. Patients treated with metronidazole have fewer spasms and require less sedation than those treated with penicillin.[31] Penicillin is similar in structure to GABA, and although it does not readily cross the blood–brain barrier, in high doses it can act as a central GABA competitive antagonist, thus exacerbating the effects of tetanus toxin.

Unbound toxin should be neutralized with antitoxin. Historically equine antitetanus serum has been used, but it is associated with a high incidence of anaphylactic reactions. In many countries it has now been replaced by the human tetanus immune globulin (HTIG). Much debate has centred on the best route of administration of antitoxin. Results of animal experiments almost 100 years ago suggested that intrathecal administration of antitoxin may be superior. Meta-analysis of the available evidence concludes uncertain benefit in humans.[32] At present, the intrathecal route of administration should not be recommended. Common formulations are unlicensed for intrathecal use and there remains concern as to the potential neurotoxicity of some of the preparations.

Good nursing care is crucial to the outcome of patients with tetanus. All patients should be nursed in quiet, dark rooms to minimize provoked spasms. Frequent turning is necessary to prevent the development of pressure sores, although truncal rigidity of the patients makes this difficult. Patients who are unable to swallow will require a nasogastric tube. Close attention should be paid to fluid balance as tetanus patients have greatly increased insensible fluid losses. Up to 3.5 litres a day of insensible losses may occur, especially in the presence of autonomic dysfunction.[33]

Benzodiazepines are the mainstay of treatment in mild to moderate tetanus. As inhibitors of an endogenous inhibitor at the $GABA_A$ receptor they oppose the effects of tetanus toxin on the GABA-ergic neurones. Diazepam is the most commonly used although its long half-life, and those of its metabolites, may cause prolonged effects. It can be given orally in mild cases, or intravenously in more severe disease. Doses up to 100 mg/hour have been reported, and up to 200 mg a day is common. Intravenous infusion of midazolam may be a preferred option by virtue of its shorter half-life, although prolonged use will still lead to accumulation. The anaesthetic agent propofol has been used to provide sedation and additional muscle relaxation. It is non-cumulative and has a short duration of action, making it an attractive adjunct.[34]

If spasms persist despite benzodiazepine therapy then paralysis and mechanical ventilation should be instituted. Non-depolarizing muscle relaxants with minimal cardiovascular effects, such as vecuronium or cisatracurium, are the muscle relaxants of choice. Older agents, such as pancuronium, may exacerbate autonomic instability. Tracheostomy is the usual means of securing the airway, allowing ventilation and secretion clearance. Patients with laryngeal spasm may require urgent tracheostomy. For this reason all tetanus patients should be nursed under close supervision with appropriately skilled personnel at hand to deal with any emergencies.

Tetanus literature contains many reports of the use of other agents[19] used to treat spasticity: dantrolene has been used to reduce spontaneous muscular spasms, but it is potentially hepatotoxic if used for prolonged periods. The $GABA_B$ agonist baclofen has successfully suppressed spasticity in cases where diazepam failed.

In patients with autonomic instability the usual manifestation is a tachycardia accompanied by hypertension.

First-line therapy in this situation is intravenous or intramuscular morphine. It inhibits sympathetically mediated vasoconstriction and induces peripheral arteriolar vasodilatation by inhibiting central sympathetic discharge. Up to 140 mg a day may be required.[35] Peripheral β-adrenoceptor blockade alone is usually insufficient to gain satisfactory cardiovascular control in severe cases of tetanus. The relatively long duration of action of most agents has been associated with subsequent refractory hypotension and cardiac arrest. The combined α- and β-blocker labetolol may confer some advantages, but its duration of action is still be too long to be a useful alternative. The new short-acting β-blocker esmolol, however, has been used successfully. Peak effects are observed within 6–10 minutes of injection, and have almost completely disappeared after 20 minutes. Chlorpromazine, clonidine and epidural bupivacaine have all been used with success in the past.[19] Recent interest has surrounded magnesium sulphate—a vasodilator and muscle relaxant that offers the potential to control both muscle spasms and autonomic instability.

Hypotension may be treated by head-down positioning, noxious stimulation or inotropic agents. Bradyarrhythmias require atropine.

Finally, the amount of toxin circulating in natural disease is insufficient to provoke an immunizing antibody response. Therefore all patients should receive a course of tetanus toxoid to prevent recurrences.

Prevention

The prevention of tetanus depends on primary immunization and the thorough management of wounds in those people who have not been immunized or whose immune status is thought to be inadequate. In addition, health education and improved socio-economic conditions are important: for example, the use of aseptic techniques in the management of the umbilical cord and the provision of adequate protective footwear.

Tetanus toxoid is produced by formaldehyde treatment of the toxin (plain toxoid). Although it is a relatively good immunogen, the duration of antibody response is much improved by adsorption with aluminium hydroxide as an adjuvant. In many countries a course of three injections of adsorbed toxoid is given for active immunization. A protective antibody level is attained after the second dose but a third dose is recommended to ensure prolonged immunity. In the UK the first dose is given at 2 months of age, followed by the second and third doses at 4-week intervals.[36] Adsorbed toxoid is available in combination with diphtheria toxoid and pertussis vaccine (DTP) for use in these immunization schedules of young children. Two booster doses of tetanus and diphtheria toxoids (DT) are given at 3–5 years of age and at 13–18 years old. In the USA an initial four-dose schedule is recommended with intervals of 4–8 weeks between the first three doses and the fourth dose 6–12 months later. A booster is given at 4–6 years old and again 10 years later.[37] Adults and older

children who have not been immunized previously should also receive a primary course of three doses of adsorbed tetanus toxoid. In the USA advice is to give additional booster doses of adsorbed tetanus toxoid every 10 years. However, in the UK more recent advice is that five doses (primary course plus two boosters) are sufficient and additional booster doses are not recommended unless a tetanus-prone wound occurs.[36] Reactions to tetanus toxoid are infrequent, and usually local and mild. They may be more severe if booster doses are given more often than outlined.

Neonatal tetanus may be prevented by immunization of women during pregnancy. Two or preferably three doses of adsorbed toxoid should be given, with the last dose at least 2–4 weeks prior to delivery. Immunity is passively transferred to the fetus and the antibodies will remain long enough to protect the baby during the neonatal period. In subsequent pregnancies a single booster can be given at 6 months gestation, but if pregnancies are frequent boosters should only be given every 5 years. Special care should be taken to ensure those with HIV or living in malaria endemic areas receive a full course of vaccination.[6,7]

One problem with these immunization schedules is their complexity. In the developing world, particularly in rural areas, people may not return for the second and subsequent doses; therefore a single-dose regimen is desirable. This has been achieved by using much larger doses of toxoid or using a different adjuvant such as calcium phosphate.[38] However, the response is delayed and if used in pregnant women it should be given 6 months prior to delivery.

Prevention of tetanus also depends on the effective management of wounds. It is most important that wounds are thoroughly cleaned, all foreign material removed and non-viable tissue debrided. Particular attention should be given to tetanus-prone wounds. These include puncture wounds, burns, animal and human bites, wounds contaminated with soil or faeces, and any wound where treatment is delayed. These wounds should not be sutured: packing, frequent inspection and delayed primary closure is preferable. Antibiotic chemoprophylaxis is of secondary importance to good surgical management and immunoprophylaxis. When indicated, a long-acting penicillin can be given. If the wound is infected with β-lactamase-producing staphylococci an appropriate alternative antibiotic such as erythromycin or flucloxacillin should be used.

A history of previous immunization should be sought as this will determine the exact type of immunoprophylaxis to be given. If the patient has received a full course or a booster of tetanus toxoid within 10 years, a further dose is not required. If the last dose was more than 10 years ago a further dose should be given. Where there is doubt about previous immunization or a full course was never completed, a full course of adsorbed tetanus toxoid should be commenced.[36]

Passive immunization with HTIG (250 units) should also be given for tetanus-prone wounds occurring in people with inadequate immunization status (i.e. incomplete, unknown or a booster more than 10 years ago). Even where immunization is adequate (the last dose within 10 years) a dose of HTIG may be given if the risk of developing tetanus is high. If HTIG is not available, equine antiserum (1500 units) is an alternative. Very high-risk wounds are those with heavy soil or faecal con- tamination, extensive burns, or where foreign material or necrotic tissue cannot be removed. In these cases the dose of HTIG should be doubled to 500 units and a further dose may be given after 4 weeks if the wound is still not clean or healed.[37] Both toxoid and immunoglobulin can be given at the same time provided that separate injection sites are used.

REFERENCES

1   Dietz V, Milstien J B, van Loon F, Cochi S & Bennett J. Performance and potency of tetanus toxoid: implications for eliminating neonatal tetanus. *Bull World Health Organ* 1996; 74(6):619–628.

2   Urwadia F E. Historical perspective. In Urwadia F E (ed.) *Tetanus*. New York: Oxford University Press, 1994: 1–6.

3   Cumberland N S, Kidd A G & Karalliedde L. Immunity to tetanus in United Kingdom populations. *J Infect* 1993; 27:255–260.

4   Progress towards the global elimination of tetanus, 1989–93. *JAMA* 1995; 273(3):196–197.

5   Eregie C O & Ofovwe G. Factors associated with neonatal tetanus mortality in northern Nigeria. *East Afr Med J* 1995; 72(8):507–509.

6   Brair M E, Brabin B J, Milligan P, Maxwell S & Hart C A. Reduced transfer of tetanus antibodies with placental malaria. *Lancet* 1994; 343:208–209.

7   De Moraes-Pinto M I, Almeida A C M, Kenj G et al. Placental transfer and maternally acquired neonatal IgG immunity in human immunodeficiency virus infection. *J Infect Dis* 1996; 173:1–8.

8   Yen L M, Doa L M, Day N P J et al. Role of quinine in the high mortality of intramuscular injection in tetanus. *Lancet* 1994; 344:786–787.

9   Cherubin C E. Epidemiology of tetanus in narcotic addicts. *NY State J Med* 1970; 15:267–271.

10 Sun K O, Chan Y W, Cheung R T F, So P C, Yu Y L & Li P C K. Management of tetanus: a review of 18 cases. *J R Soc Med* 1994; 87:135–137.

11 Ichiro S & Nishida S. Isolation of *Clostridium tetani* from soil. *J Bacteriol* 1965; 89(3):626–629.

12 Smith J W G & Collee J G. Tetanus. In Smith R S and Easmon C S F (eds) *Topley and Wilson's Principles of Bacteriology, Virology and Immunity*, vol. 3, 8th edn. London: Edward Arnold, 1990: 331–351.

13 Weller U, Dauzenroth M E, Meyer zu Heringdorf D & Habermann E. Chains and fragments of tetanus toxin: separation, reassociation and pharmacological properties. *Eur J Biochem* 1989; 182(3):649–656.

14 Eisel U, Jarausch W, Goretzki K et al. Tetanus toxin: primary structure, expression in E. coli and homology with botulinum toxins. *EMBO J* 1986; 5(10):2495–2502.

15 Blasi J, Chapman E R, Link E et al. Botulinum neurotoxin A selectively cleaves the synaptic protein SNAP-25. *Nature* 1993; 365(6442):160–163.

16 Mellanby J & Green J. How does tetanus toxin act? *Neuroscience* 1981; 6(3):281–300.

17 Li Y, Foran P, Fairweather N et al. A single mutation in recombinant light chain of tetanus toxin abolishes its proteolytic activity and removes toxicity seen after reconstitution with native heavy chain. *Biochemistry* 1994; 33(22):7014–7020.

18 Cobot J B, Mennone A, Bogan N, Carroll J, Evinger C & Erichsen J T. Retrograde trans-synaptic and transneuronal transport of fragment C of tetanus toxin by sympathetic preganglionic neurones. *Neuroscience* 1991; 40(3):805–823.

19 Farrar J J, Yen L M, Cook T et al. Tetanus. *J Neurol Neurosurg Psychiatry* 2000; 69(3):292–301.

20 Urwadia F E. Complications. In Urwardia F E (ed.) *Tetanus*. New York: Oxford University Press, 1994: 77–87.

21 Femi-Pearse D. Blood gas tensions, acid–base status and spirometry in tetanus. *Am Rev Respir Dis* 1974; 110:390–394.

22 Kerr J H, Corbett J L, Prys-Roberts C, Crampton Smith A & Spalding J M K. Involvement of the sympathetic nervous system in tetanus. *Lancet* 1968; 2:236–241.

23 De Michele D J & Da Silva A M T. Cardiovascular findings in a patient with severe tetanus. *Crit Care Med* 1983; 11(10):828–829.

24 Kelty S R, Gray R C, Dundee J W & McCullough H. Catecholamine levels in severe tetanus. *Lancet* 1968; 2(7561):195.

25 Rose A G. Catecholamine-induced myocardial damage associated with phaeochromocytomas and tetanus. *S Afr Med J* 1974; 48:1285–1289.

26 Daher E F, Abdulkader R C R M, Motti E, Marcondes M, Sabbaga E & Burdmann E A. Prospective study of tetanus- induced acute renal dysfunction: role of adrenergic overactivity. *Am J Trop Med Hyg* 1997; 57(5):610–614.

27 Antia-Obong O E, Ekanem E E, Udo J J & Utsalo S J. Septicaemia among neonates with tetanus. *J Trop Pediatr* 1992; 38:173–175.

28 Phillips L A. A classification of tetanus. *Lancet* 1967; 1(7501):1216–1217.

29 Veronsisi R & Focaccia R. The clinical picture. In Veronisi R (ed.) *Tetanus: Important New Concepts*. Amsterdam: Excerpta Medica; 1981: 183–210.

30 Illis L S & Taylor F M. Neurological and electroencephalographic sequelae of tetanus. *Lancet* 1971; 1(7704):826–830.

31 Yen L M, Dao L M, Day N P J et al. Management of tetanus: a comparison of penicillin and metronidazole. In *Symposium of Antimicrobial Resistance in Southern Viet Nam*, 1997.

32 Abrutyn E & Berlin J A. Intrathecal therapy in tetanus: a meta- analysis. *JAMA* 1991; 266(16):2262–2267.

33 Kerr J H. Insensible fluid losses in severe tetanus. *Intensive Care Med* 1981; 7:209–212.

34 Borgeat A, Popovic V & Schwander D. Efficiency of a continuous infusion of propofol in a patient with tetanus. *Crit Care Med* 1991; 19:295–297.

35 Rie M A & Wilson R S. Morphine therapy controls autonomic hyperactivity in tetanus. *Ann Intern Med* 1978; 88:653–654.

36 Department of Health. *Immunisation against Infectious Disease*. London: HMSO, 1996.

37 Centers for Disease Control. Update on adult immunization. Recommendations of the Immunization Practice Advisory Committee (ACIP). *Morbid Mortal Weekly Rep* 1991; 40:47–52, 67–71, 73, 77–81, 86–94.

38 Veronesi R. Prophylaxis. In Veronesi R (ed.) *Tetanus: Important New Concepts*. Amsterdam: Excerpta Medica, 1981: 238–263.

Chapter 63
Plague

M. D. Smith

Plague is an acute infectious disease caused by the organism *Yersinia pestis*. It is a zoonosis, transmitted mainly by the bite(s) of infected fleas. Wild rodents are the natural reservoir. In man the most common clinical presentation is bubonic plague (regional lymphadenitis) which accounts for over 90% of reported cases. Other forms include septicaemic plague without bubo, pneumonic plague (either primary or secondary to bacteraemia), meningitis and pharyngitis. Asymptomatic and minor self-limiting infections also occur.

Plague is best known as an ancient disease (pestilence), although it remains endemic in many parts of the world today. There have been three documented world pandemics. The first was in the sixth century. In the fourteenth century, the Black Death swept across Europe killing between one-quarter and one-third of the entire population. The third pandemic originated in China in 1860 and reached Hong Kong in 1894. It was here that Alexandre Yersin successfully isolated the causative organism. The pandemic spread—by rats on board ships, to South-East Asia, India, Africa and the Americas. The infection was then transmitted to sylvatic rodents, allowing it to become established in rural areas. In India there may have been up to ten million deaths by 1919. During the 1960s and early 1970s there was a resurgence of plague in Vietnam, with a peak of over 4000 cases per year.

Epidemiology

Plague is still reported consistently from several countries in Africa, Asia, South America, and the USA. During the 1990s an average of 2650 cases were reported annually to the World Health Organization (WHO). Between 1995 and 1999, half of the world total cases occurred in Madagascar (8416 cases); other leading countries during this period were Tanzania (2988 cases), Mozambique (1571 cases) and Vietnam (949 cases). In the USA a few cases continue to occur every year.[1]

Foci of infection (Figure 63.1) are maintained worldwide in natural animal reservoirs, and transmission occurs by bites of infected fleas or ingestion of infected animals. In Asia and Africa the domestic black rat *Rattus rattus* and the brown sewer rat *R. norvegicus* remain the most important animal reservoir(s) for transmission of plague to man. A sudden 'die off' in these urban rodents may presage human plague. Other rodents maintain the infection in the field, for example *R. exulans* in Asia, and *Mastomys* spp. and gerbils in Africa (Figure 63.2). The most important flea vector involved in transmission is *Xenopsylla cheopis*.

In the USA, plague is maintained in sylvatic rodents such as ground squirrels, rock squirrels and prairie dogs. These animals may enter areas of human habitation directly, or the infected fleas may be carried by domestic cats and dogs. Occasional cases of human plague have also resulted from direct contact with infected cats.[2]

A distinct seasonal pattern is seen. Most cases occur in warm dry periods when fleas are most abundant and humans are most likely to come into contact with the natural hosts. In the highland plateaus of Madagascar the plague season is September–April, whereas on the west

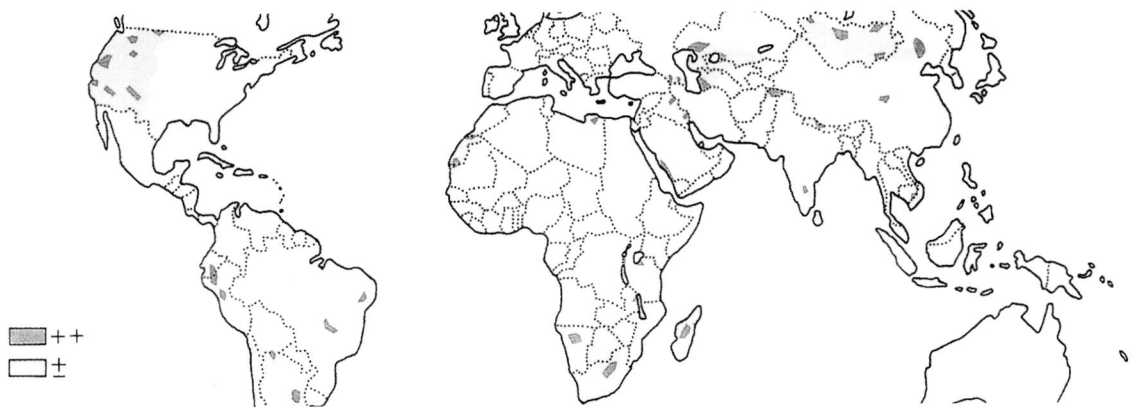

Figure 63.1: Known and probable foci of plague. ++, Frequent transmission; ±, infrequent or suspected transmission.

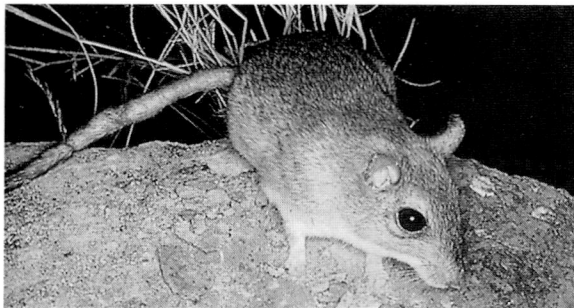

Figure 63.2: *Tatera robusta*. Several gerbils from this genus have been found infected with *Y. pestis* in East and South Africa, as well as in India where they are associated with focal outbreaks in humans.

coast it is July–November.[3] In Vietnam the peak months are March–April.

Bacteriology

Y. pestis is a small Gram-negative coccobacillus, which commonly exhibits bipolar staining and pleomorphism, particularly in clinical specimens. The genus *Yersinia* belongs to the family Enterobacteriaceae. *Y. pestis* is non-motile and non-spore forming. Both in vivo and in culture on serum agar at 37°C a capsule-like envelope may be formed. It grows aerobically on many common culture media, including nutrient agar and blood agar, and forms tiny colourless, often granular, colonies after 24 hours at 37°C; there is no haemolysis. On MacConkey agar it appears as pinpoint non-lactose fermenting colonies, which disappear after two to three days, presumably due to autolysis. Biochemically, *Y. pestis* is catalase positive, oxidase negative and reduces nitrate but does not hydrolyse urea. It does not utilize citrate or produce indole. Glucose and mannitol are fermented, but not sucrose or lactose. On triple sugar–iron agar slants it produces an acid butt and an alkaline slope. Identification of *Y. pestis* is confirmed by specific phage lysis.

The organism is susceptible to adverse conditions but can survive for many months in the cool damp conditions of the soil in rodent burrows. Organisms are killed by heating at 56°C for 15 minutes, and by exposure to sunlight for four hours. They may survive drying for a few days, but survival is prolonged in dried blood and secretions.

Pathogenesis

Y. pestis produces a number of virulence factors encoded either chromosomally or on one of three plasmids.[4] A temperature-dependent coagulase is produced during infection of the flea, which causes clotting of blood in the proventriculus. As a consequence of this blockage of the flea's foregut, blood containing many organisms is regurgitated during subsequent attempts to feed. The coagulase is most active at temperatures below 30°C but is inactive at 35°C or above. Fleas are cold blooded and

these observations may explain why transmission of plague ceases in the hot seasons in endemic areas.[5] Fraction 1 antigen is a capsular glycoprotein which enables the organism to evade phagocytosis; it is produced at 37°C but not below 27°C. Thus in the flea and when first inoculated into humans these organisms express F1 antigen poorly and are easily phagocytosed, but not killed, by neutrophils and monocytes. However, subsequent generations express F1 antigen fully, enabling them to avoid phagocytosis. The 'low calcium response', mediated by a 70 kb plasmid, occurs at 37°C but not 26°C, and is important for adaptation to an intracellular environment. This enables the bacterium to step down growth and initiate synthesis of various virulence factors under conditions of low calcium concentrations, such as found in the phagolysosome.[4] These include soluble V antigen, which is present within the cyotoplasm or secreted from the cell. V antigen is an essential virulence factor and is highly immunogenic. The exact function of V antigen is not known, but it appears to maintain bacteriostasis,[4] suppress pro-inflammatory cytokines[6] and inhibit neutrophil chemotaxis.[7] *Yersinia* outer membrane proteins (Yops) are also produced, of which type E appears to be important for virulence.[8]

Other virulence factors include pH 6 antigen, pigment production and classical lipopolysaccharide endotoxin. The largest plasmid also encodes for a murine exotoxin, which is essentially lethal for mice and rats only.[4]

Pathology

The essential feature of plague in man is the bubo—an enlarged, congested and centrally necrotic lymph node. *Y. pestis* can be demonstrated in abundance in these lesions. Congestion and haemorrhage may be seen in most organs of the body, and extensive haemorrhages may be present in

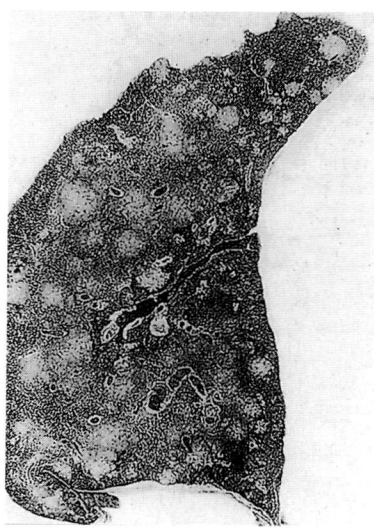

Figure 63.3: The lung from a fatal case of pneumonic plague. The lower lobe shows intense hyperaemia and haemorrhage with necrotic nodules. The upper lobe contains only necrotic nodules with compensatory emphysemal changes.

the mucosa of the gastrointestinal tract. In pneumonic plague the findings are of a haemorrhagic pneumonia and blood-stained fluid in the pleural cavities (Figure 63.3).

Clinical features

Historical accounts suggest that plague is one of the most virulent infections known to man, but subclinical cases are not uncommon and bubonic plague can be of mild or moderate severity. The incubation period is generally two to five days but may be up to 15 days. With primary pneumonia the incubation period is often short, sometimes only one day, and the disease is rapidly fatal. In a small proportion of cases there is a prodromal stage of fever, weakness and anorexia. The initial manifestations are usually due to lymphadenitis in the nodes draining the site of a flea bite.

Bubonic plague

This is the most common form of plague and has a characteristic clinical picture. Typically, bubonic plague presents with a short prodrome of fever, malaise, anorexia and headache. Sometimes there is a dull ache at the site of future buboes, which will develop within 24 hours. The primary buboes will be found in different locations depending on the site of inoculation. The most common site is the groin (70–80%), with the femoral nodes more often involved compared to inguinal nodes (Figure 63.4).[9] Other primary sites are the axilla (14–20%), the cervical and submaxillary regions, and very rarely the clavicular, popliteal and epitrochlear nodes. Cervical and submaxillary node involvement is more often present in children. Buboes usually affect only one site but very occasionally two or more may be involved.

Development of the bubo is characterized by severe pain, swelling and marked tenderness of the affected lymph node. Individual nodes may attain the size of a hen's egg; sometimes clusters of nodes form a larger, more irregular swelling. There is surrounding oedema and the overlying skin is warm, reddened and adherent. The mass is immoveable and non-fluctuant, although, particularly if not treated with antibiotics, suppuration and abscess formation will occur during later stages. The buboes are generally so tender that the patient will hold the associated limb, or head, in such a position as to relieve the pressure.

The onset of fever in plague is often abrupt with the temperature rising rapidly to 39–40°C or even higher. Prostration and lethargy is marked. Sometimes there is agitation or even delirium. Vomiting and diarrhoea occur occasionally. Hepatomegaly is common, but the spleen, although slightly enlarged, is not usually palpable.

In some patients small skin lesions such as vesicles and pustules may be seen in the region drained by the affected nodes. These may ulcerate or form an eschar (Figure 63.5), or rarely a carbuncle. *Y. pestis* can be isolated from these lesions. Although uncommon, perhaps the best-known skin manifestation is a patchy purpuric dermal necrosis, which gave rise to the popular name 'Black Death'.

Laboratory findings include an elevated leucocyte count (12,000–22,000/mm^3) and toxic granulation of neutrophils. Eosinophilia is absent in the acute phase but is often noticed during convalescence. There is also laboratory evidence of disseminated intravascular coagulation.[10] Liver enzymes and bilirubin are frequently elevated, especially in more severe cases, although clinical jaundice is rare.

Although the picture of severe bubonic plague is distinctive, other infections can cause acute lymphadenitis. Staphylococcal and streptococcal infections will usually be associated with an obvious suppurative lesion or an area of lymphangitis in the region drained by the affected lymph nodes. In the USA tularaemia may cause confusion. Lymphogranuloma venereum and chancroid also cause inguinal lymphadenopathy; however the buboes are less

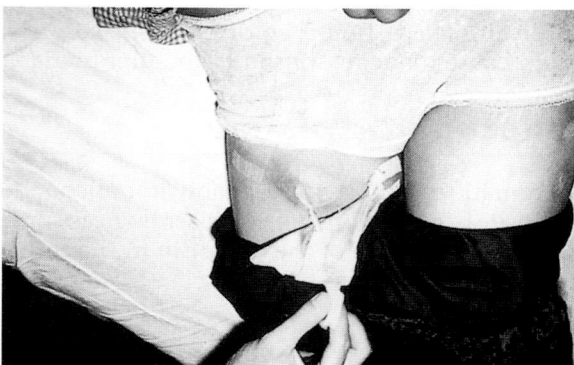

Figure 63.4: Bubonic plague. Fever and regional lymphadenopathy with suppuration, especially in the inguinal and axillary regions, commence after an incubation period of less than one week.

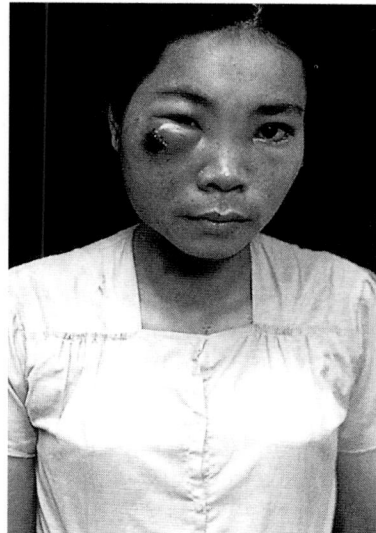

Figure 63.5: A young woman with eschar of an infected flea bite and local facial carbuncle.

painful and often fluctuant, and there are usually mild constitutional features.

Minor infections also occur and may go unnoticed. They may present with mild fever and less pronounced lymph node enlargement ('pestis minor'), which is self-limiting.

Septicaemic plague

Episodes of bacteraemia often occur in bubonic plague: in one study quantitative culture of small volumes of blood detected bacteraemia in 40% of cases.[11] Densities greater than 10^2/ml were associated with higher mortality.

The term 'septicaemic plague' denotes a severe acute illness characterized by a high density of organisms in the blood, without clinically apparent buboes. The bacteraemia may be so high (up to 10^7/ml) that organisms are detectable in a peripheral blood smear. Septicaemic plague accounted for 11% of cases in the USA during the 1970s.[12] However, in New Mexico from 1980 to 1984, 25% of the 71 cases reported were septicaemic.[13] This was more likely to occur in people aged over 40 years. Symptoms include: fever, rigors, malaise and headache and are generally indistinguishable from those of other Gram-negative septicaemias. Gastrointestinal symptoms of nausea, vomiting, diarrhoea and abdominal pain are more frequent than in bubonic plague. The duration of illness is shorter than in bubonic plague and, if not treated appropriately, the patient rapidly becomes shocked and dies within a few days.

Pneumonic plague

Pneumonia in plague can occur in two forms, either as a primary pneumonia or secondary to bacteraemic spread in bubonic plague or septicaemic plague. The illness begins with intense headache and malaise, fever, vomiting and marked prostration and clouding of consciousness. In the initial stages there may be little to suggest pneumonia, but cough and dyspnoea develop with the production of watery, bloodstained sputum. Physical signs in the lungs are slight; there are reduced breath sounds and coarse crepitations at the bases. Respiratory failure ensues and the patient rapidly dies (Figure 63.6). Chest radiography shows evidence of multilobar consolidation or broncho-pneumonia; there may be minimal pleural effusions. The discrepancy between gross radiographic abnormalities and minimal physical signs in the chest is characteristic. Pneumonia in plague has to be differentiated from the 'adult respiratory distress syndrome' that may occur in bubonic and septicaemic forms. The mortality rate in both types of plague pneumonia is extremely high, and appropriate antibiotic treatment must be given within 24 hours of onset if the mortality rate is to be reduced.

Pneumonic plague is generally very uncommon, but it is the one form that may result in human-to-human transmission via infected droplets from patients with a productive cough. Where the climate is cool and humid, allowing infectious particles to persist, epidemics

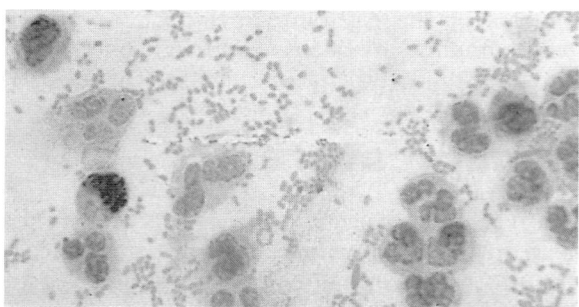

Figure 63.6: *Yersinia pestis* in cerebrospinal fluid taken from a patient with meningitis.

of pneumonic plague have occurred, such as that in Manchuria in 1910–1911. It is also a potential risk in laboratory workers handling cultures of *Y. pestis*.

Plague meningitis

Primary plague meningitis is extremely rare. Most cases of meningeal involvement have occurred as a complication of inadequately treated bubonic plague, typically after 9–15 days. There is an association between the presence of axillary buboes and the development of meningitis.[11] It is postulated that this may be due to spread by the lymphatic route, but bacteraemia is considered to be the means of spread from other sites.

Plague meningitis presents with symptoms and signs common to all types of pyogenic meningitis, including fever, headache, vomiting and neck stiffness. Examination of cerebrospinal fluid will show a predominately neutrophil leucocytosis, and *Y. pestis* may be demonstrated by Gram stain (Figure 63.6). Mortality is higher than in un-complicated bubonic plague.

Pharyngeal or tonsillar plague

This is a very rare variety of plague that possibly results from ingestion or inhalation of the organism. Usually the tonsils become swollen and inflamed. There is anterior cervical lymphadenopathy and swelling of the parotid area, with surrounding oedema. *Y. pestis* can be isolated from the throat. It should be distinguished from other common causes of acute tonsillitis and diphtheria.

Asymptomatic plague

Asymptomatic infections are probably not uncommon in endemic areas as demonstrated by serological surveys.[14] Asymptomatic carriage of the organism in the throat has also been documented.[15]

Mortality

The mortality rate from plague before the antibiotic era ranged from 50 to 95%. With the advent of effective antibiotic therapy the mortality rate fell dramatically. The overall fatality rate in cases reported to WHO during the 1990s was 7.2%.[1] In uncomplicated bubonic plague this may be as low as 5%, but in septicaemic plague documented in New Mexico the case fatality rate was 33%.[13] The prognosis is much worse in patients with pulmonary involvement and, in particular, primary pneumonia invariably remains fatal if treatment is delayed more than 24 hours.

Diagnosis

The diagnosis of plague must be considered in anyone presenting with fever and localized lymphadenitis, without another obvious cause of infection, if they live in, or have returned from, an endemic area. Once plague is suspected, laboratory confirmation should be sought as quickly as possible so that appropriate therapy is given. The definitive diagnosis of plague requires culture of *Y. pestis* from a clinical specimen, or a fourfold rise in antibody titre.[16]

In most cases aspiration of a bubo will provide material for microscopic examination and culture. If no fluid or pus is obtained a small amount of saline can be injected and reaspirated. Smears may be stained with Wayson, Giemsa or Gram stains. A presumptive diagnosis of plague is made by demonstration of bipolar staining coccobacilli, with rapid identification by immunofluorescence using F1-specific antibodies labelled with fluorescein. Blood cultures should always be taken, and in suspected pneumonic or meningeal plague specimens of sputum or cerebrospinal fluid should be processed in the same way as bubo aspirates. Specimens for culture should be inoculated on to blood agar and MacConkey agar, and may also be placed into an enrichment broth—with subculture after 24–48 hours.

Serological diagnosis is possible but antibodies may not be detectable when the patient first presents; however it is useful in culture-negative cases. Haemagglutinating antibodies to F1 antigen appear after a week and may be detected by the passive haemagglutination test (PHA). A single titre of ≥16 is very suggestive of plague, whereas a fourfold rise in paired sera is diagnostic. Enzyme immunoassays have been applied to the detection of serum antibody[17] and F1 antigenaemia.[18] Both appear to be useful diagnostic tests.

Several methods of DNA detection using polymerase chain reaction (PCR) have been developed recently. One clinical study to determine the diagnostic value of PCR on bubo aspirates found that, although very specific, it was not as sensitive as culture or F1 antigen detection.[19]

Treatment

In clinically suspected cases appropriate antibiotic therapy should be started as soon as specimens have been taken for microbiological confirmation. Even bubonic plague can evolve quickly into a life-threatening disease. Streptomycin, tetracycline and chloramphenicol are the antibiotics traditionally used in the treatment of plague, and they remain highly effective today. The response to treatment is dramatic provided the patient is not already moribund. Patients with pulmonary involvement are highly infectious and must be kept in strict isolation, with precautions against air-borne spread, until at least three days of antibiotic treatment has been given and the patient is clinically improved.

Streptomycin was established as the treatment of choice over 40 years ago; the regimen is 30 mg/kg per day in two divided doses, given intramuscularly, for 10 days. This drug is potentially ototoxic and nephrotoxic. In elderly patients and those with renal impairment, the frequency of administration and total dosage should be reduced. Renal function should be monitored and blood taken for streptomycin levels, if available. There have not been any clinical studies with the newer aminoglycosides, although gentamicin has very good in vitro and in vivo activity.[20–22]

Tetracycline (250–500mg four times daily, for 10 days) is a satisfactory alternative, especially in milder cases when an oral drug is required. Doxycycline has better in vitro activity[21] and may be preferred (100 mg twice daily). The tetracyclines are useful when prophylaxis is considered necessary. They should not be given to pregnant women or children up to 8 years of age, and should also be avoided in renal failure.

Chloramphenicol is the drug of choice for plague meningitis because it achieves good concentrations in the cerebrospinal fluid. An initial loading dose of 25 mg/kg is given intravenously, followed by 100 mg/kg per day in four divided doses. When the clinical condition permits, it can be administered orally for a total course of 10 days.

Susceptibility studies show that the fluoroquinolone compounds and third-generation cephalosporins are the most active antimicrobial agents against *Y. pestis* in vitro.[21,22] In murine models of infection the fluoroquinolones are also highly active against *Y. pestis*,[20,23,24] suggesting that they will be effective in treating human disease. However the newer cephalosporins gave conflicting results,[20,23] so they cannot be recommended for treatment until more data are available.

Until recently all strains of *Y. pestis* were remarkably sensitive to a wide range of antibiotics. In 1995 two distinct strains, with antibiotic resistance, were isolated from patients in different areas of Madagascar. One was resistant to streptomycin alone.[25] However the other strain was resistant to streptomycin, tetracycline, chloramphenicol and sulphonamides, but remained susceptible to trimethoprim, fluoroquinolones and cephalosporins.[26] In both cases, the resistance was mediated by a plasmid, which could be transferred easily to other strains of *Y. pestis*.

Prevention

Plague is subject to the International Health Regulations and confirmed cases should be reported to WHO. The control of plague depends upon public education, active surveillance, and rodent and flea control measures. During an outbreak, active case finding and follow-up of contacts are essential.[16]

Surveillance should be undertaken to assess the potential for epizootic plague and the risk of transmission to man. This includes bacteriological monitoring of dead or sick rodents and the serological testing of 'sentinel animals' such as carnivores and dogs, which are more likely to have contact with plague-infected rodents.[16] Enzyme-linked immunosorbent assay (ELISA) techniques have advantages over PHA for serological surveillance.[27] Flea indices should be established; this involves determining the number and species of fleas per host animal, as well as the percentage of hosts infested. DNA detection, using PCR, has been applied to the identification of *Y. pestis* in fleas and is more sensitive than mouse inoculation.[28]

The presence of food sources and shelter in areas of human habitation encourages rodents and may be associated with outbreaks of plague. There should be proper disposal of food and refuse; unused out-buildings, wood piles and other forms of shelter for rats should be removed.[29] People should be educated to avoid activities that will bring them into contact with rodents and their fleas. In areas of sylvatic plague, pet cats and dogs should be treated periodically with insecticides.

Specific rodent and flea control measures with the use of rodenticides and effective insecticides, although important, are most likely to be successful in the control of urban plague rather than sylvatic plague (which may cover a large area). Attempts at rodent control must be preceded by flea control measures because of the potential risk of increasing human exposure to plague-infected fleas.[16] Rat control on ships and in docks, by fumigation, poisoning and trapping, is very important in preventing the dissemination of plague.

Until recently an inactivated vaccine, consisting of formalin-killed *Y. pestis*, was available for individuals working in high-risk areas, but production has now stopped. Two initial injections were given one to three months apart, with booster doses every six months.[30] However, there were doubts about this vaccine's efficacy in preventing pneumonic plague. New subunit vaccines based on F1 and V antigens are being developed and show much greater efficacy in mice.[31]

Chemoprophylaxis with oral tetracycline, doxycycline or trimethoprim-sulphamethoxazole is recommended for persons in close contact with plague pneumonia, and individuals contaminated in laboratory accidents. Ciprofloxacin should be a suitable alternative as it has proved to be protective against experimental pneumonic infection in mice.[24]

REFERENCES

1 [Anonymous]. Human plague in 1998 and 1999. *Weekly Epidemiol Rec* 2000; 42:338–343.
2 Gage K L, Dennis D T, Orloski K A et al. Cases of cat-associated human plague in the western US, 1977–1998. *Clin Infect Dis* 2000; 30:893–900.
3 Chanteau S, Ratsifasoamanana L, Rasoamanana B et al. Plague, a reemerging disease in Madagascar. *Emerg Infect Dis* 1998; 4:101–104.
4 Brubaker R R. Factors promoting acute and chronic diseases caused by *Yersiniae*. *Clin Microbiol Rev* 1991; 4:309–324.
5 Cavanaugh D C. Specific effect of temperature upon transmission of the plague bacillus by the Oriental rat flea *Xenopsylla cheopis*. *Am J Trop Med Hyg* 1971; 20:264–273.
6 Nakajima R & Brubaker R R. Association between virulence of *Yersinia pestis* and suppression of gamma interferon and tumor necrosis factor alpha. *Infect Immun* 1993; 61:23–31.
7 Welkos S, Friedlander A, McDowell D et al. V antigen of *Yersinia pestis* inhibits neutrophil chemotaxis. *Microb Pathog* 1998; 24:185–196.
8 Straley S C, Skrzypek E, Plano G V et al. Yops of *Yersinia* spp. Pathogenic for man. *Infect Immun* 1993; 61:3105–3110.
9 Butler T. A clinical study of bubonic plague: observations of the 1970 Vietnam epidemic with emphasis on coagulation studies, skin histology and electrocardiograms. *Am J Med* 1972; 53:268–276.
10 Butler T, Bell W R, Linh N N et al. *Yersinia pestis* infection in Vietnam. I. Clinical and hematologic aspects. *J Infect Dis* 1974; 129:S78–S84.
11 Butler T, Levin J, Linh N N et al. *Yersinia pestis* infection in Vietnam. II. Quantitative blood cultures and detection of endotoxin in the cerebrospinal fluid of patients with meningitis. *J Infect Dis* 1976; 133:493–499.
12 Kaufmann A F, Boyce J M & Martone W J. Trends in human plague in the United States. *J Infect Dis* 1980; 141:522–524.
13 Hull H F, Montes J M & Mann J M. Septicemic plague in New Mexico. *J Infect Dis* 1987; 155:113–118.
14 Legters L J, Cottingham A J Jr & Hunter D H. Clinical and epidemiologic notes on a defined outbreak of plague in Vietnam. *Am J Trop Med Hyg* 1970; 19:639–652.
15 Marshall J D, Quy D V & Gibson F L. Asymptomatic pharyngeal plague infection in Vietnam. Am J Trop Med Hyg 1967; 16:175–177.
16 Dennis D T, Gage K L, Gratz N et al. *Plague Manual: Epidemiology, Distribution, Surveillance and Control*. Geneva: World Health Organization; 1999.
17 Rasoamanana B, Leroy F, Boisier P et al. Field evaluation of an immunoglobulin G anti-F1 ELISA assay for serodiagnosis of plague in Madagascar. *Clin Diag Lab Immunol* 1997; 4:587–591.
18 Chanteau S, Rabarijaona L, O'Brien T et al. F1 antigenaemia in bubonic plague patients, a marker of gravity and efficacy of therapy. *Trans R Soc Trop Med Hyg* 1998; 92:572–573.
19 Rahalison L, Vololonirina E, Ratsitorahina M et al. Diagnosis of bubonic plague by PCR in Madagascar under field conditions. *J Clin Microbiol* 2000; 38:260–263.
20 Bonacorsi S P, Scavizzi M R, Guiyoule A et al. Assessment of a fluoroquinolone, three β-lactams, two aminoglycosides, and a cycline in treatment of murine *Yersinia pestis* infection. *Antimicrob Agents Chemother* 1994; 38:481–486.
21 Smith M D, Vinh D X, Hoa N T T et al. In vitro antimicrobial susceptibilities of strains of *Yersinia pestis*. *Antimicrob Agents Chemother* 1995; 39:2153–2154.
22 Wong J D, Barash J R, Sandfort R F et al. Susceptibilities of *Yersinia pestis* to 12 antimicrobial agents. *Antimicrob Agents Chemother* 2000; 44:1995–1996.
23 Byrne W R, Welkos S L, Pitt M L et al. Antibiotic treatment of experimental pneumonic plague in mice. *Antimicrob Agents Chemother* 1998; 42:675–681.

24 Russell P, Eley S M, Green M et al. Efficacy of doxycycline and ciprofloxacin against experimental *Yersinia pestis* infection. *J Antimicrob Chemother* 1998; 41:301–305.

25 Guiyoule A, Gerbaud G, Buchrieser C et al. Transferable plasmid-mediated resistance to streptomycin in a clinical isolate of *Yersinia pestis*. *Emerg Infect Dis* 2001; 7:43–48.

26 Galimand M, Guiyoule A, Gerbaud G et al. Multidrug resistance in *Yersinia pestis* mediated by a transferable plasmid. *N Engl J Med* 1997; 337:677–680.

27 Shepherd A J, Leman P A, Hummitzsch D E et al. A comparison of serological techniques for plague surveillance. *Trans R Soc Trop Med Hyg* 1984; 78:771–773.

28 Engelthaler D M, Gage K L, Montenieri J A et al. PCR detection of *Yersinia pestis* in fleas: comparison with mouse inoculation. *J Clin Microbiol* 1999; 37:1980–1984.

29 Mann J M, Martone W J, Boyce J M et al. Endemic human plague in New Mexico: risk factors associated with infection. *J Infect Dis* 1979; 140:397–401.

30 Centers for Disease Control. Prevention of plague: Recommendations of the Advisory Committee on Immunization Practices (ACIP). *MMWR* 1996; 45:1–15.

31 Anderson G W, Heath D G, Bolt C R et al. Short- and long-term efficacy of single-dose subunit vaccines against *Yersinia pestis* in mice. *Am J Trop Med* 1998; 58:793–799.

Chapter 64
Melioidosis

D. Dance

Introduction

The term melioidosis is used to describe any infection caused by the bacterium *Burkholderia* (formerly *Pseudomonas*) *pseudomallei*. It is known to be an important cause of illness and death in some tropical and sub-tropical regions, and is probably underdiagnosed in others.[1]

History

Whitmore and Krishnaswami first described melioidosis in Rangoon, Burma, in 1912.[2] Over the next 20 years, the infection was found to be widespread amongst man and animals in British Malaya and French Indochina, where *B. pseudomallei* was shown to be a free-living environmental saprophyte.[3] Over 400 French and American soldiers contracted the disease whilst stationed in Vietnam.[4] Interest in the disease has been rekindled by the increasing recognition of indigenous cases in north-east Thailand and northern Australia.[1,5,6] More recently, *B. pseudomallei* has even been considered as a potential biological weapon.

Epidemiology

Melioidosis is known to be endemic in Thailand, Malaysia, Singapore, and northern Australia, although it is unevenly distributed within these areas. In north-east Thailand, the average annual incidence has been estimated as 4.4/100 000, although this is probably an underestimate, and *B. pseudomallei* accounts for almost 20% of community-acquired septicaemia.[6,7] Incidences of 16.5/100 000 and 1.7/100 000 have been estimated in the Northern Territory of Australia and Singapore, respectively.[5,8] It is clear that the disease is also present elsewhere in South and South-East Asia and the Caribbean, although the incidence in most countries is unknown.[9] Sporadic cases have been reported from Central Africa, Central and South America, the Pacific islands, and Iran.[1] During the 1970s an unusual epizootic also occurred in France.[1]

In endemic areas, *B. pseudomallei* is readily isolated from mud and surface water, particularly rice paddy.[3] Melioidosis is most common in people who have close contact with soil and water (e.g., rice farmers in Thailand, aboriginals in Australia), although in most cases the precise mode of acquisition is unclear. Inoculation events or near-drowning episodes can only be identified in 5–25% of cases.[5,7] One recent outbreak was traced to a contaminated potable water supply.[3] Iatrogenic and laboratory-acquired infections have occurred occasionally,[1] but the disease is rarely transmitted by contacts of infected humans or animals.[10]

Melioidosis is highly seasonal, with 75–85% of cases presenting during the rainy season,[7,11] presumably because this is when exposure to the organism in the environment is greatest. When a specific exposure can be identified, the incubation period is 1–21 days (mean 9 days).[5] However, *B. pseudomallei* has the remarkable ability to remain latent for periods of up to 29 years,[12] which has given rise to the nickname 'Vietnamese time-bomb'. The proportion of seropositive persons who are latently infected is unknown.

Aetiology

B. pseudomallei is an ovoid, oxidase-positive, motile Gram-negative bacillus which often exhibits marked bipolarity microscopically. It grows readily on most routine culture media, giving off a sweet earthy smell. Other important characteristics include arginine dihydrolase and gelatinase activity, growth at 42°C, the ability to use a wide range of carbon and energy sources, and intrinsic resistance to aminoglycosides, polymyxins and the early beta-lactams. The species is antigenically homogeneous, but a number of molecular techniques can distinguish between isolates.[13] It is closely related to *B. mallei*, the causative agent of glanders, with which it has antigenic cross-reactivity, and *B. cepacia*, with which it may occasionally be confused in culture. An avirulent organism, *Burkholderia thailandensis*, that is extremely similar to *B. pseudomallei* phenotypically, but differs in characteristics including the ability to assimilate arabinose, has been isolated from soil in South-East Asia.[14]

Pathogenesis

Although severe melioidosis may occur in apparently normal individuals, 53–80% of cases have underlying diseases, most frequently diabetes mellitus or chronic renal failure.[5,7,11] Steroid therapy, liver disease, chronic lung disease, alcohol abuse, kava consumption, malignant disease and pregnancy may also predispose to melioidosis,[5,7,11,15] but as yet there is no evidence that infection with HIV does so. Recrudescence of latent infection also usually occurs at times of intercurrent stress.[12]

The result of exposure to *B. pseudomallei* in the environment varies markedly from case to case. The possible outcomes are summarized in Figure 64.1. Which route is followed in any individual depends on a balance between the size of the inoculum and the virulence of the infecting strain on the one hand, and the host response on the other. Putative bacterial virulence factors include secreted products (e.g., protease, lipase, lecithinase, various toxins) and their secretory machinery, bacterial components such as lipopolysaccharide (LPS), one type of which (LPS II) is essential for serum-resistance, acid phosphatase (possibly an insulin receptor), an extracellular polysaccharide 'capsule, and a siderophore 'malleobactin'.[16] The ability of the organism to survive and grow intracellularly probably also contributes to the recalcitrant and persistent nature of the infection. However, the relative contributions of individual virulence factors to the disease process have not been well characterized. On the host side, cellular and innate immunity, particularly interferon-gamma production, appear important in determining resistance to overwhelming infection,[17] although an exaggerated host response may also be damaging, and levels of a number of pro-inflammatory cytokines have been associated with a fatal outcome in human melioidosis.[18] Humoral immunity clearly also plays a role, as antibodies to LPS can confer passive protection in an animal model, and levels of antibody to LPS II correlate with survival in human melioidosis.[19]

Pathology

The microscopic appearance of lesions is not pathognomonic and forms a spectrum from abscess to granuloma depending on the duration of the illness and the response of the individual. Multinucleate giant cells, often containing 'globi' of bacteria, in a background of acute necrotizing inflammation, are a characteristic feature.[20]

Clinical features

The variable course and manifestations have made it difficult to develop a satisfactory clinical classification of melioidosis. Since up to 80% of the population in endemic areas has antibodies to *B. pseudomallei* by the age of 4 years,[21] the majority of infections are presumably mild or asymptomatic. Seroconversion has been associated with a flu-like illness.[22] Some of the more common forms are described below.

Septicaemic melioidosis

Forty-six to sixty per cent of cases of culture-positive melioidosis are bacteraemic, and the majority of these are clinically septicaemic.[5,6,11] Patients usually have a short history (median 6 days; range 1 day to 2 months) of fever and rigors.[6] Some 4% of cases in Australia are thought to represent recrudescent latent infections.[5] Approximately half have evidence of a primary focus of infection, usually pulmonary or cutaneous.[6,11] Diminished consciousness, jaundice and diarrhoea may also be prominent features. Initial investigations usually reveal anaemia, a neutrophil leucocytosis, coagulopathy and evidence of renal and hepatic impairment. Deterioration is often rapid, with the development of widespread metastatic abscesses, particularly in the lungs, liver and spleen, and metabolic acidosis with Kussmaul's breathing. Cutaneous or subcutaneous abscesses occur in approximately 10% of cases and an abnormal chest radiograph is found in 80% of patients, the most common pattern being widespread, nodular shadowing (Figure 64.2). Poor prognostic features include hypotension, absence of fever, leucopenia, azotaemia and abnormal liver function tests.[6]

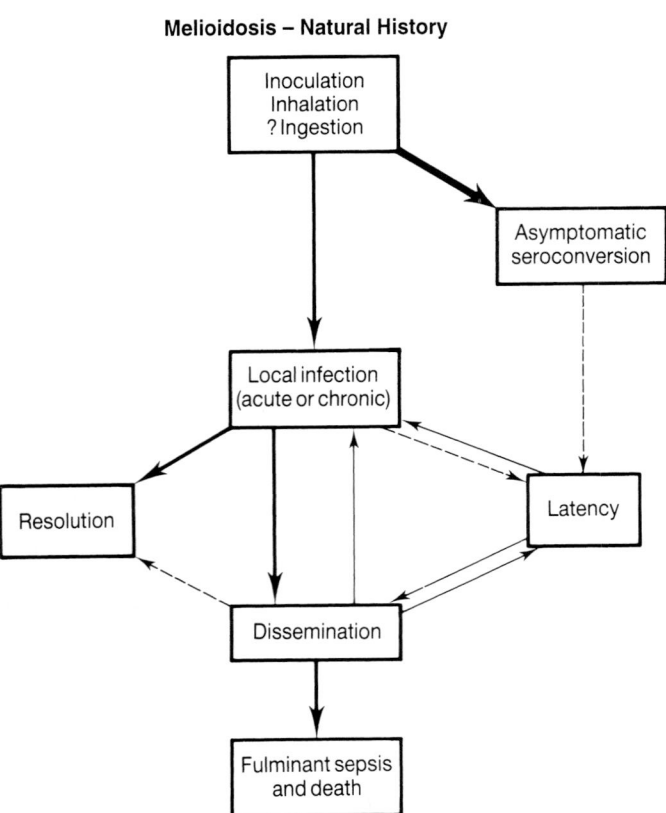

Melioidosis – Natural History

Figure 64.1: Natural history of melioidosis. The most common progression is represented by the broadest arrows. Dotted lines indicate rare or uncertain sequences of events.

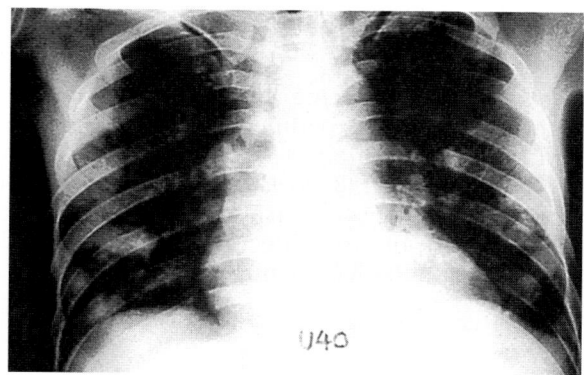

Figure 64.2: Septicaemic melioidosis. Widespread nodular shadowing representing blood-borne pneumonia.

Localized melioidosis

The lung is the most common site for localized melioidosis. The most frequent form is a cavitating pneumonia accompanied by profound weight loss, which is often confused with tuberculosis or lung abscess, although mild bronchitis or bronchopneumonia may be the only manifestations. Any lung zone may be affected, although there is a predilection for upper lobe involvement.[23] Localized complications include pneumothorax, empyema and purulent pericarditis, whilst progression to septicaemia is not uncommon.

Localized *B. pseudomallei* infection may occur in any organ. Well described presentations include: cutaneous and subcutaneous abscesses, suppurative parotitis,[24] lymphadenitis, osteomyelitis and septic arthritis, liver and/or splenic abscesses,[25] cystitis, pyelonephritis, prostatic abscesses, epididymo-orchitis, keratitis, meningo-encephalitis, and brain abscesses.[26] For reasons that have yet to be explained, parotitis in children is common in Thailand but not Australia, whereas prostatic abscesses and neurological melioidosis are reported more frequently from Australia than Thailand.[11]

Diagnosis

Melioidosis is difficult to diagnose on clinical grounds alone, so the diagnosis depends on the isolation of *B. pseudomallei* or the detection of specific antibodies. Melioidosis should be considered in any patient who has ever visited an endemic area and presents with septicaemia and/or abscesses. The index of suspicion should be particularly high in diabetics. Microscopy of pus, sputum or urine may reveal bipolar or unevenly staining Gram-negative rods, but this appearance is not specific for *B. pseudomallei*. Several methods for the detection of *B. pseudomallei* antigens and nucleic acids in clinical material are under development. Only immunofluorescent microscopy has yet found a role in routine practice in areas of high endemicity.[27]

The organism should be sought in blood, pus, urine, sputum or any other specimen indicated by the patient's clinical presentation. The laboratory should be notified when melioidosis is suspected, since selective techniques may increase the isolation rate,[28] and the organism may be overlooked or discarded as a contaminant by the unwary. Furthermore, it is classified as a 'category 3' pathogen because of the risk of infection amongst laboratory staff.

The serodiagnosis of melioidosis is fraught with problems. Numerous assays have been described, but there is no 'standard' method and none has satisfactory sensitivity and sensitivity, particularly in endemic areas where background seropositivity rates are high.[21] The indirect haemagglutination (IHA) test, which detects antibodies to heat-stable antigens (probably lipopoly-saccharide), is the test most widely used for the detection of *B. pseudomallei* antibodies, although recently developed enzyme linked immunosorbent assays (ELISAs) may give better results.[29] These tests are useful in patients from non-endemic areas in whom a single IHA titre of < 1:40 at presentation is highly suggestive of melioidosis. In patients from endemic areas, only a rising or very high titre or the presence of specific IgM can be taken as evidence of melioidosis. Although molecular assays directed at a range of targets have been developed, the results in practice have so far also been disappointing.[29,30]

Management
General

Patients with septicaemic melioidosis require aggressive supportive treatment, with particular attention to correction of volume depletion and septic shock, respiratory and renal failure, and hyperglycaemia or ketoacidosis. Severe cases should ideally be managed in an intensive care unit. Corticosteroids are of doubtful benefit, but antiendotoxin and anticytokine antibodies remain to be evaluated. Abscesses should be drained surgically whenever possible in both disseminated and localized disease.

Antimicrobial therapy

B. pseudomallei is intrinsically resistant to the combination of penicillin and gentamicin which is often used empirically to treat patients with septicaemia in the tropics, and a complete failure to defervesce on this regimen may help to suggest the diagnosis in an endemic area.

Several prospective randomized comparisons of antimicrobial therapy for melioidosis have been reported in recent years, the results of which have been summarised by Chaowagul.[31] High dose intravenous ceftazidime (120 mg/kg per day in divided doses or an equivalent dose adjusted for renal function), for at least 2 weeks or until fever has subsided, is the treatment of choice. Imipenem, meropenem, co-amoxiclav or cefoperazone-sulbactam are acceptable alternatives. Even with these regimens, severe melioidosis still has a high mortality (approximately 40%).[11,31] The question of whether co-trimoxazole (trimethoprim 10 mg/kg per day plus sulphamethoxazole 50 mg/kg per day) should be added to initial treatment remains to be answered. In beta-lactam-allergic patients, conventional drugs (chloramphenicol 100 mg/kg per day, doxycycline 4 mg/kg per day, and co-trimoxazole) should be used. Thereafter, treatment with oral agents (co-amoxiclav or the conventional combination regimen as above) should be continued for 12–20 weeks in order to prevent relapse, which occurs in up to 13% of cases and may be associated with the emergence of antibiotic resistance.[32] Mild cases may be treated with these oral drugs alone.

Prevention

No *B. pseudomallei* vaccine has been developed for human use, although experimental vaccines are under development.[16] Prevention is thus limited to the avoidance of contact with *B. pseudomallei* in the environment, particularly by 'at-risk' individuals such as diabetics. The risk of cross-infection appears to be very low, but cases may be barrier nursed where facilities are available.

REFERENCES

1 Dance D A B. Melioidosis: the tip of the iceberg? *Clin Microbiol Rev* 1991; 4:52–60.

2 Whitmore A, Krishnaswami C S. An amount of the discovery of a hitherto undescribed infective disease occurring among the population of Rangoon. *Indian Med Gazette* 1912; 47:262–267.

3 Inglis T J, Mee B J, Chang B J. The environmental microbiology of melioidosis. *Rev Med Microbiol* 2000; 12:13–20.

4 Sanford J P. *Pseudomonas* species (including melioidosis and glanders). In: Mandell G L, Bennett J E, Dolin R (eds). *Principles and Practice of Infectious Diseases*, 4th edn. New York: Churchill Livingstone; 1995:2003–2009.

5 Currie B J, Fisher D A, Howard D M et al. The epidemiology of melioidosis in Australia and Papua New Guinea. *Acta Tropica* 2000; 74:121–127.

6 Chaowagul W, White N J, Dance D A B et al. Melioidosis: a major cause of community-acquired septicemia in Northeastern Thailand. *J Infect Dis* 1989; 159:890–899.

7 Suputtamongkol Y, Hall A J, Dance D A B et al. The epidemiology of melioidosis in Ubon Ratchatani, Northeast Thailand. *Int J Epidemiol* 1994; 23:1082–1090.

8 Heng B H, Goh K T, Yap E H et al. Epidemiological surveillance of melioidosis in Singapore. *Ann Acad Med Singapore* 1998; 27:478–484.

9 Dance D A B. Melioidosis as an emerging global problem. *Acta Tropica* 2000; 74:115–119.

10 Kunakorn M, Jayanetra P, Tanphaichitra D. Man to man transmission of melioidosis. *Lancet* 1991; 337:1290–1291.

11 Currie B J, Fisher D A, Howard D M et al. Endemic melioidosis in tropical Northern Australia: a 10-year prospective study and review of the literature. *Clin Infect Dis* 2000; 31:981–986.

12 Chodimella U, Hoppes W L, Whalen S et al. Septicemia and suppuration in a Vietnam veteran. *Hosp Pract* 1997; 32:219–221.

13 Pitt T L, Trakulsomboon S, Dance D A B. Molecular phylogeny of *Burkholderia pseudomallei*. *Acta Tropica* 2000; 74:181–185.

14 Brett P J, DeShazer D, Woods D E. *Burkholderia thailandensis* sp. Nov., a *Burkholderia pseudomallei*-like species. *Int J Syst Bacteriol* 1998; 48:317–320.

15 Suputtamongkol Y, Chaowagul, Chetchotisakd P et al. Risk factors for melioidosis and bacteremic melioidosis. *Clin Infect Dis* 1999; 29:408–413.

16 Brett P J, Woods D E. Pathogenesis of and immunity to melioidosis. *Acta Tropica* 2000; 74:201–210.

17 Santanirand P, Harley V S, Dance D A B et al. Obligatory role of gamma interferon for host survival in a murine model of infection with *Burkholderia pseudomallei*. *Infect Immun* 1999; 67:3593–3600.

18 Simpson A J H, Smith M D, Weverling G J et al. Prognostic value of cytokine concentrations (tumor necrosis factor-α, interleukin-6, and interleukin-10) and clinical parameters in severe melioidosis. *J. Infect Dis* 2000; 181:621–625.

19 Charuchaimontri C, Suputtamongkol Y, Nilakul C et al. Antilipopolysaccharide II: an antibody protective against fatal melioidosis. *Clin Infect Dis* 1999; 29: 813–818.

20 Wong K T, Putucheary S D & Vadivelu J. The histopathology of human melioidosis. *Histopathology* 1995; 26:51–55.

21 Kanaphun P, Thirawattanasuk N, Suputtamongkol Y et al. Serology and carriage of *Pseudomonas pseudomallei*: a prospective study in 1000 hospitalised children in northeast Thailand. *J. Infect Dis* 1993; 167:230–233.

22 Ashdown L R, Johnson R W, Koehler J M et al. Enzyme-linked immunosorbent assay for the diagnosis of clinical and subclinical melioidosis. *J. Infect Dis* 1989; 160:253–260.

23 Dhiensri T, Puapairoj S & Susaengrat W. Pulmonary melioidosis: clinical and radiologic correlation in 183 cases in northeastern Thailand. *Radiology* 1988; 166:711–715.

24 Dance D A B, Davis T M E, Wattanagoon Y et al. Acute suppurative parotitis in children caused by *Pseudomonas pseudomallei*. *J. Infect Dis* 1989; 159:654–660.

25 Vatcharapreechasagul T, Suputtamongkol Y, Dance D A B *et al*. *Pseudomonas pseudomallei* liver abscess: a clinical, laboratory and ultrasonographic study. *Clin Infect Dis* 1992; 14:412–417.

26 Currie B J, Fisher D A, Howard D M et al. Neurological melioidosis. *Acta Tropica* 2000; 74:145–151.

27 Walsh A L, Smith M D, Wuthiekanun V et al. Immunofluorescent microscopy for the rapid diagnosis of melioidosis. *J. Clin Pathol* 1994; 47:377–379.

28 Wuthiekanun V, Dance D A B, Wattanagoon Y et al. The use of selective media for the isolation of *Pseudomonas pseudomallei* in clinical practice. *J Med Microbiol* 1990; 33:121–126.

29 Sirisinha S, Anuntagool N, Dharakul T et al. Recent developments in laboratory diagnosis of melioidosis. *Acta Tropica* 2000; 74:235–245.

30 Haase A, Brennan M, Barrett S et al. Evaluation of PCR for diagnosis of melioidosis. *J. Clin Microbiol* 1998; 36:1039–1041.

31 Chaowagul W. Recent advances in the treatment of severe melioidosis. *Acta Tropica* 2000; 74:133–137.

32 Currie B J, Fisher D A, Anstey N M et al. Melioidosis: acute and chronic disease, relapse and reactivation. *Trans R Soc Trop Med Hygiene* 2000; 94:301–304.

Chapter 65
Diphtheria

N. J. White and T. T. Hien

Definition

Diphtheria is an acute infectious disease of the tonsils, pharynx, larynx or nose, and occasionally of other mucous membranes or skin caused by *Corynebacterium diphtheriae*. The word diphtheria originates from the term 'diphtherite', which has a Greek root meaning skin or hide, and refers to the leathery appearance of the characteristic pharyngeal membrane.[1] The disease is caused by the local effects of destructive infection (usually in the nasopharynx) and the distal effects of diphtheria toxin on the heart, peripheral nerves and kidneys. Death results from airways obstruction, myocarditis or polyneuritis. Diphtheria has declined dramatically in affluent countries over the past 70 years,[2,3] but it remains an important disease in many parts of the tropics and there has been a recent resurgence of the disease in some of the former Soviet Socialist Republics and Eastern Europe.

Bacteriology

The diphtheria bacillus was first grown in pure culture by Loeffler in 1884. The causative organism, *C. diphtheriae* is a non-motile, non-capsulated, non-spore-forming aerobic bacillus. Although it is described as Gram-positive, it is easily decolorized during the staining procedure and may appear Gram-negative. On microscopy, *C. diphtheriae* exhibits considerable pleomorphism, ranging from the classical club shape to long slender bacilli. The arrangement of organisms on a smear often resembles Chinese letters. The presence of metachromatic granules when stained by Loeffler's methylene blue or Albert's stain is characteristic, although this should not be relied upon for identification.

C. diphtheriae grows well on blood agar, but tellurite blood agar (Hoyle's medium) is recommended as this inhibits other respiratory flora and allows the characteristic colonial morphology of the three biotypes (*gravis*, *intermedius* and *mitis*) to develop.[4] Although, as the name implies, toxigenic *gravis* strains are generally associated with more severe disease, in vitro *mitis* strains often produce more toxin than *gravis* or *intermedius* strains. Toxin production is very dependent on the composition of the growth medium. The iron content is particularly important. Young organisms produce more toxin than older organisms, and thus increased toxin production is associated with rapid growth. The association between biotype and severity is not constant. *C. diphtheriae* is further identified by biochemical reactions: acid is produced from glucose and maltose but only very rarely from sucrose; urea is not hydrolysed. The *gravis* biotype ferments starch.[5] Simple screening tests have been developed for identification of the pathogenic corynebacteria, which do not produce pyrazinamidase, but do produce cystinase (seen as a brown halo around colonies, when cystine is incorporated into modified Tinsdale's agar).[6]

Pathogenesis

The potentially lethal effects of diphtheria in humans are caused by an exotoxin. The toxigenicity of *C. diphtheriae* depends on the presence of a *tox*+ phage (a lysogenic β-phage) which induces the organism to produce toxin. Harmless non-toxigenic strains of *C. diphtheriae*, lacking the *tox*+ β-phage, can be converted to pathogenic toxigenic strains by infection with a lysogenic phage (in vitro). This process may also occur in vivo.[7]

Toxin production by corynebacteria is usually detected by Elek's test[5] or guinea pig inoculation, but recently enzyme immunoassays have been developed which are cheaper and easier.[8] Diphtheria toxin can also be produced by *C. ulcerans* and this has resulted in clinical diphtheria.[9]

Diphtheria exotoxin is a 62 000-Da polypeptide which includes two segments: the active toxin moiety (A) and the binding (B) segment, which binds to specific receptors on susceptible cells. The binding B portion attaches to the cell membrane, allowing the active A portion to enter the cells where it catalyses a reaction that inactivates the transfer RNA (tRNA) translocase 'elongation factor 2' (EF-2), in eukaryotic cells. This factor is essential for reactions that transfer triplet codes from messenger RNA to amino acid sequences via tRNA. Thus EF-2 inactivation stops synthesis of the polypeptide chains. The diphtheria toxin affects all human cells, but the most profound effects are on the myocardium (myocarditis), peripheral nerves (demyelination) and kidneys (acute tubular necrosis).

Epidemiology

The only known reservoir for *C. diphtheriae* is the human. Diphtheria spreads from person to person, either from acute cases or from asymptomatic carriers. The principal modes of spread are by respiratory droplets or direct contact with secretions from the respiratory tract or exudate from infected skin. Fomites and dust are not important vehicles of transmission, but the organism can resist drying and may be isolated from floor dust in a ward or a room in which an infected patient is being nursed. Epidemics have been caused by milk contaminated by a human carrier. Some patients become carriers and continue to harbour *C. diphtheriae* for weeks or months, or rarely for a lifetime.

The incidence of diphtheria in the Western world has decreased in the last 50–75 years (152 cases per 100 000 population in 1920 to 0.002 per 100 000 in 1980 in the USA). As diphtheria began to decline before the immunization programmes were instituted, and epidemics have occurred even in well immunized populations, it seems that there are additional undefined factors contributing to the low incidence of diphtheria in affluent countries. Although there has been a great decline in the disease in wealthy countries (such that most physicians in these countries have never seen a case of diphtheria), the disease is still a significant problem in many developing countries.

Clinical manifestations

Diphtheria is predominantly a disease of childhood.[10,11] After an incubation period of 2–5 days, diphtheria presents in a variety of different forms depending upon the location of the pseudomembrane. The grey-white membrane is the hallmark of the infection. It is caused by the destructive effects of the toxin on epithelial cells. The membrane is composed of a coagulum of leucocytes, bacteria, cellular debris and fibrin. It is adherent to underlying tissues and bleeds if pulled away. In clinical practice the disease can be divided into groups as follows: cutaneous, nasal, faucial, tracheolaryngeal and malignant diphtheria. Faucial diphtheria is the most common, whereas cutaneous diphtheria is relatively rare in endemic areas; however, where the disease is rare, cutaneous diphtheria is relatively more common.

Anterior nasal diphtheria

The principal symptom is nasal discharge (100%). This usually unilateral, thin at first, then purulent and bloody with excoriations of the nostril and skin above the upper lip. Nasal diphtheria is relatively common in infancy. It is often mild except when nasopharyngeal or faucial forms coexist.

Faucial diphtheria

This is the most common form of diphtheria. The onset is usually slow, with moderate fever, malaise and sore throat (80%). Other symptoms may include nausea, vomiting and painful dysphagia. There is typically a patch or patches of greyish-yellow adherent membrane with a surrounding dull red inflammatory zone on one or both tonsils. At the beginning of the illness, diphtheria can look like any type of tonsillitis, with only a small spot of membrane on one tonsil. The membrane may then extend to the uvula, soft palate, oropharynx, nasopharynx or larynx. The lymph nodes in the neck are enlarged and painful, and the neck may be slightly swollen. The fetor of diphtheria is characteristic and was once one of the four criteria for clinical diagnosis (membrane, fetor, lymphadenitis, oedema).[2]

Tracheolaryngeal diphtheria

Diphtheria of the larynx is usually secondary to faucial diphtheria (85%). Occasionally, there is no membrane on the pharynx at all. The initial symptoms include moderate fever (75%) with hoarseness (100%), unproductive cough and dyspnoea. Obstruction of breathing by the expanding membrane and associated oedema occurs gradually over about 24 hours. Sometimes the membrane detaches, causing acute respiratory obstruction. The severely affected child appears agitated, but is quiet, sweating and ominously cyanotic. The accessory muscles of respiration are used, with retraction of supraclavicular, substernal and intercostal tissues on inspiration. Without a tracheostomy the child will suffocate and die.

Malignant diphtheria

This is the most severe form of diphtheria. The onset is more acute than in other forms. The patient becomes rapidly 'toxic', with high fever, rapid pulse, low blood pressure and cyanosis. Usually, extension of the membrane is more rapid, spreading from the tonsils to the uvula, then creeping forward across the hard palate, up the nasopharynx, or sometimes down the nostrils. Cervical adenitis and oedema produce the classical 'bull neck' appearance. The patient may bleed from the mouth, nose and skin. Cardiac involvement with heart block occurs earlier, within a few days from the onset. More than one half of malignant diphtheria cases are fatal, and this high mortality rate has changed little with treatment.

Cutaneous diphtheria

Skin infections with *C. diphtheriae* are now more common than nasopharyngeal disease in the West. This particularly affects vagrants and alcoholics living in unhygienic conditions. The clinical features range from a simple pustule to a chronic non-healing ulcer with a grey, dirty, membrane. Toxic complications from these infections are infrequent, and when they do occur are more likely to manifest as neuritis than myocarditis.

Other sites

Occasionally, clinical infections with *C. diphtheriae* may occur in other sites, such as ears, conjunctiva or vagina. Swabs of ear discharge from otitis media may occasionally grow *C. diphtheriae* but toxic manifestations are rare.

Complications

Severe diphtheria is a terrible disease. Even if patients survive the acute destructive phase of the infection, they are likely to die from the remote effects of the toxin. Patients recovering from diphtheria may die suddenly up to 8 weeks following the acute disease. The most prominent toxic complications of diphtheria are myocarditis and neuritis. The risk and the severity of toxin damage correlate with the extent of the pseudomembrane and the delay in administration of antitoxin. The frequency of cardiac involvement following laryngeal and malignant diphtheria is 3–8-fold higher than for tonsillar diphtheria, and 2–3-fold higher if antitoxin is given 48 hours or more from the onset of disease. Overall, approximately 10% of patients with diphtheria develop myocarditis, although two-thirds of patients with severe infection will have some evidence of cardiac involvement. The first evidence of cardiac toxicity usually occurs after the first week of illness.[12,13] Clinical signs include soft heart sounds, a gallop rhythm, and less commonly signs of congestive heart failure. Incompetent murmurs may develop as the ventricles dilate. The mortality rate associated with diphtheritic myocarditis is approximately 50%. Echocardiography shows dilated, poorly contracting ventricles. Electrocardiographic (ECG) abnormalities are more common than clinical signs of myocarditis and include frequent supraventricular and ventricular ectopics, broadening of the QRS complex, ST and T wave changes, varying degrees of heart block, and both tachyarrhythmias and bradyarrhythmias.[13,14] The loss of anterior R waves or the development of complete heart block is an ominous sign. Patients with bundle branch block and complete heart block have a very high mortality rate (more than 80%). Levels of cardiac enzymes (creatine phosphokinase MB, myoglobin and troponins) rise in proportion to the degree of cardiac damage.

The exotoxin causes degeneration of the myelin sheath and axon cylinder of peripheral nerves. Polyneuritis is uncommon in mild diphtheria but occurs in approximately 7–10% of moderate and severe cases. Neurological complications develop late, usually between 3 and 8 weeks after the onset of local symptoms, and often when other severe manifestations are resolving.

Paralysis of the soft palate is characteristic. This results in a nasal voice and regurgitation of ingested fluids through the nose. Later, blurred vision may occur because of paralysis of the muscles of accommodation. Paralysis of the pharynx, larynx and respiratory muscles is the most common manifestation. The IXth and Xth cranial nerves are most commonly affected, followed by the VIIth nerve, the nerves to the external ocular muscles (III, IV and VI) and the IXth nerve.[15] Quadriparesis is common, and death from respiratory failure may result either from paralysis of the respiratory muscles or paralytic closure of the larynx. Sensory deficit affects proprioception in particular. Autonomic dysfunction is common, and sudden hypotension may occur between the fourth and seventh weeks of disease. The evolution of the neurological deficit is often asynchronous such that cranial nerve deficits may be improving while peripheral nerve deficits worsen.[15]

The less common complications of diphtheria include acute tubular necrosis, disseminated intravascular coagulation, endocarditis and secondary pneumonia. The overall mortality rate of diphtheria is approximately 5–10%, with a relatively higher rate in infancy and old age.

Diagnosis

In many parts of the world, especially in developing countries, diphtheria is still a common disease. It should be considered in any patient with the following symptoms: tonsillitis and/or pharyngitis with pseudomembrane, hoarseness and stridor, cervical adenopathy or cervical swelling (bull neck), unilateral bloody nasal discharge or paralysis of the palate. Direct smears of infected areas of the throat are often made, but these are unreliable. The diagnosis is confirmed by isolation and identification of *C. diphtheriae* from infected sites, but cultures are often negative, particularly if the patient has received antibiotics before admission to hospital. The differential diagnosis includes streptococcal or viral pharyngitis and tonsillitis, and Vincent's angina. Common and sometimes tragic errors are to diagnose tonsillar diphtheria as infectious mononucleosis, or a case of 'bull neck' (malignant diphtheria) as mumps.

Management

Emergency tracheostomy should be performed to anticipate or relieve respiratory obstruction in laryngeal diphtheria. The procedure must not be delayed until the patient develops cyanosis. Agitation and the use of the accessory respiratory muscles are indications for immediate tracheostomy. As the mortality rate of diphtheria increases with delay in antitoxin administration, treatment with diphtheria antitoxin should be started on clinical suspicion, without waiting for definitive laboratory confirmation. The dose of antitoxin depends on the site of primary infection, the extent of pseudomembrane, and the delay between the onset and the antitoxin administration: 20 000–40 000 units for faucial diphtheria of less than 48 hours' duration, or cutaneous infection; 40 000–80 000 units for faucial diphtheria of more than 48 hours' duration, or laryngeal infection; 80 000–100 000 units for malignant diphtheria (bull neck, toxic state). Adrenaline (epinephrine) should be available to cope with rare anaphylactic reactions to the antitoxin.

Antibiotics will stop toxin production and prevent further spread of organisms in the host. *C. diphtheriae* is susceptible to a variety of antibiotics including penicillin, cephalosporins, erythromycin and tetracycline. In a recent randomized comparison in Vietnam, the use of penicillin was associated with shorter fever clearance (median 27 hours) compared with 46 hours for erythromycin recipients and, whereas there was no penicillin resistance, 27% of the *C. diphtheriae* isolated were resistant to erythromycin.[16] The recommended antibiotic treatment regimen is therefore penicillin G, 50 000 units/kg daily in four divided doses, with erythromycin, parenterally or orally, 5 mg/kg four times daily as an alternative for penicillin-allergic patients. Antibiotic susceptibility should be checked when cultures are positive. Erythromycin is considered to be more effective in eliminating the carrier state, although there are limited data.

Bed rest is recommended during the acute phase, but there is no proof of its benefit. Close ECG monitoring is indicated, particularly after the first week, to detect cardiac involvement. Angiotensin-converting enzyme inhibitors (captopril) have been used in patients, but there have been no randomized trials. If there is high-grade or complete heart block, then temporary pacing should be performed, although again there have been no large trials to determine whether these measures influence outcome.[17] One study has suggested that carnitine may be beneficial by decreasing the incidence of myocarditis,[18] but additional evidence of its efficacy is required. The administration of corticosteroids may benefit laryngeal diphtheria by reducing swelling,[19] but otherwise is of no benefit.[20]

Prevention

Diphtheria is readily preventable by vaccine administration. This is included in the triple vaccine: diphtheria, tetanus and pertussis vaccine (DTP). The recommended primary course of immunization of children aged up to 7 years consists of three doses: the first at 6–8 weeks of age, the second at 3 months and the third at 4 months. A fourth dose is given 6–12 months after the third. A booster dose of diphtheria and tetanus (DT) vaccine is given at school entry. If primary immunization is delayed until 7 years of age, or is interrupted, a series of three doses of tetanus and diphtheria toxoid adsorbed (DT ads), which contains less diphtheria toxoid than DTP, should be completed, giving the second dose 4–8 weeks after the first, and the third 6–12 months later. Some have argued that all people should receive a DT booster in later life (55–65 years). Research continues into combination vaccines and the intranasal delivery route. Patients with diphtheria should receive active immunization after recovery. Close contacts should be screened for *C. diphtheriae* with throat swab culture. If the immunization status is unclear, they should be treated with an appropriate antibiotic if culture positive, and receive primary immunization according to their age. Immunity following immunization can be assesssed by means of the Schick test. A standardized sterile diluted filtrate from a culture of *C. diphtheriae* (the Schick test toxin) is injected intradermally (0.2 ml) into the flexor surface of the left forearm. An equal volume (0.2 ml) of heat-inactivated filtrate (Schick test control) is injected intradermally into the right forearm. The injection sites are inspected after 24–48 hours and again at 5–7 days. A lack of inflammation indicates adequate antitoxic immunity. Sometimes non-specific reactions (pseudoreactions) occur, but these are usually equal in both arms (i.e., toxin and control elicit an equal inflammatory reaction). Schick-negative patients are either resistant to disease or, with *gravis* and *intermedius* strains, they may sometimes develop mild disease.

REFERENCES

1   English P C. Diphtheria and theories of infectious disease: centennial appreciation of the critical role of diphtheria in the history of medicine. *Pediatrics* 1985; 76:1–9.

2   Kwantes W. Diphtheria in Europe. *J Hyg (Camb)* 1984; 93:433–347.

3   Dixon J M S. Diphtheria in North America. *J Hyg (Camb)* 1984; 93:419–432.

4   Noble W C & Dixon J M S. *Corynebacterium* and other coryneform bacteria. In Parker T M & Duerden B I (eds) *Topley and Wilson's Principles of Bacteriology, Virology and Immunity*, vol. 2, 8th edn. London: Edward Arnold, 1990:103–118.

5   Brooks R & Joynson D H M. Bacterial diagnosis of diphtheria. *J Clin Pathol* 1990; 43:576–580.

6   Coleman G, Weaver E & Efstratiou A. Screening tests for pathogenic corynebacteria. *J Clin Pathol* 1992; 45:46–48.

7   Pappenheimer A M & Murphy J H. Studies on the molecular epidemiology of diphtheria. *Lancet* 1983; ii:923–926.

8   Hallas G, Harrison T G, Samuel D & Coleman G. Detection of diphtheria toxin in culture supernates of *Corynebacterium diphtheriae* and *C.ulcerans* by immunoassay with monoclonal antibody. *J Med Microbiol* 1990; 32:247–253.

9   Meers P D. A case of classical diphtheria due to *Corynebacterium ulcerans*. *J Infect* 1979; 1:139–142.

10   Hong N T, Phu V T & Hien T T. A study of 2597 cases of diphtheria treated at Cho Quan Hospital during 10 years (1976–85). *Annual Scientific Report of Cho Quan Hospital, Vietnam* 1985:65–78.

11   Naiditch M J & Bower A G. Diphtheria. A study of 1433 cases observed at the Los Angeles County Hospital. *Am J Med* 1954; 17:229–245.

12   Boyer N H & Weinstein L. Diphtheritic myocarditis. *N Engl J Med* 1948; 239:913–919.

13   Loukoushkina E F, Bobko P V, Kolbasova E V et al. The clinical picture and diagnosis of diphtheritic carditis in children. *Eur J*

Pediatr 1998; 157:528–533.

14 Bethell D B, Dung M N, Loan H T et al. Prognostic value of electrocardiographic monitoring in severe diphtheria. *Clin Infect Dis* 1995; 20:1259–1265.

15 Piradov M A, Pirogov V N, Popova L M & Avdunina I A. Diphtheritic polyneuropathy: clinical analysis of severe forms. *Arch Neurol* 2001; 58:1438–1442.

16 Kneen R, Giao P N, Solomon T et al. Penicillin versus erythromycin in the treatment of diphtheria. *Clin Infect Dis* 1998; 27:845–850.

17 Stockins B A, Lanas F T, Saavedra J G & Opazo J A. Prognosis in patients with diphtheric myocarditis and bradyarrhythmias: assessment of results of ventricular pacing. *Br Heart J* 1994; 72:190–191.

18 Ramos A C M F, Elias P R D, Barrucand L & Silva J A F D. The protective effect of carnitine in human diphtheric myocarditis. *Pediatr Res* 1987; 18:815–819.

19 Havaldar P V. Dexamethasone in laryngeal diphtheritic croup. *Ann Trop Paediatr* 1997; 17:21–23.

20 Thisyakorn U, Wongvanich J & Kumpeng V. Failure of corticosteroid therapy to prevent diphtheric myocarditis or neuritis. *Pediatr Infect Dis* 1984; 3:126–128.

Chapter 66
Endemic Treponematoses

M. Kapembwa

The endemic or non-venereal treponematoses include yaws, endemic syphilis and pinta. Their causative organisms, *Treponema pertenue* for yaws, *T. pallidum* for endemic syphilis and *T. carateum* for pinta, have remained until the present time morphologically and antigenically indistinguishable from *T. pallidum*, which causes venereal syphilis (Chapter 21). Likewise, there are no differences in serology or response to penicillin. Nevertheless, there are significant clinical and epidemiological differences among these treponematoses.

The discrepant manifestations of these biologically 'similar' organisms has generated considerable interest leading to academic disputes and much speculation and argument among medical historians. Hudson[1] recognized only *T. pallidum* and believed in an all-embracing concept (unitarian theory): all the treponematoses were due to the same organism and the differences were determined by the socio-environmental conditions such as age, microclimate of skin, temperature and humidity. Others, including Hackett,[2] believe that these conditions are separate entities caused by different organisms. Whereas it is generally believed that the DNA profiles of the causative organisms of venereal syphilis, yaws and endemic syphilis are indistinguishable,[3] there may well be subtle morphological differences that remain to be characterized. In one study, *T. pertenue* and *T. pallidum* were reported to differ in at least one nucleotide.[4] The differences with regard to experimental infections by these treponemes in laboratory animals have also been described.[5] Humans are the only proven reservoirs for the non-venereal treponemes and, although similar organisms have been isolated from primates in Africa, their significance with regard to human disease is unclear.[6]

Endemic treponematoses were among the most predominant diseases in the pre-antibiotic era. Thus, in the mid-twentieth century there were an estimated 50 million cases of yaws worldwide (half in Africa), over 1 million cases of endemic syphilis (mostly in North Africa and the eastern Mediterranean basin) and about 1 million cases of pinta confined to Central and South America. Discovery of long-acting penicillin preparations, which were cheap, safe and curative with a single intramuscular injection, made a cost-effective eradication programme possible. Consequently in 1948, the World Health Organization, in conjunction with UNICEF and many national governments, established a global control programme, first against yaws and later extended to include endemic syphilis and pinta. Mobile teams were formed, and over 50 million individuals were treated of 160 million examined in 46 countries. As a result these diseases were brought under control or even eliminated from some areas. However, dismantling of the mobile teams and lack of active surveillance led to the persistence of endemic foci in some countries. From 1980, not surprisingly, reports began to appear of an alarming resurgence, notably of yaws and endemic syphilis, particularly in West Africa, Central Africa, and to a lesser extent South-East Asia and the western Pacific.[7-11] In some parts of the Central African Republic, the pygmy population has been suggested to harbour the main focus of yaws.[12] Sporadic cases were also being reported from some countries in the Americas.[13,14] The geographical distribution of the endemic treponematoses in the early 1990s is shown in Figure 66.1. In some tropical areas, when yaws came under control, venereally acquired syphilis had apparently become more prevalent, possibly because of immunological and socio-cultural factors. Thus, both yaws and venereally acquired syphilis were being encountered in these areas, giving rise to diagnostic problems.

In addition to the similarities mentioned above, the endemic treponematoses have some other common characteristics, including non-venereal transmission (mainly in childhood), a predominantly rural distribution associated with poverty, overcrowding, the absence of congenital transmission, and the lack of involvement of cardiovascular and central nervous systems. The occasional reports purporting to show evidence of involvement of cardiovascular and central nervous systems have attracted little support, and positive serological tests in the newborn may be due to passive transplacental transfer of IgG. Their differentiation, therefore, at the present time, is dependent on clinical and epidemiological aspects. The *incubation period* of endemic treponematoses is similar to that of venereal syphilis.

Yaws

The causative organism is *T. pertenue*. The disease is also known by different names; Framboesia (German), Pian (French), Buba (Spanish), Parangi and Paru (Malay).

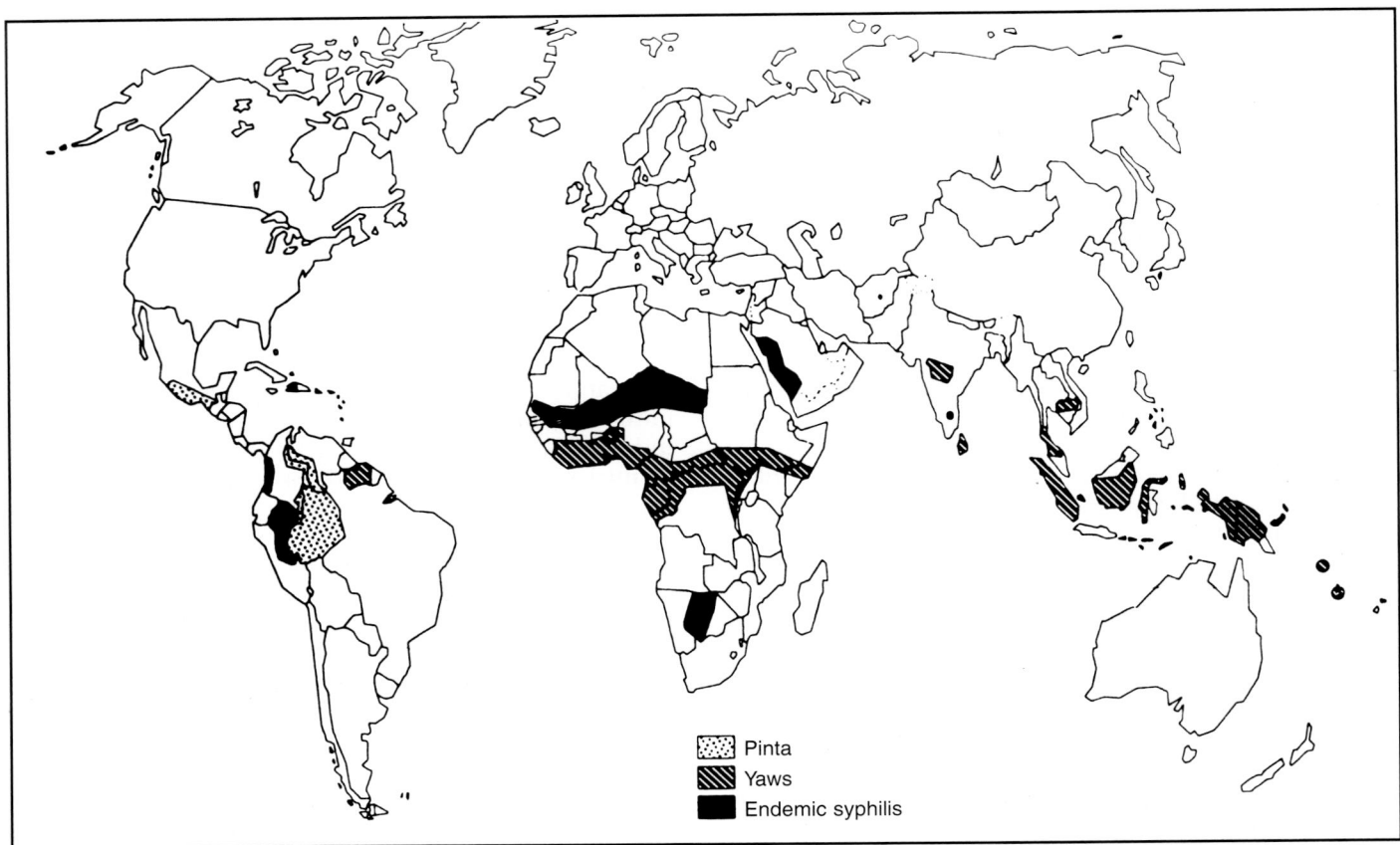

Figure 66.1: Geographical distribution of the endemic treponematoses in the early 1990s. (From *Clinics in Dermatology* 1999; 17:144; courtesy of Dr Herman Jan H. Engelkens.)

Epidemiology and mode of transmission

Yaws is found in the warm, humid, tropical, predominantly rural areas of Africa, Central and South America, the Caribbean, and equatorial islands of South-East Asia, notably Indonesia and Papua New Guinea, with a limited distribution in some remote parts of India and Thailand. In endemic areas the prevalence of infectious yaws increases during the rainy season, when skin lesions tend to be more numerous.

Yaws occurs commonly among children aged 2–15 years who live in poor, overcrowded and insanitary conditions. Direct personal skin-to-skin contact is the major route of transmission of yaws. The reproducibility of yaws in humans by inoculation with secretions from patients with framboesia was demonstrated by Paulet in 1848 and by Charlouis in 1881, well before the identification of *T. pertenue* by Castellani in 1905.[15–17] A lack of soap and water, clothes and footwear facilitates the spread of the disease. Infectivity occurs particularly under humid tropical conditions. Indirect transmission of treponemal infection by formites and insects settling on open moist lesions is theoretically possible but no evidence exists.[18] Sexual transmission does not, as a rule, play a role in endemic treponematoses.

Clinical features

The course of yaws may be divided into early, latent (during which infectious relapses may occur) and late (tertiary) non-infectious stages.

Early stage

Early yaws comprises the primary and secondary stages. After an average incubation period of 21 (range 9–90) days, the *initial* or *primary* lesion ('mother yaw') appears at the site of entry of the organisms, usually on the exposed parts of the body such as legs, arms, face and neck. The lesion manifests as a round or oval papule, 2–5 cm in diameter, and may develop into a large papilloma (Figure 66.2). Early-stage skin lesions are often itchy, leading to excoriation and ulceration. Such lesions contain numerous treponemes and are, therefore, highly infectious.

The *primary* lesion may last for 3–6 months and heal with or without scar formation. Lymphatic spread may lead to lesions in the neighbouring areas, and haematogenous spread of the organisms may produce lesions elsewhere in the body.

Secondary lesions usually appear a few weeks to up to 2 years after the appearance of the primary lesion, and

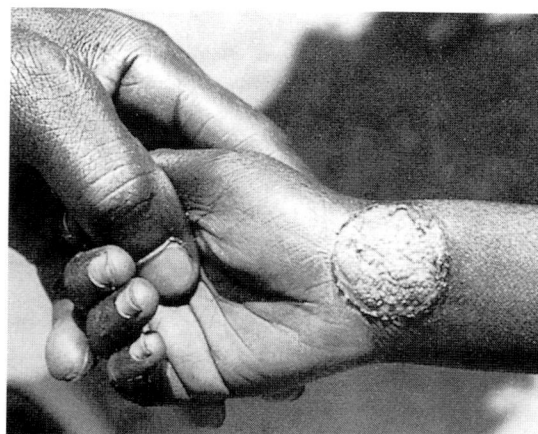

Figure 66.2: Yaws: initial lesion 'mother yaw'. (Courtesy of C. J. Hackett.)

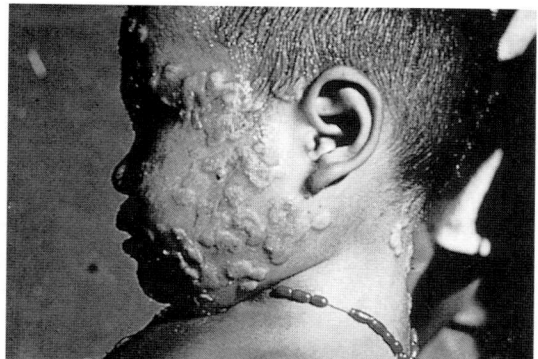

Figure 66.3: Cutaneous early yaws: papillomas. (Courtesy of C. J. Hackett.)

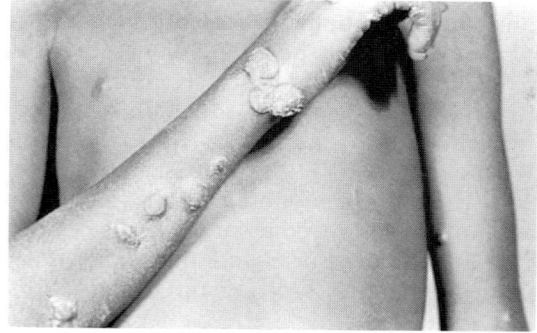

Figure 66.4: Cutaneous early yaws: papillomas. (Courtesy of C. J. Hackett.)

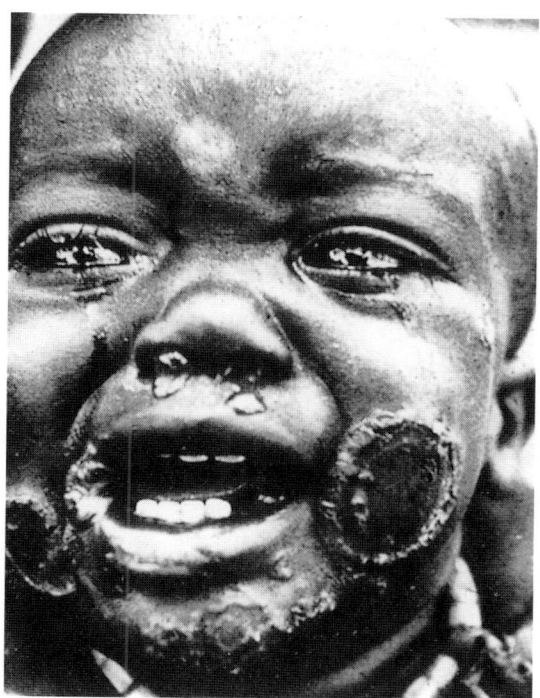

Figure 66.5: Cutaneous early yaws: papillomas. (Courtesy of C. J. Hackett.)

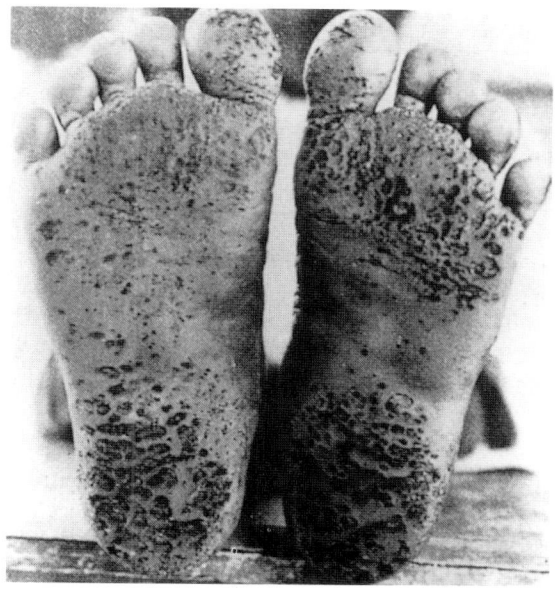

Figure 66.6: Indeterminate yaws: plantar hyperkeratosis (crab yaws).

may be preceded or accompanied by fever, malaise and generalized lymphadenopathy. The skin manifestations resemble the initial lesion but are more disseminated. They may become crusted and removal of the yellow crust reveals raspberry granulomas (framboesides) (Figures 66.3 and 66.4). Annular, discoid (Figure 66.5), crescentic or irregularly shaped papules and nodules can also be seen. The palms of the hand and soles of feet show hyperkeratosis (crab yaws). Plantar papillomas, in particular, take longer to erupt than those elsewhere on the skin and may make walking painful, resulting in a sideways crablike gait (crab yaws) (Figure 66.6). Lesions occurring on the moist areas of the body, or at the muco-cutaneous junctions, may resemble the condylomata lata of syphilis. The secondary lesions, which tend to occur in crops, may last for up to 6 months and heal without any scars except when ulcerated and secondarily infected.

Bone involvement is manifested by osteitis and periostitis; the affected bones are painful (worse at night) and tender. Dactylitis (i.e., osteoperiostitis of the proximal

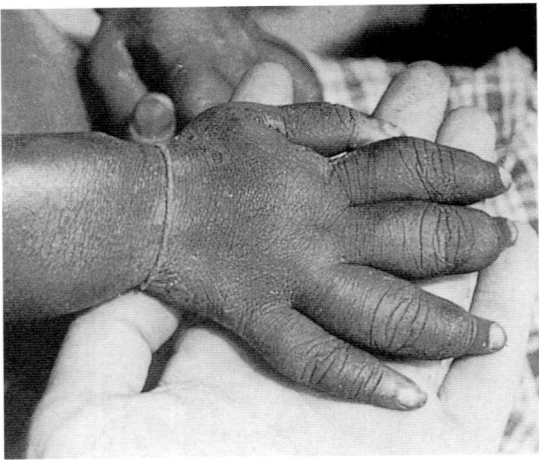

Figure 66.7: Early yaws: polydactylitis.

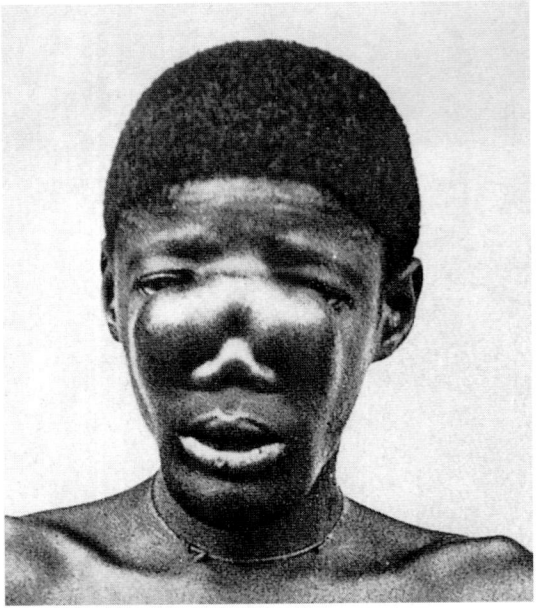

Figure 66.8: Early yaws: goundou. (Courtesy of C. J. Hackett.)

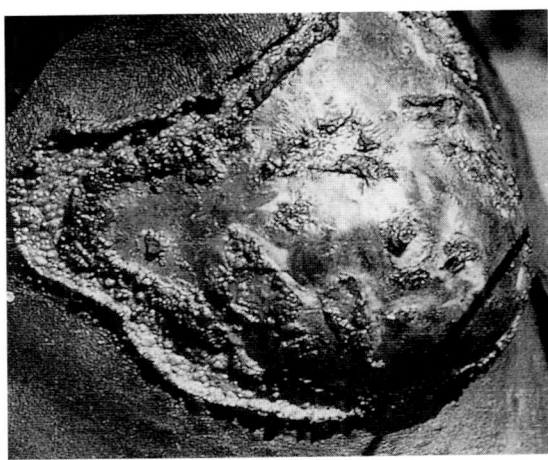

Figure 66.9: Late yaws: gumma of the right breast. (Courtesy of C. J. Hackett.)

titres. An estimated 10% of patients develop late lesions after 5 or more years of untreated infection.

Late stage

The late stage, which develops in approximately 10% of cases, is characterized by necrotic destructive lesions of the skin (Figure 66.9) and gummatous lesions of the bones (Figure 66.10) and overlying tissues, resulting in varying degrees of scarring and deformity. These lesions are similar to those of venereal syphilis (Chapter 21). The late manifestations include: hyperkeratosis of palms and soles with deep fissuring; juxta-articular subcutaneous fibrous nodules around the elbows and knees; bursitis (Figure 66.11); disfiguring lesions of the nasopharynx (rhinopharyngitis mutilans or gangosa) (Figure 66.12) as a result of ulceration of the palate or nasal septum progressing to perforation and destruction of the turbinates and pharynx, and secondary infection with offensive discharge; and sabre tibia (Figure 66.13) as a result of hypertrophic osteoperiostitis. Hyperkeratosis of palms and soles (see Figure 66.6) and *goundou* (see Figure 66.8) are much more pronounced in late yaws. The former may be accompanied by fissures and may be very painful. Eventually, there may be scarring and disfiguration of the hands and feet.

Congenital transmission does not occur, and the cardiovascular and nervous systems are considered not to be affected. However, in one study ocular and neurological abnormalities were noted in patients presumed to be suffering from late yaws.[20] Other indirect evidence of yaws causing idiopathic myeloneuropathy has led to suggestions that the potential sequelae of yaws are identical to those of venereal syphilis.[21]

Histopathology

In early yaws, papillomatous epidermal hyperplasia is the main feature and treponemes can be demonstrated in

phalanges of the fingers; Figure 66.7) and swelling of the ulna, as well as involvement of the long bones of the legs, are common in children. Plain radiography is usually sufficient to identify early bone changes.[19] In very rare cases there is hypertrophic osteitis of the nasal process of the maxillae, giving rise to the swellings on both sides of the bridge of the nose, called *goundou* (Figure 66.8). In untreated cases the swellings may grow and obstruct the nostrils.

Latent stage

The disease may then progress to latency, resulting eventually in spontaneous cure or persistent latency. Serological tests may remain positive, usually at low

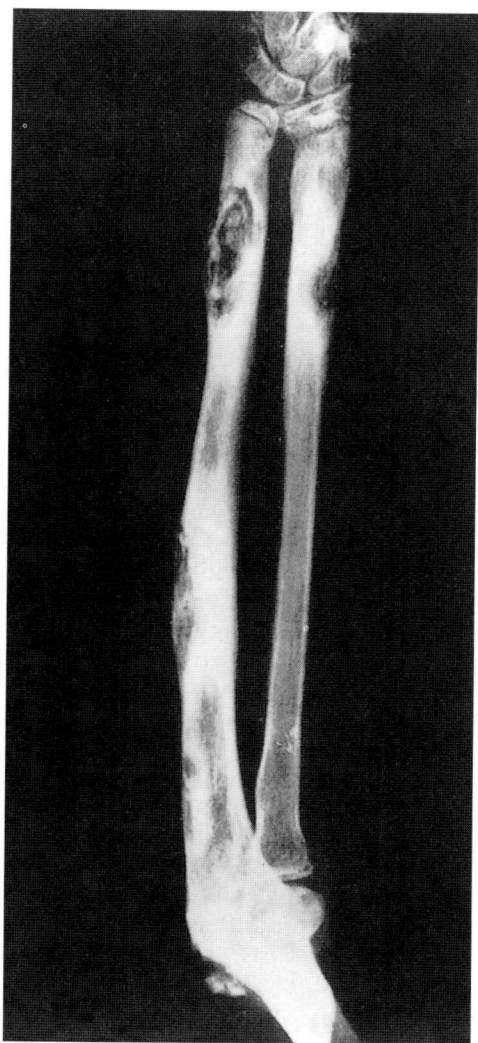

Figure 66.10: Late yaws: gummatous osteitis of radius and ulna. (Courtesy of C. J. Hackett.)

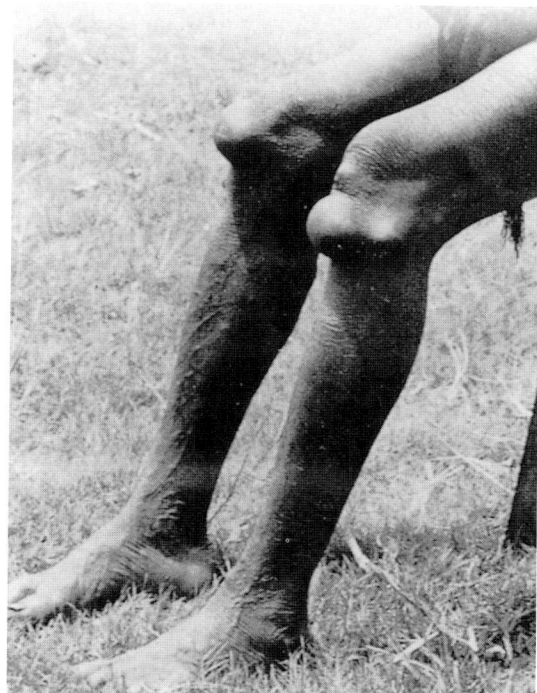

Figure 66.11: Late yaws: chronic bilateral prepatellar bursitis.

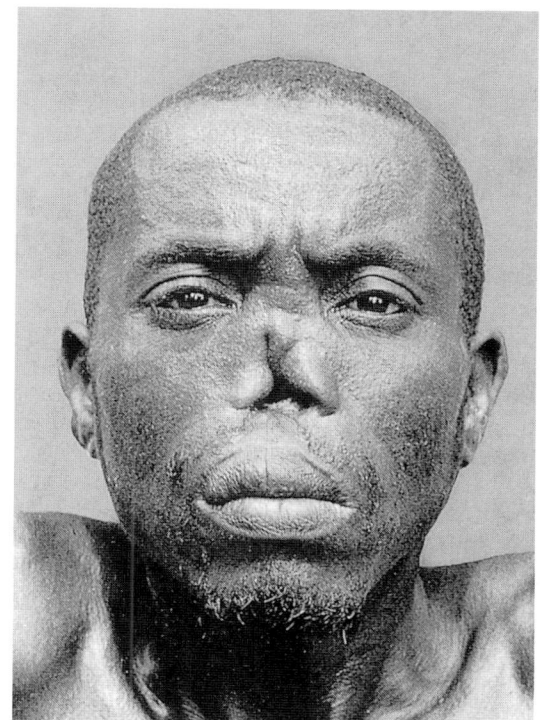

Figure 66.12: Late yaws: gangosa. (Courtesy of C. J. Hackett.)

specimens stained by silver impregnation technique[22] or immunofluorescence.[23] It is generally believed that the basic pathology in yaws is the same as that in venereal syphilis. However, in yaws, endothelial proliferation seems to be much less marked; obliterative changes in the vessels are not encountered and acanthosis is more prominent.[22]

Studies have been carried out to localize treponemes and characterize inflammatory infiltrate in skin biopsies from patients with early venereal syphilis and early infectious yaws.[24] Treponemes in yaws cases (from West Sumatra) were found to be mostly, but not exclusively, confined to the epidermis as opposed to early venereal syphilis lesions—in which the organisms were demonstrated largely in the dermal–epidermal junction as well as in the dermis. Using specific monoclonal antibodies, these same authors were also struck by the paucity of T and B lymphocytes in yaws specimens.

Diagnosis and differential diagnoses

Dark-field examination of exudates from primary and secondary skin lesions will reveal motile treponemes which

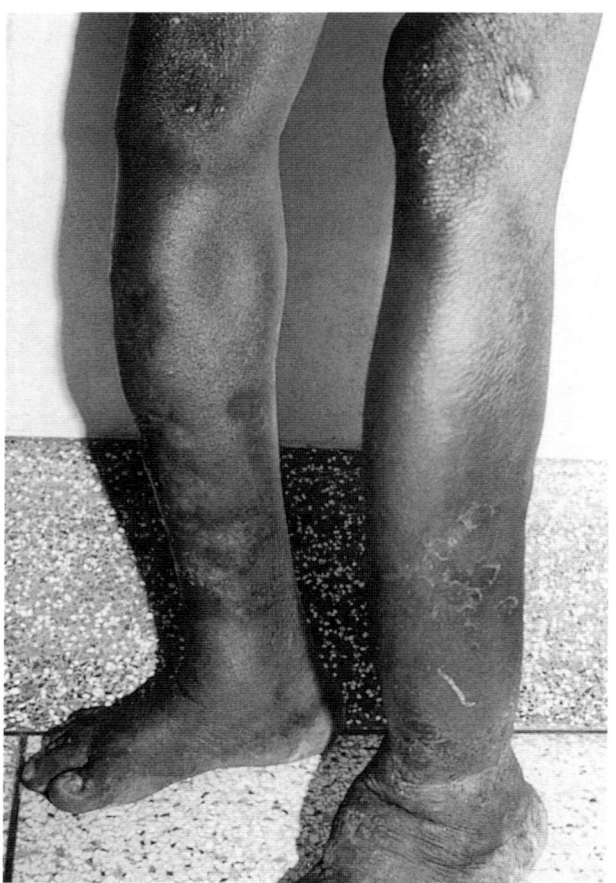

Figure 66.13: Late yaws: sabre tibia. (Reproduced with permission from Arya O P, Osoba A O & Bennett F J (eds) *Tropical Venereology*, 2nd edn. Edinburgh: Churchill Livingstone, 1988:138.)

must be differentiated from saprophytic spirochaetes. Serological tests behave as in the case of venereal syphilis (Chapter 21).

Clinical diagnosis of yaws in the presence of classical lesions is straightforward in endemic areas, but differentiation from endemic syphilis may occasionally be difficult. The common skin conditions to be differentiated include scabies, fungal infections, impetigo, lichen planus, psoriasis and tungiasis. Gummatous lesions should be differentiated from: tropical ulcer, fungating mycotic lesions, cutaneous leishmaniasis, leprosy, neoplasm(s) and possibly other conditions. Juxta-articular nodules of onchocerciasis and dactylitis of tuberculosis and sickle cell disease should be distinguished by appropriate tests. Radiography will demonstrate bone lesions but these may be identical to those of venereal and endemic syphilis.

If differentiation from venereal syphilis is difficult, especially in latent cases—as may happen when an immigrant presents at a clinic in a country with a temperate climate and the adequacy of any previous treatment is in doubt—the person should be treated as for syphilis. However, in view of the social implications, special care should be taken in communicating the diagnosis to the patient, who should be given a full explanation.

Management and control

See page 1151.

Endemic syphilis (Bejel, Firjal, Loath, Njovera, Dichuchwa, Siti)

Epidemiology and mode of transmission

Endemic syphilis is a chronic childhood infection of skin, bone and cartilage. The disease is endemic in the arid Sahelian areas of West Africa, with foci also in Zimbabwe and Botswana, and to a lesser extent among the nomadic people in the Arabian peninsula and the aborigines of central Australia. The disease primarily affects people in poor rural communities living in unhygienic and over-crowded conditions. The majority of early cases are found in children aged 2–15 years, who are the main reservoir of infection. The initial lesion is usually on the oral mucosa, and transmission is by direct contact through kissing and by indirect contact through eating and drinking utensils. The infection spreads easily among family groups and village communities from infected children to other children and previously uninfected adults. The role of flies acting as vectors remains unproven. There is no proof that congenital transmission occurs in endemic syphilis.

Clinical features

A primary lesion is rarely present in endemic syphilis. The earliest lesions encountered are the mucous patches, which are shallow painless ulcers on the lips (Figure 66.14) and in the oropharynx, when the patient may

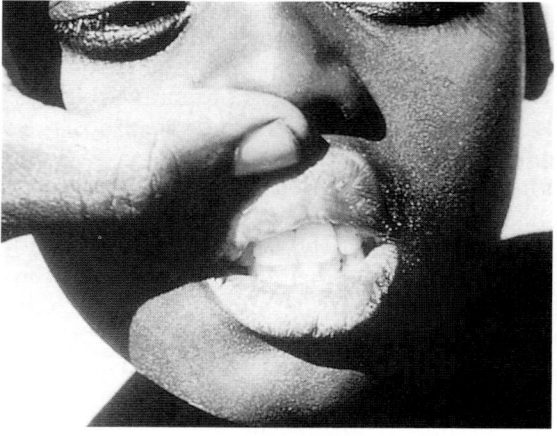

Figure 66.14: Early endemic syphilis: mucous papules on the buccal surface of the upper lip.

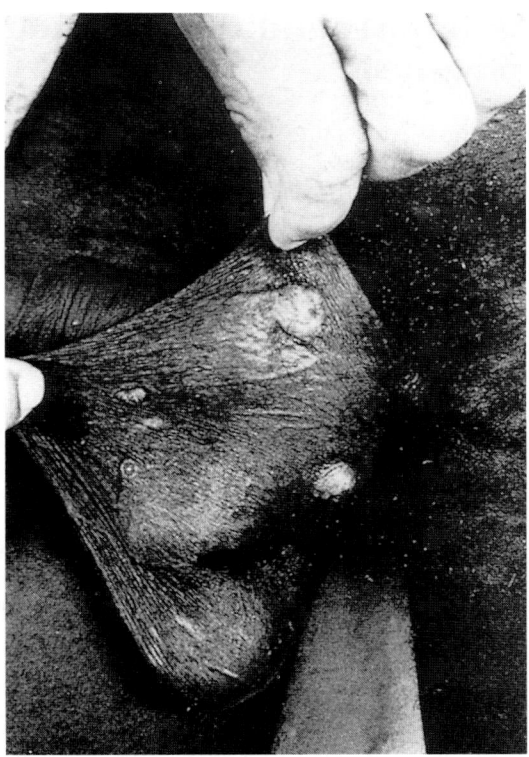
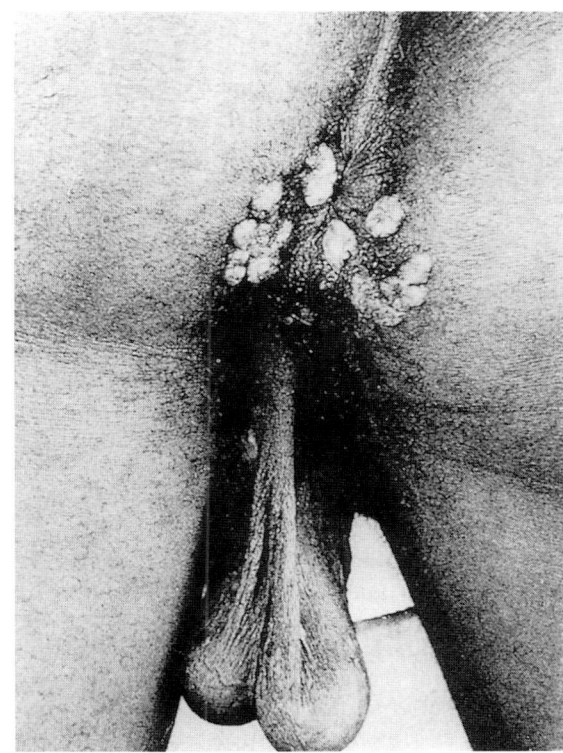

Figure 66.15: Early endemic syphilis: moist papules involving the anus and scrotum. (Courtesy of P. D. Marsden.)

complain of sore throat and hoarseness of the voice, the latter due to laryngitis. Other early manifestations of the disease are osteoperiostitis of the long bones causing nocturnal bone pains as in yaws, condylomata lata occurring in the moist areas of the body (e.g., anogenital area; Figure 66.15) and axillae, angular stomatitis and split papules, and occasionally a generalized maculopapular and other forms of rash, as in venereal syphilis. Generalized lymph gland enlargement may also be encountered.

In untreated patients the early lesions tend to undergo healing with or without scarring, and the patient passes into the latent phase of the disease. Secondary relapses are uncommon. The period of latency is usually prolonged, after which some patients develop late lesions, such as osteoperiostitis, and gummatous lesions. These result in ulceration and destruction of the skin and bones. As in yaws, destruction of the maxilla, palate and nasal bones results in 'gangosa'. Severe plantar and palmar keratosis may be encountered, with ulceration and disability. Juxta-articular nodules also occur. There is, as yet, no convincing evidence of the involvement of cardiovascular and nervous systems in endemic syphilis. Recently, ocular manifestations were described in 17 patients (age range 37–73 years) with clinical findings consistent with bejel.[25]

Diagnosis and differential diagnosis

This is essentially the same as that for yaws.

Management and control

See page 1151.

Pinta (Azul, Carate, Mal De Pinto)
Epidemiology and mode of transmission

Pinta, caused by *T. carateum*, is unique among the non-venereal treponematoses in having principally skin manifestations. The disease is confined to the under-developed rural areas of northern South America and Mexico. However, there is a paucity of data with regard to the current prevalence of pinta.

The infection is acquired in childhood or early adolescence among people living in unhygienic conditions. Those aged 15–30 years with long-standing skin lesions comprise the main reservoir. Treponemes persist in these lesions for many years. The lesions tend to be dry but are itchy, and scratching may release serum with abundant treponemes. Transmission, as in the case of yaws, is believed to be by direct lesion-to-skin contact, facilitated by a breach in the recipient's skin. As in the case of other treponematoses, the role of flies in the transmission of pinta remains uncertain.

Clinical features

The primary lesion appears at the site of entry of the organisms, usually located on the exposed parts of the body such as arms, legs or face. It starts as an itchy erythematosquamous papule which enlarges slowly and is accompanied by satellite lesions. The initial lesion may become pigmented, hyperkeratotic and scaly. The regional lymph nodes are enlarged and painless.

The secondary stage develops several months after the initial lesion, with the appearance of more extensive, often smaller, erythematosquamous plaques either around the primary lesion or disseminated to other areas. These 'pintids' are painless but itchy. They undergo a variety of colour change(s) from red to copper colour, lead-grey and bluish-black. Such lesions, which may remain present for years or reappear in recurrences, are to be found anywhere on the body.

The late lesions are characterized by varying degrees of pigmentary changes, hypochromia and atrophy around dyschromic lesions (Figure 66.16). Hyperkeratosis of the palms and soles, and juxta-articular nodes, are occasionally encountered, but some experts dispute this and consider that these patients may in fact be suffering from yaws. Leucoderma is the main complication, and this may result in social stigmas. There is no reliable evidence of systemic involvement.

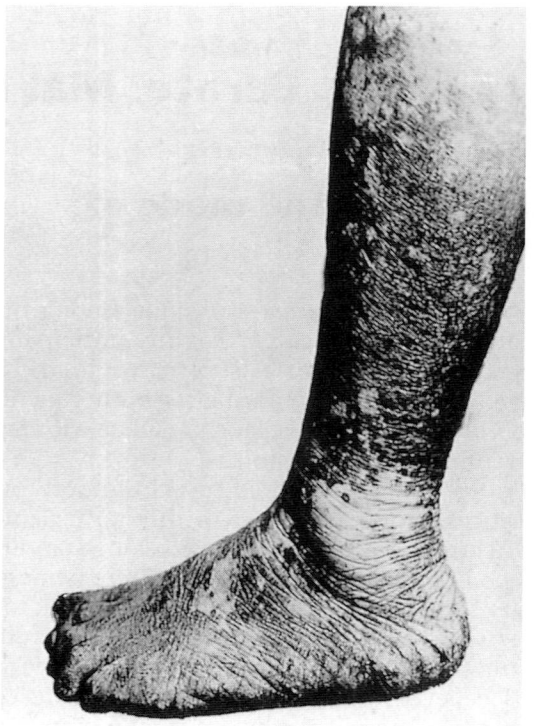

Figure 66.16: Late pinta: depigmentation of the lower leg. (Courtesy of L. A. Leon.)

Diagnosis and differential diagnosis

Diagnostic tests are the same as those for other endemic treponematoses, i.e., dark-field examination of the material from the early lesions, and serological tests. The histopathological picture is largely similar to that of yaws. In addition, the basal cells show loss of melanin and many melanophages may be present in the dermis.[26] A moderate dermal inflammatory infiltrate consisting mainly of plasma cells and lymphocytes may be present. The characteristic colour changes provide a clue to the diagnosis, but other conditions, such as vitiligo, pityriasis versicolor, leprosy, discoid lupus erythematosis, chronic pellagra, psoriasis and tinea corporis, should be excluded.

Human immunodeficiency virus infection and endemic treponematoses

No information is at present available on the relationship between human immunodeficiency virus (HIV) infection and endemic treponematoses. However, immunological abnormalities associated with HIV infection have been reported to alter the course of syphilis, albeit in a minority of patients. These abnormalities may reactivate latent infection, decrease the latent period before onset of neurosyphilis, increase the severity of manifestations, alter serological responses and render conventional therapy inadequate.[27–29] It is highly likely that HIV infection will have similar influences on endemic treponematoses. The modified clinical manifestations and serological responses may cause difficulties in diagnosis.

Ulcerative lesions caused by syphilis are believed to facilitate HIV transmission. Likewise, yaws lesions may also enhance the risk of acquiring and transmitting HIV.

Management of endemic treponematoses

A long-acting penicillin preparation is the drug of choice. Benzathine penicillin G is given as a single intramuscular injection in the upper outer quadrant of the buttock. The dose is 600 000 units for children and contacts under 6 years of age, 1.2 million units for those aged 6–15 years, and 2.4 million units for adults.

Treatment in the early stage(s) will result in cure and complete resolution of manifestations, but treatment in the late stages will not reverse the damage that has already occurred. The lesions become non-infectious within 24 hours after administration of the antibiotic.

Erythromycin or tetracycline, 500 mg by mouth four times daily for 15 days, is recommended for those allergic to penicillin. Children between the ages of 8 and 15 years should receive half that dose. Tetracycline should not be given to pregnant women or to children below 12 years of age.

Contacts

See below.

Follow-up

After adequate treatment, in the great majority of patients non-treponemal tests, namely the rapid plasma reagin (RPR) or Venereal Disease Research Laboratory (VDRL), titres either decline or become negative in due course. However, in a small proportion of patients, especially if treated in the late stages, these tests may remain positive at low titre (below 1:8). This is not an indication for further treatment. The specific tests such as *T. pallidum* haemagglutination (TPHA) or fluorescent treponemal antibody absorption (FTA-ABS), which remain reactive throughout life, play no part in assessment of the adequacy of treatment.

Control of endemic treponematoses

Following the successful mass detection and treatment campaigns of 1950s and 1960s, surveillance for the endemic treponematoses diminished and a resurgence of these infections has now been documented. Millions of people are again at risk of contracting these infections due to the ever increasing frequency of worldwide travel,

migration and poverty in the developing world. Development of a treponemal vaccine in the foreseeable future and the prospect of eradication of the non-venereal treponematoses seem unlikely. The main method of control will, therefore, lie in identification and treatment of infectious cases, including treatment of immediate contacts. There is no evidence of emergence of penicillin-resistant treponemes, but this situation could change at any time; hence, the *control* of endemic treponematoses should be a priority. Clinical surveillance (requiring dark-field microscopy and RPR or VDRL tests) to detect the prevalence of active infection is the first step. The detection of latent disease relies on serological tests.

The treatment policies recommended by the World Health Organization[30] are as follows:

1. If the prevalence of clinically active infection in the community is over 10%, give benzathine penicillin G to the entire population.
2. If the prevalence of clinically active cases is 5–10%, give benzathine penicillin G to the patients, their contacts and to all children below the age of 15 years.
3. If the prevalence of clinically active infection is under 5%, treat all active cases as well as household and other obvious contacts with benzathine penicillin G.

Economic considerations may necessitate integration of treponematosis control activities into other public health programmes.

The standards of living and personal and environmental hygiene must be improved. Sustained surveillance, integrated into existing primary health care, must be maintained to detect and treat new or missed cases including their contacts, and treatment failures. This will necessitate surveys as well as strengthening of the primary health care infrastructure.

REFERENCES

1   Hudson E H. *Non-venereal Syphilis. A Sociological and Medical Study of Bejel.* Edinburgh: Livingstone, 1958.
2   Hackett C J. On the origin of the human treponematoses. *Bull WHO* 1963; 29:7–41.
3   Norris S J. Polypeptides of *Treponema pallidum*: progress toward understanding their structure, functional and immunologic roles. Treponema Pallidum—Polypeptide Research Group. *Microb Rev* 1993; 57:750–779.
4   Noordhoek G T, Hermans P W M, Paul A N et al. *Treponema pallidum* subspecies *pallidum* (Nichols) and *Treponema pallidum* subspecies *pertenue* (CDC 2575) differ in at least one nucleotide: comparison of two homologous antigens. *Microb Pathog* 1989; 6:29–42.
5   Turner T B & Hollander D H. *Biology of the Treponematoses.* WHO Monograph Series, no. 35. Geneva: World Health Organization, 1957.
6   Fribourg-Blanc A & Mollaret H H. Natural treponematoses of the African pimate. *Primates in Medicine* 1969; 3:113–121.
7   Editorial. Yaws again. *BMJ* 1980; 281:1090.
8   Editorial. Endemic treponematoses in the 1980s. *Lancet* 1983; ii:551–552.
9   Agadzi V K, Aboagye-Atta Y, Nelson J W, Perine P L & Hopkins D R. Resurgence of yaws in Ghana. *Lancet* 1983; ii:389–390.
10 Proceedings of Inter-regional Meeting on Yaws and other Endemic Treponematoses, Cipanas, Indonesia, 22–24 July 1985. *Southeast Asian J Trop Med Public Health* 1986; 17 (Supplement 4):1–96.
11 Noordhoek G T, Engelkens H J, Judanarso J et al. Yaws in West Sumatra, Indonesia: clinical manifestations, serological findings and characterisation of new *Treponema* isolates by DNA probes. *Eur J Clin Microb Infect Dis* 1991; 10:12–19.
12 Herve V, Kassa Kelembho E, Normand P, Georges A, Mathiot C & Martin P. Resurgence of yaws in Central African Republic. Role of the pygmy population as a reservoir of the virus. *Bull Soc Pathol Exot* 1992; 85:342–346.
13 St John R K. Yaws in the Americas. *Rev Infect Dis* 1985; 7 (Supplement 2):266–272.
14 Guderian R H, Guzman J R, Calvopina M & Cooper P. Studies on a focus of yaws in the Santiago Basin, Province of Esmeraldas, Ecuador. *Trop Geogr Med* 1991; 43:142–147.
15 Paulet P. Memoire sur le yaws, pian ou framboesia; de son traitement, et des moyens de faire disparaitre cette maladie des contrees ou elle sevit. *Arch Gen Med* 1848; 17:385–405 .
16 Charlouis M. Ueber Polypapilloma tropicum (Framboesia). *Vierteljahrsschrift fur Dermatologie und Syphilis* 1881; 8:431–466.

17 Castellani A. On the presence of Spirochaeteae in two cases of ulcerated parangi (yaws). *J Trop Med* 1905; 8:253.

18 Goncalves A P, Basset A & Maleville J. Tropical treponematoses. In Canizares O & Harman R R M (eds) *Clinical Tropical Dermatology*, 2nd edn. Oxford: Blackwell Scientific, 1992: 129–150.

19 Engelkens H J H, Ginai A Z & Judanarso J et al. Radiological and dermatological findings in 2 patients suffering from early yaws in Indonesia. *Genitourin Med* 1990; 66:259–263.

20 Lawton Smith J, David N J, Indgin S et al. Neuro-ophthalmological study of late yaws and pinta: II. the Caracas project. *Br J Vener Dis* 1971; 47:226–251.

21 Román G C & Román L N. Occurrence of congenital cardiovascular, visceral, neurologic, and neuro-ophthalmologic complication in late yaws; a theme for future research. *Rev Infect Dis* 1986; 8:760–770.

22 Engelkens H J H, Vuzevski V D, Judanaso J et al. Early yaws; a light microscopic study. *Genitourin Med* 1990; 66:264–266.

23 Lever W F & Schaumburg-Lever G. Treponemal diseases. In Lever W F & Schaumburg-Lever G (eds) *Histopathology of the Skin*, 7th edn. Philadelphia, PA: J B Lippincott, 1992: 353–359.

24 Engelkens H J H, ten Kate F J W, Judanarso J et al. The localisation of treponemes and characterization of the inflammatory infiltrate in skin biopsies from patients with primary or secondary syphilis, or early infectious yaws. *Genitourin Med* 1993; 69:102–107.

25 Tabbara K F, Al Kaff A S & Fadel T. Ocular manifestations of endemic syphilis (bejel). *Ophthalmology* 1989; 96:1087–1091.

26 Marquez F. Pinta. In Canizares O (ed.) *Clinical Tropical Dermatology*. Oxford: Blackwell Scientific Publications, 1975: 86–92.

27 Johns D R, Tierney M & Felsenstein D. Alterations in the natural history of neurosyphilis by concurrent infection with the human immunodeficiency virus. *N Engl J Med* 1987; 316:1569–1572.

28 Hicks C B, Benson P M, Lupton G P & Tramont E C. Seronegative secondary syphilis in a patient infected with the human immunodeficiency virus (HIV) with Kaposi sarcoma: a diagnostic dilemma. *Ann Intern Med* 1987; 107:492–495.

29 Musher D M, Hamill R J & Baughn R E. Effect of human immunodeficiency virus (HIV) infection on the course of syphilis and on the response to treatment (review). *Ann Intern Med* 1990; 113:872–881.

30 World Health Organization. Treponemal infections. *World Health Organ Tech Rep Ser* 1982; 674:16–20.

FURTHER READING

Csonka G W. Clinical aspects of bejel. *Br J Vener Dis* 1953; 29:95–103.

Hackett C J & Loewenthal L J A. *The Differential Diagnosis of Yaws.* Monograph no. 36. Geneva: World Health Organization, 1960.

Hudson E H H. Bejel: the endemic syphilis of the Euphrates Arab. *Trans R Soc Trop Med Hyg* 1937; 37:9–46.

Perine P L, Hopkins D R, Niemel P L A, St John R K, Causse G & Antal G M. *Handbook of Endemic Treponematoses: Yaws, Endemic Syphilis and Pinta.* Geneva: World Health Organization, 1984.

Chapter 67
Other Spirochaetal Diseases (excluding *Treponema* spp. and *Leptospira* spp.)

G. C. Cook

There are several examples of tick-borne diseases of *Homo sapiens*;[1,2] the most topical at present is Lyme disease.

Lyme disease

This consists of a tick-borne zoonosis (in its natural cycle, rodents and hard ticks *Ixodes ricinus* complex are involved) caused by *Borrelia burgdorferi*;[3–5] clinical manifestations can be divided into acute and chronic forms involving the skin, joints, nervous system, and pericardium, endocardium and myocardium. Deer and other mammals form a reservoir of infection.

History

The disease was first described in the mid-1970s in the USA, following an outbreak in children at Lyme, Connecticut. However, it occurs throughout much of the northern hemisphere and in the most common 'tick-borne' diseases in Europe, Russian and, to a lesser extent, Asia (especially South-East Asia). Suspected but unsubstantiated cases of Lyme borreliosis have been documented in sub-Saharan Africa, South America and Australia. Since 1980, several outbreaks have occurred in the eastern USA, and circumstantial evidence suggests that the infection is becoming more common in both northern America and Europe, although it is impossible to exclude increased awareness and greater recognition.

Aetiology

The spirochaetes were first identified in the mid-gut of the adult black-legged tick, *Ixodes scapularis* (Figure 67.1). They were subsequently isolated from blood, skin and cerebrospinal fluid (CSF) of patients with early Lyme disease.

B. burgdorferi was taxonomically described in 1984; it is a flagellated, helical, spirochaetal bacterium. Surface membrane proteins are specific for individual strains; a prominent 41-kDa antigen is located on the flagellum. Arthropathy is more common with the predominant strain in North America, and entaneous and neurological complications with the European and Asian strains.

Humans are incidental hosts of *B. burgdorferi* and are usually infected in late spring and early summer. The ticks responsible for this infection require a shady environment of high humidity, and ready access to appropriate vertebrate hosts. These vary enormously—from the white-footed mouse in coastal north-eastern USA, the chipmunk (in the eastern USA), to deer in much of Europe and Asia. Transmission of *B. burgdorferi* to *Homo sapiens* is via saliva of feeding ticks. There is no person-to-person transmission, although there is some evidence of transplacental infection. The organism can survive for long periods in stored blood, although transfusion-acquired infection has not been recorded.

Pathology

Lyme disease consists of an inflammatory process with

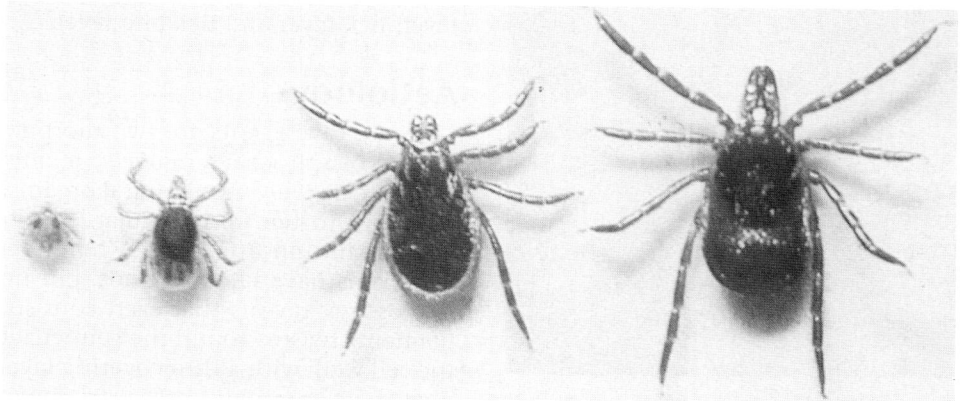

Figure 67.1: *Ixodes scapularis.* Larva, nymph, adult male and adult female. (Courtesy of Pfizer Central Research.)

non-specific histological changes; the causative agent is extremely sparse in infected tissue and is difficult to identify, even in silver-stained sections. The most striking histological changes are in joints, in both the acute and chronic stages. There is very little information on neuro-pathological changes histologically.

B. burgdorferi has been isolated from the myocardium of a patient with a long-standing cardiomyopathy; the organism has also been documented in the myocardium of a patient who suffered from both Lyme disease and babesiosis.

Clinical features

Lyme disease can affect all age groups of both sexes,[6] but highest rates have been recorded in children aged less than 15 years and in adults aged 40 years or more.

The portal of entry is the dermis; following inoculation by the infected tick, spread of infection is via cutaneous, lymphatic or haematogenous routes. The incubation period is 7–14 (3–30) days. Early infection is either localized or disseminated; in the former a slowly expanding, annular, erythematous rash (Figure 67.2) (which is not always remembered by the patient), and in the latter the skin, nervous sytem, musculoskeletal system and/or heart, are involved. Late disseminated infection occurs weeks or months after initial infection, assuming the patient has not previously received treatment. Intermittent arthropathy usually involving a large joint—often the knee—is the most common chronic manifestation. Neurological sequelae[7–10] are less common. Morbidity is severe, chronic and disabling, but only in a minority of infected individuals;[11] however, no known deaths have yet been attributable to B. burgdorferi infection alone—only when associated with other infections, such as babesiosis or ehrlichiosis.

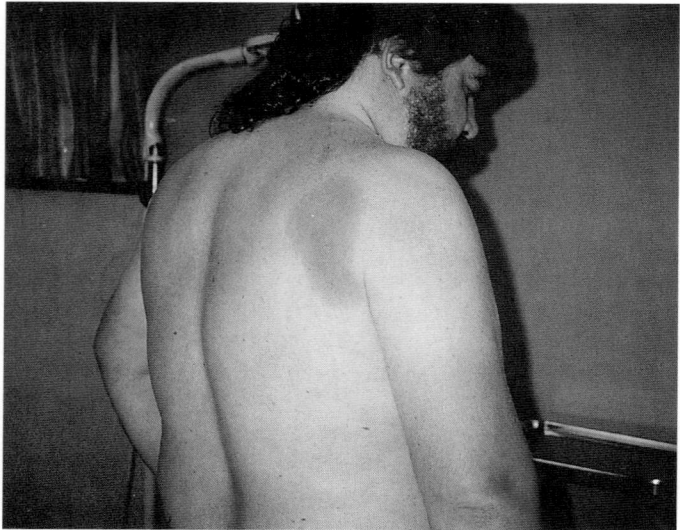

Figure 67.2: Erythema migrans. A lesion with a dusky centre, a common variant. (Courtesy of Dr Steven Luger.)

The post-Lyme syndrome (like the post-viral syndromes) seems to be a real entity; in the presence of proven disease, neurological or arthritic manifestations persist in a minority of infected individuals in spite of an adequate course of antibiotic therapy (see below).

Diagnosis

Diagnosis is usually obvious if there is a history of a tick bite in an endemic area.[12] Immunoglobulin (Ig) M antibodies to B. burgdorferi can be detected within about 2 weeks of infection; the peak usually occurs between the third and sixth week. By 6 weeks or more, the level of IgG is usually raised. An enzyme immunoassay, indirect fluorescent antibody, and/or Western immunoblot and polymerase chain reaction are also of value. Serological reactivity is usually present in disseminated infection.[13] Early (acute) lesions yield a positive result in 80% of cases, but this is not a routine diagnostic procedure.

Management

Lyme disease can be treated successfully with antibodies at all stages; amoxicillin, doxycycline, cefuroxime and erythromycin (for 14–21 days) have all been used in acute cases.[14,15] Later, a complicated disease often responds slowly or incompletely, and more than a single course of antibiotic may be necessary; parenteral cephalosporin or penicillin (for 21–28 days) are usually most effective.

Prevention

Avoidance of tick bites in an endemic area is vital;[16] protective clothing and tick repellents are of value (in the same way as mosquito bites may be prevented by a similar approach). Removal of a tick as soon as possible after attachment is obviously advisable. Vaccines against infection with B. burgdorferi have been developed for both humans and dogs;[17–19] they are safe and effective in adults, but have not yet been evaluated satisfactorily in children.

Relapsing fever

Relapsing fever is also known as recurrent fever, spirillum fever, tick fever and tick bite fever.

Aetiology

The causative agents are two morphologically indistinct species of spirochaete: *Borrelia recurrentis* and *B. duttoni*; these are actively motile spiral organisms (6–10 × 0.4 μm) with five to ten fairly regular, but loose, waves (Figure 67.3). Multiplication is by transverse fission. These organisms have tapering ends, but not flagella; electron microscopy reveals that each consists of a bundle of 12 filaments twisted round the spirochaete body, external to the cell wall, with a thin covering layer of viscid material. They have a rapid 'corkscrew' movement and can be visualized in blood films between the red cells, staining

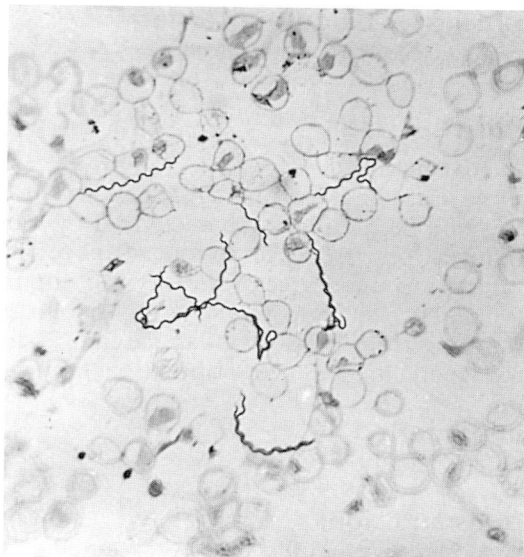

Figure 67.3: *Borrelia recurrentis* in a peripheral blood film.

pink with Giemsa or Leishman reagents, and sometimes appearing beaded or granular. The organisms may assume irregular shapes, and appear tangled together towards the end of a pyrexial attack. They can be visualized by dark-ground illumination, and grown with difficulty in enriched media[20,21] in the allantoic fluid of fertile hen's eggs, but are best demonstrated by animal inoculation. Susceptible animals include newborn rabbits, monkeys, mice,[22] rats and ground squirrels; guinea pigs are not normally susceptible.

Species differentiation

B. recurrentis infects lice (but not ticks); guinea pigs are resistant, except in East Africa. Sudanese strains are not infective to monkeys. *B. duttoni* involves soft ticks, which can infect lice and most rodents.

Pathophysiology
Human cycle

During pyrexial attacks spirochaetes appear in the blood, where they may be visualized in leucocytes; they disappear during a crisis and can be detected only by animal inoculation. Resistant spirochaetes persist in the brain and other tissues until a fresh immunologically distinct strain proliferates and reaches the bloodstream.

Pathogenesis

Borrelia spp. enter the skin and subcutaneous tissues without causing a primary lesion; from there they invade both systemic and lymphatic circulations. They multiply in blood, being phagocytosed by the reticuloendothelial system; there is no replication at extravascular sites. However, sequestration of platelets occurs in the bone marrow with thrombocytopenia; this is responsible for petechial rashes in the skin, together with haemorrhages. In the liver there is intrahepatic biliary obstruction; hepatocellular involvement results in jaundice.

Fever is caused by large numbers of *Borrelia* spp. There is no toxin production; the outer envelope is heat stable, and stimulates mononuclear cells to produce pyrogens. A Jarisch–Herxheimer reaction may occur spontaneously, or following treatment consequent on phagocytosis of a large number of *Borrelia* spp. Disseminated intravascular coagulation may also occur.

Morphology

Features at autopsy consist of jaundice and congestion of organs with petechial haemorrhages in the pleura, lungs, heart, brain, kidneys, stomach and intestine.

Borrelia spp. concentrate in the liver, where they multiply causing focal necrosis of parenchymal cells, which they invade. Fixed phagocytes do not respond to live *Borrelia* spp. but ingest dead ones. Shortly before a 'crisis' the *Borrelia* spp. 'roll up' and are taken up by endothelial cells in the liver, spleen and bone marrow. Surviving *Borrelia* spp. remain in these organs, and also the brain, until the next relapse. In the spleen *Borrelia* spp. accumulate and multiply in sinuses, causing cellular infiltration; they may enter endothelial cells, causing infarcts and necrosis; they can be demonstrated in infarcts. The spleen is large, soft and red; perisplenitis is common. *Borrelia* spp. may also be demonstrated in the kidneys. In blood vessels, damage to endothelium causes haemorrhage, which may present as petechiae. Myocardium shows 'cloudy swelling'. Bronchopneumonia is common.

A polymorphonuclear leucocytosis is present and *Borrelia* spp. may sometimes be visualized within polymorphs. The bone marrow is hyperaemic. Lymph glands may be involved.

Borrelia spp. are neurotropic, involving the meninges and central nervous system. In infected animals they may be found in the brain (in capillaries) and cerebellum as long as 1 year after infection. There are no changes in nerve cells, but intense microglial reaction in the cortex. Meningitis is sometimes present.

Immunity

Immunologically, *Borrelia* spp. behave in a way comparable with the African trypanosome. Antigenic variation overcomes specific humoral antibodies to give rise to a series of relapses. When spirochaetes first enter in the circulation, IgM antibodies (agglutinins, immobilizing antibodies, spirochaeticidine, lysins and leucostatic antibodies which promote phagocytosis) specific to the antigenic *Borrelia* spp. type overwhelm the haematological forms but do not eradicate the organisms from the tissue(s). Remaining *Borrelia* spp., which are antigencially unstable, generate new antigens—only to be removed by fresh IgM antibodies specific to that type. This process leads to 'waves' of IgM antibodies succeeding one another; it is followed by the formation of IgG antibodies that lack specificity. Lytic activity is dependent on complement. There is no significant immunity to subsequent attacks of relapsing fever.

Louse-borne relapsing fever: epidemic (cosmopolitan) type

Geographical distribution

The major endemic area lies in the highlands of Ethiopia[23–27] and in Burundi; the infection can appear anywhere in areas of low endemicity in Peru and Bolivia, north-west and East Africa, India, Asia and China—wherever environmental conditions are suitable—and also in times of social unrest and war (Figure 67.4).

Transmission

Louse transmission

Homo sapiens constitutes the only known mammalian host, and the disease is transmitted from person to person by the body (*Pediculus humanus* var. *corporis*) and head louse (*P. h.* var. *capitis*). Lice can be infected only by feeding on blood during a pyrexial episode. Spirochaetes are taken into the stomach and disappear from there in 24 hours at 28°C; they cannot be detected again until 6 days later, when they appear in the body cavity (haemocoele), where they increase rapidly in numbers to involve all organs, except the ovaries, salivary glands and intestinal tract. The louse remains unaffected; spirochaetes can escape only by injury to the body or limbs. Lice are not infective until 6 days after a feed, and humans are infected by crushing lice on the skin—not by a bite. There is no transovarian transmission.

Congenital transmission

Transplacental transmission and abortion are not uncommon.

Transmission by blood transfusion

This has been recorded, albeit rarely.

Clinical features

Natural history

Louse-borne relapsing fever can manifest as a severe disease, consisting of a febrile illness characterized by a primary attack of fever, followed by up to four relapses. There is a great variation in the degree of severity, varying from an asymptomatic parasitaemia to a severe febrile illness with death resulting from hepatic or cardiac failure. In some epidemics a mortality rate of 70% or more has been recorded.

Incubation period

This is 2–10 (usually 4–8) days.

Symptoms and signs

Onset is sudden, with chills and fever (temperature rises rapidly to 40.5°C or even higher) and the patient may become delirious.[24,25] The patients sits or lies on the bed or ground, silent, with a glazed expression and apathetic manner, and is mentally dull or confused. There is associated dizziness, severe headache,[24,25] and pain in the back, chest, abdomen, legs (especially the calves) and joints. Nausea, vomiting and dysphagia are common. Dyspnoea is often present; it is loud and hissing, and can be heard for some distance away from the patient; the diagnosis may be suspected from a distance. Cough is common; the sputum may contain *Borrelia* spp. The spleen becomes enlarged,[24] occasionally to such a degree that spontaneous rupture occurs. Hepatomegaly is present; jaundice is common. Bleeding often occurs into the skin (petechial

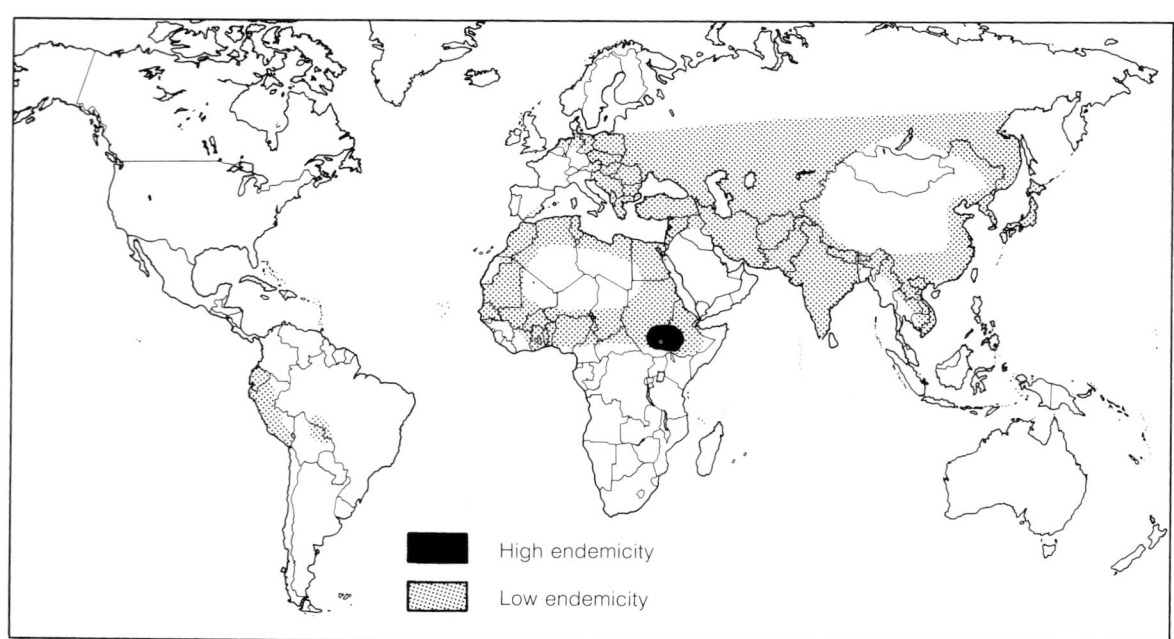

High endemicity

Low endemicity

Figure 67.4: Geographical distribution of louse-borne relapsing fever (*Borrelia recurrentis*). (Courtesy of Department of Entomology, London School of Hygiene and Tropical Medicine.)

rash),[24] over the flanks and shoulders, and into mucous membranes; epistaxis is common. During a first attack, an erythematous rash may appear over the upper part of the body, resembling that of typhoid fever (see Chapter 53). Conjunctival vessels are congested and may bleed (clumps of adherent *Borrelia* spp. become impacted in capillaries, where they enmesh red cells, causing capillary rupture followed by haemorrhage). There may be widespread intravascular coagulation. Heavy albuminuria is usually present.

Fever lasts for 5–7 days; temperature falls by crisis to 36°C or even lower (when there may be a state of collapse) and is accompanied by profuse sweating, diarrhoea, weakness and relief from associated symptoms.

Relapse occurs 5–9 days after the first attack in two-thirds of patients (Figure 67.5); it is less severe and there is no rash. A second relapse occurs in one-quarter of those infected, but more than four relapses are exceedingly unusual.

Liver function tests reflect extensive hepatocellular dysfunction.[24] Anaemia is present and a marked polymorphonuclear leucocytosis ($15–30 \times 10^9$/l) is apparent on a peripheral blood film. CSF pressure is often raised; a lymphocytic pleocytosis is common and *Borrelia* spp. may be present.

Complications

Complications include pneumonia (of lobar distribution),[24,25] which may by a major clinical feature, and nephritis, parotitis, diarrhoea, arthritis, neuropathy, acute ophthalmitis and iritis, meningoencephalitis, meningitis and meningism.

Cardiac involvement

Myocardial involvement[25] is common on the day of crisis; this is accompanied by a prolonged QTc, altered T waves, pulse greater than 100/min, systolic blood pressure of 90 mmHg or less, gallop rhythm, and reversed splitting of the second sound in the pulmonary area. A phase of critically low cardiac output (resulting from myocardial damage) may ensue; this usually resolves after treatment.

Prognosis

The case mortality rate varies; it is usually around 2–9% but occasionally reaches 12%. Death usually occurs during the first febrile attack, as a result of prothrombin deficiency, hepatic coma, myocarditis or disseminated intravascular coagulation. During the initial crisis death may result from hyperpyrexia, with convulsions, heart failure, shock or cerebral oedema. Death is usually sudden and unexpected, and may occur shortly after initiation of treatment.

Differential diagnosis

In parts of East Africa, epidemics of febrile illness in which jaundice[24] is a feature often result from louse-borne relapsing fever. During the initial attack, other causes of febrile jaundice can present similarly: yellow fever (which does not usually present with jaundice as a major feature), viral hepatitis, leptospirosis, severe *Plasmodium falciparum* infection, typhoid fever, louse-borne typhus fever (with which it sometimes coexists), trench fever and cerebrospinal meningitis (CSF has been known to reveal meningococci and *Borrelia* spp. in the same microscopical field). After the initial attack, and during relapses,[24,25] other differential diagnoses are relapsing typhoid fever, relapsing malaria (*Plasmodium vivax*), pyelonephritis, gallstones and kala-azar.

Diagnosis

Borrelia spp. are usually detected in thick blood films obtained during a febrile attack. They may be isolated at any time by inoculation of blood or CSF into young rats or white mice, in which the blood yields a positive result within 2–3 days; guinea pigs, adult rabbits and dogs are refractory.

Serological tests

These are unreliable; those for syphilis may give false-positive results. A complement fixation test has been

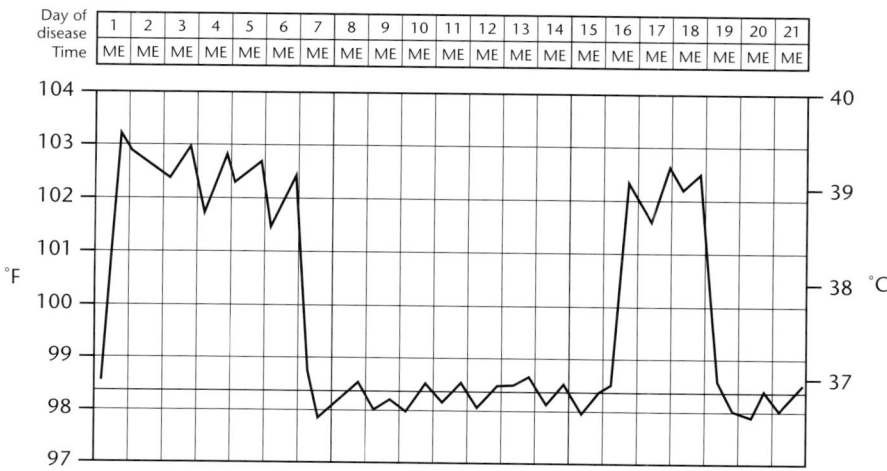

Figure 67.5: Temperature chart in a case of louse-borne relapsing fever. There is usually one relapse, and not more than four.

devised, and an immobilization test has proved sensitive; a fluorescent antibody test using *Borrelia* spp. antigen is less sensitive and cross-reacts with *Treponema pallidum*.

Management

Tetracycline, either alone or combined with penicillin,[24,25] is effective. Procaine penicillin (300 mg) plus tetracycline (500 mg) 6 hourly for 7 days is safe and effective. In Ethiopia a single 500-mg dose of tetracycline or erythromycin has proved effective. Intravenous tetracycline 250 mg is effective when oral therapy is contraindicated. A Jarisch–Herxheimer reaction[24,25] commonly occurs after administration of tetracycline and/or penicillin, especially after intravenous administration. The patient becomes restless, a rigor lasting 10–30 minutes with an abrupt temperature rise, and a rapid pulse rate, respiratory rate and raised blood pressure are accompanied by intense shivering; this is followed by a phase of flushing and profuse sweating when the blood pressure falls. The affected patient then becomes more comfortable and falls asleep; the temperature is normal the following day. *Borrelia* spp. disappear from peripheral blood about the time of the peak reaction. The mortality rate is low. Corticosteroids are ineffective, but meptazinol (an opioid antagonist with agonist properties) 300–500 mg intravenously reduces the severity of an attack. Intravenous fluid is often necessary to counteract dehydration.[25]

Epidemiology

Louse-borne relapsing fever behaves similarly to louse-borne typhus, with which it frequently coexists. It is a disease of great antiquity; epidemics have occurred in times of war. Refugees and major population migrations (with overcrowding and poor hygiene) favour epidemics. It has been estimated that there were 15 million cases in sub-Saharan Africa, Sudan, Ethiopia, eastern Europe and Russia between 1910 and 1945, with over five million deaths; the mortality rate reached up to 75%. It is a disease of overcrowding, cold and poor hygiene—conditions that lead to heavy louse infection. It is also encountered in the tropics at high altitudes, where head lice may be important in transmission.

Control

With modern delousing methods, using insecticides, epidemics should be brought immediately to a halt.[26] Insecticide powder is blown into the clothes of the at-risk population to eliminate lice; heat sterilization of clothing kills the eggs. Personal prevention may be achieved by careful delousing, without crushing the lice, and avoidance of scratching. Lice cannot transmit infection by bite or faeces (see Appendix IV).

Tick-borne relapsing fever

Geographical distribution

Tick-borne relapsing fever has a wide distribution in both Old[27] and New[28] Worlds, in five main areas (three in the Old World and two the New World); each has a specific *Borrelia* spp. tick vector complex (Figure 67.6).

Aetiology

Seven species of *Borrelia* spp. are involved (Table 67.1).

Transmission
Ticks
The major mode of transmission is by soft ticks of the genus *Ornithodoros* (see Appendix IV).

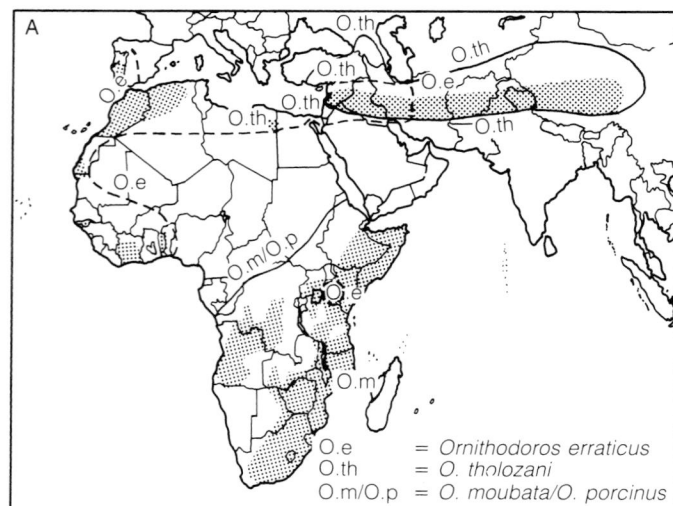
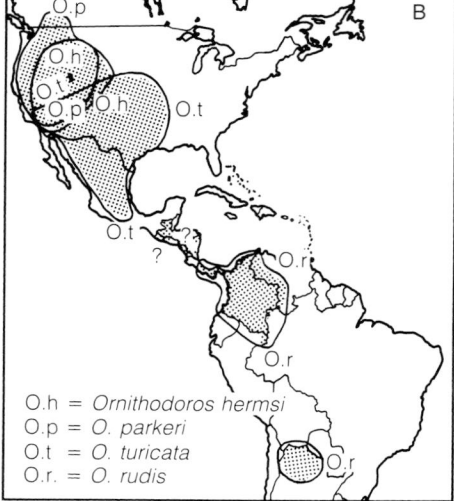

Figure 67.6: Geographical distribution of tick-borne (endemic) relapsing fever in (**A**) the Old World and (**B**) the New World. (Courtesy of Department of Entomology, London School of Hygiene and Tropical Medicine.)

Table 67.1 Species of *Borrelia* involved in tick-borne relapsing fevers

Species	Vector	Geographical area
B. duttoni	*O. moubata* (*O. m. porcinus* and *O. savignyi*)	East, central and south Africa
B. hispanica	*O. erraticus*	Mediterranean region (part), north and west Africa, Portugal and Spain
B. persica	*O. tholozani* (= papillipes) including var. *crossi*	Mediterranean region (part), Tobruk, Cyprus, Israel, through Iran to Kashmir and Sinkiang province of western China
B. parkeri	*O. parkeri*	Central and western USA, Mexico
B. turicatae	*O. turicata*	Central and western USA, Mexico
B. hermsi	*O. hermsi*	Central and western USA, Mexico
B. venezuelensis	*O. rudis* (= *venezuelensis*)	Northern, South and Central America southwards to northern Argentina

Tick cycle

Both nymphs and adults transmit infection via salivary glands (and bite), and by coxal fluid. *Borrelia* spp. penetrate the wall of the small intestine after being ingested during a blood meal; they subsequently invade the haemocoele and other organs, including salivary glands, coxal glands and ovary, where they multiply. Organisms are not found in tick faeces. Infection of a susceptible animal may take place via the bite of an infected tick—a relatively large puncture into which infective saliva is pumped, or which may be the portal of entry for coxal fluid secreted during feeding. *O. moubata* nymphs transmit by both salivary and coxal fluid, whereas those of *O. turicata, O. parkeri, O. hermsi* and *O. tholozani* do not produce coxal fluid whilst feeding. Transmission can occur in less than 1 minute after tick attachment.

Transovarian transmission is usual; a tick remains infected for many years, transmitting the infection to its offspring. The organisms can perpetuate themselves enzootically in ticks (without the requirement of another host) for at least five generations.

Other methods of transmission

Borrelia spp. can enter through intact mucous membrane and skin. Accidental infection via the conjunctiva is also possible. Transfusion, transplacental transmission and infection via intravenous drug administration are all recorded. *Borrelia* spp. can survive in lice and bed bugs; they do not develop further in these hosts.

Hosts

Homo sapiens is the only source of infection for *O. moubata*; major sources of infection for other soft ticks are rodents, which live in open country, caves and burrows, and do not infest human dwellings. Infection is transmitted to humans only incidentally. Animal hosts include monkeys, squirrels, chipmunks, rats, hedgehogs, and possibly bats and other cave-dwelling mammals.

Immunity

Tick-borne relapsing fever is more serious in expatriates than in indigenous people, who have usually been exposed to the disease previously; neurological complications are far more common in visitors to an endemic area.

Clinical features

Natural history

Tick-borne relapsing fever is usually milder than the louse-borne form. A primary bout of fever is followed by several relapses (not exceeding 11) before the infection resolves. The mortality rate is low, but neurological complications (see below) are a significant feature. Recovery is usually complete; there are no long-term sequelae.

Incubation period

Although this may be short (1–2 days has been recorded in the Spanish form), it is more often longer—up to 14 days.

Symptoms and signs

Onset

The primary attack begins abruptly with severe headache and fever of up to 40°C. It may rarely be fulminating, leading to coma and death; it can also take the form of chronic low-grade fever. During this attack the spleen enlarges (45%) and may infarct; haemorrhage may ensue. Hepatomegaly can also occur (11%), but jaundice is not as common as in the louse-borne form. There may also be diarrhoea, bronchitis and pneumonia. Massive haematuria, associated with nephritis, has been recorded in Israel.

Changes in peripheral blood

Borrelia spp. are less numerous in peripheral blood than in the louse-borne form. A polymorphonuclear leucocytosis is present. The initial attack may last for 4–5 days (shorter in the African form), ending in a 'crisis'; this can lead to 'collapse'.

Relapses

Relapses are characteristic of the tick-borne form, which may occur at intervals of a day or two, or may be separated by up to 3 weeks. Between three and six relapses are common, with up to 11 in the African form (Figure 67.7).

Complications
Neurological

Borrelia spp. causing tick-borne relapsing fever are neurotropic.[27] They may be present in CSF and can be detected by microscopic examination or animal inoculation. Various neurological syndromes may result, initially appearing at the end of the first bout of fever or during relapses.

Cranial nerve involvement

This is the most common neurological complication. The seventh nerve is most frequently involved (22% in one series in North Africa); the third, fourth, fifth, sixth (with ophthalmoplegia) and the eighth (with deafness) nerves may also be affected.

Meningitic form

Lymphocytic meningitis, and occasionally subarachnoid haemorrhage, may occur. The CSF is under pressure; a pleocytosis is frequently present. This form is not uncommon in expatriates in the Dakar area.

Other cerebral syndromes

Hemiplegia, aphasia, encephalitis, optic atrophy, iritis and iridocyclitis are by no means uncommon. The spinal nerves may be involved, especially in *O. moubata* and *O. tholozani* infections. There may be seventh nerve involvement and sciatic neuralgia, with anaesthesia. Most cerebral complications resolve without residual deficit.

Other complications

Bronchitis, hepatic failure and arthritis may occur.

Differential diagnosis

Other fevers should be distinguished, and between louse-borne relapsing fever and other relapsing fevers (rat bite fevers); major differences between the tick-borne and louse-borne forms are summarized in Table 67.2.

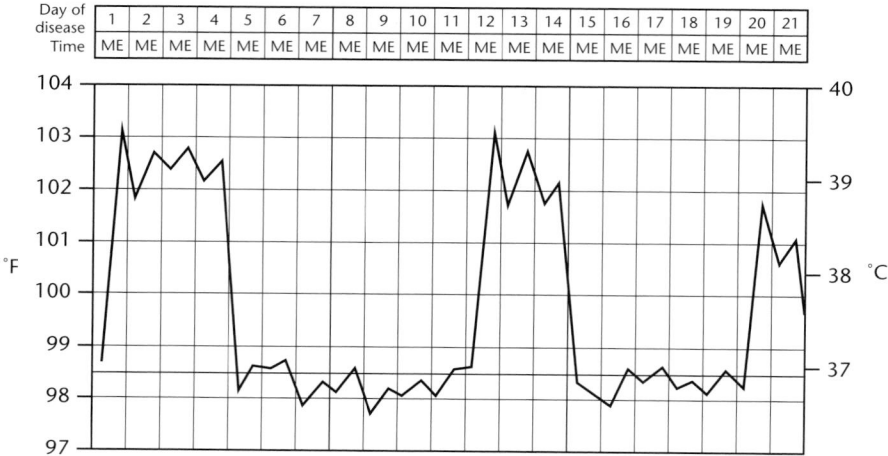

Figure 67.7: Temperature chart in tick-borne relapsing fever. There are usually three to six relapses; as many as 11 have been recorded.

Table 67.2 Major differences between tick-borne and louse-borne relapsing fevers[a]

	Tick-borne	Louse-borne
Parasites in peripheral blood	Scanty	Numerous
Paroxysms	Relatively short, not more than 5–7 days. Often chronic, irregular fever	Relatively long—up to 10 days
Relapses	Two or more	Two or fewer, often none
Vomiting	Only with meningitis	At any stage
Other symptoms	Lethargy, loss of weight, debility	Diarrhoea, jaundice, coma, severe haemorrhage
Neurological complications	Common. Cranial nerve palsies	Infrequent
Ocular complications	Papilloedema with meningitis	Infrequent
Illness	Less severe	More severe
Mortality	Less than 10%	May be high—up to 50%

[a]After Cogill N F. J R Army Med Corps 1949; 93:2.

Diagnosis

In the febrile phase, *Borrelia* spp. can be visualized in a peripheral blood film; they are fewer than in the louse-borne form, and inoculation into mice and rats may be required for demonstration. Diagnosis is often difficult in the afebrile period; a history of travel and residence in a known infected camp or village is of value, and in a subsequent relapse *Borrelia* spp. can be demonstrated at the onset and peak of the febrile episode. Serological tests may be useful, as in louse-borne relapsing fever.

Management

Treatment is the same as for louse-borne relapsing fever: tetracycline (a single 500-mg dose) or procaine penicillin (300 mg). Doxycycline has also been used.[27,28] The Jarisch–Herxheimer reaction is not a common complication, but can occur.[27]

Epidemiology

Tick-borne relapsing fever is an endemic disease found only in certain locations. In central, east and south Africa, where humans are the sole reservoir, it is present in human habitations and wherever people live collectively (i.e., in certain types of house, staging camps for migrant workers and old camping sites). In East Africa, *O. moubata* consists of two types: one preferring to feed on chickens (which are not important in transmission) living in hot humid conditions, and the other preferring humans and found in cooler, wetter locations (highlands), where it is an important vector.

O. moubata porcinus, which is widely distributed in African dwellings at all altitudes in East Africa, feeds on humans and favours a higher rainfall and a high relative humidity; it is a superior vector to *O. moubata*. *O. savignyi* prefers a hot, dry climate and infests marketplaces and cattle byres around wells; here it comes into contact with humans.

In North Africa, the eastern Mediterranean, central Asia, and North and South America, rodents constitute the major reservoir; infection is transmitted to humans incidentally. Ticks live in animal burrows and caves, and in North America in holiday homes—where chipmunks live in roofs.

Control

Control of infection (where dwellings are the source of infection) is effected by the construction of concrete floors and improved walls so that ticks lack access. Ticks can be killed by insecticides but are relatively unaffected by DDT; they are, however, susceptible to BHC (20 mg per 900 cm^2) used to dust the floor. Old camping sites and mud houses should be avoided. Travellers must never sleep on the floor.[27]

Rat bite fevers[29]

Two forms have been described: (1) sodoku (sokosha),[30,31] named by Japanese workers and caused by *Spirillum minus*

(*S. morsus-muris*); and (2) Haverhill fever (infectious erythema), named by American workers and caused by *Actinobacillus muris* (formerly *Streptobacillus moniliformis*).

These are not strictly *tropical* diseases; their inclusion here is because they are 'relapsing' diseases and may be confused with other infections.

Sodoku

Geographical distribution

Most recorded cases have occurred in Japan; the condition also occurs in Australia, Africa, the Americas and Europe.

Aetiology

Spirillum minus is a short spiral organism (2–4 μm long), rather thick, and with regular rigid spirals and pointed ends continued into one or more flagella. It moves rapidly, resembling a vibrio, and is readily stained by methylene blue or Giemsa.

S. minus can be cultivated; subcultivation has been successful. It can be grown by intraperitoneal inoculation into guinea pigs, mice and rats.

Transmission

S. minus parasitizes rats, which are healthy carriers. Transmission is from rat to human, although infection can be caused by the bite of cats, ferrets and bandicoots. Rat urine contaminating food constitutes a further vehicle of transmission.

Pathology

The organism enters at the site of the bite; local inflammation and even necrosis may be present. It is transmitted to regional lymph glands. In fatal cases neuronal degeneration has been recorded in brain, and degenerative changes in liver and kidneys.

Clinical features
Natural history
Sodoku consists of a relapsing fever that may subside spontaneously or continue for many months. It is a relatively mild disease, but the mortality rate is about 10%.

Incubation period
This varies from 5 to 30 days, the average being 5–10 days.

Symptoms and signs
There is usually a history of a bite,[30] which heals but may later break down to form an ulcer (Figure 67.8). Later, the scar and sometimes the surrounding tissues become inflamed, with formation of blebs and even necrosis. The local lymphatics are involved and regional glands become swollen and tender. Onset of fever is characterized by rigors and malaise; body temperature gradually rises in 3 days to a maximum of 39.4–40°C; after a further 3-day

period this ends in a crisis, accompanied by profuse sweating.

Following the primary attack, a quiescent interval (5–10 days) ensues. One or more relapses associated with similar symptoms and a characteristic purple popular exanthem, or urticaria, on the chest and arms have been recorded. The eruption is sometimes nodular. With each bout of fever the cicatrix at the site of the original bite becomes inflamed.

In most cases the reflexes are increased; there may be pain involving muscles and joints, and hyperaesthesiae and oedema in various parts of the body. Arthritis has been recorded. The mortality rate is about 10%. In fatal cases the terminal phase is ushered in by delirium, often followed by coma. Some cases subside spontaneously; others continue for months.

As in relapsing fever the organism can be demonstrated in peripheral blood during the febrile episode only, disappearing during apyrexial intervals. During the paroxysm there is an eosinophilia and moderate leucocytosis (e.g., $15 \times 10^9/1$). CSF pressure is increased.

Differential diagnosis

Differential diagnosis is from the different forms of relapsing and trench fevers, with which the temperature chart (Figure 67.9) has much in common. In tropical countries the possibility of coexistent *Plasmodium* spp. infection should be borne in mind. Puffiness of the face accompanying the urticarial eruption may simulate acute nephritis.

The reaction occurring around the site of the scar may be confused with erysipelas or cellulites.

Diagnosis

A diagnosis of rat bite fever can usually be established from the history, infiltration at the site of the bite, typical temperature chart, a characteristic rash and response to penicillin administration. Diagnosis can be confirmed either by dark-ground illumination (spirilla may be visualized in the exudates obtained from the site of the bite, or in serous fluid from the papule)[30] or by a Giemsa-stained smear. It is seldom possible to demonstrate spirilla in a thick blood film. If a number of relapses have occurred, the most useful investigative procedure consists of demonstrating lytic antibodies. Absolute proof of clinical diagnosis may be obtained by inoculating the patient's blood, lymph gland or wound biopsy into a guinea pig or mouse.

S. minus is not easily found in peripheral blood (although it enters the bloodstream after a few days), but is found in exudates near the bite and in 'juice' from local lymph nodes. Inoculation of infected material into a mouse or rat produces a haematological infection, and in the guinea pig a febrile disease. Infected dogs remain asymptomatic. Monkeys and rabbits are susceptible. The spirilla are present in rat tongue muscle. Rats, mice and guinea pigs may be healthy carriers.

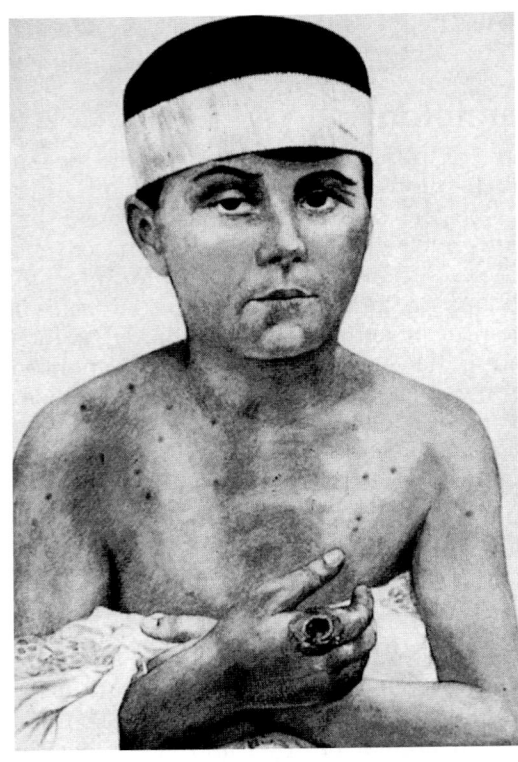

Figure 67.8: Rat bite fever produces an initial lesion at the site of the bite; this is followed by relapsing fever and rash. (Courtesy of Tropical Resources Unit.)

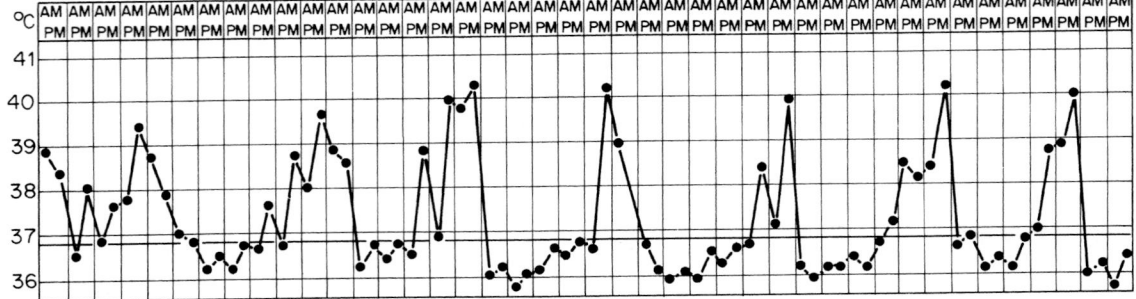

Figure 67.9: Temperature chart in rat bite fever, showing periodic relapses.

Serology

There is a weak positive treponemal serological reaction, and a positive Weil–Felix test result to proteus OXK strain.

Management

Response to penicillin is rapid; a single 300-mg injection of a repository penicillin[30,31] is adequate. Streptomycin and tetracycline are also effective.

Epidemiology

Single sporadic cases occur following a rat bite. Small epidemics can follow when contaminated raw milk is the vehicle of infection.

Haverhill fever

Geographical distribution

Haverhill fever is present in the USA, Europe and elsewhere.[32–35]

Aetiology

Actinobacillus muris (*A. moniliformis*, *Streptobacillus moniliformis*) is a natural 'parasite' of the nasopharynx of rats. It consists of a pleomorphic organism that forms slender, branching filaments ($1-3 \times 0.3-0.4$ µm); these break up to form chains of bacillus or coccoid bodies. It is a more common cause of rat bite fever than *S. minus*.

Transmission

Although infection is sometimes traced to a rat bite, transmission can occur via raw milk contaminated by rat urine; this has caused many epidemics.

Pathology

Little is known of the pathology; ulcerative endocarditis and subacute myocarditis have both been recorded. Hepatomegaly is usually present.

Clinical features

Natural history

Haverhill fever consists of a febrile illness, an erythematous rash (most prominent on hands and feet), arthralgia[32] and subsequent development of a sore throat. The fever may relapse and, untreated, may continue for months.

Incubation period

This is 3–10 days; during this time gastrointestinal symptoms may be present.

Symptoms and signs

If bitten,[32–34] the wound has usually healed; this is followed by fever, extreme prostration, severe generalized muscular pain and tenderness, headache and a generalized morbilliform rash,[34] most marked on the hands and feet. Generalized lymphadenopathy is present. Non-suppurative

Table 67.3 Differentiating features of sodoku and Haverhill fever

	Sodoku	Haverhill fever
Transmission	Bite of rat	Bite of rat or other animal. Possibly contaminated food
Incubation period (days)	5–30	3–10 (average 5)
Wound from bite	Apparent healing, followed by chancre-like ulceration	Heals promptly
Lymph glands	Regional lymphadenitis	Not involved
Systemic manifestations	Regularly relapsing fever	Intermittent, but not regularly relapsing fever
	Generalized maculopapular rash	Macular, pustular and petechial eruption
	Varying degrees of prostration and debility	Varying degree(s) of prostration
	Arthritis very rare	Metastatic arthritis fairly common
Laboratory findings	Polymorphonuclear leucocytosis	Same
	Secondary anaemia	Same
	Kahn test, usually positive	Negative
	Isolation of *Spirillum* spp. by animal inoculation of blood or infected gland	Isolation of *A. muris* by blood culture and from pustules on veal infusion broth enriched with rabbit serum
	Agglutination test negative	Agglutination test with *A. muris* positive. Serum agglutinates a polyvalent antigen of the bacillus

*After Cogill N F. J R Army Med Corps 1949; 93:2.

shifting arthropathy[32] is characteristic. In untreated cases the disease may subside spontaneously after 9–10 days; it may continue with a prolonged relapsing fever accompanied by night sweats that may recur for weeks or months at irregular intervals. The case mortality rate is about 10%, the cause usually being bacterial endocarditis and/or abscess formation.[35]

Diagnosis (Table 67.3)

Differential diagnoses include Coxsackie infection, meningococcal septicaemia and erythema multiforme. The organism can be isolated from blood by aerobic culture,[32] and subcultured on blood agar (in a carbon dioxide atmos-phere) after 48 hours. The role of imaging in spirachaetal infection has recently been reviewed.[36]

Serology

A. muris can be agglutinated by serum; a fluorescent anti-body titre (IgM) at 1:400 has been obtained using an antigen consisting of *Actinobacillus* spp.

Management

Tetracycline (250 mg 6 hourly for 2 weeks) is the antibiotic of choice. Erythromycin is also effective.[33] Penicillin has also been used,[34] although some coccobacillary variants are resistant to this agent.

REFERENCES

1 Shapiro ED. Tick-borne diseases. *Adv Pediatr Infect Dis* 1997; 13:187–218.

2 Edlow JA. Lyme disease and related tick-borne illnesses. *Ann Emerg Med* 1999; 33:680–693.

3 Evans J. Lyme disease. *Curr Opin Rheumatol* 1997; 9:328–336.

4 Nadelman R B & Wormser G P. Lyme borreliosis. *Lancet* 1998; 352:557–565.

5 Evans J. Lyme disease. *Curr Opin Rheumatol* 1999; 11:281–288.

6 Sigal LH. Lyme disease: a clinical update. *Hosp Pract (Off Ed)* 2001; 36:31–32, 35–37, 41–42, 47.

7 Haass A. Lyme neuroborreliosis. *Curr Opin Neurol* 1998; 11:253–258.

8 Kaiser R. Neuroborreliosis. *J Neurol* 1998; 245:247–255.

9 Prasad A & Sankar D. Overdiagnosis and overtreatment of Lyme neuroborreliosis are preventable. *Postgrad Med J* 1999; 75:650–656.

10 Paparone PW. Neuropsychiatric manifestations of Lyme disease. *J Am Osteopath Assoc* 1998; 98:373–378.

11 Wilke M, Eiffert H, Christen HJ & Hanefeld F. Primarily chronic and cerebrovascular course of Lyme neuroborreliosis: case reports and literature review. *Arch Dis Child* 2000; 83:67–71.

12 Rahn DW & Felz MW. Lyme disease update. Current approach to early, disseminated, and late disease. *Postgrad Med* 1998; 103:51–54, 57–59, 63–64.

13 Schmidt BL. PCR in laboratory diagnosis of human *Borrelia burgdorferi* infections. *Clin Microbiol Rev* 1997; 10:185–201.

14 Keenan GF. Lyme disease: diagnosis and management. *Compr Ther* 1998; 24:147–152.

15 Loewen PS, Marra CA & Marra F. Systematic review of the treatment of early Lyme disease. *Drugs* 1999; 57:157–173.

16 Poland GA. Prevention of Lyme disease: a review of the evidence. *Mayo Clin Proc* 2001; 76:713–724.

17 Lutwick LI & Abramson JM. Pediatric immunization for the future. Lyme disease vaccine and beyond. *Pedriatr Clin North Am* 2000; 47:465–479, viii.

18 Poland GA & Jacobson RM. The prevention of Lyme disease with vaccine. *Vaccine* 2001; 19:2303–2308.

19 Rahn DW. Lyme vaccine: issues and controversies. *Infect Dis Clin North Am* 2001; 15:171–187.

20 Morshed MG, Konishi H, Nishimura T & Nakazawa T. Evaluation of agents for use in medium for selective isolation of Lyme disease and relapsing fever *Borrelia* species. *Eur J Clin Microbiol Infect Dis* 1993; 12:512–518.

21 Cutler SJ, Fekade D, Hussein K et al. Successful *in-vitro* cultivation of *Borrelia recurrentis*. *Lancet* 1994; 343:242.

22 Cadavid D, Bundoc V & Barbour AG. Experimental infection of the mouse brain by a relapsing fever *Borrelia* species: a molecular analysis. *J Infect Dis* 1993; 168:143–151.

23 Almaviva M, Hailu B, Borgnolo G, Chiabrera F, Tolesse G & Gebre B. Louse-borne relapsing fever epidemic in Arssi Region, Ethiopia: a six months survey. *Trans R Soc Trop Med Hyg* 1993; 87:153.

24 Borgnolo G, Denku B, Chiabrera F & Hailu B. Louse-borne relapsing fever in Ethiopian children: a clinical study. *Ann Trop Paediatr* 1993; 13:165–171.

25 Borgnolo G, Hailu B, Ciancarelli A, Almaviva M & Woldemariam T. Louse-borne relapsing fever. A clinical and an epidemiological study of 389 patients in Asella Hospital, Ethiopia. *Trop Geogr Med* 1993; 45:66–69.

26 Sundnes KO & Haimanot AT. Epidemic of louse-borne relapsing fever in Ethiopia. *Lancet* 1993; 342:1213–1215.

27 Colebunders R, De-Serrano P, Van-Gompel A et al. Imported relapsing fever in European tourists. *Scand J Infect Dis* 1993; 25:533–536.

28 Spach DH, Liles WC, Campbell GL, Quick RE, Anderson DE Jr & Fritsche TR. Tick-borne diseases in the United States. *N Engl J Med* 1993; 329:936–947.

29 Dow GR, Rankin RJ & Saunders BW. Rat-bite fever. *N Z Med J* 1992; 105:133.

30 Hinrichsen SL, Ferraz S, Romeiro M et al. Sodoku—a case report. *Rev Soc Bras Med Trop* 1992; 25:135–138.

31 Bhatt KM & Mirz NB. Rat bite fever: a case report from a Kenyan. *East Afr Med J* 1992; 69:542–543.

32 Fordham JN, McKay-Ferguson E, Davies A & Blyth T. Rat bite fever without the bite. *Ann Rheum Dis* 1992; 51:411–412.

33 Konstantopoulos K, Skarpas P, Hitjazis F et al. Rat bite fever in a Greek child. *Scand J Infect Dis* 1992; 24:531–533.

34 Rygg M & Bruun CF. Rat bite fever (*Streptobacillus moniliformis*) with septicemia in a child. *Scand J Infect Dis* 1992; 24:535–540.

35 Vasseur E, Joly P, Nouvellon M, Laplagne A & Lauret P. Cutaneous abscess: a rare complication of *Streptobacillus moniliformis* infection. *Br J Dermatol* 1993; 129:95–96.

36 Kornbluth CM & Destian S. Imaging of rickettsial, spirochetal, and parasitic infections. *Neuroimaging Clin North Am* 2000; 10:375–390.

Chapter 68
Leptospirosis

G. Scott and T. J. Coleman

Leptospirosis is a zoonosis that occurs in many parts of the world but most frequently in tropical and subtropical regions. Most cases are mild or asymptomatic but the most severe illness, known as Weil's disease, characterized by a severe febrile illness with bleeding, jaundice and renal failure, may be associated with death through renal failure or pulmonary haemorrhage.[1–5] It is known by many different local names (e.g., mud, swamp, sugar cane, Fort Bragg and Japanese autumnal fevers). Overall, the major maintenance hosts are rodents and the organism is passed in their urine for long periods of time—or even for the lifetime of the animal. Leptospires can survive for up to a few weeks in fresh water depending on the pH, but they remain viable for a much shorter period in brackish water. Humans are infected through direct or indirect contact with the urine of infected animals.

Aetiology
The organism

The causative agents belong to the genus *Leptospira*, fine spiral bacteria of 0.1 μm in diameter and 6–20 μm in length.[6] The organism appears straight with one or both ends hooked (Figure 68.1). Spinning motility around their long axis may disguise the spiral nature of the organisms on dark-ground examination.[7]

Classification

Traditionally, the family of Leptospiraceae has been subdivided into two genera—the *Leptospira* and *Leptonema*. The genus *Leptospira* comprises three species: *L. interrogans* (pathogenic), *L. biflexa* (saprophytic) and *L. parva* (a single strain that is considered non-pathogenic but is serologically related to both other species).

The species *L. interrogans* is divided into many serovars, and strains are identified by cross-agglutination–absorption with known strains using homologous antisera raised in rabbits. The test is labour intensive and therefore expensive. Major and unique antigens are currently being defined by raising monoclonal antibodies and these may be applied to the identification of certain specific serovars.

Chromatography of whole-cell DNA digests may also

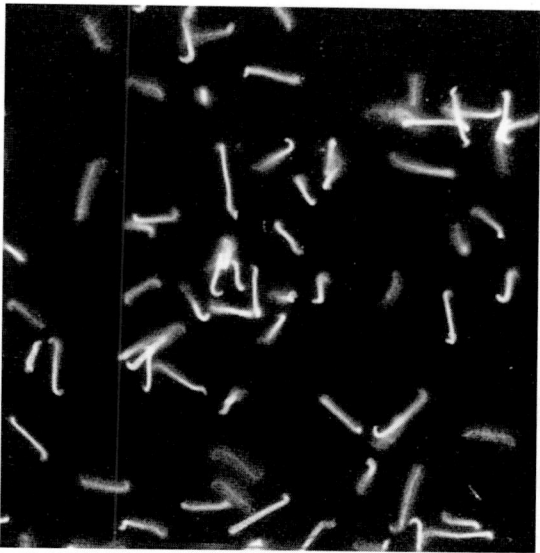

Figure 68.1: Leptospires under dark-ground illumination—characteristically hooked at both ends.

be used to show dissimilarities between strains.[8,9] This welcome move away from (potentially variable) antigen characterization may well reveal even more strains contained in what are termed 'geno' and 'subgeno' groups. However, at present, classification based on serological differences rather than DNA relatedness is often the most practical for clinical usage.

L. interrogans comprises the parasitic and pathogenic strains that can cause disease in humans and animals, whereas *L. biflexa* includes those that are considered non-pathogenic. The species *L. interrogans* can be divided into more than 200 recognized serovars. The severity of infection is probably as much to do with dose and host susceptibility as to the strain involved, because any serovar has the ability to cause mild to severe disease in different hosts. Some serovars tend to show a particular geographical distribution and differences in the major maintenance host. For example, in the UK, *L. hardjo* is particularly associated with cattle, explaining the observed increased risk of infection with this serovar in dairy farmers. Occasionally, an animal serovar unexpectedly crosses the species barrier into humans.[10]

Free-living saprophytic strains (*L. biflexa*) do not cause disease in humans but their presence in the environment indicates that conditions exist under which strains pathogenic to humans can survive. *L. biflexa* strains grow at 13°C and in the presence of β-azaguanine, both of which are inhibitory to *L. interrogans* and are not pathogenic to hamsters.

Requirements for culture

L. interrogans is an obligate aerobe that can be grown on various media that incorporate vitamins B$_1$ and B$_{12}$, long-chained fatty acids (≥ C$_{15}$) and ammonium salts. The optimal growth conditions are pH 7.2–7.6 with media enriched with fresh serum or albumin, with incubation at a temperature of 28–30°C. The organism survives in anti-coagulated (but not citrated) blood for many days and, for a few days, in some commercial blood culture bottles.[11] As most blood cultures are incubated at 37°C, leptospires are unlikely to survive for subsequent culture in the case of a late suspected diagnosis made after more frequent causes of bacteraemia have been excluded. However, it is unusual for clinicians and laboratories routinely to undertake blood culture specifically to detect leptospires, unless they are in a centre of endemic or epidemic infection.

Epidemiology and transmission

Rodents, particularly species of rat, are the most important maintenance hosts of leptospires that may infect humans. However, it is likely that every mammal has the potential to become a carrier of some serovar and is capable of spreading the disease among its own kind and to other species, including humans. In maintenance hosts, the organisms continue to replicate in the renal tubules after primary infection and may then be excreted in the urine asymptomatically for months or years.

Rural seroprevalence surveys in some developing countries indicate 15–20% of the population has been exposed. Humans acquire infection by direct or indirect contact with the urine of maintenance hosts, which include rodents and other wild animals, some domestic animals (e.g., dogs excreting *L canicola*) and farm animals (e.g., cattle excreting *L. hardjo*). Leptospires are naturally aquatic bacteria, and their prolonged survival in urine-contaminated water is an extremely important factor with regard to transmission of infection. In order for humans to be infected, the organism generally gains entry through fresh cuts or grazes on the skin and possibly through intact mucous membranes. Other routes of infection are probably of minor importance in humans. Immersion in heavily contaminated fresh water carries a high risk; the number of organisms may increase in the late summer in temperate climes, particularly in stagnant water, so bathing in canals carries a significant risk.[12] Working closely with infected animals also carries a risk, as does working in an environment heavily con-taminated with infected urine unless work practices are adopted to reduce the risk of skin contact. Sporadic cases are seen in alley dwellers in temperate urban situations.[13]

The survival of leptospires in the environment is favoured by warm, moist conditions and neutral or slightly alkaline pH. They survive in fresh water at neutral pH for up to 4 weeks but at pH 5, survival is reduced to about 2 days. Comparison of workers in two rat-infested mines in Japan showed the seroprevalence of leptospirosis to be very high in the mine where the water was alkaline but low where the water was acid. The incidence of leptospirosis relates directly to the daily maximum rainfall[14] and increases during some disasters, including floods[15] and hurricanes.[16]

Occupations associated with leptospirosis include mining, farming, animal slaughter, veterinary medicine, fish farming and processing, sewage and canal work, sugar cane harvesting and trench warfare. Leptospirosis is known by many different local names describing the likely source, location, season or occupational associations (e.g., mud, swamp, Fort Bragg, Japanese autumnal fevers, cattle-associated leptospirosis). More recently, the disease has been described in those taking part in recreational water sports such as canoeing, white-water rafting or windsurfing. Major sports events may be involved[17–19] and disease may be more severe in those who take exercise during the prodrome.[20] The sources of leptospirosis in Denmark (118 cases between 1970 and 1996) were occupational (63%), travel (8%), exposure to sewers (7%) and recreational activities (4%).[21]

Domestic animals such as dogs may be infected. Although human infection with *L. canicola* is most often contracted from dogs, the latter are more likely to develop overt disease from infection caused by *L. icterohaemorrhagiae*. This observation demonstrates that an animal may be a maintenance host for one serovar and show no evidence of disease, and yet is susceptible to other pathogenic serovars. Disease and carriage in domestic animals have no implication for human disease.

Pathology and immunology

Leptospires disseminate widely after entering the body. In the most severe cases jaundice, bleeding and renal failure occur.[22] Virulence factors are poorly understood but include hyaluronidase and a 'burrowing motility'. These could explain the ability of the organism to penetrate intact mucous membranes and perhaps the dissemina-tion, but neither explains the full pathological picture.

Whereas the first phase does not involve much inflammation, direct hepatocellular damage leads to jaundice, and tubular damage occurs by a yet undis-covered mechanism. The liver is not enlarged and micro-scopic damage ranges from no appreciable changes on light microscopy, to unicellular damage with oedema, to multiple necrotic foci, seen only in those who die soon after onset of symptoms.[23] Normally, regeneration of the liver begins rapidly and reorganization will have begun even in a patient who dies later from renal failure. Renal changes include enlargement with oedema and sub-capsular haemorrhage, and renal tubular necrosis.[24–26]

Haemorrhage may be present in any internal organ, and reflects endothelial damage and increased capillary fragility. Disseminated intravascular coagulation is not a feature.[27] The mechanism of damage in liver, kidneys and blood vessels is not known. Although much of the pathological change could be explained by cytotoxins, none has been demonstrated. Cell damage may occur by interference by glycolipoprotein fractions with Na–K ATPase, but this does not explain cross-species specificity of virulence.[28] Curiously the renal failure is accompanied by a high aldosterone concentration and hypokalaemia.[29] The second phase of the illness is characterized by the host immune response and includes immune complex glomerulonephritis and vasculitis with endothelial injury. In those who have died with pulmonary disease, histopathological examination reveals swollen capillary endothelial cells with increased pinocytotic vesicles and giant dense bodies in the cytoplasm.[30] Leptospiral antigen can be demonstrated by immunocytochemistry, but distribution and intensity are not related to the severity of the pathology seen. Platelets adhere to and aggregate at the vascular endothelium.[30]

Clinical presentation

Most people who have been infected with leptospires do not remember any illness to account for their sero-positivity. Severe infection resulting in jaundice and renal failure is rare. Of 50 cases of acute hepatorenal syndrome in central India, 17 (34%) showed good evidence for leptospirosis.[31] Although some serovars (e.g., *icterohaemorrhagiae*) tend to be associated with more serious illness, there is no 'serovar-specific presentation' in humans. Men are infected more frequently than women but this is considered to reflect increased risk of occu-pational or recreational exposure rather than increased susceptibility. In many cases, leptospirosis follows a biphasic course.

Early non-specific bacteraemic phase

The incubation period of is usually 7–12 (median 11) days, although in a very few cases it may be as short as 2 days or as long as 30 days. There follows an acute febrile, influenza-like illness with chills, sore throat, headache, myalgia, back pain, anorexia, nausea and vomiting, and herpes labialis. Sometimes the acute phase is severe, the patient is prostrate and has a persistently high fever (39–40°C) with exquisitely tender muscles, some cough and perhaps even haemoptysis, with dyspnoea and persistent vomiting. Abdominal pain is common and the patient tends to be constipated.

During this phase, leptospires may be cultured from blood and cerebrospinal fluid (CSF), but not from urine. Serological tests are negative until at least 5 days after the onset of symptoms. This so-called bacteraemic phase lasts around 4–7 days. Wide dissemination of the organism in the acute phase may result in meningeal invasion. The organism can be seen in and cultured from the CSF and tissues. There may be a transient skin rash; for example, in Fort Bragg fever there is a pretibial rash with raised erythematous patches (2–5 cm in diameter) with some induration but much less tenderness than would be expected with erythema nodosum. It seems to be more common following infection with *L. autumnalis* or *pomona* than with *L. canicola* or *icterohaemorrhagiae*. Myalgia and tender musculature, with raised serum creatine phosphokinase levels, and conjunctival suffusion are characteristic. There may be moderate hepatomegaly but splenomegaly is less common.

The platelet count may fall and thrombocytopenic purpurae and frank bleeding ensue. Urinalysis shows proteinuria but creatinine clearance usually remains normal until tubular necrosis or glomerulonephritis occurs.

Second (immune) phase

After the initial illness, a second phase begins, charac-teristically the patient having developed antibodies to the infecting organism. In mild cases the second phase may be associated with minimal symptoms and signs, but in a proportion of more severe infections meningeal or hepatorenal manifestations predominate. In the severe form of the disease, the first and second phases merge imperceptibly; with persistent high fever the patient deteriorates, becoming jaundiced and starting to bleed into the skin, mucous membranes and lungs. The liver enlargement is now more prominent. As the sclerae become icteric, the suffused vessels glow orange. Purpurae and ecchymoses are seen. Oliguric renal failure, shock and myocarditis follow and are associated with a high mortality rate. The patient develops pulmonary oedema and subpleural pulmonary haemorrhages with haemoptysis. Acute adult respiratory distress syndrome occurs occasionally and, in these cases, smoking may be an important risk factor.[32] The patient will deteriorate rapidly if significant gastrointestinal haemorrhage occurs, but pulmonary haemorrhage is an important cause of death.[33] The electrocardiogram is often abnormal, reflecting myopericarditis.

Patients who develop oliguria then anuria with rising plasma creatinine concentrations require renal dialysis. The serum potassium level is paradoxically low. The bilirubin concentration is high, but often without marked enzyme abnormalities, and the combination of high bilirubin and creatinine levels should immediately raise the question of leptospirosis. Renal failure is the usual cause of death but myocarditis, adrenal failure, haemorrhage and cerebral artery thrombosis may also be contributory. In those who are going to survive without renal support, the creatinine concentration begins to fall at the end of the second week of the illness, indicating rapid resolution of the tubular necrosis.

Abdominal pain may occur with sufficient increases in the level of amylase and lipase, despite renal failure, to suggest that pancreatitis is the cause, especially in younger patients.[34]

Central nervous system involvement

A patient may present, especially in the first phase of the illness, predominantly with meningitis; the CSF contains moderate numbers of lymphocytes and mildly raised protein levels without altered glucose concentration. The presence of myalgia, conjunctival suffusion, slight jaundice and occasional petechiae can be clues to help move the diagnosis away from enterovirus infection. Cerebral arteritis is an unusual late complication—moyamoya syndrome is caused by obstruction of the internal carotid arteries near the circle of Willis.

Eye involvement

The eyes are suffused and there may be subconjunctival haemorrhages during acute leptospirosis. Pathogenic *leptospires* may invade the eye during the acute febrile phase and this may be followed by uveitis weeks or months after recovery. More commonly a mild anterior iridocyclitis, blurring of the vitreous and haemorrhages in the retina can occur and result in disturbance to vision.

Differential diagnosis

Jaundice and renal failure with an acute febrile illness should immediately include leptospirosis in the differential diagnosis, and a full history of occupational, recreational and animal exposure must be taken. In practice, most cases of jaundice will at first be thought to be due to viral hepatitis: a raised bilirubin level with relatively unchanged enzymes and polymorphonuclear leucocytosis with negative viral serology should point away from viral infection. However, many other acute fevers are associated with jaundice (e.g., malaria, acute schistosomiasis, visceral leishmaniasis, melioidosis, plague, tularaemia and relapsing fever). The most important clinical clue is the link with renal failure. The haemolytic–uraemic syndrome may be caused by toxin produced by gut pathogens such as *Shigella* spp. and *Escherichia coli* (serotype O157), but dysentery is a prominent feature in such cases. If petechiae are present, meningococcal disease must be excluded. Examination of the CSF is, therefore, very important when there is any hint of meningitis. Any patient with acute lymphocytic meningitis must have a full history for possible exposure to leptospirosis taken.

Diagnosis

It is unlikely that the early non-specific illness of leptospirosis will be diagnosed unless there is a clear suggestion of the diagnosis in some occupational or recreational exposure, or if there is an outbreak. Clinical clues that may suggest the diagnosis of leptospirosis over other causes of acute fever are disproportionate myalgia, jaundice, conjunctival suffusion, pretibial rash and lymphocytic meningitis. If the diagnosis is suspected at this early stage, it is important to liaise with the microbiologist to arrange for appropriate specimens to be examined.[3] However, rapid results are not always possible: cultures may take 2–3 weeks to prove positive and antibodies are unlikely to be detected until at least 5–6 days after the onset of symptoms. Diagnosis using dark-field microscopy requires considerable experience; many artefacts (e.g., red blood cell membranes) may resemble leptospires when blood cultures are viewed directly. Culture into special media is more sensitive than direct microscopy. The chance of detecting leptospires in blood cultures declines rapidly when the specimen is taken after day 4 of the illness.[35]

The urine will be negative in the bacteraemic phase, so is not worth testing until the illness has been under way for some 10 days; but by then serological tests will be positive. Therefore, it is not often worthwhile to examine urine if serum is available. If urine is submitted, it must be examined fresh and the leptospires will die if it is acid. A simple way of alkalinizing the urine is to give potassium citrate mixture, for example as Cystopurin, one sachet (equivalent to 3 g) three times per day for 2 days, or sodium bicarbonate, 3 g every 2 hours, until the urine pH is greater than 7. Some confusion will occur if there are protein fibrils in the urine associated with renal tubular damage—they look surprisingly like immobile leptospires. Viability and motility of the bacteria are therefore particularly important.

When the patient is jaundiced the bilirubin level is markedly raised but transaminase and alkaline phosphatase concentrations do not rise much beyond the upper limit of normal. The urine contains bilirubin and urobilinogen with some protein. The creatine phosphokinase level is raised.[36] There is also a polymorphonuclear leucocytosis, which is useful in distinguishing leptospirosis from acute viral hepatitis. The haemoglobin level may fall, partly due to the infection and partly to haemorrhage. As the illness develops, the albumin level falls and the globulin concentration rises. The bleeding time is prolonged: the clotting is normal and bleeding is due to capillary fragility.[27] There is no consumption of clotting factors. Later a rise in prothrombin time reflects hepatocyte failure. The erythrocyte sedimentation rate rises in the second week.

Serological detection of antibodies to leptospires is usually the investigation of choice after symptoms have been present for 5–6 days.[2,37] After this, a single high titre may be of help but a rising titre is diagnostic. Reference laboratories may provide differentiation of the antibody into IgM and IgG, and perform more specific tests including one of a variety of enzyme-linked immunosorbent assay (ELISA) techniques or microscopic agglutination against live or formalized organisms (MAT), which aids differentiation between serovars.[38,39] Various assays have been compared including microscopic agglutination (MAT) versus IgM-ELISA;[40] the latter may become positive somewhat earlier than the former. Rapid latex agglutination and dipstick assays are currently under evaluation.[41–44] Crude agglutination or complement fixation tests using a standardized polyvalent antigen are performed in some local laboratories.

Syndromes associated with other serovars

There are no serovar-specific syndromes of leptospirosis. Any of the serovars of *L. interrogans* can cause any of the syndromes mentioned, and the illness can be of any seriousness. Serovar *L. lai* was first recognized in association with pulmonary haemorrhagic syndrome; this was then recognized as being an occasional feature of other serovars. Recognition of disease, dynamic epidemiology, virulence and predominant strains are all subject to variation, according to changes in climate and animal hosts. Nevertheless, there have been some striking associations with particular serovars.

Canicola fever

Serovar *canicola* is more likely to cause lymphocytic meningitis than the hepatorenal syndrome and is rarely fatal.[45] If acquired in pregnancy, the fetus may abort. The disease is usually acquired from domestic dogs, which can excrete the organism in the urine for years. Dogs may fall ill themselves on acquiring the infection and should be immunized against leptospirosis as puppies. A common symptom in the infected dog is polyuria, and the history of contact with dogs, other pets or farm animals must be sought from any patient with lymphocytic meningitis (or other symptom complex suggestive of leptospirosis). Pigs sometimes also acquire *L. canicola* but are usually asymptomatic.

Other serovars

Outbreaks of infection with other serovars are geographically focal and become well recognized locally. Most cause symptoms that are non-specific (headache, myalgia, fever, perhaps with mildly raised bilirubin levels but rarely with overt jaundice). However, *autumnalis* is particularly associated with a Fort Bragg fever: curious pretibial, raised 2–4-cm erythematous patches which are much less tender than erythema nodosum and occur at the height of the illness.[46] Pretibial fever may also occur

with other serovars (e.g., *pomona*) and there has been some confusion with legionellosis. Serovar *pomona*, a parasite predominantly of pigs, causes swineherd's disease, first described in Australia and then in Switzerland, and behaves in humans like canicola fever. Serovar *australis* group antibodies that were not cross-reactive with *canicola* and *icterohaemorrhagiae* were shown in Beagles with chronic hepatitis.[47]

Serovar *grippotyphosa* causes swamp or mud fever, and *bataviae* causes rice-field disease, described in outbreaks first in Indonesia and later in Italy.

Management

Penicillin and other related β-lactam antibiotics are active against experimental leptospirosis in animals.[48] Tetracyclines are also effective and there is some controversy as to whether penicillin is preferable to tetracyclines. However, penicillin (1.2 g benzylpenicillin intravenously or intramuscularly every 4–6 hours) is probably the drug of choice in patients suspected of having leptospirosis, yet it is a widely held view that this would be ineffective if delayed beyond the first few days of the illness.[49] This is, perhaps, explained by the fact that after this time the manifestations of the disease are immunologically mediated. However, whereas recent placebo-controlled studies suggest that there may still be a small advantage in giving penicillin late (i.e., beyond the fourth day of the illness),[50] a systematic review revealed only three trials that were acceptable for analysis that failed to prove any benefit for antibiotic treatment at all.[51] Tetracycline (e.g., doxycycline 100 mg orally every 12 hours)[52] or erythromycin (500 mg orally every 12 hours) are alternatives in patients who are allergic to penicillin, but are not more likely to be effective.

For very ill patients, intensive care support may be necessary. Specific support therapy is required for anaemia due to bleeding and for renal failure. Haemodiafiltration is now favoured if resources permit, but when resources are limited peritoneal dialysis should be instituted to tide the patient over until the tubular necrosis has begun to resolve. A tendency to bleeding is not a contraindication to instituting haemodialysis. Parenteral feeding is important because of the hypercatabolic state of the febrile patient in renal failure.[25]

There are neglible risks to health care workers of acquiring the disease from an infected patient.

Control and prevention

With more than 200 pathogenic serovars and the fact that all animals may become infected, some chronically, the eradication of leptospirosis is clearly impossible. However, there are three main ways in which the risk of leptospirosis in humans can be reduced. First, domestic farm animals and pets can be immunized. This does not completely abolish the risk of an animal acquiring infection but significantly reduces the overall risk to humans.[53] Second, risks in occupational exposure can be identified and addressed. Although classically described in sewer workers, leptospirosis is now rare in this group in many countries because protective clothing and simple hygienic precautions have been introduced. In general, farmers tend not to take similar precautions because of a misconception in some parts of the world that the disease is not particularly associated with farming. However, specific measures can be taken; for example, burning cane fields prior to harvest reduces the risk of the sharp young shoots cutting hands. Other simple measures, such as removing rubbish from work and domestic environments, will reduce the rodent population. Improved education of people at particular risk (e.g., farmers and those taking part in water sports)

and health care staff increases awareness and may enable earlier diagnosis and treatment. Third, chemoprophylaxis (e.g., with doxycycline) can be used in groups at particularly high risk.[54–56]

A Cochrane database review found only two properly controlled prophylactic trials of doxycycline (and in one of these the method of blinding was not described) involving 1022 subjects. The risk of leptospirosis in the treated groups was 0.6% (3 of 509) compared with 4.9% (25 of 513) in those who received no treatment. It was calculated that prophylaxis in 24 subjects (95% confidence intervals 17–43) was needed to prevent disease in one subject. Side effects were recorded in 3% of those receiving doxycycline, compared with 0.2% of control subjects, and this has to be taken into account when deciding on a prophylaxis strategy at times of high risk and special circumstances.[57]

REFERENCES

1   Turner L H. Leptospirosis I. *Trans R Soc Trop Med Hyg* 1967; 61:842–855.

2   Turner L H. Leptospirosis II. *Trans R Soc Trop Med Hyg* 1968; 62:880–899.

3   Turner L H. Leptospirosis III. *Trans R Soc Trop Med Hyg* 1970; 64:623–646.

4   Edwards G A & Domm B M. Human leptospirosis. *Medicine* 1960; 39:117–156.

5   Heath C W Jr, Alexander A D & Galton M M. Leptospirosis in the United States. Analysis of 483 cases in man 1949–1961. *N Engl J Med* 1965; 273:857–864.

6   Johnson R C & Faine S. *Leptospiraceae*. In Krieg N R & Holt J G (eds) *Bergey's Manual of Systemic Bacteriology*, vol. 1. Baltimore, MD: Williams & Wilkins, 1984: 62–67.

7   Cox P J & Twigg G I. Leptospiral motility. *Nature* 1974; 250:260–261.

8   Hookey J V, Waitkins S A & Jackman P J H. Numerical analysis of *Leptospira* DNA-restriction endonuclease patterns. *FEMS Microbiol Lett* 1985; 29:185–188.

9   Robinson A J, Ramadass P, Lee A & Marshall R B. Differentiation of subtypes within *Leptospira interrogans* serovars *hardjo, balcanica* and *tarassovi* by bacterial restriction-endonuclease DNA analysis (BRENDA). *J Med Microbiol* 1982; 15:331–338.

10 Peterson A M, Boyce K, Blom J, Schlichting P & Krogfelt K A. First isolation of *Leptospira fainei* serovar Hurstbridge from two human patients with Weil's syndrome. *J Med Microbiol* 2001; 50:96–100.

11 Palmer M F & Zochowski W J. Survival of leptospires in commercial blood culture systems revisited. *J Clin Pathol* 2000; 53:713–714.

12 Hutchinson J H, Pippard J S, White M H G & Sheehan H L. Outbreak of Weil's disease in the British Army in Italy. *BMJ* 1946; i:81–86.

13 Vinetz J M, Glass G E, Flener C E, Mueller P & Kaslow D C. Sporadic urban leptospirosis. *Ann Intern Med* 1996; 15:794–798.

14 Kupek E, de Sousa Santos Faversini M C & de Souza Phillippi J M. The relationship between rainfall and human leptospirosis in Florianopolis, Brazil, 1991–1996. *Braz J Infect Dis* 2000; 4:131–134.

15 Trevejo R T, Rigau-Perez J G, Ashford D A et al. Epidemic leptospirosis associated with pulmonary haemorrhage—Nicaragua, 1995. *J Infect Dis* 1998; 178:1457–1463.

16 Sanders E J, Rigau-Perez J G, Smits H L et al. Increase of leptospirosis in dengue-negative patients after a hurricane in Puerto Rico in 1996. *Am J Trop Med Hyg* 1999; 61:399–404.

17 Anonymous. Leptospirosis outbreak in Eco Challenge 2000 participants. *Commun Dis Rep CDR Wkly* 2000; 22:341.

18 Anonymous. Update: leptospirosis and unexplained acute febrile illness among athletes participating in triathlons—Illinois and Wisconsin, 1998. *MMWR Morb Mortal Wkly Rep* 1998; 47:673–676.

19 Anonymous. Outbreak of leptospirosis among white-water rafters—Costa Rica, 1996. *MMWR Morb Mortal Wkly Rep* 1997; 46:577–579.

20 Friman G & Wesslen L. Special features for the Olympics: effects of exercise on the immune system: infections and exercise in high-performance athletes. *Immunol Cell Biol* 2000; 78:510–522.

21 Holk K, Nielsen S V & Ronne T. Human leptospirosis in Denmark 1970–1996: an epidemiological and clinical study. *Scand J Infect Dis* 2000; 32:533–538.

22 Arean V M. The pathologic anatomy and pathogenesis of fatal human leptospirosis (Weil's disease). *Am J Pathol* 1962; 40:393–423.

23 Ramos-Morales F, Díaz-Rivera R S, Cintrón-Rivera A A et al. The pathogenesis of leptospiral jaundice. *Ann Intern Med* 1959; 51:861–878.

24 Sitprija V. Renal involvement in human leptospirosis. *BMJ* 1968; ii:656–658.

25 Kennedy N D, Pusey C D, Rainford D J & Higginson A. Leptospirosis and acute renal failure: clinical experiences and a review of the literature. *Postgrad Med J* 1979; 55:176–179.

26 Lai K N, Aarons I, Woodroffe A J & Clarkson A R. Renal lesions in leptospirosis. *Aust N Z J Med* 1982; 12:276–279.

27 Edwards C N, Nicholson G D, Hassell T A, Everard C O R & Callender R J. Thrombocytopenia in leptospirosis: the absence of evidence for disseminated intravascular coagulation. *Am J Trop Med Hyg* 1986; 35:352–354.

28 Younes Ibrahim M, Buffin-Meyer B, Cheval L et al. Na,K-ATPase: a molecular target for *Leptospirosis interrogans* endotoxin. *Braz J Med Biol Res* 1997; 30:213–233.

29 Abuldaker R C, Seguro A C, Malheiro P S, Burmann E A & Marconde M. Peculiar electrolyte and hormonal abnormalities in acute renal failure due to leptospirosis. *Am J Trop Med Hyg* 1996; 54:1–6.

30 Nicodemo A C, Duarte M I, Alves V A et al. Lung lesions in human leptospirosis: microscopic, immunohistochemical and ultrastructural features related to thrombocytopenia. *Am J Trop Med Hyg* 1997; 56:181–187.

31 Sharma A, Joshi S A, Srivastave S K, Bharadwaj R & Kahre P M. Leptospirosis in the causation of hepato-renal syndrome in and around Pune. *Indian J Pathol Microbiol* 2000; 43:337–341.

32 Martinez-Garcia M A, de Diego Damia A, Menendez Villanueva R & Lopez Hontagas J L. Pulmonary involvement in leptospirosis. *Eur J Clin Microbiol Infect Dis* 2000; 19:471–474.

33 Yersin C, Bovet P, Merien F et al. Pulmonary haemorrhage as a predominant cause of death in leptospirosis in Seychelles. *Trans R Soc Trop Med Hyg* 2000; 94:71–76.

34 O'Brien M M, Vincent J M, Person D A & Cook B A. Leptospirosis and pancreatitis: a report of ten cases. *Pediatr Infect Dis J* 1998; 17:436–438.

35 Smith J. Weil's disease in the north-east of Scotland. *Br J Ind Med* 1949; 6:213–220.

36 Johnson W D, Silva I C & Rocha H. Serum creatine phosphokinase in leptospirosis. *JAMA* 1975; 233:981–982.

37 Cursons R T M, Pyke P A & Penniket J. The serological diagnosis of leptospirosis. *N Z J Med* 1982; 95:26–37.

38 Pappas M G, Ballou W R, Gray M R et al. Rapid serodiagnosis of leptospirosis using the IgM-specific dot-ELISA: comparison with the microscopic agglutination test. *Am J Trop Med Hyg* 1985; 34:346–354.

39 Watt G, Alquiza L M, Padre L P, Tuazon M L & Laughlin L W. The rapid diagnosis of leptospirosis: a prospective comparison of the dot enzyme linked immunosorbent assay and the genus-specific microscopic agglutination at different stages of illness. *J Infect Dis* 1988; 157:840–842.

40 Cumberland P, Everard C O & Levett P N. Assessment of the efficacy of an IgM-ELISA and microscopic agglutination test (MAT) in the diagnosis of acute leptospirosis. *Am J Trop Med Hyg* 1999; 61:731–734.

41 Smits H L, van de Hoorn M A, Goris M G et al. Simple latex agglutination assay for rapid serodiagnosis of human leptospirosis. *J Clin Microbiol* 2000; 38:1272–1275.

42 Ramadass P, Samuel B & Nachimuthu K. A rapid latex agglutination test for detection of leptospiral antibodies. *Vet Microbiol* 1999; 70:137–140.

43 Yersin C, Bovet P, Smits H L & Perolat P. Field evaluation of a one-step dipstick assay for the diagniosis of human leptospirosis in the Seychelles. *Trop Med Int Health* 1999; 4:38–45.

44 Smits H L, Hartskeerl R A & Terpstra W J. International multi-centre evaluation of a dipstick assay for human leptospirosis. *Trop Med Int Health* 2000; 5:124–128.

45 McIntyre W I & Seiler H E. The epidemiology of canicola fever. *J Hyg (Camb)* 1953; 51:330–339.

46 Fraser D W, Glosser J W, Francis D P et al. Leptospirosis caused by serotype *Fort-Bragg. Ann Intern Med* 1973; 79:786–794.

47 Adamus C, Buggin-Daubie M, Izembart A et al. Chronic hepatitis associated with leptospiral infection in vaccinated beagles. *J Comp Pathol* 1997; 117:311–328.

48 Alexander A D & Rule P L. Penicillins, cephalosporins and tetracyclines in treatment of hamsters with fatal leptospirosis. *Antimicrob Agents Chemother* 1986; 30:835–839.

49 Christie A B. Leptospiral infections. In *Infectious Diseases*, vol. 2, 4th edn. Edinburgh: Churchill Livingstone, 1982: 1173.

50 Watt G, Padre L P, Tuazon M L et al. Placebo controlled trial of intravenous penicillin for severe and late leptospirosis. *Lancet* 1988; i:433–435.

51 Guidugli F, Castro A A & Atallah A N. Antibodies for treating leptospirosis. *Cochrane Database Syst Rev* 2000; 2:CD001306

52 McClain J B L, Ballou W R & Harrison S M. Doxycycline therapy for leptospirosis. *Ann Intern Med* 1984; 100:696–698.

53 Feigin R D, Lobes L A Jr, Anderson D & Pickering L. Human leptospirosis from immunized dogs. *Ann Intern Med* 1973; 79:777–785.

54 Takafuji E T, Kirkpatrick J W, Miller R N et al. An efficacy trial of doxycycline prophylaxis against leptospirosis. *N Engl J Med* 1984; 310:497–500.

55 Sehgal S C, Sugunan A P, Murhekar M V, Sharma S & Vijayachari P. Randomized controlled trial of doxycycline prophylaxis against leptospirosis in an endemic area. *Int J Antimicrob Agents* 2000; 13:249–255.

56 Gonsalez C R, Casseb J, Monteiro F G et al. Use of doxycycline for leptospirosis after high-risk exposure in Sao Paulo, Brazil. *Rev Inst Med Trop Sao Paulo* 1998; 40:59–61.

57 Guidigli F, Castro A A & Atallah A N. Antibiotics for preventing leptospirosis (Cochrane review). *Cochrane Database Syst Rev* 2000; 4:CD001305.

Section 9

Mycotic Infections

Fungal infections are ubiquitous and can cause a variety of clinical diseases. Superficial skin fungal infections such as ringworm and candida, have plagued *Homo sapiens* for centuries. These cause morbidity but are rarely fatal in immunocompetant individuals. Other fungal infections such as *Histoplasma capsulatum, Coccidiodes immitis* and *Cryptococcus neoformans* are responsible for causing severe pneumonia in the immunocompetant individuals and can proceed to fatal systemic disease in the immuno-suppressed. Fungal toxins such as those produced by *Aspergillus flavus* (aflatoxin) are associated with the development of hepatocellular carcinoma. This section focuses on the superficial, subcutaneous and systemic mycoses. The section also covers *Pneumocystis carinii,* the classification of which has 'yo-yoed' between a protozoan and mycosis over the past decade.

Chapter 69
Fungal Infections

R. J. Hay

The fungi are recognized causes of disease in most parts of the world. The commonest of the infections caused by these eukaryotic organisms are superficial, and include diseases such as dermatophytosis or ringworm and candidosis. However, extensive, deforming and potentially fatal deep or systemic fungal infections can also occur.[1] Fungal cells are similar to animal cells but are characterized by the presence of a polysaccharide-based cell wall. There are two principal types of fungi: the yeasts, single cells which reproduce by a process of bud formation to give rise to single daughter cells; and the mycelial or mould fungi, which form chains of contiguous cells. Some fungi, the dimorphic fungi, exist as either a yeast or mycelium at different stages of their life cycles. Examples of these organisms include most of the major respiratory pathogens such as *Histoplasma capsulatum* and *Coccidioides immitis*. The formation of specialized reproductive structures or spores (conidia) is also typical of fungi. Fungi can cause human disease in a number of different ways, through the production of toxins, sensitizing antigens (allergens) or by the invasion of tissue. Invasive diseases caused by fungi are known collectively as the mycoses: the superficial, subcutaneous or systemic mycoses.

The distribution of mycoses is affected by a number of factors: the presence of the organisms in the environment, host immunity, frequency and route of exposure and the availability of invasive or immunosuppressive medical technology. These influence the spread of fungal disease in the tropics as well as in temperate climates. The main superficial mycoses are common in the tropics. The subcutaneous infections, which occur through implantation of pathogenic organisms via injury, are largely confined to the tropics and subtropics. The main systemic mycoses due to respiratory pathogens such as *Histoplasma capsulatum* also occur in the tropics, while systemic opportunistic infections caused by organisms such as *Aspergillus* are probably more common in temperate areas where there is a greater reliance on therapeutic immunosuppression.

Superficial mycoses

Superficial infections caused by fungi are common in all environments, particularly the tropics. While, on occasions, this is due to the existence of endemic foci of specific diseases such as tinea imbricata or tinea capitis, there is also a real increase in prevalence of certain

Table 69.1 Superficial mycoses

Dermatophytosis (ringworm, tinea)
Superficial candidosis (thrush)
Malassezia infections: pityriasis versicolor, *Malassezia* folliculitis, seborrhoeic dermatitis *Scytalidium* infections
Less common: tinea nigra, white piedra, black piedra, alternariosis, onychomycosis due to mould fungi
Otomycosis
Keratomycosis

infections. Factors such as climate, humidity of the skin surface and the $P\text{CO}_2$ concentration may all affect the expression of these diseases.

The main superficial infections are dermatophytosis or ringworm, superficial candidosis and pityriasis (tinea) versicolor (Table 69.1). However, other conditions such as foot infection caused by *Scytalidium dimidiatum* as well as the hair shaft infections, white and black piedra, and tinea nigra are also seen. Otomycosis, a superficial infection of the external auditory meatus, is also common. Oculomycosis, in particular mycotic keratitis, occurs in both temperate as well as tropical environments but poses a frequent and difficult management problem in the tropics (see Chapter 18).

Dermatophytosis

The dermatophyte or ringworm fungi are common causes of superficial infections.[2] They are mould fungi which have become adapted to parasitize the skin by attacking the keratin by elaborating proteases with keratin specificity. They can invade epidermis but remain confined to the stratum corneum as well as the hair shaft or nail plate. There are three pathogenic genera of dermatophyte in humans: *Trichophyton*, *Microsporum* and *Epidermophyton*. These organisms normally cause exogenous infections originating from outside the human host. There are three main sources: other humans, animals or soil, known respectively as anthropophilic, zoophilic or geophilic. Examples of possible animal hosts are cats and dogs (*M. canis*), cattle (*T. verrucosum*), monkeys (*T. simii*) and rodents (*T. mentagrophytes*).

Pathogenesis

The fungi invade after adhering to stratum corneum cells. Factors which encourage fungal invasion include increased environmental humidity and CO_2 content, both of which may occur in a tropical environment. Less is known about those factors which determine human susceptibility; generally it is thought that most individuals are susceptible to infection.[3] The presence of medium chain length fatty acids in sebaceous material may, however, prevent hair shaft invasion by dermatophytes in postpubertal children. There is evidence that susceptibility to tinea imbricata may be mediated via an autosomal recessive gene.[4] In addition, patients with persistent treatment-unresponsive dermatophytosis affecting the palms and soles are significantly more likely to be atopic than others.[5] Resistance is largely mediated via non-specific factors such as an increase in epidermal turnover, unsaturated transferrin or by activation of T cell-mediated immunity. Patients with the acquired immune deficiency syndrome (AIDS), for instance, although not apparently showing an increased incidence of infection, may have clinically atypical and extensive lesions.[6]

Epidemiology

In most tropical countries dermatophytosis is common.[7–11] The main types of infection seen are tinea corporis, tinea cruris and tinea capitis. Tinea pedis is considered to be less common in many parts of the tropics. However, there are several features of the epidemiology of foot infections which may be relevant.[12] Occlusion of the feet with shoes or socks predisposes to infection, although a higher proportion of the populace may have asymptomatic infections of their soles. In areas of the tropics where there is industrial activity, such as in the mining or petroleum industries, the incidence of foot infections may be much higher. There are a number of different organisms which can cause this type of infection, ranging from dermatophytoses to *Candida* species, Gram-negative bacteria and erythrasma, a Gram-positive bacterial infection.[13] For instance, in eastern Saudi Arabia there is a high rate of *Candida* infection in the toe-web spaces rather than dermatophytosis.[14] Populations of organisms on the feet, particularly those affecting the interdigital spaces, may vary from time to time and one may replace another to cause infection; the term 'dermatophytosis complex' has been coined to describe this phenomenon.[13]

Laboratory diagnosis

The diagnosis of dermatophytosis can be confirmed by demonstrating the organisms in skin scrapings or hair or nail samples taken from lesions.[2,15] Scrapings are generally best removed with a blunt scalpel from the edge of lesions. They are mounted in 5–10% potassium hydroxide and are then scanned with a microscope. The organisms are seen in scrapings as chains of cells forming hyphae. In addition, they grow on simple mycological media such as Sabouraud's agar and their gross and microscopic morphology is used to distinguish the different species.

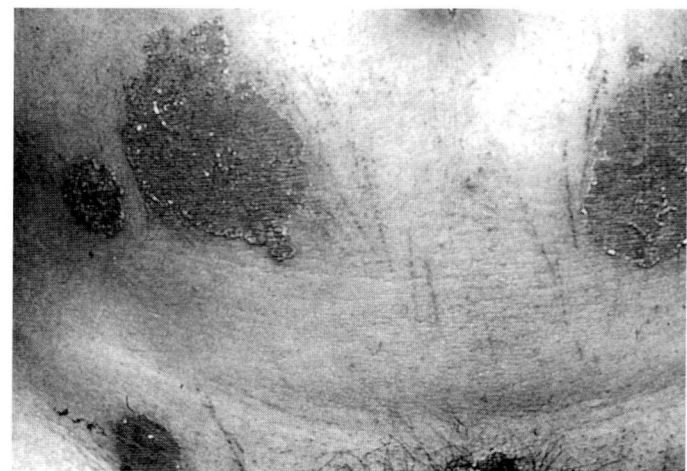

Figure 69.1: Tinea corporis due to *Trichophyton rubrum*.

Clinical features

The normal term for dermatophytosis is tinea, followed by the Latin for the appropriate part of the body affected (tinea capitis, head; tinea cruris, groin, etc.).

Tinea corporis

This presents with a scaly and itchy rash affecting the trunk or proximal limbs. The typical lesion is a circular scaling patch with some central clearance (Figure 69.1). However, in many lesions the main abnormalities, scaling or papule/pustule formation, are seen at the edge where an intact or broken rim can just be made out. Tinea corporis lesions may be very large and affect a wide area on the back and chest. In patients with AIDS the symptoms and signs may be altered considerably, with extensive or follicular forms being seen in some patients.[16]

Tinea imbricata is a specific type of tinea corporis caused by the fungus *Trichophyton concentricum*.[17] It is endemic in remote and humid tropical areas in the West Pacific and parts of Malaysia, India and South America. Lesions are characterized by the development of multiple concentric rings of scales which may cover a large area of the body from an early age (Figure 69.2). Other patterns include diffuse desquamation with large scales and lichenification. This infection is notoriously difficult to eradicate from patients who are living in endemic areas.

Localized lesions respond to one of the azole antifungals such as clotrimazole or econazole or topical terbinafine. Whitfield's ointment is also effective in many patients. Oral therapy is generally needed for extensive disease or tinea imbricata; the main choices are griseofulvin, itraconazole or terbinafine.

Tinea capitis

Tinea capitis or scalp ringworm is endemic in many developing countries. It can be caused by either anthropophilic or zoophilic fungi.[18] Generally in rural areas anthropophilic organisms are more common and this is true for large areas of India, Latin America and Africa.[19] By contrast, in the Middle East and in some

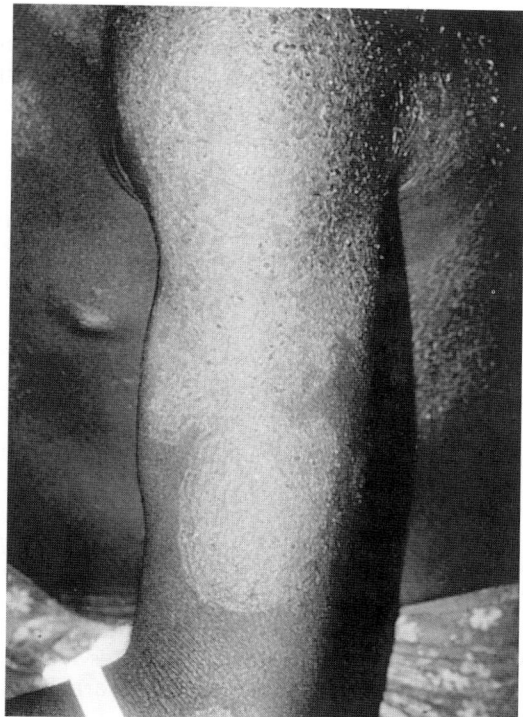

Figure 69.2: Tinea imbricata.

South American countries, particularly in cities, zoophilic infections are being seen more frequently, usually caused by *Microsporum canis*. The difference between the two types is in their transmission, with those originating from human sources being more easily transmitted from child to child, causing small or large epidemics of disease. In many communities in Africa, for instance, scalp ringworm is endemic.[20–22]

Tinea capitis is an infection generally confined to prepubertal children. With most anthropophilic fungi the infections present insidiously with diffuse or circumscribed areas of hair loss. Scaling may be minimal and hairs are broken at scalp level, leaving a swollen black dot in the hair follicle (Figure 69.3). More scaly types which resemble seborrhoeic dermatitis, but highly inflammatory lesions (kerion) are occasionally seen. The course of disease is indolent but lesions normally clear at puberty. The zoophilic organisms are generally more inflammatory, and scaling with hair loss is obvious. Lesions are often quite itchy and inflammatory crusts cover the lesions. Children (and adults) may carry the organisms without clinical lesions.[23,24] Adult tinea capitis, although rare, may be seen in patients with AIDS.

Favus is a specific form of scalp ringworm caused by *Trichophyton schoenleinii*. It is found mainly in isolated pockets in parts of North, East and South Africa, the Middle East and South America. The infection is characterized by the formation of large matted crusts—scutula—over the scalp. Hairs are often retained until late in the course of the disease but their loss may be permanent.

The diagnosis of this infection can be confirmed by examining scrapings from the patient's scalp and by

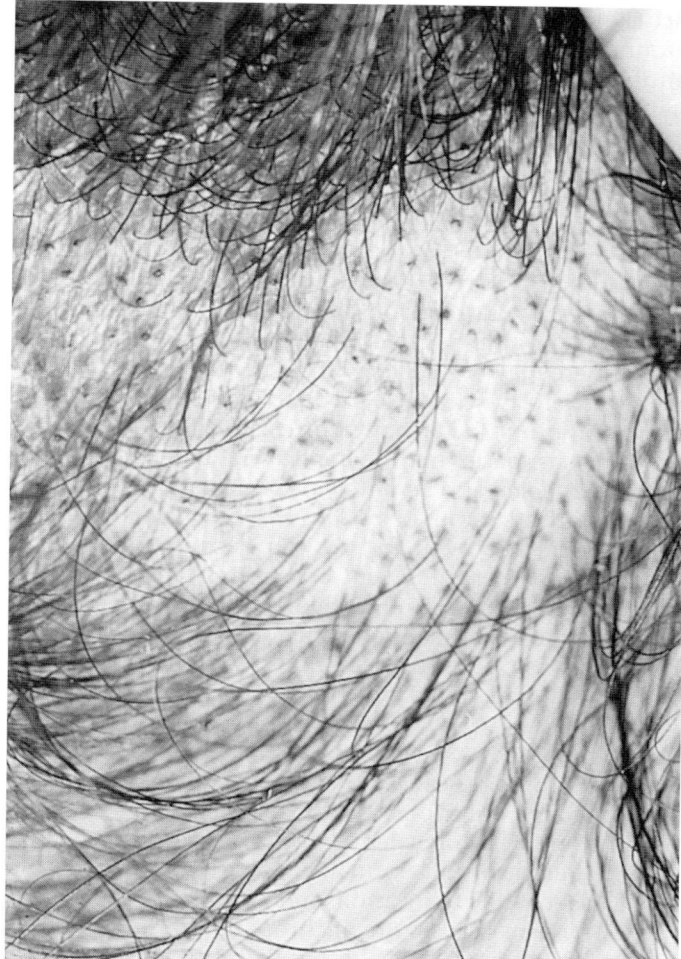

Figure 69.3: Scalp ringworm (tinea capitis) due to *Trichophyton violaceum* showing the 'black dot' appearance.

culture.[25] Some causes of dermatophytosis affecting hairs, notably those due to *Microsporum* species, produce greenish fluorescence in scalp hairs under a filtered ultraviolet (Wood's) light.

The best treatment for dermatophytosis affecting the scalp is oral; topically applied drugs are seldom effective.[22] Griseofulvin in a dose of 10–20 mg/kg daily is the usual agent.[26,27] The normal duration of therapy is 6–8 weeks. However, in some cases it is possible to use a single dose of 1 g daily, which can be given under supervision to large numbers of children in a school.[18] Terbinafine and itraconazole are also effective.

Tinea cruris

Dermatophytosis affecting the groin—tinea cruris—is common in most tropical countries. It is almost always caused by anthropophilic species of dermatophytes, mainly *Trichophyton rubrum* and *Epidermophyton floccosum*. Sometimes these infections may appear to reach epidemic proportions in certain groups such as soldiers or prisoners. The usual lesion is an itchy rash with a raised border extending from the groin down the upper thigh, and on occasions into the natal cleft. In women it may extend around the waist area. Treatment with topically applied antifungal creams such as clotrimazole or miconazole or half-strength Whitfield's ointment works well in most cases.[28]

Tinea pedis

Dermatophytosis affecting the feet is very common in most temperate climates; although less common in developing countries it none the less occurs. The most common sites of infection are the interdigital spaces or the soles. The main symptoms are itching and occasionally pain. There may be erosions affecting web spaces. If there are severe erosive changes, particularly if there is greenish discoloration of the area, Gram-negative bacteria such as *Pseudomonas* species may be implicated. Other possibilities include *Candida* and *Scytalidium* species or erythrasma, a bacterial infection caused by *Corynebacterium minutissimum*.

The usual treatment for toe-web dermatophytosis is a topically applied antifungal. Good results can be obtained with a range of compounds including Whitfield's ointment, azoles such as clotrimazole or micronazole, or terbinafine. For infections of the sole requiring treatment oral therapy with griseofulvin, terbinafine or itraconazole is preferable.

Onychomycosis

Nail plate invasion caused by dermatophytes is common in temperate countries, where it may affect 3–4% of the population. The prevalence of this infection in the tropics is unknown. It normally occurs together with sole or web-space infections and is most common on the toe-nails. The usual causes are anthropophilic fungi such as *Trichophyton rubrum*. The affected nails become thickened and opaque; distal erosion of the nail plate occurs in long-standing cases[29] (Figure 69.4). Superficial invasion of the nail plate caused by dermatophytes, such as *T. interdigitale*, or moulds such as *Acremonium* or *Fusarium* species, is seen more frequently in the tropics.[30] This is

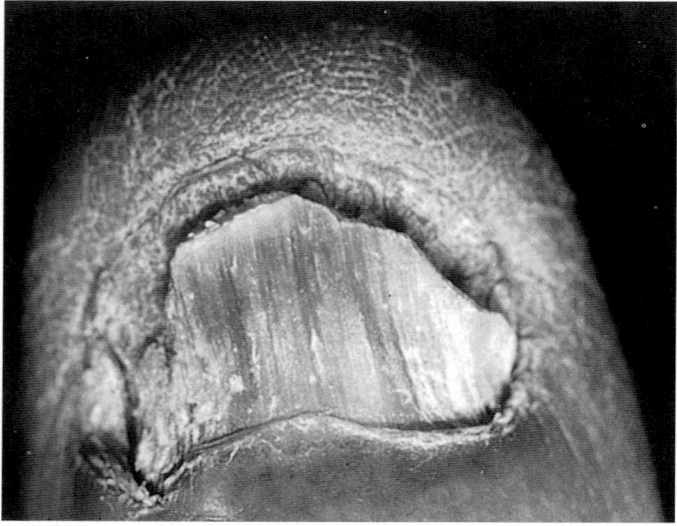

Figure 69.4: Onychomycosis due to a dermatophyte.

called superficial white onychomycosis. Therapy is difficult, with few nail infections responding to topical antifungals, although in the early stages some will clear with tioconazole or amorolfine nail solutions. The most common oral treatment, griseofulvin, is associated with a high relapse rate when toe-nails are involved. It may have to be used for 12–18 months. The newer oral drugs, terbinafine (250 mg)[31] or itraconazole (400 mg daily for 1 week per month × 3),[32] produce higher recovery rates in shorter periods (3 months). They are also more expensive than griseofulvin.

Superficial candidosis

Superficial infections due to *Candida* species are common in a tropical environment and include oral and vaginal as well as skin infections.[33] The principal pathogen is *C. albicans*, although other species such as *C. tropicalis*, *C. parapsilosis*, *C. krusei* and *C. glabrata* may also cause human infections. *C. albicans* forms filaments or hyphae during the process of tissue invasion. The disease is seen worldwide, although some clinical varieties such as inter-digital candidosis are more common in warm climates.[14]

Pathogenesis and epidemiology

Candida albicans is a normal commensal of the mouth, gastrointestinal tract and vagina. Carriage rates vary but 15–60% of normal individuals have commensal carriage in the mouth. Somewhat lower percentages have colonization of the gastrointestinal tract or vagina.[34] Survival of the organisms in these sites depends on a variety of factors, including their ability to adhere to mucosal cells and compete with commensal bacteria. Factors which disturb this balance favour either elimination or growth and subsequent invasion by the organism. They can usually be explained logically. For instance, use of antibiotics eliminates other members of the commensal flora of the mouth and bowel and allows *Candida* to invade. Depression of either T lymphocyte or neutrophil-mediated immunity allows the organisms to grow and invade following inhibition of normal control mechanisms. The main exception is vaginal candidosis, where most women with the infection have no detectable predisposition.

Clinical features

The main clinical forms of superficial disease are oropharyngeal, vaginal and cutaneous candidosis. In addition, chronic mucocutaneous candidosis is a condition which may appear as a rare chronic infection in predisposed patients. Systemic candidosis is a serious infection generally confined to compromised patients. It will be discussed elsewhere.

Oropharyngeal candidosis

Oral infection is seen in all countries, particularly in infants, the elderly and immunocompromised patients, including those with AIDS.[35] It occurs in breast-fed and bottle-fed infants and may be a complication of malnutrition, in which it can affect the reintroduction of feeding because of soreness of the mouth. As a complication of human immunodeficiency virus (HIV) infection, the appearance of oropharyngeal candidosis is a common and early manifestation of the development of AIDS.

There are a number of different clinical types of oropharyngeal candidosis.[36,37] These are largely distinguished by their chronicity and clinical appearances. Acute pseudomembranous candidosis presents with white plaques on the epithelium that are inflamed and easily detached. The scattered nature of these appearances is suggestive of the speckling on a thrush's breast, hence its common name 'thrush'. This may present as an acute infection in infants, the elderly or in patients who are immunocompromised, such as those with AIDS. In the last group and in patients with chronic mucocutaneous candidosis the condition is often persistent and refractory to therapy—chronic pseudomembranous candidosis.

In some individuals plaques are not formed but the mucosal surface appears red and glazed—acute erythematous candidosis, also known as acute atrophic oral candidosis. This may occur in patients with AIDS.[37,38] In patients presenting with inflammatory changes and oral discomfort associated with dentures (denture sore mouth), persistent erythema associated with *Candida* is a common feature—chronic erythematous candidosis. In smokers, chronic candidosis may have additional features such as the appearance of irregular white plaques, which cannot be detached, on the tongue and other areas of the mouth—chronic plaque-like candidosis. Histologically this contains epithelial atypia and, in some patients, oral carcinomas have developed. A few patients with chronic oral *Candida* infection may develop a pebbly appearance on the mucosa—chronic nodular candidosis.

Any of the above changes can be accompanied by splitting at the corners of the mouth (angular cheilitis), which in these cases may be due to *Candida* infection. This is an important and common sign of candidosis.

In most patients the main focus of infection is the buccal mucosa, but in severely infected individuals there is involvement of the tongue or pharynx, as well as the oesophagus. Oesophageal candidosis is mainly seen in patients with AIDS, leukaemia or chronic mucocutaneous candidosis. While it may present with retrosternal pain on swallowing, it is often silent. Secondary oral infection due to *Candida* may occur in patients with epithelial abnormalities such as hyperkeratosis or ulceration due to lichen planus, pemphigus and other conditions such as oral submucous fibrosis, mainly seen in Indian patients.

Vaginal candidosis

Vaginal *Candida* infection is normally caused by *C. albicans*, although other *Candida* species such as *C. glabrata* or *C. tropicalis* have also been cultured.[33] While it can occur in pregnant women or diabetic persons, one of the features of this condition is that there is usually no underlying abnormality to be found. Severely immunocompromised women do not usually show a higher frequency of persistent vaginal infections than appropriate control groups, although persistent vaginal infection has been reported in some women with AIDS.

The main clinical forms of vaginal candidosis are similar to those seen in the oral mucosa, most commonly an acute (pseudomembranous or erythematous) form.[34] However, chronic relapsing or persistent vaginal candidosis and secondary vaginal candidosis can all occur.[39] The symptoms of the acute types vary from a creamy discharge to itching and dyspareunia. Recurrent infections are unfortunately common and occasionally they are persistent. The clinical appearances are varied but the main variations are the presence or absence of soft white plaques (thrush). Secondary candidosis may occur in those with underlying mucosal disease such as pemphigoid, lichen planus or Behçet's syndrome.

Candida intertrigo

The skin is only indirectly involved in vaginal infection when there is spread of infection to the vulva and the perineum. In this case a prominent red rash in the groin and on the upper surface of the thighs may appear, together with satellite pustules and papules. The same can occur in other sites such as beneath the breasts and around the umbilicus. In some cases there is no underlying skin abnormality, although groin candidosis in males and females is more common in diabetic subjects. Eczema or psoriaris affecting the skin flexures may be accompanied by secondary candidosis.

Interdigital candidosis

Infection of the finger- or toe-web spaces by *Candida* is more common in hot climates. It may be the most common type of foot infection in army groups in the tropics. Lesions are white with soggy-looking skin which is superficially eroded. *Candida* may be a secondary invader of interdigital dermatophytosis. Lesions between the fingers are mainly seen in women and a relationship between repeated washing and cooking has been suggested; it is also more common in the overweight.

Candida infection and nappy dermatitis

Nappy rash in infants is a form of irritant eczema which is often secondarily infected with, among other organisms, *C. albicans*. The presence of yeasts may be suspected by the appearance of satellite pustules and this is confirmed by culturing the organisms from swabs of the area.

Candidosis of the nails

Paronychia are acute or chronic infections of the nail folds caused by *Candida* species such as *C. albicans* or *C. parapsilosis*.[40] These are common in the tropics. They occur in patients who are likely to immerse their hands frequently in water or whose occupations involve cooking. In addition to swelling of the nail fold, pain and intermittent discharge of pus, the lateral border of the nail may be undermined with onycholysis (Figure 69.5). Other causes of paronychia are staphylococcal and Gram-negative bacterial infections. The latter often coexist with *Candida* species.

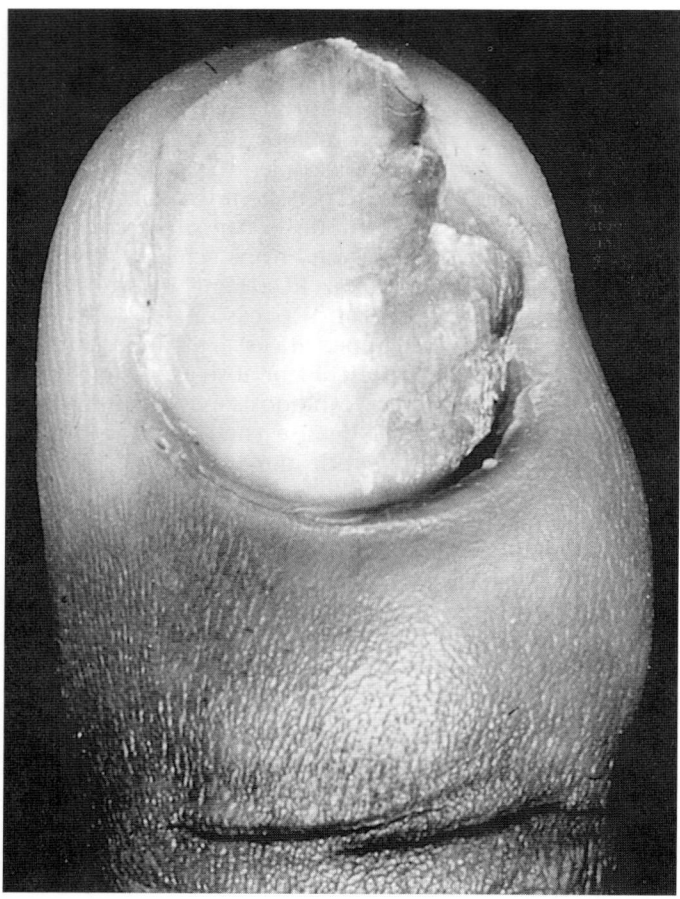

Figure 69.5: Chronic *Candida* paronychia.

Chronic mucocutaneous candidosis

The rare syndrome of chronic mucocutaneous candidosis (CMC) usually presents in childhood or infancy with oral, nail and cutaneous candidosis which recurs despite treatment.[41] Other chronic skin infections such as warts (papilloma viruses) and dermatophytosis may also appear. An adult form also exists.

The oral lesions are usually of the chronic pseudomembranous or plaque types. The skin may be covered with crusted plaques—the so-called *Candida* granulomas—particularly where the infection has spread to the face or scalp. The fingernail changes involve the nail plates, nail folds and periungual skin, all of which may be severely damaged.

A large number of immunological abnormalities have been described in association with this condition but with few exceptions these have been found to change with time and therapy. For this reason it is likely that the real defect(s) in most patients with this condition remains unknown and the immunological investigation of children with CMC is not necessary unless they have very extensive infections or a history suggestive of abnormal responses to other infections, such as chickenpox or severe staphylococcal boils. Here it is worth excluding functional leucocyte abnormalities, such as chronic granulomatous disease, although such patients usually have a history of internal infection. With the exception of bronchiectasis most patients with CMC do not have internal disease, although the most severely affected patients may later develop systemic infections such as tuberculosis.

Laboratory diagnosis

The diagnosis of superficial candidosis can be confirmed by direct microscopy (see Dermatophytosis) of skin scrapings or swabs. Both yeasts and hyphae can be seen. *Candida* species can be distinguished on culture by assimilation and fermentation reactions.[15]

Treatment

Candida infections respond well to a range of antifungals available in cream, vaginal tablet or oral pastille forms.[27] These include the polyene antifungals such as amphotericin B or nystatin and azole drugs (econazole, clotrimazole, ketoconazole, miconazole). Gentian violet is still used in some areas but the response to treatment is much slower than with the specific antifungals. Patients with AIDS may respond poorly to topical therapy and orally absorbed antifungals, such as fluconazole 100–200 mg daily),[42] ketoconazole (200–400 mg daily)[43] or itraconazole (100–200 mg daily),[44] given intermittently are used. Prolonged use of ketoconazole and fluconazole in AIDS patients may give rise to drug resistance. Oral antifungal therapy is also needed for patients with CMC.

Scytalidium infections

Scytalidium dimidiatum, a plant pathogen found in the tropics and subtropics, and *S. hyalinum*, which has only been isolated from humans, cause infections of the skin which mimic the dry-type infections caused by *Trichophyton rubrum*.[45] These infections have mainly been reported in immigrants from tropical areas to temperate countries, although infection in the tropics may be more common than previously believed.[46] Recent studies from Nigeria, for instance, have suggested that this is a common infection in both dermatological outpatients and industrial groups such as mine workers. Infections have been reported from West and East Africa, India and Pakistan, Thailand, Hong Kong and several countries in Latin America.

The infection presents with scaling of soles and palms and cracking between the toe webs (Figure 69.6). Nail dystrophy is common and onycholysis without significant thickening is often seen; some patients have nail-fold swelling. The clinical features of *S. dimidiatum* and *S. hyalinum* infections are indistinguishable.

It is important to recognize these infections because they are common in some areas and do not respond to most antifungal drugs. The laboratory diagnosis follows similar lines to that used in dermatophytosis—skin scrapings and culture.[47] The appearances of these fungi in

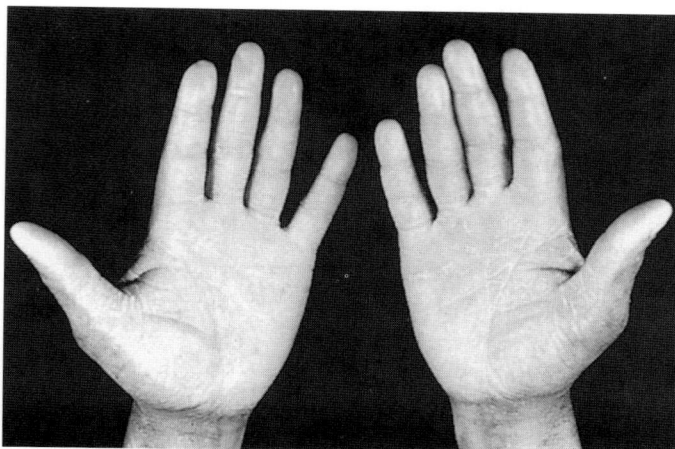

Figure 69.6: Palm infection caused by *Scytalidum*. This mimics dermatophytosis.

skin scrapings is characteristic as they are sinuous and irregular. They do not grow on media containing cycloheximide.

Treatment of these infections is difficult. Nail disease does not respond to any of the antifungal agents. Responses of skin infection have been recorded with a number of compounds such as Whitfield's ointment, econazole or terbinafine, although relapse is common.

Malassezia yeast infections

The *Malassezia* (lipophilic) yeasts are skin-surface commensals which have also been associated with certain human diseases, the most common of which are pityriasis versicolor, *Malassezia* folliculitis and seborrhoeic dermatitis and dandruff.[48] In addition these organisms rarely cause systemic infections, usually in neonatal infants receiving intravenous lipid infusions. There are a number of *Malassezia* species which are oval or round yeasts and their distribution on the skin surface differs. The formation of short stubby hyphae by round yeasts on the skin surface is a feature of the development of pityriasis versicolor.

Pityriasis versicolor

The pathogenesis of pityriasis versicolor is still ill understood. The disease occurs in young adults and older individuals but is less common in childhood.[49] Pityriasis versicolor is a common disease in the tropics and elsewhere in otherwise healthy patients and there is no evidence of immunosuppression in these groups. However, it has also been associated with Cushing's syndrome and immunosuppression associated with organ transplantation, but not with AIDS. The infection is very common in the tropics and incidence rates of over 70% have been reported in some studies. Generally this disease is associated with warm climates and sun exposure.

The rash consists of multiple hypo- or hyperpigmented, occasionally red, macules which are distributed across the upper trunk and back; with time these coalesce. The lesions are asymptomatic and scaly. The hypopigmented lesions

may be confused with vitiligo but here there is complete loss of pigmentation. The presence of scaling and partial loss of pigment is, however, typical of pityriasis versicolor.

Lesions can also be highlighted by shining a Wood's light on the area. They fluoresce with a yellowish light, although this is generally a weak response and complete darkness as well as a powerful light source are necessary. Alternatively, scrapings from the lesions will show the characteristic organisms, which consist of clusters of round yeasts closely associated with short stubby hyphae. These are normally viewed in 10% potassium hydroxide-treated mounts, although the addition of Parker Quinck ink to the potassium hydroxide is an easy stain to apply and it highlights the fungi well.

Malassezia folliculitis

A second condition associated with *Malassezia* yeasts is an itchy folliculitis on the back and upper trunk which often appears after sun exposure usually in teenagers or young adult males. Lesions are itchy papules and pustules which are often widely scattered on the shoulders and back. The condition has to be distinguished from acne as it does not respond to the same range of treatments.

Seborrhoeic dermatitis

Lipophilic yeasts of the genus *Malassezia* are part of the normal skin flora and therefore any evidence that they are either directly or indirectly implicated in the pathogenesis of common skin diseases such as dandruff (scalp scaling) or seborrhoeic dermatitis is difficult to assess. However, these yeasts are found in large quantities in the scales of seborrhoeic dermatitis and dandruff. Most patients with seborrhoeic dermatitis or dandruff respond to treatment with azole antifungal agents and this coincides with the disappearance of the yeasts. Seborrhoeic dermatitis is one of the earliest and most consistent abnormalities seen in patients with AIDS[50] but it is also common in perfectly healthy individuals.

The main clinical feature of seborrhoeic dermatitis is the appearance of erythema, together with greasy scales in the scalp, eyebrows and eye lashes, in the nasolabial folds, behind the ears and over the sternum.

Management

Treatment of *Malassezia* infection can usually be accomplished using topical azole antifungals such as clotrimazole (cream) or ketoconazole (cream or shampoo). Oral therapy with ketoconazole or itraconazole is also a possibility. Cheaper alternatives include selenium sulphide (1–2%) or 20% sodium hyposulphite solution. In the case of seborrhoeic dermatitis, topically applied azole antifungals will produce significant improvements; other possibilities include topical tar-based preparations and corticosteroids.

Rarer superficial infections

White piedra is a chronic infection of the hair shafts caused by a yeast, *Trichosporon beigelii*.[51] It is generally

Table 69.2 Causes of mycetoma

Organism	Colour of grain	Common distribution
Fungi		
Madurella mycetomatis	Black	Africa, Middle East, India
M. grisea	Black	Central and South America, Caribbean
Scedosporium apiospermum	White/yellow	Anywhere, USA and Europe
Fusarium or *Acremonium* spp.	White/yellow	Anywhere
Aspergillus nidulans	White/yellow	Sudan, elsewhere
Neotestudina rosati	White/yellow	Africa
Actinomycetes		
Actinomadura madurae	White/yellow	Africa, Middle East, elsewhere
A. pelletieri	Red	Africa, India, elsewhere
Streptomyces somaliensis	White/yellow	Africa, Middle East, elsewhere
Nocardia spp.	Small white/yellow	Americas, elsewhere

Table 69.3 Subcutaneous mycoses

Mycetoma
Chromoblastomycosis (chromomycosis)
Sporotrichosis
Lobomycosis
Subcutaneous zygomycosis
due to *Basidiobolus*
due to *Conidiobolus*

sporadic and rare and the infection is mainly seen in genital hair. It may also affect the axilla and scalp. The lesions are soft yellowish nodules around the hair shafts.[52] This disease can be seen in temperate and tropical areas. It is usually asymptomatic and is noticed on routine inspection. Trichomycosis axillaris, in which hairs in the axillae are covered with a soft yellowish coating, is caused by a bacterial infection associated with excessive sweating. It is generally easily controlled with an antiperspirant.

Black piedra caused by *Piedraia hortae* is a rare asymptomatic infection confined to the tropics. Here, scalp hairs are surrounded by a dense black concretion containing spores, thus forming a small nodule.[53] The disease has been reported in both humans and apes.

Tinea nigra is an infection of palmar or plantar skin caused by a black yeast, *Phaeoannellomyces werneckii*. It is mainly seen in the tropics but can present in Europe and the USA. The main differential diagnosis is an acral melanoma as it presents as a flat pigmented mark on the hands or feet. If the lesion is scraped with a glass slide or scalpel it can be shown to be scaly. Lesions are usually solitary. The presence of pigmented hyphae in skin scrapings is typical. Tinea nigra responds to a variety of treatments including Whitfield's ointment and azole creams.

Alternaria species cause a rare form of skin granuloma, often presenting with ulceration in normal or immuno-compromised patients. The lesions are most often located over exposed sites such as the dorsum of the hands. It has been seen in patients with AIDS.

A variety of different fungi, such as *Fusarium*, *Aspergillus* and *Pyrenochaeta*, also occasionally cause onychomycosis. *Acremonium* and *Fusarium* species, in particular, are sometimes associated with superficial nail-plate invasion (superficial white onychomycosis) in the tropics.

Otomycosis

Otomycosis or otitis externa caused by fungi is seen in most tropical areas. The most common cause is *Aspergillus niger*,[54] which forms an inflammatory mat in the external auditory meatus, with loss of hearing and serous secretion. This can be removed carefully with a wax hook through an otoscope.

Subcutaneous mycoses

Subcutaneous fungal infections are mainly confined to the tropics and subtropics (Table 69.2). While they are seldom common, their diagnosis and management are difficult and they therefore attract a disproportionate share of attention. These infections are generally caused by direct introduction of organisms through the skin into the dermis or subcutaneous tissues and for this reason they are often called 'mycoses of implantation' (Table 69.3). They generally remain confined to their site of introduction, only spreading by contiguity; however, there are rare examples where the infection disseminates beyond this area to affect distal sites. In addition, the disease sporotrichosis has both a subcutaneous and a systemic form, in the latter instance the infection spreading from a primary pulmonary focus.

Mycetoma

Mycetoma (Madura foot) is a chronic subcutaneous infection caused by actinomycetes or fungi in which the organisms form into aggregates (called grains), attracting an inflammatory response in the deep dermis and subcutaneous tissue and leading to the development of draining sinuses communicating with the overlying skin and causing osteomyelitis.[55] Those mycetomas caused by actinomycetes are called actinomycetomas; those caused by fungi, eumycetomas (mycotic mycetomas) (Table 69.4).

Epidemiology

Mycetoma is generally a disease seen in the tropics or subtropics, although cases are described from other zones.[55,56] It is more often seen in areas where there is a low annual rainfall. The main sites for this infection are Mexico, Central and northern South America, Africa, the Middle East and India. Cases are reported less frequently in the Far East. The main causes of mycetoma are shown in Table 69.3. Organisms prevalent in certain areas are shown; however, cases may rarely be seen outside these endemic zones. As a general principle the main causes of mycetoma in Central America are *Nocardia* species,[57] whereas in most African countries and the Indian subcontinent *Madurella mycetomatis* is the most common cause. The causes of mycetoma are generally classified according to organism, namely fungi (eumycetoma) or actinomycetes (actinomycetoma), and by grain colour—black, red or pale, e.g. red grain actinomycetoma is an infection caused by *Actinomadura pelletieri*. The proportion of pale grain eumycetomas is higher in temperate areas and in addition many of the fungi isolated are sterile moulds which cannot be identified because of a lack of distinguishing characteristics.

Mycetoma is more common in males than females and generally affects adults. It is also mainly seen in agricultural workers, although this is not invariable. The majority of patients appear to have no predisposing illness. There is evidence that the organisms are spread from the environment via a penetrating injury such as a thorn prick. The fungal causes of mycetoma have been isolated from plants and plant debris; *Nocardia* species have been isolated from soil. It appears that the organisms possess mechanisms for survival in the human host which allow them to evade defences. Some of the mechanisms of adapation include the deposition of intra- or extracellular melanin, cell wall thickening and immunomodulation.[58]

Clinical features

The earliest sign of a mycetoma is the appearance of a small symptom-free dermal or subcutaneous swelling.[55,56] It is difficult to give an accurate estimate of incubation periods as few patients give a history of a penetrating injury. However, it may take several years before the first sign of disease, a painless subcutaneous nodule, is seen. With time this slowly enlarges and sinuses appear on its upper surface (Figure 69.7). Pain may occur prior to rupture of sinuses on to the skin surface and in the early stages these dry up. Chronically discharging sinuses may be formed in well-established lesions. At this stage there

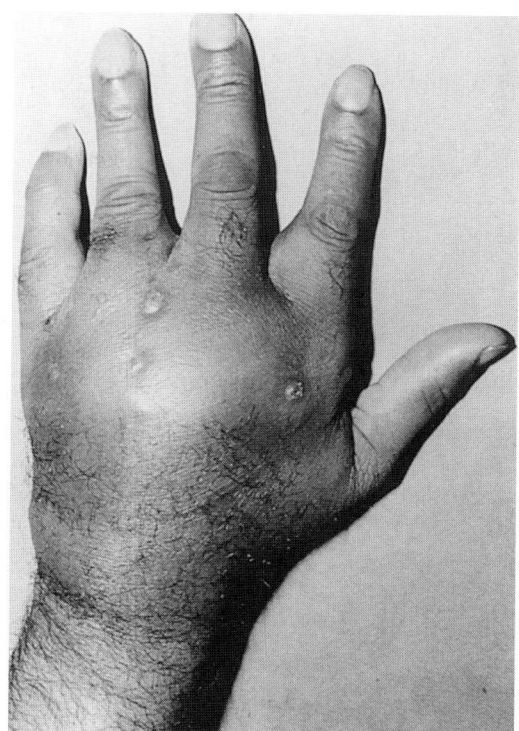

Figure 69.7: Mycetoma affecting the hand due to *Madurella grisea*.

is considerable woody swelling affecting the site, accompanied by deformity.

The main areas affected are those subject to trauma such as the feet, lower legs and hands. *Nocardia* species are prominent among causes of lesions on the chest and back; *Streptomyces somaliensis* is the most common cause of head and neck lesions. Dissemination is rare, although some infections may become very extensive and spread widely over a limb. The only threat to life is where they involve the skull.

Radiological changes include cortical thinning or hypertrophy, periosteal proliferation and lytic lesions.[59] Magnetic resonance imaging (MRI) is the best method of delineating the extent of lesions.

Differential diagnosis

Mycetomas may be mistaken for osteomyelitis caused by bacteria or actinomycosis. Actinomycosis is an infection caused by *Actinomyces israelii*, *A. bovis* or other actinomycetes such as *Arachnia propionica*. The infections are usually located close to the sites where these organisms can be carried, such as the oral cavity, chest, and within the abdominal cavity, around the caecum.

Laboratory diagnosis

The laboratory diagnosis of mycetoma depends on the demonstration of grains of the organisms.[60] These are generally obtained by opening a sinus where there is a small amount of pus beneath the skin surface, using a sterile needle. The grains can usually be seen with the

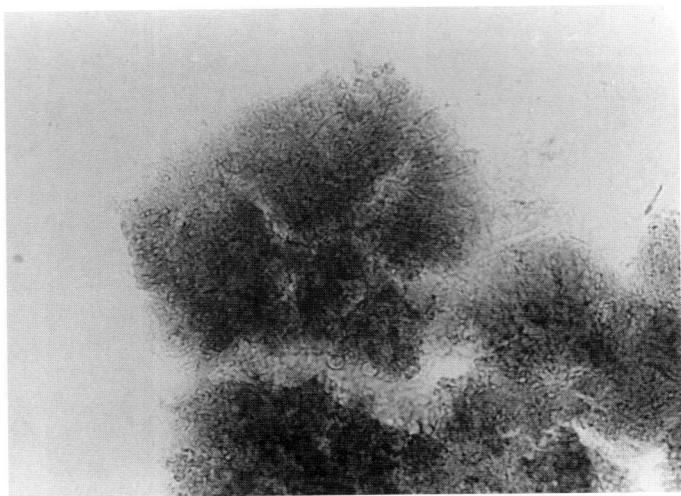

Figure 69.8: Direct microscopy in potassium hydroxide (10%) of a black grain eumycetoma. (× 40.)

naked eye in the pus and blood from the sinus tract. They can be processed as follows:

- *Direct microscopy.* Grains are mounted in 5–10% potassium hydroxide (Figure 69.8). They can gently be squashed. As a general rule if the filaments can be seen with the 40 × objective the cause is a fungus. However, if these are not visible the cause is likely to be an actinomycete.
- Grains can be taken for *histology* and embedded after formalin fixation. The pathology laboratory should be shown were the grains are, otherwise they may be discarded prior to fixation.[61] The appearance of many grains is typical in haematoxylin and eosin stained sections and the use of special fungal stains such as periodic acid–Schiff or methenamine silver is not strictly necessary.
- Grains can be *cultured* on a variety of media and the appearances of the fungi or actinomycetes is typical, although a specialist laboratory will be needed for their identification.

The main aim of laboratory diagnosis is to separate fungal and actinomycete causes because the treatment of each is different.

Management

The treatment of mycetoma depends on knowing whether the cause is an actinomycete or a fungus.[62] The actinomycetes respond to a variety of antibiotics such as sulphonamides and sulphones or co-trimoxazole. For many infections it is advisable to use a second-line drug such as rifampicin or streptomycin. Alternatives include amikacin, ciprofloxacin and imipenem for difficult cases. Most of these infections will respond to therapy although *Streptomyces somaliensis* is notoriously resistant to therapy in some cases. Here, alternative regimens include combined sodium fusidate and a sulphonamide.

Treatment of eumycetomas is more difficult. About

40–50% of infections due to *Madurella mycetomatis* respond to ketoconazole 200–400 mg daily. Other possibilities include griseofulvin (500–1000 mg daily) and itraconazole 200–400 mg daily. Although surgery remains an option the most effective approach is amputation and if the patient is not incapacitated by the infection, which is usually the case, removal of a limb, for instance, may do more harm than good. This is especially true where facilities for artificial limbs and rehabilitation are poor. Generally mycetomas are only slowly progressive and are seldom life threatening. It may be better for the patient to receive no treatment in these circumstances.

Chromoblastomycosis

There are a number of fungal infections which are caused by pigmented fungi, known as dematiaceous fungi.[63] Generally these organisms contain melanin or secrete extracellular melanin into the environment. The production of melanin is of evolutionary importance as it allows these fungi to withstand environmental changes such as drought, heat or cold. There are a number of different infections caused by dematiaceous fungi but the most common is chromoblastomycosis (chromomycosis).

Epidemiology and pathogenesis

Chromoblastomycosis is a chronic infection caused by pigmented fungi which form specialized cells, muriform or sclerotic cells, in tissue (Table 69.4).[64] It involves the dermis and epidermis where a variety of pathological changes occurs, ranging from pseudoepitheliomatous hyperplasia to granuloma formation. The organisms which cause this infection are found in the natural environment in plant debris or forest detritus. The main range of chromoblastomycosis involves the tropics and subtropics and the incidence of infection is highest in countries with a high rainfall. The disease is mainly seen in countries of Central and northern South America, parts of Africa, particularly the east coast of southern Africa, the Far East, Japan and the West Pacific.[63] The infection is most common in males and in agricultural workers.

Like mycetoma there is no evidence of underlying predisposition in those with chromoblastomycosis. The infection is believed to gain entry via an abrasion, although there are no animal models of the infection to establish this as the chief mode of entry.

Clinical features

The hallmark of chromoblastomycosis is warty proliferation

Table 69.4 Causes of chromoblastomycosis

Fonsecaea pedrosoi
F. verrucosa
Rhinocladiella aquaspersa

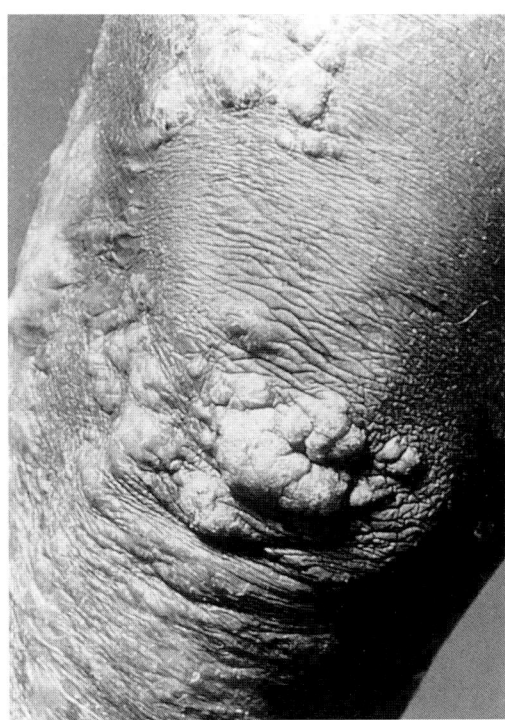

Figure 69.9: Chromoblastomycosis.

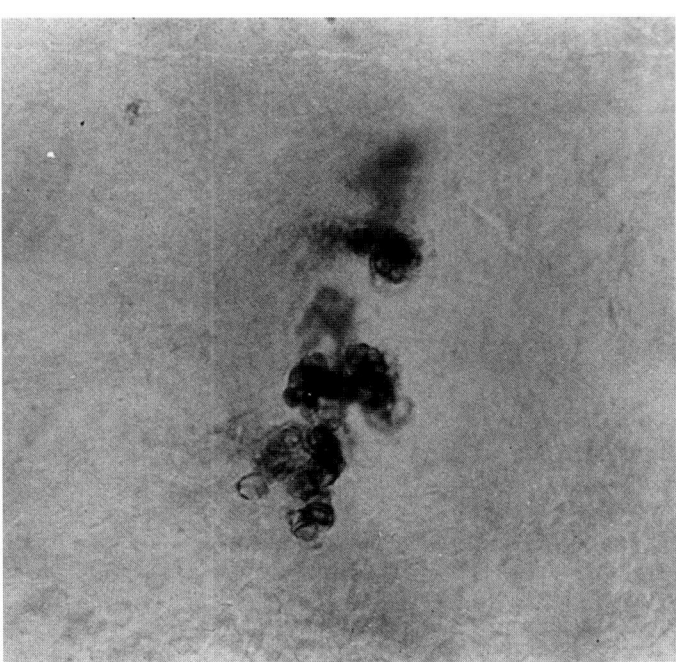

Figure 69.10: Direct microscopy in potassium hydroxide (10%) of a skin scraping from a case of chromoblastomycosis showing the muriform cells. (× 40.)

of the skin. The early lesions are small nodules or papules which slowly enlarge.[65,66] They become raised and verrucose and adjacent nodules amalgamate to form a complex of warty growth (Figure 69.9). Other lesions are flatter and plaque-like and extend slowly, sometimes healing with central scarring. Cyst-like changes and mycetoma-like lesions are also seen. The lesions are asymptomatic, although with necrosis of keratin there is often an unpleasant smell associated with them. Long-standing lesions can cause considerable deformity at the site infected and rarely squamous carcinomas can develop.

The main sites affected are those on peripheral locations such as hands, feet and lower legs. The infection spreads locally and bloodstream dissemination is very rare. Occasionally, deep infections with the same organism have been reported.

Differential diagnosis

The changes of chromoblastomycosis are typical, although there are some features which may be confused with other processes. For instance, early lesions may resemble other warty conditions such as papilloma virus infections or tuberculosis verrucosa. In extensive chromoblastomycosis the chronic changes may superficially resemble mossy foot secondary to lymphoedema. However, in the latter condition the changes are diffusely distributed over the skin surface.

Laboratory diagnosis

The process of identification of chromoblastomycosis follows standard mycological lines:

- *Direct microscopy* of skin scrapings. These should be taken from the surface of lesions. The pigmented muriform cells with transverse septa can be seen in potassium hydroxide-treated specimens (Figure 69.10).
- *Biopsy*. The histopathology of chromoblastomycosis is characteristic. The epidermis shows pseudoepitheliomatous hyperplasia with some attempt at transepidermal elimination of fungi. The latter can also be seen in granulomas or neutrophil abscesses in the dermis.
- *Culture*. Although the organisms grow readily on conventional mycological media they are black moulds which are difficult to identify because of the close resemblance of many of their specific features, such as sporulation. Often it is necessary to send cultures to specialist laboratories.[67] However, the diagnosis can be made on histopathological grounds alone.

Management

The treatment of chromoblastomycosis has changed over recent years. Generally it is inadvisable to use surgical excision unless the lesion is very small and chemotherapy is also used. The reason is that the infection may spread within the scar.

The commonly used drugs are itraconazole (100–400 mg daily), terbinafine (250 mg daily) or flucytosine 150 mg/kg in a patient with normal renal function). Thiabendazole is an alternative. A combination of flucytosine and itraconazole is probably most successful in late and extensive cases. A further approach to therapy is the use of local heat applied from heat-retaining gels or pocket hand-warmers. The heat must not be sufficient to burn the patient but high enough to be just comfortable.

Phaeohyphomycosis

Phaeohyphomycosis is another infection due to pigmented fungi in the skin. Cases are diffusely distributed through most tropical countries but are not common. Generally the infection presents with large cysts around the lower or upper limbs and these can mimic ganglia or Baker's cysts.[67]

The organisms are implanted from the environment and in some of these cysts there are fragments of plant material. Each cyst is surrounded by a fibrous capsule but contains palisading granulomas and a necrotic centre. The fungi are present as irregular mycelial fragments whose pigmentation may be very variable and sometimes it is necessary to use specific fungal stains. Occasionally this form of infection is seen in immunocompromised patients, particularly those receiving systemic corticosteroids.

The treatment is excision.

Sporotrichosis

Sporotrichosis, the infection caused by the dimorphic fungal pathogen *Sporothrix schenckii*, is widely distributed through the tropical world.[68] It may present either as a cutaneous infection or on occasion as a deep mycosis (see below). Extensive disseminated cutaneous infections are seen in patients with AIDS.[69]

Epidemiology

Sporotrichosis was first described in the USA and subsequently in Europe but although it is seen in central and southern USA the main foci of infection are in Mexico, Central and South America, Africa and Japan. Scattered cases are seen in the Far East and Australia. The organism is part of an extensive group of soil and plant pathogens, the *Sporothrix* and *Sporotrichum* species. But *Sporothrix schenckii*'s ability to invade animals is unique, as is its dimorphism whereby it exists as a mould at room temperature and in the environment but as a yeast in animal tissue.[68]

Exposure to infection is usually sporadic, although small outbreaks of infection have been described in certain occupational groups, such as florists, packers, plant workers, fishermen and armadillo hunters. There are also focal areas where the disease appears to be hyperendemic in Guatemala,[70] Peru and South Africa. In South Africa contamination of pit props has been reported to cause disease in mine workers.

Sporotrichosis affects both males and females and can also infect children and infants.

Clinical features

There are a variety of different clinical forms of sporotrichosis.[71,72] Some infections appear to resolve spontaneously, although the frequency of this occurrence is unknown. Certain patients develop fixed lesions which are usually solitary ulcerated granulomas on exposed sites, including the face. Small satellite lesions frequently develop around the edge of these larger granulomas. Ulcers enlarge slowly. A second form of cutaneous sporotrichosis is called lymphangitic because the infection spreads from a primary granuloma or ulcer along the course of local lymphatics. Secondary lesions formed along the lymphatic path may discharge or ulcerate. Other forms of infection may mimic chronic leg ulcers and lupus vulgaris. Disseminated deep lesions of sporotrichosis may affect other body sites such as the joints, lungs and meninges.[73] While most of these patients do not have major underlying conditions, alcoholism or diabetes is seen in some.

In patients with AIDS these infections may spread to involve multiple skin sites with large numbers of ulcers or nodules.[71]

Differential diagnosis

Leishmaniasis may resemble either of the two principal forms of sporotrichosis and where this condition is endemic some physicians advise using a sporotrichin intradermal skin test to orient the direction of investigation. This is read after 48 hours, like a tuberculin reaction. Atypical mycobacterial infection may cause similar changes, particularly *Mycobacterium marinum*, which spreads along lymphatics.

Laboratory diagnosis

Sporotrichosis differs from the other subcutaneous mycoses in that culture is the most reliable mode of diagnosis because there are few organisms present in lesions and these may be difficult to find.[68]

- *Direct microscopy* seldom has a role to play although it may be used to screen for amastigotes of *Leishmania* species.
- *Culture.* *Sporothrix schenckii* grows well on Sabouraud's agar and will form characteristic spores. Samples from swabs, curettings and biopsies are all suitable. They should be taken from the edge of lesions.
- *Biopsy.* The histopathology shows a mixed granulomatous and polymorphonuclear response. Organisms are scattered in this infiltrate, although some are surrounded by a refractile eosinophilic halo called an asteroid body. In some centres an immunofluorescence test is available using specific antibody conjugates for application to fixed biopsy tissue.
- *Sporotrichin* skin test. This is an intradermal reaction. The agent is prepared from polysaccharide antigens of the organism. Uninfected patients from endemic areas may also have positive responses.

Management

The treatment for sporotrichosis is potassium iodide made up in a saturated solution. The starting dose is 1–2 ml given three times daily and increased drop by drop to a maximum of 4–6 ml three times a day. The slow increase is necessary because of the unpleasant taste and the possibility of symptoms of iodism: nausea, dry mouth, altered taste, swollen salivary glands. The normal duration of therapy is at least 2 months and often up to 4 months. Alternatives are itraconazole in doses of 100–200 mg daily or terbinafine 250 mg daily.

Subcutaneous zygomycosis

Subcutaneous zygomycosis (phycomycosis) comprises two separate diseases: those caused by *Basidiobolus* and *Conidiobolus*.[74] Generally the clinical features of these infections are distinct, as are their epidemiology and age prevalence.

Subcutaneous zygomycosis due to *Conidiobolus* (conidiobolomycosis, rhinoentomophthoromycosis) is uncommon but is found in different tropical areas of the West Indies, South America, Africa and Southern India.[75,76] The causative organism is usually *C. coronatus*, a fungus which is an insect pathogen. The usual focus of infection is within the nasal cavity and the infection spreads from the turbinates to involve the subcutaneous tissues of the face and neck with a hard painless swelling. The deformity may be severe. This infection is seen mainly in adults.

Subcutaneous zygomycosis is also caused by *Basidiobolus* (subcutaneous phycomycosis, basidiobolomycosis). The usual cause of this infection is *B. ranarum*, a pathogen of amphibians and reptiles. The site of infection is usually confined to the limb girdles or proximal limbs.[77,78] It is mainly seen in Central, East and West Africa and chiefly infects children. Once again the swelling is deforming and has a woody consistency.

In both diseases the histology is similar, with a dense infiltrate of eosinophils in the subcutis and large strap-like hyphae contained in granulomas.

The treatment is either ketoconazole or itraconazole, although saturated potassium iodide can be used.

Lobomycosis

Lobomycosis is a rare infection, seen in Central and South America, caused by *Loboa loboi*, a fungus which has not been cultured to date.[79] The infection is seen in subcutaneous tissues and presents with plaques and keloid-like scars. The only treatment is excision. The epidemiology of the infection is unusual as it is seen mainly in remote areas[80] and the same infection has also been seen in sea or freshwater dolphins. Rarely squamous carcinomas may develop in long-standing lesions.

Systemic mycoses

The systemic mycoses are fungal infections which involve deep organs. While some, often referred to as the endemic mycoses, affect healthy individuals, others are opportunistic infections which occur in patients with some underlying predisposition. In recent years systemic mycoses, such as cryptococcosis and histoplasmosis, have become prominent as secondary complications in patients with AIDS, although it is of interest that other systemic mycoses have not increased in this population. Generally in most developed countries the opportunistic infections are more common but in many tropical areas the endemic systemic fungal infections are seen more frequently.

Endemic systemic mycoses

The main endemic mycoses are shown in Table 69.5. The usual route of entry of all organisms in this group is the lung, although direct implantation into the skin after an accident is also possible. Each disease has a defined endemic area and their pathogenesis is similar. The majority of people exposed to infection are merely sensitized to the organism and develop delayed-type hypersensitivity to the fungus, seen on intradermal testing with an appropriate antigen (the *asymptomatic form*). In some patients there is a primary illness which appears to follow massive exposure to the organisms (the *acute pulmonary form*). *Chronic pulmonary forms* of these diseases may also occur and they closely resemble pulmonary tuberculosis. Dissemination from the primary lung focus may also take place. It may be a rapid event followed by widespread infiltration of organs (*acute disseminated form*). The infection in such cases progresses rapidly and the disease may be fatal unless treatment is instituted. Acute disseminated forms are most likely to occur in patients who are immunosuppressed (AIDS, lymphoma) but may also be seen in infants and others. More slowly progressive forms also occur and have to be monitored carefully (*chronic disseminated forms*).

Table 69.5 Systemic mycoses

Mycosis	Organism
Endemic respiratory infections	
Histoplasmosis	*Histoplasma capsulatum* var. *capsulatum*
African histoplasmosis	*H. capsulatum* var. *duboisii*
Blastomycosis	*Blastomyces dermatitidis*
Coccidioidomycosis	*Coccidioides immitis*
Paracoccidioidomycosis	*Paracoccidioides brasiliensis*
Infection due to *Penicillium marneffei*	
Opportunistic infections	
Systemic candidosis	
Systemic candidosis	*Candida albicans, C. tropicalis, C. glabrata*, etc.
Aspergillosis	*Aspergillus fumigatus, A. flavus, A. niger*
Cryptococcosis	*Cryptococcus neoformans*
Mucormycosis	Species of *Absidia, Rhizopus* and *Rhizomucor*
Others: infections due to *Fusarium, Trichosporon*	

While generally they only spread slowly, in some situations they may begin to disseminate. In some infections, histoplasmosis and coccidioidomycosis for example, disseminated and pulmonary forms do not generally coexist. *Primary cutaneous infections* are rare and generally follow laboratory or post-mortem room accidents.

Histoplasmoses

The classification of histoplasmosis in man is somewhat complicated. There are two main types.[81] The first, sometimes called classical or small form histoplasmosis, is caused by *Histoplasma capsulatum* var. *capsulatum*. This is a dimorphic fungus whose yeast phase forms are those present in tissue. The disease is endemic throughout much of the world, with the exception of Europe, and presents with pulmonary and disseminated infection affecting the lungs, reticuloendothelial system and mucosal surfaces. The yeast forms seen in tissue are small (2–4 μm in diameter). It will be referred to hereafter as histoplasmosis. The second form, African or large-form histoplasmosis caused by *H. capsulatum* var. *duboisii*, only occurs in Africa.[82] The yeasts found in tissue are large (12–20 μm) and the main signs of infection follow dissemination to lymph nodes, skin and bones. The organisms isolated from both are identical in culture but can be differentiated by molecular genetic techniques and are regarded as variants of a single species, *H. capsulatum*.

Histoplasmosis

Histoplasmosis is an infection caused by the dimorphic fungus, *Histoplasma capsulatum* var. *capsulatum*. The organism can be found in soil or areas where large numbers of birds or bats have roosted, including barns, caves and under the eaves of houses. There is no association with any one particular bat species in the tropics. The endemic areas include parts of the USA, West Indies, Central and South America, Africa, India and the Far East.[81] Apart from the USA the endemic areas with the highest incidence of new infections occur in Central and South America. It is thought that bird or bat excreta provides the necessary milieu for growth of organisms present in the environment, although bats can also be infected. Exposure in man is usually sporadic, although occasionally the disease is seen in groups of exposed patients such as cave explorers or farm workers.

Defence against *H. capsulatum* is largely by cell-mediated responses. The organism is about 2–4 μm in diameter and can be taken up by macrophages. The infection may therefore be prolonged in individuals with defective T lymphocyte-mediated responses, including those with AIDS.

Clinical features

The majority of patients who acquire histoplasmosis remain asymptomatic, the only sign of past exposure being a positive intradermal histoplasmin test which is read after

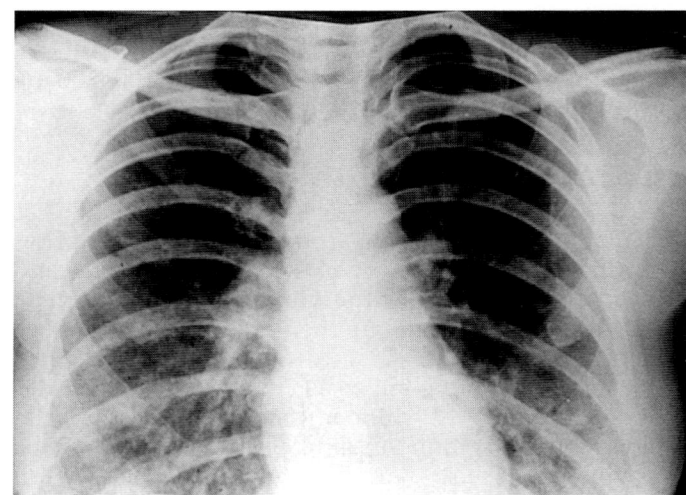

Figure 69.11: Acute pulmonary histoplasmosis.

48 hours. This test is used for studying the epidemiology of infection but has little value as a diagnostic procedure because it only indicates exposure and many patients with active infection are anergic.

The acute pulmonary form of histoplasmosis often follows exposure to a site containing numerous *Histoplasma* spores such as a cave. Patients develop an acute febrile illness 10–14 days after exposure. There is cough, chest pain, joint pains and, in some cases, erythema multiforme. Radiologically there is often diffuse mottling and in some cases hilar enlargement (Figure 69.11). Normally, spontaneous recovery occurs and no treatment is given except supportive measures. However, very rarely in some patients the disease progresses and disseminates.

Some patients may be found on routine radiography to have solitary or multiple asymptomatic pulmonary nodules, which are surgically removed in order to distinguish them from a carcinoma. These are then found to contain *Histoplasma* yeasts (Figure 69.12). Once again therapy is not necessary. A second type of chronic pulmonary disease

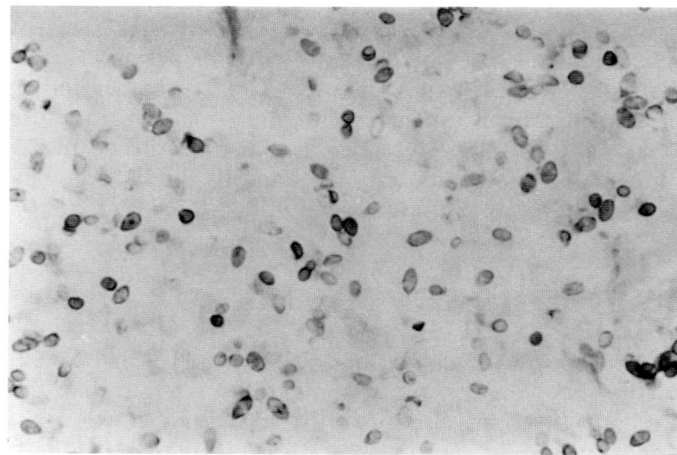

Figure 69.12: *Histoplasma capsulatum* in a lung lesion. Gomori (methenamine silver) (GMS × 100.)

produces focal consolidation and cavitation, usually in one or both apices and seen on radiography. This closely resembles pulmonary tuberculosis. The main symptoms, such as cough, chest pain and haemoptysis, are also similar. In the early stages some recovery can occur but later in established cases there is slow progression of the inflammatory lesion which can encroach on other lung areas. This form of histoplasmosis is not often seen in the tropics.

Acute disseminated histoplasmosis affects the bone marrow and lymph glands as well as the liver and spleen.[83] Patients present with fever, weight loss, malaise and hepatosplenomegaly. There may be evidence of bruising and purpura. Diffuse pulmonary infiltrates and small skin papules and ulcers can also occur. This type of histoplasmosis will progress to death if unchecked. Acute forms of disseminated histoplasmosis are seen in patients with AIDS.[84,85] In the latter groups the symptoms may be non-specific (weight loss and fever), although some clues such as hepatosplenomegaly or multiple skin lesions (nodules, papules, ulcers) may be seen. A more indolent type of disseminated histoplasmosis is seen in otherwise healthy individuals. They usually present with either oral ulceration or hypoadrenalism. The latter should be sought in such patients. Chronic disseminated histoplasmosis may present years after the patient has left an endemic area. The oral ulcers are persistent and painful. Laryngeal involvement, meningitis and endocarditis can also occur.

Laboratory diagnosis

The organisms of *H. capsulatum* are very small and difficult to visualize by direct microscopy but they can sometimes be seen in bone marrow or blood smears stained with Giemsa. They can be grown readily from sputum or other sources such as bone marrow in appropriate cases. Blood cultures are sometimes positive in patients with AIDS. The organisms grow as moulds at room temperature and have to be converted into yeast phase at 37°C. As this process is slow a more rapid test involving the detection of antigen leached from culture, the exoantigen test, is available. Serology has a useful role in diagnosis. There are complement fixation tests for histoplasmosis as well as an immunodiffusion test, both of which use standardized reagents. These tests can be used in diagnosis and as a guide to prognosis. New tests of particular value in patients with AIDS have been developed for the detection of circulating *Histoplasma* antigen, but these are not widely available. Histopathology is also useful. *Histoplasma* are small oval yeasts up to 5 μm in diameter. They are usually found intracellularly. In patients with AIDS they tend to be more pleomorphic in size and shape.

A guide to the use of diagnostic tests in the different forms of histoplasmosis is seen in Table 69.6.

Management

The asymptomatic forms of histoplasmosis do not necessarily require therapy. Therapy is also usually withheld in acute pulmonary forms, although supportive

Table 69.6 Use of laboratory tests in histoplasmosis

Type	Tests
Acute pulmonary	Serology (after 14–18 days), culture, chest radiography
Chronic pulmonary	Culture (sputum), serology, chest radiography
Acute disseminated	Culture (bone marrow, blood, sputum, skin) Serology* (including antigen detection) Histopathology†
Chronic disseminated	Culture (ulcers) Serology (often negative) Histopathology

*In acute forms of histoplasmosis titres of complement fixation test antibodies greater than 1:64 indicate a risk of dissemination. New tests of antigen detection are available in some areas
†Some laboratories can carry out immunofluorescence on fixed tissue using conjugated anti-*Histoplasma* antibodies to identify the organisms.

treatment such as bedrest and fluids may be given where necessary. The value of antifungals in these types is not known, although itraconazole would be a possible choice. Chronic pulmonary histoplasmosis and chronic disseminated histoplasmosis are usually treated with itraconazole. The role of fluconazole in this infection is not as yet clear. Itraconazole (200–400 mg daily) can also be given in more rapidly disseminating types of infection. An alternative is amphotericin B (0.6–1.0 mg/kg daily) in the disseminated types. In patients with AIDS it is necessary to use long-term suppressive therapy with itraconazole after induction of remission with amphotericin B, otherwise relapse will normally occur.

African histoplasmosis

African histoplasmosis, as the name suggests, is confined to Africa. It is caused by *H. capsulatum* var. *duboisii*, which resembles the other variant but forms larger yeasts in tissue.[82] The infection is not common but occurs in Central and West Africa south of the Sahara and north of the Zambezi River. The ecological source of this fungus is unknown. It is thought that, as with the other type of histoplasmosis, it gains entry through the lungs.

The patient usually presents with focal disease affecting the skin, bone or a lymph gland. Alternatively multiple sites may be affected, including the gastrointestinal tract, lungs and other mucosal surfaces. This form is more rapidly progressive.

The disease is diagnosed by the presence of large oval yeasts (8–14 μm) seen in direct microscopy (Figure 69.13) or histopathological examination of biopsied lesions. The organism can be isolated in culture. Serology is generally negative.

The main agents are itraconazole, ketoconazole or even amphotericin B.

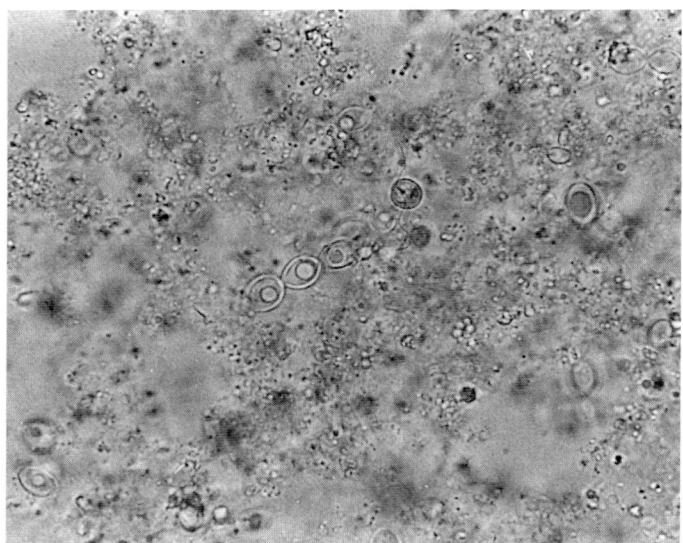

Figure 69.13: African histoplasmosis. Direct microscopy in potassium hydroxide (10%) of pus from a skin ulcer. (× 40.)

Blastomycosis

Blastomycosis is a systemic fungal infection caused by *Blastomyces dermatitidis*, a dimorphic pathogen.[86] The disease is mainly found in the USA and Canada but cases have also been seen in Africa, India and the Middle East. As with histoplasmosis the main portal of entry is via the respiratory tract. Yeast phase organisms cause disease.

Epidemiology

B. dermatitidis has only occasionally been isolated from the natural environment, usually in North America and in sites where there is a risk of flooding, such as river banks.[87] The organism has not been isolated from such sources in Africa and its ecological niche here is unknown. The infection was first described in the USA and subsequently it became known as North American blastomycosis, until the first case was described from North Africa. Since then cases have been described from a variety of African countries from the north coast (e.g. Algeria) to Namibia.[88] The largest number of cases have been seen in Zimbabwe. It is not clear whether the disease differs in different geographic areas, but in African cases the principal signs of the disease are those of disseminated infection affecting the bone or skin. There is also evidence that the organisms from African and US sources are antigenically and genetically different although morphologically identical. Other cases have been detected in the Middle East,[89] India[90] and Europe.

Clinical features

The main clinical features of infection follow a somewhat similar pattern to those seen with histoplasmosis.

There is no commercially available skin test for blastomycosis but the use of experimental antigens has suggested that subclinical exposure is present in endemic areas. There is an uncommon acute pulmonary form of the infection which presents with acute respiratory symptoms—cough, pleuritic pain and fever. This is most often seen in children and has not been described in the tropics.[86]

The chronic pulmonary type of blastomycosis presents with focal consolidation and cavitation in the chest with symptoms of cough, fever and weight loss. This may be confused radiologically with pulmonary tuberculosis. Unlike histoplasmosis this may coexist with disseminated lesions of blastomycosis. Disseminated blastomycosis is most often seen in the tropics. The main sites of dissemination are the skin and bones. Skin lesions may be ulcers, abscesses, granulomas or crusted plaques which heal with scar formation. The bones involved are principally axial skeletal bones, such as vertebrae, and spinal cord compression may occur as a result of this infection. Dissemination also occurs in the immunocompromised patient.[91]

Laboratory diagnosis

The diagnosis of this infection is based on direct microscopy at suitable sites as well as sputum and culture. *B. dermatitidis* is a dimorphic fungus which grows as a mould at room temperature but as a yeast at 37°C. Histological changes of blastomycosis are typical as the yeasts produce a characteristic broad-based bud.

Management

Therapy of blastomycosis involves the use of either itraconazole (200–400 mg daily) or ketoconazole (200–400 mg daily). Intravenous amphotericin B is an alternative (0.6–1.0 mg/kg daily).

Coccidioidomycosis

Coccidioides immitis is a soil organism, geographically confined to semi-desert areas of the New World.[92] The infection consists of a respiratory disease which may spread to other sites. Coccidioidomycosis may affect both healthy and immunocompromised patients.

Epidemiology

This infection is seen mainly in a geological zone known as the lower Sonoran life zone, where there is a low annual rainfall and a characteristic vegetation including cacti and creosote bushes. The disease is confined to the semi-desert areas of the New World in the USA, Central America (Honduras, Guatemala), Colombia, Venezuela, Argentina and Paraguay. The infecting form is an arthrospore which is inhaled but is transformed in the host into a spore-like structure, the spherule. This is a large 50–80 μm diameter spore containing small endospores which are released by rupture of the spherule; they can develop into further spores.

Clinical features

Infection follows inhalation. Once again in the endemic area a significant proportion of the populace appear to be subclinically sensitized, e.g. up to 70% in California.[93] The primary infection, when it is symptomatic, may present with fever, weight loss, cough and chest pains. Arthralgia, conjunctivitis and erythema nodosum or erythema multiforme may all develop. The radiological changes vary from minimal focal consolidation to pleural effusion to massive hilar adenopathy. This clinical type is usually self-resolving, although progression is much more likely in American Indians, Blacks or mestizos. Pregnant women are also at risk from dissemination. An extensive pneumonia may follow infection in patients with depressed T lymphocyte function, such as those who have received organ transplants. Chronic pulmonary nodules or cavitation may also occur.[92] The latter is characteristically thin-walled on radiography. Dissemination is also seen. Dissemination of coccidioidomycosis often affects the joints or meninges, but skin and other organs may also be affected. Skin changes include ulcers and granulomas as well as warty papules and nodules. Meningitis is a chronic process which clinically mimics tuberculous infection. It is notoriously difficult to treat. In patients with AIDS prolonged pneumonia and disseminated infections can both occur.[94]

Laboratory diagnosis

The diagnosis depends on the identification of spherules in smears, biopsies or sputum as well as on the growth of the organism. *C. immitis* is a white mould fungus which is easily spread by aerosol. It is therefore a potential laboratory hazard and laboratory staff should be forewarned if this is being considered diagnostically. There are also a number of useful serological tests (complement fixation, immunodiffusion and immunoelectrophoresis).

Management

The treatment of coccidioidomycosis has been changing in recent years, with an increasing reliance on the use of ketoconazole, itraconazole and fluconazole. Intravenous amphotericin B is an alternative. The responses of widely disseminated infection and meningitis to these treatments are often poor.

Paracoccidioidomycosis

Paracoccidioidomycosis or South American blastomycosis is a systemic fungal infection which is confined to Central and South America.[95] It causes a range of pulmonary and systemic symptoms but is a sporadically occurring infection caused by the dimorphic fungus *Paracoccidioides brasiliensis*. Yeast phase organisms can be found in tissue.

Epidemiology

The main areas where this disease is present are Colombia, Venezuela, Ecuador, Brazil and Argentina, but other South and Central American countries may be involved. Skin testing reveals that the distribution of sensitization in the community is patchy, and seldom more than 25% have positive skin tests. Both sexes may be sensitized but this infection is more common in men than women. The process of transformation from hyphal (environmental) phase to yeast phase *P. brasiliensis* is partly regulated by an intracytoplasmic oestrogen receptor. The natural source of the organism is unknown.

Clinical features

The presence of a small group of healthy individuals in an endemic area with positive skin test reactions suggests that there is a subclinical form of this disease.[96] The main clinical types are named after those parts of the body predominantly affected, such as pulmonary, lympho-nodular, mucocutaneous or mixed. In chronic pulmonary infection there is often widespread and extensive infiltration followed by severe fibrosis. There is also dissemination to other sites such as the oral or nasal mucosa or lymph nodes.[97] These are the mucosal (mucocutaneous) or lymphatic forms, respectively, but the most common variety is a mixed type where there are multiple foci of infection. Usually all are only slowly progressive. On mucosal surfaces this infection produces large erosions and ulcers, less commonly warty papules. All these forms of infection are virtually confined to males. While in most patients paracoccidioidomycosis is an indolent infection, an agressive widespread form of disease occurs occasionally in younger patients. Paracoccidioidomycosis is rare in patients with AIDS.

Laboratory diagnosis

The infection is diagnosed by demonstrating presence of the characteristic yeast forms in sputum, smears or biopsies. These yeasts form multiple buds, often appearing around the periphery of a parent cell. The organism is a dimorphic fungus which can be isolated in culture. At room temperature it grows as a mycelial form and has to be converted on enriched agar into the yeast phase at 37°C. Immunodiffusion and complement fixation tests are also available.

Management

The main treatments are itraconazole (100–200 mg daily) or ketoconazole (200 mg daily), but intravenous amphotericin B is an alternative. The latter may be necessary in the widespread aggressive forms of infection.

Infection due to *Penicillium marneffei*

P. marneffei is a fungus which is a pathogen of bamboo rats found in China and South-East Asia. It causes a disease which grossly resembles histoplasmosis in both otherwise healthy and immunocompromised patients.[98,99]

It is common in AIDS patients. The endemic areas extend from parts of Malaysia through Thailand to Myanmar and Assam and north to South China and Hong Kong. Infections are commoner after the rains and it is assumed that the main portal of entry is the lung.

The main sites affected are the lungs, skin, liver, spleen and bone marrow. Most patients have disseminated disease although occasionally the infection is localized. Skin lesions occur in about 60% of cases with AIDS and consist of umbilicated papules, small ulcers of nodules. They are very prominent on the face.

The organisms resemble *Histoplasma* species but do not form buds, individual cells being divided by septa. Cells may also be curved. The organism has a characteristic appearance in culture and often produces a diffusible red pigment.

The main therapeutic agents are itraconazole or amphotericin B. In AIDS patients the initial treatment is amphotericin B followed by long-term suppressive treatment with itraconazole.

Systemic opportunistic pathogens

The main opportunistic fungi are listed in Table 69.7. In industrialized countries they are a major problem in severely ill patients, particularly those with neutropenia and those receiving solid organ or bone marrow transplants. They are also seen in intensive care units. In addition to these, some infections such as cryptococcosis are present in patients with AIDS. In the tropics less attention has been paid to some of these opportunists, such as candidosis and aspergillosis, with some important exceptions;[100] by contrast, cryptococcosis is recognized to be a common and increasingly important problem everywhere. For more detailed information on these infections the reader is referred to other texts.[101]

Systemic candidosis

Systemic *Candida* infections occur in a variety of patients, particularly those who are neutropenic, such as leukaemia patients, those who have received major surgery and patients receiving long-term intravenous feeding. The importance of these infections in the tropics is largely unknown. Their management is discussed elsewhere.[101]

Table 69.7 Opportunistic systemic mycoses

Systemic candidosis
Aspergillosis
Mucormycosis
Cryptococcosis
Less common
Systemic infections due to *Trichosporon, Fusarium, Bipolaris*

Aspergillosis

Aspergillosis is a disease caused by species of the genus *Aspergillus*, principally *A. fumigatus*, *A. flavus* and *A. niger*. There are a number of different clinical syndromes caused by these fungi, which occur in temperate and tropical climates alike. Aspergilli are well-recognized causes of allergic pulmonary disease, either when inhaled as spores (extrinsic asthma) or when growing within airways where, in susceptible individuals, they may cause a form of intrinsic asthma known as allergic broncho-pulmonary aspergillosis.[102] The latter causes reversible bronchoconstriction in the early stages but thereafter irreversible pulmonary damage may occur. This type of disease has been recorded in India, among other tropical areas. A form of aspergillosis seen regularly in tropical areas is the development of a fungus ball in patients with pulmonary cavitation, usually secondary to tuberculosis.[103] This fungus ball may elicit an inflammatory response and in a minority of patients (15%) will cause severe haemoptysis.[104] The other mode of pathogenesis by *Aspergillus* is through invasion of tissue. This is mainly a problem in the severely neutropenic patient. However, there is one invasive *Aspergillus* syndrome which is mainly seen in the tropics: invasive paranasal *Aspergillus* granuloma.

Invasive *Aspergillus* granuloma of the paranasal sinuses is a slowly progressive infection affecting the sinuses, orbit and brain.[101,105] It is seen mainly in Africa and the Middle East and in most patients is caused by *A. flavus*. The patient presents with headache, nasal obstruction and orbital swelling with, in some cases, proptosis. In later stages invasion of the brain may ensue. On radiography a mass can be seen in the maxillary or ethmoid sinuses with erosion of the bones of the base of the skull and orbit. These changes can be confirmed with computed tomography. If nuclear MRI is available the infiltrated area contains a typically dense mass. If the lesions are biopsied the main change is a hard granulomatous mass with fibrosis. Scattered fungal fragments can be seen in giant cells, using specific stains, and the organism can be isolated in culture. Serology (immunodiffusion) is often positive. The main differential diagnosis consists of other *Aspergillus*-related illnesses. The presence of an intrasinus mass without bone erosion may be due to an aspergilloma or dense colonization with aspergilli. In this instance presence of the organism may not be of pathological significance. The decision is difficult as unless numerous fragments of tissue are examined the more sinister changes of fibrosis will not be seen. Aggressive paranasal sinus invasion may also occur in neutropenic patients.

The main treatment for paranasal *Aspergillus* granuloma is surgical removal of as much of the tumour as is possible, followed by long-term therapy with itraconazole (200–400 mg daily). This may have to be extended for 6–24 months and, if available, serology is a helpful way of monitoring. An alternative therapeutic option is amphotericin B but long-term therapy is not possible with this drug.

Mucormycosis

Fungi belonging to the genera *Absidia*, *Rhizopus* and *Rhizomucor*, and less commonly other groups, may cause an aggressive paranasal, pulmonary or disseminated infection in predisposed groups such as diabetic or neutropenic patients.[106] This infection, known as mucormycosis, is seen in temperate as well as tropical countries and may cause the rapid demise of a patient unless there is prompt surgical intervention and treatment with intravenous amphotericin B. It may also present with orbital cellulitis or as a necrotizing wound infection. In malnourished children it may cause a necrotizing gastrointestinal infection.

Treatment with amphotericin B combined, where possible, with surgical debridement offers the best chance of recovery.

Cryptococcosis

Cryptococcosis is a systemic infection caused by an encapsulated yeast fungus, *Cryptococcus neoformans*. Its distribution is worldwide and it generally presents with meningitis or some other manifestation of extrapulmonary dissemination. While it may cause disease in otherwise healthy individuals, it is also a pathogen of patients with defective T lymphocyte function, such as patients with AIDS, lymphoma or those receiving systemic steroid therapy.

Epidemiology and pathogenesis

There are two variants of *C. neoformans*: *C. neoformans* var. *neoformans* and *C. neoformans* var. *gattii*.[107,108] The *neoformans* variety causes disease in immunocompromised patients including those with AIDS, and is found in most countries. Its ecological niche appears to be soil or areas where there are large amounts of pigeon excreta, from which this fungus can be isolated. The presumed route of entry is via inhalation. The *gattii* form is seen mainly in tropical areas in otherwise healthy individuals. It has been reported from Africa, the Far East, Papua New Guinea and Australia. This organism has only recently been isolated from the environment from debris from certain species of *Eucalyptus*. In addition to the differences in distribution there are possible differences in their clinical behaviour apart from the predilection of the *neoformans* variety for patients with AIDS.[109] In *gattii* infections mass lesions, e.g. lung, appear to be more common.

Subclinical sensitization occurs in the general population. Infection rates in the tropics are not known and appear to be variable, even in patients with AIDS. There is evidence that in Zaire about 12% of those with AIDS have circulating cryptococcal antigen, indicating active infection. However, in AIDS patients in Ghana the incidence is lower; in Zambia the infection is again more common. The explanation for these fluctuations is unknown. However, clustering of cases may occur and has been seen for instance in Papua New Guinea, where the disease is mainly caused by *C. neoformans* var. *gattii*.

Clinical features

Cryptococcal infection may present with pulmonary infection—cough, chest pain and fever.[108] However, pulmonary lesions are more often present as an incidental, and symptomless, finding in a patient with other manifestations of cryptococcosis. The common presentation of this infection in the non-AIDS patient is with meningitis, although headache and neck stiffness may not be severe; but other signs such as confusion, drowsiness, photophobia and cranial nerve palsies may be seen. Other signs of dissemination such as papular or ulcerative skin lesions, lytic bone deposits and prostatitis may be found. In patients with AIDS the symptoms of meningitis are often minimal and fever may be the main clinical sign, together with malaise and tiredness.[110]

Laboratory diagnosis

The laboratory diagnosis of cryptococcosis is straightforward. It depends on the demonstration of the organism(s) by staining smears, cerebrospinal fluid (CSF) or sputum with Indian ink (Figure 69.14) or nigrosin. The capsule surrounding the organism displaces the opaque stain and the surrounding clear halo seen with the microscope is typical of *Cryptococcus*. The organism can be cultured readily on conventional mycological media such as Sabouraud's agar, although it may take 3–12 days for the yeasts to be recognizable. Sources of culture material include CSF, sputum and biopsies.[111] In patients with AIDS blood cultures may also be positive.

The quickest method of diagnosis is the use of the antigen detection test, which employs antibody-sensitized latex particles or an enzyme-linked immnosorbent assay test. Both are used to detect capsular antigen in serum or CSF. The tests are specific and the latex tests will produce a positive response in 30 minutes. It can also be used to follow the course of therapy. Biopsy material will also

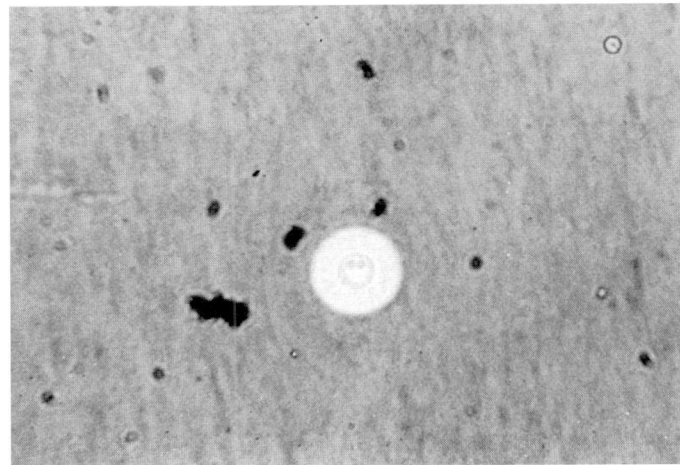

Figure 69.14: Cryptococcal cell in CSF. (India ink, × 100.)

show the large yeast cells using periodic acid–Schiff or Grocott stains; the mucicarmine stain is specific for cryptococcal capsule, which it stains pink.

Management

The main therapy in the non-AIDS patient is a combination of intravenous amphotericin B (0.4–0.8 mg/kg daily) and flucytosine (120–150 mg/kg daily divided in four doses). The response in most patients is good but therapy may have to be continued for 4–6 weeks, and sometimes longer. The treatment of the AIDS case is more complex. Few treatments can produce permanent recovery and the usual strategy is to start with a period of induction therapy followed by long-term suppression to prevent relapse. At present the best choice of drugs is still unclear. Many units will use an initial period of amphotericin (0.4–0.8 mg/ kg daily), with or without flucytosine, for 2 weeks, followed by long-term daily suppressive therapy with fluconazole (200–400 mg) or itraconazole (200–400 mg). Fluconazole may also be used to produce remission on its own, although the dose is usually 600 mg or higher.

Other mycoses

Other opportunistic infections with fungi are seen in different countries and are not specifically associated with the tropics. Again they usually occur in the neutropenic patient. They include infection with *Trichosporon*, *Fusarium* and *Bipolaris* species. These diseases are generally uncommon, but carry a high mortality.

Oculomycosis (See also Chapter 18)

Infections of the eye caused by fungi are regularly seen in the tropics. Generally they involve the cornea and follow contamination of a traumatic external injury (keratomycosis).[112] The chief causes in the tropics are filamentous fungi of the genera *Fusarium*, *Aspergillus*, *Curvularia*, *Acremonium* and *Penicillium*. Less commonly yeasts such as *Candida* species are implicated. Patients usually present with pain in the eye and photophobia. There is often an obvious ulcer, although it may be necessary to demonstrate this with slit-lamp microscopy. The ulcer may be covered with slough and with small satellite ulcers around the edge. Surrounding chemosis and a hypopyon may also be present. If the condition is not treated, severe intraocular infection followed by glaucoma, blindness and perforation of the globe will occur. Scrapings from the ulcer will readily show the presence of fungal hyphae and these can then be isolated on Sabouraud's medium. It is very important to establish the presence of fungi in such cases of keratitis because their management is very different from that used for bacteria.

Intensive application of antifungal drops such as econazole (1%) in arachis oil, clotrimazole or natamycin every few hours is advised. Oral itraconazole may help in some infections although it is seldom useful where *Fusarium* is involved. Mechanical debridement may also be useful in some cases. Keratomycosis is a preventable cause of blindness if recognized and treated as soon as possible.

REFERENCES

1 Rippon J W. *Medical Mycology*, 2nd edn. Philadelphia: W B Saunders, 1985.
2 Midgley G, Clayton Y M & Hay R J. *Diagnosis in Colour: Medical Mycology*. Mosby-Wolfe, London, 1997.
3 de Vroey C. Epidemiology of ringworm (dermatophytosis). *Semin Dermatol* 1985; 4:185–200.
4 Serjeantson S & Lawrence G. Autosomal recessive inheritance of susceptibility to tinea imbricata. *Lancet* 1977; i:13–15.
5 Hay R J. Chronic dermatophyte infections. I. Clinical and mycological features. *Br J Dermatol* 1982; 106:1–6.
6 Torssander J, Karlsson A, Morfeldt-Mason L et al. Dermatophytosis and HIV infection: study in homosexual men. *Acta Derm Venereol* 1988; 68:53–59.
7 Amer M, Taha M, Tossan Z & El-Garf A. The frequency of causative dermatophytes in Egypt. *Int J Dermatol* 1981; 20:431–434.
8 Bhardway G, Hajini G H, Khan I A et al. Dermatophytosis in Kashmir, India. *Mykosen* 1987; 30:135–138.
9 Blank H, Taplin D & Zaias N. Cutaneous *Trichophyton mentagrophtyes* infections in Vietnam. *Arch Dermatol* 1969; 99:135–144.
10 Gugnani H C & Njoku-Obi A N U. Tinea capitis in school children in East Nigeria. *Mykosen* 1986; 29:132–144.
11 Karaoui R, Selim M & Mousa A. Incidence of dermatophytosis in Kuwait. *Sabouraudia* 1979; 17:131–137.
12 Howell S A, Clayton Y M, Phan Q G & Noble W C. Tinea pedis: the relationship between symptoms and host characteristics. *Microbiol Ecol Health & Dis* 1988; 1:131–138.
13 Leyden J J & Kligman A M. Interdigital athletes foot: the interaction of dermatophytes and residual bacteria. *Arch Dermatol* 1978; 114:1466–1472.
14 Al-Sogair S M, Moawad M K & Al-Humaidan Y M. Fungal infection as a cause of skin disease in the Eastern Province of Saudi Arabia: tinea pedis and tinea manuum. *Mycoses* 1991; 34:339–344.
15 Seal D, Hay R J & Middleton K. *Infections of the Skin*. London: Martin Dunitz, 2000.
16 Pernicario C & Peters M S. Tinea faciale mimicking seborrheic dermatitis in a patient with AIDS. *N Engl J Med* 1986: 314:315–316.
17 Hay R J, Reid S, Talwat E & MacNamara K. Endemic tinea imbricata: a study on Goodenough Island, PNG. *Trans R Soc Trop Med* 1984; 78:246–251.
18 Clayton Y M. Scalp ringworm (tinea capitis). In Verbov J L (ed.) *Superficial Fungal Infections*. Manchester: MTP Press, 1986: 1–8.
19 Rippon J W. Epidemiology and emerging patterns of dermatophyte species. *Curr Top Med Mycol* 1985; 1:208–234.
20 Vanbreusegehem R. *Trichophyton soudanense* infection in and outside Africa. *Br J Dermatol* 1968; 80:140–148.
21 Verhagen A R. Distribution of dermatophytes causing tinea capitis in Africa. *Trop Geogr Med* 1973; 26:101–120.
22 Wright S & Robertson V J. An institutional survey of tinea capitis in Harare, Zimbabwe and a trial of miconazole cream versus Whitfield's ointment in its treatment. *Clin Exp Dermatol* 1986; 11:371–377.

23 Ive F A. The carrier state of tinea capitis in Nigeria. *Br J Dermatol* 1966; 78:219–221.

24 Babel D & Baughman S A. Evaluation of the adult carrier state in juvenile tinea capitis caused by *Trichophyton tonsurans*. *J Am Acad Dermatol* 1989; 21:1209–1212.

25. Elewski B. Tinea capitis: a current perspective. *J Am Acad Dermatol* 1999; 42:1–20.

26 Davies R R, Griseofulvin. In Speller D C E (ed.) *Antifungal Chemotherapy*. Chichester: Wiley, 1980: 149–182.

27 Gupta A K, Sauder D N & Shear N H. Antifungal agents: an overview. *J Am Acad Dermatol* 1994 30(Part I):677–698 (Part II):911–933.

28 Clayton Y M & Connor B L. Comparison of clotrimazole cream, Whitfield's ointment and nystatin ointment for the topical treatment of ringworm infections, pityriasis versicolor, erythrasma and candidiasis. *Br J Dermatol* 1973; 89:297–303.

29 Baran R, Hay R J, Tosti A, & Haneke E. Classification of onychomycosis. *Br J Dermatol* 1998; 139:67–71.

30 Zaias N. Superficial white onychomycosis. *Sabouraudia* 1966; 5:99–103.

31 Goodfield M J D, Rowell N R, Forster R A et al. Treatment of dermatophyte infection of the finger- and toe-nails with terbinafine (SF 86-327, Lamisil), an orally active fungicidal agent. *Br J Dermatol* 1989; 121:753–758.

32 Terrell C L. Antifungal agents. Part II. The azoles. *Mayo Clin Proc* 1999; 74:78–100.

33 Odds F C. *Candida and Candidosis*. London: Baillière Tindall, 1988.

34 Gough P M, Warnock D W, Turner A et al. Candidosis of the genital tract in non-pregnant women. *Eur J Obstet Gynecol Reprod Biol* 1985; 19:237–246.

35 Torssander J, Morfeldt-Mauson L, Biberfeld G et al. Oral *Candida albicans* in HIV infection. *Scand J Infect* 1987; 189:291–295.

36 Samaranayake L P & MacFarlane T W (eds). Oral *Candidosis*. London: Wright, 1990.

37 Pindborg J J. Classification of oral lesions associated with HIV infection. *Oral Surg Oral Med Oral Pathol* 1989; 67:292–295.

38 Greenspan D & Greenspan J S. Oral mucosal manifestations of AIDS. *Dermatol Clin* 1987; 5:733–737.

39 Sobel J D. Recurrent vulvovaginal candidiasis. *N Engl J Med* 1986; 315:1455–1458.

40 Hay R J. Yeast Infections. In Elgart M L (ed.) *Cutaneous Mycology. Dermatologic Clinics*. Philadelphia: W B Saunders, 1996: 113–124.

41 Dwyer J M. Chronic mucocutaneous candidiasis. *Annu Rev Med* 1981; 32:491–497.

42 Grant S M & Clissold S P. Fluconazole: a review of its pharmacodynamic and pharmacokinetic properties, and therapeutic potential in superficial and systemic mycoses. *Drugs* 1990; 39:877–916.

43 Jones H E (ed.). *Ketoconazole Today: A Review of Clinical Experience*. Manchester: ADIS Press, 1987.

44 Grant S M & Clissold S P. Itraconazole: a review of its pharmacodynamic and pharmacokinetic properties and therapeutic use in superficial and systemic mycoses. *Drugs* 1989; 37:310–344.

45 Hay R J & Moore M K. Clinical features of superficial fungal infections caused by *Hendersonula toruloidea* and *Scytalidium hyalinum*. *Br J Dermatol* 1984; 110:677–683.

46 Gugnani H C, Nzelibe F K & Osunkwo I C. Onychomycosis due to *Hendersonula toruloidea* in Nigeria. *J Med Vet Mycol* 1986; 24:239–241.

47 Moore M K. Morphological and physiological studies of isolates of *Hendersonula toruloidea* Nattrass cultured from human skin and nail samples. *J Med Vet Mycol* 1988; 26:25–39.

48 Midgley G The lipophilic yeasts: state of the art. *Med. Mycol* 2000; 38(Suppl. 1):9–16.

49 Roberts S O B. Pityriasis versicolor: a clinical and mycological investigation. *Br J Dermatol* 1969; 81:315–326.

50 Mathes B M & Douglas M C. Seborrheic dermatitis in patients with acquired immunodeficiency syndrome. *J Am Acad Dermatol* 1985; 13:947–951.

51 Kaiter D C A, Tschen J A, Cernoch P L et al. Genital white piedra: epidemiology, microbiology and therapy. *J Am Acad Dermatol* 1986; 14:982–993.

52 Lassus A, Kanerva L, Stubbs S et al. White piedra. *Arch Dermatol* 1982; 118:208–211.

53 Adam B A T, Soo-Hoo T S & Chong K C. Black piedra in West Malaysia. *Austr J Dermatol* 1977; 18:45–47.

54 Pahwa V K, Chamiyal P C & Suri P N. Mycological study of otomycosis. *Indian J Med Res* 1983; 77:334–338.

55 Mahgoub E S & Murray I G. *Mycetoma*. London: Heinemann, 1973.

56 Mariat F, Destombes P & Segretain G. The mycetomas: clinical features, pathology, etiology and epidemiology. *Contrib Microbiol Immunol* 1977; 4:1–39.

57 Mahe A, Develoux M, Lienhardt C, Keita S & Bobin P. Mycetoma in Mali: causative agents and geographic distribution. *Am J Trop Med Hyg* 1996; 54:77–79.

58 Wethered D B, Markey M A, Hay R J et al. Ultrastructural and immunogenic changes in the formation of mycetoma grains. *J Med Vet Mycol* 1986; 25:39–46.

59 Czechowski J, Nork M, Haas D et al. MR and other imaging methods in the investigation of mycetomas. *Acta Radiol* 2001; 42:24–26.

60 Palestine R F & Rogers R S. Diagnosis and treatment of mycetoma. *J Am Acad Dermatol* 1982; 6:107–111.

61 Destombes P. Histological diagnosis of mycetoma granules. In *Proceedings of the First International Symposium on Mycetoma*, Venezuela, 1978: 80–94.

62 Hay R J, Mahgoub E S, Leon G et al. Mycetoma. *J Med Vet Mycol* 1992; 30(Suppl. 1):41–49.

63 Bayles M A H. Chromomycosis. *Baillière's Clin Trop Med Commun Dis* 1989; 4:45–70.

64 Banks I S, Palmieri J R, Lanoie L, Connor D H & Meyers W M. Chromomycosis in Zaire. *Int J Dermatol* 1985; 24:302–307.

65 Carrion A L. Chromoblastomycosis and related infections. *Int J Dermatol* 1975; 14:27–32.

66 Esterre P, Andriantsimahavandy A & Raharisolo C. Natural history of chromo-blastomycosis in Madagascar and the Indian Ocean. *Bull Soc Pathol Exot* 1997; 90:312–317.

67 McGinnis M R. Chromoblastomycosis and phaeohyphomycosis: new concepts, diagnosis and mycology. *J Am Acad Dermatol* 1983; 8:1–16.

68 de Albornoz M C B. Sporotrichosis. *Baillière's Clin Trop Med Commun Dis* 1989; 4:71–96.

69 Bibler M R, Luber H J, Clueck H I et al. Disseminated sporotrichosis in a patient with HIV infection after treatment for acquired factor VIII inhibitor. *JAMA* 1986; 256:3125–3126.

70 Quintal D. Sporotrichosis infection on mines of the Witwatersrand. *J Cutan Med Surg* 2000; 4:51–54.

71 Kauffman C A. Sporotrichosis. *Clin Infect Dis* 1999; 29:231–236.

72 Itoh M, Okamoto S & Kanya H. Survey of 260 cases of sporotrichosis. *Dermatologica* 1986; 172:203–213.

73 Brian M & Strom R. Multiarticular sporotrichosis. *JAMA* 1978; 240:556–557.

74 Baker R D, Seabury J H & Schneidau J D. Subcutaneous and cutaneous mucormycosis and subcutaneous phycomycosis. *Lab Invest* 1962; 11:1091–1102.

75 Martinson F D. Clinical, epidemiological and therapeutic aspects of entomophthoromycosis. *Ann Soc Belg Med Trop* 1972; 52:329–342.

76 Segura J J, Gionzale K, Berrocal J et al. Rhinoentomophthoromycosis; report of the first two cases observed in Costa Rica (Central America) and review of the literature. *Am J Trop Med Hyg* 1981; 30:1078–1084.

77 Joe L K & Eng N I T. Subcutaneous phycomycosis: a new disease found in Indonesia. *Ann N Y Acad Sci* 1969; 89:4–16.

78 Kamalam A & Thambiah A S. Muscle invasion by *Basidiobolus haptosporus*. *Sabouraudia* 1984; 22:273–277.

79 Baruzzi R G & Marcopito L F. Lobomycosis. *Baillière's Clin Trop Med Commun Dis* 1989; 4:97–112.

80 Baruzzi R G, Lacaz C S & Souza F A A. Historia natural da doenca de Jorge Lobo: ocorrencia entre os indios Caiabi (Brasil Central). *Rev Inst Med Trop São Paulo* 1979; 21:302–338.

81 Goodwin R A, Loyd J E & DesPrez R M. Histoplasmosis in normal hosts. *Medicine* 1981; 60:231–266.

82 Drouhet E. African histoplasmosis. *Baillière's Clin Trop Med Commun Dis* 1989; 4:221–247.

83 Goodwin R A, Shapiro J L, Thurman G H et al. Disseminated histoplasmosis. *Medicine* 1980; 59:1–33.

84 Wheat J, Sarosi G, McKinsey D et al. Practice guidelines for the management of patients with histoplasmosis. Infectious Diseases Society of America. *Clin Infect Dis* 2000; 30:688–695.

85 Barton E N, Roberts L, Ince W E et al. Cutaneous histoplasmosis in the acquired immunodeficiency syndrome: a report of three cases from Trinidad. *Trop Geogr Med* 1988; 40:153–157.

86 Lemos L B, Guo M & Baliga M. Blastomycosis: organ involvement and etiologic diagnosis. A review of 123 patients from Mississippi. *Ann Diagn Pathol* 2000 4:391–406.

87 Klein B S, Vergeront J M, Weeks R J et al. Isolation of *Blastomyces dermatitidis* in soil associated with a large outbreak of blastomycosis in Wisconsin. *N Engl J Med* 1986; 314:529–534.

88 Emerson P A, Higgins E & Branfoot A. North American blastomycosis in Africans. *Br J Dis Chest* 1984; 78:286–291.

89 Kingston M, El-Mishad M M & Ashraf A M. Blastomycosis in Saudia Arabia. *Am J Trop Med Hyg* 1980; 29:464–466.

90 Randhawa H S, Khan Z V & Gaur S N. *Blastomyces dermatitidis* in India: first report of its isolation from clinical material. *Sabouraudia* 1983; 21:215–221.

91 Chapman S W, Bradsher R W Jr, Campbell G D Jr et al. Practice guidelines for the management of patients with blastomycosis. Infectious Diseases Society of America. *Clin Infect Dis* 2000; 30:679–683.

92 Drutz D J & Catanzaro A. Coccidioidomycosis. Parts I and II. *Am Rev Respir Dis* 1978; 117:559–585, 727–771.

93 Gifford J & Catanzaro A. A comparison of coccidioidin and spherulin skin testing in the diagnosis of coccidioidomycosis. *Am Rev Respir Dis* 1981; 124:440–444.

94 Bronniman D A, Adam R D, Galgiani J N et al. Coccidioidomycosis in the acquired immunodeficiency syndrome. *Ann Intern Med* 1987; 106:373–379.

95 Del Negro G, Lacaz C S & Fiorillo A M (eds). *Paracoccidioidomicose*. São Paulo: Sarvier, 1982.

96 Benard G, Duarte A J. Paracoccidioidomycosis: a model for evaluation of the effects of human immunodeficiency virus infection on the natural history of endemic tropical diseases. *Clin Infect Dis* 2000; 31:1032–1039.

97 Restrepo A, Robledo M, Giraldo R et al. The gamut of paracoccidioidomycosis. *Am J Med* 1976; 61:33–42.

98 Sirisanthana T & Supparatpinyo K. Epidemiology and management of penicilliosis in human immunodeficiency virus-infected patients. *Int J Infect Dis* 1998 3:48–53.

99 Sirisanthana T, Supparatpinyo K, Perriens J & Nelson K E. Amphotericin B and itraconazole for treatment of disseminated *Penicillium marneffei* infection in human immunodeficiency virus-infected patients. *Clin Infect Dis* 1998; 26:1107–1110.

100 Hay R J. Opportunistic fungal infection in the tropics. *Ballière's Clin Trop Med Commun Dis* 1989; 4:249–267.

101 Warnock D & Richardson M D (eds). *Fungal Infections in the Compromised Patient*. Chichester: Wiley, 1989.

102 Attapattu M C. Allergic bronchopulmonary aspergillosis in a chronic asthmatic. *Ceylon Med J* 1983; 28:251–270.

103 Bovornkitti S, Pacharee P, Chatvanich K et al. Aspergilloma in a bronchogenic cyst: a case report. *J Med Assoc Thai* 1984; 53:211–215.

104 Martinson F D, Ali A F & Clarke B M. Aspergilloma of the ethmoid. *J Laryngol Otol* 1970; 84:857–861.

105 Veress B, Malik O A, El Tayeb A A et al. Further observations on the primary paranasal aspergillus granuloma in the Sudan. *Am J Trop Med Hyg* 1973; 22:765–772.

106 Bahadur S, Ghosh P, Chopra P et al. Rhinocerebral phycomycosis. *J Laryngol Otol* 1983; 97:267–270.

107 Bennett J E, Kwon-Chung K J & Howard D H. Epidemiologic differences among serotypes of *Cryptococcus neoformans*. *Am J Epidermiol* 1977; 10:582–586.

108 Dupont B. Cryptococcosis. *Baillière's Clin Trop Med Commun Dis* 1989; 4:113–124.

109 Swinne D & de Vroey C. Epidémiologie de la cryptococcose. *Rev Iberica Micol* 1987; 4:77–83.

110 Kovacs J A, Kovacs A A, Polis M et al. Cryptococcosis in the acquired immunodeficiency syndrome. *Ann Intern Med* 1985; 103:533–538.

111 Odhiambo F A, Murage E M, Ngare W & Ndinya-Achola J O. Detection rate of Cryptococcus neoformans in cerebrospinal fluid specimens at Kenyatta National Hospital, Nairobi. *East Afr Med J.* 1997; 74:576–578.

112 Thomas P A. Keratomycosis. *Baillière's Clin Trop Med Commun Dis* 1989; 4:269–286.

Chapter 70
Pneumocystis carinii Infection
R. F. Miller

History

Pneumocystis carinii was first described by Chagas in 1909, but it was not until 1951 that it was identified as the cause of interstitial plasma cell pneumonitis. This had been described as an epidemic in Europe in the late 1930s and 1940s in premature and malnourished children, especially those in orphanages. In the 1960s *P. carinii* pneumonia occurred largely in children with congenital defects of the immune system and in both children and adults with acquired immune defects secondary to malignancy or its treatment.[1] With organ transplantation it became apparent that *P. carinii* pneumonia was associated with the immunosuppression used to prevent organ rejection. With prophylaxis (see below), case rates fell in those populations. In 1980, clusters of *P. carinii* pneumonia in previously healthy men precipitated a search for underlying immunosuppression and subsequently the acquired immune deficiency syndrome (AIDS) was defined.[1]

Risk factors

Most patients who develop *P. carinii* pneumonia have abnormalities of T-lymphocyte function or numbers; rarely *P. carinii* pneumonia occurs in patients with isolated B-cell defects and in persons without underlying immunosuppression[2–4] (Table 70.1). Irrespective of the nature or intensity of the underlying immunosuppression, glucocorticoid therapy is an independent risk factor for development of *P. carinii* pneumonia in non-HIV immunosuppressed individuals.[2–4]

Before the introduction of prophylaxis, attack rates for *P. carinii* pneumonia in children varied from 25% in those with rhabdomyosarcoma and 22–43% in those with acute lymphoblastic leukaemia to 27–42% in those with severe combined immunodeficiency.[2,4] After organ transplantation, attack rates in adults for *P. carinii* pneumonia vary from 4–10% following renal transplantation to 16–43% after heart or heart–lung transplantation, if prophylaxis is not given.[2,4]

The CD4+ T-lymphocyte count is used in HIV-infected patients to determine the risk of *P. carinii* pneumonia in an individual and also when to start prophylaxis (see

Table 70.1 At-risk groups for *P. carinii* pneumonia.

1. Sporadic disease
Patients receiving chemotherapy
Acute lymphoblastic leukaemia
Hodgkin's disease
Rhabdomyosarcoma
Organ transplant recipients
Allogeneic bone marrow
Heart, heart–lung
Liver
Renal
Immunosuppression for inflammatory disorders
Wegener's granulomatosis
Collagen vascular disease
Congenital immunodeficiency
Severe combined immunodeficiency syndrome
Hypogammaglobulinaemia
2. Epidemic disease
HIV infection
3. No apparent risk factors

below). The CD4+ T lymphocyte count may also be useful in determining risk of *P. carinii* pneumonia in non-HIV-infected immunosuppressed patients.[5]

P. carinii pneumonia remains a common AIDS-defining diagnosis in Europe, North America and Asia, but is largely confined to patients unaware of their HIV status at presentation and to those who are non-complaint with or intolerant of prophylaxis and antiretroviral therapy.

P. carinii pneumonia had been regarded as uncommon in HIV-infected patients in Africa,[6–10] in contrast to the high incidence reported in developed countries in the early stages of the HIV epidemic. Data emerging from central Africa about the significance of *P. carinii* pneumonia in adult patients with HIV infection yielded conflicting data.[11,12] Differences in patient selection criteria, difficulties in diagnosing *P. carinii* pneumonia or true geographical variation in the prevalence of *P. carinii* might have accounted for such differences. More recently, several studies have shown that *P. carinii* is an important pathogen causing much morbidity and mortality in African adults and children infected with HIV.[13–19]

Pathogenesis

The *P. carinii* is inhaled and deposited in the alveoli where the trophozoite form attaches to type 1 pneumocytes. The organism is eliminated by immune-competent individuals; in the immunodeficient host, *P. carinii* pneumonia will develop. The major surface glycoprotein (MSG) of *P. carinii* binds macrophages, induces proliferation of T lymphocytes and secretion of tumour necrosis factor α (TNFα), interleukin (IL) 1 and IL-2.[20] *P. carinii* induces changes in pulmonary surfactant: the phospholipid level is reduced and total cholesterol, phosphatidylglycerol and phospholipase A_2 levels are increased.[21]

Histopathology

Pulmonary infection with *P. carinii* is characterized by an eosinophilic foamy intra-alveolar exudate which is associated with a plasma cell interstitial infiltrate.[22] Two forms of *P. carinii* may be identified morphologically. By using Grocott's methaminine silver, toluidine blue O or cresyl violet stains, thick-walled cysts (6–7 μm in diameter), each containing four to eight sporozoites, are seen to lie freely within the alveolar exudate (Figure 70.1). The exudate itself consists largely of thin-walled, irregularly shaped, single nucleated trophozoites (2–5 μm in diameter) which are shown with Giemsa stain or electron microscopy. Both forms of *P. carinii* may also be

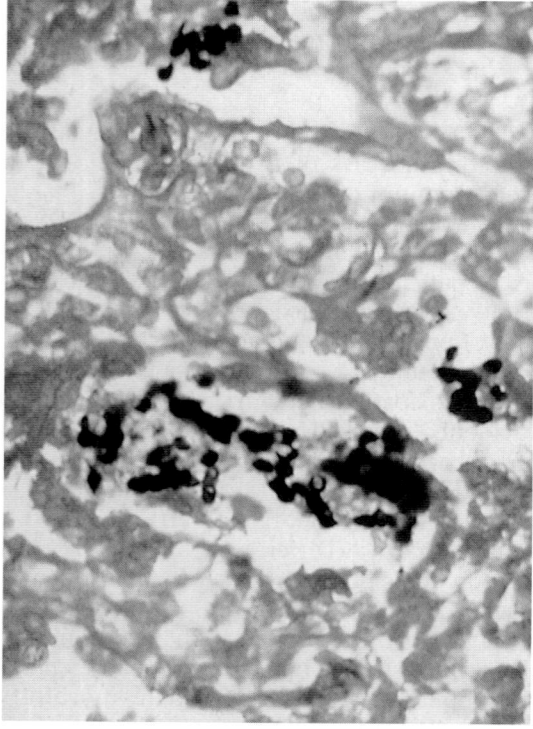

Figure 70.1: Transbronchial biopsy showing cysts of *P. carinii* (Grocott's methenamine silver, × 200).

demonstrated by use of indirect immunofluorescence with monoclonal antibodies raised against *P. carinii*. Unusually interstitial fibrosis, granulomatous inflammation, diffuse alveolar damage, cavitary lesions and pneumatocele formation may occur.[23] Rarely, *P. carinii* infection may extend beyond the alveoli and extrapulmonary pneumocystosis involving liver, spleen or gut may occur.[24]

Is *P. carinii* a fungus or a protozoan?

Based on its morphology and lack of response to antifungal drugs, *P. carinii* has, until recently, been regarded taxonomically as a protozoan. *P. carinii* cannot be cultured in vitro: molecular biological techniques show that *P. carinii* is a fungus.[25,26] *P. carinii* from humans and other mammalian host species show antigenic, karyotypic and genetic heterogenicity.[27,28] Cross-infection between host species has not been achieved, suggesting host specificity and that *P. carinii* infection in humans is not a zoonosis.[27–29] Lower levels of genetic diversity are seen among human-type *P. carinii* than occurs between *P. carinii* from different mammalian hosts.[30] There are more than 30 genotypes of human *P. carinii*—some types are associated with severe pneumonia, others with a mild pneumonia.[31]

Is *P. carinii* due to reinfection or reactivation?

The majority of healthy children and adults have antibodies to *P. carinii*, suggesting that *P. carinii* pneumonia in an immunosuppressed individual arises by reactivation of a childhood-acquired, symptomless, latent infection.[28] However, this hypothesis is challenged by the failure to find *P. carinii* in bronchoalveolar lavage fluid or autopsy lung tissue from immune-competent individuals[32] and by the observation that *P. carinii* DNA is detectable (and only at low levels) in less than 25% of HIV-positive patients with CD4+ T-lymphocyte counts lower than 200 cells per μl who present with respiratory episodes and diagnoses other than *P. carinii* pneumonia. Human *P. carinii* pneumonia is now thought to arise by de novo infection from an exogenous source;[28] this model is supported by the finding of different *P. carinii* genotypes in each episode in patients with recurrent pneumonia.[33] Recent molecular data also suggest that transmission of *P. carinii* from infected patients to susceptible immunocompromised individuals may occur, although there are insufficient data to support routine isolation of patients with suspected or proven *P. carinii* pneumonia.[34]

Clinical presentation

Patients typically present with progressive exertional

Table 70.2 Presentation of *P. carinii* pneumonia.

Typical features	Atypical features
Progressive exertional dyspnoea over days or weeks	Sudden onset of dyspnoea over hours
Dry cough ± mucoid sputum	Cough productive of purulent sputum
Inability to take in a deep breath not due to pleuritic pain	Haemoptysis
Fever ± sweats	Pleurtic chest pain
Tachypnoea	
Examination of the chest:	
Normal breath sounds or fine end-inspiratory basal crackles	Signs of focal consolidation, pleural effusion or wheeze
Chest radiography:	
Normal	
or	
perihilar haze	Early presentation
or	
bilateral interstitial shadowing or alveolar-interstitial changes or 'white out' (marked alveolar consolidation with sparing of apices and costophrenic angles)	Late presentation
Arterial blood gases:	

	Pao$_2$	Paco$_2$
Early:	Normal	Normal or hypocarbia
Late:	Hypoxaemia	Normal or hypercarbia

Reproduced from Malin A S & Miller R F. *Pneumocystis carinii* pneumonia: presentation and diagnosis. *Rev Med Microbiol* 1991; 3:80–87. © Churchill Livingstone.

dyspnoea, a non-productive cough and fever of several days' or weeks' duration which is often associated with a sensation of inability to take in a deep breath.[35] In patients immunosuppressed by HIV infection, symptoms are usually of longer duration than in patients immuno-suppressed as a result of other causes.[36] Auscultation of the chest is usually normal; rarely, fine inspiratory crackles may be heard. Table 70.2 shows typical and atypical features for patients presenting with *P. carinii* pneumonia.

Investigations

Non-invasive investigations

These investigations have moderate to high sensitivity but lack specificity.

Chest radiology

In early pneumonia the chest radiograph may be normal; with later presentations, and with more severe disease, diffuse perihilar interstitial infiltrates are seen (Figure 70.2). These appearances may progress to diffuse bilateral air space (alveolar) consolidation resembling pulmonary oedema (Figure 70.3).[35] With delayed presentation or untreated severe disease, there may be confluent alveolar shadowing ('white out') throughout both lungs, with sparing of the costophrenic angles and apices. The chest

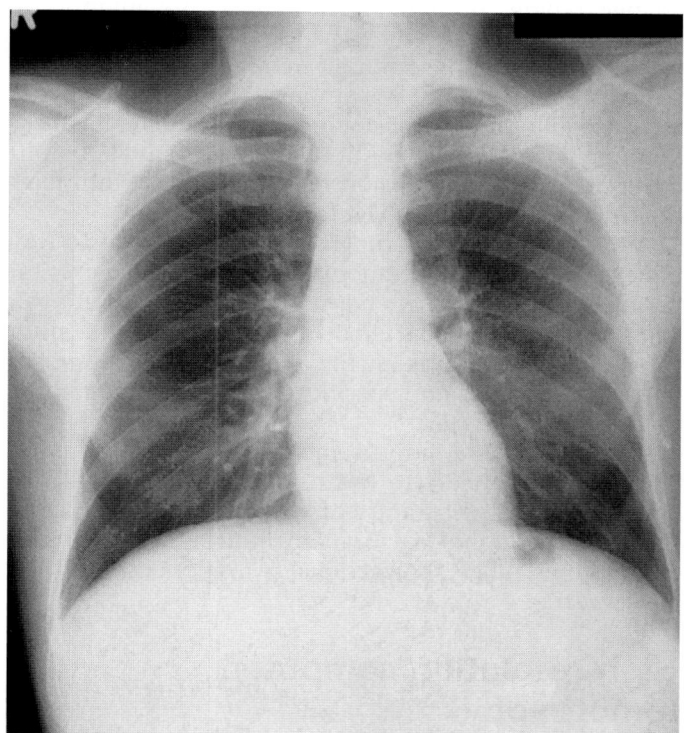

Figure 70.2: Perihilar shadowing in a patient with early *Pneumocystis* pneumonia.

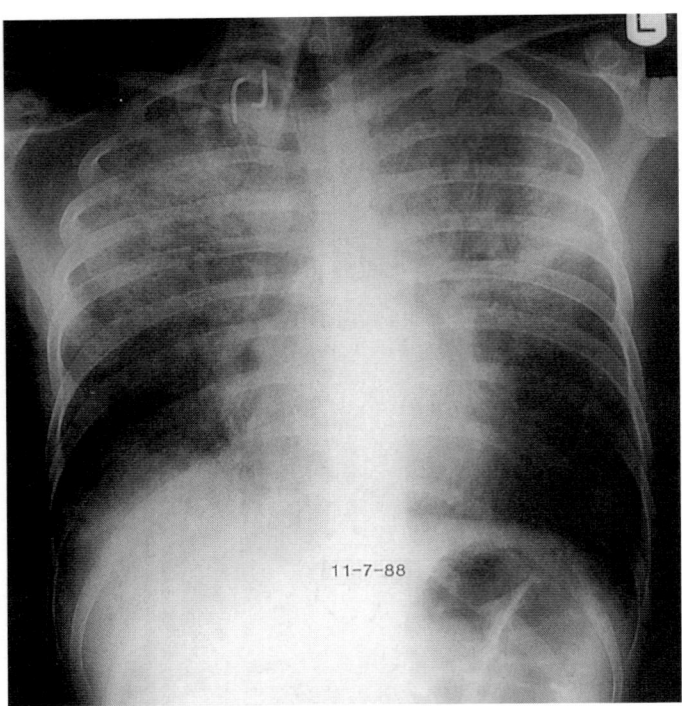

Figure 70.3: Extensive bilateral shadowing in a patient with severe *Pneumocystis* pneumonia.

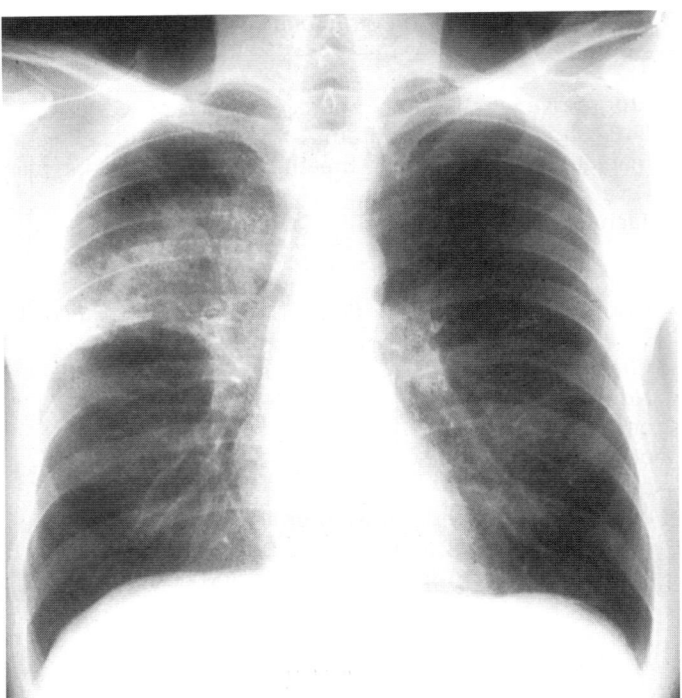

Figure 70.4: Atypical appearances of upper lobe consolidation, mimicking tuberculosis, in a patient with *Pneumocystis* pneumonia.

radiographic appearances in *P. carinii* pneumonia may change rapidly from being normal at presentation to markedly abnormal over a period of only 2–3 days.[35] Atypical radiographic features are seen in up to 20% of patients with *P. carinii* pneumonia; these include cystic air space and pneumatocele formation, unilateral consolidation, lobar infiltrates, nodules, mediastinal lymphadenopathy, pleural effusions and upper zone infiltrates resembling tuberculosis (Figure 70.4).

Although the chest radiograph is a very sensitive way of detecting *P. carinii* pneumonia, these typical and atypical radiographic appearances may also occur in other fungal, mycobacterial and bacterial infections, and in non-infectious conditions such as pulmonary Kaposi's sarcoma (KS) and non-specific interstitial pneumonitis (NIP).

With treatment, improvements in the chest radiographic appearances are not usually apparent for 7–10 days. After treatment and clinical recovery some radiographs remain abnormal for many months in the absence of symptoms; others show residual fibrosis or postinfectious bronchiectasis.

High-resolution computed tomography

This may be useful in the symptomatic patient with a normal or equivocal chest radiograph. Patches of 'ground glass' shadowing indicate active pulmonary disease caused by *P. carinii* or by cytomegalovirus or fungal pneumonia.

Arterial blood gases

In early *P. carinii* pneumonia, even though the arterial oxygen tension (Pao_2) may be normal or near normal, hypocarbia (indicating hyperventilation) may be present. With progression of the pneumonia hypoxia may occur (Table 70.2).[35] The occurrence of hypercarbia in the hypoxaemic patient with *P. carinii* pneumonia is an ominous sign and implies severe respiratory compromise. By performing arterial blood gas analysis the alveolar–arterial oxygen gradient $D(A - a)o_2$ may be calculated. The $D(A - a)o_2$ gradient is widened in over 90% of patients with *P. carinii* pneumonia. Both hypoxaemia and a widened $D(A - a)o_2$ gradient may occur in bacterial and mycobacterial infections, NIP and KS as well as in *P. carinii* pneumonia.[35]

Exercise oximetry

In immunosuppressed patients with respiratory symptoms, normal or near-normal chest radiographs and normal resting Pao_2 values, exercise-induced arterial desaturation is a sensitive and specific method of detecting *P. carinii* pneumonia. A normal exercise test (with no desaturation) virtually excludes the diagnosis.

Invasive investigations

Sputum induction

Immunosuppressed patients with suspected *P. carinii* pneumonia rarely expectorate sputum spontaneously, but sputum may be obtained by inhalation of an aerosol of hypertonic (2.7%, 0.46 mol/l) saline generated by an ultrasonic nebulizer. The success rate for this technique varies considerably between centres.[37] Careful patient preparation (in particular rigorous cleansing of the mouth before the procedure) and deployment of an experienced nurse or physiotherapist to supervise the procedure increases the success rate.[36] *P. carinii* is usually found in clear 'saliva-like' samples. Purulent samples suggest a bacterial infection. The sensitivity varies between 55% and 90%; a negative result from sputum induction for *P. carinii* should prompt referral for bronchoscopy. Some patients find sputum induction is unpleasant and experience cough, nausea and retching, or dyspnoea. Unpredictable arterial blood desaturation may occur during inhalation of saline and persist for up to 20 minutes after the procedure.[38] The patient's arterial oxygen saturation should be measured with an oximeter during sputum induction. The procedure should be carried out away from other patients, ideally in a 'negative pressure' room to avoid the risk of nosocomial transmission of tuberculosis.[39]

Fibreoptic bronchoscopy

Fibreoptic bronchoscopy with bronchoalveolar lavage (BAL) and transbronchial biopsy (TBB) have a high diagnostic yield when used in the investigation of immunocompetent and immunosuppressed patients with radiographically diffuse pneumonia. Early in the AIDS epidemic both BAL and TBB were used routinely in order to diagnose *P. carinii* pneumonia in other pathogens. With the realization that BAL alone has a sensitivity of 90% or greater for detection of *P. carinii* and that TBB adds very little additional diagnostic information, yet is associated with pneumothorax (in up to 20% of cases), haemorrhage and sudden falls in PaO_2 which occasionally requires ventilatory support, the technique has been used less frequently.[40] At bronchoscopy the majority of AIDS centres now routinely perform only BAL. Treatment should never be deferred pending results of bronchoscopy in a patient with suspected *P. carinii* pneumonia as significant clinical deterioration may occur. The yield for cysts of *P. carinii* from BAL fluid is not reduced for up to 10 days after starting antimicrobial therapy.

Open lung biopsy

The high yield from bronchoscopy and BAL for diagnosis of *P. carinii* pneumonia means that this technique is now rarely necessary. Open lung biopsy is still occasionally performed in immunosuppressed patients with diffuse pneumonia and negative results from two or more bronchoscopies, and in patients who deteriorate despite treatment for a bronchoscopically confirmed pathogen.[23,41]

DNA amplification

Detection of *P. carinii* DNA in BAL fluid and induced sputum is superior to histochemical staining.[42] *P. carinii*

DNA may also be detected in oropharyngeal samples obtained by gargling with normal saline.[43,44] Compared with conventional staining of BAL fluid, DNA detection on oropharyngeal samples has a sensitivity of 89% and a specificity of 94%.[44] Molecular diagnostic tests are not currently available commercially.

Empirical therapy

Some physicians have suggested that it is not necessary to perform invasive tests, including bronchoscopy, in HIV-infected patients presenting with symptoms, chest radiographic and arterial blood gas abnormalities typical of *P. carinii* pneumonia, and that such patients may be treated empirically, with bronchoscopy reserved for those who fail to respond by day 5 or deteriorate on therapy and for those who have presentations atypical for *P. carinii* pneumonia.[45] Others have argued strongly that bronchoscopic confirmation of the diagnosis is mandatory is every case. Both strategies appear to be equally effective in clinical practice.[46]

Prognosis

Several clinical and laboratory features are predictive of a poor outcome in an HIV-infected patient with *P. carinii* pneumonia.[35,47] These include at admission no prior knowledge of HIV status, presentation with a second or subsequent episode of *P. carinii* pneumonia, a history of respiratory symptoms of more than 4 weeks' duration, tachypnoea (more than 30 breaths/min), evidence of poor oxygenation ($PaO_2 < 7.0$ kPa or $D(A - a)O_2 \geq 4.0$ kPa), marked chest radiographic abnormalities, peripheral blood leucocytosis (white blood cell count $> 10.8 \times 10^9$/l), a low serum albumin concentration (< 35 g/l) and raised serum lactate dehydrogenase (LDH) enzyme levels (> 300 iu/l). After admission and investigation the identification of a co-pathogen in induced sputum or BAL fluid, the presence of neutrophilia greater than 5% in BAL fluid, marked interstitial oedema in TBB specimens and raised serum LDH enzyme levels (that remain increased despite treatment) are also predictive of a poor outcome.[35,47]

Management

An assessment of the severity of the pneumonia, using the history, examination findings and results of arterial blood gas estimations and the chest radiograph (Table 70.3), will enable decisions to be made about choice of therapy; some drugs are unproven or ineffective in severe disease.[47-49] Severity stratification also identifies patients who will benefit from adjunctive glucocorticoids (see below). Patients with glucose 6-phosphate dehydrogenase deficiency should not receive co-trimoxazole, dapsone and primaquine as they increase the risk of haemolysis.[48,49]

Table 70.3 Grading of severity of *P. carinii* pneumonia.

	Mild	Moderate	Severe
Symptoms and signs	Increasing exertional dyspnoea with or without cough and sweats	Dyspnoea on minimal exertion, occasional dyspnoea at rest, fever with or without sweats	Dyspnoea at rest, tachypnoea at rest, persistent fever, cough
Blood gas tensions (room air)	PaO_2 normal, SaO_2 falling on exercise	PaO_2 8.1–11 kPa	$PaO_2 < 8.0$ kPa
Chest radiograph	Normal or minor perihilar infiltrates	Diffuse interstitial shadowing	Extensive interstitial shadowing with or without diffuse alveolar shadowing ('white out'), sparing costophrenic angles and apices

SaO_2, arterial oxygen saturation, measured with a transcutaneous oximeter.
Reproduced from Miller R F & Mitchell D M. *Pneumocystis carinii* pneumonia. *Thorax* 1992; 47:305–314. © 1992 BMJ Publishing Group.

Co-trimoxazole

High-dose co-trimoxazole (100 mg/kg daily of sulfamethaxozole and 20 mg/kg daily of trimethoprim) given in two to four divided doses orally or intravenously is first choice therapy for *P. carinii* pneumonia of all grades of severity. In HIV-infected patients treatment is given for 21 days because shorter courses are associated with treatment failure.[49] In patients with other causes of immunosuppression, shorter courses (e.g., 14–17 days) are often given.[49] In patients with moderate or severe disease, co-trimoxazole is given intravenously for the first 7–10 days, then orally; in patients with mild disease oral co-trimoxazole may be given throughout. Adverse reactions to co-trimoxazole, which are usually first evident at 6–14 days of treatment, are common and include neutropenia and anaemia in up to 40% of patients, rash in 25%, fever in over 20% and abnormal liver function in approximately 10%.[49]

Co-administration of folic or folinic acid does not reduce or prevent haematological toxicity and may be associated with increased therapeutic failure. Dose reduction of co-trimoxazole, to 75% of the dose given above, is associated with a reduced toxicity profile but no reduction in efficacy.[49,50] It is not clear why there is such a high frequency of adverse reactions to co-trimoxazole in patients immunosuppressed by HIV infection compared with patients immunosuppressed by other causes, but it may

be due to HIV-induced changes in acetylator status, accumulation of toxic metabolites such as hydroxylamines, or glutathione deficiency.[49]

Alternative therapy

Several other treatments are available if co-trimoxazole is not tolerated by the patient or if treatment fails[48,49] (Table 70.4).

Clindamycin with primaquine

This combination was originally only used to 'salvage' patients with mild and moderate severity disease who failed to respond to co-trimoxazole or pentamidine. It is now used as alternative therapy in patients with *P. carinii* pneumonia of all grades of severity.[49] Clindamycin 450–600 mg four times daily with primaquine 15 mg daily (by mouth) are used. Higher doses of primaquine confer no therapeutic advantage and are associated with a greater risk of methaemoglobinaemia.[49] Treatment is for 21 days regardless of the type of underlying immunosuppression. Clindamycin is usually given intravenously for the first 7–10 days, then orally in moderate and severe disease; the treatment may be given orally throughout in patients with mild disease. Clindamycin–primaquine is as effective as co-trimoxazole or dapsone–trimethoprim (see below) when given as initial treatment for patients

Table 70.4 Treatment of *P. carinii* pneumonia.

	Mild	Moderate	Severe
First choice	Co-trimoxazole	Co-trimoxazole	Co-trimoxazole
Second choice	Clindamycin–primaquine	Clindamycin–primaquine	Clindamycin–primaquine
Alternative therapy	Dapsone–trimethoprim Atovaquone	Dapsone–trimethoprim Atovaquone Trimetrexate–folinic acid	Trimetrexate–folinic acid Intravenous pentamidine
Adjunctive glucocorticoids	No	Yes	Yes

with *P. carinii* pneumonia of mild and moderate severity.[49,51] Almost two-thirds of patients develop a rash and approximately 25% develop diarrhoea. If diarrhoea occurs during clindamycin–primaquine therapy, the stool should be analysed for the presence of *Clostridium difficile* toxin.

Dapsone with trimethoprim

In patients with mild or moderate severity *P. carinii* pneumonia, the combination of dapsone (100 mg per day) and trimethoprim (20 mg/kg daily) is as effective as co-trimoxazole (doses as above) and is better tolerated.[49,52] Rash, nausea and vomiting, and asymptomatic methaemoglobinaemia (due to dapsone) are the major side effects with this combination. Approximately 50% of patients develop mild hyperkalaemia (< 6.1 mmol/l), which is due to trimethoprim. This combination has not been shown to be of benefit in severe disease.

Atovaquone

Atovaquone 750 mg twice daily, orally for 21 days, is less effective than either oral high-dose co-trimoxazole or intravenous pentamidine for treatment of mild and moderate severity *P. carinii* pneumonia, but is better tolerated than either drug.[49,53] There are no data to support its use in patients with severe pneumonia. Common adverse reactions include rash, nausea and vomiting, and constipation. Absorption of the drug from the gastro-intestinal tract is variable; taking the suspension with food may increase its absorption.

Trimetrexate and folinic acid

Trimetrexate, a methotrexate analogue, given with folinic acid (to protect human cells from trimetrexate-induced toxicity) is less effective than co-trimoxazole for treatment of moderate and severe *P. carinii* pneumonia; the two regimens have similar rates of toxicity.[49,54] The most commonly used regimen is 45 mg/m^2 daily, given intravenously together with folinic acid 20 mg/m^2 four times daily, orally. Trimetrexate–folinic acid is also used to salvage patients who have failed to respond to co-trimoxazole; in this situation approximately two-thirds of patients respond to therapy.

Parenteral pentamidine

Intravenous pentamidine is now seldom used in mild and moderate severity disease because of its toxicity profile and because other less toxic treatments have equivalent efficacy. It continues to be used in patients with severe pneumonia.[49] It is given at a dose of 4 mg/kg daily, by intravenous infusion for 21 days. Intramuscular pentamidine is no longer used because of the risk of sterile abscess at the injection site. Compared with high-dose co-trimoxazole, intravenous pentamidine is of almost equivalent efficacy but has a greater toxicity profile. Up to 60% of patients receiving pentamidine

develop nephrotoxicity, which is usually manifested as an isolated increase in the serum creatinine level; approximately half develop leucopenia. Hypotension and nausea/vomiting both occur in up to 25% of patients.[49] Hypoglycaemia occurs in approximately 20% of patients. Reduction of the dose of pentamidine (to 3 mg/kg daily) does not compromise efficacy and reduces toxicity. There are no therapeutic advantages if high-dose co-trimoxazole and intravenous pentamidine are combined; indeed the combination has a much higher toxicity profile than when either drug is used alone.

Nebulized pentamidine

This form of therapy is no longer recommended for the treatment of mild and moderate severity *P. carinii* pneumonia; it should never be used to treat severe disease.[49] Patients given nebulized pentamidine (600 mg per day) for 21 days respond to therapy very slowly; reductions in fever and dyspnoea and improvements in radiographic appearances and blood gases may take more than 14 days.[49,55] There is a greater rate of relapse of *P. carinii* pneumonia in patients treated with nebulized pentamidine when compared to those given parenteral therapy.[55] Development of extrapulmonary pneumocystosis may not be suppressed by this form of treatment as very little of the inhaled pentamidine is absorbed systemically. If nebulized pentamidine is used to treat mild *P. carinii* pneumonia, it has been advocated that it is combined with intravenous pentamidine (doses as above) for the first 3–5 days of therapy to ensure rapid accumulation of the drug within the lungs.[39]

Corticosteroids

Adjunctive therapy with glucocorticoids for patients with moderate and severe *P. carinii* pneumonia has been shown to reduce the likelihood of respiratory failure (by half) and death (by one-third) in HIV-infected patients.[56] In the non-HIV-infected immunosuppressed population, adjuvant steroids reduce the duration of time on mechanical ventilation and overall time in the intensive care unit.[4,57] Corticosteroids probably act by reducing the body's intrapulmonary inflammatory response to *P. carinii*. It is recommended that glucocorticoids are given to HIV-infected patients with proven or suspected *P. carinii* pneumonia who have a $Pao_2 \leq 9.3$ kPa or $D(A-a)o_2 \geq 4.7$ kPa (both measured while the patient is breathing room air).[56] No specific recommendations exist for non-HIV-infected patients, but the above criteria are often used in clinical practice.

Corticosteroid treatment should begin at the start of specific antipneumocystis therapy. Clearly, in some patients treatment will begin on a presumptive basis and it is necessary to confirm the diagnosis as soon as possible. Several regimens have been used, the most common being oral prednisolone 40 mg twice daily for 5 days, thereafter 40 mg once daily for days 6–10 and then 10 further days of 20 mg daily. Intravenous methyl-prednisolone may be given at 75% of these doses;

alternatively, higher doses may be given for a shorter period of time, such as methylprednisolone 1 g once daily for 3 days and 0.5 g on days 4–6, followed by oral prednisolone 40 mg once daily reducing to zero over 10 days.[52,56] There is no evidence that adjunctive corticosteroids are of benefit in patients with mild *P. carinii* pneumonia.

General management

Patients with mild *P. carinii* pneumonia may be treated with oral co-trimoxazole as outpatients under close supervision of a physician. All patients with moderate and severe *P. carinii* pneumonia should be treated in hospital with intravenous co-trimoxazole or pentamidine and adjunctive corticosteroids. If the patient does not respond by 7–10 days, or deteriorates before this time, he or she should be switched to alternative therapy.[49]

All hypoxaemic patients with *P. carinii* pneumonia should receive supplemental oxygen therapy via a tight-fitting face mask in order to maintain the $Pa_{O_2} \geq 8.0$ kPa.[47] If an inspired oxygen concentration of 60% fails to maintain the $Pa_{O_2} \geq 8.0$ kPa, non-invasive ventilatory support with continuous positive airways pressure (CPAP) ventilation, either by nasal or face mask, may be used.[47,58] If CPAP ventilation fails to maintain oxygenation, or the Pa_{CO_2} rises, or the patient becomes tired, mechanical ventilation should be considered. The decision to carry out mechanical ventilation is not an easy one to make as the prognosis of patients with severe *P. carinii* pneumonia with respiratory failure who fail to respond to specific therapy and adjunctive steroids, and who are ventilated, remains extremely poor.[59] Most centres would mechanically ventilate patients with a first episode of *P. carinii* pneumonia and those who rapidly deteriorate following bronchoscopy.

Chemoprophylaxis

With progressive immunosuppression and falls in CD4+ T-lymphocyte counts, HIV-infected individuals are at increased risk of developing *P. carinii* pneumonia. Primary prophylaxis, to prevent a first episode of *P. carinii* pneumonia, is given when the CD4+ T-lymphocyte count falls below 200 cells/µl or the CD4 total lymphocyte ratio is less than 1 : 5, to patients with HIV-related constitutional symptoms such as unexplained fever of 3 weeks or more in duration, or oral candida regardless of CD4 count, and to patients with other AIDS-defining diagnoses, such as Kaposi's sarcoma.[49] Secondary prophylaxis is given in order to prevent a recurrence.[49] In individuals immunosuppressed by other causes, prophylaxis is given to those with high attack rates for *P. carinii* pneumonia, for example children with acute lymphoblastic leukaemia or severe combined immunodeficiency syndrome, adults with Hodgkin's disease, rhabdomyosarcoma or Wegener's granulomatosis and to individuals following organ transplantations such as allegoric bone marrow, renal, heart or heart–lung, or liver.[2,4]

Co-trimoxazole 960 mg once daily is the first-choice regimen for both primary and secondary prophylaxis. Lower doses, 960 mg three times weekly or 480 mg once daily, may be equally effective and have fewer side effects.[49] Co-trimoxazole may also protect against bacterial infections and reactivation of cerebral toxoplasmosis.[60] Rash, with or without fever, occurs in up to 20% of patients. Desensitization should be attempted in those unable to tolerate co-trimoxazole.[49] Alternatively, other less effective agents may be used for prophylaxis. These include:

- *Nebulized pentamidine*—300 mg once per month, via a jet nebulizer (once per fortnight if the CD4+ T-lymphocyte count is ≤ 50 cells/µl).
- *Dapsone*—100 mg daily with pyrimethamine 25 mg once weekly. Pyrimethamine may protect against cerebral toxoplasmosis.
- *Atovaquone*—750 mg twice daily.

Long-term effects of co-trimoxazole prophylaxis

While the efficacy of co-trimoxazole as prophylaxis for *P. carinii* pneumonia is clearly demonstrated, long-term use of this combination is associated with adverse reactions (see above) and with the development of resistance in *P. carinii* itself and in other micro-organisms.[61,62] The drug target for sulfamethoxazole and dapsone is dihydropteroate synthase (DHPS). Molecular biological techniques show that non-synonymous single nucleotide polymorphisms in the DHPS gene of human *P. carinii*, which confer resistance, occur more frequently in patients who have received prophylaxis with dapsone or co-trimoxazole and have been described in patients failing treatment of *P. carinii* pneumonia with co-trimoxazole.[61,63]

In populations exposed to co-trimoxazole used as prophylaxis, there are parallel marked increases in resistance to this drug in other micro-organisms, including Enterobacteriaceae, *Escherichia coli* and *Staphylococcus aureus*.[62] This phenomenon was first described in North America but is of relevance, particularly in Africa, where use of co-trimoxazole is increasing and few alternative regimens for prophylaxis exist.

Stopping prophylaxis

The widespread availability and uptake of highly active antiretroviral therapy (HAART) in North America, Europe and Australasia has been associated with marked reductions in incidence of many opportunistic infections, including *P. carinii* pneumonia, hospital admissions and mortality from HIV infection. In most patients, within a few weeks of starting HAART, there are rapid decreases in plasma HIV RNA and, in parallel, increases in CD4 T-lymphocyte counts. The United States Public Health Service/Infectious Disease Society of America now recommend that primary prophylaxis against *P. carinii* pneumonia may be discontinued in HIV-infected patients who respond to HAART with an increase in CD4 lymphocyte counts to above 200 cells/μl, sustained for at least 6 months.[64,65] Many of these patients will also have reduction in HIV RNA to below the limit of detection. As yet, there is insufficient evidence to recommend with-drawal of secondary prophylaxis; despite this, many clinicians do so using these criteria. If, despite HAART, the CD4 lymphocyte count falls to below 200 cells/μl and/or the HIV RNA 'load' rises, then prophylaxis should be re-instituted using the criteria for primary prophylaxis. Clearly, close patient monitoring is needed to detect any such changes rapidly.

REFERENCES

1 Hughes W T. Prologue to AIDS. The recognition of infectious opportunists. *Medicine* 1998; 77:227–232.

2 Sepkowitz K A, Brown A E & Armstrong D. *Pneumocystis carinii* pneumonia without acquired immunodeficiency syndrome: more patients, same risk. *Arch Intern Med* 1995; 155:1125–1128.

3 Arend S M, Kroon F P & Van't Wout J W. *Pneumocystis carinii* pneumonia in patients without AIDS, 1980 through 1993. *Arch Intern Med* 1995; 155:2436–2441.

4 Miller R F. *Pneumocystis carinii* infection in non-AIDS patients. *Curr Opin Infect Dis* 1999; 12:371–377.

5 Walzer P D. Editorial response: *Pneumocystis carinii* pneumonia in patients without human immunodeficiency virus infection. *Clin Infect Dis* 1997; 25:219–220.

6 Elvin K, Lumbwe C M, Luo N P et al. *Pneumocystis carinii* is not a major cause of pneumonia in HIV-infected patients in Lusaka, Zambia. *Trans R Soc Trop Med Hyg* 1989; 83:553–555.

7 Carme B, Mboussa J, Andzin M et al. *Pneumocystis carinii* is rare in AIDS in central Africa. *Trans R Soc Trop Med Hyg* 1991; 85:80.

8 Abouya Y, Beaumal A, Lucas S et al. *Pneumocystis carinii* pneumonia. An uncommon cause of death in African patients with AIDS. *Trans R Soc Med Hyg* 1992; 145:617–620.

9 Kamanfu G, Mlika-Cabanne N, Girard P M et al. Pulmonary complications of human immunodeficiency virus infection in Bujumbura, Burundi. *Am Rev Respir Dis* 1993; 147:658–663.

10 Batungwanayo J, Taelman H, Lucas S et al. Pulmonary disease associated with the human immunodeficiency virus in Kigali, Rwanda. A fiberoptic bronchoscopic study of 111 cases of undetermined etiology. *Am J Respir Crit Care Med* 1994; 149:1591–1596.

11 Machiels G & Urban M I. *Pneumocystis carinii* as a cause of pneumonia in HIV-infected patients in Lusaka, Zambia. *Trans R Soc Trop Med Hyg* 1992; 86:399–400.

12 Russian D A & Kovacs J A. *Pneumocystis carinii* in Africa: an emerging pathogen? *Lancet* 1995; 346:1242–1243.

13 Malin A S, Gwanzura L K, Klein S et al. *Pneumocystis carinii* pneumonia in Zimbabwe. *Lancet* 1995; 346:1258–1261.

14 Ikeogu M O, Wolf B & Mathe S. Pulmonary manifestations in HIV seropositivity and malnutrition in Zimbabwe. *Arch Dis Child* 1997; 76:124–128.

15 Nathoo K J, Gondo M, Gwanzura L et al. Fatal *Pneumocystis carinii* pneumonia in HIV-seropositive infants in Harare, Zimbabwe. *Trans R Soc Trop Med Hyg* 2001; 95:37–39.

16 Zar H J, Maartens G, Wood R & Hussey G. *Pneumocystis carinii* pneumonia in HIV-infected patients in Africa—an important pathogen? *S Afr Med J* 2000; 90:684–688.

17 Zar H J, Hanslo D, Tannenbaum E et al. Aetiology and outcome of pneumonia in human immunodeficiency virus-infected children hospitalized in South Africa. *Acta Paediatr* 2001; 90:119–125.

18 Graham S M, Mtitimila E I, Kamanga H S et al. Clinical presentation and outcome of *Pneumocystis carinii* pneumonia in Malawian children. *Lancet* 2000; 355:369–373.

19 Mahomed A G, Murray J, Klempman S et al. *Pneumocystis carinii* pneumonia in HIV infected patients from South Africa. *East Afr Med J* 1999; 76:80–94.

20 Benfield T L & Lundgren J D. The *Pneumocystis carinii* major surface glycoprotein (MSG): its potential involvement in the pathophysiology of pneumocystis. *FEMS Immunol Med Microbiol* 1998; 22:129–134.

21 Prevost M-C, Escamilla R, Aliouat E L M et al. *Pneumocystis* pathophysiology. *FEMS Immunol Med Microbiol* 1998; 22:123–128.

22 Foley N M, Griffiths M H & Miller R F. Histologically atypical *Pneumocystis carinii* pneumonia. *Thorax* 1993; 48:996–1001.

23 Travis W D, Pittaluga S, Lipshik G Y et al. Atypical pathologic manifestations of *Pneumocystis carinii* pneumonia in the acquired immunodeficiency syndrome. *Am J Surg Pathol* 1990; 14:615–625.

24 Coker R J, Clark D, Claydon E L et al. Disseminated *Pneumocystis carinii* infection in AIDS. *J Clin Pathol* 1991; 44:820–823.

25 Pixley F J, Wakefield A E, Banerji S et al. Mitochondrial gene sequences show fungal homology for *Pneumocystis carinii*. *Mol Microbiol* 1991; 5:1347–1351.

26 Ypma-Wong M F, Fonzi W A & Sypherd P S. Fungus-specific translation elongation factor 3 gene present in *Pneumocystis carinii*. *Infect Immun* 1992; 60:4140–4145.

27 Wakefield A E. Genetic heterogeneity in *Pneumocystis carinii*: an introduction. *FEMS Immunol Med Microbiol* 1998; 22:5–13.

28 Stringer J R & Walzer P D. Molecular biology and epidemiology of *Pneumocystis carinii* infection in AIDS. *AIDS* 1996; 10:561–571.

29 Stringer J R. *Pneumocystis carinii*: what is it, exactly? *Clin Microbiol Rev* 1996; 9:489–498.

30 Wakefield A E. Genetic heterogeneity in human-derived *Pneumocystis carinii*. *FEMS Immunol Med Microbiol* 1998; 22:59–65.

31 Miller R F & Wakefield A E. *Pneumocystis carinii* genotypes and severity of pneumonia. *Lancet* 1999; 353:2039–2040.

32 Peters S E, Wakefield A E, Sinclair K et al. A search for *Pneumocystis carinii* in post-mortem lungs by DNA amplification. *J Pathol* 1992; 166:195–198.

33 Tsolaki A G, Miller R F, Underwood A P et al. Genetic diversity at the internal transcribed spacer region of the ribosomal RNA operon among isolates of *Pneumocystis carinii* from AIDS patients with recurrent pneumonia. *J Infect Dis* 1996; 174:141–148.

34 Helweg-Larsen J, Tsolaki A G, Miller R F et al. Clusters of *Pneumocystis carinii* pneumonia: analysis of person to person transmission by genotyping. *Q J Med* 1998; 91:813–820.

35 Malin A & Miller R F. *Pneumocystis carinii* pneumonia: presentation and diagnosis. *Rev Med Microbiol* 1991; 3:80–87.

36 Kovacs J A, Heimenz J W, Macher A M et al. *Pneumocystis carinii* pneumonia: a comparison between patients with the acquired immunodeficiency syndrome and patients with other immunodeficiencies. *Ann Intern Med* 1984; 100:663–671.

37 Miller R F, Kocjan G, Buckland J et al. Sputum induction for the diagnosis of respiratory disease in HIV positive patients. *J Infect* 1991; 23:5–16.

38 Miller R F, Buckland J & Semple S J G. Arterial desaturation in HIV positive patients undergoing sputum induction. *Thorax* 1991; 46:444–451.

39 Miller R F, Escamilla R, Hermant C et al. Nebuliser use in patients with HIV infection and AIDS. *Eur Respir Rev* 2000; 10:523–526.

40 Griffiths M H, Kocjan G & Miller R F. Diagnosis of pulmonary disease in human immunodeficiency virus infection: role of transbronchial biopsy and bronchoalveolar lavage. *Thorax* 1989; 44:554–558.

41 Miller R F, Pugsley W B & Griffiths M H. Open lung biopsy for investigation of acute respiratory episodes in patients with HIV infection and AIDS. *Genitourin Med* 1995; 71:280–285.

42 Wakefield A E, Pixley F J, Miller R F et al. Detection of *Pneumocystis carinii* with DNA amplification. *Lancet* 1990; 336:451–453.

43 Wakefield A E, Miller R F, Guiver L A et al. Oropharyngeal samples for detection of *Pneumocystis carinii* by DNA amplification. *Q J Med* 1993; 86:401–406.

44 Helweg-Larsen J, Skov Jensen J, Benfield T et al. Diagnostic use of PCR for detection of *Pneumocystis carinii* in oral wash samples. *J Clin Microbiol* 1998; 36:2068–2072.

45 Miller R F, Millar A B, Weller I V D et al. Empirical treatment without bronchoscopy for *Pneumocystis carinii* pneumonia in the acquired immunodeficiency syndrome. *Thorax* 1989; 44:559–564.

46 Tu J V, Biem H J & Detsky A S. Bronchoscopy versus empirical therapy in HIV infected patients with presumptive *Pneumocystis carinii* pneumonia: a decision analysis. *Am Rev Respir Dis* 1993; 148:370–377.

47 Miller R F & Mitchell D M. *Pneumocystis carinii* pneumonia. *Thorax* 1992; 47:305–314.

48 Miller R F. Prophylaxis and treatment of *Pneumocystis carinii* pneumonia. *Drug Ther Bull* 1994; 32:12–15.

49 Miller R F, Le Noury J, Corbett E L et al. *Pneumocystis carinii* infection: current treatment and prevention. *J Antimicrob Chemother* 1996; 37 (Supplement B):33–53.

50 Sattler F R, Conwan R, Nielsen D M et al. Trimethoprim–sulfamethoxazole compared with pentamidine for treatment of *Pneumocystis carinii* pneumonia in the acquired immunodeficiency syndrome. *Ann Intern Med* 1988; 104:280–287.

51 Black J R, Feinberg J & Murphy R L. Clindamycin and primaquine therapy for mild-to-moderate episodes of *Pneumocystis carinii* in patients with AIDS: AIDS clinical trial group 044. *Clin Infect Dis* 1994; 18:9095–9098.

52 Medina I, Leoung G, Hopewell P C et al. Oral therapy for *Pneumocystis carinii* pneumonia with acquired immunodeficiency syndrome. A controlled trial of trimethoprim–sulfamethoxazole versus trimethoprim-dapsone. *N Engl J Med* 1990; 323:776–782.

53 Hughes W, Leoung G, Kramer F et al. Comparison of atovaquone (566C80) with trimethoprim–sulfamethoxazole to treat *Pneumocystis carinii* pneumonia in patients with AIDS. *N Engl J Med* 1993; 328:1521–1527.

54 Sattler F R, Frame P, Davis R et al. Trimetrexate with leucovorin versus trimethoprim–sulfamethoxazole for moderate to severe episodes of *Pneumocystis carinii* pneumonia in patients with AIDS. *J Infect Dis* 1994; 170:165–172.

55 Montgomery A B, Feigal D W, Sattler F et al. Pentamidine aerosol versus trimethoprim–sulfamethoxazole for *Pneumocystis carinii* in acquired immune deficiency syndrome. *Am J Respir Crit Care Med* 1995; 151:1068–1074.

56 National Institutes of Health. University of California Expert Panel for Corticosteroids as adjunctive therapy for *Pneumocystis carinii* in the acquired immunodeficiency syndrome. *N Engl J Med* 1990; 323:1500–1504.

57 Pareja F G, Garland R & Koziel H. Use of adjunctive glucocorticoids in severe adult non HIV *Pneumocystis carinii* pneumonia. *Chest* 1998; 113:1215–1224.

58 Miller R F & Semple S J G. Continuous positive airway pressure ventilation for respiratory failure associated with *Pneumocystis carinii* pneumonia. *Respir Med* 1991; 85:133–138.

59 Gill J K, Greene L, Miller R et al. ICU admission in patients infected with the human immunodeficiency virus: a multicentre study. *Anaesthesia* 1999; 54:727–732.

60 Schneider M M E, Hoepelman A I M, Efftinck-Schattenkesk J K M et al. A controlled trial of aerosolized pentamidine or trimethoprim–sulfamethoxazole as primary prophylaxis against *Pneumocystis carinii* pneumonia in patients with human immunodeficiency virus infection. *N Engl J Med* 1992; 327:1836–1841.

61 Kazanjian P, Armstrong W, Hossler P A et al. *Pneumocystis carinii* mutations are associated with duration of sulfa or sulfone prophylaxis exposure in AIDS patients. *J Infect Dis* 2000; 182:551–557.

62 Martin J N, Rose D A, Hadley W K et al. Emergence of trimithoprim–sulfamethoxazole resistance in the AIDS era. *J Infect Dis* 1999; 180:1809–1818.

63 Helweg-Larsen J, Benfield T L, Eugen-Olsen J et al. Effects of mutations in *Pneumocystis carinii* dihydropteroate synthase gene on outcome of AIDS-associated *Pneumocystis carinii* pneumonia. *Lancet* 1999; 354:1347–1351.

64 USPHS/IDSA. Guidelines for the prevention of opportunistic infection in persons infected with human immunodeficiency virus. *MMWR Morb Mortal Wkly Rep* 1999; 48:RR-10.

65 Miller R F. Prophylaxis of *Pneumocystis carinii* pneumonia: too much of a good thing? *Thorax* 2000; 55 (Supplement I):S15–S22.

FURTHER READING

Dei-Cas E & Calliez J C (eds) *Pneumocystis* and pneumocystosis: advances in *Pneumocystis* research. *FEMS Immunol Med Microbiol* 1998;22:1–189.

Miller R F & Lipman M C I. Pulmonary infections (AIDS). In Albert R, Spiro S & Jett J (eds) *Comprehensive Respiratory Medicine*. London: Mosby, 1999: 32.1–32.22.

Walzer P D (ed.) *Pneumocystis carinii* pneumonia. *Lung Biology in Health and Disease*, series no. 69, 2nd edn. New York: Marcel Dekker, 1993.

Section 10

Protozoan Infections

Sir Ronald Ross published his autobiography in 1923; he subtitled the work: '. . . *the great malaria problem and its solution.*' Few, if any, would then have believed that *Plasmodium* spp. infection would remain a potentially greater health problem in the tropics the better part of a century later! This disease is very far from 'solved', and with growing expanses of tropical and subtropical terrain becoming endemic to this protozoan parasitosis, together with the continuing emergence of parasite-resistance to most of the available chemoprophylactic and chemotherapeutic agents, the health problems presented by this infection worldwide are probably greater today than was the case in Ross' time. In fact, we have been forced back to the most fundamental form of prophylaxis—avoidance of mosquito bites between dusk and dawn! This section opens with a detailed account of *Plasmodium* spp. infection—dominated by *P. falciparum*—and steers the reader through the chemoprophylactic maze: efficacy *versus* safety. Chemotherapy also leaves much to be desired and the brunt of the attack is back to quinine—first listed in the London Pharmacopoeia in 1677—following its introduction into Europe from Peru. And, as with all parasitic infections—both protozoan and helminthic—a satisfactory vaccine (applicable both to the developing country scenario and the traveller) seems far away.

The trypanosomiases—both African and South American—also present major problems as they did in Manson's day. Basic research continues on *Trypanosoma brucei*, but in chemotherapy the only gleam of hope lies in eflornithine—effective in West Africa, but not East or Central Africa. *T. cruzi* infection continues to be a major problem in South America; although chemotherapy in the early stage(s) of the infection yields moderately satisfactory results, the 'end-stage' disease remains unamenable to chemotherapy (or any other effective measure). *Leishmania* spp., which also figured prominently in the first edition of this text, remains a problem in both its visceral and cutaneous forms; fortunately, chemotherapy has progressed (albeit slowly), and modern methods of management are proving promising.

A major problem worldwide involves the gastrointestinal protozoan infections (well covered in this section). Small-intestinal disease is dominated by *Giardia lamblia* (the mechanism[s] of pathogenicity remains unclear—despite an enormous amount of research), whilst colorectal disease in tropical locations is largely dominated by *Entamoeba histolytica* infection. Significant progress has been made in this latter infection; the suggestion by Emile Brumpt in 1925 of two strains of the parasite—one pathogenic and the other not—has been (largely) confirmed by recent molecular biological observations. The 5-nitroimidazole compounds have revolutionized management in both of these gastrointestinal infections.

This section also highlights several other important protozoan infections; however, very little progress has been made in *prevention*! Following his seminal work which demonstrated the complete life-cycle of avian *Plasmodium* spp. infection, Ross devoted most of energies to *prevention* of the disease; sadly, advances in this area have been exceedingly slow—not only with this protozoan infection, but with most others also.

Chapter 71
Malaria

N. J. White

Malaria is the most important parasitic disease of man. Approximately 5% of the world's population is infected, and there are approximately one million deaths each year. The human disease is a protozoan infection of red blood cells transmitted by the bite of a blood-feeding female anopheline mosquito. Malaria, or ague as it was commonly known, has been described since antiquity. Hippocrates is usually credited with the first clear description amongst occidental writers: In *Epidemics* he distinguished different patterns of fever, and in his *Aphorisms* he describes the regular paroxysms of intermittent fever. In Europe seasonal periodic fevers were particularly common in marshy areas, and were frequently referred to as 'paludial' (L. *palus* marshy ground; Fr. *paludisme*). In the early nineteenth century miasmatic influences were believed to cause a variety of diseases. Malaria was thought by Italian writers to be caused by the offensive vapours emanating from the Tiberian marshes.[1] The word 'malaria' comes from the Italian, and means literally 'bad air'. Indeed the cause of the seasonal periodic fevers was a continuous source of debate until the late nineteenth century.[2] The work of Meckel, Virchow and Frerichs had established that the pigment (mistakenly thought to be melanin) observed in the blood of some patients with periodic fever resulted from the destruction of red blood corpuscles. This same pigment caused the characteristic grey discolouration of the internal organs in patients dying from this disease. In the 1870s, medicine slowly moved towards the germ theory of disease, following the pioneering work of Koch. In 1879, Edwin Klebs and Corrado Tommasi-Crudelli reported the identification of a bacterial cause of malaria. Recovery of the 'organism', *Bacillus malariae*, from patients with malaria was confirmed by several influential Italian physicians and pathologists— and similar reports began to appear in the USA. It was not surprising, therefore, that the report of a French Army surgeon working in Algeria, claiming that malaria was caused by a parasite, was treated initially with some scepticism.[3] On the 20 October 1880 (or in a later publication he gives the date as 6 November) Charles Louis Alphonse Laveran was examining the fresh blood of a patient with ague, and observed moving bodies (he was probably watching gametocyte exflagellation) which he surmised correctly were parasites of the red blood cells. The transmissability of the infection in blood was proved four years later by Gerhardt, but the route of natural infection was not discovered until the next decade. Following the suggestion of Patrick Manson, a young Scottish physician in the Indian Medical Service, Ronald Ross, began to investigate the possibility that malaria could be transmitted by mosquitoes. In 1897, after many months of failure, he reported the presence of pigmented bodies in the gut of a certain species of brown 'dapple winged' mosquito that had fed on patients with malaria.[4] He speculated that these might represent the parasite stage in the mosquito (he was in fact describing the oocysts) but, because of difficulties in obtaining these 'unusual' mosquitoes and his transfer to Calcutta, he was unable to characterize the complete life cycle, i.e., transmission from human to mosquito to human. After many years of study, Ross finally proved the existence of the complete life cycle involving a mosquito in the malaria of canaries.[5] He identified the anopheles mosquito as the vector of human malaria, although by the time Ross finally had the opportunity to demonstrate *Plasmodium falciparum* sporogony in anopheline mosquitoes in Sierra Leone, Bignami[6] and his colleagues, following the pioneering work of Grassi, had succeeded in infecting a healthy volunteer with *P. falciparum* from mosquito bites in Rome. Both Laveran and Ross received Nobel Prizes for their respective discoveries.

Understanding of the biology of malaria was further advanced by a third Nobel-prize winning discovery. In 1883 the Viennese psychiatrist Julius Wagner-Jauregg became interested in the relationship between fever and mental illness. Between 1888 and 1917 he experimented on a number of methods of inducing fever to treat patients with general paralysis of the insane (GPI is a form of neurosyphilis). On 14 June 1917 he inoculated blood from a soldier with tertian fever into two patients with GPI.[7] So began the era of malaria therapy of neurosyphilis. This became standard practice throughout the world until the introduction of penicillin thirty years later. Overall, at a time when GPI accounted for 10% of all mental hospital patients in Europe, malaria therapy gave approximately 30% of patients a full, and 20%, a partial remission of this debilitating and ultimately lethal infection.

Until the nineteenth century malaria was found in northern Europe, North America and Russia – and transmission in Southern Europe was intense. Since then it has been eradicated from these areas, and the number of cases in the Middle East, China, and the Indian subcontinent has fallen, but elsewhere in the tropics there has been a resurgence of the disease[1] and the number of cases worldwide continues to increase. This has been associated with

Table 71.1 Human malaria parasites

	P. falciparum	P. vivax	P. ovale	P. malariae
Exoerythrocytic (hepatic) phase of development (days)	5.5	8	9	15
Erythrocytic cycle (days)	2	2	2	3
Hypnozoites (relapses)	No	Yes	Yes	No
Number of merozoites per hepatic schizont	30,000	10,000	15,000	2000
Erythrocyte preference	Young RBCs but can invade all ages[a]	Reticulocytes	Reticulocytes	Old RBCs
Maximum duration of untreated infection (years)	2	4	4	40

[a]Parasites causing severe malaria are not selective.

increasing resistance of the anopheline vector to insecticides, and of the parasite to the antimalarial drugs. Approximately 270 million people suffer from malaria, and there are between 1 and 2.5 million deaths each year. Most of these deaths are in African children. The mortality rate is rising. This is attributed directly to drug resistance.

Four species of the genus *Plasmodium* infect humans, although occasional infections with errant primate malarias may also occur.[8] The individual characteristics of the four species of human malaria parasites are shown in Table 71.1. Almost all deaths and severe disease are caused by *P. falciparum*. This parasite appears to be a relatively recent evolutionary acquisition of man (perhaps within the past 10,000 years).[9,10] In phylogenetic terms, it is closest to the avian malarias (*P. lophurae, P. gallinaceum*). Its propensity to kill has been cited as an example of evolutionary immaturity, although for such a widespread and successful infection this is debatable. The three 'benign' malarias, *P. vivax, P. ovale* and *P. malariae*, all lie close together on the evolutionary tree near the other primate malarias.[9] Severe disease with these species is very unusual, although occasionally patients will die from rupture of an enlarged spleen;[11] and these infections may also reduce birthweight which predisposes children to neonatal death.[12]

Geographical apsects
Distribution

Malaria is found throughout the tropics. In Africa, *P. falciparum* predominates, as it does in Papua New Guinea and Haiti, whereas *P. vivax* is more common in Central and parts of South America, North Africa, the Middle East and the Indian subcontinent. The prevalence of both species is approximately equal in other parts of South America, East Asia and Oceania. *P. vivax* is rare in sub-Saharan Africa, whereas *P. ovale* is relatively uncommon outside West Africa. *P. malariae* is found in most areas, but is less common outside Africa. Malaria was once endemic in Europe and northern Asia, and was introduced to North America, but it has since been eradicated from

these areas. In China and adjacent countries *P. vivax* strains (*P. vivax* hibernans) with long incubation periods and long intervals (10–12 months) between relapses may still be found.

Epidemiology

The vector

Malaria is transmitted by some species of anopheline mosquitoes. Malaria transmission does not occur at temperatures below 16°C or above 33°C, and at altitudes greater than 2000 m above sea level because development in the mosquito (sporogony) cannot take place. The optimum conditions for transmission are high humidity and an ambient temperature between 20 and 30°C. Although rainfall provides breeding sites for mosquitoes, excessive rainfall may wash away mosquito larvae and pupae.[13]

The epidemiology of malaria is complex and may vary considerably even within relatively small geographic areas. Malaria transmission to man depends on several interrelated factors.[14–16] The most important pertain to the anopheline mosquito vector and, in particular, its longevity. As sporogony (development of the sporozoite parasites in the vector) takes over a week (depending on ambient temperatures), the mosquito must survive for longer than this after feeding on a gametocyte-carrying human, if malaria is to be transmitted. MacDonald gave the following formula for the likelihood of infection based on the sporozoite rates,[14,15] i.e., the proportion of anopheline mosquitoes with sporozoites in their salivary glands:

$$S = \frac{P^n ax}{ax - \log_e P}$$

where P = the probability of mosquito survival through 1 day; n = the duration, in days, of the extrinsic cycle of the parasite in the mosquito; a = average number of blood meals on man per day, and x = the proportion of bites infective to man. The probability of a mosquito surviving n days is given by:

$$\frac{P^n}{-\log_e P}$$

The inoculation rate, or the mean daily number of bites *(h)* received by sporozoite-bearing mosquitoes is given by:

$$h = mabs$$

where m = anopheline density in relation to man, and b = proportion of bites that are infectious. The reproductive rate of the infection *(r)* or the number of secondary cases resulting from a primary case is then given by:

$$r = \frac{ma^2 bP^n}{-z\log_e P}\ (1\frac{ax}{ax - \log_e P})$$

where z is the recovery rate, or the reciprocal of the duration of human infectivity. This is usually estimated at 80 days for *P. falciparum* in a non-immune subject, i.e., $z = 0.0125$. The term:

$$1 - \frac{ax}{ax - \log_e P}$$

refers to the proportion of anopheline mosquitoes 'not yet infected'. When transmission is very low (i.e., x approaches *0*) then the basic reproductive rate (r_0) reduces to:

$$r_0 = \frac{ma^2 bP^n}{-z\log_e P}$$

Thus, as a general approximation, malaria transmission is directly proportional to the density of the vector, the square of the number of times each day that the mosquito bites man, and the tenth power of the probability of the mosquito surviving for 1 day. The model described by MacDonald has certain theoretical limitations (it has been refined in recent years to accommodate these), but it does illustrate certain fundamental points of practical relevance to control or eradication programmes. The importance of vector longevity in determining transmission is clearly important and focuses control measures on the adult mosquito. At very high levels of transmission there is considerable reserve in the system and large reductions in transmission reduce malaria by a negligible amount (e.g., a reduction in transmission of 90% from 300 infectious bites per year to 30 bites/year will make very little difference to the prevalence of malaria) – but as r_0 approaches the critical value of 1 (below which the disease dies out), small reductions in r_0 have very large effects on the amount of malaria. Control programmes can be very effective in these circumstances, and can eradicate malaria—as indeed they did in Europe where r_0 was certainly low in many areas, and the vector rested inside houses and could be attacked with residual insecticides. The precise value of r_0 has been much debated, although there is good reason to believe it is generally low (e.g., less than 10). This gives hope to those developing vaccines and other interventions aimed at reducing transmission of malaria. Vectors differ considerably in their natural abundance (particularly with season of the year), feeding and resting behaviours, breeding sites, flight ranges, choice of blood source (many anopheline vectors also bite animals), and vulnerability to environmental conditions and insecticides.

Thus there is also considerable variation in their ability to transmit malaria (the vectorial capacity). Of the nearly 400 species of anopheline mosquitoes (many of which are species complexes), approximately 80 can transmit malaria, 66 are considered natural vectors, and about 45 are considered important vectors.[13,14] Each vector has its own behaviour patterns. For example in South-East Asia mosquitoes of the *Anopheles dirus* complex are an important cause of 'forest fringe' malaria. They breed in tree collections of water, and are consequently vulnerable to deforestation, or too little or too much rainfall, but they are very difficult to attack with insecticides. *A. stephensi*, the principal vector in the Indian subcontinent, breeds in wells or stagnant water and can be controlled by treating breeding sites with insecticides or polystyrene balls. The most effective malaria vectors (such as the *A. gambiae* complex) are hardy, long lived, naturally occur in high densities, and bite humans frequently. Malaria is often seasonal, coinciding with the rainy season which provides water for mosquito breeding and increased humidity favouring mosquito survival. Other factors, which are not well understood, also influence mosquito populations and lead to fluctuations in the prevalence of malaria.

The human host

The behaviour of man also plays an important role in the epidemiology of malaria.[14–16] There must be a human reservoir of viable gametocytes to transmit the infection. In areas of high transmission rates, infants and young children are more susceptible to malaria than the more immune older children and adults. Parasite densities are higher and gametocytaemia is detected more frequently in children. The relative contribution of the younger age group versus older asymptomatic individuals who have lower parasite densities and also immunity, but who are less likely to receive antimalarial treatment, to overall transmission is unclear. The endemicity of malaria is defined traditionally in terms of the spleen or parasite rates in children aged between 2 and 9 years.[8,14]

- Hypoendemic: spleen rate or parasite rate 0–10%.
- Mesoendemic: spleen or parasite rate 10–50%.
- Hyperendemic: spleen or parasite rate 50–75% and adult spleen rate is also high.
- Holoendemic: spleen or parasite rate over 75%, and adult spleen rate low. Parasite rates in the first year of life are high.

In areas which are holoendemic or hyperendemic for *P. falciparum*, such as much of tropical Africa or coastal New Guinea, people are infected repeatedly throughout their lives.[16] There is considerable morbidity and mortality during childhood. In The Gambia, where people are infected once each year on average (a relatively low figure for the African continent),[17] malaria has been estimated to cause 25% of deaths in children between 1 and 4 years of age,[18] but eventually, if the child survives, a state of 'premunition' is achieved where infections cause little or no problems to the host. Thus a form of immunity develops which is sufficient to control, but not prevent, the infection. The slow rate at which premunition is acquired may be a function of age. Non-immune adults entering an area of intense transmission acquire premunition more rapidly than children.[19] Falciparum malaria infections are more severe in pregnancy, particularly in primigravidae,[20,21] and may be augmented by iron supplementation, although this is disputed.[22]

Clinical epidemiology

Babies develop severe malaria relatively infrequently (although, if they do, the mortality rate is high). The factors responsible for this include passive transfer of maternal immunity,[23] and the high haemoglobin F content of the infants' erythrocytes which retards parasite development.[24] In holoendemic areas the baby is inoculated repeatedly with sporozoites during the first year of life, but the blood stage infection is seldom severe.[14] Where transmission is most intense people may receive up to three infectious bites per day. In this epidemiological context the main clinical impact of falciparum malaria is to cause severe anaemia in the 1–3-year age group (Figure 71.1). With less intense or more variable or unstable transmission the age range affected by severe malaria extends to older children, and cerebral malaria becomes a more prominent manifestation of severe disease.[25-27] In hyperendemic and holoendemic areas indigenous adults never develop severe malaria, unless they leave the transmission area and return years later (and even then malaria is seldom life threatening). Immunity is constantly boosted and effective premunition prevents parasite burdens reaching dangerous levels. Nearly all infections in adults are asymptomatic. In terms of the mathematical models presented earlier, an index of malaria transmission stability is given by al-$\log_e P$; values of > 2.5 indicate stable transmission.

Where the transmission rate of malaria is low, erratic, markedly seasonal, or focal, symptomatic infections are more common. A state of premunition is often not attained. Symptomatic disease occurs at any age, and cerebral malaria is a prominent manifestation of severe disease at all ages. This is termed 'unstable' malaria.[14] In many areas the transmission of malaria varies considerably over short distances, and severe disease is common when non-immune individuals enter these areas (e.g., woodcutters in South America and South-East Asia where malaria is of the 'forest fringe' type).

Malaria is usually a 'rainy season disease' coinciding with increased mosquito abundance. However, in some areas parasite rates (i.e., the proportion of people with positive blood smears) are relatively constant throughout the year, but the majority of cases still do occur during the wet season.[28] In Europe, before eradication, falciparum malaria was common in spring and in late summer and autumn, and was termed 'aestivo-autumnal malaria'.[29] The intensity of transmission or 'endemicity' can change. For example in Africa, the sub-Sahelian drought has reduced rainfall and mosquito transmission in countries such as Senegal and The Gambia. In the 1960s transmission was intense, and severe disease was rare in children over 3 years of age.[30,31] Today, transmission has fallen to levels found in areas of unstable endemicity, such as some areas of South-East Asia[32] and cases of cerebral malaria occur occasionally in indigenous adults. Deforestation, population migration and changes in agricultural practices have profound effects on malaria transmission. Urban malaria is becoming an increasing problem in many countries.

Malaria can also behave as an epidemic disease carrying a high mortality rate.[14] Epidemics are caused by migrations (i.e., introduction of susceptible hosts), the introduction of new vectors, or changes in the habits of the mosquito vector or the human host. Epidemics have occurred in North India, Sri Lanka, South-East Asia, Madagascar, Brazil (when the formidable African vector *A. gambiae* was inadvertently imported from Africa in the 1930s), and more recently in Burundi where drug resistance was a major contributory factor.

With increasing international air travel and worsening antimalarial drug resistance, imported cases of malaria in tourists, travellers and immigrants are now common. With the recent exception of some of the former Soviet republics in East Europe and West Asia, fortunately this has not led to the reintroduction of malaria to areas from where it had earlier been eradicated (although the vector, and thus the potential, remains). Imported malaria is often misdiagnosed, and severe presentations of falciparum malaria are not uncommon. Malaria may also be transmitted by blood transfusion, transplantation, or through needle-sharing among intravenous drug addicts.

Aetiology
Pre-erythrocytic development

Infection with human malaria begins when the feeding female anopheline mosquito inoculates plasmodial

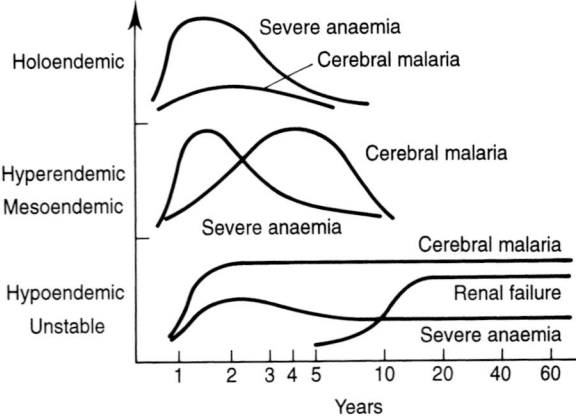

Figure 71.1: Relationship between age and the clinical presentations of severe malaria at different levels of malaria transmission.

Table 71.2 Malaria incubation periods in malaria therapy and volunteer studies

	Prepatent period (days)	Incubation period (days)
P. falciparum	11.0 (2.4)	13.1 (2.8)
P. vivax	12.2 (2.3)	13.4 (2.7)
P. malariae	32.7*	34.7*
P. ovale	12.0	14.1

Values are mean (SD).
*These data are taken from artificially induced malaria data in Boyd (1948); naturally acquired infections are considered to have an incubation period of between 13–28 days.

sporozoites at the time of feeding.[33] The small motile sporozoites are injected during the phase of probing as the mosquito searches for a vascular space before aspirating blood. In most cases, relatively few sporozoites are injected (approximately 8–15), but up to 100 may be introduced in some instances.[34,35] Most sporozoites come from the larger salivary ducts and represent only a small fraction of the total number in the salivary gland. After injection they enter the circulation, either directly or via lymph channels, and rapidly target the hepatic parenchymal cells. Within 45 minutes of the bite all sporozoites have either entered the hepatocytes or have been cleared. Each sporozoite bores into the hepatocyte and there begins a phase of asexual reproduction. This stage lasts on average between 5.5 (P. falciparum) and 15 days (P. malariae) before the hepatic schizont ruptures to release merozoites into the blood stream (Table 71.2).[8] In some instances the primary incubation period can be much longer. In P. vivax and P. ovale infections a proportion of the intrahepatic parasites do not develop, but instead rest inert as sleeping forms or 'hypnozoites', to awaken weeks or months later, and cause the relapses which characterize infections with these two species. During the pre-erythrocytic or hepatic phase of development considerable asexual multiplication takes place and many thousands of merozoites are released from each ruptured infected hepatocyte. However, as only a few liver cells are infected, this phase is asymptomatic for the human host.

Asexual blood-stage development

The merozoites liberated into the bloodstream closely resemble sporozoites. They are motile ovoid forms which rapidly invade red blood cells. The process of invasion involves attachment to the erythrocyte surface, orientation so that the apical complex (which protrudes slightly from one end of the merozoite and contains the rhoptries, the micronemes, and dense granules) abuts the red cell, and then interiorization takes place by a vigorous wriggling or boring motion inside a vacuole composed of the invaginated erythrocyte membrane. Once inside the erythrocyte the parasite lies within the erythrocyte cytosol enveloped by its own plasma membrane, and a surrounding parasitophorous vacuolar membrane. It has

been suggested that the parasite may be connected directly to the surrounding plasma by a parasitophorous duct, but this is widely disputed. The attachment of the merozoite to the red cell is mediated by a attachment of one or more of a family of erythrocyte-binding proteins, localized to the micronemes of the merozoite apical complex, to a specific erythrocyte receptor. In P. vivax this is related to the Duffy blood group antigen Fy^a or Fy^b.[36,37] The absence of these phenotypes in West Africans, or people who originate from that region, explains their resistance to infection with P. vivax, and the absence of vivax malaria in West Africa. For P. falciparum much attention has focused on the merozoite protein EBA 175, a member of the 'Duffy binding-like' (DBL) superfamily of genes encoding ligands for host cell receptors.[38] This binds to sialic acid and the peptide backbone of the red cell membrane sialoglycoprotein glycophorin A. But other, sialic acid-dependent and independent pathways of invasion also occur, indicating considerable reserve in the invasion system.[39,40] The red cell surface receptors for P. malariae and P. ovale are not known.

During the early phase of blood stage development (< 12 hours) the small 'ring forms' of the four parasite species often appear similar under light microscopy. The young developing parasite looks like a signet ring or, in the case of P. falciparum, like a pair of stereo-headphones, with darkly staining chromatin in the nucleus, a circular rim of cytoplasm, and a pale central food vacuole (Figures 71.2 and 71.3). Parasites are freely motile within the erythrocyte. As they grow they increase in size logarithmically and consume the erythrocyte's contents (most of which is haemoglobin). Proteolysis of haemoglobin within the digestive vacuole releases amino acids which are taken up and utilized by the growing parasite for protein synthesis, but the liberated haem poses a problem. When haem is freed from its protein scaffold it oxidizes to the toxic ferric form. Toxicity is avoided by spontaneous dimerization (using histidine-rich protein 2 as a scaffold) to an inert crystalline substance, haemozoin.[41] Non-polymerized haem exits the food vacuole and is degraded by glutathione.[42] The digested products, mainly the brown or black insoluble refractile pigment haemozoin, can be seen within the digestive vacuole of the growing parasite. To obtain amino acids and other nutrients and to control the electrolytic milieu in the infected erythrocyte the parasite inserts specific transporters and chemicals in the red cell membrane.[43] These and other disruptions make the red cell more permeable. The infected erythrocyte becomes progressively less elastic and deformable and more spherical as the parasite grows.[44]

At approximately 12–14 hours of development P. falciparum parasites begin to exhibit a high molecular weight strain-specific variant antigen, *Plasmodium falciparum erythrocyte membrane protein 1* (PfEMP1) on the surface of the infected red cell which mediates attachment to vascular endothelium.[45] This is associated with the formation of knob-like projections from the erythrocyte membrane. Expression increases towards the middle of the cycle (24 hours). These red blood cells then

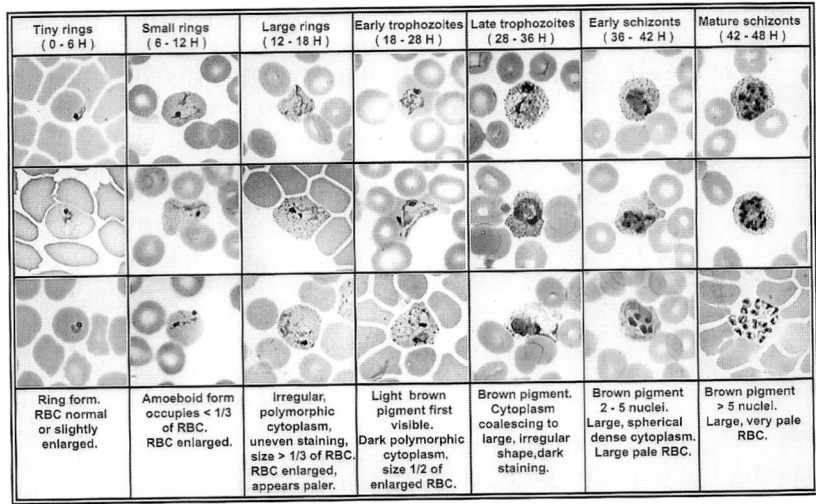

Tiny rings (0 - 6 H)	Small rings (6 - 12 H)	Large rings (12 - 18 H)	Early trophozoites (18 - 28 H)	Late trophozoites (28 - 36 H)	Early schizonts (36 - 42 H)	Mature schizonts (42 - 48 H)
Ring form. RBC normal or slightly enlarged.	Amoeboid form occupies < 1/3 of RBC. RBC enlarged.	Irregular, polymorphic cytoplasm, uneven staining, size > 1/3 of RBC. RBC enlarged, appears paler.	Light brown pigment first visible. Dark polymorphic cytoplasm, size 1/2 of enlarged RBC.	Brown pigment. Cytoplasm coalescing to large, irregular shape, dark staining.	Brown pigment 2 - 5 nuclei. Large, spherical dense cytoplasm. Large pale RBC.	Brown pigment > 5 nuclei. Large, very pale RBC.

Plasmodium vivax in vitro culture   Wellcome Unit, Bangkok 2000

Figure 71.2: Asexual life cycle of *Plasmodium falciparum*. After approximately 13–16 hours of development the parasitized erythrocytes start to adhere to the vascular endothelium lining the capillaries and venules.

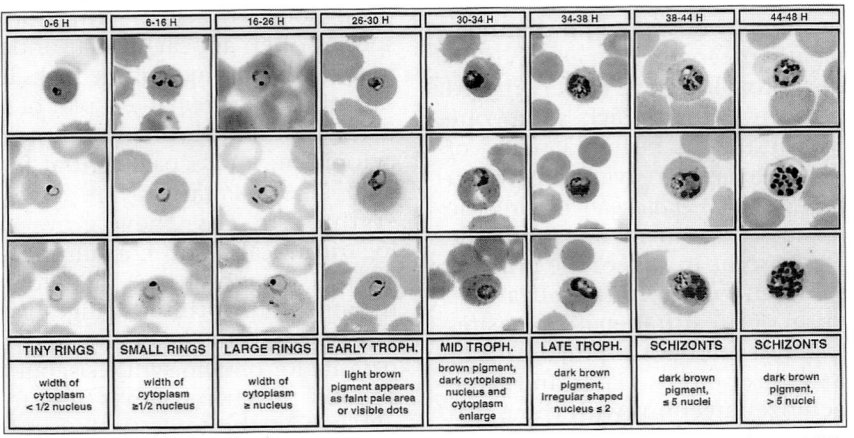

0-6 H	6-16 H	16-26 H	26-30 H	30-34 H	34-38 H	38-44 H	44-48 H
TINY RINGS	SMALL RINGS	LARGE RINGS	EARLY TROPH.	MID TROPH.	LATE TROPH.	SCHIZONTS	SCHIZONTS
width of cytoplasm < 1/2 nucleus	width of cytoplasm ≅1/2 nucleus	width of cytoplasm ≥ nucleus	light brown pigment appears as faint pale area or visible dots	brown pigment, dark cytoplasm nucleus and cytoplasm enlarge	dark brown pigment, irregular shaped nucleus ≤ 2	dark brown pigment, ≤ 5 nuclei	dark brown pigment, > 5 nuclei

P.falciparum staging (*in vitro* culture)   Wellcome unit, Bangkok 2000

Figure 71.3: Asexual life cycle of *Plasmodium vivax*.

progressively disappear from the circulation by attachment or 'cytoadherence' to the walls of venules and capillaries in the vital organs. This process is called 'sequestration'. The other three 'benign' human malarias do not cytoadhere significantly and all stages of development are seen in peripheral blood.

As *P. vivax* grows it enlarges the infected red blood cell, and red granules appear throughout the erythrocyte. These are known as Schuffner's dots. Similar dots are also prominent in *P. ovale*, which also distorts the shape of the infected erythrocyte (hence its name). *P. malariae* produces characteristic 'band forms' as the parasite grows. It is usually present at low parasitaemias. High parasitaemias (over 2%) are usually caused by *P. falciparum*.[8] Approximately 36 hours after merozoite invasion (or 54 hours in *P. malariae*) repeated nuclear division takes place to form a 'segmenter' or schizont (the term 'meront' is etymologically more correct). Eventually the growing parasite occupies the entire red cell which has become spherical, rigid, depleted

in haemoglobin and full of merozoites. This then ruptures; between 6 and 36 merozoites are released, destroying the remnants of the red cell. These rapidly reinvade other red blood cells and start a new asexual cycle. Thus the infection expands logarithmically at around tenfold per cycle.[46] The asexual life cycle is approximately 48 hours for *P. falciparum*, *P. vivax* and *P. ovale*, and 72 hours for *P. malariae*.

Sexual stages and development in the mosquito

After a series of asexual cycles in *P. falciparum*, a subpopulation of parasites develops into sexual forms (gametocytes) which are long lived and motile. This process (gametocytogony) takes about 4 days in *P. vivax* infections, and more than 7–10 days in *P. falciparum*. The male-to-female gametocyte sex ratio for *P. falciparum* is approximately 1:4.[47] Following ingestion in the blood meal of a biting female anopheline mosquito, the male and female gametocytes become activated. The male gametocytes undergo rapid nuclear division and each of the eight nuclei formed associates with a flagellum (20–25 µm long). The motile male microgametes then separate and seek the female macrogametes. Fusion and meiosis then takes place to form a zygote. For a brief period the malaria parasite is diploid. Within 24 hours the enlarging zygote becomes motile and this form (the ookinete) penetrates the wall of the mosquito mid-gut (stomach) where it encysts (as an oocyst). This spherical bag of parasites expands by asexual division to reach a diameter of approximately 500 µm, i.e., it becomes visible to the naked eye. During the early stage of oocyst development there is a characteristic pigment pattern and colour that allows speciation (it was this that caught the eye of its discoverer, Ronald Ross, in 1894), but these patterns become obscured by the time the oocyst has matured to contain thousands of fusiform motile sporozoites. The oocyst finally bursts to liberate myriads of sporozoites into the coelomic cavity of the mosquito. The sporozoites then migrate to the salivary glands to await inoculation into the next human host during feeding. The development of the parasite in the mosquito is termed sporogony, and takes between 8 and 35 days depending on the ambient temperature and species of parasite and mosquito. Obviously the longevity of the mosquito is a critical factor in determining its vectorial capacity (see above).

Molecular genetics

Inheritance in *Plasmodium* is similar to that in other eukaryotes. Haploid and diploid generations alternate. The haploid genome of *P. falciparum* is divided among 14 chromosomes and codon composition is extremely biased to adenine and thymidine. A large number of individual genes were cloned and sequenced on the long and winding road towards the development of a malaria vaccine, and in the past few years the entire genome has been sequenced.[48] *P. falciparum* has approximately 6000 genes in its 14 chromosomes and plastid-like organelle compared with the 31,000 of its natural host. There appears to be some groupings of genes related to function. For example the genes encoding the merozoite surface proteins are grouped. The many genes encoding the variant red cell surface antigens (*var* and *rif* families), which contribute to the antigenic diversity necessary for the parasite to elude the host immune system, are also located close to each other near the telomeres.[49] The *var* gene product, the variant surface protein which mediates cytoadherence, (PfEMP1) appears to be the main antigen determining the parasite population structure during chronic falciparum malaria infections.[50] Variation in surface antigenicity results from the activation of a different *var* gene. This switching occurs at over 2% per asexual cycle. It has been suggested that the diversity of these immunodominant variant antigenic repeats sequences interferes with the selection of high-affinity antibody responses, and perpetuates low affinity responses in malaria. This delays the development of effective immunity.[51] Immune selection also provides the selective pressure to maintain diversity in T- and B-cell epitopes through a high frequency of non-synonymous base mutations during the asexual development of malaria parasites.

The mechanisms maintaining genetic diversity within the parasite genome are many and complex.[52] Some of the polymorphic antigens identified are encoded by single gene copies in the haploid genome. These polypeptide antigens are characterized by tandem repeat sequences. Unequal crossing over during recombination can generate completely different sequences of these repeats. As these repeat sequences are also antibody targets, their variation provides further antigenic diversity. Another mechanism for generating antigenic diversity is intragenic recombination between two parental alleles.

The infection
Genetic factors protecting against malaria

In 1949, J.B.S. Haldane suggested that people who were heterozygous for red cell abnormalities such as thalassaemia or sickle cell disease might be protected against malaria.[53] This, he said, would explain the high gene frequencies for the haemoglobinopathies in tropical areas. A state of 'balanced polymorphism' would exist, whereby the premature loss of the disadvantaged homozygotes would be offset by the survival advantage in heterozygotes. There is now good evidence from detailed epidemiological studies that this hypothesis is correct. The greatest protection is conferred by sickle cell trait and Melanesian ovalocytosis.[54,55] These patients' cells resist parasite invasion (in the case of sickle cell trait under low oxygen tensions), and once invaded the AS cells sickle readily, facilitating clearance by the reticuloendothelial system. The protective effect conferred by the thalassaemias or glucose-6-phosphate dehydrogenase (G6PD) deficiency (which share a geographical distribution with malaria) is generally weaker.[55,56] In some epidemiological studies a protective effect has not been apparent, but recent large epidemiological studies do support the Haldane hypothesis. For example in two large African case–control studies, G6PD deficiency (both in female heterozygotes and male hemizygotes) was associated with a 46–58% reduction in the risk of severe malaria.[57] The mechanism of protection in many of these haemoglobinopathies is also less well understood. Red blood cells from patients with α-thalassaemia are invaded normally by *P. falciparum*, but they may bind greater numbers of antibody molecules to the erythrocyte surface than infected normal cells, and may therefore be cleared from the circulation more readily.[58] In addition, the rate of decline of haemoglobin F in the first year of life is slower in α- and β-thalassaemia heterozygotes. Erythrocytes containing high haemoglobin F concentrations do not support parasite growth well. But studies from Vanuatu indicate that children with α-thalassaemia actually have more malaria (both *P. falciparum* and *P. vivax*) in the early years of life than their 'normal' counterparts, suggesting a complex interaction between malaria species and haemoglobin chain synthesis.[59] Melanesian ovalocytic erythrocytes both resist invasion by malaria parasites and provide a hostile intraerythrocytic ionic milieu for development. The mechanisms whereby the other haemoglobinopathies or red cell abnormalities protect against malaria remain controversial.

Certain human leucocyte antigens (HLAs) are rare in Northern Europeans, but common in West Africans. Two of these, the class I antigen HLA-BW53 and the class II antigen HLA-DR B1* 1302, may also confer protection against severe malaria.[60] HLA molecules present processed antigenic peptides to cytotoxic T lymphocytes. HLA-B53-restricted cytotoxic T cells recognize a conserved nonamer peptide from a pre-erythrocytic (liver) stage-specific malaria antigen (LSA-1).[61] This suggests that cytotoxic T-lymphocyte responses to the pre-erythrocytic stages of malaria may be important in immunity, and would explain how possession of HLA-B53 might confer a survival advantage.

A large number of genetic polymorphisms have been associated with protection or susceptibility to severe falciparum malaria. In some cases a polymorphism has been associated with protection in one study and susceptibility in another! Three different TNF promoter polymorphisms appear independently to be associated with severe malaria in African children; Gambian children homozygous for the TNF-308A allele were at a sevenfold increased risk of dying or recovering with neurological sequelae.[62] TNF-238A was associated independently with severe anaemia,[63] and TNF-376A with susceptibility to cerebral malaria. The TNF-308A association is not found in South-East Asian adults with severe malaria. A single nucleotide polymorphism in the inducible nitric oxide synthase gene promoter region was associated with severe anaemia in Gabon and SNP in the TNF promoter region which alters OCT 1 binding has been associated with a fourfold increased risk of malaria in Gambian and Kenyan children. Recent separate case–control studies on genetic polymorphisms in CD36 and ICAM-1, two major receptors for *P. falciparum* cytoadherence, have given conflicting results. The CD36 polymorphism protected from severe malaria in one study but increased the risk in the other. An African ICAM-1 polymorphism predisposed to cerebral malaria in Kenya, was neutral in The Gambia, and protected in Gabon. In some of these associations the possibility of linkage cannot be ruled out (i.e., the polymorphic gene lies close to another gene which is cansally associated with the observed effect). For example the MHCIII region, where the TNF promoter polymorphisms are located, contains a remarkably high density of genes with probable immune functions.[64]

Expansion of the infection

When the hepatic meronts rupture, they liberate approximately 10^5–10^6 merozoites into the circulation (i.e., the

product of 5–100 successful sporozoites). These invade passing red blood cells immediately. In non-immune subjects the multiplication rate in *P. falciparum* usually exceeds 10 per cycle (i.e., >50% efficiency)[46] and may reach twentyfold per cycle during the expanding phase of the infection (Figure 71.4). For the first few cycles the host is unaware of the brewing infection. On average, parasites are detectable in the blood by microscopy on the 11th day after sporozoite inoculation (the diligent microscopist can detect 20–50 parasites/μl reliably on Giemsa-stained thick films). At this stage the host may still feel well, or may complain of vague non-specific symptoms of malaise, headache, myalgia, weakness or anorexia.[65,66] On average the fever begins two days later, but in some cases fever precedes detectable parasitaemia. The rise in parasite count is logarithmic initially, with a rising sine wave pattern of parasitaemia,[67,68] but in most cases the parasite expansion terminates abruptly to limit the infection at a parasitaemia of 10^4–10^5/μl (Figure 71.4). Only *P. falciparum* has the capacity for untrammelled multiplication, and parasitaemias may exceed 50% in some cases. Several factors converge to limit parasite multiplication. The host mobilizes specific and non-specific immune defences. The parasite meronts are also damaged by high fevers, and this alone could explain the brake on parasite expansion.[69] The availability of suitable red blood cells is exhausted: *P. vivax* and *P. falciparum* prefer younger red blood cells and *P. malariae* prefers older cells. Interestingly whereas *P. vivax* shows invasion restricted to only 13% of the red blood cell population, and *P. falciparum* causing uncomplicated malaria to 40%, *P. falciparum* parasites causing severe malaria show unrestricted invasion.[70]

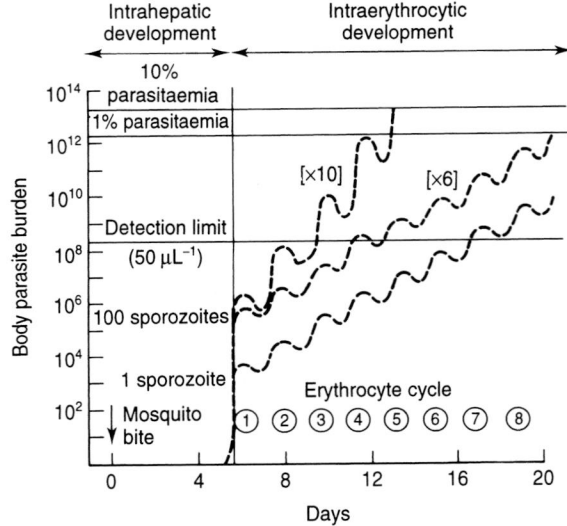

Figure 71.4: Logarithmic expansion of malaria infections in vivo. The body burden represents the total number of parasites in the body following infection of an adult of 50 kg. The infection rapidly reaches a lethal burden at high multiplication rates unless restrained. Maximum recorded multiplication rates are approximately x20 in vivo. (From White & Krishna: *Trans R Soc Trop Med Hyg*, 1989, with permission.)

Thus the untreated infection increases exponentially, the rate of expansion decelerates rapidly, and parasitaemia fluctuates, settles around a plateau, then declines and continues for several weeks or months at low levels before finally being eliminated. Although natural infections often contain two or more genetically different parasite strains, development tends to be relatively synchronous from the outset.[68] Further synchronization takes place in untreated infections in non-immune subjects, such that merogony ('sporulation') takes place within 1–2 hours. This is associated with fever and rigors (the 'paroxysm'). Although one 'brood' predominates, in *P. falciparum* there is often at least one minor 'brood' or subpopulation cycling 24 hours out of phase with the major brood.

The periodicity of malaria is enshrined in the terminology of the fever pattern. *P. malariae* has a 72–hour life cycle, and in untreated infections the paroxysm occurred on the fourth day (using the Greek system of inclusive reckoning the previous paroxysm is considered to occur on day 1). This is termed 'quartan malaria'. The other malarias are termed tertian (fever on the third day; 48-hour asexual cycle). *P. falciparum* often synchronized to a daily fever spike (quotidian fever), presumably caused by two broods of approximately equal size oscillating 24 hours out of phase, or failed to synchronize at all.[65–67] The classic descriptions of malaria symptomatology derive largely from detailed clinical observations made in the late nineteenth and early twentieth centuries, the experience with artificial infections in early chemotherapy studies, studies conducted by the military, and the extensive use of malaria therapy in the treatment of neurosyphilis.[67,71] These observations were usually made on non-immune adults. In malaria therapy patients with neurosyphilis were artificially infected, by mosquito bite or transfusion, and the infection with *P. falciparum* or *P. vivax* was left untreated so that the patient experienced recurrent high fevers, or if symptoms were severe, was judiciously titrated with quinine. Nowadays these characteristic fever charts are rarely seen because malaria is treated promptly. It was also apparent from these studies and later animal experiments[72,73] that some strains of *P. falciparum* were more virulent than others. For example, the now extinct European strains were notorious. The virulence factors of malaria parasites have not been characterized fully, but include multiplication capacity,[74] cytoadherence and rosetting ability, the potential to induce cytokine release, antigenicity, and antimalarial drug resistance.

Parasite biomass

Malaria is readily diagnosed from the blood film stained with a Romanowsky dye. In the benign malarias (where sequestration is considered not to occur) the number of parasites in the body may be estimated simply by multiplying the parasitaemia by the estimated blood volume. In *P. falciparum* the microscopist can see only the first half of the asexual life cycle. In the second half the parasitized

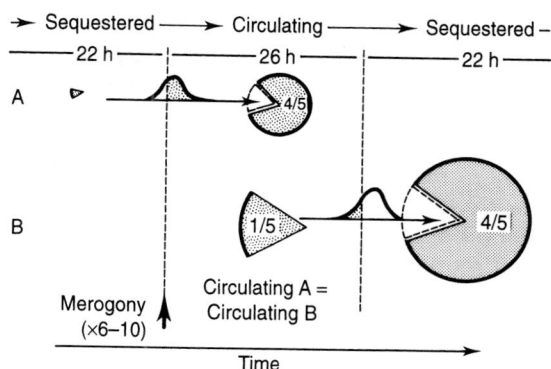

Figure 71.5: The problem of assessing the parasite burden from the peripheral parasitaemia in *P. falciparum* malaria. Sequestration hides the parasites causing harm. Two patients A and B have the same parasitaemia. In patient A, most of the parasites are circulating, and only a few from the previous cycle have yet to undergo merogony. In patient B, most of the parasites have already sequestered and only 20% of the biomass still circulates. There are over 60 times more parasites in patient B than in patient A. The clue lies in the stage distribution (shown crossing the hatched lines) of the circulating parasites which will be more mature in patient B. (From Silamut & White: *Trans R Soc Trop Med Hyg* 1993; 87:436–443.)

cells are sequestered. As a consequence there may be large discrepancies between the number of parasites in the peripheral (circulating) blood and the number of parasites in the body (the parasite burden) (Figure 71.5).[68,75] This has often puzzled and misled clinicians; some patients appear to tolerate high parasitaemia with little adverse effects, whereas others die with low parasite counts. The clue to the discrepancy lies both in the immune status of the host and in the stage of development of parasites on the peripheral blood smear.[76] A predominance of more mature parasites indicates that a greater proportion are sequestered, and carries a worse prognosis for any parasitaemia than a predominance of younger forms. Two patients with the same peripheral parasitaemia may have as much as a 100-fold difference in the total number of parasites in the body (Figure 71.5). In synchronous *P. falciparum* infections the peripheral blood parasite numbers fall at the time of sequestration, and rise abruptly at the time of merogony (when a predominance of tiny rings are seen).[68] The other explanation for the ability to tolerate high parasitaemias without apparent adverse effects relates to the development of 'antitoxic' immunity.[77] The host adapts to repeated infection by producing less cytokines for a given quantum of parasites (see below).[78] Eventually a state is reached where infections are asymptomatic. This is called premunition.

Immunity

The precise mechanisms controlling malaria infections are still incompletely understood. It was apparent from the era of malaria therapy for neurosyphilis that a strain-specific immunity developed which protected against rechallenge with the same parasite strain, but did not protect from challenge with a different strain.[71,79] Effective immunity, as distinct from premunition, may be reached when there has been exposure to all local strains of malaria parasites. This is difficult to quantify as there is no good in vitro correlate of either antitoxic or strain-specific immunity to malaria. In controlling the acute infection, non-specific host defence mechanisms and the development of more specific cell-mediated and humoral responses are both important.[80] Protective antibodies inhibit parasite expansion by agglutinating merozoites and through co-operation with the monocyte-macrophage series by binding to parasitized erythrocytes and then activating these cells' Fc receptors.[80,81] Non-specific effector mechanisms include non-opsonic phagocytosis via direct binding to monocyte-macrophage CD36, pro-inflammatory cytokine release, and the activation of phagocytic cells (including neutrophils) to release toxic oxygen species[83] and nitric oxide,[84] both of which are parasiticidal. The reaction of these oxygen intermediates with lipoproteins produces lipid peroxides. These are more stable cytotoxic molecules and are unaffected by antioxidants. There is also augmentation of splenic clearance function: both filtration[85] and Fc receptor-mediated phagocytosis are increased.[86,87] Infected erythrocytes are more rigid[44,88] and more opsonized than uninfected red blood cells as they express both host and parasite-derived neoantigens on the erythrocyte surface. However, the parasite proteins expressed on the red cell surface undergo antigenic variation,[89,90] and this is probably instrumental in avoiding complete immune clearance and sustaining the untreated infection. The systemic and splenic monocyte-macrophage series appear to be the most important immune effector cells in the direct attack on parasitized erythrocytes and merozoites, although neutrophils may also play a role.[91]

The immune response

Following natural infection there is a transient humoral response to sporozoite antigens; sporozoite antibodies decline, with a half-life of 3–4 weeks.[92] In areas with high transmission rates sporozoite antibody levels tend to plateau between 20 and 30 years of age, and do not correlate with premunition. Cytotoxic T-cell immune responses cannot be directed against the blood stage parasite as red blood cells do not express human leucocyte (HLA) antigens, but the pre-erythrocytic liver stages of the parasite are vulnerable. Several lines of experimental evidence in animal malarias, and the observation that certain HLA types are relatively protected from severe malaria, indicate that class 1 restricted CD8(+) T cells play an important role in immunity. There is evidence supporting a role for both alpha-beta and gamma-delta CD4+ cells in the immune reponse to malaria,[93] but the relatively weak interaction between malaria and the acquired immune deficiency syndrome (AIDS) in endemic areas does not suggest a major contribution in controlling malaria in immune individuals.

Strain-specific immunity to the asexual blood stage parasites develops slowly during natural untreated in-

fections, but it then provides good protection against rechallenge.[72,79] However, parasite populations are diverse, and cross-strain protection is initially weak or negligible. The development of immunity in endemic areas may represent the gradual acquisition of a repertoire of immunological memory for the range of local parasites. This involves strain transcending immunity sufficient to ameliorate disease (antitoxic immunity) and a more strain-specific immunity which protects from or attenuates the infection. The immune response to malaria is clearly very complex, and the relative importance of humoral and cellular immunity in man has not been defined clearly. Infusion of hyperimmune serum to patients with acute malaria can reduce or eliminate parasitaemia[94,95] mainly through opsonization, activation of phagocytic and cytotoxic effector functions by cytophilic IgG antibodies, and augmentation of ring-form infected erythrocyte clearance.[96] Immune serum also reduces parasite multiplication by agglutinating merozoites. Cell-mediated immunity is undoubtedly important as well, both in controlling the infection and in retaining immunological memory, but despite intensive study the complex interaction of specific and non-specific cellular immune responses[97] has yet to be unravelled in human infections.

Pathophysiology

The pathophysiology of malaria results from destruction of erythrocytes, the liberation of parasite and erythrocyte material into the circulation, and the host reaction to these events. *P. falciparum* malaria-infected erythrocytes also sequester in the microcirculation of vital organs, interfering with microcirculatory flow and host tissue metabolism.

Toxicity and cytokines

For many years malariologists hypothesized that parasites contained a toxin which was liberated at meront rupture, and caused the symptoms of the paroxysm. No toxin in the strict sense of the word has been identified, but malaria parasites do induce the release of cytokines in much the same way as bacterial endotoxin.[98,99] A glycolipid material with many of the properties of bacterial endotoxin is released on meront rupture.[100–102] This material appears to be associated with the glycosylphosphatidylinositol anchor which covalently links proteins, including the malaria parasite surface antigens, to the cell membrane lipid bilayer.[103] Malaria antigen-related IgE complexes also activate cytokine release. The limulus lysate assay, a test of endotoxin-like activity, is often positive in acute malaria. These products of malaria parasites, like the endotoxin of bacteria, induce activation of the cytokine cascade. But they are *considerably* less potent. For example an *Escherichia coli* bacteraemia of 1 bacterium/ml carries an approximate mortality rate of 20% whereas in falciparum malaria only parasitaemias of well over 10^9/ml produce such a lethal effect. Clearly compared with bacteria, malaria parasites are *not* very toxic! Cells of the macrophage-monocyte series, gamma-delta T cells, alpha-beta T cells CD14+ cells, and possibly endothelium, are stimulated to release cytokines in a mutually amplifying chain reaction. Initially tumour necrosis factor (TNF), which plays a pivotal role, interleukin (IL)-1, and gamma interferon are produced and these, in turn, induce the release of a cascade of other 'pro-inflammatory' cytokines including IL-8, IL-12, IL-18.[76] These are balanced by production of the 'anti-inflammatory' cytokines IL-6 and IL-10.[104,107] Cytokines are responsible for many of the symptoms and signs of the infection, particularly fever and malaise. Plasma concentrations of the cytokines are elevated in both acute vivax and falciparum malaria.[108,109] In established vivax malaria, which tends to synchronize earlier than *P. falciparum*, a pulse release of TNF occurs at the time of meront rupture and this is followed by the characteristic symptoms and signs of the 'paroxysm', i.e., shivering, cool extremities, headache, chills, a spike of fever, and sometimes rigors followed by sweating, vasodilatation and defervescence.[108] For a given number of parasites, *P. vivax* is a more potent inducer of TNF release than *P. falciparum* which may explain its lower pyrogenic density.

Cytokines are a subject of considerable interest, but the interpretation of blood concentration data has been difficult, and their relevance to tissue concentrations uncertain. In the case of TNF, the assays (other than bioassays) available until recently measured both bioactive and inactive forms of TNF and also TNF bound to soluble receptors. They did not assess the effects of circulating inhibitors. Cytokine levels measured by enzyme-linked immunosorbent assay (ELISA) or indirect fluorescent antibody test (IRMA) fluctuate widely over a short period of time, and are high in both *P. vivax* and *P. falciparum* malaria; indeed some of the highest TNF concentrations recorded in malaria occur during the paroxysms of synchronous *P. vivax* infections.[108] Nearly all the TNF measured in these assays is bound to soluble receptors; there is usually little or no bioactivity. Nevertheless there is a positive correlation between cytokine levels and prognosis in severe falciparum malaria.[106,109] Acute malaria is associated with high levels of most cytokines, but the balance differs in relation to severity. IL-12 and TGF-beta 1, which may regulate the balance between pro- and anti-inflammatory cytokines, are higher in uncomplicated than severe malaria.[110] IL-10, a potent anti-inflammatory cytokine, increases markedly in severe malaria,[107] but in fatal cases does not increase sufficiently to restrain the production of TNF.[111] A reduced IL-10/TNF ratio has also been associated with childhood malarial anaemia in areas of high transmission rates.[112] All this points to a disturbed balance of cytokine production in severe malaria.

The first studies to associate elevations in plasma cytokine levels with disease severity focused on TNF and cerebral malaria, and led to the suggestion that TNF played a causal role in cerebral dysfunction. More recently, genetic studies indicate that children with the (308A) TNF2 allele, a polymorphism in the TNF promoter region, have a relative risk of 7 for death or neurological sequelae from cerebral malaria in African children (but not South-East Asian adults).[62] A separate polymorphism in this region which affects gene expression was associated with a fourfold increased risk of cerebral malaria.[64] On the other hand, the clinical studies in cerebral malaria with anti-TNF antibodies, and other strategies to reduce TNF production, reported to date have shown no convincing effects other than reduction in fever.[112] Cytokines do play a causal role in the pathogenesis of cerebral symptoms in murine models of severe malaria,[109] but these models are clinically and pathologically unlike human cerebral malaria. There is no direct evidence that systemic release of TNF or other cytokines causes coma in humans (although mechanisms involving release of nitric oxide within the central nervous system and consequent inhibition of neurotransmission can be hypothesized). In a recent study of adults with severe malaria, elevated plasma TNF concentrations were associated specifically with renal dysfunction,[111] and TNF levels were actually lower in patients with pure cerebral malaria than those with other manifestations of severe disease. Severe malarial anaemia has been associated with yet another TNF promoter polymorphism (238A; odds ratio 2.5).[63] Taken together these suggest a role for TNF and other cytokines in severe disease, not encephalopathy per se, but the extent to which this is the cause or an effect of severe disease remains to be determined.

Cytokines are probably involved in placental dysfunction, suppression of erythropoiesis and inhibition of gluconeogenesis, and certainly cause fever in malaria.[112,113] Tolerance to malaria, or premunition, reflects both immune regulation of the infection and also reduced production of cytokines in response to malaria ('antitoxic immunity'). Cytokines up-regulate the endothelial expression of vascular ligands for *P. falciparum*-infected erythrocytes, notably ICAM1, and thus promote cytoadherence. They may also be important mediators of parasite killing by activating leucocytes, and possibly other cells, to release toxic oxygen species,[114] nitric oxide, and by generating parasiticidal lipid peroxides, and causing fever. Thus, whereas high concentrations of cytokines appear to be harmful, lower levels probably benefit the host.

Sequestration

The process whereby erythrocytes containing mature forms of *P. falciparum* adhere to microvascular endothelium ('cytoadherence') and thus disappear from the circulation is known as sequestration (Figure 71.6). This phenomenon is also seen in the simian malarias *P. coatneyi* and *P. fragile* that infect rhesus monkeys, but it does not occur to a significant extent with the other three human malaria parasites. Sequestration is thought to be central to the pathophysiology of falciparum malaria.[115–117] Once infected red blood cells adhere, they do not enter the circulation again, remaining stuck until they rupture at

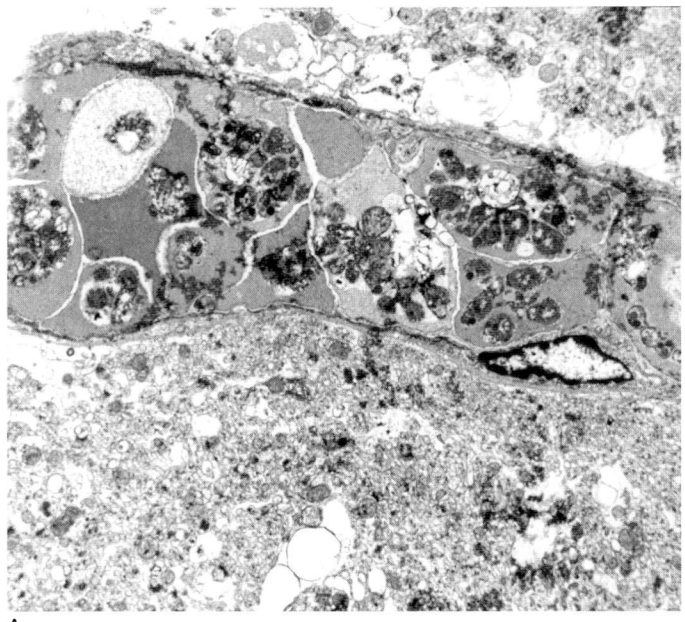

A

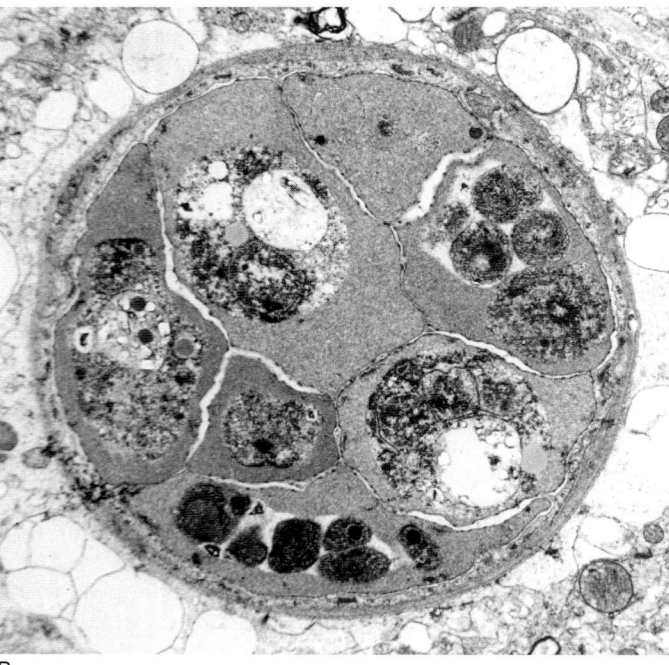

B

Figure 71.6: Two electron micrographs (x 4320) showing densely packed parasitized erythrocytes sequestered in cerebral venules of a fatal case of cerebral malaria. Note that even when no intracellular parasite is seen, electron dense deposits are evident on the cell membranes indicating the red cell does contain a parasite, but that its body has been missed in the section. The packing of red cells is much tighter than in normal conditions. (Courtesy of Emsrii Pongponratn.)

merogony (schizogony).[118] Cytoadherence begins in the first half of the parasites' 48-hour asexual life cycle. As a consequence, whereas in the other malarias of man mature parasites are comonly seen on blood smears, these forms are rare in falciparum malaria, and often indicate serious

infection.[76] It was thought that ring stage infected erythrocytes do not cytoadhere at all, but recent pathological and laboratory studies show that they do, although much less so than more mature stages.[118,119] Sequestration occurs predominantly in the venules of vital organs (Figure 71.6 and 71.7). It is not distributed uniformly throughout the body, being greatest in the brain, particularly the white matter, prominent in the heart, eyes, liver, kidneys, intestines and adipose tissue, and least in the skin.[117] Even within the brain the distribution of sequestered erythrocytes varies markedly from vessel to vessel,[118] presumably reflecting differences in the expression of endothelial receptors. Cytoadherence and the related phenomenon of rosetting lead to microcirculatory obstruction in falciparum malaria[116] (Figure 71.6). The consequences of microcirculatory obstruction are activation of the vascular endothelium, and reduced oxygen and substrate supply, which leads to anaerobic glycolysis and lactic acidosis and cellular dysfunction.

Cytoadherence

Cytoadherence is mediated by several different processes. The most important parasite ligands are a family of strain-specific, high molecular weight parasite-derived proteins termed *P. falciparum* erythrocyte membrane protein 1 or PfEMP$_1$.[120,121] These proteins (molecular mass 240–260 kDa) are encoded by *var* genes, a family of 50–150 genes distributed throughout the parasite's genome.[122] PfEMP$_1$ is transcribed, synthesized, and stored within the parasite and, beginning at around 12 hours of development, it is then exported to the surface of the infected erythrocyte.[123] There it is apposed by an electrostatic interaction through the membrane to a submembranous accretion of parasite-derived histidine-rich protein (HRP) which is, in turn, anchored to the red cell via the cytoskeleton protein ankryn.[124] These accretions cause humps or knobs on the surface of the red cell, and these are the points of attachment to vascular endothelium (Figures 71.7 and 71.8). The protuberances are not essential for cytoadherence. A small subpopulation of naturally occurring parasites do not induce surface knobs, and parasites can be selected in culture which are knob negative (K–) but still cytoadhere. However, natural parasite isolates are always knob positive (K+). PfEMP$_1$ expression is greatest at the beginning of the second half of the asexual cycle. PfEMP$_1$ also appears to be a major antigenic determinant for the blood stage parasite. As in other protozoal parasites the immuno-dominant surface antigen undergoes antigenic variation to 'change its coat' and avoid immune mediated attack. *P. falciparum* 'switches' to a new variant of PfEMP$_1$ at a rate of about 2% per cycle.[125] In the chronic phase of untreated infections this results in small waves of parasitaemia approximately every three weeks. Other gene superfamilies thought to have similar function have been revealed by genome sequencing. These are the *rifin* family in *P. falciparum* and *vir* in *Plasmodium vivax*.[126] A protein

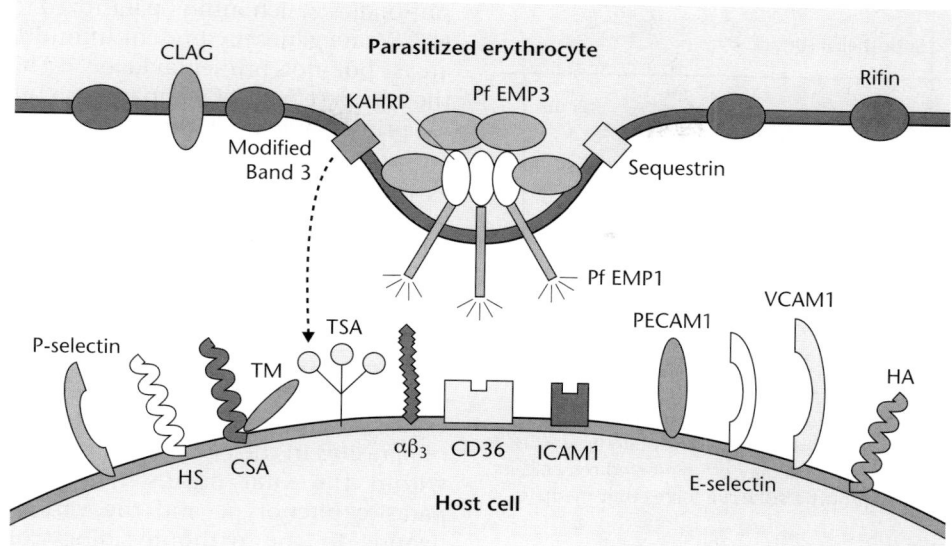

Figure 71.7: Schematic representation of cytoadherence in falciparum malaria. On the red cell side the principle ligand is the variant antigen *Plasmodium falciparum* erythrocyte membrane protein 1 (*Pf*EMP1). This is expressed on the surface of 'knobs' which protrude from the red cell surface. It is anchored beneath to the knob associated histidine rich protein (KAHRP), and stabilised by *Pf*EMP3. The *rifin* and CLAG gene products are not directly involved in adhesion but CLAG does appear to be required for cytoadherence. Parasite modified band 3 (the major anion transporter) contributes to adhesion probably by binding to thrombospondin (TSA). Sequestrin is a distinct parasite derived protein also mediating adhesion. The ring stage adhesion[119] (not shown) is distinct from *Pf*EMP1, and expressed in the first third of the asexual cycle. On the vascular endothelial side many molecules facilitate adhesion by binding *Pf*EMP1. The most important is the cellular differentiation antigen: CD36. Intercellular adhesion molecule 1 (ICAM 1) is important particularly in the brain, elsewhere it synergises with CD36. Chondroitin sulphate A (CSA) attached to thrombomodulin (TM), and hyaluronic acid (HA) are very important for placental sequestration. The other identified adhesion molecules are vascular cell adhesion molecule 1 (VCAM1), E-selectin, platelet endothelial cell adhesion molecule 1 (PECAM1), $\alpha_v \beta_3$ integrin, heparan sulphate (HS) and P-selectin.

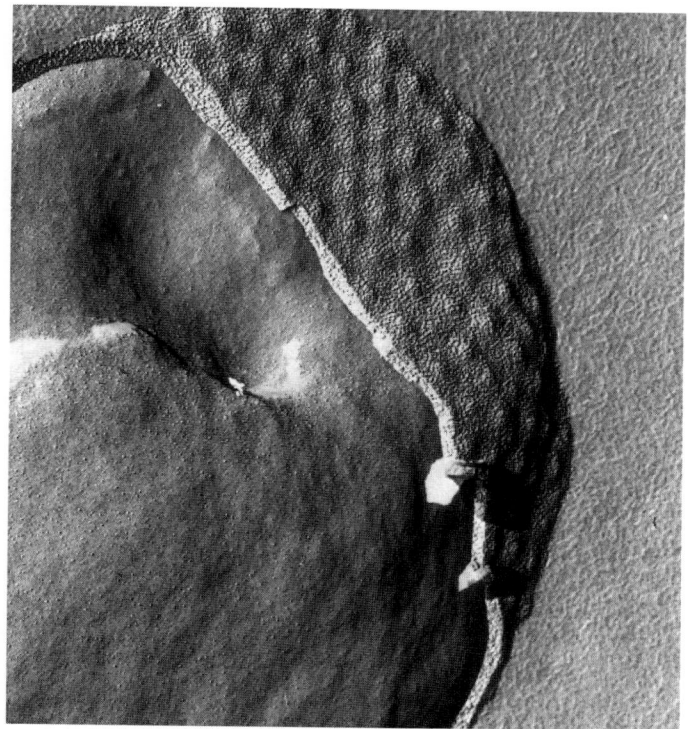

Figure 71.8: Freeze fracture electron micrograph of the membrane of a red cell containing mature *P. falciparum* showing regularly spaced knobs. (Courtesy of David Ferguson.)

similar to *Pf*EMP$_1$ named sequestrin (molecular mass 270 kDa) has been identified on the surface of infected red blood cells using anti-idiotypic antibodies raised against one of the putative vascular receptors CD36 (see below).[127] The protein MESA may also be partially expressed on the surface of the red cell and has been suggested as a contributor to cytoadherence.[128] The central role of parasite-derived proteins in cytoadherence is not accepted by all researchers. It has been suggested that cytoadherence is mediated by altered red cell membrane components such as a modified form of the red cell cytoskeleton protein band 3 (the major erythrocyte anion transporter, also called *Pf*alhesin). In culture, most parasites lose the ability to cytoadhere after several cycles of replication. In vivo, cytoadherence may be modulated by the spleen.[129] This has been shown in *Saimiri* monkeys infected with *P. falciparum*. Parasitized erythrocytes do not cytoadhere in splenectomized monkeys. In rare patients who have had a splenectomy all stages of the parasite are seen in peripheral blood smears.[130]

Vascular endothelial ligands

Several different sticky proteins present on the surface of vascular endothelium have been shown to bind parasitized red blood cells (Figure 71.7). The interaction between these proteins and the variant surface adhesin of the parasitized red cell is complex. The property of cytoadherence can be

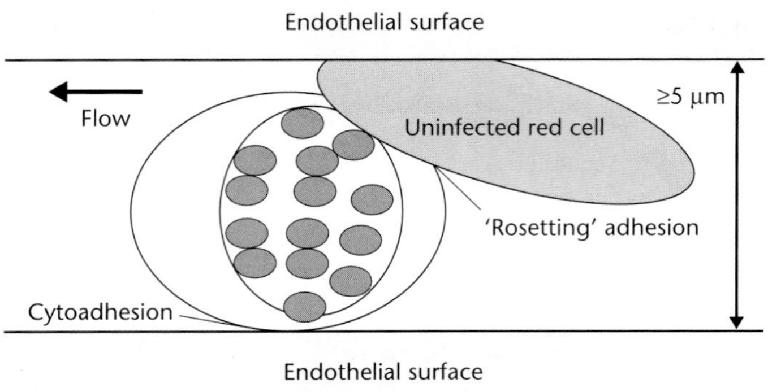

Figure 71.9: Uninfected red cells must squeeze past the static rigid, spherical cytoadherent parasitized erythrocytes to maintain flow. This is compromised by the reduced deformability of uninfected red cells in severe malaria and the intererythrocytic adhesive forces that mediate rosetting.

studied in vitro with cells expressing the potential ligands on their surface (e.g., melanoma cells, human umbilical vein endothelial cells or COS cells) or with the immobilized purified candidate ligand proteins. Probably the most important of these proteins is the leucocyte differentiation antigen CD36;[121,131] nearly all freshly obtained parasites bind to CD36.[132] Binding is increased at low pH (< 7.0) and in the presence of high calcium concentrations.[133,134] CD36 is constitutively expressed on vascular endothelium and monocytes/macrophages, although it is usually not present on the surface of cerebral vessels.[135] The intercellular adhesion molecule (ICAM1), which is also the receptor for rhinovirus attachment, appears to be the major cytoadherence receptor in the brain.[135,136] ICAM1, but not CD36, is upregulated by cytokines (notably TNF), and provides a plausible pathological scenario whereby cytokine release enhances cytoadherence. At physiological shear rates (i.e., those likely to be encountered in the human microcirculation) the binding forces (circa 10^{-10} N) are similar for CD36 and ICAM1.[137,138] For both, the forces of attachment are lower than those required for detachment, which suggests post-attachment alterations to increase adhesion. Binding to the two ligands is synergistic.[139] Flow studies show first rolling of infected red blood cells along the vascular surface followed by tethering. Once stuck the parasitized erythrocytes remain attached until schizont rupture, and then the residual ghost's membranes (sometimes with attached malaria pigment) often remain tethered within the vessel. Thrombospondin (a natural ligand to CD36) will also bind to some parasitized red blood cells (probably to modified band 3), and recently the ubiquitous proteins VCAM, PECAM, E-selectin and alpha-beta integrin have also been shown to bind in some circumstances.[140] P-selectin has been shown to mediate rolling. The relative importance of these molecules and their interactions is still not clear. Chondroitin sulphate A (CSA) appears to be the major receptor for cytoadherence in the placenta.[141,142] Recently, hyaluronic acid has also been proposed as a candidate for placental adhesion.[143]

Antibodies which inhibit parasitized red cell cytoadherence to CSA are generally present in multigravidae in endemic areas, but not primegravidae.[143] This may explain why the adverse effects of pregnancy on birth weight are greater in primegravidae. Other as yet unidentified vascular receptors are also present, as sequestration also occurs in vessels expressing none of the potential ligands identified so far. Thus ICAM1 appears to be the major vascular ligand in the brain involved in cerebral sequestration, CSA in placenta, and CD36 is probably the major ligand in the other organs. The relationship between cytoadherence, measured ex vivo, and the severity of infection or clinical manifestations has been inconsistent between studies.[144] This is not particularly surprising as all parasitized erythrocytes cytoadhere. Severity is related to the number of parasites in the body and distribution of cytoadherence within the vital organs. The relative importance of parasite phenotype and the various potential vascular ligands in the pathophysiology of severe falciparum malaria and the precise role of the spleen still remains to be determined.

Rosetting

Erythrocytes containing mature parasites also adhere to uninfected erythrocytes.[145] This process leads to the formation of 'rosettes' when suspensions of parasitized erythrocytes are viewed under the microscope (Figure 71.10). Rosetting shares some characteristics of cytoadherence.[146,147] It starts at around 16 hours of asexual life cycle development (slightly after cytoadherence begins),[123] and it is trypsin-sensitive. Parasite species which do not sequester do rosette[148,149] and, unlike cytoadherence, rosetting is inhibited by certain heparin subfractions and calcium chelators. Furthermore, whereas all fresh isolates of *P. falciparum* cytoadhere, not all rosette. Rosetting is mediated by the attachment of specific domains of *Pf*EMP$_1$ to the complement receptor CR1, heparan sulphate, blood group A antigen, and probably other red cell surface molecules. Attachment is facilitated by serum components. The forces required to separate a rosette are approximately five times greater than those required to separate cytoadherent cells. When known rosetting parasite lines (K+R+) are perfused through the rat mesocaecum, an ex vivo model for the study of vascular perfusion, they cause significantly more microvascular obstruction than isolates which cytoadhere but do not rosette (K+R–).[150] Rosetting has been associated with severe malaria in some studies but not in others.[151–154] It has been suggested that rosetting might encourage cytoadherence by reducing flow (shear rate), which would enhance anaerobic glycolysis, reduce pH and facilitate adherence of infected erythrocytes to venular endothelium. Rosetting tends to start in venules, and this could certainly reduce flow. The adhesive forces involved in rosetting could also impede forward flow of uninfected erythrocytes as they squeeze past sticky cytoadherent parasitized red blood cells in capillaries and venules[155,156] (Figure 71.8). The mechanical obstruction or 'static hindrance' would

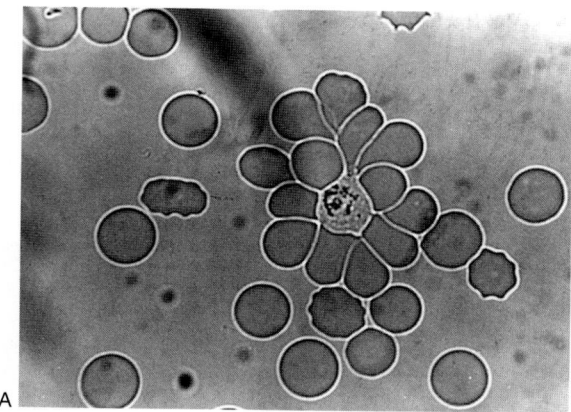

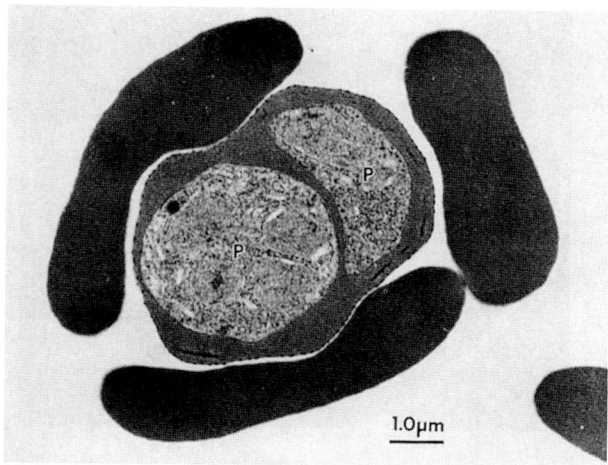

Figure 71.10: Rosetting. **(A)** Uninfected red blood cells bind to a *P. vivax*-infected erythrocyte. (Courtesy of R. Udomsangpetch.) **(B)** Transmission electron micrograph of a rosette around a *P. falciparum*-infected erythrocyte. (Courtesy of D. Ferguson.)

be compounded by the lack of deformability of the adherent, and circulating parasitized red blood cells.

Aggregation

A new adherence property of parasitized red blood cells has recently been characterized and associated with disease severity in African children.[157] This is the platelet-mediated aggregation of parasitized erythrocytes and is mediated via platelet CD36. These cells clump together in ex vivo cultures. Aggregation could also contribute to vascular occlusion.

Deformability

As the parasite matures inside the erythrocyte, the normally flexible biconcave disc becomes progressively more spherical and rigid.[44,155] The reduction in deformability results from reduced membrane fluidity, increasing sphericity, and the enlarging and relatively rigid intraerythrocytic parasite. Infected red blood cells are less filterable than uninfected cells. However, reduced infected red cell deformability alone cannot account for microvascular obstruction as it would lead to obstruction at the mid-capillary (i.e., the smallest internal diameter in the vasculature) and could not explain sequestration in venules.[116,156] Loss of *uninfected* red cell deformability has been recognized recently as a major contributor to disease severity and outcome. Increased erythrocyte rigidity measured at the low shear stresses encountered in capillaries and venules is correlated closely with outcome in severe malaria.[156,158] When assessed at the shear rates encountered on the arterial side of the circulation, and importantly in the spleen, reduced red cell deformability correlates with anaemia.[159]

Immunological processes

It has been suggested that severe malaria, and in particular cerebral malaria, results from specific immune-mediated damage. This is unlikely. In relation to the degree of parasitizd red blood cell sequestration, relatively few leuco-cytes are found in or around the cerebral vessels in fatal cases (although there are more in children than adults). Thus there is little pathological evidence in man for widepread cerebral vasculitis. Indeed, fatal falciparum malaria is remarkable for the lack of extravascular pathology. Although some glomerular abnormalities have been noted in fatal malaria,[160] the clinical and pathological findings suggest that acute tubular necrosis, and not acute glomerulonephritis, is the cause of renal dysfunction. The pathogenesis of pulmonary oedema is uncertain – as it is for the adult respiratory distress syndrome in other conditions – but it is unlikely to involve a specific immune-mediated process. Despite the enormous intravascular antigenic load in malaria, with the formation and deposition of immune complexes and variable complement depletion,[161–164] there is little evidence of a specific immuno-pathological process in severe malaria.

Acute malaria infections are associated with malaria antigen-specific unresponsiveness.[165–167] This selective paresis is one of the factors contributing to the slow development of an effective and specific immune response in malaria. Acute malaria is characterized by non-specific polyclonal B-cell activation. There is a reduction in circulating T cells with an increase in the γ/δ T-cell subset,[168] but other T-cell proportions are usually normal.[169] Although residents of hyperendemic or holoendemic malarious areas have hypergammaglobulinaemia, most of this antibody is not directed against malaria antigens.[170] In non-immune individuals, the acute antibody response to infection often comprises mostly IgM or IgG_2, isotypes which are unable to arm cytotoxic cells and thus kill asexual malaria parasites.[171] These observations have led to the suggestion that malaria induces an immunological 'smoke-screen' with broad-spectrum and non-specific activation that interferes with the orderly development of a specific cellular immune response. In severe malaria there is evidence of a broader immune suppression,[172] with defects in monocyte and neutrophil chemotaxis, reduced monocytic phagocytic function and a tendency to bacterial super-infection.[172–174]

In the nephrotic syndrome associated with chronic *P. malariae* infections, malaria antigen and immune complexes can be eluted from the kidney, indicating a role for quartan malaria in this condition.[175] Why some children are affected but the majority are not remains unresolved.

Permeability

There is evidence of a mild generalized increase in systemic vascular permeability in severe malaria.[176] In the past it was suggested that cerebral malaria resulted from an increase in cerebral capillary permeability which led to brain swelling, coma and death.[177–178] It is now clear from imaging studies that the majority of adults and children with cerebral malaria have no evidence of cerebral oedema (Figure 71.11).[179–181] However, the role of raised intracranial pressure in cerebral malaria still remains unclear. Whereas 80% of adults have opening pressures at lumbar puncture which are in the normal range (<200 mm CSF), 80% of children have elevated opening pressures (>100 mm CSF: the normal range is lower in children)[182–184] and intracranial pressure may rise transiently to very high levels. Some patients with cerebral malaria die from acute respiratory arrest with neurological signs that are compatible with brain stem compression. But these signs are also common, and may persist for many hours, in survivors. The elevation in opening pressure is usually not great (in general it is much lower than in bacterial or fungal meningitis), and there is no difference between these lumbar puncture opening pressures in surviving children and fatal cases.[184] Studies of com-

puterized tomography or magnetic resonance imaging have generally shown slight brain swelling in cerebral malaria (compatible with an increased intracerebral blood volume), but no cerebral oedema.[179–181] Immunohistochemical studies on autopsy brain tissues indicate focal disruption of endothelial junctions, and endothelial

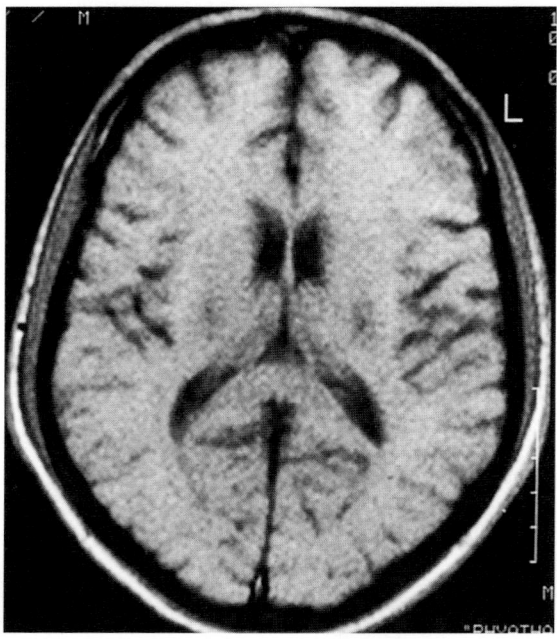

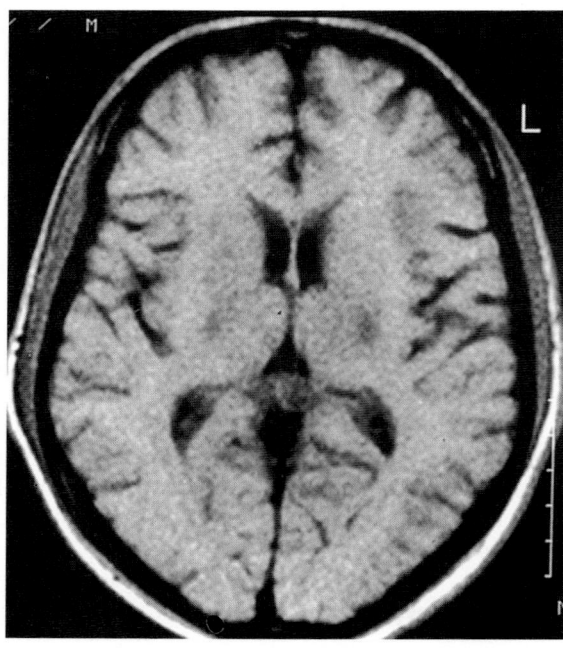

Figure 71.11: (*Cont'd*) T$_1$-weighted magnetic resonance imaging (550/25 TR/TE) of the brain in a 28-year-old man with cerebral malaria. (**B**) Following recovery of consciousness showing shrinkage. (**C**) 135 days later the brain is normal. There was no evidence of cerebral oedema on T$_2$-weighted images. The acute swelling was interpreted as representing increased intracerebral blood volume. (From Looareesuwan et al. *Clin Infect Dis* 1995; 21, with permission.)

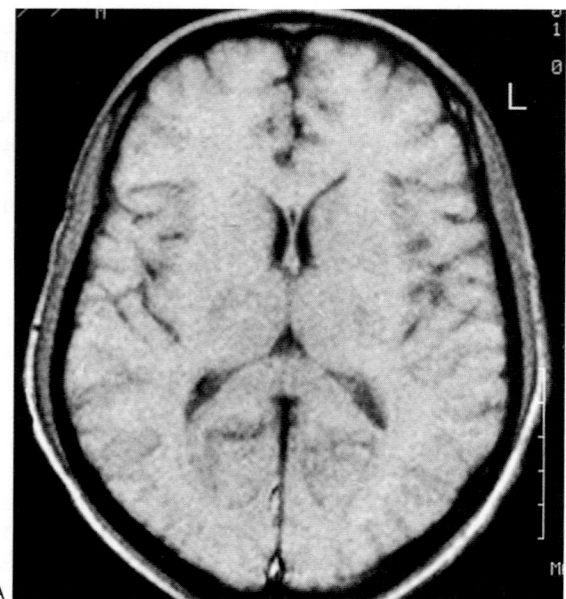

Figure 71.11: T$_1$-weighted magnetic resonance imaging (550/25 TR/TE) of the brain in a 28-year-old man with cerebral malaria. (**A**) During coma showing slight swelling.

activation in areas of intense sequestration, but clinical investigation has also failed to detect major alterations in blood–brain barrier permeability.[185–188] Thus, raised intracranial pressure probably arises from an increase in cerebral blood volume, independent of permeability.[189] This results from the circulating blood required to maintain cerebral perfusion in the presence of a considerable sequestered static biomass of intracerebral parasites. Children may be particularly vulnerable as after the skull sutures have fused, there is less space for cranial expansion than in adults. The relationship between intracerebral pressure and volume is non-linear (i.e., once the brain has expanded to fill the skull, only small further increases in volume cause large increases in intracranial pressure). The possibility that a sudden rise in intracranial pressure accounts for some deaths cannot be excluded.[189]

Pathogenesis of coma

The cause of coma in cerebral malaria is not known. There is undoubtedly an increase in cerebral anaerobic glycolysis with cerebral blood flows that are inappropriately low for the arterial oxygen content, increased cerebral metabolic rates for lactate, and increased CSF concentrations of lactate,[190,191] but these changes do not provide sufficient explanation for coma.[116,189] Presumably the metabolic milieu created adjacent to the sequestered and highly metabolically active parasites and their attachment to the activated cerebral vascular endothelium alters endothelial and blood–brain barrier function. But how this interferes with neurotransmission is not known. Cytokines increase production of nitric oxide, a potent inhibitor of neurotransmission, by leucocytes, smooth muscle cells, microglia and vascular endothelium through induction of the enzyme nitric oxide synthase. Inducible nitric oxide synthase expression is increased in the brain in fatal cerebral malaria.[192] Local synthesis of nitric oxide could well be relevant to the impairment of consciousness. Coma in malaria is not caused by raised intracranial pressure. There has been considerable interest in the mechanism of coma, and attempts to reverse it. But it should be remembered that the brain in cerebral malaria has a compromised blood supply, and waking a patient from coma may result in an increased cerebral metabolic demand. Coma in cerebral malaria could be neuroprotective.

Renal failure

There is renal cortical vasoconstriction and consequent hypoperfusion in severe falciparum malaria.[193] Renal vascular resistance is increased in patients with acute renal failure (ARF). The renal injury in severe malaria results from acute tubular neurosis.[194] The oxygen consumption of the kidneys is reduced in ARF, and it is not improved by dopamine-induced arteriolar vasodilatation and the consequent increase in renal blood flow which suggests a fixed injury.[195] Acute tubular necrosis presumably results

from renal microvascular obstruction and cellular injury consequent upon sequestration in the kidney and the filtration of free haemoglobin, myoglobin and other cellular material. Significant glomerulonephritis is very rare.[196,197] The role of systemic and local cytokine release and altered regulation of renal microvascular flow is uncertain., although in a recent study elevated plasma TNF was associated with renal impairment.[111] Massive haemolysis compounds the insult in blackwater fever complicating malaria, and haemoglobinuria may itself lead to renal impairment.[198,199] Mild renal impairment occurs in young children with severe malaria, but established acute renal failure is almost confined to older children and adults.

Pulmonary oedema

Despite intense sequestration in the myocardial vessels, the heart's pump function is remarkably well preserved in severe malaria. Pulmonary oedema in malaria results from a sudden increase in pulmonary capillary permeability that is not reflected in other vascular beds.[200–202] The pulmonary capillary wedge pressure is usually normal and the threshold for the development of pulmonary oedema is relatively low. Whereas acute renal failure, severe metabolic acidosis and coma are seen only in falciparum malaria, acute pulmonary oedema may also occur in vivax malaria. The cause of this increase in pulmonary capillary permeability is not known.

Fluid space and electrolyte changes

Following rehydration, the plasma volume is increased in moderate and severe malaria.[203–205] Total body water and extracellular volume are normal. Plasma renin activity, aldosterone and antidiuretic hormone concentrations are elevated, reflecting an appropriate activation of homeostatic mechanisms to maintain adequate circulating volume in the presence of general vasodilatation and a falling haematocrit. Mild hyponatraemia and hypochloraemia are common in severe malaria, but serum potassium concentrations are usually normal. Occasionally hyponatraemia is severe. Recent studies in Kenyan children indicate inappropriate antidiuretic hormone (arginine vasopressin) secretion in two-thirds of cases.[206]

Anaemia

The pathogenesis of anaemia is multifactorial.[207,208] There is obligatory destruction of red blood cells containing parasites at merogony, there is accelerated destruction of non-parasitized red blood cells that parallels disease severity and there is bone marrow dyserythropoeisis.[209,210] In severe malaria anaemia develops rapidly; the rapid haemolysis of unparasitized red blood cells is the major contributor to the decline in haematocrit.[211–213] Bone marrow dyserythropoeisis persists for days or weeks following acute malaria and reticulocyte counts are usually low in the acute phase of the disease.[214,215] The cause of the dyserythropoiesis is thought to be related to intra-medullary cytokine production. Severe malarial anaemia in African children has been associated with the 238A TNF promoter polymorphism and low levels of the anti-inflammatory cytokine IL-10.[63] Serum erythropoetin levels are usually elevated, although in some series it has been suggested that the degree of elevation was not sufficient for the degree of anaemia.[216–218] In falciparum malaria the entire red cell population (i.e., both infected and uninfected red blood cells) becomes more rigid. This loss of deformability correlates with disease severity and outcome[157,158] and, when measured at the high shear rates encountered in the spleen, with the degree of resulting anaemia.[159] The mechanism responsible has not been identified, although there is evidence in acute malaria for increased oxidative damage which might compromise red cell membrane function and deformability.[219] In simian malarias there is evidence of an inversion of the erythrocyte membrane lipid bilayer in uninfected erythrocytes,[220] but this has not been studied in man. The role of antibody (i.e., Coombs'-positive haemolysis) in anaemia is unresolved.[221–223] The majority of studies to date do not show increased red blood cell immunoglobulin binding in malaria, but in the presence of a lowered recognition threshold for splenic clearance, this might be difficult to detect. The splenic threshold for the clearance of abnormal erythrocytes, whether because of antibody coating or reduced deformability, is lowered.[85–87] Thus the spleen removes large numbers of relatively rigid cells resulting in shortened erythrocyte survival, particularly in severe malaria. This is unaffected by corticosteroids.[224]

In the context of acute uncomplicated malaria the anaemia is worse in younger children, and those with protracted infections. Loss of unparasitized erythrocytes accounts for approximately 90% of the acute anaemia resulting from a single infection.[211] Iron deficiency and malaria often coincide in the same patient, and in some areas routine iron supplementation following malaria promotes recovery from anaemia.

Coagulopathy and thrombocytopenia

There is accelerated coagulation cascade activity with accelerated fibrinogen turnover, consumption of anti-thrombin III, reduced factor XIII and increased concentrations of fibrin degradation products in acute malaria.[225–229] In severe infections the prothrombin and partial thromboplastin times may be prolonged, and in occasional patients (<5%) bleeding may be significant. The coagulation cascade is activated via the intrinsic pathway.[230] Intravascular thrombus formation is observed rarely at autopsy in fatal cases. Fibrin deposition is sparse and platelets are strikingly unusual.[117]

Thrombocytopenia is common to all the four human malarias and is caused by increased splenic platelet clearance.[231] This is associated with appropriately raised concentrations of thrombopoeitin (a key growth factor for platelet production). Plasma concentrations of macrophage colony stimulating factor are high, which stimulate macrophage activity and may increase platelet destruction.[232] Platelet turnover is increased. The role of platelet-bound antibody in malarial thrombocytopenia is controversial.[233–235] There has been evidence of platelet activation in some studies, but not others.[236] Erythrocytes containing mature parasites may activate the coagulation cascade directly,[237] and cytokine release is also procoagulant. The high plasma levels of P-selectin found in severe malaria may derive from platelets, but could also come from vascular endothelium, as plasma concentrations of other endothelial-derived proteins (thrombomodulin, ICAM1, VCAM) are elevated as well.[238,239] It was suggested in the past that disseminated intravascular coagulation (DIC) is important in the pathogenesis of severe malaria,[240–242] but detailed prospective clinical and pathological studies have refuted this. Coagulation cascade activity is directly proportional to disease severity,[228] but hypofibrinogenaemia resulting from DIC is significant in less than 5% of patients with severe malaria, and lethal haemorrhage (usually gastrointestinal) is very unusual.[243]

Blackwater fever (Figure 71.12)

This is a poorly understood condition in which there is massive intravascular haemolysis and the passage of 'Coca-Cola'-coloured urine.[244] Blackwater (urine) occurs

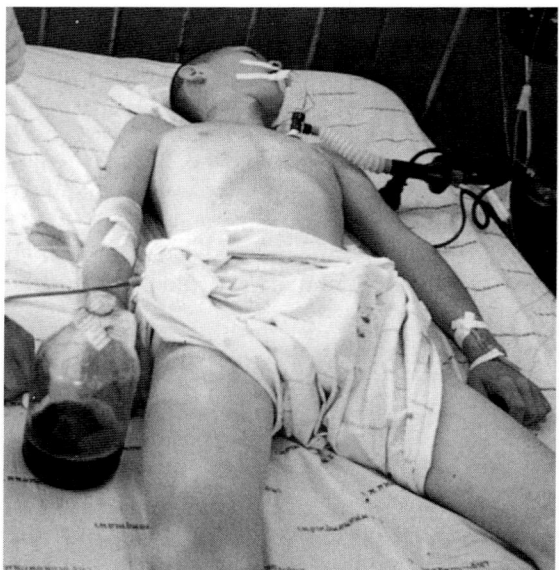

Figure 71.12: Blackwater fever. A 25-year-old male with severe malaria, pulmonary oedema, renal impairment and massive haemolysis.

in three circumstances: (1) when patients with G6PD deficiency take oxidant drugs (e.g., primaquine or sulphonamides) irrespective of whether they have malaria or not; (2) occasionally when patients with G6PD deficiency have malaria and receive quinine treatment; and (3) in some patients with severe quinine-treated falciparum malaria who have normal erythrocyte G6PD levels. How quinine causes blackwater in these last two situations is not known as it is not an oxidant drug. G6PD-deficient red blood cells are particularly susceptible to oxidant stress as they are unable to synthesize adequate quantities of NADPH through the pentose shunt. This leads to low intraerythrocytic levels of reduced glutathione, and both alterations in the erythrocyte membrane and increased susceptibility to organic peroxides. Blackwater fever may be associated with acute renal failure, although in the majority of cases renal function remains normal.[244]

The spleen

There is considerable splenic enlargement in malaria, and an increased capacity to clear red blood cells from the circulation both by Fc receptor-mediated (immune) mechanisms[86,87] and by recognition of reduced deformability (filtration).[85] The increased filtration of the spleen and the reduced deformability of the entire red cell population[159] results in the rapid development of anaemia in severe malaria. The spleen may also modulate cytoadherence.[129] It plays a central role in limiting the acute expansion of the malaria infection by removing parasitized erythrocytes, and this has led to the suggestion that a failure to augment splenic clearance sufficiently rapidly may be a factor in the development of severe malaria. The spleen is capable of removing damaged intraerythrocytic parasites and returning the once infected red blood cells to the circulation (a process known as 'pitting'),[245] where they have shortened survival.[246] This is an important contributor to parasite clearance following antimalarial drug treatment (particularly treatment with artemisinin derivatives).[247]

Gastrointestinal dysfunction

Abdominal pain may be prominent in acute malaria. Minor stress ulceration of the stomach and duodenum is common in severe malaria. The pattern of malabsorption of sugars, fats, and amino acids suggests reduced splanchnic perfusion.[248–250] This results from both gut sequestration and visceral vasoconstriction. Gut permeability is increased,[251] and this may be associated with reduced local defences against bacterial toxins, or even whole bacteria in severe disease. Antimalarial drug absorption is remarkably unaffected in uncomplicated malaria, except for those drugs which have fat (i.e., food)-dependent absorption (halofantrine, atovaquone, lumefantrine).

Liver dysfunction

Jaundice is common in adults with severe malaria, and there is other evidence of hepatic dysfunction, with reduced clotting factor synthesis, reduced metabolic clearance of the antimalarial drugs, and a failure of gluconeogenesis which contributes to lactic acidosis and hypoglycaemia. Nevertheless, true liver failure (as in fulminant viral hepatitis) is very unusual. There is sequestration in the hepatic microvasculature, and although many patients with acute falciparum malaria have elevated liver blood flow values, in very severe infections liver blood flow is reduced.[251–253] Liver blood flow values less than 15 ml/kg per minute are associated with elevated venous lactate concentrations,[253] which suggests a flow limitation to lactate clearance and thus a contribution of liver dysfunction to lactic acidosis. Recent direct measurements of hepatic venous lactate concentrations in severe malaria confirm that the hepatosplanchnic extraction ratio is inversely correlated with mixed venous plasma lactate (i.e., hyperlactataemia is associated with reduced liver clearance of lactate).[254] There is no relationship evident between liver blood flow and impairment of antimalarial drug clearance.[255] Jaundice in malaria appears to have haemolytic, hepatic, and cholestatic components. Cholestatic jaundice may persist well into the recovery period.

Acidosis

Acidosis is a major cause of death in severe falciparum malaria. This is mainly a lactic acidosis, although ketoacidosis (and sometimes salicylate intoxication) may predominate in children, and the acidosis of renal failure is common in adults.[254,256–259] In severe malaria the arterial, capillary, venous and CSF concentrations of lactate rise in direct proportion to disease severity. Indeed, the venous lactate concentration 4 hours after admission to hospital is a very good indicator of prognosis in severe malaria (the best is the simple venous plasma bicarbonate). In bacterial sepsis there is hyperlactataemia, but, unless there is profound shock, the lactate-pyruvate ratio is usually less than 15. This indicates that hypermetabolism is the source of lactate accumulation in sepsis. In severe malaria the pathogenesis is different; lactate-pyruvate ratios often exceed 30 reflecting tissue hypoxia and anaerobic glycolysis. Lactic acidosis results from several discrete processes: the tissue anaerobic glycolysis consequent upon microvascular obstruction; a failure of hepatic and renal lactate clearance; and the production of lactate by the parasite.[116,260,261] Mature malaria parasites consume up to 70 times as much glucose as uninfected cells, and over 90% of this is converted to L-lactic acid (plasmodia do not have the complete set of enzymes necessary for the citric acid cycle). Interestingly, up to 6% of the lactic acid appears as D-lactate, but this does not contribute materially to the acidosis.[262] However, calculations based on glucose and lactate turnover in man indicate that the majority of the lactic acid produced in malaria derives from host rather than parasite sources. Lactate levels also rise after generalized convulsions. Lactate turnover in both adults and children with severe malaria is increased approximately threefold compared with values obtained in healthy adults.[263,264] Studies in children using stable isotope techniques indicate that increased lactate production (resulting from anaerobic glycolysis) rather than reduced clearance is the main cause of lactate accumulation,[264] although in adults reduced clearance is certainly a contributor.[254] Hyperlactataemia is associated with hypoglycaemia and is accompanied by hyperalaninaemia and elevated glycerol concentrations reflecting the impairment of gluconeogenesis through the Cori cycle.[265–268] Lactate, glutamine, and alanine are the major gluconeogenic precursors. Triglyceride and free fatty acid levels are also elevated in acute malaria,[269] and plasma concentrations of ketone bodies are raised in patients who have been unable to eat. Ketoacidosis may be prominent in children. In severe malaria there is dysfunction of all organ systems, particularly those with obligatory high metabolic rates. The endocrine glands are no exception. Pituitary-thyroid axis abnormalities result in the 'sick euthyroid' syndrome and also parathyroid dysfunction.[270] Mild hypocalcaemia is common,[271,272] and hypophosphataemia may be profound in the very seriously ill.[271] By contrast, the pituitary-adrenal axis appears normal in acute malaria.[273]

Hypoglycaemia

Hypoglycaemia is associated with hyperlactataemia and shares the same pathophysiological aetiology: an increased peripheral requirement for glucose consequent upon anaerobic glycolysis (the Pasteur effect); the increased metabolic demands of the febrile illness,[265–268] and the obligatory demands of the parasites which use glucose as their major fuel (all of which increase demand); and a failure of hepatic gluconeogenesis and glycogenolysis (reduced supply). Hepatic glycogen is exhausted rapidly: stores in fasting adults last approximately two days, but children only have enough for 12 hours. Healthy children have approximately three times higher rates of glucose turnover compared with adults, but in severe malaria turnover is increased by more than 50% (to values five times higher than those in adults with severe malaria).[274–276] The net result of impaired gluconeogenesis, limited glycogen stores, and greatly increased demand results in hypoglycaemia in 20–30% of children with severe malaria. In patients treated with quinine, this is compounded by quinine-stimulated pancreatic β-cell insulin secretion.[265,267,277,278] Hyperinsulinaemia is balanced by a reduced tissue sensitivity to insulin,[279] which returns to normal as the patient improves. This probably explains why quinine-induced (hyperinsulinaemic) hypoglycaemia tends to occur after the first 24 hours of treatment, whereas malaria-related hypoglycaemia (with appropriate suppression of insulin secretion) is often present when the patient with severe malaria is first admitted. Hypoglycaemia contributes to nervous system dysfunction, and in cerebral malaria is associated with residual neurological deficit in survivors.

Placental dysfunction

Pregnancy increases susceptibility to malaria. This is probably caused by a suppression of systemic and placental cell-mediated immune responses.[280] There is intense sequestration of *P. falciparum*-infected erythrocytes in the placenta,[281] local activation of pro-inflammatory cytokine production, and maternal anaemia. This leads to placental insufficiency[282–286] and fetal growth retardation. Illness close to term also results in prematurity. In areas of intense transmission, a malaria-attributable reduction in birth weight (circa 170 g) is confined to primigravidae. There is no convincing evidence that malaria causes abortion or stillbirth in this context. With lower levels of transmission (i.e., less immunity) the risk extends to other pregnancies[287] and there is a propensity to develop severe malaria with a high incidence of fetal death.[288] The recent discovery that *P. vivax*, a parasite not thought to cytoadhere, also reduces birth weight (by about two-thirds the amount caused by *P. falciparum*),[12] has questioned the primary role of sequestration in the pathogenesis of placental insufficiency.

Bacterial infection

Patients with severe malaria are vulnerable to bacterial infections, particularly of the lungs and urinary tract (following catheterization). Postpartum sepsis is also common. Spontaneous bacterial septicaemia may also occur in severe malaria. This is relatively unusual in adults (probably less than 1% of cases) but is more common in young children.[289–291] In malaria endemic areas, where parasitaemia is common in children, it may be difficult to distinguish bacterial infections with *coincident* parasitaemia from infections complicating malaria. Salmonella septicaemias are an important complication of otherwise uncomplicated falciparum malaria in African children.[291]

Pathology

As the benign human malarias are rarely fatal there is very little information available on the pathology of these infections. Unfortunately this is not the case for *P. falciparum* malaria. In fatal malaria the microvasculature of the vital organs is packed with erythrocytes containing mature forms of the parasite.[292–298] There is abundant intra- and extra-erythrocytic pigment and organs such as the liver, spleen and placenta may be grey-black in colour. Sequestration is not uniformly distributed; it tends to be greatest in the brain and heart,[117,299] followed by the gut, kidney, adipose tissue, liver, lungs and least of all in bone marrow and skin. There is remarkably little extravascular pathology in malaria.

Brain

If the patient dies from the acute infection the brain is commonly slightly swollen with multiple small petechial haemorrhages throughout the white matter.[292–300] Different architectural types of haemorrhage are seen: simple petechial, zonal ring haemorrhages, and Durck's granulomata. Haemorrhages are less prominent in the grey matter. Large haemorrhages or infarcts are rare. There is usually no evidence of tentorial or foramen magnum herniation. Many capillaries and venules are packed with erythrocytes containing mature forms of the parasite (whereas these are seen rarely in peripheral blood smears).[117] This sequestration is particularly prominent in the white matter, although the tissue is much less vascular than the grey matter. The degree of cerebral sequestration and the intensity of erythrocyte packing is greater in cerebral malaria than in fatal malaria in which the patient was not comatose.[117,299] A large quantity of intra- and extra-erythrocytic pigment is evident. In the white matter, accumulations of glial cells are seen surrounding haemorrhagic foci (Durck's granuloma) where vessels appear to have been occluded by a mass of parasitized cells, and then ruptured. At the ultrastructural level the erythrocytes are seen to be packed closely together and the infected red blood cells are adherent to the vascular endothelium by attachment of knob-like surface projections to the endothelial surface.[117,299,300] Occasional fibrin strands are seen, but there are relatively few platelets[117] and usually no leucocyte aggregation, i.e., there is no evidence of thrombus formation or vasculitis. On immunofluorescent staining malarial antigens may be seen on the endothelial basement membrane,[301,302] but the significance of this observation is uncertain (i.e., does it reflect pathology in vivo or an agonal artefact?). In some cases there are only few or no parasites in the cerebral vessels. This is seen when death occurred several days after parasite clearance.

Heart and lungs

Despite intense sequestration in the myocardial microvasculature the heart is remarkably normal, although petechial epicardial haemorrhages are common and in anaemic patients the heart is commonly pale and dilated. As in all other organs, extravascular pathological changes are rare. In adults there is often evidence of pulmonary oedema. Hyaline membrane formation suggests leakage of proteinaceous fluid. There is moderate sequestration[303,304] and leucocyte aggregates are more prominent than in the brain. There may be secondary bacterial pneumonia.

Liver and spleen

The liver is generally enlarged and may be black from malaria pigment. There is congestion of the centrilobular capillaries with sinusoidal dilatation and Kupffer cell hyperplasia.[305] Sequestration of parasitized erythrocytes is associated with variable cloudy swelling of the hepatocytes and perivenous ischaemic changes, and sometimes centrizonal necrosis. Hepatic glycogen is often present despite hypoglycaemia. In uncomplicated malaria the liver histology is often normal.[306,307] The spleen is often dark or black from malaria pigment, enlarged, soft and friable. It is full of erythrocytes containing mature and immature parasites.[308] There is evidence of reticular hyperplasia and architectural reorganization.[309] The soft and acutely enlarged spleen of acute lethal infections contrasts with the hard fibrous enlargement associated with repeated malaria.

Kidneys

The kidneys are often slightly swollen. In adults there are commonly tubular abnormalities consistent with ischaemia. There is sequestration, particularly in the glomerular capillaries,[193] and sometimes mesangial and endothelial cell proliferative changes are seen. Leucocyte sequestration is similar to that in the lung and more marked than in the brain. Immunofluorescent studies show immunoglobulin deposition on the glomerular capillary basement membranes.

Alimentary tract

Upper gastrointestinal bleeding from erosions may occur in severe malaria. There is intense sequestration in the gut, and visceral ischaemia may explain the acute abdominal pain that sometimes occurs in severe malaria.[249] Despite this, drug absorption is often remarkably normal.

Bone marrow

Dyserythropoetic change is prominent in all the acute malarias.[207,212,213,310] Bone marrow macrophages contain pigment, and erythrophagocytosis may be seen. Iron is usually plentiful. The platelet and white cell series are usually normal.

Placenta

The placenta may be black from malaria pigment even if the mother is asymptomatic throughout her pregnancy. Large numbers of mature parasites are seen on crush smears,[311] although the peripheral blood smear may be negative. There is often trophoblastic thickening, macrophage infiltration and perivillous fibrin deposition. Active infection is associated with basement membrane thickening, fibrinoid necrosis and syncitial knots.[312–316]

Chronic infection is associated with marked mononuclear cell infiltration.

Clinical features

The clinical manifestations of malaria are dependent on the previous immune status of the host. In areas of intense *P. falciparum* malaria transmission, asymptomatic parasitaemia is usual in adults (premunition). Severe malaria never occurs in this age group: it is confined to the first years of life, and becomes progressively less frequent with increasing age. The rate at which age-specific acquisition of premunition occurs is proportional to the intensity of malaria transmission. In areas with a constant high-level *P. falciparum* transmission (e.g., average infected anopheline biting frequencies of daily up to monthly), severe malaria occurs predominantly between 6 months and 3 years of age; mild symptoms are seen in older children, and adults are usually asymptomatic and have low parasitaemias. Malaria is common in pregnancy, but is asymptomatic (although anaemia may be severe), but the birth weight of babies born to primagravidae is reduced significantly. Spleen rates will be high (>50%) in children between 2 and 9, corresponding with the epidemiological terms hyperendemic and holoendemic malaria. Severe anaemia in infancy is the most common presentation of severe falciparum malaria in these circumstances. With lower or more seasonal or unstable transmission patterns the age distribution of severe malaria shifts upwards; severe malaria is seen in older children as well, and cerebral malaria becomes the most prominent manifestation (Figure 71.1). Spleen rates in children are lower than 50%. With even lower or more sporadic patterns of transmission, and when non-immunes travel to endemic areas, symptomatic disease is seen at all ages. Severe malaria does not occur with *P. vivax*, *P. ovale* or *P. malariae* but acute infection in a non-immune patient is still serious and debilitating. With more intense exposure a state of premunition is also reached with these infections.

Incubation period

Precise data on the incubation period of malaria comes from the detailed studies of malaria therapy for neurosyphilis, and also the many hundreds of volunteer experiments conducted between the turn of the century and 1965 (Table 71.2).[65–67,71,72] In the majority of mosquito-transmitted infections several heavily infected anophelines were allowed to bite. The sporozoite inocula were therefore probably larger than those received in most naturally acquired (autochthonous) infections. In most cases of falciparum or vivax malaria the incubation period is approximately two weeks. The shortest incubation period documented was reported by Shute[317] in a sailor who docked briefly in West Africa and somehow developed malaria 3 days later. Primary incubation periods can be long, particularly if the infection is suppressed by partially effective chemoprophylaxis. Most tropical strains of *P. vivax* had similar incubation periods to *P. falciparum*, but some strains from cooler countries had extremely long incubation periods. The primary infection began 9–12 months after sporozoite inoculation. This coincided with the short summertime mosquito breeding season in these cold countries. These long incubation period strains of *P. vivax* (e.g., *P. vivax* var *hibernans*) acquired in northern and eastern Europe, Russia, central and northern China, are now nearly extinct but for a few areas of China, North Korea, and South Korea near the demilitarized zone.

In the artificial infection experiments the differences in recorded incubation periods between strains of the same *Plasmodium* species were small, although a negative correlation was apparent between the probable dose of sporozoites and the duration of the prepatent period (the time from sporozoite inoculation until the first positive blood film). The incubation period (time from sporozoite inoculation to fever) was prolonged by ineffective antimalarial treatment or prophylaxis—both of which reduce the effective multiplication rate.

The duration of the prepatent and incubation periods are also strongly influenced by previous exposure, i.e., 'immunity'. Effective immunity both reduces effective multiplication, which prolongs the prepatent period, and raises the threshold at which symptoms occur (premunition), which prolongs the incubation period. In vivax malaria the symptom threshold is raised disproportionately in immune individuals, i.e., the gap between the prepatent and incubation period widens.

Mixed infections

The incidence of mixed infections is nearly always underestimated. In simultaneous infection with *P. falciparum* and *P. vivax*, the former suppresses the latter, and the primary vivax malaria infection may not appear until several weeks later.[318,319] Sometimes the reverse occurs and *P. vivax* suppresses *P. falciparum*.[320] In Africa *P. falciparum* commonly occurs together with *P. malariae* or *P. ovale*. In many areas outside Africa *P. falciparum* and *P. vivax* are both common and coexistent infections are frequent but, because of mutual suppression, the incidence is considerably underestimated.[321–323] For example in Thailand approximately 30% of patients with *P. falciparum* malaria will have a subsequent symptomatic infection with *P. vivax* within two months of their primary falciparum malaria, without further exposure to malaria infection.[318] The converse *P. vivax* malaria with undiagnosed coincident *P. falciparum* infection occurs in 8% of cases.[320] Coincident infection of *P. falciparum* with *P. vivax* reduces the risk of severe malaria fourfold,[324] reduces the degree of anaemia,[211] and reduces *P. falciparum* gametocyte carriage.[325] Some researchers have said that *P. vivax* is the best falciparum malaria vaccine we have now! Mixed infections with *P. malariae* and *P. ovale* are also underestimated.[322,323]

Pyrogenic density

The parasitaemia at which fever (> 37.3°C) occurs is termed the 'pyrogenic density'. Similar estimates for both species have been derived from recent epidemiological studies. This varies widely: some non-immune patients will become febrile before parasites are visible on blood smears (i.e., the incubation period is shorter than the prepatent period), whereas immune adults can on occasions tolerate up to 100 000 *P. falciparum* parasites/μl without fever. The pyrogenic density for *P. vivax* is generally lower than that of *P. falciparum*; in 76% of cases reported by Kitchen[326] the pyrogenic density was < 100 parasites/μl. In *P. falciparum* infection average pyrogenic densities in non-immunes can be as high as 10 000/μl,[65,321] but it must be remembered that less than half the life cycle circulates in falciparum malaria.[327] The parasites in the blood smear are the circulating parasites in the generation subsequent to that which underwent pyrogenic merogony, and they are therefore an underestimate of the total parasite burden. The pyrogenic density is a marker of immunity. High pyrogenic densities indicate premunition, and a lower risk of severe disease. There are less data on pyrogenic densities in *P. malariae* infections, but it appears that they are higher than for *P. vivax*; values over 500/μl were found in 38% of Boyd's cases. There are limited data on *P. ovale*, but the available evidence suggests a pyrogenic density similar to *P. vivax*.

Uncomplicated malaria

The clinical features of uncomplicated malaria are common to all four species, although there is a suggestion that *P. vivax*, which tends to synchronize rapidly, may cause more severe symptoms early in the course of the infection. *P. malariae* and possibly *P. ovale* both have a more gradual onset than *P. vivax*. *P. falciparum* is unpredictable: the onset ranges from gradual to fulminant. The first symptoms of malaria are non-specific and resemble influenza. They are similar for all four species of *Plasmodium*. Headache, muscular ache, vague abdominal discomfort, lethargy, lassitude and dysphoria often precede fever by up to two days. The temperature rises erratically at first, with shivering, mild chills, worsening headache and malaise, and loss of appetite. Children are irritable, lethargic and anorexic. If the infection is left untreated the fever in *P. vivax* and *P. ovale* regularizes to a two-day cycle (tertian), and *P. malariae* fever spikes occur every three days (quartan pattern). *P. falciparum* remains erratic for longer, and may never regularize to a tertian pattern.[243] These terms derive from the Greek practice of inclusive reckoning, in which the beginning of the fever is considered day one. Thus, a tertian fever recurs every *third* day and a quartan fever every *fourth* day, with intervals of 2 and 3 days, respectively.

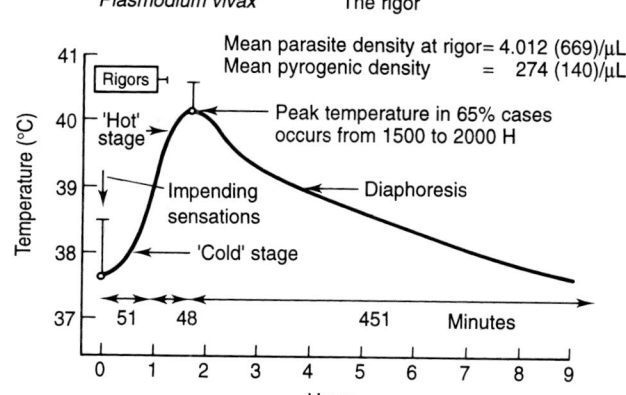

Figure 71.13: The rigor of *P. vivax* malaria. The time course of signs and symptoms is taken from Kitchen & Puttnam: *J Natl Malaria Soc* 1946; 5:57–78. True rigors are rare in *P. falciparum* malaria and occur only after the infections with the other three parasites have synchronized sufficiently.

Some infections consist of two broods cycling 24 hours out of phase and in these there is a daily fever spike (quotidian fever). Even more complex fever patterns are described in detail in the early literature.

The classical malaria fever charts (which graced earlier editions of this textbook), and the teeth-chattering rigors and profuse sweats that characterized the 'paroxysm' (Figure 71.13), are relatively unusual today as malaria therapy of neurosyphilis is no longer practised (penicillin is more effective and more pleasant), and symptomatic infections are treated as soon as they are diagnosed. In a true paroxysm the temperature usually rises steeply from a normal or slightly elevated level to exceed 39°C. As the temperature begins to rise there is intense headache and muscular discomfort. The patient feels cold, clutches at blankets, and curls up shivering and uncommunicative (the chill). There is peripheral vasoconstriction, and often 'goose-pimples'. Within minutes the limbs begin to shake and the teeth chatter, and the temperature climbs rapidly to a peak (usually between 39 and 41.5°C). The rigor usually last 10–30 minutes, but can last up to 90 minutes. By the end of the rigor there is peripheral vasodilatation and the skin feels hot. A profuse sweat then breaks out. The blood pressure is relatively low and there may be symptomatic orthostatic hypotension. The patient feels exhausted and may sleep. Defervescence usually takes 4–8 hours. Paroxysms with rigors are more common in *P. vivax* and *P. ovale* than in *P. falciparum* or *P. malariae* malaria. They may begin a relapse, or occur after several days of more chaotic fever in primary infections with these two malaria species. True rigors are unusual in naturally acquired falciparum malaria. As the infection continues the spleen and liver enlarge and anaemia develops. The patient loses weight. If no treatment is given the natural infection stabilizes for several weeks or months and then gradually resolves. The duration of illness is proportional to the level of immunity and differs between the parasite species.

Mild abdominal discomfort is common in malaria, and rarely patients may appear to have an 'acute abdomen'. Constipation or diarrhoea may occur. In some areas watery diarrhoea is a prominent manifestation. However, there is usually no difficulty distinguishing malaria from gastroenteritis. A dry cough has been reported in some series, but this is not prominent, and on chest examination there is no other clinical evidence of respiratory tract involvement. However, the respiratory rate may be raised, particularly in children, and this can give rise to diagnostic confusion in primary health care facilities where respiratory rate is used as the only criterion for the diagnosis of acute respiratory infection. In routine clinical practice in malarious areas of the tropics, malaria is the most common cause of fever in children and is the most likely diagnosis in a febrile patient with no obvious respiratory or abdominal abnormalities. In travellers returning from such areas any fever must be considered to be malaria unless proved otherwise. In semi-immune patients low-grade fever may be the only complaint in malaria. In tropical practice malaria is so common that it must be excluded in any febrile patient.

Relapse

Both *P. vivax* and *P. ovale* have a tendency to relapse after resolution of the primary infection. Relapse, which results from maturation of persistent hypnozoites in the liver, must be distinguished from recrudescence of the primary infection because of incomplete treatment. *P. falciparum* is the usual cause of recrudescent infections and these tend to arise 2–4 weeks following treatment (but this can be as long as 10 weeks following mefloquine treatment). Relapses occur weeks or months (or even years) after the primary infection. The proportion of cases relapsing and the intervals between relapses vary between strains. The pattern of relapse is determined largely by the geographic origin of the infection. The rare subtropical *P. vivax* infection tends to have long gaps between relapses, whereas tropical strains have short intervals (3–6 weeks). In Patrick Manson's famous experiment conducted in September 1900, he infected his 23-year-old son with *P. vivax* through mosquitoes sent by rail from Rome to London. His son became ill with 'double tertian fever', but was treated with quinine and recovered fully. In June 1901 he suddenly became ill again with vivax malaria, a relapse interval of nine months.[328,329] In recent years a relapse interval of six weeks has been quoted widely for tropical strains, but this is an artefact of the use of chloroquine which suppresses the first relapse (at three weeks). Blood levels have declined by the time of the second relapse at six weeks, and this is the first to manifest. The symptoms of a relapse start more abruptly than in the primary infection as the infection is more synchronous. They may begin with a sudden chill or rigor. Primaquine will eradicate hypnozoites in over 80% of patients but, if it is not given, relapse occurs in approximately half of those

infected (the proportion varies depending on the geographic region).

Malaria in pregnancy

In areas of intense transmission the principal impact of falciparum malaria in pregnancy is an increased incidence of anaemia and a reduction in birth weight (approximately 170 g on average) of babies born to primigravidae.[201] Thus a greater proportion of babies have low birth weights (<2.5 kg). Low birth weight is a major risk factor for infantile death. Malaria reduces birth weight mainly by intrauterine growth retardation (IUGR). In high transmission areas, malaria may also cause prematurity.[330] In low transmission areas prematurity is caused by symptomatic malaria close to term, not earlier in the pregnancy. The net result is an increased risk of neonatal death.[331] Despite intense sequestration of parasites in the placenta, the mothers are usually asymptomatic, although they are more likely to be anaemic. In areas with lower levels of malaria transmission (mesoendemic or hypoendemic) symptomatic disease occurs and pregnant women are at an increased risk of severe falciparum malaria, particularly in the second and third trimesters. In low transmission areas the adverse effects of malaria on birth weight extend to the first three pregnancies (and in non-immunes, to all pregnancies).[22] Again anaemia is common and there is an increased risk of developing severe malaria. Anaemia itself is a risk factor for maternal mortality; moderate anaemia (Hb4-8 g/dl) carrying a relative risk of 1.35 and severe anaemia (Hb <4 g/dl) a risk of 3.5.[331] If a pregnant woman does develop severe malaria, fetal loss is common, and the maternal mortality rate is also high. The mortality rate of cerebral malaria in pregnancy is approximately 50%, compared with 15–20% in non-pregnant adults. Acute pulmonary oedema and hypoglycaemia are particular complications of severe malaria in pregnancy. The baby is commonly stillborn. The clinical features of uncomplicated vivax, ovale or malariae malaria are similar to those of uncomplicated *P. falciparum* malaria. *P. vivax* infections also increase anaemia and they reduce birth weight by approximately 100 g. In contrast to *P. falciparum*, vivax malaria affects multigravidae more than primigravidae.[12]

Malaria in children (Figure 71.14)

The majority of childhood malaria infections present with fever and malaise, and respond rapidly to antimalarial treatment. Severe falciparum malaria is rare in infancy, although when it does occur the mortality rate is high. In young children the progression of falciparum malaria can be rapid. Generalized seizures are associated with fever, but they are more common in *P. falciparum* than *P. vivax* malaria, even in the absence of other signs of cerebral involvement. This suggests that cerebral sequestration causes significant pathology even in conscious patients. Coma, convulsions, acidosis, hypoglycaemia and severe

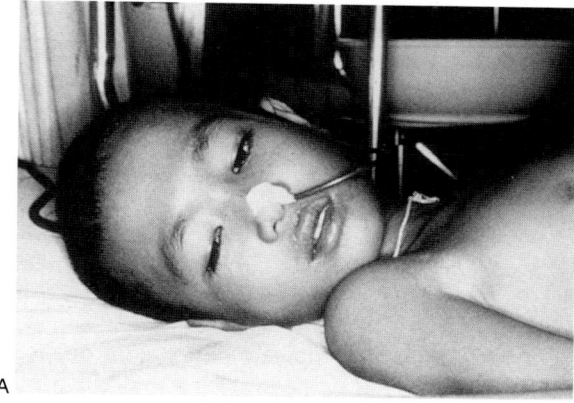

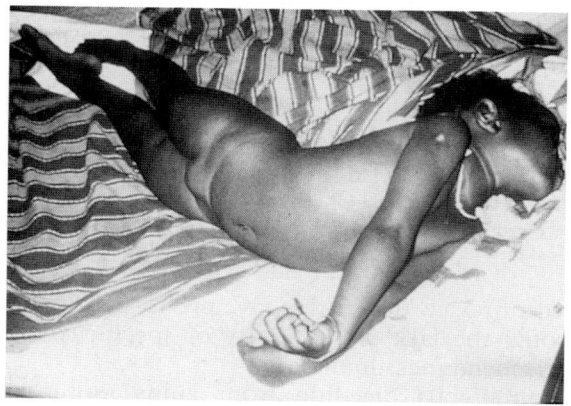

Figure 71.14: (**A**) A 6-year-old Thai boy with cerebral malaria. His father was admitted at the same time with cerebral malaria—both survived. (**B**) A 3-year-old Gambian girl with cerebral malaria and opisthotonos. (Courtesy of Jane Crawley.)

anaemia are common presenting features of severe malaria in childhood.[332–335] At the bedside, the presence of respiratory distress (acidotic breathing) or deep coma defines children at high risk of dying.[26] These two clinical syndromes account for the majority of lethal infections. In areas of intense transmission profound anaemia is the usual manifestation of severe malaria, and this occurs in the 1–3 year age group. Severe malaria is rare in older children in high transmission settings. In areas of lower, less stable transmission areas cerebral malaria becomes a predominant manifestation of severe disease, and the age range shifts upwards (Figure 71.1). Jaundice and pulmonary oedema are unusual in young children, and renal failure is very rare (a dramatic difference compared with adults). As a consequence, iatrogenic overhydration is less of a problem than in adults, although intravenous fluid administration must be carefully supervised in small children. Dehydration is more common. In cerebral malaria seizures occurs frequently, particularly in the <3-year age group, and should be treated promptly. Hypoglycaemia is common, occurring in up to 30% of children with severe malaria, and is often accompanied by lactic acidosis. The blood glucose should be checked frequently and, where possible, continuous intravenous

infusions of 5% or 10% dextrose given as a preventive measure.

In general, children tolerate the antimalarial drugs better than adults, and their symptoms resolve more quickly. The temptation to estimate body weight by 'eye' should be resisted, and all children should be weighed so that the doses of antimalarial drugs can be given on the correct mg/kg basis. (Although administration of drugs adjusted to surface area is theoretically preferable, antimalarial doses have been devised on the basis of body weight.) Children with acute malaria vomit readily, particularly if the temperature is high. Oral antimalarial treatment is more likely to be retained if it is palatable and the child is cool and calm before drug administration. In busy tropical clinics only a minority of patients can be admitted to hospital, and many children with moderately severe malaria have to be treated on an outpatient basis. It is common practice to administer a single dose of parenteral chloroquine or quinine and to send the patient home with the remainder of the oral regimen, and to give the parents advice to return if the child deteriorates further. In this situation there is a danger of significant iatrogenic hypotension if the child is kept upright (e.g., on the mother's back). If possible the child should be observed for at least 2 hours following parenteral drug administration and reassessed before discharge.

Severe malaria

Death from acute *P. vivax*, *P. ovale* or *P. malariae* infections is very rare. Occasionally already debilitated patients may succumb, and fatal haemorrhage may follow a ruptured spleen (either traumatic or spontaneous), but these events are very uncommon. There have been many case reports of 'cerebral vivax malaria' but none of these is entirely convincing, i.e., clinical details were sketchy, or coexistent falciparum malaria could not be excluded. If it does occur it must be rare. By contrast, falciparum malaria is a potentially lethal infection. The progression to severe disease can be rapid. In young children presenting with cerebral malaria a history of less than one day's illness is common. Severe malaria is rare in malnourished children and often seems to strike down the healthiest people. The great malariologist Ettore Marchiafava noted over 100 years ago how common severe malaria was in the 'hale and hearty' Italian shepherds who descended from the malaria-free mountains to the malarious valleys every autumn.[336] In adults, patients with severe malaria usually have a history of being ill for several days before admission to hospital.

Definitions of severe falciparum malaria are useful for clinical and epidemiological purposes. Definitions were proposed by working groups convened by the World Health Organization (WHO) in 1986, 1990,[243] and 2000.[333] The widely used 1990 definition was modified in a more recent series of recommendations to make it more inclusive and practical and to focus more on children (Table 71.3). Both are presented with comments.

Table 71.3 Outline classification of severe malaria in children

Group 1
Children at immediately increased risk of dying who require parenteral antimalarial drugs and supportive therapy
Prostrated children (prostration is the inability to sit upright in a child normally able to do so, or to drink in the case of children too young to sit)
Prostrate but fully conscious
Prostrate with impaired consciousness but not in deep coma
Coma (the inability to localize a painful stimulus)
Respiratory distress (acidotic breathing)
Mild—sustained nasal flaring and/or mild intercostal indrawing (recession)
Severe—the presence of either marked indrawing (recession) of the bony structure of the lower chest wall or deep (acidotic) breathing
Group 2
Children who, though able to be treated with oral antimalarial drugs, require supervised management because of the risk of clinical deterioration, but who show none of the features of group 1 (above)
Children with a haemoglobin level <5 g/dl or a haematocrit <15%
Children with two or more convulsions within a 24 h period
Group 3
Children who require parenteral treatment because of persistent vomiting but who lack any specific clinical or laboratory features of groups 1 or 2 (above)

1990 Definition

1. Cerebral malaria – unrousable coma not attributable to any other cause in a patient with falciparum malaria. The coma should persist for at least 30 minutes (one hour in the 2000 definition) after a generalized convulsion to make the distinction from transient postictal coma. Coma should be assessed using the Blantyre coma scale in children or the Glasgow coma scale in adults (see Table 71.12).

2. Severe anaemia—normocytic anaemia with haematocrit < 15% or haemoglobin < 5 g/dl in the presence of parasitaemia more than 10 000/μl. Note that finger prick samples may underestimate the haemoglobin concentration by up to 1 g if the finger is squeezed. If anaemia is hypochromic and/or microcytic, iron deficiency and thalassaemia/haemoglobinopathy must be excluded. (These criteria are rather generous; and would include many children in high transmission areas. A parasitaemia of > 100 000/μl might be a more appropriate threshold.)

3. Renal failure—defined as a urine output of less than 400 ml in 24 hours in adults, or 12 ml/kg in 24 hours in children, failing to improve after rehydration, and a serum creatinine of more than 265 μmol/l (>3.0 mg/dl). (In practice, for initial assessment, the serum creatinine alone is used.)

4. Pulmonary oedema or adult respiratory distress syndrome.

5. Hypoglycaemia—defined as a whole blood glucose concentration of less than 2.2 mmol/l (40 mg/dl).

6. Circulatory collapse or shock—hypotension (systolic blood pressure < 50 mmHg in children aged 1–5 years or < 70 mmHg in adults), with cold clammy skin or core-skin temperature difference > 10°C. (The more recent review declined to give precise definitions, but noted the lack of sensitivity or specificity of core-peripheral measurements.)

7. Spontaneous bleeding from gums, nose, gastro-intestinal tract, etc., and/or substantial laboratory evidence of DIC. (This is relatively unusual.)

8. Repeated generalized convulsions—more than two observed within 24 hours despite cooling. (In young children, these may be febrile convulsions, and the other clinical and parasitological features need to be taken into account.) Clinical evidence of seizure activity may be subtle (e.g., tonic clonic eye movements, profuse salivation, delayed coma recovery).

9. Acidaemia—defined as an arterial or capillary pH < 7.35, or acidosis defined as a plasma bicarbonate concentration < 15 mmol/l or a base excess > 10 (note temperature corrections are needed as most patients are hotter than 37°C; add 0.0147 pH unit per degree Celsius (°C) over 37°C. Operationally the clinical presentation of 'respiratory distress' or 'acidotic breathing' is focussed upon in the 2000 recommendations. Abnormal breathing patterns are a sign of severity indicating severe acidosis, pulmonary oedema or pneumonia.

10. Macroscopic haemoglobinuria—if definitely associated with acute malaria infection and not merely the result of oxidant antimalarial drugs in patients with erythrocyte enzyme defects such as G6PD deficiency. (This is difficult to ascertain in practice: if the G6PD status is checked following massive haemolysis, the value in the remaining red blood cells may be normal even in mild G6PD deficiency. This part of the definition is not very useful.)

11. Post-mortem confirmation of diagnosis. In fatal cases a diagnosis of severe falciparum malaria can be confirmed by histological examination of a post-mortem needle necroscopy of the brain. The characteristic features, found especially in cerebral grey matter, are venules/capillaries packed with erythrocytes containing mature trophozoites and schizonts of *P. falciparum*. (These features may not be present in patients who die several days after the start of treatment, although there is usually some residual pigment in the cerebral vessels.)

The 2000 WHO recommendations also include the following (Table 71.3):

1. Impairment of consciousness less marked than unrousable coma. (Any impairment of consciousness must be treated seriously. Assessment using the Glasgow Coma Scale is straightforward, but the Blantyre Scale needs careful local standardization particularly in younger children.)
2. Prostration—inability to sit unassisted in a child who is normally able to do so. In a child not old enough to sit, this is defined as an inability to feed. This definition is based on examination, not history.
3. Hyperparasitaemia—the relation of parasitaemia to severity of illness is different in different populations and age groups, but in general very high parasite densities are associated with increased risk of severe disease, e.g., > 4% parasitaemia is dangerous in non-immune children, but may be well tolerated in semi-immune children. In non-immune children studied in Thailand a parasitaemia ≥ 4% carried a 3% mortality rate (30 times higher than in all uncomplicated malaria), but in areas of high transmission values much higher may be tolerated well. Whatever the circumstances a parasitaemia ≥ 20% indicates severe malaria.

The followings were not considered criteria of severe malaria:

1. Jaundice—detected clinically or defined by a serum bilirubin concentration > 50 μmol/l (3.0 mg/dl). This is only a marker of severe malaria when combined with evidence of other vital organ dysfunction such as coma or renal failure.
2. Hyperpyrexia—a rectal temperature above 40°C in adults and children is no longer considered a sign of severity.

In severe malaria there is often evidence of multiple vital organ dysfunction, and more than one of the above criteria are fulfilled. Physicians should not worry unduly about definitions or semantics. They should treat *any patient about whom they are worried* as having severe malaria, even if they do not fall clearly into one of the above categories.

Cerebral malaria

This may be defined strictly as unrousable coma (i.e., there is a non-purposeful response or no response to a painful stimulus) in falciparum malaria. In practice any patient with altered consciousness should be treated for severe malaria. Although cerebral malaria is the most prominent feature of severe falciparum malaria, some patients with ultimately lethal infections never lose consciousness until they die. In cerebral malaria the onset of coma may be sudden, often following a generalized seizure, or gradual, with initial drowsiness, confusion, disorientation, delirium or agitation, followed by unconsciousness. Extreme agitation is a poor prognostic sign in falciparum malaria. The length of the prodromal history is usually several days in adults, but in children can be as short as 6–12 hours. A history of convulsions is common.

On examination the patient is febrile and unrousable. There may be some passive resistance to head flexion, but the board-like rigidity of meningitis is not found, and there are no other signs of meningeal irritation. There may be anaemia, which in some cases, particularly children, may be profound. Conversely, jaundice is relatively unusual in children but common in adults. Signs of bleeding are unusual and indicate a poor prognosis. The patient is usually warm, dry and well-perfused peripherally, with a low-normal blood pressure and a sinus tachycardia. Skin perfusion is variable, intermittent 'goose-pimples' are common in association with cutaneous vasoconstriction. Sustained hyperventilation is a poor prognostic sign as it indicates metabolic acidosis if the chest is clear, or pneumonia or pulmonary oedema if it is not. The liver and spleen are commonly enlarged, but soft. Massive splenomegaly is not found. There is no lymphadenopathy and no rash. The clinical features are usually of a symmetrical encephalopathy. Focal signs are unusual. On examination of the nervous system the gaze is usually normal or divergent (but there is no evidence of extra-ocular muscle paresis) (Figure 71.15). The pupils are usually mid-size and equally reactive. The fundus should be examined carefully. Five distinct fundoscopic abnormalities have been observed; retinal whitening, retinal haemorrhages, focal whitening of vessels, papilloedema and cotton wool spots.[337] Papilloedema is unusual and is a sign of poor prognosis, as is retinal oedema. Retinal haemorrhages

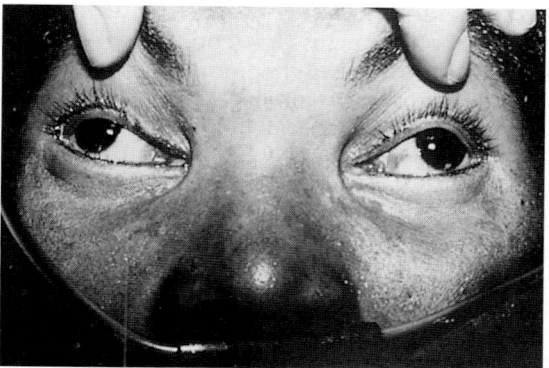

Figure 71.15: Divergent gaze in a 42-year-old Burmese woman with cerebral malaria.

have been reported in between 6 and 37% of cases.[337–339] (They are more easily identified if indirect ophthalmoscopy is used.) The haemorrhages are often flame shaped, and may have a pale centre resembling Roth spots. They rarely affect the macula. The retinal vessels should be examined for a very characteristic segmental whitening that probably reflects intense sequestration with red blood cells containing little haemoglobin and mature parasites.[340] In adult patients the corneal reflexes are usually preserved but in children with deep coma they may be lost (a poor prognostic sign). It is important to examine the eyes carefully to exclude the rapid repetitive jerky movements that indicate seizure activity. There may be forced jaw closure with repetitive spontaneous teeth grinding (bruxism). The jaw jerk is sometimes brisk and there is often a pout reflex. Other frontal release signs are very unusual. Cranial nerve abnormalities are rare. Tone may be increased, decreased or normal. Likewise the reflexes can be brisk or depressed. The abdominal reflexes are invariably absent, the cremasteric reflexes often preserved, and the plantar responses extensor in approximately half the patients. Patients may exhibit phasic increases in tone with extensor posturing of the decorticate (arm flexed, legs extended), or more usually decerebrate (arms and legs extended) types. The back may arch as in opisthotonus, with sustained, usually upward and lateral, ocular deviation. The posturing is commonly associated with noisy hyperventilation. Generalized or sometimes focal seizures may occur. The duration of coma varies considerably, but overall is shorter in children (average 1 day) than in adults (average 2–3 days). Clinical evidence for seizure activity may be very subtle (e.g., tonic clonic eye movements without limb movement), and in some children there are no signs despite electroencephalographic evidence. Aspiration pneumonia is a potentially lethal sequel.

Untreated cerebral malaria is probably uniformly fatal. The overall mortality rate of treated cerebral malaria obviously depends on the referral practices and medical facilities available, but in reported studies averages 15% in children and 20% in adults (but up to 50% in pregnancy).[333–335,341] Some series have reported lower mortality rates, but in these studies the definition of cerebral malaria has been more 'generous', i.e., they have included patients who were obtunded or delirious but not unrousable. Hospitals acting as secondary or tertiary referral centres often experience higher mortality rates as they see a residue of more severe patients. The later the patient is referred, the higher the probability of mortality. In the Vietnam war, the mortality rate of acute falciparum malaria was higher in soldiers who had returned to the USA than it was in Vietnam.[342] Obviously the diagnosis was made much more rapidly in Vietnam where physicians were well aware of malaria, than in the USA where they were not.

Case history

A 2-year-old girl is brought to a provincial African hospital by her mother in the afternoon. She has had two generalized convulsions in the morning, and she was unrousable after the first of these. Her mother noticed she did not eat the previous evening and that she had a fever, but before that she appeared to be well (although the mother had been working in the fields the previous day, and so could not be exact as to the time when symptoms began). After the first convulsion the child had been taken to a health centre where a presumptive diagnosis of malaria was made, and a single intramuscular injection of chloroquine given before the child was referred on to hospital. In the past the child had received her immunizations, and had received treatment for malaria in the previous rainy season. She had also had several febrile episodes which the mother had treated at home with chloroquine and traditional medicines, and these had resolved without complications.

On examination the child was unrousably comatose with only a non-localized motor response to a painful stimulus (Blantyre coma score 1). She was not anaemic or jaundiced, and she weighed 8 kg. The blood pressure was 85/65 mmHg, the pulse 138/min, and the rectal temperature 40.1°C. The child was not clinically dehydrated. The respiratory rate was 52/min. She was breathing deeply with use of accessory muscles of respiration, intercostals indrawing, and flaring of the alar nasae. There were coarse breath sounds, particularly over the left lung field. The spleen tip was palpable and the liver 3 cm enlarged. There was some passive resistance to head flexion, but no other evidence of meningeal irritation. On fundoscopy a flame-shaped haemorrhage with a pale centre was visible adjacent to the superior nasal artery in the left eye. The optic discs were flat. The eyes were divergent. Positive findings on examination of the central and peripheral nervous systems were a pout reflex, a symmetrical increase in tone, and extensor plantar responses. Intermittent extensor posturing of the 'decerebrate' type, with extended arms and legs, sustained upward gaze, and hyperventilation lasting 10–15 seconds, occurred every 5 minutes. Blood was taken and an intravenous infusion of 5% dextrose water was started. A glucose oxidase stick test indicated the blood glucose was only 1.1 mmol/l; 8 ml (0.5 g/kg) of 50% dextrose was given by slow intravenous injection and the infusion was changed to 10% dextrose. There was no improvement in her clinical condition. The haematocrit was read as 36% and the parasitaemia on brief microscopic examination of the thin film was heavy; a subsequent count gave a value of 136/1000 red blood cells. In 25% of the parasites pigment was evident indicating they were mature trophozoites, and 3% were schizonts. Phagocytosed pigment could be seen in 10% of the neutrophils. Chloroquine-resistant falciparum malaria is prevalent nearly everywhere in Africa, and so an infusion of quinine dihydrochloride was started. A loading dose of 160 mg (20 mg salt/kg) was drawn up (as close as possible to 0.53 ml of a 300 mg/ml solution in a 1 ml syringe) and injected into a 120 ml burette (infusion chamber) with 10% dextrose and set to run at 30 ml/hour. (The hospital was fortunate to have a stock of paediatric infusion sets, but if these had not been available the quinine could have been given by intramuscular injection.) A lumbar puncture was performed; the CSF was clear, there was clear CSF with free rise and fall with respiration, and the opening pressure was recorded as 140 mm CSF. Tepid sponging brought the rectal temperature down to 38.3°C. The posturing lessened in intensity and frequency. The vital signs remained stable over the next 4 hours and the chest remained clear, but the respiratory rate increased to 60/min. The breathing was deep and noisy. The bed was wet, indicating that urine had been passed. A repeat blood glucose at 4 hours was 3.2 mmol/l. At 5 hours the blood pressure was 80/50, pulse 150/min, temperature 37.7°C and respiratory rate 62/min. The Blantyre coma score was still 1, and the neurological signs were unchanged. Twenty minutes later the respiration became ataxic, and then stopped. She could not be resuscitated.

Comment

This child with cerebral malaria had several poor prognostic features on admission to hospital: deep coma, convulsions, extensor posturing, respiratory distress, hyperparasitaemia, a predominance of mature parasites on the peripheral blood smear, pigment in peripheral blood neutrophils and hypoglycaemia. The admitting physician was aware immediately that the outlook was bleak from the combination of coma and respiratory distress. The short history and absence of anaemia together with the high parasite count suggest a fulminant infection. The predominance of mature parasites suggests the possibility of a much greater sequestered parasite biomass than that evident from the peripheral parasitaemia. She was hypoglycaemic and almost certainly had lactic acidosis. Although the best available parenteral antimalarial treatment was started as soon as the diagnosis was made, irreversible pathological processes may already have taken place. As in many fatal cases in children, the exact cause of the final respiratory arrest was not known.

Convulsions

Seizures are common, particularly in young children. They are associated with falciparum malaria even in uncomplicated infections.[343] In the majority of cases the child recovers uneventfully following one or two generalized convulsions, but some patients do not recover consciousness rapidly (< 30 minutes) and may remain unrousable (cerebral malaria). In some cases the cause of the protracted coma is status epilepticus. Focal seizures may also occur, but they are less common. Aspiration pneumonia is a common and preventable sequel to grand mal seizures. (Repeated grand mal seizures in cerebral malaria are associated with residual neurological sequelae.)

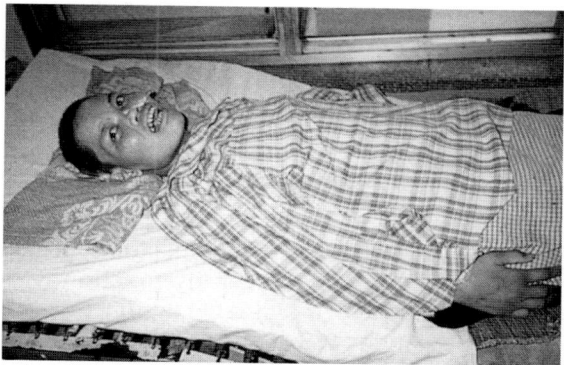

Figure 71.16: Permanent global residual neurological deficit following prolonged hypoglycaemia in a 33-year-old Vietnamese woman who had cerebral malaria in pregnancy. She had received intravenous quinine but despite parenteral glucose administration became repeatedly hypoglycaemic.

Post-malaria neurological syndromes

In approximately 3% of adults and 10–20% of children there is a persistent neurological deficit following cerebral malaria (Figure 71.16).[344-348] In children this is associated with profound and protracted coma, anaemia, and prolonged convulsions. In some studies hypoglycaemia was a risk factor, but in others it was not. In appro ximately 60% of severe cases there is a hemiparesis with variable hemisensory deficit and sometimes hemianopia.[346] Cortical blindness, diffuse cortical damage, tremor and occasionally isolated cranial nerve palsies may occur. Many of the deficits recover rapidly, and by six months only 4% of survivors have neurological abnormality.[347]

Rarely patients who recover from cerebral malaria may lapse into coma again, usually after a period of 1–2 days when they are rousable. In this condition the CSF protein may be elevated (200–300 mg/dl) and there is sometimes an increase in CSF lymphocytes. There may be residual neurological deficit on recovery. A variety of other late neurological complications may occur following recovery from cerebral malaria. These include psychosis, encephalopathy, Parkinsonian rigidity and tremor, a fine tremor and cerebellar dysfunction.[348-351] These post-malaria neurological syndromes (PMNS) may also rarely follow uncomplicated malaria, and could account for some of the cases previously attributed to mefloquine or chloroquine neurotoxicity. On the other hand, there appears to be a strong interaction between mefloquine and cerebral malaria such that 5% of patients who receive mefloquine after severe malaria develop PMNS (a risk 10–50 times higher than following mefloquine treatment of uncomplicated malaria).[349] Mefloquine should not be used following cerebral malaria. The conditions are self-limiting, but very distressing, and usually resolve over several days, or sometimes 1–2 weeks. The syndrome of cerebellar ataxia occurring 2–3 weeks after acute uncomplicated malaria appears to be relatively common in Sri Lanka.[351] It too is usually self-limiting with recovery over a few weeks. Although central nervous system recovery is remarkably good, there remains uncertainty over the extent of subtle persistent cognitive or behavioural deficits.[352,353]

Acute renal failure

In some adult patients with severe malaria acute oliguric renal failure and other vital organ dysfunction is present on admission, whereas in others renal dysfunction becomes evident as the patient recovers from the acute phase of severe disease.[191,354,355] In the former fulminant presentation there is a high incidence of associated hepatic dysfunction and metabolic acidosis, and pulmonary oedema is the usual terminal event. The blood pressure is normal. Jaundice is common and there may be a bleeding tendency. There may be slight proteinuria, but the urine sediment is unremarkable. The subacute presentation carries a better prognosis. The patient may be oliguric but is rarely anuric. The serum creatinine rises over a period of days until either dialysis is required because of hyperkalaemia or uraemic complications such as bleeding, pleural or pericardial effusions, encephalopathy or intractable vomiting, or there is gradual resolution with an increase in urine output. In the subacute presentation of acute renal failure parasitaemia may have cleared following antimalarial treatment before the patient is referred to hospital.[191] Although acute renal failure is a common complication of malaria in adults living in areas of low or unstable transmission, it is rare in children. Indeed in high-transmission areas it is almost unheard of. Renal failure is also associated with haemoglobinuria in patients with massive haemolysis[356] (see below, blackwater fever).

Metabolic acidosis

The main clinical indication of metabolic acidosis is laboured hyperventilation with increased inspiratory effort (often termed respiratory distress) and a clear chest on auscultation (Kussmaul's breathing). This usually results from lactic acidosis, but ketoacidosis may be present in children.[256–259] Hypovolaemia is an important contributor and must be corrected. In areas where aspirin is used widely salicylate intoxication should also be considered.[357] Acidosis may be associated with renal failure in adults, but in the acute infection there is also a lactic acidosis. The outlook for persistent acidosis is poor. Although blood pressure and tissue perfusion is usually adequate initially, hypotension commonly ensues.

Blackwater fever

The sinister reputation of blackwater fever derives from the high mortality rate (20–30%) documented in Europeans and Asians working in colonial Africa in the first half of the twentieth century.[244,358] Approximately half of these deaths were caused by renal failure. G.R. Ross,[358] writing from Southern Rhodesia (Zimbabwe), described blackwater fever as 'a disease to blanch the cheek of the bravest', and such was its reputation that magistrates considered it as an excuse for a felony! Today the mortality rate is much lower. Indeed the passage of black or dark-brown-red urine (blackwater) is often not associated with significant renal impairment. Blackwater is usually transient and resolves without complications, but in severe cases renal failure may develop.[244,359] This behaves as acute tubular necrosis. Blackwater results from massive haemolysis. Transfused blood is also rapidly haemolysed. The mortality rate is highest when blackwater fever is associated with severe malaria and other evidence of vital organ dysfunction. Patients with blackwater fever and severe anaemia often have a slate-grey appearance, and their plasma may be red (haemoglobinaemia).

Acute pulmonary oedema

Hyperventilation or Kussmaul's breathing (sometimes termed respiratory distress) is a poor prognostic sign in malaria. In the tachypnoea associated with high fever, breathing is shallow compared with the ominous laboured hyperventilation associated with metabolic acidosis, pulmonary oedema or pneumonia. Acute pulmonary oedema may develop at any time in severe falciparum malaria. It is particularly common in pregnant women, but rare in children. This is one form of the adult respiratory distress syndrome,[198–200,360–362] and in some cases may be difficult to distinguish clinically from aspiration pneumonia. The heart sounds are normal. The central venous pressure and pulmonary artery occlusion pressures are usually normal, the cardiac index is high, and systemic vascular resistance is low. This points to an increase in capillary permeability (unless the patient has been overhydrated). The chest radiograph shows increased interstitial shadowing and a normal heart size.

Hypotension

The majority of patients with severe malaria are febrile, with a high cardiac output, a low systemic vascular resistance, and a low-normal blood pressure. They are usually warm and well perfused. Patients with severe disease may develop sudden hypotension and become shocked. This is called 'algid malaria'.[363,364] In a proportion of cases there is bacterial septicaemia, but in the majority blood cultures are negative. Shock usually responds temporarily to saline infusion and inotropes, but pulmonary oedema may be provoked if too much salt is given and left-sided filling pressures (pulmonary artery wedge pressures) rise above 15 mmHg. The overall mortality rate is high. Orthostatic hypotension is common in acute uncomplicated malaria.[365,366] It is associated with impaired reflex cardioacceleration and is worsened by the quinoline antimalarial drugs.[367]

Hypoglycaemia

Hypoglycaemia is either asymptomatic in severely ill patients, or presents as a further deterioration in the level of coma.[265–268,368] In severe malaria the usual signs of sweating and increased sympathetic nervous system activity are commonly absent or indistinguishable from the signs of malaria. Hypoglycaemia occurs in approximately 8% of adults and up to 30% of children with cerebral malaria. It is often recurrent. The clinical response to glucose is usually disappointing. In pregnant women with uncomplicated malaria who have quinine-stimulated hyperinsulinaemic hypoglycaemia, the clinical features of hypoglycaemia are usually evident, and the patient responds dramatically to glucose. Hypoglycaemia can often be prevented by infusion of 10% dextrose but frequent monitoring is still necessary.

Anaemia

The degree of anaemia and the rate at which it develops vary enormously. The haemoglobin concentration may fall by up to 2 g/dl each day. Anaemia is a particular problem in children, where it may lead to sudden death. These complications are particularly likely with haemoglobin concentrations below 5 g/dl (15% haematocrit) and the risk rises steeply below 4 g/dl.[369] Some patients appear to tolerate severe malarial anaemia relatively well. These patients usually have an underlying chronic anaemia, and have adapted to increase oxygen carriage (right-shifted oxygen dissociation curve). Thus it is both the absolute haemoglobin concentration and the magnitude of the fall that determine the clinical consequences. In the past a syndrome of malaria associated anemic congestive heart failure was often diagnosed, and was managed by fluid restriction, and often very cautious blood transfusion. It is now clear that the majority of these children with severe anaemia, rapid deep breathing and low blood pressure are hypovolaemic and need quite the opposite treatment: intravenous rehydration and urgent blood transfusion.[370]

Persistent fever

Patients with severe malaria may have persistent fever after parasite clearance. Although a proportion of cases have an identifiable chest or urinary tract infection, or in children blood cultures may grow *Salmonella* spp., the majority of cases have no clear explanation and the fever eventually resolves in a few days without further treatment.

Laboratory findings
Haematology

There is a progressive normochromic normocytic anaemia. The white count is usually normal, but may be raised in very severe malaria, and very occasionally there is a leucoerythroblastic picture. There is slight monocytosis and eosinopenia, with reactive eosinophilia in the weeks following the acute infection.[371] The platelet count is reduced in all acute malarias, usually to around 100 000/μl, but thrombocytopenia is profound in some cases. Fibrinogen levels are usually elevated—a reduction indicates significant DIC. The fibrin degradation products are elevated. There is evidence of increased coagulation cascade activity through intrinsic pathway activation with antithrombin III depletion that is proportional to disease severity and there may be prolongation of the prothrombin and partial thromboplastin times. Polymorphonuclear leucocyte elastase levels are elevated in severe malaria, suggesting neutrophil activation.[372]

Acute phase proteins

The C-reactive protein, orosomucoid (α_1-acid glycoprotein) and fibrinogen levels are raised, and immunoglobulin levels rise while albumin falls. Cytokine levels are raised in acute malaria; there are increased concentrations of circulating cytokine receptors, and there is an increase in urinary neopterin.

Biochemistry

There may be mild hyponatraemia,[373] but the serum potassium is remarkably normal. The serum bicarbonate is often reduced and the anion gap widens in proportion to the acidosis. In adults the serum creatinine and blood urea may be raised, with an increased urea to creatinine ratio. Total and conjugated bilirubin may be elevated, the transaminase concentrations are often raised, and there may also be slight elevation of the hepatic alkaline phosphatase concentration. In children the 5-nucleotidase is raised in proportion to disease severity. Creatine phosphokinase, myoglobin and plasma urate levels are elevated in adults and children with severe malaria.[374] The serum calcium may be low and hypophosphataemia may be profound in severe infections.[271] Hypoglycaemia may occur, and in the absence of quinine treatment, this is accompanied by elevated ketones, raised plasma lactate and alanine, and low insulin levels.[265–268] Lactate levels in arterial or venous blood, or CSF, are elevated and blood bicarbonate is reduced in proportion to disease severity.[188,375]

Cerebrospinal fluid

The opening pressures at lumbar puncture in adults and

children are similar, averaging approximately 160 mm CSF. But because the normal range in children is lower (<100 mm) most values in children are elevated.[181] The CSF is usually normal in cerebral malaria, but moderately raised concentrations of protein are common (sometimes up to 200 mg/dl). There may be up to 10 cells/ml, and on occasions up to 50 are seen (all lymphocytes). The CSF lactate concentration is raised in cerebral malaria, and the glucose may be slightly low relative to blood. If the patient is deeply jaundiced the CSF may appear yellow.

Prognostic factors

The prognostic factors listed in Table 71.4 reflect vital organ dysfunction and the magnitude of the parasite burden. They are not absolute, and in fatal cases several factors

Table 71.4 Laboratory indicators of a poor prognosis in severe malaria

Biochemistry	
Hypoglycaemia	<2.2 mmol/l
Hyperlactataemia	>5 mmol/l
Acidosis	Arterial pH <7.3, venous plasma HCO_3 <15 mmol/l
Serum creatinine	>265 µmol/l[a]
Total bilirubin	>50 µmol/l
Liver enzymes	sGOT (AST) × 3 upper limit of normal
	sGPT (ALT) × 3 upper limit of normal
	5-Nucleotidase ↑
Muscle enzymes	CPK ↑
	Myoglobin ↑
Urate	>600 µmol/l
Haematology	
Leucocytosis	>12 000/µl
	Severe anaemia (PCV <15%)
Coagulopathy	Platelets <50 000/µl
	Prothrombin time prolonged >3 s
	Prolonged partial thromboplastin time
	Fibrinogen: <200 mg/dl
Parasitology	
Hyperparasitaemia increased mortality[b]	>100 000/µl – increased mortality[b]
	>500 000/µl – high mortality[b]
>20% of parasites are pigment-containing trophozoites and schizonts	
>5% of neutrophils contain visible malaria pigment	

PCV, packed cell volume; sGOT (AST), serum glutamic oxaloacetic transferase (aspartate aminotransferase); sGPT (ALT), serum glutamic pyruvic transaminase (alanine aminotransferase); CPK, creatine phosphokinase.
[a]This is the criterion for adults. Less elevated values are found in children with severe malaria.
[b]These refer to thresholds in non-immune adults. The thresholds are much higher in children in endemic areas.

usually coexist. Some of the apparently poor prognostic factors can have a benign explanation. Hyperventilation (respiratory distress) is usually a bad sign (indicating metabolic acidosis, pulmonary oedema, or pneumonia), but shallow tachypnoea can result from high fever alone (the tidal volume is lower). Upper gastrointestinal bleeding in cerebral malaria may also occur spontaneously. The prognostic implications of severe anaemia depend on the rate at which the haematocrit falls, the coexisting parasitaemia and the stage of the infection. If anaemia develops gradually then even haemoglobin values less than 7 g/dl (packed cell volume < 20%) can be surprisingly well tolerated as there is time for homeostatic adaptations such as the right shift in the oxygen dissociation curve, the increase in cardiac index and the fall in systemic vascular resistance. Hypotension is a poor prognostic sign only when associated with poor tissue perfusion. Patients, particularly children, with acute malaria often have very low blood pressures but they are warm and well perfused. The biochemical measures are in general proportional to severity, but individual abnormalities can have other explanations. For example, hypoglycaemia carries a fivefold higher mortality in severe malaria, but in pregnant women treated with quinine hypoglycaemia may occur in uncomplicated infections because of quinine-stimulated hyperinsulinaemia. The concentration of lactate in venous or arterial blood or CSF is linearly proportional to the severity of disease. In terms of predictive prognostic value the admission venous bicarbonate concentration has the best sensitivity and specificity, and it is available widely. Although deep jaundice is often a bad sign, some adult patients develop a profound cholestatic jaundice without other evidence of vital organ dysfunction.

Parasitaemia has traditionally been used as a measure of severity since the classic studies of Field and colleagues in Kuala Lumpur, Malaysia.[376,377] They established that *P. falciparum* parasite counts over 100 000/µl were associated with an increased risk of dying, and that the mortality of a count over 500 000/µl was 50%. The distribution of parasite counts in severe malaria is shifted to higher parasitaemias in children living in areas of intense transmission, compared with non-immune adults. For example, parasite counts over 200 000/µl are not uncommon in ambulant semi-immune children who are mildly ill, whereas parasitaemias in this range are usually associated with severe disease in non-immune adults (Table 71.5). The sensitivity and specificity of parasitaemia alone as a prognostic indicator is limited, but can be improved by staging parasite development (more mature parasites—worse prognosis),[378] and noting the number of polymorphonuclear neutrophil leucocytes which contain pigment (>5%—poorer prognosis).[379] For any parasitaemia the prognosis is worse if >20% of parasites contain visible pigment, and better if >50% of parasites are at the tiny ring stage. In severe malaria if >50% of neutrophils contain visible pigment the prognosis is worse.

Table 71.5 Severe manifestations of *P. falciparum* malaria in adults and children

| Prognostic value[a] | | | Frequency[a] | |
Children	Adults		Children	Adults
Clinical manifestations[b]				
+	(?)	Prostration	+++	+++
+++	++	Impaired consciousness	+++	++
+++	+++	Respiratory distress (acidotic breathing)	+++	++
+	++	Multiple convulsions	+++	+
+++	+++	Circulatory collapse	+	+
+++	+++	Pulmonary oedema (radiological)	+/–	+
+++	++	Abnormal bleeding	+/–	+
++	+	Jaundice	+	+++
+	+	Haemoglobinuria	+/–	+
Laboratory findings				
+	+	Severe anaemia	+++	+
+++	+++	Hypoglycaemia	+++	++
+++	+++	Acidosis	+++	++
+++	+++	Hyperlactataemia	+++	++
+/–	++	Hyperparasitaemia	++	+
++	++	Renal impairment	+	+++

[a]On a scale from + to +++; +/– indicates borderline prognostic value or infrequent occurrence.
[b]Anuria and hypothermia (core temperature <36.5°C) are also poor prognostic signs.

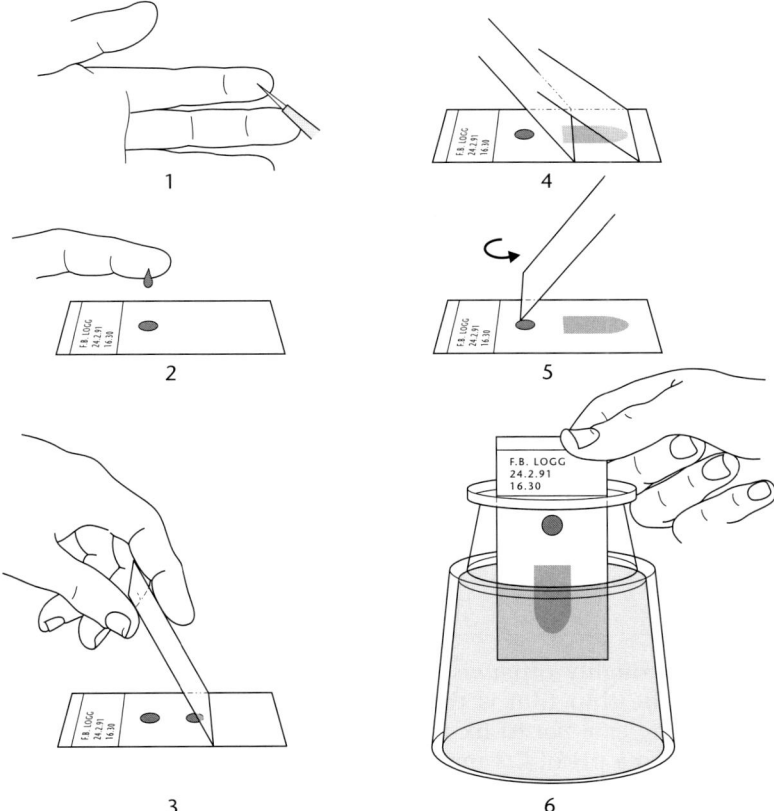

Figure 71.17: Making a peripheral blood smear.

Diagnosis

Blood smears

Malaria is diagnosed by microscopic examination of the blood. It is not a clinical diagnosis. Thick and thin blood films are made on clean, grease-free glass slides (Figure 71.17). Having written the patient's name, time and date, the glass slide can be cleaned by breathing on the surface and wiping with a clean cloth. The patient's finger should be cleaned with alcohol, allowed to dry, and then the side of the finger tip should be pricked with a sharp sterile lancet or needle. Two drops of blood are placed at one end of the slide. The thin film is made immediately by placing the *smooth* leading edge of a second (spreader) slide in the central drop of blood, adjusting the angle (less blood—more acute) and, whilst holding the edges of the slide, smearing the blood with a swift and steady sweep along the surface. If the blood drop is too large, the spreader slide should be dunked in the drop, then 'jumped' to the slide surface carrying a smaller amount of blood—and then smeared. Making good thin films requires some practice. Anaemic blood smears poorly. The thick film should be stirred in a circular motion with the corner of the second slide until clotting takes place. The thick film must be of uneven thickness, but it should be possible to read the hands, but not the figures, of a watch face through the film.

Intradermal smears

Chinese researchers have shown that smears from intra-dermal blood may contain more mature forms of *P. falciparum* than the peripheral blood.[380] This is considered to allow a more complete assessment of severe malaria. The intradermal smears may also be positive or may show pigment-containing leucocytes after the blood smear is negative. In terms of diagnostic sensitivity the intradermal smear is similar to the bone marrow (i.e., slightly more sensitive than peripheral blood). The smears are taken (Figure 71.18) from multiple intradermal punctures with a 25 G needle on the volar surface of the upper forearm. The punctures should not ooze blood spontaneously, but sero-sanguinous fluid can be expressed on to the slide by squeezing.

Staining and reading

The thick film should be dried thoroughly otherwise it may wash away during staining. The thin film is then fixed in anhydrous methanol (taking care *not* to fix the thick film). Giemsa's stain buffered to a pH of 7.2 makes the best malaria slides, but for optimum results the stain should be left on the slide for 30 minutes. Field's stain is quicker, but the thin and thick films are treated differently.[381] The thin film is immersed in the red stain (Field's B) for 6 seconds, then gently washed off for 5 seconds, then immersed in the blue stain (Field's A) for

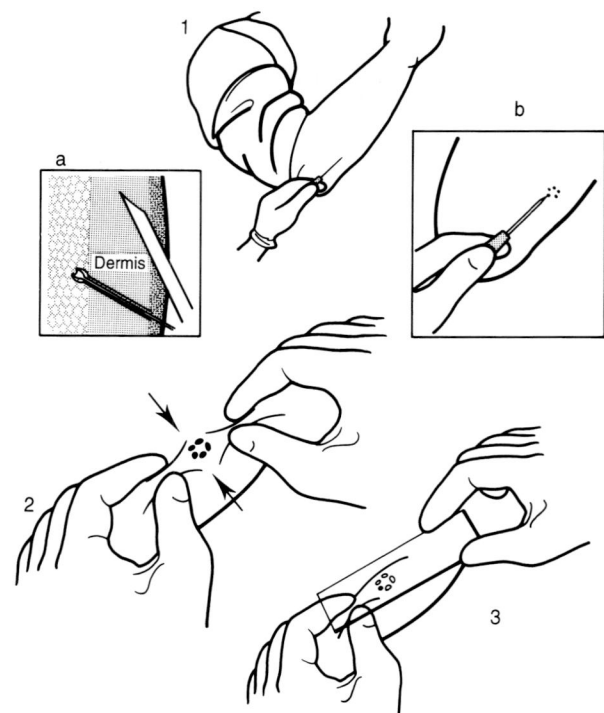

Figure 71.18: Making an intradermal smear.

3–4 seconds and then gently washed off (5 seconds). The reverse order applies to the thick film: the slide is first immersed in the blue stain (Field's A) for 5 seconds, then gently washed off (5 seconds) then the red stain (Field's B) for 5 seconds, then gently washed off (5 seconds). Slides should be dried in a slide rack before examining under oil immersion at a magnification of x 1000.

Before going to oil immersion (magnification 10×100) on the microscope, the slide should be scanned briefly under low magnification to identify the best area for detailed examination. For the thin film, the tail of the film should be examined; for the thick film the area of optimum thickness and staining and least artefact is chosen. The thick film is approximately 30 times more sensitive than the thin film, although sensitivity and specificity depend to a great extent on the experience of the microscopist, the quality of the slides, stains and microscope, and the time spent examining the slide. Artefacts are common and often confusing. Speciation of malaria at the trophozoite stage is easier on the thin film, although gametocytes and schizonts are more likely to be seen on the thick film. The thin film is more accurate for parasite counting. The number of parasitized red blood cells per 1000 red blood cells should be counted. If there are two parasites in one red cell, this is counted as one. At low parasitaemias (< 5/1000 on the thin film) the thick film should be counted; the number of parasites per 200, or preferably 500 white cells is noted. These figures can then be corrected by the total red cell and white cell counts to give the number of parasites per unit blood volume (µl). If the white count is not available then the count is assumed to be 8000 µl. An alternative is to count all parasites in a fixed volume of blood.[381] In severe malaria parasitaemias are usually high and the stage of parasite development should be assessed on the thin film. The proportion of asexual parasites containing visible pigment (i.e., mature trophozoites and schizonts) should be counted. The presence of pigment in neutrophils and monocytes should also be noted. In patients who have already received antimalarial treatment, pigment may still be present in leucocytes after clearance of parasitaemia, and this is an important clue to the diagnosis. Monocytes containing pigment are cleared more slowly than pigment containing neutrophils.

The morphological characteristics of human malaria parasites are given in Table 71.6.

Antigen detection methods

The introduction of simple, rapid, sensitive, highly specific, and increasingly affordable dipstick or card tests for the diagnosis of malaria has been a major advance in recent years. These are based on antibody detection of two malaria specific antigens in blood samples; histidine rich protein 2 (*Pf*HRP2), and parasite lactate dehydrogenase (which is antigenically distinct from the host enzyme). As the name implies *Pf*HRP2 is specific for *P. falciparum*. Current *Pf*HRP2 and *Pf*LDH tests, based on colour reactions, provide a diagnostic sensitivity similar to trained microscopists.[381–385] *Pf*LDH is cleared rapidly from blood, the test becomes negative within days of treatment, but *Pf*HRP2 is cleared very slowly from the blood, and may remain positive for up to one month after the acute infection, particularly if the parasitaemia was high.[386] This is a disadvantage in areas where transmission is high, and infections frequent, but is very useful in the diagnosis of severely ill patients who have received previous antimalarial treatment. Their parasitaemia may have cleared but the *Pf*HRP2 test will remain strongly positive. *Pf*HRP2 is present in parasitized erythrocytes, but it is also secreted into plasma, and plasma concentrations (which can be assessed semi-quantitatively from the intensity of the

Table 71.6 Morphological characteristics of human malaria parasites

	P. falciparum	*P. vivax*	*P. ovale*	*P. malariae*
Asexual parasites	Usually only ring forms seen. Fine blue cytoplasm oval, circular, comma-shaped or occasionally squeezed to the edge of the cell (appliqué form). One or two chromatin dots. Parasitaemia may exceed 2%	Irregular large fairly thick rings becoming very pleomorphic as the parasite matures. One chromatin dot	Regular dense ring enlarges to compact blue mature trophozoite. One chromatin dot	Dense thick rings, maturing to dense round trophozoites or rectangular or band-form trophozoites. Pigment associated with rings and trophozoites. Large red chromatin dot or band. Low parasitaemia usual
Meronts (Schizonts)	Rare in peripheral blood. 8–32 merozoites, dark brown-black pigment	Common. 12–18 merozoites, orange brown pigment	8–14 merozoites, brown pigment	8–10 merozoites, black pigment
Gametocytes	Banana-shaped. Male: light blue. Female: darker blue. Red-black nucleus with few scattered blue-black pigment granules in cytoplasm	Round or oval. Male: round, pale blue. Female: oval, dark blue. Triangular nucleus, few orange pigment granules	Large round dense blue like *P.malariae*, but prominent James' dots. Brown pigment	Large oval-shaped. Male: pale blue. Female: dense blue. Large black pigment granules
Red cell changes	Normal size. As parasite matures cytoplasm becomes pale, the cells become crenated, and a few small red dots appear over the cytoplasm (Maurer's clefts)	Enlarged. Pale red Schüffner's dots increase in number as parasite matures	Cells become oval with tufted ends. Prominent James' dots	Normal size and shape. No red dots

NB. Multiple invasion is often quoted as a feature of falciparum malaria. This is simply a function of higher parasite densities: At any given density multiple invasion is over three times more frequent with *P.vivax* compared to *P.falciparum*.

colour reaction) are a guide to the parasite biomass and thus severity.[387] The *Pf*HRP2 test has proved useful in detecting mixed *P. falciparum* and *P. vivax* infections where the former was not evident microscopically.[320] False positive tests may occur in patients with high concentrations of rheumatoid factor,[388] and false negative results have been reported in patients whose parasites have a rare antigenically variant form of *Pf*HRP2. Recently pan-malaria antibodies have been added to the tests. These detect all malaria parasite species. The cards or sticks then carry two band colour reactions plus a control (which should be positive). Thus a positive test with these two bands, with a negative in the *Plasmodium falciparum* test, signifies one of the other malaria species is causing the infection (and therefore chloroquine rather than another antimalarial drug is required). These tests may remain positive in patients with persistent gametocytaemia.[384]

Other techniques

Unlike mature red blood cells, malaria parasites contain DNA and RNA. This can be stained with fluorescent dyes and visualized under ultraviolet light microscopy, or, with appropriate filters, seen under ordinary light microscopy. In the QBC™ technique blood samples are taken into a specialized capillary tube containing acridine orange stain and a float. Under high centrifugal forces (14 000 g) the infected erythrocytes, which have a higher buoyant density than uninfected cells, become concentrated around the float. Using a modified lens adaptor (Paralens™) with its own light source, the acridine orange fluorescence from malaria parasites can be visualized through an ordinary microscope.[389] In some series this system has proved more sensitive than conventional light microscopy, although it does not give parasite counts or speciation with accuracy, and it is relatively expensive. It is useful for screening large numbers of blood samples rapidly. DNA probes have also been developed for malaria diagnosis, but their utility outside epidemiological surveys is uncertain. Detection of malaria antibody can be useful in some circumstances, such as confirmation of earlier infection, but has no place in acute diagnosis.

Post-mortem diagnosis

The diagnosis of cerebral malaria post-mortem can be confirmed from a brain smear. A needle aspirate or biopsy is obtained through the superior orbital foramen or the foramen magnum. A smear of grey matter is examined after staining the slide in the same way as for a thin blood film. Capillaries and venules are identified microscopically under low power, and examined under high power. If the patient died in the acute stage of cerebral malaria the vessels are packed with erythrocytes containing mature parasites and a large amount of pigment.

The antimalarial drugs
History

Extracts of the plant qinghao *(Artemesia annua)*, known as qinghaosu, have been used in traditional medical practice in China for over two millenia. In AD 340 Ge Hong described the use of qinghao infusions for the treatment of fever in the famous *Handbook of Emergency Treatments*. Thereafter qinghao is mentioned frequently in the Chinese materia medica as a treatment for agues. The antimalarial

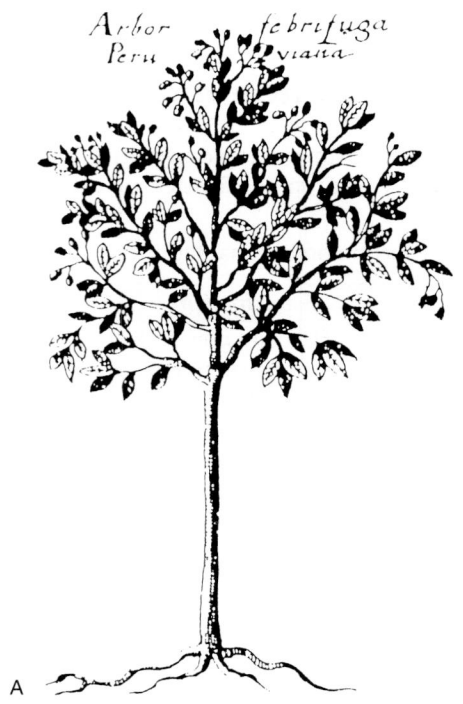

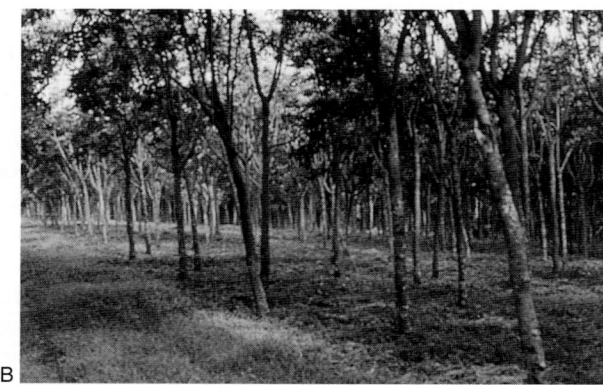

Figure 71.19: (**A**) The 'Arbor febrifuga Peruviana'. 'In the district of the city of Loja, diocese of Quito, grows a certain kind of large tree, which has a bark like cinnamon, a little more coarse and very bitter: which ground to powder is given to those who have fever, and with only this remedy, it leaves them' (Bernabé Cobo S. J. *Historia del Nuevo Mundo*; 1582-1657. (**B**) A cinchona plantation in Democratic Republic of Congo today.

properties of qinghaosu were rediscovered in 1971 when low temperature ethylether extracts of the plant were shown to have activity against experimental rodent malaria.[390] On the other side of the world another medicinal plant came to medical attention during the reign of the Count of Cinchon as Viceroy of Peru between 1628 and 1629 (Figure 71.19). Legend has it that the Viceroy's wife, the Countess, was afflicted by ague in Lima. She was a well-known and popular figure and news of her illness spread inland. It eventually reached Lloxa where a Spaniard was in governorship. He knew of a local remedy obtained from the bark of a tree and sent it to the ailing Countess. The therapeutic result was excellent; she improved rapidly, and was so impressed that she ordered the bark in quantity and dispensed it to the poor of Lima who commonly suffered from the dangerous tertian fevers. The pulverized bark became known as 'los polvos de la Condeca' or the Countess's powder, and Linnaeus subsequently named the tree from which the bark was obtained 'Cinchona' in honour of the Countess. Sadly the detective work of one A.W. Haggis, reported in 1941,[391] has shown that 'the fabulous story of the Countess of Cinchon' is almost certainly a romantic fable. Nevertheless it is likely that the bark was introduced to Europe by the Fathers of the Society of Jesus around the time of the story, or even earlier (circa 1630) and was widely promoted in Europe by the Jesuit Cardinal Juan de Hugo. For these reasons it became known as Jesuit's bark. Not everyone was convinced by the new remedy, and when in 1653 Archduke Leopold of Austria relapsed one month after being cured of double quartan fever, his personal physician Jean-Jacques Chifflet began a bitter polemic on the merits of the bark which was to last for 200 years. Much of the dispute stemmed from the fact that many considered all fevers had the same cause, and clearly not all responded to Jesuit's bark. It was probably Torti in 1712 who first stated that the bark was 'specific solely for the ague'.

Another source of debate, and one that is still active today, was dosage. Sir Robert Talbor (Talbot) was one of the few physicians who was not afraid to give the bark in large and repeated doses, and when he cured the Dauphin (the son of Louis XIV) with his 'remede anglais' his fame spread far and wide. He subsequently treated Charles II of England successfully with the same medicament. Others were less enthusiastic. Many protestants believed the bark to be a poison disseminated by the Jesuits. The dose-response question was clarified in 1768 by Lind, who demonstrated clearly that in order to get best results the bark should be given in full doses as soon as the disease was diagnosed. (Advice that has stood the test of time.)

In 1820 the French chemists Pierre Pelletier and Joseph Caventou isolated the alkaloid quinine from cinchona bark. Purification of the various cinchona alkaloids allowed standardization of dosage. Adequate doses could now be given in relatively small amounts of pure drug, but by the middle of the nineteenth century enormous doses (up to 100–150 grains over two days) were being prescribed. Toxicity was common and the popularity of the medicine

fell. Gradually, however, the diagnosis of agues and the prescription of cinchona alkaloids became more rational and logical. The new colonial powers recognized the importance of cinchona, and improved methods of horticulture resulted in better yields of the alkaloids from the cultivated trees. The Dutch took the lead and vast plantations of high yielding *Cinchona ledgeriana* were started in the East Indies (principally in Java).[392]

Laveran, having identified haematozoa as the cause of paludisme (malaria), later concluded that quinine cured the disease by killing the newly discovered parasites. This theory encountered considerable resistance in the years immediately following its publication. In 1880 Bacelli described the intravenous method of administering quinine (although there is evidence that this route had been used for 50 years before that). Laveran considered intravenous injection to be dangerous, giving rise to both local and general complications, and was only justified in 'the most grave and pernicious disease'. He also confirmed the earlier observations of Thomas Willis (1659) that cinchona cured the acute attacks of ague, but did not prevent relapses, and also appeared to have no effect on crescents (gametocytes of *P. falciparum*).[393] The eminent Italian malariologists subsequently showed that quinine prevented asexual blood-stage development but could not stop sporulation of formed segmenters (meronts).

In England in 1856 William Henry Perkin discovered analine purple (mauve) whilst attempting to synthesize quinine from coal tar products. Thus began the synthetic dye industry. Later in Germany, the antimicrobial properties of those newly discovered aniline dyes were investigated. In 1890 Ehrlich showed that methylene blue had antimalarial activity against *P. cathemerium* in canaries, but the dye proved disappointing in clinical practice, and structural modifications did not lead to compounds with improved activity. During the Great War (1914–1918) whole armies were immobilized in the Balkans because of malaria, and there were heavy losses in Mesopotamia, East Africa and the Jordan Valley. The British and French armies used quinine extensively, and despite frequent objections to the bitter medicament many lives were saved. The military and strategic importance of antimalarial drugs stimulated much research immediately after the war.[394] In the early 1920s the resurgent German chemical industry again focused its attention on new antimicrobial compounds. The first synthetic antimalarial was discovered in 1926. This was an aminoquinoline compound, pamaquine, also known as plasmoquine or plasmochin, a precursor of the 8-aminoquinoline primaquine. Pamaquine was followed by the acridine compound mepacrine (quinacrine) in 1932, and the structurally related 4-aminoquinoline, chloroquine, in 1934. Initially chloroquine was rejected as being too toxic for human use, and the research team at Bayer were asked to produce a safer compound. They then produced 3-methylchloroquine (Sontoquine) but, despite clinical studies, these compounds were generally unavailable at the outbreak of the Second World War.

Malaria research has often been tied to warfare. Armies fighting in tropical theatres of war usually lose more men to malaria than bullets.[394] At the outset of the Second World War, the Allies knew their position was precarious in the tropics as most of the world's cinchona was grown in Java,[395] and this was vulnerable to Japanese invasion. They embarked upon a tremendous combined research effort into the development and evaluation of new antimalarial drugs. In the event Java did fall to the Japanese, but widespread use of mepacrine (quinacrine) prophylaxis by the Allied soldiers proved highly effective (albeit somewhat toxic) and probably saved the day. Information on chloroquine was, in fact, available to the Allied Powers through pre-war reciprocal arrangements between the pharmaceutical companies, Bayer and Winthrop, but lay buried in documents until the defection of two French soldiers in North Africa in 1943. They brought with them a German antimalarial drug, later identified as Sontoquine. However, chloroquine was not fully evaluated until the end of the war.[396]

An entirely separate line of research in the UK led to the discovery in 1945 of the antimalarial biguanides, proguanil and subsequently chlorproguanil. These compounds were later shown to inhibit the plasmodial enzyme dihydrofolate reductase (DHFR). Researchers at the Wellcome Research Laboratories synthesizing purine analogues developed the antimitotic compound 6-mercaptopurine (and later azathioprine) and in 1952 discovered the antiprotozoal DHFR inhibitor pyrimethamine. This same line of Nobel Prize winning research later developed trimethoprim, which has considerably greater affinity for bacterial DHFR (but also inhibits the plasmodial enzyme), and also allopurinol, acyclovir and zidovudine (AZT).

By the early 1950s the 4-aminoquinolines, chloroquine, and to a much lesser extent amodiaquine, had become the treatment of choice for all malaria throughout the world. Pyrimethamine was used in treatment, and chloroquine, pyrimethamine and proguanil were used for prophylaxis. Primaquine was given to prevent relapses of *P. vivax* and *P. ovale*.[397] The cinchona alkaloids were little used outside francophone Africa, and with the discontinuation of quinine, blackwater fever became a rarity. This was the heyday of the malaria eradication era,[398] and with the tremendous successes in Europe and many urban areas of the tropics, interest in the development of new antimalarial drugs waned rapidly. But eradication in the tropics failed, and in the 1960s antimalarial drug resistance emerged as a major threat.

The expanding tide of antimalarial drug resistance, together with the looming conflict in Vietnam and the manifest failure of the eradication programme prompted a massive US army-led research effort to screen and test new antimalarial compounds. Most of the compounds developed were structurally related to the known quinoline antimalarial drugs. Mefloquine and halofantrine are the result of this effort.[399] An 8-aminoquinoline compound (tafenoquine) which is less toxic and more active than primaquine has been developed by the US army research programme in recent years and is now in phase III trials.

Since the 1960s there has been almost no research on new antimalarial drugs by the pharmaceutical industry. The exception is a naphthaquinone compound (atovaquone, a modification of a compound discovered over 40 years ago) which has been combined with proguanil in a single formulation and has been registered widely. It is a safe and very effective antimalarial drug, although very expensive to manufacture.

It is the Chinese who have given us the most important antimalarial drugs in recent years. Several very promising synthetic antimalarial compounds, structurally related to existing drugs, have been produced, evaluated, and deployed. These are lumefantrine (formerly known as benflumetol), pyronaridine, piperaquine, and naphthoquine. All are active against multi-drug resistant malaria. By far the most important development in malaria treatment in recent years has been the Chinese rediscovery and development of the drugs related to artemisinin (qinghaosu).[390,400–406] These drugs are structurally unrelated to existing antimalarial drugs. They are rapidly effective, safe, and to date no significant resistance has developed. Artemisinin and the derivatives artemether and artesunate have been used widely in China for over fifteen years. These drugs have been used extensively in Vietnam and Thailand for over a decade, and now they being used increasingly throughout the tropical world. Artemisinin and its derivatives are used in combination with other antimalarial drugs for uncomplicated malaria, and as parenteral or rectal formulations for severe disease.

Antimalarial drug resistance

The global death toll from malaria is rising, and this is attributed directly to drug resistance. *Plasmodium falciparum* has developed resistance to all classes of antimalarial drugs with the exception of the artemisinin derivatives.[407–412] The other human malarias are generally more drug-sensitive, although they have developed antifol resistance rapidly in some areas. Significant chloroquine resistance has now developed in *P. vivax* in Oceania, and parts of Indonesia.[413,414] Elsewhere *P. vivax* remains chloroquine sensitive. Quinine resistance in *P. falciparum* was first reported from Brazil in 1910,[415] but has never been high grade, and has not compromised use of the drug. Within years of the introduction of the antifols proguanil and pyrimethamine, resistance was noted in both *P. falciparum* and *P. vivax* which did compromise use of these drugs, but antimalarial resistance was not treated seriously until chloroquine resistance in *P. falciparum* developed almost simultaneously in South-East Asia and South America in the early 1960s. The selection of resistance may have resulted from the misguided use of chloroquine (and pyrimethamine)-impregnated salt as an attempt to control malaria by mass prophylaxis.[416] During the 1970s chloroquine resistance in *P. falciparum* spread from South-East Asia and South America, and fuelled the resurgence of falciparum malaria in the tropics. By the early 1980s

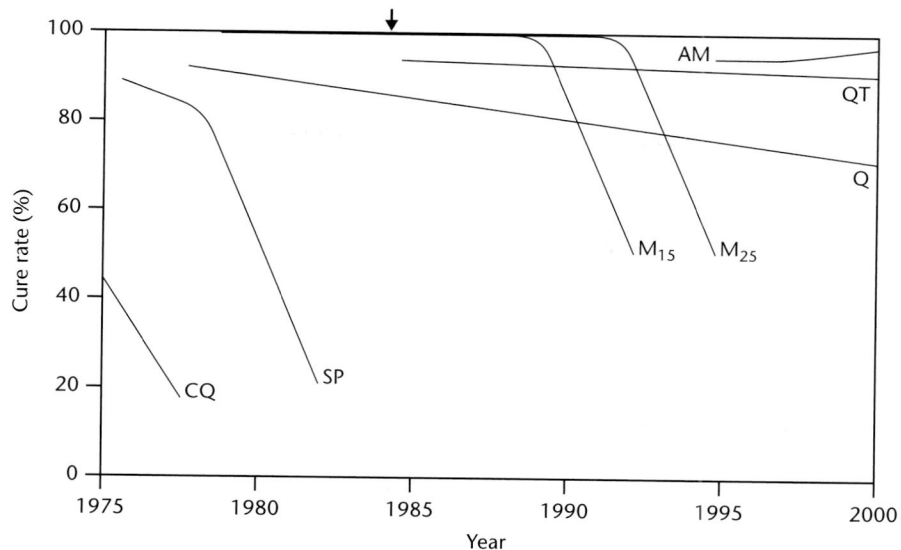

Figure 71.20: Antimalarial resistance at its most severe; the decline in antimalarial drug efficacy on the borders of Thailand. Chloroquine (CQ) and sulphadoxine-pyrimethamine (SP) were no longer effective by the beginning of the 1980s. Quinine (Q) efficacy declined slowly. Mefloquine (M) was introduced in November 1984 (arrow), at a dose of 15 mg/kg combined with SP—although SP was already useless by then. Resistance to mefloquine developed rapidly despite tight control over its use. A seven-day quinine-tetracycline regimen (QT) remained effective, but the introduction of artesunate-mefloquine (artesunate 12 mg/kg over 3 days, combined with 25 mg/kg mefloquine split dose) in 1994 has led to a remarkable reversal of the resistance trend. This regimen remains nearly 100% effective in 2002.

chloroquine was no longer effective in many countries, and the first ominous reports of resistance on the east coast of Africa appeared. Since then chloroquine resistance has spread remorselessly across Africa, and now few countries in the tropics are unaffected. Pyrimethamine resistance has also worsened rapidly, and the synergistic combination with sulphonamides (SP, sulphadoxine-pyrimethamine) is no longer effective in many areas. This is particularly alarming in Africa where, because of chloroquine resistance, the mortality rate is rising.[417] Many countries in the east and south of the continent have been forced to change their treatment policy from chloroquine to SP. The loss of SP has been more rapid, as predicted, and many countries are facing the bleak prospect of needing unaffordable treatments.

South-East Asia, and in particular Cambodia and Thailand, have traditionally had the world's most drug-resistant malaria parasites and events there act as harbingers of the development of resistance elsewhere (Figure 71.20). Chloroquine resistance spread throughout the region in the 1960s and 1970s, and SP fell rapidly to resistance in the early 1980s. In 1984 mefloquine replaced quinine as the treatment of choice for falciparum malaria in Thailand. This was the first country in which mefloquine was used widely. It was introduced in combination with sulfadoxine and pyrimethamine in order to delay the onset of resistance. However, since 1988 mefloquine resistance has developed rapidly in Thailand[410,418] and adjacent Cambodia and western Burma, and later in Vietnam, while sensitivity to quinine has declined very gradually. By 1994 high-level mefloquine resistance had developed in some areas and, on the western border of Thailand, the combination of artesunate, given for three days, and high dose mefloquine (25 mg/kg) was introduced.[419] Despite the fact that *P. falciparum* there was already mefloquine resistant, this proved remarkably effective. In the subsequent seven years cure rates have remained over 95%. There has been no further decline in mefloquine resistance,[412,420] and there was a marked decline in the incidence of falciparum malaria. These results and the dramatic decline in malaria mortality associated with artemisinin deployment in Vietnam, led to a global initiative to evaluate antimalarial drug combinations based on the artemisinin derivatives. These combinations have proved safe and effective, and it is now widely accepted that such combinations should replace existing monotherapies for the treatment of malaria to ensure sustained efficacy and prevent the emergence of resistance. This is central to the 'Roll Back Malaria' initiative. But implementing these changes is a formidable challenge. In 2002 the majority of countries affected by malaria still have, as National recommendations for treatment, drugs which are partially, or sometimes completely ineffective. This must be changed.

Antimalarial treatment

In general, the antimalarial drugs are more toxic than antibacterial drugs, i.e., the therapeutic ratio is narrower, but serious adverse effects are still rare. The available antimalarial drugs fall into three broad groups: the aryl aminoalcohols (quinoline-related or quinoline-like) compounds (quinine, quinidine, chloroquine, amodiaquine, mefloquine, halofantrine, lumefantrine, piperaquine, primaquine, tafenoquine); the antifols (pyrimethamine, proguanil, chlorproguanil, trimethoprim); and the artemisinin compounds (artemisinin, dihydroartemisinin, artemether, artesunate). Of these, the artemisinin drugs have the broadest time window of action on the asexual malarial parasites, from medium-sized rings to early schizonts, and produce the most rapid therapeutic responses.[421,422] Several antibacterial drugs also have antiplasmodial activity, although in general their action is slow, and they are used in combination with the antimalarial drugs. Those used are the sulphonamides and sulphones, tetracyclines, lincosamides, macrolides, and inadvertently, chloramphenicol. Significant resistance has been reported to the sulphonamides but not to the other classes of antibiotics. Drugs which are active against sensitive *P. falciparum* are also active against the other three malaria species.

Antimalarial pharmacodynamics

The principle effect of antimalarial drugs in the treatment of uncomplicated malaria is to inhibit parasite multiplication (by stopping parasite development). The untreated infection can multiply at a maximum rate given by the average number of viable merozoites per mature schizont (100% efficiency).[423] In non-immune subjects multiplication is often relatively efficient with multiplication rates of 6–20/cycle (30–90% efficiency). Antimalarial drugs exerting their maximum effects (E_{max}) will convert this to a negative figure from –10 to –10 000, thus reducing parasite numbers by between 10 and 10 000-fold per cycle. The E_{max} is the effect represented at the top of the sigmoid dose-response or concentration-effect relationship. Drugs differ in their E_{max}; for example, the artemisinins often produce a 10 000-fold reduction per asexual cycle, whereas antimalarial antibiotics such as tetracycline or clindamycin may achieve only at most a tenfold parasite reduction per cycle (Figure 71.21).[423] The lowest blood or plasma concentration of antimalarial drug which results in E_{max} can be considered a minimum parasiticidal concentration (MPC). Parasite reduction appears to be a first-order process throughout.[424] This means that provided that the MPC is exceeded then a fixed fraction of the population is removed each successive asexual cycle. Patients with acute malaria may have up to 10^{12} parasites in the circulation. Even with killing rates per cycle of 99.99% it will take at least three life cycles (6 days) to eradicate all the parasites. Thus antimalarial treatment must usually provide therapeutic drug concentrations for 7 days (covering four cycles) to affect a cure.[423,425] For rapidly eliminated drugs this means the course of treatment must be 7 days (Figure 71.22). Treatment responses are always better in patients with some immunity.[426] In endemic areas this means that the worst treatment results are seen in young children.

In the treatment of severe malaria the stage of antimalarial drug activity is also important as the object of treatment is to stop parasite maturation, particularly from the less pathogenic circulating ring forms to the more pathogenic cytoadherent stages. The drugs used for the treatment of severe malaria all act predominantly in the middle third of the life cycle when there is the greatest increase in parasite synthetic and metabolic activity.[421,422] The antifols act a little later, but none of the drugs will prevent rupture and reinvasion once the meront (schizont) has formed (the widely used term schizontocidal is therefore incorrect). Young rings are also relatively drug resistant (particularly to quinine and pyrimethamine). The artemisinin compounds have the broadest time window of antimalarial action, and the most rapid in vivo activity.[422,423] These compounds, and to a lesser extent chloroquine, prevent maturation of ring stages, therefore inducing accelerated clearance and reducing subsequent cytoadherence (whereas quinine does not).[247,427,428]

Mode of action and mechanisms of resistance

Resistance means that there is a shift to the right in the dose-response (concentration-effect) relationship. The shape of the relationship may also change and the E_{max} be reduced. Pyrimethamine and the antimalarial biguanides interfere with folic acid synthesis in the parasite by inhibiting the bifunctional enzyme dihydrofolate reductase—thymidilate synthase (DHFR). Sulphonamides act at the previous step in the synthetic pathway by inhibiting dihydropteroate synthase (DHPS), and there is marked synergy between the two classes of compounds. Resistance to pyrimethamine in *P. falciparum* was reported within a few years of its introduction.[430] DHFR resistance is associated with point mutations in the DHFR gene which lead to reduced affinity (100–1000 times less) of the enzyme complex for the drug.[431–433] The first mutation is usually at position 108 of *Pf*DHFR (serine to asparagine). This has little clinical relevance initially, but then mutations arise at positions 51 and 59 conferring increasing resistance to pyrimethamine. Infections with triple mutants are relatively resistant but some therapeutic response is usually seen to sulphadoxine-pyrimethamine (SP). The stage is then set for the acquisition of a fourth and devastating mutation at position 164 (isoleucine to leucine).[434] This renders the available antifols completely ineffective. This mutation is prevalent in parts of South-East Asia and South America, and sadly has just been reported in East Africa. Interestingly mutations conferring moderate pyrimethamine resistance do not necessarily confer cycloguanil resistance, and vice versa.[435,436] For example mutations at position 16 (alanine to valine) plus serine to threonine at position 108 confer high level resistance to cycloguanil but not pyrimethamine.[436] In general the biguanides (cycloguanil, chlorcycloguanil) are more active than pyrimethamine against the resistant mutants (and they are more effective clinically too), but they are ineffective against parasites with the DHFR 164 mutation. *P. vivax* shares similar antifol resistance mechanisms through serial acquisition of mutations in *Pv*DHFR. The marked synergy with sulphonamides and sulphones is important

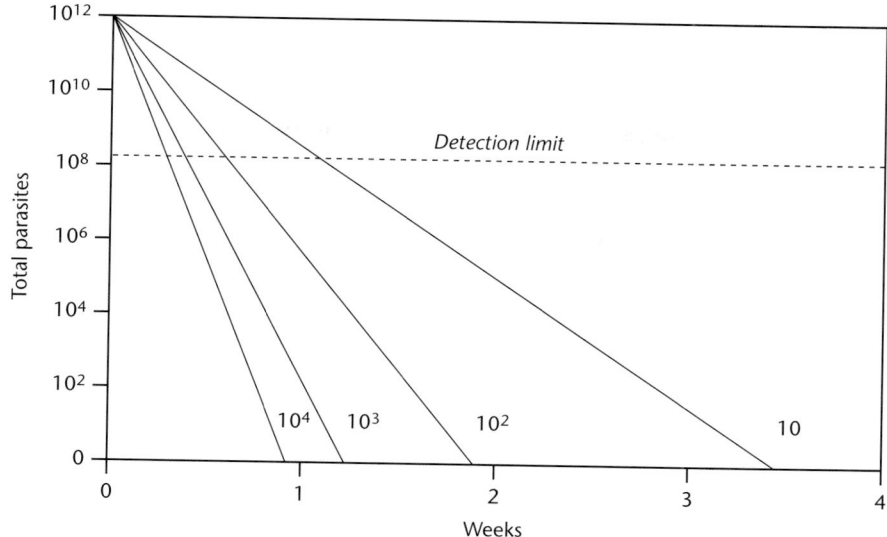

Figure 71.21: Pharmacodynamics. The effects of different rates of parasite killing on the elimination of the malaria infection. The individual parasite biomass is given on the vertical axis. 10^{12} parasites corresponds to about 2% parasitaemia in an adult who is not anaemic. The artemisinin derivatives achieve the highest parasite reduction ratios (PRR: 10^4 per asexual cycle) and eradicate the infection in 6–8 days. Most of the other antimalarials achieve PRR values of 10^2 to 10^3 per cycle. The antimalarial antibiotics alone (e.g., doxycycline) have PRR values of approximately 10 and take three weeks to cure malaria if used alone (which they clearly should not be!).

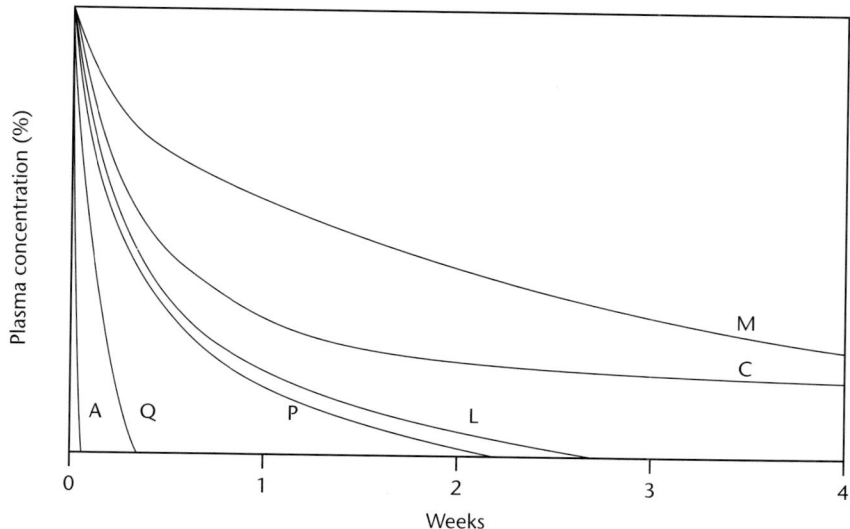

Figure 71.22: Pharmacokinetics. A comparison of the elimination profiles of the antimalarial drugs (normalized to the initial peak concentration). A, artemisinin and derivatives; Q, quinine/quinidine; P, pyrimethamine; L, lumefantrine; C, chloroquine; M, mefloquine.

for the antimalarial activity of SP or sulphone-biguanide combinations.

Sulphonamide and sulphone resistance also develops by progressive acquisition of mutations in the gene encoding the target enzyme DHPS[437,438] (which is a bifunctional protein with the enzyme PPPK). Specifically altered amino acid residues have been found at positions 436, 437, 540, 581, and 613 in the DHPS domain. The 581 and 613 mutations do not occur in isolation, but always on top of an initial mutation (usually alanine to glycine at 437).

The mode of action of the quinoline antimalarial drugs has been a source of controversy for years. These drugs are weak bases, and they concentrate in the acid food vacuole of the parasite,[439] but this in itself does not explain their antimalarial activity.[440] Chloroquine intercalates DNA, but only at concentrations (1–2 mmol/l) much higher than required to kill parasites (10–20 nmol/l). Chloroquine binds to ferriprotoporphyrin IX, a product of haemoglobin degradation,[441] and thereby chemically inhibits haem dimerization. This is an essential defence mechanism for the parasite to detoxify haem, and inhibition of this process provides a plausible explanation for the selective antimalarial action of these drugs.[41,442] Chloroquine also competitively inhibits glutathione mediated haem degradation, another parasite detoxification pathway.[42]

Chloroquine resistance is associated with reduced concentrations of drug in the acid food vacuole. Both reduced influx and increased efflux have been implicated.[442] The resistant parasites pump chloroquine out 40–50 times faster than drug-sensitive parasites. This efflux mechanism is similar to that found in multi-drug resistant (MDR) mammalian tumour cells. One of the efflux mechanisms is through an ATP-requiring transmembrane pump, *P. glycoprotein*. Genes encoding these MDR proteins have been identified in *P. falciparum (pfmdr1)*. These MDR genes are found in increased copy numbers in most quinine and mefloquine resistant parasites, and point mutations (notably asparagine to tyrosine at position 86) are associated with chloroquine resistance.[443-445] Recent transfection studies confirm a role for *pfmdr* in mediating resistance to chloroquine and mefloquine.[446] Recently point mutations in CRT (a food vacuolar membrane protein thought to have a transporter function), have been shown to mediate chloroquine resistance.[447-449] The principle correlate is a *PfCRT* mutation resulting in a change in coding from lysine to threonine at position 76.[449-450] From an epidemiological standpoint multiple unlinked mutations are probably required for the development of chloroquine resistance, and it is likely that other contributors to quinoline resistance remain to be discovered.

The chloroquine efflux mechanism in resistant parasites can be inhibited by a number of structurally unrelated drugs: calcium channel blockers, tricyclic antidepressants, phenothiazines, cyproheptadine, antihistamines, etc., whereas mefloquine resistance is reversed by penfluridol which does not reduce chloroquine efflux.[451-452] This has

given hope that chloroquine resistance might be reversed in clinical practice. Initial evaluations were uniformly disappointing, but recent studies in Nigerian children given chloroquine together with very high doses of chlorpheniramine indicate significantly improved efficacy against chloroquine resistant falciparum malaria.[453] Whether general use of resistance reversers will be a safe and feasible therapeutic option remains to be seen. In general, antimalarial drug resistance to mefloquine, quinine, lumefantrine, and halofantrine is linked, but, as suggested by their different susceptibility to reversing agents, chloroquine resistance and mefloquine resistance are not linked closely. Indeed within a particular geographic area there is a reciprocal relationship; increasing mefloquine resistance is associated with increasing susceptibility to chloroquine.[412,454,455]

Atovaquone interferes with parasite mitochondrial electron transport, and it also depolarises the parasite mitochondria thereby blocking cellular respiration.[456] High levels of resistance result from single point mutations in the gene encoding cytochrome *b*. This gene is encoded on a small extrachromosomal plastid-like DNA-containing organelle which may have an intrinsically high mutation rate.[457] Resistance mutations arise frequently (circa 1 in 10^{12} asexual divisions) (Figure 71.23).

The mechanism of action of the artemisinin drugs appears to involve the generation of carbon-centred free radicals which alkylate critical proteins.[458,459] Parasiticidal activity is dependent on the integrity of the peroxide bridge. Although in general multi-drug-resistant parasites are more artemisinin resistant, and reduced susceptibility can be induced experimentally, the degree of resistance is slight and very unlikely to be of clinical relevance. Artemisinin and its derivatives induce very rapid ring form clearance. This results from splenic removal of the

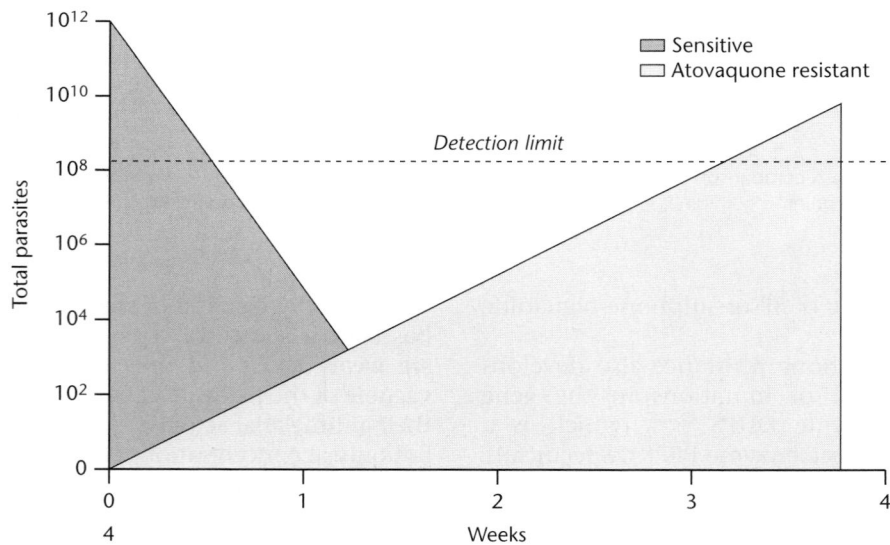

Figure 71.23: The emergence of high-evel resistance. Following atovaquone (only) treatment highly resistant recrudescent infections emerged in one-third of patients. This represented untrammelled growth of a single starting parasite; a per parasite mutation frequency of 1 in 10^{12}.

damaged intraerythrocytic parasites, and return of the once-infected red blood cells to the circulation.[247]

Resistance is thought to arise from spontaneous chromosomal point mutations or gene duplications which are independent of drug selection pressure.[460] Once formed, these more resistant mutants have a survival advantage in the presence of antimalarial drugs.[461,462] Several factors encourage the development of resistance. These are the intrinsic frequency with which the genetic changes occur, the degree of resistance conferred by the genetic change (pharmacodynamics), the proportion of all transmissible infections which are exposed to the drug, the drug concentration profile (pharmacokinetics), the pattern of drug use, and the immunity profile of the community.[460] Resistant parasites will be selected when parasites are exposed to subtherapeutic drug concentrations. Thus non-immune patients infected with large numbers of parasites who receive inadequate treatment (either because of poor drug quality, adherence, vomiting of an oral treatment etc.) are a potent source of resistance. This emphasises the importance of correct prescribing, and good adherence to prescribed drug regimens in slowing the emergence of resistance. The emergence of resistance is slower in high transmission areas, because background immunity may eliminate the resistant mutants and stop them being transmitted. The spread of resistant mutant parasites is facilitated by the use of drugs with long elimination phases which provide a 'selective filter', allowing infections by the resistant parasites while the residual antimalarial activity prevents infection by sensitive parasites.[463] Slowly eliminated drugs such as mefloquine ($T_{1/2}\beta$ 3 weeks) or chloroquine ($T_{1/2}\beta$ 2 months) persist in blood and provide such a selective filter for months after drug administration (Figure 71.22). The selection pressure can be enormous. In Africa approximately 250 000 kg or 170×10^6 adult treatment doses of chloroquine are consumed annually.

Thus in many parts of the continent the majority of the population has chloroquine in the blood at any time.

Prevention of resistance using combinations of antimalarial drugs

The emergence of resistance can be prevented by the use of combinations of drugs with different mechanisms of action, and therefore different drug targets.[426,460,464] The same rationale underlies the current treatment of tuberculosis, leprosy, HIV infections and many cancers. If two drugs are used, which do not share a common mode of action and therefore the parasite develops different mechanisms of resistance to them, then the per parasite probability of developing resistance to both drugs is the product of their individual per parasite probabilities. For example, if the per parasite probability of developing resistance to drug A and drug B are both 1 in 10^{12} then a simultaneously resistant mutant will arise spontaneously every 1 in 10^{24} parasites. As there are approximately 10^{17} malaria parasites in the entire world, and a cumulative total of less than 10^{20} in one year, such a simultaneously resistant parasite would arise spontaneously roughly once every 10 000 years—if the drugs always confronted the parasites in combination (Figure 71.24). Thus the lower the de novo per parasite probability of developing resistance, the greater the delay in the emergence of resistance. However this powerful approach has several limitations. If not everyone receives the combination, and some patients only receive one of the components, then resistance can arise (emphasizing the importance of achieving high coverage when these drugs are deployed). Combinations are also more expensive. But the increased cost is outweighed by the longer term benefits. At present there are a number of important, but unanswered, practical questions concerning resistance. We do not know the relative

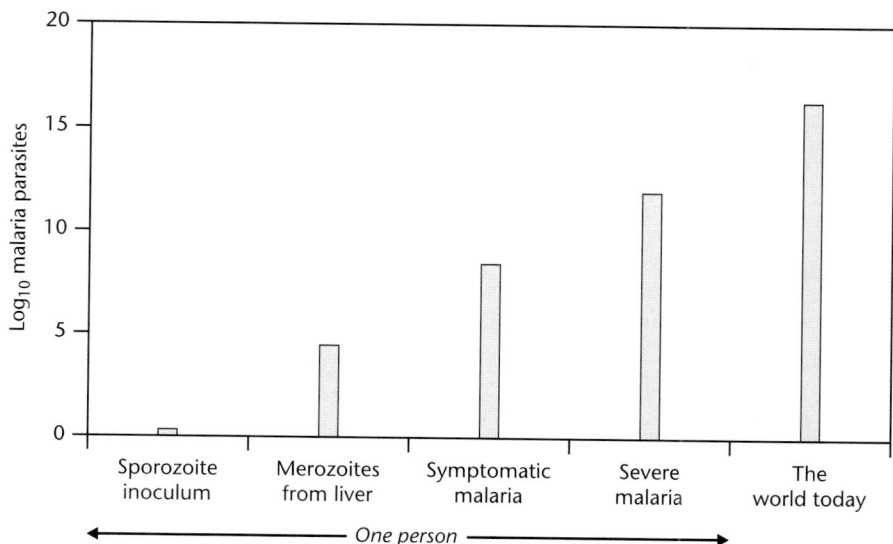

Figure 71.24: The logarithmic distribution of malaria parasites. There are probably between 10^{16} and 10^{18} parasites in the world today. The day after tomorrow there will be another 10^{16}–10^{18}!

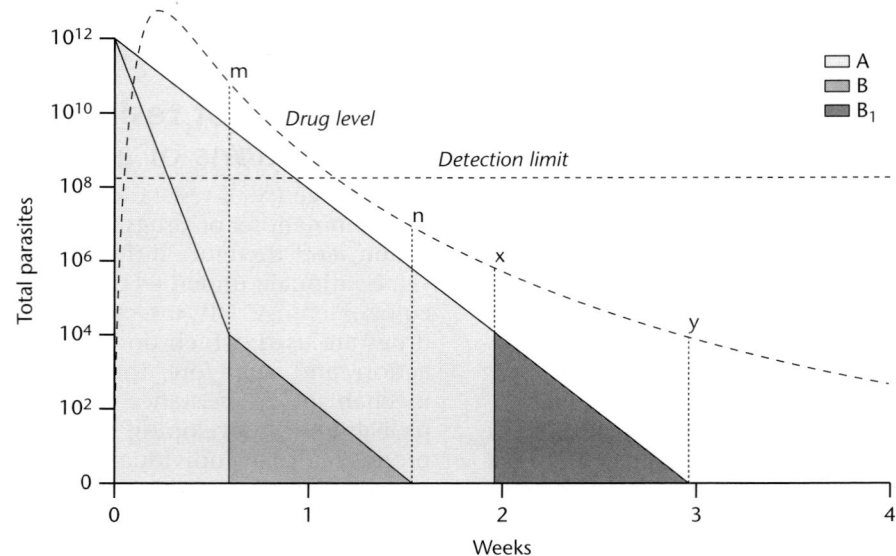

Figure 71.25: Artemisinin combination treatment. The effects of adding a three day course of artesunate to high-dose (25 mg/kg) mefloquine on malaria parasite killing in an area of pre-existing mefloquine resistance (e.g., in Thailand). Without the artesunate the parasitaemia declines 100-fold per asexual cycle, and is eliminated finally in three weeks. If artesunate is added for three days, covering two asexual cycles, then the parasite biomass is reduced 10^8-fold leaving a tail of a maximum of only 10^5 parasites remaining (and usually much fewer) for the high concentrations of mefloquine to remove (B). This offers a hundred million fold lower opportunity of selecting a resistant parasite. Note that without artesunate the corresponding number of parasites (B$_1$) 'see' much lower concentrations of mefloquine (from *x* to *y*, compared with *m* to *n*) and have therefore an increased risk of recrudescing.

importance of all the factors which contribute, and therefore the optimum strategy to prevent resistance. The most promising approach is the systematic deployment everywhere of artemisinin combinations, but which combination (Figure 71.25)? Will combinations prevent resistance in high transmission areas? Theoretically they should. Will resistance reverse if drug pressure is removed? Does widespread trimethoprim/ sulphamethoxazole use for bacterial infections encourage antimalarial antifol resistance? Unfortunately the situation is deteriorating so rapidly that we will not have sufficient time to answer all these questions satisfactorily. Radical action is needed in the near future if we are to control malaria, and protect the few antimalarial drugs available to us.[465]

Quinine

Quinine is a bitter powder obtained from the bark of the cinchona tree. It is widely used as a flavouring (tonic water, bitter lemon) and it is an effective treatment for night cramps, as well as for malaria. Contrary to widespread belief quinine is not antipyretic. Quinine is usually formulated as the dihydrochloride salt for parenteral administration, and as the sulphate, bisulphate, dihydrochloride, ethylcarbonate, hydrochloride or hydrobromide salts for oral administration. Unlike the other antimalarial drugs, and somewhat confusingly, quinine doses are usually prescribed as weights of salt rather than base (the different salts have different base contents) (Table 71.7). Quinine acts principally on the mature trophozoite stage of parasite development. It does not prevent sequestration or further development of formed meronts and does not kill the pre-erythrocytic or sexual stages of *P. falciparum*.

Pharmacokinetics (Table 71.8)

Quinine is well absorbed after oral or intramuscular administration both in adults and children.[466-471] Peak levels are usually reached within 4 hours (more rapidly if the intramuscular injections are diluted) (Figure 71.26). In acute malaria the total apparent volume of distribution

Table 71.7 Antimalarial drugs: salt-base equivalents

	Salt (mg)	Base (mg)
Chloroquine sulphate	204	150
Chloroquine diphosphate	242	150
Chloroquine hydrochloride	184	150
Amodiaquine dihydrochloride	261	200
Mefloquine hydrochloride	274	250
Quinine sulphate	363	300
Quinine bisulphate	508	300
Quinine hydrochloride	405	300
Quinine dihydrochloride	366	300
Quinine hydrobromide	366	300
Quinine ethylcarbonate	366	300
Quinidine sulphate	217	200
Quinidine bisulphate	234	200
Quinidine gluconate	289	200
Primaquine phosphate	26	15

Table 71.8 Pharmacokinetic properties of the antimalarial drugs

Drug	Absorption: Time to peak p.o.	i.m.	Oral dose (mg/kg)	Plasma peak level (mg/l)	Binding (%)	V_d/f (l/kg)	Clearance/f (ml/kg/min)	$T_{1/2}\beta$ (hours)	Notes
Uncomplicated malaria									
Quinine	6	1	10	8	90	0.8	1.5	16	Protein binding increased. Vd and clearance further reduced in severe malaria. Rate of i.m. absorption proportional to concentration of injectate
Quinidine	1	–	10	5	85	1.3	1.7	10	–
Chloroquine	5	0.5	10	0.12	55	10–1000	2.0	30–60 days	Concentrated in red cells, white cells and platelets. Kinetics unaffected by disease severity
Artesunate	1.5	0.5	4	0.5	–	0.15	50	0.75[a]	–
Artemether	2	3–18	4	1.5	95	2.7	54	1	–
Mefloquine	17	–	25	–	>98	20	0.35	14 days	Whole blood and plasma concentrations similar
Halofantrine	15	–	8	0.9[b]	>98[c]	–	7.5	113	Metabolized to active desbutyl metabolite which is eliminated more slowly
Lumefantrine	6	–	9	3.5[b]	>98[c]	2.7	3.0	86	Very variable bioavailability
Pyrimethamine	12	41	1.25	0.5	94	–	0.33	87	–
Atovaquone	6	–	15	5[b]	99.5	6	2.5	30	–
Healthy subjects									
Primaquine	3	–	0.6	0.15	–	3	6	6	Unidentified active metabolite
Proguanil (Chloroguanide)	3	–	3.5	0.17	75	24	19	16	Mainly a prodrug for active triazine metabolite cycloguanil which is eliminated more rapidly
Pyrimethamine	4	–	0.3	0.35	–	2.9	0.4	85	–

V_d/f is the total apparent volume of distribution divided by f, the fraction of drug absorbed.
a $T_{1/2}$ of the active metabolite dihydroartemisinin.
b Absorption increased significantly by fats.
c Binds to lipoproteins.

(V_d) is contracted and systemic clearance reduced in proportion to disease severity.[471–473] As a result blood concentrations are higher in uncomplicated malaria than in healthy subjects, and highest of all in severe malaria.[470] The elimination half-life is approximately 18–20 hours in cerebral malaria, 16 hours in uncomplicated malaria and 11 hours in health.[470,472,473] In children and pregnant women the apparent volume of distribution is relatively smaller and elimination is more rapid.[467,469,471,473,475] Quinine is a base and is bound principally to the acute phase plasma protein α_1-acid glycoprotein.[476] Plasma protein binding is increased in malaria from approximately 75–80% in healthy subjects to over 90% in severe malaria.[476–478] Red blood cell concentrations vary between one-third and one-half of the corresponding plasma concentrations,[479] and concentrations in breast milk and cord blood are approximately one-third of those in plasma.[474] The therapeutic range has not been well defined but total plasma concentrations of between 8 and 15 mg/l are certainly safe and effective.[480] Toxicity is increasingly likely with plasma concentrations over 20 mg/l (free quinine >2 mg/l). Approximately 80% of the administered drug is eliminated by hepatic bio-

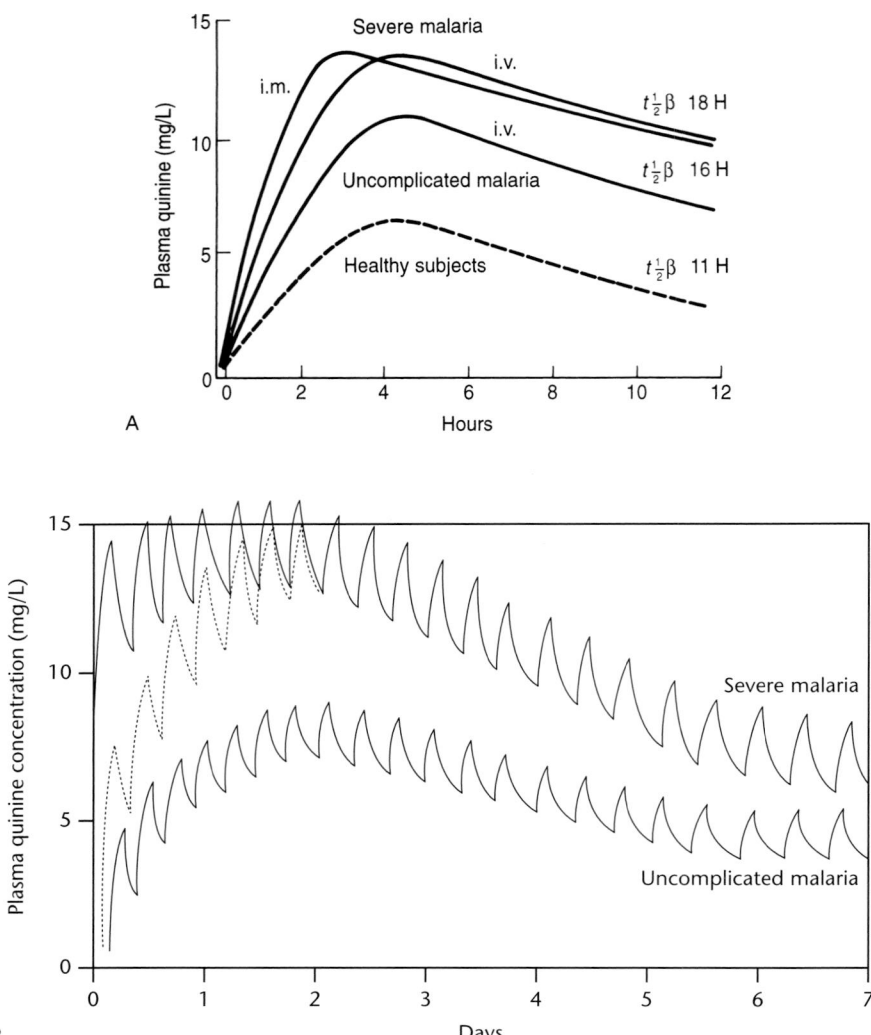

Figure 71.26: Quinine plasma concentrations. (**A**) Time profiles in malaria and in healthy subjects following a single dose of 20 mg salt/kg (from White N. J. British Journal of Clinical Pharmacology 1992; 34:1–10 with permission). (**B**) During the treatment of malaria.

transformation, and the remaining 20% is excreted unchanged by the kidney.[470] Although systemic clearance is reduced in severe malaria, this 80:20 proportion is preserved. The principal metabolite 3-hydroxyquinine is biologically active, contributing approximately 10% of the overall antimalarial activity, but more in renal failure where it accumulates.[481,482] The other more polar metabolites are either much less active, or inactive as antimalarial drugs.

Toxicity

Minor adverse effects are common with quinine but serious toxicity is remarkably rare in the treatment of malaria. Quinine is extremely bitter and therefore unpleasant to take, and regularly produces a symptom complex known as 'cinchonism'. This comprises tinnitus, high-tone hearing impairment, nausea, dysphoria and often vomiting. As a consequence compliance with the 5–7 day regimens required for cure is poor. Quinine predictably prolongs repolarization in skeletal and cardiac muscle and this is reflected in the electrocardiograph as prolongation of the QT_c interval by approximately 10% at therapeutic concentrations.[481] The effect is greater in children under 2 years of age.[475] This can be used as a pharmacodynamic measure of toxicity. However, significant conduction or repolarization abnormalities are rare and iatrogenic dysrhythmias are extremely uncommon. Quinine, like the other quinoline antimalarial drugs, exacerbates malaria-induced orthostatic hypotension,[367] but iatrogenic supine hypotension is rare. Blindness, resulting from retinal ganglion cell toxicity, and deafness are common following self-poisoning,[482,483] but rare in malaria treatment. Perhaps the most important toxic effect of quinine is its stimulatory action on the pancreatic β-cell.[265,484] This causes hyperinsulinaemic hypoglycaemia. It is particularly common in pregnant women but may occur in any severely ill patient, particularly if intravenous glucose solutions are not given.[267,277,279] Contrary to popular opinion, quinine does not induce premature labour at therapeutic doses. Quinine is rarely associated with a variety of allergic reactions, notably immune thrombocytopenia. Blackwater fever is undoubtedly associated with quinine use, but the underlying pathophysiological mechanism is still not understood.[485] Incorrect or non-sterile administration of intramuscular quinine is associated with tetanus, and this carries a very high mortality rate.[486]

Concerns over quinine cardiovascular toxicity in severe malaria are generally exaggerated in comparison to the dangers of undertreatment, and tend to arise from units in temperate countries managing occasional elderly travellers with imported malaria. Severe malaria is a potentially lethal condition. Antimalarial treatment is the only intervention proven to reduce mortality. Undertreatment may cause death—but physicians usually blame the malaria infection in a fatal case, and seldom ascribe death to their use of inadequate doses of quinine. On the other hand, cardiovascular complications are readily ascribed to the treatment rather than the fulminant disease. Large studies in endemic countries have confirmed the safety of quinine in severe malaria.[487,488] It is essential that patients receiving this drug achieve therapeutic concentrations of quinine in their blood within hours of reaching a treatment facility.[489]

Use

Parenteral quinine should be given by rate-controlled intravenous infusion in either 0.9% saline, 5 % or 10 % dextrose, or by deep intramuscular injection to the anterior thigh. It should *never* be given by intravenous injection (as it causes hypotension). The initial doses (mg/kg) in children and pregnant women are the same as in non-pregnant adults, although in areas with resistant parasites it has been recommended that the dose be increased in children to 15 mg salt/kg from day 4 to day 8 to prevent recrudescent infection.[490] In severe malaria, treatment should begin with a loading dose so that therapeutic levels are reached as quickly as possible.[491] If adequate treatment has been given before referral to hospital (i.e., >15 mg/kg in the preceding 24 hours) the loading dose is unnecessary. But if there is any doubt at all, or lower doses have been given, then the full loading dose should be given. In severe malaria, quinine doses should be reduced by one-third to one-half after 48 hours if there is no clinical improvement, or if there is acute renal failure. This prevents blood concentrations accumulating to toxic levels. Intramuscular quinine is painful and sclerosant if given undiluted (300 mg/ml). It should be diluted in sterile water 1:3 to 1:5 and given to the anterior thigh, never the buttock (to avoid the risk of sciatic nerve damage), using strict aseptic technique. Oral quinine is given in a dose of 10 mg salt/kg three times daily for 7 days (shorter courses are less effective) combined with either doxycycline or clindamycin.

Quinidine

Quinidine is the dextrorotatory diastereoisomer of quinine.

It is intrinsically more active as an antimalarial drug, but is also significantly more cardiotoxic and cardiac effects are common when it is used in treatment. There is no role for oral quinidine now in malaria, and its use for severe malaria is a last resort if quinine or an artemisinin derivative are not available.

Pharmacokinetics (Table 71.8)

Oral quinidine is well absorbed in malaria.[492] The V_d and systemic clearance are significantly greater than for quinine,[493,494] and the free fraction in plasma is approximately twice that of quinine. As for quinine, systemic clearance and V_d are reduced in malaria in proportion to disease severity.

Toxicity

Quinidine has a greater effect on the cardiovascular system, approximately equal stimulatory effect on the pancreatic β-cell, and causes less deafness than quinine. Systemic hypotension and myocardial conduction and repolarization abnormalities (widening of the QRS complex and greater than 25% prolongation of the electrocardiographic QT_c interval) are much more common in patients receiving parenteral quinidine compared with those receiving quinine treatment.[493,494] Electrocardiographic monitoring is advisable (this is not necessary for quinine). The spectrum of adverse effects is otherwise similar to quinine.

Use

Quinidine should be given for the treatment of severe chloroquine-resistant falciparum malaria only if quinine or qinghaosu derivatives are not available. It is more toxic than quinine and therefore more difficult to use. The usual salt is quinidine gluconate. It should be given by careful rate-controlled intravenous infusion with continuous electrocardiographic monitoring. The infusion should be stopped or the rate reduced if the ECG shows >25% prolongation of the QT_c interval or >50% widening of the QRS complex.[495] Hypotension usually responds promptly to saline loading. There are no data on intramuscular quinidine in malaria. Oral quinidine is given in the same doses of base equivalent as for quinine, but should only be used if nothing else is available. There has been some debate over the correct dose of intravenous quinidine in severe malaria,[496–498] largely because of the paucity of data. The doses given in Table 71.9 are higher than those recommended by some authorities.

Cinchonine and cinchonidine

These methylated natural cinchona alkaloids have no advantages over quinine and quinidine.

Chloroquine

Chloroquine is a 4-aminoquinoline. It is formulated as

Table 71.9 Antimalarial drug doses in severe malaria

	Hospital Intensive care unit (ICU)	Health clinic: No intravenous infusions possible	Rural health clinic: No injection facilities
Known chloroquine-sensitive *P.falciparum*	Chloroquine 10 mg base/kg infused intravenously at constant rate over 8 hours followed by 15 mg base/kg over 24 hours	Chloroquine 3.5 mg base/kg 6-hourly or 2.5 mg base/kg 4-hourly by i.m. or s.c. injection. Total dose 25 mg base/kg	10 mg/kg daily or nasogastric chloroquine as for oral regimen
Chloroquine-resistant *P.falciparum*	*Quinine* Quinine dihydrochloride 7 mg salt/kg infused over 30 minutes followed by immediately 10 mg/kg over 4 hours; or 20 mg salt/kg infused over 4 hours. Maintenance dose: 10 mg salt/kg infused over 2–8 hours at 8-hour intervals	Quinine dihydrochloride 20 mg salt/kg diluted 1:2 with sterile water given by split injection into both anterior thighs. Maintenance dose: 10 mg/kg 8-hourly	
	Quinidine 10 mg base/kg infused over 1–2 hours followed by 1.2 mg base/kg per hour. Electrocardiographic monitoring advisable		
	Artemisinin derivatives a) Artemether 3.2 mg/kg stat. by i.m. injection followed by 1.6 mg/kg daily; b) Artesunate 2.4 mg/kg stat. by i.v. injection followed 1.2 mg/kg daily	As for hospital ICU: artesunate can also be given by i.m. injection	Artesunate rectocap: 10 mg/kg daily Artemisinin suppository 20 mg/kg at 0 and 4 hrs. then daily.

General points:
If in doubt, consider the infection as chloroquine-resistant.
Infusions can be given in 0.9% saline, 5% or 10% dextrose/water.
Infusion rates for the quinoline antimalarials should be carefully controlled.
Oral treatment should start as soon as the patient can swallow reliably enough to complete a full course of treatment.

sulphate, phosphate and hydrochloride salts, and is prescribed in weights of base content. Various liquid formulations are available for paediatric use. Chloroquine can be given by intravenous infusion, intramuscular or subcutaneous injection, orally, or by suppository. Chloroquine acts mainly on the large ring-form and mature trophozoite stages of the parasite. It is more rapidly acting than quinine. Chloroquine is also used in the treatment of hepatic amoebiasis, and for some collagen-vascular and granulomatous diseases, notably rheumatoid arthritis (where hydroxychloroquine is preferred).

Pharmacokinetics (Table 71.8)

Chloroquine has complex pharmacokinetic properties with an enormous V_d (resulting from extensive tissue binding) and a very long elimination phase.[499,500] The terminal elimination half-life is 1–2 months. As a consequence, the blood concentration profile during malaria is determined mainly by distribution rather than elimination processes.[501,502] Chloroquine is well absorbed by mouth[503] and is very rapidly absorbed following subcutaneous or intramuscular injection, such that absorption may outpace distribution, and transiently toxic concentrations may occur.[501,502] To circumvent this, intravenous chloroquine is administered by constant-rate infusion, and subcutaneous or intramuscular chloroquine given in small (2.5–3.5 mg base/kg) frequent injections. A suppository formulation has been developed which also has good bioavailability.[504] Chloroquine is approximately 55% bound to plasma proteins. The principal metabolite of chloroquine, desethylchloroquine, has approximately equivalent antimalarial activity. This is of relevance to prophylactic, but not therapeutic efficacy.

Toxicity

Chloroquine is generally well tolerated. Oral chloroquine

may induce nausea or dysphoria and visual disturbances. Orthostatic hypotension may be accentuated. Pruritus is particularly troublesome in dark-skinned patients and may be dose limiting.[505] Very rarely chloroquine may cause an acute and self-limiting neuropsychiatric reaction. In prophylaxis cumulative doses over 100 g (> 5 years prophylaxis) are associated with an increased risk of retinopathy.[506,507] Residents on long-term chloroquine prophylaxis should probably have regular ophthalmological checks after taking the drug for 5 years, or if they experience any visual loss. Myopathy is rare at the doses used in antimalarial prophylaxis. Parenteral chloroquine may cause hypotension if administered too rapidly or a large dose (> 3.5 mg base/kg) is given by intramuscular or subcutaneous injection. In self-poisoning, chloroquine produces hypotension, arrhythmias and coma. Diazepam is a specific antidote.[508]

Use

Chloroquine is still the drug of choice for sensitive malaria parasites. It is therefore used widely for *P. vivax*, *P. malariae* and *P. ovale*, but is being progressively replaced for *P. falciparum* treatment. The time-honoured oral chloroquine regimen of 25 mg base/kg spread over three days (10, 10, 5 or 10, 5, 5, 5 mg/kg at 24-hour intervals) can be condensed into 36 hours of drug administration.[509] Intravenous chloroquine should only be used if the infusion rate can be monitored carefully, otherwise intramuscular or subcutaneous administration is safer.

Amodiaquine

Amodiaquine is also a 4-aminoquinoline with a similar mode of action to chloroquine. It is more active against resistant isolates of *P. falciparum*, and is being used increasingly now as a replacement.

Pharmacokinetics

Oral amodiaquine undergoes extensive first-pass metabolism to the biologically active metabolite desethylamodiaquine.[510] This exerts the principal antimalarial activity. The parent compound has an elimination half-life of approximately 10 hours,[511] but desethylamodiaquine, like chloroquine, is extensively distributed and eliminated slowly. Unfortunately there are inadequate data on the elimination kinetics of the metabolite. There are no parenteral formulations commercially available, although a structurally similar compound, amopyraquine, is available for intramuscular administration in some countries.

Toxicity

Prophylactic use of amodiaquine is associated with an unacceptably high incidence of serious toxicity. Approximately 1 in 2000 patients develop agranulocytosis.[512] Serious hepatotoxicity has also been reported. Agranulocytosis results from bioactivation to a reactive quinoneimine

metabolite. The incidence of these serious reactions is lower when amodiaquine is used in treatment, although precise estimates of the risk are lacking. Minor adverse effects are similar to those of chloroquine, although pruritus is less of a problem, and children find the drug more palatable.

Mepacrine (quinacrine)

Mepacrine is structurally similar to chloroquine. It has the same side chain, but is an acridine instead of a quinoline. It is more toxic and less effective than chloroquine. It should not be used as an antimalarial drug.

Mefloquine

Mefloquine is a fluorinated 4-quinoline methanol compound used for the treatment of multi-drug-resistant falciparum malaria. It has two asymmetric carbon atoms and is used clinically as a 50:50 racemic mixture of the erythroisomers. These have equal antimalarial activity but different pharmacokinetic properties.[513–515] The parasiticidal action is similar to that of quinine. Mefloquine is very insoluble in water. It is available as tablets, which should be kept dry. There are no parenteral or paediatric liquid formulations. Mefloquine has been combined with pyrimethamine and sulfadoxine, but this combination preparation offers no advantage over mefloquine alone, and carries the potential for severe sulphonamide toxicity.[516]

Pharmacokinetics (Table 71.8)

Mefloquine is moderately well absorbed, extensively distributed, and slowly eliminated.[513–520] It is highly (>98%) bound to plasma proteins. Mefloquine is cleared principally by hepatic biotransformation to inactive metabolites. The apparent volume of distribution and clearance of the (+)RS enantiomer is approximately four times higher than for the (–)SR enantiomer. The terminal elimination half-life is approximately three weeks in healthy subjects and two weeks in malaria (Figure 71.27). The absorption of mefloquine is reduced in the acute phase of illness and bioavailability of the higher 25 mg/kg dose is improved by dividing it (e.g., giving 15 mg/kg initially and 10 mg/kg 8–24 hours later) or in combination with artesunate delaying mefloquine administration until the second day of treatment.[519,520] Splitting the dose also reduces the incidence of acute adverse effects. Blood concentrations are higher in malaria than in healthy subjects and are reduced in diarrhoea (probably by interruption of enterohepatic recycling). Mefloquine clearance is increased in pregnancy.[521] The pharmacokinetics in adults and children are similar. Co-administration with artesunate results in a more rapid recovery from malaria which enhances oral bioavailability if the mefloquine dose is split.[520,521]

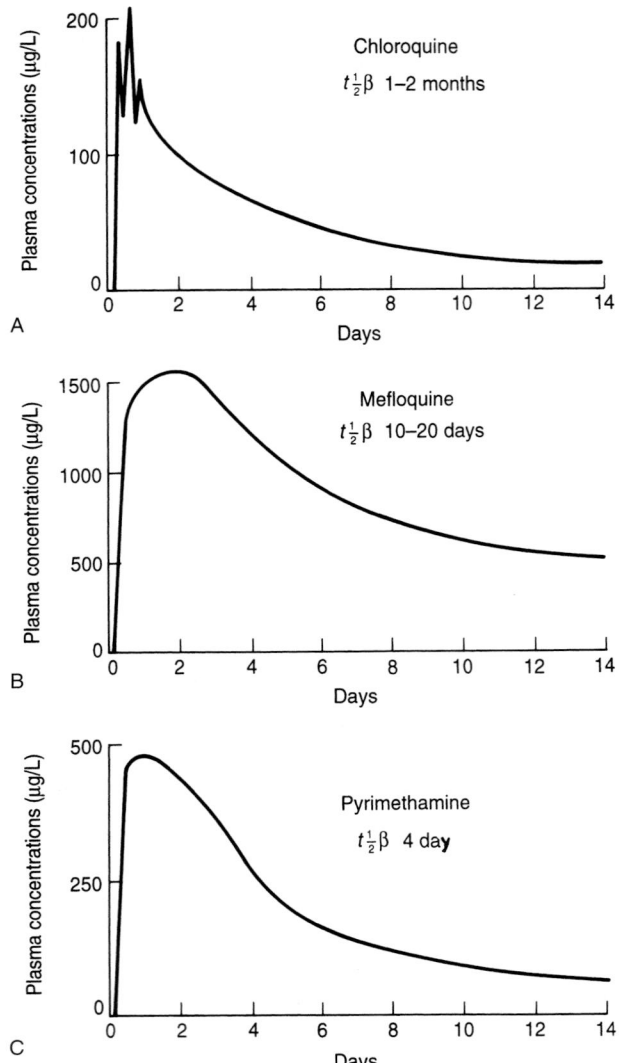

Figure 71.27: Plasma concentration time profiles following treatment doses of (**A**) chloroquine, (**B**) mefloquine, and (**C**) pyrimethamine.

Toxicity

Nausea, vomiting, dizziness, weakness, sleep disturbances and dysphoria are relatively common.[522,523] Although children are more likely to vomit immediately after receiving mefloquine, and this is a significant problem when the drug is used alone, they otherwise tolerate the drug better than adults.[523-526] Women, in particular, commonly complain of dizziness and dysphoria for up to 4 days after receiving mefloquine treatment.[523] Mefloquine exacerbates malarial orthostatic hypotension. The main serious adverse effect of mefloquine is the development of acute but self-limiting neuropsychiatric reactions (convulsions, psychosis, encephalopathy).[527] The incidence of these is approximately 1:10 000 when used as a prophylactic, but higher with treatment (1:1000 in Asian patients, 1:200 in Caucasian or African patients) and 1:20

following severe malaria.[528-532] For these reasons mefloquine should not be given following severe malaria. In one large study mefloquine treatment in pregnancy was associated with a fourfold increased risk of stillbirth, although this effect was not see in women exposed before conception (who would have had residual drug levels during early fetal organogenesis).[533]

Use

Mefloquine is used for the oral treatment of uncomplicated multi-drug-resistant falciparum malaria. It should be given in combination with an artemisinin derivative (e.g., artesunate 4 mg/kg/day for 3 days). The usual dose is 25 mg base/kg and should be split (15 mg/kg stat. followed by 10 mg/kg 8–24 hours later, or 8 mg/kg/day for three days).[419] A single dose of 15 mg base/kg is widely used in semi-immune patients, but there is theoretical evidence that this leads more rapidly to resistance.[534] The first dose should be repeated if the patient vomits (full dose if vomiting within 30 minutes, half dose 30–60 minutes, no further dose if vomiting after one hour). Mefloquine is used for antimalarial prophylaxis at a dose of approximately 4 mg base/kg once weekly for both adults and children.

Halofantrine

Halofantrine is a 9-phenanthrene methanol. It has one asymmetric carbon atom and is used as a racemate. The enantiomers have equal antimalarial activity. Halofantrine is intrinsically more potent than quinine or mefloquine, but unfortunately it is associated with rare but potentially lethal ventricular tachycardias which have curtailed its use. It is available as tablets and a suspension for paediatric use.

Pharmacokinetics (Table 71.8)

Halofantrine is poorly and erratically absorbed. Furthermore, absorption appears to be 'saturable', i.e., with individual doses over 8 mg/kg no increment in blood concentrations occurs. Absorption is increased markedly by co-administration with fats.[535] Halofantrine is extensively distributed and cleared largely by hepatic biotransformation. It is bound principally to lipoproteins in the plasma. The terminal elimination half-life is about 1–3 days in healthy subjects and approximately 4 days in patients with malaria.[536] There is significant first-pass metabolism to a biologically active desbutyl metabolite. This is eliminated more slowly ($T_{1/2}$ 3–7 days) than the parent compound and undoubtedly contributes significantly to antimalarial activity.

Toxicity

Halofantrine is very well tolerated subjectively,[537] but it carries a significant risk of sudden death, presumably resulting from ventricular tachyarrhythmias.[538-541]

Halofantrine slows atrioventricular conduction and produces the 'quinidine effect' on myocardial repolarization reflected in a significant dose-related prolongation of the electrocardiograph QT interval. This is increased by previous treatment with mefloquine.[538] This dangerous effect is a property more of halofantrine itself, than the desbutyl metabolite.[541] Diarrhoea may be provoked by high halofantrine doses. There are no data for pregnancy, so halofantrine should not be used in pregnant women.

Use

Although an intravenous preparation has been studied, halofantrine is only available for oral use. When used at standard doses (8 mg/kg given three times at 6–8 hour intervals, and repeated one week later in non-immune patients), in patients with a normal resting electrocardiogram, halofantrine is considered safe and effective in areas with fully sensitive malaria parasites. In multi-drug-resistant areas, higher total doses are required for high cure rates,[542] but these are associated with an unacceptable risk of cardiotoxicity. Halofantrine should not be used to treat recrudescent infections following mefloquine treatment as the cardiac effects are potentiated.[538]

Pyrimethamine

Pyrimethamine is a dihydrofolate reductase (DHFR) inhibitor. It is now used only together with long-acting sulphonamides such as sulfadoxine (as SP) and sulfalene which considerably potentiate its activity. SP is not a combination, in the 'resistance prevention' sense. The mechanism of action of the two drugs is linked, and so they do not protect each other from resistance to the extent unrelated drugs would. SP is used to treat chloroquine-resistant falciparum malaria, but in many areas SP resistance also occurs. *Plasmodium vivax* is also often resistant. There is an intramuscular formulation but this should not be used to treat severe malaria. The DHFR inhibitors inhibit development of the mature trophozoite stage of the asexual parasite, in addition to having pre-erythrocytic and sporontocidal activities. Pyrimethamine is also used for the treatment of toxoplasmosis.

Pharmacokinetics (Table 71.8)

Pyrimethamine is well absorbed following oral administration, and is eliminated over several days ($T_{1/2}$ 3 days; the companion sulfadoxine $T_{1/2}$ is 7 days), allowing single-dose treatment (Figure 71.27).[543] Following intramuscular injection absorption is as rapid as after oral administration but blood concentrations are lower and more variable, which suggests incomplete intramuscular bioavailability.[543]

Toxicity

Pyrimethamine is very safe and well tolerated. Occasionally megaloblastic anaemia, neutropenia or thrombocytopenia may develop in patients with pre-existing folate deficiency. The toxicity of the widely used combinations with long-acting sulphonamides (sulfadoxine, sulfalene) or sulphones (dapsone) is almost entirely related to the sulpha components.[544,545] The sulphonamides may cause severe skin reactions (at worst the Stevens–Johnson syndrome), hepatitis, blood dyscrasias and other allergic reactions. The sulphones commonly cause methaemoglobinaemia, and also rarely cause blood dyscrasias.[545] Severe reactions occurred in about 1:7000 subjects receiving prophylaxis (mortality was 1:18 000). The risk with treatment use is almost certainly much lower, but there are no precise estimates.

Use

Combinations of pyrimethamine with long-acting sulphonamides (SP) should not be used for prophylaxis, whereas the sulphone combination, which appears to be safer (at a once weekly dose), is used for prophylaxis but not treatment. Pyrimethamine alone is no longer used. SP is given in a single oral dose ensuring that this contains a minimum of 1.25 mg/kg of pyrimethamine. This may be combined with a three-day course of artesunate (4 mg/kg/day) to improve efficacy.[546] A single day of artesunate is insufficient for optimum efficacy in this combination. This is well tolerated, inexpensive, and efficient. SP is regarded as safe in pregnancy. Studies from Africa indicate that administration of SP twice during pregnancy (once in the second and once in the third trimester) has a beneficial effect on maternal anaemia and pregnancy outcome (birthweight).[547,548] HIV-positive women need monthly SP for the same effect. This approach has now been extended to infancy, and is being evaluated for possible incorporation in EPI programmes.[549] Whether other drugs are as good, whether artesunate should be added, and what to do when resistance develops, all remain to be determined.

Proguanil/chlorproguanil

Proguanil (chloroguanide) and the dichlorobiguanide chlorproguanil are considered the safest of all antimalarial drugs. Both compounds are mainly prodrugs for the active triazine metabolites cycloguanil and chlorcycloguanil. The metabolites are DHFR inhibitors. The parent compounds do possess weak antimalarial activity, with a different, as yet uncertain, mode of action.

Pharmacokinetics (Table 71.8)

Proguanil and chlorproguanil are well absorbed by mouth, and converted rapidly to the triazine metabolites. These in turn are metabolized to the inactive metabolites chloro- and dichlorophenylbiguanide, respectively.[550,551] As the parent compounds are eliminated more slowly than the metabolites the profile of antimalarial activity resulting from the cyclic metabolites is determined by the parent drug distribution and elimination. The $T_{1/2}$ of proguanil and chlorproguanil is approximately 16 hours in healthy subjects and 13 hours in malaria. Approximately 3% of Caucasian and African populations, but up to 20% of Oriental patients, fail to convert the parent compounds to their active metabolites.[552] In some parts of Micronesia the prevalence is even higher.[553] This is related to a genetic polymorphism in the 2C19 subfamily of the cytochrome P450 mixed-function oxidase system. The conversion of proguanil to the active metabolite is reduced in pregnancy.[554]

Toxicity

The antimalarial biguanides are very well tolerated. They occasionally cause mouth ulcers, and at high doses abdominal discomfort. Hair loss has been reported.[555] Two patients with renal failure, in whom the drugs may have accumulated, developed pancytopenia following prophylactic administration of proguanil.[556]

Use

Proguanil is used as a prophylactic taken once daily (3 mg/kg), often in combination with chloroquine. Chlorproguanil has been available for many years for prophylactic use, but it will be available in the future only in a fixed combination with dapsone (and probably artesunate) as a treatment of uncomplicated chloroquine resistant falciparum malaria.[557] Proguanil-dapsone and chlorproguanil-dapsone are both more active than SP against resistant *P. falciparum,* particularly the triple *dhfr* mutants currently prevalent in East Africa. The treatment doses of proguanil used are 5–8 mg/kg/day (in combination with atovaquone), and for chlorproguanil 2 mg/kg/day. As both chlorproguanil and dapsone are eliminated more rapidly than pyrimethamine and sulfadoxine, the use of this combination also provides less selective pressure for the emergence of resistance.[553,558,559]

Atovaquone-proguanil

This is a highly active new antimalarial drug, a hydroxynaphthaquinone unlike other antimalarial drugs. Atovaquone is active even against multi-drug-resistant falciparum malaria. The speed of therapeutic reponse is similar to that with mefloquine, and slower than that with artemisinin derivatives. Originally atovaquone alone was developed, but high-level resistance developed in approximately 30% of treated patients.[560] This suggested that the point mutations in *cyt b,* which conferred resistance, occurred at an approximate frequency of 1 in 10^{12} parasites[460] (Figure 71.23). The fixed combination with proguanil proved much more effective producing cure rates of nearly 100%, and emergence of resistance in less than 1:500 treated patients.[561,562] It is this combined formulation (Malarone®) which is now registered both for prophylaxis and treatment use in many countries. Nevertheless it must be considered vulnerable, and for treatment use in endemic areas should probably be combined with an artemisinin derivative. Interestingly it is the parent compound proguanil which is the important contributor to antimalarial efficacy, as atovaquone-proguanil is equally effective against highly antifol resistant parasites, and also in individuals unable to convert proguanil to cycloguanil.

Pharmacokinetics (Table 71.8)

Atovaquone is similar to halofantrine and lumefantrine in that oral absorption is augmented considerably by fats. Elimination is slower in patients of African origin ($T_{1/2}$ 70 hours)[563] than in Oriental patients ($T_{1/2}$ 30 hours). There are no significant interactions with proguanil or artesunate.

Use

Atovaquone-proguanil is becoming established as a safe, effective, and expensive antimalarial prophylactic for travellers because it is effective everywhere.[564] The adult dose is one tablet (atovaquone 250mg proguanil 100 mg) daily with food. For treatment use cost has been a major limitation to its use. In some malaria endemic countries it has been provided free through a donation programme as a third-line drug for falciparum malaria. The treatment dose is 15–20/6–8 mg/kg/day for three days, which corresponds to an adult dose of 4 tablets per day. It is equally effective and well tolerated in young children,[565] but has not been evaluated in pregnancy and therefore should not be used in pregnant women. In order to protect against resistance atovaquone-proguanil has been combined with artesunate, which accelerates the treatment response and reduces the failure rate to almost zero.

Toxicity

The combination is very well tolerated. The adverse effects are similar to those of proguanil.

Primaquine

Primaquine is an 8-aminoquinoline used for its actions against the hypnozoites of *P. vivax* (to prevent relapse) and the gametocytes of *P. falciparum* (to prevent transmission). Primaquine also has activity against liver and blood stage parasites. It is an effective prophylactic.

Pharmacokinetics (Table 71.8)

Primaquine is well absorbed. It is cleared by hepatic biotransformation[566] to the more polar metabolite carboxyprimaquine with an elimination half-life of 7 hours. It is not known whether primaquine itself or its metabolites are responsible for the action against *P. vivax* hypnozoites.

Toxicity

Nausea, headache, vomiting and abdominal discomfort are relatively common particularly if higher doses (> 30 mg) are taken on an empty stomach. Chest pain, weakness, visual disturbances and pruritus occur occasionally. Methaemoglobinaemia is rare. The principal toxicity of primaquine is oxidant haemolysis in patients with G6PD deficiency,[567,568] (indeed, this is how the enzyme deficiency was originally discovered). Primaquine is contraindicated in pregnancy.

Use

Primaquine is given once daily in a dose of 0.25 to 0.5 mg/kg (adult doses 15 to 30 mg) together with food. The usual course of treatment for the radical treatment of vivax and ovale malaria is 14 days, and there is no good evidence to support shorter courses. In patients with mild G6PD deficiency a once-weekly dose of 0.6–0.8 mg/kg (adult dose 45 mg) is given for six weeks. For *P. falciparum* gametocytocidal activity a single dose of 0.5 mg/kg (30 mg) is given. For prophylaxis the adult dose evaluated has been 30 mg daily taken with food. This has been remarkably well tolerated.[566–570]

Tafenoquine

Formerly known as etaquine or WR 238605, this slowly eliminated 8-aminoquinoline was developed by the US army. It is currently undergoing phase III trials in antimalarial prophylaxis, and for the radical treatment of vivax malaria.[571] Tafenoquine is more efficacious and less toxic than primaquine, although it still causes oxidant haemolysis in G6PD deficient subjects. Tafenoquine has a terminal elimination half-life of two weeks.[572]

Qinghaosu (artemisinin) (Figure 71.28)

Qinghaosu or artemisinin is a sesquiterpene lactone peroxide extracted from the leaves of the shrub *Artemesia annua* (Qinghao). Three derivatives are used widely: the oil-soluble methyl ether artemether (or the very similar compound arteether), the water-soluble hemisuccinate derivative artesunate, and dihydroartemisinin (DHA). Artesunate, artemether, and arteether are all synthesized from DHA, and they are converted back to it within the body. DHA is five to ten times more potent as an antimalarial drug compared with artemisinin. Artemisinin itself is available in a few countries. It is less active than the derivatives, and is not metabolized to DHA. These compounds are the most rapidly acting of known antimalarial drugs, and they have the broadest time window of antimalarial effect (from ring forms to early schizonts). They produce rapid parasite clearance and they have proved to be very safe in clinical practice.[401,406,573–576] In falciparum malaria the artemisinin derivatives effectively prevent progression to severe disease. For example in western Thailand a parasitaemia over 4% without vital

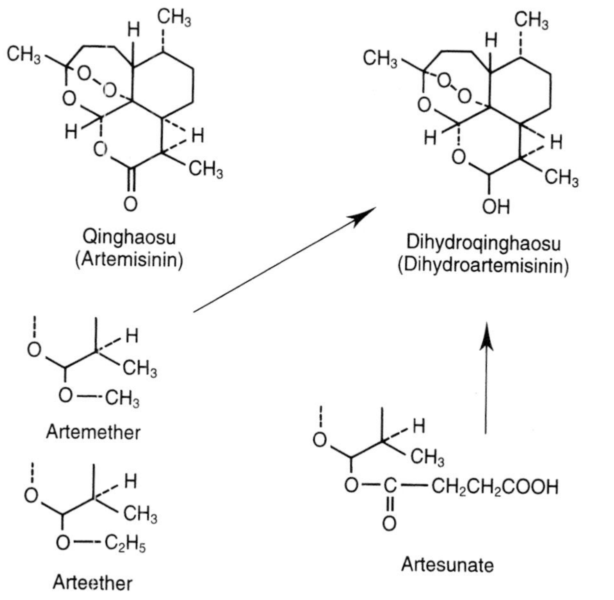

Figure 71.28: Qinghaosu: the parent compound artemisinin and the three derivatives. The oil-soluble ethers, artemether and arteether, and the water-soluble artesunate are all converted in vivo to a common biologically active metabolite dihydroartemisinin. The peroxide bridge in the sesquiterpene structure is essential for antimalarial activity. (From Hien & White: *Lancet* 1993; 341:603-608.)

organ dysfunction carries a 3% mortality rate (i.e., 30 times higher than uncomplicated malaria but less than one-fifth that of severe malaria). In this context oral artesunate produces considerably superior therapeutic responses compared with an intravenous quinine loading dose.[578] In severe malaria most trials have been conducted with artemether, although there are questions over the reliability of absorption in severe malaria. Over 1900 patients have been included in a series of randomized controlled trials in severe malaria. Compared with quinine, intramuscular artemether was associated with a significantly lower mortality in South-East Asian adults, but not in African children.[577] Artemether was not associated with more rapid clinical responses (fever clearance, coma recovery), but it did accelerate parasite clearance. Comparative studies with parenteral artesunate, which does not have the pharmacokinetic disadvantages of artemether or arteether, are now under way.

As most deaths from severe malaria occur away from facilities capable of providing injections, methods of delivering these drugs at a village or household level have been investigated. Following the promising results with artemisinin suppositories in China and Vietnam,[579–581] a rectal formulation of artesunate has been developed and is under large-scale evaluation.[582]

In clinical studies in uncomplicated falciparum malaria the artemisinin derivatives provide both more rapid parasite and fever clearance than with other treatments, and also reduce gametocyte carriage, and thus transmission.[583,584] Concerns over their neurotoxic potential, revealed in animal studies, have not been confirmed in large and detailed clinical studies.[585–587] Indeed their remarkable safety, efficacy, and lack of adverse effects[587] have led to widespread unregulated use and the manufacture of fake products.[588] Artemisinin is available as capsules of powder or as suppositories. Artemether is formulated in peanut oil, and arteether in sesame seed oil, for intramuscular injection, and in capsules or tablets for oral use. Artesunate is formulated either as tablets, in a gel enclosed in gelatin for rectal administration (called a rectocap™), or as dry powder of artesunic acid for injection, supplied with an ampoule of 5% sodium bicarbonate. The powder is dissolved in the sodium bicarbonate, to form sodium artesunate, and then diluted in 5% dextrose or normal saline for intravenous or intramuscular injection. Artelinic acid is a water-soluble second-generation compound under protracted development. It has not yet been used in treatment. The majority of clinical data pertain to the most widely used derivative artesunate.

To date there is no significant resistance to these drugs, which have become central to antimalarial treatment. Combinations of artemisinin derivatives with other antimalarial drugs result in high and sustained efficacy, rapid therapeutic responses preventing the development of severe malaria and allowing earlier return to school or work, mutual protection against resistance, and reduced gametocyte carriage which may reduce the incidence of malaria in low transmission settings.

Pharmacokinetics (Table 71.8)

The artemisinin derivatives are rapidly absorbed and eliminated.[589] Artesunate and artemether are hydrolyzed to the active metabolite dihydroartemisinin, which has an elimination half-life of approximately 45 minutes.[590,591] They are by far the most rapidly eliminated of the antimalarial drugs. Despite this they are highly effective when given once daily. Unlike some antibiotics it is not necessary to exceed the MIC throughout the dosing interval for antimalarial drugs (after all it is only necessary to kill each parasite once!). After oral or parenteral administration artesunate is hydrolysed rapidly (by stomach acid, and esterases in plasma and erythrocytes) and most of the antimalarial activity results from the DHA metabolite. Oral absorption is rapid and bioavailability is approximately 60%.[591,592] Rectal bioavailability is more variable;[582] following administration of the rectocap™ bioavailability averages 50% (although absorption is more variable).[574] As for quinine there is a contraction in the volume of distribution and reduced clearance in acute malaria, which increases blood concentrations. There may also be a malaria-related inhibition of intestinal and hepatic first-pass metabolism which improves oral bioavailability. After oral administration artemether is absorbed rapidly, but is converted more slowly (via CYP 3A4) to DHA, although the metabolite still accounts for the majority of antimalarial activity.[590] In contrast after intramuscular administration absorption of artemether and arteether is slow and erratic. Peak

concentrations are often not reached for many hours. Concentrations of the parent compound exceed those of the active DHA metabolite. In some patients with severe malaria absorption may be inadequate.[593] Oral formulations of DHA contain excipients which promote absorption and give bioavailability comparable to that of artesunate. Elimination of DHA is largely by conversion to inactive glucuronides. Artemisinin, and to 9 lesser extent artemether, induce their own metabolism. No other significant drug interactions have been identified with these compounds.

Toxicity

The artemisinin-related compounds have been remarkably well tolerated in clinical evaluations. There has been no documented significant toxicity[587,594] other than rare type 1 hypersensitivity reactions (incidence approximately 1:3000 treatments).[595] In volunteer studies a depression of reticulocyte counts has been noted, but increased anaemia has not been observed in clinical studies. In animal studies they are much less toxic than the quinoline antimalarial drugs. The principal toxicity in animals has been an unusual dose-related selective pattern of neuronal cell damage affecting certain brain stem nuclei.[596,597] This is related to the pharmacokinetic properties of the drug. Neurotoxicity is related to protracted exposure related to the sustained blood concentrations, which follow intramuscular administration of the high doses of oil-based artemether and arteether. Neuronal damage is much less following oral administration or intravenous artesunate because the drugs levels are not sustained.[598,599] Extensive clinical neurophysiological and to a lesser extent pathology studies have failed to show any evidence of neurotoxicity or cardiotoxicity in clinical use.[585,586]

Use

In severe malaria artesunate is given by intravenous or intramuscular injection. The initial dose is 2.4 mg/kg and the subsequent daily doses are 1.2 mg/kg. Artemether and arteether are given by intramuscular injection. The dose is 3.2 mg/kg initially followed by 1.6 mg/kg daily. Rectal artemisinin suppositories are very effective but they are available only in Vietnam. The artesunate rectocap is used in a dose of 10 mg/kg/day until parenteral or oral treatment can be given. For oral treatment, when used alone, the artemisinin derivatives should be given in a 7- (not 5) day course, preferably combined with doxycycline or clindamycin. The initial oral dose is 4 mg/kg followed by 2 mg/kg/day. These drugs should be combined with longer-acting drugs (e.g., mefloquine) in a three day course to accelerate the initial therapeutic response, increase overall cure rates, and protect from resistance.[460,600] Dose restrictions are not necessary in renal failure or with liver disease. The artemisinin derivatives are safe in children and studies to date in pregnancy (over 600 exposures) do not indicate any adverse effects.[601] These drugs should be used for the treatment of severe malaria in pregnancy at any gestational age as they are safer than quinine. For pregnant women presenting with uncomplicated malaria in multi-drug-resistant areas, the artemisinin derivatives should be used in the second and third trimesters and quinine given in the first trimester.

Artemisinin combinations

These are likely to be used very widely in the near future as part of the global initiative to ensure effective antimalarial treatment and thereby, we hope, to Roll Back Malaria.[602] The artemisinin derivative induces a rapid therapeutic response, with rapid resolution of fever. This may improve absorption of the combination partner (e.g., mefloquine, lumefantrine). It also protects the partner drug from the emergence of resistance and reduces gametocyte carriage. The partner drug removes the relatively few parasites remaining after the 3-day course of treatment (a hundred million times less than when treatment started), and also protects the artemisinin derivative from resistance (Figure 71.25).

Lumefantrine

Formerly called benflumetol, lumefantrine was developed by Chinese scientists. It is now available only in a fixed tablet combination with artemether. Each tablet contains artemether 20 mg and lumefantrine 120 mg. The combination is registered in many tropical countries and in Europe. It is very effective against multi-drug-resistant falciparum malaria, and it is remarkably well tolerated.

Pharmacokinetics (Table 71.8)

Lumefantrine is lipophilic and hydrophobic. Its absorption is considerably augmented by taking the drug together with food (a 16-fold increase with a fatty meal). Absorption is reduced in the acute phase of malaria, but then increases considerably as symptoms resolve and the patient starts to eat.[603] The elimination half-life is 3–4 days.[604] The pharmacokinetic properties of lumefantrine are similar in adults and children.[605] The principle pharmacokinetic variable which correlates with therapeutic response is the area under the plasma concentration curve (AUC).[605] The plasma level on day 7 after starting treatment is a good surrogate of the AUC; plasma levels of lumefantrine above 500 ng/ml on day 7 are associated with a >90% cure rate.

Use

The treatment course which has been most widely evaluated approximates to 1.5/9 mg/kg (adult dose four tablets) given at 0, 8, 24, and 48 hours. This is effective in patients with background immunity, but in non-immune patients with multi-drug-resistant infections cure rates are approximately 80%.[606] Increasing the regimen to six doses (i.e., twice daily on each day) results in >95% cure

rates.[607,608] As children in endemic areas are relatively non-immune the six-dose regimen is a preferable regimen for general use. The patient should be encouraged to take the drug with food. There is no experience in pregnancy and therefore the drug should not be used in pregnant women. There is no paediatric formulation.

Toxicity

This combination is remarkably free of adverse effects. Concerns about possible cardiotoxicity have been refuted by careful studies.[609] Lumefantrine is not cardiotoxic.

Pyronaridine

Structurally a relative of amodiaquine, pyronaridine has been developed and used in China. It is active against multi-drug-resistant *P. falciparum* malaria.[610,611] Originally pyronaridine was deployed as an enteric-coated formulation for monotherapy (which had poor oral bioavailability), and was given in a three day course of 1200 mg or 1800 mg (adult dose) over five days. It is now being developed as a fixed co-formulation with artesunate. Clinical trials should start in the near future.

Piperaquine

Also developed in China, this bisquinoline compound and its hydroxy-derivative are active against multi-drug-resistant *P. falciparum*.[612] Piperaquine is now available as a fixed combination with dihydroartemisinin (and also sometimes trimethoprim and primaquine). It is relatively inexpensive (adult doses just over US$1). These combinations are registered and used in China, Vietnam and Cambodia. Given as a four-dose (0, 8, 24, 48 hours) regimen comprising a total of 5120 mg of piperaquine for an adult, the combination is well tolerated and effective, but more clinical trial information on efficacy and safety is needed before this exciting new drug can be recommended more widely.

Antibacterial drugs with antimalarial activity

The antibacterial drugs which act on protein or nucleic acid synthesis often have significant antimalarial activity. But they are not sufficiently active to be used alone to treat malaria.[613] The sulphonamides and sulphones inhibit plasmodial folate synthesis by competing for the enzyme dihydropteroate synthetase. The sulphas are usually used in combination with pyrimethamine or the antimalarial biguanides. Trimethoprim has good antimalarial activity and shares resistance profiles with pyrimethamine. The tetracyclines are consistently active against all species of malaria. Doxycycline is the most widely used both for prophylaxis and treatment.[614] Clindamycin is as effective as the tetracyclines and has the advantage that it can be used in children and pregnant women.[615,616] The macrolides are active in vitro but are generally disappointing in vivo. Azithromycin is more active and has been evaluated both in prophylaxis and treatment. Rifampicin also has a weak antimalarial effect in vivo. Chloramphenicol also has antimalarial activity. The fluoroquinolones have some activity but, despite one promising sentinel report, subsequent clinical experience has proved uniformly disappointing. These drugs all act relatively slowly, and they are therefore used in combination with more rapidly acting agents.

Choice of drugs (Tables 71.9 and 71.10)

In severe malaria, rapidly acting parenteral treatment should be given. Rectal formulations of artemisinin or its derivatives offer the possibility of starting treatment in the home or village. Quinine is still the mainstay of parenteral treatment, although its position is increasingly challenged by the artemisinin compounds which are safer and easier to use, and may be more effective. The presence of low-grade chloroquine resistance in *P. falciparum* does not contraindicate use of chloroquine in severe malaria, but there are now very few areas where resistance is absent or low grade only. If there is any doubt then an artemisinin derivative or quinine should be used. The choice of drugs in uncomplicated malaria depends on local patterns of sensitivity, background immunity, availability, toxicity and cost. The decision of when to change drug recommendations for falciparum malaria in the face of increasing resistance is a difficult one, and a source of much debate. Figures such as a threshold of a 20% early failure rate have been suggested, but these are still unacceptable for a life-threatening infection. In fact the failure rates for chloroquine in Africa now are higher than this nearly everywhere. For the future effective drugs must be used, and this means the wide-scale deployment of artemisinin combinations. The adverse impact of antimalarial drug resistance is usually underestimated, particularly in higher transmission areas. This is because drug evaluations are often conducted in older children or sometimes adults who have significant background immunity and may respond to ineffective drugs.[409] The greatest impact is on younger children in whom infections recur with increasing frequency, anaemia does not recover, and morbidity and mortality rise. For the treatment of *P. vivax, P. malariae,* and *P. ovale* malaria chloroquine can still be relied upon almost every where except parts of Indonesia, Micronesia, and the island of New Guinea.

Case example

A medical NGO arrived to help manage an epidemic of falciparum malaria in a central African country brought about by war and population movement. Adults and children were affected, and there was considerable mortality rate. There were no recent data on antimalarial drug resistance from within the country but information from the adjoining countries (with generally higher malaria transmission) suggested high-level resistance to both chloroquine and sulphadoxine-pyrimethamine (SP). Chloroquine was the national treatment policy in the affected country. There was uncertainty how to proceed as different concerns and contradictory advice were expressed by various interested parties. One argument put forward was that the NGO should conform with national policy (i.e., chloroquine) in order for the intervention to be 'sustainable'. An international organization recommended SP as this was the traditional next step when changing national policy from chloroquine. Other advisors suggested use of artesunate-mefloquine or artemether-lumefantrine although neither was registered in the country. Initially SP was used, but the death toll mounted rapidly. Eventually the NGO managed to persuade the government authorities to import artemether-lumefantrine and this was deployed widely. The incidence of malaria and associated mortality fell abruptly.

Comments

Severe malaria was seen in adults as well as children suggesting that this epidemic involved non-immune patients. Treatment responses would therefore have been expected to be even worse than suggested by the poor results with chloroquine and SP in adjacent countries. The prior probability of chloroquine or SP working well, and controlling this epidemic was therefore very low. SP is known to increase gametocyte carriage and may even have fuelled transmission. The NGO was in a difficult position. National malaria treatment policies may be very slow to change during the emergence of drug resistance. But there was an ethical imperative to provide effective antimalarial drugs. Provision of ineffective treatments for life threatening infections by international organizations is simply wrong.

Combinations of antimalarial drugs containing artemisinin derivatives were particularly appropriate in this context of an uncontrolled epidemic. These combinations prevent the progression to severe malaria by ensuring a rapid and reliable resolution of the illness, and they prevent transmission.

Antimalarial drug interactions

Antimalarial drug interactions have not been defined adequately. Mefloquine, halofantrine, quinidine and quinine are structurally similar and may compete for blood and tissue-binding sites. Cardiotoxicity is assumed to be additive, and significant only for halofantrine, where there is a potentially dangerous interaction with mefloquine. It is also recommended that mefloquine should not be given to people also receiving quinine to avoid adverse cardiovascular effects, but no interaction has been demonstrated.[618] Inducers of CYP 3A4 such as rifampicin and anticonvulsant drugs accelerate the clearance of quinine and mefloquine resulting in lower drug levels (and a greater chance of treatment failure).[619] There is no evidence that the structurally dissimilar antimalarial drugs interact. Use of artesunate with mefloquine improves the tolerance and absorption of mefloquine presumably curing malaria rapidly.

There are many reports of synergy or antagonism between antimalarial drugs based on isobolograms drawn from in vitro observations. These are often used to justify a particular choice of antimalarial combination but, for the most part, the results are irrelevant to the clinical use of the drugs. Only when synergy or antagonism is extreme, such as the marked synergy between sulphadoxine and pyrimethamine, is this relevant clinically. There are no cases of marked antagonism between the available antimalarial drugs.

Case history

A 31-year-old married female aid worker returned to the UK from a project in rural western Cambodia. One week later she developed headache, malaise and low-grade fever. She was found to have a *P. falciparum* infection; the peripheral blood parasite count was 35 000/µl, and she was referred to hospital. She had no relevant past medical history. She had been taking chloroquine and proguanil antimalarial prophylaxis regularly since the beginning of her project two months previously. On examination she was listless and febrile (oral temperature 38.9°C) but there were no other abnormal clinical findings. As she was able to take fluids and there were no signs of severe malaria, she was given oral mefloquine (25 g base/kg) in a single dose on arrival at hospital, but 15 minutes later she vomited. The dose was therefore repeated and this time the drug was retained. The next morning her fever was higher (up to 40.4°C) and the parasite count had risen to 78 500/µl, but she remained lucid and able to sit and drink. Thereafter, the fever gradually subsided, the parasite count fell, and she felt steadily better. The fever clearance time was 84 hours and the parasite clearance time 108 hours. Eighteen days after discharge (24 days after treatment) she was readmitted with fever. A blood smear was again positive for *P. falciparum*; the count was 1800/µl. She said that her period was late, and a pregnancy test proved positive. She was treated with oral quinine sulphate 10 g salt/kg three times daily. Her fever and parasitaemia resolved within four days and she was discharged with instructions to finish a 7-day course of treatment. Three weeks later she returned to hospital with a recurrence of symptoms. On examination she was apyrexial but gave a history of fever, and she was clinically anaemic. The spleen tip was palpable.

The blood smear was again positive (count 560/µl). She admitted having taken quinine for only 5 days in total because she was continually nauseated, felt the drug gave her a constant buzzing in the ears and made her dizzy. She was readmitted to hospital and given a supervised 7-day course of quinine. Her haematocrit was 27% and the blood film was normochromic and normocytic. Iron and folic acid treatment was started. Thereafter she made an uncomplicated recovery, had no further recrudescences of malaria, and seven months later delivered a healthy baby girl weighing 3.0 kg.

Comment

This case illustrates several points.

- Chloroquine and proguanil prophylaxis are ineffective in this area of multi-drug-resistant *P. falciparum*. Chloroquine should have prevented *P. vivax* (up to 50% of the malaria infections in this area were *P. vivax*), and proguanil may have had some effect against *P. falciparum*, but protection would have been partial at best.
- Vomiting after administration of oral antimalarial drugs to patients with high fever is common. If vomiting occurs within one hour the dose should be repeated, as was done in this case. If possible the fever should have been brought down with antipyretics and tepid sponging and the patient made comfortable before being given the antimalarial treatment mefloquine. The 25 mg/kg dose should have been divided (15 mg/kg stat., 10 mg/kg 12 hours later), and preferably given on the second day of a 3-day treatment in combination with artesunate (4 mg/kg/day). But artesunate is not registered and is therefore not available in the UK!
- Parasitaemia may rise over the 24 hours following treatment with quinoline antimalarial drugs or pyrimethamine-sulfadoxine. This does not mean the infection is resistant. It is a reflection of the timing of drug administration and synchronicity of the infection. Merogony (schizogony) is not prevented if most of the parasites are mature meronts when the drugs are started. The rise in parasitaemia is expected. The blood film shows a predominance of young rings. A change to parenteral treatment is indicated only if the patient deteriorates clinically and fulfils the criteria for severe malaria, or cannot take oral medication. R_3 resistance (see below) is assessed at 48 hours.
- This patient's infection was mefloquine resistant. Blood concentrations of mefloquine would have been higher if the dose had been divided, and might have cured the infection. However, highly mefloquine-resistant strains of *P. falciparum* are now prevalent in western Cambodia and eastern Thailand. These infections respond poorly to treatment with mefloquine alone, but they do respond well to three-day courses of artesunate-mefloquine, artemether-lumefantrine, or a 7-day course of quinine and tetracycline (doxycycline) or clindamycin. However, this patient was pregnant:

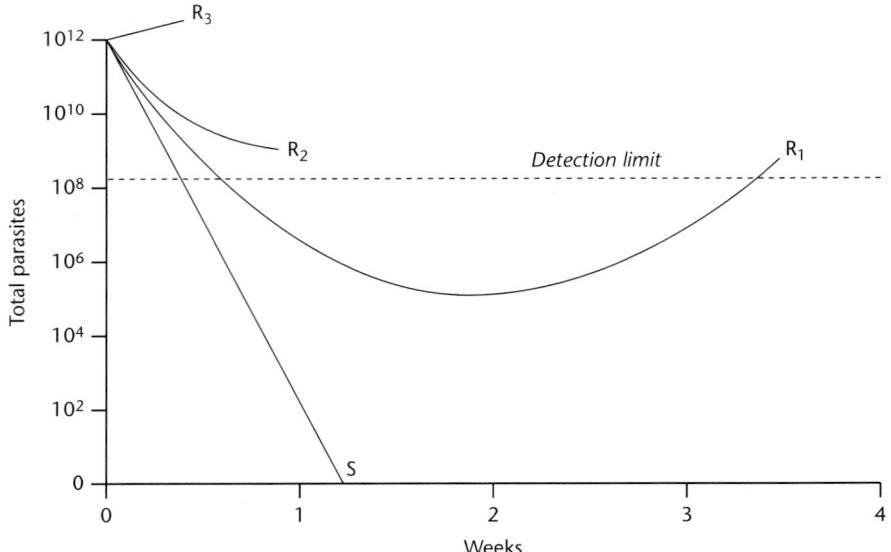

Figure 71.29: The original 1973 WHO classification of resistance. The vertical axis shows the number of parasites in the body of an adult.

quinine is the only drug recommended in this situation (although clindamycin is generally regarded as safe). The suggested treatments for recrudescent infections are shown in Table 71.10.

- Treatment failure rates with quinine alone are over 50% in non-immune pregnant women with falciparum malaria acquired in this area. Poor compliance is a major contributor to this poor therapeutic response, as in this case. A further recrudescence after the second course of quinine would not have been unexpected. The addition of clindamycin to quinine would have increased the probability of cure to over 90%.
- Anaemia is a common consequence of treatment failure in malaria, and a particular complication of malaria in later pregnancy.
- Although malaria consistently reduces birth weight, the effects in this case are difficult to assess as her infection occurred very early in pregnancy.

Table 71.10 The treatment of recrudescent falciparum malaria

Recrudescence following:		Treat with:
Chloroquine	⇘	Sulphadoxine-pyrimethamine
Sulphadoxine-pyrimethamine	→	Artesunate-mefloquine[a]
Mefloquine ± Artesunate[a]	⇘	Quinine + doxycycline or clindamycin for 7 days Artesunate + doxycycline or clindamycin for 7 days

[a]Artemether lumefantrine (AL) can substitute, although the safety and efficacy of artemether-lumefantrine retreatment of a mefloquine failure has not been evaluated.

Assessment of the therapeutic response

Generally understood and standardized definitions of antimalarial drug responses are important for epidemiological purposes, and helpful in therapeutic decision making. The definitions of severe malaria and treatment failure have both undergone changes in recent years.

Uncomplicated malaria

In uncomplicated malaria the immediate therapeutic response is usually assessed by the parasite and fever clearance times. In defining criteria for resistance to the aminoquinoline antimalarial drugs nearly thirty years ago, the WHO has described three grades of resistance following treatment (Figure 71.29):[620]

R₁: (low grade): recrudescence of the infection between 7 and 28 days of completing treatment following initial resolution of symptoms and parasite clearance.

R₂: (high grade): Reduction of parasitaemia by >75% at 48 hours, but failure to clear parasites within 7 days.

R₃: Parasitaemia does not fall by >75% within 48 hours.

These criteria are useful for all the antimalarial drugs, but have several limitations. In endemic areas it may be impossible to distinguish recrudescence from reinfection. It is often difficult to follow patients for 28 days. A simple and practical alternative in high-transmission areas is to assess after two weeks. In the newer WHO classification the therapeutic response is divided into three categories.[621]

The therapeutic response is classified as an early treatment failure (**ETF**) if the patient develops one of the following during the first three days of follow-up:

- Development of danger signs or severe malaria on day 1, day 2 or day 3, in the presence of parasitaemia;
- Axillary temperature $\geq 37.5°C$ on day 2 with parasitaemia > of day count;
- Axillary temperature $\geq 37.5°C$ on day 3 in the presence of parasitaemia;
- Parasitaemia on day 3 $\geq 25\%$ of count on day 0.

The therapeutic response is classified as late treatment failure (**LTF**) if the patient develops one of the following during the follow-up period from day 4 to day 14:

- Development of danger signs or severe malaria in the presence of parasitaemia on any day from day 4 to day 14, without previously meeting any of the criteria of early treatment failure;
- Axillary temperature $\geq 37.5°C$ in the presence of parasitaemia on any day from day 4 to day 14, without previously meeting any of the criteria of early treatment failure.

The response to treatment is classified as adequate clinical response (**ACR**) if the patient shows one of the following during the follow-up period (up to day 14):

- Absence of parasitaemia on day 14 irrespective of axillary temperature, without previously meeting any of the criteria of early or late treatment failure;
- Axillary temperature $< 37.5°C$ irrespective of the presence of parasitaemia, without previously meeting any of the criteria of early or late treatment failure.

This '14-day test' may be used to compare different drug regimens, but it is a blunt tool. It will always underestimate resistance by a considerable amount because at low levels of resistance nearly all recrudescences occur after 14 days. Unfortunately the 1996 recommendations are being applied in low-transmission areas—whereas they were clearly designed for high transmission settings.

There are several other considerations:
1973 WHO classification [620]

- R_1 resistance: Recrudescent infections may recur up to two months or more following treatment (i.e., after the 28-day 'limit') if slowly eliminated antimalarial drugs are used (particularly mefloquine).
- Therapeutic failure may result from many factors unrelated to resistance such as poor quality drugs, inadequate dosing, failure to absorb the antimalarial, vomiting or host pharmacokinetic factors.[425,621] Unless the blood concentration of antimalarial drug is measured at the time of recrudescent infection (or earlier preferably particularly in the case of rapidly eliminated drugs), these factors cannot be excluded.
- R_2 resistance: This category is very broad. Parasitaemia may clear very slowly in some patients (often a harbinger of resistance). The patient improves clinically but a few parasites may still be present at day 7. These may clear by day 9 without further treatment.[623] Alternatively, in highly resistant infections parasitaemia

may fall for 1–2 days, then rise alarmingly, with deterioration in the patient's condition.

- R_3 resistance: In occasional cases treatment is started at a time when synchronous merogony is either taking place or about to occur. The starting count is low but the parasite count rises considerably and by 48 hours has not fallen by >75% of the initial value (even though the parasites are drug sensitive) but will do so over the next few hours.

1996 WHO classification of antimalarial resistance in high-transmission areas
ETF: The development of signs of severe malaria after starting oral treatment does not necessarily mean the infection is resistant (although it does mean that parenteral treatment is needed).

In young children fever and parasite clearance times often exceed two days, even in high-transmission areas. High-level resistance will therefore be overestimated.

LTF: Low and intermediate levels of resistance manifest as recrudescences after 14 days. Therefore resistance is not detected until it has already reached a high level.

Parasite clearance time (PCT)

This is the time between beginning the antimalarial treatment and the first negative blood slide. The accuracy of the measurement depends on the frequency with which blood slides are taken and the quality of microscopy. The PCT is directly proportional to the admission parasitaemia. The time taken for parasitaemia to fall to half of the admission value (PCT_{50}) and to fall to 10% of the admission value (PCT_{90}) are also useful comparative measures.

Fever clearance time (FCT)

This is the time from beginning antimalarial treatment until the patient is apyrexial. This is easier said than read! Fever does not come down linearly—it often fluctuates erratically. The method and site of measurements should be standardized and the use of antipyretics documented. One approach is to record when temperature first falls below 37.5°C (FCT_a), and then when the temperature falls and remains below 37.5°C for 24 hours (FCT_b).

In vivo testing of antimalarial drug efficacy

Continuous assessment of antimalarial drug efficacy is needed in the face of increasing drug resistance. In comparative studies the groups should reflect the population affected by malaria. Too many trials are conducted in older children or adults in highly endemic areas. These groups have significant background immunity and a high rate of self-cure. Drug efficacy is therefore overestimated. The analysis should be age stratified if there is a wide age range included in the study. It is very important that patients, parents or guardians truly understand that participation in a drug trial is voluntary, and give informed consent. Ideally pre-treatment with another antimalarial drug is an exclusion criterion, but in some areas this is very common. In which case such patients should be included provided details are taken, and preferably a baseline blood level is taken. An adequate sample size is required. For example with a sample size of 60 studied patients and six treatment failures, the 95% confidence interval around the 90% cure rate is 82.4 to 97.6%. This study is too small as it leaves too much uncertainty as to the true cure rate in the population. Comparative studies of antimalarial drugs are often underpowered to show important differences in efficacy. For example if the cure rate with SP in an area is currently 80%, then to detect an improvement of 10% with a new drug (with 95% confidence and 80% power) requires a complete study of 352 patients (i.e., 440 patients enrolled with a 20% drop-out rate).

Data should be entered on a case record form. Baseline clinical and demographic details should be recorded and, at a minimum, the parasitaemia counted and haematocrit measured. In well-equipped sites, parasite culture to correlate the in vivo response with in vitro susceptibility can also be performed. A baseline whole blood sample (or blood spot on filter paper) should be stored for parasite genotyping. Molecular typing of P. falciparum (usually by assessment of size polymorphisms in fragments of the genes encoding MSP1, MSP2 and GLURP) has considerably improved the accuracy of drug trials conducted in endemic areas.[624,625] The genotype(s) of infections recurring within the follow-up period are compared to those in the initial isolate. If the same genotype is found the infection is considered a recrudescence (i.e., a treatment failure). A different genotype indicates a newly aquired infection. The method is not foolproof; genotypes may be difficult to ascribe in mixed infections and resistant infections might be subpatent on admission, but genotyping is a considerable advance. For studies of slowly eliminated drugs taking a blood level measurement at day 7 in all patients may help to interpret treatment failures (i.e., whether they resulted from drug resistance or low blood concentrations).

Antimalarial treatment should be observed and adverse effects recorded. The patients should be followed daily until parasite clearance then at weekly intervals. The rate of resolution of anaemia is a sensitive measure of the treatment response. The haemoglobin or haematocrit should be measured each time a parasite count is performed in therapeutic assessments. Four weeks is a minimum for accurate drug assessments. Six-week- follow-up is necessary for trials of slowly eliminated drugs in low-transmission areas (e.g., SP or artemether-lumefantrine). A minimum of 80% follow-up at six weeks should be aimed for, and sample sizes adjusted for likely 'drop-out' rates. At low levels of mefloquine resistance some P. falciparum recrudescences will occur between six and ten weeks after treatment. If parasitaemia returns, blood should be taken for parasite genotyping, and the patient treated with an effective regimen. The appearance of P. vivax, P. malariae or P. ovale malaria requires chloroquine treatment. Whether such patients should be excluded from the analysis in a falciparum malarial trial depends on the level of chloroquine resistance in P. falciparum and needs to be decided before the trial. Trials should be analysed on an intention to treat basis.

Severe malaria

In addition to parasite and fever clearance the rate of clinical recovery in survivors should be assessed. In unconscious patients the Glasgow coma scale should be assessed 4–6 hourly and the times to reach scores of 8, 11 and 15 recorded. Modified scales have been devised for children. The time to drink, sit, walk and leave hospital should also be documented. The changes in venous lactate, venous bicarbonate and, in adults, serum creatinine can also be followed and used as measures of the therapeutic response.

In vitro sensitivity testing

Both in vivo and in vitro assessments of antimalarial efficacy are needed to guide treatment recommendations and planning of policy. P. falciparum can be cultured relatively easily in vitro, whereas the other malaria parasites are more difficult to grow ex vivo. Short-term culture of P. falciparum over one cycle is relatively easy, requiring simple culture media, a candle jar and an incubator.[626] Short-term culture of P. vivax is also possible with modifications to the conditions.[627] Antimalarial drug susceptibility can be tested by measuring either the inhibition by different concentrations of drugs of parasite maturation to the schizont stage (i.e., microscopy), or the degree of inhibition of radio-labelled ^{3}H-hypoxanthine uptake, or the synthesis of parasite specific lactate dehydrogenase.[628–630] These are useful epidemiological tools, but they do not predict the clinical response to treatment in an individual because they do not take into account differences between people in antimalarial pharmacokinetics, immunity, or stage of disease.

Retreatment of recrudescent infections

A suggested algorithm is shown in Table 71.10. It is important to try and differentiate true resistance from a failure of drug adherence or absorption or inadequate dosing. Chloroquine failures will respond to sulfadoxine-pyrimethamine in some areas. In multi-drug-resistant areas failures following artemisinin combination treatment are unusual. Retreatment of a mefloquine failure with mefloquine again is associated with an increased risk of neuropsychiatric reactions. Artesunate or artemether (4 mg/kg followed by 2 mg/kg/day for a total of 7 days) or quinine (10 mg/kg three times daily) *plus* either clindamycin (10 mg/kg twice daily) or tetracycline taken properly for 7 days will cure approximately 90% of recrudescent infections.[650] Artemether-lumefantrine has not been evaluated yet in recrudescent infections following mefloquine treatment.

Management

Where possible, a definite species diagnosis should be obtained by microscopic examination of the blood smear. If there is any doubt, *P. falciparum* infection should be assumed. The management of malaria depends very much on the health facilities available and the endemicity of disease, i.e., the likely immune status of the patient. For example, in areas of intense transmission asymptomatic parasitaemia is common in older children and adults, and fever is more likely to be the result of some other infection. On the other hand, fever may precede detectable parasitaemia in non-immune adults or young children. The blood film should be rechecked in suspected cases. 'Blood smear-negative malaria' is a common diagnosis in the tropics, but one to be avoided. Other infections are more likely. In uncomplicated malaria it is safe to wait, seek other causes for the symptoms, and repeat the blood smears at 12 to 24 hour intervals. In severely ill patients antimalarial treatment should be started immediately in full doses, but other diagnoses sought. Patients may remain unconscious or develop renal failure after parasite clearance, but there is usually a clear history of previous treatment, and malaria pigment may still be found in monocytes in peripheral blood or intradermal smears,[424] and the *Pf*HRP2 dipstick will be positive.[386] If the temperature is high on admission (> 38.5°C) then symptomatic treatment with oral antipyretics (paracetamol, *not* aspirin) and tepid sponging brings symptomatic relief, and may also reduce the likelihood that the patient vomits the oral antimalarial drugs. This is particularly important for young children who are less likely to have a seizure and more likely to tolerate oral antimalarial drugs when their temperature has been lowered and they are quiet and calm. Unfortunately there are no paediatric formulations of mefloquine, artemether-lumefantrine, or the artemisinin derivatives. For young children large pills should be crushed and given as a suspension in a small volume of sweet drink or milk. A disposable syringe (*without* the needle!) may be used to draw up and give an accurate volume of the suspension into the child's mouth.

Benign malarias

Although *P. vivax*, *P. ovale* or *P. malariae* rarely kill, the disease can be moderately severe, requiring initial parenteral treatment. More usually oral treatment with chloroquine (Table 71.11) leads to resolution of the fever within 2–3

Table 71.11 Treatment of uncomplicated malaria

Malaria	Drug treatment
P. vivax, P. malariae, P. ovale, known chloroquine-sensitive *P. falciparum*[a]	Chloroquine 10 mg base/kg stat. followed by: 5 mg/kg at 12, 24 and 36 h; or 10 mg/kg at 24 h, 5 mg/kg at 48 h or amodiaquine 10 mg base/kg/day for 3 days
Chloroquine-resistant *P. falciparum*[a] known to be sensitive to sulfadoxine-pyrimethamine (SP)	Pyrimethamine 1.25 mg/kg + sulfadoxine 25 mg/kg (single dose) 3 tablets in an adult or Amodiaquine 10 mg base/kg/day for 3 days
Chloroquine-resistant *P. vivax*[b] and multi-drug resistant *P. falciparum*[a]	Oral artesunate 4 mg/kg daily for 3 days + mefloquine 25 mg base/kg (15 mg/kg on day 2, 10 mg/kg on day 3) Artemether-lumefantrine 1.5/9 mg/kg twice daily for three days with food. Quinine 10 mg salt/kg three times daily plus tetracycline 4 mg/kg four times daily or doxycycline 3 mg/kg once daily or clindamycin 10 mg/kg twice daily for 7 days[2]

[a]For acute treatment of falciparum malaria combinations containing an artemisinin-derivative are preferred. Artesunate (4mg/kg/day for 3 days) has been combined successfully with chloroquine, amodiaquine and SP.
[b]This refers to truly resistant infections, which are a significant problem only in Oceania and Indonesia, and should not be confused with relapses.

General points
Pregnancy: Mefloquine and artesunate should not be given in the first trimester. Halofantrine, primaquine, and tetracycline should not be used at any time in pregnancy, and sulfadoxine should not be used very near to term (if alternatives are available).
Vomiting is less likely if the patient's temperature is lowered before oral drug administration.
Short courses of artesunate or quinine (<7 days) alone are not recommended.
In renal failure the dose of quinine should be reduced by one-third to one-half after 48 hours, and doxycycline but *not* tetracycline should be prescribed.
The doses of all drugs are unchanged in children and pregnant women.

Specific points
Patients with *P. vivax* and *P. ovale* infections should also be given primaquine 0.25 mg base/kg daily (0.375–0.5 mg base/kg in Oceania) for 14 days to prevent relapse.
In mild G6PD deficiency 0.75 mg base/kg should be given once weekly for 6 weeks.
None of the tetracyclines should be given to pregnant women or children under 8 years of age.

days. The total dose is usually 25 mg base/kg. The initial dose is 10 mg base/kg and this is followed at 12-hour intervals with subsequent doses of 5 mg/kg or the dose is divided as 10, 10, 5 mg/kg on days 0, 1 and 2 respectively. Resistance to SP is widespread and chloroquine-resistant *P. vivax* is now a significant problem on the island of New Guinea and in parts of Indonesia. These infections respond to quinine or mefloquine. *Plasmodium vivax* responds to antimalarial drugs similarly to *P. falciparum*.[613,631] Primaquine is given to patients with *P. vivax* or *P. ovale* to prevent relapse. The usual adult dose is 15 mg base/day (0.25 mg/kg) for 14 days but 22.5 to 30 mg base/day is needed for the relatively resistant 'Chesson-like' strains (found in East Asia and Oceania).[632] Primaquine is unnecessary if the patient is going to return immediately to a highly endemic area, and should not be given to pregnant or lactating women or patients with known severe variants of G6PD deficiency. If mild variants of G6PD deficiency are known or likely then primaquine should be given in a dose of 0.75 mg/kg (45 mg) once weekly for six weeks. Primaquine does have significant activity against the asexual (blood stage) parasite and this may mask chloroquine resistance in combined treatment, but may also protect against chloroquine resistance in areas with sensitive parasites.[633]

P. falciparum malaria

In endemic areas, uncomplicated falciparum malaria is treated on an outpatient basis in the same way as the other malarias. In temperate countries imported cases should usually be hospitalized. The choice of drugs will depend on the local pattern of resistance where the infection was acquired. Because of the propensity for *P. falciparum* infections to kill, careful assessment of severity is most important. There is obviously a distribution of severity from asymptomatic parasitaemia to fulminant lethal malaria. In practice any patient who is unable to take oral medication will require parenteral treatment and careful observation, and any impairment of consciousness should be treated seriously. The progression to cerebral malaria can be rapid, particularly in young children.

Management of severe *P. falciparum* malaria

Severe malaria is a medical emergency. The airway should be secured in unconscious patients, an intravenous infusion should be started, and other resuscitation measures taken. The patient should be weighed so that the antimalarial drugs can be given on a body weight basis (for adults, a simple method is for the stretcher-bearers to stand on bathroom scales with, and without, the patient). Immediate measurements of blood glucose (stick test), haematocrit, parasitaemia (parasite count, stage of development, and proportion of neutrophils containing malaria pigment) and, in adults, renal function (blood urea or creatinine) should be taken. The degree of acidosis is an important

determinant of outcome; the plasma bicarbonate or venous lactate should be measured if possible (lactate rapid stick tests are now available). Arterial or capillary blood pH and gases should be measured in patients who are unconscious, hyperventilating or shocked. Blood should be taken for cross-match, and later (if available) full blood count, platelet count, clotting studies, blood culture and full biochemistry. Parenteral antimalarial treatment should be given as soon as possible. Where there are adequate nursing facilities the antimalarial drugs should be given by intravenous infusion. There is no specific treatment for severe malaria other than antimalarial drugs. These are potentially life saving and so it is *very* important that the dosing is correct (the first dose is by far the most important). Artesunate should be given by intravenous or intramuscular injection, and artemether by intramuscular injection only. A full loading dose (20 mg dihydrochloride salt/kg) of quinine should be given to all patients unless there is a clear history of adequate pretreatment.[333,489,634,635] The quinoline antimalarial drugs (chloroquine, quinine, quinidine) are compatible with saline or dextrose solutions. They should *never* be given by bolus intravenous injection. The assessment of fluid balance is critical in severe malaria. Overhydration may produce pulmonary oedema, whereas underhydration may contribute to shock or precipitate or worsen acidosis and renal impairment. In adults there is a very thin dividing line between the two, and careful and frequent evaluations of the jugular venous pressure, peripheral perfusion, venous filling, skin turgor and urine output should be made. Where there is uncertainty over the jugular venous pressure, and if nursing facilities permit, a central venous catheter should be inserted and the pressure (CVP) measured directly. The CVP should be maintained around 5 cm above the mid-axillary line. If the venous pressure is elevated (usually because of over-enthusiastic fluid administration), the patient should be nursed with the head at 45° and if necessary intravenous frusemide given. Children are often 'dry on admission'. Acidotic breathing or respiratory distress, particularly in severely anaemic children often indicates hypovolaemia and requires prompt rehydration and, if available, rapid blood transfusion.[370] Convulsions should be treated promptly with intravenous or rectal diazepam or intramuscular paraldehyde. The role of prophylactic anticonvulsants is unresolved (see below).

When these immediate procedures have been completed a more detailed clinical examination should be conducted, with particular note of the level of consciousness and record of the coma score. Several coma scores have been advocated. The Glasgow coma scale (GCS)[636] is suitable for adults, and the simple Blantyre modification (BCS)[332] is readily performed in children (Table 71.12). Unconscious patients must have a diagnostic lumbar puncture to exclude bacterial meningitis. The opening pressure should be recorded and the rise and fall with respiration noted. The CSF should be sent for microscopic analysis, culture, and measurement of glucose, lactate and protein. Subsequent clinical observations should be as frequent as possible and should include vital signs,

Table 71.12 Suitable coma scales to assess levels of consciousness in adults and children

The Blantyre coma scale for children		The modified Glasgow coma scale for adults	
	Score[a]		Score
Best motor response		**Best motor response**	
Localizes painful stimulus[b]	2	Obeys commands	6
Withdraws limb from pain[c]	1	Localizes pain	5
Non-specific or absent response	0	Withdraws limb from pain	4
		Flexion to pain	3
		Extension to pain	2
		None	1
Verbal response		**Verbal response**	
Appropriate cry	2	Oriented	5
Moan or inappropriate cry	1	Confused	4
None	0	Inappropriate words	3
		Incomprehensible sounds	2
		None	1
Eye movements		**Eye open**	
Directed (e.g., follows mother's face)[d]	1	Spontaneously	4
Not directed	0	To speech	3
		To pain	2
		Never	1

[a]Total score can range from 0 to 5; 2 or less indicates 'unrousable coma'.
[b]Painful stimulus: rub knuckles on patient's sternum.
[c]Painful stimulus: firm pressure on thumbnail bed with horizontal pencil.

[d]Total score can range from 3 to 15; 'Unrousable coma' reflects a score of <9.

with an accurate assessment of respiratory rate and pattern, assessment of the coma score, and urine output. The blood glucose should be checked, using rapid stick tests every four hours if possible, until recovery of consciousness. These stick tests may overestimate the frequency of hypoglycaemia so laboratory confirmation may be necessary. Important milestones on the road to recovery are the time to recover consciousness (GCS 15 or BCS 5), time to drink, and times to sit unaided and walk.

Cerebral malaria

When managing a patient who is unconscious with severe malaria, the physician must exclude, as far as possible, continuous seizure activity and hypoglycaemia as the cause. Both are more common in children than in adults. Many adjuvant therapies have been suggested, based on the prevailing pathophysiology hypothesis of the time. These include heparin, low molecular weight dextran, urea, high-dose corticosteroids, aspirin, prostacyclin, pentoxifylline (oxpentifylline), desferrioxamine, anti-TNF antibody, cyclosporin and hyperimmune serum. Unfortunately none has proved to be beneficial, and several have proved harmful.[635–643] None of these adjuvants should be used. The cornerstone of management is good intensive care and correct antimalarial treatment.

Prophylactic phenobarbitone prevents seizures in cerebral malaria. But the role of prophylactic anticonvulsants is uncertain since a recent large well-conducted double-blind trial in Kenyan children with cerebral malaria showed a doubling of mortality in children receiving a single prophylactic intramuscular injection of phenobarbitone (20 mg/kg). Mortality was increased in children who received three or more doses of diazepam (i.e., had recurrent treated seizures), which suggests a possible interaction between these two sedative drugs, and points to respiratory depression as the lethal effect.[644] Thus the standard loading dose of phenobarbitone is contraindicated unless the patient can be ventilated. Some physicians give a smaller dose of phenobarbitone in unconscious patients, others do not give any seizure prophylaxis and rely on treatment. The safety and effectiveness of phenytoin and other anticonvulsants is not known. The role of osmotic agents to treat raised intracranial pressure in cerebral malaria also remains uncertain. Although approximately 80% of children with cerebral malaria have moderately elevated pressures at lumbar puncture (whereas in adults 80% of pressures are in the normal range) and some children have very high pressures, there is no evidence that use of osmotic agents (such as mannitol) influences outcome. Those factors known to exacerbate raised intracranial pressure such as uncontrolled seizures and hypercapnoea should be treated promptly. Specific management includes care of the unconscious patient, careful fluid balance, rapid treatment of convulsions, treatment of hyperpyrexia, and early detection and treatment of other manifestations or complications of severe malaria.

Hypoglycaemia should be suspected in any patient who deteriorates suddenly, and this should be treated empirically if glucose stick tests are unavailable. Supervening bacterial infections are common, particularly chest infections and catheter-related urinary tract infections, and spontaneous septicaemia may occur. Bacteraemia is more common in African children than in adults or children studied in South-East Asia. Empirical broad-spectrum antibiotics should be given to any patient who deteriorates suddenly and in whom hypoglycaemia has been excluded. Aspiration pneumonia commonly follows generalized seizures. Patients should be nursed on their sides, and turned frequently. The role of prone positioning has not been studied. Most children will recover consciousness within two days, and most adults within three days. Rarely adults may remain unconscious for as long as ten days. Obviously with longer periods of coma complications such as pressure sores and secondary infections become increasingly likely.

Fluid balance

Children with severe malaria are often dehydrated, but renal failure and pulmonary oedema are extremely unusual in young children. A common mistake is to be too cautious in giving blood to an anaemic acidotic child for fear of precipitating 'congestive failure'. Recent studies indicate that anaemic congestive failure is uncommon, and that respiratory distress in these children represents acidosis not pulmonary oedema.[259,370] The acidosis is aggravated by anaemia and hypovolaemia. In approximately 50% of adults admitted with severe malaria there is evidence of renal impairment. In the majority of these there will be a transient period of oliguria, followed by uncomplicated recovery, but a minority will progress to established acute tubular necrosis. A polyuric phase is very unusual. Adults with severe malaria are very vulnerable to fluid overload and the physician treads a narrow path between underhydration, and thus worsening renal impairment, and overhydration, with the risk of precipitating pulmonary oedema. Following admission patients should be rehydrated carefully to a CVP of approximately 5 cm with 0.9% (normal) saline or other isotonic electrolyte solutions. Thereafter the daily fluid requirements will depend on urine output (+ diarrhoea) and insensible losses, which can be considerable in febrile patients nursed in hot environments. Water and glucose are provided by 5% or 10% dextrose solutions. It is not possible to generalize on initial fluid requirements as these can vary from deficits of several litres, to patients who are admitted oliguric and unconscious but well hydrated with a slightly elevated jugular venous pressure. Each patient's requirements should be assessed individually. If there is no CVP line it is well worth spending some time establishing clearly the level of the jugular venous pressure. If blood glucose is less than 4 mmol/l then 10% glucose should be started following saline replacement; if it is less than 2.2 mmol/l then hypoglycaemia should be treated immediately (0.3–0.5 g/kg of glucose). The fluid regimen must also be tailored around infusion of the antimalarial drugs. Some physicians prefer to put the 24-hour quinine maintenance dose in one 500 ml bottle of 0.9% saline or 5% dextrose water and infuse this at constant rate, whilst adjusting fluid balance as necessary through a separate piggy-backed line. It is rarely necessary to give potassium or other electrolyte supplements. Many patients will require blood transfusion. The exact criteria for transfusion will depend on blood availability, but in general if the haematocrit falls below 20% then blood should be given. In adults with severe malaria where there is a greater danger of precipitating pulmonary oedema, transmission of packed cells may be indicated. In practice if blood is allowed to sediment in a bag or bottle, only the cells can be given. If the patient is volume overloaded the transfusion should be stopped, or continued very slowly adding frusemide (0.3 mg/kg) to each unit.

Acute renal failure

If the patient remains oliguric (< 0.4 ml of urine/kg per hour) despite adequate rehydration, and the blood urea or creatinine are rising or already high, then fluids should be restricted to replace insensible losses only. Dialysis should be started early when there is evidence of multiple organ dysfunction. The role of dopamine and loop diuretics in preventing the progression of renal failure is controversial.[192] Renal failure is hypercatabolic in the acute phase of the disease, and once conventional indications for dialysis have been reached (i.e., metabolic acidosis, uraemic complications, volume overload, or less commonly hyperkalaemia) the patient may deteriorate quickly. An ECG should be performed if acute renal failure is suspected and an immediate blood potassium measurement is unavailable. If there are signs of hyperkalaemia (peaked T waves, widening of the QRS complex) then calcium, and glucose plus insulin, should be given immediately. The exact indications for beginning dialysis require careful clinical appraisal and some experience, but in general, if there is doubt, dialysis should be started. The tempo of disease is faster in patients with acute disease and multiple organ dysfunction, and dialysis should be started earlier than in those whose renal failure develops *after* other acute manifestations have resolved. Haemofiltration or haemodialysis are preferable to peritoneal dialysis. Haemofiltration is associated with a considerably more rapid resolution of biochemical abnormalities and a lower mortality than peritoneal dialysis. Despite the coagulopathy associated with severe malaria, bleeding problems are unusual. After the initial outlay for the pumps and balance haemofiltration is also less expensive, although well-trained nursing care is essential. When there is no alternative to peritoneal dialysis the addition of hypertonic dextrose to the peritoneal dialysate can be used to remove excess fluid, and also to provide glucose in hypoglycaemic cases. The efficiency of peritoneal dialysis often improves after the first 24 hours. Reduced peritoneal clearance is thought to be related to sequestration in the peritoneal microvasculature during the acute phase. Peritonitis (cloudy dialysis effluent) is

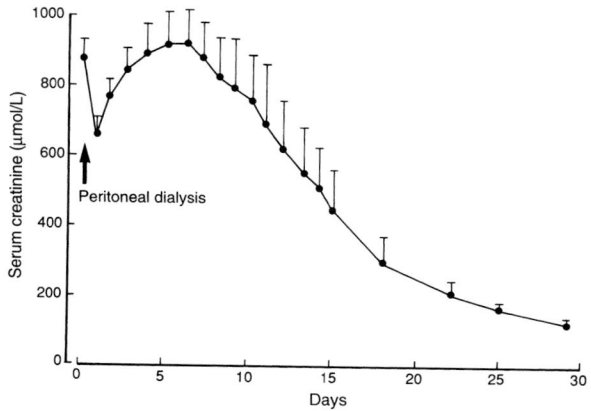

Figure 71.30: Recovery from malarial acute renal failure. This results from acute tubular necrosis. Many patients will not become oliguric, despite a rising serum creatinine in the first few days of hospitalization, and can be managed conservatively.

relatively common if dialysis is continued for more than 72 hours. The dose of quinine should be reduced by between one-third and one-half on the third day of treatment. Tetracycline is contraindicated, but doxycycline can still be given. The median time to recovery of urine flows of >20 ml/kg per 24 hours is 4 days. The overall prognosis and rate of recovery is better in oliguric than in anuric cases (Figure 71.30).

Patients with blackwater fever should be managed in the same way as other patients. Parenteral quinine should not be stopped unless an artemisinin derivative is available for substitution (both have been associated with blackwater). The preventitive or therapeutic role of urinary alkalinization has not been evaluated yet. Blood transfusion is often needed but the increase in haematocrit is often less than predicted because of the brisk haemolysis of the transfused cells. If the patient is volume overloaded, but needs blood, then dialysis or haemofiltration must be given first to create enough vascular 'space' for the blood. Packed cells should be given and the transfusion administered as slowly as possible.

Acute pulmonary oedema

This grave manifestation of severe malaria commonly co-exists with acute renal failure. The differential diagnosis includes pneumonia, if there are abnormal chest signs, and metabolic acidosis, if the chest is clear. Frothing at the mouth does not necessarily mean acute pulmonary oedema. In children it is often hypersalivation resulting from continuous seizures. Tachypnoea is a serious sign in malaria; occasionally it results from high fever alone, in which case breathing is shallow, but more usually there is noisy hyperventilation with use of accessory muscles of respiration, intercostal recession and flaring of the nostrils. Patients with acute pulmonary oedema should be nursed

upright and given oxygen, and the right-sided filling pressures should be reduced with whichever treatments are available (loop diuretics, opiates, venodilators, venesection, haemofiltration, dialysis). The right-sided pressure should be reduced to the lowest level compatible with an adequate cardiac output. Positive pressure ventilation should be started if the patient becomes hypoxic.

Hypoglycaemia

There may be no signs of hypoglycaemia in a patient already unconscious with cerebral malaria. Ideally, blood glucose should be checked 4-hourly while patients are unconscious. Hypoglycaemia should be treated by slow intravenous injection of 0.5–1 ml/kg of 50% dextrose water, and prevented by administering a 10% dextrose infusion at 1–2 mg/kg per hour. Quinine-stimulated hyperinsulinaemia may be blocked by somatostatin or its synthetic analogue, if available (they seldom are!). If possible, serum potassium should be checked frequently in hypoglycaemic patients receiving quinine and hypertonic dextrose solutions.

Lactic acidosis

Hypovolaemia should be corrected. The circulatory status is more difficult to assess in children than in adults. But in many cases the acidosis persists despite adequate blood pressure, warm peripheries, and normal jugular venous pressure. Although acidosis may result from acute renal failure, ketonaemia, and even salicylate poisoning, in most cases there is lactic acidosis. Venous, arterial and CSF concentrations of lactate rise in proportion to disease severity, and in contrast to sepsis, they are associated with an increased lactate-pyruvate ratio (often > 30) indicating anaerobic glycolysis. Lactic acid accumulation is buffered initially, but decompensation often occurs in severe malaria. The role of sodium bicarbonate in the treatment of metabolic acidosis has declined from established practice to the controversial. Now most authorities either do not give sodium bicarbonate at all, or give it once only in very severe acidosis (e.g., pH < 7.15). The pyruvate dehydrogenase activator dichloroacetate has proved promising in preliminary clinical trials, but its role in treatment remains to be defined. Haemofiltration or haemodialysis may be used to control acidosis.

Bleeding

Patients with cerebral malaria may have haematemesis or a bloody nasogastric aspirate because of acute gastric erosions. The incidence of upper gastrointestinal bleeding has declined since the discontinuation of high-dose corticosteroids in cerebral malaria. The role of prophylactic antacids, H_2 blockers, sulfacrate or proton pump inhibitors (e.g., omeprazole) has not been studied. Less than 5% of patients with severe malaria develop clinically significant DIC. These patients should be given fresh blood transfusions and vitamin K.

Bacterial superinfection/continued fever

Patients with secondary pneumonia should be given empirical treatment with a third-generation cephalosporin, unless admitted with clear evidence of aspiration, in which case penicillin or clindamycin is adequate. Children with persistent fever despite parasite clearance may have a systematic *Salmonella* infection, although in the majority of cases of persistent fever after parasite clearance no other pathogen is identified. Urinary tract infections are common in catheterized patients. Antibiotic treatments should depend on likely local antibiotic sensitivity patterns. Sustained high fever in the acute phase of severe malaria is a poor prognostic sign. Continued fever after parasite clearance is common; antibiotic treatment is only indicated if the patient becomes severely ill or there is a definite focus of infection.

Case history

A 46-year-old Brazilian forestry official was admitted to a large provincial hospital with a 5-day history of fever and malaise. Four days previously he had attended a health clinic and was told he had malaria. An intramuscular injection was given, and he was given three large white tablets to take immediately. A further six tablets were prescribed: two to be taken every 4–6 hours. On direct questioning he said that the injection was not painful (and looked like water), that the tablets were not particularly bitter, and that he did not have subsequent ringing in the ears or deafness. His symptoms did not improve, and so he left for the city. When he arrived (the previous morning), he was still febrile and felt ill so he consulted his private practitioner who gave him more white tablets (two to be taken three times daily) and red/yellow capsules (one to be taken four times daily). He found this medicine extremely bitter. By the time of admission he had taken four white tablets and two capsules, but had vomited twice the previous evening.

On examination he was lucid, but slightly agitated, jaundiced and anaemic. His oral temperature was 38.7°C. He was slightly dehydrated; the blood pressure was 100/70 and the pulse 120/min. The cardiovascular and respiratory systems were normal, but the liver and spleen were both enlarged. The haematocrit was 24%, and the thick blood film showed a heavy *P. falciparum* parasitaemia with gametocytes. The thin film count was 58/1000 red blood cells (no mature parasites with pigment were seen). An urgent serum creatinine was 4.1 mg/dl (360 µmol /l) and blood glucose 72 mg/dl (4.0 mmol/l). The admitting physician put up an intravenous infusion and, after considering the history of previous treatment, gave a loading dose of quinine dihydrochloride (20 mg salt/kg)

over 4 hours. This was followed by further infusions of 10 mg/kg 8-hourly. The next day the serum creatinine had risen to 5.5 mg/dl (485 µmol/l), with a blood urea nitrogen of 120 mg/dl, but the serum potassium was 4.6 mmol/l and the urine output 1500 ml (positive balance 1200 ml). The parasite count was 22/1000 red blood cells. The following day the serum creatinine was 6.3 mg/dl (554 µmol/l), the potassium 4.8 mmol/l and the urine output 1800 ml, but the fever had improved and the patient felt better. The quinine dose was reduced to 10 mg/kg 12-hourly. Thereafter the patient improved steadily, and the serum creatinine fell. The fever clearance time was 74 hours and parasite clearance time 82 hours. The patient was discharged after 10 days with a serum creatinine of 260 µmol/l. He was given doxycycline 100 mg daily for 7 days to take as an outpatient. One week later he was well, with a serum creatinine of 180 µmol/l.

Comment

This patient had severe malaria. The admitting physician was confronted with the common question of whether to give a loading dose of quinine or not. She could have given an artemisinin derivative in full doses without worry, but there was none available at the time. She decided that at the patient's first consultation the injection given was probably an antipyretic (and even if it had been quinine —which is painful if undiluted, and yellow in colour—it would not have altered her decision). 'Four days ago' would correspond to approximately five half-lives (5×18 hours) in severe malaria, i.e., if peak concentrations after the injection were 15 mg/l, then four days later they would be less than 1 mg/l). She thought on balance that the antimalarial treatment had probably been sulfadoxine-pyrimethamine (three tablets), and the other tablets antipyretics. On the previous day, however, he had probably been given quinine and tetracycline and, despite having vomited, he could have absorbed up to 1200 mg (four tablets) of quinine. Her decision then was difficult: the patient might have a plasma quinine concentration as high as 6 mg/l, but it was probably lower, and it could be that she was wrong about the drugs he had been prescribed. On the other hand, he was clearly sick and in need of urgent treatment. In practice, quinine toxicity is unusual in the treatment of severe malaria. If plasma quinine levels are over 3 mg/l on admission a loading dose is unnecessary and should not be given, but precise information such as this is almost never available. The admitting physician had to make an educated guess.

Although this patient's malaria infection responded well to treatment, and his urine output remained good, his renal function deteriorated initially. When renal function deteriorates steadily but there is no other evidence of vital organ failure, and urine output is adequate, then a careful 'watch and wait policy' is reasonable until an indication for dialysis arises. In the acute phase of severe malaria with multiple organ failure there should be a lower threshold for starting dialysis. In this case the patient fortunately turned the corner and made a good recovery with conservative management.

Malaria in pregnancy
Severe malaria

Pregnant women in the second and third trimesters are more likely to develop severe malaria than other adults, often complicated by pulmonary oedema and hypoglycaemia. Fetal death and premature labour are common.[288] The role of early Caesarean section for the viable live fetus is unproven, but recommended by many authorities. Obstetric advice should be sought at an early stage, the paediatricians alerted, and the blood glucose checked frequently. Hypoglycaemia should be expected and is often recurrent if the patient is receiving quinine. The antimalarial drugs should be given in full doses. Severe malaria may also present immediately following delivery. Postpartum bacterial infection is a common complication in these cases. Falciparum malaria has also been associated with severe mid-trimester haemolytic anaemia in Nigeria.[645] This often requires transfusion, in addition to antimalarial treatment and folate supplementation.

Uncomplicated malaria

Symptomatic malaria in pregnancy requires hospitalization where possible. Premature labour may occur and pregnant women receiving quinine are liable to develop hypoglycaemia. Chloroquine, pyrimethamine, proguanil and quinine are considered safe in pregnancy, and the sulphonamides are safe until term (when there is the theoretical risk of causing kernicterus in the newborn). Indeed there is now increasing use of intermittent SP for the prevention of malaria in endemic areas.[547,548] The options for treating resistant malaria in pregnancy are limited. There is increasing evidence that the artemisinin derivatives are safe,[646,647] but there is not enough experience yet to recommend them in the first trimester. Mefloquine has been associated with a fourfold increased risk of stillbirth in Thailand,[648] but not in Malawi,[649] so there is uncertainty over its safety. Halofantrine, artemether-lumefantrine, dihydroartemisinin-piperaquine, and atovaquone-proguanil have not been evaluated and should not be used. The tetracyclines and primaquine are contraindicated. Where necessary the artemisinin derivatives can be used after the first trimester. Quinine (10 mg salt/kg three times daily for 7 days) is still the treatment of choice for resistant falciparum malaria in the first trimester. The artemisinin derivatives and quinine should both be combined with clindamycin (10 mg/kg twice daily) to increase cure rates. Treatment failure rates are higher in pregnant women than in non-pregnant adults for any antimalarial regimen. Close follow-up is essential. Women in malarious areas should be encouraged to attend weekly antenatal clinics where blood smears and haematocrit can be checked, in addition to routine obstetric assessment.

Prophylaxis

If effective in the area and safe, antimalarial prophylaxis should be given during pregnancy. Chloroquine (5 mg base/kg/week) is generally still very effective in preventing *P. vivax*, *P. ovale* and *P. malariae* infections. Unfortunately *P. falciparum* is usually present at the same time and usually resistant. In areas where *P. falciparum* is still sensitive to antifols, daily proguanil (3.5 mg/kg/day) is safe and effective. There are some concerns over mefloquine in treatment use, although there is no significant evidence of an increased stillbirth risk when used as prophylaxis. Primaquine and doxycycline are contraindicated, and atovaquone-proguanil has not been evaluated yet.

Breast-feeding

Nearly all the antimalarial drugs appear in breast milk, but the actual amounts excreted are small. Primaquine should be avoided, but otherwise there seems no reason to discourage breast-feeding in women receiving antimalarial drugs.

Malaria in children

Although maternal malaria is very common, congenital malaria is surprisingly rare given the high frequency with which placental smears are positive in endemic areas, and the not infrequent finding of parasites in cord blood smears.[651] Nevertheless, it may occur with any of the four human malarias. Congenital falciparum malaria is seldom severe. Congenital *P. vivax* or *P. ovale* infections do not require radical treatment as there are no pre-erythrocytic stages in the baby; primaquine should not be given to neonates.

Severe malaria is relatively uncommon in the first six months of life, although when it does occur the mortality is high. In young children malaria presents as a febrile illness without focal signs. In *P. falciparum* infections, convulsions are an important complication in the first three years. They are twice as common as in *P. vivax* malaria, despite similar fever profiles. The progression to cerebral malaria in young children can be very rapid. Recovery is also rapid compared with adults. In areas of intense transmission, severe anaemia in the 1–3-year age group is the principal manifestation of severe falciparum malaria. A comparison of the relative frequencies of complications in adults and children is shown in Table 71.13.

Children receive the brunt of malaria's assault on humans. Most of the deaths from malaria are in children and most of those are in Africa. Malaria is also an important cause of morbidity, failure to thrive, and probably increased susceptibility to other infections. Whether cerebral malaria, malaria-associated convulsions, or the debilitating effects of repeated weakening febrile illnesses and anaemia cause developmental or intellectual retardation remains to be

Table 71.13 Relative incidence of severe falciparum malaria complications

	Non-pregnant adults	Pregnant women	Children
Anaemia	+	++	+++
Convulsions	+	+	+++
Hypoglycaemia	+	+++	+++
Jaundice	+++	+++	+
Renal failure	+++	+++	−
Pulmonary oedema	++	+++	+/−

determined. There is now some evidence for learning difficulties in cerebral malaria survivors.[352,353] In general, children tolerate the antimalarial drugs better than adults. In childhood severe malaria fluid balance is also easier as renal failure is very unusual. However, the difficulties of providing adequate nursing in the tropics, of obtaining intravenous access, and the small volumes of intravenous fluid required often mean that antimalarial drugs are given by the intramuscular, subcutaneous or suppository routes. Children may deteriorate very rapidly in severe malaria and sudden death is common in cerebral malaria but, if they survive, recovery is also more rapid than in adults.

Malaria with limited resources

The majority of patients with malaria in the world are either untreated or treated inadequately by self-medication. In many countries the private sector is the main source of antimalarial treatment. Fake or substandard drugs are common and incomplete treatment courses are often sold. Education of the public and the private commercial vendors is vitally important. Coherent and efficient schemes for the purchase and distribution of quality assured drugs are needed. In order to slow the pace of antimalarial resistance it is essential that whoever gives antimalarial treatment (parent, relative, village health worker, shop assistant) ensures a full course of treatment is administered. This is obviously much easier for single-dose antimalarial treatment, but with the exception of SP, most treatment regimens now are three-day courses.

Most patients with severe malaria are not admitted to hospital; they are treated at home or at rural health clinics. Where intravenous infusions cannot be given, intramuscular administration is acceptable for chloroquine, quinine or the artemisinin derivatives. It is essential that sterile technique is adhered to fully. Where injections are not possible then oral, suppository or, if a tube is available, nasogastric instillation should be attempted, pending transfer of the patient. Artemisinin, artesunate and chloroquine are available as suppositories or rectal formulations in some countries and these are simple and effective alternatives to parenteral administration.

The problem facing most tropical countries is serious. Their governments cannot afford to buy sufficient anti-

Table 71.14 Cost of antimalarial treatment for a 60 kg adult

Drug	US $
Atovaquone-proguanil	30.0
Halofantrine	5.0
Artemether-lumefantrine	2.4[a]
Mefloquine	2.0
Artesunate	1.2
Quinine	1.5
Amodiaquine	0.30
Sulfadoxine-pyrimethamine	0.13
Chloroquine	0.10

[a]Only through WHO approved sources.

malarial drugs for their needs and most people cannot afford to purchase effective treatments.[652] The annual per capita expenditure on antimalarial drugs in most of sub-Saharan Africa is still less than US $5. An adult (60 kg) course of chloroquine costs US $0.08, but a one-day course of halofantrine is over US $5 (Table 71.14). The target unit price for a single course of adult treatment with the new artemisinin combinations is between US $1 and US $3 (Table 71.14). This is currently unaffordable. The economic implications of deteriorating chloroquine and SP resistance in poor countries are horrendous. It is clear that if malaria is to be 'rolled back' then international financial support must be given to offset the costs of providing adequate treatment throughout the world.

Prevention
Personal prevention

The chances of being bitten by a malaria-infected female anopheline mosquito can be reduced considerably by simple measures. Covering exposed skin surfaces and remaining indoors or under a net at peak biting times will obviously reduce exposure. For example, most mosquitoes feed at night; sleeping indoors under insecticide (permethrin, deltamethrin)-treated bed-nets reduces morbidity and mortality in malarious areas. A single impregnation of a cotton or nylon mosquito net will provide protection for one year.[653] Nylon tends to retain permethrin and deltamethrin better than cotton. The impregnated bed-nets

(IBN) can be washed and can tolerate small tears or holes without markedly reducing the protective effects. The benefits conferred by bed-nets depend greatly on the biting habits of the mosquito, the size and constitution of the nets, whether they are impregnated with insecticide, the number of nets being used in the village, and a variety of sociological factors that determine actual use of the nets in practice. The protective efficacy of unimpregnated bed-nets is variable and depends very much on the way in which they are used (Do they have holes? Are they tucked under the mattress? etc.). These considerations are relatively unimportant for IBNs. In some studies unimpregnated nets have not demonstrated protective efficacy. The use of IBNs has proved remarkably effective in some areas. In a pivotal study from The Gambia, use of IBNs reduced the overall childhood mortality rate by 60%,[654] whereas earlier studies had shown malaria to account for approximately one-quarter of deaths in this age group, i.e., the reduction in mortality was over twice that expected.[655] This suggested either that malaria mortality had been seriously underestimated or that the debilitating effects of malaria may predispose to other infections, and consequent mortality. Many other studies have confirmed these findings.[656–658] As a consequence many countries have taken up IBN programmes as an important component of their antimalarial strategy. Unfortunately even in areas where striking benefits have been demonstrated the proportion of people who sleep under IBNs is still disappointingly low. This emphasises the importance of economic, educational, logistic and operational difficulties in limiting the success of proven effective antimalarial interventions. Impregnation of household curtains, or even cattle has been shown to reduce malaria.[659,660] It has been assumed that IBNs work mainly through personal protection, but their mass insecticidal effect may be more important in some contexts.[660] Thus the protection afforded by sleeping without a net in a village where IBNs are used extensively, may be greater than sleeping under an IBN in a village where no-one else uses them!

However, impregnated nets do not work in some areas, presumably because of different human and mosquito behaviour. Obviously if malaria is contracted by vectors which bite in the early evening or early morning away from human habitation then IBNs are not going to be very effective. Other simple preventive measures, including the application of permethrin or deltamethrin to clothing or the use of insect repellents such as diethyltoluamide (DEET) on exposed skin surfaces, are also effective and need not be prohibitively expensive. DEET is generally very safe, including in pregnancy.[661] Coconut oil and DEET 'soap bar' preparations are available which are cheap, stable, and readily applied. Houses can be mosquito proofed by using wire-mesh grilles over windows, and designed in such a way as to discourage mosquito ingress. All these measures reduce the chances of an infection, but they do not eliminate it.

Chemoprophylaxis

Although the early colonists devised many ingenious methods of taking quinine regularly (including 'Indian tonic water'), they were generally neither pleasant nor fully effective. Quinine (a poor prophylactic) was relied upon by armies and colonists until after the Great War. The subsequent discovery of mepacrine (quinacrine, atebrine) in 1934 gave the Allied Powers an efficacious, albeit rather toxic, prophylactic which prevented malaria effectively during the Second World War. However, it was the introduction of chloroquine, the antimalarial biguanides, and subsequently pyrimethamine after the war, that finally brought safe and effective antimalarial prophylaxis. The DHFR inhibitors (pyrimethamine, proguanil, chlorproguanil) and atovaquone inhibit parasite development in the liver (pre-erythrocytic activity) and in the erythrocyte. They are sometimes called causal prophylactics. These drugs also inhibit development in the mosquito (sporontocidal activity). Chloroquine and mefloquine inhibit asexual blood-stage development but do not prevent development of the liver stages. Thus the parasites emerge from the liver but cannot multiply in the red blood cells. They are called suppressive prophylactics. These drugs also have gametocytocidal activity against *P. vivax*, *P. malariae* and *P. ovale*, but not *P. falciparum*. Atovaquone-proguanil, doxycycline, and primaquine have been added to the list of antimalarial prophylactics. Each is active against resistant *P. falciparum* but each must be taken daily. Antimalarial prophylaxis must be taken regularly to ensure therapeutic antimalarial concentrations are maintained. Recommendations vary considerably depending on risk, prevalence and drug resistance. Up-to-date recommendations are easily obtained on the internet (e.g., http://www.who.int) (see Figure 71.31 for the current World Health Organization recommendations for antimalarial prophylaxis by region). Increasing drug resistance in recent years has meant that many prophylactic drugs can no longer be relied upon, particularly in areas of multiple drug resistance such as South-East Asia and South America.[662–664]

The recommended prophylactic drug regimens are shown in Table 71.15. When prescribing antimalarial prophylaxis to travellers, it is important to emphasize that no antimalarial is completely effective, and that a febrile illness could still be malaria. It is essential that prophylaxis is taken regularly, and for most drugs continued for four weeks after leaving the transmission area. The need to take the drugs for a month after leaving the transmission area is to 'catch' any parasites acquired shortly before departure when they leave the liver. But drugs acting on the liver stages (atovaquone-proguanil, primaquine) can be stopped immediately. This is a particular advantage for travellers visiting a malarious area for a short time. It is prudent to begin prophylaxis one week before departing for a malarious area so that tolerance to the drug regimen can be assessed, and therapeutic concentrations are present on arrival.[662–664] In anglophone countries, chloroquine is prescribed weekly, but in francophone countries it is given

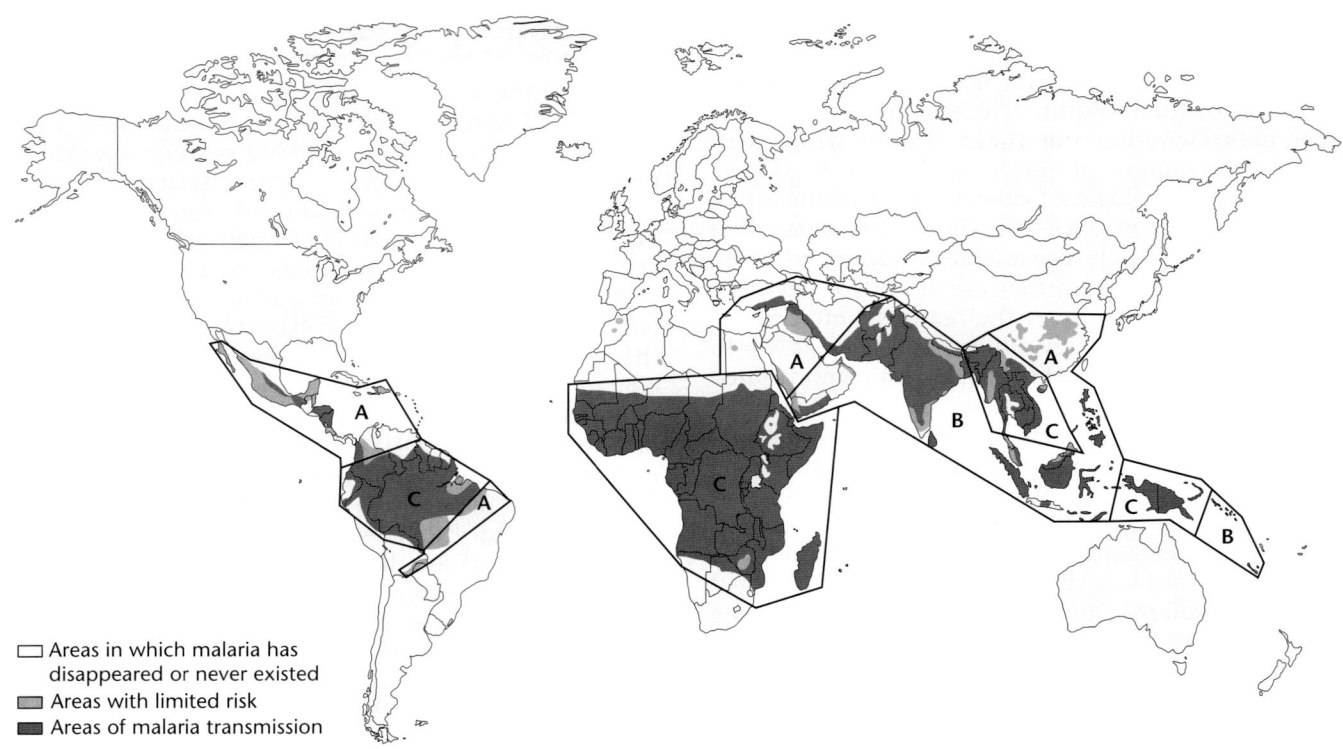

☐ Areas in which malaria has
   disappeared or never existed
▨ Areas with limited risk
■ Areas of malaria transmission

Figure 71.31: WHO recommendations for antimalarial prophylaxis: see Table 71.15.

Table 71.15 Antimalarial chemoprophylaxis*

	Weight adjusted dose for children	Adult dose
Chloroquine-sensitive malaria†		
Chloroquine[a]	5 mg base/kg weekly, or	300 mg base
	1.6 mg base/kg daily	100 mg base
and/or		
Proguanil	3.5 mg/kg daily	200 mg base
Chloroquine-resistant malaria		
Mefloquine[b]	5 base/kg/weekly	250 mg base
or		
Doxycycline[c]	1.5 mg/kg daily	100 mg
or		
Primaquine	0.5 mg base/kg daily with food	30 mg base
or		
Atovaquone-proguanil	4/1.6 mg/kg daily	250/100 mg

*Detailed local knowledge of *P. falciparum* antimalaria susceptibility and malaria risk should always be obtained.
[a]Chloroquine should not be taken by people with a history of seizures, generalized psoriasis or pruritus previously on chloroquine.
[b]Mefloquine is not recommended for babies < 3 months of age. Mefloquine should not be taken by people with psychiatric disorders, epilepsy, or those driving heavy vehicles, trains, aeroplanes etc. or deep sea diving.
[c]Doxycycline may cause photosensitivity. Use of sunscreens is recommended.

For current World Health Organisation recommendations see (http://www.who.int)
The WHO divides the world into three risk categories and makes the following recommendations:
A. Malaria risk low and seasonal, and *P. falciparum* is either absent or still sensitive to chloroquine.
This comprises Central America, north of the Panama Canal and northern Columbia, plus the southern and eastern ends of the malarious areas of Brazil, Turkey, Iraq, western Iran, and much of China (except for Yunnan, Hainan, and the areas adjoining Laos and Vietnam).
Prophylaxis: Chloroquine alone or no prophylaxis if very low risk.

B. Low malaria risk in most areas: chloroquine and proguanil still have significant efficacy.
This comprises Saudi Arabia, Yemen, the remainder of Iran, Afghanistan, Pakistan, India (except for the North East), Malaysia, Philippines, most of Indonesia, Micronesia.
Prophylaxis: Chloroquine + proguanil. 2nd choice: mefloquine.

C. Low malaria risk in Asia and most of South America, but high in most of Africa, lowland New Guinea, parts of Micronesia, and the Amazon basin. Drug resistance is more common.
Prophylaxis: 1st choice: mefloquine
            2nd choice: doxycycline. NB doxycycline is first choice for border areas of Cambodia, Myanmar and Thailand.
            3rd choice: Chloroquine and proguanil

once daily (this is theoretically preferable). Mefloquine and pyrimethamine-dapsone are taken once a week and proguanil, atovaquone-proguanil, primaquine and doxycycline daily. Amodiaquine, quinine, sulfadoxine-pyrimethamine and the artemisinin drugs should not be used for prophylaxis.

In situations where the risk of infection is low, or there are no effective antimalarial drugs available, or there is brief repeated exposure to intermediate or high transmission (e.g., aircrews), travellers can be advised to carry a treatment course of antimalarial drugs with them. If they become ill, and there are no medical facilities for malaria diagnosis and treatment, the treatment course is self-administered.

The use of antimalarial prophylaxis by the inhabitants of malarious areas remains controversial. It is generally agreed that pregnant women should take antimalarial prophylaxis if there is a significant risk of malaria, but that other adults should not. Chloroquine, pyrimethamine and proguanil are all considered safe in pregnancy. Mefloquine is considered safe, although there are uncertainties as treatment use has been associated with stillbirth in one large series. Tetracyclines and primaquine are contraindicated in pregnancy, and atovaquone-proguanil has not been evaluated. The use of antimalarial prophylaxis by children living in an endemic area has been shown to reduce mortality; in The Gambia administration of pyrimethamine and dapsone (Maloprim) in the 1–4-year age group reduced the mortality rate by 25%.[655] Despite this encouraging result, this practice has not been generally adopted.

Adverse effects

Adverse effects are a very important determinant of adherence to antimalarial prophylaxis regimens. As those taking the drugs prophylactically are healthy subjects, their tolerance of adverse effects is much lower than in treatment of malaria (where the patient often ascribes side effects to the disease, and takes the drugs only for a brief period). About 20% of patients taking prophylactic antimalarial drugs report some adverse effects. These are usually minor and do not require a change in prophylaxis. Nausea is the most common side effect. Chloroquine causes pruritus in subjects of African origin. Dizziness, dysphoria and sleep disturbances are particularly associated with mefloquine, visual disturbances with chloroquine, and photosensitivity and monilia with doxycycline. The risks of neuropsychiatric reactions or seizures are approximately 1:10 000, and appear similar for mefloquine and chloroquine.[530,531] There has been much television publicity over the CNS adverse effects of mefloquine. Minor but debilitating CNS effects are reported more commonly in travellers taking mefloquine than in other groups of subjects.[665] Mefloquine prophylaxis should not be offered to subjects with epilepsy, psychiatric disorders, or to subjects in whom any CNS disturbances could have disastrous consequences such as pilots, coach drivers etc.

Primaquine (0.5 mg/kg/day) is well tolerated if taken with food. It should not be given to subjects who are G6PD deficient. On an empty stomach it causes abdominal discomfort. Atovaquone-proguanil is remarkably well tolerated (similar adverse effects to proguanil alone).

Progress towards a malaria vaccine

Despite considerable effort and expense, a generally available and highly effective malaria vaccine is unlikely in the near future. Indeed the original goals of a vaccine producing sterile immunity (like the polio or yellow fever vaccines) without natural boosting are now considered unrealistic (and in some cases unwanted). The path of vaccine development has proved long and strewn with pitfalls, but there has been progress. Research has concentrated on all stages of the parasite life cycle: the sporozoite, the liver stage, the asexual blood stage, and the gametocyte. The most effective vaccine produced to date was produced over a quarter of a century ago and consisted of irradiated sporozoites.[666] The genes coding for the circumsporozoite protein of P. falciparum, the major surface antigen of the sporozoite, were cloned and sequenced in 1984. The central region of the protein consists of a series of tetrapeptide repeats, nearly all of which are NANP. Vaccines based on this repeat sequence have already been tried in man, but with only limited success. The early vaccines lacked T-cell epitopes and produced only transient antibody responses. Strategies to improve the immune response to these constructs included coupling the NANP repeats with known T-cell epitopes from the circumsporozoite protein, or from non-malarial proteins such as pseudomonas toxin A, or fusion with other 'boosters' such as monophosphoryl lipid A. The vehicle for vaccines also plays an important role in immunogenicity and presentation in alum or in liposomes augments the antibody response. A number of liver stage antigens, apart from CSP, have been identified and developed as vaccine candidates (LSA1, LSA3). The liver stage is important because it is the only stage in the parasite's life cycle where it inhabits cell expressing HLA antigens, and can therefore come under direct T-cell-mediated attack. For the development of a blood-stage vaccine, work has concentrated on two merozoite surface antigens (MSP_1, MSP_2,), the ring-infected erythrocyte surface antigen (RESA) and, to a lesser extent, proteins associated with the rhoptries, and the parasitophorous vacuole.[667,668] A vaccine developed in Columbia (SPf66) consisting of a combination of synthetic peptides containing a number of antigenic epitopes from the sporozoite and blood stage parasite has already been tested extensively in South America, Tanzania, The Gambia, and Thailand. It proved ineffective. Transmission blocking vaccines directed against the gametocytes and P. vivax sporozoite vaccines are also under development. Overall more than 30 distinct antigens from different stages of the parasite life cycle have been proposed as possible vaccine candidates. Future vaccines will be multi-component, multi-stage vaccines.[668] The mode of delivery is also under intense investigation; will it be the purified protein with a potent adjuvant, will the genes encoding the vaccine antigens be inserted into a viral vector (e.g., a recombinant modified poxvirus), or will the naked DNA be inoculated? The current preference seems to be to mix these such that the first immunization is given by one route and the boosters by another. At present it seems unlikely that these various vaccines will give complete or long-lasting protection. In endemic areas they will be part of the overall antimalaria strategy. Indeed, rather than preventing infection in areas of intense transmission (and thus interrupting the natural acquisition of immunity), their principal benefit may be to attenuate infection and prevent death rather than disease.

Chronic complications of malaria

Malaria is a major cause of chronic ill health in the tropics, particularly in childhood. Repeated attacks of malaria cause anaemia, failure to thrive, and probably also contribute to vulnerability to other infections and retard educational development. Chronic malaria is associated with certain specific syndromes.

Quartan nephropathy (see also Chapter 15)

The nephrotic syndrome, with albuminuria, hypo-albuminaemia, oedema and variable renal impairment, is common in the tropics.[669] Repeated or continuous *P. malariae* infection is associated with childhood nephrotic syndrome in West Africa and Papua New Guinea. In the past, quartan nephropathy was also described in eastern Asia. It has disappeared from countries where *P. malariae* has been eradicated, such as Guyana, where Giglioli first described the relationship between malaria and nephrosis. This strong epidemiological association has been supported by pathological studies,[669,670] although it is not known why certain individuals develop quartan nephropathy whereas the majority of those infected with *P. malariae* do not. The other species of malaria are also suspected of causing occasional glomerulonephritis, but the evidence is less convincing than for *P. malariae*.

Pathology

Quartan nephropathy is a chronic soluble immune complex nephropathy. Renal biopsy reveals a variety of abnormalities. There is commonly thickening of the sub-endothelial aspect of the basement membrane, giving rise to a double contour of argyrophilic fibrils. The changes are segmental initially. The capillary lumens narrow and become obliterated. On electron microscopy the basement membrane is irregularly thickened with lacunae of electron-dense material. Immunofluorescent study[669] shows IgG and IgM along the capillary walls. In two-thirds of cases this is accompanied by C3 and other complement components. Coarse granular deposits with IgG3 are more common than fine granular or linear staining, which is more associated with IgG2, and a poor response to cytotoxic therapy. In acute disease *P. malariae* antigens are demonstrable in approximately one-third of cases, but these are not evident in long-standing nephrosis. The severity of the glomerulonephritis is usually graded: <30% glomeruli involved, grade I; 30–75% glomeruli involved + tubular atrophy, grade II; and >75% of glomeruli involved, with extensive tubular pathology, grade III. Very occasionally adults develop a proliferative glomerulonephritis. This is not seen in children.

Clinical features

The pattern of renal involvement varies from asymptomatic proteinuria to full-blown nephrotic syndrome. Oedema, ascites or pleural effusions are usual presenting features. Anaemia and hepatosplenomegaly are common, and many patients have fever on admission. The blood pressure is usually normal; the urinary sediment may show granular or hyaline casts in addition to proteinuria, but haematuria or red cell casts are rare. The disease usually progresses inexorably to renal failure over 3–5 years. Spontaneous remission is rare. Antimalarial treatment does not prevent progression, and corticosteroids are usually ineffective. Some cases respond to cytotoxic therapy.

Hyper-reactive malarial splenomegaly (see also Chapters 10 and 13)

This is also known as the tropical splenomegaly syndrome. It occurs where transmission of malaria is intense and has been reported throughout the tropics.[671] The highest incidence of hyper-reactive malarial splenomegaly (HMS) yet reported is in the Upper Watut Valley of Papua New Guinea, where 80% of adults and older children have large spleens. Genetic factors undoubtedly play a role because within a malarious area the geographical distribution of HMS does not follow closely that of malaria transmission.

Pathology

There is gross splenomegaly with normal architecture, and lymphocytic infiltration of the hepatic sinusoids with Kupffer cell hyperplasia. The massively enlarged spleen leads to hypersplenism with anaemia, leucopenia and thrombocytopenia. There is a polyclonal hypergamma-globulinaemia with high serum concentrations of IgM. High titres of malaria antibodies, and a variety of auto-antibodies (antinuclear factor, rheumatoid factor) are usually present. The hypergammaglobulinaemia is believed to result from polyclonal B-cell activation in the absence of adequate numbers of CD8+ suppressor T cells,[672,673] which have been removed by an antibody-dependent cytotoxic mechanism. Cell-mediated immune responses are otherwise normal. Immunoglobulin gene rearrangements have been demonstrated in a sub-group of patients with HMS.[674] This indicates clonal lymphoproliferation and the potential for progression to malignant lymphoma or leukaemia.

Clinical features

Most patients present with abdominal swelling and a dragging sensation in the abdomen. The malaria blood slide is usually negative. HMS commonly presents in pregnancy. The large, hard spleen is vulnerable to trauma. Acute left-sided abdominal pain suggests splenic infarction. The liver is also enlarged. Anaemia is often symptomatic and associated with pancytopenia (hypersplenism), and there is an increased susceptibility to bacterial infections. The long-term prognosis of HMS is not good, with an increased mortality from infection. HMS appears to be a pre-malignant condition developing into lymphoma in some patients.

Treatment

The enlarged spleen usually regresses over a period of months with effective antimalarial prophylaxis. Most experience has been gained with chloroquine and mefloquine. The liver also returns to normal, and the IgM levels fall. Treatment is required for the duration of malaria exposure. Splenectomy is only recommended if there is an unequivocal failure of prophylaxis given for at least six months and there is severe hypersplenism.

Lymphoma (see also Chapter 44)

In some countries, Burkitt's lymphoma is the most common malignancy of childhood. It is an uncontrolled proliferation of B lymphocytes, and is associated with Epstein–Barr (EB) virus infections and malaria. The epidemiological association between malaria and Burkitt's tumour is very strong. EB virus infections are widespread in the tropics, and in most countries over 80% of children have serological evidence of infection by the age of 3 years. Normally, progression of EB virus in B lymphocytes is controlled by virus-specific cytotoxic T cells (the atypical mononuclear cells of infectious mononucleosis). This EB virus cytotoxic T-cell response is decreased significantly during acute malaria, and there is increased proliferation of EB virus-infected lymphocytes.[675] This may predispose to malignant transformation. In Ghana prospective studies of HMS and splenic lymphoma with villous lymphocytes suggest that a proportion of patients with HMS develop lymphoma.[674] The prognosis is poor.

Malaria control

In his classic work on the prevention of malaria, Ronald Ross (1910) noted that in approximately 550 BC Empedocles

rid the Sicilian town of Selinus from a pestilence by draining the nearby marshes. Hippocrates (400 BC) knew that stagnant water and marshlands were unhealthy, and that people living nearby would have enlarged spleens. The principles of drainage and land-fill to control disease have continued since Roman times. The early attempts at joining the Atlantic and Pacific oceans were thwarted by disease, of which malaria was a major contributor, but during the final building of the Panama Canal, malaria was almost eradicated from the Canal Zone by a vigorous combination of felling, drainage, house screening, pesticide use and antimalarial drugs. In recent years the practices of vector control have evolved, and environmental management and modification have come to the fore, both for disease control and for agricultural and other economic purposes.[676] This is a complex and multidisciplinary field. Only a brief outline of the various approaches to malaria control will be described here.

Water level management

The oldest method of vector control—drainage—remains the most cost effective, particularly in relatively dry areas where there is a high ratio of population to standing water. The practical aspects of drainage are beyond the scope of this book. Water level management to flush out mosquito breeding areas, and to provide a hostile aquatic environment for mosquito egg and larval development, is an alternative to drainage. Changing water salinity or allowing organic matter pollution may also reduce vector populations. As always, major alterations to the environment should not be undertaken lightly: short-term benefits may be offset by long-term problems.

Human behaviour

Mosquitoes cannot fly far; most anophelines cannot fly more than 4 km, and in general they remain within 2 km of their breeding sites. If humans do not live near breeding sites, then the chances of infection are reduced. Many vectors bite inside houses, and the design and protection offered by the dwelling are important determinants of malaria risk. Wire-mesh screens and other mosquito proofing measures are effective but expensive, and may also reduce ventilation. The use of mosquito-proof bed-nets prevents human—vector contact, but they are considerably more effective in preventing malaria when impregnated with insect repellents or insecticides. Pyrethroid insecticide (permethrin, deltamethrin)-impregnated nylon nets are best. The use of insect repellents applied to exposed skin is also effective, and can be relatively cheap (e.g., diethyltoluamide). Where domestic species of anophelines exist (e.g., *A. stephensi* in India), water jars, tanks or containers should be closed to prevent mosquito access.[676]

Imagocides

Although chemical agents, such as the larvicide Paris

green, and pyrethrum insecticides, had been widely used for vector control before the Second World War, the discovery of 2,2-bis-(*p*-chlorophenyl)-1,1,1-trichloroethane (DDT), with excellent activity against the adult mosquito (imagocidal activity), was a major advance in malaria control. DDT had residual imagocidal activity, which pyrethrum did not. It could be sprayed on the interior of houses, and would kill or deter mosquitoes for many months afterwards. DDT, along with two other chlorinated hydrocarbon residual insecticides, gamma benzene hexachloride (gamma HCH) and dieldrin, were the principal weapons in the campaign to eradicate malaria and they had a tremendous impact on health and development in the tropics. Imagocides can be classified into three general categories.

Pyrethrins and pyrethroids

The naturally occurring compounds are light sensitive and unstable, but the new synthetic pyrethroids (permethrin, deltamethrin) are both highly toxic to mosquitoes and stable, giving good residual activity. A single point mutation (resulting in phenyalanine or serine for leucine at position 1014) in the gene encoding a voltage-gated sodium channel protein is associated with pyrethroid and DDT resistance.[677,678] Known as the pyrethroid knock down resistance (kdr) mutation, it has been found at several different locations, but predominantly in *A. gambiae* in West and South Africa. Insecticide resistance is spreading and represents a serious threat to the efficacy of impregnated bed-nets and vector control.[679,680]

Chlorinated hydrocarbons

DDT, gamma HCH and dieldrin are widely used as water-dispersible powders which form an aqueous suspension suitable for spraying. Resistance, human toxicity and ecological concerns have restricted the use of DDT in recent years, but a global ban has been reversed. Used appropriately, DDT is still a very valuable malaria control tool (e.g., in KwaZulu Natal where *A. funestus* is pyrethroid resistant but DDT sensitive). Dieldrin is now considered too toxic to humans and it is no longer used.

Anticholinesterases

These comprise the organophosphorous compounds (malathion, fenitrothion) and the carbamates (propoxur, trimethacarb, bendiocarb). Although resistance to the organophosphates has limited use in some areas, these compounds are still distributed widely. Malathion is the cheapest and most widely used. The anticholinesterases pose a potential health hazard to spraying teams, despite their wide therapeutic ratios.

Imagocides are also classified either by their portal of entry to the body of the mosquito, or to the method of application. Residual insecticides are applied as a deposit on to surfaces where the mosquitoes will rest (e.g., walls, ceilings). Space sprays fill the air with a mist or fog of insecticide. The choice of insecticide and application method will be determined by the sensitivity and behaviour of the local vectors and the nature of the environment.[676] The anopheline mosquito vectors have countered these chemical assaults by changing their behaviour (resting and feeding preferences) and evolving resistance to the insecticides. This has had drastic consequences: reduced effectiveness; the necessity for more expensive replacements (to which resistance has also developed in some species); a disinclination of the chemical industry to invest further in a difficult and often unprofitable field; and as a consequence an inability of impecunious governments to pay for the new insecticides. Over 50 vector species are resistant to one or more of the organochlorine insecticides, over ten are resistant to the organophosphates, and pyrehroid resistance is spreading. Most important, *A. gambiae s.l.*, the dominant vector in Africa, has developed resistance to organochlorine insecticides in many areas. In Central America *A. albimanus* has developed multiple insecticide resistance. In India the major vectors, *A. culicifacies* and *A. stephensi*, have become resistant to the organochlorines and malathion.

Larviciding

With the problems besetting use of residual imagocidal insecticides, there has been renewed interest in methods of larval control in recent years. These include environmental and water manipulation to prevent creation of mosquito breeding sites, the use of larvivorous fish and bacterial toxins, and the application of chemical agents. Mineral oils were the first larvicides to be employed, and diesel oil is still widely used today. Many of the imagocidal compounds described above are also used for larvicides. However, the organochlorines were highly effective but are no longer recommended because of their adverse environmental impact, and the development of resistance. The organophosphorous compounds are used widely and are relatively safe; for example, compounds such as temephos are safe to warm-blooded animals and fish and can be used to treat potable water.

Overall approach

The objectives of a malaria control programme will depend on the prevailing epidemiological situation, the availability of resources, and feasibility. The first priority is the reduction of malaria mortality by making available facilities and personnel for diagnosis and effective treatment. The second priority is to reduce malaria morbidity (such programmes should focus on malaria in childhood and malaria in pregnancy), and again rely on use of effective drugs. The third priority is to try and reduce transmission in the most appropriate and cost-effective way. The fourth is to anticipate and prevent the development of epidemics. Having 'secured' the situation, it is also necessary to secure those areas free from malaria to prevent re-establishment of the infection. Finally, and in a carefully planned and multifaceted programme, work to eliminate the disease should begin.

REFERENCES

1. Bruce-Chwatt LJ. History of malaria from prehistory to eradication. In Wernsdorfer WH & McGregor I (eds) *Malaria: Principles and Practice of Malariology*. Edinburgh: Churchill Livingstone, 1988:1–59.

2. Smith DC & Sanford LB. Laveran's germ: the reception and use of a medical discovery. *Am J Trop Med Hyg* 1988; 34:2–20.

3. Laveran CLA. Note sur un nouveau parasite trouve dans le sang de plusieurs malades atteints de fievre palustre. *Bull Acad Med* 1880; 9:1235.

4. Ross R. On some peculiar pigmented cells found in two mosquitoes fed on malarial blood. *Brit Med J* 1897; 2:1786–1788.

5. Ross R. *The prevention of Malaria*, 2nd Edn. London: Murray.

6. Bignami A. Come si prendono le febbri malariche. *Boll R Acad Med Roma* 1899; 25:17–46.

7. Julius Wagner-Jauregg. *Lebenserinnerungen* L. Schönbauer und M Jantsch (eds), Wien, Springer Verlag 1950, 157.

8. Garnham PCC. *Malaria Parasites and other Haemosporidia*. Oxford: Blackwell, 1966.

9. Waters AP, Higgins DG & McCutchan TF. Plasmodium falciparum appears to have arisen as a result of lateral transfer between avian and human hosts. *Proc Natl Acad Sci USA* 1991; 88:3140–3144.

10. Conway DJ, Fanello C, Lloyd JM, et al. Origin of Plasmodium falciparum malaria is traced by mitochondrial DNA. *Mol Biochem Parasitol*. 2000; 111:163–71.

11. Covell G. Spontaneous rupture of the spleen. *Trop Dis Bull* 1955; 52:705–723.

12. Nosten F, McGready R, Simpson JA, et al. The effects of *Plasmodium vivax* malaria in pregnancy. *Lancet*. 1999; 354:546–549.

13. Gillies MT. Anopheline mosquitos: vector behaviour and bionomics. In Wernsdorfer WH & McGregor I (eds) *Malaria: Principles and Practice of Malariology*. Edinburgh: Churchill Livingstone, 1988:453–485.

14. Molineaux L, Muir DA, Spencer HC & Werndorfer WH. The epidemiology of malaria and its measurement. In Wernsdorfer WH & McGregor I (eds) *Malaria: Principles and Practice of Malariology*. Edinburgh: Churchill Livingstone, 1988:999–1090.

15. MacDonald G. *The Epidemiology and Control of Malaria*. London: Oxford University Press.

16. Cattani JA, Tulloch JL, Vrbova H et al. The epidemiology of malaria in a population surrounding Madang, Papua New Guinea. *Am J Trop Med Hyg* 1986; 35:3–15

17. Marsh K, Snow RW. Malaria transmission and morbidity. *Parasitologia*. 1999; 41:241–6.

18. Greenwood BM, Bradley AK, Greenwood AM et al. Mortality and morbidity from malaria among children in rural areas of The Gambia, West Africa. *Trans R Soc Trop Med Hyg* 1987; 81:478–486.

19. Baird JK, Jones TR, Danudirgo EW et al. Age dependent acquired protection against *Plasmodium falciparum* in people having two years exposure to hyperendemic malaria. *Am J Trop Med Hyg* 1991; 45:65–76.

20. Brabin BJ. Analysis of malaria in pregnancy in Africa. *Bull World Health Organ* 1983; 61:1005–1016.

21. Nosten F, ter Kuile F, Malankirri L et al. Malaria in pregnancy in an area of unstable endemicity. *Trans R Soc Trop Med Hyg* 1991; 85:424–429.

22. Oppenheimer SJ, Gibson FD, Macfarland SB et al. Iron supplementation increases prevalence and effects of malaria: report on clinical studies in Papua New Guinea. *Trans R Soc Trop Med Hyg* 1986; 80:603–612.

23. McGregor IA. Epidemiology, malaria and pregnancy. *Am J Trop Med Hyg* 1984; 33:517–525.

24. Pasvol G, Weatherall DJ & Wilson RJM. Effects of fetal hemoglobin on susceptibility of red cells to *Plasmodium falciparum. Nature* 1977; 270:171–173.

25. Smith TA, Leuenberger R, Lengeler C. Child mortality and malaria transmission intensity in Africa. *Trends Parasitol.* 2001; 17:145–9.

26. Marsh K, Forster D, Waruiru C, et al. Indicators of life-threatening malaria in African children. *N Engl J Med.* 1995; 332:1399–404.

27. Hendrickse RG, Hasan AH, Olumide LO & Akinkunmi A. Malaria in early childhood. An investigation of five hundred seriously ill children in whom a 'clinical' diagnosis of malaria was made on admission to the Children's Emergency Room at University College Hospital, Ibadan. *Ann Trop Med Parasitol.* 1971; 65:1–20.

28. Lindsay SW, Wilkins HA, Zieler HA et al. Ability of *Anopheles gambiae* mosquitos to transmit malaria during the dry and wet seasons in an area of irrigated rice cultivation in The Gambia. *J Trop Med Hyg* 1991; 94:313–324.

29. Marchiafava E. Pernicious malaria. *Am J Trop Med Hyg* 1932; 21:1–56.

30. McGregor IA. Consideration of some aspects of human malaria. *Trans R Soc Trop Med Hyg* 1965; 59:145–152.

31. Brewster DR & Greenwood BM. Seasonal variation of paediatric diseases in The Gambia, West Africa. *Ann Trop Paediatr.* 1993; 13:133–146.

32. Luxemburger C, Kyaw Ley Thew, White NJ, et al. The epidemiology of malaria in a Karen population on the western border of Thailand. *Trans R Soc Trop Med Hyg* 1996; 90:105–111.

33. Garnham PCC. Malaria parasites of man: life cycles and morphology. In Wernsdorfer WH & McGregor I (eds) *Malaria: Principles and Practice of Malariology*. Edinburgh: Churchill Livingstone, 1988:61–69.

34. Ponnudurai T, Lensen AHW, van-Gemart GJA et al. Feeding behaviour and sporozoite ejection by infected *Anopheles stephensi. Trans R Soc Trop Med Hyg* 1991; 85:175–180.

35. Rosenburg R & Wirtz RA. An estimation of the number of sporozoites ejected by a feeding mosquito. *Trans R Soc Trop Med Hyg* 1990; 84:209–212.

36. Miller LH, Mason SJ, Clyde DF & McGinniss MH. The resistance factor to *P. vivax* in Blacks: the Duffy blood group genotype. *N Engl J Med* 1976; 295:302–304.

37. Miller LH. Genetically determined human resistance factors. In Wernsdorfer WH & McGregor I (eds) *Malaria: Principles and Practice of Malariology*. Edinburgh: Churchill Livingstone, 1988:487–500.

38. Holder AA. Proteins on the surface of the malaria parasite and cell invasion. *Parasitology* 1994; 108 Suppl:S5–S18.

39. Mayer DC, Kaneko O, Hudson-Taylor DE, Reid ME & Miller LH.Characterization of a *Plasmodium falciparum* erythrocyte-binding protein paralogous to EBA-175. *Proc Natl Acad Sci USA.* 2001; 24; 98:5222–5227.

40. Reed MB, Caruana SR, Batchelor AH, Thompson JK, Crabb BS, Cowman AF. Targeted disruption of an erythrocyte binding antigen in *Plasmodium falciparum* is associated with a switch toward a sialic acid-independent pathway of invasion. *Proc Natl Acad Sci USA.* 2000; 97:7509–7514 .

41. Pagola S, Stephens PW, Bohle DS, Kosar AD, Madsen SK. The structure of malaria pigment beta-haematin. *Nature.* 2000; 404:307–310.

42. Ginsburg H, Famin O, Zhang J & Krugliak M. Inhibition of glutathione-dependent degradation of heme by chloroquine and amodiaquine as a possible basis for their antimalarial mode of action. *Biochem Pharmacol.* 1998; 56:1305–1313.

43. Kirk K. Membrane transport in the malaria-infected erythrocyte. *Physiol Rev.* 2001; 81:495–537.

44 Cranston HA, Boylan CW, Carroll G L et al. *Plasmodium falciparum* maturation abolishes physiologic red cell deformability. *Science* 1984; 223:400–402.

45 Leech JH, Barnwell JW, Miller LH & Howard RJ. Identification of a strain-specific malarial antigen exposed on the surface of *Plasmodium falciparum* infected erythrocytes. *J Exp Med* 1984; 159:15657–1575.

46 Simpson JA, Aarons L, Collins WE, Jeffery G, White NJ. Population dynamics of the *Plasmodium falciparum* parasite within the adult human host in the absence of antimalarial drugs. *Parasitology*, 2002; 124:247–263.

47 Read AF, Nanara A Nee S et al. Gametocyte sex ratios as indirect measures of outcrossing rates in malaria. *Parasitology* 1992; 104:387–395.

48 Fletcher C. The *Plasmodium falciparum* genome project. *Parasitol Today* 1998; 14:342–344.

49 Philips RS. Current status of malaria and potential for control. *Clin Microbial Rev* 2001; 14:208–226.

50 Gupta S & Anderson RM. Population structure of pathogens: the role of immune selection. *Parasitol Today*. 1999; 15:497–501.

51 Anders RF. Multiple cross reactivities amongst antigens of *Plasmodium falciparum* impair the development of protective immunity against malaria. *Parasite Immunol* 1986; 8:529–539.

52 Kemp DJ, Cowman AF & Walliker D. Genetic diversity in *Plasmodium falciparum*. *Adv Parasitol* 1990; 29:75–149.

53 Haldane JBS. Disease and evolution. *Ric Sci* 1949; 19 (Supplement):68–75.

54 Hill AVS. Malaria resistance genes: a natural selection. *Trans R Soc Trop Med Hyg* 1992; 86:225–226.

55 Allen SJ, O'Donnell A, Alexander ND, et al. Prevention of cerebral malaria in children in Papua New Guinea by southeast Asian ovalocytosis band 3. *Am J Trop Med Hyg* 1999; 60:1056–60.

56 Weatherall DJ. Thalassaemia and malaria, revisited. *Ann Trop Med Parasitol* 1997; 91:885–90.

57 Ruwende C, Khoo SC, Snow RW, et al. Natural selection of hemi- and heterozygotes for G6PD deficiency in Africa by resistance to severe malaria. *Nature*. 1995; 376:246–9.

58 Luzzi GA, Merry AH, Newbold CI et al. Surface antigen expression on *Plasmodium falciparum* infected erythrocytes is modified in α- and β-thalassaemia. *J Exp Med* 1991; 173:785–791.

59 Williams TN, Maitland K, Bennett S, et al. High incidence of malaria in alpha-thalassaemic children. *Nature*. 1996; 383:522–5.

60 Hill AVS, Bennett S, Allsopp CEM et al. Common West African HLA antigens are associated with protection from severe malaria. *Nature* 1991; 352:595–600.

61 Hill AVS, Elvin J, Willis AC et al. Molecular analysis of an HLA-disease association: HLA-B53 and resistance to severe malaria. *Nature* 1992; 360:434–439.

62 McGuire W, Hill AV, Allsopp CE, Greenwood BM & Kwiatkowski D. Variation in the TNF-alpha promoter region associated with susceptibility to cerebral malaria. *Nature*. 1994;371:508–510.

63 McGuire W, Knight JC, Hill AV, Allsopp CE, Greenwood BM & Kwiatkowski D. Severe malarial anemia and cerebral malaria are associated with different tumor necrosis factor promoter alleles. *J Infect Dis*. 1999; 179:287–290.

64 Kwiatkowski D. Genetic susceptibility to malaria getting complex. *Curr Opin Genet Dev* 2000; 10:320–4.

65 Kitchen SF. Symptomatology: general considerations and falciparum malaria. In Boyd MF (ed) *Malariology*, vol. 2. Philadelphia: W B Saunders, 1949:996–1017.

66 James SP, Nichol WD & Shute PG. A study of induced malignant tertian malaria. *Proc R Soc Med* 1932; 25:1153–1186.

67 Fairley NH. Sidelights on malaria in man obtained by subinoculation experiments. *Trans R Soc Trop Med Hyg* 1947; 40:521–676.

68 White NJ, Chapman D & Watt G. The effects of multiplication and synchronicity on the vascular distribution of parasites in falciparum malaria. *Trans R Soc Trop Med Hyg* 1992; 86:590–597.

69 Kwiatkowski D & Nowak M. Periodic and chaotic host parasite interaction in human malaria. *Proc Natl Acad Sci USA* 1990; 88:5111–5113.

70 Simpson JA, Silamut K, Chotivanich K, Pukrittayakamee S & White NJ. Red cell selectivity in malaria: a study of multiple infected erythrocytes. *Trans R Soc Trop Med Hyg* 1999; 93:165–168.

71 Wagner-Jauregg D. The treatment of general paresis by inoculation of malaria. *J Nerv Ment Dis* 1922; 55:369–375.

72 Jeffery GM. Epidemiological significance of repeated infections with homologous and heterologous strains and species of Plasmodium. *Bull World Health Organ* 1966; 35:873–882.

73 Schmidt LH. *Plasmodium falciparum* and *Plasmodium vivax* infections in the owl monkey (Aotus trivirgatus). 1. The course of untreated infections. *Am J Trop Med Hyg* 1978; 27:671–702.

74 Chotivanich K, Udomsangpetch R, Simpson JA, Newton P, Pukrittayakamee S, Looareesuwan S & White NJ. Parasite multiplication potential and the severity of falciparum malaria. *J Infect Dis* 2000; 181:1206–1209.

75 White NJ & Krishna S. Treatment of malaria: some considerations and limitations of the current methods of assessment. *Trans R Soc Trop Med Hyg* 1989; 83:767–777.

76 Silamut K & White NJ. The relationship of stage of parasite development to prognosis in falciparum malaria. *Trans R Soc Trop Med Hyg* 1993; 87:436–443.

77 Playfair JHL, Taverne J, Bate CAW & de Souza JB. The malaria vaccine: anti-parasite or anti-disease immunity. *Immunol Today* 1990; 11:25–27.

78 Riley EM, Andersson L, Otoo N et al. Cellular immune responses to *Plasmodium falciparum* antigens in Gambian children during and after an acute attack of falciparum malaria. *Clin Exp Immunol* 1988; 73:17–22.

79 Ciuca M, Baluf L & Chelarescu-Vierum. Immunity in malaria. *Trans R Soc Trop Med Hyg* 1934; 27:619–622.

80 Brown KN, Berzins K, Jarra W & Schetters T. Immune responses to erythrocytic malaria. *Clin Immunol Allergy* 1986; 6:227–249.

81 Bouharoun-Tayoun H, Attanath P, Sabcharoen A et al. Antibodies that protect humans against *P. falciparum* blood stages do not on their own inhibit parasite growth in vitro but act in co-operation with monocytes. *J Exp Med* 1990; 172:1633–1641.

82 McGilvray ID, Serghides L, Kapus A, Rotstein OD & Kain KC. Nonopsonic monocyte/macrophage phagocytosis of *Plasmodium falciparum*-parasitized erythrocytes: a role for CD36 in malarial clearance. *Blood* 2000; 96:3231–40.

83 Nnalue NA & Friedman MJ. Evidence for a neutrophil-mediated protective response in malaria. *Parasite Immunol* 1988; 10:47–58.

84 Rockett KA, Awburn MA & Aggarwal BB. In vivo induction of nitrite and nitrate by tumor necrosis factor, lymphotoxin and interleukin-1: possible role in malaria. *Infect Immun* 1992; 60:3725–3730.

85 Looareesuwan S, Ho M, Wattagagoon Y et al. Dynamic alterations in splenic function in falciparum malaria. *N Engl J Med* 1987; 317:675–679.

86 Lee SH, Looareesuwan S, Wattanagoon Y et al. Antibody dependent red cell removal during *P. falciparum* malaria: the clearance of red cells sensitised with IgG anti-D. *Br J Haematol* 1989; 73:396–402.

87 Ho M, White NJ, Looareesuwan S et al. Splenic Fc receptor function in host defence and anaemia in acute falciparum malaria. *J Infect Dis* 1990; 161:555–561.

88 Lee MV, Ambrus JL, De Souza JM & Lee RV. Diminished red blood cell deformability in uncomplicated human malaria. A preliminary report. *J Med* 1982; 13:479–485.

89 Marsh K & Howard R. Antigens induced on erythrocytes by *P. falciparum*. Expression of diverse and conserved determinants. *Science* 1986; 231:150–153.

90 Craig A & Scherf A. Molecules on the surface of the *Plasmodium falciparum* infected erythrocyte and their role in malaria pathogenesis and immune evasion. *Mol Biochem Parasitol* 2001; 115:129–143.

91 Good MF & Doolan DL. Immune effector mechanisms in malaria. *Curr Opin Immunol* 1999; 11:412–419.

92 Webster HK, Brown AE, Chuenchitra C et al. Characterisation of antibodies to sporozoites in *Plasmodium falciparum* malaria and correlation with protection. *J Clin Microbiol* 1988; 26:923–927.

93 Worku S, Bjorkman A, Troye-Blomberg M, Jemaneh L, Farnert A & Christensson B. Lymphocyte activation and subset redistribution in the peripheral blood in acute malaria illness: distinct gammadelta+ T cell patterns in *Plasmodium falciparum* and *P. vivax* infections. *Clin Exp Immunol* 1997; 108:34–41.

94 Cohen S, McGregor IA & Carrington S. Gamma-globulin and acquired immunity to human malaria. *Nature* 1961; 192:735–737.

95 McGregor IA, Carrington S & Cohen S. Treatment of East African *P. falciparum* malaria with West African human gamma-globulin. *Trans R Soc Trop Med Hyg* 1963; 50:170–175.

96 Sabcharoen A, Burnouf T, Ouattara D et al. Parasitologic and clinical response to immunoglobulin administration in falciparum malaria. *Am J Trop Med Hyg* 1991; 45:297–308.

97 Taliaferro WH & Mulligan MW. The histopathology of malaria with special reference to the function and origin of the macrophages in defence. *Indian Med Res Mem* 1937; 29:1–138.

98 Kwiatkowski D, Cannon J, Manogue K et al. Tumour necrosis factor production in falciparum malaria and in association with schizont rupture. *Clin Exp Immunol* 1989; 77:361–366.

99 Clark IA, Virelizier J-L, Carswell EA & Wood PR. Possible importance of macrophage-derived mediators in acute malaria. *Infect Immun* 1981; 32:1058–1066.

100 Bate CAW, Taverne J & Playfair JHL. Malaria parasites induce TNF production by macrophages. *Immunology* 1988; 64:227–231.

101 Bate CAW, Taverne J & Playfair JHL. Soluble malarial antigens are toxic and induce the production of tumour necrosis factor in vivo. *Immunology* 1989; 66:600–605.

102 Bate CAW, Taverne J, Dave A & Playfair JH. Malaria exoantigens induce T-independent antibody that blocks their ability to induce TNF. *Immunology* 1990; 70:315–320.

103 Schofield L & Hackett F. Signal transduction in host cells by a glycosylphosphatidylinositol toxin of malaria parasites. *J Exp Med* 1993; 177:145–153.

104 Kern P, Hemmer CJ, Van Damme J et al. Elevated tumor necrosis factor alpha and interleukin 6 serum levels as markers for complicated *Plasmodium falciparum* malaria. *Am J Med* 1989; 87:139–143.

105 Grau GE, Taylor TE, Molyneux ME et al. Tumor necrosis factor and disease severity in children with falciparum malaria. *N Engl J Med* 1989; 320:1586–1591.

106 Kwiatkowski D, Hill AVS, Sambou I et al. TNF concentrations in fatal cerebral, non-fatal cerebral, and uncomplicated *Plasmodium falciparum* malaria. *Lancet* 1990; 336:1201–1204.

107 Ho M, Schollaardt T, Snape S, Looareesuwan S, Suntharasamai P White NJ. Endogenous IL-10 modulates proinflammatory response in *Plasmodium falciparum* malaria. *J Infect Dis* 1998; 178:520–525.

108 Karunaweera ND, Grau GE, Gamage P et al. Dynamics of fever and serum levels of tumour necrosis factor are closely associated during clinical paroxysms in *Plasmodium vivax* malaria. *Proc Natl Acad Sci USA* 1992; 89:3200–3203.

109 Grau GE, Piguet PF, Vassalli P & Lambert PH. Tumour necrosis factor and other cytokines in cerebral malaria: experimental and clinical data. *Immunol Rev* 1989; 112:49–70.

110 Perkins DJ, Weinberg JB, Kremsner PG. Reduced interleukin-12 and transforming growth factor-beta1 in severe childhood malaria: relationship of cytokine balance with disease severity. *J Infect Dis* 2000; 182:988–992.

111 Day NPJ, Hien TT, Schollaardt, et al. The prognostic and pathophysiological role of pro- and anti-inflammatory cytokines in severe malaria. *J Infect Dis* 1999; 180:1288–1297.

112 Luty AJ, Perkins DJ, Lell B, et al. Low interleukin-12 activity in severe *Plasmodium falciparum* malaria. *Infect Immun* 2000; 68:3909–3915.

113 Clark IA & Chaudhri G. Tumour necrosis factor may contribute to the anaemia of malaria by causing dyserythropoiesis and erythrophagocytosis. *Br J Haematol* 1988; 70:99–103.

114 Malhotra K, Salmon D, Le Bras J & Vilde JL. Susceptibility of *Plasmodium falciparum* to a peroxidase-mediated oxygen-dependent microbicidal system. *Infect Immun* 1988; 56:3305–3309.

115 Raventos-Suarez C, Kaul D K, Maculuso F & Nagel R L. Membrane knobs are required for the microcirculatory obstruction induced by *Plasmodium falciparum*-infected erythrocytes. *Proc Natl Acad Sci USA* 1985; 82:3829–3833.

116 White N J & Ho M. The pathophysiology of malaria. *Adv Parasitol* 1992; 31:34–173.

117 MacPherson GG, Warrell MJ, White NJ et al. Human cerebral malaria: a quantitative ultrastructural analysis of parasitized erythrocyte sequestration. *Am J Pathol* 1985; 119:385–401.

118 Silamut K, Phu NH, Whitty C, et al. A quantitative analysis of the microvascular sequestration of malaria parasites in the human brain. *Am J Path* 1999; 155:395–410.

119 Pouvelle B, Buffet PA, Lepolard C, Scherf A & Gysin J.Cytoadhesion of *Plasmodium falciparum* ring-stage-infected erythrocytes. *Nat Med* 2000; 6:1264–1268

120 Magowan C, Wollish W, Anderson L & Leech J. Cytoadherence by *Plasmodium falciparum*-infected erythrocytes is correlated with the expression of a family of variable proteins on infected erythrocytes. *J Exp Med* 1988; 168:1307–1320.

121 Howard RJ & Gilladoga AD. Molecular studies related to the pathogenesis of cerebral malaria. *Blood* 1989; 74:2603–2618.

122 Su XZ, Heatwole VM, Wertheimer SP, et al. The large diverse gene family var encodes proteins involved in cytoadherence and antigenic variation of *Plasmodium falciparum*-infected erythrocytes. Cell. 1995; 82:89–100.

123 Treutiger CJ, Carlson J, Scholander C & Wahlgren M. The time course of cytoadhesion, immunoglobulin binding, rosette formation, and serum-induced agglutination of *Plasmodium falciparum*-infected erythrocytes. *Am J Trop Med Hyg* 1998; 59:202–7.124.

124 Magowan C, Nunomura W, Waller KL, et al. *Plasmodium falciparum* histidine-rich protein 1 associates with the band 3 binding domain of ankyrin in the infected red cell membrane. *Biochim Biophys Acta* 2000; 1502:461–470.

125 Roberts DJ, Craig AG, Berendt AR, Pinches R, Nash G, Marsh K & Newbold CI. Rapid switching to multiple antigenic and adhesive phenotypes in malaria. *Nature* 1992; 357:689–692.

126 Kyes SA, Rowe JA, Kriek N & Newbold CI. Rifins: a second family of clonally variant proteins expressed on the surface of red cells infected with *Plasmodium falciparum*. *Proc Natl Acad Sci USA* 1999; 96:9333–9338.

127 Ockenhouse CF, Klotz FW, Tandon NN & Jamieson GA. Sequestrin, a CD36 recognition protein on *Plasmodium falciparum* malaria-infected erythrocytes identified by anti-idiotype antibodies. *Proc Natl Acad Sci USA* 1991; 88:3175–3179.

128 Sherman IW, Crandall I & Smith H. Membrane proteins involved in the adherence of *Plasmodium falciparum* infected erythrocytes to the endothelium. *Biol Cell* 1992; 74:161–178.

129 David PH, Hommel M, Miller LH et al. Parasite sequestration in *Plasmodium falciparum* malaria: spleen and antibody modulation of cytoadherence of infected erythrocytes. *Proc Natl Acad Sci USA* 1983; 80:5075–5079.

130 Israeli A, Shapiro M & Ephros MA. *Plasmodium falciparum* malaria in an asplenic man. *Trans R Soc Trop Med Hyg* 1987; 81:233–234.

131 Barnwell JW, Asch AS, Nachman RL et al. A human 88-kD membrane glycoprotein (CD36) functions in vitro as a receptor for a cytoadherence ligand on *Plasmodium falciparum* infected erythrocytes. *J Clin Invest* 1989; 84:765–772.

132 Ockenhouse CF, Ho M, Tandon NN et al. Molecular basis of sequestration in severe and uncomplicated *Plasmodium falciparum* malaria. Differential adhesion of infected erythrocytes to CD36 and CD54 (ICAM-1). *J Infect Dis* 1991; 164:163–169.

133 Marsh K, Marsh VM, Brown J et al. *Plasmodium falciparum*: the behavior of clinical isolates in an in vitro model of infected red blood cell sequestration. *Exp Parasitol* 1988; 65:202–208.

134 Crandall I, Smith H & Sherman IW. *Plasmodium falciparum*: the effect of pH and Ca2+ concentration on the in-vitro cytoadherence of infected erythrocytes to amelanotic melanoma cells. *Exp Parasitol* 1991; 73:362–368.

135 Turner GDH, Morrison H, Jones M, et al. An immunohistochemical study of the pathology of fatal malaria: Evidence for widespread endothelial activation and a potential role for intercellular adhesion molecule-1 in cerebral sequestration. *Am J Pathol* 1994; 145:1057–1069.

136 Berendt AR, Simmons DL, Tansey J et al. Intercellular adhesion molecule-1 is an endothelial cell adhesion receptor for *Plasmodium falciparum*. *Nature* 1989; 341:57–59.

137 Wick TM & Louis V. Cytoadherence of *Plasmodium falciparum* infected erythrocytes to human umbilical vein and human dermal microvascular endothelial cells under shear conditions. *Am J Trop Med Hyg* 1991; 42:578–586.

138 Nash GB, Cooke BM, Marsh K et al. Rheological analysis of the adhesive interactions of red blood cells parasitised by *Plasmodium falciparum*. *Blood* 1992; 79:798–807.

139 McCormick CJ, Craig A, Roberts D, Newbold CI & Berendt AR. Intercellular adhesion molecule-1 and CD36 synergize to mediate adherence of *Plasmodium falciparum*-infected erythrocytes to cultured human microvascular endothelial cells. *J Clin Invest* 1997; 100:2521–2529.

140 Yipp BG, Anand S, Schollaardt T, Patel KD, Looareesuwan S & Ho M. Synergism of multiple adhesion molecules in mediating cytoadherence of *Plasmodium falciparum*-infected erythrocytes to microvascular endothelial cells under flow. *Blood* 2000; 96:2292–2298

141 Fried M & Duffy PE. Adherence of *Plasmodium falciparum* to chondroitin sulfate A in the human placenta. *Science* 1996; 272:1502–1504.

142 Reeder JC, Cowman AF, Davern KM, Beeson JG, Thompson JK, Rogerson SJ, Brown GV. The adhesion of *Plasmodium falciparum*-infected erythrocytes to chondroitin sulfate A is mediated by *P. falciparum* erythrocyte membrane protein 1. *Proc Natl Acad Sci USA* 1999; 96:5198–5202.

143 Fried M, Nosten F, Brockman A, Brabin BJ & Duffy PE. Maternal antibodies block malaria. *Nature* 1998; 395:851–852.

144 Ho M & White NJ. Molecular mechanisms of cytoadherence in malaria. *Am J Physiol* 1999; 276:C1231–C1242.

145 David PH, Handunnetti SM, Leech JH et al. Rosetting: a new cytoadherence property of malaria-infected erythrocytes. *Am J Trop Med Hyg* 1988; 38:289–297.

146 Handunnetti SM, David PH, Perera KLRL & Mendis KN. Uninfected erythrocytes form 'rosettes' around *Plasmodium falciparum* infected erythrocytes. *Am J Trop Med Hyg* 1989; 40:115–118.

147 Udomsangpetch R, Wahlin B, Carlson J et al. *Plasmodium falciparum*-infected erythrocytes form spontaneous erythrocyte rosettes. *J Exp Med* 1989; 169:1835–1840.

148 Angus BJ, Thanikkul K, Silamut K, White NJ & Udomsangpetch R. Rosette formation in *Plasmodium ovale* infection. *Am J Trop Med Hyg* 1996; 55:560– 561

149 Udomsangpetch R, Thanikkul K, Pukrittayakamee S & White NJ. Rosette formation by *Plasmodium vivax*. *Trans R Soc Trop Med Hyg* 1995; 89:635–637.

150 Kaul DK, Roth EF, Nagel RL et al. Rosetting of *Plasmodium falciparum* infected red blood cells with uninfected red blood cells enhances microvascular obstruction under flow conditions. *Blood* 1991; 78:812–819.

151 Carlson J, Helmby H, Hill AVS et al. Human cerebral malaria: association with erythrocyte rosetting and lack of anti-rosetting antibodies. *Lancet* 1990; 336:1457–1460.

152 Ho M, Davis TME, Silamut K et al. Rosette formation of *P. falciparum* infected erythrocytes from patients with acute malaria. *Infect Immun* 1991; 59:2135–2139.

153 Rowe A, Obeiro J, Newbold CI & Marsh K. *Plasmodium falciparum* rosetting is associated with malaria severity in Kenya. *Infect Immun* 1995; 63:2323–2326.

154 al-Yaman F, Genton B, Mokela D, et al. Human cerebral malaria: lack of significant association between erythrocyte rosetting and disease severity. *Trans R Soc Trop Med Hyg* 1995; 89:55–8.

155 Nash GB, O'Brien E, Gordon-Smith EC & Dormandy JA. Abnormalities in the mechanical properties of red blood cells caused by *Plasmodium falciparum*. *Blood* 1989; 74: 855–861.

156 Dondorp AM, Kager PA, Vreeken J & White NJ. Abnormal blood flow and red blood cell deformability in severe malaria. *Parasitol Today*, 2000; 16:228–232.

157 Pain A, Ferguson DJ, Kai O, Urban BC, Lowe B, Marsh K & Roberts DJ. Platelet-mediated clumping of *Plasmodium falciparum*-infected erythrocytes is a common adhesive phenotype and is associated with severe malaria. *Proc Natl Acad Sci USA* 2001; 98:1805–1810.

158 Dondorp AM, Angus BJ, Hardeman MR, et al. Prognostic significance of reduced red cell deformability in severe falciparum malaria. *Am J Trop Med Hyg* 1997; 57:507–511.

159 Dondorp AM, Angus BJ, Chotivanich K, et al. Red cell deformability as a predictor of anemia in severe falciparum malaria. *Am J Trop Med Hyg* 1999; 60:733–737.

160 Bhamarapravati N, Boonpucknavig S, Boonpucknavig V & Yaemboonruang C. Glomerular changes in acute *Plasmodium falciparum* infection. *Arch Pathol* 1973; 96:298–293.

161 Adam C, Geniteau M, Gougerot-Pocidalo M et al. Cryoglobulins, circulating immune complexes and complement activation in cerebral malaria. *Infect Immun* 1981; 31:530–535.

162 Neva FA, Howard WA, Glew RH et al. Relationship of serum complement levels to events of the malarial paroxysm. *J Clin Invest* 1974; 54:451–460.

163 Petchclai B, Chutanondh R, Hiranras S & Benjapongs W. Activation of classical and alternate complement pathways in acute falciparum malaria. *J Med Assoc Thai* 1977; 60:174–176.

164 Phanuphak P, Hanvanich M, Sakultamrung R et al. Complement changes in falciparum malaria infection. *Clin Exp Immunol* 1985; 59:571–576.

165 Ho M, Webster H K, Looareesuwan S et al. Antigen-specific immuno-suppressiom in human malaria due to *Plasmodium*

falciparum. J Infect Dis 1986; 153:763–771.

166 Ho M, Webster HK, Green B et al. Defective production of and response to interleukin 2 in acute falciparum malaria. *J Immunol* 1988; 141:2755–2759.

167 Riley EM, MacLennan C, Kwiatkowski DK & Greenwood BM. Suppression of in-vitro lymphoproliferative responses in acute malaria patients can be partially reversed by indomethacin. *Parasite Immunol* 1989; 11:509–517.

168 Ho M, Webster HK, Tongtawe P et al. Increased gamma/delta T cells in acute falciparum malaria. *Immunol Lett* 1990; 25:139–142.

169 Ho M & Webster HK. T cell responses in acute falciparum malaria. *Immunol Lett* 1990; 25:135–138.

170 Hogh B. Clinical and parasitological studies on immunity to *Plasmodium falciparum* malaria in children. *Scand J Infect Dis Suppl* 1996; 102:1–53.

171 Bouharoun-Tayoun H & Druilhe P. *Plasmodium falciparum* malaria: evidence for an isotype imbalance which may be responsible for delayed acquisition of protective immunity. *J Clin Microbiol* 1992; 60:1473–1481.

172 Brasseur P, Agrapart M, Ballett JJ et al. Impaired cell mediated immunity in *Plasmodium falciparum* infected patients with high parasitaemia and cerebral malaria. *Clin Immunol Immunopathol* 1983; 27:38–50.

173 Druilhe P, Brasseur P, Agrapart M et al. T-cell responsiveness in severe *Plasmodium falciparum* malaria. *Trans R Soc Trop Med Hyg* 1983; 77:671–672.

174 Ward KN, Warrell MJ, Rhodes J et al. Altered expression of human monocyte Fc receptor in *Plasmodium falciparum* malaria. *Infect Immun* 1984; 44:623–626.

175 Allison AC, Houba V, Hendrickse RG et al. Immune complexes in the nephrotic syndrome of African children. *Lancet* 1969; ii:1232–1237.

176 Davis TME, Suputtamongkol Y, Spencer JL et al. Measures of capillary permeability in acute falciparum malaria: relation to severity of infection and treatment. *Clin Infect Dis* 1992; 256–266.

177 Maegraith BG & Fletcher A. The pathogenesis of mammalian malaria. *Adv Parasitol* 1972; 10:49–75.

178 Migasena P & Areekul S. Capillary permeability function in malaria. *Ann Trop Med Parasitol* 1987; 81:549–560.

179 Looareesuwan S, Warrell DA, White NJ et al. Do patients with cerebral malaria have cerebral oedema? A computed tomography study. *Lancet* 1983; i:434–437.

180 Looareesuwan S, Wilairatana P, Krishna S, Kendall B, Vannaphon S, Viravan C & White NJ. Magnetic resonance imaging of the brain in cerebral malaria. *Clin Infect Dis* 1995; 21:300–309.

181 Newton CR, Peshu N, Kendall B, et al. Brain swelling and ischaemia in Kenyans with cerebral malaria. *Arch Dis Child* 1994; 70:281–287.

182 Newton CRJC, Kirkham F , Winstanley PA et al. Intracranial pressure in African children with cerebral malaria. *Lancet* 1991; 337:573–576.

183 Waller D, Crawley J, Nosten F et al. Intracranial pressure in childhood cerebral malaria. *Trans R Soc Trop Med Hyg* 1991; 85:362–364.

184 White NJ. Lumbar puncture in cerebral malaria. *Lancet* 1991; 338:640–641.

185 Warrell DA, Looareesuwan S, Phillips RE et al. Function of the blood-cerebrospinal fluid barrier in human cerebral malaria: rejection of the permeability hypothesis. *Am J Trop Med Hyg* 1986; 35:882–889.

186 Badibanga B, Dayal R, Depierreux M et al. Etude des principaux facteurs immunologiques et de la barriere hemato-meningee au cours de la malaria cerebrale chez l'enfant en pays d'endemie (Zaire). *Ann Soc Belg Med Trop* 1986; 66:23–27.

187 Brown HC, Chau TT, Mai NT, et al. Blood-brain barrier function in cerebral malaria and CNS infections in Vietnam. *Neurology* 2000; 55:104–111.

188 Brown H, Rogerson S, Taylor T, Tembo M, Mwenechanya J, Molyneux M & Turner G. Blood-brain barrier function in cerebral malaria in Malawian children. *Am J Trop Med Hyg* 2001; 64:207–213.

189 Newton CR, Hien TT, White NJ. Cerebral malaria. *J Neurol Neurosurg Psychiatry* 2000; 69:433–441.

190 Warrell DA, White NJ, Veall N et al. Cerebral anaerobic glycolysis and reduced cerebral oxygen transport in human cerebral malaria. *Lancet* 1988; ii:534–538.

191 White NJ, Warrell DA, Looareesuwan S et al. Pathophysiological and prognostic significance of cerebrospinal-fluid lactate in cerebral malaria. *Lancet* 1985; i:776–778.

192 Maneerat Y, Viriyavejakul P, Punpoowong B, et al. Inducible nitric oxide synthase expression is increased in the brain in fatal cerebral malaria. *Histopathology* 2000; 37:269–277.

193 Arthachinta S, Sitprija V & Kashemsant U. Selective renal angiography in renal failure due to infection. *Aust J Radiol* 1974; 18:446–452.

194 Trang TTM, Phu NH, Vinh H et al. Acute renal failure in severe falciparum malaria. *Clin Infect Dis* 1992; 15:74–880.

195 Day NP, Phu NH, Mai NT, et al. Effects of dopamine and epinephrine infusions on renal hemodynamics in severe malaria and severe sepsis. *Crit Care Med* 2000; 28:1353–1362.

196 Boonpucknavig V & Sitprija V. Renal disease in acute *Plasmodium falciparum* infection in man. *Kidney Int* 1979; 16:44–52.

197 Hartenblower DL, Kantor GL & Rosen VJ. Renal failure due to acute glomerulonephritis during falciparum malaria. Case report. *Milit Med* 1972; 137:74–76.

198 Barratt JOW & Yorke W. An investigation into the mechanism of production of blackwater. *Ann Trop Med Parasitol* 1909–1910; 3:1–256.

199 Maegraith BG. *Pathological Processes in Malaria and Blackwater Fever.* Oxford: Blackwell, 1948:348–349.

200 James MFM. Pulmonary damage associated with falciparum malaria: a report of ten cases. *Ann Trop Med Parasitol* 1985; 79:123–138.

201 Charoenpan P, Indraprasit S, Kiatboonsri S et al. Pulmonary edema in severe falciparum malaria. Hemodynamic study and clinicophysiologic correlation. *Chest* 1990; 9:1190–1197.

202 Day NP, Phu NH, Bethell DP, Mai NT, Chau TT, Hien TT & White NJ. The effects of dopamine and adrenaline infusions on acid-base balance and systemic haemodynamics in severe infection. *Lancet.* 1996; 348:219–223.

203 Brooks MH, Malloy JP, Bartelloni PJ et al. Pathophysiology of acute falciparum malaria. Correlation of clinical and biochemical abnormalities. *Am J Med* 1967; 43:735–744.

204 Chongsuphajaisiddhi T, Kasemuth R, Tajavanija S & Harinasuta T. Changes in blood volume in falciparum malaria. *Southeast Asian J Trop Med Public Health* 1971; 2:344–350.

205 Malloy JP, Brooks MH, Barry KG et al. Pathophysiology of acute falciparum malaria. II. Fluid compartmentalization. *Am J Med* 1967; 43:745–750.

206 Sowunmi A, Newton CR, Waruiru C, Lightman S & Dunger DB. Arginine vasopressin secretion in Kenyan children with severe malaria. *J Trop Pediatr* 2000; 46:195–199.

207 Zuckerman A. Recent studies on factors involved in malarial anaemia. *Milit Med* 1966; 131(supplement):1201–1216.

208 Perrin LH, Mackey LJ & Miecher PA. The hematology of malaria in man. *Semin Hematol* 1982; 19:70–82.

209 Abdallah S, Weatherall DJ, Wickramasinghe SN & Hughes M. The anaemia of *P. falciparum* malaria. *Br J Haematol* 1980; 46:171–183.

210 Looareesuwan S, Davis TME, Pukrittayakamee S et al. Erythrocyte survival in severe falciparum malaria. *Acta Trop* 1991; 48:263–270.

211 Davis TME, Krishna S, Looareesuwan S et al. Erythrocyte sequestration and anaemia in severe falciparum malaria. Analysis of acute changes in venous haematocrit using a simple mathematical model. *J Clin Invest* 1990; 865:793–800.

212 Looareesuwan S, Merry AH, Phillips RE et al. Reduced erythrocyte survival following clearance of malarial parasitaemia in Thai patients. *Br J Haematol* 1987; 67:473–478.

213 Price RN, Simpson J, Nosten F, et al. Factors contributing to anemia in uncomplicated falciparum malaria. *Am J Trop Med Hyg*, 2001; 65:614–622.

214 Phillips RE, Looareesuwan S, Warrell D A et al. The importance of anaemia in cerebral and uncomplicated falciparum malaria: role of complications, dyserythropoiesis and iron sequestration. *Q J Med* 1986; 58:305–323.

215 Knuttgen HJ. The bone marrow of non-immune Europeans in acute malaria infection: a topical review. *Ann Trop Med Parasitol* 1987; 81:567–576.

216 Vedovato M, De Paoli Vitali E, Dapporto M & Salvatorelli G. Defective erythropoietin production in the anaemia of malaria. *Nephrol Dial Transplant* 1999; 14:1043–1044.

217 Burgmann H, Looareesuwan S, Kapiotis S, et al. Serum levels of erythropoietin in acute *Plasmodium falciparum* malaria. *Am J Trop Med Hyg* 1996; 54:280–283.

218 Burchard GD, Radloff P, Philipps J, Nkeyi M, Knobloch J & Kremsner PG. Increased erythropoietin production in children with severe malarial anemia. *Am J Trop Med Hyg* 1995; 53:547–551.

219 Griffiths MJ, Ndungu F, Baird KL, Muller DP, Marsh K & Newton CR. Oxidative stress and erythrocyte damage in Kenyan children with severe *Plasmodium falciparum* malaria. *Br J Haematol* 2001; 113:486–491.

220 Joshi P, Alam A, Chandra R et al. Possible basis for membrane changes in non parasitised erythrocytes of malaria infected animals. *Biochim Biophys Acta* 1986; 862:220–222.

221 Facer CA, Bray RS & Brown J. Direct Coombs' antiglobulin reactions in Gambian children with *Plasmodium falciparum* malaria. I. Incidence and class specificity. *Clin Exp Immunol* 1979; 35:119–127.

222 Facer CA. Direct Coombs' antiglobulin reactions in Gambian children with *Plasmodium falciparum* malaria. II. Specificity of erythrocyte bound IgG. *Clin Exp Immunol* 1980; 39:279–288.

223 Merry AH, Looareesuwan S, Phillips RE et al. Evidence against immune haemolysis in falciparum malaria in Thailand. *Br J Haematol* 1986; 64:187–194.

224 Charoenlarp P, Vanijanonta S & Chat-Panyaporn P. The effect of prednisolone on red cell survival in patients with falciparum malaria. *SE Asian J Trop Med Public Health* 1979; 10:127–131.

225 Jaroonvesama N. Intravascular coagulation in falciparum malaria. *Lancet* 1972; i:221–223.

226 Horstmann RD & Dietrich M. Haemostatic alterations in malaria correlate with parasitaemia. *Blut* 1975; 51:329–333.

227 Sucharit P, Chongsuphajaisiddhi T, Harinasuta T et al. Studies on coagulation and fibrinolysis in cases of falciparum malaria. *SE Asian J Trop Med Public Health* 1975; 6:33–39.

228 Pukrittayakamee S, White NJ, Clemens R et al. Activation of the coagulation cascade in falciparum malaria. *Trans R Soc Trop Med Hyg* 1989; 83:762–766.

229 Holst FG, Hemmer CJ, Foth C, Seitz R, Egbring R & Dietrich M. Low levels of fibrin-stabilizing factor (factor XIII) in human *Plasmodium falciparum* malaria: correlation with clinical severity. *Am J Trop Med Hyg* 1999; 60:99–104.

230 Clemens R, Pramoolsinsap C, Lorenz R, Pukrittayakamee S, Bock HL & White NJ. Activation of the coagulation cascade in severe falciparum malaria through the intrinsic pathway.

Brit J Haematol 1994:87; 100–105.

231 Skudowitz RB, Katz J, Lurie A et al. Mechanisms of thrombocytopenia in malignant tertian malaria. *Brit Med J* 1973; ii:515–518.

232 Lee SH, Looareesuwan S, Chan J, Wilairatana P, Vanijanonta S, Chong SM & Chong BH. Plasma macrophage colony-stimulating factor and P-selectin levels in malaria-associated thrombocytopenia. *Thromb Haemost* 1997; 77:289–293.

233 Essien E. The circulating platelet in acute malaria infection. *Br J Haematol* 1989; 72:589–590.

234 Kelton JG, Keystone J, Moore J et al. Immune-mediated thrombocytopenia of malaria. *J Clin Invest* 1983; 71:8323–836.

235 Looareesuwan S, Davis JG, Allen DL et al. Thrombocytopenia in malaria. *SE Asian J Trop Med Public Health* 1992; 23:44–50.

236 Supanaranond W, Davis TME, Dawes J et al. In-vivo platelet activation and anomalous thrombospondin levels in severe falciparum malaria. *Platelets* 1992; 3:195–200.

237 Udeinya IJ & Miller LH. Plasmodium falciparum: effect of infected erythrocytes on clotting time of plasma. *Am J Trop Med Hyg* 1987; 37:246–249.

238 Ohnishi K. Serum levels of thrombomodulin, intercellular adhesion molecule-1, vascular cell adhesion molecule-1, and E-selectin in the acute phase of *Plasmodium vivax* malaria. *Am J Trop Med Hyg*. 1999; 60:248–250.

239 Boehme MW, Werle E, Kommerell B, Raeth U. Serum levels of adhesion molecules and thrombomodulin as indicators of vascular injury in severe *Plasmodium falciparum* malaria. *Clin Investig* 1994; 72:598–603.

240 Punyagupta S, Srichaikul T, Nitiyanant P & Petchclai B. Acute pulmonary insufficiency in falciparum malaria: summary of 12 cases with evidence of disseminated intravascular coagulation. *Am J Trop Med Hyg* 1974; 23:551–559.

241 Reid HA & Nkrumah FK. Fibrin-degradation products in cerebral malaria. *Lancet* 1972; i:218–221.

242 Borochovitz D, Crosley A & Metz J. Intravascular coagulation with fatal haemorrhage in cerebral malaria. *Brit Med J* 1970; ii:710.

243 World Health Organization, Control of Tropical Diseases. Severe and complicated malaria. 2nd ed. *Trans R Soc Trop Med Hyg* 1990; 84 (Suppl 2): 1–65.

244 Chau TTH, Day NPJ, Chuong LV, et al. Blackwater fever in Southern Viet Nam: a prospective descriptive study of 50 cases. *Clin Infect Dis* 1996; 23:1274–1281.

245 Angus B, Chotivanich K, Udomsangpetch R, White NJ. In vivo removal of malaria parasites from red cells without their destruction in acute falciparum malaria. *Blood* 1997; 90:2037–2040.

246 Newton P, Chotivanich K, Chierakul W, et al. A comparison of the in vivo kinetics of *Plasmodium falciparum* ring-infected erythrocyte surface antigen (RESA) positive and negative erythrocytes. *Blood* 2001; 98:450–457.

247 Chotivanich K, Udomsangpetch R, Dondorp A, et al. The mechanisms of parasite clearance after antimalarial treatment of *Plasmodium falciparum* malaria. *J Infect Dis* 2000; 182:629–633.

248 Karney WW & Tong MJ. Malabsorption in *Plasmodium falciparum* malaria. *Am J Trop Med Hyg* 1972; 21:1–5.

249 Olsson RA & Johnston EH. Histopathologic changes and small bowel absorption in falciparum malaria. *Am J Trop Med Hyg* 1969; 18:355–359.

250 Segal HE, Hall AP, Jewell JS et al. Gastrointestinal function, quinine absorption and parasite response in falciparum malaria. *SE Asian J Trop Med Public Health* 1974; 5:499–503.

251 Molyneux M E, Looareesuwan S. Menzies I S et al. Reduced hepatic blood flow and intestinal malabsorption in severe falciparum malaria. *Am J Trop Med Hyg* 1989; 40:470–476.

252 Pukrittayakamee S, White NJ, Davis TME et al. Hepatic blood

flow and metabolism in severe malaria: the clearance of intravenously administered galactose. *Clin Sci* 1992; 82:63–70.

253 Pukrittayakamee S, White NJ, Davis TME, Supanaranond W, Crawley J, Nagachinta B & Williamson DH. Glycerol metabolism in severe falciparum malaria. *Metabolism* 1994; 43:887–892.

254 Day NP, Phu NH, Mai NT, et al. The pathophysiologic and prognostic significance of acidosis in severe adult malaria. *Crit Care Med* 2000; 28:1833–1840.

255 Pukrittayakamee S, Looareesuwan S, Keeratithakul D, et al. A study of the factors affecting the metabolic clearance of quinine in malaria. *Eur J Clin Pharmacol* 1997; 52:487–493.

256 Taylor TE, Borgstein A & Molyneux ME. Acid-base status in paediatric *Plasmodium falciparum* malaria. *Q J Med* 1993; 86:99–109.

257 Krishna S, Waller DW, ter Kuile F, et al. Lactic acidosis and hypoglycaemia in children with severe malaria. *Trans R Soc Trop Med Hyg* 1994; 88:67–73.

258 English M, Sauerwein R, Waruiru C, Mosobo M, Obiero J, Lowe B & Marsh K. Acidosis in severe childhood malaria. *Q J Med* 1997; 90:263–270.

259 English M, Muambi B, Mithwani S & Marsh K. Lactic acidosis and oxygen debt in African children with severe anaemia. *Q J Med* 1997; 90:563–569.

260 Jensen MD, Conley M & Helstowski LD. Culture of *Plasmodium falciparum*: the role of pH glucose and lactate. *J Parasitol* 1983; 69:1060–1067.

261 Pfaller MA, Parquette AR, Krogstad DJ & Nguyen-Dinh P. *Plasmodium falciparum*: stage-specific lactate production in synchronized cultures. *Exp Parasitol* 1982; 54:391–396.

262 Vander Jagt D, Hunsaker LA, Campos N M & Baack B R. D-lactate production in erythrocytes infected with *Plasmodium falciparum*. *Mol Biochem Parasitol* 1990; 42:277–284.

263 Davis TME, Benn JJ, Suputtamongkol Y, Weinberg J, Umpleby AM, Chierakul N & White NJ. Lactate turnover and forearm lactate metabolism in severe falciparum malaria. *Endocrinol Metabol* 1996; 3:105–115.

264 Agbenyega T, Angus BJ, Bedu-Addo G, Baffoe-Bonnie B, Guyton T, Stacpoole PW & Krishna S. Glucose and lactate kinetics in children with severe malaria. *J Clin Endocrinol Metab* 2000; 85:1569–1576.

265 White NJ, Warrell DA, Chanthavanich P et al. Severe hypoglycaemia and hyperinsulinaemia in falciparum malaria. *N Engl J Med* 1983; 309:61–66.

266 White NJ, Miller KD, Marsh K et al. Hypoglycaemia in African children with severe malaria. *Lancet* 1987; i:708–711.

267 Taylor TE, Molyneux ME, Wirima JJ et al. Blood glucose levels in Malawian children before and during the administration of intravenous quinine in severe falciparum malaria. *N Engl J Med* 1988; 319:1040–1047.

268 English M, Wale S, Binns G, Mwangi I, Sauerwein H, Marsh K. Hypoglycaemia on and after admission in Kenyan children with severe malaria. *Q J Med* 1998; 91:191–197.

269 Onongbu IC & Onyeneke EC. Plasma lipid changes in human malaria. *Tropenmed Parasitol* 1983; 34:193–196.

270 Davis TME, Supanaranond W, Pukrittayakamee S et al. The pituitary-thyroid axis in severe falciparum malaria. *Trans R Soc Trop Med Hyg* 1990; 84:330–335.

271 Davis TME, Pukrittayakamee S, Woodhead JS et al. Calcium and phosphate metabolism in acute falciparum malaria. *Clin Sci* 1991; 81:297–304.

272 Petithory JC, Lebeau G, Galeazzi G & Chauty A. L'hypocalcemie palustre. Etudes des correlations avec d'autres parametres. *Bull Soc Pathol Exot Filiales* 1983; 76: 455–462.

273 Brooks MH, Barry KG, Cirksen WJ et al. Pituitary-adrenal function in acute falciparum malaria. *AM J Trop Med Hyg* 1969; 18:872–877.

274 Davis TME, Looareesuwan S, Pukrittayakamee S et al. Glucose turnover in severe falciparum malaria. *Metabolism* 1993; 42:334–340.

275 Dekker E, Romijn JA, Ekberg K, et al. Glucose production and gluconeogenesis in adults with uncomplicated falciparum malaria. *Am J Physiol* 1997; 272:E1059–1064

276 Dekker E, Romijn JA, Waruiru C, et al. The relationship between glucose production and plasma glucose concentration in children with falciparum malaria. *Trans R Soc Trop Med Hyg* 1996; 90:654–657

277 Okitolonda W, Delacollette C, Malengreau M & Henquin JC. High incidence of hypoglycaemia in African patients treated with intravenous quinine for severe malaria. *Brit Med J* 1987; 295:716–718.

278 Davis TME, Karbwang J, Looareesuwan S et al. Comparative effects of quinine and quinidine on glucose metabolism in normal man. *Br J Clin Pharmacol* 1990; 30:397–403.

279 Davis TME, Pukrittayakamee S, Supanaranond W et al. Glucose metabolism in quinine-treated patients with uncomplicated falciparum malaria. *Clin Endocrinol* (Oxf) 1990; 33:739–749.

280 Riley EM, Schneider G, Sambou I & Greenwood BM. Suppression of cell-mediated immune responses to malaria antigens in pregnant Gambian women. *Am J Trop Med Hyg* 1989; 40:131–144.

281 Archibald HM. The influence of malaria infection of the placenta on the incidence of prematurity. *Bull World Health Organ* 1956; 15:842–845.

282 Jelliffe EFP. Low birth weight and malarial infection of the placenta. *Bull World Health Organ* 1968; 38:69–78.

283 Bray RS & Sinden RE. The sequestration of *Plasmodium falciparum* infected erythrocytes in the placenta. *Trans R Soc Trop Med Hyg* 1979; 73:716–719.

284 Brabin BJ. Analysis of malaria in pregnancy in Africa. *Bull World Health Organ* 1983; 61:1005–1016.

285 McGregor IA, Wilson ME & Billewicz WZ. Malaria infection of the placenta in The Gambia, West Africa: its incidence and relationship to stillbirth, birthweight and placental weight. *Trans R Soc Trop Med Hyg* 1983; 77:232–244.

286 Bray RS & Anderson MJ. Falciparum malaria and pregnancy. *Trans R Soc Trop Med Hyg* 1979; 73:427–431.

287 Nosten F, ter Kuile F, Malankirri L et al. Malaria in pregnancy in an area of unstable endemicity. *Trans R Soc Trop Med Hyg* 1991; 85:424–429.

288 Looareesuwan S, Phillips RE, White NJ et al. Quinine and severe falciparum malaria in late pregnancy. *Lancet* 1985; ii:4–8.

289 Bygbjerg IC & Laang C. Septicaemia as a complication of falciparum malaria. *Trans R Soc Trop Med Hyg* 1982; 76:705.

290 Mabey DCW, Brown A & Greenwood BM. *Plasmodium falciparum* malaria and Salmonella infections in Gambian children. *J Infect Dis* 1987; 155:1319–1321.

291 Berkley J, Mwarumba S, Bramham K, Lowe B & Marsh K. Bacteraemia complicating severe malaria in children. *Trans R Soc Trop Med Hyg* 1999; 93:283–286

292 Marchiafava E & Bignami A. *On Summer-Autumnal Fever*. London: New Sydenham Society, 1894.

293 Dudgeon LS & Clarke C. A contribution to the microscopical histology of malaria. *Lancet* 1917; ii:153–156.

294 Dudgeon LS & Clarke C. An investigation on fatal cases of pernicious malaria caused by *Plasmodium falciparum* in Macedonia. *Q J Med* 1918; 12:372–390.

295 Gaskell JF & Millar WL. Studies on malignant malaria in Macedonia. *Q J Med* 1920; 13:381–426.

296 Kean BH & Smith JA. Death due to aestivo-autumnal malaria. A resume of one hundred autopsy cases 1925–1942. *Am J Trop Med Hyg* 1944; 24:317–322.

297 Edington GM. Pathology of malaria in West Africa. *Brit Med J* 1967; i:715–718.

298 Spitz S. Pathology of acute falciparum malaria. *Milit Med* 1946; 99:555–572.

299 Pongponratn E, Riganti M, Punpoowong B & Aikawa M. Microvascular sequestration of parasitised erythrocytes in human falciparum malaria – a pathological study. *Am J Trop Med Hyg* 1991; 44:168–175.

300 Oo MM, Aikawa M & Than T. Human cerebral malaria: a pathological study. *J Neuropathol Exp Neurol* 1988; 46:223–231.

301 Igarashi I, Oo MM, Stanley H et al. Knob antigen deposition in cerebral malaria. *Am J Trop Med Hyg* 1987; 37:511–515.

302 Boonpucknavig V, Boonpucknavig S, Udomsangpetch R & Nitiyanant P. An immunofluorescent study of cerebral malaria. *Arch Pathol Lab Med* 1990; 114:1028–1034.

303 Duarte MIS, Corbett CEP, Boulos M & Amata Neto V. Ultrastructure of the lung in falciparum malaria. *Am J Trop Med Hyg* 1985; 34:31–35.

304 Feldman RM & Singer V. Non-cardiogenic pulmonary edema and pulmonary fibrosis in falciparum malaria. *Rev Infect Dis* 1987; 9:134–139.

305 Deller JJ, Cifarelli PS, Berque S & Buchanan R. Malaria hepatitis. *Milit Med* 1967; 132:614–620.

306 De Brito T, Barone AA & Earia RM. Human liver biopsy in *P. falciparum* and *P. vivax* malaria. A light and electron microscopy study. *Virchows Arch* 1969; 348:220–229.

307 Corcoran TE, Hegstrom GJ, Zoeckler SJ & Keil PG. Liver structure in non fatal malaria. *Gastroenterology* 1953; 24:53–62.

308 Pongponratn E, Riganti M, Harinasuta T & Bunnag D. Electron microscopic study of phagocytosis in human spleen in falciparum malaria. *SE Asian J Trop Med Public Health* 1989; 20:31–39.

309 Weiss L. The spleen in malaria; the role of barrier cells. *Immunol Lett* 1990; 25:165–172.

310 Wickramasinghe SN, Looareesuwan S, Nagachinta B & White NJ. Dyserythropoiesis and ineffective erythropoiesis in *Plasmodium vivax* malaria. *Br J Haematol* 1989; 72:91–99.

311 Clark HC. The diagnostic value of the placental blood film in aestivo-autumnal malaria. *J Exp Med* 1915; 22:427–444.

312 Walter P, Gavin JF & Blot P. Placental pathologic changes in malaria. *Am J Pathol* 1982; 109:330–342.

313 Philippe E & Walter P. Les lesions placentaires du plaudisme. *Arch Fr Pediatr* 1985; 42(Supplement):921–923.

314 Galbraith RM, Fox, Hsi B et al. The human materno-fetal relationship in malaria. II. Histological, ultrastructural and immunopathological studies of the placenta. *Trans R Soc Trop Med Hyg* 1980; 74:61–72.

315 Smail MR, Ordi J, Menendez C, et al. Placental pathology in malaria: a histological, immunohistochemical, and quantitative study. *Hum Pathol* 2000; 31:85–93.

316 Mattelli A, Caligaris S, Castelli F & Carosi G. The placenta and malaria. *Ann Trop Med Parasitol* 1997; 91:803–810.

317 Shute PG. Malaria. *Brit Med J* 1951; 11:1280.

318 Looareesuwan S, White NJ, Chittamas S et al. High rate of *Plasmodium vivax* relapse following treatment of falciparum malaria in Thailand. *Lancet* 1987; ii:1052–1055.

319 Mason DP & McKenzie FE. Blood-stage dynamics and clinical implications of mixed *Plasmodium vivax-Plasmodium falciparum* infections. *Am J Trop Med Hyg* 1999; 61:367–374.

320 Mayxay M, Pukrittayakamee S, Chotivanich K, Imwong M, Looareesuwan S & White NJ. Identification of cryptic co-infection with *Plasmodium falciparum* in patients presenting with vivax malaria. *Am J Trop Med* 2000; in press.

321 Luxemburger C, Kyaw Ley Thew, White NJ, et al. The epidemiology of malaria in a Karen population on the western border of Thailand. *Trans R Soc Trop Med Hyg* 1996; 90:105–111.

322 May J, Mockenhaupt FP, Ademowo OG, Falusi AG, Olumese PE, Bienzle U & Meyer CG. High rate of mixed and subpatent malarial infections in southwest Nigeria. *Am J Trop Med Hyg* 1999; 61:339–343.

323 Zhou M, Liu Q, Wongsrichanalai C, et al. High prevalence of *Plasmodium malariae* and *Plasmodium ovale* in malaria patients along the Thai-Myanmar border, as revealed by acridine orange staining and PCR-based diagnoses. *Trop Med Int Health* 1998; 3:304–12.

324 Luxemburger C, Ricci F, Nosten F, Raimond D, Saw Bathet White NJ. The epidemiology of severe malaria in an area of low transmission in Thailand. *Trans R Soc Trop Med Hyg* 1997; 91:256–262.

325 Price RN, Nosten F, Luxemburger C, et al. Risk factors for gametocyte carriage in uncomplicated falciparum malaria. *Am J Trop Med Hyg* 1999; 60:1019–1023.

326 Kitchen SF. *Vivax malaria*. In Boyd. Ed Malariology. Vol.2 Philadephia. WB Saunders 1949: 1027–1045.

327 Marchiafava E & Bignami A. *On Summer-Autumnal Fever*. London: New Sydenham Society, 1894.

328 Manson P. Experimental proof of the mosquito-malaria theory. *Brit Med J* 1900;ii:949–951

329 Manson PT. Experimental malaria; recurrence after nine months. *Brit Med J* 1901; ii:77

330 Menendez C, Ordi J, Ismail MR, et al. The impact of placental malaria on gestational age and birth weight. *J Infect Dis* 2000; 181:1740–1745.

331 Brabin BJ, Hakimi M & Pelletier D. An analysis of anemia and pregnancy-related maternal mortality. *J Nutr* 2001; 131:604S–614S.

332 Molyneux ME, Taylor TE, Wirima JJ & Borgstein J. Clinical features and prognostic indicators in paediatric cerebral malaria: a study of 131 comatose Malawian children. *Q J Med* 1989; 71:441–459.

333 World Health Organization. Severe falciparum malaria. *Trans R Soc Trop Med Hyg* 2000; 94 Supplement 1; S1–S90.

334 Waller D, Krishna S, Crawley J, et al. The clinical features and outcome of severe malaria in Gambian children. *Clin Infect Dis* 1995; 21:577–587.

335 Jaffar S, Van Hensbroek MB, Palmer A, Schneider G & Greenwood B. Predictors of a fatal outcome following childhood cerebral malaria. *Am J Trop Med Hyg* 1997; 57:20–4.

336 Marchiafava E. Pernicious malaria. *Am J Hyg* 1931; 13:1–56.

337 Lewallen S, Harding SP, Ajewole J, et al. A review of the spectrum of clinical fundus findings in *P. falciparum* malaria in African children with a proposed classification and grading. *Trans R Soc Trop Med Hyg* 1999; 93:619–622.

338 Looareesuwan S, Warrell DA, White NJ et al. Retinal haemorrhage, a common physical sign of prognostic significance in cerebral malaria. *Am J Trop Med Hyg* 1983; 32:911–915.

339 Lewallen S, Bakker H, Taylor TE, Wills BA, Courtright P & Molyneux ME. Retinal findings predictive of outcome in cerebral malaria. *Trans R Soc Trop Med Hyg* 1996; 90:144–146.

340 Lewallen S, White VA, Whitten RO, et al. Clinical-histopathological correlation of the abnormal retinal vessels in cerebral malaria. *Arch Ophthalmol* 2000; 118:924–928.

341 Newton CR, Krishna S. Severe falciparum malaria in children: current understanding of pathophysiology and supportive treatment. *Pharmacol Ther* 1998; 79:1–53.

342 Dover A S & Western K A. Fatalities due to malaria in the United States, 1966–1969. *J Infect Dis* 1970; 121:573–575.

343 Wattanagoon Y, Srivilairit S, Looareesuwan S & White NJ. Convulsions in childhood malaria. *Trans R Soc Trop Med Hyg* 1994; 88:426–428.

344 Omanga U, Nithinyurwa M, Shako D & Mashako M. Les hemiplegies au cours de l'acces pernicieux a Plasmodium falciparum de l'enfant. *Ann Pediatr* 1983; 30:294–296.

345 Collomb H, Rey M, Dumas M et al. Les hemiplegies au cours du paludisme aigue. *Bull Soc Med Afr Noire* 1967; 12:791–795.

346 Brewster DR, Kwiatkowski D, White NJ. Neurological sequelae of cerebral malaria in children. *Lancet* 1990; 336:1039–1043.

347 van Hensbroek MB, Palmer A, Jaffar S, Schneider G Kwiatkowski D. Residual neurologic sequelae after childhood cerebral malaria. *J Pediatr* 1997; 131:125–129.

348 Newton CR, Hien TT & White N. Cerebral malaria. *J Neurol Neurosurg Psychiatry* 2000; 69:433–441.

349 Mai NTH, Day NPJ, Chuong LV, et al. Post-malaria neurological syndrome. *Lancet* 1996; 348:917–921.

350 De Silva H J, Gamage R, Herath H K N et al. A delayed onset cerebellar syndrome complicating falciparum malaria. *Ceylon Med J* 1986; 31:147–150.

351 Senanayake N. Delayed cerebellar ataxia: a new complication of falciparum malaria. *Brit Med J* 1987; 294:1253–1254.

352 Holding PA, Stevenson J, Peshu N & Marsh K. Cognitive sequelae of severe malaria with impaired consciousness. *Trans R Soc Trop Med Hyg* 1999; 93:529–534.

353 Holding PA, Snow RW. Impact of Plasmodium falciparum malaria on performance and learning: review of the evidence. *Am J Trop Med Hyg* 2001; 64(Suppl):68–75.

354 Dukes D C, Sealey B J & Forbes J L. Oliguric renal failure in blackwater fever. *Am J Med* 1948; 45:899–903.

355 Canfield C J. Renal and hematologic complications of acute falciparum malaria in Vietnam. *Bull N Y Acad Med* 1969; 45:1043–1057.

356 Blackie WK. Blackwater fever. *Clin Proc* 1944; 3:272–312.

357 English M, Marsh V, Amukoye E, Lowe B, Murphy S & Marsh K. Chronic salicylate poisoning and severe malaria. *Lancet* 1996; 347:1736–7.367.

358 Ross GR. Blackwater fever in Southern Rhodesia in retrospect. *Cent Afr Med J* 1962; 8:294–297.

359 Stone WJ, Hanchett JE & Knepshield JR. Acute renal insufficiency due to falciparum malaria. *Arch Intern Med* 1972; 129:620–628.

360 Brooks MH, Kiel FW, Sheehy TW & Barry KG. Acute pulmonary edema in falciparum malaria. *N Engl J Med* 1968; 279:732–737.

361 Gurman G, Schlaeffer F, Alkan M & Heilig I. Adult respiratory distress syndrome and pancreatitis as complications of falciparum malaria. *Crit Care Med* 1988; 16:205–206.

362 Fein LA, Rackow EC & Shapiro L. Acute pulmonary edema in *Plasmodium falciparum* malaria. *Am Rev Respir Dis* 1978; 118:425–429.

363 Sullivan J. Pernicious fever: febris algida and febris comatosa. *Med Times Gaz* 1876; 1:277–279.

364 Gage A. Algid malaria. *Ther Gaz* 1926; 50:77–81.

365 Butler T & Weber DM. On the nature of orthostatic hypotension in acute malaria. *Trans R Soc Trop Med Hyg* 1973; 22:439–442.

366 Kofi-Ekue JM, Phiri DED, Mukunyandela M et al. Severe orthostatic hypotension during treatment of malaria. *Brit Med J* 1988; 296:396.

367 Supanaranond W, Davis TME, Pukrittayakamee S et al. Abnormal circulatory control in falciparum malaria: the effects of antimalarial drugs. *Eur J Clin Pharmacol* 1993; 44:325–329.

368 Das BA, Satpathy SK, Mohanty D et al. Hypoglycaemia in severe falciparum malaria. *Trans R Soc Trop Med Hyg* 1988; 82:197–201.

369 Zucker JR, Lackritz EM, Ruebush TK II, et al. Childhood mortality during and after hospitalization in western Kenya: effect of malaria treatment regimens. *Am J Trop Med Hyg* 1996; 55:655–560.

370 English M. Life-threatening severe malarial anaemia. *Trans R Soc Trop Med Hyg* 2000 ;94:585–588.

371 Davis TME, Ho M, Supanaranond W et al. Changes in the peripheral blood eosinophil count in falciparum malaria. *Acta Trop* 1991; 48:243–245.

372 Pukrittayakamee S, Clemens R, Pramoolsinap C et al. Polymorphonuclear leukocyte elastase in *Plasmodium falciparum* malaria. *Trans R Soc Trop Med Hyg* 1992; 86:598–601.

373 Miller LH, Makaranond P, Sitprija V et al. Hyponatraemia in malaria. *Ann Trop Med Parasitol* 1967; 61:265–279.

374 Miller KD, White NJ, Lott LA et al. Biochemical evidence of muscle injury in African children with severe malaria. *J Infect Dis* 1989; 159:139–142.

375 White NJ, Miller KD, Brown J et al. Prognostic value of CSF lactate in cerebral malaria. *Lancet* 1987; i:1261.

376 Field JW & Niven JC. A note on prognosis in relation to parasite counts in acute subtertian malaria. *Trans R Soc Trop Med Hyg* 1937; 30:569–574.

377 Field JW. Blood examination and prognosis in acute falciparum malaria. *Trans R Soc Trop Med Hyg* 1949; 43:33–68.

378 Silamut K & White NJ. Relation of the stage of parasite development in the peripheral blood to prognosis in severe falciparum malaria. *Trans R Soc Trop Med Hyg* 1993; 87:436–443.

379 Phu NH, Day NPJ, Diep TS, Ferguson DJP % White NJ. Intraleukocytic malaria pigment and prognosis in severe malaria. *Trans R Soc Trop Med Hyg* 1995; 89:197–199.

380 Li QQ, Guo X, Jian N et al. Development state of *Plasmodium falciparum* in the intradermal, peripheral and medullary blood of patients with cerebral malaria. *Natl Med J Chin* 1983; 63:692–693.

381 White NJ & Silamut K. Rapid diagnosis of malaria. *Lancet* 1989; i:435.

382 Humar A, Ohrt C, Harrington MA, Pillai D, Kain KC. Parasight F test compared with the polymerase chain reaction and microscopy for the diagnosis of *Plasmodium falciparum* malaria in travelers. *Am J Trop Med Hyg* 1997; 56:44–48.

383 Tjitra E, Suprianto S, Dyer M, Currie BJ & Anstey NM. Field evaluation of the ICT malaria P.f/P.v immunochromatographic test for detection of *Plasmodium falciparum* and *Plasmodium vivax* in patients with a presumptive clinical diagnosis of malaria in eastern Indonesia. *J Clin Microbiol* 1999; 37:2412–2417.

384 Tjitra E, Suprianto S, McBroom J, Currie BJ & Anstey NM. Persistent ICT malaria P.f/P.v panmalarial and HRP2 antigen reactivity after treatment of *Plasmodium falciparum* malaria is associated with gametocytemia and results in false-positive diagnoses of *Plasmodium vivax* in convalescence. *J Clin Microbiol* 2001; 39:1025–1031.

385 Proux S, Hkirijareon L, Ngamngonkiri C, McConnell S & Nosten F. Paracheck-Pf: a new, inexpensive and reliable rapid test for *P. falciparum* malaria. *Trop Med Int Health* 2001; 6:99–101.

386 Mayxay M, Pukrittayakamee S, Chotivanich K, Looareesuwan S & White NJ. Persistence of *Plasmodium falciparum* HRP-2 in successfully treated acute falciparum malaria. *Trans R Soc Trop Med Hyg* 2001; 95:179– 182.

387 Desakorn V, Silamut K, Angus B, et al. Quantitative measurement of PfHRP2 antigen in blood and plasma; methods and applications. *Trans R Soc Trop Med Hyg* 1997; 91:479–483.

388 Iqbal J, Sher A, Rab A. Plasmodium falciparum histidine-rich protein 2-based immunocapture diagnostic assay for malaria: cross-reactivity with rheumatoid factors. *J Clin Microbiol* 2000; 38:1184–1186.

389 Rickman LS, Long GW, Oberst R et al. Rapid diagnosis of malaria by acridine orange staining of centrifuged parasites. *Lancet* 1989; i:68–71.

390 Editorial. Rediscovering wormwood, qinghaosu, for malaria. *Lancet* 1992; 339:649–651.

391 Haggis AW. Fundamental errors in the early history of Cinchona. *Bull Hist Med* 1941; 10:568–592.

392 Duran-Reynolds MG. *The Fever Bark Tree.* New York: Doubleday, 1946.

393 Dawson WT. Cinchona alkaloids and bark in malaria. *Int Clin* 1930; 2:121–149.

394 Melville CH. The prevention of malaria in war. In Ross R (ed). *The Prevention of Malaria*, 2nd edn. London: Murray, 1911:577–599.

395 Taylor N. *Cinchona in Java*. New York: Greenberg, 1945.

396 Coatney GR. Pitfalls in a discovery: the chronicle of chloroquine. *Am J Trop Med Hyg* 1963; 12:121–128.

397 Covell G. Chemotherapy of malaria. WHO Monograph Series 1967;27.

398 Pampana EJ. *A Textbook of Malaria Eradication*, 2nd edn. London: Oxford University Press, 1969.

399 Rozman R S & Canfield C J. New experimental antimalarial drugs. *Adv Pharmacol Chemother* 1979; 16:1–43.

400 Ding GS. Recent studies on antimalarials in China: a review of literature since 1980. *Int J Exp Clin Chemother* 1988; 1:9–22.

401 Qinghaosu Antimalarial Coordinating Research Group. Antimalarial studies on qinghaosu. *Chin Med J* 1979; 92:811–816.

402 Klayman DL. Qinghaosu (artemisinin). An antimalarial drug from China. *Science* 1985; 228:1049–1055.

403 Jiang JB, Li GQ, Gao XB et al. Antimalarial activity of mefloquine and qinghaosu. *Lancet* 1982; ii:285–288.

404 Lee I S & Hufford C D. Metabolism of antimalarial sequiterpene lactones. *Pharmacol Ther* 1990; 48:345–355.

405 Li GQ, Guo XB & Jiang R. Clinical studies on treatment of cerebral malaria with qinghaosu and its derivatives. *J Tradit Chin Med* 1982; 2:124–130.

406 Hien TT & White NJ. Qinghaosu. *Lancet* 1993; 341:603–608.

407 White NJ. Antimalarial drug resistance: the pace quickens. *J Antimicrob Chemother* 1992; 30:571–585.

408 Trape JF. The public health impact of chloroquine resistance in Africa. *Am J Trop Med Hyg* 2001; 64(1–2 Suppl):12–17.

409 White NJ. Antimalarial drug resistance and mortality in falciparum malaria. *Trop Med Intl Hlth* 1999; 4:469–470.

410 Nosten F, ter Kuile F, Chongsuphajaisiddhi T et al. Mefloquine-resistant falciparum malaria on the Thai-Burmese border. *Lancet* 1991; 337:1140–1143.

411 Simon F, Le-Bras J, Gaudebout C & Girard P M. Reduced sensitivity of *Plasmodium falciparum* to mefloquine in West Africa. *Lancet* 1988; i:467–468.

412 Brockman A, Price RN, van Vugt M, et al. *Plasmodium falciparum* antimalarial drug susceptibility on the northwestern border of Thailand during five years of extensive use of artesunate-mefloquine. *Trans R Soc Trop Med Hyg* 2000, 94:537–544.

413 Rieckmann KH, Davis DR & Hutton DC. *Plasmodium vivax* resistance to chloroquine? Lancet 1989; ii:1183–1184.

414 Baird JK, Sustriayu Nalim MF, et al. Survey of resistance to chloroquine by *Plasmodium vivax* in Indonesia. *Trans R Soc Trop Med Hyg* 1996; 90:409–411.

415 Nocht B & Werner H. Beobachtungen uber relative Chininresistenz bei Malaria aus Brasilien. *Dtsch Med Wochenschr* 1910; 36:1557–1560.

416 Verdrager J. Epidemiology of emergence and spread of drug-resistant falciparum malaria in Southeast Asia. *SE Asian J Trop Med Public Health* 1986; 17:111–118.

417 Trape JF, Pison G, Preziosi MP, et al. Impact of chloroquine resistance on malaria mortality. *C R Acad Sci III* 1998; 321:689–697.

418 Fontanet AL, Johnston DB, Walker AM, et al. High prevalence of mefloquine-resistant falciparum malaria in eastern Thailand. *Bull World Health Organ* 1993; 71:377–383.

419 Nosten F, Luxemburger C, ter Kuile FO, et al. Treatment of multi-drug resistant *Plasmodium falciparum* malaria with 3-day artesunate-mefloquine combination. *J Infect Dis* 1994; 170:971–977.

420 Nosten F, van Vugt M, Price R, et al. Effects of artesunate-mefloquine combination on incidence of *Plasmodium falciparum* malaria and mefloquine resistance in western Thailand; a prospective study *Lancet* 2000; 356:297–302.

421 Yayon A, Vande Waa JA, Yayon M et al. Stage dependent effects of chloroquine on *Plasmodium falciparum* in vitro. *J Protozool* 1983; 30:642–647.

422 ter Kuile F, White NJ, Holloway P, Pasvol G, Krishna S. *Plasmodium falciparum*: in vitro studies of the pharmacodynamic properties of drugs used for the treatment of severe malaria. *Exp Parasitol* 1993; 76:85–95.

423 White NJ. Assessment of the pharmacodynamic properties of the antimalarial drugs in vivo. *Antimicrob Agents Chemother*, 1997; 41:1413–1422.

424 Day NPJ, Diep PT, Ly PT, et al. Clearance kinetics of parasites and pigment-containing leukocytes in severe malaria. *Blood* 1996; 88:4696–4700.

425 White NJ. Why is it that antimalarial drugs do not always work? *Ann Trop Med Parasitol* 1998; 92:449–458.

426 York W & Macfie J W S. Observations on malaria made during treatment of general paralysis. *Trans R Soc Trop Med Hyg* 1924:12–44.

427 Watkins WM, Woodrow C & Marsh K. Falciparum malaria: differential effects of antimalarial drugs on ex vivo parasite viability during the critical early phase of therapy. *Am J Trop Med Hyg* 1993; 49:106–112.

428 Udomsangpetch R, Pipitaporn B, Krishna S, et al. Antimalarial drugs reduce cytoadherence and rosetting of *Plasmodium falciparum*. *J Infect Dis* 1996; 173:691–698.

429 Clyde D F & Shute G T. Resistance of East African varieties of *Plasmodium falciparum* to pyrimethamine. *Trans R Soc Trop Med Hyg* 1954; 48:495–500.

430 Peters W. *Chemotherapy and drug resistance in malaria*. 2nd ed. London; Academic Press, 1987

431 Peterson DS, Walliker D & Wellems T. Evidence that a point mutation in dihydrofolate reductase-thymidylate synthase confers resistance to pyrimethamine in falciparum malaria. *Proc Natl Acad Sci USA* 1988; 85:9114–9118.

432 Foote SJ & Cowman AF. The mode of action and the mechanism of resistance to antimalarial drugs. *Acta Trop* 1994; 56:157–171.

433 Mberu EK, Mosobo MK, Nzila AM, Kokwaro GO, Sibley CH & Watkins WM.The changing in vitro susceptibility pattern to pyrimethamine/sulfadoxine in *Plasmodium falciparum* field isolates from Kilifi, Kenya. *Am J Trop Med Hyg* 2000; 62:396–401

434 Biswas S, Escalante A, Chaiyaroj S, Angkasekwinai P & Lal AA. Prevalence of point mutations in the dihydrofolate reductase and dihydropteroate synthetase genes of *Plasmodium falciparum* isolates from India and Thailand: a molecular epidemiologic study. *Trop Med Int Health* 2000; 5:737–743.

435 Peterson DA, Milhous WK & Wellems TE. Molecular basis of differential resistance to cycloguanil and pyrimethamine in *Plasmodium falciparum* malaria. Proc *Natl Acad Sci USA* 1990; 87:3018–3022.

436 Foote S J, Galatis D & Cowman A F. Aminoacids in the dihydrofolate reductase-thymidylate synthase gene of *Plasmodium falciparum* involved in cycloguanil resistance differ from those involved in pyrimethamine resistance. Proc *Natl Acad Sci USA* 1990; 87:3014–3017.

437 Wang P, Lee CS, Bayoumi R, et al. Resistance to antifolates in *Plasmodium falciparum* monitored by sequence analysis of dihydropteroate synthetase and dihydrofolate reductase alleles in a large number of field samples of diverse origins. *Mol Biochem Parasitol* 1997; 89:161–177.

438 Hyde JE & Sims PF. Sulfa-drug resistance in *Plasmodium falciparum*. *Trends Parasitol* 2001; 17:265–266.

439 Krogstad D & Schlesinger P H. Acid vesicle function, intracellular pathogens and the action of chloroquine against *Plasmodium falciparum*. *N Engl J Med* 1987; 317:542–549.

440 Krugliak M & Ginsburg H. Studies on the antimalarial mode of action of quinoline-containing drugs: time dependence and irreversibility of drug action, and interactions with compounds that alter the function of the parasite's food vacuole. *Life Sci* 1991; 49:1213–1219.

441 Chou AC, Chevli R & Fitch CD. Ferriprotoporphyrin IX fulfills the criteria for identification as the chloroquine receptor of malaria parasites. *Biochemistry* 1980; 19:1543–1549.

442 Bray PG, Mungthin M, Ridley RG, Ward SA. Access to hematin: the basis of chloroquine resistance. *Mol Pharmacol* 1998; 54:170–179.

443 Foote SJ, Thompson JK, Courman AF & Kemp DJ. Amplification of the multidrug resistance gene in some chloroquine-resistant isolates of *Plasmodium falciparum*. *Cell* 1989; 57:921–930.

444 Price RN, Cassar C, Brockman A, et al. The pfmdr1 gene is associated with a multidrug resistance phenotype in *Plasmodium falciparum* from the western border of Thailand. *Antimicrob Agents Chemother* 1999; 43:2943–2949.

445 Duraisingh MT, Jones P, Sambou I, von Seidlein L, Pinder M & Warhurst DC. The tyrosine-86 allele of the pfmdr1 gene of *Plasmodium falciparum* is associated with increased sensitivity to the anti-malarials mefloquine and artemisinin. *Mol Biochem Parasitol* 2000; 108:13–23.

446 Reed MB, Saliba KJ, Caruana SR, Kirk K & Cowman AF. Pgh1 modulates sensitivity and resistance to multiple antimalarials in *Plasmodium falciparum*. *Nature*. 2000; 403:906–909.

447 Korsinczky M, Chen N, Kotecka B, et al. Fidock DA, Nomura T, Talley AK, Cooper RA, Dzekunov SM, Ferdig MT, Ursos LM, Sidhu AB, Naude B, Deitsch KW, Su XZ, Wootton JC, Roepe PD & Wellems TE. Mutations in the *P. falciparum* digestive vacuole transmembrane protein PfCRT and evidence for their role in chloroquine resistance. *Mol Cell*. 2000; 6:861–871.

448 Djimde A, Doumbo OK, Cortese JF, et al. A molecular marker for chloroquine-resistant falciparum malaria. *N Engl J Med* 2001; 344:257–263.

449 Durand R, Jafari S, Vauzelle J, et al. Analysis of PfCRT point mutations and chloroquine susceptibility in isolates of *Plasmodium falciparum*. *Mol Biochem Parasitol* 2001; 114:95–102.

450 Warhurst DC. A molecular marker for chloroquine-resistant falciparum malaria. *N Engl J Med* 2001; 344:299–302.

451 Martin SK, Oduola AMJ & Milhous WK. Reversal of chloroquine resistance in *Plasmodium falciparum* by verapamil. *Science* 1987; 235:899–901.

452 Oduola AM, Omitowoju GO, Gerena L, Kyle DE, Milhous WK, Sowunmi A & Salako LA. Reversal of mefloquine resistance with penfluridol in isolates of *Plasmodium falciparum* from south-west Nigeria. *Trans R Soc Trop Med Hyg* 1993; 87:81–83.

453 Sowunmi A, Oduola AM, Ogundahunsi OA, Falade CO, Gbotosho GO & Salako LA. Enhanced efficacy of chloroquine-chlorpheniramine combination in acute uncomplicated falciparum malaria in children. *Trans R Soc Trop Med Hyg* 1997; 91:63–67.

454 Brasseur P, Kouamouo J & Brandicourt O. Patterns of in-vitro resistance to chloroquine, quinine, and mefloquine of *Plasmodium falciparum* in Cameroon 1985–1986. *Am J Trop Med Hyg* 1988; 39:166–172.

455 Warsame M, Wernsdorfer WH, Payne D & Bjorkman A. Susceptibility of *Plasmodium falciparum* in vitro to chloroquine, mefloquine, quinine and sulfadoxine/ pyrimethamine in Somalia: relationship between the responses to different drugs. *Trans R Soc Trop Med Hyg* 1991; 85:565–569.

456 Srivastava IK, Rottenberg H & Vaidya AB. Atovaquone, a broad spectrum antiparasitic drug, collapses mitochondrial membrane potential in a malarial parasite. *J Biol Chem* 1997; 272:3961–3966.

457 Korsinczky M, Chen N, Kotecka B, et al. Mutations in *Plasmodium falciparum* cytochrome b that are associated with atovaquone resistance are located at a putative drug-binding site. *Antimicrob Agents Chemother* 2000; 44:2100–2108.

458 Meshnick SR. Artemisinin antimalarials: mechanisms of action and resistance. *Med Trop* (Mars) 1998; 58(3 Suppl):13–17.

459 Olliaro PL, Haynes RK, Meunier B & Yuthavong Y. Possible modes of action of the artemisinin-type compounds. *Trends Parasitol* 2001; 17:122–126.

460 White NJ. Antimalarial drug resistance and combination chemotherapy. *Phil Trans R Soc Lond B* 1999; 354:739–749.

461 Curtis CF & Otoo LN. A simple model of the build up of resistance to mixtures of antimalarial drugs. *Trans R Soc Trop Med Hyg* 1986; 80:889–892.

462 Hastings IM & D'Alessandro U. Modelling a predictable disaster: the rise and spread of drug-resistantmalaria. *Parasitol Today* 2000; 16:340–347.

463 Watkins, WM & Mosobo M. Treatment of *Plasmodium falciparum* malaria with pyrimethamine-sulphadoxine: selective pressure for resistance is a function of long elimination half-life. *Trans R Soc Trop Med Hyg* 1993; 87:75–78.

464 Peters W. The prevention of antimalarial drug resistance. *Pharmacol Ther* 1990; 47:499–508.

465 White NJ, Nosten F, Looareesuwan S, et al. Averting a malaria disaster. *Lancet* 1999; 353:1965–1967

466 Supanaranond W, Davis T M E, Pukrittayakamee S et al. Disposition of oral quinine in acute falciparum malaria. *Eur J Clin Pharmacol* 1991; 40:49–52.

467 Waller D, Krishna S, Craddock C et al. The pharmacokinetic properties of intramuscular quinine in Gambian children with severe falciparum malaria. *Trans R Soc Trop Med Hyg* 1990; 84:488–491.

468 Mansor SM, Taylor TE, McGrath CS, Edwards G, Ward SA, Wirima JJ & Molyneux ME. The safety and kinetics of intramuscular quinine in Malawian children with moderately severe falciparum malaria. *Trans R Soc Trop Med Hyg* 1990; 84:482–487.

469 Sabcharoen A, Chongsuphajaisiddhi T & Attanath P. Serum quinine concentrations following the initial dose in children with falciparum malaria. *SE Asian J Trop Med Public Health* 1989; 13:689–692.

470 White NJ, Looareesuwan S, Warrell DA et al. Quinine pharmacokinetics and toxicity in cerebral and uncomplicated falciparum malaria. *Am J Med* 1982; 73:564–572.

471 Krishna S, Nagaraja NV, Planche T, et al. Population pharmacokinetics of intramuscular quinine in children with severe malaria. *Antimicrob Agents Chemother* 2001; 45:1803–1809.

472 White NJ, Chanthavanich P, Krishna S et al. Quinine disposition kinetics. *Br J Clin Pharmacol* 1983; 16:399–404.

473 Krishna S, White NJ. Pharmacokinetics of quinine, chloroquine and amodiaquine. Clinical implications. *Clin Pharmacokinet* 1996; 30:263–299.

474 Phillips RE, Looareesuwan S, White NJ et al. Quinine pharmacokinetics and toxicity in pregnant and lactating women with falciparum malaria. *Br J Clin Pharmacol* 1986; 21:677–683.

475 van Hensbroek MB, Kwiatkowski D, van den Berg B, Hoek FJ, van Boxtel CJ & Kager PA. Quinine pharmacokinetics in young children with severe malaria. *Am J Trop Med Hyg* 1996; 54:237–242.

476 Silamut K, Molunto P, Ho M et al. Alpha-one acid glycoprotein (orosomucoid) and plasma protein binding of quinine in

falciparum malaria. *Br J Clin Pharmacol* 1991; 32:311–315.

477 Silamut K, White N J, Warrell D A & Looareesuwan S. Binding of quinine to plasma proteins in falciparum malaria. *Am J Trop Med Hyg* 1985; 34:681–686.

478 Mansor SM, Molyneux ME, Taylor TE et al. Effect of *Plasmodium falciparum* malaria infection as the plasma concentration of alpha acid glycoprotein and the binding of quinine in Malawian children. *Br J Clin Pharmacol* 1991; 32:317–325.

479 White NJ, Looareesuwan S & Lavansiri K. Red cell quinine concentrations in falciparum malaria. *Am J Trop Med Hyg* 1983; 32:456–460.

480 White NJ. Antimalarial pharmacokinetics and treatment regimens. *Brit J Clin Pharmacol* 1992; 34:1–10.

481 White N J, Looareesuwan S & Warrell D A. Quinine and quinidine: a comparison of EKG effects during the treatment of malaria. *J Cardiovasc Pharmacol* 1983; 5:173–177.

482 Dyson EH, Proudfoot AT, Prescott LF & Heyworth R. Death and blindness due to overdose of quinine. *Brit Med J* 1985; 291:31–33.

483 Boland ME, Brennand-Roper SM & Henry JA. Complications of quinine poisoning. *Lancet* 1985; i:384–385.

484 Henquin JC, Horeman B, Henquin M et al. Quinine-induced modifications of insulin release and glucose metabolism by isolated pancreatic islets. *FEBS Lett* 1975; 57:280–284.

485 Bruce-Chwatt LJ. Quinine and the mystery of blackwater fever. *Acta Leiden* 1987; 55:181–196.

486 Yen LM, Dao LM, Day NPJ, et al. Role of quinine in the high mortality of intramuscular injection tetanus. Lancet 1994; 344:786–787.

487 Hien TT, Day NPJ, Phu NH, et al. A controlled trial of artemether or quinine in Vietnamese adults with severe falciparum malaria. *N Engl J Med* 1996; 335:76–83.

488 van Hensbroek MB, Onyiorah E, Jaffar S, et al. A trial of artemether or quinine in children with cerebral malaria. *N Engl J Med* 1996; 335:69–75.

489 White NJ. Controversies in the management of severe falciparum malaria. In Pasvol G (ed.) *Bailliere's Clinical Infectious Diseases* 2nd edn. Balliere Tindall. London. 1995; 309–330

490 Chongsuphajaisiddhi T, Sabcharoen A & Attanath P. In-vivo and in-vitro sensitivity to quinine in Thai children. *Ann Trop Paediatr* 1981; 1:21–26.

491 White NJ, Warrell DA, Looareesuwan S et al. Quinine loading dose in cerebral malaria. *Am J Trop Med Hyg* 1983; 32:1–5.

492 White NJ, Looareesuwan S, Warrell DA et al. Quinidine in falciparum malaria. *Lancet* 1981; ii:1069–1072.

493 Phillips RE, Warrell DA, White NJ et al. Intravenous quinidine for the treatment of severe falciparum malaria. Clinical and pharmacokinetic studies. *N Engl J Med* 1985; 312:1273–1278.

494 Karbwang J, Davis TME, Looareesuwan S et al. A comparison of the pharmacokinetic and pharmacodynamic properties of quinine and quinidine in healthy Thai males. *Br J Clin Pharmacol* 1993; 35:265–271.

495 Miller KD, Greenberg AE & Campbell CC. Treatment of severe malaria in the United States with a continuous infusion of quinidine gluconate and exchange transfusion. *N Engl J Med* 1989; 321:65–70.

496 Kain KC, Gadd ED, Gushulak B, McCarthy A & MacPherson D. Errors in treatment recommendations for severe malaria. Committee to Advise on Tropical Medicine and Travel (CATMAT) *Lancet* 1996; 348:621–622.

497 Krogstad DJ, Pearson RD, Bennett JE, Dolin R & Mandell GL. Dosage for malaria treatment. *Lancet* 1996; 348:1311–1312.

498 White NJ & Warrell DA. Dosage for malaria treatment. *Lancet* 1996; 348:1312.

499 Gustafsson LL, Walker O, Alvan G et al. Disposition of chloroquine in man after single intravenous and oral doses. *Br J Clin Pharmacol* 1983; 15:471–479.

500 Frisk-Holmberg M, Bergqvist Y, Termond E & Domeij-Nyberg B. The single dose kinetics of chloroquine and its major metabolite desethylchloroquine in healthy subjects. *Eur J Clin Pharmacol* 1984; 26:521–530.

501 White NJ, Watt G, Bergqvist Y & Njelesani E. Parenteral chloroquine in the treatment of falciparum malaria. *J Infect Dis* 1987; 155:192–201.

502 White NJ, Miller KD, Churchill FC et al. Chloroquine treatment of severe malaria in children: pharmacokinetics, toxicity, and revised dosage recommendations. *N Engl J Med* 1988; 319:1493–1500.

503 Walker O, Daurodu AH, Adeyokunnu AA et al. Plasma chloroquine and desethylchloroquine concentrations in children during and after chloroquine treatment for malaria. *Br J Clin Pharmacol* 1983; 16:701–705.

504 Minker F & Iran J. Experimental and clinicopharmacological study of rectal absorption of chloroquine. *Acta Physiol Hung* 1991; 77:237–248.

505 Mnyika KS & Kihamia CM. Chloroquine-induced pruritus: its impact on chloroquine utilization in malaria control in Dar es Salaam. *J Trop Med Hyg* 1991; 94:27–31.

506 Easterbrook M. Ocular effects and safety of antimalarials. *Am J Med* 1988; 85 (supplement 4a):23–29.

507 Peruval SPB & Meancock I. Chloroquine: ophthalmological safety and clinical assessment in rheumatoid arthritis. *Brit Med J* 1968; 3:579–584.

508 Riou B, Barriot P, Rimailho A & Band FJ. Treatment of severe chloroquine poisoning. *N Engl J Med* 1988; 316:1–6.

509 Pussard E, Lepers JP, Clavier F et al. Efficacy of a loading dose of oral chloroquine in a 36-hour treatment schedule for uncomplicated *Plasmodium falciparum* malaria. *Antimicrob Agents Chemother* 1991; 35:406–409.

510 Winstanley P. Edwards G, Orme ML'E & Breckenridge A M. The disposition of amodiaquine in man after oral administration. *Br J Clin Pharmacol* 1987; 23:1–7.

511 White NJ, Looareesuwan S, Edwards G et al. Pharmacokinetics of intravenous amodiaquine. *Br J Clin Pharmacol* 1987; 23:127–135.

512 Hatton CS, Peto TEA, Bunch C et al. Frequency of severe neutropenia associated with amodiaquine prophylaxis against malaria. *Lancet* 1986; i:411–414.

513 Gimenez F, Pennie RA, Koren G, Crevoisier C, Wainer IW & Farinotti R. Stereoselective pharmacokinetics of mefloquine in healthy Caucasians after multiple doses. *J Pharm Sci* 1994; 83:824–827.

514 Hellgren U, Jastrebova J, Jerling M, Krysen B & Bergqvist Y. Comparison between concentrations of racemic mefloquine, its separate enantiomers and the carboxylic acid metabolite in whole blood serum and plasma. *Eur J Clin Pharmacol* 1996; 51:171–173.

515 Bourahla A, Martin C, Gimenez F, et al. Stereoselective pharmacokinetics of mefloquine in young children. *Eur J Clin Pharmacol* 1996; 50:241–244.

516 White NJ. Combination treatment for P. falciparum prophylaxis. *Lancet* 1987; i:680–681.

517 Karbwang J & White NJ. Clinical pharmacokinetics of mefloquine. *Clin Pharmacokinet* 1990; 19:264–279.

518 Looareesuwan S, White N J, Warrell D A et al. Studies of mefloquine bioavailability and kinetics using a stable isotope technique: a comparison of Thai patients with falciparum malaria and healthy Caucasian volunteers. *Br J Clin Pharmacol* 1987; 24:37–42.

519 Price RN, Simpson JA, Teja-Isavatharm P, et al. Pharmacokinetics of mefloquine combined with artesunate in children with acute falciparum malaria. *Antimicrob Agents Chemother* 1999; 43:341–346.

520 Simpson JA, Price RN, ter Kuile FO, Teja-Isvadharm P, Nosten F, Aarons L & White NJ. Population pharmacokinetics of

mefloquine in patients with acute falciparum malaria. *Clin Pharmac Ther* 1999; 66:472–484.

521 Nosten F, Karbwang J, White N J et al. Mefloquine antimalarial prophylaxis in pregnancy: dose finding and pharmacokinetic study. *Br J Clin Pharmacol* 1990; 30:79–85.

522 ter Kuile F, Nosten F, Thieren M et al. High-dose mefloquine in the treatment of multidrug-resistant falciparum malaria. *J Infect Dis* 1992; 166:1393–1400.

523 ter Kuile FO, Nosten F, Luxemburger C et al. Mefloquine treatment of acute falciparum malaria: A prospective study of non-serious adverse effects in 3673 patients. *Bull WHO* 1995; 73:631–642.

524 Nosten F, ter Kuile F, Chongsuphajaisiddhi T et al. Mefloquine pharmacokinetics and resistance in children with acute falciparum malaria. *Br J Clin Pharmacol* 1991; 31:556–559.

525 Slutsker LM, Khoromana CD, Payne D et al. Mefloquine therapy for *Plasmodium falciparum* malaria in children under 5 years of age in Malawi: in vivo/in vitro efficacy and correlation of drug concentration with parasitological outcome. *Bull World Health Organ* 1990; 68:53–59.

526 Luxemburger C, Price RN, Nosten F, ter Kuile F, Chongsuphajaisiddhi T & White NJ. Mefloquine in infants and young children. *Ann Trop Paediatr* 1996; 16:281–286.

527 Weinke T, Trautman M, Held T et al. Neuropsychiatric side effects after the use of mefloquine. *Am J Trop Med Hyg* 1991; 45:86–91.

528 Luxemburger C, Nosten F, ter Kuiile F, Frejacques L, Chongsuphajaisiddhi T & White NJ. Mefloquine for multidrug-resistant malaria. *Lancet.* 1991; 338:1268.

529 Bem JL, Kerr L & Stuerchler D. Mefloquine prophylaxis: an overview of spontaneous reports of severe psychiatric reactions and convulsions. *J Trop Med Hyg* 1992; 95:167–179.

530 Steffen R, Fuchs E, Schildknecht J, et al. Mefloquine compared with other malaria chemoprophylactic regimens in tourists visiting east Africa. *Lancet* 1993; 341:1299–1303.

531 Lobel HO, Miani M, Eng T, et al. Long-term malaria prophylaxis with weekly mefloquine. *Lancet.* 1993; 34:848–851.

532 Phillips-Howard PA, ter Kuile FO. CNS adverse events associated with antimalarial agents. Fact or fiction? *Drug Saf* 1995; 12:370–383.

533 Nosten F, Vincenti M, Simpson JA, et al. The effects of mefloquine treatment in pregnancy. *Clin Infect Dis* 1999; 28:808–815.

534 Simpson JA, Watkins ER, Price RN, Aarons L, Kyle DE & White NJ. Mefloquine pharmacokinetic-pharmacodynamic models: implications for dosing and resistance. *Antimicrob Agents Chemother* 2000; 44:3414–3424.

535 Milton KA, Edwards G, Ward SA et al. Pharmacokinetics of halofantrine in man: effects of food and dose size. *Br J Clin Pharmacol* 1989; 28:71–77.

536 Veenendaal JR, Parkinson AD, Kere N et al. Pharmacokinetics of halofantrine and n-desbutylhalofantrine in patients with falciparum malaria following a multiple dose regimen of halofantrine. *Eur J Clin Pharmacol* 1991; 41:161–164.

537 Watkins WM, Oloo JA, Lury JD et al. Efficacy of multiple dose halofantrine in treatment of chloroquine resistant falciparum malaria in children in Kenya. *Lancet* 1988; ii:247–250.

538 Nosten F, ter Kuile FO, Luxemburger C, Woodrow C, Kyle DE, Chongsuphajaisiddhi T, White NJ. Cardiac effects of antimalarial treatment with halofantrine. *Lancet* 1993; 341:1054–1056.

539 Malvy D, Receveur MC, Ozon P, et al. Fatal cardiac incident after use of halofantrine. *J Travel Med* 2000; 7:215–216.

540 Akhtar T & Imran M. Sudden deaths while on halofantrine treatments—a report of two cases from Peshawar. *J Pak Med Assoc* 1994; 44:120–121.

541 Wesche DL, Schuster BG, Wang WX & Woosley RL. Mechanism of cardiotoxicity of halofantrine. *Clin Pharmacol Ther* 2000; 67:521–529.

542 ter Kuile FO, Dolan G, Nosten F, et al. Halofantrine versus mefloquine in the treatment of multi-drug resistant falciparum malaria. *Lancet* 1993; 341:1044–1049.

543 Winstanley P, Watkins WM, Newton CRJC et al. The disposition of oral and intramuscular Pyrimethamine/sulphadoxine in Kenyan children with high parasitaemia but clinically non-severe falciparum malaria. *Br J Clin Pharmacol* 1992; 33:143–148.

544 Miller K D, Lobel H O, Satriale R F et al. Severe cutaneous reactions among American travellers using pyrimethamine-sulfadoxine (Fansidar™) for malaria prophylaxis. *Am J Trop Med Hyg* 1986; 35:451–458.

545 Bjorkman A & Phillips-Howard P A. Adverse reaction to sulfa drugs: implications for malaria chemotherapy. *Bull World Health Organ* 1991; 69:297–304.

546 von Seidlein L, Milligan P, Pinder M, et al. Efficacy of artesunate plus pyrimethamine-sulphadoxine for uncomplicated malaria in Gambian children: a double-blind, randomised, controlled trial. *Lancet* 2000; 355:352–357.

547 Rogerson SJ, Chululuka E, Kanjala M, Mkundika P, Mhango C & Molyneux ME. Intermittent sulfadoxine-pyrimethamine in pregnancy: effectiveness against malaria morbidity in Blantyre, Malawi, in 1997–99. *Trans R Soc Trop Med Hyg* 2000; 94:549–553.

548 Wolfe EB, Parise ME, Haddix AC, Nahlen BL, Ayisi JG, Misore A & Steketee RW. Cost-effectiveness of sulfadoxine-pyrimethamine for the prevention of malaria-associated low birth weight. *Am J Trop Med Hyg* 2001; 64:178–186.

549 Schellenberg D, Menendez C, Kahigwa E, et al. Intermittent treatment for malaria and anaemia control at time of routine vaccinations in Tanzanian infants: a randomised, placebo-controlled trial. *Lancet* 2001; 357:1471–1477.

550 Wattanagoon Y, Taylor RB, Moody RR et al. Single dose pharmacokinetics of proguanil and its metabolites in healthy adult volunteers. *Br J Clin Pharmacol* 1987; 24:775–780.

551 Winstanley P, Watkins W, Muhia D, Szwandt S, Amukoye E, Marsh K. Chlorproguanil/dapsone for uncomplicated *Plasmodium falciparum* malaria in young children: pharmacokinetics and therapeutic range. *Trans R Soc Trop Med Hyg* 1997; 91:322–327

552 Helsby NA, Ward SA, Edwards C et al. The pharmacokinetics and activation of proguanil in man: consequences of variability in drug metabolism. *Br J Clin Pharmacol* 1990; 30:593–598.

553 Kaneko A, Kaneko O, Taleo G, Bjorkman A & Kobayakawa T. High frequencies of CYP2C19 mutations and poor metabolism of proguanil in Vanuatu. *Lancet* 1997; 349:921–922.

554 Wangboonskul J, White N J, Nosten F et al. Single dose pharmacokinetics of proguanil and its metabolites in pregnancy. *Eur J Clin Pharmacol* 1993; 44:247–251.

555 Harries AD, Forshaw AI & Friend H M. Malaria prophylaxis among British residents of Lilongwe and Kasungu districts, Malawi. *Trans R Soc Trop Med Hyg* 1988; 82:690–692.

556 Boots M, Phillips M & Curtis J R. Megaloblastic anaemia and pancytopenia due to proguanil in patients with chronic renal failure. *Clin Nephrol* 1982; 18:106–108.

557 Watkins WM, Brandling-Bennett D, Nevill CG, et al. Chlorproguanil/dapsone for the treatment of non-severe *Plasmodium falciparum* infection in Kenya. *Trans R Soc Trop Med Hyg* 1988; 82:398–403.

558 Amukoye E, Winstanley PA, Watkins WM, et al. Chlorproguanil-dapsone: effective treatment for uncomplicated falciparum malaria. *Antimicrob Agents Chemother* 1997; 41:2261–2264.

559 Nzila AM, Nduati E, Mberu EK, et al. Molecular evidence of greater selective pressure for drug resistance exerted by the long-acting antifolate Pyrimethamine/Sulfadoxine compared with the shorter-acting chlorproguanil/dapsone on Kenyan *Plasmodium falciparum. J Infect Dis* 2000; 181:2023–2028.

560 Looareesuwan S, Viravan C, Webster HK, Kyle DE, Hutchinson DB & Canfield CJ. Clinical studies of atovaquone, alone or in combination with other antimalarial drugs, for treatment of acute uncomplicated malaria in Thailand. *Am J Trop Med Hyg* 1996; 54:62–66.

561 Looareesuwan S, Wilairatana P, Chalermarut K, Rattanapong Y, Canfield CJ & Hutchinson DB. Efficacy and safety of atovaquone/proguanil compared with mefloquine for treatment of acute *Plasmodium falciparum* malaria in Thailand. *Am J Trop Med Hyg* 1999; 60:526–532.

562 Bustos DG, Canfield CJ, Canete-Miguel E & Hutchinson DB. Atovaquone-proguanil compared with chloroquine and chloroquine-sulfadoxine-pyrimethamine for treatment of acute *Plasmodium falciparum* malaria in the Philippines. *J Infect Dis* 1999; 179:1587–1590.

563 Hussein Z, Eaves J, Hutchinson DB & Canfield CJ. Population pharmacokinetics of atovaquone in patients with acute malaria caused by *Plasmodium falciparum. Clin Pharmacol Ther* 1997; 61:518–530.

564 Hogh B, Clarke PD, Camus D, et al. Atovaquone-proguanil versus chloroquine-proguanil for malaria prophylaxis in non-immune travellers: a randomised, double-blind study. Malarone International Study Team. *Lancet* 2000; 356:1888–1894.

565 Sabchareon A, Attanath P, Phanuaksook P, et al. Efficacy and pharmacokinetics of atovaquone and proguanil in children with multidrug-resistant *Plasmodium falciparum* malaria. *Trans R Soc Trop Med Hyg* 1998; 92:201–206.

566 Mihaly GW, Ward SA, Edwards C et al. Pharmacokinetics of primaquine in man: identification of the carboxylic acid derivative as a major plasma metabolite. *Br J Clin Pharmacol* 1984; 17:441–446.

567 Carson PE, Flangan CL, Ickes CE & Alving AS. Enzymatic deficiency in primaquine sensitive erythrocytes. *Science* 1956; 124:484–485.

568 Chan TK, Todd D & Tsao SC. Drug-induced haemolysis in glucose-6-phosphate dehydrogenase deficiency. *Brit Med J* 1976; ii:1227–1229.

569 Fryauff DJ, Baird JK, Basri H, et al. Randomised placebo-controlled trial of primaquine for prophylaxis of falciparum and vivax malaria. *Lancet* 1995; 346:1190–1193.

570 Soto J, Toledo J, Rodriquez M, et al. Double-blind, randomized, placebo-controlled assessment of chloroquine/primaquine prophylaxis for malaria in nonimmune Colombian soldiers. *Clin Infect Dis* 1999; 29:199–201.

571 Lell B, Faucher JF, Missinou MA, et al. Malaria chemoprophylaxis with tafenoquine: a randomised study. *Lancet* 2000; 355:2041–2045.

572 Brueckner RP, Lasseter KC, Lin ET & Schuster BG. First-time-in-humans safety and pharmacokinetics of WR 238605, a new antimalarial. *Am J Trop Med Hyg.* 1998; 58:645–649.

573 Li G Q. Clinical studies on artemisinin suppository and on artesunate and artemether. In Shen J X (ed). *Antimalarial Drug Development in China*. Beijing: National Institute of Pharmaceutical Research and Development, 1989:69–73.

574 Li G Q, Guo X B, Fu L C & Jian H X. A summary of clinical studies on the treatment of malaria with qinghaosu suppositories. In Li G Q, Guo X B & Yang F (eds) *Clinical Trials on Qinghaosu and its Derivatives*, Vol 1. Guangzhou: College of Traditional Chinese Medicine, Sanya Tropical Medicine Institute, 1990:17–22.

575 McIntosh HM & Olliaro P. Treatment of uncomplicated malaria with artemisinin derivatives. A systematic review of randomised controlled trials. *Med Trop* (Mars). 1998;58(3 Suppl):57–58.

576 McIntosh HM, Olliaro P. Treatment of severe malaria with artemisinin derivatives. A systematic review of randomised controlled trials. *Med Trop* (Mars). 1998; 58(3 Suppl):61–62.

577 The Artemether-Quinine Meta-analysis Study Group. A meta-analysis of trials comparing artemether with quinine in the treatment of severe falciparum malaria using individual patient data. *Trans R Soc Trop Med Hyg,* 2001; 95:637–650.

578 Luxemburger C, Nosten F, Shotar RD, Chongsuphajaisiddhi T & White NJ. Oral artesunate in the treatment of uncomplicated hyperparasitemic falciparum malaria. *Am J Trop Med Hyg* 1995; 53:522–525.

579 Hien TT, Arnold K, Vinh H, et al. Comparison of artemisinin suppositories with intravenous artesunate and intravenous quinine in the treatment of cerebral malaria. *Trans R Soc Trop Med Hyg* 1992; 86:582–583.

580 Phuong CXT, Bethell DB, Phuong PT, et al. Comparison of artemisinin suppositories, intramuscular artesunate, and intravenous quinine for the treatment of severe childhood malaria. *Trans R Soc Trop Med Hyg* 1997; 91:335–342.

581 Nosten F, van Vugt M & White NJ. Intrarectal artemisinin derivatives. *Med Trop* (Mars) 1998; 58(3 Suppl):63–64.

582 Krishna S, Planche T, Agbenyega T, et al. Bioavailability and preliminary clinical efficacy of intrarectal artesunate in Ghanaian children with moderate malaria. *Antimicrob Agents Chemother* 2001; 45:509–516.

583 Price RN, Nosten F, Luxemburger C, ter Kuile F, Paiphun L, Chongsuphajaisiddhi T & White NJ. The effects of artemisinin derivatives on malaria transmissability. *Lancet* 1996; 347:1654–1658.

584 Targett G, Drakeley C, Jawara M, et al. Artesunate reduces but does not prevent posttreatment transmission of *Plasmodium falciparum* to *Anopheles gambiae. J Infect Dis* 2001; 183:1254–1259.

585 van Vugt M, Angus BM, Price RN, et al. A case-control auditory evaluation of patients treated with artemisinin derivatives for multi-drug resistant *Plasmodium falciparum* malaria. *Am J Trop Med Hyg* 2000; 62:65–69.

586 Kissinger E, Hien TT, Hung NT, et al. Clinical and neurophysiological study of the effects of multiple doses of artemisinin on brain-stem function in Vietnamese patients. *Am J Trop Med Hyg* 2001; 63:48–55.

587 Price RN, van Vugt M, Phaipun L, et al. Adverse effects in patients with acute falciparum malaria treated with artemisinin derivatives. *Am J Trop Med Hyg* 1999; 60:547–555.

588 Newton P, Proux S, Green M, et al. Fake artesunate in SE Asia. *Lancet* 2001; 357:1948–1950

589 Navaratnam V, Mansor SM, Sit NW, Grace J, Li Q & Olliaro P. Pharmacokinetics of artemisinin-type compounds. *Clin Pharmacokinet.* 2000; 39:255–270.

590 Teja-Isavadharm P, Nosten F, Kyle DE, et al. Comparative bio-availability of oral, rectal and intramuscular artemether in healthy subjects-use of simultaneous measurement by high performance liquid chromatography with electro-chemical detection and bioassay. *Brit J Clin Pharmacol* 1996; 42:599–604.

591 Batty KT, Thu LT, Davis TM, et al. A pharmacokinetic and pharmacodynamic study of intravenous vs oral artesunate in uncomplicated falciparum malaria. *Br J Clin Pharmacol* 1998; 45:123–129.

592 Newton P, Suputtamongkol Y, Teja-Isavadharm P, et al. Antimalarial bioavailability and disposition of artesunate in acute falciparum malaria. *Antimicrob Agents Chemother* 2000; 44:972–977.

593 Murphy SA, Mberu E, Muhia D, et al. The disposition of intramuscular artemether in children with cerebral malaria; a preliminary study. *Trans R Soc Trop Med Hyg* 1997; 91:331–334.

594 Ribeiro IR & Olliaro P. Safety of artemisinin and its derivatives. A review of published and unpublished clinical trials. *Med Trop* (Mars) 1998;58(3 Suppl):50–53.

595 Leonardi-Nield E, Gilvary G, White NJ & Nosten F. Severe allergic reactions to oral artesunate: a report of two cases. *Trans R Soc Trop Med Hyg* 2001; 95:182–183.

596 Brewer TG, Peggins JO, Grate SJ, et al. Neurotoxicity in animals due to arteether and artemether. *Trans R Soc Trop Med Hyg* 1994 Jun;88 Suppl 1:S33–S36.

597 Genovese RF, Newman DB, Petras JM & Brewer TG. Behavioral and neural toxicity of arteether in rats. *Pharmacol Biochem Behav* 1998; 60:449–458

598 Nontprasert A, Nosten-Bertrand M, Pukrittayakamee S, Vanijanonta S, Angus BJ & White NJ. Assessment of the neurotoxicity of parenteral artemisinin derivatives in mice. *Am J Trop Med Hyg* 1998; 59:519–522.

599 Nontprasert A, Pukrittayakamee S, Nosten-Bertrand M, Vanijanonta S & White NJ. Studies of the neurotoxicity of oral artemisinin derivatives in mice. *Am J Trop Med Hyg* 2000; 62:409–412.

600 White NJ. Preventing antimalarial drug resistance through combinations. *Drug Res Updates* 1998; 1:3–9.

601 McGready R, Cho T, Keo, NK, et al. Artemisinin antimalarials in pregnancy: a prospective treatment study of 539 multidrug resistant *P. falciparum* episodes. *Clin Infect Dis*, in press.

602 Brundtland GH. Reaching out for world health. *Science* 1998; 280:2027

603 Ezzet F, Mull R, Karbwang J. Population pharmacokinetics and therapeutic response of CGP 56697 (artemether + benflumetol) in malaria patients. *Br J Clin Pharmacol* 1998; 46:553–561.

604 Ezzet F, van Vugt M, Nosten F, Looareesuwan S & White NJ. The pharmacokinetics and pharmacodynamics of lumefantrine (benflumetol) in acute uncomplicated falciparum malaria. *Antimicrob Agents Chemother* 2000; 44:697–704.

605 White NJ, van Vugt M & Ezzet F. Clinical pharmacokinetics and pharmacodynamics of artemether-lumefantrine. *Clin Pharmacokinet* 1999; 37:105–125.

606 van Vugt M, Brockman A, Gemperli B, et al. Randomised comparison of artemether-benflumetol and artesunate-mefloquine in the treatment of multi-drug resistant falciparum malaria. *Antimicrob Agents Chemother* 1998; 42:135–139.

607 van Vugt M, Wilairatana P, Gemperli B, et al. Efficacy of six doses or artemether-benflumetol in the treatment of multi-drug resistant falciparum malaria. *Am J Trop Med Hyg* 1999; 60:936–942.

608 van Vugt M, Looareesuwan S, Wilairatana P, et al. Artemether-lumefantrine for the treatment of multidrug resistant falciparum malaria.. *Trans R Soc Trop Med Hyg* 2000; 94:545–548.

609 van Vugt M, Ezzet F, Nosten F & White NJ. No evidence of cardiotoxicity during antimalarial treatment with artemether-lumefantrine. *Am J Trop Med Hyg* 1999; 61:964–967.

610 Looareesuwan S, Kyle DE, Viravan C, Vanijanonta S, Wilairatana P & Wernsdorfer WH. Clinical study of pyronaridine for the treatment of acute uncomplicated falciparum malaria in Thailand. *Am J Trop Med Hyg* 1996; 54:205–209.

611 Ringwald P, Bickii J, Basco LK. Efficacy of oral pyronaridine for the treatment of acute uncomplicated falciparum malaria in African children. *Clin Infect Dis* 1998; 26:946–953.

612 Chen L. Recent studies on antimalarial efficacy of piperaquine and hydroxypiperaquine. *Chin Med J* 1991; 104:161–163.

613 Pukrittayakamee S, Clemens R, Chantra A, et al. Therapeutic responses to antibacterial drugs in vivax malaria. *Trans R Soc*

Trop Med Hyg 2001; in press.

614 Taylor WR, Widjaja H, Richie TL, et al. Chloroquine/doxycycline combination versus chloroquine alone, and doxycycline alone for the treatment of *Plasmodium falciparum* and *Plasmodium vivax* malaria in northeastern Irian Jaya, Indonesia. *Am J Trop Med Hyg* 2001; 64:223–238.

615 Kremsner PG, Zotter GM, Feldmeier H et al. A comparative trial of three regimens for treating uncomplicated falciparum malaria in Acre, Brazil. *J Infect Dis* 1988; 158:1368–1371.

616 Pukrittayakamee S, Chantra A, Vanijanonta S, Clemens R, Looareesuwan S & White NJ. Therapeutic responses to quinine and clindamycin in multidrug-resistant falciparum malaria. *Antimicrob Agents Chemother* 2000; 44:2395–2398.

617 Zucker JR, Lackritz EM, Ruebush TK II et al. Childhood mortality during and after hospitalization in western Kenya: effect of malaria treatment regimens. *Am J Trop Med Hyg* 1996; 55:655–660.

618 Supanaranond W, Suputamongkol Y, Davis TME, Pukrittayakamee S, Teja-Isavadharm P, Webster HK, White NJ. Lack of a significant adverse cardiovascular effect of combined quinine and mefloquine therapy for uncomplicated malaria. *Trans R Soc Trop Med Hyg* 1997; 91:694–696.

619 Ridtitid W, Wongnawa M, Mahatthanatrakul W, Chaipol P & Sunbhanich M. Effect of rifampin on plasma concentrations of mefloquine in healthy volunteers. *J Pharm Pharmacol* 2000; 52:1265–1269.

620 World Health Organization. Chemotherapy of malaria and resistance to antimalarials. Report of a WHO Scientific Group. WHO Tech Rep Ser 1973; 529:30–35.

621 World Health Organization. Assessment of therapeutic efficacy of antimalarial drugs for uncomplicated falciparum malaria in areas with intense transmission. WHO/MAL/96.1077. 1996

622 Looareesuwan S, Charoenpan P, Ho M et al. Fatal *Plasmodium falciparum* malaria after an inadequate response to quinine treatment. *J Infect Dis* 1990; 161:577–580.

623 Nosten F, Imvithaya S, Vincenti M, et al. Malaria on the Thai-Burmese border: treatment of 5182 patients with mefloquine- sulfadoxine-pyrimethamine combination. *Bull WHO* 1987; 65:891–896.

624 Farnert A, Arez AP, Babiker HA, et al. Genotyping of Plasmodium falciparum infections by PCR: a comparative multicentre study. *Trans R Soc Trop Med Hyg* 2001; 95:225–232.

625 Brockman A, Paul REL, Anderson TJC, et al. Application of genetic markers to the identification of recrudescent *Plasmodium falciparum* infections on the northwestern border of Thailand. *Am J Trop Med Hyg* 1999; 60:14–21.

626 Trager W & Jensen JB. Continuous culture of *Plasmodium falciparum*: its impact on malaria research. *Int J Parasitol* 1997; 27:989–1006.

627 Chotivanich K, Silamut K, Udomsangpetch R, Stepniewska K, Pukrittayakamee S, Looareesuwan S & White NJ. Ex-vivo short term culture and developmental assessment of *Plasmodium vivax*. *Trans R Soc Trop Med Hyg* in press.

628 Rieckmann KH. Visual in-vitro test for determining the drug sensitivity of *Plasmodium falciparum*. *Lancet* 1982; 1:1333–1335.

629 Webster HK, Boudreau EF, Pavanand K et al. Antimalarial drug susceptibility testing of *Plasmodium falciparum* in Thailand using a microdilution radioisotope method. *Am J Trop Med Hyg* 1985; 34:228–235.

630 Druilhe P, Moreno A, Blanc C, Brasseur PH & Jacquier P. A colorimetric in vitro drug sensitivity assay for *Plasmodium falciparum* based on a highly sensitive double-site lactate dehydrogenase antigen-capture enzyme-linked immunosorbent assay. *Am J Trop Med Hyg* 2001; 64:233–241.

631 Pukrittayakamee S, Chantra A, Simpson JA, Vanijanonta S, Clemens R, Looareesuwan S & White NJ. Therapeutic responses to different antimalarial drugs in vivax malaria. *Antimicrob Agents Chemother* 2000; 44:1680–1685.

632 Arnold J, Alving AS, Hockwald RS et al. The effect of continuous and intermittent primaquine therapy on the relapse rate of Chesson strain vivax malaria. *J Lab Clin Med* 1954; 43:429–438.

633 Pukrittayakamee S, Vanijanonta S, Chantra A, Clemens R & White NJ. Blood stage antimalarial efficacy of primaquine in *Plasmodium vivax* malaria. *J Infect Dis* 1994; 169:932–935.

634 White NJ. Optimal regimens of parenteral quinine. *Trans R Soc Trop Med Hyg* 1995; 89:462–463.

635 van der Torn M, Thuma PE, Mabeza GF, et al. Loading dose of quinine in African children with cerebral malaria. *Trans R Soc Trop Med Hyg* 1998; 92:325–331.

636 Teasdale G & Jennett B. Assessment of coma and impaired consciousness. A practical scale. *Lancet* 1974; 2:81–84.

637 Punyagupta S, Srichaikul T, Nitiyanant P & Petchclai B. Acute pulmonary insufficiency in falciparum malaria: summary of 12 cases with evidence of disseminated intravascular coagulation. *Am J Trop Med Hyg* 1974; 23:551–559.

638 Warrell D A, Looareesuwan S, Warrell M J et al. Dexamethasone proves deleterious in cerebral malaria. A double blind trial in 100 comatose patients. N *Engl J Med* 1982; 306:313–319.

639 Hoffman S L, Rustama D, Punjabi N H et al. High-dose dexamethasone in quinine-treated patients with cerebral malaria: a double-blind, placebo-controlled trial. *J Infect Dis* 1988; 158:325–331.

640 Taylor TE, Molyneux ME, Wirima JJ, et al. Intravenous immunoglobulin in the treatment of paediatric cerebral malaria. *Clin Exp Immunol* 1992; 90:357–362.

641 van Hensbroek MB, Palmer A, Onyiorah E et al. The effect of a monoclonal antibody to tumor necrosis factor on survival from childhood cerebral malaria. *J Infect Dis* 1996; 174:1091–1097.

642 Thuma PE, Mabeza GF, Biemba G et al. Effect of iron chelation therapy on mortality in Zambian children with cerebral malaria. *Trans R Soc Trop Med Hyg* 1998; 92:214–218.

643 White NJ. Not much progress in treatment of cerebral malaria (editorial). *Lancet* 1998; 352:594–595.

644 Crawley J, Waruiru C, Mithwani S, et al. of phenobarbital on seizure frequency and mortality in childhood cerebral malaria: a randomised, controlled intervention study. *Lancet* 2000; 355:701–706.

645 Fleming AF. Tropical obstetrics and gynaecology. 1. Anaemia in pregnancy in tropical Africa. *Trans R Soc Trop Med Hyg* 1989; 83:441–448.

646 McGready R, Brockman A, Cho T et al. Randomized comparison of mefloquine-artesunate versus quinine in the treatment of multi-drug resistant falciparum malaria in pregnancy. *Trans R Soc Trop Med Hyg* 2000; 94:689–693.

647 McGready R, Cho T, Keo, NK et al. Artemisinin antimalarials in pregnancy: a prospective treatment study of 539 multidrug resistant *P. falciparum* episodes. *Clin Infect Dis* in press.

648 Nosten F, Vincenti M, Simpson JA, et al. The effects of mefloquine treatment in pregnancy. *Clin Infect Dis* 1999; 28:808–815.

649 Steketee RW, Wirima JJ, Slutsker L et al. Malaria treatment and prevention in pregnancy: indications for use and adverse events associated with use of chloroquine or mefloquine. *Am J Trop Med Hyg* 1996; 55 (1 Suppl):50–56.

650 Price RN, van Vugt M, Nosten F et al. Artesunate versus artemether for the treatment of recrudescent multi-drug resistant falciparum malaria. *Am J Trop Med Hyg* 1998; 59:883–888.

651 Fischer PR. Congenital malaria: an African survey. *Clin Pediatr* (Phila) 1997; 36:411–413.

652 Foster SD. Pricing, distribution and use of antimalarial drugs. *Bull World Health Organ* 1991; 69:349–363.

653 Lindsay SW & Gibson ME. Bednets revisited – old idea, new angle. *Parasitol Today* 1988; 4:270–272.

654 Alonso PL, Lindsay SW, Armstrong JRM et al. The effect of insecticide-treated bed nets on mortality of Gambian children. *Lancet* 1991; 337:1499–1502.

655 Greenwood BM, Greenwood AM, Bradley AK, Snow RW, Byass P, Hayes RJ & N'Jie AB. Comparison of two strategies for control of malaria within a primary health care programme in the Gambia. *Lancet* 1988; 1:1121–1127.

656 Snow RW, Lengeler C, de Savigny D & Cattani J. Insecticide-treated bed nets in control of malaria in Africa. *Lancet* 1995; 345:1056–1057.

657 Lengeler C. Insecticide-treated bednets and curtains for preventing malaria.

658 Lengeler C. Comparison of malaria control interventions. *Bull World Health Organ* 2001; 79:77.

659 Rowland M, Durrani N, Kenward M et al. Control of malaria in Pakistan by applying deltamethrin insecticide to cattle: a community-randomised trial. *Lancet* 2001; 357:1837–1841.

660 Curtis CF, Mnzava AE. Comparison of house spraying and insecticide-treated nets for malaria control. *Bull World Health Organ* 2000; 78:1389–1400.

661 McGready R, Simpson JA, Htway M et al. A double-blind randomized therapeutic trial of insect repellents for the prevention of malaria in pregnancy. *Trans R Soc Trop Med Hyg* 2001; 95:137–138.

662 Lobel HO & Kozarsky PE. Update on prevention of malaria for travelers. *JAMA.* 1997; 278:1767–1771.

663 Kramer MH & Lobel HO. Antimalarial chemoprophylaxis in infants and children. *Paediatr Drugs* 2001; 3:113–121.

664 Evans MR, Day JH & Behrens RH. Prevention and treatment of malaria in UK travellers. *Hosp Med* 2000; 61:162–166.

665 Davis TM, Dembo LG, Kaye-Eddie SA, Hewitt BJ, Hislop RG & Batty KT. Neurological, cardiovascular and metabolic effects of mefloquine in healthy volunteers: a double-blind, placebo-controlled trial. *Br J Clin Pharmacol* 1996; 42:415–421.

666 Clyde DF, McCarthy VC, Miller RM, Hornick RB. Specificity of protection of man immunized against sporozoite-induced malaria. *Am J Med Sci* 1973; 266:398–401.

667 Genton B, Al-Yaman F, Anders R, et al. Safety and immunogenicity of a three-component blood-stage malaria vaccine in adults living in an endemic area of Papua New Guinea. *Vaccine* 2000; 18:2504

668 Anders RF & Saul A. Malaria vaccines. *Parasitol Today* 2000; 16:444–447.

669 Hendrickse R G, Adeniyi A, Edington G M et al. Quartan malarial nephrotic syndrome. Collaborative clinicopathological study in Nigerian children. *Lancet* 1977; i:1143–1149.

670 Gilles HM & Hendrickse RG. Nephrosis in Nigerian children: role of *Plasmodium malariae* and effect of antimalarial treatment. *Brit Med J* 1963; ii:27–31.

671 Crane G. Tropical splenomegaly. Part II Oceania. *Clin Haematol* 1981; 10:976–982.

672 Piessens WF, Hoffman SL, Wadee AA et al. Antibody mediated killing of T suppressor lymphocytes as a possible cause of macroglobulinaemia in the tropical splenomegaly syndrome. *J Clin Invest* 1985; 75:1821–1827.

673 Hoffman SL, Piessens WF, Ratiwayanto S et al. Reduction of suppressor T-lymphocytes in the tropical splenomegaly syndrome. *N Engl J Med* 1984; 310:337–341.

674 Bate I, Bedu-Addo G, Bevan H & Rutherford TR. Use of immunoglobulin gene rearrangements to show clonal lymphoproliferation in hyper-reactive malarial splenomegaly. *Lancet* 1991; 337:505–507.

675 Lam KMC, Syed N, Whittle H & Crawford DH. Circulating Epstein-Barr virus-carrying B cells in acute malaria. *Lancet* 1991; 337:876–879.

676 Rozendaal J. *Vector Control; methods for use by individuals and communities.* World Health Organization, Geneva, 1997.

677 Martinez-Torres D, Chandre F, Williamson MS et al. Molecular characterization of pyrethroid knockdown resistance (kdr) in the major malaria vector *Anopheles gambiae* s.s. *Insect Mol Biol* 1998; 7:179–184

678 Ranson H, Jensen B, Vulule JM, et al. Identification of a point mutation in the voltage-gated sodium channel gene of Kenyan *Anopheles gambiae* associated with resistance to DDT and pyrethroids. *Insect Mol Biol* 2000; 9:491–497.

679 Hargreaves K, Koekemoer LL, Brooke BD et al. *Anopheles funestus* resistant to pyrethroid insecticides in South Africa. *Med Vet Entomol* 2000; 14:181–189.

680 Chandre F, Darrier F, Manga L et al. Status of pyrethroid resistance in *Anopheles gambiae* sensu lato. *Bull World Health Organ* 1999; 77:230–234.

Chapter 72
Babesiosis

P. L. Chiodini

Babesia spp. are protozoan parasites of domestic and wild animals. They are members of the phylum Apicomplexa, order Piroplasmida, family Babesiidae.

Most human cases of babesiosis are due to *Babesia bovis*, *B. divergens* or *B. microti*. *B. caucasica* has also been reported to infect humans, but Hoare[1] considered it to be synonymous with *B. bovis*. He also regarded *B. divergens* as a synonym of *B. bovis* but this has not been adopted; thus Kakoma and Mehlhorn[2] recognize *B. divergens* and *B. bovis* as separate species. There is one case reportedly due to *B. canis*,[3] and a new *Babesia*, known as WA1, was isolated from a patient in Washington State, USA.[4] Parasites isolated from cases of human babesiosis in California, USA, known as CA1–CA4, have been shown to be closely related to WA1 by molecular criteria.[4] A *Babesia divergens*-like parasite, MO1, has been isolated from a fatal case of babesiosis from Missouri, USA,[5] and a *Babesia microti*-like organism has caused human infection in Taiwan.[6]

Life cycle

Human babesiosis is a zoonosis acquired by tick bite when individuals accidentally interact with the natural life cycle of the parasite. Humans represent dead-end hosts for *Babesia* spp.

Bovine babesias

Sporozoites are injected into the bloodstream by tick bite and penetrate erythrocytes. In contrast to the malaria life cycle, no tissue stage has ever been demonstrated for *B. bovis* or *B. divergens*. Within the erythrocyte the parasites vary in appearance, being oval, round or pear shaped.

Ring forms, especially, may be confused with malaria parasites, especially *Plasmodium falciparum*. However, *Babesia* does not form pigment and does not cause alterations in red cell morphology or staining, such as the Maurer clefts of *P. falciparum*, the Schüffner dots of *P. vivax* or the James dots of *P. ovale*. *Babesia* multiplies in the red cell by budding (*Plasmodium* by schizogony). Release of daughter parasites is followed by reinvasion of fresh erythrocytes and further asexual multiplication.

Some of the sporozoites injected by the tick vector follow a different path of intraerythrocytic development, growing slowly and 'folding' to form accordion-like structures, thought to be gametocytes[2] that are destined to undergo further development in the tick vector.

Within the gut of the tick the accordion-like stage is able to resist digestion and eventually fuses with another, to form a zygote. Further development outside the intestine occurs in a variety of tissues, the salivary glands and ovaries being especially important for transmission.

Sporozoites in tick salivary glands are injected into the mammalian host at the next blood meal. Transovarial transmission of *B. bovis* also takes place so that newly hatched larvae are already infected. Trans-stadial transmission to nymph and then to adult stages can then take place.

Babesia microti

In the small mammal host of *B. microti*, sporozoites from the tick vector first enter lymphocytes and undergo merogony, the daughter parasites of which then enter erythrocytes.[2] There is no published report of this intra-lymphocytic stage in human *B. microti* infections.

B. microti does not undergo transovarial transmission,[2] but once a larva has become infected from a mammalian host it is able to pass on the infection trans-stadially to the nymph.

Epidemiology

Human infection follows tick bite or, rarely, blood transfusion or transplacental/perinatal infection. Each *Babesia*–vector–mammalian host system has its own characteristics, and the ecology and bionomics of the vector tick define the pattern of risk for the human population.

European cases

Twenty-two cases of human infection with *B. divergens* have been reported in Europe since 1957.[7] European cases reportedly due to *B. microti* and to *B. canis* have also been recorded.[3] The vector of *B. divergens* is *Ixodes ricinus* and that of *B. microti* in England is *I. trianguliceps*, in contrast to the situation in the USA where *B. microti* is transmitted by *I. dammini*. Previous splenectomy had been undertaken in 84% of European cases of *B. divergens* infection.[8] One patient with *B. microti* infection had an intact spleen.[3]

There is an association of human *B. bovis* infection with exposure to land grazed by infected cattle for occupational or recreational purposes.

North American cases

Almost all the cases have been due to *B. microti*. Most reports have come from the north-eastern coastal region of the USA,[9] with some from Wisconsin[10] and sporadic reports from California, Georgia and Missouri.[5,11]

B. microti infects the mouse *Peromyscus leucopus*, the preferred host for the larva of *I. dammini*. Nymphs of this tick feed either on *Peromyscus* or on the deer *Odocoileus virginianus*, which does not appear to be susceptible to *B. microti*. Adult *I. dammini* prefer to feed on *Odocoileus*. Humans appear to become infected via nymphs and the peak month for transmission is June, which coincides with their active feeding period.

The vector for *B. microti* in North America is *I. dammini*, which is also the vector for *Borrelia burgdorferi*, the causative agent of Lyme disease. Co-infection of the same patient can occur and, in such cases, there are more symptoms and greater duration of illness than in patients with either infection alone.[12]

B. microti in North America can infect previously healthy individuals with intact spleens. The infection is more severe in splenectomized individuals. Benach and Habicht[13] studied common risk factors for babesiosis in 17 patients. They found no association with a particular blood group. Age was an important risk factor. The presence of a significant medical history (including splenectomy, cancer, cancer therapy, autoimmune disease, endocrinopathy and previous parasitic disease) was noted in 10 of the 17 cases. The mean age of patients with a significant medical history (47.7 years) was significantly less than of those who were previously healthy (63.4 years).

B. microti infection has been reported from human immunodeficiency virus (HIV)-positive patients, in whom persistent parasitaemia and severe disease have occurred.[14,15]

Pathology

Haemolytic anaemia, jaundice due to unconjugated hyperbilirubinaemia, frank haemoglobinuria and acute renal failure due to acute tubular necrosis are all features of *B. bovis* infection in splenectomized individuals.[16] Thrombocytopenia has been recorded.[17]

B. microti infection also results in haemolytic anaemia, which may last for several days to a few months.[18] Its presence in splenectomized as well as intact patients indicates that hypersplenism alone cannot explain the occurrence of haemolytic anaemia. Scanning electron microscopy of human blood infected with *B. microti* has revealed substantial damage to the erythrocyte membrane, with protrusions, inclusions and perforations evident, suggesting that red cell destruction is parasite mediated.[19] C3 and C4 levels were suppressed in acute *B. microti* infections.[20] Thrombocytopenia and raised levels of liver enzymes occur in severe cases.[21] Immunity to babesiosis depends upon humoral and cellular factors, although current opinion regards the humoral component of limited importance, the role of antibodies being restricted to a period when the parasites have entered the bloodstream but not yet become intracellular.[18] T cells are regarded as vital in developing resistance to *Babesia* and CD4+ T helper cells appear to be the subpopulation mainly responsible.[18] Non-specific responses via natural killer cells and macrophages are also important in resistance to babesial infection.[18]

Clinical features
Babesia bovis/divergens

The incubation period varies from 1 to 4 weeks. The patient may feel vaguely unwell at first, but by the time the diagnosis has been made is usually very ill, with fever, prostration, myalgia, jaundice, anaemia and haemoglobinuria. Nausea, vomiting and diarrhoea are also recorded.[16] Hepatomegaly, signs of pulmonary oedema and oliguric renal failure may occur. Finding an operation scar gives a clue to previous splenectomy. Infection is sometimes unsuspected and, given the fulminant nature of this condition, may not be confirmed until after the patient has died or the diagnosis is considered to be *P. falciparum* malaria when intraerythrocytic parasites are seen in the blood film. Other misdiagnoses include leptospirosis and viral hepatitis. Thus, for the diagnosis to be made early, babesiosis should be considered in the differential diagnosis of any splenectomized patient in whom exposure to tick bites is a possibility.

Babesia microti

Most human infections are subclinical.[22] Where clinical illness develops, the incubation period is 1–3 weeks, occasionally up to 6 weeks, for tick-transmitted infections and 6–9 weeks for post-transfusion cases. The illness usually begins gradually, with anorexia and fatigue, plus fever (without periodicity), sweating, rigors and generalized myalgia. Physical examination may reveal only fever, but may also show mild splenomegaly and sometimes mild hepatomegaly.[11] In a series of 34 patients with severe babesiosis requiring hospitalization, 41% developed complications which included the adult respiratory distress syndrome, disseminated intravascular coagulation, congestive heart failure and renal failure. Complicated babesiosis was more often associated with the presence of severe anaemia (haemoglobin concentration < 10 g/dl).[21]

Given the non-specific nature of the clinical findings, human infection with *B. microti* cannot be diagnosed with certainty on clinical grounds alone. In a series of severe babesiosis, the average time from onset of symptoms to diagnosis was 15 days.[21] A history of tick bite is helpful but is not elicited in most cases.[13] However, public knowledge of Lyme disease, which shares the same vector with *B. microti* in the USA, can raise awareness of tick-transmitted disease. The relatively localized geographical distribution of human *B. microti* infections in the USA means that local physicians may become very aware of the infection but it may be missed by those practising in non-endemic areas in other countries.

Laboratory diagnosis

Definitive diagnosis depends upon finding parasites on blood film examination. The use of the polymerase chain reactin (PCR) is increasing and serodiagnosis is also helpful. Hamster inoculation is very seldom indicated.

Blood film examination

Babesia bovis/divergens (Figure 72.1)

B. divergens was separated from *B. bovis* as a result of the predominance of paired forms, diverging at a wide angle of up to 180°, situated on the periphery of the red cell.[1] In addition, *B. divergens* is smaller (0.4 × 1.5 μm) than *B. bovis* (2.4 × 1.5 μm). However, the parasites are pleomorphic and their size can vary depending upon the host they infect.[1]

    B. bovis/divergens are pear shaped, oval or round and may exist in pyriform pairs. In fulminant human cases *B. divergens* takes the form of rings, loops, clubs, rods, pyriform and amoeboid shapes. Occasional divergent forms are seen. There may be one to eight parasites per red cell. Parasitaemia as high as 70% has been reported from a fatal case.[16] The 'Maltese cross' form is unique to *Babesia* among members of the Apicomplexa, but in its absence it may be very difficult to distinguish young ring forms of *Plasmodium* spp., especially *P. falciparum*. The absence of pig-

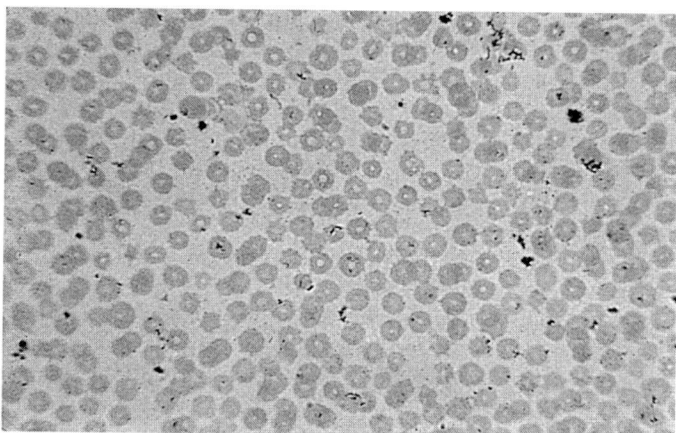

Figure 72.1: *Babesia divergens* in calf blood.

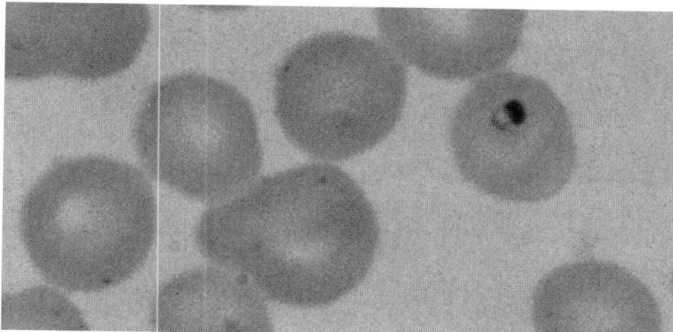

Figure 72.2: *Babesia microti* in human blood.

ment cannot be relied upon as young rings of *Plasmodium* spp. do not exhibit pigment. If cultured in vitro, *P. falciparum* will develop pigment, but *Babesia* will not. *Babesia* is smaller than malaria parasites, and in some of the larger rings there is a white vacuole, instead of the pink vacuole containing erythrocyte stroma seen in malaria. *Babesia* does not form schizonts.

Babesia microti (Figure 72.2)

Ring, rod-shaped, pyriform, amoeboid and 'Maltese cross' forms are seen.[1] In heavy infections different stages may be noted in the same red cell. Intraerythrocytic stages measure approximately 2 × 1.5 μm. In very high parasitaemias extracellular merozoites with plentiful cytoplasm were found singly or as a syncytial structure.[19]

    Peak parasitaemia varies between less than 1% to approximately 10%,[11] but a splenectomized patient who was also taking systemic steroids developed a *B. microti* parasitaemia of 85%.[19]

Other laboratory findings

Babesia bovis/divergens

Anaemia, leucocytosis, haemolysis, unconjugated hyperbilirubinaemia and raised blood urea levels are found. Reticulocytosis occurs in response to the haemolytic anaemia. Frank haemoglobinuria is evident.[16]

Babesia microti

Anaemia may be mild to moderately severe, ranging from 5.8 to 11.6 g/dl in one series.[11] Serum haptoglobin levels may be reduced and the reticulocyte count increased, supporting the view that most of the anaemia is due to haemolysis. Total white blood cell counts are low or normal and there may be thrombocytopenia.[11]

    Mean and differential lymphocyte counts and percentages of B lymphocytes and levels of T lymphocytes with the immunoglobulin (Ig) G Fc receptor were raised in acute infection. Polyclonal hypergammaglobulinaemia was found. Levels of serum IgG, IgM and C1q binding were significantly increased; C3 and C4 levels and haemolytic activity were reduced in acute-phase sera.[20]

There may be a mild increase in serum glutamic oxaloacetic transaminase (aspartate aminotransferase), alkaline phosphatase and bilirubin concentrations.[11]

Electron microscopy

This technique is not helpful for routine diagnosis of human babesiosis but may provide useful confirmation of the nature of the infection. Transmission electron microscopy of *B. microti* from a splenectomized patient also receiving systemic steroids showed considerable pleomorphism. All developmental stages were seen in both reticulocytes and mature erythrocytes. The same study identified convoluted cells with many free ribosomes, thought to represent an early gametocyte stage.[19]

Serodiagnosis

The indirect fluorescent antibody test (IFAT) is available for bovine babesia and for *B. microti*. However, serology should not be seen as an alternative to blood film examination, especially in view of the fulminant nature of bovine babesia infection in splenectomized patients. Demonstration of parasites in a blood film provides unequivocal proof of current infection. Some *B. microti* infections may have low level or transient parasitaemia,[22] and serology, with PCR testing of seropositive individuals,[18] has a useful part to play in establishing the diagnosis. Ruebush et al.[22] defined individuals with IFAT titres to *B. microti* of 64 or greater as seropositive. In patients with acute *B. microti* infection, IFAT titres were greater than or equal to 1 in 1024, and fell to 1 in 256 or 1 in 64 over 8–12 months. The possibility of cross-reaction with antimalarial antibody must be borne in mind when serological results are interpreted. The *B. microti* IFAT has a reported 88–96% sensitivity and 90–100% specificity.[23]

Polymerase chain reaction

This technique has been applied to the diagnosis of *B. microti*, with a reported limit of detection of approximately three merozoites.[24] It is deployed increasingly to confirm infection in antibody-reactive individuals and to monitor the response to treatment.[18]

Animal inoculation

This is not used for routine diagnosis of individual cases, but *B. microti* from human cases can be isolated in hamsters,[11] and *B. divergens* from a fatal human case was successfully passaged to gerbils and to a splenectomized calf.[16]

Clinical course and management
Babesia bovis/divergens

If untreated, infection of splenectomized humans with bovine babesias leads to fulminant illness and death. Specific treatment is based upon anecdotal case reports. Diminazene (Berenil) is active against *Babesia* in animals and was used in a case of human *B. divergens* infection, but the patient died.[25] Successful treatment of *B. divergens* (5% parasitaemia) in a splenectomized patient with pentamidine plus co-trimoxazole has been recorded.[25] Quinine and chloroquine plus pyrimethamine have proven ineffective.[16]

Brasseur and Gorenflot[26] reported successful treatment of three cases with massive exchange blood transfusion (2–3 blood volumes) followed by intravenous clindamycin and oral quinine.

Atovaquone is effective against *B. divergens in vitro*.[27]

In the absence of data from randomized controlled trials, current therapy should consist of exchange blood transfusion plus intravenous clindamycin and intravenous or oral quinine, depending upon the patient's condition.

Babesia microti

In most instances patients suffer a mild illness from which they recover spontaneously. Recovery may be prolonged, with several months of fatigue and malaise.[11] Where treatment is required, oral quinine 650 mg every 8 hours plus clindamycin 300–600 mg intravenously or intramuscularly every 6 hours (adult doses) for 7–10 days has been regarded as the treatment of choice,[3,28] although it is not universally effective.[29] Paediatric dosage is oral quinine 25 mg per kg per day and intravenous or intramuscular clindamycin 20 mg per kg per day. Krause et al.[30] compared atovaquone 750 mg every 12 hours plus azithromycin 500 mg on day 1 and 250 mg daily thereafter for 7 days with clindamycin 600 mg every 8 hours and quinine 650 mg every 8 hours for 7 days, all drugs being given orally. Atovaquone plus azithromycin proved to be as effective as clindamycin plus quinine and had fewer adverse reactions. The authors recommended that atovaquone plus azithromycin be considered for the treatment of non-life-threatening babesiosis in immunocompetent adult patients and in others who cannot tolerate clindamycin and quinine.[30] Weiss et al.[31] reported the successful use of azithromycin 12 mg per kg per day and atovaquone 40 mg per kg per day in neonates without toxic effects, and had used a higher dose of azithromycin (600 mg per day) in combination with atovaquone (750 mg twice daily) in adults. They reported that the 600-mg daily dose of azithromycin led to earlier resolution of fever and rapid clearance of parasites from the blood.[31] Ranque[32] has suggested that a trial of atovaquone plus clindamycin should be performed.

Chloroquine is unhelpful. Diminazene was used in one case and the patient recovered but developed neurological complications resembling the Guillain–Barré syndrome.[33]

Whole blood or red cell exchange transfusion has produced a rapid and substantial fall in parasitaemia and its use as an adjunct to chemotherapy should be considered in severely ill patients with high parasitaemia.[34]

Prevention

There is no vaccine licensed for human use. Prevention of human babesiosis depends upon avoidance of tick bite:

avoidance of tick habitats; wearing appropriate clothing to cover the lower part of the body; use of insect repellent (e.g., diethyltoluamide and permethrin-impregnated clothing); and prompt removal of ticks found on the person. In endemic areas, awareness of the possibility of transfusion-transmitted *Babesia* infection should be maintained so that those thought to be potentially infected with *Babesia* can be excluded from donation, although routine screening of donor blood is not yet established.

REFERENCES

1 Hoare C A. Comparative aspects of human babesiosis. *Trans R Soc Trop Med Hyg* 1980; 74:143–148.
2 Kakoma I & Mehlhorn H. *Babesia* of domestic animals. In Kreier J P (ed.) *Parasitic Protozoa 7*, 2nd edn. San Diego: Academic Press, 1994:141–216.
3 Telford S R III, Gorenflot A, Brasseur P & Spielman A. Babesial infections in man and wildlife. In Kreier J P & Baker J R (eds) *Parasitic Protozoa 5*, 2nd edn. San Diego: Academic Press, 1993:1–47.
4 Thomford J W, Conrad P A, Telford S R et al. Cultivation and phylogenetic characterisation of a newly recognised human pathogenic protozoan. *J Infect Dis* 1994; 169:1050–1056.
5 Herwaldt B, Persing D H, Precigout E A et al. A fatal case of babesiosis in Missouri: identification of another piroplasm that infects humans. *Ann Intern Med* 1997; 124:643–650.
6 Shih C M, Liu L P, Chung W C, Ong S J & Wang C C. Human babesiosis in Taiwan: asymptomatic infection with a *Babesia microti*-like organism in a Taiwanese woman. *J Clin Microbiol* 1997; 35:450–454.
7 Berry A, Morassin B, Kamar N & Magnaval J-F. Clinical picture: human babesiosis. *Lancet* 2001; 357:341.
8 Kjemtrup A M & Conrad P A. Human babesiosis: an emerging tick-borne disease. *Int J Parasitol* 2000; 30:1323–1337.
9 Meldrum S C, Birkhead G S, White D J, Benach J L & Morse D L. Human babesiosis in New York State: an epidemiological description of 136 cases. *Clin Infect Dis* 1992; 15:1019–1023.
10 Steketee R W, Eckman M R, Burgess E C et al. Babesiosis in Wisconsin: a new focus of disease transmission. *JAMA* 1985; 253:2675–2678.
11 Ruebush T K II. Human babesiosis in North America. *Trans R Soc Trop Med Hyg* 1980; 74:149–152.
12 Krause PJ, Telford SR III, Spielman A et al. Concurrent Lyme disease and babesiosis. Evidence for increased severity and duration of illness. *JAMA* 1996; 275:1657–1660.
13 Benach J L & Habicht G S. Clinical characteristics of human babesiosis. *J Infect Dis* 1981; 144:481.
14 Ong K R, Stavropoulos C & Inada Y. Babesiosis, asplenia and AIDS. *Lancet* 1990; 336:112.
15 Falagas M E & Klempner M S. Babesiosis in patients with AIDS: a chronic infection presenting as fever of unknown origin. *Clin Infect Dis* 1996; 22:809–812.
16 Williams H. Human babesiosis. *Trans R Soc Trop Med Hyg* 1980; 74:157.
17 Uhnoo I, Cars O, Christensson D & Nystrom Rosander C. First documented case of human babesiosis in Sweden. *Scand J Infect Dis* 1992; 24:541–547.
18 Homer M J, Aguilar-Delfin I, Telford S R III, Krause P J & Persing D H. Babesiosis. *Clin Microbiol Rev* 2000; 13:451–469.
19 Sun T, Tenenbaum M J, Greenspan J et al. Morphologic and clinical observations in human infection with *Babesia microti*. *J Infect Dis* 1983; 148:239–248.
20 Benach J L, Habicht G S & Hamburger M I. Immunoresponsiveness in acute babesiosis in humans. *J Infect Dis* 1982; 146:369–380.
21 Hatcher J C, Greenberg P D, Antique J & Jimenez-Lucho V E. Severe babesiosis in Long Island: review of 34 cases and their complications. *Clin Infect Dis* 2001; 32:1117–1125.
22 Ruebush T K II, Juranek D D, Chisholm E S, Snow P C, Healy G R & Sulzer A J. Human babesiosis on Nantucket Island. Evidence for self-limited and subclinical infections. *N Engl J Med* 1977; 297:825–827.
23 Krause P J, Telford S R, Ryan R et al. Diagnosis of babesiosis: evaluation of a serologic test for the detection of *Babesia microti* antibody. *J Infect Dis* 1994; 169:923–926.
24 Persing D H, Mathiesen D, Marshall W F, Telford S R & Spielman A. Detection of *Babesia microti* by polymerase chain reaction. *J Clin Microbiol* 1992; 30:2097–2103.
25 Raoult D, Soulayrol L, Toga B, Dumon H & Casanovna P. Babesiosis, pentamidine and cotrimaxozole. *Ann Intern Med* 1987; 107:944.
26 Brasseur P & Gorenflot A. Human babesiosis in Europe. *Mem Inst Oswaldo Cruz* 1992; 87:131–132.
27 Pudney M & Gray J S. Therapeutic efficacy of atovaquone against the bovine intraerythrocytic parasite, *Babesia divergens*. *J Parasitol* 1997; 83:307–310.
28 Gelfand J A & Poutsiaka D. Babesia. In Mandell G L, Bennett J E & Dolin R (eds) *Principles and Practice of Infectious Diseases*, 5th edn. Philadelphia. Churchill Livingstone, 2000; 2899–2902.
29 Anonymous. Clindamycin and quinine treatment for *Babesia microti* infections. *MMWR Morb Mortal Wkly Rep* 1983; 32:65–71.
30 Krause P J, Lepore T, Sikand V K et al. Atovaquone and azithromycin for the treatment of babesiosis. *N Engl J Med* 2000; 343:1454–1458.
31 Weiss L M, Wittner M & Tanowitz H B. The treatment of babesiosis. *N Engl J Med* 2001; 344:773.
32 Ranque S. The treatment of babesiosis. *N Engl J Med* 2001; 344:773–774.
33 Ruebush T K II, Rubin R H, Wolpow E R, Cassady P B & Schultz M G. Neurologic complications following the treatment of human *Babesia microti* infection with diminazene aceturate. *Am J Trop Med Hyg* 1979; 28:184–189.
34 Evenson D A, Perry E, Kloster B, Hurley R & Stroneck D F. Therapeutic apheresis for babesiosis. *J Clin Apheresis* 1998; 13:32–36.

Chapter 73
Human African Trypanosomiasis
C. Burri and R. Brun

Historical background

David Livingstone (1813–1873) had been convinced in the mid-nineteenth century that the tsetse fly was responsible for the tansmission of 'nagana', a disease that affected cattle in central Africa. This is clearly recorded in his classic *Missionary Travels*, first published in 1857; there is, in this work, an accurate drawing of the tsetse fly. It seems probable that Livingstone had in fact associated the bite of *Glossina palpalis* with 'nagana' as early as 1847. It was not until 1894, however, that the causative role of *Trypanosoma* (later designated *T. brucei*) was delineated in nagana, and this resulted from the brilliant work of David Bruce (Figure 73.1) in Zululand, where he had been posted from military duty in Natal. Shortly before this, animal trypanosomes had been visualized, and in 1878 Timothy Lewis had first indicated that trypanosomes could cause infection in mammals.

A febrile illness associated with cervical lymph-adenopathy and lethargy had been clearly recorded in Sierra Leone by T. M. Winterbottom (1765–1859) in 1803. In 1902, Joseph Dutton (1874–1905) and John Todd (1876–1949) demonstrated that *Trypanosoma* spp. were responsible for this condition, then named 'trypanosome fever' in West Africa; their observations were made on an Englishman who had been infected in The Gambia. Studies were carried out in both The Gambia and Liverpool. This work was published in 1902 with a full clinical description, accompanied by temperature charts.

Early in the twentieth century an outbreak that was described at the time as 'negro lethargy' swept central Africa; this involved the northern shores of Lake Victoria in Nyanza. No one, it seems, equated the disease with 'trypanosome fever'. In 1902, the Royal Society sent a Sleeping Sickness Expedition, consisting of Low, Castellani (1877–1971) and Christy (1864–1932), in an attempt to determine the aetiological agent responsible for this disease. Manson was of the opinion that *Filaria perstans* was responsible; he had visualized this parasite in three cases of sleeping sickness investigated in London, at the London and Charing Cross Hospitals. After a great deal of painstaking work, Castellani concluded that the disease was caused by a streptococcus. He reported his finding to the Royal Society's Malaria Committee, chaired by Joseph Lister (1827–1912), but they were far from enthusiastic. In the meantime, Castellani had visualized *Trypanosoma*

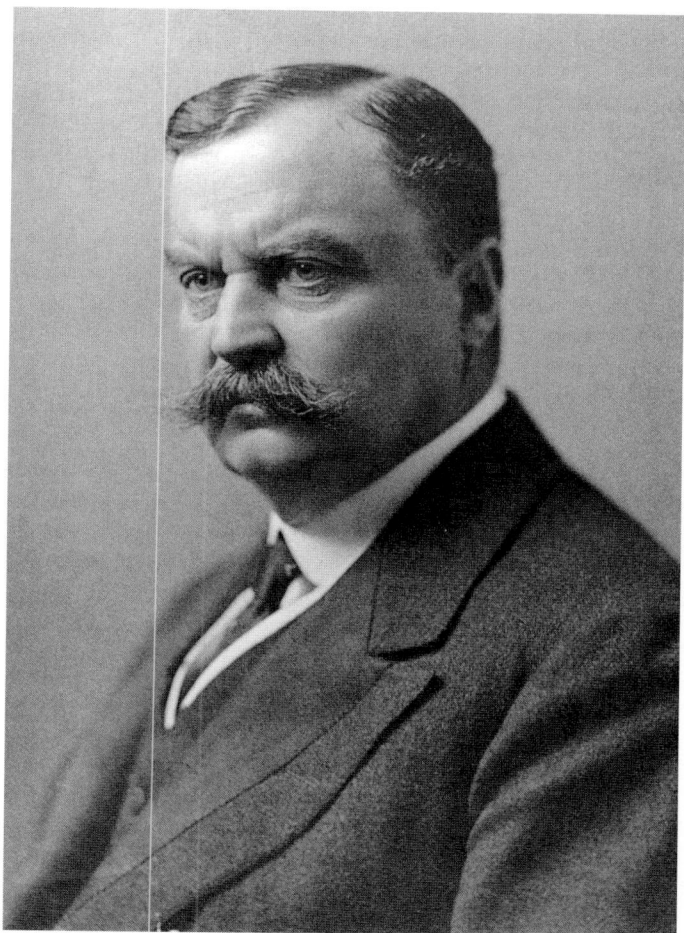

Figure 73.1: David Bruce (1855–1931) established the causes of nagana in Zululand and of 'negro lethargy' in Uganda. From Gillespie S H et al. (eds) *Principles and Practice of Clinical Parasitology*. Wiley, 2001.

spp. in the cerebrospinal fluid (CSF) of a single patient with 'negro lethargy'; however, he disregarded this organism, and favoured the streptococcal theory. The Royal Society proceeded to send a second team to Uganda in 1903, consisting of Bruce (Figure 73.1) and David Nabarro (1874–1958). They demonstrated *Trypanosoma* spp. in numerous cases of sleeping sickness (in both CSF and blood) and, furthermore, were able to transmit *T. gambiense* to monkeys via the bite of infected *Glossina palpalis* (the local species of tsetse fly); this work clinched the aetiological agent responsible for this disease.

Castellani remained convinced, however, that he should be given credit for discovering the cause of sleeping sickness, now correctly attributed to Bruce and Nabarro. Acrimonious correspondence emerged, some being recorded in *The Times* for 1908. In retrospect, it seems likely that Castellani was unduly influenced by a report from some Portuguese workers which concluded that a diplo-streptococcus was responsible for the disease; Castellani, a trained bacteriologist, was clearly far more impressed with this organism than with *Trypanosoma* spp.!

Several years were to pass before the animal reservoirs of African trypanosomiasis were delineated. Was the causative organism of nagana identical with that which caused African trypanosomiasis? It was not until 1910 that J. W. W. Stephens (1865–1946) and H. B. Fantham (1875–1937) discovered *T. rhodesiense* in Nyasaland (now Malawi) and northern Rhodesia (now Zimbabwe). In 1911, Allan Kinghorn (?–1955) and Warrington Yorke (1883–1943) demonstrated the transmission of *T. rhodesiense* to humans by *Glossina morsitans*.

It is now known that human African trypanosomiasis ('sleeping sickness') is caused by the protozoan parasites *Trypanosoma brucei gambiense* in west and central Africa, and by *Trypanosoma brucei rhodesiense* in eastern Africa. By the end of the 1960s the disease had been almost eliminated by means of large-scale control and intervention programmes. However, the situation has deteriorated since and today the number of prevalent cases is estimated at 300 000 to 500 000 with about 60 million people at risk, but fewer than 4 million under appropriate surveillance. Major outbreaks have been reported from the Democratic Republic of Congo, Angola, Sudan and Uganda.

The causative organisms are flagellated protozoa of the genus *Trypanosoma* (subgenus *Trypanozoon*), classified in the subkingdom Protozoa, the phylum Sarcomastigophora, order Kinetoplastida. The organisms responsible for human trypanosomiasis in Africa belong to the species *Trypanosoma brucei*, a complex of organisms transmitted to humans by the bite of tsetse flies (*Glossina*). *T. cruzi* (Chagas' disease) and *Leishmania* are relatives classified in the same order.

Fever, headache, adenopathy, joint pains and pruritus are the most common early symptoms, while severe neurological symptoms such as mental alterations, abnormal movements, sensory problems and sleep disturbances characterize the second stage of the disease after the parasites have invaded the central nervous system (CNS). The disease is fatal if untreated, and only a few drugs are available for cure.

Geographical distribution

Sleeping sickness is endemic only in areas where *Glossina* species are found. The ecological limit of *Glossina*

distribution is approximately a line from 14°N from Senegal in the west to 10°N in southern Somalia in the east, and 20°S corresponding to the northern fringes of the Kalahari and Namibian Deserts. The distribution of *Glossina* is determined by climatic factors (temperature and humidity) through its effects on vegetation. It is anticipated that satellite technology will be of increasing use in defining fly distribution in relation to habitats.[1] Comparison of such images over time will, in association with geographical information system (GIS) techniques, be of value in predicting tsetse distribution in relation to changes in ecology. Rogers and Williams[2] examined how GIS can contribute to studies of human and animal trypanosomiasis and how data from meteorological satellites help to understand the spatial distribution of vectors and disease.

There are 23 species of *Glossina* and a number of subspecies, most of which are capable of acting as vectors of trypanosomes that cause human sleeping sickness (as well as animal disease). Two groups of flies transmit sleeping sickness: the *G. palpalis* group transmits *T. b. gambiense*, which is responsible for the chronic form of the disease; and the *G. morsitans* group transmits *T. b.*

Table 73.1 Major vectors of *T. b. gambiense* and *T. b. rhodesiense* and geographical distribution

T. b. gambiense
G. palpalis palpalis, G. palpalis gambiensis
Angola, Benin, Burkina Faso, Cameroon, Central African Republic, Congo, Democratic Republic of Congo, Gabon, Gambia, Ghana, Guinea, Guinea-Bissau, Ivory Coast, Liberia, Mali, Nigeria, Senegal, Sierra Leone, Togo
G. tachinodes
Benin, Burkina Faso, Cameroon, Central African Republic, Chad, Ethiopia, Ghana, Guinea, Ivory Coast, Mali, Niger, Nigeria, Sudan, Togo
G. fuscipes quanzensis, G. fuscipes martinii
Angola, Congo, Democratic Republic of Congo
G. fuscipes fuscipes
Cameroon, Central African Republic, Chad, Congo, Democratic Republic of Congo, Sudan, Uganda
T. b. rhodesiense
G. morsitans morsitans, G. morsitans centralis
Angola, Botswana, Burundi, Malawi, Mozambique, Rwanda, Tanzania, Zambia, Zimbabwe
G. pallidipes
Burundi, Ethiopia, Kenya, Malawi, Mozambique, Rwanda, Sudan, Tanzania, Uganda, Zambia, Zimbabwe
G. swynnertoni
Kenya, Tanzania
G. fuscipes fuscipes
Ethiopia, Kenya, Tanzania, Uganda

rhodesiense, which causes a more acute disease. In Uganda, epidemic *T. b. rhodesiense* is transmitted by the riverine tsetse fly *G. fuscipes*. The major vectors and their geographical distribution are listed in Table 73.1. The current distribution of sleeping sickness in Africa is shown in the map (Figure 73.2). Jordan[3] provides an up-to-date summary of *Glossina* biology and control.

Glossina spp. infest approximately 10 million km² or about one-third of the African continent. Sleeping sickness is endemic in 36 countries with a prevalence of 300 000 to 500 000 patients and over 50 000 new cases annually. These figures might be underestimates, particularly because surveillance has been reduced due to economic constraints, and priority has been given to other problems such as malaria and the HIV/AIDS epidemics. This situation was highlighted by the last World Health Organization (WHO) Expert Committee report.[4] The report details up-to-date country information in active foci of the disease and provides numbers of reported cases and recent documented trends. It is emphasized that current figures suffer from reduced surveillance in over 200 known foci, inadequate reporting when passive detection systems are used, shortage of trained personnel, and the logistic and financial constraints that prevent endemic foci from being surveyed regularly. Since the WHO report,[4] the continued deterioration of health services suggests that sleeping sickness will be an increasing public health problem. The number of deaths has been estimated in the World Health Report 2000 as 66 000 per year.[5] Death from sleeping sickness is inevitable if the disease is untreated. The economic and social impact of sleeping sickness has not been studied in great detail. However, the World Health Report 2000 calculated that the disability of adjusted life-years (DALYs) lost is 2.05×10^6 DALYs, combining healthy life-years lost through premature death with those of disability. This figure places African sleeping sickness as the third most important contributor to the global burden of parasitic disease after malaria (45 million) and lymphatic filariasis (4.9 million).

Biology

T. brucei subspecies trypanosomes of the subgenus *Trypanozoon* are morphologically indistinguishable. However, since the 1970s much research has been undertaken to find biochemical and molecular markers that might define clinical disease and epidemiology. The problems that these extensive studies have addressed are the identity and potential infectivity to humans of trypanosomes circulating in domestic and game animals, and those isolated from *Glossina*.

The morphology of *T. brucei* is described by Hoare[6] (Figure 73.3). Parasites are pleomorphic, extracellular in the blood and tissues, and vary in length from 12 to 42 µm; they have a small subterminal kinetoplast and a free flagellum. Parasite multiplication is impaired by specific antibodies produced by the host, resulting in a decrease in the parasitaemia. However, some parasites escape the immune response by the mechanism of antigenic variation, a mechanism that enables the trypanosomes to produce a surface coat composed of a different glycoprotein.[7] The result is a fluctuating parasitaemia with multiple progressive pathological changes, which vary in pattern and intensity with the different parasite strains and host.

T. brucei organisms are infective to laboratory animals: inoculation of infective material from human, animal reservoir and *Glossina* produces infection in a range of laboratory animals. *T. b. rhodesiense* can be propagated in mice, rats, rabbits and guinea pigs. However, *T. b. gambiense* infections are less infective and can be propagated only in the multimammate rat (*Mastomys natalensis*), *Grammomys* spp. (P. Büscher, personal communication) or in mice with severe combined immune deficiency (SCID).[8] *T. b. gambiense* in humans from some locations (in particular Cameroon) have not proved infective to a range of hosts. The development of a kit for in vitro isolation of trypanosomes, known as KIVI,[9] enables the isolation of procyclic (insect gut) forms and the characterization of such isolates using polymerase chain reaction (PCR), molecular and isoenzyme analysis. However, to study the human serum resistance or drug resistance, bloodstream forms are required. Those can be obtained only from procyclic forms after a full passage through the tsetse vector.[10]

It is generally recognized that *T. b. brucei* is the animal infective form of the subgenus *Trypanozoon*, which is not infective to humans because of its human serum sensitivity. *T. b. brucei* is lysed by human serum; this is associated with high-density lipoprotein molecules, which are

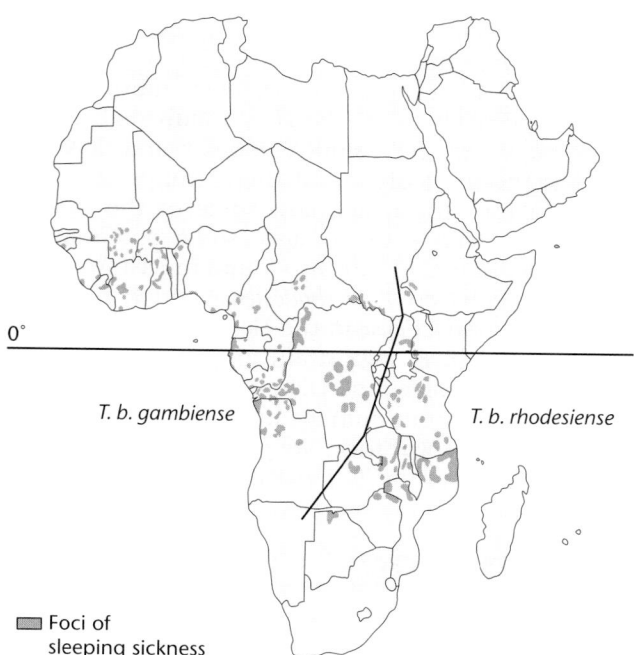

T. b. gambiense   T. b. rhodesiense

▭ Foci of
sleeping sickness

Figure 73.2: Distribution of human African trypanosomiasis. Reproduced with permission from the World Health Organization.[4]

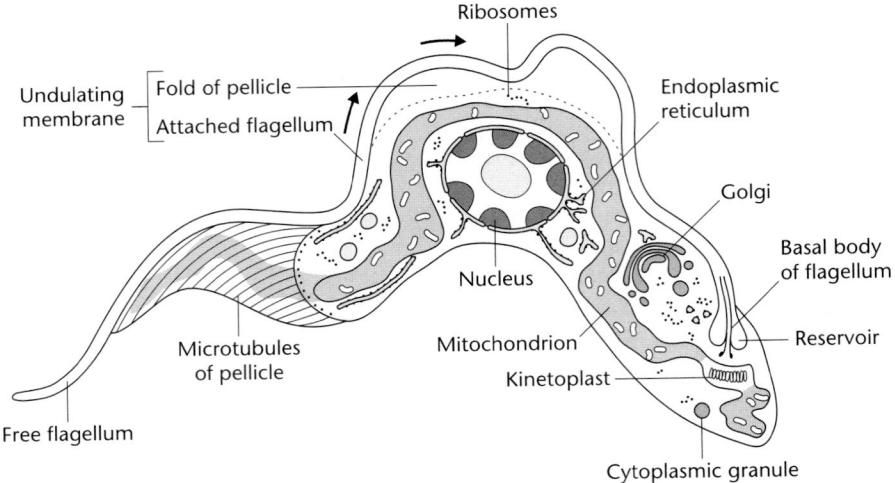

Figure 73.3: Morphology of *Trypanosoma brucei*. Reproduced with permission from Allen and Unwin.

trypanocidal.[11] The lytic effect of human serum was the basis for the development of the blood incubation infectivity test (BIIT).[12] This test involved incubation of trypanosomes in human serum before inoculation into rats. Potentially human-infective trypanosomes developed infection, whereas *T. b. brucei* was lysed by human serum and did not develop infection in recipient rats. The BIIT was modified for studies in *T. b. gambiense* by the use of *Mastomys natalensis* as a recipient animal because it is more easily infected with avirulent parasite stocks.[13] The most recent development of BIIT was by Jenni and Brun,[14] who introduced an in vitro test in which the viability of the test organism is compared in parallel cultures containing 20% human serum or 20% heat-inactivated horse serum as control. The method can detect single serum-resistant forms in a population of sensitive forms.

The analysis of parasite populations using modern technologies revealed the diversity and complexity of the trypanosomes infective to humans. The problem of understanding the relationships between different demes or populations has been compounded by the demonstration that *T. brucei* can hybridize in *Glossina* in the laboratory.[15] Markers for identification of parasite stocks in hybridization studies are isoenzymes and restriction fragment length polymorphisms of endonuclease-digested DNA. It could also be shown that human serum resistance can be passed on from a parent to the offspring of a cross *T. b. rhodesiense* × *T. b. brucei*.[16] Neither the frequency of hybridization in the wild nor its significance in terms of epidemiology and patterns of drug resistance is yet known.

These studies have provoked extensive discussion on the genetics of wild populations of parasites and the relative importance of clonality[17] and sexuality in such populations. The application and use of modern techniques in the epidemiology of trypanosomiasis are described by Gibson and Miles.[18] Extensive studies of nearly 1000 parasite stocks have been undertaken. Several reviews summarize the results[19,20] and attempts to reduce the number of enzymes used to identify sub-

species and strain groups.[21] Although there is a tendency to remain with *T. b. rhodesiense* and *T. b. gambiense* as nomenclature, it may be appropriate to consider recognizing strain groups if an association between geographical distribution, clinical features and particular zymodemes becomes apparent. Strain groups are made up of zymodemes characteristic of specific localities which, when subjected to numerical taxonomic analysis, cluster in dendrograms which provide an indication of the degree of genetic identity. The groupings proposed by Stevens and Godfrey[21] are corroborated by DNA methods,[18,22] while similar results were obtained using two different methods (the Jaccard coefficient and the Nei method) to construct a dendrogram of relationships. The groupings of the subgenus *Trypanozoon*, after over a decade of molecular and biomedical studies, suggest that *T. b. gambiense* and *T. evansi* (the equine and camel parasite) can be regarded as distinct subspecies and species respectively. *T. b. brucei* is subdivided into the strain groups 'bouaflé', 'sindo', 'kiboko' and 'kakumbi'. Bouaflé is the most diverse of these groups and is also found in West African animals. Some of the stocks of bouaflé are infective to humans, some potentially so; some isolates of bouaflé are also found in East Africa. The relationship between *T. b. rhodesiense* and *T. b. brucei* is complex. *T. b. rhodesiense* in the classical sense is divided into Zambezi and Busoga strain groups with characteristic isoenzyme profiles and DNA banding.[21] The Zambezi group of isolates from humans in Zambia is of relatively low virulence; Busoga stocks are from people in northern and central areas of the *T. b. rhodesiense* distribution.

Epidemiology
T. b. gambiense

T. b. gambiense is endemic throughout West and Central Africa, and is frequently associated with foci of infection,

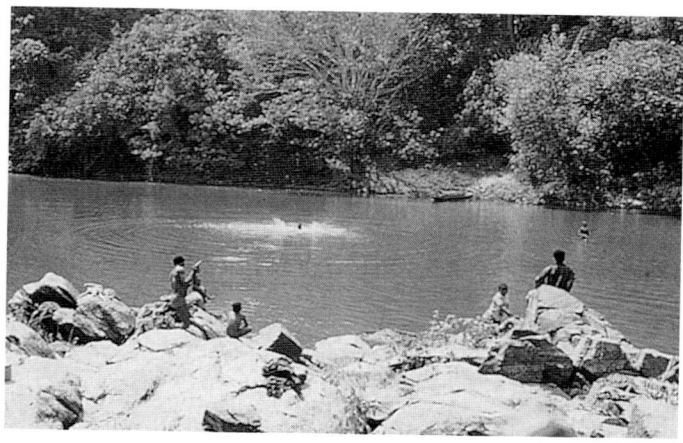

Figure 73.4: Typical site of transmission of *T. b. gambiense* where human–fly contact is high; habitat of *G. palpalis*.

which historically were recognized as areas where prevalence was often tenfold higher. Transmission of *T. b. gambiense* is associated with particular sites, usually near riverine vegetation, river crossings, water collection points, washing sites, sacred forests and villages adjacent to rivers or lakes (Figure 73.4). *T. b. gambiense* transmission is 'site associated', and intense transmission was considered to occur particularly at the end of the dry season when contact between humans and *G. palpalis* was most frequent. Flies require regular blood meals and humans are always available at these particular sites. In more humid forest regions, however, *G. palpalis* distribution is more widespread and hence transmission sites are less well localized. Human–fly contact is less intense and *Glossina* can live for several weeks. Once infected, a fly can transmit trypanosomes each time it bites; hence a single infected *Glossina* could infect many individuals at a particular site.

The most recent categorization of *T. b. gambiense* places this organism in a particular strain group. All isolates from humans in West and Central Africa in this group are comprised of six zymodemes (stocks with characteristic isoenzyme profiles). There are, however, chronic infections of humans from the Ivory Coast, the most sampled area, which are now placed in the bouaflé strain group and which belong to the same zymodeme as stocks isolated from a range of wild and domestic animals.[23] This suggests that classical *T. b. gambiense* of humans is not normally associated with animals. However, a pig isolate from Liberia and a sheep isolate from Congo are biochemically similar to *T. b. gambiense*, although a second 'non-gambiense' organism[24] causing chronic infections of humans with an animal reservoir also occurs in West Africa. Animal reservoirs of the bouaflé strain group, consisting of some 16 zymodemes, are pigs, dogs and cattle. Most isolations have been made from pigs. Game animal species that are hosts of bouaflé parasites are kob (*Kobus kob*) and hartebeest (*Alcelaphus buselaphus*); isolates of bouaflé have also been obtained from *G. palpalis*. Early experimental studies demonstrated that a range of domestic and wild animals was capable of being infected with isolates of *T. b. gambiense* from humans,

although the strain group to which these isolates belonged is not known. Recent decades have seen a considerable increase in our understanding of the complex interrelationships of the subgenus *Trypanozoon*. Earlier studies were handicapped by a lack of methods for parasite isolation and identification. Isoenzymes and DNA methods have provided a strong base for future detailed epidemiological studies, particularly using PCR, to identify precisely the strain group from small amounts of parasite material from humans, mammals or *Glossina*.

T. b. rhodesiense

The endemic situation

T. b. rhodesiense is the causative agent of the acute form of sleeping sickness. It is distributed from Uganda and Kenya in the northern part of East Africa to Botswana in the south. Recent biochemical and molecular studies have identified two main strain groups associated with acute sleeping sickness, Zambezi and Busoga, the strain groups representing the southern and northern limits of distribution respectively. Zambezi strains from Zambia and Malawi are often less virulent than the Busoga strain group.[25]

Sleeping sickness is endemic throughout eastern and south-eastern Africa, and humans are infected by the bite of *Glossina* spp. associated with woodland savannah habitats (Figure 73.5). The *G. morsitans* group, particularly *G. pallidipes* and *G. swynnertoni*, as well as *G. morsitans* itself, are the vectors; these species are preferentially bovid feeders and are not attracted to humans. Savannah *Glossina* spp. therefore feed on humans only when other hosts are not available. The classical view of the epidemiology of *T. b. rhodesiense* trypanosomiasis is that specific groups of people are more at risk of becoming infected—usually those whose activities or occupations bring them into more frequent contact with *Glossina*. Examples of such groups are honey gatherers, fishermen,

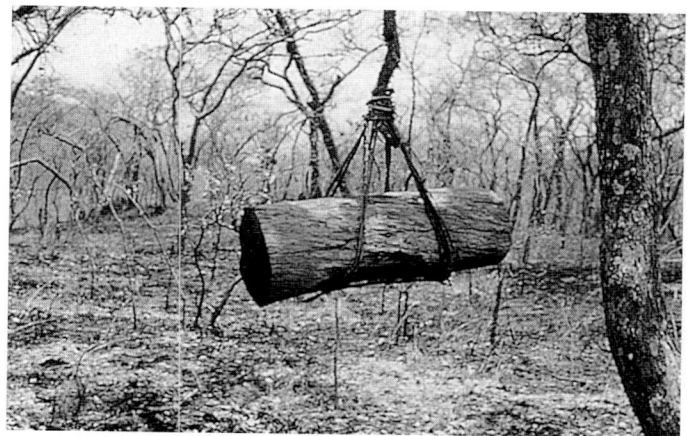

Figure 73.5: Savannah woodland in Malawi showing a beehive used by honey gatherers, who are regarded as a high-risk group because of frequent contact with *G. morsitans*.

game wardens, poachers and firewood collectors. *T. b. rhodesiense* is a zoonosis; the known reservoir hosts are domestic animals such as cattle, sheep and goat, and a variety of game animals including carnivores.[26] The difference between *T. b. brucei* and *T. b. rhodesiense* is the sensitivity or resistance to human serum. Responsible is a human serum resistance gene, which is coexpressed with the variant surface antigen in *T. b. rhodesiense* stocks.[27,28]

Analysis of the zymodemes of *T. brucei* from the Lambwe Valley, Kenya, by Cibulskis,[29] using a contingency table approach, has suggested that particular zymodemes are associated with particular mammalian hosts and that such relationships are stable, at least over a 32-month period. Earlier studies in this locality showed that the *T. brucei* population changed during the sleeping sickness outbreak in 1980,[30,31] showing that outbreaks arose from within the locality rather than through the introduction of strains from outside. In the context of the experimental finding of sexual recombination in *T. brucei*, Cibulskis[29] suggested that genetic exchange has an important role in the macroevolution of *T. brucei* populations. This view differs from that of Tibayrene et al.,[17] who consider sexual reproduction predominant in establishing clones stable in space and time.

Epidemic *T. b. rhodesiense*

Epidemics of acute disease have been observed over many decades, but most recently in Busoga, Uganda. This epidemic involved around 8000 cases per year in the mid-1980s but now is under control through a combination of interventions: intense surveillance, diagnosis and treatment, and vector control. The epidemic in Busoga was believed to be caused by a change in the agriculture of the area when cotton and coffee production ceased and the land was not cultivated, allowing the weed *Lantana camara* to become abundant. This shrub provided a suitable habitat for *G. f. fuscipes* to invade Busoga from the lakeside where it was characteristically found. A similar invasion of *G. f. fuscipes* occurred in Alego, Kenya,[32] and was associated with an earlier epidemic. In both of these epidemics cattle have been implicated as reservoir hosts.[30–32] Detailed analysis of zymodemes has allowed the characterization of these parasites into the strain group Busoga, with a smaller number of isolates belonging to the Zambezi strain group which is more characteristic of Zambia. *G. f. fuscipes* flies can be found in peridomestic situations in East Africa, associated with cattle and pigs as a reservoir. This situation parallels peridomestic populations of West African riverine flies where, in humid areas, peridomestic *G. palpalis* group flies are associated with domestic pig populations living close to or within villages.[33]

Transmission

T. brucei subspecies are transmitted to mammalian hosts by the bite of tsetse flies (*Glossina* spp.). A complex developmental cycle in the fly ends with the infective metacyclic stage in the lumen of the salivary glands (Figure 73.6). Metacyclic trypanosomes are injected into the skin of the mammalian host during the probing and feeding process. Development in the tsetse fly involves a complex series of changes in the morphology and biochemistry of the parasite. The factors influencing the development of the trypanosome in *Glossina* are complex. These mechanisms involve lectins present in *Glossina* midgut and haemolymph, the presence of *Rickettsia*-like organisms, and molecular signals that influence parasite transformation, establishment and maturation.[34] Lectins in the tsetse midgut kill incoming trypanosomes. Feeding lectin-inhibitory sugars or procyclin to flies significantly increased the midgut infection rates. While lectins are detrimental for the establishment of a midgut infection, the same lectins are required for maturation to the infective metacyclic stage. Female tsetse produce less salivary gland infections due to a product that is linked to the X gene. Knowledge of the parasite–vector interactions could eventually lead to novel control strategies to interrupt transmission.

The possibility of mechanical (non-cyclical) transmission by biting insects or *Glossina* has been suggested, although there is only circumstantial evidence to support the idea. Mechanical transmission has been suggested as the reason for the clustering of cases in a household or where cases are found outside the normal range of *Glossina*.

Diagnosis

A sequential approach for diagnosis of *T. b. gambiense* sleeping sickness is generally followed: suspected cases detected by serological methods (usually the card agglutination test for trypanosomiasis; CATT) undergo parasitological diagnosis by investigation of the blood and/or lymph (Figure 73.7). In case of a positive result, examination of the CSF has to follow for stage determination.[4]

T. b. rhodesiense is usually directly detected in the blood.

Immunodiagnostic methods

The most frequently used test for mass screening for *T. b. gambiense* sleeping sickness is the CATT.[35] This is a serological test which uses a reagent composed of stained freeze-dried trypanosomes of selected variable antigen types (VATs), which can be obtained from the Institute of Tropical Medicine, Antwerp, Belgium. The CATT is an agglutination test of high sensitivity and specificity, and is easy to perform in the field. A drop of heparinized whole blood is mixed with a drop of the reagent on a card and, in the presence of specific antibodies, the trypanosomes in the reagent will agglutinate. It is inexpensive and results are obtained within 5 minutes.[4]

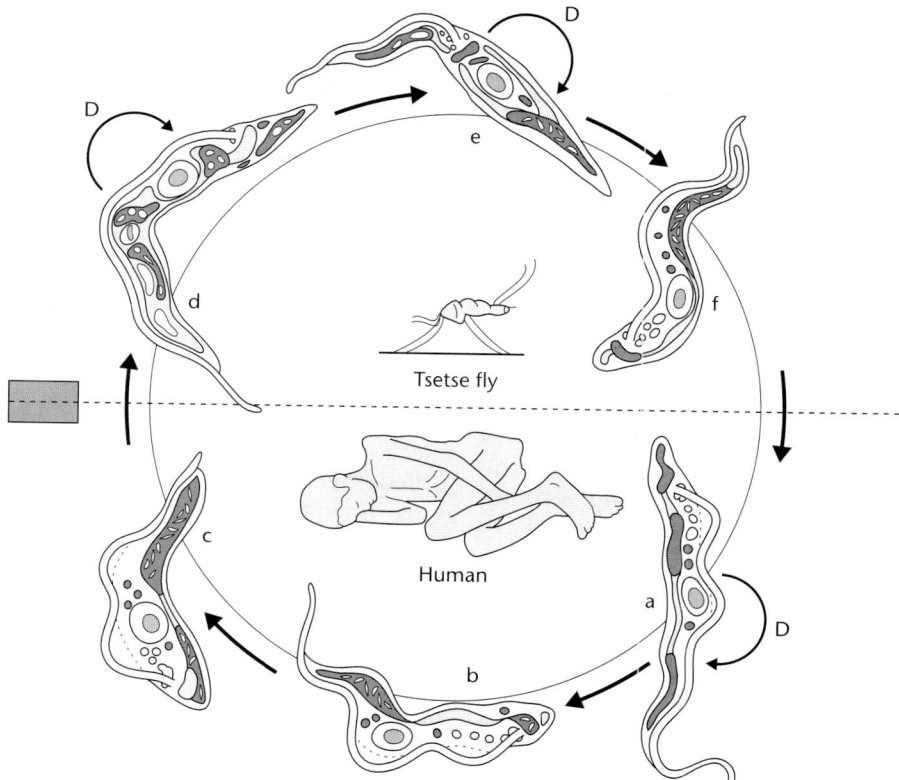

Figure 73.6: Cycle of *T. brucei* spp. showing the different morphological forms in the human and in the tsetse fly. In the blood and lymphatic system of humans (**a**) slender, (**b**) intermediate and (**c**) short stumpy forms are present. Stumpy forms differentiate in the fly midgut to (**d**) procyclic forms, then to (**e**) epimastigote forms and finally in the salivary glands to (**f**) infective metacyclic forms. Bloodstream forms (a–c) and metacyclic forms are covered by the variable surface glycoprotein (VSG) coat. D indicates the capability to undergo cell division. Reproduced from Brun R. Sleeping sickness in Africa; on the rise again. *Karger Gazette* 1999; 63:5–7, with permission from Karger, Basle.

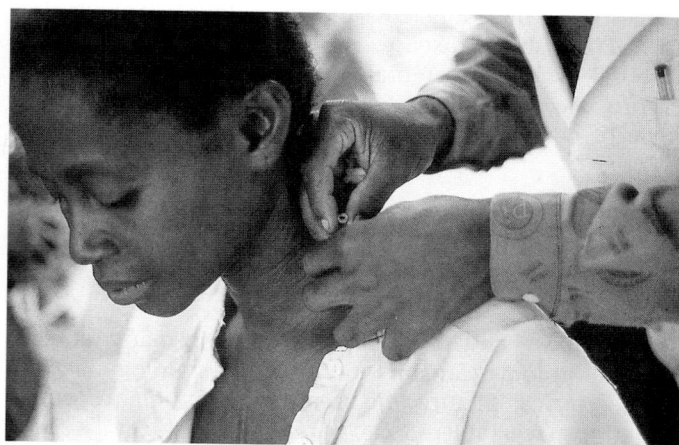

Figure 73.7: Lymph node aspiration for diagnosis. Source: J. Blum (Swiss Tropical Institute); Vanga, Democratic Republic of Congo.

the use of serial dilutions of patient serum, and specificity by the addition of ethylenediamine tetra-acetic acid (EDTA).[36]

Alternative tests, such as the card indirect antigen test for trypanosomiasis (CIATT), in which specific antibodies are coupled to latex beads and used to trap antigens in serum or whole blood,[37] or the rapid latex agglutination test (LATEX/*T. b. gambiense*) for detection of antibodies against *T. b. gambiense* in which the reagent is coated with a mixture of three variable surface antigens of bloodstream-form trypanosomes,[38] have recently been proposed. The results on the performance of these tests are ambiguous and they will be further evaluated.

For laboratory use other methods, such as immuno-fluorescence (IF), indirect haemagglutination (IHA), enzyme-linked immunosorbent assay (ELISA) and different PCR methods, have been described.

Parasitological methods

Serological indication of a trypanosome infection alone does not justify treatment because of the relative toxicity of all drugs in use. Therefore, the detection of the parasite is of great importance.

Use of the CATT has considerably increased the detection rate in active surveys compared with the sole use of parasitological assays. No such test exists presently for *T. b. rhodesiense*, although parasite detection in the blood is much easier in this form of the disease. Refinements of the CATT allowed a considerable increase in specificity by

The body fluids that are most commonly examined for the presence of trypanosomes are blood, lymph node aspirates and CSF. Trypanosomes may also be detected in bone marrow aspirates and ascites fluid.

Different techniques are used for diagnosis in blood:

- Blood films (thin, thick or wet) can be used for direct detection of trypanosomes. Wet blood films are used for the detection of motile trypanosomes, whereas thin and thick blood films are fixed in methanol and Giemsa stained.
- Concentration methods increase the chances for detection of the parasite because the parasitaemia, especially in *T. b. gambiense* infections, is usually very low.
- The microhaematocrit centrifugation technique (m-HCT)[39] is based on microscopic examination of the buffy coat zone of blood cells using a long working distance objective following centrifugation in microhaematocrit capillaries. This method is used widely in the field.
- The miniature anion-exchange centrifugation technique (m-AECT)[40] is based on the detection of trypanosomes in the eluate after the passage of infected blood through an anion-exchange (diethylaminoethyl cellulose) column followed by centrifugation in microhaematocrit capillaries. This method has proven to be more sensitive under field conditions than other methods.
- The quantitative buffy coat (QBC) technique, originally developed for the diagnosis of malaria, uses a glass haematocrit tube precoated with acridine orange and anticoagulant.[41] A float forces the sedimentation of red blood cells on centrifugation. Motile fluorescent trypanosomes are found in the buffy coat around the float.
- For analysis of the lymph, a wet preparation of the aspirate from enlarged lymph nodes is examined at a magnification of 400×.[4]
- In vivo inoculation of biological material from humans, animal hosts or vectors into susceptible animals has been used to detect trypanosomes. Mice and rats are used for detecting *T. b. rhodesiense*, whereas *Mastomys natalensis*, guinea pigs and suckling rats should preferably be used for *T. b. gambiense*.
- In vitro culture systems can be used for isolating trypanosomes from infected patients.

Determination of the stage of the disease

Chemotherapy, especially the use of melarsoprol for second-stage disease, bears a significant risk. Therefore, a correct determination of the stage is crucial before commencing treatment.

Examination of the CSF is used to determine the stage of the disease. Parasites can sometimes be seen during white cell counting, but detection after concentration by single or, better, double centrifugation is substantially more sensitive.

The criteria for second-stage infection are: trypanosomes found in the CSF and/or a raised leucocyte count of more than 5 cells/mm^3. This cut-off is similar to that currently used in neurology.[4] Recent findings indicated that infections of up to 20 cells/mm^3 may be treated with the first-stage drug pentamidine with only a minor increase in the relapse rate.[42] Based on these results Angola has changed the national criteria for second-stage treatment accordingly. Results of large-scale application are awaited.

An increased protein content of the CSF was used as an additional criterion for staging, but due to the frequent lack of materials, variability of the results and the lesser predictive value compared with white blood cell counting, this method is only rarely used today.

A recently published latex agglutination field test for quantification of immunoglobulin (Ig) M in CSF may, when fully evaluated, become useful for determination of the stage.[43]

Differential diagnosis

Owing to the many clinical variations of sleeping sickness, it is difficult to describe a 'typical' case of the disease; differential diagnosis might therefore be of unusual importance. In first-stage human African trypanosomiasis, other causes of protracted febrile illness such as drug-resistant malaria, typhoid fever and viral hepatitis should be considered. The prominent lymphadenopathy can be suggestive of mononucleosis or tuberculous lymphadenitis. In second-stage disease, syphilitic meningomyelitis, cerebral tumour, cerebral tuberculosis, HIV-associated cryptococcal meningitis and chronic viral encephalitis must be considered.

Clinical symptoms and signs

T. b. gambiense and *T. b. rhodesiense* differ in many respects, such as biology, transmission and epidemiology, as well as the clinical picture and treatment of their respective infections (see Table 73.2).

T. b. gambiense

T. b. gambiense infections run a chronic course of years from infection to extensive nervous system involvement and the classical picture of sleeping sickness. The symptoms and signs described in the literature, especially for second-stage disease, vary considerably. This is in part explainable by the largely varying status of the patient at hospital admission, which depends on the social status of

Table 73.2 Differences between *T. b. gambiense* and *T. b. rhodesiense* sleeping sickness. Adapted after[45].

	West African (Gambian)	East African (Rhodesian)
Parasite	*T. b. gambiense*	*T. b. rhodesiense*
Main vectors	*G. palpalis* group	*G. morsitans* group
Main habitat	Near water	Savannah, cleared bush
Highest incidence	Congo (DRC), Angola, South Sudan, North Uganda	South-east Uganda, Tanzania
Main reservoir	Humans Pig, dog	Antelope and cattle
Disease type	Chronic (years)	Acute (months)
Parasitemia	Low	Moderate
Diagnosis	Lymph node aspiration CSF (lumbar puncture)	Blood CSF (lumbar puncture)
Serology	CATT	None
Treatment		
Early stage	Pentamidine	Suramin
Late stage	Melarsoprol	Melarsoprol
Alternative treatment	Eflornithine Melarsoprol & Eflornithine Melarsoprol & Nifurtimox	Melarsoprol & Nifurtimox
Disease control	Active case search & Tsetse trapping	Tsetse trapping

the local population, nutrition and transport facilities, and the virulence of the trypanosome strain. A typical list of signs and symptoms observed is given in Table 73.3.

First-stage illness

The incubation period is usually 2–3 weeks. The onset of the disease is very unspecific; the only sign may be irregular fever, varying in cycles of one to several days and not responding to antimalarials. This scheme reflects the stimulation of the immune system by changing variant surface glycoproteins (VSGs; see Immunopathology). Lymphadenopathy, headache, myalgia, fatigue and general malaise may accompany this phase. The initial phase may be followed by a relatively asymptomatic phase lasting for several months to, sometimes, a few years.

The posterior cervical lymph nodes are enlarged in as many as 85% of hospitalized patients (classic Winterbottom's sign) (Figure 73.8). Pruritus and transient oedema (mostly of the face) are also frequently observed (Figure 73.9). Cutaneous eruptions of the papulo-erythematous type may be found, but are very difficult to spot on the trunk of dark-skinned individuals, and generally resolve spontaneously.

With progress of the disease, the symptoms associated with the waves of parasitaemia become less frequent, and parasites become difficult to find in the blood. Endocrine dysfunctions occur at a more advanced phase and may manifest as amenorrhoea, reduced libido, impotence and a high abortion rate. Profound anaemia is another feature that may be observed at this stage of infection.

Table 73.3 Typical symptoms and signs of *T. b. gambiense* sleeping sickness. Compiled from data of 500 late-stage patients enrolled in a controlled clinical trial on sleeping sickness treatment with melarsoprol in Angola[69].

	n/N[1]	%
Lymphadenopathy	425	85.0
Headache	349	69.8
General motor weakness	256	51.2
Menstruation absent[2]	66/214	30.8
Diurnal somnolence	143	28.6
Nocturnal insomnia	143	28.6
Aggressiveness	116	23.2
Tremors	95	19.0
Pruritus	87	17.4
Disturbed appetite	51	10.2
Unusual behaviour	48	9.6
Fever (temp. > 37.5°C)	47	9.4
Hepatomegaly	35	7.0
Abnormal movements[3]	29	5.8
Splenomegaly	25	5.0
Epileptiform attacks[4]	14	2.8
Impaired speech	7	1.4
Inability to walk unaided	6	1.2

[1]If not indicated N is 500
[2]Considers only women who have not yet reached menopause
[3]Preventing the patient from performing daily tasks
[4]History reported by patient

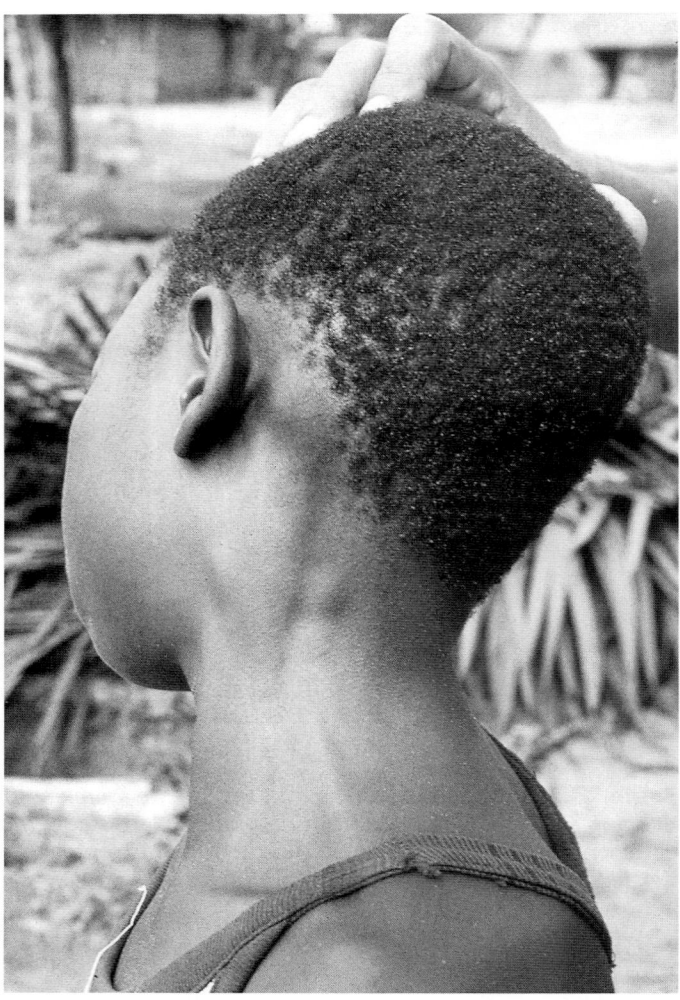

Figure 73.8: Winterbottom's sign; enlarged cervical lymph nodes in a patient with *T. b. gambiense* infection. Source: J. Blum (Swiss Tropical Institute); Vanga, Democratic Republic of Congo.

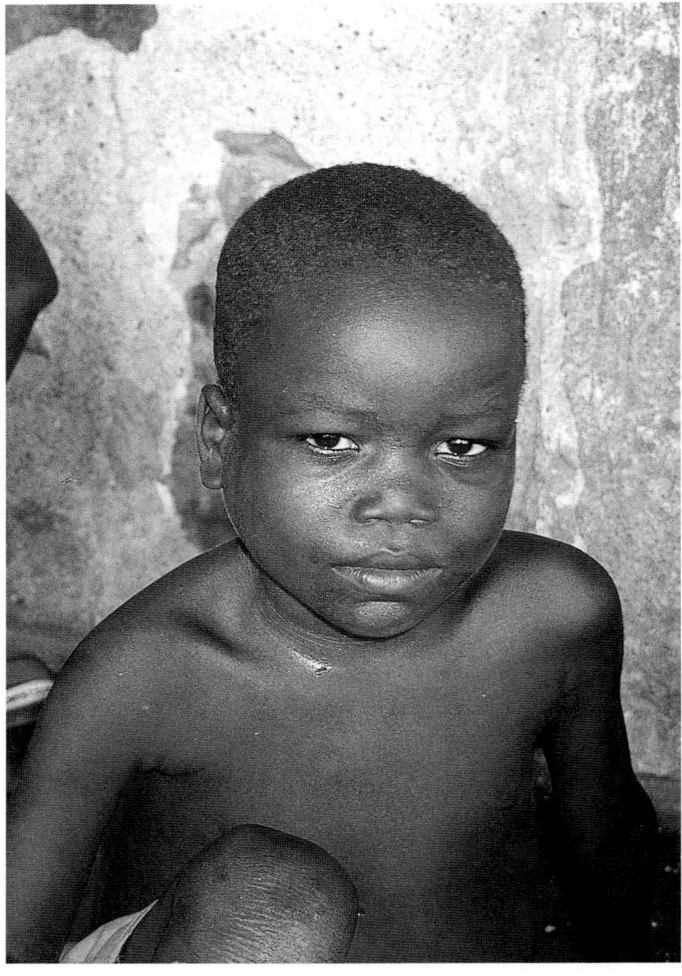

Figure 73.9: Facial oedema in a patient with first-stage *T. b. gambiense* infection. Source: C. Burri (Swiss Tropical Institute); Dondo, Angola.

Second-stage illness

Invasion of the trypanosomes into the CNS marks the onset of the second stage of the infection. It occurs first in the least protected areas such as the choroid plexus, thalamus, area postrema, median eminence, and pineal and hypophysal regions. This localization may explain in part the principal clinical and neurological signs observed.

The second stage is the result of a chronic meningo-encephalitis, with characteristic symptoms such as progressive mental deterioration proceeding to coma.

The interval between the start of the infection and the second, encephalitic, stage is in the order of several months to 2 years, but much longer periods have been observed. The average duration of this stage is from 4 months to 1 year.

Headaches become constant and may be unresponsive to analgesics. Motor functions become seriously impaired, and the patient may only be able to walk aided. Speech becomes slurred and abnormal movements and tremor occur; the picture may resemble Parkinsonism. At this stage mental changes of considerable variation may become obvious. The pattern ranges from basic lethargy with bouts of mania, to delirium, paranoia, aggressive behaviour and schizoid attacks. Involvement of sleep-regulating regions such as the thalamus, area postrema, median eminence and the pineal region cause sleep derangements characteristic for *T. b. gambiense* infection. They are generally described as daytime somnolence and sometimes restlessness at night. However, recent investigations have shown that the total sleeping duration of the subject remains unchanged, while the sleep cycles are divided, shorter and spread out over 24 hours.[44] Patients are is generally indifferent to activities going on around them (Figure 73.10). General pruritus and bedsores are a frequent feature at this stage, as well as weight loss and substantial wasting. It is generally accepted that sleeping sickness is ultimately fatal in all patients, if left untreated. The patient finally becomes comateous and will die,

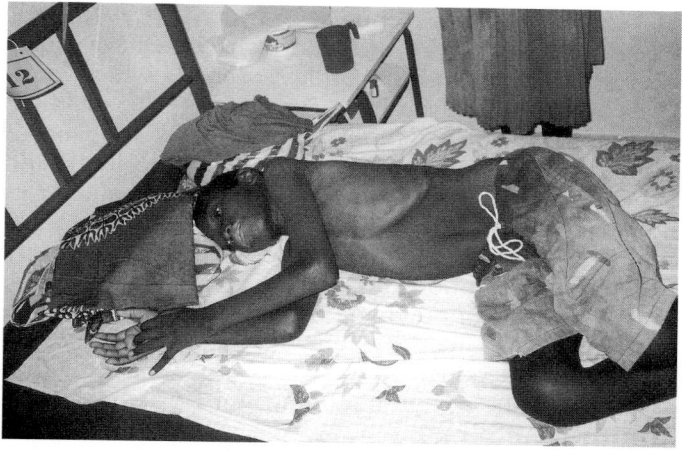

Figure 73.10: Patient with late-stage *T. b. gambiense* infection.
Source: C. Burri (Swiss Tropical Institute); Viana, Angola.

often from bacterial superinfections such as aspiration pneumonia. Most of the neurological signs described above remain reversible with treatment for a long time, confirming the predominance of potentially reversible inflammatory processes over destructive lesions.

T. b. rhodesiense

The East African form of the disease is a much more acute infection: the incubation period, the early stage, and the late stage with CNS involvement develop over a few weeks.

First-stage illness

An inoculation chancre, which often remains invisible in Africans, develops 5–15 days after the bite. It is a painful, circumscribed, indurated dusky-red papule 2–5 cm in diameter, which disappears after 2–3 weeks. Regional lymphadenopathy or adjacent cellulitis occurs. Fever and parasitaemia appear hours to days later or, in the absence of a chancre, within 1–3 weeks of the infective bite.[45] Generally, the parasites are far more numerous in the blood than in the *gambiense* form of the disease. Cervical lymphadenopathy (Winterbottom's sign) is less common than in Gambian human African trypanosomiasis, but submandibular, axillary or inguinal lymph nodes may be enlarged. Keratitis and conjunctivitis have been observed.

Second-stage illness

The disease progresses much more rapidly than for *T. b. gambiense*, causing the death of the patient within 6–9 months. Symptoms and signs of CNS involvement may be absent, except for drowsiness and tremors. Pericardial effusion and congestive heart failure have been described in *T. b. rhodesiense* infection, and in one-third of patients abnormal electrocardiograms were found.[46]

Pathology and pathogenesis

Sleeping sickness produces multiple pathological changes that involve most organs and systems. The changes are progressive and their anatomy, histology, physiology, biochemistry and immunology have been described extensively. The damage results from a complex interplay of factors between the different systems.

Pathology

A local inflammatory response with oedema and mononuclear infiltration occurs at the site of infection. The trypanosomes then spread to the lymphatic system and glands, and to the bloodstream. The lymph glands become enlarged and trypanosomes can be found in lymph gland aspirates. Microscopically the follicles are enlarged with prominent reactive centres and many plasma cells in the sinuses. The main feature of the pathological change is a vasculitis.

The spleen is slightly enlarged. The malpighian follicles are few and inconspicuous. There is a general proliferation of the reticuloendothelium, congestion at the periphery of the splenic sinuses, often focal necrosis with endothelial macrophages and ingested red corpuscles.

The liver may be slightly enlarged in some cases; there is infiltration with mononuclear cells in the periportal tracts and microscopical mononuclear cell granulomas.

In *T. b. rhodesiense* infections there is a pancarditis involving all layers of the heart including mural and valvular endocardium. In experimental infections in monkeys, myocarditis with trypanosomes in the interstitial tissues, especially the endocardium, was observed. Histologically there is a marked interstitial infiltration with plasma and morular cells, with disappearance of muscle fibres and fibrosis.

Proliferative glomerulonephritis leading to fibrosis has been observed.

The bone marrow is hypercellular with areas of gelatinous degeneration.

The lesions in the lungs are characterized by intravascular proliferation of the reticuloendothelium, which may block the capillaries with fibrosis, and collapse of the alveoli.

Localized oedema due to collections of lymphocytes may be observed in the eyelids, perineum and the skin of the back.

Typical pathological lesions of the CNS are seen only after invasion of the trypanosomes. No gross lesions of the nerve centres are present, but there is progressive chronic leptomeningitis, especially in the Virchow–Robin spaces (where the pia sheathes the blood vessels and the fluid acts as lymph) and also on the vertex (Dürck's nodes).

The dura may be adherent to the skull and to the arachnoid. The brain itself is congested and oedematous, the surface smooth, with convolutions flattened by increased pressure. The consistency of the brain tissues is unaltered except for softening around any haemorrhages that may occur. The ventricles are distended with fluid. In all cases there is perivascular round-cell infiltration (perivascular cuffing) throughout the brain tissue and meninges, varying in amount and in different anatomical regions. The invading cells are glia cells, lymphocytes, the morular (Mott) and Marhalko cells. The two latter types are degenerative plasmocytes. Trypanosomes have been found in the brain, mainly in frontal lobe, pons and medulla. Demyelination and neuronal damage have been described. The organisms also invade the CSF, which they enter by the canal from the choroidal plexus.[46]

Patients have markedly altered plasma albumin: globulin ratios; the macroglobulinaemia is characteristic of both the Gambian and Rhodesian forms. The increases are highest for IgM with the first parasitaemia, whereas IgG responses are not so marked. This is followed by a progressive suppression, which is selective for the IgG production, with IgM levels remaining high. Another obvious change in plasma is the increase in total lipid content, which in rabbits may be up to four times that of uninfected animals. Large amounts of cholesterol and β-lipoprotein(s) are present, together with increased amounts of free fatty acids (e.g., linoleic, oleic, palmitic and stearic). Disturbances of other plasma constituents (e.g., decrease of calcium and bicarbonate, increase of phosphate, urea and creatinine levels) indicate renal damage. Gross pathological changes to the kidney are not a usual feature of patients with sleeping sickness, but glomerulonephritis has been observed in experimental animals.

The aetiology of the anaemia in sleeping sickness is multifactorial, with haemolysis, haemodilution and disordered and/or non-compensatory erythropoiesis having continued with variable contributions during the infection. Haemolysis is largely responsible, with phagocytosis of red cells that have become coated with immune complexes in the spleen sinusoids and by the Kupffer cells of the liver. The haemolysis may also result in part from haemolytic factors liberated by trypanosomes. As infection progresses the blood and plasma volumes become progressively enlarged, thus causing a haemodilution effect. Red cell production by the bone marrow is significantly reduced. The defect here is associated with a failure of iron incorporation into the red cell precursors, with a large excess of storage iron not employed for haemoglobin synthesis.

Patients may also have a moderate leucocytosis; differential counts regularly show monocytosis, lymphocytosis and plasmacytosis, and large Mott morular cells may also be found.

Blood homeostasis becomes seriously disturbed. The disease is commonly associated with minor haemorrhages and multiple petechiae, although these are rarely sufficiently severe to be life threatening. The pathogenesis is associated with vascular injury, coagulopathy with increased fibrinolysis, and thrombocytopenia. The coagulopathy is most common in acute *T. b. rhodesiense* disease and consists of thrombosis, haemorrhage, tissue necrosis and microangiopathic anaemia, which have been attributed to the condition termed disseminated intravascular coagulation. Fibrinogen and fibrin degradation products are present at increased levels and may be detected in the urine if there is renal damage. In both types of the disease there are decreased platelet numbers, platelet clumping and altered aggregatory responses. In addition the blood becomes hyperviscous. The mechanisms underlying those complex changes are not well investigated.[47]

A recent detailed summary of the pathology of sleeping sickness can be found in Kristensson and Bentivoglioi.[48]

Immunopathology

The major protein on the surface of bloodstream trypanosomes is the variant surface glycoprotein (VSG). Approximately 10^7 molecules of a single VSG are normally found on the surface of one parasite, protecting invariant constituents of its outer membrane from the immune system. Each parasite genotype contains a repertoire of more than 100 (*T. b. gambiense*) to 1000 (*T. b. rhodesiense*) different VSG genes, distributed throughout the genome as basic copy genes. At any time, only a single VSG gene is actively transcribed at a telomeric expression site. Antigenic conversion may happen by three main processes: (1) duplicative transposition (gene conversion), (2) reciprocal recombination (non-duplicative transposition) and (3) in situ telomeric activation by rearrangement of upstream promoters. Variant antigen switching occurs in a spontaneous non-programmed manner at a rate of 10^{-4} to 10^{-5} per cell division.

The primary component of the antibody response to VSG is a T cell-independent IgM response. However, T cell-dependent B-cell responses are also involved in eliciting VSG-specific IgG. The VSG coat on intact trypanosomes acts as a T cell-independent antigen, while non-variant buried T-cell epitopes are presented to T cells only after phagocytosis of dying or opsonized trypanosomes. This T cell-mediated response plays a significant role in the cytokine response profile in trypanosome infections. In conclusion, the successive peaks of the recurring parasitaemia are due to trypanosomes expressing immunologically different VSGs.[49]

The immune responses to a trypanosome infection are dominated by two main phenomena: a prominent non-specific polyclonal activation of B cells and a generalized suppression of some humoral (B cell) and cellular (T cell) immune functions. The polyclonal B-cell activation results in a large production of IgM, not directed solely to VSG and other trypanosome antigens, but also against the proteins and nucleic acids of the host. In the CNS, autoantibodies against nervous tissue elements, such as myelin basic protein, cerebrosides and gangliosides, have been reported.[50] Increased major histocompatibility complex (MHC) class II expression, nitric oxide and prostaglandin (PG) E_2 production are characteristics typical of macrophage activation, and suppressor macrophages were found to be closely associated with the occurrence of immunosuppression. However, an array of other factors is also involved in a complex interplay. Tumour necrosis factor (TNF) α is released in significant quantities and may cause the pronounced loss of weight and cachexia during the course of trypanosome infection. A macrophage-activating factor that is significantly upregulated during infections in rodent models and humans is interferon (IFN) γ, produced mainly by CD4+ and CD8+ cells.[49] The CD8+ T-cell population is activated directly by a trypanosomal factor, the trypanosome-derived lymphocyte triggering factor (TLTF), which is a 42–45-kDa polypeptide of which the gene sequence was recently identified.[51] In contrast to TNFα, which has been found to be inhibitory to the growth of trypanosomes, IFNγ has a proliferative effect on trypanosomes, and it was proposed to be a component of a bidirectional pathway in which TLTF triggers CD8+ cells to release IFNγ. There is evidence for the synthesis of nitric oxide by activated macrophages, and it was suggested to be significantly involved in immunosuppression. However, its growth inhibiting effect on trypanosomes found in vitro may not play a role in vivo because of the protective effect of haemoglobins in the blood, which acts as a sink for nitric oxide. The cytokine interactions during trypanosome infection are depicted in Figure 73.11.

Another, as yet uncharacterized, trypanosome-secreted factor, trypanosomal macrophage-activating factor (TMAF), was recently shown directly to co-stimulate macrophage activation in the presence of IFNγ.[49]

The processes in the CNS are not fully understood. Astrocyte activation is a known feature of late-stage sleeping sickness, and attention has been given to the involvement of cells that are involved in the control of inflammatory responses in nervous tissue. Astrocytes are capable of secreting an array of cytokines, prostaglandins and mediator substances, but the detailed role has yet to be established. An increased expression of TNFα, interleukin (IL) 1 and IL-4 has been reported in a murine model.[52] In humans IL-1 was not increased significantly, but high levels of one of the major sleep-regulating substances, PGD_2, as well as PGE_2 and PGF_2, were reported.[53]

Recently, the early production by rat astrocytes and resident microglia brain cells of chemokines—macrophage inflammatory protein (MIP) 2, RANTES (regulated on activation normal T cell expressed and secreted), MIPα and monocyte chemotactic protein (MCP) 1—after infection with trypanosomes was demonstrated.[54] Based on their functions as chemoattractants of diverse cell types, it was speculated that these mediators were involved in the attraction of infiltrating cells from the circulation to the brain. This finding supports the view that astrocyte activation precedes the inflammatory process in the brain and is not a secondary process.

Detailed summaries on the immunology, immuno-pathology, involvement of cytokines and hormonal changes during the course of sleeping sickness have been published.[49,53,55–57]

Management of sleeping sickness

Treatment of first stage

The use of trypanocidal drugs that do not cross the blood–brain barrier sufficiently to reach adequate drug levels in CSF to eliminate trypanosomes in this compartment is limited to the first stage of the disease. Drugs restricted to this phase are pentamidine and suramin.

Pentamidine

Pentamidine, introduced in 1940, became the drug of first choice for first-stage *gambiense* sleeping sickness. Cure rates are 93–98% and have not decreased over the decades.[4] Failures in *Rhodesiense* sleeping sickness, however, are quite frequent.[58]

The most commonly used dosage regimen is pentamidine isethionate 4 mg per kg body weight daily or on alternate days, so that seven to ten injections are given. Because of the frequent occurrence of hypotension after intravenous application, the drug is usually given as deep intramuscular injection in the treatment of sleeping sickness.

Generally, pentamidine is well tolerated, although minor adverse reactions are common. Immediate adverse drug reactions include hypotension in about 10% of the patients, with dizziness, sometimes collapse and shock; after intravenous injection the frequency of a hypotensive reaction can be as high as 75%. Other adverse drug reactions occasionally observed are nausea and/or vomiting, and pain. Sterile abscesses or necroses may occur at the site of intramuscular injection. Systemic reactions reported include acotaemia due to a nephrotoxic effect, leucopenia, abnormal findings in liver function tests, and hypoglycaemia and hyperglycaemia. Persistent manifestation of diabetes is a rare, but feared, event.[59] In Africa about 1% of the patients die in temporal relation with pentamidine treatment; the precise cause of death is usually difficult to determine.[45]

The maximum plasma levels in patients treated for *T. b. gambiense* with 10 intramuscular injections of pentamidine methanesulfonate were generally reached within 1 hour after injection and varied extensively (214–6858 ng/ml). The median plasma concentration after the last dose was about five times higher than after the first. The median half-life associated with the first, second and third phase of elimination was 4 minutes, 6.5 hours and 512 hours, respectively.[60] Pentamidine is converted to at least seven primary metabolites by the cytochrome P-450-dependent oxygenases in rat liver homogenates and rat liver microsomes.[61]

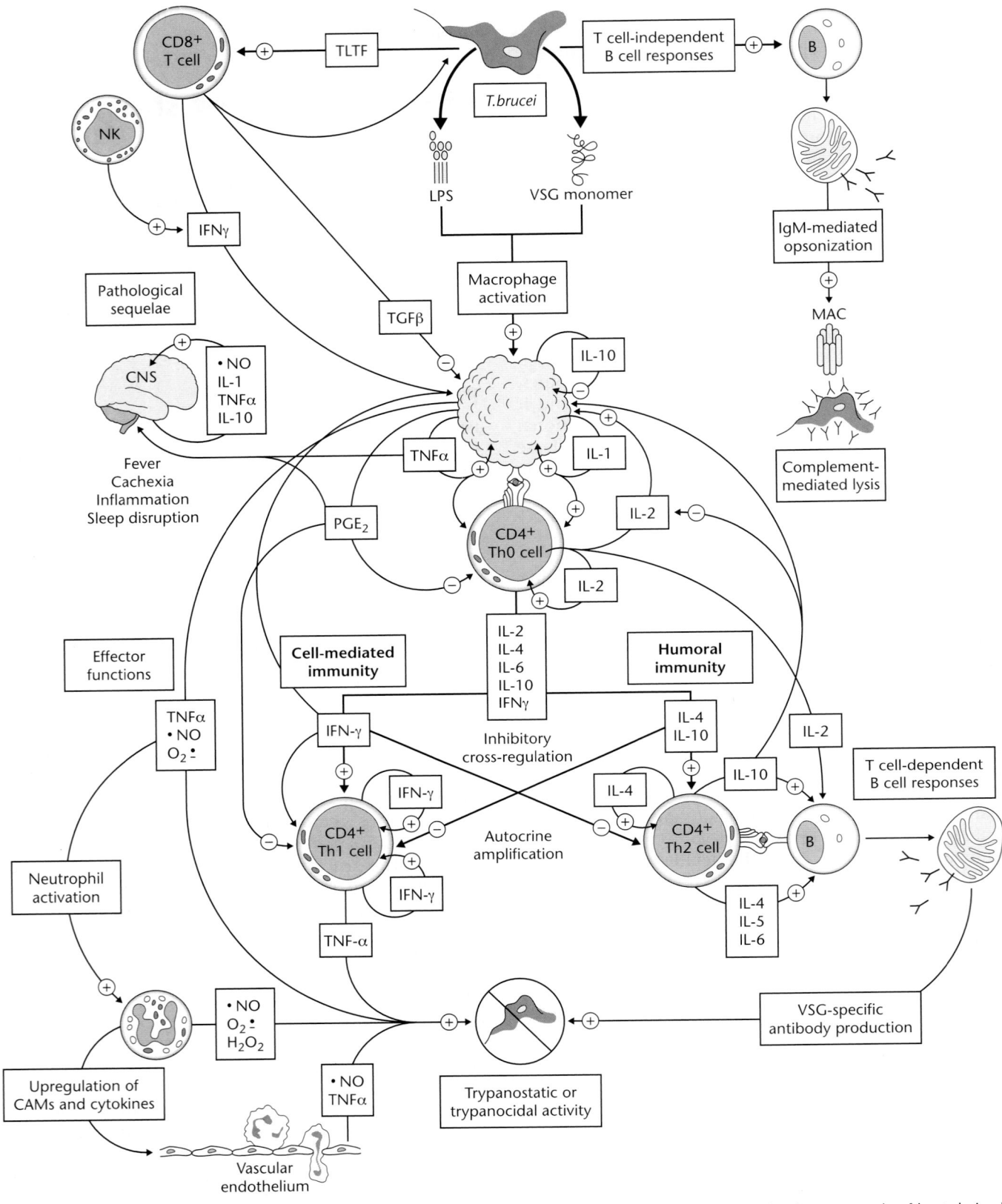

Figure 73.11: Activation of the cytokine network during African trypanosomiasis infections. Trypanosomes stimulate a cascade of host-derived cytokines by IFNγ-activated macrophages (MΦ) and T helper (Th) cell subsets. Both specific and non-specific defences are activated and can lead to host protection or pathology. B, B cell; H_2O_2, hydrogen peroxide; IFN, interferon; Ig, immunoglobulin; IL, interleukin; NO, nitric oxide; PGE_2, prostaglandin E_2; O_2^-, superoxide; TLTF, trypanosome-released lymphocyte triggering factor; TNF, tumour necrosis factor; VSG, variable surface glycoprotein; +, stimulation; –, inhibition. Reproduced from Rhind and Shek,[56] with permission from Springer, Paris.

The mode of action is unknown. Binding to nucleic acids, disruption of kinetoplast DNA, inhibition of RNA editing in trypanosomes, and inhibition of messenger RNA trans-splicing have been suggested to be involved.[62]

Suramin

Suramin was introduced in 1920 in Germany for the treatment of trypanosomiasis. It is effective against the first stage of both forms of the disease, but pentamidine is generally preferred today for treatment of *T. b. gambiense*.

The most commonly used dosage regimen consists of a test dose of suramin 4–5 mg per kg body weight on day 1, followed by five injections of 20 mg per kg body weight of suramin every 7 days (e.g., days 3, 10, 17, 24, 31).[4] The maximum dose per injection is 1 g. Suramin is injected intravenously after dilution in distilled water. Intramuscular injection is very irritant.

Some degree of kidney damage is common, but nephrotoxicity is usually mild and reversible.[63] The first symptoms of renal impairment are albuminuria, later cylinduria and haematuria. Regular urine checks during the course of treatment are therefore recommended. Other adverse drug reactions reported are early hypersensitivity reactions such as nausea, circulatory collapse and urticaria, and late hypersensitivity reactions such as exfoliative dermatitis and haemolytic anaemia, peripheral neuropathy, and bone marrow toxicity with agranulocytosis, thrombocytopenia. Pruritus is more frequent with concomitant filariasis.

Some 99.7% of the drug is bound to plasma proteins (e.g., albumin, globulins, fibrinogen), which places suramin in the class of the most extensively bound drugs. Consequently suramin has one of the longest half-lives of all drugs given to humans. In patients with HIV/AIDS who were given suramin once weekly for 5 weeks, the drug accumulated during the time of administration and then diminished, with a half-life of 44–54 days. Total plasma levels remained above 100 µg/ml for several weeks. The volume of distribution was 38–46 litres, and total clearance was less than 0.5 ml/min.[64] The renal clearance contributed essentially to the removal of the drug from the body.

Suramin inhibits, rather non-specifically, numerous enzymes including L-α-glycerophosphate oxidase, glycerol-3-phosphate dehydrogenase, RNA polymerase and kinases, thymidine kinase, dihydrofolate reductase, hyaluronidase, urease, hexokinase, fumarase, trypsin, reverse transcriptase and the receptor-mediated uptake of low-density lipoprotein by trypanosomes. Suramin is taken up by trypanosomes by pinocytosis, as a plasma protein-bound complex.[65] The accumulation of suramin in the trypanosomes was hypothesized to be one of the reasons for the differential toxicity between the host and the parasite.

Diminazene aceturate

Diminazene aceturate (Berenil) was developed for use in animal trypanosomiasis, and it is not registered for sleeping sickness therapy. However, it has been used in case of lack of other drugs in several instances. No clinical trials have compared its safety and efficacy with those of pentamidine, but preliminary data suggest an inferior efficacy for diminazene. In preclinical investigations severe cerebral haemorrhages were observed in dogs,[66] but not in other animal species. The use of diminazene in humans should at this point be limited to strictly controlled investigational settings.

Treatment of second stage

Melarsoprol

The organo-arsenical drug melarsoprol, Mel B (Arsobal®, Aventis), was developed 1949 by the addition of the heavy metal chelator dimercaptopropanol (British Anti-Lewisite; BAL) to the trivalent arsenic of melarsen oxide.[67] Despite the high frequency of severe adverse drug reactions and an increasing number of patients refractory to treatment, the drug still is the first choice for treatment of second-stage sleeping sickness owing to a lack of valid alternatives.

A wide range of different empirically derived treatment regimens has been used in the past. These schedules share application of the drug in repeated series of three to four injections every 24 hours, spaced by 7–10 days (for details see Figure 73.12). None of the schedules has proved to be of significant advantage.[4] Recently acquired knowledge about the pharmacokinetics of the drug led to the suggestion of a new, concise treatment schedule, which is currently being evaluated in multinational clinical trials.[68,69]

Owing to irritating properties of the solvent propylene glycol, melarsoprol has to be given strictly as an intravenous injection; a paravasal deposition of the drug has to be avoided.

Adverse drug reactions of melarsoprol may be severe and life threatening. The most important is an encephalopathic syndrome, which occurs in 5–10% of all treated cases, and which is fatal for about 10–70% of those patients.[4,70] Clinically, the syndrome has been defined either as convulsions, the rapid deterioration of neurological symptoms and progressive coma, or psychotic reactions/abnormal behaviour.[70]

The cause of the reaction to melarsoprol and the influence of the treatment schedule on its frequency have been discussed extensively during the past decade. An immune reaction is generally thought to underlie the syndrome,[4,70,71] but the detailed mechanisms remain unknown. Trypanosome antigens can be excluded as a unique trigger, because identical encephalopathic syndromes were also observed in patients treated experimentally with melarsoprol for advanced leukaemia.[72] The temporal distribution of the occurrence of the syndrome was virtually identical under standard treatment interrupted with breaks compared with the continuous daily application for 10 days in a large-scale controlled clinical trial.[69] As the drug pressure in the CSF during the

Day of drug application

| 1 | 2 | 3 | 4 | 5 | 6 | 7 | 8 | 9 | 10 | 11 | 12 | 13 | 14 | 15 | 16 | 17 | 18 | 19 | 20 | 21 | 22 | 23 | 24 | 25 | 26 | 27 | 28 | 29 | 30 | 31 | 32 | 33 | 34 | 35 |

Schedule used in Angola

Days 1–4: M¹ M² M³ M³; Days 11–14: M¹ M² M³ M³; Days 23–26: M¹ M² M³ M³

Schedule used in Côte d'Ivoire

Days 1–4: M⁴ M⁵ M³ M³; Days 11–13: M⁴ M⁵ M³; Days 23–25: M⁴ M⁵ M³

Schedule used in the Democratic Republic of Congo

Days 1–3: M³ M³ M³; Days 10–12: M³ M³ M³; Days 19–21: M³ M³ M³

Schedule used Uganda (adapted)

Days 1–3: Mˣ Mˣ Mˣ; Days 9–11: Mˣ Mˣ Mˣ; Days 17–19: Mˣ Mˣ Mˣ

Former schedule used in Côte d'Ivoire

Days 1–2: P P; Days 3–6: M¹ M² M³ M³; Days 15–18: M¹ M² M³ M³; Days 31–34: M¹ M² M³ M³

Concise schedule under investigation [Burri, 2000 #23]

Days 1–10: M⁶ M⁶ M⁶ M⁶ M⁶ M⁶ M⁶ M⁶ M⁶ M⁶

M¹ = melarsoprol 1.2 mg/kg bw; M² = melarsoprol 2.4 mg/kg bw; M³ = melarsoprol 3.6 mg/kg bw (max. 5 ml)
M⁴ = melarsoprol 1.08 mg/kg bw; M⁵ = melarsoprol 2.52 mg/kg bw; M³ = melarsoprol 3.6 mg/kg bw (max. 5 ml)
Mˣ = one series of 1.8, 2.16, 2.52 mg/kg bw, one series of 2.52, 2.88, 3.52 mg/kg bw, one series of 3.6, 3.6, 3.6 mg/kg bw (max. 5 ml)
P = pentamidine 4 mg/kg
M⁶ = melarsoprol 2.16 mg/kg bw (max. 5 ml)

Figure 73.12: Examples of different schedules for treatment of patients with late-stage *T. b. gambiense* sleeping sickness.

continuous new treatment schedule is uninterrupted and constantly increasing until the end of treatment, another postulated reason, namely non-curative treatment leading to a reaction against recurrent trypanosomes in the CSF, can also be excluded. Another possible target for stimulating a delayed immune reaction not yet investigated is the hapten consisting of one of the melarsoprol metabolites and plasma proteins.[73] In a large-scale clinical trial the concomitant application of prednisolone at 1 mg per kg body weight has been shown to reduce the incidence of encephalopathic syndromes by two-thirds (i.e., 11.4% to 4.1%; difference in percentage –7.3% (C.I.₉₅ – 11.7% to –2.7%)) and the mortality rate by one-third (i.e., 7.5% to 5.2%; difference in percentage – 2.3% (C.I.₉₅ – 6.3% to + 1.7%)).[74] It is possible that two different reactions lead to the syndrome: the prognosis of patients with a single convulsion is reasonably good, whereas 50–70% of those rapidly developing coma die within 3 days.[75]

Management of encephalopathic syndromes is attempted by the application of anticonvulsants (diazepam, phenobarbital, phenytoin) and high-dose parenteral steroids (dexamethasone, hydrocortisone) to reduce cerebral oedema. Adrenaline (epinephrine) is often given, but its beneficial use has not been proven, and dimercaprol is contraindicated.

Other frequent adverse drug reactions to melarsoprol are pyrexia, headache, general malaise and thrombophlebitis at the sites of injection. Skin reactions such as pruritus and maculopapular eruptions are quite common, but severe complications such as bullous eruptions occur only in less than 1% of cases.[4] Other occasional adverse reactions are peripheral motoric or sensorial (paraesthesia) neuropathy, cardiac failure, renal dysfunction (proteinuria and hypertension) as well as hepatotoxicity (raised levels of liver enzymes, bilirubinaemia).[76]

Serum concentrations of melarsoprol determined by biological assay and atomic absorption spectrometry were, respectively, in the range of 2.5–6 µg/ml at 5 minutes and 220 (±80) ng/ml at 120 hours after the fourth injection of the therapy courses. Melarsoprol is rapidly metabolized to melarsen oxide with a half-life of 0.5 hours; melarsen oxide decays with a half-life of 3.9 hours, not solely due to a rapid elimination but also because of irreversible binding to plasma proteins of more than 20 kDa in size.[73] The mean terminal elimination half-life of melarsoprol determined as total trypanocidal activity by bioassay is approximately 35 hours, the volume of distribution is about 2 l/kg and total clearance is 1 ml per min per kg.[77] CSF samples are obtained by spinal tap, and therefore only marginal information about this compartment is available from humans. The CSF drug levels are generally very low, in the range of 2% of those in the serum in humans and monkeys, and the half-life of activity in this compartment was about 5 days in a monkey model.

The mechanisms of action of melarsoprol are not completely understood. Trypanothione (N^1,N^8-bis(glutathionyl)-spermidine), which plays a major role in the dithioldisulfide redox balance in trypanosomes and forms an adduct with melarsen oxide (MelT), was proposed as the primary target of melarsoprol. However, this idea was contested based on the high K_i value required for this target, and a modest decrease in intracellular levels of reduced trypanothione and glutathione.[62] Additionally, melarsen oxide was found inside treated trypanosomes and inhibited pyruvate kinase, phosphofructokinase and fructose-2,6-biphosphatase. In summary, melarsoprol appears to be a highly non-discriminating inhibitor of a large number of mammalian and trypanosomal enzymes that contain dithiols.

Eflornithine

In 1990 the US Food and Drug Administration (FDA) approved eflornithine (α-difluoromethylornithine; DFMO) for the treatment of *gambiense* sleeping sickness. The most commonly used dosage regimen consists of 100 mg of eflornithine per kg body weight at 6-hour intervals for 14 days (150 mg per kg body weight in children) by short infusions over a period of at least 30 minutes. Currently the oral application of the compound is being reinvestigated.

Adverse drug reactions are frequent and the characteristics are similar to those of other cytotoxic drugs. Their occurrence and intensity increases with the duration of treatment and the severity of the general condition of the patient.[78] The most frequent adverse effects are bone marrow toxicity (anaemia, leucopenia, thrombocytopenia) in 25–50% of treated patients.[79] Gastrointestinal symptoms such as nausea, vomiting and diarrhoea can be observed in about 10%, alopecia, usually towards the end

of the treatment, is seen in about 5–10%, and neurological symptoms such as convulsions in 7% of treated patients. Generally, adverse drug reactions of eflornithine are reversible after the end of the treatment course.

After low oral doses (5–10 mg/kg), peak plasma concentrations were reached 1.5–6 hours later. The mean half-life was 3.3 hours and the volume of distribution in the range of 0.35 l/kg. Renal clearance was about 2 ml per min per kg (after intravenous application) and accounted for more than 80% of drug elimination. Bioavailability of an orally administered 10 mg/kg dose was estimated at 54%. Eflornithine produces CSF : plasma ratios of between 0.13 and 0.51.[79]

Ornithine decarboxylase (ODC) catalyses the conversion of ornithine to putrescine, the first and rate-limiting step in the synthesis of putrescine and of the polyamines spermidine and spermine.[80] Polyamines are involved in nucleic acid synthesis, contribute to the regulation of protein synthesis and are essential for the growth and multiplication of all eukaryotic cells.[81] Trypanosomes are more susceptible to the drug than human cells, possibly because of the slow turnover of this enzyme in *T. b. gambiense*.[80] The rapid turnover is also responsible for the innate resistance of *T. b. rhodesiense* to eflornithine.[82]

Table 73.4 Treatment of *T. b. gambiense* and *T. b. rhodesiense* sleeping sickness

	West African (*T. b.* gambiense)	East African (*T. b.* rhodesiense)
Early stage	Endemic countries: According to National legislation or guidelines	
	Other countries: Pentamidine (pentamidine isethionate) 4 mg kg^{-1} body weight daily or on alternate days for 7 to 10 i.v.[a] or i.m.	Suramin Test dose of 4–5 mg kg^{-1} body weight at day 1, followed by five injections of 20 mg kg^{-1} body weight every 7 days (e.g. day 3, 10, 17, 24, 31). The maximum dose per injection is 1 g
Late stage	Endemic countries: According to National legislation or guidelines	
	Other countries: If available: Eflornithine 100 mg kg^{-1} body weight at 6 hourly intervals for 14 days (150 mg kg^{-1} body weight in children) by short infusions over a period of at least 30 minutes Alternative: Melarsoprol[b] 3 series of 3.6 mg kg^{-1} body weight at 24 hourly intervals for 3 days; The series spaced by intervals of 7 days	Eflornithine not recommended (Low efficacy; Ref 82) Melarsoprol[b,c] 1 series of 1.8, 2.16, 2.52 mg kg^{-1} body weight at 24 hourly intervals; 1 series of 2.52, 2.88, 3.25 mg kg^{-1} body weight at 24 hourly intervals; 1 series of 3.6, 3.6, 3.6 mg kg^{-1} body weight at 24 hourly intervals; The series spaced by intervals of 7 days (The maximum dose is 5 ml)

No firm recommendations exist for the use of the trypanocidal drugs; the schedules indicated are those most commonly used
A concise treatment schedule for treatment of *T. b. gambiense* sleeping sickness consisting of 10*
2.2 mg/kg body weight is under final evaluation (ref 69). Results can be expected at the end of 2002. **Note**: This schedule must not be used for treatment of *T.b. rhodesiense* sleeping sickness, since there are no data available.
[a]Very slow i.v. injection or short infusion, only under well controlled circumstances
[b]The concomitant application of 1 mg kg^{-1} body weight prednisolone has been shown to reduce the incidence of encephalopathic syndromes in one large scale clinical trial (Ref 70).
[c]A single dose of Suramin is often applied prior to the stage determining lumbar puncture

Therapy for treatment failures and relapses

Background

The relapse rate after melarsoprol treatment was generally in the range of 3–10% for both forms of human African trypanosomiasis. Only recently has this proportion increased in some areas with epidemic *T. b. gambiense*, to 30% in north-west Uganda,[83] 21% in south Sudan and 25% in north Angola.[84] Reasons for these treatment failures might be: (i) the parasite (drug-resistant trypanosomes, pronounced tissue tropism that allows the trypanosomes to escape to niches inaccessible to the drug) or (ii) the host (altered drug metabolism resulting in changed pharmacokinetics). A Ugandan *T. b. rhodesiense* isolate from 1960–1961 was recently reanalysed and found to have a 10-fold decreased melarsoprol sensitivity in vitro and to behave resistant in the mouse model at 20 mg/kg for four consecutive days (R. Brun, unpublished results). However, no drug-resistant *T. b. gambiense* isolates have yet been described, although trypanosome populations from relapse patients were examined. Studies in north Angola[85] and north-west Uganda (R. Brun, unpublished results) indicated that melarsoprol levels were identical in relapsing patients and those who could be cured.

Melarsoprol is transported into the trypanosomes by an adenosine transporter. The gene for this transporter has been cloned and the structure of the protein elucidated. The transporter of a laboratory-induced arsenical-resistant trypanosome population was found to be mutated (six different point mutations in the protein) and thus to have lost its capacity to transport arsenicals.[86] It has yet to be established to what extent this mutated adenosine transporter is involved in melarsoprol refractoriness in the field.

Nifurtimox

Nifurtimox (Lampit®; Bayer) is a drug that was introduced in the late 1960s for use in patients with Chagas' disease.[87] It is not registered for use in sleeping sickness, and its use is currently restricted to the compassionate treatment in combination with melarsoprol of patients not responding to melarsoprol if eflornithine is not available.

For treatment schedules, see Combination treatment.

Nifurtimox is generally not well tolerated, and only about one-third of the patients remain free from adverse drug reactions,[88] but generally adverse effects are not severe, very rarely fatal, and dose related.[74] Gastrointestinal disturbances with nausea, abdominal pains and vomiting are very frequent, and neurological adverse reactions with general convulsions, tremor or agitation may occur. The development of peripheral polyneuropathy and generalized skin reactions were seen as occasional events. All adverse reactions were rapidly reversible after discontinuation of the drug.

In healthy human volunteers given a single oral dose of 15 mg/kg nifurtimox average peak plasma levels of 751 (range 356–1093) ng/ml were reached within 2–3 hours. The drug has an apparent volume of distribution of about 755 litres (approximately 15 l/kg) and a high apparent clearance of 193 l/h (about 64 ml per min per kg). Nifurtimox is quickly eliminated with an average plasma elimination half-life of 3 (range 2–6) hours.[89]

The mechanism of action of nifurtimox is not completely elucidated. Its trypanocidal action may be related to its ability to undergo partial reduction to form chemically reactive radicals causing the production of superoxide anions, hydrogen peroxide and hydroxyl radicals. These free radicals may react with cellular macromolecules and cause membrane injury, enzyme inactivation, damage to DNA and mutagenesis.[90]

Combination treatment

The increasing number of patients refractory to treatment made necessary the consideration of drug combinations. Preliminary laboratory results suggest a certain degree of synergism between the drugs, especially melarsoprol with eflornithine or nitro-compounds,[91,92] but detailed in vitro and in vivo investigations are lacking.

To overcome the precarious field situation, a preliminary clinical trial combining melarsoprol and nifurtimox indicated the potential usefulness of the approach,[93] and detailed trials on the combinations of melarsoprol and nifurtimox or eflornithine, and eflornithine and nifurtimox, are planned.

Different treatment schedules are in use, all developed on an empirical basis. Based on pharmacokinetic considerations and the preliminary results of ongoing trials, a schedule of melarsoprol 1.8 mg/kg plus nifurtimox 15 mg/kg for 10 days was selected for further investigation in patients with melarsoprol-refractory sleeping sickness.

In all combinations under investigation melarsoprol is applied according to the new 10-day treatment schedule, in some instances with slightly decreased doses, considering the supposed synergistic action.

Treatment follow-up

Because of the increasing frequency of treatment-refractory infections, the policy to perform a confirmatory lumbar puncture 1 day after the last drug application of each late-stage case should be recommended. The CSF should be analysed with a sensitive method for parasite detection (any concentration technique). The white cell count is not a helpful criterion at this point, because it may remain raised for several weeks. All patients should be monitored for 2 years, with lumbar punctures performed every 6 months. Early-stage patients should be considered to have relapsed if they present at any examination with a white cell count greater than 20 cells/mm^3 and should be retreated with melarsoprol. In case of equivocal results the patient should be seen again after 1–2 months. A relapse is confirmed if trypanosomes can be found in the CSF at any follow-up examination. There is no analytical method for distinguishing between relapse and reinfection. A relapse is suspected if the CSF white cell count is 50 cells/mm³ or more, and has doubled since the previous examination, or 20–49 cells/mm³ with recurrence of symptoms. Retreatment with melarsoprol may be attempted once in regions with a low relapse rate, but drug combinations are recommended in regions where treatment failure is common.

Disease control

Infected persons are contagious, but may remain almost asymptomatic for long periods before they develop signs of sleeping sickness. Therefore, the most important control measure for *gambiense* trypanosomiasis is active case finding followed by treatment of the identified infected subjects. Populations of endemic areas (foci) with a prevalence of over 1% should be examined once a year by mobile teams. In areas with a prevalence below 1%, active case detection may be maintained with a reduced periodicity.[4] The use of the CATT has become a routine tool, and its increased sensitivity over lymph node aspiration has partially made up for the lower participation of the population today compared with that in colonial times. CATT-positive patients should be subjected to the diagnostic path described in the section on diagnosis.

In highly endemic areas, the additional use of tsetse fly traps placed in spots of high risk of transmission supports the control of the disease.

For *T. b. rhodesiense* generally, a fixed post-surveillance approach is chosen because the symptoms are severe and patients tend to volunteer for treatment.[4]

Chemoprophylaxis is no longer in use because of the poor risk : benefit ratio owing to the adverse effects of the drugs in use.

Indicators for monitoring the efficacy of national control programmes have been suggested and may assist in improvement of the activities.[94]

REFERENCES

1   Program Against African Trypanosomiasis Information System. Available: http://www.fao.org/paat/html/gis.htm. 2001.
2   Rogers D J & Williams B G. Monitoring trypanosomiasis in space and time. *Parasitology* 1993; 106 (Supplement):S77–S92.
3   Jordan A M. *Trypanosomiasis Control and African Rural Development*. London: Longman, 1986.
4   World Health Organization. *Control and Surveillance of African Trypanosomiasis*. Geneva: WHO, 1998.
5   World Health Organization. *Health Systems: Improving Performance (World Health Report 2000)*. Geneva: WHO, 2000.
6   Hoare C A. *The Trypanosomes of Mammals (A Zoological Monograph)*. Oxford: Blackwell Scientific, 1972.
7   Vickerman K. Antigenic variation in trypanosomes. *Nature* 1978; 273(5664):613–617.
8   Inoue N, Narumi D, Mbati P A et al. Susceptibility of severe combined immuno-deficient (SCID) mice to *Trypanosoma brucei gambiense* and *T. b. rhodesiense*. *Trop Med Int Health* 1998; 3(5):408–412.
9   Truc P, Aerts D, McNamara J J et al. Direct isolation in vitro of *Trypanosoma brucei* from man and other animals, and its potential value for the diagnosis of gambian trypanosomiasis. *Trans R Soc Trop Med Hyg* 1992; 86(6):627–629.
10 Dukes P, Kaukas A, Hudson K M et al. A new method for isolating *Trypanosoma brucei gambiense* from sleeping sickness patients. *Trans R Soc Trop Med Hyg* 1989; 83(5):636–639.
11 Tomlinson S & Raper J. Natural human immunity to trypanosomes. *Parasitol Today* 1998; 14(9):354–359.
12 Rickman L R & Robson J. The blood incubation infectivity test: a simple test which may serve to distinguish *Trypanosoma brucei* from *T. rhodesienses*. *Bull World Health Organ* 1970; 42(4):650–651.
13 Mehlitz D. Investigations on the susceptibility of *Mastomys natalensis* to *Trypanosoma (Trypanozoon) brucei gambiense*. *Trop Med Parasitol* 1978; 29(1):101–107.
14 Jenni L & Brun R. A new in vitro test for human serum resistance of *Trypanosoma (T.) brucei*. *Acta Trop* 1982; 39(3):281–284.
15 Jenni L, Marti S, Schweizer J et al. Hybrid formation between African trypanosomes during cyclical transmission. *Nature* 1986; 322(6075):173–175.
16 Gibson W C & Mizen V H. Heritability of the trait for human infectivity in genetic crosses of *Trypanosoma brucei* ssp. *Trans R Soc Trop Med Hyg* 1997; 91(2):236–237.
17 Tibayrenc M, Kjellberg F & Ayala F J. A clonal theory of parasitic protozoa: the population structures of *Entamoeba*, *Giardia*, *Leishmania*, *Naegleria*, *Plasmodium*, *Trichomonas*, and *Trypanosoma* and their medical and taxonomical consequences. *Proc Natl Acad Sci U S A* 1990; 87(7):2414–2418.
18 Gibson W & Miles M A. Application of new technologies to epidemiology. *Br Med Bull* 1985; 41(2):115–121.
19 Gibson W C, de C Marshall T F & Godfrey D G. Numerical analysis of enzyme polymorphism: a new approach to the epidemiology and taxonomy of trypanosomes of the subgenus *Trypanozoon*. *Adv Parasitol* 1980; 18:175–246.
20 Godfrey D G, Baker R D, Rickman L R et al. The distribution, relationships and identification of enzymic variants within the subgenus *Trypanozoon*. *Adv Parasitol* 1990; 29:1–39.
21 Stevens J R & Godfrey D G. Numerical taxonomy of *Trypanozoon* based on polymorphisms in a reduced range of enzymes. *Parasitology* 1992; 104:75–86.
22 Paindavoine P, Pays E, Laurent M et al. The use of DNA hybridization and numerical taxonomy in determining relationships between *Trypanosoma brucei* stocks and subspecies. *Parasitology* 1986; 92:31–50.
23 Stevens J R, Lanham S M, Allingham R et al. A simplified method for identifying subspecies and strain groups in *Trypanozoon* by isoenzymes. *Ann Trop Med Parasitol* 1992; 86(1):9–28.
24 Gibson W C. Will the real *Trypanosoma brucei gambiense* please stand up. *Parasitol Today* 1986; 2:255–257.
25 Buyst H. The epidemiology of sleeping sickness in the historical Luangwa valley. *Ann Soc Belg Med Trop* 1977; 57(4–5):349–359.
26 Geigy R, Mwambu P M & Kauffmann M. Sleeping sickness survey in Musoma district, Tanzania. IV. Examination of wild mammals as a potential reservoir for *T. rhodesiense*. *Acta Trop* 1971; 28(3):211–220.
27 De Greef C, Imberechts H, Matthyssens G et al. A gene expressed only in serum-resistant variants of *Trypanosoma brucei rhodesiense*. *Mol Biochem Parasitol* 1989; 36(2):169–176.

28 Xong H V, Vanhamme L, Chamekh M et al. A VSG expression site-associated gene confers resistance to human serum in *Trypanosoma rhodesiense. Cell* 1998; 95(6):839–846.

29 Cibulskis R E. Genetic variation in *Trypanosoma brucei* and the epidemiology of sleeping sickness in the Lambwe Valley, Kenya. *Parasitology* 1992; 104(Pt 1):99–109.

30 Gibson W C & Gashumba J K. Isoenzyme characterization of some *Trypanozoon* stocks from a recent trypanosomiasis epidemic in Uganda. *Trans R Soc Trop Med Hyg* 1983; 77(1):114–118.

31 Gibson W C & Wellde B T. Characterization of *Trypanozoon* stocks from the South Nyanza sleeping sickness focus in western Kenya. *Trans R Soc Trop Med Hyg* 1985; 79(5):671–676.

32 Onyango R J, van Hoeve K & de Raadt P. The epidemiology of *T. rhodesiense* sleeping sickness in Alego location, central Nyanza, Kenya. I. Evidence that cattle may act as reservoir hosts of trypanosomes infective to man. *Trans R Soc Trop Med Hyg* 1966; 60:175.

33 Baldry D A T & Chaudhuri M F B. Epidemiology of African trypanosomiasis. *Insect Sci Appl* 1980; 1(1):85–93.

34 Welburn S C & Maudlin I. Tsetse–trypanosome interactions: rites of passage. *Parasitol Today* 1999; 15(10):399–403.

35 Magnus E, Vervoort T & Van Meirvenne N. A card agglutination test with stained trypanosomes (CATT) for the serological diagnosis of *T. b. gambiense* trypanosomiasis. *Ann Soc Belg Med Trop* 1978; 58:169–176.

36 Pansaerts R, Van Meirvenne N, Magnus E et al. Increased sensitivity of the card agglutination test CATT/*Trypanosoma brucei gambiense* by inhibition of complement. *Acta Trop* 1998; 70(3):349–354.

37 Nantulya V M. TrypTect CIATT—a card indirect agglutination trypanosomiasis test for diagnosis of *Trypanosoma brucei gambiense* and *T. b. rhodesiense* infections. *Trans R Soc Trop Med Hyg* 1997; 91(5):551–553.

38 Buscher P, Lejon V, Magnus E et al. Improved latex agglutination test for detection of antibodies in serum and cerebrospinal fluid of *Trypanosoma brucei gambiense* infected patients. *Acta Trop* 1999; 73(1):11–20.

39 Woo P T. The haematocrit centrifuge for the detection of trypanosomes in blood. *Can J Zool* 1969; 47(5):921–923.

40 Lumsden W G R, Kimber C D, Evans D A et al. *Trypanosoma brucei*: miniature anion exchange centrifugation for detection of low parasitemias: adaptation for field use. *Trans R Soc Trop Med Hyg* 1979; 73:313–317.

41 Bailey J W & Smith D H. The use of the acridine orange QBC technique in the diagnosis of African trypanosomiasis. *Trans R Soc Trop Med Hyg* 1992; 86(6):630.

42 Doua F, Miezan T W, Sanon Singaro J R et al. The efficacy of pentamidine in the treatment of early-late stage *Trypanosoma brucei gambiense* trypanosomiasis. *Am J Trop Med Hyg* 1996; 55(6):586–588.

43 Lejon V, Buscher P, Sema N H et al. Human African trypanosomiasis: a latex agglutination field test for quantifying IgM in cerebrospinal fluid. *Bull World Health Organ* 1998; 76(6):553–558.

44 Dumas M & Bisser S. Clinical aspects of human African trypanosomiasis. In Dumas M, Bouteille B & Buguet A (eds) *Progress in Human African Trypanosomiasis, Sleeping Sickness.* Paris: Springer, 1999:215–233.

45 Pepin J. African trypanosomiasis. In Strickland G T (ed.) *Hunter's Tropical Medicine and Emerging Infectious Diseases*, 8th edn. Philadelphia: Saunders, 2000:643–654.

46 Manson-Bahr P E C & Bell D R. African trypanosomiasis. In *Manson's Tropical Diseases*, 19th edn. London: Baillère Tindall, 1987:54–73.

47 Molyneux D H, Pentreath V & Doua F. African trypanosomiasis in man. In Cook G C (ed.) *Manson's Tropical Diseases*, 20th edn. London: WB Saunders, 1996:1171–1196.

48 Kristensson K & Bentivoglio M. Pathology of African trypanosomiasis. In Dumas M, Bouteille B & Buguet A (eds) *Progress in Human African Trypanosomiasis, Sleeping Sickness.* Paris: Springer, 1999:157–182.

49 Sternberg J M. Immunobiology of African trypanosomiasis. *Chem Immunol* 1998; 70:186–199.

50 Hunter C & Kennedy P. Immunopathology in central nervous system human African trypanosomiasis. *J Neuroimmunol* 1992; 36(2–3):91–95.

51 Vaidya T, Bakhiet M, Hill K L et al. The gene for a T lymphocyte triggering factor from African trypanosomes. *J Exp Med* 1997; 186(3):433–438.

52 Hunter C A, Jennings F W, Kennedy P G E et al. Astrocyte activation correlates with cytokine production in central nervous system of *Trypanosoma brucei brucei* infected mice. *Lab Invest* 1992; 67(5):635–642.

53 Pentreath V & Bentivoglio M. Cytokines and the blood brain–brain barrier in human and experimental African trypanosomiasis. In Dumas M, Bouteille B & Buguet A (eds) *Progress in Human African Trypanosomiasis, Sleeping Sickness.* Paris: Springer, 1999:105–118.

54 Sharafeldin A, Eltayeb R, Pashenkov M et al. Chemokines are produced in the brain early during the course of experimental African trypanosomiasis. *J Neuroimmunol* 2000; 103(2):165–170.

55 Vincendeau P, Jaubertau M O, Daulouede S et al. Immunology of African trypanosomiasis. In Dumas M, Bouteille B & Buguet A (eds) *Progress in Human African Trypanosomiasis, Sleeping Sickness.* Paris: Springer, 1999:137–156.

56 Rhind S G & Shek P N. Cytokines in the pathogenesis of human African trypanosomiasis: antagonistic roles of TNF-α and IL-10. In Dumas M, Bouteille B & Buguet A (eds) *Progress in Human African Trypanosomiasis, Sleeping Sickness.* Paris: Springer, 1999:119–136.

57 Radomski M W & Brandenberger G. Hormones in human African trypanosomiasis. In Dumas M, Bouteille B & Buguet A (eds) *Progress in Human African Trypanosomiasis, Sleeping Sickness.* Paris: Springer, 1999:183–190.

58 Apted F I C. Present status of chemotherapy and chemoprophylaxis of human trypanosomiasis in the eastern hemisphere. *Pharmacol Ther* 1980; 11:391–413.

59 Doua F & Yapo F B. Human trypanosomiasis in the Ivory Coast—therapy and problems. *Acta Trop* 1993; 54(3–4):163–168.

60 Bronner U, Doua F, Ericsson O et al. Pentamidine concentrations in plasma, whole blood and cerebrospinal fluid during treatment of *Trypanosoma gambiense* infection in Côte d'Ivoire. *Trans R Soc Trop Med Hyg* 1991; 85(5):608–611.

61 Berger B J, Lombardy R J, Marbury G D et al. Metabolic N-hydroxylation of pentamidine in vitro. *Antimicrob Agents Chemother* 1990; 34(9):1678–1684.

62 Wang C C. Molecular mechanisms and therapeutic approaches to the treatment of African trypanosomiasis. *Annu Rev Pharmacol Toxicol* 1995; 35:93–127.

63 Apted F I C. Treatment of human trypanosomiasis. In Mulligan H W (ed.) *The African Trypanosomiasis.* London: Allen & Unwin, 1970:684–710.

64 Collins J M, Klecker R W J, Yarchoan R et al. Clinical pharmacokinetics of suramin in patients with HTLV-III/LAV infection. *J Clin Pharmacol* 1986; 26:2–26.

65 Fairlamb A H & Bowman B R. Uptake of the trypanocidal drug suramin by bloodstream forms of *Trypanosoma brucei* and its effect in respiration and growth rate in vivo. *J Biochem Pathol* 1980; 1:315–333.

66 Losos G J & Crockett E. Toxicity of Berenil in the dogs. *Vet Rec* 1969; 85:196.

67 Friedheim E A H. Mel B in the treatment of human trypanosomiasis. *Am J Trop Med Hyg* 1949; 29:173–180.

68 Burri C, Blum J & Brun R. Alternative application of melarsoprol for treatment of *T. b. gambiense* sleeping sickness. Preliminary results. *Ann Soc Belg Med Trop* 1995; 75(1):65–71.

69 Burri C, Nkunku S, Merolle A et al. Efficacy of new, concise treatment schedule for melarsoprol in treatment of sleeping sickness caused by *Trypanosoma brucei gambiense*: a randomised trial. Lancet 2000; 355:1419–1425.

70 Pepin J & Milord F. The treatment of human African trypanosomiasis. *Adv Parasitol* 1994; 33:1–47.

71 Haller L, Adams H, Merouze F et al. Clinical and pathological aspects of human African trypanosomiasis (*T. b. gambiense*) with particular reference to reactive arsenical encephalopathy. *Am J Trop Med Hyg* 1986; 35:94–99.

72 Soignet S L, Tong W P, Hirschfeld S et al. Clinical study of an organic arsenical, melarsoprol, in patients with advanced leukemia. *Cancer Chemother Pharmacol* 1999; 44(5):417–421.

73 Keiser J, Ericsson O & Burri C. Investigations of the metabolites of the trypanocidal drug melarsoprol. *Clin Pharmacol Ther* 2000; 67(5):478–488.

74 Pepin J, Milord F, Mpia B et al. An open clinical trial of nifurtimox for arseno-resistant *Trypanosoma brucei gambiense* sleeping sickness in central Zaire. *Trans R Soc Trop Med Hyg* 1989; 83(4):514–517.

75 Blum J, Nkunku S & Burri C. Clinical description of encephalopathic syndromes and risk factors for their occurrence and outcome during melarsoprol treatment of human African trypanosomiasis. *Trop Med Int Health* 2001; 6:390–400.

76 Van Nieuwenhove S. Present strategies in the treatment of human African trypanosomiasis. In Dumas M, Bouteille B & Buguet A (eds) *Progress in Human African Trypanosomiasis, Sleeping Sickness*. Paris: Springer, 1999:253–280.

77 Burri C, Baltz T, Giroud C et al. Pharmacokinetic properties of the trypanocidal drug melarsoprol. *Chemotherapy* 1993; 39(4):225–234.

78 Milord F, Pepin J, Loko L et al. Efficacy and toxicity of eflornithine for treatment of *Trypanosoma brucei gambiense* sleeping sickness. *Lancet* 1992; 340(8820):652–655.

79 Marion Merrell Dow. *Ornidyl*. Ornidyl Patient Information, 1991.

80 Bacchi C J, Nathan H C, Hutner S H et al. Polyamine metabolism: a potential therapeutic target in trypanosomes. *Science* 1980; 210(4467):332–334.

81 Pegg A E & McCann P P. Polyamine metabolism and function. *Am J Physiol* 1982; 243(5):C212–C221.

82 Iten M, Mett H, Evans A et al. Alterations in ornithine decarboxylase characteristics account for tolerance of *Trypanosoma brucei rhodesiense* to D,L-alpha-difluoromethylornithine. *Antimicrob Agents Chemother* 1997; 41(9):1922–1925.

83 Legros D, Evans S, Maiso F et al. Risk factors for treatment failure after melarsoprol for *Trypanosoma brucei gambiense* trypanosomiasis in Uganda. *Trans R Soc Trop Med Hyg* 1999; 93:439–442.

84 Stanghellini A & Josenando T. The situation of sleeping sickness in Angola: a calamity. *Trop Med Int Health* 2001; 6:330–334.

85 Burri C & Keiser J. Pharmacokinetic investigations on patients from northern Angola refractory to melarsoprol treatment. *Trop Med Int Health* 2001; 6:412–420.

86 Maser P, Sutterlin C, Kralli A et al. A nucleoside transporter from *Trypanosoma brucei* involved in drug resistance. *Science* 1999; 285(5425):242–244.

87 Gonnert R. Nifurtimox: causal treatment of Chagas' disease. *Drug Res* 1972; 22(9):1563.

88 Wegner D H & Rohwedder R W. Experience with nifurtimox in chronic Chagas' infection. Preliminary report. *Drug Res* 1972; 22(9):1635–1641.

89 Paulos C, Paredes J, Vasquez I et al. Pharmacokinetics of a nitrofuran compound, nifurtimox, in healthy volunteers. *Int J Clin Pharmacol Ther Toxicol* 1989; 27(9):454–457.

90 Docampo R & Moreno S N. Free radical metabolism of antiparasitic agents. *Fed Proc* 1986; 45(10):2471–2476.

91 Jennings F W. The potentiation of arsenicals with difluoromethylornithine (DFMO): experimental studies in murine trypanosomiasis. *Bull Soc Pathol Exot* 1988; 81:595–607.

92 Jennings F W. Chemotherapy of CNS-trypanosomiasis: the combined use of the arsenicals and nitro-compounds. *Trop Med Parasitol* 1991; 42(2):139–142.

93 Bisser S, Van Nieuwenhove S, Lejon V et al. New therapeutic regimen for sleeping sickness. Description, results and lessons from the clinical trial established in Bwamanda (Equateur, RDC). *COST B9 Meeting*, Bruges, Belgium: 2000.

94 Bouchet B, Legros D & Lee E. Key indicators for the monitoring and evaluation of control programmes of human African trypanosomiasis due to *Trypanosoma brucei gambiense*. *Trop Med Int Health* 1998; 3(6):474–481.

Chapter 74
American Trypanosomiasis (Chagas Disease)

M. A. Miles

History

American trypanosomiasis, which results from infection with the protozoan parasite *Trypanosoma cruzi*, is justly referred to as Chagas disease in homage to the great discoveries of the Brazilian scientist Carlos Chagas. In 1907 Carlos Chagas left the beautiful city of Rio de Janeiro to work at Lassance in the state of Minas Gerais as a malaria control officer. The local inhabitants who lived in poor-quality housing complained that they were attacked at night by a large blood-sucking insect, the triatomine bug (Hemiptera, Reduviidae). Carlos Chagas immediately suspected that such blood-sucking insects might transmit a human infectious disease. He collected examples of the bug (*Panstrongylus megistus*; Figure 74.1) and found abundant protozoan flagellates in the bug faeces. He sent specimens of the insect back to Rio de Janeiro, to his mentor, Oswaldo Cruz. Marmosets exposed to infected bugs developed a circulating trypanosome which Chagas named *Trypanosoma cruzi*. Back in Lassance he began to look for human infections and found the same organisms circulating in the blood of children with an acute febrile illness (Figure 74.2). As far as I am aware, this discovery is unique as the disease agent was first found in the insect vector and only subsequently in patients.

Carlos Chagas went on to describe all the major features of the *T. cruzi* life cycle in experimental animals and to

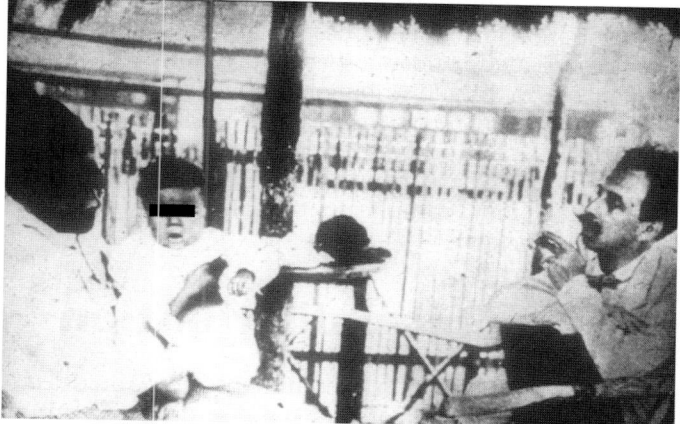

Figure 74.2: Carlos Chagas in Lassance, Minas Gerais State, Brazil, with one of the first infants with diagnosed Chagas disease.

discover natural reservoir hosts, such as the armadillo. The mechanism of transmission from the vector was hotly debated but was finally proven in 1912, by Emile Brumpt, to be by contamination with infected bug faeces, rather than directly through the bite of the triatomine bug.

The clinical and public health significance of Chagas disease remained controversial for several years, until its widespread distribution in Latin America became recognized. A more detailed account of the discovery of Chagas disease is given by Miles.[1]

Serological surveys throughout Latin America eventually revealed that up to 18 million people might carry *T. cruzi*. At its peak, it was estimated that up to 90 million people might be exposed to infection. Of those infected up to 10%, especially children, might be expected to die in the initial acute phase of infection. In some regions up to 30% of those surviving the acute phase might suffer the chronic consequences: chagasic heart disease and, more rarely, enlargement and dysfunction of the oesophagus and colon.[2]

Vector-borne Chagas disease is essentially a disease of poverty and poor housing. As we shall see, in the last decade enormous progress has been made through national and international control programmes, in reducing the incidence of infection. *T. cruzi* can also be transmitted by blood transfusion, and screening of donor blood is thus an essential part of prevention. Congenital

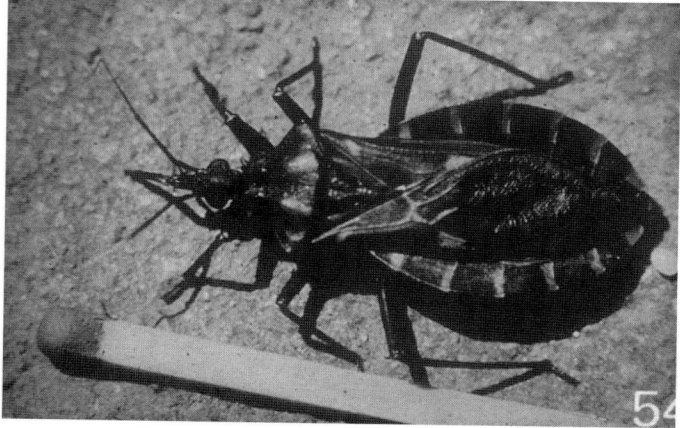

Figure 74.1: The triatomine bug *Panstrongylus megistus,* female with egg. (Courtesy of T. V. Barrett.)

transmission and oral transmission, usually via food contaminated with infected bug faeces, are also known. An infected individual retains low-level infection for life. An immunocompromised state, as in human immunodeficiency virus (HIV) infection or in organ recipients, can reactivate the acute infection.

Like other trypanosomatids (trypanosomes and leishmanias), *T. cruzi* has generated intense research interest because of its molecular biology and the uncertain pathogenesis of Chagas disease. Epidemiologically the disease is enigmatic because the prognosis is unpredictable and many of those infected remain healthy for life. Fundamental to the understanding of Chagas disease has been the demonstration that *T. cruzi* has remarkable heterogeneity, with at least two major subspecific divisions, which have distinct geographical distributions and epidemiologies.[3]

A second human trypanosomiasis can be found in the New World, resulting from *Trypanosoma rangeli* infection. *T. rangeli*, however, is considered to be non-pathogenic, although it may complicate the diagnosis of Chagas disease (see below).

Geographical distribution

Human *T. cruzi* infection is confined to the Americas. It extends from approximately 40° 45′ south in Argentina into the southern states of the USA. Human infection is rare in the USA and still relatively uncommon in the vast Amazon basin of South America, for reasons that will be explained (see Epidemiology). Natural cycles of *T. cruzi* infection, involving many different triatomine bug species and mammal hosts, are much more widespread than the human infection, from southern Argentina and Chile (46° south) to northern California (42° north). Rarely, locally acquired infection might be anticipated outside

the normal geographical distribution if infected donor blood is transfused into a naive recipient. Further details of the geographical distribution are given in conjunction with the description of the epidemiology (see below).

Aetiology

T. cruzi is a eukaryotic, single-celled, protozoan parasite of the order Kinetoplastida and the family Trypanosomatidae. Like other kinetoplastid organisms, *T. cruzi* has mitochondrial DNA in the form of a discrete organelle, the kinetoplast. The kinetoplast can be seen by light microscopy in stained blood films or tissue sections and is an important diagnostic feature (Figure 74.3).

The morphological stages in the life cycle of *T. cruzi* are defined by the position of the kinetoplast relative to the

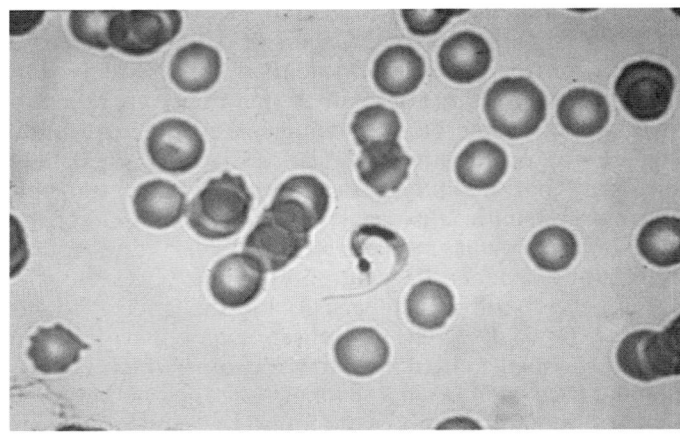

Figure 74.3: Typical trypomastigote of *Trypanosoma cruzi* in blood, showing C shape and large posterior kinetoplast.

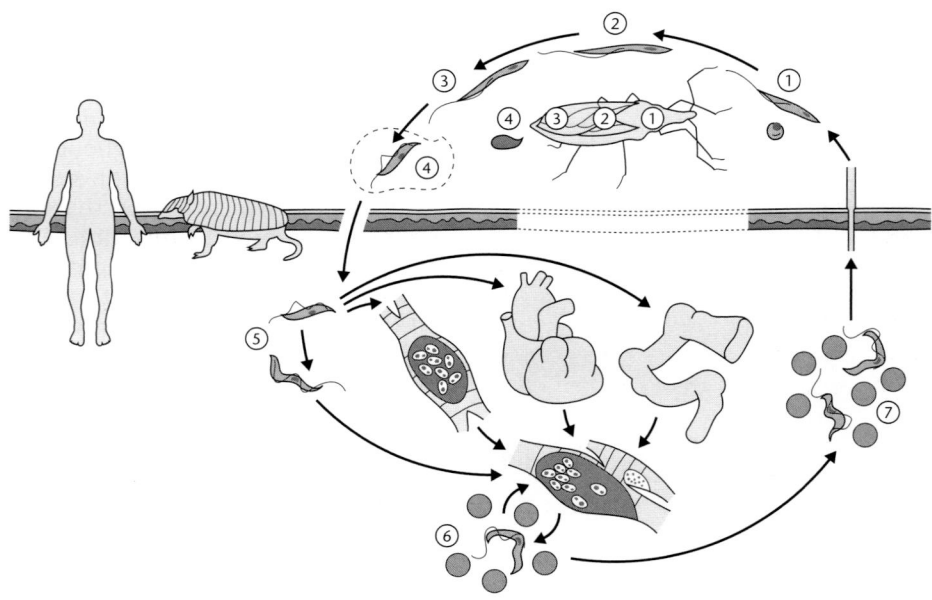

Figure 74.4: Summary of the life cycle of *Trypanosoma cruzi*, in the vector (1–4) and mammalian host (5–7). (Courtesy of Meddia.)

nucleus and by the presence and extent of the free flagellum[4] (Figure 74.4). Unlike the African trypanosome, *Trypanosoma brucei*, *T. cruzi* does not divide in the blood of the mammalian host, but divides intracellularly in non-phagocytic and phagocytic cells. Thus *T. cruzi* is predominantly an intracellular parasite in mammals, and this influences the pathogenesis of the disease and the nature of the immune response to infection. In the triatomine bug vector, *T. cruzi* divides solely within the intestinal tract and does not escape into the haemocoel. Division is by binary fission in the lumen of the gut largely as *epimastigotes*, which have the kinetoplast adjacent to the nucleus. In the rectum of the triatomine bug, epimastigotes attach by the flagellum to the epithelium of the rectum wall and transform to infective (metacyclic) *trypomastigotes*. When the bug takes a blood meal, metacyclic trypomastigotes are released with the faeces and urine, and can establish infection in the mammalian host either by crossing mucous membranes, such as the conjunctiva, nasal or oral mucosae, or through abraded skin such as the wound made by the bite of the bug. Trypomastigotes cannot cross the barrier of intact skin, however, and once the bug faeces is dry it is no longer infective. Bugs acquire infection by feeding on the blood of an infected mammal or, rarely, by piercing the intestinal tract of another recently fed, infected bug, or by probing freshly deposited faeces of an infected bug (coprophagy). There is no transmission of *T. cruzi* infection from the bug through its egg stage to its offspring (transovarial transmission).

The infective metacyclic trypomastigotes in bug faeces are slender and highly motile. Inside the mammal they can penetrate non-phagocytic cells, particularly muscle cells, but also phagocytic cells and a wide variety of cell types. Inside the cell, *T. cruzi* escapes from the cell vacuole (phagolysosome) to lie free in the cytoplasm. There it loses its flagellum and transforms to a small oval *amastigote* stage which multiplies by binary fission, forming a false cyst or pseudocyst. After about 5 days the amastigotes in the mature pseudocyst transform to small C-shaped trypomastigotes which are released when the pseudocyst ruptures. Multiplication may occur locally at the initial site of infection, causing a cutaneous or ocular lesion, before systemic spread of the organism (see Clinical features). Trypomastigotes released from pseudocysts are of two types: a slender, highly active trypomastigote, which can be found in the blood only in severe acute infections, and a smaller, broader, less motile trypomastigote, which is the most common form found circulating in the blood. It is thought that these two forms have distinct functions. The slender form may be designed to re-establish the next intracellular cycle, whereas the short broad forms are more usually taken up by the insect vector. Pseudocysts may be very widely distributed among tissues of an infected mammal but they are frequently abundant in heart muscle, skeletal muscle or smooth muscle of the alimentary tract, in accord with the pathology of chronic Chagas disease. Microscopically patent blood parasitaemia, if present, is usually transient in the acute phase of infection. Nevertheless low numbers of circulating trypomastigotes usually remain for life and the host is a lifelong potential source of infection to triatomine bugs. If the host is attacked by bugs, trypomastigotes transform in the bug foregut to amastigotes and sphaeromastigotes (with a free flagellum) and begin to multiply by binary fission, which continues in the midgut as the epimastigote stage, thus completing the cycle. Bugs become infective 10–15 days after taking the infected blood meal.

All stages of the life cycle can be readily reproduced in tissue culture. Thus epimastigotes can be grown in liquid media or in liquid overlay above blood agar base. Transformation to metacyclic trypomastigotes may occur in older cultures but is not guaranteed with all strains. Intracellular amastigotes can be grown in many different mammalian cell lines: small, motile trypomastigotes can be seen in vitro in infected mammalian cells ('boiling cells') just before rupture, which releases trypomastigotes into the liquid overlay.

As already noted, there are important secondary methods of transmission in addition to vector-borne transmission. Of these, blood transfusion transmission has been particularly important epidemiologically (see below). Congenital transmission is also well documented (Figure 74.5). Reported congenital transmission rates vary, but around 1% of infants born to seropositive mothers may acquire infection in utero. Oral outbreaks may occur from food contaminated by triatomine faeces, or through consumption of raw infected meat of a reservoir host. Sexual transmission is not known but may rarely occur. Milk transmission from mother to child occurs rarely. Oral transmission may be important in sustaining zoonotic *T. cruzi* infection among reservoir hosts, many of which eat insects. Anal gland infections occur in the opossum (*Didelphis*) with the glands containing life-cycle stages typically found in the insect vector. It is not known whether this represents a primitive or a secondary stage of the life cycle, but anal gland secretions are presumably highly infective.

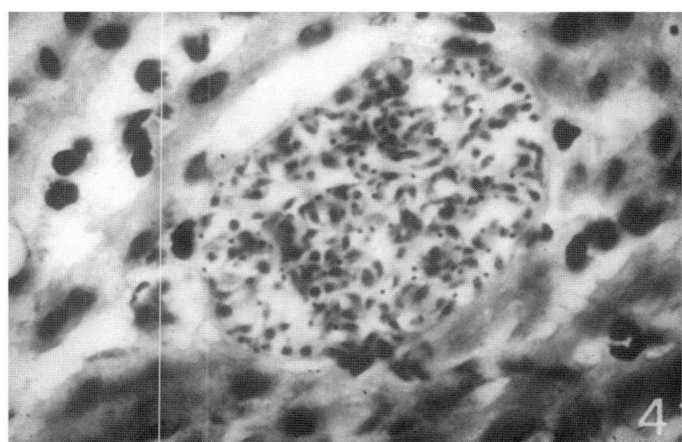

Figure 74.5: Mature pseudocyst of *Trypanosoma cruzi* in umbilical cord, from a congenital case of Chagas disease. (Courtesy of Hipolito de Almeida.)

Clinical features

The acute phase

The initial acute phase of *T. cruzi* infection may be asymptomatic or undetected because of the lack of specific signs and symptoms. There may be a lesion at the portal of entry of the organism. If this is the skin, an oedematous cutaneous lesion (chagoma) reminiscent of the chancre seen in African trypanosomiasis may be present. If the portal of entry is the eye, unilateral peri-ophthalmic oedema with conjunctivitis—the so-called Romana's sign—may be present (Figure 74.6). There may be regional lymphadenopathy adjacent to cutaneous or ocular lesions. Other clinical signs in the acute phase may include generalized lymphadenopathy, fever, myalgia, headache, hepatosplenomegaly, facial or generalized oedema, rash, vomiting, diarrhoea and anorexia. In infants there may be multiple cutaneous chagomas during the acute phase of infection. The incubation period may be only 2 weeks, or up to several months if contaminated transfusion blood is the source of the

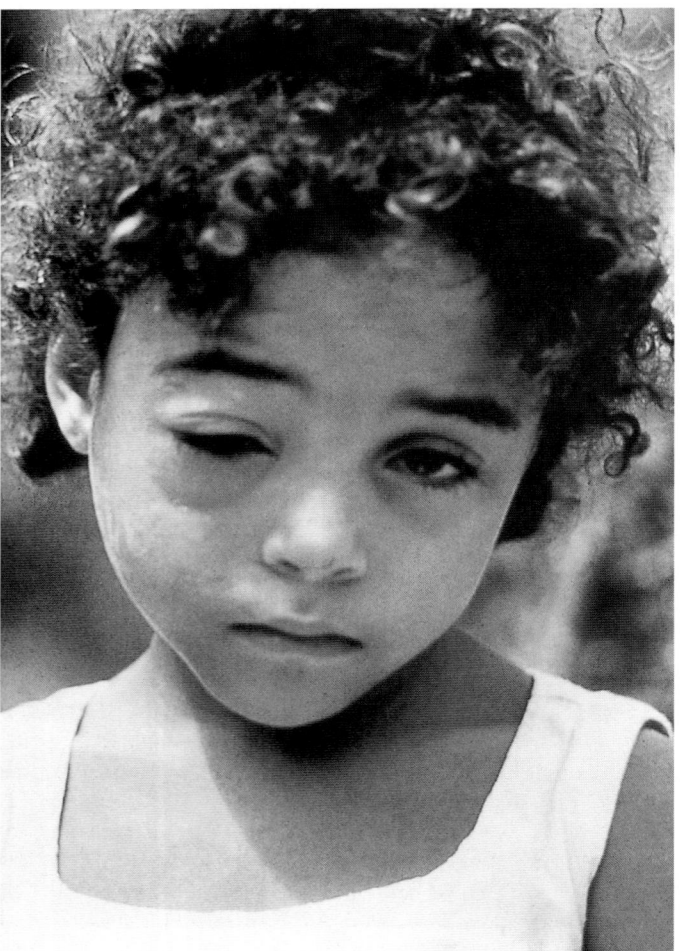

Figure 74.6: Romana's sign, unilateral oedema and conjunctivitis at the portal of entry in acute Chagas disease.

infection. There may be early electrocardiographic (ECG) changes such as sinus tachycardia, increased P-R interval, T-wave changes and low QRS voltage. Acute myocarditis may be fatal. Meningoencephalitis is a rare complication in adults. In congenital infections, however, or in immuno-compromised adults, meningoencephalitis is more common and carries a very poor prognosis. The T helper cell type 1 (Th1) arm of the cell-mediated immune response is important in controlling *T. cruzi* infection. Impairment of the Th1 response in patients with acquired immune deficiency syndrome (AIDS) explains the reactivation of acute Chagas disease in *T. cruzi*–HIV co-infections.

Hepatosplenomegaly is frequent in congenital Chagas disease. There may also be fever, oedema, neurological signs such as convulsions, tremors and weak reflexes, metastatic chagomas and apnoea. The ECG is not often changed but there may be low-voltage complexes, decreased T-wave height and increased atrioventricular (AV) conduction time. Congenital Chagas disease associated with premature birth carries a poor prognosis.[5]

Chronic phase

Asymptomatic or symptomatic acute-phase *T. cruzi* infection may be followed by an indeterminate phase with no clinical indications of infection. The indeterminate phase may last for the life of the patient, even though the parasite can be isolated repeatedly by sensitive diagnostic methods. In a proportion of patients, however, chronic-phase symptoms arise. In particular, up to 30% of patients who survive the acute phase may develop ECG abnormalities attributable to Chagas disease. Typical ECG abnormalities include right bundle branch block (RBBB) and left anterior hemiblock (LAH). There may also be AV conduction abnormalities such as AV block. Arrhythmias such as sinus bradycardia, sinoatrial block, ventricular tachycardia, primary T-wave changes and abnormal Q waves may be present. Other cardiac symptoms may include palpitations, chest pain, oedema, dizziness, syncope and dyspnoea. The severity of heart involvement is usually graded by the degree of ECG disturbance. Mega-cardia may be seen on radiography of the thorax. Embolism may occur and death may be sudden.[5]

A small proportion of patients with chagasic heart disease may have associated abnormalities of the alimentary tract. The oesophagus and colon are most commonly affected with regurgitation and dysphagia, loss of peristalsis or severe constipation, and faecaloma. The severity of involvement may be graded clinically according to the degree of dilatation detected by radiography. Dysfunction may also affect other hollow organs. The severity of chronic involvement varies regionally (see Epidemiology).

Pathology and pathogenesis

At the level of gross pathology, cardiac changes may

include notable enlargement of the heart (megacardia), detectable by radiography, or obvious at autopsy in situ. Further signs are focal thinning of the myocardium in the form of aneurysms, which may occur anywhere in the heart but are typically described at the apex of the left ventricle in the form of an apical aneurysm (Figure 74.7). Such an apical aneurysm is considered to be a pathognomonic indication of chronic chagasic myocardiopathy. Trans-illumination is a convenient method of detecting inapparent cardiac aneurysms.

Intestinal complications of chronic Chagas disease include megaoesphagus (Figure 74.8) and, less commonly, megacolon[2] (Figure 74.9). In both cases there is dilatation

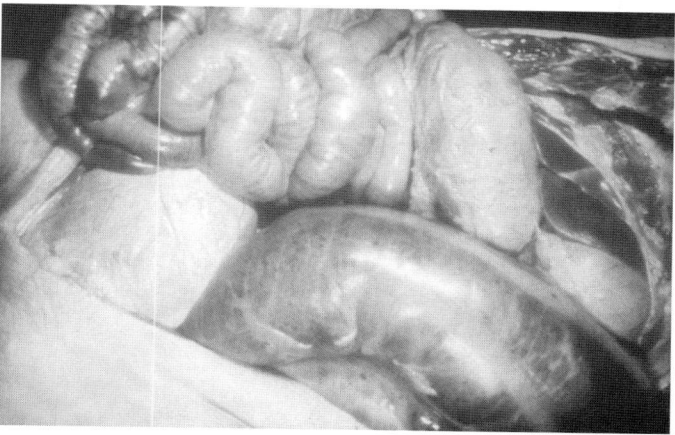

Figure 74.9: Megacolon in chronic Chagas disease. (Courtesy of J. S. de Oliveira.)

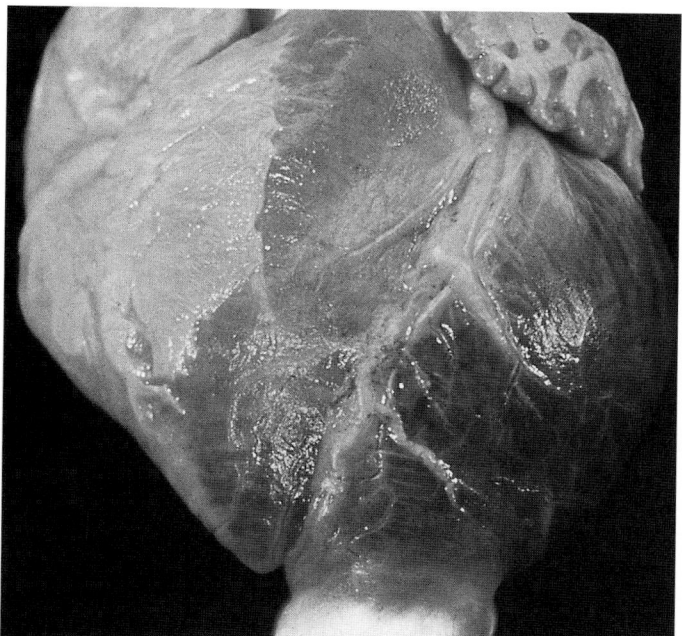

Figure 74.7: Apical aneurysm in chronic Chagas disease. (Courtesy of J. S. de Oliveira.)

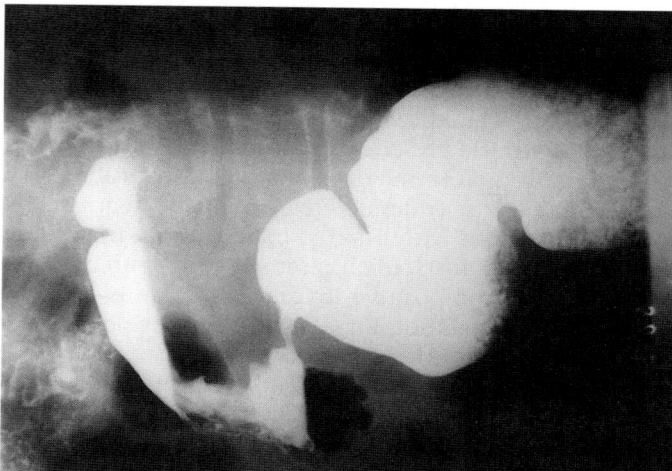

Figure 74.8: Radiograph showing megaoesophagus in chronic Chagas disease. (Courtesy of J. S. de Oliveira.)

of the hollow organ and thinning of the wall, classified according to degree of severity, and associated with a failure of peristalsis. Each of these signs is frequently associated with chagasic cardiopathy and both may occur in the same individual. Rarely megaoesophagus or megacolon may occur in infants following congenital infection. Megaoesophagus may be a prelude to carcinoma. Both megasyndromes may be detected by radiography; megacolon may be apparent externally. In extreme cases a wide variety of other organs may be affected, and enlarged.

Histopathological examination of Romana's sign or cutaneous chagoma shows infiltration of lymphocytes and monocytes. In the heart, unruptured pseudocysts appear to generate no inflammatory response (Figure 74.10A). Pseudocyst rupture gives rise to infiltration of lymphocytes, monocytes and/or polymorphonuclear cells (Figure 74.10B).

Pseudocysts may be very widespread, particularly in congenital cases, although they are still found most commonly in cardiac and skeletal muscle or reticuloendothelial cells. In meningoencephalitis, parasites may be found in perivascular spaces or in glial and neuronal cells. The histopathological picture is typical of acute meningoencephalitis.

The pathogenesis of chronic Chagas disease is still far from fully understood, and is much debated.[6] In particular, the role that continued infection, albeit at very low levels, plays in the progression and prognosis of chronic Chagas disease is controversial. Several aspects of the pathogenesis of chronic Chagas disease are, however, beyond doubt. Thus detailed follow-up of patients with ECG abnormalities and subsequent autopsy demonstrates a close correlation between the nature of the ECG changes and the location of focal lesions in the conducting system of the heart. Experimental studies in dogs, with precise post-mortem reconstruction of three-dimensional histopathology, show similar correlations between ECG abnormalities and the distribution of lesions. Furthermore it is quite clear that there is a marked loss of ganglion cells in megacardia, megaoesophagus and megacolon.

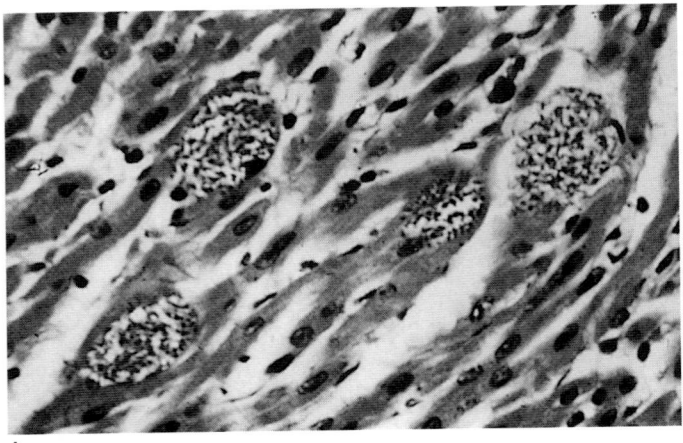
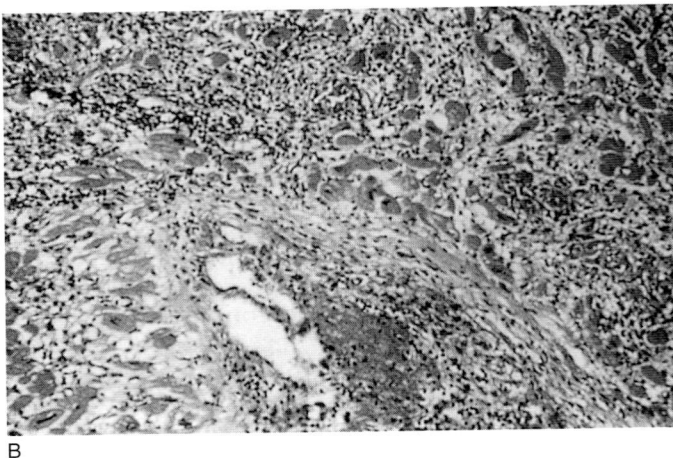

A

B

Figure 74.10: (**A**) Early acute-phase *Trypanosoma cruzi* infection: myocardium showing unruptured pseudocysts with no inflammatory reaction. (**B**) Later infection showing destruction of myocardium and inflammatory response.

This appears primarily to affect the parasympathetic innervation, leading to a sympathetic overload. The frequency of right bundle branch block (RBBB) in chronic Chagas disease is thought to be due to the fact that the right conducting system of the heart is less diffuse and more vulnerable to focal lesions than the bifascicular left conducting system. The pathogenesis of 'neurogenic' Chagas disease is thus partially explained in terms of: (1) pseudocyst rupture which deposits antigens on uninfected cells around the site of the pseudocyst; (2) focal immunological destruction of uninfected cells carrying adsorbed *T. cruzi* antigens, including ganglion cells; (3) further loss of ganglion cells with age; and (4) dysfunction and enlargement of the affected organs when the loss of ganglion of cells crosses a critical threshold. The latter may occur at any time after the acute phase, or not at all during the life of the infected individual. The majority of neurological damage is thought to occur in the acute phase of the infection and to be related to the level of parasitaemia. The sympathetic overload can be mimicked in experimental rats by the inoculation of catecholamines, and this alone may induce apical aneurysm.[7]

The inflammatory response in the tissues normally subsides after the acute phase of the infection. In some patients this inflammatory response appears to be renewed, leading to a progressive myocarditis and a slow decline in cardiac function. This 'myogenic' picture is thought to have an autoimmune component. Cross-reactive antibodies between *T. cruzi* and normal host tissues can be generated experimentally, and tissue cross-reactive antibodies have been reported in patients with chronic Chagas disease. Some reports show that heart transplants from normal mice into syngeneic chagasic mice suffer autoimmune rejection. In contrast, conflicting reports show the survival of such syngeneic transplants without autoimmune rejection unless the heart is parasitized.[8] Hence, it is uncertain whether the continued presence of a small number of parasites, which are difficult to eliminate by chemotherapy, is relevant to the prognosis of chronic Chagas disease.

Note that much of the pathogenesis of Chagas disease has been worked out by studies in Brazil. It is notable that megasyndromes are said to be less common in the north of South America and Central America, although fewer studies have been undertaken. It has been suggested that regional differences in the pathology of Chagas disease may be related to radically distinct subspecific strains of *T. cruzi* (see Epidemiology).

Diagnosis

In a known endemic area of Chagas disease, Romana's sign is suggestive of acute infection, although there are other potential causes of unilateral conjunctivitis such as insect bite or injury. Many of the systemic signs of early Chagas disease are not specific and could be confused with other febrile illnesses. In chronic disease, particular ECG abnormalities (e.g., RBBB) are highly indicative if associated with positive serological findings. Hirschsprung's megacolon can be distinguished from chagasic megacolon because the former is rare in adults; if necessary, radiography or electromanometry can be used for differential diagnosis.[2] For immigrants or travellers returning from Latin America who have symptoms that might be attributable to Chagas disease, it is essential to investigate thoroughly for the presence of a supporting history, such as exposure to triatomine bugs or blood transfusion. Very rarely infection in endemic areas might be acquired by food contaminated with infected material from triatomine bugs or reservoir hosts. In all cases serology, correctly performed, should be positive if Chagas disease is present. Exhaustive investigation for Chagas disease is pointless if serology is consistently negative.

Parasitological examination may reveal the presence of trypanosomes in peripheral blood during the acute phase of infection. In some acute cases direct microscopy of unstained wet blood films may be positive. Methods for detecting scanty trypomastigotes include: (a) microscopy of thick blood films; (b) microscopy of the buffy coat layer after haematocrit centrifugation (be careful to avoid exposure to infection if tubes are inadequately sealed); (c) searching for trypomastigotes in centrifuged serum after blood coagulation (Strout's method); and (d) centrifugation of blood after lysis of red cells with 0.87% ammonium chloride. Note that *T. cruzi* is a relatively fragile organism and if thin films are prepared a high angle between the lower slide and smearing slide is required or the organisms disintegrate.

All of these concentration methods may fail to detect trypomastigotes in some acute cases. After the acute-phase infection the parasitaemia subsides to very low levels that are usually subpatent to all these direct techniques. Patent parasitaemia may reoccur in immuno-compromised patients.

The only parasitological techniques that may be effective in the chronic phase are xenodiagnosis or blood culture.[9] In xenodiagnosis, triatomine bugs from laboratory colonies reared by feeding on birds (which are insusceptible to *T. cruzi* infection) are fed on the patient. Some 20–25 days later the intestinal tract of each triatomine bug is removed, mixed with sterile physiological saline (using a blunt spatula) and observed microscopically for the presence of epimastigotes. Care must be taken to avoid exposure to infective metacyclic trypomastigotes in bug faeces. Bugs are usually fed on the underside of the patient's forearm, enclosed in plastic pots within black bags. Xenodiagnosis is quite sensitive, with up to 50% of seropositive patients yielding a positive xenodiagnosis when 10 or 20 bugs are used. It is essential to use sterile saline for the dissection or contaminants may confuse diagnosis; if *Triatoma infestans* is used for xenodiagnosis, examination for colonies must be carried out beforehand to detect the presence of *Blastocrithidia triatomae*, which is a natural invertebrate parasite of this species. Local triatomine bug species should be used as susceptibility to different strains of *T. cruzi* varies. Delayed hypersensitivity reactions may require treatment. Anaphylactic reactions are extremely rare, but two cases are known. Multiple cultures using a sensitive blood agar base with physiological saline overlay may, under ideal conditions, be as sensitive as xenodiagnosis. Contamination of cultures, particularly in the field, may interfere. Through-the-cap inoculation of cultures reduces contamination. Xenodiagnosis is generally the preferred method rather than blood culture because it is so robust. Adult bugs are not recommended because they are less resistant to starvation. Normally, starved fourth or fifth instars are used as they can be kept unfed for weeks and transported easily, as long as they are protected from high temperatures.

Theoretically detection of parasite DNA by the polymerase chain reaction (PCR) is a reliable alternative to detect intact trypomastigotes. PCR methods are available but are not yet sufficiently practical or of sufficently low cost to replace parasitological diagnosis.

In the absence of effective treatment, *T. cruzi* infection and antibodies are almost always retained for life. Many serological tests have been described since the development of the complement fixation test in 1913. The most reliable and frequently applied are the indirect immunofluorescent antibody test (IFAT) and the enzyme-linked immunosorbent assay (ELISA). The IFAT requires a fluorescent microscope; results must be interpreted with care, positive and negative controls should be run on each slide, and serum dilutions of less than 1:80 may give false-positive results. The ELISA requires careful standardization and the inclusion of positive and negative controls on every plate but, once established, has the advantages that very large numbers of samples may be screened simultaneously and positives and negatives may be distinguished by eye, as well as by measurement of light absorption in a spectrophometer. A commercial indirect haemagglutination test (IHAT) is available but is expensive and thought to be somewhat less sensitive than IFAT or ELISA. Blood spots can be used in place of serum, but serum samples give accurate measurement of antibody titre. Cross-reactions may occur, for example with visceral or cutaneous leishmaniasis. Ideally a proportion of serum samples should be referred to reference centres for checking. Children born of seropositive mothers may be antibody positive for up to 9 months because IgG crosses the placenta. The presence of IgM antibodies to *T. cruzi* in a newborn child is usually indicative of congenital infection. Such antibodies may be detected with an IgM-specific conjugate.

Management

Only two effective drugs have been developed for the treatment of *T. cruzi* infection. Nifurtimox is a synthetic nitrofuran given orally. Although still in production (Bayer), it is not readily available. Nifurtimox is given in three divided daily doses at 8–10 mg/kg for 90 days. Double doses are recommended for infected children. There are many potential side effects that could lead to interruption of treatment. Hospitalization is usually recommended to monitor side effects and ensure compliance. Nifurtimox may act by increasing oxidative stress on *T. cruzi* through the production of free radicals. The present drug of choice is benznidazole (Rochagan; Roche) which is a nitroimidazole. The dosage is 5–7 mg/kg in two divided daily doses for 60 days, or 10 mg/kg for children. As with nifurtimox there are many potential side effects. Benznidazole metabolites may act on *T. cruzi* by interaction with DNA.

Acute cases should always be treated with benznidazole, as this may be life saving and may drastically reduce the parasite load or eliminate the infection. As there are fewer side effects in children, recent recommendations are that children in the chronic phase should also be treated.[10] The value of treatment for the chronic phase in adults is debated because of side effects and treatment failure, and also because the role of continued low-level infection in the pathogenesis of the disease is still uncertain. High doses are used to treat congenital cases: up to 25 mg/kg nifurtimox daily for 30 days or up to 10 mg/kg benznidazole daily for 30–60 days. Immunocompromised patients must be treated. Double or even higher doses are recommended for treatment if meningoencephalitis is present. Indicators of cure are persistently negative xenodiagnosis or, for acute cases, serological reversion within 1 year.

Supportive chemotherapy is vital for treatment of acute symptoms and for heart failure in patients with chronic Chagas disease. Chagasic heart disease may be treated by restricted sodium intake, diuretics, vasodilatation (angiotensin-converting enzyme inhibitors) and maintenance of serum potassium concentratiaon. Digitalis may be recommended in acute Chagas disease with heart involvement, but is a last resort in those with chronic heart disease because it can make arrhythmias worse by causing premature ventricular beats or impeding AV conduction. Acute meningoencephalitis may be managed with anticonvulsants, sedatives and intravenous mannitol. Pacemakers may be fitted if bradycardia does not respond to atropine, or for complete AV block or for atrial fibrillation with a slow ventricular response that does not improve with vagolytic drugs. Lidocaine (lignocaine), mexiletine, propafenone, flecainide, β-adrenoreceptor antagonists and amiodarone are effective for the treatment of ventricular extrasystoles; the most effective drug in the management of arrhythmias is amiodarone. Treatment of arrhythmias may prolong the life expectancy of patients but may also aggravate symptoms.

In emergencies lidocaine may be used intravenously. Experienced physicians and expert reports, for example from the World Health Organization,[5] should be consulted to ensure optimal case management.

Surgery is a vital part of the treatment of chronic Chagas disease, particularly for megaoesphagus and megacolon.[11] Mild megaoesphagus can be treated by control of diet or balloon dilatation of the cardiac sphincter. In more severe megaoesphagus, a section of muscle is removed surgically from the junction of the oesophagus and stomach, which alleviates the condition and retains muscle control of the stomach (the Heller–Vasconcelos procedure). As a last resort, partial surgical removal of the distal oesophagus may be required, followed by replacement with a section from elsewhere in the alimentary tract, such as the jejunun. Less severe megacolon can be treated with laxatives, colonic lavage or manual evacuation, if necessary with laparotomy. Decompressing intubation before surgery can release sigmod volvulus. Surgery may be simplified by initial sigmoidostomy as subsequently more of the colon may be retained. Severe megacolon may be corrected effectively by the modified Duhamel–Haddad operation which consists of resection of the sigmoid loop, closing the rectal stump, and bringing the descending colon into the rear wall of the rectum (Figure 74.11). The operation is performed in two stages, the first of which leaves a perineal colostomy, and

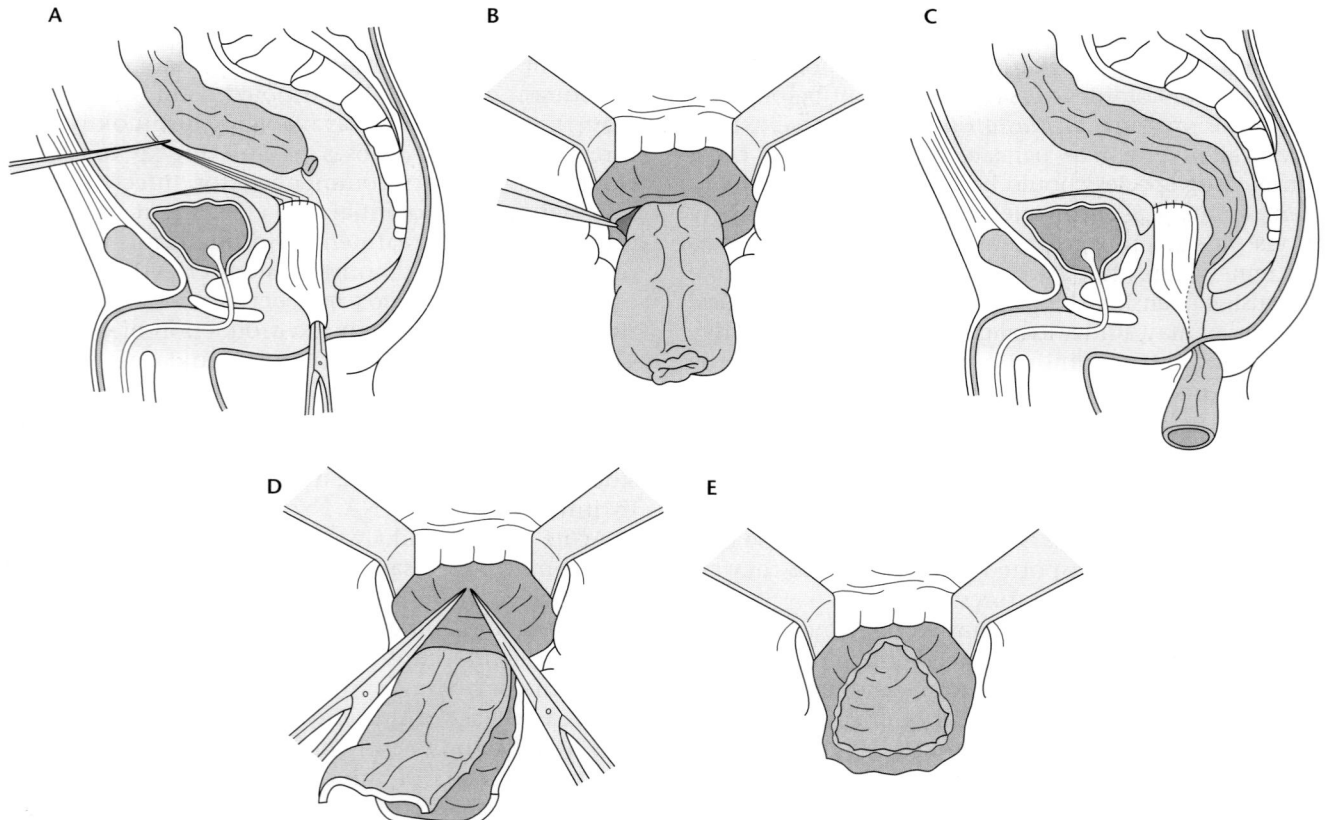

Figure 74.11: Modified Duhamel–Haddad procedure for surgical correction of megacolon in chronic Chagas disease. (See text for details.)

the second in which a wide join is made between the colon and the rectal stump, with peridural anaesthesia. Surgical resection may also be part of treatment of chagasic heart disease to remove aneurysms or arrhythmic regions.

Epidemiology

The natural habitats of triatomine bugs are the nests and resting sites of mammals and birds, particularly palm trees, hollow trees, tree cavities, burrows and rock crevices. The vast majority of approximately 130 species are confined to the New World.[12,13] Eight of 13 Old World species are closely related to *Triatoma rubrofasciata,* which has been disseminated around the world by shipping, in association with the rat (*Rattus rattus*). *T. rubrofasciata* transmits *Trypanosoma conorhini* to rats by the contaminative route. The strange Old World genus *Linshcosteus* has five species. An unidentified trypanosome species similar to *T. conorhini* has recently been isolated from *Linshcosteus* in India.

Five species of triatomine bug have become notorious vectors of Chagas disease because they have adapted so well to colonize human dwellings. *T. infestans* is the main vector in the southern cone countries of South America (Argentina, Bolivia, Brazil, Chile, Paraguay and Uruguay). *Rhodnius prolixus* and *T. dimidiata* are the principal vectors in northern South America and Central America. *Panstrongylus megistus* is an important vector in central and eastern Brazil, and *Triatoma brasiliensis* in north-east Brazil. There are several other domestic vector species of secondary importance in different geographical areas. Some silvatic species also rarely form domestic colonies or invade houses as flying adults, causing sporadic cases of Chagas disease. Male and female bugs are obligatory blood-feeders and they require at least one blood meal before moulting to the next of their five instars. Fifth-stage nymphs have rudimentary wing lappets; only adults are fully winged. One species, *Triatoma spinolai,* has wingless females and winged or wingless males. While virtually all species feed on mammal, bird or reptilian blood, a few species have also been reported to take invertebrate blood.

All mammal species are considered to be susceptible to *T. cruzi,* and more than 150 species of 24 families have been reported as infected. Birds and reptiles are not susceptible to *T. cruzi* infection, but chickens are nevertheless particularly important epidemiologically as they may sustain large colonies in chicken houses. Guinea pigs that are bred within or adjacent to houses, dogs, cats, rats and mice may carry *T. cruzi* and be attacked by triatomine bugs. Cats probably acquire infection by the oral route through eating mice and infected bugs. *T. cruzi* prevalence rates in pigs, goats, cattle and horses are usually very low. The mammal reservoir host first decribed by Carlos Chagas was the armadillo, *Dasypus novemcinctus;* the most commonly infected silvatic mammal is the common opossum, *Didelphis* species.

Serological surveys have been used to establish the prevalence of Chagas disease in South America. The prevalence of human infection in endemic areas rises with age, as is to be expected because the contamination route of transmission is precarious. Locally acquired Chagas disease is very rare in North America as the local bug species rarely colonize houses, although adult bugs occasionally fly into campsites, attracted to light. Similarly in the vast Amazon basin no triatomine bug species has yet adapted well to colonize houses. Most of the 200 or so cases of Chagas disease known from the Amazon basin are due to adult bugs flying into houses, to oral outbreaks through contaminated food or *to Rhodnius brethesi,* a silvatic species that attacks gatherers of piassaba palm fronds. *Panstrongylus geniculatus* has been found in peridomestic pigs in the Amazon basin.[14] Silvatic *T. cruzi* infection where human Chagas disease is rare, such as in the Amazon basin or the USA, is referred to as enzootic transmission. The regional distribution of chronic Chagas disease does not correspond with the prevalence of *T. cruzi* infection. Thus mega-syndromes are reported as common in the southern cone countries but much less so in northern South America and Central America, although studies there have been less intense.

The disparate distribution of chronic Chagas disease and many other factors relating to the biology of *T. cruzi* led to the suggestion that *T. cruzi* was not a single entity but a diverse species. Thus response to chemotherapy, infectivity to triatomine bug species, behaviour in experimental animals, morphology, antigenic profiles and biochemical characteristics suggested heterogeneity within the species. This was proven in the 1970s by phenotyping *T. cruzi* strains using isoenzyme electrophoresis. In particular, the first of these studies noted that strains of *T. cruzi* from domestic and silvatic transmission cycles in eastern Brazil were radically distinct (more so than recognized species of *Leishmania*) and involved different triatomine vector species. This approach strengthened the concept that in some localities domestic and silvatic transmission cycles are separate, or overlapping, as may be the case in Venezuela where the domestic vector is *R. prolixus* and where *R. prolixus* also infests palm trees. The distinction between transmission cycle types is vital for planning control programmes.[15]

The heterogeneity of *T. cruzi* has been reaffirmed many times by many methods, including profiles of randomly amplified polymorphic DNA (RAPD), microsatellites and diversity of 24S alpha, miniexon, 18S, and pteridine reductase DNA. Isoenzyme electrophoresis originally classified *T. cruzi* into principal zymodemes Z1, Z2 and Z3.[15] Many different studies over several decades have shown that there are at least two major subspecific divisions within the species. These are named by international consensus simply as *T. cruzi* I and *T. cruzi* II (*T. cruzi* I corresponding with Z1 and *T. cruzi* II encompassing Z2).[16] This is, however, an oversimplification; for example, there are at least five notable subdivisions within *T. cruzi* II.[17] The terms discrete typing unit (DTU), lineage and sublineage have been used to indicate subgroups within the species, although there has been some conflicting use of the latter term, lineage.

There can be no doubt that such marked diversity in the disease agent must have an impact on the epidemiology of Chagas disease. *T. cruzi* II predominates throughout the southern cone countries of South America where *T. infestans* is the main domestic vector and where Chagas disease is said to be most severe. *T. cruzi* I predominates in the Amazon basin, north of the Amazon basin, and in some silvatic cycles further south. Nevertheless, proof of the link between the genotype of the disease agent and the outcome of human infection is difficult to obtain. Furthermore, multiple *T. cruzi* genotypes may be isolated from one patient, with different tissue distributions between the infected organs.[18] It has been suggested that *T. cruzi* I has an ancient evolutionary history with the opossum (*Didelphis*) and tentatively with the triatomine genus *Rhodnius* and the palm tree habitat. The evolutionary history of *T. cruzi* II is uncertain. An ancient association with armadillos has been suggested and subsequent transfer to rodents through shared ecotopes (for a review see Gaunt and Miles[3]).

The propagation of *T. cruzi* appears to be predominantly clonal. Nevertheless there is some evidence of extant capacity for genetic recombination. Thus putative parental and hybrid phenotypes have been recorded among sympatric natural populations of *T. cruzi* and it has been possible to produce such hybrid forms experimentally in the laboratory. This was done by genetically transforming putative parental isolates to resistance to different drug markers and by co-passaging such transformed biological clones through the life cycle. Dual drug-resistant clones obtained in this way carried phenotypic and genotypic markers characteristic of both parental clones.[19] Theoretically, genetic recombination may have epidemiological implications in producing new virulent or drug-resistant genotypes.

Prevention and control

Transmission by blood transfusion contributes significantly to the public health problem of Chagas disease.[20] Congenital transmission and oral transmission are important for the unfortunate few infected by these routes. Nevertheless the overwhelming majority of cases of Chagas disease are disseminated by triatomine bugs. When I first set foot in South America in 1971, I was dismayed to see the way in which triatomine bugs multiplied unimpeded in poor-quality housing. Chagas disease is thus largely a disease of poverty. There is no chemoprophylaxis. There is no vaccine. It is unlikely that there will ever be a vaccine as induction of autoimmunity[21] must be reliably excluded from any candidate vaccine preparation, and vaccine trials are difficult to envisage when chronic side effects might be revealed decades later. Fortunately there are proven, highly effective, methods for controlling both triatomine bugs and blood transfusion transmission of Chagas disease.

Many attempts have been made to devise strategies for controlling triatomine bugs. Most, such as juvenile hormone mimics to prevent development, household traps and release of parasitic wasps that grow in triatomine eggs, have been abandoned. Effective control depends on insecticide spraying (Figure 74.12), supported by health education, community participation and house improvement[22] (Figure 74.13). The insecticides of choice are synthetic pyrethroids. Effective control campaigns have three phases: preparatory, attack and vigilance. In the *preparatory phase*, the distribution of all dwellings is mapped, the abundance of triatomine infestation assessed, and the attack and vigilance phases are planned and costed. In the *attack phase*, all houses and peridomestic buildings are sprayed irrespective of whether bugs have been found. Chicken houses or other peridomestic infestations that are missed may lead to rapid reinvasion. In the *vigilance phase*, appropriate sections of the community report residual infestations, which brings in a rapid response team to spray such dwellings and surrounding sites.

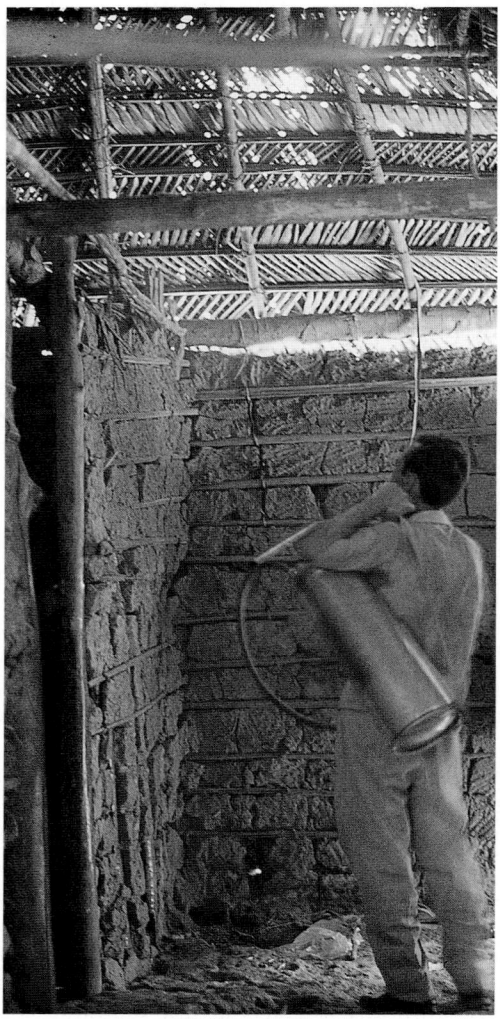

Figure 74.12: Spraying a triatomine-infested house.

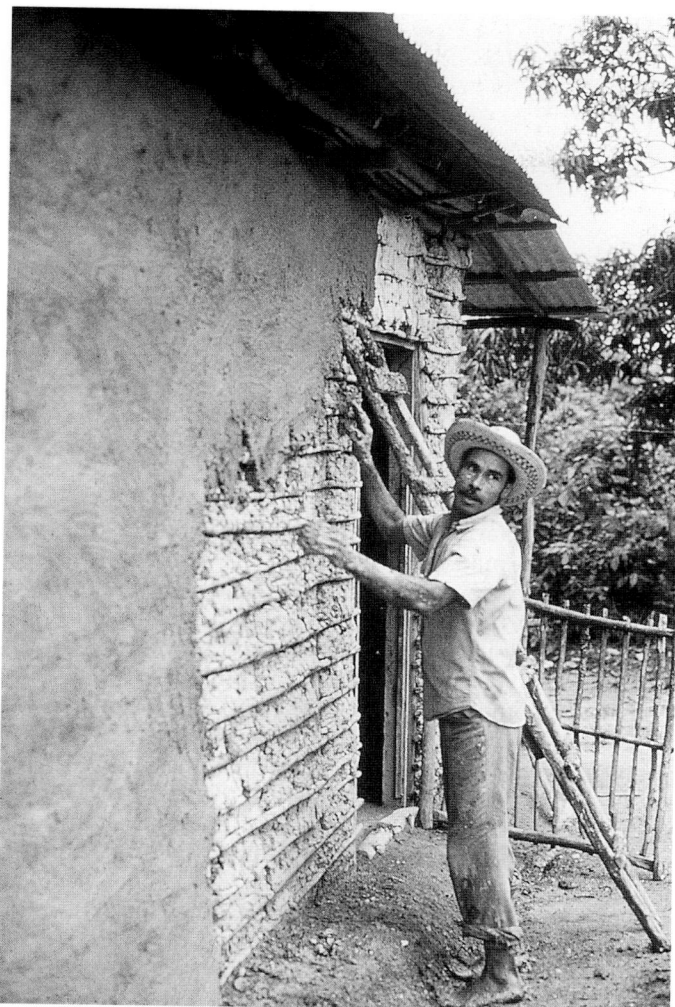

Figure 74.13: A new roof and plastered walls to combat *Rhodnius prolixus* infestation in Venezuela.

Serological testing is an essential part of monitoring the success of vector control. All children born after the beginning of a vector control campaign should be sero-negative except for those less than 9 months of age and born of seropositive mothers, who will have acquired IgG transplacentally, and except for occasional congenital cases. Thus, tracing seropositive children will reveal residual triatomine infestations. Low-cost assays, such as the ELISA, allow entire endemic regions to be screened. In addition, serological testing provides a means of screening blood donors, organ donors and organ recipients. In highly endemic areas contaminated blood can be treated with crystal violet (250 mg/litre) and stored at 4°C for at least 24 hours to kill *T. cruzi*. Prophylactic benznidazole should be given to immuno-supressed organ recipients.

The enormous economic burden of chronic Chagas disease is much greater than the cost of prevention and control. This has stimulated national and international campaigns. In the southern cone countries of South America, virtually the only important domestic triatomine vector is *T. infestans*. This species is thought to have spread from silvatic habitats in Bolivia as elsewhere it has been found only in domestic and peridomestic sites. The realization that reinvasion should not be a significant problem in southern cone countries led to the launch of the southern cone programme, to eliminate *T. infestans* from Argentina, Bolivia, Brazil, Chile, Paraguay, Uruguay and southern Peru.[23] Although not yet complete or uniformly adopted, the programme has been a resound-ing success. It is reported that 85% of domestic trans-mission has been eliminated from Brazil. Chile and Uruguay are essentially free of domestic transmission, which is also much reduced in the remaining countries. The southern cone programme provides a model for international collaboration in disease control.

New international control programmes are planned for the Andean Pact countries and for Central America. Here control may be less straightforward as the geographical distribution of *R. prolixus* in palm trees is not clear, and thus the extent of reinvasion of houses from the silvatic habitat is not known (Figure 74.14). Palm trees around

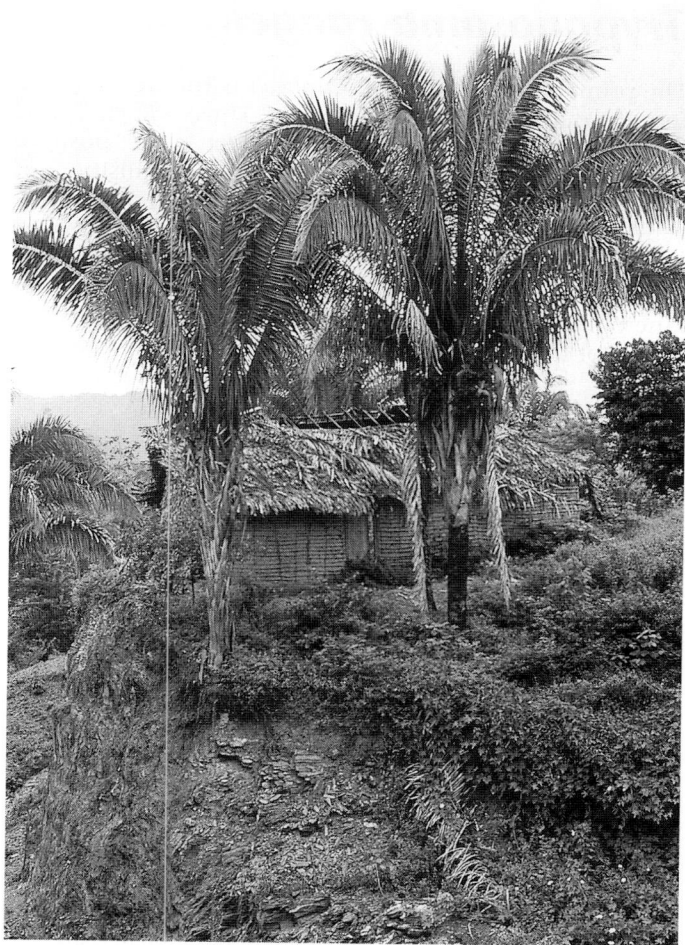

Figure 74.14: Palms adjacent to a house in Venezuela, where it is suggested that *Rhodnius prolixus* replenishes the domestic cycle from the sylvatic habitat.

dwellings may now be surveyed by a new triatomine bug trap, the Noireau trap, in which bugs are trapped on adhesive tape around a plastic vessel containing a sentinel mouse. Effective methods for insecticide treatment of infested palms need to be devised. Secondary domestic species may also emerge as complications for vector control. In the Amazon basin a diligent surveillance programme is required to respond rapidly to any domestic bug species brought in from outside endemic areas. Furthermore some Amazonian species, such as *P. geniculatus*, reported from peridomestic pigsties, may adapt to live in human dwellings. In addition, food preparation plants such as palm or sugar-cane presses should be protected from contamination by triatomine bugs attracted to artificial light.

The molecular biology of *T. cruzi* and other trypanosomatids is of immense research interest.[24] The full genome sequence of *T. cruzi* will shortly be available and may help to identify new drug targets.[25] A low-cost, nontoxic, oral drug is needed to eliminate the reservoir of human infection. Further research is also required to elucidate the epidemiological significance of subspecific diversity.

Trypanosoma rangeli

The primary importance of *T. rangeli* is that it may confuse the diagnosis of Chagas disease. Thus, if *R. prolixus* is used for xenodiagnosis of a suspect case, positive xenodiagnosis bugs may be due to the acquisition of *T. rangeli* infection and not *T. cruzi*, or to both organisms. With appropriate training, *T. rangeli* in triatomine bugs can be distinguished from *T. cruzi* by the presence of epimastigotes of up to 80 µm in length, by the smaller kinetoplast, or by the fact that *T. rangeli* escapes from the lumen of the intestinal tract to reach the haemocoel and

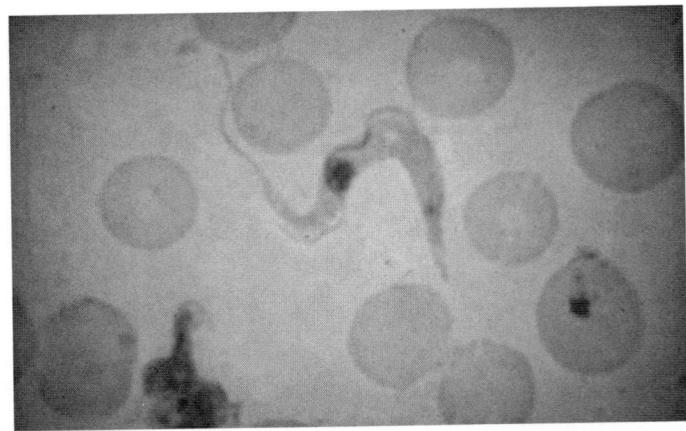

Figure 74.15: Trypomastigote of *Trypanosoma rangeli* in blood.

the salivary glands in some infected bugs. A drop of haemolymph may be removed for microscopic examination by severing one of the bug legs and extruding the haemolymph under a coverslip placed on a microscope slide. *T. rangeli* may be pathogenic to *Rhodnius*.

T. rangeli is very rarely seen in human blood (Figure 74.15). Trypomastigotes of *T. rangeli* in blood are much larger than those of *T. cruzi*, and they also have a smaller subterminal kinetoplast. The main natural host of this appears to be the common opossum (*Didelphis*). *T. rangeli* is thought to divide in peripheral blood, but the full life cycle in the mammalian host is uncertain. Transmission is by triatomine bite. Antibodies to *T. rangeli* may be fairly prevalent where *R. prolixus* is the domestic triatomine vector. Theoretically such antibodies may cross-react with *T. cruzi*, although the extent of this problem is not clear. It is certain that antibodies to *T. cruzi* in chronic Chagas disease, which may have titres excess of 1 in 10[6], do cross-react with *T. rangeli*.

REFERENCES

1. Miles M A. New World trypanosomiasis. In Cox F E G (ed.) *The Wellcome Trust Illustrated History of Tropical Diseases*. London: Wellcome Trust; 1996:192–205.
2. Miles M A. Chagas' disease and chagasic megacolon. In Kamm M A & Lennard-Jones J E (eds) *Constipation*. Petersfield, UK: Wrightson Biomedical; 1994:205–210.
3. Gaunt M & Miles M A. The ecotopes and evolution of triatomine bugs (Triatominae) and their associated trypanosomes. *Mem Inst Oswaldo Cruz* 2000; 95:557–565.
4. Hoare C A. *The Trypanosomes of Mammals*. Oxford: Blackwell; 1972.
5. World Health Organization. *Control of Chagas Disease*. WHO Technical Report Series 811. Geneva: WHO, 1991.
6. Pan American Health Organization. *Chagas' Disease and the Nervous System*. Scientific Publication no. 547. Washington, DC: PAHO; 1994.
7. Miles M A. New World trypanosomiasis. In Cox F E G, Kreier J P & Wakelin D (eds) *Topley & Wilson's Microbiology and Microbial Infections*, vol. 5. London: Arnold, 1997:283–302.
8. Tarleton R L, Zhang L & Downs M O. 'Autoimmune' rejection of neonatal heart transplants in experimental Chagas disease is a parasite-specific response to infected host tissue. *Proc Natl Acad Sci USA* 1997; 94:3932–3937.
9. Miles M A. Culturing and biological cloning of *Trypanosoma cruzi*. In Hyde J E (ed.) *Protocols in Molecular Parasitology*. Humana Press, 1993:15–28.
10. Estani S S, Segura E L, Ruiz A M et al. Efficacy of chemotherapy with benznidazole in children in the indeterminate phase Chagas' disease. *Am J Trop Med Hyg* 1998; 59:526–529.
11. Raia A A. *Manifestaçoes Digestivas da Moléstia de Chagas*. São Paulo: Sarvier Brasil, 1983.
12. Lent H & Wygodzinsky P. Revision of the Triatominae (Hemiptera, Reduviidae), and their significance as figures of Chagas disease. *Bull Am Mus Nat Hist* 1979; 163:123–520.
13. Schofield C J. *Triatominae: Biology and Control*. UK, Eurocommunica Publications, 1994.
14. Valente V C, Valente S A S, Noireau F et al. Chagas disease in the Amazon Basin: association of *Panstrongylus geniculatus* (Hemiptera: Reduviidae) with domestic pigs. *J Med Entomol* 1998; 35:99–103.
15. Miles M A. Transmission cycles and the heterogeneity of *Trypanosoma cruzi*. In Lumsden W H R & Evans D A (eds) *Biology of the Kinetoplastida*, vol. 2. London: Academic Press, 1979:117–196.

16 Anonymous. Recommedations from a satellite meeting. *Mem Inst Oswaldo Cruz* 1999; 94:429–432.

17 Brisse S, Barnabe C & Tibayrenc M. Identification of six *Trypanosoma cruzi* phylogenetic lineages by random amplified polymorphic DNA and multilocus enzyme electrophoresis. *Int J Parasitol* 2000; 30:35–44.

18 Vago A R, Andrade L O, Leite A A, et al. Genetic characterisation of *Trypanosoma cruzi* directly from tissues of patients with chronic Chagas disease: different distribution of genetic types into diverse organs. *Am J Pathol* 2000; 156:1805–1809.

19 Stothard J R, Frame I A & Miles M A. Genetic diversity and genetic exchange in *Trypanosoma cruzi*: dual drug-resistant 'progeny' from episomal transformants. *Mem Inst Oswaldo Cruz* 1999; 94:189–193.

20 Shulman I A, Appleman M D, Saxena S et al. Specific antibodies to *Trypanosoma cruzi* among blood donors in Los Angeles, California. *Transfusion* 1997; 37:727–731.

21 Kali J & Cunha-Neto E. Autoimmunity in Chagas disease cardiomyopathy: fulfilling the criteria at last. *Parasitol Today* 1996; 12:396–399.

22 Dias J C P. Control of Chagas disease in Brazil. *Parasitol Today* 1987; 3:336–341.

23 Schofield C J & Dias J C P. The southern cone initiative against Chagas disease. *Adv Parasitol* 1998; 2:2–22.

24 Frasch A C. Functional diversity in the trans-sialidase and mucin families in *Trypanosoma cruzi*. *Parasitol Today* 2000; 16:282–286.

25 Andersson B, Aslund L, Tammi M et al. Complete sequence of a 93.4-kb contig from chromosome 3 of *Trypanosoma cruzi* containing a strand-switch region. *Genome Res* 1998; 8:809–815.

Chapter 75
Leishmaniasis

J. P. Dedet and F. Pratlong

Leishmaniases are parasitic diseases caused by protozoan flagellates of the genus *Leishmania*, parasites infecting numerous mammal species, including humans, and transmitted through the infective bite of an insect vector, the phlebotomine sandfly.

The leishmaniases are threatening 350 million people in 88 countries of four continents. The annual incidence of new cases is estimated between 1.5 and 2 million.[1] In numerous underdeveloped countries, they remain a major public health problem.

The genus *Leishmania* includes around 30 different taxa, the majority of which commonly infect humans, in whom they are responsible for various types of disease: visceral, cutaneous (of localized or diffuse type) and muco-cutaneous leishmaniases. This variability of the clinical features results from both the diversity of the *Leishmania* species and the immune response of the hosts.

Parasite

Leishmania are protozoa belonging to the order Kineto-plastida and the family Trypanosomatidae, which includes other parasites of mammals, including humans (genus *Trypanosoma*), of plants (*Phytomonas*) and of insects (*Leptomonas*, *Crithidia*, etc.).

Description

Leishmania are dimorphic parasites which present as two principal morphological stages: the intracellular amastigote, within the mononuclear phagocytic system of the mammalian host, and the flagellated promastigote within the intestinal tract of the insect vector and in culture medium.

The amastigote stage is a round or oval body about 2–6 μm in diameter, containing a nucleus, a kinetoplast and an internal flagellum seen clearly in electron micrographs. The amastigotes multiply within the parasitophorous vacuoles of macrophages.

The promastigote stage has a long and slender body (about 15–30 μm by 2–3 μm), with a central nucleus, a kinetoplast and a long free anterior flagellum.

Identification

Since the creation of the genus *Leishmania* by Ross,[2] the number of species described has constantly increased. As the different species are indistinguishable by their morphology, other criteria have been used for their identification. Lumsden distinguished between extrinsic characters (such as clinical features, geographical distribution, behaviour in culture, laboratory animals or vectors) and intrinsic ones (such as immunological, biochemical or molecular criteria).[3] Among them, isoenzyme electrophoresis remains the current gold standard technique, while DNA-based techniques are being used increasingly. Applied to *Leishmania* initially by Gardener et al.,[4] isoenzyme analysis has been widely developed for the study of these parasites. Its success principally results from the existence of a high degree of polymorphism, expressed as stable and relatively specific electromorphs. These have permitted characterization of the strains by their enzymatic profiles and their grouping in homogeneous electrophoretic taxonomic units termed zymodemes.[5]

Isoenzyme characterization is currently the reference technique for *Leishmania* identification at specific and infra-specific levels, and for classification of the genus.[6]

Classification

Various types of classification have been successively applied to the genus. Those proposed between 1916 and 1987 were monothetic Linnean classifications based on few hierarchical characters. Lainson and Shaw are the authors who worked the most on these types of classification and who made them evolutive. Their last classification[7] divided the genus *Leishmania* into two subgenera: *Leishmania* sensu stricto, present in both Old and New Worlds, and *Viannia*, restricted to the New World. Within these two subgenera various species complexes were individualized.

Since the 1980s, Adansonian phenetic classifications have been employed. They are based on a number of similarly weighted characters (absence of hierarchy) used simultaneously (polythetic classification) without a prior hypothesis. They were at first phenetic. Isoenzymes are considered as different allelic forms of a gene, and enzymatic variation at a given locus can be interpreted as a mutation occurring during evolution. Subsequently, phylogenetic classification revealed a parental relationship between the different species of *Leishmania*[6,8] (Table 75.1).

Table 75.1 Classification of the genus *Leishmania*. Simplified classification derived from the phylogenetic analysis of Rioux et al. based on isoenzymes.[6]

I. Sub-genus *Leishmania* Ross, 1903

L. donovani complex
    L. donovani (Laveran & Mesnil, 1903)
    L. archibaldi Castellani & Chalmers, 1919

L. infantum complex   *L. infantum* Nicolle, 1908 (syn. *L. chagasi* Cunha & Chagas, 1937)
L. tropica complex   *L. tropica* (Wright, 1903)
L. killicki complex   *L. killicki* Rioux, Lanotte & Pratlong, 1986
L. aethiopica complex   *L. aethiopica* Bray, Ashford & Bray, 1973
L. major complex   *L. major* Yakimoff & Schokhor, 1914
L. turanica complex   *L. turanica* Strelkova, Peters & Evans, 1990
L. gerbilli complex   *L. gerbilli* Wang, Qu & Guan, 1964
L. arabica complex   *L. arabica* Peters, Elbihari & Evans, 1986
L. mexicana complex   *L. mexicana* Biagi, 1953 (syn. *L. pifanoi* Medina & Romero, 1959)

L. amazonensis complex
    L. amazonensis Lainson & Shaw, 1972 (syn. *L. garnhami*, Scorza et al., 1979)
    L. aristidesi Lainson & Shaw, 1979

L. enriettii complex   *L. enriettii* Muniz & Medina, 1948

L. hertigi complex
    L. hertigi Herrer, 1971
    L. deanei Lainson & Shaw, 1977

II. Sub-genus *Viannia* Lainson and Shaw, 1987

L. braziliensis complex
    L. braziliensis Vianna, 1911
    L. peruviana Velez, 1913

L. guyanensis complex
    L. guyanensis Floch, 1954
    L. panamensis Lainson & Shaw, 1972
    L. shawi Lainson et al., 1989

L. naiffi complex   *L. naiffi* Lainson & Shaw, 1989
L. lainsoni complex   *L. lainsoni* Silveira et al., 1987

The phenetic, and especially the cladistic classifications confirmed the majority of the taxonomic groups previously established by the Linnean classifications, and particularly that of Lainson and Shaw.[7] The concordance between them mutually validated the extrinsic and intrinsic identification criteria. However, cladistic analysis allowed a more detailed study of some groups and led to the establishment of new complexes (*L. infantum*, *L. turanica* and *L. guyanensis*), and also to the grouping in the same complex of taxa previously separated (*L. guyanensis*, *L. panamensis* and *L. shawi*).

Epidemiology

The *Leishmania* species circulate in natural infection foci where a haematophagous insect acting as a vector, the phlebotomine sandfly, and a mammal reservoir coexist.

Vector

Sandflies are Diptera of the family Psychodidae, subfamily Phlebotominae. Their life cycle includes two different biological stages: the flying adult and the development phase, which includes egg, four larval stages and pupa, and which occurs in wet soil rich in organic material.[9]

The adults are small flying insects of about 2–4 mm in length, with a yellowish hairy body. During the day, they rest in dark and sheltered places (resting sites). They are active at dusk and during the night. Both sexes feed on plants, but females also need a blood meal before they are able to lay eggs. Reptiles, amphibia, birds and mammals are potential hosts. Feeding habits depend on the sandfly species, and the nature of the host on which it takes its blood meal is a key point for *Leishmania* transmission.

When engorged, a female lays 50–100 eggs, from which hatches the first larval stage. The larvae are cylindrical, dirty white in colour, with a distinct dark head, and long caudal setae. Larval development may take 30–60 days, depending on species, prevailing temperature and food supplies. They breed in soil, on decaying organic matter. The precise localization of sandfly breeding sites remains unknown for the majority of the species, which is a limiting factor for sandfly control. The fourth larval stage attaches itself to the substrate and transforms into the pupa, from which the adult emerges after 7–8 days.

About 800 species of sandflies have been described, and they are divided into five widely accepted genera: *Phlebotomus* and *Sergentomyia* in the Old World, and *Lutzomyia*, *Brumptomyia* and *Warileya* in the New World.[10] Among these species, about 70, belonging to the genera *Phlebotomus* and *Lutzomyia*, are proven or suspected vectors of *Leishmania*, and a certain level of specificity between *Leishmania* and sandfly species exists.[11] Some *Leishmania* species are restricted to a single sandfly species (*L. amazonensis* to *Lutzomyia flaviscutellata*, *L. tropica* to *Phlebotomus sergenti*) or to close species of a same subgenus (*L. major* transmitted by *P. papatasi* or by *P. duboscqi*, two species of the *Phlebotomus* subgenus). For other species the host specificity seems less strong; for example, the vectors of *L. donovani* are included in various subgenera of the *Phlebotomus* genus (*Euphlebotomus* for *P. argentipes* in India, *Larroussius* for *P. orientalis* in Sudan, or *Synphlebotomus* for *P. martini* in Kenya). Similarly the main vectors of *L. infantum* include species of the *Larroussius* (*P. perniciosus* and *P. ariasi* in the Mediterranean basin) or of the *Adlerius* (*P. chinensis* in China) subgenus of *Phlebotomus*, but also of the *Lutzomyia* subgenus and genus in the New World (*Lu. longipalpis*).

Reservoir

Most leishmaniases are zoonoses and the reservoir hosts are various species of mammals which are responsible for the long-term maintenance of *Leishmania* in nature.[12] Depending on the focus, the reservoir can be either a wild or a domestic mammal, or even in particular cases human beings. In the case of visceral leishmaniasis, these different types of reservoir represent different evolutive steps on the path towards anthropization of a wild zoonosis.[13] Most reservoir hosts are well adapted to *Leishmania* and develop only mild infections which may persist for many years, an important exception being the dog, which commonly develops a generalized and fatal disease.

The reservoirs are included in seven different orders of mammals: marsupials, primates, edentates, rodents, carnivores, hyraxes and perissodactyls.

In the Old World, rodents and hyraxes are reservoirs of wild zoonotic cutaneous leishmaniases due respectively to *L. major* and *L. aethiopica*. Various rodent species are the main reservoirs of *L. major*, as the great gerbil *Rhombomys opimus* in the arid regions of Central Asia or the fat sand jird *Psammomys obesus* in the Near East and North Africa. Hyraxes are the main reservoir hosts of *L. aethiopica* in Ethiopia and Kenya.

In the New World, various sylvatic mammals are reservoirs of American cutaneous leishmaniases. They include mammals of the forest canopy, such as the sloths *Choleopus didactylus* for *L. guyanensis* and *C. hoffmanni* for *L. panamensis*, and ground-level rodents, such as the spiny rat *Proechimys guyannensis* and *P. cuvieri* for *L. amazonensis*, the climbing rat *Ototylomys phyllotis* for *L. mexicana*, the paca *Cuniculus paca* for *L. lainsoni* and the armadillo *Dasipus novemcinctus* for *L. naiffi*.

Dogs have been found infected with *L. infantum*, *L. tropica*, *L. peruviana* and *L. braziliensis*, but are currently considered as true reservoirs of *L. infantum* and *L. peruviana*, two species which have peri-domestic or even domestic transmission. Some wild carnivores, such as foxes *Vulpes* species and *Cerdocyon thous*, jackals *Canis aureus*, wolves *C. lupus* and racoon dogs *Nyctereutes procyonoides*, were found harbouring *L. infantum*, and could be considered as ancestral hosts of a wild zoonotic leishmaniasis according to the Garnham hypothesis.[13]

Humans are the commonly recognized reservoir host of *L. donovani* visceral leishmaniasis and *L. tropica* cutaneous leishmaniasis. The life cycles of these two species correspond to the tertiary epidemiological type. The elective localization of *L. donovani* to skin (post-kala-azar dermal leishmaniasis) makes man a genuine reservoir

for this species in India and East Africa. *L. tropica* is basically anthroponotic, but has been isolated from dogs in some countries, where the role of dogs as a reservoir has been discussed.

Life cycle

In nature, *Leishmania* are alternatively hosted by the insect (flagellated promastigote) and by mammals (intracellular amastigote stage) (Figure 75.1). When a female sandfly takes a blood meal from a *Leishmania*-infected mammal, intracellular (and maybe also extracellular) amastigotes are ingested by the insect. Inside the blood meal, amastigotes transform into motile promastigotes, which escape through the peritrophic membrane enveloping the blood meal. The promastigotes multiply intensively inside the intestinal tract of the sandfly, successively as free elongated promastigotes (nectomonads) or as attached pro- and paramastigotes (haptomonads).[14] This intraluminal development occurs in the midgut (*Leishmania* subgenus, previously section Suprapylaria according to Lainson and Shaw[15]), or in the hindgut and the midgut (*Viannia* subgenus, previously section Peripylaria). Whatever the multiplication site, the parasites subsequently migrate to the anterior part of the sandfly midgut, where they change into free-swimming metacyclic promastigotes, the stage infective for the vertebrate host.

The bite of an infected sandfly deposits infective metacyclic promastigotes in the mammal's skin, which are rapidly phagocytosed by cells of the mononuclear phagocyte system. The intracellular parasites change into amastigotes, which multiply by simple mitosis. The molecular aspects of the parasite–cell interaction in the mammalian host are briefly summarized below (see Pathology section).

Transmission

The inoculation of metacyclic promastigotes through the sandfly bite is the usual method of leishmaniasis transmission. Other routes remain exceptional.

In visceral leishmaniasis (VL), a few cases of congenital and of blood transfusion transmission have been reported. A case of direct transmission by sexual contact has been reported.[16] Exchange of syringes has been incriminated to explain the high prevalence of *L. infantum*/HIV co-infection in intravenous drug-users in southern Europe.[17]

In cutaneous leishmaniasis (CL), contact with the active lesion is innocuous; infection should require inoculation of material from active sores, as was carried out in ancient times by various populations of endemic areas as a crude form of vaccination.

Geographical distribution

Leishmaniases are widely distributed around the world. They range over the intertropical zones of America and

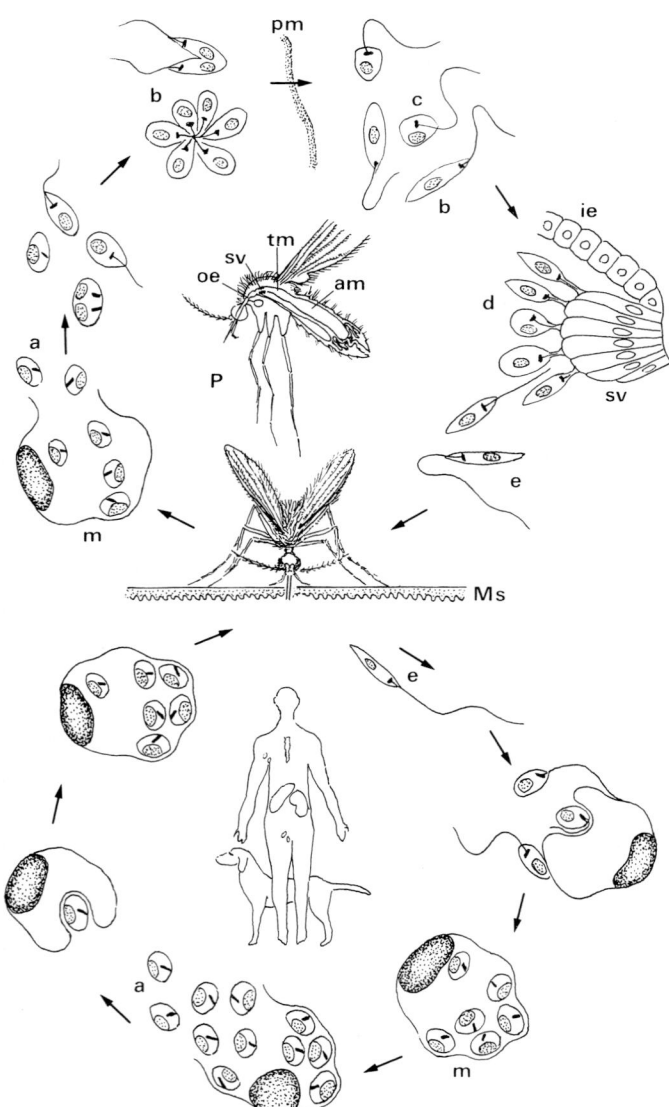

Figure 75.1: Life cycle of the *Leishmania* parasites. P: phlebotomine sandfly; pm: peritrophic membrane; am: abdominal midgut; tm: thoracic midgut; oe: oesophagus; sv: stomodeal valve; ie: intestinal epithelium; Ms: mammal skin ; m: macrophage. a: amastigotes; b: nectomonad promastigotes; c: paramastigotes; d: attached haptomonads; e: metacyclic promastigotes. (Original drawing by D. M. Jarry.)

Africa, and extend into temperate regions of South America, southern Europe and Asia. Their extension limits are latitude 45° north and 32° south. Geographical distribution of the diseases is related to that of the sandfly species acting as vectors, their ecology and the conditions of internal development of the parasite.

Leishmaniases are present in 88 countries in four continents, of which 16 are industrialized and 72 developing countries, 13 of them among the poorest in the world. There are an estimated 12 million cases in a worldwide population of exposed at risk estimated at 350 million people. One-and-a-half to two million new cases occur each year.[1]

VL is found in 47 countries and its mean annual incidence is estimated around 500 000 new cases. The main historical foci of endemic VL are located, east to west, in China, India, Central Asia, East Africa, the Mediterranean basin and Brazil (Figure 75.2). The anthroponotic species *L. donovani* is restricted to China, India and East Africa, while the zoonotic species *L. infantum* extends from China to Brazil. India is certainly the biggest focus of VL in the world. Between 1875 and 1950, the disease there took on an epidemic feature, with three severe outbreaks in Assam and a subsequent extension to other Indian states.[18]

At the present time, 90% of the VL cases in the world are in Bangladesh, India and Nepal, Sudan and Brazil. Bihar State in India experienced a dramatic epidemic, with more than 300 000 cases reported between 1977 and 1990 and a mortality rate over 2%.[19] In southern Sudan, an outbreak was responsible for 100 000 deaths from 1989 to 1994, in a population of Upper Nile Province of less than 1 million.[20] Population movements, such as rural to suburban migration in north-eastern Brazil,[21] are factors for VL extension, by exposing thousands of non-immune individuals to the risk of infection.

The large majority of Old World CL (Figure 75.3) are due to the two species *L. major* and *L. tropica* and proceed from countries of the Near and Middle East: Afghanistan, Iran, Saudi Arabia and Syria. *L. major*, the species responsible for zoonotic CL, has a large distribution area, including West, North and East Africa, the Near and Middle East and Central Asia. Economic developments have been accompanied by movement of populations which have caused dramatic epidemic outbreaks of this species in several countries of the Middle East, but also in Algeria and Tunisia. The anthroponotic species *L. tropica* is present in various cities of the Near and Middle East, but extends also to Tunisia and Morocco, where an animal reservoir is suspected in some foci. Other species have restricted distribution areas: *L. aethiopica* to Ethiopia and Kenya, *L. arabica* to Saudi Arabia and *L. killicki* to Tunisia. *L. turanica* and *L. gerbilli* are Central Asian species restricted to rodents.

In the New World (Figure 75.4), *L. braziliensis* is the species with the widest distribution area. It extends from south of Mexico to north of Argentina. *L. amazonensis* has a large distribution in South America, but human cases of this rodent enzootic species are unusual. Other species have more restricted areas: *L. guyanensis* (north of the Amazonian basin), *L. panamensis* (Colombia and Central America), *L. mexicana* (Mexico and Central America), and lastly *L. peruviana*, which is restricted to the Andean valleys of Peru. With the exception of this latter species, all other American dermotropic species are responsible for wild zoonoses of the rainforest.

Pathology

The bite of an infected sandfly results in the intradermal inoculation of metacyclic leishmaniae. Their establishment

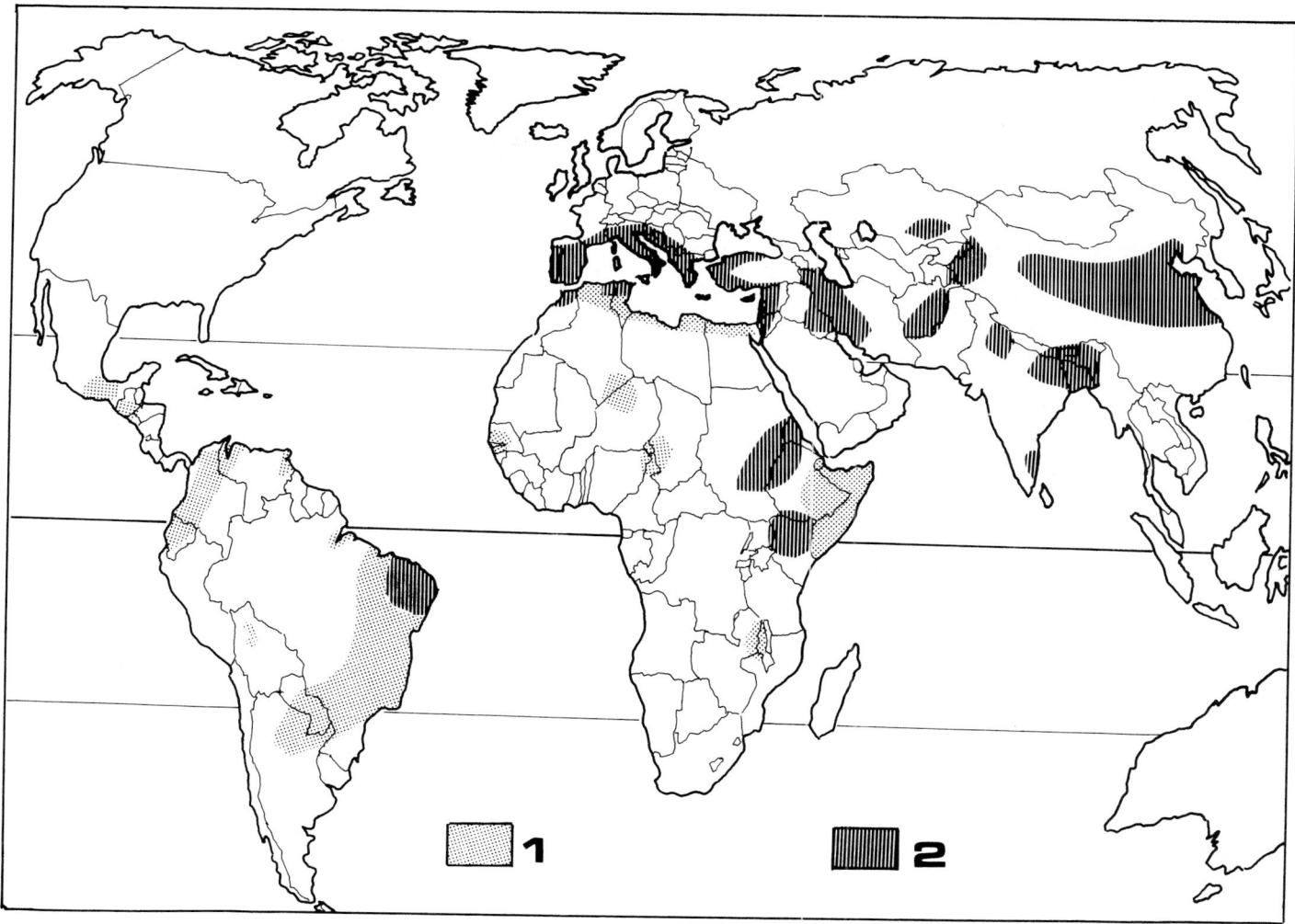

Figure 75.2: Geographical distribution of visceral leishmaniasis. 1: Low-endemicity areas. 2: High-endemicity areas.

in the mammalian host is facilitated in a remarkable way by the sandfly saliva delivered at the same time, which enhances *Leishmania* infectivity.[22] Sandfly saliva contains various pharmacologically active substances, which globally prevent haemostatic mechanisms of the host, and cause vasodilatation and local immuno-suppression.[23]

Within the dermis of mammalian skin, the metacyclic promastigotes escape complement activation, thanks to their surface components, mainly lipophosphoglycan and glycoprotein (63 kDa). They are then phagocytosed by macrophages within which they transform into amastigotes, and have the capacity to resist intracellular digestion. Their survival in these cells is the result of several factors related to the cell itself (decrease in the production of oxidative and nitrogenic derivatives triggered by the presence of the parasite) and to the amastigote's ability to resist lysosomal hydrolases, a property probably related to surface glyco-inositol-phospholipids.[24]

When the intracellular development of the amastigotes remains localized at the inoculation site, various cyto-

kines are released and cell reactions are generated, resulting in the development of a localized lesion of CL.[25] In other instances, the parasites spread to the organs of the mononuclear phagocytic system, giving rise to VL. Amastigotes may also spread to other cutaneous sites, as in diffuse cutaneous leishmaniasis (DCL), or to mucosae in the case of mucocutaneous leishmaniasis (MCL).

The localization of the parasite to the various organs of the patient results in the clinical expression of the disease. It is directly related to the tropism of the parasite species (Table 75.2). In that sense, the genus *Leishmania* can be divided broadly into viscerotropic (*L. donovani*, *L. infantum*) and dermotropic species (roughly all other species). *L. braziliensis*, and more rarely *L. panamensis*, are known for their secondary mucosal spread.

In spite of this general tropism of the species some exceptions occur, which are independent of the clinical status of the patient harbouring the parasite. Thus, well-established viscerotropic species can occasionally be responsible for limited cutaneous lesions without signs or symptoms of any visceral involvement. One of the best examples are dermotropic enzymatic variants of the

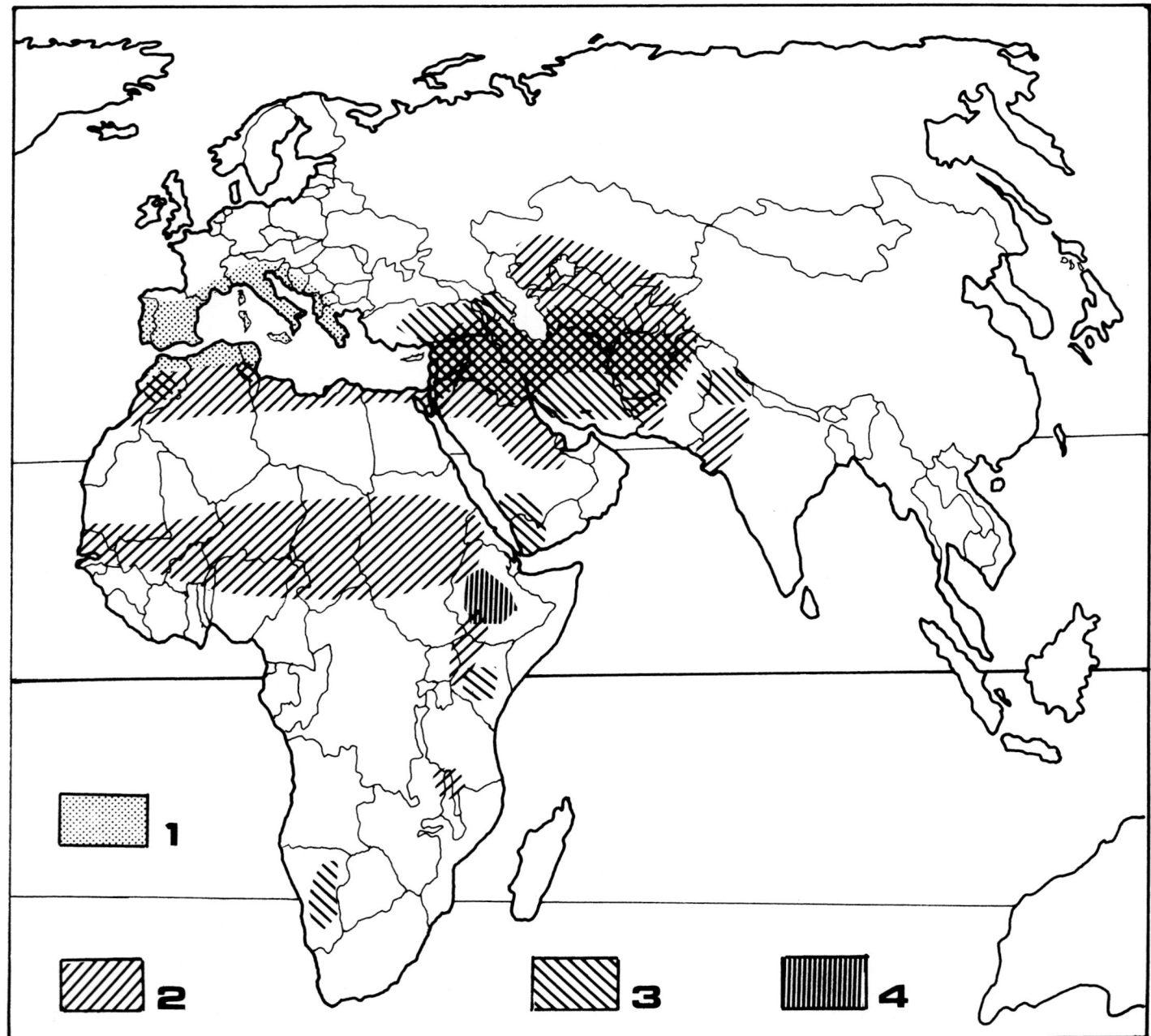

Figure 75.3: Geographical distribution of Old World CL. 1: *L. infantum* CL. 2: Zoonotic CL caused by *L. major*. 3: *L. tropica* CL. 4: *L aethiopica* CL.

normally visceralizing species *L. infantum* in the Mediterranean basin.[26] This unusual tropism of certain populations of a species may be explained by intraspecific variation of the parasite genome, the markers of which remain unknown.

The clinical expression of the leishmaniases depends not only on the genotypic potential of the different parasites but also on the immunological status of the patient. For many years, *L. aethiopica* and *L. amazonensis* were known to be responsible for localized cutaneous leishmaniasis (LCL) in immunocompetent patients, but for DCL in anergic individuals. Since infection with the human

immunodeficiency virus (HIV) has spread to areas where leishmaniasis is endemic, DCL has been found with species which were never previously known to cause this form of disease (e.g. *L. major* and *L. braziliensis*). In immunodeficient patients, particularly those with HIV infection, the dermotropic variants of the viscerotropic species are responsible for VL[27] (Table 75.2).

In CL, interactions of the patient's cell-mediated immune response with the parasites result in a spectrum of clinical and pathological changes. The histological patterns range from a diffuse granuloma containing large numbers of macrophages full of amastigotes, while

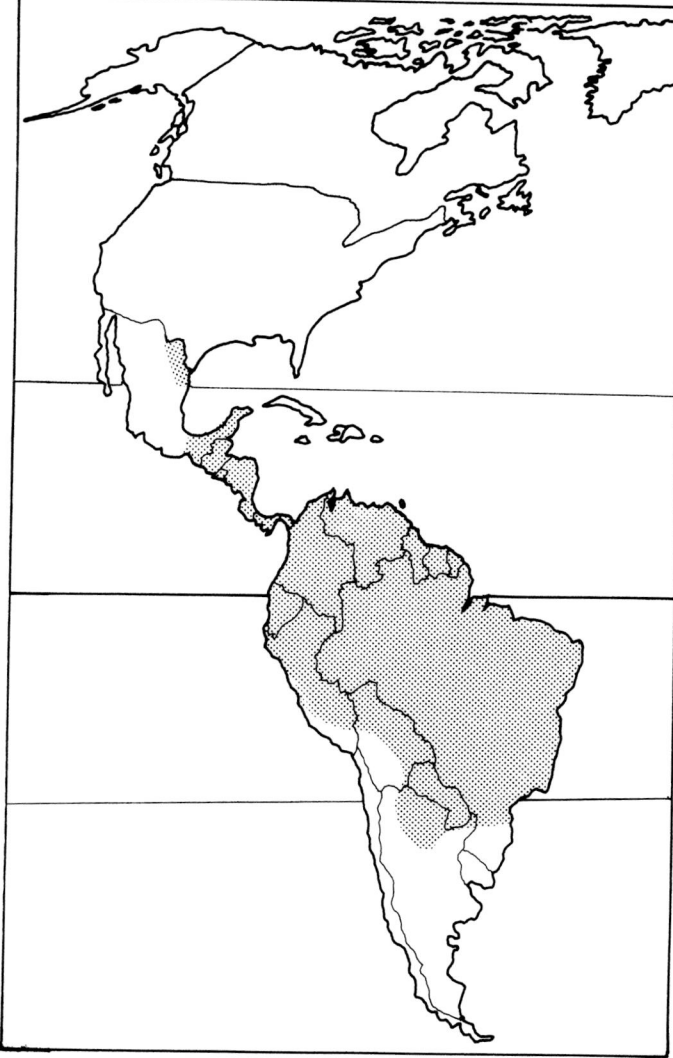

Figure 75.4: Global geographical distribution of New World cutaneous and mucocutaneous leishmaniasis.

Table 75.2 Usual tropism and clinical expression of the anthropophilic species of *Leishmania*

Usual tropism	Species	Clinical expression	
		Usual	Exceptional
Viserotropic species	*L. donovani*	VL	LCL
	L. infantum	VL	LCL, DCL*
Dermotropic species	*L. aethiopica*	LCL	DCL
	L. killicki	LCL	
	L. major	LCL	DCL*
	L. tropica	LCL	VL
	L. amazonensis	LCL	DCL, VL
	L. colombiensis	LCL	–
	L. guyanensis	LCL	MCL
	L. lainsoni	LCL	–
	L. mexicana	LCL	DCL, VL*
	L. naiffi	LCL	–
	L. peruviana	LCL	–
	L. shawi	LCL	–
	L. venezuelensis	LCL	–
Dermo-mucotropic species	*L. braziliensis*	LCL, MCL	DCL*, VL*
	L. panamensis	LCL	MCL, DCL*

VL: visceral leishmaniasis; LCL: localized cutaneous leishmaniasis; DCL: diffuse cutaneous leishmaniasis; MCL: mucocutaneous leishmaniasis.
*during immunosuppression

Clinical features

Visceral leishmaniasis

VL was described at the end of nineteenth century in India, under the name of kala-azar (black fever). Its parasite was discovered in 1903,[29,30] described by Laveran and Mesnil,[31] and named *Leishmania donovani* the same year.[2]

The two *Leishmania* species usually considered as responsible for VL are *L. donovani* and *L. infantum*. *L. archibaldi*, related to *L. donovani* by some authors, occurs in East Africa. *L. chagasi*, agent of New World VL, is currently considered as a synonym of *L. infantum*. Unusual cases of VL have been attributed to *L. tropica*,[32] *L. mexicana*[33] and *L. amazonensis*.[34]

Symptoms

The incubation period is difficult to evaluate precisely. It is generally 2–6 months, but can range from 10 days to many years. Long incubation periods, up to 10 years, have been occasionally reported,[35,36] related to clinical outcome of asymptomatic infection following immune system alteration.

The onset of the disease may be sudden or gradual. In sudden onset, there is a rapid rise in temperature, with continuous or high remittent fever persisting for several days. The overall condition of the patient is usually good in the early stages. The gradual insidious onset includes

lymphocytes are scarce or absent (DCL), to hypersensitive tuberculoid granuloma, with many Langhans giant cells but small numbers of lymphocytes and plasma cells (leishmaniasis recidivans). Between these two special, non-healing, forms of CL, the common localized self-healing lesions are characterized by an epidermal and dermal infiltrate consisting of histiocytes containing amastigotes, lymphocytes and plasma cells (Figure 75.5A, B, C).[28]

VL is a disease of the mononuclear phagocytic system, commonly affecting the spleen, liver, lymph nodes and bone marrow. But other organs (intestine, lung) and tissues (skin) may also become involved, as they contain elements of the mononuclear phagocytic system. In immuno-suppressed patients and in advanced cases, all body organs are involved. The presence of amastigotes within macrophages remains the hallmark of *Leishmania* infection. The histological aspects depend on the organs, their specific structure and cellular make-up (Figure 75.5 D, E, F).

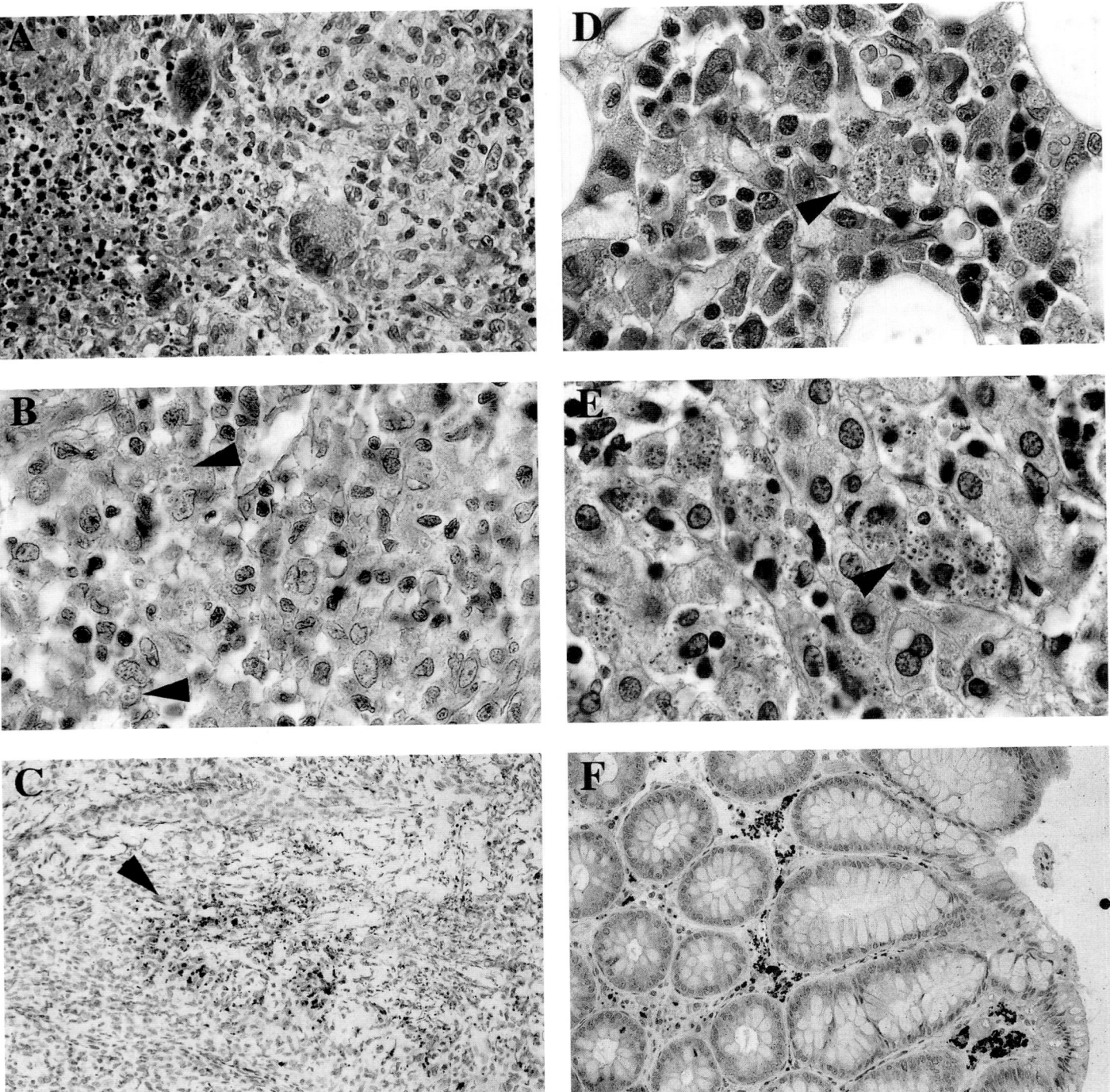

Figure 75.5: Cutaneous and visceral leishmaniasis: histopathology. (A) Skin: CL due to *L. major*. Mature granuloma and giant cells; no parasite detected (haematoxylin and eosin staining, × 250). (B) Skin: CL. Infiltrate by histiocytes, lymphocytes and plasma cells; numerous amastigotes in histiocytes (haematoxylin and eosin staining, × 400). (C) Skin: CL. Amastigotes of *L. major* detected by immunohistochemistry using a mouse anti-*L. amazonensis* immune serum (streptavidin peroxidase method and amino-ethyl carbazole (AEC) as chromogen, ×250). (D) Bone marrow: VL due to *L. infantum* (haematoxylin and eosin staining, × 400). (E) Liver: VL due to *L. infantum*. Numerous parasitized histiocytes (haematoxylin and eosin staining, × 400). (F) Colon: HIV/*Leishmania* co-infection. Amastigotes in the submucosae (immunohistochemistry: streptavidin peroxidase and AEC, × 400). Arrowheads indicate the presence of parasites. (M. Huerre and J. C. Antoine, Institut Pasteur, Paris, France, reproduced with permission.)

irregular fever, slowly increasing, with sometimes a transitory fall to subfebrile levels, which can delay the diagnosis.

In well-established VL, the patient presents a protuberant abdomen and muscle wasting of limbs. A general syndrome including fever, asthenia, weight loss, anaemia, splenomegaly, hepatomegaly and sometimes adenopathia dominates the classical presentation (Figures 75.6 and 75.7).

Fever is the major symptom in acute presentations as well as in the chronic insidious forms. It is intermittent and irregular, with a double or triple rise per day, usually to 38–39°C, but possibly reaching 40–41°C. It lasts for some weeks followed by an apyrexial period. But all types of fever have been described: continuous, undulant and remittent.

Splenomegaly appears early and is almost invariably present. It is firm, smooth, mobile and painless. Spleen size increases regularly, in relation to the duration of the disease. Eventually the spleen may extend down into the left hypochondrium.

Hepatomegaly is less frequent and occurs later than splenomegaly. The liver is generally slightly enlarged and

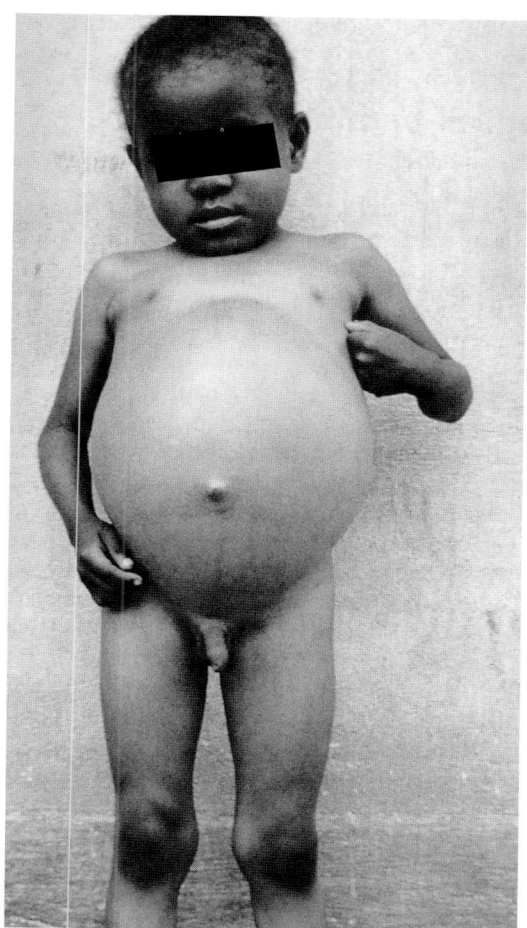

Figure 75.7: Visceral leishmaniasis: protuberant abdomen caused by voluminous enlargement of spleen and liver. (IRD, INSERM and P. Desjeux, reproduced with permission from LePont et al. Leishmaniases et phlebotomes in Bolivie. Editions ORSTOM et INSERM, © 1992.)

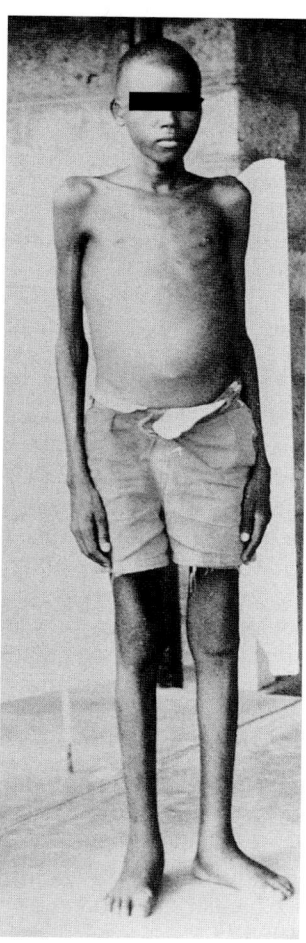

Figure 75.6: General presentation of visceral leishmaniasis: weight loss and splenomegaly in an East African patient. (J.P. Dedet.)

painless. Rarely jaundice appears in late stages and is considered of poor prognosis. Discrete superficial lymph node enlargement can appear during evolution. The nodes are small, firm painless and mobile.

Anaemia is responsible for an extreme paleness of skin and mucosa. In India, patient skin has a greyish pigmentation, which gives rise to the local name of the disease (kala-azar). Other symptoms can be found, such as digestive, pulmonary and bleeding manifestations.

Diarrhoea is frequently reported and is related to ulcerations of the digestive mucosa. Pulmonary involvement can occur, with a dry, non-productive cough. Episodes of bleeding are principally epistaxis, and more rarely bleeding from the gums, purpura, petechiae and menorrhagia.

During evolution, the clinical presentation progressively worsens, with amplification of the above-described symptoms. Ascites is considered as a late sign of bad prognosis, sometimes associated with oedema and pleural effusion. These unusual signs are more common in Indian kala-azar. As a result of albuminuria and immune complex deposition, renal involvement may occur as a late complication.

Biological parameters

VL is characterized by haematological as well as plasmatic protein alterations.

Anaemia is the major and most frequent haematological sign. Generally of normochromic and normocytic type, it progressively and regularly increases until becoming intense (haemoglobin levels are around 7–10 g/dl, and can decrease down to 4 g/dl). Leucopenia (1–3000/mm^3) with neutropenia is frequently reported, and can, when severe, be responsible for numerous associated infections. Platelet numbers are occasionally decreased. Severe thrombopenia (below 40 000/mm^3), when associated with alterations of hepatic coagulation factors, is responsible for haemorrhages, which can be quite dramatic. The decrease of the three blood cell lines corresponds to the classical picture of pancytopenia, commonly associated with VL.

The inflammation syndrome includes a raised erythrocyte sedimentation rate and increase of C reactive protein. The plasma protein profiles are disturbed, with low albumin levels and hypergammaglobulinaemia (up to 20 g/litre), corresponding to overproduction of polyclonal immunoglobulins, mainly IgG.

Evolution

VL is a chronic disease, evolving slowly over many months or even a few years. The clinical and biological signs are progressively aggravated: body wasting reaching cachexia, anaemia, leucopenia and splenomegaly. Spontaneous evolution is fatal in 90% of cases, mainly caused by intercurrent infection or haemorrhages. When administered in time, specific treatment generally leads to patient cure. However, relapses are more and more frequently reported and attributed to the emergence of resistant parasite strains and/or to host characters such as immunosuppression.

Clinical forms

Asymptomatic and subclinical infections

Leishmanial infection does not lead to clinical disease in all cases: asymptomatic and subclinical forms are frequent, as shown during field epidemiological surveys in various foci, for example in Italy,[37] Brazil,[21,38] Kenya[39] and France.[40]

These infections may lead to subsequent patent clinical disease, when the immune status of the patient changes (see below). They can therefore present a therapeutic dilemma for the clinician.

Infantile visceral leishmaniasis due to *L. infantum*

This form is predominant in the Mediterranean basin, where it was described in 1908.[41] In North Africa, the prevalence in young children remains high (85–94% of cases[42]), while over the last 20 years in southern European countries the number of infected adults has equalled, or even exceeded, that of children.[43] Affecting principally

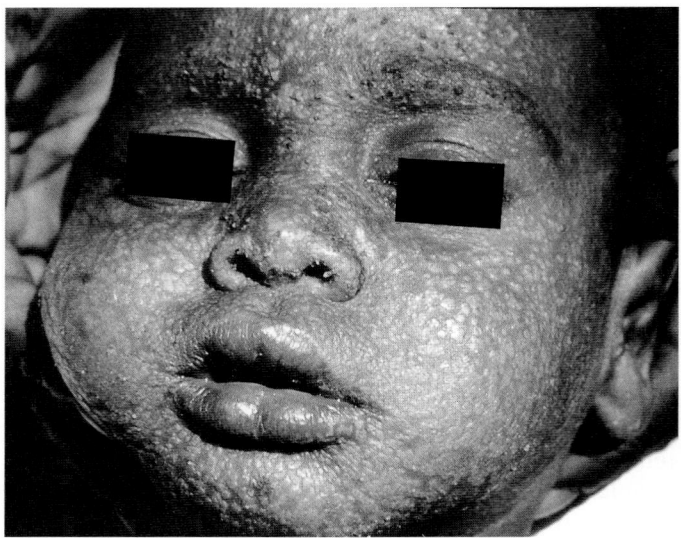

Figure 75.8: Post-kala-azar dermal leishmaniasis: multiple nodular eruption in a Sudanese patient. (Ellipses and E. E. Zijlstra, reproduced with permission.)

young children (3–5 years), it is characterized by the classical symptomatic triad: fever, anaemia and splenomegaly. When diagnosed in time it responds favourably to antileishmanial drugs.

L. donovani visceral leishmaniasis

This form occurs in India, where it was first described in 1903,[29,30] and also in East Africa. The clinical picture is that of the classical presentation given above. A particularity in India is the skin pigmentation starting in the early stage and enhancing during evolution. Skin lesions have been recorded in East Africa.

In both areas, a special form frequently occurs: post-kala-azar dermal leishmaniasis, currently known as PKDL. It was reported as occurring in 20% of cases in India[19] and 56% in Sudan.[44] In India, PKDL appears after a latent period of approximately 1 year after kala-azar cure, while in Sudan it can start before symptoms of kala-azar have completely subsided. Beginning as depigmented macules, the PKDL skin lesions turn into papular, then nodular eruptions. Located initially on the face (Figure 75.8) and the tips of upper limbs, they can extend to the whole body surface. The lesions may self-cure within 6 months (India) or last for many months or years. They contain numerous parasites whatever their stage, and can play an important role in sandfly transmission and parasite dissemination.

Cutaneous leishmaniases

CL is a dermatological disease known since earliest antiquity, and reported at the end of the nineteenth century to be caused by a parasitic protozoon.[45,46] Wright named the parasite in 1903.[47]

CL presents as skin lesions, which are generally localized, without the involvement of mucosae, and not generalized infections. They occur on exposed parts of the body surface accessible to sandflies, principally on the face, hands, forearms and lower limbs. Rarely, dermotropic parasites may give rise to DCL, with multiple nodules on large areas of the skin.

Localized cutaneous leishmaniasis

All anthropophilic species of *Leishmania* (Table 75.2), including the usually viscerotropic species *L. donovani* and *L. infantum*, can be responsible for LCL, a mild self-healing infection.

The incubation period depends on the infecting species and the size of the inoculum, and varies between a week and several months, the mean duration being around 1 month.

The cutaneous lesion starts as an erythematous papule, similar to an insect bite. It regularly enlarges, reaching its definitive size in a few weeks.

The mature lesion is well defined, with a regular outline, and generally round or oval in shape (Figure 75.9); it is rarely of geographical shape. Its dimensions are variable, usually in the range 0.5–10 cm in diameter. Depending on the number of infecting bites, the lesions can be single or multiple, 2–10 usually, but occasionally more. The lesions are painless unless secondarily infected.

The clinical types of cutaneous lesions are variable, depending on the species of parasite and on the genetic, immunological and cultural background of the patient. A single *Leishmania* species can be responsible for lesions of different morphology; the same morphological type of lesion can also be produced by different *Leishmania* species. The common ulcerative clinical type will be described first, followed by the other possible clinical forms.

Ulcerative lesion

This is the most common clinical feature of LCL. It resembles a volcano with sloping sides and a central ulcer, which has a variable depth and a sanious bottom.

A scab resulting from the coagulation of exudates can cover the ulceration (Figure 75.10). The outline of the

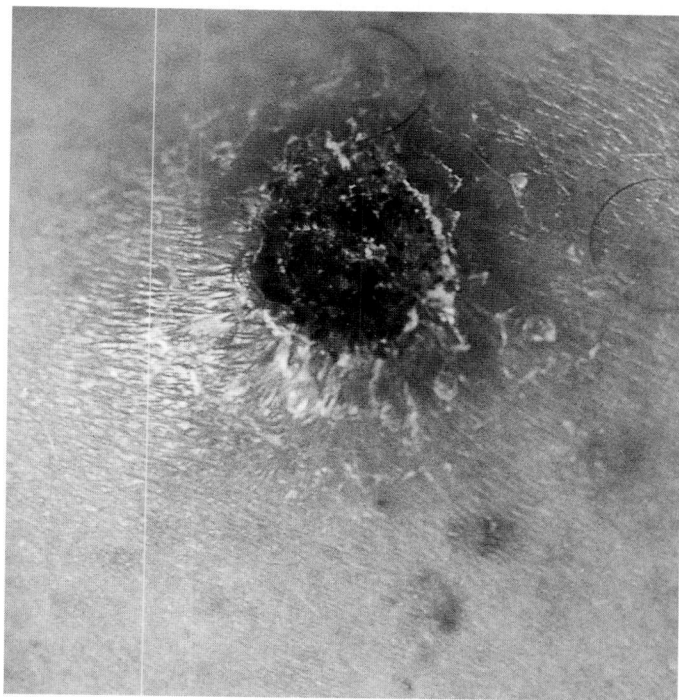

Figure 75.10: Localized cutaneous leishmaniasis. Typical volcano-like lesion with sloping sides and a central ulcer covered with a scab (J. P. Dedet.)

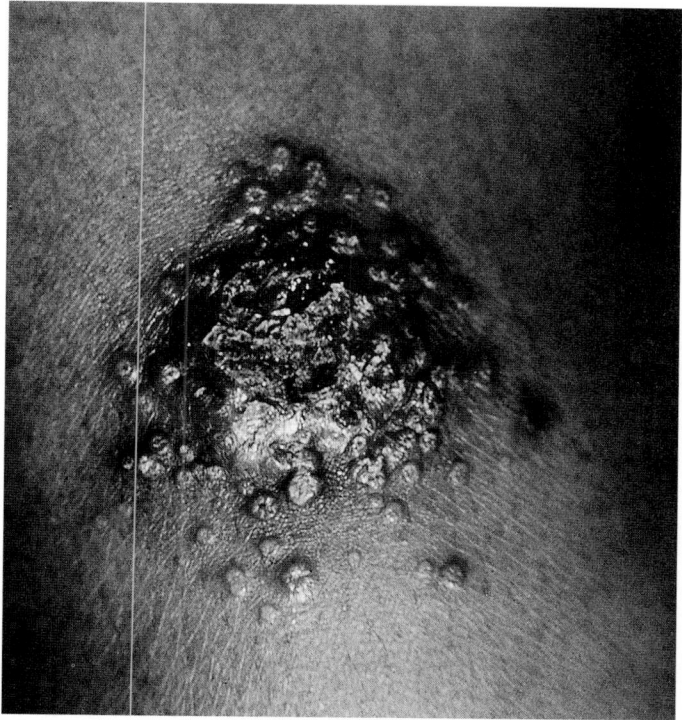

Figure 75.11: Localized cutaneous leishmaniasis. The lesion is sometimes surrounded by smaller daughter papules containing parasites (J. P. Dedet.)

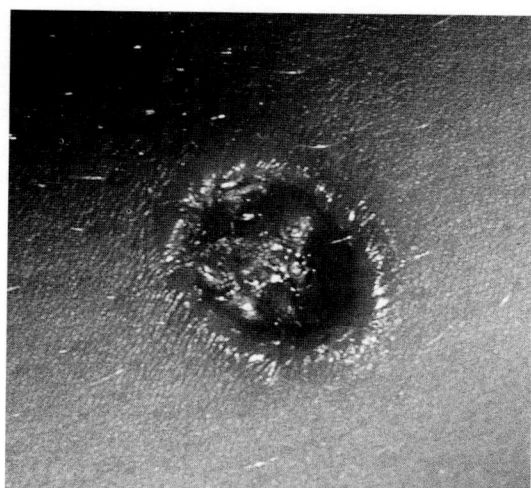

Figure 75.9: Localized cutaneous leishmaniasis. The lesion is typically ulcerated with a raised inflammatory outline (J. P. Dedet.)

lesion is more or less elevated, inflammatory, of reddish or purplish colour on pale skin but hyperpigmented on darker skin. It can sometimes be slightly squamous and surrounded by smaller daughter papules (Figure 75.11). This type of lesion, classically known as 'wet form', corresponds to the majority of the lesions of zoonotic CL, principally due to *L. major* (oriental sore, Biskra boil, Gafsa boil), *L. mexicana* (chiclero's ulcer), *L. guyanensis* (pian bois), *L. peruviana* (uta) and *L. braziliensis* (cutaneous lesion).

Dry type

This presents as a papulo-nodular lesion, covered by superficial scales. It can enlarge to form a large plaque. It is the current clinical type of anthroponotic CL due to *L. tropica*.

Other types of lesions

More rarely, other clinical types of lesions are encountered: closed nodular type, infiltrative plaques, eczematoid, warty and pseudo-tumoural. This clinical polymorphism of the lesions is unrelated to species.

Lymphangitic dissemination

Solitary or multiple subcutaneous nodules in the draining territory are sometimes associated with a cutaneous lesion (Figure 75.12). Palpation easily detects a lymphangitic cord, regularly enlarged in small round and painless nodules, containing parasites. They can occasionally become open to the skin and transform into secondary lesions. This type of dissemination ('sporotrichoid spread') is mainly reported with *L. major*, *L. braziliensis*, *L. guyanensis* and *L. panamensis*.

Evolution

Whatever the clinical type of lesion, the evolution is chronic and leads most often to spontaneous cure, after a time varying according to the *Leishmania* species from a few months (about 6 months for *L.major*, *L. mexicana* or *L. peruviana*) to a few years (more than 1 year for *L. aethiopica*, *L. infantum*, *L. tropica* or *L. guyanensis*). The cure, either spontaneous or following treatment, results in an indelible scar, pinkish or whitish on pale skin and hyperpigmented on dark skin. Depending on the clinical feature of the lesion, the scar is generally depressed (ulcerative lesion). The evolution of CL does not generally lead to mutilations, with the exception of chiclero's ulcer, which is occasionally responsible for partial amputation of the ear auricle.

Clinical cure does not always lead to a complete disappearance of the parasites. In about 10% of cases it is followed by the resurgence of an active lesion on the scar. This reactivation can occur between a few months to a few years following the initial cure. This secondary lesion will also spontaneously cure.

Diffuse cutaneous leishmaniasis

This particularly severe form of CL was described from Venezuela.[48] It is a peculiar and scarce clinical form, resulting from the parasitism of particular *Leishmania* species, *L. amazonensis* and occasionally *L. mexicana*[49] in

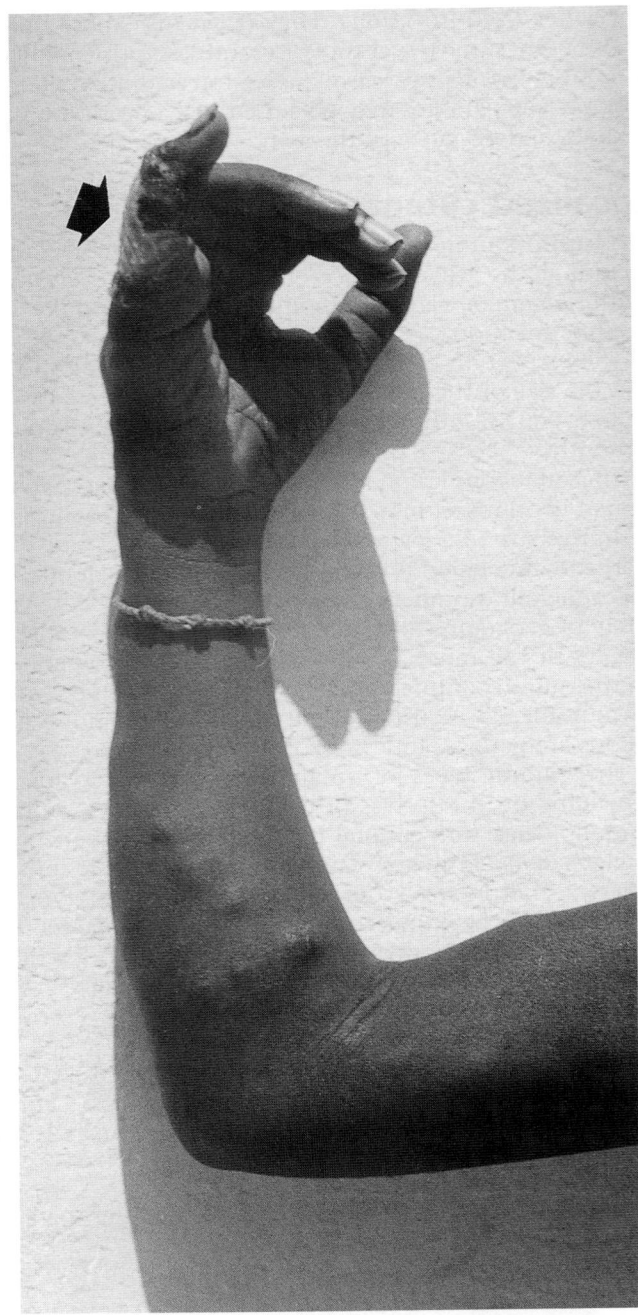

Figure 75.12: Lymphangitic extension along the forearm and the arm, from a finger-localized cutaneous lesion (arrow). (Société de Pathologie Exotique, reproduced with permission.)

the New World, and *L. aethiopica* in the Old World, in patients with an antileishmanial specific defect in cell-mediated immunity.[50] Since HIV infection has spread to leishmaniasis endemic areas, DCL cases have been occasionally reported due to unusual species, such as *L. braziliensis* in the New World[51] and *L. infantum*[52] and *L. major*[53] in the Old World.

A non-ulcerated nodule rich in parasites represents the basic cutaneous lesion of this form of disease. The nodules are numerous, at first isolated, then joining to form large patches, disseminated to the whole of the body, to the face, as well as to the trunk and limbs. The general appearance of the patient mimics the presentation of lepromatous leprosy, with 'leonine' facies. The pathology of the lesion is characteristic, with a homogeneous epidermal and dermal infiltrate of vacuolized macrophages full of *Leishmania* amastigotes. The leishmanin skin test is consistently negative.

During the development of this condition there is no ulceration, nor mucosal or visceral involvement, but a slow constant aggravation by successive relapses, interrupted with phases of remission. This form is resistant to therapy by classical antileishmanial drugs, and especially to pentavalent antimonials, and never cure spontaneously.

Leishmaniasis recidivans

This is a chronic form of leishmaniasis, due essentially to *L. tropica* in the Old World and occasionally to *L. braziliensis* in the New World.[54] The lesion is located on the face and follows an acute lesion, after numerous months of evolution. The lesion shows a peripheral active zone, constantly enlarging, around a central healing part (Figure 75.13). The presentation mimics that of lupus vulgaris. The lesion contains a small number of parasites and corresponds to an exaggerated cell-mediated immune response on the part of the host.

Mucocutaneous leishmaniasis

MCL, also named 'espundia' since its early description,[55] is a particular nosological entity mainly due to the species

L. braziliensis, and occasionally to *L. panamensis*.[56] It is a wild zoonosis, of which the natural reservoirs remain unknown. It occurs from southern Mexico to the north of Argentina.

This form of leishmaniasis evolves in two stages: a primary cutaneous lesion, eventually followed, after a variable time of latency, by secondary mucosal involvement.

The initial cutaneous lesion does not fundamentally differ from the localized lesions occurring during infection by other *Leishmania* dermotropic species (see above), and its evolution generally leads to spontaneous cure. Once the primary cutaneous lesion(s) cure, the leishmanial infection remains for a variable period of time, which can be very long, sometimes indefinite. The frequency of occurrence of secondary mucosal involvement appears variable, according to foci considered and authors. The period of time between cutaneous lesion and subsequent appearance of the mucosal involvement extends from several weeks to many years. Very long time intervals have been occasionally observed by several authors.[57,58]

If it occurs, the mucosal involvement starts on the nasal mucosa. The patient suffers with nasal congestion (Figure 75.14), which causes nocturnal discomfort.

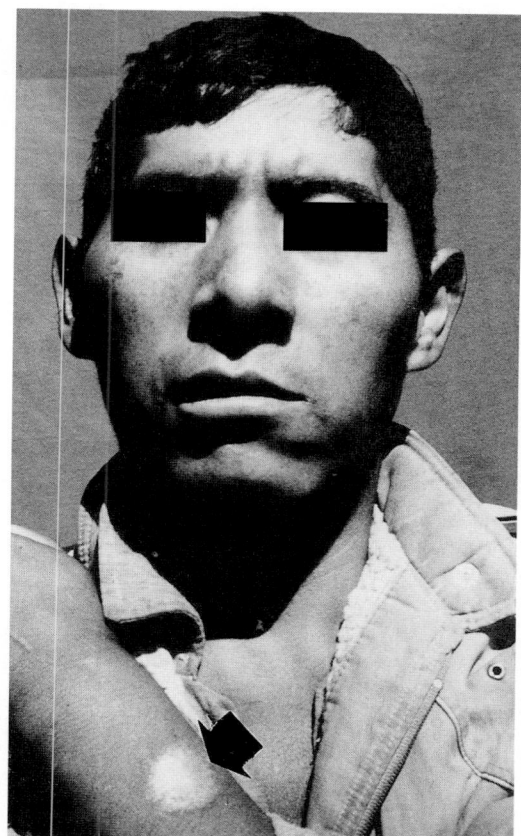

Figure 75.14: Mucocutaneous leishmaniasis. Classical presentation of the patient harbouring the scar of the initial cutaneous lesion (arrow), and consulting for congestion and oedema of the nasal pyramid. (L. Valda Rodriguez, reproduced with permission.)

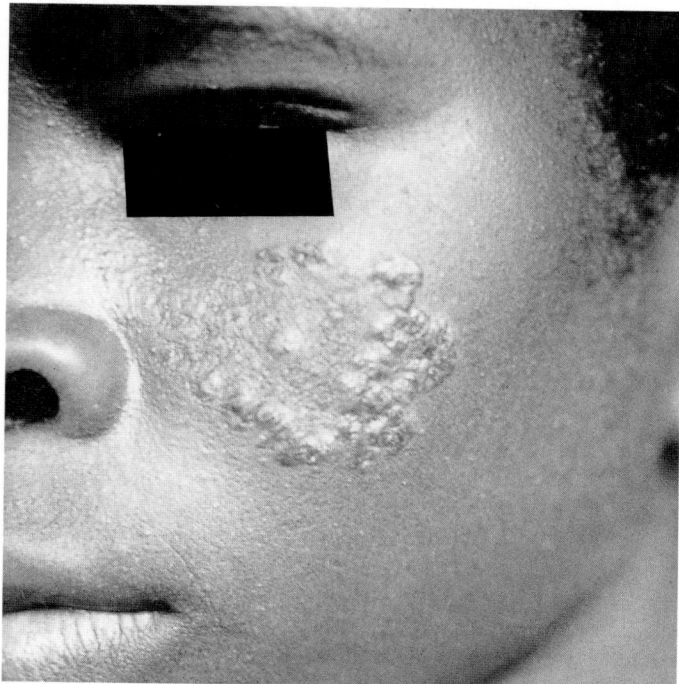

Figure 75.13: Leishmaniasis recidivans. (P. Desjeux, reproduced with permission.)

Epistaxis can also be the initial symptom.[57] The initial nasal lesion is generally localized to the anterior, cartilaginous part of the nasal septum. It appears as a small-sized hyperaemic inflammatory granuloma, rapidly evolving to an ulcer.[59] The septum is rapidly invaded and destroyed, which leads to the perforation of the nasal septum in its anterior part, which is generally considered a symptom pathognomonic of MCL[57] (Figure 75.15). The involvement of nasal mucosa can be apparent from the exterior, even as early as the initial inflammatory stage, and manifests as congestion and oedema of the nasal pyramid (Figure 75.14). At the stage of septum destruction, the nose shape is flattened and weighed down, and is classically described as 'tapir nose' (Figure 75.16).

The buccal mucosa is commonly affected at a later stage of the disease, with or without contiguous spread from the nasal lesions. The mucosae of the palate and of the interior lips are the most frequently involved, while the tongue generally remains uninjured. The palatal lesions are granulomatous and extensive, and reach the velum (Figure 75.17). They produce the classical 'Escomel cross'. The lip lesions are inflamed and ulcerated,

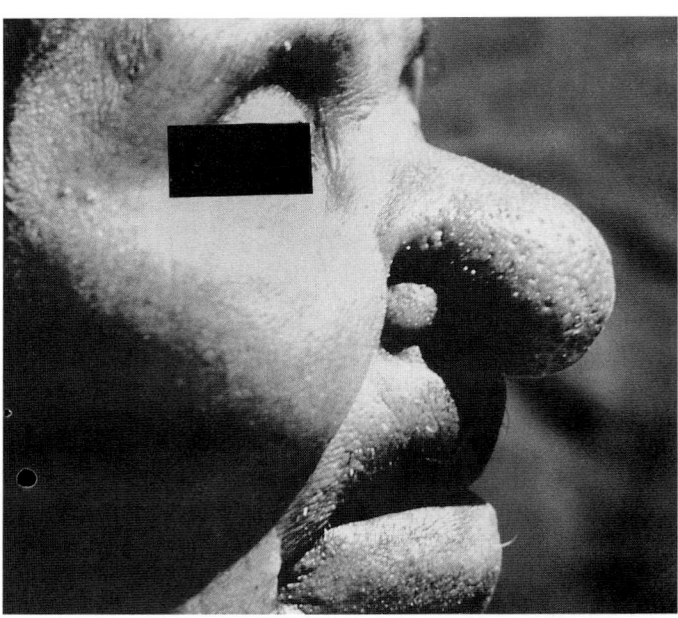

Figure 75.16: Mucocutaneous leishmaniasis: 'tapir nose'. (L. Valda Rodriguez, reproduced with permission.)

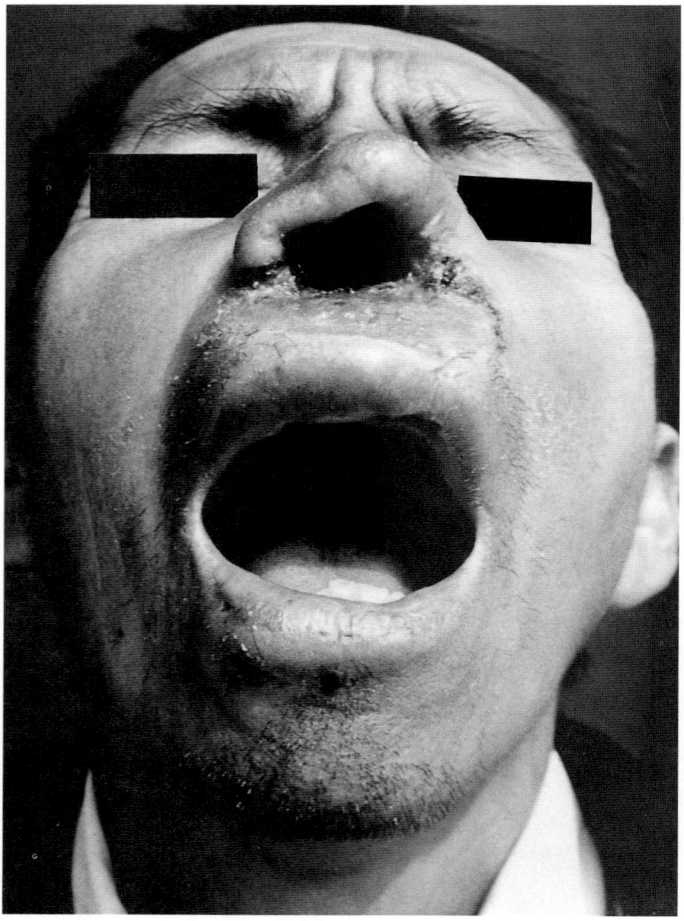

Figure 75.15: Mucocutaneous leishmaniasis. Localization and development of the mucosal involvement to the nasal septum, eventually leading to its destruction. (L. Valda Rodriguez, reproduced with permission.)

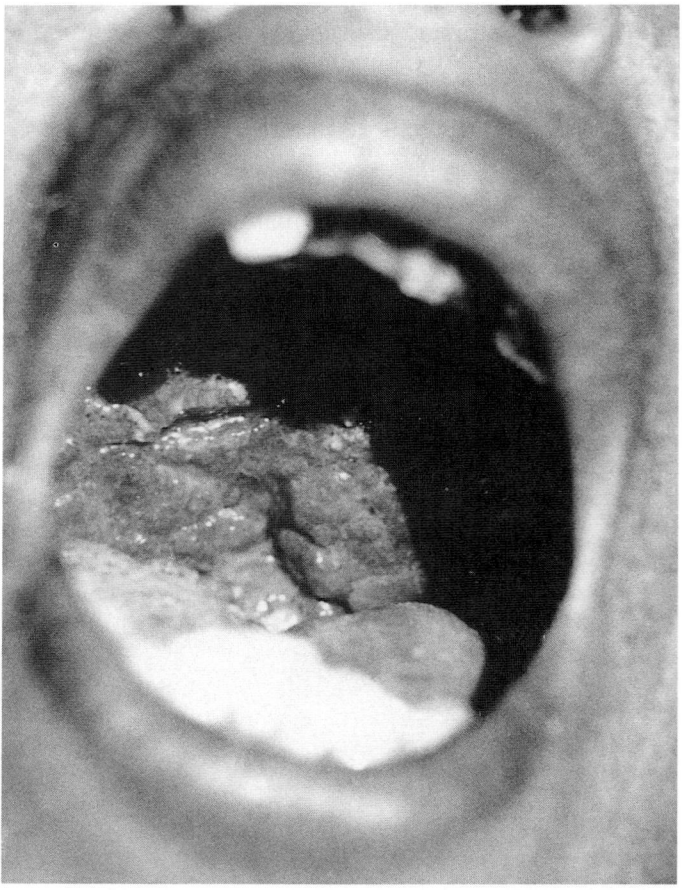

Figure 75.17: Mucocutaneous leishmaniasis. Granulomatous and extensive lesion of the palate. (L. Valda Rodriguez, reproduced with permission.)

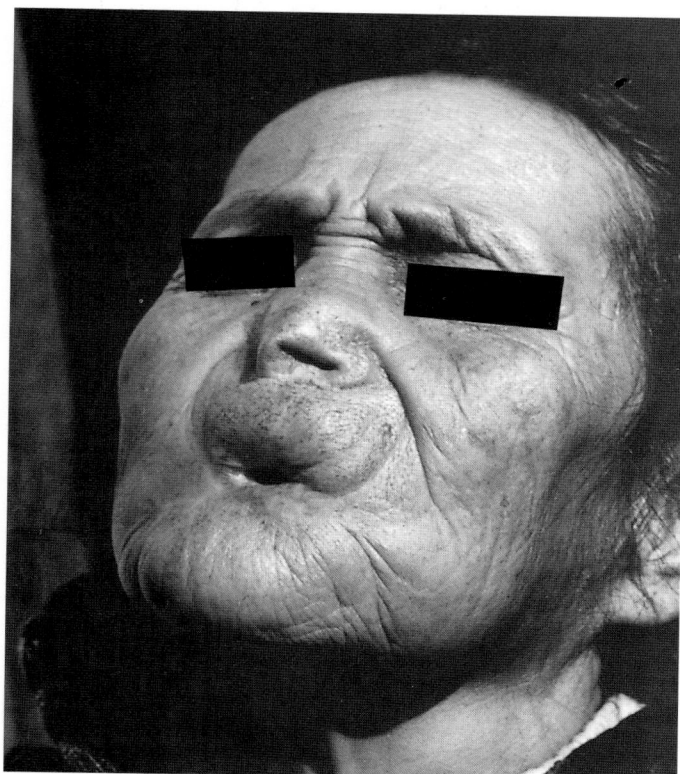

Figure 75.18: Mucocutaneous leishmaniasis. Disfiguring retractile cured lesions. (P. Desjeux, reproduced with permission.)

sometimes extending to the external part, with frequent tissue destruction. A palatal perforation can occur in the later stages and results in the nasal fossae and mouth cavity becoming interconnected.

Laryngeal extension follows the rhino-buccal–pharyngeal localization of the parasite. The lesion is firstly infiltrative and manifests as dysphonia and metallic cough. When granulomatous, the laryngeal lesion can cause obstruction of the respiratory tract, with possible fatal consequences due to acute respiratory distress. Dysphagia and the resulting undernutrition have serious consequences for the physical condition of the patient.

Tissue necrosis and disfigurement appear in the advanced stage of the condition and can be extremely severe. They result in disfiguring mutilations: the nose and lips can totally disappear, at which time the mouth and nasal cavity become connected by a single hole. Socio-psychological consequences are considerable for the patient, often leading to suicide.

Death can occur following pulmonary super-infections consecutive to false alimentary passage or for acute respiratory obstruction. When treated and cured, patients exhibit disfiguring, sometimes retractile, scars (Figure 75.18).

Leishmaniasis and immunosuppression

The number of leishmaniasis cases, particularly of the visceral form, associated with immunosuppression has increased regularly over the past 15 or so years. Immunosuppression related to HIV infection or to an immunosuppressive treatment for organ transplantation or neoplastic disease is especially important.

Cases of VL during HIV infection have regularly been recorded in various foci in the world, particularly in southern Europe.[1] For the period 1990–1998, there were a total of 1616 cases reported, 87% of which were located in the Mediterranean basin: Spain 56.7%, southern France 17.7%, Italy 14.9% and Portugal 8.1%. Cases were also reported from countries of North Africa. In the southern European countries, the prevalence of VL during HIV infection was around 2%.[43,60] The spread of AIDS to rural areas where visceral leishmaniasis is endemic, and the spread of VL to suburban areas, has resulted in a progressively increasing overlap between the two diseases, not only in the Mediterranean basin but also in the historical foci of VL, such as East Africa, India and Brazil.

In southern Europe, co-infected patients are mainly young adults, 86% are 20–40-year-olds, while 71% of the total cases belong to the risk group of intravenous drug users.[61] The predominance of the co-infected cases in the intravenous drug user group has led to the postulate that direct inter-human transmission may occur via syringe sharing, an element with important epidemiological implications.[17] This hypothesis is supported by two additional epidemiological arguments. Co-infected patients harbour parasites in blood and normal skin: parasites can be isolated from peripheral blood in 88% of the patients at initial diagnosis.[62] Moreover, during co-infection, particular species or zymodemes were found outside their usual endemic areas; for example, *L. donovani* MON-18 has been found in an HIV patient in Portugal, where only *L. infantum* is present.[63]

In cases of HIV/*Leishmania* co-infection, long duration times, up to 5 years, have been reported between the stay in the endemic area and development of the disease. The diagnosis of VL during HIV infection coincides with a serious state of immunosuppression, as 90.4% of patients have less than 200 CD4/ml.[61] The clinical features are typical of VL in 84.2% of cases, but atypical symptoms are found in 15.8% of cases; these unusual symptoms are commonly of a cutaneous, pulmonary or digestive nature with the presence of parasites in lung, pleura, oesophagus, stomach, duodenum, jejunum, colon, rectum and healthy skin.[61] The classical haematological abnormalities associated with VL in the immunocompetent host are frequently absent. These signs interfere with the alterations specific to AIDS and to other opportunistic infections, often associated with, or induced by, antiretroviral treatment.

Diagnosis is essentially parasitological, as the circulating antibodies are only detectable in about half of the HIV-infected patients. The most efficient method of immunological diagnosis in an immunocompromised patient is undoubtedly the Western blot.[64]

Dermal leishmaniases are less frequently found during immunosuppression. Few cases have been reported.[65] Within these cases, DCL has been described during infections by *L. infantum*, *L. major* and *L. braziliensis*. During HIV/*Leishmania* co-infection, the immunocompromised patients infected with dermotropic *Leishmania* tend usually to develop directly a VL without cutaneous stage.[27]

Other immunosuppressive states, resulting from the pathological process itself or from the use of immunosuppressive treatment, in the case of systemic diseases or organ transplantation, favour the development of VL. The main aetiologies are: haemopathia, acute lymphoblastic leukaemia, chronic myeloid leukaemia, Hodgkin's disease, systemic lupus erythematosus, Crohn's disease, sarcoidosis and typhoid fever.

Diagnosis

Primarily based on clinical presentation, epidemiological elements and non-specific biological parameters, the diagnosis of leishmaniasis is confirmed by direct detection of parasites and/or presence of specific antibodies.

Parasitological and molecular diagnosis

Definitive diagnosis is based on the detection of the parasite or its DNA in samples, the nature of which depends on the type of leishmaniasis: visceral or tegumentary.

Sample collection
Visceral leishmaniasis
Bone marrow and spleen aspirations, in spite of their inconvenience, are the most commonly used. Splenic puncture is considered the most sensitive method but must be only performed when haematological examinations are normal. Bone marrow material is obtained by sternal (adults) or iliac crest aspiration (children). Lymph node aspiration is a safer and simpler method, and less traumatic for the patient; however, it can be used only in foci where lymphadenopathy is frequent (e.g. Sudan). Liver aspiration is not frequently used. Parasite detection in peripheral blood has been updated since the development of HIV/*Leishmania* co-infection; it is a relatively non-invasive method and, as such, much appreciated by HIV co-infected as well as in immunocompetent patients, and its sensitivity seems comparable in both groups.

Parasites have been found in a variety of unusual sites, such as cerebrospinal fluid, normal skin, digestive mucosa, bronchiolo-alveolar fluid and pleural liquid. These sites of parasite research are not included in the current diagnosis route, but have been fortuitously used in immunocompromised HIV patients.

Cutaneous and mucocutaneous leishmaniasis
The circumstances in which parasites are found in the skin are: CL of Old and New Worlds, PKDL in India and East Africa, and even in healthy skin during *Leishmania*/HIV co-infection. Skin material is obtained by superficial scraping with a scarifier or a Brock curette, by needle aspiration, or by tissue collection made with a dental broach or biopsy punch. The site from which diagnostic material is collected is the determining factor in the discovery of the parasite and depends on the clinical type of the lesion. For example, the inflammatory edge of an ulcerative cutaneous lesion is the elected place for parasite detection. In the particular case of mucosal lesions, material is collected with biopsy forceps.

Detection methods
Collected material can be smeared on to a microscope slide, cultured, fixed for pathological examination or more recently, submitted to the polymerase chain reaction (PCR) technique. Inoculation into laboratory animals is rarely performed.

The staining method most appropriate for *Leishmania* detection is one employing panoptic May Grünwald–Giemsa stain. Amastigotes are typically intramonocytic, but frequently extracellular in smears, the nucleus and kinetoplast staining characteristically purple (Figure 75.19). Direct examination of smears may give a rapid diagnosis if carefully practised, but has a limited sensitivity, inferior to that of culture and particularly that of new PCR techniques. Specific staining of biopsy material using mouse anti-*Leishmania* immune serum and peroxidase conjugate can be used for an easy detection of the parasites, the immune serum cross-reacting with various taxa of *Leishmania* (Figure 75.5 C, F).

Culture has a higher sensitivity than direct detection of parasites on smears, and is a useful complement to parasitological diagnosis. In addition, isolation of the parasite strain allows parasite drug sensitivity testing and parasite identification, by isoenzyme electrophoresis, monoclonal antibodies or specific probes hybridization. The classical blood agar NNN medium[66] is the most currently used, but numerous diphasic and liquid media are presently available. The ease with which parasites may be established in culture varies according to species, and even to strains, some being difficult to cultivate in vitro (*L. venezuelensis*, *L. braziliensis*). Guidelines for

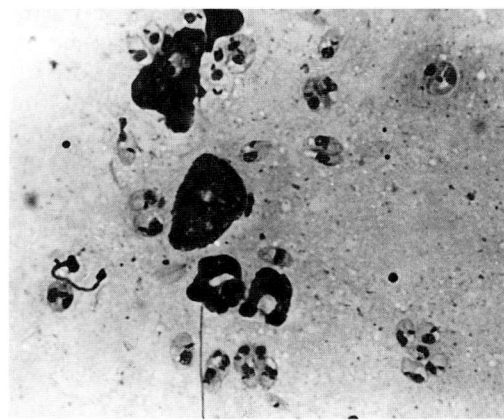

Figure 75.19: *Leishmania* amastigotes stained by May Grünwald–Giemsa technique on smears prepared from a cutaneous lesion.

Leishmania culture and isolation can be found in Evans et al.[67] *Leishmania* cultures are incubated at 24–26°C. The parasite develops as a mobile promastigote stage, and grows slowly with a doubling time of about 48–72 hours.

Animal inoculation into the golden hamster, one of the most susceptible laboratory animals, is an alternative to in vitro cultivation, but is not really practical in current diagnosis.

Molecular diagnosis has been developed during recent years, and can be applied to various types of sample, including bone marrow, spleen, blood and skin. DNA repetitive sequences are the preferential probes used. Direct detection of parasite DNA can be achieved by in situ hybridization or on filters. PCR allows the detection of parasite DNA thanks to the production of several million or billion copies of a precise DNA sequence. Its theoretical advantage consists of a high sensitivity, allied to a quasi absolute specificity. In reality, the tests are not standardized and use in-house methods, and few comparative studies have been carried out.

Molecular diagnosis has been successfully applied by various authors to the diagnosis of VL[68–70] and of CL.[71–73] In VL, PCR has been found to be more sensitive than other diagnostic procedures, including culture, particularly in HIV co-infected patients, in which it is highly appreciated as a relatively non-invasive diagnostic method.[74]

Immunological diagnosis

During VL and DCL, the immune response of the patient is of humoral type, with the development of high levels of specific circulating antibodies in serum which, however, can be absent in immunocompromised patients. During CL and MCL, the preponderant immune response is of cell-mediated type, which can be explored by a delayed hypersensitivity test.

Various serological tests have been developed to detect circulating specific antibodies for the diagnosis of VL.[75] The techniques proposed are numerous and differ in their sensitivity and specificity, and their use depends on their cost and reagent availability: indirect fluorescent antibody technique (the most commonly used), immuno-enzymatic techniques, counter-current immuno-electro-phoresis, indirect haemagglutination test and immunoblot. There are a few which are relatively easy to practise in field conditions: direct agglutination test, latex particle agglutination, dot-ELISA and fast-ELISA. According to the antigen used, cross-reactions may occur with other infectious diseases, such as malaria, trypanosomiasis, mycobacteriosis and schistosomiasis. Immunological diagnosis is a relatively non-invasive approach, and useful to combine with direct demonstration of the parasite, which, of course, remains the reference technique. The presence of specific antibodies is not necessarily correlated to an active disease and can reveal a subclinical infection. The immunological diagnosis has some limits, particularly for post-treatment follow-up (specific antibodies remain present for a long time after treatment) and in immunocompromised patients, in which the immune response can be weak or even negative.

The leishmanin skin test[76] measures delayed-type hypersensitivity. It consists of an intradermal injection of a suspension of promastigotes killed by heat and phenol; the test is read 48–72 hours later; only an induration of at least 5 mm is considered positive. It is usually positive during LCL and MCL. It is always negative during DCL. It is currently negative during acute VL, in which it usually turns positive several months after clinical cure. The leishmanin skin test is useful for epidemiological studies, during which it reveals asymptomatic infections.

Treatment

There have been no significant changes in the treatment of leishmaniases for many years. Since the 1920s, treatment has been based on pentavalent antimonial compounds. Following the increasing incidence of VL cases in immuno-compromised patients and the rise of acquired resistance to antimonials, amphotericin B, mainly in its liposomal form, has joined the antimonials as a first-line drug for leishmaniasis. Alternative drugs are investigated for many years without passing the step of clinical trials. Miltefosine, a new oral compound tested during the last few years, has shown promising results, and could change completely the therapy of leishmaniases in the near future.

Products

Antimonials

Two closely related pentavalent antimonials are currently used: sodium stibogluconate (Pentostam®, GlaxoSmithKline), available in English-speaking countries, and meglumine antimoniate (Glucantime®, Aventis), available in France, Latin America and Francophone countries. Chemically close, they have distinct antimony rates of respectively 100 and 85 mg Sb/ml. When properly manufactured and stored, they have comparable efficacy and toxicity.

Antimonials have proven to be efficient in leishmaniasis treatment through a century of use. However, the mechanism of action as antileishmanial agents remains unclear. They may involve inhibition of ATP synthesis. It might be possible that antimonial salts have to be concentrated within the macrophage or parasite and transformed into active trivalent metabolites to be efficient. Antimonials have poor oral absorption and therefore are administered by the parenteral route. They are rapidly excreted by the kidneys.

In spite of numerous side effects attributed to anti-monials, the scarcity of reported accidents allows their continued use, since no alternative efficient and non-toxic drug is available. The side effects of pentavalent antimonials can be categorized into intolerance signs and toxic effects. The intolerance side effects include shivers, fever, arthralgias, myalgias, skin rashes, abdominal symptoms and headache. The stibo-intoxication signs occur at the end of treatment. They include reversible elevation of hepatocellular enzymes, subclinical pancreatitis, and decrease in haemoglobin level and platelet count. Cardiac side effects are the most worrisome. Several electrocardiogram (ECG) changes occur, of which flattening and/or inversion of T waves is the most common. Patients can develop prolongation of the corrected QT interval, concave ST abnormality and prolongation of PR interval. These ECG changes are transient; they gradually approach normal in a 1–3-week period after patients complete therapy. Exceptional sudden deaths have been reported for a few patients who received more than the recommended dose of Sb^V.

Sodium stibogluconate is supplied in multi-dose 100 ml bottles (100 mg Sb^V/ml), while meglumine antimoniate is supplied as 5 ml ampoules (85 mg Sb^V/ml). They are administered on the basis of their Sb^V content. The recommended dosage of Sb^V is 20 mg/kg per day, for 20 days in CL and 28 days in VL and MCL.[77,78] They are currently injected by intravenous (i.v.) or intramuscular (i.m.) route. The i.v. route is preferred when the volume of drug is high, as it is for most adults. The appropriate volume of drug is mixed with 50 ml of 5% dextrose in water and infused over at least a 10-minute interval. In the case of a few localized cutaneous lesions, intralesional injections are used.

Where resources permit, an ECG, serum chemistries and a complete blood count should be obtained for all patients before therapy is begun and weekly during therapy. The drug should be given on consecutive days throughout the course of therapy. The course is often started with progressive doses of antimonials, full dosage being reached by day three. It is not absolutely clear if the administration of antimonials every 8 or 12 hours should be clinically more efficient. However, tradition and practicality have preserved the once-daily regimen.

Amphotericin B

Amphotericin B is a polyene antibiotic isolated in 1955 from a soil *Streptomyces*. It is currently used in the treatment of systemic fungal infections. The use of amphotericin B for treatment of leishmaniases is biochemically rational because its target is ergosterol-like sterols, which are the major membrane sterols of *Leishmania* as well as fungi. It is therefore a powerful antileishmanial used in the treatment of severe leishmaniases (VL, MCL) or of forms resistant to antimonials. During the last 15 years it has become an alternative first-line drug.

Amphotericin B binds to sterols in the plasma membrane, forming pores that leak ions. It can also stimulate cytokine production of macrophages, and enhance their phagocytic capacities. Efficient plasma concentrations are rapidly reached, and even exceeded, from the beginning of the infusion, and persist beyond 24 hours. The product has slow renal elimination.

Amphotericin B side effects are of two types. Intolerance signs occur during infusion and include chills, headache, cramps, hypotension, vertigo, paraesthesias, vomiting and, exceptionally, anaphylactic shock or cardiogenic shock. These manifestations are usually controlled by addition of corticoids within the liquid of suspension, or by slowing down the infusion duration. Nephrotoxicity is the most important of the toxic effects of amphotericin B.

Amphotericin B deoxycholate is formulated as a colloidal suspension (Fungizone®, Bristol Myers Squibb), which is administered as a slow (6–8 hours) i.v. infusion (0.5–1 mg/kg dissolved in 500 ml dextrose 5%) on alternate days. The common regimens range from 14 to 20 infusions, for a total dose of 1.5–2 g. Mixing the drug in lipid solutions designed for parenteral feeding (Intralipid®, KabiVitrum) has the objective of reducing its toxicity, but the recent major advances have been in new lipid formulations of amphotericin B.

Lipid-associated amphotericin B

When associated with lipids, amphotericin B is delivered at the site of intracellular infection, which leads to more drug accumulation in infected cells, thereby increasing the therapeutic index.

The three existing formulations are similar in some respects, and globally less toxic than amphotericin B, but have different tolerability and kinetics. Liposomal amphotericin B (AmBisome®, Nexstar) is a unilamellar formed from a variety of phospholipids in a membrane bilayer containing amphotericin B. This compound has a licence for VL treatment in Europe and the USA. The two other formulations—Amphotericin B phospholipid complex (Abelcet®, Wyeth-Lederle) and amphotericin B cholesterol dispersion (Amphocil®, Liposome technology Inc.)—are not yet licensed for VL.

Liposomal amphotericin B has been used in several countries for VL treatment and shown to be less toxic than conventional amphotericin B, and more efficient in immunocompetent and immunocompromised patients.[79,80] Short-course treatment is now currently used, including five daily injections of 3–4 mg/kg, plus a further injection of the same dose on the 10th day (total dose 18–20 mg/kg). For immunocompromised patients the number of injections is increased to 10.

Pentamidine

Pentamidine is an aromatic diamine and was first synthesized in the late 1930s. It has been used as an alternative drug to treat antimonial-resistant VL in India and Kenya, and infantile VL in alternative course with antimonials in several countries of the Mediterranean basin. At present, the isethionate salt (Pentacarinat®, Aventis) is the only form available for human use and is restricted to treatment of CL.

Pentamidine inhibits the synthesis of parasitic DNA, by blocking thymidine synthase and fixation of transfer RNA. In the absence of oral absorption the drug is administered by the parenteral route, which provides a transient blood concentration, with rapid subsequent distribution and high tissue fixation. It is excreted slowly by the kidney.

Pentamidine can be responsible for immediate side effects, mainly in the case of rapid i.v. injection (hypotension, tachycardia, nausea, vomiting, facial erythema, pruritus, syncope). Local reactions can also occur (urticaria, abcess formation, phlebitis). Toxic side effects depend upon the dose and can affect pancreas, kidney and blood cell lines. Alterations of glucose metabolism are directly linked to the product toxicity to pancreatic cells, and can result in diabetes mellitus induction.

Pentamidine is given in doses of 4 mg/kg per injection. The i.m. or slow i.v. injections are made on alternate days, on patients confined to bed and having eaten nothing. Short courses (four doses) are currently used for treatment of CL. Long courses of over a period of weeks, suggested for treatment of resistant VL, have significant potential side effects.

Alternative products

Various molecules already known and used against other infectious agents were tested during recent decades for leishmaniasis treatment. None is yet recognized as a genuine antileishmanial. The most promising seems to be miltefosine.

Miltefosine

This alkyl phospholipid is an oral antineoplastic agent, which is a phosphocholine analogue affecting cell signalling pathways and membrane synthesis. It proved to be efficient in the treatment of experimental murine leishmaniasis. Several phase II studies carried out in India showed a remarkable efficacy of the product, with 100% cure with an optimal dose of 100 mg/day over 4 weeks.[81] The side effects are minor with this dose, limited to digestive troubles. An extensive phase III trial has been completed in India, and will determine if miltefosine is the orally efficient low-toxic drug expected for many years for the treatment of VL.

Aminosidine

Aminosidine (paromomycin) is a wide-spectrum antibiotic of the aminoglycoside family—the same family as monomycin, used for several years by Soviet clinicians to treat Central Asian CL. It showed powerful antileishmanial activity in vitro and in animal models.[82] Like other aminoglycosides, paromomycin has renal and eighth cranial nerve toxicity. It is available as an injectable formulation which can be administered by i.m. injection or i.v. infusion. The recommended dose is 15 mg/kg per day, given for 10 days.

Paromomycin has been efficiently used for VL treatment as monotherapy and in combination with pentavalent antimonials,[83,84] but is no longer available in parenteral formulation. It exists only in topical formulation for treatment of CL.[85]

Interferon γ

Interferon γ (IFNγ) is a macrophage-activating cytokine, endowed with various host defence-enhancing properties, with antimicrobial and antitumour activities. Within the clinical applications of IFNγ, leishmaniasis is of interest since the defect of macrophage activation is the key point in the development of leishmanial infection.

IFNγ was successfully used in combination with pentavalent antimonials in the treatment of VL[86,87] and MCL.[88] But in spite of a relevant rationale and efficient clinical trials, the use of IFNγ remains limited to date.

Imidazoles

The antifungal azoles inhibit the sterol synthesis pathway of *Leishmania*. Some of them (ketoconazole, itraconazole) have been tested in the treatment of CL, with contradictory results. In spite of their low toxicity and the comfort of oral administration, these products are of low interest in leishmaniasis treatment.

Allopurinol

This purine structural analogue has the capacity to be incorporated into *Leishmania* RNA, with a lethal effect on the parasite. It is orally administered and rapidly metabolized and eliminated by renal route. Its side effects are limited to digestive troubles and cutaneous intolerance. Limited clinical trials showed its efficiency in CL[89] and VL,[90] with a synergistic activity with pentavalent antimonials.

Treatment regimens according to clinical features

The large variability of clinical forms of leishmaniasis, with their distinct evolution processes and different levels of gravity, lead to a decision on the drug regimen from case to case. This strategy is all the more relevant since the available classical antileishmanial drugs are not devoid of toxicity.

Visceral leishmaniasis

VL may be treated as soon as diagnosis is completed. The efficiency of treatment is dependent on the evolution duration, advanced stages responding less to antileishmanial drugs. Treatment requires confirmed first-line products, principally antimonials and amphotericin B.

The conventional treatment is based on a 28-day course of pentavalent antimonial at a dose of 20 mg Sb^V/kg per day. A single course is not always sufficient to obtain a complete cure, and should be repeated after a pause. Due to its excellent results, liposomal amphotericin B tends to be used in first intention, with five daily injections (3 mg/kg per injection), and a final injection on the 10th day (total dose 18 mg/kg). Its use is limited by cost in poor countries.

Management of VL cases includes correcting nutritional deficiencies in patients severely wasted, blood transfusion in case of dramatic anaemia, and treating with appropriate antibiotics any secondary bacterial infection.

Clinical response is slow, the patient becoming afebrile in 4–5 days, other clinical symptoms and biological parameters slowly regressing and evolving to normal. Circulating antibodies progressively decrease and disappear in the end, 6–8 months after patient cure. Relapses are uncommon in immunocompetent patients.

Clinical antimony resistance is increasing in one geographical focus, Bihar State of India, where antimony primary resistance occurs in about 10% of cases.[91] Various alternative treatments were tested in such a situation, including amphotericin B,[92] liposomal amphotericin B,[93] pentamidine,[91] aminosidine[84] and more recently miltefosine.[81]

VL occurring in HIV-infected patients appears globally as non-responsive to the classical antileishmanial drugs, with incomplete cure and frequent relapses. Amphotericin B is usually used first in these cases. In immunocompromised patients, the side effects of antileishmanial drugs are more frequent and serious than in immunocompetent patients.

VL following organ transplantation poses apparent therapeutic problems resulting from the toxicity of the main antileishmanial drugs for transplanted organs. In reality these cases need to be treated, as they are fatal in the absence of specific treatment. The best results were obtained by treating patients successively with both antimonials and amphotericin B.

Once the antileishmanial treatment has been concluded, the problem with immunocompromised patients is that of secondary prophylaxis for prevention of relapses. Numerous schemes have been proposed, of which available data are insufficient for evaluating the respective efficiency: monthly injections of antimonial, twice-monthly injections of liposomal amphotericin B or of pentamidine, daily allopurinol or itraconazole.[94] The most frequently adopted maintenance treatment is pentamidine 4 mg/kg every 2 weeks. All these protocols, however, need to be validated.

Localized cutaneous leishmaniasis

Management of patients with LCL depends on the type and characters of the lesion(s), the *Leishmania* species involved, the risk of extension and the opinion of the patient. Briefly, three options are possible: therapeutic abstention, or local or general treatment.

Mild, rapidly self-healing forms of CL, such as those due to *L. major* or *L. peruviana*, can ultimately remain untreated, if the patient wishes. Belazzoug and Neal[95] showed that, out of two groups of patients with *L. major* CL, the group receiving distilled water as placebo was more rapidly cured than that receiving pentavalent antomonial.

Various local treatments have been proposed, including diverse physical means (diathermy, cryotherapy, radiotherapy, laser), surgical excision or local applications of ointments. They were all limited trials, made without control groups, the results of which were inconclusive. These procedures cannot be generalized.

Local infiltrations of pentavalent antomonials are recommended for the treatment of small numbers of lesions. Various protocols have been proposed consisting of a course of 5–10 infiltrations of 1–5 ml of antimonial,

often accompanied by a local anaesthetic in order to avoid pain, associated or not with cryotherapy. Infiltrations are done two or three times a week.

Systemic treatment is recommended for CL with large and/or multiple lesions, with lymphangitic dissemination, those of recidivans type or with a risk of mucosal involvement. CL of immunocompromised patients should also be treated by systemic treatment. The currently used systemic treatment is that of a course of 20 days of pentavalent antimonial, at a dose of 20 mg Sb^V/kg per day. As alternatives to antimonials, oral ketoconazole or itraconazole is proposed for *L. major* or *L. mexicana* CL. A course of four to five i.m. injections of pentamidine (4 mg/kg per injection) on alternate days is used for various types of lesions, including those due to *L. guyanensis*, with variable results.

Diffuse cutaneous leishmaniasis

Once established, DCL is resistant to treatment. Systematic pentavalent antimonials can improve the clinical evolution temporarily. Pentamidine showed some efficacy, but with high doses close to toxicity. There is a need for testing various new molecules or formulations (liposomal amphotericin B, IFNγ). But the scarcity of cases does not allow randomized clinical trials with control groups.

Mucocutaneous leishmaniasis

Systemic treatment of the primary cutaneous lesion is recommended, with the hope of avoiding parasite extension to facial mucosae. The treatment currently used in endemic areas is pentavalent antimonial, a 20-day course of i.m. injections, 20 mg Sb^V/kg per day. However, it has been shown that a correct treatment does not consistently prevent the development of secondary mucosal lesions.

The treatment of mucosal lesions should be as early as possible, in order to avoid the extension of lesions and subsequent mutilations. The antimonials, at standard doses, are injected daily over 28 days. The level of cure is variable according to country and the evolution grade of the lesions. Amphotericin B has been currently used for cases with long evolution or poorly responding to antimonials. Cure was sometimes obtained from 1 g, but superior doses (2–3 g) were often necessary. Amphotericin B was used as first-line drug during a mass campaign in Bolivia.[96] Cases of resistance seem to exist, but few documented observations are available. Liposomal amphotericin B and association of IFNγ or paromomycin to antimonials can be an alternative solutions.

Prophylaxis

Intervention strategies for prevention or control are hampered by the variety of the structure of leishmaniasis foci, with many different animals able to act as reservoir hosts of zoonotic forms and a multiplicity of sandfly vectors, each with a different pattern of behaviour. In 1990, a WHO Expert Committee described no less than

11 distinct eco-epidemiological entities and defined control strategies for each of them.[97]

The aim of prevention is avoiding host infection (human or canine) and its subsequent disease. It includes means to prevent intrusion of people into natural zoonotic foci and ways to protect against infective bites of sandflies. Prevention can be at an individual or collective level.

Control programmes are intended to interrupt the life cycle of the parasite, to limit or, ideally, to eradicate, the disease. The two main targets in control programmes are the vector and the reservoir, which are not mutually exclusive. As the majority of the leishmaniases are zoonoses, control programmes are generally limited and rarely pass beyond the experimental stage. In the New World, almost all the leishmaniases are sylvatic, and control is not usually feasible. Even removal of the forest itself may not reach the objective, as various *Leishmania* species have proved to be remarkably adaptable to environment degradation. For example, *L. braziliensis* survived the great deforestation of eastern Brazil.

Whatever type of intervention strategy is selected, an active participation of the population is essential to success. Public information on the natural history of the parasite, transmission and the disease is a prerequisite for any prevention measure or development of a control programme.

Prevention

Prevention includes all individual or collective measures aimed at preventing infection of the human or canine population.

Individual prevention

Numerous individual protective means are available but are not equally feasible. The simplest measure is avoiding exposure to risk. Other means include mechanical, chemical or therapeutic measures.

Avoiding risk exposure
The risk of infection is geographically and temporally localized. A simple preventive measure is, therefore, to avoid the vicinity of sandlfy development or resting sites in endemic areas during critical periods (seasons and activity cycles of the vector). This is less feasible in tropical than temperate regions where transmission seasons are limited, but occasionally it can be applicable elsewhere. However, this way of avoiding risk is not applicable to the general situation of many developing countries where regular migration leads to human settlements inside the heart of natural foci. This results in a high exposure to risk by non-immune, uninformed populations.

Mechanical means
Mechanical means have the objective of protection from sandfly bites. They include wearing clothes that cover as much skin as possible and using bed-nets.

Sandflies bite uncovered skin and do not have the ability to bite through clothes, even thin material like cotton. Wearing full clothes during the hours of sandfly activity is a good preventive measure which can decrease the number of cutaneous lesions, even if it does not avoid all contamination.[98]

Sandflies can generally pass through the mesh of mosquito bed-nets, and therefore it is generally recommended to use fine bed-nets of Terylene. A disadvantage of these nets is that they impede air circulation, and are thus uncomfortable in hot weather. The present trend is to use conventional mosquito bed-nets impregnated with various insecticides, including the pyrethroids permethrin (300 mg/m^2), deltamethrin ($15-25 \text{ mg/m}^2$) and lambdacyhalothrin (10 mg/m^2). They have been found to be efficient because of both their repellent and residual killing effects. But the intrinsic limitation of bed-nets is related to the behaviour of the people who tend to be at greatest risk between sunset and bedtime. This method therefore provides more protection for women and children than for male adults.[99] Pilot control programmes with impregnated bed-nets are ongoing in Bolivia, Afghanistan, Iran, Sudan and Syria.

Chemical means
Sandflies are sensitive to various repellents used against mosquitoes. They are sprayed or spread on uncovered skin before the hours of sandfly activity (dusk and night). The duration of efficacy depends not only on the product but also on the climatic conditions, mainly heat and humidity. It is generally considered that protection is limited to 2–6 hours.

Permethrin-treated uniforms tested in Colombian soldiers on patrol resulted in a fall in the number of infections.[100]

For dogs, delthametrin-impregnated collars developed for protection against ticks were previously tested against sandflies in the South of France[101] and were found to be repellents. Trials in other countries confirmed that this simple device provides an effective long-term protection for dogs against the bites of sandflies.

Self-protection insecticides can reduce man–vector contact. Mosquito coils containing pyrethroid insecticides provide good protection during the time of combustion (6–8 hours). Electrically heated fumigation mats are also efficient, but need electricity, which is often unavailable in developing countries. Insecticide spraying has a good but temporary efficacy.

Chemo-prophylaxis and vaccine
Neither chemo-prophylaxis nor vaccines are available against leishmaniasis.

Various vaccines have been made and experimentally tested in different animal models, but none has prevented human or canine leishmaniasis. Putative vaccines include live, irradiated or killed parasites, parasitic crude fractions and recombinant parasitic antigens.[102]

The first vaccines contained live *L. major* promastigotes and were empirically used in the past in Central Asia republics of the former USSR, Israel and later intensively in Iran during the war against Iraq. Similar vaccines were developed in Brazil for American CL. Vaccines containing killed promastigotes, with or without BCG as an adjuvant, were then used in field trials in several countries including Brazil, Venezuela and Iran.

A variety of second-generation vaccines are at different developmental stages and include recombinant *Leishmania*, bacteria or viruses expressing leishmanial antigens, and defined recombinant subunits and synthetic peptides. But none of them is presently available for human or canine use.

Collective measures

Independently of an established control programme, the human population can be collectively protected through a few measures to keep sandflies away from people. To reduce peridomestic transmission, environmental changes have been proposed in particular situations, such as forest clearings around human settlements. Insecticide application inside houses is also occasionally recommended.

Forest clearance
The establishment of human settlements in South American primary forest results in outbreaks of CL.[103] In such situations, a high level of human infection is related to domestic or peridomestic transmission by sandflies flying from the neighbouring forest. Establishment of a forest-free zone of about 400 m around a human settlement in French Guiana resulted in a dramatic decrease in human cases during the following years.[104] Such changes in the environment must, however, be maintained, as secondary forest appeared to favour an increase in *Lutzomyia flaviscutellata* and rodent populations, leading to an increase in enzootic rodent leishmaniasis.[105]

Indoor residual spraying
This is a simple, cost-effective method for controlling endophilic vectors which can have a long-lasting effect depending on the insecticide. Sandflies are sensitive to all classes of insecticides: organochlorines, organophosphates, carbamates or pyrethroids.[106] Vectors of VL remain sensitive to DDT even in places where *P. papatasi* shows some level of resistance.[107] It is therefore the first-line insecticide for indoor spraying owing to its low cost and long residual action.

Control

The structure and dynamics of natural foci of leishmaniasis are so diverse that a standard control programme cannot be defined and control measures must be adapted to local situations. The strategy depends on the ecology and behaviour of the main targets: the reservoir hosts and the vector(s). Control measures will be totally different depending on whether the disease is anthroponotic or zoonotic. Case detection and treatment are recommended when the reservoir is man or dog, while massive destruction may be the chosen intervention if the reservoir is a wild animal. As far as vectors are concerned, control of breeding sites is limited to the few instances where they are known (rodent burrows for *P. papatasi* and *P. duboscqi*). Anti-adult measures consist of insecticide spraying. In practice, control programmes include several integrated measures targeted not only to the reservoir and/or vector, but also associated environmental changes. Health education campaigns can considerably improve the efficacy of control programmes.

National leishmaniasis control programmes have been developed in various countries to face endemics or epidemics (India, China and Brazil for VL, Central Asia republics of the former USSR and Tunisia for CL).

Case detection and treatment
Case detection and treatment is the basic intervention measure when the reservoir is man. It requires diagnostic facilities and the permanent availability of drugs in health centres based in endemic areas, both of which should be easily accessible and free of charge. Passive case detection can be considerably improved by active surveillance. In 1976–1978, this proved to be more efficient in a village in Bihar State, India, than insecticide spraying in other areas.[108] It has, however, the disadvantage of the high cost, limited number and toxicity of antileishmanial drugs.

When dogs are reservoir hosts, an active case detection is based on a house-to-house sampling of dogs, the sera of which are tested by antileishmanial antibodies. Due to the limited efficiency of antileishmanial drugs in canine leishmaniasis, the positive animals are culled, not treated. Such measures showed only a limited efficacy in China[109] and in Brazil.[110] With a mathematical model, Dye predicted that neither killing nor treating seropositive dogs were efficient measures for controlling the incidence of human VL with a canine reservoir.[111]

Wild reservoir control
Generally, no control measures are applicable to wild mammals. An exception, however, concerns rodents which, as they live in burrows, can be destroyed by chemical means or by environmental changes, or a combination of both. For example, the great gerbils destruction, by poisoning their burrows with zinc phosphide or by ploughing to a depth of 50 cm, was the basis of the control programme in the Central Asian republics of the former USSR, to eradicate zoonotic CL caused by *L. major*.[112]

Sandfly control
Destruction of breeding sites
Only a few breeding sites of sandfly species are known: *P. papatasi* and *P. duboscqi* in rodent burrows are the best example. The destruction of these burrows, combined with both reservoir and vector elimination, and has shown to be an efficient control method in Central Asia.[112] DDT dust injected into rodent burrows had only a transitory effect.

Insecticide spraying

Malaria control programmes based on indoor residual insecticide spraying have had a side benefit for leishmaniasis incidence in several countries where a resurgence of leishmaniasis was observed in numerous areas after cessation of these campaigns: India,[113] Italy, Greece and the Middle East [112] and Peru.[114]

In 1977, following the reappearance of VL, DDT was sprayed twice annually with the specific purpose of controlling the disease. But it is difficult to assess the contribution of sandfly reduction to the decrease in the number of cases, as this measure was currently associated with case detection and treatment and, because DDT was in short supply, only half the target areas were covered. In contrast, in Ceara State in Brazil, a 58% decrease in the incidence of human VL was obtained over 4 years by spraying DDT in houses and animal pens.[115] In areas of Uta in Peru, peridomestic applications of DDT controlled the vectors *Lutzomyia verrucarum* and *Lu. peruensis* and was followed subsequently by a marked decline in human cases.[116]

For peridomestic vectors, house spraying should include external as well as internal walls, and adjacent animal dwellings (chicken houses, cattle sheds, etc.). In peri-urban rainforest, Ready et al. sprayed the lower part of trees with DDT and reported the subsequent disappearance of sandflies for 11 months.[117]

The resistance of sandflies to insecticides is not the limiting factor for use during control programmes, but more their acceptance by the population. Resistance by sandflies to insecticides was first reported with *P. papatasi* in Bihar State in India,[118] but it has not been demonstrated with other species. In particular, the vector of VL in India, *P. argentipes*, seems until now to be susceptible to all insecticides, including DDT.[106,107]

In conclusion, leishmaniases are diseases widely distributed around the world, and include visceral and tegumentary forms. Over the past century, advances in treatment and prophylaxis were limited, which consequently has led to their persistence as an important public health problem in various countries.

Acknowledgements

The authors express their warmest thanks to S. Croft, D. A. Evans and R. Killick-Kendrick for revision of the manuscript.

REFERENCES

1. Desjeux P. Global control and *Leishmania*/HIV co-infection. *Clin Dermatol* 1999; 17:317–325.
2. Ross R. Note on the bodies recently described by Leishman and Donovan. *Br Med J* 1903; 2:1261–1262.
3. Lumsden W H R. Biochemical taxonomy of *Leishmania*. *Trans R Soc Trop Med Hyg* 1974; 68:74–75.
4. Gardener P J, Chance M L & Peters W. Biochemical taxonomy of *Leishmania*. II. Electrophoretic variation of malate dehydrogenase. *Ann Trop Med Parasitol* 1974; 68:317–325.
5. Godfrey D G. The zymodemes of trypanosomes. In *Problems in the Identification of Parasites and their Vectors. Symp Br Soc Parasitol* 1979; 17:31–53.
6. Rioux J A, Lanotte G, Serres E et al. Taxonomy of *Leishmania*. Use of isoenzymes. Suggestions for a new classification. *Ann Parasitol Hum Comp* 1990; 65:111–125.
7. Lainson R & Shaw J J. Evolution, classification and geographical distribution. In Peters W & Killick-Kendrick R (eds). *The Leishmaniases in Biology and Medicine*, vol. 1. London: Academic Press, 1987: 1–120.
8. Rioux J A & Lanotte G. Apport de la cladistique à l'analyse du genre *Leishmania* Ross, 1903 (Kinetoplastida, Trypanosomatidae). Corollaires épidémiologiques. *Biosystema* 1993; 8:79–90.
9. Ward R D. Vector biology and control. In Chang K P & Bray R S (eds) *Leishmaniasis*. Amsterdam: Elsevier, 1985: 199–212.
10. Lewis D J. The biology of Phlebotomidae in relation to leishmaniasis. *Annu Rev Entomol* 1974; 19:363–384.
11. Killick-Kendrick R. Phlebotomine vectors of the leishmaniases: a review. *Med Vet Entomol* 1990; 4:1–24.
12. Ashford R W. Leishmaniasis reservoirs and their significance in control. *Clin Dermatol* 1996; 14:523–532.
13. Garnham P C C. The Leishmanias, with special reference of the role of animal reservoirs. *Am Zool* 1965; 5:141–151.
14. Walters L L. *Leishmania* differentiation in natural and unnatural sandfly hosts. *J Eukaryot Microbiol* 1993; 40:196–206.
15. Lainson R & Shaw J J. The role of animals in the epidemiology of South American leishmaniasis. In Lumsden W H R & Evans D A (eds) *Biology of the Kinetoplastida*, vol. 2. London: Academic Press, 1979: 1–116.
16. Symmers W S C. Leishmaniasis acquired by contagion: a case of marital infection in Britain. *Lancet* 1960; 1:127–132.
17. Alvar J & Jimenez M. Could infected drug-users be potential *Leishmania infantum* reservoirs? *AIDS* 1994; 8:854.
18. Dye C & Wolpert D M. Earthquakes, influenza and cycles of Indian kala-azar. *Trans R Soc Trop Med Hyg* 1988; 82:843–850.
19. Thakur C P & Kumar K. Post kala-azar dermal leishmaniasis: a neglected aspect of kala-azar control programmes. *Ann Trop Med Parasitol* 1992; 86:355–359.
20. Seaman J, Ashford R W, Schorscher J et al. Visceral leishmaniasis in southern Sudan: status of healthy villagers in epidemic conditions. *Ann Trop Med Parasitol* 1992; 86:481–486.
21. Badaro R, Jones T C, Carvalho E M et al. New perspectives on a subclinical form of visceral leishmaniasis. *J infect Dis* 1986; 154:1003–1011.
22. Titus R G & Ribeiro J M C. Salivary gland lysates from the sandfly *Lutzomyia longipalpis* enhance *Leishmania* infectivity. *Science* 1988; 239:1306–1308.
23. Kamhawi S. The biological and immunomodulatory properties of sandfly saliva and its role in the establishment of *Leishmania* infections. *Microbes Infect* 2000; 14:1765–1773.
24. Antoine J C, Lang T & Prina E. Biologie cellulaire de *Leishmania*. In Dedet J P (ed.) *Les Leishmanioses*. Paris: Ellipses, 1999: 41–58.
25. Barral-Netto M, Machado P & Barral A. Human cutaneous leishmaniasis: recent advances in physiopathology and treatment. *Eur J Dermatol* 1995; 5:104–113.
26. Gradoni L & Gramiccia M. *Leishmania infantum* tropism: strain genotype or host immune status? *Parasitol Today* 1994; 10:264–267.
27. Pratlong F, Dedet J P, Marty P et al. *Leishmania*–human immunodeficiency virus coinfection in the Mediterranean

Basin: isoenzymatic characterization of 100 isolates of the *Leishmania infantum* complex. *J Infect Dis* 1995; 172:323–326.

28 Ridley D S. Pathology. In Peters W & Killick-Kendrick R (eds) *The Leishmaniases in Biology and Medicine* vol. 2. London: Academic Press; 1987; 665–729.

29 Donovan C. A possible cause of kala-azar. *Indian Med Gaz* 1903; 38:478.

30 Leishman W B. On the possibility of the occurrence of trypanosomiasis in India. *Br Med J* 1903; 2213:1252–1254.

31 Laveran A & Mesnil F. Sur un protozoaire nouveau (*Piroplasma donovani* Laveran et Mesnil), parasite d'une fièvre de l'Inde. *CR Acad Sci* 1903; 137:957–961.

32 Sacks D L, Kenney R T, Kreutzer R D et al. Indian kala-azar caused by *Leishmania tropica*. *Lancet* 1995; 345:959–961.

33 Ramos-Santos C, Hernandez-Montes O, Sanchez-Tejeda G et al. Visceral leishmaniasis caused by *Leishmania (L.) mexicana* in a Mexican patient with human immunodeficiency virus infection. *Mem Inst Oswaldo Cruz* 2000; 95:733–737.

34 Barral A, Badaro R, Barral-Netto M et al. Isolation of *Leishmania mexicana amazonensis* from the bone marrow in a case of American visceral leishmaniasis. *Am J Trop Med Hyg* 1986; 35:732–734.

35 Ma D D F, Concannon A J & Hayes J. Fatal leishmaniasis in a renal transplant patient. *Lancet* 1979; 2:311–312.

36 Wright M I. Kala-azar of unusual duration, associated with agammaglobulinaemia. *Br Med J* 1959; 1:1218–1232.

37 Pampiglione S, Manson-Bahr PEC, La Placa M et al. Studies on Mediterranean leishmaniasis. 3. The leishmanin skin test in kala-azar. *Trans R Soc Trop Med Hyg* 1975; 69:60–68.

38 Carvalho E M, Barral A, Pedral-Sampaio D et al. Immunologic markers of clinical evolution in children recently infected with *Leishmania donovani chagasi*. *J Infect Dis* 1992; 165:535–540.

39 Ho M, Siongok T K, Lyerly W H et al. Prevalence and disease spectrum in a new focus of visceral leishmaniasis in Kenya. *Trans R Soc trop Med Hyg* 1982; 76:741–746.

40 Meller-Melloul C, Farnarier C, Dunan S et al. Evidence of subjects sensitized to *Leishmania infantum* on the French Mediterranean coast: differences in gamma interferon production between this population and visceral leishmaniasis patients. *Parasite Immunol* 1991; 13:531–536.

41 Nicolle C. Sur trois cas d'infection splénique infantile à corps de Leishman observés en Tunisie. *Arch Inst Pasteur Tunis* 1908; 3:1–26.

42 Dedet J P & Belazzoug S. Leishmaniasis in North Africa. In Chang K P & Bray R S (eds) *Leishmaniasis*. Amsterdam: Elsevier, 1985: 353–375.

43 Marty P, Le Fichoux Y, Pratlong F et al. Human visceral leishmaniasis in Alpes-Maritimes, France: epidemiological characteristics for the period 1985–1992. *Trans R Soc Trop Med Hyg* 1994; 88:33–34.

44 Zijlstra E E, El-Hassan A M, Ismael A et al. Endemic kala-azar in eastern Sudan: a longitudinal study on the incidence of clinical and subclinical infection and post-kala-azar dermal leishmaniasis. *Am J Trop Med Hyg* 1994; 51:826–836.

45 Firth R H. Notes on the appearances of certain sporozoid bodies in the protoplasm of an 'oriental sore'. *Br Med J* 1891; 1567:60–62.

46 Borovsky P F. On Sartov ulcer. *Voenno-Med Zh* 1898; 195:925–941.

47 Wright J H. Protozoa in a case of tropical ulcer ('Delhi sore'). *J Med Res* 1903; 10:472–482.

48 Convit J & Lapenta P. Sobre un caso de leishmaniasis tegumentaria de forma diseminada. *Revta Policlin Caracas* 1948; 17:153–158.

49 Velasco O, Savarino S J, Walton B C et al. Diffuse cutaneous leishmaniasis in Mexico. *Am J Trop Med Hyg* 1989; 41:280–288.

50 Bryceson A D M. Diffuse cutaneous leishmaniasis in Ethiopia. III. Immunological studies. *Trans R Soc Trop Med Hyg* 1970; 64:380–393.

51 Rodrigues Coura J, Galvao-Castro B & Grimaldi G Jr. Disseminated American cutaneous leishmaniasis in a patient with AIDS. *Mem Inst Oswaldo Cruz* 1987; 82:581–582.

52 Jimenez M I, Guttierrez-Solar B, Benito A et al. Cutaneous *Leishmania (L.) infantum* zymodemes isolated from bone marrow in AIDS patients. *Res Rev Parasitol* 1991; 51:91–94.

53 Gillis D, Klaus S, Schnur L F et al. Diffusely disseminated cutaneous *Leishmania major* infection in a child with acquired immunodeficiency syndrome. *Pediatr Infect Dis J* 1995; 14:247–249.

54 Salman S M, Rubeiz N G & Kibbi A. Cutaneous leishmaniasis: clinical features and diagnosis. *Clin Dermatol* 1999; 17:291–296.

55 Escomel E. La Espundia. *Bull Soc Pathol Exot* 1911; 4:489–492.

56 Corredor A, Kreutzer R D, Tesh R B et al. Distribution and etiology of leishmaniasis in Colombia. *Am J Trop Med Hyg* 1990; 42:206–214.

57 Walton B C. American cutaneous and mucocutaneous leishmaniasis. In Peters W & Killick-Kendrick R (eds) *The Leishmaniases in Biology and Medicine*, vol. 2. London: Academic Press, 1987: 637–664.

58 Desjeux P. Leishmaniose cutanée et cutanéo-muqueuse. Etude de 113 cas observés en Bolivie. Doctoral thesis, Paris, 1974.

59 Marsden P D & Nonata R R. Mucocutaneous leishmaniasis: a review of clinical aspects. *Rev Soc Bras Med Trop* 1975; 9:309–326.

60 Alvar J. Leishmaniasis and AIDS co-infection: the Spanish example. *Parasitol Today* 1994; 10:160–163.

61 Desjeux P, Alvar J, Gradoni L et al. Epidemiological analysis of 692 retrospective cases of *Leishmania*/HIV co-infections. WHO/LEISH 1996; 39:11p.

62 Dereure J, Pratlong F, Reynes J et al. Haemoculture as a tool for diagnosing visceral leishmaniasis in HIV-negative and HIV-positive patients: interest for parasite identification. *Bull World Health Organ* 1998; 76:203–206.

63 Campino L, Santos-Gomes G, Pratlong F et al. The isolation of *Leishmania donovani* MON-18 from an AIDS patient in Portugal: possible needle transmission. *Parasite* 1994; 1:391–392.

64 Mary C, Lamouroux D, Dunan S et al. Western-blot analysis of antibodies to *Leishmania infantum* antigens: potential of the 14-kD and 16-kD antigens for diagnosis and epidemiologic purposes. *Am J Trop Med Hyg* 1992; 47:764–771.

65 Pratlong F, Lambert M, Bastien P et al. Leishmanioses et immunodépression: aspects biocliniques actuels. *Rev Fr Lab* 1997; 291:161–168.

66 Nicolle C. Isolement et culture des corps de Leishman. *Arch Inst Pasteur Tunis* 1908; 2:55–56.

67 Evans D A, Godfrey D, Lanham S et al. *Handbook on Isolation, Characterization and Cryopreservation of Leishmania*. Geneva: WHO, 1989.

68 Mathis A & Deplazes P. PCR and in vitro cultivation for detection of *Leishmania* spp. in diagnostic samples for humans and dogs. *J Clin Microbiol* 1995; 33:1145–1149.

69 Osman O F, Oskam L, Zijlstra E E et al. Evaluation of PCR for diagnosis of visceral leishmaniasis. *J Clin Microbiol* 1997; 35:2454–2457.

70 Lachaud L, Dereure J, Chabbert E et al. Optimized PCR using patient blood samples for diagnosis and follow-up of visceral leishmaniasis, with special reference to AIDS patients. *J Clin Microbiol* 2000; 38:236–240.

71 Lopez M, Inga R, Cangalaya M et al. Diagnosis of *Leishmania* using the polymerase chain reaction: a simplified procedure for field work. *Am J Trop Med Hyg* 1993; 49:348–356.

72 Belli A, Rodriguez B, Aviles H et al. Simplified polymerase

chain reaction detection of New World *Leishmania* in clinical specimens of cutaneous leishmaniasis. *Am J Trop Med Hyg* 1998; 58:102–109.

73 Pirmez C, Silva Trajano V, Paes-Oliveira Neto M et al. Use of PCR in diagnosis of human American tegumentary leishmaniasis in Rio de Janeiro, Brazil. *J Clin Microbiol* 1999; 37:1819–1823.

74 Costa J M, Durand R, Deniau M et al. PCR enzyme-linked immunosorbent assay for diagnosis of leishmaniasis in human immunodeficiency virus-infected patients. *J Clin Microbiol* 1996; 34:1831–1833.

75 Zijlstra E E & Modabber F. The leishmaniases: diagnosis. In Gilles H M (ed.) *Protozoal Diseases*. Oxford: Arnold, 1999: 425–440.

76 Montenegro J. A cutis reaçao na leishmaniose. *Ann Fac Med Sao Paulo* 1926; 1:323–330.

77 Herwaldt B L & Berman J D. Recommendations for treating leishmaniasis with sodium stibogluconate (Pentostam©) and review of pertinent clinical studies. *Am J Trop Med Hyg* 1992; 46:296–306.

78 World Health Organization. *WHO Model Prescribing Information, Drugs Used in Parasitic Diseases*. Geneva: WHO, 1997.

79 Davidson R N, Di Martino L, Gradoni L et al. Short-course treatment of visceral leishmaniasis with liposomal amphotericin B (AmBisome). *Clin Infect Dis* 1996; 22:938–943.

80 Berman J D, Badaro R, Thakur C P et al. Efficacy and safety of liposomal amphotericin B (AmBisome) for visceral leishmaniasis in endemic developing countries. *Bull World Health Organ* 1998; 76:25–32.

81 Sundar S, Makharia A, More D et al. Short-course of oral miltefosine for treatment of visceral leishmaniasis. *Clin Infect Dis* 2000; 31:1110–1113.

82 Neal R A. Experimental chemotherapy. In Peters W & Killick-Kendrick R (eds). *The Leishmaniases in Biology and Medicine*, vol. 2. London: Academic Press, 1987: 793–845.

83 Chunge C N, Owate J, Pamba H O et al. Treatment of visceral leishmaniasis in Kenya by aminosidine alone or combined with sodium stibogluconate. *Trans R Soc Trop Med Hyg* 1990; 84:221–225.

84 Thakur C P, Kanyok T P, Pandey A K et al. A prospective randomized, comparative, open-label trial of the safety and efficacy of paromomycin (aminosidine) plus sodium stibogluconate versus sodium stibogluconate alone for the treatment of visceral leishmaniasis. *Trans R Soc Trop Med Hyg* 2000; 94:429–431.

85 El-On J, Halevy S, Grunwald M H et al. Topical treatment of Old World cutaneous leishmaniasis caused by *Leishmania major*: a double-blind control study. *J Am Acad Dermatol* 1992; 27:227–231.

86 Badaro R, Falcoff E, Badaro F S et al. Treatment of visceral leishmaniasis with pentavalent antimony and interferon gamma. *N Engl J Med* 1990; 322:16–21.

87 Squires K E, Rosenkaimer F, Sherwood J A et al. Immunochemotherapy for visceral leishmaniasis: a controlled pilot trial of antimony versus antimony plus interferon-gamma. *Am J Trop Med Hyg* 1993; 48:666–669.

88 Falcoff E, Taranto N J, Remondegui C E et al. Clinical healing of antimony-resistant cutaneous or mucocutaneous leishmaniasis following the combined administration of interferon-gamma and pentavalent antimonial compounds. *Trans R Soc Trop Med Hyg* 1994; 88:95–97.

89 Martinez S & Marr J J. Allopurinol in the treatment of American cutaneous leishmaniasis. *N Engl J Med* 1992; 326:741–744.

90 Chunge C N, Gachihi G, Muigai R et al. Visceral leishmaniasis unresponsive to antimonial drugs. III. Successful treatment using a combination of sodium stibogluconate plus allopurinol. *Trans R Soc Trop Med Hyg* 1985; 79:715–718.

91 Thakur C P, Kumar M & Pandey K. Comparison of regimes of treatment of antimony-resistant kala-azar patients: a randomized study. *Am J Trop Med Hyg* 1991; 45:435–441.

92 Thakur C P, Sinha G P, Pandey A K et al. Amphotericin B in resistant kala-azar in Bihar. *Nat Med J India* 1993; 6:57–61.

93 Thakur C P, Pandey A K, Sinha G P et al. Comparison of three treatment regimens with liposomal amphotericin B (AmBisome) for visceral leishmaniasis in India: a randomised dose-finding study. *Trans R Soc Trop Med Hyg* 1996; 90:319–322.

94 Davidson R N. Practical guide for the treatment of the leishmaniases. *Drugs* 1998; 56:1009–1018.

95 Belazzoug S, Neal R A. Failure of meglumine antimoniate to cure cutaneous lesions due to *Leishmania major* in Algeria. *Trans R Soc Trop Med Hyg* 1986; 80:670–671.

96 Dedet J P, Melogno R, Cardenas F et al. Rural campaign to diagnose and treat mucocutaneous leishmaniasis in Bolivia. *Bull World Health Organ* 1995; 73:339–345.

97 World Health Organization. Control of the leishmaniases. Report of a WHO Expert Committee. 1990 Technical Report Series 793.

98 Dedet J P, Esterre P & Pradinaud R. Individual clothing prophylaxis of cutaneous leishmaniasis in the Amazonian area. *Trans R Soc Trop Med Hyg* 1987; 81:748.

99 Elnaiem D A, Elnahas A M & Aboud M A. Protective efficacy of lambdacyhalothrin-impregnated bednets against *Phlebotomus orientalis*, the vector of visceral leishmaniasis in Sudan. *Med Vet Entomol* 1999; 13:310–314.

100 Soto J, Medina F, Dember N et al. Efficacy of permethrin-impregnated uniforms in the prevention of malaria and leishmaniasis in Colombian soldiers. *Clin Infect Dis* 1995; 21:599–602.

101 Killick-Kendrick R, Killick-Kendrick M, Focheux M et al. Protection of dogs from bites of phlebotomine sandflies by deltamethrin collars for control of canine leishmaniasis. *Med Vet Entomol* 1997; 11:105–111.

102 Modabber F. Vaccines against leishmaniasis. *Ann Trop Med Parasitol* 1995; 89:83–88.

103 Barrett T V & Senra M S. Leishmaniasis in Manaus, Brazil. *Parasitol Today* 1989; 5:255–257.

104 Esterre P, Chippaux J P, Lefait J F et al. Evaluation d'un programme de lutte contre la leishmaniose cutanée dans un village forestier de Guyane française. Bull World Health Organ 1986; 64:559–565.

105 Ready P D, Lainson R & Shaw J J. Leishmaniasis in Brazil. XX. Prevalence of 'enzootic rodent leishmaniasis' (*Leishmania mexicana amazonensis*), and apparent absence of 'pian bois' (*Le. braziliensis guyanensis*), in plantations of introduced tree species and other non-climax forests in eastern Amazonia. *Trans R Soc Trop Med Hyg* 1983; 77:775–785.

106 Mazzarri M B, Feliciangeli M D, Maroli M et al. Susceptibility of *Lutzomyia longipalpis* (Diptera: Psychodidae) to selected insecticides in an endemic focus of visceral leishmaniasis in Venezuela. *J Am Mosq Control Assoc* 1997; 13:335–341.

107 Mukhopadhyay A K, Hati A K, Chakraborty S et al. Effect of DDT on *Phlebotomus* sandflies in Kala-azar endemic foci in West Bengal. *J Commun Dis* 1996; 28:171–175.

108 Sanyal R K, Alam S N, Kaul S N et al. Some observations of epidemic of current outbreaks of kala-azar in Bihar. *J Commun Dis* 1979; 11:170–182.

109 Guan L R. Current status de kala-azar and vector control in China. *Bull World Health Organ* 1991; 69:595–601.

110 Lacerda M M. The Brazilian leishmaniasis control programme. *Mem Inst Oswaldo Cruz* 1994; 89:489–495.

111 Dye C. The logic of visceral leishmaniasis control. *Am J Trop Med Hyg* 1996 ; 55:125–130.

112 Saf'janova V M. Leishmaniasis control. *Bull World Health Organ* 1971; 44:561–566.

113 Sanyal R K, Banjerjeeb D P, Ghosh T K et al. A longitudinal review of kala-azar in Bihar. *J Commun Dis* 1979; 11:149–169.

114 Davies C R, Llanos-Cuentas A, Canales J et al. The fall and rise of Andean cutaneous leishmaniasis: transient impact of the DDT campaign in Peru. *Trans R Soc Trop Med Hyg* 1994; 88:389–393.

115 Alencar J E de. Profilaxia do calazar no Ceara, Brasil. *Rev Inst Med Trop Sao Paulo* 1961; 3:175–180.

116 Hertig M & Fairchild G B. The control of *Phlebotomus* in Peru with DDT. *Am J Med* 1947; 28:207–230.

117 Ready P D, Arias J R & Freitas R A. A pilot study to control *Lutzomyia umbratilis* (Diptera, Psychodidae), the major vector of *Leishmania braziliensis guyanensis*, in a peri-urban rainforest of Manaus, Amazonas State, Brazil. *Mem Inst Oswaldo Cruz* 1985; 80:27–36.

118 Joshi G C, Kaul S M, Wattal B L. Susceptibility of sandflies to organochlorine insecticides in Bihar, India: further report. *J Commun Dis* 1979; 11:209–213.

Chapter 76
Toxoplasmosis

R. E. Holliman

Toxoplasma gondii is an obligate intracellular parasite that causes infection in most mammals worldwide. Human infection is usually mild or asymptomatic but toxoplasmosis represents a life-threatening disease in the immunocompromised patient.

History

The organism was first described when Nicolle and Manceaux[1] found the parasite in the liver and spleen of a North African rodent, the gondii (*Ctenodactylus gundi*) in 1908. An association was made with human disease when Jankû[2] observed parasitic cysts in the retina of a child with hydrocephalus and microphthalmia. Wolf and Cowen[3] demonstrated the significance of congenital toxoplasmosis, while the discovery by Pinkerton and Weinman[4] of postnatal infection followed in 1940. Sabin and Feldman[5] developed the first reliable serological assay, the dye test, in 1948. This test allowed studies to establish the prevalence and clinical spectrum of the infection.

Epidemiology

The prevalence of antibodies specific to *T. gondii* is directly proportional to the age of the population, indicating that infection is acquired throughout life. The incidence of infection shows marked geographical variation: less than a quarter of pregnant women in England will have serological evidence of exposure to the parasite, whereas three-quarters of pregnant French women will have been infected.[6] These differences are associated with diet, climate and cat contact, so that toxoplasmosis is most common in warm, wet areas with a large cat population where meat is eaten lightly cooked or raw. Recent studies indicate that the relative importance of these routes of transmission may vary by region. Ingestion of raw, undercooked or cured meats is the primary risk factor in Europe.[7] Many developed countries have noted a decline in the prevalence of the disease in recent years which may be associated with the practice of freezing meat and the introduction of intensive farming techniques which separate cats from livestock.

Aetiology

T. gondii is a coccidian parasite which has a sexual cycle in the intestinal epithelium of the definitive host, members of the cat family and an asexual cycle in secondary hosts, such as birds, rodents and other mammals (including man).

Parasitology

The characteristic form of toxoplasma is the crescent-shaped trophozoite, 6 μm in length and 3 μm wide, containing a single nucleus (Figure 76.1). *Toxon*, the Greek word for an arc or bow, the incidence of parasitaemia and the original animal source provide the derivation of the proper name *Toxoplasma gondii*.

Sexual and asexual multiplication of toxoplasma occurs in the enterocytes of felids and leads to the excretion of oocysts in their faeces. The oocysts sporulate within 3–4 days to form the infectious sporocyst. The sporocyst can retain viability for over 1 year in moist soil. Ingestion of the sporocyst by a secondary host is followed by release of tachyzoites which disseminate via the blood and lymphatic system and by active cell invasion. Asexual multiplication of tachyzoites occurs in all nucleated cells, leading to disruption and invasion of adjoining cells. Eventually a tissue cyst forms, consisting of a cyst wall (partly parasite, partly host in origin), and up to several

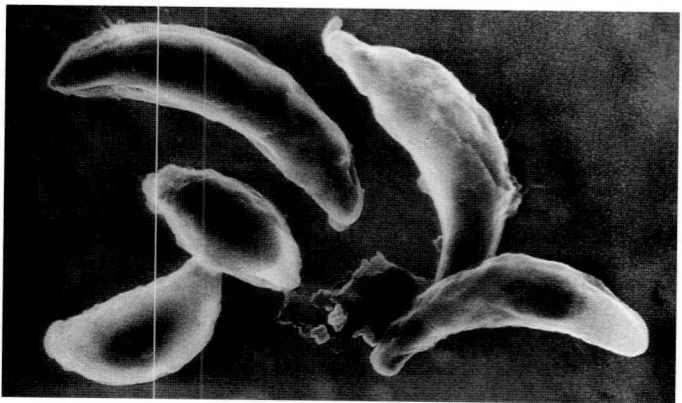

Figure 76.1: Trophozoites of *T. gondii* (scanning electron micrograph).

thousand bradyzoites. The bradyzoite is morphologically similar to the tachyzoite but shows greatly reduced metabolic activity. Predation of the secondary host completes the life cycle. Tissue cysts release their contents in the gut lumen of the cat and the active tachyzoites invade the intestinal epithelium.[6,8]

Transmission (Figure 76.2)

Human infection is acquired by ingestion of tissue cysts in raw, poorly cooked or cured meat, notably lamb and pork, or ingestion of sporocysts derived from cat faeces contaminating soil or inadequately washed vegetables. Rarely, infection can be acquired via an organ transplant.

Pathogenesis

The tachyzoite actively invades the cell and generates the formation of a parasitophorous vacuole which does not fuse with intracellular organelles, thereby avoiding destruction.[9] The tachyzoites divide by binary fission, forming an intracellular pseudocyst which distorts the host cell and ultimately leads to cellular disruption. The tachyzoites released in this process invade adjacent cells. Eventually tissue cysts form, containing quiescent bradyzoites. Periodic excystation occurs, controlled by mechanisms which are not established. Release of toxoplasma results in cellular destruction due to invasion and disruption by tachyzoites as well as damage associated with the host immune response.

Immunity is predominantly cell mediated. Activated macrophages and T cells play a central role, while interferon γ and other cytokines induce an effective immune response.[10] Specific antibody in the presence of complement eliminates extracellular parasites.

Pathology

Lesions observed at histopathological examination result from the dissemination of the parasite in the circulation, cytolytic action of the organism and the immune response of the host. Tissue necrosis is associated with thrombosis of small vessels.

Lymphadenopathy in the immunocompetent individual shows follicular hyperplasia and collections of mononuclear cells, usually at the periphery of the node. The normal tissue architecture is preserved and the parasites are rarely identified unless immunohistochemical stains are used.[11] The immunosuppressed patient, by contrast, may have abundant toxoplasma in the tissues. In cases of toxoplasmic encephalitis with the acquired immune deficiency syndrome (AIDS), cerebral tissues show central necrosis with surrounding astrocytosis. Pseudocysts are seen at the necrotic margins.[12] Necrosis, thrombosis and pseudocysts are present in the heart, liver, lung and brain of immunosuppressed patients with disseminated toxoplasmosis.

Transmission of Toxoplasmosis

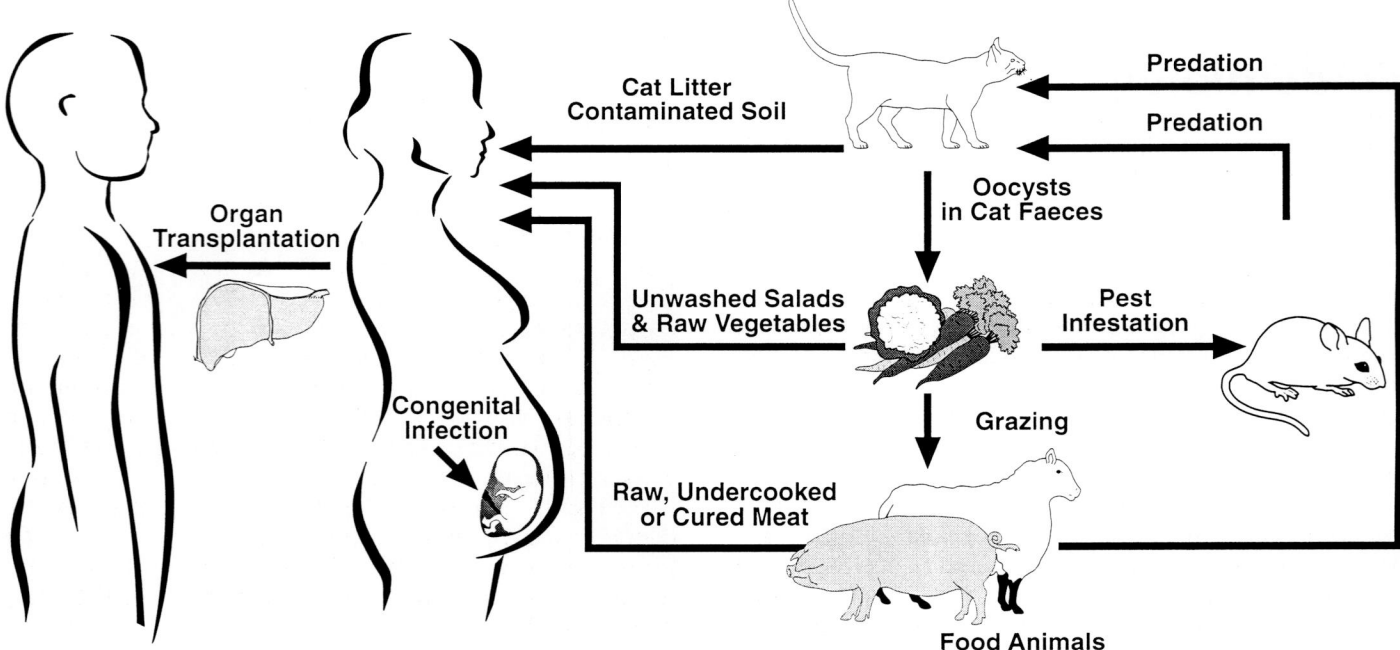

Figure 76.2: Transmission of toxoplasmosis.

Congenital toxoplasmosis can be generalized or predominantly localized in the CNS. Brain tissue shows encephalitis with multiple infarcts and necrosis, particularly in the cortex, basal ganglia and periventricular areas. Characteristic glial nodules are formed. Focal calcification with zones of necrosis are present in severe disease of prolonged duration. Hydrocephalus results from obstruction of the aqueduct of Sylvius or cerebral tissue destruction.[13] The infected placenta has chronic inflammation in the decidua and focal reaction within the villi.[14] Infected ocular tissue shows destruction of areas of the retina, with proliferation of pigment at the borders of lesions during healing. Occasionally parasites may be seen at the margins.[15]

Clinical features

The immunocompetent patient

In most cases of toxoplasmosis the source of infection cannot be identified but the usual incubation period is between 1 and 3 weeks. The majority of individuals suffer no discernible illness and the acute infection passes unnoticed. The most common presentation of symptomatic toxoplasmosis is painless cervical lymphadenopathy, which may be accompanied by fever. Fewer persons experience generalized lymphadenopathy with malaise and myalgia which follows a course of relapse and remission over several weeks or months. The differential diagnosis includes lymphoma and infectious mononucleosis. Rarely, cutaneous rash, arthralgia, pericarditis or acute chorioretinitis may be associated with postnatal toxoplasma infection.[16] Some studies have suggested a link between hepatitis and toxoplasmosis but this remains contentious.[17]

Congenital infection

The incidence and presentation of acute toxoplasmosis in the pregnant woman does not differ from that of the population as a whole. Consequently, most infections pass unrecognized unless systematic screening is undertaken. The primary risk of congenital toxoplasmosis is associated with maternal parasitaemia and subsequent placentitis. As parasitaemia is normally limited to less than 20 days' duration, the greatest risk of fetal infection is associated with maternal infection acquired during pregnancy. A number of cases of congenital toxoplasmosis have been reported where the mother acquired the infection well before conception, but this is likely to be a rare event.[18] The rate of maternal–fetal transmission of infection rises as the gestational age at the time of maternal infection progresses. If left untreated the risk of fetal infection is 25% when the mother acquires her infection during the first trimester, and 65% if maternal infection is acquired in the third trimester. Conversely, the risk of severe fetal damage is highest if the infection crosses the placenta in early pregnancy.[19]

The features of congenital toxoplasmosis range from a severely damaged infant, with death in the perinatal period, to an infected but clinically unaffected child. Severe congenital toxoplasmosis presents with hydrocephalus, mental retardation, cerebral calcification and retinochoroiditis. Skin rash, hepatitis, pneumonia, myocarditis and myositis may be present.[20] Only 10% of all congenitally infected infants suffer such severe disease. Studies suggest some children born with congenital infection will develop ocular disease in later life, regardless of the clinical status at birth.[21]

Ocular toxoplasmosis

Most cases of ocular toxoplasmosis are thought to result from periodic reactivation of infection established in the prenatal period. Excystation of the parasite is associated with acute inflammatory episodes and progressive retinal damage occurs. Retinal lesions may be apparent at birth but most often present as late sequelae in the second and third decades of life. Severe congenital disease is associated with microphthalmia, cataract, strabismus and nystagmus. The characteristic lesion is that of necrotizing retinitis, which appears as yellow-white 'cotton-wool' patches in the fundus during acute episodes. The lesions appear 'punched out' and pigmented when quiescent. The degree of visual disturbance depends on the location of the lesions within the retina. The differential diagnosis of ocular toxoplasmosis includes: colobomatous defect, intraocular haemorrhage, defects of retinal blood vessels, retinoblastoma and glioma.[22] The relative importance of postnatal infection as a cause of ocular disease is uncertain. Some recent studies have proposed that most cases of ocular toxoplasmosis are associated with postnatal rather than congenital infection.[23]

Toxoplasmosis and AIDS

In the absence of effective antiviral therapy, toxoplasmosis is the most common cause of focal brain lesions and one of the most frequent opportunistic infections in patients with AIDS. Most cases result from secondary reactivation of a chronic, previously quiescent infection associated with impairment of the individual's immune function. Features of cerebral infection predominate and the characteristic presentation is that of fever, persistent headache, deterioration of mental status and focal neurological signs. Retinochoroiditis, following extension of CNS infection, and pulmonary disease (presenting with cough and dyspnoea) are also described. Disseminated infection involving the heart, liver, CNS and lungs may be found at post-mortem.[24] The differential diagnosis of cerebral toxoplasmosis with AIDS includes lymphoma, cryptococcal infection and bacterial brain abscess. Human immunodeficiency virus (HIV)-infected patients with residual cell-mediated immune function (pre-AIDS) may present with an indolent illness comprising malaise, chronic headache and lymphadenopathy, usually associated with primary toxoplasma infection.

Toxoplasmosis and organ transplantation

Toxoplasmosis represents a life-threatening complication to organ graft recipients. Severe toxoplasma infection in association with solid organ transplantation (heart, heart–lung, liver and kidney) is restricted to the recipient without pre-existing immunity to toxoplasma (sero-negative) who is given an organ containing viable cysts of the parasite (seropositive donor). The frequency of infection in such 'mismatches' reflects the likelihood of the organ transplant containing cysts. Consequently, infection is most frequent after cardiac transplant and least common in association with renal transplantation. The infected recipient develops fever, deterioration of consciousness and signs of respiratory failure—reflecting disseminated disease, usually 3–6 weeks after the operation.[25] Such complications are effectively prevented by routine co-trimoxazole prophylaxis for solid organ graft recipients.

As the duration of parasitaemia following acute infection is limited, blood transfusion will rarely transmit toxoplasmosis. The risk is greater after granulocyte transfusion. Toxoplasmosis associated with bone marrow transplant is a rare event and is usually due to reactivation of the recipient's previously quiescent, chronic infection. Fever, CNS signs and pulmonary dysfunction are characteristic findings 15–150 days after transplantation.[26]

Diagnosis

In most instances the non-specific nature of the signs and symptoms of toxoplasmosis do not permit reliable diagnosis based solely on the clinical findings. However, due to the diversity of toxoplasma infection, investigations must be selected which are appropriate to that patient group.[27] Suitable test selections are given in Table 76.1.

Isolation

T. gondii can be isolated from infected tissues by animal inoculation or tissue culture. Intraperitoneal injection into mice is a highly sensitive diagnostic method but results are only available 3–6 weeks after inoculation. Tissue culture is less sensitive but produces a result within 10 days.[28]

Parasite detection

Histological examination can be helpful, particularly following excision of enlarged lymph nodes or biopsy of a cerebral lesion in AIDS. The sensitivity of these investigations is improved if immunohistochemical studies are employed.[29] A number of antigen detection methods have been developed utilizing enzyme-linked immunosorbent assay (ELISA) and agglutination systems.[30] Antigen detection is most valuable when investigating

Table 76.1 Investigation of toxoplasmosis

	Parasite isolation	Histology	Parasite detection	Serology	Other
Immunocompetent patient					
Lymphadenopathy	—	Excision biopsy	—	IgG, IgM	—
Pregnancy	—	—	Amniotic fluid	IgG, IgM, IgA, avidity tests	—
Ocular disease	—	—	Ocular fluid	IgG, local antibody production	—
Immunosuppressed patient					
Fetus	Amniotic fluid, blood cells	—	Amniotic fluid, blood cells	IgM, IgA	Total IgM, liver function tests
Neonate	Placenta, blood cells	—	Blood cells Western blot	Sequential IgG assessment IgM, IgA	Radiology of brain, ocular examination
AIDS	Brain biopsy	Brain biopsy	Brain biopsy	IgG	Radiology of brain, therapeutic trial
Organ transplant					
Heart/lung/liver/kidney	Tissue biopsy, bone marrow	Tissue biopsy	—	IgG, IgM	—
Bone marrow	Bone marrow, blood cells	—	Bone marrow	—	Therapeutic trial

the immunocompromised when the serological response is altered. The limitation of antigen detection has been the relative lack of sensitivity of the assay. Methods based on the detection of toxoplasma DNA by hybridization with specific probes or amplification using the polymerase chain reaction represent a considerable advance,[31] particularly when applied to testing amniotic fluid in suspected toxoplasmosis during pregnancy.[32]

Serology

A wide range of antibody detection methods are available and serology is often the investigation of choice. *T. gondii* contains a large number of membranous and cytoplasmic antigens which are incorporated into the different serological assays in variable proportions. It is not possible to compare antibody levels recorded by different tests. Whole organisms are used as the antigen source in the dye test, direct agglutination test and fluorescent antibody assay. Disrupted organisms are fixed to carrier particles in the indirect haemagglutination test and latex agglutination test and provide the antigen source for ELISA-based systems.[27]

The presence of specific IgG indicates prior exposure to the parasite and the potential for reactivation in the immunocompromised. Specific IgM, IgA or low-avidity IgG is associated with more recent infection of the immunocompetent individual. The dye test remains the 'gold standard' test but the availability of this bioassay is restricted.

Other methods

Cell-mediated immunity can be measured by a skin test or in vitro assays but has limited clinical applications. Computed tomography of the brain is useful in the investigation of patients with congenital toxoplasmosis and AIDS (Figure 76.3). Therapeutic trials of antiparasite drugs may be required to confirm the diagnosis of toxoplasmosis in the profoundly immunosuppressed.[24]

Management

None of the agents currently available for clinical use shows activity against the encysted form of the parasite. Consequently, treatment is directed against the active tachyzoite form and complete eradication of the parasite is not attempted.[33]

Immunocompetent patients

Specific therapy has *not* been shown to be effective in otherwise healthy individuals and is rarely indicated in view of the potential toxicity of antitoxoplasma agents. Therapy may be considered when the illness is protracted or unusually severe. Sulfadiazine (2 g/day) with pyrimethamine (25 mg/day) is given by the oral route.

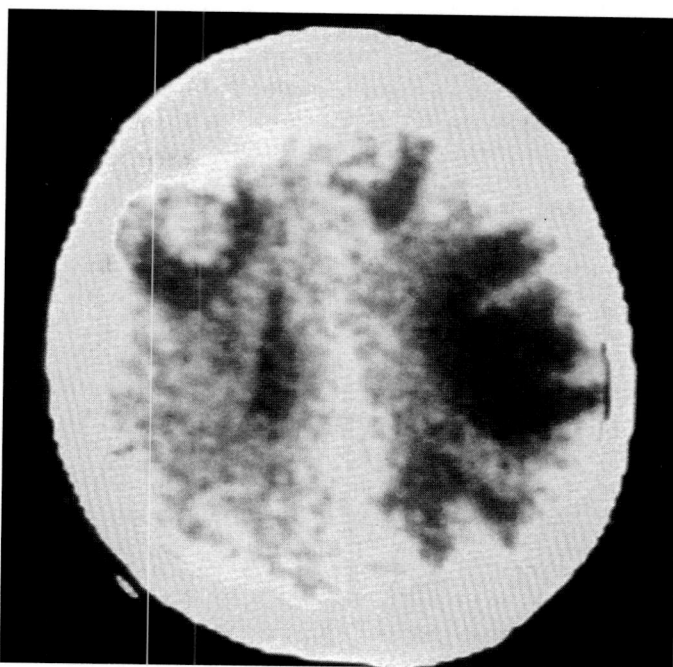

Figure 76.3: Computed tomography of the brain in cerebral toxoplasmosis associated with AIDS.

Sulfadimidine may be substituted for sulfadiazine. Vitamin supplementation consisting of folinic acid (15 mg twice weekly) or yeast tablets BPC (8 tablets twice weekly) is given to prevent bone marrow toxicity.[34] Increasingly, azithromycin (3 g/day for 10 days) is used to avoid sulfonamide toxocity.

The pregnant woman

The macrolide antibiotic spiramycin should be given at a dose of 3 g/day throughout the confinement in an attempt to reduce the risk of transplacental passage of the parasite. If fetal infection is confirmed by amniocentesis or ultrasound investigation, antiparasite therapy is given to reduce the severity of congenital disease. Sulfadiazine (50–100 mg/kg per day)–pyrimethamine (0.5–1.0 mg/kg per day) with vitamin supplement is given for 3 weeks, followed by a further 3 weeks' therapy consisting of spiramycin (3 g/day). Alternating 3 weeks' drug courses are given until delivery. The frequency of pyrimethamine dosing is reduced if bone marrow toxicity is demonstrated.[35]

Congenital infection

All infected infants are given specific therapy until the age of 1 year, irrespective of the severity of the disease. Rotating 3-week courses of sulfadiazine with pyrimethamine and folinic acid (doses as for the pregnant woman) followed by spiramycin (100 mg/kg per day) are given.[36] The role of corticosteroids is not fully established but these are often given when ventricular dilatation is noted.

Ocular disease

Quiescent lesions recognized beyond the age of 1 year require observation only. When active inflammation is noted sulfadiazine (2 g/day) or clindamycin (1.2 g/day) given with pyrimethamine (25 mg/day) and vitamin supplementation is advised. Treatment is continued for 10 days after inflammation subsides. Systemic corticosteroids are usually administered during the antiparasite therapy.[37] Laser or cryotherapy was previously used in an attempt to limit the spread of a lesion across the retina but this approach has been shown to be ineffective.[38]

Toxoplasmosis with AIDS

Acute therapy comprises sulfadiazine (4–8 g/day)–pyrimethamine 50–75 g/day) with vitamin supplements continued for 6 weeks. Clindamycin (2.4–4.8 g/day) can be substituted if severe sulfonamide toxicity is experienced. Reduced dose maintenance therapy is given after an acute episode to prevent relapse.[39] Dapsone (200 mg/day) is less effective for this purpose.

Organ transplant recipients

Seronegative recipients of a seropositive heart, heart–lung or liver donor should be given pyrimethamine (2.5 mg/day) prophylaxis for 6 weeks after the operation to prevent primary infection.[40] When significant disease is established in any organ graft recipient high-dose therapy, similar to that given in AIDS, is indicated. Maintenance therapy is not required unless the period of immunosuppression is likely to be prolonged.

Prevention and control
Health education

Women contemplating pregnancy or shown to be seronegative after conception should be given guidance to reduce the risk of acquiring toxoplasmosis during pregnancy. Foods eaten without further preparation, such as vegetables and fruit, should be washed to remove contaminating soil and sporocysts. Gloves should be worn when gardening or emptying cat litter trays. Meats that might contain tissue cysts should be cooked until well done and hand-washing after preparing raw meat should be emphasized.[41] Similar advice can be given to HIV-infected individuals.

Previously, deliberate exposure to the parasite prior to puberty was encouraged in some areas by the habit of eating raw meat. This practice is no longer considered ethical due to the risk of reactivated infection should the individual later become immunosuppressed.

Vaccination

Short-lived immunity can be induced when using nonviable toxoplasma, while viable organisms of reduced pathogenicity are associated with chronic infection and potential reactivation.[42] A non-cyst-forming strain of *T. gondii* is available for sheep[43] but there is presently no vaccine suitable for humans.

Antenatal screening

Any screening programme should be evaluated in four main areas: frequency and severity of the disease; sensitivity, specificity, performance and cost of diagnosis; effectiveness of management; administrative structure.[44] In France, a programme based on IgG seroconversion is in operation and similar schemes have been promoted in other countries.[45] Further research is required to establish the harm:benefit ratio of screening for toxoplasmosis in pregnancy before the diversion of scarce funds from other health projects can be justified.

REFERENCES

1   Nicolle C & Manceaux L. Sur une infection à corps de leishman (où organisme voisins) du gondii. *CR Acad Sci* 1908; 147:763–766.
2   Jankû J. Pathogensa a pathologiká anatomie tak nazvaného vrozeného kolobomu zluté skurny v oku normálne velikém a mikrophthalmickém s nálezem parazitu v sítnici. *Cas Lék Ces* 1923; 62:1021–1027.
3   Wolf A & Cowen D. Granulomatous encephalomyelitis due to an encephalitozoan (encephalitozoic encepholomyelitis): a new protozoan disease of man. *Bull Neurol Inst NY* 1937; 6:306–371.
4   Pinkerton H & Weinman D. Toxoplasma infection in man. *Arch Pathol* 1940; 30:374–392.
5   Sabin A B & Feldman H A. Dyes as microchemical indicators of a new immunity phenomenon affecting a protozoan parasite. *Science* 1948; 108:660–663.

6   Remington J S & Desmonts G. In Remington J S & Klein J O (eds) *Infectious Diseases of the Fetus and Newborn Infant.* London: W B Saunders, 1990: 89–195.
7   Cook A J, Gilbert R E, Buffolano W et al. Sources of toxoplasma infection in pregnant women: European multicentre case–control study. *Br Med J* 2000; 321:142–147.
8   Dubey J P & Beatie G P. *Toxoplasmosis of Animals and Man (Homo sapiens).* Boca Raton, FL: CRC Press, 1988: 41–60.
9   Joiner K. Cell attachment and entry by *Toxoplasma gondii. Behring Inst Mitt* 1991; 88:20–26.
10 Suzuki Y, Orellana M A, Schreiber R D & Remington J S. Interferon gamma, the major mediator of resistance against *Toxoplasma gondii. Science* 1988; 240:516–518.
11 Fleck D G & Kwantes W. *The Laboratory Diagnosis of Toxoplasmosis.* Public Health Laboratory Service Monograph 13. London: HMSO, 1980.

12 Luft B J, Brooks R G, Conley F K, McCabe R E & Remington J S. Toxoplasmic encephalitis in patients with acquired immune deficiency syndrome. *JAMA* 1984; 257:913–917.

13 Frenkel J K. Toxoplasma: mechanisms of infection, laboratory diagnosis and management. *Curr Top Pathol* 1971; 54:27–75.

14 Elliot W G. Placental toxoplasmosis: report of a case. *Am J Clin Pathol* 1970; 53:413–417.

15 Hogan M J. *Ocular Toxoplasmosis.* New York: Columbia University Press, 1951: 86.

16 Kean B H. Clinical toxoplasmosis—50 years. *Trans R Soc Trop Med Hyg* 1972; 66:549–571.

17 Weitberg A B, Alper J C, Diamond I & Flegiel Z. Acute granulomatous hepatitis in the course of acquired toxoplasmosis. *N Engl J Med* 1979; 300:1093–1096.

18 Holliman R E. Clinical sequelae of chronic maternal toxoplasmosis. *Rev Med Microbiol* 1994; 5:47–55.

19 Carter A O & Frank J W. Congenital toxoplasmosis: epidemiological features and control. *Can Med Assoc J* 1986; 135:618–623.

20 Eichwald H. *A Study of Congenital Toxoplasmosis.* Munksgaard: Copenhagen, 1960: 41–49.

21 Koppe J G, Loewer-Sieger D H & de Roever-Bonnet H. Results of 20 year follow-up of congenital toxoplasmosis. *Lancet* 1986; 1:254–255.

22 de Jong P T. Ocular toxoplasmosis: common and rare symptoms and signs. *Int Ophthalmol* 1989; 13:391–397.

23 Gilbert R E & Stranford M. Is ocular toxoplasmosis caused by prenatal or postnatal infection? *Br J Ophthlmol* 2000; 84:224–226.

24 Holliman R E. Toxoplasmosis and the acquired immune deficiency syndrome. *J Infect* 1988; 16:121–128.

25 Wreghitt T G, Hakim M, Gray J J et al. Toxoplasmosis in heart and heart and lung transplant recipients. *J Clin Pathol* 1987; 42:194–199.

26 O'Driscoll J C & Holliman R E. Toxoplasmosis and bone marrow transplantation. *Rev Med Microbiol* 1991; 2:215–222.

27 Holliman R E. The diagnosis of toxoplasmosis. *Serodiagn Immunother Infect Dis* 1990; 4:83–93.

28 Hughes H P, Hudson L & Fleck D G. In vitro culture of *Toxoplasma gondii* in primary and established cell lines. *Int J Parasitol* 1986; 16:317–322.

29 Conley F K & Junkins K A. Immunohistological study of the anatomic relationship of toxoplasma antigens to the inflammatory response in the brains of mice chronically infected with *Toxoplasma gondii. Infect Immun* 1981; 31:1184–1192.

30 van Knapen F & Panggabean S O. Detection of circulating antigens during acute infections with *Toxoplasma gondii* by enzyme-linked immunosorbent assay. *J Clin Microbiol* 1977; 6:545–547.

31 Savva D, Morris J C, Johnson J D & Holliman R E. Polymerase chain reaction for detection of *Toxoplasma gondii. J Med Microbiol* 1990; 32:25–31.

32 Forestier F, Hohfeld P, Sole Y & Daffos F. Prenatal diagnosis of congenital toxoplasmosis by PCR: extended experience. *Prenat Diagn* 1998; 18: 405–415.

33 McCabe R E & Oster S. Current recommendations and future prospects in the treatment of toxoplasmosis. *Drugs* 1989; 38:973–987.

34 Krick J A & Remington J S. Toxoplasmosis in the adult: an overview. *N Engl J Med* 1978; 298:550–553.

35 Couvreur J & Desmonts G. Toxoplasmosis. In MacCleod C L (ed.) *Parasitic Infections in Pregnancy and the Newborn.* Oxford: Oxford University Press, 1988: 112–142.

36 Holliman R E. Uncommon infections: toxoplasmosis, toxocariasis and cryptosporidiosis. *Prescribers J* 1992; 32:127–132.

37 Dutton G N. Recent developments in the prevention and treatment of congenital toxoplasmosis. *Int Ophthalmol* 1989; 13:407–413.

38 Desmettre T, Labalette P, Fortier B, Mordon S & Constantinides G. Laser photocoagulation around the foci of toxoplasma retinochoroiditis: a descriptive statistical analysis of 35 patients with long-term follow-up. *Ophthalmologia* 1996; 210:90–94.

39 Navia B A, Petito C K, Gold J W, Cho E S, Jordan B D & Price R W. Cerebral toxoplasmosis complicating the acquired immune deficiency syndrome: clinical and neuropathological findings in 27 patients. *Ann Neurol* 1986; 19:224–238.

40 Holliman R E, Johnson J D, Adams S & Pepper J R. Toxoplasmosis and heart transplantation. *J Heart Lung Transplant* 1991; 10:608–610.

41 Carter A O, Gelmon S B, Wells G A & Toepell A P. The effectiveness of a prenatal education programme for the prevention of congenital toxoplasmosis. *Epidemiol Infect* 1989; 103:539–545.

42 Overnes G, Nesse L L, Waldeland H, Lougren K & Gudding R. Immune response after immunisation with an experimental *Toxoplasma gondii* ISCOM vaccine. *Vaccine* 1991; 9:25–28.

43 Buxton D & Innes E A. A commercial vaccine for ovine toxoplasmosis. *Parasitology* 1995; 110:S11–S16.

44 Wilson J M & Junger G. Principles and practice of screening for disease. *Public Health Papers* No. 34. WHO: Geneva, 1968.

45 McCabe R E & Remington J S. Toxoplasmosis: the time has come. *N Engl J Med* 1988; 318:313–315.

Chapter 77
Intestinal Protozoa

M. J. G. Farthing, A. M. Cevallos and P. Kelly

Human intestinal protozoan infections are found worldwide in both developing countries and the industrialized world. Pathogenic intestinal protozoa produce disease by infecting the small or large intestine, or both. Intestinal protozoa are found in highest prevalence in developing countries, where they are responsible for a substantial burden of disease. The small intestinal protozoa *Giardia lamblia* and *Cryptosporidium parvum* have their major impact in children, while the large bowel pathogen *Entamoeba histolytica* infects all age groups but has its most profound effects in adults. The epidemiology of intestinal protozoan infection has developed rapidly with the increase in acquired immunodeficiency states, particularly that relating to cytotoxic chemotherapy for cancer and human immunodeficiency virus (HIV) infection and the acquired immune deficiency syndrome (AIDS). Interestingly, some of the protozoa, particularly *Cryptosporidium* and *Isospora belli*, have a profoundly increased morbidity in immunodeficiency states, whereas the severity of disease due to giardiasis and amoebiasis is little affected.

The world of human intestinal pathogenic protozoa continues to expand. Human infection with *Cryptosporidium parvum* was first recognized in 1976, since when several new pathogenic protozoa have been discovered in humans, namely the microsporidia (*Enterocytozoon bieneusi, Encephalitozoon intestinalis*) and *Cyclospora cayetanensis*. As methods of detection improve, it seems likely that other human protozoan pathogens will emerge.

Despite the prevalence of human protozoan enteropathogens, their history has evolved gradually during the nineteenth and twentieth centuries, with major advances occurring since the 1970s when it has been possible to culture some in the laboratory. The coccidia, however, have largely resisted attempts at in vitro culture, presumably because of their more complex life cycle. The pathogenic potential of these protozoa has been debated vigorously; during the first half of the twentieth century, for example, the clinical importance of *Giardia lamblia* was still seriously questioned, even by eminent parasitologists such as Dobell. The fact that these infections are responsible for significant intestinal disease in humans, with profound morbidity, and in some cases mortality, is now well established, although parasite biology and mechanisms of pathogenesis are still not clearly established. For many of the protozoa the host immune response remains poorly defined, as are the mechanisms involved

in eradication and the development of protective immunity. As yet there is no candidate vaccine for any of the intestinal protozoa. It is likely that the next decade will produce great advances in our understanding of many of these questions, with commensurate progress in treatment and prevention.

The Sarcodina (amoebae)

The subphylum Sarcodina is characterized by organisms that move by pseudopodia or by locomotive protoplasmic flow without discrete pseudopodia; flagella, when present, are usually restricted to developmental or other temporary stages. Most species are free living, such as *Acanthamoeba* and *Naegleria*. However, many species such as *Entamoeba histolytica, E. coli, E. hartmanni, E. gingivalis, Dientamoeba fragilis, Endolimax nana* and *Iodamoeba bütschlii* have been definitely established as parasites of humans. All live in the large intestine, except *E. gingivalis*, which is found in the mouth.

Entamoeba histolytica

Amoebiasis, the infection caused by the parasitic protozoan, *E. histolytica*, is responsible for 70 000 deaths per annum.[1] It was Fedor Löch in St Petersburg in 1875[2] who first described the clinical and autopsy findings of a case of fatal dysentery and identified the amoeba. Although he was able to infect a dog with this organism, he was not able to mimic the disease produced in his patient and failed to recognize the relationship. In 1890, William Osler[3] reported the case of a young man who contracted dysentery and developed an hepatic abscess that led to his death. One year later, Councilman and Lafleur[4] conducted a detailed study of patients with amoebic dysentery and hepatic abscess. They confirmed the pathogenic role of amoebae and created the terms 'amoebic dysentery' and 'amoebic liver abscess'. Schaudinn[5] differentiated *E. histolytica* from *E. coli* in 1903. In 1913, Walker and Sellards[6] definitively established the pathogenicity of *E. histolytica* by feeding cysts to volunteers. Brumpt[7] in 1925 was the first to suggest that the differences in symptomatology and in the global distribution of invasive amoebiasis were due to the presence of two species of amoeba, morphologically indistinguishable one from another, but with different pathogenic potential. He distinguished the two species based on their pathogenicity in humans and in experimentally infected kittens. He suggested the term *E. dysenteriae* for the pathogenic amoeba and *E. dispar* for the non-pathogenic amoeba. Because Brumpt was unable to distinguish morphologically between the two proposed species and because there was growing evidence that cysts obtained from asymptomatic carriers could produce experimental infection, his explanation gained little support. It regained favour only after Sargeaunt and associates[8,9] were able to distinguish pathogenic strains of *E. histolytica* from non-pathogenic strains on the basis of isoenzyme typing. Since then, many other markers that allow the discrimination between both groups have been identified. In 1993, Diamond and Clark,[10] using all the biochemical, immunological and genetic evidence for distinguishing pathogenic from non-pathogenic strains of *E. histolytica*, redescribed *E. histolytica* Schaudinn, 1903, formally separating it from *E. dispar* Brumpt, 1925. In 1997 a World Health Organization (WHO) expert committee met in Mexico City and endorsed the separation of pathogenic and non-pathogenic strains into two separate species.[11,12]

The organism
Taxonomy
The systematics of amoeboid eukaryotes is in a state of flux. *E. histolytica* was considered by some authors to be an early branching of the eukaryotic lineage, as it appeared to lack mitochondria, peroxisomes, rough endoplasmic reticulum and Golgi system, and has an unusual glycolytic metabolism. Many of these features are shared with other amitochondriate protists known as Archezoa.[13] However, small-subunit ribosomal RNA-based phylogenetic trees placed *E. histolytica* in a branch that arises more recently than several lineages with typical eukaryotic organelles and metabolism.[13,14] The demonstration that *E. histolytica* has a cryptic organelle that corresponds to a rudimentary mitochondria[15,16] and the identification of genes involved in vesicular transport[17] have seriously undermined the hypothesis that *Entamoeba* represent early branching eukaryotes. In 1998, Cavalier-Smith revised the position of *E. histolytica* and placed it in the kingdom Protozoa, subkingdom Neozoa, infra-kingdom Sarcomastigota, phylum Amoebozoa, subphylum Conosa.[18]

Structure
The trophozoite is distinguished from other intestinal amoebae by morphological characteristics of diagnostic importance. It ranges in size from 20 to 40 μm. Two zones can be recognized within the cytoplasm: an outer zone, or ectoplasm, and an inner zone, or endoplasm. The ectoplasm is clear, refractive and sharply separated from the endoplasm. The endoplasm contains abundant vesicles embedded in a cytoplasmic matrix, which gives them the appearance of ground glass. The cytoplasmic vesicles sometimes contain ingested red blood cells in

various stage of disintegration. Using DNA-specific stains it is possible to identify a small spherical DNA-containing body 1–2 μm in size that corresponds to rudimentary mitochondria.[19] Ribosomes appear to be ordered in helical arrays. The cytoskeleton is characterized by micro-filaments, generally found immediately below the plasma membrane at the sites of attachment of the amoeba to the substrate and where phagocytic channels are formed. The nucleus is not usually visible, although it may be faintly discerned as a finely granular ring in the unstained amoeba. When stained with haematoxylin, trichrome or Lawless stain, details of nuclear structure may be observed. The nucleus is spherical and 4–7 μm in diameter. The nuclear membrane is clearly defined; its inner surface is lined with uniform and closely packed fine granules of chromatin. In the centre of the nucleus is a small mass of chromatin, the karyosome. A clear halo surrounding the karyosome and a 'linin' network giving a 'cartwheel' appearance has been described, but these probably represent fixation artefacts. The presence of a rough endoplasmic reticulum or Golgi system has not been demonstrated. However, the presence of genes encoding proteins involved in vesicular transport and translational machinery suggest that functional equivalents may exist.[17]

In fresh isolates, *E. histolytica* can move as fast as 5 μm per second. Trophozoites move by means of pseudopodia, cytoplasmic protrusions that may be formed at any point on the surface of the organism. Actively moving trophozoites have a well-defined morphological polarity. The clear glass-like ectoplasm flows out to form the pseudopodium, slowly followed by the more granular endoplasm as the amoeba moves in the direction in which it was extruded. The pseudopodial extension is accompanied by recycling of the cytoplasm and the formation of a posterior appendix, commonly referred to as the uroid. The uroid accumulates capped ligands as bacteria, lectins or antibodies and, by an unknown mechanism, is detached from the amoeba without damaging the parasite.

The precyst amoebae are colourless, round or oval cells that are smaller than the trophozoite but larger than the cyst. They may be distinguished by a rounded single nucleus, absence of ingested material and lack of a cyst wall. The cytoplasm usually contains deposits of diffuse glycogen and, occasionally, chromatoid bodies are seen. The nuclear morphology is often confusing at this stage and it is best to rely upon either trophozoites or cysts for specific identification.

The cysts are round or oval, slightly asymmetrical hyaline bodies, 10–16 μm in diameter, with a smooth, refractive, non-staining wall about 0.5 μm thick. The immature cyst has a single nucleus, about one-third of its diameter, whereas the mature infective cyst contains four smaller nuclei, rarely more. The nuclei may at times appear as small refractive spheres within the cytoplasm of the unstained cyst, but more often they are not visible. The cytoplasm of the young cysts contains vacuoles with glycogen and chromatoid bodies. These chromatoid bodies, so named because they stain with haematoxylin like the chromatin of the nucleus, are reported to contain ribonucleic and deoxyribonucleic acids and phosphates, and tend to disappear as the cyst matures, so that they may be absent in about half of the cysts. When stained with iodine, the cytoplasm of the cyst will be yellow-green to yellow-brown in colour; the nuclear membrane and karyosome are distinct and light brown. Chromatoidal bars do not stain and appear as clear spaces in the cytoplasm. If glycogen is present in the cytoplasm, it will stain a dark yellow-brown.

Microbiology

The main reservoir of *E. histolytica* is the human, although morphologically similar amoebae may be found in primates, dogs and cats. The complete life cycle of *E. histolytica* consists of four consecutive stages: the trophozoite, precyst, cyst and metacyst. The cyst is resistant to gastric acid, and on ingestion it passes into the small intestine. The amoeba within the cyst becomes active in the neutral or alkaline environment of the small intestine. The cyst wall is digested, probably by the digestive enzymes within the lumen of the gut. The encysted amoeba becomes very active and each of the four nuclei in the emerging *E. histolytica* undergoes one round of division, thus forming eight amoebae, smaller than the trophozoites seen in the colon, from a single cyst. They are carried into the caecum where they complete their maturation. They multiply by binary fission, the nucleus dividing by modified mitosis. As the amoebae pass down the colon they become dehydrated and assume a spherical shape known as a precyst. A thin cyst wall is secreted, forming an unripe cyst. Two mitotic divisions occur, resulting in a cyst that contains four nuclei. They are evacuated in the stool and discharged into the environment. Cysts remain viable and infective for several days in faeces and water, but are easily killed by desiccation.

Diamond's[20] medium allows the cultivation of *E. histolytica* without bacteria or other living organisms (i.e., axenically). Optimal growth occurs at 35–37°C, at pH 7.0, and under reduced oxygen tension.

Metabolism

Carbohydrates are the main source of energy for the parasite. The uptake of glucose involves a specific transport system that provides approximately 100 times the amount incorporated by endocytosis. Glucose is degraded to pyruvate via the Embden–Meyerhof pathway. The principal end-products of the anaerobic carbohydrate metabolism are ethanol and carbon dioxide; lactate is not produced and lactate dehydrogenase has not been reported. In many of the glycolytic reactions inorganic pyrophosphate, rather than adenosine triphosphate (ATP), is used as an energy source. Amoeba are obligate fermenters that lack pyruvate dehydrogenase and the enzymes for oxidative phosphorylation and Krebs cycle.[21] The fermentation enzymes include the pyruvate : ferredoxin oxidoreductase, ferredoxin and alcohol dehydrogenase, which are most similar to the equivalent enzymes in anaerobic bacteria.[22] Alcohol dehydrogenase and ferredoxin are found throughout the cytosol.[15] In contrast, pyruvate : ferredoxin oxidoreductase is located in the plasma membrane and in a cytoplasmic structure that most likely corresponds to the rudimentary mitochondria.[23]

Synthesis of nucleic acids depends on the salvage of preformed purines as *E. histolytica* lacks a de novo purine pathway. It is also able to salvage pyrimidine bases, although it is able to synthesize them de novo.

Genetics

E. histolytica has a complex molecular karyotype composed of six linear DNA molecules of 227, 366, 631, 850, 1112 and 1361 kilobaes (kb),[24] circular DNA molecules ranging from 5 to 50 kb and extranuclear DNA in the rudimentary mitochondria.[15,16,25] The estimated genome size based on the DNA content per cell is between 2×10^7 kb and 3.7×10^8 kb depending on the methodology employed.[26] This difference may be due to various factors including repetitive DNA (which may be about 20% of the total genome in *Entamoeba*), the level of ploidy and multinucleate cells often seen in axenic cultures. The total genome G + C content is low (about 24%), with a G + C content of coding regions approximately 33% higher. Several copies of ribosomal DNA (rDNA) are present as extrachromosomal circular elements. The number of copies in the different strains varies. These circular rDNA molecules contain two large repetitive regions. A number of other circular DNA molecules have been observed in *Entamoeba*, but their function or coding potential is not known. The physiological importance and biogenesis of these molecules needs to be investigated.

The more widely used system to characterize *E. histolytica* strains was based on the migration of six isoenzymes (hexokinase, phosphoglucomutase, aldolase, acetylglucosaminidase, peptidase and nicotinamide–adenine dinucleotide (NAD) diaphorase). Its popularity was based on its ability to divide *E. histolytica* into two distinct groups: pathogenic and non-pathogenic (Figure 77.1).[8] Further study of the biological, genetic and immunological differences between these groups led to the formal separation of the non-pathogenic strains into a different species, *E. dispar*.[10] This separation was supported by the WHO in 1997.[11] As all the research efforts to characterize *E. histolytica* strains were geared towards the separation of pathogenic and non-pathogenic strains, there is little information of differences between 'pathogenic' strains. There is no doubt that diversity does exist as they can be classified into at least 10 different zymodemes, but clearly more studies are needed.

Epidemiology

E. histolytica has a worldwide distribution and is endemic in most countries with low socioeconomic conditions. Before the separation of the 'non-pathogenic strains' into

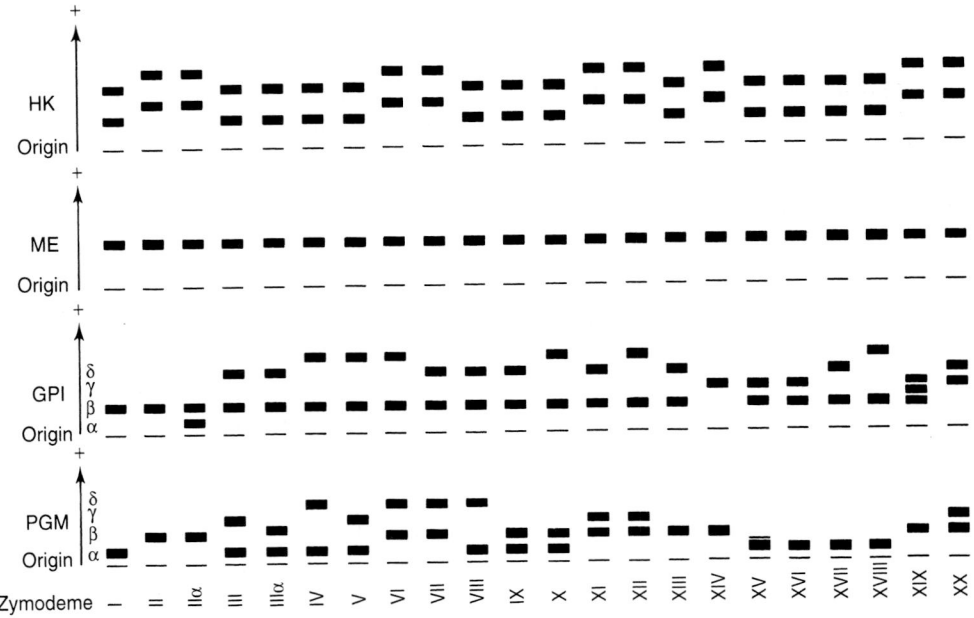

Figure 77.1: Zymodemes of *E. histolytica* identified by using GPI (EC 5.3.1.9), L-malate:NADP⁺ oxidoreductase (ME; oxaloacetate decarboxylating) (EC 1.1.1.4.0), PGM (EC 2.7.5.1) and HK (EC 2.7.1.1). Pathogenic zymodemes include II, IIα, VI, VII, XI, XII, XIII, XIV, XIX and XX. Non pathogenic zymodemes include I, III, IIIα, IV, V, VIII, IX, X, XV, XVI, XVII, XVIII and (not shown) XXI. From Bruckner D A. Amebiasis. *Clin Microbiol Rev* 1992; 5:356–369.

a different species, it was estimated that approximately 480 million people, or 12% of the world's population, were infected and 40 000–110 000 persons died anually.[27] In endemic areas, it is now clear that *E. dispar* is the more prevalent species, by a ratio of up to 10 : 1. The risk of asymptomatic carriers of *E. histolytica* developing invasive disease is estimated at about 10%.[28] In Europe and North America, where invasive amoebiasis is rare, almost all infections previously ascribed to *E. histolytica* were in fact due to *E. dispar*. When these data are taken into account, it is more likely that only 10% of the 480 million infections (approximately 48 million people) are infected with *E. histolytica*, whereas the rest have infections with *E. dispar*. However, global mortality is still estimated to be at about 70 000 deaths per annum.[1]

Infection occurs via the faecal–oral route, food and drink becoming contaminated through exposure to human faeces. Food-borne outbreaks of disease are due to insanitary handling of food and its preparation by infected individuals. Therefore, it is not surprising that prevalence is high in places where human faeces are used for fertilizer. Cyst carriers are the main reservoir of infection. Epidemics occur when raw sewage contaminates water supplies. Sexual transmission also occurs. Recognized high-risk groups include travellers, immigrants, migrant workers, immunocompromised individuals, individuals in mental institutions, prisons and, possibly, children in day-care centres. Severe infections occur in very young children, pregnant women, the malnourished and individuals taking corticosteroids. Patients with AIDS do not have an increased risk of severe infection.

Pathogenesis

E. histolytica has the capacity to destroy almost all tissues of the human body. The intestinal mucosa, the liver and, to a lesser extent, the brain and skin are affected most commonly. Even cartilage and bone can be eroded by *E. histolytica* trophozoites. Several virulence factors have been identified, such as adhesion molecules, contact-dependent cytolysis, proteases, haemolysins and phagocytic activity.

To produce damage, trophozoites must first colonize the colon. The presence of bacteria is essential for colonization as they provide an environment with low oxygen tension and probably supply other metabolic needs. Trophozoites must then penetrate through the mucus layer and adhere to the host cells. *E. histolytica* enhances mucus secretion, alters its composition and depletes goblet cells of mucin, thereby making epithelial surfaces more vulnerable to invasion.

Once the mucus barrier has been broken down, *E. histolytica* reaches the luminal surface of enterocytes and initially produces a contact-dependent focal and superficial epithelial erosion. Trophozoites adhere to colonic mucins and host cells through the *N*-acetyl-D-galactosamine-inhibitable lectin, a 260-kDa protein also known as the Gal/GalNAc adherence lectin, composed of a 170-kDa and a 35/31-kDa subunit. The 170-kDa subunit is immunologically similar to the integrins.[29] Other molecules involved in adhesion include a 220-kDa lectin, a 112-kDa adhesin and a surface lipophosphoglycan. They also possess several receptors that recognize proteins in the extracellular matrix; two of these receptors recognize fibronectin and a futher three recognize collagen.[30]

Although there is evidence to suggest that *E. histolytica* can induce apoptosis of host cells,[31,32] cell damage is primarily contact dependent. The Gal/GalNAc adherence lectin is not directly cytotoxic but it is required for cytolysis as target cell lysis is reduced in the presence of galactose. Furthermore, a monoclonal antibody against the heavy subunit is capable of partially inhibiting cytolysis without blocking adherence. It has been suggested that cell lysis is produced through the channel-forming peptides of *E. histolytica* (amoebapores). Three isoforms have been identified, amoebapores A, B and C, which are present in a ratio of 35 : 10 : 1, with the genes showing 35–57% deduced amino acid sequence identity. Like other pore-forming peptides, amoebapores are readily soluble but are capable of changing rapidly into a membrane-inserted stage. It has been hypothesized that amoebapores bind to negatively charged phospholipids via protonated lysine residues, followed by insertion of the peptide into the lipid bilayer driven by the negative membrane potential of the target membrane.[33] Oligomerization occurs by formation of a channel through the plasma membrane, allowing the passage of water, ions and other small molecules, and thus lysing the target cell. Amoebapore C seems to be the most effective, while amoebapore A is not efficient in lysing erythrocytes. Amoebapores are found in cytoplasmic vesicles and show maximum activity in acidic pH, which is consistent with previous observations that lysis of target cells by *E. histolytica* required a pH of 5.0 within amoebic vesicles. In spite of all the advances in the characterization of amoebapores, their participation in the cytolytic event produced by *E. histolytica* has not yet been demonstrated. Amoebapores are not spontaneously secreted from viable trophozoites. The presence of pore-forming activity in the non-pathogenic *E. dispar,* although 60% less potent, suggests that the primary function of amoebapores is to destroy phagocytosed bacteria.

During the invasion to deeper layers of the mucosa, trophozoites must lyse surrounding cells and degrade the extracellular matrix. Contact of trophozoites with the extracellular matrix induces the formation of adhesion plaques, containing actin filaments, vinculin, α-actinin, tropomyosin and myosin I. Binding to the extracellular matrix occurs through a 37-kDa fibronectin-binding protein and a 140-kDa integrin-like receptor, inducing a sustained rise of intracellular calcium concentration needed to reorganize the trophozoite cytoskeleton to form the adhesion plaque. In the absence of calcium, adhesion is poor. Contact of trophozoites with the extracellular matrix also induces the release of cysteine proteinases and the content of electron-dense granules, which includes collagenase, two proteases and at least 25 other polypeptides.[34,35] There are at least seven genes (*EhCP1–EhCP6* and *EhCP112*) encoding for cysteine proteinases in *E. histolytica*.[36] The majority of the proteinase activity can be attributed to the expression of four of these genes, *EhCP1–3* and *EhCP5*. Cysteine proteinases are synthesized as precursors proteins with a 12–14-amino-acid hydrophobic predomain signal peptide, a 78–82-amino-acid prodomain, a 216–225-amino-acid catalytic domain, and no C-terminal extension. The predominant mature forms are 27–30 kDa in size and are able to cleave collagen, elastin, fibrinogen and laminin, that is, the elements of the extracellular matrix that trophozoites must penetrate to cause invasive disease.[37] The cytopathic effect correlates with the amount of cysteine proteinase activity released into the medium by clinical isolates of *E. histolytica* and can be inhibited by specific peptide inhibitors. A number of haemolysins, which are encoded by plasmid rDNA and are cytotoxic to an intestinal mucosal cell line (Caco.2), have been identified.

Invasion of the colonic and caecal mucosa by *E. histolytica* begins in the interglandular epithelium. This is a site of low resistance where intestinal cells are normally shed as the final stage in the renewal of the epithelium. Cell infiltration around invading amoebae leads to rapid lysis of inflammatory cells and tissue necrosis; thus, acute inflammatory cells are seldom found in biopsy samples or in scrapings of rectal mucosal lesions. Ulceration may deepen and progress under the mucosa. Further progression of the lesion may produce loss of the mucosa and submucosa, and eventually perforation of the colon.

Amoebae probably spread from the intestine to the liver through the portal circulation. The presence and extent of liver involvement bears no relationship to the degree of intestinal amoebiasis, and these conditions do not necessarily coincide. The early stages of hepatic amoebic invasion have not been studied in humans. In experimental animals, inoculation of *E. histolytica* trophozoites into the portal vein produces multiple foci of neutrophil accumulation around parasites, followed by focal necrosis and granulomatous infiltration. As the lesions extend in size, the granulomas are gradually substituted by necrosis, until the lesions coalesce and necrotic tissue occupies progressively greater portions of the liver. Hepatocytes close to the early lesions show degenerative changes that lead to necrosis, but direct contact of liver cells with amoebae is rarely observed. It is thought that liver damage is not caused directly by the amoebae but rather by the lysosomal enzymes of lysed polymorphonuclear neutrophils (PMNs) and monocytes that accumulate around the parasite. During experimental infection, hypocomplementaemic and leucopenic animals demonstrate reduced amoebic-induced liver damage when compared with normal animals.

In severe cases, especially in patients treated with corticosteroids, amoebic trophozoites can be found in virtually every organ of the body, including the brain, lungs and eyes.

Immunity

The first contact of the trophozoite with the immune system is through the epithelial intestinal cells. *E. histolytica* stimulates human intestinal epithelial cells to secrete interleukin (IL) 8 and tumour necrosis factor (TNF) α.[38,39] Neutrophils are rapidly recruited and activated in response to the proinflammatory cytokine

IL-8. Cell infiltration around invading amoebae leads to rapid lysis of inflammatory cells followed by tissue necrosis.

E. histolytica in axenic culture is susceptible to complement lysis, whereas when grown in the presence of human serum or after passage through animals they become resistant. E. histolytica activates the complement system by both classical and alternative pathways. Complement resistance is mediated in part by the Gal/GalNAc adherence lectin. The adhesin binds to C8 and C9, inhibiting their assembly and therefore C5b–9-mediated lysis. The immune complex disappears from the amoebic surface, probably by capping, as the biochemical analysis of the uroid reveals the presence of complement components. The resistance to complement-mediated lysis decreases after incubation of the trophozoite with either cytochalasin B or trypsin, and after glutaraldehyde fixation. This suggests that intact membrane mobility and a trypsin-sensitive surface component are necessary to inhibit the activation of the alternative complement pathway. Inactivation of the anaphylotoxins C3a and C5a by secreted cysteine proteases of E. histolytica may also play a role in mediating resistance to complement lysis.[40]

Invasive infection with E. histolytica produces a marked immune response which results in the development of protective immunity. Recurrence of amoebic colitis or abscess is unusual. De Leon[41] monitored more than 1000 patients with amoebic liver abscess for 5 years and found a recurrence rate of 0.29%. The risk of recurrence is increased if treatment fails to eradicate the pathogenic amoeba from the colon.[42] Patients with AIDS, surprisingly, do not appear to be more susceptible to amoebic disease than those without AIDS; amoebic lesions in patients with AIDS do not differ from those in non-AIDS patients. Intestinal invasion by E. histolytica results in a prompt local secretory antibody response followed by a systemic antibody response. Circulating antibodies can be demonstrated as early as 1 week after the onset of invasive amoebiasis in humans and experimental animals. All immunoglobulin classes are involved, but there seems to be a predominance of IgG_2 antibodies. However, it has been demonstrated that the cysteine proteinases of E. histolytica can degrade both IgA[43] and IgG[44] antibody, which may limit the effectiveness of the host humoral response.

Clinical features (see also Chapter 10)

The clinical spectrum of intestinal E. histolytica infection ranges from asymptomatic carrier state or acute colitis, to fulminant colitis with perforation.

Asymptomatic infection

Asymptomatic cyst carriage of E. histolytica is well documented. The majority will clear the infection spontaneously. An epidemiological study in a semirural area in South Africa showed that 90% of asymptomatic carriers of E. histolytica cleared the infection within a year; the remaining 10% developed amoebic colitis.[28]

Intestinal amoebiasis (Table 77.1)

The onset is insidious, except in fulminating cases, with abdominal discomfort, loose motions or frank diarrhoea, not necessarily with blood or excessive mucus. In more severe cases the stools rapidly become bloodstained with mucus. Tenesmus occurs in half of the patients and is always associated with rectosigmoid involvement. Constitutional symptoms are not prominent. On physical examination tenderness may be localized anywhere in the lower abdomen but is usually over the caecum, transverse colon or sigmoid. The liver may be slightly enlarged and tender. Rectosigmoidoscopy and colonoscopy of mild or moderate cases usually reveals the presence of small ulcers (3–5 mm in diameter) which most frequently involve the caecum and rectum but may be scattered throughout the colon and are especially numerous in the region of the flexures. Rarely, the disease may involve the terminal ileum. The ulcers are initially superficial with hyperaemic borders and a necrotic base covered with a yellowish exudate. There is normal mucosa between sites of invasion. However, diffuse inflammation has also been described, making firm diagnosis on gross appearance difficult. On rare occasions involvement of the blood vessels at the base of the ulcer may produce brisk bleeding. More rarely, an ucler may perforate and the patient may die from peritonitis. Extensive inflammatory polyposis has been demonstrated as a complication of amoebic colitis and this may be a source of confusion with idiopathic inflammatory bowel disease. Acute amoebic dysentery must be differentiated from bacterial colitis caused by Shigella spp., Salmonella spp., Campylobacter jejuni, enteroinvasive and enterohaemorrhagic Escherichia coli, and Yersinia enterocolitica.

In surgical specimens ulcers look flat and oval in shape, without induration of the underlying bowel wall. Histologically, there is non-specific diffuse inflammation around the superficial ulcerations. As the disease advances, the classically described flask-shaped ulcers with undermined edges are formed. The lamina propria is infiltrated

Table 77.1 Symptoms and findings in acute colitis

	%
Symptoms	
Duration of symptoms (weeks)	
0–1	48
2–4	37
> 4	15
Diarrhoea	100
Dysentery	99
Abdominal pain	85
Low back pain	66
Physical findings	
Fever	38
Abdominal tenderness	83

Source: Adams E B & MacLeod I N. Invasive amebiasis. I. Amebic dysentery and its complications. *Medicine* 1977; 56:315–323.

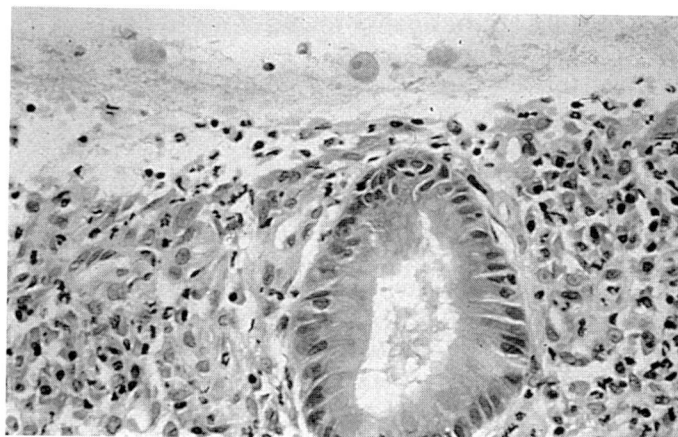

Figure 77.2: Colonic mucosa showing superficial ulceration with amoebic invasion. (Haematoxylin and eosin stain; magnification × 400.) (Courtesy of Paola Domizio, Department of Morbid Anatomy, St Bartholomew's Hospital, London.)

Table 77.2 Symptoms and findings in amoebic liver abscess

	%
Symptoms	
Duration of symptoms (weeks)	
< 2	37–66
2–4	20–40
4–12	16–42
> 12	5–11
Pain	90
Diarrhoea and/or dysentery	14–66
Weight loss	33–53
Cough	10–32
Dyspnoea	4
Physical findings	
Localized tenderness	80–95
Enlarged liver	43–93
Fever	75–98
Rales, rhonchi	8–47
Localized intercostal tenderness	40
Epigastric tenderness	22
Swelling over the liver	10
Jaundice	10–25
Laboratory findings	
Increased bilirubin	10–25
White blood cell count > 10×10^9/l	63–94
Raised transaminases	26–50
Raised alkaline phosphatase	38–84
Increased erythrocyte sedimentation rate	81

Source: Martinez-Palomo A. *The Biology of Entamoeba histolytica.* Chichester: University Research Press/Wiley, 1982.

by plasma cells, lymphocytes, neutrophils and eosinophils. There is oedema and focal haemorrhage. The infiltrate also involves the surface epithelium, and frequently there is an overlying exudate within which trophozoites may be found (Figure 77.2).

Fulminant colitis is the result of confluent ulceration and necrosis of the colon. The clinical picture is virtually indistinguishable from that of fulminant ulcerative colitis. The bowel is dilated, particularly in its transverse portion. The patient is extremely febrile and toxic, and shows signs of hypovolaemia and electrolyte imbalance. Despite the severity of the illness, amoebae may not be readily recovered from the stools of these patients. Surgical specimens reveal extensive areas of necrosis within which some patches of intact hyperaemic mucosa are found.

An amoeboma, or amoebic granuloma, may result from repeated invasion of the colon by *E. histolytica*, complicated by pyogenic infection. Amoebomas may be found anywhere in the colon but are more frequent at the caecum (40%) and rectosigmoid junction (20%). Lesions are usually single and involve a short segment of the colon. These mass lesions are often mistaken for malignancy and may occasionally be palpable. Histologically the amoeboma is non-fibrotic and contains granulation tissue with lymphocytes, plasma cells, eosinophils and giant cells. There is remarkably little inflammation and most of the swelling is due to oedema. Amoebae are scanty and difficult to demonstrate. Fibrous tissue is formed later.

Amoebic liver abscess (Table 77.2)
This is the most common extraintestinal form of invasive amoebiasis. Amoebic abscesses may be found in all age groups, but are 10 times more frequent in adults than in children, and are more frequent in males than in females. They are more common in the poorest sectors or urban populations. Approximately 20% of patients have a past history of dysentery. About 10% of patients have diarrhoea

or dysentery at the time of diagnosis of amoebic liver abscess. The parasite can be detected in faeces in less than 50% of cases if standard microscopy is used; the prevalence rises to 75% if culture is used.[42] The onset of symptoms is usually abrupt, with pain in the upper abdomen and high fever. The pain is intense and constant, radiating to the scapular region and right shoulder; it increases with deep breathing or coughing, or when the patient rests on the right side. When the abscess is localized on the left lobe, pain occurs on the left side of the abdomen and may radiate to the left shoulder. Localized tenderness in the region of the abscess, most commonly at the lower right intercostal spaces, is frequent even in the absence of diffuse liver pain. Fever is present in most cases; it varies between 38° and 40°C, frequently in spikes but sometimes constant over several days, with rigors and profuse sweating. Anorexia, weight loss, nausea, vomiting and fatigue may all be present. On physical examination the cardinal sign of amoebic liver abscess is painful hepatomegaly. Digital pressure and fist percussion will often produce intense pain in the liver region. On palpation the liver is soft and smooth. Hepatomegaly may not be detected in patients with amoebic abscess of the dome of the liver because the enlargement is upward. Mild jaundice is quite common, but severe obstructive jaundice is rare. Amoebic abscess and cirrhosis may coexist, so a hard liver does not exclude the diagnosis. Movement of the right side of the chest and diaphragm is restricted and there is hypoventilation of the right lower lobe of the lung. This is frequently associated with atelectasis or effusion in the right chest. The presentation may be so abrupt that it can be confused with an acute surgical abdomen. The usual clinical diagnosis in such a case is acute cholecystitis or appendicitis. Differential diagnosis with pyogenic liver abscess should be established, particularly in non-endemic areas.

Lesions are usually single and most are found in the right lobe of the liver in the posterior, external and superior portions. The incidence of amoebic abscess of the left lobe ranges from 5 to 21%. The liver abscess has a thin capsular wall with a necrotic centre composed of a thick fluid, an intermediate zone of coarse stroma and an outer zone of nearly normal tissue. Typically, abscess fluid is odourless, resembling 'chocolate syrup' or 'anchovy paste', and bacteriologically sterile, although secondary bacterial invasion may occur. Microscopic examination of the abscess fluid reveals granular eosinophilic debris with no or few cells; amoebae tend to be located at the periphery of the abscess. Liver abscesses may heal, rupture or disseminate. The mortality rate has been estimated to be around 0.2–2.0% in adults and up to 26% in children.[45]

Invasive amoebic lesions in humans, whether localized in the large intestine, liver or skin, almost invariably heal without the formation of scar tissue, if treated properly. The absence of fibrotic tissue following necrosis is particularly striking in the liver. The complete anatomical and functional restitution of liver integrity after treatment of liver abscess has been assessed by scintillography.

Peritoneal amoebiasis

This is caused by the rupture of a hepatic liver abscess or, less frequently, by perforation of the caecum. It is characterized by a sudden increase in abdominal pain, frequently generalized, which resembles that of septic peritonitis. A plain abdominal radiograph will reveal the presence of free air in the peritoneal cavity. In some instances the perforation may be smaller and the abdominal signs are more localized.

Pericardial amoebiasis

Pericardial involvement is the most serious complication of an amoebic liver abscess. It occurs in less than 1% of all amoebic liver abscesses, especially of the left lobe. Although there may be a presuppurative stage that is associated with a sterile effusion, perforation of the abscess into the pericardium is usually followed by progressive tamponade or the sudden development of shock. Although the mortality rate from pericardial involvement has decreased from more than 90% to less than 40%, it is still frequently necessary to perform open drainage because of the development of loculations and thickened pericardium.

Pleuropulmonary amoebiasis

Invasion of the pleural cavity or the lung parenchyma is most commonly due to extension from a liver abscess and occurs in less than 1% of those with amoebic dysentery, in 3% of all autopsies on people dying from amoebiasis and in 15% of patients with liver abscess. Haematogenous spread is rare. The first clinical symptoms are those of the liver abscess, followed by severe pain in the lower chest, often radiating to the right shoulder. There may be dyspnoea and non-productive cough. Bronchohepatic fistulas are characterized by expectoration of large amounts of dark brown material. Superimposed bacterial infections are common.

Cerebral amoebiasis

Cerebral involvement has been documented in 1.2–2.5% of patients who have amoebiasis at autopsy, but in less than 0.1% of patients whose cases are reported in studies of large clinical series. Although the symptoms of cerebral amoebiasis depend on the site and size of the lesion, as many as 50% of patients may have abrupt onset of symptoms and die from cerebellar involvement or rupture within 12–72 hours. The availability of metronidazole, which penetrates the blood–brain barrier, should greatly improve the prognosis of this unusual complication.

Genitourinary amoebiasis

Renal amoebiasis, a rare complication of amoebic liver abscess, is thought to occur by rupture of a hepatic abscess, haematogenous spread from lesions in the liver or lungs, or extension through the lymphatics. Patients who have renal amoebiasis usually respond well to aspiration and medical therapy. Genital lesions also occur infrequently and are usually caused by fistulas from a liver abscess or rectocolitis. Typically, lesions are painful punched-out ulcers with profuse discharge. Medical treatment is usually sufficient for resolution of the lesions.

Cutaneous amoebiasis

This results from perforation of an abscess or intestine into the skin. It may also develop from surgical wounds infected secondarily with an internal amoebic lesion or in the perineal–genital area. Histologically there is ulceration with extensive necrosis in the base, pseudo-epitheliomatous hyperplasia at the margins, and a non-specific inflammatory infiltrate extending into the deep dermis and subcutaneous tissues beneath the ulcer base. Sometimes there is extensive pseudoepitheliomatous hyperplasia involving much of the lesion with only small punctate areas of ulceration. This may resemble verrucous carcinoma. *E. histolytica* may be found in the overlying exudate.

Diagnosis and differential diagnosis

Detection of the parasite (see also Appendix II)

Amoebiasis, although often suspected clinically, requires confirmation in the laboratory by finding cysts and trophozoites in the stools (which need to be

Table 77.3 Laboratory diagnosis of *E. histolytica*

Sample	Fixative	Examination	Stain
Stool	PVA, 10% formalin, Schaudinn's fixative, sodium acetate–acetic acid formalin	Concentrate, permanently stained slide	Gomori trichrome, iron haematoxylin
Sigmoid colon	PVA, Schaudinn's fixative	Permanently stained slide	Gomori trichrome, iron haematoxylin
Aspirate			
Direct	None	Wet mount with or without enzyme digest	
Fixed	PVA, Schaudinn's fixative	Permanently stained slide	Gomori trichrome, iron haematoxylin, periodic acid
Biopsy	Formalin	Routine histology	Schiff, haematoxylin and eosin

PVA, polyvinyl alcohol with either $HgCl_2$ or $CuSO_4$; with periodic acid–Schiff organism stains intensely pink and has a distinct outline, but cytoplasmic and nuclear details are obscured. Haematoxylin and eosin stain cytoplasm pink and nucleus blue; in sections the nucleolus may not always be present.
Source: Bruckner D. A. Amebiasis. *Clin Microbiol Rev* 1992; 5:356–369.

differentiated by special tests from those of *E. dispar*) or trophozoites in the various tissues. The detection of the organism depends on appropriate specimen collection, processing and examination by trained personnel (Table 77.3).

Stools

The diagnosis of invasive intestinal amoebiasis is based on the identification of *E. histolytica* trophozoites in rectal smears or recently evacuated stools and on the results of rectosigmoidoscopy. Fresh samples should be examined for detection of trophozoites containing erythrocytes. However, the test is useful only if the sample is examined within 30 minutes of the passage of the specimen. Three types of wet mount preparation should be made from each specimen: mounts in saline solution (to observe amoebic motility in a warm specimen); mounts in saline plus iodine (to differentiate *E. histolytica* cysts from other amoebic species and helminth ova); and mounts in saline plus methylene blue (to distinguish cysts from leucocytes, which stain blue). It is advisable always to confirm the diagnosis by using a permanent-stained slide (iron haematoxylin or trichrome). The presence of trophozoites containing ingested red blood cells is strongly suggestive of *E. histolytica* and invasive disease.

Examination of material scraped or aspirated from mucosal surfaces during sigmoidoscopy may reveal the presence of trophozoites. Microscopic examination of wet preparations may be difficult because of the need for low light intensity and difficulties in differentiating the unstained *E. histolytica* from other amoebae and from inflammatory cells (Table 77.4). The mucosal material may also be smeared, fixed and stained with trichrome stain. Fixation of stool smears can be achieved by immersion of the slide in Schaudinn's solution or by adding two or three drops of polyvinyl alcohol to the mucosal material directly on the slide, mixing it, and allowing the slide to air dry.

Examination for ova and parasites in a minimum of three stool specimens, using concentration and permanent stain techniques, is the standard method of detection and identification of cysts of the organism. If possible, the stools should be examined before the administration of antimicrobial, antidiarrhoeal and antacid preparations or barium because all these agents may interfere with the recovery of amoebae. However, the cysts of *E. dispar* are indistinguishable from those of *E. histolytica* and, therefore, positive stools should be reported as containing *E. histolytica/E. dispar*.[11] Many research techniques have been used to differentiate between both species but only one of them has achieved commercialization. The *Entamoeba histolytica* II kit (TechLab, Blacksburg, Virginia, USA) is based on the detection of epitopes of the 170-kDa adhesin, present only in *E. histolytica*. The specificity and sensitivity of the assay for detection of *E. histolytica* in stool is 93% and 95%, respectively.[46] However, its high cost limits its use, particularly in the developing world where *E. histolytica* is endemic. A differential diagnosis should also be made with *E. hartmanni* which is morphologically identical to *E. histolytica* and can be positively identified only by measuring its size.

Sigmoidoscopy

This is of value in symptomatic cases. The mucosal lesions should be aspirated and the material examined for trophozoites. Biopsies may be taken from the edge of the ulcers and stained with periodic acid–Schiff solution.

Liver aspirate

This should be collected in a number of different containers as it is obtained from the abscess. The amoebae are sparse in necrotic material from the centre of the abscess, but they are more abundant on the marginal walls and are therefore more commonly found in the last portions of aspirated material. Demonstration of the

Table 77.4 Differential characteristics of host cells, *E. coli* and *E. hartmanni*, commonly mistaken for *E. histolytica*, in wet preparations

Cell	Diameter or length (μm)	Motility	Nucleus		Cytoplasm appearance (stained)	Inclusions
			No.	Visibility Nucleus: cytoplasm ratio		
E. histolytical/E. dispar						
Trophozoites	20–40	Progressive with hyaline fingerlike pseudopodia; may be rapid	1	Hard to see in unstained preparations (1:10–1:12)	Ground glass appearance. Clear differentiation of ectoplasm and endoplasm; vacuoles usually small.	Presence of erythrocytes diagnostic
Cysts	10–20	None	1–4	1:2–1:3	Clear	Chromidial bodies (stained) may be present; usually elongate with blunt, smooth rounded edges; round or oval
E. coli						
Trophozoites	15–50	Sluggish. non-directional; blunt, granular pseudopodia	1	Often visible in unstained preparation	Granular, little differentiation into ectoplasm and endoplasm; usually vacuolated	Bacteria, yeast cells other debris
Cysts	10–35	None	1–8	≥ 16 nuclei seen occasionally	Clear	Chromidial bodies (stained) may be present, less frequently than in *E. histolytica/ E. dispar*; splinter shape with rough pointed ends
E. hartmanni						
Trophozoites	6–10	Progressive, with hyaline finger-like pseudopodia; may be rapid	1	Hard to see in unstained preparations 1:10–1:12	Ground glass appearance. Clear differentiation of ectoplasm and endoplasm; vacuoles usually small	Can only be differentiated from *E. histolytica* by direct measurement of either trophozoite or cyst
Cysts	5–8	None	1–4	1:2–1:3	Clear	–

Table 77.4 (*Cont'd*)

Cell	Diameter or length (µm)	Motility	No.	Nucleus Visibility Nucleus: cytoplasm ratio	Cytoplasm appearance (stained)	Inclusions
Host cells						
PMNs	Average 16	None	1	2–4 segments; if lobed, nucleus fragments may mimic the four nuclei found in *E. histolytica* cyst (1:1).	Granular	None
Macrophages	20–60; may be 5–10	Sluggish	1	Large, may be irregular in shape (like monocyte); may mimic *E. histolytica* trophozoite; can also ingest erythrocytes	Coarse; may be highly vacuolated	Usually contain ingested debris, PMNs and erythrocytes

Source: Bruckner D A. Amebiasis. *Clin Microbiol Rev* 192; 5:356–369.

organism is often extremely difficult because trophozoites may be trapped in viscous pus or debris and will not exhibit typical motility.

Laboratory investigations (see also Appendix I)

In mild cases of colitis laboratory tests are normal. With severe disease leucocytosis is present. About 75% of patients with amoebic liver abscesses have a white blood cells count greater than 10 000/mm³. The occasional patient with leucopenia will usually have long-standing disease and may have underlying alcoholism or folate deficiency. Eosinophilia is not associated with extra-intestinal amoebiasis. Anaemia is common, particularly in patients who have chronic amoebic liver abscesses. The level of alkaline phosphatase is raised in more than 75% of patients, particularly in those with long-standing disease. Levels of transaminases may be increased in 50% of cases, especially in patients with acute disease or complications. The levels of transaminases usually return to normal soon after therapy is initiated, although alkaline phosphatase concentration may remain raised for several months. In extraintestinal amoebiasis, organisms may or may not be found in the stool; therefore, the presence of antibodies against *E. histolytica* may be useful. Serology can be useful in the diagnosis of amoebiasis, particularly in non-endemic areas. Antibody response is present in 85–95% of patients with invasive disease. Virtually all known serological tests have been employed to detect antiamoebic antibody, including immuno-fluorescent antibody tests, indirect haemagglutination assays (IHAs), radio-immunoassay, countercurrent immuno-electrophoresis and enzyme-linked immunosorbent assays (ELISAs). ELISAs are the most sensitive and do not give false-negative results in patients with amoebic liver abscesses. ELISA is also specific, giving only 3.6% false-positive results in controls living in endemic areas. The

results of serological tests may be negative in patients who present acutely and should be repeated in 5–7 days. Serological responses measured by agar gel diffusion, countercurrent immunoelectrophoresis and ELISA usually become negative within 6–12 months, although they may persist for more than 3 years. However, results of IHAs may remain positive for more than 10 years after clinical and parasitological cure, even in the absence of reinfection. Therefore these tests should be interpreted with caution as antibody may be present for prolonged periods, and in areas of high endemicity a high prevalence of seropositivity already exists. Clinical laboratories should check with their local health authorities for guidelines for use and interpretation of serological tests.

Radiology

Radiological changes in the colon consist of mucosal oedema, haustral blunting and ulceration, usually localized to one part of the colon. Ulcers are initially shallow but may deepen and assume a 'collar-button' or flasked-shaped appearance. There may be toxic dilatation of the colon. Amoebomas manifest as an intraluminal mass, an annular lesion or irregularity of the bowel wall with lack of normal distensibility. Differential diagnosis with carcinoma may be difficult; rapid disappearance of the lesion after treatment favours the diagnosis.

In patients with hepatic involvement, plain radiography of the thorax may reveal elevation of the right hemi-diaphragm, pleural reaction obscuring the right cost-ophrenic angle. Radiologically, unruptured abscesses do not show a fluid level, and calcification of the liver parenchyma is rare. Non-invasive radiographic studies have dramatically increased early diagnosis of amoebic liver abscesses and their potential complications. The isotope liver scan is very useful as it becomes positive within the first days of illness, often before other imaging techniques. Presumably these early changes reflect either a focal decrease in blood supply or injury to the Kupffer cells rather than liquefaction necrosis. Ultrasonography of an amoebic liver abscess typically reveals a round or oval hypoechoic area that is contiguous to the liver capsule and without significant wall echoes (Figure 77.3). Computed tomography and magnetic resonance imaging are also sensitive studies for demonstrating amoebic liver abscesses (Figure 77.4). More than 80% of patients who have symptoms of an abscess for more than 10 days have a single lesion of the right lobe of the liver, while 50% of patients who present acutely may have multiple lesions. Abscesses resolve slowly and may increase in size during

the first few weeks after therapy, even with successful treatment. The ultrasonographic abnormalities resolve within 6 months in two-thirds of the patients with amoebic liver abscess; however, 10% remain abnormal for more than 1 year after treatment. The differential diagnosis includes pyogenic liver abscess, gallbladder disease and sepsis.

Management

Two classes of drugs are used in the treatment of amoebic infections. Luminal amoebicides, such as diloxanide furoate and iodoquinol, act on organisms in the intestinal lumen and are not effective against organisms in tissue. Tissue amoebicides, such as metronidazole, dehydroemetine and chloroquine, are effective in the treatment of invasive amoebiasis but less effective in the treatment of organisms in the bowel lumen (Table 77.5).

Asymptomatic patients
The WHO has suggested that, in asymptomatic individuals, treatment is not appropriate when *E. histolytica/E. dispar* has been detected but *E. histolytica* has not been identified with specific tests, unless there are reasons to suspect infection with *E. histolytica*, including high specific antibody titres, a history of close contact with a case of invasive amoebiasis, or an outbreak of amoebiasis.[11] Patients with demonstrated *E. histolytica* infection can be treated with diloxanide furoate, paromomycin or iodoquinol. Iodoquinol and its analogue iodochlor-hydroxyquin are effective against intraluminal amoebae but have been reported to cause myelo-optic neuropathy after long-term use.

Intestinal infection
Metronidazole or tinidazole are the drugs of choice for amoebic colitis as they are very effective against the trophozoite; however, they have little effect on the cyst and therefore treatment should be followed by a luminal agent such as diloxanide furoate. Other imidazol compounds such as ornidazole may be used.

Liver abscess
Metronidazole or tinidazole followed by diloxanide furoate is the treatment of choice. The potential cardio-vascular and gastrointestinal adverse effects of dehydro-emetine and emetine limit their use, and they are used only as second-line treatment. Higher relapse rates are associated with chloroquine than with other therapeutic agents.

Aspiration of the abscess may be necessary in some cases (Table 77.6).[47] However, the need for open surgical drainage has decreased since the success of percutaneous drainage. Surgery should be reserved for patients with rupture of the abscess, with bacterial superinfection, or when an abscess that needs drainage cannot be approached.

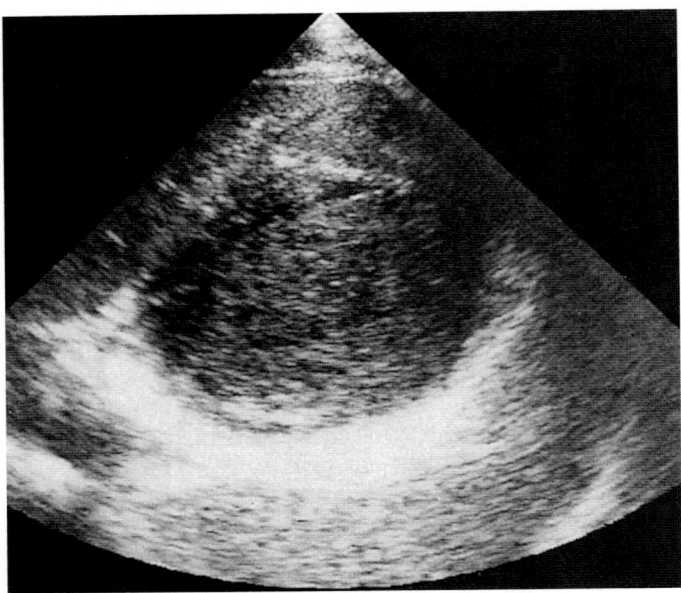

Figure 77.3: Liver ultrasonogram demonstrating an amoebic hepatic abscess. (Courtesy of Alison McLean.)

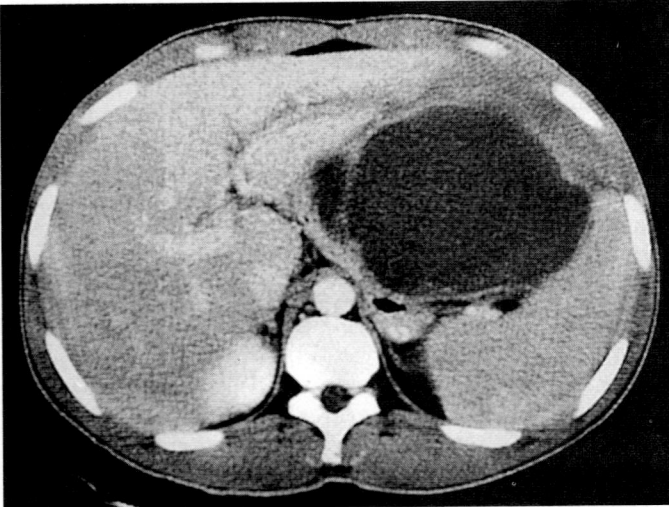

Figure 77.4: Computed tomogram of the liver demonstrating a left lobe amoebic abscess. (Courtesy of Alison McLean.)

Table 77.5 Treatment of amoebiasis

		Adult dosage	Paediatric dosage (mg/kg daily)
Asymptomatic intestinal carrier			
1st choice	diloxanide furoate	500 mg t.i.d. × 10 days	20 (divided in 3 doses × 10 days)
2nd choice	paromomycin	25–30 mg/kg daily in 3 doses × 7–10 days	25–30 (divided in 3 doses × 7–10 days)
	or iodoquinol	650 mg t.i.d. × 20 days	20–40 (divided in 3 doses × 20 days)
Intestinal infection			
1st choice	metronidazole followed by	750–800 mg t.i.d. × 10 days	35–50 (divided in 3 doses × 10 days)
	diloxanide furoate[a]	500 mg t.i.d. × 10 days	20 (divided in 3 doses × 10 days)
	tinidazole followed by	2 g/day × 2–3 days	50–60 (× 3 days)
	diloxanide furoate[a]	500 mg t.i.d. × 10 days	20 (divided in 3 doses × 10 days)
2nd choice	paromomycin	25–30 mg/kg daily in 3 doses × 7–10 days	25–30 (divided in 3 doses × 7–10 days)
Amoebic liver abscess			
1st choice	metronidazole followed by	750–800 mg t.i.d. × 10 days	35–50 (divided in 3 doses × 7–10 days
	diloxanide furoate[a]	500 mg t.i.d. × 10 days	20 (divided in 3 doses × 10 days)
	or tinidazole followed by	2 g/day × 3–5 days	50–60 (× 5 days)
	diloxanide furoate[a]	500 mg t.i.d. × 10 days	20 (divided in 3 doses × 10 days)
2nd choice	dehydroemetine followed by	1–1.5 mg/kg daily (max. 90 mg/day) i.v. × 5 days	1 (× 10 days maximum)
	diloxanide furoate[a]	500 mg t.i.d. × 10 days	20 (divided in 3 doses × 10 days)

[a]Paromomycin or iodoquinol may be used as an alternative to diloxanide furoate.

Table 77.6 Indications for aspiration of amoebic liver abscess

Formal indications
To rule out a pyogenic abscess, particularly with multiple lesions
As adjunct to medical therapy (no response after 72 hours)
If rupture is believed to be imminent
Abscess in the left lobe where the risk of rupture is increased
Possible indications
To reduce the period of disability[47] (further trials are necessary to confirm this indication)

Prevention

The control of invasive amoebiasis could be achieved through improvement of living standards and the establishment of adequate sanitary conditions in countries where the disease is prevalent. Methods of attack should aim at: (1) the community, through the improvement of environmental sanitation including water supply, adequate disposal of faeces, food safety and health education to prevent faecal–oral transmission; and (2) the individual, through early detection and treatment in cases of infection and disease.

Cysts remain viable and infective for several days in faeces and may survive in soil for at least 8 days at 34–38°C, and for 1 month at 10°C. They also remain infective in fresh water, sea water, sewage and wet soil. Cysts survive for up to 45 minutes in faecal material lodged under the fingernails but are killed within 1 minute by desiccation on the surface of the hands. Amoebic cysts are destroyed by exposure to 200 parts per 10^6 of iodine, 5–10% acetic acid, and heating at a temperature above 68°C. They can be removed from water by sand filtration but are not killed by the quantity of chlorine ordinarily used to purify water; therefore chlorination alone cannot prevent epidemics originating from faecal contamination of water. In places where purification of water supplies is inadequate, boiling for 10 minutes will kill all cysts.

There is no vaccine available against amoebiasis. Several antigens of *E. histolytica* have been developed as possible immunogens. These have different degrees of purity and are used in conjunction with a variety of adjuvants. As yet these have been tried only in animal models. Individual chemoprophylaxis for travellers is not indicated because the possibility of acquiring the infection has been shown to be very low (0.3%).[48]

Entamoeba dispar (formerly known as non-pathogenic *E. histolytica*)

E. dispar is the most frequently found *Entamoeba* both in humans and primates. It is morphologically identical to *E. histolytica* and is its closest genetic relative in the genus *Entamoeba*. Unlike *E. histolytica*, *E. dispar* does not cause disease in humans. However, there is some evidence to suggest that *E. dispar* is capable of inducing focal surface erosion of the colonic mucosa without invading the submucosa or causing ulcers.[49] Although up to 20% of *E. dispar* infections may lead to seropositivity for standard immunodiagnosis of *E. histolytica*, the antibody levels during *E. dispar* infection never approach those seen with *E. histolytica*. Infection is asymptomatic and does not require treatment.[11]

Several biological differences have been described between *E. dispar* and *E. histolytica*, but none of them fully explains why *E. dispar* is unable to produce invasive disease. *E. dispar* produces less protease,[50] does not bind to target cells as strongly and is less cytotoxic, has a thinner glycocalyx, higher surface charge and has less phagocytic activity than *E. histolytica*.[51] In vitro, *E. dispar* is less likely to be lysed by complement.[52] The study of the cell biology of *E. dispar* has been hindered by the difficulty of growing *E. dispar* without bacteria. The successful axenization of one strain in 1995[53] will allow for more detailed studies of the interaction of *E. dispar* with its host.

Entamoeba moshkovskii ('E. histolytica-like' amoebae)

E. moshkovskii was originally isolated from sewage in Moscow and subsequently reported in many parts of the world. *E. moshkovskii* is described as morphologically indistinguishable from *E. histolytica* but is isolated from free-living sources, usually in the sediment of sewage-polluted waters. Similar amoebae have been isolated from humans and were grouped under the name of 'E. histolytica-like amoebae'. The best known of these is the 'Laredo' strain. Initially, they were thought to represent atypical *E. histolytica*. Numerous studies revealed differences between these strains and true *E. histolytica*, including a lack of serological cross-reactivity, dissimilar DNA base composition and distinctive isoenzyme profiles. Recently, analysis of the small subunit rRNA gene has suggested that these amoebae are strains of *E. moshkovskii* and are not closely related to *E. histolytica*. This amoeba has a wide temperature tolerance, multiplying at 10–37°C. It produces contractile vacuoles in hypotonic media and is highly resistant to amoebicidal drugs.

Entamoeba chattoni

This amoeba frequently infects apes and monkeys, in which it causes no clinical symptoms. Asymptomatic infection in individuals who are in close contact with monkeys has been reported.[54]

Endolimax nana

Endolimax nana is a cosmopolitan and common intestinal amoeba of humans, primates and pigs which can be confused with *E. histolytica*. *Endolimax nana* is non-pathogenic. The trophozoites are small (6–15 µm in diameter). Movement is by pseudopodia but this fails to produce directional locomotion. The cysts are 8–10 µm in diameter and have a refractile cyst wall. The details of nuclear structure and the appearance of the cytoplasm closely resemble those of *Iodamoeba bütschlii*. Usually there is only one nucleus in trophozoites, but there are four nuclei in immature cysts. *Endolimax nana* has no chromidial body in stained samples, and the nuclear membrane appears to be devoid of peripheral chromatin.

Iodamoeba bütschlii

Iodamoeba bütschlii is the most common amoeba of swine, and the pig was probably its original host. It is also frequently found in humans and monkeys. Trophozoites vary greatly in size, ranging from 6 to 20 µm in diameter. The cytoplasm contains one or more glycogen mass(es) that may be seen after iodine staining, as well as bacteria, yeasts and debris; red blood cells are never ingested. The nucleus is usually not visible but permanent stains will reveal a characteristic appearance with a large central karyosome surrounded by a ring of small chromatin granules. Cysts of *I. bütschlii* are 8–15 µm in diameter, commonly ovoidal or irregularly pyriform in shape. The cysts are distinctive in preparations stained with iodine because of the constant presence of the large, sharply outlined and dense glycogen-containing vacuole. Only one nucleus is found in most cysts.

I. bütschlii is non-pathogenic; only exceptionally has the presence of this parasite been linked to symptomatic infection in humans. As is the case with other amoebae commonly found in the human colon, *I. bütschlii* has a distinct isoenzyme profile.

Dientamoeba fragilis

According to morphological[55] and molecular[56] evidence, *Dientamoeba fragilis* is now considered to be an aberrant trichomonad flagellate, not an amoeba. Infection with this organism may be associated with gastrointestinal symptoms, such as diarrhoea and abdominal pain, but most cases are asymptomatic. *D. fragilis* is a small (6–12 µm) cosmopolitan parasite. Only trophozoites are known; they can be differentiated from other intestinal amoebae by the presence of two nuclei in the majority of them. However, around 30–40% of organisms are mononucleate and may be confused with *Blastocystis hominis*, which is more common. Trichrome stains should always be performed. Culture is possible and the parasite can be differentiated by its distinct isoenzyme profile. Polymerase chain reaction (PCR)–restriction fragment length polymorphism analysis of its ribosomal genes suggests the presence of two genetically distinct forms.[57] Further studies are needed to determine whether there is a correlation between these genetic groups and virulence.

The Mastigophora (flagellates)
Giardia intestinalis

Giardia intestinalis (syn. *lamblia, duodenalis*) is the most common human protozoan enteropathogen and there is now compelling evidence to indicate that infection with this parasite can cause both acute and chronic diarrhoea.[58,59] Intestinal malabsorption may be severe, such that chronic infection in children may be associated with retardation of growth and development. Molecular and genetic analysis of the parasite has shown that *Giardia* has a unique place in evolution as it is probably the first organism to emerge from the prokaryotic to the eukaryotic state.[60] Our knowledge of this parasite has expanded rapidly since it was first cultured in the 1970s, but many aspects of its biology and interactions with its mammalian hosts remain unanswered. There is no unifying explanation for the diverse clinical spectrum seen in giardiasis, which ranges from asymptomatic carriage to persistent diarrhoea with malabsorption. As yet no classical virulence factors have been identified and thus a clear explanation of pathogenesis is lacking. In addition, despite extensive investigation in animal models and to some extent during human infection, the key immunological determinants for clearance of acute infection and the development of protective immunity remain only partially defined. There is now good evidence that this infection is a zoonosis that can be transmitted through domestic water supplies; control within the environment is therefore an important public health issue.

The organism
Taxonomy
Giardia is in the subphylum Sarcomastigophora, the superclass Mastigophora and the order Diplomonadida.[61] *Giardia* belongs to the family Hexamitidae which contains six genera, three of which, including *Giardia*, are exclusively parasitic. Members of the genus *Giardia* have an adhesive disc on the ventral surface, unlike other members of the family Hexamitidae. There are three major morphological subtypes of *Giardia*: *G. agilis* from amphibians, *G. muris* from mice and *G. intestinalis* from humans and some other vertebrates (Figure 77.5). These different types can be distinguished by the overall shape and dimensions of the trophozoite body and also by the distinctive shapes of the median bodies. Two other *Giardia* isolates have been described: *G. psittaci* isolated from a budgerigar and *G. ardeae* from the great blue heron. Again, these can be distinguished from the other subtypes by an absence of the ventrolateral flange in the

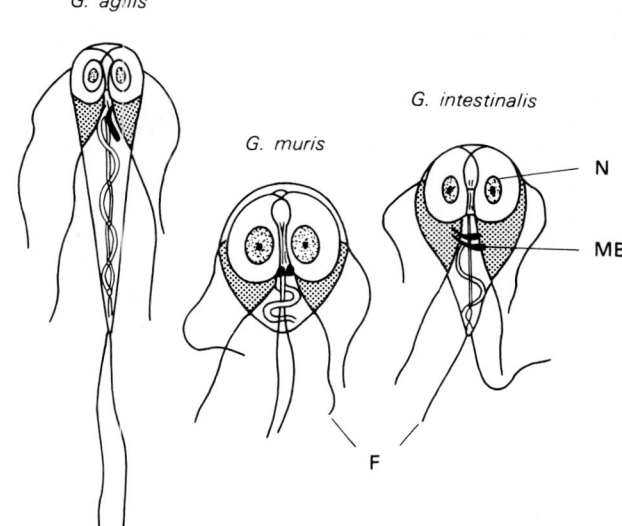

Figure 77.5: *G. agilis, G. muris* and *G. intestinalis*. N, nucleus; MB, median body; F, flagellum.

former and a single (rather than a double) caudal flagellum in the latter.

The chemotaxonomy of *Giardia* has been explored using a variety of techniques, including antigen, isoenzyme and DNA analysis. These approaches have clearly shown that *Giardia* isolates differ from one to another, although the sensitivity of the techniques varies. Molecular genetic approaches have shown that human *Giardia* isolates may be subdivided into two major genotypes, types I and II.[62] Some animal isolates have been identified to possess the same genotype providing further evidence that giardiasis is a zoonosis.

Structure
Giardia exists as a trophozoite, which colonizes the proximal small intestine and is responsible for the production of diarrhoea and malabsorption, and as a cyst, which is able to exist outside the host in a suitable environment and is the form of the parasite by which giardiasis is usually transmitted.

The trophozoite, when fixed for light microscopy, is 12–15 μm long and 5–9 μm wide (Figure 77.6). It has two nuclei and four symmetrically placed flagella originating from basal bodies at the anterior pole of the nuclei. The median body is found posteriorly and varies in shape according to subtype (see Figure 77.5). A median body contains cytoskeletal proteins, including the giardins, actin and α-actinin. The trophozoite has a convex dorsal surface and a concave ventral surface containing the ventral disc. This organelle is unique to *Giardia* and is a rigid structure consisting of microtubules, cross-bridges attached to microtubules and microribbons which run perpendicularly to both the microtubules and the cross-bridges. The disc contains a variety of cytoskeletal proteins, including the family of giardins, actin, α-actinin, myosin and tropomyosin. α₁-Giardin has recently been identified

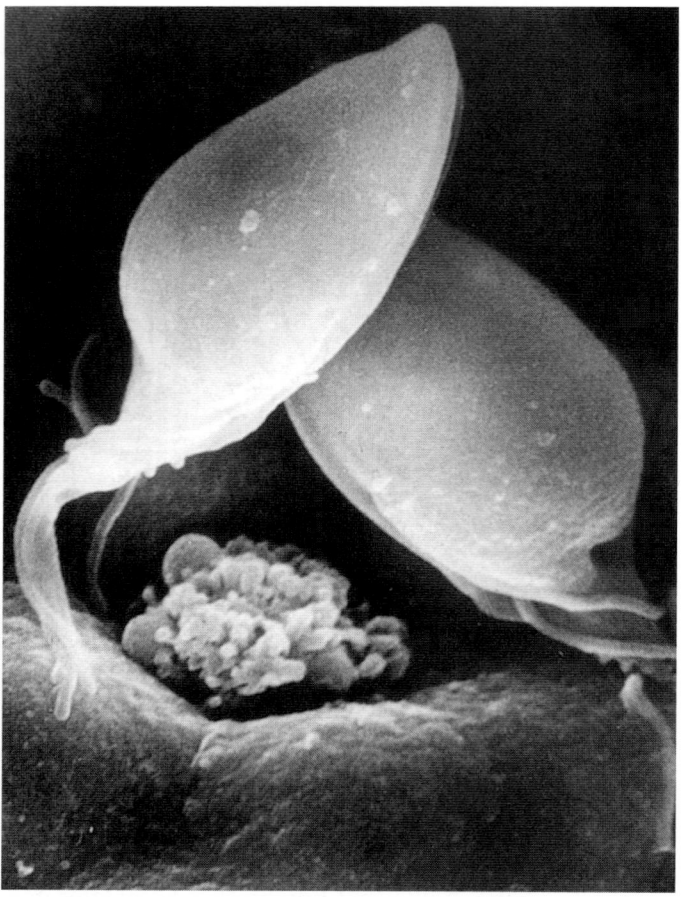

Figure 77.6: Scanning electron micrograph showing two *G. intestinalis* trophozoites.

structurally and functionally to be an annexin with a typical calcium-binding domain.[63] These proteins give the disc flexibility and allow it to change shape, a process that is thought to be important for attachment. The flagella have the usul eukaryotic structure consisting of nine pairs of microtubules with two central single microtubules.

Giardia trophozoites are largely devoid of cytoplasmic organelles, the major structure being multiple ovoid vacuoles which appear to resemble lysosomes, containing a variety of hydrolases, including acid phosphatase, proteinases and DNases and RNases. Other structures include what may be a primitive Golgi apparatus that is involved in protein sorting, bacterial endosymbionts and a 35-nm double-stranded RNA virus. The role of these organisms in the life cycle of *Giardia* has not been established.

Cysts are ovoid or elliptical, approximately 7–10 μm in length. The cyst wall is composed of a layer of fibrils arranged as a felt-like web. There is controversy as to whether *N*-acetylglucosamine or galactosamine is the major cyst wall sugar, although recent work indicates that the former is most important.[64] The cyst contains two or four nuclei; a median body and cytoskeletal components can usually be identified. The cyst is able to survive in a cool, moist environment for weeks or even months.

Microbiology

The life cycle of *Giardia* is simple, involving the ingestion of cysts in contaminated water or food or through direct person-to-person contact, infection being initiated with as few as 10 to 100 cysts. Excystation occurs in the proximal small intestine where the trophozoite multiplies. The cycle is completed when encystation occurs in the distal small intestine and colon, and cysts are excreted again into the environment in faeces at a concentration of approximately 150 000 to 20 000 cysts per gram of faeces.

Colonization involves three processes: excystation, attachment to the intestinal epithelium, and multiplication. Excystation is thought to be triggered by low pH and duodenal and pancreatic secretions. The intracellular vacuoles have been observed to discharge their contents during excystation, suggesting that hydrolases are required to complete the process.[65]

Giardia attaches to the intestinal epithelium, probably by a variety of mechanisms, although it seems likely that the ventral disc plays a major part, either by flagella-generated hydrodynamic forces beneath the disc or by direct disc movement mediated by its contractile proteins, particularly those in the peripheral regions of the disc. Pharmacological disruption of microfilament function inhibits attachment, supporting a central role for the ventral disc. However, like many micro-organisms, *Giardia* possesses a mannose-binding surface lectin that appears to exist as a prolectin in the cytoplasm and is activated by trypsin. This lectin has been purified and shown to have a molecular weight of 28–30 kDa. Experiments in attachment models using mammalian intestinal epithelial cells or culture cell lines suggest that both disc and lectin-mediated mechanisms are important, at least in vitro.

Giardia trophozoites divide by binary fission but the mechanisms by which growth is controlled and the factors that are essential for growth remain poorly defined. Bile has been shown to promote growth of *Giardia* both in vivo and in vitro.[66] This probably relates to *Giardia*'s absolute requirement for preformed phospholipid, uptake being facilitated by the presence of conjugated bile salts. Bile salt uptake has been shown to occur by an active transport process, suggesting that a specific carrier may be present in the surface membrane. Other factors that are known to be essential for growth include a carbohydrate source, usually glucose, and a low partial pressure of oxygen.

The final stage of the life cycle, encystation, can also be completed in vitro following exposure of trophozoites to high concentrations of conjugated bile salts and myristic acid at neutral pH. Thus, bile and bile salts may have a dual role in the parasite life cycle, on one hand promoting growth and multiplication, while at the same time ensuring that the parasite completes its life cycle by encystation. An encystation-specific promoter for glucosamine-6-phosphate isomerase, the first enzyme required for *N*-acetylgalactosamine synthesis, has recently been identified.[67]

None of these in vitro studies of the parasite life cycle would have been possible without the ability to culture the parasite in vitro. This was first achieved axenically in 1970 by Meyer[68] using a complex, undefined medium containing serum. This medium has been modified slightly since then; the most widely used medium is TYI-S-33 which includes casein digest (typticase), yeast extract, iron as ferric ammonium citrate, dextrose, bovine serum, ascorbic acid, bile salts and cysteine. *Giardia* may be cultured in screw-capped glass tubes or flasks, ensuring only a small air space to maintain a low oxygen concentration.

Metabolism

Following the development of methods for axenic cultivation of *Giardia*, knowledge of the parasite's biochemistry and metabolism expanded rapidly. *Giardia* lacks mitochondria and mitochondrial enzymes, and respires in the presence of oxygen by a flavin, iron–sulphur protein-mediated electron transport system. Glucose is the major energy source, and is converted to pyruvate by Embden–Meyerhof and hexose monophosphate shunt pathways. Glucose is metabolized incompletely to carbon dioxide, ethanol and acetate. In strictly anaerobic environments, alanine is produced from pyruvate and ketoglutarate, whereas in the presence of low oxygen concentrations ethanol production increases and alanine production is reduced.

Giardia predominantly acquires membrane and other lipids from the culture medium and has little or no capacity for in vivo synthesis. Phosphotidylglycerol has been identified as a major phospholipid of *Giardia* and is probably esterified by parasite phospholipases. Trophozoites can use exogenous arachidonic acid for phosphatidylinositol synthesis.

Giardia is unable to synthesize purines and pyrimidines, which distinguishes it from most other eukaryotes. *Giardia* relies therefore on salvage pathways for both of the nucleic acids which must be synthesized exogenously. Pyrimidines are taken up by active transport processes, one for uridine and cytosine and another for thymidine.

The calcium-binding protein calmodulin has been detected in *Giardia* trophozoites and probably has a similar function in maintaining intracellular calcium homeostasis as it does in other eukaryotes.

Genetics

Restriction fragment length polymorphism analysis and DNA fingerprinting have demonstrated marked genetic heterogeneity in *Giardia* isolates from animals and humans. A stable transformation with foreign DNA is also not easy to achieve in protozoa. Information on the genetics of *Giardia* derives predominantly from analysis of the few genes that have been cloned. A variety of molecular genetic approaches has been used to identify two major human genotypes, which have also been isolated in some animals.[69,70]

Giardia has five chromosomes with four or as many as eight copies in each nucleus.[71] Chromosome size varies between 1 and 4×10^6 base pairs (bp), giving a total of 1.2×10^7 bp for the five chromosomes. Densitometric scanning of restriction endonuclease digests of *Giardia* DNA produce a similar genome size. *Giardia* nuclei appear to be haploid, and thus genetic diversity is explained on the basis of clonal divergence.

The G + C content of the *G. intestinalis* genome has been estimated to be 42–48%, that of the protein-coding gene sequences to be from 49% to more than 60%, and that of the rDNA gene to be 75%.[71] The non-coding regions are relatively A + T rich. *Giardia* rRNAs are smaller than other eukaryotes and eubacteria. The rDNA gene is only 5566 bp in *G. intestinalis* and slightly larger in *G. muris* and *G. ardeae*. Sequence analysis of the 16S-like RNA has demonstrated *Giardia*'s intermediate position between prokaryotes and eukaryotes.

Epidemiology

Giardiasis is found worldwide but in high prevalence in the developing world, where prevalence rates can reach 20–30%. Prevalence rates can often underestimate the overall impact of a pathogen. In rural Guatemala 45 children were followed from birth through the first 3 years of life; all were found to have giardiasis during this period and many had recurrent and prolonged infections with the parasite. Prevalence in Peruvian children reached 40% by the age of 6 months, and stool examination confirmed prevalence rates of about 20% in children in Zimbabwe and Bangladesh. Age-specific prevalence rises throughout infancy and childhood, declining only in adolescence. In the industrialized world, prevalence varies between 2% and 5%, although within these low prevalence areas there may be localized regions of higher prevalence.

Age appears to be a risk factor for susceptibility to giardiasis, infection being more common in infants and young children, although giardiasis is rare during the first 6 months of life, particularly where breast-feeding is practised. Undernutrition may increase the susceptibility to infection, as indicated by a study in Gambian children with chronic diarrhoea and malnutrition of whom 45% had giardiasis compared with only 12% of healthy age- and sex-matched controls.[72]

Giardiasis is well recognized to occur in travellers, although overall it accounts for no more than 5% of cases of traveller's diarrhoea. However, 30% of travellers to the former Soviet Union were positive for *Giardia* in one study and more than 40% of Scandinavian visitors to St Petersburg acquired the infection.[73] Travelling within the USA may be hazardous, particularly for skiers in Colorado and visitors to National Parks, especially if they drink the apparently clean surface water.

Individuals with hypogammaglobulinaemia or agammaglobulinaemia are at risk of chronic giardiasis, but individuals with HIV and AIDS do not seem to be at particularly increased risk of developing symptomatic disease, although carriage rates are generally higher than in the general population. These observations are consistent with the view that secretory immunity in the intestinal lumen is more important for clearance than cell-mediated responses within the intestinal mucosa.

A key factor in transmission of giardiasis is the ability of the cyst to survive for long periods in a suitable environment outside the host. Surface water in many parts of the world, including North America and Europe, are contaminated with *Giardia* cysts, which are not inactivated by chlorination alone. Interruption of the ancillary water purification procedures can lead to contamination of municipal water supplies and has been shown to account for many of the reported epidemics of water-borne giardiasis.[74,75] A recent survey in the USA suggested that there may be as many as 2.5 million cases of giardiasis each year.[76] Water-borne transmission has also been shown to occur in swimming pools. Despite these epidemics, water-borne transmission probably represents a relatively small proportion of the total infections worldwide. Food has also been shown to be a vehicle for transmission of giardiasis, although again this is probably a relatively uncommon route of transmission.

Direct person-to-person spread by faecal–oral transmission certainly accounts for the high prevalence of giardiasis in day-care centres, schools and residential institutions, where prevalence may be as high as 35%. Person-to-person spread is also known to occur as a result of sexual contact.

The major reservoirs of *Giardia* cysts are the human host and contaminated surface water. There is increasing evidence that a variety of domestic and wild animals carry *Giardia* spp. that are genotypically indistinguishable from human isolates. Although there is as yet no direct evidence that transmission has occurred from animals to humans, the higher prevalence of *Giardia* in companion animals that are in close contact with humans, particularly children in the home, makes this a strong possibility.

Pathogenesis

As yet no specific virulence factors have been identified in *Giardia* and thus no unifying hypothesis for pathogenesis has yet emerged. Current evidence suggests that *Giardia* is able to perturb mucosal structure and function; at the same time there may be additional factors operating in the intestinal lumen which may also contribute to diarrhoea and malabsorption (Table 77.7).[77,78]

Mucosal factors
Disruption of intestinal structure
In human giardiasis the full spectrum of abnormalities of villous architecture has been described, ranging from normal to subtotal villous atrophy (Figure 77.7). A majority of infected individuals have relatively mild abnormalities of villous architecture, with associated crypt hyperplasia. Infections in experimental models produce similar changes but, as in human infection, the abnormalities are generally mild. The gerbil provides a good model for studying small intestinal structure and function as weanling gerbils develop diarrhoea and by the sixth day of infection have villous shortening in the duodenum and crypt hyperplasia throughout the small intestine. However, as with murine giardiasis there is no associated mucosal inflammation.

Even in the absence of gross changes in villous architecture, ultrastructural abnormalities such as shortening and disruption of microvilli have been described in both humans and the gerbil model. Recent work in a neonatal rat model of giardiasis confirmed the reduction in villous height and an increase in crypt depth.

These morphological abnormalities are associated with reduction in disaccharidase activity. In animal models diarrhoea is at its peak when disaccharide activities are most profoundly reduced.

Intestinal dysfunction
Intestinal solute and electrolyte absorption is impaired in gerbil and neonatal rat models of infection. Perfusion of a lactose-containing solution in neonatal rats exaggerated the abnormalities of water and electrolyte absorption and

Table 77.7 Pathogenesis of giardiasis: possible mechanisms

Mucosal factors
Direct damage by trophozoites
Microvilli
Disaccharidases
Transport proteins
Parasite products
Proteases
Lectin
Immune mediated
T-cell activation
Luminal factors
Bacterial overgrowth
Inhibition of digestive enzymes
Bile salt deconjugation
Bile salt uptake by trophozoites

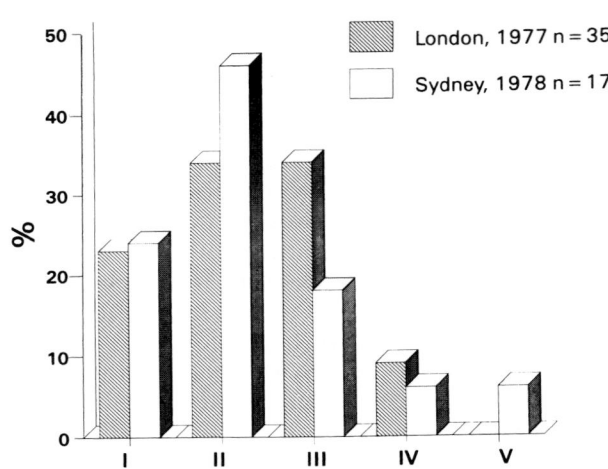

Figure 77.7: Percentage of patients with giardiasis with normal (I), mild (II), moderate (III) and severe (IV) partial villous atrophy, and subtotal villous atrophy (V).

also showed impaired glucose absorption compared with non-infected controls. In vitro studies in Ussing chambers and brush-border membrane vesicles from infected mice provide further support for an impairment of glucose and amino acid transport.

Mechanisms of mucosal injury

A variety of mechanisms has been proposed to explain these structural and functional abnormalities of the intestinal mucosa.[77,78] Attachment of *Giardia* trophozoites to the epithelium can disrupt and distort microvilli, particularly in murine giardiasis. It seems unlikely that this degree of disruption can account for the widespread changes of microvillous membrane surface area and other abnormalities of villous architecture observed in the small intestine.[77,78] However, recent work in tissue culture cell lines has shown that *Giardia* trophozoites induce localized condensation of F-actin and loss of perijunctional α-actinin. These cytoskeletal rearrangements could account for early changes in epithelial cell function.[79]

There is some evidence to suggest that *Giardia* trophozoites produce cytopathic substances that might be responsible for this disruption of epithelial structure and function. *Giardia* is known to produce a variety of proteinases that could find cleavage sites in proteins of the microvillous membrane. *Giardia* also has a mannose-binding surface lectin, which could interact with mannose residues on relatively immature enterocytes and again contribute to epithelial damage. Other dietary plant lectins are known to be able to produce substantial abnormalities of villous architecture.

There is increasing evidence to suggest that T-cell activation within the intestinal mucosa can produce villous atrophy.[80,81] This mechanism is thought to operate in graft-versus-host disease and in coeliac disease. T-cell activation in normal human fetal small intestinal explants with pokeweed mitogen or with an anti-CD3 antibody results in villous atrophy, crypt hyperplasia and increased IL-2 production, confirming T-cell activation. Further support for this hypothesis has been obtained from studies of experimental *G. muris* infection in athymic nu/nu mice. Despite prolonged infection the alteration of villous : crypt cell ratio is less severe in T cell-deficient mice compared with immunocompetent controls.[80] When lymphocytes from the spleen of immunologically intact mice are injected into athymic infected mice, histological abnormalities in the small intestine become more apparent. Reduction in the villous : crypt cell ratio does occur to some extent in immunocompromised mice before reconstitution, and thus it seems likely that T cell-independent mechanisms are also involved.

Luminal factors
Bacterial overgrowth

Giardiasis has been associated with increased numbers of aerobic and/or anaerobic bacteria in the upper small intestine of the indigenous Indian population or in travellers to the Indian subcontinent. Bacterial over-growth can produce architectural abnormalities in the small intestine similar to those seen in giardiasis and thus may have a role in the pathogenesis of mucosal damage.

Bile salt deconjugation

Conjugated bile salts have an important role in dietary fat absorption, but if deconjugated by luminal bacteria they lose their detergent properties and may damage cell membranes. One study in Indian patients with giardiasis showed evidence of bile salt deconjugation, although this was not confirmed by a further study of patients in the UK. *Giardia* itself does not have the ability to deconjugate bile salts.

Bile salt uptake

As discussed above, bile salts have an important role in the life cycle of *Gardia*. There is evidence to suggest that the organism takes up bile salts during growth by an energy-requiring active transport process, possibly involving a membrane carrier.[82] Although the precise metabolic advantages to the parasite have not been defined, a secondary effect of this process could be the depletion of intraluminal bile salt, thus impairing micellar solubilization of dietary fats and at the same time inhibition of pancreatic lipase, which is dependent on bile salts for full expression of hydrolytic activity.

Pancreatic enzyme inhibition

Several studies have suggested that concentrations of pancreatic enzymes in the duodenum are reduced in patients with giardiasis. Although there is no evidence of primary pancreatic failure in giardiasis, *Giardia* trophozoites are able to inhibit trypsin and lipase activity in vitro.[83] The precise mechanisms by which the organism achieves this have not been established, although it seems likely that this may relate to a direct effect of *Giardia* proteinases on the secreted pancreatic proteins.

Until specific virulence factors have been identified it is unlikely that the relative importance of these mucosal and luminal mechanisms in pathogenesis will be established. At present it seems reasonable to assume that the process is multifactorial, involving a combination of varying degrees of mucosal injury combined with disruption of the luminal phases of digestion and absorption.

Immunity

Studies in experimental models and limited studies in human giardiasis have made it possible to attribute essential roles to the immune system in the eradication of acute infection and to determine, at least in part, the determinants of persistent infection in an otherwise immunocompetent host.[84] There is increasing evidence to suggest that immunological factors are important in protecting mammalian hosts from reinfection, and thus the development of protective immunity. It seems unlikely that a single infection provides long-lasting protective immunity because age-specific prevalence increases throughout childhood and into early adolescence, suggesting that multiple exposures to the parasite are required before protection is achieved.

Giardia antibodies
Serum antibody
Anti-*Giardia* IgG can be detected in more than 80% of patients with symptomatic infection; antibody titres may remain raised for months or even years after primary infection. In endemic areas anti-*Giardia* IgG titres are increased in individuals without infection, suggesting widespread previous exposure to the parasite. Anti-*Giardia* IgM titres increase early in infection and then decline rapidly. Studies in India and The Gambia indicate that only 30% of patients with infection have detectable anti-*Giardia* IgA. Giardiasis has also been associated with raised total serum IgE, although in one case where this was investigated in depth this was not directed towards *Giardia* but possibly to food antigens as a result of increased intestinal permeability following acute giardiasis.[85] Similar patterns in antibody responses have been demonstrated in murine and neonatal rat models of giardiasis.

Secretory antibody
The secretory (s) IgA response in giardiasis is likely to be the most important aspect of immune response for parasite clearance. This is probably the reason why individuals with immunoglobulin deficiency have persistent giardiasis which is often refractory to treatment. Specific sIgA has been detected on the surface of *G. lamblia* trophozoites in human jejunal biopsies and in human jejunal fluid. Anti-*Giardia* sIgA has also been detected in human milk and saliva, and epidemiological evidence suggests that the presence of these antibodies may contribute to protection from giardiasis in breast-fed infants.

Experimental infections in mice and neonatal rats support a role for sIgA and IgG antibodies in parasite clearance. Administration of anti-IgM to mice produces a profound reduction in sIgA and results in chronic giardiasis. Protective effects of immune milk have also been demonstrated experimentally in mice. However, anti-*Giardia* sIgA is clearly not the only determinant of chronic infection, as C3H/He mice develop persistent infection despite normal concentrations of anti-*Giardia* sIgA. The human secretory response is directed to a range of *Giardia* membrane antigens.

Giardia antigens
The surface antigen profile varies between *Giardia* isolates and this may be one contributory factor to the delay in achieving protective immunity to this parasite. Thus, ideally all studies seeking to identify immunodominant antigens should relate to the serum or secretory antibody responses to the particular isolate in each given infection. This is extremely difficult and probably impossible to achieve on a wide scale. A variety of antigens (24–225 kDa) has been detected by immunoprecipitation and immunoblotting techniques using polyclonal antisera, mono-clonal antisera and monoclonal antibodies. Some antigens have been studied in more depth, particularly a 170-kDa surface antigen which has been partly cloned and sequenced. This is one of a series of cysteine-rich proteins that appear to be immunogenic, although their role in the parasite clearance of protective immunity has not been established.

An 82–88-kDa surface antigen has also been studied by several groups and is known to be a target for the immune response in human giardiasis. Recently a *Giardia* heat shock antigen has also been shown to be important in human giardiasis, and failure to produce an antibody response to this antigen may be an important factor leading to persistent infection. Expression of this antigen is now known to occur not only following a temperature shift but also on exposure to the physical and chemical environment found in duodenal fluid. This antigen has been recently identified to be homologous with hsp70, a highly conserved family of heat shock proteins found throughout the animal kingdom and shown to be important determinants of the host immune response in other bacterial and parasitic infections.

Giardia has also been shown to be able to vary expression of certain of its surface antigens in both experimental and human infection, and this may be a way in which the parasite evades immune clearance. These variant-specific surface proteins (VSPs) constitute a family of related proteins, the expression of which is regulated by the organism. Expression of individual VSPs appears to be related to the stage of differentiation and genotype.[86,87] Further evidence is required before it can be established whether this mechanism is relevant in humans in vivo.

Cell-mediated immunity
Cellular immune responses are thought to be important in the immune response to this parasite, although evidence stems largely from work in animal models. Increased numbers of lamina propria and intraepithelial lymphocytes have been reported in both experimental giardiasis and in human infection, although an increase in absolute lymphocyte numbers does not appear to be a prerequisite for parasite clearance. There have, however, been no detailed studies on lymphocyte phenotype in human giardiasis.

T lymphocytes
The most compelling evidence of a role for T lymphocytes in parasite clearance has been obtained from the natural history of murine giardiasis in the athymic nu/nu T cell-deficient mouse.[80] Infection is prolonged in this strain but can be eradicated by reconstitution with lymphocytes from syngeneic mice with normal immune function. These experiments have suggested that CD4 cells are critically important for the ability of mice to clear *G. muris* infection and may be involved in switching B-cell IgM to IgA production during infection. Recent work in B cell-deficient mice has clearly shown the importance of T cells in controlling acute *Giardia* infection.[88] Genetic factors are also important because immunocompetent

mice with different genetic backgrounds vary in their susceptibility to infection with *G. muris* and in their ability to eradicate infection.

B lymphocytes

Total B-cell numbers increase in human small intestinal mucosa infected with *G. intestinalis*, IgM-bearing cells being the predominant subtype. IgM cells are prominent early in infection and in nodular lymphoid hyperplasia of the small intestine, which occurs in some patients with giardiasis. A further study found only IgA and IgG cells, although this may reflect differences in sampling time because it would be expected that, during the later stages of infection, IgM-producing cells would switch to IgA production.

Mast cells, macrophages and polymorphonuclear leucocytes

Mast cell deficiency prolongs experimental infection in mice but the role of mast cells in human infection has not been established. Macrophages may also act as effector cells, their phagocytic activity for *Giardia* trophozoites being increased in the presence of specific antibodies. Neutrophils from patients with giardiasis also exhibit antibody-dependent cell-mediated cytotoxicity (ADCC) against *Giardia* trophozoites in vitro.

Integrated immune response in giardiasis

The immune system, particularly T cells, has a major role in parasite clearance during acute infection, the control of mucosal invasion and ultimately the development of protective immunity. Current evidence suggests that anti-*Giardia* sIgA also has a role in clearing *Giardia* from the gut lumen, possibly by trophozoite agglutination and/or inhibition of flagella motility.[89] Monoclonal antibodies have been shown to be directly cytotoxic to *Giardia* trophozoites and it is likely that ADCC may occur within the intestinal lumen.

Invasion of the intestinal epithelium by *Giardia* trophozoites is a rare event but a variety of mechanisms is available within the mucosa to inhibit this process; these include cytotoxic intraepithelial lymphocytes, ADCC and the complement system.

The immunological determinants of long-term protective immunity remain to be discovered. Clinical and experimental evidence suggests that secretory antibody in the intestinal lumen is likely to be important, although the antigenic determinants are as yet not defined. Preliminary evidence suggests that *Giardia* heat shock antigen, one of the family of hsp70 proteins, may be involved.

Clinical features (see also Chapter 10)

The most common form of giardiasis is asymptomatic carriage. This is common in highly endemic areas in the developing world, although it also occurs in Europe and North America. Such individuals appear to suffer no ill effects from the parasite, although there have been no systematic studies of the subclinical impact of such an infection. It is unclear whether asymptomatic infections

Table 77.8 Symptoms of acute giardiasis in travellers

Clinical features	Patients (%)
Diarrhoea	95
Weakness	76
Weight loss	68
Abdominal pain	69
Nausea	60
Steatorrhoea	56
Flatulence	35
Vomiting	29
Fever	17

relate to carriage of 'non-pathogenic' strains or whether the host is able to maintain parasite numbers at a level below expression of clinical disease without complete clearance of the infection.

Acute giardiasis has been well characterized in individuals travelling from areas of low to high endemicity.[59] Symptoms usually begin within 3–20 (mean 7) days of arrival within a high-risk area and in the vast majority recovery occurs within 2–4 weeks. In up to 25% of travellers with giardiasis, symptoms may persist for 7 weeks or more. Diarrhoea is the major symptom and is usually watery initially but subsequently develops the features of steatorrhoea, often associated with nausea, abdominal discomfort, bloating and weight loss (Table 77.8).

Although giardiasis is self-limiting in the majority of healthy immunocompetent individuals, a proportion, possibly 30–50%, goes on to have persistent diarrhoea, usually with features of steatorrhoea.[59] Weight loss can be profound, with losses of 10–20% of the usual or ideal body weight. In symptomatic patients with persistent diarrhoea, 50% will have biochemical evidence of fat malabsorption and possibly of other nutrients, including vitamin A and vitamin B_{12} (Table 77.9). Secondary lactase deficiency is well recognized to occur in human giardiasis and in experimental models, and patients may take many weeks to recover even after clearance of the parasite.

Clinical complications of giardiasis

Retardation of growth and development

A series of hospital-based studies has clearly shown the potential of giardiasis to impair growth and development in infants and young children.[90] This is a highly selected population, biased towards more severely affected children, and thus gives no indication as to the impact of giardiasis in the community. Several studies from Central America and West Africa suggest that giardiasis does have an independent inhibitory effect on child growth, but it is difficult to arrive at firm conclusions because within these populations many other factors contribute to undernutrition and impaired development.

Allergic and inflammatory conditions

Lymphoid nodular hyperplasia has been associated with chronic giardiasis and immune deficiency. There is no

Table 77.9 Intestinal malabsorption in giardiasis

Study	Location	No. of subjects	Subjects with normal results (%)				
			D-*xylose*	Lactose	Fat	Vitamin B$_{12}$	Vitamin A
Veghelyi, 1939	Hungary	14	–	–	71	–	–
Katsampes, 1944	USA	15	–	–	–	–	100
Cantor, 1967	Argentina	20	–	–	25	–	–
Hoskins, 1967	USA	6	50	100	40	100	–
Alp, 1969	Australia	5	20	20	100	–	–
Barbieri, 1970	Brazil	11[a]	27	–	82	–	–
Ament, 1972	USA	77	–	–	66	100	–
Cowen, 1973	USA	3	100	–	60	100	–
Tewari, 1974	India	30	23	–	50	6	–
Rabassa, 1975	Cuba	50	62	27	34	–	–
Wright, 1977	UK	40	45	–	35	–	–
Tandon, 1977	India	63	4	–	27	0	–
Hartong, 1979	USA	12	55	–	64	60	–
Mahalanabis, 1979	India	4	79	–	50	–	100
Mean (%)			47	49	55	61	100

[a]Asymptomatic children.

clear indication as to the precise pathogenetic relationship between these phenomena, although there is some evidence to suggest that a common feature may be a predominance of IgM-producing B cells, possibly as a result of the failure to switch from IgM to IgA production within the intestine. IgE-mediated allergic phenomena are uncommon in giardiasis, unlike many helminth infections, although occasional cases have been described.

Protein-losing enteropathy
This is a rare occurrence in giardiasis but has been described in children in West Africa and may contribute to undernutrition.[91]

Diagnosis
Clinically, giardiasis is often suggested by a typical history which often includes a period of recent foreign travel. The main differential diagnoses include other causes of intestinal malabsorption such as tropical sprue and coeliac disease. Other infective causes of persistent diarrhoea include strongyloidiasis, cryptosporidiosis, microsporidiosis and cyclosporiasis. Many clinicians treat giardiasis empirically with a nitroimidazole derivative, even without achieving a firm microscopic diagnosis.

Microscopy
Giardia cysts and occasionally *Giardia* trophozoites are detected in faecal specimens by light microscopy, which continues to be the gold standard for the diagnosis of giardiasis. Faecal specimens are examined, either fresh or fixed with polyvinyl alcohol formalin, and then stained with trichrome or iron haematoxylin. Cyst detection can be improved by concentration techniques using formalin–ethyl acetate or zinc sulphate. Immunofluorescent anticyst antibodies have been used to assist the detection of cysts in faecal specimens. Examination of multiple faecal specimens increases the chances of making a positive diagnosis, with up to 70% of positive stools detected following examination of a single faecal specimen, rising to 85% when at least three separate stool specimens are examined. Trophozoites are usually found only in freshly passed watery diarrhoea. Trophozoites can also be detected microscopically in duodenal fluid and, although overall this technique has a lower sensitivity than faecal microscopy, it does complement the latter, in that some patients with negative stool microscopy will have a positive duodenal aspirate.[92] Trophozoites may also be detected by endoscopic brush cytology or in mucosal impression smears of small intestinal biopsies.

Faecal antigen ELISA
Sensitive and specific ELISAs for *Giardia* antigens have been developed and some of these assays are now marketed commercially.[93,94] Sensitivity and specificity are reported to be 87–100%.[95,96] However, further studies are awaited to determine whether their use can be widely recommended in routine diagnostic laboratories. False positives, however, are almost always reported in these assays and the interpretation of these findings is difficult. Enthusiasts for the test will regard this as 'microscopy-negative' giardiasis, but the pessimist will merely regard this as a true false positive, possibly due to the presence of cross-reacting faecal antigens. It seems likely, however,

that microscopy-negative cases of giardiasis do exist and the more sensitive methods of detection such as ELISA or DNA-based diagnostic techniques will eventually prove the case.[97,98]

Serology

Anti-*Giardia* IgG titres are not helpful in diagnosis because they are commonly found to be increased in non-infected individuals in endemic areas. Anti-*Giardia* IgM titres are usually inceased only in infected individuals and have been shown to be useful in a research setting for detecting individuals with acute giardiasis in endemic areas such as India and The Gambia. Sensitivity and specificity decrease, however, in children with persistent diarrhoea, in some of whom anti-*Giardia* IgM titres persist for several months.

DNA-based techniques

Specific DNA probes for *Giardia* are now available, although preliminary studies suggest that there may be difficulties in liberating DNA from *Giardia* cysts.[98] A PCR-based assay that amplifies the intergenic spacer region of multicopy rRNA gene followed by nested PCR appears to be a rapid and reliable technique for detecting Giardia in stool.[99]

Management

In many healthy immunocompetent individuals giardiasis is a self-limiting illness, with the parasite being eradicated by host defence mechanisms without specific treatment. Administration of an antigiardial drug will generally reduce the severity of symptoms and the duration of the illness.[100] Although symptomatic patients with giardiasis are generally offered antimicrobial chemotherapy, the question as to whether asymptomatic patients, particularly those in an endemic area, should be treated continues to be discussed. Since the development of in vitro culture techniques for *Giardia* isolates, methods have been developed to assess drug sensitivity in vitro. However, the precise relationship between indices of drug susceptibility in vitro and the subsequent behaviour of the drug in vivo has not been clearly established. Treatment failures do occur and it is thought that at least some of these episodes are related to drug resistance.

Three classes of drugs are commonly used to treat giardiasis: the nitroimidazole derivatives, the acridine dyes, such as mepacrine, and the nitrofurans such as furazolidone. Some commonly used treatment regimens for adults and children are shown in Table 77.10. Nitroimidazole derivatives are probably the drugs of choice, particularly when used as short-course regimens. Mepacrine has a similar efficacy but is generally less well tolerated. Furazolidone has a lower efficacy but is popular for the treatment of giardiasis in childhood as it has relatively few adverse effects and is available as a suspension. The adverse effects of these agents are summarized in Table 77.11.

A variety of other chemotherapeutic agents has been assessed in vitro and some have also been used in the clinical setting. The benzimidazole drugs appear to have some antigiardial activity, which almost certainly relates to their ability to inhibit cytoskeletal function. Albendazole has been shown to have antigiardial activity in vitro[101] and recent clinical trial data support its value in human infection. Other drugs such as sodium fusidate, D- and DL-propranolol, mefloquine, doxycycline and rifampicin have all been shown to have antigiardial activity,[102] although the majority have not been subjected to rigorous evaluation in clinical practice.

Prevention

It seems highly unlikely that *Giardia* spp. will ever be eliminated from the environment, as they can survive for weeks or months outside the host in water or a moist environment and it is now well established that surface water in many parts of the world is contaminated with *Giardia* cysts. This reservoir could potentially maintain the animal reservoir of *Giardia*, which is increasingly thought to be another potential source of human infection. Despite vigilance about water quality, it is vital to ensure that contaminated surface water collecting grounds are appropriately treated before water enters the public water supply. Attention to personal hygiene in order to break the faecal–oral cycle is also important, particularly in residential institutions and day-care centres.

There is compelling evidence that breast-feeding protects against giardiasis; this can be partly attributed to passive immunization. Whether active immunization in

Table 77.10 Drug treatment of giardiasis

Drug	Adults	Children	Efficacy (%)
Metronidazole	2 g (single dose) daily for 3 days or 400 mg three times daily for 5 days	15 mg/kg per day (max. 750 mg) for 10 days	> 90
Tinidazole	2 g single dose	50–75 mg/kg single dose	> 90
Mepacrine (quinacrine)	100 mg three times daily for 5–7 days	2 mg/kg three times daily for 5–7 days	> 90
Furazolidone	100 mg four times daily for 7–10 days	2 mg/kg three times daily for 7–10 days	> 80

Table 77.11 Adverse effects of antigiardial drugs

Drugs	Adverse effects
Metronidazole and tinidazole	Nausea, vomiting, metallic taste, gastrointestinal disturbances, rashes, urticaria and angioedema *Rarely* drowsiness, headache, dizziness, ataxia *Prolonged* use, peripheral neuropathy Disulfiram-like reaction with alcohol *Avoid* in pregnancy and breast-feeding
Mapacrine (quinacrine)	Gastrointestinal disturbances, dizziness, headache, nausea and vomiting Occasionally toxic psychosis *Prolonged* use, yellow discoloration of skin, sclerae and urine, chronic dermatoses, hepatitis and aplastic anaemia *Avoid* in pregnancy, hepatic impairment, psoriasis, the elderly and history of psychosis
Furazolidone	Nausea, vomiting Haemolysis in glucose-6-phosphate dehydrogenase deficiency

the form of a vaccine is feasible, or even appropriate, continues to be evaluated. Parenteral immunization with adjuvants can protect experimental animals from challenge with *G. intestinalis*, and the epidemiological evidence in humans that protective immunity does eventually develop, probably over a number of years, suggests that immunological approaches to prevention are feasible. However, it is unclear as to why the development of protective immunity following natural infection appears to require repeated exposure to the organism. It is possible that this is related, at least in part, to the variable antigenic profiles of different *Giardia* isolates. In addition, it is known that the expression of certain *Giardia* antigens can vary during both experimental and human infection, thus providing a way in which the organism may evade the host immune response. Failure to mount an antibody response to *Giardia* heat shock antigen in children with chronic diarrhoea in The Gambia suggests that impaired response may also be a factor. Clearly all of these issues need to be taken into account in planning a vaccine development strategy. Preliminary studies in animal models of giardiasis suggest that a trophozoite-derived vaccine can provide some measure of protection in dogs and cats.[103,104]

Non-pathogenic flagellates

There are a number of other flagellates found in humans that do not appear to cause disease. *Trichomonas hominis* is commonly found in faeces of individuals living in the developing world. Only the trophozoite form is recognized; it varies from 5 to 14 μm in length. There is a single nucleus, anterior to which are basal bodies from which arise three to four flagella.

Chilomastix mesnili occurs as both cysts and trophozoite and is larger than *Trichomonas hominis*, being usually 10–15 μm in length, although it may occasionally be as large as 20 μm. The trophozoite has a large spiral longitudinal cleft anteriorly and an anterior single nucleus.

Basal bodies at the anterior pole of the nucleus give rise to three anterior flagella, two fibrils that support the margins of the longitudinal cleft (the mouth), and a fourth flagellum which moves within the longitudinal cleft. There are no cytoskeletal elements, the parasite maintaining its shape by a pellicle. The cyst is pear-shaped and approximately 18 μm in length. Internal structures are apparent in the stained cyst in which one or two nuclei may be observed.

Rare non-pathogenic flagellates include *Embadomonas intestinalis* and *Enteromonas hominis*.

The Ciliophora

Members of this class are all relatively large in size and covered by short hair-like organelles called cilia, which give the organism its motility. They have two nuclei, one somatic and one germinal. Reproduction is by binary fission, although conjugation does occur when nuclear material is exchanged between parasites. The only ciliate that is pathogenic to humans is *Balantidium coli*.

Balantidium coli

Balantidium coli is the largest and probably least common protozoan pathogen of humans.[105] It can cause a severe life-threatening colitis which is potentially avoidable by appropriate antibiotic therapy. Fatalities are almost invariably due to diagnostic imprecision.

The organism

B. coli exists as a trophozoite (usually found in stools of acute infection) and cysts, which become more apparent in chronic infection or asymptomatic carriers. The trophozoite is oval in shape, about 17 μm long and 15 μm wide. In its favoured host, the pig, trophozoites may reach 200 μm in length, when they can be seen with the aid of a hand lens or in some cases with the naked eye.

The trophozoite is covered with cilia which propel the organism through the fluid contents of the intestinal lumen. At the anterior end of the trophozoite there is a cytostome (a mouth) leading into the cytopharynx, which extends approximately one-third of the body length. Posteriorly there is a cytopyge (anus).

There are two nuclei, a larger macronucleus and a smaller micronucleus which lies in the concavity of the macronucleus. There are two contractile vacuoles connected by a canal. Intracellular organelles are limited, the major features being food vacuoles which circulate through the endoplasm. The trophozoite multiplies by lateral transverse fission, which may be preceded by conjugation, in which nuclear material is exchanged between trophozoites.

B. coli forms a large spherical cyst which may reach 60 µm in diameter. Cysts can survive outside the mammalian host for several weeks in moist conditions but are rapidly destroyed in hot, dry conditions. Infection is usually transmitted by the cyst.

Epidemiology

The parasite is found in northern and southern hemispheres, although it is most commonly reported in tropical and subtropical regions, particularly Central and South America, Iran, Papua New Guinea and the Philippines. Prevalence is usually less than 1%, although higher rates are reported in hyperendemic areas and some residential institutions. *B. coli* is found in many mammals other than humans, particularly pigs and monkeys. Swine appear to be the most important animal reservoir for human disease, although enteric disease does not seem to occur in this host. The largest reported endemic of balantidiasis, involving 110 persons, resulted from gross contamination of ground and surface water supplies by pig faeces after a severe typhoon.[106] Communities that live in close association with swine tend to have increased prevalence of the disease because carriage by pigs has been estimated to be 40–90%.

Pathogenesis

The trophozoite is able to invade the distal ileal and colonic mucosa to produce intense mucosal inflammation and ulceration. The mechanisms involved are not clearly understood, although it is considered that the motile trophozoite is able to penetrate the mucosa and submucosa, and even in some instances the muscle layers of the colon. Invasion is thought to be facilitated by the enzyme hyaluronidase, produced by the parasite. The resulting inflammation may be mediated partly by other products liberated by the parasite and possibly by recruitment of mucosal inflammatory cells, particularly neutrophils.

Clinical features

In many respects the illness produced by infection with *B. coli* closely resembles amoebic colitis. Clinical presentation occurs in three forms: (1) the asymptomatic carrier state, most commonly seen in persons in institutional care and possibly accounting for up to 80% of all infections; (2) acute and acute fulminant colitis; and (3) chronic infection. In the acute form, diarrhoea with blood and mucus begins abruptly and may be associated with nausea, abdominal discomfort and marked weight loss. Proctosigmoidoscopy reveals inflammatory changes, including discrete ulceration, although the rectum is not invariably involved. The illness can progress rapidly, accompanied by fever and prostration, and lead to death, usually due to peritonitis from colonic perforation. A protracted course with intermittent diarrhoea but only occasional blood in the stools is typical of the chronic form of the disease. A few cases of balantidial appendicitis have been reported.

Diagnosis and differential diagnosis

The large motile trophozoites are the predominant form of the parasite excreted in faeces and these can often be seen with the aid of a hand lens. Trophozoites may also be obtained from material from the margins of ulcers seen in the rectum at proctosigmoidoscopy. The macroscopic appearances at sigmoidoscopy do not, however, distinguish balantidiasis from other forms of infective or non-specific inflammatory bowel disease. Specific antibody responses to the parasite can be detected in serum but the value of serological tests in clinical diagnosis has not been clearly determined.

Management

The most commonly used treatment is tetracycline 500 mg four times daily for 10 days. The parasite is also sensitive to bacitracin, ampicillin, metronidazole and paramomycin. Surgery may be required in fulminant disease, as in amoebiasis, although a conservative approach should be taken wherever possible.

The Coccidia
Cryptosporidium parvum

Tyzzer,[107] in 1907, was the first to describe an organism of this genus with a short account of *Cryptosporidium muris* in the gastric mucosa of laboratory mice. He identified the mode of transmission as faecal–oral, and provisionally classified the organism with the coccidia. A further report in 1912 by the same author demonstrated a similar parasite in the small intestine; as he was unable to cross-infect from one site to the other with the two organisms, he recognized that they were different species. This latter organism is *C. parvum*.

Following this early description, the organism was regarded as non-pathogenic until 1955, when a syndrome of fatal diarrhoea in turkeys was described, and then in 1971 a similar disorder in calves was recognized. The first report in humans was in 1976,[108] and its identification in patients with AIDS in the 1980s cast it firmly in the role of an 'opportunist'. It is now recognized to represent a substantial threat to HIV-infected individuals, with a lifetime risk of infection of around 10%, but it is also responsible for substantial outbreaks of water-borne diarrhoea in the immunocompetent, and for diarrhoea in travellers and in children.

The organism

Taxonomy

C. parvum is a protozoan, of the phylum Apicomplexa, class Sporozoasida, subclass Coccidiasina, order Eucoccidiorida. There are four other species in the genus: *C. muris*, which parasitizes rodents, some cattle and a gazelle; *C. nasorum*, which affects fish; two avian species, *C. meleagridis* and *C. baileyi*; *C. serpentis*, which infectes reptiles; *C. wrairi*, which infects guinea pigs; and *C. felis*, which infects cats. *C. parvum* infects humans, cattle, sheep, goats, deer, horses, buffaloes, cats and other non-mammalian vertebrates.

Structure and ultrastructure

It is characteristic of these coccidia that the life cycle (Figure 77.8) includes merogony, gametogony and sporogony, and takes place within a vertebrate host. The ingested form is the oocyst, which has probably already sporulated before shedding. Excystation takes place in the small intestine, with four sporozoites being released from each oocyst. These are actively motile and penetrate the enterocyte. Electron micrographs show that the

trophozoite takes up an intracellular but extracytoplasmic position (Figure 77.9). Merogony or schizogony leads to the liberation of eight merozoites from the cell in the first cycle and four in the second, and direct invasion of neighbouring enterocytes takes place, magnifying the infection. Sexual multiplication takes place, leading to the formation of the zygote, and subsequently to the development of thin-walled oocysts (20%) and thick-walled oocysts (80%). Thick-walled oocysts are excreted in the faeces, but it is thought that thin-walled oocysts may lead to autoinfection.[109]

Genetics

Scanty information is available on the genetic make-up of *C. parvum* as there is no way of amplifying parasite material in vitro for analysis. However, some progress has been made, largely through the use of genomic libraries.[110] The genes that encode actin, tubulin, thymidylate synthase, topoisomerase, 18S rRNA and a few surface proteins (of unknown function) have been isolated. As yet there are no data on genes responsible for pathogenicity or virulence.

Restriction fragment length polymorphism (RFLP) analysis was the first technique to show variation between isolates of *C. parvum*, and this has subsequently been confirmed by a variety of other techniques, including isoenzyme analysis, random amplification of polymorphic DNA (RAPD) by PCR, sequence analysis (especially of the rRNA gene loci, the oocyst outer wall protein and the thrombospondin-related adhesion

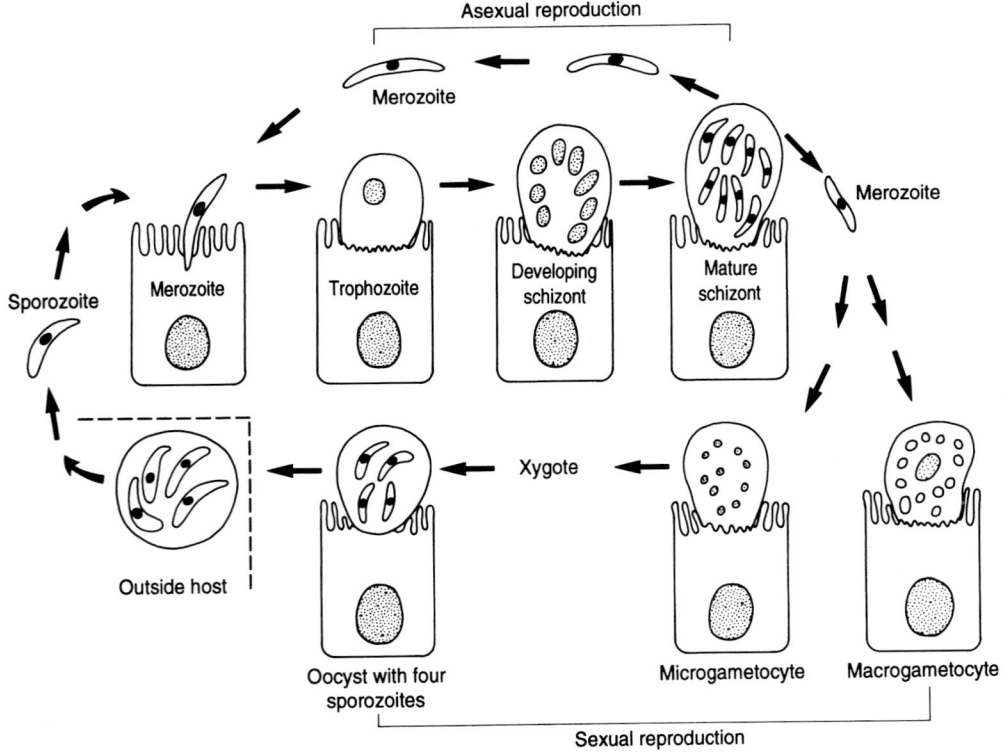

Figure 77.8: Life cycle of *C. parvum*.

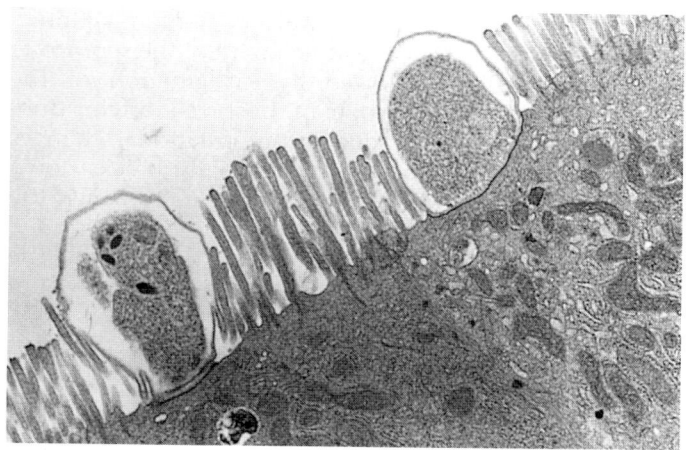

Figure 77.9: Transmission electron micrograph of *C. parvum* trophozoites in distal duodenal mucosa. The trophozoites occupy an intracellular but extracytoplasmic position. (Magnification × 20 000.) (Courtesy of Graham McPhail.)

protein). These techniques broadly confirm that the species *C. parvum* comprises at least two major genotypes, one of which infects humans exclusively and the other with a broader range of host specificity infecting animals as well as humans.[111,112] There is early evidence that immunocompromised hosts may be infected by a wider range of *C. parvum* genotypes than immunocompetent hosts.[113]

Epidemiology

Immunocompetent individuals

Substantial evidence has accumulated implicating *C. parvum* in outbreaks of water-borne diarrhoea[114] and in stable endemic childhood diarrhoea among the poor of the developing world. Travellers' diarrhoea may result from infection with this parasite. The evidence for the water-borne nature of the infection comes from epidemics that have occurred along water distribution patterns and the finding that oocysts can be detected in the water supply by filtration of large volumes through 1-μm pores. As cryptosporidiosis is a common pathogen in calf and lamb diarrhoea, it is probably a zoonosis, transmitted in surface run-off water contaminated by calf faeces. Chlorination of water at usual levels fails to inactivate oocysts. It is probably this resistance to chlorination that allowed transmission of 70 cases following contamination of a swimming pool in the UK, and in a similar outbreak reported from California.

Data from the Public Health Laboratory Service in north Wales,[115] based on diagnostic laboratory returns, show an age distribution of infection, with a peak between 1 and 5 years, and a marked reduction over the age of 35 years. The incidence is seasonal and varies with rainfall. Cryptosporidial infection is a common cause of diarrhoea outbreaks in children, and these may cluster in nurseries. The spring peak in incidence in the UK closely parallels that observed for lambs, according to reports

from the Central Veterinary Laboratories. Cases have been identified in which the only apparent transmission opportunity has been exposure to horse manure used as garden fertilizer. Veterinary students have an increased risk of infection, as do dairy farmers compared with other farming groups. Indirect transmission has occurred to young urban children from the clothing of mechanical digger operators returning home with boots and clothes soiled by farm manure.[115]

Cryptosporidiosis is an important contributor to childhood diarrhoea, with a prevalence among children with diarrhoea of 1–3% in the industrialized world and 4–17% in developing countries. Values of 1–13% have been reported in several studies from China.[116] In the developed world cryptosporidiosis is found in outbreaks clustered around day-care nurseries. In a careful prospective study in Guinea-Bissau, cryptosporidia were found in 6.1% of patients with acute (less than 2 weeks) diarrhoea and in 15% of those with chronic diarrhoea, with a relative mortality in children with cryptosporidial diarrhoea in the first year of life of 2.9.[117]

Serological studies show that exposure to cryptosporidial infection is common. In a study of IgM and IgG antibody responses to the parasite, Ungar et al.[118] found IgG-specific antibodies in 13 of 15 immunocompetent individuals with cryptosporidiosis, and in 26 of 26 patients with cryptosporidiosis and AIDS. Presumed uninfected individuals were negative in 57 of 60 cases. Serum from 9 (20%) of 44 Ecuadorian children with diarrhoea was positive, as were almost 50% of serum samples taken from adults with other parasitic diseases.

Insight into the transmission and pathobiology of the infection arises from the report of an outbreak of cryptosporidiosis in Denmark in 1990.[119] The setting was an infectious disease ward with a mixed population of HIV-seropositive and -seronegative patients; the index case was a demented seropositive man with cryptosporidial diarrhoea who contaminated an ice machine with faeces. None of the 73 HIV-seronegative inpatients became infected, but 18 (32%) of 57 HIV-positive patients developed infection, 17 of whom had AIDS. The mean incubation time was at least 13 days.

Immunodeficient individuals

Infection is acquired by the faecal–oral route. The course of the illness is variable and depends largely, but not entirely, on the degree of immune deficiency, as measured by the CD4 cell count in the peripheral blood.[120]

Cryptosporidiosis first came to prominence as a problem in the context of AIDS, to the extent that chronic cryptosporidial diarrhoea is a case-defining diagnosis for AIDS. Table 77.12 gives a summary of the studies that have examined relative contributions of protozoal infection to AIDS-related diarrhoea. Infections other than protozoa have been described, particularly salmonellae, shigellae and, in Africa, *Strongyloides stercoralis*. The contribution of viruses to the diarrhoea is uncertain at present. Differences in the proportions of specific infections found in patients in Africa and in patients in

Table 77.12 Summary of studies of prevalence of protozoa in HIV-related diarrhoea in different geographical areas

	Percentage of cases in which protozoan identified	
	Africa + Caribbean[a]	Industrial countries[b]
C. parvum	27	12
I. belli	13	0.5
Microsporidia	5[c]	27[d]
G. intestinalis	2	5
E. histolytica	2	5

[a]Means of 11 studies from Haiti, Zaire, Uganda, Burundi, Zambia and Mali.
[b]Means of 15 studies from UK, USA, France, Germany, Holland and Australia.
[c]Only two studies included a search for microsporidia.
[d]Some of these studies were of selected patients and the prevalence is raised artefactually.

developed countries may reflect the more advanced stage of immune deficiency in the latter group before death, as well as the overall prevalence of the infection in the environment. Given the number of cases in which no infection is found, the significance of any coprodiagnostic finding is uncertain, and there are those who believe that many intestinal infections are incidental, and that the real culprit is 'HIV enteropathy'.

Pathogenesis

Human studies on the distribution of infection are limited. Blanshard et al.[120] showed that C. parvum is detected less frequently in duodenal and rectal biopsies than in faeces. In children with normal immune function, Phillips et al.[121] found trophozoites in jejunal biopsies by light or scanning electron microscopy in seven of nine patients with chronic diarrhoea (defined as diarrhoea for more than 14 days) and malnutrition due to cryptosporidiosis. Goodgame et al.[122] studied 12 patients with AIDS-related intestinal cryptosporidiosis and found no parasites on duodenal biopsy in four; in two patients the entire biopsy surface was covered; in the remainder, a partial covering was observed. They found that the total daily count of shed oocysts varied by only one order of magnitude and correlated significantly with the proportion of duodenal biopsy surface covered. There was no relationship between oocyst shedding rate and stool volume. In their study, most duodenal biopsy specimens showed normal villous architecture.

Studies in piglets have suggested that the infection moves along the gut in a caudal direction. The heaviest infections were seen in the distal jejunum and ileum, moving to the colon with time, and were associated with partial villous atrophy, crypt hyperplasia and an inflammatory infiltrate in the lamina propria.

Electron microscopy of the infection shows that the presence of the trophozoites leads to destruction of the microvilli (Figure 77.9), which is associated with a reduction in disaccharidase activity.[121] Detailed ultra-structural work in a guinea pig model of infection[110] shows the initial event to be attachment of the sporozoite to the microvillus, followed by invagination of the protozoan into an envelope of host cell origin. Subsequently the parasite induces conformational changes in the host membrane, which eventually breaks down with the formation of a 'feeder organelle' by which the parasite communicates directly with host cytoplasm.

Experiments in germ-free lambs showed that the villous architecture was normal in jejunum and ileum during colonization, until the appearance of sexual stages of the life cycle. At this point the villi were reduced in height and became fused, an inflammatory infiltrate appeared in the lamina propria and diarrhoea commenced.[110]

Cryptosporidial infection has been associated with increased numbers of mitotic figures in the crypts and with villous atrophy. In the normal human intestine, cell maturation takes place during migration up the crypt and along the length of the villus. This process is accompanied by the change from a crypt cell generating net water and salt secretion to a villous cell with net salt and water absorption. Maturation is also accompanied by the synthesis of a normal complement of brush-border enzymes, including disaccharidases, lipases and alkaline phosphatase. According to the 'enterocyte immaturity hypothesis',[123] the repopulation of the villus with immature enterocytes leads to the failure of digestion and absorption seen in many protozoal small bowel parasitoses.

It has been assumed that, because some conspicuous individuals have high sodium and water losses in stool, often quoted at up to 20 litres per day, the principal mechanism of diarrhoea must be a cholera-like jejunal secretory state: 'diarrhoea in the human appears to be mostly due to hypersecretion of fluid and electrolytes from the proximal small intestine into the gut lumen'.[124] Animal perfusion studies in a neonatal piglet model of cryptosporidiosis do not support this hypothesis; nor do studies in humans using a jejunal perfusion technique.[125] It has been suggested that ileal malabsorption of bile salts may have a role in the pathogenesis of the diarrhoea.

Immunity

Studies on the gastrointestinal specific immune responses to cryptosporidial infection in humans are limited. Immunoblotting using postinfection serum, hyperimmune bovine colostrum and monoclonal antibodies has identified a range of antigens on the surface of the oocyst and the sporozoite. Various techniques reveal around 17 proteins on the surface of the oocyst, and between 20 and 40 antigens on the surface of the sporozoite. Most of these potential antigens are glycoproteins, with a molecular weight range between 15 and more than 900 kDa, and a dense cluster in the range 20–25 kDa. One of these glycoproteins, GP900, appears to be the target of protective antibodies in hyperimmune bovine colostrum.[110] Intra-epithelial lymphocytes (CD4 positive) are important in eradication of infection in a mouse model.

The majority of cases of chronic cryptosporidiosis occur in patients with HIV-induced immunosuppression. Chronic diarrhoea has been reported in congenital hypogammaglobulinaemia and in IgG_2 deficiency,[126] and in severe combined immune deficiency.[124] Chronic diarrhoea may also follow the administration of immunosuppressive drugs, and usually resolves on withdrawal. There is evidence that innate immunity plays a role in controlling infection, and individuals deficient in mannose-binding lectin appear to be more susceptible to persistent infection.[127]

Clinical features

Early reports considered the infection in the context of AIDS as 'unremitting, profuse diarrhoea lasting for months', but this is an oversimplification. The clinical picture of infection is variable, and there is variation in disease severity even after accounting for the degree of immune deficiency by blood CD4 cell count. It is now established that patients with AIDS may carry heavy parasite burdens asymptomatically, and transient infection is not uncommon. However, a substantial proportion of patients present with diarrhoea, abdominal cramps and vomiting. About 8% of patients in London had fulminant diarrhoea, with collapse and severe dehydration due to the passage of high volumes of diarrhoea. The majority of patients in this study had stool volumes of 500–1500 ml per 24 hours, with stool frequency of 2 to 10 per day.[128] There is no way of clinically distinguishing patients with cryptosporidiosis from those with any other chronic diarrhoeal illness. The natural history of the infection in the West is that of a remitting and relapsing diarrhoea. In one study, 11 of 38 patients with HIV-related cryptosporidiosis underwent spontaneous remission lasting for more than 2 months. These patients had higher peripheral blood CD4 cell counts than those who did not.[129] In a series of patients in Lusaka, Zambia, the median duration of diarrhoea at presentation with cryptosporidiosis was 5 months, with 60% admitting to intermittent diarrhoea (P. Kelly, personal observations). Among the patients studied by Colebunders et al.,[130] in a series of Zairean patients, 89% had intermittent diarrhoea and the mean duration was 9 months; no difference was demonstrated between patients with cryptosporidiosis and those with other forms of HIV-related diarrhoea.

Patients in all areas of the globe show considerable wasting as AIDS progresses, but it is difficult to discern how much can be attributed to any particular infection. There is certainly anorexia in AIDS, and oral and oesophageal candidiasis exacerbate the problem. There is no evidence that cryptosporidiosis is associated with a greater degree of nutritional impairment than any other enteric manifestation of AIDS. Phillips et al.,[121] however, showed an association between cryptosporidial infection and nutritional impairment in immunocompetent children. Children in Guinea-Bissau who were undernourished were not more likely to develop the infection.[117]

Some patients develop small bowel disease alone, while others may also have involvement of the biliary tract. The first large study of biliary disease in AIDS[131] described a syndrome of sclerosing cholangitis, sometimes associated with cholecystitis. This may be associated with cryptosporidial infection of the biliary tract, with microsporidiosis (see below) or with cytomegalovirus, or it may be impossible to identify a cause. The disorder usually occurs in patients with chronic diarrhoea and is associated with progressive right upper quadrant abdominal pain. The patients tend to have had other opportunistic infections by this stage of the HIV infection. Biochemical tests of hepatic damage usually show raised serum levels of alkaline phosphatase and γ-glutamyltransferase in the absence of jaundice. Transaminase concentrations may or may not be increased. Ultrasonographic examination of the liver may show irregularly dilated intrahepatic bile ducts. The definitive test is endoscopic retrograde cholangio-pancreatography, which shows this distortion of the biliary anatomy, with or without papillary stenosis. Forbes et al.[132] found cryptosporidia in 13 of 20 cases, and estimated that up to one in six of all cases of AIDS-related cryptosporidiosis may also have sclerosing cholangitis. This sort of study is unlikely to be carried out in the tropics, but there may be undiagnosed cases amongst patients with AIDS, usually presenting with chronic right upper quadrant pain.

Cryptosporidiosis is associated with malnutrition and increased mortality in children in developing countries.[133,134] Longitudinal studies in Guinea-Bissau have demonstrated that cryptosporidiosis precedes the development of growth failure.[134] In malnourished children with persistent diarrhoea in Zambia, cryptosporidiosis was associated with higher mortality independently of HIV infection.[135]

Diagnosis

Current diagnostic methods rely heavily on the identification of the oocysts in faeces. Three staining methods are in common use: auramine staining, modified Ziehl–Neelsen staining and immunofluorescence using monoclonal antibodies to oocysts. These techniques are relatively insensitive. The threshold of reliable (100%) detection was found to be 10 000 cysts/g in watery stool, but in formed stool thresholds were 50 000/g by immunofluorescence and 500 000/g by acid-fast staining.[136]

ELISAs that incorporate anti-oocyst antibodies to detect cryptosporidial antigen in faeces have been developed. There is a problem in knowing what to use as a reference standard, but two analyses have suggested sensitivities of 82.3%[137] and 93%.[138] The specificity of such assays (which would be expected to be more sensitive than the reference standard, i.e., microscopy) is difficult to interpret. Several different assays using PCR have been published for detection of DNA in stool or biopsies.[139]

Serological tests have been described, but have not reached the stage of routine use. The ELISA technique has been mentioned above, and an indirect fluorescent antibody test (IFAT) has been developed that will detect serum antibodies to oocyst antigens. The IFAT was positive in 50% of patients with AIDS and gastrointestinal complaints, and in 24.6% of patients without AIDS.

Management

There is no effective treatment that will eradicate cryptosporidial infection in all cases; over 80 drugs have been tested. Paromomycin is of some value but the consensus seems to be that its effect is modest. Most studies that suggest benefit have been small and uncontrolled. Several controlled trials have now confirmed that nitazoxanide is effective against *C. parvum* in well-nourished and malnourished children. A 3-day course is effective: children under 4 years receive 100 mg twice daily and those over 4 years 200 mg twice daily, orally. Early data indicate that HIV-positive adults or children require a longer course, but the duration is as yet uncertain. The most important aspect of treatment is fluid and electrolyte replacement with oral rehydration solutions, although intravenous therapy may be necessary. Symptomatic treatment with codeine phosphate or powerful opiates should be given readily, according to resources, and nutritional support is probably beneficial.

Prevention

When dealing with a disease affecting mainly the immunocompromised, it is difficult to evaluate measures directed at reduction of incidence. On the basis of what little we know about transmission, it would seem prudent to advise those at risk, including HIV-infected individuals, to boil all drinking water and to avoid swimming in public water. There is no immediate prospect of effective immunization against the infection.

Prevention of nosocomial or laboratory-acquired infection requires strict attention to containment and generous washing of any contaminated areas. Disposables should be used where possible. The oocysts are resistant to many disinfectants, but are reliably inactivated by boiling, freezing, drying and 3% hydrogen peroxide.[140]

Isospora belli

This coccidian was first described in 1915 but has received much less attention in the world literature than cryptosporidia, probably because of its comparative rarity in the developed world. It has recently attracted interest because of its identification in patients with AIDS. The infective form of the parasite is the oocyst, which releases sporozoites, leading to a small bowel infection. The parasite there takes up an intracellular location and undergoes merogony and sporogony.

Epidemiology

The route of transmission of the parasite is not established but faecal–oral spread seems likely. Infection is uncommon in the developed world, as reflected by the prevalence in European and North American patients with AIDS (compared with Africans) shown in Table 77.12. In Paris, in a series of 3500 patients from the tropics studied before the HIV pandemic, only five (0.1%) cases of isosporiasis were found. A survey of 55 421 stool specimens in Chile over a 10-year period revealed only 452 (0.8%) positives.[141]

Pathogenesis

Isosporiasis is associated with mild to a subtotal villous atrophy. This is seen in patients with AIDS, but was also reported before the HIV pandemic.[142] Inflammatory cells and eosinophils are seen in the lamina propria.

Clinical features

As with cryptosporidiosis, isosporiasis leads to a self-limiting diarrhoea in the immunocompetent, and to chronic diarrhoea in the immunocompromised. The illness in the apparently immunocompetent may be prolonged, extending to 20 years in one report.[143] There is little evidence regarding the frequency with which isosporiasis spontaneously remits in patients with AIDS. In AIDS, isosporiasis is associated with wasting and dehydration. The most thorough analysis is that of De Hovitz et al.,[144] in which 15 patients with *Isospora belli* were identified among 131 Haitian patients with AIDS; their main complaints were watery diarrhoea, cramping abdominal pain and nausea.

Diagnosis

Diagnosis rests on stool examination using wet preparations and modified Ziehl–Neelsen acid-fast stained smears. The oocysts appear oval, larger than cryptosporidial oocysts (20–30 × 11–19 μm); some oocysts are sporulated before leaving the host and have two easily identified sporoblasts. The oocysts fluoresce with the phenol auramine stain under ultraviolet light. The parasites may also be recognized in small bowel biopsies, visible within enterocyte cytoplasmic vacuoles under electron microscopy and light microscopy.[142]

Management

Treatment with oral co-trimoxazole (sulfamethoxazole 800 mg and trimethoprim 160 mg) four times daily for 10 days eliminated the parasite from stool in most cases, with an interruption in diarrhoea.[144] Unfortunately this was followed by relapse in 50%, usually within 12 weeks. Retreatment was usually effective. Prophylactic co-trimoxazole may be necessary. Pyrimethamine–sulphonamide combinations are also effective.[143,145] There is little information on the regimen of choice for those who are intolerant of sulphonamides.

Sarcocystis species

Infection with this coccidian, formerly known as *Isospora hominis*, is uncommonly recognized. The parasite is similar to *I. belli* in its biology,[141] but the life cycle requires alternating infection of intermediate hosts, such as cattle and pigs, and definitive hosts, such as humans. In Strasbourg the infection was present in 286 patients over a 5-year period, representing 0.4–1.5% of all stool specimens. The infection has not so far been recognized in AIDS. In the Strasbourg series, 30% of patients had peripheral eosinophilia. Biopsy specimens may show an eosinophilic infiltrate. Sporocysts are recognized in stool with the same stains as are used for isosporiasis, but the cysts are smaller (15 × 10 μm).

Cyclospora cayetanensis

During the mid-1980s a new intestinal pathogen was identified in the stools of individuals with persistent diarrhoea; these were initially known as cyanobacterium-like bodies. It has subsequently become evident that this organism is a member of the coccidia, of the genus *Cyclospora*. The organism was tentatively named *Cyclospora cayetanensis*,[146] which now appears to have been formally adopted.

The organism

Until the recent reports in humans, organisms of the genus *Cyclospora* have been identified only in reptiles, myriapods, insectivores and rodents. Oocysts of the human parasite differ morphologically from oocysts in these animal species, and it thus appears that the human isolate is a new species. Each oocyst has two sporocysts. Sporulation has been effected in vitro after 7–13 days in culture. Excystation results in the liberation of two sporozoites which are crescent shaped, approximately 9 μm in length and 1.2 μm in width.[146] The ultrastructural characteristics of the oocysts are entirely consistent with those of other members of the coccidia. The parasite life cycle would appear to have both sexual and asexual components. The asexual stages of sporozoite, trophozoite, schizont and merozoite have been identified by electron microscopy in human duodenal biopsies.[147] However, it was assumed that the sexual cycle had also taken place because oocysts were also detected in the patient's stool. It was concluded, therefore, that *Cyclospora* requires only a single host to complete its entire life cycle in humans. Recent molecular phylogenetic analysis indicates that *Cyclospora* is closely related to *Eimeria* species.[148]

Epidemiology

Cyclospora spp. were first identified in individuals with a history of foreign travel and those infected with HIV. Seasonal outbreaks were described in Nepal among foreign residents and travellers, and a small outbreak has been reported in medical staff in a Chicago hospital. Since these initial observations a more detailed study in Nepal has revealed new information about the infection. As yet the global prevalence of the infection is unknown,

although a prevalence of 4–7% has been reported in foreign residents in Nepal, with peak prevalence rates occurring during the warmer months with higher rainfall.[149] *Cyclospora* diarrhoea has now been described in the Americas, the Caribbean, Africa, Bangladesh, South-East Asia, Australia, England and Eastern Europe. The incubation period is quite short, ranging from 1 to 7 days. Transmission appears to be by the faecal–oral route, with water being the most important vehicle. The first waterborne outbreak in the USA was reported in 1995.[150] However, in 1996 a major outbreak of cyclosporiasis was investigated in the USA which was found to be due to the ingestion of Guatemalan raspberries.[151] Several further outbreaks have been documented in the USA and Canada, which again were thought to be associated with the consumption of berries.

Pathogenesis

The mechanism by which this organism produces diarrhoea has not been clearly established. However, the organism takes up an intracellular location within enterocytes, and histological examination of small intestinal biopsies has demonstrated mild reduction in villous height, with associated mucosal inflammation and increased numbers of intraepithelial lymphocytes.[152] No specific virulence factors have yet been identified. *Cyclospora* diarrhoea has been associated with the development of the Guillain–Barré syndrome.

Clinical features

There is increasing epidemiological evidence that *C. cayetanensis* is responsible for persistent diarrhoea in both immunocompetent and immunocompromised individuals. Diarrhoea can last for 1–8 weeks and may be associated with abdominal pain, nausea, vomiting and anorexia. Abdominal gas and bloating are also commonly associated features.[146,149] In prolonged infection weight loss can be profound. Other than the persistence of symptoms there are no specific features that can distinguish *Cyclospora* diarrhoea from other causes of persistent diarrhoea.

Diagnosis

Oocysts can be detected in stool by light microscopy and can be induced to sporulate in the presence of 5% potassium dichromate solution.[146] Cyst concentration techniques can be used to increase the chances of cyst identification and typical features of the *Cyclospora* spp. can be detected by transmission electron microscopy. Parasites can also be detected in small intestinal biopsies by transmission electron microscopy.

Differential diagnosis includes other parasitic infections such as giardiasis, cryptosporidiosis, microsporidiosis and tropical sprue. A careful search for these parasites in faeces and in small intestinal biopsies is required to identify these infective agents.

Management

The treatment of choice for *C. cayetanensis* infection is trimethoprim–sulfamethoxazole (TMP-SMX) 160–800 mg twice daily for 7 days.[153] This results in the eradication of infection in more than 90% of individuals; continuation of treatment for a further 3 days will cure the majority of remaining patients. Ciprofloxacin is less effective but is suitable for patients who cannot tolerate TMP-SMX.[154]

Prevention

Epidemiological studies suggest that the major vehicle for the transmission of *Cyclospora* spp. oocysts is in water. Travellers should be advised to heed the usual advice regarding the drinking of tap water in tropical and sub-tropical climates. As yet there are no data on the susceptibility of sporocysts to chlorination, although it is likely that, like other members of the protozoa, this is an unreliable way of inactivating cysts. However, boiling water for 10 minutes should lead to their destruction.

TMP-SMX is effective for chemoprophylaxis but is usually indicated only in immunocomprised patients who experience frequent reinfections or in those who fail to clear the infection following the standard treatment regimen.

The Microspora

Microsporidia fall into the phylum Microspora.[155] Known to be parasites of vertebrates and invertebrates for many years, it is only since the outbreak of the HIV epidemic that they have been found to infect humans. Two species cause intestinal disease in humans: *Enterocytozoon bieneusi* and *Encephalitozoon intestinalis*.

Enterocytozoon bieneusi

Infection with this organism was first reported in 1985 by Modigliani et al.,[156] who found the parasite in electron micrographs of small intestinal biopsies. Infection in humans had not been reported before the syndrome of AIDS-related diarrhoea was recognized, but various microsporidia infect other species of vertebrates and invertebrates. Since the first report, many cases have been identified, and microsporidial infection is prominent among those infections to which the HIV-infected individual is susceptible.

The organism

Microsporidia constitute their own phylum within the protozoa, distinct from the coccidia which are part of the phylum Apicomplexa. They are obligate intracellular spore-forming organisms with a wide range of hosts.

Infection is acquired via the spore. Following ingestion, the spore extrudes a polar tube (possibly through increased intracellular pressure), through which sporoplasm is passed, infecting any enterocytes penetrated by the tube.[157] This infection of the enterocyte is followed by proliferation by binary fission (merogony), with the meront in an intracytoplasmic position, surrounded by a simple membrane. Microsporidia have a few elements of endoplasmic reticulum but no mitochondria.[158] Ribosomal molecular analysis indicates that the ribosomes are of prokaryotic size (70S), and RNA sequence analysis demonstrates considerable divergence from the ribosomal structure of most eukaryotes, suggesting that, like *G. intestinalis*, microsporidia evolved early along a divergent path from other protozoa. Merogony overlaps with sporogony, which leads to the development of spores. These are about 1.5 × 0.9 μm in size, and are shed in the faeces.

Epidemiology

The prevalence of infection with microsporidia in studies of patients with AIDS diarrhoea is shown in Table 77.12. It is important to note that different diagnostic tools were used and that some of the patient series were subject to selection. There are a few reports of the infection in patients without HIV infection, but overall there is little information on the epidemiology of microsporidiosis. Infection has been diagnosed in immunocompromised organ transplant recipients, and in one child with a congenital thymic immunodeficiency. Early data from longitudinal studies of intestinal infection in Lusaka, Zambia, indicate that microsporidiosis can affect both HIV-seropositive and HIV-seronegative adults, although persistent diarrhoea is more likely in patients with advanced immunodeficiency.

Pathogenesis

Morphological studies of biopsies of infected small bowel reveal multiple meronts and sporonts in the host cell, often around the nucleus. Cells thus infected are apparently healthy at first, but the development of the later stages of sporogony is associated with enterocyte degeneration, vacuolation and loss of the brush border. These cells are subsequently sloughed off into the lumen, where the spores are liberated after cytolysis. Adjacent uninfected cells are not apparently damaged.[159] Infection of enterocytes with microsporidia is seen only on the villi, not in the crypts. Villous atrophy occurs, possibly through increased enterocyte loss.[158] It is not known whether adjacent spread of infection occurs from cell to cell. There is no synchrony of life cycles amongst different organisms parasitizing the same cell.

Infection is confined to the small bowel, principally from the distal duodenum to the ileum.[160] One study demonstrated an equal prevalence of microsporidial infection in biopsies from HIV-infected homosexual men without diarrhoea as in a group with diarrhoea, casting doubt on the causal association of the parasite and diarrhoea.[161] Another study showed microsporidia only in patients with diarrhoea.[162] Studies in patients have demonstrated diminished D-xylose absorption compared with patients with AIDS-related diarrhoea without microsporidiosis, but serum vitamin B_{12} concentrations were not reduced.

Immunity

There are few data regarding immune responses to microsporidia, and serological studies are very limited.

Clinical features

E. bieneusi infection is most frequently diagnosed in patients with AIDS and persistent diarrhoea. Among 38 HIV-seropositive patients with the infection, only one did not have diarrhoea,[163] and most series do not report any asymptomatic infections. Patients in this Australian study had a mean duration of diarrhoea of 7 months and a mean peripheral blood CD4 cell count of 40×10^6/l. The volume of the diarrhoea is variable, and is associated with anorexia, nausea and crampy abdominal pain.[161] This is probably true of all forms of AIDS-related diarrhoea.

There are several reports in the literature of a sclerosing cholangitis-like syndrome,[163,164] indistinguishable from that associated with cryptosporidiosis.

Diagnosis

The original and 'gold standard' technique for diagnosis is electron microscopy of small bowel biopsies. Early meronts are recognized by the paler appearance of the cytoplasm relative to that of the host cell (Figure 77.10). The hallmark of the late meront or sporont is the development of the characteristic electron-dense polar tube, which has about 5 to 7.5 coils. Other characteristics include the presence of electron-lucent inclusions (ELIs) and electron-dense discs (EDDs). Spores are identifiable by their intensely osmophilic walls.

Light microscopic diagnosis of histological sections of small bowel biopsy material is possible using careful scanning of sections stained with Giemsa,[159] Brown–Brenn or Unna blue. Biopsies obtained from the distal duodenum are perfectly adequate, and either light or electron microscopy provides a more sensitive diagnostic tool than stool examination.[165]

Detection of spores in stool has become possible by the use of a chromotrope.[166]

Management

Albendazole is the treatment of choice.[167] Albendazole inhibits microtubule formation, and thus reduces cell division and possibly polar tube action. The usual dose is 400 mg twice daily for 4 weeks, but there is evidence that *E. bieneusi* responds much less satisfactorily than *E. intestinalis*.[168]

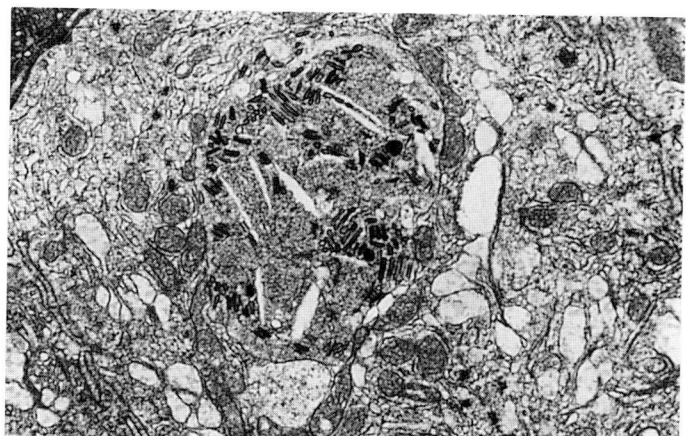

Figure 77.10: Meront of *Enterocytozoon bieneusi*, showing EDDs. (Magnification × 20 000.) (Courtesy of Graham McPhail.)

Encephalitozoon spp.

Unlike *Enterocytozoon bieneusi*, *Encephalitozoon* spp. are widespread amongst other vertebrates. *Encephalitozoon cuniculi* is the best known, and differs from *Enterocytozoon bieneusi* in that all stages lie within a parasitophorous vacuole, and it does not cause enteropathy. Five human cases have been recorded, three with neurological disorders, one with hepatitis and one with peritonitis in a patient with AIDS.[157] However, serological testing for *Encephalitozoon cuniculi* indicates that exposure to this microsporidian may in fact be quite common.[169]

Recently, infection with *Enterocytozoon hellem* has been described in patients with AIDS, with corneal infection and disseminated disease involving lungs and kidneys, but not the gastrointestinal tract.

Another microsporidian, *Encephalitozoon intestinalis*, has been reported in patients with AIDS in developed countries and in Africa. The first case was of chronic diarrhoea due to an organism resembling, but distinct from, *Encephalitozoon cuniculi*. Subsequently it has become apparent that this microsporidian is capable of dissemination, leading to an interstitial nephritis. The microsporidia may be found in lamina propria macrophages, and free spores can be found in the renal vasculature and portal vein. The spores are then shed in the urine. One of the characteristics of this organism is its development within a parasitophorous vacuole which is septated. For this reason, it was originally given the name *Septata intestinalis*. Most series report that it is less common in patients with AIDS and persistent diarrhoea than *E. bieneusi*, but it is more sensitive to albendazole.[170]

REFERENCES

1   World Health Organization. The World Health Report 1998. *Life in the 21st Century: A Vision for All.* Geneva: WHO, 1998.

2   Löch F D. Massive development of amebas in the large intestine. Translated and reprinted in *Am J Trop Med Hyg* 1875; 24:383–392.

3   Osler W. On the Amoeba coli in dysentery and in dysenteric liver abscess. *Johns Hopkins Hosp Bull* 1890; 1:53–54.

4   Councilman W T & Lafleur H A. Amoebic dysentery. *Johns Hopkins Hosp Rep* 1891; 2:395–548.

5   Schaudinn F. Untersuchungen über die Fortpflanzung einiger Rhizopoden (Vorläufige Mittheilung). Arb Kaiserlichen *Gesundheitsamte* 1903; 19:547–576.

6   Walker E L & Sellards A W. Experimental entamoebic dysentery. *Philippine J Sci B Trop Med* 1913; 8:253–330.

7   Brumpt E. Etude sommaire de l' 'Entamoeba dispar' n. sp. Amibe à kystes quandrinuclées, parasite de l'homme. *Bull Acad Med* (Paris) 1925; 94:943–952.

8   Sargeaunt P G, Williams J E & Grene J D. The differentiation of invasive and non-invasive *Entamoeba histolytica* by isoenzyme electrophoresis. *Trans R Soc Trop Med Hyg* 1978; 72:519–521.

9   Sargeaunt P G & Williams J E. Electrophoretic isoenzyme patterns of the pathogenic and non-pathogenic intestinal amoebae of man. *Trans R Soc Trop Med Hyg* 1979; 73:225–227.

10   Diamond L S & Clark C G. A redescription of *Entamoeba histolytica* Schaudinn, 1903 (Emended Walker, 1911) separating it from Entamoeba dispar Brumpt, 1925. *J Eukaryot Microbiol* 1993; 40:340–344.

11   WHO/PAHO/UNESCO. A consultation with experts on amoebiasis. Mexico City, Mexico 28–29 January, 1997. *Epidemiol Bull* 1997; 18:13–14.

12   WHO. Amoebiasis. *Wkly Epidemiol Rec* 1997; 72:97–99.

13   Cavalier-Smith T. Kingdom protozoa and its 18 phyla. *Microbiol Rev* 1993; 57:953–994.

14   Silberman J D, Clark C G, Diamond L S & Sogin M L. Phylogeny of the genera *Entamoeba* and *Endolimax* as deduced from small-subunit ribosomal RNA sequences. *Mol Biol Evol* 1999; 16:1740–1751.

15   Mai Z, Ghosh S, Frisardi M, Rosenthal B, Rogers R & Samuelson J. Hsp60 is targeted to a cryptic mitochondrion-derived organelle ('crypton') in the microaerophilic protozoan parasite *Entamoeba histolytica. Mol Cell Biol* 1999; 19:2198–2205.

16   Tovar J, Fischer A & Clark C G. The mitosome, a novel organelle related to mitochondria in the amitochondrial parasite *Entamoeba histolytica. Mol Microbiol* 1999; 32:1013–1021.

17   Azam A, Paul J, Sehgal D, Prasad J, Bhattacharya S & Bhattacharya A. Identification of novel genes from *Entamoeba histolytica* by expressed sequence tag analysis. *Gene* 1996; 181:113–116.

18   Cavalier-Smith T. A revised six-kingdom system of life. *Biol Rev Camb Philos Soc* 1998; 73:203–266.

19   Ghosh S, Field J, Rogers R, Hickman M & Samuelson J. The *Entamoeba histolytica* mitochondrion-derived organelle (crypton) contains double-stranded DNA and appears to be bound by a double membrane. *Infect Immun* 2000; 68:4319–4322.

20   Diamond L S. Techniques of axenic cultivation of *Entamoeba histolytica* Schaudinn, 1903 and E. histolytica-like amebae. *J Parasitol* 1968; 54:1047–1056.

21   Reeves R E. Metabolism of *Entamoeba histolytica* Schaudinn, 1903. *Adv Parasitol* 1984; 23:105–142.

22   Rosenthal B, Mai Z, Caplivski D et al. Evidence for the bacterial origin of genes encoding fermentation enzymes of the amitochondriate protozoan parasite *Entamoeba histolytica.*

23   *J Bacteriol* 1997; 179:3736–3745. Rodriguez M A, Garcia-Perez R M, Mendoza L, Sanchez T, Guillen N & Orozco E. The pyruvate : ferredoxin oxidoreductase enzyme is located in the plasma membrane and in a cytoplasmic structure in Entamoeba. *Microb Pathog* 1998; 25:1–10.

24   Riveron A M, Lopez-Canovas L, Baez-Camargo M et al. Circular and linear DNA molecules in the *Entamoeba histolytica* complex molecular karyotype. *Eur Biophys J* 2000; 29:48–56.

25   Orozco E, Gharaibeh R, Riveron A M et al. A novel cytoplasmic structure containing DNA networks in *Entamoeba histolytica* trophozoites. *Mol Gen Genet* 1997; 254:250–257.

26   Bhattacharya A, Satish S, Bagchi A & Bhattacharya S. The genome of *Entamoeba histolytica. Int J Parasitol* 2000; 30:401–410.

27   Walsh J A. Problems in recognition and diagnosis of amebiasis: estimation of the global magnitude of morbidity and mortality. *Rev Infect Dis* 1986; 8:228–238.

28   Gathiram V & Jackson T F. A longitudinal study of asymptomatic carriers of pathogenic zymodemes of *Entamoeba histolytica. S Afr Med J* 1987; 72:669–672.

29   Adams S A, Robson S C, Gathiram V et al. Immunological similarity between the 170 kD amoebic adherence glycoprotein and human beta 2 integrins. *Lancet* 1993; 341:17–19.

30   Guillén N. Cell signalling and motility in *Entamoeba histolytica. Parasitol Today* 1993; 9:364–369.

31   Seydel K B & Stanley S L Jr. *Entamoeba histolytica* induces host cell death in amebic liver abscess by a non-Fas-dependent, non-tumor necrosis factor alpha-dependent pathway of apoptosis. *Infect Immun* 1998; 66:2980–2983.

32   Huston C D, Houpt E R, Mann B J, Hahn C S & Petri W A Jr. Caspase 3-dependent killing of host cells by the parasite *Entamoeba histolytica. Cell Microbiol* 2000; 2:617–625.

33   Andra J & Leippe M. Pore-forming peptide of *Entamoeba histolytica*. Significance of positively charged amino acid residues for its mode of action. *FEBS Lett* 1994; 354:97–102.

34   Munoz M L, Lamoyi E, Leon G et al. Antigens in electron-dense granules from *Entamoeba histolytica* as possible markers for pathogenicity. *J Clin Microbiol* 1990; 28:2418–2424.

35   Leon G, Fiori C, Das P et al. Electron probe analysis and biochemical characterization of electron-dense granules secreted by *Entamoeba histolytica. Mol Biochem Parasitol* 1997; 85:233–242.

36   Que X & Reed S L. Cysteine proteinases and the pathogenesis of amebiasis. *Clin Microbiol Rev* 2000; 13:196–206.

37   Schulte W & Scholze H. Action of the major protease from *Entamoeba histolytica* on proteins of the extracellular matrix. *J Protozool* 1989; 36:538–543.

38   Yu Y & Chadee K. *Entamoeba histolytica* stimulates interleukin 8 from human colonic epithelial cells without parasite–enterocyte contact. *Gastroenterology* 1997; 112:1536–1547.

39   Seydel K B, Li E, Swanson P E & Stanley S L Jr. Human intestinal epithelial cells produce proinflammatory cytokines in response to infection in a SCID mouse–human intestinal xenograft model of amebiasis. *Infect Immun* 1997; 65:1631–1639.

40   Reed S L, Ember J A, Herdman D S, DiScipio R G, Hugli T E & Gigli I. The extracellular neutral cysteine proteinase of *Entamoeba histolytica* degrades anaphylatoxins C3a and C5a. *J Immunol* 1995; 155:266–274.

41   De Leon A. Pronóstico tardío en el absceso hepático amibiano. *Arch Invest Med* 1970; 1:205–206.

42 Irusen E M, Jackson T F & Simjee A E. Asymptomatic intestinal colonization by pathogenic *Entamoeba histolytica* in amebic liver abscess: prevalence, response to therapy, and pathogenic potential. *Clin Infect Dis* 1992; 14:889–893.

43 Kelsall B L & Ravdin J I. Degradation of human IgA by *Entamoeba histolytica*. *J Infect Dis* 1993; 168:1319–1322.

44 Tran V Q, Herdman D S, Torian B E & Reed S L. The neutral cysteine proteinase of *Entamoeba histolytica* degrades IgG and prevents its binding. *J Infect Dis* 1998; 177:508–511.

45 Carrada-Bravo T. [Invasive amebiasis as a public health problem]. *Bol Med Hosp Infant Mex* 1989; 46:139–148.

46 Haque R, Neville L M, Hahn P & Petri W A Jr. Rapid diagnosis of Entamoeba infection by using Entamoeba and *Entamoeba histolytica* stool antigen detection kits. *J Clin Microbiol* 1995; 33:2558–2561.

47 Freeman O, Akamaguna A & Jarikre L N. Amoebic liver abscess: the effect of aspiration on the resolution or healing time. *Ann Trop Med Parasitol* 1990; 84:281–287.

48 Weinke T, Friedrich-Janicke B, Hopp P & Janitschke K. Prevalence and clinical importance of *Entamoeba histolytica* in two high-risk groups: travelers returning from the tropics and male homosexuals. *J Infect Dis* 1990; 161:1029–1031.

49 Vohra H, Bhatti H S, Ganguly N K & Mahajan R C. Virulence of pathogenic and non-pathogenic zymodemes of *Entamoeba histolytica* (Indian strains) in guinea-pigs. *Trans R Soc Trop Med Hyg* 1989; 83:648–650.

50 Bruchhaus I, Jacobs T, Leippe M & Tannich E. *Entamoeba histolytica* and *Entamoeba dispar*: differences in numbers and expression of cysteine proteinase genes. *Mol Microbiol* 1996; 22:255–263.

51 Espinosa-Cantellano M, Gonzales-Robles A, Chavez B et al. *Entamoeba dispar*: ultrastructure, surface properties and cytopathic effect. *J Eukaryot Microbiol* 1998; 45:265–272.

52 Walderich B, Weber A & Knobloch J. Sensitivity of *Entamoeba histolytica* and *Entamoeba dispar* patient isolates to human complement. *Parasite Immunol* 1997; 19:265–271.

53 Clark C G. Axenic cultivation of *Entamoeba dispar* Brumpt 1925, *Entamoeba insolita* Geiman and Wichterman 1937 and *Entamoeba ranarum* Grassi 1879. *J Eukaryot Microbiol* 1995; 42:590–593.

54 Sargeaunt P G, Patrick S & O'Keeffe D. Human infections of *Entamoeba chattoni* masquerade as *Entamoeba histolytica*. *Trans R Soc Trop Med Hyg* 1992; 86:633–634.

55 Camp R R, Mattern C F & Honigberg B M. Study of *Dientamoeba fragilis*. I. Electron microscopic observations of the binucleate stages. II. Taxonomic position and revision of the genus. *J Protozool* 1974; 21:69–82.

56 Silberman J D, Clark C G & Sogin M L. *Dientamoeba fragilis* shares a recent common evolutionary history with the trichomonads. *Mol Biochem Parasitol* 1996; 76:311–314.

57 Johnson J A & Clark C G. Cryptic genetic diversity in *Dientamoeba fragilis*. *J Clin Microbiol* 2000; 38:4653–4654.

58 Farthing M J G. Host–parasite interactions in human giardiasis. *Q J Med* 1989; 70:191–204.

59 Farthing M J G. Giardiasis as a disease. In Reynoldson J A, Thompson R C A & Lymbery A J (eds) *Giardia: From Molecules to Disease and Beyond*. London: CAB International, 1993:15–37.

60 Kabnick K S & Peattie D A. *Giardia*: a missing link between prokaryotes and eukaryotes. *Am Sci* 1991; 79:34–43.

61 Meyer E A. Taxonomy and nomenclature. In Meyer EA (ed.) *Giardiasis*. Amsterdam: Elsevier, 1990; 51–60.

62 Carnaby S, Katelaris PH, Naemm A, Farthing MJG. Genotypic heterogeneity within *Giardia lamblia* isolates demonstrated by M13 DNA fingerprinting. *Infect Immun* 1994; 62:1875–1880.

63 Bauer B, Engelbrecht S, Bakker-Grunwald T & Scholze H. Functional identification of alpha 1-giardin as an annexin of

Giardia lamblia. *FEMS Microbiol Lett* 1999; 173:147–153.

64 Van Keulen H, Steimle P A, Bulik D A, Borowiak R K & Jarroll E L. Cloning of two putative *Giardia lamblia* glucosamine 6-phosphate isomerase genes only one of which is transcriptionally activated during encystment. *J Eukaryotic Microbiol* 1998; 45:637–642.

65 Hetsko M L, McCaffery J M, Svard S G, Meng T C, Que X & Gillin F D. Cellular and transcriptional changes during excystation of *Giardia lamblia* in vitro. *Exp Parasitol* 1998; 88:172–183.

66 Farthing M J G, Keusch G T & Carey M C. Effects of bile and bile salts on growth and membrane lipid uptake by *Giardia lamblia*: possible implication for pathogenesis of intestinal disease. *J Clin Invest* 1985; 76:1727–1732.

67 Knodler L A, Svard S G, Silberman J D, Davids B J & Gillin F D. Developmental gene regulation in *Giardia lamblia*: first evidence for an encystation-specific promoter and differential 5′ mRNA processing. *Mol Microbiol* 1999; 34:327–340.

68 Meyer E A. *Giardia lamblia*: isolation and axenic cultivation. *Exp Parasitol* 1976; 39:101–105.

69 Lu S Q, Baruch A C & Adam R D. Molecular comparison of *Giardia lamblia* isolates. *Int J Parasitol* 1998; 28:1341–1345.

70 Thompson R C, Hopkins R M & Homan W L. Nomenclature and genetic groupings of *Giardia* infecting mammals. *Parasitol Today* 2000; 16:210–213.

71 Adam R D. The *Giardia lamblia* genome. *Int J Parasitol* 2000; 30:475–484.

72 Sullivan P B, Marsh M N, Phillips M B et al. Prevalence and treatment of giardiasis in chronic diarrhoea and malnutrition. *Arch Dis Child* 1991; 66:304–306.

73 Jokipii L & Jokipii A M. Giardiasis in travelers: a prospective study. *J Infect Dis* 1974; 30:295–299.

74 Craun G F. Waterborne outbreaks of giardiasis. Current status. In Erlandsen S L & Meyer E R (eds) *Giardia and Giardiasis*. New York: Plenum Press, 1984:243–261.

75 Jephcott A E, Begg N T & Baker I A. Outbreak of giardiasis associated with mains water in the United Kingdom. *Lancet* 1986; i:730–732.

76 Furness B W, Beach M J & Roberts J M. Giardiasis surveillance—United States, 1992–1997. *Morbid Mortal Weekly* 2000; 49:1–13.

77 Katelaris P H & Farthing M J G. Diarrhoea and malabsorption in giardiasis: a multifactorial process. *Gut* 1992; 33:295–297.

78 Farthing M J G. Diarrhoeal disease: current concepts and future challenges. Pathogenesis of giardiasis. *Trans R Soc Trop Med Hyg* 1993; 87 (Supplement 3):17–21.

79 Teoh D A, Kamieniecki D, Pang G & Buret A G. *Giardia lamblia* rearranges F-actin and alpha-actinin in human colonic and duodenal monolayers and reduces transepithelial electrical resistance. *J Parasitol* 2000; 86:800–806.

80 Roberts-Thomson I C & Mitchell F G. Giardiasis in mice. I. Prolonged infections in certain mouse strains and hypothymic (nude) mice. *Gastroenterology* 1978; 75:42–46.

81 Scott K G, Logan M R, Klammer G M, Teoh D A & Buret A G. Jejunal brush border microvillous alterations in *Giardia muris*-infected mice: role of T lymphocytes and interleukin-6. *Infect Immun* 2000; 68:3412–3418.

82 Das S, Schteingart C D, Hofmann A F, Reiner D S, Aley S B & Gillin F D. *Giardia lamblia*: evidence for carrier-mediated uptake and release of conjugated bile acids. *Exp Parasitol* 1997; 87:133–141.

83 Seow F, Katelaris P H & Ngu M. The effect of *Giardia lamblia* trophozoites on trypsin, chymotrypsin and amylase in vitro. *Parasitology* 1993; 106:233–238.

84 Faubert G. Immune response to *Giardia duodenalis*. *Clin Microbiol Rev* 2000; 13:35–54.

85 Farthing M J G, Chong S & Walker-Smith J A. Acute allergic phenomena in giardiasis. *Lancet* 1984; ii:1428.

86 Svard S G, Meng T C, Hetsko M L, McCaffery J M & Gillin F D. Differentiation-associated surface antigen variation in the ancient eukaryote *Giardia lamblia*. *Mol Microbiol* 1998; 30:979–989.

87 Nash T E. Antigenic variation in *Giardia lamblia* and the host's immune response. *Philos Trans R Soc Lond* [Biol] 1997; 352: 1369–1375.

88 Singer S M & Nash T E. T-cell-dependent control of acute *Giardia lamblia* infections in mice. *Infect Immun* 2000; 68:170–175.

89 Char S, Cevallos A M, Yamson P, Sullivan P B, Neale G & Farthing M J G. Impaired IgA response to *Giardia* heat shock antigen in children with persistent diarrhoea and giardiasis. *Gut* 1992; 34:38–40.

90 Farthing M J G, Mata L J, Urrutia J J & Kronmal R A. Giardiasis: impact on child growth. In Walker-Smith J A & McNeish A S (eds) *Diarrhea and Malnutrition in Childhood*. London: Butterworth, 1986:68–78.

91 Sullivan P B, Lunn P G, Northrop-Clewes C A & Farthing M J G. Parasitic infection of the gut and protein-losing enteropathy. *J Pediatr Gastroenterol Nutr* 1992; 15:404–407.

92 Goka A K J, Rolston D D K, Mathan V I & Farthing M J G. The relative merits of faecal and duodenal juice microscopy in the diagnosis of giardiasis. *Trans R Soc Trop Med Hyg* 1990; 84:66–67.

93 Green E L, Miles M A & Warhurst D C. Immunodiagnostic detection of *Giardia* antigen in faeces by a rapid visual enzyme-linked immunosorbent assay. *Lancet* 1985; ii:691–693.

94 Addiss D G, Sanders C A, Sonnad S S et al. Stool diagnosis of giardiasis using a commercially available enzyme immunoassay to detect *Giardia*-specific antigen 65 (GSA 65). *J Clin Microbiol* 1989; 27:1137–1142.

95 Aldeen W E, Carroll K, Robison A, Morrison M & Hale D. Comparison of nine commercially available enzyme-linked immunosorbent assays for detection of *Giardia lamblia* in fecal specimens. *J Clin Microbiol* 1998; 36:1338–1340.

96 Fedorko D P, Williams E C, Nelson N A, Calhoun L B & Yan S S. Performance of three enzyme immunoassays and two direct fluorescence assays for detection of *Giardia lamblia* in stool specimens preserved in ECOFIZ. *J Clin Microbiol* 2000; 38:2781–2783.

97 Char S & Farthing M J G. DNA probes for diagnosis of enteric infection. *Gut* 1991; 32:1–3.

98 Butcher P D & Farthing M J G. DNA probes for the faecal diagnosis of *Giardia lamblia* infections in man. *Biochem Soc Trans* 1988; 17:363–364.

99 Ghosh S, Debnath A, Sil A, De S, Chattopadhyay D J & Das P. PCR detection of *Giardia lamblia* in stool: targeting intergenic spacer region of multicopy rRNA gene. *Mol Cell Probes* 2000; 14:181–189.

100 Davidson R A. Issues in clinical parasitology: the treatment of giardiasis. *Am J Gastroenterol* 1984; 79:256–261.

101 Meloni B P, Thompson R C A, Reynoldson J A & Seville P. Albendazole: a more effective antigardial agent in vitro than metronidazole or tinidazole. *Trans R Soc Trop Med Hyg* 1990; 84:375–379.

102 Crouch A A, Seow W K, Whitman L M & Thong Y H. Sensitivity in vitro of *Giardia intestinalis* to dyadic combinations of azithromycin, deoxycline, mefloquine, tinidazole and furazolidone. *Trans R Soc Trop Med Hyg* 1990; 84:246–248.

103 Olson M E, Morck D W & Ceri H. Preliminary data on the efficacy of a Giardia vaccine in puppies. *Can Vet J* 1997; 38:777–779.

104 Olson M E, Ceri H & Morck D W. Giardia vaccination. *Parasitol Today* 2000; 16:213–217.

105 Arean V M & Koppisch E. Balantidiasis: a review and report of cases. *Am J Pathol* 1956; 32:1089–1115.

106 Walzer P D, Judson F N, Murphy K B, Healy G R, English D K & Schultz M G. Balantidiasis outbreak in Truk. *Am J Trop Med Hyg* 1973; 22:33–41.

107 Tyzzer E E. A sporozoan found in the peptic glands of the common mouse. *Proc Soc Exp Biol Med* 1907; 5:12–13.

108 Nime F A, Burek J D, Page D L & Hoescher M A. Acute enterocolitis in a human being infected with the protozoan *Cryptosporidium*. *Gastroenterology* 1976; 70:592–598.

109 Angus K W. Cryptosporidiosis and AIDS. *Baillieres Clin Gastroenterol* 1990; 4:425–440.

110 Petersen C. Cellular biology of *Cryptosporidium parvum*. *Parasitol Today* 1993; 9:87–91.

111 Morgan U M, Xiao L, Fayer R, Lal A A & Thompson R C A. Epidemiology and strain variation of *Cryptosporidium parvum*. In Petry F (ed.) *Cryptosporidiosis and Microsporidiosis. Contributions to Microbiolog*y, vol. 6. Basel: Karger, 2000:116–139.

112 McLauchlin J, Pedraza-Diaz S, Amar-Hoetzeneder C & Nichols G L. Genetic characterization of *Cryptosporidium* strains from 218 patients with diarrhea diagnosed as having sporadic cryptosporidiosis. *J Clin Microbiol* 1999; 37:3153–3158.

113 Sulaiman I M, Xiao L, Yang C et al. Differentiating human from animal isolates of *Cryptosporidium parvum*. *Emerging Infect Dis* 1998; 4:681–685.

114 Smith H V & Rose J B. Waterborne cryptosporidiosis. *Parasitol Today* 1990; 6:8–12.

115 Casemore D P. Epidemiological aspects of human cryptosporidiosis. *Epidemiol Infect* 1990; 104:1–28.

116 Zu S X, Zhu S Y & Li J F. Human cryptosporidiosis in China. *Trans R Soc Trop Med Hyg* 1992; 86:639–640.

117 Molbak K, Hojlyng N, Gottschau A et al. Cryptosporidiosis in infancy and childhood mortality in Guinea-Bissau, West Africa. *BMJ* 1993; 307:417–420.

118 Ungar B L P, Soave R, Fayer R & Nash T E. Enzyme immunoassay detection of IgM and IgG antibodies to *Cryptosporidium* in immunocompetent and immunocompromised persons. *J Infect Dis* 1986; 153:570–577.

119 Ravn P, Lungren J D, Kjaeldgaard P et al. Nosocomial outbreak of cryptosporidiosis in AIDS patients. *BMJ* 1991; 302:277–280.

120 Blanshard C, Jackson A M, Shanson D C, Francis N & Gazzard B. Cryptosporidiosis in HIV seropositive patients. *Q J Med* 1992; 85:813–823.

121 Phillips A D, Thomas A G & Walker-Smith JA. *Cryptosporidium*, chronic diarrhoea and the proximal small intestinal mucosa. *Gut* 1992; 33:1057–1061.

122 Goodgame R W, Genta R M, White A C & Chappell C L. Intensity of infection in AIDS associated cryptosporidiosis. *J Infect Dis* 1993; 167:704–709.

123 Buret A, Gall D G, Nation P N & Olson M E. Intestinal protozoa and epithelial cell kinetics, structure and function. *Parasitol Today* 1990; 6:375–380.

124 Tzipori S. Cryptosporidiosis in perspective. *Adv Parasitol* 1988; 27:63–129.

125 Kelly P, Thillainayagam A V, Smithson J et al. Jejunal water and electrolyte transport in human cryptosporidiosis. *Dig Dis Sci* 1996; 41:2095–2099.

126 Jacyna M R, Parkin J, Goldin R & Baron J H. Protracted enteric cryptosporidial infection in selective immunoglobulin A and saccharomyces opsonin deficiencies. *Gut* 1990; 31:714–716.

127 Kelly P, Jack D, Naeem A et al. Mannose binding lectin is a contributor to mucosal defence against *Cryptosporidium parvum* in AIDS patients. *Gastroenterology* 2000; 119:1236–1242.

128 Connolly G M, Dryden M S, Shanson D C & Gazzard B G. Cryptosporidial diarrhoea in AIDS and its treatment. *Gut* 1988; 29:593–597.

129 McGowan I, Hawkins A & Weller I. The natural history of cryptosporidial diarrhoea in HIV infected patients. *AIDS* 1993; 7:349–354.

130 Colebunders R, Francis H, Mann J M et al. Persistent diarrhea, strongly associated with HIV infection in Kinshasa, Zaire. *Am J Gastroenterol* 1987; 82:859–864.

131 Teixidor H S, Godwin T A & Ramirez E A. Cryptosporidiosis of the biliary tract in AIDS. *Radiology* 1991; 180:51–56.

132 Forbes A, Blanshard C & Gazzard B. Natural history of AIDS related sclerosing cholangitis: a study of 20 cases. *Gut* 1993; 34:116–121.

133 Molbak K, Hojlyng N, Gottschau A et al. Cryptosporidiosis in infancy and childhood mortality in Guinea-Bissau, West Africa. *BMJ* 1993; 307:417–420.

134 Molbak K, Andersen M, Aaby P et al. *Cryptosporidium* infection in infancy as a cause of malnutrition: a community study from Guinea-Bissau, West Africa. *Am J Clin Nutr* 1997; 65:149–152.

135 Amadi B C, Kelly P, Mwiya M et al. Intestinal and systemic infection, HIV and mortality in Zambian children with persistent diarrhoea and malnutrition. *J Pediatr Gastroenterol Nutr* 2001; 32:550–554.

136 Weber R, Bryan R T, Bishop H S, Wahlquist S P, Sullivan J J & Juranek D D. Threshold of detection of *Cryptosporidium* oocysts in human stool specimens: evidence for low sensitivity of current diagnostic methods. *J Clin Microbiol* 1991; 29:1323–1327.

137 Ungar B L P. ELISA for detection of cryptosporidial antigens in faecal specimens. *J Clin Microbiol* 1990; 28:2491–2495.

138 Chapman P A, Rush B & McLauchlin J. An EIA for detecting cryptosporidia in faecal and environmental samples. *J Med Microbiol* 1990; 32:233–237.

139 Webster K. Molecular methods for detection and classification of *Cryptosporidium*. *Parasitol Today* 1993; 9:263–266.

140 Casemore D P, Blewett D A & Wright S E. Cleaning and disinfection of equipment for gastrointestinal flexible endoscopy: interim recommendations of a working party of the British Society of Gastroenterology. *Gut* 1990; 31:1156–1157 (letter).

141 Stürchler D. Parasitic diseases of the small intestinal tract. *Baillieres Clin Gastroenterol* 1987; 1:397–424.

142 Brandborg L L, Goldberg S B & Breidenbach W C. Human coccidiosis—a possible cause of malabsorption. *N Engl J Med* 1970; 283:1306–1313.

143 Trier J S, Moxey P C, Schimmel E M & Robles E. Chronic intestinal coccidiosis in man: intestinal pathology and response to treatment. *Gastroenterology* 1974; 66:923–935.

144 De Hovitz J A, Pape J W, Boncy M & Johnson W D. Clinical manifestations and therapy of *Isospora belli* infection in patients with AIDS. *N Engl J Med* 1986; 315:87–90.

145 Pape J W, Verdier R I & Johnson W D. Treatment and prophylaxis of *Isospora belli* infections in patients with AIDS. *N Engl J Med* 1989; 320:1044–1047.

146 Ortega Y R, Sterling C R, Gilman R H, Cama V A & Diaz F. *Cyclospora* species—a new protozoan pathogen of humans. *N Engl J Med* 1993; 328:1308–1312.

147 Sun T, Hardi C F, Asnis D et al. Light and electron microscopic identification of *Cyclospora* species in the small intestine: evidence of the presence of asexual life cycle in human host. *Am J Clin Pathol* 1996: 105:215–220.

148 Relman D A, Schmidt T M, Gajadhar A et al. Molecular phylogenetic analysis of *Cyclospora*, the human intestinal pathogen, suggests that it is closely related to *Eimeria* species. *J Infect Dis* 1996; 173:440–445.

149 Hoge C W, Shlim D R, Rajah R et al. Epidemiology of diarrhoeal illness associated with coccidian-like organism among travellers and foreign residents in Nepal. *Lancet* 1993; 341:1175–1179.

150 Huang P, Weber J T, Sosin D M et al. The first reported outbreak of diarrheal illness associated with *Cyclospora* in the United States. *Ann Intern Med* 1995; 123: 409–414.

151 Herwaldt B I, Ackers M-L, Farrar J et al. An outbreak in 1996 of cyclosporiasis associated with imported raspberries. *N Engl J Med* 1997; 336:1548–1556.

152 Bendall R P, Lucas S, Moody A, Tovey G & Chiodini P L. Diarrhoea associated with cyanobacterium-like bodies: a new coccidian enteritis of man. *Lancet* 1993; 341:590–592.

153 Hoge C W, Shlim D R, Ghimire M et al. Placebo-controlled trial of co-trimoxatole for *Cyclospora* infections among travellers and foreign residents in Nepal. *Lancet* 1995; 345:667–668, 691–693.

154 Verdier R-I, Fitzgerald D W, Johnson W D Jr & Paper J W. Trimethoprim–sulfamethoxazole compared with ciprofloxacin for treatment and prophylaxis of *Isopora belli* and *Cyclospora cayetanensis* infection in HIV-infected patients. A randomized, controlled trial. *Ann Intern Med* 2000; 132:885–888.

155 Desportes-Livage I. Biology of microsporidia. In Petry F (ed.) *Cryptosporidiosis and Microsporidiosis. Contributions to Microbiology*, vol. 6. Basel: Karger, 2000:116–139.

156 Modigliani R, Bories C, le Charpentier Y et al. Diarrhoea and malabsorption in AIDS: a study of four cases with special emphasis on opportunistic protozoan infections. *Gut* 1985; 26:179–187.

157 Canning E U & Hollister W S. *Enterocytozoon bieneusi* (Microspora): prevalence and pathogenicity in AIDS patients. *Trans R Soc Trop Med Hyg* 1990; 84:181–186.

158 Cali A & Owen R L. Intracellular development of *Enterocytozoon*, a unique microsporidian found in the intestine of AIDS patients. *J Protozool* 1990; 37:145–155.

159 Peacock C S, Blanshard C, Tovey D G, Ellis D S & Gazzard B G. Histological diagnosis of intestinal microsporidiosis in patients with AIDS. *J Clin Pathol* 1991; 44:558–563.

160 Orenstein J M, Tenner M & Kotler D P. Localization of infection by the microsporidian *Enterocytozoon bieneusi* in the gastrointestinal tract of AIDS patients with diarrhoea. *AIDS* 1992; 6:195–197.

161 Rabeneck L, Gyorkey F, Genta R M, Gyorkey P, Foote L W & Risser J. The role of microsporidia in the pathogenesis of HIV-related chronic diarrhea. *Ann Intern Med* 1993; 119:895–899.

162 Eeftinck-Shattenkerk J K M, Van Gool T, Van Ketel R J et al. Clinical significance of small intestinal microsporidiosis in HIV-1 infected individuals. *Lancet* 1991; 337:895–898.

163 Field A S, Hing M C, Millikan S T & Marriott D J. Microsporidia in the small intestine of HIV-infected patients. A new diagnostic technique and a new species. *Med J Aust* 1993; 158:390–394.

164 Pol S, Romana C A, Richard S et al. Microsporidia infection in patients with HIV and unexplained cholangitis. *N Engl J Med* 1993; 328:95–99.

165 Beauvais B, Sarfati C, Molina J M, Lesourd A, Lariviere M & Derouin F. Comparative evaluation of five diagnostic methods for demonstrating microsporidia in stool and intestinal biopsy specimens. *Ann Trop Med Parasitol* 1993; 87:99–102.

166 Weber R, Bryan R T, Owen R L, Wilcox C M, Gorelkin L & Visvesara G S. Improved light microscopical detection of microsporidia spores in stool and duodenal aspirates. *N Engl J Med* 1992; 326:161–166.

167 Blanshard C, Ellis D S, Tovey D G, Dowell S & Gazzard B. Treatment of intestinal microsporidiosis with albendazole in patients with AIDS. *AIDS* 1992; 6:311.

168 Weber R, Deplazes P & Schwartz D. Diagnosis and clinical aspects of human microsporidiosis. In Petry F (ed.) *Cryptosporidiosis and Microsporidiosis. Contributions to Microbiology*, vol. 6. Basel: Karger. 2000:116–139.

169 Hollister W S & Canning E U. An ELISA for detection of antibodies to *Encephalitozoon cuniculi* and its use in determination of infections in man. *Parasitology* 1987; 94:209–219.

170 Molina J M, Oksenhendler E, Beauvais B et al. Disseminated microsporidiosis due to *Septata intestinalis* in patients with AIDS: clinical features and response to albendazole therapy. *J Infect Dis* 1995; 171:245–249.

Chapter 78
Potentially Pathogenic Free-living Amoebae

D. C. Warhurst

For many years the only amoeba thought to be of significance in human disease was the obligate parasite *Entamoeba histolytica*. It is now recognized that facultatively parasitic free-living amoebae, normally found in soil and water, cause three important diseases in man: primary amoebic meningoencephalitis (PAM), granulomatous amoebic encephalitis (GAE) with invasion of other tissues, and chronic amoebic keratitis (CAK). Both PAM and CAK occur in healthy individuals, while GAE and related diseases are generally associated with immuno-deficient states.[1]

The free-living amoebae concerned belong to three groups: amoeboflagellates, Acanthamoebidae and Leptomyxida.

Amoeboflagellates

Naegleria fowleri, which causes PAM, is found worldwide in warm fresh water, normally feeding on bacteria. Its life cycle has three stages: the feeding, growing, multiplying form or trophozoite found on surfaces of vegetation and mud; the rapidly motile biflagellate form (Figure 78.1) found in the surface layers of water; and the dormant cyst form found in the same locations as the trophozoite.

Experimental and epidemiological evidence supports the infectivity to man of the trophozoite and flagellate. Infection takes place through the olfactory epithelium of the nose when the organisms are inhaled in contaminated water, usually during swimming, penetrate the epithelium and pass along the olfactory nerve branches in the cribriform plate to enter the meninges, where they multiply in the perivascular Virchow–Robin spaces. Trophozoites penetrate the substance of the brain, ingesting cerebral tissue (Figure 78.2). The symptoms and features of the CSF are characteristic of a purulent bacterial meningitis, but there is no response to antibacterials. Coma culminates in death. The application of specific therapy after early diagnosis of the condition has led to recovery in only four of more than 172[2] recorded cases. Although relatively few cases of PAM are recorded, the disease is significant among those associated with recreational water use because of its almost invariably fatal outcome. In the 10 years from 1989, 22 cases of PAM caused by *N. fowleri* were reported in the USA, all fatal. Cases of illness associated with recreational water use totalled 7359 (omitting

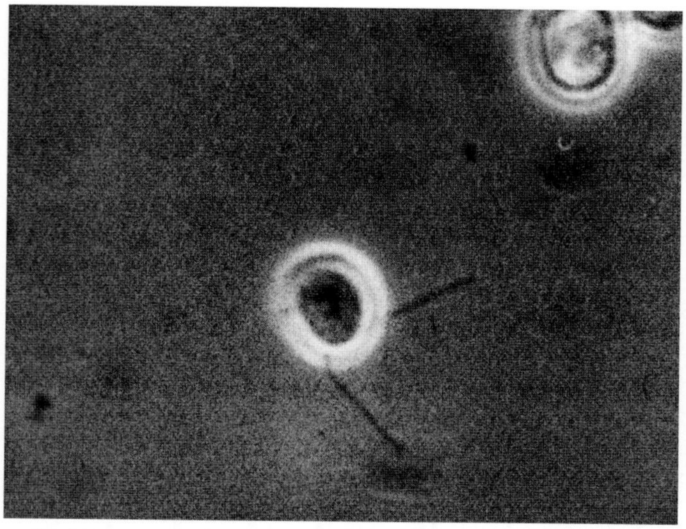

Figure 78.1: Flagellate stage of *Naegleria fowleri*. (Environmental isolate; organism fixed with osmic acid vapour and examined under phase contrast.)

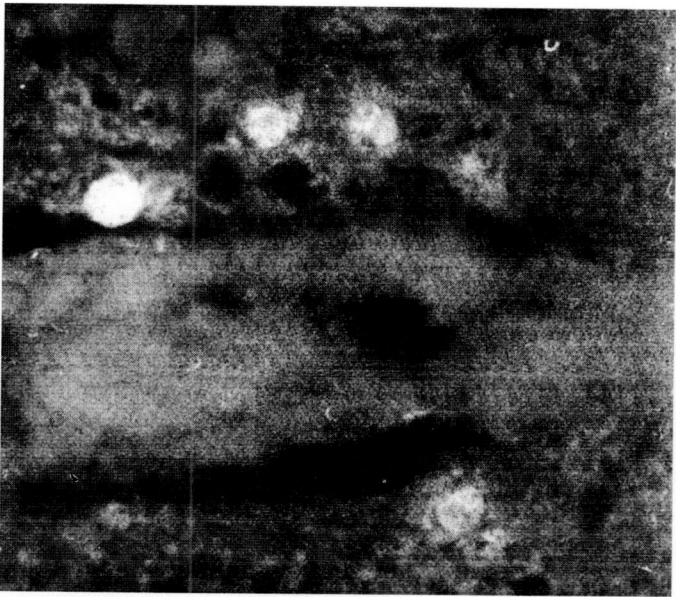

Figure 78.2: *Naegleria fowleri* in human brain section. (Stained by specific fluorescent antibody test. This shows a cerebral vessel, and *Naegleria* trophozoites invading the brain tissue from the perivascular CSF.)

two large outbreaks of recreational water-associated cryptosporidiosis occurring in 1995–6): *N. fowleri* was responsible for 0.3% of these non-cryptosporidial cases. Since only one other cause of death in recreational water-associated illness was reported over the period (*E. coli* 0157), *N. fowleri* was responsible for 96% of the deaths.[3]

Acanthamoebidae

Acanthamoeba species which cause GAE and CAK are found worldwide and also feed on bacteria. They are not necessarily associated with warm fresh water, and can also multiply in brackish conditions. The life cycle consists only of the trophozoite and cyst forms, and either of these can be a source of infection for man. Several species of the genus have been isolated from human tissue, and the ubiquitous distribution of these organisms means that human exposure is widespread. For example, it is estimated that humans inhale one of the resistant cysts every day.[4] As a corollary of this wide exposure, the organism finds it difficult to colonize man, and infections are generally restricted to the immunodeficient or to immunoprivileged sites, the most common of which is the cornea (Figures 78.3 and 78.4). Infections are generally of a chronic type and there is a marked granulomatous tissue reaction. Treatment by medical or surgical means is usually successful in ocular infection, but a few successes have been reported in systemic infection.

Acanthamoeba and upper respiratory infection

Association of *Acanthamoeba* with upper respiratory infections was suspected in the 1960s[5] and the organism has been regularly isolated from oronasal swabs. Several strains isolated from room and outside air using a slit sampler were found to be cytopathic to mammalian cell cultures.[4] Although there is a suggestive link between the isolation of *Acanthamoeba* from the upper respiratory tract and nose bleeding, rhinitis and upper respiratory infections, the connection has not yet been convincingly

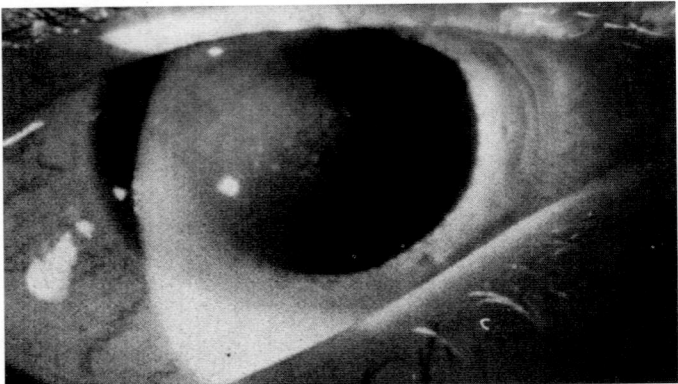

Figure 78.3: *Acanthamoeba* species keratitis. Corneal ulceration, hypopyon, conjunctival hyperaemia and radial neuritis are visible in this photograph of an infected eye.

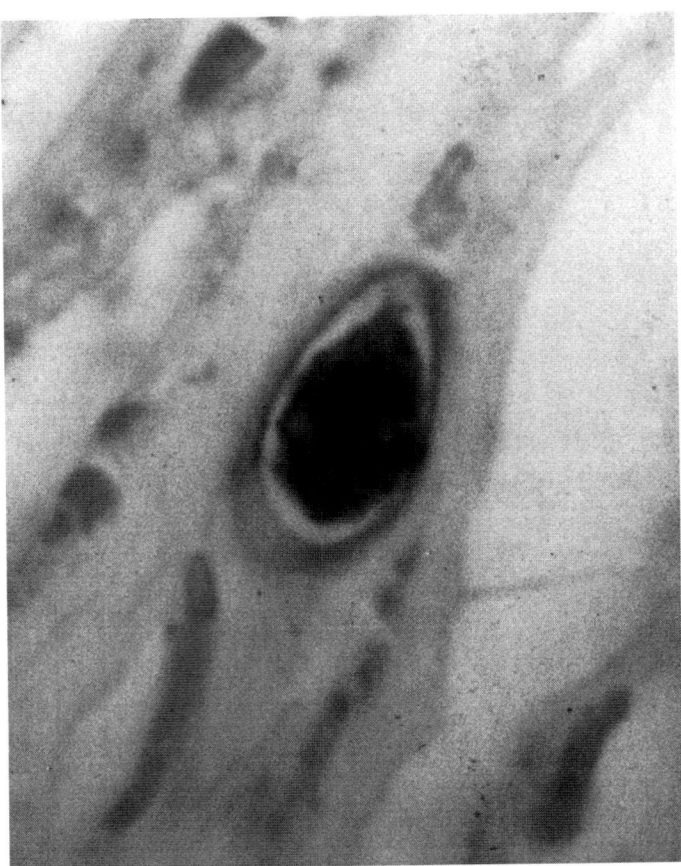

Figure 78.4: Encysting trophozoite of *Acanthamoeba* species in corneal laminae. (Stained with immunoperoxidase using rabbit anti-*Acanthamoeba* serum. Note cellular infiltration and the heavily stained amoebic trophozoite.)

drawn. It may be argued that, in some cases at least, isolations from the nose represent trapped airborne cysts, and not active infections.

Leptomyxida

Among more than 56 case reports of GAE, mainly due to infection with *Acanthamoeba* species, are a few cases of infection with leptomyxid free-living amoebae (now designated *Balamuthia mandrillaris*). The predisposing factors are apparently similar to those for systemic *Acanthamoeba* infection, and the life cycle of the leptomyxids also resembles that of these amoebae. Nothing is yet known about treatment, and diagnosis may prove difficult. These amoebae are not known to cause CAK.[6] A recent molecular study has produced evidence that the Leptomyxida are polyphyletic, and that *B. mandrillaris* does not belong in the order.[7]

Association of free-living amoebae with *Legionella* and other bacteria

Acanthamoeba species and *Naegleria* species can harbour

pathogenic micro-organisms such as *Legionella*[8,9] and the cholera vibrio[10] and are thought capable of serving as chlorine-resistant infection reservoirs for these organisms in water supplies. The short incubation period, non-pneumonic form of legionellosis, 'Pontiac fever', and 'humidifier fever', are both thought to be linked to hypersensitivity reactions to free-living amoebae in air-conditioning systems.[11,12]

Primary amoebic meningoencephalitis
Clinical features[13]

In the first documented case of infection, *Naegleria* was found disseminated in many tissues,[14,15] but this is the only such report and the patient was severely malnourished. *N. fowleri* is normally restricted to the central nervous system.

The illness begins 3–7 days after exposure to contaminated water, in patients previously of good health, with headache and slight pyrexia, in some cases associated with sore throat and rhinitis. Over the next 3 days the disease progresses, with rising fever and increasing headache, vomiting and stiff neck. The severely disoriented or comatose patient is admitted to hospital with a diagnosis of acute pyogenic meningitis. Lumbar puncture reveals a purulent cerebrospinal fluid (CSF) but no bacteria are demonstrated. The CSF pressure is generally raised. No response is noted to antibacterials. Deep coma is followed by cardiorespiratory failure and death ensues.[16] Haemorrhagic pulmonary oedema may develop during the course of the disease and this is thought to be neurogenic.[17] In addition, myocarditis may be detected at post-mortem.[18]

Although involvement with water sports antecedes most cases, some fatal infections reported from Australia have been acquired from the mains water supply. In one US case,[15,19] the patient, a narcotic addict, who had recently had teeth extracted, had no history of water contact other than with public water supplies; and a Nigerian farmer is thought to have become infected after ritual nose rinsing with water from a local pond.[20]

Diagnosis

The major problem in diagnosis of PAM is to distinguish between it and other encephalitides of rapid onset such as meningococcal, acute tubercular and viral meningitis. Distinction from all but non-tubercular bacterial meningitis is relatively straightforward because on CSF examination there is a markedly raised cell count, mainly polymorphonuclear cells. In tubercular or viral meningitis the cellular increase, when present, is composed mainly of mononuclear cells. The presence of erythrocytes in CSF has been suggested as characteristic of PAM, but evidence so far does not confirm its specificity and, in addition,

erythrocytes may accidentally contaminate CSF during the lumbar puncture procedure. CSF protein is generally above 1 g/l and may be up to 10 g/l, and this contrasts with viral meningitis where low values are usually found. Glucose may be lower than normal, as in bacterial meningitis, but this is not a useful diagnostic feature.

It is recommended that in investigation of CSF from meningitis cases a fraction of the CSF should be put on one side while the film is being stained for bacteria, so that if bacteria are not seen the CSF can be examined in wet film in more detail. Observation of the CSF under a coverslip is a procedure which may give much information. First, in the case of bacterial meningitis, the presence of bacteria may be observed directly, before cultures have grown. If no bacteria are seen, amoebic trophozoites may be discovered. Here there is scope for error. Highly active mononuclear or other white cells may be found in the CSF, and unless careful observation is made to detect the large granular nucleus and the non-progressive movement of the mammalian cells, the cells may be mistaken for amoebae. In CSF, *Naegleria* moves actively at a rate of one to three body lengths per minute. The movement is progressive and the body is elongated like a slug during movement, with characteristic explosive protrusion of a clear pseudopodium on alternate sides of the anterior. Warming the wet preparation may be a useful method of stimulating movement.

As well as wet microscopy, examination of cytospin films stained by a Romanovsky stain should be carried out. An acridine orange stain with examination under the fluorescent microscope[17] may also be useful to differentiate the amoebae from leucocytes, the small nucleus and large area of reddish foamy cytoplasm of the amoebae being particularly noteworthy.[21]

To confirm the diagnosis after treatment has been instituted, cultures of the CSF sample upon 1.5% non-nutrient agar coated with washed *E. coli* bacteria and maintained in a moist box at 37°C overnight should be examined. The agar may be made up in distilled water or ideally in the dilute amoeba saline solution of Page:[22]

NaCl	0.12 g
$MgSO_4.7H_2O$	0.004 g
$CaCl_2.2H_2O$	0.004 g
Na_2HPO_4	0.14 g
KH_2PO_4	0.136 g

in 1 litre distilled water, autoclaved in 100 ml aliquots and stored at room temperature.

N. fowleri will grow in cell cultures used in the usual virus isolation techniques, and these may be used as an isolation method. It is important to ensure that antifungals such as amphotericin (Fungizone) are not included in the cultures.

N. fowleri-specific monoclonal antibodies have been developed which are likely to prove valuable in diagnosis,[23,24] and isoenzyme,[25] restriction digestion[26] and polymerase chain reaction (PCR) techniques for identification of *N. fowleri* from environmental and pathological material have been described.[27]

Management

There is a shortage of successful treatments on which to base recommendations. However, in all except one of four successfully treated cases, success followed the institution of a high-dose regimen of amphotericin B after early diagnosis of the infection.

It is informative to compare two case histories in female children of 9 (case 2, Table 78.1) and 11 years of age.[29,32] A mild headache was the first indication of the disease, with no upper respiratory symptoms noted. Treatment in the former case was successful. The patient had been swimming in a hot spring where a fatal case of PAM had been acquired in 1971.[33] Before admission the patient had a 3-day history of symptoms, initially headache, followed by nausea, vomiting and increasing lethargy. On the morning of admission she was unresponsive. A diagnosis of bacterial meningitis was made on the cell count and chemical features of the CSF. Cells with amoeboid movement were observed in the CSF and in stained preparations[34] in the County Hospital to which she was transferred, and a diagnosis of PAM was made. The treatment was begun while the patient was responsive to pain and to tactile stimulation. Although nuchal rigidity and diffuse papilloedema were present, muscle tone and deep tendon reflexes were normal. Serum electrolytes, blood urea nitrogen and glucose were within normal limits and, significantly, computed tomography showed cerebral oedema was mild. Combination drug treatment was successful in achieving removal of detectable amoebae from the CSF and stabilization of the patient's condition after 3 days. During the remainder of her stay in hospital the patient's condition continued to improve, although after discharge some decrease in pain sensation in the left leg was noted, which resolved within 2 months, while the CSF remained abnormal for several months. Subsequent cases in the USA treated with a similar though not identical regimen have not survived.[35]

Table 78.1 Details of four successfully treated cases of primary amoebic meningoencephalitis

Location	Culture proof	Delayed (cerebral oedema, coma, etc.)	Antiamoebic drug treatment
Case 1			
S. Australia[28]	Yes	>3 days (coma, responding to painful stimuli)	Amphotericin B: 1.0 mg/kg per day i.v. × 5, then 0.5 mg intrathecally and a ventricular reservoir fitted to allow 10 doses of 0.1 mg on alternate days, with Stemetil premedication. The intraventricular amphotericin dose was mixed with CSF prior to administration (K. Anderson, personal communication)
Case 2			
California[30]	Yes	3 days (mild: coma, responding to painful stimuli)	Amphotericin B: 1.5 mg/kg per day i.v. in 2 divided doses for 3 days then 1 mg/kg per day for 6 days. For the first 2 days 0.15 mg amphotericin was given per day intrathecally and then 0.1 mg every other day for 8 days; miconazole intravenously 350 mg/m² of body surface per day in 3 divided doses for 9 days; miconazole intrathecally, 10 mg/day and then 10 mg every other day for 8 days, and rifampicin orally at 10 mg/kg per day in 3 divided doses for 9 days. Dexamethasone and phenytoin were given respectively for increased intracranial pressure and for seizures
Case 3			
Pennsylvania[31]	No	<13 hours (mild)	Amphotericin B: 75 mg/day i.v. (weight not given, but adult male). Oral rifampicin by nasogastric tube, 600 mg twice a day. In addition on the next day, an Ommaya reservoir was fitted to give intrathecal amphotericin B: 0.1 mg with 0.25 mg dexamethasone in 0.4 ml dextrose and water, on every other day. Therapy continued for 10 days
Case 4			
Northern Thailand[32]	No, on six occasions	1–2 days (purposefully responsive to painful stimuli. No evidence of cerebral oedema)	Amphotericin B: 0.5 mg/kg per day i.v. for 14 days, rising from 10 to 50 mg/day; oral rifampicin (600 mg/day) and oral ketoconazole (800 mg/day) for 1 month cured the patient, with no recurrence

The second patient, at Bath Spa, UK, was also admitted to hospital with a 3-day history of headache and a 1-day history of pyrexia, vomiting and blurred vision. She had swum in a warm mineral water pool 6 days previously. The patient was drowsy, with slight neck stiffness. Eye movements and fundi were normal. Thus the clinical condition on admission to hospital was apparently no worse than in the first case. On the basis of purulent CSF and other characteristic features a diagnosis of pyogenic meningitis was made, and treatment with antibacterial antibiotics was instituted. The condition of the patient deteriorated during the next few hours, and convulsions began to occur which were controlled with phenytoin, diazepam and intramuscular paraldehyde. The optic fundi remained normal, but cerebral oedema was assumed to be present, and mannitol was given intravenously. Respiratory arrest occurred 20 hours after admission, and at 36 hours identification of amoebae was made in the CSF, followed by culture, and antiamoebic therapy (amphotericin B 0.5 mg/kg per day by single 6-hourly intravenous infusion, concurrently with sulfadimidine and rectal metronidazole) was begun. Amphotericin B (0.15 mg) was administered through a ventricular catheter. Although it had been planned to increase the intravenous amphotericin dose to 1 mg/kg per day, poor urinary output and rising blood urea led to only 0.6 mg/kg being achieved. On day 3, 0.05 mg amphotericin was given, and on day 4, 0.1 mg intraventricularly. Although amoebae were then absent from the CSF (and not detected by culture), the patient did not wake from her coma and died on day 5 after cardiac arrest.

A significant difference between the two cases is that the clinicians and laboratory staff in the first were aware of the possibility of PAM, having seen an earlier fatal case acquired from the same stream, and identification of amoebae in the CSF was made soon after the patient was admitted to hospital. Differences in the treatment may also have been significant, in particular the initial lower intravenous dose of amphotericin in the fatal case, but early diagnosis is clearly to be aimed at. It is, however, important to note that studies on DNA from the isolate from the Californian case indicate that the *N. fowleri* involved was an unusual variety which had a restriction pattern that diverges most from all other strains tested.[24]

Recommendations for treatment were made by Duma.[36] The administration of amphotericin B should not be delayed once diagnosis of the condition has been made. In addition, the approach that is normally made to intravenous amphotericin treatment for other conditions, that is, to start at a lower dose (0.25–0.5 mg/kg per day) and increase it cautiously to detect idiosyncrasy and delay kidney damage, is inappropriate. After a low trial dose the maximum dose possible should be given immediately, by slow intravenous infusion. Judging by the intrathecal dose of amphotericin B used in case 1, it appears that there is some scope for increase. It is recognized that children can tolerate higher doses of amphotericin B than adults (see also references 37 and 38). The Thai report, however, maintains that a gradual increase in amphotericin dose is best. An argument maintained by Ferrante[39] is that too high a dose of the drug leads to lysis of amoebae and an adverse immunological reaction to the released foreign protein. However, it may be relevant to point out that the Thai case is abnormal in several respects. No history of swimming or exposure to water could be elucidated, although as the patient was a gardener, hose-pipe spray exposure might have been responsible. Also the patient was older than usual (61 years) and may have acquired some immunity. Another significant point is that six unsuccessful attempts were made to culture the amoebae. However, the prompt institution of rifamycin and ketoconazole oral therapy may be significant. Ferrante's point is probably best addressed by the judicious use of corticosteroids to moderate the inflammatory reaction, as in cases 2 and 3.

It is important to monitor the blood urea nitrogen value daily during amphotericin treatment, and the manufacturers recommend that if this rises above 17.8 mmol/litre (50 mg/dl), or the creatinine above 310 μmol/litre (3.5 mg/dl), one day of therapy should be omitted and the next dose lowered. Amphotericin B methyl ester, a less toxic modification of the drug, though active in vitro, has not been found effective in protecting experimental mice.[40]

The use of drug combinations

In in vitro and animal studies a potentiative synergism of amphotericin with tetracycline,[41,42] miconazole[43] and rifampicin[44] has been reported. The rationale for using combination drug treatment with miconazole is supported by in vitro studies carried out on the strain of *N. fowleri* isolated from the CSF in the Californian case, since synergism was seen with amphotericin. Synergism was not demonstrated between rifampicin and amphotericin, but there was clearly an additive effect, while the effects of rifampicin and miconazole were apparently mildly antagonistic. In the view of the present author there is still some doubt as to whether combination drug treatments are really necessary, but provided there is no evidence of antagonism with amphotericin B there seems no reason not to try them. It is worth noting that for *Candida albicans* miconazole is antagonistic to amphotericin B,[45] but this was not seen for *N. fowleri*. Ketoconazole appears to be an alternative to miconazole and potentially less toxic.

Pathology and pathogenesis

N. fowleri injures nerve cells by two alternate mechanisms: trogocytosis (ingestion of the cytoplasm through a feeding cup), and contact-dependent lysis due to alteration of the permeability of the target cell by lytic proteins. Cell death is due to the release of ions, followed later by the loss of large macromolecules.[46]

The pathogenic process in the brain is probably similar to that in bacterial meningitis. An inflammatory reaction develops in the meninges and the cellular influx leads to damage of the cellular functions of the blood–brain barrier. In addition there is damage to the integrity of the barrier due to direct invasion of amoebae into the brain tissue, which occurs without obvious cellular reaction.

Although it probably has no relevance to the pathogenesis of PAM, it is interesting to note that even non-pathogenic species of *Naegleria* harbour an agent capable of causing cytopathic changes in cultured vertebrate cells. The agent is termed NACM (*Naegleria* amoeba cytopathic agent) and is a protein of 35 kDa. NACM shows the features of an infectious agent, with some similarity to a prion.[47]

Immunology

Reciprocal titres in the indirect fluorescent antibody test of 5 to 20 were found in a survey of normal human sera in New Zealand.[48] It will probably be concluded that for such low titres to be found in such a sensitive test indicates little exposure and probable cross-reactivity with antigens from related or unrelated species. The disease course is too rapid in the majority of clinical cases for humoral antibody to be stimulated, but it has been demonstrated in a recovered case. Although a low total serum IgA level has been postulated to be a predisposing factor in infection,[49] this has not been confirmed.[50] Evidence has been obtained experimentally in BALB/c mice that immunity can be transferred by immune spleen cells but not by immune serum.[51] However, an earlier study did show transfer by immune serum.[52] There is experimental evidence that immunity is manifested at the nasal mucosa by polymorphonuclear leucocytes, which kill the amoebae, and also by the shedding of necrotic epithelium.[53]

Although the amoebae are unaffected by recombinant human interleukin 1 or tumour necrosis factor,[54] the latter stimulates the adherence of neutrophils to *N. fowleri*, with destruction of the amoeba. This is independent of complement or specific immunoglobulin. Ingestion of neutrophils by trophozoites was observed following more prolonged incubation, particularly in the absence of tumour necrosis factor. Ability of trophozoites to ingest host neutrophils may represent a virulence factor.[55]

The trophozoites are killed by complement[56] in the bloodstream, and this probably explains the usual restriction to the CNS.

Epidemiology

N. fowleri has been isolated from thermally elevated aquatic environments worldwide, but temperature factors associated with occurrence of the amoeba remain relatively undefined. It is interesting that, although *N. fowleri* will grow well at temperatures up to 45°C, cysts are not readily produced at high temperatures, in contrast to the non-pathogenic species *N. lovaniensis*,[57] which also grows at 45°C. This may perhaps explain the persistence of *N. fowleri* in areas of fluctuating temperature or exposure to a temperature gradient. At Bath Spa[58] *N. fowleri* was isolated from water in an area where warm water mixed with cool, and only *N. lovaniensis* in a site where the water was uniformly at a high temperature. In a study of a newly created cooling reservoir (Clinton Lake, Illinois) before and after thermal additions from a nuclear power plant, *N. fowleri* was isolated from the thermally elevated arm but not from the ambient-temperature arm of the reservoir. The probability of isolating thermophilic *Naegleria* and pathogenic *N. fowleri* increased significantly with temperature. Repetitive DNA restriction fragment profiles of the *N. fowleri* Clinton Lake isolates and a known *N. fowleri* strain of human origin were homologous.[59] This suggests that even in temperate areas we can expect *N. fowleri* colonization of any newly introduced heated freshwater habitats, such as warm pools. Isolation of the amoebae from environmental sources is difficult since overgrowth of non-pathogenic species such as *N. lovaniensis* readily takes place. To avoid this it is recommended that multiple small water samples of 10 ml should be collected, concentrated by gentle centrifugation, and each sediment cultured on a different culture plate.[60] The use of swab samples from surfaces has also been reported to increase success in isolating pathogenic free-living amoebae.[61]

Prevention

In the North Island of New Zealand the bathing places fed by hot springs are generally lined with earth, and the only preventive measures which are applicable are warnings not to immerse the head. These are presented to the public in graphic notices around the pools. In the UK, the contaminated pools associated with the Bath Spa mineral spring have been closed for bathing, and a borehole has been drilled into the aquifer, allowing hot water to reach the surface uncontaminated.

Water treatment
Filtration
Treatment of raw water to be used for drinking purposes by coagulation and filtration is generally effective for removal of organisms which do not multiply in the environment, such as bacterial pathogens, *Entamoeba histolytica* and *Giardia*. In the case of the potentially pathogenic free-living amoebae, even one organism which passes through the filter is significant, since unlimited multiplication is possible in the 'purified' water provided a suitable bacterial food source is present. Chemical or physical disinfection is therefore the only suitable approach.

Physical treatment
N. fowleri is not usually isolated from waters at temperatures below 25°C. The cysts and trophozoites are killed by temperatures above 60°C. Attractive recreational waters generally exceed 25°C and are at well below amoebicidal

temperatures. The amoebae will grow at a wide range of pH in culture, although growth halts below pH 4.6 and above pH 9.5. Ultraviolet radiation appears ineffective in preventing *Naegleria* or bacterial contamination of swimming pools.[62]

Chemical treatment

N. fowleri will not grow in brackish water. Concentrations of sodium chloride of more than 0.75% will inhibit growth. It has also been shown experimentally that high concentrations of calcium (40–60 mmol/l) are inhibitory.[63]

The cysts of *N. fowleri*, like those of *E. histolytica* and *Giardia*, need a free chlorine residual concentration (mg/l) × time (minutes) factor (CT factor) in the region of 40 for 99.9% inactivation,[64] i.e. 4 mg/litre for 10 minutes or 2 mg/litre for 20 minutes. (Depending on the amount of organic material capable of reacting with chlorine present in the water, an initial quantity of chlorine added will produce different residual concentrations of chlorine available for microbial inactivation. In any experimental study it is therefore important to determine the residual concentration of chlorine which remains after the experiment. This level only is relevant in determination of microbial sensitivity. The pH of the water is also relevant, since the active chemical species HOCl, hypochlorous acid, decreases in concentration as pH is raised.) However, the trophozoites are killed by lower chlorine residuals in the antibacterial region of 0.5–1 mg/l. Disinfection efficiency of chlorine is inversely related to pH, and these values are valid up to pH 7.5, but not higher. It is also important to note that chlorination is less efficient at lower temperatures. If bacterial growth is prevented, and this can be confirmed in water masses by a low or nil total plate count, growth of the amoebae should not be possible. It is still possible, however, that bacteria and amoebae may be growing on and in surfaces not adequately in contact with the disinfectant. For example, in the Czechoslovakian series of infections associated with a chlorinated swimming pool, the amoebae were being harboured in unchlorinated water behind a false wall at one end of the pool.[65] In the Bath Spa episode there was a channel of communication between contaminated unchlorinated warm spring water flowing under the swimming pool and the chlorinated contents. The South Australian series of PAM cases were apparently infected from the public water supply, which was piped over desert after chlorination and thus lost its chlorine content and allowed amoebae to grow. The problem was solved by introducing supplementary chlorination points along the desert pipeline.[66] In addition, the disinfectant monochloramine has been used because it is more persistent than chlorine itself.[67] Ozonation has been tested with some success.[68]

Although the problem of eliminating *Naegleria* from swimming pools seems immense, this is a much more serious problem for natural waters than for artificial pools, where careful design and proper maintenance should be able to achieve effective control.[69]

Granulomatous amoebic encephalitis

The first evidence for involvement of *Acanthamoeba* in human cerebral granulomatous disease was reported in the early 1970s.[70,71] Several species of the genus have now been identified in human pathological material. The organism produces infections in various tissues in the immunocompromised or debilitated, including those with the acquired immune deficiency syndrome (AIDS).

Clinical features

The incubation period is generally prolonged. The signs and symptoms are typical of a variety of conditions resulting from space-occupying lesions in the brain and include hemiparesis, seizures and, in about 70%, altered mental ability (stupor or lethargy, and later disorientation, irritability and combativeness). The predisposing factors include use of corticosteroids (42%), antibiotics, chemotherapy, alcoholism, AIDS, diabetes and pregnancy.[13] Although the disease is generally found in immunocompromised states and is prolonged and chronic, acute *Acanthamoeba* meningoencephalitis has been seen associated with *Acanthamoeba* keratitis and uveitis in a child.[72]

Martinez[73] reviewed 15 cases of GAE known or assumed to be due to *Acanthamoeba*. The patients, six female and nine male, were aged from 5 to 58 years, 11 were white and four black, and their illnesses lasted from 7 to 120 days. In six cases there was a history of chronic skin ulceration or other visceral or superficial lesion. The symptoms were those of a focal or diffuse encephalopathy, with meningeal irritation. Fever, mental abnormalities, seizures, headache and hemiparesis were predominant. On admission to hospital none of these patients was in coma, in contrast to the situation often found with PAM. Cirrhosis or other liver disease was also present in 3/15 patients; pneumonitis, diabetes, Hodgkin's disease and glucose-6-phosphate dehydrogenase deficiency were also seen. Apart from antibiotic treatment, eight (53%) had been given corticosteroids. Six had been given cancer chemotherapy, three radiation therapy, three were alcoholic and two of the four females of child-bearing age were pregnant. More than 56 cases have now been reported as due either to *Acanthamoeba* or some other free-living amoeba causing GAE[6] and there have been at least two cases following bone marrow transplantation.[74]

No patient in this series had any recent history of swimming or water sports.

Leptomyxid amoebae

The involvement of this soil amoeba group in disease was not discovered until 1989, when Visvesvara was able to detect and culture an unusual amoeba[75] in the brain of a baboon showing symptoms similar to those of meningoencephalitis and GAE, and it soon became clear that several human GAE cases which had been thought to be caused by *Acanthamoeba*, but where the amoebae in sections did not stain with *Acanthamoeba*- or *Naegleria*-specific serum were in fact of leptomyxid origin. Subsequently, an infection was seen in an AIDS case.[76]

Clinical features and diagnosis of GAE

The disease can mimic a deep mycosis with systemic dissemination. In five cases reviewed by Jager and Stamm there was frontal headache, fluctuating coma, with or without significant history of a predisposing disease. The route of infection of the brain in the Hodgkin's lymphoma case they reviewed is thought to have been intranasal, since there were basal cortical changes in the brain, with the olfactory lobes affected. Presence of amoebae in the vessel walls gives rise to a vasculitis of an allergic type. Dead and dying organisms and cysts are found, and there is evidence of a foreign body giant cell reaction. It is noteworthy that amoebic cysts are seen in the tissues in GAE and CAK, unlike the situation in *Naegleria* PAM.

The CSF cell count was raised in all patients, lymphocytes being markedly elevated, composing 19–100% of the cells present. Glucose concentrations, where measured, were not appreciably lowered, as would be found in bacterial meningitis or PAM.

Although amoebic trophozoites have been reported in CSF in a few cases of GAE, there is no doubt that this is an extremely unusual finding, which may, however, be more frequent in AIDS.[77]

Further clarification on the clinical features of *B. mandrillaris* infection is developing. An initial lesion of the skin is often seen, sometimes in the nasal pyramid, which may be compact, firm and well delineated. This may or may not ulcerate, and can persist for several months before cerebral symptoms develop.[78] The cerebral lesions are characterized by angeitis/vasculitis, which leads to thrombosis and infarct, when the brain tissue is then locally infiltrated by amoebae to give granulomatous lesions (Figure 78.5).[79] In Peru, the disease has been diagnosed in cases of stroke in immunocompetent children. Headaches, lethargy and coma may supervene. In one patient with neutropenia, CSF glucose was extremely low or unmeasurable.[80] Survival after development of cerebral symptoms is generally a matter of days or weeks.

In view of the chronic nature of the infection with *Acanthamoeba* and *Balamuthia* and the invasive character of attempts to obtain biopsy specimens, the ideal initial investigation would seem to be serological. For *Acanthamoeba*, Kenney[70] examined 1000 sera collected on a routine basis from patients in a New York hospital and found two which reacted at a high titre with *A. culbertsoni* antigen in a complement fixation test. One of the patients had suffered from gastrointestinal problems, and there was little other evidence to incriminate amoebae. (It is

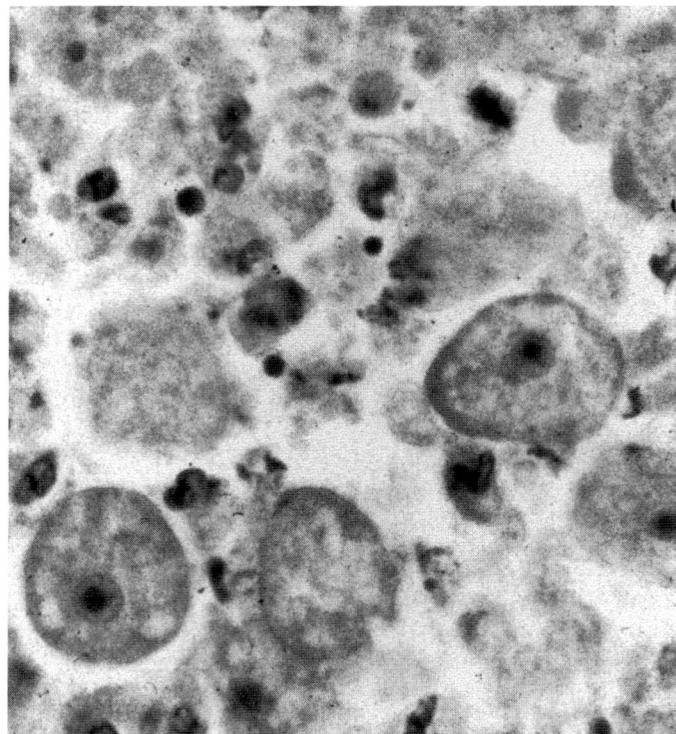

Figure 78.5: Section of brain from AIDS patient showing necrotic granuloma containing trophozoites of *Balamuthia mandrillaris*, showing typical nuclear features of free-living amoebae (haematoxylin and eosin).

interesting to note that we have recently seen a case of *A. culbertsoni* infection in the small intestinal wall of a Malaysian patient.) The other died of a cerebrovascular accident, and amoebae similar to *Acanthamoeba* were demonstrated at post-mortem histological examination of the brain. This case illustrates the probable usefulness of antibody tests in the diagnosis of systemic *Acanthamoeba* infections.

Cerebral biopsy is not an uncommon procedure, and specific polyclonal antibody has been used on wax-embedded sections in immunofluorescence[81] or immuno-peroxidase techniques. *Acanthamoeba*-specific monoclonal antibodies which are likely to prove valuable in diagnosis have been developed.[23]

Cultures (as above for *Naegleria*) may be made from (ideally unfrozen) biopsy material and incubated at 37°C for up to a week under humid conditions. Leptomyxid amoebae apparently do not grow well under these conditions, but they, *Naegleria* and *Acanthamoeba* can be isolated in cell cultures. Attempts at culture from CSF can also be made.

PCR techniques for the identification of axenic *Acanthamoeba* isolates at the generic and specific level have been described[82] but these are not currently suitable for detection of the organism in clinical material. However, rhodamine- and fluorescein-labelled probes have been developed, the former reacting with RNA and DNA of the genus *Acanthamoeba* and the latter with type T4 (most often associated with amoebic keratitis) of 12 ssu-rRNA subgeneric sequences.[83,84] Because samples containing only cysts may be difficult to grow, and amoebae may be very scanty and need culture amplification before detection, the best system for diagnosis would be to divide the sample, to probe one portion, and to culture the other, repeating the probing on the culture.

Management

There are reports of the successful use of rifampicin and of paromomycin in treatment of *Acanthamoeba* infections in mice.[85] Experience is being gained in the treatment of *Acanthamoeba* GAE in humans.[86] A case is known to the reviewer of successful treatment using rifampin, of a brain infection in a liver transplant patient, and successful treatment of a solitary *Acanthamoeba* brain lesion in AIDS by excision and fluconazole/sulfadiazine has recently been reported.[87]

Pathology and pathogenesis

Acanthamoeba probably injures cells by two mechanisms: trogocytosis (ingestion of the cytoplasm through a feeding cup), and contact-mediated lysis of cellular components due to secreted enzymes. Much of the pathology is probably related to attraction of a granulomatous cellular response. It has been shown that collagenase, for example, is effective in attracting cells into the cornea (see below, Chronic *Acanthamoeba* keratitis).

Immunology

Reciprocal titres of up to 80 in the indirect fluorescent antibody test were found in a survey of normal human sera in New Zealand.[48]

Chronic *Acanthamoeba* keratitis

Acanthamoeba is present in all types of environments throughout the world. Since its cysts are resistant to drying, the chance of cyst inoculation into a mucous surface is high. The cornea is an immunoprivileged site, because there is no direct contact with the blood, and it is possible for cysts or trophozoites of this organism to infect corneal stroma.

Acanthamoeba keratitis or keratouveitis presents a serious diagnostic and treatment problem to ophthalmologists. Since the first reports from the UK and the USA in the early 1970s, many further cases have been seen in Europe, the USA and other countries. The major part of the increase in developed countries is probably related to contact lens use and is related to direct inoculation of amoebic trophozoites or cysts into the cornea during insertion of the contaminated lens.

Clinical features

The first ocular infections[88,89] were thought to be associated with trauma to the cornea, leading to invasion of the amoebae, and were not linked to contact lens use. However, 85% of *Acanthamoeba* eye infections in a US survey were in hard or soft contact lens wearers.[90]

Symptoms characteristically mimic those of herpes keratitis, although the condition is generally more painful than the viral disease.

Retrospective studies of keratitis material in London prior to 1973 failed to reveal any earlier cases.[91]

Lang and von Heimburg-Elliger[92] in 1991 reviewed 108 literature case reports: eight (7%) patients were wearing hard contact lenses; 19 (17%) remembered trauma; four (4%) had visited a hot tub; 61 (56%) needed penetrating keratoplasty, 11 (10%) rekeratoplasty; five (5%) eyes were enucleated; in 21 (19%) of the patients the diagnosis was made on histological grounds.

Acanthamoeba keratitis has occurred in both male and female patients aged from 23 to 67 years. Inflammation of the cornea (keratitis) is seen, generally with a larger or smaller epithelial defect. Accumulation of pus in the anterior chamber (hypopyon) is a common feature, together with a ring infiltrate. Following erosion of the cornea the posterior membrane (Descemet's membrane) may bulge forwards (descemetocele) and may perforate, releasing the aqueous humour. There may also be secondary infection with bacteria, graft rejection, swelling of the conjunctiva (chemosis) or accumulation of blood in the anterior chamber (hyphema). Secondary glaucoma (increased intraocular tension related to inflammation of the ciliary body) may complicate the disease.[93] Radial neuritis is reported to be a pathognomonic sign.[94]

The disease runs a slow relapsing course; often a ring abscess is persistent, epithelial breakdown is recurrent, and the hypopyon waxes and wanes.

Diagnosis[95]

Clinical signs have been confused not only with those of other infective entities but also with those due to topical anaesthetic abuse.[96]

Diagnosis may be made by observation of characteristic cysts in wet mounts (10% KOH wet mount is reported to be satisfactory[97]) of corneal ulcer scrapings, and subsequent culture. Cultures made from superficial scrapings of the cornea, or from punch biopsies,[98] are valuable. Suggestive but not conclusive evidence for the infection is obtained when the amoeba is isolated from the contact lenses themselves, the cases or washing fluid. The fluorescent dye Calcofluor has been used to stain the cysts in smears, but it does not detect the trophozoites well.

The temperature of the eye is lower than that of the rest of the human body; therefore *Acanthamoeba* strains that grow at lower temperatures may also contribute to infection. This should be taken into account in cultivation, and a sample should always be cultured at 30°C and at 37°C if there is sufficient material. Recent evidence indicates that perhaps only a limited number of species cause ocular disease. Delineation of the exact species of *Acanthamoeba* which cause keratitis is a prerequisite for the study of the ecology of the keratitis-producing amoebas.[2] Further comments on the value of nucleic acid-based diagnosis and cultures will be seen above in the section on Diagnosis of GAE.

Epidemiology

Acanthamoeba is ubiquitous in air,[4] soil and water. In a study of the moist areas in physiotherapy departments of 10 hospitals, 61% of the swabs taken in those areas were positive for one or several species of amoebae cultivated on non-nutrient agar according to Page. Forty-seven strains of *Acanthamoeba* and only two non-pathogenic strains of *Naegleria* were isolated. Six of the 47 strains of *Acanthamoeba* isolated revealed pathogenic characters in mice.[99]

Management

The most effective therapeutic drugs so far examined have been the diamidines: propamidine and dibromo-propamidine.[100] It is important to remember that *Acanthamoeba*, unlike *Naegleria*, encysts in infected tissues. Clinical cure generally utilizes medication in combination with surgical procedures, such as keratoplasty or, sometimes, debridement.[101] Anti-inflammatory corticosteroids are thought to increase the susceptibility of the eye to *Acanthamoeba* infection, but their judicious use in conjunction with drug treatment has been valuable in many cases. This problem is discussed with respect to several eye infections by Stern and Buttross.[102]

The first patient treated successfully at Moorfields Eye Hospital[100] had a 4-month history of suppurative keratitis, associated with an epithelial defect, hypopyon and secondary glaucoma. *Acanthamoeba* was isolated from the eye on three occasions. Intensive therapy with propamidine isethionate (0.1%) drops hourly by day and night, with dibromopropamidine ointment (0.15%) 4-hourly, was instituted. After 9 days, although corneal improvement was noted, signs of toxicity, including reddening of the eye and swelling of the lids, were seen. The intensive propamidine treatment was discontinued, neomycin drops were instilled 4-hourly day and night, and the 4-hourly dibromopropamidine treatment was continued. After a month the epithelium had healed and 4-hourly prednisolone drops were added, with steady improvement in the corneal inflammation. The treatment was tapered off over a further month, leaving only the neomycin drops, which were continued for 1 year, when some toxic signs developed (limbal follicles, with some increased palpebral conjunctival hyperaemia and cellularity, but no signs of skin irritation). Following cessation of all topical therapy, 4 months elapsed, with disappearance of limbal and conjunctival signs and no recurrence of the disease.

Twenty-two months after initial presentation a penetrating keratoplasty (corneal graft) was carried out. The excised corneal disc showed no special changes and no morphologically identifiable *Acanthamoeba* on light and electron microscopical examination. Using the indirect fluorescent antibody technique and rabbit anti-*Acanthamoeba* serum it was possible to see small curved arcs, which probably represented fragments of cyst wall.

Propamidine isethionate drops were instilled four times a day for 2 months, in addition to the usual post-operative topical steroids and antibiotics. There was no evidence of adverse effect(s) on the graft or the remainder of the eye. The graft remained clear for a further 9 months, when a rejection episode developed which was readily controlled with topical corticosteroids. Because of persisting secondary glaucoma, the intraocular pressure needed to be controlled using timolol maleate (0.25%) drops twice daily.

The initial intensive treatment probably need not be continued for more than 1 week because intensive therapy with propamidine may give rise to corneal toxicity.[103] More recent observations confirm the effectiveness of propamidine (or dibromopropamidine) and neomycin.[104] However, one case was successfully treated with propamidine isethionate and 'Neosporin' (neomycin/polymyxin/gramicidin) at 30-minute intervals for 11 and 9 days,[105] whereas in seven other cases 1% miconazole topically was used successfully in triple therapy with a less intensive course of the other two agents.[106] Earlier studies at Moorfields and in my laboratory showed that the gramicidin component of 'Neosporin' was irritating and relatively non-toxic to amoebae. A successful regimen used neomycin, polymyxin and dibromopropamidine together with gentamicin.[107]

An early report of the efficacy of oral ketoconazole (200 mg twice a day) and topical miconazole[108] encouraged the use of these antifungals, which have shown some success. Miconazole or ketoconazole drops have been used, with or without 'Neosporin' drops.[109] In a more recent study the new antifungal itraconazole was used orally with topical 0.1% miconazole hourly during the day. The therapy was successful after 5, 8 and 9 weeks in three patients.[110]

Resistance to topical dibromopropamidine was observed in a case of bilateral keratitis. Eradication of amoebae was finally achieved following prolonged topical therapy and two corneal grafts in each eye. Paromomycin, benzethonium chloride, clotrimazole and R11/29 (a phenanthridinium compound) were continued topically for 3 months postoperatively. There were no further recurrences during a 14-month follow-up. Drug sensitivities were performed for three isolates of *Acanthamoeba* species (group II), which demonstrated the development of resistance to dibromopropamidine. In addition the resistant isolates were temperature-sensitive mutants which would not grow at temperatures above 30°C.[111]

A novel treatment with a polyhexamethylene biguanide (PHMB) biocide, first shown to be active on free-living amoebae in the early 1970s,[112] 'Baquacil' or 'ReNu', has recently shown promise in the elimination of *Acanthamoeba* from the human eye. It is active at low concentrations against the cysts,[113] unlike most other agents, and this means that it attacks one of the main sources of treatment failure because drug treatment may stimulate encystment.[114,115] Chlorhexidine, another biguanide, is now regularly used with success, alone or in combination with other agents.[116]

Animal models of *Acanthamoeba* keratitis have recently been developed and will be important in understanding the pathogenic mechanisms involved in the disease and in testing new drug treatments. It may be that improvements will be possible when the host response is better understood.[117,118]

Pathology and pathogenesis

Parasite-conditioned medium contains both collagenase and lower concentrations of other proteolytic enzymes. However, most of the collagenolytic and pathogenic activity is directly attributable to specific collagenase. Intrastromal injection of sterile, *Acanthamoeba*-conditioned culture medium into naive Lewis rats produces corneal lesions clinically similar to and closely resembling those found in biopsy specimens of human patients diagnosed with acanthamoebic keratitis. There is moderate to severe neutrophil infiltration, disruption of stromal lamellae and oedema. Identical pathological sequelae have been produced by intrastromal injection of purified collagenase (25 units/ml).[119]

In acanthamoebic keratitis the organisms apparently depend on the cellular components of the cornea as substrates for growth.[120]

Commensal bacteria on the eyelids, conjunctiva and tear film may have a role in pathogenesis.[121] This may also be the case for viruses. Many cases of human keratitis due to *Acanthamoeba* species have a pseudoherpetic appearance and the infection is known to have followed herpes infection in some cases. After herpetic and amoebic co-infection rabbits show severe corneal lesions, and when the viral infection is treated the amoebic co-infection progresses unchecked with severe lesions until day 37 post infection, with numerous trophozoites and cysts.[122] This may have significant implications in human disease. However, experimental infections have also been established in the rabbit without co-infection with herpes,[123] and several rat models have now been described.[124] In the Wistar rat model the inflammatory cell profile was observed to change at intervals. In tissue sections the cellular response consisted of neutrophils on the first day but predominantly macrophages on the following days. Some T lymphocytes but no B lymphocytes were observed.[125]

Immunology

Immunity against these amoebae involves a combination of complement, antibody and cell-mediated immunity. Evidence suggests that the major mechanism is activation of phagocytic cells, especially neutrophils, by lymphokines and opsonization of the amoebae by antibody, which promotes an antibody-dependent cellular destruction of the organism.[126]

Prevention of contact lens-related *Acanthamoeba* eye infection

There can be little doubt that the reason for the increase in case numbers of *Acanthamoeba* keratitis in the developed world since the 1970s has been the introduction of contact lenses, and of soft contact lenses in particular.[127] The type of lens and the way the lenses are handled by the patient may be crucial in raising the risk of infection. Adequate means for lens cleaning, disinfection, rinsing and storage need to be available. In addition, for patients who are careless or persist in using non-sterile rinsing solutions, user-friendly and foolproof adequate methods of disinfection will be of great help in prevention.[128]

When storage cases for contact lenses of 102 asymptomatic lens wearers were tested for contamination by bacteria and free-living amoebae, 43 had significant counts of viable bacteria. Seven had contamination by acanthamoebae.[129] In a recent study, infection of the eye by *Acanthamoeba* has been conclusively linked to the contact lens storage container, the home-made saline solution and the kitchen cold water tap. The authors recommend that the use of home-made saline solutions and the rinsing of contact lenses in tap water be strongly discouraged.[130]

Unfortunately, many contact lens users receive poor lens care instructions or cannot be relied on to follow appropriate routines. Finding a foolproof means of lens disinfection for them is critical. Recently, several disinfection systems were tested against *A. castellanii* and *A. polyphaga* cysts and trophozoites to see which might prove most effective. Effective systems included heat disinfection at 70–80°C for 10 minutes, 3% hydrogen peroxide for 2–3 hours, 0.001% thimerosal with edetate for 4 hours, 0.005% benzalkonium chloride with edetate for 4 hours, and either 0.001% chlorhexidine for 4 hours or 0.004% chlorhexidine for 1 hour.

Problems associated with chemical disinfection (with, for example, 3% hydrogen peroxide) of plastic contact lenses include lens fit alterations, which may lead to epithelial trauma. In addition, antimicrobial chemicals need to be rinsed, neutralized or degraded after use, as they can injure the corneal and conjunctival epithelium.[131] In a study of contamination of lenses in 101 users,[132] 81% of cases were found to be microbiologically contaminated. While 75% used hydrogen peroxide solution for de-contamination, all contaminating organisms were catalase positive. Where the lens material will resist it, heat disinfection at 70–80° C for 10 minutes, or 3% hydrogen peroxide for 2–3 hours, is recommended. A neutralization step should follow exposure to the peroxide.[131]

Adherence of cysts and trophozoites to the contact lens is probably important in mediation of infection.

Trophozoites of *A. polyphaga* adhered in vitro to low and high water content non-ionic soft contact lenses. Adherence was greater to high water content soft lenses. Cyst attachment occurred only to the soft lenses, and was higher for the high water content lenses. Attachment of cysts to each lens tested was significantly lower than that of trophozoites. Recommended cleaning procedures using two commercial solutions (10% sodium tridecyl ether sulphate for rigid gas-permeable lenses; EDTA and sorbic acid for soft contact lenses) removed all adherent trophozoites and cysts from lenses. Correctly applied lens cleaning agents which remove adherent trophozoites, cysts and epithelial cells from the lenses and cases may reduce the risk of infection.[133]

The use of disposable hydrogel contact lenses, which are worn continuously and then discarded, is thought to protect against lens-related infection. But if lenses are removed during the period of use, or rinsed or stored in tap water or well water, this protective effect may be lost.[134]

REFERENCES

1 Warhurst D C. Pathogenic free-living amoebae. *Parasitol Today* 1985; 1:24–28.

2 Warhurst D C. Potentially pathogenic free-living amoebae. Chapter 18 In Gilles H M (ed.) *Protozoal Diseases*. London: Arnold, 1999: 647–666.

3 Barwick R S, Levy D A, Craun G F, Beach M J & Calderon R L. Surveillance for waterborne-disease outbreaks: United States, 1997–1998. *MMWR* 1991; 40:1–21. (See also previous reports in the same journal).

4 Kingston D & Warhurst D C. Isolation of amoebae from the air. *J Med Microbiol* 1969; 2:27–36.

5 Warhurst D C. Ryan virus and the lipovirus: examples of *Acanthamoeba* (*Hartmannella*) contamination of cell cultures. *Parasitol Today* 1989; 5:161–162.

6 Visvesvara G S & Stehr-Green J K. Epidemiology of free-living ameba infections. *J. Protozool* 1990; 37:25S–33S.

7 Amaral Zettler L A, Nerad T A, O'Kelly C J, Peglar M T, Gillevet P M, Silberman J D & Sogin M L. A molecular reassessment of the Leptomyxid amoebae. *Protist* 2000; 151:275–282.

8 Rowbotham T J. Preliminary report of the pathogenicity of *Legionella pneumophila* for freshwater and soil amoebae. *J Clin Pathol* 1980; 33:1179–1183.

9 Kilvington S & Price J. Survival of *Legionella pneumophila* within cysts of *Acanthamoeba polyphaga* following chlorine exposure. *J Appl Bacteriol* 1990; 68:519–525.

10 Thom S, Warhurst D C & Drasar B S. Association of *Vibrio cholerae* with fresh water amoebae. *J Med Microbiol* 1992; 36:303–306.

11 Rowbotham T J. Pontiac fever explained. *Lancet* 1980; ii:969.

12 Humidifier fever: report of MRC Symposium 1976. *Thorax* 1977; 32:635–663.

13 Martinez A J. Clinical manifestations of free-living amoeba infections. In Rondanelli E G (ed.) *Amphizoic Amoebae: Human Pathology*. Padua: Piccin Press, 161–177.

14 Derrick E H. A fatal case of generalized amoebiasis due to a protozoon closely resembling if not identical to *Iodamoeba buetschlii*. *Trans R Soc Trop Med Hyg* 1948; 42:191–198.

15 Stamm W P. The staining of free-living amoebae by indirect immunofluorescence. *Ann Soc Belg Med Trop* 1974; 54:321–325.

16 Carter R F. Primary amoebic meningoencephalitis: an appraisal of present knowledge. *Trans R Soc Trop Med Hyg* 1972; 66:193–213.

17 Miller G, Cullity G, Walpole I, O'Connor J & Masters P. Primary amoebic meningoencephalitis in Western Australia. *Med J Aust* 1982; 1:352–357.

18 Markowitz S M, Martinez A J, Duma R J & Shiel F O M. Myocarditis associated with primary amebic meningoencephalitis. *Am J Clin Pathol* 1974; 62:619–628.

19 Patras D & Andujar J. Meningoencephalitis due to *Hartmannella* (*Acanthamoeba*). *Am J Clin Pathol* 1966; 46:226–233.

20 Lawande R V, MacFarlane J T, Weir W C & Awunor-Renner C. A case of primary amebic meningoencephalitis in a Nigerian farmer. *Am J Trop Med Hyg* 1980; 29:21–25.

21 Medley S. Acridine orange: method for diagnosis of amoebic meningitis? *Med J Aust* 1980; 2:635.

22 Page F C. Taxonomic criteria for limax amoebae, with descriptions of 3 new species of *Hartmannella* and 3 of *Vahlkampfia*. *J. Protozool* 1967; 14:499–521.

23 Flores B M, Garcia C A, Stamm W E & Torian B E. Differentiation of *Naegleria fowleri* from *Acanthamoeba* species by using monoclonal antibodies and flow cytometry. *J Clin Microbiol* 1990; 28:1999–2005.

24 Reveiller F L, Marciano-Cabral, F, Pernin P, Cabanes P A & Legastelois S. Species specificity of a monoclonal antibody produced to *Naegleria fowleri* and partial characterization of its antigenic determinant. *Parasitol Res* 2000; 86:634–641.

25 Kilvington S, Mann P G & Warhurst D C. Differentiation between *Naegleria fowleri* and *N. lovaniensis* using isoenzyme electrophoresis of aspartate aminotransferase. *Trans R Soc Trop Med Hyg* 1984; 78:562–563.

26 De Jonckheere J F. Characterization of *Naegleria* species by restriction endonuclease digestion of whole-cell DNA. *Mol Biochem Parasitol* 1987; 24:55–66.

27 McLaughlin G L, Vodkin M H & Huizinga H W. Amplification of repetitive DNA for the specific detection of *Naegleria fowleri*. *J Clin Microbiol* 1991; 29:227–230.

28 Anderson K & Jamieson A. Primary amoebic meningoencephalitis. *Lancet* 1972; ii:379.

29 Seidel J S, Harmatz P, Visvesvara G S, Cohen A, Edwards J & Turner J. Successful treatment of primary amebic meningoencephalitis. *N Engl J Med* 1982; 306:346–348.

30 Brown R L. Successful treatment of primary amebic meningoencephalitis. *Arch Intern Med* 1991; 151:1201–1202.

31 Poungvarin N & Jariya P. The fifth nonlethal case of primary amoebic meningoencephalitis. *J Med Assoc Thai* 1991; 74:112–115.

32 Cain A R R, Wiley P E, Brownell B & Warhurst D C. Primary amoebic meningoencephalitis. *Arch Dis Child* 1981; 56:140–143.

33 Hecht R H, Cohen A H, Stoner J & Irwin C. Primary amebic meningoencephalitis in California. *Calif Med* 1972; 117:69–73.

34 Boyle A L, Friedman T A, Braustein H & Tomasulo M. Rapid diagnosis of primary amoebic meningoencephalitis due to *Naegleria*: detection of organisms with bacterial stains. *J Clin Pathol* 1979; 32:306–307.

35 Stevens A R, Shulman S T, Lansen T A, Cichon M J & Willaert E. Primary amebic meningoencephalitis: a report of two cases and antibiotic and immunologic studies. *J Infect Dis* 1981; 143:193–199.

36 Duma R J. Disease caused by free-living amoebae. *Infect Dis Newslett* 1989; 8:25–32.

37 Drutz D J. Rapid infusion of amphotericin B: is it safe, effective and wise? *Am J Med* 1992; 93:119–121.

38 Cruz J M, Peacock J E, Loomer L et al. Rapid intravenous infusion of amphotericin B: a pilot study. *Am J Med* 1992; 93:123–130.

39 Ferrante A. Free living amoebae: pathogenicity and immunity. *Parasite Immunol* 1991; 13:31–47.

40 Ferrante A. Comparative sensitivity of *Naegleria fowleri* to amphotericin B and amphotericin B methyl ester. *Trans R Soc Trop Med Hyg* 1982; 76:476–478.

41 Thong Y H, Rowan-Kelly B, Ferrante A & Shepherd C. Synergism between tetracycline and amphotericin B in experimental amoebic meningoencephalitis. *Med J Aust* 1978; 1:663–664.

42 Thong Y H. Delayed treatment of primary amoebic meningoencephalitis with amphotericin B and tetracycline. *Trans R Soc Trop Med Hyg* 1979; 73:806–808.

43 Thong Y H. Chemotherapy for primary amebic meningoencephalitis. *N Engl J Med* 1982; 306:1295–1296.

44 Thong Y H, Rowan-Kelly B & Ferrante A. Treatment of experimental *Naegleria* meningoencephalitis with a combination of amphotericin B and rifamycin. *Scand J Infect Dis* 1979; 11:151–153.

45 Schachter L P, Owellen R J, Rathbun H K & Buchanan B. Antagonism between miconazole and amphotericin-B. *Lancet* 1976; ii:318.

46 Marciano-Cabral R, Zoghby K L & Bradley S G. Cytopathic action of *Naegleria fowleri* amoebae on rat neuroblastoma target cells. *J Protozool* 1990; 37:138–144.

47 Dunnebacke T H & Dixon J S. NACM, a cytopathogenic protein from *Naegleria gruberi*, EGs: purification, production of monoclonal antibody, and immunoidentification of a product that develops in NACM-treated vertebrate cell cultures. *J Protozool* 1990; 37:11S–16S.

48 Cursons R T M, Brown T J, Keys E A, Moriarty K M & Till D. Immunity to pathogenic free living amoebae: role of humoral antibody. *Infect Immun* 1980; 29:401–407.

49 Cursons R M, Keys E A, Brown T M, Learmonth J, Campbell C & Metcalf P. IgA and primary amoebic meningoencephalitis. *Lancet* 1979; i:223–224.

50 Cain A R R, Mann P G & Warhurst D C. IgA and primary amoebic meningoencephalitis. *Lancet* 1979; i:441.

51 Ahn M H & Min D Y. [Resistance to *Naegleria fowleri* infection passively acquired from immunized splenocyte, serum or milk.] *Kisaengchunghak Chapchi* 1989; 27:79–86.

52 Thong Y H, Ferrante A, Shepherd C & Rowan-Kelly B. Resistance of mice to *Naegleria* meningoencephalitis transferred by immune serum. *Trans R Soc Trop Med Hyg* 1978; 72:650–652.

53 Thong Y H, Carter R F, Ferrante A & Rowan-Kelly B. Site of expression of immunity to *Naegleria fowleri* in immunized mice. *Parasite Immunol* 1983; 5:67–76.

54 Fischer-Stenger K, Cabral G A & Marciano-Cabral F. The interaction of *Naegleria fowleri* amoebae with murine macrophage cell lines. *J Protozool* 1990; 37:168–173.

55 Michelson M K, Henderson W R Jr, Chi E Y, Fritsche T R & Klebanoff S J. Ultrastructural studies on the effect of tumor necrosis factor on the interaction of neutrophils and *Naegleria fowleri*. *Am J Trop Med Hyg* 1990; 42:225–233.

56 Rowan-Kelly B, Ferrante A & Thong Y H. Activation of complement by *Naegleria*. *Trans R Soc Trop Med Hyg* 1980; 74:333–336.

57 Aufy S, Kilvington S, Mann P G & Warhurst D C. Improved selective isolation of *Naegleria fowleri* from the environment. *Trans R Soc Trop Med Hyg* 1986; 80:350–351.

58 Kilvington S, Mann P G & Warhurst D C. *Pathogenic Naegleria Amoebae in the Waters of Bath: A Fatality and its Consequences.* Bath: Bath City Council, 1991, 89–96.

59 Huizinga H W & McLaughlin G L. Thermal ecology of *Naegleria fowleri* from a power plant cooling reservoir. *Appl Environ Microbiol* 1990; 56:2200–2205.

60 Pernin P, Pelandakis M, Rouby Y, Faure A & Siclet F. Comparative recoveries of *Naegleria fowleri* amoebae from seeded river water by filtration and centrifugation. *Appl Environ Microbiol* 1998; 64: 955–959.

61 John D T & Howard M J. Techniques for isolating thermotolerant and pathogenic freeliving amebae. *Folia Parasitol (Praha)* 1996; 43: 267–271.

62 De Jonckheere J F. Hospital hydrotherapy pools treated with ultraviolet light: bad bacterial quality and presence of thermophilic Naegleria. *J Hyg (Camb)* 1982; 88:205–214.

63 Brown T M & Cursons R T M. Prophylaxis. In E G Rondanelli (ed.) *Amphizoic Amoebae: Human Pathology.* Padua: Piccin Press, 1987: 217–236.

64 Chang S L. Resistance of pathogenic *Naegleria* to some common physical and chemical agents. *Appl Environ Microbiol* 1978; 35:368–375.

65 Kadlec V, Cerva L & Skvarova J. Virulent *Naegleria fowleri* in an indoor swimming pool. *Science* 1978; 201:1025.

66 Dorsch M M, Cameron A S & Robinson B S. The epidemiology and control of primary amoebic meningoencephalitis with particular reference to South Australia. *Trans R Soc Trop Med Hyg* 1983; 77:372–377.

67 Esterman A, Roder D M, Cameron A S, Robinson B S, Walters R P, Lake J A & Christy P E. Determinants of the microbiological quality of South Australian swimming pools. *Appl Env Microbiol* 1984; 47: 325–328.

68 Cursons R T M, Brown T J & Keys E A. Effect of disinfectants on pathogenic free-living amoebae: in axenic conditions. *Appl Environ Microbiol* 1980; 40:401–407.

69 Lyons T B & Kapur R. Limax amoebae in public swimming pools of Albany, Schenechtady and Rensselaen counties, New York: their concentration, correlations and significance. *Appl Environ Microbiol* 1977; 33:551–555.

70 Kenney M. The Micro-Kolmer complement fixation test in routine screening for soil ameba infection. *Health Lab Sci* 1971; 8:5–10.

71 Jager B V & Stamm W P. Brain abscesses caused by free living amoeba probably of the genus *Hartmannella* in a patient with Hodgkin's disease. *Lancet* 1972; ii:1343–1345.

72 Jones D B, Visvesvara G S & Robinson N M. *Acanthamoeba polyphaga* keratitis and Acanthamoeba uveitis associated with fatal meningoencephalitis. *Trans Ophthalmol Soc UK* 1975; 95:221–232.

73 Martinez A J. Is Acanthamoeba encephalitis an opportunistic infection? *Neurology* 1980; 30:567–574.

74 Anderlini P, Przepiorka D, Luna M et al. Acanthamoeba meningoencephalitis after bone-marrow transplantation. *Bone Marrow Transplant* 1994; 14: 459–461.

75 Visvesvara G S, Martinez A J, Schuster F L et al. Leptomyxid ameba, a new agent of amebic meningoencephalitis in humans and animals. *J Clin Microbiol* 1990; 28:2750–2756.

76 Anzil A P, Rao C, Wrzolek M A, Visvesvara G S, Sher J H & Kozlowski P B. Amebic meningoencephalitis in a patient with AIDS caused by a newly recognized opportunistic pathogen, leptomyxid ameba. *Arch Pathol Lab Med* 1991; 115:21–22.

77 Hawley H B, Czachor J S, Malhotra V, Funkhouser J W & Visvesvara G S. *Acanthamoeba* encephalitis in patients with AIDS. *AIDS Reader* 1997; 7:137–144.

78 Deol I, Robledo L, Meza A, Visvesvara G S & Andrews R J. Encephalitis due to a free-living amoeba (Balamuthia mandrillaris): case report with literature review. *Surg Neurol* 2000; 53:611–616.

79 Recavarren-Arce S, Velarde C, Gotuzzo E & Cabrera J. Amoeba angeitic lesions of the central nervous system in *Balamuthia mandrillaris* amoebiasis. *Hum Pathol* 1999; 30:269–273.

80 Katz J D, Ropper A H, Adelman L, Worthington M & Wade P. A case of *Balamuthia mandrillaris* meningoencephalitis. *Arch Neurol* 2000; 57:1210–1212.

81 Warhurst D C. *Naegleria* and *Acanthamoeba* in tissue sections. In J M B Edwards, C E D Taylor & A H Tomlinson (eds) *Immunofluorescence techniques in Diagnostic Microbiology*. London: HMSO, 1982: 46–48.

82 Vodkin M, Howe D K, Visvesvara G S & McLaughlin G L. Identification of *Acanthamoeba* at the generic and specific levels using the polymerase chain reaction. *J Protozool* 1992; 39:378–385.

83 Stothard D R, Hay J, Schroeder-Diedrich J M, Seal D V & Byers T J. Fluorescent oligonucleotide probes for clinical and environmental detection of *Acanthamoeba* and the T4 18S rRNA gene sequence type. *J Clin Microbiol* 1999; 37:2687–2693.

84 Stothard D R, Schroeder-Diedrich J M, Awwad M H, Gast R J, Ledee D R, Rodriguez-Zaragoza S, Dean C L, Fuerst P A & Byers T J. The evolutionary history of the genus *Acanthamoeba* and the identification of eight new 18S rRNA gene sequence types. *J. Eukaryotic Microbiol* 1998; 45:45–54.

85 Mazur T, Kasprzak W & Zagarska-Nowak G. Sensitivity of limax amoebae to some antiparasitic drugs II activity in vivo. *Wiadomosci Parazitologiczne* 1983; 29:271–272.

86 Slater C A, Sickel J Z, Visvesvara G S et al. Brief report: successful treatment of disseminated acanthamoeba infection in an immunocompromised patient. *N Engl J Med* 1994; 331:85–87.

87 Seijo-Martinez M, Gonzalez-Medeiro G, Santiago P, Rodriguez de Lope A, Diz J, Conde C & Visvesvara G S. Granulomatous amebic encephalitis in a patient with AIDS: isolation of *Acanthamoeba* sp. group II from brain tissue and successful treatment with sulfadiazine and fluconazole. *J Clin Microbiol* 2000; 38:3892–3895.

88 Nagington J, Watson P G, Playfair T J, McGill J, Jones B R & Steele A D McG. Amoebic infection of the eye. *Lancet* 1974; ii:1537–1540.

89 Visvesvara G S, Jones D B & Robinson N M. Isolation, identification, and biological characterization of *Acanthamoeba polyphaga* from a human eye. *Am J Trop Med Hyg* 1975; 24:784–790.

90 Stehr-Green J K, Bailey T M & Visvesvara G S. The epidemiology of *Acanthamoeba keratitis* in the United States. *Am J Ophthalmol* 1989; 107:331–336.

91 Ashton N & Stamm W P. Amoebic infection of the eye: a pathological report. *Trans Ophthalmol Soc UK* 1975; 95:214–220.

92 Lang G E & von Heimburg-Elliger A. [Acanthamoeba keratitis in hard contact lens wearers. Case report and review of the literature of 108 cases.] *Klin Monatsbl Augenheilkd* 1991; 198:290–294.

93 Hirst L W, Green W R, Merz W et al. Management of *Acanthamoeba* keratitis: a case report and review of the literature. *Ophthalmology* 1984; 91:1105–1111.

94 McCulley J P, Alizadeh H & Niederkorn J Y. *Acanthamoeba* keratitis. *CLAO J* 1995; 21:73–76.

95 Visvesvara G S. Acanthamoebiasis and naegleriosis. In Balows A, Hausler W J, Ohashi M & Turano A (eds) *Laboratory Diagnosis of Infectious Disease*. New York: Springer, 1988: 723–730.

96 Rosenwasser G O, Holland S, Pflugfelder S C et al. Topical anesthetic abuse. *Ophthalmology* 1990; 97:967–972.

97 Sharma S, Srinivasan M & George C. Diagnosis of acanthamoeba keratitis: a report of four cases and review of literature. *Indian J Ophthalmol* 1990; 38:50–56.

98 Lee P & Green W R. Corneal biopsy: indications, techniques, and a report of a series of 87 cases. *Ophthalmology* 1990; 97:718–721.

99 Michel R & Menn T. [*Acanthamoeba, Naegleria* and invertebrates in wet areas of physiotherapy equipment in hospitals.] *Zentralbl Hyg Umweltmed* 1991; 191:423–437.

100 Wright P, Warhurst D C & Jones B R. *Acanthamoeba* keratitis successfully treated medically. *Br J Ophthalmol* 1985; 69:778–782.

101 Osato M S, Robinson N M, Wilhelmus K R & Jones D B. In vitro evaluation of antimicrobial compounds for cysticidal activity against *Acanthamoeba*. *Rev Infect Dis* 1991; 13(Suppl.):S431–S435.

102 Stern G A & Buttross M. Use of corticosteroids in combination with antimicrobial drugs in the treatment of infectious corneal disease. *Ophthalmology* 1991; 98:847–853.

103 Johns K J, Head W S & O'Day D M. Corneal toxicity of propamidine. *Arch Ophthalmol* 1988; 106:68–69.

104 Maudgal P C. Acanthamoeba keratitis: report of three cases. *Bull Soc Belg Ophthalmol* 1989; 231:135–148.

105 John T, Lin J & Sahm D F. Acanthamoeba keratitis successfully treated with prolonged propamidine isethionate and neomycin–polymyxin–gramicidin. *Ann Ophthalmol* 1990; 22:20–23.

106 Berger S T, Mondino B J, Hoft R H et al. Successful medical management of *Acanthamoeba* keratitis. *Am J Ophthalmol* 1990; 110:395–403.

107 Beattie A M, Slomovic A R, Rootman D S & Hunter W S. Acanthamoeba keratitis with two species of *Acanthamoeba*. *Can J Ophthalmol* 1990; 25:260–262.

108 Hirst L W, Green W R, Merz W et al. Management of *Acanthamoeba* keratitis: a case report and review of the literature. *Ophthalmology* 1984; 91:1105–1111.

109 Sharma S, Srinivasan M & George C. Acanthamoeba keratitis in non-contact lens wearers. *Arch Ophthalmol* 1990; 108:676–678.

110 Ishibashi Y, Matsumoto Y, Kabata T et al. Oral itraconazole and topical miconazole with debridement for *Acanthamoeba* keratitis. *Am J Ophthalmol* 1990; 109:121–126.

111 Ficker L, Seal D, Warhurst D & Wright P. Acanthamoeba keratitis: resistance to medical therapy. *Eye* 1990; 4:835–838.

112 Warhurst D C & Singer M. Inhibition of growth of Naegleria by a swimming pool additive. *Trans R Soc Trop Med Hyg* 1975; 69:7.

113 Kilvington S. Activity of water biocide chemicals and contact lens disinfectants on pathogenic free-living amoebae. *Int Biodeterioration* 1990; 26:127–138.

114 Kim B G, McCann P P & Byers T J. Inhibition of multiplication of *Acanthamoeba castellanii* by specific inhibitors of ornithine decarboxylase. *J Protozool* 1987; 34:264–266.

115 Byers T J, Kim B G, King L E & Hugo E R. Molecular aspects of the cell cycle and encystment in Acanthamoeba. *Rev Infect Dis* 1991; 13:S378–S384.

116 Hay, J, Kirkness, C M, Seal, D V et al. Drug resistance and *Acanthamoeba* keratitis: the quest for alternative antiprotozoal chemotherapy. *Eye* 1994; 8:555–563.

117 Badenoch P R. The pathogenesis of *Acanthamoeba* keratitis. *Aust NZ J Ophthalmol* 1991; 19:9–20.

118 He Y G, Niederkorn J Y, Alizadeh H et al. A pig model of Acanthamoeba keratitis: transmission via contaminated contact lenses. *Invest Ophthalmol Vis Sci* 1992; 33:126–133.

119 He Y G, Niederkorn J Y, McCulley J P et al. In vivo and in vitro collagenolytic activity of *Acanthamoeba castellanii*. *Invest Ophthalmol Vis Sci* 1990; 31:2235–2240.

120 Stopak S S, Roat M I, Nauheim R C et al. Growth of acanthamoeba on human corneal epithelial cells and keratocytes in vitro. *Invest Ophthalmol Vis Sci* 1991; 32:354–359.

121 Larkin D F & Easty D L. External eye flora as a nutrient source for *Acanthamoeba*. *Graefes Arch Clin Exp Ophthalmol* 1990; 228:458–460.

122 Paniagua-Crespo E, Tsouria-Belaid A, Bellon C, Jacquemin J L & Simitzis-Le-Flohic A M. [Amoebic keratitis caused by

Acanthamoeba sp. May HSV1 infection play a role?] *J Fr Ophthalmol* 1991; 14:25–31.

123 Cote M A, Irvine J A, Rao N A & Trousdale M D. Evaluation of the rabbit as a model of *Acanthamoeba* keratitis. *Rev Infect Dis* 1991; 13(Suppl.):S443–S444.

124 Larkin D F & Easty D L. Experimental *Acanthamoeba* keratitis: I. Preliminary findings. *Br J Ophthalmol* 1990; 74:551–555.

125 Larkin D F & Easty D L. Experimental *Acanthamoeba* keratitis: II. Immunohistochemical evaluation. *Br J Ophthalmol* 1991; 75:421–424.

126 Ferrante A. Free living amoebae: pathogenicity and immunity. *Parasite Immunol* 1991; 13:31–47.

127 Meisler D M & Rutherford I. Acanthamoeba and disinfection of soft contact lenses. *Rev Infect Dis* 1991; 13(Suppl.):S410–S412.

128 Moore M B. Acanthamoeba keratitis and contact lens wear: the patient is at fault. *Cornea* 1990; 9(Suppl.):S33–S35.

129 Larkin D F, Kilvington S & Easty D L. Contamination of contact lens storage cases by *Acanthamoeba* and bacteria. *Br J Ophthalmol* 1990; 74:133–135.

130 Kilvington S, Larkin D F, White D G & Beeching J R. Laboratory investigation of *Acanthamoeba* keratitis. *J Clin Microbiol* 1990; 28:2722–2725.

131 Chandler J W. Biocompatibility of hydrogen peroxide in soft contact lens disinfection: antimicrobial activity vs. biocompatibility—the balance. *CLAO J* 1990; 16(Suppl.):S43–S45.

132 Gray T B, Cursons R T M, Sherwan J F et al. *Acanthamoeba*, bacterial and fungal contamination of contact lens storage cases. *Br J Ophthalmol* 1995; 79:601–605.

133 Kilvington S & Larkin D F. Acanthamoeba adherence to contact lenses and removal by cleaning agents. *Eye* 1990; 4:589–593.

134 Heidemann D G, Verdier D D, Dunn S P & Stamler J F. *Acanthamoeba* keratitis associated with disposable contact lenses. *Am J Ophthalmol* 1990; 110:630–634.

Chapter 79
Trichomonal Infection

G. C. Cook

Trichomonas vaginalis is a pathogenic protozoan with a high degree of site specificity—affecting predominantly the lower female genitourinary tract.[1] Infection may or may not be symptomatic; it can be sexually transmitted. In women <10^4, and in men 4×10^6 organisms produce an infection. Related organisms are: *T. tenax* and *Pentatrichomonas hominis*; whilst both colonize the gums and colon, respectively, neither is of proven pathogenicity.

First visualized by Donné in 1836, *T. vaginalis* was first shown in the early twentieth century, as a result of inoculation studies, to be pathogenic. It is an ovoid organism, 10–20 mm wide; 'twitching' motility is brought about by four anterior flagella and a recurrent flagellum (embedded in an undulating membrane, which runs along two-thirds of the cell). It is actively phagocytic, optimal growth occurring under moderately anaerobic conditions. Reproduction is by binary fission; unlike many pathogenic protozoa, cysts are not formed. When subjected to either in vitro or in vivo study, a strain variation in virulence is apparent.

Distribution and epidemiology

Infection occurs worldwide—in both urban and rural settings.[1] In the 1970s, the World Health Organization estimated an annual world incidence of 180 million cases; however, *T. vaginalis* infection is not notifiable, and data on prevalence tends therefore to be highly unreliable. In sexually transmitted disease (STD) clinics, overall figures varying from 7 to 32% have been recorded. Highest prevalence rates are in groups with a high level of sexual activity. In female prostitutes figures of up to 80% have been noted. In tropical populations, recorded prevalence has varied from 3% in Manila university students, to 15–20% in clinic populations studied in Asia and Africa. Three studies from Nigeria give an insight into the prevalence of infection in West Africa.[2–4] Infection was detected in 505 (24.7%) out of 2048 urine specimens submitted by students at a 'higher institution'; 374 (74%) occurred in women, and 131 (26%) in men.[2] At Jos, infection rates of 37.6% and 24.8% were recorded in groups (250 were examined in each group) of urban and rural women, respectively.[3] Specimens from 2224 adult women examined at the cytology clinic at University College Hospital, Ibadan, revealed an infection rate of 9.8%. In Turkish women with a vaginal discharge, a 13% incidence has been recorded.[5] Infection tends to be high in human immunodeficiency virus (HIV)-infected individuals.[6–8] At Dar-es-Salaam, Tanzania, an investigation of 359 gynaecological inpatients revealed that those infected with *T. vaginalis* had an almost threefold higher risk of being infected with HIV.[9] In men (in whom the disease is usually asymptomatic and self-limiting [see below]), meaningful prevalence figures are virtually non-existent. The organism is frequently coexistent with another infection, e.g., candidiasis, gonorrhoea, syphilis or HIV infection; it is therefore important to screen an infected woman for another STD(s), which often has a greater medical significance. Although non-venereal transmission of *T. vaginalis* is rare, the organism can survive for several hours in a moist environment. Perinatal infection in about 5% of female babies born (vaginally) to infected mothers has been recorded.

Pathogenesis and pathology

The organism involves squamous (rather than columnar) epithelium; only rarely can it be isolated from the endocervix, but the urethra is involved in 90% of infected cases. Rarely, it has been demonstrated in the epididymis and prostate, and occasionally causes non-gonococcal (tetracycline-resistant) urethritis (NGU). *T. vaginalis* infection is accompanied by large numbers of polymorphonuclear neutrophils (PMNs) (which together with macrophages kill the organism) and a consequent vaginal discharge. The organism is *not* invasive, existing either free in the vaginal cavity or adherent to epithelium; in about 50% of cases microscopic haemorrhage is apparent using an appropriate technique. Local IgA is usually detectable (see below); however, serum antibody concentration remains low, and is of no use diagnostically (see below).

Clinical aspects

Classical presentation consists of vulvo-vaginitis.[10–13] In an experimentally induced infection the incubation period ranges from 3 to 28 days. Although 50–90% of infected women are symptomatic, it is frequently difficult to attribute symptoms directly to *T. vaginalis*, because another organism(s) is coexistent. In 50-75% of those infected a vaginal discharge (often frothy and greenish-yellow,[3,5] and sometimes odorous) is present; 25–50% of women infected suffer from vulval irritation,[2,3] while 50% experience dyspareunia; mild dysuria is sometimes present. Lower abdominal discomfort is described by 10% of infected women; it may be accompanied by salpingitis, although this may have a different aetiology—possibly another STD. A yellowish vaginal discharge is present in 50–75% of those infected, whilst vulval erythema is present in less than one-third. It is probably a cause of female infertility.[14]

In men, NGU may be present,[15-20] but the majority of cases are asymptomatic. When symptomatic, infection may resemble NGU of another aetiology;[17,18] it is usually recognized following failure of response to standard chemotherapeutic regimens. *T. vaginalis* can be detected in 70% of men who have experienced sexual intercourse with an infected woman within the previous 48 hours. It is one of several STDs to affect male homosexuals.[21] Involvement of the epididymis and prostate are rare events.

A small percentage of female infants born to infected mothers may be infected (see above), but a *T. vaginalis* infection in older children may indicate sexual abuse.

In the long term *T. vaginalis* infection is benign. There is no evidence that it directly predisposes to cervical carcinoma; an associated organism(s), e.g., a papillomavirus,[12] may, however, be implicated in this pathology.

Diagnosis

Definitive diagnosis depends on demonstration of the parasite in a specimen from a symptomatic woman (see above)—who in many cases has recently had sexual intercourse with a 'new' partner. Recent use of antibiotic(s) suggests the possibility of a *Candida* spp. infection. Presence of another STD should be sought by careful examination of the vulva using a speculum; further examination after trichomoniasis has been treated may also reveal an associated (coexistent) infection. Vaginal inflammation is present with both *T. vaginalis* and *Candida* spp. infection, but not usually in bacterial vaginosis.[10,12,22,23] The cervix should be examined for evidence of cervicitis and a purulent or mucopurulent discharge.

T. vaginalis can be demonstrated using a vaginal swab. The specimen can either be transferred directly to a microscope slide, or the swab agitated in a tube containing about 1 ml saline.[24] The organism can be cultured using a variety of media.

Normal vaginal pH is ≤4.5; this is maintained in most women suffering from vulvovaginal candidiasis. However, more than 75% of women with a *T. vaginalis* infection, accompanied by bacterial vaginosis,[1,15] have a pH >4.5. Cervical discharge has an elevated pH; therefore, that in vaginal material may be artificially elevated; recent coitus also significantly elevates pH (semen is significantly more alkaline than vaginal secretion). Following determination of pH, several drops of 10–20% potassium hydroxide can be added to the discharge obtained during speculum examination; a pungent, fishy, amine-like odour is present in 75% of women with a *T. vaginalis* infection,[5] and most of those with bacterial vaginosis;[22] this test is negative in vulvovaginal candidiasis.

For a definitive diagnosis, microscopic examination of vaginal discharge is mandatory; a drop of wet-mount preparation should be examined under a coverslip.[24,25] In a *T. vaginalis* infection the flora consists of rods or coccobacilli, while epithelial cells are unaltered and PMNs plentiful; motile *T. vaginalis* (decreasing in older, cooled preparations) can be visualized in 40–80% of those infected. Gram staining is virtually useless for recognition of *T. vaginalis*; Giemsa staining is 50%, and an acridine orange technique about 60% sensitive. Use of a routine Papanicolaou technique[25] on a cervical specimen detects *T. vaginalis* in 60–70% of cases. Newer fluorescent antibody techniques[24] possess a sensitivity of 80-90% when compared with culture. In bacterial vaginosis the normal flora consisting of rods is replaced by coccobacilli (which encrust the epithelial cells); few PMNs are present.

In men, diagnosis is usually more difficult;[26] occasionally a wet-mount preparation of urethral discharge will reveal motile organisms. The most effective means of diagnosis is by culture (see below) of a urethral specimen or sample of urine sediment following prostatic massage.[16]

Culture techniques (with a sensitivity of >95%) are not widely used, but these increase the detection rate.[27,28] *T. vaginalis* grows best on a suitable medium in an anaerobic environment at 37°C; selective growth can be achieved by addition of an appropriate antibiotic(s). Recently, an enzyme-linked immunosorbent assay has been compared with wet-mount and culture techniques for detecting *T. vaginalis*;[28-31] culture proved to be more sensitive. Other recently developed techniques include: employment of monoclonal antibodies;[24] a molecular probe for identification of *T. vaginalis* DNA;[29] a polymerase chain reaction (PCR);[23] and detection of anti-*T. vaginalis* antibodies in cervical secretions and serum samples.[31-37]

Local IgA is detectable in most infected women (see above);[28,31,32] however, there is not a significant elevation of the serum concentration.

Treatment

T. vaginalis is usually highly sensitive (minimal inhibitory concentration ≤1 μg/ml) to the 5-nitroimidazole compounds,[38] but *not* to most other antimicrobial agents. Recently, however, relative resistance in some strains has been demonstrated.[13,24,39,40]

In women, metronidazole is most widely used[10,13,21,22,41–43] with a recommended dose regimen of 2.0 g as a single dose; this cures 85% of cases, and when the sexual partner is treated simultaneously the success rate rises to 95%. Another regimen utilizes a single-day divided dose of 1.6 g. A regimen using 250 mg three times a day for 7 days, probably gives a comparable result. In men, a 7-day course is of proven efficacy, while the single-dose regimen has not been adequately assessed. Metronidazole possesses significant side effects (Chapter 00), including the development of a *Candida* spp. infection. Although there is no evidence of teratogenicity in *Homo sapiens*, metranidazole should, if possible, be avoided during the first trimester of pregnancy.[24] Experience with tinidazole is limited,[24,38,44,45] but results using a single-dose regimen are encouraging; it has the advantage of being significantly less expensive, and possesses minimal side effects. A 100% cure rate has been recorded using nimorazole (4 g in two equally divided doses 24 hours apart).[38] Clotrimazole 100 mg intra-vaginally at night usually relieves symptoms, but a 7-day course cures only about 20%. Clindamycin is also an alternative.[22] Mebendazole, furazolidone and anisomycin may all be effective in 5-nitroimidazole-resistant *T. vaginalis*;[46] however, 'prospective, randomized, double-blind, active-control comparative studies' are required.[47] More recently, paromomycin has proved effective in metronidazole-resistant infection.[48,49]

Use of condoms is effective in prevention of infection.[2] A spermatocide, nonoxynol 9—which is present in many vaginal preparations—possesses significant tricho-monacidal properties.[46]

REFERENCES

1   Hook E W. Trichomonas vaginalis—no longer a minor STD. *Sex Transm Dis* 1999 Aug; 26(7):388–389.
2   Anosike J C, Onwuliri C D, Inyang R E et al. Trichomoniasis amongst students of a higher institution in Nigeria. *Appl Parasitol* 1993; 34:19–25.
3   Ogbonna C I, Ogbonna I B, Ogbonna A A & Anosike J C. Studies on the incidence of Trichonomas vaginalis amongst pregnant women in Jos area of Plateau State, Nigeria. *Angew Parasitol* 1991; 32:198–204.
4   Konje J C, Otolorin E D, Ogunniyi J D, Obisesan K A & Ladipo G A. The prevalence of *Sardnerella vaginalis*, *Trichomonas vaginalis* and *Candida albicans* in the cytology clinic at Ibadan, Nigeria. *Afr J Med Sci* 1991; 20:29–34.
5   Yereli K, Balcioglu I C, Degerli K, Ozbilgin A & Daldal N. Incidence of *Trichomonas vaginalis* among women having vaginal discharge, in Manisa, Turkey. *J Egypt Soc Parasitol* 1997; 27:905–911.
6   Jackson D J, Rakwar J P, Bwayo J J, Kreiss J K & Moses S. Urethral *Trichomonas vaginalis* infection and HIV-1 transmission. *Lancet* 1997; 350:1076.
7   Press N, Chavez V M, Ticona E, Calderon M et al. Screening for sexually transmitted diseases in human immunodeficiency virus-positive patients in Peru reveals an absence of *Chlamydia trachomatis* and identifies *Trichomonas vaginalis* in pharyngeal specimens. *Clin Infect Dis* 2001; 32:808–814.
8   Niccolai L M, Kopicko J J, Kassie A, Petros H, Clark R A & Kissinger P. Incidence and predictors of reinfection with *Trichomonas vaginalis* in HIV-infected women. *Sex Transm Dis* 2000; 27:284–288.
9   Meulen J ter, Mgava H N, Chang-Claude J et al. Risk factors for HIV infection in gynaecological inpatients in Dar es Salaam, Tanzania, 1988-1990. *East Afr Med J* 1992; 69:688–692.
10   Kent H L. Epidemiology of vaginitis. *Am J Obstet Gynecol* 1991; 165:1168–1176.
11   Sobel J D. Vulvovaginitis. *Dermatol Clin* 1992; 10:339–359.
12   Hatch K D. Vulvar and vaginal disorders. *Curr Opin Obstet Gynecol* 1992; 4:904–906.
13   Heine P & McGregor J A. Trichomonas vaginalis: a reemerging pathogen. *Clin Obstet Gynecol* 1993; 36:137–144.
14   el-Sharkawy I M, Hamza S M & el-Sayed M K. Correlation between *Trichomonas vaginalis* and female infertility. *J Egypt Soc Parasitol* 2000; 30:287–294.
15   Fowler J E Jr. Urethritis in men. *Semin Urol* 1991; 9:15–27.
16   Saxena S B & Jenkins R R. Prevalence of *Trichomonas vaginalis* in men at high risk for sexually transmitted diseases. *Sex Transm Dis* 1991; 18:138–142.
17   Krieger J N, Jenny C, Verdon M et al. Clinical manifestations of trichomoniasis in men. *Ann Intern Med* 1993; 118:844–849.
18   Krieger J N, Verdon M, Siegel N & Holmes K K. Natural history of urogenital trichomoniasis in men. *J Urol* 1993; 149:1455–1458.
19   Bakare R A, Ashiru J O, Adeyemi-Doro F A, Ekweozor C C et al. Non-gonococcal urethritis (NGU) due to *Trichomonas vaginalis* in Ibadan. *West Afr J Med* 1999; 18:64–68.
20   el-Seoud S F, Abbas M M & Habib F S. Study of trichomoniasis among Egyptian male patients. *J Egypt Soc Parasitol* 1998; 28:263–270.
21   Levine G I. Sexually transmitted parasitic diseases. *Prim Care* 1991; 18:101–128.
22   Majeroni B A. New concepts in bacterial vaginosis. *Am Fam Physician* 1991; 44:1215–1218.
23   Hart G. Factors associated with trichomoniasis, candidiasis and bacterial vaginosis. *Int J STD AIDS* 1993; 4:21–25.
24   Lossick J G & Kent H L. Trichomoniasis: trends in diagnosis and management. *Am J Obstet Gynecol* 1991; 165:1217–1222.
25   Weinberger M W & Harger J H. Accuracy of the Papanicolaou smear in the diagnosis of asymptomatic infection with *Trichomonas vaginalis*. *Obstet Gynecol* 1993; 82:425–429.
26   Krieger J N, Verdon M, Siegel N, Critchlow C & Holmes K K. Risk assessment and laboratory diagnosis of trichomoniasis in men. *J Infect Dis* 1992; 166:1362–1366.
27   Boeke A J, Dekker J H & Peerbooms P G. A comparison of yield from cervix versus vagina for culturing *Candida albicans* and *Trichomonas vaginalis*. *Genitourin Med* 1993; 69:41–43.
28   Sharma P, Malla N, Gupta I, Ganguly N K & Mahajan R C. A comparison of wet mount, culture and enzyme linked immunosorbent assay for the diagnosis of trichomoniasis in women. *Trop Geogr Med* 1991; 43:257–260.
29   Rubino S, Muresu R, Rappelli P et al. Molecular probe for identification of *Trichomonas vaginalis* DNA. *J Clin Microbiol* 1991; 29:702–706.
30   Riley D E, Roberts M C, Takayama T & Krieger J N. Development of polymerase chain reaction-based diagnosis of *Trichomonas vaginalis*. *J Clin Microbiol* 1992; 30:465–472.
31   Romia S A & Othman T A. Detection of antitrichomonal antibodies in sera and cervical secretions in trichomoniasis. *J Egypt Soc Parasitol* 1991; 21:373–381.
32   Bhatt R, Pandit D & Deadhar L. Detection of serum antitrichomonal antibodies in urogenital trichomoniasis by immunofluorescence. *J Postgrad Med* 1992; 38:72–74.
33   Okuyama T, Takahashi R, Mori M, Osaka M, Kobayashi T K & Maeda S. Polymerase chain reaction amplification of

Trichomonas vaginalis DNA from Papanicolaou-stained smears. *Diagn-Cytopathol* 1998; 19:437–440.

34 Madico G, Quinn T C, Rompalo A, McKee K T & Gaydos C A. Diagnosis of *Trichomonas vaginalis* infection by PCR using vaginal swab samples. *J Clin Microbiol* 1998; 36: 3205–3210.

35 van Der Schee C, van Belkum A, Zwijgers L, van Der Brugge et al. Improved diagnosis of *Trichomonas vaginalis* infection by PCR using vaginal swabs and urine specimens compared to diagnosis by wet mount microscopy, culture, and fluorescent staining. *J Clin Microbiol* 1999; 37:4127–4130.

36 Ryu J S, Chung H L, Min D Y, Cho Y H et al. Diagnosis of trichomoniasis by polymerase chain reaction. *Yonsei Med J* 1999; 40: 56–60.

37 Mayta H, Gilman R H, Calderon M M, Gottlieb A et al. 18S ribosomal DNA-based PCR for diagnosis of *Trichomonas vaginalis*. *J Clin Microbiol* 2000; 38:2683–2687.

38 Chunge C N, Kangethe S, Pamba H D & Dwate J. Treatment of symptomatic trichomoniasis among adult women using oral nitroimidazoles. *East Afr Med J* 1992; 69:398–401.

39 Sobel J D, Nagappan V & Nyirjesy P. Metronizadole-resistant vaginal trichomoniasis—an emerging problem. *N Engl J Med* 1999; 341:292–293.

40 Snipes L J, Gamard P M, Narcisi E M, Beard C B, Lehmann T & Secor W E. Molecular epidemiology of metranizadole resistance in a population of *Trichomonas vaginalis* clinical isolates. *J Clin Microbiol* 2000; 38:3004–3009.

41 Hager W D & Rapp R P. Metronizadole. *Obstet Gynecol Clin North Am* 1992; 19:497–510.

42 Drug-resistant *Trichomonas vaginalis*. *Commun Dis Rep CDR Weekly* 1993; 3:141.

43 Ikeh E I, Bello C S & Ajayi J A. In vitro susceptibility of *Trichomonas vaginalis* strains to metronizadole—a Nigerian experience. *Genitourin Med* 1993; 69:241–242.

44 Hamed K A & Studemeister A E. Successful response of metronizadole-resistant trichomonal vaginitis to tinidazole. A case report. *Sex Transm Dis* 1992; 19:339-340.

45 D-Prasertsawat P & Jetsawangsri T. Split-dose metronizadole or single-dose tinidazole for the treatment of vaginal trichomoniasis. *Sex Transm Dis* 1992; 19:295–297.

46 Livengod C H & Lossick J G. Resolution of resistant vaginal trichomoniasis associated with the use of intravaginal nonoxynol-9. *Obstet Gynecol* 1991; 78:954–956.

47 McCutchan J A, Ronald A R, Corey L & Handsfield H H. Evaluation of new anti-infective drugs for the treatment of vaginal infections. Infectious Diseases Society of American and the Food and Drug Administration. *Clin Infect Dis* 1992; 15 (supplement 1):S115–S122.

Section 11

Helminthic Infections

Helminthic infections traditionally dominated the discipline of tropical medicine; this followed Manson's great interest in and seminal work on lymphatic filariasis. It is not therefore inappropriate that the first contribution to this section should address the filariases. Soil-transmitted helminthiases (also nematode infections) are extremely common in a tropical context and their true importance is undoubtedly underrated as far as clinical manifestations, morbidity and socioeconomic sequelae are concerned.

Schistosomiasis is a disease of colossal relevance worldwide; one estimate is that over 200 million individuals suffer from hepatosplenic disease caused by this group of trematodes (flukes)—involving the gastrointestinal (and liver) and urinary tracts. Numerically, other trematodes are of lesser importance; the majority of these are localized to South-East Asia.

Intestinal cestode (tapeworm) infections are by and large benign, but when they assume the role of systemic infections—caused by the larval stages (most importantly hydatidosis and neurocysticerosis)—significant pathology frequently ensues.

This section illustrates very clearly how writing and teaching of the traditional discipline followed upon parasitological and hence taxonomic classification(s).

The filariases and schistosomiases, for example, both consist of several divergent *clinical* entities. To a physician it makes little or no sense to group gastrointestinal and urinary forms of schistosomiasis together. Similarly, do lymphatic filariasis, onchocerciasis, loiasis, dracontiasis and *Mansonella perstans* infections have anything in common to the clinician? Surely the time has come for a reorientation!

Diagnosis and management of helminthic infections has advanced almost beyond recognition since the early 1970s. Improved serological techniques have simplified the diagnosis of several of these—including filariasis, schistosomiasis, hydatidosis and neurocysticercosis; regrettably such techniques are not yet available for most of the intestinal infections (with the exception of strongyloidiasis), and a search for adult worms and/or their eggs remains the sole method for diagnosis. In chemotherapy, the newer bensimidazoles (for most nematode infections) were introduced in the 1960s, praziquantel (for schistosomiasis and other trematode and cestode infections) in the 1970s, and ivermectin (for onchocerciasis and to a lesser extent, other filariases) in the 1980s. Much remains to be accomplished, however, in preventive strategies for this extremely important group of human infections.

Chapter 80
Schistosomiasis

A. Davis

The term human schistosomiasis indicates a complex of acute and chronic parasitic infections caused by mammalian blood flukes (*Schistosoma*). These infections are transmitted by specific aquatic or amphibious snails in a wide variety of freshwater habitats.

The various species of the genus *Schistosoma* are members of the family Schistosomatidae—dioecious digenean parasites whose habitat is the blood-vascular system of vertebrates. The family is divided into three, the Schistosomatinae, Bilharziellinae and Gigantobilharziinae, and contains 12 genera, of which several are confined to birds and five to mammals; only *Schistosoma* is associated with humans.

A general feature of the family is that the female is longer and more slender than the male and is normally carried in a ventral groove, the gynaecophoric canal, formed by ventrally flexed lateral outgrowths of the male body. Of all the mammalian blood flukes, the genus *Schistosoma* has achieved the greatest geographical distribution and diversification.[1]

Of the 16 species of schistosome known to infect humans or animals, only five are responsible for the overwhelming proportion of human infections: *Schistosoma haematobium*, *S. intercalatum*, *S. mansoni*, *S. japonicum* and *S. mekongi*. Rarely, other zoophilic species or hybrids may be found in humans.[2]

The five principal species infecting humans are subdivided into three groups characterized by the size and appearance of the eggs produced by the female schistosome:

- Eggs with a terminal spine—*S. haematobium*, *S. intercalatum*.
- Eggs with a lateral spine—*S. mansoni*.
- Rounded or ovoid minutely spined eggs—*S. japonicum* and *S. mekongi*.

History

S. haematobium

Chronic haematuria and various bladder disorders occurred in Egypt and Mesopotamia from the earliest times in association with the agricultural civilizations of the great river valleys. Haematuria was described in the Gynaecological Papyrus of Kahun, written in the mid-XII dynasty period, about 1900 BC. Many remedies for haematuria were recorded from the time of the Ebers Papyrus and it can be assumed that the condition was widespread.[3] Calcified ova of the parasite were demonstrated in the kidneys of two Egyptian mummies of the XXth dynasty (1250–1000 BC).[4] During the Napoleonic invasion of Egypt (1799–1801), symptoms of the disease in troops were rife,[5] yet it was not until 1851 that the causal agent (*Distoma haematobium*, now *Schistosoma haematobium*), a blood fluke, was found by Theodor Bilharz in a mesenteric vein during a post-mortem examination at the Kasr el Aini Hospital in Cairo.[6]

S. mansoni

In 1902 Manson[7] found lateral spined eggs in the faeces of a West Indian patient in London and postulated the existence of a second species of blood fluke. Subsequent controversy between A. Looss and L. W. Sambon, eminent scientists of the day, was resolved by the work of Leiper[8] at El Marg, a village in the present Qualyubia Governorate, just north of Cairo, in 1915; Leiper established beyond doubt the existence of two distinct species of schistosome and the presence of snail intermediate hosts belonging not only to two different genera but also to two different subfamilies. In the New World, eggs with a lateral spine were found in Bahia (Brazil) in 1904 and described in 1908[9] and in Venezuela in 1906.[10]

S. japonicum

In 1847 the clinical entities 'Kabure itch' and 'Katayama syndrome' were described in a village in the Hiroshima Prefecture in Japan,[11] while in 1904 Katsurada[12] recovered worms from the portal system of a cat and named the species *Schistosomum japonicum*. From 1909 to 1915 the biology of this parasite, its life cycle and the pathology it caused were elucidated and described by Japanese and other investigators.[13–16]

The investigation was recognized clinically in both China[17] and the Philippines in the early years of the twentieth century[18] and in Sulawesi, Celebes, in the 1930s.[19]

In China the *Oncomelania* intermediate hosts were discovered in 1924[20] and in the Philippines in 1932.[21]

S. intercalatum

Suspicion arose in 1923 that, because some cases of human 'intestinal' schistosomiasis in the Yakusu area near Kisangani in present-day Zaire showed an atypical clinical picture and possessed an unusual egg morphology, a species distinct from *S. haematobium* was involved.[22] Follow-up of this work led to a description in 1934 of a new species, *S. intercalatum*, of which the snail intermediate host was a member of the *Bulinus africanus* group.[23]

S. mekongi

Described initially in 1978,[24] the parasite causes human schistosomiasis in an, as yet, restricted area in Laos and Kampuchea (Cambodia). The intermediate host, *Tricula aperta*, is aquatic and is not susceptible to strains of *S. japonicum*.[25] A monograph provides the most authoritative account of the species to date.[26]

Geographical aspects

(Figures 80.1 and 80.2)

Schistosomiasis is now endemic in 76 countries and territories;[27] *S. mansoni* is found in 55 countries, ranging from the Arabian peninsula, numerous countries in the African continent and, of the Indian Ocean islands, solely in Madagascar. High-prevalence endemicity exists in the Nile valley, particularly the neighbours Sudan and Egypt. In the New World, the infection exists in Brazil, Surinam, Venezuela and several islands in the Caribbean. Brazil stands out, with 25 million people resident in endemic areas and 3 million infected.

S. haematobium is now endemic in 53 countries in the Middle East, most of the African continent and some islands in the Indian Ocean: Mauritius (although now near to extinction), Madagascar, Zanzibar and Pemba. In India, a focus of urinary schistosomiasis was described at Gimvi, in the Ratnagiri district, Maharashtra State.[28] A re-examination in 1981 was confirmatory,[29] but a combined Indian government/World Health Organization (WHO)/ World Bank mission in 1985 found only two persons infected of 352 examined by Nuclepore filtration of urine. The presumed intermediate host, a freshwater limpet, *Ferrissia tenuis*, was found in all water bodies of major human water contact.[30] This ill-defined focus still excites scientific interest but should soon be controlled absolutely.

In 40 countries, double infections with *S. mansoni* and *S. haematobium* are endemic.[31]

S. japonicum infection in humans is found only in mainland China, Indonesia (Lindu Lake valley and the Napu valley in central Sulawesi) and the Philippines. There is no evidence of recent tranmission in Thailand,

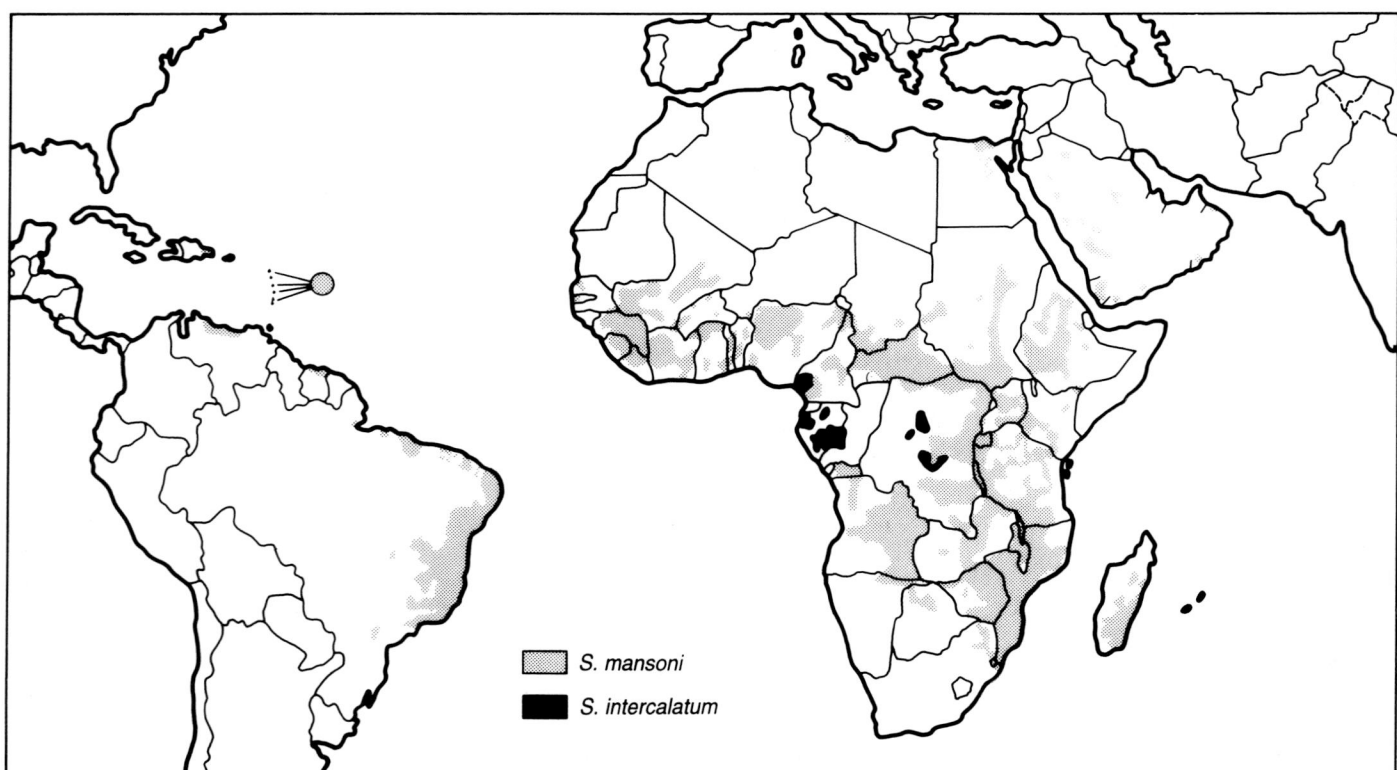

Figure 80.1: Global distribution of schistosomiasis due to *Schistosoma mansoni* and *S. intercalatum*, 1985.

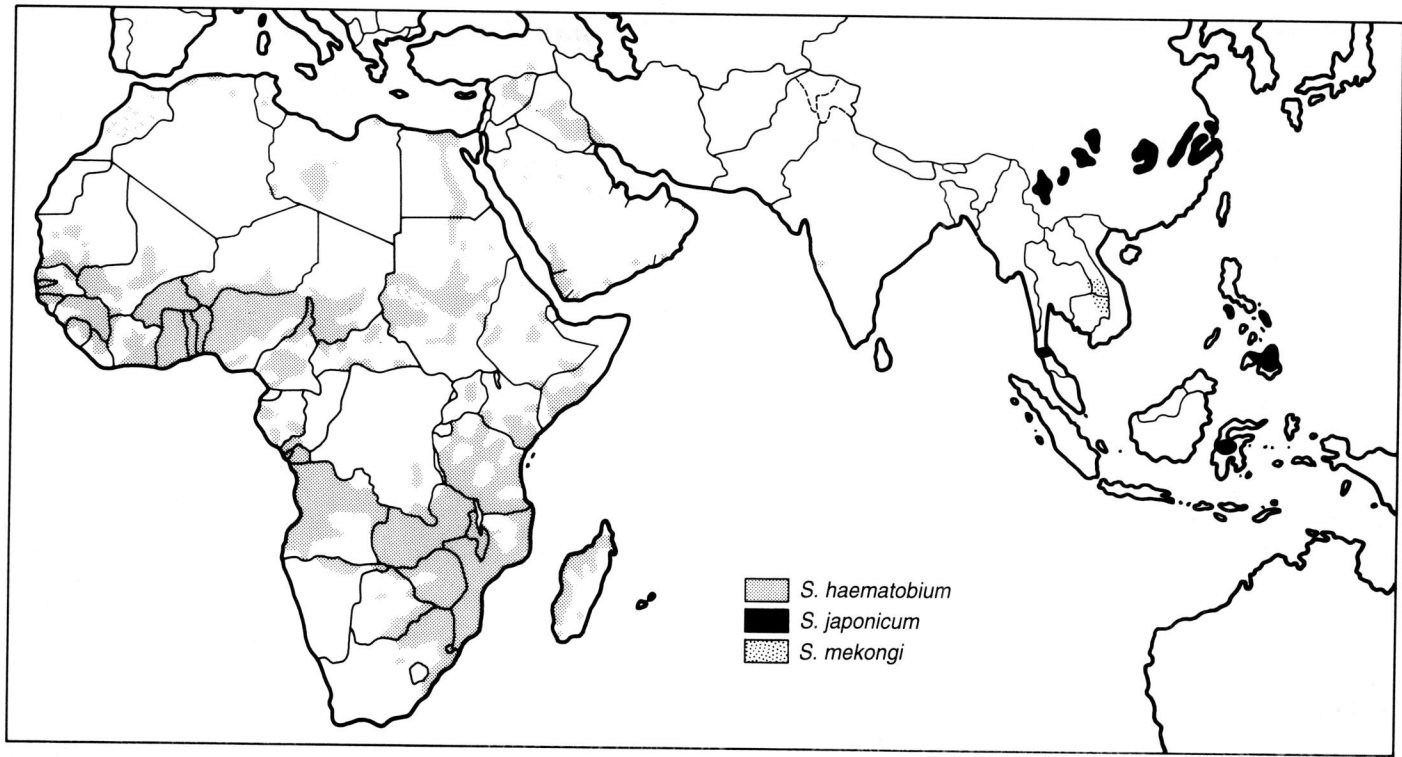

Figure 80.2: Global distribution of schistosomiasis due to *Schistosomiasis haematobium* and *S. japonicum*, 1985.

and schistosomiasis was eradicated in Japan some three decades ago.

A parasite resembling *S. japonicum* (*S. malayensis*), transmitted by *Robertsiella kaporensis*, has been found in humans in Pahang State, Malaysia.[32] Wild rats are the only known natural hosts and it is thought that the human is not an important host for this parasite.

S. intercalatum is endemic in 10 countries in central and west Africa.[27,33]

S. mekongi is endemic on Khong Island, Lao People's Democratic Republic, and in some areas of Democratic Kampuchea.[27]

Aetiology

Of the five species of the genus *Schistosoma* responsible for most human infections, *S. mansoni*, *S. japonicum* and *S. mekongi* inhabit the pericolonic venules within the distribution of the portal venous system. The eggs of *S. mansoni* are characterized by a laterally placed spine; those of *S. japonicum* and *S. mekongi* are smaller and are round or ovoid with a rudimentary spine. All of these species produce 'intestinal' or 'rectal' schistosomiasis.

S. haematobium inhabits the terminal venules in the wall of the bladder, the genitourinary system and the pelvic plexus within the distribution of the inferior vena cava; its eggs have a terminal spine and it causes 'urinary' or 'vesical' schistosomiasis.[34]

Neither *S. haematobium* nor *S. mansoni* is restricted exclusively in their anatomical vascular habitats within the respective distributions of the inferior vena caval or the portal venous systems. *S. haematobium* can exist in the perirectal venules and its eggs may be found in the stools, although almost invariably they are dead. *S. mansoni* may live in the pelvic plexus and its eggs can be detected in urine ('mansonuria'), although this is an uncommon finding during epidemiological surveys.

Much less is known on human infection with *S. intercalatum* than is the case with the other species. Two geographical strains ('Cameroon' and 'Zaire') have been described,[35,36] each with distinct and different intermediate snail hosts and patterns of egg distribution within the host. *S. intercalatum* appears to be a species distinct from *S. haematobium*; it produces terminal-spined eggs of characteristic morphology and the clinical syndrome of infection is that of a lower bowel colitis, i.e., lower abdominal discomfort or pain with either dysentery or diarrhoea. This should be qualified with the reminder that many cases are asymptomatic. Its geographical distribution is restricted to central and west Africa. Natural hybridization has been described.[37–39] Experimentally, hybridization between *S. mansoni* and *S. intercalatum* in a monkey (*Erythrocebus patas*) from Nigeria has been reported.[40]

S. mekongi is, as yet, confined to Laos and Kampuchea (Cambodia), is transmitted by an aquatic intermediate host, *Tricula aperta*, and is also found in dogs.

Infrequently, humans are infected by schistosomes that normally live in other mammalian hosts,[34] for example

S. bovis, a member of the *S. haematobium* complex and a common parasite in cattle and sheep; *S. mattheei*, which has multiple hosts in both domestic and wild animals in southern Africa, and *S. margrebowiei*, a parasite frequent in antelopes in central Africa. Such infections in humans are seldom of pathological significance but suggestions have been advanced that they may confer a relative type of immunity (heterologous immunity) against *S. mansoni* and *S. haematobium* infections in areas where all species coexist.[41,42]

The cercariae of certain avian blood flukes, *Trichobilharzia*, *Gigantobilharzia* and *Ornithobilharzia*, may penetrate human skin producing cercarial dermatitis or 'swimmer's itch'. Outbreaks may occur in either tropical or temperate climates but development of cercariae into adult schistosomes does not occur in humans. Even less frequently, cercariae of adult schistosomes normally parasitic in mammals (e.g., *S. douthitti* from rodents and *S. spindale* from water buffaloes) may produce a similar syndrome.

Parasitology and biology of the stages of the parasite

(Table 80.1)

Adult worms

In nature, a population of schistosomes in the final definitive host usually comprises both male and female worms (Figure 80.3). Since the genus *Schistosoma* differs from most digenetic trematodes in being dioecious, a consequence of heteromorphic chromosomes in the ovum,[43] a population could conceivably be unisexual (male or female worms only). Under laboratory conditions, single miracidial snail infections carried through to cercarial infections of the final host result in either populations of unisexual males or unisexual females.[44]

Table 80.1 Comparison of principal features of *Schistosoma* spp. infecting humans.

	S. japonicum	S. mekongi*	S. mansoni	S. haematobium	S. intercalatum
Adult worms					
Location of adult in host	Mesenteric veins	Mesenteric veins	Mesenteric veins	Vesical plexus	Mesenteric veins
Length of posterior gut caecum	Medium	Medium	Very long	Short	Short
Male					
Length (mm)	10–20	115	6–13	10–15	11–14
Width (mm)	0.55	0.41	1.10	0.90	0.3–0.4
No. of testes	6–7	6–7	4–13 (6–9)[†]	4–5	2–7 (4–5)[†]
Tubercles	Absent	Absent?	Coarse	Fine	Fine
Female					
Length (mm)	20–30	112	10–20	16–26	10–14
Width (mm)	0.30	0.23	0.16	0.25	0.15–0.18
Ovary: position in body	Middle	Rear half	Front third	Rear third	Rear half
Uterus: position in body	Front half	Front half	Front half	Front two-thirds	Front two-thirds
Length	Short	Short	Very short	Long	Long
No. of eggs	50–200	10+	1–2	10–50	5–60
Mature egg					
Shape	Round	Round	Ovoid	Ovoid	Ovoid
Size (µm)	6×100	57×66	61×140	62×150	61×176
Spine	Lateral (reduced)	Lateral (reduced)	Lateral (prominent)	Terminal (prominent)	Terminal (prominent)
Normally passed in	Faeces	Faeces	Faeces	Urine	Faeces (and urine)
Eggs per female per day	3500	?	100–300	20–300	150–400
Reaction of egg shell to Ziehl–Neelsen stain[‡]	+ve	?	+ve	-ve	+ve
Intermediate host snail	Oncomelania	Tricula	Biomphalaria	Bulinus	Bulinus

*From experimental animal infections. †Usual range. ‡In histological sections. Courtesy of R. F. Sturrock, Department of Medical Parasitology, London School of Hygiene and Tropical Medicine.
Reproduced with permission from Jordan P, Webbe G & Sturrock R F (eds) *Human Schistosomiasis*. Wallingford: CAB Inernational, 1993.

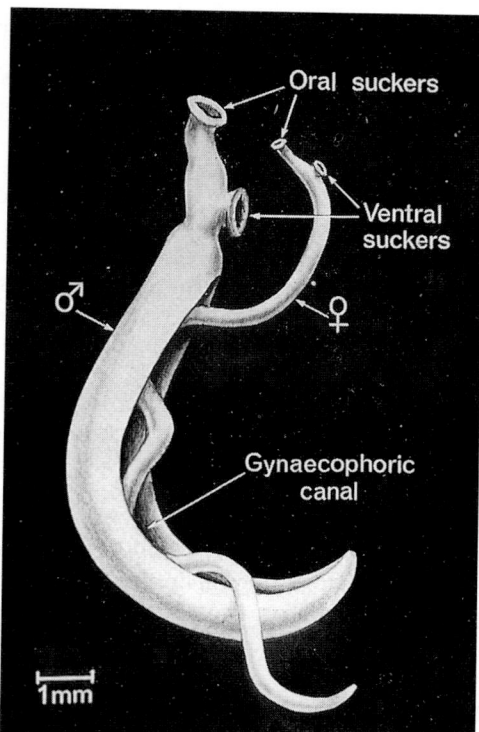

Figure 80.3: Male and female schistosomes. (Courtesy of Tropical Resources Unit.)

Adult worms, of separate sex, are small, with a species variation in length of 6–28 mm and in breadth of 0.25–1 mm. In all species the outer tegument of the female is smooth, whereas that of the male *S. haematobium* and *S. mansoni* is covered with minute spines or tubercles. The outer surface of the male *S. japonicum* is non-tuberculated.[34] The tegument of the adult parasite, derived from that of the skin-penetrating cercarial stage, has unusual structural features, of great significance in the ability of the fluke to withstand immunological attacks by the host.[44]

Adult worms possess an oral sucker opening into the alimentary tract, and a more posteriorly situated sucker used for the attachment to the endothelium of blood vessels. In the male, a distinctive large ventral groove, the gynaecophoric canal, encloses the female during pairing.

The digestive system consists of a short oesophagus opening into an intestine that divides anteriorly to the ventral sucker and reunites behind the gonads as a blind posterior gut caecum.[45] The black gut contents contain haematin derived from ingested blood.

The excretory system consists of flame cells, collecting tubules and an excretory bladder with a terminal pore.

The male reproductive system comprises four or five pairs of dorsally situated testes opening to the exterior through a vas deferens and seminal vesicle through an infolded cirrus.[44]

In females the reproductive system consists of a pear-shaped ovary in the mid-body line from which the oviduct runs anteriorly to join the common reproductive

duct formed after fusion with a vitelline duct. The common duct enters the ootype, which in turn opens into the uterus which eventually opens to the exterior just below the ventral sucker.[44]

The lifespan of the adult worm in humans is not known accurately. In the past, stress was laid on evidence of longevity with periods quoted ranging from 18 to 28 years[46] to more than 30 years.[47] Since the 1970s, epidemiological studies of the excretal egg outputs of groups of infected people, in the absence of treatment or in the absence of reinfection after successful treatment, have suggested that a proportion of children, in particular, cease to pass eggs in the excreta within a relatively short time. This has been interpreted as indicative of the mortality of established worm burdens and has led to the popular (but not necessarily correct) current concept of the mean length of life of the female schistosome being of the order of 3–8 years.[48]

Detailed reviews of the somewhat fragmentary knowledge of the physiology, biochemistry and genetic constitution are given in specialist publications.[49,50] A later—most useful—review of advances in cell biology and mechanisms of protective immunity together with prospects for the advancement of vaccine studies is available.[51]

Eggs

A general description of egg morphology is given in the section on Aetiology; the microscopic appearance is diagnostic of the parent schistosome species (Figure 80.4) and the eggs are laid by fertilized female schistosomes

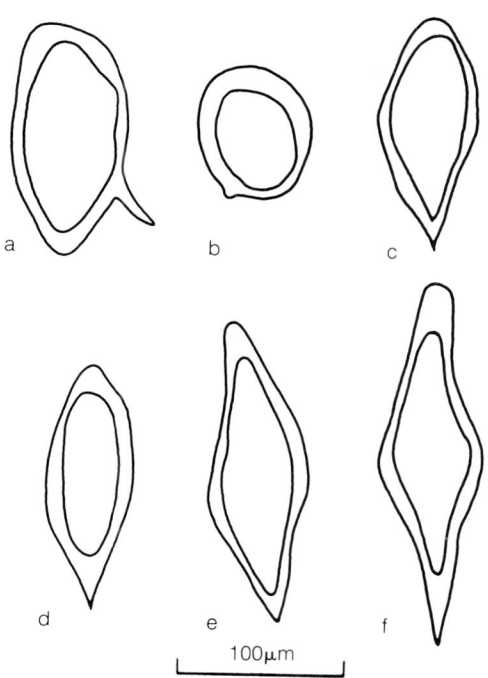

Figure 80.4: Eggs of Schistosoma spp. (a) *S. mansoni*; (b) *S. japonicum*; (c) *S. haematobium*; (d) *S. intercalatum*; (e) *S. mattheei*; (f) *S. bovis*.

intravascularly towards the periphery of the capillary venules. Eggs are non-operculate, possess a spine and contain an embryo, the miracidium, which develops inside the egg within a period of some 16 days. As a rough generalization it is supposed that approximately 50% of eggs pass through the walls of the bladder, the genitourinary apparatus or the colon to be excreted in urine or faeces and the remainder are retained within the tissues. The latter die about 21 days after oviposition. Excreted eggs usually contain embryos seen to be viable by observation of flame cell, ciliary or whole-body movement on microscopy. In a suitable environment of fresh water and warmth (10–30°C), the embryos (miracidia) hatch and leave the egg through slits induced partly by their own activity and partly by osmotic effects.

An adult *S. haematobium* female produces 20–200 terminal-spined eggs per day, *S. mansoni* produces 100–300 or more lateral-spined eggs per female per day and *S. japonicum* produces 500–3500 ovoid eggs with a rudimentary lateral 'knob' per female per day.[2] The fecundity of *S. intercalatum* (another terminal-spined species and *S. mekongi* (ovoid eggs with a rudimentary lateral spine) is unknown.[2]

Miracidia

Although miracidia of different species differ in size, they have similar morphological features and behavioural patterns. Details are given in specialist texts.[52]

On hatching from an egg in appropriate conditions, miracidia swim actively (at 2 mm/s), have behavioural patterns similar to those of the molluscan intermediate hosts and are infective to snails for 8–12 hours.

Intramolluscan development

There appear to be two main mechanisms by which miracidia locate the intermediate snail host: miracidial responses to the main physical variables present in the environment and also their responses to the chemical stimuli originating from snail hosts. The considerable amount of published experimental work on these topics is reviewed in specialist texts.[45,52]

After contact, miracidia penetrate the body surface of the snail through a secretion from the apical gland cells; penetration is initiated by the papilla, the miracidial boring movement probably being assisted by lytic enzymes secreted from the gut.[45] Penetration occurs via the foot of the snail in 70%, other points of entry being the tentacle or the edge of the mantle.[52] In *S. japonicum* infections, penetration points are found over the whole of the cephalopedal area.[52]

After penetration, the ciliated surface of the miracidium disappears and, in an appropriate species of snail, a mother sporocyst develops near the entry site. If the snail is not a potential host, miracidia are destroyed by phagocytic action. Only a small proportion of entering miracidia develop to mature mother sporocysts.

At 96 hours the mother sporocyst is an elongated sac filled with germinal cells and small, centrally located, vacuoles; at 8 days it has undergone further considerable growth. Germ cells are budded off from the epithelial lining; these develop into daughter sporocysts which migrate to other parts of the body of the snail, mainly through the loose connective tissue, to the digestive gland. Further germ ball production ensues, resulting in the final form of the larvae, the cercariae.

As a result of this asexual multiplication process within mother and daughter sporocysts, thousands of cercariae are formed, all of the same sex, and all originating from a single miracidium.

A proportion of infected snails have a shortened lifespan or become sterile. Some exhibit self-cure and their egg laying returns to normal; some die.

From the time of miracidial penetration, production of mature cercariae occurs after 4–5 weeks in *S. mansoni* infection, 5–6 weeks in *S. haematobium* and 7 weeks or longer in *S. japonicum*. Numerous physical, environmental and biological factors account for these variations in time.[45]

Cercariae

All cercariae originating from one miracidium are of the same sex; when mature, they emerge from the snail as a free-swimming stage adaptable to invasion of the definitive host (Figure 80.5).

Cercariae are furcocercous (brevifurcate), have no eye spots or pharynx, are less than 1 cm in length, have an oral muscular sucker occupying about one-third of the body, and a small ventral sucker or acetabulum. Their trilaminar tegument is covered with minute spines and hairs; the digestive system has a mouth in the centre of the oral sucker, an oesophagus and a pair of dorsally

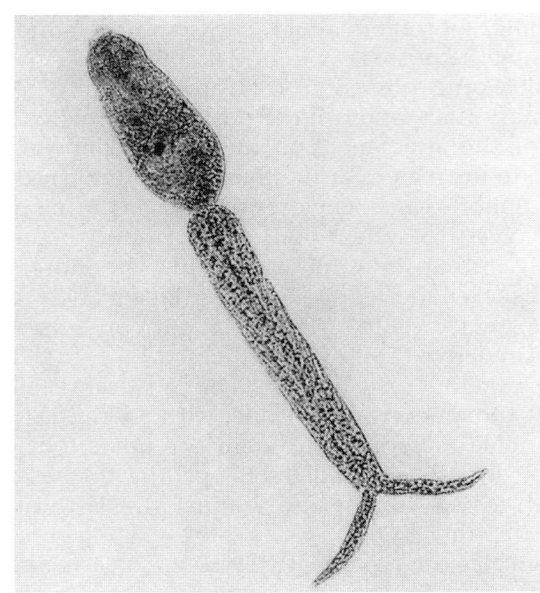

Figure 80.5: Schistosome cercaria. (Courtesy of O. D. Standen.)

placed caeca; behind the oral sucker is a mass of nerve fibres from which three pairs of nerves emerge; the excretory system consists of flame cells, collecting tubules, an excretory bladder and one pair of protonephridia in the tail. Six pairs of cephalic glands subserve the emergence from the snail and penetration of the host skin, aided by enzymatic secretions which have an adhesive function as the cercariae move over the skin in host location.

Cercarial production

In *S. haematobium* and *S. mansoni* the main stimulus for the release of cercariae is light, usually at temperatures between 10 and 30°C. Cercariae can, however, be shed in small numbers in the dark. In the laboratory, marked differences in shedding patterns are seen between the two species. Patterns of shedding in the field are, as might be anticipated, variable and reference should be made to biology texts.[45,52]

In *S. japonicum* infections in the field, cercarial numbers are maximal during the early night; minimal concentrations were recorded at 15.00 hours and maxima at 23.00 hours. Prolonged exposure to light seems to be essential in this species.[53]

Cercarial production varies daily. Correlated with the susceptibility of a snail to infection, a small number excreted initially rises to a peak and then falls to a relatively constant level throughout the life of the snail or until spontaneous cure occurs. The size of the intermediate snail host is probably the most important variable determining cercarial output; other things being equal, large snails shed more than small snails; high cercarial outputs from *Biomphalaria glabrata* are common: 1000–3000 cercariae per day; African *Biomphalaria* spp. shed some 500 cercariae daily and rarely exceed 1500; among the larger *Bulinids*, similar numerical shedding occurs but rarely is 2000 cercariae per day exceeded.

In *S. japonicum* infections, the snail hosts are much smaller and estimates of natural shedding in *Ocomelania hupensis quadrasi* were as low as 15 per day, although, under particular conditions, 160 per day were obtained.[53] In Japan, *O. h. nosophora* is thought to produce many more cercariae than *O. h. quadrasi*.

Cercarial lifespan is short: 36–48 hours. As they are non-feeding organisms dependent on their large glycogen reserves, adverse environmental variables that stimulate glycogen usage reduce cercarial viability.

Water velocity studies relating cercarial penetration and infection rates have produced anomalous results; patently, most cercariae are infective to vertebrate hosts under field conditions.

Schistosomula

After cercariae have penetrated human skin (or pharyngeal mucosa), a rapid process aided by lytic substances from the penetration glands, they lose their tails and become schistosomula. A remarkable additional transition is from a 'freshwater environment' to a 'saltwater environment' within the body.

Schistosomula are thus tailless and worm-like in appearance, shed the glycocalyx, and the skin becomes the seven-layered of the adult worm, consisting of two closely opposed lipid bilayers.[52,54] They then traverse the subcutaneous tissues within 48 hours, penetrate the peripheral or venous channels, and are transported to the right side of the heart and lungs, where the peak concentration is attained in 5–7 days. Further developments in length and surface area occur. Whilst controversy on the route of migration of schistosomula from the lungs to the hepatic portal system has existed for 60 years,[54] more recent evidence suggests that lung development adapts schistosomula for intravascular migration and the parasites exit the lungs in the direction of blood flow, pass to the left side of the heart, and are then distributed to system organs in proportion to cardiac output—a totally intravascular route.

Those parasites entering splanchnic organs penetrate capillary networks rapidly, enter the hepatic portal venous system and most are trapped in the liver. The parasites distributed to organs supplied by the systemic circulation eventually return to the lungs in venous blood.[54] This implies that individual organisms may make repeated circuits of the pulmonary-systemic circulation before entering a blood vessel leading to the hepatic portal system. On arrival in the hepatic portal system, the majority of schistosomula begin to feed on blood, increase in mass and, from a primary location in the smallest hepatic portal distributaries, grow and move upstream into larger vessels.[54] The parasites shorten in dimension, experience a marked loss in motility and undergo various metabolic changes, and, once schistosomula have transformed to adult worms in the liver, lose their ability to undertake intravascular migration.[55]

In experiments with *S. mansoni* pairing occurred 28–35 days after infection. This was succeeded by migration of paired adults to egg-laying sites in the distribution of the mesenteric superior and inferior veins, or the veins of the vesical and pelvic plexus.

Life cycle

The life cycle of all species of schistosome that infect humans has a common pathway from a sexual generation of adult schistosomes within the vascular system of the definitive host, an asexual phase in the freshwater intermediate snail host and a return to the human via cercarial invasion of the skin or mucosa on a host's exposure to cercaria-infested water (Figure 80.6).

Adult schistosomes, living as pairs within capillary blood vessels, the slender females held in the gynaecophoric canal of the male, copulate and the females produce eggs daily throughout their life, the numbers varying with the species (see section on Eggs above).

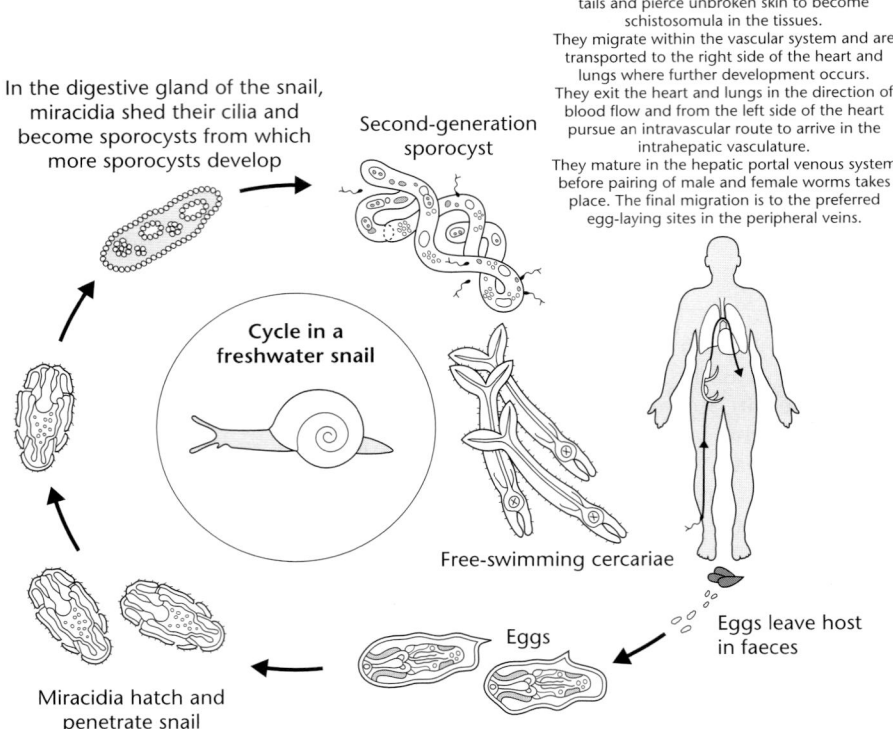

In the digestive gland of the snail, miracidia shed their cilia and become sporocysts from which more sporocysts develop

Second-generation sporocyst

Cycle in a freshwater snail

Person infested by cercariae which shed their tails and pierce unbroken skin to become schistosomula in the tissues.
They migrate within the vascular system and are transported to the right side of the heart and lungs where further development occurs.
They exit the heart and lungs in the direction of blood flow and from the left side of the heart pursue an intravascular route to arrive in the intrahepatic vasculature.
They mature in the hepatic portal venous system before pairing of male and female worms takes place. The final migration is to the preferred egg-laying sites in the peripheral veins.

Free-swimming cercariae

Eggs

Eggs leave host in faeces

Miracidia hatch and penetrate snail

Figure 80.6: Life cycle of *S. mansoni*. (Courtesy of Tropical Resources Unit.)

Eggs, the microscopic appearance of which is diagnostic of the parent schistosome species, are laid intravascularly toward the peripheral branches of the capillary venules. Partly mature at oviposition, some eggs pass through the vessel wall, aided by their spine and cytolytic secretions, into the lumen of the genitourinary tract (*S. haematobium*) or the bowel (*S. mansoni, S. japonicum, S. mekongi, S. intercalatum*) and reach the external world in the excreta (urine and/or faeces). Other eggs, which are the immune-stimulating and pathogenic agents in the tissues, embolize from their intravascular origin to liver, lung and many other sites.

When viable schistosome eggs are excreted and reach fresh water, either by direct deposition or by being washed in from a neighbouring site, in a suitable environment of warmth and light, the larvum within each egg becomes active and, aided by osmosis, the egg ruptures or 'hatches'; the larvum, now termed a miracidium, emerges. Miracidia are mobile organisms swimming actively by means of ciliary movements. Miracidial behaviour is related in a general way to the ecology of the snail intermediate host, and adaptive behavioural patterns have been described. During a short lifespan, miracidia are infective to snail intermediate hosts for some 8–12 hours, and must find a suitable freshwater snail for continuance of their life cycle; such snails (intermediate hosts) are specific for each species of schistosome.

Miracidia then penetrate the soft tissues of the snail, influenced by numerous variables, including chemotaxis, the relative number of larvae and snails within a water body, length of contact time and physical characteristics of the surrounding medium, i.e., water temperature, velocity of flow, turbulence and the presence of ultraviolet light.

Usually, only one or two miracidia undergo further intramolluscan development, producing a sacculate mother sporocyst that in turn produces daughter sporocysts. This is followed by migration to the digestive gland of the snail and subsequent cercarial development.

After an incubation period within the snail, the time of which varies with the species and the surrounding physical environment, cercariae escape from the daughter sporocysts and emerge from the snail under suitable conditions of temperature, light and pH.

Free-swimming fork-tailed cercariae, less than 1 cm in length, penetrate human skin or mucosa (Figure 80.7) when a person is exposed to infested water and, after passage as schistosomula through the tissues, lymphatics and venules, will develop into a male or female schistosome.

Throughout their long life snails continue to produce a reasonably constant output of cercariae; many thousands can originate from a single miracidium.

After migration of schistosomula to the portal vascular system, further growth occurs in the intrahepatic vessels. Pairing of male and female schistosomes takes place on sexual maturity, with subsequent migration to the preferred sites of egg deposition: *S. mansoni* and *S. intercalatum* in the distribution of the inferior mesenteric veins; *S. japonicum* and *S. mekongi* in the distribution of the superior

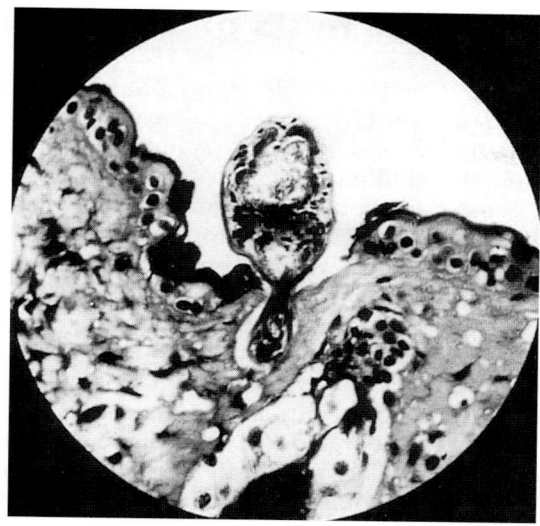

Figure 80.7: Cercarial penetration in schistosomiasis. (Courtesy of O. D. Standen.)

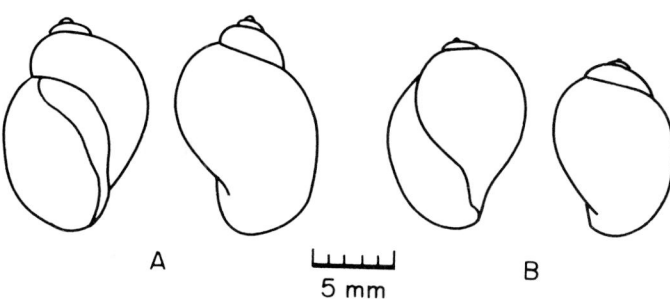

Figure 80.8: Snails of the *Bulinus* genus hosts of *S. haematobium*. A, *Bulinus truncatus* group. B, *B. africanus* group.

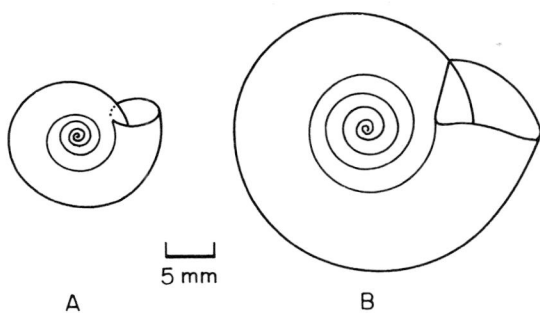

Figure 80.9: Snails of the *Biomphalaria* genus hosts of *S. mansoni*. A, *Biomphalaria alexandrina*. B, *B. glabrata*.

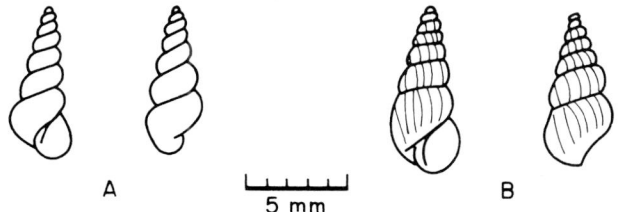

Figure 80.10: Snails of the *Oncomelania* genus host of *S. japonicum*. A, *Oncomelania hupensis nosophora*. B, *O. h. hupensis*.

and inferior mesenteric veins; and *S. haematobium* in the distribution of the vesical veins and the pelvic plexus. Egg deposition and excretal egg excretion begins.

Intermediate hosts

(Figures 80.8–80.10)

The biology of the intermediate snail hosts of the schistosomes is a complex subject covered in numerous specialist texts to which reference should be made for specific details.[2,56–63]

The snail host range of schistosomes is comparatively limited. Successful parasitism of the approximately 18 recognized species of schistosome depends on the ability of the parasite to develop in a small number of species of intermediate hosts within only 10 genera.[61]

Although the schistosomes and their intermediate hosts can be divided roughly into groups reflecting their zoogeographical distribution and host specificity, the situation is complicated because the distribution of schistosomes does not exactly match that of the potential intermediate hosts.[61]

Intermediate hosts of *S. haematobium*

S. haematobium is transmitted by some 30 nominal species of the genus *Bulinus*, classified into four species-groups: *Bulinus africanus*, an important group medically as species within the group are intermediate hosts of *S. haematobium* in Africa south of the Sahara and, additionally, some cattle schistosomes; the *B. forskalli* group is distributed in a pan-African fashion with representatives found in Arabia and in some Indian Ocean islands; the *B. truncatus/tropicus* complex, again of pan-African distri-

bution, extends from Malawi to east, west and north Africa and the Middle East as far as Iran; a small group *B. reticulatus* is found patchily in Africa (e.g., in Ethiopia) and in isolated habitats in the Arabian peninsula.

Intermediate hosts of *S. intercalatum*

Of the two biologically distinct strains of *S. intercalatum* known to exist, one is transmitted by snails of the *Bulinus africanus* group and occurs in a restricted area of northeast Zaire; the other is transmitted by *B. forskalli* and occurs in Cameroon and Gabon. Each strain is unable to develop in a snail with which the other is compatible and, additionally, there are differences in prepatent periods and in certain enzyme patterns of the parasite.[2]

Intermediate hosts of *S. mansoni*

S. mansoni is transmitted by species of the genus *Biomphalaria*, widely distributed in the Old World throughout Africa, the Nile valley and the Arabian peninsula but not in Iraq or Iran. In the New World the genus is found in the southern USA, several Caribbean islands (notably Puerto Rico, St Lucia, Guadeloupe and the Dominican Republic) and on the South American continent in Brazil, Surinam and Venezuela.

The framework for the taxonomic status was described in 1978[63] and four species-groups are still recognized. In the Old World the *Biomphalaria pfeifferi* group has several forms and is found in all parts of Africa south of the Sahara, the Malagasy Republic, in Aden, Yemen and Saudi Arabia; the *choanomphala* group has only a few forms restricted to certain of the great natural African lakes; the *alexandrina* group has a scattered distribution in Africa and is common in the Sudan and Egypt. *B. sudanica* has both east and west African species components.

In the New World, the genus *Biomphalaria* is represented by some 20 species but, of these, only *B. glabrata* (Say), *B. straminea* (Dunker) and *B. tenagophila* (Orbigny) have been found to be naturally infected with *S. mansoni*.

Parasite–intermediate host relationships

There are many complex and complicated variations in the relationships between schistosomes and their intermediate hosts; parasite infectivity is as important as intermediate host susceptibility and differences in relationships occur even within limited geographical areas. Both environmental and genetic factors play a part in influencing the transmission of a schistosome through a particular species of snail.

The genera *Bulinus* and *Biomphalaria* are aquatic snails and are identified on a basis of various conchological, anatomical and biological characteristics. This is a highly specialized field and requires biological expertise. The snails are found in many different habitats including permanent or semipermanent small ponds, marshes, swamps, rivers and streams, and large permanent water bodies such as lakes, dams, irrigation channels and rice fields. Their biology varies with their environment and lengthy studies are required to elucidate the details.

Cross-fertilization is usual in aquatic snail intermediate hosts but they are in fact hermaphrodites and capable of self-fertilization. Ova are laid in water as egg masses some 5–10 mm in diameter. Hatching of free-living snails occurs in 1–2 weeks; a steady growth ensues, and maximal size and maturity is seen in 3–6 months. Snail intermediate hosts have an enormous reproductive potential because egg laying continues throughout life and lifespans have wide variations in the different species; for example, *Bulinus globosus* infected with *S. haematobium* lived for 400 days[64] and *Biomphalaria pfeifferi* infected with *S. mansoni* survived for 213 days.[65]

Intermediate hosts of *S. japonicum*

S. japonicum is transmitted by amphibious snails, populations of polytypic *Oncomelania hupensis*, of which there six subspecies: *O. h. hupensis* in mainland China; *O. h. quadrasi* in the Phillipines; *O. h. nosophora* in Japan; *O. h. lindoensis* in Sulawesi, Indonesia; and *O. h. formosana* and *O. h. chiui* in Taiwan, where schistosomiasis is confined to animals and does not exist in humans.[59] A genus *Tricula aperta* from the subfamily Triculinae transmits *S. mekongi*.

The oncomelanid shell differs markedly in size and shape from those of the aquatic snails (Figure 80.10) and oncomelanid snails have very different biological characteristics. They are dioecious and lay their eggs mainly at night and above the water on a solid-phase location. The separate sexes copulate repeatedly and the female is able to lay eggs more than 3 months after isolation from the male.[53] In the Philippines the average longevity is 66 days but in other endemic areas they may survive for 12 months or longer. Egg laying and hatching are continuous throughout the year.

Aestivation

Both aquatic and amphibious snails have the capacity to survive out of water for weeks, or in some cases, for months; this phenomenon—'aestivation'—has important consequences on the epidemiology of the infection and its control; immature infections of both *S. mansoni* and *S. haematobium* can be carried through from one wet season to another season, thus perpetuating the transmission cycle.

Epidemiology of human schistosomiasis

The epidemiology and epidemiological dynamics of schistosomiasis are heterogeneous and complicated, involving a definitive host in the human, an intermediate host in various species of aquatic or amphibious snail, a freshwater environment that humans contaminate with excreta through unsanitary habits, and from which infection is also acquired through repeated water contact by means of many occupational and recreational activities.[34]

The parasites need the internal environment of the two hosts, definitive and intermediate, to complete the sexual and asexual phases of the life cycle respectively, and the free-living larval stages present in the common aquatic environment are the linking infective factors.[66]

Transmission is influenced by numerous variables, the major ones being:

1. The distribution, biology and population dynamics of the intermediate snail host(s).
2. The patterns and extent of environmental contamination with human excreta, which in turn depend on

the prevalence and intensity of human infection and the socio-economic and hygienic backgrounds.
3. Human water contact activities, patterns and duration.
4. The host–parasite relationship in both snail and human, and the role of protective mechanisms in the human host.[67]

Of all the parasitic infections of humans, schistosomiasis is one of the most widespread, as illustrated by data advanced by the WHO.[2] The disease ranks second only to malaria in terms of socio-economic and public health importance in many tropical and subtropical areas. It is second to none in prevalence among the water-borne diseases, and is most common in rural areas of developing countries. The latest WHO estimates, extrapolated from the world atlas of schistosomiasis[31] and applied to 1995 population estimates, gave figures of 652 million at risk of infection from the five schistosome species commonly infecting humans and a global prevalence of 193 million. Of more crucial importance, 85% of infected people are on the African continent.[27] The background is one of low socio-economic status on a base of poverty and ignorance, with resultant poor housing, lack of potable water, inadequate hygienic conditions, few if any sanitary facilities, and a multitude of activities bringing a population into contact with water into which eggs are passed and in which are found intermediate snail hosts. Obligatory human water contact may be of domestic, hygienic, occupational, recreational or religious origin. Thus transmission begins. Children are particularly important as reservoirs of infection because of their indiscrimate excretory habits, especially urination when swimming, and their unrivalled opportunities for water contact in hot climates.

Schistosomiasis is not invariably a rural disease: expanding populations in periurban fringes of cities overwhelm the available sanitation and are thus at risk of transmission; examples are not infrequent within the boundaries of the modern cities of Africa. The infection also arises as a result of the movement of infected people into refugee camps, where endemic foci may be initiated.

Major factors associated with the spread and intensification of schistosomiasis are its links with water development projects, particularly human-made lakes and irrigation schemes because these are often sites of population immigrations for farming and fishing, so much a feature of the present tropical scene.

In many countries schistosomiasis is not a notifiable disease and prevalence estimates (i.e., the proportion of subjects infected at a given point in time) are frequently gross underestimates. The advanced clinical symptoms, signs and complications known to occur do not represent the full picture of infection in a community. Moreover, the intensity of infection (i.e., measures of worm burdens in a group or in a community, usually inferred by the surrogate technique of quantitative egg counting in stools or urine) is extremely variable. Whilst in general there is a good correlation between intensity of infection and the pathology produced, expressed as morbidity, exceptions

occur and many cases of schistosomiasis are uncovered only during a purposive survey or incidentally in the investigation of another complaint.

This generalized correlation between prevalence and intensity of infection means that, for all practical purposes, the higher the prevalence, the greater the mean intensity of infection in a sample.

The epidemiology of schistosomiasis shows wide variations within any endemic country. Focality is a major feature of the epidemiology and surprising differences in prevalence and intensity of infection occur between neighbouring geographical environments. This makes broad generalized descriptions of the status of the infection within a country different and renders many comparisons between countries invalid. The epidemiology can change rapidly in any endemic area, or in any previously uninfected area, as a result of water resource development projects of any type.

Community-based studies of schistosomiasis usually demonstrate that age-specific prevalences and intensities are highly positively skewed, this phenomenon being more marked in *S. haematobium* infections than for *S. mansoni*, and even less so for *S. japonicum*, while data for *S. intercalatum* and *S. mekongi* are as yet too fragmentary to allow definitive statements.

In urinary schistosomiasis (*S. haematobium*), the prevalence rises rapidly from the age when youngsters begin to wander afield.[34] The peak prevalence and intensity of infection occur in children aged 10–14 years, and thereafter successive decades see a progressive lowering of prevalence to much reduced levels. Some 60–70% of all infected persons lie within the age range of 5–14 years and the heaviest infections occur similarly in this same age range.

In areas endemic for *S. mansoni*, prevalences and intensities of infection are maximal in the 10–24 years age group. Although reductions occur with increasing age, prevalence levels remain at higher levels than those seen in *S. haematobium* infections. Some 5–25% of the infected population excretes at least 50% of the total number of eggs contaminating the environment, and the majority of heavily infected children lie in the 10–14 years age group. In a high proportion of those with over 800 eggs per gram of faeces, an enlarged liver and spleen are present.[2]

The explanation for the reduction of prevalence and intensity of infection in older age groups in areas endemic for *S. haematobium* and *S. mansoni* depends on multiple factors: immune mechanisms certainly contribute; tissue fibrosis prevents eggs from reaching the exterior; and a proportion of the body population of infecting worms will have died. Apart from occupational water contact, exposure to cercaria-infested waters is likely to be less with increasing age.[34]

The exact roles played by immune, pathological, parasitological and environmental, ecological and human behavioural mechanisms and their possible interactions are uncertain and remain a topic for constant debate among various 'lobby protagonists'.

In *S. japonicum* infection, 'typical' age distribution and intensity patterns do not seem to occur. This doubtless reflects epidemiological variations between areas within a country and also between countries, and perhaps the many animals that can act as reservoir hosts.

Bimodal prevalence peaks in the 10–14 years grouping and those aged 36–44 years have been documented.[2]

Animal reservoirs

Some 31 wild mammals and 13 domestic animals have been shown to be infected with *S. japonicum* in China,[68] but only rarely has their role in transmission been evaluated. However, animals cannot be considered negligible for, based on the total animal populations, prevalence, mean daily egg output and hatchability, the dog, cow, pig, rat, carabao (water buffalo) and goat were, in decreasing order of magnitude, estimated to be responsible for some 25% of the total potential environmental contamination, while humans were thought to provide 75% in the Philippines.[53]

In striking contrast, the human is the only definitive host of *S. haematobium*. The few infections with this parasite reported in primates, Arteridactyla or Rodentia can be considered as incidental and of no epidemiological importance.

Many reports exist of infection with *S. mansoni* in a wide range of mammals (Primates, Insectivora, Arteriodactyla, Marsupilia, Rodentia, Carnivora, Edentata). Evidence implicating their role in maintenance of transmission of the parasite is, with two exceptions, lacking. In Tanzania, it was considered that baboons were maintaining the parasite among themselves[69] and there is good reason to believe that *S. mansoni* is maintained by both rats (*Rattus rattus*—a known reservoir host) and humans in a natural habitat in Guadeloupe[70,71] and in some areas of Brazil.[1]

In *S. mekongi* infections, dogs are known to be a reservoir host.[26]

Immunity

Neither sex nor age confers immunity and all races are susceptible to infection. The female adult schistosomes lay eggs after pairing and deposit them in the capillary habitat for many years. Thus schistosomiasis is a chronic disease with morbidity produced by granulomatous reactions to eggs deposited in the tissues. Primary infections occur early in life. Although the host is presented with new and heavy antigenic burdens when cercariae invade and schistosomula are maturing, few infected persons are diagnosed as having the clinical picture of the acute febrile illness known as 'acute toxaemic' schistosomiasis or 'Katayama syndrome'.

The development of acquired immunity in schistosomal infections is slow and inefficient, and differs from the immediate and complete immunity of the type occurring after common childhood viral or bacterial infections.[72] The reasons for this are unclear but IgG and IgM antibodies antagonize the protective effects of the immune system in young children and may be related to the slow development of immunity faced with a number of potentially protective responses.[73–77]

After the primary infection in childhood, numerous reinfections occur in subsequent years and are largely unopposed. As schistosomes do not replicate within the human host, this results in a rapid acquisition of high worm loads, high egg outputs, and resultant pathology and morbidity. Yet it is well known from community-based surveys that the prevalence and intensity of infection progressively decrease in the teenage years, and that successive decades see a decline in prevalence to much lower levels. One theory advanced to explain the age distributions of prevalences and intensities in whole populations was that the decreases in older age groups might be due to changing social habits resulting in decreased human water contact.[78] Other factors involved may be tissue fibrosis, preventing eggs from reaching the exterior, and the death of various proportions of the body population of infecting worms, which, additionally, would account for the phenomenon of 'loss of infection' encountered during epidemiological surveys, i.e., the failure to detect eggs in excreta on successive surveys in persons who were previously egg positive.[66]

Despite enormous amounts of recent experimental, immunological and clinicoepidemiological research inputs into the explanation of acquired resistance or anti-schistosome resistance in schistosomiasis, a wide variety of basic questions remain.[79]

A high proportion of adults in endemic areas who acquired the primary infection in childhood possess immunity to superinfection and usually show few clinical signs. Although this immunity is protective against schistosomula and adult worms, it causes characteristic lesions of the infection when directed against eggs.

Protective immunity directed against cercariae and schistosomula reduces the numbers surviving to adulthood. Two mechanisms are involved: an antibody-dependent cell-mediated cytotoxicity process, itself dependent on eosinophils and IgG; and a process involving IgE and macrophages.

Concomitant immunity, in experimental terms, describes the resistance, partial or total, of an actively infected host to a subsequent challenge infection by the same type of organism. Adult worms evade the immune responses by adding a layer of host-specific antigens to their tegmental membranes. Adult worms of a primary infection are unharmed by cercarial challenge but the invading forms of the challenge infection tend to be destroyed.[72] Concomitant immunity occurs in schistosome infections and challenges in many experimental hosts and in humans.[79]

Further exploratory progress was made through longitudinal field studies involving detailed quantitation of egg outputs and water contact in children, allied to the technique of reinfection studies. Chemotherapy is given to remove existing infections; the levels of newly acquired infections (reinfections) are observed, quantitated, and related to water contact and degree of exposure. These techniques produced strong evidence that age-dependent resistance to reinfection is distinct from age-dependent exposural change, in two areas, The Gambia and Kenya, for both *S. haematobium* and *S. mansoni* infection. For example, in The Gambia, changes in intensity of infection with time were compared in two communities, in one of which transmission had been interrupted by mollusciciding. In this area, the mean lifespan of the worms was 3–4 years, allowing the comparison in the untreated area (control) area of the numbers of eggs deposited by worms over the same 3-year period. The acquisition of new infections by adults over 25 years of age was 1000-fold less than that of 5–8-year-old children. This difference could not be attributed to a 1000-fold reduction of water contact in the adults, thus suggesting age-dependent acquisition of immunity to superinfection.[80–83]

Thus the role of immunity in limited schistosome infections in communities in two areas endemic for *S. haematobium* and *S. mansoni* was placed on a firmer footing. However, the immunity is probably not absolute, is evident only after years of exposure to infection, and some data suggest that it occurs earlier in areas of high prevalence and intensity.

The balance of the immune response in the early years of exposure to infection is directed towards production of blocking antibodies, which may be of IgM, IgG or IgG$_4$. Protective antibodies, IgE or other immunoglobulin isotypes, are detected in both older children and adults who appear to be resistant to infection.[84]

Later data led to a surmise that 'resistance' to acquired infection, or reinfection after successful chemotherapy, is multifactorial and compartmentalized. It may involve both humoral and cellular responses at different stages of parasitic invasion. Known influencing variables are an IgE response, high levels of interferon γ (IFNγ) and tumour necrosis factor α (TNFα) and peripheral blood mononuclear cell (PBMC) responses involving different groups of cells and various cytokines, allied to a possible genetic factor on chromosome 5q31-q33. Further molecular exploration is ongoing.[85]

Pathogenesis

The lesions that occur during this long-lived infection are caused largely by schistosome eggs. Adult worms are impervious to the immune system of the host and by themselves cause little or no pathology, although they excrete antigens, such as the gut-associated soluble antigens found in the sera of patients with schistosomiasis and which are now used both as a marker for infection and as an indicator of therapeutic success through estimation of the cathode- and anode-associated antigens.[86]

Schistosome eggs cannot traverse capillary beds unaided because they measure up to 70 µm in width. Slightly less than half of the eggs are laid into the lumen of the gut or urinary tract. The remainder are laid in the walls of the organ or embolize into the portal radicles or lung arterioles. Collateral vascular bypasses enable eggs to reach many other organs in the body.

At oviposition, eggs are immature but miracidial maturation takes place within a few days. Soluble egg antigens (SEAs) originating from the secretory glands of miracidia enclosed within eggs diffuse out though submicroscopic pores in the eggshell and induce a host hypersensitivity response. The immunopathology of schistosomiasis is considered to be due to granuloma formation around tissue-deposited eggs and is a manifestation of delayed hypersensitivity through a T cell-mediated immune response.

During an active infection, a range of early, mature and involuting granulomas is present.[87] Granulomas vary with the immune status of the host: in primary infections with marked reactions to soluble egg antigens, large florid granulomas occur with some central necrosis. The florid granuloma is composed of the schistosome egg surrounded by cellular aggregates of eosinophils, mononuclear phagocytes, lymphocytes, neutrophils, plasma and fibroblasts. Activated macrophages cluster close to the eggshell, while lymphocytes and plasma cells are peripherally placed. Fibroblasts appear early and throughout the lengthy involution process replace other cell types.[87] Many granulomas are of sizes much greater than those of schistosome eggs.

After the acute phase of some 3 months, modulation of host immune responses to SEAs results in relatively small granulomas which have fewer surrounding cells.

There are consistent and strong correlations of high organ and tissue egg loads and severe pathology in quantitative autopsy studies in *S. haematobium* and *S. mansoni*;[88,89] clinicoepidemiological findings are in agreement. Other factors may operate, such as direct and indirect fibroblastic proliferation and induced abnormalities of types I and III collagen.

Thus the pathology of schistosomiasis results from collections of granulomas, from fibroblastic lesions obstructing vessels and fibroinflammatory swellings containing millions of eggs.[87] Unlike early granulomas, these late and obstructive and fibrous lesions respond poorly to antischistomal chemotherapy.

There is a plethora of systemic host responses to schistosome infection, as cercariae, schistosomula, adult worms and eggs all generate multiple antigens to which the host immune system responds through immunocompetent cells. Antibodies specific to each stage are long lived and persist after successful chemotherapy. Several defined schistosome antigens have been detected; the most useful in clinical work is the cathode-associated antigen. Other antigens are complexed to immunoglobulins and can be found at various sites, e.g., schistosomal nephropathy.[90]

Von Lichtenberg[87] has strikingly contrasted the pathogenetic variables and prognosis in the hepatosplenomegaly of the early infection resulting from cell proliferation with florid granulomas, reticuloendothelial hyperplasia and diffuse inflammatory infiltrates, all reversible by specific chemotherapy, with the hepatosplenomegaly of the advanced disease induced by fibrovascular pathology with periportal fibrosis, portal hypertension and its associated effects on the spleen in which the prognosis is far less dependent on chemotherapy but more on surgical alleviation of a mechanical obstructive condition.

The influence of genetic factors on immunopathology and on protective immunity remains unclear. While two studies in Egypt[91] and the Philippines[92] suggested a relationship between severe disease and specific human leucocyte antigen (HLA) haplotypes, the association was not found in Brazil.[93] However, a more recent Brazilian study demonstrated that host genetic factors were implicated in human resistance to *S. mansoni* in one specific focus.[94] No firm generalizations can yet be made.

Pathology

It is useful to consider the pathology and pathophysiology of the various schistosome infections within the stages of the life cycle and their time frames:

- Cercarial invasion and schistosomular migration.
- Maturation of schistosomes, pairing and commencement of egg laying.
- Established infection with continuous egg laying.
- Late stages and complications.

Attempts to link discrete clinical entities with these stages should be made only with the realization that the apparently endless series of epidemiological, immunological and physiological interactions encountered, particularly in endemic areas, make resultant associations and correlations less than clearcut.

Frequently, much clearer relationships between clinical expressions and pathophysiological derangements are seen in non-immune visitors, transients or immigrants who become infected in endemic areas. In parallel, infected travellers or holiday-makers returning to temperate locations may present clear pictures of infections acquired in endemic zones.

Cercarial invasion of the skin or mucosal penetration on exposure to infested water, particularly when the quantum of infection is high, can occur in less than 15 minutes; the clinical complement of cercarial dermal invasion is a schistosome (cercarial or allergic) dermatitis lasting for some 24–48 hours.

The pathophysiological response is the initiation of the first mechanisms of the immune response with marked eosinophilia and an antibody-dependent cell-mediated cytotoxic response involving IgG.

At widely different times, ranging from 2 to 16 weeks after cercarial invasion, during the migration of schistosomula, their maturation, pairing and initiation of egg laying, the clinical manifestations of acute toxaemic schistosomiasis or Katayama syndrome may arise. Worm and/or egg antigens produce a marked antigenic stimulus with rapidly rising antibody levels and an increase in

serum IgG, IgA and IgM levels. Circulating antigen–antibody complexes are found and may be deposited in glomeruli, producing immune complex glomerulopathy. The whole clinical picture is one resembling the acute serum sickness syndrome.

At variable times after infection, from some 2 months onwards, the stage of established infection occurs, with continuous egg laying associated with the 'classical' symptoms and signs of established schistosomiasis. SEAs from miracidia in the eggs provoke a T lymphocyte-mediated host response which, in time, results in the characteristic granuloma with eosinophils prominent in the destruction of the eggs.

After some years, changes in clinical symptoms and physical signs appear, and there is superimposition of late-stage complications such as obstructive uropathy, hydronephrosis and pyelonephritic renal failure in *S. haematobium* infection, or portal hypertension which may be 'compensated' or 'decompensated' with ascites, and hepatospenomegaly with or without gastrointestinal bleeding in *S. mansoni*, *S. japonicum* and *S. mekongi* infections. Modulation by T suppressor lymphocytes and antibody blockade diminish the host immune response over time; fibroblasts stimulate collagen production and fibrotic complications involving a variety of anatomical sites (e.g., periportal hepatic fibrosis and obstructive uropathy) ensue.

Pathology of established infection

S. haematobium
Urinary bladder
The urinary bladder is the most frequently affected organ. Cystoscopy, surgery or autopsy reveals the gross lesions, which are often multiple. A hyperaemic mucosa on cystoscopy is universal. 'Sandy patches' occur in one-third; these are raised greyish-yellow mucosal irregularities associated with heavy egg deposition and surrounded by dense fibrous tissue. Calcification may occur. They are sited most commonly at the trigone and near the ureteric orifices.[95]

Other raised lesions are granulomas, nodules and polyps which may be sessile or pedunculated and are related to local heavy tissue egg loads. Focal granulomas are of pin-head size with the customary histological appearances.

Vesical ulcers are less common and can vary in size from a small irregular defect to an irregular deep transverse fissure. They occur mainly on the posterior wall of the bladder.

Many degrees of bladder muscle hypertrophy are found at autopsy but specific associations with tissue egg loads or local lesions are lacking; muscle hypertrophy appears to be more frequent in cases with obstructive uropathy. Obstructive lesions from fibrosis of the neck of the bladder in periurethral granulomatous reactions are a common complication, as are bladder calculi.

Bladder calcification is common and is often encountered both in clinical practice and in radiological surveys.

Calcification is linear, occurring along lines of deposited eggs. Calcified bladders usually retain normal elasticity.

Ureters

Although the ureters are less frequently affected than the bladder, their involvement is important for it leads to morbidity and is the forerunner of obstructive uropathy. Tissue egg loads in the ureters are greater in cases with obstructive uropathy than in those without.[95,96] Arguments on whether unilateral disease predominates more on the left than on the right side have continued for at least a decade. In a quantitative analysis, tissue egg burdens were much higher in the right lower ureter than in the left, but unilateral obstructive uropathy occurred equally on both sides.[95,96] Bilateral ureteric involvement is the rule.

The histopathological appearance of the ureteric lesions resembles that of bladder lesions. Granulomatous lesions resolve and lead to ureteral fibrotic stenosis. Rising back pressure leads to hydroureter, with or without hydronephrosis, the collective title of which is obstructive uropathy. This condition predisposes to *Escherichia coli* or *Salmonella* urinary tract infection, which can lead to chronic pyelonephritis and Gram-negative septicaemia.[97,98]

Genital organs

Because *S. haematobium* parasitizes the vesical plexus, eggs are not uncommonly found in both male and female genital organs, but the long-running debate of their functional significance has not yet been concluded.

In males, the mean *S. haematobium* egg count per gram of seminal vesicle tissue was 20 000 in one investigation.[95] The resultant enlargement, muscular hypertrophy and fibrosis produced an increase in weight of the seminal vesicles that correlated with the presence of obstructive uropathy.[95] Much less commonly affected were the prostate, testes, epididymis and penis. A causal role for these lesions in the production of male infertility has not been substantiated.

In females, the finding of eggs in the female genital organs is similarly frequent; eggs may be found in the vulva, vagina and cervix, where ulcerating, polypoid or nodular lesions may be seen. Nodules in the perianal skin are not rare. The internal female genital organs—ovaries, Fallopian tubes and uterus—are much less commonly affected. In Malawi, gynaecological complications of schistosomiasis were considered a significant cause of female morbidity, particularly when the lower genital tract was involved; ovarian, uterine and tubal pathologies were not major causes of morbidity, but diagnosis was difficult.[99] There is a dearth of recent reports associating ectopic pregnancy or infertility and *S. haematobium* infection.[100]

Schistosomiasis has little impact on female infertility and rarely renders a woman anovulatory despite the proximity of eggs to the gonads, tubes and uterus.[87]

Gastrointestinal tract

S. haematobium eggs are found frequently in the gastrointestinal tract, their density being highest in the appendix with a gradual decrease in density down to the distal tract. Polyps have been recorded in the rectosigmoid colon in an autopsy study of *S. haematobium* cases; the polyps were inflammatory and were often ulcerated.[101]

S. haematobium eggs are often seen in rectal biopsy material but are usually dead.

Kidney

Although schistosomal granulomas are rare in the parenchyma, renal lesions occur as a sequel of obstructive uropathy and are manifest as pyelonephritis.

Schistosomal antigens in mesangial areas of the glomeruli in uncomplicated cases of *S. haematobium* infection have been observed by immunofluorescent microscopy as well as granular deposits of IgG, IgM and C3, yet there was a lack of basement membrane changes, an absence of clinical renal disease and normal renal function.[102] There remains doubt about whether *S. haematobium* causes a specific nephropathy in the face of other mechanisms of renal failure.[103] A reversible nephrotic syndrome in *S. haematobium* complicated by *Salmonella* infection has been described.[104]

Lung

Pulmonary arteritis and cor pulmonale are rare in pure *S. haematobium* infection, yet egg granulomas are frequently encountered at autopsy.[100]

Ectopic lesions

Migration of *S. haematobium* within the vascular system and subsequent egg laying may produce a variety of ectopic lesions.

It was formerly considered that *S. haematobium* in Egypt was not a cause of Symmer's periportal hepatic fibrosis (despite the common finding of *S. haematobium* granulomas in the liver). More recent studies, and in particular those using ultrasonography, have shown that *S. haematobium* in Egypt does indeed cause schistosomal hepatic fibrosis, hepatic granulomas, cellular infiltration of the portal tracts, and obstruction and substitution of portal radicles by granulomas.[105,106]

Cutaneous deposition of *S. haematobium* eggs is not uncommon and has been recognized for decades.[107] Papular or nodular lesions occur in many sites, most frequently in the genital and perigenital areas but also in the neck, chest and abdominal wall.[108–112]

Other sites of ectopic lesions are the central nervous system (CNS), an occurrence less frequent than in infections due to *S. japonicum* or *S. mansoni*.

The finding of eggs of *S. haematobium* in the CNS without clinical sequelae is not rare; eggs appear to produce minimal or no histological reaction, in contrast to the production of inflammatory responses when laid elsewhere.[113] The spinal cord is affected more often than the brain.[100,113]

Rare and curious lesions have been described, such as multiple *S. haematobium* egg deposition in the pericardium, causing a fibrous pericarditis,[114] and the demonstration of an adult *S. haematobium* worm in the choroid plexus.[115]

Bladder cancer and *S.haematobium* infection

Despite at least 14 reviews of the relationship between bladder cancer and *S. haematobium* infection published since the early 1980s, the aetiological significance of the parasite in the causation of this cancer remains a topic for argument.[100]

In Egypt, where *S. haematobium* has been hyper-endemic for centuries and despite the fact that the prevalence and intensity of infection has decreased rapidly and substantially since the 1960s, cancer in a bladder infected with schistosomiasis occupies the primary rank among all recorded cancers.[116]

In certain other countries, for instance Iraq, coastal Kenya, Ghana, Malawi, Mozambique, Zambia and Zimbabwe, a consistent association between the presence of *S. haematobium* and bladder carcinoma seems to exist. However, in Nigeria, South Africa and Saudi Arabia, all countries with a moderate or high prevalence of *S. haematobium*, the association is not present: bladder cancer is no more frequent than in non-endemic countries.

When cancer is associated with urinary schistosomiasis, the tumour may occur at any site in the bladder, yet it rarely originates in the trigone, a frequent site of origin in non-schistosomal cancers and the commonest site of 'sandy patches' and heavy egg deposition.

Schistosomal bladder cancer occurs in an age group significantly younger than that in which cancer occurs in non-schistosomal areas. In the Nile delta, where men do most of the agricultural work, which involves repeated exposure to cercaria-infested waters, the ratio of male : female bladder cancer with histological evidence of past schistosomal infection is as high as 12 : 1,[117] whereas the sex ratio among those with no such evidence approximates the 4 : 1 ratio seen in the UK.[118]

The histopathology of cancer in association with schistosomiasis is dominated by squamous cell tumours, in contrast to the commoner transitional cell carcinoma encountered in non-schistosomal areas.[88,100,119]

Most squamous cell cancers in schistosomal bladders are fairly well differentiated, largely indolent and localized, spreading directly through the bladder wall with late and infrequent lymphatic spread. Bloodstream metastasis is rare. This picture contrasts sharply with that of transitional cell carcinoma.

Bladder cancer has been produced experimentally in monkeys and baboons infected with *S. haematobium*,[120,121] species not known for the common occurrence of bladder tumours. However, two large consecutive autopsy studies conducted in Cairo showed no differences of significance in the frequency or type of urothelial malignancies in patients with or without urinary schistosomiasis.[95,101]

Several mechanisms have been suggested to explain the suspected role of *S. haematobium* in bladder cancer, none of which is proven; for example, fibrosis induced by schistosome eggs may induce proliferation, abnormal hyerplasia and metaplasia, all possible precancerous changes, in epithelial cells;[122] chronic urinary bacterial infection and the production of nitrosamines (well-known bladder carcinogens) from their precursors in urine;[123] urinary stasis allowing concentration of endogenous carcinogens leading to their absorption from urine and exposure of the bladder epithelium;[124,125] raised urinary β-glucuronidase levels originating from miracidia and adult schistosomes liberating carcinogenic amines in urine.[120]

In summary, carcinogenic change associated with *S. haematobium* occurs only after many years of infection. The schistosomal infection is considered to be a tumour promoter, potentiating carcinogenesis, rather than a direct inducer. The various cofactors necessary for malignant neoplasia are not known with certainty.

However, arguments against an association between urinary schistosomiasis and bladder cancer still remain.[126] Possibly, the next few decades will provide clarification of the relationship. Large-scale population-based chemotherapy directed at the control of morbidity would be expected to lower cancer incidence rates in the most badly affected endemic countries, and studies to this end are in place in Egypt. The critical problem will be the acquisition of accurate and acceptable population-based incidence estimates of bladder cancer.

Should this prove to be the case, it will validate the most penetrating report to date on the relationship between *S. haematobium* and bladder cancer from the International Agency for Research on Cancer[127] (IARC), which concluded that there is sufficient evidence in humans for the carcinogenicity of infection with *Schistosoma haematobium* and arrived at the overall evaluation that infection with *Schistosoma haematobium* is carcinogenic to humans.

S. mansoni

A range of chronic lesions is found, from scattered granulomas of the intestinal tract to gross hepatic periportal fibrosis (Symmer's pipe-stem fibrosis; bilharzial clay-pipe stem fibrosis).

Focal granulomas and fibrosis may occur in any part of the intestinal tract, most frequently in the rectosigmoid colon because the preferred habitat of adult *S. mansoni* is in the tributaries of the inferior mesenteric vein. These lesions rarely lead to gross clinical symptoms. Pathology in the small bowel is not as severe as that in the large gut, even though in late-stage infections, particularly in Egypt and Brazil, there was a shift in egg deposition from the colon to the small intestine at autopsy.[89]

Colonic polyposis, a syndrome peculiar but not exclusive to Egypt, occurs in young patients and is related directly to the intensity of infection. The colon and rectum are the sites of multiple pedunculated polyps with associated mucosal swelling, hyperaemia and oedema. The concentration of eggs within the polyps is much higher than at other sites in the intestine. The clinical accompaniments are significant blood and protein losses producing anaemia, chronic diarrhoea, tenesmus and a protein-losing enteropathy.

Occasionally pseudotumours of schistosomal eggs surrounded by extensive fibrous tissue occur in *S. mansoni*

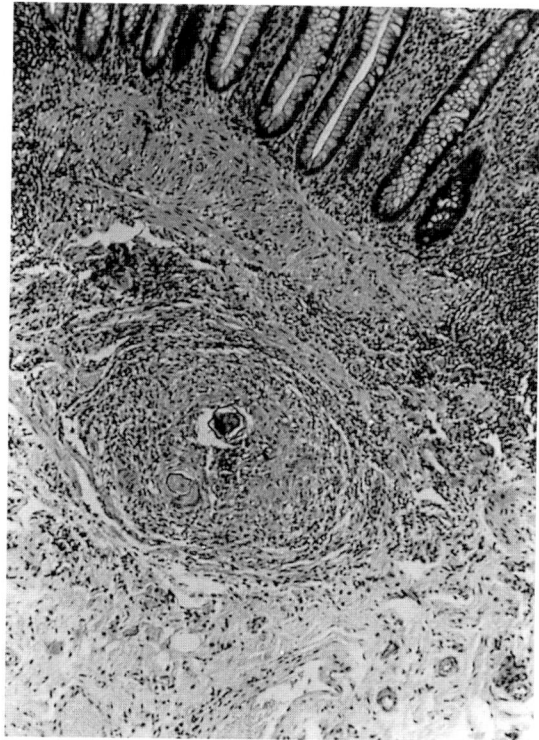

Figure 80.11: Schistosomal granuloma (*S. mansoni*) of bowel. The structureless mass at the centre is an egg.

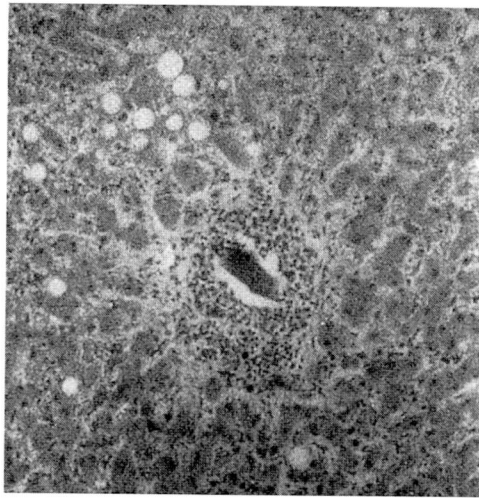

Figure 80.12: Schistosomal granuloma (*S. mansoni*) in liver. The structureless mass at the centre is an egg. (Courtesy of B. H. Kean.)

infection and are termed 'bilharziomas'. Sites of predilection are the omentum, mesenteric lymph nodes, paracaecal region and infrequently the wall of the gut.

Schistosomal granulomas in bowel and liver are illustrated in Figures 80.11 and 80.12.

Hepatosplenic schistosomiasis

The major, and undoubtedly the most important, complication of chronic *S. mansoni* infection is periportal hepatic fibrosis; because the basic pathology is sited in and around the portal tracts and the hepatic parenchyma is normal in uncomplicated cases, the term cirrhosis is inappropriate. A cut section of the liver, which may or may not be enlarged, shows macroscopic wide bands of fibrosis around portal tracts, resembling the stems of a number of clay pipes (see Figure 80.19). The surface of the liver may be smooth, granular or nodular. Between portal fields, the hepatic parenchyma does not exhibit the nodularity of Laënnec's cirrhosis.

Deposited eggs produce granulomas with surrounding inflammatory infiltrates in the connective tissue that surrounds the hepatic veins, proximal to presinusoidal vessels. Affected portal tracts become blocked with granulomas and disorganized by inflammation, fibrosis and pyelophlebitis.[87] Eggs, an eosinophilic infiltrate, schistosomal pigment and/or organizing thrombi are found. The accumulation of egg granulomas around sites of blockage leads to further portal enlargement, and simultaneously the hepatic arteries enlarge and push out new branching capillaries. Thus the presinusoidal portal hypertension produces a compensatory arterial flow. Total intrahepatic blood flow remains within normal limits, with maintenance of hepatocellular integrity.

The diminished portal blood flow from portal hypertension is compensated for by the increase in hepatic arterial supply and the rich capillary arterial network around the portal branches which communicates with the portal vein.[128] There remain unexplained discrepancies between clinical and pathological interpretations of the arterial origin of the hepatic capillary network.[128]

Hepatic fibrosis results from the accumulation of collagen in the liver[129] and may originate in the proliferation of collagen-synthesizing cells, increased synthesis by existing cells or deficiency in collagen degradation.[130] In experimental animals, the amount of collagen in the liver increases in parallel with egg granuloma formation;[131] in human hepatic schistosomiasis there is increased collagen content and marked collagen synthesis in wedge liver biopsy material when compared with control tissue.[132]

The natural course of pure periportal fibrosis is slow and is termed 'compensated' because liver cell function tests show only slight abnormalities, if any. Over time, the consequences of portal hypertension with splenomegaly and/or variceal haemorrhage, with or without ascites, appear, although hepatic decompensation does not develop until an advanced stage of the process. In countries where there is a high prevalence of viral hepatitis (hepatitis B, C, D or E), these may coexist with hepatosplenic schistosomiasis, and the clinical progression of decompensated hepatic fibrosis presents a much more rapid progress because hepatocellular pathology is much more severe than in the 'pure' state of schistosomal hepatic fibrosis.

Spleen

Splenomegaly is the usual accompaniment of hepatic schistosomiasis and is due to portal venous hypertension, chronic passive congestion and reticuloendothelial hyperplasia. Focal infarcts and trabecular haemorrhages may occur and the spleen is tough and fibrotic. Hypersplenism may produce a pancytopenia or a leucoerythroblastic anaemia. The spleen may become enormously enlarged (Egyptian splenomegaly or Banti's syndrome in the older literature), as in kala azar (visceral leishmaniasis) or the myeloproliferative syndromes.[87] Lymphomas have been reported occasionally.[133]

Lungs and heart
Pulmonary hypertension caused by granulomatous pulmonary arteritis originating from large-scale embolization of eggs is commonly the result of hepatic pipe-stem fibrosis with extensive portocaval shunts occurring in *S. mansoni* or *S. japonicum* infections. This may produce schistosomal cor pulmonale. Strangely, and despite a direct access to the lungs via the inferior vena cava, cor pulmonale occurs less frequently in pure or mixed *S. haematobium* infection than would be anticipated.[100] There are fewer reports of cor pulmonale in *S. japonicum* than in *S. mansoni* infection despite the similar pathogenetic mechanisms.[128]

Granulomatous inflammation occludes distal pulmonary arterial branches and eventually produces a rise in pulmonary arterial pressure with right ventricular hypertrophy and strain; the smaller arterioles show fibrointimal sclerosis; fibrinoid necrosis and angiomatoid formation is widespread in alveolar tissue. This complication arises in long-standing cases of heavy infection and presents clinically as congestive heart failure arising in chronic cor pulmonale.

Kidney
Renal lesions (schistosomal nephropathy; glomerulonephritis), consisting of deposition of immune complexes of host immunoglobulins with adult worm or egg antigens in the glomerular mesangium and basement membrane, occur in *S. mansoni* infection. A variety of glomerular lesions has been found at autopsy in hepatosplenic patients.[134] Mild proteinuria is common in chronic *S. mansoni* infection, and in hepatosplenic cases progressive nephropathy leading to renal failure occurs in a small proportion, although the clinical course is slow and the greater risks are from the hepatic complications.[87]

Amyloidosis has been demonstrated in renal biopsy material from patients with the nephrotic syndrome and schistosomiasis in Egypt.[135]

Egg deposition in the kidney is rare and is not thought to be responsible for serious renal pathology.

Central nervous system
Various forms of 'neurological schistosomiasis' occur in infections due to *S. mansoni*, *S. japonicum* and *S. haematobium*. Yet, in view of the global total of infected people, CNS localization is rare. Eggs of all three species have been found in the brain and spinal cord, and adult worms have been demonstrated at various sites.

'Cerebral' schistosomiasis has traditionally been associated with *S. japonicum* infection, but eggs of *S. mansoni*

and *S. haematobium* have also been found in the brain, rather more frequently with *S. mansoni*. The route of infection is thought to be via Batson's valveless intervertebral plexus or by arterial egg embolism.[136] Eggs may be present in the CNS with little or no histological reaction and, in a randomly selected series of hepatosplenic cases of schistosomiasis coming to autopsy, one-quarter had *S. mansoni* eggs in the brain;[136] these cases may be symptom free.

Myelopathy with various motor and/or sensory presentations occurs, more commonly in *S. mansoni* than in *S. haematobium* infection, and cord transection with paraparesis is well known. Not infrequently, spinal cord schistosomiasis is recognized in the acute toxaemic stages that occur in tourists and transient visitors to endemic areas on their return to temperate climates after a short tropical stay.

Other ectopic lesions
Cutaneous lesions due to *S. mansoni* are rare, although papular or nodular lesions at different sites are known.

In Egypt, genital lesions are not uncommonly found at autopsy.[128] Placental schistosomiasis has been reported from Brazil.[137]

S. japonicum
The intestinal and hepatic lesions of *S. japonicum* are in general similar to those occurring in *S. mansoni* infection but with several specific differences. The primary lesion is a T cell-mediated granuloma formation around the eggs, but modulation of the granuloma size is largely antibody mediated, whereas in *S. mansoni* infection cell mediation is the dominant mechanism.

The adult worms are located in the branches of the inferior mesenteric vein and in the superior haemorrhoidal vein,[138] and an adult female deposits 1000–3500 eggs per day in highest density in the large intestine and, in descending order, in the rectum, sigmoid and descending colon. The small intestine is relatively lightly infected.[139]

Knowledge of the pathological anatomy (gross and microscopic), of *S. japonicum* lags behind that of *S. mansoni* infection because autopsy studies are fewer, are currently seldom performed in the countries endemic for *S. japonicum* and, in the broad public health sense, schistosomiasis has been declining progressively as a cause of death for some decades.[140]

Gastrointestinal lesions in experimental animals are focal and isolated, and are interspersed with normal bowel. Segmental lesions occur in humans and multiple lesions are common, including mucosal hyperplasia, pseudo-polyposis, ulceration and thickening of the intestinal wall.

Gastric schistosomiasis is seen frequently in surgical or biopsy specimens. Subclinical cases are probably common but unrecognized, owing to non-diagnostic symptoms and insensitive diagnostic techniques.

Macroscopic hepatic changes in the chronic phase parallel those in *S. mansoni* infection. The liver is frequently enlarged with an irregular surface. On cross-section the characteristic wide bands of fibrous tissue surrounding the larger portal tracts are seen and Symmer's periportal (clay-pipe stem) fibrosis is found at autopsy. Microscopically the picture is one of chronic pseudotubercles with chronic inflammation, cellular infiltrates around eggs, extensive fibrosis and neo-vascularization in the portal tracts. The accompanying manifestations of portal hypertension (i.e., splenomegaly with or without gastrointestinal varices, with or without bleeding) are to be anticipated.

Although *S. japonicum* eggs are often found in the lung and obliterative pulmonary arteritis is similar to that seen in *S. mansoni*, clinical cor pulmonale has not been reported as in *S. mansoni* infection.[141]

In contrast to *S. mansoni* and *S. haematobium*, the brain is more commonly affected in *S. japonicum* infection, although spinal cord involvement appears to be less frequent. The cerebral lesions are held to be caused by intracranial egg deposition or embolism via a vascular route.

In the first half of the 20th century, schistosomal dwarfism with retardation of growth and sexual development was recognized as a not uncommon occurrence in China. This syndrome is rare in modern times.

Cancer and *S. japonicum* infection

Epidemiological studies have not demonstrated any direct relationships between gastric cancer and *S. japonicum* infection.[127]

The situation regarding a relationship between colonic or rectal cancer and *S. japonicum* is much more complex. Case–control studies in China and the Philippines, and an epidemiological cross-sectional survey in China, have suggested both positive and negative associations. One case–control study in China showed a strong association between *S. japonicum* infection and rectal cancer but no association between colonic cancer and a history of *S. japonicum* infection.[140]

No definitive conclusions can be reached from the studies to date. Improved designs of further studies are essential for clarification.

A similar position exists regarading the presence or absence of a relationship between primary liver cell cancer and schistosomiasis. The ubiquity of hepatitis B infection, a known precancerous condition, in areas endemic for *S. japonicum*, has complicated study designs. Again, the correlation is speculative. The authoritative IARC monograph[127] concluded that there is limited evidence in humans and experimental animals for the carcinogenicity of infection with *S. japonicum*, although the overall evaluation was that infection with *S. japonicum* is possibly carcinogenic to humans. Simultaneously the evaluation concluded that infection with *S. mansoni* is not classifiable with regard to its carcinogenicity to humans.

S. mekongi

Although the clinical manifestations of *S. mekongi* infection are similar to those of *S. japonicum*, the morbidity and pathology resulting from the former is compounded by the presence of *Opisthorcis viverrini* in areas endemic for *S. mekongi*. Objective descriptions of detailed pathology in humans are lacking.

S. intercalatum

The distribution of *S. intercalatum* is restricted in 10 countries in central and west Africa, and more information exists on experimental infection than does pathological description.[142]

The disease is mild, and in proctoscopy in hospital inpatients the rectal and colonic mucosa was considered abnormal in 47 of 85 patients. Non-specific lesions predominated: mucosal congestion, oedema, bleeding and/or ulceration. In liver biopsies, granulomatous lesions, of a size smaller than those seen in *S. mansoni* infection, were seen in the portal tracts. Tissue reaction to eggs was slight or absent in some patients. No portal hypertension was seen.[143]

Clinical features
General

To the clinician, particularly in the tropics, schistosomiasis can be a frustrating infection. With the exception of haematuria in urinary schistosomiasis, there is no one diagnostic symptom or sign; even the commonly described various symptoms and signs are rarely pathognomic. Schistosomiasis is a collection of infections of protean manifestations.

Whereas clinical medicine is taught in the context of classical descriptions of symptoms and signs, these were, in the past, culled from classical and advanced cases. This is rarely the rule in practice, for classical and advanced cases represent only a small proportion of an extensive frequency distribution of clinical syndromes. 'Classical' cases of schistosomiasis are in a minority: many patients have non-specific symptoms and many are symptom free or ignore their symptoms, and infection is discovered only on purposive surveys or during investigation for some unrelated complaint. This is due to the biological phenomenon of the overdispersed distribution of parasites within hosts; this aggregated distribution means that, in any population of hosts, there exists only a small proportion of 'heavy' infections with 'typical' symptoms, and the majority of cases are moderate or light infections with a corresponding freedom from symptoms—or even a complete lack of symptoms.

While it is useful to consider schistosomiasis within the 'classical' stages of the life history—i.e., cercarial invasion, transformation of schistosomula and maturation of adults, established infection, late stages and complications—in an attempt to link clinical pointers to these stages, it should be realized that the stages merge into one another and are rarely clearcut, especially in endemic areas in those who are semi-immune. Non-immune visitors to endemic areas or transients who become infected often provide a clearer clinical description than residents of endemic zones.

Syndromes common to all schistosome infections

Cercarial dermatitis

Seldom, if ever, described in indigenous inhabitants of endemic areas, especially in Africa, and only rarely in non-immune visitors, cercarial dermatitis occurs more commonly on exposure to avian cercariae where symptoms are more intense than in cases exposed to human schistosomal cercaria-infested waters.

Arising within a few minutes of exposure and receding within 24–72 hours, itching (pruritus) of the skin is the prime symptom, accompanied in some cases by erythema and/or a papular eruption. The condition can occur after exposure to any of the five common schistosomes infecting humans.

Acute schistosomasis

Also termed acute toxaemic schistosomiasis, Katayama syndrome or Katayama fever, after the Katayama region in Hiroshima prefecture, Japan, where it was originally described, this acute illness can be found after exposure to any of the schistosomes infecting humans but is most marked in primary infections in non-immune individuals.

Recent reports from China indicate that this acute syndrome due to S. japonicum is not limited to uninfected individuals living in an endemic area at the time of first exposure, but may occur even in those with an active chronic infection or in persons with a recent history of infection and documented treatment and cure.[140]

In the acute syndrome due to S. mansoni infection, a diminution in transmission produced by control measures has led to a relative increase in reports of acute cases, and this phenomenon has been observed in Puerto Rico and Venezuela.

Acute schistosomiasis is much less commonly reported for S. haematobium infection and there are no data on its occurrence with S. intercalatum or S. mekongi.

As the incubation periods of the different schistosome infections are not known accurately and have been the subject of numerous estimates, only broad descriptions of the time phases of the occurrence of the syndrome after initial cercarial exposure can be given.

In S. japonicum infection, the mean period between exposure and the onset of fever in 105 people with no previous history of infection and with only a single day's exposure to cercaria-infested water was 41.5 (range 14–84) days.[140] For S. mansoni, the incubation period of the Katayama syndrome ranges from 4 to 87 days, but is generally between 3 and 7 weeks.[128]

Surprisingly short incubation periods may be encountered in non-immunes who became infected in endemic areas. For example, within 35 days of returning from Botswana, symptoms occurred in 12 of 13 US travellers with a history of water contact; symptoms lasted for 1–30 (mean 8) days, and 9 of 11 had eggs of S. mansoni in the stools during the symptomatic period.[144] Three Dutch non-immunes infected in Mali developed illness within 1–4 weeks of exposure and all had eggs of both S. mansoni and S. haematobium in the stools at 12 weeks.[145]

The clinical picture is one of an acute pyrexial illness; continuing fever is a prime characteristic; the patient feels ill and may have rigors, sweating, general myalgia and headache. An urticarial skin rash may appear and lymphadenopathy or other non-specific signs may occur. Anorexia, nausea, abdominal discomfort and loose stools or diarrhoea, sometimes with blood and mucus, is not rare. The liver is frequently slightly enlarged and tender, and a slightly enlarged spleen occurs in about one-third of patients.

A cough with, on physical examination, dry or moist rales, is frequent, and an intense eosinophilia is almost invariable present.

Cerebral symptoms may appear and the occurrence of spinal cord syndromes or suggestive initial symptoms is an indication for urgent investigative measures.

Established infections

S. haematobium (urinary schistosomiasis)

With the proviso that many patients will have minimal symptoms, the cardinal complaint is recurrent painless haematuria. Other urinary tract symptoms may precede or be associated, for instance burning on micturition, frequency, suprapubic discomfort or pain. Bladder involvement may lead to precipitancy, dribbling or incontinence. In fact, in an endemic area, any urinary tract symptom is an indication to explore for the presence of S. haematobium. However, in many countries in Africa, in the young age groups and early teenagers, macroscopic haematuria may be virtually universal; in boys it provokes little comment and is regarded as a natural sign of puberty and an approach to manhood.

In the phase of established infection it is common practice to recognize two stages: (1) an active stage in children, adolescents and young patients, with egg deposition in many organs and egg excretion in the urine with proteinuria and haematuria, macroscopic or microscopic; and (2) in older patients, urinary egg excretion is sparse or absent but extensive pathology has developed. Even in the later stages of obstructive uropathy, symptoms may be absent or minimal. Chronic bladder lesions may produce persistent urinary dribbling and occasionally multiple fistulas in the perineum, with the picture of the 'watering-can scrotum'; this is also seen in areas of heavy transmission in children and young teenagers where exposure is maximal, but the phenomenon is much rarer nowadays than in the past, coincidental with the widespread use of chemotherapy at the peripheral and school level of health care.

Surveys have shown wide regional variation in coexistent bacteriuria; when present, the predominant organisms are *E. coli*, *Klebsiella* spp., *Pseudomonas* spp. and *Salmonella* spp.

In Egypt, recurrent *Salmonella* bacteraemia is a well recognized complication of *S. haematobium* infection. Patients with urinary schistosomiasis presenting with a recurrence of salmonellosis should first be treated for the *S. haematobium* infection.[146]

In the later stages of obstructive uropathy, hydronephrosis may develop and cause renal parenchymal dysfunction which, added to urinary tract infection, leads to impaired kidney function.[147] The ominous relationship between bilateral schistosomal uropathy, bacteriuria with impairment of hydrogen ion excretion, non-functioning kidneys and death has been well described.[147]

S. intercalatum (intestinal or urinary schistosomiasis)

In comparison with *S. haematobium* or *S. mansoni* infection, clinical symptoms of disease are commonly mild or absent in *S. intercalatum* infection and it is not regarded as a serious public health problem.[148,149] Active infection is seen in children and adolescents, and pathology is detected only in those with egg excretion in excess of 400 eggs per gram of faeces.

The usual clinical presentation is one of diarrhoea, often with blood in the faeces, and lower abdominal pain or discomfort. However, some patients may present with haematuria and, in a report from Nigeria, *S. intercalatum* eggs were found in the urine, but not in faeces, in 6% of 1709 people surveyed.[150] The known existence of natural hybridization between *S. intercalatum* and *S. haematobium* can produce atypical clinical pictures with ectopic localization of worms.[151]

S. mansoni, *S. japonicum* and *S. mekongi* (intestinal schistosomiasis)

The wide spectrum of clinical presentations has been emphasized in recent decades by the increasing use of community-based surveys as a tool of investigation, in contrast with the customary descriptions of infection and disease rooted in hospital patients. Many, if not the majority, of persons infected with *S. mansoni* or *S. japonicum* are symptom free or have minimal and non-specific symptoms, findings again in agreement with the known epidemiological and biological distribution of the parasite within the human host.

Clinical features are encountered in only a small proportion of patients with persistent or heavy infections. Intestinal disease is shown by a chronic or intermittent diarrhoea with blood in the stools, abdominal discomfort or pain, and colicky cramps. Severe dysentery is rare but certainly does occur. Secondary symptoms of fever, weakness, fatigue, anorexia and weight loss are frequent.

In epidemiological surveys there are significant correlations between visible or occult blood in the stools, abdominal pain and diarrhoea.

Hepatomegaly, often of the left lobe, and splenomegaly are frequent accompaniments. In the later stages of infection, there occurs a chronic catarrhal state of the intestine with a swollen, granular mucosa and loose stools with blood and/or mucus or an intermittent dysenteric syndrome.

The primary complications of polyposis and hepatosplenic schistosomiasis have their own symptomatology; polyposis produces what is in effect a severe chronic dysentery with blood and protein loss. Intussusception and/or rectal prolapse may occur.

Hepatosplenic schistosomiasis, often remarkably symptom free, presents as upper abdominal discomfort, left upper abdominal pain or a swelling of the abdomen. Physical signs include a firm enlargement of the liver, often with splenomegaly. The spleen may become greatly enlarged, sometimes extending downwards past the umbilicus into the left iliac fossa, and may even at times fill most of the abdomen. Ascites may be present, but the classical signs of hepatocellular disease, spider-web angiomata, gynaecomastia, palmar erythema, jaundice and alterations in hair distribution are not present in 'pure' schistosomal disease. They may, however, be found where hepatitis B, C, D or E coexists with schistosomal periportal fibrosis and lead to posthepatitic hepatocellular damage. In advanced cases, endocrine changes can be found—growth retardation, infantilism, retarded bone age—all probably due to hypopituitarism. Amenorrhoea, early menopause, infertility and loss of libido have been attributed to a similar cause.[128]

A not uncommon primary presenting sign of hepatosplenic disease in schistosomiasis is haematemesis from gastro-oesophageal varices. This may occur without warning or may be preceded by a feeling of weakness or upper abdominal discomfort; patients have classical signs of acute blood loss with sweating, pallor, thirst, somnolence and a lowered blood and pulse pressure. In many cases melaena follows, and this acute episode may precipitate ascites and/or peripheral oedema. Fatalities may occur with the primary haemorrhage if treatment is not available; recurrent multiple haemorrhagic episodes are usual. Unless complicated by hepatitis B, C, D or E, liver function and hepatic encephalopathy does not develop. Where mixed infections of *S. mansoni* or *S. japonicum* and the various hepatitis viruses coexist, the downhill clinical course is correspondingly rapid and the typical signs of hepatocellular failure appear with, in parallel, a poor prognosis.

S. japonicum and *S. mekongi*

While infections with the oriental schisosomes follow a broadly similar clinical course to that of *S. mansoni*, several distinct differences emerge. In general, infection with *S. mekongi* is milder than that with *S. japonicum*. Hepatosplenomegaly is common but cerebral and cardiopulmonary complications are not reported.

In the past there have been more hospital-based clinical studies of *S. japonicum* than community-based investigations. Hence the clinical descriptions have been slanted towards advanced cases. In fact, at least half of patients infected with *S. japonicum* are asymptomatic. General symptoms, fatigue, weakness, non-specific abdominal discomfort, and irregular bowel movements or intermittent diarrhoea are frequent. Chronic diarrhoea is said to be a common complaint and lower abdominal pain is a frequent symptom.[139]

The later signs of hepatosplenic schistosomiasis evolve as do those of those in *S. mansoni* infection. Although schistosomal dwarfism was not uncommon in China in the first half of the twentieth century, it has become a rarity nowadays. Cardiopulmonary and renal complications are well known.

The main difference clinically is the occurrence of cerebral schistosomiasis in *S. japonicum* infection. Spinal cord involvement appears less frequently than with *S. mansoni*, but such generalizations are difficult, if not impossible, to confirm scientifically.

In the acute phase of cerebral schistosomiasis, the presenting symptoms and signs are those of a meningo-encephalitis, with pyrexia, headache, vomiting, blurred vision and disturbed consciousness. In the established or chronic phase of the infection, several distinct neurological presentations are recognized; most common is epilepsy which may be generalized but is more frequently jacksonian in type; signs suggestive of a space occupying lesion or a stroke are also described. Advances in neuroradiology, with or without operational biopsy, are diagnostic.

Differential diagnosis

In an infection of such diverse clinical manifestations it is scarcely surprising that schistosomiasis in any of its forms can be confused with many other disease processes. Acute schistosomiasis (Katayama syndrome) must be differentiated from typhoid (leucopenia, no eosinophilia), brucellosis, malaria, leptospirosis and numerous other causes of pyrexia of uncertain origin (PUO). Pyrexia and eosinophilia occur in trichinosis, tropical eosinophilia, visceral larva migrans and infections with *Opisthorcis*, *Paragonimiasis* and *Clonorchis* spp.

In the established stage, *S. haematobium* must be distinguished from haemoglobinurias, cancer of the urogenital tract, other infections such as acute nephritides, and rarer conditions such as renal tuberculosis with haematuria.

S. mansoni, with its common presentation of non-specific abdominal symptoms, may suggest peptic ulcer, biliary disease or pancreatitis; in such cases, symptoms disappear after specific antischistosomal treatment.

Lower abdominal conditions to be excluded are the various forms of dysentery, particularly amoebic dysentery, ulcerative colitis and non-schistosomal polyposis.

The differential diagnosis of hepatosplenic schistosomiasis is wide and embraces all causes of hepatomegaly and splenomegaly, separately and combined. The marked splenic enlargement of portal hypertension due to periportal fibrosis must be distinguished from kala-azar (visceral leishmaniasis), certain of the chronic leukaemias or myeloproliferative syndromes, some of the haemoglobinopathies (e.g., thalassaemias) and the tropical splenomegaly syndrome.

In endemic areas, schistosomiasis must always be considered as one of the causes of cor pulmonale and virtually any neurological presentation, but particularly the various forms of epilepsy and the different types of myelopathy or spinal cord compression syndromes.

A sound knowledge of local or regional epidemiological patterns of parasitic and other infectious diseases and a high index of diagnostic suspicion contribute greatly to the avoidance of diagnostic error.

Diagnosis

A definitive diagnosis is made by the direct visual demonstration of the eggs of the parasite in body excretions or secretions, overwhelmingly stool and urine (Figures 80.13–80.16); or alternatively in material from rectal biopsy or biopsies from liver or surgically removed tissue. A sensitive direct diagnosis can also be made by hatching tests in which swimming miracidia originating from excreted eggs can be seen with the naked eye. This is an indication beyond doubt that the eggs are viable and have originated from living fertilized female schistosomes.

A recent addition to direct diagnostic techniques is the detection of schistosome antigens in serum or urine: circulating anodic antigen (CAA) and circulating cathodic antigen (CCA). These two glycoprotein circulating antigens associated with the gut of the adult worm are well characterized, are genus specific and their presence

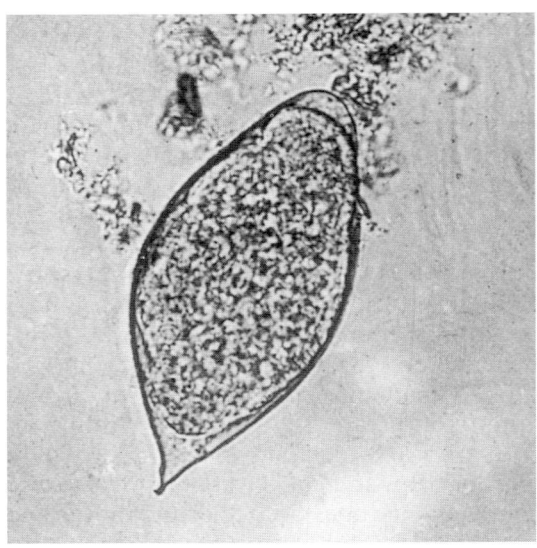

Figure 80.13: Egg of *S. haematobium*. (Courtesy of Tropical Resources Unit.)

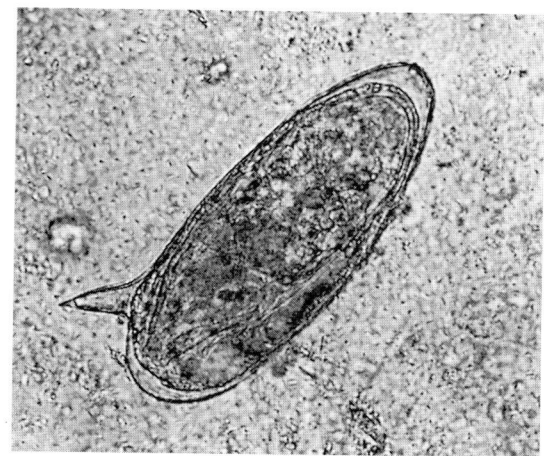

Figure 80.14: Egg of *S. mansoni*. (Courtesy of O. D. Standen.)

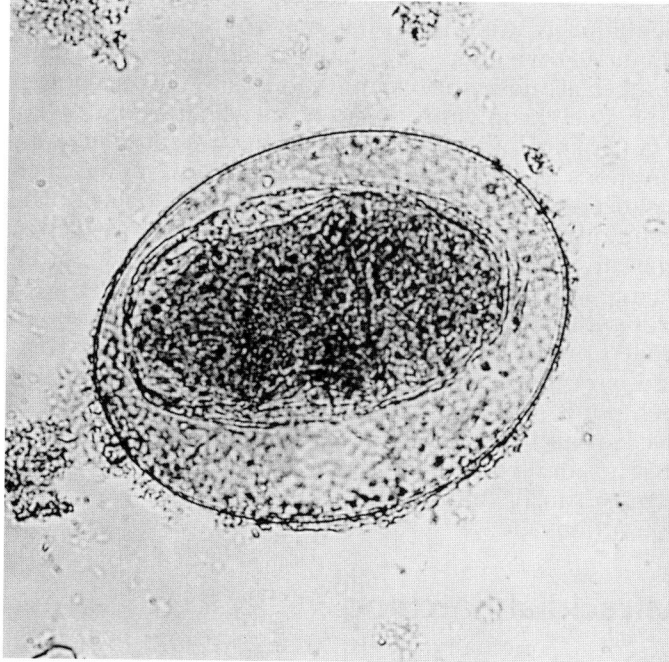

Figure 80.15: Egg of *S. japonicum*. (Courtesy of Tropical Resources Unit.)

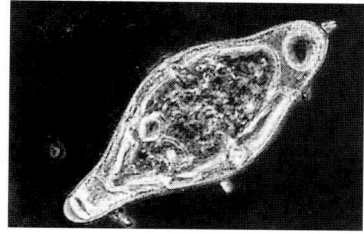

Figure 80.16: Egg of *S. intercalatum*. (Courtesy of V. R. Southgate.)

indicates active infection in persons of *S. mansoni*, *S. haematobium* or *S. intercalatum* infection. They are detected by enzyme immunoassay and have virtually 100% specificity and very high sensitivity. Patently they offer new possibilities for epidemiological and post-

chemotherapeutic monitoring, but are expensive, are 'high technology', need complex reagents and require standardization and controlled trials before operational use in control programmes. At present, they are used at the research level in individual patients or in small groups[152–156] (see Immunodiagnosis below).

All other methods of diagnosis, whether clinical, immunological, radiological (see Figures 80.17 and 80.18), ultrasonographic (see Figures 80.19 and 80.20) or endoscopic without biopsy, are essentially indirect.

Direct diagnostic techniques

Parasitological diagnosis

No single optimal technique applicable to all situations exists. Most of the current techniques can be interpreted qualitatively or quantitatively depending on the diagnostic setting. Quantitative techniques are virtually always used in research, in experimental chemotherapy and clinical trials, in epidemiological surveys and in the evaluation of intervention measures.

In an individual clinical setting it is customary to examine repeated specimens of excreta parasitologically (in practice, three specimens) before declaring a patient to be 'negative'. Confirmation of a diagnosis by hatching tests demonstrates that the eggs are viable and an active infection exists; the finding of dead eggs only in the excreta is not an indication for chemotherapy.

Egg counting

The direct demonstration of eggs represents an enormous advantage over all other diagnostic measures because specificity is obviously maximal, yet a slavish belief in the absolute virtues of quantitative diagnosis is scarcely justified. Egg counts are merely indirect estimates of worm loads; they vary in time and place and with technicians, and the assumed Poisson distribution of eggs in the excreta may not hold.[157] Conclusions on chemotherapeutic efficacy of drugs based on single post-treatment examinations should be viewed with cynicism; coefficients of variation of daily egg output are very high and in *S. haematobium* infections egg output is subject to a circadian rhythm: it peaks and is least variable from 10.00 to 14.00 hours.

Diagnosis of *S. haematobium* infection

Ova of *S. haematobium* are usually detected easily in the urine. A qualitative diagnosis is made by the microscopic examination of a sedimented or centrifuged urine specimen. Exercise before specimen collection is unnecessary. Eggs of *S. mansoni* or *S. intercalatum* are found not infrequently in the urine. In one series, 15% of patients with a sole *S. mansoni* infection had 'mansonuria', but this is an unusually high rate.[158]

Nowadays, filtration techniques, giving a quantitative estimation of egg excretion, have tended to replace simple sedimentation and/or centrifugation and are certainly the 'norm' in epidemiological studies. Currently, urine samples are passed through filter paper,[159,160] polycarbonate[161,162] or a polyamide material[163,164] by a variety of syringes or pumps. The principle common to all is that eggs are retained on the filter and can be counted with or without staining. Many different stains are in use and preferences are largely personal; eggs may be 'stored' in preservative or a preservative–stain mixture.[160] As with all techniques, problems arise during field usage. False epidemiological results may occur from loss of eggs during bulk transport of dried filter papers,[165] and, in a small but significant proportion, eggs are retained on polyamide filters (Nytrel) even after careful attempts to reuse them. As a general rule, any filter should be used once only and then discarded.

Diagnosis of intestinal dwelling schistosomes

In infections with *S. mansoni, S. japonicum, S. mekongi* and *S. intercalatum,* where eggs are excreted in the faeces, simple comminution of the stool and sedimentation before microscopy is a reliable diagnostic technique. Direct saline microscopy of stool has a very low diagnostic sensitivity owing to the small amount of the faecal sample examined.

Many concentration techniques have been described.[166–170] All involve removal of fat, faecal debris and mucus, and of necessity require more sophisticated laboratory facilities. They find their optimal use in the detection of 'light' infections where egg excretion is of a low intensity or is intermittent.

In South Africa, a popular and efficient technique for egg recovery from stools in both medical and veterinary practice is based on twin nylon gauze filters and the use of water pressure to break up faecal material. Claims of high sensitivity have been advanced.[171]

Nowadays, the cellophane thick faecal smear, the Kato technique or one of its numerous modifications[172,173] has become a standard diagnostic tool in both clinical and epidemiological studies. Essentially a semi-concentration–clearing–staining process, it is a simple microscopic method examining 20–50 mg of stool, depending on the template used, and is quantitative, thus permitting the comparisons of internationally acquired data. It can be performed in the field and may be used at the primary health care level. The prepared slide takes some time to clear; this varies with ambient temperature and humidity. Slides can be stored for at least 1 week, often longer, the time again being variable, so that assessments of technicians' counts can be incorporated into a system of quality control. A further advantage lies in its use in the diagnosis and counting of eggs of many intestinal nematodes or cestodes (e.g., *Ascaris lumbricoides, Trichuris trichuria, Taenia* spp. and hookworms), although to assess hookworm egg excretion counts must be made 15–30 minutes after slide preparation because hookworm eggs disappear after this

period owing to solution from the Kato slides, and assessment is useless after 1 hour. A historical fact of interest is that the original Kato technique was invented and adopted during the major national ascariasis control campaigns conducted in Japan after the Second World War, directed against the public health problems existing in the country at that time. The exact details of the procedure must be calibrated for each working location, taking into account environmental variables, resources and locally available material and human skills. Disadvantages of the Kato technique are that watery or diarrhoeal stools cannot be processed and dietary habits may result in hard fibrous stools that are difficult to process. Additionally, there is a definite lower limit of sensitivity of 50–100 eggs per gram of stool detectable by a single smear. Numerous variants of the technique exist and it is common practice to examine two or three subsamples of single faecal specimen. Whichever technique is used, it is vital that the amount of stool examined, whether in a single examination or by a number of subsample examinations, should be reported so that valid comparisons can be made between areas.

A variant of the thick smear technique for *S. mansoni* infections is the glass sandwich technique[174,175] which has been used widely in the Sudan and Malawi. The technique requires no reagents and it has been suggested that it is more cost-effective than other similar quantitative methods. A small-scale experiment showed no significant differences in egg recovery or in methods, readers or slides prepared from the same stool specimens and processed by either the Kato or glass sandwich technique.[176] Further comparisons on a larger scale are needed, and a major disadvantage of this technique is that it is limited to use in restricted endemic areas; hence comparison of findings with other endemic areas is, at present, invalid.

Miracidial hatching

Described originally by Fulleborn in 1921,[177] and in routine use in biological and chemotherapeutic studies for decades, it is surprising that more attention has not been given to this technique in clinical medicine because hatching is generally accepted as the most sensitive of all parasitological methods in all forms of schistosomiasis. The method remains essential for adequate post-treatment evaluation in clinical trials. However, adaptation to field studies has been uncommon because standardization and quantification are more difficult than in techniques where eggs can simply be counted. Nevertheless it is salutary to recall that diagnosis and follow-up of treated patients in the huge Chinese control programmes of the 1960s and 1970s were based on a 'nylon network running water sedimentation technique'—essentially a field-adapted miracidial hatching process.[178,179]

The relative ease of isolation of eggs from urine led to many more attempts to quantify hatching procedures in *S. haematobium* than in *S. mansoni* infections. As a rough estimate of the numbers of hatchable eggs, the miradiascope was used as a macroscopic technique routinely for surveys in southern Africa.[180–182] More sensitive and accurate hatching techniques have followed[183,184] and further refinements are appearing;[185–187] undoubtedly the use of 'wet' preparations has complicated field standardization, but hatching retains its primacy as the most sensitive diagnostic tool in *S. haematobium* infections.

In *S. mansoni* infections, many variants of hatching techniques exist, some semiquantitative and all possessing high sensitivity.[188–190] In *S. japonicum* endemic areas in China, miracidial hatching is widely and routinely used for both epidemiological surveys and as an indicator of parasitological cure after chemotherapy.[140]

Rectal biopsy

Used for decades as a simple direct diagnostic technique at the individual clinical level, rectal biopsy may be employed in addition to faecal examination and provides an effective way of visualizing eggs. Small biopsy specimens of mucosa are soaked in water and examined microscopically as a crush preparation. In the intestinal dwelling species, egg viability can often be determined by observation of flame cell or miracidial movement within the eggshell. Biopsies may be taken from rectal valves via a crocodile forceps or—a much simpler procedure—with a curette and proctoscope; the mucosa is pulled over the end of the proctoscope and cut off with the curette.[188]

Ova of *S. haematobium* in rectal snips are usually non-viable and black.

In Brazil, the oogram technique (a quantitative rectal biopsy with division of eggs into devlopmental stages) is commonly used. If an oogram is used in addition to faecal examination in an assessment of the effects of antischistosomal drugs, it can be confidently predicted that estimates of 'cure rates' based solely on excretal examination will be considerably reduced.[191]

Other biopsy sites

As expected, schistosome ova are frequently found in other biopsy locations, such as liver, bladder, cervix, vagina, perineum and skin, and indications for a biopsy of such sites lie at the individual clinical level.

Indirect diagnostic techniques

A high index of epidemiological suspicion with appropriate physical or radiological signs, sero-immunological assessment of antibody levels by a variety of assays and, in *S. haematobium* infections, the detection of red blood cells and protein in the urine in subjects in endemic areas all remain indirect diagnostic techniques.

Chemical reagent strips

Indirect diagnostic techniques are used most frequently in *S. haematobium* infections. The application of chemical reagent strips (CRSs) in a semiquantitative fashion is highly useful as a diagnostic surrogate in endemic areas of the disease; a positive result is interpreted as indicating active infection.

Reagent strips in current use have ranges of sensibility of 5–15 red blood cells per microlitre and 0.015–0.03 mg of haemoglobin per 100 ml urine. They use a peroxide compound and orthotolidine as a chromogen. The colour distinction between negative and the first level of reactivity on the strips is well defined, and in the presence of blood the colour indicators show distinct changes from yellow or pale orange to green or blue.[192] False-positive reactions occur in myoglobinuria and in the presence of bacterial peroxidases resulting from heavy bacteriuria, and inhibition of the reactions may occur if urinary ascorbic acid levels exceed 10 mg per 100 ml urine.

CRSs that measure levels of proteinuria semi-quantitatively use tetrabromophthalein ethylester with a buffer. The colour discrimination between negative and the first level of proteinuria is, however, not well defined. Precise assessment of colour change from yellow-green to green-blue is difficult. False positives occur in alkaline urines or when quinine or a quinine derivative is present. False negatives have occurred in strongly acid urine with Bence Jones proteinuria and in urine containing predominantly γ-globulin.

Many experiences of the use of CRSs in areas endemic for *S. haematobium*[193–196] have confirmed the consistent and significant correlation between reagent strip reactions indicating haematuria and/or proteinuria and increasing intensity of egg output.

Good predictive values resulting from high sensitivity and specificity emphasize the limitations of conventional single microscopic examinations at very low egg output levels and confirm the validity of CRSs in detecting those with a 'high' egg output (i.e., over 50 eggs per 10 ml urine in this case).[197] CRSs can be used in areas of both high and low transmission patterns and find an optimal use in the detection of those with 'heavy' infections who are a priority for chemotherapy. The use of CRSs can be expected to increase at primary health care levels in programmes of morbidity control in *S. haematobium* infection.

Immunodiagnosis

Serodiagnostic techniques are used for the detection of either specific antibodies or genus-specific antigens.

Antibodies to adult worm, schistosomular, cercarial or egg antigens are detected by a multiplicity of procedures including the various forms of enzyme-linked immunosorbent assay (ELISA), radioimmunoassay (RIA), indirect immunofluorescence tests (IFAT), gel precipitation techniques (GPT), indirect haemagglutination (IHA), latex agglutination (LAT) and circumoval precipitin tests (COPT) that have superseded the older Cercarienhüllen reactions (CHR) and complement fixation tests (CFT).

In general, antibody detection techniques have been less useful to the practising physician and epidemiologist than the techniques of direct parasitological diagnosis. Their basic disadvantage is that they all point to past exposure to mammalian or, in rare instances, avian schistosomes without indicating the duration, activity or quantum of infection. Further disadvantages are an absence of globally agreed criteria of performance and standards; the necessity for expensive equipment, costly or labile reagents; the need for skilled technical personnel; and the slow diminution of specific antibody level after treatment, thus reducing their value as a marker of chemotherapeutic success. Each laboratory in endemic or non-endemic areas has tended to use its own particular antigen and assay procedure. The WHO has conducted several collaborative studies[198,199] in attempts to improve the technology and to standardize both antigens and procedures. Agreement is not yet in sight. A most useful review of the present position has been produced.[200]

In striking contrast, very real advances have been made in antigen detection. Improvements in the production of monoclonal antibodies has led to new diagnostic tests of CAA and CCA in serum and urine.

A recent review details the technological advances made in one leading research centre,[201] compares the efficacy of antigen detection with both parasitological and antibody determinations in a range of clinicoepidemiological situations, and summarizes the 'pros' and 'cons' of these techniques. It appears that no single method can be optimal in all circumstances and the availability of laboratory facilities, the need for a rapid diagnosis and the local logistical frame, plus, of course, the overall costs, will determine whether antigen detection, antibody detection or parasitological examination will be dominant in practical usage. This seems to point to a north–south divide in the provision of laboratory facilities.

Radiology (Figures 80.17 and 80.18)

As a form of indirect diagnosis, various radiological procedures for detecting morbidity from schistosomal infection have long been in use in hospital practice and have included plain abdominal radiography to detect calcification, intravenous pyelography to detect bladder and ureteral changes or obstructive uropathy, isotope renography, computed tomography for cerebral schistososomiasis, myelography for suspected cord damage, and portal venography for hepatosplenic schistosomiasis with portal venous hypertensive changes. Complications such as gastrointestinal bleeding may require the use of specialized techniques, such as abdominal ultrasonography, splenoportography and nuclear isotopic studies of hepatic blood flow. The rapidly advancing techniques in radiology make this an area which is becoming a specialist zone.

The indications for a particular investigation lie at the individual patient level and are the joint responsibilities of the physician and the radiologist.

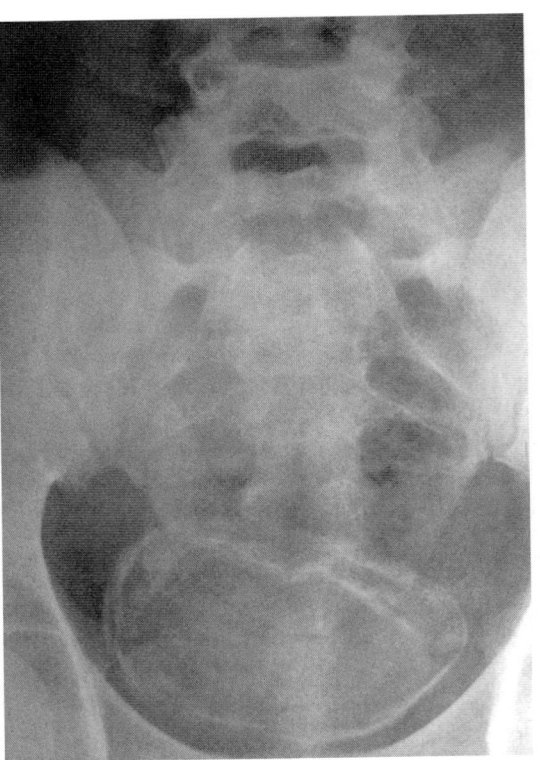

Figure 80.17: Calcification of the bladder in late *S. haematobium* infection.

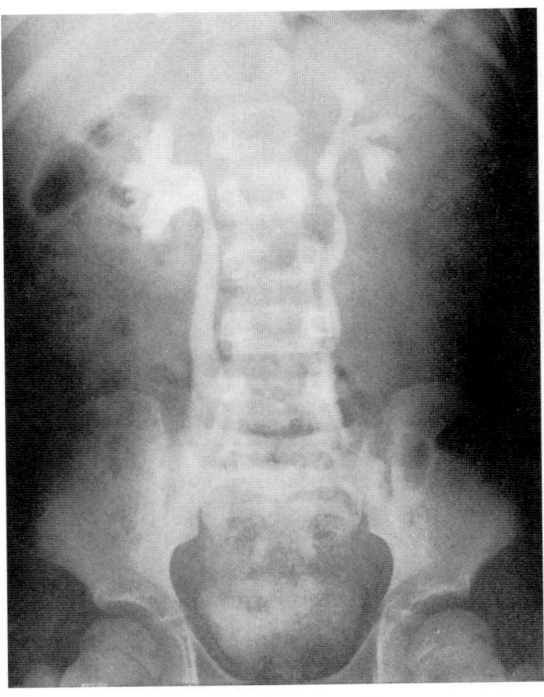

Figure 80.18: Dilated ureters, calcified bladder and hydronephrosis caused by *Schistosoma* infection. (Courtesy of D. M. Forsyth.)

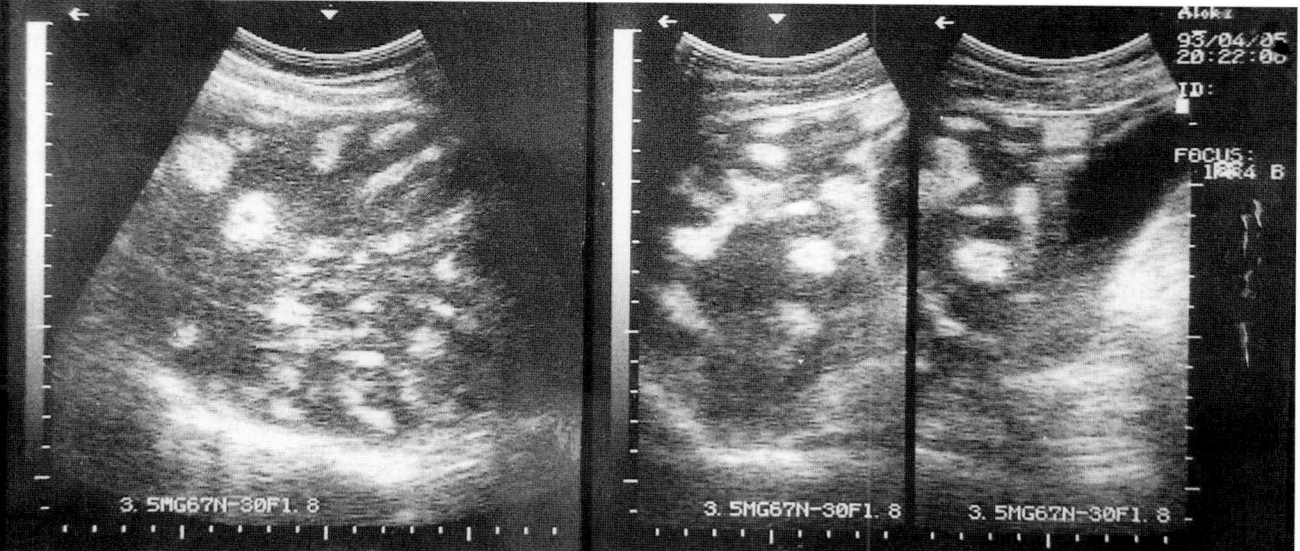

Figure 80.19: Symmer's periportal fibrosis in *S. mansoni* infection (Courtesy of Dr Ashraf Omar, Department of Tropical Medicine, Cairo University.)

Ultrasonography (Figures 80.19 and 80.20)

Major changes in the diagnostic approach in individual patients and in the epidemiological assessment of morbidity in communities have occurred in parallel with the introduction and expanded use of ultrasonography. The technique is non-invasive, simple, portable, has no biological hazard to the patient or the operator and either complements or is an alternative diagnostic method to many invasive techniques. With the exception of

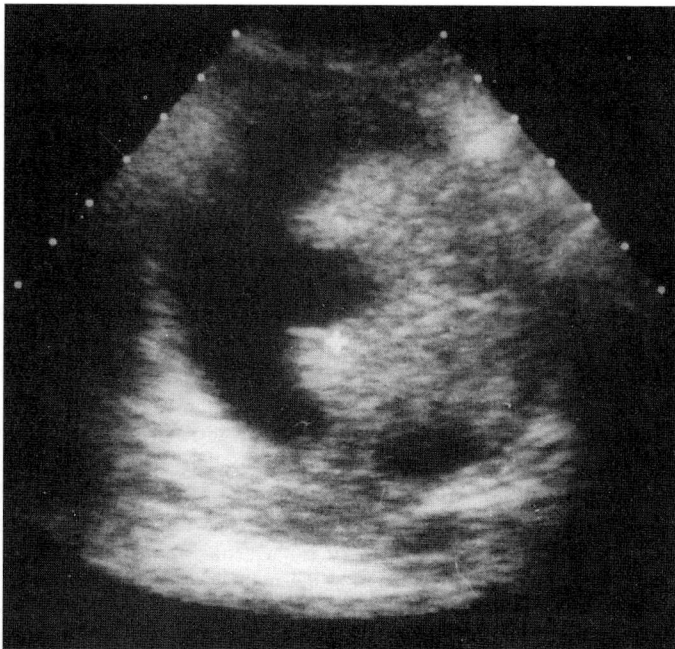

Figure 80.20: Carcinoma of the bladder in *S. haematobium* infection (Courtesy of Dr Ashraf Omar, Department of Tropical Medicine, Cairo University.)

hydroureter, ureteral calculi and bladder calcification, it has, in comparison with other diagnostic procedures, high specificity and sensitivity, is superior to physical examination in measuring liver and spleen size, and is the best technique for grading schistosomal periportal fibrosis, portal hypertension, hydronephrosis, urinary bladder wall lesions and renal and bladder stones.[202] An extensive review of technical and clinical experience is available.[203]

Following field use of portable ultrasonography, particularly in Egypt, where it is widely used, an agreed protocol for standardized investigations and methods of reporting was produced by the WHO.[204]

It has been demonstrated in community studies that sonographic lesions of periportal fibrosis in *S. mansoni* infection, with thickening of portal tracts and portal vein walls, correlated with the number of eggs in the stool.[205] Fine measurements of hepatic pathology are possible and are superior to clinical examination.[206] Where available, ultrasonography should replace clinical grading and physical examination as a preferred method of assessing liver and spleen enlargement.[206]

The sonographic patterns of schistosomal hepatic fibrosis are characteristic and are distinct from those of other hepatic diseases. Schistosomiasis can now be distinguished from cirrhosis with confidence.[207]

Additionally, an ultrasonographic scoring system is of clinical use in the prediction of both oesophageal varices and the likelihood of bleeding from them.[208]

An interesting outcome of ultrasonographic studies has been the demonstration that *S. haematobium* can cause mild degrees of schistosomal periportal fibrosis in an area where *S. mansoni* does not exist;[105] this confirms an observation, first made in 1974 in Upper Egypt, that hepatosplenic disease caused by *S. haematobium* is a distinct entity.[106]

The use of abdominal ultrasonography to determine the decrease in morbidity following population-based chemotherapy programmes can be expected to grow dramatically.

Management

For no other parasitic diseases have there been such major advances in chemotherapy as have occurred since the 1960s in the treatment of schistosomiasis. The introduction and widespread use, at both the individual patient level and in large-scale community-based operations, of the current highly effective, orally administered, well tolerated, antischistosomal drugs have provided physicians, epidemiologists and public health practitioners with therapeutic opportunities not in existence at the end of the 1960s.

The primary objective of chemotherapy is cure of the individual patient by eradication of the infection (or the infection with two species) from which he or she suffers. Cure leads to cessation of egg deposition, the pathogenic agent in the tissues, and this prevents additional organ damage; existing lesions will, in the vast majority of cases, regress. In large-scale community-based chemotherapy programmes, where compromises on dosage may have to be made to ensure a viable delivery system and optimal population coverage, the main aim is to reduce the community egg load and excretion by the greatest amount possible. Individual 'cure' may or may not occur; the community benefits as a whole by the block of the egg–miracidium–snail stage of the biological cycle, which reduces transmission by minimizing excretal pollution of water supplies and thus diminishes cercarial contamination of human water contact sites. Of even greater importance is the reduction of community morbidity caused by schistosomiasis; nowadays this can be measured and the success of interventions can be evaluated with some accuracy and precision.

Since the last edition of this book, major changes in the outlook for antischistosomal chemotherapy have taken place.[209] Whereas three antischistosomal compounds were used globally and were all on the WHO List of Essential Drugs, the position now is totally different. Metrifonate has been withdrawn from the market and pursues, under a different nomenclature and with pharmacological refinements, a role in the treatment of dementia.

Oxamniquine is available currently in only very few countries, but its manufacturer has assured the WHO that production will continue for the foreseeable future.[210]

Praziquantel

Praziquantel is the drug of choice, and is effective against all schistosome species that occur in humans. It is also effective in the other snail-borne trematode infections—clonorchiasis, paragonimiasis and opisthorciasis—and in

infections due to the adult cestodes, *Taenia solium*, *T. saginata*, *Hymenolepis nana* and *Diphyllobothrium* spp. It is active against the secondary larval stages of *T. solium* in humans, dermal cysticercosis and neurocysticercosis, but has little or no effect in ocular cysticercosis. Praziqantel is not active in the human secondary larval stages of *Echinococcus* spp. and is generally ineffective in *Fasciola hepatica* infections. There is no therapeutic activity in protozoan or nematode infections including the filariae.

Originally formulated as 600-mg tablets, the expiry of patent has led to many suppliers and marked reductions in price, which is expected to level off at approximately US$0.09 per tablet.[210]

Although dosage is standardized in large-scale epidemiologically based morbidity control programmes, there is frequently a variation in dose in the treatment of the individual patient.

In field programmes, a single oral dose of 40 mg/kg is effective in *S. haematobium*, *S. mansoni* and *S. intercalatum* infections.

For *S. japonicum* infection the dosages employed originally were a total dose of 60 mg/kg, given at 4-hourly intervals as three 20-mg/kg doses or two 30-mg/kg doses, but present field practice, since the mid-1980s, has been to use a single oral dose of 40 mg/kg.[211]

The usual total dose for *S. mekongi* is 60 mg/kg, although there is evidence that repeated treatment at this dosage may be necessary for cure of this species.[212–215]

For treatment of individual patients with heavy infections with *S. mansoni* (over 800 eggs per gram of stool), a total dose of 50 or 60 mg/kg, given in two equally divided doses 4–6 hours apart, may be needed; single doses are best given after food and, if possible, in the evening.

Patient tolerance is extremely good and virtually all trials have confirmed the absence of toxicity in the liver, kidney, haematopoietic system, or other body organs and functions. However, minor side effects do occur; those related to the gastrointestinal tract are epigastric or generalized abdominal pain or discomfort, nausea, rarely vomiting, anorexia and loose stools. These side effects are mild, transient and, even if their incidence is high, rarely if ever require medication. A rare event in patients heavily infected with *S. mansoni* or *S. japonicum* is the passage of blood in the stools after praziquantel treatment. The explanation is unknown; it occurs a few hours after dosage but recovery is rapid and without clinical sequlae.

Headache and dizziness may be encountered, as may fever, pruritus or a transient skin eruption, none of which is serious or lasting. Side effects that occur in field treatments tend to be more frequent in foci of intense transmission, and should not be used as an argument for reduction of the dose.

'Cure rates' are high; it can be expected that with the appropriate dosage they will be around 80% in small groups. In large-scale field operations, where supervision is of necessity less stringent and where total compliance may be difficult to ensure, rates of 50–60% will be found when a single oral dose of 40 mg/kg is used; egg output reduction in those not 'cured' should exceed 90% of pretreatment output.

A disturbing trend has appeared in field programmes of control in recent years. 'Resistance' or 'tolerance' to praziquantel has been claimed and documented on several occasions in the treatment and control of S. mansoni,[216,217] and resistance can be induced in laboratory studies.[218]

Cure rates after praziquantel treatment in a new highly endemic focus of intense transmission of S. mansoni in northern Senegal in the early 1990s were alarmingly low.[219–221] However, a WHO consultation decided that the intensity of transmission in this focus was such as to cause the initially observed low cure rates,[27] because praziquantel is ineffective or at least less effective against maturing worms. In a new focus in non-immunes with a high intensity of transmission, these would be present in the majority of infections.

There is good evidence from Egypt that in the delta some 2–3% of patients were still excreting eggs after two or three praziquantel treatments. Some 20% of field isolates showed a normal susceptibility to praziquantel, but some of the remaining sampled isolates required two to six times the normal dose to achieve a 50% reduction in worm numbers in laboratory studies. However, this reduced susceptibility was not increased upon repeated passages under drug pressure. Thus evidence exists that certain schistosome isolates or strains of the parasite are inherently less susceptible to praziquantel. Persistent monitoring and surveillance is obviously essential to detect the emergence of true drug resistance. The picture is not clear, and the story unfolds.[209] The recent introduction of a simple new technique for assessing praziquantel effect on miracidia hatched from eggs may, if confirmed in different species, offer an affordable surveillance device to predict praziquantel 'resistance' or 'tolerance'.[222]

Although this 'resistance–tolerance' phenomenon has been reported in human S. mansoni infections, no evidence exists at present of 'resistance' in S. japonicum or S. haematobium infections. Field trials of praziquantel treatment monitored over many years in China[211] and in Kenya[223] have produced consistent 'cure rates' year on year during annual treatments of both S. japonicum and S. haematobium infections. In the latter case, theoretical mathematical modelling suggested that the emergence of resistance might take some 7 years on an annual treatment coverage of 100% of an infected population. As this coverage is rarely, if ever, obtained in field practice, where a range of 25–75% compliance is more usual, emergence of resistance may take 10–15 years.[223]

Oxamniquine

A tetrahydoquinoline compound distantly related to hycanthone, oxamniquine is effective only against S. mansoni. In animal models it proved inactive against S. japonicum and early trials in humans showed virtually no activity against S. haematobium or S. matthei.

In the animal studies one peculiarity was that male worms proved more susceptible than female worms. Egg laying by surviving females ceased in the absence of males after successful treatment, thus removing the basic pathogenetic mechanism in S. mansoni infection.[224,225]

Oxamniquine is available as capsules of 250 mg or as a syrup containing 50 mg/ml, and is marketed as Mansil® in South America and as Vansil® in Africa. In the USA, capsules have a yellow body marked PFIZER 641 with a dark green cap marked VANSIL. The shelf life is 5 years for capsules and 3 years for the syrup.

Oxamniquine is used at all stages, from acute toxaemic to chronic and complicated S. mansoni infections, with good results.

Advanced S. mansoni infection with hepatosplenomegaly, portal hypertension and/or ascites responds well, and in schistosomal polyposis there are great improvements in both the associated anaemia and protein-losing enteropathy.[226–228]

High cure rates (60–90% in different samples) are seen after oxamniquine treatment of uncomplicated S. mansoni infections.

From 1975 to 1979 oxamniquine was used in a major control campaign in Brazil when some 5 million doses were given in the field programmes with high cure rates and very good tolerance.[229]

The dose of oxamniquine varies with the geographical origin of the S. mansoni infection, the age and hence the surface area of the patient. In South America, adults are given 15 mg/kg of body weight as a single oral dose; in children 20 mg/kg is preferred, given in two divided portions each of 10 mg/kg with an interval of 4–6 hours between doses. If practicable, the drug should be given after food or just before sleep.

With S. mansoni occurring on the African continent only those with strains of West African origin are given the same doses as in South America. In Egypt, Sudan and southern Africa, a total dose of 60 mg/kg body weight is used, either as 15 mg/kg for 2 days or as 20 mg/kg once daily for 3 days. In East Africa, a total dose of 30–40 mg/kg is given in a split regimen over 1 or 2 days.

In general, oxamniquine is well tolerated. There are virtually no contraindications but classes of patients exist who require close monitoring. Patients with a history of any form of epilepsy must be supervised for 48 hours after treatment because a small number of epileptiform convulsions have been reported, as have generalized seizures after the drug, fortunately without sequelae and with clinical and electroencephalographic recovery.[230]

As with many other drugs, treatment should not be given during the first 4 months of pregnancy.

Any patient whose occupation involves care of heavy machinery or who is employed in the transport industry (e.g., pilots, truckers, dockers, crane drivers) should be placed off work for 48 hours after treatment.

Side effects are uncommon; dizziness, drowsiness and headache are most frequent but last for some 4–6 hours only. Hallucinations and a state of excitement are very rare events. Although abdominal discomfort, vomiting and diarrhoea do occur, there is no constant statistical correlation and, in practice, adverse effects have had no influence on compliance in field programmes.

A harmless orange-red discoloration of the urine may occur but is transitory, and a syndrome of peripheral blood eosinophilia, scattered pulmonary infiltrates and increased immune complexes in serum with urinary excretion of schistosomal antigens is known in Egypt but has not been described in other locations.[231]

An eosinophilia after treatment occurs commonly and is maximal in 7–10 days; it represents a reaction to dead or dying schistosomes. Changes in hepatic enzyme levels may be seen but no constant pattern exists.

In summary, oxamniquine is a highly useful drug for treatment of all forms of *S. mansoni* infection, including many advanced and complicated syndromes. Resistance to oxamniquine is known in South America but is not yet a public health problem as such patients are treated successfully with praziquantel.[232]

The future of chemotherapy

Regrettably, for economic reasons there appears to be little possibility of major pharmaceutical industry investment in exploration of new antischistosomal compounds. Cost recovery in Third World endemic countries is highly questionable even disregarding the profit motive.[209] Thus the importance of monitoring control programmes for true 'drug resistance' cannot be overemphasized, although at present there are lamentably few such efforts.

The recent introduction of a simple new technique for assessing the effects of praziquantel on miracidia hatched from eggs may, if confirmed in different species, offer an affordable surveillance device to predict praziquantel 'resistance' or 'tolerance'.[222]

It is known that artemisinin derivatives, by killing immature worms, have preventive effects in *S. japonicum* infections in animal models.[233,234] This action was confirmed in humans in randomized double-blind placebo-controlled trials in China during recent floods where the incidence and intensity of infection in endemic areas was reduced significantly.[235]

The preventive effects were confirmed in *S. mansoni* in animal experiments[236,237] and a well conducted field trial of oral artemether against *S. mansoni* infections in humanas showed a very useful prophylactic effect.[238]

However, because artemisinin derivatives are one of the current mainstays in antimalarial chemotherapy and because endemic malaria and endemic schistosomiasis coexist in numerous areas, especially in Africa, wider use of these derivatives must await the clarification of several epidemiological and public health issues. There may be a risk of selecting schistosome strains less sensitive to praziquantel if artemether is given at an early stage after infection when maturing schistosomes are known to be

insensitive to praziquantel. Furthermore, the effects of repeated doses of artemether (or other derivatives) on the biology and local epidemiology of malaria is as yet unknown. Much further work remains before these problems are clarified in many areas of Africa.

Assessment of chemotherapy

Assessment of patients treated for schistosomiasis is conducted by repeated clinical observation, evaluation of symptomatic improvement, and diminution or disappearance of physical, radiological, particularly ultrasonographic, and endoscopic signs.

Direct parasitological examination of urine, stool or rectal biopsy is essential and should be performed on repeated (three) specimens of excreta at about 6–8 weeks and 4–6 months after treatment, by a selection of appropriate techniques detailed above.

Follow-up is simple if no reinfection risk is present; the explanation of viable eggs in the excreta at 4–6 months is less clear in endemic areas where transmission persists. It may be due to a maturing prepatent infection unaffected by chemotherapy, a true reinfection or a therapeutic failure. It is not always easy to decide which event, or even combination of events, is responsible. Increased use of antigen detection techniques (e.g., CAA, CCA) offer real possibilities for clarification of these problems.

Special clinical syndromes and management

Neurological schistosomiasis

The efficacy and safety of modern antischistosomal drugs has led to early treatment of encephalopathies, myelopathies or other spinal cord syndromes, reasonably suspected, even if not proven, to be due to schistosomiasis. This improves prognosis as cord damage in myelopathy is closely related to time of diagnosis.

An ELISA using keyhole limpet haemocyanin is said to distinguish between antibody responses in acute and chronic schistosomal infection,[239] and CAA can be diagnostic where eggs are not yet excreted. These two diagnostic techniques should be used when available; unfortunately they are, as yet, restricted to certain high-technology centres.

The use of corticosteroids remains controversial. Laminectomy is an important technique in acute paraplegia with spinal compression or block, or in deteriorating clinical circumstances during conservative treatment.

In *S. japonicum*, suspected cerebral schistosomiasis should be localized with modern imaging techniques and treated with praziquantel, which is safe and effective. Computed tomography demonstrates resolution of intracerebral masses, regression of cerebral oedema and the subsequent disappearance of epilepsy.[240] Appropriate neurosurgical supervision should be on hand.

Acute toxaemic schistosomiasis (Katayama syndrome)

Early diagnosis of a suspicious clinical presentation can now be made with the keyhole limpet haemocyanin antibody assay and CAA antigen detection techniques. Disputes remain whether steroids should be added to specific drug treatment with praziquantel or oxamniquine, and the position has not yet been resolved. As a general principle, patients should be treated with praziquantel, which is effective against all species.

Associated salmonellosis

The chronic bacteraemia due to *Salmonella typhi* or *S. paratyphi* is due to the attachment of the bacteria to the integument or in the gut of the adult schistosome. Although clinical response to antibiotics is good, bacteraemia will recur unless the underlying schistosomiasis is treated. The therapeutic response to antischistosomal drugs is good.

Associated hepatitis

Even if, in hepatosplenic schistosomiasis, there is serological or other evidence of an associated hepatitis B infection (or C, D or E), and activity of schistosomiasis is still present, it is worthwhile treating the later with praziquantel.

Portal hypertension

Chemotherapy is but one part of patient care as complications are mainly due to the mechanical obstructive pathology resulting from periportal fibrosis. Where eggs are still found in the excreta, treatment with praziquantel or oxamniquine is indicated and gives the usual response.

Gastrointestinal bleeding

Admission to a specialized centre is essential because that is where skills in assessment, immediate resuscitation, fibreoptic endoscopy, balloon tamponade and/or endoscopic sclerotherapy are present. The treatment of this complication is beyond the scope of the general physician and is preferably a matter for specialists in this area of intensive care. Emergency portocaval shunts have fallen into disrepute as a high proportion of operative deaths may occur and, in the survivors, there is frequently a loss of shunt patency and/or encephalopathy. A selective distal splenorenal shunt has been claimed to offer a lower haemorrhage recurrence rate and an improved survival rate.[241]

The clinical application of β-adrenergic blockade using non-selective beta-blockers (e.g., propranolol) for the prevention of an initial gastrointestinal haemorrhage in either cirrhosis or portal hypertension from schistosomal periportal fibrosis is ambiguous. It is not yet clear which clinical variables are the best predictors of response to beta-blockers.

In endemic rural areas, the major difficulty is diagnosing the presence of oesophageal varices in the absence of a history or an actual bleed, for the necessary diagnostic facilities are not there. Thus referral to a specialized centre possessing the essential facilities is the optimal, if Elysian, form of management.

Schistosomiasis without eggs

This title describes cases where no ova can be found on investigation but there exists a high index of clinical suspicion of schistosomal infection, usually based upon an epidemiological history of exposure, existing cases in fellow members of a group, an unexplained eosinophilia in a presenting suspect and/or a suggestive or suspicious seroimmunodiagnostic test result.

In areas endemic for *S. haematobium*, the presence of a positive test for microhaematuria on CRS examination is taken as indicative of infection.

Again, the simplicity of use of modern drugs has clarified many difficult diagnostic situations and frequently treatment is undertaken on 'suspicion alone', a practice justifiable only when exhaustive efforts to reach a parasitological or serological diagnosis have failed.

Detailed monographs on the properties of anti-schistosomal drugs and their use in clinical and field practice have been produced.[242–245]

Prevention and control

Both prevention and control depend on an area-specific, species-specific and epidemiologically specific mixture of intervention methods. The characteristics of endemic areas, the transmission patterns, the infecting parasite species and strains, the intermediate snail host(s), the availability or otherwise of water supplies and sanitary facilities, the behavioural customs of the human communities, especially their water contact patterns and above all the socio-economic background, all contribute to a multiplicity of interactions to produce a vast mosaic of transmission and epidemiological pictures. An accurate diagnosis of all of these variables, quantitative when possible, is necessary before entering into prevention and control programmes. The aims of both prevention and control are:

1. The reduction in the number of eggs excreted from infected people reaching waters harbouring the intermediate snail host(s); this is dependent on health education, the provision and use of adequate sanitary facilities, and specific antischistosomal chemotherapy for infected communities and individuals.
2. The reduction in the probability of miracidial/snail contact; this relies on all factors in (1), appropriate modifications of the aquatic environment and reduction of intermediate snail host numbers by application of chemical molluscicides or the use of suitable biological control means.

3. The reduction of cercarial densities, which will occur as a result of all of the preceding actions but overwhelmingly from the employment of molluscicides.
4. The reduction of the probability of cercariae locating a definitive host, again due to the cumulative effects of all of the preceding factors plus the reduction of human water contact with infected water bodies by the provision of adequate domestic or peridomestic water supplies and the substitution of safe recreational water sites.
5. The reduction of the longevity of the adult worms in the human host, a function of chemotherapy.

Multiple overlaps are obvious in these processes and, conventionally, stress in 'prevention' is directed towards health education and the provision of adequate water supplies and sanitation supplemented by environmental improvements. 'Control' is dominated by chemotherapy and molluscicides, yet integration of these interventions is essential for success and each endemic focus or region requires an individual clinicoepidemiological, zoogeographic, sociological and environmental approach based on the common principles listed above.

In the past, emphasis was given to 'transmission control', largely through repetitive mollusciciding. This was expensive; molluscicides did not achieve total kills of snails and their eggs in operationally difficult terrains, and the techniques require skilled biologists and technical personnel. Epidemiological extrapolation of the successes of modern chemotherapy and the employment of simple low-cost diagnostic techniques led inevitably to a reappraisal of the strategy and tactics of control. Many schistosomiasis control operations operated through a single disease control mechanism are simply beyond the financial and human resources of the great majority of endemic countries in Africa, where 85% of the global prevalence exists. A strategy of control has now evolved that stresses repetitive population-based chemotherapy, aimed at 'morbidity control' rather than 'transmission control'. It is implemented through the peripheral health care workers in the primary health care system adopted by all countries, and many successes have been documented that have been evaluated by epidemiological, parasitological and ultrasonographic tools. However, the naïve supposition that chemotherapy alone will provide the definitive answer to schistosomiasis control is not substantiated. In such a multifaceted socio-economic, biological and clinical syndrome, 'control' needs population-based chemotherapy as a spearhead but also needs to be reinforced by such snail control measures as required by epidemiological criteria. Reinfection after chemotherapy is a risk that is ever present against a backdrop of unchanging socio-economic conditions, because the constraints of achieving total population coverage with drugs and the less than absolute cure rates mean that egg deposition continues, albeit at a much lower level, and therefore transmission persists.

Add to this the difficulties in environmental improvement, the provision of sanitation and water supplies[209]

and the deployment of continuing health education, and the 'control' of schistosomiasis implying a permanent cessation of transmission is clearly a herculean task. Patently the constraining factors are political and economic, not technical.

A summary of the current rationale for control and data on its employment are provided in the last two reports of the WHO Expert Committee.[2,246]

Mollusciciding

The use of molluscicides in the control of schistosomiasis is a highly specialized field. Synthetic chemical molluscicides are virtually restricted nowadays to one compound, niclosamide (Bayluscide; Bayer) and, although other chemicals lethal to snails exist, their practical use is minimal. Although many molluscicides of plant origin are known,[247] the eventual outlook for the isolation, characterization, toxicological screening, large-scale production and distribution of their active ingredients for use in endemic countries is blurred.

A useful specialist text on indications, technical use, application in different habitats and evaluation of molluscicides has been produced by the WHO.[248]

Molluscicides will continue in use as one of the integral specific control tools, but techniques have changed markedly from the old 'blanket application' to a much more focused approach guided by the epidemiological criteria of high prevalence, high intensity and rapidity of reinfection rates in any particular focus or area of infection.

Vaccines and vaccination

The limitations of current control measures have changed the old aims of 'transmission control', with implied eradication after cessation of transmission, to the current strategy of 'morbidity control', with an uncertain diminution of transmission but recognition that some residual infection will continue.

These factors, added to the virtually unchanging socio-economic circumstances in many countries, especially in Africa where 85% of current prevalence is found, and added to the recent explosion of new techniques in biotechnology, led to a huge rise in research aimed at the production of vaccines against the invasive stages of schistosomiasis or the pathology produced. Whilst advances in molecular biology have led to the identification and characterization of an impressive number of schistosome antigens, progress in human vaccination studies has lagged behind those in animal models. One view emerging is that a vaccine, even with a long-term protective effect, would probably be insufficient as a sole control mechanism but would need to be given in conjunction with chemotherapy and other control methods.[72,249]

The antigenic identities of the biologically active molecules selected as candidates for schistosomal vaccine development are: a variant of the isoenzyme glutathione *S*-transferase (Sm28GST); paramyosin (Sm97); an irradiation-associated vaccine antigen (IrV-5); the glycolytic enzyme triose-phosphate isomerase (TPI); and the membrane antigen Sm23 and a fatty acid-binding protein (FABP) 14 (Sm14).[250] However, further testing of these six antigens in mice by two independent laboratories experienced in experimental schistosomiasis research showed that a stated goal of consistent induction of 40% protection or better was not reached with any of the molecules tested.[250]

Currently the only vaccine candidate molecule with what appeared to be satisfactory antigenic properties is a glutathione *S*-transferase (Sh28GST) in *S. haematobium* infections. Preliminary phase 1a safety trials in humans have been conducted in France and Senegal, and are leading to efficacy studies. Results might be anticipated in 1–2 years' time.[251]

The case for the sceptics of the feasibility or even utility of a vaccine in schistosomiasis has been argued recently and persuasively by Gryseels.[252] It was pointed out that, apart from the complex technical problems to be met and solved, there were marked difference from the campaigns with vaccines against the childhood viral and bacterial diseases, and there were fundamental differences in the public health concepts involved.

While a vaccine programme of sequential steps of preclinical development, independent testing of antigens at all stages, human correlate studies, scale-up, subsequent field trials and large-scale production have been initiated by the UNDP/World Bank/WHO Tropical Diseases Research Programme (TDR), many problems exist.[250] There remain many unanswered questions on the immunology of schistosomiasis and on the mechanisms of protection when it exists, and formidable challenges lie ahead regarding large-scale antigen production and the improvement of the current modest levels of protection achieved to date in animal models.

It has been estimated that a vaccine development and scale-up programme leading to market availability will take some 10 years—not dissimilar to a drug development schedule.[253] It will be some years before vaccines in humans evolve from the present enthusiastic hopes to realistic practical usage in the field, and the methodological difficulties in assessing their possible application in the numerous epidemiological mosaics of schistosomiasis transmission foci will be profound.

REFERENCES

1   Rollinson D & Southgate V R. The genus *Schistosoma*: a taxonomic appraisal. In Rollinson D & Simpson A J G (eds) *The Biology of Schistosomes. From Genes to Latrines*. London: Academic Press, 1987: 1–4.

2   World Health Organization. The control of schistosomiasis. *World Health Organ Tech Rep Ser* 1985; 728:1–49.

3   Farooq M. Historical development. In *Epidemiology and Control of Schistosomiasis (Bilharziasis)*. Basle: Karger, 1973: 1–16.

4   Ruffer M A. Note on the presence of *Bilharzia haematobia* in Egyptian mummies of the 20th dynasty 1220–1000 BC. *BMJ* 1910; I:16.

5   Larrey D J. *(Haematurie) Mémoires de Chirurgie Militaire et Campagnes*. Paris: Smith, 1812–1817.

6   Bilharz T M. Fernere Beobachtungun uber das die Pfortader des Menschen bewohnende Distomum haematobium und sein verhaltniss zu gewissen pathologischen Bildungen aus brieflichen Mitheilungen an Professor v. Siebold vom 29 Marz 1852. *Zeitschrift für Wissenschaftliche Zoologie Leipzig* 1852; 4:72–76.

7   Manson P. Report of a case of bilharzia from the West Indies. *BMJ* 1902; ii:1894–1895.

8   Leiper R T. *Researches on Egyptian Bilharziosis*. (A report to the War Office on the results of the Bilharzia Mission in Egypt, 1915). London: John Bale Sons and Danielson, 1918:1–140. Reprinted from *J R Army Medical Corps* 1915; XXV:1, 147, 253; 1916; XXVII:171; 1918; XXX:235.

9   Silva M Piraja da. La schistosomose à Bahia. *Arch Parasitol* 1908; 13:231–302. Contribution to the study of schistosomiasis in Bahia, Brazil (English translation of original paper). *J Trop Med Hyg* 1909; 12:159–164.

10 Soto V R. *Naturateza de la disenteria en Caracas*. Doctoral thesis no. 63, 1906.

11 Fujii Y. *Chugai Iji Shimpo*. 1847; 691:55 (in Japanese).

12 Katsurada F. *Schistosomum japonicum*, a new parasite of man by which an endemic disease in various areas of Japan is caused. *Annot Zool Japan* 1904; 5:146–160.

13 Miyagaawa Y. *Mitte Med Fak Univ Tokyo* 1913; 1383:1–3 (in Japanese).

14 Miyairi K & Suzuki M. *Tokyo Iji Shinshi* 1913; 1386:1 (in Japanese).

15 Miyairi K & Suzuki M. *Mitte Med Fak Kais Univ Kyushu (Fukuoka)* 1914; 1:187.

16 Leiper R T & Atkinson E L. Observations of the spread of Asiatic schistosomiasis. *Chin Med J* 1915; 29:143–149.

17 Logan O T. Three cases of infection with *Schistosoma japonicum* in Chinese subjects. *J Trop Med Hyg* 1906; 9:294–296.

18 Woolley P G. The occurrence of schistosomiasis japonicum vel cattoi in the Phillipine islands. *Phillipine J Sci* 1906; 1:83–90.

19 Brug S L & Tesch J W. Parasitic worm infestations in inhabitants around Lake Lindoe, Celebes. *Geneeskd T Ned Ind* 1937; 77:2151–2158.

20 Faust E C & Meleney H E. Studies on schistosomiasis japonica. With a supplement on the molluscan hosts of the human blood fluke in China and Japan, and species liable to be confused with them, by Nelson Anandale. *Am J Hyg (Monogr Ser)* 1924; 3:1–139.

21 Tubangui M A. The molluscan intermediate host in the Phillipines of the oriental blood fluke *Schistosoma japonicum*. *Phillipine J Sci* 1932; 49: 295–304.

22 Chesterman C C. Note sur la bilharziose dans la region de Stanleyville (Congo belge). *Ann Soc Belg Méd Trop* 1923; 3:73.

23 Fisher A C. A study of the schistosomiasis of the Stanleyville district of the Belgian Congo. *Trans R Soc Trop Med Hyg* 1934; 28:277–306.

24 Voge M, Bruckner D & Bruce J I. *Schistosoma mekongi* sp.n from man and animals compared with four geographic strains of *Schistosoma japonicum*. *J Parasitol* 1978; 64:577–584.

25 Liang Y S & Kitikoon V. Susceptibility of *Lithoglyphopsis aperta* to *Schistosoma mekongi* and *Schistosoma japonicum*. In Bruce J I, Sornmani S, Asch H L et al. (eds) The Mekong schistosome. *Malacol Rev* 1980; Supplement 2:53–60.

26   Bruce J I, Sornmani S, Asch H L et al. (eds) The Mekong schistosome. *Malacol Rev* 1980: Supplement 2:1–282.

27   World Health Organization. *Report of the WHO Informal Consultation on Schistosomiasis Control*, Geneva, 2–4 December 1998. WHO/CDS/CPC/SIP/99.2. Geneva: WHO, 1999.

28   Gadgie R K & Shah S N. Human schistosomiasis in India. Discovery of an endemic focus in the Bombay state. *Indian J Med Sci* 1952; 6:760–763.

29   Sathe D B, Mukerji S, Gaitonde B B et al. Reinvestigation of an old focus of schistosomiasis in Gimvi village, District Ratnagiri, in Maharashtra State, India. *Bull Haffkine Inst* 1981; 9:34–37.

30   World Health Organization. Assessment of the risk of introduction of schistosomiasis in water resources development projects and a survey of schistosomiasis in Gimvi, Ratnagiri District, Mararashtra State, India. A report of joint mission. British Museum (Natural History), Haffkine Institute, Maharashtra State Directorate of Health, National Institute of Communicable Diseases, World Bank, World Health Organization, 13–22 November 1985. *Wkly Epidemiol Rec* 1985; 60:43.

31   Doumenge J P, Mott K E, Cheung C et al. *Atlas de la Répartition Mondiale des Schistosomiases*. Talence, CEGET-CRNS. Geneva: WHO; Talence PUB, 1987:400.

32   Davis G M & Greer G J. A new genus and two new species of Triculinae (Gastropoda Prosobranchia) and the transmission of a Malaysian mammalian *Schistosoma* sp. *Proc Acad Nat Sci Philadelphia* 1980; 132:245–276.

33   Chitsulo L, Engles D, Montresor A & Savioli L. The global status of schistosomiasis and its control. *Acta Tropica* 2000; 77(1):41–51.

34   Davis A. Schistosomiasis. In Robinson D (ed.) *Epidemiology and the Community Control of Disease in Warm Climate Countries*, 2nd edn. Edinburgh: Churchill Livingstone, 1985: 389–412.

35   Browne D S, Sarfati C, Southgate V R et al. Observations on *Schistosoma intercalatum* in southeast Gabon. *Z Parasitenkd* 1984; 70:243–253.

36   Wolfe M S. *Schistosoma intercalatum* infection in an American family. *Am J Trop Med Hyg* 1974; 23:45–50.

37   Wright C A, Southgate V R, van Wijk H B et al. Hybrids between *Schistosoma intercalatum* and *S. haematobium* in Cameroon. *Trans R Soc Trop Med Hyg* 1974; 68:413–414.

38   Burchard G D & Kern P. Probable hybridization between *S. intercalatum* and *S. haematobium* in Western Gabon. *Trop Geogr Med* 1985; 37:119–123.

39   Southgate V R, van Wijk H B & Wright C A. Schistosomiasis at Loum, Cameroon: *Schistosoma haematobium*, *S. intercalatum* and their natural hybrid. *Z Parasitenk* 1976; 49:145–159.

40   Kuntz R E, McCullough B, Huang T C et al. *Schistosoma intercalatum*, Fisher 1934 (Cameroon) infection in the patas monkey. (*Erythrocebus patas*, Schreber, 1775). *Int J Parasitol* 1978; 8:65–68.

41   Nelson G S, Amin M A, Saoud M F A et al. Studies on heterologous immunity in schistosomiasis. 1. Heterologous schistosome immunity in mice. *Bull World Health Organ* 1968; 38:9–17.

42   Amin M A, Nelson G S & Saoud M F A. Studies on heterologous immunity in mice. 2. Heterologous schistosome immunity in rhesus monkeys. *Bull World Health Organ* 1968; 38:19–27.

43   Short R B. Sex and the single chromosome. *J Parasitol* 1983; 69:3–22.

44   Erasmus D A. The adult schistosome; structure and reproductive biology. In Rollinson D & Simpson A J G (eds) *The Biology of Schistosomes. From Genes to Latrines*. London: Academic Press, 1987: 51–82.

45   Webbe G. The life cycle of the parasites. In Jordan P & Webbe G (eds) *Schistosomiasis, Epidemiology, Treatment and Control*. London: Heinemann, 1982: 50–78.

46   Christopherson J B. Longevity of parasitic worms. The term of living existence of *Schistosoma haematobium* in the human body. Lancet 1924; i:742–743.

47   Chabasse D, Bertrand G, Leroux JP et al. Bilharziose à *Schistosoma mansoni* evolutive découverte 37 ans après l'infection. *Bull Soc Pathol Exot Filiales* 1985; 78:643–647.

48   World Health Organization. Immunology of schistosomiasis. *Bull World Health Organ* 1974; 51:553–595.

49   Simpson A J G. Schistosome molecular biology. In Rollinson D & Simpson A J G (eds) *The Biology of Schistosomes. From Genes to Latrines*. London: Academic Press, 1987: 147–161.

50   Rumjanek F D. Biochemistry and physiology. In Rollinson D & Simpson A J G (eds) *The Biology of Schistosomes. From Genes to Latrines*. London: Academic Press, 1987: 163–183.

51   Capron A. Schistosomiasis. Forty years War on the Worm. *Parasitol Today* 1998; 14:379–384.

52   Jourdane J & Théron A. Larval development; eggs to cercariae. In Rollinson D & Simpson A J G (eds) *The Biology of Schistosomes. From Genes to Latrines*. London: Academic Press, 1987: 83–113.

53   Pesigan T P, Farooq M, Hairston N et al. Studies on *Schistosoma japonicum* in the Philippines. 1. General considerations and epidemiology. *Bull World Health Organ* 1958; 18:345–455.

54   Wilson R A. Cercariae to liver worms: development and migration in the mammalian host. In Rollinson D & Simpson A J G (eds) *The Biology of Schistosomes. From Genes to Latrines*. London: Academic Press, 1987: 115–146.

55   Miller P & Wilson R A. Migration of the schistosomula of *Schistosoma mansoni* from the lungs to the hepatic portal system. *Parasitology* 1980; 80:267–288.

56   Wright W H. Geographical distribution of schistosomes and their intermediate hosts. In Ansari N (ed.) *Epidemiology and Control of Schistosomiasis (Bilharziasis)*. Basle: Karger, 1973: 32–249.

57   Hairston N G. The dynamics of transmission. In Ansari N (ed.) *Epidemiology and Control of Schistosomiasis (Bilharziasis)*. Basle: Karger, 1973: 250–336.

58   Browne D S. *Freshwater Snails of Africa and their Medical Importance*. London: Taylor & Francis, 1980: 1–488.

59   Webbe G. The intermediate hosts and host–parasite relationships. In Jordan P & Webbe G (eds) *Schistosomiasis, Epidemiology, Treatment and Control*. London: Heinemann, 1982: 16–49.

60   Malek E A. *Snail Hosts of Schistosomiasis and Other Snail-Transmitted Diseases in Tropical America: A Manual*. Scientific Publication no. 478, Pan American Health Organization, World Health Organization. Geneva: WHO, 1988:1–316.

61   Southgate V R & Rollinson D. Natural history of transmission and interactions. In Rollinson D & Simpson A J G (eds) *The Biology of Schistosomes. From Genes to Latrines*. London: Academic Press, 1987:347–378.

62   Sobhon P & Upatham E S. *Snail Hosts, Life-Cycle and Tegmental Structure of Oriental Schistosomes*. UNDP/World Bank/WHO Special Programme for Research and Training in Tropical Diseases. Geneva: WHO, 1990:1–321.

63   Mandahl-Barth G. *An Appraisal of the Present Taxonomic Status of* Biomphalaria *and* Bulinus *in Africa and the Near East*. SCHISTO/WP 78:5.Geneva: WHO, 1978 (unpublished document).

64   Fryer S E. Studies on the epidemiology of a Nigerian strain of *Schistosoma haematobium* with particular reference to the molluscan hosts. PhD thesis, University of Wales, 1986.

65   Meulemann E A. Host–parasite relationships between the freshwater pulmonate *Biomphalaria pfeifferi* and the trematode *Schistosoma mansoni*. *Neth J Zool* 1972; 22:355–427.

66 Jordan P & Webbe G. Epidemiology. In Jordan P & Webbe G (eds) *Schistosomiasis: Epidemiology, Treatment and Control.* London: Heinemann, 1982: 227–292.

67 Wilkins H A. Epidemiology of schistosome infections in man. In Rollinson D & Simpson A J G (eds) *The Biology of Schistosomes. From Genes to Latrines.* London: Academic Press, 1987: 379–397.

68 Cheng T H. Schistosomiasis in mainland China. A review of research and control programs since 1949. *Am J Trop Med Hyg* 1971; 20:26–53.

69 Fenwick A. Baboons as reservoir hosts of *Schistosoma mansoni. Trans R Soc Trop Med Hyg* 1969; 66:557–567.

70 Combes C & Delattre P. Principaux paramétrès de l'infestation des rats (*Rattus rattus* et *Rattus norvegicus*) par *Schistosoma mansoni* dans un foyer de schistosomiase intestinale de la region caraibe. *Oecol Appl* 1981; 2:63–79.

71 Rollinson D, Imbert-Establet D & Ross G C. *Schistosoma mansoni* from naturally infected *Rattus rattus* in Guadeloupe: identification, prevalence and enzyme polymorphism *Parasitology* 1986; 93:39–53.

72 Bergqvist R. Prospects of vaccination against schistosomiasis. *Scand J Infect Dis* 1990; 76:60–71.

73 Butterworth A E. Immunity in human schistosomiasis. In Prospects for immunological intervention in human schistosomiasis. Proceedings of a Meeting of the Scientific Working Group on Schistosomiasis 26–28 May 1986, Geneva. *Acta Trop* 1987; Supplement 12:31–40.

74 Khalife J, Capron M, Grzych J-M et al. Immunity in human schistosomiasis. Regulation of protective immune mechanisms by IgM blocking antibodies. *J Exp Med* 1986; 164:1626–1640.

75 Butterworth A E, Bensted-Smith R, Capron A et al. Immunity in human schistosomiasis mansoni: prevention by blocking antibodies of the expression of immunity in young children. *Parasitology* 1987; 94:281–300.

76 Butterworth A E, Fulford A J C, Dunne D W et al. Longitudinal studies on human schistosomiasis. *Philos Trans R Soc Lond [Biol]* 1988; 321:495–511.

77 Capron A, Dessaint J P, Capron M et al. Immunity to schistosomes: progress toward vaccine. *Science* 1987; 238:1065–1072.

78 Dalton P R. A sociological approach to the control of *Schistosoma mansoni* in St Lucia. *Bull World Health Organ* 1976; 54:587–595.

79 Colley D G & Colley M D. Protective immunity and vaccines to schistosomiasis. *Parasitol Today* 1989; 5:350–354.

80 Wilkins H A, Goll P H, Marshall T F de C et al. Dynamics of *Schistosoma haematobium* infection in a Gambian community. The patterns of human infection in the study area. *Trans R Soc Trop Med Hyg* 1984; 78:216–221.

81 Goll P H, Wilkins H A & Marshall T F de C et al. Dynamics of *Schistosoma haematobium* infection in a Gambian community. 2. The effect on transmission of control of *Bulinus senegalensis* by the use of niclosamide. *Trans R Soc Trop Med Hyg* 1984; 78:222–226.

82 Wilkins H A, Goll P H, Marshall T F de C et al. Dynamics of *Schistosoma haematobium* infection in a Gambian community. 3. Acquisition and loss of infection. *Trans R Soc Trop Med Hyg* 1984; 78:227–232.

83 Butterworth A E & Hagan P. Immunity in human schistosomiasis. *Parasitol Today* 1987; 3:11–16.

84 Hagan P. Reinfection, exposure and immunity in human schistosomiasis. *Parasitol Today* 1992; 8:12–16.

85 Corrêa-Oliveira R, Caldas I R & Gazzinelli G. Natural versus drug-induced resistance in *Schistosoma mansoni* infection. *Parasitol Today* 2000; 16:397–399.

86 De Jonge N, Gryseel B, Hilberath G W et al. Detection of circulating anodic antigen by ELISA for seroepidemiology of schistosomiasis mansoni. *Trans R Soc Trop Med Hyg* 1988; 82:591–594.

87 von Lichtenberg F. Consequences of infections with schistosomes. In Rollinson D & Simpson A J G (eds) *The Biology of Schistosomes: From Genes to Latrines.* London: Academic Press, 1987: 185–232.

88 Smith J H & Christie J D. The pathobiology of *Schistosoma haematobium* in humans. *Hum Pathol* 1986; 17:333–345.

89 Cheever A W, Kamel I A, Elwi A M et al. *Schistosoma mansoni* and *S. haematobium* infections in Egypt. II. Quantitative parasitological findings at necropsy. *Am J Trop Med Hyg* 1977; 26:702–716.

90 Hoshino-Shimizu B, Brito T & Kanamura H Y. Human schistosomiasis. *Schistosoma mansoni* antigen detection in renal glomeruli. *Trans R Soc Trop Med Hyg* 1976; 70:492–496.

91 Abdel-Salam E, Ishaak S & Mahmoud A A F. Histocompatibility linked susceptibility for hepatosplenomegaly in human schistosomiasis mansoni. *J Immunol* 1979; 123:1829–1851.

92 Sazazuki T, Ohuta N, Kanoeoka R et al. Association between an HLA haplotype and low responsiveness to schistosomal worm antigen in man. *J Exp Med* 1979; 152:314–318.

93 Pereira D M da S M. *Sistemas HLA, ABO e Rhe caracteristicas racais em patientes com hepatosplomegalia equistossomitca.*Thesis, University of Brazilia, 1979.

94 Abel L, Demenais F, Prata A et al. Evidence for the segregation of a major gene on human susceptibility/resistance to infection by *Schistosoma mansoni. Am J Hum Genet* 1991; 48:959–970.

95 Smith J H, Kamel I A, Elwi A et al. A quantitative post mortem analysis of urinary schistosomiasis in Egypt. I. Pathology and pathogenesis. *Am J Trop Med Hyg* 1974; 23:1054–1071.

96 Smith J H, Elwi A, Kamel I A et al. A quantitative post mortem analysis of urinary schistosomiasis in Egypt. II. Evolution and epidemiology. *Am J Trop Med Hyg* 1975; 24:806–822.

97 Farid Z. Chronic urinary *Salmonella* carriers with intermittent bacteraemia. *J Egypt Public Health Assoc* 1970; 45:157–160.

98 Farid Z, Trabolsi B & Hafez A. *Escherichia coli* bacteraemia in chronic schistosomiasis Ann. *Trop Med Parasitol* 1984; 78:661–662.

99 Wright E D, Chiphangi J & Hutt M S R. Schistosomiasis of the female genital tract. A histopathological study of 176 cases from Malawi. *Trans R Soc Trop Med Hyg* 1982; 76:822–829.

100 Chen M G & Mott K E. Progress in the assessment of morbidity due to *Schistosoma haematobium.* A review of recent literature. In Progress in Assessment of Morbidity due to Schistosomiasis. *Trop Dis Bull* 1989; 86:R1–R36.

101 Cheever A W, Kamel I A, Elwi A M et al. *Schistosoma mansoni* and *S. haematobium* infections in Egypt. III. Extrahepatic pathology. *Am J Trop Med Hyg* 1978; 27:55–75.

102 Higashi G I, Abdel-Salam E, Soliman M et al. Immunofluorescent analysis of renal biopsies in uncomplicated *Schistosoma haematobium* infections in children. *J Trop Med Hyg* 1984; 87:123–129.

103 Sadigursky M, Andrade Z A, Danner R et al. Absence of schistosomal glomerulopathy in *Schistosoma haematobium* infection in man. *Trans R Soc Trop Med Hyg* 1976; 70:322–323.

104 Farid Z, Higashi G I, Bassily S et al. Chronic salmonellosis, urinary schistosomiasis and massive proteinuria. *Am J Trop Med Hyg* 1972; 21:578–581.

105 Nafeh M A, Medhat A, Swifae Y et al. Ultrasonographic changes of the liver in *Schistosoma haematobium* infection. *Am J Trop Med Hyg* 1992; 47:225–230.

106 Nooman Z M, Nafeh M A, El-Kateb H et al. Hepatosplenic disease caused by *Bilharzia haematobium* in Upper Egypt. *J Trop Med Hyg* 1974; 77:42–48.

107 Girges R. *Schistosomiasis (Bilharziasis)*. London: John Bale Sons & Danielson, 1934.

108 Adeyemi-Doro F A B, Osoba A O & Junaid T A. Perigenital cutaneous schistosomiasis. *Br J Vener Dis* 1979; 55:446–449.

109 Develoux M, Blanc L, Veller J M et al. Bilharziose cutanée thoracique. *Ann Dermatol Vener* 1987; 114:695–697.

110 Hull P R & Hay I T. Peri-umbilical cutaneous schistosomiasis. *S Afr Med J* 1979; 53:654.

111 Macdonald D M & Morrison J G L. Cutaneous ectopic schistosomiasis. *BMJ* 1976; ii:619–620.

112 Obasi O E. Cutaneous schistosomiasis in Nigeria. An update. *Br J Dermatol* 1986; 114:597–602.

113 Scrimgeour E M & Gajdusek D C. Involvement of the central nervous system in *Schistosoma mansoni* and *S. haematobium* infection, a review. *Brain* 1985; 108:1023–1038.

114 van der Horst R. Schistosomiasis of the pericardium. *Trans R Soc Trop Med Hyg* 1979; 73:243–244.

115 Chitiyo M E. Schistosomal involvement of the choroid plexus. *Centr Afr J Med* 1972; 18:45–47.

116 Isebai I. Parasites in the aetiology of cancer: bilharziasis and bladder cancer. *CA Cancer J Clin* 1977; 27:100–106.

117 Makhyoun N A, El-Kashlan K M, Al-Ghorab M M et al. Aetiological factors in bilharzial bladder cancer. *J Trop Med Hyg* 1971; 74:73–78.

118 Prates M D & Gillman J. Carcinoma of the urinary bladder in the Portuguese East Africa with special reference to bilharzial cystitis and preneoplastic reactions. *S Afr Med Sci* 1959; 24:13–40.

119 Lucas S B. Squamous cell carcinoma of the bladder and schistosomiasis. *East Afr Med J* 1982; 59:345–351.

120 Kuntz R E, Cheevers A W & Myers B J. Proliferative epithelial lesions of the urinary bladder of nonhuman primates infected with *Schistosoma haematobium*. *J Natl Cancer Inst* 1972; 48:223–235.

121 Hicks R M, James C & Webbe G. Effect of *S. haematobium* and *N*-butyl-*N*-(4-hydroxy butyl)nitrosamine on the development of urothelial neoplasia in the baboon. *Br J Cancer* 1980; 42:730–755.

122 Brand K G. Schistosomiasis-cancer: etiological considerations. *Acta Trop* 1979; 36:203–214.

123 Hicks R M, Ismael M M, Walters C L et al. Association of bacteriuria and urinary nitrosamine formation with *Schistosoma haematobium* infection in the Qualyub area of Egypt. *Trans R Soc Trop Med Hyg* 1982; 76:519–528.

124 Bhagwandeen S B. Schistosomiasis and carcinoma of the bladder in Zambia. *S Afr Med J* 1976; 50:1616–1620.

125 Cheever A W. Schistosomiasis and neoplasia. *J Natl Cancer Inst* 1978; 61:13–18.

126 Attah E B & Nkposong E O. Schistosomiasis and carcinoma of the bladder: a critical review of causal relationship. *Trop Geogr Med* 1976; 28:268–272.

127 World Health Organization. *Schistosomes, Liver Flukes and Helicobacter pylori*. IARC Monographs on the Evaluation of Carcinogenic Risks to Humans, vol. 61. Geneva: WHO, 1994.

128 Chen M G & Mott K E. Progress in assessment of morbidity due to *Schistosoma mansoni* infection. In *Progress in assessment of morbidity due to schistosomiasis. Reviews of recent literature.* From *Trop Dis Bull* 1988; 85:R1–R56.

129 Warren K S. The kinetics of hepatosplenic schistosomiasis. *Semin Liver Dis* 1984; 4:293–300.

130 Dunn M A & Kamel R. Hepatic schistosomiasis. *Hepatology* 1981; 1:653–661.

131 Warren K S. The relevance of schistosomiasis. *N Engl J Med* 1980; 303:203–206.

132 Dunn M A, Kamel R, Kamel I A et al. Liver collagen synthesis in schistosomiasis mansoni. *Gastroenterology* 1979; 76:978–982.

133 Andrade Z A & Abreu W N. Follicular lymphoma of the

134 Andrade Z A, Andrade S G & Sadigursky M. Renal changes in patients with hepatosplenic schistosomiasis. *Am J Trop Med Hyg* 1971; 20:77–83.

135 Barsoum R S, Bassily S, Soliman M M et al. Renal amyloidosis and schistosomiasis. *Trans R Soc Trop Med Hyg* 1979; 73:367–374.

136 Pitella J E H & Lana-Peixoto M. Brain involvement in hepatosplenic schistosomiasis mansoni. *Brain* 1981; 104:621–632.

137 Bittencourt A L, Almeida M A C, Inues M A F et al. Placental involvement in schistosomiasis mansoni; report of four cases. *Am J Trop Med Hyg* 1980; 29:571–575.

138 Chen M G. Relative distribution of *Schistosoma japonicum* eggs in the intestine of man: a subject of inconsistency. *Acta Trop* 1990; 48:163–171.

139 Mao S P, He Y X, Yang Y Q et al. *Schistosoma japonicum* and schistosomiasis japonica. In Wu Z J, Mao S P & Wang J W (eds) *Chinese Medical Encyclopaedia, Parasitology and Parasitic Diseases*. Shanghai: Shanghai Publishing House for Sciences and Technology, 1984:44–55 (in Chinese).

140 Cheng M G & Mott K E. Progress in assessment of morbidity due to *Schistosoma japonicum*. A review of recent literature. In *Progress in Assessment of Morbidity due to Schistosomiasis*. From *Trop Dis Bull* 1988; 85:R1–R45.

141 Santos A T. The present status of schistosomiasis in the Philippines. *Southeast Asian J Trop Med Public Health* 1984; 15:439–445.

142 Garin D, Chapalain J C, Thierry J et al. Le point sur *Schistosoma intercalatum*. *Med Trop* 1990; 50:433–440.

143 van Wijk H B & Elias E A. Hepatic and rectal pathology in *Schistosoma intercalatum* infection. *Trop Geogr Med* 1975; 27:237–248.

144 Centers for Disease Control. Acute schistosomiasis in US travelers returning from Africa. *MMWR* 1990; 39:141–148.

145 Stuiver P C. Acute schistosomiasis (Katayama fever). *BMJ* 1984; 288:221–222.

146 Farid Z, Bassily S, Kent D C et al. Chronic urinary salmonella carriers with intermittent bacteraemia. *Am J Trop Med Hyg* 1970; 73:153–156.

147 Farid Z, Kilpatrick M E & Ishak E A. *S. haematobium* and *S. intercalatum*. Clinical and pathological aspects. In Jordan P, Webbe G & Sturrock R F (eds) *Human Schistosomiasis*, 3rd edn. Wallingford: CAB International, 1993: 159–193.

148 Simarro P P, Sima F O & Mir M. African trypanosomiasis and *Schistosoma intercalatum* infection in Equatorial Guinea: comparative epidemiology and feasibility of integrated control. *Trop Med Parasitol* 1989; 40:159–162.

149 Simarro P P, Sima F O & Mir M. Urban epidemiology of *Schistosoma intercalatum* in the city of Bata, Equatorial Guinea. *Trop Med Parasitol* 1990; 41:254–256.

150 Arene F O, Ukpeibo E T & Nwanze E A. Studies on schistosomiasis in the Niger Delta; *Schistosoma intercalatum* in the urban city of Port Harcourt, Nigeria. *Public Health* 1989; 103:295–301.

151 Corachan M, Escosa R, Mass J et al. Clinical presentations of *Schistosoma intercalatum* infestation. *Lancet* 1987; I:1139.

152 Deelder A M, De Jonge N, Boerman O C et al. Sensitive determination of circulating anodic antigen in *Schistosoma mansoni* infected individuals by an enzyme-linked immunosorbent assay using monoclonal antibodies. *Am J Trop Med Hyg* 1989; 40:268–272.

153 De Jonge J, Fillié Y E, Hilberath G W et al. Presence of the schistosome circulating anodic antigen (CAA) in urine of patients with *Schistosoma mansoni* or *S. haematobium* infections. *Am J Trop Med Hyg* 1989; 41:563–569.

154 De Jonge N, Schommer G, Krikger F W et al. Presence of

circulating anodic antigen in serum of *Schistosoma intercalatum*-infected patients from Gabon. *Acta Trop* 1989; 46:115–120.

155 De Jonge N, Rabello A L T, Krijger F W et al. Levels of the schistosome circulating anodic and cathodic antigens in serum of schistosomiasis patients from Brazil. *Trans R Soc Trop Med Hyg* 1991; 85:756–759.

156 Kremsner P G, De Jonge N, Simarro P P et al. Quantitative determination of circulating anodic and cathodic antigens in serum and urine of individuals infected with *Schistosoma intercalatum*. *Trans R Soc Trop Med Hyg* 1993; 87:167–169.

157 Braun-Munzinger R A & Southgate B A. Repeatability and reproducibility of egg counts of *Schistosoma haematobium* in urine. *Trop Med Parasitol* 1992; 43:149–154.

158 Cook J A & Jordan P. Excretion of *Schistosoma mansoni* eggs in the urine. *Trans R Soc Trop Med Hyg* 1970; 64:793–794.

159 Bell D R. In *East African Institute for Medical Research: Annual Report 1961–1962*. Kenya: Government Printer, 1962:24.

160 Dazo B C & Biles J E. Two new field techniques for detection and counting of *Schistosoma haematobium* eggs in urine samples. *Bull World Health Organ* 1974; 51:399–408.

161 Peters P A, Warren K S & Mahmoud A A F. Rapid accurate quantification of schistosome eggs via nuclepore filters. *J Parasitol* 1976; 62:154–155.

162 Peters P A, Mahmoud A A F, Warren K S et al. Field studies of rapid accurate means of quantifying *Schistosoma haematobium* eggs in urine samples. *Bull World Health Organ* 1976; 54:159–162.

163 Mott K E, Baltes R, Bambahga J et al. Field studies of a reusable polyamide filter for detection of *Schistosoma haematobium* eggs by urine filtration. *Trop Med Parasitol* 1981; 33:227–228.

164 Mott K E. A reusable polyamide filter for diagnosis of *S. haematobium* infection by urine filtration. *Bull Soc Pathol Exot* 1983; 76:101–104.

165 Braun-Munzinger R A & Rohde R. False epidemiological results from the bulk transport of dried filter paper in urinary schistosomiasis. *Trop Med Parasitol* 1986; 37:286–289.

166 Ritchie L S. An ether sedimentation technique for routine stool examination. *Bull US Army Med Dept* 1948; 8:326.

167 Hunter G W III, Hodges E P, Jahnes W G et al. Studies on schistosomiasis. II. Summary of further studies on methods of recovering eggs of *S. japonicum*. *Bull US Army Med Dept* 1948; 8:128–131.

168 Blagg W, Schaegel E L & Mansour N S. A new concentration technique for the demonstration of protozoa and helminthic eggs in the faeces. *Am J Trop Med Hyg* 1955; 4:23–28.

169 Knight W B, Hiatt R A, Cline B L et al. A modification of the formol-ether concentration technique for increased sensitivity in detecting *Schistosoma mansoni* eggs. *Am J Trop Med Hyg* 1970; 25:818–823.

170 Allen A V H & Ridley D S. Further observations on the formol-ether concentration technique for faecal parasites. *J Clin Pathol* 1970; 23:545–546.

171 Visser P S & Pitchford R J. A simple apparatus for rapid recovery of helminthic eggs from excreta with special reference to *Schistosoma mansoni*. *S Afr Med J* 1972; 46:1344–1346.

172 Komiya Y & Kobayashi A. Evaluation of Kato's thick smear with a cellophane cover for helminth eggs in faeces. *Jpn J Med Sci Biol* 1966; 19:59–64.

173 Katz N, Chaves A & Pellegrino J. A simple device for quantitative thick smear technique in schistosomiasis mansoni. *Rev Inst Med Trop São Paulo* 1972; 14:397–400.

174 Teesdale C H & Amin M A. Comparison of the Bell technique, a modified Kato thick smear technique and a digestion method for the field diagnosis of schistosomiasis mansoni. *J Helminthol* 1976; 59:17–20.

175 Teesdale C H & Amin M A. A simple thick smear technique for the diagnosis of *Schistosoma mansoni* infection. *Bull World Health Organ* 1976; 54:703–705.

176 Chitsulo L, Teesdale C H & Dixon H. Comparison of the Teesdale glass sandwich and Kato–Katz techniques for the diagnosis of *Schistosoma mansoni*; a double-blind study. *Trop Med Parasitol* 1990; 41:447–449.

177 Fulleborn F. Über den Nachweis der Schistosomum mansoni: Eir in Stuhle. *Arch Schiffs Tropenkr Hamburg* 1921; 25:334–340.

178 Fun-Zhi. *Schistosomiasis Shou Chai*, 2nd edn. (Prevention and control of schistosomiasis handbook compiled by the Revolutionary Committee of Shanghai Schistosomiasis Research Institute.) Shanghai: People's Press, 1971 (in Chinese).

179 Shanghai Municipal Institute for Prevention and Treatment of Schistosomiasis. *Handbook on the Prevention and Treatment of Schistosomiasis* (translated by the US Department of Health, Education and Welfare, Public Health Service, National Institutes of Health). DHEW publication no. (NIH) 77-1290. 1977:61–69.

180 Gorman S, Ross W F & Blair D M. The macroscopic diagnosis of urinary schistosomiasis. *S Afr Med J* 1947; 21:853–854.

181 Meeser S V, Ross W F & Blair D M. Further observations on the macroscopic diagnosis of urinary schistosomiasis. *J Trop Med Hyg* 1948; 51:54–59.

182 Weber M C. Miracidial hatching. *Centr Afr J Med* 1973; 19 (Supplement 9):11–14.

183 Davis A. Field trials of 'Ambilhar' in the treatment of urinary bilharziasis in schoolchildren. *Bull World Health Organ* 1966; 35:827–835.

184 Davis A. Comparative trials of antimonial drugs in urinary schistosomiasis. *Bull World Health Organ* 1968; 38:197–227.

185 Braun-Munzinger R A & Southgate B A. Egg viability in urinary schistosomiasis. I. New methods compared with available methods. *J Trop Med Hyg* 1993; 96:22–27.

186 Braun-Munzinger R A & Southgate B A. Egg viability in urinary schistosomiasis. II. Simplifying modifications and standardization of new methods. *J Trop Med Hyg* 1993; 96:71–75.

187 Braun-Munzinger R A & Southgate B A. Egg viability in urinary schistosomiasis. III. Repeatability and reproducibility of new methods. *J Trop Med Hyg* 1993; 96:179–185.

188 Newsome J. Recent investigations into the treatment of schistosomiasis by Miracil D in Egypt. *Trans R Soc Trop Med Hyg* 1951; 44:611–634.

189 Upatham E S, Sturrock R F & Cook J A. Studies on the hatchability of *Schistosoma mansoni* from a naturally infected human community on St Lucia, West Indies. *Parasitology* 1976; 73:253–264.

190 Zicker F, Katz N & Wolf J. Availaçao do teste de ecloso de miracidios na equistossoma mansonica. *Rev Bras Malariol Doencas Trop* 1977; 30:65–75.

191 Da Cunha A S. A availiaçao terapéutica da oxamniquine na equistossomose mansoni humana pelo metodo do oograma per biopsia de mucosa rectal. *Rev Inst Med Trop São Paulo* 1982; 24:88–94.

192 World Health Organization. *Diagnostic Techniques in Schistosomiasis Control*. WHO/SCHISTO/83.69 Parasitic Diseases Programme. Geneva: WHO, 1983:1–36 (unpublished document).

193 Briggs M, Chatfield M, Mummery D et al. Screening with reagent strips. *BMJ* 1971; iii:433–434.

194 Wilkins H A, Goll P, Marshall T F de C & Moore P J. The significance of proteinuria and haematuria in *Schistosoma haematobium* infection. *Trans R Soc Trop Med Hyg* 1979; 73:74–80.

195 Pugh R N H, Bell D R & Gilles H M. Malumfashi endemic diseases research project. XV. The potential medical importance of bilharzia in northern Nigeria: a suggested

rapid cheap and effective solution for control of *Schistosoma haematobium* infection. *Ann Trop Med Parasitol* 1980; 74:597–613.

196 Feldmeir H, Doehring E & Dafallah A A. Simultaneous use of a sensitive filtration technique and reagent strips in urinary schistosomiasis. *Trans R Soc Trop Med Hyg* 1982; 76:416–421.

197 Savioli L, Hatz C, Dixon H et al. Control of morbidity due to *Schistosoma haematobium* on Pemba Island: egg excretion and haematuria as indicators of infection. *Am J Trop Med Hyg* 1990; 43:289–295.

198 Mott K E & Dixon H. Collaborative study on antigens for immunodiagnosis of schistosomiasis. *Bull World Health Organ* 1981; 60:729–753.

199 Mott K E, Dixon H, Carter C E et al. Collaborative study on antigens for immunodiagnosis of *Schistosoma japonicum* infections. *Bull World Health Organ* 1987; 65:233–244.

200 Bergquist R. In Bergquist R (ed.) *Immunodiagnostic Approaches in Schistosomiasis.* Chichester: Wiley, 1992: 1–8.

201 van Lieshout L, Polderman A M & Deelder A M. Immunodiagnosis of schistosomiasis by determination of the circulating antigens CAA and CCA, in particular in individuals with recent or light infection. *Acta Trop* 2000; 77:69–80.

202 Abdel-Waheb M F & Strickland G T. Abdominal ultrasonography for assessing morbidity from schistosomiasis. 2. Hospital studies. *Trans R Soc Trop Med Hyg* 1993; 87:135–137.

203 Hatz C, Jenkins J M & Tanner M. Ultrasound in schistosomiasis. *Acta Trop* 1992; 51:1–97.

204 World Health Organization. *Meeting on Ultrasonography in Schistosomiasis.* UNDP/World Bank/WHO Special Programme for Research and Training in Tropical Diseases. TDR/SCH/ULTRASON/91.3, CTD/91.3. Geneva: WHO, 1991:1–32 (unpublished document).

205 Abdel-Wahab M F, Esmat G, Narooz S I et al. Sonographic studies of schoolchildren in a village endemic for *Schistosoma haematobium. Trans R Soc Trop Med Hyg* 1990; 84:69–73.

206 Abdel-Waheb M F, Esmat G, Farrag A et al. Grading of hepatic schistosomiasis by the use of ultrasonography. *Am J Trop Med Hyg* 1992; 46:403–408.

207 Abdel-Wahab M F, Esmat G, Milad M et al. Characteristic sonographic patterns of schistosomal hepatic fibrosis. *Am J Trop Med Hyg* 1989; 40:72–76.

208 Abdel-Waheb M F, Esmat G, Farrag A et al. Ultrasonographic prediction of esophageal varices in schistosomiasis mansoni. *Am J Gastroenterol* 1993; 88:560–563.

209 Davis A. The Professor Gerald Webbe Memorial Lecture. Global control of schistosomiasis. *Trans R Soc Trop Med Hyg* 2000; 94:609–615.

210 Doenhoff M J, Kimani G & Cioli D. Praziquantel and the control of schistosomiasis. *Parasitol Today* 2000; 16:364–366.

211 Liang Y S, Dai J R, Ning A et al. Susceptibility of *Schistosoma japonicum* to praziquantel in China. *Trop Med Int Health* 2001 6(9):707–714.

212 Ajana F, Dei-Cas E, Colin J J et al. La bilharziose humaine à *Schistosoma mekongi*; problèmes diagnostiques et thérapeutiques. *Méd Mal Infect* 1986 3:141–146.

213 Chidiac C, Beaucaire G, Mouton Y et al. Echecs au praziquantel dans le traitement des bilharzioses; intéret de la biopsie de muqueuse rectale et du suivi prolonge. *Méd Mal Infect* 1986; 5:380–384.

214 Duong T H, Furet Y, Lorett G et al. Traitement de la bilharziose à *Schistosoma mekongi* par le praziquantel. *Méd Trop* 1988; 48:39–43.

215 Manoury V, Guillemot F, Mathieu-Chandelier C et al. Bilharzioses à *Schistosoma mekongi* diagnostiquées par biopsie rectale et traitées par praziquantel; à propos de 5 cas. *Gastroenterol Clin Biol* 1990; 14:1032–1033.

216 Ismael M, Metwally A, Farghaly A et al. Characterization of isolates of *Schistosoma mansoni* from Egyptian villagers that tolerate high doses of praziquantel. *Am J Trop Med Hyg* 1996; 55:212–218.

217 Ismael M, Botros S, Metwally A et al. Resistance to praziquantel. Direct evidence from *Schistosoma mansoni* isolated from Egyptian villagers. *Am J Trop Med Hyg* 1999; 60:932–935.

218 Fallon P G & Doenhoff M J. Drug resistant schistosomiasis: resistance to praziquantel and oxamniquine induced in *Schistosoma mansoni* in mice is drug specific. *Am J Trop Med Hyg* 1994; 51:83–89.

219 Gryseels B, Stelma F F, Talla I et al. Epidemiology, immunology and chemotherapy of *Schistosoma mansoni* infections in a recently expressed community in Senegal. *Trop Geogr Med* 1994; 46:209–219.

220 Stelma F F, Talma I, Sow S et al. Efficacy and side effects of praziquantel in an epidemic focus of *Schistosoma mansoni. Am J Trop Med Hyg* 1995; 53:167–170.

221 Guissé F, Polman K, Stelma F F et al. Therapeutic evaluation of two different dose regimens of praziquantel in a recent *Schistosoma mansoni* focus in northern Senegal. *Am J Trop Med Hyg* 1997; 56:511–514.

222 Liang Y S, Coles G C & Doenhoff M J. Detection of praziquantel resistance in schistosomes. *Trop Med Int Health* 2000; 5:72.

223 King C H, Muchiri E M & Ouma J H. Evidence against rapid emergence of praziquantel resistance in *Schistosoma haematobium*, Kenya. *Emerg Infect Dis* 2000; 6(6):585–593.

224 Foster R & Cheetham B L. Studies with the schistosomicide oxamniquine (UK-4721). 1. Activities in rodents and in vitro. *Trans R Soc Trop Med Hyg* 1973; 67:674–684.

225 Foster R, Cheetham B L & King D F. Studies with the schistosomicide oxamniquine (UK-4271). II. Activity in primates. *Trans R Soc Trop Med Hyg* 1973; 67:685–693.

226 Bassily S, Farid Z, Higashi G I et al. Treatment of complicated schistosomiasis mansoni with oxamniquine. *Am J Trop Med Hyg* 1978; 27:1284–1286.

227 Farid Z, Higashi G I & Bassily S. Treatment of advanced hepatosplenic with oxamniquine. *Trans R Soc Trop Med Hyg* 1980; 74:400–401.

228 Abaza H H, Hammouda N, Abd Rabbo H et al. Chemotherapy of schistosomal polyposis with oxamniquine. *Trans R Soc Trop Med Hyg* 1978; 72:602–604.

229 Machado P A. The Brazilian control programme for schistosomiasis control 1975–1979. *Am J Trop Med Hyg* 1982; 31:76–86.

230 Stokvis H, Bauer A G C, Stuiver P C et al. Seizures associated with oxamniquine therapy. *Am J Trop Med Hyg* 1986; 35:330–331.

231 Higashi G I & Farid Z. Oxamniquine fever: drug induced or immune complex reaction. *BMJ* 1979; 2:830.

232 Katz N, Rocha R S, De Souza C P et al. Efficacy of alternating therapy with oxamniquine and praziquantel to treat *Schistosoma mansoni* in children following failure of first treatment. *Am J Trop Med Hyg* 1991; 44:509–512.

233 Xiao S H, You J Q, Yang Y Q et al. Experimental studies on early treatment of schistosomal infection with artemether. *Southeast Asian. J Trop Med Public Health* 1995; 26:306–318.

234 Xiao S H, You J Q, Mei J Y et al. Preventive effect of artemether in rabbits infected with *Schistosoma japonicum* cerariae. *Acta Pharmacol Sin* 1998; 19:63–66.

235 Xiao S H, Booth M & Tanner M. The prophylactic effect of artemether against *Schistosoma japonicum* infections. *Parasitol Today* 2000; 16:122–126.

236 Xiao S H & Catto B A. *In vitro* and *in vivo* studies of the effect of artemether on *Schistosoma mansoni. Antimicrob Agents Chemother* 1989; 33:1557–1562.

237 Xiao S H, Chollet J, Weiss N A et al. Preventive effect of artemether in experimental animals infected with *Schistosoma mansoni*. *Parasitol Int* 2000; 49:19–24.

238 Utzinger J, N'Goran E K, N'Dri A et al. Oral artemether for prevention of *Schistosoma mansoni* infection: randomised controlled trial. Lancet 2000; 355:1320–1325.

239 Mansour N M, Omer Ali P, Farid Z et al. Serological differentiation of acute and chronic schistosomiasis mansoni by antibody responses to keyhole limpet haemocyanin. *Am J Trop Med Hyg* 1989; 41:338–344.

240 Watt G, Adapon B, Long G W et al. Praziquantel in treatment of cerebral schistosomiasis. *Lancet* 1986; ii:529–532.

241 Ezzat F A, Abu-Elmagd K M, Aly M A et al. Selective shunt versus nonshunt surgery for management of both schistosomal and nonschistosomal variceal bleeders. *Ann Surg* 1990; 212:97–108.

242 Davis A. Metriphonate. In Dollery C (ed.) *Therapeutic Drugs*, vol. 2. Edinburgh: Churchill Livingstone, 1991: M164–M170.

243 Davis A. Oxamniquine. In Dollery C (ed.) *Therapeutic Drugs*, vol. 2. Edinburgh: Churchill Livingstone, 1991: O42–O45.

244 Wegner D H G. Praziquantel. In Dollery C (ed/) *Therapeutic Drugs*, vol. 2. Edinburgh: Churchill Livingstone, 1991: P189–P195.

245 Davis A. Antischistosomal drugs and clinical practice. In Jordan P, Webbe G & Sturrock R F (eds) *Human Schistosomiasis*, 3rd edn. Wallingford: CAB International, 1993: 367– 404.

246 World Health Organization. The control of schistosomiasis. Second Report of the WHO Expert Committee. *WHO Tech Rep Ser* 1993; 830:1–86.

247 Mott K E (ed.) *Plant Molluscicides.* Published on behalf of the UNDP/World Bank/WHO Special Programme for Research and Training in Tropical Diseases. Chichester: Wiley, 1987.

248 McCullough F S. *The Use of Mollusciciding in Schistosomiasis Control.* WHO/SCHISTO/92.107 Geneva: WHO, 1992 (unpublished document).

249 Bergquist N R. Controlling schistosomiasis by vaccination: a realistic option? *Parasitol Today* 1995; 11:191–194.

250 Bergquist N R & Colley D G. Schistosomiasis vaccines: research to development. *Parasitol Today* 1998; 14(3):99–104.

251 Capron A, Rriveau G & Capron M. Vaccine strategies against schistosomiasis: from concepts to clinical trials. In Conference and abstract book *New Challenges in Tropical Medicine and Parasitology*, Oxford, UK, 18–22 September 2000:58–59 (Abstract PL10.2).

252 Gryseels B. Schistosomiasis vaccines: a devil's advocate view. *Parasitol Today* 2000; 16(2):46–47.

253 Stuck M-M. Chances and risks of developing vaccines. *Vaccine* 1996; 14(14):1301–1302.

Chapter 81
Food-borne Trematodes

M. R. Haswell-Elkins and E. Levri

The liver flukes (*Fasciola, Opisthorchis, Clonorchis*), lung flukes (*Paragonimus*) and intestinal flukes (*Fasciolopsis, Echinostoma, Heterophyes*) are important causes of human disease.[1] Although these are commonly thought of as 'tropical' parasites, some species are not limited to hot climates. An extreme example is *Opisthorchis felineus* which is commonly acquired through the consumption of raw frozen fish in Siberia. The availability of freshwater flora and fauna and a preference for eating them raw or incompletely cooked are the most important factors determining their distribution in man.

All food-borne trematodes are hermaphroditic and have oral and ventral suckers for attachment. Their life cycles are complex and involve one or more intermediate hosts (the first always being a snail) and several morphological stages (Figure 81.1). Although differing in anatomical location in

the final host and therefore causing different diseases, transmission to man occurs almost exclusively through the consumption of raw foods harbouring the infective stage. In contrast, schistosomes have two sexes and enter their final hosts by active penetration.

Among the thousands of food-borne trematodes, hundreds may infect man, and new species are still being discovered.[1-3] Because most species also parasitize other animals and are of veterinary importance, the term 'accidental' is sometimes used to describe human infections. The term is appropriate for some representatives, such as *Fasciola*, which in most endemic areas occurs in isolated cases or outbreaks, or for flukes rarely reported in humans, e.g. *Watsoni, Dicrocoelium, Eurytrema*. However, estimates that 40 million people harbour food-borne trematodes[4] argue against a major role of chance in most infections.

The endemic areas of these parasites often overlap, since people often enjoy many kinds of raw food. For example, adult worms of 13 food-borne trematode species (plus *Taenia saginata*) were found among 224 residents of a single village in north-east Thailand.[3] Up to seven species have been reported in a single individual.[2] Some authors have reported an association between 'tastiness' of fish and the season or species with the highest intensity of infective stages.[5] This may reflect an influence of human taste preference on parasite life cycles.

Food-borne trematodes have received less attention than other helminth infections, perhaps because of their focal distribution and lack of acute symptoms. However, some authors have mistakenly reported them as comparatively benign, which is certainly not the case for the liver flukes and *Paragonimus*, as reviewed here. Severity of disease is associated with worm burden, except perhaps in the case of ectopic infections.

Due to increasing tourism and migration, infections previously confined to endemic areas are increasingly being reported in non-endemic countries.[6] There is also evidence that some endemic areas are expanding due to domestic migration, environmental changes that favour snail proliferation, declining economic conditions and sanitation, and increasing availability of contaminated foods through wider distribution networks and lack of food inspections.[7-12] On the other hand, as newly industrialized countries alter their natural environment and pollute their river systems, native snail, crustacean and fish fauna decline. Night-soil and manure, potentially containing fluke eggs, are being replaced by chemical

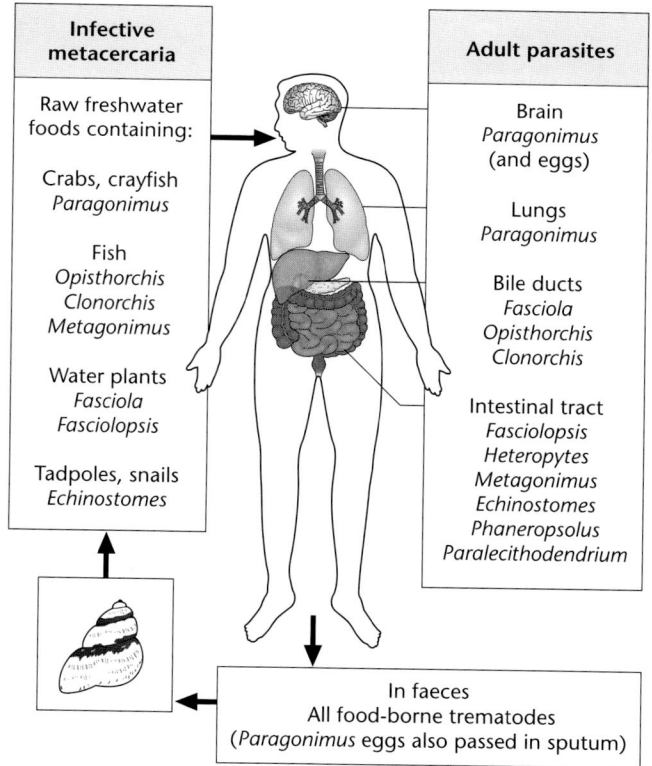

Infective metacercaria	Adult parasites
Raw freshwater foods containing:	Brain *Paragonimus* (and eggs)
Crabs, crayfish *Paragonimus*	Lungs *Paragonimus*
Fish *Opisthorchis Clonorchis Metagonimus*	Bile ducts *Fasciola Opisthorchis Clonorchis*
Water plants *Fasciola Fasciolopsis*	Intestinal tract *Fasciolopsis Heteropytes Metagonimus Echinostomes Phaneropsolus Paralecithodendrium*
Tadpoles, snails *Echinostomes*	

In faeces
All food-borne trematodes
(*Paragonimus* eggs also passed in sputum)

Figure 81.1: Diagrammatic representation of the life cycle of the major food-borne trematode infections of man. (Drawn by Banchob Sripa.)

fertilizer. Thus risk of infection by eating raw 'wild' foods might be gradually replaced by risk of exposure to potentially hazardous chemicals.

Efforts to control food-borne parasites were revolutionized by the drug praziquantel, which is now inexpensive and widely available. However, in addition to anthelmintic treatment to cure current infection, improvements in sanitation and health promotion to encourage the cooking of foods involved in transmission are important components of control to prevent re-infection. Eating habits have cultural and social significance and often are difficult to change.[12–14]

Liver flukes
Opisthorchiasis and clonorchiasis

Aetiology

The human liver flukes, *Clonorchis sinensis*, *Opisthorchis viverrini* and *O. felineus*, remain important public health problems in many endemic areas, where they infect approximately 17 million people.[4,8,10,12,15] *O. guayaquilensis* has been reported in a small human focus in Ecuador.[1] In addition to their association with hepatobiliary disease, *O. viverrini* and *C. sinensis* are major aetiological agents of bile duct cancer.[16–23] This is a leading cause of death in north-east Thailand.[18]

The three major flukes have similar adult and egg morphologies, life cycles and pathogenesis (Figures 81.1 and 81.2). Distinction between them is generally based on the flame cell pattern of the adult worms.

History and seminal discoveries

Human infection with these flukes was first discovered in 1875 (*C. sinensis*), 1892 (*O. felineus*) and the early 1900s (*O. viverrini*).[1] The close association between bile duct carcinoma and *O. viverrini* and *C. sinensis* was first researched by Hoeppli,[19] Viranuvatti and Mettiyawongse[20] and Hou.[21] Thamavit et al. established a laboratory model of cholangiocarcinoma in hamsters exposed to *O. viverrini* infection and low doses of *N*-dimethylnitrosamine.[22] The very high incidence of this cancer in an endemic area of Thailand is documented by Vatanasapt et al.[18] In 1994, the International Agency for Research on Cancer classified *O. viverrini* and *C. sinensis* as human carcinogens.[23]

Life cycle

The adult parasites live in the smaller intrahepatic bile ducts of their final hosts, which include humans, cats, dogs and other wild and domestic fish-eating mammals. Eggs pass down the bile duct and into the faeces and can also be found in the gallbladder. Eggs are fully embryonated upon excretion, and hatch into miracidia after being ingested by snails. Generally fewer than 1–2% of snails are infected.[15] The miracidia transform into sporocysts and rediae which multiply, then become free-swimming cercaria which exit the snail and attach, penetrate and encyst in susceptible species of fish. Most belong to the

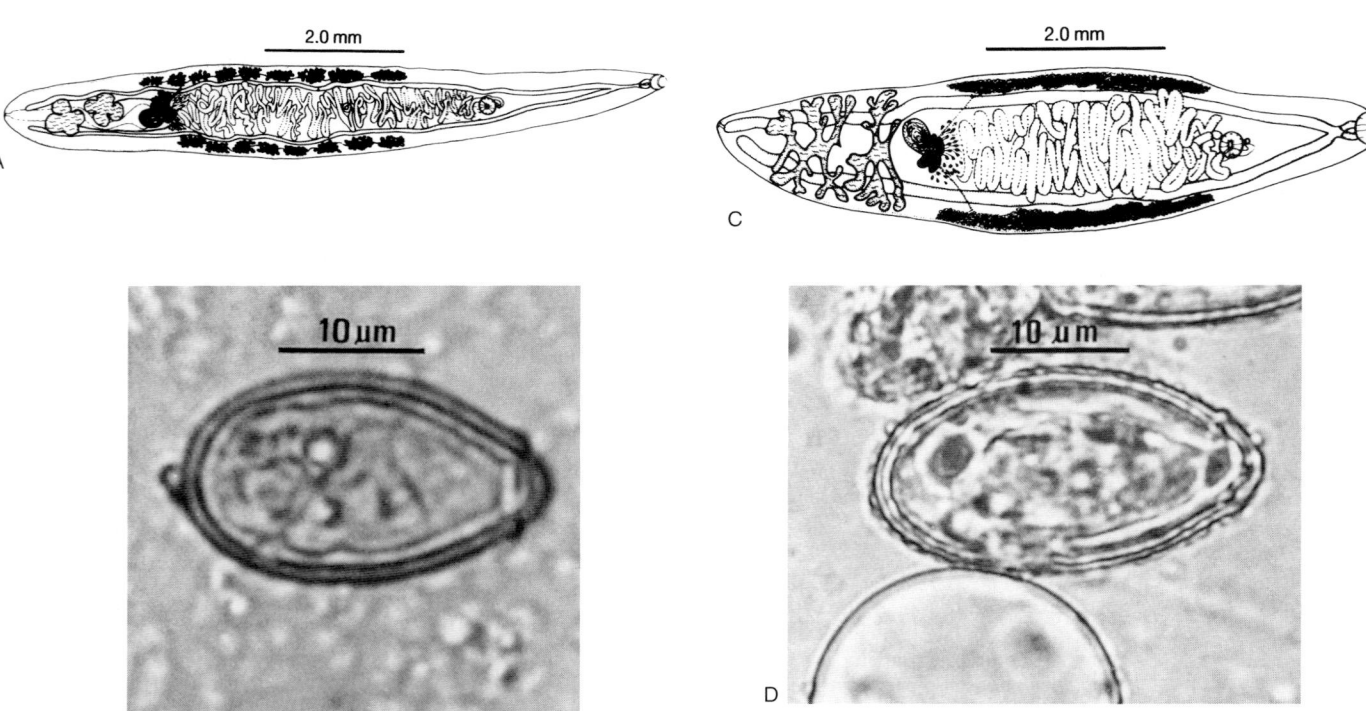

Figure 81.2: (**A**) Adult stage worm of *Opisthorchis viverrini*. (Drawn by Sasithorn Kaewkes.) (**B**) Egg of *O. viverrini*. (Photograph by Sasithorn Kaewkes.) (**C**) Adult stage worm of *Clonorchis sinensis*. (Drawn by Sasithorn Kaewkes.) (**D**) Egg of *C. sinensis*. (Photograph by Sasithorn Kaewkes.)

family Cyprinidae. Wide variation in the prevalence (up to 100%) and intensity of metacercaria is found between seasons, types of water bodies and species of fish.[15,24] Metacercaria are infective to humans and other mammals if consumed uncooked. The metacercaria excyst, migrate up the duodenum through the ampulla of Vater and the extrahepatic biliary system to the intrahepatic bile ducts, where they mature. The prepatent period is about 1 month and the adults may live many years.[1,15]

Epidemiology

Humans become infected with *Opisthorchis* and *Clonorchis* through the consumption of raw or undercooked cyprinoid fish containing metacercariae. Geographical and age-related patterns of human infection therefore overlap with this dietary habit.

O. felineus is prevalent in animals throughout Europe, and has been reported in humans from eastern Germany, Poland, Kazakhstan, Russia and the Ukraine.[1,4,15,23] Most recent information comes from Siberia, notably the Tyumen and Khanty regions, where high prevalences and intensities are reported.[25] Residents and immigrants to the endemic focus in Siberia enjoy eating thinly sliced frozen or lightly salted cyprinoid fish.

Control efforts in north-east Thailand have led to a drop in the prevalence of *O. viverrini* infection among the population of 20 million from approximately 35% in 1981, to 24 to 30% in 1992 and 18.6% in 1994.[12] The infection remains common in Laos. Reports also suggest an increase in the average prevalence of infection in central and northern Thailand: up to 26% in 1992.[12] However, studies in northern Thailand collecting adult worms post treatment and examining metacercariae in fish have suggested that the observed increase may be partly due to misdiagnosis of minute intestinal fluke infections.[26]

Raw fish dishes are a well-established dietary tradition of Laos people and the ethnic Laos in north-east Thailand. Fresh fish dishes may contain large numbers of metacercariae and are eaten occasionally. Uncooked fermented fish, which is eaten daily, also contain metacercariae, but its importance as a source of infection is unclear.

C. sinensis, although largely eliminated from Japan and drastically reduced in Korea, remains prevalent and may be increasingly common in parts of Taiwan, Hong Kong, Vietnam, Macao and China.[7,8,10,15] Human infection occurs in 24 Chinese provinces, with one major focus in the south (especially Guangdong and Guangsxi provinces) and another in the north-east (Henjian). Some Chinese people enjoy eating raw fish dipped in hot rice porridge, or children catch and eat them during play. This latter practice results in an unusual age-related pattern of infection, whereby most infection occurs in children.

Generally, prevalence and intensity of infection rise with age, with most initial infections occurring in the early teens, and may be higher in males than females.[15,17]

Thus despite widespread availability of praziquantel and massive control efforts, these liver flukes remain common and a major public health problem in endemic areas.

Clinical features

Most chronically infected individuals have few specific signs or symptoms, except an increased frequency of palpable liver, as shown in community-based studies using physical examination.[15,23,25,27,28] Haematological and biochemical features are unremarkable, even in heavy infections. Ultrasonography, however, reveals a high frequency of gallbladder enlargement, sludge, gallstones and poor function in asymptomatic individuals.[28,29]

Symptomatic cases of *Opisthorchis* and *Clonorchis* infection generally experience pain in the right upper quadrant, diarrhoea, loss of appetite, indigestion and fullness. Severe cases may present with weakness, lassitude, weight loss, ascites and oedema.[30] Complications may include cholangitis, obstructive jaundice, intra-abdominal mass, cholecystitis and gallbladder or intrahepatic stones.[15,27,30] Such stones are particularly frequent in clonorchiasis.

The most important clinical manifestation of liver fluke infection is an enhanced susceptibility to cholangiocarcinoma. Case-control studies in Thailand suggest a fivefold increased risk during infection of any intensity, while heavily infected people may face a 15-fold risk.[31] This is reflected in a sixfold and 10-fold higher incidence of cholangiocarcinoma (in females and males, respectively) in an endemic province of Thailand above that of a non-endemic area.[18] While such a dramatic increase is not reported for *Clonorchis* infection, there is ample evidence that this fluke is also strongly associated with cholangiocarcinoma.[15,23,32]

A special feature of *O. felineus* infection, not often reported for the other species, is acute opisthorchiasis.[25] This is characterized by hepatosplenomegaly and tenderness, eosinophilia up to 40%, and chills and fever. It occurs early in infection and may be associated with primary exposure to a large dose of metacercaria.

Pathology and pathogenesis

Liver enlargement and dilated subcapsular bile ducts with thick fibrotic walls can be seen grossly in heavily infected cases.[1,15–17,19,21,33] Microscopically, bile duct pathology is characterized by desquamation of epithelial cells of secondary and tertiary ducts and chronic inflammation with infiltration of lymphocytes, monocytes, eosinophils and plasma cells. Epithelial hyperplasia may lead to the formation of glands lined with columnar epithelial cells beneath the epithelial lining. In severe cases, adenomatous hyperplasia, periductal fibrosis and goblet cell metaplasia may be seen. Inflammation, necrosis and atrophy of hepatic cells have also been reported.

The pathology of fluke-associated cholecystitis consists of fibrosis, infiltration of mast cells and eosinophils and mucosal hyperplasia of the gallbladder wall.[34] Parasites and eggs have been observed in the nidus of gallbladder and intrahepatic stones.[15]

It remains unclear whether liver flukes mediate tissue damage directly via mechanical or chemical irritation, or whether the pathogenesis is immune mediated.[35,36] A 24 kDa antigen of *Clonorchis* is thought to be a major cytotoxic protease causing direct pathology.[35] Inflammatory changes associated with excretory and secretory antigens can be found throughout the intrahepatic and extrahepatic bile ducts in animals experimentally infected with *Opisthorchis*.[36] Ultrasonography reveals enhanced echoes of the portal veins in heavily infected people and these may result from heavy chronic inflammation and fibrosis of the bile ducts.[28] Increased endogenous production of *N*-nitroso compounds and enhanced hepatic activation of carcinogens in these areas of fibrosis may create highly mutagenic conditions for the chronically proliferating bile duct epithelium, and an ideal environment for cancer development.[16,17,22,37,38]

Diagnosis and investigations

Egg counts have traditionally been used to diagnose liver fluke infection, most often using the Kato thick smear, Stoll's dilution or quantitative formalin ethyl acetate concentration technique. All three techniques effectively detect moderate and heavy infections. However, comparative studies in low-intensity areas have shown that a single reading of the concentration and dilution techniques detect about 70% of infections, while the sensitivity of Kato is considerably lower (45%). Worm burden and egg count correlate closely, with an estimated egg output of 53 per gram of faeces per worm (using Stoll's dilution technique).[39] Stoll's egg counts tend to be higher than those of the concentration technique.

Although egg detection is almost always used in surveys and treatment programmes, several immunodiagnostic tests have been described for *Opisthorchis* and *Clonorchis* infections.[15,40,41] While most antigens are non-specific and antibodies persist long after treatment, good results have been gained from new serological tests using individual antigens and detecting isotype-specific antibodies. Faecal antigen detection by enzyme-linked immunosorbent assays (ELISAs) using monoclonal antibodies against secretory antigens and DNA probes also shows promise.[42]

Management

Treatment with praziquantel at 40 mg/kg body weight in a single dose is effective against opisthorchiasis and clonorchiasis.[15,43,44] This regimen has been used most commonly in large-scale treatment programmes. Reports from China, however, indicate that higher doses (120 mg/kg over 2 days) are needed to cure heavy *Clonorchis* infections.[44] Side effects, such as dizziness, vomiting and abdominal pain, occur frequently but are transient and rarely severe. Most abnormalities of the gallbladder are also eliminated by elimination of the parasite.[29] Praziquantel may be dangerous for people with early cholangiocarcinoma, since the sudden expulsion of many worms may aggravate obstruction. No such cases have been reported, but

caution should be exercised. The drug hexachloroparaxylol (Chloxyle) has also been used extensively for the treatment of *O. felineus*, but it may be less effective than praziquantel.

Prevention and control

Prevention of human liver fluke infection can be facilitated by treatment (to reduce the excretion of eggs), sanitation (to prevent eggs from reaching water sources) and health education (to discourage the eating of raw fish).[12,13] The application of Hazard Analysis Critical Control Point principles and procedures during fish farming can reduce metacercarial contamination of fish.[45] Treatment of raw fish by freezing, irradiation and chemical treatment have also been suggested.[46] Control of snail vectors by molluscicides is not considered feasible because of their widespread distribution and resistance to adverse conditions. To be most effective, health education should be designed and delivered in a culturally sensitive manner with the aim of effecting behaviour change as well as simply providing information. Large-scale efforts in endemic areas by public health ministries have probably had a major impact on the intensity of all three infections.

Fascioliasis

There are an estimated 2.4 million people infected with the two larger human liver flukes, *Fasciola hepatica* and *Fasciola gigantica*, often causing serious acute and chronic morbidity.[4,47,48] These parasites commonly infect domestic ruminants and wildlife throughout the world and indirectly impact on human well-being through massive economic loss in the livestock industry. Humans usually become infected by eating aquatic plants grown in water that is contaminated with faeces from animals harbouring *Fasciola*.

History and seminal discoveries

Fasciola hepatica was the first trematode to be described—500 years before most others (de Brie, 1379; cited in reference 1). Its complete life cycle was identified by Leuckart (1882) and Thomas (1883); this greatly facilitated the elucidation of other trematode life cycles. The successful search for effective veterinary vaccines through elegant immunological and molecular biochemistry studies has greatly increased our understanding of host and trematode parasite relationships.[49]

Aetiology and life cycle

F. hepatica (the sheep liver fluke) and *F. gigantica* (mainly of cattle) cause human fascioliasis. The parasites vary in adult and egg size and shape (Figure 81.3) and species of the snail host of the family Lymnaeidae. *F. hepatica* is common in temperate and subtropical areas, especially in sheep-raising areas. Human infections are relatively common in Europe (especially France, Spain, UK and

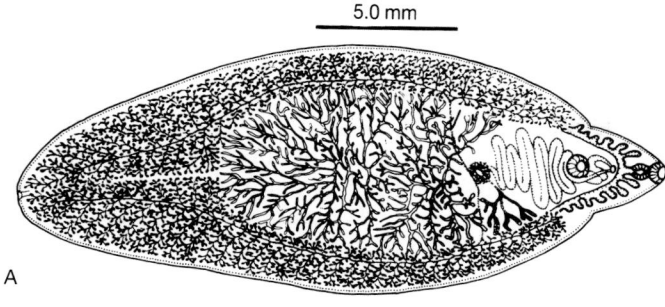

A

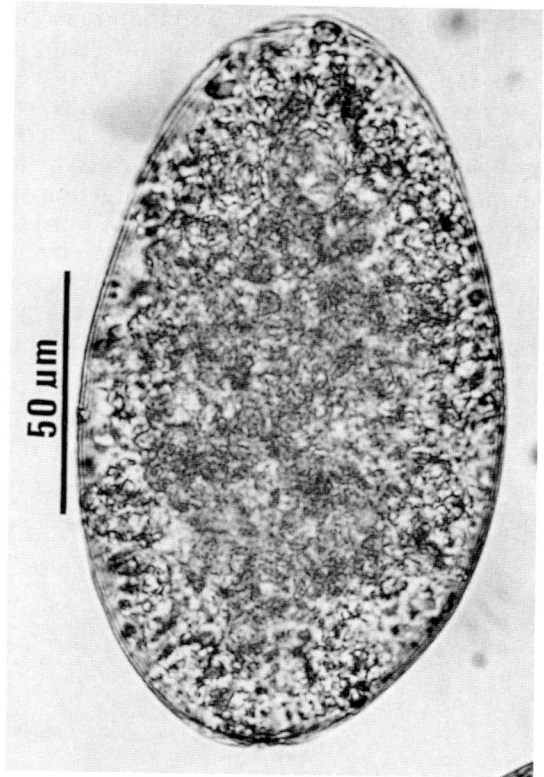

B

Figure 81.3: (**A**) Adult stage worm of *Fasciola hepatica*. (Drawn by Sasithorn Kaewkes.) (**B**) Egg of *F. hepatica*. (Photograph by Sasithorn Kaewkes.)

Portugal), the Middle East (particularly Egypt and Iran), Central and South America (Cuba, Peru, Ecuador and Bolivia) and Africa.[47,48,50] *F. gigantica* occurs in South and South-East Asia and Africa. The two coexist in some countries, and differentiation is difficult.

The adult worm lives in the bile duct of the final host, which may be sheep (*F. hepatica*), cattle/buffalo (*F. gigantica*) or humans. Eggs are excreted in the faeces. The eggs undergo further development upon reaching a water body; miracidia then hatch and penetrate a suitable snail host. After multiplication as sporocysts and rediae, free-swimming mature cercariae exit the snail, attach to aquatic vegetation and become metacercarial cysts. These cysts establish infection upon ingestion by man and other mammals. They excyst in the duodenum, then migrate through the intestinal wall, into the body cavity,

through Glisson's capsule across the liver parenchyma and into the bile ducts, where they may live for many years. Eggs are excreted 3–4 months after ingestion, and the entire cycle is completed in 4–6 months. High humidity, moderate temperatures and rainfall favour transmission.[50]

Epidemiology

Human infection with *Fasciola* is most common in villages and larger towns within rural areas, especially sheep- and cattle-grazing areas.[51] Levels of infection depend on the frequency of humans eating plants (mainly watercress in Europe, morning glory in Asia) from water bodies contaminated with animal faeces.[52] In most endemic areas, human infection is relatively rare, even where prevalence among domestic animals is high. Outbreaks of *F. hepatica* occur in households and communities, and are often traced to consumption of wild, rather than cultivated, watercress.[51,52] A high proportion of exposed people become infected but some do not have symptoms. Infection might also occur from contaminated drinking water or cooking utensils.[53]

Fasciola infection as reported in general parasite surveys is undoubtedly underestimated since eggs are often not detected by faecal examination.[11,48,54] Community-based studies using improved diagnostic methods have demonstrated areas with very high prevalence and intensity of infection in Bolivia and Egypt.[50,55] Heavy infections found in the high altitudes of the Bolivian Altiplano region result from frequent consumption of kjosco (raw water-plant salad) by children tending their grazing animals.[11,50]

Pathogenesis

These parasites cause considerable mortality in sheep and cattle, and human morbidity which is dependent on the number of worms and stage of infection.[47,48,56,57] The acute phase occurs during migration of the immature flukes through the liver. Severe pathology results from parasite ingestion and destruction of parenchymal tissue, haemorrhage, parasite death and inflammatory responses largely mediated by eosinophils. Repair mechanisms can lead to extensive fibrosis, increased pressure atrophy of the liver and periportal fibrosis.

The chronic phase, during which parasites are present in the bile ducts, tends to be less severe. Tissue change, including bile duct proliferation, dilatation and fibrosis, is largely caused by mechanical obstruction of the ducts, inflammatory responses and the activity of proline, which the fluke excretes in large quantities.[55] Proline may facilitate movement of the parasite through the narrow ducts. Anaemia may result from blood loss through bile duct lesions. Death is uncommon, but is usually caused by haemorrhaging in the bile duct and case reports suggest it occurs more frequently in children.[47,48]

Flukes that migrate out of the intestine but do not locate in the liver can form ectopic lesions in many tissues.[48,56] These nodules, granulomas or migration tracts are often misdiagnosed as malignant tumours or gastric ulcers.

Pathology

Multiple yellow nodules of necrotic tissue (1–4 mm in diameter) and linear lesions through the parenchyma infiltrated with eosinophils and Charcot–Leyden crystals can be observed, probably as a result of inflammatory reaction(s) to dead parasites and migration, respectively.[47,48,56] Proliferation, dilatation, fibrosis and calcification of the bile ducts, plus sequelae of partial obstruction, may occur during the chronic phase of infection. Dead flukes are sometimes observed inside calcified areas of tissue, and granulomas and abscesses can form around eggs trapped in the parenchymal tissue. Eosinophils may infiltrate the gallbladder wall, which may be thickened and oedematous with perimuscular fibrosis. Stones are often present in the gallbladder during infection. Self-cure occurs frequently and may result from inflammation and calcification.

Clinical features

Where cases are symptomatic, diarrhoea, upper abdominal pain or pain in the right costal margin, urticaria, malaise, weight loss, coughing, fever and night sweats may begin approximately 2 months following ingestion of metacercaria and 1–2 months prior to the onset of egg excretion.[52,53,56] The signs of this acute phase of infection are hepatomegaly, splenomegaly, anaemia, weakness and marked peripheral eosinophilia, up to 80%.

Adult flukes in the bile ducts may be associated with cholangitis and calculous or acalculous cholecystitis. Through their large size and the inflammatory and fibrotic response, the infection may cause obstruction leading to cholestatic jaundice, nausea, pruritus, abdominal pain and tenderness, hepatomegaly and fatty food intolerance.[48,56,57] Ultrasonography may reveal impaired contraction, debris, calculi and thickening of the gallbladder, dilation of the bile ducts and, in some cases, the flukes themselves.[58] In severe cases, ascites with blood and severe anaemia may ensue. Since these moderate signs and symptoms do not differ from cholangitis and cholecystitis from other causes, the infection often goes unnoticed until worms are observed at surgery or histopathology.

Diagnosis and investigations

Fascioliasis has been diagnosed by observation of eggs during faecal examination, by parasite-specific antibody detection in a variety of immunodiagnostic assays, by radiological methods and by laparotomy. Dietary history is helpful for differential diagnosis and in investigating outbreaks.

Examination of faeces for eggs is of limited use since eggs are not excreted during the invasive stage of infection, when many patients present with severe symptoms.[47,48,52,53,56] Often eggs are undetectable during the chronic phase, but it is unclear whether the techniques used are insensitive for very low egg outputs in light infections (< 100 eggs per gram) or if eggs are not being produced. If eggs are present, sensitivity of stool examination can be increased by using an optimum technique (Weller–Dammin's modification and the AMS III technique) and examining many fields for eggs and several faecal samples.[48] Differentiation of eggs from *F. hepatica*, *F. gigantica*, echinostomes and *Fasciolopsis* is difficult (see Figures 81.3b, 81.4b and 81.5b,d). Eggs can also be found in duodenal contents, bile and histological sections.

A further problem with faecal examination is that eggs may be passed after eating liver from infected animals. This does not indicate infection; thus positive cases should be reconfirmed if liver has been eaten recently.[1]

Immunodiagnostic tests using every available technique have been reported in the literature, from skin tests to antibody and antigen detection assays targeting somatic and excretory/secretory antigens of adult worms.[48,59–61] Most claim excellent sensitivity (>90%), and problems with cross-reactivity with other trematode infections are avoided by using purified specific antigens, cystatin-treated plates or specific antibody subclasses.

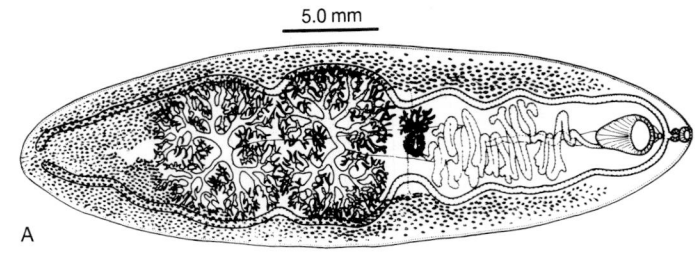

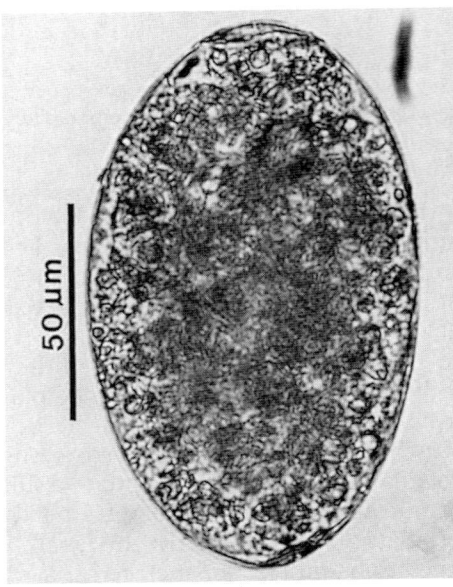

Figure 81.4: (**A**) Adult stage worm of *Fasciolopsis buski*. (Drawn by Sasithorn Kaewkes.) (**B**) Egg of *F. buski*. (Photograph by Sasithorn Kaewkes.)

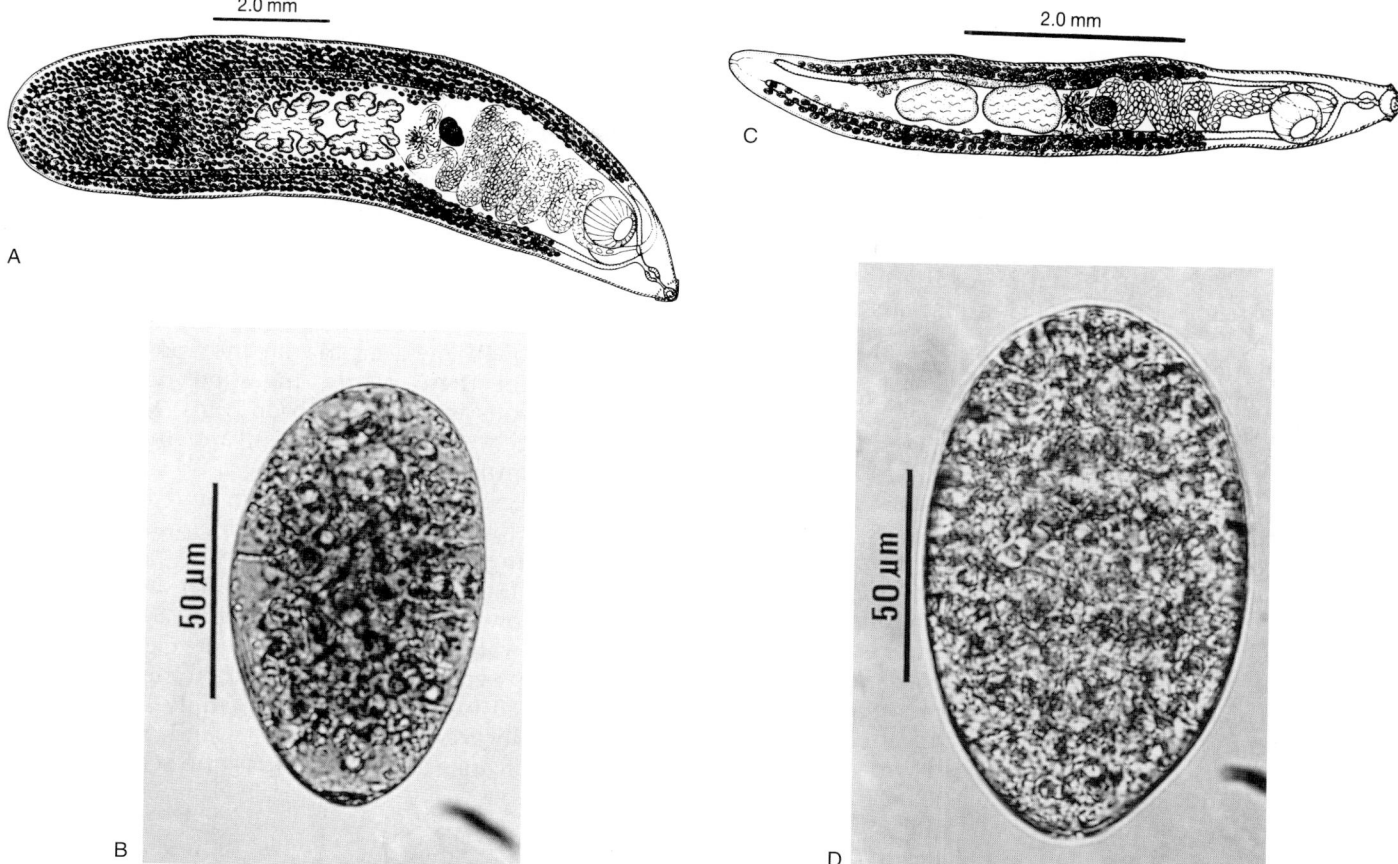

Figure 81.5: (**A**) Adult stage worm of *Echinostoma ilocanum*. (Drawn by Sasithorn Kaewkes.) (**B**) Egg of *E. ilocanum*. (Photograph by Sasithorn Kaewkes.) (**C**) Adult stage worm of *E. malayanum*. (Drawn by Sasithorn Kaewkes.) (**D**) Egg of *E. malayanum*. (Photograph by Sasithorn Kaewkes.)

The advantage of immunodiagnosis over parasitological techniques is that they can detect early, prepatent infections as well as chronic stages with little or no egg output. In contrast to other infections, antibodies drop rapidly after successful treatment, so the assays tend to detect only active infection and can be used to assess treatment efficacy.

Biochemical tests can also support diagnosis. Acute-phase proteins, serum bile acids and some liver enzymes, notably alkaline phosphotase, may be elevated.[62] Eosinophilia is common.

Clinical diagnosis is often difficult because presentations are not markedly different from hepatobiliary disease of other origin(s).[48,53,57] Clinicians may not think about fascioliasis where human infections are uncommon. In temperate climates, outbreaks are almost invariably associated with eating wild watercress. The finding of multiple, related cases with similar diet histories and high-risk occupation (e.g. sheep farmers) may provide supporting evidence. In tropical areas where people consume water plants daily, this may be of limited use.

Laparotomy and radiological imaging by ultrasonography, endoscopic retrograde cholangiopancreatography and percutaneous cholangiography may be useful.[57,58,63] These allow visualization of the lesions of acute and chronic fascioliasis and sometimes eggs (by laparotomy) or worms in the hepatobiliary system.

Management

The treatment of fascioliasis remains highly problematic, in contrast to other trematode infections, requiring high or multiple doses of drugs with significant side effects.[57,58] Praziquantel is not effective against fascioliasis even at high doses. Efficacy is often variable and difficult to assess. These problems result from differing sensitivities of the adult and migrating worms, the size and thick tegument of *Fasciola*, impaired hepatic function and varying clinical presentations.

Triclabendazole at a dose of 10 or 20 mg/kg has been shown to be effective against *Fasciola* infection and without serious side effects, although two treatments are often required.[58,64,65] Although treatment is usually recommended after overnight fasting, absorption may be enhanced by taking the drug with meals.[65]

Previously, the drug bithionol was most often used against fascioliasis at a dose of 30–50 mg/kg body weight per day in three divided doses on alternate days for a duration of 10–15 days.[66] Success against acute infection has been reported for dehydroementine at a dose of 1 mg/kg daily for 10 days given intramuscularly or subcutaneously.[48,52] Moderate to severe side effects have been observed; both drugs and multiple courses are often required.

Nitazoxanide has been found to be effective in some clinical trials, with one study reporting 97% of patients free of *Fasciola* eggs in stool samples after 30 days of treatment. However, further studies are needed.[67]

Depending on the presentation of the patient, other drugs given before the fasciolicide may assist recovery. Prednisolone (5–10 mg/day) may alleviate toxaemia, while antibiotics are often used to treat acute cholangitis due to secondary bacterial infection. Chloroquine was previously used because it rapidly relieves symptoms of acute disease but does not kill the flukes.[48,52]

Prevention and control

Ultimate control of *Fasciola* must focus on strategic treatment or immunization of livestock and other herbivorous animals that maintain the life cycle.[47,48] Advances in the development of veterinary vaccines are very encouraging.[49] Widespread livestock immunization is being considered by some countries to reduce human infection and economic loss to the parasite. Control of the snail vectors using molluscicides is not considered practical in most situations. Health education to discourage human consumption of raw wild watercress and other edible water plants may be effective in areas where the disease is prevalent. Strict controls on commercial production of water plants, as has been instituted in some Western countries, would help to prevent the expansion of endemic areas in developing countries. Increased awareness by clinicians of the problem and its diagnostic difficulties, plus data from community-based studies assessing seroprevalence, will help quantify the extent to which fascioliasis affects human health.

Intestinal flukes

Fasciolopsiasis

Fasciolopsiasis is caused by the giant intestinal fluke, *Fasciolopsis buski*.[1] It is in the same family as *Fasciola*, and its life cycle and morphology are similar (Figure 81.4). However, *Fasciolopsis* infection is largely confined to Asian countries, namely southern China, India, Bangladesh, Thailand, Malaysia, Borneo, Sumatra and Myanmar, and may reach high prevalences within endemic areas. The parasite attaches to the intestinal wall of man and pig. Light infections are less pathogenic than those of *Fasciola* and more easily diagnosed and treated. Heavy infections can be severe.

History and seminal discoveries

The life cycle was first described by Nakagawa (1921) and Barlow (1925).[1] Detailed studies were done in Thailand by Sadun and Maiphoom[68] and Manning et al.[69] Jaroonvesama et al.[70] identified many important factors which determine fasciolopsiasis endemicity.

Life cycle

In contrast to *Fasciola*, the final host range of *F. buski* is limited and many mammals are refractory.[1,71] Humans and pigs become infected through the consumption of viable metacercaria attached to the seed pods of water plants. These include the water caltrops, water hyacinth, water chestnut, water bamboo, lotus roots and wild rice shoots. Although metacercaria are not present on the edible seed of these plants, ingestion occurs during removal of pods with the teeth and lips. Metacercariae also float freely on pond surfaces, and infection may occur from drinking water.[72]

F. buski excysts in the duodenum and the escaping larvae attach to the duodenal and jejunal wall. The larvae become mature adults in 3 months and produce large numbers (an estimated 10 000–25 000 per day per worm) of large, yellow, operculated eggs (Figure 81.4). If these eggs reach water sources, further development and embryonation occur over 3–7 weeks, then miracidia hatch and enter snail intermediate hosts (family Planorbidae). After multiplication as sporocysts and rediae, free-swimming cercariae attach and encyst on seed pods.

Epidemiology

In Thailand, infection was largely confined to low-lying areas in the central region(s) with heavy rainfall and extensive flooding, which leads to faecal contamination of the water.[68–71] Elsewhere the use of pig or human faeces for fertilization is associated with endemicity.[72] The highest prevalence occurs in areas with cultivation or year-round availability of water caltrops and other aquatic vegetation and where people enjoy eating the nuts raw. Chinese investigators have emphasized the importance of contaminated drinking water as a source of infection.[72]

Community-based prevalences generally reach 20%, with a typical peak in children over 5 years of age and little difference between sexes.[68–70,73,74] Children are often more frequently and heavily infected than adults since they enjoy gathering and eating water plants during play.[73–75]

There is little recent information on the existing prevalence of this infection in the published literature, but its absence in national surveys suggests it may be eradicated from most areas.

Pathogenesis and pathology

Eosinophils accumulate at the site of parasite attachment on the jejunal or duodenal wall, where mechanical injury and inflammation lead to ulcer formation.[1,56,71] These ulcers sometimes bleed due to capillary damage or become abscesses. Mild infection in healthy people is associated with lower haematocrit and serum levels of vitamin B_{12}, but no apparent change in other nutrients.[70,76] This may result from parasite sequestering of vitamin B_{12} or its impaired absorption from the damaged intestinal mucosa.

Although a few parasites cause little damage, the presence of many (hundreds to thousands) is associated with severe pathology and sometimes acute intestinal obstruction. Extensive intestinal ulceration may interfere with digestion, and cause malabsorption, leading to severe malnutrition and wasting. Oedema also occurs in severe cases; it may result from toxic parasite metabolites, allergic reactions or from hypoalbuminaemia secondary to electrolyte and protein imbalance from chronic malabsorption.

Clinical features

Symptoms are generally absent or mild, and may include diarrhoea, hunger pains, flatulence, poor appetite, mild abdominal colic, vomiting, eosinophilia and fever.[1,56,68,71] The abdominal pain may mimic that of peptic or duodenal ulcer. Late, severe cases present with ascites or oedema of the face, abdomen and legs, anaemia, anorexia, weakness and vomiting and patients may pass stools containing large amounts of undigested material. Deaths have been reported.

Diagnosis and investigations

Diagnosis by faecal examination is not difficult, given the large quantity and large size of the eggs. Stoll's dilution, formalin ether concentration, direct smears and Kato techniques have been used successfully. Differentiation from *Fasciola* eggs is difficult (Figures 81.3b and 81.4b), so that a dietary and clinical history should also be considered.

Management

In the past, hexylresorcinol crystoids, tetrachloroethylene and dichlorophen were used for treatment of fasciolopsis with varying effectiveness.[71,75] Praziquantel is now the treatment of choice, with high efficacy at a dose of 15 mg/kg body weight.[71-75] In heavily infected cases there may be some danger of exacerbating obstruction or acute toxaemia with treatment, such that conservative treatment is advised.

Prevention and control

In Indonesia, community-based praziquantel treatment has been used to control infection.[73,74] However, migration and rapid reinfection after treatment (prevalence approached pretreatment levels within 12 months) confounded efforts to control infection by chemotherapy alone.

Weng et al.[72] advocate the use of fermented, instead of fresh, silage for feeding pigs in endemic areas since metacercariae are sensitive to both heat and salt. Drying the plants may also be effective. Sterilizing or prohibiting the use of human and pig faeces for fertilizer and improved sanitation would help interrupt the life cycle. Refraining from using the mouth to peel vegetables, then boiling for a few seconds, or careful washing after peeling them with hands or knife would reduce human infection. Filtering drinking water may prevent some infection. Health education should help people recognize the problem as well as indicate acceptable ways to avoid infection, since most infections are mild.

Successful control efforts in one Chinese county reduced the prevalence from 76% in 1951 to 24% in 1976.[72]

Echinostomiasis

Sixteen species of echinostomes have been recorded in man, and the most common appear to be *E. ilocanum*, *E. revolutum*, *E. malayanum*, *E. echinatum* and *E. hortense* (Figure 81.5).[1,9,77-80] Although they are considered of minor medical importance, infections with these parasites reach high prevalences in endemic areas. The literature on human infections is limited and has been reviewed.[9,77,79]

Life cycle

These parasites have a highly variable and wide host range. Humans become infected with echinostomes through the consumption of raw or incompletely cooked freshwater snails, clams, fish and tadpoles harbouring metacercaria. The parasite lives in the intestine of the definitive host, and eggs are excreted in faeces. Snails are the first intermediate host, then after a brief free-swimming stage cercariae encyst within a second intermediate host which may be another mollusc, fish or amphibian larva. Aquatic birds are the most important final host of most species.

Epidemiology

Most human infections occur in Asia in areas where raw or incompletely cooked molluscs and fish are eaten. Infection is common in Korea, Indonesia, the Philippines, Malaysia, Taiwan and Thailand.[1,77-83] Reported prevalences in endemic communities generally range from 1% to 50%.[9,80,82] Infections are most prevalent in poor rural areas and may be clustered in families who prefer raw foods.[9,75]

Diagnosis

The large, unembryonated, operculated eggs of echinostomes can be observed in faeces and are difficult to differentiate from those of *Fasciola* and *Fasciolopsis* (Figures 81.3b, 81.4b and 81.5b,d). Adult worms can be recovered from faeces following treatment.[78,83] This allows for positive differentiation based on morphology, of which the predominant feature is the collar of spines around the oral sucker[1,77,78] (Figure 81.5a,c). It should be noted that the morphology may be altered by the drug.[78,81]

Pathogenesis, pathology and clinical features

Like *F. buski*, the major pathological lesions of echinostomes are associated with parasite attachment deep between the villi of the jejunal wall.[56,77,79,80] There may be inflammation and ulceration of the mucosa where the parasites locate. However, echinostomes are not highly pathogenic to humans and there are only a few reports of clinical aspects of this infection. While light burdens are asymptomatic, heavy infections may cause diarrhoea, eosinophilia, abdominal discomfort and anorexia. These symptoms apparently do not develop into the life-threatening presentations that are described (albeit rarely) in fasciolopsis infection.

Management, prevention and control

Infections are relatively easily cured with mebendazole, albendazole, praziquantel, bithionol, hexylresorcinol crystoids and niclosamide.[79,80] Treatment with praziquantel at 15 mg/kg is recommended in areas where other trematodes are present, due to its broad efficacy, safety and ease of use.[77–79,82,83] In these areas, drug application may be provided to facilitate control of echinostomiasis together with other trematode infections.

Prevention can be supplemented by health education to discourage the consumption of raw or incompletely cooked fish and molluscs, as for other fish-borne infections. However, programmes to control echinostomiasis have had limited success compared to other helminthiases owing to several factors. Among these are the broad specificity for the second intermediate host and the existence of reservoir final hosts.[9] Also, demanding too many dietary changes at one time from a population may jeopardize the successful control of the medically most important parasites. This should be kept in mind when designing health promotion strategies.

Heterophyiasis

There are a large number of small or minute intestinal flukes, measuring less than 2.5 mm in length and just visible to the eye, which parasitize man, birds and other mammals[1,78] (Figure 81.6). These include members of the families Heterophyidae, Plagiorchiidae, Lecithodendridae and Microphallidae. The examination of faeces passed after treatment with praziquantel or bithionol has shown that these parasites, previously considered 'rare', may be common and very numerous in people who live in areas where raw aquatic foods and/or insect larvae are eaten.[2,3,26,84–86] Species of *Heterophyes*, *Haplorchis*, *Metagonimus* and *Carneophallus* may cause disease in man.[1,56,84] Because of their similarity these parasites are covered here under the term 'heterophyids'.

Aetiology and life cycle

Heterophyes heterophyes, *Metagonimus yokogawai*, *Haplorchis*

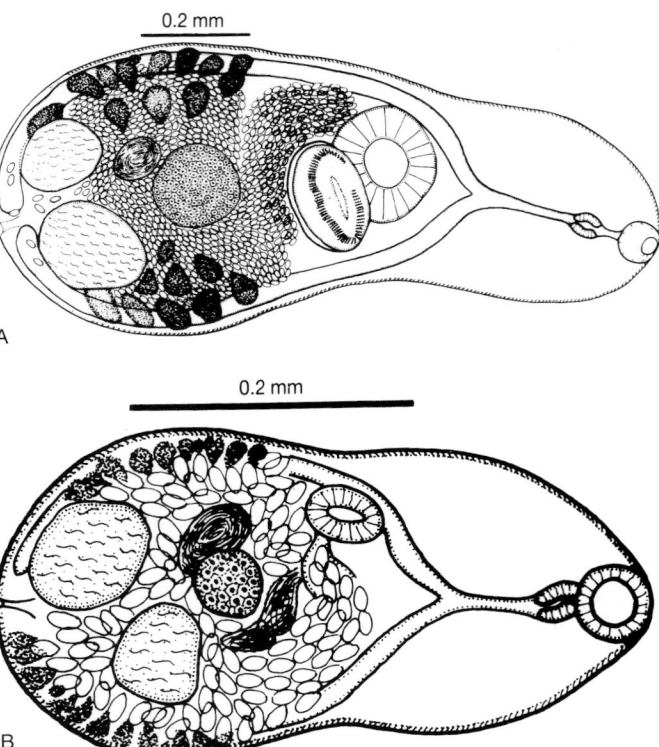

Figure 81.6: (**A**) Adult stage worm of *Heterophyes heterophyes*. (Drawn by Sasithorn Kaewkes.) (**B**) Adult stage worm of *Metagonimus yokogawai*. (Drawn by Sasithorn Kaewkes.)

taichui, *Haplorchis pumilio* and *Stellantchasmus falcatus* are a few of the many heterophyids known to infect man.[1,78,84] The first two species are thought to be the most important medically.

Adult heterophyids live deeply embedded in the intestinal mucosa of mammals and birds where they produce fully embryonated eggs which are excreted in faeces. Upon ingestion by a freshwater snail (*Melania*, *Semisulcospira* and others), the larvae escape, undergo multiplication, then exit as cercariae. The cercariae penetrate and encyst within many species of fresh and brackish water fish or shrimps.[78] Humans become infected while eating fish or shrimps harbouring viable metacercariae, which become mature adults within 5–10 days. An average of 10 000 metacercariae of *Metagonimus yokogawai* are found in the sweetfish (*Plecoglossus altivelis*) during the 'eating season' in Korea.[5]

Epidemiology

Heterophyids are mainly found in Asia (Japan, Korea, Laos, Thailand, Taiwan, Philippines, China), Hawaii, Siberia, Turkey and the Balkans.[1–3,26,78,84–86] The use of expulsion chemotherapy to recover adult worms has revealed the enormous number and remarkable variety of flukes that can be harboured by a person. Food habits and access to rich aquatic fauna are the important determinants of human infection.

Metagonimus yokogawai infects 1.2% of the Korean population, and is common (5–20% prevalence) in riverside communities where raw sweetfish is enjoyed.[5] One study found infection rates to be as high as 29.7%, with a striking difference between males (46.6%) and females (16.3%).[85] Over 100 000 adults were found in a single person. Large numbers of another species, *Heterophyes nocens*, which utilizes brackish water intermediate hosts, was found in 42% of residents from a Korean island and in 75% in some coastal areas.[86]

Pathogenesis, pathology and clinical symptoms

These are similar for different species. Most infections are asymptomatic or accompanied by mild intestinal discomfort, which may include mucous diarrhoea, colicky pains, intermittent neurasthenia and lethargy.[1,56,84] These probably result from mild inflammation with mainly eosinophils, superficial necrosis, excessive mucus secretion and bleeding at the site of attachment. Movement of the parasite's spiny surface may contribute to ulceration, and hyperplasia in the mesenteric lymph nodes may also cause abdominal pain.

Symptoms are most frequent in heavy infections, but they subside spontaneously after approximately 1 month, although the flukes remain.[5] Upon further infection, symptoms may recur, giving rise to occasional episodes of diarrhoea in endemic areas.

One special aspect of heterophyid pathogenesis is the involvement of eggs. These embed deeply in the intestinal wall, eliciting eosinophil and neutrophil infiltration. The eggs (and sometimes adult worms) may then enter nearby lymphatics or blood vessels and be transported to other sites—notably the heart, spinal cord or brain, lungs, liver and spleen.[56,84,87] Eggs become trapped and elicit granulomatous lesions and fibrosis. Signs of heterophyid myocarditis may include cardiac enlargement, cough, dyspnoea, cyanosis, fatigue, oedema and ascites, palpitation, loss of reflexes and abnormal heart sounds. Eggs or worms in the spinal cord or brain may cause neurological disease, transverse myelitis and loss of sensory and motor function.

Diagnosis

Diagnosis is usually based on the recovery of eggs in faeces, but there are many problems. The daily egg output is low (35–45) and light infections (< 100 worms) are easily missed. Extraintestinal cases of heterophyiasis may be discovered at surgery or autopsy, and then only after careful searching. Distinction between species of heterophyids and *Clonorchis* and *Opisthorchis* by egg is exceedingly difficult. However, recent publications have helped establish criteria for differentiation.[3,88,89] The recovery of adult worms from post-treatment stools allows a definitive diagnosis, but this procedure is extremely tedious due to their minute size.[2,3]

Antibodies against heterophyids cross-react with those against *O. viverrini* in ELISA.[90] However, antibody recognition patterns visualized by immunoblotting may differ and help to distinguish liver fluke from heterophyid infections.

Management

Niclosamide, bithionol and tetrachloroethylene were previously used, but praziquantel is now the drug of choice. A single dose of 10–20 mg/kg is highly effective.[84-86]

Prevention and control

Like other fish-borne trematodes, treatment with praziquantel, combined with health education to encourage cooking of fish and other aquatic foods, is important. More studies are required on the frequency and spectrum of clinical consequences in order to assess the amount of resources that should be allocated for control. Although the ability of the parasites to cause fatal disease is clear, the actual frequency of this has recently received very little attention.

Lung flukes
Paragonimiasis

These flukes are distributed widely, and infect an estimated 10 million people in China alone and about 20 million worldwide.[4,91-100] Infection can cause severe respiratory or cerebral disease, depending on intensity, duration and site where the parasites become lodged.

Aetiology

Although there are many lung flukes of mammals, only *Paragonimus* species infect man. Their taxonomy is unclear, but it is generally agreed that seven or eight species are of major medical importance in fairly distinct geographic areas[91,100] (Figure 81.7). These include *P. westermani*, *P. miyazakii*, *P. skrjabini* and *P. heterotremus* in Asia, *P. africanus* and *P. uterobilateralis* in Africa and *P. mexicanus* (and *P. ecuadoriensis*) in Latin and South America. Countries with significant numbers of cases include China, Taiwan, Thailand, Japan, Korea, Nigeria, Cameroon, Peru, Guatemala and Ecuador.[91-104]

Life cycle

Paragonimus lives in the lungs of some mammals: mainly wild and domestic cats, but also dogs, monkeys and humans. Parasite eggs are coughed up from the lungs and either expectorated in the sputum, or swallowed and excreted in the faeces. When these eggs reach water, further development occurs until miracidia hatch; they then penetrate a snail host (mainly species of Thiaridae and Pleuroceridae). Multiplication and development occur in the snail until cercariae are produced. These may enter

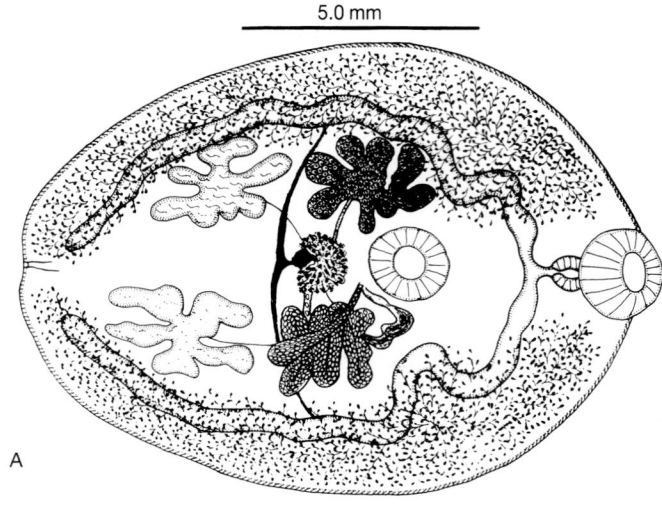

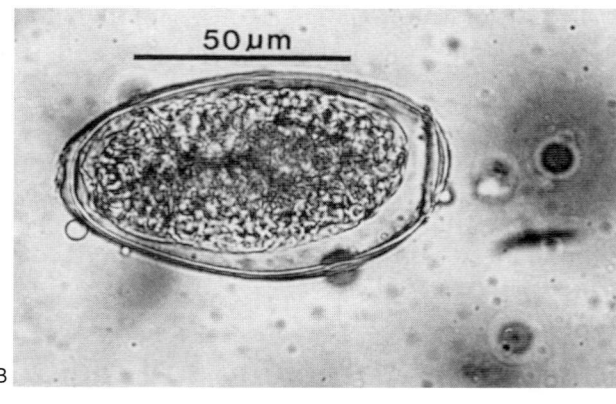

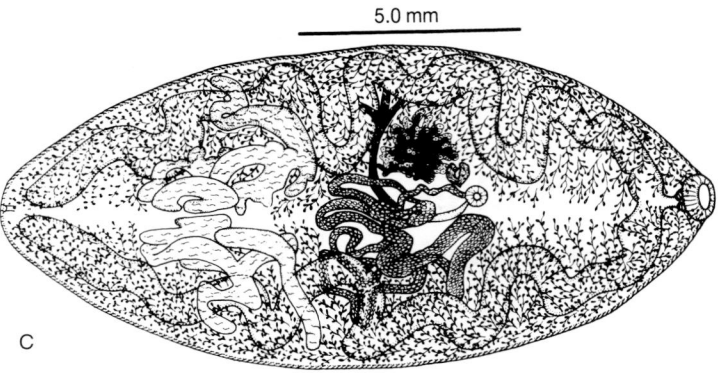

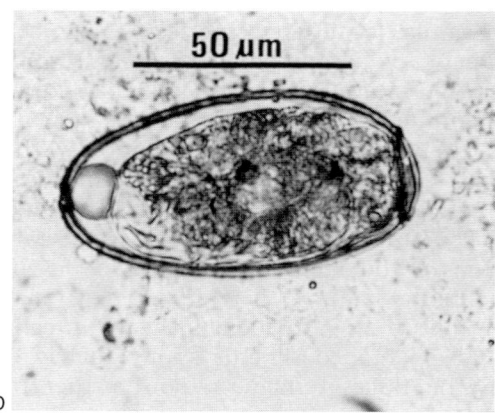

Figure 81.7: (**A**) Adult stage worm of *Paragonimus westermani*. (Drawn by Sasithorn Kaewkes.) (**B**) Egg of *P. westermani*. (Photograph by Sasithorn Kaewkes.) (**C**) Adult stage worm of *P. heterotremus*. (Drawn by Sasithorn Kaewkes.) (**D**) Egg of *P. heterotremus*. (Photograph by Sasithorn Kaewkes.)

the second intermediate host, namely potamid or other crabs, crayfish and one species of shrimp, while free-swimming or during consumption of the snail by the crustacean. The cercariae encyst in the gills, liver and muscle tissue of the crab and require about 2 months to become infective metacercariae. When the crabs are eaten by a final mammalian host, the cysts excyst in the small intestine, penetrate the intestinal wall, travel from the peritoneum to the subperitoneal tissue, passing through the diaphragm to the lungs—where they mature in 2 months. Adult worms may live for 20 years. Due to aberrant migration, larvae sometimes become lodged in ectopic sites, e.g. brain, abdomen, groin, skin or heart.

In some mammals which serve as paratenic hosts, the larvae exit the small intestine and lodge without further development in muscle tissue.[91–95] When a final mammalian host consumes the paratenic host, the larvae survive passage through the stomach and escape through the intestinal wall. Migration to the lungs then results in maturation and egg excretion.

Epidemiology

Human infection most often results from consumption of raw or incompletely cooked pickled, wine- or brine-soaked crabs, crayfish and shrimps harbouring metacercariae.[91–96,100] Alternatively, transmission may occur via eating wild boar, pigs, or small animals harbouring pre-adult worms. Metacercariae may also be ingested during preparation of these foods via contamination of hands or utensils. In addition to dietary preferences, raw crab meat and juice are thought to have medicinal properties for enhancing fertility, reducing fever and treating measles.[94] This last practice once caused high levels of infection in Korean children, while Philippine children enjoy eating incompletely roasted crabs.[93]

Although endemic pockets are still being discovered in Korea, the number infected has dropped dramatically in recent years.[94] High prevalences of infection (up to 45%) were observed during a skin test survey in endemic communities in Korea in 1959. Infection levels have also significantly dropped in Japan in the past 50 years. However, changing dietary practices and reluctance to stop eating raw crabs are leading to increased infection levels in some areas.[96,103] The infection is endemic throughout China, although again, vigorous control efforts have successfully reduced prevalences in some areas.[95,97] Surveys in the Philippines found prevalences of 0.5–12% in human communities, while 50–100% of crabs in endemic areas harbour *Paragonimus*.[93] Significant prevalences have been reported recently from parts of Nigeria (16.8%) and Cameroon (2.1–28.6%).[98] Although eating raw food is not a widespread habit in India, 39 cases of *Paragonimus* were reported from Manipur State.[99]

Pathogenesis and pathology

The site of pathology of paragonimiasis depends upon the migratory route of the larvae and the tissue in which they lodge.[1,56,91,92,105] Inflammatory responses to the adult worms, immature worms and eggs are similar, regardless of location. Resulting lesions are granulomatous, beginning with leucocyte (mainly eosinophil) infiltration and finally resulting in thick cysts or abscesses and ultimately calcification. The parasites live within these fibrotic, greyish-white capsules (1.5–5 cm in diameter) in pairs or triplets, surrounded by thick, blood-streaked fluid and numerous eggs. Later, the capsules may be empty or fluid filled. Eggs trapped in the tissue may also provoke granulomas at the periphery of the necrotic area. The capsules occur most frequently in the upper right quadrant of the lungs and, in the fewer cases of cerebral involvement, the posterior portion of the brain is usually affected.

In both human and experimental infections there appears to be a subsidence of inflammation in later periods. This may be due to modulation of the immune response.

Clinical features

Pulmonary infection is accompanied by a chronic productive cough, with brownish purulent sputum containing streaks of blood and parasite eggs in *P. westermani*, *P. heterotremus* and African and American paragonimiasis. Chest pain and night sweats may also occur. The signs mimic bronchiectasis, bronchopneumonia, or tuberculosis not responding to antibiotics. Eosinophilia of 20–25% is common.

Pleural effusion and pneumothorax with marked eosinophilia in the exudate and peripheral blood occur particularly frequently in *P. miyazakii* infections in Japan. Although there may be a persistent cough, neither brownish sputum nor eggs are expelled in *P. skrjabini* and *P. miyazakii* infections.

Cerebral paragonimus may cause eosinophilic meningitis, which is characterized by headache, convulsions of the focal Jacksonian type, hemiplegia and visual impairment with insidious onset.[56,92,106] Most cases involve males under 10 years of age. Flukes in the spinal cord may cause spastic paraplegia. Pulmonary symptoms (cough with brownish sputum) usually accompany cerebral disease. Cutaneous paragonimiasis occurs when the parasites lodge in subcutaneous tissue, forming painless, mobile swellings which may contain immature worms. The patient may also exhibit mild pulmonary abnormalities. This manifestation occurs frequently in *P. skrjabini* infection, which does not localize to the lungs.

Sometimes the flukes migrate through the peritoneal cavity eliciting the formation of multiple nodules (abdominal paragonimiasis) which often appear similar to malignant tumours.

Mortality has been reported, either due to parasites and resulting abscesses in the heart or to fulminating infection in the abdominal cavity.

Diagnosis and investigations

The clinical signs are fairly pathognomonic, particularly when diet history and residence in an endemic area are known, but misdiagnosis is commonly due to unfamiliarity with the disease.[6,99] Tests to rule out tuberculosis, skin tests and sputum smear and culture are helpful in differentiation. Eggs of *Paragonimus* may be found in the faeces, sputum, gastric washings or tissue. Blood in the sputum contains sufficient eggs to be visualized by direct smear. Sputum without blood should be collected over 24 hours, centrifuged and the sediment dissolved in 3% sodium hydroxide for examination for eggs.[93] Eggs may not be present in the sputum of infected children or elderly people, but faecal examination using a concentration technique may reveal eggs. Adult worms might be expectorated after treatment or found in skin lesions.

Skin and immunodiagnostic tests using parasite antigens are highly sensitive and useful for surveys and in diagnosing the infection(s).[92,99,107] Complement fixation tests and ELISA detect early as well as chronic infection and titres decline rapidly (becoming negative in 1–2 months) after cure. These tests therefore assist in assessing cure following treatment.

Radiological investigations, particularly plain radiography and computed tomography, are useful in diagnosing pulmonary disease. Lesions typically show a nodular or ring shadow, patchy infiltration and cavities.[99,105] In eosinophilic meningitis, computed tomography reveals a 'soap bubble appearance' of dilated ventricles and multiple dense calcification and calcified cystic lesions.[106]

Management

Long regimens of bithionol, totalling 10–15 doses of 30 mg/kg body weight on alternate days, and niclofan (2 mg/kg, single dose) are effective and have been used widely. Praziquantel has been the drug of choice, with a course of 3 × 25 mg/kg body weight for 3 days being nearly 100% effective against all species.[95–98,108,109] Side effects are usually mild and pulmonary abnormalities decrease within 4 months. Caution is required in the treatment of cerebral disease; one such patient became comatose for 48 hours, while others showed no severe effects.[44,109] Recent studies have also shown triclabendazole to be effective.[100,110] Doses ranging from 5 mg/kg body weight once daily for 3 days, 10 mg/kg twice on one day, to 10 mg/kg in a single dose have been found to be better tolerated and as effective as praziquantel in eliminating infection of *Paragonimus mexicanus*.[110]

Prevention and control

In addition to drug treatment, health education to discourage the consumption of raw crustaceans is recommended, particularly addressing the special danger of infection to children. Increased recognition of the problem by health workers and the population may facilitate earlier treatment and dietary change. Folk beliefs regarding medicinal properties of raw crabs, plus the inability of rapid dry cooking or soaking in brine, soy sauce or alcohol to kill the parasites, may require special attention in health promotion messages.

REFERENCES

1 Beaver P C, Jung R C & Cupp E W. *Clinical Parasitology*, 9th edn. Philadelphia: Lea & Febiger, 1984: 406–414.

2 Radomyos P, Bunnag D & Harinasuta T. Worms recovered in stools following praziquantel treatment. *Drug Res* 1984; 34:1215–1217.

3 Kaewkes S. The epidemiology and taxonomy of minute intestinal flukes in Northeast Thailand. PhD thesis, University of Queensland, 1993.

4 World Health Organization. Control of food-borne trematode infections. *WHO Tech Rev Serv*, 1995.

5 Cho S Y, Kang S Y & Lee J B. Metagonimiasis in Korea. *Drug Res* 1984; 34:1211–1213.

6 Johnson J R, Boeck R, Paulson D & Godes J. Paragonimiasis in Hmong refuges—Minnesota. In Hillyer G V and Hopla C E (section eds) *Section C: Parasitic Zoonoses*, vol. III. Boca Raton, FL: CRC Press, 1982: 165–166.

7 Cross J H. Changing patterns of some trematode infections in Asia. *Drug Res* 1984; 34:1224–1126.

8 Ooi H K, Chen C I, Lin S C, Tung K C, Wang J S & Kamiya M. Metacercariae in fishes of Sun Moon lake which is an endemic area for Clonorchis sinensis in Taiwan. *Southeast Asian J Trop Med Public Health* 1997; 28(Suppl 1): 222–223.

9 Graczyk T K & Fried B. Echinostomiasis: a common but forgotten food-borne disease. *Am J Trop Med Hyg* 1998, 58:501–504.

10 Xu L, Jiang Z, Yu S, Xu S et al. [Characteristics and recent trends in endemicity of human parasitic diseases in China]. *Chung Kuo Chi Sheng Chung Hsueh Yu Chi Sheng Chung Ping Tsa Chih* 1995; 13:214–217 (in Chinese).

11 Mas-Coma M S, Esteban J G & Bargues M D. Epidemiology of human fascioliasis: a review and proposed classification. *Bull WHO* 1999; 77:340–346.

12 Jongsuksuntigul P & Imsomboon T. The impact of a decade long opisthorchiasis control program in northeastern Thailand. *Southeast Asian J Trop Med Public Health* 1997; 28:551–557.

13 Seo B S. Socio-economic and cultural aspects of human trematode infections in Korea. *Drug Res* 1984; 34:1116–1118.

14 Eckert J. Workshop summary: food safety: meat- and fish-borne zoonoses. *Vet Parasitol* 1996; 64:143–147.

15 Rim H J. The current pathobiology and chemotherapy of clonorchiasis. *Korean J Parasitol Suppl* 1986; 24:1–141.

16 Kim Y I. Liver carcinoma and liver fluke infection. *Drug Res* 1984; 34:1121–1126.

17 Haswell-Elkins M R, Satarug S & Elkins D B. Liver fluke infection and cholangiocarcinoma in Northeast Thailand. *J Gastroenterol Hepatol* 1992; 7:538–548.

18 Vatanasapt V, Uttaravichien T, Mairiang E, Pairojkul C, Chartbanchachai V, Haswell-Elkins M R. Northeast Thailand: a region with a high incidence of cholangiocarcinoma. *Lancet* 1990; 1:116–117.

19 Hoeppli R. Histological changes in the liver of sixty-six Chinese infected with *Clonorchis sinensis*. *Chin Med J* 1933; 47:1125–1141.

20 Viranuvatti V & Mettiyawongse S. Observation of two cases of opisthorchiasis in Thailand. *Ann Trop Med Parasitol* 1953; 47:291–293.

21 Hou P C. The relationship between primary carcinoma of the liver and infestation with *Clonorchis sinensis*. *J Pathol Bact* 1956; 72:239–246.

22 Thamavit W, Bhamarapravati N, Sahaphong S, Vajrasthira S & Angsubhakorn S. Effects of dimethylnitrosamine on induction of cholangiocarcinoma in *Opisthorchis viverrini* infected Syrian golden hamsters. *Cancer Res* 1978; 38:4634–4639.

23 Working Group of the International Agency for Research on Cancer. Infection with liver flukes. *Monographs on the Evaluation of Carcinogenic Risks to Humans. Volume 61: Some Bacterial and Parasitic Infections.* International Agency for Research on Cancer, 1994, Lyon, France: 121–175.

24 Sithithaworn P, Pipitgool V, Srisawangwong T, Elkins D B & Haswell-Elkins M R. Seasonal variation of *Opisthorchis viverrini* infection in cyprinoid fish in north-east Thailand: implications for parasite control and food safety. *Bull World Health Organ* 1997; 75:125–131.

25 Bronshtein A M. [Communication 2. Morbidity of opisthorchiasis and diphyllobothriasis in the indigenous population of the Kyshik village in the Khanty-Mansiisk Autonomic region]. *Med Parazit* (Mosk) 1986; 3:44–48 (in Russian, cited in *Helminthol Abstr*).

26 Radomyos B, Wongsaroj T, Wilairatana P et al. Opisthorchiasis and intestinal fluke infections in northern Thailand. *Southeast Asian J Trop Med Public Health* 1998; 29:123–127.

27 Upatham E S, Viyanant V, Kurathong S et al. Relationship between prevalence and intensity of *Opisthorchis viverrini* infection, and clinical symptoms and signs in a rural community in northeast Thailand. *Bull WHO* 1984; 62:451–461.

28 Elkins D B, Mairiang E, Sithithaworn P et al. Cross-sectional patterns of hepatobiliary abnormalities and possible precursor conditions of cholangiocarcinoma associated with Opisthorchis viverrini infection in humans. *Am J Trop Med Hyg* 1996; 55:295–301.

29 Pungpak S, Viravan C, Radomyos B et al. Opisthorchis viverrini infection in Thailand: studies on the morbidity of the infection and resolution following praziquantel treatment. *Am J Trop Med Hyg* 1997; 56:311–314.

30 Pungpak S, Riganti M, Bunnag D & Harinasuta T. Clinical features in severe opisthorchiasis viverrini. *Southeast Asian Trop Med Public Health* 1985; 16:405–409.

31 Haswell-Elkins M R, Mairiang E, Mairiang P et al. Cross-sectional study of *Opisthorchis viverrini* infection and cholangiocarcinoma in communities within a high risk area in Northeast Thailand. *Int J Cancer* 1994; 58:1–5.

32 Shin H R, Lee C U, Park H J et al. Hepatitis B and C virus, *Clonorchis sinensis* for the risk of liver cancer: a case–control study in Pusan, Korea. *Int J Epidemiol* 1996; 25:933–940.

33 Pairojkul C, Sithithaworn P, Sripa B et al. Risk groups for opisthorchiasis-associated cholangiocarcinoma indicated by a study of worm burden-related biliary pathology. *Kan Tan Sui* 1991; 22:111–120.

34 Kim Y H. Eosinophilic cholecystitis in association with clonorchis sinensis infestation in the common bile duct. *Clin Radiol* 1999; 54:552–554.

35   Park H, Ko M Y, Paik M K et al. Cytotoxicity of a cysteine proteinase of adult Clonorchis sinensis. *Korean J Parasitol* 1995; 33:211–218.

36   Sripa B & Kaewkes S. Localisation of parasite antigens and inflammatory responses in experimental opisthorchiasis. *Int J Parasitol* 2000; 30:735–740.

37   Satarug S, Lang M A, Yongvanit P et al. Induction of cytochrome P450 2A6 expression in humans by the carcinogenic parasite infection, opisthorchiasis viverrini. *Cancer Epidemiol Biomarkers Prev* 1996; 5:795–800.

38   Satarug S, Haswell-Elkins M R, Sithithaworn P et al. Relationships between the synthesis of N-nitrosodimethylamine and immune responses to chronic infection with the carcinogenic parasite, Opisthorchis viverrini, in men. *Carcinogenesis*, 1998; 19:485–491.

39   Sithithaworn P, Tesana S, Pipitgool V et al. Relationship between faecal egg count and worm burden of *Opisthorchis viverrini* in humans. *Parasitology* 1991; 102:277–281.

40   Hong S T, Lee M, Sung N J et al. Usefulness of IgG4 subclass antibodies for diagnosis of human clonorchiasis. *Korean J Parasitol* 1999; 37:243–248.

41   Yong T S, Yang H J, Park S J et al. Immunodiagnosis of clonorchiasis using a recombinant antigen. *Korean J Parasitol* 1998; 36:183–190.

42   Sirisinha S, Chawengkirttikul R, Haswell-Elkins M R, Elkins D B, Kaewkes S & Sithithaworn P. Evaluation of a monoclonal antibody-based enzyme linked immunosorbent assay for the diagnosis of *Opisthorchis viverrini* infection in an endemic area. *Am J Trop Med Hyg* 1995; 52:521–524.

43   Pungpak S, Radomyos P, Radomyos B E, Schelp F P, Jongsuksuntigul P & Bunnag D. Treatment of *Opisthorchis viverrini* and intestinal fluke infections with praziquantel. *Southeast Asian J Trop Med Public Health* 1998; 29:246–249.

44   Sui F, Shu-hua X & Catto B A. Clinical use of praziquantel in China. *Parasitol Today* 1988; 4:312–315.

45   Khamboonruang C, Keawvichit R, Wongworapat K et al. Application of hazard analysis critical control point (HACCP) as a possible control measure for *Opisthorchis viverrini* infection in cultured carp. *Southeast Asian J Trop Med Public Health* 1997; 28(Suppl 1):65–72.

46   Fan P C. Viability of metacercariae of Clonorchis sinensis in frozen or salted freshwater fish. *Int J Parasitol* 1998; 28:603–605.

47   Boray J C. Fascioliasis. In Hillyer G V & Hopla C E (section eds) *Section C: Parasitic Zoonoses*, Vol III. Boca Raton, FL: CRC Press, 1982: 71–88.

48   Chen M G & Mott K E. Progress in assessment of morbidity due to *Fasciola hepatica* infection: a review of recent literature. *Trop Dis Bull* 1990; 87:R1–R38.

49   Spithill T W, Piedrafita D & Smooker, P M. Immunological approaches for the control of fasciolosis. *Int J Parasitol* 1997; 27:1221–1235.

50   Mas-Coma S, Angles R, Esteban J G et al. The Northern Bolivian Altiplano: a region highly endemic for human fascioliasis. *Trop Med Int Health* 1999; 4:454–467.

51   Rondelaud D, Dreyfuss G, Boutielle B et al. Changes in human fasciolosis in a temperate area: about some observations over a 28-year period in central France. *Parasitol Res* 2000; 86:753–757.

52   Hardman E W, Jones R L H & Davies A H. Fasciliasis: a large outbreak. *BMJ* 1970; 3:502–505.

53   Chen M G. *Fasciola hepatica* infection in China. In Cross J H (ed.) *Emerging Problems in Food-Borne Parasitic Zoonosis: Impact on Agriculture and Public Health.* Thai Watana Panich Press, 1991:356–360.

54   Hassan M M, Farghaly A M, Gaber N S et al. Parasitic causes of hepatomegaly in children. *J Egyptian Soc Parasitol* 1996; 26:177–189.

55   Wolf-Spengler M L & Isseroff H. Fasciliasis: bile duct collagen induced by proline from the worm. *J Parasitol* 1983; 69:290–294.

56   Gutierrez Y. *Diagnostic Parasitology of Parasitic Infections with Clinical Correlations.* Philadelphia: Lea & Febiger, 1990: 359–392.

57   Patrick K M & Isaac-Renton J. Praziquantel failure in treatment of Fasciola hepatica. *Can J Infect Dis* 1992; 3:33–36.

58   Richter J, Freise S, Mull R et al. Fasciliasis: sonographic abnormalities of the biliary tract and evolution after treatment with triclabendazole. *Trop Med Int Health* 1999; 4: 774–781.

59   Shehab A Y, Abou Basha L M, El-Morshedy H N et al. Circulating antibodies and antigens correlate with egg counts in human fascioliasis. *Trop Med Int Health* 1999; 4: 691–694.

60   Ikeda T. Cystatin capture enzyme-linked immunosorbent assay for immunodiagnosis of human paragonimiasis and fascioliasis. *Am J Trop Med Hyg* 1998; 59:286–290.

61   Osman M M, Shehab A Y, Masry S A et al. Evaluation of Fasciola excretory–secretory (E/S) product in diagnosis of acute human fasciolosis by IgM ELISA. *Trop Med Parasitol* 1995; 46:115–118.

62   Osman M M, Ismail Y & Aref T Y. Human fascioliasis: a study on the relation of infection intensity and treatment to hepatobiliary affection. *J Egyptian Soc Parasitol* 1999; 353–363.

63   Uribarren R, Borda F, Munoz M & Riveropuente A. Laparoscopic findings in eight cases of liver fascioliasis. *Endoscopy* 1985; 17:137–138.

64   Apt, W, Aguilera, X, Vega F et al. Treatment of human chronic fascioliasis with triclabendazole: drug efficacy and serologic response. *Am J Trop Med Hyg* 1995; 52:532–535.

65   Lecaillon J B, Godbillon J, Campestrini J et al. Effect of food on the bioavailability of triclabendazole in patients with fascioliasis. *Br J Clin Pharmacol* 1998; 45:601–604.

66   Farag H F, Salem A, Al-Hifni S A & Kandil M. Bithionol (Bitin) treatment in established fascioliasis in Egyptians. *J Trop Med Hyg* 1988; 91:240–245.

67   Kabil S M, Ashry E E & Ashraf N K. An open-label clinical study of nitazoxanide in the treatment of human fascioliasis. *Curr Ther Res* 2000; 61(6):339–345.

68   Sadun E H & Maiphoom C. Studies on the epidemiology of the human intestinal fluke, *Fasciolopsis buski* (Lankester) in central Thailand. *Am J Trop Med Hyg* 1953; 2:1070–1084.

69   Manning G S, Sukhawat K, Viyanant V, Subhakul M & Lertprasert P. *Fasciolopsis buski* in Thailand, with comments on other intestinal parasites. *J Med Assoc Thailand* 1969; 52:905–913.

70   Jaroonvesama N, Charoenlarp K, Areekul S, Aswapokee N & Leelarasmee A. Prevalence of *Fasciolopsis buski* and other parasitic infection in residents of three villages in Sena District, Ayudhaya Province, Thailand. *J Med Assoc Thailand* 1980; 63:493–499.

71   Rim H J. Fasciolopsiasis. In Hillyer G V & Hopla C E (section eds) *Section C: Parasite Zoonoses*, vol. III. Boca Raton, FL: CRC Press, 1982: 89–97.

72   Weng Y L, Zhuang Z L, Jiang H P, Lin G R & Lin J J. [Studies on ecology of *Fasciolopsis buski* and control strategy of fasciolopsiasis]. *Chinese J Parasitol Parasit Dis* 1989; 7:108–111 (in Chinese, cited in *Helminthol Abstr*).

73   Handoyo I, Ismuljowono B, Darwis F & Rudiansyah. Evaluation of post-treatment control of fasciolopsiasis in Sei Papuyu village of Babirik Subdistrict, Hulu Sungai Utara Regency, South Kalimantan Province, Indonesia. *Trop Biomed* 1987; 4:125–127.

74   Handoyo I, Ismuljowono B, Darwis F & Rudiansyah. Further survey of fasciolopsiasis in Babirik Subdistrict, Hulu Sungei Utara Regency, South Kalimantan Province. *Trop Biomed* 1986; 3:119–123.

75 Bunnag D, Radomyos P & Harinasuta T. Field trial on the treatment of fasciolopsiasis with praziquantel. *Southeast Asian J Trop Med Public Health* 1983; 14:216–219.

76 Jaroonvesama N, Charoenlarp K & Areekul S. Intestinal absorption studies in *Fasciolopsis buski* infection. *Southeast Asian J Trop Med Public Health* 1986; 17:582–586.

77 Rim H J. Echinostomiasis. In Hillyer G V & Hopla C E (section eds) *Section C: Parasitic Zoonoses*, vol. III. Boca Raton, FL: CRC Press, 1982: 53–69.

78 Waikagul J. Intestinal fluke infections in Southeast Asia. In Cross J H (ed.) *Emerging Problems in Food-Borne Parasitic Zoonosis: Impact on Agriculture and Public Health*. Thai Watana Panich Press, 1991: 158–162.

79 Huffman J E & Fried B. Echinostoma and echinostomiasis. *Adv Parasitol* 1990; 29:215–269.

80 Carney W P. Echinostomiasis: a snail-borne intestinal trematode zoonosis. In Cross J H (ed.) *Emerging Problems in Food-Borne Parasitic Zoonosis: Impact on Agriculture and Public Health*. Thai Watana Panich Press, 1991: 206–211.

81 Tangtrongchitr A & Monzon R B. Eating habits associated with *Echinostoma malayanum* infections in the Philippines. In Cross J H (ed.) *Emerging Problems in Food-Borne Parasitic Zoonosis: Impact on Agriculture and Public Health*. Thai Watana Panich Press, 1991: 212–216.

82 Phathihutthagon W, Sornmani S, Imphan P & Srithabut P. [Studies on the prevalence and reinfection rate of *Echinostoma* spp in an irrigated area]. *J Parasit Trop Med Assoc Thailand* 1984; 7:12–16 (in Thai).

83 Radomyos P, Bunnag D & Harinasuta T. *Echinostoma ilocanum* (Garrison, 1908) Odhner, 1911, infection in man in Thailand. *Southeast Asian J Trop Med Public Health* 1982; 13:265–269.

84 Velasquez C C. Heterophyidiasis. In Hillyer G V & Hopla C E (section eds) *Section C: Parasitic Zoonoses*, vol. III. Boca Raton, FL: CRC Press, 1982: 99–107.

85 Chai J Y, Han E T, Park Y K, Guk S M, Kim J L & Lee S H. High endemicity of *Metagonimus yokogawai* infection among residents of Samchok-shi, Kangwon-do. *Korean J Parasitol* 2000; 38(1):33–36.

86 Chai J Y, Kim I M, Seo M, Guk S M, Kim J L, Sohn W M & Lee S H. A new endemic focus of *Heterophyes nocens*, *Pygidiopsis summa*, and other intestinal flukes in a coastal area of Muan-gun, Chollanam-do. *Korean J Parasitol* 1997; 35(4):233–238.

87 Africa C, Leon W D E & Garcia E Y. Intestinal heterophyidiasis with cardiac involvement: a contribution to etiology of heart failure. *J Philippine Islands Med Assoc* 1935; 15:358–361.

88 Lee S H, Hwang S W, Chai J Y & Seo B S. Comparative morphology of eggs of heterophyids and *Clonorchis sinensis* causing human infections in Korea. *Korean J Parasitol* 1984; 22:171–180.

89 Ditrich O, Giboda M, Scholz T & Beer S A. Comparative morphology of eggs of the Haplorchiinae (Trematoda: Heterophyidae) and some other medically important heterophyid and opisthorchiid flukes. *Folia Parasitol* 1992; 39:123–132.

90 Ditrich O, Kopacek P, Giboda M, Gutvirth J & Scholz T. Serological differentiation of human small intestinal fluke infections using *Opisthorchis viverrini* and *Haplorchis taichui* antigens. In Cross J H (ed.) *Emerging Problems in Food-Borne Parasitic Zoonosis: Impact on Agriculture and Public Health*. Thai Watana Panich Press, 1991: 174–178.

91 Miyazaki I. Paragonimiasis. In Hillyer G V & Hopla C E (section eds) *Section C: Parasitic Zoonoses*, vol. III. Boca Raton, FL: CRC Press, 1982: 143–164.

92 Yokogawa M. Paragonimiasis. In Hillyer G V & Hopla C E (section eds) *Section C: Parasitic Zoonoses*, vol. III. Boca Raton, FL: CRC Press, 1982: 123–142.

93 Cabrera B D. Paragonimiasis in the Philippines: current status. *Drug Res* 1984; 34:1188–1192.

94 Choi D W. Paragonimus and paragonimiasis in Korea. *Korean J Parasitol* 1990; 28:79–102.

95 Zhi-Biao X. Studies on clinical manifestations, diagnosis and control of paragonimiasis in China. In Cross J H (ed.) *Emerging Problems in Food-Borne Parasitic Zoonosis: Impact on Agriculture and Public Health*. Thai Watana Panich Press, 1991: 345–348.

96 Gyoten J. Changes of living habits related to the infection in human paragonimiasis in Japan, based on the epidemiological data. *Japan J Parasitol* 1994; 43(6):462–470.

97 Lien-Yin H E. Advance in studies of *Paragonimus* and paragonimiasis in China. In *Abstracts Vol. 1 of the XIIIth International Congress for Tropical Medicine and Malaria*, Pattaya, 1992: 58–59.

98 Pozio E. Current status of food-borne parasitic zoonoses in Mediterranean and African regions. In Cross J H (ed.) *Emerging Problems in Food-Borne Parasitic Zoonosis: Impact on Agriculture and Public Health*. Thai Watana Panich Press, 1991: 85–87.

99 Singh T S, Mutum S S & Razaque M A. Pulmonary paragonimiasis: clinical features, diagnosis and treatment of 39 cases in Manipur. *Trans R Soc Trop Med Hyg* 1986; 80:967–971.

100 Blair D, Xu Z B & Agatsuma T. Paragonimiasis and the genus *Paragonimus*. *Adv Parasitol* 1998; 42:113–222.

101 Hatsushika R. Human cases of infection with *Paragonimus miyazakii* (Trematoda: Troglotrematidae) in Japan: a bibliographical review. *Kawasaki Igakkai Shi* 2000; 26:65–82.

102 Kobayashi M, Yokogawa M, Tongu Y, Pinto M R & Tsuji M. Epidemiological survey for parasitic diseases, especially for paragonimiasis, Guatemala. *Japan J Parasitol* 1996; 45(3):207–214.

103 Uchiyama F, Morimoto Y & Nawa Y. Re-emergence of paragonimiasis in Kyushu, Japan. *Southeast Asian J Trop Med Public Health* 1999; 30:686–691.

104 Nishimura K & Hung T P. Current views on geographic distribution and modes of infection of neurohelminthic diseases. *J Neurol Sci* 1997; 145:5–14.

105 Vanijanonta S, Bunnag D & Harinasuta T. Radiological findings in pulmonary paragonimiasis heterotremus. *Southeast Asian J Trop Med Public Health* 1984; 15:122–128.

106 Jaroonvesama N. Differential diagnosis of eosinophilic meningitis. *Parasit Today* 1988; 88:262–266.

107 Maleewong W. Recent advances in diagnosis of paragonimiasis. *Southeast Asian J Trop Med Public Health* 1997; 28(Suppl 1):134–138.

108 Udonsi J K. Clinical trials of praziquantel in pulmonary paragonimiasis due to *Paragonimus uterolateralis* in endemic populations of the Igwun Basin, Nigeria. *Trop Med Parasitol* 1989; 40:65–68.

109 Vanijanonta S, Bunnag D & Harinasuta T. *Paragonimus* spp. in Thailand: pathogenesis, clinic and treatment. *Drug Res* 1984; 34:1186–1188.

110 Calvopina M, Guderian R H, Paredes W, Chico M & Cooper P J. Treatment of human pulmonary paragonimiasis with triclabendazole: clinical tolerance and drug efficacy. *Trans R Soc Trop Med Hyg* 1998; 92(5):566–569.

Chapter 82
Filariases

P. E. Simonsen

The filariases result from infection with vector-borne tissue-dwelling nematodes called filariae. Depending on the species, adult filariae may live in the lymphatics, blood vessels, skin, connective tissues or serous membranes. The females produce larvae (microfilariae) which live in the bloodstream or skin. All true filariae that infect humans (superfamily Filarioidea; family Onchocercidae) are transmitted by dipteran vectors. The guinea worm (superfamily Dracunculoidea) is not a true filaria, but is included in this section as a related nematode transmitted by arthropod vectors. A summary of the common filarial worms infecting humans and the common disease symptoms is shown in Table 82.1. A few species of animal filariae may accidentally infect humans. The transmission of human filariae is confined to warm climates, a high temperature being necessary for the parasites to develop in the vectors.

The pattern of the life cycle of all species of filariae is shown in Figure 82.1. Detailed life cycles of the species infecting humans are given in Appendix III. The infective form is the third-stage larva which is transmitted by the vector. The rate of growth and differentiation of worms and longevity of both microfilariae and adult worms differ markedly between different species. Some adult worms may live as long as 20 years. A high specificity of the filaria–vector and the filaria–host relationships has evolved over a long period of time.

From the public health point of view onchocerciasis and lymphatic filariasis are the most important filarial infections. Dracunculiasis (guinea worm infection) results in severe ulceration, and Calabar swellings and other clinical manifestations of loiasis may have severe consequences for the patient.

Lymphatic filariasis

Three species of lymphatic dwelling filarial worms, *Wuchereria bancrofti*, *Brugia malayi* and *B. timori*, cause lymphatic filariasis in humans. The vectors are species of

Table 82.1 Characteristics of filarial parasites and guinea worm and common clinical manifestations in humans.

Species	Distribution	Vectors	Main location of adults	Main location of microfilariae	Common disease symptoms
Wuchereria bancrofti	Tropics	Mosquito spp.	Lymphatics	Blood	Lymphangitis Elephantiasis Hydrocele
Brugia malayi	South, East and South-East Asia	Mosquito spp.	Lymphatics	Blood	Lymphangitis Elephantiasis
Brugia timori	Indonesia	Mosquito spp.	Lymphatics	Blood	Lymphangitis Elephantiasis
Loa loa	Central and west Africa	*Chrysops* spp.	Connective tissue	Blood	Calabar swellings
Mansonella perstans	Africa, Central and South America	*Culicoides* spp.	Body cavities Serous membranes	Blood	Usually symptomless
Mansonella streptocerca	Central and west Africa	*Culicoides* spp.	Skin	Skin	Usually symptomless
Mansonella ozzardi	Central and South America	*Culicoides* spp. *Simulium* spp.	Peritoneal cavity Serous membranes	Blood and skin	Usually symptomless
Onchocerca volvulus	Africa, Central and South America	*Simulium* spp.	Skin	Skin	Dermatitis Nodules Eye lesions
Dracunculus medinensis	Africa	Copepods	Connective tissue including skin	–	Ulceration

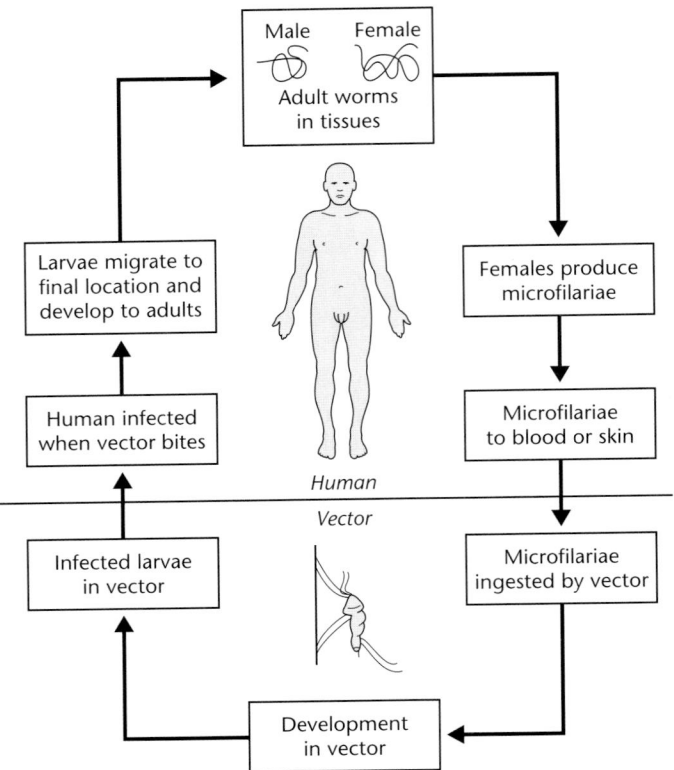

Figure 82.1: General life cycle of filariae.

mosquitoes (*Anopheles*, *Culex*, *Aedes* and *Mansonia* spp). Infection with *W. bancrofti* is sometimes called bancroftian filariasis, while brugian filariasis refers to infection by the other two species. *W. bancrofti* is geographically much more widespread than the *Brugia* spp. Lymphatic filariasis is a major cause of debilitating and disfiguring chronic disease manifestations (especially lymphoedema, elephantiasis and hydrocele) in endemic areas.[1]

Historical background

Our present knowledge of filariasis owes much to investigations carried out towards the end of the nineteenth and the beginning of the twentieth centuries. Microfilariae, recovered in hydrocele fluid from a Cuban patient, were first described by Jean-Nicolas Demarquay in Paris in 1863.[2] Three years later, microfilariae were found in chylous urine in a patient in Brazil by Otto Wucherer, who was unaware of the earlier French report.[3] Timothy Lewis, working in India, first reported the finding of microfilariae in human blood in 1872.[4] Adult worms were recovered by Joseph Bancroft in Australia in 1876 and named *Filaria bancrofti*.[5] In 1921 this species was included in the genus *Wuchereria*.

The distinguished pioneer of tropical medicine, Sir Patrick Manson, while working in Amoy in China, made several contributions to the understanding of the biology of *W. bancrofti*.[6] Thus, in 1877 he observed the development of the parasite in mosquitoes fed on the blood of

his microfilaraemic gardener, and he speculated that it was transmitted by mosquitoes. He also noticed that microfilariae could not always be found in the blood of infected patients. By serial blood examinations every few hours, he then revealed the nocturnal periodicity of the microfilariae.

Examination of specimens of adult worms revealed two new species, subsequently called *Brugia malayi* (1960) and *B. timori* (1977). A detailed history of lymphatic filariasis has been written.[7]

Geographical distribution

The distribution of the three causal parasites of lymphatic filariasis, *W. bancrofti*, *B. malayi* and *B. timori*, is shown in Figure 82.2. *W. bancrofti* is distributed throughout the tropical regions of Asia, Africa, the Americas and the Pacific, and is particularly prevalent in areas with hot and humid climates. *B. malayi* is found in South-East Asia, and in areas of south-west India and of south and central China, whereas *B. timori* occurs only on some small islands in Indonesia.

It is difficult to estimate the total world prevalence of lymphatic filariasis, because in many countries accurate information is not available. It is estimated that at least 128 million individuals are infected, 115 million with *W. bancrofti* and 13 million with the *Brugia* spp.[9] India (48 million cases) and sub-Saharan Africa (51 million cases) account for most of this burden. Lymphatic filariasis has disappeared from North America, Japan and Australia, and in some countries, especially China, recent control programmes have greatly decreased the prevalence. It continues to be a major public health problem in most of southern and South-East Asia, in Africa, and in a number of Caribbean and Pacific islands. In recent years the amount of urban filariasis has increased due to an increase in both human and vector populations in these areas.

Life cycle and transmission

The adult worms reside in the lymphatics of the human host. Female *W. bancrofti* measure 80–100 × 0.25 mm and the male 40 × 0.1 mm. The adult *Brugia* spp. have only half of this dimension. Microfilariae are produced from ova in the uterus of the female worm. They are sheathed and measure on average 260 × 8 μm (Figures 82.3 and 82.4). Microfilariae are ingested by the vector female mosquito during a blood meal. They exsheath in the mosquito stomach, becoming first-stage larvae which penetrate the stomach wall of the mosquito and migrate to the thorax muscles. There they develop through two moults to the infective third-stage larvae (1500 × 20 μm). The development in the mosquito takes a minimum of 10–12 days. Mature infective larvae then migrate to the mouthparts of the mosquito from where they enter the skin of the human host, probably through the puncture site made by the proboscis of the vector when it takes its blood meal. The larvae migrate to the lymphatics and develop to adult worms. Microfilariae appear in the blood

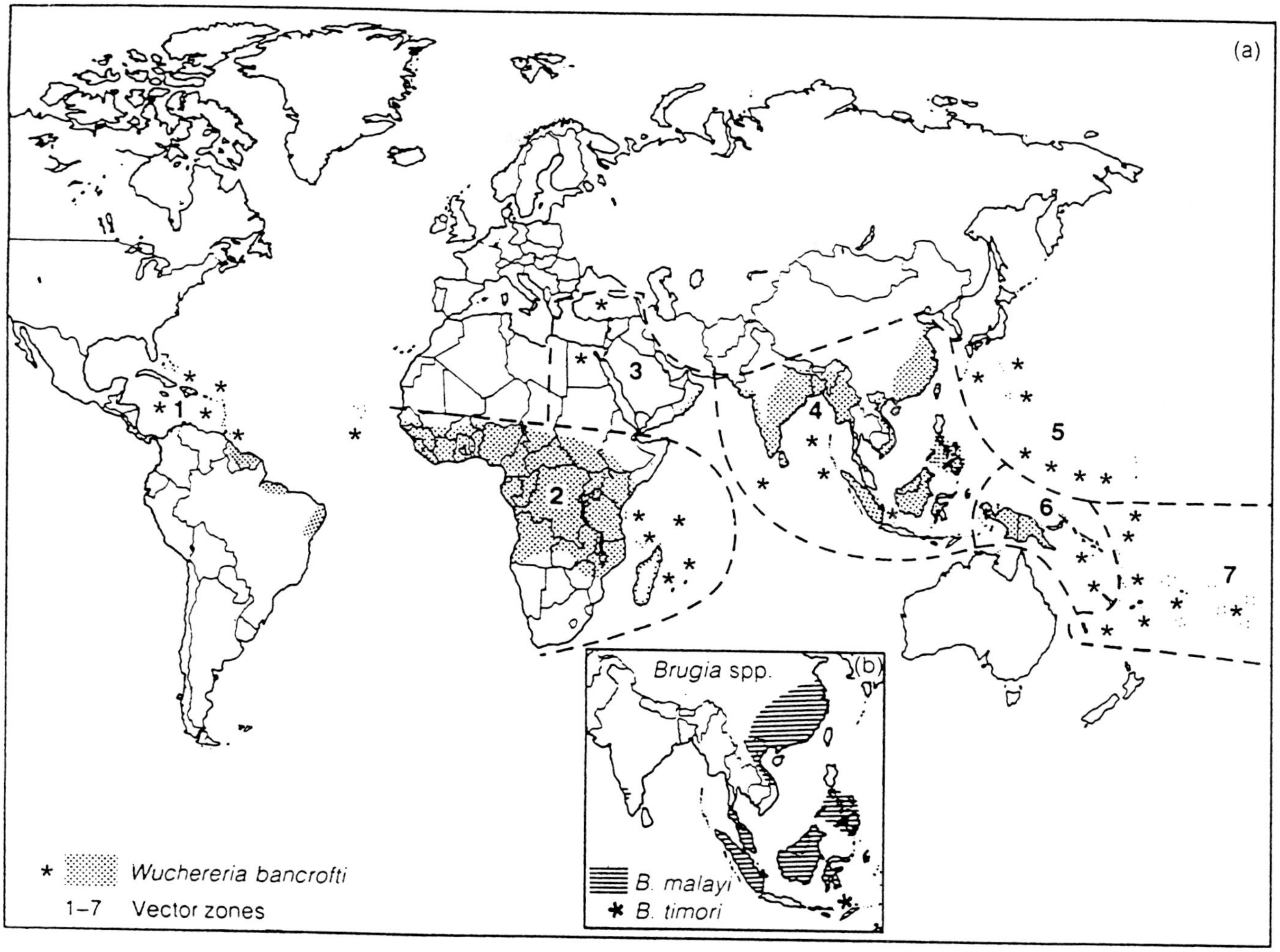

Figure 82.2: Geographical distribution of human lymphatic filariasis. (**A**) Bancroftian filariasis. (**B**) Brugian filariasis. For vector species in the different zones, see Appendix IV. (After WHO.[8])

after a minimum of 8 months in *W. bancrofti* and 3 months in *B. malayi*. The adult worms may live and produce microfilariae for more than 20 years, but on average the lifespan is shorter. Microfilariae have a lifespan of approximately 1 year. Microfilarial densities may reach 10 000 per ml of blood or more, but are usually lower.

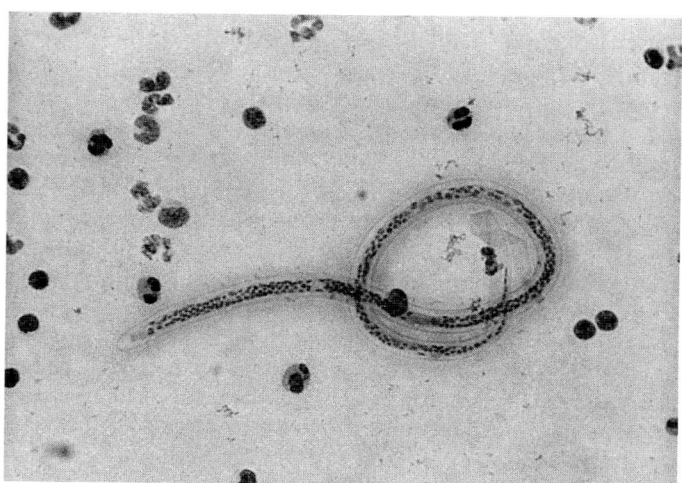

Figure 82.3: Microfilaria of *W. bancrofti* in thick blood film.

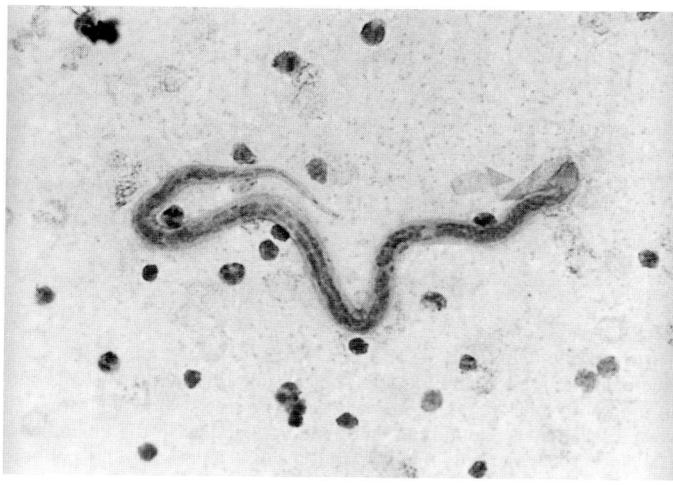

Figure 82.4: Microfilaria of *B. malayi* in thick blood film.

For details of the life cycles of the three causal parasites of lymphatic filariasis and of the mosquito vectors transmitting this infection in different geographical zones, see Appendices III and IV.

Microfilarial periodicity

Like many filarial species, *W. bancrofti, B. malayi* and *B. timori* exhibit a daily periodicity in the concentration of microfilariae in the peripheral blood of the host. The different periodicities of microfilariae correspond with the biting habits of their principal vector. This adaptation enhances their chances of onward transmission. The details of microfilarial periodicity are discussed in Appendix III.

Depending on whether the highest microfilarial density over a 24-hour period occurs during the night or the day, periodicity is termed nocturnal or diurnal (Figure 82.5). In most areas the periodicity of both *W. bancrofti* and *B. malayi* is nocturnal, with peak concentrations in the blood around midnight, and none or very few at midday.[10] In these areas, the parasites are transmitted by night-biting mosquitoes. There are also diurnally subperiodic and nocturnally subperiodic forms of *W. bancrofti*, where microfilariae are present continuously in the peripheral blood but where the concentrations are higher than average during day and night, respectively. A strain of *B. malayi* also exhibits nocturnal sub-periodicity (Figure 82.5).

The periodicity is due to a biological rhythm inherent in the microfilariae but influenced by the circadian rhythm of the host. Microfilaraemia of nocturnally periodic *W. bancrofti* ceases to be periodic in persons who start work at night and sleep during the day, and in patients who have been hospitalized for long periods.

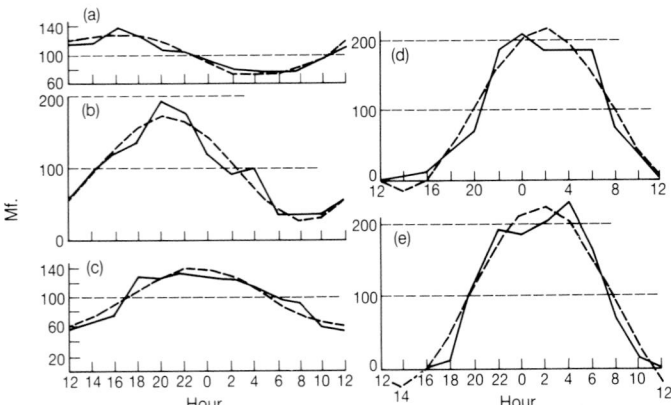

Figure 82.5: Observed (–) and theoretical (- - -) periodicity of microfilariae in peripheral blood. (**A** Diurnally subperiodic *W. bancrofti* in the South Pacific. (**B**) Nocturnally subperiodic *W. bancrofti* from west Thailand. (**C**) Nocturnally subperiodic *B. malayi* in the Philippines. (**D**) Nocturnally periodic *B. malayi* in Malaysia. (**E**) Nocturnally periodic *W. bancrofti* in Malaysia. (Reproduced from *Control of Lymphatic Filariasis. A Manual for Health Personnel.* WHO, Geneva, ©1987.)

Clinical features

Lymphatic filariasis is characterized by a wide range of clinical presentations.

One group of individuals in the endemic community shows no clinical manifestations or microfilariae (asymptomatic amicrofilaraemia). This includes individuals who have not been sufficiently exposed to be infected, individuals with prepatent infection or adult worm infection without microfilaraemia, and individuals who have cleared the infection. It is possible that some of the asymptomatic amicrofilaraemics are immune or partially immune to infection.

Another group of individuals in the endemic community shows microfilariae in their blood but no obvious clinical manifestations (asymptomatic microfilaraemia). Some of these may remain microfilaraemic and asymptomatic for years or even for the rest of their lives.

Through the use of ultrasonography and lymphoscintigraphy it has been recognized that most infected but apparently asymptomatic individuals (with or without microfilaraemia) suffer from subclinical lymphatic abnormalities, especially dilatation of the vessels (lymphangiectasis).[11-13]

Obvious symptomatic filarial disease manifests itself in both acute and chronic forms, and may be with or without microfilaraemia.

Bancroftian filariasis

Common clinical manifestations of bancroftian filariasis are acute adenolymphangitis, hydrocele, lymphoedema and elephantiasis, chyluria, and tropical pulmonary eosinophilia. Although common in males, genital manifestations do not appear to be a substantial problem in females.[14]

Acute manifestations

Manifestations of acute filarial disease ('filarial fever'), often described as adenolymphangitis (ADL), are characterized by episodic attacks of malaise, fever and chills, and by the appearance of enlarged painful lymph nodes draining the affected part, usually the lower limb, followed by an acute, warm and tender swelling. The episodes usually resolve spontaneously after about a week, and may recur several times within a year. Regression of the swelling after an ADL attack of the leg is commonly followed by excessive skin exfoliation.[15] In males the genitals are frequently affected and attacks may present as acute funiculitis or epididymo-orchitis. Acute attacks may be unilateral or bilateral, and commonly occur also in individuals with chronic manifestatons.[16]

Two distinct syndromes of acute filarial attacks in the extremities have recently been recognized.[17] One, called acute filarial lymphangitis (AFL), is caused by the death of adult worms, either spontaneously or after treatment. It presents as a circumscribed inflammatory nodule or cord centred around degenerating adult worms, with lymphangitis spreading in a descending (centrifugal) fashion. It usually has a mild clinical course and rarely causes residual lymphoedema. The other syndrome, acute dermatolymphangioadenitis (ADLA) is not caused by filarial worms per se, but probably results from secondary bacterial infections in the legs with compromised lymphatics. It is characterized by diffuse subcutaneous inflammation with or without ascending lymphangitis, and is often accompanied by oedema in the affected leg. It is believed to be the common cause of chronic lymphoedema and elephantiasis.

Hydrocele

Hydrocele is the most common chronic manifestation in bancroftian filariasis. It results from the accumulation of clear straw-coloured fluid in the sac surrounding the testicles. The onset may be silent, i.e., without accompanying acute episodes, or it may be preceded by one or more attacks of funiculitis or epididymo-orchitis. Following early acute episodes, the swelling around the testis usually disappears completely, but over the years the tunica vaginalis becomes thickened and there is progressive enlargement of the hydrocele (Figure 82.6). Most cases are unilateral, but bilateral hydrocele, often with different sizes on the two sides, is not uncommon.[18] Rarely, the fluid may have a milky appearance if lymph from a ruptured lymphatic vessel pours into the hydrocele to form a chylocele.

In clinical surveys, hydrocele is graded according to developmental stage and size. A commonly used scale records swelling of the spermatic cord as hydrocele grade I, and true hydroceles are classified from their length as grade II (6.0–8.0 cm), III (8.1–11.0 cm), IV (11.1–15.0 cm) and V (> 15 cm).[19,20]

Lymphoedema and elephantiasis

Chronic lymphoedema progressing to elephantiasis most commonly affects the legs (Figure 82.7). The arms (Figure 82.8), scrotum (Figure 82.9), penis, vulva and breasts may also more rarely be affected. Following recurrent episodes of acute attacks in the limbs, first pitting oedema and then chronic non-pitting oedema with loss of skin elasticity and fibrosis develops. The development of elephantiasis may be arrested at any stage. It commences in one leg but often becomes bilateral.

In the leg, loss of contour is first observed around the ankles. Following initial attacks the limb returns to normal. Over several years the oedema becomes non-pitting with thickening and loss of skin elasticity. Further progression leads to evident elephantiasis with skin folds, dermato-sclerosis and papillomatous lesions.[21] Secondary bacterial and fungal infections are common in the lymph-oedematous skin, and probably exacerbate the progression of elephantiasis. In severe cases pus may ooze from chronic ulcerations in the affected part, which may also emanate a foul smell. Scarification, a common traditional treatment for body swellings in many filariasis endemic areas (see Figure 82.8), has been recognized as a risk factor for rapid progression of filarial elephantiasis.[22]

In clinical surveys, leg lymphoedemas are commonly classified as grade I: pitting lymphoedema spontaneously reversible on elevation, loss of contour; grade II: non-pitting lymphoedema not spontaneously reversible on elevation, loss of skin elasticity; and grade III: evident elephantiasis with skin folds and papules.[19,20]

Chyluria

Chyluria, the presence of chyle in the urine, follows the

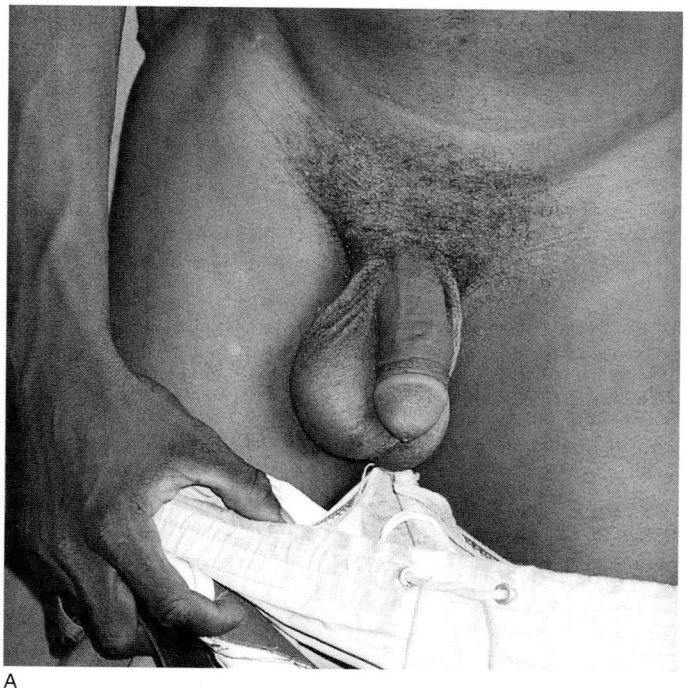
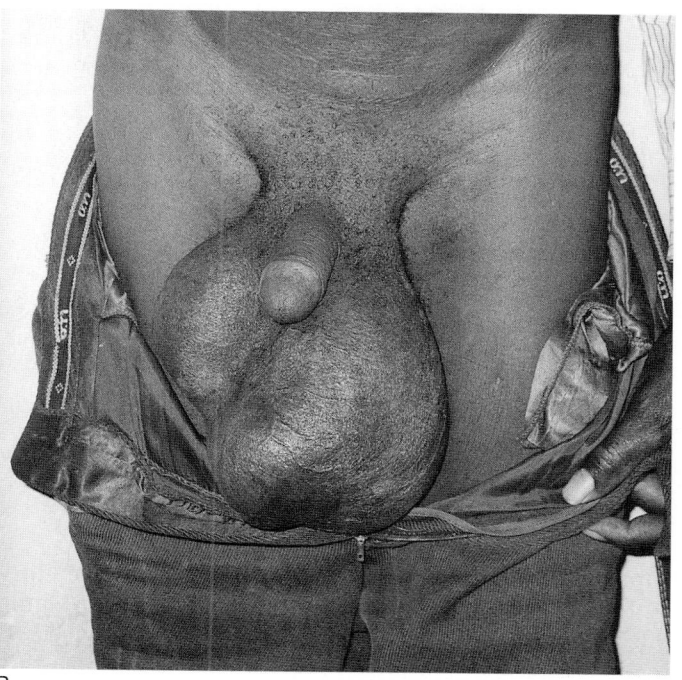

A B

Figure 82.6: Lymphatic filariasis: hydrocele. (**A**) Early; (**B**) advanced.

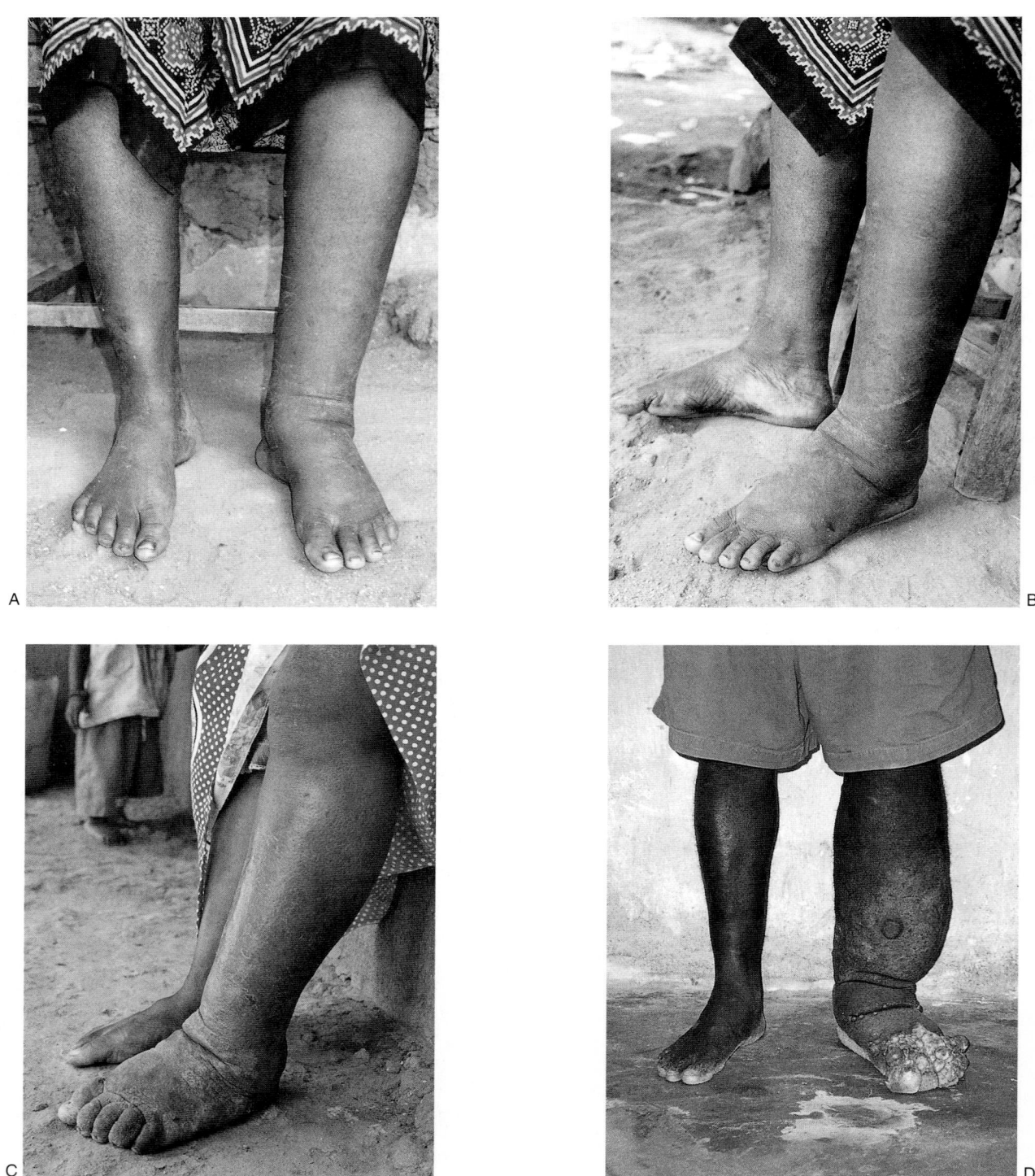

Figure 82.7: Lymphatic filariasis: elephantiasis of the leg. (**A, B**) Early stage lymphoedema of left leg; (**C, D**) advanced stage elephantiasis of left leg.

rupture of dilated lymphatics into the urinary excretory system. Chylous urine is milky in appearance (Figure 82.10). Blood may sometimes be present. Chyluria is frequently a recurrent phenomenon, with episodes lasting for days or weeks. The onset may be insidious or sudden. Retention of urine from the presence of chylous or blood clots may occur. Chyluria is more pronounced in the morning and after a heavy meal containing fat. Prolonged chyluria may result in loss of weight and subcutaneous fat, hypoproteinaemia, lymphopenia and anaemia. In most areas endemic for filariasis, the prevalence of chyluria is low.

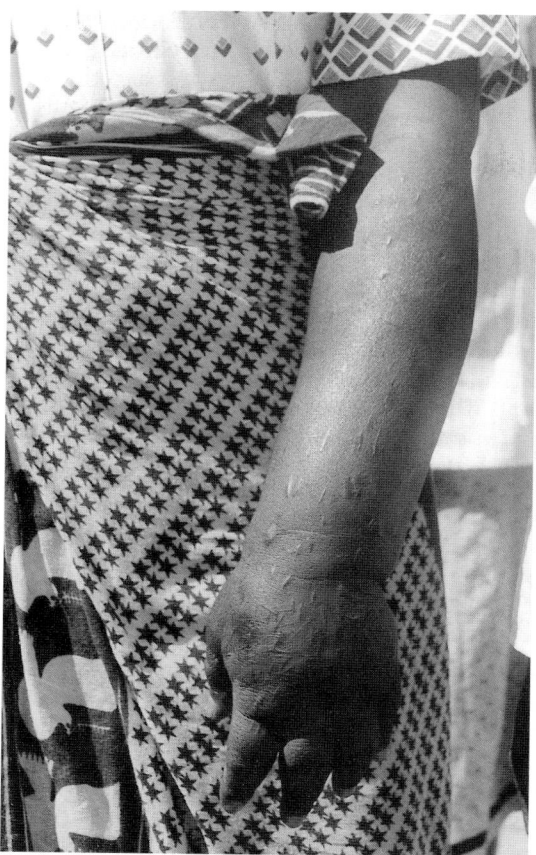

Figure 82.8: Lymphatic filariasis: elephantiasis of the arm, with visible scarification marks.

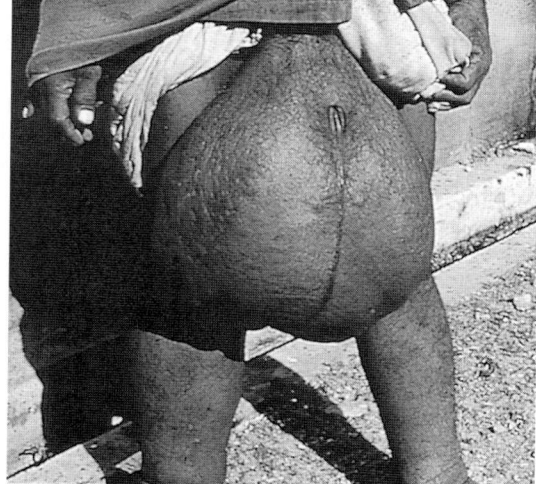

Figure 82.9: Lymphatic filariasis: elephantiasis of the scrotum.

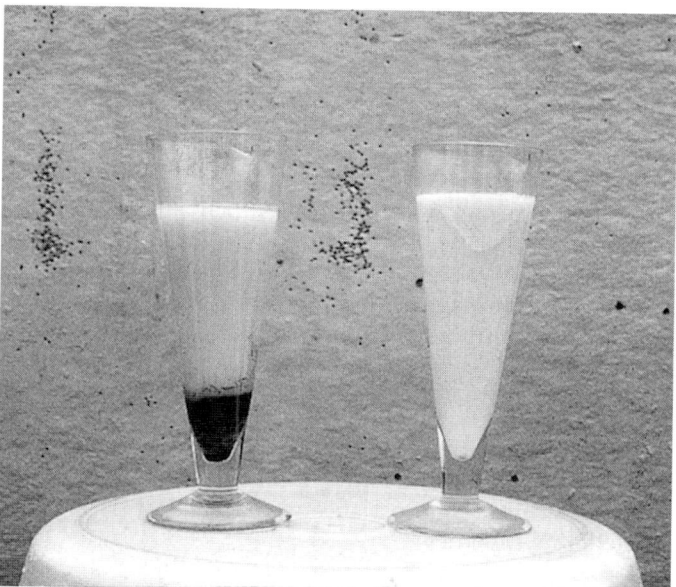

Figure 82.10: Lymphatic filariasis: chyluria—milky urine with sedimented blood.

Tropical pulmonary eosinophilia

Tropical pulmonary eosinophilia (TPE) is a syndrome of immunological hyperresponsiveness to microfilariae in the lungs.[23] It occurs with low frequency in most areas endemic for lymphatic filariasis. It is more common in males than in females. Microfilariae are absent from the blood but have been recognized in lung biopsies, and adult worms have been seen on ultrasonography.[24]

Patients present with paroxysmal coughing and wheezing that is worse at night, and extreme blood eosinophilia with eosinophil counts above 3000 cells/mm³ of blood. This hypereosinophilia, and a therapeutic response to diethylcarbamazine (DEC) treatment, is the most constant feature of the syndrome. The level of eosinophilia is not related to the severity of symptoms. Patients have extremely high titres of filarial antibodies. There is radiological evidence of diffuse miliary lesions. Extrapulmonary manifestations occur in some patients and include splenomegaly, lymphadenopathy and hepatomegaly. In most cases of TPE lung function is impaired, with a reduction in the vital capacity, total lung capacity and residual volume. If left untreated, TPE may progress to a chronic stage with interstitial fibrosis and permanent loss of lung function.

TPE is a classical example of occult filariasis (filarial infection where microfilariae are not found in the blood, but where adult worms, microfilariae or other larval stages may be seen in the tissues).

Other conditions

Monoarthritis is common in filarial endemic areas, and a possible association has long been recognized.[24] The knee joint is most frequently affected, followed by the ankle. The joint becomes painful, warm and tender, and the condition is indistinguishable from other forms of arthritis. A rapid cure follows treatment with DEC.

Haematuria (usually microscopic) and proteinuria occur in many microfilaraemic persons.[24] The pathogenesis probably relates to immune complexes deposited on the basement membrane of the renal glomeruli.

Scattered reports associate endomyocardial fibrosis, tenosynovitis, thrombophlebitis, nerve palsies and dermatoses with filariasis. These conditions sometimes coexist with filariasis and may be atypical manifestations of other diseases conditioned by pre-existing filarial infection.

Brugian filariasis

The main difference in the clinical manifestations between brugian and bancroftian filariasis is the rarity of hydroceles and other genital lesions in areas endemic for *B. malayi*. Chyluria is another sign not associated with *B. malayi*. Elephantiasis of the legs in *B. malayi* infections is often confined to below the knee, whereas in infections with *W. bancrofti* the lower leg as well as the thigh is frequently involved.

B. timori infections produce similar clinical manifestations to those seen in infections due to *B. malayi*, i.e., scrotal lesions are almost absent and elephantiasis tends to be below the knee.

Geographical variation in clinical picture

Clinical manifestations of lymphatic filariasis have been reported in the past to differ considerably between geographical zones. However, as examination and grading procedures become more standardized, differences appear to be less marked.

Most cases of TPE and chyluria have been reported from south and South-East Asian countries. In Africa, the prevalence of both chyluria and TPE is low. At a weekly filariasis clinic conducted over a 5-year period on the East African coast, only five cases of chyluria and two of TPE were seen (J E McMahon, personal communication). A recent search for TPE cases in a highly endemic lymphatic filariasis area of Tanzania confirmed the rarity of this syndrome in the population.[25]

In *W. bancrofti* endemic areas of Papua New Guinea, microfilarial prevalences can be exceedingly high, reaching 60–80% for the overall population, whereas clinical sign rates for hydrocele and elephantiasis tend to be similar or even lower than those seen in highly endemic areas (overall 20–30% microfilarial prevalence) elsewhere in the world.[26]

Diagnosis

Clinical diagnosis

Acute or chronic manifestations resembling those described above in individuals who live in or who have visited areas endemic for transmission of *W. bancrofti*, *B. malayi* or *B. timori* are indicative of lymphatic filariasis.

A sudden onset of fever, accompanied by acute groin pain with swollen tender lymph glands and/or oedematous swelling of the leg distinguishes an acute attack of filarial ADL from the many other causes of fever and adenitis that occur in tropical countries. Filarial funiculitis needs to be differentiated from funiculitis due to bacterial infection.

Inguinal hernia is the most common scrotal swelling that needs to be distinguished from hydrocele. If the hernia is irreducible then the translucency test and the inability of the examiner to get above the swelling distinguish it from hydrocele. Both irreducible hernias and hydroceles often exist in the same patient. Obstructed hernias, tumours of the testis, tuberculosis and other bacterial infections of the epididymis, *Schistosoma haematobium* of the cord and acute lymphadenitis of the groin glands need to be distinguished from genital lesions of filarial origin.

Common conditions that need to be distinguished from filarial lymphoedema are swollen limbs due to congestive cardiac failure, subacute nephritis or blockage of venous (thrombosis) or lymphatic (tuberculosis, leprosy) systems, and Kaposi's sarcoma. In all these conditions the patient's history greatly assists in differentiating them from filarial elephantiasis. The oedema of cardiac failure and subacute nephritis has a painless onset and is bilateral. Secondary carcinoma of lymph glands and surgical ablation may also result in elephantiasis of the limbs.

An endemic form of leg elephantiasis occurs in many parts of Africa at altitudes that preclude a filarial aetiology. Mineral particles from volcanic soils, absorbed through the plantar skin of bare-footed peoples, are believed to be the causative agents (see Chapter 30). Non-filarial tropical elephantiasis has also been reported from South and Central America.

Early stages of scrotal elephantiasis need to be distinguished from other conditions that affect the scrotal skin, such as fungal infections, scrotal oedema due to onchocerciasis and the thickened skin that results from the intense itching and scratching in scabies infections.

TPE should be differentiated from bronchial asthma and other allergic conditions, tuberculosis and eosinophilic leukaemia. TPE must also be distinguished from helminth infections that have a stage of the life cycle that involves lung tissue: *Ascaris*, *Strongyloides*, *Schistosoma* spp. and trichinosis. Confusion may also arise with visceral larva migrans caused by *Toxocara*. A rapid beneficial response to DEC therapy distinguishes TPE from the above-mentioned conditions.

Parasitological diagnosis

Adult worms are recovered only rarely from the tissues, and parasitological diagnosis is usually based on recovery of microfilariae from the patient's blood. Amicrofilaraemia does not exclude filarial disease, nor does microfilaraemia denote it. Blood samples taken from patients with clinical manifestations, whether acute or chronic, are often negative for microfilariae. In individuals there is no relationship between microfilarial density and severity of disease. Microfilariae frequently occur in hydrocele fluid and may occasionally be seen in urine or other body fluids.

For parasitological diagnosis of lymphatic filariasis, a blood specimen should be obtained at the time of the day when the peak concentration of microfilariae is expected (e.g., between 21.00 and 03.00 hours for nocturnally periodic forms).[10]

Many techniques have been described for demonstrating microfilariae in blood samples (see also Appendix V). The counting chamber technique is fast, quantitative and cheap.[27] An aliquot of 100 µl of finger-prick blood is added to a tube containing 0.9 ml of 3% acetic acid. Microfilariae are counted in a counting chamber under the low power of a compound microscope. If only one species of filaria is present in the area, this technique is the most suitable for routine hospital diagnosis as well as for field surveys. Species identification of the microfilariae may be difficult with the counting chamber technique.

In areas where more than one species of blood microfilaria exists, staining techniques are recommended. These are simple to perform but sensitivity is rather low owing to the small amount of blood examined and loss of microfilariae during the staining procedure. Microfilariae of *W. bancrofti*, *B. malayi* and *B. timori* have sheaths (see Figures 82.3 and 82.4). Microfilariae of *W. bancrofti* measure on average 260 × 8 µm, whereas those of *B. malayi* are slightly shorter and can be distinguished from microfilariae of *W. bancrofti* by the two isolated nuclei at the tip of the tail and the absence of nuclei in the cephalic space (see Appendix III). Microfilariae of *B. timori* are longer than those of *B. malayi*. Apart from microfilariae of *W. bancrofti*, two other species of microfilariae found in the blood in parts of Africa are those of *Loa loa* and *Mansonella perstans*. Staining with Giemsa or haematoxylin enables microfilariae of these species to be differentiated morphologically. *M. perstans* and *M. ozzardi* microfilariae also occur in the blood in South America and the West Indies.

The membrane (Nuclepore) filtration techniques are sensitive and excellent if the high cost of filters can be afforded. Staining of filters enables identification of the microfilariae. The techniques are impractical for field surveys because venous blood is needed. If filters are not available for examination of large quantities of blood, the Knott concentration technique may be used as an alternative, highly sensitive test (see Appendix V).

Diethylcarbamazine provocative day test
Nocturnally periodic microfilariae of *W. bancrofti* and *B. malayi* may be provoked, by the administration of DEC, to enter the peripheral blood in the daytime. Between 30 and 60 minutes is the optimum time for blood examination after the administration of a dose of 2 mg/kg of DEC (usually 100 mg of DEC is given to adults and 50 mg to children below 12 years of age).[28] The DEC provocative day test results in a significant long-term reduction of microfilaraemia, and therefore should not be used for diagnosis in follow-up studies on microfilaraemia.[29]

In contrast to its daytime action on nocturnally periodic *W. bancrofti*, the administration of DEC at night reduces the microfilaraemia. A similar reduction occurs following the daytime administration of the drug to diurnally subperiodic *W. bancrofti*. In persons with normal daily activity, the daytime DEC provocative method is as sensitive a method for detecting microfilariae of the

nocturnally periodic *W. brancrofti* as examination of night blood.[28] In hospitalized patients and others whose sleep rhythms have been altered, the test is of little use.

The test has an important practical use in obtaining a clear reflection of the prevalence and density of the microfilaraemia in a community in areas where it is difficult to obtain the cooperation of the population for night blood surveys. Because of the risk of a severe Mazzotti reaction, the test is contraindicated in onchocerciasis endemic regions. A similar provocative effect is not exerted by daytime administration of ivermectin or albendazole.[30]

Immunological and polymerase chain reaction (PCR)-based diagnosis
Filarial worms induce a wide range of immune responses in the host, and several immunodiagnostic techniques for lymphatic filariasis, based on the detection of specific antibodies in the patients serum, have been devised in the past. These have generally been of limited value in endemic areas, because most individuals are positive for antibodies to crude filarial antigens as a result of constant exposure. Tests have furthermore suffered from cross-reactions to other nematode infections, and from being unable to distinguish past and present infection.

The development of new, specific and sensitive immunodiagnostic tests has been a priority in lymphatic filariasis research. Cross-reactions have been reduced through detection for specific IgG4 antibodies, and specific IgG4 has been reported to be a good marker of active infection. Such tests may be of particular value in brugian filariasis,[31,32] for which progress in development of circulating antigen detection-based diagnosis has been limited. They may also be of value in diagnosing visitors to endemic areas who develop symptoms of lymphatic filariasis but have no microfilaraemia.

Highly sensitive and specific tests for detection of specific circulating filarial antigens (CFAs) have been produced for bancroftian filariasis. These tests rely on the capture of filarial antigens in serum, plasma or blood specimens by use of specific monoclonal antibodies. Two different test principles have been utilized by two companies in the manufacture of test kits, which are now commercially available.[33,34] The TropBio-test (TropBio Pty Ltd, Australia) is a semiquantitative sandwich enzyme-linked immunosorbant assay (ELISA) for detection of CFA in serum or plasma specimens. A sub-version of this test is adapted for analysis of finger-prick blood collected on filter paper discs. The ICT-test (Amrad ICT, Binax Inc., USA) is an immunochromatographic card test that in a few minutes can provide a yes/no answer for serum or fresh finger-prick blood specimens. In contrast to the parasitological tests, the CFA-based tests diagnose adult worm infection and not just microfilaraemia. Their specificity appears to be greater than 99%, and only a few individuals with undetectable or ultra-low microfilaraemia are missed.[35] As the tests are not dependent on the microfilarial periodicity, blood specimens can be collected and examined at any time of the day. No such test is currently available for brugian filariasis.

Polymerase chain reaction (PCR) assays for the detection of microfilarial infections in humans have been developed for both *W. bancrofti*[36,37] and *B. malayi*.[38] The techniques need at least one microfilaria in the volume of blood used for DNA extraction, and therefore are not more sensitive than microscopic blood examination for microfilariae. In contrast, these tests appear to be powerful tools for detection of infection in vectors and to monitor transmission.[36]

Ultrasonography

Adult *W. bancrofti* can be detected by ultrasonography in lymphatic vessels of the scrotal area of infected males.[11,39] The live worms move actively inside the lymphatic vessel ('filarial dance sign'). Live adults of *W. bancrofti* have also been detected by ultrasonography in the female breast.[40] Attempts to detect adult *B. malayi* in the scrotal lymphatics of infected males have failed, perhaps because this species occupies a different location in the human body.[41]

Pathology and immunology

Most of the pathology in lymphatic filariasis is associated with the adult worms and their location in the lymphatics. A spectrum of manifestations is seen in endemic regions[42] (Figure 82.11). On one hand are people with no obvious signs of infection or disease and asymptomatic microfilaria-carriers, and on the other are those who develop signs of lymphatic responsiveness to adult worms, with fever, and who later develop chronic lymphatic pathology. In the case of TPE there is a vigorous immune response directed against the microfilariae, with consequent pathology. The pathogenesis in lymphatic filariasis has long been a matter of debate.

The majority of individuals in endemic areas mount an immunological response to filarial antigens as a result of the constant exposure. Polarization of the antibody and T-cell responses towards a T helper cell (Th) type 2 response in microfilaraemic individuals, as opposed to a Th1-type response in patients with chronic disease, has been recognized.[43] A relative Th1-type hyporesponsiveness in infected individuals appears to be limited to filarial antigens, and its existence is presumably important for the successful persistence of the parasites within the host.

When examining patients with filariasis in studies on pathogenesis, a common approach has been to compare and contrast two poles in the clinical spectrum, namely individuals with detectable microfilaraemia but with no evident clinical manifestations, and individuals with chronic lymphatic disease who have generally been assumed to be amicrofilaraemic.[43] A hypothesis claiming a developmental sequence from the first to the second of these categories has been supported by the observation of more vivid immunological sensitization to filarial antigen in patients with chronic disease than in those with asymptomatic microfilaraemia. According to this hypothesis, microfilaraemic individuals are in a state of immunological tolerance. Breakdown of tolerance (for whatever reason) and activation of host protective responses would lead to clearing of the parasites but would at the same time have detrimental immunopathological effects.

This hypothesis of a basically immune-mediated pathogenesis of lymphatic disease has recently been challenged by observations from several lines of research. Analysis of epidemiological data has shown that in most endemic communities microfilaraemia is equally likely to occur in individuals with or without chronic pathology.[18,20,44] Use of strict classification criteria based on circulating antigenaemia, microfilaraemia and clinical status has furthermore indicated that host immune responses are more related to infection status than to disease status in the endemic population.[45,46]

Further evidence for a different pathway of disease development in lymphatic filariasis comes from studies applying the new imaging techniques of ultrasonography and lymphoscintigraphy in the assessment of lymphatic damage, and from detailed clinical, microbiological and histological observations.[45,47,48] According to these, it appears that dilatation of the lymphatics (lymphangiectasia) is the basic lesion in the natural history of disease development. Lymphangiectasia is present in virtually all individuals with adult worms whether or not they are microfilaraemic or have obvious signs of clinical disease. Apparently the adult worms themselves are capable of inducing endothelial cell proliferation and lymphatic dilatation via mechanisms that do not involve lymphatic obstruction or involvement of the host immune responses. Death of the adult worms may result in formation of granulomatous nodules or episodes of acute filarial lymphangitis (AFL), with activation of host inflammatory reactions. More seriously, however, lymphangiectasia impairs lymphatic function and predisposes to microbial infection that may result in the more common and more severe pathological syndrome of acute dermato-lymphangioadenitis (ADLA). This is frequently accompanied by oedema in the affected part, and repeated attacks of ADLA might lead the way to chronic lymphoedema.[17] Recurrent secondary bacterial infections thus appear to

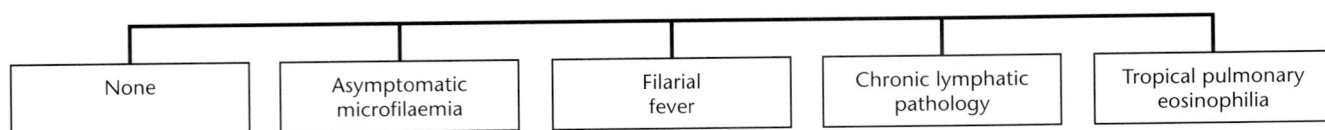

Figure 82.11: Spectrum of clinical manifestations of lymphatic filariasis in endemic areas. (After Ottesen.[42])

be important co-factors in the development of filarial lymphoedema and elephantiasis.[47,48] Acute hydrocele may result from an AFL attack in the intrascrotal lymphatics, but most of these disappear within a short time. The pathogenesis of most cases of chronic hydrocele is still unclear.

Patients with TPE are immunologically hyperresponsive to filarial antigens.[23] Laboratory studies demonstrate high serum levels of filaria-specific IgG and IgE, and marked peripheral blood eosinophilia. The manifestations of TPE are most marked in the lungs. Recent findings have implicated immunological cross-reactions between parasite allergens and host compounds located in lung epithelial cells in the pathogenesis.[49] Lung biopsies have shown inflammatory foci around degenerating microfilariae. These findings, together with the absence of circulating microfilariae, suggest that an antibody-mediated mechanism of microfilaria destruction occurs in the lungs of these patients.

Protective immunity has not been proved in lymphatic filariasis. However, there is evidence that some individuals in endemic areas develop resistance to the microfilarial or the infective larval stages of the parasite. In filarial endemic areas, a proportion of the amicrofilaraemic individuals (with or without symptoms) produces antibodies to the microfilarial sheath. A close correlation between positivity for anti-sheath antibodies, a negative microfilaraemia status and a negative CFA status suggests that these individuals may have developed a resistance mechanism against the microfilarial stage of the parasite.[50,51] In Papua New Guinea, protection against reinfection was seen to correlate with the presence of an antibody binding to the surface of the infective-stage larvae.[52] Epidemiological analysis of observed age–infection patterns in endemic communities has suggested an increasing proportion of resistant individuals with increasing age, with the reached level of resistance being related to the community transmission intensity.[53]

Visitors to endemic from non-endemic areas only rarely develop microfilaraemia, but they may acquire adult worms. Expatriates, exposed to intense transmission, may develop symptoms faster than is the case with resident natives of the endemic area. During the Second World War 40 000 American service personnel were exposed to infection with *W. bancrofti*. More than 10 000 cases of disease were diagnosed, but microfilaraemia developed in fewer than ten of these. In a study of expatriate mineworkers with a length of exposure ranging from 1 to 8 years, some were positive for specific IgG1 and IgG4 antibody responses to the parasite but none was positive for specific circulating antigens.[54]

The effects of human immunodeficiency virus (HIV) infection on concurrent lymphatic filariasis, and vice versa, are largely unknown, but peripheral blood mononuclear cells from individuals with filarial infection appear to have enhanced susceptibility to HIV infection *in vitro*.[55]

Management

Individual treatment of filariasis aims to prevent or reverse progression of disease. A detailed account of current knowledge and experience on the treatment and management of lymphatic filariasis in its different clinical forms has been given.[56]

Antifilarial drugs

For almost half a century, the drug most commonly used has been diethylcarbamazine citrate (DEC; Hetrazan, Banocide, Notezine). DEC is a microfilaricidal agent also capable of killing a proportion of the adult *W. bancrofti*, *B. malayi* and *B. timori* (Table 82.2). Ivermectin (Mectizan) is a potent microfilaricide, but has no macrofilaricidal effect.

Diethylcarbamazine

DEC exerts no direct lethal action on the microfilariae but apparently modifies them so that they are removed by the host's immune system. The lethal effect of DEC on adult worms in vivo can be directly monitored by ultrasonography.[57]

DEC treatment of microfilaraemic patients (and amicrofilaraemic circulating antigen-positive patients) may prevent development of lymphatic damage by eliminating adult worms. It apparently has little or no effect on already induced lymphatic damage, or on chronic obstructive disease.[58] Dying adult worms following DEC treatment may trigger transient attacks of acute

Table 82.2 Effect of diethylcarbamazine and ivermectin on microfilariae and adults of human filarial parasites.

Drug	Stage	Wuchereria bancrofti and Brugia spp.	Loa loa	Mansonella perstans	Mansonella streptocerca	Mansonella ozzardi	Onchocerca volvulus
Diethylcarbamazine	Microfilaria	++	++*	–	++	–	++*
	Adult	+	+	–	++	–	–
Ivermectin	Microfilaria	++	++*	–	++	++	++
	Adult	–	?	?	?	?	–

–, No effect; +, few/some are eliminated; ++, most are eliminated; ?, unknown; *, severe side effects may occur.

filarial lymphangitis.[17] DEC treatment is not recommended during acute episodes because it may provoke additional adult worm death and exacerbate the inflammatory response.

DEC is administered orally. The recommended therapeutic dose is 6 mg/kg body weight daily, in three divided doses after food, for 12 days. The number of microfilariae in the blood usually decreases rapidly after the start of treatment and then increases, usually at reduced intensity, after some months. Clearance of circulating filarial antigen is highly variable, probably because some living adult worms persist after treatment.[59] Drug reactions, due to dying parasites, may commence a few hours after the start of treatment. They are less severe in bancroftian filariasis than in brugian filariasis. There are two groups of reactions: systemic and local.[60] Systemic reactions include headache, joint and body pain, dizziness, anorexia, malaise and vomiting. Fever and systemic reactions tend to be related to the intensity of infection. Localized reactions include lymphadenitis, abscess formation and transient lymphoedema. In bancroftian filariasis funiculitis, epididymitis and hydrocele formation also occur. These local reactions tend to occur later and last longer than the systemic effects. Interruption of treatment is not usually necessary. Side effects of DEC therapy are reduced, and efficacy increased, when treatment is spaced, for example when single doses (6 mg/kg) are given weekly or monthly. The passing of *Ascaris* worms is often a beneficial side effect of DEC therapy.

Treatment may be repeated every 6 months for as long as the person remains microfilaraemic or has symptoms. There may be severe reactions to DEC in persons infected with *Onchocerca volvulus* or *Loa loa*. Therefore, special care must be taken in areas where these two parasites occur.

The recommended treatment for TPE is a 3-week course of DEC. Following DEC therapy most patients show rapid improvement. Repeat treatment may be necessary.

Ivermectin

Owing to its efficacy in killing microfilariae of *O. volvulus*, studies were initiated to test the efficiency of ivermectin against *W. bancrofti* and *B. malayi* (Table 82.2). Results indicated that a single oral dose of ivermectin (150 μg/kg body weight) effectively removes microfilariae of *W. bancrofti*,[61] but microfilariae reappear in the blood faster than after treatment with a dose of DEC and there is no evidence of a macrofilaricidal effect.[62] In brugian filariasis the fall in microfilaraemia is more gradual than is the case in bancroftian filariasis. Side effects of ivermectin therapy are generally similar to those mentioned above for DEC. A comparative evaluation of efficacy and tolerability of a single dose of the two drugs has been carried out.[63] Ivermectin should not be used in pregnant women or in children below 5 years of age.

The major role of ivermectin in lymphatic filariasis is for treatment and control of infection in areas that are co-endemic for onchocerciasis and/or loiasis (i.e., many parts of Africa). Since it has no macrofilaricidal effect,

repeated half-yearly or yearly treatments are needed to keep the microfilaraemia at a low level. Ivermectin also has an effect against *Ascaris*, hookworm and scabies infection.

Symptomatic treatment

It has increasingly been recognized that microbial co-infections play an important role in the aetiology of most ADL attacks, and that foot care combined with antibiotic and antifungal therapy can play an important role in their prevention and cure.[64,65]

Chronic lymphoedema and elephantiasis can also benefit greatly from prevention and treatment of superficial bacterial and fungal infections. Patient education should emphasize the importance of hygiene and skin care to reduce the number of acute attacks and thereby to prevent progression of the disease. Wearing of shoes, made to fit the often deformed feet, is an important way to limit the risk of skin lesions. Physiotherapy and bandaging are more professional approaches which can be very helpful to alleviate and reduce the lymphoedema. Elevation of the affected limb during rest and sleep may also be beneficial.

Surgical management

Before any surgical procedure, a course of DEC is recommended. Chronic hydroceles require excision and eversion of the sac. In scrotal elephantiasis the surgical removal of the grossly elephantoid skin and scrotal tissues with preservation of the penis and testicles has proved worthwhile. Surgical treatment of limb elephantiasis has generally proved unsuccessful. Earlier techniques involving the excision of redundant tissue from severely affected limbs generally led to long-term results that were unsatisfactory. More beneficial responses have been obtained recently with lymphovenous procedures, followed by removal of excess subcutaneous and fatty tissue from the affected extremities and adequate postural drainage and physiotherapy. In chyluria, if conservative approaches using DEC therapy and restriction of dietary fats are not helpful, then surgery is indicated.

Epidemiology

Humans are infected by mosquitoes carrying infective larvae. There is no evidence for animals being infected with *W. bancrofti* under natural conditions. The nocturnally periodic form of *B. malayi* has been reported only in humans, but the subperiodic form is found also in a wide variety of domestic and wild animals (monkeys, cats). There appears to be no animal reservoir of *B. timori*.

Microfilariae of all species can be transmitted in blood transfusions and will circulate in the recipient's blood for weeks. Congenital transmission of microfilariae has been reported but seems to be of little significance, and these microfilariae do not undergo further development.

Infection and disease in the endemic community

Characteristic patterns of microfilaraemia, circulating antigenaemia and disease are seen in affected populations in endemic areas.[18,20,66] An example of this pattern in a highly *W. bancrofti* endemic East African village is seen in Figure 82.12. Usually, microfilaraemia starts to appear in children of about 5 years of age. The prevalence then rises with increasing age and commences to level out above the age of 30 years. The prevalence rarely goes above 40–50% in any age group. It may decrease slightly in older persons. The prevalence of specific circulating antigenaemia is higher than that of microfilaraemia in all age groups. Signs of disease begin to develop around the onset of puberty or in early adult life, with recurrent ADL attacks. Hydroceles also begin to appear around this age. The prevalence of signs rises steadily, and in highly endemic areas the majority of elderly males may have hydroceles. In stable endemic communities elephantiasis is seen mainly in older people, but younger persons may also be affected. The overall burden of infection and disease in the endemic community is proportional to the intensity of transmission.

Cross-sectional surveys, although providing important information on the distribution of infection and disease in the affected population, give only a static view of the situation. In reality there is a dynamic sequel in development of infection and disease. Many of the people who are amicrofilaraemic during the survey have tested positive for microfilariae previously, or will become so later. Also, clinical manifestations often develop late in the course of infection, when some people have already reached an amicrofilaraemic stage. In many surveys the prevalence and intensity of microfilaraemia has been slightly higher in males than in females, and this appears to be especially significant for those aged 15–40-years. It has been suggested that hormonal factors in females of reproductive age make them more resistant to infection than males of the same age group.[67]

Exposure to intense transmission over long periods is necessary before a patent infection with microfilariae is acquired, and visitors to endemic areas rarely acquire microfilaraemia. Prenatal exposure to parasite antigens may explain why children born to microfilaraemic mothers appear to have a higher chance of developing microfilaraemia later, than do those born to amicrofilaraemic mothers,[20,68] but increased household exposure may also be a contributing factor.[69]

Geographical variation in transmission

The epidemiology of *W. bancrofti* and *B. malayi* infections varies in different geographical areas, especially with respect to the prevalence and intensity of infection, the transmission pattern and the clinical manifestations. Differences in vectorial capacity and density are

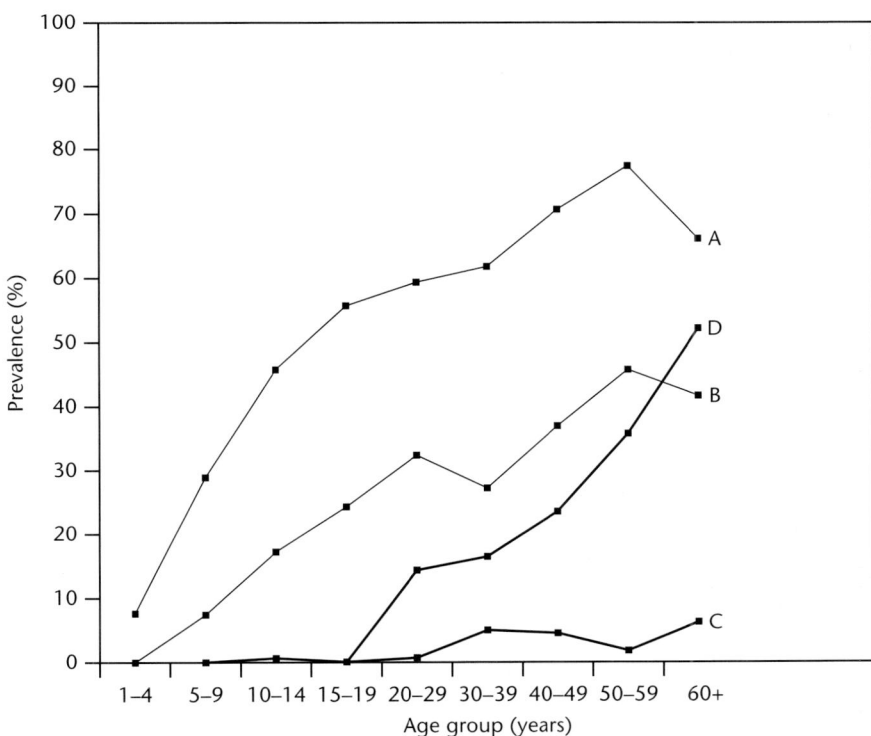

Figure 82.12: *W. bancrofti* infection and chronic disease in an endemic village on the coast of north-east Tanzania. Prevalence of (**A**) circulating filarial antigenaemia, (**B**) microfilaraemia and (**C**) elephantiasis in the whole population and (**D**) the prevalence of hydrocele grade 2 and above among the males. (Based on Simonsen et al.[66])

important factors influencing these epidemiological parameters in different endemic areas. There are also inherent differences in the parasite; for example, three strains of *W. bancrofti* and two strains of *B. malayi* have been recognized on the basis of differences in periodicity of the microfilariae. It is possible that variation in worm habitat preferences within the host's lymphatic system may contribute to differences in clinical manifestations.

In most areas the microfilariae of *W. bancrofti* are nocturnally periodic, being adapted to transmission by night-biting *Culex* and *Anopheles* mosquitoes. A diurnal subperiodic form is found in the South Pacific and in the Andaman and Nicobar Islands (India), whereas a nocturnally subperiodic form is found in Thailand. *B. malayi* occurs both in a nocturnal periodic and a nocturnal subperiodic form, whereas *B. timori* is nocturnally periodic. The subperiodic forms are transmitted by vectors that bite mainly during the daytime.

For details of the vector species and their bionomics, see Appendix IV. The different geographical vector zones are also shown in Figure 82.2. *Culex quinquefasciatus* is the principal vector of *W. bancrofti* in urban and semiurban areas of southern and South-East Asia, East Africa and America. Increased pollution of freshwater bodies and the introduction of pit latrines, which favour breeding of this mosquito, has led to increased transmission in many areas. *C. quinquefasciatus* is an endophilic night-biter. There is no evidence that it is transmitting filariasis in West Africa. In rural areas of Asia and Africa, *Anopheles* spp. are the main vectors, with the *A. gambiae* complex and *A. funestus* being the most important vectors in Africa. The main vectors of the *Anopheles* spp. bite indoors at night and breed in open, rather clean, water.

In the South Pacific islands the predominant vectors of *W. bancrofti* belong to day-biting *Aedes* spp., especially *A. polynesiensis*. The majority of these mosquitoes bite outdoors and breed in small temporary water collections: tree holes, empty cans and bottles, coconut shells, plant axils and crab holes. In Papua New Guinea night-biting *Anopheles* spp. are the principal vectors.

The nocturnally subperiodic form of *B. malayi* is transmitted by *Mansonia* mosquitoes in dense swamp forest areas. This form is commonly found also in wild monkeys. Nocturnally periodic *B. malayi* has been reported only from humans. It is transmitted in open plains and agricultural areas, mainly by *Mansonia* spp. mosquitoes, although in some areas species of *Anopheles* and *Aedes* also play a role. The larvae and pupae of *Mansonia* mosquitoes obtain their oxygen directly from the cells of certain species of aquatic plants present in clean waterbodies. Survival of the *Mansonia* spp. is dependent on the association with the plants. Increased pollution has in some places led to a decrease in breeding of *Mansonia*, with a subsequent drop in transmission of *B. malayi*. *Mansonia* spp. prefer to feed outside and biting usually commences shortly after dusk. *A. barbirostris* is the only mosquito to date to have been identified as a vector of *B. timori*.

Control

In communities endemic for lymphatic filariasis the disfiguring and debilitating clinical manifestations result in much suffering and have severe socio-economic and psychological consequences for those affected.[70,71] The objective of control is to reduce transmission and morbidity, thereby eliminating lymphatic filariasis as a public health problem. Successful programmes for the control of lymphatic filariasis must be based on a thorough understanding of the distribution and dynamics of the disease in the targeted population. The diverse characteristics of communities in endemic foci, as well as differences in vector, parasite and disease parameters, emphasize the importance of having multiple measures and approaches for control.

The main method used in the control of lymphatic filariasis is mass chemotherapy. It may be supplemented by mosquito control. Morbidity control through patient management (hygiene, antimicrobial treatment, physiotherapy) and establishment of self-help groups is recommended, but experience is limited. To achieve success in a control programme it is necessary for the community to be actively involved. Community leaders and motivated persons should be identified and approached for the purpose of obtaining their cooperation. Adequate health education should be given regarding the nature of the disease and on the methods used for its control.

Before starting a control programme, knowledge of the geographical delimitation of the disease is essential. Rapid assessment procedures are based on examination of specific age–sex groups in selected populations to determine the prevalence of easily recognizable signs such as hydrocele or circulating antigenaemia.[72,73] Geographical information system (GIS) has been utilized for large-scale mapping of the disease, for instance in Africa and India.[74,75] All areas with indigenously acquired infections are considered to be endemic. Criteria for distinguishing different levels of endemicity have so far not been established.

Mathematical models of lymphatic filariasis transmission, infection and disease within the endemic community have been developed and are being validated.[76,77] It is hoped that such models can be used to predict the outcome of control based on different measures, and thus can provide guidance towards the most cost-effective control strategies in specific settings.

Chemotherapeutic control

Chemotherapeutic control of lymphatic filariasis is generally based on mass treatment, i.e., the drug is administered to the total population in the community (except individuals in whom it is contraindicated). In mass treatment campaigns there is no need to conduct parasitological or other diagnoses before treatment. Thus cost is reduced. The amicrofilaraemic infections and persons who may have been falsely negative in a diagnostic test are included for treatment. A continued high population treatment coverage is essential for a mass treatment programme to produce sustained reduction in transmission.[78]

Chemotherapeutic regimens of DEC have been used for several decades for the control of bancroftian and brugian filariasis. DEC is relatively cheap, it rapidly reduces the prevalence and intensity of microfilaraemia, and it also kills a proportion of the adult worms. The efficacy and side effects of the normal 12-day standard regimen of DEC are discussed above under Management. This regimen, however, is not feasible for use on a mass scale because of the many daily dosages. Rather, the drug may be administered in widely spaced doses, in regularly repeated low doses, or it may be added to salt. These regimens effectively reduce microfilaraemias and have fewer and less severe side effects than the more intensive regimens. Control programmes with DEC-medicated salt have successfully controlled lymphatic filariasis in parts of China and Taiwan. Recent comparative trials in Tanzania have shown that a semi-annual single dose of DEC (6 mg/kg body weight), a monthly low dose of DEC (100 mg to adults and 50 mg to children), or administration of medicated cooking salt (0.3% DEC) were more effective in reducing microfilaraemias over a 4-year follow-up period than the standard 12-day intensive regimen.[79] The low-dose and the medicated salt strategies were by far the most effective.

Owing to the risk of inducing severe adverse reactions in individuals with onchocerciasis, DEC should not be used on a mass scale for control of lymphatic filariasis in areas co-endemic for *O. volvulus* infection. For these areas, ivermectin is the drug of choice. When distributed in a dose of 150 μg/kg body weight it effectively reduces microfilaraemias. Side effects are few and comparable to those of DEC. Adult worms are not affected by the ivermectin treatment, and regularly repeated treatments (half-yearly or yearly) are therefore even more important in control programmes based on ivermectin than for those based on DEC, to gain a long-term effect on transmission. Since 1998, ivermectin has been available free of charge for control of lymphatic filariasis in countries of Africa with endemic onchocerciasis, through the Mectizan Donation Program. Combinations of DEC and ivermectin have proved even more effective in lymphatic filariasis than any of the drugs alone but, because ivermectin is currently available only in countries where the use of DEC is contraindicated, this increased effect is of mainly theoretical interest.

The combination of albendazole with either ivermectin or DEC appeared in recent studies to give a considerably more effective and sustained reduction in lymphatic filariasis microfilaraemia than ivermectin or DEC alone.[73,80] Macrofilaricidal properties of albendazole apparently prolonged and reinforced the microfilaricidal suppression produced by the other two drugs. Following these promising findings it was recommended that DEC and ivermectin should be given in combination with albendazole in programmes for lymphatic filariasis control. The effect of albendazole on intestinal helminth infections would be an additional benefit of the combi-

nation treatments.[81] Other recent studies have failed to provide clear evidence for the superiority of these combinations in the clearing of microfilaraemias.[82,83]

Mosquito control

Vector control can provide a useful supplement to chemotherapy in control of lymphatic filariasis. Effective vector control rapidly reduces transmission but, because it is slow to reduce the prevalence of filariasis in a population, it should be combined with chemotherapy. The feasibility and value of vector control as one of the components of filariasis control depends upon the local epidemiological conditions, including the species of vectors, their biting, resting and breeding habits, and the type of environment (e.g., rural or urban).

The main antivector measures that have been used in the control of filariasis are environmental control of breeding sites, larviciding, and the use of insecticides against adult mosquitoes. Environmental management varies from the filling in of temporary pools and clearing of refuse that collects water, to the construction of drainage systems in urban areas. *C. quinquefasciatus* breeds in highly polluted water and plays a major role in the transmission of *W. bancrofti* in urban and semi-urban areas. A new method, aimed at controlling *C. quinquefasciatus* in stagnant water, especially cesspits and latrines, utilizes a layer of expanded polystyrene beads that float on the water surface and prevent the mosquito larvae from breathing (Figure 82.13). This method has proved to be long lasting and has been successful in filariasis control in Zanzibar.[84] The usefulness of *Bacillus sphaericus*, a toxin-producing bacteria, as a biological agent for control of *C. quinquefasciatus* is also being assessed.

Anopheles vectors are responsible for transmission of much rural filariasis. In areas where malaria and filariasis transmission depends on the same *Anopheles* species or

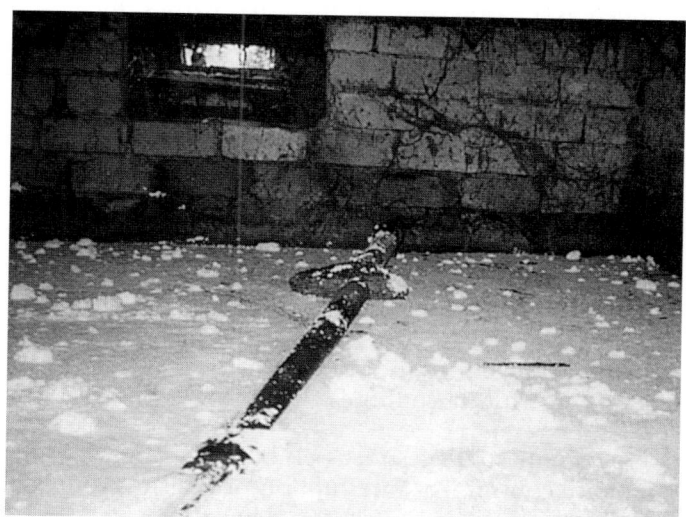

Figure 82.13: Flooded cellar (heavily infested with *C. quinquefasciatus*) in Zanzibar after treatment with polystyrene beads. (Courtesy of C. Curtis.)

vectors with similar bionomics, filariasis control may benefit from malaria vector control programmes. In the Solomon Islands, bancroftian filariasis was eliminated as a result of a malaria control programme utilizing residual insecticides against *Anopheles* mosquitoes. Because of variability in feeding behaviour and resting places of *Mansonia* mosquitoes, control using insecticides is not very effective. *Mansonia* larvae are best controlled by destruction of the host plants. *Aedes* vectors have scattered and inaccessible breeding sites, and vector control is not easily accomplished.

Disadvantages of using chemical insecticides in control schemes may include their high cost, development of resistance by the target organisms and environmental damage. Despite these problems insecticides remain the major weapon in the control of vectors. The use of pyrethroid-impregnated bed nets can significantly reduce morbidity due to malaria and has recently been shown to have a strong suppressive effect on the transmission of lymphatic filariasis.[85]

Programme for global elimination

Increased awareness of the public health burden of lymphatic filariasis combined with development of better tools for diagnosis, development of effective mass drug treatment strategies, and improved knowledge on disease development processes has greatly stimulated political interest and commitment towards its control. Compared with many other vector-borne diseases, a number of biological features furthermore favours the control of lymphatic filariasis, namely its almost exclusive human reservoir, its inability to multiply in the vectors and its inefficiency of transmission.

In 1997, the World Health Assembly called for a strengthening of activities to eliminate lymphatic filariasis as a public health problem. Subsequently, the Global Programme to Eliminate Lymphatic Filariasis was founded as a partnership of interested parties, including ministries of health from endemic countries, international and national development agencies and academic institutions, and with the World Health Organization (WHO) serving as the secretariat.[86] In essence, the programme assists in the preparation of national plans of actions for individual endemic countries, and coordinates and advises on financial, technical and managerial matters. The programme is supported by a large-scale donation of albendazole for worldwide elimination of lymphatic filariasis (from Glaxo SmithKline), and by an expansion of the Mectizan Donation Program for onchocerciasis to include free ivermectin for elimination of lymphatic filariasis in African countries where the two infections coexist.

Programme strategies focus on both transmission and morbidity control. For interruption of transmission, it is recommended that the entire population at risk be treated once yearly with single-dose two-drug regimens (albendazole 400 mg plus ivermectin 150 µg/kg in countries of Africa co-endemic for onchocerciasis; albendazole 400 mg plus DEC 6 mg/kg in other parts of the world). Treatment should continue until the level of microfilariae in the blood is below the level required for transmission (estimated at 4–6 years). Alternatively, daily treatment for a 6–12-month period with DEC-medicated salt is recommended. Morbidity control focuses on improved hygiene, treatment of secondary infections and proper limb care to alleviate suffering and decrease disability among those already affected. To ensure sustainability of programme activities, the design of filariasis control programmes emphasizes their integration into existing national health structures and facilities.

Onchocerciasis

Onchocerciasis (river blindness) results from infection with *Onchocerca volvulus*. Humans are the natural hosts and the vectors are species of blackflies (*Simulium* spp.). In endemic regions it is a major cause of severe disfiguring skin changes and damaging eye lesions.

Historical background

In 1875, in the Gold Coast (now Ghana), John O'Neill described microfilariae recovered from the skin of Africans suffering from 'craw-craw'.[87] Later (1893) Rudolf Leuckart described the adult worms and named the parasite *Filaria volvulus*. Rodolfo Robles,[88] working in Guatemala, first associated subcutaneous nodules with eye lesions. The pioneer studies of Donald Blacklock[89] in Sierra Leone culminated in the discovery of the life cycle of *O. volvulus*. A detailed history of onchocerciasis has been written.[7]

Geographical distribution

It is estimated that about 17.5 million individuals worldwide are infected with *O. volvulus*, of whom some 270 000 are blind and 500 000 are severely visually disabled[90] (Figures 82.14 and 82.15). More than 99% of all cases are in Africa in a zone that spreads from west to east. This band extends between 15° N and 15° S in the west, widening slightly towards the east.

Foci in Guatemala and Mexico of about 90 000 infected individuals exist mainly on the Pacific slope of the Sierra Madra between altitudes of 500 and 1500 m. Northern Venezuela has a focus with about 40 000 infected individuals. Smaller foci have been found in southern Venezuela, Columbia, Brazil, Ecuador and Yemen.[90]

Life cycle and transmission

The general filarial life cycle is shown in Figure 82.1. For details of the life cycle of *O. volvulus*, see also Appendix III.

Adult worms live mainly in subcutaneous nodules or are free in the skin. The ratio of adult females : males in

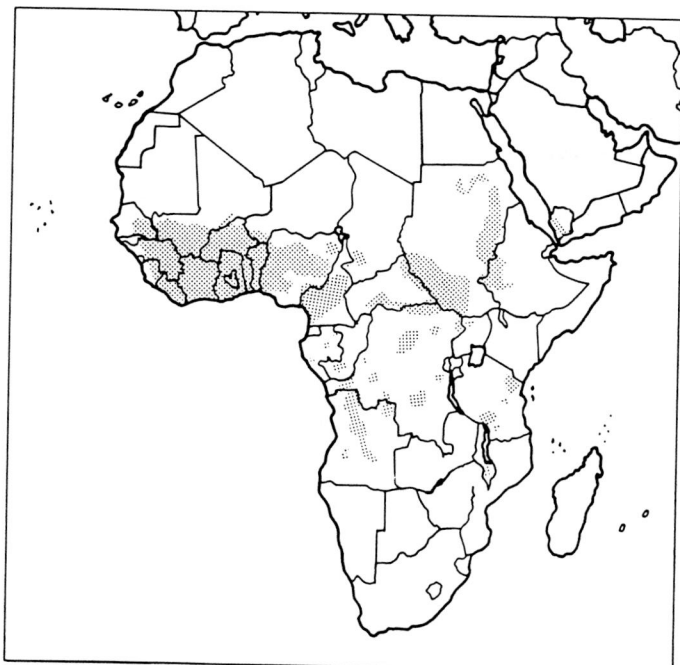

Figure 82.14: Geographical distribution of onchocerciasis in Africa and the Arabian peninsula.

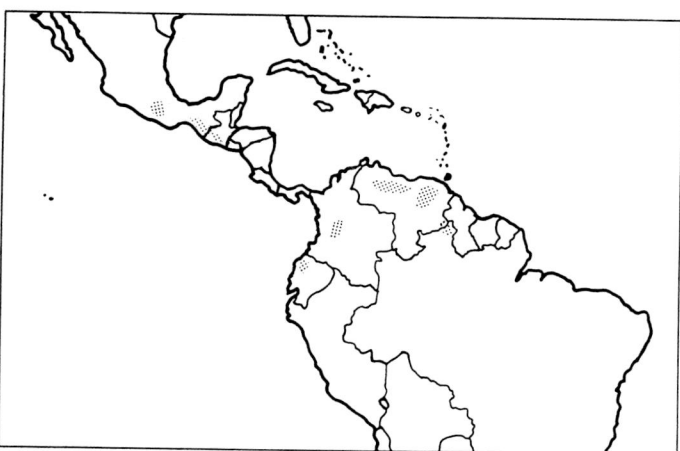

Figure 82.15: Geographical distribution of onchocerciasis in Central and South America.

nodules is about 3 : 1. The adults are slender white worms, the male being 2–5 cm × 0.2 mm and the females 35–70 cm × 0.4 mm. The female produces sheathless microfilariae measuring 300 × 8 μm with an expanded head free of nuclei and a sharply pointed tail (Figure 82.16A).

Microfilariae are found mainly in the upper dermis and in nodules but may also appear in blood, urine or any body fluid, particularly after treatment with DEC. They are common in the eye, with direct spread from adjacent skin appearing to be their main mode of entry. Microfilarial loads can be as high as 2000 per mg of skin, and heavily infected individuals may harbour more than 100 000 000 microfilariae.[91] The microfilariae have a lifespan of 1–2 years.

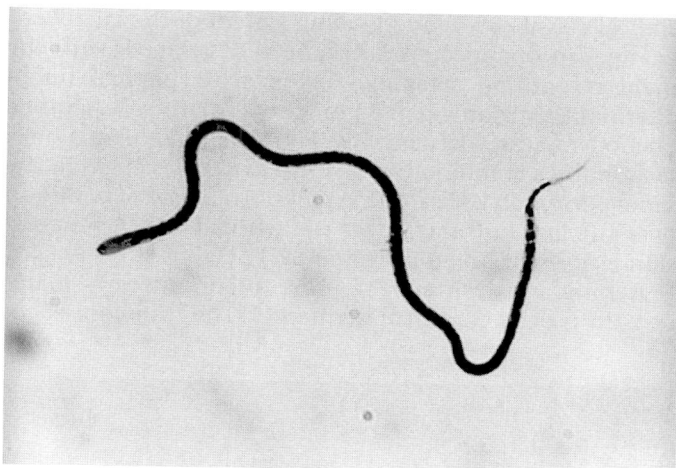

Figure 82.16: Skin microfilaria of *O. volvulus.*

Microfilariae present in the skin are ingested by the *Simulium* vector when feeding. Some of the ingested microfilariae migrate from the gut of the blackfly into the thoracic muscles and develop via two moults into infective larvae over a period of 6–12 days (for a description of the development in the fly see Appendix III, and for the life history of *Simulium* see Appendix IV). Transmission of infective larvae to humans occurs when the fly takes its next blood meal. The larvae migrate to the subcutaneous tissues, moult twice, and then develop over several months to adult worms. The gravid female releases microfilariae, which may appear in the skin after a prepatent period of 10–15 months after the introduction of infective larvae. Some 500–1500 microfilariae are released per female per day, and the mean duration of female reproductive life has been estimated at 9–11 years.

Simulium flies can breed only in well oxygenated water. The gravid female oviposits into free-flowing rivers and streams, particularly in rapids, and transmission takes place mainly near these locations, hence the name 'river blindness'.

Transmission in utero of microfilariae of *O. volvulus* has been reported. These microfilariae do not undergo further development.

Clinical features

The main clinical manifestations of onchocerciasis are skin lesions, eye lesions and nodule formation. In general, clinical manifestations develop after long exposure to infection, and their severity depends on the intensity of infection. Many individuals who have microfilariae in the skin, especially those with light infections, have no symptoms or signs.

Skin lesions

Dermal changes occur when the microfilariae undergo destruction in the skin and vary from a few papules to the extensive pigmentary and chronic atrophic changes.[92] A clinical classification and grading system of the cutaneous changes in onchocerciasis has been developed, with the main recognized categories being acute papular onchodermatitis, chronic papular onchodermatitis, lichenified onchodermatitis, skin atrophy, and skin depigmentation.[93] Frequently a combination of these categories exists in the same person. In Africa, the skin lesions are most common over the legs but may cover the whole body. A range of skin lesions is shown in Figure 82.17.

Itching and rash are the most important early manifestations of onchocercal dermatitis. The rash consists of many raised papules, which are due to microabscess formation, and may disappear within a few days or may spread. Often the rash is confined to one anatomical quarter of the body. The resulting pruritus can be very intense ('gale filarienne', filarial itch), and the skin often becomes secondarily infected following scratching. In the later stages there may be heavy lichenification and thickening of the skin (lizard skin).

The more chronic changes are probably related to the repeated occurrence of local pathology around dying parasites. There is skin atrophy with loss of elasticity,

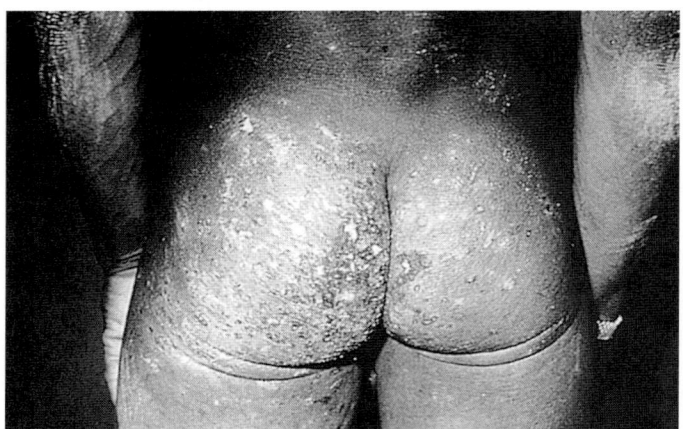

A

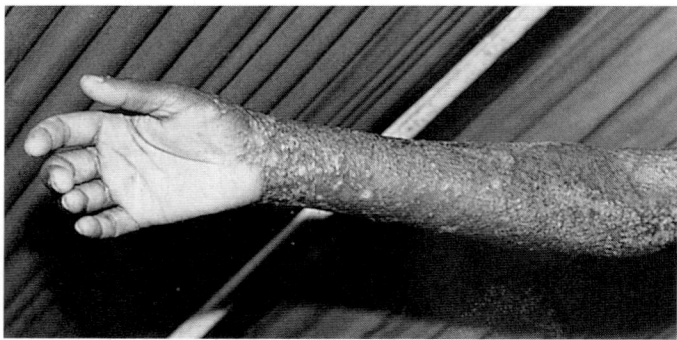

C

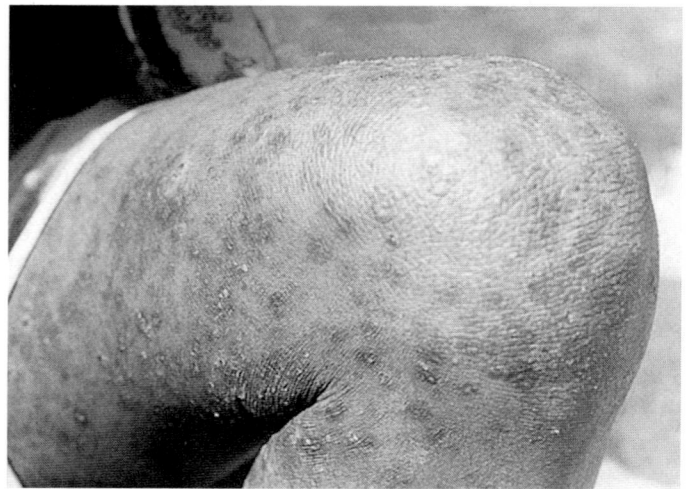

D

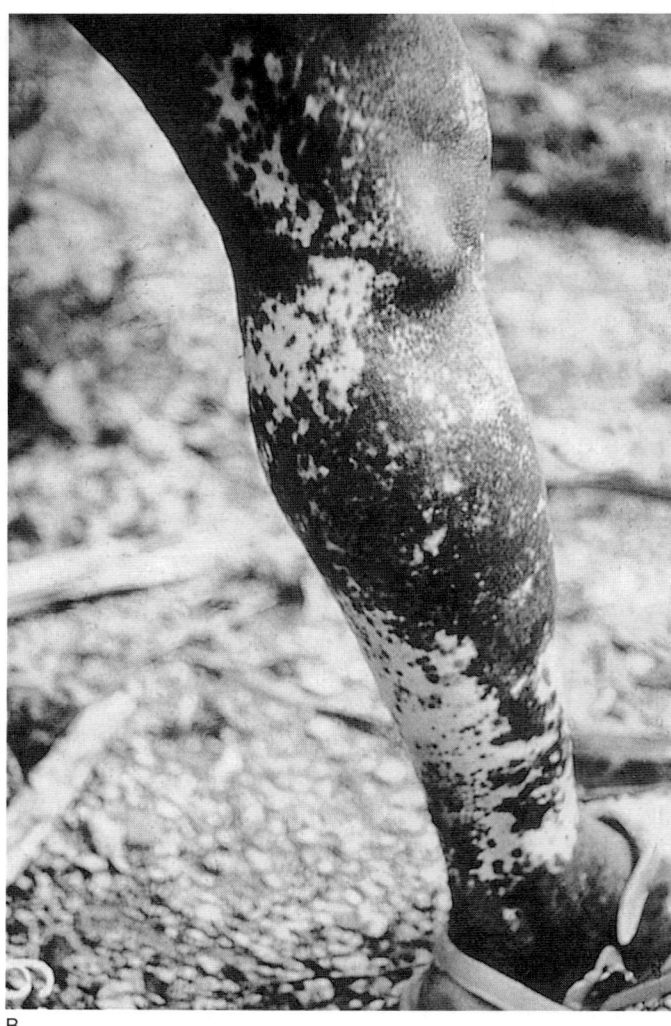

B

Figure 82.17: Onchocerciasis: skin lesions. (**A**) Papule formation and scratching (courtesy of WHO); (**B**) depigmentation and leopard skin (courtesy of WHO); (**C**) lichenified eczematoid dermatitis of the arm and (**D**) of the leg (courtesy of D. Morgan).

giving a prematurely aged appearance (presbyderma). Loss of elastic fibres in the skin of the groin may lead to hernia, and to the classical 'hanging groin' with inguinal and/or femoral glands contained in pendulous folds.

A condition called leopard skin (Figure 82.17B) may occur. This results from loss of pigment, degeneration of the dermal collagen and thinning of the epidermis. Leopard skin particularly affects the pretibial regions, where trauma or scratching following the bites of *Simulium* flies may exacerbate, or even cause, the depigmentation of this condition.

Sowda

Sowda (Figure 82.18), from the Arabic for black or dark, is a localized form of onchodermatitis. It is common in the Yemen, but is also found in the northern Sudan and in West Africa. It has also been described from Guatemala.

Sowda is the result of a strong immune response on the part of the host. The condition is usually localized to one limb but both legs and/or arms or the trunk may be involved. It is characterized by intense itching. The involved skin becomes swollen and darkened, and covered with scaly papules. Local lymph glands are enlarged. Microfilariae are extremely difficult to find in skin snips.

Nodules

Nodules (onchocercomata) are subcutaneous granulomas resulting from a tissue reaction around adult worms. They are most often located in the subcutaneous tissues. They are painless, round to oval, firm, smooth, vary in

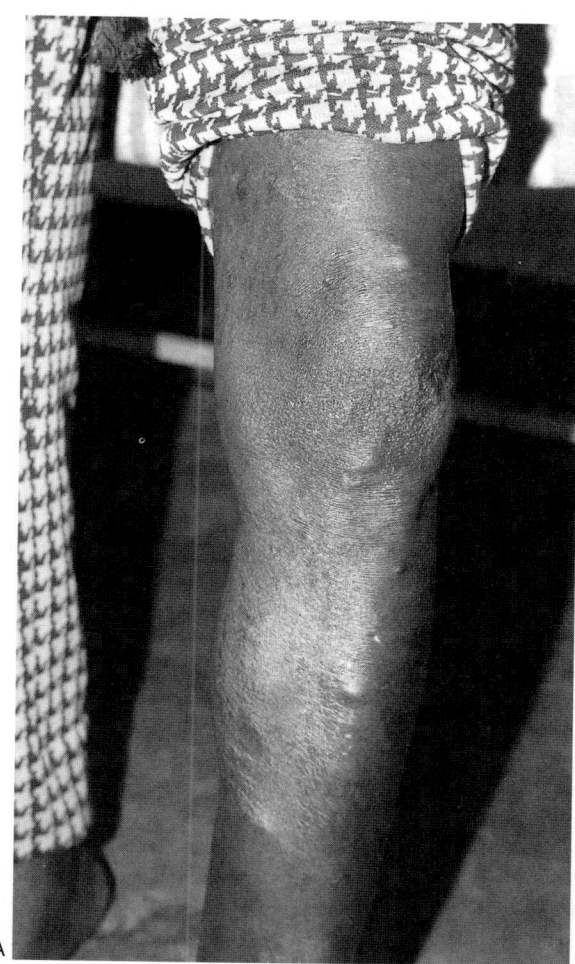

A

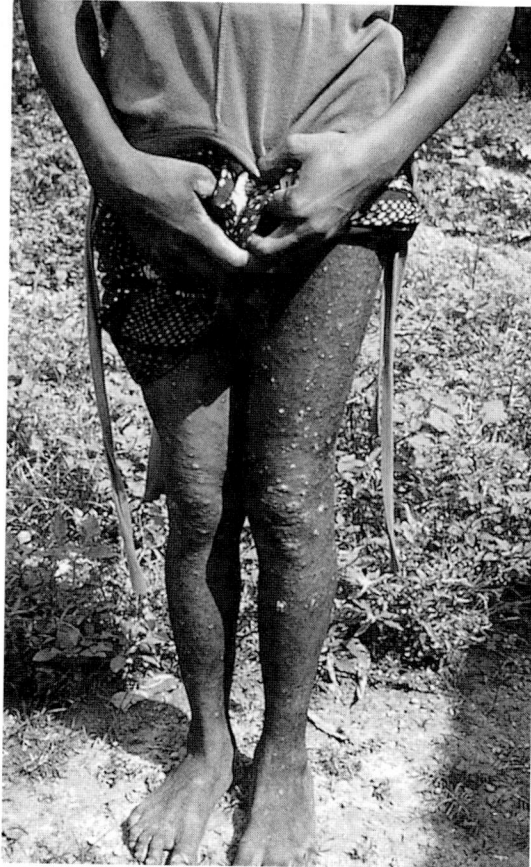

Figure 82.18: Onchocerciasis: Sowda. (Courtesy of D. Morgan.)

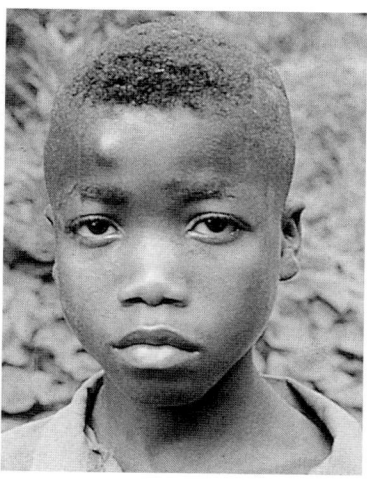

B

Figure 82.19: Onchocerciasis: nodules: (**A**) on leg; (**B**) on head. (Courtesy of D. Morgan.)

size from a few millimetres to several centimetres and are often matted together in clumps (Figure 82.19).

Some, perhaps one-quarter of nodules, are found in deeper tissues and are not palpable. In Africa 80% of palpable nodules occur on the body prominences of the pelvic girdle. Others occur on the abdomen, chest wall, head or limbs. In Central America, palpable nodules are commonly found on the head. It is believed that the location of the nodules reflects the biting habits of the vector flies. Nodules do not cause medical problems unless they press on vital areas. Large clumps are often aesthetically displeasing to the patient.

Eye lesions

Many changes in both anterior and posterior segments can occur in the eyes of infected individuals.[94] The more serious lesions may progress to blindness (see also Chapter 18).

Anterior segment lesions

Punctate keratitis (snowflake opacities) occurs as an acute inflammatory reaction around microfilariae (Figure 82.20). It appears to be the corneal equivalent of the discrete papule reactions seen in the skin. Punctate keratitis is more common in the younger age groups. These lesions are reversible. In sclerosing keratitis, vascular infiltrates begin at the limbus and pass inwards, resulting in a cellular organization and excessive scarring of the cornea, which causes blindness.

Microfilariae dying in the ciliary body give rise to iridocyclitis and the formation of synechiae. Inflammation of the uveal tract also contributes to iridial pathology.

Posterior segment lesions

Both optic nerve atrophy and choroidoretinitis of the posterior segment may result in blindness. Lesions of choroidoretinitis range from unequivocal inflammatory processes to exclusively atrophic lesions with atrophy

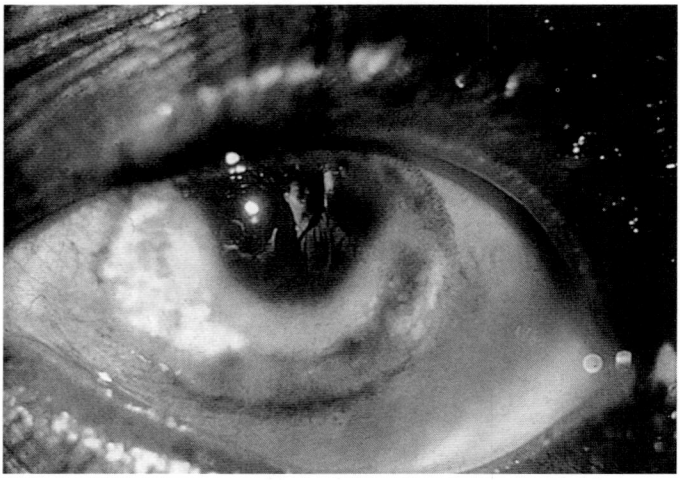

Figure 82.20: Onchocerciasis: punctate keratitis.

of the retinal pigment epithelium and of the chorio-capillaris and hyperpigmentation of the pigment epithelial layer.

Optic nerve atrophy rather than choroidoretinal degeneration is considered to be an important cause of both decreased visual acuity and visual field constriction. Acceleration of optic nerve damage may follow treatment with DEC. In fact, with any of the eye lesions, exacerbation associated with the death of microfilariae may be a complication of drug therapy.

Other conditions

Onchocerciasis has been associated with weight loss and musculoskeletal pain. Several reports have indicated a higher than normal frequency of epilepsy in onchocerciasis hyperendemic areas, but a recent case–control study in the Central African Republic found no statistical significant association.[95] Onchocerciasis has also been associated with a syndrome of growth arrest and delayed sexual development (the Nakalanga syndrome) seen in Uganda and Burundi.[96]

Geographical variation in clinical picture

Clinical manifestations (skin and eye lesions) are known to differ widely in varied endemic geographical areas.[97] Surveys in Cameroon showed the prevalence of sclerosing keratitis and blindness to be much higher in savannah than in forest areas.[98] This picture appeared to be valid for most of West Africa, with a gradation from very severe ocular lesions in the dry (Sudan type) savannah, to moderately severe in wet savannah areas, to a much lower prevalence of eye lesions in forest zones. The pattern in Sierre Leone is different from this more general observation, in that the prevalence of blindness and sclerosing keratitis is higher in the forest than in the savannah areas (Figure 82.21).[99]

In East and Central Africa the clinical picture of onchocerciasis is generally less severe, and eye manifestations are rare in most parts. In the Yemen, and in some parts of the Sudan, a severe form of Sowda occurs. The proportion of head nodules in Mexico and Guatemala is much higher than in Africa, and these may be associated with a high prevalence of severe ocular onchocerciasis.

Pathology and immunology

Large numbers of live microfilariae may be present in the skin without inducing any tissue reaction (Figure 82.22). Pathology in the skin and in the anterior segment of the eye is caused mainly by dying and dead microfilariae.

The initial lesions comprise foci of inflammatory reactions around degenerating microfilariae, composed mainly of eosinophils, neutrophils and macrophages.[100–102] Antibodies, immune complex formation and complement activation on the surface of the microfilariae may be microsporidiosis, but serum vitamin B$_{12}$ concentrations were not reduced.

Immunity

There are few data regarding immune responses to microsporidia, and serological studies are very limited.

Clinical features

E. bieneusi infection is most frequently diagnosed in patients with AIDS and persistent diarrhoea. Among 38 HIV-seropositive patients with the infection, only one did not have diarrhoea,[163] and most series do not report any asymptomatic infections. Patients in this Australian study had a mean duration of diarrhoea of 7 months and a mean peripheral blood CD4 cell count of 40×10^6/l. The volume of the diarrhoea is variable, and is associated with anorexia, nausea and crampy abdominal pain.[161] This is probably true of all forms of AIDS-related diarrhoea.

There are several reports in the literature of a sclerosing cholangitis-like syndrome,[163,164] indistinguishable from that associated with cryptosporidiosis.

Diagnosis

Definitive diagnosis relies on electron microscopy. Early meronts are recognized by the paler appearance of the cytoplasm relative to that of the host cell (Figure 77.10). The hallmark of the late meront or sporont is the development of the characteristic electron-dense polar tube, which has about 5 to 7.5 coils. Other characteristics include the presence of electron-lucent inclusions (ELIs) and electron-dense discs (EDDs). Spores are identifiable by their intensely osmophilic walls.

Light microscopic diagnosis of histological sections of small bowel biopsy material is possible using careful scanning of sections stained with Giemsa,[159] Brown–Hopps or Warthin–Starry. Biopsies obtained from the distal duodenum are perfectly adequate, and either light or electron microscopy provides a more sensitive diagnostic tool than stool examination.[165]

Detection of spores in stool has become possible. The use of chromotrope 2R[166] may be the most practical approach.

Management

Albendazole is the treatment of choice.[167] Albendazole inhibits microtubule formation, and thus reduces cell division and possibly polar tube action. The usual dose is 400 mg twice daily for 4 weeks, but there is evidence that *E. bieneusi* responds much less satisfactorily than *E. intestinalis*.[168]

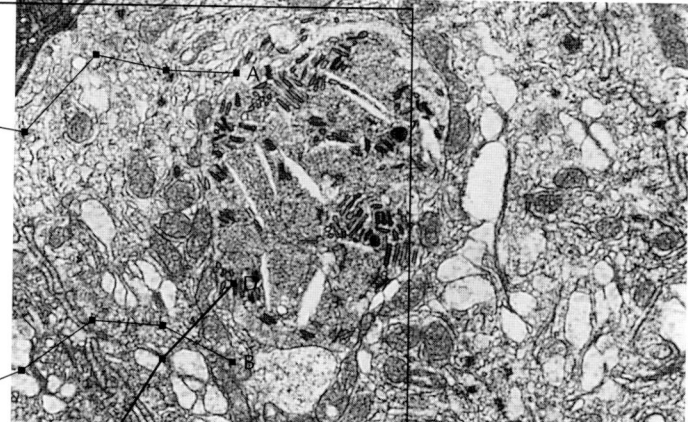

Figure 77.10: Meront of *Enterocytozoon bieneusi*, showing EDDs. (Magnification × 20 000.) (Courtesy of Graham McPhail.)

Encephalitozoon spp.

Unlike *Enterocytozoon bieneusi*, *Encephalitozoon* spp. are widespread amongst other vertebrates. *Encephalitozoon cuniculi* is the best known, and differs from *Enterocytozoon bieneusi* in that all stages lie within a parasitophorous vacuole and it does not cause enteropathy. Five human cases have been recorded, three with neurological disorders, one with hepatitis and one with peritonitis in a patient with AIDS.[157] However, serological testing for *Encephalitozoon cuniculi* indicates that exposure to this microsporidian may in fact be quite common.[169]

Recently, infection with *Enterocytozoon hellem* has been described in patients with AIDS, with corneal infection and disseminated disease involving lungs and kidneys, but not the gastrointestinal tract.

Another microsporidian, *Encephalitozoon intestinalis*, has been reported in patients with AIDS in developed countries and in Africa. The first case was of chronic diarrhoea due to an organism resembling, but distinct from, *Encephalitozoon cuniculi*. Subsequently, it has become apparent that this microsporidian is capable of dissemination, leading to an interstitial nephritis. The microsporidia may be found in lamina propria macrophages, and free spores can be found in the renal vasculature and portal vein. The spores are then shed in the urine. One of the characteristics of this organism is its development within a parasitophorous vacuole which is septated. For this reason, it was originally given the name *Septata intestinalis*. Most series report that it is less common in patients with AIDS and persistent diarrhoea than *E. bieneusi*, but it is more sensitive to albendazole.[170]

Figure 82.21: Onchocercal skin and ocular disease. Age-related prevalence for (A) blindness and/or severe eye lesions, (B) canthus skin snips, (C) in the cornea, and (D) in small bowel biopsies in rainforest villages of Sierra Leone. (After McMahon.)

Figure 82.22: Onchocercal microfilariae in the subcutaneous tissue.

infiltration of onchocercomata. The tissue between the early focal lesions shows no changes. Later, dermal fibroblasts increase in numbers, leading to fibrosis, and the normal collagen and elastic fibres of the dermis are gradually replaced by hyalinized scar tissue. There may also be loss of pigment in the skin. The histological appearance of the skin in advanced cases closely resembles that of very old subjects (i.e. presbyderma). Some of the skin damage observed in onchocerciasis patients may also be caused by the mechanical effects of scratching, by toxins inoculated when blackflies take a blood meal or by secondary infections.

In the skin condition Sowda, there is immunological hyperactivity, and the most striking histopathological feature is the presence of an extensive inflammatory cell infiltrate of the upper dermis. Identification of *O. volvulus* collagen as a principal antigen recognized by antibodies

posterior segment lesions is less clear. Autoantibodies against retinal proteins, cross-reacting with antibodies against *Onchocerca* antigens, were thought to be involved, but a more recent study showed no relationship between the antiretinal antibody levels and the occurrence of chorioretinitis in ocular onchocerciasis.

Some adult worms are found free in the subcutaneous tissues, but most are contained in nodules. Nodules are essentially granulomatous reactions around adult worms. They often have separate chambers containing several worms. Nodules have thick fibrous walls and a variable degree of cellular infiltration (Figure 82.23) with macrophages being the predominant cell type.[102] Calcification may occur in older nodules and in dead worms.

Specific humoral immune responses of individuals living in areas endemic for onchocerciasis are usually marked. Most infected individuals have a diminished

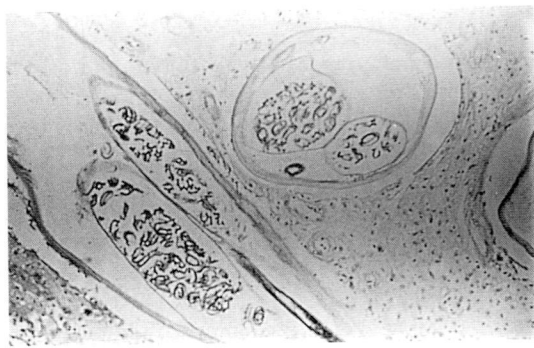

Figure 82.23: Onchocerciasis: adult *O. volvulus* in nodule. (Courtesy of H. Zaiman.)

cellular responsiveness to *O. volvulus* antigens in comparison to apparently uninfected persons from the same endemic areas and to patients with the more localized Sowda.[102] A major role of immune responses appears to be to contain or limit inflammation around dying or dead microfilariae. Antibodies mediating cellular killing of microfilariae and infective larvae in vitro have been observed in sera from some persons living in endemic areas.[103] The presence of such antibodies may indicate that immune elimination of larval stages occurs in some infected individuals, although protective immunity has not been proved in onchocerciasis. In utero exposure to *O. volvulus* antigens may affect the child's immune responses and perhaps his or her susceptibility to *O. volvulus* infection later in life.[106]

In individuals from non-endemic areas who become infected during visits to endemic areas, infections are usually mild and the most common clinical presentation is dermatitis.[107] Microfilaraemia may be of low density or absent. Nodules or eye lesions are rare. The patients usually have specific antibody responses to *O. volvulus* and raised eosinophil levels.

Immune responses to mycobacterial infections[108] and to tetanus vaccination[109] are downregulated in *O. volvulus*-infected individuals. HIV-infected onchocerciasis patients exhibit significantly impaired antibody responses to *O. volvulus* antigens and tend to loose their reactivity to these antigens over time.[110]

Diagnosis

Clinical diagnosis

Skin lesions, eye lesions and/or subcutaneous nodules resembling those described in the clinical section and presented by individuals who live in or have visited areas with transmission of *O. volvulus* may be indicative of onchocerciasis.

The pruritic onchodermatitis (filarial itch) must be distinguished from: infection with *Mansonella streptocerca*, in which the legs are rarely affected; scabies, where the typical burrows and mites can be found between the fingers; reactions to insect bites that come on early after residence in the tropics; prickly heat; and contact dermatitis. In heavy infections of long standing, the skin changes must be differentiated from tertiary yaws, superficial mycoses, leprosy and chronic eczema.

Painlessness, firmness and extreme mobility are characteristic of onchocercomas. However, some nodules, particularly those on the head, become fixed due to adherence to underlying tissues. Nodules must be distinguished from enlarged lymph glands, lipomas, dermal cysts, ganglia and neurofibromas.

For the diagnosis and differential diagnosis of onchocercal eye lesions, see Chapter 18.

Ultrasonography

Ultrasonography has proved capable of distinguishing onchocercal nodules in the tissues of patients.[111] This technique may be especially useful for detecting deep non-palpable nodules.

Mazzotti test

This test involves the administration of a small dose (usually 50 mg for an adult) of DEC by mouth. The death of microfilariae in the skin results in a reaction between 20 minutes and 24 hours later of intense pruritus, with the appearance of a skin rash or the exacerbation of an existing one. The test may precipitate serious complications and is not recommended as a routine diagnostic procedure. Either false-negative or false-positive results may also occur. The Mazzotti test can assist diagnosis when onchocerciasis is suspected in persons with a negative skin snip. A Mazzotti patch test using a topical application of DEC in lotion form on the skin has also been devised.

Parasitological diagnosis

The diagnosis is made by demonstrating microfilariae that have emerged from bloodless skin snips. Although most persons with clinical signs have positive skin snips, this is not always the case. The optimal site for the biopsy depends on the geographical area. In Africa, the preferred body site is from the iliac crest or below, whereas in Mexico the skin over the scapula or deltoid region is favoured. Two to four skin snips are taken. When epidemiological and clinical studies of onchocercal eye lesions are being conducted, it is important to take a skin snip from the outer canthus.

After cleaning the skin with spirit and allowing it to dry, a razor blade can be used to shave off the tip of a dome of skin that has been elevated with a needle. Alternatively a Walser corneoscleral punch is used to produce skin snips with an average weight of 1.0 mg. Punches must be very carefully sterilized before reuse. Snips are immersed in isotonic saline, for instance in wells of a microtitration plate. Microfilariae that have emerged after 0.5–24 hours are counted under the low power of a compound microscope. Teasing of the skin is unnecessary. The sensitivity of skin snips to diagnose infection depends upon the number of skin snips taken and on the intensity of infection. Microfilariae of *O. volvulus* are 270–320 µm long, unsheathed, and have a characteristic head and a pointed tail (see Figure 82.16). They must be differentiated from the smaller skin-dwelling microfilariae of *M. streptocerca* in

Africa and *M. ozzardi* in South America. Blood microfilariae—*W. bancrofti, Loa loa* and *M. perstans*—occasionally appear in skin snips contaminated by blood.

Immunological and PCR-based diagnosis

Several immunodiagnostic tests have been devised for onchocerciasis.[112] Adult *O. volvulus* isolated from nodules, or adult worms or microfilariae of *O. gibsoni* or *O. gutturosa* from cattle, have frequently been used as the source of antigen. Generally, immunodiagnosis based on detection of antibodies to crude antigens is of limited practical use owing to the low specificity and sensitivity of the tests. Cross-reactions to other nematode infections are common and the tests cannot distinguish between past and present infections. In endemic areas, where the population is continuously exposed to infection, most people are positive to the tests. Such tests may be of value in the diagnosis of onchocerciasis in persons from non-endemic areas who have visited an endemic area.

The development of specific and sensitive immunodiagnostic tests has been a priority in onchocerciasis research. The specificity of tests has been improved by the detection of specific IgG4 antibodies[113] and by the identification and use of specific antigens. Tests utilizing specific recombinant antigens have been developed, and an ELISA with a cocktail made from three of these antigens has shown a high sensitivity and 100% specificity.[114] Recently, a rapid-format card test that detects IgG4 to a recombinant antigen in serum or blood specimens has proved to be sensitive and specific.[115] Tests for detection of specific circulating antigens in onchocerciasis have given mixed results, and in general have not been as successful as in lymphatic filariasis.

A PCR technique with high specificity for *O. volvulus* DNA has recently been developed.[116] In addition to identifying worm DNA in skin snips from infected humans, this technique is capable of distinguishing between various strains of the parasite and of detecting *O. volvulus* larvae in extracts of blackfly vectors.[112]

Management

Drug treatment

For more than 40 years, DEC was the drug of choice for the treatment of onchocerciasis. It has now been replaced by ivermectin (Mectizan).[90] Both of these drugs have a strong microfilaricidal effect, whereas adult worms remain essentially unaffected (see Table 82.2).

Suramin, although largely used as a macrofilaricide, also has some microfilaricidal effects. Fatalities due to drug toxicity may occur and its use is not recommended. The macrofilaricidal effects of benzimidazoles are being investigated. Endosymbiontic rickettsia (*Wolbachia* spp.), recently discovered in *O. volvulus*, may be potential new targets for chemotherapy.[117]

Diethylcarbamazine

In 1947, DEC was found to be an effective microfilaricide in onchocerciasis. Adverse reactions, subsequently known as Mazzotti reactions, have been used diagnostically to detect the presence of *O. volvulus* infection.

Adverse reactions associated with DEC therapy may be local (pruritus, skin rash, exacerbation of eye lesions) or systemic (fever, headache, joint and muscle pains, postural hypotension, collapse, respiratory distress or vertigo). The reactions occur especially in heavily infected patients but can also be seen in some lightly infected individuals. DEC may also aggravate existing ocular lesions or precipitate new lesions. Because of the severity of some of the reactions, DEC has largely been replaced by ivermectin as the microfilaricide of choice in onchocerciasis.

If DEC is administered, the clinical severity of reactions can be reduced by starting treatment with very low doses, which are then gradually increased, and by the use of anti-inflammatory drugs. The initial dose of DEC recommended for the first 1–2 days is 25 or 50 mg for an adult (0.5–1.0 mg/kg). This is increased to 100 mg (2.0 mg/kg) twice daily for 5–7 days so that the total drug dose given is approximately 1.3 g (30 mg/kg). Betamethazone is the drug of choice for damping down inflammatory reactions. Aspirin can be very useful for the treatment of severe side effects of DEC.

Ivermectin

Ivermectin in a single oral dose of 150 μg/kg body weight causes a rapid elimination of microfilariae from the skin.[118] More than 80% of skin microfilariae are eliminated in the first 48 hours and this then slowly increases to 97%. The low level of microfilaraemia is maintained over a period of several months, after which there is a gradual increase. Retreatment may be necessary and follow-up skin snips should be examined 6–12 months after the initial treatment. Treatment is contraindicated in pregnant women, breast-feeding women with infants below 1 week old, children below 5 years of age, or individuals with serious acute or chronic illnesses.

Adverse reactions resemble, but appear to be much less severe than, those associated with DEC therapy. In a study in Sierra Leone[119] the most common side effect of ivermectin was the passing of *Ascaris* worms! Other effects in descending order of frequency were itching and/or rash, muscle and/or joint pains, fever, headache, swelling of the limbs, joint or face, dizziness, tender lymphadenopathy, conjunctivitis and tender nodules. Other investigators have noted severe postural hypotension and bronchoconstriction to be side effects of ivermectin therapy. These conditions are reported to be transient and to respond to symptomatic management. The single-dose ivermectin regimens have no known long-lasting effect on mature worms, but the drug causes intrauterine degeneration and temporary sequestration of unborn microfilariae.

The disappearance of microfilariae from the eye is much more gradual than microfilarial reduction in the skin. Available data on the impact of repeated doses of ivermectin on ocular onchocercal disease indicate regression of early lesions of the anterior segment, including iridocyclitis and sclerosing keratitis. It also appears to have a beneficial effect on optic nerve disease and visual field loss, but not on chorioretinitis.[91,120]

Nodulectomy

Nodulectomy has only limited use because many worms are present outside the nodules and some nodules are not palpable. Head nodules should be excised because their presence increases the risk of blindness.

Epidemiology

O. volvulus is transmitted between humans and the vectors. The infection is not a zoonosis. Many species and subspecies of *Simulium* flies can act as vectors. Despite geographical variation in pathogenicity, *O. volvulus* parasites are morphologically indistinguishable throughout their range of distribution.

Infection and disease in the endemic community

The epidemiology of onchocerciasis varies throughout its distribution. Different patterns of infection and disease are associated with differences in the abundance, vector competence and feeding characteristics of the local blackfly populations, differences in parasite strains and differences in the human host response to the parasites. Other human host factors that may affect the epidemiology are occupation, seasonal migration, concomitant or social standing, concurrent infections and racial group.

The prevalence and intensity of infection and the amount of clinical disease within the endemic community are generally low in the young children and increase gradually with age (Figure 82.2; Table 82.3). The overall burden of infection and disease in the population is proportional to the intensity of transmission. In

Table 82.3 Prevalence of microfilaraemia (iliac crest), pruritus and nodules by age in a rainforest village of Sierra Leone endemic for onchocerciasis. (After McMahon et al.[127])

Age group (years)	No. examined	Microfilariae (%)	Pruritus (%)	Nodules (%)
1–4	70	5.9		0.0
5–9	82	26.8	2.4	8.5
10–14	67	50.8		20.9
15–19		71.4		
20–29	68	61.9		
30–39	73	73.6		44.1
40–49	99	93.6	46.8	54.8
50–59	59	91.5	50.8	89.9
60+	71	87.3	50.7	85.9
Total	598	63.1	26.6	46.3

hyperendemic communities almost all adult individuals are infected and have clinical disease. Males and females generally appear to be affected by infection and disease to a similar extent.

Available quantitative data on the transmission, infection and disease in endemic populations have been used to develop mathematical models describing the population biology of human onchocerciasis.[121,122] Analysis of these models is useful for understanding the transmission dynamics and disease processes and for assessing the potential effect of control measures.

Endemicity

Different criteria have been used to define the level of endemicity of onchocerciasis in a population. Most commonly used today is a classification of levels as hypoendemic, mesoendemic or hyperendemic, on the basis of the population microfilarial prevalence being less than 40, 40–59 and 60% or more, respectively. In hyperendemic areas, blindness rates can exceed 10%, the disease is socially intolerable and fertile lands are often abandoned. In hypoendemic areas, the blindness rate is generally below 1% and the disease has few or no social effects.

In the course of the development of a programme for onchocerciasis control the endemicity should be mapped, to help to focus efforts where most needed. Methods for rapid epidemiological mapping have been developed which depend on determining the prevalence of nodules in a specific age-sex group of selected communities. The current standard practice is to examine a sample of 50 males per community for nodules. Nodule prevalence of less than 20%, 20–39% and 40% or more correspond approximately to the hypoendemic, mesoendemic and hyperendemic levels based on microfilarial detection. Other methods with less sensitivity and specificity have utilized the prevalence of leopard skin or blindness.

African onchocerciasis

Members of the *Simulium damnosum* complex are the

87 Nash T E. Antigenic variation in *Giardia lamblia* and the host's immune response. *Philos Trans R Soc Lond [Biol]* 1997; 352:1369–1375.

88 Singer S M & Nash T E. T-cell-dependent control of acute *Giardia lamblia* infections in mice. *Infect Immun* 2000; 68:170–175.

90 Farthing M J G, Mata L J, Urrutia J J & Kronmal R A. Giardiasis: impact on child growth. In Walker-Smith J A & McNeish A S (eds) *Diarrhea and Malnutrition in Childhood*. London: Butterworth, 1986:68–78.

91 Sullivan P B, Lunn P G, Northrop-Clewes C A & Farthing M J G. Parasitic infection of the gut and protein-losing enteropathy. *J Pediatr Gastroenterol Nutr* 1992; 15:404–411.

93 Green E L, Miles M A & Warhurst D C. Immunodiagnostic detection of *Giardia* antigen in faeces by a rapid visual enzyme-immunoassay. *Lancet* 1985; 2:691–693.

94 Addiss D G, Sanders C A, Sonnad S S et al. Stool diagnosis of giardiasis using a commercially available enzyme immunoassay to detect *Giardia*-specific antigen 65. *J Clin Microbiol* 1991; 29:1137–1142.

95 Aldeen W E, Carroll K, Robison A, Morrison M & Hale D. Comparison of nine commercially available enzyme-linked immunosorbent assays for detection of *Giardia lamblia* in fecal specimens. *J Clin Microbiol* 1998; 36:1338–1340.

96 Hanson K L & Cartwright C P. Use of an enzyme immunoassay does not eliminate the need to analyze multiple stool specimens for sensitive detection of *Giardia lamblia*. *J Clin Microbiol* 2001; 39:474–477.

97 Char S & Farthing M J G. DNA probes for diagnosis of enteric infection. *Gut* 1991; 32:1–5.

98 Butcher P D, Farthing M J G. DNA probes for the faecal diagnosis of *Giardia lamblia*. *Acta Trop Suppl* 1989; 2:93–95.

99 Mahbubani M H, Bej A K, Perlin M et al. Detection of *Giardia lamblia* in stool: targeting intergenic spacer region of multicopy rRNA gene. *Mol Cell Probes* 2000; 14:189.

101 Meloni B P & Thompson R C A. Simplified methods for obtaining purified oocysts from mice and for growing *Giardia* axenically. *J Parasitol* 1987.

101 Crouch A A, Seow W K, Whitman L M & Thong Y H. Sensitivity in vitro of *Giardia intestinalis* to dyadic combinations of azithromycin, deoxycline, mefloquine, tinidazole and furazolidone. *Trans R Soc Trop Med Hyg* 1990; 84:246–248.

103 Olson M E, Morck D W & Ceri H. Preliminary data on the efficacy of a Giardia vaccine in puppies. *Can Vet J* 1997; 38:777–779.

106 Olson M E, Ceri H & Morck D W. Giardia vaccination. *Parasitol Today* 2000; 16:213–217.

107 Tyzzer E E. A sporozoan found in the peptic glands of the common mouse. *Proc Soc Exp Biol Med* 1907; 5:12–13.

108 Klinc F A, Burst J P, Page D L & Hoescher M A. Acute *Cryptosporidium* infection in a human being. *Gastroenterol* 1980; 78:1156–1160.

110 Petersen C. Cellular biology of *Cryptosporidium parvum*. *Parasitol Today* 1993; 9:87–91.

111 Morgan U M, Xiao L, Fayer R, Lal A A & Thompson R C A. Epidemiology and strain variation of *Cryptosporidium parvum*. In Petry F (ed.) *Cryptosporidiosis and Microsporidiosis*. Contributions to Microbiology, vol. 6. Basel: Karger, 2000:116–139.

112 McLauchlin J, Pedraza-Diaz S, Amar-Hoetzeneder G & Nichols G L. Genetic characterization of *Cryptosporidium* strains from 218 patients with diarrhea diagnosed as having sporadic cryptosporidiosis. *J Clin Microbiol* 1999; 37:3153–3158.

115 Casemore D P. Epidemiological aspects of human cryptosporidiosis. *Epidemiol Infect* 1990; 104:1–28.

116 Zu S, Zhu S & Warhurst D C. Intestinal cryptosporidiosis in China. *Trans R Soc Trop Med Hyg*.

118 Ungar B L P, Soave R, Fayer R & Nash T E. Enzyme immunoassay detection of IgM and IgG antibodies to *Cryptosporidium* in immunocompetent and immunocompromised persons. *J Infect Dis* 1986; 153:570–578.

120 Blanshard C, Jackson A M, Shanson D C, Francis N & Gazzard B. Cryptosporidiosis in HIV seropositive patients. *Q J Med* 1992; 85:813–823.

121 Phillips A D, Thomas A G & Walker-Smith JA. *Cryptosporidium*, chronic diarrhoea and the proximal small intestinal mucosa. *Gut* 1992; 33:1057–1061.

122 McMahon S, Kelly P et al. Intensity of infection in AIDS associated cryptosporidiosis. *J Infect Dis* 1993; 167:704–709.

123 Buret A, Gall D G, Nation P N & Olson M E. Intestinal protozoa and epithelial cell kinetics, structure and function. *Parasitol Today* 1990; 6:375–380.

124 Tzipori S. Cryptosporidiosis in perspective. *Adv Parasitol* 1988; 27:63–124.

125 Kelly P, Thillainayagam A V, Smithson J et al. Jejunal water and electrolyte transport in human cryptosporidiosis. *Dig Dis Sci* 1996; 41:2095–2099.

126 Jacyna M R, Parkin J, Goldin R & Baron J H. Protracted enteric cryptosporidial infection in selective immunoglobulin A and saccharomyces opsonin deficiencies. *Gut* 1990; 31:714–716.

127 Kelly P, Jack D, Naeem A et al. Mannose binding lectin is a contributor to mucosal defence against *Cryptosporidium parvum* in AIDS patients. *Gastroenterology* 2000; 119:1236–1242.

128 Connolly G M, Dryden M S, Shanson D C & Gazzard B G. Cryptosporidial diarrhoea in AIDS and its treatment. *Gut* 1988; 29:593–597.

predominant vectors in most of the endemic areas of Africa (see Appendix IV). In parts of East and Central Africa species of *S. neavei* group also transmit the infection.

Flies of the *S. damnosum* complex breed in large rivers or small streams where there is an adequate velocity of water, adequate food supplies and suitable attachment sites (rocks, sticks, trailing vegetation). Primary larval habitats are rivers in which exposed rocks create white water rapids. Female blackflies generally restrict their flight to within a few kilometres of breeding sites and most intensely in the immediate vicinity. However, with the assistance of prevailing winds, they may migrate several hundred kilometres from one river basin to another.

The female flies feed mainly on humans but in some areas blood meals are also taken from animals, particularly bovines, horses and small ruminants. *S. damnosum* s.l. is a complex of numerous sibling species that differ in bionomics and vectorial capacity. They are very similar morphologically but can be distinguished by the banding patterns of their larval salivary gland chromosomes.

West Africa

The main West African onchocerciasis vectors of the *S. damnosum* complex can be grouped in three pairs: the *S. damnosum* s.s.–*S. sirbanum* pair, the *S. sanctipauli*–*S. leonense* pair and the *S. squamosum*–*S. yahense* pair. The geographical distribution of these species is considerably influenced by local climatic and ecological characteristics. The first two are termed 'savannah' species, and the other four 'forest' species. The *S. damnosum* s.s.–*S. sirbanum* pair occupies the savannah zone as far as 14° N, which is also the northern limit of the endemic area for onchocerciasis. These species may find their way into forest areas along the major water courses. The *S. sanctipauli*–*S. leonense* pair is forest dwelling but spreads into the savannah up to 10° N. *S. squamosum* has a focal distribution in forest and savannah with a preference for small or medium-sized rivers in hilly and mountainous areas, and *S. yahense* is limited to small forest water courses.

Experimental infection studies have indicated that the different sibling species of *Simulium* allow development of the savannah and forest strains of *O. volvulus* with widely different efficiency and have suggested that separate vector–parasite complexes exist in West Africa. However, use of new DNA techniques to identify the strain of parasite in the vector, has not supported this hypothesis.

Blinding lesions are much more severe in the dry savannah than in forest areas, and there is evidence that two different strains of *O. volvulus* are transmitted in these areas. However, when considering the pathogenicity of eye lesions as well as possible strain difference of the parasite, it is also important to consider environmental factors — a dry atmosphere, photophobic effects, dust exposure to higher levels of ultraviolet radiation — that may in combination or separately result in damage to the cornea. All of these factors are likely to be higher in dry savannah than in rainforest zones.

In the dry savannah, transmission of onchocerciasis is

East and central Africa

The most important vectors in East and Central Africa belong to the *S. damnosum* complex, but vectors of the *S. neavei* group also transmit onchocerciasis in Ethiopia, Tanzania, Malawi, Uganda, and parts of Zaire. This group includes all *Simulium* species with larvae and pupae that become attached to riverine crabs of the genus *Potamonautes*. In Tanzania, *S. woodi* is the most important vector within the *S. neavei* group. In the Tukuyu valley and Mahenge mountains transmission is by *S. damnosum* s.l. In East Africa onchocerciasis rarely causes blindness, but itching and dermatitis may be severe.

Central and South American onchocerciasis

Onchocerciasis is believed to have been introduced recently to the New World, possibly as a result of the slave trade. In America, the parasites have adapted to transmission by local species of *Simulium* flies.

In Mexico and Guatemala, the principal vector is *S. ochraceum* s.l., which breeds in small streams at altitudes between 500 and 1500 m. Transmission is mainly confined to the dry season. In some foci there are many head nodules and eye involvement is common.

In Venezuela, clinical manifestations are in northern and eastern foci. The *S. metallicum* s.l. is the principal vector. In the south, onchocerciasis occurs in both highland and lowland areas, being hyperendemic in some groups of Yanomama Indians. *S. guianense* s.l. is the main vector in the highlands and *S. oyapockense* in the lowlands.

In the western Andes in Colombia, where SR *exiguum* s.l. is the vector, lesions are mild. In Ecuador, onchocerciasis occurs in the north-western coastal province of Esmeraldas, and in particular it affects both Chachi Indians and the Black population of the Santiago River Basin. Owing to the presence of an efficient vector (*S. exiguum* s.l.) and the migration of infected individuals, onchocerciasis is increasing in prevalence and becoming more widespread. Severe skin and eye lesions exist in both races. In Brazil, onchocerciasis occurs in the north in the Amazonia, in a focus bordering Venezuela. The prevalence of onchocerciasis in the focus is not known.

Control

Onchocercal skin and eye lesions can have serious social and socio-economic consequences in the affected communities, especially in areas of high endemicity. Considerable efforts have been made in the last decades to establish control programmes, aiming at eliminating onchocerciasis as a public health problem.

Antivector control, particularly larviciding of breeding sites, was previously the main control measure used in onchocerciasis. To date, no macrofilaricidal drug of low toxicity is available for mass drug treatment against the parasite, and the microfilaricide DEC has not been widely used in control schemes, as side effects may also be severe. In the late 1980s, mass chemotherapy with ivermectin proved to be a practical and feasible alternative to vector control.

Vector control

Since 1974, the Onchocerciasis Control Programme (OCP) has been engaged in a large-scale attempt to control the savannah species of the vectors of onchocerciasis in seven West African countries (Burkina Faso, Benin, Ivory Coast, Ghana, Mali, Niger and Togo) in the Volta River Basin area. In 1986 the programme expanded its operations and included four additional countries (Guinea, Guinea-Bissau, Senegal and Sierre Leone). Successful vector control by aerial larviciding of *Simulium* breeding sites has reduced the parasite to such a level that it is close to being eliminated from the hyperendemic foci of the core area of the programme.[136–138] The campaign has markedly reduced the incidence of skin and eye lesions.

The emergence of resistance to larvicides being applied and the reinvasion of treated areas from non-controlled areas are major problems that have been encountered. Attempts to counter the resistance problem have involved alternating the larvacides being used, whilst extension of the programme into countries to the west and south has reduced the reinvasion problem. The cost of such a large control scheme is high. During wet seasons, a fleet of up to 11 helicopters and two fixed-wing aircraft operated over 23 000 km of rivers. In later years, the programme has included mass treatment with ivermectin as an important additional intervention measure, and vector control activities have been considerably reduced.

Vector control programmes of a much smaller scale than the OCP have been conducted in several African countries. *S. neavei* has been entirely eradicated from Kenya by larvicidal treatments, except for a small focus on the Ugandan border. Transmission has been completely interrupted and no new cases of onchocerciasis have been reported in any of the districts since the elimination of the vector.

Chemotherapeutic control

Community trials in several endemic areas have shown that ivermectin is acceptable for mass treatment,[139,140] and annual mass treatment with ivermectin has now become the principal control strategy for onchocerciasis control. It reduces the microfilarial burden and thus transmission in the community.[141] Since ivermectin is only microfilaricidal, treatments should continue for a period equivalent to the reproductive lifespan of the adult female worms, in order to halt transmission. Currently a dose of 150 µg/kg body weight every 6 months

or once yearly is being encouraged. Children under the age of 5 years should not be treated.

Repeated treatments with ivermectin result in significant improvement of itching and severe onchocercal skin disease[142] and in regression of both early and advanced lesions of the anterior segment of the eye.[94,120] As an additional benefit ivermectin reduces the prevalence and intensity of *Ascaris* infections.

Following the initial field testing of ivermectin, the OCP started large-scale distribution for transmission and morbidity control in the programme area.[136,137] Nigeria has initiated a nationwide onchocerciasis control programme with large-scale ivermectin treatment.[143] Numerous smaller control programmes utilizing mass treatment have been started in endemic areas. Partnerships of non-governmental organizations involved in blindness prevention, international organizations (including the WHO and the World Bank) and governments of endemic countries have established the African Programme for Onchocerciasis Control (APOC) and the Onchocerciasis Elimination Program in the Americas (OEPA) for the promotion and coordination of control activities on the African and American continents, respectively. APOC will take over as the leading coordinating body of onchocerciasis control in Africa when the OCP is scheduled to end its activities in 2002.

Serious reactions, including death, after mass ivermectin treatment for onchocerciasis have recently been reported in individuals with high-intensity *Loa loa* microfilaraemia,[144] and call for caution when using ivermectin in loiasis endemic areas. Most of these reactions have been observed in Cameroon.

To date, resistance of *O. volvulus* to ivermectin has not been observed.

The manufacturer of Mectizan (Merck) has made this product available free of charge through the Mectizan Donation Program to governmental and non-governmental healthcare organizations involved in onchocerciasis control programmes.

Nodulectomy

Nodulectomy campaigns have been encouraged in some countries, especially in those where head nodules are common. The impact of such campaigns on ocular disease can be difficult to assess. In Guatemala, for example, where systematic campaigns have been associated with decreased blindness, other factors, particularly changes in socio-economic conditions, may have decreased human–vector contact.

Other filarial infections

In addition to the filarial worms resulting in human lymphatic filariasis and onchocerciasis, four other species of filariae commonly infect humans. These are *Loa loa*, *Mansonella perstans*, *M. streptocerca* and *M. ozzardi* (see

Table 82.1). A few species of animal filariae cause rare zoonotic infections in humans.

Loa loa

Loa loa is a filarial parasite of humans in parts of West and Central Africa.[145] It is commonly known as the 'eye-worm', because adult worms are occasionally seen to move across the eye of the patient.

Life cycle and transmission

Adult *L. loa* live and move around in the connective tissues of humans. They frequently wander through the subcutaneous tissues and may sometimes pass beneath the conjunctiva of the eye. The females measure $50–70 \times 0.5$ mm and the males $30–35 \times 0.4$ mm. More detailed morphology is given in Appendix III. The sheathed microfilariae circulate in the blood and measure $230–300 \times 6–8$ µm (Figure 82.24).

Human *L. loa* is transmitted by tabanid flies of the genus *Chrysops*. The microfilarial periodicity is adapted to the day-biting habits of the vectors. It is diurnal, with peak concentration in the peripheral blood around noon (Figure 82.25). Microfilariae ingested by the vectors during feeding penetrate the stomach wall of the flies and migrate to the fat body where they develop in 8–12 days. Infective larvae (2 mm $\times 25$ µm) then move via the thorax to the proboscis. The larvae burrow into the skin of the human host when the vector feeds. The minimum prepatent period (until appearance of microfilariae) is 5–6 months, but it can be much longer, and adult worms may live for 17 years or more.

Clinical features

The most common clinical manifestations of loiasis are Calabar swellings and pruritus. Adult worms may be noticed when they pass under the conjunctiva of the eye (Figure 82.26) or under the skin (Figure 82.27).[146–148] They

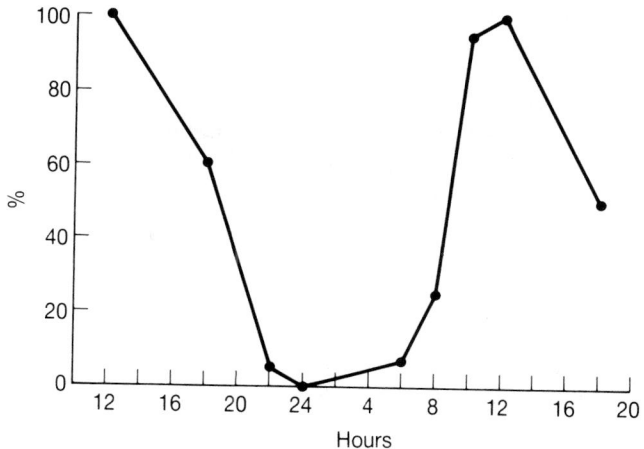

Figure 82.25: Periodicity of *L. loa* microfilariae in the peripheral blood.

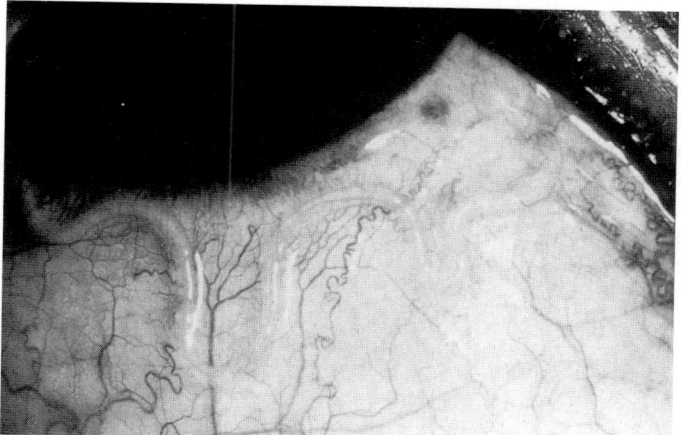

Figure 82.26: Transocular migration of adult *L. loa*. (Courtesy of J. Anderson.)

usually appear and then disappear within 10–15 minutes, leaving no trace behind. Hypereosinophilia, especially in expatriates, is common. Calabar swellings (Figure 82.28) are most commonly observed on the hands, wrists and forearms, but they may appear anywhere on the body. The swellings are painless, and do not pit on pressure. They may last from a few hours to several days. Usually one swelling occurs at a time, and may recur at irregular intervals for years after the patient has left the endemic area. Calabar swellings probably reflect the host's response to parasite antigens at the site of the swellings. Other common symptoms include generalized pruritus, fatigue and arthralgia. The death of an adult worm may occasionally cause a localized abscess. Dead worms sometimes calcify and are then easily seen on radiography.

More serious complications can occur when *L. loa* invade the central nervous system and other vital organs. An epidemiological correlation has been observed between loiasis and the occurrence of endomyocardial fibrosis, and it is possible that hypereosinophilia induced by the infection may lead to the cardiac damage.[149] Nephropathy

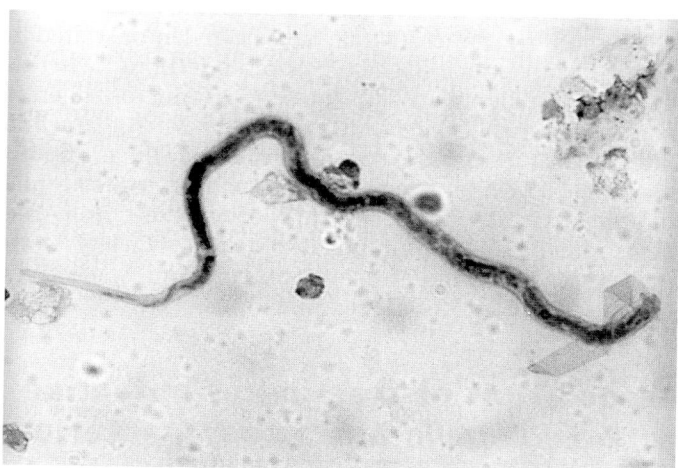

Figure 82.24: Microfilaria of *L. loa*.

two large outbreaks of recreational water-associated cryptosporidiosis occurring in 1995–6): *N. fowleri* was responsible [illegible] of these non-cryptosporidial cases. Since only [illegible] cause of death in recreational water-associated [illegible] was reported over the period (*E. coli* 0157), *N. fowleri* was responsible for 96% of the deaths.[3]

Acanthamoebidae

Acanthamoeba species which cause GAE and CAK are found worldwide and also feed on bacteria. They are not necessarily associated with warm fresh water, and can also multiply in brackish conditions. The life cycle consists only of the trophozoite and cyst forms, and either of these can [illegible] of infection. Several species of the genus have been isolated from human tissue, and the ubiquitous distribution of these organisms means that human exposure is widespread. For example, it is estimated that humans inhale one of the resistant cysts every day.[4] As a corollary of this wide exposure, the organism finds it difficult to colonize man, and infections are generally restricted to the immunodeficient or to immunoprivileged sites, the most common of which is the cornea (Figures 78.3 and 78.4). Infections are generally of a chronic type and there is a marked granulomatous tissue reaction. Treatment by medical or surgical means is usually successful in ocular infection but a few [illegible] have been reported in systemic infection.

Acanthamoeba and upper respiratory infection

Association of *Acanthamoeba* with upper respiratory infections was suspected in the 1960s and the organism has been regularly isolated from oronasal swabs. Several strains isolated from room and outside air using a [illegible] sampler were found to be cytopathic to mammalian cell cultures.[4] Although there is a suggestive link between the isolation of *Acanthamoeba* from the upper respiratory tract and nose bleeding, rhinitis and upper respiratory infections, the connection has not yet been convincingly drawn. It may be argued that, in some cases at least, isolations from the nose represent trapped airborne cysts, and not active infections.

Leptomyxida

Among more than 56 case reports of GAE, mainly due to infection with *Acanthamoeba* species, are a few cases of infection with leptomyxid free-living amoebae (now designated *Balamuthia mandrillaris*). The predisposing factors are apparently similar to those for systemic *Acanthamoeba* infection, and the life cycle of the leptomyxids also resembles that of these amoebae. Nothing is yet known about treatment, and diagnosis may prove difficult. These amoebae are not known to cause CAK.[6] A recent molecular study has produced evidence that the Leptomyxida are polyphyletic, and that *B. mandrillaris* does not belong in the order.[7]

Association of free-living amoebae with *Legionella* and other bacteria

Acanthamoeba species and *Naegleria* species can harbour

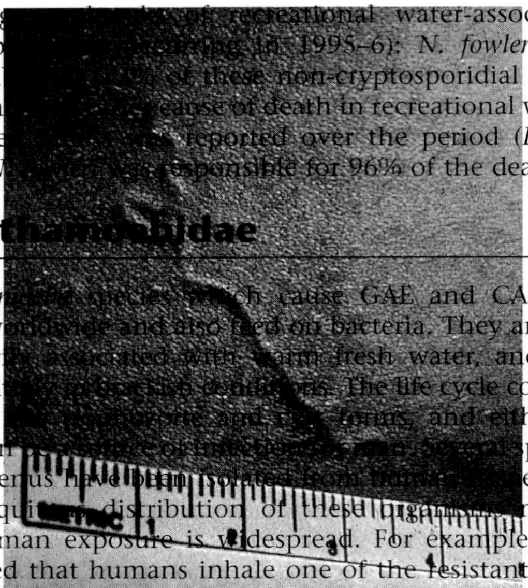

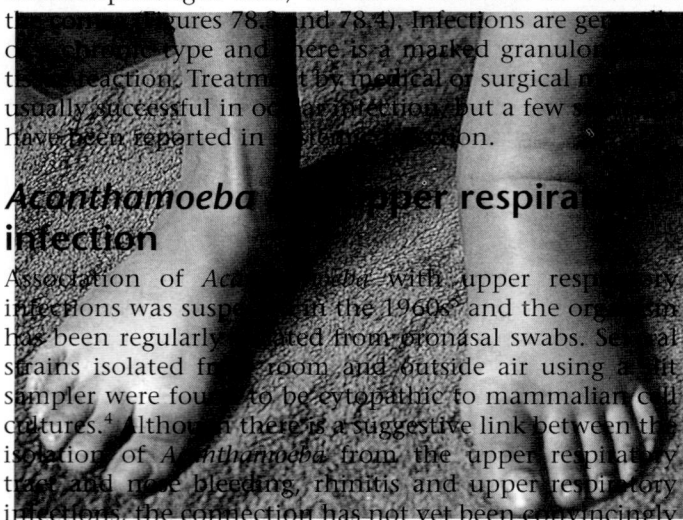

Figure 82.27: *L. loa* migrating under the skin. (Courtesy of P. G. P. Manson-Bahr)

Figure 82.28: Calabar swelling.

Figure 78.3: *Acanthamoeba* species keratitis. Corneal ulceration, hypopyon, conjunctival hyperaemia and radial neuritis are visible in this photograph of an infected eye.

Figure 78.4: Encysting trophozoite of *Acanthamoeba* species in corneal laminae. (Stained with immunoperoxidase using rabbit anti-*Acanthamoeba* serum. Note cellular infiltration and the heavily stained amoebic trophozoite.)

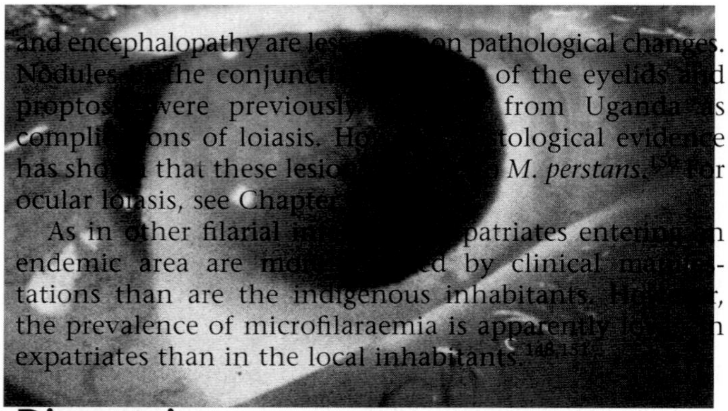

and encephalopathy are less common pathological changes. Nodules of the conjunctiva [illegible] of the eyelids and proptosis were previously [illegible] from Uganda as complications of loiasis. However, histological evidence has shown that these lesions [illegible] *M. perstans*.[159] For ocular loiasis, see Chapter [illegible]

As in other filarial infections expatriates entering an endemic area are more affected by clinical manifestations than are the indigenous inhabitants. However, the prevalence of microfilaraemia is apparently lower in expatriates than in the local inhabitants.[148,151]

Diagnosis

The appearance of characteristic Calabar swellings in persons who live in an endemic area or who have visited such an area, or a history by the patient of a worm having crossed the eye, is strongly suggestive of *L. loa* infection.

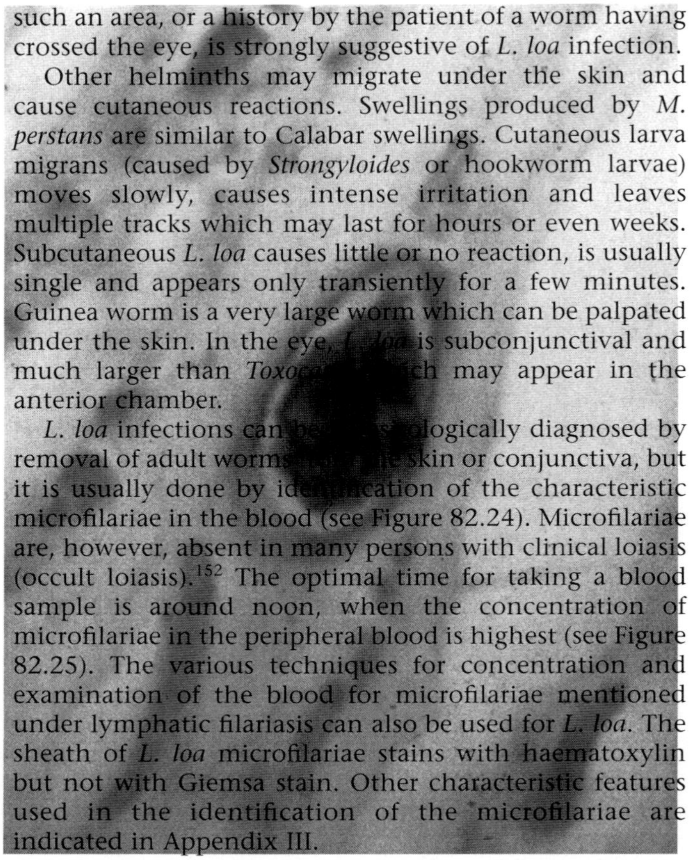

Other helminths may migrate under the skin and cause cutaneous reactions. Swellings produced by *M. perstans* are similar to Calabar swellings. Cutaneous larva migrans (caused by *Strongyloides* or hookworm larvae) moves slowly, causes intense irritation and leaves multiple tracks which may last for hours or even weeks. Subcutaneous *L. loa* causes little or no reaction, is usually single and appears only transiently for a few minutes. Guinea worm is a very large worm which can be palpated under the skin. In the eye, *L. loa* is subconjunctival and much larger than *Toxocara* which may appear in the anterior chamber.

L. loa infections can be parasitologically diagnosed by removal of adult worms from the skin or conjunctiva, but it is usually done by identification of the characteristic microfilariae in the blood (see Figure 82.24). Microfilariae are, however, absent in many persons with clinical loiasis (occult loiasis).[152] The optimal time for taking a blood sample is around noon, when the concentration of microfilariae in the peripheral blood is highest (see Figure 82.25). The various techniques for concentration and examination of the blood for microfilariae mentioned under lymphatic filariasis can also be used for *L. loa*. The sheath of *L. loa* microfilariae stains with haematoxylin but not with Giemsa stain. Other characteristic features used in the identification of the microfilariae are indicated in Appendix III.

Immunodiagnosis on its own is of limited value because of low sensitivity and cross-reactions with other filarial species. Detection of specific IgG4, using a crude extract of *L. loa* microfilariae or adult worms in ELISA, can be useful for confirming the diagnosis of *L. loa* in amicrofilaraemic individuals with clinical signs suggesting loiasis.[153] A PCR assay with 100% specificity and 95% sensitivity for microfilaraemia and occult loiasis has been developed.[154]

Immunology

Most infected individuals show high antibody titres to filarial antigen.[148,153] Antibodies recognizing a surface antigen on *L. loa* microfilariae have been demonstrated in persons with amicrofilaraemic adult infections, whereas these antibodies were not present in microfilaraemic persons from the same endemic area.[155] Microfilaraemic individuals furthermore have diminished cellular responsiveness to specific antigens compared with amicrofilaraemic individuals.[156] Occult loiasis may thus result from the development of an immune response specifically eliminating the microfilarial stage of the parasite. Some cases may also be due to single sex infections.

Management

DEC rapidly eliminates microfilariae of *L. loa* from the blood (see Table 82.2) in dosages varying from 3 to 10 mg/kg body weight divided daily into three doses for 2–4 weeks. DEC has some effect on adult worms, but

complete cure may require repeated treatment with the usual regimen.[10,13,21,22,41-43] Side effects may include severe vomiting as a single dose, but this subsides if used when the meal, and side effects are commonly less than the excess risk of severe neutropenia. Another regimen, using a divided dose of infection, a regimen using 25 mg the first time a day for 7 days, probably gives a down gradual escalation of steroid dosage is of danger of efficacy, while the single-dose regimen best taken be an adequate assessment. Metronidazole possesses significant side effects (Chapter 00), including the development of expatriate visitors to infection. Although there is no evidence of teratogenicity in *Homo sapiens*, dosages of 200-400 μg/kg body weight avoided during the treatment of a risk stand of efficacy in my experience[58,159] with. However, recent reports of serious reactions using a single-dose regimen in overdose imaging do-based the for loiasis call for caution.[144] Reactions are perhaps due to the high *L. loa* microfilarial counts.

Mebendazole in low doses has been shown to reduce microfilaraemia significantly in persons with heavy *L. loa* infection. Side effects were low. A recent study indicated that albendazole therapy may be useful for the treatment of symptomatic loiasis in cases when DEC is ineffective.[161]

REFERENCES

1 Hook E W. Trichomonas vaginalis - no longer a minor STD. *Sex Transm Dis* 1999; Aug: 26(7):388-389.

2 Anosike J C, Onwuliri C D, Inyang R E et al. Trichomoniasis amongst students of a higher institution in Nigeria. *Appl Parasitol* 1993; 34:19-25.

3 Ogbonna C I, Ogbonna I B, Ogbonna A A & Anosike J C. Studies on the incidence of Trichomonas vaginalis amongst pregnant women in Jos area of Plateau State, Nigeria. *Angew Parasitol* 1991; 32:198-204.

4 [entry illegible]

5 Yereli K, Balcioglu I C, Degerli K, Ozbilgin A & Daldal N. Incidence of Trichomonas vaginalis among women having vaginal discharge, in Manisa, Turkey. *J Egypt Soc Parasitol* 1997; 27:905-911.

6 Jackson D J, Rakwar J P, Bwayo J J, Kreiss J K & Moses S. Urethral Trichomonas vaginalis infection and HIV-1 transmission. *Lancet* 1997; 350:1076.

7 Press N, Chavez V M, Ticona E, Calderon M et al. Screening for sexually transmitted diseases in human immunodeficiency virus-positive patients in Peru reveals an absence of Chlamydia trachomatis and identifies Trichomonas vaginalis in pharyngeal specimens. *Clin Infect Dis* 2001; 32:808-814.

8 Niccolai L M, Kopicko J J, Kassie A, Petros H, Clark R A & Kissinger P. Incidence and predictors of reinfection with Trichomonas vaginalis in HIV-infected women. *Sex Transm Dis* 2000; 27:284-288.

9 Meulen J ter, Mgaya H N, Chang-Claude J et al. Risk factors for HIV infection in gynaecological inpatients in Dar es Salaam, Tanzania, 1988-1990. *East Afr Med J* 1992; 69:688-692.

10 Kent H L. Epidemiology of vaginitis. *Am J Obstet Gynecol* 1991; 165:1168-1176.

11 Sobel J D. Vulvovaginitis. *Dermatol Clin* 1992; 10:339-359.

12 Hatch K D. Vulvar and vaginal disorders. *Curr Opin Obstet Gynecol* 1992; 4:904-906.

13 Heine P & McGregor J A. Trichomonas vaginalis: a reemerging pathogen. *Clin Obstet Gynecol* 1993; 36:137-144.

14 el-Sharkawy I M, Hamza S M & el-Sayed M K. Correlation between Trichomonas vaginalis and female infertility. *J Egypt Soc Parasitol* 2000; 30:287-294.

15 Fowler J E Jr. Urethritis in men. *Semin Urol* 1991; 9:15-27.

16 Saxena S B & Jenkins R R. Prevalence of Trichomonas vaginalis in men at high risk for sexually transmitted diseases. *Sex Transm Dis* 1991; 18:138-142.

17 Krieger J N, Jenny C, Verdon M et al. Clinical manifestations of trichomoniasis in men. *Ann Intern Med* 1993; 118:844-849.

18 Krieger J N, Verdon M, Siegel N & Holmes K K. Natural history of urogenital trichomoniasis in men. *J Urol* 1993; 149:1455-1458.

19 [entry illegible]

20 el-Seoud S F, Abbas M M & Habib F S. Study of trichomoniasis among Egyptian male patients. *J Egypt Soc Parasitol* 1998; 28:263-270.

21 Levine T J. Sexually transmitted parasitic diseases. *Prim Care* [illegible]

22 [entry illegible] Bouree [illegible]

23 Hay [illegible] Factors associated with trichomonas, candidiasis and bacterial vaginosis. *Int J STD AIDS* 1993; 4:21-25.

24 Lossick J G & Kent H L. Trichomoniasis: trends in diagnosis and management. *Am J Obstet Gynecol* 1991; 165:1217-1222.

25 [illegible] M W & Harger J H. Accuracy of the Papanicolaou smear in the diagnosis of asymptomatic infection with Trichomonas vaginalis. *Obstet Gynecol* 1993; 82:423-429.

26 Krieger J N, Verdon M, Siegel N, Critchlow C & Holmes K K. [illegible] of trichomoniasis in men. *J Infect Dis* 1992; 166:1362-1366.

27 [illegible] yield from cervix versus vagina for culturing Candida albicans and Trichomonas vaginalis. *Genitourin Med* 1993; 69:41-43.

28 Sharma P, Malla N, Gupta I, Ganguly N K & Mahajan R C. A comparison of wet mount, culture and enzyme linked immunosorbent assay [illegible] of trichomoniasis.

29 Riley [illegible] identification of Trichomonas vaginalis DNA. *J Clin Microbiol* 1991; 29:702-706.

30 Riley D E, Roberts M C, Takayama T & Krieger J N. Development of polymerase chain reaction-based diagnosis of [illegible] *Microbiol* 1992; 30:465-472.

31 Romia S A & Othman T A. Detection of antitrichomonal antibodies in sera and cervical secretions in trichomoniasis. *J Egypt Soc Parasitol* 1991; 21:371-381.

32 Bhatt R, Pandit S & Deodhar L. Detection of serum antitrichomonal antibodies in urogenital trichomoniasis. *J [illegible]* 1992; 35:[illegible]

33 Ohkawa T, Bekku H [illegible] Makino [illegible] Maeda S. Polymerase chain reaction amplification [illegible]

advantage from being significantly less expensive and possesses a proven safety. A 100% cure rate has been recorded using ivermectin in two equally divided doses of 4 flies of the genus *Chrysops* orally 100 mg and vaginally at night, especially if symptoms of local and day-course, especially in about 20% only in the transmission alternative. Metronidazole and tinidazole can cause nitroimidazoles. They have respective advantages but both active centres operate the studies are required. More recently development is slow, and effective or metronidazole-resistant in stage. Transmission takes place mainly during the wet season by more information to the *Aspergillus* and chromosomes which is Appendix IV. Many vaginal parasites are similar reservoir for *L. loa* than social properties extensively. Species of forest-dwelling primates, including the mandril and several species of *Cercopithecus*, harbour filariae that closely resemble *L. loa*. The periodicity of these parasites is nocturnal. Monkeys can be infected with the human parasite, which retains its diurnal periodicity in the new host. The non-human primate *L. loa* are transmitted by species of *Chrysops* which are feeding only at night on monkeys living in the canopy, whereas blood-meal analyses have shown that *C. silacea* and *C. dimidiata* do not feed on non-human primates. Thus it appears that in nature, human and monkey *L. loa* comprise two distinct transmission complexes, and that the parasite is not a zoonosis.

The microfilaria rate in children tends to be low. In adults, it gradually rises with age, but even in old age rarely exceeds 20%. Despite the lack of microfilaraemia, many children harbour the adult parasites, which occasionally cross the eye. Within an endemic community, microfilarial prevalence is commonly higher in males than females.

Control

Methods to control loiasis include environmental modifications, personal protection and vector control. No large-scale control programmes have been conducted in these areas. New housing and rubber plantations should be established some distance from the forest edge and swamps where the vectors breed. The larvae of *Chrysops* live in the mud and can be destroyed there with insecticides. However, this method is impractical.

The wearing of light-coloured clothing and frequent application of insect repellent reduces the risk of bites by the flies. Personal prophylaxis with 300 mg dose of DEC once a week has been shown effective in expatriates working in endemic areas.[163]

Mansonella perstans

M. perstans is a human filarial parasite, widely distributed in Africa as well as in parts of Central and South America and in the Caribbean (Figure 82.30). It is transmitted by tiny biting midges of the genus *Culicoides*. Rarely have adult worms been recovered from man. They live in the serous cavities, mainly the peritoneal cavity, and usually

Epidemiology

Human loiasis occurs only in Africa, where transmission is confined to the tropical forest and swamps of West and Central Africa (Figure 82.29). The vectors breed in these areas. It is estimated that 20-30 million people reside in endemic areas. The parasite was previously also observed in the more western rainforests of Sierra Leone, Liberia, Ivory Coast and Ghana, but it has not been [illegible]

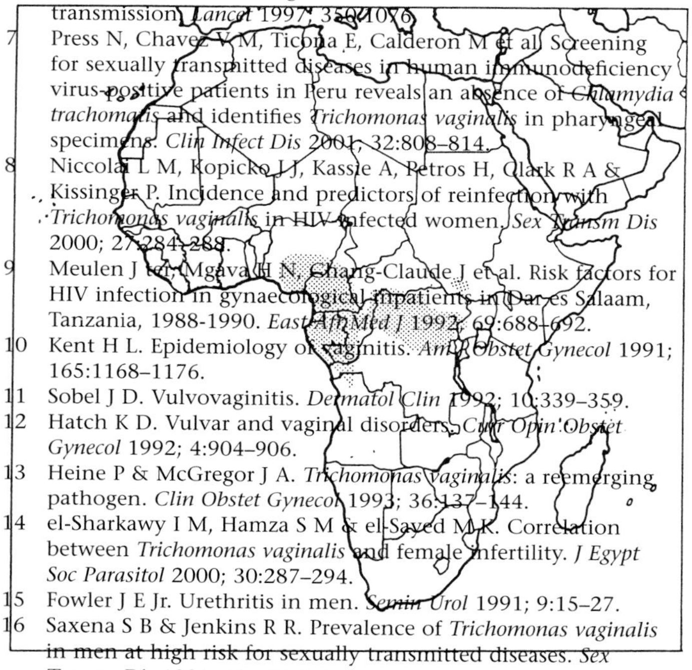

Figure 82.29: Geographical distribution of *L. loa*.

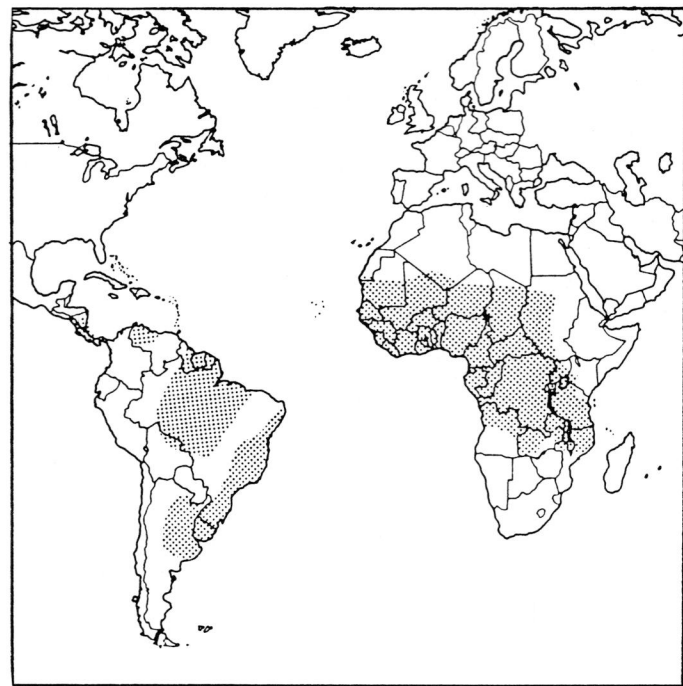

Figure 82.30: Geographical distribution of *M. perstans*.

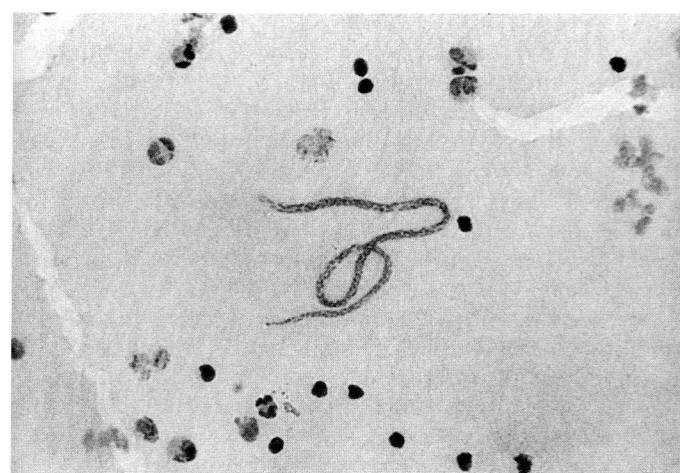

Figure 82.31: Microfilaria of *M. perstans*.

cause no symptoms. Occasionally they have been found subcutaneously. The adult female measures 70–80 × 0.1 mm and the male 35–45 × 0.06 mm. Microfilariae (200 × 4.5 μm) are unsheathed, non-periodic, and circulate in the blood (Figure 82.31).

In the vector, following a blood meal, the ingested microfilariae develop to the infective stage. Infective larvae penetrate the skin of humans when the vector feeds again. The time from infection until appearance of microfilariae in the blood of humans is unknown.

M. perstans infections are largely non-pathogenic, but a variety of clinical manifestations can occur in some infected individuals. Symptoms are more common in expatriates coming to endemic areas from non-endemic ones. Transient swellings resembling the Calabar swellings of loiasis occur. Other manifestations are pruritus, fever, and pain or ache in bursae and/or joint synovia. Severe abdominal pain, especially in the liver region, may occur. Nodules in the conjunctiva, swelling of the eyelids and proptosis have also been attributed to *M. perstans* infections.[150] Eosinophilia is present in many cases of infection. It is likely that some of the pathological changes observed are induced by immune responses to the infection.

Diagnosis is by recovering the microfilariae (Figure 82.31) from the blood. Blood samples may be obtained at any time of the day, and techniques similar to those used for concentration and examination of blood samples for the diagnosis of lymphatic filariasis are utilized. For morphological features of the microfilariae, see Appendix III.

DEC and ivermectin have little or no effect on *M. perstans* infections (see Table 82.2). Mebendazole has

proved effective in eliminating the microfilariae in a dose of 100 mg two to three times daily for 28–45 days.[160] Albendazole (400 mg twice daily) given for 10 days resulted in a slow but significant decrease in *M. perstans* microfilaraemia after 1–3 months.[164] It is possible that the drug is mainly macrofilaricidal. The treatment was well tolerated.

Very few studies have been carried out on the epidemiology of *M. perstans* infections. In some localities a high prevalences and intensity of microfilaraemia are found. The microfilarial prevalence is generally lower in children than in adults, and males are usually more frequently infected than females.[162,165] Microfilarial prevalences can reach more than 80% in adults in highly endemic areas.

The main vector in Africa is *C. grahami*, but other species of *Culicoides* also play a role. The species of *Culicoides* transmitting *M. perstans* in the Americas have not been identified. *M. perstans* is found commonly in chimpanzees and gorillas, but it is also widespread in areas where there are no large apes.

Mansonella streptocerca

M. streptocerca is a filarial parasite of humans, having a limited distribution in Central and West Africa (Figure 82.32). A new focus in Uganda was described recently.[166] The adult worms inhabit the dermis of the upper thorax and shoulders, but they have rarely been recovered and very few have been examined in detail. The adult female measures 27 × 0.075 mm and the male 17 × 0.05 mm. The microfilariae (Figure 82.33) also inhabit the dermis. They are unsheathed, measure 180–240 × 3–5 μm and exhibit no periodicity.

M. streptocerca is transmitted by tiny biting midges of the genus *Culicoides*, the most common vector probably being *C. grahami*. Complete development in the vector has been observed experimentally to take 9 days. Infor-

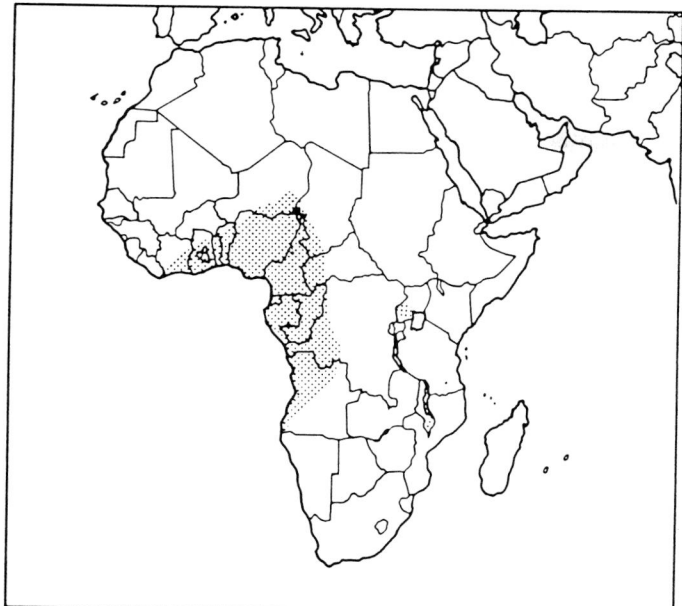

Figure 82.32: Geographical distribution of *M. streptocerca*.

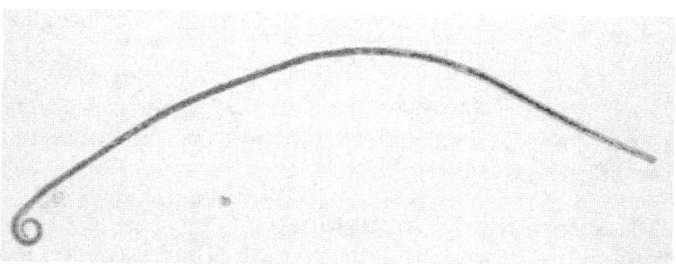

Figure 82.33: Microfilaria of *M. streptocerca*. (Courtesy of P. Fischer.)

mation on the development of *M. streptocerca* in the human host is lacking, and the prepatent period is unknown.

The infection generally causes few clinical manifestations. Dermatitis is the most common sign and is most marked over the thorax and shoulders.[166, 167] It is characterized by pruritus, hypopigmented macules and papules. Microscopically, infected skin shows dilated dermal lymphatics, and it has been suggested that *M. streptocerca* might be a cause of lymphoedema and elephantiasis. Clinically the infection must be distinguished from onchocerciasis and leprosy.

Diagnosis is made by finding the unsheathed microfilariae of *M. streptocerca* in skin snips (for the technique, see Onchocerciasis). The microfilariae have a characteristic 'shepherd's crook' tail. Other distinguishing features of the microfilariae are shown in Figure 82.33 and mentioned in Appendix III. A sensitive and specific PCR assay for specific detection of *M. streptocerca* DNA in skin biopsies has been developed.[168]

DEC eliminates both microfilariae and adults (see Table 82.2) of *M. streptocerca* when given in a dosage of 2–6 mg/kg body weight for 21 days. In most patients, the DEC treatment causes intense pruritus and development

of cutaneous papules in which degenerating adult worms may be found.[169] Other side reactions similar to the Mazzotti reaction during DEC treatment of onchocerciasis may occur but are not common. Ivermectin in a single dose of 150 µg/kg body weight leads to sustained suppression of microfilaraemia in the skin.[170] Common short-term adverse reactions are increased pruritus and dermatitis.

Adults and microfilariae of *M. streptocerca* are found in the skin of chimpanzees, but whether the infection is a zoonosis is not known.

Mansonella ozzardi

M. ozzardi is a human filarial parasite found only in the New World. Foci exist in Central America, in northern South America and in some Caribbean islands (Figure 82.34). A new focus in Bolivia was described recently.[171] Few adult female worms (65–80 × 0.25 mm) have been recovered from the peritoneal cavity of humans. The microfilariae (Figure 82.35) measure 200 × 4.5 µm. They are unsheathed, non-periodic, and are found in both blood and skin.

Two groups of vectors have been shown to transmit *M. ozzardi* infections. In the Caribbean islands the vectors are biting midges of the genera *Culicoides*, whereas in the Amazon basin *Simulium* blackflies have been incriminated. The development of the parasite has been studied in the vectors and in experimental infections in patas monkeys. In the monkeys the prepatent period was 5–6 months.

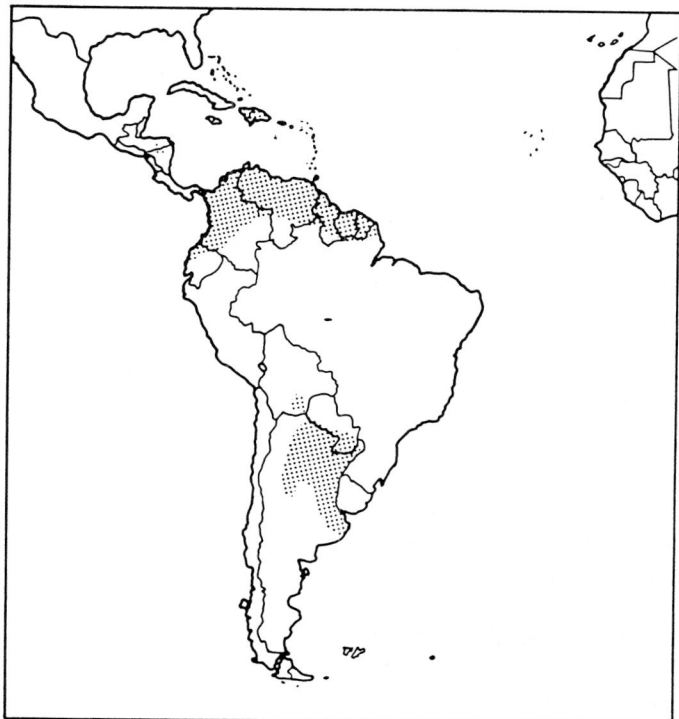

Figure 82.34: Geographical distribution of *M. ozzardi*.

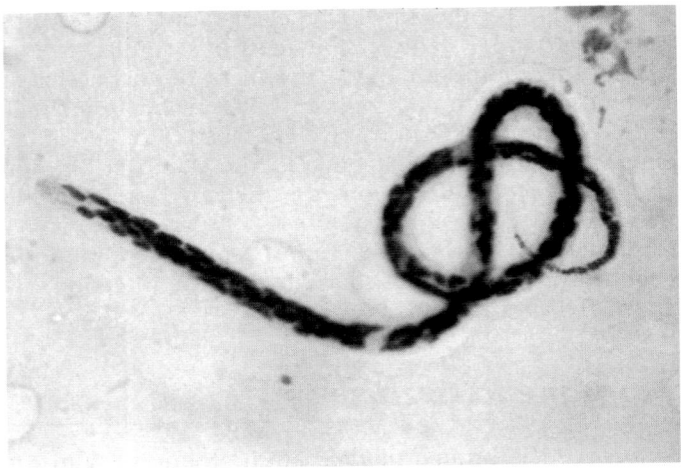

Figure 82.35: Microfilaria of *M. ozzardi*. (Courtesy of M. Eberhard.)

Natural *M. ozzardi* infections have not been reported from animals. In endemic foci, human infections tend to be highly prevalent, with the microfilarial infection rates increasing with age.[171,172]

Most people infected with *M. ozzardi* are symptomless. Symptoms of severe articular pain, headache, fever and pruritus have been reported, but these have generally not been closely associated to infection.[171,173] Eosinophilia is common. Individuals in endemic areas have high titres of antibodies against filarial antigens.[174]

The infection is diagnosed by finding the microfilariae in blood or in skin biopsies.[175] The techniques described under Lymphatic filariasis and Onchocerciasis can be used. For characteristics of the microfilariae, see Figure 82.35 and Appendix III. DEC has little or no effect on *M. ozzardi* infections (see Table 82.2), but a single dose of 6 mg ivermectin has been reported to provide significant long-term reduction in microfilaraemia.[176]

Rare filarial infections

Humans occasionally become infected with species of filariae normally found in animals.[150] Among these zoonotic infections, those due to *Dirofilaria* spp. are the most frequently reported and the most widespread.

Dirofilariasis

Dirofilaria spp. are natural parasites of various species of carnivores. In these hosts, the microfilariae circulate in the blood. Transmission is by mosquitoes. In human infections, parasite development is impaired and no microfilariae are produced.[177]

Pulmonary dirofilariasis

D. immitis is a filarial parasite of dogs. It is transmitted worldwide, except in cold climates. In the dog, adult *D. immitis* inhabit the right ventricle of the heart, where they may occur in large coiled masses. Pulmonary dirofilariasis in humans results from infection with *D. immitis*. In humans, the parasite may develop partially in the right ventricle of the heart before being swept into the pulmonary artery. Typically a spherical nodule 1–3 cm in diameter is discovered in the lungs on routine radiography (a 'coin lesion') or at autopsy. A single worm, usually necrotic and sometimes calcified, is present in the lumen of the artery. Most patients are asymptomatic. When present, symptoms include cough, chest pain, eosinophilia, haemoptysis and fever. Diagnosis is usually based on biopsy. Serological diagnosis has not been very successful. The only treatment is surgical excision.

Subcutaneous dirofilariasis

D. repens is a natural parasite of dogs and cats in warmer climates of the Old World. It has not been reported from America. In the normal hosts, adult worms are located in the subcutaneous tissues. In humans, occasional infections may result in the formation of subcutaneous nodules consisting of a degenerating immature worm surrounded by granulomatous tissue.[178] Nodules occur in many parts of the body, especially the breasts, arms, legs, scrotum, eyelid and conjunctiva. The nodules may occasionally be slowly migrating. Immunodiagnosis has not proved useful, and diagnosis is by biopsy. Treatment is by surgical removal of the nodule.

In North America, other species of *Dirofilaria*, especially *D. tenuis* and *D. ursi* (natural parasites of racoons and bears, respectively), have been reported to cause subcutaneous dirofilariasis in humans.

Other rare filarial infections

Human infections with *Brugia* parasites have occasionally been reported from countries where transmission of human *Brugia* spp. does not occur. This includes infections acquired in Africa and America. These *Brugia* parasites are believed to be of animal origin.[1]

Microfilariae with no resemblance to those of human filarial species have been reported from humans.[150] Cases of encephalopathy with microfilariae found in the cerebrospinal fluid were described from Zimbabwe. The microfilariae were shown to be *Meningonema peruzzi*, a filarial parasite of cercopithecus monkeys. Microfilariae similar to *Microfilaria rodhaini* from chimpanzees were recovered in skin biopsy specimens from humans during a survey in Gabon. Microfilariae of unknown species found in the blood of native South Americans in a remote jungle area in Venezuela were named *Microfilaria bolivarensis*. In a survey in north-western Zaire, many villagers had microfilariae of unknown species in the blood. These were named *Microfilaria semiclarum*.

Dracunculiasis (guinea worm)

Dracunculiasis or guinea worm disease in humans results from infection with *Dracunculus medinensis*.

Chapter 80

Schistosomiasis

A. Davis

The term human schistosomiasis indicates a complex of acute and chronic parasitic infections caused by mammalian blood flukes (*Schistosoma*). These infections are transmitted by specific aquatic or amphibious snails in a wide variety of freshwater habitats.

The various species of the genus *Schistosoma* are members of the family Schistosomatidae—dioecious digenean parasites whose habitat is the blood-vascular system of vertebrates. The family is divided into three, the Schistosomatinae, Bilharziellinae and Gigantobilharziinae, and contains 12 genera, of which several are confined to birds and five to mammals; only *Schistosoma* is associated with humans.

A general feature of the family is that the female is longer and more slender than the male and is normally held in a ventral groove, the gynaecophoric canal, formed by ventrally flexed lateral outgrowths of the male body. Of all the mammalian blood flukes, the genus *Schistosoma* has achieved the greatest geographical distribution and diversification.[1]

Of the [illegible] species of schistosome known to infect [illegible] mammals, only five are responsible for the overwhelming proportion of human infections: *Schistosoma haematobium*, *S. intercalatum*, *S. mansoni*, *S. japonicum* and *S. mekongi*. Other zoophilic species or hybrids may be found [illegible]

The five schistosome species infecting humans are subdivided into groups characterized by the size and appearance of eggs produced by the female schistosome:

- eggs with a terminal spine—*S. haematobium*, *S. intercalatum*
- eggs with a lateral spine—*S. mansoni*.
- rounded or ovoid minutely spined eggs—*S. japonicum* [illegible]

History

S. haematobium

Chronic haematuria and various bladder disorders occurred in Egypt and Mesopotamia from the earliest times in association with the agricultural civilizations of the great river valleys. Haematuria was described in the Gynaecological Papyrus of Kahun, written in the mid-XII dynasty period, about 1900 BC. Many remedies for haematuria were recorded from the time of the Ebers Papyrus and it can be assumed that the condition was widespread.[6] Calcified ova of the parasite were demonstrated in the kidneys of two Egyptian mummies of the XXth dynasty (1250–1000 BC). During the Napoleonic invasion of Egypt (1799–1801), symptoms of the disease in troops were rife, yet it was not until 1851 that the causal agent (*Distoma haematobium*, now *Schistosoma haematobium*), a blood fluke, was found by Theodor Bilharz in a mesenteric vein during a post-mortem examination at the Kasr el Aini Hospital in Cairo.[6]

S. mansoni

In 1902 Manson found lateral spined eggs in the faeces of a West Indian patient in London and postulated the existence of a second species of blood fluke. Subsequent controversy between A. Looss and L. W. Sambon, eminent scientists of the day, was resolved by the work of Leiper at El Marg, a village in the present Qualyubia Governorate, just north of Cairo, in 1915. Leiper established beyond doubt the existence of two distinct species of schistosome and the presence of small intermediate hosts belonging not only to two different genera but also to two different subfamilies. In the New World, eggs with a lateral spine were found in Bahia (Brazil) in 1904 and described in 1908[9] and in Venezuela in 1906.[10]

S. japonicum

In 1847 the clinical entities 'Kabure itch' and 'Ka[illegible] syndrome' were described in a village in the Hiro[illegible] Prefecture in Japan,[11] while in 1904 Katsurada[12] re[illegible] worms from the portal system of a cat and [illegible] species *Schistosomum japonicum*. From 190[illegible] biology of this parasite, its life cycle and the patholo[illegible] it caused were elucidated and described by Japanese and other investigators.[13–16]

The investigation was recognized clinically in both China[17] and the Philippines in the early years of the twentieth century[18] and in Sulawesi, Celebes, in the 1930s.[19]

In China the *Oncomelania* intermediate hosts were discovered in 1924[20] and in the Philippines in 1932.[21]

Life cycle and transmission

D. medinensis is a nematode parasite related to filarial worms. [illegible] copepods (water fleas), which are tiny free-swimming crustaceans usually found in abundance in natural freshwater bodies. Humans acquire the infection by drinking water containing the vectors infected with guinea worm larvae. The presence of guinea worm in an area is therefore essentially due to the poor quality of drinking water.

Adult female *D. medinensis* (up to 60–80 cm long and 1.5–2.0 mm in thickness) inhabit the subcutaneous connective tissues of humans. They may be located anywhere on the body but in the late stage of infection they are usually attracted to the legs and feet. At this stage most of the interior of the worm is occupied by the uterus, which contains thousands of first-stage larvae. A blister (Figure 82.36) is formed on the skin of the host around the anterior end of the worm, and when exposed to water the blister ruptures. The female guinea worm protrudes its anterior end from the ulcer and discharges first-stage larvae (640 × 23 µm) into the water. It remains protruding for the following 2–6 weeks, releasing larvae each time it is immersed in water. After this period it dies.

The larvae are infective in freshwater for 5–6 days, and for further development must, within this period, be swallowed by a copepod of the right species. The larva penetrates the gut wall, and in the haemocoel it moults twice. It can reach the infective third stage (450 × 14 µm) in about 2 weeks. Vectors that contain third-stage larvae become sluggish and sink to the bottom of a pond. Many species of cyclopoid copepods have been found naturally infected in various parts of the world, mainly being of the genera *Mesocyclops* and *Thermocyclops*.[179]

In humans, vectors ingested in drinking water are dissolved by the gastric juice. The guinea worm infective larvae are released and penetrate the stomach or intestine of the new host. After a period in the abdominal cavity, the larvae enter the connective tissues, where they develop to mature worms. Mating occurs about 3 months after the initial infection, and the males, which are much smaller than the females (1–4 cm × 0.4 mm), die shortly thereafter. The females move about in the connective tissues and usually reach the lower extremities between 8 and 10 months after infection.

Clinical features

There are usually no symptoms in the prepatent period. The first sign appears a few days before the worm pierces the skin. The dermis becomes elevated and a blister develops (Figure 82.36). The patient feels a burning sensation and itching, which he or she tries to relieve by placing the affected part in water. On exposure to water the blister ruptures, the anterior part of the worm protrudes and *Dracunculus* larvae are discharged into the water.

The worm is most frequently located in the foot or lower leg (Figure 82.37), but may appear on arms, breasts, head, back, scrotum or anywhere on the body surface. When it is close to joints it may cause arthritis. Further inflammation, or the calcification of worms, may cause

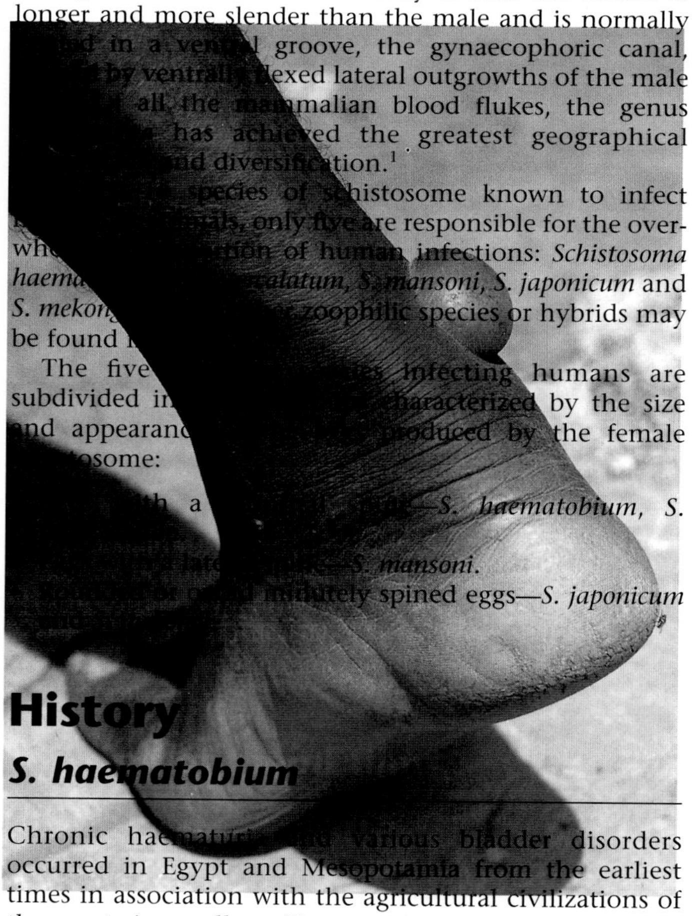

Figure 82.36: Blister on the skin prior to the appearance of guinea worm. (Courtesy of P. Bloch.)

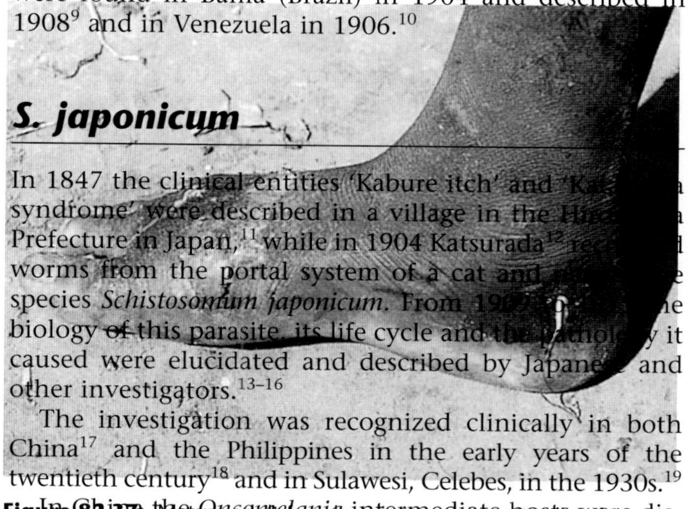

Figure 82.37: Mature adult female guinea worm protruding from a foot. (Courtesy of P. Bloch.)

joints of legs and feet to become stiff, thereby crippling the patient. In many cases (sometimes 50% or more), the ulcer caused by the parasite becomes secondarily infected with bacteria, and a spreading cellulitis may develop. Tetanus infection is a serious complication of guinea worm infection.

Inflammation around it makes the whole worm difficult to extricate before the uterus is empty of larvae. Provided there is no secondary infection, the ulcer heals spontaneously after extrication of the empty worm. If broken, the remainder of the worm withdraws into the host tissue, causing a severe inflammatory reaction followed by an ulcer and later scar tissue. Usually only a single worm appears in the patient annually, but up to 20 or more can appear at the same time in one individual.

Some female worms fail to emerge and die in the body. Usually they become encysted and calcify, and are then only apparent on radiography. Dead or ruptured worms may lead to formation of a sterile subcutaneous abscess. Migration of worms to vital organs can cause serious consequences. Such migrations are rare.

Diagnosis

Guinea worm infections cannot be diagnosed in the prepatent period, i.e., for the first 8–10 months of infection. Shortly before appearance the adult female worm can sometimes be seen or palpated under the skin. A clinical diagnosis is made by examining the guinea worm ulcer and observing the female protruding from the blister (see Figure 82.37). The appearance of the blister, with local itching and burning pain, makes diagnosis simple, even for the sufferer. Active larvae can be obtained by immersing the protruding adult female in a small tube or container with water. The first-stage larvae, with their characteristic pointed tails (see Appendix III), can then be observed under the microscope.

Serology is of no practical use in diagnosis. The finding of a high specificity of IgG4 antibodies[180] should assist in the development of more specific tests, including tests for prepatent infection. Attempts to identify specific circulating antigens have not been successful.[181] High eosinophilia is commonly observed in guinea worm infections. Dead calcified worms are easily seen on radiological examination.

Immunology

Owing to constant exposure, all persons in endemic areas usually have high antibody titres. These responses vary with infection status and transmission season.[182,183] There is no evidence of acquired immunity: people in endemic areas suffer from infections year after year. Whether the vigorous antibody response has any effect on the course of the infection is unknown.

Management

The traditional method of slow extraction of the emergent

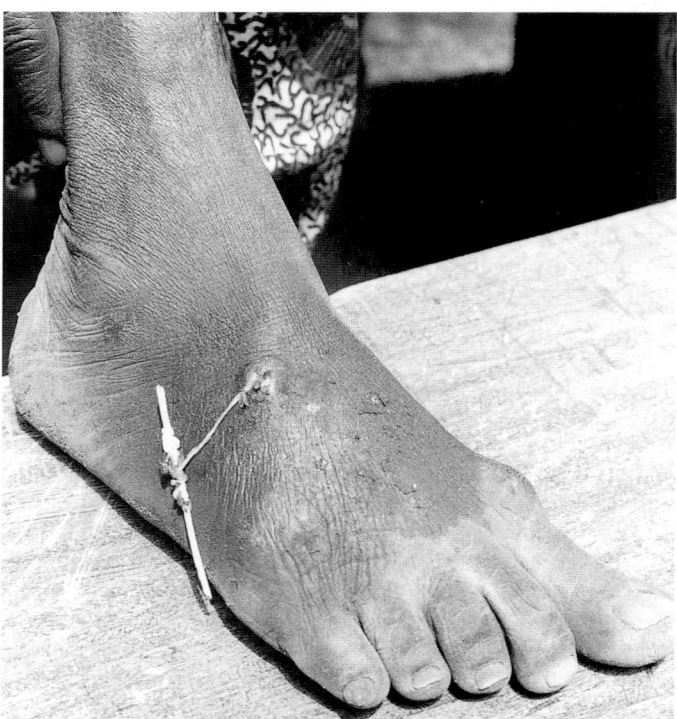

Figure 82.38: Traditional method of removal of guinea worm. (Courtesy of P. Bloch.)

guinea worm is usually the most effective. The protruding part of the female worm is attached to a small stick which is twisted a small amount each day until the worm has been removed (Figure 82.38). Care should be taken not to break the worm. Administration of antibiotics and cleaning and dressing of the ulcers are important in reducing secondary infections, and tetanus vaccination is recommended.

A technique for surgical extraction of the guinea worm prior to eruption through the skin has been described.[184] In the field, surgical removal of unerupted worms resulted in a significant decrease in guinea worm associated disability.

No anthelmintic treatment is available. Some drugs, especially niridazole (given orally at 12.5 mg/kg body weight daily) have been reported to reduce inflammation around the worm, thereby allowing easier extraction. Treatment of prepatent guinea worm infections with ivermectin had no effect.[185]

Epidemiology

Human guinea worm infections were previously much more widespread, but as a result of extensive control efforts (see below) the distribution is now limited to the Sahelian and sub-Sahelian areas of Africa (Figure 82.39).

The occurrence of guinea worm infection is associated with the use of small sources of water in semi-arid countries. Humans contract the infection by drinking the water containing infected cyclopoid copepods, and again

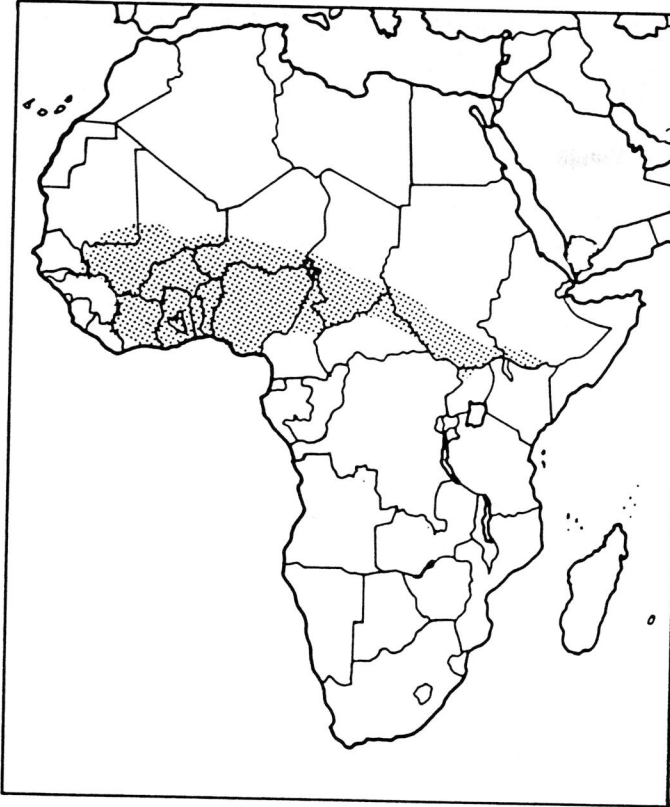

Figure 82.39: Geographical distribution of guinea worm.

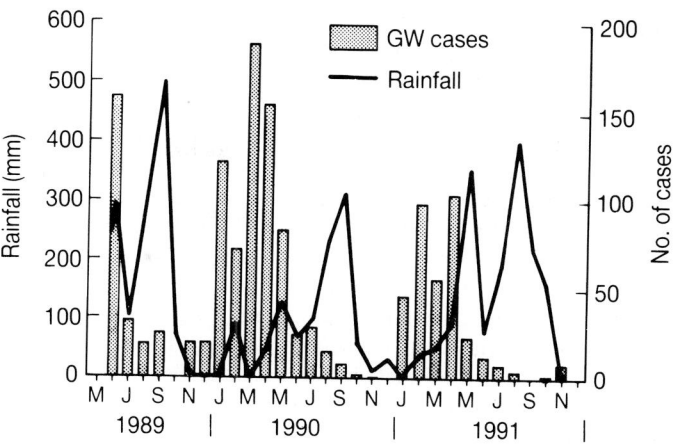

Figure 82.40: Seasonal variation in rainfall and number of guinea worm ulcers in a village in the northern region of Ghana. (Courtesy of P. Magnussen.)

contribute to transmission by immersing the guinea worm ulcer in water, thereby allowing the release of first-stage larvae. In the Sahelian region of Africa, transmission occurs mainly in small surface water pools used for collecting drinking water and for washing.

The transmission of guinea worm is frequently seasonal, with the majority of patent infections and infected copepods occurring within a few months of the year (Figure 82.40). The seasonality is closely related to the rainfall. In the arid areas the transmission usually coincides with the rainy season, when surface water is available, whereas in wet areas transmission is most intense in the dry season, when drinking water sources are few. The incidence of infection varies from area to area, but where endemicity is high, 50% or more of the population may be affected by the infection every year. However, even in highly endemic areas, some people never experience guinea worm infections, although they use the same drinking water source as the rest of the population. There is considerable variation in sex prevalence between different endemic areas. Persons aged between 15–40 years are mostly affected. The transmission season often coincides with the peak period of agricultural work. Because a large proportion of the farmers may be incapacitated, guinea worm infection can severely reduce agricultural output.

Parasites resembling *D. medinensis* are seen in animals, especially in dogs, but there is no evidence that they are a reservoir of infection for humans.

Control

Owing to its simple life cycle, and the apparent lack of an animal reservoir, the elimination of guinea worm appears feasible. The United Nations-supported International Drinking Water and Sanitation decade (1981–1990) raised global attention to the possibility of eradicating the infection by improving the quality of human drinking water, and in 1986 the WHO declared guinea worm the next human infection to be eradicated. Many organizations are currently involved in programmes to reach this goal.[186] By the end of 1998, Asia was declared free of transmission, and the global incidence had been reduced by more than 97%, from an estimated 3.2 million cases in 1986 to less than 80 000 cases. Dracunculiasis is now confined to 13 countries in Africa, with most of the remaining cases in the Sudan, Nigeria and Ghana.

Provision of safe drinking water in the form of bore-holes is the most expensive, but also the most effective, measure and has been shown to result in a dramatic reduction in the incidence of guinea worm infection.[187] As well as efforts being made to improve drinking water sources, other measures to control guinea worm transmission are health education and chemical vector control. Health education focuses on drinking water as the source of infection and on the importance of boiling or filtering the water before use. Special monofilament nylon material has been produced for filtering water, but effective and less expensive filters can be made from polyester cloth[188] or even from a layer of tightly woven cotton cloth. To prevent infestation of the water with guinea worm larvae, health education also emphasizes the reasons why people with guinea worm ulcers should avoid entering water sources. Vector control can be achieved in ponds and wells by applying the insecticide temephos (Abate). In the later stages of control, active surveillance on the increasingly smaller number of infected villages is being adopted, with the aim of implementing all possible control measures around each case immediately (case containment).

REFERENCES

1. World Health Organization. Lymphatic filariasis: the disease and its control. Fifth report of the WHO expert committee on filariasis. WHO Tech Rep Ser 1992; 821.

2. (text obscured)

3. Wucherer O E. Noticia preliminar sobre vermes de una especie ainda não descripta, encontrados na urina de doentes de hematuria intertropical no Brazil. Gaz Med Bahia 1868; 1:889-890.

4. (text obscured)

5. Cobbold T S. Discovery of the adult representative of microscopic filariae. Lancet 1877; ii:70-71.

6. McGregor I A. The Third Manson Oration. Patrick Manson 1844-1922. The birth of the science of tropical medicine. Trans R Soc Trop Med Hyg 1995; 89:...

7. Grove D I. A History of Human Helminthology. London: CAB International, 1990.

8. World Health Organization. Lymphatic filariasis. Fourth report of the WHO expert committee on filariasis. WHO Tech Rep Ser 1984; 702.

9. ... E C, Rupprecht D A. Of global patterns of Schistosomiasis/filariasis. Parasitol Today 1997; 13:472-476.

10. Simonsen P E, Niemann L & Meyrowitsch D W. Wuchereria bancrofti in Tanzania: microfilarial periodicity and effect of blood sampling time on microfilarial intensities. Trop Med Int Hlth 1997; 2:153-158.

11. Amaral F, Dreyer G, Figueredo-Silva J et al. Adult worms detected by ultrasonography in human bancroftian filariasis. Am J Trop Med Hyg 1994; 50:753-757.

12. Norões J, Addiss D, Santos A, Medeiros Z, Coutinho A & Dreyer G. Ultrasonographic evidence of abnormal lymphatic vessels in young men with Wuchereria bancrofti infection in the scrotal area. J Urol 1996; 156:409-412.

13. ... Filho P J A, Besh ..., Silva M C M, Brag... & Dreyer ... lymphoscintigraphic abnormalities in symptomatic and asymptomatic human filariasis. J Infect Dis 1994; 70:927-933.

14. Bernhard P, Makunde R W, Magnussen P & Lemnge M M. Genital manifestations and reproductive health in female residents of a Wuchereria bancrofti endemic area in Tanzania. Trans R Soc Trop Med Hyg 2000; 94:...

15. Dunyo S K, Nkrumah F K, Ahorlu C K & Simonsen P E. Exfoliative skin manifestations in acute lymphatic filariasis. Trans R Soc Trop Med Hyg 1998; 92:539-540.

16. Gasarasi D B, Premji Z G, Mujinja P G M & Mpembeni R. ... adenolymphangitis due to bancroftian filariasis in ... district, south east Tanzania ... Trop 2000; 75:...

17. ... Medeiros Z, Netto M J, ... Castro L G ... Piessens W F. Acute attacks in the extremities of persons living in an area endemic for bancroftian filariasis: differentiation of two syndromes. Trans R Soc Trop Med Hyg 1999; 93:413-417.

18. Simonsen P E, Meyrowitsch D W, Makunde W H & Magnussen P. ... pattern of microfilaraemia and ... of ... three endemic communities of ... Tanzania. Acta Trop 1995; 60:179-187.

19. McMahon J E, Magayuka S A, Kolstrup N et al. Studies on the transmission and prevalence of bancroftian filariasis in four coastal villages of Tanzania. Ann Trop Med Parasitol 1981; 75:415-431.

20. Meyrowitsch D W, Simonsen P E & Makunde W H. Bancroftian filariasis: analysis of infection and disease in five ... communities ... Trop Med Parasitol 1995; 89:653-663.

21. Burri H, Loutan L, Kumaraswami V & Vijayasekaran V. Skin changes in chronic lymphatic filariasis. Trans R Soc Trop Med Hyg 1996; 90:671-674.

22. Dunyo S K, Ahorlu C K & Simonsen P E. Scarification as a risk factor for rapid progression of filarial elephantiasis. Trans R Soc Trop Med ...

23. ... Ann Rev Med 1993; 43:417-424.

24. Dreyer G, Dreyer P & Piessens W F. Extralymphatic disease due to bancroftian filariasis. Braz J Med Biol Res 1999; 32:1467-1472.

25. Magnussen P, Makunde W, Simonsen P E, Meyrowitsch D & Jakobsen ... pulmonary disorders ... results ... bronchial ... Tanzania. Trans R Soc Trop Med Hyg 1995; 89:406-409.

26. Kazura J W, Bockarie M, Alexander N et al. Transmission intensity and its relationship to infection and disease due to Wuchereria bancrofti in Papua New Guinea. J Infect Dis 1997; 176:242-246.

27. McMahon J E, Marshall T F C, Vaughan J P & Abaru D E. Bancroftian filariasis: a comparison of microfilariae counting ... counting chamber, standard slide and membrane (nuclepore) filtration. Ann Trop Med Parasitol ...:457-464.

28. McMahon J E, Marshall T F C, Vaughan J P & Kolstrup N. Tanzania filariasis project: a provocative day test with diethylcarbamazine for the detection of microfilariae of nocturnally periodic Wuchereria bancrofti in the blood. Bull World Health Organ 1979; 57:759-765.

29. Simonsen P E, Meyrowitsch D W & Makunde W H. Bancroftian filariasis: long-term effect of the DEC provocative day test on microfilaraemia. Trans R Soc Trop Med Hyg 1997; 91:290-293.

30. Dunyo S K, Nkrumah F K & Simonsen P E. A study on the provocative day test effect of ivermectin and albendazole on nocturnal periodic Wuchereria bancrofti microfilaraemia. Trans R Soc Trop Med Hyg 1999; 93:608-610.

31. Haarbrink M, Terhell A, Abadi K, Beers S, Asri M & Yazdanbakhsh M. IgG4 antibody assay in the detection of filariasis. Lancet 1995; 346:853-854.

32. Rahmah N, Anuar A K, Ariff R H T et al. Use of antifilarial ... to detect ... malayi infection ... endemic area of Malaysia. Trop Med Int Hlth 1998; 3:184-188.

33. Weil G J, Lammie P J & Weiss N. The ICT filariasis test: a rapid-format antigen test for diagnosis of bancroftian filariasis. Parasitol Today 1997; 13:401-404.

34. Simonsen P E & Dunyo S K. Comparative evaluation of three tools for diagnosis of bancroftian filariasis based on detection of specific ... antigens. Trans R Soc Trop Med Hyg 1999; 93:278-282.

35. Rocha A, Addiss D, Ribeiro M E et al. Evaluation of Og4C3 ELISA in Wuchereria bancrofti infection: infected persons with undetectable or ultra-low microfilarial densities. Trop Med Int Hlth 1996; 1:859-864.

36. Zhong M, ... Farid ..., ... Kamal I H et al. A ... chain reaction-based assay for detection of Wuchereria bancrofti in human blood and Culex pipiens. Trans R Soc Trop Med Hyg 1997; 91:156-160.

37. Dissanayake S, Rocha A, Norões J, Medeiros Z, Dreyer G & Piessens W F. Evaluation of PCR-based methods for the diagnosis of infection in bancroftian filariasis. Trans R Soc Trop Med Hyg 2000; 94:526-530.

Parasitology and biology of the stages of the parasite

(Table 80.1)

Adult worms

In natural populations of schistosomes in the final definitive host usually comprises both male and female worms (Figure 80.3). Since the genus Schistosoma differs from most digenetic trematodes in being dioecious, a consequence of heteromorphic chromosomes in the ovum, a population could conceivably be unisexual (male or female worms only). Under laboratory conditions, single-miracidium infections carried through to cercarial infections in the final host result in either populations of unisexual males or unisexual females.[44]

Table 80.1 Comparison of principal features of Schistosoma spp. infecting humans

	S. japonicum	S. mekongi*	S. mansoni	S. haematobium	S. intercalatum
Adult worms					
Location of adult in host	Mesenteric veins	Mesenteric veins	Mesenteric veins	Vesical plexus	Mesenteric veins
Length of posterior gut	Medium	Medium	Very long	Short	Short
Male					
Length (mm)	10-20	15	10-15	11-14	
Width (mm)	0.95	0.41	0.90	0.3-0.4	
No. of testes	6-7	6-7	4-13(6-9)	4-5	2-7(4-5)
Tubercles	Absent	Absent?	Coarse	Fine	Fine
Female					
Length (mm)	20-30	12	10-20	16-26	10-14
Width (mm)	0.30	0.23	0.16	0.25	0.15-0.18
Ovary position in body	Middle	Rear half	Front third	Rear third	Rear half
Uterus position in body	Front half	Front half	Front third	Front two thirds	Front two thirds
No. of eggs	Many	Short	Short	Long	Long
		10+		5-60	
Mature egg					
Shape	Round	Round	Ovoid	Ovoid	Ovoid
Size (μm)	65 × 100	57 × 66	65 × 140	62 × 150	61 × 176
Spine	Lateral (reduced)	Lateral (reduced)	Lateral	Terminal	Terminal (prominent)
Normally passed in	Faeces	Faeces	Faeces	Urine	Faeces (and urine)
Eggs per female per day	3500		100-300	20-300	150-400
Reaction of eggshell to Ziehl-Neelsen‡					
Intermediate host snail	Oncomelania	Tricula	Biomphalaria	Bulinus	Bulinus

*From experimental animal infections. †Usual range. ‡In histological sections. Courtesy of R. F. Sturrock, Department of Medical Parasitology, London School of Hygiene and Tropical Medicine.
Reproduced with permission from Jordan P, Webbe G & Sturrock R F (eds) Human Schistosomiasis. Wallingford 2000; 1:1-526. 1993.

38 Fischer P, Supali T, Wibowo H, Bonow I & Williams S A. Detection of DNA of nocturnally periodic *Brugia malayi* in night and day blood samples by a polymerase chain reaction-ELISA-based method using an internal control DNA. *Am J Trop Med Hyg* 2000; 62:291–296.

39 Dreyer G, Santos A, Norões J, Amaral F & Addiss D. Ultrasonographic detection of living adult *Wuchereria bancrofti* using a 3.5-MHz transducer. *Am J Trop Med Hyg* 1998; 59:399–403.

40 Dreyer G, Brandão C A, Amaral F, Medeiros Z & Addiss D. Detection by ultrasound of living adult *Wuchereria bancrofti* in the female breast. *Mem Inst Oswaldo Cruz* 1996; 91:95–96.

41 Shenoy R K, John A, Hameed S, Suma T K & Kumaraswami V. Apparent failure of ultrasonography to detect adult worms of *Brugia malayi*. *Ann Trop Med Parasitol* 2000; 94: 77–82.

42 Ottesen E A. Immunopathology of lymphatic filariasis in man. *Springer Semin Immunopathol* 1980; 2:373–385.

43 Maizels R M, Sartono E, Kurniawan A, Partono F, Selkirk M E & Yazdanbakhsh M. T-cell activation and the balance of antibody isotypes in human lymphatic filariasis. *Parasitol Today* 1995; 11:50–56.

44 Michael E, Grenfell B T & Bundy D A P. The association between microfilaraemia and disease in lymphatic filariasis. *Proc R Soc Lond B Biol Sci* 1994; 256:33–40.

45 Freedman D O. Immune dynamics in the pathogenesis of human lymphatic filariasis. *Parasitol Today* 1998; 14:229–233.

46 Nicolas L, Langy S, Plichart C & Deparis X. Filarial antibody responses in *Wuchereria bancrofti* transmission area are related to parasitological but not clinical status. *Parasite Immunol* 1999; 21:73–80.

47 Dreyer G, Norões J, Figueredo-Silva J & Piessens W F. Pathogenesis of lymphatic disease in bancroftian filariasis: a clinical perspective. *Parasitol Today 2000*; 16:544–548.

48 Olszewski W L, Jamal S, Manokaran G et al. Bacteriological studies of blood, tissue fluid, lymph and lymph nodes in patients with acute dermatolymphanioadenitis (DLA) in course of 'filarial' lymphedema. *Acta Trop* 1999; 73:217–224.

49 Lobos E, Zahn R, Weiss N & Nutman T B. A major allergen of lymphatic filarial nematodes is a parasite homolog of the γ-glutamyl transpeptidase. *Mol Med* 1996; 2:712–724.

50 Simonsen P E & Meyrowitsch D W. Bancroftian filariasis in Tanzania: specific antibody responses in relation to long-term observations on microfilaraemia. *Am J Trop Med Hyg* 1998; 59:667–672.

51 Ravindran B, Satapathy A K, Sahoo P K & Geddam J J B. Protective immunity in human bancroftian filariasis: inverse relationship between antibodies to microfilarial sheath and circulating filarial antigen. *Parasite Immunol* 2000; 22:633–637.

52 Day K P, Gregory W F & Maizels R M. Age-specific acquisition of immunity to infective larvae in a bancroftian filariasis endemic area of Papua New Guinea. *Parasite Immunol* 1991; 13:277–290.

53 Michael E & Bundy D A P. Herd immunity to filarial infection is a function of vector biting rate. *Proc R Soc Lond [Biol]* 1998; B265:855–860.

54 Melrose W, Usurup J, Selve B, Pisters P & Turner P. Development of anti-filarial antibodies in a group of expatriate mine-site workers with varying exposure to the disease. *Trans R Soc Trop Med Hyg* 2000; 94:706–707.

55 Gopinath R, Ostrowski M, Justement S J, Fauci A S & Nutman T B. Filarial infections increase susceptibility to human immunodeficiency virus infection in peripheral blood mononuclear cells *in vitro*. *J Infect Dis* 2000; 182:1804–1808.

56 Addiss D G & Dreyer G. Treatment of lymphatic filariasis. In: Nutman T B (ed.) *Lymphatic Filariasis*. London: Imperial College Press, 2000: 151–199.

57 Norões J, Dreyer G, Santos A, Mendes V G, Medeiros Z & Addiss D. Assessment of the efficacy of diethylcarbamazine on adult *Wuchereria bancrofti in vivo*. *Trans R Soc Trop Med Hyg* 1997; 91:78–81.

58 Freedman D O, Bui T, Filho P J A et al. Lymphoscintigraphic assessment of the effect of diethylcarbamazine treatment on lymphatic damage in human bancroftian filariasis. *Am J Trop Med Hyg* 1995; 52:258–261.

59 Eberhard A L, Hightower A W, Addiss D G & Lammie P J. Clearance of *Wuchereria bancrofti* antigen after treatment with diethylcarbamazine or ivermectin. *Am J Trop Med Hyg* 1997; 57:483–486.

60 Dreyer G, Pires M L, Andrade L D et al. Tolerance of diethylcarbamazine by microfilaraemic and amicrofilaraemic individuals in an endemic area of bancroftian filariasis, Recife, Brazil. *Trans R Soc Trop Med Hyg* 1994; 88:232–236.

61 Cao W, Ploeg C P B, Plaisier A P, Sluijs I J S & Habbema J D F. Ivermectin for the chemotherapy of bancroftian filariasis: a meta-analysis of the effect of single treatment. *Trop Med Intl Hlth* 1997; 2:393–403.

62 Dreyer G, Addiss D, Norões J, Amaral F, Rocha A & Coutinho A D. Direct assessment of the adulticidal efficacy of repeat high-dose ivermectin in bancroftian filariasis. *Trop Med Int Hlth* 1996; 1:427–432.

63 Reddy G S, Vengatesvarlou N, Das P K, Vanamail P, Vijayan A P, Kala S & Pani S P. Tolerability and efficacy of single-dose diethylcarbamazine (DEC) or ivermectin in the clearance of *Wuchereria bancrofti* microfilaraemia in Pondicherry, south India. *Trop Med Int Hlth* 2000; 5:779–785.

64 Shenoy R K, Suma T K, Rajan K & Kumaraswami V. Prevention of acute adenolymphangitis in brugian filariasis: comparison of the efficacy of ivermectin and diethylcarbamazine, each combined with local treatment of the affected limb. *Ann Trop Med Parasitol* 1998; 92:587–594.

65 Shenoy R K, Kumaraswami V, Suma T K, Rajan K & Radhakuttyamma G. A double-blind, placebo-controlled study of the efficacy of oral penicillin, diethylcarbamazine or local treatment of the affected limb in preventing acute adenolymphangitis in lymphoedema caused by brugian filariasis. *Ann Trop Med Parasitol* 1999; 93:367–377.

66 Simonsen P E, Meyrowitsch D W, Jaoko W G et al. Bancroftian filariasis infection, disease and specific antibody response patterns in a high and a low endemicity community in east Africa. *Am J Trop Med Hyg* 2001; in press.

67 Alexander N D E & Grenfell B T. The effect of pregnancy on *Wuchereria bancrofti* microfilarial load in humans. *Parasitology* 1999; 119:151–156.

68 Lammie P J, Hitch W L, Allen E M W, Hightower W & Eberhard M L. Maternal filarial infection as risk factor for infection in children. *Lancet* 1991; 337:1005–1006.

69 Das P K, Sirvidya A, Vanamail P et al. *Wuchereria bancrofti* microfilaraemia in children in relation to parental infection status. *Trans R Soc Trop Med Hyg* 1997; 91:677–679.

70 Dreyer G, Norões J & Addiss D. The silent burden of sexual disability associated with lymphatic filariasis. *Acta Trop* 1997; 63:57–60.

71 Ahorlu C K, Dunyo S K, Koram K A, Nkrumah F K, Aagaard-Hansen J & Simonsen P E. Lymphatic filariasis related perceptions and practices on the coast of Ghana: implications for prevention and control. *Acta Trop* 1999; 73:251–264.

72 Gyapong J O, Adjei S, Gyapong M & Asamoah G. Rapid community diagnosis of lymphatic filariasis. *Acta Trop* 1996; 61:65–74.

73 Ottesen E A, Duke B O L, Karam M & Behbehani K. Strategies and tools for the control/elimination of lymphatic filariasis. *Bull World Health Organ* 1997; 75:491–503.

74 Sabesan S, Palaniyandi M, Das P K & Michael E. Mapping of lymphatic filariasis in India. *Ann Trop Med Parasitol* 2000; 94:591–606.

75 Lindsay S W & Thomas C J. Mapping and estimating the population at risk from lymphatic filariasis in Africa. *Trans R Soc Trop Med Hyg* 2000; 94:37–45.

76 Chan M S, Srividya A, Norman R A et al. Epifil: a dynamic model of infection and disease in lymphatic filariasis. *Am J Trop Med Hyg* 1998; 59:606–614.

77 Plaisier A P, Subramanian S, Das P K et al. The LYMFASIM simulation program for modeling lymphatic filariasis and its control. *Methods Inf Med* 1998; 37:97–108.

78 Plaisier A P, Stolk W A, Oortmarssen G J & Habbema J D F. Effectiveness of annual ivermectin treatment for *Wuchereria bancrofti* infection. *Parasitol Today* 2000; 16:298–302.

79 Meyrowitsch D W & Simonsen P E. Long-term effect of mass diethylcarbamazine chemotherapy on bancroftian filariasis: results at four years after start of treatment. *Trans R Soc Trop Med Hyg* 1998; 92:98–103.

80 Ottesen E A, Ismail M M & Horton J. The role of albendazole in programmes to eliminate lymphatic filariasis. *Parasitol Today* 1999; 15:382–386.

81 Beach M J, Streit T G, Addiss D G, Prospere R, Roberts J M & Lammie P J. Assessment of combined ivermectin and albendazole for treatment of intestinal helminth and *Wuchereria bancrofti* infections in Haitian schoolchildren. *Am J Trop Med Hyg* 1999; 60:479–486.

82 Shenoy R K, Dalia S, John A, Suma T K & Kumaraswami V. Treatment of the microfilaraemia of asymptomatic brugian filariasis with single doses of ivermectin, diethylcarbamazine or albendazole, in various combinations. *Ann Trop Med Parasitol* 1999; 93:643–651.

83 Dunyo S K, Nkrumah F K & Simonsen P E. A randomized double-blind placebo-controlled field trial of ivermectin and albendazole alone and in combination for the treatment of lymphatic filariasis in Ghana. *Trans R Soc Trop Med Hyg* 2000; 94:205–211.

84 Maxwell C A, Mohammed K, Kisumku U & Curtis C F. Can vector control play a useful supplemantary role against bancroftian filariasis? *Bull World Health Organ* 1999; 77:138–143.

85 Mukoko D A N, Pedersen E M, Masese N N et al The effect of permethrin impregnated bednets on the transmission of bancroftian filariasis in Kwale District in the coastal region of Kenya. *Am J Trop Med Hyg* 2002; in press.

86 Ottesen E A. The global programme to eliminate lymphatic filariasis. *Trop Med Int Hlth* 2000; 5:591–594.

87 O'Neill J. On the presence of a filaria in 'craw-craw'. *Lancet* 1875; i:265–266.

88 Robles R. Enfermedad nueva en Guatemala. *Juventud Med* 1917; 17:97–115.

89 Blacklock D B. The development of *Onchocerca volvulus* in *Simulium damnosum*. *Ann Trop Med Parasitol* 1926; 20:1–48.

90 World Health Organization. Onchocerciasis and its control. Report of a WHO expert committee on onchocerciasis control. *WHO Tech Rep Ser* 1995; 852.

91 Duke B O L. The population dynamics of *Onchocerca volvulus* in the human host. *Trop Med Parasitol* 1993; 44:61–68.

92 Hagan M. Onchocercal dermatitis: clinical impact. *Ann Trop Med Parasitol* 1998; 92 (Supplement 1):S85–S96.

93 Murdoch M E, Hay R J, Mackenzie C D et al. A clinical classification and grading system of the cutaneous changes in onchocerciasis. *Br J Dermatol* 1993; 129:260–269.

94 Abiose A. Onchocercal eye disease and the impact of Mectizan treatment. *Ann Trop Med Parasitol* 1998; 92 (Supplement 1):S11–S22.

95 Druet-Cabanac M, Preux P-M, Bouteille B et al. Onchocerciasis and epilepsy: a matched case–control study in the Central African Republic. *Am J Epidemiol* 1999; 149:565–570.

96 Kipp W, Burnham G, Bamuhiiga J & Leichenring M. The Nakalanga syndrome in Kabarole District, western Uganda. *Am J Trop Med Hyg* 1996; 54:80–83.

97 Kale O O. Onchocerciasis: the burden of disease. *Ann Trop Med Parasitol* 1998; 92 (Supplement 1):S101–S115.

98 Anderson J, Fuglsang H, Hamilton P J S & Marshall T F de C. Studies on onchocerciasis in The United Cameroon Republic. II. Comparison of onchocerciasis in rain-forest and Sudan-savanna. *Trans R Soc Trop Med Hyg* 1974; 68:209–222.

99 McMahon J E, Sowa S C I, Maude G H, Hudson C M & Kirkwood B R. Epidemiological studies of onchocerciasis in forest villages of Sierra Leone. *Trop Med Parasitol* 1988; 39:251–259.

100 Pearlman E. Immunopathology of onchocerciasis: a role for eosinophils in onchocercal dermatitis and keratitis. *Chem Immunol* 1997; 66:26–40.

101 Mackenzie C D, Williams J F, Sisley B M, Steward M W & O'Day J. Variations in host responses and the pathogenesis of human onchocerciasis. *Rev Infect Dis* 1985; 7:802–808.

102 Ottesen E A. Immune responsiveness and the pathogenesis of human onchocerciasis. *J Infect Dis* 1995; 171:659–671.

103 Greene B M, Taylor H R & Aikawa M. Cellular killing of microfilariae of *Onchocerca volvulus*: eosinophil and neutrophil-mediated immune serum-dependent destruction. *J Immunol* 1981; 127:1611–1618.

104 Garate T, Conraths F J, Harnett W, Büttner D W & Parkhouse R M E. Identification of *Onchocerca volvulus* collagen as an antigen mainly recognized by antibodies in chronic hyperactive onchodermatitis (Sowda). *Am J Trop Med Hyg* 1996; 54:490–497.

105 Van der Lelij A, Rothova A, Stilma J S, Vetter J C M, Hoekzema R & Kijlstra A. Humoral and cell-mediated immune response against retinal antigens in relation to onchocerciasis. *Acta Leiden* 1990; 59:271–283.

106 Soboslay P T, Geiger S M, Drabner B et al. Prenatal immune priming in onchocerciasis—*Onchocerca volvulus*-specific cellular responsiveness and cytokine production in newborns from infected mothers. *Clin Exp Immunol* 1999; 117:130–137.

107 McCarthy J S, Ottesen E A & Nutman T B. Onchocerciasis in endemic and nonendemic populations: differences in clinical presentation and immunologic findings. *J Infect Dis* 1994; 170:736–741.

108 Stewart G R, Boussinesq M, Coulson T, Elson L, Nutman T & Bradley J E. Onchocerciasis modulates the immune response to mycobacterial antigens. *Clin Exp Immunol* 1999; 117:517–523.

109 Cooper P J, Espinel I, Wieseman M et al. Human onchocerciasis and tetanus vaccination: impact on the postvaccination antitetanus response. *Infect Immunol* 1999; 67:5951–5957.

110 Tawill S A, Gallin M, Erttmann, K D, Kipp W, Bamuhiiga J & Büttner D W. Impaired antibody responses and loss of reactivity to *Onchocerca volvulus* antigens by HIV-seropositive onchocerciasis patients. *Trans R Soc Trop Med Hyg* 1996; 90:85–89.

111 Leichenring M, Tröger J, Nelle M, Büttner D W, Darge K & Doehring-Schwerdtfeger E. Ultrasonographical investigations of onchocerciasis in Liberia. *Am J Trop Med Hyg* 1990; 43:380–385.

112 Bradley J E & Unnasch T R. Molecular approaches to the diagnosis of onchocerciasis. *Adv Parasitol* 1996; 37:57–106.

113 Weil G J, Ogunrinade A F, Chandrashekar R & Kale O O. IgG4 subclass antibody serology for onchocerciasis. *J Infect Dis* 1990; 161:549–554.

114 Bradley J E, Trenholme K R, Gillespie A J et al. A sensitive serodiagnostic test for onchocerciasis using a cocktail of recombinant antigens. *Am J Trop Med Hyg* 1993; 48:198–204.

115 Weil G J, Steel C, Liftis F, Mearns G, Lobos E & Nutman T B. A rapid-format antibody card test for diagnosis of onchocerciasis. *J Infect Dis* 2000; 182:1796–1799.

116 Zimmerman P, Guderian R H & Araujo E. Polymerase chain-reaction based diagnosis of *Onchocerca volvulus* infection; improved detection of patients with onchocerciasis. *J Infect Dis* 1994; 169:686–689.

117 Hoerauf A, Volkman L, Hamelmann C et al. Endosymbiotic bacteria in worms as targets for a novel chemotherapy in filariasis. *Lancet* 2000; 355:1242–1243.

118 Awadzi K, Dadzie K Y, Klager S & Gilles H M. The chemotherapy of onchocerciasis. XIII. Studies with ivermectin in onchocerciasis patients in northern Ghana, a region with long lasting vector control. *Trop Med Parasitol* 1989; 40:361–366.

119 Whitworth J A, Morgan D, Maude G H & Taylor D W. Community-based treatment with ivermectin. *Lancet* 1988; ii:97–98.

120 Mabey D, Whitworth J A, Eckstein M, Gilbert C, Maude G & Downham M. The effects of multiple doses of ivermectin on ocular onchocerciasis. *Ophthalmology* 1996; 103:1001–1008.

121 Habbema J D F, Alley E S, Plaisier A P, van Oortmarssen G J & Remme J H F. Epidemiological modelling for onchocerciasis control. *Parasitol Today* 1992; 8:99–103.

122 Basáñez M-G & Boussinesq M. Population biology of human onchocerciasis. *Philos Trans R Soc Lond [Biol]* 1999; 354:809–826.

123 Duke B O L, Lewis D J & Moore P J. Transmission of forest and Sudan-savanna strains of *Onchocerca volvulus* from Cameroon by *Simulium damnosum* from various west African bioclimatic zones. *Ann Trop Med Parasitol* 1966; 60:318–336.

124 Toé L, Tang J, Back C, Katholi C R & Unnasch T R. Vector–parasite transmission complexes for onchocerciasis in West Africa. *Lancet* 1997; 349:163–166.

125 Zimmerman P A, Dadzie K Y, De S G, Remme J, Alley E S & Unnasch T R. *Onchocerca volvulus* DNA probe classification correlated with epidemiological patterns of blindness. *J Infect Dis* 1992; 165:964–968.

126 Ogunrinade A, Boakye D, Merryweather A & Unnasch T R. Distribution of blinding and nonblinding strains of *Onchocerca volvulus* in Nigeria. *J Infect Dis* 1999; 179:1577–1579.

127 McMahon J E, Davies J B, White M D, Goddard J M, Beech-Garwood P A & Kirkwood B R. Onchocerciasis in Sierra Leone 1: studies on the prevalence and transmission in Gbaiima village. *Trans R Soc Trop Med Hyg* 1986; 80:802–809.

128 Pedersen E M & Maegga B T. Quantitative studies on the transmission of *Onchocerca volvulus* by *Simulium damnosum* s.l. in the Tukuyu Valley, south west Tanzania. *Tropenmed Parasitol* 1985; 36:249–254.

129 Makunde W H, Salum F M, Massaga J J & Alilio M S. Clinical and parasitological aspects of itching caused by onchocerciasis in Morogoro, Tanzania. *Ann Trop Med Parasitol* 2000; 94:793–799.

130 Zimmerman P A, Katholi C R, Wooten M C, Lanf-Unnasch N & Unnasch T R. Recent evolutionary history of American *Onchocerca volvulus*, based on analysis of a tandemly repeated DNA sequence family. *Mol Biol Evol* 1994; 11:384–392.

131 Botto C, Gillespie A J, Vivas-Martinez S et al. Onchocerciasis hyperendemic in the Unturán Mountains: the value of recombinant antigens in describing a new transmission area in southern Venezuela. *Trans R Soc Trop Med Hyg* 1999; 93:25–30.

132 Corredor A, Nicholls R S, Duque S et al. Current status of onchocerciasis in Columbia. *Am J Trop Med Hyg* 1998; 58: 594–598.

133 Guderian R H & Shelley A J. Onchocerciasis in Ecuador: the situation in 1989. *Mem Inst Oswaldo Cruz* 1992; 87:405–415.

134 Evans T G. Socioeconomic consequences of blinding onchocerciasis in West Africa. *Bull World Health Organ* 1995; 73:495–506.

135 Vlassoff C, Weiss M, Ovuga E B L et al. Gender and the stigma of onchocercal skin disease in Africa. *Soc Sci Med* 2000; 50:1353–1368.

136 Boatin B, Molyneux D H, Hougard J M et al. Patterns of epidemiology and control of onchocerciasis in West Africa. *J Helminthol* 1997; 71:91–101.

137 Molyneux D H & Davies J B. Onchocerciasis control: moving towards the millennium. *Parasitol Today* 1997; 13:418–425.

138 Hougard J-M, Yaméogo L, Sékétéli A, Boatin B & Dadzie K Y. Twenty-two years of blackfly control in the Onchocerciasis Control Programme in West Africa. *Parasitol Today* 1997; 13:425–431.

139 Remme J, Baker R H A, De Sole G et al. A community trial of ivermectin in the onchocerciasis focus of Asubende, Ghana. I. Effect on the microfilarial reservoir and the transmission of *Onchocerca volvulus*. *Trop Med Parasitol* 1989; 40:367–374.

140 De Sole G, Awadzi K, Remme J et al. A community trial of ivermectin in the onchocerciasis focus of Asubende, Ghana. II. Adverse reactions. *Trop Med Parasitol* 1989; 40:375–382.

141 Boatin B A, Hougard J-M, Alley E S et al. The impact of Mectizan on the transmission of onchocerciasis. *Ann Trop Med Parasitol* 1998; 92 (Supplement 1):S47–S60.

142 Brieger W R, Awedoba A K, Eneanya C I et al. The effects of ivermectin on onchocercal skin disease and severe itching: results of a multicentre trial. *Trop Med Int Hlth* 1998; 3:951–961.

143 Edungbola L D. Onchocerciasis control in Nigeria. *Parasitol Today* 1991; 7:97–99.

144 Gardon J, Gardon-Wendel N, Demanga-Ngangue, Kamgno J, Chippeaux J-P & Boussinesq M. Serious reactions after mass treatment of onchocerciasis with ivermectin in an area endemic for *Loa loa* infection. *Lancet* 1997; 350:18–22.

145 Boussinesq M & Gardon J. Prevalence of *Loa loa* microfilaraemia throughout the area endemic for the infection. *Ann Trop Med Parasitol* 1997; 91:573–589.

146 Noireau F, Apembet J D, Nzoulani A & Carme B. Clinical manifestations of loiasis in an endemic area in the Congo. *Trop Med Parasitol* 1990; 41:37–39.

147 Carme B, Mamboueni J P, Copin N & Noireau F. Clinical and biological study of *Loa loa* filariasis in Congolese. *Am J Trop Med Hyg* 1989; 41:331–337.

148 Klion A D, Massougbodji M, Sadeler B-C, Ottesen E A & Nutman T B. Loiasis in endemic and non-endemic populations: immunologically mediated differences in clinical presentation. *J Infect Dis* 1991; 163:1318–1325.

149 Andy J J, Bishara F F & Soyinka O O. Relation of severe eosinophilia and microfilariasis to chronic African endomyocardial fibrosis. *Br Heart J* 1981; 45:672–680.

150 Orihel T C & Eberhard M L. Zoonotic filariasis. *Clin Microbiol Rev* 1998; 11:366–381.

151 Churchill D R, Morris C, Kakoya A, Wright S G & Davidson R N. Clinical and laboratory features of patients with loiasis (*Loa loa* filariasis) in the UK. *J Infect* 1996; 33:103–109.

152 Dupont A, Zue-N'dong J & Pinder M. Common occurrence of amicrofilaraemic *Loa loa* filariasis within the endemic region. *Trans R Soc Trop Med Hyg* 1988; 82:730.

153 Touré F S, Egwang T G, Millet P, Bain O, Georges A J & Wahl G. IgG4 serology of loiasis in three villages in an endemic area of south-eastern Gabon. *Trop Med Int Hlth* 1998; 3:313–317.

154 Touré F S, Mavoungou E, Kassambara L et al. Human occult loiasis: field evaluation of a nested polymerase chain reaction assay for the detection of occult infection. *Trop Med Int Hlth* 1998; 3:505–511.

155 Pinder M, Dupont A & Egwang T G. Identification of a surface antigen on *Loa loa* microfilariae the recognition of which correlates with the amicrofilaraemic state in man. *J Immunol* 1988; 141:2480–2486.

156 Baize S, Wahl G, Soboslay P T, Egwang T G & Georges A J. T helper responsiveness in human *Loa loa* infection; defective specific proliferation and cytokine production by CD4+ T cells from microfilaraemic subjects compared with amicrofilaraemics. *Clin Exp Immunol* 1997; 108:272–278.

157 Klion A D , Ottesen E A & Nutman T B. Effectiveness of diethylcarbamazine in treating loiasis acquired by expatriate visitors to endemic regions: long-term follow-up. *J Infect Dis* 1994; 169:604–610.

158 Martin-Prevel Y, Cosnefroy J Y, Tshipamba P, Ngari P, Chodakewitz J A & Pinder M. Tolerance and efficacy of single high-dose ivermectin for the treatment of loiasis. *Am J Trop Med Hyg* 1993; 48:186–192.

159 Duong T H, Kombila M, Ferrer A, Bureau P, Gaxotte P & Richard-Lenoble D. Reduced *Loa loa* microfilaria count ten to twelve months after a single dose of ivermectin. *Trans R Soc Trop Med Hyg* 1997; 91:592–593.

160 Hoegaerden M V, Ivanoff B, Flocard F, Salle A & Chabaud B. The use of mebendazole in the treatment of filariases due to *Loa loa* and *Mansonella perstans*. *Ann Trop Med Parasitol* 1987; 81:275–282.

161 Klion A D, Horton J & Nutman T B. Albendazole therapy for loiasis refractory to diethylcarbamazine treatment. *Clin Infect Dis* 1999; 29:680–682.

162 Noireau F, Carme B, Apembet J D & Gouteux J P. *Loa loa* and *Mansonella perstans* filariasis in the Chaillu mountains, Congo: parasitological prevalence. *Trans R Soc Trop Med Hyg* 1989; 83:529–534.

163 Nutman T B, Miller K D, Mulligan M et al. Diethylcarbamazine provides effective prophylaxis for human loiasis. *N Engl J Med* 1988; 319:752–756.

164 Duong T H, Kombila M, Ferrer A, Nguiri C & Richard-Lenoble D. Decrease in *Mansonella perstans* microfilaraemia after albendazole treatment. *Trans R Soc Trop Med Hyg* 1998; 92:459.

165 Fischer P, Kilian A H D, Bamuhiiga J, Kipp W & Büttner D.W. Prevalence of *Mansonella perstans* in western Uganda and its detection using the QBC-fluorescence method. *Appl Parasitol* 1996; 37:32–37.

166 Fischer P, Bamuhiiga J & Büttner D W. Occurrence and diagnosis of *Mansonella streptocerca* in Uganda. *Acta Trop* 1997; 63:43–55.

167 Meyers W M, Connor D H, Harman L F, Fleshman K, Moris R & Neafie R C. Human streptocerciasis. A clinico-pathologic study of 40 Africans (Zairans) including identification of the adult filaria. *Am J Trop Med Hyg* 1972; 22:528–545.

168 Fischer P, Büttner D W, Bamuhiiga J & Williams S A. Detection of the filarial parasite *Mansonella streptocerca* in skin biopsies by a nested polymerase chain reaction-based assay. *Am J Trop Med Hyg* 1998; 58:816–820.

169 Meyers W M, Moris R, Neafie R C, Connor D H & Bourland J. Streptocerciasis: degeneration of adult *Dipetalonema streptocerca* in man following diethylcarbamazine therapy. *Am J Trop Med Hyg* 1978; 27:1137–1147.

170 Fischer P, Tukesiga E & Büttner D W. Long-term suppression of *Mansonella streptocerca* microfilariae after treatment with ivermectin. *J Infect Dis* 1999; 180:1403–1405.

171 Bartoloni A, Cancrini G, Bartalesi F et al. *Mansonella ozzardi* infection in Bolivia: prevalence and clinical association in the Chaco Region. *Am J Trop Med Hyg* 1999; 61:830–833.

172 Raccurt C, Lowrie R C & McNeeley D F. *Mansonella ozzardi* in Haiti. I. Epidemiological survey. *Am J Trop Med Hyg* 1980; 29:803–808.

173 McNeeley D F, Raccurt C P, Boncy J & Lowrie R C. Clinical evaluation of *Mansonella ozzardi* in Haiti. *Trop Med Parasitol* 1988; 40:107–110.

174 Katz S P, Raccurt C P, Lowrie R C, Boncy J & Leiva L M. *Mansonella ozzardi* in Haiti. IV. Evaluation of antibody reactivity to heterologous antigens. *Am J Trop Med Hyg* 1986; 35:303–307.

175 Raccurt C, Lowrie R C, Boncy J & Katz S P. *Mansonella ozzardi* in Haiti. III. A comparison of the sensitivity of four sampling methods in detecting infections. *Am J Trop Med Hyg* 1982; 31:275–279.

176 González A A, Chadee D D & Rawlins S C. Single dose of ivermectin to control mansonellosis in Trinidad: a four-years follow-up study. *Trans R Soc Trop Med Hyg* 1998; 92:570–571.

177 Boreham P F L. Dirofilariasis in man. In Boreham P F L & Atwell R B (eds) *Dirofilariasis*. Boca Raton: CRC Press, 1988: 218–226.

178 Pampiglione S, Trotti G C & Rivasi F. Human dirofilariasis due to *Dirofilaria (Nochtiella) repens*: a review of world literature. *Parassitologia* 1995, 37:149–193.

179 Yelifari L, Frempong E & Olsen A. The intermediate hosts of *Dracunculus medinensis* in Northern Region, Ghana. *Ann Trop Med Parasitol* 1997; 91:403–409.

180 Bloch P & Simonsen P E. Studies on immunodiagnosis of dracunculiasis. I. Detection of specific serum antibodies. *Acta Trop* 1998; 70:73–86.

181 Bloch P, Vennervald B J & Simonsen P E. Studies on immunodiagnosis of dracunculiasis. II. Search for circulating antigens. *Acta Trop* 1998; 70:303–315.

182 Bloch P & Simonsen P E. Immunoepidemiology of *Dracunculus medinensis* infections. I. Antibody responses in relation to infection status. *Am J Trop Med Hyg* 1998; 59:978–984.

183 Bloch P & Simonsen P E. Immunoepidemiology of *Dracunculus medinensis* infections. II. Variation in antibody responses in relation to transmission season and patency. *Am J Trop Med Hyg* 1998; 59:985–990.

184 Rohde J E, Sharma B L, Patton H, Deegan C & Sherry J M. Surgical extraction of guinea worm: disability reduction and contribution to disease control. *Am J Trop Med Hyg* 1993; 48:71–76.

185 Issaka-Tinorgah A, Magnussen P, Bloch P & Yakubu A. Lack of effect of ivermectin on prepatent guinea-worm: a single-blind, placebo-controlled trial. *Trans R Soc Trop Med Hyg* 1994; 88:346–348.

186 Hopkins D R, Ruiz-Tiben E, Ruebush T K, Diallo N, Agle A & Withers Jr. P C. Dracunculiasis eradication: delayed, not denied. *Am J Trop Med Hyg* 2000; 62:163–168.

187 Hunter J M. Bore holes and the vanishing of guinea worm disease in Ghana's Upper Region. *Soc Sci Med* 1997; 45:71–89.

188 Olsen A, Magnussen P & Anemana S. The acceptability and effectiveness of a polyester drinking-water filter in a dracunculiasis-endemic village in Northern Region, Ghana. *Bull World Health Organ* 1997; 75:449–452.

Chapter 83
Soil-transmitted Helminths (Geohelminths)

H. M. Gilles

These are intestinal nematodes, part of the development of which takes place outside the body—in the soil.

Soil-transmitted nematodes are of great importance in the health of many populations in developing countries where the frequency of infection is a general indication of the local level of development of hygiene and sanitation. These nematodes are usually found as multiple infections and measures against and treatment of one closely affect the others. They may be divided into three types according to their life cycle.

Type 1: direct

Embryonated eggs are passed; they hatch and reinfect within 2–3 hours by being carried from the anal margin to the mouth and either do not reach the soil or, if they do, do not require a period of development there. This group includes *Enterobius vermicularis* (threadworm) and *Trichuris trichiura* (whipworm).

Type 2: modified direct

Eggs are passed out in the stool and undergo a period of development in the soil before being ingested, where they hatch, releasing larvae which penetrate the mucous membrane(s) of the stomach and enter the circulation to reach the lungs, passing up the respiratory tract to enter the oesophagus, reaching the intestine where they become adult. These include *Ascaris lumbricoides* (roundworm) and *Toxocara canis*.

Type 3: penetration of the skin

In this group eggs are passed in the stools to the soil, where they hatch into larvae which undergo further development before they are ready to penetrate the skin and reach the circulation and lungs, which they penetrate to enter the respiratory tract; they move up to enter the oesophagus and reach the small intestine, where they become adult. *Ancylostoma* (hookworm) and *Strongyloides stercoralis* belong to this group, but differ in that *Strongyloides* larvae are passed in the stool and autoinfection can occur at the anal margin, or independent development takes place in the soil, where they can exist in the absence of any further cycle through man.

Type 1: direct (*Enterobius, Trichuris*)

Enterobiasis (threadworm, Pinworm, Oxyuriasis)

Geographical distribution

Enterobius vermicularis has a worldwide distribution.

Aetiology

The adult *Enterobius vermicularis* (Figure 83.1, Chapter 11 and Appendix III) are small and white with a double bulb oesophagus and a mouth surrounded by a cuticular expansion; the skin is transversely striated. The female (9–12 mm) has a long, pointed tail and a slit-like vulva in the anterior quarter of the body. The male, which is much smaller (2.5 mm), has a posteriorly curved third and a blunt caudal extremity. The egg (Figure 83.2) measures 50–54 × 20–27 mm and has a characteristic shape, flattened on one side. It is almost colourless, with a bean-shaped double contour shell containing a fully formed embryo.

Life cycle (see Appendix III)

There is no multiplication inside the body. The mature female has a life duration of 37–93 days and when the

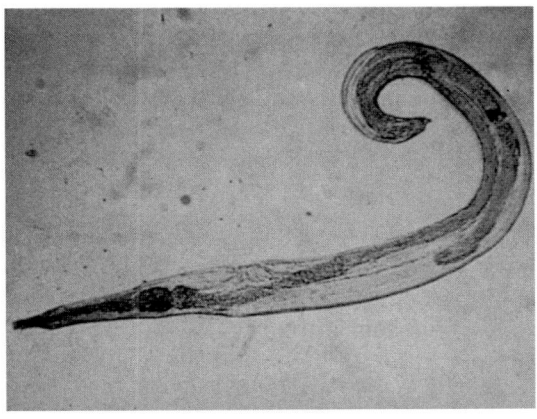

Figure 83.1: Adult *Enterobius vermicularis* (threadworm, pinworm).

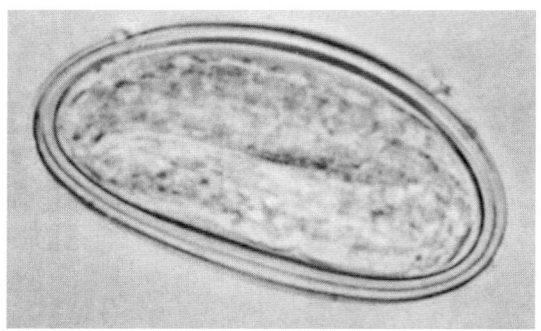

Figure 83.2: Egg of *Enterobius vermicularis*, as laid partially embryonated.

ovary is full of eggs she migrates down to the anus, from which she emerges to lay the eggs on the perianal skin and on the perineum. The eggs, which are ingested in faecal material lodged under the fingernails, hatch in the stomach and larvae emerge which rapidly grow to 140–150 μm in length. They pass through the intestine to the caecum and appendix, where they invade the glandular crypts and mature. The whole cycle takes 2–4 weeks.

Transmission

There are four possible methods of transmission; the most common is by direct transmission from the anal and perianal region to the mouth by fingernail contamination and by soiled nightclothes. A second way is by exposure to viable eggs on soiled bed linen and other contaminated objects in the environment. A third way is via the mouth or nose from contaminated dust in which embryonated eggs have been detected. The fourth way is by retroinfection in which eggs hatch on the anal mucosa and larvae migrate up the bowel.

Pathology

The adult worm lives in the upper part of the colon, especially the caecum and lower ileum, where minute ulcerations may develop at the site of attachment of the adult worms to the caecal and appendiceal mucosa. At times haemorrhages occur and secondary infection causes ulcers and submucosal abscesses. Symptoms are caused when gravid females migrate out of the anus on to perianal skin to deposit eggs, where they cause pruritus.

Ectopic lesions

Occasionally *Enterobius* is found in the female genital organs and more rarely in the ear and nose. Rarely worms can invade the abdominal cavity and cause threadworm granulomas of the liver, ovary, kidney, spleen and lung. Chronic pelvic peritonitis and ileocolitis have been described.[1] The route by which *Enterobius* gains access to these organs is not clear but may be via the Fallopian tubes or haematogenous spread. Direct infection following

abdominal operations may also occur. The granuloma which forms around the female and eggs consists chiefly of lymphocytes with a few eosinophils but no giant cells. Four cases of eosinophilic granuloma of the large bowel and omentum have been ascribed to *Enterobius*.

Clinical features

Natural history

In the majority of infections *Enterobius* lives out its normal life span in the caecum and appendix, migrates down to the anus and deposits its eggs, and the larvae re-establish themselves in the host, causing few or no symptoms.

Symptoms and Signs

Pruritus ani is the main symptom and varies from mild itching to acute pain, which occurs mainly at night. The pruritus produces scratching of the perianal region resulting in excoriation and secondary infection.

Vulvitis may be caused by pinworms entering the vulva, causing a mucoid discharge and *pruritus vulvi*.

General symptoms are insomnia and restlessness, and a considerable proportion of children show loss of appetite, loss of weight, irritability, emotional instability and enuresis. There is usually no eosinophilia or anaemia.

Diagnosis

The diagnosis is made by finding the characteristic eggs (see Figure 83.2) in the faeces (5% only), perianal scrapings or swabs from under the fingernails, or by finding adult worms round the anus, usually at night.

Faecal examination (See also Appendix I)

Eggs are present in the faeces of no more than 5% of infected individuals.

A Sellotape swab has been devised with which it is possible to obtain eggs by scraping the perianal area. Enclosed in a container, it may be sent through the post and examined at leisure. The Sellotape is mounted in water or 0.1 mol sodium hydroxide on a slide, covered with a coverslip and examined.

The Scotch tape method, in which eggs adhere to a sticky surface, is very popular (see Appendix I).

Treatment

The whole family must be treated to avoid reinfection. Chemotherapy must be combined with education, and personal hygiene aimed at preventing autoinfection. Although it is simple to effect a temporary cure, eradication may prove difficult because of reinfection from the contaminated environment or from asymptomatic members of the same household. Eradication may necessitate repeated courses of treatment for up to a year or more.

Chemotherapy

Abendazole is the treatment of choice, as a single oral dose of 400 mg or 10–14 mg/kg for children.

Mebendazole is as effective in a single oral dose of 100 mg. It is available 'over the counter'.

Pyrantel pamoate (Combantrin) 10 mg/kg may be given as a single oral dose and repeated every 6 weeks until the environment is clear.

During treatment it is important to prevent reinfection. The child must sleep in cotton clothes and gloves and the fingernails must be kept short and scrubbed. Other members of the family or school should also be treated.

Epidemiology

Enterobiasis is worldwide in distribution and is a group infection, more common in children than adults. It occurs in family groups or institutions, such as asylums and schools, especially under crowded conditions. When one infection is found it is likely that there are others also. Although it is a human infection, chimpanzees, gibbons and marmosets can all be infected.

Trichuriasis (*Trichuris trichiura*) (Whipworm)

Geographical distribution

Trichuris trichiura occurs worldwide. It is estimated that 46 million people in the world are infected with associated morbidity, resulting in an annual mortality of 60 000.[2]

Aetiology

Trichuris trichiura is a greyish-white worm, often slightly pink, which lives in the caecum and appendix. The male

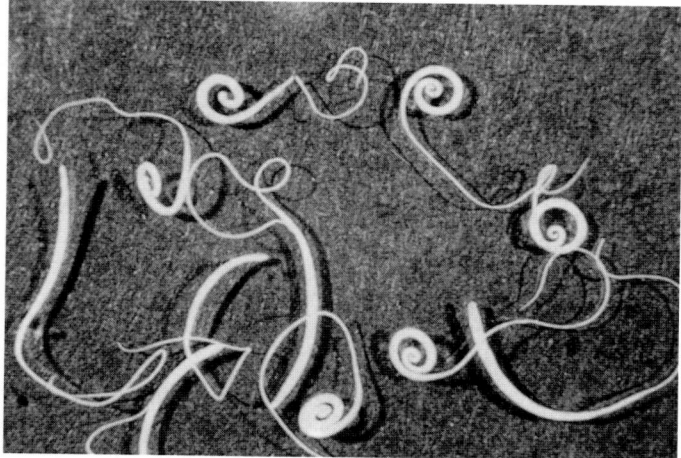

Figure 83.3: Adult *Trichuris* worms (whipworms), male and female. (Courtesy H. Zaiman.)

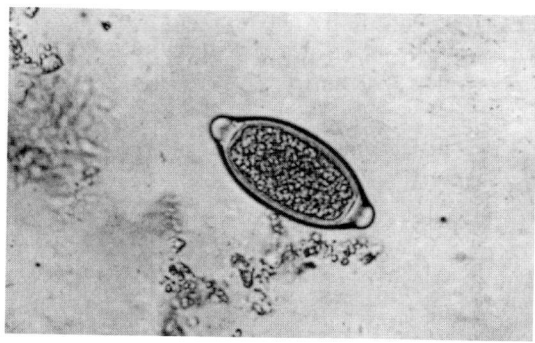

Figure 83.4: Egg of *Trichuris*. (Courtesy of Tropical Resources Unit.)

(30–45 mm long) has an attenuated anterior portion containing a cellular oesophagus which is half as long again as the thicker posterior portion, and a caudal extremity curved through 360° with a single spicule in the sheath which is studded with spines (Figure 83.3). The female (30–35 mm long) has the posterior half occupied by a stout uterus packed with eggs. The egg (50 × 22 μm) is brown with a characteristic band shape and a single cell with a plug at each end; it contains a single embryo (Figure 83.4).

Life cycle (See Appendix III)

The worms live in the caecum, where they maintain their position by transfixing a superficial fold of mucosa and lie embedded in mucus between the intestinal villi. The egg is laid unsegmented, and embryonation takes at least 21 days. It can withstand low temperatures but not desiccation. Infection is direct from stale faeces. The egg hatches after being swallowed in the intestine, where the shell is digested by intestinal juices and the larva emerges in the small intestine; it penetrates the villi and develops for a week until it re-emerges and passes to the caecum and colorectum, where it attaches itself to the mucosa and becomes adult.

Transmission

Transmission is direct from mature eggs to the mouth via fingers contaminated from infected soil.

Pathology

When there are only a few worms there is little damage but with heavy infections they spread throughout the colon to the rectum. They cause haemorrhages, muco-purulent stools and symptoms of dysentery with rectal prolapse.[3]

There is an acute-phase response and a specific elevation of plasma fibronectins and plasma viscosity,[4] as well as low admission plasma levels of insulin growth factor-1 ((IGF-1), low type of procollagen and high serum levels of tumour necrosis factor α which may contribute to the understanding of growth failure in children with *Trichuris* dysentery syndrome.[5]

Trichuris is frequently associated with *Ascaris* and hookworm and a secondary infection with *Entamoeba histolytica* causes further ulceration.

Clinical features

Natural history

In the vast majority of infections, which are light, the worms live harmlessly in the caecum and appendix but when the infection is heavy (more than 10 000/g of faeces) there can be marked symptoms and signs. In children, however, even symptomless geohelminth infections have been shown to affect growth.[6]

Incubation period

The prepatent period from ingestion of eggs to the appearance of eggs in the stool is 60 days.

Symptoms and signs

In light infections there are no symptoms, but when associated with *Ascaris* or hookworm mild symptoms occur. Epigastric pain, vomiting, distension, flatulence, anorexia and weight loss may occur. Pain in the epigastrium and right iliac fossa is common. When associated with *Entamoeba histolytica*, *Balantidium coli* or shigellosis, symptoms are highly aggravated and dysenteric symptoms occur. Anaemia and low serum albumin is more pronounced in double infections with *Trichuris* than in amoebic infection alone. There is usually no eosinophilia which, if pronounced, usually denotes a concurrent *Toxocara* infection, with which it is often associated.

In heavy infections, as seen in the southern USA, the West Indies and South-East Asia, infection may extend from the caecum to the rectum and there may be quite a severe dysentery with blood and mucus in the stools (Figure 83.5) and prolapse of the rectum (Figure 83.6). These infections, which are sometimes associated with

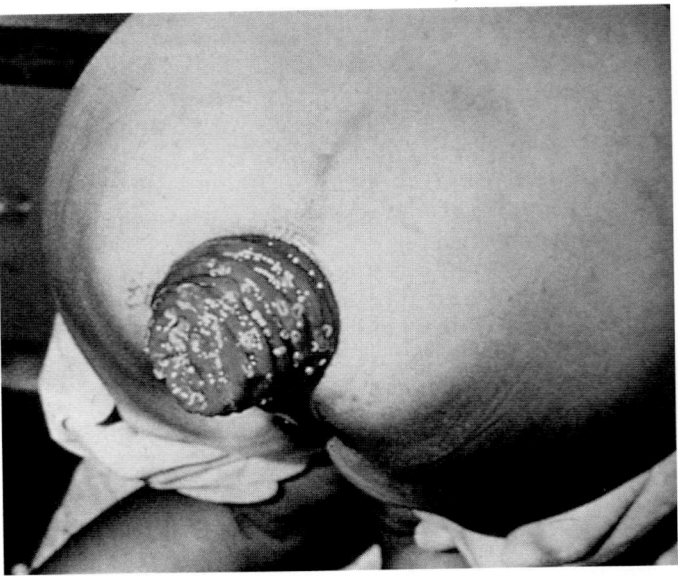

Figure 83.6: Prolapse of the rectum in *Trichuris* dysentery.

amoebiasis, respond well to anthelmintic treatment. In severe massive infantile trichuriasis digital clubbing, hypoproteinaemia, severe anaemia and growth retardation are common.[7]

Differential diagnosis

In severe infection the clinical picture may resemble hookworm disease, acute appendicitis or amoebic dysentery.

Diagnosis

The diagnosis is made by finding the characteristic eggs in the stool (see Figure 83.4) by direct smear or by concentration methods (see Appendix I). An egg count (see Appendix I) will reveal the degree of infection and 30 000 eggs/g of faeces or more is a heavy infection[5] which would indicate the presence of several hundred worms and the production of symptoms.

Proctoscopy in cases of dysentery will show numerous worms attached to the mucosa, which is reddened and ulcerated where they are responsible for the dysentery.

Radiological

In some cases a 'honeycomb' appearance of the small intestine has been seen with the appearances of Crohn's disease; deformity of the intestine is most marked in the proximal colon but also present in the ileum and appendix.

Treatment

Albendazole and mebendazole 400 mg and 500 mg respectively as a single dose are highly effective, as is a combination of albendazole 400 mg with ivermectin 200 µg/kg.[8]

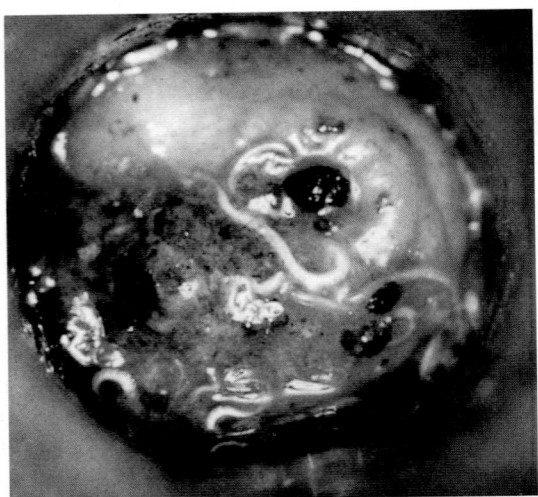

Figure 83.5: Protoscopic view of *Trichuris* worms causing dysentery.

Epidemiology

Trichuris trichiura is primary a human infection but *Trichuris suis* of pigs is indistinguishable from the human species and can infect man. There is an increased incidence of *Trichuris* infection in people handling pigs.

Trichuris infection is common in areas of high rainfall, high humidity, dense shade and poor sanitation and contaminated soil. It is the most common soil-transmitted helminthic infection in Malaysia. The greatest prevalence is in children of primary school age who pollute the soil around the house and who develop heavy worm burdens. *Trichuris* infection is often associated with *Ascaris* and *Toxocara*, the epidemiology of which is similar.

Control is the same as that for *Ascaris*: avoidance of soil pollution and periodic mass chemotherapy (see pp. 1550–1552). Regional differences in susceptibility of *Trichuris trichiura* to albendazole seem to occur and it would therefore be prudent to evaluate local sensitivity when planning mass chemotherapy.

Type 2: modified direct (*Ascaris, Toxocara*)

Ascaris

Geographical distribution

Ascaris lumbricoides (roundworm) is one of the most common and most widespread human infections. Over 250 million people with associated morbidity are infected, resulting in an annual mortality of 60 000.

The prevalence of *Ascaris* varies in different parts of the world. In China and South-East Asia it is highly prevalent. In the Central Asian republics of the former USSR it is common in humid areas. In Central and South America the average rate of infection is 45%, and in parts of Africa 95%. In Europe and the southern USA it is low.

Aetiology and life cycle (Figure 83.7)

Ascaris lumbricoides (Figure 83.8) is a comparatively large worm (female 20–25 cm × 3–6 mm; male 15–31 cm × 2–4 mm) which inhabits the small intestine (the morphology is described in Appendix III). Eggs (Figure 83.9) are laid in the small intestine and are passed out as immature ova containing no segmented or differentiated embryo. In damp soil an embryo develops at 36–40°C in 2–4 months (at the optimum of 25°C in 3 weeks); it lies coiled up in the egg, undergoing one moult before being hatched as an infective second stage rhabditiform larva in the small intestine when the egg is swallowed (see Appendix III). Here the rhabditiform larva penetrates the mucous membrane and enters the bloodstream, reaching the lungs via the right heart where it cannot pass through the lung capillaries, so that it burrows through the alveolar wall to

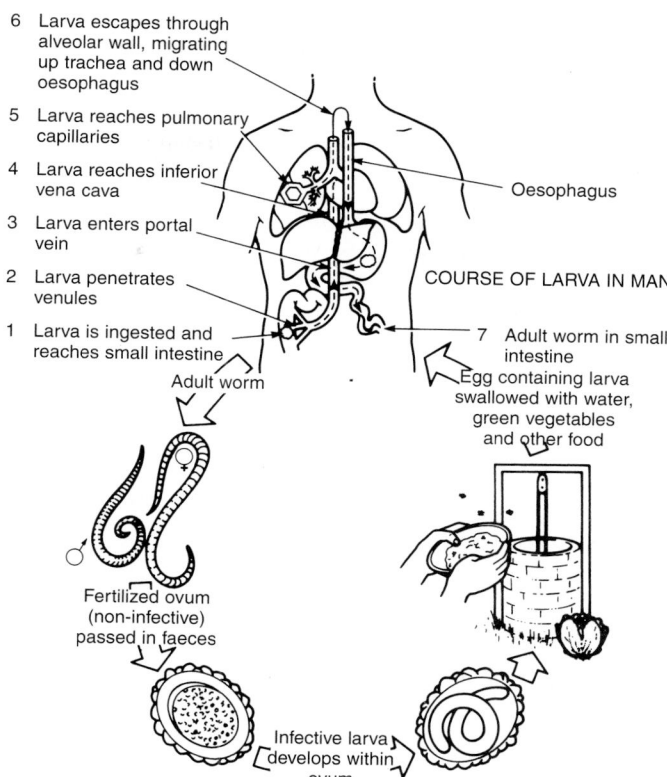

6 Larva escapes through alveolar wall, migrating up trachea and down oesophagus
5 Larva reaches pulmonary capillaries
4 Larva reaches inferior vena cava
3 Larva enters portal vein
2 Larva penetrates venules
1 Larva is ingested and reaches small intestine
Oesophagus
COURSE OF LARVA IN MAN
Adult worm
7 Adult worm in small intestine
Egg containing larva swallowed with water, green vegetables and other food
Fertilized ovum (non-infective) passed in faeces
Infective larva develops within ovum

Figure 83.7: Life cycle of *Ascaris lumbricoides* (roundworm). (Courtesy of Tropical Resources Unit.)

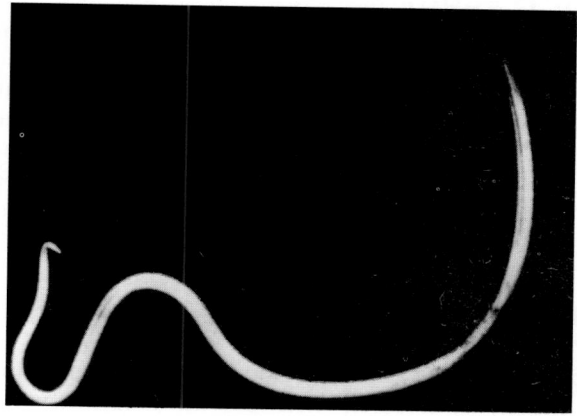

Figure 83.8: Adult *Ascaris* worm (roundworm). (Courtesy of Tropical Resources Unit.)

enter the respiratory tract. From here it is carried up the trachea to the larynx, where it moves over the epiglottis and enters the oesophagus, and is swallowed a second time to reach the small intestine. The whole process takes 10–14 days, during which time the larva moults twice, the fourth moult taking place between the 25th and 29th days. Larvae may reach the intestine as early as the fifth day. In man the period from infection to the first passage of ova in the stool is 60–70 days.

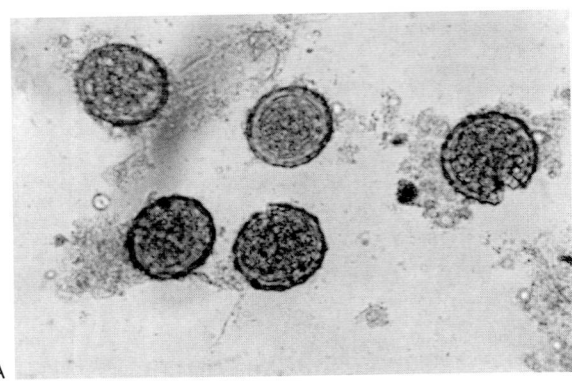

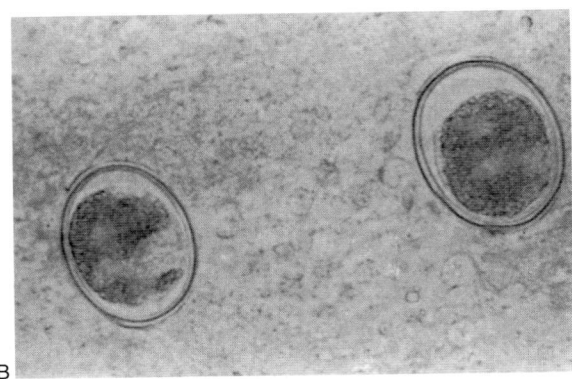

Figure 83.9: Eggs of *Ascaris lumbricoides* (roundworm). (**A**) Fully formed, fertile, in stool. (Courtesy of Tropical Resources Unit.) (**B**) Decorticated from liver abscess. (Courtesy M. L. Chu).

Ascaris suum

Ascaris suum is almost indistinguishable from human *Ascaris* and man is not a normal host but *Ascaris* pneumonia is common in pigs and a proportion of similar respiratory troubles in people associated with pigs may be due to *Ascaris suum*. Although *Ascaris suum* can infect humans, man is not its normal host; double infections may occur and eosinophilic granuloma of the bowel may be caused by *Ascaris suum*.

Transmission

Infection is acquired from ingestion of eggs in contaminated soil, usually by children when playing around the house situated in suitable soil.

Pathology

Pathology may be caused by migrating larvae or adults.

Migrating larvae (larval ascariasis)

Migrating larvae cause symptoms from their actual physical presence and the immune reactions they elicit.

Pneumonia
Damage to the lungs occurs during the migration of larvae on their way to the intestine. 'Löffler's syndrome' may be produced with fever, cough, sputum, asthma, eosinophilia and radiological pulmonary infiltration. In 1956 it was concluded that the majority of cases of Löffler's syndrome were due to larval ascariasis.[9] Segments of fourth-stage larvae can be seen in the bronchioles associated with infiltration with polymorphonuclear and eosinophilic leucocytes with scattered Charcot–Leyden crystals usually associated with lysed eosinophils.

Small areas of necrosis with eosinophils may be found in the liver. Migrating larvae have been recovered from aspirated gastric juice and sputum. If the larvae reach the general circulation they may cause localized symptoms resembling those of visceral larva migrans caused by *Toxocara canis*. Larvae may wander into the brain, eye or retina, causing granulomas simulating *Toxocara canis*. In small children ascariasis is frequently associated with *Toxocara*. Hundreds of larvae have been removed from a swelling in the neck (but see Lagochilascariasis, p. 1538).

Adults worms

Adults worms by themselves cause little pathology in their normal habitat (small intestine). Heavy infections can cause intestinal colic, which is the most important complaint. Aggregate masses of worms may cause volvulus, intestinal obstruction (Figure 83.10) or intussusception.

Wandering ascarids

Wandering ascarids may reach abnormal situations and cause acute symptoms: ileus from mechanical obstruction, perforation of the bowel in the ileocaecal region, acute appendicitis from a worm blocking the lumen, diverticulitis, gastric or duodenal trauma, blocking of the ampulla of Vater with pancreatic necrosis, blocking of the common bile duct with obstructive jaundice, entry into the liver parenchyma and liver abscess, invasion of the genital tract and oesophagel perforation.

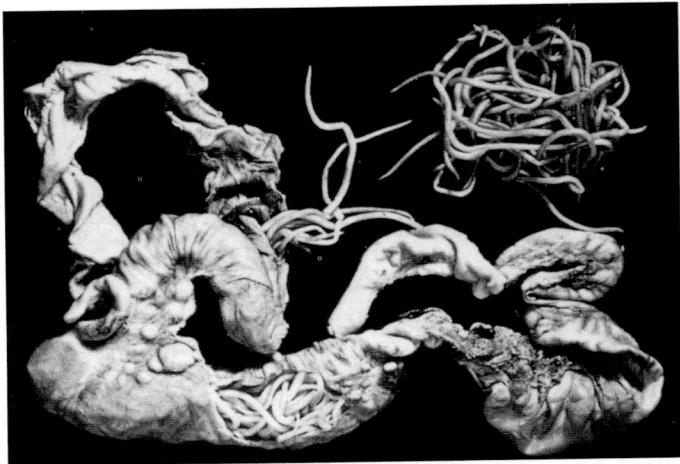

Figure 83.10: Impacted mass of adult *Ascaris* worms in the small intestine causing fatal intestinal obstruction.

Liver

Ascaris liver abscess is caused by female *Ascaris* worms migrating up the common bile duct into the liver where they die, releasing eggs. Histologically there is a granulomatous reaction round the dead worm with release of the eggs, which can be demonstrated in the abscess as smooth, oval bodies from which the outer coat has been digested (see Figure 83.9b). In some parts of the world *Ascaris* liver abscess is more common in young children than amoebic abscess.

Granulomatous masses may form around the eggs released from the female worms which have escaped into the peritoneum and mimic tuberculous peritonitis. An eosinophilic granuloma of the bowel may be caused by *Ascaris suum*.

Biliary ascariasis is not uncommon in the Philippines, where 20% of patients treated surgically for biliary disease are found to have live or dead *Ascaris* worms in the biliary tract; and in South Africa it is common in children.[10] The symptoms are acute onset of right upper abdominal pain, sometimes with fever and jaundice from recurrent cholangitis. Adult worms may be demonstrated on plain radiographs, by barium meal, by intravenous cholangiography, ultrasonography, computed tomography or magnetic resonance imaging.[12] At post-mortem cholangitis or liver abscess may be found. Adult worms, larvae and ova may all initiate stone formation and can be found in the core of many bile duct stones. The management of biliary ascariasis is primarily medical, including analgesics and anthelminthic therapy. If medical treatment fails endoscopic extraction using biopsy forceps is successful.[13]

Immunopathological effects

Many infected individuals manifest a sensitivity to the antigens of *Ascaris*, and entry to a laboratory where worms are being dissected is enough to cause conjunctivitis, urticaria and asthma. The skin of these people is extremely sensitive to minimal doses of *Ascaris* antigen and gives an immediate hypersensitivity reaction, often with urticaria and erythematous lesions.

The passage of adult worms in sensitive persons may give rise to intense anal pruritus, vomiting of worms and oedema of the glottis.

Indirect effects

Micro-organisms may be carried by adult worms on their migration from the bowel and a relationship between *Ascaris* infection and the incidence of poliomyelitis has been suggested.

Nutritional relationships

Ascariasis may contribute to protein–energy malnutrition. From calculations in an experimental study in man it has been estimated that in children infected with 13–40 worms approximately 4 g of protein are lost per day from a daily diet containing 35–50 g of protein.[14] Kwashiorkor

has been associated with *Ascaris* infection from the time when it was first recognized as a nutritional syndrome. *Ascaris* infection may contribute to vitamin A deficiency and children suffering from night blindness have shown rapid improvement in their eye symptoms within a few days of therapeutic elimination of the worms. Deworming of children has been shown to increase serum retinol concentration.[15] Ascariasis can also adversely affect normal growth and educational achievement.[16–18] However, a low level of helminth infection did not affect significantly the energy metabolism of Gambian children.[19]

Immunity

Man acquires only partial immunity to reinfection, and animals can be protected using extracts of adults and larvae. The main immune reaction is humoral and is directed against the migrating larval stage. The reaction to adult worms in unusual locations is cellular.

Larval migratory stages

The antigens which elicit antibodies are released at the moulting period between the second and third larval stages when there is a great increase in IgE. A further response is elicited in the bowel between the fourth and fifth stages, at which time there may be a marked loss of worm burden; this may be a regulatory mechanism in natural infections.

Adult stage

Adult worms in the bowel elicit no response but when they wander into tissues the reaction is cellular and results in a granuloma. Immediate hypersensitivity to adult *Ascaris* antigens develops in some people.

Clinical features

Natural history

Most *Ascaris* infections are symptomless but heavy infections in childhood give rise to symptoms. These heavy infections are controlled by immunity, or by diminished exposure, so that adults have much lighter infections, although reinfection can occur throughout life.

Incubation period

The incubation period from infection after swallowing eggs to the first appearance of eggs in the stools is 60–70 days. In larval ascariasis pulmonary symptoms occur 4–6 days after infection.

Symptoms and signs

Light infections do not usually cause symptoms, though a single adult worm can cause a liver abscess or block the common bile duct. Acute manifestations are roughly proportional to the number of worms harboured and serious disease may be caused when the burden amounts to 100 worms or more.

Ascariasis
Ascaris

During the migratory stages the larvae cause a pneumonitis 4–16 days after infection, with fever, cough, sputum and radiological infiltration of the lungs. There is a high eosinophilia and larvae can be found in the sputum or gastric juice, especially if a quantity is collected, digested with trypsin and centrifuged. Seasonal attacks of *Ascaris* pneumonia have occured in Saudi Arabia following the onset of spring rains and the restarting of transmission.[20] The pneumonitis is of short duration—about 3 weeks (in contrast to tropical pulmonary eosinophilia (TPE), which lasts for many months). There may be asthma, which can be so intense as to cause status asthmaticus, and the liver may be affected, becoming enlarged and tender.

On reaching the general circulation larvae may cause symptoms similar to those of *Toxocara canis*. Neurological disorders including convulsions, meningism and epilepsy, palpebral oedema, insomnia and tooth grinding during the night may occur. When the larvae wander into the brain they cause granulomas, presenting as small tumours in the eye, retina or brain.

The major manifestation of adult ascariasis is small bowel obstruction (Figure 83.10), which usually occurs in children, and as many as 1000 worms have been removed from one patient. Gastrointestinal discomfort, colic and vomiting are quite common. Ascariasis is a common cause of abdominal surgical emergency in children in South Africa and Rangoon. Plain abdominal radiography and abdominal ultrasonography featuring the characteristics 'railway track' sign and 'bull's eye' appearance help to confirm the diagnosis.[21]

Adult worms tend to migrate when their environment is disturbed. In the presence of tetrachloroethylene, anaesthetics or fever they migrate and wander into the bile ducts, ampulla of Vater, appendix, perineal sinuses and Eustachian tubes. They can cause volvulus and gangrene of the bowel, intestinal perforation and peritonitis, acute pancreatitis, suppurative cholangitis, liver abscess, acute cholecystitis and obstructive jaundice.

For these reasons it is important not to give tetrachloroethylene when there is a possibility of *Ascaris* infection and to deworm children when they are ill and febrile or before giving an anaesthetic. With advent of the imidazoles and other anthelmintics the use of tetrachloroethylene is virtually extinct.

Diagnosis

A diagnosis can be made from passage of worms in the stool or by finding eggs in faeces.

Fertile eggs are oval and measure about $60 \times 45\ \mu m$. The shell is transparent, is surrounded by an outer mamillated shell stained by bile pigments and contains an unsegmented embryo (see Figure 83.9a).

Unfertile eggs are longer and narrower ($90 \times 40\ \mu m$), have a thinner shell, more irregular outer covering and are found in about two-thirds of infections, due either to a shortage or absence of males. In male infections no eggs are passed in the stool.

Decorticated eggs are usually found in ectopic sites where they have had the outer shell removed and present as smooth oval objects (see Figure 83.9b).

Eosinophilia

In larval ascariasis there is a high eosinophilia but in adult infections there is little or none. If a marked eosinophilia occurs in adult infections then an associated *Toxocara* or *Strongyloides* infection must be suspected.

Adult worms

Sometimes the passage of an adult worm from the nose, mouth or anus will be reported and causes distress. The size and shape will distinguish it from other worms, especially tapeworms, which may be noticed by patients.

Radiography

Radiographic examination 4–6 hours after an opaque meal displays the worms as cylindrical filling defects or as string-like shadows produced by the opaque substance which the worms have ingested. Modern imaging techniques are now increasingly available.[11,12]

Serological diagnosis

Since there is much cross-reactivity with other helminthic antigens, immunodiagnosis is of little help in *Ascaris* infection, either adult or larval.

Differential diagnosis

The syndrome of pulmonary symptoms, radiological lung infiltration and hypereosinophilia is common to a number of helminthic and other infections.

Larval ascariasis must be distinguished from *Toxocara*, hookworm, *Strongyloides*, schistosomiasis and TPE. Essentially, larval ascariasis is a short-term illness lasting 2–3 weeks with a rapidly falling eosinophilia.

Toxocara

Often associated with *Ascaris*, *Toxocara* causes the visceral larva migrans (VLM) syndrome which persists for many months with a persistently high eosinophilia, and lung symptoms are not prominent. Wandering *Toxocara* larvae cause almost identical lesions of the brain and eye as *Ascaris* and can be diagnosed by specific serological tests.

The invasive stage of hookworm lasts 2–3 months, subsiding gradually, ova being found in the stool from 42 days onwards. It may be preceded by a localized eruption on the legs (ground itch).

The invasive stage of schistosomiasis (Katayama syndrome) can last 2–3 months. There is usually splenomegaly and specific serology is available for diagnosis.

TPE may closely resemble *Ascaris* pneumonia. It occurs mainly in adults, has a much longer duration and specific filarial serological tests will be positive (older tests using less specific antigens cross-reacted with *Ascaris*). It responds rapidly to diethylcarbamazine.

Pulmonary aspergillosis, drug reactions and eosinophilic leukaemia are all more chronic.

Management

Treatment is effective only against the adult worms. Although the vast majority of *Ascaris* infections cause few, if any, symptoms it is easy to treat and it is wise to treat any established infection. The drugs of choice are as follows:

- *Albendazole*: for children 2–5 years a single dose of 200 mg; for older children and adults, one dose of 400 mg is given.
- *Mebendazole*: a single dose of 500 mg.
- *Levamisole*: a single dose of 2.5 mg/kg body weight.
- *Pyrantel pamoate* (Combantrin): a single dose of 10 mg/kg body weight.

They are best given between meals, without any special diet, fast or use of purgatives before or after therapy. They should be avoided in the first trimester of pregnancy.

Treatment of complications[22]

This responds dramatically to prednisolone therapy. Anthelmintics should be given 2 weeks after lung involvement.

Conservative treatment—antispasmodics, analgesics, gastric decompression via a nasogastric tube, administration of intravenous fluids—is usually successful. An anthelmintic, preferably in soluble form and quick-acting (levamisole, pyrantel) is given when the acute phase of the illness is over and intestinal function restored. If this fails, surgical removal is needed.[13]

Here again, conservative treatment is the first choice—antispasmodics, gastric decompression, intravenous fluids, liquid paraffin and anthelmintics—and is usually successful. If surgical intervention is decreed necessary because of fever, tachycardia, visible peristalsis, severe pain or lack of remission within 48 hours of conservative treatment, this should be as conservative as possible, e.g. careful unknotting of the worm bolus and milking of the worms into the colon. Rarely is enterotomy required.

Epidemiology

Ascaris eggs develop best in shady, damp soil. They are resistant to cold and to disinfectants in the strengths normally used. They are killed by direct sunlight and by temperatures above 45°C. Infection is spread by faecal pollution of the soil.

In endemic areas three distinct trends in the prevalence and intensity of endemic ascariasis in man have been observed:[23]

1. High prevalence (over 60%) in the whole population over 2 years, with the intensity of infection lower in adults; a common and constant exposure to invasive *Ascaris* eggs by dirty hands and contaminated food.
2. Moderate prevalence (below 50%) with its peak at preschool or early school ages and low values in adults; a household or family type of transmission probably prevails.
3. Overall prevalence low (below 10%) and infections tend to have a focal distribution related to particular housing and sanitary conditions or agricultural and behavioural practices.

Ascariasis is spread countrywide in a few regions where climatic and social conditions are almost uniform; in many other countries, its distribution is stratified. Thus, in the overcrowded 'shanty' towns of non-industrialized societies with poor hygiene prevalence may be higher in urban than in rural areas. In drier areas of the tropics, transmission is limited to the short rainy season. Coprophagous arthropods, e.g. dung beetles, cockroaches and animals can spread the infection widely by ingesting and excreting viable eggs.

Apart from the spatial differences in *Ascaris* prevalence at the level of country, village and family, there is considerable difference in intensity of infection among individuals, giving a negative binomial distribution.[24] The reasons for such individual predisposition—spatial, behavioural, genetic—are still unknown.

Epidemic ascariasis caused by the use of raw sewage for agricultural purposes, waste-water irrigated vegetables and contaminated imported vegetables has been reported.

Sporadic ascariasis as a result of holiday travel to endemic areas, association with infected immigrants and infection from imported fresh vegetables and fruits has been described.

Although the basic epidemiology of the geohelminths is relatively straightforward, their *quantitative epidemiology* is more complex. Some of the important features can be summarized as follows:

- The distribution of worm numbers per person tends to be highly aggregated in form. Thus, most individuals harbour a few parasites, while only a few harbour heavy burdens.[25]
- Worm fecundity appears to decline as the burden within an individual increases.[26]
- For *Ascaris* and *Trichuris*, changes in the average intensity of infection with age tend to be convex, with infection rising in childhood and declining in adulthood, while in *hookworm* there is a steady rise in intensity with age.[27]
- Predisposition of heavily infected individuals within a community due to a variety of possible factors, e.g. behavioural, social, nutritional or genetic.[28–30]

The complex interplay of these aspects has been addressed mathematically in order to predict the results of intervention by chemotherapy.[31,32] Several studies have now confirmed the association between a broad range of nematodal species and growth in children, in various parts of the world.[33–38] The immunoepidemiology of intestinal helminthic infections has recently attracted the attention of several scientists.[39–43]

Control

Control is based on a combination of personal hygiene, proper disposal of faeces, health education and chemotherapy (see pp. 1550–1552).

Toxocariasis

Toxocariasis in man is the result of infection with the dog *Ascaris*—*Toxocara canis*—which does not undergo normal development in man but is arrested at the larval stage, causing toxocariasis, VLM or ocular toxocariasis.

Geographical distribution

Toxocara canis infection in dogs has a worldwide distribution rates vary from 2% to 90%.

Visceral larva migrans, which was first described in the southern USA,[44] has been recognized mainly in the southern and eastern USA but also in Europe, the Caribbean, Mexico, Hawaii, the Philippines, Australia, South Africa and Eastern Europe.

Ocular toxocariasis (granulomatous ophthalmitis), first described in the USA,[45] has been recognized in many parts of the world and serological surveys have shown many cases of ocular toxocariasis in Britain.[46]

Aetiology

Toxocara canis is a roundworm infection in dogs. The morphology resembles that of *Ascaris lumbricoides* (see p. 1531), the males being 4–6 cm long and the females 6.5–10 cm long. The eggs, which are pitted superficially, measures 85 × 75 μm, being larger than those of *Ascaris*. They are not found in man, only in dog faeces and contaminated soil.

Life cycle

In the dog the life cycle is similar to that of *Ascaris* in man except that transplacental infection of puppies takes place in pregnant bitches and the puppies born with a patent infection shed numerous eggs from birth. In contrast, adult dogs excrete few eggs. Dogs are infected by ingesting the eggs from soil or as puppies at birth so that the whole cycle may be maintained in a small flat without any access to the outside.

In man, who is not the normal lost, the eggs hatch in the stomach and second-stage larvae penetrate the mucosa to enter the circulation via the mesenteric vessels, reaching the intestinal viscera and liver where they are held up in the capillaries, but may pass into the general circulation through the lungs and end up in the brain, eye and other organs. In these organs, as well as the liver, the larvae are eventually held up and destroyed by a granulomatous reaction which blocks their further migration and causes pathology. In the human host the larvae do not grow or moult but can remain alive for as long as 11 years, as has been show experimentally.

Transmission

The main source of infection is puppies, which excrete large numbers of eggs. Infection is acquired by children playing in contaminated soil or in playgrounds—as in *Ascaris* infection—and is encouraged by the habit of earth eating (pica). Direct infection from handling puppies in the household is not considered a major risk because embryonation of excreted *Toxocara* ova requires a minimum of 2 weeks.[47]

Pathology

The pathology depends on the density of infection. In heavy infections in childhood the syndrome of VLM is produced, whereas lighter infections cause ocular toxocariasis, found in later life.

Visceral larva migrans

In heavy infections in children the second-stage larvae, which are 450 μm × 16–20 μm in diameter, are arrested mostly in the liver, where they cause few or many miliary lesions.[54] These lesions are composed of granulomas which can be seen as white subcapsular nodules the size of millet seeds. Other sites are the lungs, kidneys, heart, striated muscle, brain and eye. Microscopically the granulomas contain a centre of closely packed eosinophils and histiocytes surrounded by larger histiocytes with pale vesicular nuclei, sometimes arranged in a palisade-like manner. Occasionally there is an atypical multinucleate giant cell. Living second-stage larvae may sometimes be demonstrated in recent granulomas but more usually only the remains can be seen. Less commonly they reach the lungs or brain, where similar lesions can be seen.

Ocular toxocariasis

In the eye the granulomatous reaction forms a large subretinal mass with a superimposed patch of choroiditis which can closely resemble a retinoblastoma (for further details see Chapter 18).

Immunity

In the abnormal host (man) the larvae elicit both a humoral and cellular response. Antibodies are formed which cause a quantitative rise in immunoglobulins—mostly IgG but also IgM (the globulin may be so elevated that a positive formol gel test can be shown) and IgE—and there is a peripheral eosinophilia. The larvae themselves elicit a cell-mediated granulomatous response causing the granulomas so typical of the infection. In the dog immunity to reinfection develops so that adult dogs pass few or no eggs.

Clinical features

Natural history

Following infection from ingested eggs which hatch in the stomach the larvae migrate to the liver, where they may be arrested, or continue and reach other organs. In most cases the larva is destroyed without causing any trouble but in some cases it can survive for many years, and on its wanderings may eventually cause a lesion. Unless the infection is heavy and the VLM syndrome is produced, most cases of infection never cause any trouble. Heavy infections cause VLM, which can be self-limiting or cause death in a few cases. Lesions in the eye can produce severe loss of vision and even complete loss of sight in the affected eye.

Incubation period

An incubation period cannot be determined but in heavy infections (VLM) it is similar to that of *Ascaris*. In light infections many years may pass before the ocular granuloma presents itself.

Symptoms and signs

There are two main clinical presentations: VLM and ocular toxocariasis (granulomatous ophthalmitis).

This is seen most commonly in younger children. The child becomes unwell with an enlarged liver, fever and asthma. There is a marked hypereosinophilia and there can be pulmonary signs (radiological mottling), cardiac dysfunction, nephrosis and neurological lesions (fits, epilepsy, pareses and transverse myelitis). There is a great increase in the serum globulin and the eosinophil count is raised to $10–20 \times 10^9$/litre. In many urban areas where lead paint is used this is ingested with soil and the habit of pica and signs of lead poisoning may accompany VLM (blue lines on the gums and anaemia).

Most cases of VLM recover naturally after 2 years but some die, and post-mortem examination will reveal extensive lesions in the liver and sometimes the brain.

The retinal lesion presents as a solid retinal tumour often at or near the macula. In the early stages it is raised above the level of the retina and closely mimics a retinal neoplasm. Later when the acute phase has subsided the lesion remains a clear-cut circumscribed area of retinal degeneration. Formerly these lesions were designated tuberculous, exanthematous or neoplastic. If the lesion is central the visual acuity is reduced or central vision may be lost.

Strabismus due to macular damage is often the presenting symptom. Low-grade iridocyclitis with posterior synechiae may develop and progress to general endophthalmitis and detachment of the retina. The second-stage larva may rarely be seen with a slit-lamp microscope in the anterior chamber of the eye. Secondary glaucoma may result. An extensive review of the ocular manifestations of toxocariasis has recently appeared.[49]

Differential diagnosis

VLM must be distinguished from other migrating helminths, larval ascariasis (much shorter duration), strongyloidiasis (much longer duration) and TPE (pulmonary symptoms are more marked and found in adults).

Ocular toxocariasis must be distinguished from a retinal tumour (retinoblastoma) and other causes of choroiditis (toxoplasmosis). All cases of retinoblastoma in children should have a serological test to exclude toxocariasis. Enzyme-linked immunosorbent assay (ELISA) has a sensitivity of 90% and a specificity of 91% at a diagnostic titre of 1:8 in ocular toxocariasis. Vitreous *Toxocara* antibody can also be measured.

Diagnosis

A history of exposure to infected soil by puppies and pica is important. The most consistent laboratory findings in VLM are: eosinophilia, leucocytosis, a decreased albumin: globulin ratio and an increase in IgG, IgH, anti-A or anti-B isohaemagglutinin titres. High-resolution ultrasonography reveals hypoechoic areas in the liver and, being non-invasive, is preferable to liver biopsy.[50]

Demonstration of larvae

This is very difficult and seldom achieved. Larvae or portions of degenerate larvae may be seen at the centre of the granuloma in liver biopsy or post-mortem material. A larva has been demonstrated in the cerebrospinal fluid in a case of meningitis.

Liver biopsy may show a granuloma containing many eosinophils which can be suggestive but which must be distinguished from a *Schistosoma mansoni* granuloma. In biopsy and post-mortem material *Ancylostoma braziliense* and *Ancylostoma caninum*, which usually invade the skin, can occasionally enter man via the intestinal tract and form granulomas in the viscera. Autoinfection with *Strongyloides* may cause a similar picture. Immunofluorescent staining of histological sections may be necessary to differentiate them.

Serology

The difficulty with serological diagnosis has always been to obtain an antigen specific to *Toxocara* second-stage larvae which does not cross-react with other tissue helminths. A specific antigen has been obtained from the secretory/excretory products of second-stage *Toxocara canis* larvae which is both sensitive and specific. It has been used in ELISA, which is the test of choice.

Using larval antigens the sensitivity of ELISA is 78% and specificity is 93% in VLM, provided the serum is first absorbed with *Ascaris suum* to remove cross-reacting antibodies.[52] A strong positive results is greater than 1.5 times screening level.

Other tests which have been used are passive haemagglutination and immunofluorescence. A radioallergosorbent test has been used to detect larva-specific IgE.[53] An indirect antibody competition ELISA (IACE) has been developed.[54]

Ocular toxocariasis

In addition to serum and vitreous *Toxocara* antibody determinations, fluorescein angiography, ultrasonography or computed tomography should be carried out to differentiate retinoblastoma from ocular larva migrans.

Management

Two drugs are used in treatment: diethylcarbamazine and thiabendazole.

Diethylcarbamazine

This is the drug of choice. Diethylcarbamazine is given orally: 3 mg/kg body weight three times daily for 21 days.

Thiabendazole

Thiabendazole is given orally 50 mg/kg body weight daily in three divided doses for 7–28 days depending upon the tolerance shown to the drug.

In VLM the high eosinophilia may persist for months after clinical cure, which is shown by subsidence of the fever and hepatomegaly. Once overcome, relapses do not occur and second infections are unlikely. In ocular toxocariasis the addition of corticosteroids may be needed (see Chapter 10). Loss of vision can be arrested but lost vision not restored.

Epidemiology

Toxocara canis is a common inhabitant of adult dogs and puppies. Puppies are infected by second-stage larvae in utero and are born with established intestinal infection. The puppies excrete eggs on to the ground which are ingested by small children along with *Ascaris* and *Trichuris* ova and, in urban areas in the USA, lead products found in old paint. Toxocariasis is often associated with *Ascaris* and *Trichuris* infection, and in urban areas with signs of lead poisoning. The most common age of infection is around $2\frac{1}{2}$ years and the infection is patent for about 3 to 5 years of age. It is uncommon at a later age unless an unusual habit of dirt eating is present, as in mental defectives. Ocular toxocariasis is found at a later age.

Control

Control rests upon control of infection in dogs, especially puppies, which are the main agents of infection, and regular treatment of dogs and bitches as well as newborn puppies with anthelmintics is essential when there are children in the house. Dogs should be denied access to sandpits in the backyard and children's playgrounds.

Lagochilascariasis
Geographical distribution

Lagochilascariasis is a rare infection of man, who is an accidental host. Cases have been described from South and Central America and the Caribbean.

Aetiology

Lagochilascaris minor is a parasite of the opossum (see below). The adult worms live in cavities in the submucosa of the small intestine and eggs containing infective larvae pass out in the stool, where they are ingested by mice and other small mammals. The larvae hatch in the intestine and migrate to skeletal muscle, where they mature and wait to be ingested by the definitive host, the opossum.

Transmission

Man becomes infected either by ingesting eggs from the soil or eating the intermediate host. A case reported from Tobago was thought to have acquired the infection through eating the raw meat of the manakou opossum.

Pathology

In man, *Lagochilascaris* causes subcutaneous abscesses on the head and neck, and lesions in the nasopharynx. The tonsils and lymphoid tissue are replaced by granulomatous tissue containing epithelioid granulomas with larvae and eggs. Absceses form in the neck and discharge pus.

Clinical features

Early symptoms are recurrent tonsillitis, a feeling of worms crawling at the back of the throat and even discharge of small white worms from the mouth. Tender tumours which swell and eventually burst discharging pus and worms form in the cervical region.

Diagnosis

Adult worms can be recognized by a longitudinal furrow along the lateral line (see Appendix III).

Management

Albendazole 400 mg/day for 30 days or ivermectin

300 µg/kg weekly for 10 weeks results in regression of the lesions with or without surgical resection.[55]

Type 3: penetration of the skin (*Ancylostoma, Strongyloides, Trichostrongylus*)

Ancylostomiasis (hookworm disease)

Hookworm disease (ancylostomiasis) is caused by two hookworms, *Ancylostoma duodenale* and *Necator americanus*, and is an extremely common infection; in many cases the nematodes, which are often present in huge numbers attached to the small intestine, suck blood and protein, causing disease (hookworm anaemia, hookworm disease).

Geographical distribution

Hookworm occurs in all tropical and subtropical countries.

A. duodenale is essentially a parasite of southern Europe, the north coast of Africa, northern India, northern China and Japan. It was introduced by migration into Paraguay around 3000 BC by Japanese fishermen and is the predominant hookworm in coastal Peru and Chile. It has been introduced into Western Australia and into areas where *N. americanus* is the predominant human hookworm, southern India, Myanmar, Malaya, the Philippines, Indonesia, Polynesia, Micronesia and Portuguese West Africa.

N. americanus is the predominant hookworm of western, central and southern Africa, southern Asia, Melanesia and Polynesia. It is widely distributed in the islands of the Caribbean, Central America and northern South America, where it was introduced by slaves from Africa. It is still occasionally found in the southern USA.

Aetiology

Two species of hookworm, *A. duodenale* and *N. americanus*, infect man.

Ancylostoma duodenale

A. duodenale is a small cylindrical white, grey or reddish-brown (from ingested blood) thread-like worm (Appendix II). Both male and female worms have a buccal capsule containing two pairs of teeth (cf. *N. americanus*) for attaching to the small intestinal mucosa. The male (0.8–1.1 × 0.4–0.5 cm) has a copulatory bursa at the rear end consisting of an umbrella-like expansion of the cuticle (Appendix III). The female (1–1.3 × 0.6 cm) is slightly larger and has the body cavity occupied by the

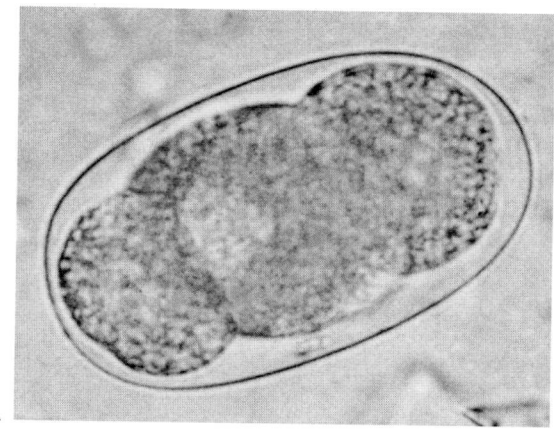

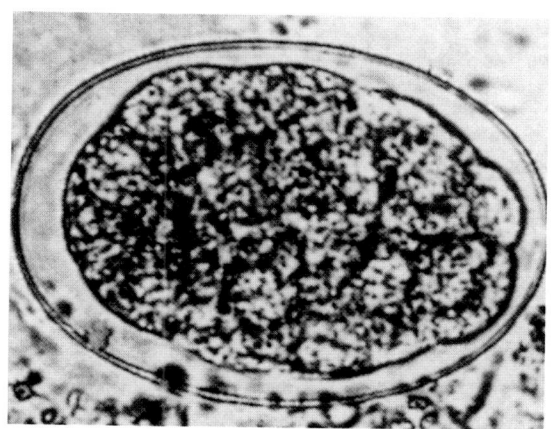

Figure 83.11: Hookworm eggs. (**A**) Immature egg showing developing larva. (Courtesy J. S. Tatz). (**B**) Mature egg. (Courtesy of Tropical Resources Unit.)

ovary and coiled uterine tubes packed with eggs. The vulva is in the posterior third of the body. The maximum egg output occurs 15–18 months after infection; the interval between infection and final disappearance of eggs from the stool with death of the worm averages 6 years. The female produces 25 000–35 000 eggs each day and some 18–54 million during its lifetime. (For full morphological description, see Appendix III.) The eggs (50–60 µm × 35–40 µm) are elliptical with a transparent shell and when freshly laid contain two to four segments (blastomeres) (Figure 83.11).

Necator americanus

N. americanus closely resembles *A. duodenale* but it is shorter and more slender (0.9–1.1 × 0.4 cm) and can be distinguished from *A. duodenale* by the position of the vulva in the female, which is in the anterior third of the body (Appendix III) and the buccal capsule, which is smaller than that of *A. duodenale*, has cutting plates instead of teeth. The egg is slightly larger than that of *A. duodenale* (64–75 × 36–40 µm). The female necator lays 6000–20 000 eggs daily and has a life duration on average of 5 years.

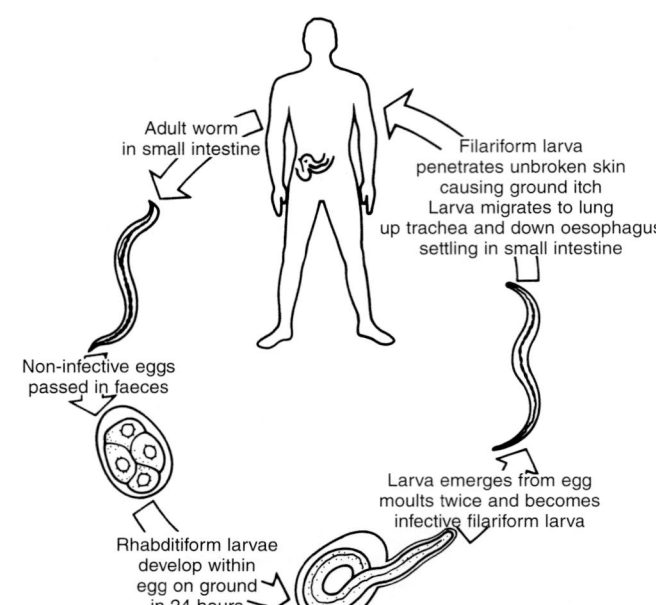

Figure 83.12: Life cycle of hookworm. (Courtesy of Tropical Resources Unit.)

Life cycle (Figure 83.12)

The eggs are deposited into the lumen of the intestine containing two, four or eight blastomeres and are passed out in the faeces where, if deposited in damp shaded soil, they hatch into *rhabditiform* (first-stage) larvae (Figure 83.12), which are free living and have a bulbed oesophagus. They feed avidly on bacteria. The larva moults on the third day and the oesophagus disappears on the fifth day, the larva becoming elongated and fully developed at 20–30°C. It then moves away from the faeces into the soil and moults to form a *filariform* (infective) larva (Figure 83.12), which has a simple muscular oesophagus and a protective sheath. The larva moves towards oxygen and cannot survive in water. The larvae are most numerous in the upper 2.5 cm of soil but can ascend from deeper layers. Protected from desiccation they can live in warm damp soil for 2 years. Direct sunlight, drying or salt water are fatal. When the filariform larva comes into contact with the skin of the host it penetrates it and enters the bloodstream, reaching the lungs on the third day. Breaking through the alveoli it enters the bronchioles, moves up the trachea, down the oesophagus to the stomach and small intestine. During this migration the third moult takes place and the buccal capsule is formed. It arrives in the intestine on the seventh day and a fourth moult takes place, the buccal capsule assumes the adult form and the worm attaches to the mucosa of the small intestine, where it can be seen at post-mortem as a small thread-like structure containing a red lining of ingested blood. In 3–5 weeks it becomes sexually mature and the female produces fertile eggs. Adult worms live from 1 to 9 years and produce 30 000 eggs per day (necator 9000 eggs daily).

The life cycles of *Ancylostoma* and *Necator* are similar except that:

- *A. duodenale* can infect by ingestion as well as via the skin.
- *N. americanus* infects only through the skin.
- Migrating larvae of *N. americanus* grow and develop in the lungs, whereas those of *Ancylostoma* do not.

Transmission

Infection is normally acquired via the skin (percutaneous route) from *filariform* (infective) larvae in the soil contaminated by human faeces; or orally via the ingestion of contaminated food. However, other methods of transmission which are comparatively unimportant have been suggested:

- Through eating uncooked meat containing the larvae of *A. duodenale* which have migrated into the muscles of the animal, where they can survive for 26–34 days.
- Via human milk (hypobiosis as in *A. caninum* in puppies).

The migrating infective filariform larvae of *A. duodenale* are arrested in their development and migrate to the mammary gland, where they are excreted in the milk and infect the child. Third-stage infective filariform larvae of *N. americanus* have been found in the milk but none of the infected mothers was found to have infected babies.

A. duodenale further differs from *N. americanus* in possessing the ability to remain within the host as a larval stage for many months before finally developing to an adult, thus bridging seasons which are inappropriate for transmission.[68]

Pathology

Ancylostoma causes pathology at three stages of infection (the first two caused by larval hookworms usually seen only in expatriates who receive a primary infection):

1. Vesiculation and pustulation at the site of entry (ground itch). This is usually mild or absent in the tropics except in expatriates.
2. Asthma and bronchitis during migration through the lungs with small haemorrhages into the alveoli and eosinophilic and leucocytic infiltration.
3. *Established infection*, seen in the inhabitants of endemic areas, leading to hookworm anaemia and hookworm disease.

Hookworm anaemia

The classical anaemia of hookworm infection is a hypochromic anaemia, the result of chronic blood loss, depletion of iron stores and deficiency of iron intake.

Hookworms have been shown to produce active suction impulses 120–200 times per minute and evidence indicates that the hookworm is indeed an habitual bloodsucker and needs serum. The blood loss has been estimated as 0.03 ml/day per worm in *N. americanus* and 0.15 ml/day per worm in *A. duodenale* infections.[57] There is a significant relationship between the level of haemoglobin and the worm burden, which depends upon the level of iron stores in the body. A significant negative correlation between plasma ferritin levels and hookworm burden, using the worm expulsion method, has been reported.[58] Hookworm anaemia is of the iron deficiency type and responds dramatically to iron salts by mouth and also to removal of the hookworm burden, but after a much longer period. Light infections may cause anaemia where the iron intake is deficient and anaemia may also be caused in spite of the presence of an adequate iron intake, provided that the worm burden is heavy enough.[59] A folate deficiency may be present, masked by the severe iron deficiency anaemia, and becomes overt only when this has been corrected. In a study in pre-school children in Kilifi, Kenya, the prevalence of heavy infection with hookworm and mean intensity were markedly age-dependent. The application of attributable morbidity methods confirmed the contribution of hookworm infection to anaemia.[60] Similar findings were reported in Zanzibari school children.[61]

Little is known about the anemia which develops in light primary infections. It may be related to that which develops in pups infected with *A. caninum* and be of immunological origin.

Hypoproteinaemia

Loss of protein is an important feature of hookworm anaemia, which is a cause of protein-losing enteropathy and the oedema of hookworm disease which does not respond to diuretics. The protein loss, which is in excess of the red cell loss and is closely related to the hookworm load, is caused by a limited capacity for albumin synthesis as well as loss caused by anaemia and other factors such as liver disease.

Hookworm enteropathy

There have been conflicting reports on the role of hookworm in tropical malabsorption states. Structural abnormalities of the villi reverting to normal after deworming have been shown in Puerto Rico and India,[62] but no changes were reported from Africa.[59] It has been suggested that it is the associated hypoalbuminaemia which is the cause of the enteropathy.

Pathological anatomy

In fatal cases the pathological changes are those of severe anaemia. There is plenty of fat in the usual situations. The appearance of plumpness is further increased by a greater or lesser amount of generalized oedema. There may be an effusion in one or more of the serous cavities. The heart is dilated and flabby. The liver is fatty and the kidneys and all other organs are pale.

If the post-mortem examination has been made within an hour or two after death the hookworms, in numbers ranging from a few dozen up to many hundreds, will be found attached by their mouths to the mucous surfaces of the lower part of the duodenum, jejunum and perhaps the upper part of the ileum. If the examination has been delayed for some time the parasites will have loosened their hold and are then found in the mucus coating the bowel. Many small extravasations of blood, some fresh, others of long standing, are seen in the mucous membranes and a minute wound in the centre of each extravasation represents the point at which a hookworm had been attached. Old extravasations are indicated by punctiform pigmentation. Occasionally streaks or large clots of blood are found in the lumen of the bowel and severe melaena may occur in children. The hookworms secrete some anticoagulant substance and may move from spot to spot, thereby increasing the damage and blood loss. The worms themselves may be seen in situ to show thin red streaks from fresh red blood in the intestinal canal; at other times they will be iron grey owing to the deposition of haemosiderin granules in the intestine.

Immunity

Dogs develop partial protective immunity towards *A. caninum* which in endemic areas can cause a 50% mortality from anaemia in early life. Pups that survive to adult life retain only minimal intestinal infection. After a single infection with 1000 irradiated *A. caninum* larvae significant immunity can be demonstrated by worm counts following challenge with unirradiated larvae, but there was no evidence of protective immunity in a volunteer repeatedly exposed to infection with *N. americanus* and no evidence of protective immunity in a field study.[59] Primary infections in man may cause fever, eosinophila and a moderate anaemia, even when the infection is light. Such light infections do not cause symptoms of anaemia in the indigenous inhabitants of endemic areas, suggesting that a partial immunity has developed.

Whereas there is good evidence that immunity plays a role in controlling infections with *A. caninum* and *A. ceylanicum*[63] in dogs, observations in communities living in endemic areas are not compatible with the existence of a vigorous, long-lasting protective immunity to hookworm infections. There is, in fact, little to indicate that infections in man are curtailed by immune phenomena.[59]

Clinical features

Natural history

After the establishment of adult worms in the intestine the females start to lay eggs. The number of eggs passed bears a direct relation to the number of female worms. The higher the worm load the greater the blood loss, so that where iron intake it satisfactory up to 100 worms may cause no symptoms. With worm loads of 500–1000 significant blood loss and anaemia will result, even in the presence of an adequate iron intake. It has been suggested that the relative freedom from hookworm anaemia shown by the African population of West, South and Central Africa is due to the use of iron cooking pots, which is also responsible for haemosiderosis, whereas in East Africa, where aluminium pots are mostly used, haemosiderosis is not found but hookworm anaemia is common. Light infections cause little trouble, but in a minority symptoms result from heavy infections.

Incubation period

In larval ancylostomiasis symptoms appear 1–2 weeks after the primary infection, and in established infection eggs appear from the 42nd day onwards after infection.

Symptoms and signs

This is seen in a primary infection, most usually in non-immune expatriates. It is not so common or so marked as *larval ascariasis*.

At the site of entry of the infective larvae there is a 'ground itch', which consists of an irritating vesicular rash limited to the exposed portion(s) of the body, usually the soles of the feet or the hands. After 1–2 weeks pulmonary symptoms develop with a dry cough and asthmatic wheezing. Fever and a high degree of eosinophilia are found. These symptoms gradually disappear and ova of hookworm can be seen on or about day 42 after infection. The whole episode is self-limiting, lasting not more than 2–3 months. Sometimes, if many larvae enter simultaneously, symptoms are quite alarming and steroid therapy may be needed.

The main effects of light infections may be seen in Europeans and other expatriates who have arrived recently in an endemic area. The practitioner in the tropics should always be on the lookout for these cases, especially in children. Minor degrees of anaemia induce a tendency to fatigue and lassitude and digestive disturbances are common. Any of these symptoms in the presence of an eosinophilia should lead to the suspicion of infection. In indigenous people most light infections are asymptomatic.

The essential symptoms of hookworm infection are connected with progressive iron deficiency anaemia associated with gastric and intestinal dyspepsia but not wasting. An early symptom is epigastric pain or discomfort which may be relieved by food and may be mistaken for duodenal ulcer. Although many people who suffer from irregular abdominal pain may possess hookworm ova in their stools it does not necessarily follow that hookworm infection is the cause of the abdominal pain.

The taste may be perverted, some patients exhibiting and persistently gratifying an unnatural craving for such things as earth, mud or lime (pica or geophagy). The stools may contain blood, and frank melaena may occur in children. The occult blood test is always positive in the stools in cases where symptoms are caused by hookworm.

When the iron deficiency anaemia develops then symptoms of anaemia occur. The mucous surfaces and the skin become pale. The face is puffy and the feet and ankles swollen and there may be generalized oedema caused by the hypoalbuminaemia. There is lassitude, breathlessness, palpitations, tinnitus and vertigo, mental apathy, depression and liability to syncope. There is often koilonychia. There is a high output failure and haemic murmurs can be heard over the heart, which is seen to be enlarged on radiographic examination. A minority of patients have a slow pulse, collapsed veins, severe oedema that often affects the face and arms, and ascites. They look ill, continuously feel cold and are hypothermic (body temperature less than 36°C).[59] Hookworm anaemia is a common cause of heart failure in the tropics and may easily be confused with rheumatic carditis. Ophthalmoscopic examination may reveal retinal haemorrhages. An irregular fever may be found in any severe anaemia.

The anaemia is typical of iron deficiency (see Chapter 13). The haemoglobin is reduced to a greater degree than the red cell count. The mean corpuscular volume is decreased and the mean corpuscular haemoglobin concentration may fall to as low as 22. The red cells show microcytosis and severe hypochromia. The serum iron is greatly reduced and the total iron-binding capacity of the serum greatly raised, indicating that iron stores are very low. There is no marked poikilocytosis or leucocytosis, although there may be an eosinophilia of 7–14%. The serum albumin is reduced in heavy infections. Because of the persistent anaemia, growth and development become stunted in children.

The rate of progress varies in different cases. In some a high degree of anaemia and even death may result within a few weeks or months of the appearance of the first symptoms. More frequently the disease is chronic, ebbing and flowing or slowly progressing over a number of years.

Infantile hookworm disease

Most cases of hookworm in infants have been reported from China and the majority have been caused by *A. duodenale*.[65] The clinical features include diarrhoea with bloody stools, melaena, anorexia, vomiting, pallor and massive haemorrhage. The mortality is up to 12%.

Transmission occurs in a variety of ways: transmammary, laying infants on contaminated soil, infected diapers consisting of a cloth bag stuffed with soil-containing hookworm larvae, and rarely transplacental infection.

Differential diagnosis

In countries where hookworm infection is endemic, eggs may be found in faeces in any number of conditions which are not causally relayed. In these conditions an egg count is essential to determine the worm load (see below). Light infections in expatriates associated with moderate eosinophilia and mild anaemia must be differentiated from other helminth infections: *Schistosoma mansoni*, *Fasciola hepatica* and other liver flukes and *Strongyloides*. The epigastric pain associated with hookworm infection may suggest duodenal ulcer or pancreatitis and any patient from an endemic area with epigastric symptoms who has hookworm ova in the stool should be treated, since in many cases the symptoms will disappear without the need for any further investigation.

Severe hookworm anaemia must be distinguished from other iron deficiency anaemias, and generalized anasarca from kwashiorkor and the nephrotic syndrome.

Diagnosis

The diagnosis is made by finding eggs in the stool (see Figure 83.11). Rhabditiform larvae may be found in stale stools and be mistaken for *Strongyloides* in which larvae only and not eggs are found in the stool (see pp. 1545–1549). The eggs may be confused with those of *Trichostrongylus*, which are more translucent and smaller. In light infections concentration methods are necessary, such as zinc sulphate concentration, formol ether or the Kato smear (see Appendix I). The worm load can be estimated by an egg count (Stoll egg count method, see Appendix I). Since *A. duodenale* lay an average 25 000 eggs per day, the number of eggs in a gram of stool multiplied by the daily stool weight in grams divided by 25 000 will give the estimated worm load. An egg count of 2500/g is significant and will be associated with symptoms. Less than 25 worms is insignificant, while 500–1000 worms invariably cause disease.

Management

Treatment consists of elimination of the parasites and treatment of the anaemia, if present. Treatment of the anaemia is the first priority but there is no reason why both objectives should not be proceeded with concurrently if non-toxic anthelmintics are used. Suggestions in the past that one drug might be best for one species and another for the other do not apply to modern drugs. Light asymptomatic infections in children should be treated if possible. In adults they are often left untreated, especially if reinfection is probable.

Treatment is usually directed against the adult stages but there is evidence that albendazole in a single dose of 400 mg is active against the pre-intestinal larval stages of *N. americanus*.[66]

Elimination of adult parasites

In the past it was necessary to examine post-treatment stools for 48 hours and examine any worms passed to determine whether the infection in the area was *A. duodenale* or *N. americanus*, since the latter was much more resistant to treatment. With the more modern drugs that is no longer necessary. It is not usually necessary to remove all worms but to reduce the worm load significantly. The drug of choice is albendazole.

- *Albendazole*: This is effective against both *A. duodenale* and *N. americanus*. A single dose of 400 mg will produce an 80% reduction in egg count and 200 mg daily for 3 days will give 100% cure. It is also highly effective against *Ascaris* and is therefore especially suitable for mass treatment.
- *Mebendazole*: A single dose of 500 mg is highly effective against both *A. duodenale* and *N. americanus*.
- *Levamisole*: A single dose of 150 mg orally or 2.5 mg/kg body weight is less effective against *N. americanus*.
- *Pyrantel pamoate (Combantrin)*: A single dose of 10 mg/kg body weight is given. In some areas, e.g. north-western Australia, it is not effective.[67]

Treatment of anaemia

The anaemia is treated by the administration of iron by mouth, in the form of ferrous sulphate or gluconate, 200 mg three times daily, which should be continued for 3 months after a normal haemoglobin level has been achieved. This will restore the iron reserves to normal.

After starting iron therapy, a reticulocyte response may be seen in about 1 week. In most cases the haemoglobin will rise by 1.0 g per week. Folic acid, 5 mg daily, should be given for at least 1 month to cover the erythopoeitic response. Many patients in the tropics fail to correct the haemoglobin fully and develop macrocytosis if this is not done.

Parenteral iron—iron–dextran complex or iron–poly (sorbitol gluconic acid) complex—may be used in patients who cannot tolerate oral iron, in patients where compliance is in doubt or in patients in whom regular follow-up is difficult or unlikely.

Epidemiology and control

The only reservoir of infection is man and the propagation of hookworm infection depends upon an adequate source of infection in the human population, the deposition of eggs in a favourable environment for extrinsic development of the parasite, appropriate conditions of the soil (moisture and warmth) to allow larvae to develop and suitable conditions for the infective larvae to penetrate the skin. In many tropical and subtropical countries transmission is perennial but in cooler and drier climates transmission may take place in the warmer or wet seasons. In some temperate climates local environmental conditions may allow transmission, as in the Cornish tin mines in the past and in the Rand in South Africa today. Cultural and agricultural practices such as the use of human faeces for fertilizer provide good opportunities for infection.

The methods which are employed to determine the amount of hookworm in a community are determination of the *prevalence* and *intensity* of infection by stool surveys and egg counts from which the worm burden can be calculated. These surveys will show whether the infection in the community is low grade; moderate or severe; soil pollution in the area must also be studied and filariform larvae of hookworm can be demonstrated in soil by the

Baermann method or they can be cultured (see Appendix I). Studies of the nutritional level of the community, especially the haemoglobin level, must also be undertaken.

Because of logistic and social difficulties, estimates of worm numbers by chemotherapeutic expulsion in an age-stratified host population have been very few, most studies having relied on an indirect measure of parasite abundance: the density of eggs in the stools. A recent study in Zimbabwe,[25] in which the intensity of infection was measured directly by parasite expulsion, showed a steady rise in intensity with age, resembling those previously reported with a similar technique from India and Papua New Guinea. I believe that a similar pattern will also be found in areas where worm loads are appreciably higher.[59]

The basis of prophylaxis and control is described on pp. 1550–1552.

Cutaneous larva migrans (creeping eruption, sandworm, plumber's itch, duckhunter's itch)

Cutaneous larva migrans is a cutaneous eruption resulting from exposure of the skin to the infective filariform larvae of non-human hookworm (A. braziliense, A. caninum) and Strongyloides of the nutria and racoon. The infective larvae cannot complete their normal life cycle in the human host but persist under the skin, without developing further, where they cause cutaneous larva migrans.

Geographical distribution

Creeping eruption occurs in most warm, humid, tropical and subtropical areas, being especially common in the southern USA, along the coast of the Gulf of Mexico and Florida. It is also common on the coast of West, South and East Africa, South-East Asia, India, Malaysia, Sri Lanka and Thailand.

Aetiology

Ancyclostoma

A. braziliense is the hookworm of dogs and cats. It is smaller than A. duodenale (female 1 cm and male 8.5 mm long), the internal pair of ventral teeth are smaller and the dorsal rays in the copulatory bursa are distinctive (Figure III.62). The eggs are indistinguishable from those of human hookworms. The life cycle is similar to that of A. duodenale but man is an unsuitable host and the third-stage larva does not enter the bloodstream but wanders under the skin, causing cutaneous larva migrans.

A. caninum is the dog hookworm. Its life history is similar to that of A. braziliense.

Strongyloides

Filariform larvae of S. stercoralis can re-enter the skin as part of autoinfection around the anus and buttock, where they cause 'larva currens', a rash rather like that of cutaneous larva migrans.

S. myopotami (nutria) and S. procyornis (racoon) all produce similar lesions in the human host, in which they cannot complete their normal life cycle. The lesions are more persistent.

Transmission

Infection is acquired from damp contaminated soil through the skin of that part of the body in contact with the soil (foot, abdomen, buttock).

Pathology

The filariform larvae are unable to penetrate below the stratum germinativum of human skin, where they form a tunnel with the corium as a floor and the stratum granulosum as a roof. Local eosinophilia and round cell infiltration occur round the tunnel and may persist for months. Rarely the larvae reach the lungs, where they cause transitory pulmonary symptoms and eosinophilia and may be recovered from bronchial washings. They do not mature in the intestine.

Immunity

Little is known about immunity. There is no protective immunity and people can be infected more than once.

Clinical features

Natural history

The larvae wander under the skin and can persist for months before they eventually die.

Incubation period

Symptoms start immediately after penetration of the skin, a matter of a few hours only.

Symptoms and signs

There is a red itchy papule at the site of entry, which becomes elevated and vesicular. The larvae move several millimetres to a few centimetres each day and leave tunnels which become dry and crusted. The track is linear and twists and turns (Figure 83.13). It causes an intense pruritus and the skin is scratched and becomes secondarily infected. The lesions may be single or multiple. The most common sites are the hands and feet with

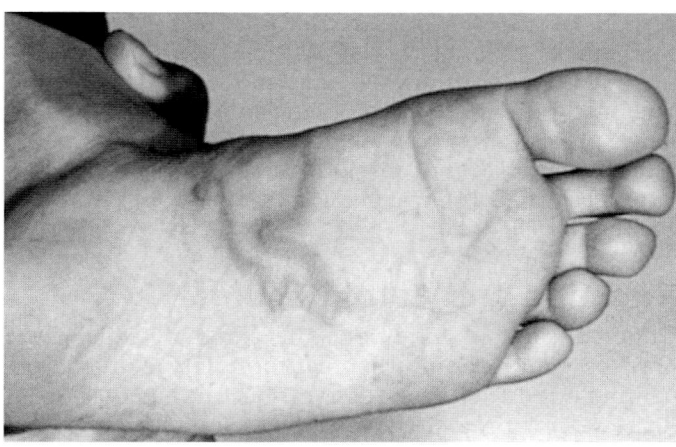

Figure 83.13: Cutaneous larva migrans (*A. braziliense*).

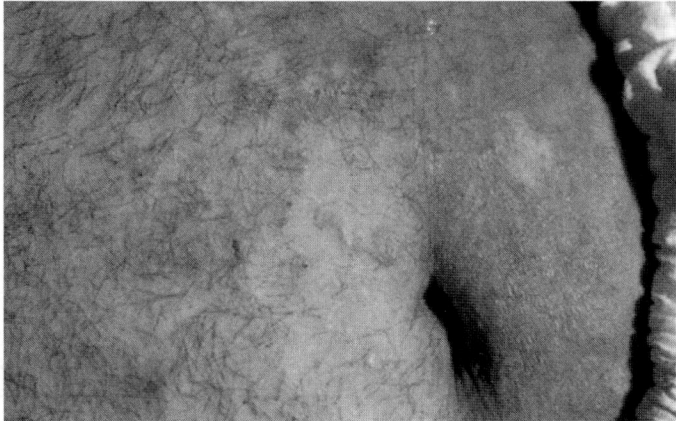

Figure 83.14: Multiple burrows of cutaneous larva migrans (creeping eruption).

A. braziliense but the abdomen is often infested in plumber's itch and the lesions may be very numerous indeed (Figure 83.14).

The lesions produced by non-human hookworms (cutaneous larva migrans) are well defined, move very slowly and persist for months. There is little surrounding flare and the track is indurated. In contrast, the lesions produced by *Strongyloides* (larva currens) are less well defined, have a red flare on the outside, move much more rapidly and persist for a few hours only.

Diagnosis

Creeping eruptions can be caused by *Strongyloides stercoralis* (larva currens), *Gnathostoma spinigerum*, cutaneous myiasis (*Hypoderma bovis* and *Hypoderma lineatum*), warble fly maggots (*Gasterophilus*) and cutaneous *Fasciola hepatica*.

The diagnosis is clinical. *Ancylostoma* larva migrans is usually situated on the foot or toe (see Figure 83.13) and lasts for months, moving very slowly. *Strongyloides* (larva currens) is situated on the buttocks and trunk and lasts

for hours only, moving comparatively quickly. Non-human *Strongyloides* is usually situated on the trunk and abdomen and can persist for many months. *Loa loa* causes no cutaneous reaction and appears and disappears in a matter of minutes. There is usually no eosinophilia but if there is then internal migration of the larvae can be suspected. It is not possible to retrieve the larva since it is invariably in advance of its track and impossible to isolate. There are no serological tests.

Management

Treatment with a single dose of 400 mg oral albendazole gives cure rates of 46–100%, while a single oral dose of 12 mg of ivermectin gives cure rates of 81–100%.[68] A 7-day course of 400 mg daily of oral albendazole results in fewer recurrences than single-dose treatment.

Oral and topical thiabendazole are also effective.[70]

Epidemiology

The source of infection is soil contaminated with dog and cat faeces underneath beach houses on stilts, exposure taking place when people crawl underneath to repair facilities (plumber's itch) or bathe with bare feet and walk along the sand above the high water mark (sandworm) or expose themselves to mounds contaminated by nutria and racoons in the marshes (duckhunter's itch). In subtropical countries exposure is most common during the summer months and early autumn.

Control

Little can be done to control dogs and cats but infection can be prevented by wearing sandals above the high water mark and protective clothing when underneath houses in hot areas.

Strongyloidiasis
Geographical distribution

S. stercoralis has a worldwide distribution in the tropics and subtropics. It is highly prevalent in parts of tropical Brazil, Colombia and South-East Asia. In temperate climates it is not uncommon in inmates of institutions, such as mental hospitals, prisons and the mentally retarded children's homes. It has become a serious problem in individuals receiving suppressive treatment.

Aetiology

Strongyloidiasis is caused by *S. stercoralis* (see Appendix III), a nematode worm which has two forms: one parasitic and the other free living. There are three developmental forms: adult, rhabditiform larva and filariform (infective) larva.

Life cycle (Figure 83.15)

There are two life cycles in which reproduction takes place: an internal sexual cycle involving parasitic worms and the external sexual cycle involving free-living worms.

Internal sexual cycle

The adult female parasitic worm (2.5 × 0.034 mm) tapers anteriorly and ends in a conical tail. There is an oesophagus occupying a quarter of the body which has two bulbs divided by a constriction. The vulva lies in the posterior third of the body and there is a prominent uterus containing 50 eggs (50–58 × 30–34 μm) (Appendix III). The male exists but disappears from the bowel soon after oviposition and eggs can be produced parthenogenetically (as happens with *S. ratti*). The eggs hatch immediately in the bowel into male and female rhabditiform larvae, which pass out in the faeces to continue the external sexual cycle.

External sexual cycle

The free-living rhabditiform larvae develop into free-living adults which copulate in the soil and produce eggs. The free-living forms have a double-bulbed muscular oesophagus. The free-living female is smaller (1 × 0.05 mm) than the parasitic female, the vulva lies posteriorly and the uterus contains eggs measuring 70 × 40 μm (Appendix III). The male form measures 0.7 × 0.035 mm. The rhabditiform larvae produced by both parasitic and free-living forms are indistinguishable and develop into filariform (infective) larvae (Figure 83.16), which can remain alive in the soil for many weeks.

Infection and autoinfection

Under unsuitable conditions the external sexual cycle may be omitted and the filariform larvae infect the definitive host via the skin or buccal mucosa, as in *Ancylostoma* or *Necator*. The larvae travel up to the lungs, enter the bronchi, cross over the glottis and pass to the small intestine, where they mature into parasitic adults.

Autoinfection

Autoinfection, which results in multiplication in the host indefinitely, arises in one of two ways. The filariform larvae do not pass out in the stools but reinvade the bowel or skin. The other way is when the filariform larvae lodge in the bronchial epithelium and produce further

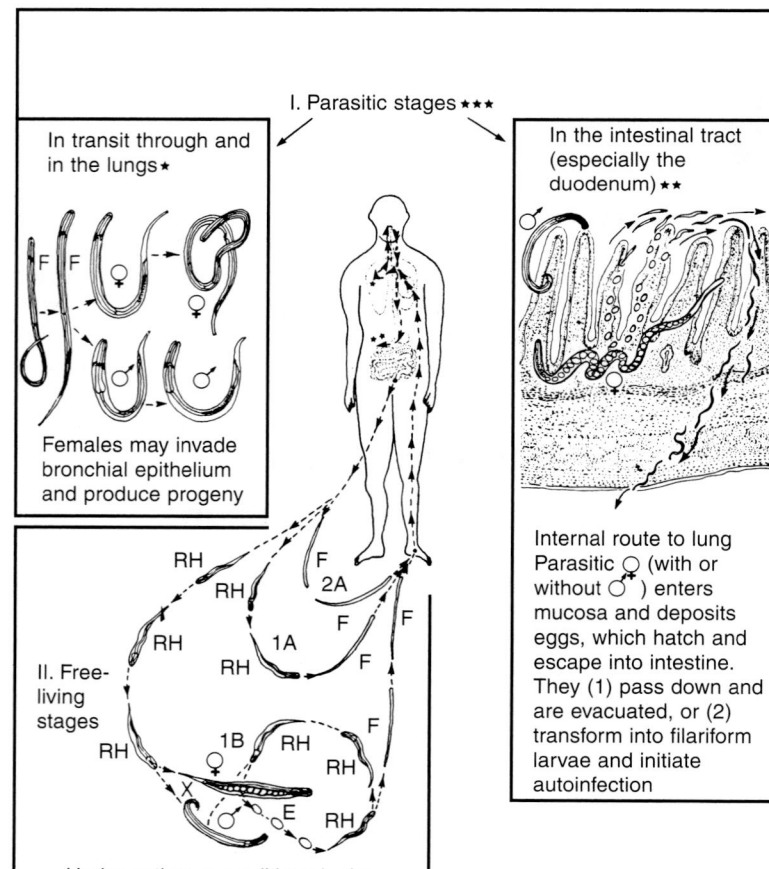

Figure 83.15: Life cycle of *Strongyloides stercoralis*.

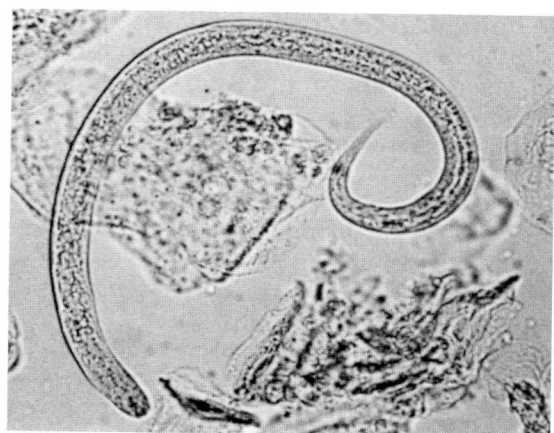

Figure 83.16: *S. stercoralis.* Rhabditiform larva in stool. (Courtesy J. S. Tatz.)

progeny. Autoinfection leads to a build-up in the body of the population so that the worms can maintain themselves in the absence of any further infection from an external source, and results in the intermittent recurrence of symptomatic episodes. In the case of any breakdown in the immune defences a rapid increase in the worm burden results in hyperinfection.

Pathology

The pathogenic effects begin with the entry of the infective larvae into the skin. The filariform larvae cause petechial haemorrhages at the site of invasion accompanied by intense pruritus, congestion and oedema. The larvae migrate into cutaneous blood vessels and are carried to the lungs. In the lungs they enter the alveoli and pass up the respiratory tree, where they may be delayed by the host response, become adults and invade the bronchial epithelium. Passing through the lungs the young worms may cause symptoms resembling those of broncho-pneumonia with some lobular consolidation.

When they have become lodged in crypts in the intestine the females mature and invade the tissues of the bowel wall but rarely penetrate the muscularis mucosae, and move in tissue channels beneath the villi, where the eggs are deposited. The eggs hatch out and first-stage larvae work towards the lumen of the bowel and are passed out in faeces.

In heavy infections the first-stage larvae, instead of passing out in the faeces, develop in the intestine, bore into the wall of the duodenum and jejunum and develop to the adult stage, producing ova, while encysted in the bowel. From here they spread throughout the lymphatic system to the mesenteric lymph glands and can enter the general circulation and be found in the liver, lungs, kidneys and gallbladder wall. The ileum, appendix and colon are sites of reinvasion and here the worms cause granulomas with a central necrotic area often containing a degenerate larva. The mesenteric glands may be similarly affected. The lungs may show abscesses and the liver may be enlarged with small pinpoint larval

granulomas. The larvae may carry micro-organisms and an overwhelming septicaemia caused by *Escherichia coli* has been caused in this way. In light infections jejunal biopsy has shown oedema, cellular infiltration and eosinophilic infiltration of the mucosa with partial villous atrophy. At post-mortem, ulceration and atrophy of the mucosa are seen with numerous adult worms in the wall of the duodedum and jejunum. At times filariform larvae fail to break out of the alveoli, gain access to the general circulation and can invade the brain, intestine, lymph glands, liver, lungs and, rarely, myocardium.

Transmission

Infection is acquired originally from contaminated soil via free-living filariform infective larvae. Once established further infection may be acquired from the colon or anal skin from parasitic infective larvae. The transmission of *Strongyloides* through the milk has been demonstrated in several animal species and it is possible that this occurs in man.

Immunity

Immunity to reinfection develops in most individuals after a primary infection and the *Strongyloides* adults and larvae are confined to the small intestine and the worm load is controlled. Immunity is both antibody and cell mediated.

Humoral antibody-mediated immunity is elicited by the secretions of the infective larvae with a Type I response, an eosinophilic tissue response, and a peripheral eosinophilia—often with urticarial rashes. Antibodies are produced which cross-react with many other helminths, including filariae.

Cell-mediated immunity is elicited by adult and larval worms in the tissues, which are localized and destroyed by a cell-mediated granulomatous reaction. If cell-mediated immunity is depressed for any reason, such as immuno-depressive states of drugs, then a generalized hyperinfection results, causing massive strongyloidiasis.

Clinical features

Natural history

In the majority of cases a small population of adult worms maintains itself in the small intestine for many years (30 or more) in the absence of any further infection from the outside causing recurrent symptoms when filari-form larvae enter the perianal skin, and cause a recurrent rash—'larva currens'—associated with urticaria. In a small minority of cases the defences of the body break down and a generalized severe infection ensues.

Incubation period

The prepatent period from infection to the appearance of rhabditiform larvae in the stools is 1 month.

Symptoms and signs

The vast majority of infections in endemic areas are symptomless. When for various reasons the number of *Strongyloides* present in the intestine increases then symptoms develop.

Primary infection

This is rarely seen in endemic areas and descriptions are based on self-induced experimental infections. A pruritic erythematous eruption, which lasts about 3 weeks, occurs at the site of entry of the larvae. A dry cough or sore throat appears on the 6th–9th day together with abdominal fullness, aching in the right lower quadrant of the abdomen and a watery diarrhoea alternating with constipation. Larvae are first detected in the stools 27 days after infection. A severe cough may occur lasting over a month.

Chronic uncomplicated strongyloidiasis

This is characterized by epigastric and right upper quadrant pain together with nausea, chronic diarrhoea and weight loss.

Skin rashes

There are two types of skin rashes. One, occurring around the anus and anywhere on the trunk, is a linear eruption—'larva currens'—in which the larvae migrate under the skin causing an itching rash with a larval track which is not indurated and has a red flare at the edge which moves quite rapidly (2–10 cm per hour), disappearing in a few hours (Figure 83.17), in contrast to the more indurated and persistent track of non-human hookworm (cutaneous larva migrans). The second form is urticaria caused by allergy to the larvae penetrating the skin in an individual who has already been sensitized. It occurs predominantly in the buttocks with pruritus ani and around the waist, lasts 1–2 days and recurs at regular intervals. The creeping type of eruption, which is seen mainly in infections from Indo-China and was common in prisoners of war in the Far East in the 1939–45 war, can last for 30 years or more. A strongyloides-related glomerulonephritis has been reported.[71]

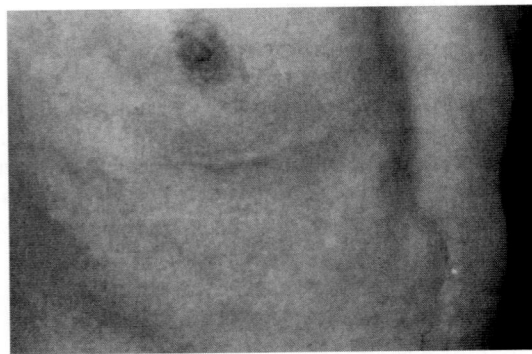

Figure 83.17: Skin rash (larva currens) of *Strongyloides stercoralis*.

Severe complicated strongyloidiasis[72,73]

In persons debilitated by disease, malnutrition or serious illness, severe complications and sometimes death may result from massive invasion of the tissues by strongyloides.[92] Treatment with immunosuppressive drugs for lymphoma, organ transplantation and other conditions may produce the same results. First-stage larvae develop in the duodenum and jejunum, bore into the bowel wall, become adult and produce ova. In this way the number of strongyloides is immensely increased and infective larvae invade the tissues and circulate, causing massive strongyloidiasis. Severe abdominal pain, vomiting and diarrhoea together with a sprue-like syndrome may develop: a protein-losing enteropathy, hypoalbuminaemea and generalized oedema occur. Fever, hypertension, abdominal tenderness and distension, reduced bowel sounds, paralytic ileus and a necrotizing jejunitis have been reported.

In the lungs, pulmonary symptoms resembling tropical pulmonary eosinophilia with hypereosinophilia, pneumonitis, diffuse crepitations, scattered bronchi, pleural effusion and pulmonary abscess and gross respiratory failure may occur.[74]

Neurological complications with headache, convulsions, confusion, stupor, meningitis and focal neurological signs occur. In 30% of immunocompromised patients, a Gram-negative (*E. coli*) meningitis is found.

Other complications include a septicaemia with enteric organisms, shock, multiple petechiae on the chest and abdomen and peri-umbilical purpura.

Laboratory findings

Raised serum IgE levels are found. Towards the end of the early stage of infection there is a high leucocytosis of up to 25×10^9/litre; an eosinophilia of 10–12×10^9/litre is characteristic. Later when the infection is chronic there is a moderate eosinophilia which may persist for years. In severe complicated strongyloidiasis the eosinophilia disappears and is an indication of poor prognosis.

Differential diagnosis

Strongyloidiasis must be differentiated from other tissue-invading helminths: *Ascaris*, ancylostomiasis and liver flukes. Disseminated strongyloidiasis may closely resemble tropical pulmonary eosinophilia, especially since serology cross-reacts. 'Larva currens' resembles cutaneous larva migrans but in distinction from it in 'larva currens' the rash is situated mainly round the buttocks and on the trunk, lasts only a few hours and may occur intermittently for many years.

Diagnosis

Only adults or rhabditiform larvae (Figure 83.16) appear in the stools, duodenal aspirate or by the Entero test capsule. They can be demonstrated by the formol ether method or cultured in charcoal at 26°C for a week (see Appendix III).

A modified agar plate method has been developed which is considered to be superior to the filter method in detecting *Strongyloides*.[75]

The differentiation of the rhabditiform larvae from hookworm and *Trichostrongylus* is shown in Appendix III. Radiological diagnosis is not much used but the appearances have been described by Louisey and Barton.[76] Other methods of diagnosis are a modified Baermann technique; the agar plate culture method; ELISA and serum IgG reactivity to larval proteins of *Strongyloides stercoralis*.[77,78]

There is considerable cross-reaction with other helminths and filariae. The filarial complement fixation test is positive in 45% of 'larva currens'[79] and in 65% of uncomplicated cases but may be negative in massive strongyloidiasis. A modified ELISA test for estimating parasite-specific serum IgG has been developed.[80]

A gelatin particle indirect agglutination test is considered to be more convenient than the micro-ELISA for mass screening for strongyloidiasis.[81]

Recombinent cDNA clones have been characterized.[82]

Management

Strongyloides should usually be treated whether or not the infection is giving rise to symptoms. It should be looked for and treated especially in immunosuppressed patients, for example those on corticosteroid therapy, immunosuppressive drugs, HIV, or persons from endemic areas in whom transplantation is being contemplated. Ivermectin using a single oral dose of 200 μg/kg repeated after 1 week or 200 μg/kg daily for 3 days has given good results. Albendazole, 400 mg daily for 3 days repeated 2 weeks later, is also very effective.[83] Mebendazole and thiabendazole can also be used.

Epidemiology

Man is the most important host of *Strongyloides* but dogs and chimpanzees have been found infected with strains indistinguishable from those of man. Larvae are unable to survive temperatures below 8°C or above 40°C or desiccation. Strongyloidiasis thrives in conditions of overcrowding on damp soil in tropical conditions such as in rural villages in South-East Asia. It was very common among prisoners of war in Burma and Indo-China in the Second World War, but it may also become established in deep mines in cold climates.

Control

Control methods are the same as for other soil-transmitted helminths (see pp. 1550–1552).

Strongyloides fülleborni

Strongyloides fülleborni is widely distributed in tropical forest regions of Central and East Africa. The main source of infection is monkey faeces, although human-to-human transmission may occur. In most cases there are no symptoms; 24% of pygmies in Zaire were found to be passing ova and very heavy infections were found without any evidence of disease.

Aetiology

S. fülleborni can be distinguished from *S. stercoralis* by the prominent vulvar lips, narrowing behind the vulva and a prominent oesophagus. Eggs are passed in the stool in contrast to *S. stercoralis* and resemble those of hookworm, for which they are commonly mistaken. Treatment is as for *S. stercoralis*.

Strongyloides fülleborni Kellyi [85]

This is a subspecies of *S. fülleborni* confined mainly to forested areas in western Papua New Guinea, along the Fly River in the Eastern Highlands.

In low prevalence areas 20% of children and 5–10% of adults are infected and transmission is percutaneous. In high-prevalence areas 100% of children aged 3–5 years are infected and 15–20% of adults. Peak intensity of infection occurs around 12 months with egg counts averaging 100 000 eggs/mg of faeces; the highest recorded was 928 000 eggs/mg in a 10-month-old patient. In these high-prevalence areas transmission is percutaneous and possibly transmammary.

The eggs are similar to those of *S. fülleborni*. Mothers carry their children in string bags lined with dried banana leaves and/or cloth which are infrequently changed and in which eggs and free-living larvae have been found.

Clinical manifestations are seen most frequently in children 2–6 months of age who present with abdominal distension, mild diarrhoea, a protein-losing enteropathy resulting in oedema and low serum protein levels—'swollen-belly disease'. Respiratory distress may occur with a characteristic high-pitched cry. Treatment is as for *S. stercoralis* supplemented by plasma infusion, if the hypoproteinaemia is severe.

Trichostrongyliasis
Geographical distribution

Normally a parasite of sheep and goats, human infection with *Trichostrongylus* is widespread in Central Africa, Egypt and in Asia and India, Assam, Indonesia and Japan.

Aetiology

Three species can infect man: *Trichostrongylus colubriformis*,

T. orientalis and, more rarely, *T. probulurus*. The female worm (5–8 × 0.07 mm) is slender and pink with a posterior vulva (Appendix III); the male (4–5 × 0.07 mm) has a bilobed copulatory bursa and two spicules. The mouth is unarmed. The parasites are situated in the duodenum and jejunum where they are not attached to the bowel but are a half to a third buried in mucus. The eggs, which have a transparent hyaline shell and resemble those of hookworm but are larger (85 × 115 µm), are passed in the stool in the morula stage and are remarkably resistant to desiccation and cold. The life cycle is similar to that of hookworm but they do not migrate through the lungs. Adults mature in the intestine within 25–30 days.

Transmission

Infection is acquired through the skin or mouth from contaminated food or drink.

Pathology

Little is known about pathology and none has been observed, even in individuals with heavy egg counts.

Symptoms and signs

These are few but mild anaemia and general ill health may result.

Diagnosis

Diagnosis is made by finding eggs in faeces and adults after treatment.

Management

Levamisole is the drug of choice and is given as a single oral dose of 2.5 mg/kg. Thiabendazole is less effective.

Epidemiology

Trichostrongylus colubriformis is a parasite of sheep and goats and is common in some areas where sheep and goats are kept: up to 70% of the inhabitants may be infected.

Trichostrongylus orientalis is common among people who look after donkeys and goats; the use of human excreta as fertilizer in Asia is responsible for the high level of infection.

Diagnosis of geohelminths

Coprological examination is still the method best suited to the resources and skills available in most of the developing countries where the infections are endemic. The procedure most commonly used is the Kato–Katz method.[86]

Efforts to develop specific and sensitive serological tests as well as to detect antigens by molecular techniques[87] continue to take place in sophisticated laboratories, but few of these are likely to be generally available in countries where geohelminths occur endemically.

Modern imaging procedures are only likely to be available in maximal care or teaching hospitals in the tropics, as are delicate surgical techniques by well-trained gastroenterologists.[88]

The effects of larval migration are identified by pulmonary opacities in chest radiographs, periperial blood eosinophilia and larvae in respiratory and gastric secretions.[89]

Community control of geohelminths

The five basic essentials needed for controlling geohelminth infections at the community level are: (1) chemotherapy; (2) sanitation; (3) health education; (4) community participation; and (5) monitoring and evaluation.

It is now generally accepted that in most areas of the tropics geohelminths not only cause specific morbidity but also result in insidious effects on nutritional status[90] and on physical and intellectual development.[91] They also interfere with the efficacy of supplementation programmes by reducing the absorption of nutrients such as vitamin A and oral iodized oil.[92]

Periodic chemotherapy should ideally be implemented in the context of ongoing improvement of sanitation and health education.[93]

School-based programmes have been shown to be a cost-effective approach for controlling the intensity of intestinal helminth infection even in environments where transmission is high.[94] However, it must be realized that this strategy alone is unlikely to be successful in areas where adults, non-enrolled school-aged children and pre-school children represent a substantial proprotion of helminth-infected persons and egg excretors. In these areas school-based programmes must be complemented by community-based helminth control.[95–97]

Critical evaluation of the above community-based programmes concluded that the current public health investments in this intervention are not based on consistent or reliable evidence.

Chemotherapy

There are now several anthelmintics active against the geohelminths. They have a broad spectrum of activity, which makes them particularly useful for community control, since polyparasitism is more common than monoparasitism in most countries where geohelminths are endemic. They are relatively non-toxic, they can be given orally, and are effective in a single dose if reduction in intensity of infection rather than absolute cure is the main objective.

For countries that adopt a national 'essential drugs' policy and take advantage of the joint UNICEF–WHO initiative for the procurement of 'essential drugs', the cost is now low. The clinical pharmacology of the most commonly used broad-spectrum anthelmintics is given on pp. 1552–1553.

Unless specifically indicated, pregnant women and children under 2 years of age or weighing under 10 kg should not be included in community control chemotherapeutic campaigns. These are high-risk groups in the tropics, and a fatality occurring within days of drug administration, even if unrelated, is frequently attributed to the event and can adversely affect community participation.

In countries where transmission of soil-transmitted helminths is seasonal, the time of the campaign is important. In these circumstances, two treatments, the first after the start of the wet season, e.g. 8 weeks, and the second after the end of the rains, e.g. 8 weeks, will reduce the risk of reinfection during the subsequent dry season. In countries where transmission is perennial, more frequent treatments may be required, e.g. three or four times yearly, which would naturally increase the cost of the campaign.

The strategy of chemotherapeutic interventions should be integrated with the other activities of the local health services: for example, primary health care programmes; immunization programmes; child health programmes; family planning programmes; school health programmes; and in *appropriate circumstances*, e.g. when age/infection of intensity distribution overlap, in a multiple-infection delivery approach.

Since reduction in morbidity is the primary objective of chemotherapy the limitations of the multiple-infection delivery approach are obvious when it is appreciated that the age distribution of infection intensity varies substantially between the parasite species:[98–100] the peak intensities of *Ascaris* and *Trichuris* occur in children under 10 years of age; of schistosomes in the age group 10–20 years; and of hookworms in adults over 20 years of age.

Three chemotherapeutic strategies can be used: *mass chemotherapy*, i.e. treatment of all persons if the prevalence of infection is 50% or over; *selective population chemotherapy*, i.e. treatment of *all* infected persons at the time of a survey; *targeted chemotherapy*, i.e. treatment of specific groups likely to suffer the greatest morbidity.

Resistance to anthelmintics drugs

Resistance is now widespread in the gastrointestinal nematodes of ruminants, particularly sheep and goats. Although resistance by human nematodes has rarely been reported, managers of control programmes should be alerted to the possibility, particularly since the current assays do not detect resistance until at least 25% of the worm population is affected.[101] A possible genetic marker for resistance to treatment of *S. stercoralis* has been identified.[102]

Mebendazole-resistant *N. americanus* in Mali[103] and pyrantel-resistant *A. duodenale* in Western Australia have been reported.[104]

Careful monitoring of mass treatment programmes is therefore essential, and it is very important that the available anthelmintics are used in ways that will delay or prevent drug resistance, possibly by combination therapies as is advocated for malaria.

Sanitation

Marked improvements in environmental hygiene are the ultimate answer to the control and elimination of geohelminth infections, but for many countries in the tropics these are relatively expensive and long-term objectives.

In the medium term, however, many varieties of affordable latrines are available, e.g. ventilated improved pit latrines and double-vault latrines. These have proved to be culturally acceptable in many countries; they are easy to install, operate and maintain. Further, they allow adequate composting of human excretion as fertilizer.

The impact of the water sanitation decade in several countries should play an important role in the control of geohelminths. It must be appreciated that the effect of sanitation is slow to develop, and that therefore periodic anthelmintic treatments should be maintained until sanitation has had an impact on transmission.[105]

Health education

Human behaviour is of great importance in the transmission of geohelminths and the success or failure of control programmes often hinges on the modification of behavioural patterns. Health education must target its activities on this crucial criterion, aiming to determine which local culture and practices are conducive to the transmission of infection and need to be modified to reduce the risk. If beneficial cultural practices are identified, these should be reinforced to enhance compliance. As many people as possible should be involved in the planning process, particularly women, who in the past have often been ignored. Improvements in personal hygiene should be actively encouraged. Modern audiovisual technology may be used when appropriate.

Community participation

This is crucial for the success of any control programme. Active participation of the community in the planning and execution of any intervention is mandatory. The schedule should suit the convenience of the community and be discussed and agreed by them. As with all the diseases of poverty, economic development is mandatory for effective community involvement.

Monitoring and evaluation[106]

Monitoring and evaluation are mandatory and should be used to review or revise any control programme. In view

Table 83.1 Spectrum of activity of antinematode drugs

	Albendazole	Pyrantel	Mebendazole	Levamisole
Ascaris lumbricoides	+++	+++	+++	+++
Trichuris trichiura	++	++	++	+
Necator americanus	+++	++	++	++
Ancyclostoma duodenale	+++	++	+++	+++
Strongyloides stercoralis	++	+	+	+

+++, High; ++, moderate; +, low.

of the severe financial constraints for health care in most developing countries, the cost-effectiveness of any strategy used should be determined wherever possible.

Targeted chemotherapy implemented within an existing health infrastructure has been shown to achieve an overall reduction in the prevalence and intensity of *Ascaris* and *Trichuris* infection in children aged 2–15 years at one-fifth of the drug purchase cost of mass chemotherapy, and with few of the attendant costs of drug delivery.[107]

A sustained community-based control programme that used albendazole, combined with continued health education and environmental management for a period of 6 years, effectively controlled *A. duodenale* in an isolated Australian community.[108]

Clinical pharmacology of anthelmintic drugs[109,110]

The drugs most commonly used for the community control of the soil-transmitted helminths are albendazole, mebendazole, pyrantel and levamisole. They are all broad-spectrum anthelmintics, although their efficacy against individual geohelminths varies. Their spectrum of activity against the various nematodes is shown in Table 83.1. These safe and orally administered, single-dose broad-spectrum anthelmintics have revolutionized our concepts for the community control of the geohelminths.

Albendazole

This is now the most widely used anthelmintic for the community control of multiple geohelminth infections and is the newest of the benzimidazole derivatives. It is poorly absorbed from the gastrointestinal tract and is rapidly and extensively metabolized by the liver to sulphoxide and sulphone metabolites. The sulphoxide metabolite is an active anthelmintic and may be responsible for most of the drug effects in vivo.

Albendazole is not detectable in plasma after oral administration. It is known to be teratogenic and embryotoxic in some animals. It should not be adminstered during confirmed or suspected pregnancy. In women of child-bearing age albendazole should be administered no more than 7 days after the start of the last menstrual period.

Adverse effects are mild and transient. They include epigastric pain, diarrhoea, headache, nausea, vomiting, dizziness, constipation, pruritus and dry mouth.

Mebendazole

Mebendazole is effective against adult worms and larval stages. It selectively inhibits glucose uptake in nematodes; this results in increased utilization of helminth glycogen and deprivation for the worms of their main source of energy. Oral absorption is limited by its poor solubility. The small amount absorbed is metabolized extensively by the liver to inactive compounds. Teratogenic and embryotoxic effects in animals have been recorded; it is therefore not recommended in pregnancy.

Adverse effects include transient gastrointestinal discomfort and headache.

Mebendazole sometimes stimulated *Ascaris* worms to emerge from the mouth and nostrils, which alarms the patients unless they are forewarned.

Pyrantel

Pyrantel owes its activity to its action on the neuromuscular system of the worms. It paralyses the worms, which are then expelled in the faeces. It is poorly absorbed from the gastrointestinal tract, with less than 15% excreted in the urine as unchanged drug and metabolites and 70% excreted unchanged in the faeces. It should be stored in tight, light-resistant containers.

Adverse effects include mild gastrointestinal discomfort, headache, dizziness, drowsiness, insomnia and skin rash.

Pyrantel and piperazine are antagonistic and should not be administered concurrently.

Levamisole

Levamisole causes a spastic paralysis of susceptible nematodes, resulting in their elimination from the intestine. It is rapidly absorbed from the gastrointestinal tract, achieving peak plasma levels within 2 hours, and is eliminated within 3 days. Much of the absorbed drug is metabolized in the liver.

Adverse effects include abdominal pain, nausea, vomiting, dizziness and headache.

Nitazoxanide[111,112] (Cryptaz®)

Nitazoxanide is a new class of anthelminth active against ascariasis, trichuriasis and hookworm. Pharmaceutical compositions of nitazoxanide include both nitazoxanide and its derivative tizoxanide, as active ingredients with particle sizes of the active drug substance ranging from 5 to 200 μm. In humans, the drug is heavily concentrated in the intestinal tract with approximately 32% of the oral dose excreted in urine and 66% in faeces. Adverse effects are mild and transient and include abdominal pain, nausea, vomiting and diarrhoea. The dose ranges from 100 mg to 400 mg twice daily for 3 days.

Other nematodes for whom man is not the normal host

Trichinosis (*Trichinella spiralis*)

Geographical distribution (Figure 83.18)

Trichinosis has a worldwide distribution and is important as an infection of man in Europe and the USA. It is less important in the tropics but occurs in both east and west sub-Saharan Africa. It is an important cause of disease and death in the Arctic, where polar explorers have died as a result of trichinosis. *It is not a soil-transmitted helminth infection.*

Aetiology

Trichinella spiralis occurs in two forms: adult and cystic.

The adult *T. spiralis* (Appendix III) is a white worm just visible to the naked eye and inhabits the small intestine. The male (1.6 × 0.04 mm) has a cloaca situated posteriorly between two caudal papillae. The female (3–4 × 0.06 mm) has a vulva in the anterior fifth, an ovary in the posterior half of the body and a coiled uterine tube in the anterior portion.

Life cycle (See Appendix III)

The female lives for 30 days and is viviparous. The eggs (20 μm) live in the upper uterus and the larvae (100 × 6 μm) break out, living free in the uterine cavity. One female produces more than 1500 larvae. The larvae, which emerges as early as 4–7 days after infection, continue to be produced for 4–16 weeks. They make their way via the lymphatics and blood circulation to the right heart and lungs, enter the arterial circulation and reach striated muscle, where they encyst.

Cystic stage

The cyst is formed by the larva encapsulated by the host tissue. The capsule is an adventitious ellipsoidal sheath with blunt ends resulting from cellular reaction around the tightly coiled larva (Figure 83.19). The long axis parallels that of the muscle fibres and host amino acids nourish it so that it can remain alive for many years. In

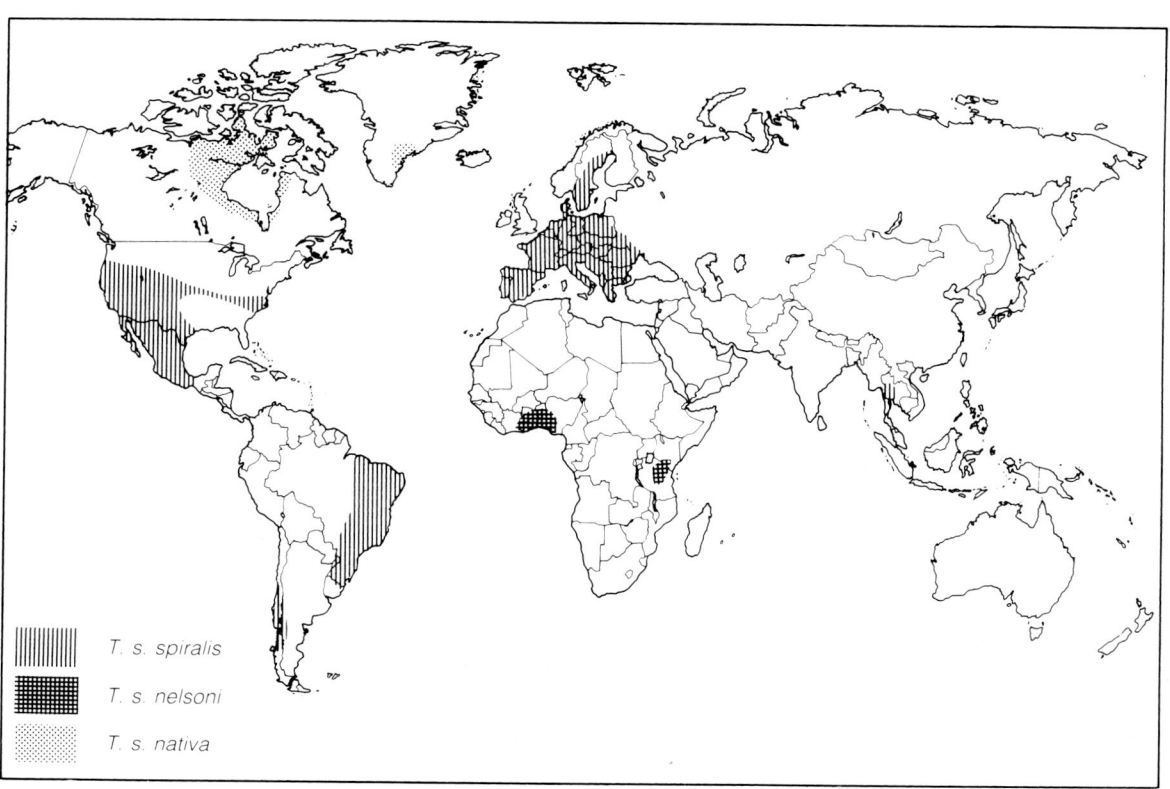

T. s. spiralis

T. s. nelsoni

T. s. nativa

Figure 83.18: Geographical distribution of trichinosis.

1554 Soil-transmitted Helminths (Geohelminths)

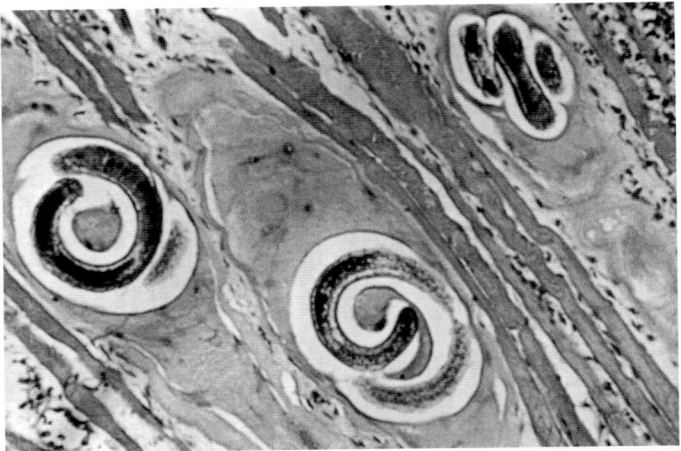

Figure 83.19: Larvae of *T. spiralis* in muscle.

man calcification may take place after 6 months and lead to death of the larva. When consumed by a carnivorous host the cysts are digested in the stomach and after encysting the larvae, which are resistant to gastric juice, invade the duodenal and jejunal mucosa, where they penetrate the columnar epithelium and develop into adults after 36 hours. The period between infection and the encysting stage in the muscles is 17–21 days.

Species and strains of *Trichinella*

T. spiralis contains three subspecies which can infect man. They are indistinguishable morphologically but vary in their host specificity and can be distinguished enzymatically:[119]

- *T. spiralis spiralis* of temperate regions, with domestic pigs the source of human infection.
- *T. spiralis nativa* of the Arctic regions; a parasite of carrion feeding carnivores; polar bears and walruses are the main sources of human infection.
- *T. spiralis nelsoni* in Africa and southern Europe in wild carnivores, with wild pigs the source of human infection.

   T. s. nativa is very resistant to freezing and *T. s. nelsoni* and *T. s. nativa* have a low infectivity for domestic pigs and rats.

Transmission

Transmission is by mouth from eating undercooked meat.

T. s. spiralis

Human infection is acquired from eating undercooked pork from infected pigs. The pigs are infected from eating raw garbage or perhaps from eating rats which themselves become infected from garbage. An epidemic due to *T. pseudospiralis* was reported from Thailand, affecting 59 individuals, all of whom ate raw pork from a wild pig that was distributed to villagers by a local hunter.[113]

T. s. nativa

Human infection is acquired from eating bear meat (the top predator), polar bear in the Arctic and brown bears in sub-Arctic regions of the former USSR and North America. Walrus meat can also be infective. Polar explorers have died as a result of eating polar bear meat.

T. s. nelsoni

Human infection results from eating bush pig or wart-hog meat which are themselves infected from carrion.

Pathology

The capsule of the infective larva is digested in the intestine since it is resistant to the gastric juice and penetrates the duodenal and jejunal mucosa, where the amount of trauma and irritation depend on the number of larvae. This will cause the symptoms of the *enteric phase*.

   After 5–7 days the worms mature and the female discharge larvae to the tissues, causing symptoms of the *migratory* or *invasive* stage. Later the larvae encyst, causing symptoms of the *encystment* stage. Larvae only encyst in striated muscle but travel through the brain and heart muscle, where they are unable to encyst.

Striated muscle

Larvae, after travelling through the circulation, encyst in muscles of the diaphragm, masseters, intercostals, laryngeal, tongue and ocular muscles. At first there is a basophilic degeneration of the muscle fibres followed by formation of a hyaline capsule around the larva with an inflammatory infiltrate of lymphocytes and a few enosinophils (Figure 83.19). Foreign body giant cells may be present. The infiltrate subsides and fat is deposited at the poles and after 6 months calcification takes place, eventually leading to death of the larva.

Brain

Larvae migrate through the brain and meninges causing leptomeningitis, granulomatous nodules in the basal ganglia, medulla and cerebellum and perivascular cuffing in the cortex. They can be found in the cerebrospinal fluid with a raised cell count and increased protein.

Heart

The larvae cause considerable damage on passage through the myocardium, cellular infiltration and necrosis with subsequent fibrosis of the myocardial bundles.

Immunity

Natural immunity

Natural immunity is confined to cold-blooded animals with a temperature below 37°C.

Acquired immunity

A well-marked immunity to reinfection develops after the first infection but it is necessary for the infective larvae to develop through to the adult stage before immunity is produced, which is both antiadult and antilarval. Cell-mediated immunity is largely responsible but humoral antibodies develop. Immunized mice respond rapidly to challenge infections with an inflammatory reaction in the bowel and the elimination of adult worms. Cellular immunity can be transferred by cellular elements and diminished by corticosteroids, adrenalectomy and whole body irradiation.

A Type I hypersensitivity reaction is responsible for most of the pathology of the migratory or invasive phase, fever, oedema, rash, hypereosinophilia and tissue damage. Immune complexes are apparently not important. Humoral antibodies develop and are used in diagnosis. Cellular immunity is responsible for sealing off the cysts during the stage of encystment. Both immediate and delayed hypersensitivity can be demonstrated by skin tests.

Clinical features

Natural history

Trichinosis is a self-limiting infection lasting in light infections 2–3 weeks and in heavy ones at the most 2–3 months. Except in heavy infections mortality is low. Light infections are often asymptomatic and routine examination of diaphragms at autopsy have shown a significant number containing calcified cysts in endemic areas.

Incubation period

From eating infected meat the development of symptoms during the enteric phase is up to 7 days after infection and for the migratory phase from 7 to 21 days.

Symptoms and signs

The symptomatology depends on the level of infection and can be related to the number of larvae per gram of muscle: light infections (subclinical) up to 10 larvae, moderate 50 to 500 larvae and severe and possibly fatal infections more than 1000. In symptomatic cases symptoms develop in three stages: enteric (invasion of the intestine) phase, migration of the larvae (invasive phase) and a period of encystation in the muscles.

Enteric phase

Irritation and inflammation of the duodenum and jejunum where the larvae penetrate cause nausea, vomiting, colic and sweating, resembling an attack of acute food poisoning. There may be a maculopapular skin rash, and in a third of cases symptoms of a pneumonitis occur between the second and sixth day, lasting about 5 days.

Migratory (invasion) phase

The cardinal symptoms and signs of this phase are severe myalgia, periorbital oedema and eosinophilia. There is difficulty in mastication, breathing and swallowing due to the involvement of the muscles and there may be some muscular paralysis of the extremities. There is a high remittent fever with typhoidal symptoms, splinter haemorrhages under the nails and in the conjunctivae and blood and albumin in the urine. Characteristically there is a hypereosinophilia from the 14th day which decreases after a week and persists at a lower level. An absence of eosinophilia denotes a poor prognosis. The lymph glands may be enlarged as well as the parotid and submental glands. Occasionally there is splenomegaly. In severe cases there may be subpleural, gastric and intestinal haemorrhages.

Myocardial complications[115]

Myocardial complications are lower than previously reported but they may lead to congestive heart failure 4–8 weeks after infection; between the second and fifth week sudden death from dysrhythmia or congestive heart failure with peripheral oedema may occur. Pericardial effusion is the most common manifestation. Most cases recover completely but a few continue with chronic cardiac disability.

Neurological complications[116]

These may occur in about 10–20% of patients. During the passage of larvae through the central nervous system symptoms of meningitis, meningoencephalitis and focal cerebral lesions may develop. Ocular disturbances, diplegia, deafness and a syndrome resembling motor neurone disease, epileptiform attacks and coma may occur in very heavy infections.

Encystment phase

This is the third stage and may be severe. There may be cachexia, oedema and extreme dehydration. During the second month after infection there is a decrease in muscle tenderness, fever and itching subside and congestive heart failure may appear. Damage to the brain may persist with protean neurological signs which may clear up later or persist. Gram-negative septicaemia from organisms introduced by the larvae, permanent hemiplegia and Jacksonian epilepsy 10 years after an attack of trichinosis have been described.

Prognosis

Death is unusual except in cases of heart failure when it occurs during the sixth and seventh week from exhaustion, heart failure, pneumonitis, peritonitis or nephritis. Persistent leakage of larval antigen leads to a continued low eosinophilia and circulating antibody with positive serology and immediate and delayed hypersensitivity.

Differential diagnosis

Trichinosis resembles many conditions: typhoid,

encephalitis, myositis and tetanus; due to the association with a high eosinophilia it closely resembles the tissue stages of schistosomiasis (Katayama syndrome), hookworm, *Strongyloides* and other helminthic infections. Trichinosis may also resemble collagen disorders such as periarteritis nodosa and acute rheumatoid arthritis.

Diagnosis

Diagnosis is made by demonstrating larvae, by immunological and molecular methods.

Demonstration of larvae

Larvae have been isolated from peripheral blood in the early stages of the migration phase by mixing blood with dilute acetic acid and centrifuging. Larvae may be demonstrated in muscle by trichinoscopy.

Trichinoscopy

This can only be used when the encystment phase has started from 7 days after infection onwards. Samples (1 cm^2) of deltoid, biceps, gastrocnemius or pectoralis major are digested with 1% pepsin and 1% hydrochloric acid for several hours at 37°C, filtered or centrifuged and the number of larvae per gram of muscle estimated. Larvae can also be seen on muscle pressed between two slides, which is more useful in the first 3 weeks of the disease.

Xenodiagnosis can be performed by feeding diaphragmatic tissue to uninfected albino white rats and examining them 1 month later.

The following immunological and antigen detection tests have been used: indirect immunofluoresence (IIF); an enzymatic immunohistochemical technique (EIT); colorimetric sandwich ELISA; microfluorescence (ELFA); enhanced chemiluminescence (ECIA); dissociated enhanced lanthemide fluoroimmunoassay (DELFIA); Western blot test. DELFIA is the most sensitive for detecting antigen.[117–119]

Management

Treatment is directed against the larvae and the immune reaction they invoke.

Larvicidal

Mebendazole

Ten days of oral mebendazole (200 mg twice a day) or thiabendazole 25 m/kg twice a day for 10 days are both effective, although the former is better tolerated by patients.[120]

Immunosuppression

In severe life-threatening infections the immune response must be controlled, and prednisone 20 mg three times daily is given, initially reducing and finally discontinuing over a period of 2–3 weeks. Some cases are resistant to prednisone. Old calcified larvae do not need treatment.

Epidemiology (Figure 83.20)

Man is not the normal host of *T. spiralis* and becomes infected only after eating raw or undercooked flesh. The usual type, *T. s. spiralis*, found in Europe and North America, is an infection of the black and brown rats by which it is propagated. These rats are cannibalistic and may be eaten by domestic pigs which infect man when raw or undercooked pork is eaten. This type is common wherever uncooked sausage is eaten, especially in Germany and other areas of the world to which Germans have travelled, for example, North America and Chile.

Clinical illness is most likely to occur when sausage prepared from a single heavily infected pig is eaten by a family or community. Where the meat has been diluted by uninfected meat then the disease is mild or subclinical. In the USA two outbreaks occurred in 1956 and one in 1957 and a severe epidemic occurred in England in Liverpool in 1953. Under the conditions developed by man for raising and fattening pigs, garbage which contains unsterilized pig scraps and other trimmings is the most common source of infection in pigs in the USA at

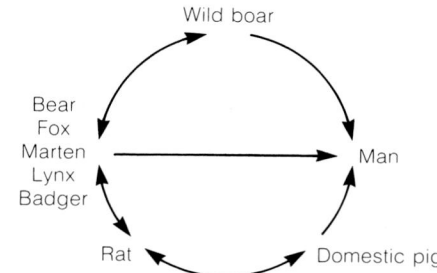

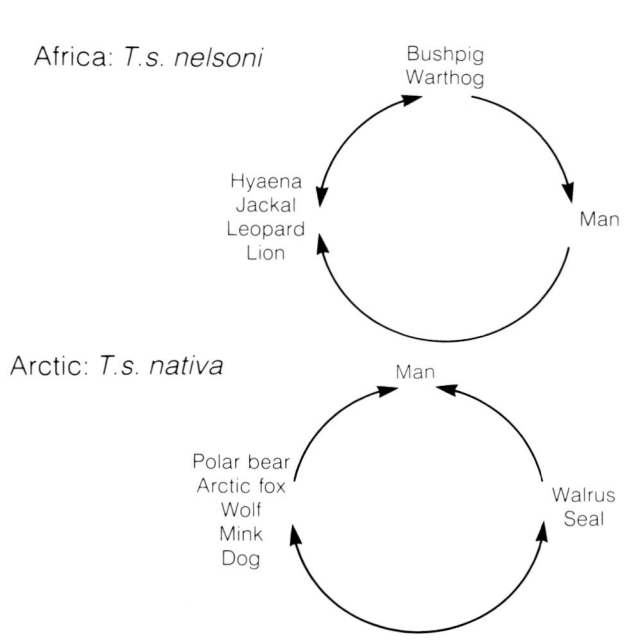

Figure 83.20: Epidemiology of *T. spiralis*.

the present time. Another possible source is the ingestion of faeces of other infected animals, mice, rats, foxes and other pigs at a time when mature larvae are becoming established in the intestinal wall. The majority of infections are symptomless and Link[121] has estimated 350 000 new infections in the USA annually, of which only 16 000 produced symptoms. It is estimated that subclinical trichinosis can be demonstrated in 20% of the population in the USA and 1% in England by digestion of material obtained at autopsy.

T. s. nativa is found mainly in Alaska and the northern regions of the world. Here trichinosis is found in the white whale, walrus, hair seal, tree squirrel, black and white polar bear, dog, wolf, fox and wolverine. The polar bear, which is at the top of the Arctic food pyramid, is usually heavily infected and is the usual source, along with black and brown bear, of human infections. Bear meat is eaten as a luxury and as an essential food in polar regions and whole expeditions have died of trichinosis after eating polar bear meat. Two epidemics have been reported from Alaska as a result of the consumption of black bear meat. In 1947 an epidemic occurred in Greenland with 300 cases and 33 deaths caused by eating walrus meat.

T. s. nelsoni is found in Africa south of the Sahara, where it has been described from East Africa[122] and Senegal.

The infection is found in bush pigs (*Potamochoerus porcus*) and in the lion, leopard, cheetah and hyena. Man is infected by eating bush pig; domestic pigs are not infected.

One of the most extensive, single-source outbreaks ever recorded in China, involving more than 600 infections and over 300 clinical cases, was reported in 1997. The entire episode was attributed to the infection of undercooked pork dumplings at one restaurant.[123] An exhaustive review on trichinellosis has been been published.[124]

Prevention

The main method of prevention is thorough cooking of all meat and regular meat inspection by means of trichinoscopy of all pork. Effective treatment of pork may be instituted by means of refrigeration. Storage of pork in deep freeze units at –18°C to –15°C is effective. The cysts are destroyed by storage at –15°C for 20 days, –20°C for 10 days, –25°C for 6 days and immediately by quick freezing at –37°C.

Cooking of all garbage will prevent the infection in pigs and dressed pork may be irradiated by cobalt-60 or caesium-137, which kills the cysts. In the Arctic and sub-Arctic regions bear meat should be avoided.

REFERENCES

1 Macedo T & MacCarty R L. Eosinophilic ileocolitis secondary to *Enterobius vermicularis*: case report. *Abdominal Imaging* 2000; 25:530–532.

2 Montresor et al. Guidelines of the evaluation of soil-transmitted helminthiasis and schistosomiasis at community level. *WHO/CDS/SIP/98.1.*

3 Jung R & Beaver P C. Clinical observations on *Trichocephalus trichuris* (whipworm) infestation in children. *Pediatrics* 1952; 8:548–557.

4 Cooper E S, Ramdath D D, Whyte-Alleng C, Howell S & Serjent B E. Plasma proteins in children with trichuris dysentery. *J Clin Pathol* 1997; 50:236–240.

5 Duff E M, Anderson N M & Cooper E S. Plasma insulin-like growth factor-1, type 1 procollagen, and serum tumour necrosis factor alpha in children recovering from *Trichuris* dysentery syndrome. *Paediatrics* 1999; 103:69.

6 Bundy D A P. The global burden of intestinal nematode disease. *Trans R Soc Trop Med Hyg* 1994; 88:259–261.

7 Callender J et al. Development levels and nutritional status of children with the *Trichuris trichiura* dysentery syndrome. *Trans R Soc Trop Med Hyg* 1993; 87:528–529.

8 Ismail M M & Jayakody R L. Efficacy of albendazole and its combinations with ivermectin or diethylcarbamazine (DEC) in the treatment of Trichuris trichiura infections in Sri Lanka, *Ann Trop Med Parasitol* 1999; 93:501–504.

9 Löffler P. Transient lung infiltrations with blood eosinophilia. *Arch Int Allergy* 1956; 8:54–59.

10 Louw J H. Biliary ascariasis in childhood. *S Afr J Surg* 1974; 4:219–225.

11 Khari A et al. Sonographic diagnosis of intestinal ascariasis. *Tropical Doctor* 1998; 28:117–118.

12 NgKK Wong et al. Biliary ascariasis: CT, MR cholangiopancreatography, and navigator endoscopic appearance: report of a case of acute biliary obstruction. *Abdominal Imaging* 1999; 24:470–472.

13 Beckingham I J et al. Management of hepatobiliary and pancreatic ascaris infection in adults after failed medical treatments. *Br J Surg* 1998; 85:907–910.

14 Venkatachalam P S & Patwardhan V N. The role of *Ascaris lumbricoides* in the nutrition of the host: effect of ascariasis on digestion of protein. *Trans R Soc Trop Med Hyg* 1976; 47:169–176.

15 Jalal F et al. Serum retinal concentrations in children are affected by food sources of beta-carotene, fat intake and anthelmintic drug treatment. *Am J Clin Nutr* 1998; 68:623–629.

16 Stephenson L S, Crompton D W T, Latham M C et al. Relationship between *Ascaris* infection and growth of malnourished pre-school children in Kenya. *Am J Clin Nutr* 1980;33:1165–1172.

17 Thein-Hlaing, Thane-Toe, Than-Saw & Myint-Luin. A controlled chemotherapeutic intervention trial on the relationship between *Ascaris lumbricoides* infection and malnutrition in children. *Trans R Soc Med Hyg* 1991; 85:523–528.

18 Hadidjaja P et al. The effect of intervention methods on nutritional status and cognitive function of primary school children infected with Ascaris. *Am J Trop Med Hyg* 1998; 59:791–795.

19 Stettler N, Schultz Y & Jequier E. Effect of low-level pathogenic helminth infection on energy metabolism in Gambian children. *Am J Trop Med Hyg* 1998; 58:476–479.

20 Gelpi A P & Mustafa A. Seasonal pneumonitis with eosinophilia: a study of larval ascariasis in Saudi Arabia. *Am J Trop Med Hyg* 1967; 16:646–657.

21 Wasadiker P P & Kulkarni A B. Intestinal obstruction due to ascariasis. *Br J Surg* 1997; 84:410–412.

22 Pawlowski Z S. Ascaris. In Pawlowski Z S (ed.) *Intestinal Helminthic Infections*, vol. 12, no. 3. London: Baillière Tindall, 1987: 595–615.

23 Crompton D W T & Pawlowski Z S. Life history and development of *Ascaris lumbricoides* and the persistence of human ascariasis. In Crompton D W T, Neisheim M C & Pawlowski Z S (eds) *Ascariasis and its Public Health Significance*. London: Taylor & Francis, 1985: 9–23.

24 Croll N A & Ghadirian E. Wormy persons: contributions to the nature and patterns of overdispersion with *Ascaris lumbricoides, Ancylostoma duodenale, Necator americanus* and *Trichuris trichiura*. *Trop Geogr Med* 1981; 33:241–248.

25 Anderson R M & Schad G A. Hookworm burdens and faecal egg counts: an analysis of the biological basis of variation. *Trans R Soc Trop Med Hyh* 1985; 79:812–825.

26 Schad G A & Anderson R M. Predisposition of hookworm infection in humans. *Science* 1985; 228:1537–1540.

27 Bradley M, Chandiwana S K, Bundy D A P & Medley G F. The epidemiology and population biology of *Necator americanus* infection in a rural community in Zimbabwe. *Trans R Soc Trop Med Hyg* 1992; 86:73–76.

28 Wakelin D. Genetics, immunity and parasitic survival. In Rollinson D & Anderson A M (eds) *Ecology and Genetic of Host–Parasite Interactions*. London: Academic Press, 1985: 39–54.

29 Chan L, Bundy D A P & Kan S P. Aggregation and predisposition to *Ascaris lumbricoides* and *Trichuris trichiura* at the familial level. *Trans R Soc Trop Med Hyg* 1994; 88:46–48.

30 Chan L, Kan S P & Bundy D A P. The effect of repeated chemotherapy on age-related predisposition to *Ascaris lumbricoides* and *Tichuris trichiura*. *Parasitology* 1992; 38:323–326.

31 Anderson R M & May R . *Helminth* infections in humans: mathematical models, population dynamics and control. *Adv Parasitol* 1985; 24:1–101.

32 Thein-Hlaing, Than-Saw & Myat-Lay-Kyin. The impact of three monthly age-targeted chemotherapy on *Ascaris lumbricoides* infection. *Trans R Soc Trop Med Hyg* 1991; 85:519–522.

33 Linillater J M et al. Absorption of carbohydrate from rice in *Ascaris lumbricoides* infected Burmese village children. *J Trop Paediatr* 1992; 38:323–326.

34 Theine-Hlaing et al. A controlled chemotherapeutic intervention trial on the relationship between *Ascaris lumbricoides* infection and malnutrition in children. *Trans R Soc Trop Hyg* 1991; 85:523–528.

35 Medley G, Gayeth A L & Bundy D A P. A quantitative framework for evaluating the effect of community treatment on the morbidity due to ascariasis. *Parasitology* 1993; 106:211–221.

36 Crompton D W T. Ascariasis and childhood malnutrition. *Trans R Soc Trop Med Hyg* 1992; 86:577–579.

37 Hall A. Intestinal parasitic worms and the growth of children. *Trans R Soc Trop Med Hyg* 1993; 87:241–242.

38 Thein H Laing. The effect of targeted chemotherapy against ascariasis on the height of children in rural Myanmar. *Trans R Soc Trop Med Hyg* 1994; 88:433.

39 Brophy P M & Pritchard D I. Immunity to helminths: ready to tip the biochemical balance? *Parasite Immunol* 1992; 8:419–422.

40 Woodhouse M E J. A theoretical framework for the immunoepidemiology of helminth infection. *Parasite Immunology* 1992; 14:563–578.

41 Bundy D A P. Immunoepidemiology of intestinal helminthic infections. 1. The global burden of intestinal nematode disease. *Trans R Soc Trop Med Hyg* 1994; 88:259–261.

42 Needham C S & Lillywhite J. E. Immunoepidemiology of intestinal helminthic infections. 2. Immunological correlates with patterns of *Trichuris* infection. *Trans R Soc Trop Med Hyh* 1994; 88:262–264.

43 MacDonald T T et al. Immunoepidemiology of intestinal helminthic infections. 3. Mucosal monophases and cybolline production in the colon of children with *Trichuris trichiura* dysentery. *Trans R Soc Trop Med Hyg* 1994; 88:265.

44 Beaver P C, Synder C H, Carrera G M et al. Chronic eosinophilia due to visceral larva migrans: report of 3 cases. *Pediatrics* 1952; 9:7–19.

45 Wilder H C. Nematode endophthalmitis. *Trans Am Acad Ophthalmol* 1950; 55:99–109.

46 Ree G H, Voller A & Rowland H A K. Toxocariasis in the British Isles 1982–3. *BMJ* 1984; 288:628–629.

47 Overgaauw P A. Aspects of Toxocara epidemiology: human toxocariasis. *Crit Rev Microbiol* 1997; 23:215–231.

48 Beaver P C. The nature of visceral larva migrans. *J Parasitol* 1969; 55:3–12.

49 Lamparielle D A & Primo S A. Ocular toxocariasis. *J Am Optometric Assoc* 1999; 70:245–252.

50 Gonzalez M T et al. Toxocariasis with liver involvement. *Acta Gastroenterol Latinoam* 2000; 30(3):187–190.

51 Savigny D H, Voller A & Woodruff A W. Toxocariasis: serological diagnosis by enzyme immunoassay. *J Clin Pathol* 1979; 32:284–288.

52 Glickman L T, Schanz P M, Dombroske R et al. Evaluation of serodiagnostic tests for visceral larva migrans. *Am J Trop Med Hyg* 1978; 27:492–498.

53 Brunello F, Genchi C & Falangiani P. Detection of larva-specific IgE in human toxocariasis.*Trans R Soc Trop Med Hyg* 1983; 77:279–280.

54 Nunes C M et al. Toxocariasis: serological diagnosis by indirect antibody competition ELISA. *Rev Inst Med Trop Sao Paulo* 1999; 41:95–100.

55 Viera M A et al. Treatment of human lagochilascariasis with ivermectin: first case report from Ecuador. *Trans R Soc Trop Med Hyg* 1998; 92:223–224.

56 Schad G A, Chowdhury A B, Dean C G et al. Arrested development in human hookworm infections: an adaptation to a seasonally unfavourable external environment. *Science* 1973; 180:52–54.

57 Roche H & Layrisse M. The nature and causes of 'hookworm anaemia'. *Am J Trop Med Hyg* 1966; 15:1031–1102.

58 Pritchard D I, Quinnell R J, Mousafa M et al. Hookworm (*Necator americanus*) infection and storage iron depletion. *Trans R Soc Trop Med Hygi* 1991; 85:235–238.

59 Gilles H M, Watson-Williams E J & Ball P A J. Hookworm infection and anaemia: an epidemiological, clinical and laboratory study. *Q J Med* 1964; 331:1–24.

60 Brooker S et al. The epidemiology of hookworm infection and its contribution to anaemia among pre-school children on the Kenyan coast. *Trans R Soc Trop Med Hyg.* 1999; 93:240–246.

61 Stoltzfus R J et al. Epidemiology of iron deficiency anaemia in Zanzibari schoolchildren: the importance of hookworms. *Am J Clin Nutr* 1997; 65(1):153–159.

62 Burman N N, Sehgal A K, Chakravarti R N et al. Morphological and absorption studies of small intestine in hookworm infestation (ankylostomiasis). *Indian J Med Res* 1970; 58:317–325.

63 Carroll S M & Grove D I. Resistance of dogs to reinfection with *Ancylostoma ceylanicum* following anthelmintic therapy. *Trans R Soc Trop Med Hyg* 1985; 79:519–523.

64 Behnke J M. Immunology. In Gilles H M & Ball P A J (eds) *Hookworm Infections*. Amsterdam: Elsevier, 1991: 93–155.

65 Wang Chang-i. Parasitic diarrhoeas in China. *Parasitol Today* 1988; 10:284–287.

66 Cline B L, Little M D, Bartholomew R K et al. Larvicidal activity of albendazole against *Necator americanus* in human volunteers. *Am J Trop Med Hyg* 1984; 33:387–394.

67 Reynoldson J A et al. Failure of pyrantel in treatment of human hookworm infections (Ancylostoma duodenale) in

the Kimberley region of north west Australia. *Acta Trop* 1997; 68:301–312.

68 Caumes E. Treatment of cutaneous larva migrans. *Clin Infect Dis* 2000; 30: 811–814.

69 Veraldi S & Rizzitelli G. Effectiveness of a new therapeutic regimen with albendazole in cutaneous larva migrans. *Eur J Dermatol* 1999; 9:352–353.

70 Tremblay A et al. Outbreak of cutaneous larva migrans in a group of travelers. *Trop Med Int Health* 2000; 5:330–334.

71 Wong T Y et al. Nephrotic syndrome in strongyloidiasis: remission after eradication with anthelmintic agents. *Nephron* 1998; 79(3):333–336.

72 Cook G C. *Strongyloides stercoralis* hyperinfection syndrome: how often is it missed? *Q J Med* 1987; 64:625–629.

73 Genta R M. Global prevalence of strongyloidiasis: critical review with epidemiologic insights into the prevention of disseminated disease. *Rev Infect Dis* 1989; 11:755–767.

74 Wehner J H & Kirsch C M. Pulmonary manifestations of strongyloidiasis. *Semin Respir Infect* 1997; 12:122–129.

75 Koga K, Kasura S, Khamboomuang C et al. A modified agar plate method for detection of *Strongyloides stercoralis*. *Am J Trop Med Hyg* 1991; 45:518–521.

76 Louisey C L & Barton C J. The radiological diagnosis of *Strongyloides stercoralis* enteritis. *Radiology* 1971; 98:535–541.

77 Convey et al. Serum IgG reactivity with 41-, 31- and 28-kDa larval proteins of *Strongyloides stercoralis* in individuals with strongyloides. *J Infect Dis* 1993; 168:784–787.

78 Girud de Kaminsky R. Evaluation of three methods for laboratory diagnosis of *Strongyloides stercoralis* infection. *J Parasitol* 1993; 79:277–280.

79 Gill G V & Bell D R. *Strongyloides stercoralis* infection in former Far East prisoners of war. *BMJ* 1979; ii:572–574.

80 Conway D J et al. Towards effective control of *Strongyloides stercoralis*. *Parasitol Today* 1995; 11:420–423.

81 Sato Y, Toma H, Kiyuna S & Shiroma Y. Gelatin particle indirect agglutination test for mass examination for strongyloidiasis. *Trans R Soc Trop Med Hyg* 1991; 85:515–518.

82 Ramachandran S et al. Recombinant cDNA clones for immunodiagnosis of strongyloidiasis. *J Infect Dis* 1998; 177(1):196–203.

83 Hiromu Toma et al. Comparative studies on the efficacy of 3 anthelminthics on treatment of human strongyloides in Okinawa, Japan. *SE Asian J Trop Med Hyg* 2000; 31:147–151.

84 Pampiglione S & Riccardi M. The presence of *Strongyloides fülleborni* von Linstow, 1905 in man in Central and East Africa. *Parassitologia* 1971; 13:257–269.

85 Ashford R W, Barnish G & Viney M E. *Strongyloides fülleborni Kellyi*: infection and disease in Papua New Guinea. *Parasitol Today* 1992; 8:314–318.

86 WHO. Bench aids for the diagnosis of intestinal parasites. Geneva: *World Health Organization*, 1994.

87 Monti J R et al. Specific amplification of Necator americanus or Ancylostoma duodenale DNA by PCR using markers in ITS-1 rDNA, and its implications. *Mol Cell Probes* 1998; 12:71–78.

88 Sharma B C et al. Diagnostic value of push-type enteroscopy: a report from India. *Am J Gastroenterol* 2000; 95:137–140.

89 Sarinas P S & Chilkara R K. Ascaris and Hookworm. *Semin Respir Infect* 1997; 12:130–137.

90 Forrester J E et al. Randomised trial of albendazole and pyrantel in symptomless trichuriasis in children. *Lancet* 1998; 352:1103–1108.

91 Simeon D T et al. Treatment of Trichuris trichiura infections improves growth, spelling scores and school attendance in children. *J Nutr* 1999; 125:1875–1883.

92 Furnee C A et al. Effect of intestinal parasite treatment on the efficacy of oral iodized oil for correcting iodine deficiency in schoolchildren. *Am J Clin Nutr* 1997; 66:1422–1427.

93 Albonico M & Savioli L. Hookworm infection and disease: advances for control. *Ann Inst Sup Sanita* 1997; 33: 567–679.

94 Albonico M et al. A controlled evaluation of two school-based anthelminthic chemotherapy regimens on intensity of intestinal helminth infections. *Int J Epidemiol* 1999; 28(3):591–596.

95 Olsen A. The proportion of helminth infections in a community in Western Kenya which would be treated by mass chemotherapy of school children. *Trans R Soc Trop Med Hyg* 1998; 92:144–148.

96 Ananthakrishnan S, Nalini P & Pani S P. Intestinal geohelminthiasis in the developing world. *Nat Med J India* 1997; 10:67–71.

97 Albonico M, Crompton D W & Savioli L. Control strategies for human intestinal neomatode infections. *Adv Parasitol* 1999; 42:277–341.

98 Booth M, Mayombana C & Kilima P. The population biology and epidemiology of schistosome and geohelminth infections among schoolchildren in Tanzania. *Trans R Soc Trop Med Hyg* 1998; 92:491–495.

99 Needham C et al. Epidemiology of soil-transmitted nematode infections in Ha Nam Province, Vietnam. *Trop Med Int Health* 1998; 3:904–912.

100 Bundy D A P, Chandiwana S K, Homeida M M A et al. The epidemiology implications of a multiple-infection approach to the control of human helminth infections. *Trans R Soc Trop Med Hyg* 1991; 85:274–276.

101 WHO. Report of WHO informal consultation on monitoring drug efficacy in the control of schistosomiasis and intestinal nematodes. *WHO/CPC/SIP/1.1*

102 Satoh M et al. Production of a high level of specific IgG4 antibody associated with resistance to abendazole treatment in HLA-DRB1*0901-positive patients with strongyloidiasis. *Am J Trop Med Hyg* 1999; 61:668–671.

103 Declerq D et al. Failure of mebendazole in treatment of human hookworm infections in Mali. *Am J Trop Med Hyg* 1997; 57:25–30.

104 Reynoldson J A et al. Failure of pyrantel in treatment of *Ancylostoma duodenale* in North West Australia. *Acta Trop* 1997; 68:301–312.

105 Bradley M, Chandivana S K & Bundy D A P. The epidemiology and control of hookworm infection in the Burma Valley area of Zimbabwe. *Trans R Soc Trop Med Hyg* 1993; 87:145–147.

106 Montresor et al. Guidelines for the evaluation of soil-transmitted helminthiasis at community level. *WHO/CIDS/SIP/98.1*.

107 Bundy D A P, Wong M S, Louis L L & Horton J. Control of geohelminths by delivery of targeted chemotherapy through schools. *Trans R Soc Trop Med Hyg* 1990; 84:115–120.

108 Thomson R C A et al. Towards the eradication of hookworm in an isolated Australian community. *Lancet* 2001; 357:770–771.

109 James D B & Gilles M. *Human Antiparasitic Drugs: Pharmacology and Usage*. Chichester: Wiley, 1985.

110 Georgie V S. Parasitic infections: treatment and developmental therapeutics 1. Necatoriasis. *Curr Pharm Design* 1999; 5:545–554.

111 Romero Cabello R et al. Nitazoxanide for the treatment of intestinal protozoan and helminthic infections in Mexico. *Trans R Soc Trop Med Hyh* 1997; 91:701–703.

112 Brockhuysen J et al. Nitazoxanide pharmacokinetics and metabolism in man. *Int J Clin Pharmacol Ther* 2000; 38:387–394.

113 Jongwutiwes S et al. First outbreak of human trichinellosis caused by Trichinella pseudospiralis. *Clin Infect Dis* 1998; 26:111–115.

114 Kapel C M. Trichinella in arctic, subarctic and temperate regions: Greenland, the Scandinavian countries and the Baltic States. *SE Asian J Trop Med Public Health* 1997, 28(suppl. 1):14–19.

115 Lazarevic A M et al. Low incidence of cardiac abnormalities in treated trichinosis: a prospective study of 62 patients from a single outbreak. *Am J Med* 1999; 107:18–23.

116 Nikolic S et al. Neurologic manifestations in trichinosis. *Srpski Arhiv Za Celokupno Lekarstvo* 1998; 126:209–213.

117 Ben G J M et al. Evaluation of an enzymatic immunohistochemical technique in human trichinellosis. *J Helminthol* 1997; 71:299–303.

118 Ko R C. A brief update on the diagnosis of trichinellosis. *SE Asian J Trop Med Public Health* 1997; 28(suppl. 1):91–98.

119 Rodriguez-Osorio M et al. Human trichinellosis in Southern Spain: serologic and epidemiologic study. *Am J Trop Med Hyg* 1999; 61:834–837.

120 Watt G et al. Blinded, placebo-controlled trial of antiparasitic drugs for trichinosis myositis. *J Infect Dis* 2000; 182:371–374.

121 Link V B. Trichinosis: a health and economic problem. *Public Health Rep Wash* 1953; 68:417–418.

122 Forrester A T T, Nelson G S & Sander G. The first record of an outbreak of trichinosis in Africa and south of the Sahara. *Trans R Soc Trop Med Hyg* 1961; 33:503–513.

123 Cui J et al. Epidemiological and clinical studies on an outbreak of trichinosis in central China. *Ann Trop Med Parasitol* 1997; 91:481–488.

124 Bruschi F & Pozio E. Trichinellosis approaching the year 2000. *Parassitologia*. 1997; 39:77–79.

Chapter 84
Echinococcosis/Hydatidosis

B. Gottstein and J. Reichen

Echinococcus species are cestode parasites commonly known as small tapeworms of carnivorous animals. The medical relevance lies in their infection of humans by predominantly two species. *Echinococcus granulosus* is the causative agent of cystic echinococcosis (CE), also called cystic hydatid disease; *Echinococcus multilocularis* causes alveolar echinococcosis (AE), also called alveolar hydatid disease. CE and AE differ pathologically and clinically so much that they will be considered separately in this chapter. Two other species, namely *E. vogeli* and

E. oligarthrus, are rarely found in humans and will thus only be covered as a small third section.

Cystic echinococcosis (*Echinococcus granulosus*)
Biology

E. granulosus is a small cestode tapeworm living firmly attached to the mucosa of the small intestine of predominantly dogs and other canids (Figure 84.1). Shedding of gravid proglottids or eggs in the faeces occurs within 4–5 weeks of prepatency. *E. granulosus* eggs are infective for intermediate hosts immediately after their

Figure 84.1: Life cycle of *Echinococcus granulosus*. Adult tapeworms parasitize in the small intestine of definitive hosts, mainly dogs (**1**). Parasite eggs (**2**) are shed with the faeces, being infectious for intermediate hosts including man (**3**) and predominantly ungulated animals. Hydatid cyst formation occurs predominantly in the liver (**4**), but also in lungs and other organs. Histologically, the cyst by itself consists of a very thin inner germinal layer, externally protected by an acellular laminated layer of variable thickness. The endogenous formation of brood capsules and protoscolices is a prerequisite for termination of the life cycle, which occurs when definitive hosts ingest protoscolex-containing hydatid cysts.

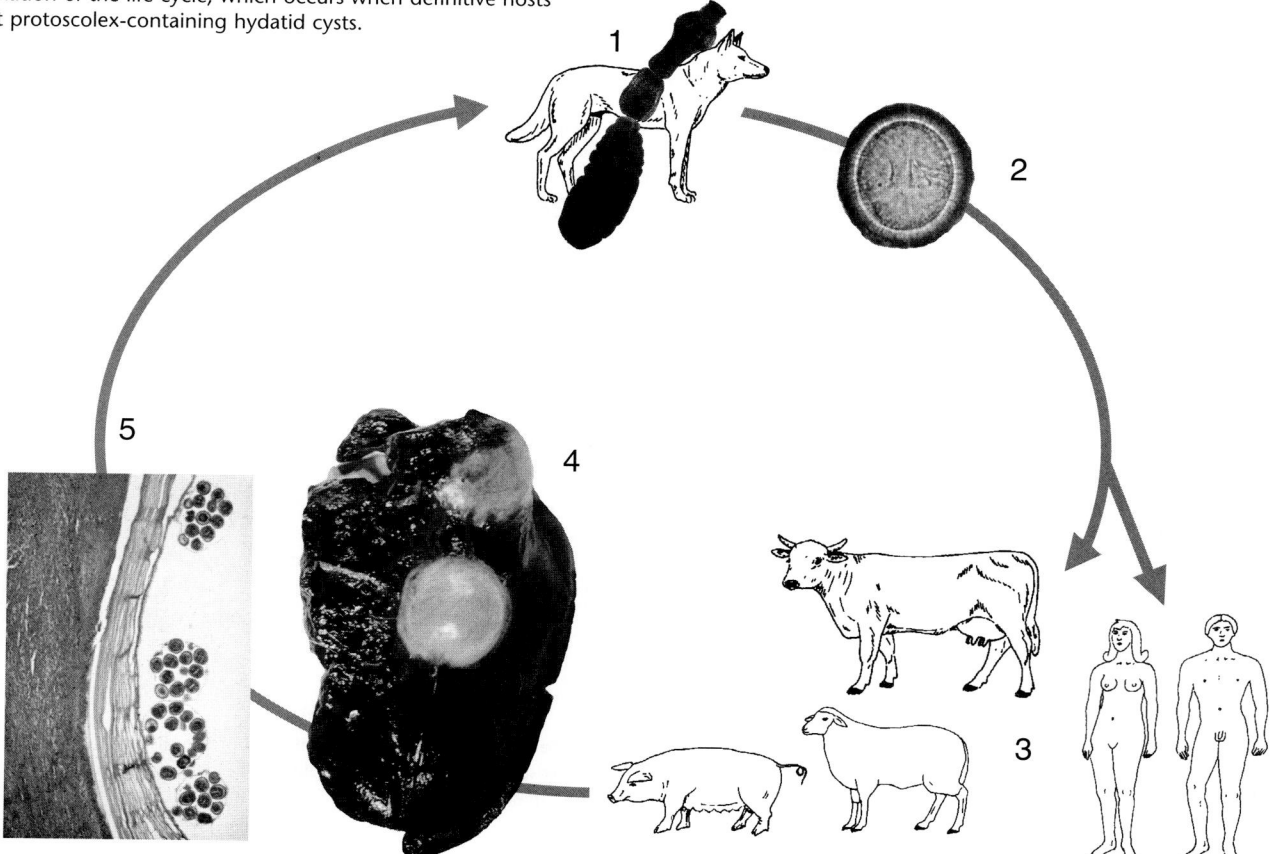

release into the surroundings. Ingestion of such *Echinococcus* eggs by susceptible intermediate animal hosts or humans results in the release of an early-stage larva, the oncosphere, into the intestinal tract. This oncosphere migrates through blood or lymph vessels to primary target organs such as liver and lungs. At this location the oncosphere matures into a vesicle, which grows expansively by concentric enlargement. The final result is a fully mature hydatid cyst, which is usually fluid filled and unilocular. The cyst consists of an inner germinal and nucleated syncytial layer supported externally by a carbohydrate-rich acellular laminated layer of variable thickness, surrounded by a host-produced fibrous adventitial layer. Occasionally, cysts may abut and coalesce, forming groups or clusters of cysts of variable size. In humans especially, where unusually large cysts may develop, daughter cysts can form within the primary cyst, including multiple, communicating chambers. The endogenous formation of brood capsules and protoscolices is a prerequisite for termination of the life cycle. Protoscolices will grow to the adult stage once ingested by a definitive host.

Distribution and epidemiology

Infections with *E. granulosus* occur worldwide; relevant public health problems focus predominantly on countries of South and Central America, the European and the African part of the Mediterranean area, the Middle East and some sub-Saharan countries, Russia and China. Annual incidence rates of diagnosed human cases per 100 000 inhabitants vary widely, e.g. 13 in Greece, 143 in some provinces of Argentina, 197 in the Hinjang province of China and 220 in the Turkana district of Kenya.[1] Most cases observed in Central Europe and the USA are related to immigration of persons from highly endemic areas. In a case–control study in a highly endemic area, risk was mainly conferred by the number of dogs and time of exposure in particular if the dogs were fed uncooked viscera.[2] Various strains of *E. granulosus* have been described so far, differing especially also in infectivity to humans. The most relevant for human infection are the sheep and the cattle strains. Another 'northern' strain, prevalent in northern parts of the North American continent and Eurasia (tundra and taiga areas), appears less virulent for humans. Epidemiologically relevant is the fact that there is no crowding effect or parasite-induced host mortality in animals, and the respective numerical distribution does not contribute to the regulation of either adult or larval parasite populations.

Measurement of the socio-economic impact of echinococcosis/hydatidosis represents an important challenge, which frequently becomes highly relevant for calculating the cost:benefit ratio of possible activities for the control or eradication of *Echinococcus* species. In humans, the quantifiable items are those connected with preoperative diagnosis, surgical treatment, hospitalization, postsurgical examination and drugs. In some countries the cost of hospitalization alone involves 45 patient-days, at an estimated cost of US $2000.[3,4] This is bound to increase in cases complicated by infection, rupture or unusual localizations or in patients with relapse. In such complicated cases—given that the site and treatment involved could mean the loss of an organ, cause irreversible sequelae or even threaten the life of the patient—the cost can be comparable with that of surgical treatment of cancer.[5] The convalescent period should also be considered as an economic loss in view of the well-documented fact that a high proportion of cases occur in actively working persons, which means that the contribution of their labour to the economy of their countries is lost.

Pathogenesis

CE is clinically related to the presence of a well-delineated spherical primary cysts, most frequently formed in the liver (60% of cases) and the lungs (20%) (Figure 84.2). Cysts at less usual localizations include the kidneys, bones, heart, spleen, pancreas, and organs of the head and neck including the brain. Pathogenetically, tissue damage and organ disfunction result mainly from this gradual process of space-occupying repression or displacement of vital host tissue or whole organs. The histology of a typical hydatid cyst, which can develop pressures of up to 80 cmH$_2$O,[6] demonstrates the germinal layer as primary site of parasite development, surrounded by a parasite-derived thick laminated layer strongly stainable with periodic acid–Schiff solution (PAS). The germinal layer forms protoscolices and brood capsules within the cyst lumen. Granulae, calcareous corpuscles and occasionally free daughter cysts are often observed. The parasite evokes an immune response which will be involved in the formation of a host-derived adventitious capsule, which often calcifies uniquely in the periphery

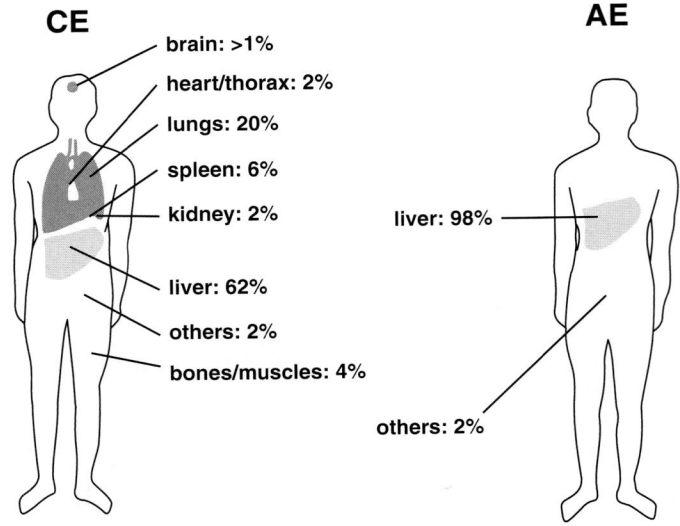

Figure 84.2: Schematic presentation of the distribution of *E. granulosus* (CE) and *E. multilocularis* (AE) cysts or metacestodes, respectively, as a percentage.

of the cyst as seen in imaging procedures. Cholestasis may be present in the liver. There is often pressure atrophy of the surrounding parenchyma. Accidental rupture of cysts can be followed by a massive release of cyst fluid and dissemination of protoscolices, resulting occasionally in anaphylactic reactions and in multiple secondary CE, as protoscolices have the potential to develop into secondary cysts within the intermediate host.

Immunology

The primary site of the host–parasite interaction is the host's gastrointestinal mucosa. Little information is available on the immune response in man against migrating and subsequently established oncospheres and their development to the hydatid cyst of *E. granulosus*. Diagnosis of CE is usually achieved at a stage where a fully developed and still proliferating hydatid cyst has already induced a respective immune response in the host.[7]

At an early stage of CE, the parasite activates complement and hence complement-dependent inflammatory responses. However, on differentiation into the hydatid cyst, the parasite exposes to the host its laminated layer, which does not activate complement strongly.[8] Mechanisms inhibiting complement activation on the cyst wall have been elucidated, contributing to the understanding of how the inflammatory response is controlled during CE. Basically, the host–parasite relationship is sustained as a dynamic equilibrium between parasite growth and acquired immunity, the balance being subject to mutual regulation and including the possibility of spontaneous rejection of the parasite.[9] Immunoregulatory events have been linked to the generation of T-suppressor populations and to impairing the accessory action of macrophages in lymphoproliferative responses. Local immune modulation by the parasite has been shown to enhance susceptibility to mycobacterial infections close to the site of parasite lesions.[10] The coexistence of elevated quantities of interferon γ (IFNγ), interleukin (IL)-4, IL-5, IL-6 and IL-10 observed in most of hydatid patients supports Th1 and Th2 cell activation in CE. In particular, Th1 cell activation seems to be more related to protective immunity, and Th2 cell activation to susceptibility to disease.[11]

Clinical features

The early phase following primary infection is always asymptomatic. Dependent upon the size and the site of the developing hydatid cyst, the infection can remain asymptomatic for months, years or even longer. After a highly variable incubation period, the infestation may become symptomatic owing to a range of different events:

(a) The growing cyst exerts pressure on or induces dysformation of adjacent tissues, thus inducing dysfunction of the affected organ or vascular compromise. In case of hepatic CE, signs and symptoms may include hepatomegaly with or without a palpable mass in the right upper quadrant, right epigastric pain, nausea, vomiting and occasionally cholestatic jaundice. In inoperable cases, hepatic compromise may lead to biliary cirrhosis and the Budd–Chiari syndrome.[12]

Infestation of the lungs may present with chronic cough, hemoptysis, bilioptysis, pneumothorax, pleuritis, lung abscess and parasitic lung embolism.

Rare but often catastrophic infestations can affect the heart or the brain. In the heart this can present as tumour, pericardial effusion up to tamponade,[13] complete heart block[14] and sudden death.[15]

In the spine and brain presentation is as a tumour with the respective neurological symptoms. Hydatid disease should be considered as a cause of stroke in young patients.[16]

(b) A cyst may rupture and spill its contents into the adjacent site. Rupture into the biliary tree will mimic biliary colic or result in cholestatic jaundice and cholangitis or pancreatitis. This is the presenting symptom in 5–25% of patients. Ruptures in the liver but also in the lungs and other organs may result in acute anaphylactic shock reactions, which usually represent the first initial and life-threatening manifestation.

(c) The cyst can become superinfected; in hepatic hydatid disease this occurs in about 9% of patients and is an indication for rapid surgical intervention.[17]

The majority of patients with CE have single organ involvement with solitary cysts (Figure 84.3). Simultaneous involvement of two or more organs is observed in 10–15% of patients, dependent on the geographical origin of the patient and the strain of the parasite. In hepatic CE, the right lobe is more frequently affected than the left lobe. Cyst size varies usually between 1 and 15 cm in diameter. Cyst growth ranges between a size increase of a few millimetres (one-third of patients) to approximately 10 mm (most patients); one-tenth of patients exhibit a rapid increase with an annual average of 30 mm. Approximately 10% of CE cases occur in children, and the rate of lung affection is significantly increased among this group of young patients. Pulmonary cysts are often infected and this is best detected by computed tomography (CT) scanning.[18] The ratio of males to females may vary dependent on the geographical area but is statistically not significant overall.

Clinical diagnosis

Symptoms are most often related to the expansive growth of the cysts. In most cases, imaging procedures together with serology will yield the diagnosis. Sonography is the diagnostic procedure of choice; however, false positives can occur in up to 10%, the main confusion arising in the differentiation between hydatid and benign congenital cysts.[19] Diagnostic features of hydatid disease include separation of the parasite germinal/laminated layer from the surrounding host capsule, daughter cysts and collapsed

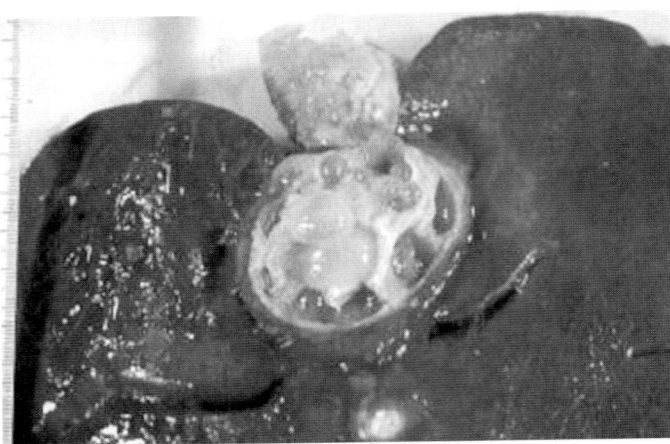
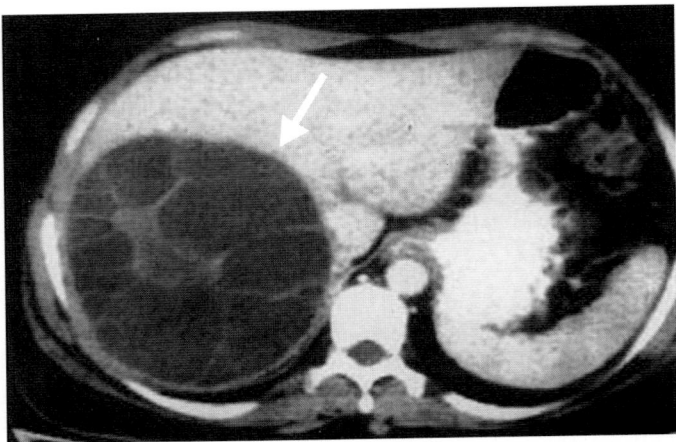

Figure 84.3: *Echinococcus granulosus* liver lesions. Left: macroscopical presentation of a cross-sectioned hepatic hydatid cyst; note the internal septation of the cyst, exhibiting multiple daughter cysts. Right: visualization of a similar lesion, marked with arrow, by CT. Note here again the septation of the hypodense hydatid lesion due to the presence of daughter cysts.

cysts.[19,20] In contrast, hydatid 'sand', often described as pathognomonic, can also be found in simple hepatic cysts.[19] An international classification system of ultrasonographic CE images has been elaborated for application in clinical and field epidemiological settings and will soon be published by the WHO. The recommendations basically refer to those published previously.[21,22] Briefly, group 1 includes various types of developing cysts and which are usually fertile; a transition group 2 includes cysts starting to degenerate, but usually still containing viable protoscoleces; group 3 includes inactive degenerated or totally calcified cysts, very unlikely to be fertile. CT, where available, is superior for the detection of extra-hepatic disease,[23] while nuclear magnetic resonance imaging (NMR) appears to add diagnostic benefit for cysts especially at difficult sites (such as spinal vertebrae, see Figure 84.4).

If a connection between the biliary system and the hydatid cyst is suspected, or even the complication of an intrabiliary hydatid cyst rupture, endoscopic retrograde cholangiopancreaticrography (ERCP) may provide useful respective information. Conversely, percutaneous transhepatic cholangiography is absolutely contraindicated, due to the potential anaphylactic shock upon cyst fluid leakage. Ultrasonography is very helpful in following treated patients, successfully treated cysts becoming

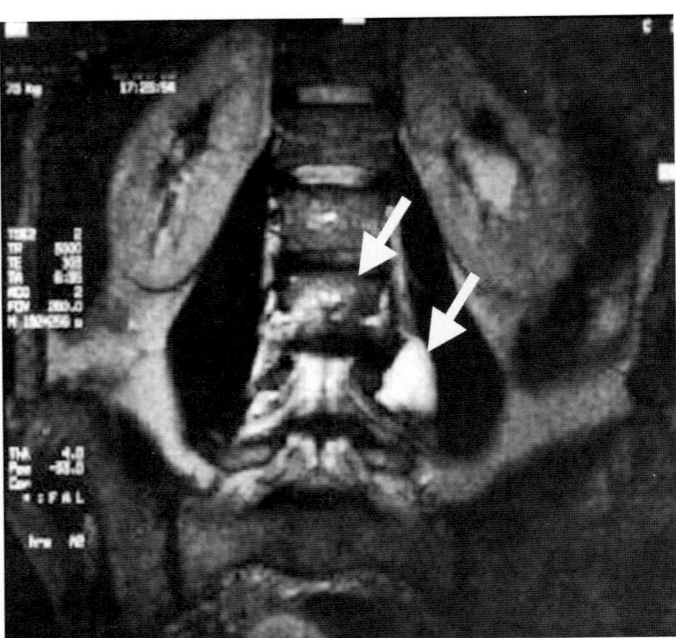
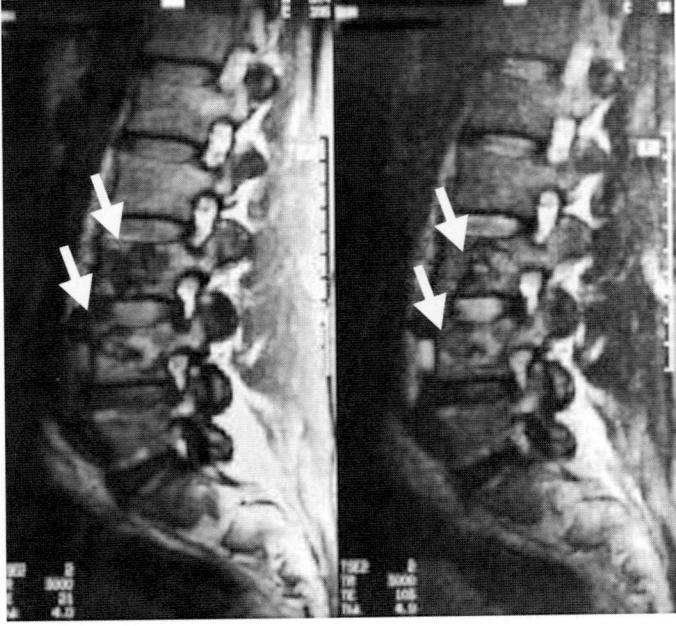

Figure 84.4: MRI of *E. granulosus* hydatid cysts located retroperitoneally, extending into the foramen intervertebrale and eroding the lateral vertebral wall L4. This patient had been surgically treated 3 years ago, and now presents a relapse of cyst growths, again surgically treated following MRI diagnosis.

hyperechogenic.[24] Calcification of variable degree in the peripheral cyst wall occurs in about 10% of cysts.

If aspiration cytology is performable, trichrome staining of the filtrated aspirate reveals the acid-fast hooklets.[25] Cytology appears particularly helpful in detecting pulmonary[26] and renal[27] involvement. Excretion of scolices into the urine is observed in 28% of cases with renal cysts.[28] Viability of aspirated protoscolices can be determined by microscopic demonstration of flame cell activity and Trypan Blue dye exclusion.

Immunodiagnosis will be considered in the next section. Otherwise, laboratory examinations are not particularly helpful in establishing the diagnosis, with the exception of determination of IgE and eosinophilia in cases of ruptured cysts presenting with allergic symptoms.

Serological and molecular diagnosis

Immunodiagnostic tests for the detection of serum antibodies or circulating antigens are used to support the clinical diagnosis of CE.[7] The indirect haemagglutination test (IHAT) and enzyme-linked immunosorbent assay (ELISA) using *E. granulosus* hydatid fluid antigen are diagnostically relatively sensitive for hepatic cases (85–98%). For pulmonary cyst localization the diagnostic sensitivity is markedly lower (50–60%), for multiple organ localization very high (90–100%). These tests are usually used for a primary serological screening. However, specificity of such tests is low with regard to other cestode infection and some other non-cestode helminthoses. In order to increase specificity, primary seropositive sera are retested in a confirmation test such as antigen 5 precipitation (arc-5 test) or immunoblotting for a relatively specific 8 kDa/12 kDa hydatid fluid polypeptide antigen.[29,30]

The demonstration of parasite-specific IgE has attracted particular attention owing to its well-known relevance in helminthic diseases[31,32] but has exhibited no significant immunodiagnostic advantage in CE. Beside problems of diagnostic sensitivity and specificity due to cross-reactions, there is accumulating evidence for false-positive antibody reactions not related to infections with heterologous helminth species, but to malignancies,[30,33,34] the presence of anti-P1 antibodies[35] and liver cirrhosis.[36]

With regard to the differential diagnosis between hepatic CE and cancer, immunoblotting has demonstrated the best respective performance so far.[30] One characteristic of CE serodiagnosis is the relatively high proportion of patients with undetectable antibody levels in their sera. Such patients were shown to produce no IL-5 and scarce IL-4 and IL-10 (Th2 type), conversely to seropositive CE patients.[37] The authors suggested that seronegativity arises because of an inadequate Th2 cell activation required for immunoglobulin expression in CE.

MAbs generated against different parasite antigens have been used for the diagnosis of CE by detection of circulating antigens in patients' sera or of native proteins in biopsies. Such MAbs have been mainly directed against two major *E. granulosus* antigens, named antigen 5 (Ag5) and antigen B (AgB).[38,39] Principally, detection of circulating antigens by the use of Mabs has been proposed as an early marker for hydatid infection, being also relevant as a method for postsurgical follow-up of patients, and to monitor the growth dynamics or/and activity of cysts.[39] Anti-Ag5 MAbs were also used for the detection of the respective antigen in diagnostic fine-needle aspiration biopsies (FNAB) from patients with suspected CE.[40]

In order to provide a practical overview and suggestions about the procedure of laboratory tests that can be used for the diagnosis and follow-up of human CE patients, we included respective recommendations in Box 84.1.

Early diagnosis of persons with asymptomatic echinococcosis is a prerequisite for efficient management of the disease. Consequently, screening may be offered to populations at risk. The currently optimal epidemiological tool to be used includes ultrasonographic examination for abdominal cystic echinococcosis combined with immunodiagnosis.[7,41,42]

The application of molecular biological techniques such as the polymerase chain reaction (PCR) has been developed for the identification of *Echinococcus*-specific nucleic acids in the last few years. For CE, molecular tools in general have been mainly used for the primary diagnostic identification of parasite materials in biological specimens resected or biopsied from patients. In many cases, ribosomal parasite DNA has been the target to develop species-specific PCR. Diagnostic applicability, however, was limited by the fact that restriction digestion of the corresponding PCR products had to be performed. Similarily, random amplified polymorphic DNA PCR (RAPD-PCR)[43] or single-stranded polymorphism PCR (SSCP-PCR)[44] was used for the characterization of *Echinococcus* isolate-specific amplification patterns, rather than for diagnostic application. Consequently, clinically well-characterized and specific molecular tests for CE are still lacking to date.

Management

It remains unclear what to do with asymptomatic patients detected at screening or with imaging for unrelated medical problems. In one small series of 28 patients followed for over 10 years, 75% of patients remained free of symptoms.[45]

Surgery

Surgery remains the mainstay in the treatment of hepatic hydatid disease. Cystectomy and pericystectomy offer a good chance for cure and should be undertaken wherever possible.[46] Occasionally, formal hepatic resection will be required.[47] Radical surgery—either pericystectomy or resection—is possible in 50–85% of cases.[46,48,49] In the absence of complications this can be achieved with little mortality and an acceptable morbidity. Recently, laparoscopic pericystectomy has been demonstrated to be as

BOX 84.1 Recommendations for the laboratory diagnosis and follow-up of human CE.

Primary diagnostic approach (screening and confirmation)
Serum antibody detection* and/or imaging procedure

Seronegative samples AND negative imaging results	**Seronegative samples AND 'positive' imaging results**	**Seropositive samples AND 'positive' or negative imaging results**
(Persons with documented infection risk only); serological and imaging follow-up every 6 months for 2 years	Differential diagnosis†	*Asymptomatic AND symptomatic cases* Species-specific (secondary) serology with:
	Asymptomatic cases	▪ ELISA using appropriately purified antigens
Differential diagnosis†	Extended/advanced imaging procedures; repeat serodiagnosis;	▪ Immunoblot for the detection of the 8/12 kDa or other specific bands[29,30]
	FNAB[40] for PCR (tissue) or antigen detection (fluid)	
	If lesions are fully calcified: serological and imaging follow-up after 6 months to confirm parasite inactivity	
	Symptomatic cases	
	Consideration of percutaneous drainage or surgical intervention and/or chemotherapy without serodignostic confirmation	

Postsurgical and/or chemotherapeutic follow-up

Postsurgical follow-up
▪ CT and/or MRI and/or ultrasound
▪ Serum antibody detection by ELISA
▪ Serum antigen detection by ELISA‡

Chemotherapeutic follow-up (assessing viability)
▪ CT and/or MRI and/or ultrasound
▪ Serum antibody detection by ELISA
▪ Serum antigen detection by ELISA‡

*ELISA for IgG detection, IHAT and latex agglutination test (LAT) with crude parasite antigen, alone or in combination, are commonly used.
†Differential diagnosis for AHD (in some cases for cysticercosis) and neoplasies may be required.[29,30,33,35]
‡Only in those patients with initially detectable circulating antigens.[39]

safe and effective as open laparatomy in selected cases with hepatic and/or splenic involvement.[50,51]

If coventional surgical cyst removal is not possible, treatment of CE has several alternatives such as PAIR (Puncture, Aspiration, Injection of a helminthicide and Reaspiration), chemotherapy or 'wait and observe' approach.

Basically, indications for hepatic surgery include large liver cysts with putatively multiple daughter cysts; single liver cysts, situated superficially which may rupture spontaneously or as a result of trauma; bacterially super-infected cysts; cysts communicating with biliary tree and/or exerting pressure on adjacent vital organs; brain, heart and kidney cysts; spinal and bone cysts.[52] Relative contraindications are inoperable cases as defined for surgical procedures in general, patients with cysts difficult to access, and abortive cysts either partly or totally calcified.

Whatever surgical procedure is chosen, care has to be taken to avoid spillage of cyst content, which is the main predictor of recurrent disease. To achieve this, the peritoneal cavity should be carefully protected, and the cyst evacuated and sterilized with scolicidal agents. The use of formalin and hypertonic saline should be abandoned since they can induce caustic injury to the biliary tree.[53,54] Formalin and hypertonic saline have also been associated with severe acidosis and hypernatraemia, respectively.[55] Currently used scolicidal agents include chlorhexidine, hydrogen peroxide, cetrizamide and, most preferably, ethanol.[46,55] Pretreatment with benzimidazole compounds—optionally complemented with praziquantel—has been proposed to avoid the use of dangerous scolicidal agents and to decrease the rate of recurrence.[56–58]

Radical surgery—hepatectomy or pericystectomy—has relatively low relapse rates, ranging from 8.5% to 22%,[46,47,52,55,59,60] whereas relapse occurs in up to 75% after non-radical surgery[49] (Table 84.1). Local recurrence has been ascribed to the formation of exogeneous daughter cysts which are left behind in the case of non-radical surgery.

Rupture into the biliary tree has been successfully treated with choledochojejunostomy or T-tube drainage;[61,62] in a comparative series, choledochojejunostomy was

Table 84.1 Selection of recurrence rates (as a percentage of the total series) after surgery for CE

Authors	n	Radical* (%)	Non-radical† (%)	PAIR° (%)
Akhan et al.[194]	31	–	–	3.2
Behrns and van Heerden[49]	23	0	50.0	–
Magistrelli et al.[70]	119	16.9	4.2	–
Morel et al.[47]	42	2.4	27.3	–

*Includes formal hepatic resections and total pericystectomy.
†Includes different procedures such as capitonnage or partial pericystectomy.
°PAIR: Puncture, aspiration, inoculation and reaspiration (see text)

found to result in fewer instances of recurrent jaundice than T-tube drainage.[62] Endoscopic sphincterotomy with or without nasobiliary drainage has been successfully used in the treatment of obstructive jaundice due to biliary rupture.[63,64] Sphincterotomy is also useful in case of postoperative biliary leaks.[64]

In selected cases, in particular where radical surgery has not been possible, liver transplantation may have to be considered and has been successfully carried out.[12]

Pulmonary cysts are often the result of infected or ruptured hepatic cysts. About 40% of patients present with complications, mainly infection but also pneumothorax.[65] In these cases, surgical treatment is mandatory. Treatment consists of wedge resection or lobectomy,[66] a two-stage procedure sometimes being necessary.[65] Recurrence of pulmonary disease appears to be rare.[60,65,66] A placebo controlled trial of albendazole in pulmonary hydatid disease showed cure in 45% in the verum group as opposed to 0 in the placebo group; thus, primary pharmacotherapy can be considered in uncomplicated cases.[67] Cardiac involvement necessitates surgery using bypass.[68]

Surgery is also the treatment of choice for renal involvement, nephrectomy being necessary only in about 15%, the others being able to be treated with pericystectomy alone.[69,70]

PAIR, once a rather controversial procedure, is now becoming well justified in selected cases but it still needs to be practised by experienced specialists. In a randomized trial comparing pericystectomy with PAIR plus albendazole, hospital stay was shorter and complications fewer in the patients treated with PAIR compared to the surgical group.[71] PAIR is indicated for:[52] patients refusing surgery; infected cysts not communicating with the biliary vessel system; inoperable patients (see contraindications for surgery); pregnant patients; children > 3 years; anechoic lesion ≥ 5 cm in diameter; cysts with a regular double laminated layer; cysts with multiple septal divisions of more than five; multiple cysts (≥ 5 cm in diameter) in different liver segments; relapse after surgery; and failure to respond to chemotherapy. Relative contraindications for PAIR are inaccessible or risky location of

the cyst in the liver; multiple septal divisions; cysts with echogenic lesions; inactive cysts or calcified lesions; communicating cysts; cysts located in the lung and bones and some others. It should not be performed when exophytic cysts or dilated bile ducts are observed on preoperative imaging.[72] A multicentric study, based on the use of 95% ethanol as a scolicidal agent, reported the successful treatment of 231 cysts in 163 Italian and Kenyan patients with abdominal, mainly hepatic CE.[73] More recent experiences with PAIR were obtained in 61 patients with 84 hepatic hydatid cysts.[74] In this study, hydatid cysts were sterilized by the injection of one of two scolicidal agents: 20% hypertonic saline solution (38 patients) or 0.5% silver nitrate (23 patients), respectively. All patients underwent follow-up examinations for 1 month to 6 years after PAIR: serial sonographic examinations revealed a heterogeneous echo pattern in 78 cysts (93%); a progressive decrease in diameter in 76 cysts (90%); calcification of the cyst wall, cystic contents or both in 10 cysts (12%); and complete disappearance of one cyst (1%) in a patient who had been monitored for over 6 years. Similar results were reported by Men and colleagues.[75] However, complications are not infrequent after PAIR. No recurrence of CE after PAIR was observed in Odev's series[74] over the follow-up period of 72 months, while there were three local recurrences and one rupture into the biliary tree in the series by Men et al.[75] and 2.8% in another Turkish series.[76]

Pharmacotherapy

Two benzimidazole compounds—mebendazole and albendazole—and praziquantel have activity against *E. granulosus* in vitro and in animal models.[77,78] No controlled studies have ever been performed in man but large series with the benzimidazoles have been published (see Table 84.2). Albendazole appears preferable to mebendazole because of its better bioavailability.[79,80] Both drugs penetrate into the cysts,[81,82] but sometimes heroic doses are needed to achieve a therapeutic plasma concentration of mebendazole.[83] Mebendazole should be given after a fat-rich meal and levels monitored 4 hours after the morning dose.[81] Plasma levels of mebendazole are unrelated to dose;[82,83] the generally accepted therapeutic levels are around 250 nmol/litre. The therapeutic level of albendazole sulphoxide, the major active metabolite in serum,[84] has not been defined in vivo yet. Better absorption of albendazole when given with a fatty meal has also been reported.[85] Cholestasis increases the blood levels of both drugs.[86] The former use of albendazole in cycles of 4 weeks, followed by a drug-free interval of 2 weeks, has been increasingly replaced by a continuous treatment.[52,87] The initial idea for the cyclic treatment had been to diminish toxicity and to avoid autoinduction of its metabolism.[84] However, more recently continous administration was found to be more efficacacious in a small comparative study than administration in cycles: 6/6 patients on continous therapy showed cyst involution, while relapse occurred in the cycling group.[88]

Table 84.2 Effect of benzimidazole treatment in CE

Authors	n (patients)	Dose per day	XR (mos)	Follow-up	Success (%)*
Mebendazole					
Davis et al.[89]	22	4.5 g	6	1 yr	78
Franchi et al.[95]	70	–	–	6 months	64
Messaritakis et al.[92]	39	200 mg/kg	3	5 yrs	51
Schantz et al.[172]	127	Variable	Variable	–	74
Todorov et al.[94]	44	50 mg/kg	6–24	30 months	48
Albendazole					
Erzurumlu et al.[195]	22	12–15 mg/kg	3–7	21	100
Morris et al.[93]	22	10 mg/kg	–	–	68
Nahmias et al.[196]	68	800 mg/d	Variable	3–7 years	58
Saimot et al.[96]	10	14 mg/kg	Variable	–	50
Todorov et al.[94]	35	10 mg/kg	4	33 months	74

*Success is defined as either disappearance or clear-cut regression of cysts, assessed by sonography. The remainder were failures, defined as unchanged or progressive radiological appearance.

Side effects of the two drugs appear to be similar and include mainly leucopenia, hair loss and hepatotoxicity.[86,89] For both benzimidazoles it appears likely that they act not truly parasiticidally in vivo but rather parasitostatically. Thus, in those treated with mebendazole for 1 year, viable scolices could be found in at least 50% of patients in spite of therapeutic drug levels.[83] The performance appears somewhat better for albendazole because prior to surgical excision only one of 14 patients had viable protoscolices when treated for longer than 1 month, as opposed to two patients treated only for a few weeks.[56] Short-term treatment is clearly inadequate since also with albendazole treatment for 3 weeks 50% viable cysts were found in a prospective study.[90] In a large multi-centre report viable cysts were found at surgery in 11% of patients treated with albendazole for an average of 2.5 cycles.[87] On the other hand, in the only randomized study published so far, 50%, 72% and 94% of cysts were non-viable after no, 1 month or 3 months treatment with albendazole, respectively.[91]

In a comparative multi-centre trial albendazole appeared to be slightly superior to mebendazole, in particular for extrahepatic sites.[89] In this trial, 68 of 112 patients were followed for at least 1 year; 39% and 14% of patients treated with albendazole (10 mg/kg per day) or mebendazole (increasing dose up to 4.5 g/day), respectively, were deemed to be treatment successes, as judged by disappearance or a major decrease in cyst size. The corresponding figures for favourable effects (meaning a decrease in cyst size or disappearance of some but not all cysts) were 39% and 64%, while treatment failures were 22% and 23%, respectively. Tolerance of the drugs was similar, side effects occurring in 18% and 20% of patients treated with mebendazole and albendazole, respectively. This trial suffers from the fact that mebendazole levels were not measured and therefore the dose was not adjusted in the individual patients. The World Health Organization

(WHO) trial and other series evaluating mebendazole and/or albendazole are summarized in Table 84.2; this table should be read with some caution since it is possible that collaborators of the WHO trial published part or all of their patients independently. Therapeutic failures have clearly been described with both drugs; combining all the studies in Table 84.2, a slight advantage seems to emerge in favour of albendazole. The data concerning mebendazole may have been biased for comparative purposes due to the fact that most investigators used fixed dosing and did not adjust for blood levels. Given the slow growth of *E. granulosus* cysts, a follow-up of at least 1 year is required to assess the value of any pharmacological treatment of this disease. The drug has also been used in children[92] and the response rate of 51% is comparable with that seen in adult series. The summarized success, as defined above, after albendazole ranges from 66% to 100%. Complete cyst disappearance was observed in 22% of patients with hepatic cysts.[93] Serum levels were not monitored and from the compilation in Table 84.2 it remains unclear whether higher doses of albendazole could increase the response rate.

Cyst size is a main determinant for response to either benzimidazole, small cysts responding better than large cysts, while cyst location, with the exception of bone, appears not to be major determinant.[94] Franchi et al.[95] observed relapse in 25% of patients after 6 months treatment; there was no difference between mebendazole and albendazole. Type II cysts tended to relapse more frequently. Bone cysts appear to be a problematic indication for pharmacological therapy in the experience of different investigators.[94,96]

The beneficial effects of praziquantel medication (additional to benzimidazoles) have been suggested and discussed.[58,78,97] The combination may be of particular interest since it appears more potent than either agent alone in an animal model of peritoneal spillage in vivo.[77]

However, Piens et al.[98] treated nine patients prior to surgery with two 10-day courses of praziquantel. The drug could not be detected in the cyst fluid and as many cysts remained vital as in an untreated control group, shedding doubt on the efficacy of praziquantel alone as a scolicidal agent. This may be due to the fact that praziquantel acts on protoscolices but not on the germinal layer.

In an uncontrolled study, the combination of albendazole and praziquantel was slightly superior to monotherapy with albendazole. In 19 patients treated with the combination, cysts disappeared in 47% and regressed >50% in 37%. In contrast, in 22 historical controls treated with albendazole alone, 36% only disappeared.[99]

Prognosis

Life expectancy in successfully operated patients appears to be normal; patients with extrahepatic disease seem to fare no worse than those with hepatic disease.[100] However, when patients present with complications, in particular cholangitis, there is an appreciable mortality.[55] Most hydatid cysts grow slowly; the best data on their natural evolution have been generated by Romig et al.;[101] these authors have followed 36 patients sonographically over a year. Of particular interest is the fact that 13.6% of cysts either disappeared or collapsed spontaneously. This has to be taken into account when evaluating results of chemotherapy, although special attention should be given to the biological particularities of the parasite strain present in the Turkana district.

Alveolar echinococcosis (*Echinococcus multilocularis*)
Biology

The natural life cycle of *E. multilocularis* involves predominantly red and arctic foxes as definitive hosts (Figure 84.5); domestic dogs or house cats can also become infected and—due to their close contact with human beings—may represent an important infection source in highly endemic areas. In the definitive host, egg production starts as early as 28 days after infection. Eggs released into the environment show a high degree of longevity and resistance to degradation, e.g. up to 2 years when they reside under humid conditions and moderate temperatures. Following egg ingestion by a rodent or a human, digestive processes and other factors in the host gut result in hatching and release of the oncosphere, which subsequently becomes activated—probably by the surface active properties of bile. The activated oncosphere penetrates the epithelial border of the intestinal villi and enters venous and lymphatic vessels, followed by distribution to other anatomical sites. Most of the oncospheres develop in the liver; some may reach the lungs or other organs. Maturation to the asexually proliferating metacestode includes degeneration of the oncospheral tissue, cellular proliferation, vesicularization and creation of a germinative membrane with formation of a central cavity and a peripheral laminated layer, followed later by endogenous and exogenous proliferation of metacestode tissue. AE will occur within the liver tissue in more than 98% of cases; subsequent metastasis formation may occur in adjacent or distant tissues (observed in approximately 20% of AE cases). Parasite tissue growth occurs by exogenous budding of metacestode tissue with a progressive, tumour-like expansion. Production of protoscolices may take place within 2–4 months in rodent hosts, but is lacking in more than 95% of human AE cases.

For completion of the life cycle, definitive hosts must ingest the mature infective metacestode containing protoscolices. Digestion of the infected tissue is followed by liberation of protoscolices with invaginated scolex. Pepsin and bile salts stimulate rapid evagination of the scolex, which is then able to attach firmly to the intestinal mucosa.

Distribution and epidemiology

The geographical distribution of *E. multilocularis* is restricted to the Northern Hemisphere. In North America, the cestode is present in subarctic regions of Alaska and Canada. The parasite in its wildlife cycle has been discovered in Manitoba, North Dakota, and more recently in another seven states including South Carolina, thus indicating an apparent expansion of the focus within the north-central American continent.[102] In Europe, relatively frequent reports of alveolar echinococcosis in humans focus on central and eastern France, Switzerland, Austria and Germany. The Asian areas with *E. multilocularis* include the whole zone of tundra, from the White Sea eastwards to the Bering Strait, covering large parts of the former Soviet Union. Large foci are found in China and northern Japan.[103]

At the global level scant data exist on the overall prevalence of human alveolar echinococcosis. The annual incidence of the populations at risk in western Alaska, including St Lawrence Island, averages 28 new cases per 100 000 inhabitants;[104] this is much lower in Switzerland, with an annual incidence of 0.18/100 000.[105] Similar data were reported from France, Germany and Austria.[106,107] In contrast to the relatively stable prevalence and incidence in Europe and Alaska, Japan reported spread of both parasite and disease in its northern areas: between 1937 and 1982, 129 cases of alveolar echinococcosis had been reported on Rebun Island; since then, the disease has spread to Hokkaido and Honshu Islands with a total of 264 and 60 new cases, respectively, registered up to 1988.[108] One of the highest incidences has been reported from China with an 8.8% seroprevalence.[109]

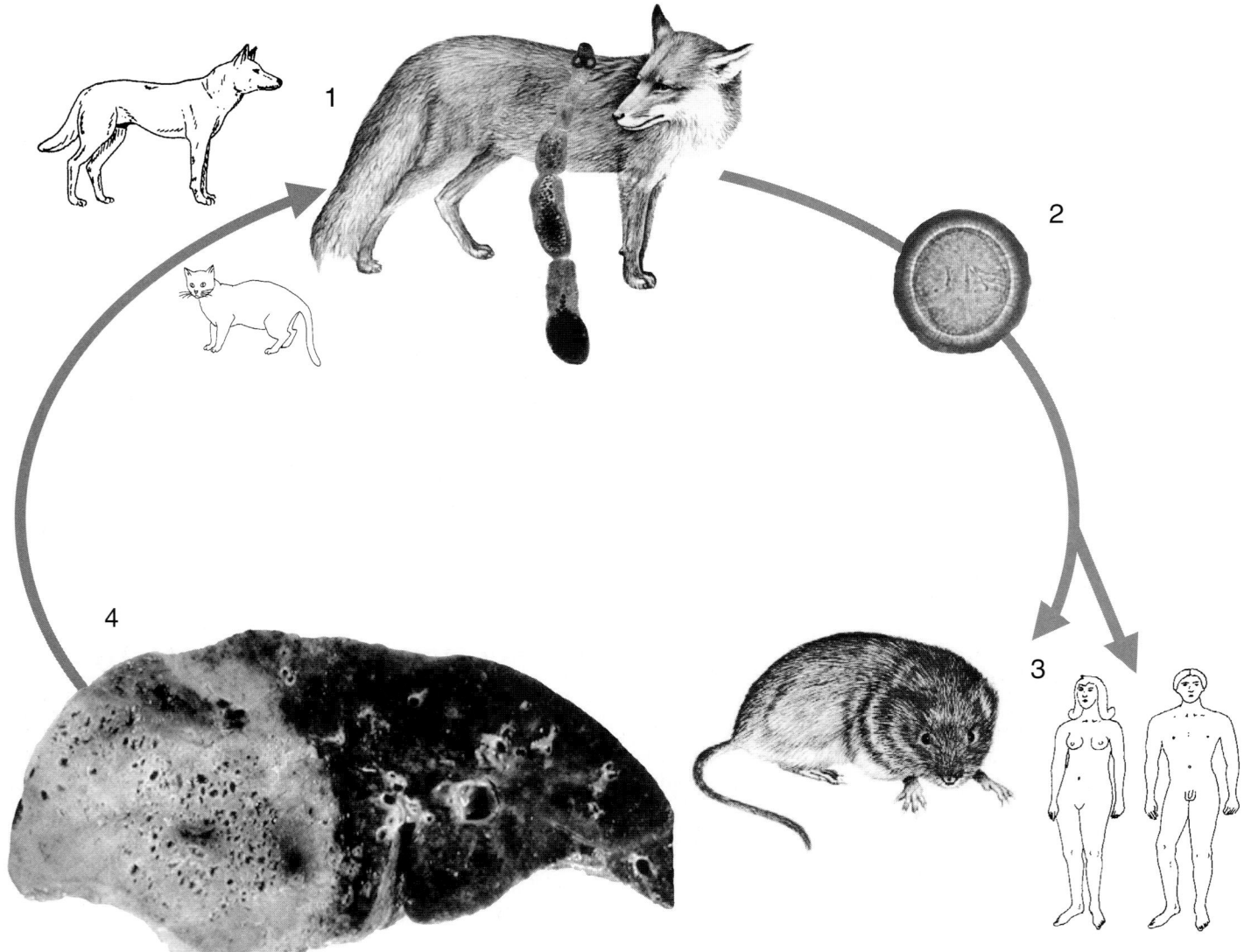

Figure 84.5: The life cycle of *E. multilocularis* involves predominantly foxes as definitive hosts (**1**), occasionally other carnivores such as domestic dogs or house cats. When parasite eggs (**2**) are ingested by a suitable intermediate host (**3**) including man and various rodents, the parasite metacestode will primarily become established in the liver (**4**). Macroscopically, the typical lesion is characterized by a dispersed mass of fibrous tissue with a multitude of interconnected vesicles ranging from a few millimetres to centimetres in size. The peroral uptake of protoscoleces-containing metacestodes by definitive hosts, e.g. when eating infected mice, terminates the life cycle.

Pathogenesis and immunology

The *E. multilocularis* metacestode (larva) will develop in infected human patients primarily in the liver (Figure 84.2). Occasionally, secondary lesions may form metastases in the lungs, brain and other organs. The typical lesion appears macroscopically as a dispersed mass of fibrous tissue with a conglomerate of scattered cavities, each ranging from a few millimetres to centimetres in size.[110] In advanced chronic cases, a central necrotic cavity can be formed which contains a viscous fluid with, rarely, a bacterial superinfection. The lesion often contains focal zones of calcification localized within the metacestode tissue. Histologically, the hepatic lesion is characterized by a conglomerate of small vesicles and cysts demarcated by a thin laminated layer with or without an inner germinative layer. Parasite proliferation is usually accompanied by a granulomatous host reaction including a vigorous synthesis of fibrous and germinative tissue in the periphery of the metacestode, but also of regressive changes centrally. In contrast to infection in susceptible rodent hosts, lesions from infected human patients rarely exhibit protoscolex formation within vesicles and cysts. Immunogenetic and immunological host factors proved responsible for phenomena of resistance shown in some patients exhibiting an early 'dying out' or 'abortion' of the metacestode[111] (see Figure 84.6). Thus, after infection with *E. multilocularis*, not every person is susceptible to

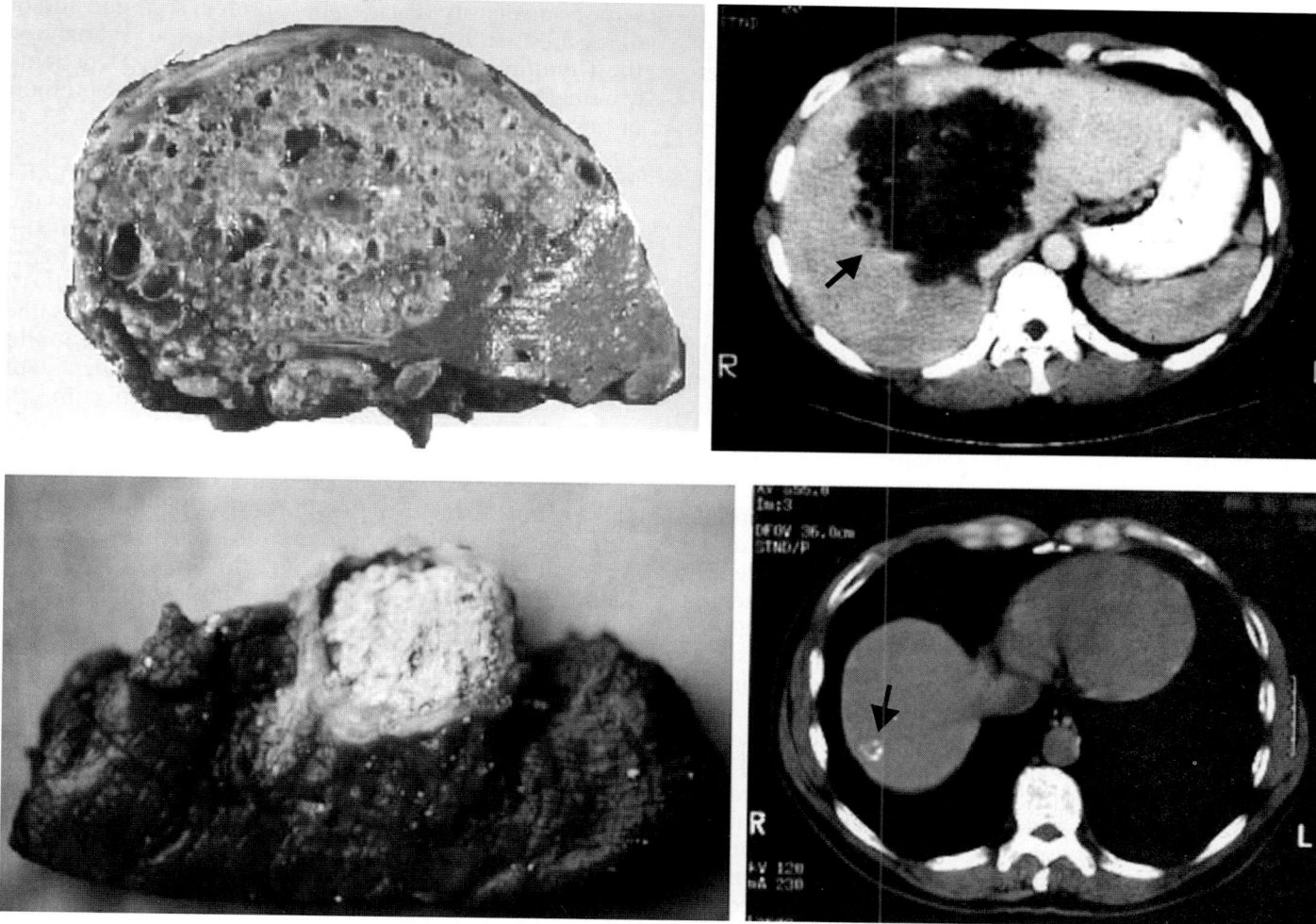

Figure 84.6: In the first row, an *E. multilocularis* active liver AE lesion is shown, while the second row presents a 'died-out' lesion. Left column: macroscopic presentation of resected and cross-sected liver lesion; right column: CT visualization of similar lesion type, parasitic mass denoted by arrow. Note in the CTs the hypodensity of the large lesions in active AE, while the 'died-out' lesion (second row) will appear as a small fully calcified white mass.

unlimited metacestode proliferation and will become actual patients within 5–15 years following infection.[112] The host mechanisms modulating the course of infection are most likely of immunological nature, including primarily T cell interactions. Thus, the periparasitic granuloma, mainly composed of macrophages, myo-fibroblasts and T cells, contains a large number of CD4$^+$ T cells in patients with abortive or died-out lesions, whereas in patients with active metacestodes the number of CD8$^+$ T cells is increased;[113] a immunosuppressive process is assumed to downregulate the lymphoid macro-phage system. Conversely, the status of cured AE is generally reflected by a high in vitro lymphoproliferative response. The cytokine mRNA levels following *E. multilocularis* antigen stimulation of lymphocytes shows an enhanced production of Th2 cell cytokine transcripts IL-3, IL-4 and IL-10 in patients, including a significant IL-5 mRNA expression in patients and not in healthy control donors.[114] The phenomenon of immunological or constitutional resistance may be dependent upon a

potential immunogenetic predisposition with the potential of an HLA-DR type association.[115,116] Conversely, lack of Th cell activity such as in advanced AIDS is associated with a rapid and unlimited growth and dissemination of the parasite in AE, as exemplified by a young AIDS patient who died from AE at the age of 6 years.[117]

As for *E. granulosus*, the primary site of interaction between *E. multilocularis* and its host is the mucosa of the gastrointestinal tract. Scarce information is available on the immune response against migrating and subsequently established oncospheres and their development into larvae of *E. multilocularis* in humans. Therefore, the following considerations will focus on the immune response to fully developed and progressively proliferating meta-cestodes. Many patients with AE respond with a marked synthesis of parasite-specific antibodies, including all isotypes of immunoglobulins. There is no evidence that specific antibodies have a direct restricting role on the growth of the metacestode. However, protoscolices and oncospheres of *E. multilocularis* can be lysed by antibody mediated complement inactivation. Antibodies appear to be involved in the rare chronic granulomatous course of the disease. In contrast to antibodies, T lymphocyte interactions appear to be of immunopathophysiological significance. The concept that T lymphocytes are the main determinant of host response is supported by different findings in animal models of alveolar echinococcosis. Thus, depletion of T cells enhances metastasis formation in mice, and in congenitally athymic nude mice *E. multilocularis* develops very rapidly, and the host tissue reaction is much less than in heterozygote mice.[118] Activated macrophages appear to be key participants in the immune response as they could be seen to adhere to the metacestode.[119] Conversely, peritoneal macrophages also contribute significantly to NO-mediated periparasitic immunosuppression.[120]

In 'resistant' human AE patients—as mentioned above—mass proliferation of the intrahepatic metacestode is putatively inhibited by an appropriate host immune response. The process finally results in the early 'dying out' of the metacestode. This was initially suggested by the identification of individuals (upon serological screening by an Em2-ELISA; for more information on Em2 see below) in Alaska,[111] France,[106] and recently also in Switzerland,[121] in whom the lesions had 'aborted'. Lesions are considered to be aborted when they have completely calcified and no viability can be observed after surgical resection of the parasite lesion and subsequent transplantation into susceptible laboratory rodents. Histological and immunological examinations revealed that in these cases the parasite material remaining within the lesion consisted largely of debris of the laminated layer.[122] Surgical removal of the died-out lesion, and thus of the immunostimulating Em2 source, resulted immediately in seronegativity with regard to anti-Em2 antibodies.[123] The inability of the patients to eliminate the Em2-positive laminated layer indicated a very low degradability of the material, and pointed towards the crucial role it may play in protecting the parasite from host effector mechanisms.

Consequently, with regard to *E. multilocularis* infection in human beings, one can discriminate between two populations. One is comprised of individuals who developed disease (AE), thus reflecting susceptibility to unlimited metacestode proliferation, and another group exhibits ceased metacestode proliferation. According to epidemiological indications, resistance to disease appears to be the predominant feature among affected humans. Thus, the basic question is how the parasite survives in those cases where AE becomes clinically manifest, especially in relation to the host cell-mediated immunity. The molecular basis of the cellular immunoregulation in AE patients is still relatively poorly understood. Bresson-Hadni et al.[124] localized the transcription of the pro-inflammatory cytokines IL-1β, IL-6 and tumour necrosis factor α (TNFα) mRNA in human livers infected with *E. multilocularis*. They showed that pro-inflammatory cytokines may be consistently produced by macrophages at the periphery of the periparasitic granuloma and could serve as mediators of acute-phase protein secretion and of fibrogenesis in that location. Kilwinski et al.[125] analysed the T lymphocyte cytokine profile in human AE patients at a single cell level. They found that the specific expression of the early activation marker CD69 was induced in CD4[+] T lymphocytes as well as in CD8[+] T lymphocytes. FACS for intracellular cytokines showed that IL-2, IL-5 and IL-10 were expressed in CD4[+] as well as in CD8[+] lymphocytes. Most notably, there was a definite increase in the expression of IL-10 in CD8[+] lymphocytes from patients suffering from AE. Serum levels of IL-4, IL-10 and IL-12 were assessed in AE patients and controls by the same group.[126] Significantly higher levels of IL-10 were found in AE patients than in controls, with a tendency to increased concentrations in progressive cases. In contrast, IL-4 could be detected only in a minority of patients and controls. IL-12 levels were comparable between AE patients and controls and showed a similar distribution pattern to IL-10 with regard to disease progression. The authors concluded that the immune response in human AE leading to disease may be Th2 driven. Godot et al.[127] found that IL-10 production was significantly higher in patient PBMC culture supernatants than in control group supernatants. Semi-quantification of IL-10 mRNA revealed a significantly higher transcript level in unstimulated-CD8+ T cells from AE patients than from healthy donors. PBMC from patients produced very low levels of IL-4 but the production of IFNγ was not significantly depressed compared to the controls. Based on the preliminary knowledge on the putative role of cytokines in human AE, patients were experimentally treated with rec IFNγ over a 3-day period once a month.[128] In the treated patients, disease progression was not detected during the observed period of 18 months. The authors claimed that bolus therapy with IFNγ may have some clinical effect; however, treatment did not result in a change in the T helper 2 lymphocyte-dominated immune response during AE. Conversely, treatment of a patient with IFNα seemed to drive the patient from a Th2 to a Th1 cytokine profile.[129]

Clinical features

The initial phase of primary *E. multilocularis* infection is always asymptomatic. The percentage of asymptomatic patients being detected owing to improved epidemiological tools[130] has increased lately, including persons harbouring 'died-out' lesions (Figure 84.6). Dependent upon the size and the site of the developing parasite lesion, the infection may remain asymptomatic for years or even decades. In Europe, the average age of AE patients at diagnosis is 55 years; young children are rarely affected. The ratio of males to females may vary dependent on the geographical area but is statistically not significant overall. After a highly variable incubation period (on average between 5 and 15 years), the infection may become symptomatic due to a range of different events: the growing parasite tissue exerts pressure on or induces dysformation of adjacent tissues and induces complication by dysfunction of the affected organ. In the case of AE, this may include hepatomegaly–cholestasis–jaundice, secondary biliary cirrhosis, liver abscess, portal hypertension and Budd–Chiari syndrome. The disease starts frequently with non-specific symptoms such as epigastric pain or cholestatic jaundice. The AE liver lesions range between 5 and 90 cm at the time when patients come to diagnosis.[1] Typical calcifications occur in 70% of cases; central or peripheral necrotic cavities are found in approximately 70% of cases. The growth rate of the parasite tissue is usually slow in immunocompetent patients. Voluminometric analysis by CT indicated an average volume increase of 15 ml per year in progressive forms of AE. In complicated cases, evidence of secondary biliary cirrhosis and/or cholangitis will be found. Amyloid has been described in two out of two kidneys and two of six livers.[131] Eosinophilia is quite rare, occurring in only 10% of patients.[132] Evidence of cholestasis is frequently present, while transaminases are only rarely and moderatley elevated, in particular when there is central necrosis.[132] One of the most feared complications is infection of a necrotic cavity and/or obstructed bile ducts, which is associated with very high mortality due to development of septic shock.[133] Distant metastases can occur late in the disease; these have been described in brain,[1,133,134] spine,[133] lung,[1,104,133,135] bone[133,134] and eyes.[136] Metastatic disease occurs in approximately 10–20% of patients. Growth can also be expansive, invading the lungs through the diaphragm, the porta hepatis and the peritoneal space and retroperitoneum, which can extend as far down as the testes, encasing the ureters in the process.[137]

Clinical diagnosis

The primary manifestations of *E. multilocularis* are related to the liver, which is affected in 92–100% of cases. The most frequent presenting symptoms include non-specific abdominal pain, hepatomegaly and jaundice. In about 15% the parasite is incidentally discovered in asymptomatic patients, or there are only unspecific symptoms such as fatigue and weight loss.[135] As a result of screening programmes since 1983, more asymptomatic patients are being discovered in France,[106] Alaska,[111] Switzerland[105,121] and Germany.[107] Occasionally, portal hypertension, either variceal bleeding and/or ascites, is the first manifestation.[133]

Among the imaging procedures, ultrasonography, CT and MRI are of greatest diagnostic value, none of those being uniquely superior.[138] Calcifications on plain abdominal radiographs may give the first clue as to the aetiology of the disease; the percentage of calcified lesions increases from 33% to 100% as the disease progresses.[139,140] On sonography, hyperechogenic and hypoechogenic zones are found in the lesion(s).[141] Due to the vesicular structure of the parasitic mass, no cystic appearance can be expected, with the exception of central necrotic cavities. Similar findings can be found on CT (Figure 84.6): the lesions are typically not enhanced with contrast medium; the characteristic lesion has been called a 'geographic map', with irregular contours and alternating hypodense and hyperdense areas, reflecting necrosis and calcification, respectively. CT is felt by some authors to be superior to ultrasonography in delineating the anatomy of parasite localization and visualization of micro-calcifications.[142] Hilar involvement can lead to liver atrophy, which is easily visualized by CT.[143] Ultrasonography is 84% sensitive and specific in areas of high prevalence and is the preferred imaging procedure for mass screening programmes.[109,142] As with *E. granulosus*, MRI adds to diagnosis in particular in cases with appropriate organ localization such as brain and bone, and to visualize pathologically altered microstructures in certain affected organs, thus allowing a precise analysis of the different components of the parasitic lesions such as necrosis and fibrosis.[143] However, in contrast to CT micro-calcifications are not visualized by MRI.[144,145]

Histopathological and immunohistochemical procedures to analyse surgically resected samples or biopsies obtained by FNAB include the use of species-specific MAbs such as MAbG11 or molecular techniques such as PCR (both methods are discussed in the section below), beside conventional histology, with PAS being the best staining method to characterize the typical laminated layer of the parasite.[146]

Assessing the parasite viability in vivo following therapeutical interventions may be of tremendous advantage when compared to the invasive analysis of resected or biopsied samples. Such alternatives may be offered by magnetic resonance spectrometry (MRS)[147] or the positron emission tomography (PET).[148] The PET technique has been recently used for assessing the efficacy of chemotherapy in AE.[148] Evaluation of the disappearance of metabolic activity detected in the parasite lesions with [^{18}F]fluorodeoxyglucose–PET is still costly and not ubiquitarily available. In vivo MRS may also complement conventional CT or MRI to provide more detailed information on the viability or metabolic activity of metacestode cysts.[147]

Serological and molecular diagnosis

Complementary to imaging procedures, immunodiagnosis represents a valuable secondary diagnostic tool to confirm the nature (and species) of the aetiological agent.[7,149,150] In general, serological tests are more reliable in the diagnosis of AE than CE. The use of purified *E. multilocularis* antigens (such as the Em2-antigen, the Em18-antigen or recombinant antigens II/3-10 or EM10-antigen) exhibit diagnostic sensitivities ranging between 91% and 100%, with overall specificities of 98–100%. These antigens allow discrimination between AE and CE with a reliability of 95%.[7,151,152]

Early diagnosis of persons with asymptomatic AE is a prerequisite for efficient management of the disease in highly endemic areas. Consequently, screening may be offered to populations at risk. The currently optimal epidemiological tools to be used include species-specific immunodiagnosis, which may be complemented by ultrasonographic examination. Specific serological tests such as discussed below exhibit operating characteristics which allow reliable seroepidemiological studies. The aim of such studies is to detect asymptomatic preclinical cases of human AE as well as those cases in which the metacestode lesion had died out at an apparently early stage of infection.[106,107,111,121]

Methodically, immunodiagnosis of AE was substantially improved by the production of new specific tools such as MAbs and recombinant antigens. Two *E. multilocularis* specific antigens, the antigen II/3-10, localized in protoscolices and brood capsules,[153] and the antigen Em2, localized in the laminated layer of the cyst,[154] were combined and successfully used in an ELISA test as a standardized hybrid antigen. The resulting Em2plus-ELISA exhibited a diagnostic sensitivity of 97% and a specificity of 99% for diagnosis of AE patients.[151] The recombinant II/3-10-encoding molecule was also cloned by others and called EM10, besides another clone called EM13.[155,156] Both recombinant antigens exhibited high sensitivity and specificity performance. Another *E. multilocularis* antigen—EM18—appeared to be a relatively good marker for differentiation of active and inactive cases of AE.[157] Comparative assessment of Em18-ELISA and the Em2plus-ELISA demonstrated a good congruence of results.[158] *E. multilocularis* alkaline phosphatase (EmAP) proved valuable for serodiagnosis and serological follow-up of treated AE patients.[159] Both diagnostic sensitivity and specificity appeared to be high.[160] In order to provide a practical overview and suggestions concerning the procedure of laboratory tests which can be used, for the diagnosis and follow-up of human AE patients, we included respective recommendations in Box 84.2.

Serological methods have been assessed for their value in the surveillance of operated or pharmacologically treated patients. Conventional serological tests (such as in Em2-ELISA or Em18), although exhibiting generally a decrease in serum antibody concentration after radical surgery, were of limited clinical use for patients with partial, palliative or no surgery.[161,162]

BOX 84.2 Recommendations for the laboratory diagnosis and follow-up of human AE.

Primary diagnostic approach (screening and confirmation)
Serum antibody detection (ELISA with crude or purified/specific parasite antigen) and/or imaging procedure

Seronegative samples AND negative imaging results	**Seronegative samples AND 'positive' imaging results**	**Seropositive samples AND 'positive' or negative imaging results**
(Persons with documented infection risk only); serological and imaging follow-up every 6 months for 2 years Differential diagnosis†	Differential diagnosis† *Asymptomatic cases* Extended/advanced imaging procedure; repeat serodiagnosis; PCR and/or immunohistochemistry from biopsies[146] If lesions are fully calcified: serological[157,170] and imaging follow-up after 6 months to confirm inactivity *Symptomatic cases* Consideration of surgical intervention and/or chemotherapy without confirmation by serodiagnosis	*Asymptomatic AND symptomatic cases* Species-specific (secondary) serology with: ■ Em2-ELISA[151] ■ Em2plus-ELISA[151] ■ Em10- or EMII/3-10-ELISA[146] ■ EmAP-ELISA[160] ■ Em18-ELISA[152] Species-specific circulating antigen detection

Postsurgical and/or chemotherapeutic follow-up

Postsurgical follow-up (radical surgery)
■ Serum antibody detection by Em2-. Em10-, EMII/3-10-, EmAP- or EM18-ELISA[157,160,162,170]
■ Specific RT-PCR from FNAB samples‡

Chemotherapeutic follow-up (assessing viability)
■ Imaging (CT or MRI) and/or PET[147,148]
■ Serum antibody detection by EM18-ELISA[152]
■ Specific RT-PCR from FNAB samples‡

†Differential diagnosis for CHD (in rare cases for cysticercosis) and some neoplasies may be required.[146,151,152]
‡FNAB only useful for RT-PCR when obtaining positive results.[167]

An exceptional immunological situation was found in patients receiving orthotopic liver transplantation:[163] serum antibodies were immediately eliminated by abundant blood transfusions coupled to immunosuppressive therapy. Patients with remaining residual foci of extrahepatic parasite tissue had extremely high recurrence rates due to immunosuppression and interruption of chemotherapy with antiparasitic benzimidazoles; this was accompanied by reappearance of anti-*Echinococcus* serum antibodies.[164]

Molecular biological techniques such as PCR have been developed and introduced for the diagnostic identification of *E. multilocularis*-specific nucleic acids in the last few years. The primary diagnostic identification of parasite materials in biological specimens (resections or biopsies) and also the assessment of the viability of parasite samples following chemotherapy or other treatment were both addressed. The *E. multilocularis* nucleic acid sequence pAL1 served to derive oligonucleotide primers suitable for use in PCR amplification,[165] allowing differentiation between *E. multilocularis* and *E. granulosus* and other parasite material of any stage and origin. These primers have been diagnostically used to detect *E. multilocularis* DNA in hepatic lesions from different intermediate hosts, including rodents,[121] but especially also in complicated cases of extrahepatic AE, e.g. pancreatic AE[146] or AE of other sites.[166] Determination of not only the presence of the parasite but also of its viability has also been attempted by PCR, as well as assessment of the efficacy of antiparasitic therapy. Kern et al.[167] used a variant of the technique, called reverse transcription PCR (RT-PCR), to detect minute amounts of parasite messenger RNA in FNABs from the liver. They used species-specific primers derived from the above-mentioned EM10-gene.[155] A positive RT-PCR result was claimed to reflect viability of the parasite and thus failure of an antiparasitic therapy. However, a negative RT-PCR result would not prove efficacy, as the biopsied sample does not cover the whole metacestode tissue, such tissue being very inhomogeneous with regard to viable, necrotic or degenerating zones. Because, for technical and anatomical reasons, whole lesions cannot be assessed by RT-PCR, new basic approaches will have to be developed for the purpose.

Management

The mainstay of treatment remains surgical; in contrast to *E. granulosus*, interventional radiology and endoscopic procedures are rarely used.

Surgery

The following strategies are commonly accepted for treatment of alveolar hydatid disease: (i) the first choice of treatment is radical surgical resection of the entire parasitic lesion from the liver and other affected organs in all operable cases. Excision of the parasitic lesion has to follow the rules of radical tumour surgery; (ii) concomitant chemotherapy in all cases after radical surgery or after non-surgical interventional procedures; (iii) long-term chemotherapy of inoperable or only partially resectable cases and all patients after liver transplantation. Presurgical chemotherapy is not indicated in cases of alveolar hydatid disease.

Radical hepatic resection is possible only in 15–58% of cases.[130,132,133,139,140] Due to earlier diagnosis, the incidence of radically resectable cases has increased from 10% to 40% in a recent series.[104] Even in presumed radical surgery, recurrences can occur in 10–20%.[133,168] In patients where eradication is impossible, a good quality of life can be achieved when adequate biliary drainage is provided.[130,132]

Among palliative procedures, marsupialization[133,139] and biliary–digestive anastomoses or T-tube drainage for intrabiliary rupture[133] and cholangitis[168] have been used with success. Portal hypertension occasionally requires treatment with portosystemic shunt.[113] Metastatic disease, in particular in the brain, is sometimes amenable to surgical resection.[169]

Recently, hepatic transplantation has been proposed for patients with inoperable disease;[163] in this series of 17 patients, actuarial survival was 75% at 15 months; the operation was felt to be radical in nine patients but serological and radiological recurrence was later reported in three of these patients, one succumbing to recurrent disease.[164]

An ELISA directed against Em2 has been reported to reliably predict radical surgery.[162] However, anti-Em2 antibodies correlate with the presence of parasite only, not with its viability[111] (see above). Promising results, however based on peliminary findings,[170] indicated that the detectability of anti-EmII/3–19 antibodies correlates with the presence of an active metacestode. It thus appears that the combination of both tests may provide useful prognostic information to assess the clinical course of AE. Similar results were reported by Ito et al.[157]

Pharmacotherapy

In animal models the same three drugs discussed in the preceding section, namely mebendazole, albendazole and praziquantel, have some activity against *E. multilocularis*.[171] Although praziquantel was the most effective scolicidal agent, it did not inhibit metacestode growth and did not affect germinal layer activity. Albendazole was the most active agent in inhibiting metacestode growth.[171]

The daily dosage for albendazole and mebendazole treatment is the same as for CE. For mebendazole, plasma drug levels should reach > 250 nmol/litre (= 74 ng/ml). Generally, duration of treatment is at least 2 years in cases after radical surgery or continuously for many years in inoperable cases or in cases with incomplete resection.

The results of some clinical studies with mebendazole[133,172–175] and albendazole[84,86,87,176–178] are reported in Table 84.3; for the earlier trials, the reader is referred to the reports of a workshop.[172] Assessing efficacy in treatment of *E. multilocularis* is even more difficult than in *E. granulosus* since viability of the parasite cannot easily be judged in vivo; spontaneous death of parasite

Table 84.3 Effect of benzimidazole treatment in AE

Authors	n	Daily dose	Follow-up (years)	Failure (%)*
Mebendazole				
Akinoglu et al.[133]	19	50 mg/kg	1–6	63
Ammann et al.[134]	57	Variable†	1–9	33
Davis et al.[89]	54	40 mg/kg	1–12	22
Kern[174]	8	50 mg/kg	–	13
Rausch et al.[175]	8	40 mg/kg	10	50
Reuter et al.[178]	17	40–50 mg/kg	3	29
Albendazole				
Horton[87]	35	800 mg/d	1	11
Liu et al.[177]	15	20 mg/kg	1–5‡	13
Reichen et al.[184]	12	600 mg/d	1–5‡	17
Reuter et al.[178]	18	10–15 mg/kg	3	22
Wilson[104]	2	800 mg/d	< 1	0

*Failure is defined as either radiological progression, development of metastatic disease or death.
†Mebendazole dose adjusted individually to reach therapeutic levels.
‡Updated from the preliminary report.[125]

has been described[111] and radiological regression is rare.[179] Therefore, radiological progression and/or death are the only hard end-points as treatment failures;[134] these are recorded in Table 84.3. With regard to respective assessments, a preliminary but promising approach has been described by Reuter et al.,[178] who were measuring pericystic metabolic activity by PET to assess and follow up patients with AE. Convincing evidence that mebendazole affects the growth rate of *E. multilocularis* has been provided by Luder et al.[179] and Rausch et al.[175] in long-term follow-up of AE patients. In a prospective Swiss chemotherapy trial covering 20 years of investigation, a total of 110 patients had been included in the study.[144] From these patients 74 had inoperable or palliatively operated AE (average observation time 12.8 years). The efficacy of long-term chemotherapy was documented by increase of 10-year survival compared to historical (untreated) AE cases (80% versus 6%) and by reduction or stabilization of the liver lesions in 83% of cases during long-term chemotherapy. A comparative assessment of the efficacy of albendazole versus mebendazole has been reported by Reuter et al.[178] In this study, 35 patients were started on either mebendazole or albendazole at the beginning of 1992 and followed for an average of 39 months (range 12–79 months). The overall success rate was 97%. An initial regimen for cases of AE was recurrence free in 71% of those treated with mebendazole and in 78% of those treated with albendazole. Seven patients received a continuous regimen with albendazole. These patients were observed over an average of 28 months (range 13–50 months) without signs of progression or significant side effects. This study had demonstrated the high therapeutic efficacy of both mebendazole and albendazole with similar response rates in the treatment of AE. Albendazole reduced costs by > 40% and was easier for patients to take, further arguing in favour of its preferred use.[178] For albendazole, recent experience indicated that continuous treatment was well tolerated for about 1–6 years, and proved to be superior to discontinuous treatment for AE associated with obstructive jaundice.[180]

Prognosis

Mortality of untreated *E. multilocularis* has been reported to be 63–93% at 10 years.[1,140] It remains unclear whether any of the benzimidazoles are truly parasitostatic or—under certain not yet defined conditions—parasitocidic.[181] Recurrence after discontinuation of mebendazole treatment was observed in 7 of 19 patients.[182] Inoculation of autopsy material from two patients treated with mebendazole failed to demonstrate growth, while growth was observed in 8 of 11 untreated patients; however, duration of treatment of at least 2 years is needed to observe such favourable effects, and viable material was found in patients treated for up to 48 months.[181] In contrast, in two patients treated for a short time with albendazole no growth could be observed,[176] which is in contrast to our own experience.[183] Finally, benzimidazole treatment has been found to render some patients—initially judged to be unresectable—fit for radical surgery.[184]

Other *Echinococcus* species
Echinococcus vogeli

E. vogeli is maintained primarily in a silvatic predator–prey cycle which includes the bush dog and occasionally domestic dogs as definitive host and pacas as intermediate hosts. Humans are rarely infected. The metacestode of *E. vogeli* is polycystic and fluid filled, with a tendency to form multi-chambered conglomerates; the predilection site in the intermediate host is the liver. Endogenous proliferation and convolution of both germinal and laminated layers lead to the formation of secondary subdivisions of the primary vesicle, including production of brood capsules and protoscolices.[185] The geographical distribution of *E. vogeli* includes the northern half of South America.

Polycystic hydatid disease due to *E. vogeli* in humans has been reported from Argentina, Brazil, Colombia, Ecuador, Panama and Venezuela. While the most frequent primary site is the liver, primary polycystic infections have also occurred elsewhere in the abdominal cavity, in the lungs and in other thoracic organs.[186,187] Patients with polycystic echinococcosis usually present with a painful right hypochondrial mass, jaundice or an hepatic abscess, rarely with signs and symptoms of pulmonary disease—in particular cough and haemoptysis.[187] Commonly, the evolution of the disease is rather benign; recovery was reported following surgical resection, and sometimes spontaneously. Diagnostic imaging is hampered

especially with regard to the differentiation from CE and AE. Laboratory tests rarely reveal eosinophilia; antibodies against homologous antigens, determined by ELISA and immunoblot, help in diagnosis.[188] In inoperable cases, albendazole yields much the same result(s) as in *E. granulosus*, with cure or improvement observed in four of six patients in a recent small series.[189]

Echinococcus oligarthrus

E. oligarthrus infects only felids (mainly the cougar, the jaguar, the ocelot, the jaguarundi and Geoffroyi's cat) as definitive hosts, with the larval stage occurring in subcutaneous muscles of large South American rodents such as agoutis and pacas. The metacestode is, like *E. vogeli*, polycystic and fluid filled. There is less subdivision into secondary chambers and the laminated layer is significantly thinner than that of *E. vogeli*. So far very few infections with larval *E. oligarthrus* have been reported in humans, e.g. in Venezuela,[190] Brazil,[191] Surinam[192] and India.[193]

REFERENCES

1. Ammann R W & Eckert J. Cestodes: *Echinococcus*. *Gastroenterol Clin North Am* 1996; 25:655–689.
2. Campos-Bueno A, Lopez-Abente G & Andres-Cercadillo A M. Risk factors for *Echinococcus granulosus* infection: a case–control study. *Am J Trop Med Hyg* 2000; 62:329–334.
3. Commission of the European Community. *Disease in Farm Livestock: Economics and Policy.* Report EUR 11285. Luxembourg, 1987.
4. Food and Agriculture Organization of the United Nations. *Cost/Benefit Analysis for Animal Health Programmes in Developing Countries.* Report of FAO Expert Consultation, 1990.
5. Attanasio E, Ferretti G & Palmas C. Hydatidosis in Sardinia: review and recommendations. *Trans R Soc Trop Med Hyg* 1985; 79:154–158.
6. Yalin R, Aktan A O, Yegen C & Doeslueoglu H H. Significance of intracystic pressure in abdominal hydatid disease. *Br J Surg* 1992; 79:1182–1183.
7. Gottstein B. Molecular and immunological diagnosis of echinococcosis. *Clin Microbiol Rev* 1992; 5:248–261.
8. Ferreira A M, Irigoin F, Breijo M, Sim R B & Diaz A. How *Echinococcus granulosus* deals with complement. *Parasitol Today* 2000; 16:168–172.
9. Dixon J B. Echinococcosis. *Comp Immunol Microbiol Infect Dis* 1997; 20:87–94.
10. Ellis M E, Sinner W, Asraf A M & Hussain Q S M. Echinococcal disease and mycobacterial infection. *Ann Trop Med Parasitol* 1991; 85:243–251.
11. Rigano R, Profumo E & Siracusano A. New perspectives in the immunology of *Echinococcus granulosus* infection. *Parassitologia* 1997; 39:275–277.
12. Moreno-Gonzalez E, Segurola C L et al. Liver transplantation for *Echinococcus granulosus* hydatid disease. *Transplantation* 1994; 58:797–800.
13. Yagmur O, Demircan O, Atilla E et al. Cardiac tamponade due to rupture of hydatid cyst into the pericardium. *Dig Surg* 1992; 9:329–331.
14. Agarwal D K, Agarwal R & Barthwal S P. Interventricular septal hydatid cyst presenting as complete heart block. *Br Heart J* 1996; 75:266.
15. Sinha P R, Jaipuria N & Avasthey P. Intracardiac hydatid cyst and sudden death in a child. *Int J Cardiol* 1995; 51:293–295.
16. Benomar A, Yahyaoui M, Birouk N, Vidailhet M & Chkili T. Middle cerebral artery occlusion due to hydatid cysts of myocardial and intraventricular cavity cardiac origin: 2 cases. *Stroke* 1994; 25:886–888.
17. Salinas J C, Torcal J, Lozano R, Sousa R, Morandeira A & Cabezali R. Intracystic infection of liver hydatidosis. *Hepatogastroenterology* 2000; 47:1052–1055.
18. Kervancioglu R, Bayram M & Elbeyli L. CT findings in pulmonary hydatid disease. *Acta Radiol* 1999; 40:510–514.
19. Harris K M, Morrisl D L, Tudor R, Toghill P & Hardcastle J D. Clinical and radiographic features of simple and hydatid cysts of the liver. *Br J Surg* 1986; 73:835–838.
20. Lewall D B & McCorkell S J. Hepatic echinococcal cysts: sonographic appearance and classification. *Radiology* 1985; 155:773–775.
21. Gharbi H A, Hassine W, Brauner M W & Dupuch K. Ultrasound examination of the hydatic liver. *Radiology* 1981; 139:459–463.
22. Perdomo R, Carbo A, Alvarez C & Monti J. Asymptomatic hepatic cystic echinococcosis (hydatidosis) diagnosed by ultrasonography. *Echinomed* 1995; 19:2–3.
23. El Tahir M I, Omojola M F, Malatani T, al Saigh A H & Ogunbiyi O A. Hydatid disease of the liver: evaluation of ultrasound and computed tomography. *Br J Radiol* 1992; 65:390–392.
24. Bezzi M, Teggi A, De Rosa F et al. Abdominal hydatid disease: US findings during medical treatment. *Radiology* 1987; 162:91–95.
25. Hira P R, Lindberg L G, Francis I, Shweiki H, Shaheen Y & Leven B K. Diagnosis of cystic hydatid disease: role of aspiration cytology. *Lancet* 1988; ii:655–657.
26. Frydman C P, Raissi S & Watson C W. An unusual pulmonary and renal presentation of echinococcosis: report of a case. *Acta Cytol* 1989; 33:655–658.
27. Gogucs O, Beduk Y & Topukccu Z. Renal hydatid disease. *Br J Urol* 1991; 68:466–469.
28. Horchani A, Nouira Y, Kbaier I, Attyaoui F & Zribi A S. Hydatid cyst of the kidney: a report of 147 controlled cases. *Eur Urol* 2000; 38:461–467.

29 Liance M, Janin V, Bresson-Hadni S, Vuitton D A, Houin R & Piarroux R. Immunodiagnosis of *Echinococcus* infections: confirmatory testing and species differentiation by a new commercial Western blot. *J Clin Microbiol* 2000; 38:3718–3721.

30 Poretti D, Felleisen E, Grimm F et al. Differential immunodiagnosis between cystic hydatid disease and other cross-reactive pathologies. *Am J Trop Med Hyg* 1999; 60:193–198.

31 Wattal C, Mohan C & Agarwal S C. Evaluation of specific immunoglogulin E by enzyme-linked immunosorbent assay in hydatid disease. *Int Arch Allergy Appl Immunol* 1987; 87:98–100.

32 Pinon J M, Poirriez J, Lepan J, Geers R, Penna R & Fernandez D. Value of isotypic characterization of antibodies of *Echinococcus granulosus* by enzyme-linked immuno-filtration assay. *Eur J Clin Microbiol* 1987; 6:291–295.

33 Dar F K, Buhidma M A & Kidwai S A. Hydatid false positive serological test results in malignancy. *BMJ* 1984; 288:1197.

34 Ben-Ismail R, Rouger P, Carme B, Gentilini M & Salmon C. Comparative automated assay of anti-P1 antibodies in acute hepatic distomiasis (fasciolasis) and in hydatidosis. *Vox Sang* 1980; 38:156–168.

35 Pfister M, Gottstein B, Cerny T & Cerny A. Immunodiagnosis of echinococcosis in cancer patients. *Clin Microbiol Infect* 1999; 5:693–697.

36 Iacona A, Pini C & Vicari G. Enzyme-linked immunosorbent assay (ELISA) in the serodiagnosis of hydatid disease. *Am J Trop Med Hyg* 1980; 29:95–99.

37 Rigano R, Profumo E, Ioppolo S, Notargiacomo S, Teggi A & Siracusano A. Cytokine patterns in seropositive and seronegative patients with *Echinococcus granulosus* infection. *Immunol Lett* 1998; 64:5–8.

38 Lightowlers M W, Liu D, Haralambous A & Rickard M D. Subunit composition and specificity of the major cyst fluid antigens of *Echinococcus granulosus*. *Mol Biochem Parasitol* 1989; 37:171–182.

39 Ferragut G, Ljungstrom I & Nieto A. Relevance of circulating antigen detection to follow-up experimental and human cystic hydatid infections. *Parasite Immunol* 1998; 20:541–549.

40 Stefaniak J. Fine needle aspiration biopsy in the differential diagnosis of the liver cystic echinococcosis. *Acta Trop* 1997; 67:107–111.

41 MacPherson C N L, Romig T, Zehyle E, Rees P H & Were J B O. Portable ultrasound scanner versus serology in screening for hydatid cysts in a Nomadic population. *Lancet* 1987; ii:259–261.

42 Shambesh M A, Craig P S, Macpherson C N, Rogan M T, Gusbi A M & Echtuish E F. An extensive ultrasound and serologic study to investigate the prevalence of human cystic echinococcosis in northern Libya. *Am J Trop Med Hyg* 1999; 60:462–468.

43 Siles-Lucas M, Felleisen R, Cuesta-Bandera C, Gottstein B & Eckert J. Comparative genetic analysis of Swiss and Spanish isolates of *Echinococcus granulosus* by southern hybridization and Random Amplified Polymorphic DNA technique. *Appl Parasitol* 1994; 35:107–117.

44 Haag K L, Araujo A M, Gottstein B, Siles-Lucas M, Thompson R C & Zaha A. Breeding systems in *Echinococcus granulosus* (Cestoda; Taeniidae): selfing or outcrossing? *Parasitology* 1999; 118:63–71.

45 Frider B, Larrieu E & Odriozola M. Long-term outcome of asymptomatic liver hydatidosis. *J Hepatol* 1999; 30:228–231.

46 Langer J C, Rose D B, Keystone J S, Taylor B R & Langer B. Diagnosis and management of hydatid disease of the liver: a 15-year North American experience. *Ann Surg* 1984; 119:412–417.

47 Morel P, Robert J & Rohner A. Surgical treatment of hydatid disease of the liver: a survey of 69 patients. *Surgery* 1988; 104:859–862.

48 Elhamel A. Pericystectomy for the treatment of hepatic hydatid cysts. *Surgery* 1990; 107:316–320.

49 Behrns K E & van Heerden J A. Surgical management of hepatic hydatid disease. *Mayo Clin Proc* 1991; 66:1193–1197.

50 Khoury G, Abiad F, Geagea T, Nabout G & Jabbour S. Laparoscopic treatment of hydatid cysts of the liver and spleen. *Surg Endosc* 2000; 14:243–245.

51 Seven R, Berber E, Mercan S, Eminoglu L & Budak D. Laparoscopic treatment of hepatic hydatid cysts. *Surgery* 2000; 128:36–40.

52 WHO. Guidelines for tretament of cystic and alveolar echinococcosis in humans. *Bull WHO* 1996; 74:231–242.

53 Kehila M, Korbi S, Tlili K et al. Les cholangites sclérosantes secondaires et les séquelles biliaires fibrosantes du kyste hydatique du foie. *Med Chir Dig* 1989; 18:467–476.

54 Belghiti J, Benhamou J P, Houry S, Grenier P, Huguier M & Fekete F. Caustic sclerosing cholangitis: a complication of the surgical treatment of hydatid disease of the liver. *Arch Surg* 1986; 121:1162–1165.

55 Schaefer J W & Khan M Y. Echinococcosis (hydatid disease): lessons from experience with 59 patients. *Rev Infect Dis* 1991; 13:243–247.

56 Morris D L. Pre-operative albendazole therapy for hydatid cyst. *Br J Surg* 1987; 74:805–806.

57 French C M. Mebendazole and surgery for human hydatid disease in Turkana. *East Afr Med J* 1984; 61:113–119.

58 Cobo F, Yarnoz C, Sesma B et al. Albendazole plus praziquantel versus albendazole alone as a pre-operative treatment in intra-abdominal hydatisosis caused by *Echinococcus granulosus*. *Trop Med Int Health* 1998; 3:462–466.

59 Little J M, Hollands M J & Ekberg H. Recurrence of hydatid disease. *World J Surg* 1988; 12:700–704.

60 Cangiotti L, Giulini S M, Muiesan P, Begni A & Tiberio G. Hydatid disease of the liver: long-term results of surgical treatment. *J Chir* 1991; 12:501–504.

61 Alper A, Ariogul O, Emre A, Uras A & Oekten A. Choledocho-duodenostomy for intrabiliary rupture of hydatid cysts of liver. *Br J Surg* 1987; 74:243–245.

62 Xynos E, Zoras O-J L, Pechlivanidis G, Neonakis E & Vassilakis J S. Intrabiliary rupture of hydatid cyst of the liver. *Dig Surg* 1990; 7:148–152.

63 Leong S, Kim Y I, Gray R, Kortan P & Haber G. Endoscopic and surgical management of intrabiliary rupture of hydatid liver cyst. *Can J Gastroenterol* 1992; 6:135–139.

64 Iscan M & Duren M. Endoscopic sphincterotomy in the management of postoperative complications of hepatic hydatid disease. *Endoscopy* 1991; 23:282–283.

65 Safioleas M, Misiakos E P, Dosios T, Manti C, Lambrou P & Skalkeas G. Surgical treatment for lung hydatid disease. *World J Surg* 1999; 23:1181–1185.

66 Novick R J, Tchervenkov C I, Wilson J A, Munro D D & Mulder D S. Surgery for thoracic hydatid disease: a North American experience. *Ann Thorac Surg* 1987; 43:681–686.

67 Keshmiri M, Baharvahdat H, Fattahi S H et al. A placebo controlled study of albendazole in the treatment of pulmonary echinococcosis. *Eur Respir J* 1999; 14:503–507.

68 Miralles A, Bracamonte L, Pavie A et al. Cardiac echinococcosis: surgical treatment and results. *J Thorac Cardiovasc Surg* 1994; 107:184–190.

69 Horchani A, Nouira Y, Kbaier I, Attyaoui F & Zribi A S. Hydatid cyst of the kidney: a report of 147 controlled cases. *Eur Urol* 2000; 38:461–467.

70 Magistrelli P, Masetti R, Coppola R, Messia A, Nuzzo G & Picciocchi A. Surgical treatment of hydatid disease of the liver. *Arch Surg* 1991; 126:518–523.

71 Khuroo M S, Wani N A, Javid G et al. Percutaneous drainage compared with surgery for hepatic hydatid cysts. *N Engl J Med* 1997; 337:881–887.

72 Lewall D B & Nyak P. Hydatid cysts of the liver: two cautionary signs. *Br J Radiol* 1998; 71:37–41.

73 Filice C & Brunetti E. Use of PAIR in human cystic echinococcosis. *Acta Trop* 1997; 64:95–107.

74 Odev K, Paksoy Y, Arslan A et al. Sonographically guided percutaneous treatment of hepatid hydatid cysts: long-term results. *J Clin Ultrasound* 2000; 28:469–478.

75 Men S, Hekimoglu B, Yucesoy C, Arda I S & Baran I. Percutaneous treatment of hepatic hydatid cysts: an alternative to surgery. *AJR* 1999; 172:83–89.

76 Ustunsoz B, Akhan O, Kamiloglu M A, Somuncu I, Ugurel M S & Cetiner S. Percutaneous treatment of hydatid cysts of the liver: long-term results. *AJR* 1999; 172:91–96.

77 Chinnery J B & Morris D L. Effect of albendazole sulphoxide on viability of hydatid protoscolices in vitro. *Trans R Soc Trop Med Hyg* 1986; 80:815–817.

78 Taylor D H & Morris D L. Combination chemotherapy is more effective in postspillage prophylaxis for hydatid disease than either albendazole or praziquantel alone. *Br J Surg* 1989; 76:954.

79 Braithwaite P A, Roberts M S, Allan R J & Watson T R. Clinical pharmacokinetics of high dose mebendazole in patients treated for cystic hydatid disease. *Eur J Clin Pharmacol* 1982; 22:161–169.

80 Marriner S E, Morris D L, Dickson B & Bogan J A. Pharmacokinetics of albendazole in man. *Eur J Clin Pharmacol* 1986; 30:705–708.

81 Luder P J, Witassek F, Weigand K, Eckert J & Bircher J. Treatment of cystic echinococcosis (*Echinococcus granulosus*) with mebendazole: assessment of bound and free drug levels in cyst fluid and of parasite vitality in operative specimens. *Eur J Clin Pharmacol* 1985; 28:279–285.

82 Morris D L, Chinnery J B, Geogiou G, Stamatakis G & Golematis B. Penetration of albendazole suphoxide into hydatid cysts. *Gut* 1987; 28:75–80.

83 Luder P J, Siffert B, Witassek F, Meister F & Bircher J. Treatment of hydatid disease with high oral doses of mebendazole: long-term follow-up of plasma mebendazole levels and drug interactions. *Eur J Clin Pharmacol* 1986; 31:443–448.

84 Steiger U, Cotting J & Reichen J. Albendazole treatment of echinococcosis in humans: effects on microsomal metabolism and drug tolerance. *Clin Pharmacol Ther* 1990; 47:347–353.

85 Lange H, Eggers R & Bircher J. Increased systemic availability of albendazole when taken with a fatty meal. *Eur J Clin Pharmacol* 1988; 34:315–317.

86 Cotting J, Zeugin T, Steiger U & Reichen J. Albendazole kinetics in patients with echinococcosis: delayed absorption and impaired elimination in cholestasis. *Eur J Clin Pharmacol* 1990; 38:605–608.

87 Horton R J. Albendazole in treatment of human cystic echinococcosis: 12 years of experience. *Acta Trop* 1997; 64:79–93.

88 Luchi S, Vincenti A, Messina F, Parenti M, Scasso A & Campatelli A. Albendazole treatment of human hydatid tissue. *Scand J Infect Dis* 1997; 29:165–167.

89 Davis A, Dixon H & Pawlowski Z S. Multicentre clinical trials of benzimidazole carbamates in human cystic echinococcosis (phase 2). *Bull World Health Organ* 67:503–508.

90 Aktan A O & Yalin R. Preoperative albendazole treatment for liver hydatid disease decreases the viability of the cyst. *Eur J Gastroenterol Hepatol* 1996; 8:877–879.

91 Gil-Grande L A, Rodriguez-Caabeiro F, Prieto JG et al. Randomised controlled trial of efficacy of albendazole in intra-abdominal hydatid disease. *Lancet* 1993; 342:1269–1272.

92 Messaritakis J, Psychou P, Nicolaidou P, Karpathios T, Syriopoulou B & Fretzayas A. High mebendazole doses in pulmonary and hepatic hydatid disease. *Arch Dis Child* 66:532–533.

93 Morris D L, Dykes P W, Marriner S et al. Albendazole: objective evidence of response in human hydatid disease. *JAMA* 1985; 253:2053–2057.

94 Todorov T, Mechkov G, Vutova K et al. Factors influencing the response to chemotherapy in human cystic echinococcosis. *Bull World Health Organ* 1992; 70:347–358.

95 Franchi C, Di Vico B & Teggi A. Long-term evaluation of patients with hydatidosis treated with benzimidazole carbamates. *Clin Infect Dis* 1999; 29:304–309.

96 Saimot A G, Cremieux A C, Hay J M et al. Albendazole as a potential treatment for human hydatidosis. *Lancet* 1983; ii:652–656.

97 Henrikson T H, Klungsoyr P & Zerihun D. Treatment of disseminated peritoneal hydatid disease with praziquantel. *Lancet* 1989; i:272.

98 Piens M A, Persat F, May F & Mojon M. Praziquantel in human hydatidosis: evaluation by preoperative treatment. *Bull Soc Pathol Exot Filiales* 1989; 82:503–512.

99 Mohamed A E, Yasawy M I & Al Karawi MA. Combined albendazole and praziquantel versus albendazole alone in the treatment of hydatid disease. *Hepatogastroenterology* 1998; 45:1690–1694.

100 Sullivan M, Delbridge L, Reeve T S & Crummer P. Hydatid disease at Royal North Shore Hospital: results of surgical treatment. *Aust NZ J Surg* 1987; 57:177–180.

101 Romig T, Zeyhle E, Macpherson C N L, Rees P H & Were J B O. Cyst growth and spontaneous cure in hydatid disease. *Lancet* 1986; i:861.

102 Kazakos K R & Schantz P M. In *Proceedings of the International Workshop on Alveolar Hydatid Disease*. Atlanta, GA: Department of Health and Human Services, 1990: 13–14.

103 WHO. *Guidelines for Diagnosis, Surveillance and Control of Echinococcosis*. WHO/VPH/ECH.92. Geneva, 1992.

104 Wilson J F & Rausch R L. Alveolar hydatid disease: a review of clinical features of 33 indigenous cases of *E. multilocularis* infection in Alaskan Eskimos. *Am J Trop Med Hyg* 1980; 29:1340–1355.

105 Gottstein B, Lengeler C, Bachmann P et al. Seroepidemiologic survey for alveolar echinococcosis (by Em2 ELISA) of blood donors in an endemic area of Switzerland. *Trans R Soc Trop Med Hyg* 1987; 81:960–964.

106 Bresson-Hadni S, Laplante J, Lenys D et al. Seroepidemiologic screening of *Echinococcus multilocularis* infection in a European area endemic for alveolar echinococcosis. *Am J Trop Med Hyg* 1994; 51:837–846.

107 Romig T, Kratzer W, Kimmig P et al. An epidemiological survey of human alveolar echinococcosis in southwestern Germany. *Am J Trop Med Hyg* 1999; 6:566–573.

108 WHO. *Report of the WHO Informal Consultation on Echinococcus multilocularis research*. WHO/CDS/VPH/88.78. Geneva, 1988.

109 Craig P S, Deshan L, Macpherson C N L et al. A large focus of alveolar echinococcosis in central China. *Lancet* 1992; 340:826–831.

110 Gottstein B & Felleisen R. Protective immune mechanisms against the metacestode of *Echinococcus multilocularis*. *Parasitol Today* 1995; 11:320–326.

111 Rausch R L, Wilson J F, Schantz P M & McMahon B J. Spontaneous death of *Echinococcus multilocularis*: cases diagnosed serologically by Em2-ELISA and clinical significance. *Am J Trop Med Hyg* 1987; 36:576–585.

112 Gottstein B & Hemphill A. Immunopathology in echinococcosis. In Freedman D O (ed.) *Immunopathogenetic Aspects of Disease Induced by Helminth Parasites*. Basel: Karger, 1997: 177–208.

113 Vuitton D A, Bresson-Hadni S, Laroche L et al. Cellular immune

response in *Echinococcus multilocularis* infection in humans. II. Natural killer cell activity and cell subpopulations in the blood and in the periparasitic granuloma of patients with alveolar echinococcosis. *Clin Exp Immunol* 1989; 78:67–74.

114 Sturm D, Menzel J, Gottstein B & Kern P. Interleukin-5 is the predominant cytokine produced by peripheral blood mononuclear cells in alveolar echinococcosis. *Infect Immun* 1995; 63:1688–1697.

115 Gottstein B & Bettens F. Association between HLA-DR13 and susceptibility to alveolar echinococcosis. *J Infect Dis* 1994; 169:1416–1417.

116 Eiermann T H, Bettens F, Tiberghien P et al. HLA and alveolar echinococcosis. *Tissue Antigens* 1998; 52:124–129.

117 Sailer M, Soelder B, Allerberger F, Zaknun D, Feichtinger H & Gottstein B. Alveolar echinococcosis of the liver in a six-year-old girl with AIDS. *J Pediatrics* 1997; 130:320–323.

118 Kamiya H, Kamiya M, Ohbayashi M & Nomura T. Studies on the host resistance to infection with *E. multilocularis*. 1. Difference of susceptibility of various rodents, especially of congenitally athymic nude mice. *Jpn J Parasitol* 1980; 29:87–100.

119 Baron R W & Tanner C E. *Echinococcus multilocularis* in the mouse: the in vitro protoscolicidal activity of peritoneal macrophages. *Int J Parasitol* 1977; 7:489–495.

120 Dai W J & Gottstein B. Nitric oxide-mediated immunosuppression following murine *Echinococcus multilocularis* infection. *Immunology* 1999; 97: 107–116.

121 Gottstein B, Saucy F, Deplazes P et al. Is a high prevalence of *Echinococcus multilocularis* in wild and domestic animals associated with increased disease incidence in humans? *Emerg Infect Dis* 2001; 7:408–412.

122 Condon J, Rausch R L & Wilson J F. Application of the avidin–biotin immunohistochemical method for the diagnosis of alveolar hydatid disease from tissue sections. *Trans R Soc Trop Med Hyg* 1988; 82:731–735.

123 Lanier A P, Trujillo D E, Schantz P M, Wilson J F, Gottstein B & McMahon B. Comparison of serologic tests for the diagnosis and follow-up of alveolar hydatid disease. *Am J Trop Med Hyg* 1987; 37:609–615.

124 Bresson-Hadni S, Petitjean O, Monnot-Jacquard B, Heyd B, Kantelip B, Deschaseaux M, Racadot E & Vuitton D A. Cellular localisations of interleukin-1 beta, interleukin-6 and tumor necrosis factor-alpha mRNA in a parasitic granulomatous disease of the liver, alveolar echinococcosis. *Eur Cytokine Network* 1994; 5:461–468.

125 Kilwinski J, Jenne L, Jellen-Ritter A, Radloff P, Flick W & Kern P. T lymphocyte cytokine profile at a single cell level in alveolar echinococcosis. *Cytokine* 1999; 11:373–381.

126 Wellinghausen N, Gebert P & Kern P. Interleukin (IL)-4, IL-10 and IL-12 profile in serum of patients with alveolar echinococcosis. *Acta Trop* 1999; 73:165–174.

127 Godot V, Harraga S, Deschaseaux M, Bresson-Hadni S, Gottstein B, Emilie D & Vuitton D A. Increased basal production of IL-10 by peripheral blood mononuclear cells in human alveolar echinococcosis. *Eur Cytokine Network* 1997; 8:401–408.

128 Jenne L, Kilwinski J, Radloff P, Flick W & Kern P. Clinical efficacy of and immunologic alterations caused by interferon gamma therapy for alveolar echinococcosis. *Clin Infect Dis* 1998; 26:492–494.

129 Harraga S, Godot V, Bresson-Hadni S, Pater C, Beurton I, Bartholomot B & Vuitton D A. Clinical efficacy of and switch from T helper 2 to T helper 1 cytokine profile after interferon alpha2a monotherapy for human echinococcosis. *Clin Infect Dis* 1999; 29:205–206.

130 Bresson-Hadni S, Vuitton D A, Bartholomot B et al. A twenty-year history of alveolar echinococcosis: analysis of a series of 117 patients from eastern France. *Eur J Gastroenterol Hepatol* 2000; 12(3):327–336.

131 Ali Khan Z & Rausch R L. Demonstration of amyloid and immune complex deposits in renal and hepatic parenchyma of Alaskan alveolar hydatid disease patients. *Ann Trop Med Parasitol* 1987; 81:381–392.

132 Bresson-Hadni S, Miguet J P, Vuitton D et al. L'échinococcose alvéolaire hépatique humaine. *Sem Hôp Paris* 1988; 64:2692–2701.

133 Akinoglu A, Demiryurek H & Guzel C. Alveolar hydatid disease of the liver: a report on thirty-nine surgical cases in eastern Anatolia, Turkey. *Am J Trop Med Hyg* 1991; 45:182–189.

134 Ammann R, Tschudi K, von Ziegler M et al. Langzeitverlauf bei 60 Patienten mit alveolaerer Echinokokkose unter Dauertherapie mit Mebendazol (1976–1985). *Klin Wochenschr* 1988; 66:1060–1073.

135 Etievent J P, Vuitton D, Allemand H, Weill F, Gandjbackhch I & Miguet J P. Pulmonary embolism from a parasitic cardiac clot secondary to hepatic alveolar echinococcosis. *J Cardiovasc Surg* 1986; 27:671–674.

136 Williams D F, Williams G A, Caya J G, Werner R P & Harrison T J. Intraocular *Echinococcus multilocularis*. *Arch Ophthalmol* 1987; 105:1106–1109.

137 Strohmaier W L, Bichler K H, Wilbert D M & Seitz H M. Alveolar echinococcosis with involvement of the ureter and testis. *J Urol* 1990; 144:733–734.

138 Reuter S, Nüssle K, Kolokythas O, Haug U, Rieber A, Kern &, Kratzer W. Alveolar liver echinococcosis: a comparative study of three imaging techniques. *Infection* 2001; 29:119–125.

139 Kasai Y, Koshino I, Kawanishi N, Sakamoto H, Sasaki E & Kumagai M. Alveolar echinococcosis of the liver: studies on 60 operated cases. *Ann Surg* 1980; 192:145–152.

140 Ammann R W, Hoffmann A F & Eckert J. Swiss study of chemotherapy of alveolar echinococcosis: review of a 20-year clinical research project. *Schweiz Med Wochenschr* 1999; 129:323–332.

141 Didier D, Weiler S, Rohmer P et al. Hepatic alveolar echinococcosis: correlative US and CT study. *Radiology* 1985; 154:179–186.

142 Choji K, Fujita N, Chen M et al. Alveolar hydatid disease of the liver: computed tomography and transabdominal ultrasound with histopathological correlation. *Clin Radiol* 1992; 46:97–103.

143 Rozanes I, Acunacs B, Celik L, Minareci O & Gokmen E. CT in lobar atrophy of the liver caused by alveolar echinococcosis. *J Comput Assist Tomogr* 1992; 16:216–218.

144 Claudon M, Bessieres M, Regent D et al. Alveolar echinococcosis of the liver: MR findings. *J Comput Assist Tomogr* 1990; 14:608–614.

145 Duewell S, Marincek B, von Schulthess G K & Ammann R. MRT and CT in alveolar echinococcosis of the liver. *ROFO* 1990; 152:441–445.

146 Diebold-Berger S, Khan H, Gottstein B, Puget E, Frossard J L & Remadi S. Cytologic diagnosis of isolated pancreatic alveolar hydatid disease with immunologic and PCR analyses: a case report. *Acta Cytol* 1997; 41:1381–1386.

147 Kreis R, Bigler P, Gottstein B & Boesch C. 1H-MRS of *Echinococcus granulosus* cysts: succinate, not pyruvate is the characteristic marker substance. In *Proceedings of the VIth Scientific Meeting of the International Society of Magnetic Resonance in Medicine*, Sydney, 18–24 April 1998.

148 Reuter S, Schirrmeister H, Kratzer W, Dreweck C, Reske S N & Kern P. Pericystic metabolic activity in alveolar echinococcosis: assessment and follow-up by positron emission tomography. *Clin Infect Dis* 1999; 29:1157–1163.

149 Lightowlers M & Gottstein B. Immunodiagnosis of echinococcosis. In Thompson R C A & Lymbery A J (eds) *Echinococcus and Hydatid Disease*. Wallingford: CAB International, 1995.

150 Gottstein B. *Echinococcus multilocularis* infection: immunology and immunodiagnosis. *Adv Parasitol* 1992; 31:321–380.

151 Gottstein B, Jacquier P, Bresson-Hadni S & Eckert J. Improved primary immunodiagnosis of alveolar echinococcosis in humans by an enzyme-linked immunosorbent assay using using the Em2plus-antigen. *J Clin Microbiol* 1993; 31:373–376.

152 Ito A, Ma L, Schantz P M et al. Differential serodiagnosis for cystic and alveolar echinococcosis using fractions of *Echinococcus granulosus* cyst fluid (antigen B) and *E. multilocularis* protoscolex (EM18). *A J Trop Med Hyg* 1999; 60:188–192.

153 Felleisen R & Gottstein B. *Echinococcus multilocularis*: molecular and immunochemical characterization of diagnostic antigen II/3-10. *Parasitology* 1993; 107:335–342.

154 Gottstein B, Deplazes P & Aubert M. *Echinococcus multilocularis*: immunological study on the 'Em2-positive' laminated layer during in vitro and in vivo post-oncospheral and larval development. *Parasitol Res* 1992; 78:291–297.

155 Frosch P M, Frosch M, Pfister T, Schaad V & Bitter-Suermann D. Cloning and characterization of an immunodominant major surface antigen of *Echinococcus multilocularis*. *Mol Biochem Parasitol* 1991; 48:121–130.

156 Frosch P M, Geier C, Kaup F J, Muller A & Frosch M. Molecular cloning of an echinococcal microtrichal antigen immunoreactive in *Echinococcus multilocularis* disease. *Mol Biochem Parasitol* 1993; 58:301–310.

157 Ito A, Schantz P M & Wilson J F. Em18, a new serodiagnostic marker for differentiation of active and inactive cases of alveolar hydatid disease. *Am J Trop Med Hyg* 1995; 52:41–44.

158 Ma L, Ito A, Liu Y H et al. Alveolar echinococcosis: Em2plus-ELISA and Em18-western blots for follow-up after treatment with albendazole. *Trans R Soc Trop Med Hyg* 1997; 91:476–478.

159 Lawton P, Hemphill A, Deplazes P, Gottstein B & Sarciron M E. *Echinococcus multilocularis* metacestodes: immunological and immunocytochemical analysis of the relationships between alkaline phosphatase and the Em2 antigen. *Exp Parasitol* 1997; 87:142–149.

160 Sarciron E M, Bresson-Hadni S, Mercier M et al. Antibodies against *Echinococcus multilocularis* alkaline phosphatase as markers for the specific diagnosis and the serological monitoring of alveolar echinococcosis. *Parasite Immunol* 1997; 19:61–68.

161 Lanier A P, Trujillo D E, Schantz P M, Wilson J F, Gottstein B & McMahon B. Comparison of serologic tests for the diagnosis and follow-up of alveolar hydatid disease. *Am J Trop Med Hyg* 1987; 37:609–615.

162 Gottstein B, Tschudi K, Eckert J & Ammann R. Em2-ELISA for the follow-up of alveolar echinococcosis after complete surgical resection of liver lesions. *Trans R Soc Trop Med Hyg* 1989; 83:389–393.

163 Bresson-Hadni S, Franza A, Miguet J P et al. Orthotopic liver transplantation for incurable alveolar echinococcosis of the liver: report of 17 cases. *Hepatology* 1991; 13:1061–1070.

164 Bresson-Hagni S, Miguet J-P, Lenys D et al. Recurrence of alveolar echinococcosis in the liver graft after liver transplantation. *Hepatology* 1992; 16:279–280.

165 Gottstein B & Mowatt M R. Sequencing and characterization of an *Echinococcus multilocularis* DNA probe and its use in the polymerase chain reaction. *Mol Biochem Parasitol* 1991; 44:183–194.

166 Reuter S, Seitz H M, Kern P & Junghanss T. Extrahepatic alveolar echinococcosis without liver involvement: a rare manifestation. *Infection* 2000; 28:187–192.

167 Kern P, Frosch P, Helbig M et al. Diagnosis of *Echinococcus multilocularis* infection by reverse-transcription polymerase chain reaction. *Gastroenterology* 1995; 109:596–600.

168 Partensky C, Landraud R, Valette P-J, Bret P & Paliard P. Radical and nonradical hepatic resection for alveolar echinococcosis: report of 18 cases. *World J Surg* 1990; 14:654–659.

169 Aydin Y, Barlas O, Yolacs C et al. Alveolar hydatid disease of the brain: report of four cases. *J Neurosurg* 1986; 65:115–119.

170 Gottstein B, Bettens F, Parkinson A J & Wilson F. Immunological parameters associated with susceptibility or resistance to alveolar hydatid disease in Yupiks/Inupiats. *Arctic Med Res* 1996; 55:14–19.

171 Taylor D H, Morris D L, Reffin D & Richards K S. Comparison of albendazole, mebendazole and praziquantel chemotherapy of *Echinococcus multilocularis* in a gerbil model. *Gut* 1989; 30:1401–1405.

172 Schantz P M, Van den Bossche H & Eckert J. Chemotherapy for larval echinococcosis in animals and humans: report of a workshop. *Z Parasitenkd* 1982; 67:5–26.

173 Davis A, Pawlowski Z S & Dixon H. Multicentre clinical trials of benzimidazolecarbamates in human echinococcosis. *Bull World Health Organ* 1986; 64:383–388.

174 Kern P. Human echinococcosis: follow-up of 23 patients treated with mebendazole. *Infection* 1983; 11:17–24.

175 Rausch R L, Wilson J F, McMahon B J & O'Gorman M A. Consequences of continuous mebendazole therapy in alveolar hydatid disease: with a summary of a ten-year clinical trial. *Ann Trop Med Parasitol* 1986; 80:403–419.

176 Wilson J F, Rausch R L, McMahon B J, Schantz P M, Trujillo D E & O'Gorman M. Albendazole therapy in alveolar hydatid disease: a report of favorable results in two patients after short-term therapy. *Am J Trop Med Hyg* 1987; 37:162–168.

177 Liu Y H, Wang X G & Chen Y T. Preliminary observation of continuous albendazole therapy in alveolar echinococcosis. *Chin Med J [Engl]* 1991; 104:930–933.

178 Reuter S, Jensen B, Buttenschoen K, Kratzer W & Kern P. Benzimidazoles in the treatment of alveolar echinococcosis: a comparative study and review of the literature. *J Antimicrob Chemother* 2000; 46:451–456.

179 Luder P J, Robotti G, Meister F P & Bircher J. High oral doses of mebendazole interfere with growth of larval echinococcus multilocularis lesions. *J Hepatol* 1985; 1:369–377.

180 Wang X, Liu Y & Yu D. Continuous therapy with albendazole for hepatic alveolar echinococcosis associated with obstructive jaundice. *Chung Hua Nei Ko Tsa Chih* 1996; 35:261–264.

181 Wilson J F, Rausch R L, McMahon B J & Schantz P M. Parasiticidal effect of chemotherapy in alveolar hydatid disease: review of experience with mebendazole and albendazole in Alaskan Eskimos. *Clin Infect Dis* 1992; 15:234–249.

182 Ammann R W, Hirsbrunner R, Cotting J, Steiger U, Jacquier P & Eckert J. Recurrence rate after discontinuation of long-term mebendazole therapy in alveolar echinococcosis (preliminary results). *Am J Trop Med Hyg* 1990; 43:506–515.

183 Reichen J, Cotting J & Steiger U. Pharmaco-therapy of hepatic hydatid disease. In Bianchi L, Gerok W, Maier K P & Deinhardt F (eds) *Infectious Diseases of the Liver*. Dordrecht: Kluwer, 1990: 235–245.

184 Ammann R W. Improvement of liver resectional therapy by adjuvant chemotherapy in alveolar hydatid disease. Swiss Echinococcosis Study Group (SESG). *Parasitol Res* 1991; 77:290–293.

185 Rausch R L & D'Alessandro A. Histogenesis in the metacestode of Echinococcus vogeli and mechanism of pathogenesis in polycystic hydatid disease. *J Parasitol* 1999; 85:410–418.

186 D'Alessandro A, Rausch R L, Cuello C & Aristizabal N. *Echinococcus vogeli* in man, with a review of polycystic hydatid disease in Colombia and neighbouring countries. *Am J Trop Med Hyg* 1979; 28:303–317.

187 Meneghelli U G, Martinelli A L C, Llorach V M A, Bellucci A D, Magro J E & Barbo M L P. Polycystic hydatid disease (*Echinococcus vogeli*): clinical, laboratory and morphological findings in nine Brazilian patients. *J Hepatol* 1992; 14:203–210.

188 Gottstein B, D'Alessandro A & Rausch R L. Immunodiagnosis of polycystic hydatid disease/polycystic echinococcosis due to *Echinococcus vogeli*. *Am J Trop Med Hyg* 1995; 53:558–563.

189 Meneghelli U G, Martinelli A L C, Bellucci A D et al. Polycystic hydatid disease (*Echinococcus vogeli*): treatment with albendazole. *Ann Trop Med Parasitol* 1992; 86:151–156.

190 Lopera R D, Melendez R D, Fernandez I, Sirit J & Perera M P. Orbital hydatid cyst of *Echinococcus oligarthrus* in a human in Venezuela. *J Parasitol* 1989; 75:467–470.

191 D'Alessandro A, Ramirez L E, Chapadeiro E, Lopes E R & de Mesquita P M. Second recorded case of human infection by *Echinococcus oligarthrus*. *Am J Trop Med Hyg* 1995; 52:29–33.

192 Basset D, Girou C, Nozais I P, D'Hermies F, Hoang C, Gordon R & D'Alessandro A. Neotropical echinococcosis in Suriname: *Echinococcus oligarthrus* in the orbit and *Echinococcus vogeli* in the abdomen. *Am J Trop Med Hyg* 1998; 59:787–790.

193 Sahni J K, Jain M, Bajaj Y, Kumar V & Jain A. Submandibular hydatid cyst caused by *Echinococcus oligarthrus*. *J Laryngol Otol* 2000; 114:473–476.

194 Akhan O, Özmen M N, Dincer A, Sayek I & Göçmen A. Liver hydatid disease: long-term results of percutaneous treatment. *Radiology* 1996; 198:259–265.

195 Erzurumlu K, Hokelek M, Gonlusen L, Tas K & Amanvermez R. The effect of albendazole on the prevention of secondary hydatidosis. *Hepatogastroenterology* 2000; 47:247–250.

196 Nahmias J, Goldsmith R, Soibelman M & Elon J. Three- to 7-year follow-up after albendazole treatment of 68 patients with cystic echinococcosis (hydatid disease). *Ann Trop Med Parasitol* 1994; 88:295–304.

Chapter 85

Other Cestode Infections: Intestinal cestodes, cysticercosis, other larval cestode infections

G. G. Baily

Tapeworms or cestodes are an ancient class of highly specialized flatworm parasites. Their ancestors diverged from free-living flatworms to parasitize the earliest vertebrates in Cambrian times, and subsequently followed all the complexities of vertebrate evolution so that there are now innumerable species subtly adapted to the behaviour, diet and immunology of their hosts. Most cestodes require at least two host species to support the different stages of their life cycles. Adult tapeworms inhabit the gut of a vertebrate animal (the definitive host), with four species adapted specifically to humans. The tapeworm consists of a scolex equipped with suckers, grooves (bothria) or hooks which are the means of attachment to the intestinal wall. This is connected by an actively growing neck region (the strobila) to a chain of a variable number of segments or proglottides which are progressively more mature towards the distal end of the worm. The mature proglottides, which form the bulk of the worm, are largely composed of hermaphrodite sexual organs and generate large numbers of eggs. A single *Taenia saginata* adult, for example, may produce 50 000 eggs daily for 10 years or more.

Cyclophyllidean cestodes typically have an exclusively terrestrial life cycle with a single intermediate host, which may be vertebrate or invertebrate. The intermediate host is infected by ingesting eggs which hatch into invasive larvae (oncospheres) in the gut, migrate into the host tissues and develop into one of the many distinctive, often cyst-like, morphologies of cestode larvae. The life cycle is completed when the intermediate host is eaten by a suitable definitive host in which the protoscolex of the larva can develop in the gut into a new adult tapeworm.

The pseudophyllidean cestodes have a more complex life cycle. The first intermediate host is typically an aquatic invertebrate which is infected by the procercoid larval stage of the parasite. When the invertebrate is ingested by a suitable second intermediate host, likely to be a fish or reptile, the parasite develops into an invasive, worm-like, plerocercoid larva. This may then ascend the food chain through a series of further second intermediate hosts until finally reaching a suitable carnivorous vertebrate definitive host in which it can develop into an adult tapeworm. Tapeworms and larvae from both these cestode families can infect humans.

Because the relationship between the parasite and its host is central to the survival and propagation of the worm, but likely to be of more marginal significance to the host population, phenomena related to this ancient and highly adapted parasitism tend to have evolved predominantly according to the needs of the worm. Thus it is in the interests of the propagation of the worm that its definitive host should be long lived and active, disseminating eggs as widely as possible. Tapeworm infections tend, therefore, to be of trivial importance to the health of the host. In contrast, the worm's life cycle is completed only when the infected intermediate host is eaten, which may well occur more readily if the function of the intermediate host is disrupted. Larval cestode infections are consequently amongst the most serious helmintic diseases.

Cysticercosis

Transmission

Cysticercosis consists of infection with the small, bladder-like larvae of the pork tapeworm, *Taenia solium*. The life cycle of this parasite is maintained between the human, the only definitive host able to harbour the adult tapeworm, and pigs infected with cysticerci (Figure 85.1). Unfortunately humans can also readily be infected with cysticerci and this is the cause of all the significant morbidity associated with the parasite. The tapeworms are acquired through eating undercooked pork containing cysticerci. Human cysticercosis, however, is a faecal–oral infection acquired by ingesting eggs excreted in the faeces of a human tapeworm carrier. Individuals harbouring an adult *T. solium* are at high risk of acquiring cysticercosis, probably through faecal–oral autoinfection. It has long been hypothesized that internal autoinfection might also occur as a result of reverse peristalsis, allowing taenia eggs to travel from the small bowel to the stomach and thus become activated and invasive. Little evidence has emerged to support this.

Cysticercosis was originally a ubiquitous disease occurring wherever pigs and humans existed in association, and is probably of great antiquity: Aristotle gives a clear description of the condition in pigs. It was once common in central Europe, with autopsy rates of 2% in Berlin[1] in the first half of the nineteenth century, coinciding closely with the 1.9% now described in Mexico City, an area of current high prevalence.[2] The parasite has

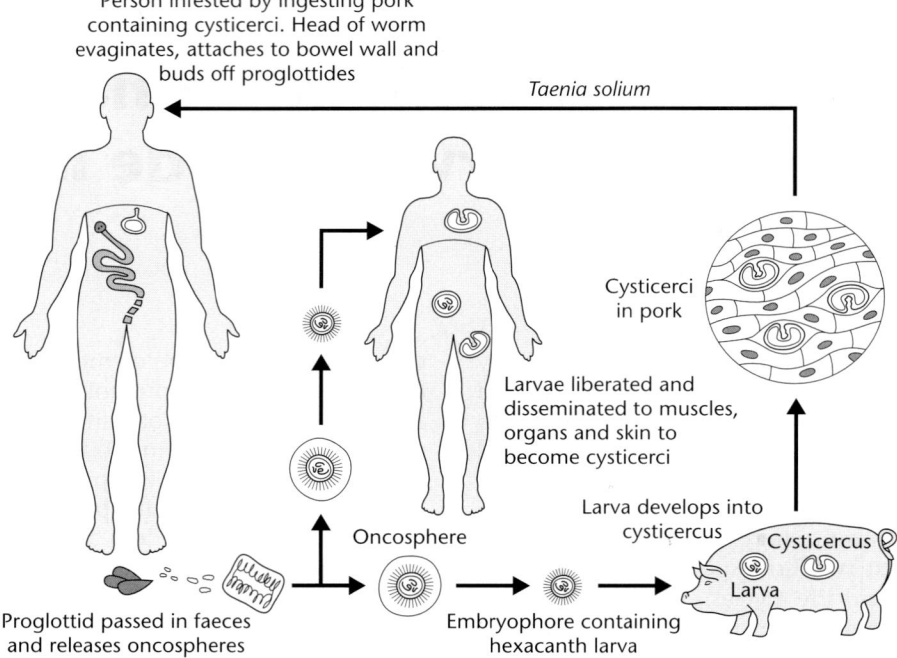

Person infested by ingesting pork containing cysticerci. Head of worm evaginates, attaches to bowel wall and buds off proglottides

Taenia solium

Cysticerci in pork

Larvae liberated and disseminated to muscles, organs and skin to become cysticerci

Larva develops into cysticercus

Cysticercus

Larva

Oncosphere

Proglottid passed in faeces and releases oncospheres

Embryophore containing hexacanth larva

Figure 85.1: The life cycle of *T. solium*. (Courtesy of Tropical Resources Unit, Wellcome Trust.)

long since been all but eradicated from the most developed countries but it remains common in Central and South America, southern Asia and China. It appears to have a patchy distribution in Africa, with some areas of very high prevalence, but is rare in the Islamic countries of North Africa and south-west Asia. In the 1970s an epidemic of cysticercosis occurred amongst the highland people of Irian Jaya[3] after the introduction of the parasite into a culture where pigs are of central importance and hygiene is primitive. The problem was first identified because of a dramatic increase in the incidence of severe burns related to individuals falling into domestic fires whilst fitting.

Pathology

Ingested taenia eggs, activated by gastric and duodenal environments, develop into invasive larvae, termed oncospheres, in the small intestine. These migrate across the intestinal wall and are probably carried by the bloodstream to the sites at which they eventually settle and mature into cysticerci, a process that takes approximately 2 months. Although cysticerci may occur anywhere in the body, the distribution is not random. There is a preference for subcutaneous tissues, muscle and the central nervous system. The basis of this tropism, as with other migratory larval helminths, is not understood. Cystercerci vary from a few millimetres to 2 cm or more across, but are typically a little less than 1 cm, the largest cysts tending to be intracranial, particularly in the ventricles and the larger subarachnoid spaces. Established cysticerci that are neither actively growing nor degenerating elicit very little host immune response. The typical

appearances in the brain is of the cyst surrounded by compressed, laminated host tissue with only a slight inflammatory infiltrate.[4] Dead, calcified or hyalinized cysts may be surrounded by a similar host-derived capsule. However, new, very large or degenerating cysts may all be associated with a much more extensive inflammatory response.

Clinical features

The morbidity of cysticercosis is almost entirely due to central nervous system disease. Subcutaneous cysts are of only cosmetic significance. A heavy parasite load in muscle may give rise to some aching,[5] but this is not common. Serious problems are confined to those anatomical sites where a small space-occupying lesion, with or without some inflammation, can give rise to a major disturbance in function. Such sites include the eye and, very rarely, the conducting system of the heart, but overwhelmingly neurocysticercosis is the principal clinical problem.

Neurocysticercosis

Although autopsy rates for neurocysticercosis in areas of high prevalence may approach 2%, the majority of these cases have had no symptoms in life attributable to the infection.[2] When symptoms do occur, much the most common manifestation is epilepsy. Studies from endemic areas suggest that cysticercosis is a major cause of epilepsy, accounting for up to a half of late-onset cases,[6–8] and it is particularly prominent as a cause of focal epilepsy in children. However, any neurological syndrome attributable to one or more small space-occupying lesions can occur, including focal weakness and extrapyramidal disorders. Changes in mental state, including cognitive impairment and psychiatric disease, are also very common.[9]

Meningitis
Careful dissection in post-mortem series has shown that 80% of intracranial cysticerci are in contact with the meninges.[4] As they are often sited deep in the cerebral sulci, this may not be apparent from in vivo imaging. It is not, therefore, surprising that some abnormality of the cerebrospinal fluid (CSF) is found in approximately 50% of cases of neurocysticercosis—usually a mild pleocytosis or raised protein level. However, in a minority of cases the clinical presentation may fall within the territory of chronic meningitis, with headache and global changes in cerebral function associated with markedly abnormal CSF findings. Fever, neck stiffness and cranial nerve palsies are not features. Thus, more than 5% of cases of chronic or subacute meningitis in childhood were attributed to cysticercosis in a series from southern India.[10] A persistently high CSF protein concentration is associated with a poor prognosis, often with progression to hydrocephalus and, without surgical intervention, consequent dementia and blindness.

Encephalitis
When there are many lesions in the brain, and particularly if the inflammatory response is brisk, the presentation may resemble subacute encephalitis.[11] In children, in particular, the inflammatory response may dominate the clinical picture, with a rapidly progressive illness over a few weeks characterized by fitting, a variety of focal neurological abnormalities, deteriorating cognitive function and raised intracranial pressure.

Ventricular disease
Intraventricular cysts occur in about 15% of cases[4] and can cause diagnostic difficulties. They give rise to episodes of obstructive hydrocephalus which may spontaneously remit and recur as a result of the ball-valve effect of cysticerci intermittently occluding the ventricular outlet foramina. Untreated, however, most cases will progress to sustained hydrocephalus.

Spinal disease
A variety of spinal cord syndromes has been reported in association with cysts in and around the cord and the cauda equina. The most common presentation is of progressive paraplegia developing over a period of weeks.

Disappearing lesions
There have been reports, mainly from India, of single small enhancing lesions on computed tomography (CT), seen commonly in patients presenting for the first time with epilepsy but disappearing within a few months of follow-up. Many causes have been suggested for these lesions, including tuberculosis, but it seems from both serological evidence and a limited series of excision biopsies[12] that cysticerci are most often responsible.

Ocular cysticercosis
The parasite appears to have a tropism for the eye, although estimates of the incidence of ocular disease vary widely. Shanchez Fontan has described a series of 70 cases of ocular disease from Mexico.[4] The great majority of cysts were subretinal or in the vitreous humour, but they could occur at any site. The initial presentation is most often as a scotoma but, if the inflammatory reaction is marked, vision may be lost.

Diagnosis
The clinical diagnosis of neurocysticercosis is often difficult as there is nothing specific about the neurological presentation. The presence of extracranial cysticerci may provide an important clue to the diagnosis. Subcutaneous cysts (Figure 85.2) can be palpated and, if in doubt, excised for histological examination. Cysts in striated muscle are in a more stressful environment than those in the central nervous system, and die and calcify more rapidly. Spindle-shaped calcifications, particularly in the large proximal muscles (Figure 85.3), may be visible on radiography. However, such clues are often absent. Spinal cysticerci may be demonstrated on myelography (see Figure 85.5). Otherwise, support for the diagnosis must be obtained from serology or by imaging the parasites within the brain.

Serological diagnosis
Many serological methods have been described for cysticercosis using most of the conventional

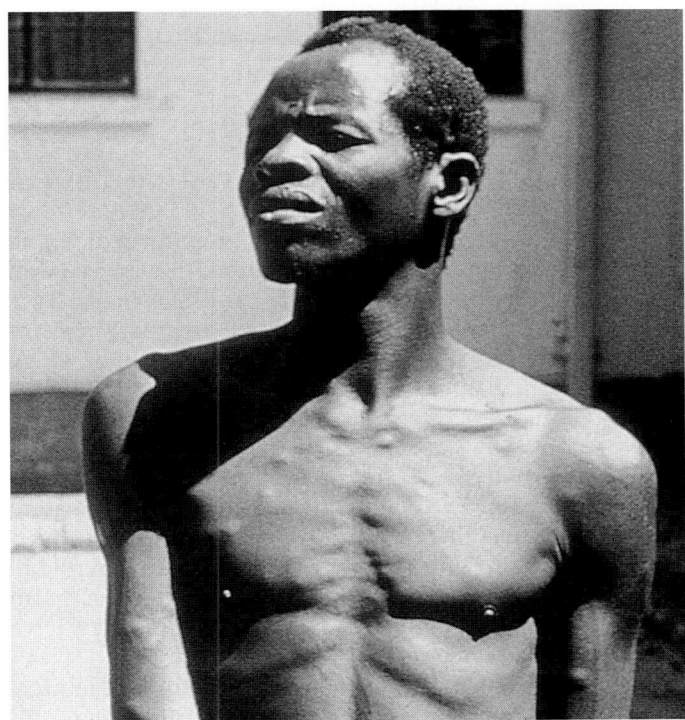

Figure 85.2: Readily visible subcutaneous cysticerci. (Courtesy of Tropical Resources Unit, Wellcome Trust)

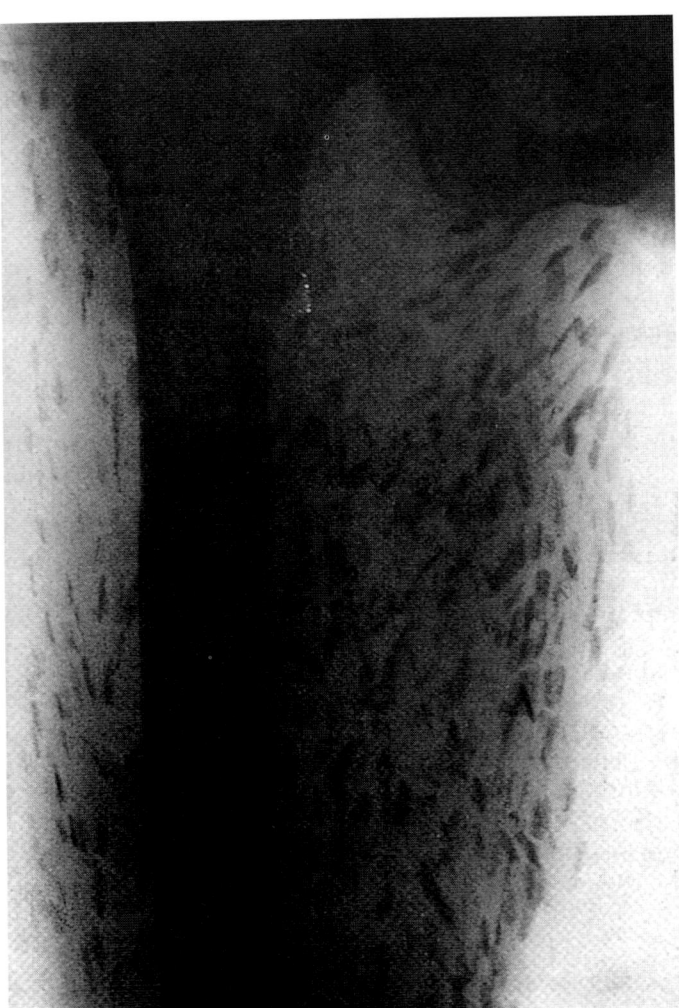

Figure 85.3: Very large numbers of calcified cysticerci in thigh muscle.

serodiagnostic techniques and a wide variety of antigens. Enzyme-linked immunosorbent assays (ELISAs) are most widely used. Antigens have varied from extracts of whole *T. solium* cysts or cyst fluid[13] to purified fractions[14] and recombinant proteins.[15] Sensitivity and specificity vary according to the population studied, the performance being less impressive in areas of high endemicity or where other helminths are prevalent. Sensitivity with present ELISA techniques exceeds 80% even in endemic areas. Cross-reactivity with other helmintic infections, particularly hydatidosis and taeniasis, remains a problem but has been reduced with the careful selection of more refined antigens.[14] The detection of antibodies or antigen in the CSF in combination with conventional serology marginally improves overall sensitivity. Antigen can also be detected in the blood, and declining serum levels have been associated with successful treatment.[16]

Even the simpler serological tests are a valuable clinical tool. In endemic areas they can be used to screen epileptic and other neurological patients. Positive cases can be confirmed by imaging and may then benefit from specific treatment. In a series of 630 patients seen at neurology clinics in Zimbabwe, 12% had antibodies detected by ELISA. The test had a positive predictive value of 87% and a negative predictive value of 85% for active neurocysticercosis potentially amenable to treatment.[17]

Imaging

Modern imaging techniques have proved very powerful in demonstrating the presence of cysticerci in the brain and have also taught us a good deal about the natural history of the disease. A number of appearances have been described on CT (Figure 85.4):

- Calcified lesions.
- Small (< 2 cm) hypodense lesions.
- Similar hypodense lesions with a bright central spot representing the protoscolex within the cyst. This is visible in a little under half of such lesions.
- Similar-sized lesions showing ring or disc enhancement. The natural history of these enhancing lesions is that they are likely to disappear from the CT image within 12 months.
- Occasionally there may be much larger cysts, up to 6 cm across, in which case other cestode larvae such as hydatid and coenurosis as well as racemose cysticercosis (see below) should be considered.

Magnetic resonance imaging has also proved valuable,[18] particularly, as with other pathologies, in demonstrating posterior fossa and spinal lesions. It is also superior for imaging ventricular cysts which, having a

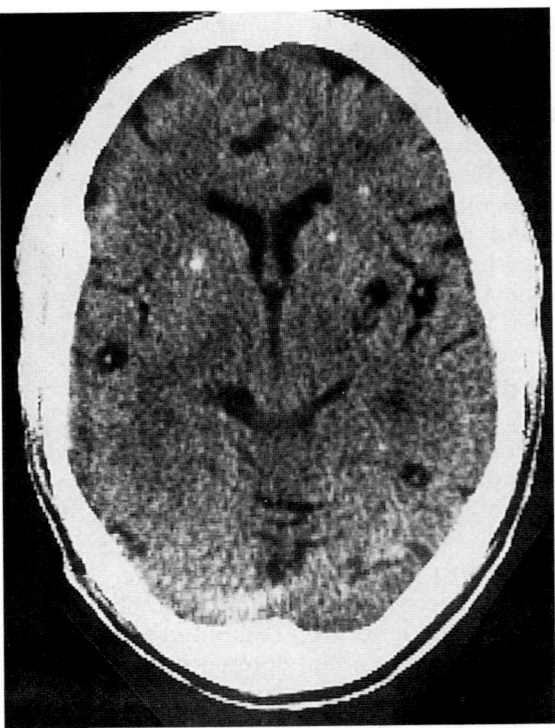

Figure 85.4: CT image of the head showing calcified and viable cerebral cysticerci, some with the protoscolex visible as a central opacity.

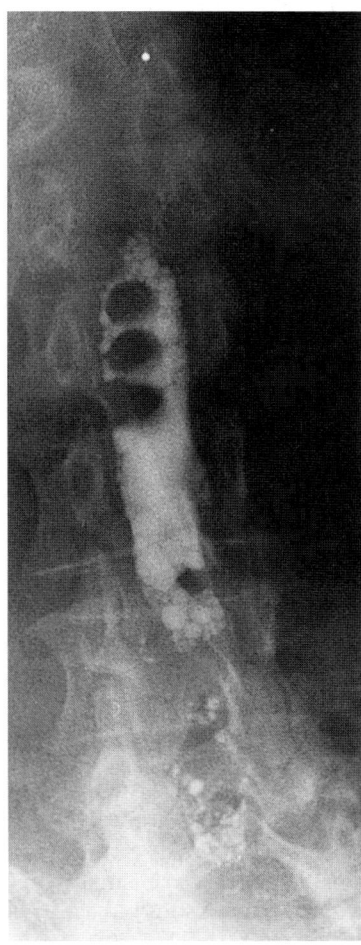

Figure 85.5: Cysticerci around the cauda equina on myelography.

similar radiodensity to CSF, are not easily visualized by means of CT.

Management

Until the 1980s there was no drug therapy that was known to be effective against cysticercosis. Treatment was therefore mostly symptomatic, although surgical inter-vention to remove cysts or to deal with their con-sequences, such as hydrocephalus, was sometimes appropriate. Since that time it has been shown that anthelmintics can be effective both in reducing the number of cysts present on CT[19] and in eliminating subcutaneous cysts.[20] The extent to which this leads to clinical benefit is more problematical and the exact role of anthelmintics remains the subject of debate. In adults with parenchymal cysts demonstrated by CT which do not show significant enhancement, there is evidence of both radiographical and clinical improvement after anthelmintic treatment.[19] In almost all other groups of patients, however, information is either contradictory or lacking. Patients with calcified cysts on CT, even though they may persist in having epilepsy, are unlikely to gain any benefit from anthelmintic treatment. Markedly enhancing parenchymal lesions, which constitute the

most common appearance in children, have been shown to disappear spontaneously from the CT image within a year.[21] From this observation it has been suggested that children can generally be managed with symptomatic treatment and corticosteroids to reduce the local inflammatory response and that anthelmintics are unnecessary.[22] This very benign view of childhood cysticercosis reflects experience with imported disease in North America. In contrast, reports from tropical countries have shown that a proportion of children have chronic disease and frequently relapsing symptoms; some of these develop severe neurological consequences such as hydrocephalus.[23] Whether enhancing lesions that disappear from the CT image have truly gone or have simply ceased to be visible because of a decrease in the inflammatory response is also a matter for debate.[23] Each case must be judged on its merits but on the available evidence it would seem reasonable that enhancing parenchymal lesions present in a child can be managed without specific anticysticercal therapy but with close follow-up.

The first drug to be shown to be effective was praziquantel, given at a dose 50 mg/kg daily for 15 days.[19] Albendazole has also been used extensively, and in substantial doses (15 mg/kg daily for 1 month) appears to have at least an equivalent effect on reducing cysts present on CT.[24,25] The ideal dose of both drugs remains uncer-tain. Eight days of albendazole appears to be of equivalent efficacy to the original 1 month[24] and has been widely adopted. Much shorter courses of praziquantel (e.g., 50 mg/kg daily for 8 days or even three doses of 25 mg/kg at 2-hourly intervals on a single day)[26] have been shown to be effective in small numbers of cases. These shorter courses of anthelmintics, repeated after a period of months if necessary, offer the promise of a less expensive regimen for developing countries.

The significant adverse effects of anticysticercal therapy are similar for the two drugs. They appear to be related directly to the damage inflicted on cysticerci and the consequent acute inflammatory response. This may result in cerebral oedema and raised intracranial pressure, particularly if there are many cysts. Typically, a severe headache arises—sometimes within a few hours of com-mencing therapy but more often after 2–4 days. If treated symptomatically most of these will resolve without sequelae but a minority of patients develop a severe acute illness. Cerebral infarction and death has been reported.[20] Concomitant use of corticosteroids in substantial doses is effective in suppressing this in most (although not all) cases. Steroids also have the unwanted effect of decreasing levels of praziquantel, although not the level of albendazole.[27] Although it has not been universally adopted, on balance the use of high-dose corticosteroids with anticysticercal treatment appears to be the safest option.

Surgical excision is still conventionally recommended for intraventricular cysts, although reports exist of success-ful medical treatment.[28] Information on the use of anthel-mintics in meningeal and spinal disease remains limited.

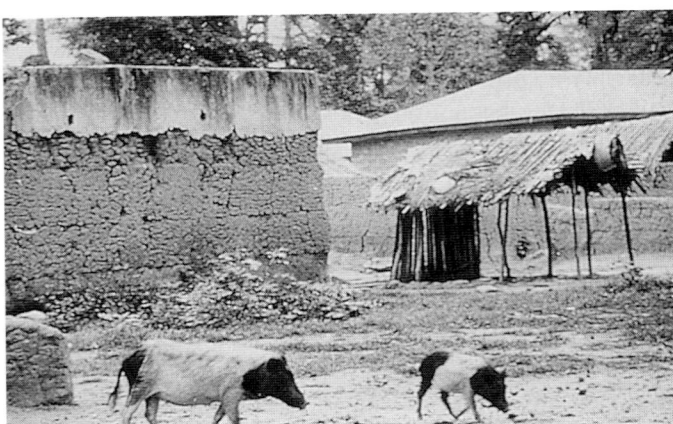

Figure 85.6: Pigs scavenging for food in an African village. (Courtesy of Tropical Resources Unit, Wellcome Trust.)

Control

Control of the parasite has been achieved in developed countries by the interruption of its life cycle at two points. The systematic inspection of pork meat and the removal of infected carcasses from the food chain effectively prevent human tapeworm infection. In addition, improvements in public health have ensured the sanitary disposal of human faeces, and eliminated the source of infection for both human and porcine cysticercosis. In contrast, in developing countries pigs often live in close association with humans, rooting around for food within village compounds (Figure 85.6), and in some areas are deliberately fed human faeces. Animals are likely to be slaughtered within the village and there may be no understanding of the health significance of 'measely' pig meat. The difficulties of introducing good sanitation and modern abattoir practices into poor communities are considerable. An alternative strategy has been to reduce tapeworm carriage by mass chemotherapy and this has been shown to reduce both human taeniasis and porcine cysticercosis.[29] In Africa there is hope that transmission could be reduced as a byproduct of mass treatment campaigns using praziquantel directed against schistosomiasis.

Racemose cysticercosis

Occasionally cestode larvae that are not easily ascribed to any particular parasite are found in the human brain. One characteristic appearance is of a cluster of interconnected grape-like cysts that have no identifiable protoscolex; they are usually situated in the cisterna magna or the ventricles and are often of considerable bulk. This is known as racemose cysticercus. As it is the protoscolex that provides much of the basis for the identification of larval cestodes, it has been difficult to be certain from which parasite racemose cysticerci are derived. Some appear to resemble cases of proven human coenurosis due to T. multiceps,[30] except for the absence of scolices. A similar sterile budding coenurus has been observed in an immunosuppressed mouse deliberately infected with T.

serialis.[31] However, circumstantial evidence suggests that most cases of racemose cysticercosis are due to the aberrant development of T. solium cysticerci. Pathological series show that typical T. solium cysticerci and racemose cysticerci are often found in the same individual, and occasionally intermediate forms with a single bud and a degenerating scolex can be found.[2]

Racemose cysticercosis is a serious condition frequently leading to hydrocephalus, as well as producing local inflammatory and mass effects. Limited experience with praziquantel suggests that medical therapy is difficult and that surgery may retain a place in management.[32]

Other larval cestode infections

Coenurosis

Taenia multiceps is a parasite of dogs, with sheep being the principal intermediate host. The larval metacestode takes the form of a coenurus, a single cyst with multiple invaginated protoscolices which may grow to be several centimetres in diameter. In sheep these often develop in the hindbrain, giving rise to the condition known as 'staggers'. Other closely related Taenia species also give rise to a coenurus which may be morphologically indistinguishable. Human coenurosis is a rare but often serious condition. The parasite has a tropism for the brain and eye, although many extracranial sites have also been described.

Prevalence and distribution

Cases have been reported from a wide geographical area but are nowhere other than rare. Most reports have been from Africa and South America, although there have also been cases in Europe (notably Sardinia) and North America. Extracranial localization has been most frequent in reports from tropical Africa, whilst reports from South Africa and elsewhere have been almost entirely of central nervous system involvement, giving rise to the suspicion that there is some heterogeneity amongst the causative parasites.[33]

Clinical features

Neurological features are those of a substantial intracranial mass lesion accompanied by varying degrees of inflammation. The cisterna magna is a particularly common site, and is associated with basal arachnoiditis and hydrocephalus. Untreated, there is usually progressive neurological disease and a poor outcome. Eye involvement may result in loss of vision.

Diagnosis and management

Intracranial lesions appear on CT as clear cysts 2 cm or more in diameter without a discernable internal structure. Definitive diagnosis can be made only by histological examination; it is distinguished from cysticercosis and hydatidosis by the presence of both multiple protoscolices and a ridged cuticle. Occasionally the protoscolices may have degenerated, in which case the condition is difficult to distinguish from racemose cysticercosis. Surgical excision has been curative in some cases. Although praziquantel appears to be effective against the parasite, the clinical benefits are less clear.[34]

Taenia crassiceps cysticercosis

Rodents are the preferred host for the cysticerci of this parasite but rare human infections have been reported, most recently in association with acquired immune deficiency syndrome (AIDS). A developing soft tissue mass is found to contain numerous cysticerci. Continuous treatment for 6 months with praziquantel and albendazole, both in high doses, gave clinical remission in one reported case, but relapse occurred on cessation of therapy.[35]

Sparganosis

Plerocercoid larvae of the *Spirometra* genus of pseudo-phyllidean cestodes are capable of infecting humans. These organisms resemble *Diphyllobothrium* spp. in their life cycles, with canines or other terrestrial carnivores as definitive hosts, a procercoid larval stage in the water flea *Cyclops*, and plerocercoids naturally infecting reptiles, amphibians and small mammals. Human sparganosis has been attributed to several species, including *S. mansoni, S. mansonoides* and, in Africa, *S. theileri*. Human infection occurs either by the ingestion of procercoid-infected invertebrates in drinking water, by ingestion of plerocercoids through eating uncooked frogs or snakes or possibly by direct transfer of a plerocercoid from fresh frog or snake tissue applied to wounds or inflamed eyes, as is the custom in some parts of eastern Asia. The plerocercoid, or sparganum, is a motile worm of very variable size (between 1 and 50 cm) but is more typically a few centimetres in length and 1–2 mm in width (Figure 85.7). It excites a brisk inflammatory response as it migrates through host tissues; in some instances it is found to be contained within a cyst or abscess cavity. Multiple infections occur.

Prevalence and distribution

This is an uncommon condition but has been recorded very widely in the tropics and subtropics. South-East Asia and East Africa are the areas of highest prevalence. Autochthonous cases are reported from North and South America.

Clinical features

The typical history is of inflammatory, sometimes migratory, subcutaneous swellings. These may break down to discharge the worm. Eosinophilia is common

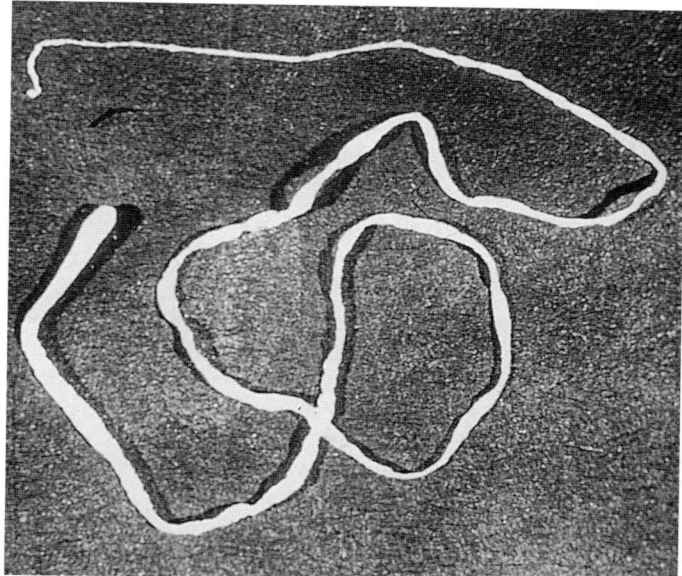

Figure 85.7: *Spirometra mansonoides.* Plerocercoid larva. (Courtesy of H. Zaiman.)

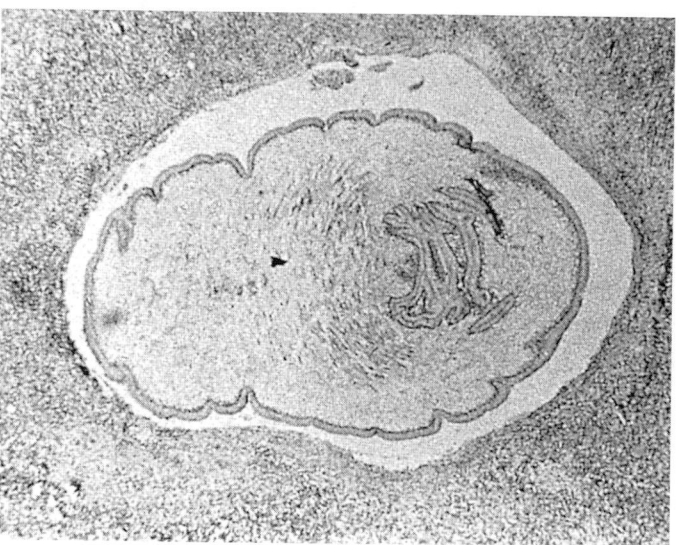

Figure 85.8: Sparganosis. Cross-section showing typical tapeworm morphology. A dense eosinophilic infiltration is present in the adjacent muscle. (Courtesy of H. Zaiman.)

but not invariable (Figure 85.8). The most frequently described sites are the chest and legs. Involvement of the periorbital tissues may cause damage to the eye. Penetration of larvae into the brain—where they cause an intense local inflammatory lesion with invariably major neurological consequences—is uncommon but well described.[36]

Diagnosis and management

The condition must be distinguished from that caused by other migratory helminths producing swellings, such as in gnathostomiasis and loiasis. Serological methods have been developed but they are not specific. Excision and identification of the worm remains necessary for a clear diagnosis. Excision is also the only effective treatment of the parasite, wherever situated, including the brain. No drug therapy has been shown to be beneficial and the killing of the worm within the tissues may not in any case be a desirable goal as it is likely to lead to much more intense inflammation in the short term.

Proliferative sparganosis

A very rare variant of sparganosis has been described, from both Asia and the Americas, in which the parasite buds and proliferates, either as an expanding mass or as multiple small disseminated lesions. Clinically there may be numerous small cutaneous nodules or larger painful tumours. The lesions contain worm-derived structures, some clearly resembling a typical sparganum but of very variable morphology. The condition is slowly progressive, with death resulting from deep organ involvement. There is no known treatment; praziquantel and mebendazole failed in one case.[37]

Tapeworms of humans

Taenia saginata

T. saginata is the beef tapeworm (Figure 85.9). The human is the only definitive host, and cattle are the significant intermediate hosts (Figure 85.10), although a variety of ungulates have been reported as being infected. The larval stage is a translucent fluid-filled bladder or cysticercus between 5 and 10 mm in diameter but, unlike the *T. solium* cysticercus, it has never been described reliably in a human. The adult is a large, white tapeworm that can reach 10 m in length, although more typically 2–5 m, weighing around 20–30 g. The scolex is equipped with suckers but not hooks (Figure 85.11). Mature proglottides detached from the distal end of the worm are highly motile and their independent emergence from the anus is the principal cause of symptomatology. An infected individual commonly harbours more than one worm. Human infection is acquired by eating undercooked beef. Cattle are infected when their feed or grazing is contaminated by human faeces.

Prevalence and distribution

Originally a ubiquitous parasite, transmission has been prevented in developed countries by the sanitary disposal of human faeces and the detection of infected meat at abattoirs. *T. saginata* remains common elsewhere, especially in poorer communities where raw or undercooked beef is traditionally eaten. Highland Ethiopia is an area of intense transmission.

Clinical features

T. saginata carriers are often aware of motile proglottides which can be felt emerging from the anus unbidden and

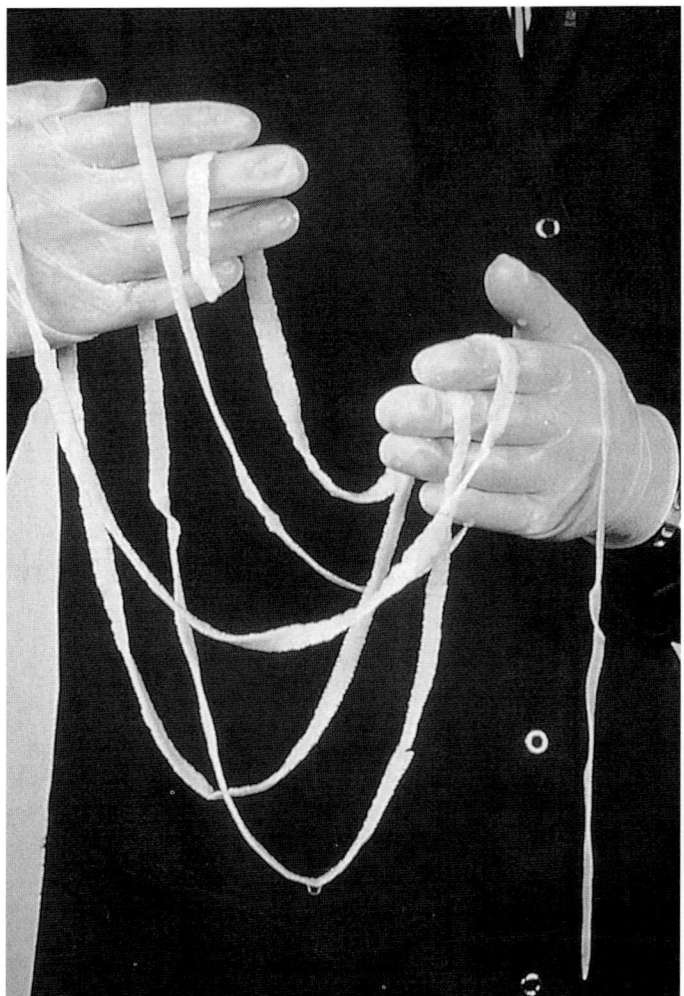

Figure 85.9: Adult beef tapeworm (*T. saginata*). (Courtesy of G. S. Nelson.)

may cause some distress. They are also conspicuous in the faeces because of their motility. Otherwise infection is largely asymptomatic. A number of 'irritable bowel-type' symptoms, particularly abdominal pain but also nausea, distension and anorexia, have been attributed to the parasite but these are so common in the general population that causality is difficult to prove. Occasionally segments of worm may be vomited. Eosinophilia is not a feature of established infection.

Diagnosis and management

Taenia eggs have a characteristic appearance (Figure 85.12) and can be detected by faecal microscopy. As all *Taenia* ova are very similar they are not easily speciated, although they may be distinguished on Ziehl–Neelsen staining, or by the use of monoclonal antibodies[38] or molecular techniques. Soluble *Taenia* antigens can be detected in faeces, but current methods tend to be cross-reactive between species and the value of this is principally for epidemiological surveillance.[39] Intact proglottides in reasonable condition can be speciated by the number of

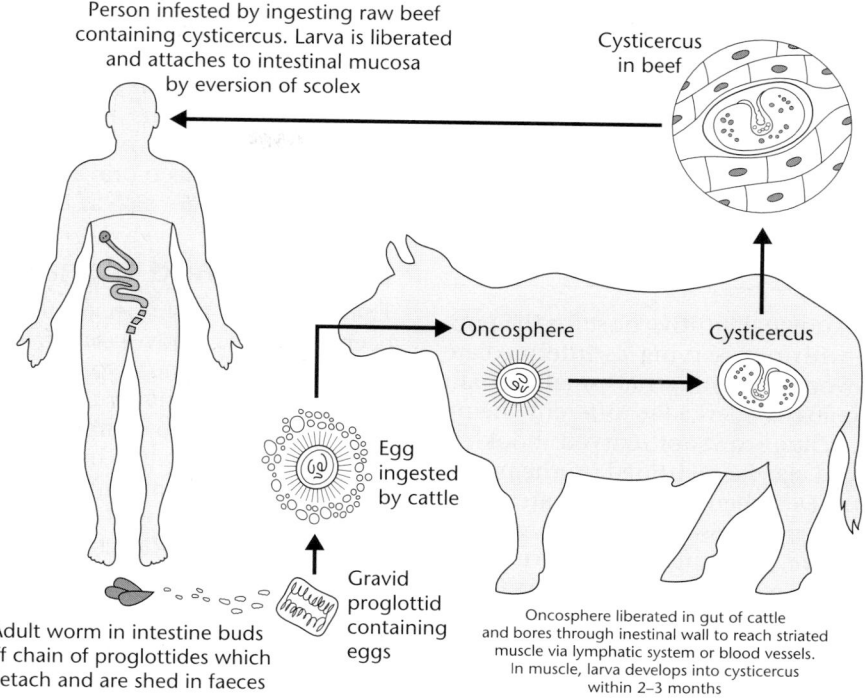

Person infested by ingesting raw beef containing cysticercus. Larva is liberated and attaches to intestinal mucosa by eversion of scolex

Cysticercus in beef

Oncosphere

Cysticercus

Egg ingested by cattle

Gravid proglottid containing eggs

Adult worm in intestine buds off chain of proglottides which detach and are shed in faeces

Oncosphere liberated in gut of cattle and bores through inestinal wall to reach striated muscle via lymphatic system or blood vessels. In muscle, larva develops into cysticercus within 2–3 months

Figure 85.10: Life cycle of *T. saginata*. (Courtesy of Tropical Resources Unit, Wellcome Trust.)

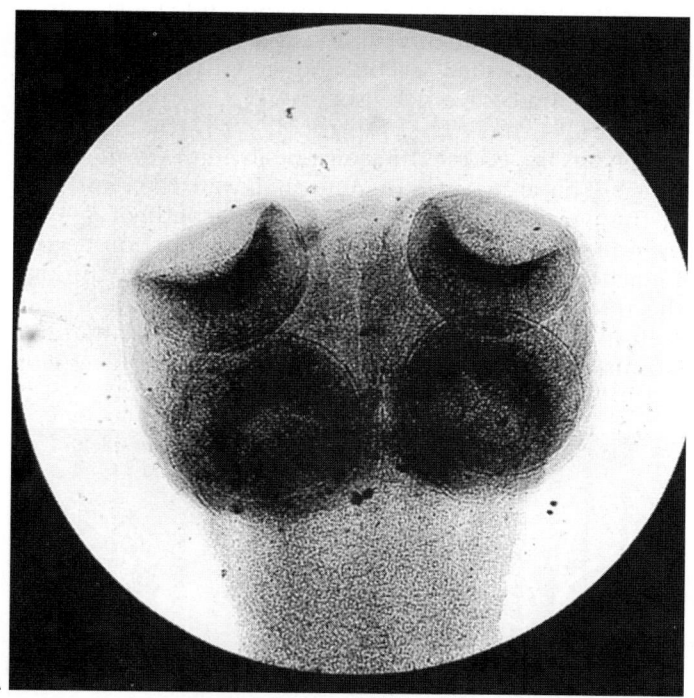

A

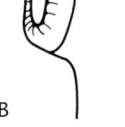

B

Figure 85.11: (**A**) *T. saginata* (unarmed tapeworm) scolex. Suckers without hooklets. (Courtesy of Tropical Resources Unit, Wellcome Trust.) (**B**) *Taenia saginata* head, showing suckers.

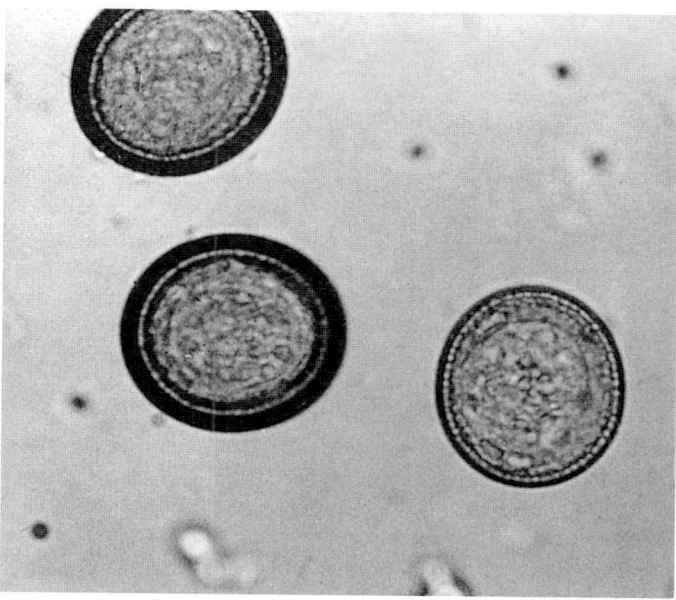

Figure 85.12: *Taenia* ova. (Courtesy of Tropical Resources Unit, Wellcome Trust.)

uterine branches. A single dose of praziquantel at 10 mg/kg is effective therapy. Niclosamide has also been used extensively.

Taenia saginata asiatica

An adult *Taenia* morphologically identical to *T. saginata* was discovered in indigenous highland people in Taiwan in areas where there are no cattle. The cysticerci, a little smaller than those of *T. solium* or *T. saginata,* are found in a number of mammalian species, including pigs, in which they have a strong tropism for the liver.[40] Molecular genetic studies show the parasite to be closely related to, but distinct from, *T. saginata.*[41] It has now been identified in other parts of east Asia, including Korea and Indonesia. It does not appear to cause human cysticercosis.

Taenia solium

The human is the only known definitive host for the pork tapeworm, *T. solium*—with pigs serving as intermediate host. The adult tapeworm is somewhat smaller than *T. saginata* and the scolex is markedly different, being armed with two encircling rows of curved hooklets (Figure 85.13), which can also be identified on the protoscolex of the cysticercus. Detached proglottides are much less motile and consequently less likely to be noticed than are those of *T. saginata.* The chief significance of the parasite is that humans are readily infected by the larval cysticerci as well as the adult worm, giving rise to human cysticercosis. This is discussed above, together with the transmission, prevalence and control of the parasite.

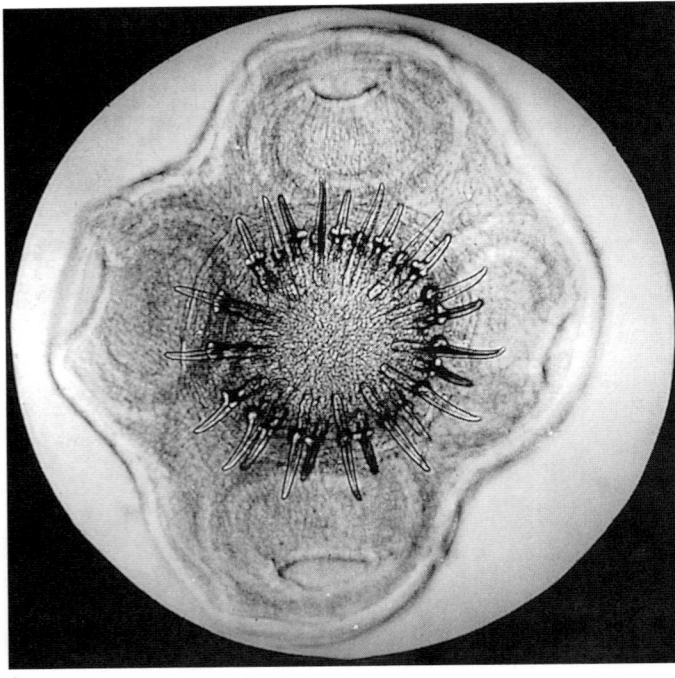

A

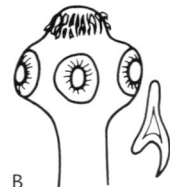

B

Figure 85.13: (**A**) *T. solium* (pig tapeworm) (armed tapeworm) scolex showing hooklets. (Courtesy of Tropical Resources Unit, Wellcome Trust) (**B**) *T. solium* head, showing suckers and the arrangement of the hooklet.

Clinical features

The great majority of *T. solium* carriers are unaware of their infection and it is detected only by screening. Minor abdominal symptoms may occur, as with *T. saginata.* However, carriers carry a substantial risk of acquiring cysticercosis by faeco-oral autoinfection and members of their household are also at increased risk.[42]

Diagnosis and management

The detection and speciation of *Taenia* infections has been discussed above—under *T. saginata.* Treatment is also similar for the two infections, with praziquantel 10 mg/kg being the drug of choice. It was previously common practice to combine anthelmintic therapy for *T. solium* with a purgative because eggs of the dying worm were believed to constitute a risk of cysticercosis through internal autoinfection. No evidence has ever emerged to support this hypothesis and purgation is no longer regarded as necessary.

Hymenolepis nana

The dwarf tapeworm *H. nana* (Figures 85.14 and 85.15) is unique amongst cestodes in that the life cycle is maintained between humans without the necessity for any other host species; indeed, the same individual acts as intermediate and definitive host. Ingested ova (Figure 85.16) are activated by the gut and invade the small intestinal mucosa where they encyst within a villus. Within 3–4 days the protoscolex of this cercocyst evaginates to become the scolex of an adult worm (Figure 85.17). This attaches to the intestinal wall, the remainder of the worm developing to a mature length of 3–4 cm over about a month, after which egg production begins. Detached proglottides degenerate during passage through the intestine, releasing their cargo of ova, and are not seen in the faeces. Infections involving several hundred worms are common. Spread is by faecal–oral transmission

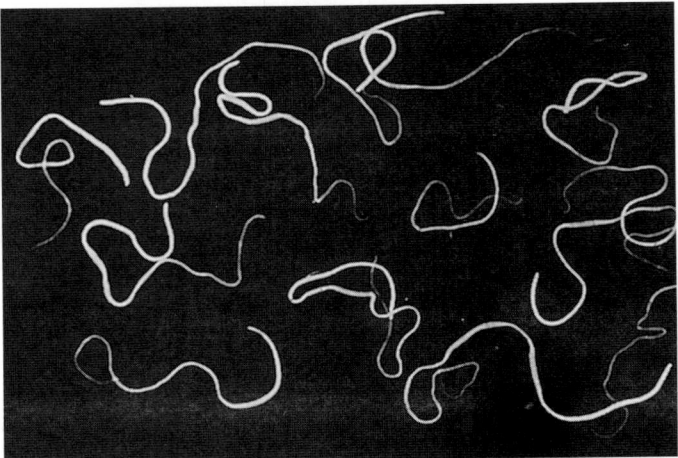

Figure 85.14: *H. nana* (dwarf tapeworm). (Courtesy of Tropical Resources Unit, Wellcome Trust.)

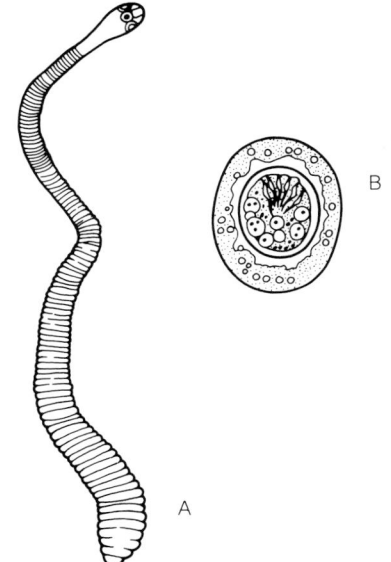

Figure 85.15: *H. nana* (dwarf tapeworm). Magnified.(**A**) adult, (**B**) egg.

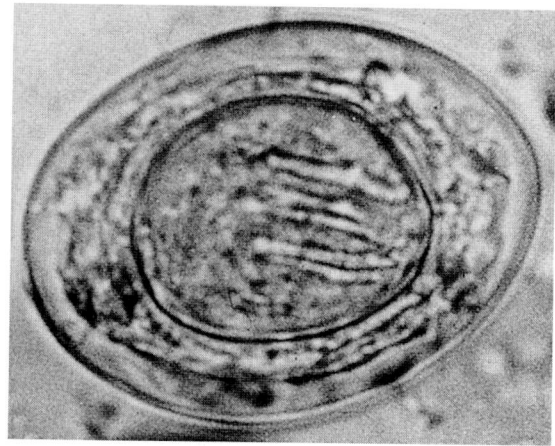

Figure 85.16: *H. nana* (dwarf tapeworm). Ovum. (Courtesy of Tropical Resources Unit.)

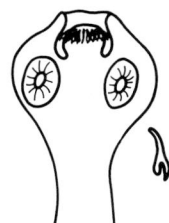

Figure 85.17: The suckers and the arrangement of the hooklets of *Hymenolepsis nana*.

with autoinfection, particularly amongst children, amplifying the intensity of infection. Rodents may act as an alternative definitive host and insects are capable of infection with the larval stage but neither of these appear to be important in parasite transmission.

Prevalence and distribution

H. nana is a very common parasite in warm climates where sanitation is poor, particularly in children, amongst whom prevalences often exceed 10%.

Clinical features

A variety of symptoms has been attributed to *H. nana* infection, including abdominal pain and anorexia as well as systemic complaints such as irritability and headache. Eosinophilia is common. Several reports have associated infection with growth retardation.[43] It is difficult to be certain whether these features are truly a direct result of the parasite or whether it is acting as a marker of faecal–oral infection, insanitation and poverty, but heavy infections probably do have significant clinical consequences.

Diagnosis and management

Diagnosis is by detecting the characteristic ova on faecal microscopy. The cercocyst stage is in contact with the host immune system and consequently, unlike other tapeworm infections, there is a sufficiently predictable humoral response for serology to be of some diagnostic value. An ELISA has been developed with sensitivity of about 80%.[44] There is extensive cross-reaction with other cestode infections. A single dose of praziquantel is effective therapy. At least 20 mg/kg is recommended. Niclosamide has also been widely used. Mebendazole gives cure rate of only around 50%.

Control

As with other faecal–oral infections, control depends on sanitation and education.

Diphyllobothrium latum

Humans can act as definitive host for a variety of pseudophyllidean tapeworms of the genus *Diphyllobothrium* (Table 85.1). Various tiny aquatic invertebrates, especially *Cyclops* water fleas, are the first intermediate host for these parasites (Figure 85.18). The plerocercoid larvae ascend to the apex of the aquatic food chain, with species specificity in their adaptation to particular larger fish. Definitive hosts include birds and marine and terrestrial mammals. *D. latum*, the fish tapeworm, is the species adapted to humans; bears and other terrestrial carnivores may act as paratenic hosts but the human is generally the host that is significant in transmission. It is a large (up to 10 m), slightly translucent tapeworm (Figure 85.19) inhabiting the small intestine, where it attaches by means of two longitudinal slit-like suckers or bothria (Figure 85.20). Infections are commonly multiple and occasionally there may be more than 100 individual worms. The largest recorded total length of *D. latum* tapeworm(s) expelled from one patient is 330 m.[45] The preferred second intermediate hosts are temperate freshwater fish, especially pike, perch and burbot.[46] Human

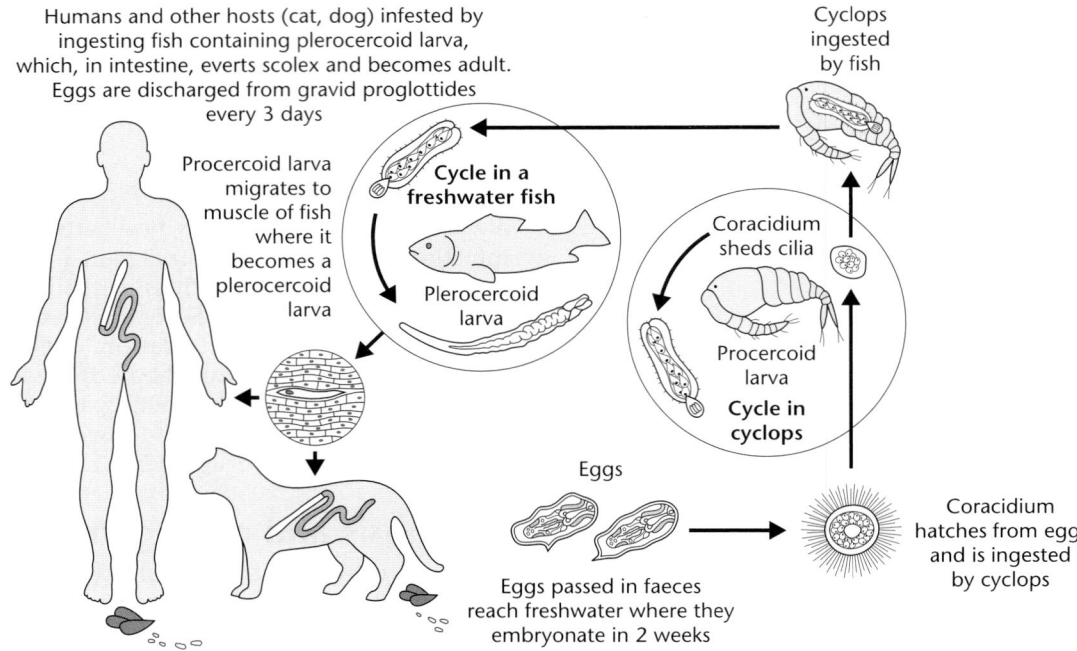

Humans and other hosts (cat, dog) infested by ingesting fish containing plerocercoid larva, which, in intestine, everts scolex and becomes adult. Eggs are discharged from gravid proglottides every 3 days

Cyclops ingested by fish

Procercoid larva migrates to muscle of fish where it becomes a plerocercoid larva

Cycle in a freshwater fish

Plerocercoid larva

Coracidium sheds cilia

Procercoid larva

Cycle in cyclops

Eggs

Eggs passed in faeces reach freshwater where they embryonate in 2 weeks

Coracidium hatches from egg and is ingested by cyclops

Figure 85.18: Life cycle of *D. latum*. (Courtesy of Tropical Resources Unit, Wellcome Trust.)

infection is acquired by eating undercooked fish. Both freezing and cooking effectively destroy the parasite.

Prevalence and distribution

Although the disease is reported from many parts of the world, most transmission occurs in Russia. The original heartland of *D. latum* infection extended from eastern Scandinavia across northern Russia and into western Siberia. Historically there have also been intense foci of transmission in the Danube delta in Romania and in the lakes of northern Italy and western Switzerland. Transmission no longer occurs in Western Europe and has been successfully controlled in Finland, where more than 20% of the entire nation was infected as recently as 1950.[47] In Russia there have been control programmes but also setbacks so that transmission continues to be common, with some extension of the range of the parasite resulting from changes to the river systems by engineering projects. The parasite has also been spread very widely by human migration so that low-intensity transmission has been recorded from many parts of the world, including the smaller lakes of central North America and several parts of South America.

Clinical features

As with other tapeworm infections, carriers experience few if any symptoms. A controlled study in Finland showed that some of the minor symptoms traditionally attributed to infection—including abdominal pain—were not significantly associated with carriage, although diarrhoea, headache and non-specific malaise all appeared to

be somewhat more common.[47] Proglottides are seldom noticed in the faeces, but occasionally carriers may become aware of their infection through the spontaneous expulsion of a whole worm.

Tapeworm anaemia

In the nineteenth century a condition was first described in which pernicious anaemia, at that time a fatal disease, was associated with *D. latum* infection and in some instances improved dramatically after eradication of the worm. In the twentieth century the condition was described exclusively from Finland and by the time that the modern understanding of the pathogenesis of megaloblastic anaemias had become established, tapeworm anaemia was already rapidly disappearing there. Our understanding of this disease is therefore tentative and, as there has been no recognized case for more than 20 years, will probably remain so. It seems clear that tapeworm anaemia was caused by vitamin B_{12} deficiency. It was strongly associated with gastritis and achlorhydria, but neither of these was a necessary condition for its development, and levels of intrinsic factor, as demonstrated by the earliest physiological methods, does not seem to have been deficient.[47] It is most probable that worms were simply competing with the host for vitamin B_{12}, with clinical consequences most likely to follow when absorption was already marginal. There is also some evidence of a familial predisposition.

Diagnosis and management

Ova (Figure 85.21) are detected by faecal microscopy with an estimated sensitivity of 95% for a single examination. *Diphyllobothrium* ova are morphologically similar and

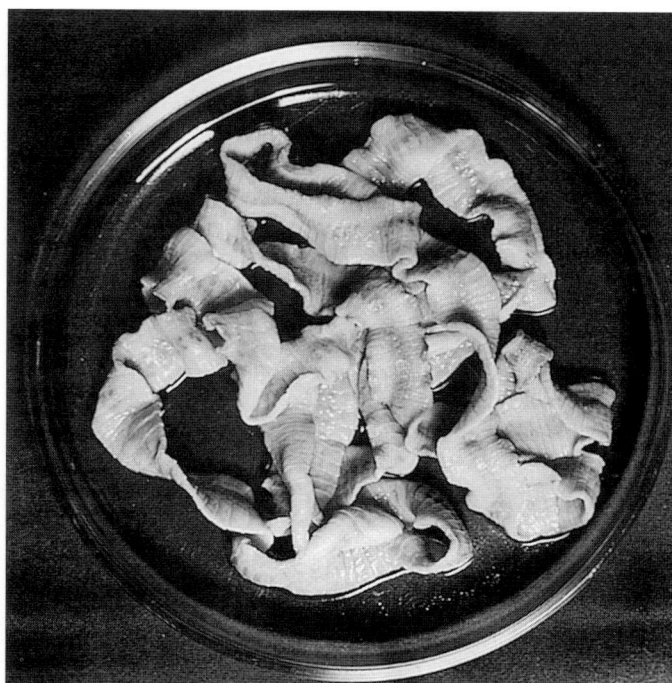

Figure 85.19: *D. latum* (fish tapeworm). Adult. (Courtesy of Tropical Resources Unit, Wellcome Trust.)

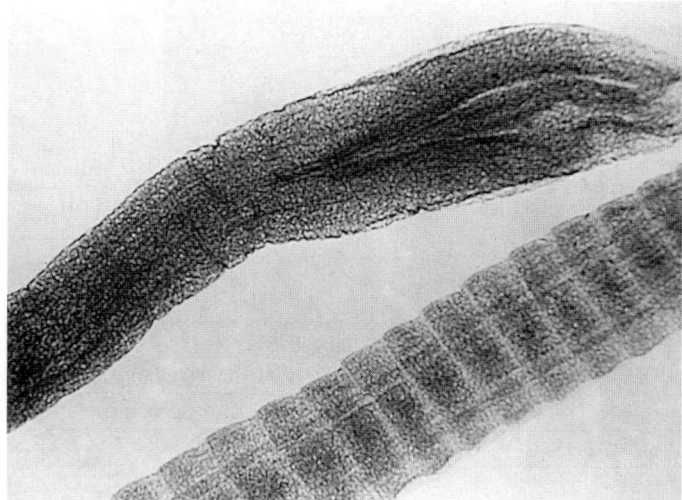

Figure 85.20: *D. latum* (fish tapeworm). Scolex without suckers or hooks but two grooves (bothria) that attach to the mucosa. (Courtesy of Tropical Resources Unit, Wellcome Trust.)

cannot be speciated by microscopy. Praziquantel is the preferred therapy, a single dose of 10 mg/kg being effective. Niclosamide has been extensively used in the past.

Control

Control has been achieved effectively in many areas by the detection and treatment of human cases, improved sanitation and education with regard to dietary habits.

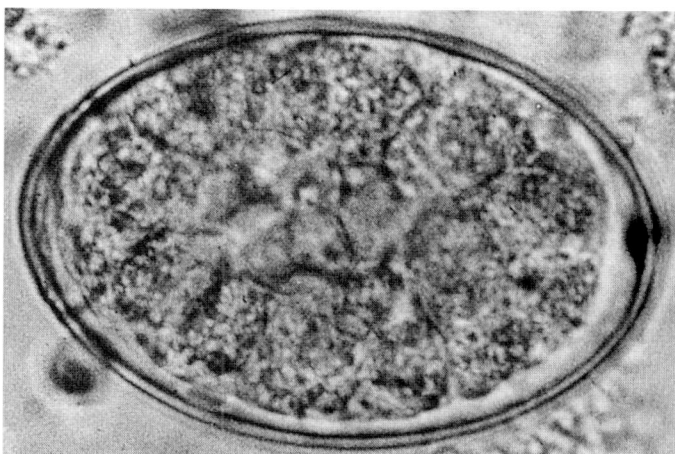

Figure 85.21: *D. latum* (fish tapeworm). Ovum. (Courtesy of D. S. Ridley.)

Zoonotic tapeworms
Hymenolepis diminuta

Rats are the definitive host for this parasite, with insects, principally fleas, acting as intermediate hosts. Humans, usually children, are infected by accidentally ingesting infected fleas. Adult worms can then develop to egg-producing maturity in the human gut, reaching a length of up to 6 cm. Human infection is uncommon but

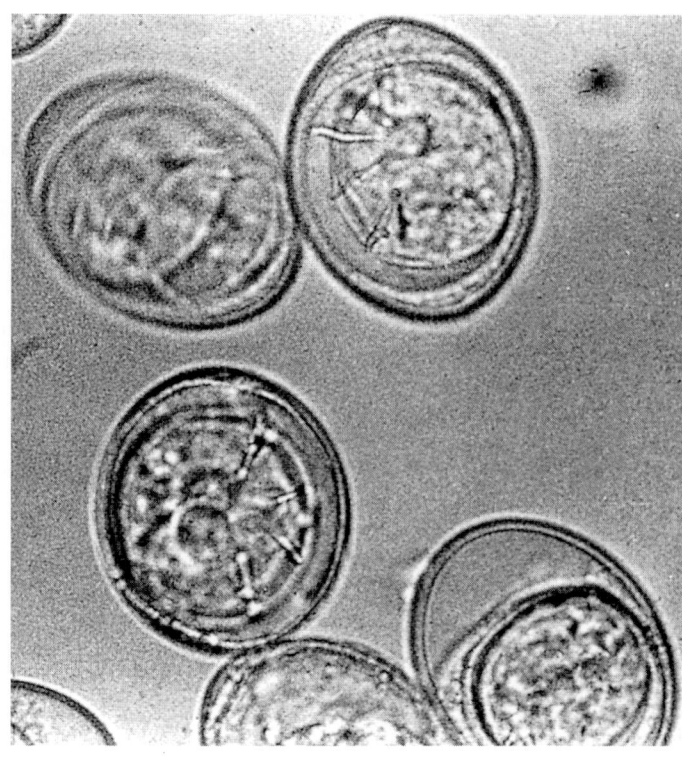

Figure 85.22: *H. diminuta* (rat tapeworm). Ova. (Courtesy of H. Zaiman.)

probably worldwide. Known clinical consequences are limited to eosinophilia and minor abdominal pain. Diagnosis is by stool microscopy, the ova (Figure 85.22) differing slightly from those of *H. nana*. Praziquantel is said to be effective.

Dipylidium caninum

A ubiquitous tapeworm of dogs, with their fleas acting as the intermediate host, this parasite is very similar to *H. diminuta*, as an uncommon zoonotic infection of children who have accidently ingested dog fleas. A medium-sized tapeworm, up to 40 cm, can develop to maturity in the human gut (Figure 85.23). Motile proglottides, the size of rice grains, are passed intact in the stool; free ova (Figure 85.24) are difficult to detect. Infection is most often asymptomatic and there are no known serious consequences. Treatment is with praziquantel.

Diphyllobothrium species

A number of species of *Diphyllobothrium* other than *D. latum* have been reported as infecting humans (Table 85.1). *D. dendriticum* is the cause of human diphyllo-bothriasis amongst the indigenous people of the subarctic region where it infects salmonid fish, especially arctic char.[46] Gulls are the most significant definitive hosts. Prevalences of 30% and more have commonly been recorded in Canadian Inuit communities. Several other parasites infect humans around the northern Pacific, through Pacific salmon,[48] including *D. klebanovskii* which is the principal parasite in the Russian Far East. The clinical consequences of these infections have not been well studied but are considered to be minor.

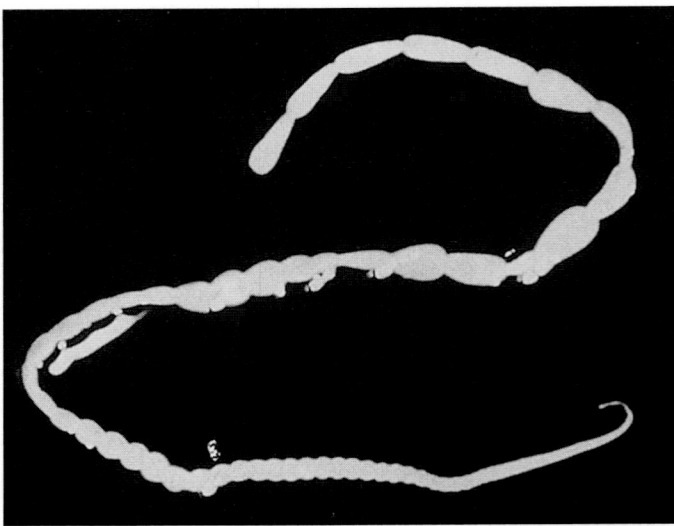

Figure 85.23: *Dipylidium caninum* (dog tapeworm). Adult. (Courtesy of Tropical Resources Unit, Wellcome Trust.)

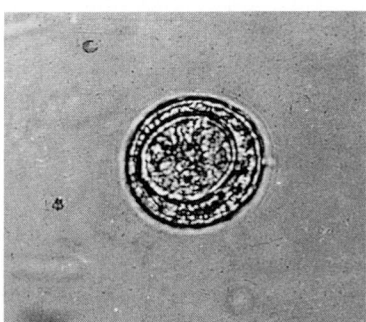

Figure 85.24: Egg of *Dipylidium caninum*.

Table 85.1 Species of *Diphyllobothrium* infecting humans.

Species	Second intermediate host	Principle definitive host	Known range
D. latum	Pike, perch, etc.	Man	Widespread, but especially Russia
D. dendriticum	Char. salmon, trout	Gulls	Throughout subarctic region
D. klebanovskii	Pacific salmon	Marine mammals	Eastern Siberia
D. cordatum	?	Bearded seal	Greenland, Alaska
D. dalliae	Blackfish	Canines?	Alaska, eastern Siberia
D. ursi	Pacific salmon	Bears	Alaska, Canada
D. nihonkaiense	Pacific salmon	Marine mammals?	Japan

REFERENCES

1 Henneberg R. Die tierischen Parasiten des Zentralnervensystem. In Lewandowsky M (ed.) *Handbuch der Neurologie*. Berlin: Springer, 1912.

2 Mahajan R C. Geographical distribution of human cysticercosis. In Flisser A, Willms K, Laclette J P, Larralde C, Ridaura C & Beltran F (eds) *Cysticercosis. Present State of Knowledge and Perspectives*. New York: Academic Press, 1982: 39–46.

3 Gajdusek D C. Introduction of *Taenia solium* into west New Guinea with a note on an epidemic of burns from cysticercus epilepsy in the Ekari people of the Wissel Lakes area. *Papua New Guinea Medical Journal* 1978; 21(4):329–342.

4 Rabiela-Cervantes M T, Rivas-Hernandez A, Rodriguez-Ibarra J, Castillo-Medina S & Cancino F de M. Anatomopathological aspects of human brain cysticercosis. In Flisser A, Willms K, Laclette J P, Larralde C, Ridaura C & Beltran F (eds) *Cysticercosis. Present State of Knowledge and Perspectives*. New York: Academic Press, 1982: 179–200.

5 McGill R J. Cysticercosis resembling myopathy. Lancet 1948; ii:728–730.

6   Medina M T, Rosas E, Rubio-Donnadieu F & Sotelo J. Neurocysticercosis as the main cause of late-onset epilepsy in Mexico. *Arch Intern Med* 1990; 150(2):325–327.

7   Chopra J S, Kaur U & Mahajan R C. Cysticerciasis and epilepsy: a clinical and serological study. *Trans R Soc Trop Med Hyg* 1981; 75(4):518–520.

8   van As A D & Joubert J. Neurocysticercosis in 578 black epileptic patients. *S Afr Med J* 1991; 80(7):327–328.

9   Forlenza O V, Filho A H, Nobrega J P et al. Psychiatric manifestations of neurocysticercosis: a study of 38 patients from a neurology clinic in Brazil. *J Neurol Neurosurg Psychiatry* 1997; 62(6):612–616.

10 Chandramuki A & Nayak P. Subacute and chronic meningitis in children—an immunological study of cerebrospinal fluid. *Indian J Pediatr* 1990; 57(5):685–691.

11 Rangel R, Torres B, Del Bruto O & Sotelo J. Cysticercotic encephalitis: a severe form in young females. *Am J Trop Med Hyg* 1987; 36(2):387–392.

12 Chandy M J, Rajshekhar V, Ghosh S et al. Single small enhancing CT lesions in Indian patients with epilepsy: clinical, radiological and pathological considerations. *J Neurol Neurosurg Psychiatry* 1991; 54(8):702–705.

13 Baily G G, Mason P R, Trijssenar F E & Lyons N F. Serological diagnosis of neurocysticercosis: evaluation of ELISA tests using cyst fluid and other components of *Taenia solium* cysticerci as antigens. *Trans R Soc Trop Med Hyg* 1988; 82(2):295–299.

14 Yang H J, Chung J Y, Yun D et al. Immunoblot analysis of a 10 kDa antigen in cyst fluid of *Taenia solium* metacestodes. *Parasite Immunol* 1998; 20(10):483–488.

15 Hubert K, Andriantsimahavandy A, Michault A, Frosch M & Muhlschlegel F A. Serological diagnosis of human cysticercosis by use of recombinant antigens from *Taenia solium* cysticerci. *Clin Diagn Lab Immunol* 1999; 6(4):479–482.

16 Garcia H H, Parkhouse R M, Gilman R H et al. Serum antigen detection in the diagnosis, treatment, and follow-up of neurocysticercosis patients. *Trans R Soc Trop Med Hyg* 2000; 94(6):673–676.

17 Mason P, Houston S & Gwanzura L. Neurocysticercosis: experience with diagnosis by ELISA serology and computerised tomography in Zimbabwe. *Centr Afr J Med* 1992; 38(4):149–154.

18 Dumas J L, Visy J M, Belin C et al. Parenchymal neurocysticercosis: follow-up and staging by MRI. *Neuroradiology* 1997; 39(1):12–18.

19 Sotelo J, Escobedo F, Rodriguez-Carbajal J, Torres B & Rubio-Donnadieu F. Therapy of parenchymal brain cysticercosis with praziquantel. *N Engl J Med* 1984; 310(16):1001–1007.

20 Pham H T & van Knapen F. Preliminary report of praziquantel treatment of cysticercosis patients in Vietnam. *Acta Leidensia* 1989; 57(2):229–233.

21 Mitchell W G & Crawford T O. Intraparenchymal cerebral cysticercosis in children: diagnosis and treatment. *Pediatrics* 1988; 82(1):76–82.

22 Moodley M & Moosa A. Treatment of neurocysticercosis: is praziquantel the new hope? Lancet 1989; i:262–263.

23 Lopez-Hernandez A & Garaizar C. Analysis of 89 cases of infantile cerebral cysticercosis. In Flisser A, Willms K, Laclette J P, Larralde C, Ridaura C & Beltran F (eds) *Cysticercosis. Present State of Knowledge and Perspectives.*New York: Academic Press, 1982: 127–137.

24 Sotelo J, Del Brutto O H, Penagos P et al. Comparison of therapeutic regimen of anticysticercal drugs for parenchymal brain cysticercosis. *J Neurol* 1990; 237(2):69–72.

25 Cruz M, Cruz I & Horton J. Albendazole versus praziquantel in the treatment of cerebral cysticercosis: clinical evaluation. *Trans R Soc Trop Med Hyg* 1991; 85(2):244–247.

26 Corona T, Lugo R, Medina R & Sotelo J. Single-day praziquantel therapy for neurocysticercosis. *N Engl J Med* 1996; 334(2):125.

27 Sotelo J & Jung H. Pharmacokinetic optimisation of the treatment of neurocysticercosis. *Clin Pharmacokinet* 1998; 34(6):503–515.

28 Allcut D A & Coulthard A. Neurocysticercosis: regression of a fourth ventricular cyst with praziquantel. *J Neurol Neurosurg Psychiatry* 1991; 54(5):461–462.

29 Allan J C, Velasquez-Tohom M, Fletes C et al. Mass chemotherapy for intestinal *Taenia solium* infection: effect on prevalence in humans and pigs. *Trans R Soc Trop Med Hyg* 1997; 91(5):595–598.

30 Jung R C, Rodriguez M A, Beaver P C, Schenthal J E & Levy R W. Racemose cysticercus in human brain. A case report. *Am J Trop Med Hyg* 1981; 30(3):620–624.

31 Lachberg S, Thompson R C & Lymbery A J. A contribution to the etiology of racemose cysticercosis. *J Parasitol* 1990; 76(4):592–594.

32 Baily G G & Levy L F. Racemose cysticercosis treated with praziquantel. *Trans R Soc Trop Med Hyg* 1989; 83(1):95–96.

33 Templeton A C. Anatomical and geographical location of human coenurus infection. *Trop Geogr Med* 1971; 23(1):105–108.

34 Ing M B, Schantz P M & Turner J A. Human coenurosis in North America: case reports and review. *Clin Infect Dis* 1998; 27(3):519–523.

35 Maillard H, Marionneau J, Prophette B, Boyer E & Celerier P. *Taenia crassiceps* cysticercosis and AIDS. *AIDS* 1998; 12(12):1551–1552.

36 Holodniy M, Almenoff J, Loutit J & Steinberg G K. Cerebral sparganosis: case report and review. *Rev Infect Dis* 1991; 13(1):155–159.

37 Torres J R, Noya O O, Noya B A, Mouliniere R & Martinez E. Treatment of proliferative sparganosis with mebendazole and praziquantel. *Trans R Soc Trop Med Hyg* 1981; 75(6):846–847.

38 Montenegro T C, Miranda E A & Gilman R. Production of monoclonal antibodies for the identification of the eggs of *Taenia solium*. *Ann Trop Med Parasitol* 1996; 90(2):145–155.

39 Allan J C, Velasquez-Tohom M, Torres-Alvarez R, Yurrita P & Garcia-Noval J. Field trial of the coproantigen-based diagnosis of *Taenia solium* taeniasis by enzyme-linked immunosorbent assay. *Am J Trop Med Hyg* 1996; 54(4):352–356.

40 Fan P C & Chung W C. *Taenia saginata asiatica*: epidemiology, infection, immunological and molecular studies. *J Microbiol Immunol Infect* 1998; 31(2):84–89.

41 Zarlenga D S, McManus D P, Fan P C & Cross J H. Characterization and detection of a newly described Asian taeniid using cloned ribosomal DNA fragments and sequence amplification by the polymerase chain reaction. *Exp Parasitol* 1991; 72(2):174–183.

42 Diaz-Camacho S, Candil-Ruiz A, Uribe-Beltran M & Willms K. Serology as an indicator of *Taenia solium* tapeworm infections in a rural community in Mexico. *Trans R Soc Trop Med Hyg* 1990; 84(4):563–566.

43 Khalil H M, el Shimi S, Sarwat M A, Fawzy A F & el Sorougy A O. Recent study of *Hymenolepis nana* infection in Egyptian children. *J Egypt Soc Parasitol* 1991; 21(1):293–300.

44 Castillo R M, Grados P, Carcamo C et al. Effect of treatment on serum antibody to *Hymenolepis nana* detected by enzyme-linked immunosorbent assay. *J Clin Microbiol* 1991; 29(2):413–414.

45 Ostling G. Treatment of tapeworm infection with desaspidin, a new phloroglucinol derivative isolated from Finnish fern. *Am J Trop Med Hyg* 1961; 10:855–858.

46 Curtis M A & Bylund G. Diphyllobothriasis: fish tapeworm disease in the circumpolar north. *Arctic Med Res* 1991; 50(1):18–24.

47 von Bonsdorff B. *Diphyllobothriasis in Man*. London: Academic Press, 1977.

48 Rausch R L, Scott E M & Rausch V R. Helminths in Eskimos in western Alaska, with particular reference to *Diphyllobothrium* infection and anaemia. *Trans R Soc Trop Med Hyg* 1967; 61:351–357.

Section 12

Ectoparasites

Parasitic infections/infestations of the skin and tissues are common worldwide, but are particularly prevalent in the tropics. This section deals with common important human ectoparasites: (a) leeches; (b) myiases; (c) jigger fleas, scabies; and (d) louse infections.

Chapter 86

Ectoparasites: Leeches and Leech Infestation, Myiasis, Jigger Fleas, Scabies, Louse Infestation

G. B. White

Leeches and leech infestation

Geographical distribution

Land leeches are common in South-East Asia, the Pacific islands, the Indian subcontinent and South America. Aquatic leeches have a worldwide distribution.

Aetiology

Leeches that attack humans have the following position in the animal kingdom:

Phylum   Annelida
Class   Hirudinea
Order   Gnathobdellida
Family   Hirudinidae

Gnathobdellid leeches are invertebrates, having a smooth cuticle, a mouth lacking a proboscis but with three jaws, two suckers (one surrounding the mouth, the other at the posterior end) and powerful muscles, circular and longitudinal. They attach themselves by the posterior sucker, the anterior end moving about freely. When unfed, they are usually about 2.5 cm long and 5 mm thick; some are bigger. When full of blood they are dark, bloated objects.

The muscular jaws are covered with chitin and produce a characteristic triradiate wound in the skin of the victim. The mouth leads to a pharynx, with salivary glands that secrete the anticoagulant hirudin, a crop in which ingested blood can be stored, a stomach, intestine, rectum and anal pore near the posterior sucker. The excretory system consists of 17 pairs of nephridia. There is a vascular system and a nervous system.

Leeches are hermaphrodites, each one possessing testes and ovaries. The spermatozoa of one individual are deposited during copulation on the cuticle (to migrate through the tissues to reach the ovary) or into the vagina of the other member of the copulating pair. Some leeches deposit egg masses on objects submerged in water; others form a cocoon to be deposited in water or mud, from which the young hatch and attach themselves to water plants. Others carry their young until they are able to suck.

Leeches that attack humans may be divided into two classes: *land leeches*, which have powerful jaws that can penetrate the skin so that they can attach anywhere on the external surface of the body, and aquatic leeches, which have weak jaws and require soft tissues to feed on. They gain entrance to orifices such as the pharynx and vagina.

Land leeches

Land leeches live in the vegetation of tropical rainforests and tend to breed near springs, streams and wells frequented by cattle, horses and other vertebrates. The species noted for attacks on humans include *Haemadipsa zelanica*, *H. sylvestris* and *H. picta*. Land leeches attach themselves to the skin and feed; when fed, they fall off on to the ground, having remained attached for a comparatively short time.

Clinical features

The punctures made in the skin by land leeches are painless, and remain open and bleeding after the leech has gone; healing is slow. Leeches take much more blood than they need and if they remain attached, or are numerous, they can take so much that the person becomes seriously anaemic and may die from loss of blood.

Management

Leeches that attach themselves to the skin must be induced to detach; however, they must not be simply pulled off because they may then leave behind their jaws, which could become the starting point of destructive ulceration. Drops of strong salt solution, alcohol or strong vinegar applied around the mouth, or heat from a lighted match or cigarette applied to the body, will cause the leech to release its hold. The wound can then be treated with a styptic and an antiseptic agent.

Prevention

People in countries where land leeches are common should, when travelling in infested country, wear boots and trousers thick enough to prevent access by the leeches to the skin. Additional protection is afforded if the garments or the skin are treated with repellents such as diethyl toluamide

(DEET), dimethyl or dibutyl phthalate (DMP, DBP) or indalone. DEET and DBP last longer on clothing and, if applied about once every 2 weeks at the rate of 28 ml per set of garments, or about 4 ml per 30 cm^2, are good repellents. On the skin, repellents are effective for only 3–5 hours—less if sweating is excessive. These repellents should not be used on synthetic fabrics, which they can dissolve.

Aquatic leeches

Aquatic leeches live exclusively in fresh water. Species that feed on humans include *Limnatis nilotica*, which is large and haunts quiet water and ponds, and *L. maculosa*. *Phytobdella catenifera*, *Dinobdella ferox* and *Myxobdella africana* occur in sub-Saharan Africa.[1] Aquatic leeches deposit their eggs on water plants, and the young may be seen in the water. They do not all require a mammalian host, and can exist on amphibians. Young leeches enter orifices such as the nose and pharynx where they attach themselves for prolonged periods until they become adult, when they drop off into the water. They are more dangerous than land leeches because they are more likely to cause severe anaemia.

Clinical features
Aquatic leech infestation is less common than land leech infestation, but may be much more harmful. Aquatic leeches can enter the mouth or nostrils during drinking or washing, and may also attack the conjunctiva, vulva, vagina and urethra in persons bathing in infested water. Having entered the mouth or nostrils, the leech can quickly pass to the nasopharynx, epiglottis or oesophagus, and even to the trachea and bronchi. When attached to the mucous membrane, the leech secretes anticoagulant and engorges. The result is bleeding, according to the site of attachment—epistaxis, haemoptysis or haematemesis—which may lead to severe anaemia. A leech in the nares may also give prolonged headache; if in the larynx, there is a cough with bloody discharge, hoarseness, dyspnoea, pain and even suffocation. Leeches in the pharynx or oesophagus may cause difficulty in swallowing.

Management
In treating leech infestation of the upper respiratory passages, an attempt should be made to see the leech. If it is in the posterior pharynx, larynx, trachea or bronchus, the patient should be positioned so that the leech cannot fall back and block the lower passages. If it is in the nares or upper pharynx, it can be paralysed with cocaine and extracted directly. If lower down, a pair of long hooked forceps can be introduced through a laryngoscope and the leech pulled out gently, although tracheostomy may be necessary. If in the oesophagus, the leech should be visualized through an oesophagoscope and treated with cocaine; it will then fall into the stomach where the gastric juice will kill it. For a leech in the genitourinary tract, irrigation with strong salt solution may make it release its hold.

Prevention
To avoid attack by aquatic leeches it is necessary to wear appropriate clothing and apply repellents, and to drink only water that has been filtered, strained through fine gauze or boiled.

Although they suck blood, leeches have not been incriminated in transmitting infection.

Myiasis

Myiasis is caused when fly maggots (larvae of Diptera) invade living tissue or when they are harboured in the intestine or bladder.

Clinically, maggots that cause myiasis may attack three parts of the body.

1. *Cutaneous tissue*. Some species of maggots cause furuncles (subcutaneous myiasis), invade sores and wounds (wound myiasis), burrow under the skin (dermal myiasis, a cause of creeping eruption) or suck blood.
2. *Body cavities*. Other species invade the nasal passages (nasal myiasis), mouth, ears and accessory passages, enter the orbit of the eye (ocular myiasis), or penetrate the anus or vagina.
3. *Gut lumen*. If accidentally ingested, fly eggs or larvae may survive passage through the stomach and bowel to emerge in the stool (intestinal myiasis).

Parasitologically, myiasis-producing flies can be divided into three categories (see also Appendix IV):

1. *Obligatory myiasis producers*. For some fly species, it is essential for the larvae to develop in living tissue because they are unable to develop elsewhere. These obligate parasites are highly specialized insects, the larvae of which have developed highly sophisticated mechanisms to avoid the host's immune system.
2. *Facultative myiasis producers*. These larvae usually develop on carrion but may invade wounds. They may be primary invaders which initiate myiasis; secondary invaders, entering tissue only when the animal has become infested; or tertiary, which become involved later, only once decomposition is advanced.
3. *Accidental myiasis producers*. These eggs or larvae are accidentally ingested and are not killed in the intestine.

Cutaneous tissue myiasis

Blood suckers (Congo floor maggot)
(see also Appendix IV)

Geographical distribution
The adult fly *Auchmeromyia luteola* (see Appendix IV) is widely distributed throughout tropical Africa from 18°N to 26°S, from northern Nigeria and southern Sudan to Natal, from sea level to 2250 m in both dry and wet climates.

Aetiology

The Congo floor maggot is the larval stage of *A. luteola* (see Appendix IV), an orange-buff coloured 'blowfly' covered with numerous small hairs which give it a smoky look. It has a stoutly built body, 10–12 mm long.

Life cycle

The adult fly sits motionless among the thatch, beams and cobwebs of the roof of huts where it is protected by its colour and is difficult to see. Human faeces are its most important source of food. It lays eggs in the crevices of mud floors, favouring those contaminated by urine, 3 weeks after its emergence from the pupa. The larva that emerges from the egg is dirty white, semi-transparent, 15 mm long and composed of 11 segments. This stage is known as the Congo floor maggot (see Appendix IV). The larva is mobile and merges from its hiding place to take blood meals from the host, which must be hairless and immobile, such as a sleeping human, aardvark or nestling bird. It feeds by scraping with its mouth hooks until it reaches a blood vessel. The first segment then retracts and its sucker is applied. After feeding, it becomes conspicuously red as it is filled with blood, and retreats into a crack in the floor, under the mats on which people sleep, or burrows in the earth to a depth of up to 8 cm. Congo floor maggots feed mainly at night and drop off at once if disturbed. They can be recognized by the characteristic shape of the spiracles (see Figure IV.17A). When ready to pupate, the larva selects a suitable place and lies dormant. The pupa is dark reddish-brown with an oblong body 9–10 × 4.5 mm; this stage lasts for 2–3 weeks.

Clinical features

The bite is painless. Blood loss has never been found sufficient to cause anaemia. No infections are known to be transmitted by its bite.

Prevention

Sleeping on a bed raised above the floor is sufficient to prevent attack. House-spraying with residual insecticide should be applied to eliminate infestations.

Subcutaneous myiasis

The maggot penetrates the skin; no previous lesion is necessary. Two species of fly are the cause; both are obligatory myiasis producers: *Cordylobia anthropophaga* (family Calliphoridae) in Africa and *Dermatobia hominis* (family Cuterebridae) in South America.

1. *Cordylobia Anthropophaga* (tumbu fly, putsi fly, ver du cayor) (see also Appendix IV)

Geographical distribution

The tumbu fly occurs throughout sub-Saharan Africa, and has been recorded from southern Spain.

Aetiology

C. anthropophaga (see Appendix IV) is a large, robust, yellow-brown fly, 7–12 mm long, resembling the adult of the Congo floor maggot (*A. luteola*) and difficult to distinguish from numerous other species of flies. *C. anthropophaga* is an obligate parasite. Adults are active in the early morning and late afternoon, laying eggs on sandy ground or contaminated clothing. The eggs hatch and the larvae that emerge invade the subcutaneous tissue and undergo three moults or instars (see Appendix IV); complete development in the subcutaneous tissues takes 8–12 days. The larvae emerge and fall to the ground, where they pupate in 24 hours, and the adult hatches after 10–20 days, according to temperature. The pupa has a characteristic shape with a truncated end. Rodents and dogs are the usual larval hosts, and humans are infected only accidentally.

Transmission

The female fly lays its eggs in two batches on sandy ground contaminated with urine or faeces, and also on clothing (although such clothing may appear clean). Clothing laid on the ground to dry is affected, but not clothing hanging in bright sunlight, because the eggs are laid only in shaded areas. The eggs are not laid directly on the skin.

On hatching, the small first-stage larvae hold themselves erect and can remain alive without food for about 9 days. The larvae, which are sensitive to both heat and vibration, become attached to a host and immediately begin to penetrate the unbroken skin, taking about 1 minute. Penetration, which is painless, may involve any part of the body but most commonly occurs on the back, head and neck in humans. Larvae are acquired from lying on the ground or from clothing, and infection is more common in children. Dogs are an important domestic reservoir.

Immunity

There is a localized degree of immunity which has been produced experimentally in guinea pigs. There are no antibodies and no general immunity. Larvae penetrating the immune area die in 40 hours, and grafted skin retains its immunity.

Clinical features

Initially, the lesion starts as a small papule containing the larva, and which may be itchy or pricking at intervals. As the papule increases in size, the symptoms recur and may keep the person awake at night. Serous fluid may be exuded and local lymphadenopathy may occur. There may be fever and general malaise. The lesion, which resembles a boil, grows over a period of 6 days, the larva being noticed by the time the third stage has been reached. While in the host (8–12 days), the larva has its posterior segment (bearing the respiratory spiracles) protruding from the aperture, but this may be withdrawn when touched. There may be numerous lesions resembling boils situated on the arms, scrotum and other parts of the body, coinciding with areas of contact with contaminated clothing. Close inspection of the lesions will reveal that, instead of a

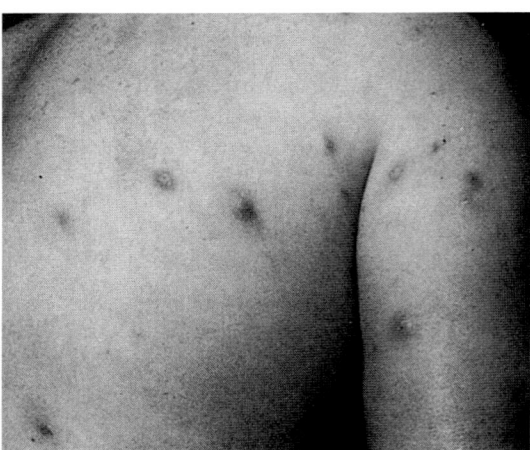

Figure 86.1: Lesions of tumbu fly (*Cordylobia anthropophaga*).

pustular head, the lesions terminate in a 1–3-mm dark line, the site of the respiratory spiracles of the larva (Figure 86.1).

Diagnosis

C. anthropophaga causes less pain than an ordinary boil, and the appearance of the spiracles is diagnostic. In case of doubt, the surface of the lesion should be covered with petroleum jelly (Vaseline), glycerine or oil. The appearance of bubbles clinches the diagnosis.

Management

The larvae can be removed by squeezing the boil, assisted by first covering the spiracles with a layer of paraffin oil to stop the oxygen supply. Mature larvae will then wriggle partly out, and can finally be removed by exerting firm digital pressure on each side. Early lesions are best left to develop for a few days, as immature larvae are reluctant to emerge. Rupture of the larvae by injudicious attempts at extraction may cause a severe inflammatory response.

Prevention

All clothing and towels should be ironed on *both* sides, and drip-dry clothes should be hung indoors with the windows closed[2] to prevent contact with the flies.

2. *Dermatobia Hominis* (ver macaque, berne, el tórsalo, beefworm, human bot fly) (see Appendix IV)

Geographical distribution

D. hominis is widely distributed throughout Central and South America, from Mexico to Argentina and Chile. It is especially common on the forested eastern slopes of the Andes in Colombia. It attacks a wide range of hosts and is a devastating pest of livestock in some areas.

Aetiology

The adult fly is a large bluish-grey fly, 1.5 cm long (see Appendix IV), with a strong flight, found primarily on the edge of tropical forests, particularly hilly areas of secondary forest between 160 and 3000 m. The adult *D. hominis*, on attaining maturity, lays its eggs directly on other insects or foliage, but especially on day-flying mosquitoes such as *Psorophora*, flies (*Sarcophaga*, *Musca* and *Stomoxys*) and ticks (*Amblyoma*). The packets of eggs adhere to the insect's thorax and are thus conveyed to the new host (usually cattle, dogs or humans). This characteristic is called phoresis or 'hitch-hiking'.

The larva remains in the egg until it senses warmth, whereupon it rapidly 'hatches' and penetrates the host's skin in 5–10 minutes, remaining at the site of penetration. Each larva penetrates individually and a small nodule develops around it with a central pore through which the larva breathes. The second-stage larva has a characteristic shape which makes it difficult to remove. The duration of larval development is uncertain but probably lasts from 6 to 12 weeks in humans, during which it grows slowly feeding on tissue exudate. It then emerges, drops to the ground and pupates.

Clinical features

Cutaneous swellings, each harbouring one larva, usually occur on exposed areas (although the flies can penetrate clothing), and are found most commonly on the head but also elsewhere on the body. In the orbit the larva can cause serious pathology and is a cause of ophthalmomyiasis (see Chapter 18). Lesions can be multiple, and 12 have been reported on one individual. The lesion is an inflamed swelling 2–3 cm in diameter, at the apex of which can be seen the small black spiracles from which exudes a seropurulent fluid containing the dark faeces of the larva. The lesions are very painful and itchy, but do not suppurate because the bacteriostatic activity of the gut of the larva prevents undesirable overgrowth of pyogenic bacteria.

Diagnosis

Diagnosis is made by examining the lesion for the characteristic spiracles and the faecal-stained serous exudate.

Complications

Loss of the eye can occur in ophthalmomyiasis. A fatal cerebral myiasis can occur in children, but is rare.

Management

Occasionally the first-stage larva can be removed (as in *Cordylobia*), but more often surgical removal is necessary with second- and third-stage larvae. The larvae are best removed by means of a cruciate incision, and care must be taken not to go through the central hole and damage the larva, portions of which must not be left in the wound.

Control

In Brazil, *D. hominis* has been controlled with insecticides including DDT, pyrethroids and Toxaphene. In Curaçao, males sterilized by radiation were released to render the females sterile after mating (females mate only once). After 2 years of the sterile male release programme, the fly was exterminated in a similar manner to the cattle screw-worm, *Callitroga hominivorax*, which has been eradicated from North America by this method.

Dermal myiasis or creeping eruption

Dermal myiasis is caused by the maggots of horse and cattle bot flies which are obligatory myiasis producers (whereas in humans the maggots cannot develop further), producing tunnels in the epidermis in which they may wander for some time.

Aetiology

Gasterophilus spp. (horse bots, warble flies) (see also Appendix IV)
Gasterophilidae are common parasites of horses, and sometimes of humans, especially people who look after horses. The eggs are laid on the hair of the host or on grasses. On contact with skin, the larvae promptly penetrate, but do not develop beyond the first instar, causing a swelling and a wandering tunnel in the lower epidermis in which they may wander for a long time.

Hypoderma spp. (cattle bots) (see also Appendix IV)
Hypoderma ovis and *H. lineatum* (Oestridae) are parasites of cattle and cause creeping eruption in persons connected with cattle. The eggs are deposited on the hair of cattle and hatch within a week. The larvae penetrate more deeply into the subcutaneous tissues than those of *Gasterophilus* spp., and have been reported to have invaded the nervous system.

Clinical features

The tunnels caused by *Gasterophilus* spp. maggots resemble the lesions caused by *Ancylostoma braziliense* (cutaneous larva migrans). They itch but do not discharge unless infected. Lesions caused by *Hypoderma* are deeper, producing a swelling that resembles a boil. The maggots migrate slowly for considerable distances. *H. ovis* has been reported to invade the central nervous system.

Differential diagnosis

Other causes of a creeping eruption are cutaneous larva migrans caused by *Ancylostoma*, *Strongyloides* (see Chapter 83), *Gnathostoma* (see Chapter 16) and *Fasciola hepatica* (see Chapter 81). *Strongyloides* is transient and very fast moving (hence 'larva currens'), whereas *Gnathostoma* and *Fasciola* larvae do not usually tarry in the skin for long before moving deeper.

For veterinary diagnosis, an increasing number of specific enzyme-linked immunosorbent assay (ELISA) tests are becoming available for identification of the presence and identity of bot and warble flies causing myiasis.

Gasterophilus larvae may be identified by smearing a small amount of clear mineral oil over the lesion. The larva can then be seen and identified by the black transverse bands of spines on its body.

Management

Gasterophilus larvae, when identified, may be removed with a needle. *Hypoderma* larvae may be removed through a cruciform incision.

Body cavity myiasis

Nasal myiasis

Geographical distribution
Nasal myiasis occurs most commonly in Asia, less commonly in Africa.

Aetiology
Chrysomyia beziana (Old World screw fly) is the most common cause, but *Oestrus ovis* (sheep nasal bot fly), *Rhinoestrus purpureus* (Russian gadfly), *Callitroga hominivorax* and *C. americana* (New World screw fly) are other causes (see Appendix IV).

Pathology
The flies are obligatory myiasis producers. The female flies lay eggs in the nasal cavity, especially where there is a chronic nasal discharge. The larvae require living tissue in which to develop. After the eggs have hatched, the larvae burrow into the tissue—even to the nasal bone—within a few hours.

Clinical features
The initial symptoms are tickling, sneezing, pain and nasal obstruction. Epistaxis is common, but the discharge soon becomes purulent and fetid. Destruction and erosion of the nose or mouth may facilitate larval migration to the brain, with meningitis and death. A mortality rate of 8% has been recorded in cases of *C. hominivorax* nasal infection.

Diagnosis
The maggots can be seen with a nasal speculum and extracted for examination. They should be preserved in 70% alcohol and sent to a laboratory to be identified by their spiracles (see Appendix IV), or kept alive and hatched to permit identification. Precise identification is academic unless control measures are intended, and is of no practical importance to the patients.

Management
A few drops of 15% chloroform in light vegetable oil applied to the nasal passages will cause the larvae to appear, when they can be removed with forceps. In advanced cases the nasal sinuses may have to be opened surgically.

Control
C. hominivorax has been eradicated from some areas by means of the large-scale release of male flies sterilized by γ radiation.

Myiasis of the ear

The same species may invade the ear, causing pain and

discomfort accompanied by deafness and tinnitus, and the drum may be perforated.

Ocular myiasis (ophthalmomyiasis) (see also Chapter 18)

External ophthalmomyiasis, which involves only conjunctivitis, is caused by *Oestrus* spp. (sheep bots) or *Wohlfahrtia* spp.

Internal ophthalmomyiasis may be caused by *Dermatobia hominis*, *Oestrus ovis* (sheep bots), *Gasterophilus* spp., *Rhinoestrus* spp. (horse bots) and *Hypoderma* spp. (cattle bots). However, *O. ovis* mainly attacks the conjunctivae (external ophthalmomyiasis). The female fly strikes the eye, depositing eggs almost instantaneously while on the wing. Larvae are deposited on the conjunctiva at the inner canthus of the eye, the nasal openings or the lips. The larvae, which do not survive for more than 10 days, developing no further, are actively motile and possess characteristic hooks which cause conjunctival irritation. They may be removed under direct vision after applying topical anaesthetic.

Internal ophthalmomyiasis involving the orbit and eye can be very destructive, leading to the loss of the eye (see Chapter 18).

Myiasis of the anus and vagina

Wohlfahrtia spp. (flesh fly) (see Appendix IV) can lay their eggs in large numbers around the anus and vagina of adults and children in poor hygienic circumstances where there are soiling and sores in the anogenital region. Large numbers of maggots may develop within a few hours.

Wound myiasis
Aetiology
This includes myiasis produced by both obligatory and facultative myiasis producers. Larvae of several groups of flies usually associated with carrion have been found in wounds and gangrenous tissues, where they act as facultative parasites feeding on necrotic tissue, although occasionally they may attack living tissues.

Larvae of the facultative parasites *Calliphora*, *Lucilia*, *Phormia*, *Musca* and *Fannia* spp. are found living in moist folds of skin and enter sores and wounds. At one time the larvae of carefully cultivated *Lucilia* were used to cleanse wounds by removal of infected tissue, and this practice may still be appropriate for cases where antibiotics are ineffective and surgery impractical.[3]

In southern Europe, Russia, the Middle East and Africa *Wohlfahrtia mangnifica* (Old World flesh fly or sheep maggot) is the common species, and *W. vigil* (New World flesh fly) in the New World. In India, the Far East and sub-Saharan Africa *Chrysomyia bezziana*, and in the New World *Callitroga hominivorax* (see above), are the most frequent agents of wound myiasis. These flies are obligatory myiasis producers, relying on living tissue for their survival.

Urogenital myiasis
Mistaken diagnosis of urinary myiasis is not uncommon, due to a larva from a contaminated vessel in which urine has been collected, or which has been introduced into the urine after it was passed; however, there have been genuine cases in which larvae have been passed via the urethra from the bladder. If the vulva or vaginal area in women is infested, there are obvious opportunities for larvae to enter the bladder. The flies concerned are usually of the genera *Psychoda*, *Musca*, *Calliphora* and *Sarcophaga*.[4]

Intestinal myiasis

Eggs, and sometimes larvae, of many species of flies are deposited on foodstuffs, and sometimes survive the journey down the intestinal tract. They may then develop in the folds of mucous membrane, even causing some irritation (pain, vomiting, diarrhoea) or even ulceration before being evacuated. If deposited around the anus, such larvae may crawl into the rectum to complete their feeding inside the body. This kind of infestation may persist for months, producing severe anxiety as well as internal irritation. The larvae can be recognized in the faeces, sometimes in vomit.

The flies that are usually implicated include species of *Musca*, *Fannia*, *Chrysomyia*, *Calliphora* and *Lucilia*. Prevention entails the careful covering of food. Treatment with purgatives will aid elimination, and ivermectin is worth a trial.

Jigger fleas

Geographical distribution
Originally found in Central and South America, the jigger has now spread to West and East Africa and to parts of the Indian subcontinent.

Aetiology (see Appendix IV)
Tunga penetrans (the sand flea, jigger flea, chigoe, chique) is the cause, the female being adapted for an intracutaneous permanent attachment to the host (human, pig, poultry and other animals). As with other fleas, the larvae are free living, dusty or sandy soil being best for *T. penetrans*. Adults are also free living at first, when copulation occurs. The fertilized female then finds a suitable host and tries to penetrate crevices in the skin, such as cracks in the soles of the feet (Figure 86.2), between the toes and especially around the toenails. Any part of the human anatomy can be affected. By means of the mouthparts, the female *Tunga* becomes firmly attached and soon swells to the size and shape of a small white pea. Somehow, the host skin envelops the jigger, which lies below the stratum corneum but above the stratum granulosum, leaving only the posterior spiracles exposed to the air. Only when the jigger is almost mature and distended, after 8–12 days, does the infection begin to irritate. Severe inflammation and ulceration ensues, so that scratching helps to expel

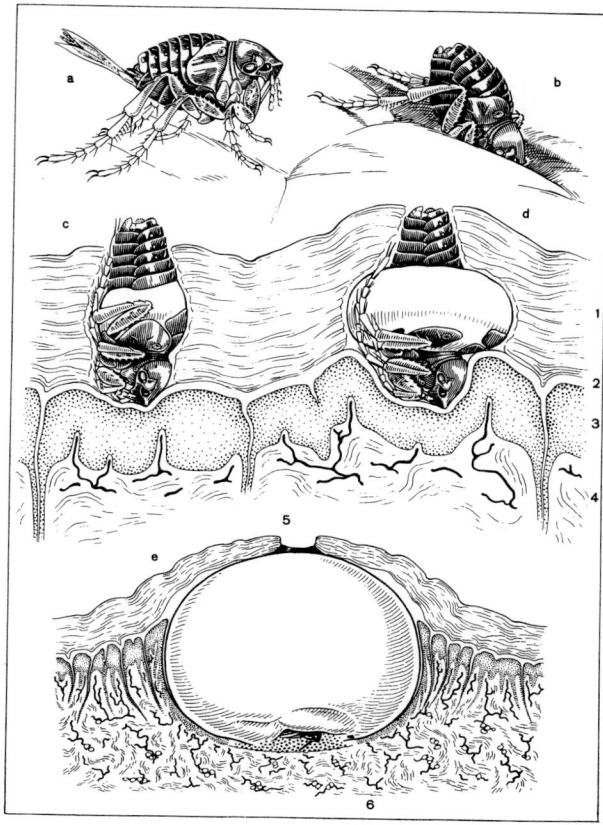

Figure 86.2: The sand flea or jigger.

large numbers of white eggs from the jigger (see also Appendix IV).

Clinical features

The jigger seldom attacks the leg above the dorsum of the foot, but no part of the body escapes. The soles (Figure 86.3), the skin between the toes and that of the roots of the nails are favourite situations. Usually only one or two jiggers are found at a time, but occasionally they are present in hundreds, the little pits left after extraction or expulsion being sometimes so closely set that parts of the surface may look like a honeycomb. During her gestation the jigger causes a considerable amount of irritation. Pus may form around her distended abdomen, which now raises the integument into a pea-like elevation. After the eggs have been laid, the skin ulcerates and the jigger is expelled, leaving a small sore which may become seriously infected or lead to tetanus. Ulceration is common and may follow removal of the jigger or natural extrusion of the egg sac. The ulcer commences as a tiny pit and, as it extends, the sloping edge may develop into a septic ulcer. It remains more or less circular in outline, except under the nail or nail margin, where the outline is more irregular and a pocket of pus forms beneath it.

Management

The mature female jigger should be removed carefully using a sterile needle, so as to pick out the jigger without

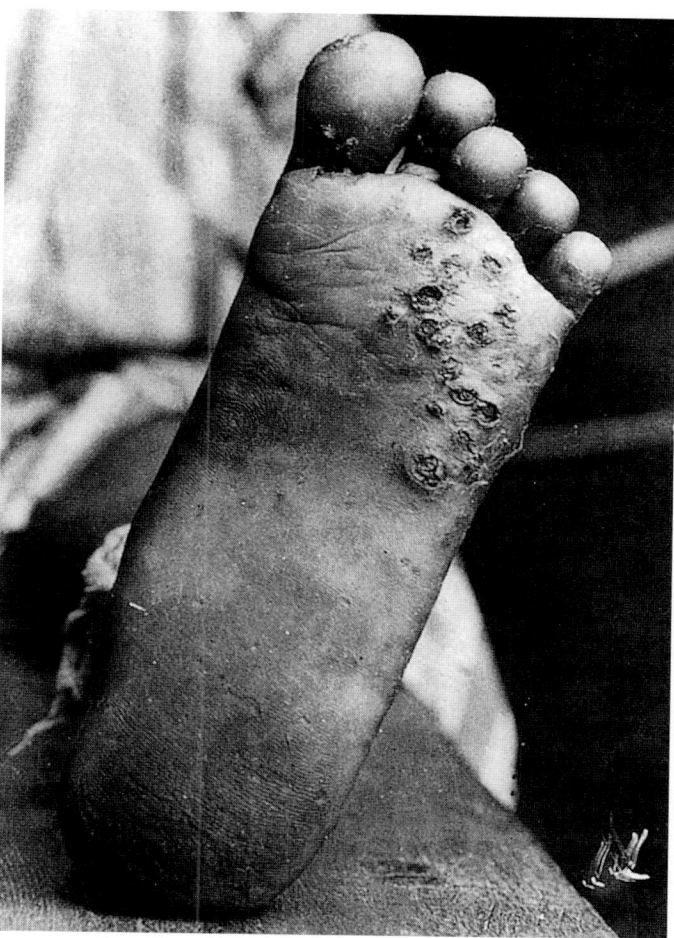

Figure 86.3: Jiggers in the sole of the foot.

bursting it. Inexpert attempts at removal may lead to severe secondary infection.

Prevention (see Appendix IV)

Affected areas of soil may be burnt off in an effort to kill the fleas, or residual insecticide applied to infested areas. As female jiggers are not good jumpers, human infestation is normally confirmed to the feet. Daily inspection of the interdigital clefts, roots of nails and soles of feet should cause freshly burrowing female jiggers to be detected and removed before they have grown much. To prevent attack, foot-enveloping shoes (non 'flip-flops' or sandals) are effective—and a more sensible solution than repellents.

Scabies

Geographical distribution

Scabies is a worldwide infection generally associated with an unhygienic lifestyle, owing to shortage of washing water, irrespective of climate.

Aetiology

Sarcoptes scabiei, the itch or scabies mite (Acari: Sarcoptidae), causes human scabies. The same species is the aetiological agent of sarcoptic mange in dogs, horses and other animals.[5]

The female *S. scabiei* (0.3–0.4 mm) is twice the size of the male (0.2 mm) (see Appendix IV). The gravid female lays her oval eggs (15 × 100 μm) in a burrow in the skin. The eggs give rise to adults 10–14 days later, after passing through the larval and one or two nymphal stages. The nymphs moult, become sexually mature, and pair off on the surface of the skin. The adults live for 4–5 weeks.

Transmission

Transmission is from person to person by direct skin contact and through bedding and clothing. Scabies is often transmitted sexually. The newly fertilized female is the infective agent.

Pathology

Both males and females of *S. scabiei* make short burrows, but it is only the fertilized female that makes a permanent burrow in the horny layers of the skin, with the female at the end (see Appendix IV). Pathology is the result of sensitization of the host to the mites and their excretions.

A vesicle is present at the entry point of the tunnel in which eggs and faeces are deposited. The larvae hatch out after 3–4 days, when they leave the burrow for the skin surface for food and shelter in the hair follicles. After 4–5 days the adults mate and the female burrows into the cuticle of the skin to complete the cycle.

The population of mites builds up over 2–4 months and a fully developed case of scabies may have no more than 20 adult mites, often less. When sensitization of the host occurs, a generalized rash develops. Infiltration with eosinophils is found round the burrows, and foci of lymphocytes and histiocytes can be found deep in the corium after cure.

Clinical features (see also Chapter 19)
Incubation period
There is an incubation period of 6–8 weeks before symptoms appear.

Symptoms and signs
The first stage is a small (1–3 mm), slightly raised, itchy papule which develops at the site of each mite. Scratching may destroy the mote and convert the papule into a pustule. Local sensitization is followed by the appearance of a rash.

The generalized rash of scabies is an itchy erythematous rash, the distribution of which does not correspond to the site of the mites. It is a phenomenon of hypersensitivity in which it may be impossible to demonstrate mites. The eruption occurs most commonly in the axillae, around the waist, at the inner aspect of the thighs and at the back of the legs, from which it may spread all over the body. It commonly occurs in reinfection, and the number of mites present may be small.

Immunosuppression and crusted scabies
Evidence for acquired immunity to scabies comes from the finding that, in immunosuppressed persons, the mites

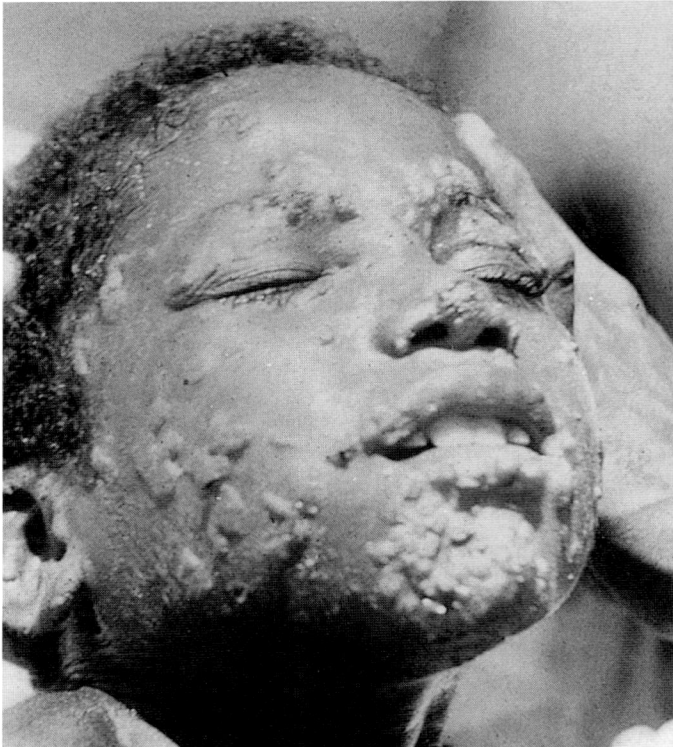

Figure 86.4: Crusted scabies. (Courtesy of P. Rotmil.)

escape control and multiply considerably, leading to encrustation of the skin, a condition known as crusted or Norwegian scabies. Steroid therapy to control undiagnosed itching may change ordinary into crusted scabies.

This is a severe type of scabies accompanied by profuse crusting and hyperkeratotic plaques (Figure 86.4). It is common in the tropics and used to be common in leprosy. Burrows are not formed and a large number of scabies mites may be present on the surface of the skin.

Scabies in children
Scabies in children is atypical. During the first year of life the lesions are general and resemble pemphigus, the buttocks and perineum being most often severely affected. Burrows are often impossible to find, and secondarily infected excoriations and scattered pustules are the most characteristic lesion (Figure 86.5).

Sarcoptic mange (animal scabies)
This is sometimes contracted by people following contact with dogs, cats and cattle infested with zoonotic races of *Sarcoptes*. It may be distinguished from human scabies by the distribution of papules and vesicles on the arms, shoulders, trunks and thighs, and by the absence of burrows on the hands. Sarcoptic mange responds rapidly to treatment with ivermectin or sulphur.

Important complication: nephritis
Secondary infection of scabies lesions is very common, especially in children. Scabies infected with nephritogenic

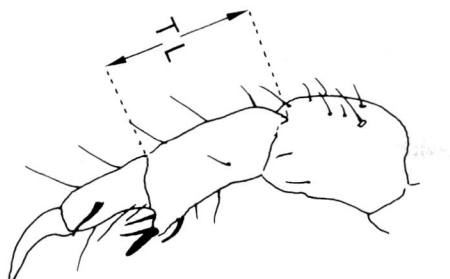

Figure 86.5: The second leg of *Pediculus*, showing the length of the tibia (TL). In *P. capitis* TL = approximately 0.3 mm, and in *P. humanus* TL = approximately 0.4 mm.

strains of β-haemolytic streptococci is an important cause of glomerulonephritis, and in some parts of the world may be a more frequent cause of nephritis than streptococcal throat infection. Secondarily infected scabies should always be treated with a course of antibiotics at the same time as antiscabetic treatment.

Differential diagnosis

Scabies in the tropics is atypical in appearance, especially in children, in whom crusted scabies may be difficult to distinguish from eczema and pyoderma. Itching is severe in scabies, in which it may be possible to identify burrows. In adults, onchocerciasis (also intensely pruritic) and lepromatous leprosy (with which scabies may coexist) must be thought of.

Diagnosis

Scabies burrows between the fingers may be seen with a magnifying glass. After opening a burrow, the mite at the end can be extracted with a needle and examined under mineral oil. Scrapings from ulcers may reveal mites or eggs.

Management (see also Chapter 19)

All members of the family in contact with the patient should be treated at the same time. In addition to affected areas of the head, it is important to treat the whole body from the neck down. Mites are found only above the neck in infants.

Benzyl benzoate 20% emulsion should be applied from the neck down after a bath and allowed to dry, when the clothes may be put on again. After 24 hours a second bath should be taken, and the clothes and bedclothes washed in the meantime. A second treatment should be given 1 week later. Crusted lesions should first be removed with a mixture of sulphur and salicylic acid. Secondary infection is treated with a 5-day course of penicillin.

NBIN emulsion concentrate consists of 68% benzyl benzoate, 6% DDT, 12% benzocaine and 14% polysorbate 80. This requires a dilution of 1:15 in water before use.

Tetmosol (tetraethylthiuram monosulphide) in a 5% solution can be used as benzyl benzoate. In soap form it is of little value.

Crotamiton (Eurax) is applied daily for 5 days and is suitable for infants. It is more expensive but has powerful antipruritic properties.

Lotions of 0.5% malathion or 1% BHC are also effective, and sting less than benzyl benzoate.

Epidemiology and control

Human scabies waxes and wanes in incidence over 15–20-year cycles, probably as a result of changing immunity patterns. Scabies is widespread in the tropics, especially among children. Infection is associated with poor hygiene—the result of inadequate water supply.

Good personal hygiene, plus the search for and treatment of infected families, is the best form of control in the community.

Prevention is by avoidance of skin contact with infected persons and clothing. People able to wash themselves frequently do not suffer much from scabies.

Louse infestation

Three species of louse are parasitic to humans:

- *Pediculus humanus* (body louse).
- *Pediculus capitis* (head louse).
- *Phthirus pubis* (crab louse).

Pediculus humanus and *P. capitis* are morphologically similar but have different habits. Although experimental interbreeding is possible, this does not happen in nature. The majority of lice are host specific, and although lice from domestic animals may be found on humans they do not persist. Most lice do not survive for long when removed from the host.

Pediculus humanus (body louse)

Aetiology

P. humanus is larger (0.4 mm) than *P. capitis* (0.3 mm) and there are minor morphological differences (Figures 86.5 and 86.6). The female *P. humanus* sometimes attaches her eggs (nits) to body hair, but more often cements them to cloth fibres, usually along seams and folds in garments. The female lice produce an average of four to five eggs per day during their life of up to 1 month. The nymphs hatch in 8 days, becoming adult after three moults in 18 days. Nymphs and adults take blood meals two to five times a day throughout life.

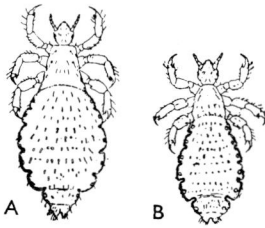

Figure 86.6: (**A**) Female *Pediculus humanus*. (**B**) Female *Pediculus capitis*.

Transmission

Pediculus infestation is usually acquired through close contact with lousy persons, shared clothes and bedding. Lice tend to leave patients with fever and sweating, thus promoting the spread of disease. They avoid light and leave a corpse as it becomes cold.

Clinical features

Body lice cause itching and a generalized red maculopapular rash. Scratching may cause secondary infection and impetigo may result. *P. humanus* is the sole transmitter of louse-borne typhus (*Rickettsia prowazeki*), trench fever (*Rickettsia quintana*) (see Chapter 50) and louse-borne relapsing fever (*Borrelia recurrentis*) (see Chapter 66).

Diagnosis

Eggs (nits) should be searched for on body hair. Adults, nymphs and eggs should be looked for in the seams and folds of clothing.

Pediculus capitis (head louse)

P. capitis females cement their eggs (nits) to the base of head hairs, and growth of the hair eventually brings the empty egg cases into view after the eggs have hatched. They are confirmed to the scalp.

Transmission

This is by close contact, usually head-to-head transfer.

Clinical features

Head lice seldom cause noticeable signs or symptoms, and infestation is principally a hygienic and aesthetic nuisance. In heavy infections some dermatitis of the scalp can result from scratching. *P. capitis* is not known to be a vector for any disease.

Diagnosis

Diagnosis is by searching for the presence of 'nits' in the hair or observing the lice themselves.

Phthirus pubis (crab louse)

Crab lice occur worldwide, and are found exclusively on humans.

Aetiology

Phthirus is shorter and broader then *Pediculus* and has massive claws on the second and third legs by which it clings to hair (Figure 86.7). It is found most commonly in the genital and inguinal regions, but may be found on any of the body hair except that of the scalp, including

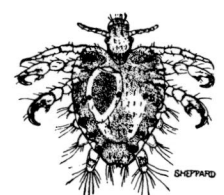

Figure 86.7: Female *Phthirus pubis*, showing the contained ovum. (12 ×.)

the beard, chest hair and eyelashes. It cannot survive off the host for more than 24 hours.

Transmission

This is by sexual and close personal contact.

Clinical features

Infection is normally noticed following irritation caused by the bite. Sometimes a characteristic small 'blue spot' (2–3 mm across) may result from the bite, different from the red spot caused by pediculid lice. *P. pubis* is not known to be the vector of any disease.

Control of lice and the treatment of lousy patients

Pediculus

Destruction of the lice and eggs on clothes is achieved most efficiently by heating to 60°C for 30–40 minutes. For practical purposes, 70°C for 30 minutes is recommended. Particular attention should be paid to folds and pleats, and the application of a hot iron to these is useful. Head lice may be removed by combing with a fine louse-comb, used with soft soap to remove nits. The most efficient comb of this type (Sacker patent) is now in short supply, but others are available, although for best effect they should be used in conjunction with chemical treatments. Chemical methods of control (both species) include the application of DDT or permethrin dusts, or malathion, carbaryl and other insecticides prepared as suitable lotions or shampoos that are commercially available. As insecticide resistance is becoming a problem in many areas, World Health Organization susceptibility tests should be made before widespread application of an insecticide. Such tests should be made on the target population. Resistance in one of the pediculids in a given area does not imply similar resistance in the other.

Phthirus

Chemical methods, as outlined above, are normally used for this species. Resistance to insecticides is rare.

REFERENCES

1 Cundall D B, Whitehead S M & Hechtel F O P. Severe anaemia and death due to the pharyngeal leech *Myxobdella africana*. *Trans R Soc Trop Med Hyg* 1986; 80:940–944.
2 Radcliffe W. *BMJ* 1972; ii:164.
3 Sherman R A & Pechter E A. Maggot therapy: a review of the therapeutic applications of fly larvae in human medicine, especially for heating osteomyelitis. *Med Vet Entomol* 1988; 2:225–230.
4 Lane R P & Crosskey R W (eds) *Medical Insects and Arachnids*. London: Chapman & Hall, 1993.
5 Arlian L G. Biology, host relations, and epidemiology of *Sarcoptes scabei*. *Annu Rev Entomol* 1989; 34:139–161.

Chapter 87
Arthropod Dermatoses, Stings, Bites, Allergies and Neuroses

G. B. White

Acarine dermatosis

Intense irritation and dermatitis, somewhat resembling that produced by scabies, can result from various mites (Acari) living as temporary ectoparasites on the skin of humans. The most common occurrence of such infestation is among workers associated with stored food products in which the mites occur as pests. The more familiar of these are grocer's itch caused by *Glycyphagus domesticus*, baker's itch (*Acarus siro*) and copra itch (*Tyrophagus putrescentiae*). *Pyemotes tritici* (= *ventricosus*), the grain or straw itch mite (Figure 87.1), causes an urticarial and papular eruption of exposed parts of the body in those who handle grain, cottonseeds, beans and especially straw.

These mites give rise to a severe pruritus, especially on the trunk. A lotion of warm water and vinegar or a saturated solution of picric acid in 90% alcohol will relieve the irritation. An application of 5% betanaphthol ointment is a preventive treatment, and a dilute phenol solution will kill the mites. *Dermatophagoides* mites have been recorded as causing an unusually severe dermatitis in humans. In one case, infestation of the scalp persisted for 7 years. Among the constituents of house dust it has been found that *Dermatophagoides* produces the most potent allergen. Bites of thrombiculid mites, or chiggers, cause a parasitic dermatitis known as trombidiosis or scrub-itch. This condition is an allergic reaction to the saliva of the mite and can be caused by about 15 species, mostly belonging to the genera *Eutrombicula*, *Schoengastia* and *Neoschoengastia*. Trombiculid bites can be prevented by mite repellents such as diethyltoluamide (see also Chapter 19).

Ticks

Extensive subcutaneous haemorrhages can be caused by the anticoagulant inoculated with the saliva of ticks.

Butterfly and moth dermatoses

Various moth and butterfly caterpillars, usually of the families Arctiidae, Lymantriidae, Saturniidae, Megalopygidae, Notodontidae and Nymphalidae, possess urticating hairs that can cause dermatitis. These hairs penetrate the skin, and poison may be injected through them from attached glands. The poisons include histamine and cause irritation which can be severe if mucous membranes are affected, for example when detached hairs enter the eye and give rise to nodular conjunctivitis.[1] Both larvae and adults can be involved.

In Papua New Guinea and northern Australia, the moth *Ochrogaster lunifer* has caused epidemics of urticaria among troops. In Brazil, flannel moths (Megalopygidae) are well known urticators. In the Panama Canal zone, the urticating caterpillars of *Megalopyge lanata* produce rapidly developing eosinophilia (8–22%), numbness and vesication. The 'puss caterpillar', *Megalopyge opercularis*,

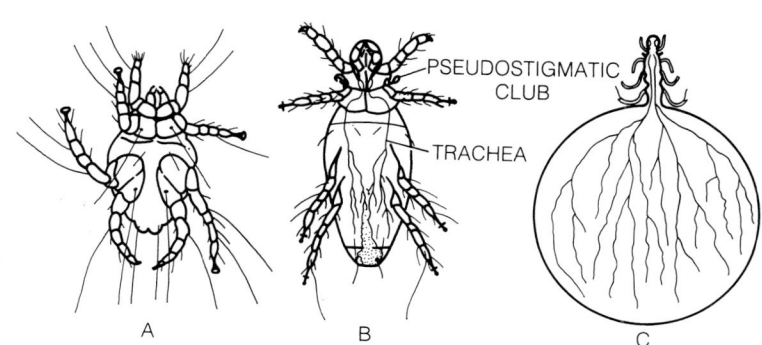

Figure 87.1: *Pyemotes tritici*. (**A**) Male. (**B**) Female. (**C**) Pregnant female with brood sac. (80 ×.)

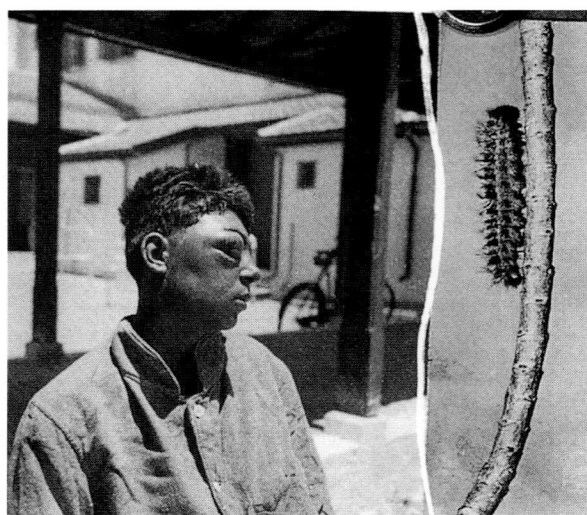

Figure 87.2: Urticating dermatitis caused by contact with a processionary caterpillar of the moth *Thaumetopoea wilkinsoni*.

causes thousands of cases of dermatitis in children in Texas, necessitating the closure of schools. In Japan, some 300 000 people were affected by the moth *Euproctis flava*. In Israel *Thaumetopoea pinivora* causes trouble every year in February and May, and caterpillar dermatitis is also common in northern Kenya (Figure 87.2).

Urticating hairs may become detached from the caterpillar and the cocoon spun by the caterpillar before pupation. Such detached hairs may retain their urticating properties for a long time. If inhaled these hairs may cause dyspnoea, and if ingested they may give rise to stomatitis. In Africa *Anaphe renata* (Notodontidae) and related moths have both imago and larva clothed with detachable irritating hairs.

Caterpillars of the Venezuelan saturniid moth *Lonomia achelous* inject, through their hairs, a powerful anti-coagulant if handled or even brushed against, and long-lasting fibrinolytic bleeding results.[2]

In Africa and Asia some adult moths of the families Pyralidae, Geometridae and Noctuidae feed upon the eye discharges of various mammals, including humans. Although their proboscces cannot penetrate living tissue, they may well be vectors of mammalian epidemic keratoconjunctivitis and other eye diseases. In Malaya one noctuid fruit-piercing moth *Calyptra eustrigata* can penetrate mammalian skin and suck blood, and must therefore be considered a potential vector of disease or producer of allergic reactions.[3]

Beetle dermatitis

Beetle larvae of the family Dermestidae have urticating hairs that produce a dermatitis. As these beetles are pests of stored products, dockers unloading ships' cargoes have developed dyspnoea and erucic stomatitis from the inhalation and ingestion of detached hairs.

The family Meloidae contains some species known as blister beetles because their body fluids contain cantharidin, a cytotoxic principle that causes vesicular dermatitis when applied to the skin. The best known species is the so-called Spanish fly *Lytta vesicatoria*, and in India *Mylabris cichorii* and *Epicauta hirticornis* are troublesome. In the Gilbert Islands severe blistering is caused by the coconut beetles *Sessinia collaris* and *Ananca decolor* of the family Oedemeridae. The bushmen of South Africa use body fluids from the larvae of the chrysomelid beetle *Diamphidia nigroornata* as a lethal arrow poison which causes death from a general paralysis. Staphylinid beetles of the genus *Paederus* cause urticaria and blistering, and minute species of the genera *Atheta* and *Oxytelus* fly in numbers and may enter the eye, causing a burning sensation.

Other insects

Other insects that cause dermatitis are ceratopogonid flies (biting midges) of the genus *Culicoides*. In Brazil *C. paraensis* is a public health problem in this way, and in El Salvador an increase in biting *Culicoides* was correlated with decreasing standards of sanitation and the cessation of a control campaign against the breeding sites of the mosquito *Aedes aegypti*. In Japan there are records of eczema following the bites of *C. erairai*, and long-lasting sores (3–4 months) following bites by *C. obsoletus*. Mosquito bites in persons sensitized to their saliva can cause troublesome chronic ulcers which will respond dramatically to topical steroids. Sandflies and black flies can similarly cause quite severe reactions in sensitized persons which will respond fairly readily to steroid ointment such as betamethasone valerate. An irritant vesicular rash, superficially resembling scabies, can be caused by Thysanoptera (see also Appendix IV).

Bee and wasp stings

The stings of bees, wasps and hornets may produce a mild reaction that is easily soothed with an ice-pack, diluted vinegar or antihistamine ointment. They may be very serious in the case of multiple stinging or stings in the mouth. Some people react violently to bee stings and may become increasingly hypersensitive with each successive sting. In such cases anaphylaxis may result, which can be fatal. Massive anaphylaxis causes muscular paralysis and suggests a curare-like action on synapses of muscle end-plates. The antidote is an injection of adrenaline (epinephrine).

People who are extremely sensitive to bee stings should always have access to a pressurized bronchodilator spray and use two puffs while breathing in; this procedure can be repeated in 15 minutes. Such patients, however, may quickly become faint and lose consciousness, and should be taken immediately into medical care.[4,5]

Bee and wasp venoms contain histamine, acetylcholine and enzymes (phospholipase A and hyaluronidase); the more superficial aspects of a sting are due to the histamine. The Africa honey bee *Apis mellifica adansonii* is abundant in equatorial and warm temperate southern Africa, and is a fairly aggressive species. In 1956 this species was introduced into South America and hybridization with local bees has produced an extremely aggressive race of Brazilian honey bees. The spread of these bees has been very rapid from South America to the USA. A number of fatalities has resulted from the abundance and special behavioural characteristics of the bee. The slightest disturbance near the hive can cause hundreds of bees to become airborne; they may then sting any animal or human within 100 m of the apiary and may pursue fleeing victims for over 1 km.[6,7]

In the honey bee, the sting is torn out by the act of stinging, but the poison gland, (which is attached to the sting) continues to inject venom into the wound. For this reason the sting should be carefully removed as soon as possible and the remaining venom expressed from the gland with forceps.

Sometimes stingless social bees (*Melipona*, etc.) are prone to aggressive mass biting, and some neotropical species squirt caustic fluid, but these insects are rarely more than a nuisance. Some tiny stingless sweat bees (*Trigona*) can be annoying in the African savannah regions and, because of their numbers and persistence, are sometimes mistaken for *Simulium* (black flies).

Wasps (*Vespula*) and hornets (*Vespa*) can sting repeatedly because, unlike the honey bee, the sting is not torn out by the action of stinging. Wasp venom contains a higher proportion of histamine and 5-hydroxytryptamine (serotonin), which is distinctly more active than that of the honey bee. *Scleroderma nipponensis* (Bethylidae), in one incident in Japan, attacked 340 people, who were left with reddish swellings and injuries leading to suppuration and lymphangitis. Some parasitic wasps of the family Ichneumonidae, such as *Ophion*, *Netelia* and *Ichneumon*, can inflict painful stings. Sensitive patients may be ill for some weeks following these stings.

Paper-wasps of the genus *Polistes* also cause many fatalities in the New World. These wasps build their nests under the eaves of houses or in ornamental shrubs and trees where people are likely to be exposed to their stings.

Arthropod venoms are considered in Chapter 32, and by Beard[8] and Bucherl and Buckley.[9]

Poisonous honey

Occasionally the honey produced by hive bees, wild honey bees, bumble-bees and stingless bees may be toxic if particular plants are foraged or if polluted liquid resources are used in the absence of clean drinking water (which should be provided in the case of honey bees).

Ants

Ants can bite, sting and squirt formic acid. Mostly, the attacks of ants produce only mild effects, but, as in wasps,

the stinging apparatus is a modified ovipositor that can be extracted after each sting and used repeatedly; multiple stinging may induce an anaphylactic response. Some ants may also be mechanical transmitters of disease; for example, Pharoah's ants (*Monomorium pharaonis*) have been found to carry *Salmonella*, *Pseudomonas*, *Staphylococcus*, *Streptococcus* and *Clostridium* spp. in hospitals.[10]

The venom of ants is largely proteinaceous but in the south-eastern USA *Solenopsis richteri* is a dangerous fire ant in which the venom is non-proteinaceous and exhibits necrotic activity resembling the bites of *Loxosceles* spiders. When a colony is disturbed, the ants erupt in thousands and 3000–5000 stings may be administered in a matter of seconds. Allergic reactions to such stings, and anaphylactic shock, may sometimes result in the death of sensitive individuals. The subject is reviewed by Gurney.[11]

Other bites and allergies

Skin reactions of both immediate and delayed hypersensitivity type were common following the bite of *Triatoma infestans* and *T. maxima* in Brazil, where the former was the major human-biting triatomid (Hemiptera). The reactions were sufficiently severe to prevent the use of these bugs for xenodiagnosis.[12]

Other orders that contain insects capable of inflicting bites or stings include other Hemiptera (plant bugs) and some Orthoptera. Chicken bugs in Mexico (*Haematosiphon inodorus*) and Brazil (*Ornithocoris toledo*) attack poultry, but may incidentally bite humans and may produce a polymorphous dermatitis with pustules, scabs and linear scars. The bite of the giant water-bugs (Belostomatidae) may be nearly as severe as a bee sting. Many other bugs will bite if handled incautiously. The larger coreid and pentatomid bugs can squirt a jet of irritant fluid from the metathoracic glands into the eye of the beholder, which may cause a very painful reaction for a day or two.

The bites of several insects not mentioned above may also produce allergic reactions. Recorded cases involve adult flies of the rhagionid genus *Symphoromyia* and larvae of Therevidae[13] and Tabanidae[14] (Diptera), and the possibility of such reactions following the bite of almost any insect must be considered; if possible, suspected specimens should be collected and identified by a specialist.

In addition to bites, other allergic reactions are not uncommon. Inhalant allergens may be acquired from acarine sources in house dust (especially from *Dermatophagoides pteronyssinus*) or among stored products from the grain weevil *Sitophilus granarius* or the Mexican bean weevil *Zabrotes subfasciatus*.

Some aquatic insects such as Ephemeroptera and Trichoptera emerge in vast numbers, and their cast exuviae are fragmented and windborne and become inhalant allergens. Chironomidae ('green nimitti') have also been associated with asthma and other allergic symptoms along the Nile.[15] Terrestrial counterparts that cause similar allergies are the prolific aphids.

Allergic reactions to the bites and stings of insects and other arthropods have been considered by Frazier[16] and Frazier and Brown.[17] Tu[18] has surveyed the whole field of arthropod poisons, allergens and venoms.

For the identification of arthropods of medical importance, Lane and Crosskey[19] should be consulted.

Neuroses

Many people have a morbid fear of insects. The extreme manifestation of this is in delusory parasitosis (Ekbom's syndrome), also loosely referred to as parasitophobia, acarophobia or entomophobia. In these cases patients suffering from dermatitis artefacta, usually of emotional origin, believe that they are infested with insects or other parasites which cause the itching. They then scratch the affected parts until the skin breaks down. Further skin damage may be caused by the overuse of disinfectants or insecticides. Such cases are difficult, and best treated by a psychiatrist, but every effort should be made to establish that there are in fact no minute biting insects such as *Culicoides* or allergen-producing mites or insects, particularly of the type bearing or shedding urticating hairs. The possibility of inanimate allergens such as paint should also be investigated carefully. Cases of delusory parasitosis may follow an actual infestation by fleas or other arthropods, by seeing or reading about ectoparasites in the popular media,[20,21] or as a result of emotional disturbances.[22] Some success in treating this difficult condition has recently been claimed from use of the drug pimozide. A common feature of these cases is that the persistence of the sufferer often results in a second member of the household presenting with similar symptoms, which adds credence to their claims.

Sometimes there are group outbreaks of imagined biting insects, a phenomenon that has only received attention in the 1980s.[22] In these cases 'phantom biters' may persist for 2–3 years in offices or small factories where several people work together. The causative agent may be carpet fibres, fragments of glass-fibre lampshades, or the coverings of wires on telephone switchboards. Spraying *during working hours* (even with water) has sometimes proved effective in these cases. Here again, extreme care should be taken that an actual infestation of mites or minute insects is not the cause.

REFERENCES

1   Watson P G & Sevel D. *Br J Ophthalmol* 1966; 50:209–217.
2   Arocha-Pinango C L & Layrisse M. *Lancet* 1969; i:810–812.
3   Bänziger H. *Mitt Schweiz Ent Ges* 1980; 53:127–142.
4   Frankland A W. Bee sting allergy. *Bee World* 1976; 57:145–150.
5   Hoffman D R. *Cutis* 1977; 19:763–767.
6   Michener C D. The Brazilian bee problem. *Annu Rev Entomol* 1975; 20:399–416.
7   Taylor O R. *Bee World* 1977; 58:19–30.
8   Beard R L. *Annu Rev Entomol* 1963; 8:1–18.
9   Bucherl W & Buckley E E. *Venomous Animals and Their Venoms. III. Venomous Invertebrates.* London: Chapman & Hall, 1971.
10 Beatson S H. *Lancet* 1972; i:425–427.
11 Gurney A B. Some stinging ants. *Insect World Digest* 1975; Sept/Oct:19–25.
12 Costa C H N, Costa M T, Weber J N et al. *Trans R Soc Trop Med Hyg* 1981; 75:405–408.
13 Smith K G V. *Lancet* 1979; i:391–392.
14 Otsuru M & Ogawa S. *Acta Med Biol* 1959; 7:37–50.
15 Crranston P S, Gad-El-Rab M & Kay A B. *Trans R Soc Trop Med Hyg* 1981; 75:1–4.
16 Frazier C A. *Insect Allergy. Allergic and Toxic Reactions to Insects and Other Arthropods.* St Louis: WH Green, 1969.
17 Frazier C A & Brown F K. *Insects and Allergy.* Norman: University of Oklahoma Press, 1980.
18 Tu A T (ed.) *Handbook of Natural Toxins,* vol. 2. *Insect Poisons, Allergens and Other Invertebrate Venoms.* New York: Marcel Dekker, 1984.
19 Lane R P & Crosskey R W. *Medical Insects and Arachnids.* London: Chapman & Hall, 1993.
20 Busvine J R. *Insects and Hygiene,* 3rd edn. London: Chapman & Hall, 1980.
21 Mester H. Das Syndrom des wahnhaften Ungezieferbefalls. *Agnew Parasitol* 1977; 18:70–84.
22 Lyell A. *Br J Dermatol* 1983; 108:485–499.

Appendix I
Clinical Laboratory Diagnosis

A. H. Moody

Health and safety[1]

Laboratory safety

Great care must be taken to provide a safe working environment for laboratory staff when handling infective material in order to prevent contamination of the area and infection of the laboratory staff.

The laboratory should be constructed with adequate impervious benching and good lighting. Protective clothing for staff should be provided and hand-washing facilities made available.

Under no circumstances should food or drink be prepared or consumed in the laboratory area.

Laboratory training

Technical staff should be well trained for the tasks they are to perform and supervised before being allowed to handle clinical samples. Training should include knowledge of potential hazards that various clinical samples present including the risk of aerosols and droplet formation. Microbiological samples should be processed away from other laboratory areas, particularly samples that carry a risk of viral transmission or tuberculosis.

Standard operating procedures (SOPs)

Each method used in the laboratory should be written into an SOP with additional information on interpretation of the results obtained and any special precautions necessary for handling the reagents or chemicals made available.

Written instructions on how to deal with breakage or spillage involving specimens should be clearly available and a suitable laboratory disinfection procedure followed.

Apparatus used in the laboratory should have clear written instructions for proper use and maintenance.

Instructions for disinfection and disposal of clinical specimens by incineration should be available.

A procedure for disposing of needles and other 'sharps' into a suitable impervious pot, with appropriate provision for incineration, should be in place.

Using the laboratory

The laboratory is an essential tool for the diagnosis of infectious diseases in most countries and much of the work is still performed manually, requiring good observation skills. Parasitic organisms are recognized by their size, colour and morphological appearance, often with the assistance of stains and in the case of scanty infections, after concentration to increase the numbers of parasite stages present. In chronic infection, active stages of a parasite may not be found easily and diagnosis may be made more appropriately by serological means. In a few cases the diagnosis may be made by only histological examination. Molecular techniques, notably using the polymerase chain reaction (PCR), are becoming important tools for diagnosis of viral (human immunodeficiency virus; HIV) and microbiological (*Mycobacterium tuberculosis*)[2] infections. Their use for the routine diagnosis of parasites is still at an early stage. The introduction of rapid diagnostic tests using labelled monoclonal antibody tests based on immunochromatography has improved the ability to screen for several important infections at clinic or small laboratory level.

Clinical parasitology diagnosis

Essential equipment for routine diagnosis of intestinal and blood parasites includes a microscope, preferably equipped with a binocular head and 10x eyepiece. A good quality substage Abbe condenser with a diaphragm to control the entry of light and objectives with 10x, 40x and 100x magnification are most suitable. Substage illumination using electric lighting is the better option, although several microscopes are available that give the alternative option of using reflected sunlight.

A calibrated graticule should be available for one of the eyepieces. The graticule can be left in situ or inserted as required. It should be calibrated for each objective using a slide micrometer.

Faecal concentration

When parasite ova, larvae or protozoan cysts are present in very low numbers, faecal concentration may be necessary. Several methods are available, depending on resources, and two methods are described below.

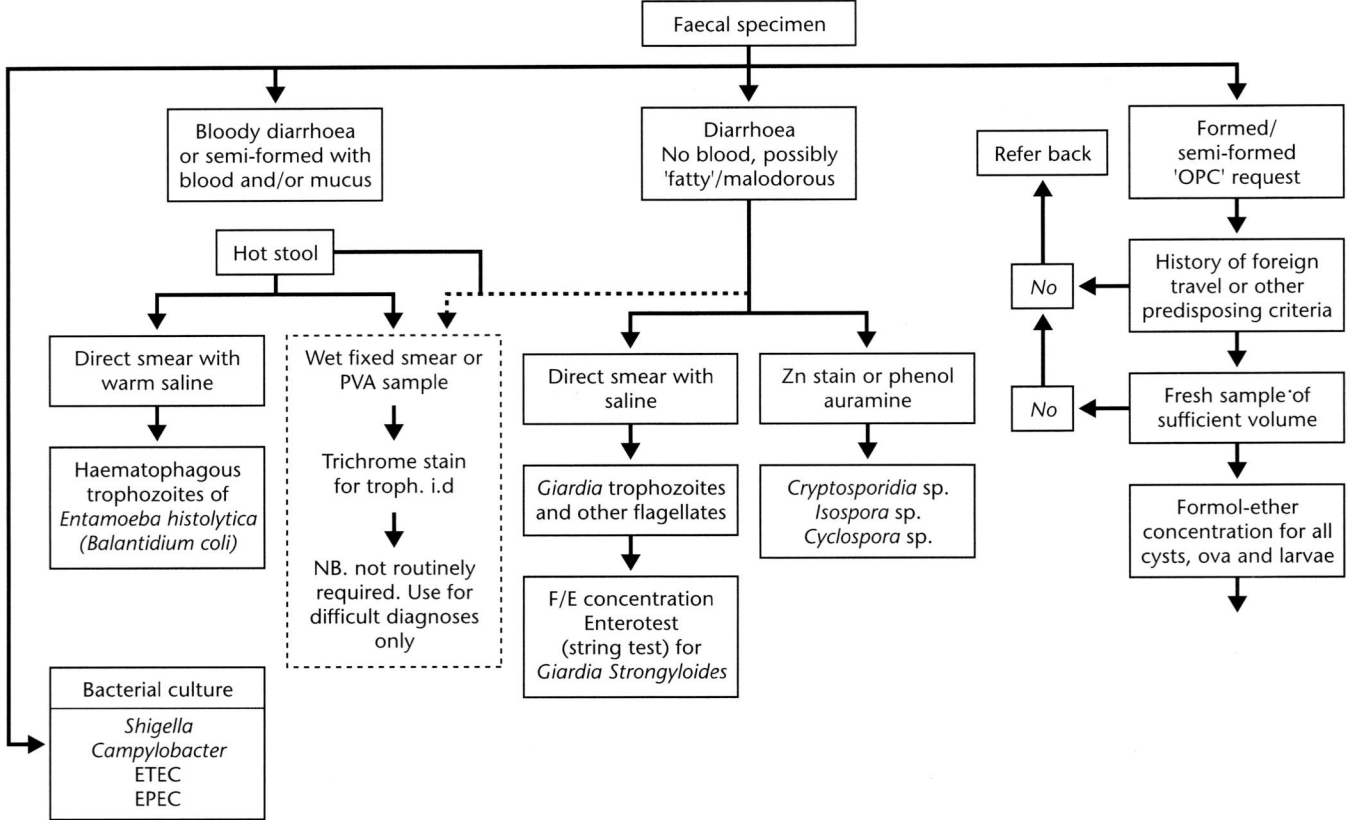

Figure I.1: Flow diagram for the laboratory investigation of causes of diarrhoea. OCP, ova, cysts, parasites; Zn, Ziehl–Neelsen; Troph, trophozoite; i.d. identification; ETEC, enterotoxigenic *Escherichia coli*; EPEC, enteropathogenic *E. coli*.

Investigation of the causes of diarrhoea (Figure I.1)

Diarrhoea may be defined as a change in bowel habits different to that normally experienced. Faecal appearance can be categorized as solid, unformed or liquid, depending on its consistency.

Causes of diarrhoea may be bacterial, parasitic[3], viral or dietary, and specific procedures may be needed to determine the cause including, enzyme-linked immunosorbent assay (ELISA)[4] and molecular methods.[5]

Direct examination of faeces

Direct examination of a suspension of fresh faeces in warm saline enables the presence of motile trophozoites of protozoa to be seen (*Entamoeba histolytica, Giardia lamblia, Chilomastix mesnilli, Trichomonas hominis*). It will also show protozoan cysts and helminth larvae and ova, when present in sufficient numbers. The presence of cellular exudate can be seen and described. The presence of white blood cells, red blood cells and macrophages may help to confirm a diagnosis of amoebic or bacillary dysentery.

Excess fat globules may be apparent in cases of malabsorption seen in parasitic or viral infections of the small bowel (*G. lamblia, Cyclospora cayetanensis, Isospora belli, Cryptosporidium parvum, Rotavirus*, etc.).

Faecal smears may be prepared and stained to show the characteristic morphological features of trophozoites[6] or spores of *Microsporidia* spp.[7] and to describe the exudate content.

Preparation of direct faecal smear

Materials
- Physiological saline (0.9% sodium chloride).
- Lugol's iodine.

Method
1. Take a microscope slide and label one end with the patient's name.
2. Place a drop of warm saline (37°C) at each end of the slide.
3. Using an applicator stick, select a small piece of faecal material and emulsify the faeces into the two drops of saline on the slide. If the faeces contains any blood or mucus, prepare a separate slide for this. Add a drop of Lugol's iodine solution to the right-hand suspension.
4. Place a 22-mm coverslip on to each preparation and view the slide using the 10x and 40x objectives.

Motile organisms will be identified by characteristic movement and appearance; confirmation can be made with one of the staining methods described.

Other parasites can be seen at lower power. Staining with Lugol's iodine solution enhances the internal structure of protozoan cysts but will kill active trophozoites. Cells present can be stained and identified by running a little 1% methylene blue stain beneath the coverslip.

Faecal concentration methods

Concentration methods are necessary when cysts and ova are present in low numbers; these methods do not show motile trophozoites (Figures I.2–I.9).

Method 1: Formol–ether/ethyl acetate concentration for ova and cysts

Materials
• 10% v/v formalin (100 ml formaldehyde + 900 ml distilled water).

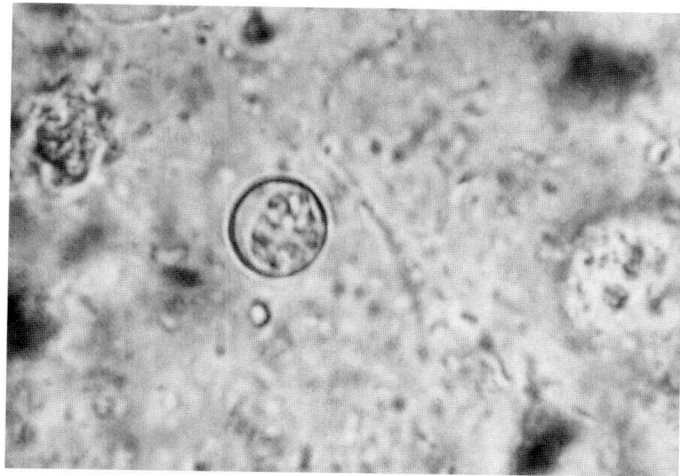
Figure I.4: Oocyst of *Cyclospora cayetanensis*.

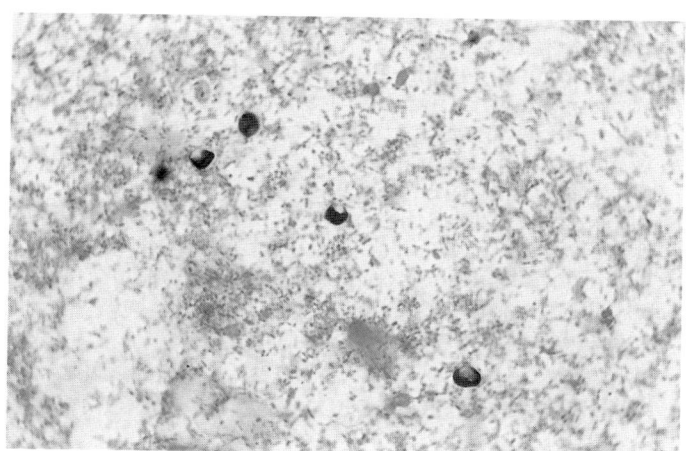
Figure I.2: Oocysts of *Cryptosporidium parvum*.

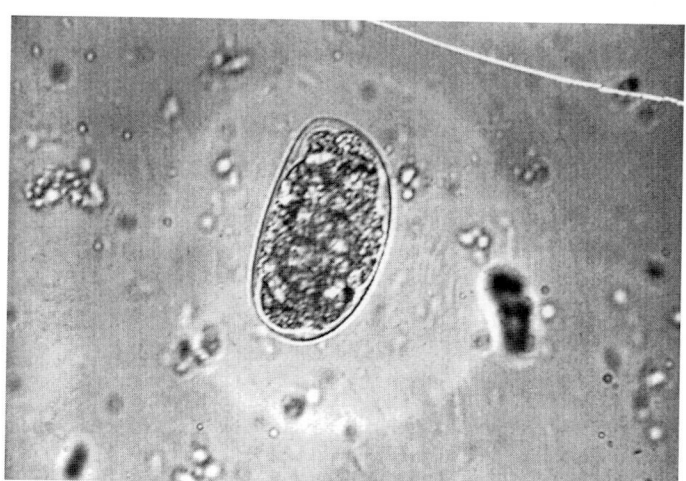
Figure I.5: Ovum of hookworm.

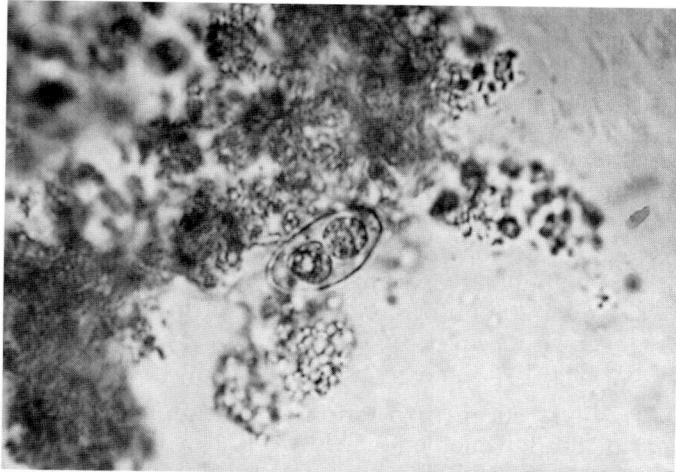
Figure I.3: Oocyst of *Isospora belli*.

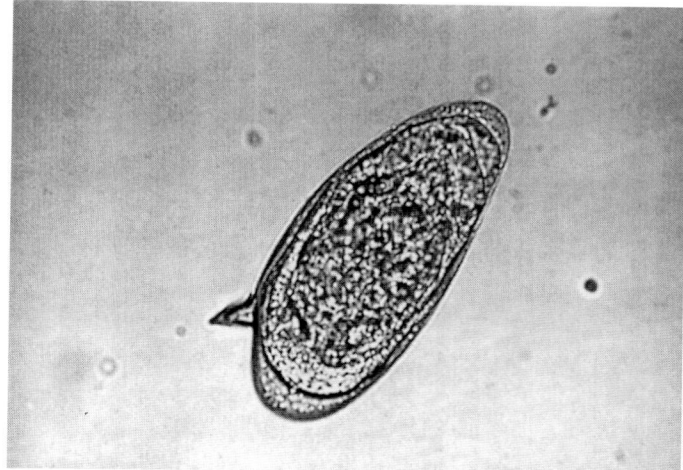
Figure I.6: Ovum of *Schistosoma mansoni*.

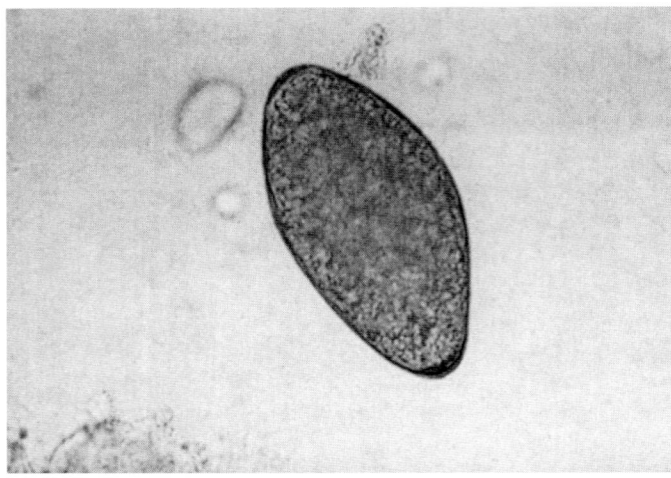

Figure I.7: Ovum of *Fasciola hepatica*.

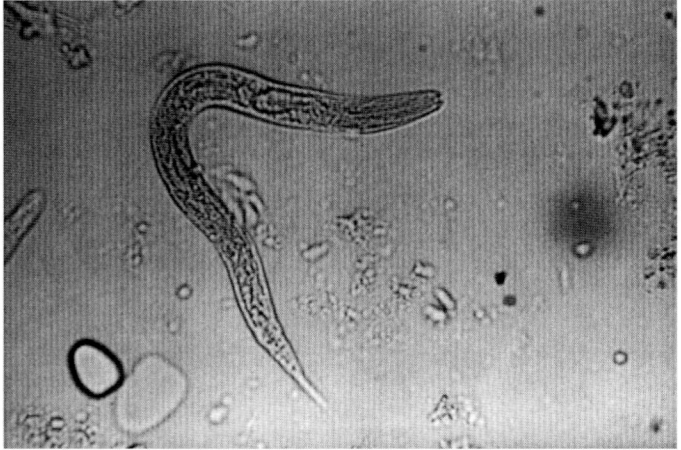

Figure I.8: Larva of *Strongyloides stercoralis*.

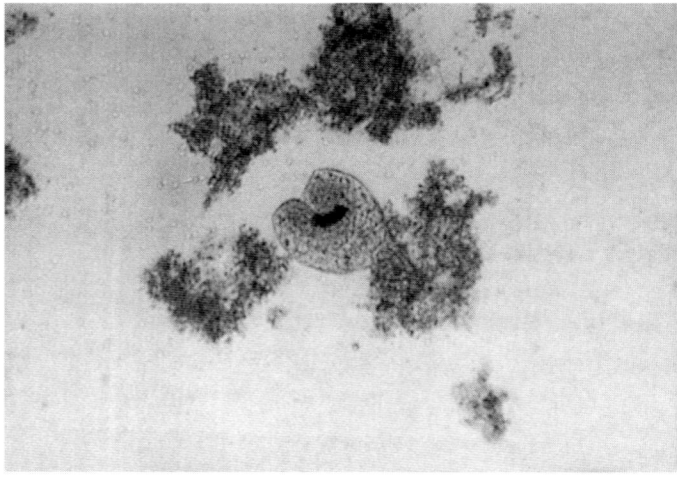

Figure I.9: Protoscolice of *Echinococcus granulosus*.

- Diethyl ether or ethyl acetate.
- 40 Mesh (425 μm) brass wire filter, 3 inches (7.5 cm) in diameter—a nylon coffee strainer (600-μm mesh) can also be used satisfactorily. Commercial versions of these filters that provide an enclosed system, adding safety to the use of flammable solvents, are available (Diassys/Intersep).
- Small 3-inch (7.5 cm) dish or beaker.

A vortex mixer and electric or battery-powered centrifuge capable of receiving 15-cm centrifuge tubes and operating at 1000 g may also be required.

Method
1. Using applicator sticks, select a quantity of faeces (approximately 1 g) to include external and internal portions.
2. Place in a centrifuge tube containing 7 ml of 10% formalin.
3. Emulsify the faeces in the formalin and filter through the brass/plastic filter into the dish.
4. Wash the filter and discard any lumpy residue.
5. Transfer the filtrate to a boiling tube; add 3 ml of ether and mix well on a vortex mixer for 15 s or by hand for 1 min.
6. Transfer back to the centrifuge tube and centrifuge at 3000 r.p.m. for 1 min.
7. Loosen the fatty plug with an orange stick and pour the supernatant away by quickly inverting the tube. It is necessary to dispose of ether/ethyl-acetate safely as these are flammable items.
8. Allow the fluid on the side of the tube to drain on to the deposit; mix well, and transfer a drop to a slide for examination under a coverslip.
9. Use the 10x and 40x objectives to examine the *whole* of the deposit for ova and cysts.

Method 2: Saturated salt flotation method

1. Coarse granular sodium chloride in excess is boiled in water to produce a saturated solution which, when cooled, has a relative density (specific gravity) of 10.18–10.20.
2. Half-fill a wide-mouthed flat-bottomed container with the saturated salt solution.
3. Emulsify 1 g of faeces in the solution and remove the larger debris from the surface.
4. Fill the container to the top with saturated salt solution until a convex meniscus forms.
5. Lay a glass slide or coverslip over the top, making sure that no bubbles are trapped.
6. Leave for 20 min before quickly inverting the slide.
7. Cover with a coverslip/slide and scan for ova using the 10x objective.

This is a cheap preparation using simple apparatus, and is ideally suitable for field work. It will concentrate nematode ova well, but does not concentrate protozoan trophozoites or cysts.

'Enterotest' capsule (the string test)

This procedure utilizes a length of thread in a weighted gelatin capsule. The end of the string is taped to the patient's face and the capsule is swallowed. The patient lies on the right side so that the capsule will travel to the duodenum. After 4 hours the string is pulled up (the weight is passed out in the faeces). The string will be stained yellow with bile and mucus where it has been in the duodenum. If no part of the string is yellow, the test should be repeated. The string is placed in a pot and covered with 5 ml of saline.

1. Agitate the string and saline, preferably using a vortex mixer, to remove mucus from the string.
2. Wind the string around an applicator stick, pressing it against the side of the container to remove mucus and excess saline, and then discard it.
3. Centrifuge the saline at 2000 r.p.m. for 2 min.
4. Discard the supernatant and transfer the deposit to a microscope slide and examine using the 10x and 40x objectives for trophozoites of *G. lamblia* and active larvae of *Strongyloides* spp. Ova from flukes in the biliary tract may also be found.

Staining methods for intestinal protozoa

Table I.1 lists the identifying features of common protozoan cysts. Particular stains can be used to identify these features,[4] the stains may be applied to the wet suspension or to an air-dried, fixed faecal smear.

Temporary stains

These stains are applied to wet preparations after concentration by the formol–ether/ethyl acetate method.

Lugol's iodine solution (double strength)

Reagent 1
- Potassium iodide   20 g
- Iodine   10 g
- Distilled water   100 ml

Add potassium iodide to the distilled water; when dissolved, add the iodine crystals. Store in a brown bottle. Remains stable for many weeks.

Reagent 2
- 25% glacial acetic acid

Method
Mix equal parts of reagents 1 and 2 for use.

Results
Iodine stains glycogen brown and the nuclear chromatin of amoebic cysts brown/black.

Burrows' stain for chromatoid inclusion of *Entamoeba* cysts

Thionin	20 mg
Acetic acid	3 ml
Ethanol	3 ml
Distilled water	94 ml

Method
Add an equal volume of the stain to the faecal concentrate and allow to stand for 12–18 hours. After this period, examine one drop of the stained deposit under the microscope.

Results
Chromidial bars within the cysts of *Entamoeba* spp. stain deep blue.

Table I.1 Identification of cysts of common protozoa.

Protozoan cyst	Size	Nuclear pattern	Inclusions
Entamoeba histolytica/dispar	1–4 Nuclei, 9–14 μm	Fine chromatin, central karyosome	Diffuse glycogen, chromidial body
Entamoeba hartmanni	1–4 Nuclei, 7–9 μm	Fine chromatin, central karyosome	Diffuse glycogen, chromidial body
Entamoeba coli	1–8 Nuclei, 14–30 μm	Fine chromatin, eccentric karyosome	Diffuse glycogen, chromidial body rare
Iodamoeba bütschlii	1 Nucleus, 9–15 μm	Coarse chromatin, no karyosome	Compact glycogen vacuole
Endolimax nana	3–4 Nuclei, 6–9 μm	3–4 granules forming refractile nuclei	Nil
Giardia lamblia	Oval, 4 nuclei, 8–12 μm (not obvious unless stained)	No diagnostic significance	Refractile axoneme and flagellar remnants
Chilomastix mesnilii	Lemon-shaped, 1 nucleus, 5–6 μm	Fine chromatin	Refractile axoneme

Permanent stains

Trichrome stain

The trichrome method for staining protozoa is especially recommended for identifying features of amoebic cysts and trophozoites.

Formula: Trichrome stain (modified)

- Chromotrope 2R   1 g
- Analine blue   0.5 g
- Phosphotungstic acid   0.7 g

Mix the components together with 3 ml glacial acetic acid in a flask and allow to stand for 30 min.
Add 100 ml distilled water and mix well.
(A pink/red granular aggregate may be found; this is not important.)

Acid alcohol decolourizer

- 4.5 ml glacial acetic acid in 995.5 ml 95% industrial methylated spirit.

Fixation

Most smears from faeces or pus can be fixed by placing immediately into methanol for 5 minutes.

Staining

1. Methanol   5 min
2. Wheatley's formula trichrome stain   30 min
3. Rinse in tap water
4. Acid alcohol decolourizer   2–3 s
5. 95% Ethanol   Dip twice
6. 95% Ethanol   5 min
7. 95% Ethanol   5 min
8. 100% Ethanol   3 min
9. Xylene or substitute   5 min
10. Mount with DPX mountant—do not allow xylene to dry on the slide.

Results

Nuclei, chromidial bars, chromatin, red cells and bacteria stain red. Cytoplasm stains blue-green. Background and yeasts stain green.

Modified trichrome formulation for spores of microsporidia

- Chromotrope 2R   6 g
- Analine blue   0.5 g
- Phosphotungstic acid   0.7 g

Mix the components together with 3 ml glacial acetic acid in a flask and allow to stand for 30 min.
Add 100 ml distilled water and mix well.
(A pink/red granular aggregate may be found; this is not important.)

Method

1. Suspend approximately 1 mg of faecal material in a drop of 10% formalin at a ratio of 1 : 3.
2. Using an applicator stick in a rolling motion, spread a drop of the faecal suspension very thinly over two-thirds of the slide surface.
3. Dry the smear and fix in methanol for 5 min.
4. Stain with modified trichrome stain for 90 min at room temperature, or for 30 min at 50°C in a waterbath.
5. Rinse in acid alcohol decolourizer for 3–5 s.
6. Rinse in 95% ethanol until excess stain has washed off the slide.
7. Dehydrate in two changes of 99% ethanol.
8. Clear in xylene or substitute for 10 min and mount in DPX mountant.
9. Examine with the oil immersion objective.

Results

Spores of microsporidia species appear pinkish red and are 1.0×0.5 μm, and oval in appearance. They frequently exhibit a central band-like structure flanked on either side by non-staining areas (polar vacuoles).

Modified Field's stain

This is a useful stain for flagellates in faecal smears.

- Field's stain A.
- Field's stain B (diluted 1 : 4 with distilled water).

Method

1. Prepare thin faecal smears and air dry.
2. Fix with methanol for several minutes.
3. Remove the methanol and flood the slide with 1 ml of diluted Field's stain B.
4. Immediately add 1 ml of undiluted Field's stain A and mix the two stains.
5. Stain for 1–2 min before rinsing in water and allowing to drain dry.

Results

Nuclei and flagella stain red; cytoplasm stains blue. Morphological features of inflammatory cells can be seen by means of this method.

Laboratory investigation for blood and tissue parasites

The blood or tissue parasites are transmitted during vector insect blood feeds and usually continue their life cycle in the human host. The common blood or tissue parasites found belong to the genus of *Plasmodium* (Table I.2), *Trypanosoma* (African and South American trypanosomes), spirochaetes, *Babesia* and the *Leishmania* complex.

Table I.2 Identification of malaria parasites.

	Plasmodium falciparum	*Plasmodium vivax*	*Plasmodium ovale*	*Plasmodium malariae*
Red blood cell	Normal size and shape	Enlarged	Enlarged, fimbriate, oval	Small, older
Inclusions	Maurer's clefts in mature trophozoite	Schüffner's dots, fine stippling	James' dots, coarse stippling	Ziemann's dots, not seen unless overstained
Trophozoite	Delicate fine rings, accolé forms	Larger, thicker rings	Thick compact rings	Small compact rings
Developing trophozoites	Compact ring, cytoplasm vacuolated	Large amoeboid parasite with central vacuole	Slightly amoeboid but smaller than *P. vivax*	Sometimes seen as a band across red cell
Schizont	2–24 merozoites; single, large, brown pigment clump	12–24 merozoites almost filling red blood cell	8–12 merozoites fill three-quarters of red blood cell	6–12 merozoites around central pigment mass
Gametocyte	Crescent-shaped aggregated chromatin and pigment in centre	Large, round, almost fills red blood cell	Smaller, round, fills half red blood cell	Round, may fill between one-half and two-thirds of red blood cell
Pigment	Single clump in schizont	Several fine clumps from late trophozoites	Coarse granules from late trophozoites	Dark fine granules at all stages

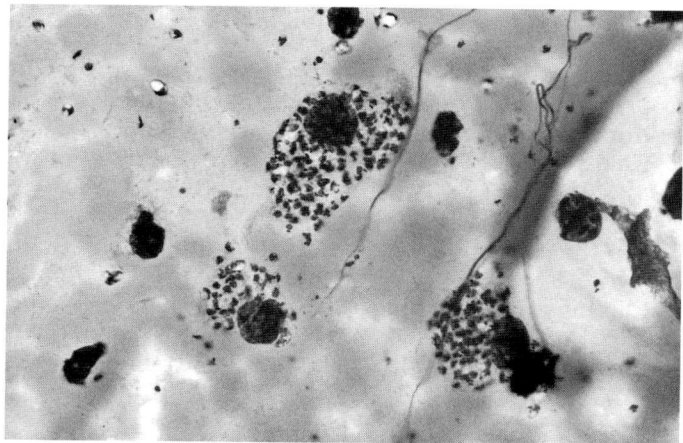

Figure I.10: Amastigotes of *Leishmania* in the bone marrow aspirate.

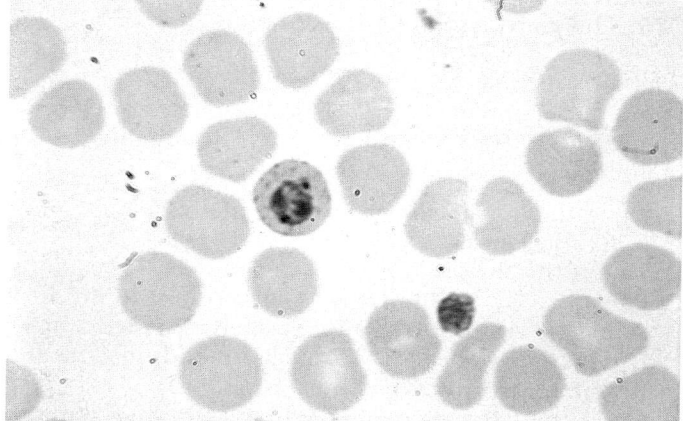

Figure I.11: Schizont of *Plasmodium falciparum* in peripheral blood.

Blood parasites can be identified from peripheral blood, bone marrow aspirate, splenic aspirate and gland aspirate, or from tissue biopsy material (Figures I.10–I.13). Routine procedures for identification include:

- Direct staining of blood or impression smears.
- Culture of appropriate sample.
- Concentration methods.
- Detection of parasite DNA using PCR.[8]
- Immunochromatographic rapid tests for the detection of parasite antigen.[9–11]

Staining of blood films

Giemsa stain

Giemsa stain is a Romanovsky stain and stains chromatin material red and cytoplasm blue. Inclusion bodies within the cell stains red or blue according to their origin.

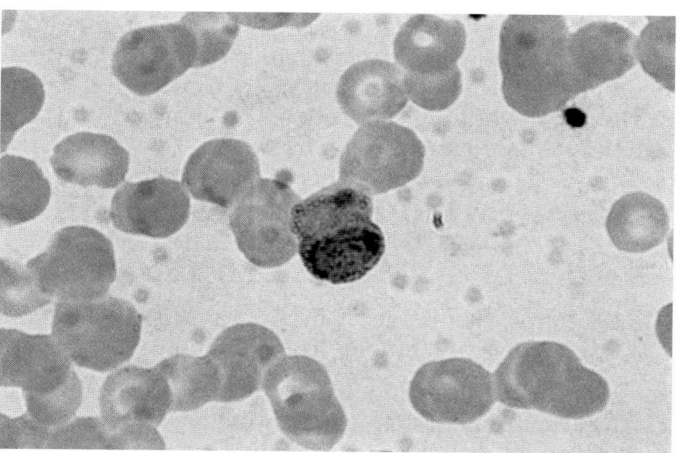

Figure I.12: Gametocyte of *Plasmodium vivax*.

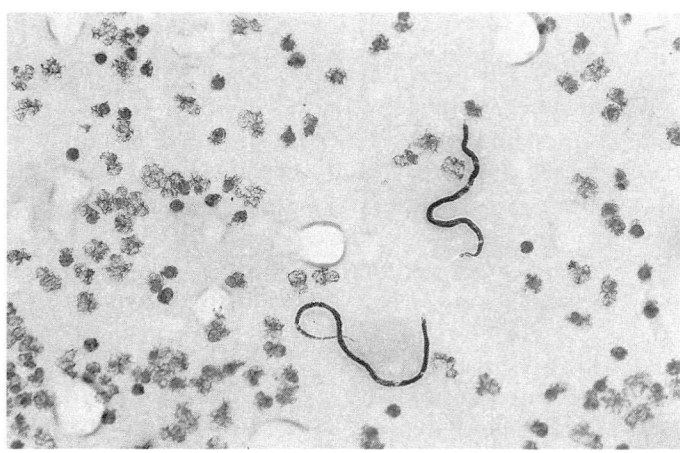

Figure I.13: Microfilaria of *Loa loa*.

Materials

- Giemsa stain; a good quality stain is necessary (e.g., Gurr's R66 formulation, E. Merck/BDH, Poole, UK).
- Solvent methanol.
- Buffered water pH 6.8 and pH 7.2; tablets are available for the preparation of 1-litre volumes.

Method

Allow smears prepared from blood, aspirates or cerebrospinal fluid (CSF) deposits to dry thoroughly before staining.

1. Flood the dry smear with solvent methanol and allow to fix for 1 min.
2. Tip off the alcohol.
3. Prepare a 1 : 10 dilution of Giemsa stain (5 drops of stain and 45 drops of appropriately buffered water). Use buffered water pH 7.2 for staining for malaria and pH 6.8 for the other blood parasites.
4. Flood the fixed slide with diluted stain and allow to stain for 30 min.
5. At the end of this time, rinse the stain from the slide with buffered water and allow the slide to drain dry.

Results

Parasite nuclear chromatin stains red, cytoplasm stains blue, and cellular inclusions stain red. Red cell nuclear remnants (Howell–Jolly bodies) stain deep blue, the nucleus of white blood cells stain purple, and the granules red.

Concentration of parasites from blood

Parasites that are scanty can be concentrated before staining by several methods. These include:

- Thick blood film—suitable for concentrating malaria parasites, trypomastigotes and spirochaetes.
- 'Buffy coat'—suitable for concentrating malaria parasites, trypomastigotes and spirochaetes.

- Mini anion exchange column—suitable for concentrating trypomastigotes.

Thick blood films

Preparation

Using an applicator stick to remove blood from an anticoagulated tube or directly from a finger prick, place two or three drops of blood on to one end of a slide. Using the applicator stick or the edge of a glass slide, spread the blood over an area of 1 cm² and allow to dry thoroughly.

Do not fix the slide with methanol.

Field's stain for thick blood films

Field's stain consists of the two components of the Romanovsky stains in separate solutions. These are called Field's stain A and Field's stain B. Used to stain *unfixed* thick blood films, the procedure will stain white blood cells, platelets and parasites but will *haemolyse* the red blood cells. It is a useful method for the concentration of malaria parasites, *Trypanosoma* sp. and *Borrelia* sp.

Materials

- Field's stain A solution (purchased as prepared stain or prepared as 2.5 g% (25 g/l) in distilled or filtered water from the powder form).
- Field's stain B solution (prepared as for Field's stain A).

Method

1. Dip the unfixed, dried, thick blood film in Field's stain A for 3 s.
2. Carefully rinse the slide in tap or buffered water for 3 s.
3. Dip the slide in Field's stain B for 3 s.
4. Rinse the slide in water again and then stand vertically to dry.

Results

Parasite chromatin stains red and cytoplasm blue; inclusion dots (Schuffner or James), if seen, stain red.

Buffy coat examination

Method

1. Collect peripheral blood into capillary tubes containing ethylenediamine tetra-acetic acid (EDTA) anticoagulant, filling the tube three-quarters full with blood and rotating to mix the anticoagulant. Seal the end with plasticine and place the tube in a micro-haematocrit centrifuge with a corresponding balance tube opposite.
2. Secure the lid and centrifuge the blood at 10 000 r.p.m. for 5 min.
3. Remove the tube and using an ampoule blade or a diamond marker, score the tube just below the layer of white cells and platelets (buffy coat) at the junction of the plasma layer. Break the tube at this point and expel the buffy coat by tapping on to the end of several slides.

4. Prepare a thin slide from the buffy coat.
5. When dry, fix the slide in methanol for 5 min and stain with Giemsa stain, as described previously.

Results

The buffy coat will contain malaria parasites, spirochaetes and trypanosomes, and may demonstrate parasites when none can be seen in the thick or thin film. It may also concentrate abnormal white blood cells which are too few to see in the peripheral blood.

When applied to the peripheral blood of immuno-compromised patients, amastigotes of *Leishmania* sp. can sometimes be found.

Mini anion exchange column technique

This is a useful concentration technique where other investigations for trypanosomes in the blood have proved negative. Blood is passed through a column of cellulose. Erythrocytes are retained in the column and trypanosomes pass out into a collecting tube.

Method

1. Place a piece of dry sponge into a 2-ml syringe barrel. (This is now termed the column.)
2. Add four drops of phosphate-buffered saline (PBS) to dampen the sponge and allow to drain out of the column.
3. Shake the cellulose (DEAE 52—diethylaminoethyl cellulose) thoroughly to resuspend, and pour into the column up to the 2-ml mark. Allow to stand so that excess PBS will drain out.
4. Add a few millilitres of PBS plus glucose (PBSG) to the top of the column and allow it to drain through.
5. Take 150–200 µl of blood (from a finger prick) and drop on to the top of the column. Allow the blood to soak into the column. Attach a collecting pipette to the base of the column.
6. Pipette a few drops of PBSG on top of the blood and *immediately* attach the reservoir and fill with PBSG (approximately 1.5 ml). This will drip slowly on to the column.
7. Leave until all the PBSG has washed through the column. (This should take approximately 4 min.)
8. The collecting pipette will now be full of PBSG plus any trypanosomes that were present in the blood.
9. Centrifuge the collecting pipette (in its plastic cover) at 2000 r.p.m. for 10 min.
10. Place the pipette on a slide or viewing chamber and, using the 20x objective, examine its tip within 20 min for motile trypanosomes.

Dipsticks for parasite antigen detection

These are rapid diagnostic tests that use gold-labelled monoclonal antibodies to capture parasite antigen from

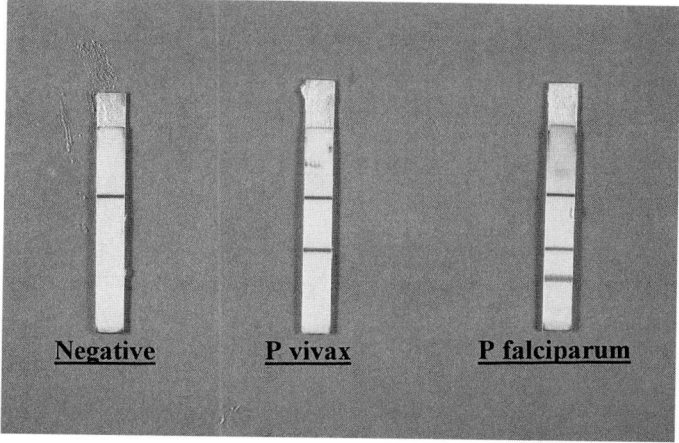

Figure I.14: Dipstick used as a rapid diagnostic test (RDT) for detection of the malaria antigen plasmodium lactate dehydrogenase (PLDH).

blood, transport it along cellulose nitrate membranes by immunochromatography where it is captured again by immobilized stripes of monoclonal antibody and can be visualized[8] (Figure I.14).

Laboratory diagnosis of the filaria parasites

Filariasis is diagnosed either serologically[12] or by finding the L3 microfilariae in peripheral blood, urine, hydrocele fluid or skin snips. Occasionally adult worms can be removed as they cross the eye (*Loa loa*) or from a subcutaneous nodule (*Onchocerca volvulus*).

Because of the periodic appearance of microfilariae, peripheral blood samples are collected between 10.00 and 14.00 hours (day blood) and between 22.00 and 02.00 hours (night blood). An early morning sample of urine is most suitable for examination. Urine may show a milky appearance, called chyluria, if filariasis is present.

Examination of blood for microfilariae

Filtration method

1. Collect 20 ml blood into sodium citrate anticoagulant at the appropriate time.
2. Draw the blood up into a syringe and connect it to a Swinnex holder containing the 5-µm pore size Nuclepore® polycarbonate membrane (Figure I.15).
3. Gently push the blood through the membrane, collecting the filtrate into a container of disinfectant.
4. Draw up 10 ml normal saline into the syringe and push this through the membrane in a similar manner.
5. Draw several millilitres of air into the syringe and push this through to clear the membrane.
6. Carefully dismantle the holder and, using forceps, remove the membrane and place it on to a slide.
7. Add a drop of normal saline to the membrane and cover with a coverslip.

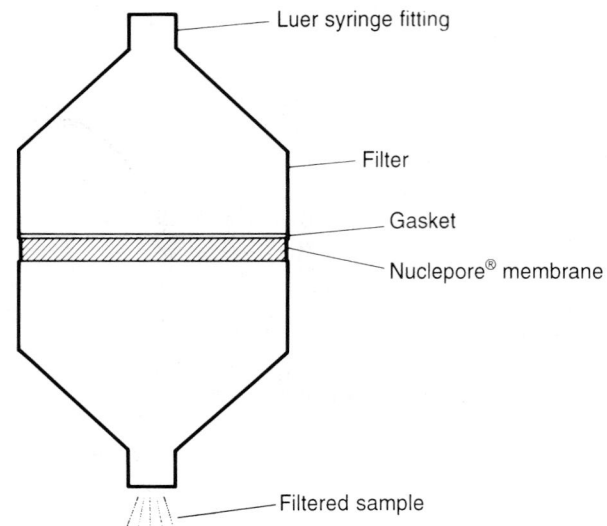

Figure I.15: Swinnex filter for membrane filtration.

8. Scan the whole area of the coverslip using the 10x objective to search for the motile microfilariae.

9. Closer inspection using the 40x objective and by allowing a drop of 1% methylene blue dye to run under the coverslip will help to show whether the microfilariae has a sheath.

Modification of Knott's method for examining blood for microfilariae

1. Collect 20 ml blood into sodium citrate anticoagulant, as described above.

2. Add the blood to an equal volume of 1% saponin in saline (or 2% formalin if saponin is not available).

3. Mix well and allow to stand for 15 min before transferring to centrifuge tubes and centrifuging for 20 min at 2000 r.p.m.

4. Pour off the supernatant into a container of disinfectant and mix the deposit well before transferring a drop to a slide, covering with a coverslip, and scanning for microfilariae. The saponin preparation will show actively moving larvae; those in the formalin preparation will not be moving.

Examination of urine and hydrocele fluid

Urine and hydrocele fluid can be filtered in a similar manner to blood to show any microfilariae present. Alternatively they can be put into a clean centrifuge tube and centrifuged at 2000 r.p.m. for 5 minutes, the supernatant discarded and a drop of the deposit transferred to a slide. Cover with a coverslip and examine in the same way as for blood above.

Identification of microfilariae (Table I.3)

Staining

Reagents
• Giemsa stain
• Delafield's haematoxylin

If sufficient microfilariae are present, films prepared directly from peripheral blood can be used. If not, the blood can be prepared as a thick film or microfilariae can be washed from the membrane filter by placing it into a small pot of saline and agitating. The saline can then be centrifuged at 2000 r.p.m. for 5 minutes and the deposit pipetted on to a slide and dried.

Method
Fix the thin blood film or the film prepared from the deposit with methanol for 5 minutes. If a thick blood film is used, it is necessary first to haemolyse the dried slide by placing it vertically in water for 5 minutes. Dry the slide well before fixing in methanol for 5 minutes.

1. Stain the slides with Giemsa stain diluted 1 : 10 with buffered water pH 6.8 for 20 min.

2. Wash the stain from the slide with the buffered water, then 'differentiate' the stain by leaving the water on the slide for 5 min. At the end of this period look at the slide to see whether the nuclei of the microfilariae are clear and discrete. If not, repeat the process, reducing the time of 'differentiation' until nuclei are clearly seen.

3. Tip the buffer from the slide and flood the slide with undiluted Delafield's haematoxylin for 15 min.

Table I.3 Identification of microfilariae.

Microfilariae	Sheath	Tail	Other features
Loa loa	Yes, stains pale blue	Blunt, large nuclei to tip	Found in peripheral blood 10.00–12.00 hours
Wuchereria bancrofti	Yes, stains pink, lies in gentle curves	Pointed, nuclei small, discrete; stop short of tail	Nocturnal, found in peripheral blood 22.00–02.00 hours
Brugia malayi	Yes, stains deep pink, lies in sharp angles	Blunt, with two large discrete nuclei in tail	Nocturnal
Mansonella perstans	No	Blunt, one large nucleus in tail	
Mansonella ozzardi	No	Pointed, nuclei stop short of tail	

4. Wash the stain from the slide using buffered water and allow the slide to remain in the water for 5 min to reach the maximum intensity of staining (called 'blueing' the slide).

Results

Giemsa stain will stain the nuclei of the microfilariae purple and the haematoxylin will stain the sheath grey.

Examination of skin snips for microfilariae of *Onchocerca volvulus*

Onchocerca volvulus is a filaria worm found in subcutaneous tissue nodules. The discharge of microfilariae into the surrounding tissue occurs. Laboratory diagnosis is made by examining small pieces of skin tissue taken from various parts of the body which contain the migrating larvae.

Method

1. Using a corneal punch, collect small pieces of skin and subcutaneous tissue to a depth of 1 mm. Alternatively use a needle point to lift the skin and cut it using a sharp scalpel blade.
2. Place the skin snips into a microtitre tray containing a few drops of saline. Alternatively, place them individually on to a slide with a drop of saline and cover with a coverslip.
3. Leave the snips in the saline for at least 4 h and examine under the microscope using the low-power (10x) objective or by using an inversion or dissecting microscope, looking for microfilariae that swim out from the snips.
4. Areas of the body that can be 'snipped' are usually the back, buttocks and calves of the legs, but any area exhibiting urticaria or itching should be included.

Laboratory diagnosis of leishmaniasis

The *Leishmania* genus comprises intracellular organisms that include a wide range of species responsible for a variety of clinical responses from self-healing ulcers to deep cutaneous or mucocutaneous invasion and visceral infection. Laboratory diagnosis is made by identifying the organism in tissue or from cells of the reticulo-endothelial system. *Leishmania* is categorized into complex groups of organisms. *L. donovani* complex and *L. brazilienses* complex are the biggest groups. Other groups include *L. tropica*, *L. major* and *L. aethiopica*, and *L. mexicana* in South America.[13] An important subgroup of organisms called the *Viannia* subgroup are found in South America and are primarily responsible for mucocutaneous leishmaniasis.

Confirmation of the organism is made in the laboratory using direct smear examination from an ulcer, culture and molecular identification of specific DNA

using the PCR.[14] Serology is applicable only to the widely disseminated visceral infection[15,16] as insufficient antibodies are produced by the localized ulcers.

Culture is an important diagnostic aid; culture media are varied but NNN media, a rabbit blood–agar base using a salt-based (e.g., Locke's solution) or water overlay and a liquid tissue culture medium (e.g., Schneider's *Drosophila* medium) with added fetal calf serum, are useful. Cultures are incubated at 23°C for up to 28 days with weekly subculture. On examination they will show a conversion from amastigote stage to motile promastigote stage. Detection of specific antibodies is really useful only in visceral leishmaniasis when high titres of antibody can be detected using the direct agglutination test (DAT).

Methods of identification

Cutaneous leishmaniasis

- *Slit-skin smears from an ulcer edge*: The edge of the ulcer is compressed to provide a blood-free area, then, using a fine point (no. 15) scalpel blade, a slit is made into the subcutaneous tissue and the base is gently scraped. The tissue juice and cells are transferred to a slide and smeared over an area of 1 cm². The preparation is allowed to dry before being fixed in methanol and stained with Giemsa stain (see above). Cultures can also be made from the slit-skin smear.
- *Biopsies* of the ulcer edge are taken and divided into two parts. One part is fixed in buffered formalin for histopathology. The second piece is aseptically cut into small pieces for culture and to make impression smears. If PCR is available, a small piece of the biopsy can be frozen at –20°C for future DNA extraction and PCR.
- *Impression smears* are made by dabbing the tissue several times on to a slide to deposit the cells. These are then dried and fixed in methanol before staining with Giemsa stain.

Visceral leishmaniasis

- Bone marrow, splenic aspirate and lymph node aspiration are the tissues used to demonstrate *Leishmania* spp. in this clinical form. Peripheral blood buffy coat may yield parasites in the immunocompromised host.
- Smears are made and fixed in methanol before being stained with Giemsa stain.
- Cultures are also made into NNN and Schneider's media and incubated at 24°C for up to 21 days.

Identifying the species of *Leishmania*

Identification of specific species of *Leishmania* can be made using two principal techniques:

1. Zymodeme: using the isoenzyme pattern.
2. Polymerase chain reaction (PCR) using complex specific primer sets for the organism's minicircle DNA.

Examination of cerebrospinal fluid

The examination of CSF to search for parasites or bacteria causing meningitis is an important diagnostic procedure. The procedures attempt to identify the causative organisms of cerebral malaria or trypanosomiasis, or to demonstrate bacteria causing meningitis. CSF is collected into two clean sterile containers; one sample is sent for bacteriological culture, the second sample is used for (a) cell count, (b) examination of stained deposit after centrifugation, and (c) biochemical tests on the supernatant, if possible.

Method
1. Examine the CSF visually and report one of the following appearances:
   (a) Clear.
   (b) Opalescent or cloudy—this specimen is likely to have a raised cell count.
   (c) Blood-stained—red blood cells that have disintegrated as a result of age may give a yellow tinge to the fluid, known as xanthochromia.
2. Note any fibrin clot that may form on standing.
3. Remove the clot carefully using a small wire loop and spread it over a small area of a slide. Allow to dry and, after fixation, stain the slide by the Ziehl–Neelsen method for *Mycobacterium*.
4. Transfer the CSF to a centrifuge tube and centrifuge at 2000 r.p.m. for 5 min.
5. Carefully tip off the supernatant into a second tube for biochemical analysis (glucose, protein).
6. Mix the deposit well by tapping the tube and use a clean Pasteur pipette to transfer a drop to each of three slides.
7. Spread the drops over a small area and allow the slides to dry well.

Staining

Stain one slide with Giemsa stain in order to differentiate any blood cells or parasites present.

Stain the second with Gram stain to detect any microorganisms present.

Stain the third with Ziehl–Neelsen stain for *Mycobacterium tuberculosis*.

Giemsa stain

Result
Normally the CSF has no more than five white blood cells per microlitre; these are usually lymphocytes. Increased numbers of white blood cells are seen in bacterial infections. Pyogenic meningitis will give an increase in polymorphonuclear cells, and tubercular meningitis gives an increase in lymphocytes. Red blood cells are not a normal finding and indicate an accidental traumatic tap or bleeding into the subarachnoid space.

Malaria parasites or *Trypanosoma* are also found in the Giemsa-stained preparation.

Gram stain

Materials
- Gram stain—1 g gentian or crystal violet dissolved in 100 ml distilled water.
- Lugol's iodine (see above).
- Acetone or methylated spirit.
- Neutral red—0.5 g neutral red dissolved in 100 ml distilled water.

Method
1. Fix the slide by passing it quickly through the flame of a spirit lamp.
2. Place the slide on a rack and flood with Gram stain for 1 min.
3. Wash the stain from the slide.
4. Flood the slide with Lugol's iodine for 1 min.
5. Tilt the slide and pour on acetone or alcohol to decolourize; allow the decolourizing agent to stay on the slide for a short time only (5–10 s) before washing off with tap water.
6. Flood the slide with the neutral red counterstain for 30 seconds.
7. Wash the stain from the slide with water and stand the slide vertically to dry.

Results
Although almost any group of bacteria can be responsible for meningitis, some are seen more commonly:

- Pneumococci—Gram-positive cocci in pairs (diplococci).
- *Haemophilus influenzae*—small, slender, Gram-negative bacilli.
- Meningococci—Gram-negative intracellular diplococci seen inside the polymorphonuclear cells.

Other bacteria will vary in morphological shape and Gram-stained appearance. *Cryptococcus neoformans*, a capsulated yeast organism seen frequently as an opportunistic organism in the immunocompromised patient, may also be seen.

Ziehl–Neelsen stain

Materials
- Strong carbol fuchsin stain.
- 1% Acid alcohol (1 ml concentrated hydrochloric acid in 99 ml methylated spirit).
- 0.5% Malachite green (0.5 g malachite green dissolved in 100 ml distilled water).

Method
1. Fix the smear by passing it through the flame of a spirit lamp.

2. Flood the slide with carbol fuchsin and, using the spirit lamp, gently warm the slide until the surface begins to steam.
3. Stain for 15 min.
4. Wash the slide with water.
5. Flood the slide with 1% acid alcohol and gently rock until no more colour will come out.
6. Wash the slide with water.
7. Flood the slide with malachite green counterstain for 1 min.
8. Wash the slide with water and drain dry.

Results

Mycobacteria are acid-fast bacilli and stain as red bacilli against a green background. (This stain can also be used to demonstrate *Cryptosporidia* oocysts in faecal smears.)

Examination of sputum

Sputum is commonly examined for parasites of the respiratory tract and for bacteria causing pulmonary infections such as tuberculosis or pneumonia. Sputum is usually described by its appearance as:

* Salivary—frothy, white and watery.
* Purulent—thicker consistency, often with a greenish colour.
* Mucopurulent—thick, sticky consistency, containing pus; may be blood stained.

Examination for parasites

Paragonimus westermani and other *Paragonimus* species discharge ova with the sputum and usually cause 'rusty' blood-stained sputum.

Ova can be recovered after dissolving mucus in the sputum by mixing a portion with an equal portion of 10% potassium hydroxide or other mucus-dissolving reagent, and, after mixing thoroughly, standing for 15 minutes before centrifuging at 2500 r.p.m. for 5 minutes. The deposit is examined for ova under the microscope using the 10x objective.

The sputum can also be concentrated after dissolving the mucus, using the formol–ether method as described.

Pneumocystis carinii. Although now reclassified as a fungal organism, demonstration of this parasitic organism of the immunocompromised host requires specialized laboratory techniques. Grocott's silver stain or PAP stains are commonly used, but a fluorescent method using specific labelled monoclonal antibodies is available.

Strongyloides stercoralis larvae (seen in wet preparation) and oocysts of *Cryptosporidium parvum* (seen by Zeihl–Neelsen stain) may be found in sputum in patients with severe immunosuppression.

Examination for bacteria

Two thin smears of sputum are made using a wire loop that can be sterilized in a flame afterwards, or an applicator stick that can be burned. The smears can then be fixed when dry by passing the back of the slide through a flame twice.

One smear is stained for acid-fast bacilli using the Ziehl–Neelsen method (see above). The second is stained for other bacteria using the Gram stain (see above).

Sputum should be sent for routine culture if available, and for culture for *Mycobacterium tuberculosis* if required.

Examination of blood for haematological assessment

Haematological values are necessary in the diagnosis of infection or anaemia. The most useful criteria include:

* Total white cell count.
* Differential white blood cell count.
* Haemoglobin.
* Haematocrit.
* Mean corpuscular haemoglobin concentration (MCHC) and mean corpuscular volume (MCV).
* Platelet count.
* Examination of the blood picture.

The *blood picture* can give much useful information even when other parameters are not available.

Method
1. Fix thin blood films in methanol and stain with Giemsa stain.
2. Examine the slide under the microscope using the oil immersion objective (100x).

Observations

Red blood cells

1. Note the *size*: a normal erythrocyte measures 7 μm in diameter. The cell may be enlarged (macrocyte), or appear smaller (microcyte).
2. Note the *colour*: in a normal erythrocyte the haemoglobin is stained pink with a small area of pallor in the centre. An enlarged area of central pallor (hypochromia) indicates an iron deficiency.
3. Note the presence of any *abnormal* erythrocytes. Target cells or sickle cells may indicate an abnormal haemoglobin type.
4. Note any *inclusions* of the erythrocytes; basophilic stippling and nucleated cells, or spherocytes may indicate a haemolytic process.
5. Note any intracellular or extracellular *parasites* which may be present (malaria, *Trypanosoma*, *Babesia*, *Borrelia*, microfilariae).

White blood cells

An impression of the *number* of white cells present can be gained from the thin blood film, an average of 1–2 cells in each field is normally seen. A differential count will indicate the *types* of cells present.

Note the *morphological appearance* of the cells. Neutrophils may show a shift to the left or to the right. Mononuclear cells may be 'atypical', and any primitive cells must be recorded.

Platelets

These are normally seen in every field, either singly or in small clumps. A decrease in platelets (thrombocytopenia) is noted when platelets are scanty and only seen in every 3–5 fields.

REFERENCES

1   Health and Safety Commission's Health Service Advisory Committee. *Safety in Health Service Laboratories: Safe Working and the Prevention of Infections in Clinical Laboratories*. London: Health and Safety Executive, 1991.

2   Soini H & Musser J M. Molecular diagnosis of mycobacteria. *Clin Chem* 2001; 47(5):809–814.

3   Gascon J, Alvarez M, Valls E M, Bordas M J & Jimenez De Anta T M. Cyclosporiasis: a clinical and epidemiological study in travellers with imported *Cyclospora cayetanensis* infection. *Med Clin (Barc)* 2001; 116(12):461–464.

4   Haque R, Mollah N U, Ali I K et al. Diagnosis of amoebic liver abscess and intestinal infection with the TechLab *E. histolytica* II antigen detection and antibody tests. *J Clin Microbiol* 2000; 38(9):3235–3239.

5   Haque R, Ali I K, Akther S & Petri W A Jr. Comparison of PCR, isoenzyme analysis, and antigen detection for diagnosis of *E. histolytica* infection. *J Clin Microbiol* 1998; 36(2):449–452.

6   Clarke S C & McIntyre M. Acid-fast bodies in faecal smears stained by the modified Ziehl–Neelsen technique. *Br J Biomed Sci* 2001; 58(1):7–10.

7   Muller A, Bialek R, Kamper A, Fatkenheuer G, Salzberger B & Franzen C. Detection of microsporidia in travellers with diarrhoea. *J Clin Microbiol* 2001; 39(4):1630–1632.

8   Srinivasan S, Moody A H & Chiodini P L. Comparison of blood-film microscopy, the OptiMAL dipstick, Rhodamine 123 staining and PCR, for monitoring antimalarial treatment. *Ann Trop Med Parasitol* 2000; 94(3):227–232.

9   Moody A H & Chiodini P L. Methods for the detection of blood parasites. *Clin Lab Haematol* 2000; 22(4):189–201.

10 Mills C D, Burgess D C, Taylor H J & Kain K C. Evalution of a rapid and inexpensive dipstick assay for the diagnosis of malaria. *Bull World Health Organ* 1999; 77(7):553–559.

11 Kaur H & Mani A. Evaluation and usefulness of immunochromatographic tests for rapid detection of *P. falciparum* infection. *Indian J Med Sci* 2000; 54(10):421–424.

12 Schuetz A, Addiss D G, Eberhard M L & Lammie P J. Evaluation of the whole blood filariasis ICT test for short-term monitoring of treatment. *Am J Trop Med Hyg* 2000; 62(4):502–503.

13 Sanchez-Tejeda G, Rodriguez N, Parra C I, Hernandez-Montes O, Barker D C & Monroy-Ostria A. Cutaneous leishmaniasis caused by members of *Leishmania braziliensis* complex in Nayarit, State of Mexico. *Mem Inst Oswaldo Cruz* 2001; 96(1):15–19.

14 Hernandez-Montes O, Monroy-Ostria A, McCann S & Barker D C. Identification of Mexican *Leishmania* species by analysis of PCR amplification. *Acta Trop* 1998; 71(2):139–153.

15 Zijlstra E E, Daifalla N S, Kager P A et al. rK39 enzyme-linked immunosorbent assay for diagnosis of *Leishmania donovani* infection. *Clin Diagn Lab Immunol* 1998; 5(5):717–720.

16 Zijlstra E E, Nur Y, Desjeux P, Khalil E A, El-Hassan A M & Groen J. Diagnosing visceral leishmaniasis with the recombinant rK39 strip test: experience from the Sudan. *Trop Med Int Health* 2001; 6(2):108–113.

Appendix II
Parasitic Protozoa

J. R. Baker

Protozoa can be broadly defined as single-celled organisms which have animal-like nutrition (i.e., they do not contain photosynthetic pigment). Structurally, protozoa are equivalent to a single animal cell; functionally, they are equivalent to a whole animal. Each protozoan cell potentially possesses all the normal metazoan cellular organelles: nucleus, mitochondria, ribosomes, Golgi apparatus, etc., although some may have been lost in certain specialized organisms. Many protozoa also possess unique organelles not found in metazoa.

Parasites can, equally broadly, be defined as organisms which live within organs or tissues of other organisms during some or all stages of their life cycle, and obtain nutrients either from the host organism's food supply or from its tissues. The processes by which these nutrients are digested, and the processes of respiration by which protozoa obtain their energy, do not differ fundamentally from those operating in other animal cells.

All protozoa reproduce asexually, by various forms of division—binary or multiple—or by budding; some also reproduce sexually, usually by division after some form of genetic exchange. Some parasitic protozoa utilize only one species of host in their life cycle; others require two. If only asexual reproduction occurs in one host, and sexual reproduction in the other, the former is termed the intermediate host and the latter is called the definitive host. Irrespective of this terminology, if one host is much smaller than the other it is often referred to as the vector. This is especially true, anthropocentrically, in human medicine, when the mosquito (for example) which infects a human being with malaria is referred to as the vector even though, on the preceding definition, it is also the definitive host. Non-human (usually mammalian) hosts which may be infected with the same stages of a parasite as the human, and from which the latter may acquire infection either directly or via a vector, are termed reservoir hosts.

An attractively simple taxonomic scheme for parasitic protozoa, which takes account of modern developments in tracing relationships between groups, is that devised by Cox[1] (Table II.1).

Most parasites are rarely, if ever, significantly harmful to their hosts. These are of marginal importance in human medicine, except in so far as they may be mistaken for other, potentially more harmful, forms. Even those which are capable of causing severe illness or death of the host do not necessarily always do so. The host–parasite

Table II.1 Classification of protozoan parasites of humans (based on that of Cox[1])

Flagellates (locomotion by flagella)
    Phylum Metamonada: *Giardia, Trichomonas*
    Phylum Kinetoplasta: *Leishmania, Trypanosoma*
    Incertae sedis*: *Naegleria*
Amoebae (locomotion by pseudopodia)
    Phylum Rhizopoda: *Acanthamoeba, Balamutha, Entamoeba*
Sporozoa (locomotion by 'gliding'—no obvious locomotory organelle)
    Phylum Apicomplexa (or Sporozoa)
        Class Coccidea: *Cryptosporidium, Cyclospora, Isospora, Sarcocystis, Toxoplasma*
        Class Haemosporidea: *Plasmodium*
        Class Piroplasmea: *Babesia*
Microsporidia (with unicellular resistant spores)
    Phylum Microsporea: *Encephalitozoon, Enterocytozoon, Nosema, Pleistophora, Thelohania, Trachipleistophora, Vittaforma*
Ciliates (locomotion by cilia)
    Phylum Ciliophora: *Balantidium*

*Of uncertain taxonomic position.

relationship can be thought of as a delicate balance which may easily be tipped in favour of one partner or the other.

Malaria parasites (See also Chapter 70)

Four species of the genus *Plasmodium* infect humans: *P. falciparum, P. malariae, P. ovale* and *P. vivax*; the diseases they cause are known, respectively, as malignant tertian malaria, quartan malaria, ovale tertian malaria and benign tertian malaria.

Life cycle and morphology

The life cycle of *P. vivax* is shown in Figures II.1 and II.2. When an infected mosquito bites a human, malaria sporozoites are injected with the insect's saliva. Within 30 minutes they have entered liver parenchyma cells (possibly via the Kupffer cells). *P. vivax* and *P. ovale* produce two kinds of sporozoites: those which continue their

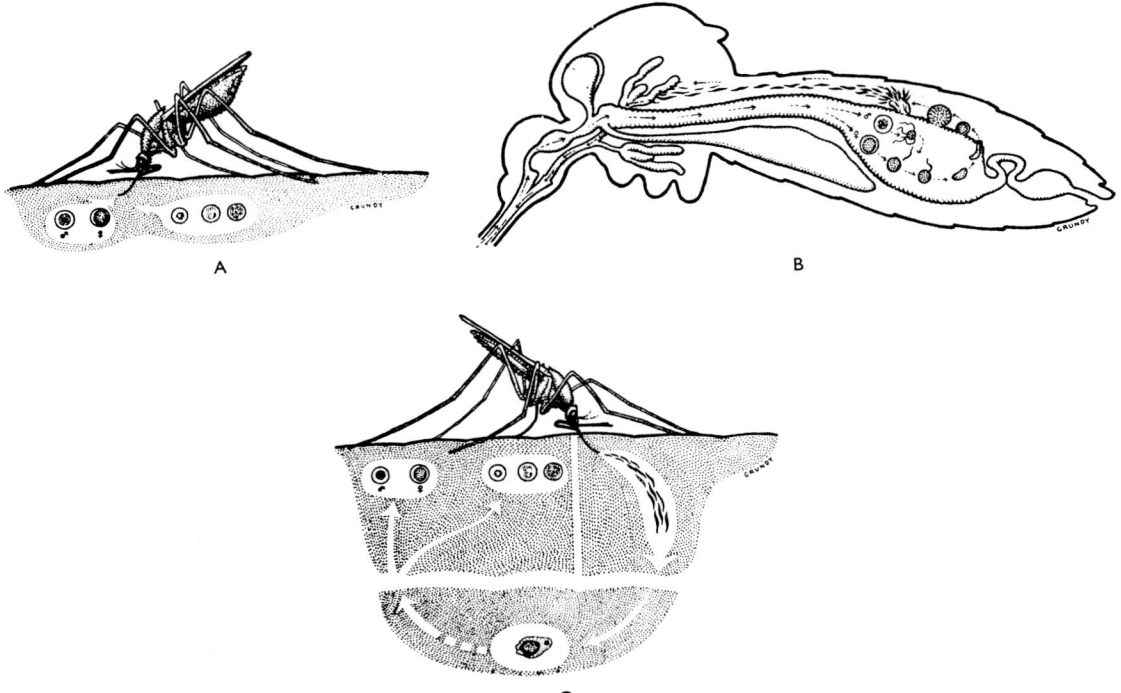

Figure II.1: Life cycle of the malaria parasite. **A**, Female *Anopheles* ingests gametocytes while feeding on the blood of an infected person; **B**, gametogony and sporogony occur within and on the stomach of the mosquito, culminating in the appearance of sporozoites in the salivary glands 1 week or more later (see Figure II.2); **C**, the infective mosquito injects sporozoites into the blood of the next person on whom it feeds. The sporozoites then enter the liver cells, within 30 minutes or so, to commence exoerythrocytic merogony (schizogony), unless they are dormant hypnozoites of *P. vivax* or *P. ovale* (see text). Depending on the species, exoerythrocytic merogony is completed in $5\frac{1}{2}$–15 days (see Table II.2), and the emerging merozoites enter erythrocytes to initiate the erythrocytic phase of the life cycle; in non-immune subjects, a clinical attack of malaria usually develops within 2–5 days. (The diagrams of mosquitoes and parasites are not to scale.) (Drawing by J. Hull Grundy.)

PRE–ERYTHROCYTIC AND
RELAPSE STAGES IN LIVER

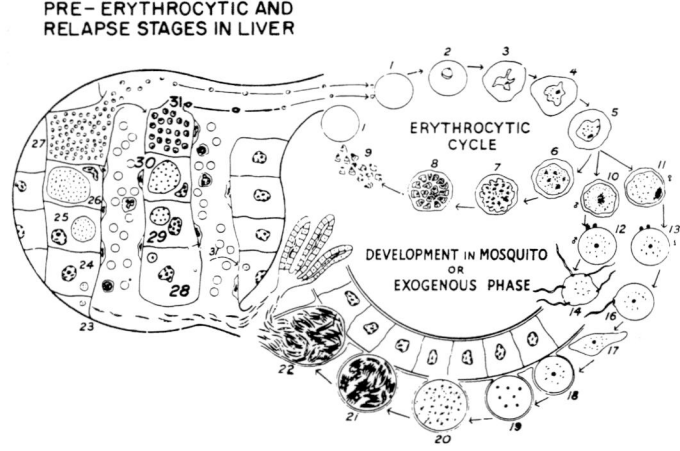

Figure II.2: Diagrammatic representation of the life cycle of a malaria parasite (*Plasmodium vivax*). **1**, Normal erythrocytes; **2–5**, erythrocytes containing young parasites (trophozoites); **6–8**, erythrocytic merogony (schizogony); **9**, rupture of cell containing mature meront (schizont) with release of merozoites into the plasma and subsequent reinvasion of other erythrocytes. **10, 11**, microgametocyte (male) and macrogametocyte (female) within erythrocytes; **12, 13**, extracellular gametocytes in the stomach of a female *Anopheles*; **14**, production of eight male microgametes by the microgametocyte ('exflagellation'); **15**, the macrogametocyte matures into a macrogamete; **16**, one microgamete fertilizes the macrogamete; **17**, the resulting motile zygote (ookinete) penetrates the wall of the mosquito's stomach; **18–21**, the ookinete encysts on the outer surface of the stomach to form an oocyst, which undergoes sporogony to produce hundreds of sporozoites. **22**, The mature oocyst ruptures, releasing the sporozoites into the mosquito's haemocoel, where they enter the cells and ducts of the salivary glands. When the mosquito next feeds, sporozoites are injected with the saliva into the host's bloodstream. **23–27**, The sporozoites enter hepatocytes and commence exoerythrocytic merogony, culminating in the release of merozoites back into the bloodstream, where they enter erythrocytes (1,2) to start the erythrocytic merogony cycle. With *P. vivax* and *P. ovale*, some sporozoites are of a special type (hypnozoites); these remain dormant as unicellular bodies within hepatocytes for up to many months. **28**, Liver cell containing a hypnozoite; **29–31**, subsequent exoerythrocytic merogony of the hypnozoite, with release of merozoites into the blood to initiate a relapse.

development inside the hepatic cells immediately, and others (hypnozoites) which remain dormant for some time before doing so (see below). Sooner or later the sporozoites commence nuclear division, and are then known as meronts (or schizonts). After producing several thousand nuclei, the meront undergoes cytoplasmic division to form a large number of small, uninucleate merozoites. Mature liver (exoerythrocytic) meronts may be as large as 50–60 μm in diameter. The merozoites are freed by the rupture of the meront and enter the circulation, where they become attached to the membranes of erythrocytes and penetrate them. They are now known as trophozoites. Very young trophozoites consist of a small hollow sphere of cytoplasm with a central vacuole and one small nucleus; when viewed through a microscope in optical section they resemble a tiny signet ring, and hence are often referred to as 'ring forms' (Figure II.3A). Electron microscopy has shown that the trophozoites are contained within a parasitophorous vacuole, the limiting membrane of which is formed, at least in part, by the erythrocyte's surface membrane, which is invaginated by the entering merozoite and then becomes separated from the cell surface. As the trophozoite grows, the central vacuole disappears and the characteristic black or brown malarial pigment begins to appear. This pigment is formed by the insoluble iron-containing part of the haemoglobin molecule, ingested by the parasite as it feeds on its host cell's cytoplasm.

As the trophozoite continues to grow, its nucleus begins to divide: it, too, becomes a meront but this time the division process (merogony or schizogony) produces only 24 (or fewer) merozoites. The number depends on the species (Table II.2, which also lists other characteristics of the exo- and intra-erythrocytic forms of the four species). When these intra-erythrocytic merozoites are released by the rupture of the containing erythrocyte, they rapidly enter other erythrocytes and the cycle of erythrocytic merogony is repeated, unless terminated by the host's immune response or its death, or by chemotherapy. *P.*

vivax and, to a lesser extent, *P. ovale* cause the host red blood cell to enlarge and, in the case of *P. ovale*, it seems to become easily deformed; during the making of a thin blood film, the host cell may be drawn out into an irregular oval, hence the parasite's specific name. Other changes may become apparent in the host cell: marks (visible when stained) appear on the surface membrane. These may be very fine and faint (Ziemann's stippling), fine but more distinct (Schüffner's dots), or relatively large and coarse and fewer in number (Maurer's clefts) (Table II.2).

Not all the merozoites develop into another generation of meronts. Some grow into the sexual cells or gametocytes. The male or microgametocyte has paler cytoplasm and a larger, less intensely staining nucleus than the female macrogametocyte. The latter (Figure II.3B) has cytoplasm which stains more intensely blue with Romanovsky stains (Field's, Giemsa's, Leishman's) because it contains a much larger number of ribosomes than does the male. The gametocytes do not develop any further in the human host; under natural conditions their continued development depends on their being ingested by a feeding female mosquito of the genus *Anopheles* (male mosquitoes do not feed on blood).

In the mosquito's stomach the mature gametocytes leave their host red cells and become gametes. This process is imperceptible in the female, but the male gametocyte produces eight long motile male gametes (microgametes) by a rapid process known as 'exflagellation'. Within a few minutes at most, the male nucleus has divided into eight, and eight lashing flagella erupt from the gametocyte's surface. One nucleus enters each flagellum, which possibly also possesses a mitochondrion, and the 'flagella' (now uninucleate microgametes) break free and swim through the blood meal in search of a female. All stages of *Plasmodium* within the vertebrate host are haploid, as are the gametes. After fertilization of a macrogamete by one microgamete, within the mosquito's midgut, a diploid zygote is formed. This zygote elongates and glides (in a fashion not fully understood) through

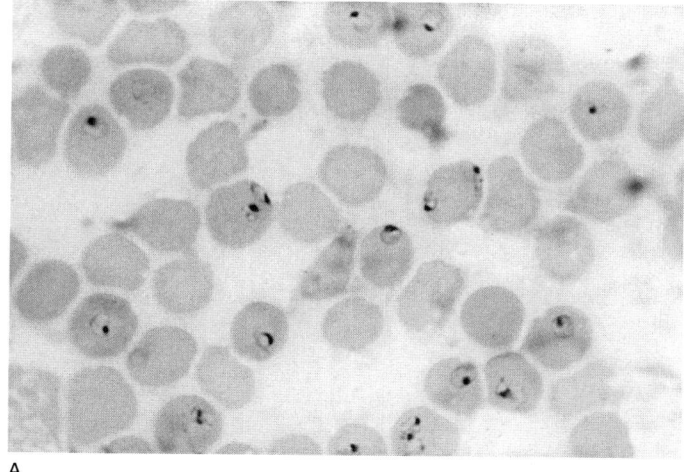

A

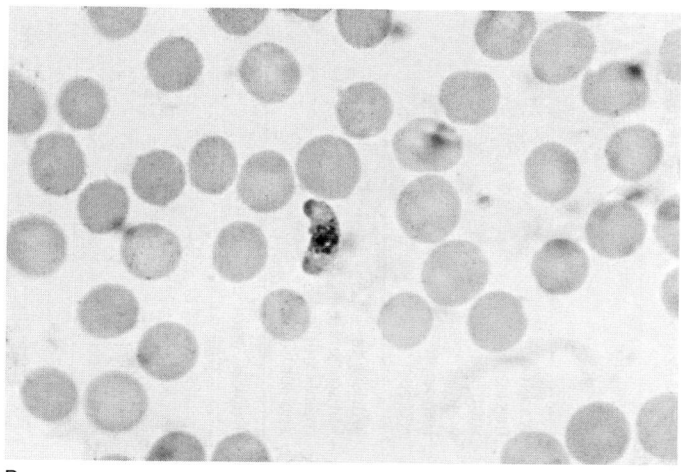

B

Figure II.3: *Plasmodium falciparum.* (**A**) Ring forms and (**B**) female (macro-) gametocyte in Giemsa-stained blood films. (From Muller R & Baker J R. *Medical Parasitology.* London: Gower Medical Publishing,1990.)

Table II.2 Species of *Plasmodium* which infect humans

Species	Geographical distribution	Duration of merogony		No. of merozoites per meront		Main morphological characteristics of erythrocytic forms				
		Exoerythrocytic (days)	Erythrocytic (hours)*	Exoerthrocytic	Erythrocytic	'Ring' form	Trophozoite	Meront	Gametocyte	Host erythrocyte*
P. vivax	Worldwide, in tropical, subtropical and warmer temperate regions	8	48	~10 000	12–24	At least one-third diameter of erythrocyte	Amoeboid	10 µm diameter	Round or ovoid, male: 9 µm, female: 10–11 µm	Enlarged, stippled ('Schüffner's dots')
P. malariae	Worldwide but scattered, mainly tropical and subtropical	14–15	72	~15 000	6–12	At least one-third diameter of erythrocyte	Compact, often bandlike	7 µm diameter	Round or ovoid, 7 µm	Not enlarged; very faint ('Ziemann's) stippling after prolonged staining only
P. ovale	Tropical Africa: also occasionally in other parts of tropics and subtropics (possibly of exogenous origin)	9	48	~15 000	6–12 (12–24 in relapses)	At least one-third diameter of erythrocyte	Compact	7 µm (larger in relapses)	Round or ovoid, 9 µm	Slightly enlarged, stippled ('Schüffner's dots'); may be distorted and elongated
P. falciparum	Worldwide, in tropics, subtropics and warmer temperate regions	5½	48	~30 000	8–24	Very small at first; two nuclei commonly; some apparently on edge of cell (accolé forms)	Compact; rarely seen in peripheral blood	5 µm; rarely seen in peripheral blood	Crescentic, male: 9–11 µm long, female: 12–14 µm	Not enlarged; often with fewer larger dots ('Maurers clefts')

*These alterations do not develop until some growth of the parasite has occurred.

the blood meal and into one of the cells of the midgut wall, in which it rounds up and secretes a thin cyst wall around itself. The motile zygote is called an ookinete, but once it has encysted it becomes an oocyst. The oocyst enlarges considerably, bulging outwards into the mosquito's haemocoel but still remaining within the basement membrane of the midgut wall. At the same time it undergoes a series of nuclear divisions, the first of which is a reduction (meiotic) division, followed by cytoplasmic cleavage in a fashion similar to that undergone by the exoerythrocytic meront. The process within the oocyst, however, is termed sporogony and the resulting small, elongate, uninucleate cells are the sporozoites; several thousand are produced within each oocyst.

The sporozoites are then liberated from the rupturing oocyst into the mosquito's haemocoel, from where some, at least, find their way to the salivary glands in the insect's thorax. They penetrate the salivary gland lumen, and are injected into the bloodstream of the next vertebrate on which the mosquito feeds. The developmental cycle in the mosquito takes between about 1 and 4 weeks, depending on the ambient temperature (the higher the temperature, the shorter the cycle).

Geographical distribution

P. falciparum is the most common species in tropical and subtropical areas, and may sometimes be found in warmer temperate regions. *P. malariae* is also distributed in the tropics and subtropics, but is less common than *P. falciparum* and its distribution tends to be patchy. *P. ovale*, the least common malaria parasite of humans, is probably restricted to Africa; the few cases reported from the western Pacific region may have been introduced or the result of a chance transmission from an imported case.

P. malariae is the only human malaria parasite to have another natural vertebrate host, the chimpanzee (*Pan troglodytes*), but this is of little, if any, epidemiological significance. The other species can experimentally infect splenectomized chimpanzees and monkeys (e.g. *Aotus* and *Macaca*).

Pathogenesis

The characteristic fever peaks of malaria result from synchronization of the intra-erythrocytic merogony cycle. Simultaneous rupture of many erythrocytes, with the concomitant release of parasite debris and malarial pigment, causes a rise in fever. Destruction of the erythrocytes also leads to anaemia. Hepatic meronts do not seem to be pathogenic.

Erythrocytes infected with *P. falciparum* adhere to the walls of capillaries, possibly due to their developing knoblike protrusions which are visible by electron microscopy only, and also to other, uninfected, erythrocytes (rosetting).[2] This can lead to capillary blockage and rupture, with haemorrhage into the surrounding tissue. Another consequence of this adhesion of infected cells is that it is rare for stages of *P. falciparum* other than ring-form trophozoites and gametocytes to be seen in films of peripheral blood, as the older trophozoites and meronts are sequestered in the small blood vessels.

Cerebral malaria, the most severe complication of *P. falciparum* infection, is a consequence, at least in part, of hypoxia resulting from capillary occlusion in the brain due to this adhesion and rosetting. However, evidence has been accumulating over the past decade of the involvement also of inflammatory cytokines and nitric oxide.[3]

Untreated malaria (if not fatal) is notoriously persistent, with recurring bouts of fever sometimes lasting for many years. In infections with *P. vivax* or *P. ovale* these recurrences may result from the reactivation of dormant hypnozoites lying within the hepatocytes, even when parasites have been eliminated from the blood by chemotherapy or the host's immune response. In a subspecies of *P. vivax*, *P. v. hibernans*, all the sporozoites are hypnozoites. The first clinical attack of malaria therefore does not occur until several months after the infective mosquito bite. This was an adaptation for survival of the parasite in a cooler climate, in which adult mosquitoes did not survive through the winter and so the parasite could not be transmitted to another host. *P. v. hibernans* is now restricted to temperate zones around the Mediterranean Sea, in the Middle East and parts of China, but its range used to extend as far north as the Netherlands and southern England (the malaria parasite which existed in England was certainly *P. vivax*, but it is only assumed that it was *P. v. hibernans*).

Hypnozoites do not exist in *P. falciparum* or *P. malariae*. Recurrences of clinical malaria in patients infected with these species are due to the survival of small numbers of erythrocytic parasites, which persist at a low level until the host's immune response wanes sufficiently to permit their multiplication to a level sufficient to cause clinical illness once more. There is evidence that at least some species of *Plasmodium* can undergo antigenic variation— a structural change in their surface antigen—rather like the process in trypanosomes (see below), but it is less well understood in malaria parasites.

Diagnosis

A clinical diagnosis, based on recurrent fever and splenomegaly, needs confirmation by the finding of parasites in stained thin or (usually) thick blood films. Serodiagnosis is also used, especially in surveys, but again needs confirmation by blood film examination as a positive serological test does not necessarily indicate active infection. The tests used include indirect immunofluorescence (IFAT), enzyme-linked immunosorbent assay (ELISA) and indirect haemagglutination (IHA). Several commercial 'dipstick' antigen capture test kits are available.

Trypanosomes

(See also Chapters 73 and 74)

Trypanosomes (genus *Trypanosoma*) are elongated protozoa

with a single flagellum. They share with the leishmanial parasites (see below) the possession of an unusually large amount of mitochondrial DNA, which forms a structure called the kinetoplast lying within the mitochondrion and, measuring from one to several micrometres in diameter, easily visible by light microscopy. The ordinal name, Kinetoplastida, is derived from the name of this organelle.

Life cycle and morphology

Like malaria parasites, trypanosomes have two hosts in the course of their life cycle: a vertebrate and an invertebrate vector. In the vertebrate host trypanosomes can exist in two forms (Figure II.4). The first is elongate, motile and extracellular; the origin of the flagellum is near the posterior end of the cell and the flagellum emerges through the flagellar pocket to run forwards along the margin of the cell, to which it is attached by a series of hemidesmosomes. As the flagellum undulates, it pulls out the surface membrane of the cell into a thin membrane-like structure called the undulating membrane. At the anterior end of the cell the flagellum may terminate or it may extend further forward. This form is called a trypomastigote. The second form is a non-motile, intracellular, more or less spherical cell called an amastigote (or micromastigote), which has at the most a very short, rudimentary flagellum.

Other stages may develop in the invertebrate host (Figure II.4). These include epimastigotes, in which the flagellar origin is close to the nucleus near the centre of the elongate cell, from whence it extends forward to form, as in the trypomastigote, an undulating membrane, and promastigotes, in which the flagellar origin is

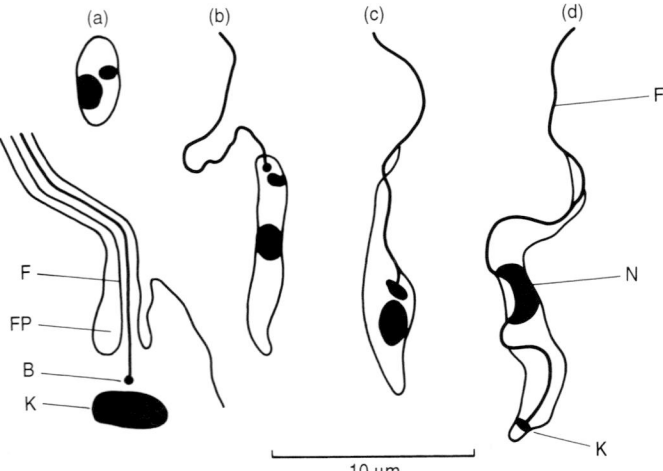

Figure II.4: The various forms which may develop in the life cycle of species of *Leishmania* and *Trypanosoma*. (**a**) Amastigote (= micromastigote), (**b**) promastigote, (**c**) epimastigote, (**d**) trypomastigote (only the first two occur in *Leishmania*). B, basal body; F, flagellum; FP, flagellar pocket; K, kinetoplast; N, nucleus. (Slightly modified from J. R. Baker. *Companion to Microbiology* (Bull A T & Meadow P M editors) London: Longman; 1987: 431–457.)

anterior and there is consequently no undulating membrane. In some species sphaeromastigotes also develop; these are small and spherical, but differ from amastigotes in having a flagellum coiled around the outside of the cell.

As far as is known, trypanosomes reproduce only by binary fission; they are uninucleate except when in the process of division. There is good evidence that some form of genetic exchange occurs, at least in the species *T. brucei*, during the course of development in the vector, but this appears to be an occasional process and details are completely unknown.

Three species of *Trypanosoma* can infect humans: *T. brucei*, *T. cruzi* and *T. rangeli*; the first two are classified in distinct subgenera: *Trypanozoon* and *Schizotrypanum*, respectively. The subgeneric assignment of *T. rangeli* is uncertain. It has been variously placed in the subgenera *Herpetosoma* and *Tejeraia* (of which it was the only member), but recent study of small subunit ribosomal RNA genes aligns it with *T. cruzi* in the subgenus *Schizotrypanum*.

Trypanosoma brucei

Life cycle and morphology

In the vertebrate host (humans and other mammals), only trypomastigotes occur. These are variable in form (pleomorphic) (Figure II.5); long, slender cells with a considerable length of free anterior flagellum appear to be those which undergo longitudinal binary fission in the blood and tissue fluids of the host, while shorter, broader ('stumpy') forms, with little or no free anterior flagellum, do not divide while in the vertebrate but remain in the G0 phase of the cell cycle until ingested by the vector, a large blood-sucking dipteran fly of the genus *Glossina*.[5] There are intermediate forms between these two extremes, although it is probable that, while slender forms transform into the broader forms, the reverse does not occur.

Once ingested with its blood meal by a *Glossina* (tsetse fly), both sexes of which feed exclusively on blood, the 'stumpy' trypomastigotes elongate to form the so-called procyclic trypomastigotes. These forms undergo binary fission, and have a fully active, large single mitochondrion and a functional Krebs cycle, as do the subsequent stages which develop in the vector, apart from the final, metacyclic forms. The stages occurring in the mammal, however, possess only an inactive mitochondrion and their respiration, though aerobic, is glycolytic and proceeds only as far as the production of pyruvate.

The procyclic trypomastigotes are at first confined within the peritrophic membrane, a chitinous tube which lines the tsetse's midgut and surrounds its blood meal, but they later appear outside this membrane but still within the midgut, presumably to prevent their being expelled with the fly's faeces. They move to the anterior portion of the midgut (the proventriculus), elongate to produce mesocyclic forms and migrate via the lumen of the alimentary tract to the salivary glands. In the lumen

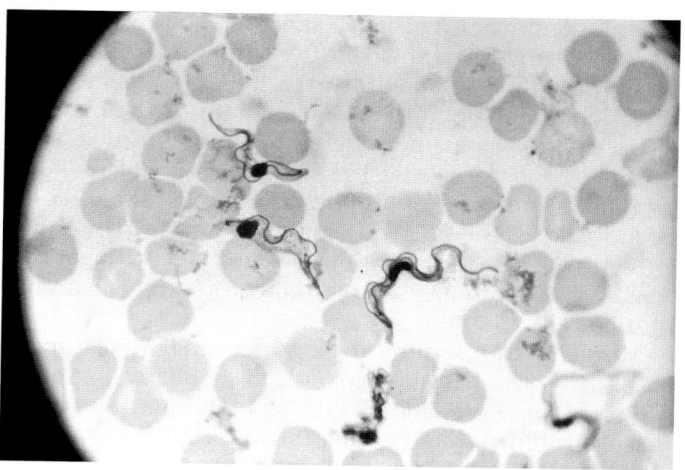

Figure II.5: *Trypanosoma brucei* in peripheral blood of an experimentally infected mouse; long slender form on the right and short stumpy forms on the left. (Giemsa stain.) (From Muller R & Baker J R. *Medical Parasitology*. London: Gower Medical Publishing, 1990.).

of the salivary glands, they develop into epimastigotes, attached by their flagella to the wall of the glands. The epimastigotes eventually change again into short trypomastigotes, with at most a very short, free flagellum—the infective metacyclic trypomastigotes. These are also in the G0 phase and do not divide until they have been injected with the fly's saliva into the next mammal on which it feeds.[5] Metacyclic trypomastigotes respire in a similar fashion to the forms which live in the mammal, without participation of the single mitochondrion. Another way in which the metacyclic forms resemble those in the vertebrate is in their possession of the variable surface glycoprotein (VSG) coat on the outer surface of the cell membrane (which is not present on procyclic trypomastigotes or epimastigotes). The life cycle in the tsetse fly takes about 2–3 weeks from ingestion of trypomastigotes to the appearance of metacyclic forms in the salivary glands.

Under natural conditions, for reasons not fully understood, the life cycle is completed in fewer than 1% of flies which ingest trypanosomes. However, once a fly does become infective (with trypomastigotes in its salivary glands), it appears to remain so for the rest of its life.

After injection into a susceptible mammal by the feeding fly, the metacyclic trypomastigotes transform into slender forms and commence division. At first they are more or less restricted to the tissue fluid around the site of the bite, where they cause the development of an inflamed trypanosomal chancre, but after a few days they spread throughout the body via the bloodstream and ultimately penetrate the central nervous system (CNS) and appear in the cerebrospinal fluid (CSF).

In the vertebrate host's bloodstream, antibodies are produced against the trypanosomes' VSG coat and these antibodies, in the presence of complement, lyse the parasites. However, the molecular architecture of the coat is genetically controlled and, by complex processes of gene rearrangement and deregulation, it is repeatedly changed. The 'new' coat is not recognized by the host's antibodies, and parasites bearing it can continue to multiply until fresh antibody specific for the restructured coat appears. Parasitaemia thus occurs in a series of waves, each consisting of a different variant antigenic type (VAT) of trypanosome. The process of changing the VSG can occur at least 100 times, but it is probably not limitless. This antigenic variation does not occur in a rigidly fixed sequence, but neither is it entirely random; much has been learned about the details of the process, but much remains to be elucidated.[5] Its occurrence, needless to say, bedevils attempts to develop an effective antitrypanosome vaccine.

Geographical distribution

T. brucei is restricted to tropical Africa because its vectors, *Glossina* species, are similarly restricted. Within these limits, however, it is by no means evenly distributed. *Glossina* and, therefore, *T. brucei*, do not occur at altitudes above about 1800 m at most, almost certainly due to the temperature.

The infraspecific taxonomy of *T. brucei* has been the subject of much debate over the last few decades. The 'classical' view was that there were three species of tsetse-transmitted trypanosomes in Africa: *T. brucei*, *T. rhodesiense* and *T. gambiense* (with only the latter two infecting humans). This has long been discarded, the three categories being reduced to subspecies of *T. brucei*.[4] The most homogeneous of these appears to be *T. brucei gambiense*, a subspecies essentially confined to west and central Africa. Infective to humans and other mammals, it produces in the former a relatively chronic disease that (if untreated) results in death only after many months or even years. Occasional reports of self-curing infections are not generally thought to have been fully substantiated. There is some evidence for the existence of two 'groups' within the subspecies, one more virulent than the other. *T. b. gambiense* is transmitted by tsetse flies of the *G. palpalis* group mainly from human to human, though reservoirs of infection exist among domestic animals (e.g. pigs) and wild ungulates. Since *G. palpalis* usually inhabits vegetation fringing rivers, transmission of the trypanosomes to humans commonly occurs at places where they come into frequent contact with the tsetse—at village watering places, fords, etc. Because of this, infection tends to be equally common in men, women and children.

In east Africa, *T. brucei rhodesiense* causes a more acute disease in humans who, unlike the situation in West Africa, are only 'accidental' hosts of a parasite which predominantly infects wild and domestic ungulates. The subspecies is sympatric with *T. brucei brucei* which is, by definition, infective to wild mammals but not to humans (and occurs throughout the range of *Glossina*). Infectivity to humans, and therefore presumably the distinction between *T. b. brucei* and *T. b. rhodesiense*, appears to be controlled by a single gene which determines resistance or sensitivity to a lytic factor in human serum associated with high-density lipoprotein. It is likely that there is considerable gene flow between these two subspecies, which is probably responsible for their considerably greater heterogeneity compared with *T. b. gambiense*.[6]

T. b. rhodesiense is therefore less focally distributed than *T. b. gambiense*, and may be found across wide areas of the east African savanna; it is predominantly associated with tsetse of the *G. morsitans* group, which can survive under much drier conditions than can *G. palpalis*. Transmission of *T. b. rhodesiense* to humans is less 'domestic' than that of *T. b. gambiense*, and infection is usually commoner in men than in women and children.

Strains of the *T. b. gambiense* type seem to have spread eastward across Africa and there is an area of overlap between them and those of the *T. b. rhodesiense* type around the northern and eastern shores of Lake Victoria.

Pathogenesis

The types of disease produced in humans by *T. b. gambiense* and *T. b. rhodesiense* are essentially very similar, although the latter produces a much more acute disease, and both can be described together.

After initial restriction to the chancre, the trypanosomes spread throughout the blood and lymph systems and give rise to a more or less acute febrile illness. Lymphadenopathy is common, and swollen cervical lymph glands constitute 'Winterbottom's sign', a classic indication of *T. b. gambiense* infection. After a period of weeks (*T. b. rhodesiense*), months or even years (*T. b. gambiense*), the parasites penetrate the CNS and multiply there in the capillaries, tissue fluid and CSF. At no stage of the infection do they enter cells of the host (except when ingested by phagocytes, in which they do not survive). Presumably in response to the repeated antigenic challenge resulting from the parasites' antigenic variation, large amounts of IgM are secreted into the blood plasma in the early stage of infection and, after invasion of the CNS, IgM also appears in the CSF. In the brain tissue there is massive lymphocytic infiltration in the arachnoid membrane and the pia mater which, in section, appears as a characteristic perivascular cuff around the brain capillaries. In addition to small round cells, the cuff often contains large plasma cells in the final stage of immunoglobulin secretion, the so-called morula (= mulberry) or Mott cells.

It is this meningoencephalitis which is responsible for the somnolence and coma which gave the disease its name 'sleeping sickness', and which is ultimately responsible for the death of the untreated patient.

Diagnosis

Clinical diagnosis may be supported by a range of immunological tests, including IFATs, complement fixation tests, ELISAs and agglutination procedures. Several commercial 'card' and 'dipstick' tests for trypanosomal antigens and antibodies are available.

Final confirmation of active infection, however, depends on demonstration of the parasites, either microscopically or by isolation in laboratory rats or mice. In the early infection, blood or lymph gland exudate is examined; the latter is likely to be more helpful in the chronic disease caused by *T. b. gambiense*. In the later stage, CSF obtained by lumbar puncture should be examined; if the CNS has been invaded, the CSF will contain scanty trypanosomes (which can sometimes be visualized by centrifugation), an increased number of lymphocytes (> 5 cells/mm^3), morula cells and IgM.

Motile trypanosomes can be seen at magnifications of 400× or more in fresh preparations of blood, lymph or CSF, or stained preparations (thick blood films are better than thin films) may be examined at a magnification of 1000×. Isolation by inoculation of blood, lymph or CSF into laboratory rats or mice is reliable for *T. b. rhodesiense*, but less so for *T. b. gambiense*, which does not readily infect rodents; unweaned rats should be used, if possible, if isolation of *T. b. gambiense* is attempted.

A micro-anion exchange centrifugation technique for isolation of *T. brucei* subspecies from blood and a kit for the cultivation in vitro of *T. b. gambiense* directly from blood or CSF have been developed for use in the field.

Trypanosoma cruzi

Life cycle and morphology

Both trypomastigotes and intracellular amastigotes develop in infected mammals, the former in the bloodstream and the latter mainly in macrophages and muscle cells. The trypomastigotes do not multiply but disseminate the infection around the body of the mammalian host and also serve to infect the vectors (large blood-sucking bugs of the subfamily Triatominae, family Reduviidae (Hemiptera); both sexes feed exclusively on blood). Trypomastigotes ingested by a feeding bug change into epimastigotes in the midgut, undergo division, and are moved back along the bug's gut as the blood meal is digested. In the hindgut they transform into small metacyclic trypomastigotes (which do not divide); these forms are expelled when the bug defecates while, or just after, feeding, and enter through the wound made by the bug's proboscis. The insects often feed on sleeping persons, and faecal matter may be transferred by the scratching or rubbing fingers of a sleepy child (or adult) to the eye; the trypomastigotes may then penetrate the conjunctiva.

T. cruzi can infect many mammals in addition to humans; dogs and cats, and wild animals living in or near houses such as rodents, armadillos, racoons, opossums and vampire bats may serve as reservoirs of human infection.

A range of molecular techniques, culminating in random amplification of polymorphic DNA (RAPD), has indicated the existence of two major groups within *T. cruz*: *T. cruzi* 1 and *T. cruzi* 2 (sometimes roman numerals, I and II, are used; unfortunately, in an earlier attempt to delineate these groupings, the terms 'lineage 1' and 'lineage 2' were used for what are now known as group 2 and group 1, respectively). Both groups infect humans, but the reservoir hosts of the former are primarily opossums, unlike those of the latter which are mainly rodents.[4]

Once within a mammal the metacyclic trypomastigotes enter the host's cells, either actively or by being phagocytosed. If they are phagocytosed, the phagosome membrane seems to disintegrate, freeing the trypanosome, which thus evades digestion within a phagolysosome. The trypomastigotes then become rounded amastigotes (sometimes, perhaps more correctly, called micromastigotes, as they do possess a rudimentary intracellular flagellum) and divide by repeated binary fission until they fill, and then rupture, the host cell. Before its rupture, however, the contained parasites have retransformed into small trypomastigotes, which elongate after their liberation into trypomastigotes which are about 20 μm long and have a sharply pointed posterior end and an anterior extension of the flagellum beyond the end of the cell (Figure II.6). On stained blood films these trypomastigotes often adopt a curved C shape. Marked pleomorphism, as in *T. brucei*, is not seen, though some workers believe that two forms can be distinguished: slender forms destined to reinvade host cells and broader forms which infect the vectors. There is as yet no firm evidence of genetic exchange in *T. cruzi*.[6]

Geographical distribution

T. cruzi is widely distributed throughout continental South America and in Central America and the southern USA, between about latitudes 25°N and 38°S, although progress is being made in its eradication from many of the 'southern cone' countries of South America.[7] The parasite has been isolated from wild mammals in the southern USA but few, if any, indigenous human cases have been reported. The disease is essentially one of poverty, poor-quality housing being associated with bug infestation and, therefore, the risk of infection.

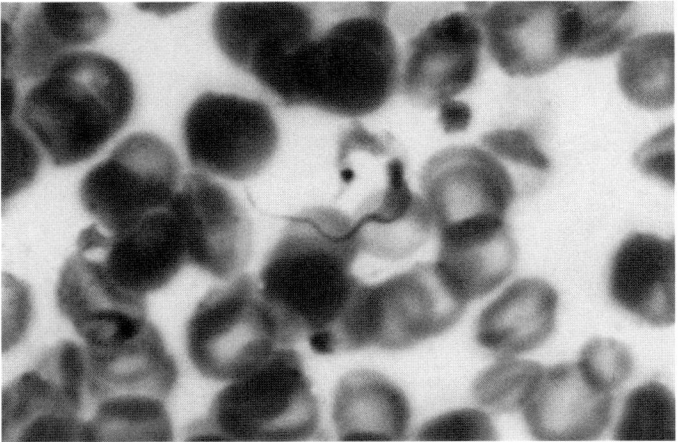

Figure II.6: Bloodstream form of Trypanosoma cruzi. (Giemsa stain). (From Muller R & Baker J R. *Medical Parasitology*. London: Gower Medical Publishing; 1990.)

Pathogenesis

The initial sign of infection is often a swelling (chagoma) at the portal of entry of the trypanosomes. When this is the conjunctiva, and the swelling involves the eye, it is known as Romaña's sign. A more or less acute, rarely fatal, febrile illness is followed by the chronic phase, during which repeated intracellular multiplication cycles continually destroy the host's cells. Not only the cells containing amastigotes are destroyed, but also neighbouring cells, probably as part of an autoimmune phenomenon; neurones are particularly vulnerable. If the intracellular groups of amastigotes (pseudocysts) are concentrated in the oesophagus or colon, peristalsis may be interfered with and gross distension of the organ ensues; the condition is known as megaoesophagus or megacolon. The pseudocysts of some strains of *T. cruzi* are particularly prone to congregate in the heart muscle, when the resulting neuronal and muscle cell destruction may lead to thinning and weakening of the wall of the heart.

Diagnosis

Clinical signs are inconclusive. Various immunological tests (IFAT, ELISA and complement fixation) are used. Confirmatory diagnosis by parasite isolation can be attempted in three ways. (1) Blood films: however, as parasitaemia is intermittent and the organisms may be scanty, this is not a reliable method. (2) Cultivation in vitro: *T. cruzi* grows readily in many nutrient media, including blood–agar media. (3) Cultivation in vivo: the parasites readily infect laboratory mice. An often used, simple diagnostic procedure is to allow uninfected reduviid bugs, laboratory reared, to feed on the patient and then to examine the bugs' faeces or gut contents for the presence of trypanosomes 3–4 weeks later; this procedure is known as xenodiagnosis. The possibility of infection (or double infection) with *T. rangeli* should be borne in mind when using any of these techniques.

Trypanosoma rangeli

T. rangeli occurs in South America but its distribution is more patchy than that of *T. cruzi*. Although it infects humans, it is apparently entirely non-pathogenic and its only medical importance lies in the possibility of its being mistakenly diagnosed as *T. cruzi*, either in human or insect hosts, as it also shares reduviid bugs as vectors. The forms seen in humans are trypomastigotes only; they are longer than those of *T. cruzi*, measuring about 30 μm (Figure II.7). In bugs the parasite differs from *T. cruzi* by completing its development into metacyclic trypomastigotes in the haemolymph and salivary glands, from whence it is transmitted to mammals by direct inoculation in the insect's saliva, as well as in the hind gut. The infective metacyclic trypomastigotes are longer than those of *T. cruzi*. Unusually amongst trypanosomes, *T. rangeli* is pathogenic to its invertebrate host.

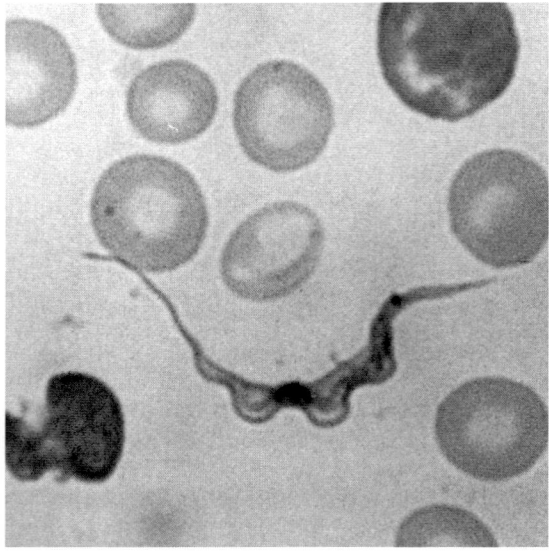

Figure II.7: Giemsa-stained bloodstream form of *Trypanosoma rangeli*. (Photograph by Nester Añez, Imperial College of Science, Technology and Medicine, University of London.)

T. rangeli can also be distinguished from *T. cruzi* with the aid of monoclonal antibodies (although the two species have some common antigens), differential complement-mediated lysis, isoenzyme electrophoresis and polymerase chain reaction amplification of kinetoplast DNA.[8]

Leishmanial parasites

(See also Chapter 75)

These parasites, species of the genus *Leishmania*, are classified in the same family (Trypanosomatidae) as the trypanosomes. Like them, they alternate between two hosts: a vertebrate and an invertebrate; however, the only forms which develop in the former are intracellular amastigotes, and those which develop in the invertebrate (insect) vector are promastigotes (Figure II.8). Promastigotes are elongate, motile flagellates with the flagellar origin and kinetoplast at the anterior end of the cell and the nucleus more or less in the middle. Both forms divide by binary fission and there is no firm evidence yet of sexual reproduction, although naturally occurring apparently 'hybrid' populations have been reported.[6]

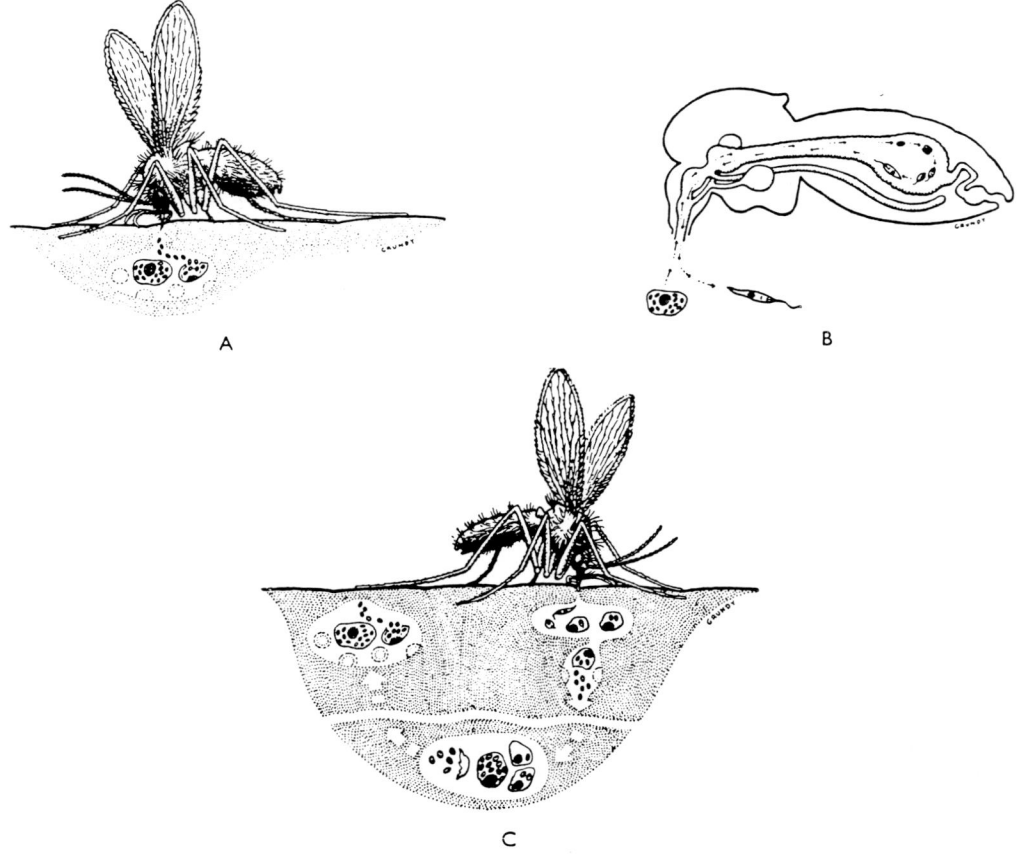

Figure II.8: Life cycle of *Leishmania* species. **A**, Feeding female sand fly ingests amastigotes from an infected vertebrate. **B**, The amastigotes develop into promastigotes, undergo division and migrate forwards to the pharynx of the sand fly. **C**, When the sand fly next feeds on blood it injects promastigotes into the wound. The developmental cycle in the sand fly takes about 10 days. (The diagrams of sand flies and parasites are not to scale.) (Drawing by J. Hull Grundy.)

The vectors of all the species of *Leishmania* which infect humans are small insects (sand flies) of the genera *Phlebotomus* (in Africa, Asia and Europe) and *Lutzomyia* and *Psychodopygus* (in South and Central America); as with mosquitoes, only female sand flies feed on blood. The species of *Leishmania* which infect humans can be divided into two major groups on the basis of their pathological behaviour: those which infect internal organs (liver, spleen, bone marrow) and cause visceral leishmaniasis (the *L. donovani* complex) and those which are restricted to the skin (dermis), causing cutaneous leishmaniasis (the *L. mexicana* and *L. braziliensis* complexes and three ungrouped species, *L. tropica*, *L. major* and *L. aethiopica*).[9]

Recent phylogenetic studies based on analysis of ribosomal RNA genes have suggested a neotropical origin for the genus,[4] but this is not universally accepted.

Life cycle and morphology

All the species infecting humans are very similar morphologically. The rounded or oval amastigotes are smaller than those of *T. cruzi*, about 2–4 μm in diameter, and the promastigotes vary considerably in length from about 15 μm to 30 μm (Figure II.9). After a feeding sand fly ingests amastigotes (presumably within monocytes or macrophages), the parasites escape from the cell and transform into promastigotes, which colonize the insect's midgut. In one subgenus of *Leishmania*, *Viannia*, there is also a phase of promastigote development in the sand fly's hindgut. Finally, the promastigotes spread forward into the foregut and proboscis of the vector, where the so-called metacyclic promastigotes are formed. These are injected with the fly's saliva when it next feeds on a mammal.

In the mammalian host the promastigotes enter phagocytes, either actively or passively, and transform into amastigotes. Unlike those of *T. cruzi*, the amastigotes remain enclosed within a phagosome which fuses with a lysosome but they somehow resist digestion by the lysosomal enzymes (or inhibit their production) and survive and multiply within the phagolysosome. When the host cell is full, it ruptures and the released amastigotes re-enter other phagocytes to continue the process. In the *L. donovani* complex the fixed liver phagocytes known as Kupffer cells also become infected.

Visceral leishmaniasis

Geographical distribution

Visceral leishmaniasis (sometimes known, particularly in India and Africa, as kala-azar) occurs in South America in the southern tropical zone, in tropical east Africa, the north African littoral and the Mediterranean coastal region of southern Europe, and in parts of India and central Asia. In South America, it is caused by *L. chagasi*, which also infects dogs and wild Canidae, which may act as reservoir hosts; the vectors are sand flies of the genus *Lutzomyia*. In Asia and sub-Saharan Africa the causative species is *L. donovani* and the vectors are species of

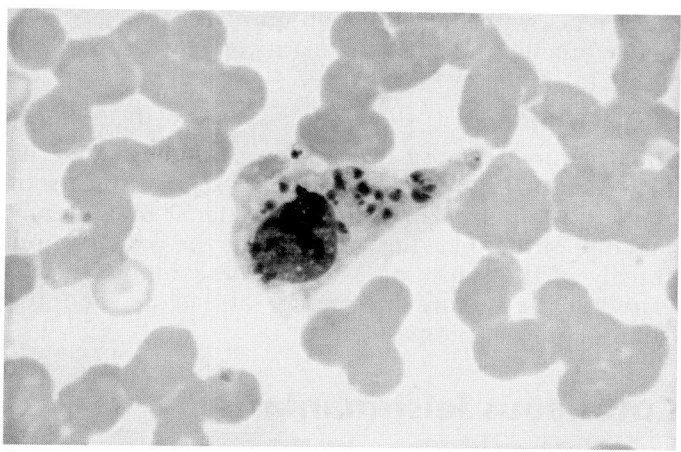

A

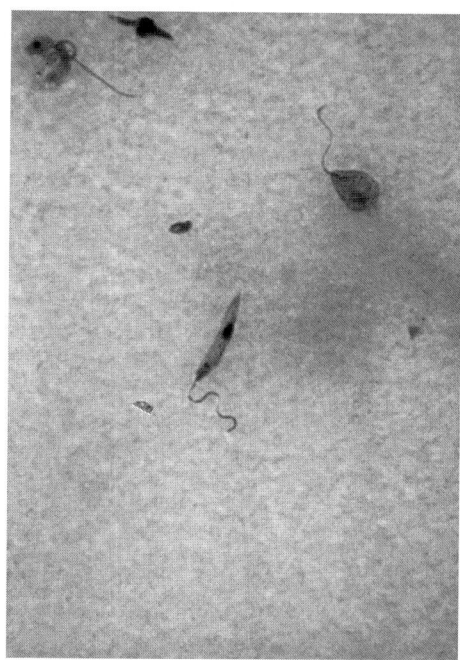

B

Figure II.9: *Leishmania*. (**A**) Amastigotes of *L. donovani* in a bone marrow macrophage and (**B**) promastigotes from a culture in vitro. (From Muller R & Baker J R. *Medical Parasitology.* London: Gower Medical Publishing, 1990).

Phlebotomus; in parts of Africa the parasite also infects dogs and certain rodents, while in India it seems that humans are the only vertebrate hosts. In countries bordering the Mediterranean Sea, visceral leishmaniasis is caused by another, closely related species: *L. infantum*; this species is also transmitted by *Phlebotomus* species, and dogs are important reservoirs of infection. All these species of *Leishmania* belong to the subgenus *Leishmania*.

Pathogenesis

Infection of cells of the monocyte/phagocyte system leads to extensive hyperplasia of the system, with gross enlargement of the liver and spleen and progressive interference with their function and with the haemato-poietic functions of the bone marrow (Figure II.9A).

Diagnosis

Confirmatory diagnosis depends on parasite isolation by microscopical examination of Giemsa-stained smears, or by cultivation in vitro of biopsy material obtained by puncture of the spleen or, more safely, the bone marrow (usually of the sternum). Most of the common blood–agar diphasic culture media are satisfactory, and the parasites grow as promastigotes.

Cutaneous leishmaniasis

Geographical distribution

L. major causes cutaneous leishmaniasis in Asia and tropical Africa, and possibly also in parts of north Africa; its vectors are *Phlebotomus* species and its reservoir hosts are rodents of various species (usually the gerbil *Rhombomys opimus* in Asia). *L. aethiopica* occurs only in east and north-east Africa, with hyraxes (*Procavia* and *Heterohyrax* species) as the main reservoir hosts and *Phlebotomus* species as vectors. *L. tropica* infects humans (and possibly dogs) in parts of Asia (the Middle East and north-eastern India), and probably also in parts of north Africa and southern Europe (including Greece) around the Mediterranean Sea; it is transmitted by *Phlebotomus*.

In Central and South America cutaneous leishmaniasis is caused by a range of species, some as yet ill defined and unnamed; the more important species are listed in Table II.3.

The African and Asian species, and all those in South America, which cause cutaneous leishmaniasis are members of the subgenus *Leishmania* except for the *L. braziliensis* complex of species (Table II.3), which are classified in the subgenus *Viannia*. All the South American species except *L. braziliensis* are transmitted by species of *Lutzomyia*; *L. braziliensis* is transmitted by *Psychodopygus*.

Pathogenesis

In the cutaneous leishmaniases, parasitized macrophages are normally restricted to the dermis and mucous membranes. Lesions may range from a single, self-healing ulcer to widespread ulceration over much of the body surface (diffuse cutaneous leishmaniasis or DCL), which sometimes results from infection with *L. aethiopica* or *L. pifanoi* (the latter having been isolated only from cases of DCL, although it presumably causes ordinary cutaneous leishmaniasis as well). *L. braziliensis* has a tendency to invade mucocutaneous junctions, particularly those of the nasopharynx and palate, where it causes the disfiguring lesions of mucocutaneous leishmaniasis or espundia. *L. peruviana* occurs at high altitudes in the Peruvian Andes; it causes cutaneous leishmaniasis with a characteristic dry sore on the skin, called uta.

Infection with human immunodeficiency virus (HIV) and the ensuing development of the acquired immune deficiency syndrome (AIDS) markedly reduces or destroys the immunological response to infection with *Leishmania*, leading to widespread dissemination of skin lesions and even invasion of the viscera by *Leishmania* species which have hitherto caused inapparent or localized infections.

Diagnosis

As with visceral leishmaniasis, confirmatory diagnosis depends on detection of the parasites either by microscopical examination of Giemsa-stained slides or by

Table II.3 Main species of *Leishmania* causing human cutaneous leishmaniasis in Central and South America (based on Lainson and Shaw[9])

Parasite	Locality	Reservoir hosts
Subgenus *Leishmania*		
L. mexicana complex		
L. mexicana	Central America	Rodents
L. amazonensis	Northern Brazil	Rodents
L. venezuelensis	Venezuela	–
*L. pifanoi**	Venezuela	–
Subgenus *Viannia*		
L. braziliensis complex		
L. braziliensis†	Brazil, Venezuela	?Rodents, opossum,‡ sloth§
L. guyanensis	South America, north of the Amazon river	Sloth,§ anteater¶
L. panamensis	Panama, Costa Rica, Colombia	Sloth‖
L. peruviana	Peru, Argentina	Dog

*So far known only from cases of diffuse cutaneous leishmaniasis; identity uncertain.
†Causes cutaneous and mucocutaneous leishmaniasis.
‡*Didelphis marsupialis*.
§*Choloepus didactylus*.
¶*Tamandua tetradactylus*.
‖*C. hoffmanni*.

cultivation in vitro. Suitable material can be obtained by puncture of the margin of a suspect lesion with a hypodermic needle attached to a syringe containing a small amount of physiological saline. The aspirate contained in the needle is then expelled on to a microscope slide or into a tube of culture medium (usually blood–agar).

Entamoeba histolytica

(See also Chapter 77)

Life cycle and morphology

E. histolytica inhabits the lumen of the large intestine of humans (and other primates, dogs, cats, pigs and rodents), where it may cause amoebic dysentery. The parasite also sometimes invades the mucosa and other viscera. The trophozoite (Figure II.10A) is motile, irregular in shape, measures about 10–40 μm in diameter, and reproduces by binary fission. Sexual reproduction is unknown, but there is some evidence of genetic exchange. The trophozoites may contain red blood cells in food vacuoles. Transmission is by ingestion of the resistant cyst, which is excreted in the host's faeces, with contaminated food or water. The mature cyst (Figure II.10B) is 9.5–15.5 μm in diameter, spherical, and contains four nuclei; often, but not always, it also contains paracrystalline aggregations of ribosomes, the 'chromatoid bodies', which appear as rods with blunt, rounded ends. They stain with iodine or haematoxylin stains, but appear glass-like in fresh specimens. Cysts develop only in the intestinal lumen, not within the tissues.

It has long been suspected, and more recently conclusively demonstrated, that two morphologically identical parasites exist: *E. histolytica*, which can invade tissues and hence become pathogenic; and *E. dispar*, which cannot.[10] Therefore many persons with intestinal amoebae which are morphologically indistinguishable from *E. histolytica* may show no sign or symptom of amoebiasis. Such persons may be found in all countries, tropical and temperate, while clinical amoebiasis is more or less restricted to the tropics.

Pathogenesis

Amoebae in the gut lumen are not significantly harmful, but if, for reasons unknown, they penetrate the intestinal mucosa they multiply within flask-shaped ulcers and lead to haemorrhage and mucosal damage. When this occurs, the amoebae feed on red blood cells, which may be seen within the organisms. Bloody dysentery (amoebic dysentery) ensues, which can be differentiated from the bloody dysentery resulting from bacterial infection by the absence of the large numbers of pus cells characteristic of the latter.

The amoebic ulcers erode blood vessels (hence the haemorrhage), and thus amoebae may enter the circulation and be carried to other organs. Here they may become established, and form so-called amoebic 'abscesses', which are not true abscesses since they are bacteriologically sterile. The liver is the organ most commonly affected in this way, but the lungs and (rarely) brain may also be invaded.

Diagnosis

Confirmatory diagnosis by identification of amoebae may be made either by direct microscopical examination of faecal specimens (fresh or concentrated) or by cultivation of the organisms in suitable media. Serological techniques can be used to detect tissue invasion, but rarely if ever detect infection with parasites living in the gut lumen only.

Non-pathogenic intestinal amoebae (See also Chapter 77)

In addition to *E. dispar*, five other well-defined species of amoebae, none of which is pathogenic, may inhabit the human alimentary canal. Their only medical significance is that they may be mistaken for *E. histolytica*; these five species are listed below (Figure II.11):

- *E. coli*: cysts larger than those of *E. histolytica*, with eight nuclei when mature; chromatoid bars are rarely present but, when they are, they are thin and splinter-like, with pointed ends.
- *E. hartmanni*: cysts smaller than those of *E. histolytica*, but with four nuclei and chromatoid bodies of the *E. histolytica* type.
- *Endolimax nana*: small, oval cysts with four nuclei but no chromatoid bars.
- *Iodamoeba buetschlii*: uninucleate cyst, often containing a large glycogen vacuole which stains dark brown with iodine but appears clear in fresh specimens.
- *E. gingivalis*: unlike all the above-mentioned species, this amoeba inhabits the mouth (and so should not be

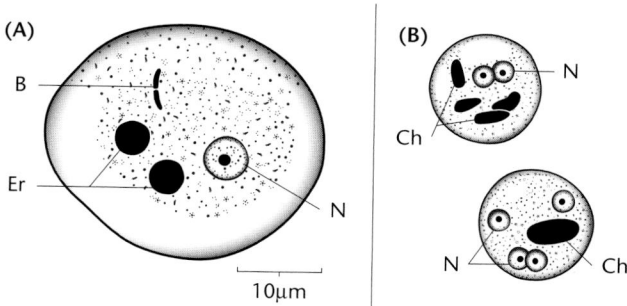

Figure II.10: *Entamoeba histolytica.* (**A**) Trophozoite with ingested erythrocytes (Er) and bacterium (B); the nucleus (N) is also visible. (**B**) Cysts with two and four nuclei (N) and chromatoid bodies (Ch; semicrystalline ribosomal masses). (Human faecal smears; iron haematoxylin stain.) (From Baker J R. *Parasitic Protozoa.* London: Hutchinson, 1969.)

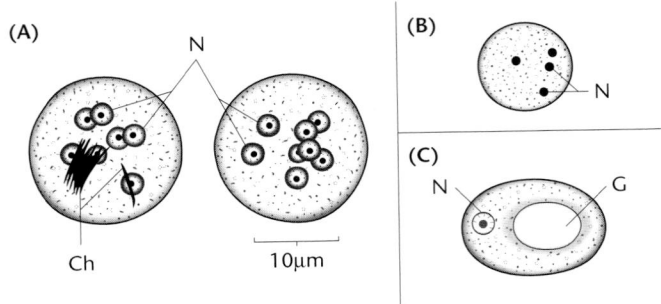

(A)
N
Ch
10µm
(B)
N
(C)
N
G

Figure II.11: Cysts of non-pathogenic intestinal amoebae. (**A**) *Entamoeba coli*; the cyst on the left contains chromatoid bodies (Ch). (**B**) *Endolimax nana*. (**C**) *Iodamoeba buetschlii*; the glycogen vacuole (G) is visible. N = nuclei. (Human faecal smears; iron haematoxylin stain.) (From Baker J R. *Parasitic Protozoa*. London: Hutchinson, 1969.)

confused with *E. histolytica*); it forms no cyst, transmission presumably being by direct contact or by the sharing of drinking vessels, etc.

The aberrant flagellate *Dientamoeba fragilis* (see p. 1643) resembles an amoeba as it lacks a flagellum, but it is binucleate and does not produce a cyst.

Giardia duodenalis

(See also Chapter 77)

Life cycle and morphology

The motile trophozoite has two nuclei, four pairs of flagella, and one or two curved median bodies of unknown function (sometimes incorrectly called parabasal bodies) (Figure II.12A); it is 10–20 µm long, 5–10 µm broad and 2–4 µm thick. Reproduction is by binary fission; no sexual process is known.

The infective stage is an oval cyst, 6–10 × 8–14 µm (Figure II.12B), which is excreted in the faeces and ingested with contaminated food or water. The cyst contains four small nuclei, grouped at one end, and a confused jumble of flagella, median bodies etc. in the centre.

Giardia has a worldwide distribution; the species infecting humans is also known as *G. intestinalis* or *G. lamblia*, though *G. duodenalis* appears to be zoologically correct.[11]

Pathogenesis

Trophozoites are attached to the mucosal surface of the duodenum or upper ileum by an oval, ventral anterior disc or 'sucker'; they do not penetrate the mucosa but may damage it if they are numerous, leading to villous atrophy and acute watery (not bloody) diarrhoea.

Diagnosis

Giardiasis can be confirmed by demonstrating cysts in faecal specimens; they are often numerous, and usually

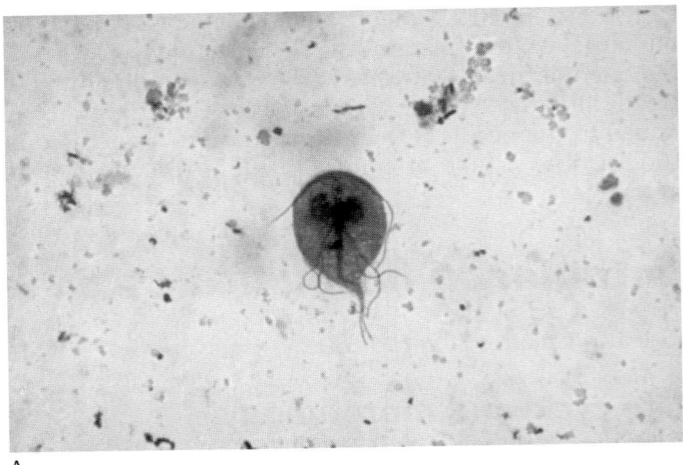

A

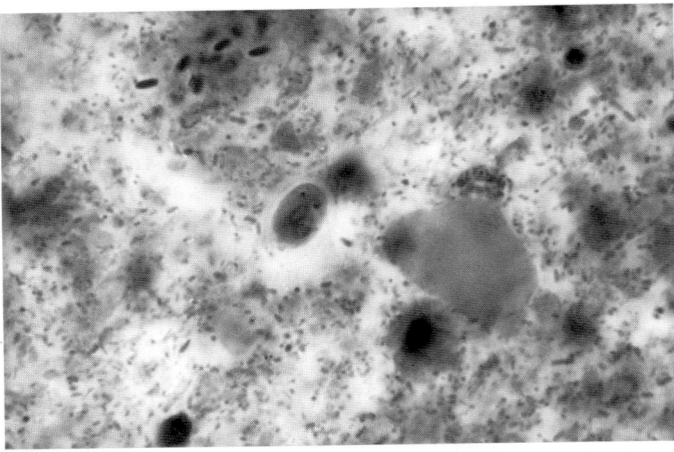

B

Figure II.12: *Giardia duodenalis*. (**A**) Trophozoite (human faecal smear, Giemsa stain). (**B**) Cyst (human faecal smear, iron haematoxylin stain). (From Muller R & Baker J R. *Medical Parasitology*. London: Gower Medical Publishing, 1990.)

easily recognizable even in unstained saline preparations, but iodine staining makes the internal structure more easily visible.

Trichomonas vaginalis

(See also Chapter 79)

Life cycle and morphology

The trophozoites are oval, 14–17 × 5–15 µm, and have a single nucleus, four anterior flagella and a single lateral flagellum which runs back along the surface of the cell, to which it is attached to form a conspicuous undulating membrane supported by a marginal filament (Figure II.13). The lateral flagellum ends about halfway along the cell, which also contains a prominent central rod or axostyle. Multiplication is by binary fission, with no sexual process.

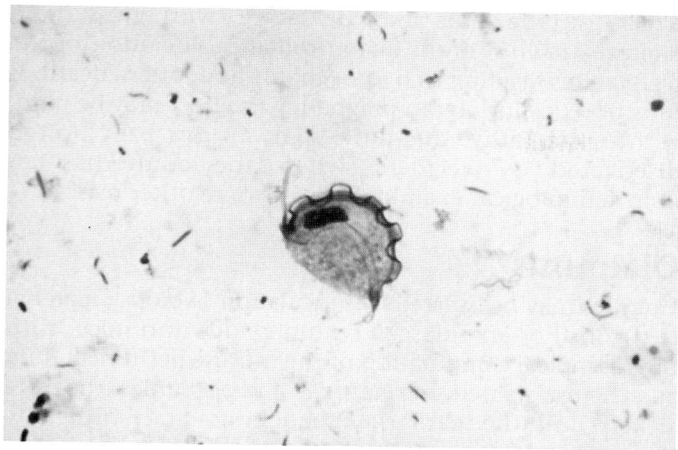

Figure II.13: Trophozoite of *Trichomonas muris* (Giemsa stain). In the human parasite *T. vaginalis*, the conspicuous lateral flagellum ends about halfway along the cell. (From Muller R & Baker J R. *Medical Parasitology*. London: Gower Medical Publishing, 1990.)

No cyst is formed, the trophozoite being transmitted directly during sexual intercourse.

Pathogenesis

T. vaginalis inhabits the vagina and urethra. It is more commonly pathogenic in women than in men, though it may cause mild urethritis or prostatitis.

Diagnosis

Clinical diagnosis may be confirmed by demonstration of the trophozoites in Giemsa-stained smears made from swabs of vaginal (or urethral) discharge. If they are not readily found, the swab can be placed in a tube of medium for cultivation of the parasites in vitro.

Non-pathogenic intestinal flagellates (See also Chapter 77)

As with the amoebae, there are other, non-pathogenic flagellates which may inhabit the human alimentary tract and which may be confused with *Giardia duodenalis*.

One of these species, *Trichomonas tenax*, inhabits the buccal cavity, but the others all live in the intestine. *Dientamoeba fragilis* is an aberrant flagellate which looks like an amoeba; it is binucleate but lacks a flagellum and median bodies. The other non-pathogenic flagellates (*Chilomastix mesnili*, *Enteromonas hominis*, *Retortamonas intestinalis* and *Pentatrichomonas hominis*) all have between one and six flagella and a single nucleus; *P. hominis* looks rather like *T. vaginalis* but can be distinguished from it by the difference in habitat.

All these species except *T. tenax*, *P. hominis* and *D. fragilis* form cysts, which can be distinguished from those of *G. duodenalis* by their round shape and lack of the remains of flagella, etc., which are so characteristic of the cyst of *G. duodenalis*. The cysts of all except *E. hominis* have only one nucleus; *E. hominis*, like *G. duodenalis*, has four, but—unlike *G. duodenalis*—these are not usually grouped at one end of the cyst.

Toxoplasma gondii

(See also Chapter 76)

T. gondii has two distinct life cycles which usually take place in vertebrate hosts belonging to different genera. The 'normal' apicomplexan life cycle of merogony, gametogony and sporogony occurs only in domestic cats and a few closely related species, within epithelial cells of the small intestine; the cat is therefore the 'definitive' host. Oocysts, measuring about $11 \times 13\,\mu m$, are voided in the cat's faeces and, when mature, contain two spherical sporocysts, each containing four elongate sporozoites.

If a mature oocyst is swallowed by another susceptible animal (the 'intermediate' host), which can be any warm-blooded vertebrate (mammal or bird), the sporozoites are liberated by the action of the host's digestive juices and the secondary life cycle commences. (This also can occur in cats.)

The sporozoites emerge from the oocyst in the intermediate host's small intestine, pass through the mucosa and enter (either actively or passively) macrophages. The macrophage's lysosomes are inhibited from fusing with the phagosomes containing the parasites, which thus survive and begin to divide rapidly until the host cell is filled with small, crescentic, uninucleate parasites known as tachyzoites or endozoites, each measuring about 5×1–$2\,\mu m$ (Figure II.14A). The infected macrophage, referred to as a pseudocyst, eventually disintegrates and the liberated tachyzoites enter other macrophages and repeat the process. This constitutes the acute phase of the infection. Unless the host dies or is treated, the acute phase is immunologically controlled and the infection moves into the chronic phase. The parasites invade cells other than macrophages (including muscle cells and neurones) and secrete a thin but tough cyst wall, within which they continue to divide, though more slowly; the organisms within this cyst are called bradyzoites or cystozoites; the cyst may attain a diameter of $60\,\mu m$ (Figure II.14B).

If a non-feline host eats uncooked meat or prey containing these tissue cysts, the bradyzoites are liberated in the duodenum and repeat the extraintestinal cycle after passing through the mucosal wall. However, if a cat ingests tissue cysts in its prey, or if infected raw meat or offal is fed to it, the cystozoites enter duodenal cells and begin the 'normal' apicomplexan life cycle. This intestinal cycle consists of a limited number of merogony cycles, with each batch of merozoites entering other duodenal cells to repeat the process, until the final generation of merozoites commences the sexual cycle of gametogony and fertilization within the duodenal cells, culminating with sporogony within the developing oocyst (which is

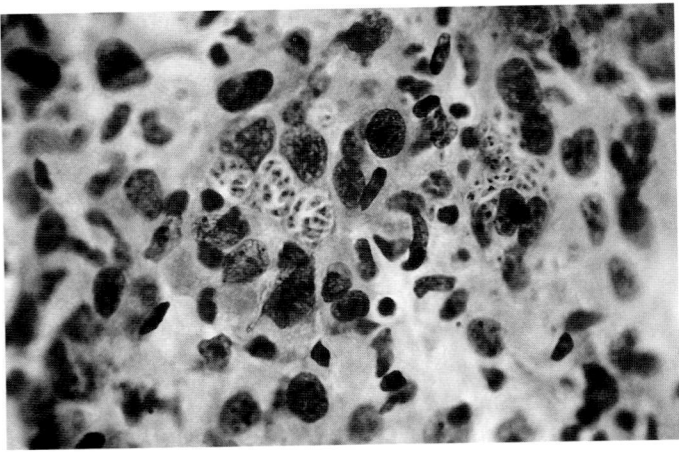

A

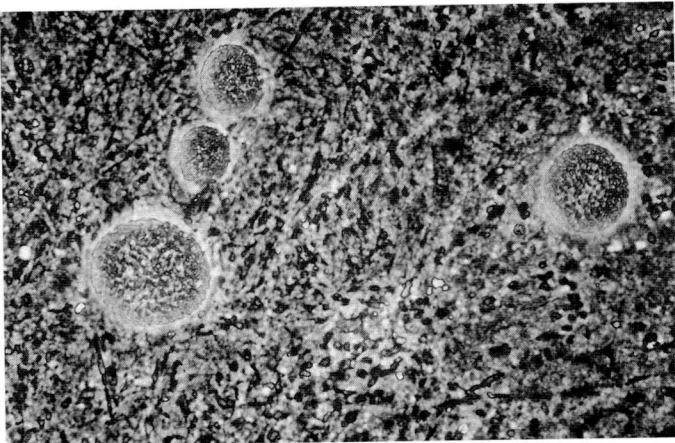

B

Figure II.14: (**A**) *Toxoplasma gondii*: intracellular groups (pseudocysts) of parasites in macrophages in a smear of mouse peritoneal fluid (Giemsa stain). (**B**) Tissue cysts in emulsified brain of mouse (phase contrast illumination). (From Muller R & Baker J R. *Medical Parasitology*. London: Gower Medical Publishing, 1990.)

secreted around the fertilized zygote). Sporogony is completed, with the production of two sporocysts each containing four sporozoites, as the oocyst passes down the cat's gut and in the expelled faeces. Oocysts can survive in the external environment for at least 1 year.

Pathogenesis

Infected cats show no obvious sign of illness. In humans the acute phase of infection (tachyzoites multiplying in macrophages) usually results in mild to moderate febrile illness with lymphadenopathy, except in immuno-compromised persons (e.g. those with AIDS), in whom the infection may become generalized and fatal. The chronic phase is symptomless and, unless the patient becomes subsequently immunocompromised, appears to remain active but quiescent for the rest of the individual's life.

T. gondii is one of the few parasites that can cross the placenta, though only if the pregnant woman has an acute infection. Infection in utero is uncommon (probably fewer than 1 case per 1000 live births), but its effects on the fetus may be severe, with gross brain damage resulting from uncontrolled proliferation of the tachyzoites, leading to hydrocephaly and, often, death. If infection occurs later in pregnancy its effect may be mild, with retinopathy the only sign in the baby (often discovered by accident when the adult has an ophthalmological examination for some other reason).

Diagnosis

Parasites may be isolated by inoculation of biopsy material (e.g. tonsil or an enlarged lymph gland) into mice, with microscopical examination of the murine peritoneal fluid as a Giemsa-stained smear after 3–4 weeks (unless the mice sicken and die earlier). Pseudocysts and artificially liberated tachyzoites will be seen. There are several sero-logical tests for anti-*Toxoplasma* antibodies, but these remain positive throughout the chronic phase of infection and so do not necessarily indicate acute infection unless two similar tests, performed a few weeks apart, reveal a sharply rising titre. The tests used include complement fixation, agglutination (of killed tachyzoites), and IFAT.

Serological evidence indicates that between 25% and 35% of the population of so-called 'developed' countries have anti-*Toxoplasma* antibodies, indicative of past infection. Reactivated acute toxoplasmosis is one of the more common, often fatal, complications of AIDS.

Sarcocystis (See also Chapter 77)

Sarcocystis species, though common parasites of herbivores and rodents, are not significant as parasites of humans. *Sarcocystis* is related to *Toxoplasma* and has a similar life cycle, though it differs in that each species has only a very limited range of intermediate hosts and extraintestinal development does not occur in the definitive host. The zooites are larger than those of *T. gondii*, being 10–15 μm long, and the tissue cysts, which occur only in muscle cells, may be very long—even visible macroscopically.

Humans are definitive hosts of *S. bovihominis* and *S. suihominis*, the intermediate hosts of which are oxen and pigs, respectively (as the specific names indicate). A few early records of human infection with tissue cysts (sarcocysts) suggest that humans can rarely, perhaps accidentally, act as intermediate hosts for one or more other species of *Sarcocystis*.

Pathogenesis

Infection of the human intestine with *S. bovihominis* or *S. suihominis* may cause moderately severe diarrhoea, which is, however, self-limiting. Infection of the muscle with sarcocysts is usually symptomless but may, if intense, lead to some muscular weakness.

Babesia (See also Chapter 72)

Species of *Babesia*, commonly known as piroplasms, are

small intraerythrocytic apicomplexan parasites which occur commonly in cattle, sheep, horses, insectivores and rodents in many parts of the world but do not normally infect humans; they are transmitted by ticks (Arthropoda, Acarina), usually members of the family Ixodidae ('hard' ticks).

The small parasites (1–2 μm) multiply within red blood cells by binary fission, and some species (e.g. *B. microti* of voles) may also invade lymphocytes for one merogonic cycle before entering red cells.

A very few (perhaps 100 or so) cases of *Babesia* infection have been reported in humans in North America and Europe. North American infections have all been due to *B. microti* of voles (insectivores of the genus *Microtus*), and the patients have recovered. In Europe, all the (few) infected persons had previously undergone splenectomy at some time, and most of them died; some (perhaps all) of the infections acquired in Europe were due to the cattle parasite *B. divergens*. No successful treatment is known for human babesiosis.

Diagnosis depends on recognizing the parasites in stained blood films, where they may be difficult to distinguish from young trophozoites of *Plasmodium*, though *Babesia* never contains pigment. Serological tests can differentiate the two genera.

Pneumocystis carinii

(See also Chapter 70)

The taxonomic position of *Pneumocystis* is uncertain. 'Molecular' studies, especially of ribosomal RNA, strongly suggest its fungal nature. It has been recorded in humans, dogs and rodents in all continents (except Antarctica); in Africa it appears to be uncommon.

The parasites are about 5–6 μm in diameter, uninucleate and spherical; they live extracellularly in lung alveolae (Figure II.15). Binary fission has been described, though details of the life cycle are sparse and somewhat conflicting. Cyst-like, spherical bodies about 10 μm in diameter are formed in the lung alveolae, and are thought to be the infective phase. Transmission presumably occurs by droplet infection.

Infection is probably common but symptomless, unless the parasites become sufficiently numerous to block the alveolae with a foamy mass composed of plasma cells, parasites and mucus. This may occur in immunologically incompetent or immunocompromised persons, such as sickly or premature babies, persons receiving immunosuppressive therapy or those afflicted with AIDS; *Pneumocystis carinii* pneumonia (PCP) is perhaps the commonest cause of death of patients with AIDS.

Facultatively parasitic amoebae (See also Chapter 78)

Three species of amoebae which normally live in water or

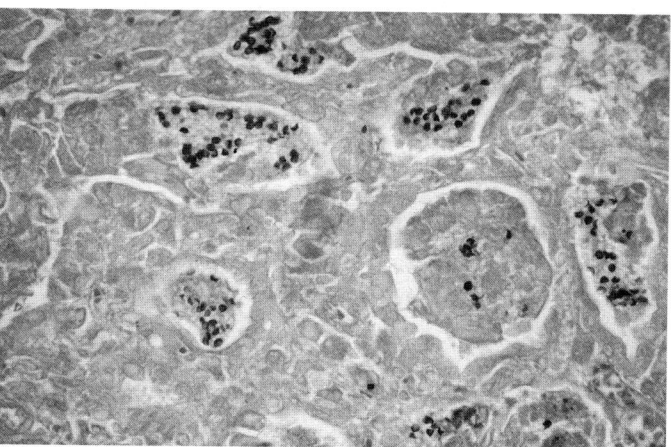

Figure II.15: *Pneumocystis carinii* within alveolae of a section of human lung. (Grocott's silver stain, methyl green counterstaining.) (From Muller R & Baker J R. *Medical Parasitology.* London: Gower Medical Publishing, 1990.)

mud occasionally infect human patients, and a fourth species is suspected of doing so.

Naegleria fowleri inhabits warm, fresh water, and has three stages in its life cycle: amoeboid form, flagellate form and cyst. Human infections with *N. fowleri* are due, apparently, to amoebae being forced up the patient's nose while he or she is swimming or jumping in infected water, and then penetrating the nasal mucosa and migrating up the olfactory nerve to the brain. In the brain they multiply extensively (as amoeboid trophozoites only) and cause considerable damage, which is usually fatal. The condition is known as primary amoebic encephalitis (PAM). PAM is more common in tropical and subtropical areas, but infection can occur in artificially (or naturally) heated waters in colder countries; overall, however, it is rare (probably fewer than 200 cases are known). A related species, *N. australiensis*, can cause experimental PAM in mice and is therefore also suspected of being a potential, if not actual, facultative parasite of humans. Another amoeba, *Balamutha mandrillaris*, has been isolated from some human cases of PAM.

Acanthamoeba culbertsoni rarely causes infection of the brain in humans. The parasite has no flagellated stage, and normally lives in damp soil or, as the cyst, in dry and dusty soil. Infection probably occurs when trophozoites in mud, or perhaps cysts in dry, dusty soil, are ingested or inhaled through the mouth. The most common manifestation of *Acanthamoeba* infection is relatively mild pharyngitis, which has been reported in a limited number of young children and even fewer adults in the USA. It is thought the children may have acquired the infection while crawling or playing with soil. In a very few individuals, *Acanthamoeba* infection of the brain has been reported post-mortem; most of these persons were immunocompromised in some way, and probably amoebae from an initial pharyngeal infection were able to penetrate the mucosa and find their way to the brain; the resulting condition is known as granulomatous amoebic encephalitis (GAE).

Acanthamoeba species can infect the cornea of persons using soft contact lenses, presumably as a result of contamination of the wash solutions. There have also been a few cases of keratitis due to *Acanthamoeba* infection apparently unassociated with the use of contact lenses.

Balantidium coli (See also Chapter 77)

Life cycle and morphology

B. coli is the only known ciliate parasite of humans. Its natural habitat is the large intestine of domestic pigs and its distribution is worldwide. The large, oval, flattened trophozoites (60–70 × 40–60 μm; Figure II.16) are covered with short, hair-like cilia, by means of which they swim; they reproduce both asexually by transverse binary fission and sexually by the complicated process known as conjugation (unique to ciliates). Like almost all ciliates, *B. coli* has two nuclei: a large, polyploid macronucleus and a small, haploid micronucleus which is involved in sexual reproduction (during which process the macronucleus degenerates, to be reformed by one of the progeny of the micronuclear fusion and subsequent fission which occurs during conjugation). Large, spherical cysts (50–60 μm in diameter) are formed and excreted in the faeces. Human infection presumably usually results from ingestion of cysts with contaminated food or water; person-to-person transmission has never been conclusively demonstrated.

Pathogenesis

Normally the ciliate lives harmlessly in the lumen of the pig's large intestine. Sometimes, however, perhaps as a result of concomitant infection with some other pathogen such as *Salmonella*, the trophozoites penetrate the submucosa and form large, flask-shaped ulcers like those caused by *E. histolytica*. Bloody dysentery then ensues. A similar sequence of events probably occurs in humans, although symptomless infections of the gut lumen only have not yet been reported from humans (perhaps because no one has looked for them).

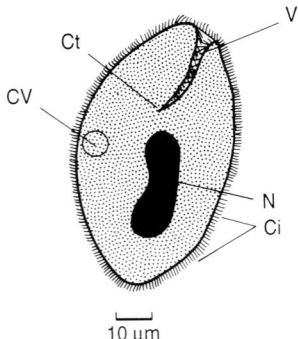

10 μm

Figure II.16: *Balantidium coli*: trophozoite from a culture in vitro (the micronucleus is not visible in this specimen). Ci, cilia; Ct, cytosome (mouth); CV, contractile vacuole; N, macronucleus; V, vestibule. (From Baker J R. *Parasitic Protozoa* London: Hutchinson, 1969.)

Diagnosis

The large cysts, with their correspondingly large macronucleus, are easily recognized in fresh or stained faecal preparations. *B. coli* grows in most of the common culture media used for *Entamoeba*, but recourse to this technique is seldom necessary.

Cryptosporidium species

(See also Chapter 77)

Life cycle and morphology

Cryptosporidium muris is an apicomplexan parasite of the group known as coccidia. It was thought to be restricted to non-human mammals, but is now recognized to be one of the commonest human enteric infections. It may be found throughout the world, more commonly in children and immunocompromised adults. The species usually found in humans is *C. parvum*, which also infects ruminants. *C. muris*, a parasite of rodents, may occur, less frequently, in humans.[12]

Cryptosporidium is transmitted by a resistant oocyst in the faeces of infected persons or animals, ingested with contaminated food or water. Four sporozoites emerge from the oocyst in the small intestine, enter cells of the microvillous border, and undergo merogony. The parasites remain intracellular, though they lie very superficially just below the host cell's plasmalemma. Sexual forms (gametocytes) also develop and form male and female gametes. The gametes fuse to form a diploid zygote, which encysts to become an oocyst, only 4–6 μm in diameter, the contents of which divide to form four sporozoites. Unlike many coccidia, sporocysts are not formed within the oocyst.

Some oocysts, with thin walls, apparently mature and 'hatch' while still within the first host's intestine, which the emergent sporozoites then reinfect, enabling the infection to build up to a very high level unless it is controlled immunologically. Other oocysts, with thicker walls, are excreted (Figure II.17) and serve to transmit the infection orally to a fresh host. Human infections usually result from person-to-person transmission, but domestic animals and rodents may sometimes act as reservoir hosts.

Pathogenesis

Damage to the small intestinal mucosa, resulting from the successive cycles of merogony, leads to diarrhoea which, in immunologically competent persons, is usually self-limiting; neither blood nor pus cells are present in the stool. In immunodeficient persons (including patients with AIDS), the infection may progress unchecked, and severe, intractable and even life-threatening diarrhoea may result, with stool volumes up to 25 litres per day. Pulmonary cryptosporidiosis has occasionally been recorded, possibly as a result of inhalation of oocysts in vomit.

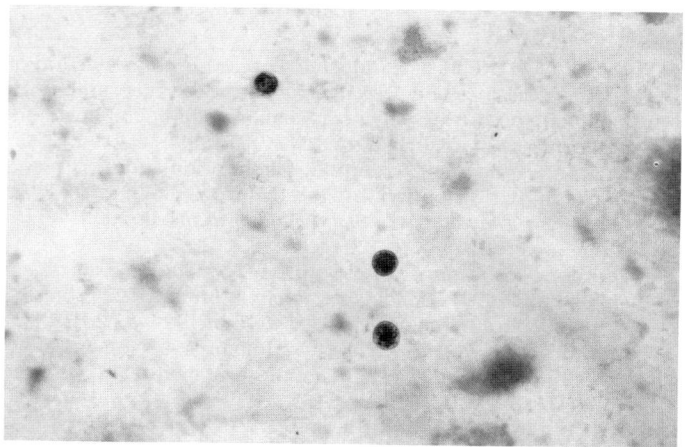

Figure II.17: *Cryptosporidium* oocysts in human faecal specimen. (Modified acid-fast stain.) (From Muller R & Baker J R. *Medical Parasitology.* London: Gower Medical Publishing, 1990. Photograph by courtesy of Dr S. Tzipori.)

Diagnosis

Confirmation of diagnosis depends on recognition of oocysts in faeces. The small size of the oocysts makes this difficult; they may be more readily found after concentration of faeces by flotation techniques followed by staining with acid-fast stains such as Ziehl–Neelsen.

Cyclospora cayetanensis

Cyclospora cayetanensis is a coccidian parasite of humans which may cause protracted watery diarrhoea and other intestinal disturbances, especially in AIDS patients.[12] It, or similar organisms (sometimes referred to as CLBs—originally 'cyanobacter-' or 'coccidia-like bodies', now '*Cyclospora*-like bodies') have been reported from tropical and temperate zones of all continents. The parasites inhabit the intestinal enterocytes and undergo a life cycle similar to that of *Cryptosporidium*. The small spheroidal oocysts (8–10 μm in diameter) contain two sporocysts, each with two sporozoites. Transmission depends on ingestion of the oocysts, which are passed out in faeces. The sporozoites emerge in the intestine of the new host, and invade enterocytes. Diagnosis depends on detection of the oocysts in stool.

Isospora belli

Isospora belli is another coccidian parasite which inhabits enterocytes of the human small intestine. The oocyst is ovoid and larger (mean diameters 30 × 12 μm) than those of the two previous species and contains two sporocysts, each with four sporozoites. The life cycle is similar. In immunocompetent hosts, *I. belli* causes relatively mild, self-limiting diarrhoea. In immunosuppressed persons, the diarrhoea may be very severe and long-lasting. As

with the others, diagnosis depends on recognizing the oocysts in faeces.

Microsporidia (See also Chapter 77)

Microsporidia are predominantly parasites of fish and insects, to which they may be very pathogenic; a few species are known to infect mammals.

The number of reports of microsporidial infection in humans, usually in those who are immunocompromised (e.g. by HIV), and the number of species involved, is increasing. Seven genera are known to infect mammals (*Encephalitozoon*, *Enterocytozoon*, *Nosema*, *Pleistophora*, *Thelohania*, *Trachipleistophora* and *Vittaforma*); it seems likely that all seven can infect immunodeficient humans and that some, at least, can infect those who are immunocompetent (at least in privileged sites). Vittaforma corneae is known only from the cornea of an immunocompetent individual.

Life cycle and morphology

The infective stages of microsporidia are small spores, about 5 × 2 μm in size, which are usually ingested orally. The ingested spore ejects a hollow, tubular polar filament which introduces (rather in the manner of a hypodermic syringe) the infective contents of the spore, the sporoplasm (which is believed to be uninucleate, although this has not been conclusively demonstrated), into the cytoplasm of a host cell. Within the host cells (which may be of many different types), successive cycles of merogony, followed by sporogony, occur, resulting in the production of many more spores.

Pathogenesis

Human infection with *Encephalitozoon* and *Enterocytozoon* involves the intestine, as the parasites invade enterocytes, and villous loss may result. Invasion of the bile duct may cause hepatobiliary disease. *Enterocytozoon* may disseminate more widely. It is likely that asymptomatic infections with microsporidia may occur, particularly in immunocompetent persons. Many of the cases of human infection are probably 'accidental' infections with species normally resident in other mammals, although *Enterocytozoon*, of which only one species—*E. bieneusi*—is known, may be a 'genuine' parasite of humans.

Serological surveys have revealed a high prevalence (up to about 40%) of positive reactions to *Encephalitozoon cuniculi* antigen among persons with tropical experience, and particularly those with malaria or tuberculosis. (*E. cuniculi* commonly infects rodents and lagomorphs (rabbits).) The significance of this is not clear.

Diagnosis

Diagnosis of infection with microsporidia is, at present, based on detection of the parasites in biopsy material.

REFERENCES

1   Cox F E G. Systematics of parasitic protozoa. In Kreier J P & Baker J R (eds) *Parasitic Protozoa*, 2nd edn, vol. 1. San Diego: Academic Press 1991: 55–80.

2   Cooke B M, Mohandas N & Coppel R. The malaria-infected red blood cell: structural and functional changes. *Adv Parasitol* 2001; 50 (in press).

3   Clark I A & Rockett K A. Nitric oxide and parasitic disease. *Adv Parasitol* 1996; 37:1–56.

4   Stevens J R, Noyes H A, Schofield C J et al. The molecular evolution of Trypanosomatidae. *Adv Parasitol* 2001; 48:1–56.

5   Barry J D & McCulloch R. Antigenic variation in trypanosomes: enhanced phenotypic variation in a eukaryotic parasite. *Adv Parasitol* 2001; 49:1–70.

6   Gibson W & Stevens J. Genetic exchange in the Trypanosomatidae. *Adv Parasitol* 1999; 43:1–46.

7   Schofield C J & Dias J C P. The Southern Cone initiative against Chagas disease. *Adv Parasitol* 1999; 42:1–27.

8   Vallejo G A, Guhl F, Chiari E et al. Species specific detection of *Trypanosoma cruzi* and *Trypanosoma rangeli* in vector and mammalian hosts by polymerase chain reaction amplification of kinetoplast minicircle DNA. *Acta Trop* 1999; 72:203–212.

9   Lainson R & Shaw J J. Evolution, classification and geographical distribution. In Peters W & Killick-Kendrick R (eds) *The Leishmaniases in Biology and Medicine*. London: Academic Press, 1987: 1–120.

10 Petithory J-C, Brumpt L C & Poujade F. *Entamoeba histolytica* (Schaudinn 1903) et *Entamoeba dispar* E. Brumpt 1925 sont deux espèces différentes. *Bull Soc Path Exot* 1994; 87:231–237.

11 Thompson R C A, Hopkins R M & Homan W L. Nomenclature and genetic groupings of *Giardia* infecting mammals. *Parasitol Today* 2000; 16:210–213.

12 Tzipori S (ed.). Opportunistic protozoa in humans. *Adv Parasitol* 1998; 40:1–430.

FURTHER READING

Gilles H M (ed.). *Protozoal Diseases*. London: Edward Arnold, 1999.

Hide G, Mottram J C, Coombs G H et al. (eds). *Trypanosomiasis and Leishmaniasis: Biology and Control*. Wallingford, UK: CAB International, 1997.

Kreier J P (and, for vols 1–3, Baker J R) (ed.). *Parasitic Protozoa*, 2nd edn, vols 1–10. San Diego: Academic Press, 1991–1995.

Orihel T C & Ash C R. *Parasites in Human Tissues*. Chicago: ASCP Press, 1995.

Peters W & Pasvol G. *Tropical Medicine and Parasitology*, 5th edn. London: Mosby, 2001.

Peters W & Killick-Kendrick R (eds). *The Leishmaniases in Biology and Medicine*, vols 1 & 2. London: Academic Press, 1987.

Ravdin J I (ed.). *Amebiasis*. London: Imperial College Press, 2000.

Rondinelli E G & Scaglia M. *Atlas of Human Protozoa*. Milan: Masson, 1993.

Taylor E R & Baker J R (eds). *In vitro Methods for Parasite Cultivation*. London: Academic Press, 1987.

Wernsdorfer W H & McGregor I (eds). *Malaria: Principles and Practice of Malariology*. Edinburgh: Churchill Livingstone, 1989.

Appendix III
Medical Helminthology

V. R. Southgate and R. A. Bray

Trematodes (See also Chapters 80 and 81)

Subclass Digenea (Carus, 1863)

Fasciola hepatica

Fasciola hepatica (Linnaeus, 1758) is a parasite of sheep and cattle causing 'liver rot'. It is also found in various species of domesticated and wild herbivores.[1]

Distribution
Worldwide.

Parasitology (Figure III.1)
Pale grey with dark borders, it measures 2.3 cm × 8–13 mm. The anterior extremity is narrow, containing the oral sucker; the ventral sucker is larger than the oral and situated 3 mm from the anterior extremity. Branched intestinal caeca with diverticula are present. The ovary is racemose, placed anterior to the testes in the posterior end of the body. The uterus is short and anterior to the ovary. An exsertile cirrus is present and the genital pore is median.

The *egg* (Figure III.2) is operculated, 130–140 × 63–90 μm, ovoid, brown and tanned and contains the ovum and yolk cells. A ciliated eye-spotted *miracidium* develops in about 3 weeks at temperatures of about 23–26°C and enters freshwater amphibious lymnaeid snails (see below).

Life cycle (Figure III.3)
Snail hosts
Lymnaea truncatula (Europe, western Asia and highland southern Africa), *L. viator*, *L. diaphana* (South America), *L. bulimoides*, *L. humilis* (North America), *L. columella* (Africa, also occasionally North and South America, Australia), *L. cubensis* (Caribbean) and *L. tomentosa* (Australasia). *L. columella* is a proven host for both *F. hepatica* and *F. gigantica* and, in recent years, *L. columella* has become established in South Africa, Australia, New Zealand and Hawaii. In these it becomes a sporocyst, giving rise to rediae (named after the Italian zoologist Redi) and cercariae. Development takes 1–2 months, depending upon temperature. The cercaria is leptocerous (simple-tailed) and gymnocephalous. The cercaria is

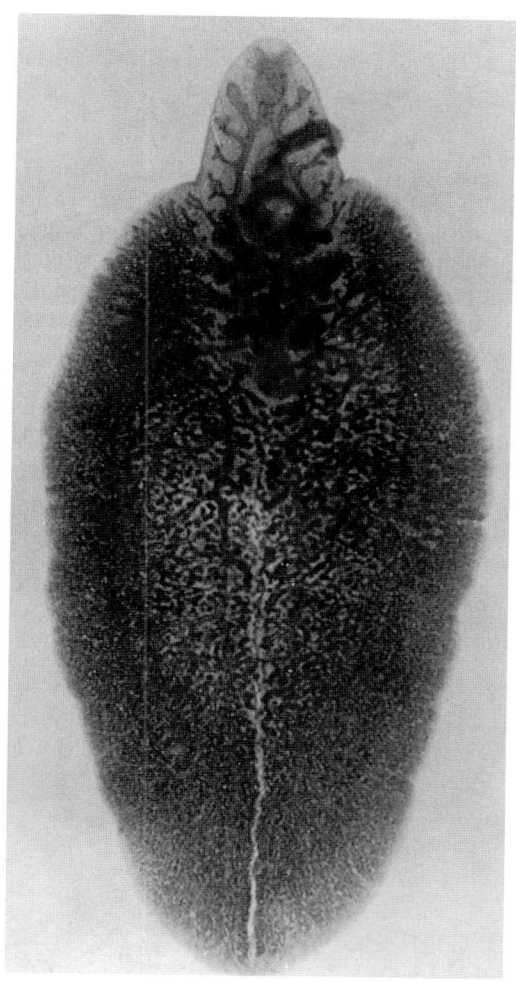

Figure III.1: Adult *Fasciola hepatica*. (Courtesy of H. Zaiman.)

positively phototactic and negatively geotactic, and encysts on aquatic vegetation to form the metacercaria. The outer cyst is composed of an external layer of tanned protein with an underlying fibrous layer of mucoprotein, the inner cyst has a complex mucopolysaccharide layer subdivided into three, and an additional layer of keratinized protein. A region of the innermost keratinized layer forms the ventral plug. Survival of metacercariae for long period depends upon temperature and sufficient moisture. When metacercariae are eaten by the mammalian host excystation occurs in two phases: a

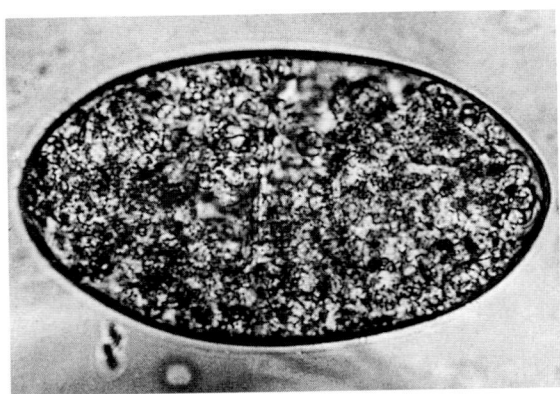

Figure III.2: Egg of *Fasciola hepatica*. (Courtesy of Tropical Resources Unit.)

passive activation phase in the stomach or rumen is followed by an active emergence phase in the small intestine, migration through the intestinal wall into the body cavity, then to the liver. The young fluke burrows through the liver in about 6–7 weeks to reach the bile ducts, where it grows to maturity. From about 8 weeks following infection, eggs are found in the faeces.

F. gigantica, a liver fluke, similar but larger, is now known to cause human infections in the former Soviet Union, Indo-China, West Africa and Hawaii. It develops in fully aquatic lymnaeid snails, such as *Lymnaea auricularia*, *L. natalensis* and *L. rufescens*.

Fasciolopsis buski (Lankester, 1857) (Odhner, 1902)

Fasciolopsis buski (Figure III.4) is a parasite of the pig and dog; they constitute a reservoir for humans.

Parasitology

F. buski inhabits the small intestine, rarely the stomach; only a small number of those infected show symptoms. This is the largest human trematode, measuring 3 cm × 12 mm, and 2 mm thick. It is flesh coloured, elongated and oval, with transverse rows of spines, especially numerous near the ventral sucker. The oral sucker is subterminal but ventral in position, and is only a quarter of the size of the ventral sucker, which is placed close to the oral, and prolonged into the cavity dorsally and backwards, a feature peculiar to this species. (For details of the anatomy see Figure III.4.) The intestinal caeca are simple with two characteristic curves towards the midline. The genital pore is median, placed anterior to the ventral sucker. Branched testes are found in the posterior half of the body; there is a branched ovary and a fine, tortuous, Laurer's canal.

Development in the freshwater snail resembles that of *F. hepatica*.

The egg is operculated and yellow, measuring 130–140 × 80–85 μm (Figures III.5,1 and III.6B). Eggs are found in large numbers in the faeces, the egg capacity of each fluke being about 25 000 per day.

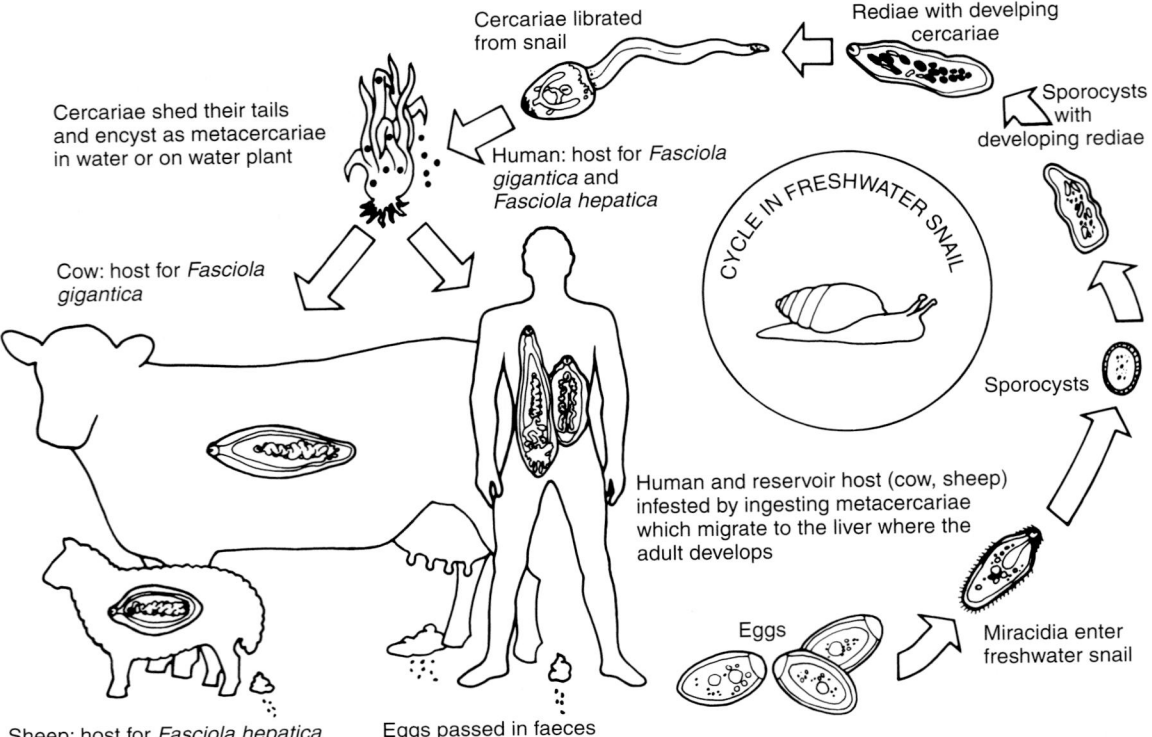

Figure III.3: Life cycle of *Fasciola hepatica* and *F. gigantica*. (Courtesy of Tropical Resources Unit.)

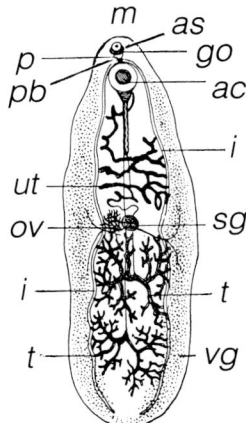

Figure III.4: *Fasciolopsis buski*. The following key is used for the terminology of the anatomy of the trematodes in this and subsequent illustrations.

ac	acetabulum or ventral sucker	ov	ovary
		ovd	oviduct
as	oral sucker	p	pharynx
exp	excretory pore	pb	pharyngeal bulb
go	genital opening	rs	receptaculum seminalis
gp	genital pore	sg	shell gland
i	intestine	t	testis
ic	branch intestine	ut	uterus
lc	Laurer's canal	va	vagina
m	mouth	vd	vas deferens
nc	nerve cord	vg	vitelline glands
oes	oesophagus	vs	vesicula seminalis
oo	ootype		

Life cycle (Figure III.7)

After 3–7 weeks in water, the eggs hatch a ciliated miracidium which develops in freshwater snails— *Segmentina hemisphaerula*, *Hippeutis umbilicalis* (Far East), *Hippeutis cantori* (Far East) and *Segmentina trochoidens* (India) (Figure III.8). A sporocyst is formed in 3 days, followed by the rediae and daughter rediae, which eventually produce cercariae (the whole cycle takes 2 months).

The cercariae, resembling those of *F. hepatica*, are oval, short lived and lophocercous, and measure 0.7 mm; they have a well developed digestive tract with a muscular bladder and collecting tubules. They encyst, as *metacercariae*, on freshwater plants, especially the outer cuticle of the water calthrop, *Trapa (Salvinia) natans* in China, *T. bicornis* in India, *T. bisponosa* in Taiwan. As many as 20 encysted metacercariae may be found on a single leaf. In south China the most important plant is the water chestnut, *Eliocharis tuberosa*, and water bamboo, *Zigania aquatica*, in Chekiang and Canton, and the water hyacinth, *Eichornia crassipes*, in Taiwan. The outer layers of the plants are torn off by the teeth. All the plants are grown in ponds in China and fertilized by human faeces, thus affording an opportunity for infection; *F. buski* is therefore limited in distribution to that of these plants. The cysts when taken into the mouth pass through the stomach, excyst in the duodenum and become attached to the intestinal wall.

Superfamily: Opisthorchioidea

Genus: *Clonorchis*

Clonorchis sinensis (Figures III.9 and III.10)

Distribution

Far East, especially China (Kwangtung province in south China, Indo-China and Okayama, Japan).

Parasitology

This is a common parasite of humans and also of the biliary passages of the dog, cat, pig, rat, mouse, camel and badger. It is found rarely in the gallbladder of humans, but often in the bile ducts, pancreas, pancreatic ducts and duodenum. It is spatulate, tapering anteriorly, reddish, semitransparent and measures 10–25 × 2–5 mm. The tegument is smooth; the oral sucker is larger than the ventral; the intestinal caeca are simple.

The genital pore is median and placed anterior to the ventral sucker. The testes are branched and situated posteriorly one behind the other. The ovary is trilobate with coils anterior to the genital glands. Vitelline glands are moderately developed in the mid-third of the body. Cross-fertilization occurs; the spermatozoa develop before the ova; the sperms enter the female genital pore, pass into the immature uterus and thence to the *spermatheca* (Figure III.10) where they are stored; the ova are fertilized in the spermatheca and then pass on.

The egg measures 20–30 × 14–17 μm; it is operculated, yellow-brown and one of the smallest trematode eggs found in humans (Figures III.5,5 and III.11). It is fully embryonated when discharged. It resembles an electric light bulb with the knob at the bottom. It withstands desiccation but not decomposition.

Life cycle (Figure III.12)

The egg can remain viable in water for 5 weeks and is ingested by the snail before the escape of the miracidium, which has a lifespan of 20 minutes. Development continues in bythinid snails. The miracidium pierces the oesophagus of the mollusc, casts its cilia and soon becomes a sporocyst; later, the elongated rediae grow within the sporocysts and burst into the peri-oesophageal sinus and move tailwards into the liver, the whole process taking 3–4 weeks.

The cercariae (Figure III.10B), 450–550 × 100–120 μm, escape from the rediae from the birthpore; they have two pigmented eyespots and a lophocercous blunt-ending tail, and burst through the space between the upper body surface and the shell, emerging into water. Within 24–48 hours they encyst as metacercariae in the muscles and underscales of freshwater fish of families Cyprinidae and Anabantidae. Cercarial glands excrete a histolytic substance which dissolves the skin of the fish, thus admitting percolating water. The metacercariae secrete a viscous fluid which forms an inner true cyst, which in turn is

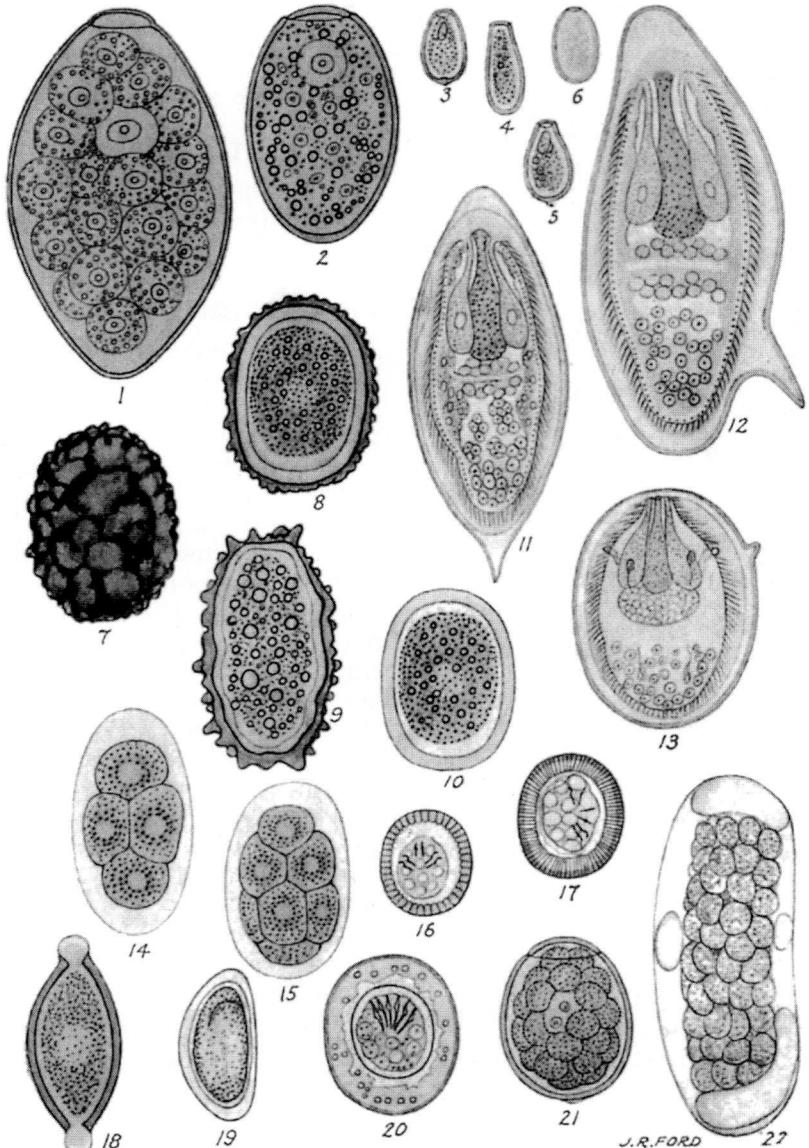

Figure III.5: 1, *Fasciolopsis buski.* 2, *Paragonimus westermani.* 3, *Heterophyes heterophyes.* 4, *Opisthorchis felineus.* 5, *Clonorchis sinensis.* 6, *Metagonimus yokogawai.* 7, 8, *Ascaris lumbricoides,* external aspect. 9, *Ascaris lumbricoides,* unfertilized egg. 10, *Ascaris lumbricoides,* decorticated egg. 11, *Schistosoma haematobium.* 12, *Schistosoma mansoni.* 13, *Schistosoma japonicum.* 14, *Ancylostoma duodenale.* 15, *Trichostrongylus colubriformis.* 16, *Taenia solium.* 17,*Taenia saginata.* 18, *Trichuris trichiura.* 19, *Enterobius vermicularis.* 20, *Vampirolepis nana.* 21, *Diphyllobothrium latum.* 22, *Heterodera radicicola*, non-parasitic, ingested with vegetables.

encapsulated by a fibrous layer formed by the tissues of the fish. These are eaten half raw, or pickled in soy sauce by the Chinese. The adolescercaria, the fully developed cyst, possesses a capsule protective against the gastric juice. In some species of fish—*Carassius auratus* (golden carp)—the parasite is found under the scales; in others it is in the flesh so that domestic animals which eat the offal may become heavily infected while humans escape. The cysts withstand a temperature of 50–70°C for 15 minutes. The cyst wall is digested by the succus entericus in the duodenum near the ampulla of Vater, and the adolescercariae escape and attach themselves to the mucosa. The young distomes at first have spines but these are soon lost. They attain maturity in 26 days. Attracted by positive chemotaxis, a small proportion of them reach the bile ducts, but 95% are digested and destroyed. The size of the resulting fluke is determined by the calibre of the bile duct. Egg production is very large; in the cat 2400 eggs are produced daily, but fewer in dogs. As many as 9400 adults have been found at autopsy. Lifespan is 12 years. Adult men are infected more than women.

The following is a list of the molluscs and fishes that may be intermediaries.

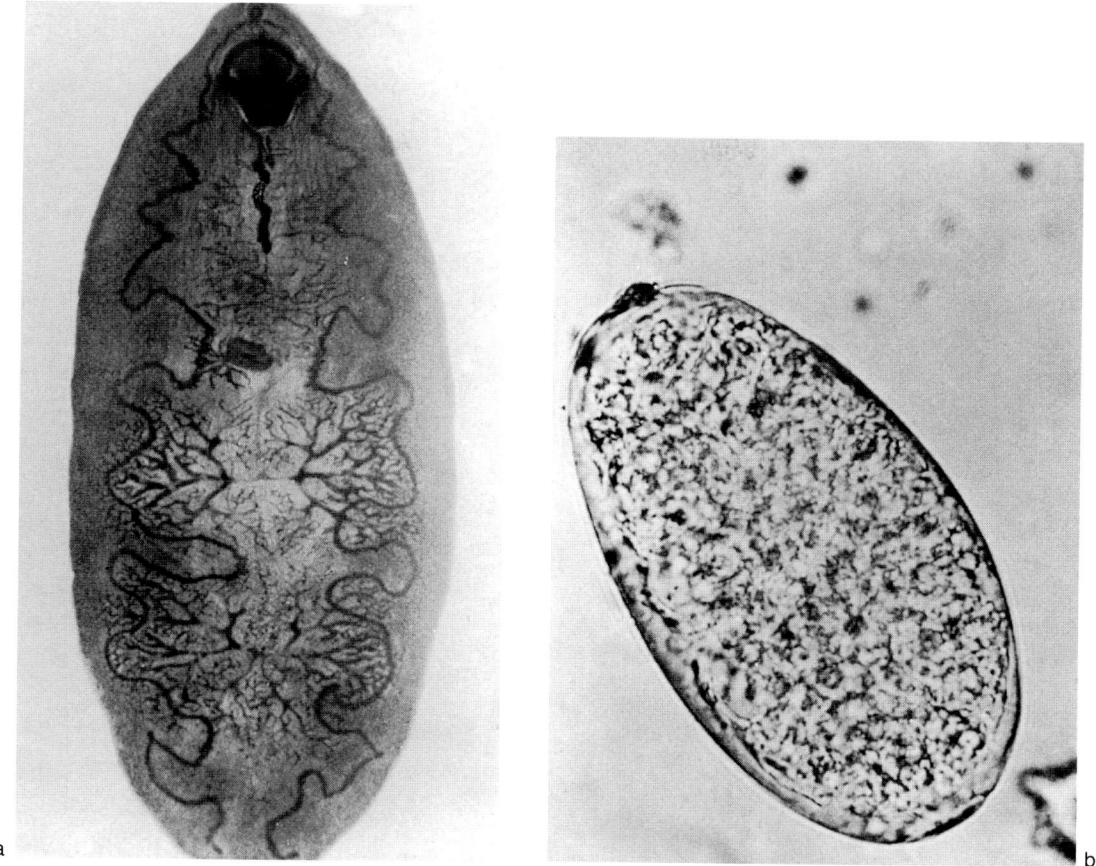

Figure III.6: (**A**) Adult *Fasciolopsis buski*. (**B**) Egg of *F. buski*. (Courtesy of Tropical Resources Unit.)

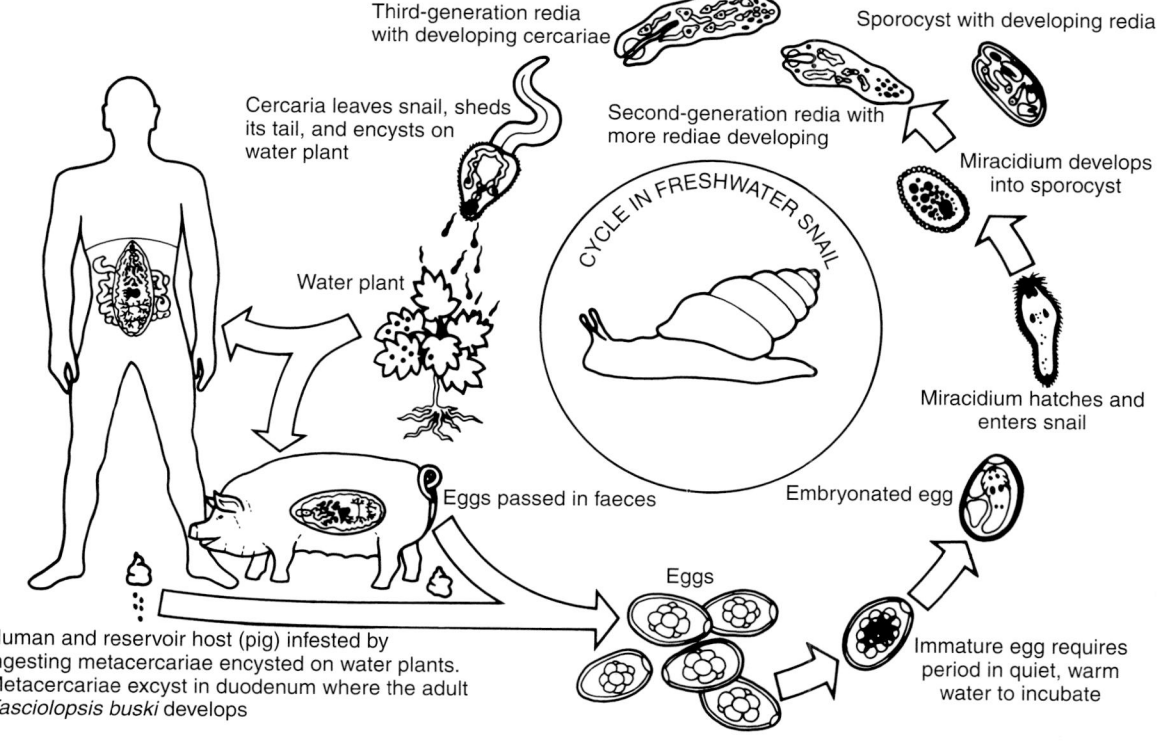

Third-generation redia with developing cercariae

Sporocyst with developing redia

Cercaria leaves snail, sheds its tail, and encysts on water plant

Second-generation redia with more rediae developing

Miracidium develops into sporocyst

Water plant

CYCLE IN FRESHWATER SNAIL

Miracidium hatches and enters snail

Eggs passed in faeces

Embryonated egg

Eggs

Immature egg requires period in quiet, warm water to incubate

Human and reservoir host (pig) infested by ingesting metacercariae encysted on water plants. Metacercariae excyst in duodenum where the adult *Fasciolopsis buski* develops

Figure III.7: Life cycle of *Fasciolopsis buski*. (Courtesy of Tropical Resources Unit.)

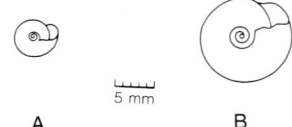

Figure III.8: Molluscan hosts of *Fasciolopsis buski*. (**A**) *Segmentina hemisphaerula*. (**B**) *Hippeutis cantori*.

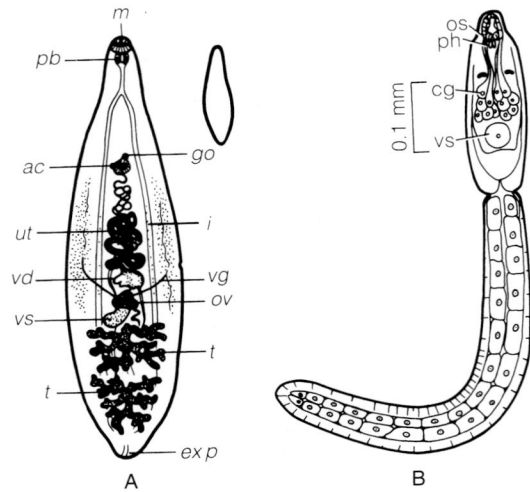

Figure III.10: (**A**) *Clonorchis sinensis*, magnified and natural size. (**B**) Cercaria of *C. sinensis*.

cg   cephalic secretory gland
os   oral sucker
ph   pharynx
vs   ventral sucker

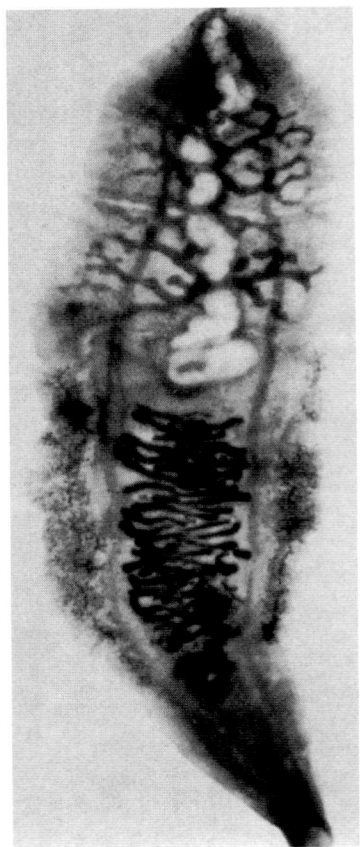

Figure III.9: Adult *Clonorchis sinensis*.

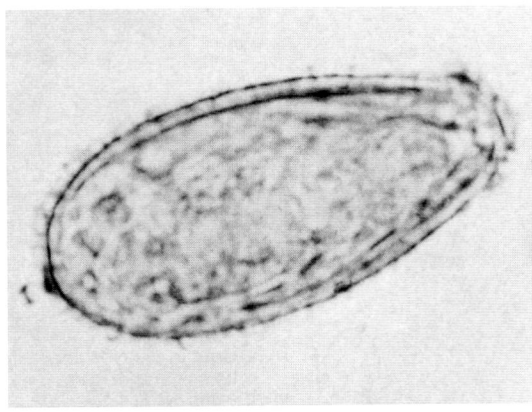

Figure III.11: Egg of *Clonorchis sinensis*.

Hosts

First intermediate hosts (molluscs) (Figure III.13)
The most important first intermediate (snail) hosts are: *Parafossarulus manchouricus* and *Bulimus fuchsiana*. Additional first intermediate hosts are *Bythinia longicornis*, *Assiminea lutea* and *Melanoides tuberculata*.

Second intermediate hosts (fish)
About 80 species of fish have been incriminated: 71 species of Cyprinidae; two species of Eleotridae; one species each of Bagridae, Cyprinodontidae, Clupeidae, Osmeripae, Cichlidae, Ophiocephalidae and Gobiidae. The most important cyprinoid fish are *Mylopharyngodon aethiops*, *Ctenopharyngodon idella* (Canton), *Cultur recurviceps* (Peking) and *Carassius auratus* (golden carp).

Major additional fish hosts are *Tribolodon hakonensis*, *Hemibarbus labes*, *Acanthorhodeus asmussi*, *Pungtungia herzi*, *Pseudogobio esocinus*, *Gnathopogon atromaculatus*, *Cultriculus kneri*, *Macropodus chinensis* and *Opsariichthydis bidens*.

In addition, in Fukien, China, freshwater shrimps (*Caridinia nilotica*, *Macrobrachium superboum*, *Palaeomonetes sinensis*) are incriminated as sources of infection in children.

Other fish hosts are *Hemicultur leucisculus*, *H. b. leekeri*, *Acanthorhodeus chankaensis*, *A. gracilis*, *Abbotina rivularis*, *Pseudorasbora parva*, *Hyspeleotris swinhoensis*, *Philypus potamophilus*, *Rhodeus sinensis*, *Sarcocheilichthys nigripennis*, *S. sinensis*, *S. variegatus*, *Macropodus opercularis*, *Biwia zezera*, *Xenocypris davidi*, *Pseudiperilampus typus*, *Abbotina psegma*, *Paraleucogobio strigatus*, *Acheilognathus rhombea*, *A. lanceolata*, *A. limbata*, *A. cyanostigma*, *Lakeo jordani* and *Hypophalmichthys nobilis*.

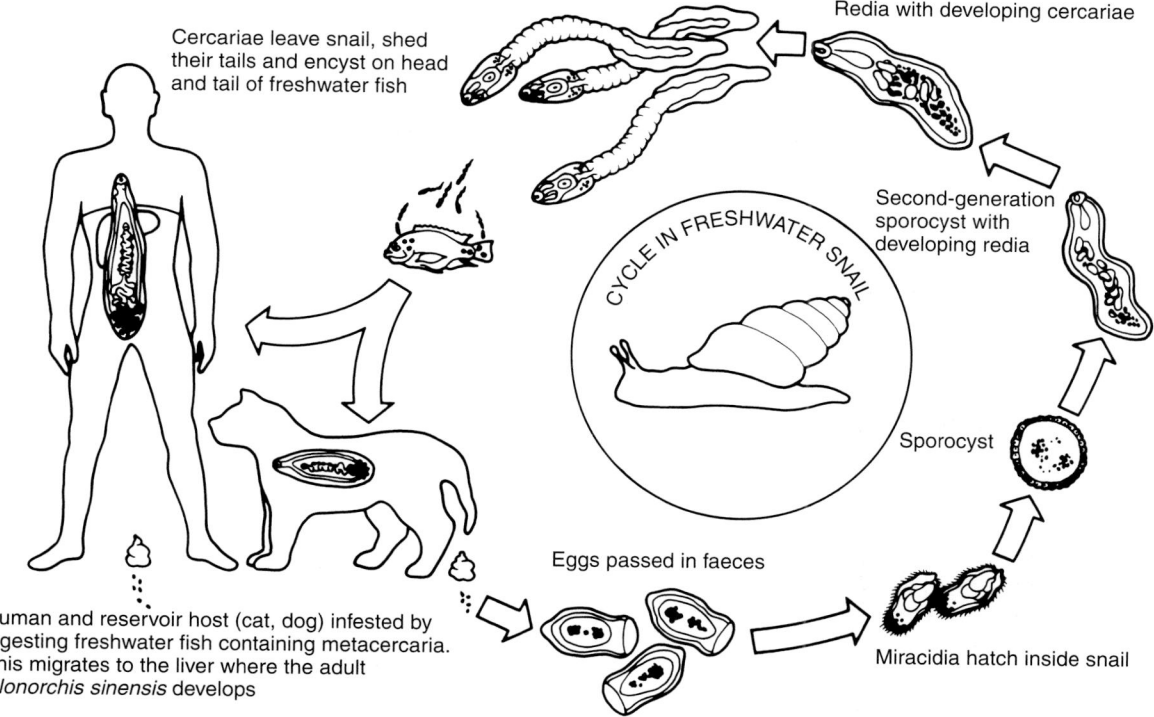

Figure III.12: Life cycle of *Clonorchis sinensis*. (Courtesy of Tropical Resources Unit.)

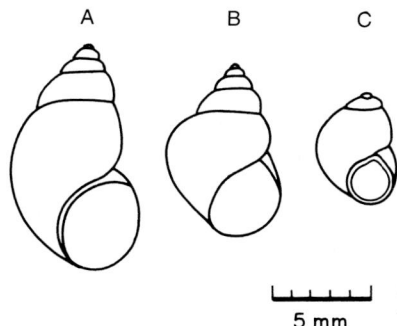

5 mm

Figure III.13: Molluscan hosts of *Clonorchis sinensis*. (**A**) *Parafossarulus manchouricus*. (**B**) *Bythinia fuschiana*. (**C**) *Bythinia longicornis*.

Genus: *Opisthorchis* (cat liver fluke)

There are two species of cat liver fluke: *Opisthorchis felineus* (Rivolta, 1884), eastern Europe and CIS and *O. viverrini* (Poirier, 1886) north-east Thailand, Laos.

Parasitology (*Opisthorchis felineus*)

Cat liver fluke inhabits the liver, pancreas, bile ducts and lungs (in Russia). It is lanceolate and measures 8–11 × 1.5–2 mm. The tegument is smooth; the suckers are equal in size and separated by 2 mm (Figure III.14). The egg measures 30 × 12 μm and is yellowish-brown with an operculum. At the posterior end there is a minute tubercular thickening (Figure III.5,4).

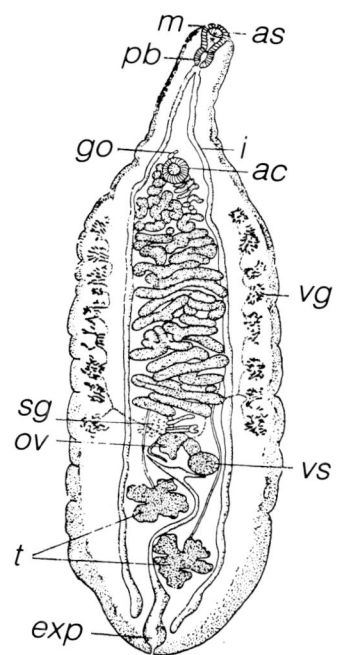

Figure III.14: *Opisthorchis felineus*. (9×.)

Life cycle (similar to *C. sinensis*, Figure III.12)

The definitive hosts are the human and wild and domestic felines. The first intermediary host is a snail, usually *Bythinia leachi* (Figure III.15); an additional snail

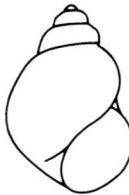

Figure III.15: *Bythinia leachi*, the molluscan host of *Opisthorchis felineus*.

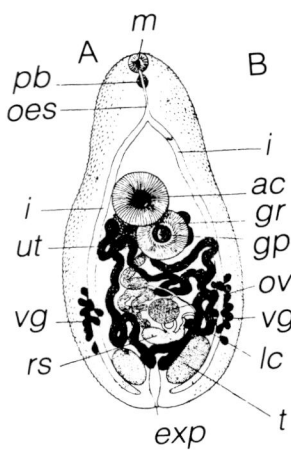

Figure III.16: *Heterophyes heterophyes*, greatly magnified.

host is *Bythinia tentaculata*. The miracidium is fully formed in the egg and hatches in the snail, forming a sporocyst in the intestine measuring 1.2–1.85 mm. Rediae are formed in 1 month and then cercariae, which mature in 4 months.

Cercariae, 430–670 × 40–50 μm, which leave the snail in daylight, are phototactic and stimulated by agitation.

The second intermediary hosts are fish—the tench (*Tinca tinca*), the ide (*Leuciscus idus*), the barbel (*Barbus barbus*) and the roach (*Rutilus rutilus*). Additional second intermediary hosts are *Idus melanotus, Abramis brama, A. sapa, Cyprinus carpio, Blicca bjorkna, Alburnus lucidus, Aspilus aspilus, Scardinus erythrophthalmus*. The cercariae penetrate in 15 minutes and grow to three or four times their original size, forming metacercariae 220 × 160 μm. When ingested by a person, they pass through the stomach, are freed by the succus entericus, attracted by the bile and travel up the bile duct in 5 hours. Infection is therefore contracted by eating raw fish. The entire life cycle requires a minimum of 4 months. This fluke is not specially pathogenic, although 200 or more have been found in the body at autopsy.

Opisthorchis viverrini is the other species and is of importance in Thailand and India. It is morphologically similar.

Life cycle of *O. viverrini* (similar to *C. sinensis*, Figure III.12)

The normal definitive hosts are the dog and civet cat. First intermediate hosts are snails. *Bythinia funiculata, B. siamensis, B. goniomphales* and *B. laevis*. Second intermediate hosts are fish, *Cyclocheilichthys siaja, Hampala dispar, Puntius orphoides, P. gonionotus, P. poctozyron, Labiobarbus lineatus* and *Osteochilus* spp.

Genus: *Heterophyes*

Heterophyes heterophyes (Siebold, 1852)

Distribution

Egypt, China, Japan, Brazil, Korea, Spain, France and Greece.

Characters

Heterophyes heterophyes (Figures III.16 and III.17) inhabits the small intestine of the human in large numbers and

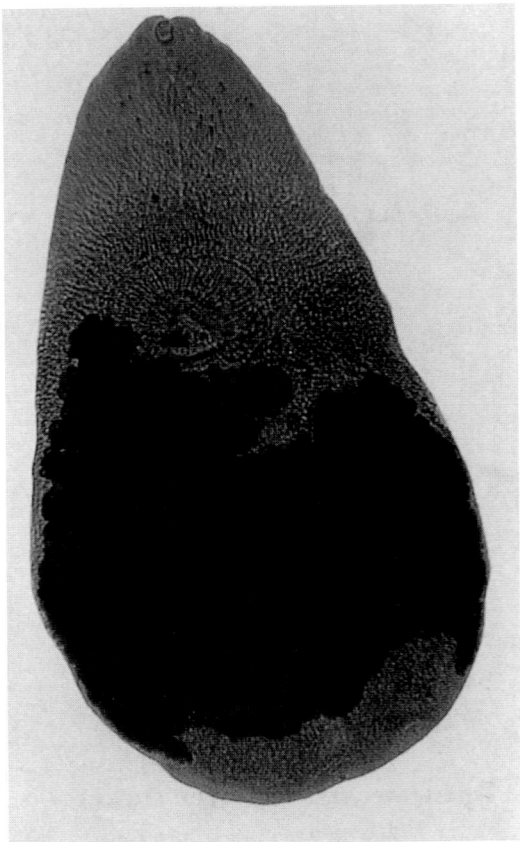

Figure III.17: Adult *Heterophyes heterophyes*. Cuticle covered by fine spines and oral sucker less conspicuous than ventral sucker. (Courtesy of Tropical Resources Unit.)

also that of the rat, fox, dog, wolf, jackal and cat; it also lives in the black kite (*Milvus migrans aegyptius*) and a bat (*Rhinolophus divosus acrotis*) in the Yemen. It imparts a 'coffee grounds' appearance to the intestinal wall. It is pyriform, grey and very small, measuring 1–1.7 × 0.3–0.7 mm. The uterus forms a brown patch in the centre. The oral sucker is subterminal and the ventral sucker is three times the size of the oral sucker. The tegument is thickly set with quadrate scales measuring 5 × 4 μm. There is a short prepharynx and long oesophagus. The intestinal caeca extend to the posterior extremity, converging close to the excretory vesicle. The vitelline glands are posterior, situated in two clumps; the genital pore is posterolateral in the vicinity of the ventral sucker and consists of a muscular ring armed with 70 chitinous cuticular teeth. The testes are oval and posterior, the ovary globular and median. There is a receptaculum seminis as large as the ovary; uterine coils are not numerous. A seminal vesicle and Laurer's canal are present.

The egg measures 20–30 × 15–17 μm, being the same size as that of *C. sinensis* (Figure III.5,3). Its greatest breadth is across the centre. There is no special ring to the operculum, the egg is light-brown and contains a ciliated miracidium when deposited. It hatches after ingestion by the appropriate snail.

Life cycle

H. heterophyes develops in brackish water snails. The proven hosts are *Pirinella conica* in the Middle East (Figure III.18A), *Cerithidea cingulata* and *Tympanotomus micropterus* in the Far East. Additional recorded hosts include *Melanoides tuberculata* and *Cleopatra bulimoides*. The cercaria, which is eyed and has a membranous tail, enters the second intermediate host—a freshwater fish, the mullet (*Mugil cephalus*), or in Japan a species of *Acanthogobius* in which metacercariae develop and encyst under the scales. Infection is acquired from eating raw fish.

Related species include: *Heterophyes continua, Haplorchis pumilio, H. vanissimus* and *Procerovum calderon*. In Japan in the vicinity of Kobe a closely related species (or synonym of *Heterophyes heterophyes*), *H. katsuradai*, is recognized which is stouter and has a relatively enormous acetabulum. The eggs are smaller, measuring 25–26 × 14–15 μm.

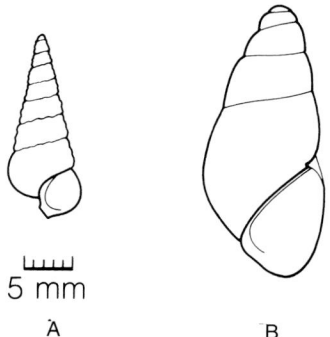

Figure III.18: **(A)** *Pirinella conica*, the molluscan host of *Heterophyes heterophyes*. **(B)** *Semisulcospira libertina*, the molluscan host of *Metagonimus yokogawai*.

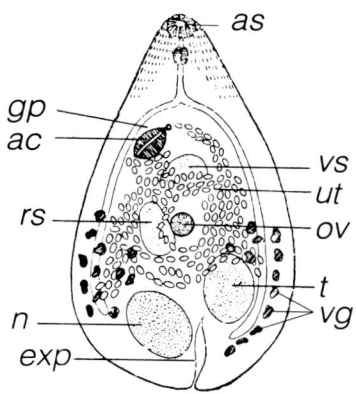

Figure III.19: *Metagonimus yokogawai*. (45×.)

Genus: *Metagonimus*

Metagonimus yokogawai (Katsurada, 1912)

Distribution

Korea, Taiwan, China, Japan, Philippines and Ukraine. Very common in the Far East.

Parasitology

Metagonimus yokogawai (Figure III.19) is found in the small intestine of humans, higher up than *H. heterophyes*, and also in the cat, dog, pig and fish-eating birds, such as the pelican. It is the smallest fluke parasitic in man with a mean size of 1.4 × 0.6 mm. The tegument is covered with small spines; the ventral sucker is deflected to the right with its long axis in the diagonal phase. There is a genital pore in front; the ovoid testes are posterior; the ovary and receptaculum seminis are situated medially in front of the testes. The yolk glands are found in clumps in the posterior third. The uterus lies between the testes and the ventral sucker, and the seminal vesicle in front of the ovary (Figure III.19).

The egg measures 27–28 × 16–17 μm and resembles that of *C. sinensis* but is more regularly ovoid (Figure III.5,6).

Life cycle

The first intermediate hosts are molluscs—*Semisulcospira libertina* (Figure III.18B) and *S. coreana*. Sporocysts, rediae and cercariae are formed; the last have an anterior end provided with armament. The tail is long and membranous with lateral flutings and is discarded on entering the fish host. *Plecoglossus altivelis* is regarded as the most important source of infection of *M. yokogawai* in Japan. Other freshwater fish hosts recorded include: *Carassius auratus, Cyprinus carpio, Zacco temminckii, Photimus steindachneri, Acheilognathus lanceolata* and *Pseudorasbora parva*. The metacercariae measure about 150 × 100 μm and encyst under the scales; infection results from eating raw fish.

Superfamily: Plagiorchidea

Genus: *Paragonimus*

Many species of *Paragonimus* are found in nature and can be divided into four main groups by the nature of the cuticular spines and the ovary.

1. Westermani: *P. westermani, P. pulmonalis.*
2. Compactus: *P. compactus, P. siamensis.*
3. Kellicotti–miyazaki: *P. kellicotti, P. miyazakii, P. heterotremus, P. caliensis, P. amazonicus, P. mexicanus (peruvianus).*
4. Ohirai–ilokstuenensis: *P. ohirai, P. ilokstuenensis.*

   Other species include: *P. tuanshenensis, P. szechuanensis, P. hueitungensis, P. bangliokensis, P. philippinensis, P. sadoensis, P. skrjabini* and the African species *P. africanus* and *P. uterobilateralis.*

Distribution

The Far East from Japan to India, Indonesia, the Pacific Islands, West and Central Africa, and central South America.

Parasitology

P. westermani measures 8–20 × 5–9 mm and is oval (almost round in section), reddish-brown and translucent. The anterior extremity is rounded. The oral sucker is subterminal; the ventral sucker larger and placed anterior to the centre of the body. The pharynx and oesophagus are short and the bifurcation of the intestine is anterior to the ventral sucker (Figures III.20 and III.21). The intestinal caeca run a zigzag course; the common genital pore lies close to the posterior margin of the ventral sucker. The body is bisected by a large excretory vesicle. The testes are tubular and racemose; the branched ovary may be to either the right or the left of the midline and posterior to the ventral sucker. The uterus is short, sac-like and lies opposite the ovary. The vitellaria are well

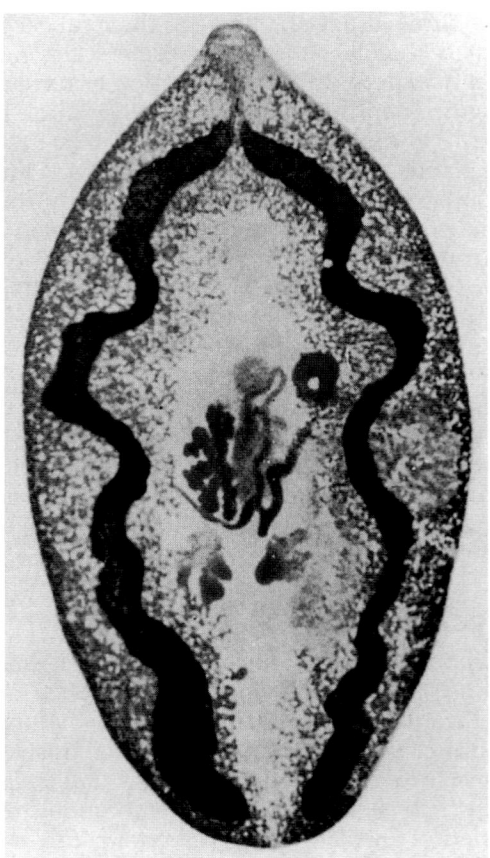

Figure III.21: Adult *Paragonimus westermani*. (Courtesy of Tropical Resources Unit.)

developed, extending through the whole body. Laurer's canal and shell gland are present. The tegument is studded with wedge-shape spines which with the ovary are used to differentiate the four main types:

1. Westermani: tegumentary spines singly spaced and ovary simply branched into four to six lobes.
2. Compactus: tegumentary spines in groups and ovary simply branched into four to six lobes.
3. Kellicotti–miyazaki: tegumentary spines singly spaced, ovary profusely branched.
4. Ohirai–ilokstuenensis: tegumentary spines in groups, ovary profusely branched.

   The egg is brown and operculated, measuring 90 × 55 µm. It shows a thickening at the pole opposite the operculum. The egg of *P. compactus* is smaller, 75 × 48 µm (Figures III.5,2 and III.22).

Life cycle (Figures III.23 and III.24)

The lung fluke can remain viable in the human body for 20 years. The eggs are first voided into cystic pockets in the lungs and then escape into water in the sputum and also in faeces from swallowed sputum. A ciliated

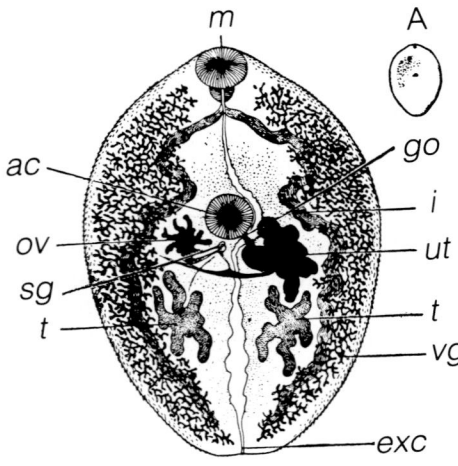

Figure III.20: *Paragonimus westermani (ringeri)*, natural size (**A**) and magnified.

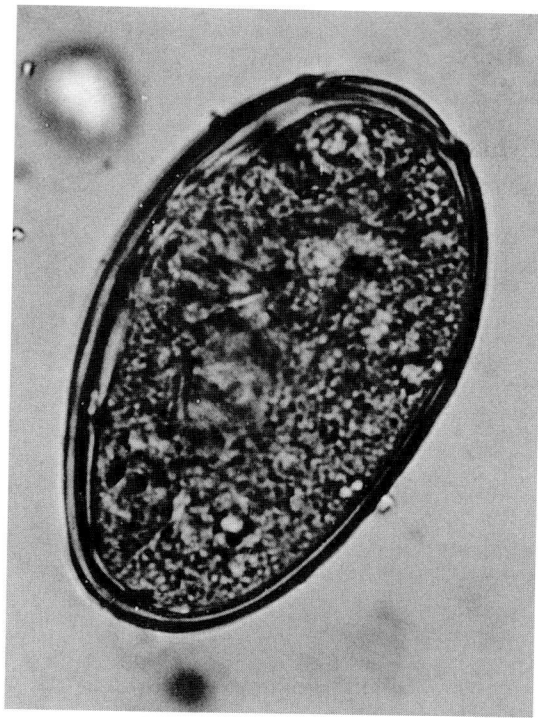

Figure III.22: Egg of *Paragonimus westermani*. (Courtesy of Tropical Resources Unit.)

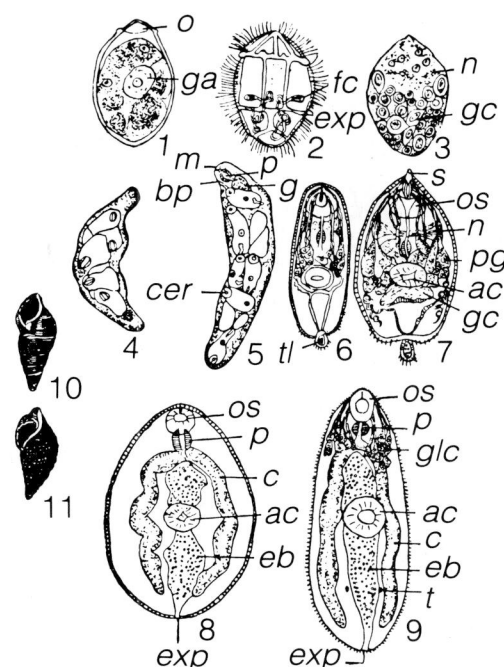

Figure III.23: Life cycle of *Paragonimus westermani* (1–9, 15×;10 and 11, half natural size). 1, Egg showing yolk cells and germinal area. 2, Miracidium with excretory system and flame cells. 3, Miracidium with ganglionic mass and germ cells. 4, Mature sporocyst in snail containing well developed first-generation rediae. 5, Mature second-generation rediae. 6 and 7, Stages of microcercous cercariae after emergence from the snail. 8, Metacercariae from the crab; the cyst wall is not shown. 9, Mature encysted metacercaria. 10, *Semisulcospira libertina*. 11, *Thiara granifera*.

bp	birth pore	n	nervous system
c	caeca	o	operculum
cer	cercaria	os	oral sucker
eb	excretory bladder	p	pharynx
fc	flame cell	pg	periacetabular glands
g	gut	s	stylet
ga	germinal area	tl	tail
gc	genital cells		

miracidium hatches in 16 days to 7 weeks and has distinctive characters. There is a ciliated covering in four rows at the anterior cone. The excretory pore forms a rosette. It enters the snail hosts (Table III.1). It develops in about 60 days into sporocysts and rediae, each containing about 20 cercariae; the latter, ellipsoid and microcercous, have a short knob-like tail and measure 200×70–80 μm with an anterior stylet and body covered with spines. The cercariae bore into freshwater crabs and become metacercariae in the crabs and crayfish shown in Table III.1.

In the crustacean (the second intermediate) the metacercariae encyst in the liver, muscles and gills. In Japan crabs are eaten but in Korea and Taiwan they are not eaten; the supposition is that the crustacean phase is not always a biological necessity. In Venezuela the appropriate snails and crustacea are present and 30% of dogs are infected, but humans are not. When the metacercariae enter the stomach of the human their cyst wall is digested and the adolescent cercariae emerge, pass through the jejunum, traverse the abdominal cavity, penetrate the diaphragm, pleura and lungs, and reach the bronchioles forming cystic cavities.

Genus: *Dicrocoelium*

Dicrocoeliosis is caused by two species of the genus: *D. dentriticum* and *D. hospes*. *D. dendriticum* is a widely distributed parasite, mainly of ruminants but also of humans, occurring in all the European countries, European and Asian parts of the former Soviet Union,

China, Japan, Indo-Malayan region, USA and Canada, Cuba and parts of South America (e.g., Brazil, Colombia). *D. hospes* has been recorded from many African countries, including Tanzania, Uganda, Sudan, Chad, Ghana and Sierra Leone. The eggs passed in faeces are fully embryonated, resist desiccation and do not hatch in water. They are ingested by land snails. Over 50 species have been recorded as hosts for *D. dendriticum* including: *Theba carthusiana*, *Zebrina detrita*, *Helicella candidula*, *H. itala*, *Cepaea memoralis*, *Helix vulgaris*, *Eulota lantzi*, *E. ruben* and others (Table III.1).

Life cycle (Figure III.25)

The miracidium is released in the digestive tract of the snail host, penetrates the glandular intestinal epithelium and finally migrates to the hepatopancreas. The mother sporocyst gives rise to daughter sporocysts, which in turn

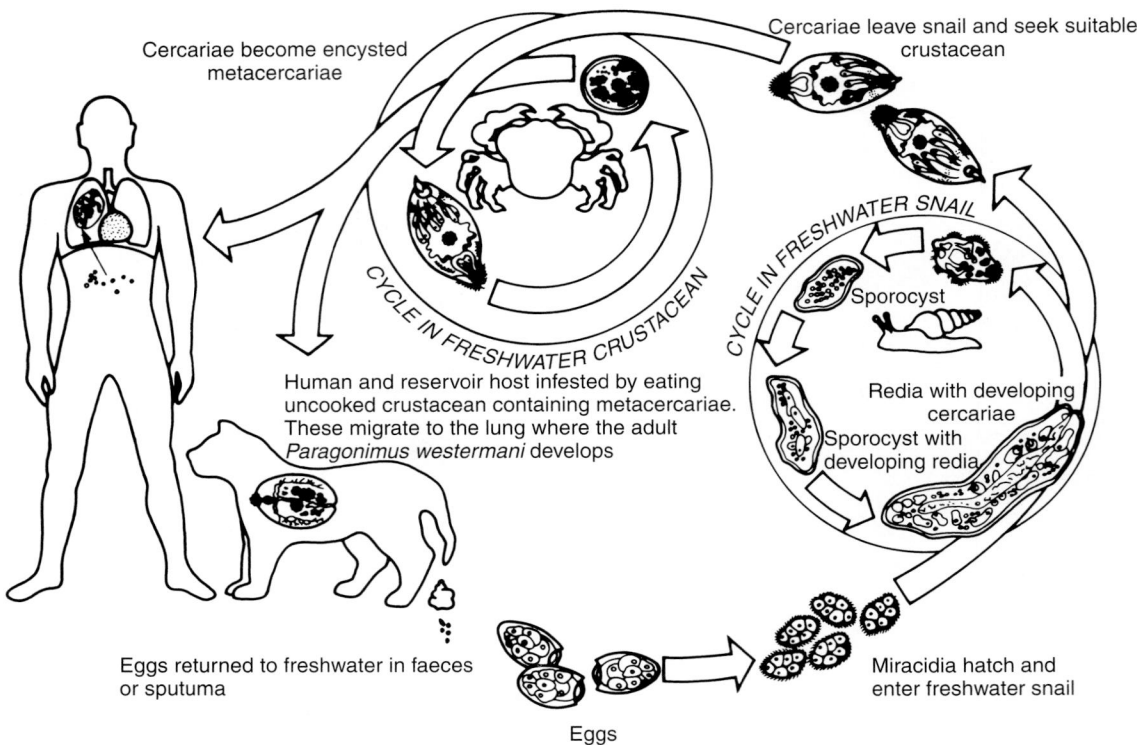

Cercariae become encysted metacercariae

Cercariae leave snail and seek suitable crustacean

CYCLE IN FRESHWATER CRUSTACEAN

CYCLE IN FRESHWATER SNAIL

Sporocyst

Redia with developing cercariae

Sporocyst with developing redia

Human and reservoir host infested by eating uncooked crustacean containing metacercariae. These migrate to the lung where the adult *Paragonimus westermani* develops

Eggs returned to freshwater in faeces or sputuma

Eggs

Miracidia hatch and enter freshwater snail

Figure III.24: Life cycle of *Paragonimus westermani*. (Courtesy of Tropical Resources Unit.)

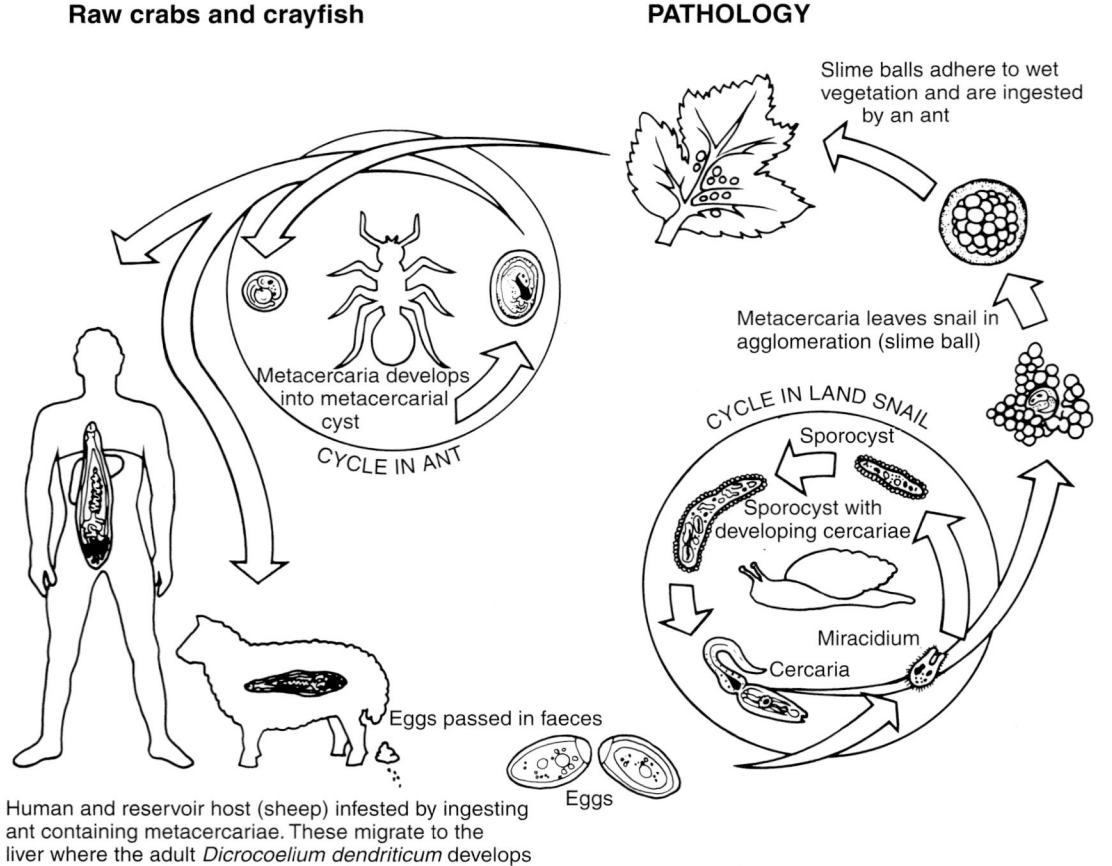

Raw crabs and crayfish

PATHOLOGY

Slime balls adhere to wet vegetation and are ingested by an ant

Metacercaria leaves snail in agglomeration (slime ball)

Metacercaria develops into metacercarial cyst

CYCLE IN ANT

CYCLE IN LAND SNAIL

Sporocyst

Sporocyst with developing cercariae

Miracidium

Cercaria

Eggs passed in faeces

Eggs

Human and reservoir host (sheep) infested by ingesting ant containing metacercariae. These migrate to the liver where the adult *Dicrocoelium dendriticum* develops

Figure III.25: Life cycle of *Dicrocoelium dendriticum*.

Table III.1 Trematode flukes that can infect humans.

Adult fluke	Morphology	Egg	Site	Vertebrate hosts	First intermediate host	Second intermediate host	Geographical distribution	Clinical features
LIVER FLUKES								
Fasciola hepatica (Figure III.1)	Large, leaf-shaped, 2–3 × 1.5 cm	130–140 × 63–90 μm (Figure III.2)	Biliary tract	Sheep, cattle, human, many other herbivores, including marsupiala	Freshwater snails: *Lymnaea truncatula* *L. viridis* *L. viatrix* *L. bulimoides* *L. humilis* *L. columella* *L. tomentosa* Other *Lymnaea* spp. *Austropeplea* spp. *Fossaria* spp. and others Land snail: *Practicoella gresicola*	Aquatic vegetation: Watercress	Europe, western Asia, highlands South Africa, Far East, South America, North America, Caribbean, Australasia	Transient hepatic disturbance with jaundice and fever
Fasciola gigantica	Larger, up to 7.5 cm long	–	Biliary tract	Sheep, cattle, other herbivores and humans	Fully aquatic lymnaeid snails	Vegetation	Africa, Asia, eastern Europe North and South America, Hawaii	–
Dicrocoelium dendriticum	Small, 1.5 × 2 mm	40 × 25 μm	Biliary tract	Herbivorous animals	Land snails: *Helix vulgaris* *Cochlicopa lubrica* *Lacinaria varnensis* *Theba carthusiana* *Zebrina detrita* *Helicella candidula* *H. itala* *Cepaea nemoralis* *Eulota lantzi* *E. rubens* *Cernuella* spp. Many others	Brown ants: *Formica fusca* *F. rufibarbi* other *Formica* spp. *Proformica nasuta* *Catagliphis bicolor* *C. aenescens* *C. albicans*	Cosmopolitan in animals. Human cases in Europe, Near East, Africa, China, North and South America, Australia	Dyspepsia and hepatomegaly with eosinophilia

Table III.1 Continued

Adult fluke	Morphology	Egg	Site	Vertebrate hosts	First intermediate host	Second intermediate host	Geographical distribution	Clinical features
Clonorchis sinensis (Figure III.9)	10–25 × 2.5 mm	20–30 × 15–17 μm (Figure III.11)	Biliary tract	Human, dog, pig, cat, mouse, camel, badger, mink, weasel, *Viverricula indica*	Freshwater snails: *Parafossarulus manchouricus* Other *Parafossarulus* spp. *Bythinia fuchsiana* *B. misella* *Alocinma longicornis* *Assiminea lutea* *Bulimus striatulus* *Melanoides tuberculata* *Semisulcospira* spp.	Carp species: *Most important:* Golden carp (*Carassius curatus*) *Ctenopharyngodon idella* *Mylopharyngodon aethiops* *Culter recurviceps* and more than 80 other species plus some freshwater shrimps (see Appendix IV)	China, Taiwan, Indo-China, Korea, Japan, south China	Recurrent cholangitis with jaundice, pancreatitis and cholangiocarcinoma
Opisthorchis felineus (*tenuicollis*)	8–11 × 1.5–2 mm	30 × 12 μm	Biliary tract	Human, dog, fox, cat, pig, seals, porpoise	*Bythinia leachi* *B. tentaculata*	Freshwater fish: Tench, ide, barbel, roach, bream	Eastern Europe, Russia and India	Recurrent cholangitis
Opisthorchis viverrini	8–11 × 1.5–2 mm	30 × 12 μm	Biliary tract	Civet cat, cat, dog, human	*Bythinia funiculata* *B. siamensis* *B. goniomphalus* *B. laevis*	Freshwater fish of the genera: *Cyclocheilicthyus* *Hampala* *Puntius* *Labiobarbus* *Osteochilus* *Barbodes* *Esomus* *Puntioplites* *Labiobarbus* *Thynnichthys*	Thailand, Laos	Recurrent cholangitis

Table III.1 Continued

Adult fluke	Morphology	Egg	Site	Vertebrate hosts	First intermediate host	Second intermediate host	Geographical distribution	Clinical features
INTESTINAL FLUKES								
Fasciolopsis buski (Figure III.6a)	3 cm × 12 cm × 2 mm	130–140 × 80–85 µm (Figure III.6b)	Small intestine	Pig and human	Freshwater snails: *Segmentina hemisphaerula* *S. trochoideus* *Hippeutis umbilicalis* *H. cantori* *Gyraulus chinensis* *C. convexiusculus* *Helicorbis umbilicalis*	Aquatic vegetation: Water calthrop (*Trapa natans*) *T. bicornis* *T. bispinosa* Water chestnut (*Eliocharis tuberosa*) Water bamboo (*Zigania aquatica*) Water hyacinth (*Eichornia crassipes*)	China, Taiwan, Laos, Vietnam, Cambodia, Thailand, India, Myanmar, Malaysia, Borneo	Chronic diarrhoea, preprandial pain, oedema of face and trunk, malabsorption
Heterophyes heterophyes (Figure III.17)	Small, 1–1.7 × 0.3–0.7 mm	20–30 × 15–17 µm	Small intestine	Human, rat, fox, dog, wolf, jackal, cat, bat	Brackish water snails: *Pirinella conica* *Cerithidea cingulata* *C. djadjariensus* *Tympanotonus micropterus*	Freshwater fish: *Mugil cephalus* *Gambusia affinis* *Acanthogobius* sp. *Tilapia nilotica* *Aphanius, Liza, Tridentiger, Glossoglobus, Sarotherodon* and	Middle East, Far East, Japan, Egypt, France	Diarrhoea and preprandial pain

Table III.1 Continued

Adult fluke	Morphology	Egg	Site	Vertebrate hosts	First intermediate host	Second intermediate host	Geographical distribution	Clinical features
Metagonimus yokogawai	Small, 1.1 × 0.42–0.7 mm	27 × 16 µm	Small intestine	Human, cat, dog, fox, rat, pig, pelican, heron, gull, piscivorous birds of prey	Freshwater snails: *Semisulcospira libertina* Other *Semisulcospira* spp. *Thiara granifera* *Fagotia* spp. *Juga* spp.	Freshwater fish: *Plecoglossus altivelus* (ayu) *Carassius auratus* (golden carp) *Cyprinus carpio* (common carp) Freshwater fishes of the genera: *Acheilognathus* *Erythroculter* *Oncorhynchus* *Photimus* *Pseudorasbora* *Tribolodon* *Zacco* Numerous other spp. and genera	Korea, Formosa and Japan, Balkan states; common in Far East	Occasionally temporary abdominal pain and watery diarrhoea
Gastrodiscoides hominis	5–8 × 3–5 mm	150–170 × 60–70 µm	Large intestine	Human, many herbivores including rodents, monkeys, orang-utan	Freshwater snail: *Helicorbis coenosus* *H. umbilicalis* *Anisus acronius* *Lymnaea stagnalis*	Aquatic plants	Assam, Bangladesh, Malaysia, Thailand, Philippines, Indonesia, Vietnam, Pakistan	Diarrhoea in heavy infections
Echinostoma lindoensis	1 cm × 1 mm	83–116 × 58–69 µm	Small intestine	Human, rat, pig and other mammals	Freshwater snails: *Anisus sarasinorum* *Gyraulus convexiusculus* *Biomphalaria glabrata*	Freshwater snail: *Vivipara javanica* Freshwater mussels: *Corbicula lindoensis* *C. subplanta* *C. celebensis* *C. javanica*	Japan, Philippines, Indonesia, Malaysia	Mostly symptomless. Heavy infections: diarrhoea, abdominal pain and eosinophilia

Table III.1 Continued

Adult fluke	Morphology	Egg	Site	Vertebrate hosts	First intermediate host	Second intermediate host	Geographical distribution	Clinical features
Echinostoma Malayanum	1 cm × 1 mm	83–116 × 58–69 μm (Figure III.26)	Small intestine	Human, rat, pig and other mammals	Freshwater snail: Lymnaea luteola	Snails: *L. luteola* *G. convexiusculus* *Bellamya ingallsiana* *Indoplanorbise xustus* *Pila scutata* Fish: *Barbus stigma*	Malaysia, Indonesia, Singapore, Thailand, India, Sino-Tibetan border	Mostly symptomless. Heavy infections: diarrhoea, abdominal pain and eosinophilia
Euparyphium ilocanum	1 cm × 1 mm	83–116 × 58–69 μm	Small intestine	Human, rat, pig and other mammals	Snails: *Gyranulus convexiusculus* (Philippines and Indonesia) *G. prashddi* and *Hippeutis umbilicalis* (Philippines)	14 Species of snail: *Gyraulus prashadi* *Vivipara* spp. *Planorbis umbilicatus* *Pila* spp.	Philippines, Celebes, Indonesia, China, Malaysia	Mostly symptomless. Heavy infections: diarrhoea, abdominal pain and eosinophilia
LUNG FLUKES								
Paragonimus westermani (Figure III.21) (ringeri, edwardsi macacae, asymmetricus, pulmonalis, filipinus, philippinensis)	8–20 × 5–9 mm Cuticular spines, singly spaced. Ovary simply branched (4–6 lobes)	90 × 55 μm (Figure III.22)	Cystic cavities in lungs	Human, wild and domestic felines, red panda, binturong, dog, wolf, fox, monkeys, mongooses, mustelids, rodents, raccoon-like dog, civets, wild pigs, potential paratenic hosts may include birds	Freshwater snails: *Simisulcospira libertina* (optimum host) Other *Semisulcospira* spp. *Tarebia granifera* *Melanoides tuberculata* *Brotia* spp. *Juga buettneri* *J. tegulata*	Crustaceans of the genera: *Cambaroides* *Candido-potamon* *C. eylon-thelphusa* *Eriocheir* *Geothelphusa* *Irmengardia* *Isolapotamon* *Huananpotamon* *Johora* *Macrobrachium* *Malayopotamon* *Nanhai* *Nanhaipotamon* *Oziothelphusa* *Parapotamon*	Japan, China, Korea, Taiwan, Philippines, Thailand, India, Laos, Vietnam, Cambodia, Indonesia, Malaysia, Myanmar, Nepal, Papua New Guinea, Sri Lanka, far eastern Russia, Pakistan	Pulmonary symptoms, cough and haemoptysis. Cerebral complications. Occasionally eggs in skin

Table III.1 Continued

Adult fluke	Morphology	Egg	Site	Vertebrate hosts	First intermediate host	Second intermediate host	Geographical distribution	Clinical features
						Parathelphusa Potamiscus Potamon Procambarus Ranguna Sesarma Sesarmops Siamthelphusa Sinolapotamon Sinopotamon St oliczia Sudanthelphusa Varuna		
Paragonimus miyazakii	Cuticular spines, singly spaced. Ovary profusely branched	–	Lungs	Human, dog, cat, raccoon-like dog, wild boar, mustelids	Bythinella nipponica B. kubotai Akiyoshia kawannensis Oncomelania hupensis Saganda spp.	Crab: Geothelphusa dehaani	Japan	
Paragonimus ohirai			Lungs	Human, dog, raccoon-like dog, cat, mustelids, pigs, rodents	Snails of the genera: Angustassiminea Assiminea Oncomelania Pomatiopsis	Crabs of the genera: Chasmagnathus Helice sesarma Sesarmops Geothelphusa	Japan, China, Korea, Taiwan	
Paragonimush heterotremus (tuanshenensis)	Cuticular spines singly spaced. Ovary profusely branched	–	Lungs	Human, dog, cat, rodents, monkeys	Neotricula aperta Assiminea spp. Oncomelania hupensis O. chiui	Crabs of the genera: Esanthelphus Larnaudia Malayopotamon Parathelphusa Potamiscus Potamon Ranguna Siammannia-thelphusa Siamthelphusa Sinolapotamon Sinopotamon Tiwaripotamon	China, Laos, Thailand, Vietnam	Pulmonary signs. Cerebral involvement and migratory subcutaneous swellings

Table III.1 Continued

Adult fluke	Morphology	Egg	Site	Vertebrate hosts	First intermediate host	Second intermediate host	Geographical distribution	Clinical features
Paragonimus skrjabini (*hueitungensis, szechuanensis, Pagumogonimus veocularis*)	Cuticular spines in groups. Ovary profusely branched	–	Does not develop to maturity. Immature flukes only. No eggs	Human, dog, fox, cats, raccoon-like dog, civets, rodents, monkeys, mustelids	Freshwater snail: *Tricula* spp. *Akiyoshia chinensis Assiminea lutea Erhaia* spp. *Neotricula* spp. *Oncomelania hupensis Semisulcospira libertina*	Freshwater crabs of the genera: *Aparapotamon Huanpotamon Isolapotamon Malayopotamon Nanhaipotamon Potamon Sinalopotamon Sinopotamon Tenuilapotamon*	China, Thailand	Immature flukes only, which migrate through body. Subcutaneous swellings (cutaneous larva migrans). Eosinophilic granuloma in brain. Cerebral lesions. Hepatic lesions
Paragonimus africanus	Cuticular spines in groups. Ovary simply branched	67–113 × 42–56 μm	Lungs	Human, mangooses, dog, cat, monkeys, potto, civets	Unknown, may be freshwater snail of genus *Potadoma* or terrestrial snail of family Achatinidae	Crabs: *Sudanautes* spp. *Liberonautes latidactylus*	Cameroon, Nigeria, Equatorial Guinea, Ivory Coast	Mild pulmonary symptoms. No radiological signs. No cerebral lesions. Retroauricular cysts
Paragonimus uterobilateralis	Double uterus; one on each side	–	Lungs	Human, civet, dog, mandrill, potto, shrew, mongoose, otter, murid rodents	Unknown, may be *Homorus striatellus*	*Liberonautes* spp. *Sudanonautes* spp.	Nigeria, Cameroon, Liberia, Gabon	Pulmonary symptoms only

Table III.1 Continued

Adult fluke	Morphology	Egg	Site	Vertebrate hosts	First intermediate host	Second intermediate host	Geographical distribution	Clinical features
Paragonimus mexicanus (*peruvianus, ecuadorensis*)	–	–	Lungs	Human, domestic cats and dogs, wild felines, monkeys (exp), opossums, skunk, coati, raccoon, peccary, grey fox	Freshwater snails: *Aroapyrgus allei A. colombiensis A. costaricensis Oncomelania hupensis Pomiatopsis lapidaria*	Crabs of the genera: *Hypolobocera Odonto-thelphusa Potamocarcinus Pseudothelphusa Ptychophallus Raddaus Tehuana Zilchiopsis*	Mexico, Peru, Ecuador, Costa Rica, Panama, Guatemala	Pulmonary signs and cerebral complications
Paragonimus kellicotti	–	–	Lungs	Human, dog, foxes, lynx, opossum, pig, raccoon, muskrat	*Pomatiopsis cincinnatiensis P. lapidaria* Exp. in *Oncomelania hupensis*	Freshwater crayfish of the genera: *Cambarus Orconectes Procambarus*	USA, Canada	

give rise to cercariae, the whole process taking 3–5 months. The cercariae leave the sporocyst and migrate to the respiratory chamber of the snail. They leave the host via the respiratory opening in the form of slime balls, cemented by mucus originating from glands located in the posterior region of the cercariae. The slime balls are released from the snails individually or in clusters of 4–16; for the life cycle to continue the slime balls must be eaten fairly quickly by an ant, e.g., *Formica fusca* (17 species have been recorded as secondary intermediate hosts, 14 species belonging to the genus *Formica*, plus *Proformica nasuta*, *Catagliphis bicolor* and *C. aenescens*). Penetration of the intestine occurs and metacercariae are formed in the abdominal cavity. If the infected ant is swallowed by a human the cyst wall is disrupted and the young flukes migrate to the bile system and the flukes mature in about 50 days.

Superfamily: Echinostomatoidea

Genus: *Echinostoma*

A trematode of minor importance is *Echinostoma lindoensis*. Until recently it was quite commonly found in humans in the environs of Lake Lindoe, Celebes, but not now as a result of changes in diet. Mice, rats, ducks and pigeons have been infected experimentally. *E. lindoensis* causes diarrhoea, abdominal pains and eosinophilia.

Life cycle

The first intermediate hosts are planorbid snails (*Anisus sarasinorum* and *Gyraulus convexiusculus*); second intermediate hosts (metacercariae) are the snail *Vivipara javanica rudipellis* and four species of mussel (*Corbicula lindoensis*, *C. subplanta*, *C. celebensis* and *C. javanica*) (Table III.1). Additional secondary intermediate hosts experimentally are snails and frogs, and *E. lindoensis* has been reported in *Biomphalaria glabrata* in Brazil. The cercariae have simple tails and a body resembling in miniature that of the adult worm. The eggs are straw coloured, operculate and measure 92–124 × 65–76 μm (Figure III.26). Immature when passed in the faeces, they mature in 6–15 days.

Euparyphium ilocanum is found in humans in the Philippines, Celebes and Indonesia. The first intermediate hosts are *Gyraulus convexiusculus* in the Philippines and Indonesia, and *G. prashadi* and *Hippeutis umbilicalis* in the Philippines. Fourteen species of snail act as second intermediate hosts, e.g., *G. prashadi*, *Vivipara burranghina*, *Planorbis umbilicatus* and *V. rudipellis* (Table III.1). Human cases arise from people eating snails.

Echinostoma malayanum (syn. *Paryphostomum sufrartyfex*) is found in Malaysia, Thailand, India and the Sino-Tibetan border. The natural hosts are pigs and rats. The first intermediate host is the snail *Lymnaea luteola*. The second intermediate hosts are snails (e.g., *L. luteola*, *G. convexiusculus* and *Indoplanorbis exustus*) or the fish *Barbus stigma* (Table III.1).

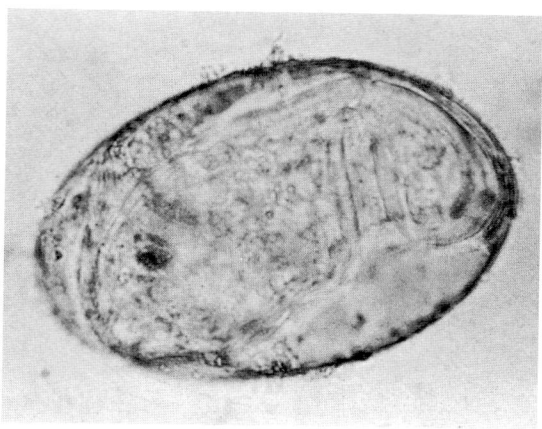

Figure III.26: Egg of *Echinostoma malayanum* containing a fully grown miracidium. (Courtesy of Lie Kan Joe.)

Euparyphium jassyense is found in Romania and has been reported from the USA. The first intermediate host is *Stagnicola emargilatus* and the second intermediate host is a tadpole in Romania and China. Normally the definitive hosts are mink, and trout are the second intermediate hosts.

Echinoparyphium recurvatum was once found in a Japanese person who had lived in Taiwan. The natural hosts are ducks, etc.

Echinostoma revolutum is found in people in Thailand. The natural hosts are ducks and geese. At least 14 species of snail are known to act as first intermediate hosts (e.g., *Indoplanorbis exustus*, *Lymnaea rubiginosa* and *L. stagnalis*). Numerous snails of the same species and others (including *Vivipara vivipara*, *Sphaerium corneum* and *Corbizula fluminea*), along with bivalves and tadpoles, are the second intermediate hosts. It is cosmopolitan in distribution in nature and is found in people in Taiwan and Indonesia where human infections result from eating salted or inadequately cooked clams.

The natural hosts of *Echinostoma hortense* are rats and mice in China, Korea and Japan. About 20 cases have been recorded in humans in Japan and Manchuria. The first intermediate hosts are lymnaeid snails (*L. japonica*, *L. pervia* and *L. ollula*). Second intermediate hosts are tadpoles (frogs and newts) and fish (e.g., *Carassius* and *Cyprinus*).

Other human echinostomes are:

E. cinetorchis—in Japan (?syn. of *revolutum*).
E. macrorchis—in Japan (normally rats, *Capella*).
Echinochasmus perfoliatus—in Japan, Taiwan (normally cats, dogs).
E. japonicus—in Japan, China, Taiwan (normally birds).
E. jiufoensis—in China.
Himasthla muehlensis—a German who had lived 6 years in Columbia picked up this worm, but probably from raw clams (*Vems merceneria*) consumed in New York.
Episthmium caninum—in Thailand (normally dogs).
Euparyphium melis—in China, Romania.
Hypodereum conoideum—in Thailand, Taiwan (normally birds).

Superfamily: Schistosomatoidea (Stiles & Hassal, 1926) Family: Schistosomatidae (Looss, 1899; Poche, 1907)

Genus: *Schistosoma* (Weinland, 1858)

The schistosomes commonly infecting humans are:

Schistosoma haematobium (Bilharz, 1852) Weinland, 1858.
Schistosoma mansoni Sambon, 1907.
Schistosoma japonicum Katsurada, 1904.
Schistosoma intercalatum Fisher, 1934.
Schistosoma mekongi Voge, Bruckner & Bruce, 1978.

Differentiation of these five species is shown in Table III.2. Human infections have also been reported with:

Schistosoma mattheei Veglia & Le Roux, 1929.
Schistosoma bovis (Sonsino, 1876) Blanchard, 1895;.
Schistosoma curassoni Brumpt, 1931.
Schuistosoma malayensis Greer, Ow Yang & Hoi-Sen Yong, 1988.

Natural hybrids of *S. haematobium* and *S. intercalatum* and of *S. haematobium* and *S. mattheei* are known to occur in humans in Cameroon and South Africa, respectively.[2,3] Although unequivocal evidence exists of *S. mattheei* in humans,[2] the evidence for human infection with *S. bovis* and *S. curassoni* is less convincing.

The schistosomes are digenetic trematodes, their life histories consisting of alternating generations, each with its own range of hosts. The adult worms inhabit vertebrates; the larval stages inhabit snails which, in the case of schistosomes pathogenic to humans, are freshwater snails.

The schistosomes are dioecious organisms (i.e., the sexes are separate). Adult schistosomes live in the veins of vertebrates; there is an oral cavity but no muscular pharynx; the eggs have no operculum; there is no encysted or metacercarial stage; the cercariae enter the definitive hosts through the skin.

Parasitology (Figures III.27–III.29)

Like other digenetic trematodes, the schistosomes are equipped with suckers. The *oral sucker* surrounds the mouth and is prehensile; the *ventral sucker (acetabulum)* is more posterior, on the ventral surface. With these suckers the worms can attach themselves to the walls of the vessels in which they live. The *mouth* itself is usually near the anterior extremity. The alimentary system consists of an *oral cavity* leading to the *oesophagus* and thence to the *gut*, which soon divides into two *caeca* that reunite more posteriorly to form the *single posterior caecum* which ends blindly; there is no anus.

Nutrition is derived from blood in which the worms live; schistosomes consume large amounts of glucose; unused material is rejected through the mouth as adult worms do not possess an anus. Despite having access to relatively unlimited supplies of oxygen, the metabolism is primarily anaerobic with lactate as the major end-product.

Table III.2 Differentiation of various species of *Schistosoma*.

Character	S. haematobium	S. mansoni	S. japonicum	S. intercalatum	S. mekongi	S. malayensis
Habitat of adult	Vesical veins; occasionally veins of rectum and portal systems	Inferior mesenteric and portal venous system	Superior and inferior mesenteric and portal venous system	Mesenteric and portal venous system	Superior mesenteric and portal veins	–
Adult male	10–15 × 0.75–1.0 mm	6–13 × 1.0 mm	12–20 × 0.5–0.55 mm	11–14 × 0.3–0.4 mm	6–15 mm	43–9.2 mm
Tegument	Tubercles and fine spines	Conspicuous tubercle and microscopic tufts of hair	No tubercles; small acuminate spines	Tubercles and fine spines	No tubercles; spined from anterior level of gynaecophoric canal to posterior end of body	–
Oesophagus	Single bulb	Single bulb	Double bulb	Single bulb	Double bulb	–
Caeca	Unite in anterior half; posterior caecum short, one-third of body length	Unite in anterior half; posterior caecum long, two-thirds of body length	Unite in posterior half; posterior caecum medium, one-half of body length	Unite in posterior half; posterior caecum one-fifth to one-quarter of body length	Unite in posterior half; posterior caecum, one-fifth to one-quarter of body length	Unite in posterior half of body
Testes	4 or 5	2–14	6–8	4–6	6–7	–
Adult female	20–26 × 0.25 mm	7–17 × 0.25 mm	12–28 × 0.3 mm	10–14 × 0.15–0.18 mm	6–20 mm	6.5–11.3 mm
	Darker than male, more blood pigment in gut	Darker than male, more blood pigment in gut	Darker than male, more blood pigment in gut	Darker than male, more blood pigment in gut	Darker than male, more blood pigment in gut	
Tegument	Transverse striations. Small tubercles at extremity	Transverse striations. Small tubercles at extremity	Transverse striations. Minute spines	Transverse striations, smooth	Transverse striations	Transverse striations
Ovary	In posterior third	In anterior half	Central	In posterior half	In anterior 5/8	In anterior half
Uterus	Anterior, long. Holds 10–100 eggs at one time. Produces 20–290 daily	Anterior, short. Holds 1–2 eggs only at one time. Produces 100–300	Anterior, long. Holds 50 or more eggs at one time. Produces 1500–3500 daily	Anterior, long. Holds 5–50 eggs at one time	Anterior, long	Contains many eggs
Eggs	83–187 × 60 μm (Figure III.30c,3) Terminal spine. Pass through bladder wall. Discharged in urine	112–175 × 45–70 μm (Figure III.30a) Lateral spine. Pass through bowel wall. Discharged in faeces	70–100 × 50–65 μm (Figure III.30b) Rudimentary lateral spine. Pass through bowel wall. Discharged in faeces	140–240 × 50–85 μm (Figure III.30d) Long terminal spine. Pass through bowel wall. Discharged in faeces	30–55 × 50–65 μm Small lateral knob. Pass through bowel wall. Discharged in faeces	52–90 × 33–62 μm Small knob, usually located laterally, occasionally near end of egg
Shell	Non-acid fast with Ziehl–Neelsen stain in tissues	Acid fast with Ziehl–Neelsen stain in tissues	Acid fast with Ziehl–Neelsen stain in tissues	Acid fast with Ziehl–Neelsen stain in tissues	Acid fast with Ziehl–Neelsen stain in tissues	–
Animal hosts	Occasionally baboons, monkeys, rats, pigs	(Occasional) baboons, rats	Rodents, dogs, cats, cattle, water buffalo, pigs, horses, sheep, goats	Sheep, goats in the laboratory	Dogs	*Rattus muelleri* *R. tiomanicus*

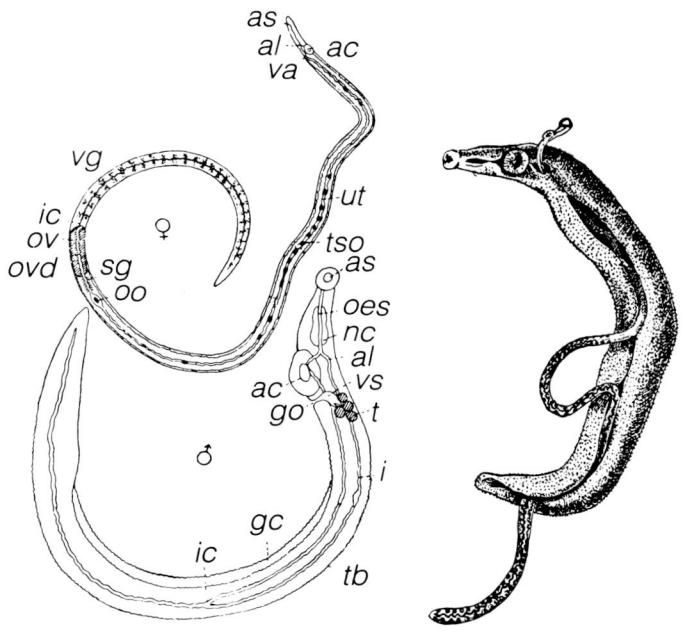

Figure III.27: *Schistosoma haematobium.* (10×.)

al	bifurcation of the alimentary canal
ac	acetabulum
as	oral sucker
gc	gynaecophoric canal
go	gonopore
ic	union of intestinal caeca
nc	nerve cord
oes	oesophagus
oo	ootype
ov	ovary
ovi	oviduct
ps	posterior sucker
sg	shell gland
t	testis
tb	tubercules
tso	terminal spined ovum
ut	uterus
va	vagina
vg	vitelline gland
vs	seminal vesicle

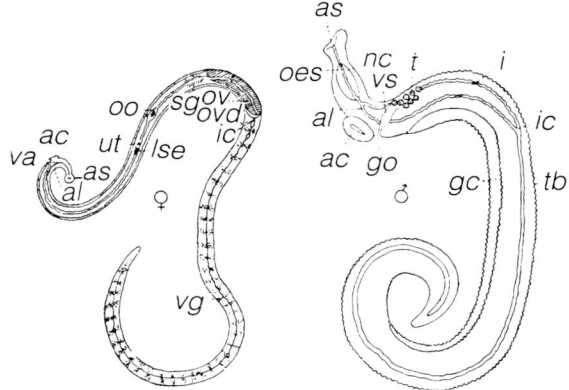

Figure III.28: *Schistosoma mansoni.* (10×.) Key as for Figure III.27. lse, Lateral spined egg.

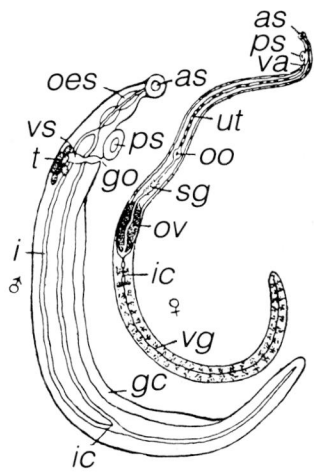

Figure III.29: Male and female *Schistosoma japonicum.* (10×.) Key as for Figure III.27.

The excretory system consists of two longitudinal canals opening posteriorly and fed by collecting tubules. There are flame cells whose function is to fan fluid wastes into the tubules by means of the vibratile cilia with which they are equipped.

There is a rudimentary *nervous system* with an oesophageal ganglion and commissure encircling the oesophagus, and two longitudinal nerve cords running to the posterior end and intercommunicating by lateral branches.

The *male reproductive organs* consist of testes dorsal to and posterior to the ventral sucker. Each testis discharges via a *vas efferens*; these unite to form the *vesicula seminalis* at the *genital pore* situated in the midline posterior to the ventral sucker.

The male worm is flat and leaf-like but is folded to form the *gynaecophoric canal*, enfolding the very slender female for almost its entire length (Figure III.27).

The *female reproductive organs* consist of an elongated *ovary* in the posterior half, from which the *oviduct* passes forward, to be joined by the *vitelline duct* from the *vitellaria (yolk glands)* to form the *common reproductive duct*. The *common reproductive duct* passes forward, entering the *ootype*, a large egg-shaped chamber which receives the ducts of the *Mehlis gland (shell gland)*, at its posterior end. Anteriorly the *ootype* opens into the uterus which passes forward and opens at the *genital pore* on the median surface posterior to the ventral sucker.

Life cycle (Figure III.30)

The eggs of the schistosomes are passed by the definitive hosts (vertebrates) in urine (*S. haematobium*; Figure III.30C) or faeces (*S. mansoni* (Figure III.30A), *S. japonicum* (Figure III.30B), *S. mekongi, S. intercalatum* (Figure III.30D)) but this is not an absolute rule as eggs of *S. haematobium* may occasionally be found in faeces and commonly in biopsy specimens of rectal mucosa, and eggs of *S. mansoni* may be found in urine samples, especially in heavy infections. *S. mattheei* (Figure III.30E) is a parasite of sheep

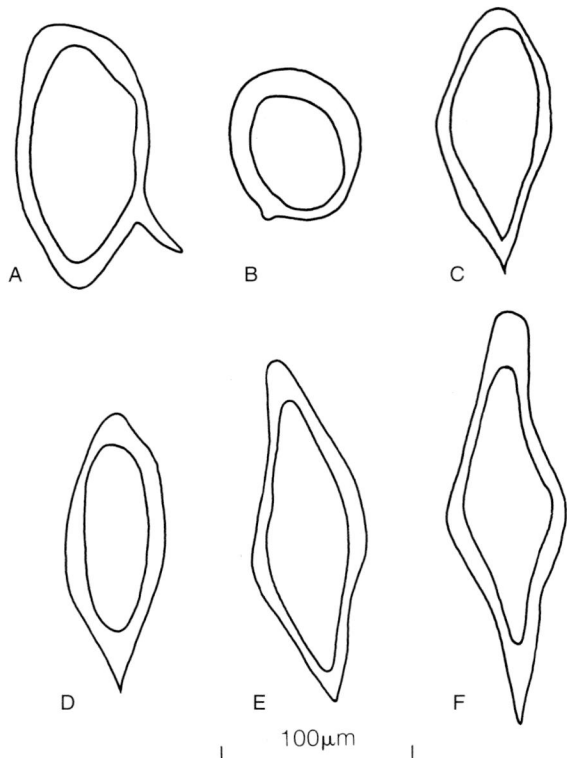

Figure III.30: Eggs of *Schistosoma* spp. (**A**) *S. mansoni.*
(**B**) *S. japonicum.* (**C**) *S. haematobium.* (**D**) *S. intercalatum.*
(**E**) *S. mattheei.* (**F**) *S. bovis.*

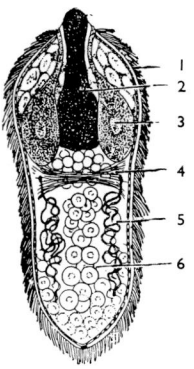

Figure III.31: Miracidium of *Schistosoma haematobium.* 1, Cilia.
2, Apical papilla. 3, Lateral gland. 4, Neural mass. 5, Excretory tubules.
6, Germinal cells.

and cattle, but *S. mattheei*-shaped eggs have been
recorded from the urine of humans in South Africa.
Subsequent analyses have demonstrated these eggs to
result from *S. haematobium* male × *S. mattheei* female.

Eggshells of *S. mansoni, S. japonicum* and *S. intercalatum*
(but not *S. haematobium* or *S. mattheei*) are acid fast when
stained by means of the Ziehl–Neelsen method.

When an egg reaches freshwater it contains a fully
embryonated miracidium which hatches within a few
minutes, partly as a result of osmosis, partly owing to its
own movements. The miracidium swims actively by
means of its ciliated epidermis for 8–12 hours, searching
for a snail host. Miracidia tend to move to the upper
layers of water where many of their snail hosts live, but
in some circumstances they can infect snails inhabiting
the bottom of canals or lakes (e.g., Lake Victoria). These
snails, however, frequently move up and down from the
depths to the surface of such waters and miracidia have
the opportunity of infecting them in the upper reaches.

The miracidium (Figure III.31) has a complex array of
sensory receptors which are considered to aid it in
locating a snail host. Also the miracidium is endowed
with a muscular apical papilla, apical gland and a pair of
lateral glands, all of which are considered to play a role in
effecting penetration of the snail's epidermis. Miracidia
do not appear to discriminate between species of snail
and will sometimes enter the incorrect host, thereby preventing further development. However, if a miracidium

enters a compatible intermediate host, metamorphosis
into the next stage—the mother sporocyst—takes place:
the ciliated epidermis is cast off and is replaced by a
syncytial tegument with numerous microvilli.

Within the elongated sac of the mother sporocyst
germinal cells develop into daughter sporocysts. These
leave the mother sporocyst after about 8 days and
migrate to the digestive gland (liver) of the snail host,
and within them further germinal cells develop into the
next stage, the cercaria. Thousands of cercariae may result
from one miracidium and all of these will be of the same
sex. Recent studies[4] have shown that the total production
of cercariae per snail of *Biomphalaria pfeifferi* Senegal
exposed to one miracidium of *S. mansoni* Senegal ranged
from 18 703 to 73 446 with a mean of 51 692. The cycle
from penetration by the miracidium to the production of
mature cercariae takes about 3–4 weeks for *S. intercalatum*,
about 4–5 weeks for *S. mansoni*, 5–6 weeks for *S. haematobium* and *S. mekongi*, and 7 weeks or more for *S.
japonicum.*[5] The snails are damaged in the process and
their lifespan is shortened. In laboratory experiments it
was demonstrated that *Biomphalaria pfeifferi* Senegal
exposed to one miracidium of *S.mansoni* Senegal showed
no mortality up to 57 days post infection, after which
mortality gradually evolved. The maximum lifespan of an
infected snail was 239 days following infection.[4]

The mature cercaria (Figure III.32) escapes from the
daughter sporocyst, migrates through the tissues of the
snail, and finally emerges to swim free in the water by
means of its muscular, bifurcated tail, usually tail first.
The data from chronobiology experiments show that, for
schistosomes that infect humans, there is usually one
peak of cercarial emission, around mid-day. Cercarial
emergence rhythms are considered as adaptive behaviours
of the parasite, under genetic control, shaped under the
selective pressures exerted by the behaviours of the
definitive host. The cercaria is approximately 0.5 mm in
length, with an oral organ and a smaller ventral sucker, a
mouth, oesophagus and a pair of short caeca, and an
excretory system of flame cells, tubules and excretory
ducts leading into an excretory bladder at the posterior
end of the body. It has three types of gland: head glands,

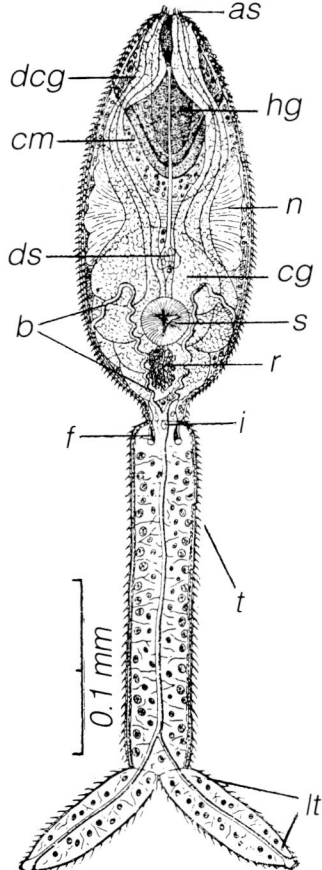

Figure III.32: Cercaria of *Schistosoma japonicum*, ventral view. (240×.)

as	anterior spines	hg	head gland
b	excretory bladder	i	island excretory bladder
cg	cephalic glands	lt	lobe of tail
cm	circular muscles	m	mouth
dcg	ducts of cephalic glands	n	nervous system
ds	digestive system	r	rudimentary genital cells
exp	excretory pore	t	tail
f	flame cell	s	ventral sucker

four preacetabular and six postacetabular glands. The secretion from the postacetabular glands is thought to help the cercaria attach itself to the skin of the vertebrate host, and the secretion of the preacetabular glands together with that of the postacetabular glands helps to break down the skin barrier.

A snail may shed up to 3000 cercariae per day when in peak production (e.g., *Biomphalaria glabrata* shedding *S. mansoni*). However, the number does vary from day to day and some host–parasite relationships are less productive: *Oncomelania hupensis* produces 15–160 cercariae per day of *S. japonicum*. Cercariae tend to swim up to the surface of water, sinking from time to time, and returning. They are influenced by the effect of light, gravity, agitation and touch. They are non-feeding and depend entirely upon their glycogen reserves when free-swimming; consequently their lifespan is short, up to 48 hours, although this depends upon external factors such

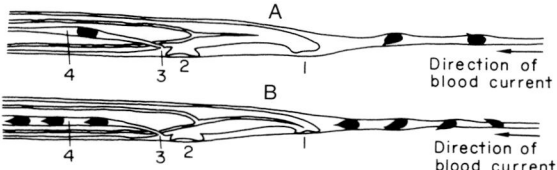

Figure III.33: The deposition of eggs by (**A**) *Schistosoma mansoni* and (**B**) *S. haematobium* in the blood vessels and their passage to the exterior. 1, Anterior sucker. 2, Posterior sucker. 3, Vaginal orifice. 4, Uterus containing eggs.

as turbulence and temperature. In many transmission areas the lifespan will be only 8–12 hours.

A cercaria can penetrate the skin of a definitive host within a few minutes. In doing so it sheds its tail and in the tissues becomes a *schistosomulum*. The trilaminate surface of the cercaria is replaced by a multilaminate surface of the schistosomulum and adult. The schistosomulum leaves the skin after about 2–4 days by the venous or lymphatic systems, to be transported to the lungs. In the lungs the schistosomulum becomes longer and thinner, and then leaves the lungs via the pulmonary veins and passes through the heart to the systemic circulation. An individual schistosomulum may make several circuits of the pulmonary–systemic circulation before finding its way to the hepatic portal system. Growth takes place in the liver and paired worms may be found after about 26 days. Most worms leave the liver when they are sexually mature and have mated, and migrate to the veins of the vesical plexus (*S. haematobium*) or the mesenteric veins (*S. mansoni, S. japonicum, S. mekongi* and *S. intercalatum*) where they begin to lay eggs. The period between penetration by the cercariae and egg-laying may be 30–50 days or more.

The mated worms move as far as possible towards the fine terminal vessels and the female then leaves the male, progressing to the finest vessels where she deposits her eggs, retracting after having done so (Figure III.33). The eggs escape from the venules into the tissues—those of *S. haematobium* largely into the wall of the bladder but occasionally into the wall of the colorectum; those of *S. mansoni, S. japonicum, S. mekongi* and *S. intercalatum* largely into the wall of the colorectum. Many pass through the mucosa to be excreted in urine or faeces but some remain trapped in the tissues where they give rise to tissue reactions. Some eggs of all species are usually also found in the liver, genital tract, lungs, central nervous system and other organs. Eggs are responsible for most of the pathological effects of the infection (see Chapter 80).

Intermediate hosts (snails)

Strains of schistosomes that infect humans vary in their ability to infect snail hosts. Usually this variation is associated with geographical area, but the subject is complex. The following lists of proved and potential snails hosts have been constructed from Jordan et al.[5] and Brown.[6]

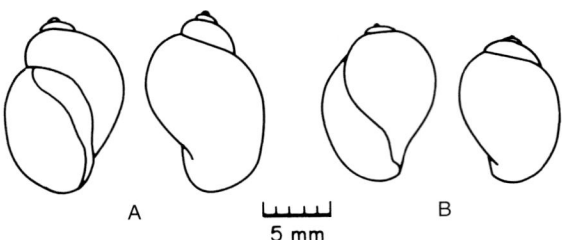

Figure III.34: Molluscan hosts of *Schistosoma haematobium*. (**A**) *Bulinus truncatus*. (**B**) *B. africanus*.

Snail hosts of *S. haematobium* (Figure III.34)

S. haematobium is a species complex and is transmitted throughout most of its range by species of the genus *Bulinus*. There are two possible exceptions: at Gimvi about 250 km south of Bombay, a schistosome considered to be *S. haematobium* is transmitted by *Ferrissia tenuis*, but clearly further studies are required on this particular focus; recent laboratory studies have demonstrated that *Planorbarius metidjensis* is compatible with an isolate of *S. haematobium*, but as yet the epidemiological significance of this observation remains enigmatic. The limited distribution of *P. metidjensis* to north-west Africa and the Iberian peninsula reduces the significance of this observation from a practical point of view. A list of hosts and their distribution is given in Table III.3.

Table III.3 Snail hosts of *S. haematobium*.

Snail species	Locality
Truncatus/tropicus complex	
Bulinus truncatus	Iran, Iraq, Near East, Yemen, North Africa, West Africa, (East Africa, potential) Egypt
B. coulboisi (potential)	East Africa
Reticulatus group	
B. reticulatus (potential)	East, central and southern Africa
B. wrighti	Saudi Arabia, South Yemen
Forskalii group	
B. forskalii	Malagasy Republic
B. bavayi (potential)	Malagasy Republic
B. beccarii	North and South Yemen, Saudi Arabia
B. camerunensis	Cameroon
B. cernicus	Mauritius
B. senegalensis	Senegal, Gambia, Nigeria
Africanus group	
B. africanus	South and east Africa
B. globosus	Afrotropical region
B. nasutus	East Africa
B. abyssinicus	Ethiopia, Somalia
B. obtusispira	Malagasy Republic
B. hightoni (potential)	North-east Kenya
B. umbilicatus	Senegal
Ferrissia tenuis	India

Table III.4 Snail hosts of *S. intercalatum*.

Snail species	Locality
Bulinus globosus *B. forskalii*	Democratic Republic of Congo Cameroon, Equatorial Guinea, Gabon, Nigeria São Tomé
Most species of the *forskalii* and *reticulatus* groups are capable of acting as hosts for the Lower Guinea strain of *S. intercalatum*, but so far none has been implicated as a natural host apart	

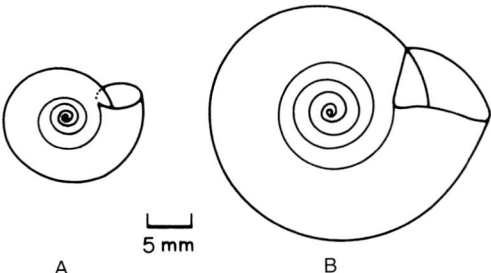

Figure III.35: Molluscan hosts of *Schistosoma mansoni*. (**A**) *Biomphalaria alexandrina*. (**B**) *B. glabrata*.

Snail hosts of *S. intercalatum*
These are shown in Table III.4.

Snail hosts of *S. mansoni* (Figure III.35)
These are shown in Table III.5.

Snail hosts of *S. japonicum* (Figure III.36)
Breeding experiments and detailed cytogenetic and biochemical studies in recent years have indicated that all of the proven hosts for *S. japonicum* should now be regarded as subspecies of a single widespread species, *Oncomelania hupensis*. A distinctive species in Japan, *O. minima*, appears to be resistant to infection. The hosts are listed in Table III.6.

Snail host of *S. mekongi*
The only recorded host is *Neotricula aperta*, which is endemic in the Mekong River, Laos and Cambodia. Three races of *N. aperta* are known: α, β and γ, which is considered to be the most important in transmission. The γ-strain of *N. aperta* is responsible for endemic transmission of *S. mekongi* in southern Laos and at Kratié.

Interspecific interaction between trematodes in snails

It has been reported[7] that, if albino *Biomphalaria glabrata* is infected with *S. mansoni* and also with *Paryphostomum segregatum* (an echinostome from Brazil), the rediae of *P. segregatum* will attack and breach the thin wall of the

Table III.5 Snail hosts of *S. mansoni.*

Snail (*Biomphalaria*) species	Locality
Biomphalaria pfeifferi	West, east and southern Africa, Arabian Peninsula, Malagasy Republic
B. choanomphala *B. smithi*[a] *B. stanleyi*[a]	Great lakes of east Africa
B. alexandrina	Egypt
B. angulosa	East and central Africa
B. sudanica	East and central Africa
B. camerunensis	West and central Africa
B. salinarum[a]	South-western Africa
B. glabrata	West Indies, Venezuela, Surinam, French Guyana, Brazil
B. tenagophila	Brazil, Bolivia, Peru, Paraguay, Uruguay, Argentina
B. straminea	Venezuela, Surinam, French Guyana, Brazil
The following neotropical species have been successfully infected with *S. mansoni* in the laboratory and must, therefore, be regarded as potential hosts	
B. chilensis	Chile
B. havanensis	Antilles, Mexico, Central America, northern South America
B. helphila	Puerto Rico, Cuba, Peru
B. peregrina	Ecuador, Bolivia, Chile, Paraguay, Argentina, Uruguay, Brazil
B. sericea	Ecuador

[a]Successfully infected in the laboratory with *S. mansoni.*

Table III.6 Snail hosts of *S. japonicum.*

Snail species	Locality
Oncomelania hupensis hupensis	China
O. h. formosana	Taiwan[a]
O. h. chiui	Taiwan
O. h. nosophora	Japan
O. h. quadrasi	Philippines
O. h. lindoensis	Celebes

[a]The Taiwanese strain is not pathogenic to humans.

early mother sporocyst of *S. mansoni* and ingest and destroy the daughter sporocysts within it. They fail, however, to destroy mature daughter sporocysts, but may cause degeneration of the schistosome sporocysts by

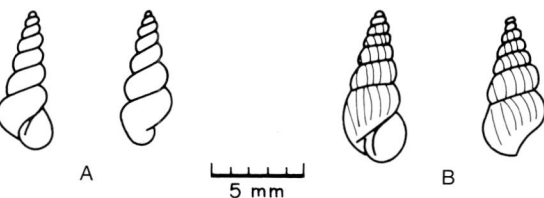

Figure III.36: Molluscan hosts of *Schistosoma japonicum.* (**A**) *Oncomelania hupensis nosophora.* (**B**) *O. h. hupensis.*

other means. They can ingest whole cercariae. However, the use of echinostomes as a form of biological control for schistosomiasis is not considered practical for field use: the necessarily high infection rates would not be achieved because of parasite overdispersion. Repeated release of echinostome eggs would be required and the costs of such operations and their evaluation would be high. Both field data and laboratory experiments have shown that *Bulinus tropicus*, which is incompatible with *S. bovis*, becomes compatible when infected with an amphistome parasite, *Calicophoron microbothrium.*[8] The recognition of non-self by the snail is suspected to be mediated by lectins or other humoral factors which potentially fuction as opsonins that promote encapsulation by haemocytes. Therefore, it is possible that the amphistome parasites secrete factor(s) that somehow alter the behaviour of the *Bulinus* haemocytes, preventing them from recognizing and encapsulating the *S. bovis* sporocysts.

Superfamily: Paramphistomatoidea (*Amphistome trematodes*)

Genus: *Gastrodiscoides*

Gastrodiscoides hominis (Lewis & McConnell, 1876; Leiper, 1913)

Distribution

Malaysia, Assam, India, Pakistan, Philippines, Myanmar, South Vietnam, Guyana, CIS. In Kamrup district, Assam, 41% of the population is infected; in Burma 5%. The normal host is the pig or the mouse deer.

Characters

The fluke is reddish from haemoglobin pigment. When alive, it is very expansile and can elongate to 1 cm. Preserved specimens measure 5–7 × 3–4 mm at the widest point. The anterior end is conical, and the posterior discoidal, flattened ventrally to form a concave disc. Prominent genital papillae are seen and the common genital pore is 2.5 mm from the oral sucker. The ventral sucker (acetabulum) is ventrally situated in the caudal portion and measures 2 mm in diameter. The tegument is smooth. The alimentary canal consists of a pharynx with two pear-shaped pharyngeal pouches. The oesophagus is 1 mm in length and ends in a muscular bulb, where the bifurcation of the intestine takes place and caeca run back to the edge of the acetabulum. There are two

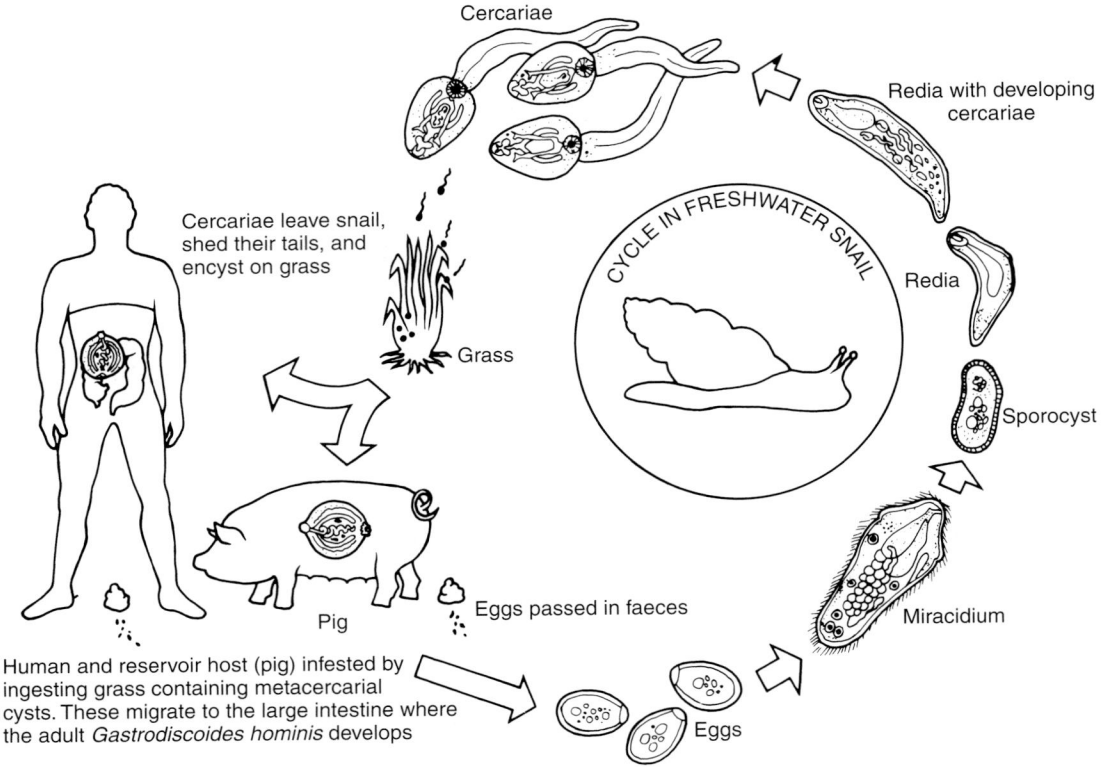

Figure III.37: Life cycle of *Gastrodiscoides hominis*.

lobulated testes placed diagonally between the intestinal caeca. A seminal vesicle is present but no cirrus. The ovary lies in the midline, posterior to the testes. An ovoid shell gland is placed near the ovary with a receptaculum seminis anterior to it. The uterus is short. Laurer's canal is present. The vitellaria lie in the middle third. The ovoid egg measures 152 × 60 μm and has an operculum.

Life cycle (Figure III.37)

The adult lives in the caecum and colon of the definitive host (pig, deer, human). Eggs are passed in the stool and hatch into miracidia. These enter a freshwater snail, *Helicorbis coenosus*, where they develop into sporocysts, and rediae are subsequently formed. Cercariae form within the rediae, and when mature leave the rediae and then the snail host to encyst on vegetation as metacercariae, which are then eaten by the definitive host.

Genus: *Watsonius*

Watsonius watsoni has been found in large numbers in an African person in south-west Africa. Its normal hosts are monkeys of the genera *Cercopithecus* and *Papio* (baboon).

Cestodes (see also Chapters 84 and 85)

Class Cestoidea or tapeworms

The name cestode is derived from 'kestos' (Gk. a girdle).

There is a head or *scolex*, and the *strobila* or segments have their own musculature which relieves the strain on the head. The worms can live for several years and absorb nutriment through the tegument. They are hermaphroditic, normally with male and female in each segment, the male fertilizing the adjacent female (with very few exceptions). Male organs often develop before the female. Human cestodes occur in two orders.

1. Pseudophyllidea with slit-like bothria, oval head (two long grooves with muscular walls), no hooks and the genital orifice on the flat surface.
2. Cyclophyllidea, cup-like or round suckers; genital orifice marginal.

Order: Pseudophyllidea

Genus: *Diphyllobothrium*

Diphyllobothrium latum (Linnaeus, 1785)

D. latum is greyish and more translucent and less fleshy than *Taenia* and may attain a length of 3–10 m, lying coiled up in the small intestine. Multiple infections are common. The scolex (3 mm) has no rostellum or hooklets but two slit-like suckers with longitudinal grooves (bothridia). The neck is thin; the proglottids number 3000 to 4000. The number of worms corresponds to the individual plerocercoids swallowed. Mature segments are more broad than long. A single worm may discharge as many as 36 000 to 1 million eggs each day. The worm may be discharged from the bowel naturally

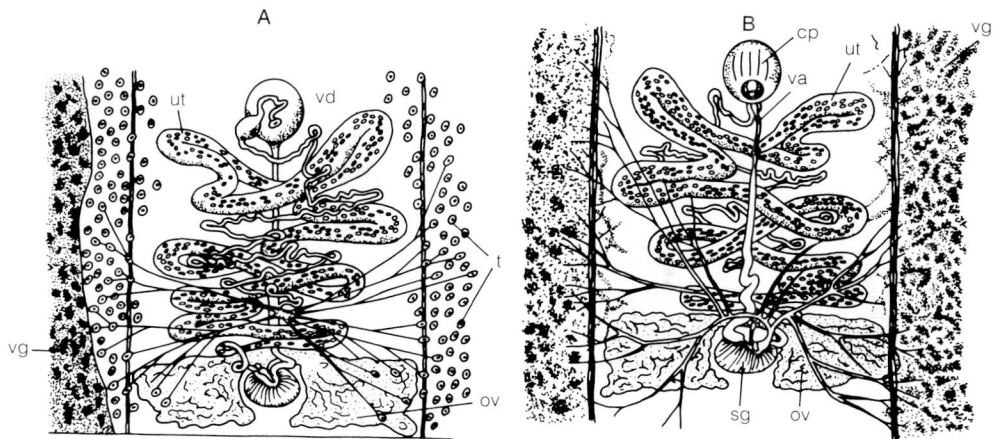

Figure III.38: Mature segment of *Diphyllobothrium latum*. (**A**) Dorsal or male aspect. (**B**) Ventral or female aspect.

cp	cirrus pouch	ov	ovary	sg	shell gland	t	testes
ut	uterus	va	vagina	vd	vas deferens	vg	vitelline glands

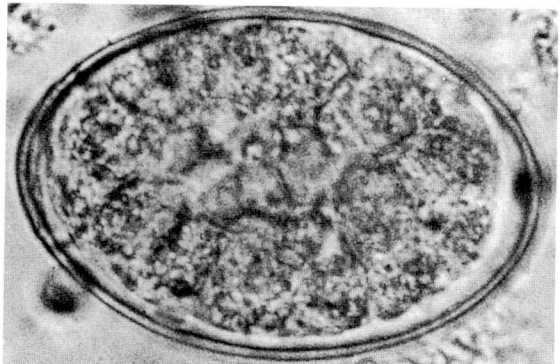

Figure III.39: *Diphyllobothrium latum* (fish tapeworm). Ovum. (Courtesy of D. S. Ridley.)

without treatment. (For details of anatomy of male and female elements, see Figure III.38.)

The egg is operculated with a brown shell measuring 70 × 45 μm (Figures III.5 and III.39). No segments are passed in faeces (unlike *Taenia*).

Life cycle (Figures III.40 and III.41)

If the egg is passed in water the operculum is lifted, the ciliated six-hooked coracidium emerges (Figure III.40C); spherical (22.30 μm), it swims by means of its cilia but dies after 12 hours to 5 days depending on temperature. Normally it is swallowed by freshwater crustacea, the first intermediate host—*Cyclops strenuus, Diaptomus gracilis, D. graciloides* or *D. oregonensis, Cyclops brevisponosus*, and *C. prasenus* in the USA. The outer layer is then digested. The hooks tear a hole in the gut wall; the larva passes into the body cavity and may kill the cyclops. Lying outside the gut wall it becomes the *proceroid larva* (Figure III.40D–G) which is ovoid, 50–60 μm long, with a terminal spherical appendix bearing six hooklets. At most two of these are found in one *Cyclops*, which is then

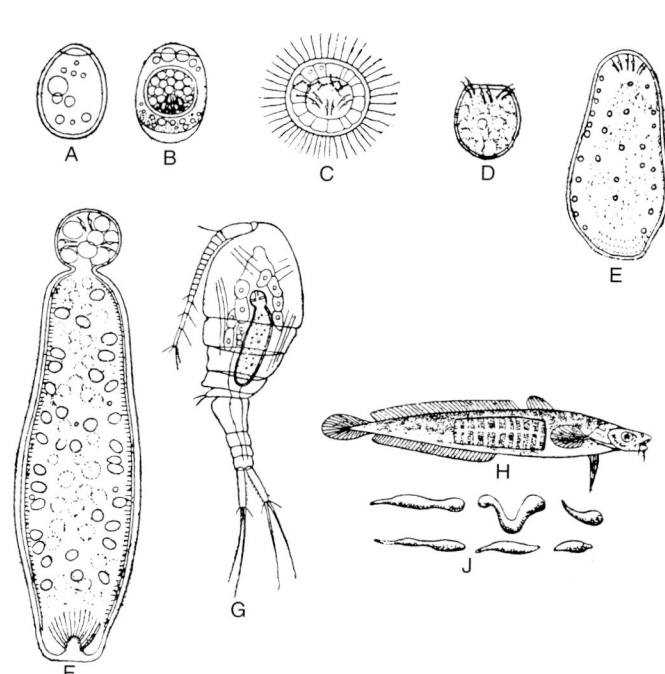

Figure III.40: Life cycle of *Diphylobothrium latum* (not to scale). (**A**) Egg of *D. latum*. (**B**) Hexacanth embryo. (**C**) Ciliated oncosphere or coracidium. (**D, E** and **F**) Development of larvae or procercoids in *Cyclops*. (**G**) Procercoid in the body cavity of *Cyclops*. (**H**) Development of plerocercoids in fishes. (**J**) Plerocercoids of different shapes ingested by a human, dog or cat.

swallowed by freshwater fishes of many species (the second intermediate hosts) such as pike, perch, salmon, trout and grayling—in Africa, the barbel; in the USA the pike, wall-eye and burbot. Reaching the stomach of the fish, the procercoid penetrates to the body cavity and after 3–4 days there encysts as a plerocercoid or *Spirometra* larva (6 mm) in the muscular and connective tissues (Figure III.40H). Bothria, nervous and excretory systems are developed. It is then ingested by a human with raw

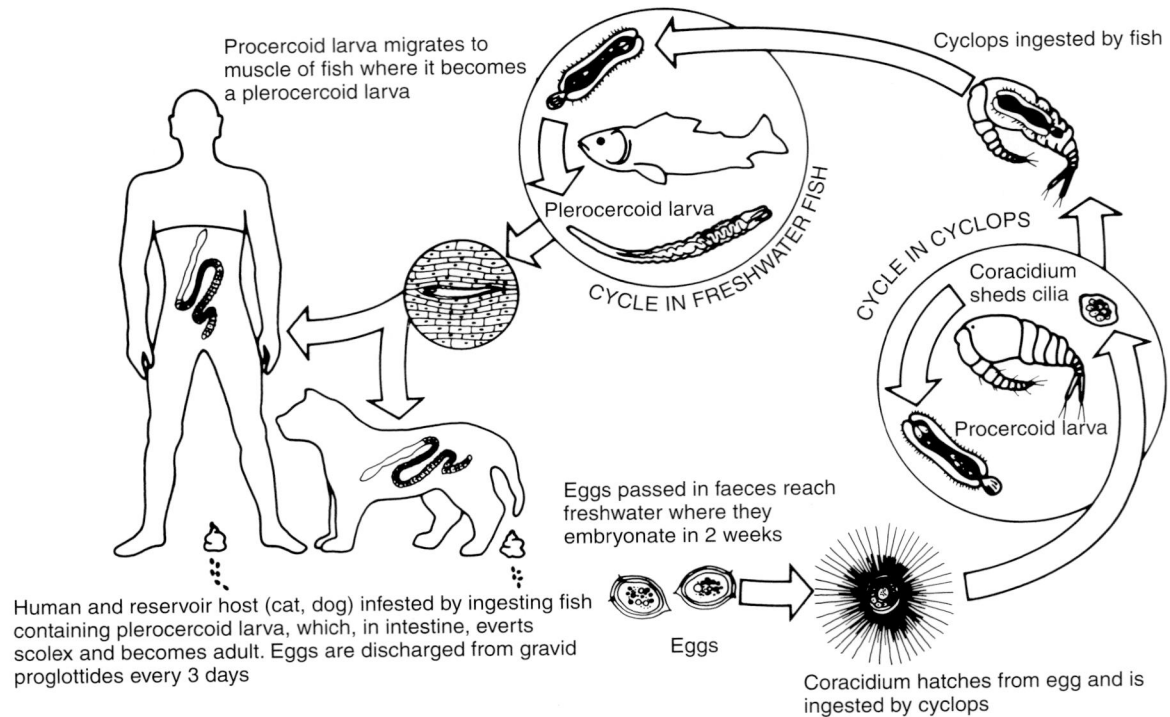

Procercoid larva migrates to muscle of fish where it becomes a plerocercoid larva

Cyclops ingested by fish

Plerocercoid larva

CYCLE IN FRESHWATER FISH

CYCLE IN CYCLOPS

Coracidium sheds cilia

Procercoid larva

Eggs passed in faeces reach freshwater where they embryonate in 2 weeks

Eggs

Human and reservoir host (cat, dog) infested by ingesting fish containing plerocercoid larva, which, in intestine, everts scolex and becomes adult. Eggs are discharged from gravid proglottides every 3 days

Coracidium hatches from egg and is ingested by cyclops

Figure III.41: Life cycle of *Diphyllobothrium latum*. (Courtesy of Tropical Resources Unit.)

roe (caviar) or insufficiently cooked fish, and the *plerocercoid* develops in 5–6 weeks into an adult *Diphyllobothrium*.

Freshwater fishes harbour other *Diphyllobothrium* larvae which are difficult to differentiate at this stage. The process of 'kippering' does not kill the plerocercoids and ordinary smoking is ineffectual, but brine saturation is effective. The adult tapeworm can live as long as 29 years. *Diphyllobothrium dendriticum (minus)* is a small variety found in Lake Baikal and has a similar history. The second intermediate hosts are various species of salmon and grayling which are eaten frozen or salted by Mongolian peoples. *D. alascense* is a species found in Eskimos and can be differentiated by the form of the scolex. The plerocercoids occur in two species of fish: *Pungitus* and *Dallia*.

Spirometrea mansoni (erinacei) (Diphyllobothrium, Dibothriocephalus mansoni)

Parasitology

This organism resembles *D. latum*, is 6–10 m long and has a more delicate structure with a narrower and more ellipsoid egg than *D. latum*.

Life cycle

The adult stage occurs in the dog and other animals, the plerocercoid (sparganum) under natural conditions in frogs or snakes. The procercoid in *Cyclops leuckarti* shows the same stages as in *D. latum*.

The human is infected by accidentally swallowing a procercoid while drinking, thus becoming a second intermediary. The Chinese custom of applying raw split frogs to sores on the hands or to inflamed eyes may afford entry. The sparganum in humans measures 8–36 cm × 0.1–12 mm × 0.5–1.75 mm thick (Figure III.42). Its body is flat and transversely wrinkled with a longitudinal median groove. It is found in many parts of the body: kidneys and iliac fossae, pleural cavities, urethra and subcutaneous tissues.

S. mansonoides (probably = *erinacei*) was formerly thought to be the parent form of *Sparganum proliferum*. It is found in the intestine of the cat in the southern USA and is separable from *D. latum* and *D. cordatum* by the scolex, uterine characteristics and smaller size. Specimens vary from 20 to 60 cm in length but may attain 1 × 8 mm. Immature proglottids number 200 to 300. The egg is pointed, 65 × 37 µm, with a conical operculum. The life cycle is as for *S. mansonoides*.

The plerocercoids (spargana) measure 3–12 × 2.5 mm (Figures III.42 and III.43) and are contained in cysts which are found in humans in Japan and Florida. The body contains calcareous corpuscles. The cysts may be disseminated throughout the body in subcutaneous tissues, intramuscular fasciae, walls of the alimentary canal, mesentery, kidney, lung, heart and brain. The prognosis in the human is grave. Similar plerocercoids have been reproduced in macaque monkeys.

Sparganosis has been found in Korea and spargana, 23–50 cm in length, were removed from the muscles of the abdomen and chest. All patients had eaten raw snakes—*Dinodon rufozonatum*. It has also been found in

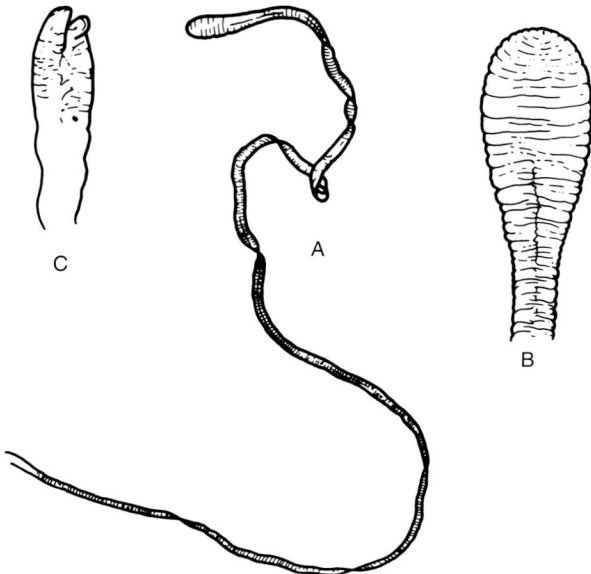

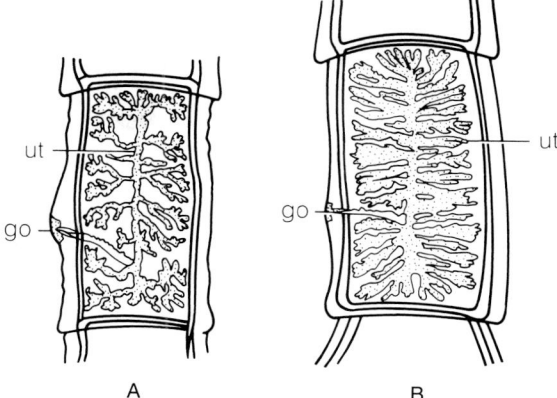

Figure III.44: Segments of tapeworms, showing the characteristic branching of the uterus as seen in mature segments. (**A**) *Taenia solium*. (**B**) *T. saginata*. go, Genital opening; ut, uterus.

Figure III.42: *Diphyllobothrium mansoni* plerocercoid, extracted from an abscess in a Masai. (**A**) Natural size. (**B**) Anterior extremity. (**C**) Posterior extremity.

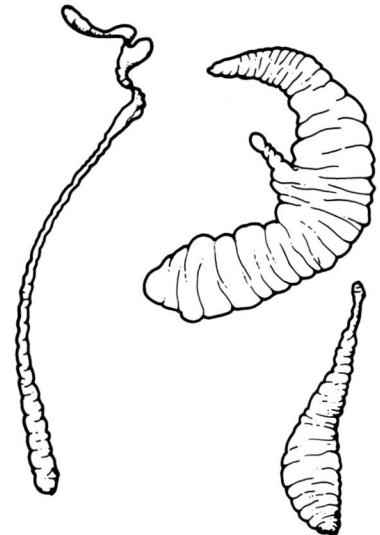

Figure III.43: Different forms of *Sparganum proliferum*.

abscess(es) of the leg. The adult form is probably *Spirometra erinacei*. Spargana are found near the central African lakes (generally in swellings in the chest), and also in Rwanda and Burundi. The adults are probably *S. theileri* or *S. pretoriensis*.

Order: Cyclophyllidea

Genus: *Taenia*

Taenia solium (Linnaeus, 1758) (pork tapeworm)

Parasitology

T. solium (Figure III.44) lives in the upper third of the small intestine. The name 'solium' is derived from the resemblance of the rostellum to the conventional figure of the sun. It attains a length of 2–3 m (exceptionally 8 m), having 800–1000 segments. The head is globular, quadrangular, 1 mm in diameter, and the rostellum is short and pigmented, with a double row of 20–50 hooklets (Figure III.45C). The four suckers project slightly and are circular, measuring 0.5 mm in diameter. The anterior proglottids are small, broader than they are long, the more mature ones measuring 12 × 6 mm. Each proglottis has a marginal genital pore with thick lips; its situation alternates irregularly between the right and left margins. The uterus is median with seven to 13 stout diverticula (Figure III.44A). The testes consist of 150–200 follicles, distributed throughout the dorsal plane. Proglottids number less than 1000. Terminal ripe segments pass out in the faeces and have an independent movement which enables them to migrate outside the anus. Each gravid segment contains 30 000–50 000 eggs.

The egg measures 31–56 µm in diameter and is round with no operculum (Figures III.5, and III.46B). It has two radially striated shells, the inner formed by the embryo (thus differing from Pseudophyllidea), and a vitelline membrane when it is in the segment which is lost in the faeces. Small numbers of eggs are found in the faeces when the segments break. They contain the six-hooked oncosphere.

Life cycle (Figure III.47)

Mature segments are detached and pass out with the faeces; they disintegrate and the eggs are set free and eaten by the intermediate host (the pig). Humans are occasionally infected by cysticerci (cysticercosis), as are other primates (macaque monkeys), occasionally sheep or dogs. The oncosphere penetrates the gut wall and enters the bloodstream, settling in the muscles, especially the heart, and becomes a *cysticercus* (5–20 mm) known as cysticercus cellulosae. Infected pork is popularly known

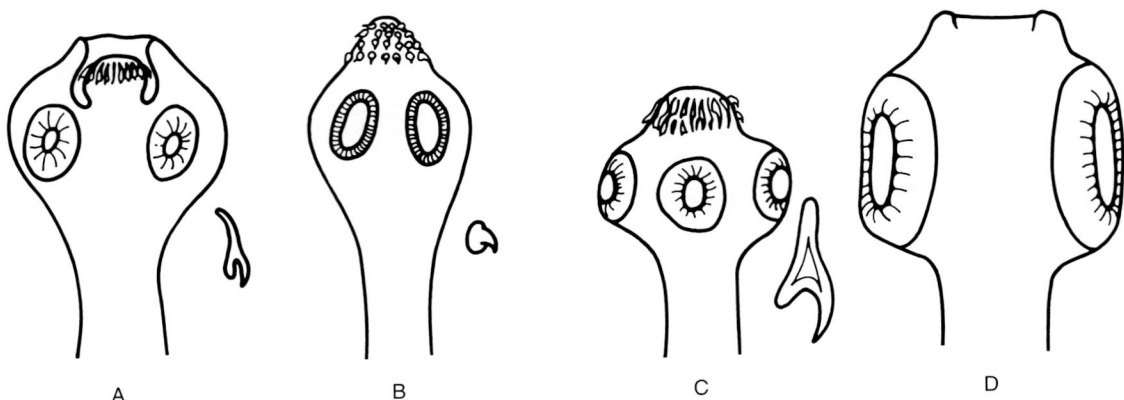

Figure III.45: Heads of human cestodes, showing suckers and, when present, the arrangement of the hooklets. (**A**) *Hymenolepis nana.* (**B**) *Dipylidium caninum.* (**C**) *Taenia solium.* (**D**) *T. saginata.*

Figure III.46: Eggs of *Taenia saginata* (**A**) and *T. solium* (**B**) showing hooklets.

as 'measly pork'. At 0°C the cysticerci can persist for 70 days.

In the alimentary tract of the human or other definitive host, the bladder of the cysticercus is absorbed by the digestive juices; the scolex and head are evaginated and then pass to the small intestine, where the scolex fixes itself to the gut wall and forms proglottides.

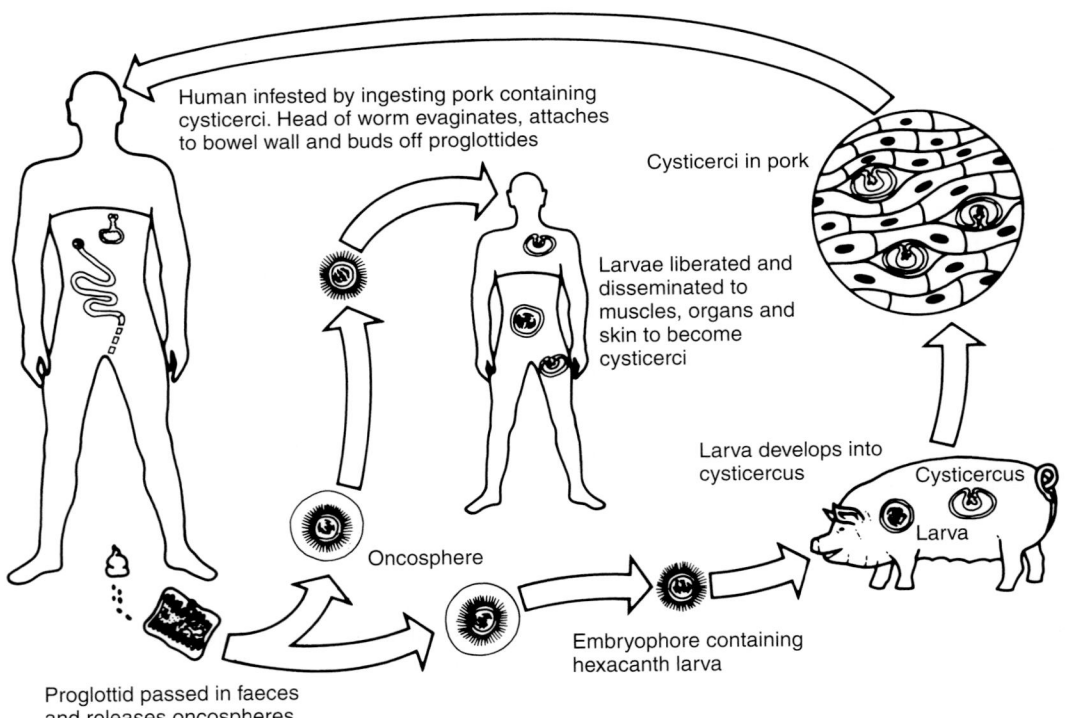

Figure III.47: Life cycle of *Taenia solium.* (Courtesy of Tropical Resources Unit.)

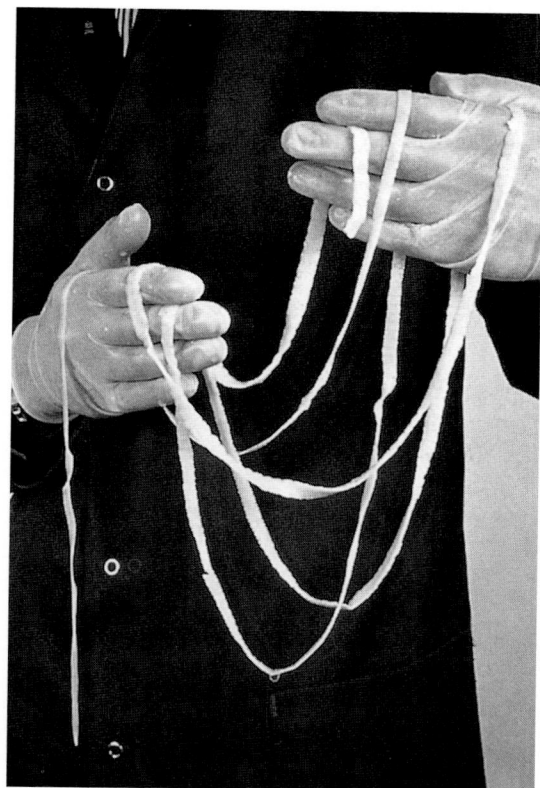

Figure III.48: Adult beef tapeworm (*Taenia saginata*). (Courtesy of G. S. Nelson.)

Taenia saginata goeze (1782) (beef tapeworm)

Parasitology

T. saginata (Figures III.44B, III.45D and III.48) is whitish and semitransparent, measuring 4–10 m; when fully adult it may contain 20–2000 segments. The scolex is pear shaped, cubical and 1–2 mm in diameter, with four lateral suckers but no rostellum or hooks. The suckers and sucker-like organ (Figure III.45D) at the apex are frequently pigmented. The neck is long and half the width of the scolex. The older proglottides are elongated; gravid individuals are three to four times longer than they are broad. The genital pore is single, marginally placed at the hind end of the proglottis, alternating regularly between the right and left margins. There are 20–35 lateral branches on each side of the uterus, which may ramify (Figure III.44B). The genital organs in the mature proglottid differ from those of *T. solium* in having about twice the number of testes (300–400) and in lacking the accessory ovarian lobe. Each gravid segment contains about 97 000 eggs. The total output per year is reckoned at 594 million.

T. saginata (like *Enterobius vermicularis*), oviposits on the perianal skin. The ova are expelled when the proglottid has detached itself from the strobila. The gravid uterus carries lateral branches terminating in blind club-shaped sacs. There they form a separate organ resembling a tassel (*thysanus*) which, when it disintegrates, leaves behind a mass of ova. The thysanus

then becomes an aperture for oviposition (*protocostoma*). The stimulus is provided by thousands of eggs compressed within the uterus. The yolk mass that envelops the embryophores of the ova causes them to adhere to the perianal skin.

The egg is globular, 30–40 × 20–30 µm, with a double-shelled striated embryophore, which contains the oncosphere consisting of an outer shell, chorionic membrane and two oncospheral membranes (Figures III.5, and III.46A). *T. saginata* embryophores stain well with Ziehl–Neelsen stain, whereas those of *T. solium* do not.[9]

Life cycle (Figure III.49)

Gravid proglottids emerge in faeces or pass to the exterior independently; they then creep into grass or herbage, where they disintegrate. When the eggs are eaten by the ox, the oncospheres are set free and pass into the small intestine, where they bore through the wall and are carried to the muscles, especially the pterygoids and the fatty tissues round heart, diaphragm and tongue. Then cysticerci (cysticercus bovis) are formed, measuring 7.5–9 × 5.5 mm. They can be distinguished from other cysticerci by the absence of hooks on the scolices, other cysticerci having large hooks. They live for 8 months in the ox and develop further in the human, who constitutes the normal definitive host. The bladder is digested and the liberated scolex, passing to the small intestine, affixes itself by suckers to the gut wall. The cysts die at 48°C. Infected meat is known to inspectors as 'measly beef'. In Egypt and Morocco the camel is the most important intermediate host.

Cysticercus

The cysticercus has a small invaginated scolex (and a neck resembling that of an adult *Taenia*). The external tissue consists of hair-like processes, a peripheral collagenous fibrous layer, two muscle layers, peripheral cells, calcareous corpuscles, flame cells, a duct system embedded in a loose fibrous net and a central band of muscles. The different cestode larvae can be distinguished in human tissues by variations in these structures (Table III.7).[9]

Genus: *Echinococcus* (see also Chapter 84)

Echinococcus granulosus (Batsch, 1786) *E. multilocularis* (Leuckart, 1863) (Vogel, 1955) *E. ologarthrus* (Diesing, 1863) *E. vogeli* (Rausch & Bernstein, 1972) (*Taenia echinococcus* or hydatid)

Parasitology

E. granulosus is very small, 3–8.5 mm long, with a pyriform scolex, 0.3 mm in diameter, provided at the apex with a projecting rostellum, four suckers and two circular rows of hooks, varying in size and number

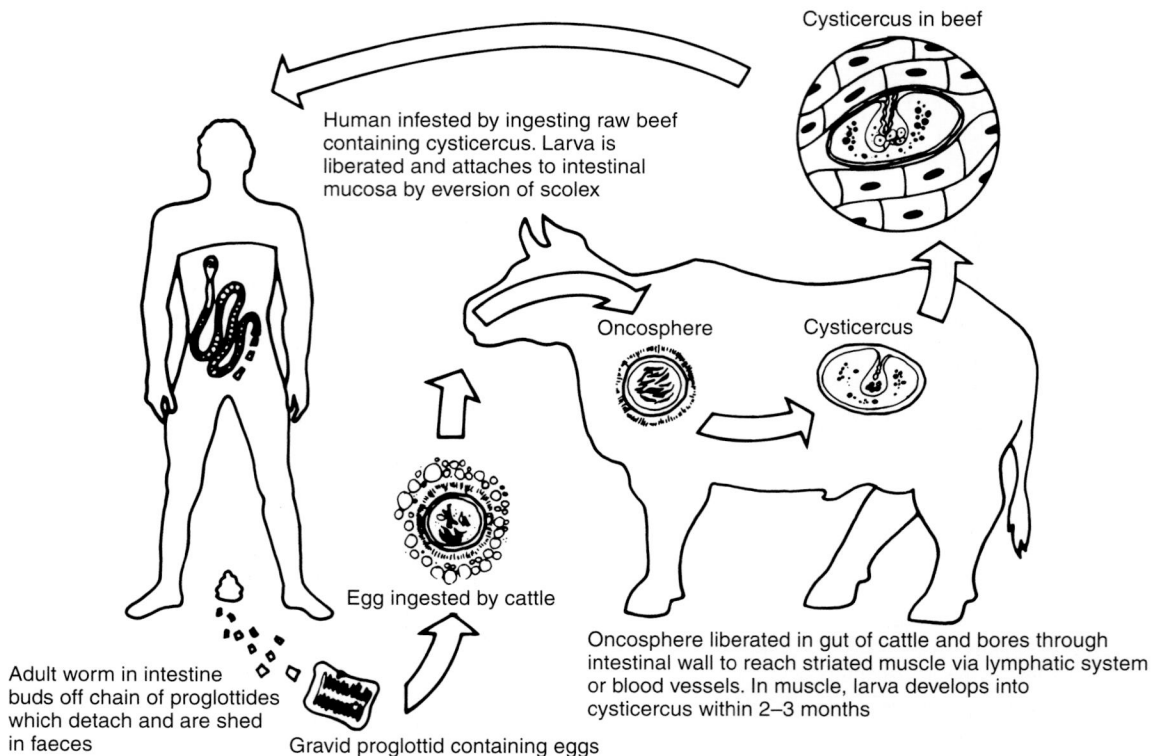

Cysticercus in beef

Human infested by ingesting raw beef containing cysticercus. Larva is liberated and attaches to intestinal mucosa by eversion of scolex

Oncosphere

Cysticercus

Egg ingested by cattle

Oncosphere liberated in gut of cattle and bores through intestinal wall to reach striated muscle via lymphatic system or blood vessels. In muscle, larva develops into cysticercus within 2–3 months

Adult worm in intestine buds off chain of proglottides which detach and are shed in faeces

Gravid proglottid containing eggs

Figure III.49: Life cycle of *Taenia saginata*. (Courtesy of Tropical Resources Unit.)

Table III.7 Diagnostic characteristics of cestode larvae found in humans.

	Cysticercus cellulosae	Cystecercus bovis	Cysticercus cerebralis	Echinococcus granulosus
Scolex	One	One	Several	Many
Hooks	Present	Absent	Present	Present
Bladder surface	Cuticle	Cuticle	Cuticle	Stratified hyaloidine material
Superficial hair-like extensions	Ranging from <1 Mm to 2.5 μm	3–6 μm	1–2 μm	None
Subcuticular groups of muscles	Present	Absent	Absent	Absent
Make-up of wall	Wart-like processes	Rugae	Smooth and also rugose	Smooth
Base of superficial protuberances	27–38 μm	50–70 μm	28–46 μm	None
Height of superficial protuberances	15–27 μm	23–27 μm	15–22 μm	None

After Slais.[11]

(Figure III.50).[10] The neck is short and thick; the proglottids usually four in number. The last one is the longest (2–3 mm); only one is sexually mature and this contains up to 5000 eggs. The genital apertures are marginal, one to each proglottis, in an alternating arrangement. The testes are spherical and numerous. The cirrus pouch is large and pear shaped. The uterus is tubular and median with short unbranched lateral diverticula. The

adult is difficult to remove from the small intestine of the dog without breaking its head. Eggs appear in dog faeces. Sometimes the fourth segment also comes away. The human is probably not a suitable intermediate host but is, of course, quite susceptible to hydatid infection.

The egg is spherical, 32–38 × 21–30 μm, and is double-shelled, the inner shell being thick. The egg is so similar to that of other tapeworms that it cannot be distinguished

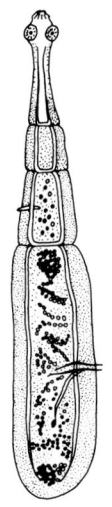

Figure III.50: *Echinococcus granulosis.* (15×.)

from them. The oncosphere contains three pairs of embryonal hooklets.

Two biological forms of *E. granulosus* are recognized on the basis of host specifity in the larval stage: the northern biotype and the European biotype. The reindeer and elk are the principal intermediate hosts in the northern biotype, whereas domestic ungulates of various species are the intermediate hosts of the European biotype. The application of molecular studies has allowed recognition of at least eight strains of *E. granulosus*: camel strain, buffalo strain, pig strain, horse strain, sheep strain, tasmanian sheep strain, cattle strain and cervid strain, all of which have known distributions.

Life cycle

The egg is passed out in the dog's faeces and is ingested by the intermediate host (sheep or human), by eating either contaminated grass or contaminated food. In the stomach the shell of the egg is digested and the oncosphere escapes. After 8 hours embryos can be found in the portal vein and liver, whence they are filtered out. The next filter is the lung, where a small number lodge. In 3 weeks the larval worm becomes vesicular and visible to the naked eye; in 3 months it attains a diameter of 5 cm and 5 weeks later has doubled that size. The hydatid cyst wall is composed of a fibrous laminated layer formed by the host, a thick median striated layer secreted by the cyst, and an inner 'germinal' layer from which the brood capsules and daughter cysts arise. There are two types of proliferation: endogenous and exogenous. In the former, proliferation is inwards towards the cyst cavity; in the latter it is outwards. The varieties of hydatid are so striking that alveolar hydatid (*E. multilocularis*) has now been recognized as a distinct entity which has a limited geographical distribution (see Chapter 84).

The brood capsules are formed from small nuclear masses of the parenchymatous germinal layer; later, they become vacuolated to form vesicles. Larval scolices arise

from a local thickening of the wall of the brood capsule; the wall evaginates to form a protective cup for the growing scolex. Near the head end the cuticle thickens and a circle of hooklets develops. The contractile part of the body of the scolex is capable of invaginating the head so that in the typical resting position the scolex has the hooklets inside. These hooklets may be strongly acid fast, a characteristic that can be recognized in histological sections and reveals that the structure is a dead hydatid cyst. Free brood capsules and free scolices in the hydatid cyst cavity are known as 'hydatid sand'. In other cysts the brood capsules never produce scolices and are known as acephalocysts.

Daughter cysts may be produced by injury or by mechanical interference with the mother cyst, inside which they arise from the detached germinal layer and also from the brood-capsule cells, rarely by vesicular changes from the detached scolices. In the liver the daughter cysts are bile stained. Intramuscular injection of scolices causes formation of new cysts and this accounts for the dissemination of hydatid cysts throughout the body, which sometimes occurs after operation.

Exogenous daughter cysts in the omentum and bones are secondary, caused by herniation or rupture of both germinal and laminated layers through weakened parts of the adventitia from intracystic pressure. By final exclusion of these herniations new cysts form.

Alveolar hydatid (*Echinococcus multilocularis*) (see Chapter 84)

In the adult worm the differences are the position of the genital pore in front of the middle of the proglottis. The number of testes is 21–29 (compared with 45–65). These lie behind the posterior end of the proglottis in the region of the cirrus sac. The uterus has no lateral branches. The length of the mature worm is 1.4–3.4 mm (versus 5–8 mm). The alveolar cyst grows by exogenous pro-liferation, invading the surrounding tissues and metastasizing. The cyst is solid with small irregular vesicles containing fluid and, very rarely, scolices.

Life cycle

The definitive hosts of *E. multilocularis* are dogs and foxes, and the intermediate hosts rodents, commonly of the family Arvicolidae.

E. oligarthrus and *E. vogeli* are about half the size of the other echinococci and the rostellar hooks are a means of identification of the protoscolices.

Genus: *Multiceps*

Multiceps multiceps. The adult worm is 40–60 cm in length, about 5 mm wide, and has a pyriform scolex of about 1 mm in diameter with four suckers and a rostellum armed with a double rank of 22–32 large and small hooks.
Multiceps brauni. The adult worm has a scolex armed with 30 rostellar hooks. The coenurus differs from that of *M. multiceps* in its larger hooks.

Life cycle

The definitive hosts of *Multiceps* are canines and the intermediate hosts sheep and other herbivorous animals.

Genus: *Vampirolepis*

Vampirolepis nana (Siebold, 1852) (*Hymenolepis nana, Taenia nana, H. murina,* dwarf tapeworm)

Distribution

This organism is found more commonly in warm countries: Egypt, Sudan, Thailand, India, Japan, South America (Brazil, Argentina and especially Cuba) and southern Europe (Portugal, Spain and Sicily, where it affects 10% of the children). It lives in the small intestine (Figure III.51).

Parasitology

H. nana is 25–45 mm long by 0.5–0.9 mm and has 100–200 proglottids. The scolex measures 139–480 μm, is subglobular with a well developed rostellum, a single crown with 20–30 hooks (14–18 μm) and four globular suckers (80–150 μm) (Figures III.45A and III.51). The neck is long; the proglottids are short anteriorly but the posterior ones increase in size and are broader than they

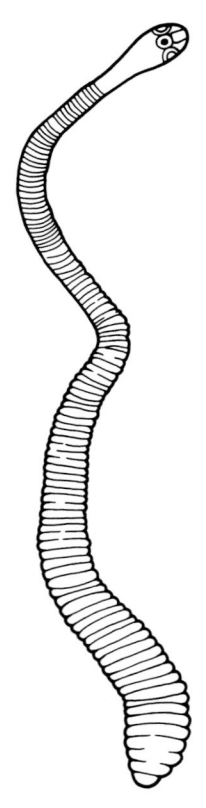

Figure III.51: *Hymenolepis nana.* Magnified.

are long. The genital pores are marginal and placed near the anterior border. There are three testes. The vas deferens widens into the seminal vesicle and the gravid uterus occupies the entire segment.

The egg is oval and there are up to 180 in each segment. It has two membranes: outer (vitelline) 40–60 μm, and inner 20–30 μm. There is a conspicuous mammillate projection at each pole, enclosing an oncospere there with three pairs of hooklets.

The segments, when freed, are partially digested and the eggs, set free in the faeces, are easily detected.

Life cycle (Figure III.52)

This worm forms an exception to other members of the group and does not necessarily have an intermediate host; the larva enters the villus of the intestine to become a cerocyst. In 40–70 hours after infestation the scolex appears; in 80–90 hours the rostellum has hooklets and then passes into the lumen of the intestine attached to the epithelium of the villus by a short neck. The rapidity of development varies greatly. Strobilization is rapid; the proglottids mature in 10–12 days and after 30 days eggs appear in the faeces to be ingested by another human host. *H. fraterna* of the rat is morphologically identical but its intermediate hosts are beetles and fleas (*Nosopsyllus fasciatus* and *Xenopsylla* spp).

Genus: *Hymenolepis*

Hymenolepis diminuta (Rudolphi, 1819)

This is a parasite of rats (*Rattus norvegicus (decumanus), R. alexandrinus*) and mice (*Mus musculus* and *Apodemus sylvaticus*); it is found as an occasional parasite of humans throughout the world.

It measures 20–60 × 3.5 mm. The head is small and cuboidal. At the apex is a rudimentary rostellum with four small, unarmed suckers. The neck is shorter than the head. The proglottides increase in size as the tail is approached and are broader than they are long.

The egg is circular or ovoid, measuring 60–80 μm; its outer shell is yellowish and thickened with indistinct radiations with a thin colourless, inner membrane, a granular intermediate layer, containing a hexanth oncosphere.

Life cycle (Figure III.53)

The cysticercus stages occur in the body cavity of insects and fleas during their larval stages: *Nosopsyllus (Ceratophyllus) fasciatus*; *Xenopsylla cheopis*; *Leptopsylla segnis* (mouse flea); *Pulex irritans*; in coleoptera and lepidoptera such as *Asopia farinalis, Anisolabis annulipes, Tinea pellionella, Akis spinosa* and *Scaurus striatus*; also in South America, in *Dermestes vulpinus, D. peruvianus, Ulosonia parvicornis* and *Embia argentina* (etc.).

The rat becomes parasitized by eating infected fleas or other insects. The cysticercoids, when ingested by the definitive host, become adult in 17 days.

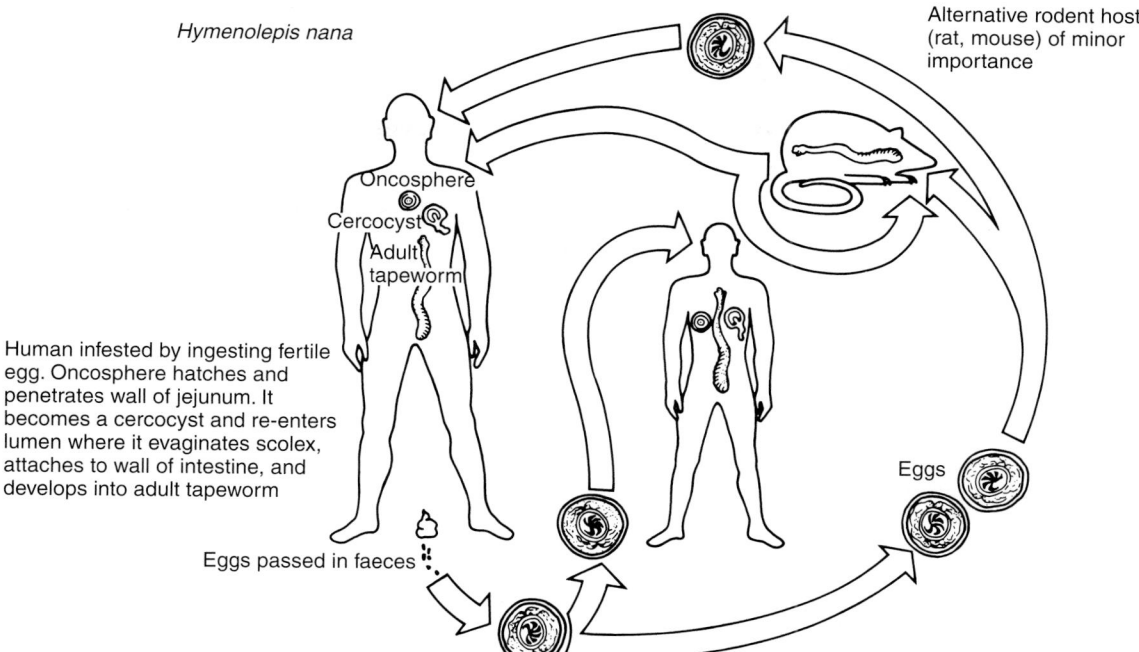

Hymenolepis nana

Alternative rodent host (rat, mouse) of minor importance

Oncosphere

Cercocyst

Adult tapeworm

Human infested by ingesting fertile egg. Oncosphere hatches and penetrates wall of jejunum. It becomes a cercocyst and re-enters lumen where it evaginates scolex, attaches to wall of intestine, and develops into adult tapeworm

Eggs passed in faeces

Eggs

Figure III.52: Life cycle of *Hymenolepis nana*.

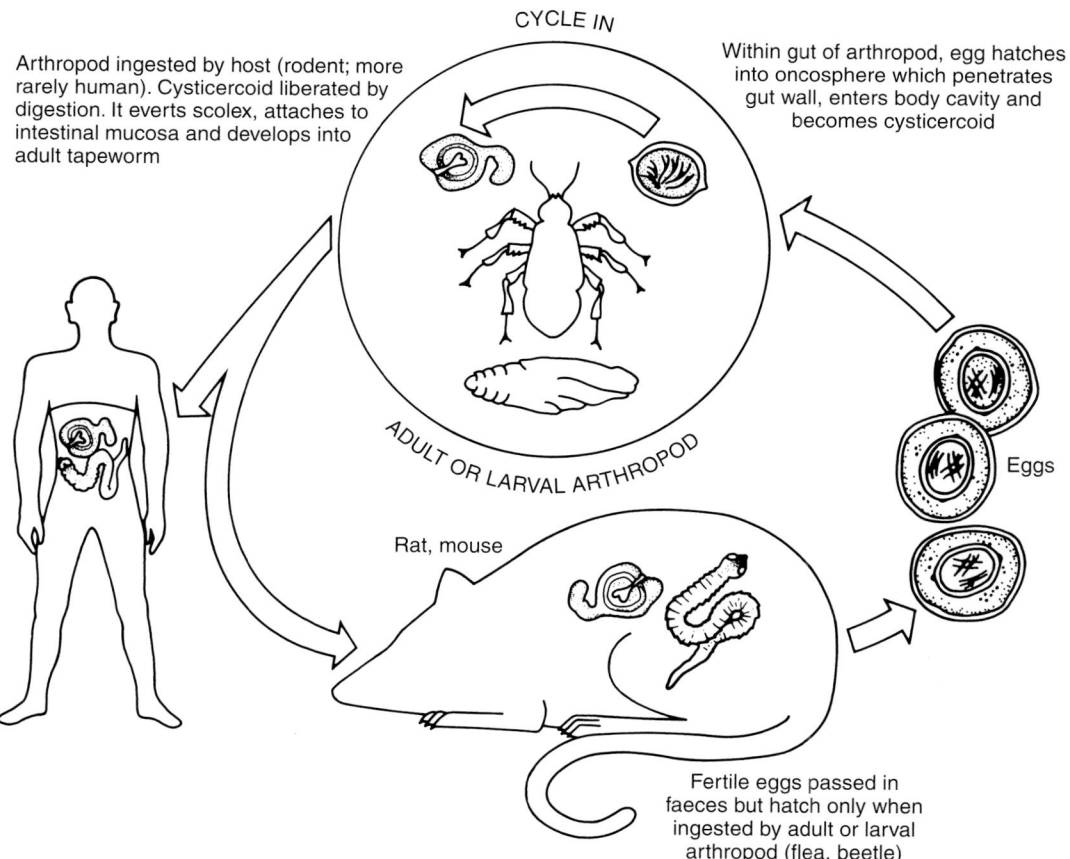

CYCLE *IN*

Arthropod ingested by host (rodent; more rarely human). Cysticercoid liberated by digestion. It everts scolex, attaches to intestinal mucosa and develops into adult tapeworm

Within gut of arthropod, egg hatches into oncosphere which penetrates gut wall, enters body cavity and becomes cysticercoid

ADULT OR LARVAL ARTHROPOD

Rat, mouse

Eggs

Fertile eggs passed in faeces but hatch only when ingested by adult or larval arthropod (flea, beetle)

Figure III.53: Life cycle of *Hymenolepis diminuta*.

Genus: *Dipylidium*

Dipylidium caninum (Linnaeus, 1758)

This is a common parasite of the dog, cat and jackal. There are many records of its occurrence in humans worldwide, especially in children in European countries.

It lives in the small intestine and measures 15–40 cm × 2–3 mm. The scolex is small and globular, 0.55 mm in diameter. The rostellum has three or four circles consisting of 28–30 hooks (14–18 μm) of 'rose-thorn' shape and four elliptical suckers (Figure III.45B). The proglottides are narrow; there are 200 or more of them. The segments measure 6–7 × 2.3 mm. Two sets of genital apparatus are found in each segment; the genital pores are placed symmetrically at the lateral margins. The uterine cavities contain egg nests, each consisting of 8–15 eggs. Mature proglottides leave the intestine. The egg is round, 35–40 μm across.

The cysticercoid stage is passed through in the dog louse (*Trichodectes canis*), dog flea (*Ctenocephalides canis*), cat flea (*C. felis*) and human flea (*Pulex irritans*). Eggs are eaten by the larval flea and the hexacanth embryo develops in the adipose tissue and muscles, first appearing as a procercoid and later as a cysticercoid larva. Infection of humans is accidental, as results from swallowing infected fleas.

Genus: *Raillietina*

R. madagascariensis (formerly *Taenia madagascariensis*), *R. demerariensis*, *R. celebensis*, etc.

These worms are found in Asia, Oceania and South America, and *R. demerariensis* has been reported in Ecuador and Australia from *Rattus fuscipes*. Two cases were reported from Thailand as *R. siviragi*. They are characterized by numerous hooks of 'coal-hammer' shape on the suckers and rostellum, and by unilateral genital pores on the proglottides. Ripe segments contain egg capsules. The ovoid eggs possess conspicuously large hooklets. Usually they are parasites of birds, more rarely of rats. Their intermediate hosts are probably flies.

Genus: *Bertiella*

Bertiella studeri has often been found in humans, and cases of infection with *Bertiella mucronata*, a tapeworm of monkeys, in Central and South America have been reported.[8]

Genus: *Inermicapsifer*

This genus closely resembles the foregoing and cannot be distinguished from it by the ripe proglottides, and, like *Bertiella*, the scolex and suckers are unarmed. *I. arvicanthidis*, a parasite normally of the field rat, was found in a European child from Kenya; since then others have been reported in Ruanda-Burundi and Arusha, Tanzania. It is suggested that it is more common than has

been supposed. No fewer than 12 species of *Inermicapsifer* are parasites of hyraxes and rodents in Africa. *I. cubensis* appears to be common in Cuba, where 76 cases in humans have been described. It is identical with the foregoing; *I. madagascariensis* is also identical.

Nematodes Phylum: Nemathelminthes Class: Nematoda or roundworms

The sexes of these worms are separate. They are cylindrical, non-segmented, and taper at both ends. They are white or yellow, sometimes semitransparent, and their eggs are characteristic.

Superfamily: Ascaridoidea

Genus: *Ascaris*

Ascaris lumbricoides (Linnaeus, 1758) (roundworm)

Characters

Ascaris lumbricoides inhabits the intestine of humans, and allied species are found in the pig, cat, dog and horse.

The adult female worm measures 20–35 cm × 3–6 mm, the male 15–31 cm × 2–4 mm (Figure 83.8). Both are pale and brown with whitish longitudinal lines and round tapering ends. The mouth is at the anterior end and is guarded by thin lips with finely denticulated ridges (Figure III.54). The anus is subterminal. In the female the vulva is anterior to the middle of the body. The vagina is directed backward and there are paired genital tubes each containing the uterus, receptaculum seminis, oviduct and ovary. The tubules and ducts attain a length of 12 cm and the capacity at any one time is 27 million eggs, the average daily output being 200 000. The male tail is conical without caudal alae and is curved in a semicircle with two rows of tactile papillae, mostly preanal but a few postanal. There are two chitinous spicules. The adults have a life span of 10–12 months.

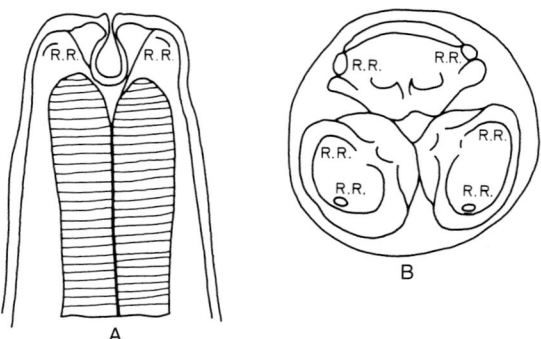

Figure III.54: Head of *Ascaris lumbricoides*. **(A)** Ventral view. **(B)** Anterior view, showing the oral labia.

The egg measures 50–70 × 40–50 μm and is elliptical; it is encased in a rough albuminous coat, giving it a mamillated appearance. It is usually stained by faecal pigments (Figure III.5).

Life cycle

When the eggs are passed in the faeces there is no segmentation or differentiated embryo. In water or in moist earth at 36–40°C within 2–4 months the embryo is seen coiled up and moving inside the eggshell. The larva undergoes a moult before hatching and must be transformed into a second-stage larva of the 'rhabditoid' type before it is infective. The embryo does not emerge from the egg until it is swallowed. The eggshell is then softened by the digestive juice and hatches in the small intestine. The rhabditiform larva penetrates the mucous membrane, enters the blood via the heart and lungs, and reaches the alveolar capillaries where it has a 'bloodbath'. As the larvae cannot pass through they burrow through the wall of the alveolus and enter the respiratory tree, finally being carried up the trachea by ciliary action. Eventually, on reaching the vocal cords, the majority of the larvae are swallowed for the second time and reach the small intestine. The second invasion is often accompanied by severe allergic phenomena, urticarial reactions and a fall in blood pressure. The whole process occupies 10–14 days. During this time the larva moults twice (once after 5 or 6 days and the second time after the tenth day). The larvae measure 1.3–2 mm on the 10th day (Figure III.55) and 1.75–2.37 mm on the fifteenth. Larvae may reach the intestine as early as the fifth day. The fourth ecdysis takes place in the intestine between days 25 and 29. In humans the incubation period (to time of first oviposition) occupies a period of 60–70 days. The diameter of the migrating larvae from the pulmonary capillaries to the terminal airspaces is considerably larger than that of the capillaries.[12]

Ascaris suum (Goeze, 1782)

Ascaris suum of the pig is almost morphologically identical with *A. lumbricoides* except that the denticular ridges in the mouth are larger and have straight edges, but these differences are not constant. It has occasionally been reported in humans, but has been shown to be a distinct species.[13]

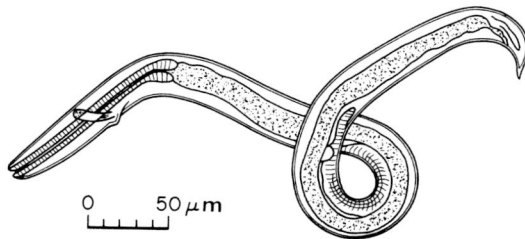

Figure III.55: Larva of *Ascaris lumbricoides* recovered from the trachea of a rat 8 days after ingestion of the eggs.

Genus: *Toxocara*

Toxocara canis (Werner, 1782)

Toxocara canis (the dog ascarid) is a cosmopolitan infection of dogs. The morphology is similar to that of *Ascaris*. The male worms are 4–6 cm long and the females 6.5–10 cm. In addition to the three characteristic lips of ascarids, there are distinct cervical alae or wings that are much longer than they are broad and extend some distance from the anterior extremity along the lateral margins. The perianal papillae of the male worms are characteristic. The ova are pitted superficially and measure 85 × 75 μm. They are dark or greyish brown and unembryonated when passed.

The life cycle is similar to that of *A. lumbricoides* with four larval stages. In pregnant bitches the pups are infected transplacentally and are born infected with adult worms laying eggs. They may die within the first few weeks of life, but, if they survive, acquire some immunity. Puppies are the main source of infection for children who develop toxocariasis.

Toxocara cati (Schrank, 1788)

This worm is the common ascarid of the domestic cat and some of its wild relatives. The male worms are 4–6 cm long and the females 4–12 cm. The anterior end has characteristic ascarid lips and is provided with a pair of broad lateral cervical alae or wings which give a pyriform outline to the anterior end of the body. The eggs are similar to those of *T. canis*, as is the life cycle.

Genus: *Lagochilascaris*

Lagochilascaris minor (Leiper, 1909)

The usual host of *Lagochilascaris minor* is unresolved. Adult males measure 5–17 × 0.19–0.6 mm, females measure 20–60 × 0.2–0.81 mm. They are ascarid in morphology but the lips bear no denticles and they have a keel-like cuticular ledge along the entire extent of the lateral line. The eggs are spherical or slightly ovoid and measure 50 × 65 μm.

Life cycle

Adult worms live in cavities in the submucosa of the small intestine of the opossum, and eggs are passed out in the stool containing infective larvae, which wait until they are ingested by mice and other small mammals when they hatch in the intestine and migrate to skeletal muscle to wait until the definitive host eats its prey.

Superfamily: Spirudoidea

Genus: *Gnathostoma*

Gnathostoma spinigerum (Owen, 1838)

The adult worms are parasites of both wild and domestic felines and canines. Cats and dogs are important reservoirs.

Parasitology

The adult worms in the feline host vary in length from 11 to 25 mm for males and 25–54 mm for females. They are stout, reddish-coloured, slightly transparent nematodes with a subglobose cephalic swelling separated from the remainder of the worm by a cervical constriction. The anterior half of the nematode is covered with leaf-like spines which are broader and tridented just behind the cervix, and narrower and single-pointed more equatorially. These spines are characteristic of the species.

The cephalic portion of the body is covered with four to eight transverse rows of sharp recurved hooks. Four conspicuous cervical glands, arranged symmetrically around the oesophagus, fuse in pairs and open through two ducts which perforate the lips. The male has a pseudobursa which is provided with four pairs of perianal papillae. The copulatory spicules are chitinoid rods measuring 1.1 and 0.4 mm, respectively. The vulva of the female is slightly postequatorial in position. The vagina is long and anteriorly directed. The other genital tubes are paired.

The eggs (Figure III.56F) are ovoid and 65–70 × 38–40 μm in size. They are transparent, superficially pitted, have a mucoid plug at one end and are unembryonated when laid.

The adult lives in tumours in the stomach wall of felines and dogs. Eggs are extruded from lesions and evacuated via the faeces into water, where they embryonate and hatch.

A motile first-stage larva, measuring 223–275 × 13.4–17.4 μm and having a rounded anterior end provided with spines, emerges from the shell and actively enters a species of *Cyclops*, bores its way into the haemocele and metamorphoses in 10–14 days into a second-stage larva (350–450 × 60–65 μm), which is provided with a head bulb armed with four rings of spines and two pairs of cervical glands.

The *third-stage larva* (Figure III.56) develops in a second intermediate host which can be a snake (rock python, cobra in India), freshwater fish (Philippines) or frog (Thailand), crayfish, crabs, amphibia, reptiles, mammals and chickens (Thailand) as well as humans, in whom complete maturation does not take place, the larva wandering around the body causing pathological damage. Complete maturation to the felines is in about 6.5 months.

Four species of *Cyclops* can act as the first intermediate host and 28 species of fish and vertebrates as the second intermediate host: two species of freshwater fish, three species of amphibian, five species of reptile, three species of fowl, two species of crab and 13 species of rodents and monkeys.

Genus: *Physaloptera*

Physaloptera caucasica (von Linstow, 1902) (*P. mordens*) (Leiper, 1907)

Normal hosts are monkeys. In humans it has been found in central Africa, Mozambique, Uganda and Malawi. It lives in the oesophagus, stomach, small intestine and occasionally the liver.

The female (2.4–10 cm × 1.14–2.8 mm) has a posterior end tapering to a sharp point, two ovaries, a single uterine tube, and a vulva in the anterior part of the body. The male (1.4–5 cm × 0.7–1 mm) has two lateral alae on the tail, formed by expansion of the cuticle, four pairs of pedunculated papillae—six pairs sessile—one unpaired postanal papilla, and two spicules of unequal length. In both sexes the mouth is guarded by two large lips, armed with two papillae and rows of teeth, which serve to grip the mucous membrane (Figure III.57).

The egg (45 × 35 μm) has a double contour, smooth, thick, colourless shell.

The life cycle is unknown; insects possibly act as intermediate hosts. The clinical symptoms are indeterminate. The worms live with heads embedded in the digestive tract from the oesophagus to the ileum.

Genus: *Anisakis*

Anisakis simplex (Rudolphi, 1809)

This is an ascarid parasite of herrings and marine animals. Its larval stages have caused symptoms in humans.

The adult form inhabits the intestine of sea mammals (whales, dolphins and porpoises) and the larval stages are found in a wide variety of fishes (haddock, mackerel, cod, pike, herring, bonito, salmon and Alaskan pollack) and squid.

The infective larva, as seen in the infective stage, is slender and thread-like, measuring 1.5–2.6 cm long and 0.1 cm in diameter. Its outer surface is somewhat striated and there is a ventriculus between the oesophagus and the intestine, with the latter two structures meeting on an oblique plane. There is an excretory pore in the anterior part of the head, ventral to a small larval tooth, and there are three anal glands near the rectum. Transverse section shows the lateral cords arranged in a Y-shaped structure along the upper intestine or oesophagus. The cuticle consists of three layers and shows no alae.

Genus: *Gonglyonema*

Gonglyonema pulchrum (Molin, 1857)

This spirurate nematode occasionally infects humans and pigs, but its optimum hosts are ruminants.

The worm lives most commonly in the upper portion of the digestive tract where it forms sinuous galleries in the mucosa and submucosa of the oesophagus, buccal cavity and tongue.

The male is 62 × 0.15–0.3 mm and the female much larger, 145 × 0.2–0.5 mm. The anterior extremity is covered with a variable number of bosses or scutes arranged in eight longitudinal series.

The transparent thick-shelled oval eggs are embryonated when laid and are 50–70 μm in length by 25–37 μm. Development takes place in dung beetles of

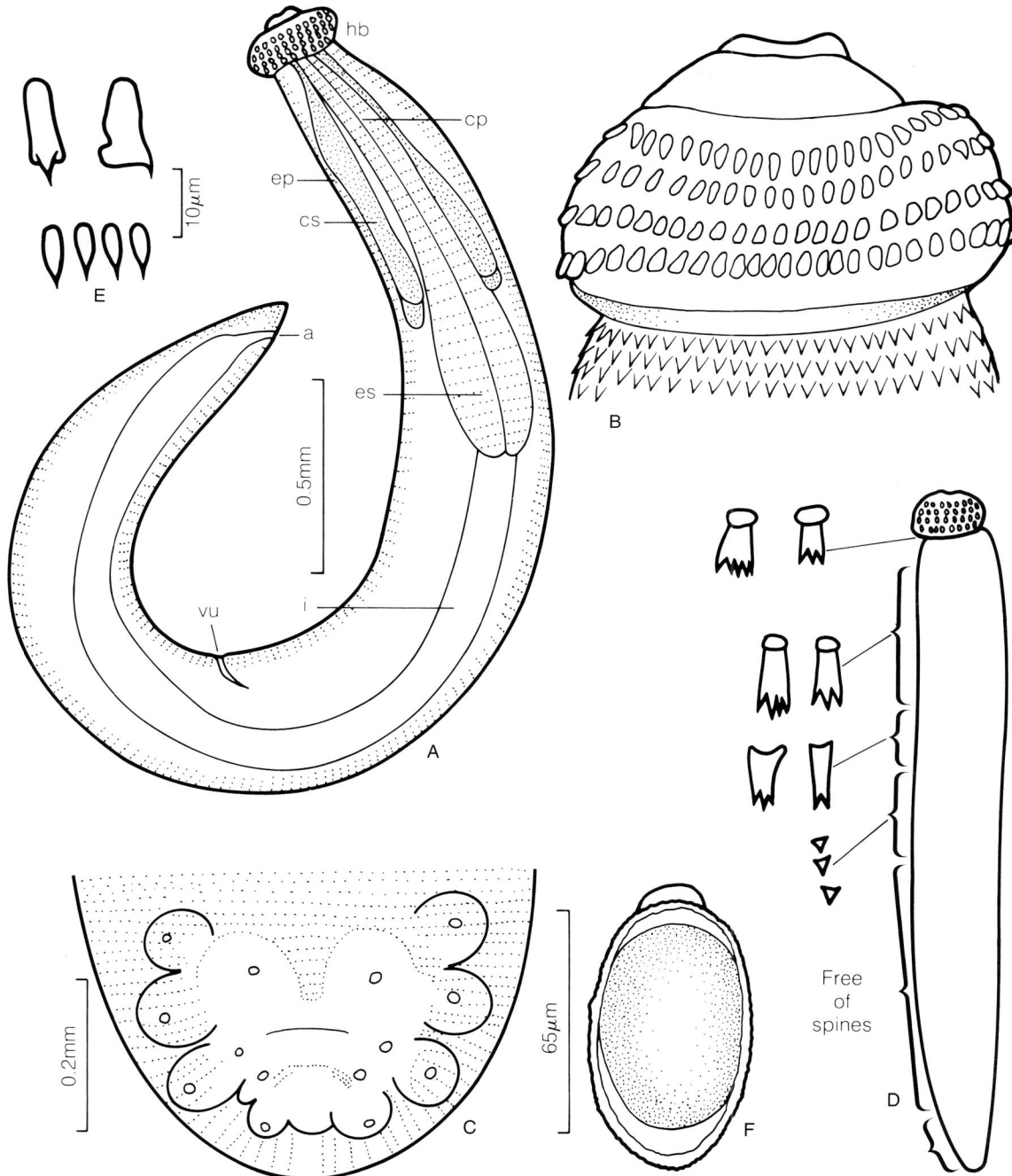

Figure III.56: *Gnathostoma spinigerum*. (**A**) Lateral view of third-stage larva. (**B**) Head bulb of third-stage larva with four rows of hooklets. (**C**) Posterior end of male, ventral view, with minute cuticular spines omitted. (**D**) Diagram of the types of spines at different levels of the body. (**E**) Detail of the spines on the head bulb. (**F**) Fertilized egg.

a	anus
cp	cervical papilla
cs	cervical sac (gland?)
ep	excretory pore
es	oesophagus
hb	head bulb
i	intestine
vu	vulva

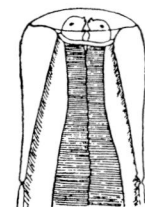

Figure III.57: The head of *Physaloptera caucasica*.

genera *Apodius* and *Onthophagus*, as well as in a small cockroach.

Superfamily: Strongyloidea

Genus: *Ancylostoma*

Ancylostoma duodenale (Dubini, 1843) (Old World hookworm, Miner's worm) (Figure III.58)

Both sexes are cylindrical, white, grey or reddish-brown (from ingested blood). The female (1–1.3 cm × 0.6 mm) is cylindrical and slightly expanded posteriorly. The vagina is in the posterior third. The body cavity is occupied by the ovary and coiled uterine tubes packed with eggs. The maximum egg output occurs 15–18 months after infection. The male (0.8–1.1 cm × 0.4–0.5 mm) has a copulatory bursa consisting of an umbrella-like expansion of the cuticle; the dorsal ray is divided towards the distal end into smaller rays, which again divide into three unequal portions (Figure III.59). There are two long delicate spicules. The genital papillae are tactile, finger-like projections near the anogenital opening. Owing to the situation of the genital openings in both sexes, the worms in copulation assume a Y-shaped figure.

Two well marked cephalic glands occupy the anterior third in both sexes and secrete an anticoagulating agent. The mouth end is bent dorsally. The excretory pore is ventral, placed at the level of the oesophagus. The buccal capsule is lined with chitin and contains two pairs of sharp teeth on its ventral aspect (Figure III.60). The worm lives mostly in the jejunum and to a lesser extent in the duodenum, but not in the ileum. The egg is ovoid (Figures III.5,14 and III.61) measuring 60 × 40 μm; the shell is thin and hyaline and is passed in the early cleavage stage (Figure III.61A–C). Outside the body it rapidly develops to the morula stage (Figure III.61D) and hatches in 1–2 days.

At autopsy 500–1000 or more worms may be found. They have a lifespan of 4–7 years. The interval between active infection and the final disappearance of eggs from the faeces may be 76 months. The female produces 25 000–35 000 eggs each day and some 18–54 million eggs during its lifetime.

Ancylostoma braziliense (De Faria, 1910)

This organism is found in dogs and cats in Brazil. In Sri Lanka *A. ceylanicum*, a closely related form from the civet cat, is reported.

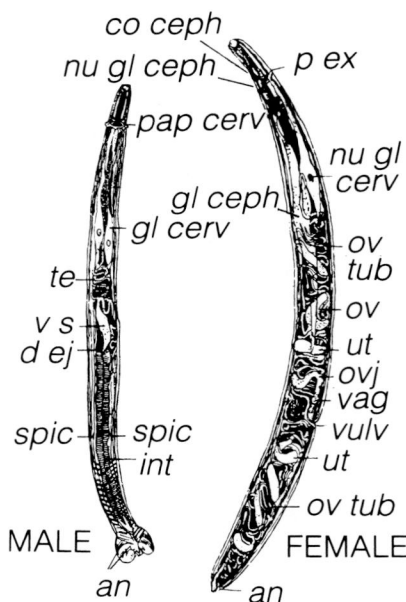

Figure III.58: Male and female *Ancylostoma duodenale*. (14×.)

an	anus
co ceph	cephalic nerve commissure
d ej	ejaculatory duct
gl	cervical gland
int	intestine
nu gl cerv	nucleus of cervical gland
ov	ovary
ovj	ovejector
ov tub	ovarian tubules
p ex	excretory pore
pap cerv	cervical papilla
spic	spicules
te	testes
ut	uterus
vag	vagina
vs	vesicula seminalis
vulv	vaginal opening

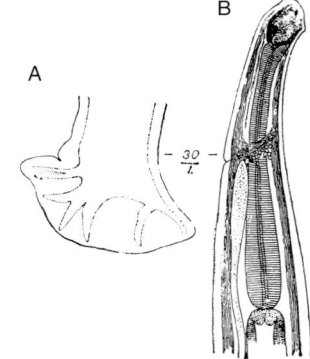

Figure III.59: (**A**) Bursa and (**B**) head of male *Ancylostoma duodenale*.

It is rarely found in the small intestine and then is part of a mixed hookworm infection in people in India, Malaysia and Thailand. It is smaller than *A. duodenale* and the internal pair of ventral teeth are smaller than the corresponding teeth of that species. The female is 1 cm

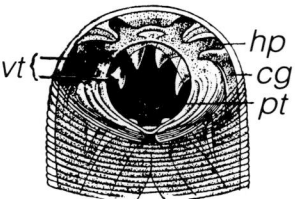

Figure III.60: Head of *Ancylostoma duodenale,* showing the hook-like teeth. (50×.)
cg cephalic gland
hp head papillae
pt pharyngeal teeth
vt ventral teeth

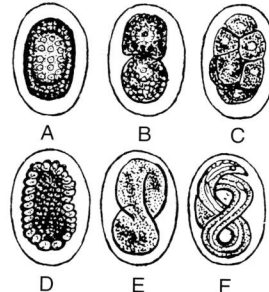

Figure III.61: Development stages of *Ancylostoma duodenale* of the larva in eggs; (**A–C**) are seen in fresh stools, and (**D–F**) when the stools are stale. (300×.)

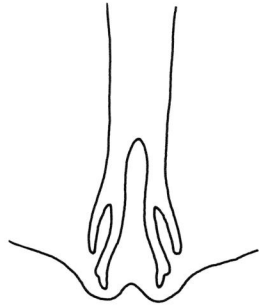

Figure III.62: Dorsal ray of *Ancylostoma braziliense.*

long and the male 8.5 mm. The rays in the copulatory bursa (Figure III.62) differ from those of *A. duodenale* and are distinctive.

The egg is indistinguishable from that of *A. duodenale.*

The life cycle is the same as that of *A. duodenale.* The human is apparently an unsuitable host. The larva does not penetrate into the bloodstream easily but wanders under the skin causing irritation (larva migrans; see Chapter 19).

Genus: *Necator*

Necator americanus (Stiles, 1902), New World hookworm (Figure III.63)

This is found in the small intestine of humans and also of the gorilla, chimpanzee, patas monkey, rhinoceros,

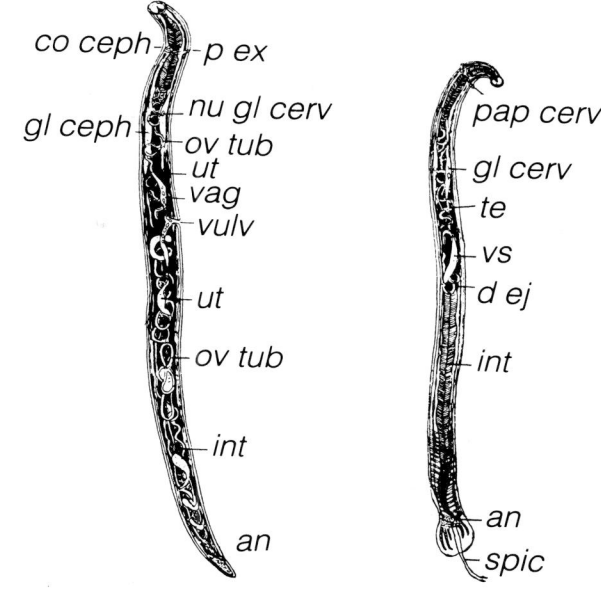

Figure III.63: *Necator americanus.* (12×.) Key as for Figure III.58.

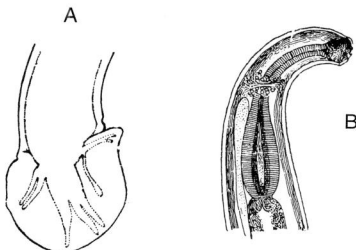

Figure III.64: (**A**) Bursa and (**B**) head of *Necator americanus.*

pangolin and a porcupine (*Coendou*), and develops also in puppies. On the whole, *N. americanus* is a shorter and more slender worm than *A. duodenale.* The female (0.9–1.1 cm × 0.4 mm) has the vulva placed slightly in front of the middle of the body so that it copulates at a Y-shaped angle, as in *A. duodenale.* The male (7–9 × 0.3 mm) has the copulatory bursa closed and blunt, and a short dorsomedian lobe which appears as if divided. The dorsal ray branches at the base into divergent arms with bipartite tips (tridigitate in *A. duodenale*). The base of the dorsal and dorsolateral rays is short (Figure III.64). Two separate spicules unite to form a single terminal 'fish-hook' barb. The living worms are greyish-yellow, at times reddish.

The sudden dorsal bend of the head, especially in the female, is distinctive (Figure III.64B). The buccal capsule is smaller than in *A. duodenale,* with an irregular border. In place of four hook-like teeth there is a ventral pair of cutting plates (Figure III.65). The first pair of dorsal teeth are represented by chitinous plates, The outlet of the dorsal gland constitutes a 'dorsal rib' or tooth which projects into the oral cavity. Deeply placed in the capsule are one pair of dorsal and one pair of submedian lancets.

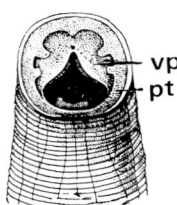

Figure III.65: The head of *Necator americanus*, showing the pharyngeal teeth (pt) and ventral plates (vp). (50×.)

The egg is slightly larger than that of *A. duodenale* (64–75 × 36–40 μm), but otherwise similar. The infective (third-stage) larva can be differentiated from that of *Strongyloides stercoralis* by the larger buccal vestibule and the intervening space between the oesophagus and midgut, and from *A. duodenale* as shown in Table III.8. The presence of 44 eggs per gram of faeces is reckoned to represent one female worm. The female lays from 6000 to 20 000 eggs per day. The estimated duration of life is about 5 years.

The life cycle is identical to that of *A. duodenale* except that *Necator* infective larvae enter through the skin only, whereas *Ancylostoma* can enter through the buccal mucous membrane as well, and that the migrating larvae of *Necator* grow and develop in the lungs in contrast to those of *Ancylostoma*.

Life cycle of hookworms

The eggs are deposited in the lumen of the intestine with two, four or eight blastomeres. They develop and hatch after expulsion in the faeces if they are deposited in damp, shaded soil.

The embryo moves about inside the shell and alters its shape, then escapes and gives rise to the rhabditiform larva which burrows into the faeces and feeds, especially on bacteria. At first it has a double-bulbous oesophagus (Figure III.66B). Feeding voraciously, it stores oil globules in its intestinal wall. It moults on the third day; on the fifth the oesophageal bulb disappears and the larva becomes elongated and fully developed at 20–30°C; the larva on the third day is 400 μm and on the fifth it is 500–700 μm long. It then moves away from the faeces into the earth, moults again and becomes the infective filariform, or third-stage larva, with a well developed mouth capsule, a simple muscular oesophagus and protective sheath, the walls of which are seen as two bright lines in the living specimen. It moves towards the oxygen

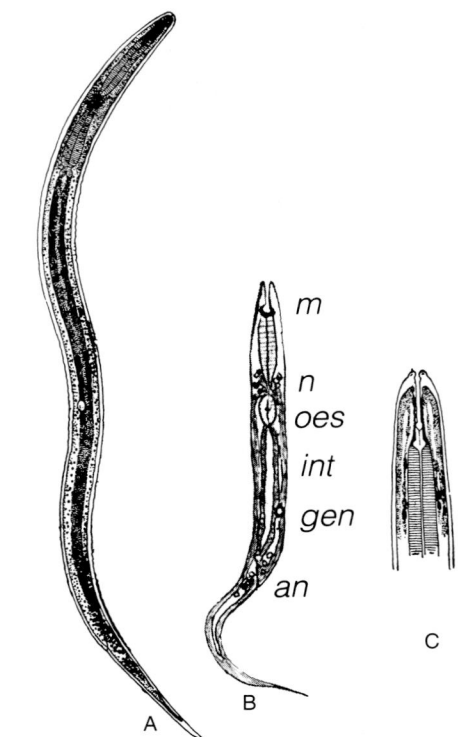

Figure III.66: *Ancylostoma duodenale*. (**A**) Mature infective larva. (**B**) Rhabditiform larva. (120×.) (**C**) Head of larva.

supply but cannot swim in water. The larvae are most numerous in the upper 2.5 cm of the soil. They can ascend from deeper layers but lateral movements are limited. Attracted by warmth, the larva is quiescent in the cold; it moves along a thin film of water as well as in the earth. Enabled by the sheath to withstand a certain degree of desiccation, the infective stage can live in warm damp soil under optimum conditions for 2 years (Figure III.66A). Direct sunlight, drying, flooding or salt water are fatal.

On penetrating the skin of the host, the sheath is left behind and the larva enters the lymphatics, then the bloodstream, and reaches the lungs on the third day. If pyogenic bacteria enter the skin with the larvae, an open lesion may develop, producing 'ground itch'. *A. duodenale* can infect via the mucous membrane of the mouth, as well as the skin, whereas *N. americanus* infects via the skin. Breaking through the alveoli of the lungs, it enters the bronchioles and travels via trachea and oesophagus to the stomach. During this migration the third moult takes place and the buccal capsule is formed. Migrating

Table III.8 Differentiation of third-stage larvae of *Necator* and *Ancylostoma*.

	Necator	Ancylostoma
Oral capsule	Sharply defined; visible dorsally and ventrally	Hardly visible; more marked dorsally than ventrally
Tail	Rather blunt	Pointed
Zone of closing cells	Leaves only small space between oesophagus and intestine	Leaves considerable space

larvae of *Necator* grow and develop in the lungs, whereas those of *Ancylostoma* do not. On arrival in the intestine on the seventh day it undergoes its fourth moult; the terminal buccal capsule is changed into the 'provisional buccal capsule' with the mouth opening directed dorsally, as in the adult, but without teeth. On the fifteenth day the 'provisional buccal capsule' is cast off and it then assumes the adult form with adult buccal capsule and bursa in the male. In 3–5 weeks it becomes sexually mature, copulates and produces fertile eggs. Adult worms live for 1–9 years and a female *Necator* lays 9000 eggs per day, and *Ancylostoma* 30 000.

Hypobiosis

A phenomenon known as hypobiosis has been observed[14] in which there is arrested development of migrating *A. duodenale* larvae, which migrate to the mammary gland, are secreted in milk and infect the child. This is similar to that seen in *A. caninumi*, which infects puppies in the same way.

Cultivation of hookworm larvae

A small portion of faeces is rubbed over a Petri dish with warm water, making a uniform layer like pea soup. Inside the cover is placed a circle of wet blotting paper. This is kept moist and incubated at 23.9°C under a shade. If there is too much water, the eggs will not develop. The larvae climb up the sides of the dish on to the blotting paper, where they can be studied.

Differentiation of hookworms

The striation of the sheath is indistinct in *A. duodenale* but very clear in *A. braziliense*. Rhabditiform ancylostome larvae are similar to those of *S. stercoralis* but are slightly more attenuated posteriorly and possess a much longer buccal vestibule. Infective (third-stage) *A. duodenale* larvae are differentiated from *Necator* by the oesophageal shears, which are unequal in thickness in *Ancylostoma* but equal in *Necator*, and by the features shown in Table III.8.

Genus: *Oesophagostomum*

Oesophagostomum apiostomum (Willach, 1891)

The female (1 cm × 0.325 mm) terminates posteriorly in a sharp point and has a vulva in its anterior half. The male (0.8–1 cm × 0.35 mm) has a copulatory bursa with a dorsal ray bifurcating into branches and forming a horseshoe-shaped structure, each limb giving off a short lateral horn near its base (Figure III.67).

The egg (60 × 40 µm) closely resembles that of *Ancylostoma* but is passed in an advanced stage of development.

The larvae hatch from the eggs in the soil. When mature, they are unsheathed. The rhabditiform stage is swallowed and passes through the stomach and intestine. Then it invades the wall of the caecum where it forms nodules and, on occasions, may penetrate the intestine

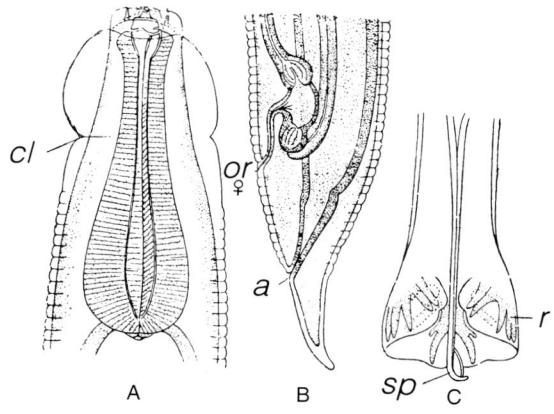

Figure III.67: *Oesophagostomum apiostomum (brumpti).* (**A**) Head, showing cuticular expansion and the oral vestibule. (**B**) Tail of the female. (**C**) Tail of the male, showing copulatory bursa.

a   anus
cl   ventral cleft
or   vaginal orifice
r   characteristic rays of bursa

and form intraperitoneal abscesses. The immature worms break out into the lumen, attach themselves to mucosa and become adult.

Oesophagostomum stephanostomum (Railliet & Henry, 1909)

This is a common parasite of monkeys (*Cercopithecus callitrichus*), gorillas and chimpanzees. The first case reported in humans was in Brazil; the patient died from dysenteric symptoms and peritonitis. It has also been reported in French Guiana and in northern Nigeria.

The morphology resembles that of *O. apiostomum*, but both sexes are larger and it is distinguished by a corona radiata with 38 leaf-like spines.

The eggs in the faeces resemble those of *Ancylostoma*.

The life history is probably similar to that of *O. apiostomum*.

Genus: *Ternidens*

Ternidens diminutus (Railliet & Henry, 1905)

The female (14–16 × 0.73 mm) has a genital orifice posterior and subterminal, and a short vagina opening into two uterine tubes (Figure III.68). The male (9.5 × 0.56 mm) has the dorsal ray of the copulatory bursa dividing into two distal extremities and each branch bifurcates again (Figure III.69).

The worm resembles a female ancylostome; its anterior extremity is not bent and the mouth capsule is terminal with a corona of setae. At the base of the cup-like buccal capsule, three serrated teeth guard the entrance to the oesophagus; this is characteristic of the genus *Ternidens* (Figure III.68).

The egg (84 × 40 µm) is delicate and transparent, and in an advanced stage of segmentation resembles that of an ancylostome.

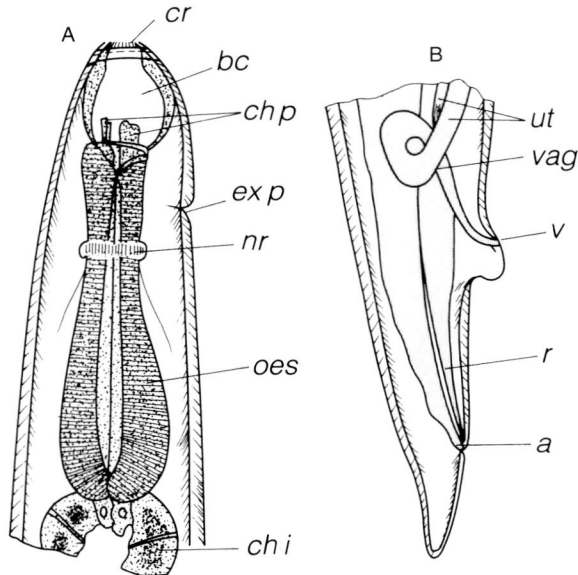

Figure III.68: Female *Ternidens diminutus*. (**A**) Anterior extremity. (**B**) Posterior extremity.

a	anus	oes	oesophagus
bc	buccal cavity	r	rectum
ch i	chyle intestine	ut	uterus
ch p	chitinous plates	v	vaginal opening
cr	corona radiata	vag	vagina

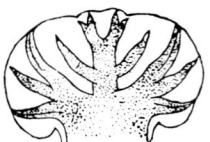

Figure III.69: Bursa of male *Ternidens diminutus*.

The rhabditiform larva (0.3 mm) with flagellar tail, hatches from the egg in soil, becomes sheathed and the infective filariform larva (0.6–0.7 mm) is formed. These can survive desiccation, reviving in water; thus they withstand drought.

The filariform infective larvae fail to penetrate human skin but gain entrance through the stomach and intestinal tract after the eggs are swallowed with soil-contaminated food or water.

Superfamily: Metastrongylidae

Genus: *Parastrongylus*

Parastrongylus cantonensis (Chen, 1935) (*Angiostrongylus cantonensis*)

The male is 15.5–22.0 mm in length by 0.25–0.35 mm in breadth. It is transparent and smooth with faint transverse striae. The head is smoothly rounded and the mouth is without lips. There are four pairs of minute,

submedian papillae which are sometimes visible en face, and two clearly defined minute triangular teeth present at the base of the oral cavity. There may possibly be a third, which is difficult to distinguish. The oesophagus is 0.29–0.33 mm long by 0.05 mm at maximum breadth at the posterior end. The intestine is a wide thin-walled tube. The excretory pore opens just posterior to the oesophageal–intestinal junction. The spicules are unequal, flexible and striated rods 1.2 mm in length. The bursa is well developed but the gubernaculum is absent and there is one pair of large adanal papillae.

The female is 18.5–33 mm long by 0.28–0.5 mm in maximum breadth. Cuticle, head, papillae, oesophagus and intestines are as in the male. In life, the spirally wound, milky white uterine tubules and the blood-filled intestine can be seen through the transparent cuticle and form a striking 'barber's pole' pattern. The uterine tubules unite about 2 mm from the posterior end to form the thin-walled vagina. The vulva is a transverse slit. The tail is obliquely truncated. The anus is 0.06 mm and the vulva 0.25–0.28 mm from the tip of the tail, which bears a minute terminal projection. The male : female length ratio is usually 2 : 3.

The eggs are ovoid with a thin hyaline shell measuring 46–48 × 68–74 μm. They are passed unembryonated.

The adult *P. cantonensis* lives in the pulmonary arteries of rats. Unsegmented ova are discharged into the bloodstream and lodge as emboli in the smaller vessels. The first-stage larvae, which hatch from these eggs, break through the respiratory tract, migrate up the trachea and eventually pass out of the body in the faeces. In Hawaii, the land snail *Achatina fulica*, the slug *Veronicella leydigi* and the land planarian *Geoplana septemlineata* have been found naturally infected.

Slugs (*Agriolimax laevis*) act as intermediate hosts. Two moults occur in the slug on about the 17th day. The slugs are then eaten by rats (*R. rattus*) and the larvae remain in their cast skins until freed in the stomach of the rat by digestion. They then pass quickly along the gut as far as the ileum, where they enter the bloodstream and congregate in the central nervous system some 17 hours after ingestion. The anterior part of the cerebrum is the favourite site and there the third moult takes place on the sixth or seventh days, with the final one on days 11–13. Young adults emerge on the surface of the brain from days 12–14 and spread during the next 2 weeks on the arachnoid surface. From the days 28–31 they migrate to the lungs via the venous system, passing through the right side of the heart to their definitive site in the pulmonary arteries. The prepatent period in the rat usually lies between days 42 and 45.

Parastrongylus costaricensis (Morera & Cespedes, 1971) (*Angiostrongylus costaricensis*)

P. costaricensis is larger than *P. cantonensis*. The male measures 22 mm × 140 μm and the female 42 mm × 350 μm, and the morphology is similar. The eggs are ovoid and measure 90 μm with a thin hyaline shell, and are passed unembryonated.

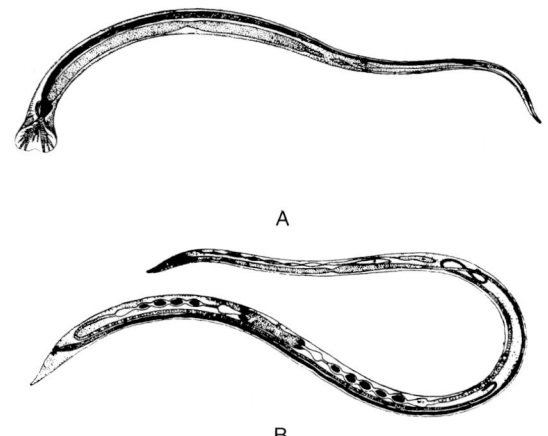

Figure III.70: *Trichostrongylus colubriformis.* (**A**) Female. (**B**) Male. (25×.)

Superfamily: Trichostrongyloidea

Genus: *Trichostrongylus*

Trichostrongylus colubriformis (Giles, 1892) and allied species

Normally this is a parasite of the upper small intestine of the sheep and goat; it is not infrequently found in the duodenum and upper jejunum of people in agricultural districts of India, central Africa, Egypt, Java, Australia, Japan, Korea and especially in Abadan (Iran), where 70% of inhabitants are infected. It has been found in Java in scrapings from the duodenum where the adults live with head embedded in the mucosa. By a flotation technique the eggs of this species can be found in the faeces, together with ancylostomes, fairly frequently in India and Assam.

The females (4–6.5 mm) (Figure III.70A) usually outnumber the males. They are very slender and pink with an attenuated anterior extremity and the vulva in the posterior quarter. The males (4–5 × 0.07 mm) have a bilobed copulatory bursa and two spicules (Figure III.70B). These parasites are found a third to a half buried in mucus. When scraped on to a slide they appear as delicate red streaks. When the slide is shaken in saline in a Petri dish, they can be seen against a dark background. The adult worms are never found in faeces. The mouth is unarmed.

The egg (85 × 115 µm) is relatively large, oval, thin shelled and contains a morula when deposited. It is apt to be mistaken for that of *Ancylostoma duodenale*; it is longer and narrower with more pointed ends.

The eggs hatch outside the body; the rhabditiform larvae metamorphose into infective filariform in 6 days at 22–25°C and can be distinguished from similar stages in *Strongyloides* and *Ancylostoma* by the bead-like swelling at the tip of the tail. The semifilariform third-stage larvae are very resistant to desiccation. These enter the body via the skin or mouth, undergoing two ecdyses.

T. orientalis (Jimbo, 1914) is commonly found in people who look after donkeys and goats in Japan, China,

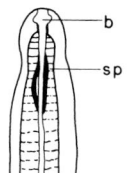

Figure III.71: *Strongyloides stercoralis.* Anterior end of the parasitic male. b, Buccal chamber; sp, buccal spears.

Taiwan and Iran. *T. probolurus* (Railliet, 1896) is rarely seen in humans; it is a natural infection of the gazelle and camel.

Superfamily: Rhabditoidea

Genus: *Strongyloides*

Strongyloides stercoralis (Bavay, 1876)

Parasitology

Formerly it was thought that embryos were produced by a parasitic, parthenogenetic female, in the absence of a male, but it is now known that a parasitic male exists, shorter and broader than the female. The oesophagus is characteristic, with a club-shaped anterior part and a postcentral constriction and a posterior bulb (Figure III.71). Later, two copulatory spicules and a gubernaculum are said to become apparent and, when developed, the adult male resembles the free-living form (Figure III.72,C). Parasitic males are found in experimentally infected dogs but not in human infections owing to the fact that they do not invade the intestinal wall and so are eliminated from the intestine soon after the females begin to oviposit. Although adolescent parasitic females may be inseminated, probably the majority are parthenogenetic. This is a process of *reversive metamorphosis*, in which the organisms loses the ability of penetrating tissues and remains a lumen parasite.

The female (2.5 × 0.034 mm) (Figure III.72,D) tapers anteriorly and ends in a conical tail. The mouth has three small lips and leads to an oesophagus occupying a quarter of the length of the body. The vulva lies in the posterior third. There is a prominent uterus containing 50 eggs (50–58 × 30–34 µm), which are laid in the lumen of the bowel in an advanced stage of development and may occasionally be found in the faeces. They hatch immediately to embryos (0.2–0.3 × 0.013 mm), which have a double-bulb oesophagus, and are apt to be confused with the rhabditiform stage of *Ancylostoma* and *Necator* (Figure III.66B,C). They are passed active in faeces and in 3–5 days are converted into free-living male and female forms, both of which have a rhabditiform, double-bulb muscular oesophagus (Figure III.72,B). The male is a free-living form (0.7 × 0.035 mm) (Figure III.72,C) with the tail curved ventrally, two spicules and an accessory piece. The free-living form of the female measures 1.0 × 0.05 mm. The vulva lies behind the middle of the body. The uterus contains thin-shelled eggs, measuring 70 × 40 µm (Figure III.72,D).

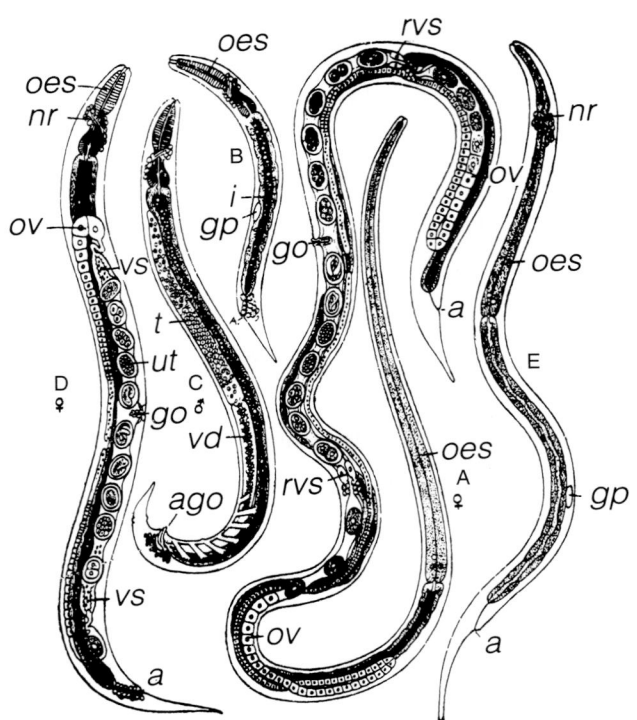

Figure III.72: Life history of *Strongyloides stercoralis*. (**A**) Parasitic female. (**B**) Rhabditiform larva. (**C**) Fully grown male. (**D**) Fully grown female. (**E**) Fully developed filariform larva. (30×.) (After Looss.)

a	anus
ago	combined anus and genital pore
go	genital opening
gp	primitive genital organs
i	intestine
nr	nerve ring
oes	oesophagus
ov	ovary
rvs	rudimentary vesicula seminalis
t	testes
ut	uterus
vd	vas deferens
vs	vesicula seminalis

Copulation between the sexes takes place in faeces. The rhabditoid larvae produced are indistinguishable from those derived from the parasitic female. After 3 or 4 days they develop into host-feeding, mature filariform larvae, which are the infective stage, and re-enter the definitive host via the skin or buccal mucosa, as in *Ancylostoma* or *Necator*, but remain alive in the soil for many weeks. The distinguishing feature is that the oesophagus in filariform larvae is half the length of the body (Figure III.72,E); in *Ancylostoma* and *Necator* it occupies about a quarter. Filariform larvae find their way into the small intestine and develop into female parasitic forms. Under unsuitable climatic conditions the sexual phase in the faeces may be omitted and rhabditiform embryos produced by the parasitic female may develop directly into filariform larvae capable of infecting the definitive host (Figure III.72,E). The larvae of *S. stercoralis* may be confused with those of *Rhabditis hominis*, a free-living worm that may gain entry by accident to the

human digestive tract. These larvae measure 240–360 μm in length by 12 μm in diameter and resemble the parent worm in shape and structure of the oesophagus and filariform larvae of *Ancylostoma duodenale*. The distinguishing features are given in Figure III.73.

Life cycle

There are two stages: parasitic and free-living in soil.

Parasitic stage

1. *Filariform* (infective) larvae from infective soil penetrate exposed skin or the mouth.
2. They may travel to the lungs via the intestine and copulate as male and female. Filariform larvae enter the human by penetrating the skin or through the mouth, and migrate through the lungs to the oesophagus; on arrival in the pulmonary capillaries the larvae produce haemorrhages, which form the avenue of escape into the alveoli, followed by cellular infiltration into the respiration passages with output of eosinophil cells. The changes result in *Strongyloides* pneumonitis. These develop in 2 weeks.
3. Females, with or without males, enter the mucosa (especially of the duodenum) and lay eggs.
4. Eggs hatch and larvae escape into the intestine. They may either (a) pass down and be evacuated or (b) become filariform larvae (infective) and re-enter the mucosa or perianal skin (autoinfection) and pass to the organs (e.g., lungs).

Free-living stage

Larvae from faeces in soil are either rhabditoid or filariform (infective). Rhabditoid larvae can either become filariform and invade exposed skin, or become male and female and produce rhabditoid larvae which continue the cycle indefinitely.

Strongyloides fuelleborni (von Linstow, 1905)

S. fuelleborni is a common parasite of monkeys and apes widely spread in human populations in tropical Africa, common in the rainforest and sporadic in the savannah, and a similar form is found in Papua New Guinea. It may be identified by prominent vulvar lips and narrowing behind the vulva in the free-living females. The prominent oesophagus in the free-living stages is also characteristic. The eggs are passed in the stools, in contrast to *S. stercoralis*, and resemble hookworm ova, for which they are commonly mistaken.

Superfamily: Oxyuroidea

Genus: *Enterobius*

Enterobius vermicularis (Linnaeus, 1758) (threadworm or pinworm, *Oxyuris vermicularis*)

This is the only nematode of humans with a double-bulb oesophagus in the adult. It is small and white, its mouth

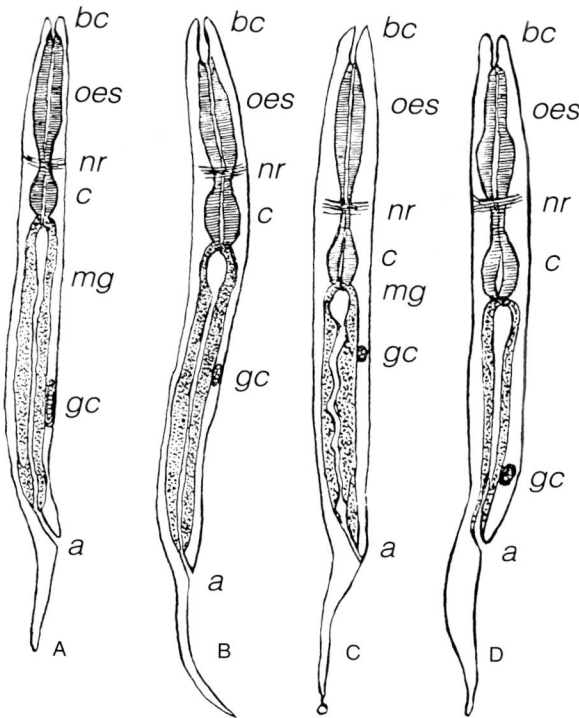

Figure III.73: Distinguishing features of nematode larvae in the faeces. (**A**) *Strongyloides stercoralis*. (**B**) *Ancylostoma duodenale*. (**C**) *Trichostrongylus colubriformis*. (**D**) *Rhabditis hominis*.

a	anus
mg	midgut
bc	buccal cavity
nr	nerve ring
c	cardiac oesophageal bulb
oes	oesophagus
cg	genital cells

Characters	*Strongyloides*	*Ancylostoma*	*Trichostrongylus*	*Rhabditis*
Average size	225 × 16 μm	275 × 17 μm	275 × 15 μm	240 × 12 μm
Posterior tip	Blunt	Sharp	Sharp with bead-like swelling	Sharp
Buccal chamber	Shorter than width at tip of head	Longer than width at tip of head	Longer than width at tip of head	Longer than width at tip of head

surrounded by a cuticular expansion and its skin transversely striated. The male is seldom seen and does not migrate like the female. Much smaller than the female (2.5 mm), its posterior third is curved spirally and its caudal extremity blunt, with six sensory papillae and a single spicule, 70 μm (Figure III.74B,C). The female (9–12 mm) has a long pointed tail, the anus 2 mm from the posterior extremity, and a transverse, slit-like vulva in the anterior fourth of the body (Figure III.74A). The gravid female lays eggs in a stream of 10 000–15 000 in a few minutes and dies when egg-laying is completed.

The egg (50–54 × 20–27 μm) (Figure III.5) has a characteristic shape, flattened on one side, and is almost colourless, with a bean-shaped double-contour shell, which contains a more or less fully formed embryo.

Life cycle (Figure III.75)

There is no multiplication of worms inside the body. The eggshell is weakened by the digestive juices and the larva breaks out of the shell. Soon afterwards it invades the glandular crypts and penetrates into the glands and stroma, where it coils up, causing some liquefaction of the tissues, but no cellular reaction.

The lifespan of *E. vermicularis* ranges from 37 to 93 days. As soon as the ovary becomes packed with eggs the female worm loosens her hold on the intestinal wall and lies passive in the faecal stream. The fertilized female migrates out of the anus to deposit her eggs in the perianal skin and perineum. The crawling of the gravid females produces intense pruritus. After a few hours the embryo develops rapidly and attains a length of 140–150 μm. The egg is ingested, generally as a result of deposits of faeces under the fingernails, conveyed to the mouth, and hatches in the digestive juices. Liberated larvae after two moults pass from the small into the large intestine, where they become mature. The whole cycle takes 2–4 weeks. Eggs can be inhaled through the nose from infected garments at some distance, and embryonated eggs have been found in dust. Damp conditions

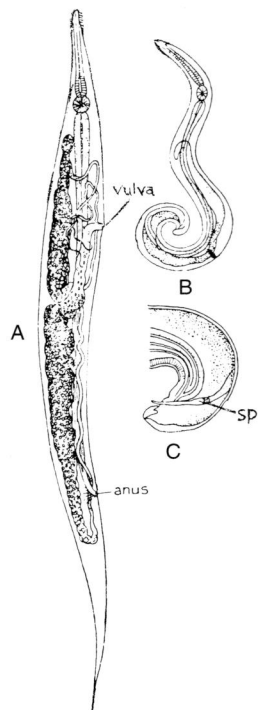

Figure III.74: *Enterobius vermicularis.* (**A**) Female. (**B**) Male, (**C**) Caudal extremity of male. (12×.)

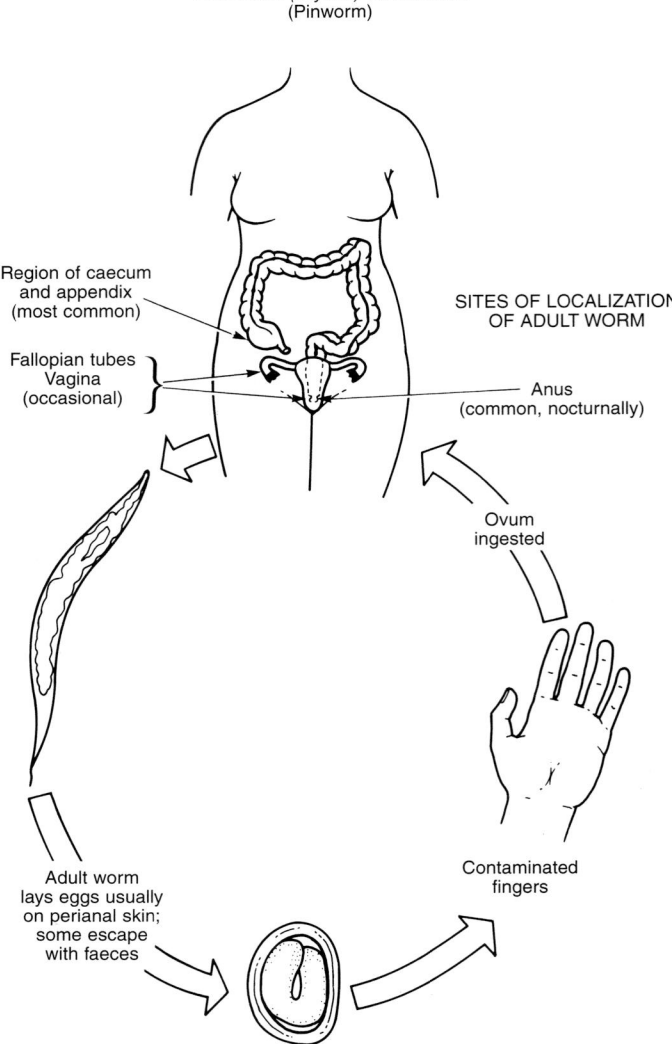

Enterobius (oxyuris) vermicularis
(Pinworm)

Region of caecum and appendix (most common)

SITES OF LOCALIZATION OF ADULT WORM

Fallopian tubes Vagina (occasional)

Anus (common, nocturnally)

Ovum ingested

Contaminated fingers

Adult worm lays eggs usually on perianal skin; some escape with faeces

Figure III.75: Life cycle of *Enterobius vermicularis.*

with minimal ventilation are necessary for survival. The eggs require a 6-hour exposure to air before they can hatch.

Superfamily: Trichinelloidea

Genus: *Trichuris*

Trichuris trichiura (Linnaeus, 1771) (*Trichocephalus dispar*, whipworm)

The male (30–45 mm) (Figure III.76,A) has an anterior attenuated portion, containing the cellular oesophagus, which is half as long again as the thicker posterior portion. The caudal extremity is curved ventrally through 360° and there is a single spicule in the sheath, studded with spines (Figure III.76,C).

The female (30–35 mm) (Figure III.76,B) has an anterior attenuated portion, twice as long as the posterior half, which is occupied by a stout uterus, tightly packed with eggs. A sacculate tubular ovary runs forward from the posterior end for over half the thick part of the body. Females preponderate over males in a proportion of over 400 to 1.

The egg (50 × 22 μm) is brown and has a characteristic barrel shape and a single shell with a plug at each end. It contains an unsegmented embryo (Figure III.5).

The worm is greyish-white or slightly pink and lives in the caecum where it maintains its position by transfixing a superficial fold of mucous membrane with its slender

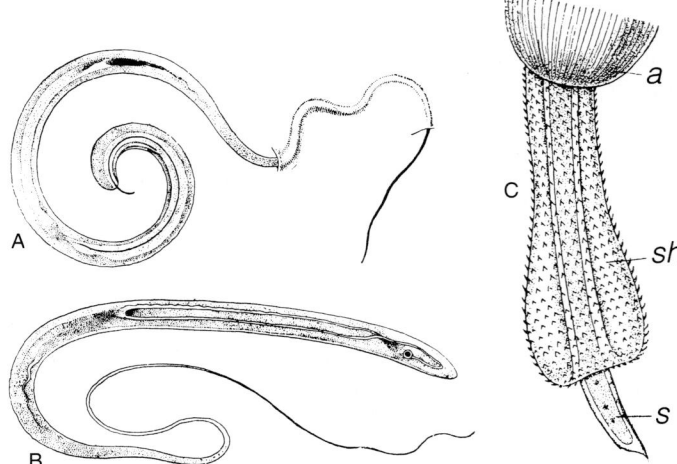

Figure III.76: *Trichuris trichiura.* (**A**), Male partly embedded in the mucous membrane of the intestine. (**B**) Female. (**C**) Copulatory apparatus, greatly magnified. (3×). a, Posterior extremity of body; s, spicule; sh, sheath.

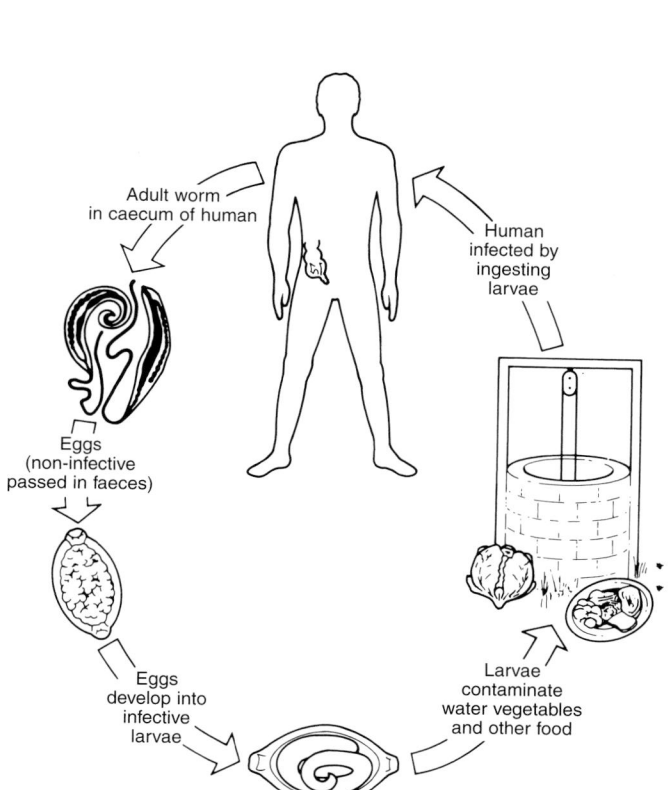

Trichuris trichiura
(Whipworm)

Adult worm
in caecum of human

Human
infected by
ingesting
larvae

Eggs
(non-infective
passed in faeces)

Eggs
develop into
infective
larvae

Larvae
contaminate
water vegetables
and other food

Figure III.77: Life cycle of *Trichuris trichiura*.

neck, and lying embedded in mucus between the intestinal villi.

Life cycle (Figure III.77)

Infection is spread chiefly by stale faeces. The egg is unsegmented; embryonation takes at least 21 days. It can withstand a low temperature owing to its thick shell. Moisture is necessary and it cannot withstand desiccation. Development is direct. The embryo hatches only when the egg is swallowed: the eggshell is digested by the digestive juices, the larva emerges in the small intestine, penetrates the villi where it develops for a week and re-enters the lumen. It then passes to the caecum or colorectum, where it attaches itself to the mucosa and becomes adult.

Trichuris suis of the pig, with eggs that are indistinguishable from those of *T. trichiura*, has been transmitted to a human in an experiment in which 1000 infective eggs were swallowed. The volunteer had no symptoms, but eggs appeared in the faeces in about 60 days and continued to be excreted for at least 10 weeks after maturation. *T. suis* may therefore be a cause of trichuriasis in humans, especially if in contact with pigs.[15]

Genus: *Calodium*

Calodium hepaticum (Bancroft, 1893) (*Capillaria hepatica*, *Trichocephalus hepaticus*, *Hepaticola hepatica*)

Calodium hepaticum is a parasite of the liver of the rat. The adult worms are very similar to *Trichuris*; the female measures 2 × 10 mm, the male being half as long. The eggs resemble those of *T. trichiura* but have an outer shell that is distinctly pitted and measures 51–67.5 × 30–35 μm. It has a direct life cycle like that of *Trichuris*.

Genus: *Aonchotheca*

Aonchotheca philippinensis (Chitwood et al., 1968) (*Capillaria philippinensis*)

The adult worms resemble *C. hepatica*. The male worm measures 2.1–3.7 mm in length and the female worm 2.6–4.9 mm. The eggs measure 45 × 21 μm and are of two types: one typical bioperculate, with a thick shell resembling a *Trichuris* ovum which is passed out in the stool unembryonated, and the other atypical, with a thin shell and embryonated resembling a *Strongyloides* ovum.

Life cycle

The typical eggs pass out in the stool where they are taken up by an intermediate host (small fish) in which they hatch and localize in the mucosa of the small intestine. The atypical eggs hatch in the host's intestine and the larvae reinvade the intestine giving rise to intestinal autoinfection.

Genus: *Trichinella*

Trichinella spiralis (Owen, 1835)

Trichinella spiralis (Figure III.78) is a white worm, just visible to the naked eye, which inhabits the small intestine. The male (1.6 × 0.04 mm) has a cloaca situated posteriorly between two caudal appendages and two pairs of papillae. The female (3–4 × 0.06 mm) has a vulva in the anterior fifth, an ovary in the posterior half, and an anterior portion occupied by a coiled uterine tube. The anus is terminal. Normally the female lives for 30 days and produces 1500 or more larvae which measure 100 × 6 μm.

Life cycle (Figure III.79)

The egg (20 μm in diameter) lies in the upper uterus, but the embryo soon breaks out from the shell and lives free in the uterine cavity.

The larvae are shed mainly into the lymphatics and bloodstream, reaching all parts of the body and encysting.

The cyst (Figure III.80) is formed by a larva encapsulated by the host tissues. The capsule is an adventitious ellipsoidal sheath with blunt ends which results from round cell and eosinophilic infiltration round the tightly

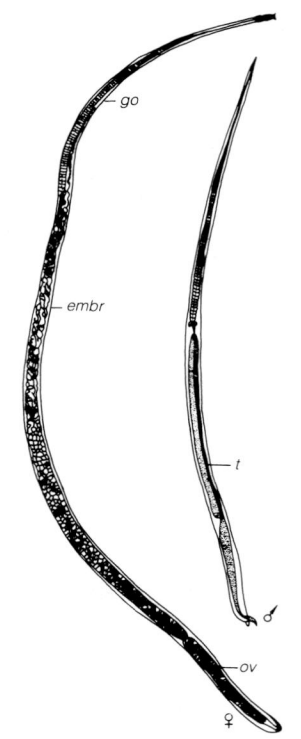

Figure III.78: Female and male *Trichinella spiralis*. (45×.)

embr	embryos
go	genital opening
ov	ovary
t	testes

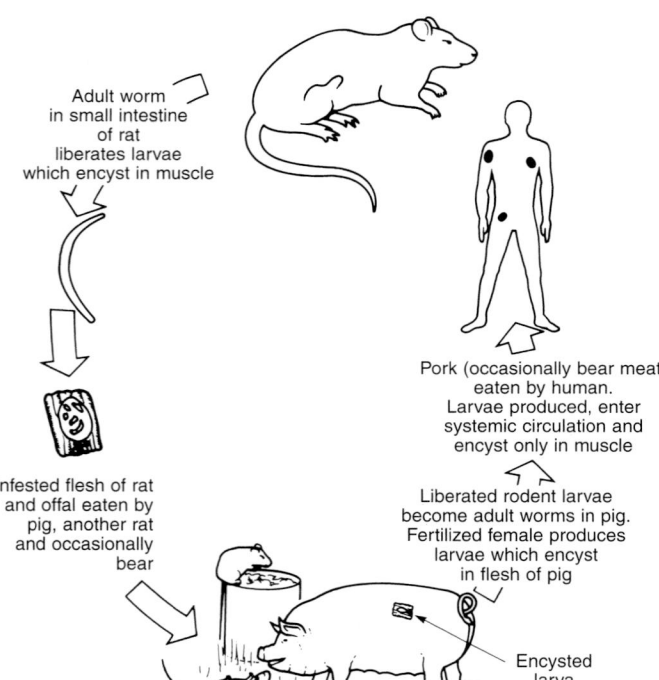

Adult worm in small intestine of rat liberates larvae which encyst in muscle

Infested flesh of rat and offal eaten by pig, another rat and occasionally bear

Pork (occasionally bear meat) eaten by human. Larvae produced, enter systemic circulation and encyst only in muscle

Liberated rodent larvae become adult worms in pig. Fertilized female produces larvae which encyst in flesh of pig

Encysted larva

Figure III.79: Life cycle of *Trichinella spiralis*.

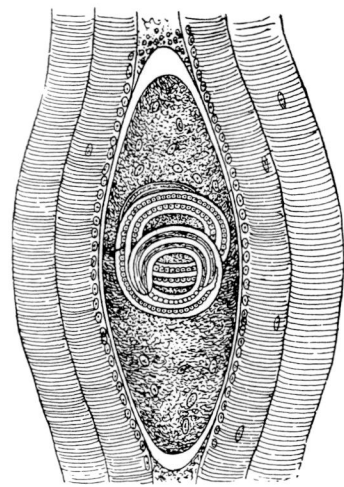

Figure III.80: Encysted larva of *Trichinella spiralis* 15 days after entering muscle. (300×.)

coiled larva. The long axis parallels that of the muscle fibres. Host amino acids can be transferred into the cyst and converted into larval protein so that an encysted larva remains viable for many years.

When consumed by a carnivorous host, the cysts are digested in the stomach and, after excysting, the larvae invade the duodenal and jejunal mucosa and develop through four ecdyses into adult males and females, which then enter the lumen of the bowel. Later they re-enter the mucosa and penetrate the villi, even reaching the mesenteric glands. Larviposition takes place over a period of 4–16 weeks or more. The larvae are carried through the right heart and lungs to the arterial circulation which they reach between day 9 and day 13, finally reaching the striated muscles where they encyst.

The number of recognised species of *Trichinella* has increased recently; they have been distinguished by morphological and molecular characters as well by by geography and ecology, and include:

1. *T. spiralis* (Owen, 1835): cosmopolitan; involving wild and domestic pigs and predators—domestic dog, cat, also bear and racoon.
2. *T. nelsoni* (Britov & Boev, 1972): Europe and Africa; involving pig, bush-pig, wart-hog and predators—dog, fox, wolf, hyena, leopard, lion.
3. *T. nativa* (Britov & Boev, 1972): arctic and subarctic America; probably involving fish and predators—walrus, seal, polar bear, fox.
4. *T. pseudospiralis* (Garkavi, 1972): Asia, Europe, Australia, one record from North America; involving marsupials, raccoon-like dog, raccoon, pig, bandicoot rat.
5. *T. britovi* (Pozio, La Rosa, Murrell & Lichtenfels, 1992): Palaearctic; involving rodents, insectivores, wild and domestic canids and felids, mustelids, bears, pigs, raccoon-like dog.
6. *T. papuae* (Pozio, Owen, La Rosa, Sacchi, Rossi & Corona, 1999): Papua New Guinea; involving domestic and wild pigs (not yet reported from humans).

7. *T. murrelli* (Pozio & La Rosa, 2000): North America; involving bears, raccoon, fox, coyote and bobcat.

Superfamily: Filarioidea

This group includes spirurate filiform nematodes adapted to inhabit the deeper tissues, such as the circulatory, lymphatic and connective tissue layers. Some insect intermediate host is necessary to complete their development.

Genus: *Wuchereria*

Wuchereria bancrofti (Cobbold, 1877) (*Filaria bancrofti*)

Parasitology

Adult filaria

This is a thread-like white worm found in lymphatic vessels and glands. The sexes are coiled together and can be separated with difficulty. The cuticle is adorned with small cuticular bosses.

The male (4 × 0.1 mm) is coiled with a corkscrew-like tail and two spicules, the larger of which measures 500 μm. The smaller spicule (300 μm) is grooved on its ventral aspect. There is a short, thick proximal and a whip-like distal portion, ending in a hook, and 15 pairs of minute sensory caudal papillae (Figure III.81A,B). A saddle-shaped thickening of the cuticle on the posterior wall of the cloaca forms a shield, and there is an accessory piece peculiar to *W. bancrofti*. There are 12 pairs of circumanal papillae of which eight are preanal and four postanal in position. There are also two pairs of large sessile papillae and at the tail a solitary pair of minute size. The female (6.5 × 0.2–2.8 mm) has a tapering anterior end with a rounded swelling (Figure III.82). There are sessile papillae on the head and an oral aperture leading to a cylindrical oesophagus. The mid-intestinal tube is one-third to one-fifth of the total diameter and opens into the rectum posteriorly. The caudal extremity is narrow and abruptly rounded (Figure III.81C). The vulva is 0.8 mm behind the anterior extremity. A swollen vagina (0.25 mm in length) leads into the uterus, which divides into two tubuli, which are much coiled, occupying the greater portion of the body with a

diameter three times that of the mid-intestine (Figure III.82). Two ovaries and ducts extend to within 1 mm of the tail.

The eggs lie in the upper uterus enclosed in a chorionic membrane, which becomes a sheath to the living embryos (microfilariae) (Figure III.83). They are emitted by the viviparous female and travel via the lymphatics into the bloodstream, whence they are abstracted by various species of mosquito. Their size in the distal part of the uterus is 38 × 25 μm, but as they are pushed to the vagina they become more elongated. The microfilaria develops from an oval egg and measures at first 216 μm. The embryo often lies curled up in its shell which becomes lobed, resembling a Dutch twist or pretzel.

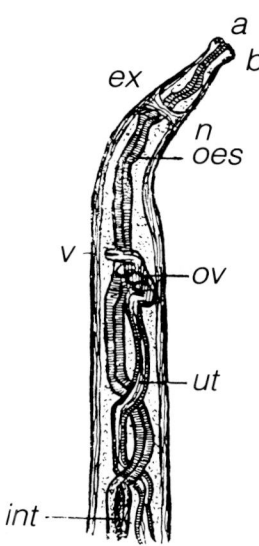

Figure III.82: The head of *Wuchereria bancrofti*, female. (50×.)

a	mouth
b	circumoral papillae
ex	excretory pore
int	intestine
n	nerve ring
oes	oesophagus
ov	oviduct
ut	uterus
v	vulva

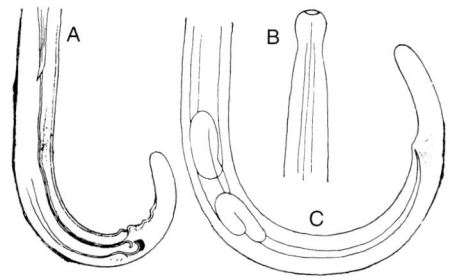

Figure III.81: *Wuchereria bancrofti*. Magnified. (**A**) Tail of male. (**B**) Head and neck. (**C**) Tail of female.

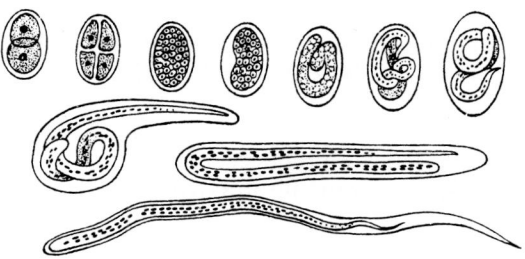

Figure III.83: Evolution of sheathed microfilaria from the ovum in the uterus of the parent worm. The later stages may occasionally take place after emission from the vagina.

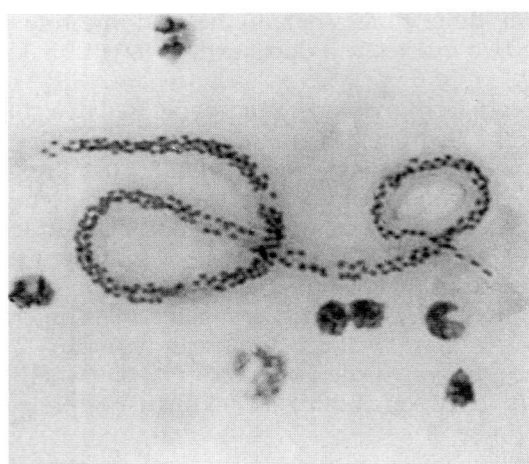

Figure III.84: Sheathed microfilaria of *Wuchereria bancrofti* in a blood film. (Courtesy of W. O'Connor.)

Microfilaria

The microfilaria (280 × 7 μm) (Figures III.84, III.85 and III.93 below) in the living state appears structureless. With higher magnification the entire microfilaria is seen to be enclosed in a sheath that is longer than the enclosed microfilaria and stains pale mauve with Giemsa, in contrast to microfilaria of *Loa loa*, the sheath of which does not stain with Giemsa. In this sheath it can move backwards and forwards and the collapsed portion trails after the head or tail. The sheath has been the subject of controversy. It is generally held to be the outstretched vitelline membrane but in the microfilariae of *Litomosoides carinii* of the cotton rat it has been found that a true larval sheath is developed during its sojourn in the blood. In the middle third is some granular material or primitive gut (*Innenkörper*). There is transverse striation of the muscular layer throughout. At one-seventh of the length from the head there is a break which denotes the nerve ring (nr) and at one-fifth of the length there is a triangular V-shaped patch, demonstrated by light staining with dilute haematoxylin, known as the 'anterior V spot', or the excretory pore and excretory cell (ep and ec). A short distance from the tail a second pore represents the anus, cloaca or terminal part of the primitive alimentary canal and is known as the 'posterior V spot'. Deeply staining cells are known as genital cells (g¹–g⁴) (Figure III.85). When stained, the body of the embryo is seen to be composed of closely packed cells and, by focusing when the movements of the living microfilaria have subsided, the head appears to be covered by a delicate prepuce. A short fang is from time to time shot out from the uncovered cephalic end and suddenly retracted.

Microfilariae pass with difficulty through the peripheral capillaries and they are less active in day than in night blood. They are capable of movement and of transit from place to place.

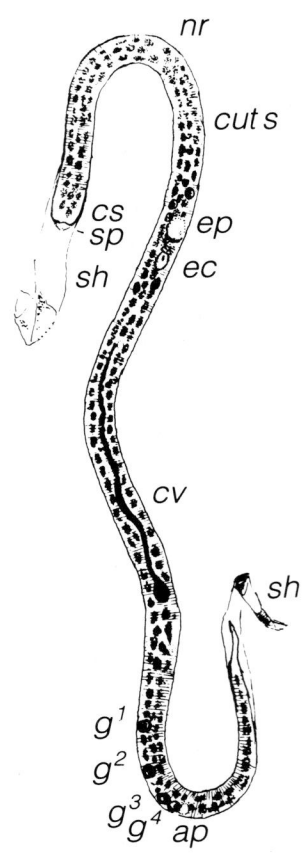

Figure III.85: Morphology of microfilaria of *Wuchereria bancrofti*.

ap	anal pore
cs	cephalic space
cuts	cuticular striations
cv	central viscus
ec	excretory cell
ep	excretory pore
g¹–g⁴	'genital cells' of Rodenwaldt
nr	nerve ring
sh	sheath
sp	spicule and prepuce

Periodicity (Figure III.86)

Microfilariae of *W. bancrofti* exhibit a nocturnal periodicity in certain parts of the world—in the West Indies, South America, north, West and East Africa, China, Indonesia, Papua New Guinea and Melanesia, i.e., they are present in peripheral blood in larger numbers during the night than during the day. The maximum concentration is from 22.00 to 02.00 hours. It occurred to Manson that this nocturnal periodicity was an adaptation to the habits of night-biting mosquitoes—*Culex quinquefasciatus, C. pipiens* and certain Anophelines. The numbers of the microfilariae are influenced by sleeping, and respond to waking and bodily activity. By reversing the hours of sleeping and waking, the periodicity is disturbed for 3 days and then reversed to diurnal periodicity. Periodicity can be easily converted by a change in the rhythm of day and night, and was found in emigrants from Okinawa

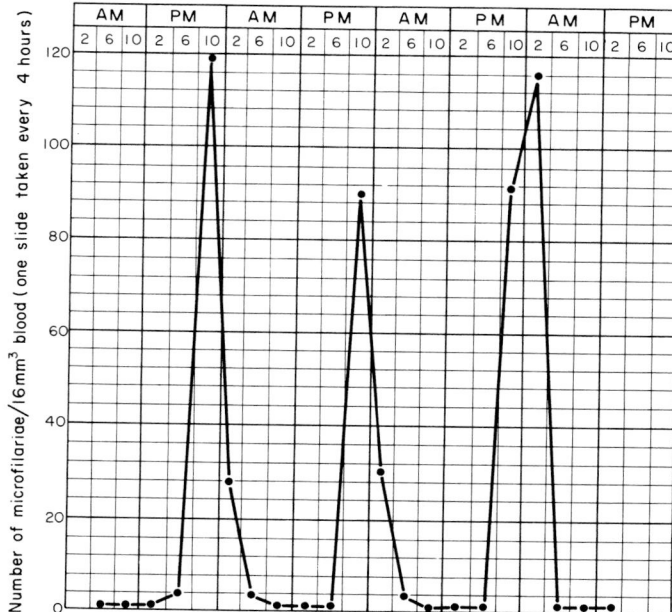

Figure III.86: Filariasis due to *Wuchereria bancrofti*, showing nocturnal periodicity.

(127° 40′ E, 28° 30′ N) to Bolivia (63° 30′ W, 17° 50′ S) to take 116 days.[16] Observations on microfilariae of animals (*Dirofilaria repens* of dog, filaria of American crow and that of Malayan monkey, *Macaca speciosa*) show that they also maintain nocturnal periodicity and reversal is easily established. Periodicity is probably a quality inherent in the microfilaria itself and persists unchanged in transfused blood. This was demonstrated in a patient injected with blood containing microfilariae and in whom a nocturnal periodicity was maintained for 14 days.

In 1897, Manson had an opportunity of ascertaining that during their diurnal absence from the peripheral circulation the microfilariae retire principally to the larger arteries and to the lungs where, during the daytime, they may be found in enormous numbers. Two mechanisms for periodicity have been suggested: alteration in oxygen tension of the blood and phototaxis on the part of the microfilariae.

Considerable light has been shed upon the mechanism of periodicity in general by the discovery of a nonsheathed microfilaria in a monkey (*Macaca speciosa*). In this animal, as in humans, the curve of microfilarial density in the venous blood follows closely that of the capillary blood. An increase of microfilariae in the blood at night is due to the periodic liberation from accumulations in the small blood vessels of the lungs.

McFadzean and Hawking[17] proved that the microfilariae of *W. bancrofti* are affected by the oxygen concentration in inspired air and by muscular exercise. The periodicity of *W. bancrofti* and *Brugia malayi* may depend on changes in the difference of oxygen tension between venous and arterial blood by day and night. During the daytime the microfilariae accumulate in the lungs where the oxygen tension is high. They manage to hold them-

selves in the pulmonary capillaries by some force that is increased by the rise in the oxygen tension and decreased by its fall. This force seems to be switched on and off every 12 hours by an unknown mechanism inside the microfilariae.[18] A curious agglutinative phenomenon has been described following the injection of anticoagulant (heparin) to the drawn blood. Intravenous injection of heparin during daytime releases microfilariae of *W. bancrofti* into the peripheral blood for a short period. It is presumed that microfilariae gather together in the capillaries and other vessels of the lung during their absence from the peripheral blood by the power of agglutination and thigmotaxis. A different mechanism for periodicity has been suggested,[16] in which the microfilariae possess a photosensitive substance containing a vitamin A-like carotenoid, similar to visual pigments in fluorescent granules in the epidermis, which causes them to leave the peripheral circulation in daylight and collect in the lungs. Periodic microfilariae possess numerous granules, in contrast to subperiodic and aperiodic forms, which have few or none.

A general anaesthetic does not affect the periodicity of *W. bancrofti* but markedly reduces the numbers of *L. loa* microfilariae in the peripheral blood.[18]

Formerly it was thought that nocturnal periodicity was uniformly observed by the microfilariae of *W. bancrofti* the world over, but in 1896 it was demonstrated that in Tonga and Fiji the microfilariae were abundant in the blood both by day and by night; those in the western Pacific, the Solomon Islands, Papua New Guinea and Bismarck Archipelago are nocturnally periodic, but in New Caledonia the microfilariae are non-periodic. The demarcating line between the two (Buxton's line) lies in longitude 170° E and this also coincides with the distribution of malaria. To the west of this line there are *Anopheles* and malaria; to the east there is neither. It was originally demonstrated that in immigrants in Fiji from India and the Solomon Islands these microfilariae maintain their nocturnal periodicity amongst the non-periodic Fijians but, if they and the Europeans also contract the infection in Fiji, the microfilariae are non-periodic. An attempt was made to explain this anomaly by the day-biting habits of the mosquito's intermediate hosts, *Aedes scutellans pseudoscutellaris* and *Ae. s. polynesiensis*, which have a regional distribution in the Pacific corresponding to that of the non-periodic filariae. As the microfilariae remain true to type after transfusion, it was suggested that they are the progeny of a parent distinct from *W. bancrofti*: this has been named *W. bancrofti* var. *pacifica*. The microfilariae of both varieties are morphologically indistinguishable. The non-periodic Pacific type in Fiji differs from that of periodic African *W. bancrofti* in that increased oxygen content of the blood brings about a *slight rise* in the microfilarial count.

Periodicity is a biological rhythm inherent in the microfilariae but influenced by the rhythm of the host, which itself is influenced by the changes in body temperature that occur every 24 hours.

The two forms of *B. malayi* from Malaysia exhibit

different periodicities which correspond with the biting habits of their chief vectors. Therefore, attempts have been made to see whether it is possible to change periodicity by feeding mosquitoes by day on a nocturnal periodic infection and transmitting the few filarial larvae that develop in them to experimental animals. Thus, when a human infection was transmitted to a cat it was found that the nocturnally periodic microfilariae became semiperiodic. By altering the feeding time and selective breeding of mosquitoes, successive transmission experiments have shown that it is possible to change the periodicity of the mosquito–filarial complex in a relatively small number of generations.

Life cycle (Figure III.87)

The life cycle was first worked out by Manson in *Culex quinquefasciatus* in China in 1878. Within 1 hour of entering the mosquito's stomach the microfilariae cast the sheaths and bore through the stomach wall. At this stage the microfilariae may be damaged by the buccopharyngeal armature of the mosquito, which may explain the differing infection rates of these vectors.[19] At the end of an infective feed the embryos collect at the anterior end of the stomach and then enter the anterior cylindrical portion of the midgut. Forward transportation is effected by reversed peristalsis until they are distributed over the whole of this cylinder. At the end of 16 hours they form a writhing mass behind the valve, which prevents their progress into the foregut. The proboscis of the mosquito exerts positive chemotaxis upon microfilariae. Therefore vector female mosquitoes can abstract more embryos than would be present in a similar quantity of circulating blood. The mosquito abstracts 1 mm^3 of blood at each feed and, in so doing, concentrates the embryos tenfold. They next enter the thorax, where they lie between the muscular fibres of the indirect

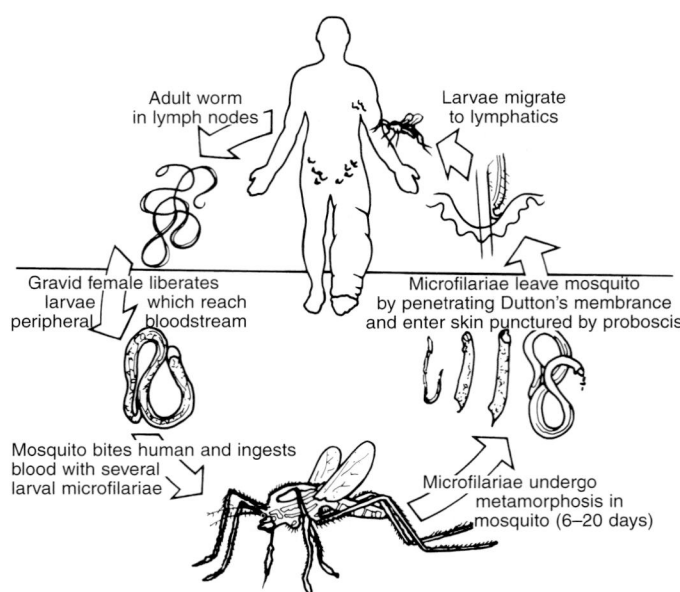

Figure III.87: Life cycle of lymphatic filariasis (*Wuchereria bancrofti*).

or fibrillar flight muscle of the thorax and pharyngeal muscle of the head of the mosquito[20] (Figure III.88). Within 2 days they increase in girth, the 'posterior V spot' (or anal pore) enlarges, and the excretory vesicle becomes more prominent. By rapid nuclear proliferation, the larval filaria now assumes a squat 'sausage' form, the tail shrinks and is then absorbed (Figure III.89). Mouth and oesophagus are apparent from the fifth day onwards. The g^2 and g^3 cells (Figure III.85) divide several times and give rise to a column of cells which form the mid-intestine (large gut). The posterior intestine (rectum) is formed from four cells derived from the g^4 cell. The genital primordium is formed from the g^1 cell.

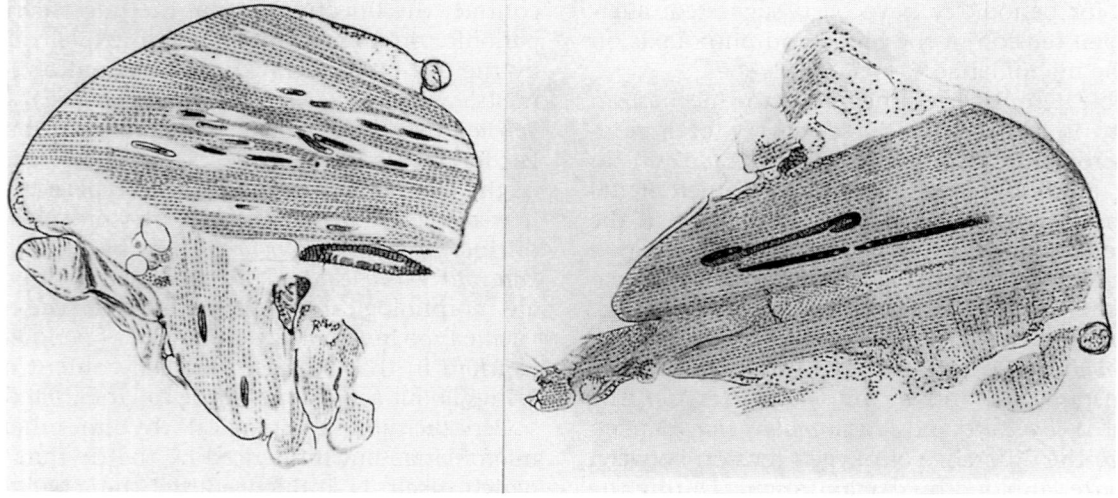

Figure III.88: Section of the thoracic muscles of *Aedes pseudoscutellaris*. Left, The second day after feeding on a filaraemic patient. Right, The second week after feeding on a filaraemic patient.

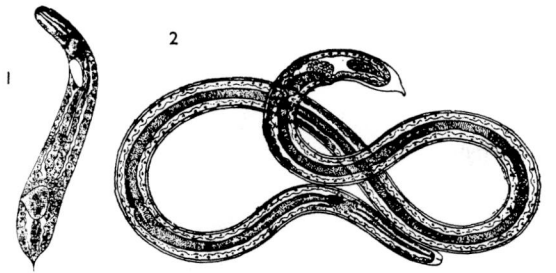

Figure III.89: Stages of the larval forms of *Wuchereria bancrofti* from the thoracic muscles of *Culex quinquefasciatus*. (150×.)

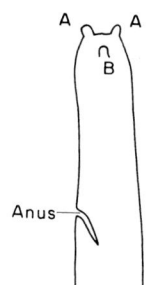

Figure III.90: Larval filaria from the proboscis sheath of *Aedes pseudoscutellaris*. A, Terminal papilla. B, Postanal papilla.

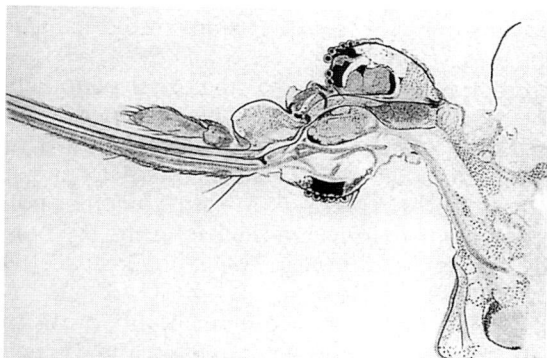

Figure III.91: *Wuchereria bancrofti* in the head and proboscis of the mosquito.

When the larva is 0.5 mm in length, a bulbar oesophagus appears at the first and second fourths of the alimentary canal. Now elongated and worm-like, the larva moves sluggishly about. Three caudal papillae develop which function in progression and facilitate penetration of human skin (Figure III.90). About the 10th day (in favourable circumstances) the larval filaria, 1.4 mm long, travels forward into the head of the mosquito where it coils up and enters the proboscis sheath (Figure III.91), but occasionally it may penetrate into the abdominal cavity and legs. Two or more ecdyses take place. At high temperatures and in moisture, the complete cycle occupies 10–14 days but it is retarded to 6 weeks by cold. Sometimes the larvae die in the thoracic muscles and are enclosed in chitin, producing a curious mummy-like structure. When an infected mosquito bites

a human, the larvae, attracted by warmth, break through the terminal portion of the proboscis sheath in the ligula at the central point of 'Dutton's membrane', wriggle out on to the skin, which they penetrate near the seat of the puncture caused by the stylets of the mosquito. A list of vectors is given in Appendix IV.

In the human host the infective larvae pass through the peripheral blood vessels to the lymphatics where they become mature in an estimated period of 3 months to 1 year. The human is the only known definitive host.

In view of the fact that considerable confusion has been generated by the discovery of larval filariae in wild-caught mosquitoes, in the course of surveys upon the natural infection rate it has become necessary to differentiate between the larval characters of human and allied species of animal origin. It has to be realized that the filariae of some animals, fruit bats and birds develop in species of mosquitoes that normally transmit human filariasis.

The infective larva of *B. malayi* is 1–2 mm in length and has three poorly defined caudal papillae; that of *B. patei* is about the same length and has a marked dorsal protuberance resembling a dog's head, in lateral position. The larva of *Dirofilaria corynodes* of monkeys (*Cercopithecus* and *Colobus*) from *Aedes pembaensis* has the typical cigar-shaped tail but less pronounced narrowing between the anus and the extremity, with three small papillae. The larva of *D. repens* of the dog and cat resembles the foregoing but with only one terminal papilla: it develops in *Aedes aegypti*, *Ae. pembaensis* and *Mansonia africanus*; that of *D. immitis* of the dog, from *Ae. aegypti* and *Culex quinquefasciatus*, cannot be distinguished from that of *D. repens*. The larva of *Setaria equina* of the horse, mule and donkey in *Ae. aegypti*, *Ae. pembaensis* and *Culex quinquefasciatus* is about the same length but can easily be distinguished by one large terminal papilla and two subterminal ones, looking like little ears. Distinguishing features are illustrated in a key by Nelson.[21]

Wuchereria bancrofti var. *pacifica* (Manson-Bahr, 1941)

It has been suggested that the filaria found in the central and southern Pacific might be a separate species. As far as can be ascertained, embryos (microfilariae) are morphologically identical to those of *W. bancrofti*. Certain small differences have been noted in the adult morphology. The average length is smaller: females 58 mm, males 27 mm. The tail of the female lacks the bulbous swelling that characterizes those from Guyana. The anterior end of the Fijian specimens is oval in outline.

Microfilariae in Polynesians (Fiji, Samoa, Tonga, Cook Islands, New Caledonia) are non-periodic. In these islands, as well as in Tokelau, Wallis, Ellice, Gilberts, Marquesas and those beyond 'Buxton's line' (longitude 170° E), they do not exhibit nocturnal periodicity but occur in equal numbers in the blood by day and night. Development of this filaria is confined to mosquitoes indigenous to the South Pacific islands of the *Aedes kochi*,

Ae. vigilax and *Ae. scutellaris* groups which are adapted to coconut palms and bite by day (see Appendix IV). The non-periodic microfilaria does not develop readily in *C. quinquefasciatus*, which is the optimum host for the nocturnally periodic *W. bancrofti*.

Genus: *Brugia* (Buckley, 1959)

The genus *Brugia* contains nine representatives: *B. malayi, B. pahangi, B. patei, B. beaveri, B. buckleyi, B. ceylonensis, B. guyanensis, B. tupiae* and *B. timori.*[22]

Brugia malayi (Brug, 1927)

Distribution

This is the common form in Malaysia, Indonesia, Timor, central India, Sri Lanka, south China, Korea, Indo-China and Koshima Island (Japan). It has not been found in Africa, America, Australia or the Pacific Islands. *B. timori* is found in Timor and islands in south-east Indonesia (Sunda group).

Parasitology

The adults are practically identical to *W. bancrofti* in nearly all characters; the females are indistinguishable. The female measures 55 mm in length by 160 μm. The vulva is situated 0.92 mm from the anterior extremity. The caudal end is bluntly rounded. The male is 22–23 mm in length by 88 μm in diameter. The posterior extremity has about three turns and the anus is 0.1–0.14 mm from the tip of the tail. One pair of large papillae are just in front of the cloaca and one behind. There are also two smaller pairs. There is a small naviculate gubernaculum and two spicules which are unlike in size and structure: the longer is 0.34–0.36 mm, the shorter 0.11–0.12 mm in length. There are morphological differences in the microfilariae and the mosquito intermediate host is distinct—*Mansonia annulifera*. It is identical with the microfilaria of the 'kra' monkey (*Macaca irus*) which is transmitted by the same mosquitoes. It is common in domestic dogs and cats in Malaysia and has been found also in the slow loris (*Nycticebus coucang*), the banded leaf monkey (*Presbytis melalophos*) as well as in the pangolin (*Manis javanica*).

The microfilaria of *B. malayi* was first discovered by Lichtenstein in Celebes and studied further by Brug in 1927. Brug and de Rook found natural infection in the mosquitoes *Mansonia longipalpis* (also known as *dives*) and *M. annulata*.

Although the human form of *B. malayi* is common in dogs and cats in Malaysia and Indonesia, there is a species, *B. pahangi*, that is confined to these animals and has distinctive morphological characters.

The human form of *B. malayi* can be transmitted to cats by the bite of *Mansonia longipalpis*. The period of full development of the adult filaria in this animal is about 65 days before microfilariae appear in the blood. The adult forms recovered from the cat correspond to the descrip-

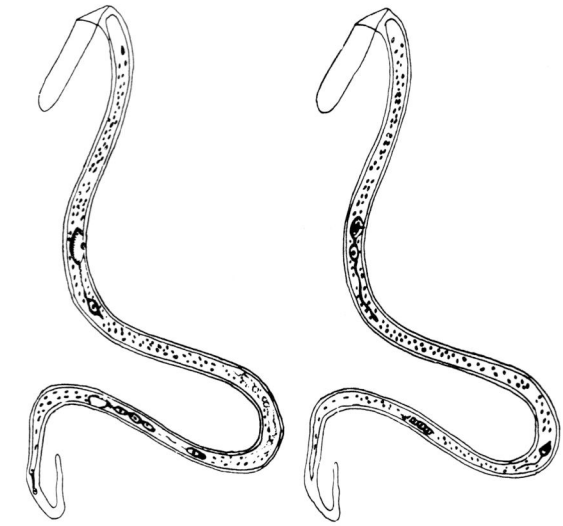

Figure III.92: Comparative morphology of the microfilariae of *Wuchereria bancrofti* (right) and *Brugia malayi* (left).

tions of *B. malayi* in humans. *B. patei* microfilariae have been found in cats in Orissa, India, and in dogs and genet cats in Pate Island, Kenya. The nocturnal periodic form in Malaysia does not develop well in cats and is transmitted by species of *Anopheles* and *Mansonia*. A semiperiodic form occurs in humans and commonly in cats, in freshwater swamps and forest. It is transmitted by *Mansonia annulata* and *M. uniformis*.

Microfilaria *B. malayi* has a nocturnal periodicity like that of *W. bancrofti* or may be semiperiodic. It is nocturnal on the west coast of the Malaysia peninsula but non-periodic in the Huantan district on the east coast. It measures 200–250 × 5–6 μm. Its chief points of distinction are the elongated nucleus at the top of the tail and the absence of nuclei in the cephalic space (Figures III.92 and III.93).

Table III.9 summarizes the main points of distinction between the microfilariae of *B. malayi* and *W. bancrofti*, and Figure III.93 (with key) shows the differences in the microfilariae of medical importance.

Life cycle

The most favoured mosquito intermediate hosts belong to the genus *Mansonia*, which are crepuscular or nocturnal feeders. Development in the mosquito is similar to that of *W. bancrofti* but more rapid, in 6–8½ days. Difficulties have been encountered in Malaysia in distinguishing larval forms of ornithofilariae of birds from those of human *B. malayi* in the routine dissection of mosquitoes.

The larval forms of *B. malayi* in *Mansonia* undergo two ecdyses. The buccal cavity is formed from the cephalic space; the oesophagus from the nuclei of the anterior part of the nuclear column; the rectum and anus from the four G cells of Rodenwaldt and the anal pore. The premature genital pore mass is derived from the nuclei of *Innenkörper* and the muscles of the body wall from the

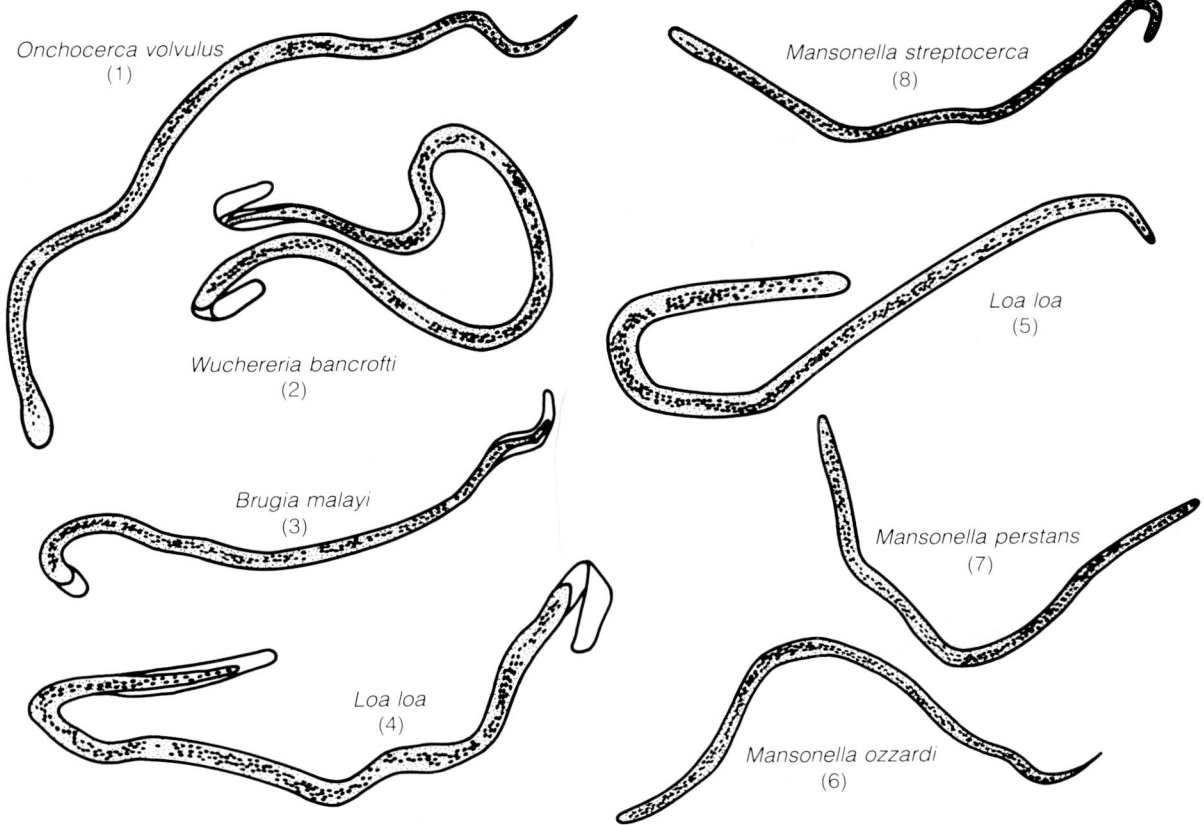

Figure III.93: Microfilariae of medical importance. (Courtesy of D. A. Denham.)

Key to microfilariae found in human blood
Method 1. After staining with Mayer's haemalum
1(a) Sheath present—*W. bancrofti*
 (b) Sheath absent—*Loa loa* (5)
2(a) Nuclei to tip of tail—*B. malayi*
 (a) Nuclei not in tip of tail—*W. bancrofti*
3(a) Two isolated nuclei in tail—*B. malayi*
 (b) Solid column of nuclei in tail—*Loa loa* (4)
4(a) Sheath loosely applied, worm over 250 μm long—*Loa loa* (4)
 (b) Sheath very small, worm under 250 μm long—*Meningonema peruzzi*
5(a) More than 275 μm in length—*M. ozzardi*
 (b) Less than 250 μm in length—*M. perstans*
6(a) Cephalic space longer than twice width of body—*O. volvulus*
 (b) Cephalic space about width of body—*W. bancrofti* (with no sheath)
7(a) Nuclei to tip of tail—*M. streptocerca*
 (b) Nuclei not to tip of tail—*M. ozzardi*
8(a) Tail straight with prominent terminal nucleus—*Dipetalonema perstans*
 (b) Tail bent into crook shape—*Dipetalonema streptocerca*

Method 2. After staining with Giemsa
1(a) Sheath present—*W. bancrofti*
 (b) Sheath absent—*B. malayi*
2(a) Sheath stained red, nuclei in tip of tail—*Brugia* spp.
 (b) Sheath stained pale mauve, no nuclei in tip of tail—*W. bancrofti*
3(a) Nuclei not extending to tip of tail—*Loa loa* (4)
 (b) Nuclei to tip of tail—*M. ozzardi*

4(a) Microfilariae about 300 μm long—*Loa loa* (5)
 (b) Microfilariae 200–225 μm long—*M. ozzardi*
5(a) Cephalic space more than 1? times diameter of head—*O. volvulus*
 (b) Cephalic space less than or equal to diameter of head—*W. bancrofti* (with no sheath)
6(a) Microfilariae at least 260 μm long—*M. perstans*
 (b) Microfilariae 200–225 μm long—*M. streptocerca*
7(a) Tail with complete column of microfilariae—*Loa loa*
 (b) Tail with two isolated nuclei—*Brugia* (with no sheath)
8(a) Tail with prominent nucleus—*Dipetalonema perstans*
 (b) Tail with crook-shaped bend—*Dipetalonema streptocerca*

Notes 1 The sheath of *Loa loa* does not stain with Giemsa.
 2 Although *O. volvulus* is normally in the skin, appreciable numbers can be detected in the blood.
 3 *B. malayi* periodic strain usually loses its sheath in blood smears.
 4 Any sheathed microfilaria may lose its sheath.
 5 The part of the tail of *M. ozzardi* that is free of nuclei is very fine and may not stain but there is no terminal nucleus as in *D. perstans*.

Table III.9 Differentiation between microfilariae of *B. malayi* and *W. bancrofti*.

	Microfilaria malayi	Microfilaria bancrofti
General	Often found closely folded with head close to tail and irregularly disposed with, typically, major curves and minor kinks	Usually seen lying with head and tail well separated and commonly shows three or four major curves of graceful appearance
Nuclei	Blurred and intermingled so that they cannot be counted easily	Well defined and spaced, and can be counted easily
Tail	Tapers to a fine point; continues as a fine thread. *Typically* one nucleus at the extremity of the tapered portion and two in the terminal thread	Tapers to a point and the terminal portion contains no nuclei
Cephalic space	Twice as long as broad	As long as broad
Excretory pore and cell	Separated	Close together. A thread of protoplasm runs posteriorly from the latter
Anal pore	Clear space about 40 μm from the tail end	
Sheath	Well stained	Hardly visible

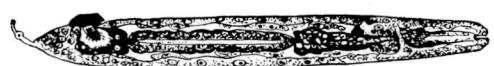

Figure III.94: Developmental stage of *Brugia malayi* showing the terminal nucleus in the tail.

'subcuticular cells' of Rodenwaldt. The tail of the microfilaria, with its two nuclei (terminal nucleus in the tail; Figure III.94), is shed with the first moult. As in the case of *W. bancrofti*, the larva, when in the thoracic muscles, feeds by absorbing food through the cuticle. It does not feed at the expense of these muscles, as has been stated.

Brugia timori (Partono, Purnomo, Dennis, Atmosoedjono, Oemijati & Cross, 1977)

The adult male *B. timori* differs from other *Brugia* spp. (except *B. malayi*) in having a spicular ratio of 3 : 1; it differs from *B. malayi* in having greater numbers of subventral adanal papillae (up to five on each side) which are loosely spaced and irregularly positioned about the cloaca, a greater diameter of the capitulum of the left spicule and greater length of the proximal section of the right spicule. The adult female has an ovejector of greater length and width than that of *B. malayi*. Microfilariae typical of the *B. timori* have a greater length than other *Brugia* spp., length : width cephalic space ratio of 3 : 1 and a sheath that does not stain bright pink with Giemsa.[23] The vector is *Anopheles barbirostris*.

Figure III.95 shows the differences between *Wuchereria* and *Brugia* forms of filaria.

Genus: *Onchocerca*

Onchocerca volvulus (Leuckart, 1893)

Parasitology

The body is white and filiform, tapering at both ends. The head is rounded. The cuticle is marked by transverse ridges and raised with prominent angular and oblique thickenings, more distinct posteriorly. It is usually found in nodules but can reproduce outside them (Figure III.96). The male (2–4 cm × 0.2 mm) has a straight alimentary canal ending in a subterminal anus. The tail ends in a slight spiral and is bulbous at the tip. There are two pairs of preanal, two postanal, an intermediate large papilla and two unequal spicules (82 μm, 77 μm) protruding from the cloaca (Figure III.97); the former has a fluted end and the latter a narrow neck and knob. The female normally measures 60–70 cm × 0.4 mm but is often smaller, 35–40 cm. The head is round and truncated (0.04 mm), the vulva 0.85 mm from the anterior extremity, and the tail curved. Cuticular striations are not so marked as in the male and the presence of two striae in the inner layer of the cuticle is a distinguishing feature of *Onchocerca* in tissue sections.[24] Usually males outnumber females by two to one (four males and two females in each tumour). The female is ovoviviparous and the egg has a striated shell with a pointed process at each pole (like an orange wrapped in tissue paper) measuring 30–50 μm in diameter. The microfilariae (300 × 8 μm) are sheathless and are found in the fluid of the nodule cavity and in the surrounding skin. The body tapers from the last fifth and ends in a sharply pointed, recurved tail (Figure III.93,1). In the anterior fifth is a marked anterior 'V spot'. The cephalic cone is thickened at the commencement of the nuclear column. This microfilaria is non-periodic; it is found in skin in the femoral, inguinal and cervical lymph glands, and in the expressed juice of 'tumours' but sometimes in blood (2%) and also in urine. It is also present in the skin of widely separated portions of the body in apparently healthy people, without producing any nodules or tumours. Microfilariae are easily demonstrated in the skin by biopsy. They are often associated with eye symptoms in the absence of tumours and, by aid of the slit lamp, may be seen in the cornea.

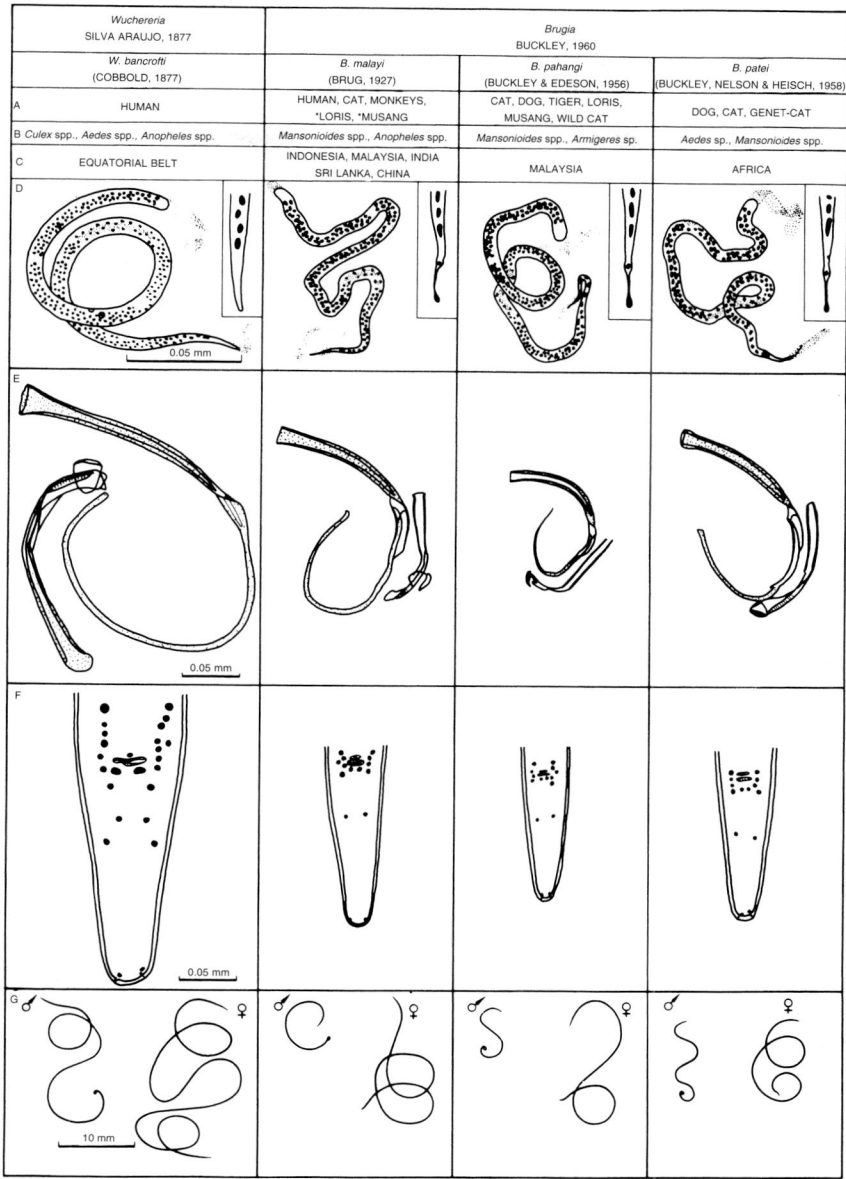

Wuchereria SILVA ARAUJO, 1877	*Brugia* BUCKLEY, 1960		
W. bancrofti (COBBOLD, 1877)	*B. malayi* (BRUG, 1927)	*B. pahangi* (BUCKLEY & EDESON, 1956)	*B. patei* (BUCKLEY, NELSON & HEISCH, 1958)
A HUMAN	HUMAN, CAT, MONKEYS, *LORIS, *MUSANG	CAT, DOG, TIGER, LORIS, MUSANG, WILD CAT	DOG, CAT, GENET-CAT
B *Culex* spp., *Aedes* spp., *Anopheles* spp.	*Mansonioides* spp., *Anopheles* spp.	*Mansonioides* spp., *Armigeres* sp.	*Aedes* sp., *Mansonioides* spp.
C EQUATORIAL BELT	INDONESIA, MALAYSIA, INDIA SRI LANKA, CHINA	MALAYSIA	AFRICA

Figure III.95: Morphological distinctions between the genera *Wuchereria* and *Brugia*. A, Definitive hosts. B, Intermediate hosts. C, Geographical distribution. D, Microfilariae and (inset) tail nuclei of microfilariae. E, Spicules of male, lateral view. F, Tails of males, ventral view. G, Adult worms, actual size. *Indicates experimental infection only. (After Bradley; by permission of *Annals of Tropical Medicine and Parasitology*.)

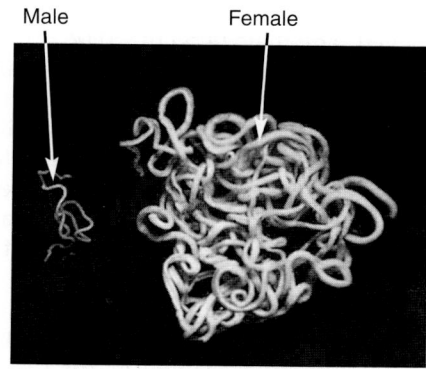

Figure III.96: Adult *Onchocerca volvulus*: male on left, female on right.

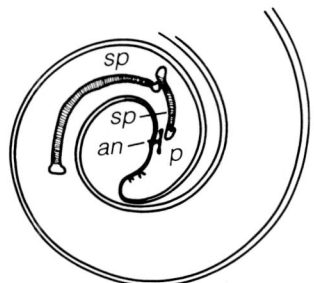

Figure III.97: The caudal extremity of a male *Onchocerca volvulus*. an, anus; p, papillae; sp, spicules.

Life cycle

The life cycle was worked out in Sierra Leone. Development takes place in 'black fly' or 'buffalo gnat' of the *Simulium damnosum* complex in Africa and other *Simulium species* in South and Central America (see Appendix IV). The fly abstracts microfilariae from the deeper layers of the skin; they then enter the stomach, pierce its walls and pass to the thoracic muscles where they undergo further development. During growth two moults take place. At the seventh day the larva measures 0.65 mm. Development has been traced to the 10th day when the larva escapes from the proboscis; *Simulium* is a day-biting fly (06.00–18.00 hours) and 2.6% may be naturally infected. They probably attract and then abstract microfilariae by scraping the skin with their prestomal teeth.

In the South American form, development is similar to that in central Africa, but occurs in *Simulium metallicum (avidum)*, *S. exiguum*, *S. ochraceum* and *S. callidum (mooseri)*, which are common in endemic areas in Central America and other vectors in South American foci. Developing larvae are frequently found in the abdomen and malpighian tubules of these flies. Two caudal papillae are seen in fully developed larvae, which measure 0.45–1.14 mm. In Guatemala 11% of *Simulium* are naturally infected. Non-human filariae can occur in *Simulium*, and a key to their identification and distinction from human *Onchocerca* is given by Nelson and Pester.[25]

Although there are no morphological differences in the various geographical forms of *Onchocerca*, there are at least six different *Onchocerca–Simulium* complexes which have their own clinical and biological attributes. Enzyme staining for the presence of acid phosphatase was found to show four distinct patterns in microfilariae from West Africa, suggesting that a number of biological strains did exist in West Africa.[26]

Onchocerca gutturosa

O. gutturosa is a parasite of cattle and has occasionally been shown to cause skin nodules in humans.[27]

Genus: *Mansonella*

Mansonella ozzardi (Manson, 1897) (*Tetrapetalonema ozzardi, Filaria ozzardi*)

Morphology[28]

The male is 24–28.4 mm long by 0.07–0.08 mm in diameter. It is coiled in one and a half to two turns and has two spicules and caudal alae. The female is twice as long, 32.2–61.5 × 0.13–0.16 mm in diameter and has a vulva 0.76 mm from the caudal extremity. The vagina leads to paired uteri filling the body cavity with highly coiled ovaries in the posterior part of the body. The adult worms live in body cavities embedded in adipose tissues and in the mesentery. The microfilariae, which are unsheathed, are 207–232 µm long by 3–4 µm in diameter. The anterior end is round and they have an attenuated tail resembling *M. perstans*, but pointed and ending in a hook (Figure III.93,6).

Transfusion experiments have shown that they can live in the blood of the recipient for more than 2 years.

Life cycle

There are two forms of *M. ozzardi*, one in the Caribbean and the other in Brazil and Venezuela. The insect vectors are a midge and a simulium. Microfilariae are ingested with blood from a blood meal and the larvae migrate within 24 hours to the muscles of the thorax where two ecdyses occur, and the third-stage infective larva, measuring 0.7 mm in length, migrates forward to the head to emerge from the proboscis in 8 days from the time of the infective blood meal.

In the Caribbean

Culicoides furens is a vector in St Vincent and Haiti, *C. paraensis* in Antigua and northern Argentina, and *C. phlebotomus* in Trinidad.

In Brazil

The main vector is *Simulium amazonicum* but *Culicoides insinuatus* may also play a part.

Microfilaria bolivarensis[29]

Microfilaria of *M. bolivarensis* has been described in the blood of Amerindians in Bolivar state in Venezuela. The microfilaria measures 256–300 × 7–8 µm and differs from *M. ozzardi*. It superficially resembles microfilaria volvulus but has a greater diameter and a straighter tail.

Mansonella (Esslingeria) perstans (Manson, 1891) (*Dipetalonema perstans, Filaria perstans, Acanthocheilonema perstans, Tetrapetalonema perstans, Tetrapetalonema berghei, Dipetalonema berghei*)

Parasitology

This organism has a long cylindrical, smooth body and a simple, unarmed mouth. The tail in both sexes is characteristic: incurvated, with a chitinous covering at the extreme tip split into two minute appendages, giving a mitred appearance. The female possesses four cuticular appendages at the posterior extremity, not two as hitherto believed. The male (4.5 cm × 0.06 mm) is smaller than the female. The head is 0.04 mm in diameter and the cloaca has four pairs of preanal and one pair of postanal papillae, and two unequal spicules (Figure III.98). The female (7–8 cm × 0.12 mm) has a club-shaped head 0.07 mm in diameter, and a vulva situated 1.2 mm from the head. The anus opens at the apex of a papilla in the concavity of the curve formed by the tail; its diameter is 0.02 mm.

The microfilaria (200 × 4.5 µm) is unsheathed (Figure III.93,7). It possesses to a remarkable degree the power of elongation and contraction. Therefore the measurements vary considerably. Long and short forms (90–110 × 4 µm)

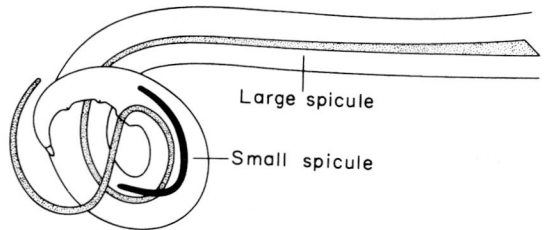

Figure III.98: The tail of *Mansonella perstans*, showing two unequal spicules and papillae. (After Leiper.)

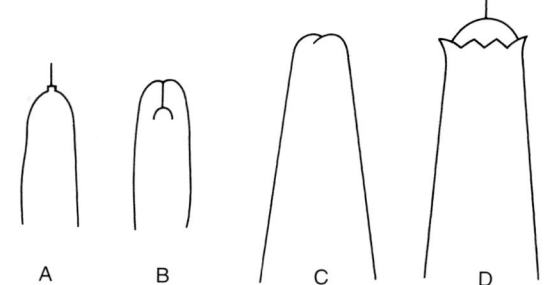

Figure III.99: Structure of the head of microfilaria perstans (**A, B**) and microfilaria bancrofti (**C,D**).

Figure III.100: Microfilaria of *Mansonella streptocerca*, showing the characteristic curvature of the tail. (200×.)

have been described. It is smaller than that of *W. bancrofti* or *L. loa* and its caudal end is truncated and abruptly rounded (Figure III.99). The tapering tail extends two-thirds of the entire length. The anterior 'V spot' is 30 μm from the anterior extremity. There is no marked tail spot, no central granular mass, and no cephalic prepuce. It moves freely in the blood.

The embryos occur in equal numbers both by day and night; according to the self-inflicted experiment of Gönnert, this embryo can persist in the recipient for 3 years after blood transfusion.

Life cycle

The insect vectors are species of *Culicoides*. Microfilariae are ingested and the larvae penetrate the stomach to develop in the thoracic muscles. Within 6–9 days third-stage infective larvae 0.7 mm long emerge from the proboscis. Prior to emerging they cause a globular expansion of the labrum which then collapses, allowing the larvae to escape. There is confusion over the identity of the vector in Africa; originally it was described as *C. austeni* but it is more likely that *C. inornatipennis* and possibly *C. grahami* are the vectors. Transmission takes place at night.

Mansonella (Esslingeria) streptocerca (Macfie & Corson, 1922) (*Dipetalonema streptocerca, Agamofilaria streptocerca, Acanthocheilonema streptocerca*)

This sheathless microfilaria is found commonly in the corium of the skin but not in the blood of people in Ghana (22 of 50 in Accra). It has a wide distribution especially in Cameroon and other West African countries.

The microfilaria (Figures III.93,8 and III.100) is 215 μm in length and is distinguished by the 'walking stick handle' of the tail extremity and an arrangement of nuclei in the head, and four prominent ones in the tail, which has a bifid end[30] that distinguishes it from the microfilariae of *O. volvulus* and *M. perstans*.

Life cycle

The vector is *Culicoides grahami* in which development takes place similar to that in *M. perstans*. Transmission takes place during the day.

Microfilariae were found in the skin of 6 of 11 bonobos and chimpanzees (*Pan paniscus* and *P. troglodytes*) in Zaire.

Two adult female worms found in the connective tissue were very similar to *M. perstans*. The microfilariae of this species, *D. vanhoofi*, closely resemble those of the latter. The incubation period of *D. streptocerca* is 3–4 months.

Meningonema peruzzii (Orihel & Esslinger, 1972)

Adults are found in the subarachnoid space of *Cercopithecus* monkeys trapped in equatorial Guinea. The microfilariae resemble those of *M. perstans* but have an inconspicuous sheath. This worm is the same as that described by Peruzzi in 1928 in monkeys in Uganda and causes cerebral filariasis in Zimbabwe.

Genus: *Loa* (eye worm)

Loa loa (Cobbold, 1864)

Adult *Loa loa* worms inhabit the subcutaneous connective tissues. Diurnal periodic sheathed microfilariae are shed into the peripheral blood.

Parasitology

The body is filiform, cylindrical, whitish and semi-transparent with numerous round, smooth, translucent protuberances of the cuticle, 12–16 μm in diameter, and 9–11 μm above the surface. These chitinous bosses are more numerous in females. Their distribution is irregular. In the male they are absent at the extremities; in the female they extend to the tail and also the cephalic end. The mouth is unarmed and destitute of papillae; there is no distinct neck, but a shoulder 0.15 mm from the mouth where there are two papillae, one dorsal, the other ventral. The alimentary canal commences at a funnel-shaped mouth as a slender straight oesophagus, going on to an intestine 65 μm wide and a short attenuated rectum. The male (3–3.4 cm × 0.35–0.43 mm) (Figure III.101) has its maximum breadth anteriorly; posteriorly

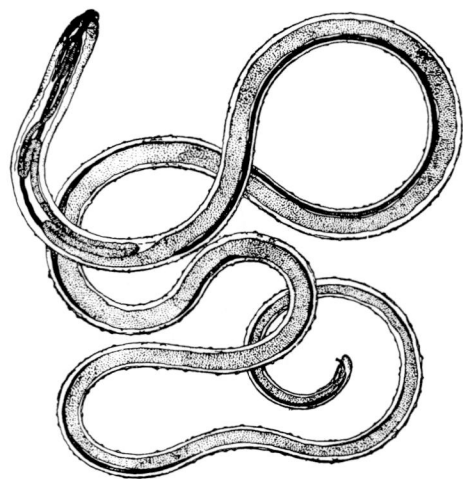

Figure III.101: Male *Loa loa*. (10×.)

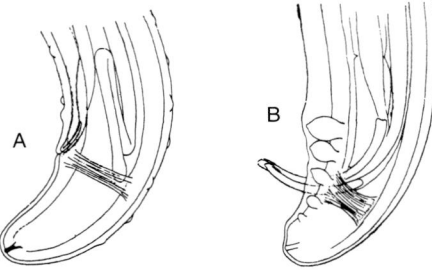

Figure III.102: Posterior extremity of *Loa loa*. (**A**) Female. (**B**) Male.

it tapers to a tail which is curved ventrally with two lateral expansions of the cuticle (0.7 × 0.029 mm) (Figure III.102B). In the middle, 0.08 mm from the tail-tip, is the opening of the anogenital orifice with two unequal spicules (123–176 µm and 88–113 µm) surrounded by thick labia. There are four large globular, pedunculated papillae, decreasing in size anteroposteriorly, and a fifth pair of small postanal papillae. The female (5–7 cm × 0.5 mm) (Figure III.103) has a straight, attenuated, broadly rounded posterior extremity and a vulva 2.5 mm from the anterior extremity placed on a small eminence (Figure III.102A). The vagina, 9 mm long, branches off into long uterine tubes extending through the length of the body. At the narrow end are the ovaries with eggs at all stages. Reproduction is ovoviviparous; the embryos develop within the egg envelope, and uncoil themselves on expulsion from the vagina. When dead the adult worm often becomes calcified.

The microfilaria (Figure III.93,4 and 5) is similar in size (298 × 7.5 µm) and structure to that of *W. bancrofti* but its sheath does not stain with Giemsa. In fresh blood it may be impossible to distinguish them. In dried stained films it assumes a stiff angular attitude, the tail end is disposed in a series of sharp flexures, giving it a corkscrew appearance, with the extreme tip flexed; the nuclei of the central column of cells of microfilaria *L. loa* are larger and less deeply stained, and the cephalic end of the column is more abruptly terminated (Figure III.93,2 and 4). By

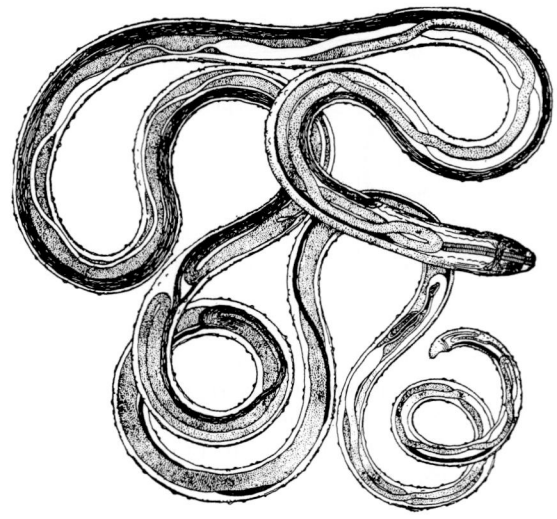

Figure III.103: Female *Loa loa*. (10×.)

special staining methods a large genital cell at the beginning of the posterior third constitutes a marked feature. Microfilaria *L. loa* takes up methylene blue (1 in 5000) in 10 minutes. In microfilaria of *W. bancrofti*, absorption it is much slower but it shows up the excretory pore. Microfilaria of *L. loa* may not be found in the peripheral blood early after infection. It is strictly diurnal, from 08.00 to 20.00 hours—the reverse of microfilaria of *W. bancrofti*. Inversion of periodicity takes place very gradually as, for instance, when daily observations are made on a voyage round the world. The periodicity of microfilaria of *L. loa* is under circadian control by temperature and not by oxygen tension as in periodic *W. bancrofti*.

Life cycle

There are two parallel and sympatric but ecologically separate cycles of *Loa loa* transmission in the West African rainforest. One cycle is that of human *Loa loa* (*L. loa loa*) which is slightly smaller than the simian *L. loa* and has strictly diurnally periodic microfilariae with day-biting vectors (*Chrysops silacea* and *C. dimidiata*). The slightly larger simian parasite of drills *L. loa papionis* has nocturnally periodic microfilariae with tree-top *Chrysops* (*C. langi* and *C. centurionis*) vectors which feed early in the night.

Development in *Chrysops*

(Figure III.104)

Microfilariae are taken up with the blood meal and, on entering the stomach, the microfilaria casts its sheath in 3 hours and, piercing the stomach wall, enters the thoracic muscles and fat body of the thorax, but principally that of the abdomen. Development is complete in 10 days. In 3 days it becomes broad and torpedo shaped; on the fourth and fifth days the squat

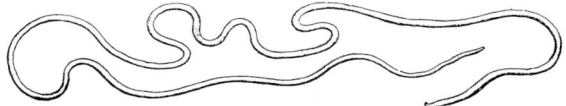

Figure III.105: Female *Dracunculus medinensis*. One-third of natural size.

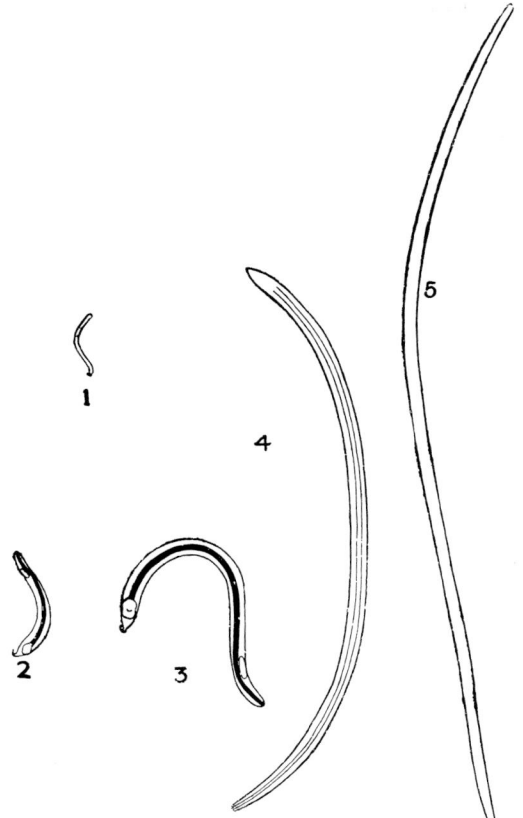

Figure III.104: Development of *Loa loa* in *Chrysops*. (30×.) 1, Larva, 24 hours old. 2, Fourth day, length 390 μm. 3, Fifth day. 4, Seventh day. 5, Tenth day, third-stage infective larva (2 × 0.025 mm).

form lengthens to 0.8–1 mm; on the sixth day the corkscrew-like appearance is replaced by gentle curves. Then the first ecdysis occurs and the sharp tail is replaced by a rounded, trilobed extremity. By the 10th day it measures 2 × 0.025 mm and two moults have occurred, and infective third-stage forms migrate forward into the head where they accumulate in large numbers, the majority at the root of the proboscis. At the next feed they break out of the labium and make their way on to the surface of the skin, which they penetrate, and migrate along the interfascial planes.

Development of *L. loa* in *Chrysops* generally takes 10–12 days from the original infecting feed. *Chrysops* feeds to repletion once every 14 days and the gestation period is 12 days. It is a pool feeder, straining the blood from the subcutaneous haemorrhages caused by its bite.

Superfamily: Dracunculoidea

Genus: *Dracunculus*

Dracunculus medinensis (Linnaeus 1758) (guinea-worm)

Parasitology

The female is the thickness of a knitting needle and usually 60 cm in length (60 cm × 1.5–1.7 mm; 90 cm is

probably exceptional but 120 cm has been recorded). It lives in connective tissue and does not harm its host until about to produce its young when it exhibits 'geotropism', i.e., it is drawn towards earth, towards the limbs—to the fingers, if in the arms; to the scrotum or penis, if in the abdomen; to the breasts in the female, although 90% migrate to the legs and feet, especially behind the outer malleolus.

The body is cylindrical, white and smooth (Figure III.105). The tip of the tail is pointed forming a blunt hook which was formerly thought to be used for holding firm in tissues, but this is not correct. The head is rounded, terminating in a thickened cuticle cap or 'cephalic shield'. The mouth is triangular, small and surrounded by six papillae and an outer circle of four double papillae. A lateral pair of cervical papillae is situated behind the nerve ring (Figure III.106A). There is a single-bulb oesophagus. The secretion from the head glands is very irritating and histiolytic. The alimentary canal is small and is thrust to one side by the branched uterus. There is no definite anus. The vulva is difficult to see and has been discovered only recently as a very small tube in the centre of the worm. The whole worm is occupied by the double uterus packed with embryos (Figure III.107). The coiled uteri, distended by three million larvae, fill the body. There is a double ovary and double oviducts at the posterior extremity (Figure III.106B). When douched with water, waves of contraction force the uterine contents forward, the thickened cuticle gives way and the 'cap' is blown off. The uterus is extruded up to a length of 1.25 cm; this also bursts and the contained embryos are shed into the water. The worm dies when its nervous system is destroyed. The sinus containing the dead worm easily becomes septic, but may coil itself round tendons and, if pulled upon, may break. It often becomes calcified and can then be demonstrated on radiography.

Males recovered from experimental infections in animals measure 15–40 × 0.4 mm. The male has subequal spicules (490–750 μm long) and a gubernaculum (about 117 μm). The posterior end is coiled on itself one or more times. There are three to six (usually four) preanal and four to six postanal caudal papillae. After copulation, the male dies and is absorbed. It lives between the muscles of the groin. Copulation probably takes place in the deeper tissues.

The embryo (Figure III.108) measures 500–750 × 17 μm and shows transverse striations of the cuticle. It is flattened, not cylindrical, with a long, slender tail and a rounded head. The alimentary canal has a rudimentary anus and a bulbous oesophagus. There are two glands at the root of the tail. In water the embryos cannot swim

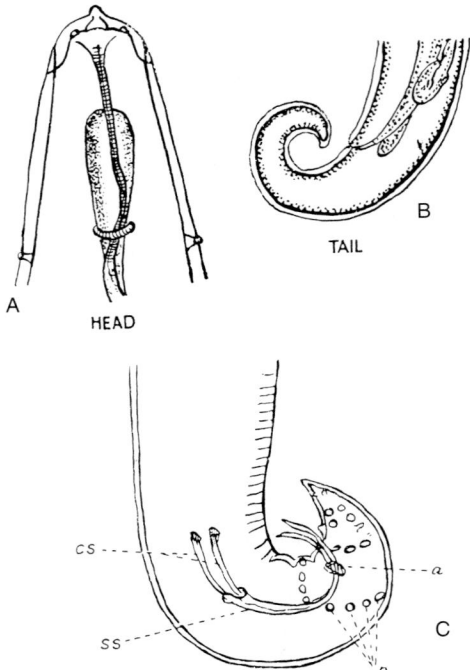

Figure III.106: *Dracunculus medinensis.* (**A**) Anterior end of female. (**B**) Tail of female. (**C**) Posterior end of male. Ventrolateral aspects. (10×.)

a   anus
cs   copulatory spicules
p   preanal and postanal papillae

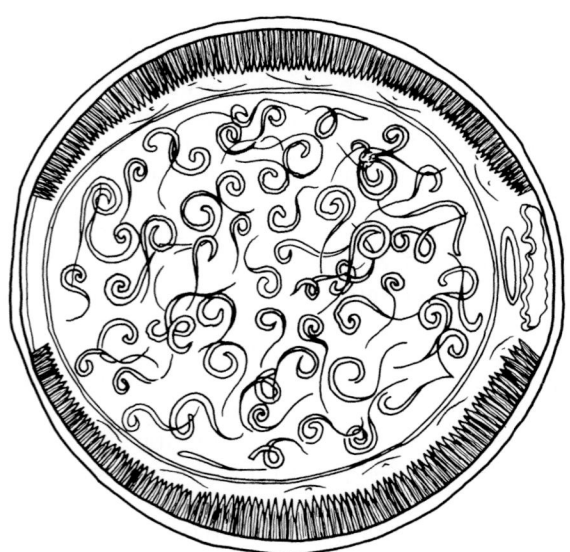

Figure III.107: Transverse section of *Dracunculus medinensis*, showing the contained embryos.

but sink and coil up and release again, moving by side-to-side lashing of the tail and tadpole-like movement of the body. Abnormal embryos, with prominences on the dorsal and ventral caudal surfaces, are not uncommon, but do not survive long.

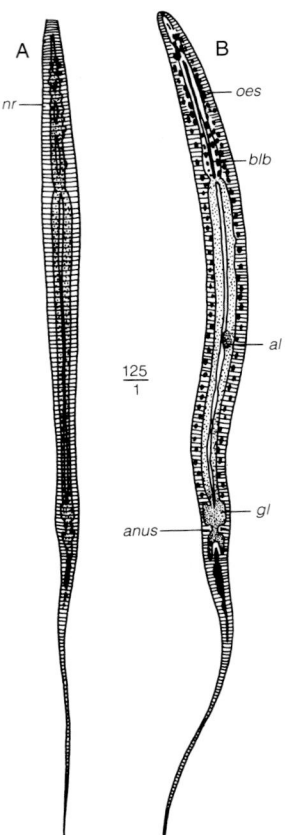

Figure III.108: Embryo of *Dracunculus medinensis*. (**A**) Side view. (**B**) Front view.

al   alimentary canal
blb   bulb
gl   glands
nr   nerve ring
oes   oesophagus

Life cycle (Figure III.109)

In water they live for 6 days; in muddy water or moist earth for 2–3 weeks. If slowly desiccated they can be revived by water. They are swallowed by *Cyclops* (*Cyclops* has a very small mouth). The efficient intermediate hosts are *Cyclops quadricornis* or allied species (*C. strenuus, C. viridis, C. coronatus, C. bicuspidatus, Mesocyclops leuckarti* and *M. hyalinus*) but, in the true tropics, *Tropocyclops multicolor* and other species; in south Nigeria it is *Thermocyclops nigerianus*. Jerky movements of the embryos attract *Cyclops* as a trout is attracted by a fly. As many as 20 may be found in one crustacean but usually they die out when there are more than four (Figure III.110). The pointed tail penetrates the gut wall; they then migrate into the body cavity and feed on the ovary or testes of the cyclops. There is no growth in size but two or three ecdyses take place. The tail is absorbed and they become cylindrical and the posterior extremity trilobed. Development takes 4–6 weeks but the larva may survive for 4 months. When 1 mm in length they acquire a simple muscular oesophagus (Figure III.108) and the tail is truncated. This distinguishes the infective stage.

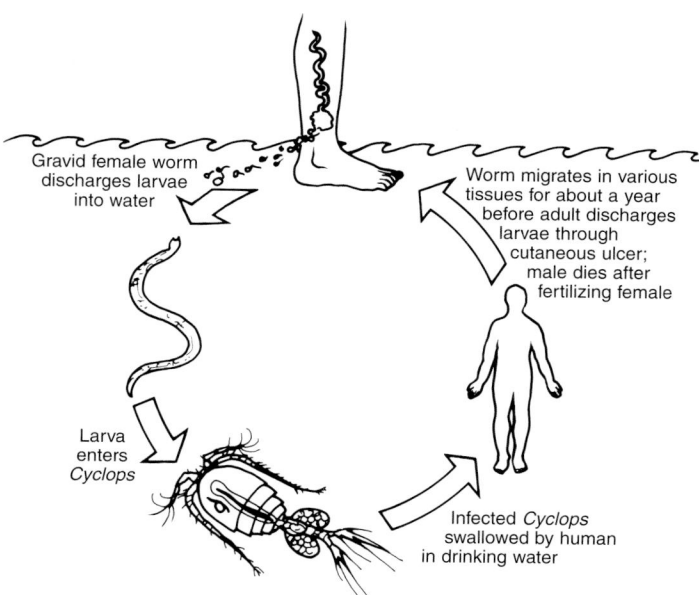

Figure III.109: Life cycle of *Dracunculus medinensis*.

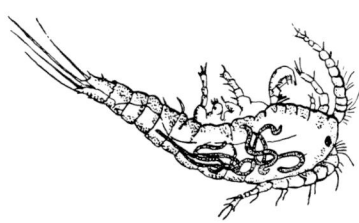

Figure III.110: Larvae of *Dracunculus medinensis* in the body cavity of *Cyclops*.

Cyclops is swallowed by humans; in the gastric juice the body of the cyclops is dissolved and the larvae become active and burst out. The migration of the early stages in the mammalian host has been clarified.[31] It takes 3–4 months for the full development of both sexes.

Immature stages were recovered at 43–48 days, while undergoing the fourth ecdysis. The route of the larvae from the alimentary canal to the subcutaneous tissues of the mammalian host takes place via the lymphatic system. The worms reach the subcutaneous tissues by day 43. In this situation the sexes live in equal numbers and sexual differentiation is distinct, although the males have not developed spicules. The final ecdysis takes place in the subcutaneous tissues. The adult worm takes exactly 1 year to develop.

Superfamily: Spiruroidea

Genus: *Thelazia*

Thelazia callipaeda (Railliet & Henry, 1910) (oriental eye worm)

This nematode is a parasite of the conjunctiva of the dog, rabbit and humans in China, Japan, Korea, India, Myanmar and European CIS.

The adult is a white thread-like worm (males 4.5–13 × 0.25–0.75 mm; females 6.2–17 × 0.3–0.85 mm). The oral end has a chitinized capsule with two circles of sessile papillae. The male has a recurved posterior end. The vulva of the female opens ventrally in the anterior half of the body. There is a single uterus which bifurcates into two ovaries.

The egg is ovoid and measures 60 × 34–37 μm, is hyaline, thin-shelled and laid fully embryonated.

Life Cycle

Dipteran flies are utilized as intermediate hosts. In China *Amiota variegata* was found as a natural and experimental host, but *Musca* spp. were not susceptible to infection.[31]

Thelazia californiensis (Price, 1930)

T. californiensis has been found in humans in California, the intermediate hosts of which include *Fannia benjamini* and *Musca autumnalis*.

REFERENCES

1 Dalton J P (ed.) *Fasciolosis*. Wallingford: CABI Publishing, 1998.
2 Southgate V R, Van Wijk H B & Wright C A. *Zeitschr für Parasitol* 1976; 49:145–159.
3 Wright C A & Ross G C. *Trans R Soc Trop Med Hyg* 1980; 74:326–332.
4 Tchuem Tchuenté L A, Southgate V R, Théron A et al. *Parasitology* 1999; 118:593-603
5 Jordan P, Webbe G & Sturrock R F. *Human Schistosomiasis*. Wallingford: CABI Publishing, 1993.
6 Brown D S. *Freshwater Snails of Africa and their Medical Importance*. London: Taylor & Francis, 1994.
7 Kian Joe Lie, Basch P W, Heynemann D et al. *Trans R Soc Trop Med Hyg* 1968; 62:299.
8 Southgate V R, Brown D S, Warlow A et al. *Parasitol Res* 1989; 75:381–391.
9 Brygoo E R & Randrimalala J C. *Bull Soc Pathol Exot* 1959; 52:26.
10 Thompson R C A & Lymbery A J. Echinococcus *and Hydatid Disease*. Wallingford: CABI Publishing, 1995.
11 Slais J. Cited in Dawes B. *Advances in Parasitology*. London: Academic Press, 1972.
12 Khera S. *Ascaris (The Intestinal Roundworm.)* New Delhi: Shree Books, 1999.
13 Peng W, Anderson T J C, Zhou X & Kennedy M W. *Parasitology* 1998; 117:355–361.
14 Schad G A et al. *Science* 1973; 180:502.
15 Beer R J S. *BMJ* 1971; ii:44.
16 Masuya T. *Jpn J Parasitol* 1976; 25:283.
17 McFadzean J S & Hawking F. *Trans R Soc Trop Med Hyg* 1956; 50:543.
18 Hawking F. *Trans R Soc Trop Med Hyg* 1956; 50:397.
19 Bryan J H, Oothman P, Andrews B J et al. *Trans R Soc Trop Med Hyg* 1974; 68:14.
20 Laurence B R. *Trans R Soc Trop Med Hyg* 1985; 79:690–699.
21 Nelson G S. *J Helminthol* 1959; 33:233.
22 David L & Edeson J F B. *Ann Trop Med Parasitol* 1964; 59:103.
23 Partono F, Purnomo A S & Dennis D T. *J Parasitol* 1977; 63:540.

24 Beaver P C, Horner G S & Bilos J Z. *Am J Trop Med Hyg* 1974; 23:595.

25 Nelson G S & Pester F N R. *Bull World Health Organ* 1962; 27:473.

26 Braun-Munziger R A & Southgate B A. *Bull World Health Organ* 1977; 55:569.

27 Collins R C. *J Parasitol* 1973; 59:1016.

28 Orihel T C & Eberhard M L. *Am J Trop Med Hyg* 1982; 31:1142–1147.

29 Godoy G A, Godoy G, Oriheltic C & Volcan G S. *Am J Trop Med Hyg* 1980; 29:545–547.

30 Orihel T C. *Am J Trop Med Hyg* 1984; 33:1278.

31 Onobamiro S D. *Ann Trop Med Parasitol* 1956; 50:157.

Appendix IV
Medical Acarology and Entomology

Edited by G. B. White

Most types of zoological organism (more than 90% of all known species) belong to the phylum Arthropoda, having an exoskeleton. Arthropods of medical interest belong to three classes: Arachnida (ticks, mites, scorpions and spiders; see below), Crustacea (crabs, crayfish, copepods, etc.) and especially the Insecta (insects), characterized by having the body subdivided as head (with antennae), thorax with legs and segmented abdomen.

Ticks and mites

M. G. R. Varma

Class: Arachnida

The arachnids differ from insects by lacking antennae and wings, and in having an unsegmented body. During the life cycle they undergo incomplete metamorphosis; the eggs hatch into six-legged larvae which develop through the nymphal stage to adults. The nymphs and adults have four pairs of legs.

Subclass: Acari; Order: Acarina (ticks and mites)

The acarine body is typically composed of an anterior gnathosoma or capitulum and a posterior idiosoma. The gnathosoma represents the head of a generalized arthropod and carries the paired palps, which are sensory in function, the paired chelicerae and the single, ventrally situated, hypostome, which together make up the cutting and blood-sucking apparatus. The idiosoma carries the paired legs.

There are about 30 000 species of acarines belonging to more than 2000 genera. The mites are usually much smaller than ticks. Of more than 200 families of mite that have been described, only a few contain species that affect humans.

Family: Sarcoptidae

Sarcoptes scabiei (itch mite, scabies mite)

Sarcoptes scabiei causes scabies in humans and mange in a variety of wild and domestic animals. Scabies mites of dogs and horses, which differ physiologically rather than morphologically from human scabies mites, can establish themselves briefly on humans and cause skin problems similar to scabies. Such infestations are usually mild and cure spontaneously. An increased incidence of human scabies tends to occur in 15–20-year cycles and the cycling is most probably due to changing levels of immunity in the human population. Scabies is widespread in the tropics, although by no means confined there. It may disappear from one area for many years, only to reappear. It is thought that the recent resurgence in scabies is due to large population movements, insufficient or incorrect diagnosis by the medical profession and an altered lifestyle among younger persons in the developed Western countries, resulting in close personal contact. Infestation levels are highest in poorer communities and in children. Even in developed countries, infestation in schoolchildren can reach 5%.

The female *S. scabiei* (0.3–0.4 mm) is bigger than the male (0.2 mm) (Figure IV.1).[1] The first and second pairs of legs of the female and the first, second and fourth pairs of legs of the male carry suckers. The surface of the female is covered with fine transverse striations and the dorsal surface bears a number of specialized spines and conical setae.

Both males and females make short burrows but it is only the fertilized females that make permanent winding burrows in the horny layers of the skin, with the female at the end (Figure IV.2). The burrows contain faeces and relatively large eggs. The majority of mite burrows are found in the interdigital skin, bends of the knees and elbows, the penis and breasts. The eggs hatch into larvae which find shelter and presumably food in the follicles. The larval stage is followed by two nymphal stages before the adult stage is reached. The whole life cycle from egg to egg takes about 10–14 days, during which there may be a mortality rate of about 90%. (For clinical features and treatment see Chapter 19.)

Family: Demodicidae

Demodex (follicle mites)

These extremely small mites, 0.1–0.4 mm long (Figure IV.3), have a worm-like transversely striated body with four pairs of stubby legs anteriorly. They infest a wide

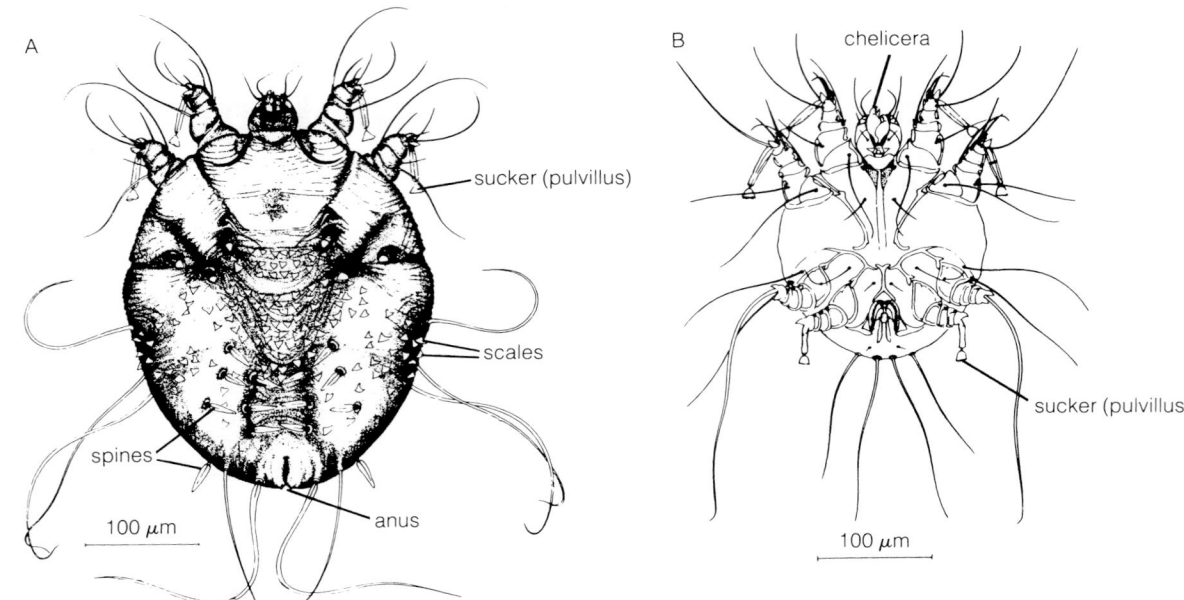

Figure IV.1: A, Dorsal view of female *Sarcoptes scabiei*. **B,** Ventral view of *Sarcoptes scabiei*. (Reproduced from Kettle.[1])

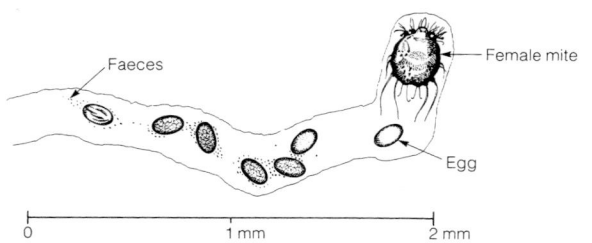

Figure IV.2: Burrow of *Sarcoptes scabiei* with female mite and eggs.

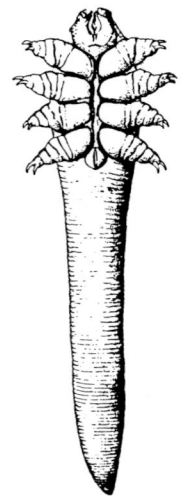

Figure IV.3: *Demodex folliculorum* the follicle mite. Ventral view. (Reproduced from Kettle.[1])

variety of mammalian hosts but are highly host-specific. More than one species may occur on the same host but in different tissues. For example, *D. folliculorum* lives in the hair follicles of humans and the stubby *D. brevis* is found in the sebaceous glands. The entire life cycle occurs in the follicles. In humans, infestations occur mainly in the region of the eyelids, nose and facial area. Infestations are usually higher in aged persons, in whom they may reach 100%. Diagnosis is by expressing sebum and examining it for mites. Infestations are usually benign, but dry erythema with follicular scaling, particularly in the region of the eyelids, may give rise to blepharitis. In the facial area there may be granulomatous acne. Gammexane (gamma benzene hexachloride) 0.5% in vanishing cream is effective.

Family: Trombiculidae

Of more than 1200 described species of trombiculid mite, only about 50 are known to attack humans or livestock. Only the larvae, popularly known as chiggers, are parasitic on vertebrates. They are widely distributed and in many countries cause a dermatitis in humans, although not all chiggers cause an itchy reaction.

Trombiculid larvae (Figures IV.4 and IV.5) normally parasitize rodents and birds but, given the opportunity, will feed readily on humans. The non-parasitic female lays eggs in damp but well drained soil. Typical breeding places are cultivated alluvial river banks in Japan, scrub jungle, grassy fields or untended gardens with a rank growth of grass and other vegetation.

Life cycle (Figure IV.6)

On hatching, the six-legged larvae, which are creamy-white to bright red in colour and 0.25 mm long, ascend grass stems or the tips of fallen leaves and wait in clusters until carbon dioxide from a passing host activates them. The round or oval-shaped larvae have a prominent gnathosoma at the anterior end. The paired toothed

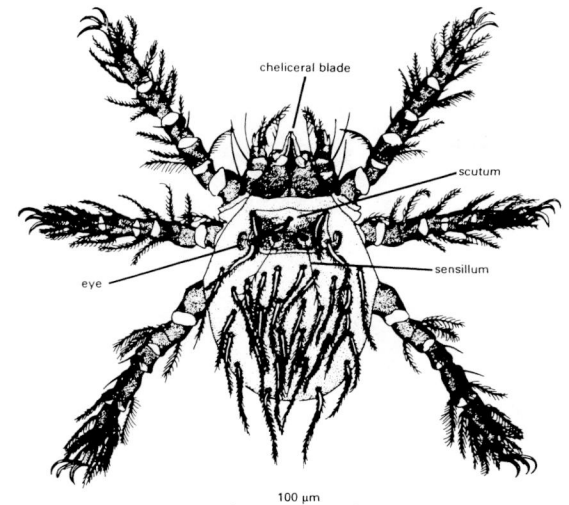

Figure IV.4: Dorsal view of *Leptotrombidium deliense*. (Reproduced from Kettle.[1])

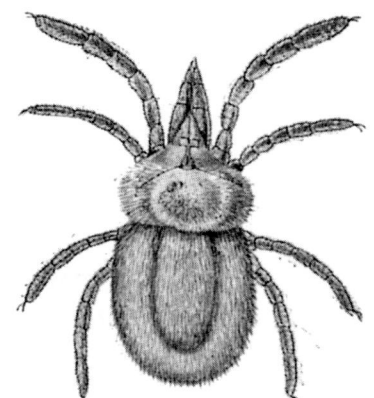

Figure IV.5: Fully grown imago of *Leptotrombidium akamushi*.

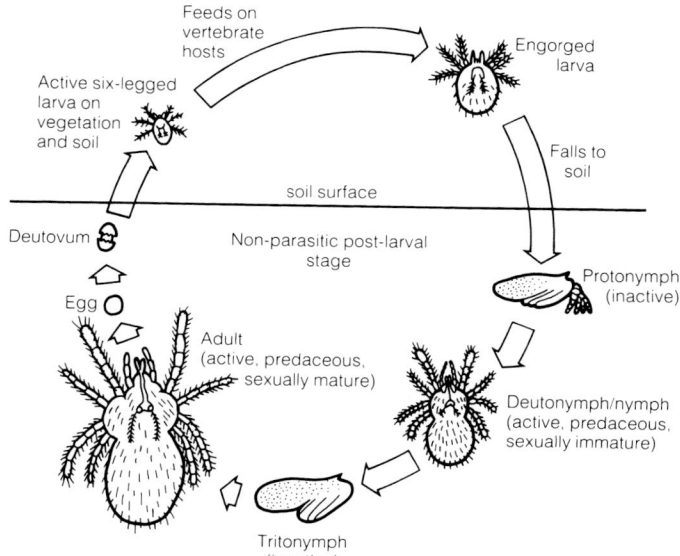

Figure IV.6: Summarized life cycle of trombiculid mites.

chelicerae are flanked by stout palps. The penultimate segment of the palp has a claw which can be apposed to the last segment. Posterior to the gnathosoma on the dorsal side is a chitinized plate or scutum. The shape of the scutum and the shape and disposition of the setae (usually seven) are important characters in the generic and specific identification of the larvae.

The larvae attach in clusters and start feeding on the host's tissues by partially digesting them with saliva and sucking it up. The continual feeding leads to the formation of a feeding tube or stylostome at the point of attachment. The most common sites of attachment are inside the ears of rodents and around the eyes of birds. On humans they tend to attach where clothing is tight, i.e., around the waist and on the scrotum. The larvae do not burrow into the skin, nor do they feed on blood, although a few blood cells may be ingested. After feeding for several days (minimum 3 days), the larvae fall from the host and enter a quiescent stage before moulting into nymphs. The eight-legged nymphs have a figure-of-eight shape and a dense covering of red hairs which gives them a velvety appearance and the name 'velvet mites'. They are non-parasitic predators and feed on insect eggs or small inactive soil invertebrates. The nymph enters a further quiescent phase from which the adult moults. The adults are larger (about 1 mm long) than nymphs but resemble them in shape and habits. The males deposit stalked spermatophores containing sperms on the substrate and the females are inseminated by walking over them. In tropical regions the life cycle may take about 40 days and breeding occurs continuously throughout the year. In temperate regions there is usually only one generation per year and the chiggers are seasonal, during summer and early autumn.

Chiggers and dermatitis

In parts of the world where the mites are present, persons who have been walking in vegetated areas may suffer from a severe itchy dermatitis consisting of pustules and wheals, 3–6 hours after exposure. The sudden appearance of these lesions should suggest attack by chiggers.

Neotrombicula autumnalis is the harvest mite, 'aoutat' or '*lepte autumnal*' of Europe. The larvae normally parasitize voles, rabbits and hares as well as ground-frequenting birds, and are active in summer and early autumn—hence the name 'harvest mite'.

Eutrombicula alfreddugesi, the common American chigger, feeds readily on humans and is also known as '*thalzahuatl*' and '*bicho colorado*'. It extends from continental USA to South America and is most abundant in second-growth, cut-over areas. Humans are frequently attacked although the usual hosts are domestic and wild animals and birds.

Eutrombicula batatas ranges from the warmer southern states of the USA to Central and South America. It is not a serious pest of humans in the USA but commonly attacks people in Panama and other tropical areas of its distribution.

Chiggers and scrub typhus

The vectors of scrub typhus (caused by *Rickettsia tsutsugamushi*) are trombiculid mites. The larvae usually infest rodents (*Rattus* spp.) and insectivores, which are the vertebrate reservoirs of the rickettsiae. The distribution of the mites on the ground is dependent on the home range of the hosts and, because the home ranges do not usually overlap, mite colonies have a restricted distribution and tend to be isolated from one another in the form of 'mite islands'. Humans become infected by intrusion into a rodent–mite cycle in infected 'mite islands'. Bird hosts of the larval mites can, however, disperse the mites into new areas, where a fresh colony could be established.

The habits and life cycle of scrub typhus vectors are similar to those of other trombiculid mites. The parasitic larvae attack humans but seldom produce any noticeable itching or skin reaction; however, the bite of an infected larva can produce a lesion—the *eschar*. Because only the larvae are parasitic and feed only once, the infection can be acquired and transmitted only at this stage. This means that trans-stadial (stage to stage; i.e., from larva to nymph to adult) and transovarial (through eggs to larvae of the next generation) transmission are obligatory for maintenance of the infection in nature. Trombiculid mites are therefore the main reservoirs of scrub typhus rickettsiae. In the mites, the rickettsiae eventually localize in the larval salivary glands and transmission is by bite. All the important scrub typhus vectors belong to the genus *Leptotrombidium*, although the genus *Ascoschoengastia* may be involved in transmission among rodents.

L. akamushi is the vector in the classical areas of the disease (tsutsugamushi disease) in Japan. It is found in the cultivated flood plains of rivers.

L. deliense is the main—or an important—vector over most of the distribution of the disease, from coastal Queensland in the south-east through Papua New Guinea, the Philippines, China, South-East Asia, Sri Lanka and India to Pakistan in the west. Over most of its range, *L. deliense* and the disease are associated with ecologically disturbed vegetation, such as secondary scrub and grass, the result of slash-and-burn cultivation of virgin forest. In South-East Asia and tropical Queensland the coarse fire-resistant kunai grass (*Imperata cylindrica*) is the typical habitat of the mite and its rodent hosts. The mites and the disease are also more likely to occur at the fringes of forests or scrub.

L. fletcher is an important vector in Malaysia, Borneo, New Guinea and the Philippines.

Other important vectors are *L. arenicola* on sandy beaches in Malaysia; *L. pallidum* in limited areas of Japan, Korea and the Primorye region of Russia; *L. pavlovskyi* in Siberia and the Primorye region of Russia; and *L. scutellare* in the Mount Fuji area of Japan.

Protection against chigger mites

Personal protection is the best method of preventing attack by the mite larvae. If a person has to go into mite-infested areas, impregnation of socks and trouser legs

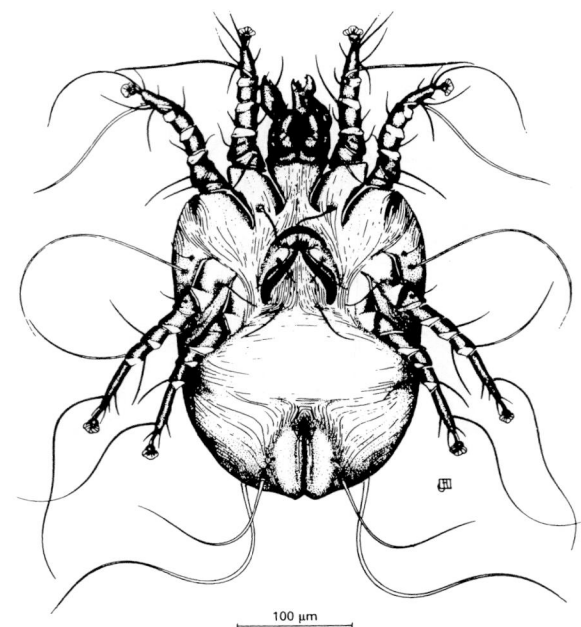

Figure IV.7: *Dermatophagoides pteronyssinus*, the house dust mite. Ventral view. (Reproduced from Kettle.[1])

with a repellent, such as permethrin, benzyl benzoate, dimethylphthalate (DPM) or diethyltoluamide (DEET) will prevent mite attack.

Other mites of medical importance

House dust mites, e.g., *Dermatophagoides pteronyssinus* (family Pyroglyphidae) (Figure IV.7)

Many mite species are commonly found in house dust, in the tropics and temperate regions. These mites can, in sensitized individuals, cause bronchial asthma, as well as extensive dermatitis. In house dust they feed mainly on desquamated skin scales. The mites become airborne during bed-making and could then be inhaled; not only the living mites but also dead ones and mite faeces contain potent allergens. The best method of controlling the mites would appear to be treatment of carpets, beds and settees with insecticides, followed by thorough vacuum cleaning to remove dead mites and faeces, as these cause symptoms.

Domestic mites causing dermatosis: *Dermanyssus gallinae* (chicken mite), (Dermanyssidae); *Ornithonyssus bacoti* (tropical rat mite), *O. sylviarum* (bird mite) and *O. bursa* (tropical poultry mite) (Macronyssidae)

These blood-sucking mites can cause dermatitis in humans. In the absence of their natural hosts they will readily attack humans. Rat mites are associated with groceries and warehouses. Bird mites are often found in the eaves of houses and in air-conditioning ducts, and may be blown into houses when the air-conditioning is switched on.

Forage mites, e.g., *Tyrophagus* (Acaridae)

These are pests of stored food products such as cheese, copra, vanilla pods, flour and macaroni. Persons handling such materials may be bitten or suffer from simple contact allergy, and various names, such as grocer's itch, copra itch and baker's itch, indicate the occupational nature of these dermatoses. Some forage mites may be swallowed or inhaled and can cause gastric disturbances or respiratory symptoms. The mites do not breed in the body but may be recovered from faeces or sputum (see Acarine dermatosis, Chapter 32).

Suborder: Ixodida; superfamily: Ixodoidea (ticks)

Ticks are larger (adult body length 3–20 mm) and lack the prominent hairs found on mites. All species are obligate blood-sucking ectoparasites of vertebrates. Originally parasites of reptiles, ticks adapted over the last 200 million years to the newly evolving warm-blooded bird and mammals, but some ticks have retained a predilection for cold-blooded vertebrates. The gnathosoma or capitulum is well developed and the prominent ventrally situated median hypostome bears on its underside rows of backwardly directed teeth which help the tick in attaching firmly to the host and prevent it from being easily dislodged by the grooming activities of the host (Figure IV.8).

There are two basic types of tick: the soft ticks (family Argasidae) and the hard ticks (family Ixodidae). Most people are familiar with the slow-feeding ixodid ticks found on dogs, cattle and other domestic animals, and which remain attached for several days. The argasids are rapid feeders, usually at night, returning quickly to their hiding places. Primarily parasites of wild animals, about 10% of tick species feed on domestic animals and many will feed opportunistically on humans. The soft tick *Ornithodoros moubata* of east, central and south Africa is probably the only true human-biting tick; it is found in huts and feeds readily on humans and chickens. Ticks parasitize a wide range of wild and domestic hosts, and many appear to have a preferred host, although this

apparent preference may be due to availability rather than choice. Both male and female adult ticks ingest considerable quantities of blood: a fully engorged female ixodid may reach a length of over 20 mm and weigh 2.0 g or more. Because of this, they threaten the health of domestic livestock with very heavy infestations. Control of veterinary pest species with insecticides is being superseded by the development of antitick vaccines. Apart from causing blood loss, ticks transmit a variety of pathogens among animals and are therefore important in veterinary medicine. However, because of their indiscriminate feeding habits, ticks acquire infection from animals and transmit it to humans during the next blood feed.

Movement of tick-infested animals, particularly of domestic livestock, has resulted in the introduction and establishment of exotic tick species in new areas. The cosmopolitan dog tick *Rhipicephalus sanguincus* is a carnivore parasite from Africa, now a worldwide parasite found in kennels and households. Many tick-borne diseases exist as silent foci where the pathogen, vertebrate host (usually a wild animal) and the tick have evolved to form a balanced relationship. Human population increase and economic pressure have led to ecological changes brought about by clearance of forests for cultivation, or the growing of cash crops. The intrusion of humans into such tick-infested areas and suburban encroachment into tick habitats with silent foci of infection have resulted in closer tick–human contact and an increase in the incidence of tick-transmitted diseases such as Rocky Mountain spotted fever in the eastern USA, tick-borne encephalitis in Europe, and the emergence of apparently 'new' diseases in humans such as Kyasanur Forest disease in India and Lyme disease in the USA and Europe.

There are several factors that make ticks efficient vectors of pathogenic organisms. Firm attachment to the host prevents them from being dislodged easily. The slow feeding of ixodids not only gives them ample time to ingest large numbers of pathogens from an infected host and ample time to transmit them to a new host, but also allows dispersal of infected ticks into new areas while still attached to a host. The multiple blood feeds during the life cycle and the wide host range ensure more opportunities to acquire and transmit infections, and makes a blood meal more certain. Many ixodids have a high reproductive potential, laying several thousands of eggs, but this is to offset the very considerable mortality during the life cycle. Some argasids can live for many years and starve for prolonged periods. This is of great survival value and gives them more opportunities to acquire and transmit pathogens during their long life. Transovarial transmission of many pathogens in ticks makes them true reservoirs of infection, and some tick-borne infections can be maintained in nature in the absence of vertebrate hosts by transovarial passage through several generations of ticks.

The Argasidae has about 150 species in three genera, of which *Argas* and *Ornithodoros* are the most important. The Ixodidae has about 800 species in 13 genera, of which *Ixodes*, *Amblyomma*, *Hyalomma*, *Haemaphysalis*, *Dermacentor* and *Rhipicephalus* transmit diseases to humans, and *Boophilus*

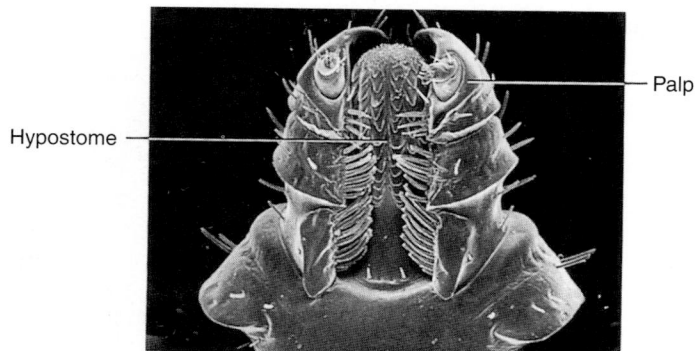

Figure IV.8: Electron micrograph view of ventral capitulum of ixodid tick. (Courtesy of M. Nawar.)

Hypostome — Palp

Table IV.1 Differences between argasid ticks and ixodid ticks.

	Argasidae	Ixodidae
Morphology		
Scutum	Absent	Present; anterior in larva, nymph and female, covering dorsal side in male
Capitulum	Ventral, not visible from above	Anterior, visible from above
Palps	Long, movable	Short, rigid
Life cycle	Several nymphal stages	One nymphal stage
	Multiple batches of eggs: 100–200 per blood meal	One batch of eggs (several 1000)
Habits	Rapid feeders, usually nocturnal; male and female feed repeatedly	Slow feeders, day and night, several days; only females feed once
	Restricted habitat, burrows or nests of hosts	Diffuse habitat, pasture, etc., where hosts forage

cattle ticks are important ectoparasites of domestic livestock. Morphological and biological differences which distinguish the two families are summarized in Table IV.1.

Family: Argasidae

These are tough, leathery ticks; the females range in size from small (4 mm) to large (15 mm), and the males are smaller but otherwise very similar. In nymphs and adults the capitulum is ventral and not visible from above; in larvae, the capitulum projects anteriorly. The jointed palps are long and movable, and in some species may be mistaken for an extra pair of legs. The surface of the integument is covered with mammillae or radially arranged depressions and discs, but the dorsal plate or scutum, characteristic of the Ixodidae, is absent (Figure IV.9)—hence the name 'soft ticks'. Eyes, when present, are simple and situated laterally. Spiracles or breathing holes are present ventrally between the first segments (coxae) of the third and fourth pairs of legs. The genital opening is anterior and ventral, behind the capitulum, and the anal opening is median and about one-third of the distance from the posterior margin. Between the first and second pairs of legs are the external openings of the coxal glands which help to concentrate the blood meal by filtering off fluid from the blood and excreting it as two drops of coxal fluid. In many *Ornithodoros* vectors of relapsing fever and arboviruses

the coxal glands are infected. Coxal fluid is excreted just before termination of a feed and pathogens in the fluid enter the bite wound. The glands therefore have an important role in disease transmission (Figures IV.10 and IV.11).

Argasids are rapid feeders, the larvae of some species taking only 2–3 minutes to engorge, those of the genus *Argas* remaining attached to their hosts for several days. The six-legged larvae feed once; larvae of *Ornithodoros* do not feed but moult straight into nymphs. Soft ticks are usually nocturnal feeders and the house-haunting *O. moubata* are not unlike bed bugs in their feeding and sheltering habits. Habitats of other Argasids include cracks and crevices in wood, stone or mud, nesting or resting places of the host animals, birds' nests in trees or

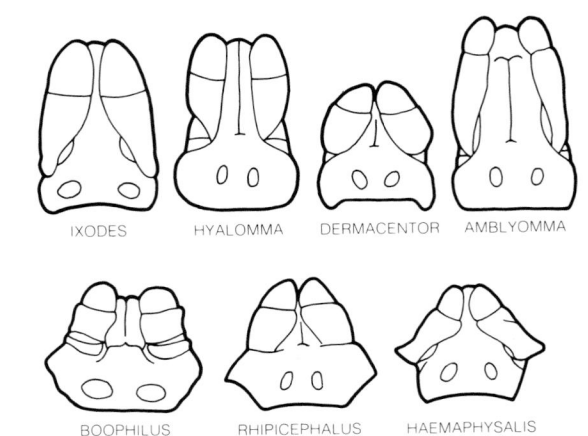

Figure IV.9: Dorsal view of capitulum of Ixodidae, showing characteristics of seven genera.

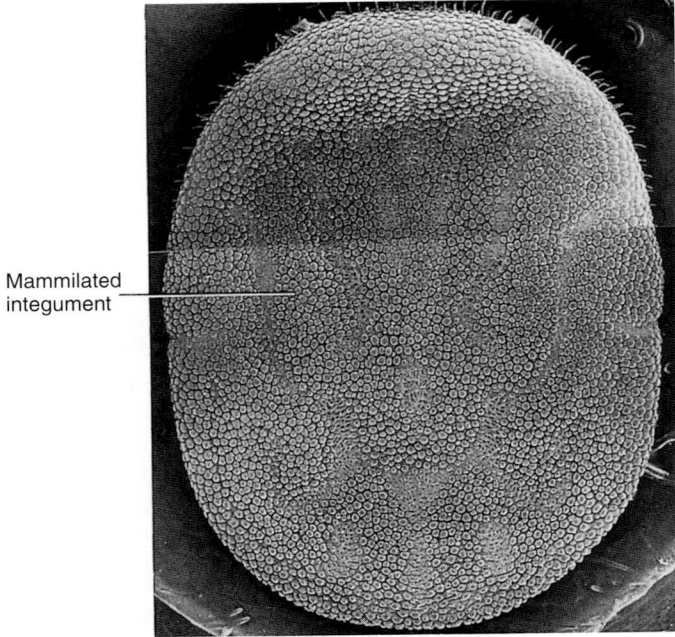

Mammilated integument

Figure IV.10: Dorsal view of adult female *Ornithodoros moubata*. (Courtesy of M. Nawar.)

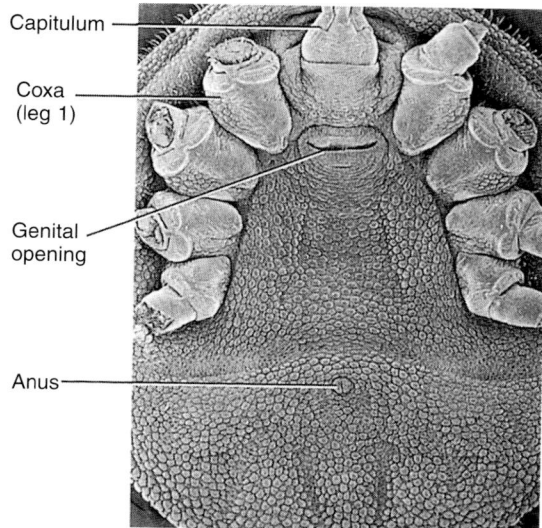

Capitulum

Coxa
(leg 1)

Genital
opening

Anus

Figure IV.11: Ventral view of adult female *Ornithodoros moubata*. (Courtesy of M. Nawar.)

Table IV.2 Human tick-borne relapsing fever: *Borrelia* spirochaetes and the *Ornithodoros* vectors which transmit them.

Tick vector	Spirochaete	Locality
O. moubata	B. duttoni	E., C. & S. Africa
O. erraticus	B. hispanica	W. Mediterranean, North Africa
O. tholozani	B. persica	E. Mediterranean eastwards through central Asia to western China
O. turicata	B. turicatae	USA, Mexico
O. parkeri	B. parkeri	N., C. & S. America
O. hermsi	B. hermsii	
O. rudis	B. venezuelensis	
O. talajae		
O. turicata		

on the ground, caves, burrows, deer beds, huts, log cabins, chicken coops, pigeon lofts, sheds and pigsties. Access to a blood meal is therefore easy and the hazards of finding a host considerably reduced. There are two to five or more nymphal stages; each stage feeds once and moults to the next stage. Adults mate off the host. Both males and females feed repeatedly, the females ovipositing after each blood meal, laying a batch of 100–200 eggs (Figure IV.12). The genera *Argas* and *Ornithodoros* can be separated by the distinct flattened lateral margin of the body in *Argas*, which is evident even when the tick is fully fed.

Argas spp. feed on birds or bats and may attack humans, causing painful bites. *Ornithodoros* spp. transmit *Borrelia* spp. spirochaetes, causing relapsing fever in humans (Table IV.2 and see Chapter 67). Foci of infection are usually restricted to caves, animal shelters, huts or resort cabins. There is a high rate of trans-stadial and transovarial

transmission of *Borrelia* among ticks; this and the longevity and ability of the vector to starve for long periods lead to the perpetuation of natural foci in the absence of vertebrate hosts. Ticks are the main reservoirs of infection, while other animals, such as rodents, probably serve only as amplifiers of infection. Following an infecting feed, the ticks have a disseminated infection of practically all the internal organs. Transmission is usually through salivary secretion containing *Borrelia* and/or contamination of the bite wound through infective coxal fluid.

Ornithodoros moubata, the 'eyeless' tampan tick, transmits relapsing fever (*Borrelia duttoni*) in tropical Africa. The integument is mammillated and greenish-brown. The absence of eyes distinguishes this species from the closely related and widely distributed sand tampan, *O. savignyi*, which has two pairs of eyes on the sides of the body. Both species are night feeders. *O. moubata* inhabits the floor of huts, animal shelters and the burrows of warthogs. There are two subspecies: *O. moubata moubata* feeds predominantly on humans and chickens, *O. m. porcinus* on warthogs, antbears and porcupines. In the cool wet habitats of the Kenya highlands and north-west Tanzania, 94% of *O. m. moubata* feed on humans and 2% on chickens, but in hot moist habitats these proportions are reversed. Both subspecies have domestic and wild populations, and it is the domestic populations that are important in disease transmission: no infected ticks have been found in wild populations. *O. moubata* is common on travel routes and may be carried long distances in mats and bed rolls. Rest houses are usually infested. To prevent the risk of infection with relapsing fever, old camping sites and mud houses should be avoided and it is advisable not to sleep on the floor. As the ticks find shelter in cracks and crevices in mud walls and floors, better housing and the use of concrete and plaster in buildings will help to control the ticks. They can also be controlled by treating the floors and walls of huts with insecticidal powder or spray.

O. savignyi, the eyed or sand tampan, is widely distributed in arid and semi-arid areas from Sri Lanka westwards

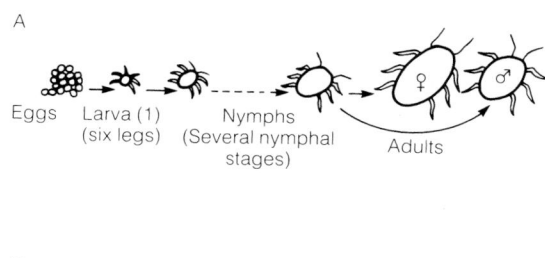

A

Eggs   Larva (1)   Nymphs   Adults
(six legs)   (Several nymphal
stages)

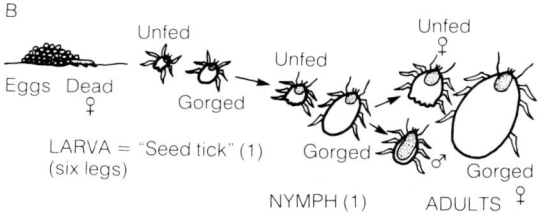

B

Unfed   Unfed ♀

Eggs Dead   Unfed
♀   Gorged

LARVA = "Seed tick" (1)   Gorged ♂
(six legs)
Gorged ♀

NYMPH (1)   ADULTS ♀

Figure IV.12: Tick life cycles: **A**, Argasidae; **B**, Ixodidae.

through India, Arabia and Africa, where the distributions of *O. savignyi* and *O. moubata* overlap. It is an outdoor tick found near the soil surface in the resting places of cattle, camels and other livestock in the shade of trees and stone fences. It will attack humans, given the opportunity, and can transmit relapsing fever in the laboratory.

O. erraticus occurs in north-west Africa, Spain and Portugal. It usually lives in burrows feeding on rodents but considerable populations exist in pigsties, where they feed on pigs. It is an important vector of relapsing fever (*B. hispanica*) in north-west Africa and Spain.

O. tholozani (=*O. papillipes*) has a widespread distribution: Libya, north-east Africa, the Mediterranean islands, northern Arabia, south-eastern Europe, southern CIS, northern India and western provinces of China. It is an important vector of relapsing fever (*B. persica*). Typical habitats are caves and large burrows but the tick has adapted successfully to stables and rest houses. *O. tholozani* feeds on domestic livestock, birds and people.

O. lahorensis occurs in Tibet, southern CIS Republics, Pakistan, Turkey, Greece, the Balkans and Bulgaria. It is found in stables and human habitations and is suspected of transmitting relapsing fever.

O. talaje is a South and Central American species extending northwards to the southern states of the USA. It feeds on wild rodents and domestic livestock as well as humans, inflicts a very painful bite and transmits relapsing fever in Guatemala, Panama and Colombia.

O. rudis (=*O. venezuelensis*) transmits *B. venezuelensis* in Panama, Colombia, Venezuela and Ecuador. It usually lives in the walls of huts and will feed avidly on humans.

O. hermsi is widespread in the Rocky Mountain and Pacific coast states of the USA. It is essentially a rodent parasite. It shelters in summer cabins at higher elevations and transmits relapsing fever (*B. hermsi*) to people occupying the cabins.

O. parkeri and *O. turicata* have similar distributions in the western USA, and the range of *O. turicata* extends southwards into Mexico. They feed primarily on rodents and are vectors of relapsing fever (*B. parkeri* and *B. turicatae* respectively) to humans.

O. coriaceus extends from California to Mexico. Known as the 'tlaaja' and the 'pajaroello', it is a large argasid, notorious for attacking humans, cattle and deer in their bedding areas. The bites are painful, but it is not a natural vector of relapsing fever.

O. rostratus, the 'quanco', occurs in southern Brazil, Bolivia, Paraguay and north-eastern Argentina. It is an avid biter of humans, domestic animals and wild animals, particularly peccaries. The bites are painful and are followed by pruritus and inflammation, and may become secondarily infected. It is not a natural vector of relapsing fever.

O. muesebecki is associated with marine birds on islands in the Arabian Gulf. The tick eagerly attacks humans and some dexterity is required to avoid being bitten. The bites may be numerous, and irritant bullae develop at the bite sites with intense pruritus, headache and fever. Zirqa virus (Bunyaviridae, Nairovirus) isolated from *O. muesebecki* may be the cause of the illness associated with the bites.

Family: Ixodidae

Hard ticks are readily distinguished from soft ticks by the presence of the prominent capitulum, projecting anteriorly, visible from above in all stages (Figure IV.13A). The mouthparts of some (*Ixodes* and *Amblyomma*) are long and can produce deep penetrating wounds in animals and humans (Figure IV.13B). The shape of the basal plate of the capitulum is an important character in generic identification (see Figure IV.9). The hard shiny scutum is present in all stages; it is small and restricted to the anterior dorsum in larvae, nymphs and adults, but large and covers the entire dorsal surface in males. The scutum of some ixodids (e.g., *Amblyomma* spp.) has a colourful pattern; such ticks are called *ornate* ticks. Those in which

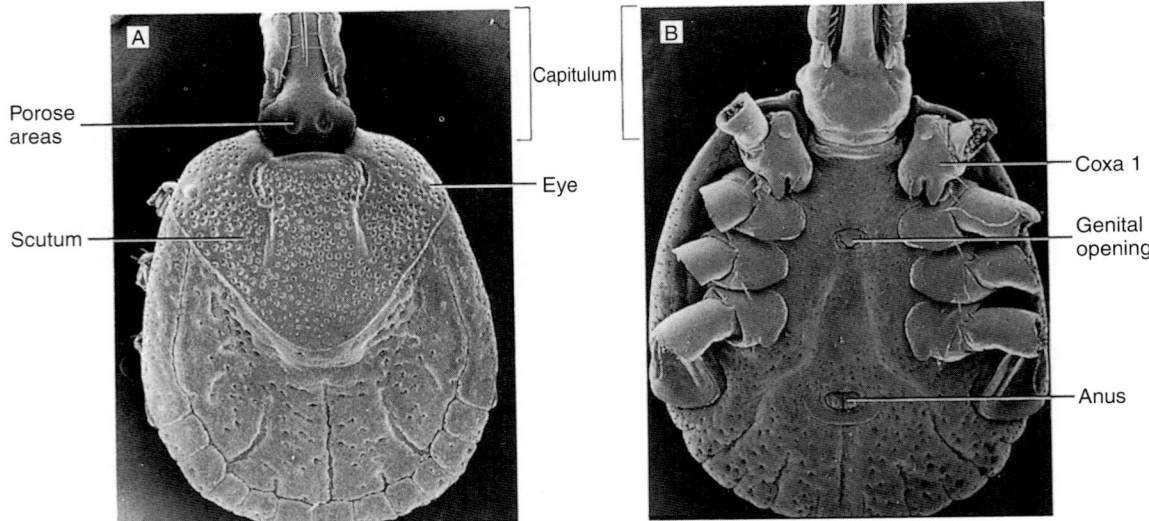

Figure IV.13: Dorsal (**A**) and ventral (**B**) views of *Amblyomma variegatum*. (Courtesy of M. Nawar.)

the scutum is not ornamented are called *inornate* ticks. Paired eyes, when present, are situated on either side of the scutum. Coxal glands are absent in ixodid ticks and the ingested blood is concentrated during the slow feeding by passage of fluid from the stomach into the body cavity, from where it is processed through the salivary glands back into the host. During their slow feeding, ixodid ticks remain attached for several days, anchoring themselves firmly with the chelicerae and hypostome, helped by 'cement' from the salivary glands. Once attached, great care should be taken in removing a tick because the mouthparts may be left behind in the host tissue and may become a source of irritation and secondary infection.

A few ticks (e.g., *Boophilus* cattle ticks) are host-specific, but most utilize a wide range of hosts. Adult ixodids usually parasitize large mammals, whereas the immature stages (larvae and nymphs) feed on smaller mammals such as rodents and ground-frequenting birds. Humans are seldom bitten by the adult ticks, but the larvae or 'seed ticks' of some ixodids feed avidly on people and are a bothersome nuisance in some outdoor areas in America and Africa.

The life cycle of Ixodidae has four stages (see Figure IV.12): the egg, followed by three mobile stages of larva, nymph and adult. The fertilized and engorged female drops off the host on to the ground and lays a mass of several thousand eggs. The female dies after oviposition. After hatching, the six-legged larvae climb to the tips of leaves, blades of grass or other vegetation to certain heights and gather in clusters questing for a host. They climb on to a passing host, feed for 4–6 days, drop to the ground and moult to the nymphal stage. Unlike the argasid ticks, ixodids have only one nymphal stage. The unfed nymphs quest for hosts like the larvae and after a blood meal (5–8 days) drop to the ground and moult into adults. Adults quest usually at a height greater than that of larvae and nymphs. Mating takes place on the host and the engorged female, after feeding for 6–12 days, drops off to lay a single batch of eggs.

The males may remain attached to the host for many weeks or months, mating with several females. The whole life cycle may take only 2–4 months in warm climates, with continuous breeding throughout the year. In cold or temperate climates the life cycle may take 3–5 years, the ticks being active or developing only in the warmer months. During the colder months and winter, one or more stages enter a diapause of several weeks or months. The parasitic feeding period of the different stages lasts from 4 to 12 days. Most ixodid ticks (e.g., *Amblyomma*, *Dermacentor*, *Ixodes*) have a three-host cycle in which each active stage (larva, nymph, adult) parasitizes a different animal of the same or different species. *Boophilus* cattle ticks have only a one-host cycle. A few species of *Hyalomma* and *Rhipicephalus* have a two-host cycle: the fed larva moults on the host (not on the ground), becoming a nymph which drops to the ground, moults to adulthood and then seeks a second host for a blood meal.

Ixodes scapularis (=*I. dammini*) (American deer tick) is widely distributed in the USA and adjacent Canada; the range appears to be extending, probably due to proliferation of deer, hosts of the adult ticks. Larvae and nymphs parasitize rodents (particularly the white-footed mouse) as well as humans. The adult ticks feed mostly on white-tailed deer, or occasionally on humans. *I. scapularis* is the vector of human babesiosis (*Babesia microti*) and Lyme disease (a spirochaetal infection caused by *Borrelia burgdorferi*) in eastern USA.

I. ricinus (European sheep tick or castor bean tick) is distributed widely in rough pasture and woodland across Europe to the Caspian Sea and northern Iran. *I. ricinus* is the vector of three human flaviviruses: louping ill (primarily of sheep and cattle but affecting humans also) in the British Isles (see Chapter 49), tick-borne viral encephalitis (TBE) in central Europe, and Lyme disease (*Borrelia burgdorferi*) (see Chapter 67), which is becoming increasingly widespread in areas with deer populations as hosts for adult *I. ricinus*. Immature ticks are found on rodents and birds; adults attack deer, sheep, cattle and also humans. The life cycle takes 2–4 years to complete.

I. persulcatus (the taiga tick) is widepread from the Baltic to Japan, its distribution overlapping with that of *I. ricinus*. It is more cold-hardy than *I. ricinus*. In Russia, *I. persulcatus* is associated with the taiga forest. The life cycle extends over 2–4 years. It is the chief vector of Russian spring–summer encephalitis (flavivirus). Transovarial transmission occurs, but the rate is variable.

I. holocyclus occurs in the humid densely vegetated coastal areas of Queensland and New South Wales in Australia where it infests a variety of mammalian hosts. Its bites may cause tick paralysis in dogs and humans. It is the vector of Queensland tick typhus (*Rickettsia australis*).

Haemaphysalis spinigera occurs in Sri Lanka and south India, most abundantly where cattle have been introduced into cleared forests. It is the chief vector of Kyasanur Forest disease (flavivirus). Immatures feed on small forest rodents, monkeys and humans. Exposure of humans to the ticks and risk of infection are highest in the dry pre-monsoon period when villagers go into the forest to gather firewood. Transmission of infection to humans is by bite by infected nymphs. There is no transovarial transmission in vector ticks.

H. leachi is widespread on carnivores. In South Africa urban cases of boutonneuse fever (*Rickettsia conori*) are associated with contamination of skin or eyes from infected ticks crushed while de-ticking dogs.

Rhipicephalus appendiculatus parasitizes cattle and wild game animals in wooded and shrubby grassland from southern Sudan to South Africa, but is absent from West Africa. In East Africa it is the vector of the protozoan disease East Coast fever (babesiosis) in cattle. In the South African veld it is the chief vector of African tick typhus (*Rickettsia*) and an avid human-biter.

R. sanguineus is a carnivore tick originating from Africa but now a cosmopolitan tick of dogs. In the Mediterranean basin it is the chief vector of boutonneuse fever to humans.

Dermacentor andersoni (Rocky Mountain wood tick) is widespread in the western USA and Canada, where it transmits Rocky Mountain spotted fever (*Rickettsia rickettsi*). Larvae and nymphs feed on practically every rodent; adults parasitize wild and domestic herbivores and eagerly bite humans. Transmission of the rickettsiae is by bite, and trans-stadial and transovarial transmission occur. There may be an interval of some hours or a day before the attached tick can transmit the rickettsiae. If the tick is removed within a few hours the risk of infection is considerably reduced. This tick also transmits Colorado tick fever virus to humans.

D. variabilis (American dog tick) occurs from Mexico to Canada, being particularly abundant along the east coast of the USA. Immatures feed on rodents, adults on wild and domestic carnivores, including dogs and also humans. It is the vector of Rocky Mountain spotted fever in the eastern USA. Infestation of dogs with *D. variabilis* brings the disease close to homes, and infections occur among women and children.

D. marginatus, *D. silvarum* and *D. nuttalli* are the chief vectors of Siberian tick typhus (*Rickettsia sibirica*). *D. marginatus* is found in shrubby areas and lowland forests from northern Kazakstan to central Europe. *D. silvarum* extends from the eastern limits of *D. marginatus* to western Siberia. *D. nuttalli* is widely distributed in central and eastern Siberia, Mongolia and China southwards to central Asia and Tibet. *R. sibirica* can survive for long periods in the ticks. Transmission is by bite, and both trans-stadial and transovarial transmission have been demonstrated.

D. pictus has the same distribution as *D. marginatus* in mixed and deciduous forests. Omsk haemorrhagic fever arbovirus has been isolated from it, but transmission to humans is believed to be by contact with, or drinking water infected with, the urine and faeces of muskrats.

Amblyomma hebraeum (the South African bont tick) extends from South Africa and Zimbabwe and Mozambique. It is the vector of boutonneuse fever in the South African veld, where immatures swarm and feed avidly on humans. *Rickettsia conori* can be maintained for several generations in *A. hebraeum* by hereditary transmission. Apart from humans, immature stages feed on birds and small and large mammals, while adults feed on large wild and domestic mammals.

A. americanum (lone-star tick) is widely distributed from South America into central and eastern USA. All stages attack people. It is the vector of Rocky Mountain spotted fever in the USA. The attached feeding ticks are difficult to remove because of the long mouthparts. Application of 0.6% pyrethrin in methyl benzoate or of camphorated phenol to the skin makes detachment easier.

A. cajennense (Cayenne tick) extends from South America and the Caribbean to southern Texas. Immatures attack humans. It is the vector of Rocky Mountain spotted fever to people in Mexico, Panama, Colombia and Brazil.

Hyalomma marginatum is a hardy tick adapted to living under arid or semi-arid conditions in Eurasia. Birds are important hosts of the immature stages and the ticks have been carried to many parts of Europe and Africa by migrating birds. It is the vector of Crimean–Congo haemorrhagic fever arbovirus.

Pentastomids

J. Riley

Pentastomids, sometimes called linguatulids or 'tongue worms', possess arthropod-like characters and there is evidence to suggest that they may be highly specialized endoparasitic crustaceans.[2] Four species, belonging to two genera, may affect humans as dead-end infections: *Linguatula*, which normally infects other mammals, and *Armillifer*, which infects snakes and mammals as intermediate hosts.

Family: Linguatulidae

Linguatula serrata is found worldwide. The adults live in the nasal passages of dogs, foxes and wolves (family Canidae), which are the definitive hosts. Eggs are expelled by sneezing or in nasal discharges, or via the intestine where some premature hatching may occur. Eggs are infective to mammal intermediate hosts, including rodents and domestic animals such as sheep and goats. Primary larvae emerge, penetrate the gut wall and migrate to the viscera, particularly to the mesenteric lymph nodes, where they become encapsulated by host tissue. Within the cyst several moults eventually lead to the formation of an infective larva or nymph. Infection of the definitive host occurs when viscera containing the encysted infective stage are eaten. The epidemiology of *L. serrata* infections is complex, because both eggs and infective larvae can become established in humans. When eggs are consumed, primary larvae encyst in the viscera, producing visceral linguatulosis, whereas ingested infective larvae attempt to migrate to the nasal passages producing nasopharyngeal linguatulosis or halzoun (Chapter 81).

The body of adult *Linguatula* (Figure IV.14) is club-shaped, flattened ventrally, convex dorsally and transversely striated into about 90 superficial annulations. The

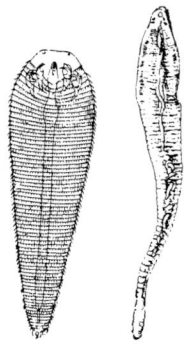

Figure IV.14: *Linguatula serrata*. Left, nymph (6 ×). Right, adult (natural size).

cephalothorax bears the quadrangular mouth, which is flanked by two pairs of simple retractile hooks. Females are 80–130 mm in length, tapering from 8–10 mm anteriorly to 2 mm posteriorly. The uterine coils, full of reddish-brown eggs, occupy the median line of the body, and the translucent flared lateral extensions of the anterior abdomen mould to the contours of the nasal sinuses. Living males are transparent in life but become white when fixed, measure 18–27 mm in length and are 3 mm wide anteriorly to 0.5 mm posteriorly. The oval eggs, measuring 70 × 100 μm are loosely enveloped by a thin hyaline outer capsule and contain mature primary larvae which have an anterior penetration stylet and four stumpy legs terminating in double claws. Infective nymphs (Figure IV.14) are worm-like, flattened and 4–6 mm in length; the posterior edge of each body annulus carries a row of prominent backward-pointing spines which are sufficient to distinguish *Linguatula* spp. in tissue section.

Clinical effects (halzoun; marrara syndrome) (see Chapter 81)

Encysted infective nymphs are well tolerated and are frequently encountered in the mesenteric glands of domestic animals, as well as in rabbits and hares. Data on human infections arise only from incidental findings during autopsy; in the few instances where sample sizes were large, nymphs were not uncommon.[3] Nymphs developing on visceral organs cause no symptoms but occasionally they penetrate the anterior chamber of the eye, causing monocular uveitis. Following surgical removal of these parasites, patients recover fully.

In tissue sections, infective larvae of *Linguatula* are enclosed within a thin fibrotic capsule lined by the preceding cast nymphal cuticle. The spinous cuticle is distinctive and the spacious body cavity contains an obvious intestinal tract flanked by a pair of prominent glands composed of large individual gland cells. These characteristics serve to distinguish them from sparganum (Appendix III).

Family: Armilliferidae

Armillifer armillatus infects humans in tropical Africa. In Oriental regions *A. moniliformis* is the usual cause of human infection, which has been recorded from Malaysia, Java, Manila, Sumatra and China.

Adult parasites inhabit the lungs of pythons, and in Africa large vipers; the larval forms encyst in the tissues of many mammal species, including monkeys and humans. The parasite is cylindrical, vermiform, yellowish and translucent with conspicuous opaque annulated rings around the body, 1–2 mm apart (Figure IV.15). In females the uterine coils, filled with white or yellowish eggs, are easily visible through the cuticle. The female of *A. armillatus* is 70–140 mm long and 5–9 mm wide, the male 30–50 mm long and 3–4 mm wide; females possess up to 22 annuli and males up to 24. Both sexes of *A.*

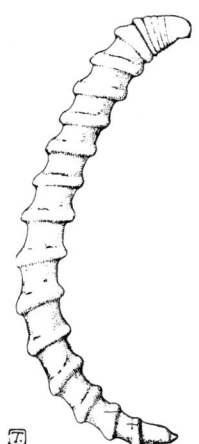

Figure IV.15: *Armillifer armillatus* (natural size).

moniliformis are more slender and have more annuli (26 and above) than *A. armillatus*. The nymphs lie coiled within their cysts in a flat spiral, with the ventral surface corresponding to the convexity of the curve. In shape and structure they resemble the adult. A third species of *Armillifer* (*A. grandis*) has been reported from humans in central Africa where nymphs are smaller (9–15 mm long) than those of *A. armillatus* (13–23 mm); *A. moniliformis* nymphs are intermediate in size (12–20 mm).

The life history of *Armillifer* is broadly similar to that of *Linguatula*, although humans can act only as an intermediate host. Eggs remain viable on soil for at least 3 months and, when ingested, hatch in the intestine; the larvae immediately bore through the intestinal wall to lodge in any tissue. At least six moults occur over a period of 6 months to 1 year, to form infective nymphs. Humans acquire the infection by eating poorly cooked snake meat, or by drinking water contaminated by snake faeces. In humans the infection comes to a dead end and the nymphs commonly encyst in or on the liver, intestinal tract and lungs.

Flies causing myiasis

G. B. White

Class: Insecta; order: Diptera (two-winged flies)

Myiasis covers a variety of associations between dipterous larvae and mammals. The most comprehensive definition is 'the infestation of live human and vertebrate animals with dipterous larvae which, at least for a certain period, feed on the host's dead or living tissue, liquid body-substance, or ingested food'.[4] Such associations vary from complete endoparasitism, via casual or accidental myiasis, to the bizarre predation on human blood by free-living larvae. A wide range of families of flies is involved, mostly 'higher flies' (Cyclorrhapha) of which the larvae are either specialized endoparasites in other mammals or are scavengers and carrion feeders.

Myiasis can be classified on the basis of either clinical or parasitological criteria. From a medical standpoint, the clinical classification is more important because it aids diagnosis and identification of the species responsible. Parasitological classification, based on the host–parasite relationship, assists in understanding the biological background and hence possible methods of prevention or control. Whilst a single incident can be remedied (e.g., by surgical removal) and the larva identified, prevention of further attacks relies on a knowledge of the insect's biology.

Myiasis in humans concerns a few common flies (e.g., *Cordylobia, Dermatobia, Chrysomya*) and a large number of uncommon or rare examples. Numerous cases of myiasis have been published in which the identification of the larva responsible is doubtful.

Clinically, myiasis-producing larvae attack three main parts of the body:

1. Cutaneous tissue, usually invading wounds or sores, producing furuncles, roving swellings or creeping myiasis. 'Sanguinivorous larvae' of the Congo floor maggot (*A. luteola*) are free-living (see Chapter 86).
2. Body cavities such as the nasopharynx, eyes and auditory canal.
3. Organs of the body, principally the gut lumen and urogenital system.

Parasitologically, myiasis producers can be divided into three other categories.

1. Obligate parasites: larvae develop in living tissue; they are unable to develop elsewhere. Larvae are endoparasitic, avoiding the host's immune system. The adults do not normally feed.
2. Facultative myiasis producers, whose larvae usually develop on carrion but may invade wounds. Primary flies initiate myiasis (e.g., *Cochliomyia hominivorax*); secondary flies enter the body only when an animal has prior infestation (e.g., *Cochliomyia macellaria*); tertiary flies become involved at a late stage of necrosis (e.g., many carrion-breeding blowflies).[1]
3. Accidental myiasis producers, whose eggs or larvae are ingested accidentally and are not killed in the intestine.

Larvae causing myiasis are essentially hydrostatic bags against which the muscles work to produce movement. The cephalopharyngeal skeleton has a pair of mouth-hooks to tear at the host's tissues, and a structure to anchor the muscles operating the mouth-hooks. They do not have a recognizable head capsule (except *Psychoda*). The overall shape of the larvae varies from the wedge shape of blow flies (*Calliphora, Lucilia*, etc.), through the ovoid tumbu fly (*Cordylobia anthropophaga*) to the pyriform *Dermatobia hominis*. There is often a change of shape during larval development. Some species possess rows of hooks or spines to prevent their expulsion from the host. The distribution and shape of such spines, together with

details of the spiracles and cephalopharyngeal skeleton, are used to identify the different species.

Myiasis of cutaneous tissue (see Chapter 86)

Larvae living in the skin and producing furuncles

These are usually specially adapted endoparasites and are the most commonly encountered by clinicians. Antibiotic prophylaxis is advisable before attempting to remove myiasis larvae from their lesions.

Cordylobia anthropophaga (Figure IV.16) (the African tumbu fly, mango fly or ver du cayor) is a large, robust, yellow-brown fly, 7–12 mm long. Adults of *C. anthropophaga* are difficult to distinguish from numerous other species of the family Calliphoridae, where the larva can be identified by its posterior spiracles (Figure IV.17B).[5]

C. anthropophaga is an obligate parasite found throughout Africa south of the Sahara, although some areas are free from the fly. As a result of air travel, people infested with *C. anthropophaga* arrive in many parts of the world. Recently this species was recorded from a patient in southern Spain who had never visited Africa, thus indicating that it might be possible for *C. anthropophaga* to establish foci outside endemic areas. Adults are active in the early morning and late afternoon and can be found resting in dark places—huts, etc.

The white, banana-shaped eggs of *C. anthropophaga* are laid in two batches of 100 to 300. The female oviposits preferentially on sandy ground, particularly if contaminated with urine or faeces, but can also lay on clothing if similarly contaminated (although such clothing may appear clean to the human eye). Clothing laid on the ground to dry may be affected, but not clothes hanging in bright sunlight because the eggs are laid only in shaded areas. Eggs are not laid directly on to skin, hairs or vegetation. On hatching, the minute first instar larvae hold themselves erect, while waving the anterior part in search of a host, and can remain alive without food for about 9 days. Larvae are sensitive to both heat and vibration and, once they become attached to a host, immediately begin to penetrate the unbroken skin, taking approximately 1 minute. Penetration is usually painless and may involve any part of the body, particularly the back, neck and head of humans. Larvae are acquired from lying on the ground

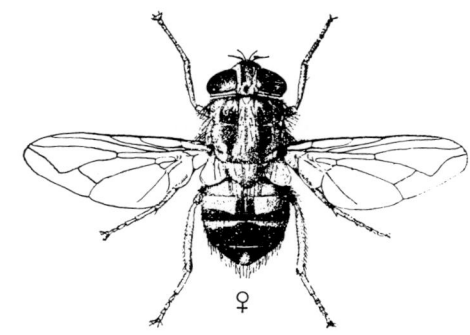

Figure IV.16: *Cordylobia anthropophaga* (twice natural size).

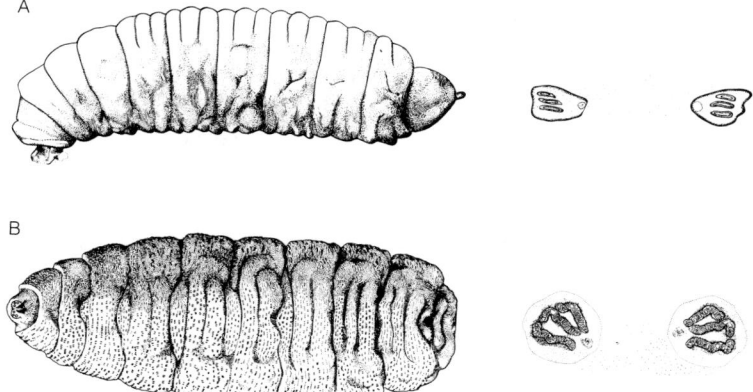

Figure IV.17: Third instar larva and posterior spiracles of (**A**) *Auchmeromyia luteola* and (**B**) *Cordylobia anthropophaga*. (Reproduced from Smith,[5] courtesy of the British Museum (Natural History), London.)

or from clothing. They are more common in children. *Cordylobia* breeds all the year round but human cases are more common in the wet season.

Initially, the small papule containing the larva of *C. anthropophaga* may be itchy or pricking at intervals. As the papule increases in size the symptoms recur and may be painful enough to interfere with sleep. Serous fluid may be exuded and gland enlargement may occur, or even febrile reactions and malaise. The larvae are usually noticed when the third stage has been reached. During the time for which the larva is in the host (8–12 days) it has its posterior segment, bearing the respiratory spiracles, protruding from the aperture; this may be withdrawn when touched. The cavity containing the larva breaks down to form a swelling, resembling a boil, which bursts without much inflammation. Larvae emerge from the swellings, fall to the ground and pupate within 24 hours. Pupal cases are commonly found in holes of black or brown rats which, together with dogs, are the principal hosts other than humans. The adult fly hatches 10–20 days (according to temperature) after pupation.

Larvae can be extracted by manipulation, if mature, or by inducing them to exit of their own accord by covering their respiratory aperture with petroleum jelly. The larvae die when covered with adhesive dressing. To prevent infestation, clothes should be ironed on both sides before

wearing and should be hung indoors for drying with the windows closed or screened to exclude the adult flies.

Dermatobia hominis (the American human bot fly, ver macaque, Berne, el tórsalo, beefworm) (Figure IV.18) is widely distributed in the Americas, from Mexico to Argentina and Chile. It attacks a wide range of hosts, including fowls, and is a devastating pest of livestock in some areas. The adult is a large bluish-grey fly, 1.5 cm long, with a strong flight. *D. hominis* is found primarily on the edge of tropical forests, particularly hilly areas of secondary forest 160–3000 m above sea level.

D. hominis is remarkable for the unique manner of delivering eggs to a new host, by using other insects as carriers. The adult female *Dermatobia* catches and firmly holds a day-flying mosquito or muscoid fly and attaches up to 30 eggs on to its abdomen (Figure IV.19). The larva remains in the eggshell until it senses proximity to a warm-blooded host, whereupon it rapidly 'hatches' and penetrates the host's skin within 5–10 minutes, remaining at the site of penetration. Each larva penetrates individually and a small nodule develops around it with a central pore through which the larva breathes. Close examination of

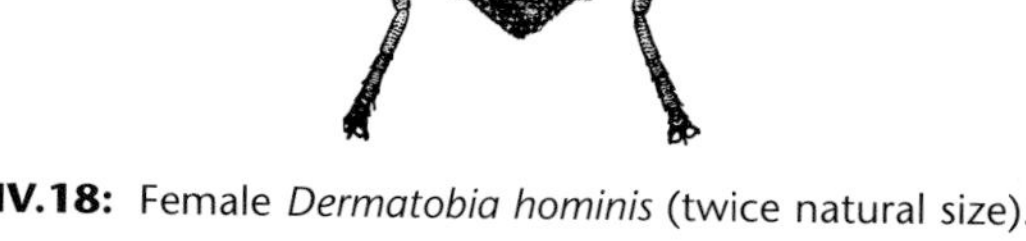

Figure IV.18: Female *Dermatobia hominis* (twice natural size).

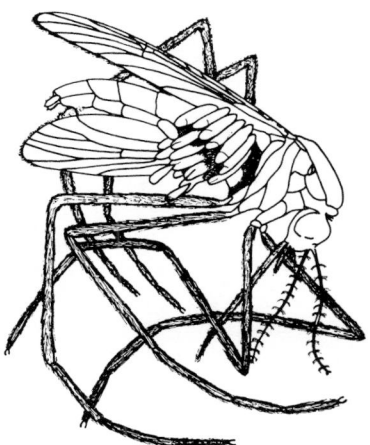

Figure IV.19: The mosquito *Psorophora lutzi* carrying eggs of *Dermatobia hominis*.

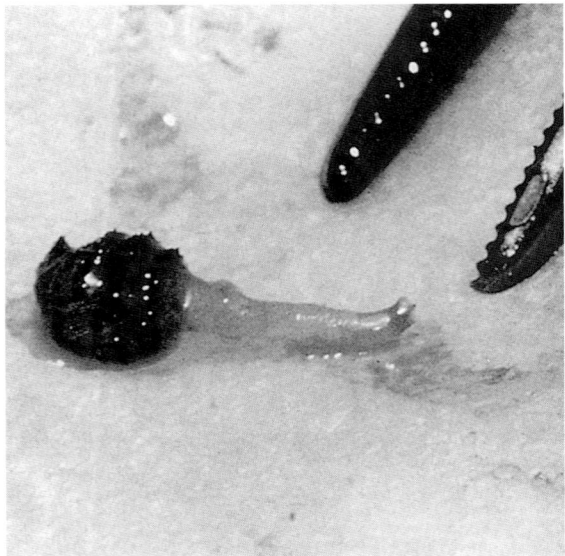

Figure IV.20: Second-stage instar of *Dermatobia hominis*.

a lesion containing a larva will reveal its posterior end bearing two small dark brown spots which are the spiracles. The first instar is subcylindrical with circlets of small spines. The second stage (Figure IV.20) is pyriform, with stronger, stout spines on the globular portion and none on the narrow posterior part, which acts like a respiratory siphon. At this stage the larva is difficult to dislodge by virtue of its shape and the numerous concentric rows of backward-projecting spines. During larval life the wound oozes serous fluid or pus continually, but bacteriostatic activity in the gut of the larva seems to prevent undesirable overgrowth of pyogenic bacteria in its environment,[6] although in some cases sécondary infection does occur.

The duration of larval development of *D. hominis* in humans is 6–12 weeks, during which it grows slowly,

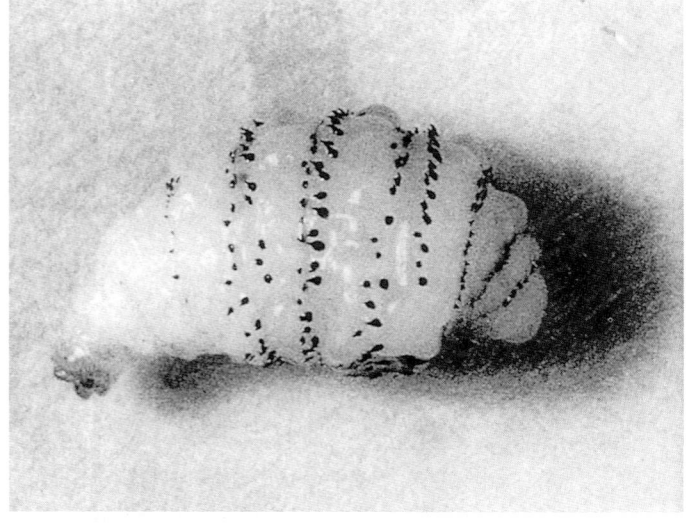

Figure IV.21: Third-stage instar of *Dermatobia hominis*.

feeding on tissue exudate. The mature larva (Figure IV.21) leaves the host and burrows into the soil to pupate, emerging after 4–11 weeks. The adults live for 8–9 days, never feed and are sexually mature about 3 hours after emergence.

Cutaneous swellings harbouring larvae usually occur on exposed areas, although larvae can penetrate clothing and may therefore be found on any part of the body. They are often single, but up to 12 have been reported on one individual. It is a common cause of ocular myiasis in Colombia (see Chapter 18). Rarely, serious complications occur, such as fatal cerebral myiasis in children. Most infestations by *Dermatobia* are painful, so larvae are removed in the first or second stages by the methods described for *Cordylobia* or surgically via a cruciate incision, taking care not to course the central hole as this may result in damage to the larva and give rise to septicaemia.

Creeping myiasis and roving swellings
(see Chapter 86)
Species that cause this syndrome are usually specialized endoparasites of other animals which are unable to develop fully in humans. It is important to distinguish them from *Ancylostoma* (nematodes), which produce similar effects.

Hypoderma bovis and *H. lineatum* cause creeping swellings and eruptions, especially in persons associated with cattle. On hatching, the larvae penetrate into the subcutaneous tissues, more deeply than *Gastrophilus*, producing a painful inflamed swelling that resembles a boil. They migrate, sometimes for considerable distances, and may invade the nervous system. The larva can be extracted through a cruciform incision.

Gastrophilus spp. are common parasites of horses and occasionally affect humans. The larvae penetrate the skin but do not develop beyond the first instar, causing a swelling and a wandering tunnel in the lower epidermis, in which they may progress for long periods.

Larvae that attack wounds and sores
(see Chapter 86)
Larvae of flies usually associated with carrion (*Galliphora, Lucilia, Phormia, Musca, Fannia*; Figure IV.22) have been found in wounds and gangrenous tissue, where they act as facultative parasites feeding on necrotic tissue and occasionally attacking healthy tissue. Pre-existing lesions may also serve as entry points for larvae of the obligate myiasis flies *C. anthropophaga* in Africa and *D. hominis* in the Americas, as described above. Occasionally, larvae are found living in soiled folds of the skin. Species that are usually found infesting soiled areas around the anus or genitalia may exceptionally enter the rectum or vagina to become internal parasites. At one time it was practice to use larvae of carefully cultivated *Lucilia* (sheep blowflies) to clean septic wounds by removal of infected tissue, but this has now been abandoned.

Cochliomyia (=*Callitroga*) *hominivorax* (New World screw-worm fly) is an obligate parasite in the Americas, affecting mainly cattle but also causing serious cases of human myiasis. Clean wounds are attacked, sometimes

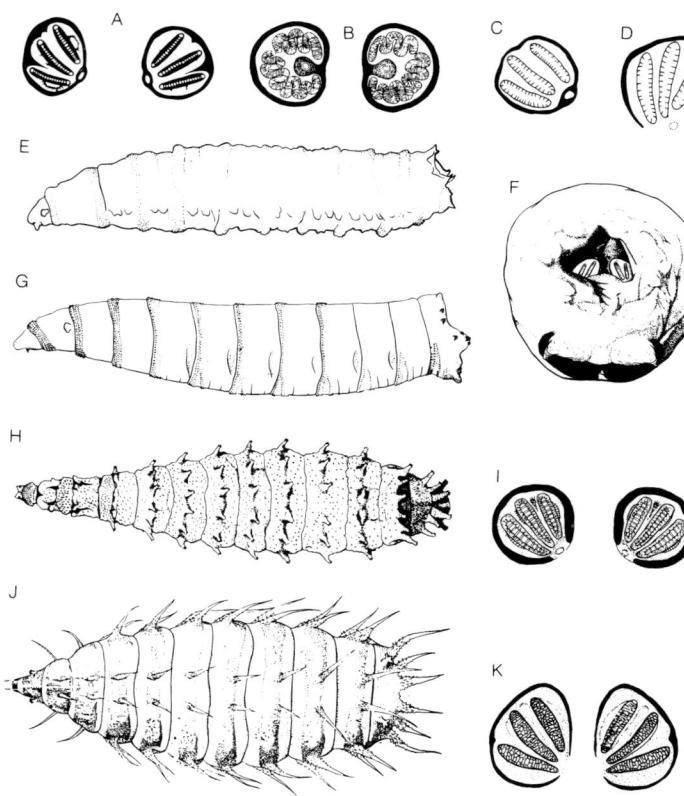

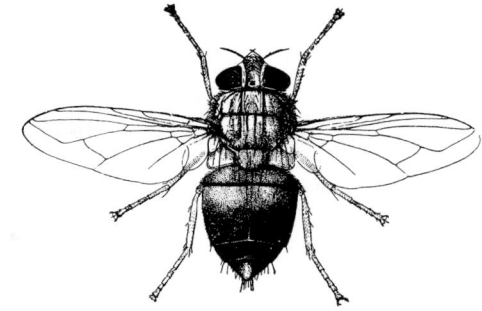

Figure IV.23: Female *Auchmeromyia luteola* (twice natural size).

Figure IV.22: General views of mature (third instar) larvae of myiasis-causing flies (Diptera) to show range in form and posterior spiracles used in identification. **A**, *Lucilia serricata*; **B**, *Musca domestica*; **C**, *Calliphora* sp.; **D**, *Wohlfahrtia* sp.; **E** and **F**, *Sarcophaga* spp.; **G** and **I**, *Callitroga macellaria*; **H** and **K**, *Chrysomyia albiceps*; **J**, *Fannia* sp. (Reproduced from Smith,[5] courtesy of the British Museum (Natural History) London.)

the smallest abrasions: even a scratch or stubbed toenail can become affected. The fly lays eggs on dry skin and the larvae subsequently invade the wound and feed rapaciously on healthy tissue, usually in groups to produce characteristic pocket-like injuries. Eggs may be deposited in the ears and nasal passages, and even in the vulva and vagina. Larvae grow rapidly and reach maturity in 4–8 days. A case mortality rate of 8% has been reported, and people in close contact with infested cattle are particularly at risk. This species gained recognition for its efficient control in North America by the release of radiation-sterilized males. A related American species, *C. macellaria*, is a facultative parasite responsible for the secondary invasion of wounds as well as scavenging on dead tissues.

Wohlfahrtia magnifica (Old World flesh fly) occurs in the warmer parts of Eurasia where it deposits its larvae in skin lesions, nasal sinuses, ears, sore eyes and vagina, producing serious disfigurement. Like the larvae of *W. vigil* and *Chrysomya bezziana*, these larvae rely on living tissue for development and do not feed on carrion or excreta.

Wohlfahrtia vigil (Nearctic flesh fly) in North America deposits its larvae in lesions of the skin or mucous

membranes, or even on uninjured skin. It is attracted by foul odours from secretions of the ear, eye or nose and possibly from the soiled nappies of babies. Young children are particularly attractive to the flies. The flies do not enter houses. Other species of *Wohlfahrtia* that cause cutaneous myiasis are widespread in the northern hemisphere.

Sanguinivorous larvae (see Chapter 86)

The larvae of several fly genera are obligatory parasites living free in the nests of birds and mammals, feeding on the blood of their hosts. Only *Auchmeromyia luteola* (Figure IV.23) (the Congo floor maggot) has been reported as attacking humans. This species is widely distributed in Africa, from Nigeria to Natal, in wet and dry climates. The larva is dirty white, about 15 mm long and has three short, fleshy lobes bearing spines on the posterior portion of each segment. The spiracles are distinctive. After feeding with its mouth-hooks, the conspicuously red larva (see Figure IV.17A) retreats to cracks in the floor. Larvae of *A. luteola* are frequently found under sleeping mats and in the earth to a depth of 7.5 cm. They feed mainly at night and drop off immediately they are disturbed. The yellowish adults can be found resting in dark areas of huts.

Myiasis of body cavities (see Chapter 86)

Several species that attack wounds and sores (discussed above) are also involved with myiasis of the eye, orbit, nasal cavities and ear canal. In nasal myiasis the initial symptoms are tickling pain and nasal obstruction. Epistaxis is common, but the discharge soon becomes purulent and fetid. Inhalation of chloroform or packing with chloroform gauze, or the careful local use of weak carbolic acid and turpentine, have been advocated, but the nasal sinuses may need to be opened.

Chrysomya bezziana (Old World screw-worm) is a large metallic-blue fly with a bright green thorax, found throughout Asia and Africa south of the Sahara. Unlike other species of this genus, it is an obligate parasite. Several other species of *Chrysomyia* have been incriminated as facultative myiasis agents, usually in wounds, but their identification in both the larval and adult stage is difficult.

The females of *C. bezziana* lay numerous eggs in the nasal cavities, especially where there is chronic nasal

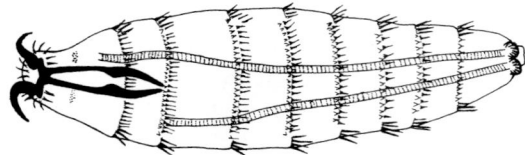

Figure IV.24: First instar larva of *Oestrus ovis*—a common cause of ophthalmomyiasis in North Africa.

discharge, or in ulcers or skin wounds (for instance in leprosy), or even in the gums, conjunctiva, ears or vagina. The larvae require living tissue in which to develop; they hatch in a few hours and burrow into the tissues, even to the bones of the nose, producing foul, infected, discharging and disfiguring lesions. These can be treated with a douche of 15% chloroform in light vegetable oil. A few drops of the mixture applied to an infested wound will cause the larvae to appear, and they can be removed with sinus forceps.

Ophthalmomyiasis is the presence of larvae in the orbit and in the accessory glands of the eye and eyeball. Infections may be quite common (10 per 100 000 population[7]) in some parts of Asia and north Africa, involving obligatory or facultative parasite species. The most common cause of ophthalmomyiasis is first-stage larvae of the sheep nasal bot fly (*Oestrus ovis*) (Figure IV.24), which drop their eggs into the orbit, and rarely the mouth or outer ear. Typically patients report being struck in the eye by an insect or foreign object. Within a few hours painful inflammation occurs, which may last for a few days as the larvae cannot develop any further in humans. Occasionally larvae reach the nasal cavities (its natural habitat in sheep and goats), where they cause swelling and pain as well as frontal headache, but do not live longer than 10 days. Other obligatory parasites of domestic animals, such as the horse bot fly (*Rhinoestrus purpureus* in Europe, Near East and North Africa), cattle warble fly (*Hypoderma*) and in parts of tropical Africa *Gedoelstia*, may affect humans by invading the orbit and (especially in *Hypoderma*) penetrating the eyeball. Rarely, carcass-breeding species such as *Lucilia serricata* (sheep blowfly) cause myiasis of the eye, but only when a pre-existing putrefying wound exists near the orbit, and this is therefore typical wound myiasis.

Myiasis of organ systems (see Chapter 86)

In the majority of cases this is due to accidental 'parasitism'.

Intestinal myiasis

This type of myiasis is usually diagnosed from the presence of larvae in vomit or faeces. Obligatory gut parasites of animals will not develop in humans and therefore species that cause intestinal myiasis are facultative or accidental parasites. About 50 species have been recorded; many cases of suspected gut myiasis have in fact resulted from contamination of samples after collection, as some species

(e.g., *Sarcophaga* spp.) can develop to the third larval stage in 24 hours, and others will lay larvae (larviposition) on faeces as they are being deposited. Occasionally, previously contaminated collection vessels have been responsible for a mistaken report.

Larvae may be swallowed in contaminated food and pass through the intestine unaffected by the extreme environment (e.g., *Piophila*—cheese skipper). However, this is unusual as most ingested larvae die and may be passed dead or, exceptionally, live if there is a concurrent intestinal infection. Even under these circumstances, larvae may cause intestinal lesions, damage to mucous membranes or haemorrhagic infiltrations—demonstrated by severe gastrointestinal disturbances (vomiting, diarrhoea, nausea). Reports of larvae developing in the anterior and median gut in humans, and even becoming paedogenic, are highly doubtful.[8]

Flies that are normally attracted to faeces may, under particularly poor standards of hygiene, deposit their eggs on or near the anus, and the larvae then penetrate into the posterior part of the rectum. Several authentic cases caused by *Eristalis* (Syrphidae), which commonly lives in sewage, have been reported.

Urogenital myiasis

Larvae of facultative parasites may be excreted in the urine or found in the vagina. The flies concerned are usually of the families Psychodidae, Muscidae, Calliphoridae and Sarcophagidae. A mistaken diagnosis of urinary myiasis due to a larva from a contaminated vessel in which urine has been collected, or introduced into the urine after it has been passed, is not uncommon, but there have been cases in which the larvae have undoubtedly been passed via the urethra from the bladder. If the vulva or vagina is infested there are obvious opportunities for larvae to enter the bladder.

Collection and preservation of larvae

After removal of myiasis larvae from the host by irrigation, manipulation or surgery, the larvae should be killed in hot water to retain their overall shape. The posterior respiratory spiracles are an important means of identification. The spiracles can be seen under a high-power dissecting microscope, but it may be necessary to remove, macerate and slide-mount them for detailed examination. Larvae should be preserved in 80% alcohol. Identification of accidental or facultative parasites is often difficult, as many species may be involved. In contrast, the identification of obligate parasites is easier as fewer species are involved, although the superficial similarity of flies of widely separated genera makes it necessary to submit specimens for identification by a specialist whenever a precise identification is required. Identification is facilitated if larvae are reared to adults on small pieces of meat. Smith[5] gives details for identification.

Phlebotomine sandflies

R. P. Lane

Family: Psychodidae; subfamily: Phlebotominae

Important genera: *Phlebotomus* (Old World) and *Lutzomyia* (New World)

Phlebotomine sandflies are small, delicate, hairy flies (1.5–3.5 mm long) with long, slender legs and filamentous antennae. Both sexes of adult sandflies feed frequently on nectar and other juices from plants. Female sandflies are also haematophagous: they feed regularly on the blood of vertebrates to obtain nutrition for egg production. Of the 700 species found throughout the tropics and subtropics, only a small proportion (*c.* 70 species) are thought to be involved in the transmission of disease to humans.

Sandflies are easily distinguished from other small Diptera when alive by the characteristic manner in which they hold their pointed wings above their body (like a vertical V; Figure IV.25). In other blood-sucking Diptera the wings are held flat over the abdomen, either one on top of the other (Culicidae, Simuliidae, *Culicoides*) or outspread (Glossinides, Tabanidae). It is important to differentiate phlebotomine sandflies from other small flies known locally as 'sandflies', i.e., midges of the genus *Culicoides* and blackflies of the family Simuliidae.

There is relatively little morphological difference between sandfly males and females, except that the males have elaborate external genitalia terminalia (see Figure IV.26). Human-biting (anthropophagous) species of sandflies belong to two genera: *Phlebotomus* in the Old World and *Lutzomyia* in the New World. In Africa, some species of the genus *Sergentomyia*, which feed principally on reptiles, occasionally bite humans also, but are not regarded as vectors of any human or zoonotic pathogen(s).

Phlebotomine sandflies are vectors of visceral leishmaniasis (VL: kala-azar; see Chapter 75), the various forms of cutaneous leishmaniasis (CL: oriental sore, espundia, etc.; see Chapter 75), bartonellosis (Oroya fever, Carrión's disease; see Chapter 61) and sandfly fever (papataci or papatasi fever, 3-day fever, etc.; see Chapter 41). Transmission of pathogens takes place during blood feeding.

Sandflies are not easy to study in relation to disease, as the adults are small and unobtrusive, while finding larvae is almost impossible. This has made the incrimination of vectors during epidemiological studies particularly difficult and, therefore, the vector status of many species remains uncertain.[9] (See also Epidemiology of leishmaniasis; Chapter 75.) Compared with other vector groups (e.g., Culicidae and Simuliidae), the biology of sandflies is poorly known. However, a thorough understanding of the natural history of sandflies is essential, because the epidemiology of the diseases they transmit is largely determined by the ecology and behaviour of the vectors.

Distribution and ecology

Sandflies are found mainly in the tropics and subtropics, with a few species penetrating into temperate regions in both the northern (to 50°N) and southern (to about 40°S) hemispheres. The distribution of leishmaniasis is not as extensive as that of sandflies, for reasons that are not entirely known; for instance, no human leishmaniasis has been recorded from South-East Asia and Australasia, although several potential vectors are present.

In the Old World, human-biting sandflies are confined to the subtropics, there being very few anthropophilic

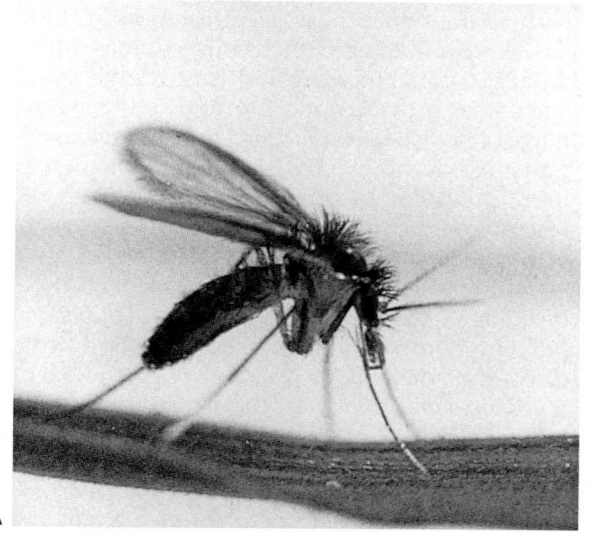
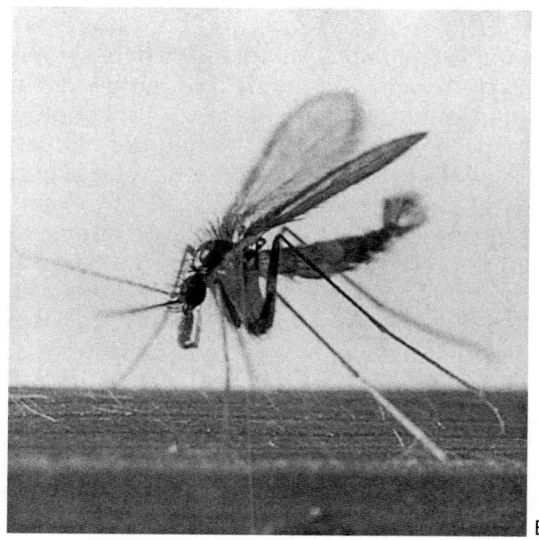

Figure IV.25: Living female (**A**) and male (**B**) phlebotomine sandflies (*Lutzomyia longipalpis*), showing the hairy body and wings, the generally mosquito-like stance and appearance except for the characteristic position of the wings, held in a V over the back. (Courtesy of C. J. Webb.)

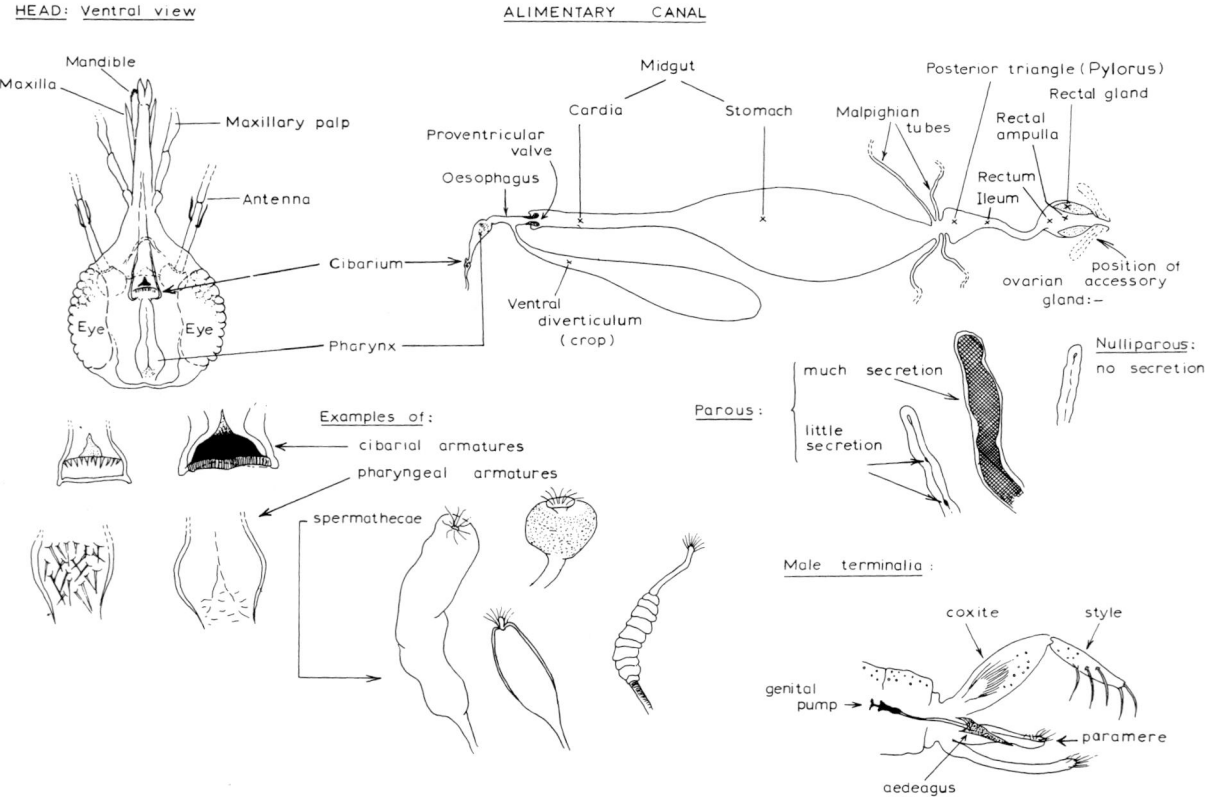

Figure IV.26: The anatomy of the alimentary canal of sandflies, showing the ovarian glands and features of taxonomic importance.

species in tropical Africa. Even in foci of visceral leishmaniasis (e.g., in Kenya) human biters are not conspicuous. In contrast, the transmission of leishmaniasis in the New World is principally in the tropics.

Sandflies occur in a very wide range of habitats, from sea level (a major focus of leishmaniasis around the Dead Sea is below sea level) to altitudes of 2800 m or more in the Andes and Ethiopia, and from hot dry deserts, through savannahs and open woodland to dense tropical rainforest. Each species of sandfly has rather distinct ecological requirements. If these encompass the conditions in and around the dwellings of humans or domestic animals, the species becomes peridomestic. The majority of peridomestic sandfly species are vectors of infections to humans. The highly focal nature of many leishmaniases is undoubtedly a result of ecological constraints on the vectors and probably, to a lesser extent, on the mammalian reservoirs. In central Asia, sandflies are localized, restricted to the natural foci of gerbil colonies and by soil texture and moisture. Even in tropical rainforests, sandflies are not uniformly distributed.

In the Old World most foci of cutaneous leishmaniasis are in dry, semi-arid areas, in contrast to the New World where it is transmitted mainly in forests (Figure IV.27). Hence occupational differences exist between those acquiring infections. Cutaneous disease in Central and South America is associated primarily with working in or modifying the forest environment, whereas in the Old

World the disease affects those in rural savannah and urban areas. The open nature of the savannah and steppe environments and the patchy distribution of suitable microclimates for sandflies, has prompted the application of landscape epidemiology in the investigation of many Old World foci of cutaneous leishmaniasis.

The distribution and abundance of sandflies can alter with changing land use. Deforestation in the New World has led to a marked reduction in cutaneous leishmaniasis (after the initial increase in disease during land clearance). Such areas provide opportunities for the extension in the range of the VL vector *Lutzomyia longipalpis* and subsequent transmission of visceral leishmaniasis which has become more prevalent in urban areas of Brazil in recent years, resembling the urban foci of VL with dogs as the reservoir of *Leishmania infantum* in the Old World. By raising the water-table, irrigation projects considerably increase the breeding of some vector species (e.g., *Phlebotomus papatasi*) but, in some circumstances at least, this may also discourage the rodent reservoir (e.g., the deeply burrowing *Rhombomys opimus* in the steppes of southern Eurasia). In the Middle East there has been a marked increase in cutaneous leishmaniasis due to *L. major* associated with development programmes.

When they are not active, sandflies seek out cool and relatively humid (but not wet) dark niches. Resting sites such as caves, tree holes, tree trunks, cavities between boulders, fissures in the ground, buildings, termite hills

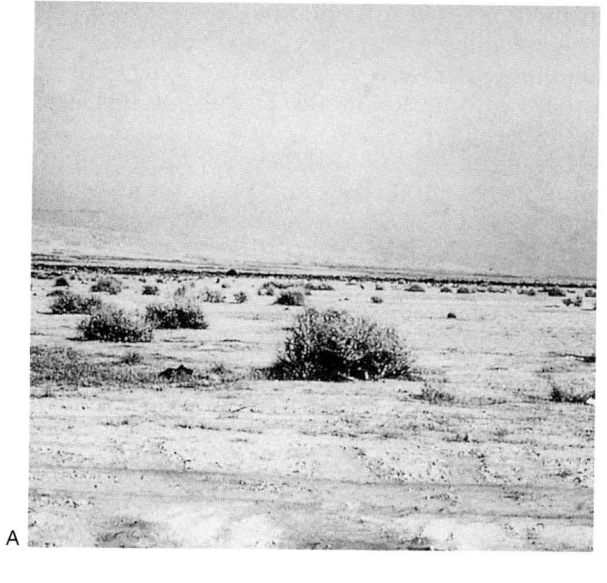
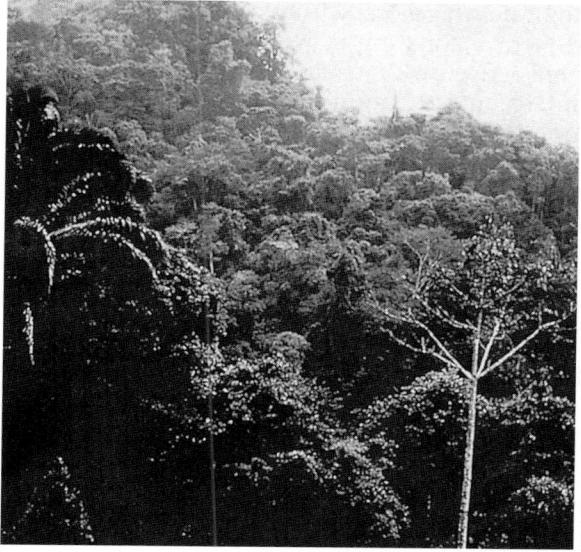
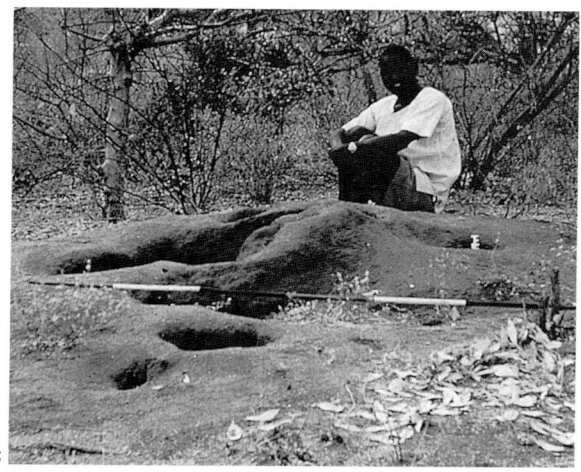
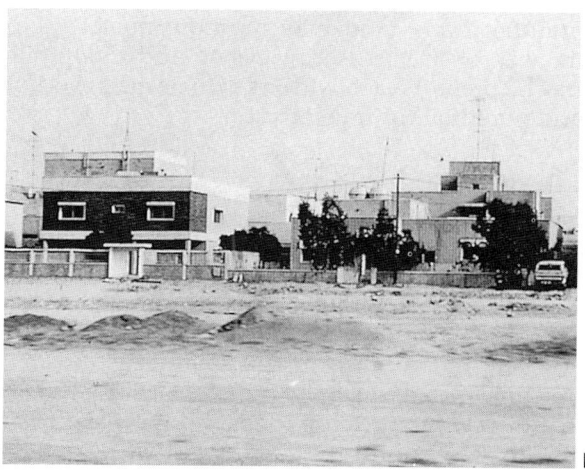

Figure IV.27: A, A typical arid habitat of *Phlebotomus papatasi* (Jordan Valley), where this species transmits *L. (L.) major* from the fat sand rat (*Psammomys obesus*) to humans and causes cutaneous leishmaniasis. **B**, Cutaneous leishmaniasis due to *L. (L.) mexicana* is transmitted from tree rats to humans by *Lutzomyia olmeca olmeca* in wet forests of Central America (Belize). **C**, Eroded termite hills are the preferred resting sites of the visceral leishmaniasis vector *Phlebotomus martini* in some areas of East Africa. (Courtesy of D. M. Minter.) **D**, Occupants of modern housing developments around expanding towns may become infected with visceral leishmaniasis by the bites of peridomestic sandflies, for example in Brazil and the Middle East.

and animal burrows are commonly used. By withdrawing to these day-time sites, sandflies are able to survive in very hot and dry climates, in conditions that would otherwise rapidly kill them, emerging at night when the ambient temperature drops and the humidity rises. Such resting sites are very important in the study of sandflies, as their availability determines the ecological distribution of different species: various traps are used to intercept sandflies moving to and from such places.

Behaviour of sandflies

Sandflies usually have a short hopping flight, especially when close to prospective hosts. Little is known of their long range movements (e.g., dispersal from breeding sites), although they can fly up to 2.2 km over a period of

a few days in open habitats. They fly only at night and in a single night they may fly several hundred metres in their search for a host and subsequent resting and breeding sites. Climatic factors affect activity markedly; biting does not usually take place below 20°C in tropical species; *P. papatasi* is active between 45 and 60% relative humidity, whereas other species require 75–85% relative humidity, and the flight range of some species (e.g., *P. sergenti*) is greater in humid than in dry climates. Although slight air movement aids the detection of hosts along odour plumes, wind speeds of greater than 1.5 m/s inhibit flight, which ceases altogether in light winds of 4–5 m/s. Forest sandflies, such as the Amazonian *Lutzomyia umbratilis*, often exhibit regular vertical movements in addition to horizontal patterns. The flies rest in the tree buttresses during the day, migrating to the canopy in search of a host at night. Furthermore, within a forest, there is often a marked vertical zonation in which different species of sandflies are active, so that some species remain close to the ground, feeding on ground-dwelling rodents (e.g., the South American vectors *Luzomyia flaviscutellata* and *Lutzomyia olmeca* feeding on the rodents *Proechimys* and *Oryzomys*). For these reasons, the transmission of some parasites between the normal animal hosts is predominantly at ground level (e.g., *L. amazonensis*) and some in the canopy (e.g., *L. panamensis*), although humans usually acquire infection at ground level.

Seasonal distribution

Several abiotic factors affect sandfly numbers, but temperature and rainfall are the most important. Some species in temperate regions may have only one generation per year, and consequently a single peak of activity and transmission. However, such species may have two or three generations per year in climatically more favourable areas. In tropical countries, species react more to rainfall cycles and may be more prevalent in either the wet or dry season. Several anthropophilic species may be present, each with its own annual cycle of activity and potential for transmission.

Blood feeding

Sandfly females feed on blood, using the nutrients to develop eggs. Feeding takes place on exposed parts of the body by thrusting the tiny mouthparts (0.15–0.57 mm) into the skin and, using minutely serated mandibles in a scissor-like manner, to create a small pool from which the blood is sucked. Blood taken in this manner is directed into the midgut. Liquids taken by other means (e.g., sugar feeding) are directed to the crop for sterilization and then to the midgut; infection of the sandfly gut with bacteria or yeasts appears to depress *Leishmania* development. Both males and females feed on sugars, which they obtain as honeydew or from plants, either passively (extrafloral nectaries, fallen fruits, etc.) or actively by piercing leaves or stems. The presence of sugars is essential for the full development of *Leishmania* (see section on invertebrate life cycles of *Leishmania*; Chapter 75).

The site of a bite determines the situation of primary lesions in cutaneous leishmaniasis, and may be influenced as much by the presence of clothes as by the intrinsic preferences of a vector. Consequently, sleeping outside in hot weather without bed-nets, or working in forests during the day without suitable clothing, increases the risk of acquiring an infection.

Sandflies are crepuscular; biting takes place at different times of the night according to the species. When disturbed, sandflies in dense forests, caves or buildings may bite during the day. Only a few species are endophilic; these are mostly peridomestic species, such as *P. papatasi, P. chinensis, P. sergenti* and *Lutzomyia longipalpis*, the majority preferring to bite outside, often near their probable breeding and resting sites. It is a relatively small ecological step from rodent burrows and caves to human dwellings. The distinction between peridomestic and 'wild' species has little meaning in sparsely populated areas, where the buildings themselves are made from local materials, perhaps without solid walls. Equally, no species is entirely domestic.

The biting rates of sandflies vary greatly, up to a maximum of about 1000 per hour. Most species probably have a narrow range of preferred hosts. Species of *Sergentomyia* feed predominantly on reptiles, as do some species of *Lutzomyia* and *Phlebotomus*, but the latter genera feed mainly on mammals. Several peridomestic mammal-feeding sandflies (*P. papatasi, P. sergenti* and *Lutzomyia longipalpis*) feed readily on poultry also; chicken coops may be a source of biting sandflies.

Most species are gonotrophically concordant, taking one blood meal for each batch of eggs matured. However, autogeny (the ability to lay eggs without a blood meal) is a feature of some human-biting species. Sandflies may feed more than once per ovarian cycle, thus increasing human–fly contact. Oviposition usually takes place 5–10 days after a blood meal. The proportion of parous females within a population (i.e., those that have laid eggs and by inference have had a blood meal, with the concomitant risk of acquiring an infection) indicates the epidemiological potential of the population. The highest parous rates occur in populations towards the end of the 'sandfly season', when sandfly infection rates are maximal and subsequent transmission most likely.

Life history

Relatively little is known about the immature stages of sandflies and their breeding sites, which are terrestrial, in striking contrast to other nematocerous flies such as Culicidae, Simuliidae, Ceratopogonidae and Chironomidae. Breeding and resting often takes place in the same microhabitat, such as the soil accumulated in cracks in walls or among rocks, in animal burrows and shelters, caves, or in damp leaf litter in forests. The main requirements for breeding sites are moisture and the presence of organic detritus, etc., on which the larvae can feed.

Eggs of sandflies (less than 0.7 mm in length) are elliptical with a fine chorionic pattern. Up to 70 eggs are scattered about the potential breeding site by the ovipositing female. Hatching occurs 1–2 weeks later. The larvae are caterpillar-like and have a distinct dark head-capsule; the pale, cream-coloured body is sparsely covered with characteristic club-shaped hairs ('match-stick' hairs). There are four instars, the first with a single pair, and the remaining instars with two pairs, of long, highly characteristic, caudal bristles on the anal segment. The caudal bristles are almost as long as the body. Diapause occurs during the fourth instar of several species in areas where there are cool winters (e.g., the Mediterranean basin). The pupa is inactive and usually hatches within 5–10 days. The duration of the larval instars varies greatly, both between and within species (in the laboratory at least), as it is regulated mainly by temperature. The period from oviposition to adult eclosion takes between 20 days and several months (in temperate or diapausing species and those living at high altitudes in the tropics, such as *P. longipes*).

Emergence takes place during the hours of darkness, often just before dawn. Males usually emerge first. Little is known of mating in sandflies. Although swarming does not generally take place, males may congregate on and around prospective hosts and mate with females there. Pheromones and auditory signals from wing beats are also probably involved. The life of adult flies is unlikely to exceed a few weeks in nature. Once the female becomes infected, perhaps at the first blood meal, parasites can be transmitted to new hosts at intervals throughout the rest of her life.

Transmission of disease organisms

Sandflies transmit viruses, bacteria and protozoa (*Leishmania*), but not nematodes, to vertebrates.

Leishmania

Phlebotomine sandflies are the only vectors of *Leishmania* species to humans. Certain species are common vectors of parasites (often peridomestic species) or secondary vectors, while most sandflies rarely if ever come into contact with humans. A species may transmit a particular parasite in one area, but not in another: no two areas or foci are the same. The degree of human involvement in leishmaniasis is very variable; many cycles are of reservoir–fly–reservoir, with occasional—almost chance—infections; others cause regular zoonotic infections, and some anthroponotic cycles are thought to involve only flies and humans. It is important to understand natural transmission cycles for two reasons. First, enzootic cycles may pose an unknown threat in remote areas being developed (mining, agriculture, etc.) and, second, transmission may be maintained by several species, only one of which transmits the infection to huamns; for example, in southern Eurasia *L. major* infections are maintained among rodents by *P. mongolensis*, *P. caucasicus* and *P. andrejevi*, but only *P. papatasi* transmits the parasite to humans.

Incrimination of a sandfly species as a vector is difficult, as many criteria have to be satisfied before a species can be implicated unambiguously. These criteria are based on the discovery of natural infections in wild-caught flies, experimental transmission studies, evidence of contact between the sandfly and humans, contact between the sandfly and the reservoir host (where known), and the life cycle of the parasite in the fly. As there is often no sharp distinction between important and minor or occasional vectors, it is impossible to draw up a definitive list of vectors. Table IV.3 gives a synopsis of the 'proven' vectors of *Leishmania*; further details of suspected vectors are given in the section on the epidemiology of leishmaniaisis (see Chapter 75).

Within the genus *Phlebotomus* the majority of subgenera contain vectors or suspected vectors. Species of *Phlebotomus* (*sensu stricto*) are associated with *L. major* transmission in arid environments of East Africa, the Middle East and the

former USSR. The subgenus *Paraphlebotomus* contains many species living in rodent burrows in central Asia and transmitting *L. major* between rodents and occasionally to humans. One species, the peridomestic *P. sergenti*, is a vector of *L. tropica* in western Asia and the Middle East. Vectors of visceral leishmaniasis in the Old World are distributed through several subgenera: *Larroussius* (Mediterranean basin and Sahel); *Synphlebotomus* (East Africa); *Euphlebotomus* (India); and *Adlerius* (Near East, northern China). The genus *Lutzomyia* is much more diverse than its Old World counterpart; some subgenera contain several vector species (e.g., *Nyssomyia* and *Psychodopygus*), whereas many other subgenera and species groups contain only one or two species that are involved in the transmission of *Leishmania* spp.

Leishmania in the sandfly

After ingestion, the parasites in an infected blood meal undergo metamorphosis to the promastigote form and multiply within the sandfly gut before they become infective. The site in which this development takes place varies between different groups of *Leishmania* and is related to the micromorphology and biochemistry of the sandfly gut. The attachment mechanisms of *Leishmania* are adapted to the surface structure (chitinous or membranous) of the section of the gut to which they adhere. Enzyme activity in the midgut, following blood meals from different hosts, will differentially affect the survival of *Leishmania*.

The location of the parasites in the gut during their development (relative to the pylorus—the sphincter between the midgut and hindgut) has been used in parasite classification (Figure IV.28).[10] This subject is discussed in detail in the section on the genus *Leishmania* (see Appendix III) and may be briefly summarized as follows:

1. Peripylarian ('both sides of the gate') development takes place in the hindgut and then the parasites migrate forward before transmission by bite. Mainly parasites of New World mammals (members of the subgenus *L. (Viannia): L. braziliensis, guyanensis, panamensis* and *peruviana*). Some parasites of Old World reptiles (e.g., the former *L. adleri*), whose taxonomic status (as 'Sauroleishmania'; see Appendix III) is presently in doubt, also have a peripylarian form of development in sandflies.
2. Suprapylarian ('above the gate') development is entirely within the midgut prior to anterior migration and transmission by bite. Parasites of New and Old World mammals (members of the subgenus *Leishmania (sensu stricto): L. donovani* group, *L. mexicana* group, *L. hertigi* group and *L. major* group).

The term hypopylarian ('under the gate') development was used for parasites of some Old World lizards formerly included in the genus *Leishmania*, but which are currently referred to as *Sauroleishmania* species (of uncertain status), for example the former *L. agamae* and *L. ceramodactyli*. Hypopylarian development is confined to the hindgut and transmission is by ingestion or crushing of the

Table IV.3 Synopsis of proven vectors of leishmaniasis (see also Chapter 75).

Parasite	Vector	Animal reservoir	Principal areas
L. (Leishmania) donovani	P. (Euphlebotomus) argentipes	? Man	India
L. (L.) infantum	P. (Larroussius) ariasi	Fox, dog	Southern France
	P. (Larroussius) longicuspis	Dog	North Africa
	P. (Larroussius) major syracus	Dog	Eastern Mediterranean
	P. (Larroussius) orientalis	Rodents and carnivores	Sudan
	P. (Larroussius) perfiliewi	Fox; Rattus spp.	Italy; former Yugoslavia
	P. (Larroussius) perniciosus	Dog	Western Mediterranean
	P. (Larroussius) smirnovi	Wolves; jackals	Former USSR
	P. (Larroussius) tobbi	Dog	Eastern Mediterranean
	P. (Paraphlebotomus) alexandri	? Man	North-west China: Sinkiang (Xinjiang)
	P. (Adlerius) sichuanensis	?	South-west China: Szechwan (Sichuan)
	P. (Adlerius) chinensis	Dog; racoon dog	China
	P. (Adlerius) longiductus	Dog; jackal	Former USSR
	P. (Synphlebotomus) martini	Dog; man	East Africa
L. (L.) chagasi	Lutzomyia (Lutzomyia) longipalpis	Dog; foxes (Lycalopex, Cerdocyon)	Brazil
L. (L.) tropica	P. (Paraphlebotomus) sergenti	? Man	Middle East to Indus basin
L. (L.) major	P. (Phlebotomus) papatasi	Burrowing rodents	North Africa, Middle East: former USSR, north-west India
	P. (Phlebotomus) duboscqi	Rodents	African Sahel (Senegal to East Africa)
	P. (Phlebotomus) salehi	Rodents	North-west India
L. (L.) aethiopica	P. (Larroussius) pedifer	Hyrax	Ethiopia, Kenya
L. (L.) maxicana	Lutzomyia (Nyssomyia) olmeca olmeca	Forest rodents	Central America
L. (L.) amazonensis	Lutzomyia (Nyssomyia) flaviscutellata	Forest rodents; agouti, opossum	Amazon basin (Brazil)
L. (Viannia) braziliensis	Lutzomyia (Psychodopygus) wellcome	?	Brazil
L. (V.) panamensis	Lutzomyia (Nyssomyia) trapidoi	Sloth (Choloepus hoffmani)	Panama
L. (V.) guyanensis	Lutzomyia (Nyssomyia) umbratilis	Sloth (Choloepus didactylus)	Northern Brazil, Guyanas
L. (V.) peruviana	?	? (Dog; as secondary host)	Western Andes (South America)

For further details, and for numerous species incriminated, but not conclusively proved as vectors, see also section on epidemiology of the leishmaniases, Chapter 75.

infected fly, when fed upon by lizards or other insectivorous vertebrates.

Although transmission occurs through the bite of a sandfly, the exact mechanism by which parasites are taken up or deposited in the skin of a new host is unclear (see section on vector–parasite interactions, below). Infection with parasites changes the behaviour of a sandfly; a heavily infected fly probes much more frequently than an uninfected fly, in a manner analogous to a flea with *Yersinia*. *Leishmania* can be transmitted readily during each probe, which may last for only a few seconds, and this is probably the origin of the multiple lesions seen in some patients (particularly those with *L. major* infections). Infection does not alter the dispersal of sandflies appreciably.

Vector–parasite specificity of sandflies and the *Leishmania* spp. they transmit is affected by several factors, including behaviour (e.g., propensity of a vector to bite a particular species of reservoir host), ecological factors and biochemical factors (e.g., enzyme activity) operating in the sandfly gut. Natural infection rates in wild flies are usually very low (below 1%), but may be exceptionally high in some foci (e.g., up to 20% in the Jordan Valley).

Viruses

Sandfly fever (papataci or papatasi fever, 3-day fever) is caused by two distinct virus serotypes (Naples and Sicilian) and results in an acute febrile illness in humans, lasting 2–4 days, although incapacitation may extend for much longer periods.[11] It is common during the summer

Section of a Phlebotomine sandfly to show the different regions of the alimentary canal

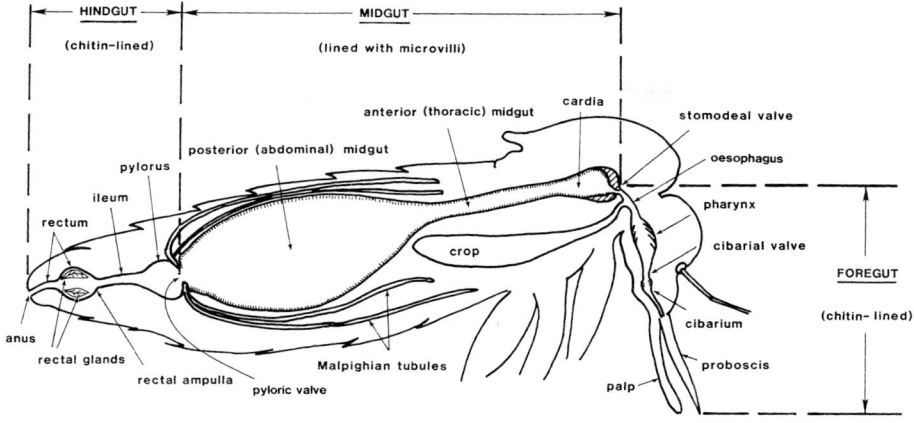

Section SUPRAPYLARIA ('above the gate')

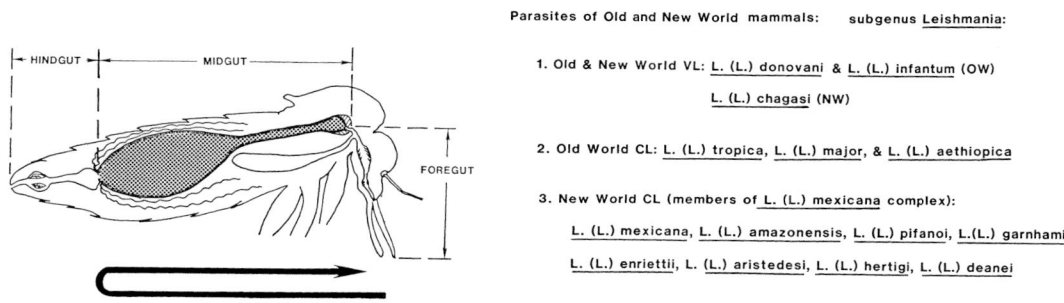

Development in midgut only (no hindgut development). Transmission by bite

Parasites of Old and New World mammals: subgenus Leishmania:

1. Old & New World VL: L. (L.) donovani & L. (L.) infantum (OW)

L. (L.) chagasi (NW)

2. Old World CL: L. (L.) tropica, L. (L.) major, & L. (L.) aethiopica

3. New World CL (members of L. (L.) mexicana complex):

L. (L.) mexicana, L. (L.) amazonensis, L. (L.) pifanoi, L.(L.) garnhami,

L. (L.) enriettii, L. (L.) aristedesi, L. (L.) hertigi, L. (L.) deanei

Section PERIPYLARIA ('on all sides of the gate')

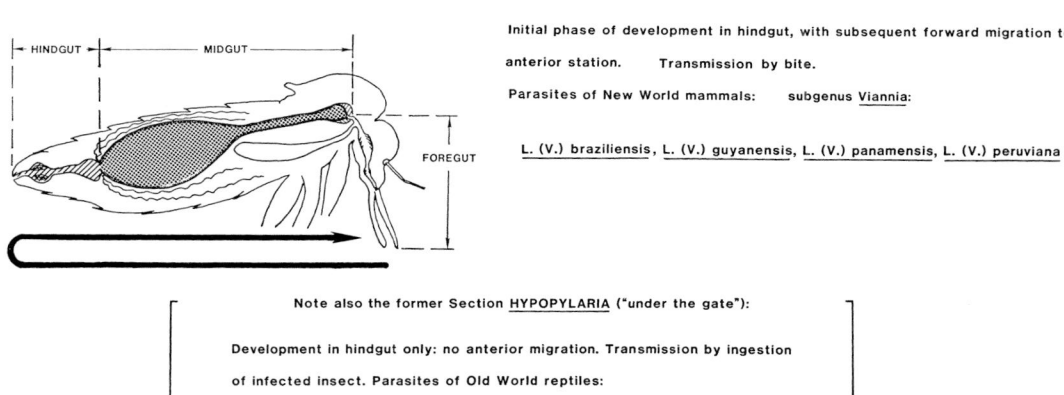

Initial phase of development in hindgut, with subsequent forward migration to

anterior station.   Transmission by bite.

Parasites of New World mammals: subgenus Viannia:

L. (V.) braziliensis, L. (V.) guyanensis, L. (V.) panamensis, L. (V.) peruviana

Note also the former Section HYPOPYLARIA ("under the gate"):

Development in hindgut only: no anterior migration. Transmission by ingestion

of infected insect. Parasites of Old World reptiles:

subgenus Sauroleishmania: (*) L. (S.) agamae, L. (S.) ceramodactyli

Figure IV.28: Classification of the *Leishmania* species based on their site of development in the phlebotomine host. (After Lanson and Shaw.[10])

months throughout the Mediterranean basin, the Middle East, Pakistan and parts of India, and Central America. The disease is of considerable military importance because up to 75% of non-immune individuals who arrive in an endemic area may be affected. In Mediterranean areas where the disease is endemic, most of the population is

thought to be infected during childhood, possibly suffering only a mild illness (see Chapter 41).

Phlebotomus papatasi was incriminated as the vector in Egypt and is generally thought to transmit sandfly fever throughout the Old World range of the disease (i.e., except Central America). Natural infection rates of sandflies are between 0.015 and 0.5%. No natural vertebrate reservoir is known, although infected humans can infect flies, and thus have some amplifying effect during epidemics. It is most likely that the principal maintenance mechanism is by transovarial transmission along genetically susceptible lines of the vector.

Sandflies transmit several other phleboviruses; *Phlebotomus perniciosus* transmits Toscana virus in the northern Mediterranean, and in the New World *Lutzomyia trapidoi* and *L. ylephiletor* transmit Chagres' and Punta Toro viruses. Viruses have been isolated from several other species.

Bacteria

Infections due to *Bartonella bacilliformis* (Oroya fever, verruga peruana) are found only in the central Andean Cordilleras of Peru, Colombia and Ecuador. The disease is endemic in valleys between 750 and 2700 m in altitude, apparently restricted by the ecological requirements of the vectors. Little detail is known of the transmission cycle. There are no known animal reservoirs; the sandfly vector acquires the pathogen from an infected human. The lack of a development cycle of *B. bacilliformis* in the vector (it occurs in the gut and on the mouthparts) suggests that transmission may be mechanical. In Peru, *Lutzomyia verrucarum* is considered to be the vector, although the disease exists in the absence of this species. The closely related *Lutzomyia colombiana* is thought to transmit the disease in Colombia.

Reaction to sandfly bites

Persons newly exposed to the bites of *P. papatasi* and other species in parts of the Middle East often experience a severe urticarial reaction to sandfly bites after a variable time. This period of sensitization may later be followed by desensitization. Such a reaction may also occur elsewhere in the world.

Control of sandflies

There is no general method of control, for several reasons: the diversity of the habitats in which the diseases occur, behaviour of the vectors, and the public health importance of the disease they transmit. Several different strategies are used, principally aimed at reducing human–fly contact. Control of larvae is often impossible, as the breeding sites of many vectors are either unknown or inaccessible. However, in the former USSR considerable success was achieved by a combined method of pumping insecticides into rodent burrows (breeding and resting sites) with destruction of the rodent reservoirs (*Rhombomys opimus*).

Personal protection

Sandflies are able to penetrate the standard insect screens used in windows of houses and for normal bed-nets, and therefore fine sandfly bed-nets have to be used, which are uncomfortable to sleep under in humid tropical climates. Chemical repellents (DEET, DMP) applied to clothing and bed-nets are effective, but when applied to the skin are rapidly lost through perspiration. This is especially so when manual work is undertaken (agricultural labour, road building or military operations).

Insecticide control

Leishmaniasis control has occurred in some countries (e.g., India, Mediterranean) as a byproduct of antimalarial spraying, with renewed outbreaks after cessation of such spraying. Sandflies are susceptible to insecticides (only one instance of resistance to DDT has been reported) which are applied to resting and breeding sites. Control programmes based on house-spraying with residual insecticides have been directed specifically at sandflies in Egypt, China, CIS, Peru and Saudi Arabia. The use of pyrethroid-treated bed-nets and curtains against sandflies is under evaluation.

Insecticide control of adults is feasible only where peridomestic transmission occurs in discrete and well populated communities. Where sandflies are exophilic, or bite away from human habitations, insecticide control may not be effective; for example, there has been little success with attempts to control forest sandflies in the 'neotropics' by barrier spraying.

Environmental modification

This has been effective in some areas, for instance moving temporary buildings and camps away from microfoci and ploughing up breeding sites. Often, changing land use affects transmission in an unpredictable way. Sandflies in dense forest will rarely cross a clearing made around isolated houses or villages.

Collection of sandflies

The diverse biology of sandflies and their habitats means that special methods have to be used to catch them. Most methods rely on an understanding of sandfly behaviour, as they involve catching resting flies, attracting sandflies to a trap, or intercepting them during their nocturnal movements, and thus the efficiency of collection will vary between methods and individuals.

The simplest method is to collect flies during the day from their resting sites, catching them directly with either an aspirator or a fine-mesh net. This is useful for peridomestic flies and for forest flies resting on tree trunks and buttresses. Battery-operated aspirators avoid the risk of histoplasmosis (see Chapter 69). A tent-like device (Damasceno trap) can be put over animal burrows or tree buttresses to catch resting sandflies. The most widely used method of collecting sandflies, at least in the Old World where sandflies live in relatively drier habitats, is setting sticky traps. These are sheets of paper (usually 10×17 cm) thinly coated in castor oil and fixed to sticks which are then placed near resting sites. Traps are set before sunset and collected the following morning. The adhering flies are removed with a needle, cleaned in dilute detergent and stored in 70% alcohol. Sticky traps are not usually effective in areas of high humidity. Several types of light traps can be used, although they are less effective in open habitats, such as deserts, than in wood-land or forests. Similarly, a range of animal-baited traps has been devised for collecting sandflies. These traps are useful in areas where human-biting species are seldom caught by other means. Baiting such traps with a known reservoir host will help determine potential vector species. Light- and animal-bait methods are combined in the Shannon trap, a rectangular cloth trap with a central wall and an inverted box-like roof.

Human-biting catches provide an accurate method of finding which species are anthropophilic and assessing the extent of human–fly contact. The ethics of collectors being exposed to potential risks of leishmaniasis transmission may be considered acceptable if local residents are employed without substantially increasing their risk. Collecting larvae is enormously time consuming and only rarely productive.

Preparation and preservation of specimens

Because many microscopic characters are used to differentiate species of sandflies, correct preparation of specimens is of paramount importance. Flies can be cleaned in dilute detergent solutions to remove any adherent oil from sticky traps, rinsed in distilled water and mounted in Berlese medium. Other, more permanent, methods of clearing and mounting flies are also used. To display the diagnostic features most clearly, the head should be detached and mounted ventral side uppermost and the remainder of the body mounted laterally. Care must be taken in ringing such mounts to ensure they are permanent. Other mounting media based on Canada balsam are used, but do not show the spermathecae and antennal sensilla very clearly.

In the absence of proper equipment and facilities, sandflies can be preserved in a dry condition, in wisps of paper tissue (not cotton wool), loosely packed in small tubes. Specimens stored dry are, naturally, rather brittle and are easily damaged.

Classification and identification of sandflies

Among the Phlebotominae there is no universal agreement on the ranking of taxa above the species level, although the proposals of Lewis et al.[12] are generally accepted. Different taxonomic opinions may cause confusion, especially when they concern vector species; for example, the South American *Psychodopygus* is treated as a genus by some but as a subgenus of *Lutzomyia* by others. Of the five genera of Phlebotominae, only two contain vector species: *Phlebotomus* (Old World) and *Lutzomyia* (New World). The remaining genera, *Sergentomyia* (Old World), *Brumptomyia* and *Warileya* (both New World), rarely feed on humans. There is a loose association between the subgenera of sandflies and the affinities of the parasites they transmit, so that deducing potential vectors from their taxonomic relationships with known vector species

is important in the initial stages of an epidemiological study.

Identification of sandflies to species is difficult and requires specialist training. Species are differentiated by minute characters (many internal), such as details (teeth- or scale-like processes) of the cibarium and pharynx, and the structure of the spermatheca. External features of the male genitalia and the antennal sensilla are also used. There is often considerable variation within species, making it difficult to determine the limits of particular taxa and to identify some vector species. Cryptic species and complexes of sibling ones make it difficult to separate many species of sandflies. Several new techniques (morphometrics, isoenzyme electrophoresis, DNA probes) are being used to differentiate some members of taxonomically intransigent species groups or complexes of sandflies.

Mosquitoes

G. B. White

Family: Culicidae

Mosquitoes are not confined to tropical regions; the main genera *Anopheles, Aedes* and *Culex* are distributed worldwide, even within the Arctic Circle. Approximately 3300 species of Culicidae have been described, more being recognized each year. They are classified in three subfamilies and 35 genera, as shown in Table IV.4.

Adult mosquitoes of both sexes feed on nectar and other fluids. Anopheline and culicine females also suck the blood of mammals, birds, frogs, etc., each species of mosquito tending to have particular host preferences. For blood-feeding, the proboscis stylets (Figure IV.29) are pushed into a blood capillary of the host's skin. Localized sensitivity to saliva from the mosquito is what causes dermal reactions popularly known as 'mosquito bites'. Each blood meal generally provides enough nutrition for the female mosquito to produce a batch of eggs, 30 to 150 in number. Anophelines show the most regular cycles of blood-feeding and egg-laying. *Toxorhynchites* and some culicines produce eggs autogenously (i.e., without having fed on blood). Male and female mosquitoes may well live for several weeks, feeding repeatedly, under natural conditions. Through their regular attacks on humans, female mosquitoes of certain species are important carriers of human diseases. All the vectors of human malaria belong to the genus *Anopheles* (Table IV.5). The main morphological differences between anophelines and culicines are portrayed in Figure IV.30. Various anophelines and especially culicines transmit arboviruses and filariasis of humans (Tables IV.5 and IV.6). Mosquitoes also serve as the vectors of enzootic infections (i.e., restricted to animals or birds) and some zoonotic diseases due to pathogens transmitted from animals to humans (e.g., yellow fever and subperiodic Brugian filariasis).

Breeding places of mosquitoes are always in water. Eggs may be deposited on damp soil or vegetation, in moist

Table IV.4 Epidemiological zones and vectors of human malaria (see also Chapter 71).

1. North American	4. North Eurasian	7. Afrotropical	10. Malaysia
A. (A.) freeborni	A. (A.) atroparvus	A. (C.) arabiensis	A. (A.) campestris
A. (A.) quadrimaculatus	(A. (A.) messeae)	A. (C.) funestus	A. (A.) donaldi
(A. (N.) albimanus)	(A. (A.) sacharovi)	A. (C.) gambiae	A. (A.) letifer
	(A. (A.) sinensis)	(A. (C.) mascarensis)	A. (A.) nigerrimus
2. Central American	(A. (C.) pattoni)	(A. (C.) melas)	(A. (A.) whartoni)
(A. (A.) aztecus)		(A. (C.) merus)	A. (C.) aconitus
(A. (A.) punctimacula)	5. Mediterranean	(A. (C.) moucheti)	A. (C.) balabacensis
A. (N.) albimanus	A. (A.) atroparvus	(A. (C.) nili)	A. (C.) dirus
(A. (N.) albitarsis)	(A. (A.) claviger)	(A. (C.) pharoensis)	A. (C.) flavirostris
A. (N.) aquasalis	A. (A.) labranchiae		A. (C.) leucosphyrus
A. (N.) argyritarsis	(A. (A.) messeae)	8. Indo-Iranian	A. (C.) ludlowae
A. (N.) darlingi	A. (A.) sacharovi	(A. (A.) sacharovi)	A. (C.) maculatus
	(A. (C.) hispaniola)	(A. (C.) annularis)	A. (C.) minimus
3. South American	(A. (C.) pattoni)	A. (C.) culicifacies	(A. (C.) philippinensis)
A. (A.) pseudopuncipennis		A. (C.) fluviatilis	A. (C.) pseudowillmori
A. (A.) punctimacula	6. Afro-Arabian	(A. (C.) pulcherrimus)	A. (C.) subpictus
(A. (K.) bellator)	(A. (C.) hispaniola)	(A. (C.) stephensi)	A. (C.) sundaicus
(A. (K.) cruzii)	(A. (C.) multicolor)	(A. (C.) superpictus)	
(A. (K.) neivai)	A. (C.) pharoensis	(A. (C.) tessellatus)	11. Chinese
A. (N.) albimanus	A. (C.) sergentii		A. (A.) anthropophagus
A. (N.) albitarsis		9. Indo-Chinese Hills	A. (A.) sinensis
A. (N.) aquasalis		(A. (A.) nigerrimus)	
A. (N.) argyritarsis		(A. (C.) annularis)	12. Australasian
A. (N.) darlingi		(A. (C.) culicifacies)	(A. (A.) bancroftii)
(A. (N.) numeztovari)		A. (C.) dirus	A. (C.) farauti type 1
(A. (N.) oswaldoi)		A. (C.) fluviatilis	A. (C.) farauti type 2
(A. (N.) rangeli)		(A. (C.) kunmingensis)	(A. (C.) hilli)
(A. (N.) triannulatus)		(A. (C.) maculatus)	(A. (C.) karwari)
(A. (N.) trinkae)		A. (C.) minimus	A. (C.) koliensis
			(A. (C) punctulatus)
			(A. (C.) subpictus)

Zonation according to the geographical distribution of the main vector species of *Anopheles*. In each (see opposite page) behaviour and ecology of *Anopheles* spp. governs transmission characteristics, e.g., indoor or outdoor transmission. *A*, Anopheles; *C*, Celia; *K*, Kerteszia; *N*, Nyssorhynchus. Names in parentheses are those of local or secondary vectors.

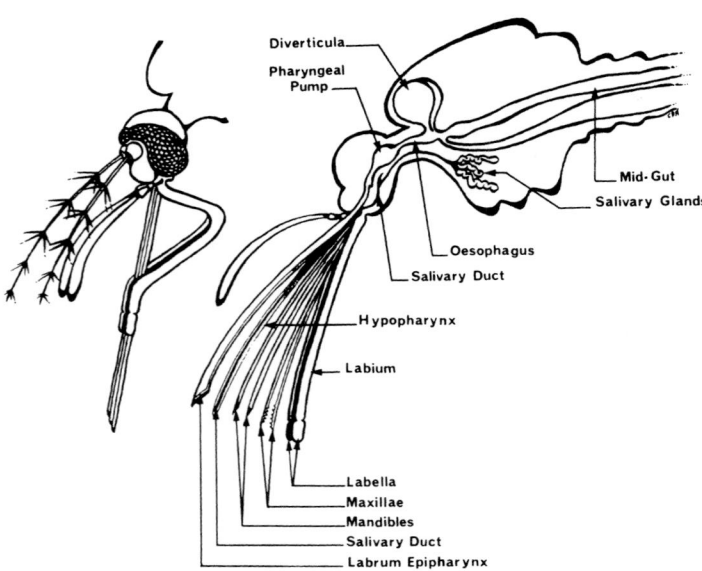

Figure IV.29: Anatomy of the proboscis of the female *Anopheles*.

tree-holes or containers, and sometimes directly on to water. It is the choice of specific oviposition sites by female mosquitoes that determines the breeding places of each species. Eggs of the Aedini usually diapause, withstanding drought or winter, whereas other kinds of mosquito eggs hatch within a few days of being laid. Flooding and decreasing oxygen concentration trigger the hatching of eggs that have undergone diapause.

Larval development takes about a week for most tropical mosquitoes, but many temperate species overwinter as larvae. The fourth stage larva moults to the pupal stage, from which the adult mosquito emerges after a few days. Larvae breathe air via a pair of posterior dorsal spiracles mounted on a characteristic 'siphon' (Figure IV.30) which is not developed in anophelines. Pupae breathe via a pair of 'trumpets' on the thorax (Figure IV.31). Although some species have predacious larvae (e.g., *Toxorhynchites*, *Aedes* subgenus *Mucidus*, *Culex* subgenus *Lutzia*), the majority of mosquito larvae have mouthparts adapted for filter-feeding. Maxillary and palatal brushes sweep small food particles from the water, or from the substrate, and pass

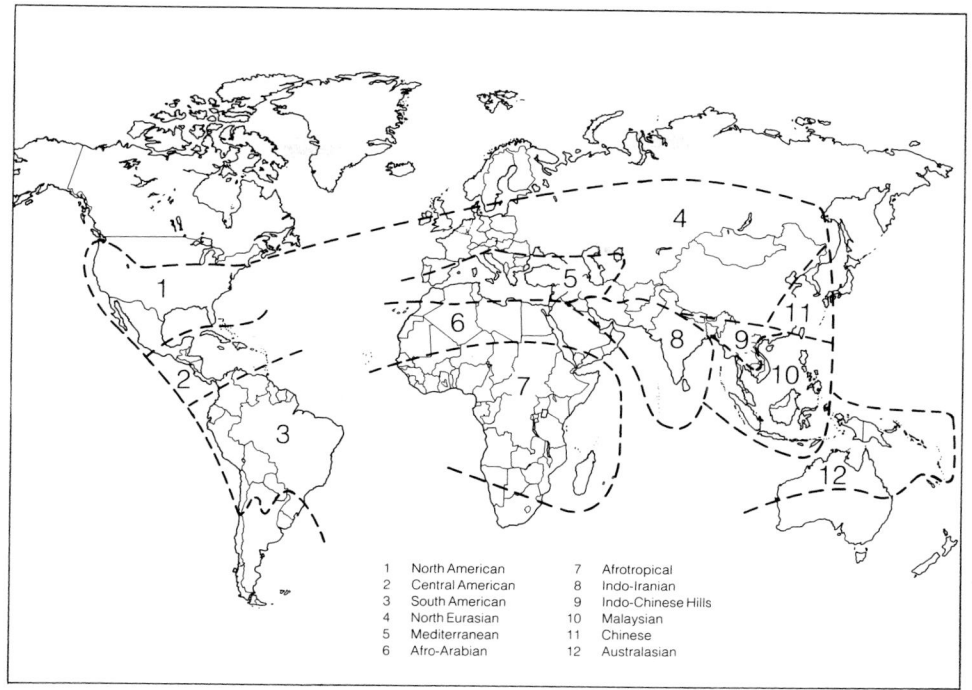

1	North American	7	Afrotropical
2	Central American	8	Indo-Iranian
3	South American	9	Indo-Chinese Hills
4	North Eurasian	10	Malaysian
5	Mediterranean	11	Chinese
6	Afro-Arabian	12	Australasian

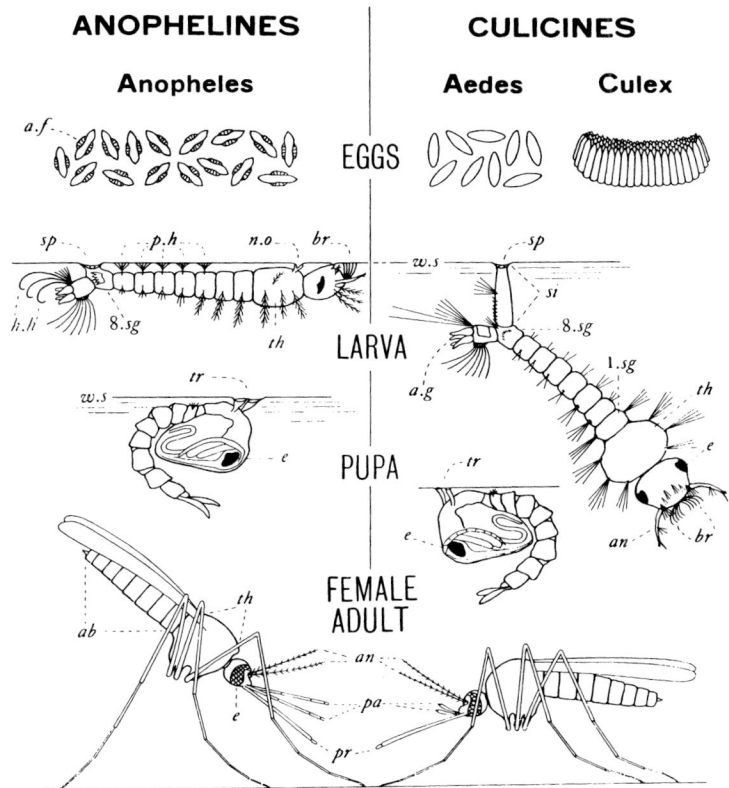

Figure IV.30: Chief distinguishing features of anophelines and culicines. *a.f.*, air floats; *a.g.*, anal gills; *ab*, abdomen; *an*, antenna; *br*, mouth brushes; *e*, eye; *h.h.*, hooked hairs or caudal setae; *n.o.*, notched organ; *pa*, palps (maxillary palpi); *p.h.*, palmate hairs or float hairs; *pr*, proboscis; 1.*sg*, first abdominal segment; 8.*sg*, eighth abdominal segment; *si*, siphon; *sp*, spiracles; *th*, thorax; *tr*, respiratory trumpets.

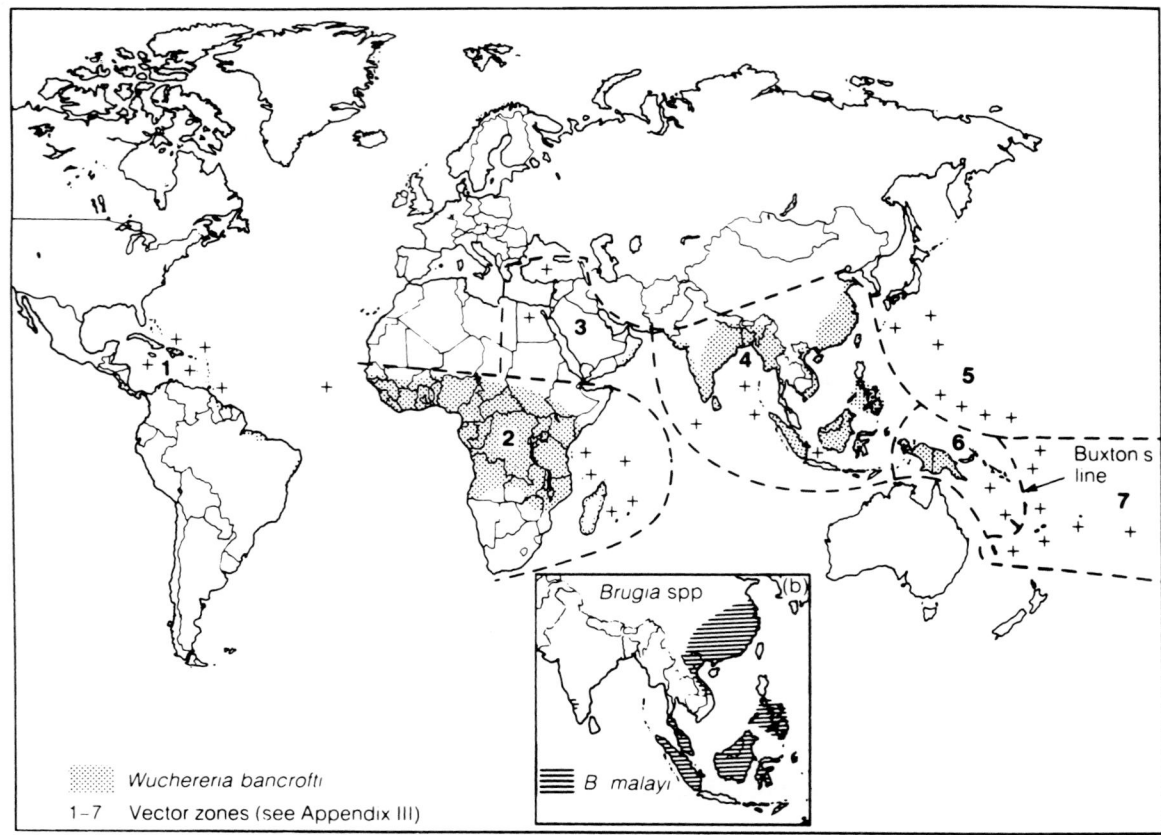

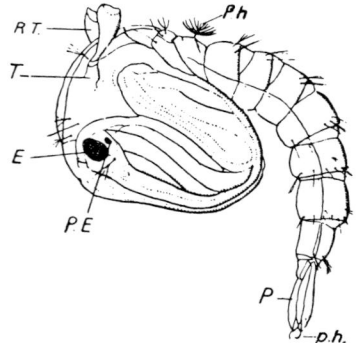

Figure IV.31: Pupa of *Anopheles maculipennis*. E, Eye of developing adult; P, paddle of pupa; PE, pupal eye; RT, respiratory trumpet; T, trachea leading to anterior thoracic spindle.

them to mandibles flanking the larval mouth. The diet of most mosquito larvae comprises micro-organisms and detritus. Rates of mosquito larval growth are influenced by such environmental factors as temperature, photoperiod, food supply and the degree of crowding. Aquatic predators, pathogenic fungi (e.g., *Coelomomyces*, *Lagenidium*) and protozoa (gregarines, microsporidians), viruses and bacteria, together with water effects such as flushing or drying out, combine to take a heavy toll of immature stages of mosquito. These natural agencies can be manipulated for mosquito control purposes.

Larvae and pupae of mosquitoes are sometimes called 'wrigglers' and 'tumblers', respectively, terms that express their vigorous movements in the water. When undisturbed, the pupa rests beneath the surface preparing for metamorphosis. Pupae do not feed. Eventually the pupal case splits along the back and the adult mosquito works its way out on to the water surface. Wings and legs become extended and the body cuticle begins to harden within half an hour of eclosion. The adult mosquito then flies to shelter and rests for several hours. Males are not able to copulate until their terminalia (external genitalia) have turned upside down, a process known as hypopygial circumversion, taking about 1 day for completion. Thereafter the males form swarms with specific characteristics at certain times daily. Female mosquitoes flying into or near a swarm are set upon by the males and copulation ensues. Once inseminated, a female mosquito carries in her spermathecae sufficient sperms for fertilization of all the eggs she may produce. Through the action of matrone, a hormone from male accessory glands, mated female mosquitoes normally become unwilling to accept sperm from additional males. Hibernation of mated females is a common way of over-wintering among temperate species of mosquito (e.g., *Culex pipiens*, *Culiseta annulata*, *Anopheles maculipennis* complex). Seasonal changes in the duriation of daylight govern the onset and end of hibernation. Tropical mosquito adults are generally incapable of long-term quiescence.

When foraging, blood-thirsty female mosquitoes fly upwind searching for the scent trail of an attractive host.

Table IV.5 The mosquito vectors of human filariasis (see map on opposite page and Chapter 82).

Mosquito groups and their general distribution	Vector species and places where incriminated	W. bancrofti np	ns	ds	B. malayi np	ns	B. timori np
ANOPHELINAE							
Anopheles (Anopheles)							
bancroftii group: Australian/Papuan areas	*bancroftii* e.g., Papua New Guinea	+					
barbirostris group: Oriental region	*barbirostris*, e.g., Malaysia; Sulawesi, Thailand; Flores	–			+	–	+
	campestris Malaysia	–			+	–	
	donaldi, e.g., Malaysia, Sarawak				+	–	
	anthropophagus, e.g., China	+			+		
	kewiyangensis, e.g., China	+					
hycanus group: Oriental and Palaearctic regions	*nigerrimus*, e.g., India, Sri Lanka, Thailand	+			+		
	sinensis complex, e.g., China, Korea, Malaysia, Thailand	+			+		
					–	–	
umbrosus group: Indomalaysian area	*letifer*, e.g., Malaysia	+			–		
	whartoni, e.g., Malaysia	+			?		
Anopheles (Cellia)							
funestus-minimus group: Afrotropical and Oriental regions	*aconitus*, Flores	+					
	flavirostris, Philippines	+					
	funestus, e.g., Ghana, Kenya, Liberia, Malagasy, Nigeria, Senegal, Sierra Leone, Tanzania, Burkina Faso, Zaire						
	minimus, Hong Kong	+					
gambiae complex: Afrotropical region	*arabiensis*, e.g., Burkina Faso, Kenya, Malagasy, Nigeria, Tanzania	+					
	bwambae, Uganda	+					
	gambiae, e.g., Ivory Coast, Kenya, Malagasy, Nigeria, Tanzania, Zaire	+					
	melas, e.g., Gambia, Guinea, Ivory Coast, Liberia, Sierra Leone	+					
	merus, e.g., Tanzania	+					
jeyporiensis: Oriental region	*candidiensis*, e.g., China	+					
leucosphyrus group: Oriental region	*balabacensis*, e.g., Indonesia	+					
	leucosphyrus, e.g., Malaysia	+					
maculatus: Oriental region	*maculatus*, e.g., Malaysia	+					
nili: Afrotropical region	*nili*, e.g., Liberia	+					
pauliani: Madagascar	*pauliani*, Madagascar	+					
philippinensis: Oriental region	*philippinensia*, e.g., India	+					
punctulatus complex: Papuan area and western Pacific	*farauti*, e.g., Solomon Islands	+					
	koliensis, e.g., Papua New Guinea	+					
	punctulatus, e.g., Papua New Guinea	+					
subpictus group: Oriental region and Papuan area	*subpictus*, Flores	+					
tessellatus: Oriental region and Papuan area	*tessellatus*, e.g., Maldives	?					
vagus: Oriental region	*vagus*, e.g., Flores	+					

Table IV.5 (*cont'd*)

Mosquito groups and their general distribution	Vector species and places where incriminated	W. bancrofti np	W. bancrofti ns	W. bancrofti ds	B. malayi np	B. malayi ns	B. timori np
Anopheles (Kerteszia) bellator: South America	bellator, e.g., Brazil	+					
Anopheles (Nyssorhynchus) albimanus group: C. & S. America	albimanus, Caribbean	?					
	darlingi, e.g., Brazil, Guyana	+					
argyritarsis group: Neotropical region	aquasalis, e.g., Brazil, Guyana	+					
CULICINAE **Aedes (Finlaya)** kochi group:	fijiensis, Fiji		+				
Indomalaysian, Papuan,	oceanicus, e.g., Samoa, Tonga				+	+	+
North Australia and	poicilius, Philippines	+					
South Pacific	samoanus, Samoa		+				+
	tutuilae, Samoa						?
niveus group: Oriental region	niveus, e.g., Philippines	+					
	harinasutai, Thailand		+				
togoi: East and S.E. Asia	togoi, e.g., China, Japan, Korea	+				+	
Aedes (Ochlerotatus) scapularis: Neotropical region	scapularis, e.g., Brazil	+					
taeniorhynchus group: USA and Neotropical region	taeniorhynchus, e.g., Virgin Islands	?					
vigilax group: East Africa, Australian, Indomalaysian, Papuan and South Pacific areas	vigilax, e.g., New Caledonia		+				
Aedes (Stegomyia) aegypti group: cosmotropical	aegypti, filaria susceptible genotypes occur at low frequency, especially in East Africa	–			–	–	
scutellaris group: North Australian,	cooki, Niue Islands		?				
	futunae, Horne Islands		+				
Indomalaysian,	kesseli, Tongo		?				
Papuan and Pacific areas	polynesiensis, central and eastern Polynesia, e.g., Fiji, Samoa, Tahiti, Tuamotu		+				
	pseudoscutellaris, Fiji		+				
	rotumae, Rotuma Island		?				
	tabu, Haapai Tongatapu Island		+				
	tongae, Haapai Islands, Vavau Island		+				
	upolensis, Samoa		+				
Culex (Culex) pipiens group:	pipiens, biotype molestus, e.g., Egypt, Turkey	+					
cosmopolitan	pipiens, form pallens, e.g., China, Japan	+					
	quinquefasciatus, tropical Africa, Asia, Caribbean and South America	+					
sitiens group:	annulirostris, e.g., West Irian	+					
Afrotropical, Australian	bitaeniorhynchus, e.g., India, West Irian	+					
and Oriental regions	gelidus, e.g., India	?					
	sitiens complex, e.g., India, Maldive Islands						
	tritaeniorhynchus, e.g., Bangladesh, India	?					
	vishnui complex, e.g., Bangladesh, India	?			?		
Mansonia (Mansonia) titillans: Neotropical region	titillans, e.g., Guyana	+					

Table IV.5 *(cont'd)*

Mosquito groups and their general distribution	Vector species and places where incriminated	Forms of filariasis					
		W. bancrofti np	ns	ds	B. malayi np	ns	B. timori np
Mansonia (Mansonioides)							
dives group:	*bonneae*, e.g., Malaysia;				–	+	
Oriental region and	Thailand				+		
Papua area	*dives*, e.g., Malaysia, Sumatra, Palawan				+	+	
uniformis group:	*annulata*, e.g., Kalimantan, Malaysia, Sri Lanka	–			+		
Afrotropical,	Sumatra, Thailand						
Australian and	*annulifera*, e.g., India, Kalimantan, Sri Lanka*,				+		
Oriental regions	Thailand						
	indiana, e.g., India, Java, Sri Lanka*, Malaysia,				+		
	Thailand						
	uniformis, e.g., Africa;	–					
	India, Kalimantan, Malaysia, Sri Lanka*;	–				+	+
	West Irian	+					

np, Nocturnally periodic; *ns*, nocturnally subperiodic or non-periodic; *ds*, diurnally subperiodic; +, proven vector, infective filarial larvae found repeatedly in wild mosquito female; –, non-vector: filarial larvae usually fail to develop; no entry, vecor status undertermined or form of filariasis absent.
Brugia malayi now virtually eradicated from Sri Lanka.

Zone 1: Neotropical: *Anopheles albimanus, aquasalis, bellator, darlingi; Aedes scapularis, taeniorhynchus; Culex quinquefasciatus; Mansonia titillans.*
Zone 2: Afrotropical: *Anopheles funestus, arabiensis, gambiae, melas, merus; Culex quinquefasciatus, sitiens.*
Zone 3: Middle Eastern: *Culex pipiens, molestus.*
Zone 4: Oriental: *Anopheles barbirostris, campestris, donaldi, nigerrimus, sinensis complex, letifer, whartoni, aconitus, flavirostris, minimus, candidiensis, maculatus, philippinensis, subpictus, tesselatus; Aedes niveus, harinasutai, togoi, poicilius; Culex bitaeniorhynchus, gelidus, sitiens complex, tritaeniorhynchus, vishnui complex; Mansonia uniformis, bonneae, annulata, annulifera, indiana.*
Zone 5: Western Pacific: *Culex pipiens; Aedes togoi.*
Zone 6: Papuan: *Anopheles bancrofti, punctulatus, farauti, koliensis, subpictus, tesselatus.*
Zone 7: South Pacific: *Aedes kochi group fijiensis, oceanicus, samoanus, tutuilae; Aedes scutellaris group cooki, futanae, kesseli, polynesiensis, pseudoscutellaris, rotumae, tabu, tongae, upolensis; Aedes vigilax.*

Table IV.6 Mosquitoes implicated as hosts involved in transmission of arboviruses affecting man (see also Chapter 41).

Arbovirus and endemic area	Natural vector (*indicates principal species)	Arbovirus and endemic area	Natural vector (*indicates principal species)
Togaviridae		*Eastern equine encephalitis (EEE)*	
ALPHAVIRUS (=GROUP A)		North America	*Aedes (Aedimorphus) vexans*
Barmah Forest Virus (BFV)			*Aedes (Ochlerotatus) atlanticus*
Australia	*Aedes (Ochlerotatus) vigilax*		*Aedes (Ochlerotatus) fulvus*
	Culex (Culex) annulirostris		*Aedes (Ochlerotatus) mitchellae*
			*Aedes (Ochlerotatus) sollicitans
Chikungunya (CHIK)			*Aedes (Ochlerotatus) sticticus*
Africa	*Aedes (Diceromyia) furcifer*		**Aedes (Ochlerotatus) taeniorhynchus*
	*Aedes (Stegomyia) aegypti		*Anopheles (Anopheles) crucians*
	Aedes (Stegomyia) africanus		*Coquillettidia (Coquillettidia)*
	Coquillettidia (Coquillettidia)		*perturbans*
	fuscopennata		*Culex (Culex) nigripalpus*
	Culex (Culex) quinquefasciatus		*Culex (Culex) quinquefasciatus*
			Culex (Culex) restuans
	Mansonia (Mansonioides) africana		*Culex (Culex) salinarius*
	Mansonia (Mansonioides) uniformis		**Culiseta (Climacura) melanura*
			*Culiseta (Culicella) morsitans
South-East Asia	**Aedes (Stegomyia) aegypti*		
	Aedes (stegomyia) albopictus?	South America	**Aedes (Ochlerotatus) taeniorhynchus*
	Culex (Culex) gelidus		*Culex (Culex) nigripalpus*
	Culex (Culex) quinquefasciatus		*Culex (Melanoconion) caudelli*
	Culex (Culex) tritaeniorhynchus		*Culex (Melanoconion) spissipes*
			Culex (Melanoconion) taeniopus
		Europe	*Culex (Culex) pipiens*

Table IV.6 (cont'd)

Arbovirus and endemic area	Natural vector (*indicates principal species)	Arbovirus and endemic area	Natural vector (*indicates principal species)
Everglades (EVE) Florida	Aedes (Ocherotatus) taeniorhynchus Aedes (Ocherotatus) crucians Culex (Culex) nigripalpus Culex (Melanoconion) spp.	Australasia	Aedes (Ochlerotatus) normanensis Aedes (Ochlerotatus) vigilax *Culex (Culex) annulirostris Mansonia (Mansonioides) septempunctata
Mayaro (MAY) South and Central America	Culex spp. *Haemagogus spp. Coquillettidia (Rhynchotaemia) venezuelensis Psorophora (Janthinosoma) ferox Sabethini spp.	Orient *Venezuelan equine encephalitis* (VEE) Tropical Americas	*Culex (Culex) bitaeniorhynchus Culex (Culex) pseudovishnui *Culex (Culex) tritaeniorhynchus about 40 species implicated, including:
Mucambo (MUC) South America	Aedes spp. Aedes (Ochlerotatus) serratus Culex spp. *Culex (Melanoconion) portesi Haemagogus spp. Sabethini spp. Wyeomyia spp.		Aedes (Ochlerotatus) angustivittatus Aedes (Ochlerotatus) scapularis *Aedes (Ochlerotatus) serratus Aedes (Ochlerotatus) sollicitans *Aedes (Ochlerotatus) taeniorhynchus Aedes (Ochlerotatus) thelcter Aedes (Stegomyia) aegypti Anopheles (Anopheles) aquasalis Anopheles (Anopheles) crucians Anopheles (Anopheles) neomaculipalpus
O'nyong-nyong (ONN) Africa	Anopheles (Cellia) funestus Anopheles (Cellia) gambiae (sensu lato)		Anopheles (Anopheles) pseudopunctipennis Anopheles (Anopheles) punctimacula Culex (Culex) corniger
Ross River (RR) Australiasia	Aedes (Ocherotatus) vigilax Culex (Culex) annulirostris		Culex (Culex) coronator Culex (Culex) nigripalpus Culex (Culex) tarsalis *Culex (Melanoconion) spp. Culex (Melanoconion) iolambdis
Semliki Forest (SF) Africa	Aedes (Aedimorphus) abnormalis group Aedes (Aedimorphus) argenteopunctatus Aedes (Aedimorphus) denatus Aedes (Neomelaniconion) palpalis Anopheles (Cellia) funestus Eretmapodites grahamii		Culex (Melanoconion) acossa/ panocossa Culex (Melanoconion) portesi Culex (Melanoconion) taeniopus Culex (Melanoconion) vomerifer Deinocerites pseudes Haemagogus spp. Limatus flavisetosus Mansonia (Mansonia) indubitans Mansonia (Mansonia) titillans
Sindbis (SIN) Africa	Aedes (Aedimorphus) cumminsi Aedes (Neomelaniconion) circumluteolus Anopheles (Celia) pharoensis Coquillettidia (Coquillettidia) fuscopennata *Culex (Culex) antennatus *Culex (Culex) perexiguus Culex (Culex) pipiens (sensu lato) *Culex (Culex) univittatus Mansonia (Mansonioides) africana		*Psorophora (Grabhamia) confinnis Psorophora (Grabhamia) discolor Psorophora (Janthinosoma) albipes Psorophora (Janthinosoma) cyanescens *Psorophora (Psorophora) ciliata Psorophora (Psorophora) cilipes Sabethes spp. Wyeomyia spp.

Table IV.6 *(cont'd)*

Arbovirus and endemic area	Natural vector (*indicates principal species)	Arbovirus and endemic area	Natural vector (*indicates principal species)
Western equine encephalitis (WEE) North and South America	mainly *Culex (Culex) tarsalis* in western USA *Culiseta (Climacura) melanura* in eastern USA occasionally *Aedes, Anopheles, Culex, Culiseta* and *Psorophora* spp.	*Japanese encephalitis (JE)* South-East Asia to India and Japan and former USSR	*Aedes (Aedimorphus) vexans* *Aedes (Cancraedes) curtipes* *Aedes (Finlaya) koreicus* *Aedes (Finlaya) togoi* *Anopheles (Anopheles) barbirostris* group *Anopheles (Anopheles) hyrcanus* group *Culex (Culex) bitaeniorhynchus* group *Culex (Culex) epidesmus* *Culex (Culex) gelidus* *Culex (Culex) pipiens* group *Culex (Culex) pseudovishnui* *Culex (Culex) tritaeniorhynchus* *Culex (Culex) vishnui (=annulus)* *Culex (Culex) whitmorei*
FLAVIVIRUS (=GROUP B) *Banzi (BAN)* Africa	*Culex (Culex) nakuruensis* *Culex (Eumelanomyia) rubinotus* *Mansonia (Mansonioides) africana*		
Bussuquara (BSQ) South and Central America	*Coquillettidia (Rhynchotaenia) venezuelensis* *Culex (Melanoconion)* spp. *Culex (Melanoconion) epanatasis (=crybda)* *Culex (Melanoconion) taeniopus* *Culex (Melanoconion) vomerifer* *Mansonia (Mansonia) titillans* *Trichoprosopon* sp.	*Kunjin (KUN)* Borneo, Australia	*Culex (Culex) annulirostris* *Culex (Culex) pseudovishnui* *Culex (Culex) squamosus*
		Murray Valley encephalitis (MVE) Australasia	*Aedes (Ochlerotatus) normanensis* *Culex (Culex) annulirostris* *Culex (Culex) bitaeniorhynchus*
Dengue (DEN) types 1–4 between 40°N and 40°S	*Aedes (Finlaya) niveus* group *Aedes (Stegomyia)* spp. *Aedes (Stegomyia) albopictus* *Aedes (Stegomyia) polynesiensis* *Aedes (Stegomyia) scutellaris*	*Septik (SEP)* Australasia	*Armigeres* sp. *Mansonia (Mansonioides) septempunctata* *Mimomyia (Mimomyia) flavens*
Ilheus (ILH) South and Central America	*Aedes (Ochlerotatus) angustivittatus* *Aedes (Ochlerotatus) fulvus* *Aedes (Ochlerotatus) scapularis* *Aedes (Ochlerotatus) serratus* *Aedes (Stegomyia) aegypti* *Coquillettidia* spp. *Culex (Culex) nigripalpus* *Culex (Culex) quinquefasciatus* *Culex (Melanoconion)* spp. *Culex (Melanoconion) caudelli* *Culex (Melanoconion) spissipes* *Culex (Melanoconion) taeniopus* *Haemagogus (Conopostegus) leucocelaenus* *Hemagogus (Haemagogus) janthinomys (=falco)* *Psorophora (Janthinosoma) albipes* *Psorophora (Janthinosoma) ferox* *Psorophora (Janthinosoma) lutzii* *Sabethes (Sabethoides) chloropterus* *Trichoprosopon* sp. *Wyeomyia* sp.	*Spondweni (SPO)* Africa	*Aedes (Aedimorphus) cumminsi* *Aedes (Aedimorphus) fowleri?* *Aedes (Neomelaniconion) circumluteolus* *Aedes (Ochlerotatus) fryeri?* *Culex (Culex) univittatus* *Eretmapodites* spp. *Eretmapodites silvestris* *Mansonia (Mansonioides) africana* *Mansonia (Mansonioides) uniformis*
		St Louis encephalitis (SLE) North America	*Aedes (Ochlerotatus) dorsalis/melanimon* *Aedes (Ochlerotatus) scapularis* *Aedes (Ochlerotatus) serratus* *Anopheles (Anopheles) crucians* *Culex (Culex) nigripalpus* *Culex (Culex) peus*

Table IV.6 (cont'd)

Arbovirus and endemic area	Natural vector (*indicates principal species)	Arbovirus and endemic area	Natural vector (*indicates principal species)
	*Culex (Culex) pipiens	Asia	Anopheles (Cellia) subpictus
	*Culex (Culex) quinquefasciatus		Culex (Culex) quinquefasciatus
	Culex (Culex) restuans		Culex (Culex) tritaeniorhynchus
	Culex (Culex) salinarius		Culex (Culex) vishnui group
	Culex (Culex) tarsalis		
		Yellow fever (YF)	
South America	*Culex (Culex) coronator	Africa	Aedes (Aedimorphus) vittatus
	Culex (Culex) declarator (as virgultus)		Aedes (Diceromyia) taylori
	Culex (Culex) nigripalpus		*Aedes (Stegomyia) aegypti
	Culex (Melanoconion) candelli		*Aedes (Stegomyia) africanus
	Culex (Melanoconion) spissipes		Aedes (Stegomyia) luteocephalus
	Culex (Melanoconion) taeniopus		Aedes (Stegomyia) metallicus
	Psorophora (Janthinosoma) ferox		*Aedes (Stegomyia) simpsoni
	Sabethes (Sabethes) belisarioi	South and	*Aedes (Stegomyia) aegypti
	Sabethes (Sabethoides) chloropterus	Central America	Haemagogus (Conopostegus) leucocelaenus
	Trichoprosopon sp.		Haemagogus (Haemagogus) janthinomys (=falco)
	Wyeomyia sp.		*Haemagogus (Haemagogus) spegazzinni
Wesselsbron (WSL)			Sabethes (Sabethoides) chloropterus
Africa	Aedes (Aedimorphus) hisutus		
	Aedes (Aedimorphus) minutus	Zika (ZIKA)	
	Aedes (Aedimorphus) tarsalis group	Africa	*Aedes (Stegomyia) africanus
	Aedes (Neomelaniconion) spp.		Aedes (Stegomyia) luteocephalus
	Aedes (Neomelaniconion) circumluteolus	Malaysia	Aedes (Stegomyia) aegypti
	Aedes (Neomelaniconion) lineatopennis	**Bunyaviridae (Bunyavirus)**	
	Aedes (Ochlerotatus) caballus	BUNYAMWERA GROUP	
	Anopheles (Cellia) gambiae (sensu lato)	Bunyamwera (BUN)	
	Anopheles (Cellia) pharoensis	Africa	*Aedes (Neomelaniconion) circumluteolus
	Culex (Culex) telesilla		Aedes (Skusea) pembaensis
	Culex (Culex) univittatus		Culex sp.
	Mansonia (Mansonioides) uniformis		Mansonia (Mansonioides) africana
			Mansonia (Mansonioides) uniformis
Thailand	Aedes (Aedimorphus) mediolineatus	Calovo (CVO)	
	Aedes (Neomelaniconion) lineatopennis	Europe	Anopheles (Anopheles) maculipennis (sensu lato)
			Coquillettidia (Coquillettidia) richiardii
West Nile (WN)		Germiston (GER)	
Africa	Coquillettidia (Coquillettidia) metallica	Africa	Aedes (Neomelaniconion) circumluteolus
	Culex (Culex) theileri		Anopheles (Cellia) arabiensis
	*Culex (Culex) univittatus		Anopheles (Cellia) funestus
	Culex (Culex) weschei		Culex (Culex) theileri?
Europe	Culex (Barraudius) modestus		*Culex (Eumelanomyia) rubinotus
Middle East	Anopheles (Anopheles) coustani	Guaroa (GRO)	
	Culex (Culex) antennatus	South America	Anopheles (Kerteszia) neivai
	Culex (Culex) perexiguus (as univittatus)	Ilesha (ILE)	
	Culex (Culex) pipiens group	Africa	Anopheles (Cellia) gambiae (sensu lato)
			Mansonia (Mansonioides) uniformis

Table IV.6 *(cont'd)*

Arbovirus and endemic area	Natural vector (*indicates principal species)	Arbovirus and endemic area	Natural vector (*indicates principal species)
Tensaw (TEN) South-east USA	*Aedes (Ochlerotatus) atlanticus* *Aedes (Ochelerotatus) infirmatus* *Aedes (Ochelerotatus) mitchellae* **Anopheles (Anopheles) crucians* *Anopheles (Anopheles) punctipennis* *(Anopheles) quadrimaculatus* *Coquillettidia (Coquillettidia) perturbans* *Culex (Culex) nigripalpus* *Culex (Culex) salinarius*	*Caraparu (CAR)* South America	*Culex (Melanoconion)* spp. *Culex (Melanoconion) caudelli* **Culex (Melanoconion) portesi* *Culex (Melanoconion) spissipes* *Culex (Melanoconion) vomerifer* *Limatus durhamii* *Wyeomyia* sp.
Wyeomyia (WYO) South and Central America	*Aedes (Howardina) septemstriatus* *Aedes (Howardina) sexlineatus* *Aedes (Ochlerotatus) fulvus* *Aedes (Ochlerotatus) scapularis* *Aedes (Ochlerotatus) serratus* *Aedes (Protomacleaya) argyrothorax* *Anopheles* spp. *Anopheles (Stethomyia) nimbus* *Coquillettidia (Rhynchotaemia) arribalzagae* *Culex (Aedinus) amazonensis* *Culex (Culex) nigripalpus* *Haemagogous (Conopostegus) leucocelaenus* *Limatus durhamii* *Limatus flavisetosus* *Psorophora (Grabhamia) cingulata* *Psorophora (Janthinosoma) albipes* *Psorophora (Janthinosoma) ferox* *Trichoprosopon (Runchomyia) leucopus* *Trichoprosopon (Runchomyia) longipes* *Trichoprosopon (Trichoprosopon) digitatum* *Wyeomyia (Dendromyia) aporonoma* *Wyeomyia (Dendromyia) complosa* *Wyeomyia (Dendromyia) melanocephala*	*Itaqui (ITQ)* Brazil	*Culex (Melanoconion)* spp. *Culex (Melanoconion) portesi* *Culex (Melanoconion) vomerifer*
		Madrid (MAD) Panama	*Culex (Melanoconion) vomerifer*
		Marituba (MTB) Brazil	*Culex (Melanoconion) ocossa/ panocossa (=aikenii)* *Culex (Melanoconion) portesi*
		Murutucu (MUR) South America	*Coquillettidia (Rhychotaenia) venezuelensis* *Culex (Melanoconion) ocossa/ panocossa (=aikenii)* *Culex (Melanoconion) portesi* other *Culex* spp. and *Sabethini*
		Oriboca (ORI) South America	*Aedes* spp. *Aedes (Ochlerotatus) taeniorhynchus* *Culex* spp. *Culex (Melanoconion) portesi* *Mansonia* sp. *Psorophora (Janthinosoma) ferox* *Sabethini*
		Ossa (OSSA) Panama	*Culex (Melanoconion) taeniopus* *Culex (Melanoconion) vomerifer*
BWAMBA GROUP *Bwamba (BWA)* Africa	*Anopheles (Cellia) funestus* *Anopheles (Cellia) gambiae (sensu lato)*	*Restam (RES)* South America	*Culex (Melanoconion) portesi*
C GROUP *Apeu (APEU)* Brazil	*Aedes (Howardina) arborealis* *Aedes (Howardina) septemstriatus* *Aedes (Ochlerotatus) serratus* *Culex (Melanoconion) acossa/ panocossa (=aikenii)*	CALIFORNIA GROUP *California encephalitis (CE)* South-western USA	*Aedes (Aedimorphus) vexans* **Aedes (Ochlerotatus) dorsalis* **Aedes (Ochlerotatus) melanimon* *Aedes (Ochlerotatus) nigromaculis* *Anopheles (Anopheles) pseudopunctipennis* *Culex (Culex) tarsalis* *Culiseta (Culex) inornata* *Psorophora (Grabhamia) signipennis*

Table IV.6 (cont'd)

Arbovirus and endemic area	Natural vector (*indicates principal species)	Arbovirus and endemic area	Natural vector (*indicates principal species)
Inkoo (INK) Finland	*Aedes (Ochlerotatus) communis/* *punctor*	**NYANDO GROUP** *Nyando (NDO)* Africa	*Anopheles (Cellia) funestus*
La Crosse (LAC) USA	*Aedes (Ochlerotatus) canadensis* *Aedes (Ochlerotatus) communis* *Aedes (Promacleaya) triseriatus* *Culex (Culex) pipiens*	**SIMBU GROUP** *Oropouche (ORO)* South America	Mainly Ceratopogonidae *Aedes (Ochlerotatus) serratus* *Coquillettidia (Rhynchotaenia)* *venezuelensis* *Culex (Culex) quinquefasciatus*
Melao (MEL) South America	*Aedes (Ochlerotatus) scapularis* *Aedes (Ochlerotatus) serratus* *Psorophora (Janthinosoma) ferox*	*Shuni (SHU)* South Africa	*Culex (Culex) theileri*
Tahyna (TAH) Africa Europe	*Aedes (Skusea) pembaensis* **Aedes (Aedimorphus) vexans* *Aedes (Ochlerotatus) cantans* *Aedes (Ochlerotatus) caspius* *Aedes (Ochlerotatus) cinereus* *Anopheles (Anopheles) hyrcanus* *(sensu lato)* *Anopheles (Anopheles) maculipennis* *(sensu lato)* *Culex (Barraudius) modestus* *Culex (Culex) pipiens (sensu lato)* *Caliseta (Culiseta) annulata*	**PHLEBOTOMUS FEVER GROUP** *Chagres (CHG)* Panama *Rift Valley fever (RVT)* Africa	*Sabethes (Sabethoides) chloropterus* and phlebotomine sandflies *Aedes (Aedimorphus) dentatus* *Aedes (Aedimorphus) tarsalis* *Aedes (Aedimorphus) triseriatus* *Aedes (Neomelaniconion)* *circumluteolus* *Aedes (Neomelaniconion)* *lineatopennis* **Aedes (Ochlerotatus) caballus* *Aedes (Ochlerotatus) juppi* *Aedes (Stegomyia) deboeri* *Aedes (Stegomyia) aegypti* *Aedes (Stegomyia) africanus* *Aedes (Stegomyia) dendrophilus* *Anopheles (Anopheles) coustani* *Coquillettidia (Coquillettidia)* *fuscopennata* *Coquillettidia (Coquillettidia)* *microbannulata* *Coquillettidia (Coquillettidia)* *versicolor* *Culex (Culex) neavei* **Culex (Culex) pipiens (sensu lato)* **Culex (Culex) theileri* *Culex (Culex) univattatus* *Culex (Culex) zombaensis* *Eretmapodites chrysogaster group* *Mansonia (Mansonioides) africana* *Mansonia (Mansonioides) uniformis?*
GUAMA GROUP *Catu (CATU)* South America	*Anopheles (Stethomyia) nimbus* *Coquillettidia (Rhynchotaemia)* *venezuelensis* *Culex (Aedinus) majuensis* *Culex (Culex) declarator (=virgultus)* **Culex (Melanoconion) portesi* *Culex (Melanoconion) vomerifer*		
Guama (GAM) South and Central America	*Aedes (Howardina) sexlineatus* *Coquillettidia (Rhynchotaenia)* *venezuelensis* *Culex (Aedinus) mojuensis* *Culex (Melanoconion) spp.* *Culex (Melanoconion) epanatasis* *(=crybda)* **Culex (Melanoconion) portesi* *Culex (Melanoconion) spissipes* *Culex (Melanoconion) taeniopus* *Culex (melanoconion) vomerifer* *Culex (Tinolestes) sp.* *Limatus durhamii* *Wyeomyia sp.*	**GANJAM GROUP** *Gamjam (GAN)* India	*Culex (Culex) vishnui group and ticks* *(Ixodidae)*

Table IV.6 (*cont'd*)

Arbovirus and endemic area	Natural vector (*indicates principal species)
ANOPHELES A GROUP *Tataguine* (TAT) Africa	*Anopheles (Cellia) funestus* *Anopheles (Cellia) gambiae (sensu lato)*
UNGROUPED *Zinga* (ZGA) Africa	*Aedes (Neomelaniconion) palpalis group* *Mansonia (Mansonioides) africana*
Poxviridae *Cotia* (COT) South America	*Aedes (Ochlerotatus) serratus* *Coquillettidia (Rhynchotaenia) venezuelensis* *Culex (Melanoconion) portesi* *Limatus pseudomethysticus* *Psorophora (Janthinosoma) ferox*

Sensilla on the palps and antennae serve to detect the host; eyes of the mosquito help to monitor ground speed, altitude, flight direction and details of host location. Intermittent downwind flights are also a feature of normal activity. The majority of mosquitoes hunt and feed at night, although many aedine mansoniine and sabethine species do so by day. Each species has a well defined activity cycle: some attack at dusk, others around midnight or at other hours. Species showing strong attraction to humans are said to be anthropophilic, or more strictly anthropophagic when the human is bitten, as opposed to zoophilic or zoophagic species which attack other creatures. Endophilic mosquitoes are those that favour houses or animal sheds for resting indoors, whereas exophilic species prefer to remain outdoors. Outdoor biting behaviour is termed exophagy, as opposed to the endophagy of mosquitoes that enter dwellings to bite people or animals. It is important to realize that mosquitoes may rest outdoors after feeding indoors, or vice versa. Male mosquitoes tend to be less endophilic than females of the same species, while many human-biting species seldom go indoors at all. Few species of mosquito have the human as their principal host. In order to quantify amounts of human–mosquito contact for epidemiological purposes, it is necessary to estimate: (1) the number of bites per person per 24 hours, (2) the percentage of mosquito blood meals obtained from human compared with other animals, and (3) the feeding interval, expressed as the mean number of days between times when successive blood meals are taken by a given species of mosquito. These data can be combined with the probability of mosquito daily survival, estimated from the proportion of parous females, in order to calculate an index of vectorial capacity.[13]

Male and female mosquitoes are good fliers and sometimes disperse over many kilometres. However, most kinds of mosquito remain in rather restricted habitats. Those breeding in salt marshes include some notorious migrants, notably *Aedes taeniorhynchus* along the American east coast. It has been suggested that *Anopheles pharoensis* occasionally travels almost 300 km over desert in the Middle East. Adult mosquitoes can be accidentally transported alive overseas in ships and aeroplanes. For instance, at least six introduced species of mosquito have recently become established on the remote Pacific island of Guam. A survey of planes arriving at Nairobi during the mid-1960s revealed mosquitoes imported from several other countries, *Culex quinquefasciatus* being most frequently encountered, and one African *Anopheles* was found returning on a flight from India. It seems that *Aedes aegypti*, *Anopheles gambiae* and possibly *C. quinquefasciatus* have been taken inadvertently by humans from the Old World to the New World, where these mosquitoes have caused inestimable trouble. *A. gambiae* was wiped out again in the 1930s before it had spread from the primary focus in Brazil, but introduced populations of *Aedes aegypti* and *C. quinquefasciatus* are continually spreading throughout the tropics. Fortunately, not many species of mosquito readily become established in fresh situations.

Identification and taxonomy of mosquitoes are matters for specialists. The morphology of hairs, scales and other body structures must be studied in precise detail on adults of both sexes and on all the immature stages. This requires specimens in perfect condition as a basis for conventional identification. Where possible the larval and pupal skins should be preserved with the adult that emerges, so that the taxonomic characteristics of all life stages can be checked. Adult mosquito specimens should be kept on micropins; larvae and skins can be preserved in 60% alcohol or permanently mounted on a microscopic slide in chloral gum or Canada balsam for examination. Many species of mosquito show few points of distinction, although the characteristics of genera and subgenera can be recognized more easily. Most medically important species of mosquito have close similarities to other species that do not bite humans. Specific identification may depend on minute features of the male, the larva or even the egg, often making it unreliable to identify individual female specimens. For some species of mosquito it may be necessary to look at their chromosomal or DNA characteristics, proteins or behaviour in order to distinguish between species that are morphologically identical, or nearly so. Groups of such closely related species are known as *sibling species complexes*. Genetic evidence shows that these biologically distinct species do not normally interbreed in nature. The significance of species complexes is that some of the species are pests and vectors of disease, whereas others are not.

Anatomy (Figures IV.29–IV.36)

The body of an adult mosquito consists of three recognizable divisions: head, thorax and abdomen. The head is rounded and attached to the thorax by a slender neck. It is provided with large eyes, antennae and mouthparts. The antennae (Figures IV.34 and IV.35) are composed of 15 segments. Each segment bears a whorl of

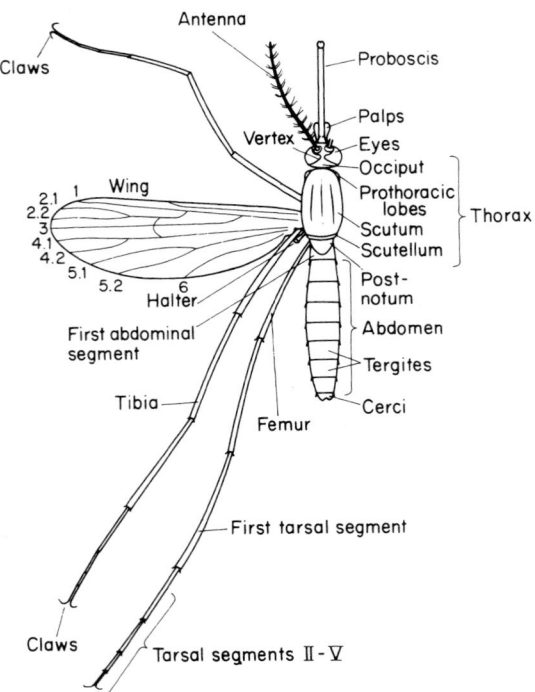

Figure IV.32: Anatomy of the female mosquito, showing wing veins 1–6.

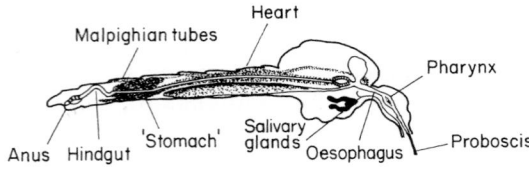

Figure IV.33: Longitudinal section of a female mosquito showing its anatomy.

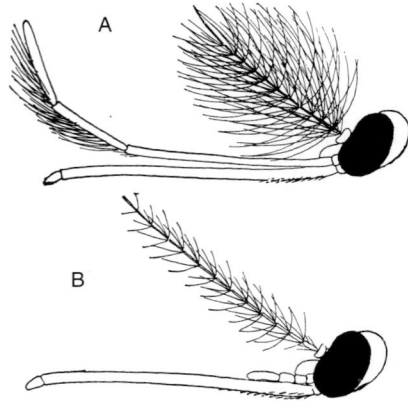

Figure IV.34: Heads of (**A**) male and (**B**) female culicine.

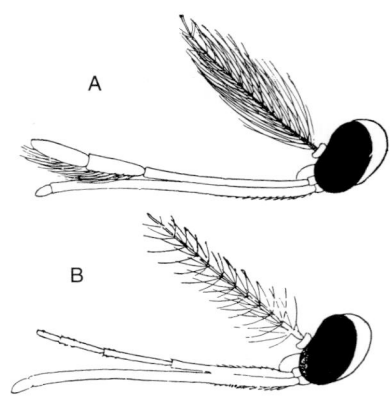

Figure IV.35: Heads of (**A**) male and (**B**) female anopheline.

hairs in the female, but in the male the hairs are profuse, giving a bristly or bottle-brush appearance. The mouthparts in the female consist of a proboscis fitted for piercing and sucking. The labium encloses the other mouthparts (Figure IV.29), except the maxillary palps, and ends distally in two pointed labella lobes clothed with scales and hairs. In the act of biting, the labellae part and are applied to the surface of the skin, forming a sheath for the delicate piercing stylets, and do not enter the wound made for obtaining blood. Within is the labrum-epipharynx, forming a V-shaped channel open on the ventral surface. This extends along the whole length of the labium and ends in a sharp point. Lying directly beneath the labrum-epipharynx, closing the ventral slit, is the hypopharynx, which consists of a thin chitinous lamella, fitting closely to the ventral surface of the labrum-epipharynx, thus forming a tube through which the blood is sucked. In the longitudinal chitinous thickening runs a very fine channel extending from the base to the tip of the hypopharynx; through this the salivary secretion is poured into the wound (Figure IV.29). The mandibles form delicate chitinous stylets at the side of the hypopharynx. The labium buckles in the act of biting and the stylets emerge. Each of these tapers slightly, ending in a sharp point. The maxillary stylets are more robustly constructed, but have the same general form; the tip is generally supplied with a row of backwardly pointing teeth. The maxillary palps consist of five partially fused segments. In the male the mouthparts are not adapted for biting. The maxillary palps are elongated, extending above the proboscis, but the mandibles and maxillae are greatly reduced and may be lacking altogether.

In female anophelines the palps are as long as the proboscis and usually closely applied, but in female culicines the palps are short. In male mosquitoes, both culicine and anopheline, the palps are as long as the proboscis. The palps of the male culicines are bushy and the two terminal segments tend to turn upwards in *Culex*, downward in *Aedes*. Those of the male anophelines are somewhat club-shaped.

The thorax is wedge-shaped in side view; the sides form the pleura, with scale patches. The various sclerites composing the side of the thorax bear stiff setae or hairs,

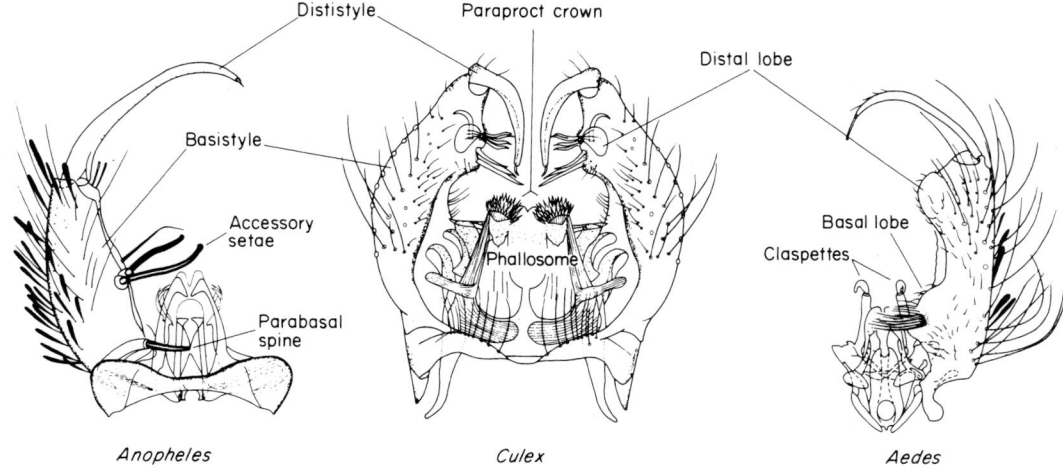

Figure IV.36: Male terminalia (external genitalia) of *Aedes*, *Anopheles* and *Culex* in ventral view, showing the main generic characteristics. These features show specific modifications that are useful for taxonomy and identification of species and genera.

arranged in definite groups. The scutellum is separated by a transverse suture from the mesonotum. In all genera except *Anopheles* it is trilobate and each lobe bears a group of stiff setae. In anophelines the scutellum is rounded and reduced. The region behind the scutellum is known as the postnotum and is generally nude. The wings are long and narrow, with venation; the scales are characteristic. Situated immediately posterior to the base of the wings is a pair of halteres or balancers, which have gyroscopic functions during flight.

The legs are long and slender, composed of coxa, trochanter, femur and tibia, as well as a tarsus of five long and slender tarsomeres. The last tarsomere bears a pair of claws (ungues), which vary greatly in size and shape; those of the hind legs are generally smaller than those of others. The abdomen is nearly cylindrical, narrow and elongated, consisting of 10 segments, the last two modified for sexual purposes. The terminal segment in the female is tapered. The ninth is reduced and in the inter-segmental area between it and the eighth lies the opening of the reproductive organs. The tenth segment is greatly reduced and bears the anal opening and paired cerci. The abdomen of the male is slightly longer than that of the female. The terminal segments are greatly modified and bear paired claspers, between which lies the aedeagus, a complex organ used in reproduction. Specific characteristics of these terminalia are the basis of much taxonomy (Figure IV.36).

Subfamily: Toxorhynchitinae

As they are larger than other mosquitoes, it is fortunate that *Toxorhynchites* cannot suck blood. The proboscis is strongly down-curved and suited only for imbibing nectar from plants or free fluids. About 60 species are known, all classified in a single genus. *Toxorhynchites* occurs in all warmer regions of the world, between 35°N and 35°S approximately. Breeding places are flooded tree-holes,

rock-holes and artificial containers such as buckets and discarded tyres. Female *Toxorhynchites* scatter their rounded buoyant eggs on to water while flying. Larvae soon hatch and become rapacious predators with mouth brushes composed of six to ten strong recurved teeth on each side for grasping prey. When the chance arises, cannibalism occurs. A relatively short, dark, strongly chitinous respiratory siphon is present at the abdominal tip, as for larval Culicinae. Populations of some dangerous container-breeding Culicinae, notably *Aedes aegypti*, can be significantly reduced through larval predation by *Toxorhynchites*. This subfamily of mosquitoes should therefore be regarded as beneficial. Adult *Toxorhynchites* are colourful as a result of their iridescent and metallic scale patterns, with patches of purple, red, orange and green ornamentation on particular species. The lateral abdominal tail tufts and large size (up to 18 mm from head to tail; wing span 12–24 mm) are distinctive. *Toxorhynchites* adults are diurnally active and sometimes venture into houses, where they may be found when trying to escape from windows.

Subfamily: Anophelinae

The palps in both sexes are as long, or nearly as long, as the proboscis. The scutellum is rounded. Wings of nearly all species have characteristic patterns of pale and dark spots of scales (Figure IV.37). The subfamily Anophelinae was divided by Edwards into three genera: *Chagasia* (scutellum slightly trilobed), *Bironella* (scutellum evenly rounded, wing with stem of median fork wavy) and *Anopheles* (scutellum evenly rounded, wing with stem of median fork straight). The genus includes more than 400 species. When settled, most *Anopheles* stand with the proboscis, head and abdomen in almost a straight line, usually resting on an upright surface at an angle of about 45°; exceptionally, as in *A. culicifacies*, the resting position adopted is more *Culex*-like (Figure IV.38). In flight the hum produced by *Anopheles* is low pitched, almost inaudible unless close to the ear. Most species require large spaces for mating flights, rendering it difficult to

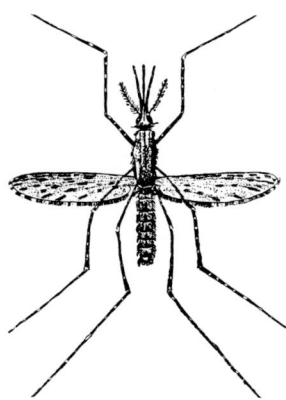

Figure IV.37: *Anopheles gambiae*. One of a series of drawings made by the late Philip Manson-Bahr, showing the wing markings characteristic of *Anopheles* (6 ×).

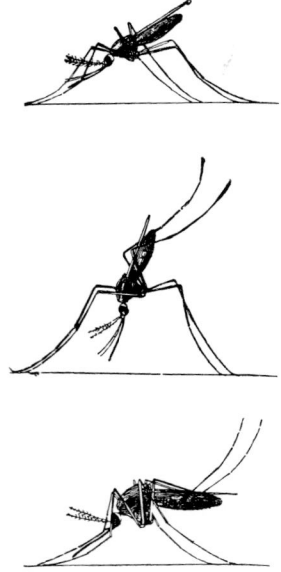

Figure IV.38: Resting positions of *Culex quinquefasciatus* (below), *Anopheles sinensis* (centre) and *Anopheles gambiae* (above).

propagate them in captivity. Overwintering females are fertilized before diapausing, but the males of temperate species cannot overwinter. For tropical species, both sexes are likely to live for several weeks, feeding intermittently. At 25–30°C tropical female *Anopheles* can be expected to suck blood and then lay eggs regularly at intervals of 2 or 3 days. The boat-shaped eggs (Figure IV.39) have an investing membrane inflated laterally to form a pair of floats. These represent air-filled spaces between the exochorion and the endochorion of the eggshell to resist submersion. Anopheline eggs are 1 mm in length. They are white when freshly laid, but tan to dull brown or black within a few hours. They are laid singly on the surface of the water, arrange themselves in a distinct pattern at that site, and hatch in 2 or 3 days. The larva feeds on small floating particles swept into its mouth by feeding brushes which can be folded under its head. When *Anopheles* larvae lie beneath the surface, the dorsal aspects of the thorax and abdomen face upward, but the head is rotated 180° so that its ventral surface lies upward. Food consists of living organisms, bacteria and protozoa obtained beneath the surface, as well as particles of floating food such as dead insect fragments. The head of the larva is complex; the central portion is known as the clypeus, the anterior plaque as the preclypus. It has a pair of short antennae, eyes, a pair of feeding brushes, and preclypeal and clypeal hairs. The respiratory opening is composed of two dorsally placed spiracles on the eighth abdominal segment. From the spiracles, the tracheae run the length of the body, conducting air to all regions for respiration.

The larva maintains itself under the surface film in a horizontal position by a row of dorsoabdominal plaques and a series of palmate hairs, known as float hairs. The terminal segment is provided with four anal papillae (gills), which have respiratory and excretory functions, but are mainly to absorb mineral salts. Above and below the anal gills are dorsal and ventral swimming brushes (Figure IV.40). The eighth segment has a chitinous plate lying between the two openings of the spiracles; just below it there is a row of teeth arising from a chitinized base, known as the pecten. Small glands secrete a waxy substance around the spiracles, which therefore cannot be wetted. (It is important to note this fact when oiling water to kill larvae.) Respiration also takes place through

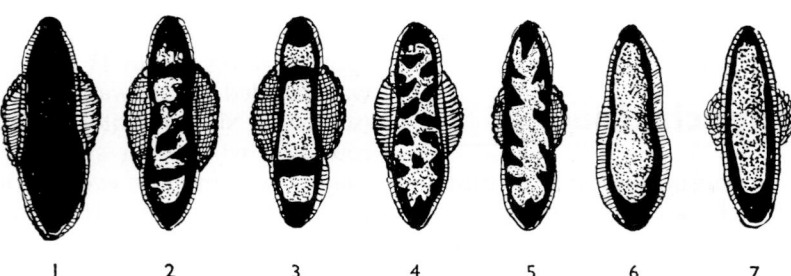

Figure IV.39: Eggs of the *Anopheles maculipennis* complex: 1, *melanoon*; 2, *messeae*; 3, *beklemishevi* or *maculipennis (sensu stricto)*; 4, *atroparvus*; 5, *labranchiae*; 6, *sacharovi* (summer); 7, *sacharovi* (winter). Species identification is based on the pattern on the deck (upper surface of egg) and the form of floats, i.e., size, number of ribs and striations.

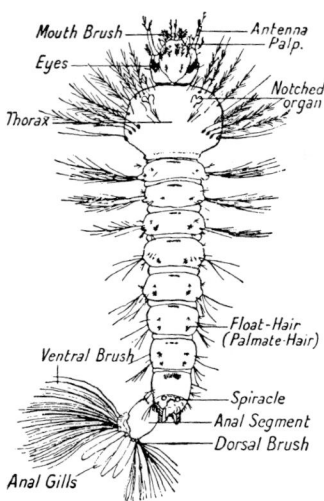

Figure IV.40: Larva of an anopheline (*A. maculipennis*) seen from above. The anal segment is twisted round to display the dorsal and ventral brushes.

the cuticle but the oxygen intake from the water is not sufficient to maintain life, except when the temperature is low and metabolism reduced.

The capability of any particular species of *Anopheles* to transmit malaria is regulated by a number of factors, such as the numbers present, the degree of anthropophily (human blood index), the probability of survival to a potentially infective age, and whether the parasites of malaria can complete their development in the mosquito. A species proved to be a natural carrier in one situation does not necessarily play an important part somewhere else. There is a striking correlation between the incidence of malaria and of *Anopheles*, as seen in the case of *A. punctulatus* complex, which occurs on some islands in the South Pacific, but not on others. Where these species occur there is malaria; where they do not, there is none. Malaria vector *Anopheles* spp. of the world are listed in Table IV.5.

Mosquito nomenclature is a vexed question. A great many species have been renamed in recent years. In case of doubt, recourse should be made to Knight and Stone.[14]

In undertaking a malaria survey, an attempt should be made to identify female anophelines; they should be collected and dissected to find out which species are infective. It is necessary to dissect at least several hundred insects and to examine the gut for oocysts and salivary glands for sporozoites. Molecular and immunological detection techniques (e.g., enzyme-linked immunosorbent assay; ELISA) are also now available for sporozoite detection. Infectivity rates are generally below 0.1%, although higher rates are often recorded, especially with *A. funestus* and the *A. gambiae* complex in Africa. Adults and larvae should be identified to determine whether known vector species are present. Any locality should be studied for at least a complete year as seasonal transmission is important: one species may be responsible in spring and another during the autumn.

Identification of the many diverse species of *Anopheles* is specialized work. The following points are of specific importance: size, general colouration, colour of erect scales on the head, pattern of pale scales on the generally dark legs, wings, and so on. The distal half of the proboscis may be pale, the palps may be smooth or shaggy, depending on the scales. The palps may be entirely dark or there may be pale bands. The general colouration of the thorax and scales on the mesonotum is helpful. These features are too intricate to be explained in detail here, and identification depends upon characters listed in the published keys.

The distribution and importance of some species of *Anopheles* have been changed in recent years as a result of malaria control or eradication programmes in which residual insecticides have been used. Formerly DDT was the insecticide of choice but, to offset DDT resistance, some more potent pyrethroids and other insecticides (e.g., carbamates, organophosphates) are increasingly being utilized for house spraying (see Table IV.13).

Some species are less responsive than others to insecticides sprayed indoors because either they tend to leave buildings after feeding, without resting on treated walls, or they tend to bite and rest in the open and therefore do not come into contact with residual insecticides.

Much success has been achieved in eradication programmes in subtropical areas and in some parts of the tropics, but even where eradication has been almost complete, there have been renewed outbreaks of malaria, as in Sri Lanka, India and Guyana. Such outbreaks can occur if surveillance is insufficient, and mosquitoes are allowed to multiply enormously if conditions change so as to stimulate breeding.

In most parts of tropical Africa malaria transmission has hardly changed. Where intensive insecticide spraying has been carried out, *A. funestus* has been eliminated, although it could re-enter the area from the periphery when spraying is discontinued. The main vectors, members of the *A. gambiae* complex (*A. gambiae, A. arabiensis, A. melas*), breed so prolifically in so many collections of water, and bite people so voraciously indoors and in the open, that control by insecticides is extremely difficult.

In addition to malaria, *Anopheles* spp. transmit *Wuchereria bancrofti*, many of the malaria-carrying species being implicated (Table IV.6). The now recognized Timor filaria parasite of humans, *Brugia timori*, has *A. barbirostris* as the only known vector, at least in the island of Flores.[15] *Anopheles* also transmit several arboviruses, for instance eastern equine encephalitis, western equine encephalitis, Venezuelan equine encephalitis, o'nyong-nyong, tataguine, and others listed in Table IV.6.

Adult anopheline mosquitoes are active only at night when the females seek avidly to feed on the blood of vertebrates. Medically important anthropophilic species belong to the subgenera *Anopheles, Cellia, Kerteszia* and *Nyssorhynchus* of the genus *Anopheles*. Neither of the other two anopheline genera, *Bironella* and *Chagasia*, nor the *Anopheles* subgenera *Lophopodomyia* and *Stethomyia* are of any applied interest. Taxonomic separation of

Table IV.7 Identification key to the genera of adult mosquitoes likely to be encountered indoors or attacking man.

1	Large iridescent mosquitoes (wing span 12–24 mm); abdominal segments VI–VIII (but not I–V) with distinctive lateral tufts of scales; proboscis curved downwards approx. 90° in middle; feeds on nectar not blood; distribution 40°N to 35°S	*Toxorhynchites*
	Typical mosquitoes of various sizes (wing span 5–16 mm); abdomen usually without distinctive lateral scale-tufts; proboscis usually straight, or curved through no more than 40° downwards or upwards; females often suck blood	2
2	Female palps as long as proboscis; male palps club-shaped (Figure IV.35); wing vein scales usually forming a conspicuous pattern of spots due to *either* clusters of scales at junctions of some veins *or* patches of pale scales and patches of dark scales alternating along some veins; scutellum evenly rounded posteriorly and lacking lateral lobes; abdomen usually not scale-covered, although some narrow scales may be mixed with the covering of fine hairs; worldwide distribution	*Anopheles*
	Female with short palps (Figure IV.34B), usually one-third to one-fifth as long as proboscis; male palps not clubbed, although often apically thickened; wing vein scales usually not forming a distinct pattern of spots or pale and dark patches, although speckling may be due to mixtures of pale and dark scales on some veins; scutellum trilobed, i.e., with large mid-lobe and smaller lateral lobes; abdomen clothed with broad scales (powdery when rubbed) above and below (Culicinae)	3
3	Female with tip of abdomen rounded, terminal segment non-retractable, cerci not conspicuous; postspiracular bristles absent (present in *Mansonia*, see no. 7)	4
	Female with tip of abdomen pointed, ending with a pair of prominent cerci, terminal abdominal segment retractable; postspiracular bristles present (Figure IV.41)	8
4	Pre-alar bristles (Figure IV.41) usually numerous and at least one lower mesepimeral bristle present; postnotum normally without apical tuft; anterior pronotal lobes small; meron well developed, so that upper edge is dorsal to the base of hind coxa	5
	Pre-alar bristles usually absent, no more than four present; no lower mesepimeral bristles; postnotum usually with an apical tuft of small setae; anterior pronotal lobes large and conspicuously ornamented with scales; meron small, so that upper edge is in line with base of hind coxa or ventral to it; essentially sylvatic mosquitoes, i.e., found in jungle	12
5	Tarsi with pulvilli (Figure IV.44) appearing as a pair of pale pads below the claws when examined at 50 × magnification or more; worldwide distribution	*Culex*
	Tarsi without pulvilli	6
6	Bristles on spiracular area (Figure IV.41) i.e., setae with roots in a vertical row just in front of the respiratory aperture on side of thorax (mesothoracic spiracle); worldwide distribution	*Culiseta*
	Spiracular bristles absent	7
7	Bristles on spiracular area (Figure IV.41); wing vein scales very broad and forming a mottled pattern on all or most veins; ornamentation without any yellow scales; worldwide distribution	*Mansonia*
	Postspiracle bristles absent; wing vein scales narrow not forming a mottled pattern on most veins; ornamentation mostly yellow, or with at least some bright yellow scales somewhere on body; worldwide distribution	*Coquillettidia*
8	Scutum covered with broad, flat, metallic green scales; legs generally dark; anterior pronotal lobes very large, almost meeting anteriorly; small species (wing span 6–9 mm) active in daytime; Caribbean, South and Central America	*Haemagogus*
	Scutum not covered with shiny green scales; legs often with pale bands, especially on tarsi anterior pronotal lobes not strongly developed; various sizes (wing span 6–16 mm), diurnal or nocturnal	9
9	Broad silver scales on back of head, sides of thorax and hind corners of abdominal tergites; thoracic cuticle orange or reddish-brown; tropical Africa only	*Eretmapodites*
	Not with silvery scales in the places specified; although some of these areas bear white scales; thoracic cuticle pale or dark, but not orange or reddish; temperate or tropical regions worldwide	10

Table IV.7 (*cont'd*)

10	Spiracular bristles present (Figure IV.41), i.e., setae with roots in a vertical row just in front of the respiratory aperture on side of thorax (mesothoracic spiracle; New World only	*Psorophora*
	Spiracular bristles absent	
11	Abdomen more than 2 × length of thorax; normally one lower mesepimeral bristle present (Figure IV.41); scales on top of head all broad, flat and decumbent; abdominal segment VIII partially retractile; distributed throughout southern Asia, from India to Japan, Philippines, Indonesia and Melanesia	*Armigeres*
	Abdomen not more than 2 × length of thorax; lower mesepimeral bristle usually absent; top of head with erect scales, seen best in side-view, forming a posterior tuft or more extensive 'crew cut' appearance (easily rubbed off), plus a layer of decumbent scales which are often curved and narrow along the midline but always broad and flat laterally; abdominal segment VIII almost completely retractile; worldwide distribution	*Aedes*
12	Spiracular area bare, i.e., no scales or bristles on the small membranous area between the posterior pronotum and the main thoracic spiracle; South-East Asia only	*Heizmannia*
	Spiracular area with scales and/or at least one bristle	13
13	Australasian or South-East Asian mosquitoes	*Tripteroides*
	New World mosquitoes	14
14	Spiracular area with broad scales only, no bristles; proboscis shorter than fore-femur, thorax with some shiny golden scales; hind tarsi with single claw	*Limatus*
	Spiracular area with at least one spiracular bristle; thoracic scales various, none golden; proboscis longer than or equal to forefemur; each hind tarsus with two claws	15
15	Scutum covered with broad, flat, shiny metallic scales; some tarsi with 'paddles' formed by inner and outer rows of long, mostly dark scales; some tarsi with 'paddles' formed by inner and outer rows of long, mostly dark scales; Central and South America	*Sabethes*
	Scutal scales usually not shiny; tarsi without paddles	16
16	Top of head often with erect scales; pronotal lobes widely separated anteriorly; membrane at wing base (squama) fringed with small setae; bristles on clypeus, i.e., bulbous area of the face between bases of antennae and palps; Central and South America	*Trichoprosopon*
	Top of head without erect scales; pronotal lobes very large and almost meeting anteriorly; membrane at wing base (squama) with more than three small fringe setae; area the face without bristles, although scales may be present; North and South America	*Wyeomyia*

Anopheles subgenera is based upon the numbers and positions of certain spines on the male basistyle (see Figure IV.36), together with other features summarized by Reid.[16]

Subgenus *Anopheles* predominates in the northern hemisphere, extending southwards with a few species found in Australia and through Africa. These mosquitoes are generally more robust and larger (wing span 8–12 mm) than those belonging to other anopheline subgenera. Taxonomists recognize six series of species within the subgenus *Anopheles*. Vectors of human diseases belong to the *Myzorhynchus* series as well as series *Anopheles (sensu stricto)*.

Series *Myzorhynchus* occurs mainly in the Oriental region, the following species groups being involved in human disease transmission. *A. hyrcanus* group, mostly zoophilic species, but including *A. sinensis* the main vector of malaria in China, also implicated as a vector of rural filariasis (both *B. malayi* and *W. bancrofti*) in parts of South-East Asia; it thrives where paddy provides suitable breeding places. The closely related *A. nigerrimus*, which breeds in more permanent ponds, also contributes to malaria and filariasis transmission in South-East Asia (see Tables IV.5 and IV.6). *A. barbirostris* group of blackish species with shaggy palps includes two important Malaysian vectors of malaria: darker *A. campestris* associated with clay but not sandy soils, especially alluvial coastal areas, where the larvae occur in lightly shaded deep waters, and paler *A. donaldi* which breeds in swampy forests. These and other members of the *A. barbirostris* group are important vectors of periodic *B. malayi*, but not of the subperiodic form or of *W. bancrofti* to which they are mostly refractory, although *A. donaldi* appears to transmit *W. bancrofti* in Borneo. The only known vector of Timor filariasis (*B. timori*) is said to be *A. barbirostris*,[15] but this mosquito might be the atypical form of *A. barbirostris (sensu lato)* regarded as a local vector of bancroftian filariasis in Sulawesi and perhaps other parts of Indonesia. In the closely related *A. bancroftii* group, the typical species transmits malaria and periodic bancroftian filariasis in Papua New Guinea and Indonesia, and formerly in Australia. Finally in this series the *A. umbrosus* group, having larvae with reduced float hairs, includes two vectors of bancroftian filariasis and malaria in Malaysia: *A. letifer* and *A. whartoni*, both of which breed in partially shaded, acidic, stagnant water. Much caution should be exercised in vector studies on mosquitoes belonging to the series *Myzorhynchus* because they are frequently infected with zoonotic parasites (e.g., monkey malarias) and the taxonomic distinctions between many of the species require expert attention.

Series *Anopheles* includes the notorious *A. maculipennis* complex of a dozen species in the northern hemisphere.[17] Specific patterns on the eggs (see Figure IV.39) are the best means of distinguishing these sibling species (i.e., morphologically similar species) which have distinctive biological characteristics despite their anatomical similarities. Differences of the chromosomes and protein electromorphs are also useful for specific identification. Typical *A. maculipennis (sensu stricto)* seldom attacks humans, so probably was never a malaria vector, although most malaria transmission in Europe was formerly due to *A. maculipennis sensu lato*, meaning all species combined in the complex. The most widespread member of the *A. maculipennis* complex is *A. messeae*, which is also mainly zoophilic. Arboviruses transmitted by the *A. maculipennis* complex (Table IV.7) are usually associated with *A. messeae*. *A. labranchiae* and *A. sacharovi* around the Mediterranean, and *A. atroparvus* in other parts of Europe, were vectors of malaria—and still are in a few places. These three species tend to breed in brackish water, although they are not confined to coastal localities. Because *A. atroparvus* females spend the winter resting indoors, periodically biting people or livestock but not producing eggs until spring, they were responsible for the phenomenon of 'winter malaria' transmission in bygone days. The disappearance of malaria from Europe has been due mainly to the decline of these mosquitoes resulting from housing improvements, draining of marshes, breeding site pollution (soaps and detergents infiltrate the larval tracheae, causing them to drown) and through the application of chemical pesticides. Former malaria vectors in North America belonging to this group are the freshwater-breeding species *A. freeborni* and the more distinctive species *A. quadrimaculatus*.[18] One more medically important species belonging to this series is *A. claviger*, which overwinters as larvae and breeds in weedy ponds throughout Europe and the Middle East, where it still transmits some malaria. *A. claviger* may also be involved with myxomatosis transmission among rabbits. Several arboviruses have been isolated from *Anopheles* spp. in Europe and North America (Table IV.7), but it is doubtful whether transmission depends upon these vectors in any case.

Subgenus *Cellia* has the majority of species in the genus *Anopheles*, with many complexes of sibling species including disease vectors that are extremely difficult to identify. The taxonomic literature is inadequate, except for the excellent monographs by Reid[16] covering Malaysian species and by Gillies and de Meillon[19] for African species. *Cellia* species are found almost exclusively in the Old World tropics, being classified into six series: *Cellia*, *Myzomyia*, *Neocellia*, *Neomyzomyia*, *Paramyzomyia* and *Pyretophorus*, according to the forms of pharyngeal teeth in females. Many *Cellia* spp. are attracted to humans for blood meals, and representatives of all six series have been implicated as vectors of human diseases.

Series *Cellia* is a group of about 10 distinctive savannah species in Africa and the Middle East. Adults differ from most other anophelines through having abdominal scales, those at the sides forming segmental tufts. The thorax and palps are unusually scaly also, the latter appearing shaggy. *A. pharoensis* is the dominant species especially in Egypt where it is the main malaria vector. It also carries arbovirus and helminth infections to animals. The closely related *A. squamosus* is an incidental malaria vector in various parts of Africa.

Series *Myzomyia* includes the *A. funestus–minimus* complex, numbering about a score of small and delicate species with varied host preferences and breeding sites. Three of the most efficient malaria vectors in the world are *A. funestus*, which breeds in African swamps and mature paddy, *A. minimus*, which breeds in streams of South-East Asia from the Himalayas to Hong Kong, with *A. flavirostris* doing likewise in the Philippines. These species are also important vectors of bancroftian filariasis. They are extremely endophilic in most areas, so usually respond well to control campaigns with residual insecticides sprayed inside houses. However, exophilic and insecticide-resistant populations of *A. minimus* are an intractable problem in Thailand. *A. fluviatilis* is another important exophilic member of this complex breeding in streams of southern Asia. *A. fluviatilis* maintains highly endemic malaria in localities where *A. minimus* has been eliminated. There is little evidence that these mosquitoes transmit arboviruses, although *A. funestus* has been involved with epidemic o'nyong-nyong fever in East Africa; *A. funestus* is also the type-host of Tanga virus. *A. aconitus* is closely related to the *A. funestus–minimus* complex, probably forming another complex of species in itself. It transmits malaria and possibly filariasis in Indonesia, but not in Malaysia. Identification of all these species presents the utmost difficulty, but is vital if effort is not to be wasted in vain attempts to control the exophilic non-vector species in the complex.

A. culicifacies also belongs to series *Myzomyia*, being an opportunistic breeder in temporary pools, wells and other clean water sites from Arabia to China. It is not an efficient malaria vector, but is the only species implicated in Sri Lanka and is clearly of importance in most parts of its range. Exophily makes control difficult and there is good evidence that several sibling species have been confused in what must therefore be regarded as the *A. culicifacies* complex. Similarly in the arid belt of North Africa and the Middle East, *A. sergentii* is an important but inefficient malaria vector, variations of which suggest that it comprises several taxonomic species.

Series *Neocellia* includes a number of oriental malaria vectors, mostly having speckled legs and hind tarsi with white tips. *A. annularis* breeds abundantly in swamps of the kind covered with *Eichornia* weed (cf. *Mansonia*) and in mature paddy, being a widespread and mainly zoophilic mosquito from India to the Philippines. In some situations *A. annularis* is a significant though inefficient malaria vector, often showing multiple resistance to insecticides. *A. karwari* is strongly zoophilic in South-East Asia, where it breeds in trickles of seepage water, but it has been reported to transmit human malaria in West Irian, Indonesia, to where it was accidentally introduced. *A. maculatus* is an unusually variable species which also breeds commonly in seepages from Pakistan to Sri Lanka, China and the Philippines. Despite being mainly exophilic and zoophilic, it serves as an important vector of malaria and contributes to *W. bancrofti* transmission in some places, especially where hilly countryside is being developed so that breeding sites for *A. maculatus* become plentiful. The African savannah species *A. rufipes* also belongs to this series and was previously regarded as a secondary vector of malaria, because sporozoite infections are frequent, but it is now known that *A. rufipes* more often transmits antelope malaria.[20] Other local vectors of malaria to be mentioned here are *A. pattoni* in China, *A. pulcherrimus* in Afghanistan, and *A. superpictus* in the eastern Mediterranean area (see Table IV.5). Finally in this series, *A. stephensi* is essentially a rural cattle-biting species in the Indian subcontinent. However, some populations have adapted to urban conditions in northern India and Pakistan, where they breed in wells and subsist largely on human blood, becoming important local vectors of urban malaria.[21]

Series *Neomyzomyia* has numerous species in Africa, Asia and Australasia, most of which are either dark and cave-dwelling or heavily spotted and forest-dwelling. *A. nili* breeds in African rivers and streams, being rather seasonal and locally important as an efficient vector of both malaria and bancroftian filariasis. *A. tessellatus* is widespread and usually zoophilic in South-East Asia, breeding in stagnant water. It transmits malaria and filariasis in the Maldive Islands, where it is the only anopheline present. The *A. leucosphyrus* group extends from India to China and the Philippines, comprising at least 12 species, several of which transmit monkey malarias (*P. cynomolgi, P. inui, P. knowlesi*, etc.) and sometimes infect humans with these zoonotic parasites. *A. leucosphyrus (sensu stricto)* is also a regular vector of human malaria in Malaysia and Indonesia. The most important component of the *A. leucosphyrus* group is the *A. balabacensis* complex, which has not yet been analysed satisfactorily. The most widespread form in South-East Asia has been named *A. dirus*, but this seems to consist of four genetic species. In forests from Assam to Indonesia and China, '*A. dirus*' (formerly known as *A. balabacensis*, or simply *A. leucosphyrus*) is an important vector of human malaria, including chloroquine-resistant *P. falciparum*, and of monkey malarias. True *A. balabacensis* is equally a vector where it occurs in Palawan and northern Borneo. Members of the *A. balabacensis* complex breed in fresh jungle pools; the adults are exophilic and elusive, but not difficult to control by home spraying with insecticides or by means of forest clearance. Their possible involvement

in transmission of arboviruses and filariae remains to be studied.

Also in series *Neomyzomyia*, the *A. punctulatus* complex comprises at least five sibling species which are vectors of malaria and nocturnally periodic bancroftian filariasis from the Moluccas, through Papua New Guinea to the Solomon Islands and formerly in northern Australia. The true *A. punctulatus* is widespread, occurring together with *A. koliensis* and *A. farauti* in some islands. *A. farauti* itself comprises three or more genetic species in Australia and Melanesia. Like the *A. balabacensis* complex, these vectors tend to rest among vegetation and to breed in small fresh pools, making it costly and difficult to attempt their control. However, house spraying with DDT has interrupted filariasis transmission in the Solomons, although malaria persists.[22]

Series *Paramyzomyia* has only four or five species, of which *A. hispaniola* and *A. multicolor* are regarded as malaria vectors in North Africa, although the evidence is equivocal. The latter species can tolerate strong salinity in its breeding places.

Series *Pyretophorus* also has several species adapted to brackish water breeding sites; the adults are characterized by banded tarsi and extensively pale wing markings. *A. sundaicus* is a mainly coastal and locally important vector of malaria in Indonesia, closely related to *A. litoralis* and *A. ludlowae* in the Philippines; the latter species extends to coastal Sulawesi where it joins in malaria transmission. *A. subpictus* ranges from the Middle East to Papua New Guinea, tending to be more anthropophilic and associated with coastal salt-water habitats eastwards; it is a secondary vector of malaria and contributes to *W. bancrofti* transmission locally in Indonesia.

Of the greatest medical importance in Africa and southern Arabia is the *A. gambiae* complex, comprising two salt-water-adapted species—*A. melas* in West Africa and *A. merus* in East Africa—*A. bwambae*, restricted to mineral spring-water sites in the Rift Valley between Uganda and Zaire, and three widespread freshwater breeding species—*A. gambiae (sensu stricto)* (species A), *A. arabiensis* (species B) and *A. quadriannulatus* (species C). The last is essentially zoophilic, so not a vector, but the other five species transmit both malaria and bancroftian filariasis.[23] High rates of female mosquito longevity, coupled with marked preferences for human blood, give very high vectorial capacities to *A. arabiensis*, *A. gambiae* and to some extent *A. melas*. Wherever these species are found, malaria is highly endemic. House spraying with residual insecticides has not reduced malaria transmission to the expected degree, because members of the *A. gambiae* complex are capable of behavioural avoidance of the sprayed surfaces. Resistance to organochlorine and organophosphate insecticides is also spreading in populations of *A. arabiensis* and *A. gambiae*. Control of the salt-water species, *A. melas* and *A. merus*, can be partially achieved by means of drainage and prevention of pool formation in coastal areas, through construction of dikes and bunds. Unfortunately, most breeding of *A. arabiensis* and *A. gambiae* occurs in temporary fresh rainwater pools, or irrigated furrows, which are impossible to prevent or treat adequately with larvicides. Separation of the six sibling species belonging to the *A. gambiae* complex depends upon the examination of chromosomal or protein characters. Adult females of *A. gambiae* (*sensu lato*) have the appearance shown in Figure IV.37, but could easily be confused with various other species in subgenus *Cellia*.

Subgenus *Kerteszia* is restricted to the American tropics, with about 10 species that breed exclusively in flooded axils of bromeliad plants or broken bamboos. As they are found only in the forests of Central and South America, their medical importance is limited, although several species are sometimes abundant and strongly attracted to humans. *A. cruzii* and *A. bellator* are significant vectors of malaria, and the latter sometimes contributes to filariasis transmission.[24]

Subgenus *Nyssorhynchus* forms the dominant anopheline fauna of the Neotropical region. Faran[25] has clarified the difficult taxonomy of the *A. albimanus* section, with species having small dark lateral scale tufts on each abdominal segment, including several vectors of disease. *A. albimanus* itself is the main malaria vector in humid lowlands from southern USA to northern South America and in Caribbean islands. It breeds in stagnant water and the adults lack scale tufts on the first full abdominal segment. *A. albimanus* is insufficiently endophilic to be readily controlled by means of house spraying and has become widely resistant to all groups of insecticides. It may contribute to filariasis transmission and has been involved with epidemics of encephalitis and perhaps other arboviruses (Table IV.7). Another malaria vector closely related to *A. albimanus* is *A. aquasalis*, which also transmits Venezuelan equine encephalitis virus, and is of importance mainly in Trinidad, Tobago, the Guianas and coastal Brazil, usually breeding in brackish water; also *A. nuneztovari* is a primary malaria vector in parts of Colombia and Venezuela, probably comprising a complex of vector and non-vector species. Another section of subgenus *Nyssorhynchus* includes the malaria vectors *A. argyritarsis* and *A. darlingi*. The latter was eradicated from coastal Guyana, but remains of major importance in places from Brazil to Mexico. Infective larvae of *W. bancrofti* have occasionally been found in *A. darlingi* and *A. aquasalis*, suggesting that these species may contribute to periodic filariasis transmission.

Subfamily: Culicinae

This large and heterogeneous subfamily of mosquitoes contains over 2500 species and some 30 genera. The scutellum is trilobed, each lobe bearing bristles. The abdomen is blunt and completely clothed with broad flat scales. The eighth segment of the larva bears a patch of comb teeth on each side, used for cleaning the mouth brushes, and is drawn out into a respiratory siphon, with well developed pecten teeth in a row on each side. There are no abdominal palmate hairs (cf. *Anopheles*). Below the

siphon the anal segment of the larva bears a chitinous saddle, four gills, caudal setae and the ventral brush for swimming. Culicine pupae are similar to those of *Anopheles*, but the respiratory trumpets are not so flared distally.

The following are the main characteristics of culicines that distinguish them from anophelines (see Figure IV.30).

1. The eggs are not provided with air floats and are either laid separately (Aedini, Sabethini) or stacked in a floating raft (Culicini, Culisetini) or in a mass on floating vegetation (Mansoniini).
2. The larval spiracles are situated at the tip of a tail-like siphon, projecting dorsally from the eighth abdominal segment. Except for *Mansonia* and some other un-important genera, which have larvae with the siphon modified for plugging into the air vessels of plants, the larvae hang head downwards from the water surface, supported by the capillary action of five hinged valves surrounding the tip of the siphon. They sweep suspended particles of food with mouth brushes below surface level (see Figure IV.30) or else dive and scavenge at the bottom.
3. The adult has an abdomen densely covered with scales. The female has short and slender palps, from one-fifth to one-half as long as the proboscis. As a rule, the male has long hairy palps which have a plume-like appearance. These mosquitoes usually rest with proboscis and abdomen more or less parallel with the supporting surface (see Figure IV.30.).

Tribe: Aedini

Genus: *Aedes*

Throughout the world, especially in temperate countries, a high proportion of mosquitoes belong to the genus *Aedes* in which there are more than 1000 species, classified as 40 subgenera. Many *Aedes* are vectors of arboviruses, including several of the most important mosquito-borne

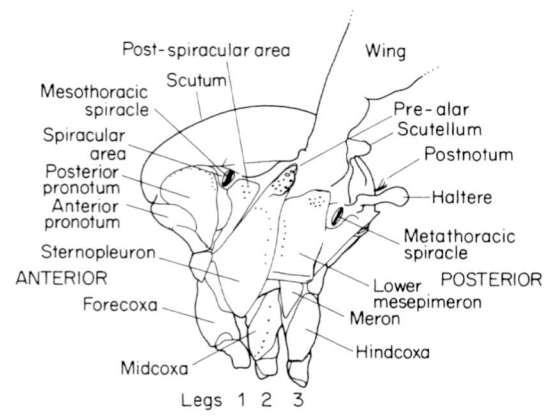

Figure IV.41: Mosquito thorax in side view, showing named components and sites of setae (bristles) referred to in the identification key (see Table IV.7).

human diseases (see Chapter 41 and Table IV.7). The genus is difficult to define precisely in morphological terms, although adults always possess bristles on the postspiracular area (Figure IV.41) and the tip of the female abdomen is retractable. Separation from other genera in the tribe Aedini depends on characters given in Table IV.8. *Aedes* larvae are characterized by having only a single pair of siphonal hairs, usually branched, in addition to pecten teeth. Many of the medically important *Aedes* spp. are active during daytime, although nocturnal activity is normal for most other species.

Aedes eggs are especially capable of withstanding desication. They are laid on damp surfaces, such as soil or around the rim of water in a hole, in situations likely to be flooded causing the eggs to hatch after adequate rainfall. Most species of *Aedes* therefore breed seasonally in swamps and pools, with some significant groups adapted to smaller containers of water such as rock-holes, rot-holes in trees, cut bamboo stumps, old snail shells, buckets and other artificial containers. Almost any kind of water can harbour some sort of *Aedes*—from sea water to melted snow. It is to be expected that, after drought or winter, rainy seasons will cause the hatching of *Aedes* broods so that blood-thirsty females of these species become prevalent early in the season.

In an increasing number of cases it has been demonstrated that arboviruses can be passed transovarially in *Aedes* (i.e., from mother to progeny via the egg). This is common with California group viruses[26] and has also been reported for yellow fever.[27] This phenomenon, a form of vertical transmission, is of great significance in epidemiology, as it can lead to long-term dormancy and reappearance of virus activity.

Representatives of three subgenera of *Aedes* are natural vectors of *Brugia malayi* and *Wuchereria bancrofti*, causing human disease. Where transmission is due to nocturnally active *Aedes* and other mosquitoes, the microfilariae are normally nocturnally periodic in the human bloodstream. In Polynesia, Melanesia and a few areas in South-East Asia (parts of Thailand, Nicobar Islands) there are diurnally active *Aedes* which transmit strains of *W. bancrofti* that are subperiodic so that microfilariae circulate in the human bloodstream during the daytime, enabling their uptake by female mosquitoes that feed by day.

The majority of taxonomic subgenera of *Aedes* have few species and no medical or veterinary significance. Subgenera *Aedes (sensu stricto)*, *Aedimorphus*, *Mucidus*, *Neomelaniconion*, *Ochlerotatus* and *Verrallina* have numerous species that breed commonly in ground water, with many arbovirus vectors included (see Table IV.7). The

Table IV.8 Diseases transmitted to man by Tabanidae (see also Chapters 30, 38 and 70).

Agent	Disease	Principal hosts	Transmission	Distribution
Loa loa	Loaiasis; Calabar swelling	Man, Drill (*Papio leucophaeus*)	Cyclical: *Chrysops* spp.	West and Central Africa
Bacillus anthracis	Anthrax	Domestic livestock (man)*	Nonc-cyclic: mechanical	Cosmopolitan
Francisella tularensis	Tularaemia	Lagomorphs, rodents, man	Non-cyclic: mechanical (esp. *Chrysops* and *Tabanus* spp.: *also* ticks)	Cosmopolitan
Borrelia burgdorferi	Lyme disease	Deer, lagomorphs, (man)*	Non-cyclic: mechanical (main vectors: Ixodid ticks)	North temperate zone (Europe, North America) and Australia
Vesicular stomatitis virus (VSV)	Sore mouth (of cattle; horses)	Equines, bovines, pigs, (man)*	Non-cyclic mechanical	North, Central and South America
Western equine encephalitis (WEE) virus		Amphibia, reptiles, birds, (man)*	Non-cyclic: mechanical	North and South America
Californian encephalitis virus (CEV) group: La Crosse (LAC) virus	—	Rodents, lagomorphs, etc., (man)*	Non-cyclic: mechanical (*also* mosquitoes)	North America (USA)
Jamestown Canyon (JC) virus	—	White-tailed deer [*Odocoileus virginianus*], (man)*	Non-cyclic: mechanical (*Chrysops*, *Tabanus* and *Hybomitra* spp.; *also* mosquitoes)	North America (Alaska, Canada, USA)

*Man an accidental host.

habit of breeding in water-filled containers, holes and plant axils is a feature of the important subgenera *Diccromyia, Howardina, Protomacleaya, Finlaya* and *Stegomyia*; arboviruses are transmitted by all five of these subgenera and the last two include filariasis vectors (see Table IV.6).

Subgenus *Stegomyia* is probably of the greatest medical interest. More than 100 species have been described, all diurnally active and having beautiful specific patterns of black and white scales, especially noticeable on the scutum and banded tarsi. They are generally exophilic species which seldom shelter indoors. The *Ae. scutellaris* group numbers approximately 35 species in South-East Asia and the Pacific, including the main vectors of subperiodic *W. bancrofti* in Polynesia: *Ae. pseudoscutellaris* in Fiji, *Ae. cooki, Ae. kesseli* and *Ae. tongae* in Tonga, *Ae. upolensis* in Samoa and *Ae. polynesiensis* generally. Adults of the *Ae. scutellaris* group are characterized by having a single white line longitudinally on the middle of the scutum. They also transmit epidemic dengue viruses on many Pacific islands and in parts of South-East Asia. However, the true *Ae. scutellaris (sensu stricto)* is confined to Seram and Papua New Guinea, where it is zoophilic and not a vector. Breeding places of the *Ae. scutellaris* group are in coconut shells, crab holes, holes in trees and coral, axils of plants such as *Pandanus* and bananas, tyres, tins and other artificial containers. All species so far mentioned have complete stripes of broad scales along each side of the thorax, ending above the wing base. This distinguishes the *Ae. scutellaris* subgroup from the *Ae. albopictus* subgroup of species having an incomplete supra-alar stripe, with only narrow scales over the wing base. Species in the latter group are widespread vectors of dengue viruses, notably dengue haemorrhagic fever in the Philippines and South-East Asian countries, but they are apparently refractory to filarial infection. These and other Pacific mosquitoes have been the subject of a monograph by Belkin[28] and a pictorial key provided by Huang.[29] A revision of Tongan species by Huang and Hitchcock[30] gives much information on bionomics and vector functions; vector genetics and speciation of *Ae. scutellaris* group have been reviewed by Macdonald.[31]

Aedes (Stegomyia) aegypti is the most widespread and dangerous species in this subgenus.[32] In African forests, non-anthropophilic populations known as *Ae. aegypti formosus* are distinguished by their lack of pale scales on the abdominal tergites (i.e., the top of the abdomen is entirely dark). Presumably from this ancestral stock, human-biting populations have adapted to domestic breeding sites and become spread throughout the tropics within the 20°C isotherms, roughly between 35°N and 35°S. The general pattern on adult *Ae. aegypti* is depicted in Fig. IV.42, showing the unique lyre-shaped pattern on the scutum, with narrow longitudinal lines flanked by curved silvery-white markings. *Ac. aegypti aegypti* has some white scales on all abdominal tergites, with *Ae. aegypti* var. *queenslandensis* having the abdomen mainly pale-scaled dorsally.[33] Populations of *Ae. aegypti* breeding indoors in water pots, especially in eastern Africa, usually have the appearance of var. *queenslandensis*, whereas peridomestic

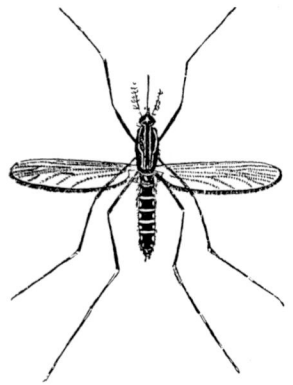

Figure IV.42: Female *Aedes aegypti* (4 ×).

populations are mainly of the type form. Evolutionary relationships among various kinds of *Ae. aegypti (sensu lato)* are still the subject of much study and debate.[34] This is relevant to the fact that *Ae. aegypti* is the principal vector of chikungunya and dengue viruses in almost every outbreak. Urban yellow fever is also transmitted mainly by *Ae. aegypti* in Central and South America and in West Africa. *Ae. aegypti formosus* is probably involved in the sylvatic cycle of yellow fever in Africa. However, other *Stegomyia* spp. have more often been implicated as vectors of African enzootic yellow fever, especially *Ae. africanus* which also transmits Zika virus. In nature, these arboviruses affect monkeys in the jungle, being transmitted by mosquito species that seldom come into contact with humans. At the forest edge, monkeys are likely to be bitten by *Aedes (Stegomyia) simpsoni* which breeds predominantly in water-filled axils of certain strains of banana plant, or rot-holes in stems of paw-paw and candelabra *Euphorbia* (e.g., in Ethiopia). People working and living among such plantations in Africa are especially likely to become infected with yellow fever and other viruses transmitted from monkeys via *Ae. simpsoni*, some populations of which are strongly attracted to humans. Human-to-human transmission may then be continued by *Ae. aegypti*. Thus the epidemiology of yellow fever in Africa conforms to the systems shown in Figure IV.43, depending on which species of *Stegomyia* and other mosquitoes are involved. Embryonated eggs of *Stegomyia* spp. can remain dormant for as long as 1 year and still hatch when flooded. The fact that *Ae. aegypti* eggs may be laid in portable containers allows this species to be inadvertently spread far and wide; continuously breeding populations often occur in water barrels on board ships and dhows.

Control of *Stegomyia* spp. presents great problems the world over, because breeding sites are small, scattered and usually inaccessible. In emergencies, as when an arbovirus epidemic is under way, periodic insecticidal space-spraying and perifocal applications (see Table IV.13) may be helpful in the vicinity of dwellings. Screening of houses and elimination of mosquito breeding places are desirable preventive measures.

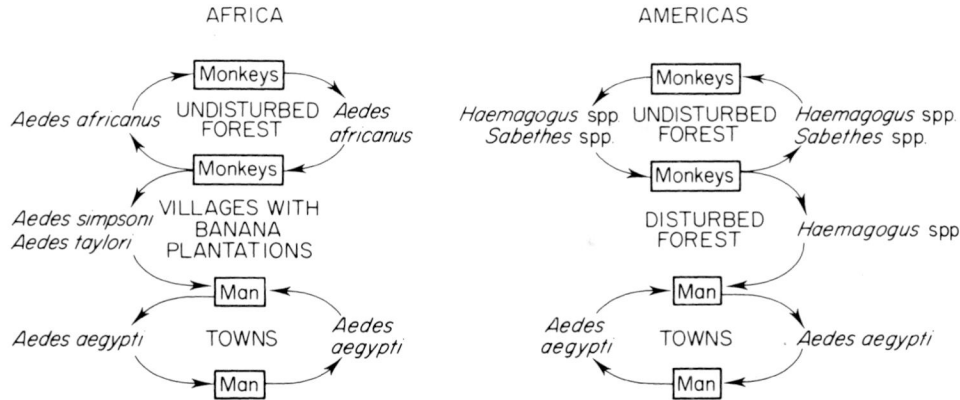

Figure IV.43: Yellow fever ecosystems in Africa and the Americas.

Subgenus *Finlaya* has females with a conspicuous ventral scale tuft on the posterior abdomen; in both sexes the wings are usually spotted. The *Ae. (F.) kochi* group includes several local vectors of periodic *W. bancrofti. Ae. poicilius* is the most widespread, in Malaysia, Indonesia and the Philippines, breeding in axils of *Colocasia, Pandanus* and bananas (*Musa sapientum*). In parts of the Philippines, where *Musa textiles* (abaca or hemp) is intensively cultivated, *Ae. poicilius* is an important rural filariasis vector. Likewise in Fiji and Samoa, bancroftian filariasis is or was transmitted by several members of the *Ae. kochi* group (see Table IV.6) which breed in plant axils. Around the coasts of South-East Asia, the large, dark-winged species *Ae. (F.) togoi* often breeds in brackish water and contributes to transmission of periodic *B. malayi* and *W. bancrofti*. Finally in this subgenus, members of the *Ae. (F.) niveus* group transmit both periodic and subperiodic strains of *W. bancrofti* locally (see Table IV.6), but are probably of wider importance as vectors of jungle dengue and perhaps other arboviruses.

Subgenus *Diceromyia* of tree-hole-breeding species resembling *Stegomyia* but having dark tarsi, includes the African *A. furcifer-taylori* group of species which have been implicated occasionally as vectors of yellow fever and chikungunya.[35]

Subgenus *Protomacleaya* has similarities in the New World, with *Ae. triseriatus* breeding in tree-holes of the eastern USA and being an important vector of California group encephalitides, with evidence of transovarial virus transmission. The closely related *Ae. hendersoni*, which may breed in the same tree-holes, is apparently incapable of virus transmission.

Subgenus *Neomelaniconion* is widespread in the Old World tropics and includes some commonly implicated vectors of arboviruses. These species are recognizable from yellowish stripes edging the scutum and some pale-scaled veins on the wings. They breed prolifically in temporary flood pans in savannahs and the adults shelter among grass. About 20 arboviruses have been isolated from *Neomelaniconion* spp., the most important to humans being Rift Valley fever transmitted by *Ae. circumluteolus* and *Ae. lineatopennis* in southern Africa and probably elsewhere.

Subgenus *Ochlerotatus* is the dominant component of *Aedes* in terms of numbers of species and their distribution. They are ground pool breeders, mostly in temperate countries. Generally they bite mammals. In North America, *Ae. atlanticus* is an important vector of *D. immitis*, a filarial parasite affecting dogs and capable of causing dog heartworm disease in humans. Rift Valley fever virus is commonly transmitted to livestock by *Ae. caballus* in southern Africa, although few *Ochlerotatus* spp. occur in Africa. *Ae. caspius* is widespread in Europe and North Africa, a fairly large speckled species that breeds commonly in brackish water, usually the vector of Inkoo virus in Scandinavia. Various North American *Ochlerotatus* spp. contribute sporadically to the transmission of encephalitides; they are beyond the reach of economical control programmes. Species such as the salt-water-breeding *Ae. detritus* in Europe and *Ae. sollicitans* and *Ae. taeniorhynchus* in America are intolerable pests, and the latter has been implicated in *W. bancrofti* transmission. *Ae. (O.) vigilax* is another salt-water-breeding species locally responsible for periodic bancroftian filariasis transmission in New Caledonia (see Table IV.6) and for Ross River virus in Australia (see Table IV.7). This species and the closely related *Ae. fryeri* are so vicious and prolific as to make many islands in the Indian and Pacific Oceans uninhabitable.

Subgenus *Aedimorphus* and other subgenera of *Aedes* also include some species that are pests and vectors of arboviruses. In particular, *Ae. vexans* is probably the second or third most widespread mosquito in the world (after *C. pipiens* and perhaps *Ae. aegypti*). Seasonal breeding in grassland follows flooding and egg-hatching of broods that are immensely troublesome when the adult females attack; they bite both day and night, being especially numerous in late spring in northern latitudes.

Genus: *Armigeres*

Widespread and common in the Australasian and Oriental regions, this genus is difficult to distinguish from *Aedes*, to which it is closely related. Development always occurs in small containers of water and the larvae grow very rapidly. *Armigeres subalbatus* (= *obturbans*) is a semidomestic species that breeds commonly in foul water, including latrines. This and several other species attack humans during night and day. It has been suggested that they may transmit *W. bancrofti* and the encephalitis virus Sepik has been isolated from *Armigeres*.

Genus: *Haemagogus*

This genus of forest mosquito is also closely related to *Aedes*. It occurs in Central and South America, breeding in flooded tree-holes. Adults are metallic blue and green due to their covering of scales on thorax and abdomen. Several species are vectors of sylvatic (jungle) yellow fever: *Haemagogus equinus*, *H. janthinomys*, *H. leucocelaenus*, *H. mesodentatus*, *H. spegazzinii* and *H. capricornii*. They are separable only on the characters of the male genitalia and not at all as larvae and pupae. The larvae of these vector species are 'hairy' and are thus distinguishable from some other species of *Haemogogus* which are not vectors. Adult females of *Haemagogus* seldom leave the forest and they attack people mainly during jungle clearance activities. Taxonomy of the genus has been revised by Arnell.[36]

Genus: *Psorophora*

Three subgenera and almost 50 species are recognized, many of them vicious human-biters. Generic characters are the presence of spiracular *and* postspiracular bristles, plus the retractable postabdomen as in other Aedini. Larvae of the typical subgenus are predacious. Eggs normally diapause before hatching and the breeding places are always in pools and marshes on the ground, not containers as used by some allied genera. Apart from their considerable significance as pests, *Psorophora* spp. are of widespread importance as vectors of arboviruses (see Table IV.7), especially Venezuelan equine encephalitis transmitted by *P. ferox* and *P. confinnis*, the latter being known as the dark rice-field mosquito. Taxonomy of this genus remains unsatisfactory, but Belkin et al.[37] and Carpenter and La Casse[18] give summaries.

Tribe: Culicini

Genus: *Culex*

About 800 species of *Culex* are known, being classified in 21 subgenera, with many species acting as the vectors of enzootic arboviruses, protozoa and filariae. They bite at night and some species have much medical significance; many species can be pests when abundant. Generic characteristics are that eggs always form a raft (see Figure IV.30), larvae have several pairs of hair tufts on the siphon, and the adults possess tarsal pulvilli (Figure IV.44) and lack postspiracular bristles, with the tip of the female abdomen being bluntly rounded. Male palps are strongly curved upwards (see Figure IV.34A). General body colouration of the adults is usually brown, with wings plain and vein scales dark. Unlike Aedini, the eggs cannot diapause, so *Culex* breeding is continuous, except

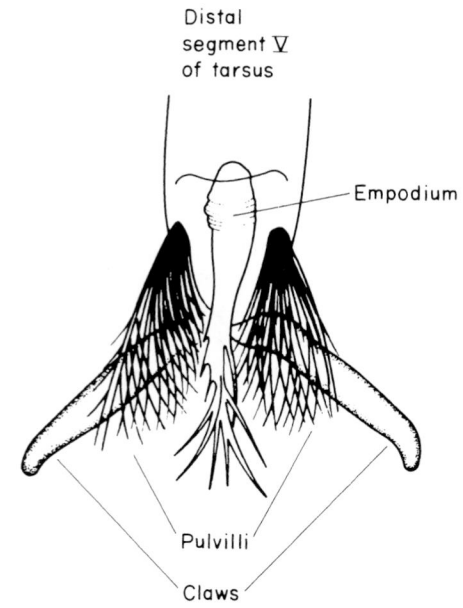

Figure IV.44: Tip of tarsus of *Culex*, showing paired pulvilli below the claws. In life these pulvilli appear as pale pads, more conspicuous than the empodium that is also present in other mosquito genera.

when fertilized females hibernate as the overwintering mechanism for species found in temperate countries.

The typical subgenus *Culex* contains the majority of species, usually with a banded proboscis and/or basal pale bands on abdominal tergites. Japanese encephalitis virus is transmitted mainly by *Culex* spp. in the Oriental region (for identification keys see Bram,[38] Sirivanakarn[39]), especially by the following species which breed prolifically in paddy and swamps: *C. tritaeniorhynchus*, *C. gelidus* and *C. vishnui*. Because they are abundant around villages wherever rice is grown in South-East Asia, and the adult females of these species attack various mammals by preference, they readily transfer Japanese encephalitis virus to humans from pigs and other amplification hosts. *C. theileri* in southern Africa and members of the *C. pipiens* complex in Egypt are important vectors of Rift Valley fever virus from livestock to humans. In Australia, *C. annulirostris* plays a similar role in the epidemiology of Murray Valley encephalitis, but the source of Murray Valley encephalitis virus remains a mystery. Like most other *Culex* spp., *C. annulirostris* feeds to some extent on birds and these may be responsible for virus dissemination. Eastern and western equine and St Louis encephalitis viruses in America are mainly found in birds (sparrows and pigeons), being transmitted by *C. nigripalpus*, *C. pipiens*, *C. restuans*, *C. salinarius*, *C. tarsalis* and other mosquitoes that occasionally pass infection to humans and other mammals that serve as dead-end hosts. *C. pipiens* serves the same function for Eastern equine encephalitis virus in Europe. West Nile virus has a similar epidemiology in Africa, being transmitted from birds to humans by members of the *C. univittatus* complex.

Culex-borne arboviruses can be carried through the winter in hibernating female mosquitoes, although the ecological importance of this remains uncertain. The arrival of virus in migratory birds may set off seasonal transmission if it coincides with high densities of bird-biting mosquitoes. Investigations of arbovirus epidemiology are frequently hampered by difficulties of distinguishing and identifying the females of *Culex* spp., taxonomy of which is based on the morphology of male terminalia in many cases.

The *Culex pipiens* complex comprises several species, subspecies and forms, with representatives in all parts of the world. Typical *C. pipiens* occurs in temperate countries of the northern hemisphere, spreading through temperate highlands to southern Africa. Closely related species or subspecies are present in temperate parts of Australia and South America, but they seldom attack humans in temperate countries. Whenever a human-biting infection occurs to the north of the Mediterranean or equivalent latitude, it is likely to be a form usually known as *molestus (autogenicus)*. This mosquito causes severe infections due to prolific breeding indoors where circumstances are suitable. Although the females are autogenous (laying one egg batch without having fed on blood) they attack humans viciously. Indoor infections of *C. p. molestus*, or autogenous *C. pipiens*, occur as far north as Moscow. It seems that incapacity to hibernate is what keeps these mosquitoes indoors, breeding in flooded basements, cess pits, etc. Southwards, especially in North Africa, such populations are more often found breeding freely outdoors and it is unclear to what extent they may interbreed with anautogenous *C. pipiens*. In Egypt, the *C. pipiens* complex is responsible for bancroftian filariasis transmission[40] and has been implicated as the main vector in outbreaks of Rift Valley fever.

C. quinquefasciatus (= *C. p. fatigans*) is the main human-biting tropical member of the *C. pipiens* complex, distributed up to 38°N in USA, 30°N in Asia, but only 24°N in Africa. In the New World it interbreeds with *C. pipiens (sensu stricto)*, but they can generally be regarded as distinct species. Bancroftian filariasis is largely maintained in tropical villages and towns by *C. quinquefasciatus* alone, although West African strains of *W. bancrofti* do not develop in this species of mosquito. Elsewhere, *C. quinquefasciatus* is an efficient vector of *W. bancrofti* but refractory to *B. malayi*.

C. quinquefasciatus (Figure IV.45) is confined to domestic habitats, breeding abundantly in heavily polluted waters occurring in ditches, village ponds, soakage pits, cess pits and the like. As these sites are inevitably associated with towns and urban development, *C. quinquefasciatus* thrives as a tropical pest in developing countries. Some breeding also occurs in rock-holes, tree-holes and artificial containers such as tins, buckets and car tyres, where larvae of *Ae. aegypti* commonly mingle with those of *C. quinquefasciatus*. Control of both is best done by elimination of breeding sites, putting covers on water pots, covering soakage pits and taking all possible precautions to prevent there being places where the female mosquitoes can lay their eggs on exposed water containing organic nutrients for the larvae. Larvicidal oils and insecticides

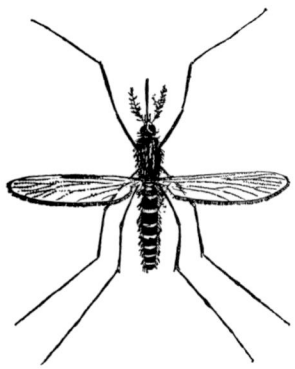

Figure IV.45: *Culex quinquefasciatus* (4 ×). The name refers to the way that, when viewed from above with the naked eye, the abdomen seems to have five broad dark bands separated by pale ones (but so do many other species). The alternative name *Culex fatigans* (the mosquito that tends to make one fatigued) has been widely used, although *quinquefasciatus* has priority and is therefore correct.

have been employed widely, but they are increasingly uneconomical and in many countries *C. quinquefasciatus* has become resistant to both organochlorines and organophosphates. Larger breeding places can be treated (see Table IV.13) with emulsions of organophosphates or the use of costly biocides or insect growth regulators (IGRs) (e.g., diflubenzuron or methoprene), the activity of which may be much reduced in polluted water. Application of a floating carpet of expanded polystyrene beads gives the most durable control of *Culex* larvae in enclosed breeding sites such as pit latrines.

As the bites of *C. quinquefasciatus* are painful, whether or not disease is likely to be transmitted, it is advisable to screen houses (plastic mesh, at least six strands per centimetre) and especially bedrooms, making them mosquito proof. Cracks around ceilings and doors should be sealed. The use of bed-nets is highly desirable wherever *C. quinquefasciatus* occurs. Although several arboviruses have been reported from *C. quinquefasciatus*, it seems that this species is not usually an important vector of such infections. Adult males and females rest both indoors and outdoors during daytime; they are naturally quite tolerant of residual insecticides.

In the Far East, *C. pipiens pallens* seems to be biologically intermediate between *C. pipiens* and *C. quinquefasciatus*. It may be a distinct species or a hybrid. Formerly a filariasis vector in Japan[41] and still a pest there, the importance and distribution of *C. p. pallens* in South-East Asian countries is not well understood.

Taxonomy of the *C. pipiens* complex is a matter of uncertainty and disagreement. Separation of species is traditionally based upon the morphology of male terminalia, as expressed by the ratio of distances between tips of the dorsal and ventral arms of the phallosome (D/V ratio) or the difference between these dimensions (D/DV ratio), as shown in Figure IV.46. General recognition of the *C. pipiens* complex depends upon the following combination of characters: proboscis dark, not banded, paler below in middle; abdominal tergites with transverse

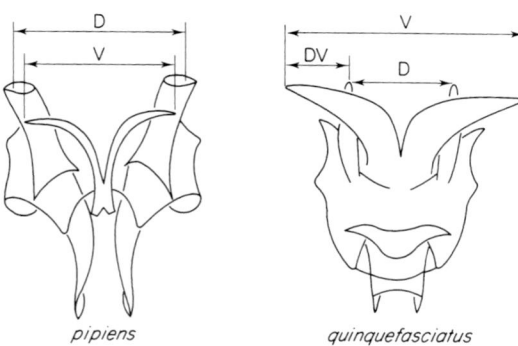

pipiens   *quinquefasciatus*

Figure IV.46: Male phallosomes of the *Culex pipiens* complex, ventral views. The shape and spread of the ventral arms is much wider in *C. quinquefasciatus* (= *C. p. fatigans*) than in typical *C. pipiens*. The ratio D/V can be used to express this contrast, sometimes given as DV/V. Members of the *C. pipiens* complex generally have the following values of D/V: *quinquefasciatus*, 0.3; *pallens*, 0.3–1.0; *pipiens*, 0.8–1.0; *molestus* (= *autogenicus*), 0.8–1.2.

pale bands basally and pale spots on hind corners; abdomen pale below, usually with median dark spots in a row; thorax reddish-brown dorsally, straw/pale brown coloured laterally without dark pleural markings, with dark bristles on scutum and whitish scales in patches on pleurae (sides) but without spiracular or postspiracular scales; usually one lower mesepimeral bristle; wings with dark scales on all veins; tarsi entirely dark; mid femur dark anteriorly, without narrow longitudinal pale stripe as in some closely related species (which may also have spiracular or postspiracular scale patches).

Apart from the species already mentioned, which all belong to subgenus *Culex*, some medically important species belong to subgenus *Melanoconion*. These small species are potent vectors of arboviruses in the American tropics (see Table IV.7). As distinct from subgenus *Culex* having narrow scales, species in subgenus *Melanoconion* have a rim of broad scales above the eyes, and wing veins 1 and 2 with broader scales distally. It is difficult to identify females of *Melanoconion* specifically and breeding places are not easy to find. Usually the larvae occupy large, quiet, non-polluted pools, often sheltering under vegetation. Control is therefore impracticable without environmental damage. Adults of *Melanoconion* spp. shelter among vegetation and their attacks may be locally reduced by insecticidal fogging during the evening flight period. They prefer to feed upon a wide range of wild creatures, but people are often bitten. Taxonomic studies by Sirivanakarn[42] should pave the way to improved understanding of the vectorial significance of the various species.

Genus: *Culiseta*

Distinctive features of this genus are the presence of spiracular bristles; the wing often has one or two dark spots in the middle (at base of vein 3 and sometimes vein 2); the siphonal tuft is large, at the extreme base of the larval siphon; eggs are usually laid as a raft which is less

well formed than in *Culex*. Approximately 35 species are classified in seven subgenera, some of which are given generic status by Maslov.[43] Most are harmless and found only in temperate countries. A few species are pests, notably *C. longiareolata* around the Mediterranean. This species inhabits arid terrain, breeding in wells and rock pools, whereas most other *Culiseta* spp. favour weedy ponds and marshes. In North America, both eastern and western equine encephalitis circulate among birds through *C. inornata*, *C. melanura* and *C. morsitans*. The latter may also be involved as a vector in Old World situations. *Culiseta* spp. breed continuously throughout the year, females of some species (e.g., *C. annulata*) sheltering indoors and feeding intermittently during winter in temperate countries.

Tribe: **Mansoniini**

Genus: *Coquillettidia*

Most of these species are mostly yellow, quite large and voracious biters, attacking by day and night. They lay egg masses on the surface of stagnant water or weedy ponds. Larvae and pupae have the respiratory siphon and trumpets pointed and strengthened for plugging into the air ducts of plant stems. The genus occurs in all continents; among 55 known species *C. perturbans* in North America and *C. venezuelensis* in South America are some of the most important pests, and the latter has been implicated as a vector of several arboviruses (see Table IV.7).

Genus: *Mansonia*

This genus differs from the preceding one by characters given in the key (Table IV.7) and because egg masses are deposited under floating leaves of certain aquatic plants. Like *Coquillettidia*, larvae and pupae of *Mansonia* breathe air from plant stems and have their respiratory appendages modified accordingly (Figures IV.47 and IV.48). Subgenus *Mansonia* has only a dozen American species, notably the widespread pest *M. titillans* which breeds in swamps and marshes with floating water lettuce (*Pistia*) and water

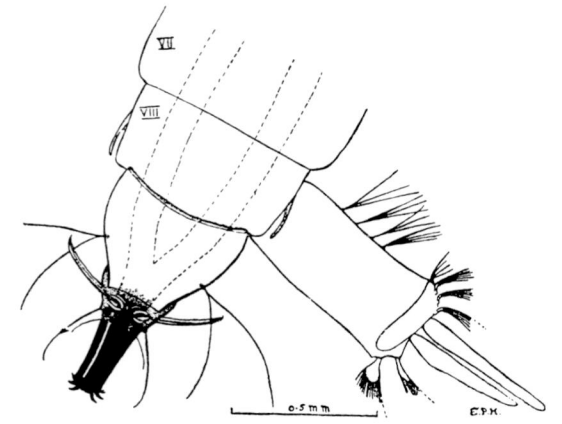

Figure IV.47: Respiratory siphon and terminal segment of the larva of *Mansonioides* (lateral view).

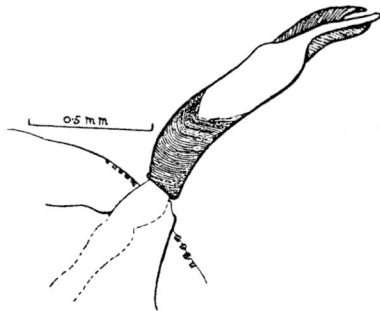

Figure IV.48: Respiratory horn of the pupa *Mansonioides*.

hyacinth (*Eichornia*) or rooted *Pontederia* and other plants favoured by the immature stages. *M. titillans* is an important vector of Venezuelan equine encephalitis and may contribute to transmission of *W. bancrofti*. As with other troublesome *Mansonia* and some *Coquillettidia*, *M. titillans* disperses far from the breeding sites in search of hosts to bite.

Subgenus *Mansonioides* also has a dozen species endemic to the Old World tropics, being pests arising from breeding sites in water with plenty of *Eichornia*, *Pistia*, rooted *Isachne* (swamp grass), *Zuzania* and other suitable vegetation. When such well-aerated plants are removed, *Mansonioides* disappears. In parts of southern India (Kerala), Sri Lanka and elsewhere, *Mansonioides* populations thrive where flooded pits for soakage of coconut husks, from which rope is made, are allowed to provide breeding sites rich in organic food for the larvae. In some areas this problem has now been controlled by keeping the water free of floating plants.

Adult *Mansonioides* are strikingly marked (Figure IV.49), with banded legs and speckled wings having very broad scales on the veins. The tip of the female abdomen is curiously boat-shaped, to facilitate oviposition under floating leaves. Some arboviruses are transmitted by *Mansonioides* spp., but these species of mosquito are generally refractory to *W. bancrofti*.

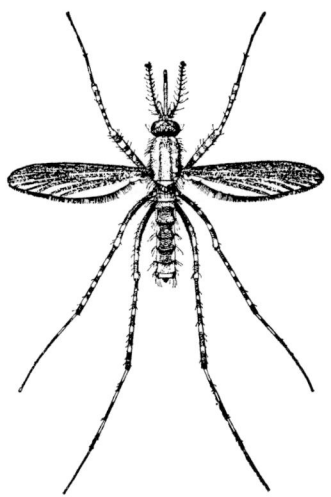

Figure IV.49: Female *Mansonia (Mansonioides) annulifera* (4 ×).

In forested localities, or when weather is overcast, the females feed by day; they attack mainly at night outdoors, coming freely into houses, but not resting indoors during the daytime. The bites are more painful than with most other mosquitoes. *Mansonioides* spp. are of particular parasitological interest because, together with *Anopheles (Anopheles)* spp., they are the vectors of brugian filariasis (see Table IV.6). In South-East Asia, according to the work of Wharton[44] in Malaysia, swamp-forest populations of *M. annulata*, *M. uniformis* and especially the sibling species *M. bonneae* and *M. dives* share the transmission of zoonotic subperiodic *B. malayi*, which they transmit to humans from leaf monkeys and other wild animals. At the same time, *M. annulata*, *M. dives* and other *Mansonioides* spp. are vectors of *B. pahangi* from animal to animal, but rarely to humans. Continuous biting activity, with peaks of attack at dusk and dawn, helps to make *Mansonioides* spp. in the forest suitable as vectors of these subperiodic parasites. In areas of paddy on the coastal plains, *M. uniformis* and *Anopheles* spp. are the principal vectors of periodic *B. malayi*, with some involvement of *M. annulata* and *M. dives*. However, *M. bonneae* is apparently refractory to the periodic strains of the parasite. In India and other parts of southern Asia, periodic *B. malayi* is or was generally transmitted by *M. annulata*, *M. annulifera*, *M. indiana* and *M. uniformis*. In eastern Africa, where *B. malayi* is absent, *M. africana* and *M. uniformis* transmit *B. patei* among dogs and cats but rarely to people.

Tribe: Sabethini

Genus: *Sabethes*

These are forest mosquitoes that transmit jungle yellow fever and other arboviruses (see Table IV.7) in South America. *S. chloropterus* is one of the most frequently involved vector species. About 30 species are known. This genus is very distinctive; its characters are given in Table IV.7. The adults have a metallic lustre. The scales of all parts of the body are flat. There is a very large pair of procumbent bristles projecting from the crown of the head and a tuft of setae on the mesonotum. The antennae are similar in both sexes; the palps are short in the female and usually also in the male. The larvae are generally predaceous and live in the water that collects in the axils and bracts of leaves, in tree-holes, or that is secreted by pitchers or other modified parts of plants. They are usually rather hairy and have smooth or stumpy antennae. A siphon is present and a single row of scales on the side of the eighth abdominal segments. The pupae are characterized by the conspicuous fan of bristles at the posterolateral angles of the eighth and ninth abdominal segments and by the small tail-fins. *Sabethes* taxonomy is unsatisfactory and their control is impractical.

Literature on mosquitoes

Information on the many species of mosquito is voluminous, with about five or six publications on Culicidae appearing daily. Much of the literature on mosquito biology and identification is now obsolete, owing to advances in knowledge. Some general references to be recommended are: Bates,[45] Gillett,[46] Harbach and Knight,[47] Harwood and James,[48] Horsfall,[49] Mattingly,[50] Service[51] and the World Health Organization.[13]

For the identification of mosquito genera and species in each part of the world, the following publications contain the most up-to-date keys and/or other information on medically important species:

Africa: Anophelinae: Gillies and de Meillon.[19] Culicinae: Edwards;[52] Hopkins;[53] Mattingly;[54] Gerberg and van Someren;[55] Cordellier et al.[56]

Americas: Lane;[57] Forrattini;[58,59] Belkin et al.,[37] Carpenter and La Casse;[18] Wood et al.;[60] Faran;[25] Darsie and Ward;[61] Sirivanakarn.[42]

Arabia: Mattingly and Knight.[62]

Australia: Lee;[63] Lee and Woodhill;[64] Dobrotworsky;[65] Marks.[66]

Cape Verde Islands: Ribeiro et al.[67]

Europe: Dahl and White.[68]

India: Anophelinae: Christophers;[69] Bhatia et al.[70] Culicinae: Barraud;[71] see also Oriental region.

Jamaica: Belkin et al.[37]

Japan: Tanaka et al.[72]

Madagascar: Grjebine;[73] Ravaon Janahary.[74]

Mediterranean: Rioux;[75] Senevet and Andarelli.[76]

Papua New Guinea: Van den Assem and Bonne-Wepster.[77]

New Zealand: Belkin.[78]

Oriental region: Anophelinae: Bonne-Wepster and Swellengrebel;[79] Reid;[16] Harrison and Scanlon;[80] Culicinae: Mattingly;[81] Bram;[38] Mattingly;[82] Reinert;[83] Sirivanakarn;[39] Huang.[84]

Pacific: Belkin;[28] Huang.[29]

Philippines: Delfinado;[85] Basio.[86]

Russia: Gutsevich et al.[87]

Seychelles: Mattingly and Brown.[88]

World: Foote and Cook;[89] Mattingly;[90] Knight and Stone.[14]

Most recent advances in mosquito control are mentioned in the two volumes edited by Laird and Miles (1983, 1985).[91]

Mosquito physiology and control

This subject is becoming more relevant to medical entomology. Some of the newer larvicides for mosquito control act as 'growth regulators'. One mode of action is to impair cuticle formation in the successive larval instars, the pupa and the adult through the application of chitin inhibitors (e.g., diflubenzuron). Another approach is to treat mosquito breeding places with compounds having activity like the juvenile hormones of insects; these 'juvenoids' (e.g., methoprene) prevent successful metamorphosis and maturation of the mosquito. So far there are no practical problems of resistance to these chemicals and there should be little cross-resistance with conventional pesticides.

As for all other insects, the mosquito body is encased in an exoskeleton made of cuticle. Insecticides that act on the nervous system (i.e., organochlorines, organophosphates, carbamates and pyrethroids) must be readily absorbed through insect cuticle, but not through human skin. Cuticular hardness depends on the degree of chitinization. Mosquito larvae have a hard head capsule, siphon and many rigid bristles or setae and spines, but the thorax and abdomen are mostly covered by a more flexible cuticle. Mosquito adults have strong and rigid cuticular plates forming the head, thorax and abdomen, with flexible joints between them, where necessary for articulation of limbs and segments. Respiratory spiracles on the larval siphon, pupal trumpets and on the adult sides (pairs on the mesothorax, metathorax and each abdominal segment) allow air to reach all internal organs via a network of tubes called tracheae. The use of larvicidal oils is intended to drown mosquito larvae by preventing them from reaching air when they try to open their spiracles at the water surface. However, Reiter,[92] working with monomolecular layers for anopheline control, has found that there may be sufficient dissolved oxygen for larval survival during much of the day and all night without access to free air. Oiling will therefore be most effective when an insecticide is included.

The body cavity or haemocoel of mosquitoes and other insects is filled with colourless haemolymph carrying haemocytes which have some of the functions of blood corpuscles. There is an open circulatory system, with a dorsal aorta and heart in the abdomen. The mosquito brain is in the head, with neurosecretory ganglia and *corpus cardiacum* for hormone production. Other important sources of hormones controlling mosquito life processes are the ovaries and the thoracic *corpora allata*. A ventral nerve cord has segmental ganglia and paired lateral branches.

The mosquito gut (Figure IV.50) passes from the proboscis to the pharynx in the head, the oesophagus in the thorax, the midgut or stomach in the abdomen and finally the rectum, where fluids are absorbed before defecation occurs through the anus below the tip of the abdomen. Within the foregut, especially of female anophelines, cuticular teeth protrude into the lumen of the gut; these are thought to have a primary function of rupturing blood corpuscles and they also inflict lethal damage on many ingested microfilariae. A large crop is formed by an oesophageal diverticulum; water and nectar are taken into the crop for digestion of sugars. Excretion is by means of a series of long white malpighian tubules in the abdomen, behind the stomach, with their ducts discharging into the midgut lumen.

When freshly engorged after biting, the abdomen of a female mosquito is swollen and reddened by the blood meal within the stomach. Paired ovaries, each with about 100 follicles for egg production, are situated posteriorly in the abdomen. In the terminal abdominal segment of females are spermathecae (three in culicines; one in anophelines) which receive and store sperms from males, so that mature oöcytes can be fertilized as eggs are laid.

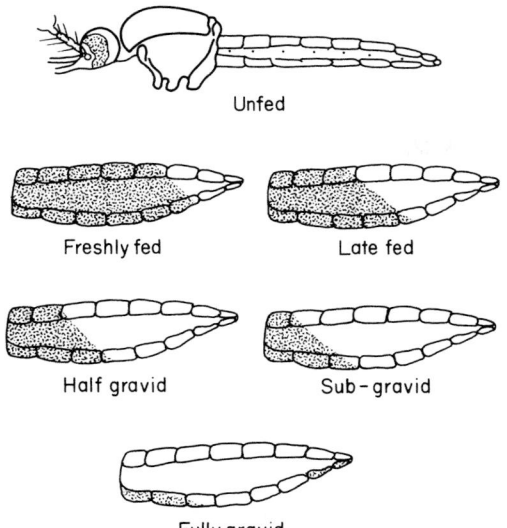

Figure IV.50: Classification in the abdominal conditions of female mosquitoes. The dark basal area of the abdomen contains the blood meal in the stomach, decreasing as digestion proceeds. The pale posterior part of the abdomen contains the developing ovaries, increasing as the gonotrophic cycle proceeds. Unfed, fed and gravid female mosquitoes may be either nulliparous or parous.

As the blood meal becomes digested during the days after blood-feeding, the ovaries develop and fill the rear abdomen with whitish eggs. Figure IV.50 shows how the changes in abdominal condition can be classified as: (1) unfed, (2) freshly fed, (3) one-third gravid or late-stage fed, (4) half gravid, (5) two-thirds gravid or subgravid, (6) fully gravid. In parallel with these abdominal stages, it is customary to assess the progress of oögenesis by classifying the development of ovarian follicles. After emergence from the pupa, the follicles pass from stage I to stage II, which is the resting stage. After blood-feeding, yolk is deposited around the oöcyte nucleus, and stage III

passes to stage IV when the clear nucleus is no longer visible when examined in saline. Finally stage V represents formation of the full-sized egg, containing the unfertilized oöcyte. These categories of ovarian development in mosquitoes are generally known as 'Christophers' stages' (Figure IV.51).

At tropical temperatures, the eggs of mosquitoes become ready to lay (laying is termed oviposition) 2 or 3 days after ingestion of the blood meal. Blood-feeding and egg-laying are the first and last steps in what is called the gonotrophic cycle. Soon after having laid a batch of eggs, the female mosquito tries to feed again on blood. Thus there are regular and usually continuous gonotrophic cycles. The feeding interval, or the duration of the gonotrophic cycle, measured in days, is an important factor affecting vectorial capacity. The more often a mosquito feeds on blood, the more likely it is to pick up infections and transmit them. Conversely, at cooler temperatures, the gonotrophic cycle takes longer—maybe 4 or 5 days—reducing the chances of transmission because: (1) occasions when parasites can be acquired or transmitted are less frequent for each female mosquito, (2) the speed of development of parasites to the infective stage in the vectors is proportional to temperature, and (3) mosquitoes are more likely to die before becoming infective. Clearly, if mosquito longevity is less than the time required for completion of parasite development, there is no likelihood of disease transmission. The aim of spraying houses with residual insecticides is to kill the majority of adult female mosquitoes before they reach the age of infectivity, and not to eliminate mosquitoes altogether. Table IV.13 summarizes the insecticidal applications used for mosquito control (see under each type of mosquito for more details of their control).

One way to monitor the age composition and life expectancy of adult mosquito populations is to determine the proportion of females that are parous (i.e., have laid eggs at least once). This involves examination of the ovaries

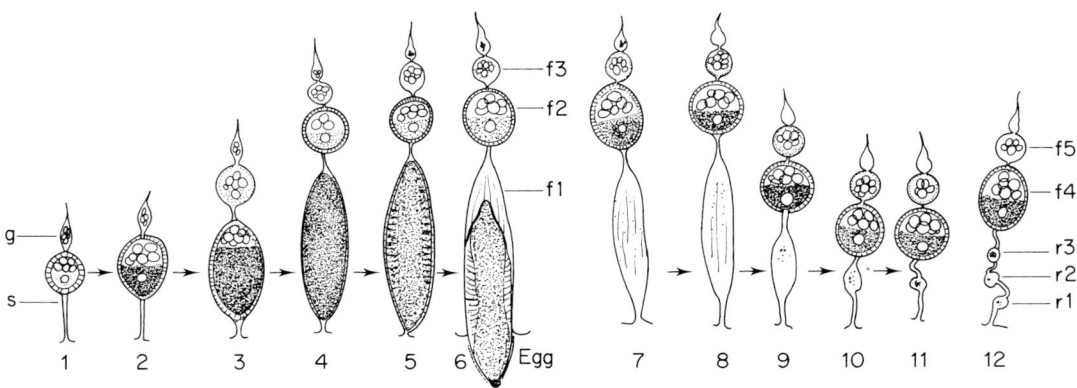

Figure IV.51: Christophers' stages of ovarian follicular development in mosquitoes. Each ovary contains approximately 100 ovarioles. Each ovariole consists of a hollow stalk (s), developing follicles (f1, f2, etc.) and a terminal germarium (g) from which successive follicles arise. Stages I–V of development of the first follicle are shown (1–5). The mature egg then passes from the stalk (6) to the common oviduct. A sac-like swelling of the ovariolar stalk contracts (7–10) to form a small persistent dilatation or follicular relic, which is slightly pigmented (11). Successive eggs formed in each ovariole leave a series of distinct relics (r1, r2, etc.) in the parous mosquito (12), from which the mosquito's age may be estimated in terms of the number of gonotrophic cycles.

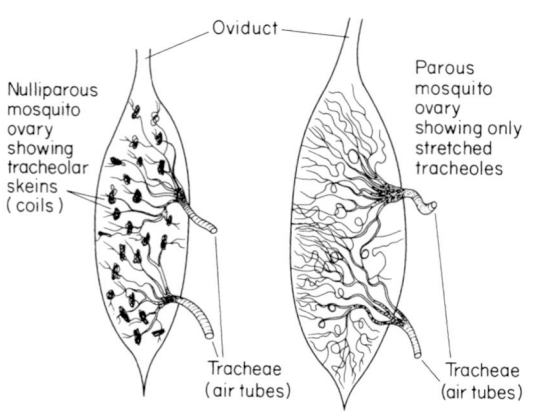

Figure IV.52: Mosquito ovaries, showing how the nulliparous female has coiled tracheolar 'skeins' in the ovary (left); tracheoles become permanently stretched in the parous ovary (right) due to previous growth of eggs. These features of the air tubes can be seen only in mosquito females with an 'unfed' abdominal condition.

to see whether tracheal skeins are present implying nulliparity, or whether follicular relics are present implying parity (Figure IV.52). It may be possible to count the number of relics on each follicular stalk in order to calculate the mosquito's age in terms of the number of gonotrophic cycles it has experienced.[13,93]

More general information on mosquito physiology has been reviewed by Clements.[94] Reviews of mosquito control methods are given by Laird and Miles.[91]

Midges

R. P. Lane

Family: Ceratopogonidae (biting midges)

Genera: *Culicoides*, *Leptoconops* and *Forcipomyia* (Subgenus *Lasiohelea*)

Biting midges are very small flies (1–4 mm long) called 'no-see-ums' in some parts of the world or, confusingly, sandflies in others such as the southern USA and Caribbean. They occur worldwide in habitats ranging from tropical forests and savannahs to agricultural districts, coastal and desert areas. The adults are compact, usually dark brown or black flies, with the wings held flat over the back at rest. Only the females suck blood and often attack in huge numbers; their bites are painful and often elicit a prolonged reaction in sensitive individuals. The males, which can be distinguished by their plumrose antennae, feed only on plant sugars. The larvae are small and worm-like, swimming in a sinusoidal manner through wet or moist habitats such as fresh or brackish water or mud, decomposing vegetation and wet bovine droppings.

The Ceratopogonidae (biting midges) are a large family of over 4000 species in 60 genera but only three contain species of medical significance: *Culicoides*, *Leptoconops* and *Forcipomyia* (subgenus *Lasiohelea*).[95] Their principal impact on humans is as biting pests but species of *Culicoides* transmit filarial nematodes and are also of veterinary importance as virus and nematode vectors.

Leptoconops

Some species are serious pests, biting during the day. The flies are shiny black with milky white wings. Species of the subgenus *Styloconops* breed in sandy beaches surrounding the India Ocean (*L. spinosifrons*; *L. holoconops*), and are coastal pests in south-east USA, eastern Central America and the Caribbean (*L. becquarti*); *Leptoconops* (*sensu stricto*) breed in fine silt soils inland in south-east USA (*L. torrens*).

A few species of *Forcipomyia* subgenus *Lasiohelea* are serious pests: *F. (L.) siberica* in central Asia, *F. (L.) taiwana* in Japan and China, and *F. (L.) townsvillensis* in Australia.

Culicoides

These have a wing length of 2 mm; those of tropical species may be only 1 mm, and usually the wings are patterned (Figure IV.53). Of the 1000 species in this genus, many are biting pests in temperate and tropical countries and may have a significant effect on tourist-based economies. Biting rates of 200–400 per hour are commonly recorded—with a maximum of 3000 per hour on a single exposed limb. Attacks may cause severe discomfort; for example, biting on the eyelids may induce sufficient swelling to prevent their opening for several days. New arrivals to tropical areas often suffer (or are worried) more than locals and subsequent scratching may produce deeply eroding secondary infections to the extent that skin grafting has been used. Dermatitis caused by *Culicoides* has been reported several times (e.g., *C. paraensis* in Bahia, Brazil).

In the Caribbean and eastern Central America, *Mansonella ozzardi* is transmitted by several species of *Culicoides*: *C. furens* in St Vincent, Haiti;[96] *C. phlebotomus* in Trinidad[97] and *C. paraensis* in Antigua and northern Argentina. Both *C. furens* and *C. phlebotomus* are coastal species, the former breeding in mangrove swamps and the latter in streams crossing beaches. *C. paraensis* is a peridomestic species breeding in decaying fruits such as calabash or cacao pods. In the Brazilian and Colombian Amazon regions, *M. ozzardi* is primarily transmitted by *Simulium*, but *C. insinuatus* may also play a role.

Culicoides are also vectors of *M. perstans* in Africa and believed to be the vector in the New World. There is considerable confusion over the identity of the species

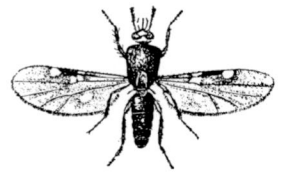

Figure IV.53: Female *Culicoides grahami* (50 ×).

incriminated as the vector of *M. perstans* in West Africa. It was originally recorded as *C. austeni* (and later as *C. milnei*), but it is more likely that *C. inornatipennis* (and possibly *C. grahami*) is responsible. The vectors breed in small pools of water in cut stems of bananas and plantains, and therefore the incidence of the disease is highest in and around plantations. Transmission takes place at night. In contrast, the transmission of *M. streptocerca* takes place during the day when the vector, *C. grahami*, bites a person.

Culicoides paraensis, a domestic pest in many parts of Brazil, has been incriminated as the vector of Oropouche virus, which causes a febrile illness in Amazonian Brazil. Several other viruses have been isolated from ceratopogonids: Japanese B encephalitis (*F. (L.) taiwana*); eastern equine encephalitis (pooled *Culicoides* in USA); Rift Valley fever (*Culicoides* in Kenya, Nigeria); and Congo and Dugbe viruses (several pools of *Culicoides* in Nigeria). Although it is most unlikely that midges transmit these viruses, the question remains open.

Control of ceratopogonids involves the use of insecticides for larviciding or space spraying, repellents and land management (draining and flooding).[98]

Blackflies, buffalo gnats, turkey gnats (see also Chapter 82)

G. B. White

Family: Simuliidae

Genus: *Simulium*

The Simuliidae, usually known as blackflies, are small, robust flies (1–5 mm long) (Figure IV.54). The females suck blood and have blade-like mouthparts; in the males these are more or less rudimentary. The flies have a characteristic humped thorax caused by the strong development of the scutum. The antennae are short and similar in both sexes. Most of what is known about blackfly biology and control has been summarized by Crosskey.[99]

Blackflies occur in enormous numbers in favourable localities during late spring and early summer in northern countries and are abundant in the north temperate and subarctic zones. They are also abundant in the tropics where human-biting species transmit *Onchocerca volvulus*. In addition to their role as transmitters of *Onchocerca*, they also act as intermediate hosts of other filariae and blood-

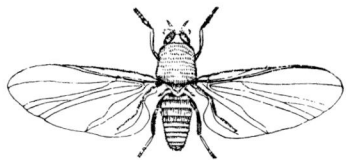

Figure IV.54: *Simulium damnosum* (10 ×).

borne protozoa of birds and mammals, and are a severe biting nuisance when the flies are numerous. The females attack viciously in the open during the day but do not enter houses. Biting activity is known to be influenced by weather conditions and older (infected) flies may differ in their behaviour from newly emerged, unfed flies.

The females lay their triangular eggs in running (and therefore oxygenated) water, in masses of 300 to 500, which are attached to rocks, grass and other objects by a gelatinous fluid. The eggs hatch in 1–2 days and the emerging larvae attach themselves by the posterior end to a pad of silk spun from the salivary glands, on to submerged leaves and stones. The larvae and pupae of most species have specialized aquatic niches on stones, twigs or other substrates. Those of the *S. neavei* complex in tropical Africa always occur on freshwater arthropods, mainly crabs, prawns or mayfly nymphs. The larvae feed by straining fine particles from the water through fan-shaped mouth brushes. There are six to eight larval instars, ending in 1–2 weeks or more. Before pupation, the larva spins a tent-like, silken coccoon which protects the pupa inside it. The pupal period is 2–10 days, and both larvae and pupae can be found in large numbers in breeding places.

The following species are actual or potential vectors of *O. volvulus* in humans.

Africa

The *Simulium damnosum* and *S. neavei* complexes are groups with sibling species that have been separated into a number of different species by biological and chromosome studies. These species differ in their ecology and feeding preferences, which affect their importance as vectors of human onchocerciasis. The *S. damnosum* complex (jinja fly) (see Chapter 82) contains at least 40 sibling species (identified chiefly by the pattern of chromosome banding), including forms found in the forest zone or in the savannah zone that are vectors only of the *O. volvulus* strain endemic to their own zones. Clinical manifestations of onchocerciasis in the savannah area are associated with lower biting densities and infection rates in the flies (annual transmission potential) compared with those found in the forest area. Different members of the complex breed in large or small rivers and in the outflow of dams, the larvae attaching to vegetation and stones in the river bed. Females are capable of long flights. In the vast Onchocerciasis Control Programme covering endemic countries of West Africa, involving regular larviciding of all waterways for 20 years, reinvasion of the controlled area was found over distances of 200–400 km owing to influx of vector females from far afield.

The *S. neavei* complex is confined to small streams in hilly forest; its flight range is limited. The larvae and pupae are found attached to crabs of the genus *Potamonautes*. The chief vector species are *S. ethiopiense* in Ethiopia, *S. neavei* in Zaire, and *S. woodi* in Tanzania. Eradication of *S. neavei* and the interruption of transmission from person to person was achieved in highland foci in Kenya by larviciding and clearance of riverine vegetation.

Central and South America

The *S. ochraceum* complex (orange-yellow species, unusual for a blackfly) are the main vectors in Mexico and Guatemala. They breed in minute trickles of water, often under leaves, and in innumerable streams in rugged country with heavy vegetational cover; hence these species are difficult to control. They also breed close to villages in irrigated coffee plantations between 500 and 1200 m.

S. metallicum, S. callidum and *S. exiguum* are considered to be minor vectors in Central America, but *S. exiguum* is the only anthropophilic species and therefore the principal vector in the endemic focus on the western slopes of the Andes in Colombia. *S. metallicum* is the main vector in Venezuela—breeding in small streams and biting humans avidly. In Mexico and Guatemala, however, this species does not feed on humans so readily and is associated with larger streams.

In recently discovered foci of onchocerciasis in Amazonia (Brazil and Venezuela) the disease is transmitted by *S. guyanense, S. limbatum* and *S. oyapockense* (formerly reported as *S. amazonicum*). The latter also transmits non-pathogenic *Mansonella ozzardi* in South America.

For control of Simuliidae, and onchocerciasis, see Chapter 82.

Horse flies, clegs, deer flies

D. M. Minter

Suborder: Brachycera; family: Tabanidae

Genera: *Tabanus, Haematopota* and *Chrysops*

The family Tabanidae includes the largest blood-sucking flies known; some have a wing span of more than 60 mm. Most species are stoutly built and robust insects, often brightly coloured in life, with large eyes and a body length of 5–25 mm. Viewed from above (Figure IV.55A), the eyes of females are widely separated (dichoptic), whereas those of males are contiguous (holoptic). In life, the eyes of both sexes are often shot with species-specific iridescent bands, chevrons or spots of brilliant colours; these colours fade soon after death.

Tabanid antennae have three segments (known as the scape, pedicel and flagellum) that differ in size and proportions in the three main genera, *Tabanus, Chrysops* and *Haematopota* (Figure IV.55B). The palps are short and consist of one or two segments only. The wing venation of tabanids is characteristic (Figure IV.55C), particularly the enclosed, almost central, hexagonal discal cell and the open branch of the radial vein which encloses, in a submarginal cell, the wing tip of most species. There is also a second, open, submarginal cell anterior to the wing tip and five open posterior cells along the hind margin of the wing. The pattern of pigmentation of the wing, or its absence, is a useful feature for identification of the three genera of medical importance, in conjunction with the shape and proportion of the antennal segments (Figure IV.55B,C). Only females bite; because of their large size they take a large blood meal, from 20 to 200 mg. The mouthparts are short and stout; they project downwards below the head and inflict a painful bite.

There are four subfamilies of Tabanidae (Scepsidinae, Pangoniinae, Chrysopsinae and Tabaninae). Medically important species are found only among the Chrysopsinae and Tabaninae. The Tabaninae is subdivided into three tribes (Haematopotini, Tabanini and Diachlorini), of which only the Haematopotini and Tabanini contain species that normally bite humans. There are about 3000 species of Tabanidae, in numerous genera, but medically important species occur only in the genera *Tabanus, Haematopota* (subfamily Tabaninae) and *Chrysops* (subfamily Chrysopsinae).

The Tabanidae are cosmopolitan; species of *Tabanus, Chrysops* and *Haematopota* occur in tropical, subtropical and temperate regions, but species of the genus *Haematopota*, although abundant in Africa, are absent from Australia and South America and are uncommon in North America.

The 'blue-tailed fly', celebrated in the well-known American ballad, is believed to be the widespread *Tabanus atratus* of eastern North America; the species is actually a uniform black colour, but there is a distinctly bluish tinge when the flies are covered with pollen or dust.

Other members of the suborder Brachycera are sometimes a severe biting nuisance, particularly in coastal and mountain regions of western North America. (They have a painful bite and are occasionally the cause of severe allergic manifestations.) These belong to the families Rhagionidae ('snipe-flies') and the closely related Athericidae. Although these two families contain blood-sucking species, none has yet been associated with the transmission of pathogens. The rhagionid genus *Symphoromyia* is a vicious biter in the western USA; in Australia, members of the genera *Spaniopsis* and *Austroleptis* are troublesome pests. As they are of no known medical (or veterinary) importance, these two families are not considered further.

Recognition of the genera: *Chrysops, Tabanus* and *Haematopota*

Chrysops (deer flies, greenheads, mango flies, mangrove flies) (Figure IV.56)

Medium size, 6–10 mm long. Wings held apart over the body, like a half-open pair of scissors. Wings usually with one or two brownish transverse bands. Antennae (see Figure IV.55B) longer than those of *Tabanus* and *Haematopota*; the three segments are of similar length and project well in front of the head. Three spot-like, light-sensitive ocelli (simple eyes) present on the top of the head, behind the compound eyes. Tibia of hind legs spurred, with paired small distal spines, as well as the more prominent pair on the tibia of the middle legs (the latter found in all three genera). Eyes in life of iridescent

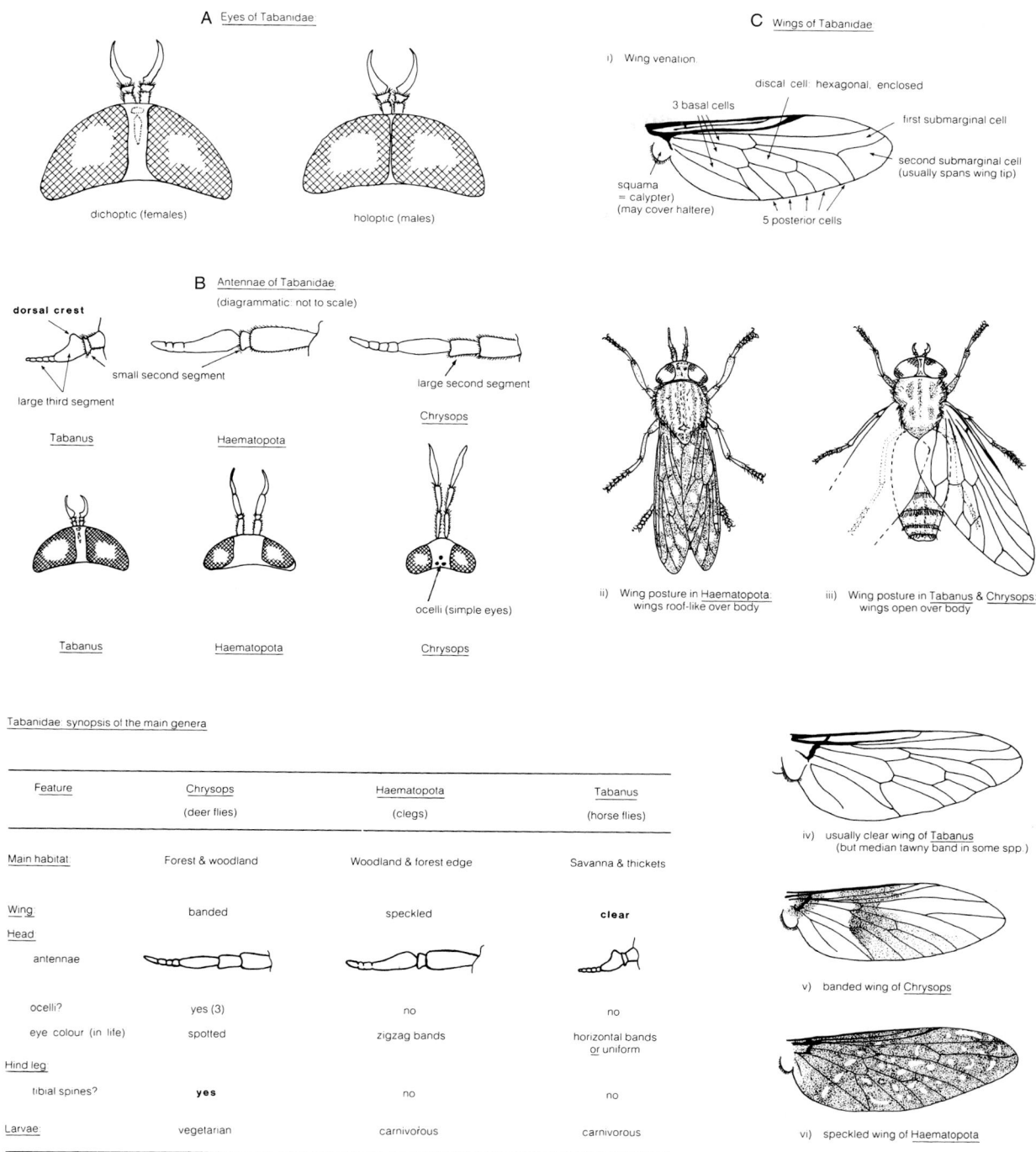

A   Eyes of Tabanidae:

dichoptic (females)   holoptic (males)

C   Wings of Tabanidae

i) Wing venation:

discal cell: hexagonal, enclosed
3 basal cells
first submarginal cell
second submarginal cell
(usually spans wing tip)
squama
= calypter)
(may cover haltere)
5 posterior cells

B   Antennae of Tabanidae
(diagrammatic: not to scale)

dorsal crest
large third segment
small second segment
large second segment

Tabanus   Haematopota   Chrysops

ocelli (simple eyes)

Tabanus   Haematopota   Chrysops

ii) Wing posture in Haematopota:
wings roof-like over body

iii) Wing posture in Tabanus & Chrysops:
wings open over body

Tabanidae: synopsis of the main genera

Feature	Chrysops (deer flies)	Haematopota (clegs)	Tabanus (horse flies)
Main habitat:	Forest & woodland	Woodland & forest edge	Savanna & thickets
Wing:	banded	speckled	**clear**
Head			
antennae			
ocelli?	yes (3)	no	no
eye colour (in life)	spotted	zigzag bands	horizontal bands or uniform
Hind leg			
tibial spines?	**yes**	no	no
Larvae:	vegetarian	carnivorous	carnivorous

iv) usually clear wing of Tabanus
(but median tawny band in some spp.)

v) banded wing of Chrysops

vi) speckled wing of Haematopota

Figure IV.55: Characteristic features of the Tabanidae. (**A**) Holoptic and dichoptic condition of the head in male and female Tabanidae. (**B**) Antennae of adult Tabanidae: antennal features in the genera *Tabanus* (horse flies), *Chrysops* (deer flies) and *Haematopota* (clegs). (**C**) Wings of Tabanidae: (**i**) wing venation of Tabanidae; (**ii**) wing posture in *Haematopota* sp.; (**iii**) wing posture in *Tabanus* and *Chrysops* spp.; (**iv**) clear wing of *Tabanus* sp; (**v**) banded wing of *Chrysops* sp.; (**vi**) speckled wing of *Haematopota* sp.

colour, often of a golden hue. Found mainly in forest and woodlands, but often also common in marshy scrub and swampy woodlands.

Tabanus (horse flies, gad flies)
Medium to large flies, 9–25 mm long, wings usually clear, held over back like a pair of half-open scissors (as in *Chrysops*). Antennae short (see Figure IV.55B); first two segments small, the third segment long, with a pronounced dorsal 'hump' and an upturned tip. No ocelli. No spines on hind tibia. In life, eyes either of uniform colour or in a series of horizontal coloured bands. Found mainly in more open habitats, such as savannah and thicket vegetation.

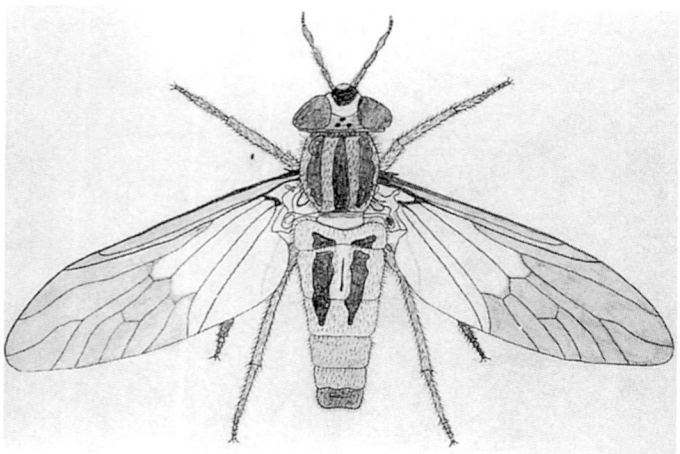

Figure IV.56: Female *Chrysops dimidiatus*. (Courtesy of D. B. Thomas.)

Haematopota (clegs, stouts)

Medium size, 6–10 mm long, wings folded over the back in a roof-like manner; in almost all species the wings have a complex mottled dark grey or brown pattern. Antennae (see Figure IV.55B) with first and third segments markedly longer than the short second segment; third segment without dorsal 'hump' or upturned end. No ocelli. No spines on hind tibia. When alive, eyes have zigzag bands of iridescent colour. Mainly flies of woodlands and forest edges.

Biology and life cycle

The family Tabanidae is believed to have evolved in close association with the ungulates, upon which they mostly feed. Other mammals are also attacked, but seldom birds or reptiles. Most species are diurnal and hunt by sight; they are most active in bright sunlight; *Tabanus paradoxus* of central and southern Europe is unusual in that it is a nocturnal species.

Most tabanids inhabit woodland and forest. Many species of *Chrysops* are found in waterlogged scrub and marshy woodlands; other species occupy more open areas of savannah woodland and grassland. Only females feed on blood; both sexes feed on sugary plant secretions. Because the female mouthparts are large and coarse, the bite is deep and painful; blood often continues to ooze from the wound for some time afterwards. Because of the painful bite, females are often forced, by defensive reactions of the human or animal host, to interrupt feeding and later resume on the same individual, or another, in order to feed to repletion. This behaviour considerably increases their efficiency as mechanical vectors of pathogens. Some individuals develop a severe allergic reaction to the large quantity of anticoagulant saliva pumped into the bite wound as the flies feed. With the exception of *Chrysops silaceus*, which will bite indoors, it is rare for tabanids to enter houses, although some species enter by accident and can be seen on windows, in an apparent attempt to escape.

The relatively short-lived adults are strictly seasonal in temperate climates, with biting confined to the warmest summer months. In tropical areas breeding is continuous, but biting activity of different species is very dependent on the rainy or dry season. The natural adult lifespan of the important tropical species *Chrysops silaceus* is thought to be about 3–4 weeks.

In this respect rather like tsetse, tabanids are attracted to large, slow-moving, dark objects including vehicles; they may enter the windows to bite the occupants, or attack the warm tyres of stationary cars and trucks.

Gravid females are selective of particular plant species or other specific oviposition sites. Females lay lozenge-shaped egg masses, firmly cemented to the underside of grasses, other vegetation, rocks or stones, where these overhang suitable larval breeding places: either shallow water, mud or damp soil (even in tree-holes high above the ground). Egg batches consist of a few dozen, or more than 1000 slender, cigar-shaped eggs—each 1–2.5 mm long (Figure IV.57). The egg batches are coated with a waterproof layer; eggs are commonly off-white in colour, sometimes grey, brownish-black or even orange. Eggs hatch after 1–2 weeks; the cream-coloured, grub-like larvae drop on to the water, mud or damp soil and soon begin to feed. Larvae of *Chrysops* feed on vegetable detritus, while those of most *Tabanus* and *Haematopota* are carnivorous; they feed on other invertebrates, including members of their own species.

Compared with the relatively short life of adults, the duration of larval life is long, for both tropical and temperate species. For most tropical species, 4–5 months is usual; 1–2 years is not uncommon, and some species in cooler climates may spend up to 3 years as larvae. When mature, after up to eight moults, larvae of different species measure 10–60 mm in length.

Larval habitats differ between the genera and species, but they are predominantly aquatic or semiaquatic. *Chrysops* larvae generally live in the wettest places, such as the muddy margins of marshes (and salt-marshes), *Tabanus* spp. usually inhabit shallow seasonal pools, mud or wet soil near water, while *Haematopota* are most often found in drier habitats, such as damp soil.

Larvae are easy to recognize (Figure IV.57). They are cylindrical, with rather pointed extremities; at one end is the small head, which can be retracted into the thorax (the head has mouth-hooks like those of the Muscidae). At the other end of the body is the slightly upturned, conical, posterior respiratory siphon. There are tyre-like rings around the body, at the leading edge of each segment, most of which have a number of ventrolateral locomotory protuberances, known as 'pseudopods'.

Graber's organ is a structure unique to larval Tabanidae and of unknown function, possibly sensory or glandular. Visible in life through the integument on the dorsal side, near the base of the respiratory siphon, is a paired row of black, rounded structures (the number of which evidently is increased in older larvae). Together with an internal pyriform sac, which opens via a narrow tube to the exterior between the last two segments, these are the

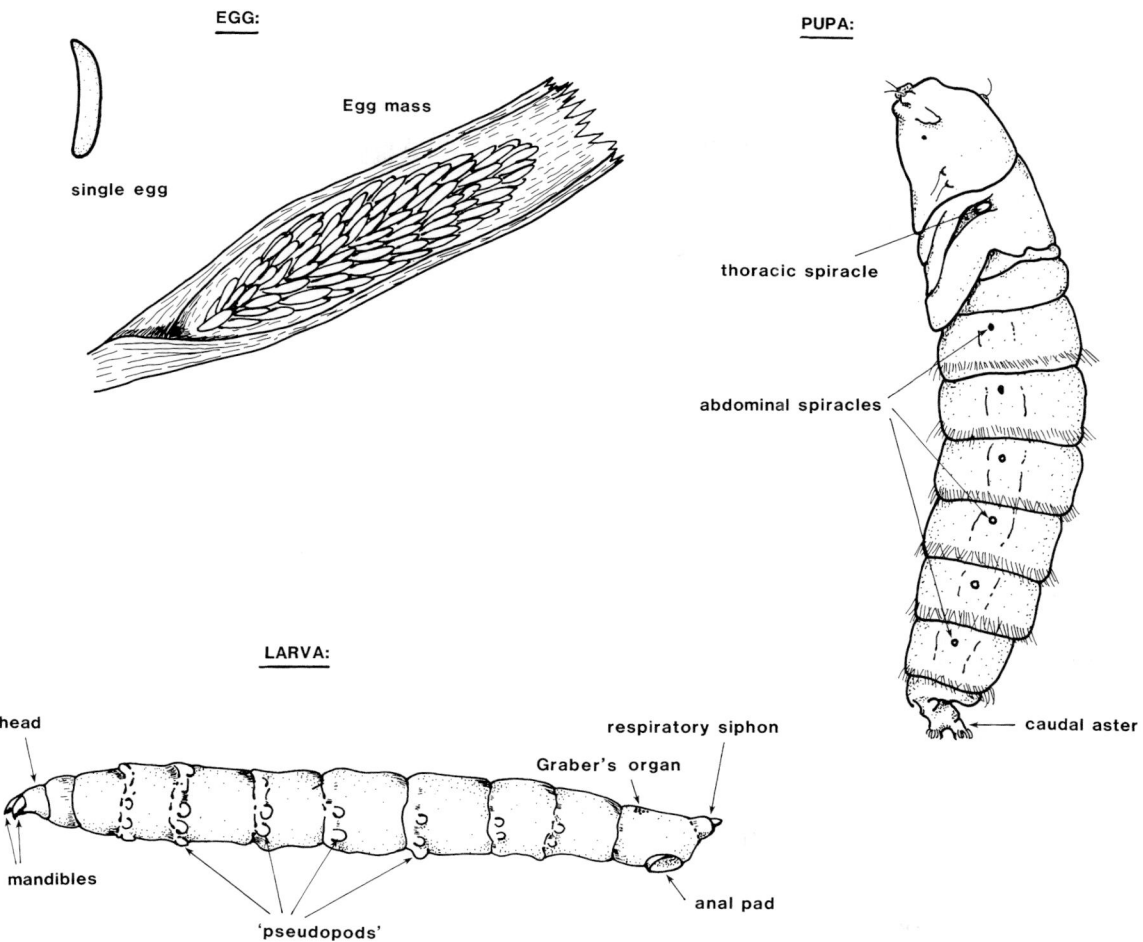

EGG:

single egg

Egg mass

PUPA:

thoracic spiracle

abdominal spiracles

caudal aster

LARVA:

head

mandibles

'pseudopods'

respiratory siphon

Graber's organ

anal pad

Figure IV.57: Egg, larvae and pupa of Tabanidae.

principal parts of Graber's organ that can be seen with a hand lens or low-power microscope.

Pupulation occurs in drier parts of the habitat; the brown-coloured pupae, 7–40 mm long (Figure IV.57), look rather similar to those of butterflies, but are partly buried, in an upright position, in soil or mud. Some *Tabanus* species whose larvae inhabit seasonal pools protect the future pupa from exposure to predators or desiccation; the mature larva excavates a vertical spiral burrow to delimit a cylinder of mud, into the centre of which it then burrows before pupation takes place. When the mud of the pool finally dries out, the cylinder cracks free from the surrounding mud and the pupa is securely housed within. The adult eventually emerges, after the pupa has partly rasped away the top of the cylinder. The pupae are provided with rings of spines on each abdominal segment, and a spiny caudal pad (known as an aster); the spines and aster facilitate limited vertical movement, whether in the substrate or in the mud cylinder. The pupal period lasts between 1 and 3 weeks until the adult emergences.

Control of Tabanidae

There are, in most instances, few or no practicable methods

of control for tabanid flies. Drainage of marshy areas would probably limit available breeding places, although this would seldom be justifiable on a cost–benefit basis.

Similarly, the use of insecticides to control likely breeding places would be difficult to justify and would be equally difficult (if not impossible) to carry out effectively, due to the practical difficulty of ensuring adequate contact of insecticide with larval or pupal stages, often buried in wet soil or mud. Tabanid breeding places are in any event generally extensive and diffuse, difficult to delimit, and would be expensive to treat with insecticides. Insecticide-impregnated plastic collars and ear-tags have been developed to protect livestock from the attacks of ticks and various Diptera; they probably help also to reduce biting of tabanids.

Some success in reducing adult numbers of pest species of *Haematopota* has been achieved by the use of dark-coloured plates (about half a metre square) coated with a sticky adhesive, placed in open habitats where the flies are troublesome and the plates visible to the flies for some distance.

The wearing of open-mesh jackets impregnated with a synthetic pyrethroid insecticide (e.g., permethrin) or a repellent such as DEET (diethyltoluamide) would afford some personal protection from the attack of tabanids in areas where they are sufficiently troublesome to warrant the inconvenience and expense of an additional garment.

Disease relationships of the Tabanidae (Tables IV.9 and IV.10)

Tabanidae can be a severe biting nuisance to people and livestock, to the extent that their attacks prevent all normal outdoor activities, affect the migration patterns of nomadic herdspeople and prevent the normal use of seasonal pastures by livestock (as in Sudan and parts of North America). In addition to the attacks of the adult flies, rice-field workers in Japan are sometimes attacked by the carnivorous aquatic larvae of *Tabanus* and *Chrysops*, which pierce feet or hands below the water surface; a severe oedematous reaction may ensue from the painful bites of the larvae.

More exceptionally, there are instances where bites of tabanid flies have resulted in the mechanical transmission of anthrax bacilli (*Bacillus anthracis*) to humans, but this evidently occurs only under very unusual circumstances, and must surely be a rare event. However, it is probable that tabanids do play a significant role in the maintenance of anthrax epizootics.

Tularaemia (see Chapter 61)

Of the two principal human diseases transmitted by tabanids, tularaemia is of lesser importance. Tularaemia is a zoonotic bacterial infection widespread in the northern hemisphere and caused by *Francisella tularensis*. In the Old World the disease occurs in most European countries, the former USSR, Iran, Turkey, Tunisia, China and Japan. Ticks are thought to be the major vectors in most affected regions, but infection is contracted also in other ways: mechanically by the bite of various arthropods, directly

Table IV.9 Animal diseases transmitted by Tabanidae which rarely or never affect man.

Agent	Disease	Principal hosts	Transmission	Distribution
Elaeophora schneideri	Arterial worm disease (sheep)	Sheep, deer, elk, moose (asymptomatic in deer)	Cyclical (*Tabanus* and *Hybomitra* spp.)	West and South-west USA; Italy
Dilofilaria roemeri	—	Wallaroo (*Macropus robustus*)	Cyclical (*Dasybasis hebes*)	Australia
Haemoproteus metchnikovi	—	Turtles	Cyclical (*Chrysops callidus*)	USA
Besnoitia besnoiti	Bovine besnoitiosis	Cattle (intermediate) Cat (definitive host)	Non-cyclic: mechanical (other mechanical vectors are *Glossina* and *Stomoxys*)	Africa, South America, Europe, former USSR, Asia
Anaplasma marginale	Anaplasmosis	Bovines	Non-cyclic: mechanical (esp. *Tabanus* spp.)	Cosmopolitan
Trypanosoma (Trypanozoon) evansi	Surra (Old World) Derrangadera, Murina (New World)	Bovines, equines, camels, dogs	Non-cyclic: mechanical	Cosmopolitan; tropics and subtropics
Trypanosoma (Trypanozoon) equinum	Mal de Caderas	Equines, bovines	Non-cyclic: mechanical	South America
Tyrpanosoma (Duttonella) vivax	Souma	Bovines, sheep, goats, equines, dogs	Non-cyclic: mechanical	Mauritius, Antilles and South America
Trypanosoma (Megatrypanum) theileri	—	Bovines, antelopes	Cyclical (?)	Cosmopolitan
Equine infectious anaemia (EIA) virus	Swamp fever	Equines, pheasants	Non-cyclic: mechanical	Cosmopolitan
Hog cholera virus (HCV)	—	Pigs	Non-cyclic: mechanical	North America
Rinderpest virus	—	Ungulates	Non-cyclic (Tabanids are unproved, but potential mechanical vectors)	Cosmopolitan

Table IV.10 Biotype, distribution and medical importance of Glossina.

Species group/subgenus	Habitat type	Distribution	Species of medical importance
fusca group (*Austenina*)	Mainly rainforest areas	Chiefly forest areas of West and Central Africa, Relict species in dry areas of East Africa	None. But several vectors of livestock trypanosomiasis
palpalis group (*Nemorhina*)	Mainly linear: shores of lakes and rivers in forested or formerly forested areas	15°N to 12°S, approx. 17°W to 40°E, approx.	*G. palpalis*, vector of *T. brucei gambiense* in West Africa
		10°N to 12°S, approx. 10°E to 40°E, approx.	*G. fuscipes* (and subspecies), vectors of *T. brucei gambiense* (West Africa, Central Africa) and *T. brucei rhodesiense* (East Africa)
		12°N to 4°N, approx. 12°W to 40°E, approx.	*G. tachinoides*, vector of *T. b. gambiense* in West Africa and of *T. b. rhodesiense* in South-west Ethiopia
morsitans group (Glossina)	'Game' tsetse of the savannah zones; open woodland ('miombo'), bushland and thicket	15°N to 20°S, approx. 17°W to 45°E, approx.	*G. morsitans* (and subspecies), vectors of *T. b. rhodesiense* in East and South-east Africa
		8°N to 20°S, approx. 25°E to 48°E approx.	
		Limited area south-east of Lake Victoria; mainly in Tanzania	*G. pallidipes*, vector of *T. b. rhodesiense* in East Africa *G. swynnertoni*, vector of *T. b. rhodesiense*

through the conjunctiva and via abrasions of the skin, and by the consumption of infected meat or contaminated water.

Tularaemia occurs also in Canada, the USA and Mexico, where it is mainly transmitted between rabbits, rodents, sheep, horses and humans, by any of the routes above, including mechanical transmission by biting arthropods, notably ticks. However, in some areas, particularly the western USA, the disease occurs in summer outbreaks (with about 200 cases annually) in circumstances where rabbits are the most important reservoir of infection, and *Chrysops discalis* is certainly implicated as a mechanical vector of infection to humans; the human disease is known locally as 'deer-fly fever'. *F. tularensis* bacteria have also been recovered from *C. fulvaster* and *C. aestuans*, but these species appear to play no part in the dissemination of tularaemia to people. (See also Chapter 61.)

Loaiasis

The principal human disease transmitted by tabanids is loaiasis, or Calabar swelling, caused by the filarial nematode *Loa loa*, and transmitted by species of *Chrysops*, notably by *C. silaceus* and *C. dimidiatus* (Bombé form), in which the worms undergo cyclical development. The disease is common and widespread in the rainforest zones of West Africa, particularly Cameroon, and occurs sporadically across central Africa to the southern Sudan, Ethiopia and western Uganda. There are features of the epidemiology of loaiasis that resemble the sylvatic cycles of yellow fever transmission.

Adult *L. loa* worms inhabit subcutaneous connective tissues; diurnal periodic sheathed microfilariae are shed into the peripheral blood, particularly during the morning hours, and are ingested by day-biting *Chrysops*. When infected people are bitten by *Chrysops*, particularly by *C. silaceus* and *C. dimidiatus* (which may enter houses to feed), a proportion of the exsheathed microfilariae survive digestion in the insect gut, penetrate into the haemocoel, and invade the abdominal and thoracic fat bodies, where they grow, moult twice and develop into infective third-stage forms; these migrate forward into the head. Here the infective stages accumulate until the fly next feeds, when they break out of the labium into the mouthparts and infect a new host via the skin. Development of *L. loa* in *Chrysops* generally takes 10–12 days from the original infecting feed.

There are two parallel and sympatric, but ecologically separate, cycles of *L. loa* transmission in the West African rainforests (Figure IV.58). One cycle is that of the slightly smaller human parasite, often given subspecific status as *L. loa loa*. This has a strictly diurnal microfilarial periodicity and day-biting *Chrysops* vectors (*C. silaceus* and *C. dimidiatus*, Bombé form). The other cycle involves the slightly larger simian parasite, *L. l. papionis*, which infects only monkeys. *L. l. papionis* is a nocturnally periodic filarial parasite of drills (forest baboons), *Papio*

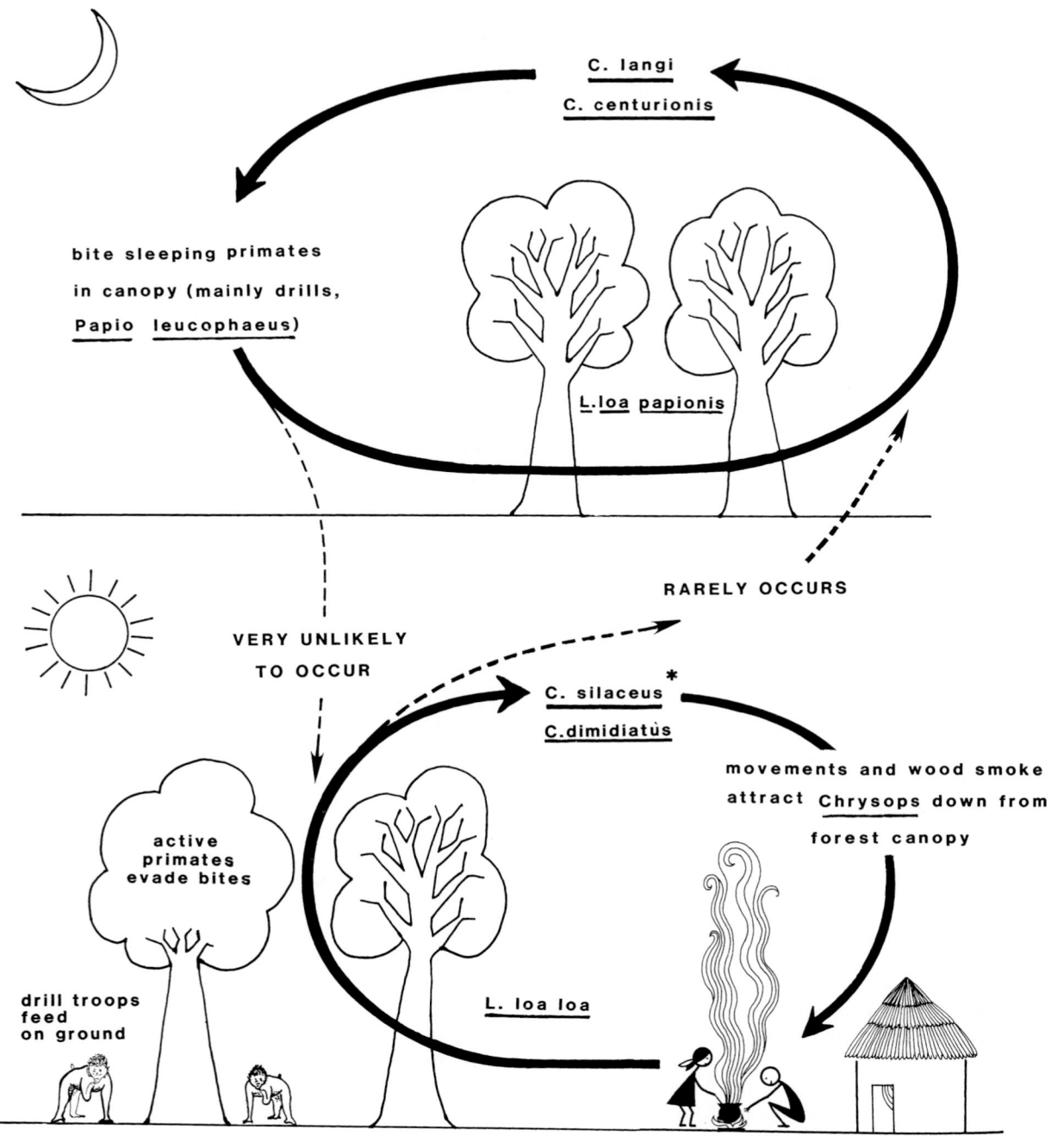

Figure IV.58: Diagram of transmission cycles in *Loa loa* to drills and to humans in West African rainforest.

(= *Mandrillus) leucophaeus* (infection rates of 96% and mean adult worm burdens of 17 have been recorded in drills). *L. l. papionis* will also naturally infect at least two cercopithecine monkeys found in the same rainforests, the putty-nosed guenon and the mona monkey, but the simian worm seems less well adapted to these two hosts.

(Infection rates and mean adult worm burdens of 24% and 6.3, and 12% and 2.4, respectively.)

The vectors of the simian parasite (*L. l. papionis*) are two tree-top *Chrysops* species, both of which are active early in the night and feed on sleeping drills and other monkeys; these are *C. langi* and *C. centurionis*. The vectors of human *Loa* (*C. silaceus* and *C. dimidiatus*) will bite both at canopy level and on the forest floor, but only in daylight hours, when they are seldom able to evade the vigorous response of the monkeys (Figure IV.58).

The obviously closely related parasites of humans and monkeys are behaviourally and ecologically distinct; additionally, they are reproductively isolated, although experimental hybrids can be produced. There is evidence which indicates that the simian *Loa* is not transmissible to humans, although drills are susceptible to experimental infection with human *Loa*, and occasional natural infections of drills with this infection are known.

The day-biting vectors of human *Loa* are active in the forest canopy, but they are especially attracted to descend to ground level both by some unknown component of wood-smoke (e.g., from cooking-fires) and by human movements. Thus human activities in general, and the scent of wood fires in particular, combine to draw these canopy-dwellers to ground level and especially into houses in the forest, in order that the females obtain a blood meal (Figure IV.58). These species will also emerge from the natural forest and enter teak or rubber plantations nearby, where there is also a high canopy.

There is at present no practicable method to reduce transmission of loaiasis by means of vector control.

Other vectors of human loaiasis

In the grassland and forest mosaic of the highland zone in the west of Cameroon, *C. zahrai* is implicated as a natural vector of local importance.

Chrysops distinctipennis and *C. longicornis* are believed to be vectors of human loaiasis in southern Sudan, beyond the eastern limits of *C. silaceus* and *C. dimidiatus*. The widespread species *C. distinctipennis* may possibly be an occasional vector elsewhere in central Africa, because the range of all three main vectors shows considerable overlap. *C. streptobalius* is the probable vector of the infections reported from Ethiopia. (See also Chapter 82.)

Tsetse flies (*Glossina*) (see also Chapter 73)

D. M. Minter

Family: Glossinidae

Genus: *Glossina* (Wiedemann 1830)

The unique viviparous genus *Glossina* contains some 30 species and subspecies of tsetse, confined to tropical Africa between latitudes 15°N and 30°S, where about 10.4×10^6 km^2 are infected—roughly half of the surface of the continent.

The tsetse flies are large, brown to greyish, narrow-bodied flies, 6–15 mm long, with a stout proboscis projecting forward well in front of the head (Figure IV.59). The proboscis is adjoined laterally, except during

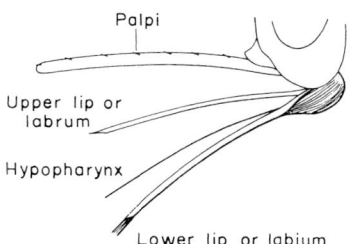

Figure IV.59: Mouth parts of *Glossina*.

the act of biting, by the paired labial palps. The mouthparts consist of a horny labrum, a slender hypopharynx (through which an anticoagulant saliva is injected into the bite wound) and a stout ventral labium (Figure IV.59). These three parts enclose a space, the food canal, through which blood is sucked by muscular action into the alimentary canal of the fly. During feeding the mouthparts, but not the palps, are lowered some 90° from the line of the body axis. Male and female tsetse feed exclusively on the blood of vertebrates.

Characteristic features that distinguish *Glossina* species (Figure IV.60) from other large biting flies, such as *Stomoxys*, *Haematobia*, *Lyperosia*, *Haematopota*, *Tabanus* and *Chrysops*, include a long straight proboscis with a basal bulb, the presence of branched hairs on the arista (Figure IV.61) (the prominent bristle on the largest, distal, segment of the antenna) and the length of the labial palps (as long as the proboscis in *Glossina*). The manner in which the wings are folded, scissor-like, over the back of the resting fly is also a very characteristic feature. The presence of the 'hatchet' or 'cleaver' cell, enclosed between the fourth and fifth longitudinal wing veins, is diagnostic of *Glossina* (Figure IV.62). This cell is clearly seen in the central area of the wings and contrasts with the triangular shape of the corresponding cell of related flies (e.g., *Stomoxys*; Figure IV.63).

The genus *Glossina* is usually divided by modern taxonomists into three species groups (Table IV.11) (sometimes given subgeneric status) as follows:

1. The *fusca* group (subgenus *Austenina*).
2. The *palpalis* group (subgenus *Nemorhina*).
3. The *morsitans* group (subgenus *Glossina*).

This taxonomic separation is reflected in the ecological requirements and distribution of the species included in each group. Characteristically, flies of the *fusca* group are associated with dense humid tropical forest or forest edges; members of the *palpalis* group are basically dependent on more or less dense riverine or lacustrine vegetation but their distribution extends into savannah zones well away from forested, or formerly forested, areas. Species of the *morsitans* group are the least hygrophilic and occupy vast areas of bushland and thicket vegetation often far from lakes and rivers. Strangely, however, one of the least hygrophilic species, occupying arid and semidesert area, is *G. longipennis*, a member of the *fusca* group. *G. brevipalpis*, also a *fusca* group species, has a

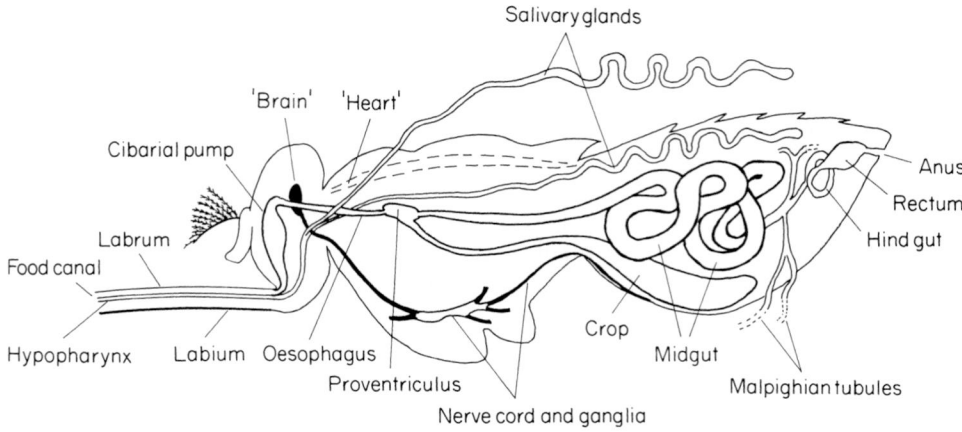

Figure IV.60: Schematic longitudinal section of *Glossina*, showing main features of the internal anatomy.

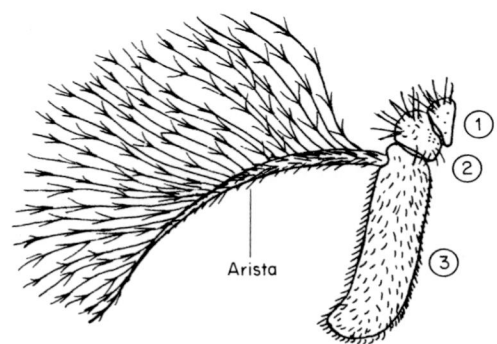

Figure IV.61: Antenna of *Glossina*, showing the dorsal arista with branched hairs, which arises from the third antennal segment. In other flies the hairs of the arista are unbranched.

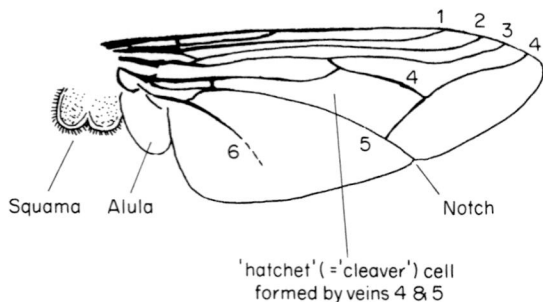

'hatchet' (='cleaver') cell
formed by veins 4 & 5

Figure IV.62: Wing of *Glossina*, showing venation and the 'hatchet' (= 'cleaver') cell enclosed between veins 4 and 5. The shape of the 'hatchet' cell is unique to *Glossina*; in all other flies the corresponding cell is triangular. *Glossina* is also unusual among higher flies in that the wings are held scissor-like over the back at rest.

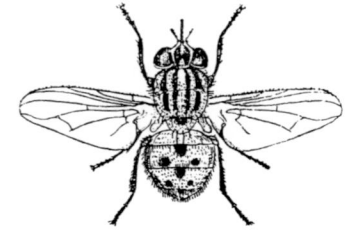

Figure IV.63: *Stomoxys calcitrans* (3 ×).

distribution that also extends into dry savannah zones. Although flies of the *fusca* group include important vectors of trypanosomes pathogenic to livestock, especially species of the *Trypanosoma vivax* (subgenus *Duttonella*) and *T. congolense* groups (subgenus *Nannomonas*), they have never been associated with the transmission of trypanosomiasis to humans and are not considered further in this section.

Figure IV.64 indicates the distribution of the groups of main medical importance and Figure IV.65 shows the general characteristics of some *Glossina* species. Mulligan[100] and Ford[101] summarize current views on the taxonomy and distribution of species and subspecies included in the *fusca*, *palpalis* and *morsitans* groups. Potts[102] gives a detailed key for the identification of all members of the genus, and Pollock[103] gives simple regional keys.

Life history

Tsetse flies, in common with a very few other Diptera, have a method of viviparous reproduction uncommon among the higher insects, by which a single larva is produced at a time and is retained and nourished within the body of the female fly. Associated with the production of single offspring is a reduction in the number of ovarioles in the two ovaries to a single pair in each, so that there are four ovarioles in all, from which fertilized eggs pass into the uterus in regular rotation. Female flies are normally fertilized only once, shortly after emergence, and store sufficient viable sperm from this single mating to last throughout life, during which, under favourable conditions, they may produce, at intervals of about 11 days, some 20 individual larvae.

Each successive fertilized egg (1.5 mm long) passes from the oviduct into the uterus where it hatches into a small, white, grub-like larva. The young larva obtains nutriment solely from the secretion of the uterine (or 'milk') glands of the mother, in which it is bathed. The larva grows, and twice moults, during the 8–12 days of intrauterine development. The mature larva, by now in the third instar, is finally extruded by the mother (by breech delivery) while she is perched on the ground, or

Table IV.11 Location of trypanosomes in tsetse flies.

Trypanosome species or group (subgenus)	Approx. time of development in Glossina	Usual range of infection rates in fly	Organs infected		
			Mouth parts	Salivary glands	Gut
T. vivax (*Duttonella*)	4–5 days	75–85%	+	–	–
T. congolense (*Nannomonas*)	8–10 days	18–25%	+	–	+
T. brucei subgroup* (*Trypanozoon*)	15–30 days	0.1–1.5%	+	+	+

*Includes the following parasites:
   T. brucei brucei—not infective to man.
   T. brucei gambiense—cause of Gambian sleeping sickness in man (chronic).
   T. brucei rhodesiense—cause of Rhodesian sleeping sickness in man (acute).

on vegetation a few centimetres above it, in a site selected for its shady situation and suitable soil texture. The newly deposited larva, creamy white in colour, with shiny black posterior polyneustic lobes through which it breathes, actively burrows below the surface soil to a depth of a few millimetres, using vigorous peristaltic movements. Having reached a point below the surface where conditions are suitable, it becomes immobile and begins to pupariate, still within the third larval skin, darkens and hardens. During emergence from the puparium, and in reaching the soil surface, the young fly is aided by an eversible bladder extruded from the front of the head and known as the *ptilinum*. During the first few days of life, this bladder can still be everted, while the body is still soft and 'soapy' in texture—if the young fly is pressed

carefully between the fingers. Flies in this stage, so far unfed, are referred to as *teneral* flies; older flies are described as *non-teneral*, as the head and body are hardened and horny and the ptilinum can no longer be everted. After the quiescent period, the young teneral flies seek their first blood meal. Flies of each sex normally feed at intervals of 3–4 days, sometimes less, and die from starvation if deprived of a blood meal for 10–12 days. The average lifespan of female *Glossina* is 2–3 months— exceptionally, up to 6–7 months. Male flies have a much shorter lifespan.

Male flies exhibit a progressive fraying of the trailing edge of the wings; this can be used to estimate the average age of *groups* of males from the same population. The wings of females also fray with age, usually less

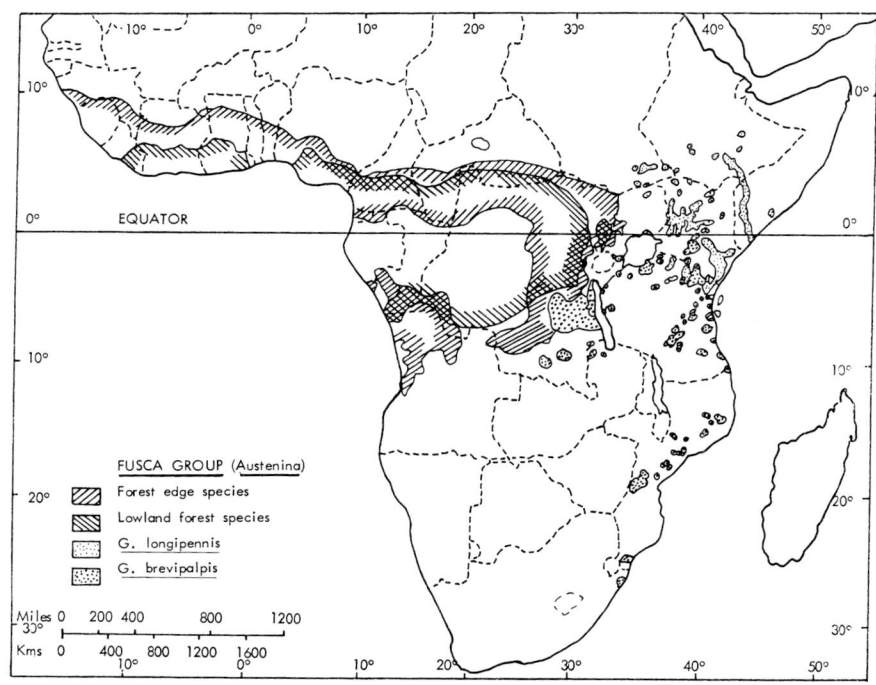

Figure IV.64: Distribution of the important species of *Glossina*. **A**, *fusca* group; **B**, *palpalis* group; **C**, *moristans* group (see also Chapter 73).

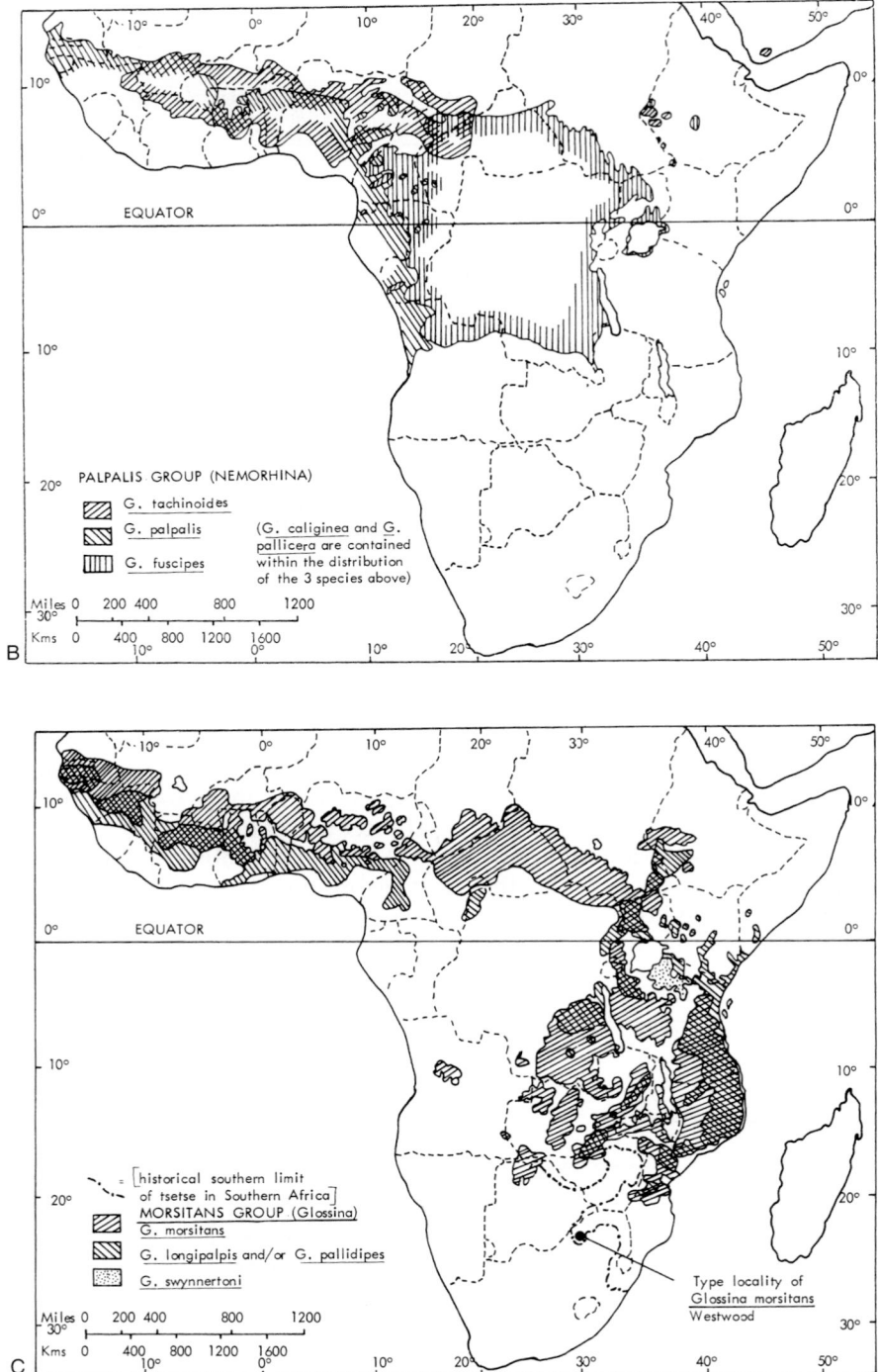

Figure IV.64: (*Cont'd*) Distribution of the important species of *Glossina*. **A**, *fusca* group; **B**, *palpalis* group; **C**, *moristans* group (see also Chapter 73).

rapidly than those of males. With females, however, careful examination of the four ovarioles enables an estimation of the age of *individual* females to be made on a physiological basis. This method of 'ovarian ageing' is accurate to within a few days up to an age of about 40 days; with older flies there is a greater margin of possible error. For a fuller discussion of ageing methods,

the reader is referred to Mulligan.[100] Figure IV.66 may be used to assess the degree of wing fray[104] and Figure IV.67 the age of individual females by examination of the ovarioles.[105,106] A new method to estimate age of *Glossina* (of both sexes) is suitable for laboratory automation, but requires sophisticated equipment. This method is based on the quantitative measurement of

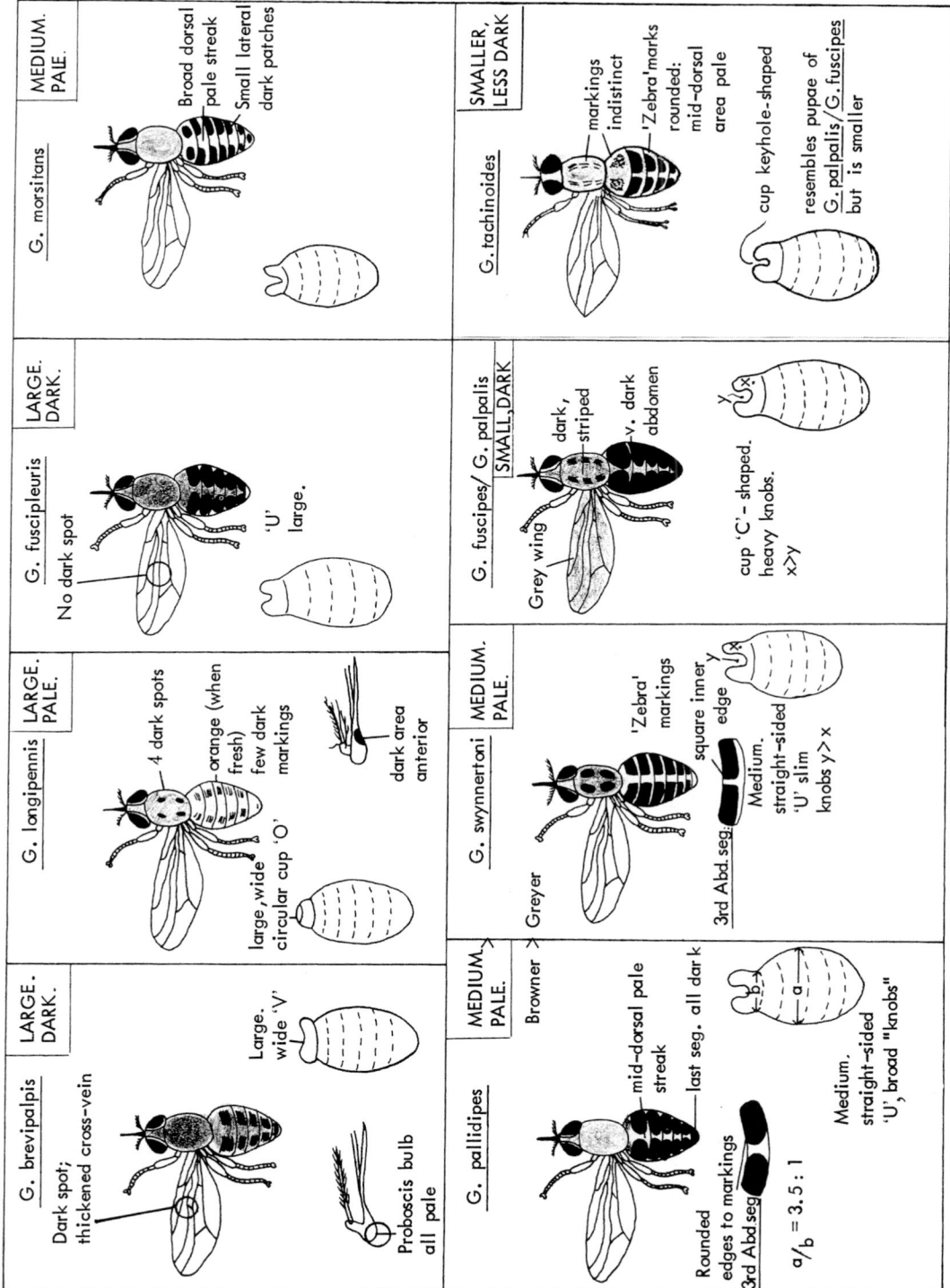

Figure IV.65: Outline guide to the identification of adults and pupae of some *Glossina* species, based on general characteristics visible to the naked eye or with the use of a simple hand-lens. The species illustrated are arranged in order of decreasing size, from top left to bottom right.

pteridine eye pigment deposition, which is correlated with age.

Female *G. fuscipes* in the field mate soon after emergence; female *G. pallidipes* are frequently fertilized near the host while seeking the first blood meal. Copulation may last from 2 to 24 hours and, at least in the laboratory, older males (about 14 days) are more potent than younger males.

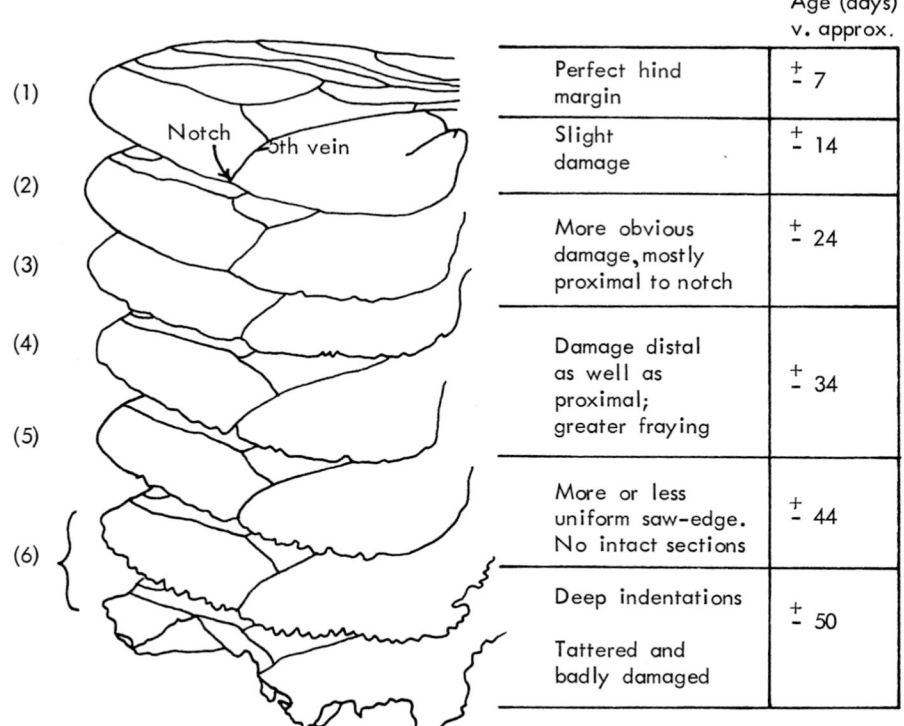

Glossina;
MALE WING FRAY DEGREES

	Age (days) v. approx.
Perfect hind margin	$\pm$ 7
Slight damage	$\pm$ 14
More obvious damage, mostly proximal to notch	$\pm$ 24
Damage distal as well as proximal; greater fraying	$\pm$ 34
More or less uniform saw-edge. No intact sections	$\pm$ 44
Deep indentations Tattered and badly damaged	$\pm$ 50

Notes:
(1) Female wings wear less rapidly
(2) The method is properly applied to find mean age for a group of males
(3) In some species (most) the wings change colour with increasing age, from a smoky brown-grey to a tawny yellow-brown.

Figure IV.66: Age estimation of *Glossina* using a wing fray chart for male flies. Wings of females wear less rapidly, but the degree of female wing fray may be used (in flies of ovarian categories IV–VII in Figure IV.67) to estimate whether flies are in an early or late stage. (Based on Jackson[104] for *G. morsitans*.)

Palpalis and *Morsitans* groups: bionomics and ecology in relation to sleeping sickness

Species of these two groups are active only during daylight hours: flight and feeding activities decrease markedly even during dull and overcast weather, and few species show evidence of purposive behaviour after dusk. Tsetse flies hunt their prey partly by sight, although scent becomes increasingly important at close range; the flies are often aware of movements at a considerable distance and will fly to investigate any large moving object in their environment. Such objects can include cars, trains, canoes and lake steamers as well as animals and people.

When not actively seeking food, the flies normally rest on woody elements of vegetation. Horizontal or inclined branches, 2–5 cm thick and 1–3 mm from the ground, are favoured resting sites during the day for most species. Resting flies are most numerous where such perches provide a good field of view, as along the edge of thickets or the margins of lakes and streams. Flies in the course of digesting a meal and females seeking to deposit larvae are found in more sheltered places. By night, both sexes of those species so far investigated change from their daytime resting sites on the larger woody elements, to spend the hours of darkness on leaves and small twigs; the change-over takes place very rapidly, during the last few moments of twilight, and a reverse movement occurs at first light in the morning. The change of resting sites has, perhaps, the function of protecting the flies from the activities of nocturnal predators. Challier[107] gives a valuable review of the ecology of tsetse; salient aspects are also considered by Molyneux and Ashford.[108]

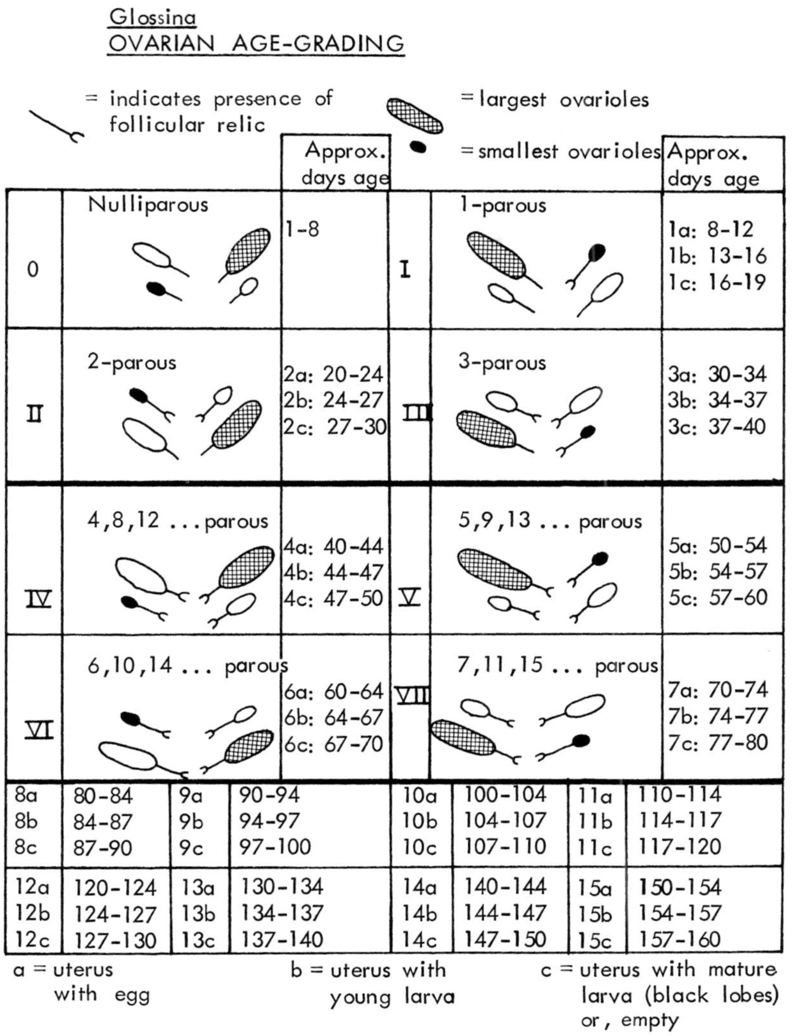

Glossina
OVARIAN AGE-GRADING

Figure IV.67: Ovarian age grading chart for female *Glossina* as seen in dorsal view. From cycles 0 to III an accurate estimation is possible; from cycles IV to VII (between the heavy lines in the figures) the estimate is subject to error because the same configuration is found in flies of different ages (e.g., 4, 8, 12 parous; 5, 9, 13 parous). The degree of wing fray (see Figure IV.66) is often a useful guide to which possible physiological age is the most probable. (Modified from Saunders[105] and Challier[106].)

Sleeping sickness vectors

G. palpalis, *G. fuscipes* and *G. tachinoides*

Until the closing years of the 1950s it was generally considered, firstly, that flies of the *palpalis* group were limited to, and dependent upon, the woody vegetation along streams and lake shores, and that the flies could not maintain themselves elsewhere except during limited sorties at favourable times of the year. Secondly, flies of the *palpalis* group were considered to be solely responsible for the transmission of Gambian sleeping sickness; while flies of the *morsitans* group transmitted only the acute, Rhodesian, type of disease. These distinctions are no longer completely tenable, although they remain as useful generalizations that apply under most circumstances. However, not only have *G. fuscipes* and *G. tachinoides* been implicated in epidemic outbreaks of the Rhodesian type of disease (*G. fuscipes* in Kenya and Uganda; *G.*

tachinoides in Ethiopia), but the same two species have been found (in Kenya and Nigeria) sometimes to live and breed in peridomestic environments far from water. It is now realized that neither species is quite so dependent upon particular vegetational associations as was formerly thought. Many instances of tsetse behaviour once labelled as atypical are now known to be quite commonplace: present-day views of the factors that influence tsetse ecology and behaviour, especially in relation to different types of vegetation, are now less rigid than was once the case.

Peridomestic pigs, sheep and dogs in West and Central Africa harbour *T. brucei* trypanosomes apparently identical to *T. b. gambiense* (on biochemical grounds, particularly isoenzymes) and appear to be significant reservoirs of the disease. Domestic pigs, moreover, are attractive to tsetse and can act as maintenance hosts for *palpalis* group flies. West African chickens are also reported naturally infected with *Trypanozoon* trypanosomes, but their importance (or otherwise) as reservoirs of human-infective organisms is unclear. In Burkina Faso (formerly Upper Volta) both hartebeest (*Alcelaphus* spp.) and kob, *Kobus* (*Adenota*) spp., harbour trypanosomes that are indistinguishable from *T. b. gambiense* by biochemical criteria. These game animals, and possibly other species, are now believed to be natural reservoirs of *T. b. gambiense* in West Africa. These recent observations, with both domestic livestock and game animals, call for a reassessment of the long-held view that there are no animal reservoirs of Gambian sleeping sickness; the evidence to the contrary is now incontrovertible and has obvious epidemiological implications.

In natural circumstances, where there is no close contact with humans and domestic animals, flies of the *palpalis* groups show a preference for feeding on large reptiles, such as monitor lizards and crocodiles. Reptiles form more than half of the feeds of wild flies in these conditions; bushbuck (*Tragelaphus scriptus*) account for about a quarter and other animals the remainder. Where humans and domestic animals are available, they too are attacked readily by species of the *palpalis* group. In circumstances where people, domestic animals and flies of the *palpalis* group come into close proximity (such as at river crossings, waterholes, etc.), people and their livestock become a major source of food for the flies, and sharp outbreaks of sleeping sickness are likely to occur, especially in the dry seasons when people, cattle and small populations of flies are likely to depend upon the same limited water sources.

G. morsitans, *G. pallidipes* and *G. swynnertoni*—the 'game' tsetse

Unlike flies of the *palpalis* group which commonly occupy waterside habitats of an essentially linear type, often intersected by patterns of human activity that may lead to close and personal contact, species of the *morsitans* group occupy vast areas of xerophytic woodland, dry bushland and thicket vegetation, particularly in the eastern parts of Africa. Under these conditions contact between humans, their livestock and the wild fly populations is seldom close and intense. Species of the *morsitans* group obtain most of their blood meals from the wild game animals, especially Bovidae and Suidae, that roam the savannahs and 'miombo' woodlands, and amongst which trypanosomes of the *T. brucei* subgroup are circulated and maintained as a zoonosis. Some of the zoonotic strains are infective to humans and give rise to symptoms, characteristically, of the acute Rhodesian type of disease. Human infections are, however, comparatively rare because of the infrequent and mainly accidental contact between the *morsitans* group and humans. The number of cases of Rhodesian sleeping sickness contracted in eastern Africa is very small in comparison with the number of mainly Gambian cases in West Africa and the Congo basin, where the human is a principal reservoir of infection, but almost certainly not the only one.

Exposure to *T. rhodesiense* strains is largely occupational: hunters, honey-gatherers, pole-cutters and charcoal-burners are among groups likely to enter fly-infested bush. In recent years the rapid growth of the tourist 'package' industry in East Africa has put another large group of itinerants at risk: the tourists themselves. Although species of the *morsitans* group are relatively little interested in people as a source of food when game animals are locally abundant, they often attack in sufficient numbers to be a considerable nuisance. Flies of the *morsitans* group are likely to acquire strains pathogenic to humans from previous feeds on bushbuck (the main proved reservoir) or other ungulates. In this latter category must be included domestic cattle; stocks of parasites that caused acute human disease in volunteers were first isolated during a localized outbreak in Kenya (Alego) some years ago. More recently, cattle isolates in Uganda (Busoga) were found to be indistinguishable from human-infective *T. b. rhodesiense* circulating in the human population during an epidemic outbreak, by isoenzymes and other intrinsic criteria. Cattle obviously act as a temporary reservoir—at any rate, under circumstances of human epidemic disease when challenge from animal trypanosomes is sufficently low to permit survival of the animals. Movement of cattle under these circumstances might also result in the dissemination of human-infective trypanosomes to new foci. Cattle can seldom be kept long in the presence of heavy or moderate fly infestations, however, because of the damaging incidence of infections with *T. vivax* and *T. congolense*.

Natural infection rates and methods of fly dissection

Infective metacyclic trypanosomes of the *T. brucei* subgroup (subgenus *Trypanozoon*) are found in the salivary glands of the tsetse fly. To reach their final station in the glands they undergo a complex migration in the fly that takes nearly 3 weeks to complete; hence it follows that only flies more than 3 weeks old can be infected with trypanosomes infective to humans. Even among older flies, infection rates with the *T. brucei* subgroup are always low (commonly 0.1% or less, rarely more than 1%), especially when compared with infection rates with the *T. vivax* (= *Duttonella*) and *T. congolense* (= *Nannomonas*) groups in the same flies. The *T. vivax* group has a short and simple life cycle in the fly; infection rates may reach 75% or more. The *T. congolense* group has a longer and slightly more complex cycle in the fly; infection rates may reach 18–25%.

The full dissection of a tsetse involves the removal and microscopic examination of the elongate salivary glands, the midgut and the mouthparts. There are several possible methods of dissection, but given some practice there is probably little to choose between them. The method preferred by the writer is as follows:

1. The fly is killed (with ether, chloroform or by judicious finger pressure against the sides of the thorax); wings and legs may be removed at this stage, or left.

Table IV.12 Haematophagous Reduviidae: tribes and genera of the subfamily Triatominae (Jeannel, 1919), with numbers of the 114 species in each genus: the most important genera are shown in bold.

Tribe	Genus	Number of species	Tribe	Genus	Number of species
Alberproseniini	*Alberprosenia*	1	Rhodniini	*Psammolestes*	3
				Rhodnius	**12**
Bolboderini	*Belminus*	4			
	Bolbodera	1	Triatomini	*Dipetalogaster*	1
	Parabelminus	2		*Eratyrus*	2
	Microtriatoma	2		*Linshcosteus*	5
				Panstrongylus	**13**
Cavernicolini	*Cavernicola*	1		*Paratriatoma*	1
				Triatoma	**66**

2. The fly is placed on a slide in a *small* amount of physiological saline (or 5% glucose solution).

3. The tough, membranous connection between head and thorax is 'frayed' carefully with the point of a needle to weaken it.

4. The proboscis is held (under a needle or with forceps) by the basal bulb and drawn slowly away from the head. With practice, the proboscis comes away from the head still attached to the salivary glands; continued slow, careful traction enables these to be pulled gradually clear of the body. If the glands break at this stage, they can be recovered later.

5. The labrum, hypopharynx and labium are preferably separated with needles and examined in saline under a coverslip. Alternatively, the intact semitransparent proboscis can be examined without separating the parts.

6. If removed with the mouthparts, the salivary glands are separated from the former and mounted in a small drop of saline under a coverslip.

7. If the salivary glands were broken during stage 4, the fly is now turned so that its abdomen lies flat on the slide, dorsal side uppermost. The thorax is pulled off and discarded, and needles are inserted through the two anterolateral corners of the abdomen, at a point roughly halfway from the corners towards the long axis of the abdomen, with sufficient pressure to pierce well below the dorsal integument. Firm traction in the direction of the forward corners of the abdomen, to tear them open, will usually result in the recovery of the glands at this stage; they may be recognized by their glass-like, refractile appearance. Continued needle traction will normally pull the glands clear of the abdomen, for examination in a separate drop of fresh saline under a coverslip.

8. With a needle or scalpel, the sides of the posterior tip of the abdomen are cut and the gut is extracted; the covering of fat body is stripped off with a needle and the gut is placed in a drop of saline, teased open and examined under a coverslip for the presence of trypanosomes.

Trypanosome infections of tsetse are identified, in the organs dissected, by reference to their location and morphology. Infections of the mouthparts only are likely to be by the *T. vivax* group; infections in the mouthparts and gut only are likely to be *T. congolense* or a mixed infection of *T. vivax* and *T. congolense* groups. Infections involving the salivary glands, gut and mouthparts certainly include the *T. brucei* subgroup but may also be complicated by the presence of *T. vivax*, *T. congolense*, or both. Gut and mouthpart infections could also include immature infections with *T. brucei* subgroup (Table IV.11).

Control of tsetse flies

The subject of tsetse control is large and complex—beyond the scope of this section. The interested reader is referred to Molyneux[109] for a useful discussion of tsetse control in relation to prevention and control of sleeping sickness generally, to Allsopp[110] for an account of insecticidal control methods, to Jordan[111] for a review of non-insecticidal methods of tsetse control, and also to Jordan.[112]

Cimicid and triatomine bugs (see also Chapter 74)

D. M. Minter

Order: Hemiptera; suborder: Heteroptera; family: Cimicidae

Genus: *Cimex*

Bed bugs (Cimicidae) have a worldwide distribution with well over 70 species; all are wingless and dorsoventrally flattened. The species parasitic on humans are: *Cimex lectularius* (Figure IV.68), the cosmopolitan bed bug, and *C. hemipterus* (= *rotundatus*), the common bed bug of the tropics, which is distinguished by its elongated narrow abdomen and the shape and proportion of the thorax (Figure IV.68). In West Africa a species of another genus, *Leptocimex boueti*, attacks humans. The body of *C. lectularius* is broad and flat, the head short and broad, attached to the thorax, the antennae four-jointed and the eyes present but reduced in size. The mouthparts consist externally of a segmented rostrum (proboscis) and are normally folded

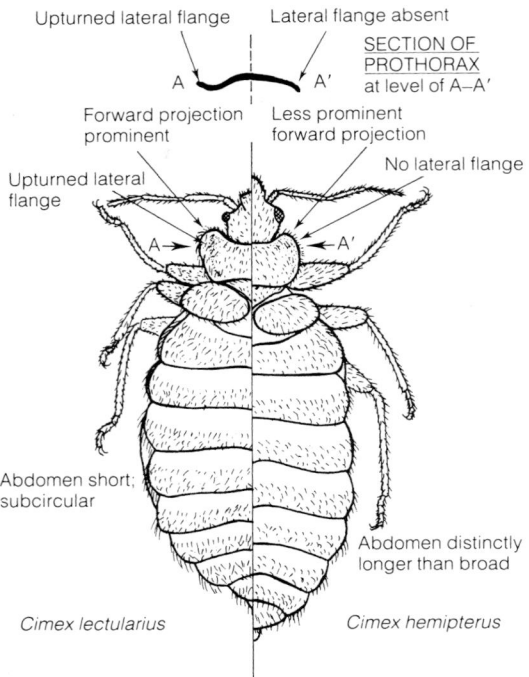

Upturned lateral flange   Lateral flange absent

SECTION OF
PROTHORAX
at level of A–A'

Forward projection prominent   Less prominent forward projection

Upturned lateral flange   No lateral flange

Abdomen short; subcircular

Abdomen distinctly longer than broad

Cimex lectularius   *Cimex hemipterus*

Figure IV.68: Comparison between *Cimex lectularius*, the common bed bug (left), and *C. hemipterus*, the tropical bed bug (right), when viewed from above.

back under the head. The maxillae are serrated at the tip. On the thorax of the adults are short pad-like hemielytra, which are vestigial forewings. Both sexes of *Cimex* feed only on blood and can resist starvation well. The labium does not pierce the skin, but buckles up during feeding like that of a mosquito. The bodies of bugs give out a nasty pungent odour. Bed bugs are nocturnal in their feeding habits, hiding in crevices during the daytime. The eggs are ovoid and operculated, and are cemented on to the surfaces of the crevices of woodwork in houses, beds, mattresses, behind pictures and in nail-holes. Aggregations of bugs can be located by finding the black faeces round holes.

The females deposit eggs in daily batches from 10 to 50, totalling 200–500. They are large, about 1 mm in diameter, yellowish-white and easily visible to the naked eye. The five successive nymphal stages resemble adults, but have no hemielytra; they mature in about 6 weeks if fed at each stage, but can resist starvation for up to 2 months. Under less favourable conditions, development may be protracted for 6 months or more. Adults may live for many months. Bed bugs are sensitive to high temperatures: even 37.8°C with a fairly high humidity will kill many. A cheap and effective control method is fumigation with sulphur. The dosage necessary varies from 0.34 to 0.74 kg/28 m³, with an exposure time of at least 6 hours. Sulphur dioxide is cheap and, owing to its smell, free from hazard(s). It kills the active stage of the bug, but a few eggs may escape, and complete combustion must be assured.

Hydrocyanic acid fumigation is very effective, but dangerous, and has been largely superseded by the use of insecticides; 5% DDT emulsion, 2% malathion, 0.5% diazinon or 0.5% dichlorvos, or 0.1–0.2% pyrethroids which act as an irritant and cause bugs to leave their hiding places.

Although bed bugs can cause a great deal of irritation by their bites, it has not actually been proved that they disseminate disease, with the possible exception of viral hepatitis (see Chapter 40).

Family: Reduviidae; subfamily: Triatominae

Triatomine bugs are also known as 'cone-nose', 'kissing' or—erroneously—'assassin' bugs; they have many local names in America, including chinchas (Mexico), chipo (Venezuela), barbeiro (Brazil) and vinchucha (Argentina). The group includes more than 100 species, divided into five tribes and 14 genera (Table IV.12). Both sexes and the five nymphal stages feed solely on vertebrate blood. The triatomine bugs are one of more than 20 subfamilies of the family Reduviidae; all the other subfamilies are predators of other insects and are the true 'assassin' bugs. Many species of the predatory Reduviidae are, however, capable of inflicting a painful bite, usually in self-defence, but they do not feed on blood. Many superficially resemble the haematophagous Triatominae but can be distinguished by the presence of a rostrum that is frequently curved and is always rigid and inflexible. The triatomines have a three-segmented rostrum that is always both straight and flexible; at rest it lies closely applied to the ventral aspect of the head and more or less parallel to it. Its extreme tip normally lies in a finely ridged stridulatory groove in the anteroventral part of the thorax. (The triatomine genera *Linshcosteus* and *Cavernicola* are unusual in that they lack this sound-producing stridulatory mechanism, in which the tip of the rostrum acts as a plectrum.)

The outer and visible part of the rostrum is the modified labium, which forms a protective sheath for the paired stylet-like mandibles and maxillae. During the act of feeding, the rostrum is swung forward (about 120°) in front of the head and is neither flexed nor telescoped; the tip of the labium rests on the surface of the skin and the apically serrate mandibles penetrate the epidermis and anchor the mouthparts in place. The smooth, lanceolate, maxillary stylets then penetrate deeply and perforate small blood capillaries. The maxillae enclose the salivary duct and the food canal and form the functional mouth. The bite of triatomines is generally painless—but by no means always. This explains why sleeping people are seldom wakened by the bite of bugs and can be bitten repeatedly in the course of the night.

In common with other Heteroptera, the adult triatomines have two pairs of functional wings; the forewings are hardened basally (the corium and clavus) and membranous distally. Thus they are referred to as hemielytra. The posterior wings are membranous throughout and lie beneath the hemielytra at rest. The wings are folded

Table IV.13 Insecticides for vector control (based on WHO[114]).

Insecticide*	Residual application			Space-spray	Larvicide
	Indoors	Perifocal	Bed-nets		
Organochlorine					
DDT	+	–	–	–	–
Organophosphate					
Temephos	–	–	–	–	+
Malathion	+	+	–	+	+
Fenitrothion	+	+	–	+	+
Pirimiphos-methyl	+	+	+	+	+
Carbamate					
Bendiocarb	+	+	+	+	–
Propoxur	+	+	–	–	–
Pyrethroid					
Bioresmethrin	+	–	–	+	–
Permethrin	+	+	+	+	–
Deltamethrin	+	+	+	+	–
Lambda-cyhalothrin	+	+	+	+	–
Cyfluthrin	+	–	+	–	–
Others					
IGRs	–	–	+	–	+
Bacterials	–	–	–	–	+

*Application rates vary according to circumstance, as per local registration authority and manufacturer's instructions.

scissor-like over the back of the bug and the lateral margins of the abdominal tergites are visible; these are often colour banded and are a useful taxonomic feature. Female bugs, viewed from above, have a broad ovate abdomen which is generally pointed posteriorly; males have a more slender abdomen with a fully rounded posterior end. The plate-like male external genitalia can easily be seen in lateral and ventral view. Female bugs are generally rather larger than males.

The visible dorsal part of the thorax consists of a large trapezoidal pronotum, usually rigid and provided with tubercles. Behind the pronotum and visible between the sclerotized bases of the hemielytra, is a triangular scutellum which is strongly pointed posteriorly. The ground colour of the triatomines is usually brownish or black, often relieved with flashes of colour (mainly shades of red, yellow or orange) on thorax and abdomen. Eyes are usually black, but white- or pink-eyed mutants are not uncommon. Adults, unlike all nymphal stages, have paired dorsal ocelli posterior to the prominent compound eyes.

The proportions of the head in lateral view are useful to separate the three genera of main medical importance (Figure IV.69). The head of *Rhodnius* is elongated with long four-jointed antennae arising close to its apical portion. In *Triatoma* the head is shorter and the antennae are inserted midway between the eye and the forward tip of the head. In the genus *Panstrongylus* the head is stouter and shorter, with the antennae arising close to the eye. See also Figures IV.70–72.

The five nymphal stages are essentially miniatures of the adult but lack wings; in the fifth nymphal stage the 'wing pads' are prominent on either side of the

scutellum. Triatomines are generally quite large insects, usually between 20 and 28 mm long in the adult female. Some genera contain species that are only about 5 mm long as adults, and the Mexican *Dipetalogaster maxima* is the giant of the triatomines, attaining a length of nearly 4.5 cm. Lent and Wygodzinsky[113] give comprehensive keys to genera and species.

Reproduction and life cycle

Female triatomines commence egg laying 10–30 days after copulation; eggs are laid singly or in small groups, either unattached or cemented to the substrate, depending on species. The ovoid, operculate, fresh eggs are whitish; in some species they later turn through pink to cherry-red; in other species the original colour is maintained. The number of eggs laid in life by a female depends upon species and external factors, but about 500 is normal and 1000 not uncommon. Virgin females will also lay eggs, but these are few in number and infertile. Eggs hatch after 10–30 days; the emerging first-stage nymph is initially pink and soft-bodied but hardens sufficiently to take its first blood meal within 48–72 hours of leaving the egg. At least one full blood meal is required by each nymphal stage, sometimes more, before the moult to the next stage can be initiated.

All triatomines have a long life cycle, even in hot climates; the average is about 300 days from egg to adult, although some species may take up to 2 years. *Rhodnius* spp. develop more rapidly than *Triatoma* and *Panstrongylus* and can reach maturity in 3–4 months.

Ocellus

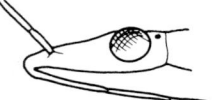

Insect-predatory reduviid
Proboscis curved (mainly)
and rigid

Haematophagous members (Triatominae):
Proboscis straight and flexible

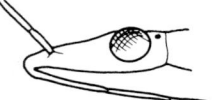

Rhodnius
Head long
Antennae forward
Examples: *R. prolixus,*
R. pallescens

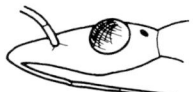

Triatoma
Head medium length
Antennae median
Examples: *T. infestans,*
T. dimidiata

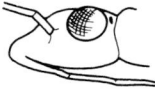

Panstrongylus
Head short
Antennae close to eye
Example: *P. megistus*

Figure IV.69: Lateral view of the head of an insect-predatory reduviid (top) with usually *curved* and always *inflexible* proboscis which serves to distinguish it from the haematophagous genera of the subfamily Triatominae, all of which have a proboscis that is *straight* and *flexible* (bottom row). The proportions of the head and the site of insertion of the antennae serve to separate members of the triatomine genera *Rhodnius*, *Triatoma* and *Panstrongylus*.

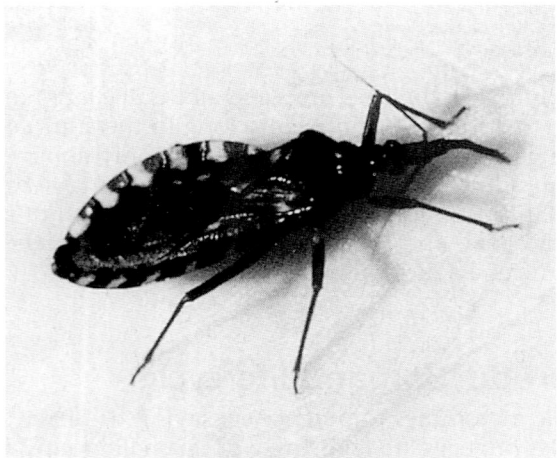

Figure IV.70: Genus *Triatoma*. Head of intermediate length, with antennae set midway between eyes and front of head. The specimen illustrated is a female *Triatoma infestans*, with its proboscis directed forwards whilst feeding. The ground colour is black with yellowish markings on the lateral edge of the abdomen, legs and hemielytra. Males are 21–26 mm long, females 26–29 mm. Nymphal stages lack the colouration seen in the adult. (Courtesy of T. V. Barrett.)

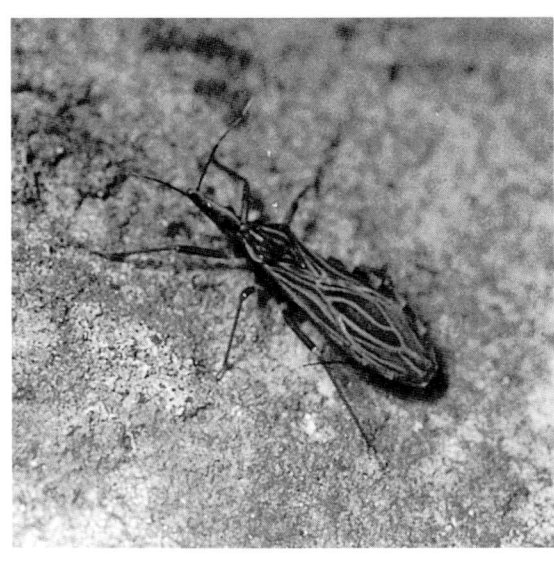

Figure IV.71: Genus *Rhodnius*. Head long, antennae set well forward. The specimen shown is an adult male *Rhodnius prolixus*, males are generally less than 20 mm in length, females up to 21.5 mm. General colour pale brown; lighter markings on thorax and forewings give the overall impression of longitudinal stripes. Nymphal stages have less obvious 'pepper and salt' markings. (Courtesy of C. J. Webb.)

Geographical distribution

The five tribes occur in tropical and subtropical areas of the neotropical region. Members of one tribe, the Triatomini, have species that are also found in the oriental region. The Triatomini also marginally enter the Australasian region. The subfamily is entirely absent from the Palaearctic and Afrotropical (= Ethiopian) regions, but *T. rubrofusciata* has been spread to all the major tropical ports by human agency. This species is always closely associated with *Rattus* spp., among which it transmits the rat trypanosome *Trypanosoma (Megatrypanum) conorhini*. Other endemic, and purely sylvatic, species of the tribe Triatomini (members of the *T. rubrofasciata* group) occur in south China, Malaysia, Indonesia, Papua New Guinea and the extreme north-east of Australia. The other group of Oriental Triatomini is the genus *Linshcosteus* (six closely related species), which occurs only in India.

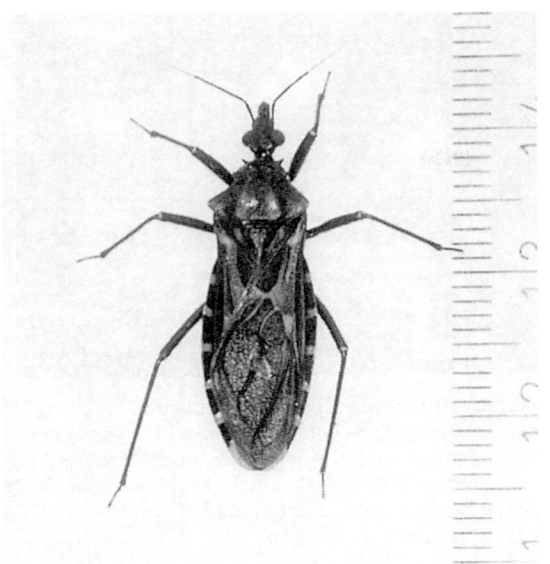

Figure IV.72: Genus *Panstrongylus*. Head short, with antennae set close to the eye. The male *Panstrongylus megistus* illustrated is black in overall colour with red, or reddish-brown, markings on the lateral margins of the abdomen, thoracic pronotum, and scutellum and hemielytra (forewings). The nymphal stages lack the prominent colouration of the adults. The specimen shown measures 25 mm; females are slightly larger.

The bulk of the Triatominae (four of the five tribes) occur exclusively in the neotropical region: the Rhodniini (the important genus *Rhodnius* and the genus *Psammolestes*) are found from Central America to Argentina; the neotropical species of Triatomini, principally the members of the genus *Triatoma*, range from the northern USA to Patagonia. The genus *Panstrongylus*, the second largest in the Triatomini, with 13 species, extends from Central America to Argentina.

Habitat of neotropical triatomines

All triatomines are dependent on the blood of vertebrates (principally mammals and birds, occasionally reptiles) for survival, development and reproduction. The primary habitat of triatomines is thus in or near the shelters, roosts, burrows and nests of a variety of wild animals, prominent amongst which are marsupials (e.g., *Didelphis* (Figure IV.73), *Marmosa*), edentates (e.g., *Dasypus*), rodents (*Rattus*, *Neotoma*), carnivores, bats and birds. Many of the animals and birds find their main shelter in palm fronds or in arboreal epiphytic bromeliads (Figure IV.74), under fallen logs or in hollow trees. Triatomines also occur under rocks, under loose bark and in stone walls, and feed on the local rodents or lizards.

A number of triatomine species have the ability to colonize the artificial habitats created by humans. Some species seldom penetrate further than the peridomestic area (stables, cattle enclosures, chicken houses, pigsties, etc.), which provide a rich food source. A relatively few species are able to colonize the extensive crevice habitat that is provided by the simple homes of the Latin American

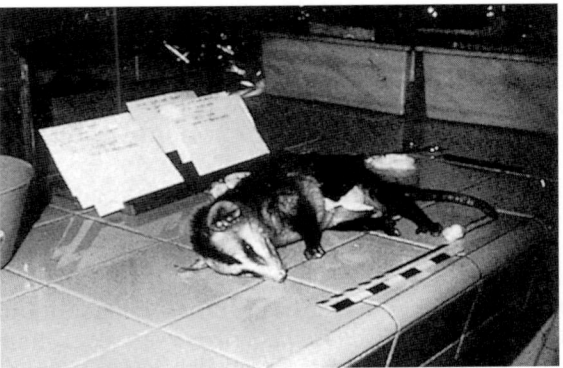

Figure IV.73: The common opossum, *Didelphis* spp., the cat-sized sylvatic marsupial most frequently naturally infected with *Trypanosoma cruzi* throughout the Americas. The animal shown is *D. albiventris* (= *D. azarae*) from Brazil and is anaesthetized whilst undergoing xenodiagnosis and collection of tail blood for microscopic and serological investigation.

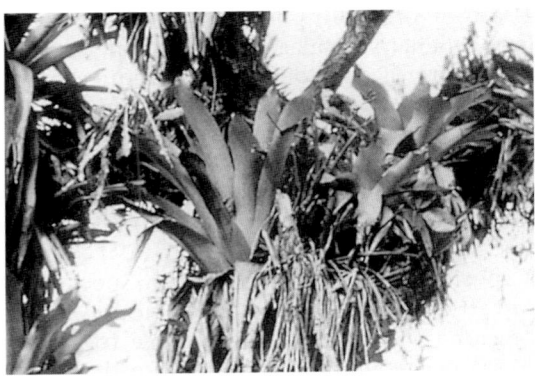

Figure IV.74: Arboreal epiphytic bromeliads (commonly species of the genera *Aechmea* and *Holmbergia*) are frequently the nesting habitat of marsupials, rodents and birds, and are thus also a natural biotope of many sylvatic triatomine species.

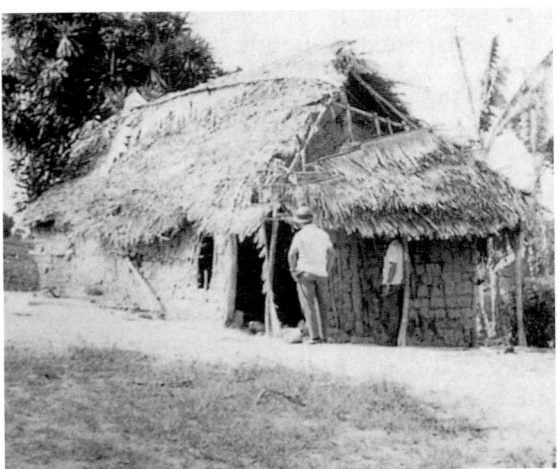

Figure IV.75: Characteristic palm-thatched, mud-and-wattle Latin American peasant house of the type often infested with domiciliary triatomine species. The deep cracks in the mud walls provide ideal harbourage for large populations of *Rhodnius*, *Triatoma* or *Panstrongylus*.

peasant majority. These houses are usually constructed from mud and wattle or unplastered adobe brick and roofed with palm fronds (Figure IV.75). More sophisticated houses with smooth plastered walls and roofs of tile or corrugated sheet are less readily and heavily colonized, often being very lightly infested or not at all. The more traditional and basic peasant house, made from local materials, may support a triatomine population that can run into thousands, particularly of *Rhodnius prolixus* or *Triatoma infestans*.

Although probably all triatomines will support the development of *Trypanosoma cruzi* (well over half the species have been found infected in the wild), it is only relatively few species that have the capacity to colonize human dwellings which are of overriding medical importance as the domiciliary vectors of Chagas disease to humans. By virtue of their wide geographical distribution and large domiciliary populations, together with the large human population in the areas they occupy, the three species *Rhodnius: prolixus*, *Triatoma infestans* and *Panstrongylus megistus* are of prime importance. Other species of the same three genera (particularly *Triatoma* spp. and especially *T. dimidiata*) are of considerable importance on a lesser geographical scale (e.g., *T. dimidiata*, *T. barberi*, *T. brasiliensis*, *T. pallidipennis*, *T. phyllosoma*, *R. pallescens* and *R. ecuadorensis*).

It is possible to divide the triatomines into convenient groups based on their association, or lack of it, with human dwellings.

Most species are fully sylvatic, a few species as flying adults are attracted by light and enter houses (when they may occasionally bite) but seem unable to colonize; an example is the geographically widespread *Panstrongylus geniculatus*, normally closely associated with the burrows of its usual host, the armadillo (*Dasypus* spp.). Others, such as *T. brasiliensis*, are attracted by lights into houses and may establish small domiciliary or peridomestic populations. Species such as the Central American *T. dimidiata* live normally in hollow trees but are often passively transported to houses (in firewood) and form large colonies. *T. sordida* is found naturally in a variety of habitats in the central and southern parts of South America, including crevices among tree bark; it readily adapts to fence-posts and timber outbuildings but never forms large domiciliary populations. This may be because it is regularly found in houses together with heavy infestations of *T. infestans*; in Venezuela and elsewhere in northern South America, *T. maculata* is in a somewhat similar situation when small populations are established in houses among heavy infestations of *R. prolixus*. Both *T. sordida* and *T. maculata* may have the potential to form epidemiologically significant domiciliary populations if and when the major domiciliary species are controlled or eradicated by insecticidal treatment. Much the same happened in southern Brazil when *T. infestans* was controlled by insecticides and within a few years large numbers of *Panstrongylus megistus* (until then a purely sylvatic species in that area) had replaced it as the domiciliary vector of *Trypanosoma cruzi*.

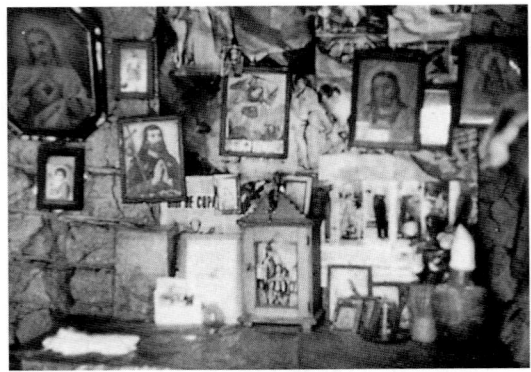

Figure IV.76: Many peasant homes incorporate a domestic shrine such as that shown here; a central case houses the family saints and the walls nearby are covered with pictures, both sacred and profane. Sites such as these are often the principal hiding places for bugs not located in the bedroom walls and furniture.

Within human habitations, triatomines prefer to hide during the day in dark and moist places; the extensive crevice habitat provided by unplastered cracked walls of mud or mud-brick can support large populations. Smaller numbers are found among furniture, boxes and, particularly, beds and bedding. Others occur among clothes hanging from pegs in the walls, or behind pictures (Figure IV.76). Some species also readily colonize palm roofs (e.g., *R. prolixus*). Other species are rarely found in the roof (e.g., *P. megistus*).

Most frequently, bugs are found by day close to the areas in which they will encounter sleeping hosts at night—bedrooms are normally the most heavily infested parts of the house. As a rule, the feeding behaviour of domiciliary triatomines is governed more by proximity to a suitable host than by specific host preference.

Some entirely or essentially sylvatic species, however, are normally associated with particular hosts: *Cavernicola pilosa* is always associated with bats, and all three species of *Psammolestes*, *T. platensis* and *T. delpontei* are found only in the nests of birds. *P. geniculatus* has a close link with burrows of armadillos; *Paratriatoma hirsuta* and species of the *T. protracta* group prey exclusively on *Neotoma* spp., the wood rat (although adults not infrequently fly into houses, attracted by lights, they never colonize; perhaps this is in some way connected with their dependence on wood rats).

All stages of triatomines, in particular the larger nymphal stages, have a remarkable ability to endure long periods of starvation (up to several months). The adults are in general poor fliers and probably take flight only when their nutritional status is poor and their weight lowest, to disperse at random to seek new habitats with new hosts on which to feed. For domiciliary species in particular, passive transport by human agency is probably responsible for nearly all house-to-house dispersal, on or in domestic goods including furniture and clothes. Triatomines of various species have been recovered from the baggage of passengers on long-distance buses and lorries, and occasionally even in aircraft. Some species of *Rhodnius* may be transported long distances as young nymphs, or as eggs, in the feathers of large migratory birds (*Jabiru mycteria* (jabiru) and *Mycteria americana* (American wood ibis)) when these leave their nests, in which bugs live and breed, on seasonal migration.

Role of triatomines as vectors of *Trypanosoma cruzi* and *Trypanosoma rangeli*

Other blood-sucking arthropods can be infected experimentally with *Trypanosoma cruzi*, but only triatomines are important in the epizootiology and epidemiology of Chagas disease (and of the less important apathogenic trypanosome affecting people in the neotropical regions, *Trypanosoma* (*Herpetosoma*) *rangeli*). Chagas disease is a zoonosis, and probably all triatomines are potential vectors of *T. cruzi*, although *T. rangeli* is naturally infective only to species of the genus *Rhodnius* (mainly *R. prolixus*, but also *R. pallescens* and *R. ecuadorensis*). Species of *Triatoma* can be infected experimentally with *T. rangeli*, but they are rarely infected in the wild. So far as the importance of triatomine species in transmission of *T. cruzi* to humans is concerned, only a relatively few species of bugs are actual and effective vectors.

Because of the contaminative (and hence inefficient) method of transmission of *T. cruzi* in the faeces of the invertebrate, only those bug species that defecate whilst feeding on the human host are able to be effective vectors. Furthermore, only in species that are capable of colonizing houses in large numbers and feeding predominantly from humans, and to a lesser extent their household animals (cats, dogs, chickens, etc.), is contaminative transmission sufficiently intense to lead to a high probability of successful infection among householders, given a high infection rate among the triatomine population. For a domiciliary vector to be of major epidemiological importance, it is also necessary for it to have a wide geographical range.

Of the relatively few triatomine species that fulfil the above criteria, *T. infestans* is the outstanding example in view of its wide occurrence in South America (from 10°N to 40°S and from Atlantic to Pacific coasts). In this extensive area it is almost exclusively a domiciliary species and the geographical range has often been extended by passive movement as a result of human agency. It is an aggressive and active species with a relatively short life cycle, which helps it to compete successfully fully with other longer-lived species (such as *P. megistus*) which are also domiciliary and which *T. infestans* tends to displace if introduced accidentally.

There are no domiciliary triatomine species in the broad expanse of the Amazon basin, but to the north of this area *R. prolixus* is the main species of epidemiological importance; it is found predominantly from about 3°N (Colombia, Venezuela, the Guyanas) from sea level to an altitude of over 2000 m, and ranges to about 20°N in Mexico. It is the major domiciliary vector of Chagas disease in Colombia and Venezuela, and is one of several important species in Central America. Throughout its range it is also the main vector of *T. rangeli* to wild and domestic animals, as well as to humans. Unlike *T. infestans*, it has an extensive extradomiciliary biotope; particularly important is its frequent occurrence in species of palm trees (where it is found in the nests of mammals and birds), which are frequently used as roofing materials for houses. Among the palms infested, the genera *Attalea* and *Acrocomia* are widespread and numerous (Figure IV.77). *R. prolixus* also occurs in the palms *Copernica* and *Leopoldina*.

In the densely populated areas of the eastern seaboard of Brazil, *Panstrongylus megistus* is the important domiciliary triatomine; in the southern part of its range, it also occurs in sylvatic foci, but further north it is confined to houses, perhaps because the almost total destruction of the original coastal forest vegetation in this area, over the past four centuries, has rendered conditions unsuitable for its survival in the wild. Alternatively, *P. megistus* may have been transported passively from south to north by human agency, but for various reasons this explanation seems less likely.

T. dimidiata is a highly variable species in colouration, etc., and was until recently divided into three subspecies (*T. d. dimidiata*, *T. d. maculipennis* and *T. d. capitata*) which are no longer recognized. The species is an important domiciliary vector in Ecuador, Peru and Central America as far as 22°N in Mexico.

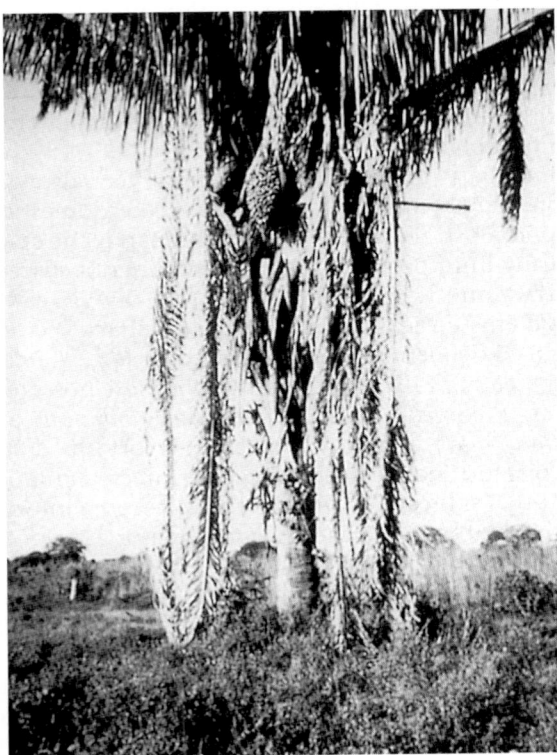

Figure IV.77: Palm tree (*Attalea humboldtiana*), sylvatic habitat of *Rhodnius prolixus* in Venezuela. Several genera and species of palm tree are a principal habitat of many triatomine species throughout Latin America, associated with the nests of various mammals and birds that inhabit the crowns and dependent fronds.

The northern limit of domiciliated triatomines, and hence essentially that of human Chagas disease, is to all intents and purposes the Tropic of Cancer: isolated cases have occurred in Texas and elsewhere in the southern USA, but none of the several sylvatic triatomines present has become domiciliated, although some are natural vectors of *T. cruzi* in wood-rat colonies. Housing standards in the areas of the USA where bugs naturally occur are such that colonization by triatomines is in any event unlikely.

Feeding behaviour of triatomines

All triatomines take large blood meals relative to their own body weight; the actual quantity varies greatly from stage to stage and from species to species; the larger bugs obviously take larger quantities.

The first-stage nymphs at their first feed take up 10 times their own body weight; successive stages take progressively less in terms of body weight, but more in actual quantity. In volumetric terms the fifth-stage nymphs take the largest feed; this represents about three to four times their body weight. Adult bugs of both sexes take less blood than at the fifth stage, but feed more often: on each occasion about two or three times their own body weight.

Blood meal identifications have been made by precipitin tests and other methods for many species of bugs in different geographical areas and variously from sylvatic, peridomestic and domestic ecotopes. In general terms, the results show that sylvatic species in the wild feed primarily on marsupials (especially the common opossum, *Didelphis* spp.), rodents, birds and edentates (e.g. armadillos, *Dasypus* spp.), bats, and occasionally reptiles and amphibians.

Domiciliary bug populations, however, always feed predominantly upon humans. Often, the domestic host fed upon most frequently after the human is the epidemiologically unimportant chicken (birds are not susceptible to *T. cruzi* infection).

Different species of important domiciliary vector may either feed frequently on cats and/or dogs (e.g., *T. infestans*, *T. dimidiata*) or feed infrequently from these hosts (e.g., *R. prolixus*, *P. megistus*). In the case of *T. infestans* and *T. dimidiata*, cats and/or dogs are important domestic reservoirs for Chagas disease, because infected animals are a perpetual source of *T. cruzi* and bugs become infected by feeding on them. Neither *R. prolixus* nor *P. megistus* in houses feeds on cats or dogs to any significant extent and these animals, even if infected, thus provide little or no feedback of trypanosomes into the domestic bug population and are thus an epidemiological dead end.

The species of domiciliary bugs so far investigated differ in the frequency with which blood from different hosts can be detected in the same individual triatomine. As blood proteins are detectable in bugs for up to 100–120 days, the occurrence of many individual meals of mixed origin in a bug population suggests that the bugs are frequently changing from one type of host to the other; a low frequency of multiple blood meals indicates that individuals are feeding repeatedly from the same host species. A high rate of feeds on humans, combined with a low rate of feeds from other sources, especially of mixed feeds, clearly indicates that bug-mediated transmission occurs from person to person, rather than from animal to human. This is the situation found with domiciliary *R. prolixus* and *P. megistus*, in Venezuela and Brazil, respectively. Domestic populations of *T. maculata* (in Venezuela) and of *T. sordida* (in Brazil) feed predominantly from the uninfectable chicken; these species are therefore of very little epidemiological importance in the domestic transmission cycle.

Triatomines can become infected with *T. cruzi* (and/or *T. rangeli*) at any stage in their life from their first feed onward. Once infected with *T. cruzi*, the infection probably almost always persists for life; infection rates found in different stages rise from a small proportion in the first-stage nymphs to levels approaching or exceeding 90% among fifth-stage nymphs and adults. Bugs appear in no way to be adversely affected by infection with *T. cruzi*. Unlike *T. cruzi*, however, *T. rangeli* is pathogenic to its invertebrate hosts and causes a disturbance in the moulting mechanism, such that the moult is delayed and the mortality rate during moulting is significantly increased. In adult bugs infected with *T. rangeli*, there is also a reduction in the number of eggs laid by females and a decrease in egg viability.

Because, particularly where *R. prolixus* is the domiciliary vector, mixed infections of bugs, animals and humans by *T. cruzi* and *T. rangeli* are common, it is frequently necessary to distinguish the two parasites, in both vertebrate and invertebrate hosts. The bloodstream stages are easily separable by their distinctive morphology; the stages in the bug can be less readily distinguished, except when trypomastigotes occur in the haemolymph and salivary glands (always *T. rangeli*). Infective forms of *T. rangeli* and *T. cruzi* in the rectum of bugs are difficult to separate without recourse to animal inoculation and study of the bloodstream stages. *T. rangeli* can certainly be transmitted to vertebrates and humans by the inoculative route when trypomastigotes occur in the salivary glands. There is controversy, however, as to whether contaminative infection by *T. rangeli* (via trypomastigote forms shed in the faeces) occurs to any significant extent, or at all (see also Chapter 74).

Transmission cycles of *Trypanosoma cruzi*

The possible cycles and their interrelationship, in bug-mediated *T. cruzi* infections of animals and humans are summarized in Figure IV.78. Zoonotic cycles involve the majority of the 114 triatomine species currently recognized and some 120 species and subspecies of mammals. Foremost among the mammalian hosts closely associated with sylvatic triatomines, and therefore frequently infected with *T. cruzi*, are the marsupials of several genera, particularly *Didelphis* spp., which occupy a range that is more than coextensive with that of *T. cruzi*: *Didelphis* spp. play a role

TRANSMISSION CYCLES OF TRYPANOSOMA CRUZI

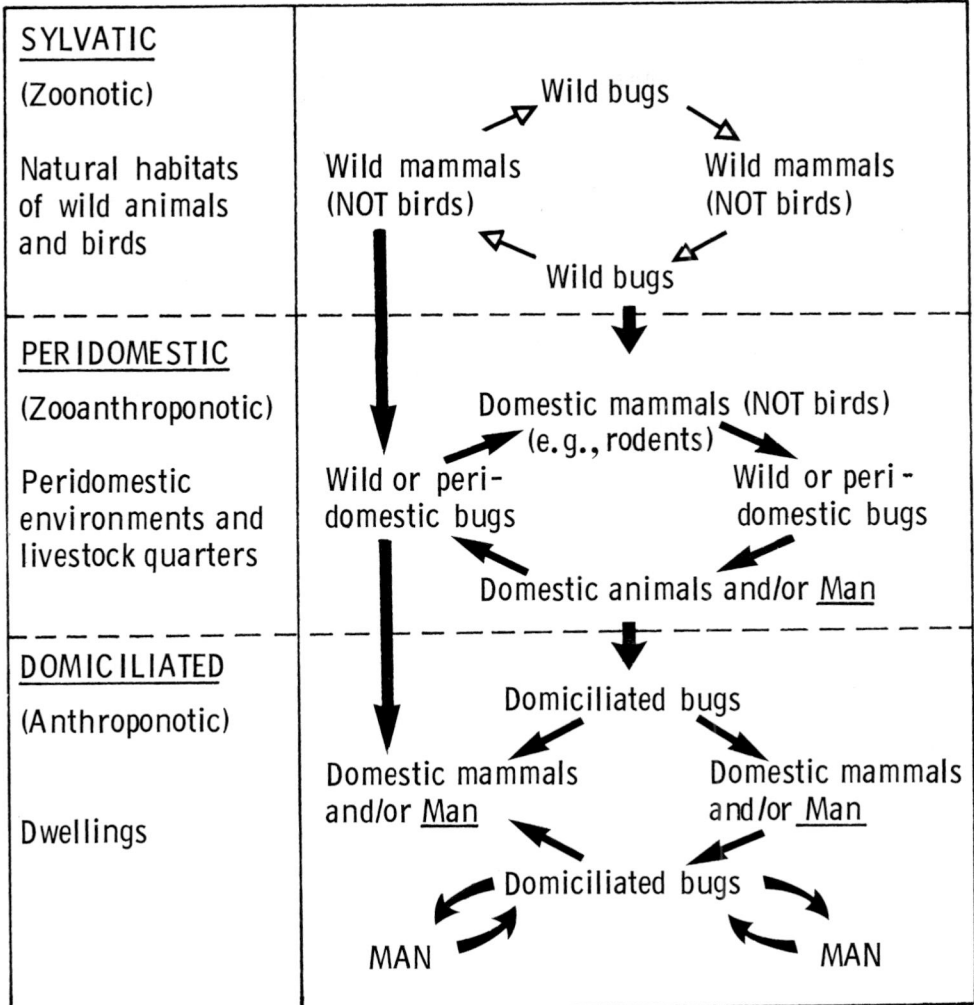

Figure IV.78: Transmission cycles of bug-mediated *Trypanosoma cruzi* infection.

in the epizootiology and epidemiology of *T. cruzi* that is in some respects reminiscent of that of the bushbuck in the case of *Trypanozoon* trypanosomes in eastern Africa. The cat-sized *Didelphis* (see Figure IV.73) are carnivorous and nocturnal, and are among the last wild animals to be disturbed by human activities. They frequently enter houses and outbuildings to search for food, steal eggs, etc., and often roost in the roofs of houses or in trees near by. They are thus well placed to introduce sylvatic *T. cruzi* strains into the peridomestic and domestic environments. Sylvatic triatomines, already infected with *T. cruzi*, may fly into houses or be carried in on palm fronds for roofing or among firewood. Strains of *T. cruzi* circulated in houses by domiciliary species are probably most frequently transferred between houses passively, either by passive transfer of infected bugs or by movement of infected people from house to house and from place to place.

Infected sylvatic rodents frequently visit outbuildings to feed on stored grain and other foodstuffs and may introduce new parasites from the wild into the peridomestic area. *Rattus* spp. and *Mus musculus* in houses are not infrequently infected with *T. cruzi*, but they probably become infected by ingesting bugs, rather than by being fed upon. In turn, rats and mice form a source of infection for cats and dogs by the oral route, and no doubt hunting dogs and foraging cats frequently eat infected sylvatic animals. It should again be emphasized, however, that neither sylvatic nor domestic birds are ever a source of *T. cruzi* because they are totally insusceptible to infection, possibly owing in part to their higher body temperature, among other factors. The role of cats and dogs within the domestic cycle has been discussed earlier in relation to the feeding behaviour of domiciliary triatomines. The role of infected rats and mice in houses can be assessed in a similar way and, from available evidence, it would seem that they are rarely of direct importance in the household epidemiology of Chagas disease. Although the larger domestic animals, such as pigs, are susceptible to *T. cruzi* and are sometimes fed upon by peridomestic/domestic triatomines (e.g., *T. infestans*, *P. megistus*, *T, dimidiata*), it is noteworthy that natural infections have been found only very rarely in pigs, rabbits and other larger domestic animals, which thus appear to play no significant role in the transmission of the parasite or in its transfer from sylvatic to peridomestic circumstances.

Once domiciliary transmission is established in the presence of large bug populations, transmission of *T. cruzi* is chiefly human–bug–human, and new human infections can occur among uninfected family members at a relatively high rate; among two families (20 persons) living in bug-infected premises in Brazil followed by serological testing and xenodiagnosis for 4 years, four new parasitologically confirmed infections occurred (a rate of 4% per annum); if two individuals with conversion to positive serology (but negative to xenodiagnosis on a single occasion) were included, the annual rate of new infections was 7.5%.

Because the contaminative method of transmission of *T. cruzi* by bugs is inherently an inefficient mechanism, a heavy trypanosome challenge over a long period from biting and defecating bugs is probably necessary for infection to occur. This is probably linked with the fact that young children are seldom infected (except congenitally or via maternal milk) until they are between 2 and 3 years of age, even under conditions of heavy challenge. Rates of infection among children are already high, however, among 5–10 year olds and rise further in older age groups.

Xenodiagnosis and epidemiology

The parasitological diagnosis of *T. cruzi* infection suggestive of present or future chagasic symptomatology can be made by conventional blood film microscopy only in the initial febrile stage of acute infection, which many infected individuals fail to experience. In the later chronic indeterminate stage of the disease, parasitological diagnosis becomes increasingly difficult, because the parasitaemia falls below the level at which it can be detected by routine methods, including standard concentration techniques. It has been shown that haemoculture is a sensitive diagnostic technique, but because only immotile amastigote stages may develop in cultures initially, much skill and experience are required to detect positive cultures in the first weeks, sometimes months, for which they need to be examined until the motile stages appear in sufficient numbers. The method of haemoculture is also difficult to use in the field.

If triatomine bugs are grown in laboratory culture under conditions that preclude the possibility of their infection with pathogenic organisms (in Latin America this is usually ensured by feeding them on pigeons or chickens), are then allowed to feed in sufficient numbers on individuals suspected to be infected with *T. cruzi*, kept for several weeks (usually about four) and examined for the presence of *T. cruzi* in their rectum, this will often

result in the unequivocal detection of parasites and is the process termed xenodiagnosis; the triatomines act as a 'living culture' for the trypanosomes. This technique is expensive, unaesthetic and time consuming, but it is effective and has the great advantage that it can be used under field conditions. Technical details (number of bugs, species and stage) vary from one laboratory or hospital to another, as does the method of examination of the bugs used (expression of a faecal drop, dissection and examination of the entire rectal contents of the individual, or pooling and maceration of batches of bugs) and there is much need for increased standardization. There is clear evidence from several sources that local 'strains' of vector are generally most susceptible to infection by the local parasite and that microscopical examination of the rectal contents of individual bugs is more sensitive than the expressed faecal drop or pooling methods; the latter, however, are often adopted for routine purposes because they save time and effort. Whenever possible it is advantageous to use fifth-stage nymphs in xenodiagnosis, because these take the largest feed and increase the possibility that a low parasitaemia may be detected. In practice, a minimum number of bugs to use would be five fifth-stage nymphs allowed to feed in the dark for about 30 minutes in a secure gauze-covered container; 10 or 20 bugs would be preferable but not always possible for logistical reasons. Repeated xenodiagnosis on several occasions also increases the number of successful diagnoses. On an experimental basis, the 'smaller' instars of the very large *Dipetalogaster maxima* gave results comparable to those with fifth-stage nymphs of the main 'standard' xenodiagnosis species (*R. prolixus* and *T. infestans*), with a saving of time and expense on colony maintenance. 'Artificial xenodiagnosis' is now widely used in Venezuela, in which bugs feed through a membrane on venous blood drawn from the patient. This is claimed to be more acceptable and equally successful as conventional xenodiagnosis.

Xenodiagnosis clearly has many disadvantages, and a better and more effective method of parasitological diagnosis is obviously desirable as a back-up for the increasingly improved serological tests now available. Serological tests, by their nature, detect antibodies to parasite antigen rather than the parasites themselves.

Not only are triatomines the principal means by which people become infected with *T. cruzi* (and *T. rangeli*), but bugs build up large domiciliary populations and these are a significant source of blood loss in many households. Calculations show that, in houses in Venezuela with heavy infestations of *R. prolixus*, monthly blood loss was in the order of $100 \, cm^3$ per person per month. Occasionally individuals become sensitized to bug bites and may suffer severe allergic reactions as a result. This phenomenon may also be a complicating factor in xenodiagnosis.

Roughly the same number of people—about 250 million in each case—live in countries affected by African trypanosomiasis and in areas of Latin America affected by Chagas disease. In Africa there are often fewer than 5000 new (treatable) infections annually. In Latin America, for diagnostic and logistical reasons, the number of new (and essentially incurable) cases each year is unknown, but crude estimates suggest up to 850 000 new infections per annum. At any one time, about 24 million people are seropositive for *T. cruzi* and a further 65 million at risk in endemic areas. Serological surveys in various countries indicate that between 5 and 10% of national populations are infected.

The magnitude of the problem which such figures suggest is immense. Unlike sleeping sickness, there is no safe and effective chemotherapy, and diagnosis of Chagas disease is more difficult; early case detection and treatment are therefore of little value. Ultimately may come the development of an effective vaccine; meanwhile, improvements in standards of new and existing houses (in the latter case, particularly by individual or community-based self-help measures), and increased public health awareness in general, would help to diminish transmission levels to a considerable degree, but alone are probably insufficient to achieve interruption of disease transmission.

Control of Chagas disease vectors

Triatomine control on a large scale must rely on house-spraying with residual insecticides (see Table IV.13).[114] Nowadays pyrethroids such as deltamethrin, cyfluthrin and lambda-cyhalothrin have become the most economical and effective products of choice, but their effects may be negated by active or passive reinvasion. Insecticide resistance has occurred (with dieldrin in Venezuela) but has not become a widespread or serious problem, although it remains a daunting threat everywhere. It is undoubtedly because of the long generation time of triatomines that resistance has yet to become a practical difficulty.

Improved cost-effectiveness of insecticidal treatments can be achieved with slow-release formulations, including paints and mastics applied to wall surfaces.

Simple and cheap methods to improve existing rural houses offer an attractive alternative to the regular use of insecticides, particularly if householders are encouraged, possibly even subsidized, to undertake the work themselves. The plastering of mud walls and/or the replacement of palm-thatched roofs by corrugated metal or plastic sheets, or locally made tiles, drastically reduces the crevice habitat available to the various domiciliary triatomine species, and hence the level of infestation. A durable and crack-resistant wall plaster can be made from sand, cattle dung, earth and lime. Lime can often be prepared cheaply from local limestone, by firing it overnight in a suitable kiln fuelled by wood or charcoal.

The mud used to build new mud-and-wattle houses can be stabilized to resist erosion, shrinkage and cracks; this can be done by adding lime, cement or bitumen (to make 'asfadobe'). Hand-operated hydraulic and mechanical rams are available which produce compressed, stabilized, soil building blocks with properties similar to those of fire bricks. The initial capital investment is relatively high (about US $2000), but the machines are rugged and durable; each family that uses the press can produce enough blocks to build a house within a week, by their own unskilled labour, and for the cost only of the small amount of lime or cement necessary to stabilize the local soil. The machines can be adapted readily to produce roof and floor tiles, or liners for pit latrines. Allied with an energetic campaign of health education, and measures to encourage community participation, much could be achieved by the application of simple house improvement measures on a wide scale, particularly if this was integrated with the use of insecticides, especially at the start. For further information, see Schofield.[115]

Fleas (see also Chapter 63)

G. B. White

Order: Siphonaptera

Fleas are small (length 1–4 mm) and wingless, with laterally compressed bodies composed of a blunt head, compact thorax and a relatively large rounded abdomen (Figure IV.79). In colour they are usually dark brown as adults. Eyes and antennae are small, the latter being modified in males for clasping the female from below during copulation. When not extended, each antenna lies in a groove on the side of the head. This groove may be extended as a strengthening bar within the head from eye to eye (e.g., in *Pulex*). Ventrally the head bears a series of appendages for sensory and feeding functions: paired maxillary palps at the front, slender epipharynx and paired maxillary laciniae form the proboscis, with basal stipes and paired labial palps posteriorly.

Within the thorax, the oesophagus leads to a crop or proventriculus with a constriction before the capacious stomach in the abdomen. Patches of strongly barbed spines protrude into the proventricular lumen so that blood

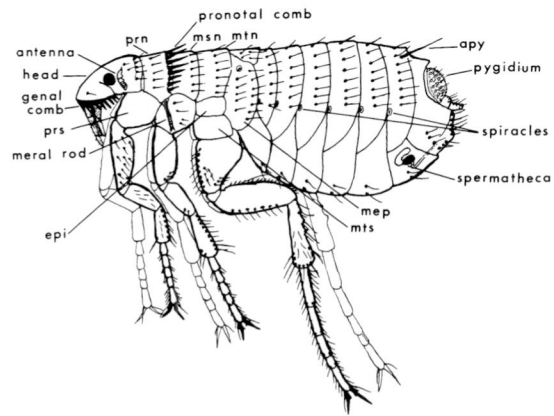

Figure IV.79: Lateral view of an adult female flea showing some of the principal taxonomic features. apy, Antepygidial bristle; epi, episternum; prn, pronotum; prs, prosternum; mep, metepimeron; msn, mesonotum; mtn, metanotum; mts, metepisternum. The meral rod (mesopleural rod) or vertical bar is present in most genera but absent from *Pulex*, the human flea.

corpuscles may be ruptured as they pass towards the stomach for digestion. Plague vectors, such as *Xenopsylla* spp., have large proventricular spines on which plague bacilli accumulate and multiply, tending to promote thrombus formation and blocking of the proventriculus. Bacilli may then be regurgitated when the flea next tries to feed, so that transmission to another host occurs.

The bodies of adult fleas bear many characteristic setae and spines. The lower margin (gena) of the head and the hind edge of the prothorax are sometimes modified to form cuticular teeth or combs (ctenidia). The size and positions of combs, spines and setae are important in relation to the taxonomy and identification of genera and species of flea. All three pairs of legs are strongly developed, the hindlegs being longest and the forelegs shortest. At the base of each midleg the mesopleuron is usually strengthened with a vertical rod of cuticle internally. Many species of flea can jump to a height of several metres for purposes of reaching hosts or escaping capture. Flea jumps are powered by a mechanism involving energy storage in the thoracic arch, which consists of cuticles impregnated with resilin, a rubbery protein. Tension is built up by the thoracic muscles and released to kick the hindlegs.[116] General information on the anatomy and biology of fleas is summarized by Smit[117] and by Traub and Starcke.[118]

Adult fleas of all species are obligate, temporary ectoparasites of birds (6%) or of mammals (94% of flea species). More than 2000 species of flea have been described and are classified into some 200 genera. They are moderately host-specific, meaning that each kind of flea tends to infest only one or a few kinds of host. Humans are frequently attacked by fleas from domestic or wild animals, as well as by the human flea *Pulex irritans*. Development takes place in the nests of particular hosts, including human dwellings. For some flea species (e.g., the European rabbit flea *Spilopsyllus cuniculi*, but not the human flea, cat flea or dog flea), host hormone levels may influence reproductive cycles of the associated fleas

so that flea breeding coincides with host nesting.[116] The period of development from egg to pupa is 2 weeks or more, depending on temperature. The active white larvae (Figure IV.80B) have sparse hairs and a small but strong head capsule. Development takes place among dust and litter in the nest of the host, or indoors among fabrics or between floorboards. Larvae feed on organic debris and may require nutrient fragments of dried blood defecated by adult fleas. There are two larval instars before the pupal stage.

Flea pupae are encased in a cocoon, loosely spun by the larva around itself. Hatching of the adult may be delayed for months until the proximity of a host (vibration, warmth) stimulates emergence. Adult fleas can survive actively and away from the host for many weeks, provided that the climate is not too harsh. In general fleas thrive at temperatures of 20–30°C and humidities of 60–90%. Host temperatures (i.e., 35–42°C) actually inhibit egg hatching and larval development, which is why breeding on the host does not normally occur. Below about 8°C development ceases and adult fleas become lethargic.

Female fleas tend to be larger than males of the same species. Both sexes feed regularly on blood and so become liable to transmit pathogens from host to host. Recognition of the female depends on presence of the

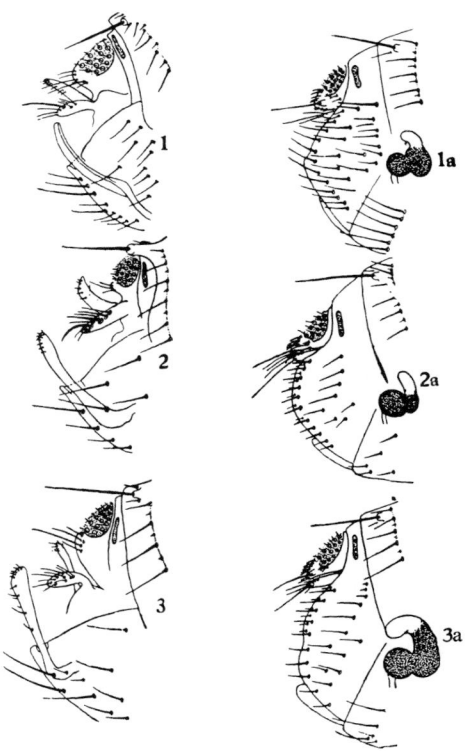

Figure IV.81: Diagnostic characters of the three widespread species of *Xenopsylla* rat fleas. 1, *X. astia*, male terminalia; 1a, *X. astia*, female terminalia with spermatheca; 2, *X. brasiliensis*, male terminalia; 2a, *X. brasiliensis*, female terminalia with spermatheca; 3, *X. cheopis*, male terminalia; 3a, *X. cheopis*, female terminalia with spermatheca. These species all possess the generic characteristics of a strong mesopleural rod, but no combs on head or pronotum.

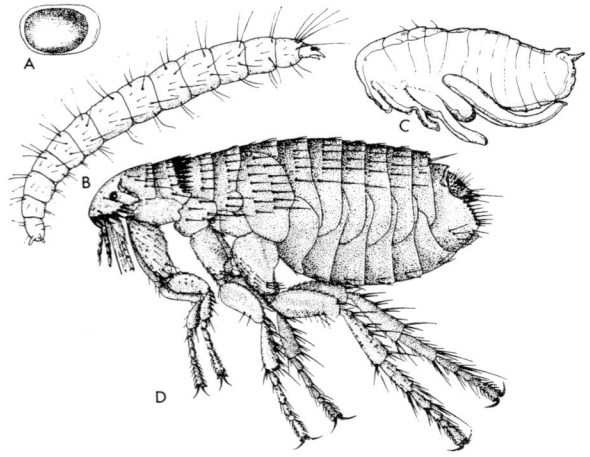

Figure IV.80: Life stages of a flea. **A**, egg; **B**, larva; **C**, pupa; **D**, adult female.

spermatheca within the posterior abdomen (see Figures IV.79 and IV.81), whereas the male abdomen includes a conspicuous, curved phallosome for eventration during copulation.

Relatively large, sticky, white eggs are produced by female fleas at a rate of 10–25 per day, being dropped indiscriminately among host fur or feathers or on the floor. In warm situations the eggs hatch within 2–3 days.

Identification keys for important genera and species of fleas in all parts of the world have been provided by Smit.[117] Specimens for identification should first be soaked for 1 or 2 days in 10% caustic soda to clear them before being washed and slide-mounted. Non-specialists should be cautious in trying to identify fleas, because many species are confusingly alike; The following guidelines may help to distinguish the genera that attack humans most frequently:

1. Head rounded, combs absent: *Pulex* or *Xenopsylla*. Mesopleural rod present: *Xenopsylla*; absent: *Pulex*. Cephalic bar present above eyes: *Pulex*; absent: *Xenopsylla*.
2. Head biangular anteriorly, combs absent: *Echidnophaga*.
3. Head sharply pointed anteriorly, combs absent, post-abdomen with large spiracles: *Tunga*.
4. Head and prothorax with combs: *Ctenocephalides*.
5. Head without comb, prothorax with comb: *Nosopsyllus*.
6. Head with comb and with two spines anteriorly, eyes absent: *Leptopsylla*.

Family: Pulicidae

The members of this family, being fleas without ctenidia (combs), include several species of medical importance both as pests and as disease vectors.

Pulex irritans, the human flea, is an ubiquitous pest of humans, prevailing in many temperate and tropical situations. It is also commonly associated with various other coarse-coated mammals, both wild and domestic, especially dogs and pigs. Occasionally suspected of bubonic plague transmission from human to human, *P. irritans* is more certainly the vector responsible for vesicular and tonsillar plague outbreaks in Ecuador. Five other *Pulex* spp. are known, of which *P. simulans* also sometimes attacks humans in North and South America and is distinguished by laciniae longer than those of *P. irritans*. Like many other fleas found in houses, *P. irritans* occasionally acts as an intermediate host of the dog tapeworm *Dipylidium caninum*, which may infect humans and is usually transmitted via *Ctenocephalides* fleas.

Xenopsylla cheopis, the oriental or black rat flea, normally infests *Rattus rattus* in urban situations throughout the world, but is scarce in parts of the northern temperature zone. It frequently attacks people in rat-infested buildings, and is the classical vector of epidemic plaque (*Yersinia pestis*) and of murine typhus (*Rickettsia mooseri*) from rat to rat and from rat to human. Other *Xenopsylla* spp. fulfil similar roles regionally, notably *X. brasiliensis* in tropical Africa where it thrives in wattle huts; the species has spread to parts of India and South America (hence its

name). The equivalent endemic Indian flea is *X. astia*. Diagnostic differences between these three common species of *Xenopsylla* are depicted in Figure IV.81. The rat tapeworm *Hymenolepis diminuta* produces eggs that may be ingested by *Xenopsylla* larvae. Intestinal infection of rodents and sometimes children results from eating adult fleas in which cysticercoids have formed. Some strains of *H. nana*, the dwarf tapeworm of humans, may also be transmitted from rat to rat via *Xenopsylla* spp.

Echidnophaga gallinacea, the sticktight flea of poultry, sometimes also infests dogs, cats, rabbits and other animals, and can be a nuisance to people. Unlike most other fleas they stay attached to the host for prolonged periods and may copulate while feeding. *E. gallinacea* tends to cluster on the head of chickens, which scratch and injure themselves to such an extent that blindness may ensue. Ulceration of the host is often caused by sticktight fleas, and the females are said to oviposit deliberately into such wounds. Usually, however, development takes place in the litter of poultry houses.

Ctenocephalides is a small genus of nine species found mainly on carnivores in Africa and Eurasia, with two species that have become generally distributed: *C. canis* and *C. felis*, the dog and cat flea, respectively. Actually, each of these species infests both cats and dogs interchangeably and *C. felis* tends to be found more often on both kinds of host. In modern centrally heated homes in temperate countries, *C. canis* and *C. felis* often thrive, sometimes in the temporary absence of cats and dogs. Recurrent infestations of these species may be more of a nuisance to humans than is *P. irritans*, especially in developed countries where intermittent domestic control cannot eliminate *Ctenocephalides* spp. Cat and dog fleas are characterized by pronounced ctenidial combs on the gena (ventral edge of head) and posteriorly on the prothorax. Figure IV.82 shows how *C. felis* has a relatively longer head than *C. canis*. The dog tapeworm *Dipylidium caninum* produces eggs that may be ingested by *Ctenocephalides* larvae. Intestinal infection of cats, dogs and sometimes of humans results from eating adult fleas carrying cysticercoids. A similar life cycle involving *Ctenocephalides* is sometimes followed by strains of

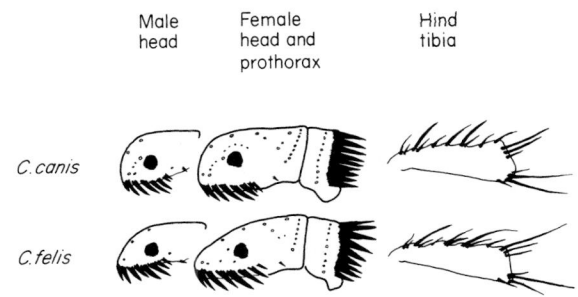

| Male head | Female head and prothorax | Hind tibia |

C. canis

C. felis

Figure IV.82: *Ctenocephalides* fleas possess rows of comb teeth (ctenidia) below the head and posteriorly on the prothorax. *C. felis*, the cat flea, has a relatively longer and more pointed head than *C. canis*, the dog flea. On the hind tibia, the number of posterior notches bearing strong setae is eight in *C. canis* and six in *C. felis*.

Hymenolepis nana, the human dwarf tapeworm, which usually does not have an intermediate host.

Family: Leptopsyllidae

Leptopsylla segnis, the European mouse flea, is frequently found indoors in various parts of the world. It also infests rats and sometimes transmits enzootic plague, but seldom bites humans.

Family: Ceratophyllidae

Ceratophyllus gallinae, the European chicken flea, has spread to many parts of the world, has a wide range of bird hosts, and occasionally invades houses and attacks people. It is a particularly large flea with a painful bite. Unlike *Echidnophaga*, it drops off the host directly after feeding. An equivalent North American species is *C. niger*, the western chicken flea. Numerous comb teeth on the pronotum facilitate the identification of *Ceratophyllus* spp.

Nosopsyllus fasciatus, the brown rat flea, has also become widespread with its main host *Rattus norvegicus*; it also infests *R. rattus* and many other small mammals and often attacks humans, but is seldom involved in plague transmission. Like *Ctenocephalides*, *N. fasciatus* serves as an intermediate host of the dog tapeworm *D. caninum* which may infect humans if infective fleas are eaten.

Family: Tungidae

Tunga penetrans, the sand flea or jigger (chigoe, chique), has females adapted for intracutaneous permanent attachment on the host. *T. penetrans* regularly infects humans, pigs, poultry and other creatures in Central America, West and East Africa, and parts of the Indian subcontinent. As for other fleas, the larvae are free-living—dusty or sandy soil being best for *T. penetrans*. Adults are also free-living at first, when copulation occurs. The fertilized female then finds a suitable host and tries to penetrate crevices in the skin, such as cracks in the soles of the feet (see Chapter 19), between the toes and especially around the toenails. Any part of the human anatomy can be affected. By means of the mouthparts, the female *Tunga* becomes firmly attached and soon swells to the size and shape of a small white pea. Somehow, the host skin envelops the jigger, which lies below the stratum corneum but above the stratum granulosum, leaving only the posterior spiracles exposed to the air. Only when the jigger is almost mature and distended, after 8–12 days, does the infection begin to irritate. Severe inflammation and ulceration ensue, so that scratching helps to expel large numbers of white eggs from the jigger. With skill and care it is possible to remove the whole insect, using a needle or forceps, but often the soft abdomen ruptures leaving the head attached in the lesion.

The jigger seldom attacks the leg above the dorsum of the foot, but no part of the body is immune. The soles (Chapter 19), the skin between the toes and that at the roots of the nails are favourite sites. Usually only one or two jiggers are found at a time, but occasionally they are present in hundreds, the small pits left after extraction or expulsion being sometimes so closely set that parts of the surface may look like a honeycomb. During her gestation the jigger causes a considerable amount of irritation. In consequence of this, pus may form around her distended abdomen which now raises the integument into a pea-like elevation. After the eggs are laid the superjacent skin ulcerates and the jigger is expelled, leaving a small sore which may become infected, sometimes causing phagedaena or even tetanus. Ulceration is common and may follow removal of the jigger or natural extrusion of the egg sac. The ulcer commences as a tiny pit and, as it extends, the sloping edge may develop into a septic ulcer. It remains more or less circular in outline, except under the nail or nail margin, where the outline is more irregular and a pocket of pus forms beneath it. Chronic absorption of pus may lead to thrombophlebitis.

Medical importance and control of fleas

More than 50 genera and numerous species of fleas have been implicated as vectors of enzootic plague in various parts of the world (Chapter 63), meaning that they maintain the transmission of *Yersinia pestis* bacilli among rodents. Humans are seldom infected primarily through the bites of such zoophilic fleas, except when infected *Xenopsylla* move on to a human after plague-stricken rats have died. Rarely are conditions conducive for person-to-person transmission by *Pulex* or *Ctenocephalides* to reach epidemic proportions. Overwintering of plague bacilli may occur in hibernating fleas.

Various flea species may also be involved in the transmission cycles of murine typhus, tularaemia, pseudotuberculosis, melioidosis, brucellosis, lymphocytic choriomeningitis and possibly other diseases.[119] Only the first depends on fleas, as well as parasitic mites and lice, as vectors. Thus the agent of murine typhus, *Rickettsia typhi* (= *R. mooseri*), is commonly transmitted by *X. brasiliensis*, *X. cheopis*, and possibly *N. fasciatus* or *L. segnis*, with a similar epidemiological picture to that of plague.[120]

As mentioned above, some fleas serve as the intermediate hosts for tapeworms usually found in animals: *Dipylidium caninum* of dogs and cats; *Hymenolepis diminuta* of rodents; *H. nana* strains endemic in rodents. These occasionally cause diarrhoea in humans, especially children who may happen to become infected by eating infective fleas.

People suffer localized dermal reactions to flea bites, which can be soothed with antihistamines. Generalized allergic sensitization is not uncommon and should be overcome by means of flea control in preference to desensitization treatment of the patient. The irritation and nuisance caused by fleas crawling on the body surface and the pain of their frequent probing and biting always justify control measures.

Simple hygienic measures of keeping houses well swept and floors washed and clean are beneficial, and the regular use of a vacuum suction cleaner is highly effective for gathering up fleas, their eggs and larvae. When flea-infested premises are re-entered after a period of disuse, newly emerged fleas may become activated and attack people in surprising numbers. Temporary relief may be gained through the use of insect repellent creams or lotions based on dimethylphthalate, diethyltoluamide, indalone and proprietary brands. Floors can be treated with a solution of naphthalenes in benzene, or simply with detergents. Synthetic chemical insecticides should be sprayed or dusted into corners, cracks and fabrics where flea larvae may be expected to occur. The value of DDT for such purposes has become diminished by the problem of insecticide resistance in many areas. Various organophosphates, carbamates and pyrethroids are ample substitutes, but compounds with high mammalian toxicity should not be used indoors. Flea-ridden domestic animals may themselves be washed thoroughly with carbolic soap, dusted with pyrethroid powder, treated with insecticidal lotion or shampoo (e.g., malathion) or fitted with a 'flea collar' made from plastic impregnated with dichlorvos which has a prolonged, localized vapour action within the fur. For direct killing of fleas it is convenient to employ spray canisters giving aerosols of synergized pyrethrins or similar quick-acting insecticides.

The particular personal problems caused by sand fleas or jiggers (*T. penetrans*) have already been mentioned. Affected areas of soil may be burnt off in an effort to kill them, and their breeding on livestock and pets should not be allowed. As female jiggers are not good jumpers, human infestation is normally confined to the feet. Daily inspection of the interdigital clefts, roots of nails and soles of feet should cause freshly burrowing female jiggers to be detected and removed before they have grown significantly. To prevent their attack, good shoes should be worn at all times. An old deterrent is to rub the feet with lysol or creosol in paraffin oil; modern repellents may be better.

In locations where *T. penetrans* is common, the local people become quite skilful at removing them with sharp instruments. The characteristic, circular, open lesions should be dressed antiseptically and protected until healed. Often they become ulcerated and secondarily infected; local pus production may occur, and be complicated by thrombophlebitis or gangrene. Timely use of antibiotics is therefore advisable and the affected limb should be rested.

REFERENCES

1 Kettle DS. *Medical and Veterinary Entomology*. London: Croom Helm, 1984.
2 Riley J. *Adv Parasitol* 1986; 15:46–128.
3 Khalil GM. *F Egyptian Public Hlth Assoc* 1972; 47:363–369.
4 Zumpt F. *Myiasis in Animals and Man in the Old World*. London, 1965.
5 Smith KGV (ed.) *Insects and Other Arthropods of Medical Importance*. London: British Museum (Natural History), 1973.
6 Landi 1960.
7 Dar MS, Ben Amer M, Dar EK et al. *Trans R Soc Trop Med Hyg* 1980; 74:303.
8 Zumpt F. *S Afr Med J* 1963; 37:305–307.
9 World Health Organization. *World Health Organ Tech Rep Ser* 1984; 701:140.
10 Lanson R & Shaw JJ. The role of animals in the epidemiology of South American leishmaniasis. In Lumsen WHR & Evans DA (eds) *Biology of the Kinetoplastida*, vol. II. New York: Academic Press, 1979:1.
11 Peters CJ & LeDuc JW. Bunyaviruses, phleboviruses and related viruses. In Belshe R B (ed.) *Textbook of Human Virology*. Littletton, MA: PSG Publishing, 1985:547–598.
12 Lewis DJ, Young DH, Fairchild GB et al. *Syst Entomol* 1977; 2:319–332.
13 World Health Organization. *Manual on Practical Entomology in Malaria*. Geneva: WHO, 1975.
14 Knight L L & Stone A. *A Catalog of the Mosquitoes of the World*. The Thomas Say Foundation, vol. VI. College Park: Entomological Society of America, 1977 (Supplement 1978).
15 Dennis PT, Partomo F, Durnomo AA et al. *Am J Trop Med Hyg* 1976; 25:797.
16 Reid JA. *Anopheline Mosquitoes of Malaya and Borneo*. Studies from the Institute for Medical Research, Malaysia, no. 31. Kuala Lumpur: Government of Malaysia, 1968.
17 White GB. *Mosquito System* 1968; 10:13.
18 Carpenter SJ & La Casse WJ. *Mosquitoes of North America*. Berkeley, CA: University of California Press, 1974.
19 Gillies MT & de Meillon B. *The Anophelinae of Africa South of the Sahara*. Johannesburg: South African Institute for Medical Research, 1968.
20 Garnham PCC. *Malaria Parasites and Other Haemosporidia*. Oxford: Blackwell Scientific Publications, 1966.
21 Kalra SL. *J Commun Dis* 1978; 10:1.
22 Webber RH. *Trans R Soc Trop Med Hyg* 1979; 73:722.
23 White GB. *Trans R Soc Trop Med Hyg* 1974; 68:278.
24 Zavortink TJ. *Contrib Am Entomol Inst* 1973; 9:1.
25 Faran ME. *Contrib Am Entomol Inst* 1980; 15:1.
26 Le Duc JW. *J Med Entomol* 1979; 16:1.
27 Dutary BE & Le Duc JW. *Trans R Soc Trop Med Hyg* 1981; 75:128.
28 Belkin JN. *Mosquitoes of the South Pacific*. Berkeley, CA: California University Press, 1962.
29 Huang YM. *Mosquito System* 1977; 9:289 (also Document WHO/VBC/76. 654, WHO/FIL/76.143).
30 Huang YM & Hitchcock JC. *Contrib Am Entomol Inst* 1980; 17:1.
31 MacDonald WW. Mosquito genetics in relation to filaria infections. *Symp Br Soc Parasitol* 1967; 14:1.
32 Christophers SR. *Aedes aegypti (L.), the Yellow Fever Mosquito*. London: Cambridge University Press, 1960.
33 McClelland GAH. *Trans R Entomol Soc Lond* 1974; 126:239.
34 Powell JR, Tabachnik WJ & Arnold J. *Science NY* 1980; 208:1385.
35 McIntosh BM. *Mosquitoes as Vectors of Viruses in South Africa*. Entomology Memoir no. 43. Pretoria: Department of Agricultural and Technical Services, 1975.
36 Arnell JH. *Contrib Am Entomol Inst* 1973; 10:1
37 Belkin JN, Heinemann S L & Page W A. *Contr Am Ent Inst* 1970; 6:1.
38 Bram RA. *Contrib Am Entomol Inst* 1967; 2:1.
39 Sirivanakarn S. *Contrib Am Entomol Inst* 1976; 12:1.

40   Southgate BA. *Trop Dis Bull* 1979; 76:1045.

41   Sasa M. *Human Filariasis*. Tokyo: University of Tokyo Press, 1976.

42   Sirivanakarn S. *Contrib Am Entomol Inst* 1982 (in press).

43   Maslov AV. *Ent Obozrenie* 1967; 43:193 (English trans. *Ent Rev, Wash*, 43:97.)

44   Wharton RH. *Bulletin No 11*. Institute for Medical Research, Federation of Malaya, 1962.

45   Bates M. *The Natural History of Mosquitoes*. New York: Macmillan, 1949.

46   Gillett JD. *Mosquitoes*. London: Weidenfeld & Nicholson, 1971.

47   Harbach RE & Knight KL. *Taxonomists' Glossary of Mosquito Anatomy*. Marlton, NJ: Plexus Publishing, 1980.

48   Harwood RT & James MT. *Entomology in Human and Animal Health*. New York: Macmillan, 1979.

49   Horsfall WR. *Mosquitoes—Their Bionomics and Relation to Disease*. New York: Ronald Press, 1955.

50   Mattingly PF. *The Biology of Mosquito-borne Disease*. Science of Biology Series, No. 1. London: Allen & Unwin, 1969.

51   Service MW. *Mosquito Ecology: Field Sampling Methods*. London: Applied Science Publishers, 1976.

52   Edwards FW. *Mosquitoes of the Ethiopian Region. III.—Culicine Adults and Pupae*. London: British Museum (Natural History), 1941.

53   Hopkins GHE. *Mosquitoes of the Ethiopian Region. I.—Larval Bionomics of Mosquitoes and Taxonomy of Culicine Larvae*. London: British Museum (Natural History), 1952.

54   Mattingly, PF. *Bull Br Mus (Nat Hist) (B)* 1952–3; 2:233; 3:1.

55   Gerberg EJ & van Someren, ECC. Document WHO/VBC/70.236, 1970.

56   Cordellier R, Germain M, Hervy JP et al. *Guide Pratique pour L'Etude des Vecteurs de Fièvre Jaune en Afrique et Méthode de Lutte*. Initiations, Documentations, Techniques, No. 33. Paris: Office de la Recherche Scientifique et Technique Oure-Mer, 1977.

57   Lane J. *Neotropical Culicidae*, vols 1 and 2. São Paulo: University of São Paulo, 1953.

58   Forratini OP. *Entomologia Médica*, vol. 1. *Anophelini*. São Paulo: E Blucher and University of São Paulo, 1962.

59   Forratini OP. *Entomologia Médica*, vol. 2. *Culicini: Culex, Aedes e Psorophora*. São Paulo: E Blucher and University of São Paulo, 1965.

60   Wood DM, Dang PT & Ellis RA. *The Mosquitoes of Canada. The Insects and Arachnids of Canada*, Part 6. Hill, Quebec: Agriculture Canada, 1980.

61   Darsie RF & Ward RA. *Identification and Geographical Distribution of the Mosquitoes of North America*. Fresno, CA: American Mosquito Control Association, 1981.

62   Mattingly PF & Knight KL. *Bull Br Mus (Nat Hist) (B)* 1956; 4:89.

63   Lee DJ. *An Atlas of the Mosquito Larvae of the Australasian Region. Tribes Megorhinini and Culicini*. Australian Military Forces, 1944.

64   Lee DJ & Woodhill AR. *The Anopheline Mosquitoes of the Australasian Region*. Department of Zoology, University of Sydney, Monograph 2, 1944.

65   Dobrotworsky N V. *The Mosquitoes of Victoria*. Melbourne: Melbourne University Press, 1965.

66   Marks EN. *An Atlas of Common Queensland Mosquitoes*. St Lucia: University of Queensland, 1973.

67   Ribeiro H, Ramos HC, Capela RA et al. *Estudios, Ensaios e Documentos, no. 135*. Lisbon: Junta de Investigacoes Cientificås do Ultramar, 1980.

68   Dahl C & White GB. In Illies J (ed.) *Limnofauna Europaea*. 1978: 390–395.

69   Christophers SR. *Fauna Br India* 1933; 4:1.

70   Bhatia ML, Kalra NL, Rao VV et al. *Vectors of Malaria in India*. Delhi: National Society of India for Malaria and Other Mosquito-Borne Diseases, 1961.

71   Barraud PJ. *Fauna Br India* 1934; 5:1.

72   Tanaka K, Mizusawa K & Saugstad E S. *Contrib Am Entomol Inst* 1979; 16:987.

73   Grjebine A. *Faune de Nadagascar, XXII. Insectes Diptères Culicidae Anophelinae*. Paris: Lahure, 1966.

74   Ravaon Janahary C. *Trav Doc Off Rech Sci Tech Outre-Mer* 1978; 87.

75   Rioux JA. *Encycl Ent B* 1958; 35:1.

76   Senevet G & Andarelli L. *Encycl Ent A* 1959; 37:1.

77   Van den Assem J & Bonne-Wepster J. *Zool Bijdr* 1964; 6:1.

78   Belkin JN. *Contrib Am Entomol Inst* 1968; 3:1.

79   Bonne-Wepster J & Swellengrebel NH. *The Anopheline Mosquitoes of the Indo-Australian Region*. Amsterdam: de Bussy, 1953.

80   Harrison BA & Scanlon JE. *Contrib Am Entomol Inst* 1975; 12:1.

81   Mattingly PF. Part I (1957) *Ficalbia*; part II (1957) *Heizmannia*; part III *Aedes* (*Paraedes*) and (*Cancraedes*); part IV *Aedes* (*Skusea*), (*Diceromyia*) (*Geoskusea*) and (*Christophersiomyia*); part V *Aedes* (*Mucidus*), (*Ochlerotatus*), and (*Neomelaniconion*); part VI *Aedes* (*Stegomyia*). London: British Museum (Natural History), 1957–65.

82   Mattingly PF. *Contrib Am Entomol Inst* 1970; 5:1.

83   Reinert JF. *Contrib Am Entomol Inst* 1973; 9:1.

84   Huang YM. *Contrib Am Entomol Inst* 1979; 15:1.

85   Delfinado MD. *Mem Am Entomol Inst* 1966; 7:1.

86   Basio RG. *Nat Mus Philipp Monogr* 1971; 4.

87   Gutsevich AV, Monchadsky AS & Stackelberg AA. *Fauna SSSR. VII (4). Family Culicidae*. Leningrad: Akad, Nauk SSSR Zool Inst (English translation (1974) Jerusalem: Keter Press), 1970.

88   Mattingly P F & Brown E S. *Bull Entomol Res* 1955; 46:69.

89   Foote RH & Cook DR. *Mosquitoes of Medical Importance*. United States Department of Agriculture, Agricultural Handbook, 1959; 152:1–158.

90   Mattingly PF. *Contrib Am Entomol Inst* 1971; 7:1. (Reproduced in Smith KGV (1973) *Insects and Other Arthropods of Medical Importance*. London: British Museum (Natural History).)

91   Laird M & Miles JW (eds) *Integrated Mosquito Control Methodologies*, 2 vols. London: Academic Press, 1983, 1985.

92   Reiter P. *Ann Trop Med Parasitol* 1980; 74:541.

93   Detinova TS. *Age-grouping Methods in Diptera of Medical Importance*. WHO Monograph Series no. 417. Geneva: WHO, 1962.

94   Clements AN. *The Physiology of Mosquitoes*. Oxford: Pergamon Press, 1963.

95   Linley JR, Hoch AL & Pinheiro FP. *J Med Entomol* 1983; 20:347–364.

96   Raccurt C, Lowrie RC & McNeeley DF. *Am J Trop Med Hyg* 1980; 29:803–808.

97   Nathan MB. *Bull Entomol Res* 1981; 71:97–105.

98   Linley JR & Davies J B. *J Econ Entomol* 1971; 64:264–278.

99   Crosskey RW. *The Biology of Blackflies*. 1993.

100   Mulligan HW. *The African Trypanosomiases*. London: George Allen & Unwin, 1970.

101   Ford J. *The Role of the Trypanosomiases in African Ecology: A Study of the Tsetse Fly Problem*. Oxford: Clarendon Press, 1971.

102   Potts.

103   Pollock JN. *Training Manual for Tsetse Control Personnel*, 3 vols. Rome: FAO, 1982.

104   Jackson CHN. *Bull Entomol Res* 1946; 37:291.

105   Saunders 1962.

106   Challier 1965.

107   Challier A. *Insect Sci Applic* 1982; 3:97–143.

108   Molyneux DH & Ashford RW. *The Biology of Trypansoma and Leishmania, Parasites of Man and Domestic Animals*. London: Taylor and Francis, 1983.

109   Molyneux DH. *Rev Infect Dis* 1983; 5:945–956.

110   Allsopp R. *Bull Entomol Res* 1984; 74:1–23.

111   Jordan AM. *Br Med Bull* 1985; 41:181–186.

112   Jordan AM. *Trypanosomiasis Control and African Rural Development*. Harlow, UK: Longman, 1986.

113   Lent H & Wygodzinsky P. *Bull Am Mus Nat Hist* 1979; 163:123.

114   World Health Organization. *Chemical Methods for the Control of Arthropod Vectors and Pests of Public Health Importance*. Geneva: WHO, 1984.

115   Schofield CJ. *Triatominae: Biology and Control*. 1993.

116   Rothschild M. *Annu Rev Entomol* 1975; 20:241.

117   Smit FGAM. Siphonaptera (fleas). In Smith KGV (ed.) *Insects and Other Arthropods of Medical Importance*. London: British Museum (Natural History), 1973:325.

118   Traub R & Starcke H. *Fleas*. Rotterdam: Balkema, 1980.

119   Bibikova VA. *Annu Rev Entomol* 1977; 22:1.

120   Traub R, Wisseman CL & Farhang-Azad A. *Trop Dis Bull* 1978; 75:237.

Appendix V
Sources of Information in Tropical Medicine

J. E. Eyers

Introduction

The literature of tropical medicine, like all clinical specialties, tends to be distributed throughout the medical literature,[1] and reliance on the specialist tropical medicine journals and books alone will not usually be sufficient to cover adequately the total literature. It is important therefore that any search of the literature will need to encompass both the general and specialist sources. This brief guide to the information sources of tropical medicine will limit itself to the main focus of this book, i.e. clinical and diagnostic aspects of tropical medicine; no attempt is made to include the wider interdisciplinary aspects of tropical medicine where it impinges on public health.

Any systematic search of the literature must use a variety of different sources including printed indexes, journals, books, databases and the Internet. Those listed below include only a selection of the most important sources, but it is often the case that most sources will lead the reader on to other resources. Where available, Internet web site addresses are given, since it is the Internet which is becoming the main vehicle for up-to-date information in medicine. Inevitably some web sites become unavailable, change URL or are not updated; see the section on Internet Web Sites for access details to updated or current web sites listed in this guide.

Guides to the literature

Deering C M. Tropical medicine. In Morton L T & Godbolt S (eds) *Information Sources in the Medical Sciences*, 4th edn. London: Bowker-Saur, 1992: 233–247.

Hague H. *Core Collection of Medical Books and Journals 2001*, 4th edn. London: Medical Information Working Party, 2000.

Textbooks and other print materials

Generally speaking, there is a dearth of texts relating to clinical and laboratory aspects of tropical and parasitic diseases, and readers will invariably have to look in textbooks of infectious diseases and other more general textbooks of medicine for current information. The texts selected below are the most well known in the field.

For students and those working in the developing world substantial price discounts are available in a student edition for many of the texts below from:

1. Tropical Health Technology
   14 Bevills Close, Doddington,
   March, Cambs PE15 0TT, UK
   Email: thtbooks@tht.ndirect.co.uk
   Website: www.tht.ndirect.co.uk

2. Teaching Aids at Low Cost (TALC)
   PO Box 49, St Albans
   Herts AL1 5TX, UK
   Email: talc@talcuk.org
   Website: www.talcuk.org

General texts

Armstrong D & Cohen J (eds). *Infectious Diseases*, 2 vols. London: Mosby, 1999.

Bell D R. *Lecture Notes on Tropical Medicine*, 4th edn. Oxford: Blackwell, 1995.

Chin J (ed.). *Control of Communicable Diseases Manual*, 17th edn. Washington, DC: American Public Health Association, 2000.

Cook G C & Zumla A (eds). *Manson's Tropical Diseases*, 21st edn. London: W B Saunders, 2002.

Eddleston M & Pierini S. *Oxford Handbook of Tropical Medicine*. Oxford: Oxford University Press, 1999.

Fernando R L, Fernando S S E & Leong A S-Y. *Tropical Infectious Diseases: Epidemiology, Investigation, Diagnosis and Management*. London: Greenwich Medical Media, 2001.

Guerrant R L, Walker D H & Weller P F (eds). *Tropical Infectious Diseases: Principles, Pathogens, and Practice*, 2 vols. Philadelphia, PA: Churchill Livingstone, 1999.

Guerrant R L, Walker D H & Weller P F (eds). *Essentials of Tropical Infectious Diseases*. Philadelphia, PA: Churchill Livingstone, 2001.

Harries J R, Harries A D & Cook G C. *Clinical Problems in Tropical Medicine*, 2nd edn. London: Saunders, 1998.

Krawinkel M & Renz-Polster H. *Medical Practice in Developing Countries*. Neckarsulm: Jungjohann, 1995.

Lucas A O & Gilles H M. *Short Textbook of Public Health Medicine for the Tropics*, 4th edn. London: Arnold, 2002.

Mandell G L, Bennett J E & Dolin R (eds). *Mandell, Douglas and Bennett's Principles and Practice of Infectious Diseases*, 5th edn, 2 vols. Philadelphia, PA: Churchill Livingstone, 2000.

Schull C R. *Common Medical Problems in the Tropics*, 2nd edn. London: Macmillan, 1999.

Strickland G T (ed.). *Hunter's Tropical Medicine and Emerging Infectious Diseases*, 8th edn. London: Saunders, 2000. [The standard US textbook of tropical medicine.]

Atlases

Chiodini P L, Moody A & Manser D W. *Atlas of Medical Helminthology and Protozoology*, 4th edn. Edinburgh: Churchill Livingstone, 2000.

Gutierrez Y. *Diagnostic Pathology of Parasitic Infections: With Clinical Correlations*, 2nd edn. Oxford: Oxford University Press, 2000.

Peters W. *A Colour Atlas of Arthropods in Clinical Medicine*. London: Wolfe, 1992.

Peters W & Pasvol G. *Tropical Medicine and Parasitology*, 5th edn. London: Mosby, 2002.

Schaller K F (ed.). *Colour Atlas of Tropical Dermatology and Venereology*. Berlin: Springer, 1994.

Spicer W J. *Clinical Bacteriology, Mycology, and Parasitology: An Illustrated Colour Text*. Edinburgh: Churchill Livingstone, 1999.

Dermatology

Arenas R & Estrada R. *Tropical Dermatology*. Georgetown, TX: Landes Bioscience, 2001.

Canizares O. *A Manual of Dermatology for Developing Countries*, 2nd edn. Oxford: Oxford University Press, 1993.

Parish L C & Millikan L E. *Global Dermatology*. New York: Springer, 1994.

Saxe N, Jessop S & Todd G. *Oxford Southern Africa Handbook of Dermatology for Primary Care*. Oxford: Oxford University Press, 1997.

Gastroenterology

Cook G C (ed.) *Tropical gastroenterology*. Oxford: Oxford University Press; 1980.

Cook G C (ed.). *Gastroenterological Problems from the Tropics*. London: BMJ Publishing, 1995.

Watters D A K & Kiire C F. *Gastroenterology in the Tropics and Subtropics: A Practical Approach*. London: Macmillan, 1995.

Laboratory techniques

Cheesbrough M. *District Laboratory Practice in Tropical Countries. Part 1: Parasitology, Clinical Chemistry, Management, Quality Control*. Doddington, UK: Tropical Health Technology, 1998.

Cheesbrough M. *District Laboratory Practice in Developing Countries. Part 2: Microbiology, Haematology, Blood Transfusion*. Doddington, UK: Tropical Health Technology, 2000.

Garcia L S. *Practical Guide to Diagnostic Parasitology*. Washington, DC: ASM Press, 1999.

Garcia L S. *Diagnostic Medical Parasitology*, 4th edn. Washington, DC: ASM Press, 2001.

Microscopical Diagnosis of Tropical Diseases. March, Cambs, UK: Tropical Health Technology, revised 1997. [Affordable series of colour laminated brochures consisting of high-quality colour plates with text for diagnosing parasitic, bacterial and viral infections, urinary tract disease, anaemia and white blood cell disorders]:

1. *Microscopical diagnosis of malaria*
2. *Microscopical diagnosis of African trypanosomiasis, South American trypanosomiasis, leishmaniasis*
3. *Microscopical diagnosis of lymphatic filariasis, Brugian filariasis, loiasis, onchocerciasis*
4. *Microscopical diagnosis of* E. histolytica/E. dispar *infection, giardiasis, cryptosporidium enteritis, isospora infection*
5. *Microscopical diagnosis of meningitis, infections associated with AIDS, gonorrhoea, syphilis, tuberculosis, leprosy, chlamydial infection*
6. *Microscopical examination of urine in bacterial urinary tract infection, urinary schistosomiasis, kidney disease*
7. *Microscopical diagnosis of blood in anaemia, sickle cell disease, leukaemias, infectious mononucleosis, lupus erythematosus, relapsing fever*
8. *Microscopical diagnosis of intestinal helminth infections, helminth eggs as seen in saline faecal preparations*
9. *Microscopical investigation of infections associated with HIV disease and AIDS*

Van Dyck E, Meheus Z A & Piot P. *Laboratory Diagnosis of Sexually Transmitted Diseases*. Geneva: WHO, 1999.

World Health Organization. *Bench Aids for the Diagnosis of Malaria Infections*, 2nd edn. Geneva: WHO, 2000.

Leprosy

Bryceson A & Pfaltzgraff R E. *Leprosy*, 3rd edn. Edinburgh: Churchill Livingstone, 1990.

Hastings R C. *Leprosy*, 2nd edn. Edinburgh: Churchill Livingstone, 1994.

Medical entomology

Eldridge B F & Edman J D (eds). *Medical Entomology: A Textbook on Public Health and Veterinary Problems Caused by Arthropods*. Dordrecht: Kluwer, 2000.

Goddard J. *Physician's Guide to Arthropods of Medical Importance*, 3rd edn. Boca Raton, FL: CRC Press, 2000.

Kettle D S. *Medical and Veterinary Entomology*, 2nd edn. Wallingford, UK: CAB International, 1995.

Service M W. *Medical Entomology for Students*, 2nd edn. Cambridge, UK: Cambridge University Press, 2000.

Neurology

Shakir R A, Newman P K & Poser C M (eds). *Tropical Neurology*. London: Saunders, 1996.

Nutrition

King F S & Burgess A. *Nutrition for Developing Countries*, 2nd edn. Oxford: Oxford University Press, 1993.

Latham M C. *Human Nutrition in the Developing World*. Rome: Food and Agriculture Organization, 1997.

Médecins sans Frontières. *Nutrition Guidelines*. Paris: MSF, 1995.

World Health Organization. *The Management of Nutrition in Major Emergencies*. Geneva: WHO, 2000.

World Health Organization. *Management of Severe Malnutrition: A Manual for Physicians and Other Senior Health Workers*. Geneva: WHO, 1999.

Ophthalmology

Sandford-Smith J. *Eye Diseases in Hot Climates*, 3rd rev. edn. Oxford: Butterworth-Heinemann, 2001.

Schwab L. *Eye Care in Developing Nations*, 3rd edn. San Francisco, CA: American Academy of Ophthalmology, 1999.

Paediatrics

Ebrahim G J. *Paediatric Practice in Developing Countries*, 2nd edn. London: Macmillan, 1993.

Seear M D. *Manual of Tropical Pediatrics*. Cambridge, UK: Cambridge University Press, 2000.

World Health Organization. *Management of the Child with a Serious Infection or Severe Malnutrition: Guidelines for Care at the First-Referral Level in Developing Countries*. Geneva: WHO, 2000.

Parasitic and vector-borne diseases

Abdi Y A, Gustafsson L L, Ericsson O et al. *Handbook of Drugs for Tropical Parasitic Infections*, 2nd edn. London: Taylor & Francis, 1995.

Bogitsh B J & Cheng T C. *Human Parasitology*, 2nd edn. San Diego, CA: Academic Press, 1998.

Cox F E G (ed.). *Modern Parasitology*, 2nd edn. Oxford: Blackwell Science, 1993.

Cox F E G, Kreier J P & Wakelin D (eds). *Topley & Wilson's Microbiology and Microbial Infections*, 9th edn, vol. 5: *Parasitology*. London: Arnold, 1998.

Cunha B A (ed.). *Tickborne Infectious Diseases: Diagnosis and Management*. New York: Marcel Dekker, 2000.

Dalton J P (ed.). *Fasciolosis*. Wallingford, UK: CABI Publishing, 1999.

Gilles H M (ed.). *Protozoal Diseases*. London: Arnold, 1999.

Gilles H M & Warrell D A (eds). *Essential Malariology*, 4th edn. London: Arnold, 2002.

Gillespie S H & Hawkey P M (eds). *Medical Parasitology*. Oxford: IRL Press, 1995.

Gillespie S & Pearson R D (eds). *Principles and Practice of Clinical Parasitology*. Chichester: Wiley, 2001

Gubler D J & Kuno G (eds). *Dengue and Dengue Hemorrhagic Fever*. Wallingford, UK: CAB International, 1997.

Jordan P, Webbe G & Sturrock R F (eds). *Human Schistosomiasis*. Wallingford, UK: CAB International, 1993.

Klei T R, Rajan T V, (eds). The Filaria. Boston MA: Kluwer Academic Publishers; 2002.

Kumar V. *Trematode Infections and Diseases of Man and Animals*. Dordrecht: Kluwer, 1999.

Mahmoud A A F (ed.). *Schistosomiasis*. London: Imperial College Press, 2001.

Markell E K, John D T & Krotoski W A. *Markell & Voge's Medical Parasitology*, 8th edn. Philadelphia, PA: Saunders, 1999.

Muller R. *Worms and Human Disease*, 2nd edn. Wallingford, UK: CABI Publishing, 2002.

Nutman T B (ed.). *Lymphatic Filariasis*. London: Imperial College Press, 2000.

Ravdin J I (ed.). *Amebiasis*. London: Imperial College Press, 2000.

Service M W (ed.). *Encyclopaedia of Arthropod-transmitted Infections of Man and Domesticated Animals*. Wallingford, UK: CABI Publishing, 2001.

Tsieh Sun. *Parasitic Disorders: Pathology, Diagnosis, and Management*, 2nd edn. Baltimore, MD: Williams & Wilkins, 1999.

Wahlgren M & Perlmann P (eds). *Malaria: Molecular and Clinical Aspects*. Amsterdam: Harwood Academic, 1999.

Wernsdorfer W H & McGregor I (eds). *Malaria: Principles and Practice of Malariology*, 2 vols. Edinburgh: Churchill Livingstone, 1988.

World Health Organization. *Dengue Haemorrhagic Fever: Diagnosis, Treatment, Prevention and Control*, 2nd edn. Geneva: WHO, 1997. [Online edition: www.who.int/emc/diseases/ebola/Denguepublication/index.html]

World Health Organization. *Management of Severe Malaria: A Practical Handbook*, 2nd edn. Geneva: WHO, 2000. [Online edition: http://mosquito.who.int/docs/hbsm.pdf]

Pathology

Meyers W M (ed.) *Pathology of Infectious Diseases*, vol. 1: *Helminthiases*. Washington, DC: Armed Forces Institute of Pathology, 2000.

Psychiatry

Tantam D, Appleby L & Duncan A (eds). *Psychiatry for the Developing World*. London: Gaskell, 1996.

Radiology

Palmer P E S & Reeder M M. *The Imaging of Tropical Diseases, with Epidemiological, Pathological and Clinical Correlation*, 2nd edn. 2 vols, Berlin: Springer, 2001.

Refugee health

Médecins sans Frontières. *Refugee Health: An Approach to Emergency Situations*. London: Macmillan, 1997.

Respiratory Medicine

Pande J N (ed.). *Respiratory Medicine in the Tropics*. Delhi: Oxford University Press, 1998.

Sharma O P (ed.). *Lung Disease in the Tropics*. New York: Marcel Dekker, 1991.

Rheumatology

McGill P E & Adebajo A O. *Tropical Rheumatology*. London: Baillière Tindall, 1995.

Sexually transmitted infections & AIDS

Arya O P & Hart C A (eds). *Sexually Transmitted Infections and AIDS in the Tropics*. Wallingford, UK: CABI Publishing, 1998.

Holmes K K, Mårdh P-A, Sparling P F et al. *Sexually Transmitted Diseases*, 3rd edn. New York: McGraw-Hill, 1999.

Surgery

Cohen R V & Aun F (eds). *Tropical Surgery*. Basel: Karger, 1997.

King M, Bewes P, Cairns J et al. (eds). *Primary Surgery*, vol. 1: *Non-Trauma*. Oxford: Oxford Medical Publications, 1993.

King M & Bewes P (eds). *Primary Surgery*, vol. 2: *Trauma*. Oxford: Oxford Medical Publications, 1993.

Rosenfeld J V & Watters D A K. *Neurosurgery in the Tropics*. London: Macmillan, 2000.

Sandford-Smith J & Hughes D. *Eye Surgery in Hot Climates*. Anstey, UK: Thorpe, 1994.

Travel medicine

Auerbach P S (ed.). *Wilderness Medicine*, 4th edn. St Louis, MO: Mosby-Yearbook, 2001.

Behrens R H & McAdam K P W J (eds). *Travel Medicine*. Edinburgh: Churchill Livingstone, 1993. [*British Medical Bulletin* 49(2).]

Centers for Disease Control & Prevention. *Health Information for International Travel 2001–2002*. Atlanta, GA: CDC, 2001.

Dupont H L & Steffen R. *Textbook of Travel Medicine and Health*, 2nd edn. Oxford: Blackwell, 2001.

Freedman D O (ed.). *Travel Medicine*. Philadelphia, PA: Saunders, 1998. [*Infectious Disease Clinics of North America* 12(2).]

Kassianos G C. *Immunization: Childhood and Travel Health*, 4th edn. Oxford: Blackwell Science, 2001.

Steffen R & Dupont H L. *Manual of Travel Medicine and Health*. Hamilton, BC: Decker, 1999.

World Health Organization. *International Travel and Health 2002*. Geneva: WHO, 2002. [http://www.who.int/ith]

Zuckerman J N (ed.). *Principles and Practice of Travel Medicine*. Chichester, UK: Wiley, 2001.

Tuberculosis

Crofton J, Horne N & Miller F. *Clinical Tuberculosis*, 2nd edn. London: Macmillan, 1999.

Crofton J, Chaulet P & Maher D. *Guidelines for the Management of Drug-Resistant Tuberculosis*. Geneva: WHO, 1997. [www.who.int/gtb/publications/gmdrt/contents.html]

Harries A D, Maher D, Raviglione M C et al. *TB/HIV: A Clinical Manual*. Geneva:WHO, 1996. [www.who.int/gtb/publications/tb_hiv/index.htm]

Journals

The following publishers make available some publications free to doctors working in selected developing countries:

1. FSG Medimedia Ltd
   Vine House
   Fair Green, Reach
   Cambridge CB5 0JD, UK
   Web: www.fsg.co.uk
   Email: info@fsg.co.uk

   Africa Health incorporating Medicine Digest. ISSN 0141-9536
   Diabetes International. ISSN 1468-6570

2. PMH Publications
   PO Box 100
   Chichester
   W. Sussex PO18 8HD, UK
   Web: www.pmh.uk.com/health/health.htm
   Email: admin@pmh.uk.com

   Postgraduate Doctor (for Africa, Middle East, Caribbean)

3. Healthlink
   Cityside, 40 Adler St
   London E1 1EE, UK
   Web: www.healthlink.org.uk
   Email: info@healthlink.org.uk

   Various newsletters and journals

Acta Tropica. Elsevier, 1944–. ISSN 0001-706X [www.elsevier.nl/locate/actatropica]
Advances in Parasitology. Academic Press, 1963–. ISSN 0065-308X [www.harcourt-international.com/serials/parasitology]
African Journal of Medicine and Medical Sciences. Spectrum Books, 1970–. ISSN 0002-0028
AIDS. Lippincott Williams & Wilkins, 1987–. ISSN 0269-9370 [www.aidsonline.com]
American Journal of Tropical Medicine and Hygiene. American Society of Tropical Medicine and Hygiene, 1921–. ISSN 0002-9637 [www.ajtmh.org/journal.html]
Annals of Tropical Medicine and Parasitology. Maney Publishing, 1907–. ISSN 0003-4983 [www.maney.co.uk/atmp.html]
Annals of Tropical Paediatrics. Maney Publishing 1981–. ISSN 0272-4936 [www.maney.co.uk/atp.html]
Bulletin de la Société de Pathologie Exotique. Société de Pathologie Exotique, 1908–. [www.pasteur.fr/sante/socpatex/pages/english/journal.html]
Bulletin of the World Health Organization. WHO, 1947–. ISSN 0043-9686 [www.who.int/bulletin]
Central African Journal of Medicine. Faculty of Medicine, University of Zimbabwe, 1955–. ISSN 0008-9176 [http://bioline.bdt.org.br/ca]
Dakar Médical. Société Médicale d'Afrique Noire de Langue Française, 1956–. ISSN 0850-797X
East African Medical Journal. Kenya Medical Association, 1923–. ISSN 0012-835X [http:\\bioline.bdt.org.br/ea]
Emerging Infectious Diseases. NCID, Centers for Disease Control & Prevention, 1995–. ISSN 1080-6040 [www.cdc.gov/eid]
International Journal of Leprosy and Other Mycobacterial Diseases. International Leprosy Association, 1933–. ISSN 0148-916X
International Journal of STD and AIDS. Royal Society of Medicine Press, 1990–. ISSN 0956-4624 [www.rsm.ac.uk/pub/std.htm]

International Journal of Tuberculosis and Lung Disease. International Union against Tuberculosis and Lung Disease, 1997–. ISSN 1027-3719 [www.iuatld.org]
Journal of Health Population and Nutrition (incorporating the *Journal of Diarrhoeal Diseases Research*). International Centre for Diarrhoeal Disease Research, Bangladesh (ICDDR,B), 1983–. ISSN 1606-0997 [http://www.icddrb.org/jhpn/]
Journal of Travel Medicine. BC Decker, 1994–. ISSN 1195-1982 [www.istm.org]
Journal of Tropical Pediatrics. Oxford University Press, 1955–. ISSN: 0142-6338 [www3.oup.co.uk/tropej]
Leprosy Review. LEPRA, 1930–. ISSN 0305-7518 [www.lepra.org.uk/review/homepage.html]
Médecine d'Afrique Noire. NG-COM, 1953–. ISSN 0047-6404 [www.santetropicale.com/Kiosque/Man/infogene_man.htm]
Médecine Tropicale. IMTSSA, 1941–. ISSN 0025-682X. [http://ifr48.free.fr/recherche/activite_sp/imtssa/rev_med_trop.html]
Memorias do Instituto Oswaldo Cruz. Instituto do Oswaldo Cruz, 1909–. ISSN 0074-0276 [www.dbbm.fiocruz.br/www-mem]
Morbidity and Mortality Weekly Report. Centers for Disease Control and Prevention, 1950–. ISSN 0149-2195 [www.cdc.gov/mmwr]
Revista Cubana de Medicina Tropical. Instituto de Medicina Tropical Pedro Kouri, 1945–. ISSN 0375-0760 [www.bvs.sld.cu/revistas/mtr/]
Revista da Sociedad Brasileira de Medicina Tropical. Sociedad Brasileira de Medicina Tropical,1968–. ISSN 0037-8682 [www.scielo.br]
Revista do Instituto de Medicina Tropical de Sao Paulo. Instituto de Medicina Tropical de Sao Paulo, 1959–. ISSN 0036-4665 [www.scielo.br]
Southeast Asian Journal of Tropical Medicine and Public Health. SEAMEO TROPMED Network, 1970–. ISSN 0038-3619
Transactions of the Royal Society of Tropical Medicine and Hygiene. Royal Society of Tropical Medicine and Hygiene, 1907–. ISSN 0035-9203 [www.rstmh.org]

Table V.1 Selected tropical medicine journals listed by impact factor* from ISI *Journal Citation Reports*[†]

Journal	Impact factor
American Journal of Tropical Medicine and Hygiene	1.765
Transactions of the Royal Society of Tropical Medicine and Hygiene	1.485
Tropical Medicine and International Health	1.350
Leprosy Review	1.343
International Journal of Leprosy	1.114
Annals of Tropical Medicine and Parasitology	0.988
Acta Tropica	0.799
Memorias do Instituto Oswaldo Cruz	0.542
Journal of Tropical Pediatrics	0.447
Annals of Tropical Paediatrics	0.413
Tropical Doctor	0.282
Bulletin de la Société Exotique	0.151

*The journal impact factor is a measure of the frequency with which the 'average article' in a journal has been cited in a particular year. Figures are for 2000—accessed March 2002.
[†]Courtesy of Institute for Scientific Information, Philadelphiia PA. ISI Journal Citation Reports & Reprints® on the web.

Tropical Doctor. Royal Society of Medicine Press, 1971–. ISSN 0049-4755 [www.roysocmed.ac.uk/pub/td.htm]
Tropical Medicine and International Health: TM&IH. Blackwell Science, 1996–. ISSN 1360-2276 [www.blackwell-synergy.com/Journals/issuelist.asp?journal=tmi]
Weekly Epidemiological Record. World Health Organization, 1925–. ISSN 0049-8114 [www.who.int/wer]

Abstracting/indexing journals

Abstracting and indexing journals list the contents and in some cases selected abstracts of specialist journals and sometimes will include books, conference proceedings, reports and other forms of publication. Most can be searched by subject and author name, but some will enable geographic and taxonomic searching. Many now have database equivalents.

African Index Medicus, WHO Regional Office for Africa, Harare, Zimbabwe. [http://whqwings.who.int/RIS/RISWEB.isa] 1990–, quarterly. Comprises medical references with selected abstracts from material published in and about Africa, and includes journals, books, reports, theses etc. It includes African medical journals not indexed in other abstracting/indexing journals. Author and subject indexes are included. Also available as a database.
Helminthological Abstracts, CABI Publishing, Wallingford, UK [http://www.cabi-publishing.org/JOURNALS/Abstract/HMA/Index.asp] 1977–, monthly. Covers all parasitic helminths including gastrointestinal nematodes, liver flukes, *Echinoccocus*, schistosomes, filaria, *Taenia* and *Trichinella*. Includes comprehensive coverage of laboratory-based and clinical aspects of diagnosis and treatment from journals, books, reports, conferences etc. Included in the CAB Health database.
Index Medicus, National Library of Medicine, Bethesda, MD, USA [www.nlm.nih.gov]. 1879–, monthly. The standard medical index, covering about 3400 journals (of which 35 are listed under the category of tropical medicine) in all areas of medicine. Important for its coverage of the general medical literature in identifying articles of relevance to tropical medicine. Contains authors and subject indexes listing references in a basic author/title/journal reference format without abstracts. The complete list of journals indexed is published annually with *Index Medicus* but is also available via the NLM website [http://www.nlm.nih.gov/tsd/serials/lji.html]. Available as the database Medline/Pubmed.
Nutrition Abstracts and Reviews—Series A: Human and Experimental, CABI Publishing, Wallingford, UK [http://www.cabi-publishing.org/JOURNALS/Abstract/NARA/Index.asp]. 1931–, monthly. Covers all aspects of clinical and laboratory-based nutrition with comprehensive coverage of the literature on malnutrition, vitamin deficiency, diarrhoea, infant feeding and the assessment of nutritional status. Author, subject and geographic indexes. Included in the CAB Health database.
Protozoological Abstracts, CABI Publishing, Wallingford, UK [http://www.cabi-publishing.org/JOURNALS/Abstract/PZA/Index.asp]. 1977–, monthly. Covers all parasitic protozoa affecting man and animals, including *Plasmodium*, *Trypanosoma, Entamoeba, Toxoplasma, Babesia*, Coccidia, *Giardia, Theileria, Leishmania*. It is particularly strong on laboratory research, diagnosis, control and treatment identified from journals, books, conference proceedings, reports etc. Included in the CAB Health database.

Review of Medical and Veterinary Entomology, CABI Publishing, Wallingford, UK. http://www.cabi-publishing.org/JOURNALS/Abstract/RMVE/Index.asp 1913–, monthly. The most important abstracting journal on insects and arthropods of medical importance to man and animals. Selecting material from journals, books, conferences and reports, it includes disease vectors, ectoparasites, venomous and toxic arthropods, and covers aspects such as physiology, taxonomy, ecology, genetics as well as disease transmission and methods for control. Included in CAB Health database.
Tropical Diseases Bulletin, CABI Publishing, Wallingford, UK [http://www.cabi-publishing.org/JOURNALS/Abstract/TDB/Index.asp]. 1912– , monthly. This is the most important abstracting journal in the field, covering all clinical and laboratory aspects of tropical medicine, and includes references from journals, books, conference proceedings, reports etc. A particular strength is its coverage of material published in the developing world (from among 130 countries), so often ignored by other indexes more focused on the Western world. Its continuous publication over nearly a century makes it an outstanding resource for historians of tropical medicine. Now also available as a subset of the CAB Health database from 1973 onwards.
Tsetse and Trypanosomiasis Information Quarterly, Food and Agriculture Organization, Rome, Italy [http://www.fao.org/ag/aga/agah/pd/Ttiqe.htm]. 1978–, quarterly. Covers all aspects of tseste and trypanosomiasis research and control and is available in both English and French versions. Includes references with abstracts from journals, books, reports, conference proceedings etc.

Databases

Many biomedical databases are now available free via the Internet. Those most useful in the field of tropical medicine are listed below with some of the more general multispecialty databases such as Medline. An understanding of database structure and indexing is an essential prerequisite of any database search if papers are not to be missed. It is therefore well worthwhile using individual database manuals and help screens before searching.[2]

CAB Health, CABI Publishing, Wallingford, UK [www.cabi.org]. 1973–. An important database for tropical medicine and parasitology incorporating many of the health-related abstracting journals from CABI (see above). Journal articles, books, reports, symposia etc from about 130 countries are included, with a strong emphasis on clinical and laboratory-based aspects of tropical medicine. Its particular strength is in infectious diseases in the developing world, but it also includes material on human nutrition, medical entomology, medicinal plants and venomous animals. A subscription-based resource is available from CABDirect [www.cabdirect.org], Silverplatter [www.silverplatter.com], Dialog [www.dialog.com], DIMDI [www.dimdi.de/engl/fr-search.htm].
Cochrane Library, Update Software Ltd, Oxford, UK [www.update-software.com]. The major resource for evidence-based medicine comprising several databases. Included is a database of systematic reviews (full-text) with an increasing number on infectious and tropical diseases, a database of abstracts of reviews of effectiveness, a comprehensive bibliography of clinical trials as well as a handbook on critical appraisal and the science of reviewing research. For further details of the Cochrane Collaboration and its specialist groups (particularly the Infectious Diseases Group) see http://www.cochrane.org

Development Databases, Institute of Development Studies, University of Sussex, UK [http://www.ids.ac.uk/ids/info/index.html]. Useful series of databases on development issues, many of which contain information on interdisciplinary aspects of health in the developing world. Some contain full-text documents. Available free.

Healthlink Online, Healthlink, London, UK [http://nt1.ids.ac.uk/data/ahrtag/ahrtag.htm]. Useful free database providing access to more than 16 000 records of materials, including books, articles, reports and training manuals, focusing on the management and practice of primary health care and disability in developing countries. It includes much material published in developing countries that is not available in other databases.

LILACS (Latin American and Caribbean Literature on Health Sciences), BIREME, Sao Paulo, Brazil [www.bireme.br/bvs/I/ibd.htm]. 1982–. Includes references from 670 of the region's medical and health journals, as well as theses, books, conferences and governmental publications. The database contains 150 000 records and is essential for the Latin American literature not indexed elsewhere. Available free on the Internet.

Medline, National Library of Medicine, Bethesda MD, USA [www.nlm.nih.gov] 1966–. The most well-known general medical database covering about 4500 journals with selected abstracts. It includes the most important journals of tropical medicine, but its main use is for information on tropical diseases which is published in general medical journals and journals of other medical specialties. Now available free from the National Library of Medicine as PubMed [http://www.ncbi.nlm.nih.gov/entrez/query.fcgi]. Also available as a subscription-based service from commercial suppliers including Silverplatter [www.silverplatter.com], Ovid [www.ovid.com], Dialog [www.dialog.com], DIMDI [www.dimdi.de/homeeng.htm].

NLM Gateway, National Library of Medicine, Bethesda MD, USA. [http://gateway.nlm.nih.gov/gw/cmd]. A database system that complements NLM's Medline/PubMed system which allows access to additional resources such as books, pre-1966 *Index Medicus* journal records and audio-visual material.

Popline, Population Information Program, Johns Hopkins School of Public Health, Baltimore, MD, USA [http://db.jhuccp.org/popinform/index.stm]. 1970–. Important database on reproductive health with excellent coverage of AIDS and other STDs and maternal and child health in the developing world, including references from books, articles and technical reports. It also includes much unpublished material and grey literature from non-governmental organizations active in the developing world. Now contains over 290 000 records and is available free on the Internet and available free to developing countries on CD-ROM [www.jhuccp.org/popline/order.stm or Popline Digital Services, 111 Market Place, Suite 310, Baltimore, MD 21202, USA].

TRIP Database [http://www.tripdatabase.com]. Searches over 75 sites of high-quality medical information, giving direct, hyperlinked access to the largest collection of 'evidence-based' material on the web (including elements of the *Cochrane Library*, such as the systematic reviews and abstracts of reviews of effectiveness), as well as articles from premier on-line journals such as the BMJ, JAMA, NEJM etc. Useful if access to the *Cochrane Library* is not available.

Web of Science (*Science Citation Index*), Institute for Scientific Information, Philadelphia, PA, USA [www.isinet.com/isi/products/citation/wos]. Subscription-based general science database series particularly useful for its facility for citation searching; this enables searching for citations to a known reference, thus giving more recent papers relating thematically to the known reference. Available via institutional subscription, commercial hosts (such as Dialog, Datastar, DIMDI or STN) as well as in CD-ROM format. Minimum delay in the indexing process, making this one of the more up-to-date online resources.

Tutorials and visual aids material

Topics in International Health [www.cabi.org]. CAB International, Wallingford OX10 8DE, UK. Email: cabi@cabi.org. CD-ROM series each containing an interactive tutorial, hundreds of photographic images and a glossary of terms: Acute respiratory infection; Diarrhoeal diseases; HIV/AIDS; Leishmaniasis; Leprosy; Malaria (2nd edn); Nutrition; Schistosomiasis; Sexually transmitted diseases; Sickle cell disease; Trachoma, Tuberculosis. Prices discounted for individuals and users from developing countries.

TALC (Teaching Aids at Low Cost). [www.talcuk.org]. PO Box 49, St Albans, Herts, AL1 5TX, UK. Slide sets for sale at low cost (See box above.)

Centers for Disease Control & Prevention. *DPDx – Identification and diagnosis of parasites of public health importance* [www.dpd.cdc.gov/dpdx].

Dermatology Online Atlas [www.dermis.net/index_e.htm].

WHO Special Programme for Research and Training in Tropical Diseases (TDR) *Image Library* [www.who.int/tdr/media/image.html].

History of tropical medicine

An extensive literature exists on the fascinating history of tropical medicine and its controversies. Much of it relates to the late nineteenth and early twentieth centuries, when many of the significant discoveries of the aetiologies of tropical and parasitic infections were first made. Listed below are a small selection of texts which will serve as an introduction to an increasingly popular subject.

Arnold D (ed.). *Warm Climates and Western Medicine: The Emergence of Tropical Medicine 1500–1900*. Amsterdam: Rodopi, 1996.

Cook G C. *From the Greenwich Hulks to Old St Pancras: A History of Tropical Disease in London*. London: Athlone Press, 1992.

Cox F E G (ed.). *The Wellcome Trust Illustrated History of Tropical Diseases*. London: Wellcome Trust, 1996.

Haynes D M. *Imperial Medicine: Patrick Manson and the Conquest of Tropical Disease*. Philadelphia, PA: University of Pennsylvania Press, 2001

Kean B H, Mott K E & Russell A J (eds). *Tropical Medicine and Parasitology: Classic Investigations*, 2 vols. Ithaca, NY: Cornell University Press, 1978.

Scott H H. *A History of Tropical Medicine*, 2 vols. London: Arnold, 1939.

Worboys M. Tropical diseases. In Bynum W F & Porter R (eds) *Companion Encyclopaedia of the History of Medicine*, vol. 1. London: Routledge, 1993: 512–536.

Schools of tropical medicine

The following are the most well-known schools of tropical medicine. Many offer postgraduate courses in clinical tropical medicine, but for a more comprehensive list of courses see the Medicus Mundi list of post-graduate training programmes in international health [www.healthtraining.org] or International Training Programs in Tropical Medicine and Health [www.astmh.org/oppor/list.html]

Bernhard Nocht Institute for Tropical Medicine, Bernhard-Nocht-Strasse 74, D-20359 Hamburg, Germany [www2.bni.uni-hamburg.de/bni/english.html]

James Cook University, Department of Public Health and Tropical Medicine, Townsville, Queensland 4811, Australia [www.jcu.edu.au/school/sphtm/phtm]

Liverpool School of Tropical Medicine, Pembroke Place, Liverpool L3 5QA, UK [www.liv.ac.uk/lstm/lstm.html]

London School of Hygiene and Tropical Medicine, Keppel Street, London WC1E 7HT, UK [www.lshtm.ac.uk]

Mahidol University Faculty of Tropical Medicine, 420/6 Rajvithi Road, Bangkok 10400, Thailand [www.tm.mahidol.ac.th]

Prince Leopold Institute of Tropical Medicine, Nationalestraat 155, B-2000 Antwerp, Belgium [www.itg.be/itg]

Swiss Tropical Institute, Socins trasse 57, Postfach CH-4002 Basel, Switzerland [www.sti.unibas.ch]

Tulane University School of Public Health and Tropical Medicine, Department of Tropical Medicine, 1430 Tulane Avenue, SL-17, New Orleans, LA 70112, USA [www.tropmed.tulane.edu]

Societies

American Society of Parasitologists [www.museum.unl.edu/asp]. Enquiries to: Dr George D. Cain, Secretary-Treasurer, ASP, Department of Cellular Biology, University of Georgia, Athens, GA 30602, USA. Tel: (706) 542-5017; Fax: (706) 542-1695; Email: gcain@cb.uga.edu

American Society of Tropical Medicine and Hygiene [www.astmh.org], 60 Revere Drive, Suite 500, Northbrook IL 60062, USA. Tel: (847) 480-9592; Fax: (847) 480-9282; Email: astmh@astmh.org

British Society for Parasitology [www.parasitology.org.uk], BSP Secratariat, Logandale Financial Services, Logandale, 12 Abington Rd, Symington, South Lanarkshire, ML12 6JX, UK; Tel/Fax: 01899-308-188; Email: bsp@parasitology.org.uk

Canadian Society for International Health [www.csih.org], 1 Nicholas Street, Suite 1105, Ottawa, Canada K1N 7B7. Tel: 613 241 5785; Fax: 613 241 3845; Email: csih@csih.org

Deutsche Gesellschaft für Tropenmedizin und Internationale Gesundheit e.V. (German Society for Tropical Medicine and International Health) [www.dtg.mwn.de/ en/index.htm], Info Service, Postfach 40 04 66, 80704 München, Germany. Tel: (89) 21 80 38 30; Fax: (89) 33 60 38; Email: dtg@lrz.uni-muenchen.de

Infectious Diseases Society of America [www.idsociety.org], 66 Canal Center Plaza, Suite 600, Alexandria, VA 22314, USA. Tel: (703) 299-0200; Fax: (703) 299-0204; Email: info@idsociety.org

International Federation for Tropical Medicine [www.iftm.org]

International Society of Travel Medicine [www.istm.org], PO Box 871089, Stone Mountain, GA 30087-0028, USA. Tel: (770) 736-7060; Fax: (770) 736-6732; Email: istm@istm.org

Royal Society of Tropical Medicine and Hygiene [www.rstmh.org], Manson House, 26 Portland Place, London W1B 1EY, UK. Tel: (0)20 7580 2127; Fax: (0)20 7436 1389; Email: mail@rstmh.org

Internet web sites

The Internet is now an indispensable source of information in medicine and has become the vehicle for making available databases, electronic journals, online textbooks, slide sets, as well as a means of communication between individuals for email and participation in professional discussion lists. However, there is evidence that the 'information gap' between the developed and developing world is increasing because telecommunication networks in the developing world are not sufficiently reliable or advanced to enable widespread access to the Internet. In time this may change and thus enable a more equitable exchange of medical information between the two worlds. The following web sites are not intended to be comprehensive, but are a representative sample of some of the Internet resources in tropical medicine currently available. A file of these web sites and others will be kept up to date during the currency of this edition and may be requested by email from the author [john.eyers@lshtm.ac.uk]. These can then be incorporated into a 'bookmarks' (Netscape) or 'favorites' (Internet Explorer) file in a personal web browser.

Guides to searching the Internet

Welsh S, Anagnostelis B & Cooke A. *Finding and Using Health and Medical Information on the Internet.* London: Aslib-IMI, 2001. An excellent and comprehensive guide with sections devoted to using search engines effectively for more focused searching, evaluating web sites for quality as well as covering subject-based searching on the Web and accessing electronic journals and full-text information.

Kiley R. *Medical Information on the Internet: A Guide for Health Professionals*, 2nd edn. London: Churchill Livingstone, 1999. [www.hbuk.co.uk/kiley/index.htm]

Health Information on the Internet. Royal Society of Medicine Press, 1998–. ISSN 1460-4140. [www.hioti.org]

Internet Medic [http://omni.ac.uk/vts/medic

Medicine on the Net. Cor Healthcare Resources, 1995–. ISSN 1085-3502 [www.corhealth.com]

Online Internet Tutorial (University of California, Berkeley) [www.lib.berkeley.edu/TeachingLib/Guides/Internet/FindInfo.html]

Prince Leopold Institute of Tropical Medicine Library (Belgium) [http://lib.itg.be/biblinks.htm#tro]. An excellent and very comprehensive starting point for searching tropical medicine sites.[3]

Free databases

African Index Medicus [http://whqwings.who.int/RIS/RISWEB.ISA]

Centre for Reviews & Dissemination Databases [UK] [http://agatha.york.ac.uk/welcome.htm]

Clinical Trials Database [USA] [http://clinicaltrials.gov/ct/gui/c/r]

Development Databases [Institute of Development Studies, University of Sussex, UK] [www.ids.ac.uk/ids/info/index.html]

Healthlink [http://nt1.ids.ac.uk/data/ahrtag/ahrtag.htm]

LILACS (Latin American databases) [www.bireme.br/bvs/I/ibd.htm]

NLM Gateway—One-stop access to US National Library of Medicine's combined journal and monograph databases [http://gateway.nlm.nih.gov/gw/Cmd]

Popline—Excellent for reproductive and sexual health issues, fertility and family planning in the developing world. [http://db.jhuccp.org/popinform/index.stm]

PubMed The standard medical database with added files from other databases [www.ncbi.nlm.nih.gov/entrez/query.fcgi]

TRIP Database—Access to 75 quality-assured Web-based sites on evidence-based practice. [http://www.tripdatabase.com]

WHO Global Database on Child Growth and Malnutrition [www.who.int/nutgrowthdb/registration_form/welcome.html]

Discussion groups/listservs

These are email-based forums for discussions and news relating to specific topics. They are usually free and are open to anyone having a professional interest in the subject; most are usually moderated in some way. Some clinical discussion lists are open only to those who are medically-qualified. All require prior subscription via email to receive and send messages. Three good directories of discussion lists are Liszt [www.liszt.com], PAML [http://paml.net] and JISCmail [www.jiscmail.ac.uk/default.htm].

African Networks for Health Research & Development – Afro-NETS [www.healthnet.org/programs/ afronets.html]
AIDS—ProCAARE [www.healthnet.org/programs/ procaare.html]
Cardiovascular health—ProCOR [www.healthnet.org/ programs/procor.html]
Essential drugs [www.healthnet.org/programs/edrug.html]
Leishmaniasis [www.bdt.org.br/listas/leish-l]
Malaria [www.wehi.edu.au/MalDB-www/discuss/listserv. html]
ProMED (Program for Monitoring Emerging Diseases) [www.promedmail.org/pls/promed/promed.home]
Travel medicine [www.istm.org]

Free electronic journals

Few electronic journals give complete full text access to all articles, but there have been recent attempts to create repositories of full text articles from a single site. These include PubMed Central (http://pubmedcentral.nih.gov), Public Library of Science (www.publiclibraryofscience.org) and BioMed Central (www.biomedcentral.com); it remains to be seen whether these are successful. At the very least most journal web sites will give tables of contents and sometimes selected full text articles. The following links give access to lists of biomedical journals:

Directory of Electronic Health Sciences Journals (Monash University) [www.med.monash.edu.au/ shcnlib/dehsj]
Free Medical Journals Site [www.freemedicaljournals.com]
Hire Wire Press [http://highwire.stanford.edu]
Prince Leopold Institute of Tropical Medicine Library [http://lib.itg.be/journals.htm#J]
PubMed-linked Journals [www.ncbi.nlm.nih.gov:80/ entrez/journals/loftext_noprov.html]

Funding agencies

Foundation Center [http://fdncenter.org/funders]
GrantsNet [www.grantsnet.org]
Internet Prospector-Foundations [http://www.internet-prospector.org/found.html]
UK Fundraising [www.fundraising.co.uk/grants.html]
Wellcome Trust [www.wellcome.ac.uk/en/1/gra.html]
Yahoo [http://dir.yahoo.com/Education/Financial_Aid/ Grants]

International organizations

Food and Agriculture Organization of the UN [www.fao.org]
International Federation of Red Cross & Red Crescent Societies [www.ifrc.org]
Médecins sans Frontières [www.msf.org]
Pan American Health Organization [www.paho.org]
UNAIDS [www.unaids.org]
UNICEF [www.unicef.org]
World Bank [www.worldbank.org]
World Health Organization [www.who.int]
World Health Organization (tropical diseases resources) [www.who.int/health-topics/idindex.htm]
WHO Regional Office for Africa [www.whoafr.org]
WHO Regional Office for the Eastern Mediterranean [www.emro.who.int/index.asp]
WHO Regional Office for South East Asia [w3.whosea.org/index.htm]
WHO Regional Office for the Western Pacific [www.wpro.who.int]

Outbreak and sentinel sites

Communicable Diseases Australia [www.health.gov.au/pubhlth/cdi/cdihtml.htm]
Disease Surveillance Online[Canada] [www.hc-sc.gc.ca/pphb-dgspsp/dsol-smed]
Eurosurveillance [www.eurosurv.org]
GeoSentinel [Global Surveillance Network of the ISTM and CDC] [www.istm.org]
Morbidity and Mortality Weekly Report [USA—CDC] [www.cdc.gov/mmwr]
ProMed [www.fas.org/promed]
Public Health Laboratory Service [UK] [www.phls.co.uk/Default.htm]
Sentiweb [France] [www.b3e.jussieu.fr/sentiweb]
Weekly Epidemiological Record [WHO] [www.who.int/wer]
WHO Communicable Disease Surveillance & Response [www.who.int/emc/index.html]

Schools of tropical medicine

Bernhard Nocht Institute of Tropical Medicine [www2.bni.uni-hamburg.de/bni/english.html]
James Cook University [www.jcu.edu.au/school/sphtm/ phtm/degrees/puawards.htm]
Liverpool School of Tropical Medicne [www.liv.ac.uk/ lstm/lstm.html]
London School of Hygiene and Tropical Medicine [www.lshtm.ac.uk]
Mahidol University Faculty of Tropical Medicine [www.tm.mahidol.ac.th]
Prince Leopold Institute of Tropical Medicine [www.itg.be/itg]
Swiss Tropical Institute [www.sti.unibas.ch]
Tulane University School of Public Health and Tropical Medicine [www.tropmed.tulane.edu]

Societies

American Society of Parasitologists [www-museum.unl.edu/asp/index1.html]
American Society of Tropical Medicine and Hygiene [www.astmh.org]
British Society for Parasitology [www.abdn.ac.uk/bsp]
Canadian Society for International Health [www.csih.org/ csihindex.html]
German Society for Tropical Medicine and International Health [www.dtg.mwn.de/en/index.htm]
International Society of Travel Medicine [www.istm.org]
Royal Society of Tropical Medicine and Hygiene [www.rstmh.org]

Specialty web sites

African trypanosomiasis
WHO [www.who.int/tdr/diseases/tryp/default.htm]

Cholera
WHO [www.who.int/emc/diseases/cholera]

Dengue
WHO [www.who.int/tdr/diseases/dengue/default.htm]

Diagnostic and infectious disease practice software
GIDEON—Global Infectious Disease and Epidemiology Network [www.cyinfo.com]

Evidence-based tropical health
Cochrane Infectious Diseases Review Group [www.liv.ac.uk/lstm/ehcap/CIDG_welcome.html]

Health data on developing countries
Demographic & Health Surveys [www.measuredhs.com/]

HIV/AIDS
Asian AIDS/HIV Information [www.utopia-asia.com/aids.htm]
HIV Insite Knowledge Base online textbook [http:// hivinsite. ucsf.edu/InSite.jsp?page=KB]
JAMA HIV/AIDS Resource Center [www.ama-assn.org/special/hiv/hivhome.htm]
UNAIDS [www.unaids.org]
    WHO [www.who.int/emc/diseases/hiv]

Leishmaniasis
WHO [www.who.int/tdr/diseases/leish/default.htm]

Leprosy
WHO [www.who.int/tdr/diseases/leprosy/default.htm]

Lymphatic filariasis
WHO [www.who.int/tdr/diseases/lymphfil/default.htm]

Malaria
Malaria database [www.wehi.edu.au/MalDB-www/who.html]
Multilateral Initiative on Malaria (MIMCOM) [www.mimcom.net]
Roll Back Malaria Programme—WHO [www.rbm. who.int]
WHO [www.who.int/tdr/diseases/malaria/default.htm]

Medical entomology
Iowa State University Entomology Resources [www.ent.iastate.edu/list/medical_entomology.html]

Meningitis
WHO [www.who.int/emc/diseases/meningitis]

Onchocerciasis
OnchoNet [http://math.smith.edu/~sawlab/OnchoNet/OnchoNet.html]
WHO [www.who.int/tdr/diseases/oncho/default.htm]

Parasitology
Karolinska Institute parasitology links [www.mic.ki.se/Diseases/c3.html]
Ohio State University Parasitology Resources [http://www.biosci.ohio-state.edu/~parasite/home.html]
Parasitology Research Groups Worldwide [www.uni-duesseldorf.de/WWW/MathNat/Parasitology/paen_ags.htm]

Reproductive health
Global Reproductive Health Forum [http://www.hsph.harvard.edu/Organizations/healthnet]
Reproductive Health Outlook [www.rho.org]

Schistosomiasis
WHO [www.who.int/tdr/diseases/schisto/default.htm]

Sexually transmitted diseases
WHO [http://www.who.int/health-topics/std.htm]
WHO Department of HIV/AIDS [http://www.who.int/HIV_AIDS/first.html]

South American trypanosomiasis (Chagas' disease)
WHO [www.who.int/tdr/diseases/chagas/default.htm]

Travel medicine
American Society of Tropical Medicine and Hygiene—Travel Clinic Directory [www.astmh.org/clinics/clinindex.html]
Canada Travel Medicine Program [www.hc-sc.gc.ca/pphb-dgspsp/tmp-pmv]
Centers for Disease Control and Prevention (USA)—Travelers' Health Pages [www.cdc.gov/travel]
Foreign and Commonwealth Office (UK)—Country Information [www.fco.gov.uk/travel/countryadvice.asp]
Hospital for Tropical Diseases (UK) [http://thehtd.org]
International Society of Travel Medicine [www.istm.org]
Medical Advisory Services for Travellers Abroad (MASTA—UK) [www.masta.org]
Public Health Laboratory Service (UK) [www.phls.co.uk/Default.htm]
State Department (USA)—Country Information [http://travel.state.gov]
Travel Health Online [www.tripprep.com]
WHO International Travel and Health: Vaccination Requirements and Health Advice [www.who.int/ith]

Tropical Diseases
Tropical Diseases Web Ring [http://myweb.worldnet.net/~ditjaste/ringform.html]

Tuberculosis
WHO [www.who.int/tdr/diseases/tb/default.htm]

REFERENCES

1   Goffman W & Warren K S. Dispersion of papers among journals based on a mathematical analysis of two diverse medical literatures. *Nature* 1969; 221:1205–1207.

2   Eyers J E. Searching bibliographic databases effectively. *Health Policy Plan* 1998; 13:339-342.
    [http://heapol.oupjournals.org/cgi/reprint/13/3/339.pdf]

3   Schoonbaert D. Tropical medicine, the Internet and current trends in biomedical communication. *Ann Trop Med Parasitol* 2000; 94:661–674.

Index

1840 Index